Principles of Pharmacology

Basic Concepts & Clinical Applications

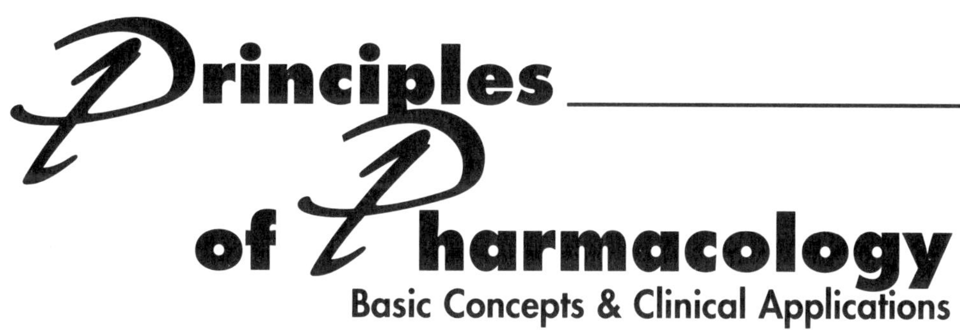

Principles of Pharmacology

Basic Concepts & Clinical Applications

Editor-in-Chief

PAUL L. MUNSON

Associate Editors-in-Chief

ROBERT A. MUELLER

GEORGE R. BREESE

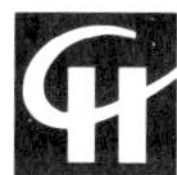

CHAPMAN & HALL

I(T)P An International Thomson Publishing Company

New York • Albany • Bonn • Boston • Cincinnati • Detroit • London • Madrid • Melbourne • Mexico City • Pacific Grove • Paris • San Francisco • Singapore • Tokyo • Toronto • Washington

Printed in the United States of America

For more information, contact:

Chapman & Hall
One Penn Plaza
New York, NY 10119

International Thomson Publishing
Berkshire House 168-173
High Holborn
London WC1V 7AA
England

Thomas Nelson Australia
102 Dodds Street
South Merlbourne, 3205
Victoria, Australia

Nelson Canada
1120 Birchmount Road
Scarborough, Ontario
Canada, M1K 5G4

Chapman & Hall
2-6 Boundary Row
London SE1 8HN

International Thomson Editores
Campos Eliseos 385, Piso 7
Col. Polanco
11560 Mexico D.F. Mexico

International Thomson Publishing Gmbh
Königwinterer Strasse 418
53228 Bonn
Germany

International Thomson Publishing Asia
221 Henderson Road
#05-10 Henderson Building
Singapore 0315

International Thomson Publishing-Japan
Hirakawacho-cho Kyowa Building, 3F
1-2-1 Hirakawacho-cho
Chiyoda-ku, 102 Tokyo
Japan

1 2 3 4 5 6 7 8 9 10 XXX 01 00 99 97 96 95

Library of Congress Cataloging-in-Publication Data

Principals of pharmacology : basic concepts and clinical applications / Paul L. Munson, editor-in-chief : Robert A. Mueller, associate editor-in-chief, George R. Breese, associate editor-in-chief : additional editors, William O. Berndt … [et al.].
p. cm.
Includes bibliographical references and index.
ISBN 0-412-04701-2
1. Pharmacology. I. Munson, Paul L., (Paul Lewis), 1910- . II. Mueller, Robert A. (Robert Arthur), 1938- . III. Breese, George R.
[DNLM: 1. Pharmacology. 2. Drugs. 3. Drug Therapy. QV 55 P957 1994]
RM300.P744 1994
615'.1—dc20
DNLM/DLC 94-41659
CIP

Please send your order for this or any Chapman & Hall book to **Chapman & Hall, 29 West 35th Street, New York, NY 10001, Attn: Customer Service Department.** You may also call our Order Department at 1-212-244-3336 or fax your purchase order to 1-800-248-4724.

For a complete listing of Chapman & Hall's titles, send your requests to **Chapman & Hall, Dept. BC, One Penn Plaza, New York, NY 10119.**

Preface

Principles of Pharmacology: Basic Concepts and Clinical Applications is the ambitious brainchild of an ad hoc committee of distinguished pharmacologists convened in Geneva by Prof. C. Liana Bolis, Founding Director of the WHO Collaborating Centre for Research and Training in Neurosciences. The members of this ad hoc committee, which after a few additions, became the Advisory Editorial Board for ***Principles of Pharmacology***, are listed in a directory following the Preface.

Subsequently, the ad hoc committee invited me to be Editor-in-Chief of their projected book. I accepted the invitation because I was intrigued by the challenge of the project and impressed by its importance and merits, the objectives of the ad hoc committee, and the eminence and promised support of these individuals. Six members of this committee became editors and/or authors of ***Principles of Pharmacology.***

Principles of Pharmacology is designed primarily as a concise reference book for medical and graduate students, residents, postdoctoral fellows, faculty members, and health professionals in medicine, pharmacy, dentistry, veterinary medicine, nursing, and public health.

This volume is divided into Sections, each the primary responsibility of a Section Editor or Coeditors. The strength of ***Principles of Pharmacology*** is based on the quality of these Section Editors, as well as on that of its authors and advisors. The Section Editors recruited the authors for their sections and reviewed and monitored the contents of the chapters. Furthermore, they were responsible for another important feature of ***Principles of Pharmacology:*** seeing to it that each chapter was expertly peer-reviewed and revised accordingly.

A major objective has been to make ***Principles of Pharmacology*** comprehensive, to give the reader a reliable overview of all aspects of pharmacology, and to present the important details about drugs necessary to understand fundamental concepts, mechanisms of action, and clinical applications.

In addition to the usual sections on general principles, neuropharmacology, both peripheral and central, cardiovascular, pulmonary, and renal pharmacology, hormones, blood, the immune system and inflammation, and chemotherapeutic agents, ***Principles of Pharmacology*** has devoted special attention to the pharmacology of nutrients and nutritional diseases, the pharmacology of skin, drugs affecting the gastrointestinal tract, and elements of toxicology. A chapter on natural medicinal products is included. Finally, there is a section on pharmacology for special patient populations, including AIDS, Alzheimer's disease, critical care, pediatrics, and geriatrics. The book also provides extensive reference lists of research reports, and of reviews, monographs, and symposia. There are also numerous illustrations.

The editors and advisors recognize the fact that Pharmacology is a world science and although many of us are from the United States and Canada, 15 other countries—Australia, Belgium, Brazil, England, France, Germany, India, Israel, Italy, Japan, Nigeria, Sweden, Switzerland, Wales, and Zaire—are represented in our group of advisors, editors, and authors.

While focusing on the drugs currently most useful in therapy, ***Principles of Pharmacology*** also provides information on promising new drugs still in the developmental stage.

Principles of Pharmacology is concluded by a paper on Scientific Responsibility and Pharmacology by Prof. Jean Bernard.

We are enormously indebted to our two broadly knowledgeable and dedicated Associate Editors-in-Chief from the University of North Carolina Chapel Hill School of Medicine, Dr. Robert A. Mueller, M.D., Ph.D., Prof. of Anesthesiology and Pharmacology, and Dr. George R. Breese, Ph.D., Prof. of Pharmacology and Psychiatry in the Brain and Development Research Center.

PAUL L. MUNSON

Table of Contents

Editors, Authors, and Advisors

Adamantidis, M.M.
Univ. du Droit et de la Santé de Lille
Faculty of Medicine

Advenier, C., M.D., Ph.D.
Prof. Ag. of Pharmacology
Institut Biomédical des Cordelliers
Faculty of Medicine
Paris-Ouest, France

Albert, Adrien (dec.), Ph.D.
Late Prof. of Chemistry
Faculty of Science
Australian National Univ.
Canberra, Australia

Anand, Nitya, M.D.
Director Em., Central Drug Research Institute
Lucknow, India

Anstey, Alex, M.D.
Consultant in Dermatology
Univ. of Wales Faculty of Medicine
Cardiff, Wales, U.K.

Antman, Elliott N., M.D.
Assoc. Prof. of Medicine
Harvard Medical School
Director, Samuel A. Levine Coronary Care Unit
Cardiovascular Division
Dept. of Medicine
Brigham and Women's Hospital
Boston, MA

Aranda, Jacob V., M.D., Ph.D.
Prof. of Pediatrics and of Pharmacology and Therapeutics
McGill Univ. Faculty of Medicine
Montreal, Quebec, Canada

Baccanari, David P., Ph.D.
Senior Research Scientist
Wellcome Research Labs.
Research Triangle Park, NC

Barnes, Peter J., D.M., D.Sc.
Prof. of Medicine
Dept. of Thoracic Medicine
National Heart and Lung Institute
London, England

Barry, David W., Ph.D.
Group Director for
Research, Development, and Medical Affairs
Burroughs Wellcome Co.
Research Triangle Park, NC

Bawden, James W., D.D.S., Ph.D.
Alumni Distinguished Prof. of Pediatric Dentistry
Univ. of North Carolina School of Dentistry
Chapel Hill, NC

Berdanier, Carolyn D., Ph.D.
Prof., Dept. of Foods and Nutrition
Univ. of Georgia
Athens, GA

Bernard, Jean, M.D.
Prof. Em. of Hematology and
Director, Institut de Recherches sur les Leucemias et les Maladies du Sang
Hôpital Saint-Louis
Past President, French Academy of Science
Paris, France

Berndt, William O., Ph.D.
Vice-Chancellor for Academic Affairs
Prof. of Pharmacology
Univ. of Nebraska Medical Center
Omaha, NE

Bogaert, M.G., M.D.
Prof. of Pharmacology
Heymans Institute of Pharmacology
Univ. of Ghent Medical School
Ghent, Belgium

Bolard, Jacques, M.D.
Univ. de Pierre et Marie Curie
Paris, France

Born, Gustav V.R., M.D.
Prof. Em. and Chairman Em. of Pharmacology
Kings College
Research Prof.
William Harvey Research Institute
St. Bartholomew's Hospital Medical College
London, England

Bowers, Cyril Y., M.D.
Prof. of Medicine and Chief, Endocrinology Division
Dept. of Medicine
Tulane Univ. School of Medicine
New Orleans, LA

Bradley, S. Gaylen, Ph.D.
Prof. of Pharmacology and Toxicology and Microbiology and Immunology
Medical College of Virginia
Virginia Commonwealth Univ.
Richmond, VA

Brater, D. Craig, M.D.
Prof. of Medicine
Univ. of Indiana and
Director, Division of Clinical Pharmacology
Wishard Memorial Hospital
Indianapolis, IN

Breese, George R., Ph.D.
Prof. of Pharmacology and Psychiatry
Brain and Development Research Center
Univ. of North Carolina School of Medicine
Chapel Hill, NC

Brown, David R., Ph.D.
Assoc. Prof.
Dept. of Veterinary Pathobiology
School of Veterinary Medicine
Univ. of Minnesota
St. Paul, MN

Burns, R. Stanley, M.D.
Head, Movement Disorders Program
Dept. of Neurology
Cleveland Clinic Foundation
Cleveland, OH

Calle, P.A., M.D.
Heymans Institute of Pharmacology
Univ. of Ghent Medical School
Ghent, Belgium

Calles-Escandon, Jorges, M.D.
Asst. Prof. of Medicine and
Director, Sims Obesity/Nutrition Research Center
Dept. of Medicine
Univ. of Vermont School of Medicine
Burlington, VT

Chaudhury, R.R., D.Phil
Scientist Em.
National Institute of Immunology
New Delhi, India

Cheng, Yung-Chi, Ph.D.
Henry Bronson Prof. of Pharmacology
Yale Univ. School of Medicine
New Haven, CT

Cohen, Myron S., M.D.
Prof. of Medicine and Microbiology
Chief, Infectious Diseases Division
Dept. of Medicine
Univ. of North Carolina School of Medicine
Chapel Hill, NC

Coleman, Rebecca, Pharm.D.
AIDS/Oncology Program
San Francisco General Hospital
San Francisco, CA

Cory, Michael, Ph.D.
Principal Scientist
Organic Chemistry Dept.
Burroughs Wellcome Co.
Research Triangle Park, NC

Crout, J. Richard, M.D.
Formerly Vice President for Medical and Scientific Affairs
Boehringer Mannheim Pharmaceutical Corp.

Davenport, Marsha I., M.D.
Assoc. Prof. of Pediatrics
Univ. of North Carolina School of Medicine
Chapel Hill, NC

Davis, Kenneth L., M.D.
Prof. of Psychiatry and Chairman, Dept of Psychiatry
Mount Sinai Medical Center
New York, NY

Davis, Mary E., Ph.D.
Prof. of Pharmacology and Toxicology
Univ. of West Virginia School of Medicine
Morgantown, WV

Davis, Vicki L., Ph.D.
Senior Staff Fellow
Receptor Biology Section
Lab. for Reproductive/Developmental Toxicology
National Institute of Environmental Health Science
National Institutes of Health
Research Triangle Park, NC

Duff, Henry J., M.D.
Prof. of Medicine
Dept. of Medicine
Univ. of Calgary Faculty of Medicine
Calgary, Alberta, Canada

Dupuis, B.A., M.D.
Prof. and Director, Lab. of Pharmacology
Faculty of Medicine
Univ. du Droit et de la Santé de Lille
Lille, France

Ebashi, Setsuro, M.D.
President
Okazaki National Research Institute
Okazaki, Japan
Prof. Em. and Chairman Em.
Dept. of Pharmacology
Univ. of Tokyo
Tokyo, Japan

Ebert, Michael H., M.D.
Prof. of Psychiatry and Pharmacology and Chairman, Dept. of Psychiatry
Vanderbilt Univ. School of Medicine
Nashville, TN

Eckel, Fred M., M.S.
Prof. of Pharmacy
Head, Division of Hospital Practice
Univ. of North Carolina School of Pharmacy
Chapel Hill, NC

Ecobichon, Donald J., Ph.D.
Prof. of Pharmacology and Toxicology
McGill Univ. Faculty of Medicine
Montreal, Canada

Egle, John L., Jr. Ph.D.
Assoc. Prof. of Pharmacology
Medical College of Virginia
Virginia Commonwealth Univ.
Richmond, VA

Ekberg-Eriksén, Kirsten
Senior Vice President for Research and Development
Coordination and European Affairs
AB Astra Pharmaceuticals
Södertalje, Sweden

Empey, D.W., M.D.
Prof. of Medicine
Dept. of Thoracic Medicine
London Hospital, Whitechapel
London, England

Ferm, Virgil H. M.D., Ph.D.
Prof. of Anatomy and Embryology
Dept. of Anatomy
Dartmouth Medical School
Hanover, NH

Feuerstein, Giora Z., M.D.
Director, Cardiovascular Pharmacology Division
SmithKline Beecham Labs.
King of Prussia, PA

Finlay, Andrew Y., M.D.
Senior Lecturer in Dermatology
Univ. of Wales Faculty of Medicine
Cardiff, Wales, U.K.

Fisher, James W., Ph.D.
Regents Prof. and Chairman
Dept. of Pharmacology
Tulane Univ. School of Medicine
New Orleans, LA

Folkers, Karl, Ph.D.
Prof. and Director
Institute for Biomedical Research
Univ. of Texas at Austin
Austin, TX

Freireich, Emil J., M.D.
Prof. of Medicine
Dept. of Developmental Therapeutics
Baylor Univ. College of Medicine
Houston, TX

Friedman, Peter A., Ph.D.
Prof. of Pharmacology and Toxicology
Dartmouth Medical School
Hanover, NH

Gaginella, Timothy S., Ph.D.
Vice-President
Dept. of Pharmacology
Aphthon Corp.
Woodland, CA

Gillenwater, Gail, Ph.D.
Director of Clinical Studies
Salk Institute Biotechnology/Industrial Associates
LaJolla, CA

Goddard, M., Ph.D.
Research Scientist
Biostatistics Division
Environmental Health Directorate
Health Canada
Ottawa, Canada

Godfraind, Théophile, M.D.
Prof. and Director, Lab. of Pharmacology
Univ. Catholique de Louvain Faculty of Medicine
Brussels, Belgium

Godin, David V.
Prof. of Pharmacology
Univ. of British Columbia Faculty of Medicine
Vancouver, B.C., Canada

Goodman, H. Maurice, Ph.D.
Prof. and Chairman
Dept. of Physiology
Univ. of Massachusetts
Worcester, MA

Hadden, Elba W., Ph.D.
Asst. Prof. of Internal Medicine
Univ. of South Florida College of Medicine
Tampa, FL

Hadden, John W. M.D.
Prof. of Medicine and
Director, Division of Immunopharmacology
Dept. of Internal Medicine
Univ. of South Florida College of Medicine
Tampa, FL

Haefely, Willy, M.D. (dec.)
Late Chief, Dept. of CNS Pharmacology
Hoffmann—LaRoche Pharmaceuticals
Basel, Switzerland

Hamilton, Holli, M.D.
Research Asst. Prof. of Medicine
Dept. of Medicine
Univ. of North Carolina School of Medicine
Chapel Hill, NC

Hauger, Richard L., M.D.
Assoc. Prof. of Psychiatry
Univ. of California at San Diego School of Medicine and
VA Medical Center
LaJolla, CA

Hay, Douglas W.P., Ph.D.
Assoc. Fellow
Dept. of Inflammation and Respiratory Pharmacology
SmithKline Beecham Pharmaceuticals
King of Prussia, PA

Hieble, J. Paul, Ph.D.
Senior Research Fellow
SmithKline Beecham Pharmaceuticals
King of Prussia, PA

Hopfer, Roy L.
Assoc. Prof. of Microbiology
Univ. of North Carolina School of Medicine
Chapel Hill, NC

Hiipakka, Richard A., Ph.D.
Senior Research Associate
Ben May Institute
Univ. of Chicago
Chicago, IL

Hirsch, Philip F., Ph.D.
Prof. Em. of Pharmacology
Univ. of North Carolina School of Medicine and Dental Research Center
Chapel Hill, NC

Hitchings, George H., Ph.D., D.Sc.
Scientist Em. and Consultant
Burroughs Wellcome Co.
Research Triangle Park, NC
Nobel Prize for Physiology and Medicine

Hollenberg, Morley D., D.Phil., M.D.
Prof. and Chairman
Dept. of Pharmacology
Univ. of Calgary Faculty of Medicine
Calgary, Alberta, Canada

Holohan, Peter D., Ph.D.
Research Prof. of Pharmacology
SUNY Health Sciences Center
Syracuse, NY

Horning, Marjorie G., Ph.D.
Prof. Em. of Biochemistry
Lipid Research Lab.
Baylor Univ. College of Medicine
Houston, TX

Izquierdo, Ivan, M.D.
Prof. of Biochemistry
Instituto de Biociências
Univ. Federal de Rio Grande de Sul
Pôrto Alegre, RS, Brazil

Janowsky, Aaron J., M.D.
Assoc. Prof. of Psychiatry and Pharmacology
Oregon Health Sciences Univ. and VA Medical Center
Portland, OR

Janssen, Paul A.
President
Janssen Research Foundation
Bearse, Belgium

Johnson, Kjel A., Pharm.D.
Asst. Prof.
Univ. of Pittsburgh School of Pharmacy
Pittsburgh, PA

Jordan, V. Craig, Ph.D., D.Sc.
Prof. of Cancer Pharmacology
Dir., Breast Cancer Research
Robert H. Lurie Cancer Center
Northwestern Univ. Medical School
Chicago, IL

Kaba Sengele, A., M.D.
Prof. of Pharmacology
Univ. of Kinshasa
Kinshasa, Zaire
Prof. of Pharmacology
Central African Republic

Kelly, Ralph A., M.D.
Asst. Prof. of Medicine
Harvard Medical School and
Dept. of Medicine
Brigham and Women's Hospital
Boston, MA

Korach, Kenneth H., Ph.D.
Chief, Receptor Biology Section
Lab. for Reproductive/Developmental Toxicology
National Institute for Environmental Health Sciences
National Institutes of Health
Research Triangle Park, NC

Krenitsky, Thomas A., Ph.D.
Vice-President for Research
Burroughs Wellcome Co.
Research Triangle Park, NC

Krewski, Daniel, Ph.D.
Chief, Biostatistics Division
Environmental Health Directorate
Health Canada
Ottawa, Canada

Lakshmanan, Mark C., M.D.
Asst. Prof. of Medicine
Metro Health Medical Center
Case Western Reserve Univ. School of Medicine
Cleveland, OH

Langer, S.Z., M.D.
Vice-President and Director
Dept. of Biology
Synthélabo LERS
Paris, France

Lechat, Philippe, M.D.
Prof. of Pharmacology
Service de Pharmacologie
Hôpital Pitié Salpétrière
Paris, France

Lee, Nancy M., Ph.D.
Prof. of Pharmacology
Univ. of Minnesota College of Medicine
Minneapolis, MN

Liao, Shutsung, Ph.D.
Prof. of Biochemistry and Molecular Biology
Ben May Institute
Univ. of Chicago
Chicago, IL

Liljestrand, Åke, Ph.D.
Prof. Em. of Pharmacotherapeutics
Univ. of Uppsala
Formerly Director, Dept. of Drugs
Swedish National Board of Health and Welfare
Gävle, Sweden

Lloyd, G. Kenneth, Ph.D.
Vice President, Pharmaceuticals: Biology
Salk Institute Biotechnology/Industrial Associates
LaJolla, CA

Loh, Horace H., Ph.D.
Stark Prof. and Head
Dept. of Pharmacology
Univ. of Minnesota College of Medicine
Minneapolis, MN

Loo, Ti Loo, D.Phil., D. Sc.
Research Prof. of Pharmacology
Dept. of Pharmacology
George Washington Univ. Medical Center
Washington, DC

Loosen, Peter T., M.D.
Prof. of Psychiatry and Medicine
Vanderbilt Univ. School of Medicine
Nashville, TN

Lovinger, David M., Ph.D.
Dept. of Molecular Biology and Biophysics
Vanderbilt Univ. School of Medicine
Nashville, TN

Lowenthal, David T., M.D., Ph.D.
Prof. of Medicine, Pharmacology, and Exercise Science
Univ. of Florida School of Medicine
Director, Geriatric Research, Education, and Clinical Center, VA Medical Center
Gainesville, FL

Lurie, Alain, M.D.
Institut de Recherche Therapeutique
Hôpital Univ. Cochain
Paris, France

MacCannell, Keith L., M.D., Ph.D.
Prof. of Pharmacology
Univ. of Calgary Faculty of Medicine
Calgary, Alberta, Canada

Marsac, J., M.D.
Prof. of Medicine
Assistance Publique—Hôpitaux de Paris
Centre Hôpitalier et Univ. Cochin
Dept. de Pneumologie et d'Asthmologie
Paris, France

Marciano-Cabral, Francine, Ph.D.
Prof. of Microbiology and Immunology
Medical College of Virginia
Richmond, VA

Marks, Ronald, M.D.
Prof. of Dermatology
Univ. of Wales Faculty of Medicine
Cardiff, Wales, U.K.

Martin, James R., Ph.D.
Head, Behavioral Pharmacology Group
Hoffmann—LaRoche Pharmaceuticals
Basel, Switzerland

Martin, Peter R., M.D.
Prof. of Psychiatry and Pharmacology
Vanderbilt Univ. School of Medicine
Nashville, TN

Mayeux, Philip R., Ph.D.
Asst. Prof. of Pharmacology and Toxicology
Univ. of Arkansas Medical Science Center
Little Rock, AR

McNamara, Dennis B., Ph.D.
Prof. of Pharmacology
Tulane Univ. School of Medicine
New Orleans, LA

Mestiri, Martine, M.D.
Institute for Therapeutic Research
Hôpital Univ. Cochain
Paris, France

Migliaccio, Silvia, M.D.
Visiting Associate
Receptor Biology Section
Lab. for Reproductive/Developmental Toxicology
National Institute of Environmental Health Sciences
National Institutes of Health
Research Triangle Park, NC

Mills, Caroline M., M.D.
Senior Registrar in Dermatology
Univ. of Wales Faculty of Medicine
Cardiff, Wales, U.K.

Montastruc, Jean-Louis, M.D.
Prof. of Medicine
Lab. of Medical and Clinical Pharmacology
INSERM U317 Faculty of Medicine
Toulouse, France

Motley, Richard J., M.D.
Consultant Dermatologist
Univ. of Wales Faculty of Medicine
Cardiff, Wales, U.K.

Mueller, Robert A., M.D., Ph.D.
Prof. of Anesthesiology and Pharmacology
Univ. of North Carolina School of Medicine
Chapel Hill, NC

Munson, Paul L., Ph.D.
Sarah Graham Kenan Prof. Em. of Pharmacology and Endocrinology and Chairman Em., Dept. of Pharmacology
Univ. of North Carolina School of Medicine
Baltimore, MD

Nicholas, Robert A., Ph.D.
Assoc. Prof. of Pharmacology
Univ. of North Carolina School of Medicine
Chapel Hill, NC

Nichols, Andrew J., Ph.D.
Asst. Director, Cardiovascular Pharmacology
SmithKline Beecham Pharmaceuticals
King of Prussia, PA

Paoletti, Rodolfo, M.D.
Prof. of Pharmacology and Director, Institute of Pharmacology and Pharmacognosy
Dean, School of Pharmacy
Univ. of Milano
Milano, Italy
Representative of Italy, NATO Scientific Council
President, Giovanni Lorenzini Medical Foundation

Olson, Robert E., M.D., Ph.D.
Prof. Em. and Chairman Em. of Biochemistry
Saint Louis Univ. School of Medicine
Prof. of Pediatrics
Univ. of South Florida School of Medicine
Tampa, FL

Ontjes, David A., M.D.
Prof. of Medicine and Pharmacology
Univ. of North Carolina School of Medicine
Chapel Hill, NC

Plaa, Gabriel L., Ph.D.
Prof. of Pharmacology and Toxicology
Univ. of Montreal Faculty of Medicine
Montreal, Quebec, Canada

Prusoff, William H., Ph.D.
Prof. Em. of Pharmacology
Yale Univ. School of Medicine
New Haven, CT

Raasch, Ralph H., Pharm. D.
Assoc. Prof. of Pharmacy
Director of Pharm. D. Program
Univ. of North Carolina School of Pharmacy
Chapel Hill, NC

Rabey, J. Martin, M.D.
Prof. of Neurology
Dept. of Neurology
Tel Aviv Univ. Sackler Faculty of Medicine
Tel Aviv, Israel

Rao, K.S., D.V.M., Ph.D.
Senior Research Scientist
DowElanco
Indianapolis, IN

Rascol, Olivier, M.D.
Lab. of Medical and Clinical Pharmacology
INSERM U317 Faculty of Medicine
Toulouse, France

Reitz, Richard H., Ph.D.
Retired Assoc. Scientist
Dow Chemical Co.
Midland, MI

Ritter, Leonard, Ph.D.
Prof. of Environmental Biology
Executive Director, Canadian Network of Toxicology Centers
Univ. of Guelph
Guelph, Ontario, Canada

Rivier, Catherine, Ph.D.
Research Prof.
Clayton Foundation Labs. for Peptide Biology
Salk Institute
La Jolla, CA

Robbins, Jacob, M.D.
Chief, Endocrine Section
Genetics and Biochemistry Branch
National Institute of Digestive Diseases and Kidney
National Institutes of Health
Bethesda, MD

Robison, G. Alan, Ph.D.
Distinguished Prof. Em. of Pharmacology
Univ. of Texas Health Sciences Center
Houston, TX

Ruffolo, Robert R., Jr., Ph.D.
Vice President and Director, Pharmacological Sciences
SmithKline Beecham Pharmaceuticals
King of Prussia, PA

Ruiz, Jorge G., M.D.
Fellow in Geriatric Medicine
Univ. of Florida School of Medicine and
VA Medical Center
Gainesville, FL

Sadoul, P., M.D.
Prof. of Medicine
Faculty of Medicine of Nancy
C.H.U. Brabois
Vandoeuvre-les-Nancy, France

Salako, L.A., Ph.D.
Prof. and Head, Dept. of Pharmacology and Therapeutics
Univ. of Ibadan College of Medicine
Ibadan, Nigeria

Sanders-Bush, Elaine, Ph.D.
Prof. of Pharmacology
Vanderbilt Univ. School of Medicine
Nashville, TN

Schiefer, H. Bruno, D.V.M., Ph.D.
Prof. of Veterinary Pathology
Director, Toxicology Research Center
Univ. of Saskatchewan
Saskatoon, Saskatchewan, Canada

Senard, Jean-Michel, M.D.
Lab. of Medical and Clinical Pharmacology
INSERM U317 Faculty of Medicine
Toulouse, France

Severson, David L., Ph.D.
Prof. of Pharmacology and Therapeutics
Univ. of Calgary Faculty of Medicine
Calgary, Alberta, Canada

Shaha, Chandrima
National Institute of Immunology
New Delhi, India

Shalton, Richard C., M.D.
Assoc. Prof. of Psychiatry
Vanderbilt School of Medicine
Nashville, TN

Silverstein, Roy L., M.D.
Assoc. Prof. of Hematology
Cornell Univ. Medical College
New York, NY

Sims, Ethan A.H., M.D.
Prof. Em. of Medicine
Univ. of Vermont School of Medicine
Burlington, VT

Sirtori, Cesare, M.D., Ph.D.
Prof. of Pharmacology and
Director, Cattedra di Chemioterapio
Univ. of Milano
Milano, Italy

Smith, Andrew P., Ph.D.
Research Assoc. in Pharmacology
Univ. of Minnesota College of Medicine
Minneapolis, MN

Smith, Roger P., Ph.D.
Irene Heinz Given Prof. of Pharmacology and Toxicology
Dartmouth Medical School
Hanover, NH

Smith, Thomas W., M.D.
Prof. of Medicine
Harvard Medical School and
Director, Cardiovascular Division
Dept. of Medicine
Brigham and Women's Hospital
Boston, MA

Spitz, Irving M., M.D.
Director, Clinical Research
Center for Biomedical Research
Population Council
New York, NY

Stern, Robert G., M.D.
Asst. Prof. of Psychiatry
Mt. Sinai School of Medicine
New York, NY and
Asst. Chief, Geropsychiatric Research Unit
FDR VA Medical Center
Montrose, NY

Strauch, Georges, M.D.
Institute for Therapeutic Research
Hôpital Univ. Cochain
Paris, France

Strum, David P., M.D.
Asst. Prof.
Dept. of Anesthesiology and Critical Care Medicine
Univ. of Pittsburgh Medical Center
Pittsburgh, PA

Sulser, Fridolin, M.D.
Prof. of Psychiatry and Pharmacology
Vanderbilt Univ. School of Medicine
Nashville, TN

Temple, Robert J., M.D.
Director, Drug Evaluation and Research
U.S. Food and Drug Administration
Rockville, MD

Toverud, Svein U., D.M.D., Ph.D.
Prof. of Pharmacology
School of Medicine and
Dental Research Center
Univ. of North Carolina
Chapel Hill, NC

Trendelenburg, Ullrich G., Dr. Med., D.Phil.
Prof. Em. and Chairman Em.
Dept. of Pharmacology and Toxicology
Univ. of Würzburg Faculty of Medicine
Tübingen, Germany

Underwood, Louis E., M.D.
Prof. of Pediatrics
Univ. of North Carolina School of Medicine
Chapel Hill, NC

Vale, Wylie W, Ph.D.
Prof. and Head
Clayton Foundation Labs. for Peptide Biology
Salk Institute
La Jolla, CA

Walker, Larry A., Ph.D.
Research Asst. Prof.
Research Institute for Pharmaceutical Science
Univ. of Mississippi School of Pharmacy
University, MS

Watanabe, Philip G., Ph.D.
Director, Health Science Toxicology Research Lab.
Dow Chemical Co.
Midland, MI

Watkins, W. David, M.D., Ph.D.
Prof. of Anesthesia
Univ. of Pittsburgh School of Medicine and
Chief, Dept. of Anesthesia
Montefiore Univ. Hospital
Pittsburgh, PA

Yaffe, Sumner J., M.D.
Director, Center for Research for Mothers and Children
National Institute for Child Health and Development
National Institutes of Health
Bethesda, MD

Yager, James D., Ph.D.
Prof. and Director
Division of Toxicological Sciences
Johns Hopkins Univ. School of Hygiene and Public Health
Baltimore, MD

Yanagita, Tomoji, M.D., Ph.D.
Central Institute for Experimental Animals
Kawasaki, Japan

Zielinski, Jean, Ph.D.
Research Scientist
Biostatistics Division
Environmental Health Directorate
Health Canada
Ottawa, Canada

Joanne Zurlo, Ph.D.
Research Associate
Dept. of Environmental Health Sciences
Johns Hopkins Univ.
Baltimore, MD

SECTION I

General Principles of Pharmacology

Section Editors:
Morley D. Hollenberg
David L. Severson
George I. Drummond (deceased)

Associate Editor:
David V. Godin

Morley D. Hollenberg

Introduction

Historical Perspective

Records dating back more than 2000 years provide good evidence of widespread knowledge of the effects of a variety of "active principles" on humans. Thus, the discipline of **pharmacology** (defined as **the interaction of biologically active agents with living systems**) has roots firmly embedded in antiquity. In Elizabethan times, it was assumed that audiences of Shakespeare's plays would have a reasonable grasp of the dynamics of action of a variety of poisons (see, for instance, *Hamlet,* Act I, Scene V; Act IV, Scene VII). Similarly, today, television commercials describing the effects of headache or cough remedies count on at least a modicum of understanding about the way drugs act. Thus, most individuals bring to their study of pharmacology a good intuitive basis for learning the principles to be outlined in this chapter. It is the object of the chapters that follow to build on that intuition so as to develop a rational basis for understanding drug action and the principles of therapeutics.

In order to develop a rational basis for therapeutics, it was essential that the discipline of pharmacology progress beyond the simple cataloguing of the actions of a variety of agents. Thus, progress did not begin until the mid-19th century, when empiric observations concerning drug action were put in the context of physiology (an approach espoused by Virchow). Not until the early 1900s, however, did the understanding of chemical structures, physiology, and biochemistry reach a level that made possible the rationalization of drug action in molecular terms. Thus, in terms of the long history of studies of drug action, the rational science of Pharmacology represents a relatively recent chapter.

Many prepared the ground for the development of modern pharmacology, including: François Magendie (1783–1855), Claude Bernard (1813–1878), Rudolf Buchheim (1820–1879), Oswald Schmiedeberg (1838–1921), and John Jacob Abel (1857–1938). However, for purposes of dealing with the principles of pharmacology, it is of importance to single out the work of: Paul Ehrlich (1854–1915: receptor concept and selective drug toxicity); John N. Langley (1852–1926: receptor concept and paradigm for drug antagonism); Alfred J. Clark (1885–1941: quantitative approach to receptor theory and drug antagonism); and Otto Loewi (1872–1961: chemical neurotransmission). The work of these individuals led to the emergence of many basic concepts of pharmacology, providing a theoretical framework for learning about a wide variety of drugs. Those beginning a study of pharmacology are strongly encouraged to consult the original publications of the above-mentioned individuals to obtain insight into the development of pharmacologic principles. Many of these references not originally written in English are now available in English translation. The emergence of these principles marked the maturation of pharmacology as a scientific discipline; furthermore, it is through a knowledge of the principles outlined in this chapter that a student of pharmacology should be able to approach with confidence and in a systematic way the enormous database relating to drug properties and drug action.

Overview of Principles

A wide variety of biologically active agents, ranging from simple ions (e.g., lithium) and low molecular weight organic molecules (caffeine and hydrocortisone) to high molecular weight polypeptides (growth hormone) can be considered as "drugs." For any of these active agents, it is important to seek answers to the questions listed in Table 1.

These questions define the general aims of most drug studies. Additionally, answers to the questions form the basic pharmacologic principles to be described in the following chapters. Furthermore, these questions have spawned the disciplines of **Toxicology** (Question 5) and **Clinical Pharmacology** (Question 8). The questions provide a convenient check-list for developing an appropriate knowledge base about any drug of interest.

Ehrlich categorically insisted that even agents acting at extremely low concentrations (like tetanus toxin) must interact by conventional physicochemical mechanisms with their target tissues or cells in order to produce a biologic effect. The binding of a drug to its target and the activation of the tissue, termed **pharmacodynamics** (i.e., the mechanisms of drug action) reflects Questions 1, 3, 5, 6, and 7 in Table 1. These subject areas are dealt with in some detail in Chapter 1. Of course, before binding to its target, any drug must first enter and disperse throughout the body. This process, termed **pharmacokinetics** (i.e., the time frame of absorption, distribution, action, and disposition of drugs) reflects Questions 2 and 4. The basic principles of pharmacokinetics are presented in Chapter 2. That chapter also shows how quantitative aspects of pharmacokinetics (concentration and time-dependence, which can be paraphrased as "how much and how often?") establishes both the magnitude and duration of drug responses, an essential feature of drug dosage regimens in successful therapeutics (Chapter 3).

In terms of the mechanisms whereby drugs act, important clues are provided by the **potencies** with which drugs act (i.e., the concentration range over which a response is observed) and the **structure-activity** relationships that govern the action of a particular class of compounds. For instance, hormonal agents such as insulin act with **high potency,** producing effects at concentrations in the range 10^{-9} to 10^{-12} M. In contrast, anaesthetic agents, including ethanol, exhibit **low potencies,** acting at concentrations greater than 10^{-3} M. In terms of the chemical requirements for the action of general anaesthetics, prime importance can be placed on physicochemical properties (principally lipid solubility and changes in membrane fluidity or polarization). In contrast, the action of epinephrine, a highly potent compound, depends dramatically on its chemical structure. For example, the D- and L-optical isomers of epinephrine differ markedly in their pharmacologic potencies.

In general it can be said that agents exhibiting high potency and chemical specificity in producing their effects do so by interacting with specialized cellular "receptive substances" (Langley's term) or **receptors,** as will be discussed in Chapter 1. The "receptor" to which an agent binds with high affinity and specificity may be an enzyme, a cell membrane-localized regulatory molecule, or a specific subcellular constituent such as DNA. A major goal of research over the past 20 years or so has been the elucidation of molecular processes triggered by drug–receptor interactions and resulting in pharmacologic responses. It can also be taken as a generalization that a number of drugs, including general anaesthetics, which act with low potencies and without a high degree of chemical specificity, do so without interacting with any specific "receptor substance" and thus are less selective in their action. A biologically active chemical (drug) can produce a biologic effect either by triggering a signal on its own (i.e., the compound is an **agonist**) or by reversing or preventing the action of some other endogenous compound (i.e. the compound can be an **antagonist**). It can be taken as a principle that selective and specific antagonists also act by binding to highly specialized cell receptors. Selective antagonism by pharmacologic agents has been of crucial historical significance in the early development of receptor theory and continues to be extensively exploited for many therapeutic applications.

(1) What is the structure of a particular drug, and what are the relationships between the chemical properties of the molecule and its biologic actions?
(2) By which routes can the drug be administered, and which of these routes is optimal for drug action?
(3) What are the dose-response relationships for the various actions of the drug?
(4) What is the time-course of drug action, and how is it eliminated from the body?
(5) What specific (i.e., desired or therapeutic) and what nonspecific (i.e., undesired or toxic) actions is the agent capable of exerting on the body?
(6) On which organs or tissues does the drug act?
(7) By what mechanism does it act?
(8) What are the therapeutic indications for the use of the drug?

Drug Action: A Duality of Perspective

The study of pharmacology often appears to involve two quite different approaches to the subject matter that relate to two of the Questions (1 and 6) posed in Table 1. On the one hand, some pharmacology textbooks seem to be an endless list of chemical structures accompanied by a description of their major actions and side-effects. On the other hand, other textbooks (as does this one) group drugs principally in terms of their effects on major target organ systems (e.g., the heart, the kidney). Both approaches illustrate the duality of perspective necessary for the study of pharmacology. An important focus must be on chemical structure and on the mechanisms of drug action (structure–activity relationships), whereas a second focus must be on the widespread influence an individual agent can have on a number of organ systems, quite apart from its main targeted therapeutic effect. This dual focus provides a rational basis for understanding the selective action and the toxicity of drugs. This essential dual perspective also renders very difficult a study of pharmacology without at least a rudimentary understanding of cell and organ system physiology. In addition, an appreciation of the widespread actions that a particular drug may have underscores the shortcoming of studying the properties of any given agent within the context of the function of only a single organ system. It is hoped that the basic principles of pharmacology outlined in this first section will serve as an organizing factor to facilitate a balanced approach to the study of pharmacology, incorporating the dual perspectives outlined above.

Therapeutic Principles and the Development of New Drugs

Until recently, discoveries of therapeutic agents (e.g., opiates, digitalis) have come from an understanding of the therapeutic properties of naturally-occurring plant or animal materials. Indeed, knowledge gained from scientific investigations of "traditional" systems of therapeutics, e.g., Chinese or American (North and South) native herbal remedies, has been and continues to be a tremendous asset in the search for new drugs. Often, it is difficult for the chemist to improve on what nature has already provided. Nonetheless, the understanding of the principles of molecular pharmacology, evolved over the past 80 years, has provided entirely novel routes for the development of new drugs. For instance, the principles of receptor specificity and selective drug toxicity have led to the development of selective adrenoreceptor and histamine receptor antagonists for use in the settings of cardiovascular disease (beta-1 and beta-2 receptor antagonists) and peptic ulcer disease (selective histamine-2 receptor antagonists). Further, the recognition that enzyme systems may function as drug targets or "drug receptors" has led to the development of purine and pyrimidine-related analogues, (6-mercaptopurine, allopurinol, acyclovir, azidothymidine) that are proving of inestimable use in the treatment of cancer, gout, herpes infection, and Acquired Immune Deficiency Syndrome (AIDS). Thus, an understanding of receptor selectivity, receptor structural and functional characteristics, and an appreciation of the basic principles of pharmacodynamics (Chapter 1) and pharmacokinetics (Chapter 2), are of importance not only theoretically in terms of understanding the mechanisms of drug action but are also of practical importance for the rational design of new drugs. With respect to rational drug design, it can be said that a new era has just begun. The procedures used in the clinical evaluation of new drugs are outlined in Chapter 3. Ultimately, knowledge concerning basic pharmacologic principles must be applied to therapeutics in order to achieve maximum benefits in the treatment of disease while minimizing toxicities. Some of the factors that influence the clinical use of drugs are presented in Chapter 3, with particular attention given to determining how pharmacokinetic parameters can be influenced by such considerations as age and pregnancy.

General References

1. Holmstedt B, Liljestrand G. Readings in Pharmacology 1981; Raven Press, New York. [*Excellent cameo portrayals of key contributors to the development of the science of pharmacology. Contains verbatim sections from many critical papers (translated into English, where appropriate) dealing with innovative concepts and discoveries that underpin current pharmacologic theories.*]
2. Temple R, Needham J. The Genius of China: 3000 Years of Science, Discovery and Invention 1986; Simon & Schuster Inc., New York. [*A highly accessible synopsis of sections from the much more extensive works of Needham and colleagues dealing with science and technology in ancient China. Highly relevant to the perspective of those who wish to trace the roots of modern therapeutics.*]

CHAPTER 1

Pharmacodynamics: Drug Receptors and Receptors/Mechanisms

Morley D. Hollenberg
David L. Severson

Development of the Receptor Concept

Historical Perspective

Although Ehrlich's pronouncement that "agents do not act unless they are bound" ("corpora non agunt nisi fixata"), may be taken today as a gratuitous conclusion, this statement, made at the turn of the century, had a considerable impact on the development of the receptor concept as we know it today. Ehrlich[r1] elaborated on this principle in his early work on the toxicity of triphenylmethane dyes in microorganisms and on the mechanism of action of tetanus toxin, wherein he explicitly developed two key concepts relating to drug action: (1) that drugs can act as chemically-related "families", where the biologic response to one member of the family (e.g., the sensitivity or resistance of a microorganism) is mirrored by responses to other chemically defined relatives; and (2) that agents can act via discrete cell surface molecules, which he termed **receptors.** The identical concept was simultaneously developed independently by Langley[1,2] who, when studying the actions of nicotine and curare at the neuromuscular junction, proposed that these agents acted directly on the "receptive substance", or **receptor** on the cell. Langley carried the concept further to encompass the phenomenon of drug antagonism (in his case, curare reversing the contractile action of nicotine on skeletal muscle), which he correctly envisioned as a mass-action competition between agonist and antagonist for binding to the receptor. Thus, by the early 1900s, the receptor paradigm of drug action was already clearly enunciated, including the concept of a discrete binding substance, the notion of structure-activity relationships and a binding-kinetic view of drug antagonism. It has taken over 70 years to elucidate in molecular terms, as outlined in the sections that follow, the receptor concept as it was first conceptualized.

Defining a Receptor

The term "receptor" as coined by Langley and Ehrlich may be employed usefully, but at times imprecisely, to describe an unknown structure by which the biologic effect of a drug on a living system is mediated. When more is known about the action of an individual agent, the "receptor" may be identified in molecular terms, for instance, as a rate-limiting enzyme of a metabolic pathway. More often than not, a **pharmacological receptor is now taken to be a cell constituent that has the dual property of (i) binding agonists with high affinity and high chemical specificity and (ii) triggering a cellular response due to an agonist-induced conformational change in the receptor.** *A priori*, however, there is no need to make any assumption about the molecular nature of a receptor in order to describe drug action both qualitatively and quantitatively according to the approaches outlined in the sections to follow. Initially, all that is required for using the receptor concept is that there be a stereochemical specificity for the triggering of the response of the system by an agonist. For example, in studying the contractile actions of a series of chemically-related catecholamines, the receptor concept is of inestimable value. In a similar vein, the actions of a large number of drugs can be described in terms of drug–receptor interactions.

Dose-Response Curves: Quantitating Drug Action

Graded Dose-Response Curves and Agonist Characterization

Much early work on drug action focused on qualitative aspects of biologic responses, such as general toxicity or antagonism. However, it was the **quantita-**

tive, not qualitative, description of drug action that was needed for further development of the understanding of pharmacology at the mechanistic level. The essence of quantifying drug response lies in the dose-response curve, illustrated in Figure 1.1. Although there are a number of ways to express the relationship between a drug concentration (or amount) and a graded response, (e.g., linear units on both abscissa and ordinate or probit plots), most commonly drug concentrations are plotted logarithmically (*abscissa*), whereas response measurements (e.g., grams of muscle tension or percent of a maximum response) are plotted linearly (*ordinate*). This manner of expressing the data has two advantages: the response to a wide concentration range of a drug may be succinctly portrayed, and the relationship between concentration and response is approximately linear over a wide portion of the curve. The essential features of the curve are: (i) the concentration at which a response is half-maximal (ED_{50} or EC_{50}); (ii) the maximum effect achieved at optimal drug concentrations (E_{max}) as the curve plateaus; and (iii) the slope of the curve in the mid-range. These three parameters are particularly useful for comparing the action of both different classes of drugs causing the same effect (e.g., muscle contraction) and the action of chemically related agents (e.g., a series of

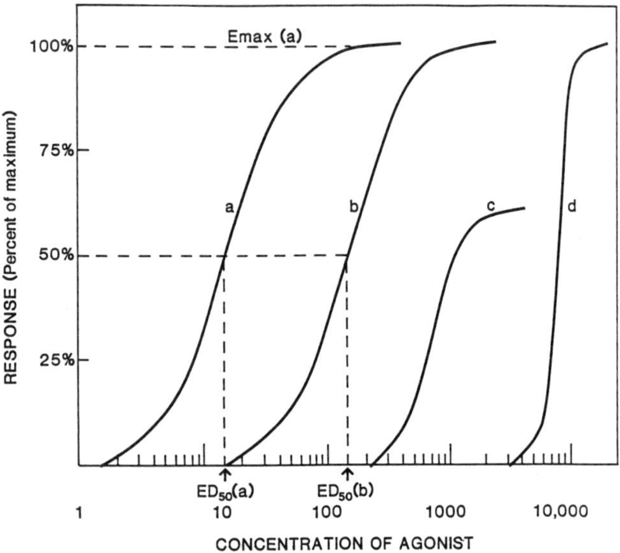

Figure 1.1 Relationship between the concentration of a drug (agonist) and the biologic effect or response: graded dose-response curves. Examples are shown for four drugs (a, b, c, and d) that differ with respect to their pharmacologic potencies (compare concentrations of drugs a and b that are required to produce a response that is 50% of maximum, ED_{50}) and their ability to produce a maximal response (Emax; compare drugs a and c). Note that the concentrations of the agonists (drugs) are plotted on a logarithmic scale.

catecholamines—see below). Further, the linear portion of the dose-response curve can be used for bioassay purposes, so that the response to known concentrations of a given agent (e.g., the contractile response of uterine muscle strips to oxytocin) can be compared with the parallel response caused by two samples of an extract containing an unknown amount of the peptide (e.g., an extract of the posterior pituitary gland). In essence the "potency" of an agent is characterized by the ED_{50} (the more potent the compound, the lower the ED_{50}); thus, in Figure 1.1, Drug a is more potent than Drug b. Agonist properties are characterized by the E_{max}. Compounds that are full agonists can cause a maximum response at sufficiently high concentrations, where the curve plateaus (e.g., curves a and b in Figure 1.1). The maximum response of a system to a series of agonists can be established by trial and error, wherein a number of compounds (full agonists) are found to cause the same maximum effect; subsequently, one of the test compounds can be used as a "standard" maximum stimulant, against which newly synthesized agents can be compared. Compounds that are "pure" antagonists cause no activation at all. However, other agents can cause an intermediate activation of a test system, even at optimal concentrations (e.g., Curve c, Fig. 1.1). Those agents that cannot fully activate a preparation are termed "partial agonists." Full and partial agonists can be distinguished from one another in terms of the degree of receptor occupation required to elicit a maximal response (see discussion of intrinsic activity, and efficacy, to follow). The slope of the dose-response curve will be the same for agonists acting on the same receptor, even though the potencies of two compounds may differ (compare curves a and b, and ED_{50} (a) and ED_{50} (b) values, Fig. 1.1). In contrast, agonists causing the same response on distinct receptors can yield dose-response curves with different slopes (Curve d, Fig. 1.1).

Partial Agonists, Spare Receptors, and the Concept of Drug Efficacy

As indicated above, two agents that act via the same receptor may or may not cause the same maximum response (e.g., curves a and c, Fig. 1.1). Originally, full agonists (curve a), partial agonists (curve c), and pure antagonists were characterized in terms of the degree (fraction of maximum) to which each agent could activate the response system, as reflected by a factor termed 'intrinsic activity.'[3] Thus, full agonists were assigned an intrinsic activity value of 1.0, whereas pure antagonists were assigned a value of zero, and agents causing an intermediate response (agent c, Fig. 1.1) were assigned a value between 0 and 1.0. This concept was elaborated upon further by Stephenson and colleagues,[4,r2] who considered the proportion of total receptors in a system that would need to be occupied to cause a maximum response. It was possible to demonstrate experimentally, using an irreversible antagonist,[5] that only a fraction of the available receptors present in a tissue might be required for a maximum effect of an agonist; that is, there were "spare receptors" present (discussed below).

Stephenson and colleagues[r2] carried the analysis of agonist action one step further than the "intrinsic activity" concept of Ariens.[3] They reasoned that even agents capable of causing a maximum response (i.e., full agonists) might do so by occupying different proportions of the available receptors. They suggested further that partial agonists causing a fraction of the maximum response might do so at very high degrees of receptor occupancy. The term "efficacy" was thus selected to reflect the efficiency with which a signal generated by a single agonist–receptor complex was amplified to evoke a tissue response. According to Stephenson's viewpoint, as with the concept of intrinsic activity, pure competitive antagonists were assigned a value of zero. However, unlike the intrinsic activity assignment, an efficacy value of 1.0 was arbitrarily given to partial agonists capable of causing maximally a response that was only 50 percent of the possible maximum caused by other agonists. Full agonists, which were then characterized in relative terms, would, therefore, have efficacies exceeding 1.0; those agonists that elicited full responses at exceedingly low degrees of receptor occupancy would be assigned quite high efficacy values (100 or greater). Although the concepts of intrinsic activity and efficacy are of interest in large part from a historical point of view, this kind of approach to characterizing agonist action was of great importance because it served to distinguish clearly between the processes of ligand binding and receptor activation, which are closely related but separate cellular events. It is only recently that ligand binding measurements (see p. 16 for experimental details) have made possible a direct estimate of the degree of receptor occupancy required for a maximum response. The ability of various agonists to cause a differential activation of a specific receptor type at equivalent degrees of receptor occupation has yet to be described systematically in molecular terms.

The concept of receptor reserve, or "spare receptors" is of sufficient importance that further discussion is warranted. Subsequent to Nickerson's observations,[5] it has become clear that most (if not all) receptor-regulated biologic systems possess some degree of "receptor reserve." For a given response, shown schematically in Figure 1.2, it is now, in many instances, possible to compare directly the dose-response curve (left-hand curve in Fig. 1.2) with the receptor binding curve measured by biochemical methods (right-hand curve, Fig. 1.2; see also, Fig. 1.7, upper). From the data in Figure 1.2, it is apparent that the maximum response is reached when only about 30 percent of the available receptor binding sites are occupied by the activating ligand. From the two curves shown in Figure 1.2, it can be appreciated that the ED_{50} determined from the dose-response curve is not equivalent to the agonist dissociation constant, which would be equal to the agonist concentration at which binding (right-hand

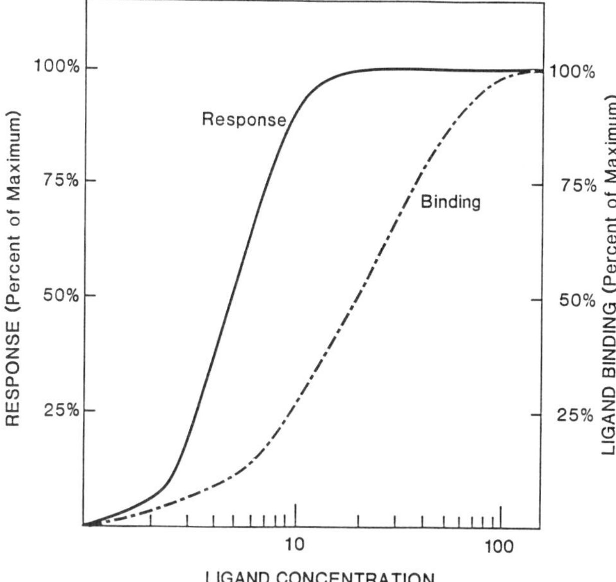

Figure 1.2 Comparison of the relationship between drug (ligand) concentration, plotted on a logarithmic scale, and either the biologic response (*solid line*) or ligand binding to receptor sites (*dashed line*). The observation that a maximal response can be obtained when only a fraction (i.e., approx. 30%) of the total number of receptors are occupied by the drug led to the concept of receptor reserve or "spare receptors."

curve) is half-maximal. This lack of correspondence between agonist ED_{50}s and dissociation constants rendered impossible early attempts to determine with accuracy the affinities of agonists for their receptors, using bioassay data alone. For direct measurements of agonist receptor affinity, a ligand binding approach was necessary (see page 16).

The existence of receptor reserve provides biologic systems with enormous flexibility. For instance, the greater the number of receptors present in a given tissue, the greater will be the ability of the tissue to detect and respond to low concentrations of an agonist in the circulation. Receptor reserve can protect an organ, enabling a full response to occur even if some of the receptors become inactivated. In such circumstances, the concentration of agonist will need to be elevated to achieve the same response. Alternatively, if the number of receptors in an organ increases, (i.e., more "spare" receptors are present), then, the tissue sensitivity will increase (i.e., the tissue will respond maximally at lower concentrations of agonist) because the same number of occupied receptors will generate the same maximum response. This kind of situation has clinical significance, for example, when hyperthyroidism causes an increase in the number of cardiac beta-receptors, so that the sensitivity of the heart to circulating catecholamines is enhanced.

The "spare receptors" in a tissue are all, in principle, equivalent and equally capable of interacting with effector systems to produce a cellular response. Thus, irrespective of the degree of receptor reserve, in theory only a fixed number of agonist-receptor complexes (for example, represented by $[AR]_n$) may be required to cause a full response. The number of occupied receptors can be expressed, according to the mass-action relationship (see page 15).

$$[AR]_n = \frac{[A][R_f]}{K_A}$$

wherein [A] = agonist concentration, $[R_f]$ = free (i.e. unbound) receptor concentration, $[AR]_n$ = concentration of agonist-receptor complex, and K_A = the agonist equilibrium dissociation constant. From the above relationship, it can be appreciated that if, as in the example of hyperthyroidism, the number of beta-adrenergic receptors **increases** (i.e. R_f goes up) then, since K_A doesn't change, the term [A] must **decrease** to maintain the equality of the mass-action equation, and hence to yield the same agonist-receptor complex concentration (and thus the same response) that was present in the euthyroid state. The system is, therefore, responsive at lower concentrations of agonist. From the above relationship, it is also evident that if the number of receptors decreases, the concentration of agonist will have to increase to maintain the level of [AR]; that is to say, a decrease in receptor numbers leads to a decrease in sensitivity. The degree to which changes in receptor number will affect the dose-response relationship will be a function of the affinity of the agonist for the receptor, reflected by the magnitude of K_A. The above relationship illustrates mechanistically, in terms of the law of mass action and the spare receptor concept, how changes in tissue receptor content can lead to changes in tissue sensitivity to an agonist.

Quantal Dose-Response Curves

The preceding sections have dealt with dose-response curves for which a graded response (e.g., muscle tension, blood pressure, or heart rate) can be monitored. A graded response can be observed for a tissue even though individual tissue elements, such as the firing of a nerve cell, can behave in an "all-or-none" fashion. Thus, from dose-response studies alone, in the absence of mechanistic information, it may not be possible to distinguish between "graded" and "quantal" responses. However, it is often the case that an over-all response of an entire system is clearly of an "all-or-none" nature (e.g., measurements of sleep-induction or lethality). In such cases, "quantal" dose-response curves can be constructed, as illustrated in Figure 1.3, where the number (or fraction) of individuals in a fixed population responding to a given dose (ordinate) is plotted (histogram) versus the dose administered (abscissa). The cumulative proportion of individuals up to and including a given dose (i.e., the area under the bell-shaped curve) can also be plotted as a function of the dose (right-hand ordinate, Fig. 1.3). For a given agent, the ED_{50} can be estimated from such curves by identifying the dose required to produce a response in 50 percent of the test population. Should the response of the population studied follow a random distribution, the histogram illustrated in Figure 1.3 would, with a sufficiently large sample size, approximate a bell-shaped curve, wherein the maximum point (mean individual effective dose, IED) would correspond exactly to the ED_{50} estimated from the cumulative frequency distribution curve. Theoretically, if all members of a population were equally responsive, the curve shown in Figure 1.3 would be a sharp step-function. The degree to which the curve is spread out reflects the heterogeneity of response within the group

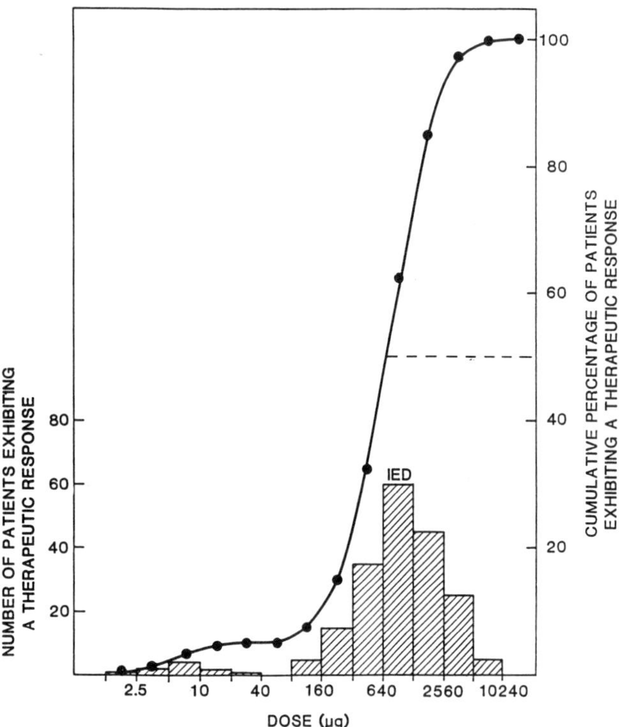

Figure 1.3 Relationship between the dose of a drug (in μg, on a logarithmic scale) and a biologic response that is quantal (number of patients exhibiting a therapeutic response), indicated by the histograms (IED, mean individual effective dose). The *cumulative percentage* of patients exhibiting a therapeutic response is also presented. In this example, a small fraction (5%) of the total patient population exhibited a particularly high sensitivity to the drug, so that the frequency distribution is bimodal.

studied. It should not be overlooked, however, that the response pattern of a population may either be skewed (for example, some individuals in a population may be resistant to very high doses of an agent, whereas most individuals might respond to low doses), or may be separated into more than one discrete population (e.g., a subpopulation consisting of 5 percent of the total population, for example, may be present exhibiting an idiosyncratically high sensitivity to an agent) (see left-hand portion of Fig. 1.3).

Dose-Response Curves and the Characterization of Antagonist Action

As indicated above, pure antagonists can reverse the action of an agonist without themselves activating the system. Langley's view of the antagonism caused by curare[1] was clearly one of competitive (or surmountable) antagonism, whereby an elevation of the amount of agonist could overcome the effect of the antagonist, as illustrated by curve a_1 in the dose-response curve shown in Figure 1.4. For truly competitive antagonists, increasing concentrations simply shift the dose-response curve in parallel to the right (e.g., a_1, a_{10}, Fig. 1.4) so that ED_{50} values increase, without a change in the maximum response. In contrast, in systems with a low degree of receptor reserve (see discussion on page 9), noncompetitive (or nonsurmountable) antagonists do not shift the dose-response curve, and thus the ED_{50} value does not change; rather, the maximum effect caused by an agonist (curves b_1 and b_{10} in Fig. 1.4) is reduced. The action of a noncompetitive antagonist may be either reversible, on removal of the antagonist from the preparation, or irreversible, as is the action of a receptor alkylating agent like dibenamine. A shift of the dose-response curve to the right may not always be taken to mean that an antagonist is of the competitive class. In situations wherein large numbers of spare receptors are present, antagonists that are really noncompetitive may first shift the dose curve in parallel to the right because enough receptors are still present to produce a maximum response; only high concentrations of the noncompetitive antagonist cause a reduction in the maximum response (curves c_1 to c_{100}, Fig. 1.4).

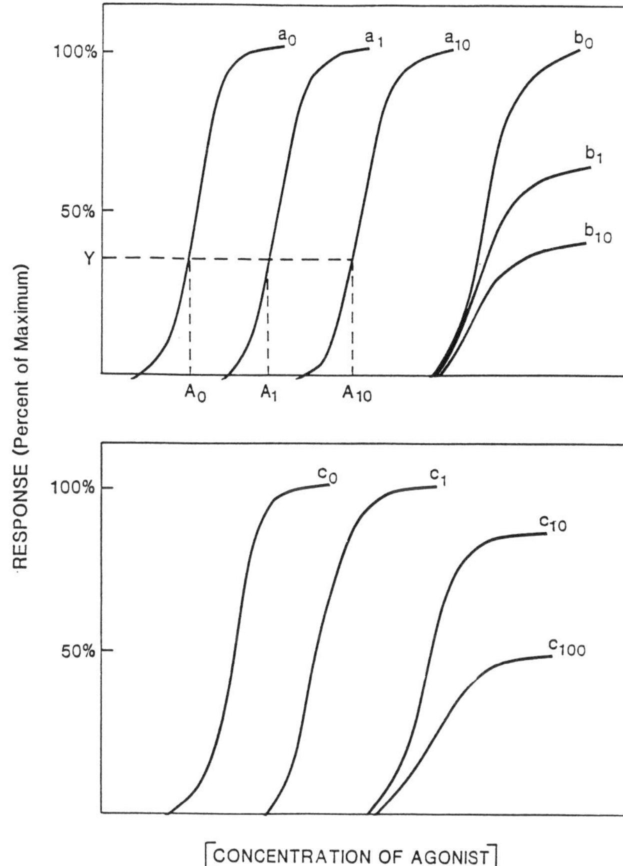

Figure 1.4 Effect of antagonists on dose-response curves. In the presence of a *competitive* antagonist (a_1), higher concentrations of the agonist can overcome the antagonism and produce a maximal response. Increasing the concentration of the *competitive* antagonist (a_{10}) shifts the dose-response curve farther to the right, so that ED_{50} values increase. A comparison of the concentrations of the agonist (A_0, A_1, A_{10}) that are required to produce any particular response (Y) can be used to obtain information about the binding of the *competitive* antagonist to the receptor (Schild plot). In contrast, a *noncompetitive* antagonist (b_1, b_{10}) results in a reduction in the maximal response without a change in ED_{50} values. In situations where "spare receptors" are present, the presence of a *noncompetitive* antagonist (c_1) will first shift the dose-response curve to the right (pseudocompetitive antagonism). Increasing the concentration of the *noncompetitive* antagonist (c_{10}, c_{100}) will eventually reduce the number of available receptors so that a maximal response cannot be obtained.

Mechanisms of Drug Antagonism

The figures portraying the different types of drug antagonism (competitive or noncompetitive: Fig. 1.4) make no assumption about the mechanism of antagonism, which can arise by a number of processes. The different ways drug action can be diminished or antagonized can be grouped under four different headings: (i) drug sequestration; (ii) pharmacokinetic antagonism; (iii) pharmacodynamic antagonism; and (iv) physiologic antagonism.

Drug sequestration represents a rather special situation in which the action of an agent can be reduced. The mechanisms are distinct from the other three mechanisms to be discussed. What can be termed "sequestration" can occur either by the direct nonmetabolic chemical reaction of a drug with another chemical (for example, oxidation or reduction of thiols) or by the direct binding of an agent to a serum protein or other constituent (e.g., binding to food or an ion exchange resin in the gastrointestinal tract) before the drug has a chance to reach its site of action. The use of metal chelating agents for antagonizing heavy metal poisoning or resins such as cholestyramine to lower blood cholesterol make use of this kind of "antagonism."

Agents that serve to increase agonist excretion or to hasten drug metabolism may appear to act as "antagonists" by altering the pharmacokinetic parameters of the agonist. For instance, alkalinization of the urine serves to hasten the excretion of weak acids, thereby diminishing the effect of agents like barbiturates. Similarly, the increase in the metabolic cytochrome P450 enzyme system caused by one drug (e.g., barbiturates) can serve to hasten the metabolism and reduce markedly the effect of a second drug (e.g., coumadin; see Chapter 2 for further details). Such effects may be termed "pharmacokinetic antagonism."

Antagonists that interfere with one or more steps in the cell activation pathway triggered by agonists (i.e., pharmacodynamic antagonists) may do so at a number of levels. At the level of the receptor itself (page 11), pharmacodynamic antagonists may act either competitively or noncompetitively to prevent agonist binding; the antagonist may or may not do so by binding directly to the agonist binding site on the receptor. Further, such antagonism at the receptor level may or may not be reversible. Alternatively, a pharmacodynamic antagonist may act at some postreceptor step in the chain of events leading to cell activation so as to abrogate agonist action. For instance, an agent that sequesters intracellular calcium or that blocks the entry of calcium into cells can antagonize the action of contractile agents like norepinephrine that cause their effects by a receptor-mediated increase in cytoplasmic calcium.

The physiologic property of integrated cell systems to respond dynamically to stimulation by initiating counterregulatory pathways (every action has an opposite reaction) provides for the ability of two drugs to antagonize each other's action by independent but counteracting pathways. For instance, the ability of one neurotransmitter to excite and another to inhibit the activity of a neuron would constitute "physiologic antagonism." Alternatively, the ability of angiotensin to increase smooth muscle contraction by elevating intracellular calcium while lowering cyclic AMP could be antagonized physiologically by the ability of isoproterenol to elevate cellular cyclic AMP. In essence, the term "physiologic antagonism" can be applied to the situation where two agents oppose one another's action by acting on separate biochemical pathways or on separate cell systems. Physiologic antagonism provides a mechanism for counteracting the effects of an irreversible (noncompetitive) pharmacologic antagonist. Importantly, physiologic antagonism (unlike competitive antagonism) can be caused by agents quite unrelated to the agonist causing the initial response. Many therapeutic regimens (e.g., the use of β-adrenergic bronchodilators in the setting of asthma) make use of the principle of physiologic antagonism.

Desensitization and Drug Resistance

One of the most intriguing types of drug antagonism stems from the ability of an individual agent, with repeated use, to abrogate its own action (see Fig. 1.5). This phenomenon is variously referred to as **desensitization** or "tachyphylaxis" and is, in the strict sense, used to refer to the reduced response over a short time frame (e.g. seconds to minutes), for a system (e.g., contracting muscle) towards one agonist (e.g., acetylcholine) but not another (e.g., bradykinin). The term **tolerance** is usually reserved for an analogous phenomenon (e.g., for opiate drugs) that develops over a longer period, e.g., hours to weeks. In the context of drug therapy, the terms **drug resistance** (especially with regard to antimicrobial agents) or drug refractoriness also can be used to describe the diminished response to a particular agent. In analyzing this phenomenon, it is important to determine whether the reduced response is either chemically *specific* or *generalized* (i.e.,

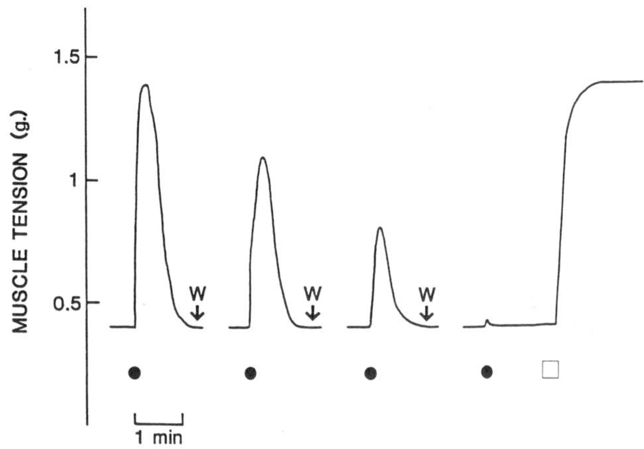

Figure 1.5 Example of desensitization. A drug results in an increase in muscle tension when injected into an organ bath (indicated by ●). After washing (W) the tissue with fresh medium, repeated administration of the drug produces a diminishing response that eventually disappears altogether. This desensitization is specific, because application of a different drug (□) still can produce muscle contraction.

whether there is cross-tolerance or cross-desensitization for other agents in a series of chemically-related compounds; heterologous desensitization). A generalized desensitization might be caused, for instance, by an agonist that acts initially by releasing a neurotransmitter, but then fails to act when all the transmitter supply has been depleted. In this situation, the system would be generally desensitized to a variety of unrelated agonists that also depend for their action on the release of the same neurotransmitter. The distinction between receptor-specific tachyphylaxis (or resistance) and generalized desensitization can be of practical value when planning therapeutic regimens that depend on the ability of drugs to act by distinct, nondesensitizing pathways.

The mechanisms that lead to desensitization can be thought of in terms of most of the same categories that were used above to explain general drug antagonism. Thus, at the pharmacokinetic level (see Chapter 2), a drug may induce its own clearance (e.g., by inducing metabolic enzymes or by blocking a reabsorption system in the kidney), thereby reducing its own activity. Alternatively, at the pharmacodynamic level, an agent, when activating a cell, may cause rapid disappearance of its own receptors (so-called "receptor down-regulation"; see page 33), resulting in a reduced response to subsequent doses of the specific agonist but not to the administration of other agents. Finally, at the physiologic level, one agonist that acts via an elevation of cellular cyclic AMP may simultaneously trigger a rise in the enzyme, cyclic AMP phosphodiesterase, that metabolizes this cellular messenger; thus all subsequent stimuli by agents that act by elevating cyclic AMP levels would be diminished. By analyzing the mechanisms whereby desensitization occurs, it should prove possible to develop rational approaches for overcoming the several types of drug resistance that can be encountered in therapeutic settings.

Dose-Response Curves: Characterizing Pharmacologic Receptors by Bioassay

Classifying Receptors According to the Selective Action of Poisons and According to a Constellation of Responses

As heralded by Ehrlich's concept of distinct drug "classes" comprising a chemical series of compounds,[r1] many drugs can now be classified according to the receptor systems with which they interact. Early work related to receptor classification depended either on the selective action of specific toxic agonists, such as nicotine (targeted to the receptor at the neuromuscular junction) and muscarine (acting selectively on glandular and smooth muscle elements) or on a constellation of distinguishable physiologic effects evoked by a single drug like epinephrine (alpha effects—in general, contractile and excitatory; beta effects—in general, inhibitory, in terms of regulating smooth muscle tension, although excitatory in the heart). In retrospect, the constellation of "alpha" effects, observed in an intact animal by monitoring responses such as an increase in blood pressure, vasoconstriction, and salivary gland secretion after epinephrine administration can now be seen as due to the concurrent activation of the same class of adrenergic receptors in a variety of tissues. Likewise, the "beta" effects (e.g., relaxation of bronchial smooth muscle, vasodilatation, relaxation of the uterus, increase in heart rate) can be seen as the activation of a receptor distinct from the "alpha" adrenergic receptor. These early insights, documenting the functional physiologic consequences of activating specific receptor systems depended on: (i) the high degree of selectivity of a number of receptors for their specific agonists, (e.g., nicotine, muscarine, norepinephrine, epinephrine) or antagonists (e.g., curare for the neuromuscular junction or atropine for glandular tissue); (ii) on the unique cellular differentiation of individual tissues such as smooth muscle or striated muscle that contain localized specific receptors at physiologically strategic anatomic sites so as to regulate over-all organ function. Thus, the actions of acetylcholine at the neuromuscular junction that mimicked the action of nicotine were said to be mediated by receptors termed "nicotinic," whereas those receptors in smooth muscle and glandular tissue that also responded to acetylcholine, but were selectively activated by muscarine, were termed "muscarinic." Further, the actions of the catecholamine, epinephrine, were subdivided into "alpha" and "beta" effects that served to define alpha and beta adrenergic receptors, as will be elaborated on below.

Receptor Classification According to the Relative Potencies of Agonists

The qualitative physiologic approach to receptor classification described above was widely applicable in many species, including humans, but met with somewhat limited success in defining discrete receptor systems. More detailed insights were obtained by the use of a quantitative analysis of agonist action in terms of the relative potencies of a series of compounds, as characterized by dose-response curves such as those illustrated in Figure 1.6. The main principle was elegantly illustrated by the landmark work of Ahlquist[6] who went far beyond the physiologic characterization of adrenergic receptors as being simply "excitatory" or "inhibitory." Using the constellation of effects (so-

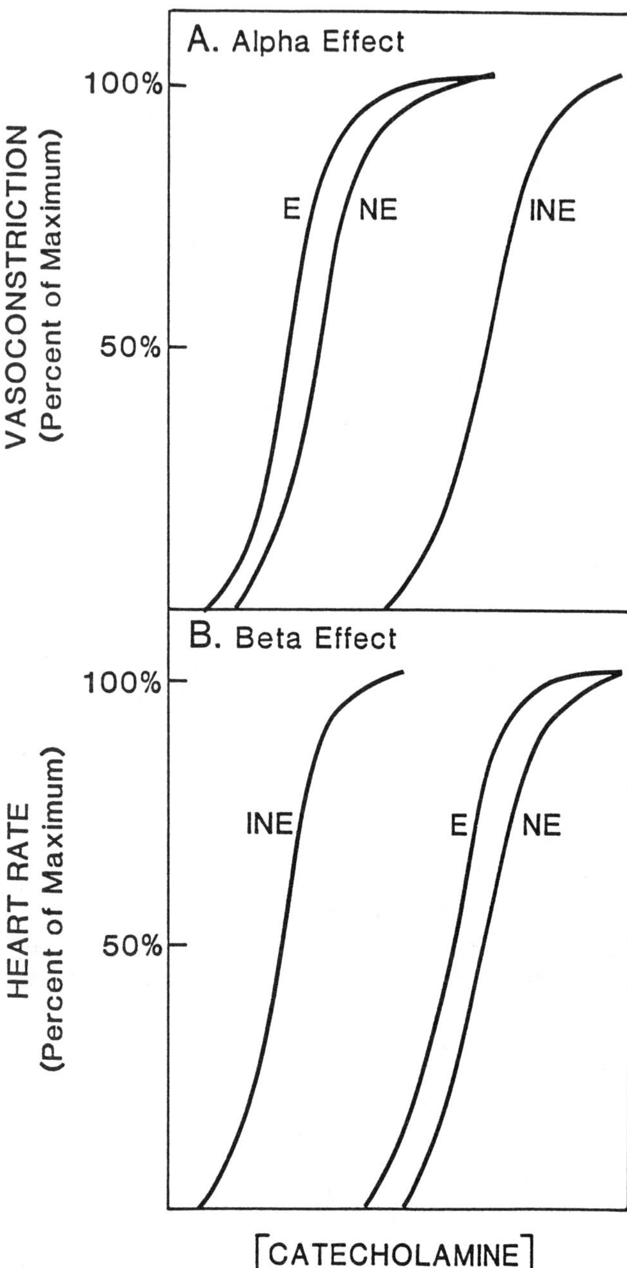

Figure 1.6 Classification of receptors according to the relative potencies of agonists. The effect of increasing concentrations of epinephrine (E), norepinephrine (NE), and isoproterenol (INE) is shown for two biologic responses: vasoconstriction (Panel A) and increasing heart rate (Panel B). Comparison of the order of potencies for the different catecholamines resulted in the classification of adrenergic receptors into alpha (A) and beta (B) subtypes by Ahlquist.[6]

called "alpha" responses) as a monitor of drug action (vasoconstriction, excitation of the uterus, contraction of the nictitating membrane of the eye, dilatation of the pupil, and inhibition of the gut), Ahlquist observed that the catecholamines norepinephrine, epinephrine, and isoproterenol had an order of potency (ED_{50}, Fig. 1.6, *A*) of: epinephrine ≥ norepinephrine >> isoproterenol. Conversely, the same series of amines had an entirely different order of potency (Fig. 1.6, *B*; isoproterenol >> epinephrine ≥ norepinephrine) when physiologically so-called "beta" responses were monitored (vasodilatation, inhibition of the uterus, and myocardial stimulation). Based on these relative orders of potencies, Ahlquist[6] postulated the existence of two distinct classes of catecholamine receptors, with the first response profile as being characteristic of the "alpha receptor" and the second, the "beta receptor." This principle of defining receptors according to the relative potencies of a series of agonists has proved to be of enormous use for the general classification of a wide variety of receptor systems (e.g., for dopamine, histamine, and serotonin), as well as for their further subclassification into subtypes (for example, the alpha 1 and 2, and beta 1 and 2 receptor systems for catecholamines). Furthermore, the use of a potency series to classify a receptor does not depend at all on the specific response used to monitor the action of a number of agonists.

Using Antagonists to Characterize Receptors

Qualitative Analysis of Antagonist Action

Perhaps one of the most clear-cut methods for the classification of receptors by bioassay procedures stems from the use of selective antagonists, employing both qualitative and quantitative approaches. It has already been mentioned that the drug curare is selective in blocking the action of acetylcholine at the neuromuscular junction, whereas atropine has no antagonist action in this system. Moreover, at the neuromuscular junction, decamethonium (C-10) optimally blocks acetylcholine action, whereas a shorter analogue, hexamethonium (C-6), is optimally active in blocking acetylcholine at ganglia. On the other hand, atropine blocks acetylcholine action in glandular tissue and in smooth muscle, whereas curare does not. Thus, by using a number of distinct antagonists that selectively block the actions of a single agonist (e.g., acetylcholine) in a variety of systems, it is possible to identify chemically distinct receptor systems. In the case illustrated above, three unique receptors for acetylcholine can be identified: two types of "nicotinic" receptors in nerve and muscle, and one type of "muscarinic" receptor in glandular and smooth muscle tissue. Similarly, the selective antagonism by the beta receptor-specific drug, propranolol, of the actions of isoproterenol in a variety of tissues can be used to identify the presence of beta-adrenergic receptors in such systems.

A key element in the use of antagonists to characterize a receptor system qualitatively lies in the demonstration that the antagonist's ability to reverse the action of an agent (either reversibly or noncompetitively, see Fig. 1.4) is agonist-specific. For instance, propranolol, an antagonist of the beta-adrenergic receptor would be expected to reverse the actions of a catecholamine, such as isoproterenol (e.g., increasing heart rate), but not to affect the chronotropic action of glucagon. It is important to appreciate that the specificity of many antagonists may be restricted to a limited concentration range (e.g., nanomolar to micromolar, but not above micromolar concentrations, where nonspecific antagonism might occur). Once the specificity of an antagonist is clearly defined in one particular system or tissue, it can be used as a qualitative tool, as outlined above for propranolol, to characterize drug receptors in other systems or tissues. For instance, knowing that the adrenergic antagonist, propranolol, at appropriate concentrations, is specific for beta receptors in the cardiovascular system, allows one to conclude that the lipolytic action of the catecholamine, isoproterenol, in adipose tissue, which is blocked by propranolol, must be mediated by an adipocyte beta-receptor.

Quantitative Analysis of Competitive Antagonist Action

Quantitative information about a competitive antagonist can also be derived from an analysis of families of dose-response curves for a given agonist measured at increasing concentrations of antagonist (e.g., curves a_1, a_{10}, Fig. 1.4), as first described by Arunlakshana and Schild.[7] In essence, the degree to which a dose-response curve shifts to the right for a given increase in competitive antagonist concentration (i.e., the magnitude of the dose-ratio, A_1/A_0, Fig. 1.4) is quantitatively related to the affinity with which the **antagonist** (but not the agonist) binds to the receptor at which the agonist is acting. That is, the shift in the response curves provide information about the affinity of the antagonist for the receptor, but not about the affinity of the agonist that is triggering the receptor. Quantitatively, the above information can be expressed by the following equations, which are based on the assumption of a reversible mass-action equilibrium of binding of the agonist, A, and antagonist, B, to a receptor, R.

The binding of an agonist, A, and an antagonist, B, to the receptor, R, can be expressed by the equations:

$$A + R \rightleftharpoons AR \text{ (AR = agonist-receptor complex)} \tag{1}$$

$$B + R \rightleftharpoons BR \text{ (BR = antagonist receptor complex)} \tag{2}$$

At equilibrium, the mass action equation for the binding of agonist in the **absence** of antagonist is given by Equation (3); and in the **presence** of antagonist, the equation for the agonist dissociation constant, K_A, is given by Equation (4)

$$K_A = \frac{([R] - [AR])\,[A_0]}{[AR]} \tag{3}$$

$$K_A = \frac{([R] - [AR] - [BR])\,[A_1]}{[AR]} \tag{4}$$

In Equations (3) and (4), $[A_0]$ and $[A_1]$ are the concentrations of agonist that are required to yield the same concentration of agonist-receptor complex [AR] either in the absence ($[A_0]$) or presence ($[A_1]$) of antagonist. [R] represents the TOTAL concentration of receptors present in the system. In the presence of agonist, the dissociation constant for the antagonist, K_B, is given by the equation:

$$K_B = \frac{([R] - [AR] - [BR])\,[B]}{[BR]} \tag{5}$$

Since the left-hand sides of Equations (3) and (4) are equal:

$$K_A = \frac{([R] - [AR])\,[A_0]}{[AR]} = \frac{([R] - [AR] - [BR])\,[A_1]}{[AR]} \tag{6}$$

canceling [AR] and rearranging Equation (6) yields Equation (7):

$$\frac{[A_1]}{[A_0]} = \frac{([R] - [AR])}{([R] - [AR] - [BR])} \tag{7}$$

The ratio, $[A_1]/[A_0]$, is defined as the "dose ratio", X, that is, the relative concentration of agonist in the presence and absence of antagonist that is required to yield the *same* amount of agonist-receptor complex. Substituting for $[A_1]/[A_0]$ by X into Equation (7) and rearranging yields the equation:

$$[BR] = \frac{([R] - [AR])\,(X - 1);}{X} \tag{8}$$

and, substituting for [BR] into Equation (5) leads to Equation (9), relating the antagonist dissociation constant, K_B, to the dose-ratio, X, and the free concentration of antagonist, [B]. In practice, the free concentration of antagonist (i.e., the concentration *not* bound to the receptor) is essentially the same as the total concentration of antagonist present in an assay system $[B_t]$. Thus, one reaches the surprisingly simple equation:

$$K_B = [B_t]/(X - 1) \tag{9}$$

Only one assumption is required to link equation (9), based on the mass-action equilibria envisioned by Langley and Ehrlich, directly to the bioassay data illustrated in Figure 1.4: that is, one must assume only that the *same* concentration of agonist-receptor complex [AR], is required to produce a response (Y in Fig. 1.4) in the presence of antagonist as is required to yield the *same* response (Y) in the absence of antagonist. This assumption allows a formal link to be made between the concentrations A_0 and A_1 shown in the dose-response curve (Fig. 1.4) and the concentrations of agonist $[A_0, A_1]$ recorded in Equations (3) to (5), wherein the concentrations of agonist-receptor complex [AR] are said to be equal. Equation (9), often referred to as the 'Schild' equation,[7,8] has proved of enormous use not only for estimating antagonist dissociation constants directly from bioassay data but also for analyzing ligand binding data for agonist-receptor interactions.[r3] From Equation (9), it can be seen that if the dose-ratio X = 2, then $K_B = [B_t]$. That is, if one can determine the concentration of antagonist for which one must double the concentration of agonist to achieve the same response, one obtains directly the antagonist dissociation constant. In practice, Equation (9) is rearranged:

$$\log (X - 1) = \log[B_t] - \log K_B \tag{10}$$

and plot of log (X – 1) versus log[B] is used to estimate the value of K_B from the abscissa intercept, equal to $-\log K_B$. For true competitive antagonists, the slope of the curve should be equal to 1.0, regardless of the concentration of antagonist. Two comments are in order regarding Equations (9) and (10), which are valid only for compounds displaying competitive antagonism. First, the equation contains information (K_B, [B]) only about the **antagonist.** Thus, the value obtained for K_B should be independent of the nature of the agonist and should be the same for experiments done with any agonist that acts on the receptor population to which the antagonist binds. Second, the dose ratio, X, makes no assumption as to the magnitude of the response that is chosen as a reference point for the measurements (i.e., Y in Fig. 1.4 may be chosen at any convenient response level). The dose-ratio relationship described by Equations (9) and (10) has proved to be valid in many studies reported in the literature, wherein dose-ratios as high as 10^4 have been used. In principle, the same receptor, if present in different tissues or even in different species should, via this approach, yield the same K_B for an antagonist and, in practice, this has been found to be the case. Few mathematical predictions of biologic behaviour can boast of such a wide-ranging success.

Quantitative Analysis of Agonist Affinity Using an Irreversible Antagonist

As illustrated by the work of Furchgott,[9] the use of a special type of irreversible antagonist that inactivates a specific receptor permanently can be used to obtain information about the affinity of the agonist for its receptor by a bioassay approach. The principles of the assay procedure are basically two-fold. First one must assume, as with the dose-ratio method, that, when the tissue response is the same, before and after antagonist treatment, then the number (or concentration) of agonist receptor complexes present, [AR], must be the same. Implicit in this assumption is the expectation that the receptor has only a single affinity state for the agonist. Secondly, one must assume that the irreversible antagonist permanently inactivates a fraction of receptors, preventing agonist binding and abrogating any response by the inactivated receptor. As with the dose-ratio method, no assumption need be made about the precise mathematical relationship between the number of occupied receptors and a tissue response. Given these two assumptions, one can use Equation (3) to express the concentration of agonist-receptor complexes, [AR], present either before (3a) or after (3b) the irreversible inactivation of a fraction of the total number of receptors present, leaving behind a fraction of the original receptors, [qR], remaining in the active state; q can assume any value between 0 and 1. Before receptor inactivation,

$$K_A = \frac{[R] - [AR])\,[A]}{[AR]};\; [AR] = \frac{[R]\,[A]}{K_A + [A]} \tag{3a}$$

After receptor inactivation, where the concentration of active receptors remaining is [qR], and the new equally effective agonist concentration is A′;

$$K_A = \frac{([qR] - [A'qR])\,[A']}{[A'qR]};\; [A'qR] = \frac{[qR]\,[A']}{K_A + [A']} \tag{3b}$$

However, if [AR] = [A′qR], when the response of the preparation is the same, before and after receptor inactivation, then one can equate Equations (3a) and (3b). Rearranging, one obtains the relationship:

$$\frac{1}{[A]} = \frac{1}{q[A']} + \frac{(1-q)}{q}\frac{1}{K_A} \tag{11}$$

In Equation 11, the concentrations of agonist, [A] and [A′], represent those concentrations causing the SAME response (i.e., same y-axis value, Fig. 1.4, lower) either before ([A]) or after ([A′]) treatment with the irreversible receptor antagonist. In practice, dose-response curves for an agonist are determined both before (e.g., curve C_0, Fig. 1.4) or after (e.g., curve C_1) irreversible inactivation of a proportion of the receptors in a preparation. According to Equation (11), a plot of 1/[A] versus 1/[A′] should yield a straight line with a slope of 1/q and an intercept of $\frac{(1-q)}{qK_A}$. The value of q is obtained from 1/slope; and the value of K_A from the expression, (slope-1)/y-intercept. The main drawback of the Furchgott approach to estimating agonist affinity relates to the necessity of synthesizing suitable irreversible antagonists that react specifically with the agonist binding site. A further drawback relates to the common use of an alkylation reaction that can modify not only the receptor to which the alkylating antagonist binds but also other important nonreceptor constituents in the plasma membrane. Further, the approach assumes equilibrium of binding between the agonist and its receptor and does not permit the measurement of multiple binding steps and multiple affinity states for the agonist-receptor complex. Thus, the use of irreversible receptor inactivation to estimate agonist affinity by bioassay with the approach of Furchgott[9] has not been as widely applied as has the dose-ratio method of Arunlakshana and Schild[7] for estimating antagonist affinity constants.

Summary

In summary, this section illustrates that it is possible to characterize a receptor system entirely by a pharmacologic approach using qualitative and quantitative bioassay systems. This approach comprises: (i) the use of system-selective agonists; (ii) the measurement of the relative potencies (ED_{50}s) of a series of chemically related agonists; (iii) the characterization of the qualitative actions of selective antagonists; and (iv) the quantitative estimate of the agonist and antagonist affinity constants for a specific receptor. This characterization of receptor systems using a bioassay approach has provided the essential basis for the biochemical characterization of receptors to be described in subsequent sections. It is important to note that the biologic approach to receptor characterization makes no assumption about either the molecular identity or the cellular location of the receptor. All that is required is a responsive system in which agonist action can be quantitated and a handful of appropriate agonists and antagonists.

Biochemical Characterization of Receptors

Measurements of Ligand Binding

By the early 1920s, the receptor concept was already firmly established and attempts were being made to develop equations relating the amount of agonist bound to the magnitude of a cellular response. For instance, Clark[10,11] established that heart tissue can respond to acetylcholine under conditions where vanishingly small numbers of agonist molecules would be bound by each heart cell. Using a bioassay for the amount of acetylcholine taken up by heart tissue exposed to the agonist at contractile concentrations, Clark performed the first "ligand binding" experiments by estimating that contraction was caused by the binding of about 20,000 molecules of acetylcholine.[10] Because of the low number of receptors present on responsive cells, little success was met in attempts to detect receptors by ligand binding methods until it became possible to synthesize radioactive receptor probes with sufficiently high specific radioactivity and with sufficient selectivity for a receptor. The requirements for the measurement of ligand binding are shown in Table 1.1. The key to the success of such studies was an understanding of the properties or characteristics of receptor binding,[r4] specifically the requirement for high affinity, reversibility, and appropriate receptor specificity in competition experiments that would be expected on the basis of the pharmacologic properties of the receptor documented by the bioassay procedures outlined earlier in this chapter. Such an approach was elegantly illustrated by the work of Paton and Rang,[12] who were the first to measure directly the binding of ^{3}H-labeled atropine to the muscarinic receptor present in guinea pig ileal smooth muscle. In their study, the high-affinity component of the atropine binding curve (dissociation constant of 1 nM) matched exactly the affinity of atropine for its receptor measured by bioassay procedures using either the rate method of Paton[13] or the dose-ratio method of Arunlakshana and Schild,[7] whereas the low-affinity site did not. It was possible to conclude, therefore, that the high-affinity binding site represented the pharmacologically relevant binding to the receptor. Thus, in measurements of ligand binding, the bioassay data provide the essential context in which the kinetic parameters of binding can be meaningfully interpreted. Such studies, integrating the previously available pharmacologic data with ligand binding measurements have, to date, provided an enormous amount of information about the numbers and affinities of a variety of receptors present in many tissue targets. An example of such a study involving the binding of the peptide growth factor, epidermal growth factor-urogastrone (EGF-URO), to its receptor in intact cultured human fibroblasts[r3,14] is shown in Figure 1.7 (upper panel). The use of an intact cell system for ligand binding studies allows for a direct comparison with the biologic response, i.e., the mitogenic action (^{3}H-thymidine incorporation) of EGF-URO, measured under comparable experimental conditions.

Table 1.1 Requirements for Measurement of Ligand Binding

1. Radioligand with appropriate specific activity
2. Availability of intact cells, isolated membranes, or soluble (detergent-solubilized) receptor preparations
3. Methodology for the rapid separation of receptor-bound and free radioligand
4. Determination of "specific" versus "nonspecific" binding, by measuring the quantity of bound radioligand in the absence (Total) and in the presence (Nonspecific) of excess unlabeled drug of known pharmacological specificity. (Total − nonspecific = specific).

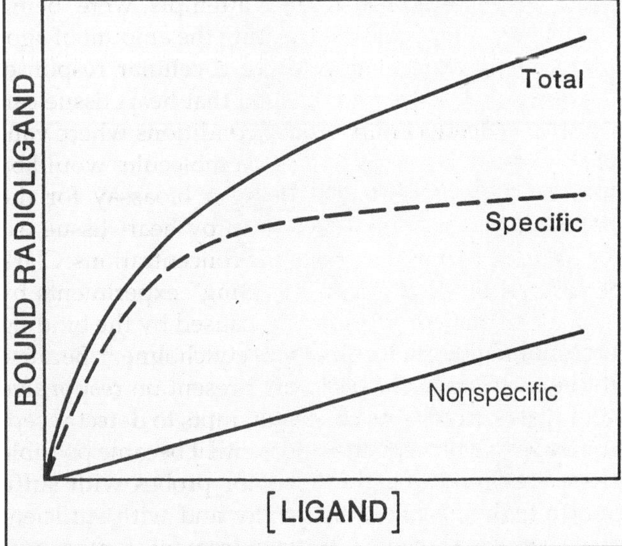

Once the specificity of binding has been established in an intact cell system (i.e., only EGF-URO and its analogues compete for the binding shown in Figure 1.7), it becomes possible to study in greater depth the cellular location and biochemical properties of the receptor. It is now a relatively straightforward procedure, using differential centrifugation and other approaches, to localize the receptor in one of several cell compartments. For instance, receptors for peptides, amines, and many other agents are now known to be localized at the plasma membrane, whereas receptors for steroids hormones are found in the cytoplasmic or nuclear compartments. As soon as the location of the receptor is known, a detailed biochemical characterization can proceed. For illustrative purposes, the discussion that follows will refer to a receptor localized in the plasma membrane. However, the general approach would be the same, irrespective of the location of the receptor.

Quantitative Analysis of Binding

Using the binding specificity of a receptor established in intact cell systems as a guide, it becomes possible to study the properties of the receptor in particulate or solubilized preparations. One question that must be answered before a receptor can be isolated from its tissue source is: does the amount of receptor present in the tissue preparation make the tissue a realistic starting material for an isolation protocol? In the literature dealing with receptor binding, the data are often analyzed according to the mass action relationship derived essentially from equations (1) and (3)

$$(A + R) \rightleftharpoons AR; \quad K_A = ([R] - [AR])\,[A]/[AR])$$

but rewritten in terms of: (i) the total number of receptor binding sites present in the system, R = Bmax; (ii) the proportion of total receptors occupied by a bound ligand, ie., B/Bmax; and (iii) the free concentration of bound ligand, A = F. K_A is the equilibrium dissociation constant for the agonist-receptor complex. Rewriting Equation (3), substituting [R] = Bmax, [A] = F, and [AR] = B, yields the relationship:

$$K_A = \frac{(\text{Bmax} - \text{B})\ (\text{F})}{\text{B}} \tag{12}$$

Rearranging Equation (12),

$$K_A\text{B} = (\text{F})\ (\text{Bmax}) - (\text{F})\ (\text{B}) \tag{13}$$

or

$$\frac{\text{B}}{\text{F}} = \frac{-\text{B}}{K_A} + \frac{\text{Bmax}}{K_A} \tag{14}$$

Equation (14) is the relationship originally discussed by Scatchard[15] for noninteracting binding sites and for which a plot of B/F versus B yields Bmax from the abscissa intercept and ($-1/K_A$) from the slope of the resulting straight line. Scatchard analysis of the binding of EGF-URO to human placental cell membranes (Fig. 1.7, lower insert) gives a receptor dissociation constant of 0.4 nM and a receptor density of 30 pmoles per mg membrane protein. This approach has been used to study the binding of a wide variety of agonists and antagonists (ranging from peptides and amines to steroid hormones) to their putative receptors. Many receptors for biologically active pharmacologic compounds have turned out to be proteins that bind their ligands via the reversible noninteractive binding mechanisms envisioned by Scatchard. The data for Scatchard analysis of a saturation isotherm (Fig. 1.7) must be obtained from equilibrium conditions of radioligand binding to the receptor preparation. Therefore, experiments to determine the rate of association must first be performed to determine the time at which saturation binding measurements can be made. The determination of both dissociation (k_{-1}) and association (k_1) rate constants for radioligand binding permits the derivation of the dissociation constant from these kinetic experiments ($K_A = k_{-1}/k_1$), which should agree with the K_A determined from Scatchard analysis of data obtained from experiments performed at equilibrium. The interpretation of data from ligand binding experiments has been facilitated by the availability of computer analysis.[16,17]

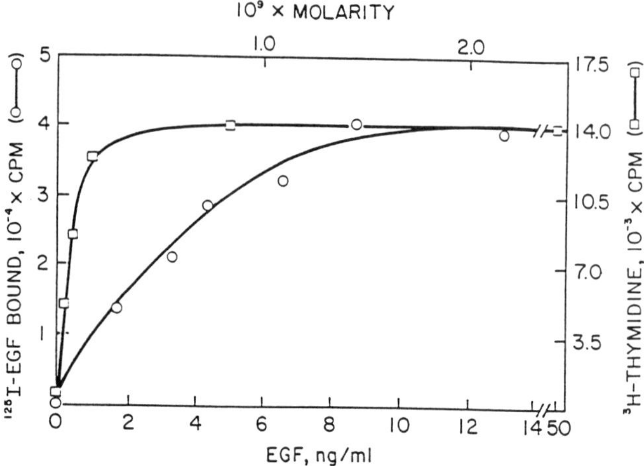

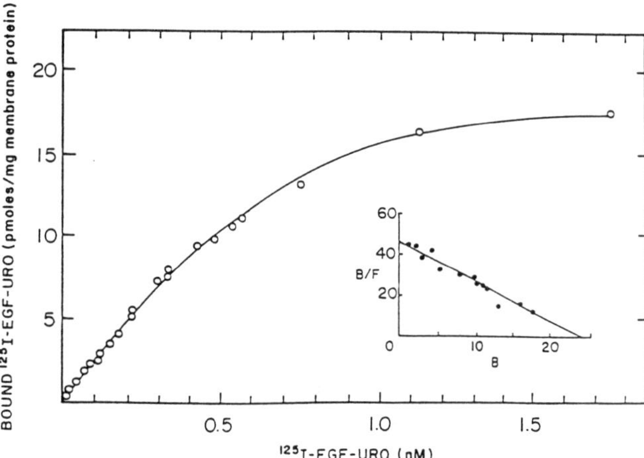

Figure 1.7 *Upper Panel*: Binding of radiolabeled epidermal growth factor-urogastrone (^{125}I-EGF-URO) and thymidine incorporation into DNA, as a function of EGF concentration in human fibroblast monolayer cultures. Note that a maximal mitogenic effect is observed at a concentration of EGF that results in occupancy of approximately 25% of the total number of receptor binding sites.

Lower Panel: Binding of epidermal growth factor-urogastrone (EGF-URO) to human placental membranes. The relationship between specific binding and the concentration of radiolabeled EGF-URO is shown, demonstrating high affinity and saturability. Scatchard analysis of this binding curve is shown in the insert (data from Cuatrecasas and Hollenberg;[r3] Hock and Hollenberg[14]).

Analysis of Covalently Attached Receptor-Ligand Conjugates

After binding to its receptor, a radioactively labeled ligand, such as ^{125}I-insulin or ^{125}I-EGF-URO, can be permanently attached to the receptor by chemical crosslinking procedures. Once crosslinked specifically to the ligand, the radioactively tagged receptor-ligand conjugate can be solubilized and analyzed by a variety of biochemical procedures (e.g., gel filtration, gel electrophoresis) that yield information about its size and subunit composition. The crosslink-labeling principle has been used for the characterization of a number of

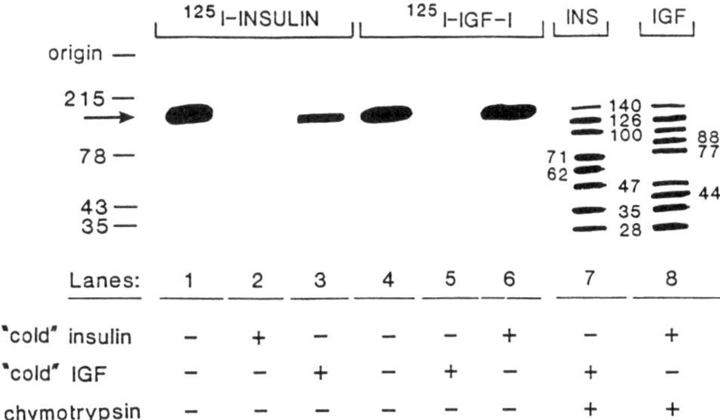

Figure 1.8 Example of chemical crosslinking to characterize receptors for insulin and insulin-like growth factor-1 (IGF-1). Receptors in placental plasma membranes were cross-linked labeled with either [^{125}I]-insulin (lane 1) or [^{125}I]IGF-1 (lane 4), using the cross-linking reagent disuccininimidyl suberate. Receptors were identified as a 140 kilodalton band (indicated by the *arrow*) on an autoradiogram following polyacrylamide gel electrophoresis. The mobilities of molecular weight markers are shown on the left (values in kilodaltons). Specificity of the cross-link labeling of the respective receptors was assessed by determining the ability of excess unlabeled "cold" insulin (lanes 2 and 6) or "cold" IGF-1 (lanes 3 and 5) to compete for radiolabeling. Thus, labeling of the IGF-1 receptor was abolished by "cold" IGF-1 (lane 5) but not by "cold" insulin (lane 6). The specifically-labeled insulin and IGF-1 receptors from lanes 3 and 6, respectively, were also subjected to proteolytic mapping with chymotrypsin (lanes 7 and 8). Both receptors had common constituents with apparent molecular weights (in kilodaltons) of 126, 100, 47, 35 and 38. The cross-link labeled insulin receptor had two unique fragments (71 and 62) whereas the IGF-1 receptor was characterized as having three (88, 77 and 44), indicating that although both receptors exhibit marked similarities in domain structure, there were subtle structural differences. (Results from Bhaumick et al.[18])

receptors, including those for peptides, amines, and steroid hormones. As an example, the receptor "footprints" derived from an autoradiogram after polyacrylamide gel electrophoresis of placental membranes cross-linked with either ^{125}I-insulin or ^{125}I-insulin-like growth factor I (^{125}I-IGF-I) are shown in Figure 1.8.[18] Although the receptors for both radioligands have an apparent Mr of 130- to 140-kdalton, the IGF-I receptor can be distinguished from the insulin receptor, based on two experimental findings. First, excess unlabeled ("cold") insulin did not abolish the labeling with radioiodinated IGF-I (Fig. 1.8, lane 6), indicating specificity of radioligand binding. And second, the peptide maps of the cross-linked receptors following proteolysis with chymotrypsin show several distinct fragments in addition to a number of common radiolabeled fragments, suggesting that the receptors for insulin and IGF-I exhibit both marked similarities in domain structure and some subtle structural differences.

Receptor Isolation

The ligand binding assay provides the essential key for receptor isolation. Indeed, the use of a binding assay that detects the soluble receptor makes it possible to characterize the hydrodynamic properties of a given receptor (e.g., behavior on gel filtration columns or in the ultracentrifuge). However, because of the low abundance of receptors in their target tissues (e.g., 10^{-12} to 10^{-15} moles/mg membrane protein), it has been necessary to develop specialized biochemical methods for use in conjunction with conventional biochemical procedures (e.g., gel filtration and ion exchange chromatography) to isolate pure receptor material for analysis. By far, the use of the technique of affinity chromatography, as adapted by Cuatrecasas and colleagues for the isolation of the insulin receptor,[r3] has proved to be the most important cornerstone for the majority of receptor isolation procedures. The principle of the affinity chromatographic approach, originally developed by Cuatrecasas and Wilchek in the Anfinsen laboratory,[19] is illustrated in Figure 1.9, wherein the insulin

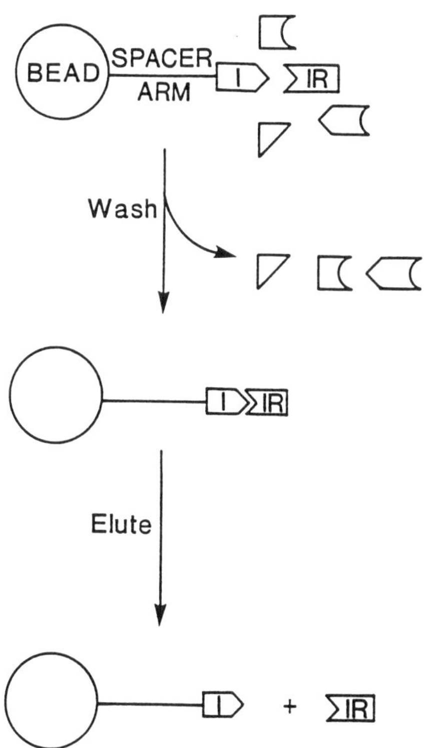

Figure 1.9 Purification of receptors by affinity chromatography. As an example, insulin can be covalently linked by a spacer arm to an agarose bead. The insulin receptor in a crude broken-cell preparation containing many other proteins will bind selectively to the insulin on the insoluble beads so that the other proteins can be washed away. Elution of the insulin receptor then results in a high degree of purification.

receptor is seen to bind specifically to the insoluble agarose support to which insulin has been covalently linked by a spacer arm. Such immobilized hormone derivatives have proved of enormous value not only because of their use for receptor isolation protocols but also because they were used to demonstrate unequivocally that an agonist (e.g., insulin) could cause its biologic effect entirely by an action at the cell surface without entering the cell.

The successful purification of the nicotinic acetylcholine receptor from the neuromuscular junction[r5] depended on two factors that emphasize some of the key features of the biochemical approaches listed above. The first was the availability of tissue from the electric organs of rays (Torpedo) and eels (Electrophorus), which are enormously enriched in receptor material. The second important factor was the use of a radiolabeled toxin from snake venom (α-bungarotoxin) as a potent and selective marker for the receptor during purification procedures. As a result, the nicotinic acetylcholine receptor was the first receptor to be isolated in sufficient amounts for the determination of its partial amino acid sequence.

Analysis of Receptor Sequence and Domain Function by Molecular Cloning

By combining conventional methods of protein purification with affinity chromatography techniques, it has become possible to isolate sufficient amounts of a number of receptors to permit the determination of partial amino acid sequences and to obtain specific antireceptor antibodies. Both the microsequence information and the antireceptor antibodies can be used to develop suitable probes (either oligonucleotide reagents for probing cDNA libraries or antibody reagents for analyzing cDNA expression systems) for the cloning of receptor cDNA and, by extension, for the determination of the entire amino acid sequence of a receptor.

As an alternative, the ability of oocyte systems to express functional receptors after the injection of receptor mRNA has provided for the expression cloning of a number of receptors that proved refractory to other approaches. One key to expression cloning has proved to be an assay of ligand-modulated ion flux. The expression cloning of the thrombin receptor, using thrombin-modulated calcium flux[20] provides an excellent example of the identification of a receptor that did not lend itself to the ligand binding and protein purification approaches outlined above.

An important feature of the receptor cloning approach relates to the ability to transfect a particular receptor cDNA so as to allow for its expression in a host cell that initially does not possess the receptor of interest. For example, each of the protein subunits of the nicotinic acetylcholine receptor at the neuromuscular junction have been cloned and sequenced.[r6] Expression of cloned subunits in frog oocytes resulted in the formation of functional ligand (acetylcholine)-gated ion channels in the cell membrane. This type of expression experiment provides the final and ultimate test of the validity of the biochemical and molecular biologic approaches to receptor characterization. Furthermore, the availability of cDNA probes for the neuromuscular nicotinic receptor, together with unique monoclonal anti-receptor antibodies, then made it possible to clone and sequence the neuronal nicotinic receptor.[r7] Sequence analysis of receptor clones, both in terms of amino acid sequence and putative membrane topology (transmembrane spanning domains), allows for comparison of homologies or structural relationships between receptors. As a result, the application of molecular cloning techniques to other ion-channel receptors (see below) that are gated by γ-aminobutyric acid (GABA)[21] and glycine[22] has revealed that these amino acid receptors share conserved sequences and domains with nicotinic acetylcholine receptors within an extended receptor superfamily.[r8,r9] Receptor cloning has also revealed unexpected homologies between the receptors for such diverse ligands as a photon of light (rhodopsin) and the sympathetic neurotransmitter norepinephrine (α- and β-adrenoceptors).[r10] As a result, the existence of a superfamily of receptors linked to GTP-binding proteins (see below) has also been discovered. Such a superfamily accounts for the observation that a receptor clone isolated by screening a human genomic library at low stringency with a full-length β_2-adrenoceptor clone was shown after transfection to have the ligand binding characteristics of a serotonin ($5HT_{1A}$) receptor subtype.[23,24]

Cloning studies have also resulted in the description of a far greater number of receptors than had been characterized previously on the basis of pharmacologic data with selective agonists and antagonists. For example, five subtypes of muscarinic receptors for acetylcholine have been cloned,[r11] whereas only three subtypes had been described from bioassay experiments with muscarinic antagonists. The availability of receptor clones coupled with the ability to express both normal and mutant clones after transfection into appropriate model cell systems permits precise structure-function relationships to be established for specific regions or domains in receptors. To illustrate, the structural features of the β-adrenergic receptor important for ligand binding (agonists and antagonists) and receptor activation have been determined by the creation and expression of deletion mutants and by site-directed mutagenesis of specific amino acid residues.[r12,r13] Furthermore, receptor constructs can be prepared in which entire regions or domains from one receptor can be spliced into domains from a second receptor to generate a receptor chimera.[25] Assessment of the function of the chimeric receptor can then provide insight about the individual domains used to synthesize the construct. Naturally occurring receptor mutations can also provide insight into receptor domain function. For instance, insulin receptor mutants obtained from patients with extreme insulin resistance have identified receptor amino acid residues that play key roles in insulin receptor function.[26,27] These transfection/reconstitution experiments, along with an evaluation of naturally occurring receptor mutants, provide for the analysis of receptor domain function at a level of sophistication that would surely have delighted Ehrlich, Langley, and Clark. Finally, knowledge concerning the structure of the genes that encode specific receptors will be an important area for future investigations. In addition, studies of the regulation of receptor gene expression may reveal how posttranscriptional editing of mRNA can generate molecular heterogeneity of receptor transcripts.

Summary

From the information discussed in this section, it can be seen that the biochemical approach to receptor characterization, begun by Clark's early measurements of acetylcholine binding, has led far beyond the pharmacologic approach outlined in the previous section, and has resulted in a description of a number of receptors in quantitative molecular terms. The general approach comprises: (i) development of a reliable and specific ligand binding assay for the compound of interest; (ii) determination of the cellular location and abundance of the receptor; (iii) characterization of the receptor properties (molecular mass, hydrodynamic parameters, subunit composition) using either a soluble receptor binding assay or a crosslink-labeling approach for receptor detection; (iv) isolation of pure receptor by conventional and affinity chromatographic procedures to allow the preparation of antireceptor antibodies and the determination of limited amino acid sequence; (v) the isolation of receptor cDNA, permitting an analysis of the entire deduced receptor amino acid sequence; (vi) expression of functional receptor clones in a transfection system; and (vii) an analysis of receptor domain function using the transfection systems along with site-directed mutagenesis or chimeric constructs of isolated receptor cDNA's. This information provides for a description of drug binding and receptor-mediated cell activation in molecular terms. The general principles of receptor characterization outlined in this section apply to any constituent that functions as a "receptor," whether it be an enzyme, a nuclear transcription factor, or a membrane-localized pharmacologic receptor, such as those to be discussed in the next section. The challenge for the future is to integrate the detailed chemical information now available for receptors and their agonists with the description, in molecular terms, of the cell signaling processes to be outlined in the sections that follow.

Biochemical Mechanisms of Cell Signaling

In general, the targets for the actions of a wide variety of drugs can be placed into two broad categories: (i) agents may interact with complex cellular enzymatic pathways (e.g., allopurinol, used in the treatment of gout, acts by inhibiting the formation of uric acid), or, more commonly; (ii) drugs may interact with regulatory proteins in communication systems that are used to convey signals (i.e., information) from one cell to another. It is the second category that will serve as the focus of this section. The receptors for drugs are usually, although not invariably, proteins, since a polypeptide structure provides for a maximization of energetically favourable interactions between active ligands and effector systems. In terms of cell-to-cell communication, two loci, the cell membrane and the nucleus, are of particular significance. Although the over-all function of the cell membrane is to maintain an effective barrier between the extracellular and intracellular milieu, it is now recognized that highly specialized membrane structures (e.g., ion channels and drug receptors) play particularly key roles in terms of selectively transmitting information from the external to the internal cell environment (and in some cases, vice versa). These membrane constituents involved in signaling serve as targets for a variety of drugs, neurotransmitters, and hormones. This section will deal in general with selected aspects of transmembrane signalling and will focus in particular on the plasma membrane-localized processes used by pharmacologic receptors.

The Plasma Membrane as a Signal Transduction Element

A great deal is now known about the membrane-localized components that participate in transmembrane signalling. In some cases, information is transmitted by highly selective transmembrane channels. In this instance, the ion or metabolite transported by the channel embodies the message that is being communicated to the intracellular space, and it is the intracellular milieu that responds to increased (or decreased) concentrations of the transported substance. It is now known that membrane constituents (e.g., voltage-dependent sodium or calcium channels) that act as selective transport molecules are highly complex oligomeric proteins that can be subject to the same kinds of allosteric regulation as are cellular enzymes. Drugs or toxins that alter the transport properties of these communication channels (e.g., dihydropyridine calcium channel blockers or sodium channel blockers such as batrachotoxin) can profoundly alter cell function.

Drug receptors situated in the plasma membrane exhibit not only the ability to recognize a ligand with high affinity and selectivity, but also the capacity, once activated by the specific ligand, to trigger a transmembrane signal. It is this dual recognition-signal triggering property, by which the receptor per se acts in part as a messenger-generating system, that distinguishes pharmacologic receptors from other cell-surface recognition/transport moieties. Thus, as opposed to channels where the transported ligand bears the message, with membrane receptors, it is the receptor itself that conveys the message, not the activating ligand. In certain instances (e.g., when antireceptor antibodies are present), a receptor can trigger a cell response in the absence of its usual activating ligand (see below). The sections that follow will deal mainly with the mechanisms whereby membrane receptors generate a cellular signal.

General Mechanisms of Receptor-Mediated Signaling

The major focus of the ensuing discussion will be on two questions: (i) how does a receptor trigger a transmembrane signal, and (ii) how is the receptor-triggered signal amplified? The answers to both questions may be found by considering a relatively small number of basic mechanisms that can account for the generation of an intracellular signal by a variety of membrane-localized receptors, and for the signal amplification process.

The key property of receptor function, irrespective of which signaling mechanism is used, lies in the ability of the ligand to act as an allosteric regulator of the receptor's activity. Thus, for membrane-localized receptors, the processes of ligand binding and receptor triggering can be seen as two distinct but related steps. Moreover, both intramolecular (i.e., ligand-modulated allosteric effects such as the activation of a receptor's enzyme activity) and intermolecular receptor dynamics (i.e., receptor mobility, aggregation, and internalization: see below) play important roles in the signal transduction process. The three basic mechanisms responsible for transmembrane signaling are shown in Figure 1.10: (i) receptors linked via GTP-binding regulatory proteins (G proteins) to effector systems that generate intracellular second messengers; (ii) receptors that are ligand-gated ion channels; and (iii) receptors that have intrinsic enzyme activity. A subset of this third class of receptor can be seen in those receptors (e.g., for cytokines) that do not of themselves possess intrinsic enzyme activity but that can rapidly activate membrane enzyme activities in a ligand-modulated manner.

G-Protein Linked Receptors that Generate Intracellular Second Messengers

A wide variety of ligands bind to membrane receptors (R_G) that are coupled to intracellular effector enzymes by G proteins. Two common effector enzymes that generate second messengers are shown in Figure 1.10. Adenylyl cyclase catalyzes the conversion of ATP into adenosine 3′, 5′-cyclic monophosphate (cyclic AMP), the original intracellular second messenger discovered by Sutherland and coworkers.[r14] The formation of cyclic AMP is translated into an appropriate cellular response by activation of a cyclic AMP-dependent protein kinase (PKA) that initiates a cascade of protein phosphorylations on serine residues. A second effector enzyme (Fig. 1.10) is the phosphoinositide-specific phospholipase C that hydrolyzes a minor membrane phospholipid, phosphatidylinositol 4,5-bisphosphate (PIP_2), into two second messengers: inositol 1,4,5-triphosphate (IP_3), which releases calcium from intracellular stores,[r15] and diacylglycerol (DAG), an activator of a calcium- and phospholipid-dependent protein kinase (PKC).[r16] Calcium will combine with calmodulin (CAM) and other calcium-binding proteins, whereas PKC will phosphorylate intracellular proteins on serine residues. Thus, phosphoinositide turnover represents an example of a bifurcating signal transduction pathway.

Receptors coupled to G proteins represent the most common mechanism for transmembrane signaling. At this time, over 100 G protein-linked receptors have been cloned and sequenced.[r13,r17] Activating ligands include neurotransmitters, autacoids, peptide hormones, and sensory stimuli,—plus a variety of other agents. A partial list of agonist-receptors that are linked to G proteins is presented in Table 1.2. Notwithstanding this amazing diversity of ligands, the proposed topologic structures of G protein-coupled receptors are remarkably similar,[r10] consisting of an extracellular N-terminal domain, seven transmembrane helices with three interconnecting intracellular and extracellular loops, and an intracellular C-terminal tail (Fig. 1.11). The function of the various receptor domains has been studied by site-directed mutagenesis and the creation of deletion mutants and receptor chimeras[r13] in order to establish the sites for agonist binding and G protein interactions.

Effector systems can be either enzymes or ion channels, so that multiple second messengers can be produced (Table 1.2). Receptors are linked to the various effector systems by distinct G proteins. The stimulation of adenylyl cyclase activity is linked to agonist activation of specific receptors by a G protein called Gs (Fig. 1.10; Table 1.2). On the other hand, activation of a different set of receptors results in inhibition of adenylyl cyclase and a fall in intracellular levels of cyclic AMP, a process mediated by a distinct G protein, Gi. Thus, the sympathetic neurotransmitter norepinephrine can either increase (β receptor) or decrease (α_2 receptor) cellular cyclic AMP levels, depending on the complement of adrenergic receptors present on the cell membrane of a particular cell.

It is apparent from the information presented in Table 1.2 that Gs and Gi can be coupled to multiple receptors. Of course, not all receptors will be present in a particular cell type. The complexity of this transmembrane signaling mechanism is increased by the fact that G proteins can regulate multiple effector systems. Thus, Gs directly stimulates voltage-gated Ca^{2+} channels in skeletal muscle,[28] and Gi opens the inwardly rectifying K^+ channel in atria in response to muscarinic (M_2) receptor stimulation.[r18]

Phosphoinositide turnover (Fig. 1.10) is also stimulated by a number of agonist-receptors (Table 1.2), including norepinephrine (α_1 receptor), through G protein activation of phospholipase C, although the precise identity of the G protein is not known in all instances (see below). The parasympathetic neuro-

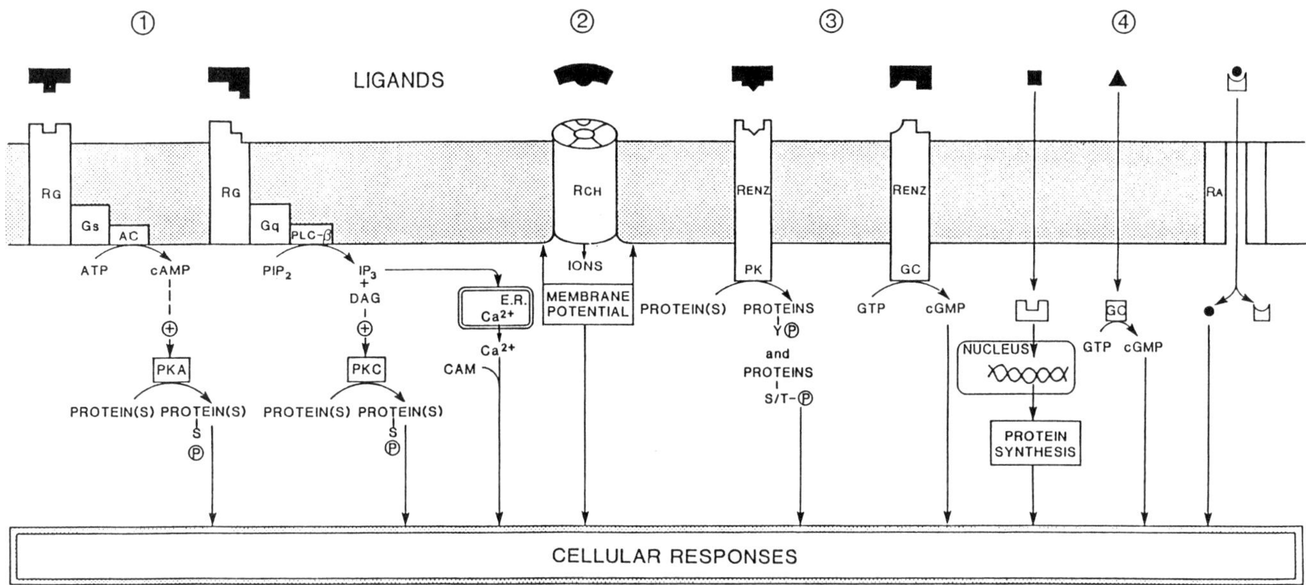

Figure 1.10 Mechanisms for transmembrane signalling (signal transduction). Ligands can interact with specific receptors in the plasma membrane that are classified according to three basic mechanisms whereby transmembrane signals are generated:

1. Receptors (R_G) linked by specific GTP-binding proteins to effector systems such as the enzymes adenylyl cyclase (AC) and phosphoinositide-specific phospholipase C (PLC-β) that generate intracellular second messengers: cyclic AMP (cAMP), inositol 1,4,5-trisphosphate (IP_3), and diacylglycerol (DAG). Cyclic AMP activates the cyclic AMP-dependent protein kinase (PKA), which catalyzes the serine phosphorylation (S-P) of cellular proteins to produce a response. IP_3 releases calcium from intracellular stores in the endoplasmic reticulum (ER), which combines with calcium-binding proteins like calmodulin (CAM) to regulate cellular function. The DAG second messenger activates protein kinase C (PKC), resulting in protein (serine) phosphorylation.

2. Receptors (R_{CH}) that are ligand-regulated ion channels where the influx of specific ions (Na^+, Cl^-) alters membrane polarization to produce a biologic response.

3. Receptors (R_{ENZ}) that are ligand-activated transmembrane enzymes with intrinsic catalytic activity. Receptors for some hormones (e.g., insulin) and polypeptide growth factors (e.g., epidermal growth factor-urogastrone) have protein (tyrosine) kinase (PK) activity, resulting in tyrosine phosphorylation (Y-P) of cellular target proteins. In contrast, other receptors (e.g., transforming growth factor-β) have protein kinase activity directed towards serine residues in proteins (S-P). A variety of extracellular peptides activate receptors that have guanylyl cyclase (GC) activity, producing cyclic GMP (cGMP).

Some ligands (■) interact with intracellular receptors (4). For example, steroid hormones bind to cytoplasmic receptors that subsequently translocate to the nucleus to regulate gene expression and the synthesis of proteins. In addition, soluble guanylyl cyclase (GC) can be activated by a diffusible ligand (▲) like nitric oxide. The plasma membrane also has specific acceptors (R_A) for substances ((●) e.g., vitamin B_{12}) bound to specific transport proteins, so that the transported substances can enter cells and regulate cellular function.

Signal amplification can result from either a change in membrane potential or from the initiation of phosphorylation-dephosphorylation cascades due to stimulation of receptor protein kinases, or from activation of protein (serine) kinases such as PKC and PKA.

transmitter, acetylcholine, stimulates phosphoinositide turnover (M_1, M_3, M_5 muscarinic receptors), inhibits adenylyl cyclase activity, and opens K^+ channels (M_2, M_4 receptors). Thus, acetylcholine represents a further example of a single ligand that can activate multiple signaling pathways. In addition to phosphoinositide turnover produced by stimulation of phospholipase C, evidence suggests that phospholipase A_2 activity and the generation of an arachidonic acid second messenger can be regulated by G proteins; but the specific G protein has not been identified.[29,r19] The arachidonic acid second messenger can be converted into prostanoids and/or leukotrienes that in turn can serve as messengers. Arachidonic acid can also directly regulate effector systems such as ion channels[r20] and modulate intracellular enzyme activities (e.g., PKC).[r16]

One of the best characterized second messenger systems involving G proteins is phototransduction.[r21] A photon of light binds to the 11-*cis* retinal chromophore in rhodopsin leading to the transducin (Gt)-mediated stimulation of cyclic GMP phosphodiesterase (cGMP-PDE) activity (Table 1.2) in the retina. The resulting fall in cyclic GMP then closes a membrane cation channel, resulting in membrane hyperpolarization and ultimately a nerve impulse that is processed by the retina before transmission to the visual cortex of the brain.

Table 1.2 Transmembrane Receptors Linked via GTP-Binding Proteins to Effector Systems that Generate Intracellular Second Messengers

Agonist (Receptor)	G-Protein	Effector(s)	Second Messengers
ACTH Adenosine (A_2) Adrenergic ($\beta_{1\text{-}3}$) Dopamine (D_1) Glucagon (G_2) Histamine (H_2) Olfactory stimuli Serotonin (5HT) Vasopressin (V_2)	Gs	Adenylyl cyclase (+) Ca^{2+} channels (+)	↑ cyclic AMP (PKA) ↑ Ca^{2+}_i
Acetylcholine (M_2,M_4) Adenosine (A_1) Adrenergic ($\alpha_{2A\text{-}D}$) Dopamine (D_2) Histamine (H_3)	Gi	Adenylyl cyclase (–) K^+ channels (+)	↓ cyclic AMP Hyperpolarization
Acetylcholine (M_1,M_3,M_5) Adrenergic ($\alpha_{1A\text{-}C}$) Angiotensin Cholecystokinin Histamine (H_1) Serotonin ($5HT_{1C}$, $5HT_2$) Thrombin Vasopressin (V_{1A}, V_{1B})	Gq/Gi	PI-phospholipase C (+)	IP_3(Ca^{2+}_i) + DAG (PKC)
Adrenergic (α_1) Purinergic (P_2) Thrombin	?	Phospholipase A_2	Arachidonic acid
Light (rhodopsin)	Gt	cGMP-PDE	↓cGMP

Models for the topologic structure of G protein-linked receptors are based on the tertiary structure of bacteriorhodopsin, a visual pigment from *Halobacterium halobium*.[r13,r22]

Receptor-coupled G proteins are heterotrimeric, consisting of α, β and γ subunits (in decreasing order by Mr).[r23] The α subunits have a high-affinity binding site for guanine nucleotides (GTP or GDP) and possess intrinsic GTPase activity. The individual classes of G proteins (Table 1.2) are defined on the basis of their unique α subunits. The heterotrimeric G proteins are part of a large superfamily of GTP binding proteins that express GTPase activity.[r24] This superfamily also includes translational factors and low-molecular weight *ras* proteins.[r25]

A general scheme for the receptor-mediated activation of the heterotrimeric G proteins and subsequent stimulation of effectors to produce intracellular second messengers is shown in Figure 1.12, based on the subunit dissociation model proposed by Gilman.[r26] In the resting or basal state, the heterotrimeric G protein has GDP bound to the α subunit. Interaction of an agonist-receptor complex with the heterotrimer facilitates dissociation of GDP and association of GTP (nucleotide exchange). The binding of GTP to the α subunit induces a conformational change that results in dissociation of the agonist-receptor complex and further dissociation of the activated heterotrimer into βγ and α-GTP subunits. The free α-GTP subunit then activates effectors (enzymes like adenylyl cyclase and cyclic GMP-phosphodiesterase) or modulates ion channel activity to produce intracellular second messengers. The intrinsic GTPase activity of the α subunit converts GTP into GDP, and thus acts as an "off-switch" by terminating the activation of the effector. Reassociation of the α-GDP subunit with βγ then completes the cycle.

There is considerable diversity in the α subunits of heterotrimeric G proteins (Table 1.3). At present, 21 distinct α subunits have been identified as the products of 17 genes.[r26] Based on sequence relationships, G protein α subunits have been subdivided into four family groupings, Gs, Gi, Gq, and G12.[r26,r27] This diversity is accentuated by distinct patterns of expression, ranging from widespread to very specific. For example, the α_{olf} subunit is closely related to αs (88 percent sequence identity) but the expression of α_{olf} is restricted solely to the olfactory epithelium, where it functions to stimulate adenylyl cyclase activity as part of an odorant signal transduction scheme.

Heterotrimeric G proteins can also be distinguished by sensitivity to bacterial toxins, specifically to cholera toxin (CTX, from *Vibrio*

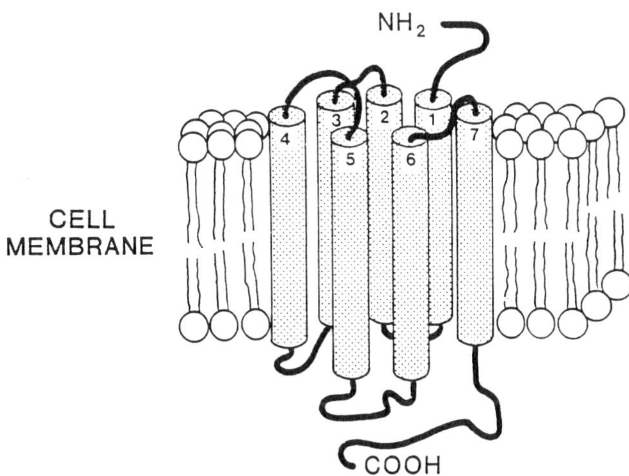

Figure 1.11 Schematic representation of receptors in the plasma membrane that are linked to GTP-binding proteins (G-proteins). Hydropathy analysis of deduced amino acid sequences[r10] has suggested that these receptors have a glycosylated NH_2-terminal domain, seven transmembrane-spanning domains (represented by the cylinders, each consisting of 20-28 hydrophobic amino acid residues) with three interconnecting intracellular and intracellular loops, and an intracellular C-terminal domain.

cholerae) and pertussis toxin (PTX, from *Bordetella pertussis*).[r28,r29] Cholera toxin catalyzes the transfer of ADP-ribose from NAD to a specific arginine residue in the α subunits of the Gs family (Table 1.3). As a consequence of ADP-ribosylation, α subunit GTPase activity is markedly reduced, thus maintaining the activation of effectors by α-GTP (Fig. 1.12). The severe diarrhea associated with *Vibrio cholerae* infections is largely due to altered water and ion transport in the small intestine because of elevated cyclic AMP.[r28] By comparison, pertussis toxin catalyzes the ADP ribosylation of a cysteine residue in the C-terminal domain of some of the α subunits in the Gi family (Table 1.3); as a result, interaction of the G protein heterotrimer with the agonist-receptor complex is blocked (Fig. 1.12). One of the symptoms associated with *Bordetella pertussis* infections (whooping cough) is hypoglycemia, because the Gi-mediated α_2-adrenergic-induced inhibition of insulin secretion is blocked.[r29] Pertussis toxin is sometimes referred to as "islet-activating protein" (IAP). Interestingly, transducin (Gt) is modified by both cholera and pertussis toxins.

A number of α subunits are not ADP-ribosylated by either toxin (Table 1.3). In the case of phosphoinositide turnover, pertussis toxin-insensitive responses are mediated by α subunits of the Gq family that specifically activate the phospholipase C-β isoenzyme.[r30] In some cells and tissues, agonist-stimulated phosphoinositide turnover is blocked by pertussis toxin, but the G protein(s) responsible for stimulating phospholipase C activity in this situation has not been identified, although Gi is a candidate.

The βγ subunits of the heterotrimeric G proteins are tightly associated. Despite some diversity in the individual β and γ proteins (Table 1.3), most studies suggest that βγ subunits are largely interchangeable among the G protein heterotrimers. The function of βγ subunits has generally been assumed to be structural, by providing a membrane anchor for the heterotrimer (perhaps as a result of prenylation of γ subunits that facilitates membrane association). But in addition, the presence of βγ in a heterotrimer is essential for

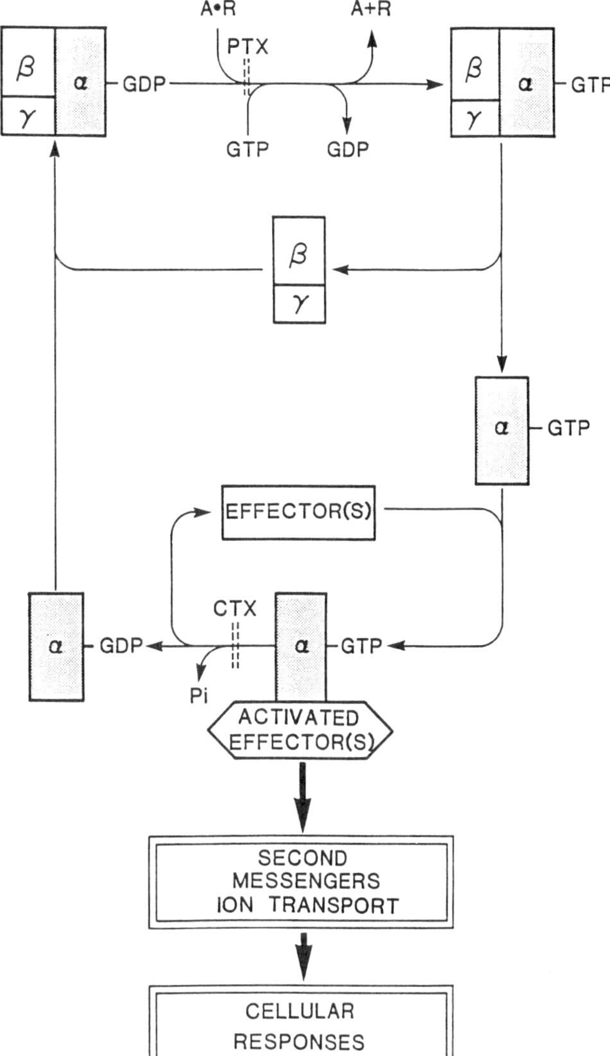

Figure 1.12 General scheme for transmembrane signalling mediated by heterotrimeric GTP-binding proteins (G proteins). G proteins consist of unique α subunits with a guanine nucleotide binding site and intrinsic GTPase activity that are combined with βγ subunits. In the basal state, the oligomeric G protein has GDP bound tightly to the α subunit. An agonist-receptor complex (A.R) facilitates nucleotide exchange (dissociation of GDP and association of GTP), producing a conformational change that then results in dissociation of the agonist-receptor complex that can then interact with another G-protein. The activated G protein oligomer also dissociates to give βγ subunits and the GTP-bound α subunit, which then activates an effector system (enzymes or ion channels) to generate intracellular second messengers. Effector activation is terminated by the intrinsic GTPase activity of the α-subunit; the α-GDP subunit then recombines with the βγ subunits to regenerate the inactive heterotrimer.

Covalent modification (ADP ribosylation) of specific α subunits by pertussis toxin (PTX) uncouples the G protein heterotrimer from interacting with receptors, thus inhibiting G protein-mediated transmembrane signalling. In contrast, cholera toxin (CTX)-catalyzed ADP ribosylation of certain α subunits inhibits their intrinsic GTPase activity; as a result, the effector system is constitutively activated.

Table 1.3 Heterotrimeric G-Proteins

A. Alpha Subunits (39-52 kDa)				
Family	**Subunit(s)**	**Toxin Sensitivity**	**Distribution**	**Effectors**
1. Gs	α_s(4)*	CTX	Widespread	adenylyl cyclase (+) Ca^{2+} channels (+) Na^+ channels(–)
	α_{olf}	CTX	Olfactory	adenylyl cyclase (+)
2. Gi	$\alpha_{i1\text{-}3}$	PTX	Widespread	adenylyl cyclase (–) K^+ channels (+) Ca^{2+} channels(–)
	α_O(2)*	PTX	Brain, others	phospholipase C(+?)
	α_{t1},α_{t2}	PTX, CTX	Retina	cGMP-PDE(+)
	α_g	PTX	Taste buds	phosphodiesterase(?)
	α_z	—	Brain, platelets	adenylyl cyclase(–)
3. Gq	α_q, α_{11}	—	Widespread	
	α_{14}	—	Liver, lung, kidney	phospholipase C-β(+)
	α_{15},α_{16}	—	Blood cells	
4. G12	α_{12},α_{13}	—	Widespread	?
B. Beta (35-36 kDa) – Gamma (7-10 kDa) Subunits				
Family	**Subunits**	**Distribution**	**Functions**	
β	$\beta_{1\text{-}4}$	Widespread	Membrane anchor for oligomer Interaction of α-subunits with receptors Inhibition of α-GTP action Direct effector regulation: —adenylyl cyclase (+/–) —phospholipase C (+) —phospholipase A_2 (+) —K^+ channels (+)	
γ	$\gamma_{1\text{-}6}$	Widespread		

*( ) = splice variants.

coupling to the receptor.[r31] Free βγ subunits would also be expected to inhibit the stimulatory effects of α-GTP subunits on effectors by promoting reassociation of the heterotrimer by mass action. Thus, inhibition of adenylyl cyclase activity by agonists acting through Gi (Table 1.2), which in theory could be due to a direct inhibitory effect of α_i-GTP on the enzyme, is thought to be mediated primarily by an indirect effect of βγ subunits, originally derived from the Gi heterotrimer, that can recombine with α_s-GTP to form an inactive Gs-GTP heterotrimer (subunit exchange).[r25] However, recently, direct effects of βγ subunits on several effectors have been reported.[r26] For example, βγ subunits released from a receptor-G protein-effector system that is separate and distinct from adenylyl cyclase could, nonetheless, modulate cyclase activity depending on specific isoenzyme expression. In addition, βγ subunits may directly regulate some phospholipases and ion channels.[r17]

Alterations in G proteins may also be a feature of certain disease states. For instance, Gs mutants (gsp oncogene product), which have reduced intrinsic GTPase activity, have been identified in human pituitary tumors;[r31] the gsp mutants cause a constitutive activation of adenylyl cyclase. In another disease entity, expression of Gs and Gi has been found to be altered in adipocyte membranes from obese and diabetic mice.[30,31] Changes in either the function or amount of heterotrimeric G proteins could thus have profound pathophysiologic effects by changing normal signal transduction pathways.

Ligand-Gated Ion Channels

A second general mechanism of transmembrane signaling is illustrated by receptors (R_{CH}) that are ligand-gated ion channels (Fig. 1.10). One of the characteristics of this signaling mechanism is the speed of the response, where alterations in ion flux can be detected in milliseconds. One of the best characterized receptors in this class is the nicotinic acetylcholine receptor from the electric organ of electric eels and rays (Table 1.4). This receptor consists of a hetero-oligo-

Table 1.4 Ligand-Gated Ion Channels

Agonist	Receptor Subtype(s)	Ion-Transport	Effect
Acetylcholine	Cholinergic (nicotinic)	Na^+	depolarization/excitation
Glutamate	NMDA	Ca^{2+}/Na^+	
	Kainate	Na^+	depolarization/excitation
	AMPA (quisqualate)	Na^+	
GABA	$GABA_A$	Cl^-	hyperpolarization/inhibition
Glycine	Glycine	Cl^-	hyperpolarization/inhibition
Serotonin	Serotonin-3	Na^+/K^+	depolarization/excitation

meric complex (α_2, β, γ, δ) of glycoprotein subunits[r9] that form a central ion channel (Fig. 1.13). Each of the subunits have the common feature of four sequences of hydrophobic amino acids arranged in α-helices that form putative membrane-spanning domains (M1-M4); the M2 segment is proposed to line the inside of the ion-conducting channel. The agonist, acetylcholine, binds to the α subunits.

Similar structural features characterize the excitatory neuronal cation channel gated by glutamate, and the inhibitory neuronal chloride channels activated by GABA and glycine (Table 1.4) Therefore, these neuronal hetero-oligomeric amino acid receptors are part of an ion channel superfamily that includes the nicotinic acetylcholine receptor.[r8] Molecular cloning studies have revealed considerable heterogeneity for each of the subunits of the amino acid receptors. The precise subunit composition and stoichiometry for the amino acid receptor-ion channels has not been determined from experiments where cDNAs for various subunits have been expressed in cells, followed by assessment of functional channel formation. Receptors that are ligand-gated ion channels are also regulated by selective antagonists. For example, strychnine selectively blocks the glycine-stimulated chloride influx in cells. In addition to selective antagonism by bicuculline at the agonist binding site, the $GABA_A$ receptor is also regulated by drugs interacting at other distinct (allosteric) sites. Of particular importance is the ability of benzodiazepines (diazepam, flunitrazepam) to potentiate the action of GABA by increasing the frequency of chloride channel opening.[r32]

In addition to the direct gating of ion channel receptors by ligands (Table 1.4), ion channels can also be modulated indirectly by ligands interacting with receptors linked to G proteins (see section on G-protein linked receptors above). In these situations, the ion channels can be regulated by G protein interactions (Fig. 1.14). This mechanism is utilized by the muscarinic (M2)-receptor to open K^+ channels in atria, a re-

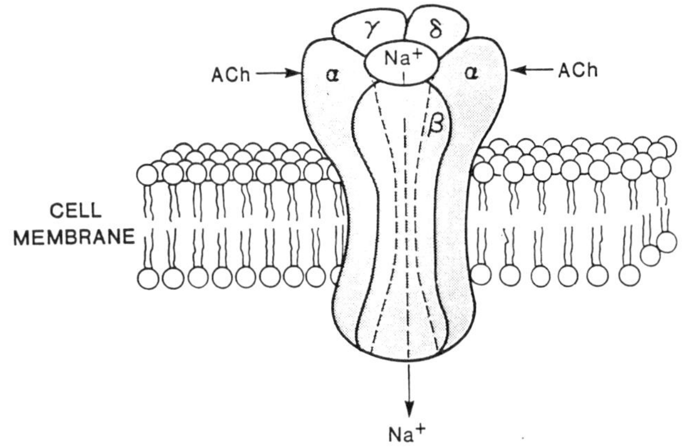

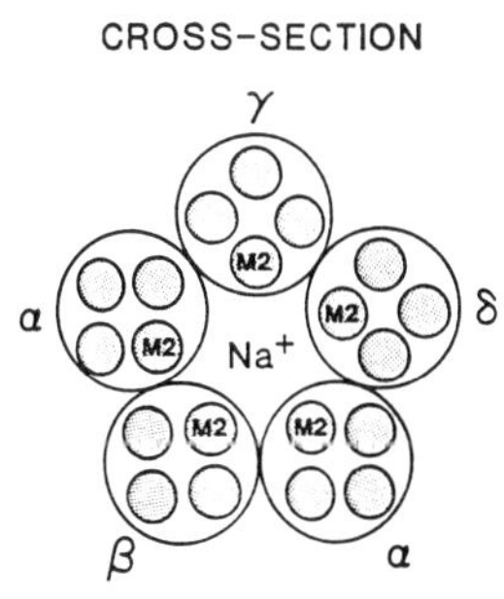

Figure 1.13 Schematic representation of the nicotinic acetylcholine receptor at the neuromuscular junction. The nicotinic receptor from the *Torpedo* electric organ is a pentameric structure consisting of four protein subunits ($\alpha_2\beta\gamma\delta$), arranged to form an ion channel for Na^+ in the plasma membrane as shown in a longitudinal view and in cross-section. Each of the four individual protein subunits have the common structural feature of four α-helical sequences of hydrophobic amino acid residues that form membrane-spanning domains (M1-M4). It is proposed that the M2 segments line the inside of the channel to form the selective ion-conducting pore. The passage of sodium ions through the ion channel is regulated by the binding of acetylcholine (ACh) to the α subunits, ultimately resulting in membrane depolarization and muscle contraction.

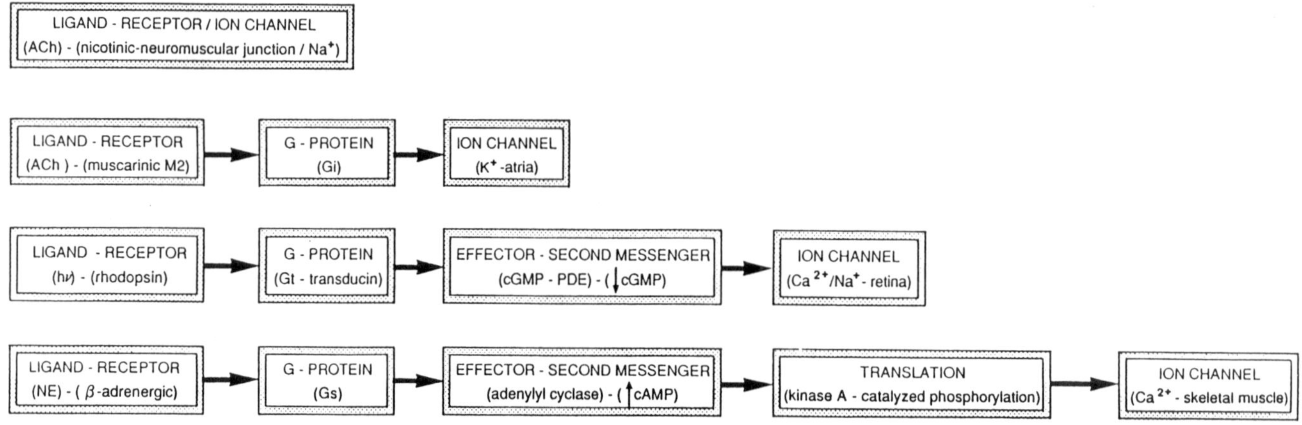

Figure 1.14 General mechanisms for the regulation of plasma membrane ion channels. Ligands may directly modulate receptors that are ion channels, such as the nicotinic acetylcholine receptor at the neuromuscular junction that regulates sodium influx into muscle cells. In addition, ion channels can be regulated by receptors linked to GTP-binding proteins (G proteins). In some instances, the ion channel can be regulated *directly* by G protein α and $\beta\gamma$ subunits (membrane-delimited mechanism); an example is the Gi-dependent opening of the inwardly rectifying K^+ channel in atrial cells as a result of muscarinic (M2) receptor stimulation. Alternatively, the G protein effect on ion channels may be *indirect*, as a consequence of the altered production of a second messenger. For example, in the phototransduction process, photoexcited rhodopsin produces a transducin-mediated activation of cyclic GMP phosphodiesterase (cGMP-PDE) that reduces cyclic GMP levels, resulting in closure of cation channels in retinal rod cells. By comparison, stimulation of β-adrenergic receptors in skeletal muscle results in the Gs-dependent stimulation of adenylyl cyclase activity. The resultant stimulatory effect of the cyclic AMP second messenger on Ca^{2+} influx is mediated by covalent modification (serine phosphorylation) of the voltage-gated calcium channel by the cyclic AMP-dependent protein kinase (kinase A).

sponse that is mediated by Gi; as a result, the atrial cell is hyperpolarized and heart rate is reduced. This direct pathway for regulation of ion channels by G protein subunits has been termed a "membrane-delimited" mechanism, since diffusible second messengers are not involved.[r33] In addition, G proteins can regulate ion channels indirectly, either through the effects of second messengers (e.g., the transducin-induced fall in cyclic GMP, which closes a cation channel in the retina) or as a consequence of covalent modification of the ion channel by the cyclic AMP-dependent protein kinase (Fig. 1.14).

Ligand-Activated Receptors with Intrinsic Enzyme Activity

The third basic transmembrane signaling mechanism (Fig. 1.10) involves receptors that are membrane-associated allosteric enzymes (R_{ENZ}), where ligand binding to the extracellular domain produces a conformational change that is transmitted via a single transmembrane domain to the intracellular domain that activates an intrinsic enzyme activity. The receptor-associated enzymes that have been documented to date comprise protein kinases (directed at either tyrosine or serine residues) and guanylyl cyclase.

To date, the most extensively studied class of receptor-enzymes is the one represented by the receptors for insulin and EGF-URO. These receptors, like the ones for a variety of other polypeptide growth and differentiation factors (e.g., fibroblast growth factor, platelet-derived growth factor, colony-stimulating factor-1), possess intrinsic tyrosine kinase activity (Table 1.5). Ligand binding to the extracellular domain results in two rapid events, oligomerization (dimerization) and activation of the cytosolic tyrosine kinase domain (Fig. 1.15).[r34,r35] As a consequence, the receptor is autophosphorylated by an intermolecular reaction. Autophosphorylation of the intracellular domain of the insulin receptor has the effect of increasing the receptor tyrosine kinase activity toward other intracellular proteins, an action that persists even in the absence of ligand as long as the receptor remains autophosphorylated.

A number of experimental approaches, including site-directed mutagenesis of receptor autophosphorylation sites, have indicated that receptor tyrosine kinase activity is essential for ligands such as insulin to produce characteristic metabolic and mitogenic responses.[32] Therefore, particular attention has been placed on the identification of the intracellular target proteins for the receptor tyrosine kinases. Autophosphorylation of the EGF-URO receptor creates binding sites for intracellular proteins that contain a specific domain (SH-2) that is also found in the *src* family of cytoplasmic (nonreceptor) tyrosine kinases.[r36] The recruitment of such SH-2-domain-containing proteins to the receptor forms a "signaling complex;" tyrosine phosphorylation of these intracellular target proteins will then presumably initiate a cascade of reactions that ultimately produces the appropriate cellular response (Fig. 1.15). One of the substrates for the EGF-URO receptor is the γ-isoenzyme of the phos-

Table 1.5 Ligand-Activated Transmembrane Receptors with Intrinsic Enzyme Activity

Agonist (Receptors)	Enzyme Activity	Effect
Insulin Epidermal growth factor Platelet-derived growth factor Fibroblast growth factor	Tyrosine Kinase	Tyrosine phosphorylation of cellular proteins
Colony stimulating factor-1 Activin Inhibin Transforming growth factor β	Serine/threonine kinase	Serine/threonine phosphorylation of cellular proteins
Natriuretic peptides (GC-A/B) Bacterial enterotoxins (GC-C) Sperm-activating peptides	Guanylyl cyclase	↑ cGMP

phoinositide-specific phospholipase C family,[r30] which is activated by tyrosine phosphorylation (Fig. 1.15). Therefore, the ability of growth factors to stimulate phosphoinositide turnover and the generation of IP_3 and DAG second messengers occurs by a mechanism that is entirely separate and distinct from that described for agonists linked to G proteins, where α_q-GTP subunits stimulate the activity of the phospholipase-β isoenzyme (Table 1.3).

The involvement of ligand-activated tyrosine kinase activity in receptor-mediated transmembrane signaling may also extend to receptors that do not, in their primary structure, possess intrinsic tyrosine kinase activity. For instance, elevated cellular tyrosine phosphorylation is an early event in cell activation by cytokines such as interleukin-2 (IL-2) and granulocyte-macrophage colony stimulating factor (GM-CSF).[r37] Although the IL-2 and GM-CSF receptors per se do not exhibit tyrosine kinase activity, it appears that ligand binding causes the formation of a complex receptor cluster, comprising at least two receptor subunits (α- and β-subunits) and possibly an associated nonreceptor tyrosine kinase, such as $p56^{lck}$ or $p59^{fyn}$. The two oncogene-related cellular tyrosine kinases, $p56^{lck}$ and $p59^{fyn}$, are also thought to play a role in the antigen-mediated activation of T-lymphocytes via the T-cell receptor oligomer, which of itself does not possess tyrosine kinase activity.[r38] The ability of receptors without tyrosine kinase activity to recruit this enzyme for the purposes of cell activation, when the ligand binds to the receptor, is entirely in keeping with the "mobile" or floating receptor paradigm to be described below (page 31).

Although receptor-tyrosine kinases were the first receptor-enzymes to be studied, it is now evident that receptors may also possess intrinsic serine/threonine kinase activity. The receptor for activin, a growth-promoting polypeptide that also regulates pituitary function, was the first receptor of this type to be cloned.[33] Receptors for other members of this polypeptide growth factor family, including the inhibins, Müllerian duct-inhibiting substance, bone morphogenetic factor, and the transforming growth factor-β group of polypeptides, are also believed to possess intrinsic serine/threonine kinase activity.

A third type of receptor with intrinsic enzyme activity is provided by the membrane-bound guanylyl cyclase[r39] (Fig. 1.10), which is stimulated by extracellular peptides (Table 1.5). Specific receptors from mammalian tissues are activated by atrial natriuretic peptides and heat-stable enterotoxins from bacteria, whereas the guanylyl cyclase receptor in sea urchin spermatozoa is activated by specific peptides from egg-conditioned medium. Therefore, the direct activation of guanylyl cyclase by ligands where the enzyme is the receptor can be contrasted with the adenylyl cyclase system with three components, where receptors are linked to the cyclase catalytic unit by heterotrimeric G proteins.

Amplification of Transmembrane Signals

Once ligand-induced receptor activation has been achieved by any of the three transmembrane signaling mechanisms outlined above, the initial signal must be greatly amplified to produce a cellular response. Signal amplification typically involves the following elements: (i) activation of G-proteins and generation of second messengers; (ii) initiation of phosphorylation-dephosphorylation cascades; and (iii) changes in membrane potential or polarization.[r40]

The general scheme for G protein activation (Fig. 1.12) has two amplification steps. First, the recycling agonist-receptor complex has a catalytic effect on activation of the heterotrimeric G protein.[r40a] For example, photoexcited rhodopsin results in the activation of hundreds of molecules of transducin. The second stage of amplification is provided by the turnover number or catalytic power of the effector enzyme. The turnover number of the intrinsic GTPase activity in α-GTP subunits is relatively slow, so that the lifetime of the activated α-GTP subunit is sufficient to produce a significant stimulation of effector systems. The activity of cGMP-PDE is increased by more than 1500-fold by α_t-GTP, so that the overall amplification in phototransduction[r20] is about 10^5.

The triggering of a phosphorylation-dephosphorylation cascade by second messengers produced by G protein activation, such as that initiated by activation of the cyclic AMP-dependent protein kinase or phospholipase C (Fig. 1.10), produces a further degree

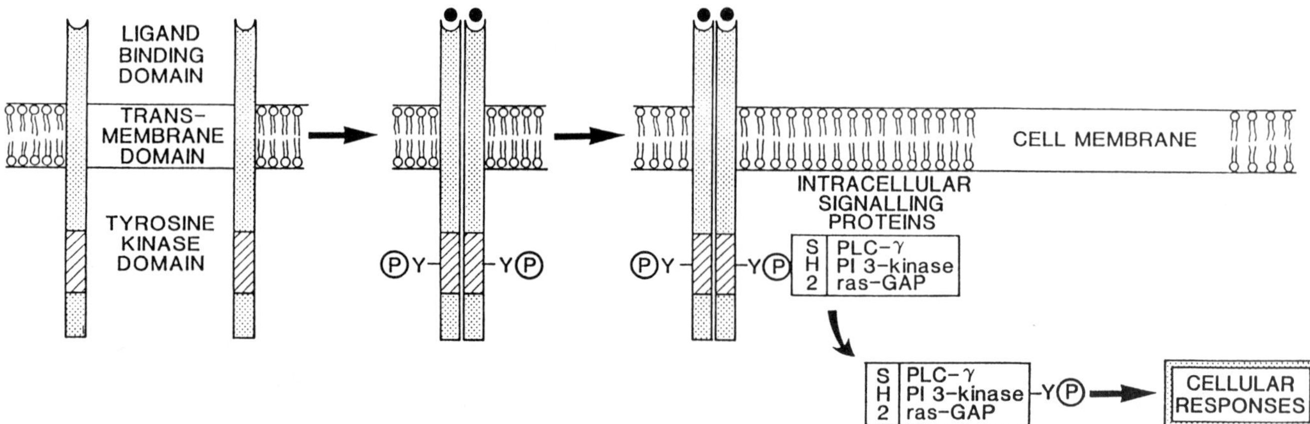

Figure 1.15 Scheme for transmembrane signaling by ligand-activated receptors with intrinsic enzyme (tyrosine kinase) activity. Ligand binding to the extracellular domain of growth factor receptors produces a conformational change that results in oligomerization (dimerization) and activation of the intracellular tyrosine kinase domain. As a result, the receptor is autophosphorylated (Y-P), thus activating the receptor tyrosine kinase activity towards intracellular signaling proteins. For example, proteins containing an SH-2 domain (found in the $pp60^{c\text{-}src}$ proto-oncogene) bind selectively to receptor autophosphorylation sites. Three examples of SH-2 domain-containing signaling proteins are the γ-isoenzyme of the phosphoinositide-specific phospholipase C (PLC-γ), a phosphatidylinositol 3-kinase (PI 3-kinase) that converts phosphatidylinositol 4,5-bisphosphate (PIP_2) to phosphatidylinositol 3,4,5-trisphosphate, and the GTPase-activating protein (*ras*-GAP) of *ras*, a low-molecular weight GTP binding protein that regulates cell growth.[r24] As a result of tyrosine phosphorylation of these proteins, their function is altered, thus initiating a series of incompletely understood events that culminates in a cellular response.

of signal amplification that ultimately results in the stimulation of processes such as glycogenolysis and muscle contraction. The stimulation of phosphoinositide turnover by the activation of phospholipase C increases the diacylglycerol second messenger that subsequently activates protein kinase C (Fig. 1.10) and thus initiates another cascade of phosphorylation reactions. Furthermore, the IP_3-induced release of Ca^{2+} can, in combination with calmodulin, activate myosin light chain kinase. As a result of this activation, myosin is phosphorylated, with an attendant increase in actomyosin ATPase activity, resulting in smooth muscle contraction. Finally, the activation of receptor tyrosine kinases in response to growth factors increases the tyrosine kinase activity toward intracellular target proteins that can continue to convey the intracellular signal, via phosphorylation-dephosphorylation cascades even in the absence of the ligand. A number of these tyrosine phosphorylated cytoplasmic target proteins are enzymes with a catalytic turnover number, providing for considerable amplification.

Small changes in ion flux produced by modulation of ion channels can cause relatively large changes in transmembrane potential, which can have an immediate and profound effect on the orientation (and presumably, therefore, on the function) of proteins situated in the plasma membrane because local changes in membrane potential are rapidly sensed by the entire membrane. Thus, small receptor-triggered changes in membrane potential can also lead to greatly amplified signals, not only by voltage-sensitive ion channels but also via changes in the activity of membrane-associated enzymes that are sensitive to changes in cell polarization.

A final signal amplification mechanism to be considered can be termed "ligand cascade", whereby the activation of one receptor system (e.g., for EGF-URO) results in the formation of extracellular mediators (e.g., prostaglandins) that in turn can activate a second cell surface receptor system. This type of cascade mechanism via the production of prostaglandins accounts for the contractile action of EFG-URO in gastric longitudinal smooth muscle.[34] In a similar vein, acetylcholine, acting via its muscarinic receptor on endothelial cells, results in the cascade production of nitric oxide (NO, the so-called endothelial-derived relaxing factor), which diffuses into the tissue to attenuate smooth muscle contractility.[35,r41,r42] The ligand-cascade signal amplification process mediated by NO represents a novel signaling mechanism triggered by a number of ligands. This NO-mediated process is of considerable importance for the control of both peripheral and central nervous system function.[r42,r43]

Summary

The previous sections have illustrated the mechanisms whereby the activation of a variety of transmembrane receptors can generate amplified cellular signals. In essence, the three main categories of receptors (G protein-linked receptors, ligand-gated ion channels, receptors that are enzymes) appear to feed into a limited number of amplification pathways, namely: (i) G-protein subunit regulatory reactions; (ii) phosphorylation-dephosphorylation networks; and (iii) change in membrane polarization. In many cases, the amplification pathways have as their targets other nonreceptor membrane constituents (e.g., ion channels) that play key roles in cell-to-cell communication. Although the general categories of receptors and the general pathways of signal amplification are relatively few in number, there are large numbers of signal messengers used by receptor activation pathways, and there is enormous potential for the many regulatory biochemical reactions set in motion by the activation of receptors to control cell function in a highly flexible manner.

Intracellular Receptors and Plasma Membrane Acceptors

Although many ligands bind to cell surface receptors and initiate transmembrane signaling mechanisms (Fig. 1.10), other agents enter the cell and interact with soluble receptors. For example, receptors for steroid hormones and thyroid hormone interact with cytosolic and nuclear receptors, respectively. The steroid hormone receptor in the cytosol following ligand binding is translocated to the nucleus. The ligand-activated nuclear receptors then bind to specific regulatory DNA elements, thus acting as transcription factors, to regulate gene expression.[r44,r45] Cis-trans experiments have provided an important molecular approach for investigations into gene regulation by nuclear receptors. Host cells are cotransfected with two plasmids, a trans-vector expressing the receptor (driven by a strong cellular promoter) and a cis-vector carrying the appropriate response element linked to a reporter gene (e.g., chloramphenicol acetyl transferase or luciferase). Analysis of the domain structure of nuclear hormone receptors has established the existence of a superfamily of this type of receptor. In addition to steroids (glucocorticoids, mineralocorticoids, sex steroids) and thyroid hormones, other ligands include vitamin D and the retinoids (vitamin A). One of the characteristics of hormone and drug effects mediated by intracellular (nuclear) receptors is a comparatively slow response time (minutes to hours) because of the requirement for new protein synthesis. It follows that the effects, once achieved, will also persist for some considerable time after removal of the agonist, determined by the turnover (degradation) rate of the newly synthesized proteins.

A second example of an intracellular receptor is the soluble form of guanylyl cyclase (Fig. 1.10),[r46] which is activated by nitric oxide (NO); soluble guanylyl cyclase is a heterodimer with heme as a prosthetic group that binds NO. Vasodilator drugs such as nitroglycerin and nitroprusside are precursors of NO. In addition, NO may function as an endogenous activator of the soluble guanylyl cyclase, either as a neurotransmitter[r43] or as the endothelium-dependent relaxing factor which mediates the vasodilatation produced by agents such as acetylcholine.[r41,r42]

Finally, substances such as cholesterol and vitamin B_{12} that are necessary for the regulation of intracellular processes are carried in the blood stream by specific transport proteins, low-density lipoprotein (LDL), and transcobalamin, respectively. These blood-borne carrier proteins are, in turn, recognized in a specific, high-affinity manner by specialized cell membrane-localized transporters or "acceptors" (R_A) that are responsible for the uptake of both the ligand and carrier protein (Fig. 1.10). Thus, as with membrane ion channels, the substance transported (cholesterol or vitamin B_{12}) is the "messenger" that is delivered to the inside of the cell. Since the cell surface "acceptor" proteins do not themselves generate a regulated transmembrane signal, they can be distinguished from transmembrane receptors that have the dual property of ligand recognition and signal generation.

Receptor Dynamics and Signaling

The previous section has summarized the basic receptor mechanisms for signal generation and signal amplification, but did not deal at all with the cellular dynamics of membrane-localized receptors. As will be seen from the discussion that follows, receptor mobility, both in the plane of the membrane and in terms of the cellular uptake of receptors, plays an important role in the overall process of cell signaling.

The Mobile Receptor Paradigm

The concept of a receptor as a "mobile" or "floating" membrane constituent has evolved with the increased understanding of the general properties of cell surface proteins. Along with investigations of immunoglobulin receptors, studies of the insulin receptor have contributed in a major way to the concept that receptor mobility and cross-linking are key factors in generating a transmembrane signal. The "mobile" or "floating" receptor model, described in more detail elsewhere,[r3,r47] permits receptors to interact with multiple effector moieties within the plane of the membrane. Some of the key observations that stimulated the development of this model relate to the ability of multiple ligands (e.g., ACTH, epinephrine, glucagon, etc.), each interacting with their specific receptors, to activate adenyl cyclase in a single target tissue such as the rat adipocyte; the data pointed to the stimulation of the same enzyme (i.e., adenyl cyclase) by each hormone acting independently via its own receptor. The key tenet of the model that emerged from the independent work of several research groups lies in the putative ability of the agonist, on binding to the receptor, to change the interaction of the receptor with other membrane components. Thus, the entity AR, resulting from the combination of a ligand, A, with its receptor, R

$$A + R \rightleftharpoons AR \rightleftharpoons AR^*$$

results in a conformationally active form of the receptor R*, that can go on to form effector complexes of the kind

$$AR^* + E \rightleftharpoons AR^*E,$$

wherein E represents an effector molecule involved in the process of cell activation. As has been alluded to in the previous section, the G-protein oligomer represents the "effector" moiety for many hormone receptor systems. In the case of receptors for cytokines, as discussed on page 28, a cytoplasmic tyrosine kinase that becomes activated by the cytokine-receptor complex may well represent an "effector" constituent. A number of variations of this model have been developed.[36–38,r48] For instance, although the above equations illustrate an association model, wherein ligand binding promotes receptor-effector coupling, an alternative possibility is a "dissociation" model: A precoupled inactive effector-receptor complex may be dissociated to yield an active effector E* when the ligand binds to the receptor

$$A + RE \rightleftharpoons AR + E^*$$

In principle, the mobile receptor model does not restrict the number of distinct effector moieties with which the ligand-receptor complex might interact. This property could readily permit a single ligand-receptor complex to trigger concurrently a variety of transmembrane signals.

Receptor Microclustering, Patching, and Internalization

Observations with a number of ligands, including insulin, EGF-URO, LDL, immunoglobulins, and transferrin have revealed that, subsequent to ligand binding, many receptors (or "acceptors," like LDL and transferrin) follow a common sequence of mobile reactions as outlined in Figure 1.16. In the absence of their specific ligands, receptors can be randomly distributed over the cell surface. However, as illustrated in Figure 1.16, at physiologic temperatures, the binding of a ligand can lead first to a rapid microclustering (receptor microclusters, containing perhaps two to ten receptors) with a reduction in receptor mobility, followed by the progressive aggregation of ligand receptor complexes into immobile patches (aggregates containing tens to hundreds of receptors) that can be visualized by fluorescence photomicrography. The microclustering event is thought to be much more rapid than the more readily detectable formation of patches that can be seen in the fluorescence microscope. Subsequent to the formation of the comparatively large receptor aggregates, the ligand-receptor complexes can either be shed into the medium or taken into the cell (internalized). Receptor internalization[r49] appears to be an ongoing process that is accelerated when a ligand such as insulin binds to its receptor. It is not clear whether receptor occupation by the ligand is a prerequisite for forming small receptor clusters in all cell types. In some cell types (adipocytes), there are data to indicate that insulin receptors exist as small clusters *prior* to the addition of insulin.[39] The mechanism(s) that lead to microclustering, aggregation, and internalization of receptors (or acceptors) are poorly understood. In many cells, such as fibroblasts, internalization appears to occur at specific sites on the cell surface, the so-called bristle-coated pit. In other cell types (e.g., adipocytes or hepatocytes), receptors may be localized and internalized at sites other than the coated pit regions. Subsequent to aggregation, the receptor can be internalized by an endocytotic process into a cellular compartment that appears to be distinct from the lysosome (Fig. 1.16). The intracellular receptor-bearing vesicles, which, in contrast to lysosomes, are not phase-dense in the electron microscope and are acid phosphatase-negative, have been termed "endosomes" or "receptosomes." The latter term emphasizes the role of these specialized endocytotic vesicles in the process of receptor-mediated endocytosis.[r49] One possible fate of such receptor-bearing endosomes is fusion with lysosomes, followed by the lysosomal degradation of the receptor (so-called receptor processing). Alternatively, the receptosome may be returned to the cell surface via a recycling process that would reintegrate the receptor into the plasma membrane. A possible fusion of the receptosome with other intracellular organelles (e.g., nuclear envelope) cannot be ruled out, but has yet to be documented. At present, little is known about the factors that control either the internalization process or the routing process that may lead on the one hand to lysosomal receptor processing or, on the other hand, to a recycling of the receptor back to the cell surface. The receptor domains that are situated at the cytoplasmic face of the plasma membrane very likely play an important role in this process. There is also little known about the possible role(s) for the degradation products (ligand or receptor fragments) that may be released into the cytoplasm as a result of the endosomal and lysosomal degradation (processing) events. In view of the peripatetic nature of the hormone-receptor complex migrating from the cell surface to the cytoplasmic space, a key question to answer is: what role (if any) do these receptor migratory pathways play in the process of transmembrane signalling? The following section will deal with this question.

Receptor Mobility and Cell Activation

It has been recognized for some time that cell surface antigens can be triggered to form patches and caps. It is now apparent that the crosslinking of cell surface receptors for immunoglobulins or for polypeptides (e.g., insulin) is a key event for cell activation. In terms of polypeptide hormone action, essential observations underlining the importance of receptor microclustering have come from work with anti-insulin receptor antibodies obtained either from insulin-resistant patients,[40] or from rabbits immunized with purified insulin receptor preparations.[41] Intact antibodies or bivalent $(Fab')_2$ antibody preparations that were able to form crosslinks between receptors were able to mimic most of the actions of insulin (e.g., stimulation of glucose and amino acid transport) in a variety of target cells except for the stimulation of DNA synthesis.[r50] The intact antibodies, like insulin, were also able to cap insulin receptors on intact cells.[42] However, monovalent Fab′ antireceptor antibody preparations that could compete effectively for insulin binding but were not able to form crosslinks between receptors were not only unable to mimic insulin action, but were also effective competitive antagonists of insulin in an adipocyte glucose oxidation assay. The biologic activity of the monovalent Fab′ fragments could be restored by the addition of a second bivalent anti-Fab′ antibody that would form crosslinks between Fab′-receptor conjugates.[r50] Results supporting the importance of receptor microaggregation for cell activation have also come from work with antibodies directed against leuteinizing-hormone-releasing-hormone (LHRH) antagonists, wherein the antagonists could be turned into agonists by dimerization (e.g., with the use of bivalent cross-linking antibodies).[43–46] The antibody-induced aggregation of the LHRH receptors could be observed at the electron

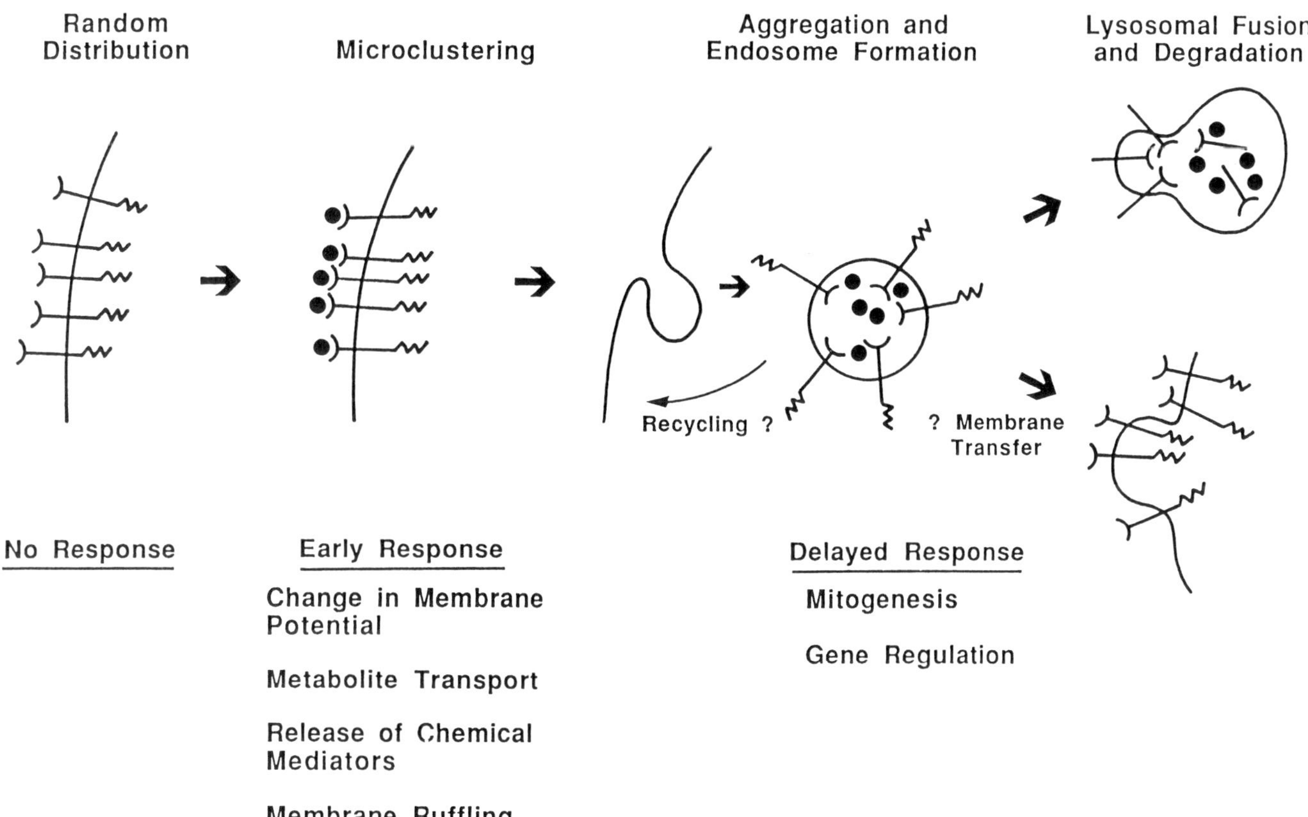

Figure 1.16 Receptor dynamics and cell activation. Rapidly regulated cell responses involve an initial microclustering event. Delayed responses may be caused by a receptor that is internalized in the endosomal organelle. The topography of the endosome would permit the intracellular domain of the receptor (*zigzag line*) to interact with intracellular constituents that may be some considerable distance from the plasma membrane. The receptor-bearing endosome may ultimately fuse with lysosomes (resulting in degradation), or with other intracellular membranes.

microscopic level.[46] Although receptor microaggregation is associated with cell activation, as mentioned above, the microclustering of adipocyte insulin receptors can be observed in the absence of insulin.[39] Thus, receptor clustering may prove to be necessary, but not necessarily sufficient, to initiate a cell response for insulin. Further, the role of receptor microaggregation in terms of activating cells by a G protein mechanism has yet to be defined adequately.

As outlined in Figure 1.16, both the ligand and the receptor can be internalized subsequent to receptor microclustering. An unresolved question is: does the internalized ligand-receptor complex play a role in cell activation? In terms of the rapid actions of hormones such as insulin (e.g., stimulation of glucose transport) or neurotransmitters such as norepinephrine (e.g. vasoconstriction), internalization per se would take place at too slow a rate to play a role in cell triggering. The internalization process might, nonetheless, function in terms of modulating over-all cell sensitivity in a tissue that possesses "spare receptors." However, in relation to some of the delayed effects of agents such as nerve growth factor (e.g., neurite outgrowth) or insulin (mitogenesis, gene regulation), a role for the internalized receptor-ligand complex has been hypothesized. The detection of the retrograde transport and nuclear binding of nerve growth factor in nerve cells and observations of the nuclear binding of EGF-URO and insulin are in keeping with this hypothesis. The demonstrated action of intracellularly administered insulin in frog oocytes also argues strongly in favour of this possibility.[37] Overall, the process of cell activation related to receptor dynamics can be viewed according to the scheme in Figure 1.16. Early responses (changes in membrane potential, metabolite transport) are thought to be triggered in concert with the microclustering of receptors. Delayed responses (mitogenesis, gene regulation) are pictured as possibly involving internalized receptor that is relocated to a specific cellular compartment (e.g., the nucleus). Thus, the temporally distinct actions of certain ligands such as insulin may relate directly to the topographically distinct dynamic events (microclustering, followed by internalization) that occur over quite different time frames subsequent to ligand binding. In this context, the continued internalization of a receptor may be required to sustain a delayed cellular response to an agent such as insulin or nerve growth factor. Thus, transmembrane signaling would involve processes that differ both in their time dependence and in their cellular localization.

Feedback Regulation

Irrespective of the pathway that triggers a cell response (either microclustering or internalization), it is now evident that the entire activation process can be subject to feedback regulation. Thus, the same receptor-triggered reactions that initiate a cell response (e.g., activation of a phosphorylation cascade), can feed back on the receptor itself to turn off a receptor-driven process. An example is provided by the process of receptor desensitization (see page 12; Fig. 1.5). Activation of a plasma membrane β-adrenergic receptor results

A. RECEPTOR PHOSPHORYLATION (SHORT-TERM)

β_2-AR
Gs
AC
ATP
cAMP
(i) PKA ⊕
(ii) β-ARK + β-arrestin
Gs
AC
S-Ⓟ

B. RECEPTOR REDISTRIBUTION AND/OR DOWN-REGULATION (LONG-TERM)

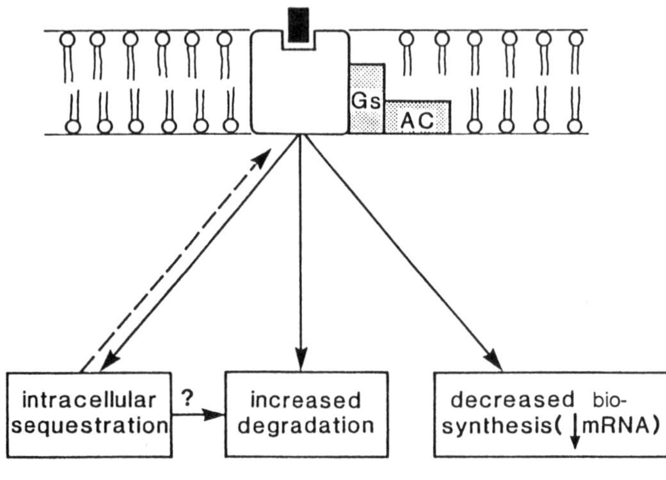

Figure 1.17 Mechanisms for receptor desensitization. *Panel A*: rapid desensitization of the β-adrenergic receptor (β_2-AR) following activation by catecholamines is due to covalent modification involving two phosphorylation reactions (S-P) that are catalyzed by: (i) the cyclic AMP-dependent protein kinase (PKA); (ii) the β-adrenergic receptor kinase (βARK) that is selective for the agonist-occupied receptor. The PKA-catalyzed phosphorylation directly uncouples the receptor from interacting with the stimulatory GTP binding protein (Gs) linked to adenylyl cyclase (AC). The β-ARK-phosphorylated receptor interacts with another protein, β-arrestin, which results in uncoupling.

Panel B: Prolonged β-adrenergic receptor stimulation results in redistribution of the receptor (sequestration) to intracellular sites where the receptor cannot interact with Gs, a process that may be reversible (*dashed lines*). This sequestration event or a separate internalization process may then lead to intracellular degradation, reducing the total number of β-adrenergic receptors. Down-regulation of β-adrenergic receptors is also caused by a reduction in receptor synthesis because of a fall in mRNA levels for the β-adrenergic receptor.

in a profound increase in intracellular cyclic AMP levels because of the Gs-dependent stimulation of adenylyl cyclase (Table 1.2). In spite of the continued presence of the β-adrenergic agonist, cyclic AMP levels generally decline within a few minutes. This rapid phase of receptor desensitization is mediated by two phosphorylation reactions[r51,r52] (Fig. 1.17*A*). At low concentrations of agonist, phosphorylation of the β-adrenergic receptor by the cyclic AMP-dependent protein kinase (PKA) directly uncouples the receptor from interacting with Gs. At higher concentrations of agonist, the agonist-occupied receptor is specifically phosphorylated by a β-adrenergic receptor kinase (βARK), resulting in the association of the phosphorylated receptor with β-arrestin and uncoupling. Interestingly, the βγ subunits of G-proteins may facilitate the localization of βARK to the plasma membrane.[48] This mechanism of receptor desensitization by phosphorylation can be rapidly reversed by a phosphatase-catalyzed dephosphorylation. In contrast, prolonged stimulation of the β-adrenergic receptor results in a redistribution or sequestration of the receptor away from functional plasma membrane sites to an intracellular location, which may subsequently lead to intracellular degradation and a down-regulation of the number of plasma membrane receptors[r52] (Fig. 1.17*B*). Long-term exposure of cells to β-adrenergic agonists also induces a decline in mRNA encoding the β-adrenergic receptor, which contributes further to the reduction in receptor numbers. Recovery from receptor desensitization produced by down-regulation will depend on new receptor synthesis, a process that may take days.

Protein kinase C-mediated phosphorylation is also believed to play a role in receptor internalization and recycling.[49,50] The protein kinase C-catalyzed phosphorylation of a specific threonine residue in the intracellular domain of the EGF-URO receptor reduces both binding affinity and tyrosine kinase activity.[r53] Further, β-adrenergic stimulation causes a downregulation of insulin receptors,[51] and elevation of cellular cyclic AMP causes a reduction in insulin receptor kinase activity.[52] Thus, in principle, the molecular processes responsible for signal generation and amplification in the various systems described in this chapter may also be targets for feedback regulation.

References

Research Reports

1. Langley JN. On the reaction of cells and of nerve-endings to certain poisons, chiefly as regards the reaction of striated muscle to nicotine and to curare. J Physiol 1905;33:374–413.

2. Langley JN. On nerve endings and on special excitable substances. Proc R Soc Lond (Biol) 1906;*78*:170–194.
3. Ariens EJ. Affinity and intrinsic activity in the theory of competitive inhibition. Arch Int Pharmacodyn 1954;*99*:32–49.
4. Stephenson RP. A modification of receptor theory. Brit J Pharmacol 1956;*11*:379–393.
5. Nickerson M. Receptor occupancy and tissue response. Nature 1956;*178*:697–698.
6. Ahlquist RP. A study of the adrenotropic receptors. Am J Physiol 1948;*153*:586–600.
7. Arunlakshana O, Schild HO. Some quantitative uses of drug antagonists. Br J Pharmacol 1959;*14*:48–58.
8. Schild HO. pAx and competitive drug antagonism. Br J Pharmacol 1949;*4*:277–280.
9. Furchgott RF. The use of β-haloalkylamines in the differentiation of receptors and in the determination of dissociation constants of receptor-agonist complexes. Adv Drug Res 1966;*3*:21–25.
10. Clark AJ. The reaction between acetylcholine and muscle cells. Part I. J Physiol (Lond) 1926;*61*:530–546.
11. Clark AJ. The reaction between acetylcholine and muscle cells. Part II. J Physiol (Lond) 1927;*64*:123–143.
12. Paton WDM, Rang HP. The uptake of atropine and related drugs by intestinal smooth muscle of the guinea pig in relation to acetylcholine receptors. Proc R Soc Lond Ser B 1965;*163*:1–44.
13. Paton WDM. A theory of drug action based on the rate of drug-receptor combination. Proc R Soc Lond Ser B 1961;*154*:21–69.
14. Hock RA, Hollenberg MD. Characterization of the receptor for epidermal growth factor-urogastrone in human placenta membranes. J Biol Chem 1980;*255*:10731–10736.
15. Scatchard G. The attraction of proteins for small molecules and ions. Ann NY Acad Sci 1949;*51*:660–672.
16. Munson PJ, Rodbard D. Ligand: A versatile computerized approach for characterization of ligand-binding systems. Anal Biochem 1980;*107*:220–239.
17. Munson PJ. Experimental artifacts and the analysis of ligand binding data: Results of a computer simulation. J Receptor Res 1983;*3*:249–259.
18. Bhaumick B, Armstrong GD, Hollenberg MD, Bala RM. Characterization of the human placental receptor for basic somatomedin. Can J Biochem 1982;*60*:923–932.
19. Cuatrecasas P, Wilchek M, Anfinsen CB. Selective enzyme purification by affinity chromatography. Proc Natl Acad Sci USA 1968;*61*:636–643.
20. Vu T-KH, Hung DT, Wheaton VI, Coughlin SR. Molecular cloning of a functional thrombin receptor reveals a novel proteolytic mechanism of receptor activation. Cell 1991;*64*:1057–1068.
21. Schofield PR, Darlison MG, Fujita N, Burt DR, Stephenson FA, Rodriguez H, Rhee LM, Ramchandran J, Reale V, Glencorse TA, Seeburg PH, Barnard EA. Sequence and functional expression of the $GABA_A$ receptor show a ligand-gated receptor superfamily. Nature 1987;*328*:221–227.
22. Grenningloh G, Rienitz A, Schmitt B, Methfessel C, Zensen M, Beyreuther K, Gundelfinger ED, Betz H. The strychnine-binding subunit of the glycine receptor shows homology with nicotinic acetylcholine receptors. Nature 1987;*328*:215–220.
23. Kobilka BK, Frielle T, Collins S, Yang-Feng T, Kobilka TS, Francke U, Lefkowitz RJ, Caron MG. An intronless gene encoding a potential member of the family of receptors coupled to guanine nucleotide regulatory proteins. Nature 1987;*329*:75–79.
24. Fargin A, Raymond JR, Lohse MJ, Kobilka BK, Caron MG, Lefkowitz RJ. The genomic clone G-21 which resembles a β-adrenergic receptor sequence encodes the $5\text{-}HT_{1A}$ receptor. Nature 1988;*335*:358–360.
25. Kobilka BK, Kobilka TS, Daniel K, Regan JW, Caron MG, Lefkowitz RJ. Chimeric α_2-, β_2-adrenergic receptors: Delineation of domains involved in effector coupling and ligand binding specificity. Science 1988;*240*:1310–1316.
26. Taylor SI. Molecular mechanisms of insulin resistance. Lessons from patients with mutations in the insulin-receptor gene. Diabetes 1992;*41*:1473–1490.
27. Flier JS. Syndromes of insulin resistance. From patient to gene and back again. Diabetes 1992;*41*:1207–1219.
28. Hamilton SL, Codina J, Hawkes MJ, Yatani A, Sawada T, Strickland FM, Froehner SC, Spiegel AM, Toro L, Stefani E, Birnbaumer L, Brown AM. Evidence for direct interaction of $G_s\alpha$ with the Ca^{2+} channel of skeletal muscle. J Biol Chem 1991;*266*:19528–19535.
29. Lowndes JM, Gupta SK, Osawa S, Johnson GL. GTPase-deficient $G\alpha_{i2}$ oncogene *gip2* inhibits adenylyl cyclase and attenuates receptor-stimulated phospholipase A_2 activity. J Biol Chem 1991;*266*:14193–14197.
30. Bégin-Heick N. Quantification of the α and β subunits of the transducing elements (G_s and G_i) of adenylate cyclase in adipocyte membranes from lean and obese (*ob/ob*) mice. Biochem J 1990;*268*:83–89.
31. Bégin-Heick N. α-Subunits of G_s and G_i in adipocyte plasma membranes of genetically diabetic (*db/db*) mice. Am J Physiol 1992;*263*:C121–C129.
32. Murakami MS, Rosen OM. The role of insulin receptor autophosphorylation in signal transduction. J Biol Chem 1991;*266*:22653–22660.
33. Mathews LS, Vale WW. Expression cloning of an activin receptor, a predicted transmembrane serine kinase. Cell 1991;*65*:973–982.
34. Yang S-G, Saifeddine M, Chuang M, Severson DL, Hollenberg MD. Diacylglycerol lipase and the contractile action of epidermal growth factor-urogastrone: evidence for distinct signal pathways in a single strip of gastric smooth muscle. Eur J Pharmacol (Mol Pharmacol) 1991;*207*:225–230.
35. Furchgott RF, Zawadzki JV. The obligatory role of endothelial cells in the relaxation of arterial smooth muscle by acetylcholine. Nature 1980;*288*:373–376.
36. Boeynaems JM, Dumont JE. The two-step model of ligand-receptor interaction. Mol Cell Endocrinol 1977;*7*:33–47.
37. DeHaen C. The non-stoichiometric floating receptor model for hormone-sensitive adenylate cyclase. J Theor Biochem 1976;*58*:383–400.
38. Levitzki A. Negative cooperativity in clustered receptors as a possible basis for membrane action. J Theoret Biol 1974;*44*:367–372.
39. Jarrett L, Smith RM. The natural occurrence of insulin receptors in groups on adipocyte plasma membranes as demonstrated with monomeric ferritin-insulin. J Supramol Struct 1977;*6*:45–59.
40. Kahn CR, Baird KL, Jarett DB, Flier JS. Direct demonstration that receptor crosslinking or aggregation is important in insulin action. Proc Natl Acad Sci USA 1978;*75*:4209–4213.
41. Jacobs S, Chang K-J, Cuatrecasas P. Antibodies to purified insulin receptor have insulin-like activity. Science 1978;*200*:1283–1284.
42. Schlessinger J, Van Obberghen E, Khan CR. Insulin and antibodies against insulin receptor cap on the membranes of cultured human lymphocytes. Nature 1980;*286*:729–731.

43. Conn PM, Rogers DC, Stewart JM, Neidel J, Sheffield T. Conversion of a gonadotropin-releasing hormone antagonist to an agonist. Nature 1982;*296*:653–655.

44. Gregory H, Taylor CL, Hopkins CR. Luteinizing hormone release from dissociated pituitary cells by dimerization of occupied LHRH receptors. Nature 1982;*300*:269–271.

45. Hazum E, Keinan D. Gonadotropin releasing hormone activation is mediated by dimerization of occupied receptors. Biochem Biophys Res Commun 1985;*133*:449–456.

46. Hopkins CR, Semoff S, Gregory H. Regulation of gonadotropin secretion of the anterior pituitary. Philos Trans R Soc Lond [Biol] 1981;*296*:73–81.

47. Miller DS. Stimulation of RNA and protein synthesis by intracellular insulin. Science 1988;*240*:506–509.

48. Pitcher JA, Inglese J, Higgins JB, Arriza JL, Casey PJ, Kim C, Benovic JL, Kwatra MM, Caron MG, Lefkowitz RJ. Role of βγ subunits of G proteins in targeting the β-adrenergic receptor kinase to membrane-bound receptors. Science 1992;*257*:1264–1267.

49. Hunter T, Ling N, Cooper JA. Protein kinase C phosphorylation of the EGF receptor at a threonine residue close to the cytoplasmic face of the plasma membrane. Nature 1984;311:*480*–483.

50. Lin CR, Chen WS, Lazar CS, Carpenter CD, Gill GN, Evans RM, Rosenfeld MG. Protein kinase C phosphorylation at Thr 654 of the unoccupied EGF receptor and EGF binding regulate functional receptor loss by independent mechanisms. Cell 1986;*44*:839–848.

51. Pessin JE, Gitomer W, Oka Y, Oppenheimer CL, Czech MP. β-adrenergic regulation of insulin and epidermal growth factor receptors in rat adipocytes. J Biol Chem 1983;*258*:7386–7394.

52. Stadtmauer L, Rosen OM. Increasing the cAMP content of IM-9 cells alters the phosphorylation state and protein kinase activity of the insulin receptor. J. Biol. Chem. 1986;*262*:3402–3407.

Reviews

r1. Ehrlich P. Nobel lecture on partial functions of the cell. In: The Collected Papers of P. Ehrlich, Vol. III. Himmelweit F, Marquardt M, Dale H (Eds.), Oxford England: Pergamon Press (1908); pp 183–194.

r2. Stephenson RP, Barlow RB. Concepts of drug action, quantitative pharmacology and biological assay. In: A Companion to Medical Studies, Vol. 2. Passmore R, Robson JS (Eds.) London: Backwell (1970); pp 3.1–3.19.

r3. Cuatrecasas P, Hollenberg MD. Membrane receptors and hormone action. Adv Protein Chem 1976;*30*:251–451.

r4. Schwarz KR. The principles of receptor binding studies. In: The Heart and Cardiovascular System, Second Edition, Fozzard HA et al (eds). New York: Raven Press Ltd. (1992); pp 483–503.

r5. Stroud RM, Finer-Moore J. Acetylcholine receptor structure, function and evolution. Ann Rev Cell Biol 1985;*1*:317–351.

r6. Numa S. A molecular view of neurotransmitter receptors and ionic channels. Harvey Lec 1989;*83*:121–165.

r7. Lindstrom J, Schoepfer R, Whiting P. Molecular studies of the neuronal nicotinic acetylcholine receptor family. Mol Neurobiol 1987;*1*:281–337.

r8. Betz H. Ligand-gated ion channels in the brain: The amino acid receptor superfamily. Neuron 1990;*5*:383–392.

r9. Stroud RM, McCarthy MP, Shuster M. Nicotinic acetylcholine receptor superfamily of ligand-gated ion channels. Biochemistry 1990;*29*:11009–11023.

r10. Dohlman HG, Caron MG, Lefkowitz RJ. A family of receptors coupled to guanine nucleotide regulatory proteins. Biochemistry 1987;*26*:2657–2664.

r11. Hosey MM. Diversity of structure, signaling and regulation within the family of muscarinic cholinergic receptors. FASEB J 1992;*6*:845–852.

r12. Ostrowski J, Kjelsberg MA, Caron MG, Lefkowitz RJ. Mutagenesis of the β_2-adrenergic receptor: How structure elucidates function. Ann Rev Pharmacol Toxicol 1992;*32*:167–183.

r13. Savarese TM, Fraser CM. *In vitro* mutagenesis and the search for structure-function relationships among G protein-coupled receptors. Biochem J 1992;*283*:1–19.

r14. Sutherland EW, Robison GA, Butcher RW. Some aspects of the biological role of adenosine 3′,5′-monophosphate (cyclic AMP). Circulation 1968;*37*:279–306.

r15. Berridge MJ. Inositol trisphosphate and calcium signalling. Nature 1993;*361*:315–325.

r16. Nishizuka Y. Intracellular signaling by hydrolysis of phospholipids and activation of protein kinase C. Science 1992;*258*:607–614.

r17. Strosberg AD. Structure/function relationship of proteins belonging to the family of receptors coupled to GTP-binding proteins. Eur J Biochem 1991;*196*:1–10.

r18. Kurachi Y, Tung RT, Ito H, Nakajima T. G protein activation of cardiac muscarinic K^+ channels. Prog Neurobiol 1992;*39*:229–246.

r19. Axelrod J. Receptor-mediated activation of phospholipase A_2 and arachidonic acid release in signal transduction. Biochem Soc Trans 1990;*18*:503–507.

r20. Clapham DE. Arachidonic acid and its metabolites in the regulation of G-protein gated K^+ channels in atrial myocytes. Biochem Pharmacol 1990;*39*:813–815.

r21. Stryer L. Visual excitation and recovery. J Biol Chem 1991;*266*:10711–10714.

r22. Hargrave PA, McDowell JH. Rhodopsin and phototransduction: a model system for G protein-linked receptors. FASEB J 1992;*6*:2323–2331.

r23. Kaziro Y, Itoh H, Kozasa T, Nakafuku M, Satoh T. Structure and function of signal-transducing GTP-binding proteins. Ann Rev Biochem 1991;*60*:349–400.

r24. Bourne HR, Sanders DA, McCormick F. The GTPase superfamily: conserved structure and molecular mechanism. Nature 1991;*349*:117–127.

r25. Satoh T, Nakafuku M, Kaziro Y. Function of ras as a molecular switch in signal transduction. J Biol Chem 1992;*267*:24149–24152.

r26. Hepler JR, Gilman AG. G proteins. Trends Biochem Sci 1992;*17*:383–387.

r27. Simon MI, Strathmann MP, Gautam N. Diversity of G proteins in signal transduction. Science 1991;*252*:802–808.

r28. Burns DL. Choleragen and *Escherichia coli* heat-labile enterotoxin: activation of adenylate cyclase by adenosine 5′-diphosphate-ribosylation of a regulatory subunit. pp 654–5. In: Moss J, moderator. Cyclic nucleotides: mediators of bacterial toxin action in disease. Ann Intern Med 1984;*101*:653–666.

r29. Hsia JA. Pertussis toxin. Toxin-catalyzed adenosine 5′-diphosphate ribosylation blocks hormonal inhibition of adenylate cyclase. pp 656–658. In: Moss J, moderator. Cyclic nucleotides: mediators of bacterial toxin action in disease. Ann Intern Med 1984;*101*:653–666.

r30. Cockcroft S, Thomas GMH. Inositol-lipid-specific phospholipase C isoenzymes and their differential regulation by receptors. Biochem J 1992;*288*:1–14.

r31. Spiegel AM, Shenker A, Weinstein LS. Receptor-effector coupling by G proteins: Implications for normal and abnormal signal transduction. Endocr Rev 1992;*13*:536–565.

r32. Sieghart W. $GABA_A$ receptors: ligand-gated Cl^-ion channels modulated by multiple drug-binding sites. Trends Biochem Sci 1992;*13*:446–450.

r33. Brown AM. A cellular logic for G protein-coupled ion channel pathways. FASEB J 1991;*5*:2175–2179.

r34. Ullrich A, Schlessinger J. Signal transduction by receptors with tyrosine kinase activity. Cell 1990;*61*:203–212.

r35. Schlessinger J, Ullrich A. Growth factor signaling by receptor tyrosine kinases. Neuron 1992;*9*:383–391.

r36. Carpenter G. Receptor tyrosine kinase substrates: src homology domains and signal transduction. FASEB J 1992;*6*:3283–3289.

r37. Miyajima A, Kitamura T, Harada N, Yokota T, Arai K-I. Cytokine receptors and signal transduction. Ann Rev Immunol 1992;*10*:295–331.

r38. Harnett M, Rigley K. The role of G-proteins versus protein tyrosine kinases in the regulation of lymphocyte activation. Immunol Today 1992;*13*:482–486.

r39. Wong SK-F, Garbers DL. Receptor guanylyl cyclases. J Clin Invest 1992;*90*:299–305.

r40. Severson DL, Hollenberg MD. The plasma membrane as a transducer and amplifier. Fundamentals of Medical Cell Biology. Volume 5A, Membrane dynamics and signaling. Greenwich, Connecticut: JAI Press (1992); pp 223–254.

r40a. Levitzki, A. From Epinephrine to Cyclic AMP. Science 1988;*241*:800–806.

r41. Furchgott RF. The role of endothelium in the responses of vascular smooth muscle to drugs. Ann Rev Pharmacol Toxicol 1984;*24*:175–197.

r42. Moncada S, Palmer RMJ, Higgs EA. Nitric oxide: Physiology, pathophysiology, and pharmacology. Pharmacol Rev 1991;*43*:109–142.

r43. Bredt DS, Snyder SH. Nitric oxide, a novel neuronal messenger. Neuron 1992;*8*:3–11.

r44. Beato M. Gene regulation by steroid hormones. Cell 1989;*56*:335–344.

r45. Wahli W, Martinez E. Superfamily of steroid nuclear receptors: positive and negative regulators of gene expression. FASEB J 1991;*5*:2243–2249.

r46. Yuen PST, Garbers DL. Guanylyl cyclase-linked receptors. Ann Rev Neurosci 1992;*15*:193–225.

r47. Hollenberg MD. Mechanisms of receptor-mediated transmembrane signalling. Experientia 1986;*42*:718–727.

r48. Boeynaems JM, Dumont JE. Outlines of receptor theory. Amsterdam, New York, Oxford:Elsevier/North-Holland Biomedical (1980).

r49. Pastan IH, Willingham MC. Receptor-mediated endocytosis of hormones in cultured cells. Ann Rev Physiol 1981;*43*:239–250.

r50. Kahn CR, Baird KL, Jarett DB, Flier JS. Direct demonstration that receptor crosslinking or aggregation is important in insulin action. Proc Natl Acad Sci USA 1978;*75*:4209–4213.

r51. Hausdorff WP, Caron MG, Lefkowitz RJ. Turning off the signal: desensitization of β-adrenergic receptor function. FASEB J 1990;*4*:2881–2889.

r52. Kobilka B. Adrenergic receptors as models for G protein-coupled receptors. Ann Rev Neurosci 1992;*15*:87–114.

r53. Iwashita S, Kobayashi M. Signal transduction system for growth factor receptors associated with tyrosine kinase activity: Epidermal growth factor receptor signalling and its regulation. Cell Signalling 1992;*4*:123–132.

General References

Clark AJ. The model of action of drugs on cells. London: Arnold (1933) [*A remarkably perceptive volume dealing with the molecular pharmacology of drug action.*]

Clark AJ. General pharmacology. Handbook of experimental pharmacology. Vol. 1 (1937) [*Provides an interesting perspective for many modern pharmacology textbooks; a revised version of Clark's 1933 text. Sections of this text are reproduced verbatim in the Holmstedt and Liljestrand reference cited above (see Introduction).*]

Linder ME, Gilman AG. G Proteins. Scientific American 1992;*267*:56–65. [*Provides a lucid description of the key experiments that led to the discovery of GTP-binding proteins as signal transduction elements.*]

CHAPTER 2

Pharmacokinetics: Disposition and Metabolism of Drugs

David V. Godin

Introduction

The actions of drugs in vivo are determined by a complex interplay between PHARMACODYNAMIC and PHARMACOKINETIC processes. As mentioned in the Introduction to this Section, **pharmacokinetics** deals with mechanisms and quantitative characteristics (time- and concentration-dependence) of drug absorption, distribution, metabolism, and excretion. These four processes (Fig. 2.1) have a direct bearing on the **magnitude** and **duration** of responses to drugs, by virtue of their overall effect on the plasma concentration of free (unbound) drug, which is able to equilibrate with the target cells at the site of drug action.[r1,r2] As also alluded to in the Introduction, the term **pharmacodynamics** refers to the mechanisms whereby the interaction of drugs at their site of action elicits a pharmacologic response. This topic was dealt with in detail in Chapter 1.

The pharmacokinetic properties of drugs depend to a large degree on bulk physicochemical characteristics, such as their molecular weight, their solubility in lipid or aqueous environment (lipophilicity or polarity, respectively) and their ionization state (only uncharged species readily cross cell membranes or other lipoidal barriers). Nonetheless, to some extent, the detailed structural features and stereochemistry of certain drugs can have an influence on their pharmacokinetic characteristics as, for example, in the case of quantitative or even qualitative differences in the metabolic disposition of R- and S-enantiomers.[r3,r4] One objective of this chapter is to point out how the general chemical features of drugs (most importantly, lipid solubility, molecular weight, and ionization state) affect the manner in which they are handled by the body.

This chapter will focus on the main pharmacokinetic principles that form the basis of all drug dosing regimens. The fundamental objective of such regimens is to achieve plasma concentrations of a drug that will produce an optimal **therapeutic** effect with minimal **toxicity** (see Chapter 3). To achieve this objective, answers to the following questions are required:

(1) By what mechanism and at what rate does the drug get into the body, and what is the optimal route of administration? In answering this question, it is important to know if the rate of drug administration or the route of administration affects its activity

(2) How is the drug distributed in the body, and what factors influence the level of free (unbound) drug at its sites of action and its sites of metabolism?

(3) How does the plasma concentration of the drug relate to its therapeutic and toxic actions?

(4) How is the drug metabolized, and how does its metabolism affect its biologic activity? In this context, the influence of illness on drug metabolism and the effect of one drug on the metabolism of a second drug are of particular importance.

(5) How is the drug eliminated from the body, and how do disease states (e.g., those involving liver or kidney) affect the elimination of the drug or its metabolites?

The answers to the above questions can, in part, be considered at two levels of complexity. On one level, the detailed properties of drug transport, serum pro-

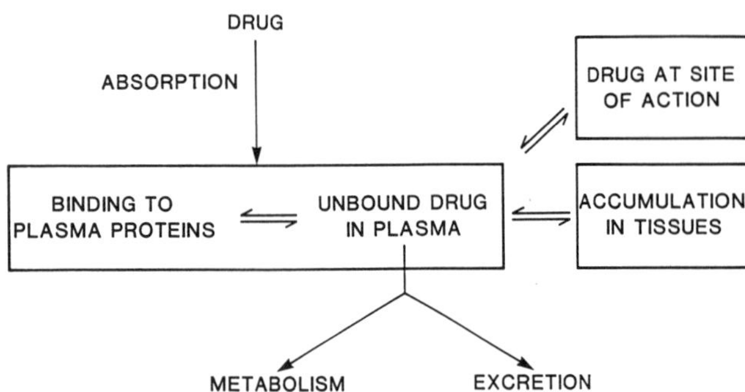

Figure 2.1 Pharmacokinetic processes: relationships between absorption, distribution, metabolism, and excretion of a drug.

tein binding, drug metabolism, and drug excretion can be examined in molecular terms. These topics are dealt with in detail throughout this chapter. On a second level, a purely empirical kinetic approach can be used to quantify the rates of drug absorption, distribution, and excretion, without making assumptions about the molecular mechanisms involved. This second approach, dealt with on page 64 (Quantitative Pharmacokinetics), yields extremely useful practical descriptive information about apparent volumes of distribution, half-lives or clearance rates, and predicted steady-state drug levels that are of key importance in planning any drug dosing regimen. For instance, the descriptive information about the apparent **volume of distribution (Vd)** of a drug, i.e., the hypothetical volume in which a dose (D) of the drug would have to be placed to yield the observed initial plasma concentration, allows one to calculate the amount of drug to be given to achieve a desired plasma concentration (Cp) according to the simple formula:

$$Cp = D/Vd$$

The **half-life (t½)** of a drug in the body (i.e., the time taken for the plasma concentration to decrease by half) provides a quantitative measure of drug elimination. Such information is used for establishing drug dosing intervals in chronic therapy, with drugs usually being given at intervals approximating the t½. Under such conditions, repeated administration of drugs leads to the development of a steady state at which the rate of drug elimination becomes equal to the rate of drug administration. As will be described on page 69, it can be shown that the time required to attain such a steady state with multiple dosing is approximately five times the t½ value.

Thus, the quantitative pharmacokinetic parameters Vd and t½ directly provide an answer to the two fundamental questions in any drug dosing regimen, namely how much and how often? Before discussing the many practical applications of pharmacokinetic principles, it will be important to consider the numerous factors that can alter the disposition (and hence Vd and/or t½ values) of drugs under various clinical conditions. Such an understanding is crucial in order that drug administration be individualized to the needs of each patient.

In the sections that follow, a number of specific drugs will be used as illustrations of pharmacokinetic principles. For instance, the effects of plasma protein binding on drug action and clearance will be illustrated using phenytoin (formerly called diphenylhydantoin) as an example. The relevance of drug metabolism to the generation of active metabolites will be illustrated with various benzodiazepines as examples. In the context of saturable metabolic pathways that have clinical relevance, salicylates (aspirin-related drugs) will be used for illustration purposes. Finally, in terms of the interplay between drug metabolism and the induction of drug-metabolizing enzymes, the ability of barbiturates to induce the metabolizing enzymes for the anticoagulant, coumadin, will be described.

The reader is asked to take a two-tiered approach when considering the examples that follow. First, it is essential to extract the basic, pharmacokinetic principles that are being illustrated. Second, it is hoped that the relevant information about each specific drug will be carried over to the more detailed sections of the text, where each of the drugs mentioned here for illustrative purposes will be dealt with more comprehensively.

Drug Absorption—Passage of Drugs Across Barriers Separating Compartments

The process of absorption involves the passage of drug molecules across single or multiple barriers interspersed between the particular site of administration and the vascular compartment. The characteristics of drug absorption are thus critically dependent on the physicochemical properties of the molecules in question and on the nature of the barrier(s) to be traversed. Depending on the route of administration, drugs may gain passage across tissue membrane barriers (that are typically lipoidal in nature) by passive diffusion based on lipophilicity (lipid solubility), by size-limited diffusion through pores of various sizes, or by carrier-mediated (facilitated) diffusion (Table 2.1). Each of these processes has important practical implications in drug administration and will therefore be discussed in some detail.

Passive Diffusion Across Lipoidal Membrane Barriers

Drugs administered by mouth or inhalation must gain access to the systemic circulation by diffusion

Table 2.1 Passage of Drugs Across Tissue Barriers

1.	Passive diffusion, dependent on (a) concentration gradient (b) lipid solubility (lipophilicity) (c) degree of ionization (pKa; weak acids and bases)
2.	Diffusion through pores (bulk flow) dependent on molecular size relative to pore dimensions in cell membranes and peripheral capillaries.
3.	Carrier-mediated transport: (a) facilitated, diffusion, requiring a concentration gradient and characterized by saturability and potential for competition by structural analogues; (b) active transport against a concentration gradient, requiring a source of energy (usually ATP).

across the epithelial or endothelial surfaces involved. Given the presence of tight (or occluded) intercellular junctions in such systems, molecules will gain passage across these barriers in proportion to their **lipid solubility**. Thus, nonpolar drugs will diffuse across membranes more rapidly than polar (charged) drugs. The rate of absorption can be expressed by the Fick equation for passive diffusion as follows:

$$\text{rate} = \frac{D\ A\ \Delta C\ K}{\Delta x}$$

where D = diffusion coefficient of the molecule in the lipid phase
A = surface area of absorption
ΔC = concentration gradient of drug across the barrier
K = drug partition coefficient
Δx = thickness of the barrier

Molecular size has little limiting effect on diffusibility for substances with molecular weights below 100,000 daltons (this mass encompasses the vast majority of therapeutic agents). Larger molecules are more likely to cross lipoidal barriers (such as cell membranes, for example) by pinocytosis rather than by simple diffusion. The relationship between surface area and absorptive capacity is well illustrated anatomically by the structural features that characterize sites of high absorptive activity in the body. The large increase in surface area in the small intestine conferred by the multiple infoldings formed by villi and superimposed microvilli structures make this the primary site of absorption for drugs administered by the oral route. Similarly, the brush border epithelial cells of the kidney are an important determinant of the crucial reabsorptive function of renal tubules. As indicated by the Fick equation, the relative proportions of diffusible solute on either side of a lipoidal surface determine the rate and direction of diffusion. The maintenance of concentration gradients favoring drug absorption *in vivo* is a dynamic process that is critically dependent on circulatory factors governing regional blood flow. Drugs are, therefore, more effectively absorbed from tissue sites of administration that are highly perfused (e.g., skeletal muscle) than from regions with a more limited blood supply (e.g., subcutaneous tissue or fat). Furthermore, delayed onset of drug action (e.g., after intramuscular administration) may be expected in states of severe circulatory impairment (e.g., shock). Finally, the previously mentioned contribution of lipophilicity to drug diffusion across lipoidal barriers is expressed quantitatively in the Fick equation in terms of the drug partition coefficient (K), a measure of drug solubility in an organic solvent (e.g., octanol) relative to that in water. It should be noted that effective drug transport *in vivo* requires a balance between lipophilicity and hydrophilicity, the latter being important for drug diffusion through aqueous interstitial spaces. Thus, the activity of various classes of pharmacologic agents *in vivo* is frequently found to be associated with optimal partition coefficient values that are characteristic both of the particular drug category and the target cell or tissue involved in the pharmacologic response. Such information has obvious applicability in the area of rational drug design.

A related consideration in the analysis of factors influencing the partitioning of drugs that are weak acids or weak bases is the degree of ionization under physiologic conditions. In general, nonionized species readily diffuse across lipoidal barriers, while charged forms are largely impermeant. The relative proportions of ionized and nonionized moieties are determined by the pH and the relative acidity or basicity of the dissociable group (i.e., its pKa value) as expressed in the following relationship derived from the law of mass action for the equilibrium: $HA - H^+ + A^-$, with HA being the protonated form (or proton donor) and A^- the unprotonated species (or proton acceptor). The equilibrium constant (Ka) for this ionization process is given by:

$$Ka = \frac{[H^+]\ [A^-]}{[HA]}$$

Taking negative logarithms of both sides of the equation and rearranging yields the relationship attributed to Henderson and Hasselbalch:

$$pH = pKa + \log \frac{A^-}{HA} = pKa = + \log \frac{[\text{proton acceptor}]}{[\text{proton donor}]}$$

In the case of a weak acid ($HA - H^+ + A^-$), the ratio in question would be $[A^-]/[HA]$ or [salt]/[acid]; for a weak base ($BH^+ - B + H^+$), the corresponding ratio is $[B]/[BH^+]$ or [base]/[salt]. The equation defines pKa as that pH at which equal amounts of ionized and nonionized forms are present (i.e., the logarithmic term becomes zero when the ratio is unity). For drugs that are either weak acids or weak bases, the extent of ionization is variable, depending on the pH of the environment (acid pH of stomach; neutral-alkaline pH of the intestine).

As an example, for a weak acid of pKa 4.4 at physiologic pH (7.4), log $[A^-]/[HA] = 7.4 - 4.4 = 3.0$. Thus, the relative proportions of ionized to nonionized forms is $10^3/1$ or 1000/1. In the case of a weakly basic drug with a pKa value of 8.4, log $[B]/[BH^+] = 7.4 - 8.4 = -1.0$, so that the ratio of nonionized/ionized species is equal to $10^{-1}/1$ or 1/10. Based on the relative preponderance of nonionized forms, one would expect that weak acids should be largely absorbed from the stomach and weak bases from the intestine. However, the extensive surface area provided by the intestine make it a major site of absorption for both acidic and basic drugs after their oral administration.

The pharmacologic activity of certain drugs is critically dependent on their ionization properties, as is well illustrated by the weakly basic tertiary amine local anesthetics. The pKa values of clinically effective agents are such that appreciable amounts of both nonionized (free base) and ionized (protonated; BH^+) forms are present at physiologic pH. The blockade of action potential-generating sodium channels is believed to result from the interaction of the positively charged (protonated) form of the anesthetic at the inner surface of the neuronal membrane, but the drug gains access to this intracellular site of action by passive diffusion of the nonionized free base into the nerve terminal.[r5] The rate of this uptake process, which is a major determinant of the time required for the onset of neuronal conduction blockade, increases with the relative abundance of the nonionized (diffusible) form of the local anesthetic. On this basis, the Henderson-Hasselbalch equation would predict that the higher the pKa value for a local anesthetic the slower would be its onset of action, since for pKa values greater than the physiologic pH of 7.4 the proportion of the charged form of these drugs will increase. This prediction is borne out clinically, as shown by a comparison of lidocaine (pKa = 7.7), bupivacaine (pKa = 8.1), and procaine (pKa = 8.9), which exhibit fast, intermediate, and slow onset rates of local anesthesia, respectively.[r6] A related clinical phenomenon is the reduced efficacy of local anesthetics injected into regions of infection, which characteristically are associated with a localized decrease in pH. Under these conditions, the increased proportion of the protonated (nondiffusible) form of the anesthetic would limit access to the intraneuronal site of action.

Diffusion Through Porous Lipoidal Barriers

The movement of drugs across lipoidal surfaces containing discontinuities or pores is determined primarily by factors relating to **size**, namely the dimensions of the pore and the molecular weight of the drug in question. Cell membranes contain small (approximately 8 A in diameter) aqueous pores that allow the passage of polar substances with molecular weights less than 100–150 daltons. In contrast to the tight intercellular junctions that exist in various epithelial barriers (e.g., the lung, skin, cornea, gastrointestinal tract, and urinary bladder), the endothelial network of peripheral capillaries (e.g., in subcutaneous or intramuscular tissue) contains discontinuities that are sufficiently large (60–80 A in diameter) to permit the permeation of substances with molecular weights below 50–60,000 daltons (which encompasses most therapeutic agents) independently of their lipophilicity, polarity, or degree of ionization. This permits the effective administration by intramuscular or subcutaneous routes, for example, of drugs showing poor absorption from the gastrointestinal tract because of limited lipid solubility.

An important exception to the generalization that capillaries show a low resistance to solute permeation exists in cerebral capillaries. Rather than the leaky intercellular junctions present in capillaries of the peripheral vasculature, brain capillaries are characterized by endothelial cell junctions of the tight (or occluded) variety, similar to epithelial cells. Furthermore, pinocytotic vesicles that are involved in the transendothelial movement of substances with molecular weights in excess of 100,000 daltons are also less abundant in capillaries of brain as compared with those elsewhere in the body. These structural features of brain capillaries are important determinants of the so-called "blood-brain barrier." Thus, drugs in the systemic circulation generally gain access to the central nervous system (CNS) in direct proportion to their lipid solubility. In a few areas of the CNS, however, the typical tight junction arrangement of capillaries is largely absent, accounting for the central effects of various circulating polar drugs and toxins. One such region of particular significance is the area postrema that contains the vomiting center.

Although most highly polar or charged drugs are largely excluded from the central nervous system, a few, by virtue of their close structural resemblance to naturally occurring compounds, may be actively transported into the brain by specific carrier-mediated processes (see below) normally used in the transport of endogenous substances. It has been suggested, for example, that the centrally-acting antihypertensive-methyl-dihydroxyphenylalanine (methyl dopa) can enter the brain by an amino acid transporting system. In most cases, however, hydrophilic drugs must be injected directly into the cerebrospinal fluid (CSF) (that is, they must be administered intrathecally) in order to obtain adequate therapeutic responses, as in the treatment of certain central nervous system infections with antibiotics that penetrate the blood-brain barrier poorly. Drugs administered intrathecally are readily accessible to brain tissue because the epithelial cells lining the cerebral ventricles are not connected by tight junctions, resulting in a highly permeable CSF - brain barrier. Certain drugs (such as penicillin) may, however, show inadequate therapeutic responses after intrathecal injection because of the presence in choroid epithelium of a carrier-mediated system capable of actively secreting organic ions from the CSF into the blood.[r7]

The permeability characteristics of the blood-brain barrier are influenced by a variety of factors. Vasoactive substances (e.g., histamine, serotonin, and bradykinin), released from cerebral endothelial cells by pathophysiologic conditions, such as hypoxia, increase the leakiness of the blood-brain barrier. Other pathologic conditions affecting the central nervous system, such as tumors, infarcts, or infections, may also be associated with an increased permeability of the blood-brain barrier. Incomplete formation of the blood-brain barrier in the newborn predisposes to the development of kernicterus ("yellow brain"), a form of neurologic damage caused by bilirubin deposition in the basal ganglia, when newborns are exposed to agents (notably sulfonamide antibiotics) that increase free circulating levels of bilirubin by competition for common binding sites on plasma albumin (see page 49). Reversible increases in blood-brain barrier permeability can be induced pharmacologically in order to facilitate drug permeation into the CNS.[r8] The intracarotid administration of hypertonic mannitol, for example, has been found to cause a 10–50-fold increase in the brain levels of the antineoplastic drug methotrexate after its systemic administration. Although it has previously been suggested that such osmotic opening of the blood-brain barrier involved the transient separation of cerebral capillary tight junctions, the importance of increased pinocytotic activity with resultant enhancement of transendothelial transport has been emphasized more recently.[r9]

Carrier-Mediated (Facilitated) Diffusion

The passage of some naturally occurring polar substances (e.g., sugars, amino acids) across lipoidal tissue (membrane) barriers can occur at rates greatly exceeding those expected for simple diffusion. Typically, such processes exhibit saturability and competition by structural analogues, indicating the presence within the lipoidal membrane of mobile carriers capable of binding in a structurally specific manner with the ligand to be transported, thereby facilitating its translocation across the membrane. If the transport process requires a concentration gradient, it is referred to as **facilitated diffusion.** By comparison, the energy-dependent transport of substances against a concentration gradient is termed **active transport.** Examples of well-characterized carrier-mediated processes include glucose entry into cells (e.g., erythrocytes), the absorption of certain products of digestion from the gut, the secretion of drug metabolites into bile, the recovery of glomerular filtrate constituents by renal tubules, as well as the weak acid and weak base tubular secretion systems mediating the excretion of drugs by the kidney. The saturability of such carrier-mediated transport processes is well illustrated by the uncontrolled diabetic state in that high levels of glucose in the glomerular filtrate exceed the reabsorptive capacity of renal tubules, resulting in the loss of glucose in the urine (glycosuria). Competition by structural analogues for transport sites may have either desirable or undesirable pharmacologic consequences. Examples of the former would be the use of probenecid (an inert organic acid) in the treatment of hyperuricemia to reduce the tubular reabsorption of uric acid, thereby enhancing its excretion. Alternatively, probenecid has been used to decrease the renal tubular secretion of penicillin, resulting in a prolongation of its antibacterial actions. On the other hand, hyperuricemia may arise as an undesirable complication of therapy with weakly acidic drugs (such as salicylates and a number of commonly used diuretics) as a consequence of competition for urate secretion at the level of the renal tubular weak acid carrier. In a similar fashion, salicylate administration can reduce the renal excretion of methotrexate (an anticancer agent), resulting in increased blood levels and an enhanced risk of serious toxicities. Finally, competitive interactions at transport sites involving dietary protein derived amino acids can reduce the intestinal absorption of levodopa after its oral administration, thus contributing to the variable therapeutic responses sometimes seen in patients treated with this drug for Parkinson's disease.

Routes of Drug Administration

A variety of routes can be used for the administration of drugs. These can be divided into two categories—**oral** and **parenteral** (nongastrointestinal). It should be clear from the previous section that the physicochemical properties of the drug (particularly its lipophilicity) will be crucial in determining the route(s) by which absorption can most effectively and conveniently be achieved. Stability of the drug to enzymatic degradation may also be a factor, most notably in the case of oral administration. Finally, the choice of the optimal route of drug administration will be influenced by general considerations such as the urgency of the clinical situation, the clinical status of the patient, and the relationship of drug plasma concentrations to the desired therapeutic effect. Some of the characteristics of the different routes of administration are summarized in Table 2.2.

Oral

Drugs administered orally account for approximately 80 per cent of all prescriptions. Despite the convenience and relative safety of the oral route, a number of inherent limitations exist, and drug absorption may be both slow and highly variable. The term "**bioavailability**" refers to the rate and extent of oral absorption of drugs. The poor absorption of drugs administered orally can be advantageous when local effects mainly on the gastrointestinal tract are desired. Examples include agents used in diarrhea or constipation and the aminoglycoside antibiotics used to sterilize the bowel prior to abdominal surgery.

The oral administration of drugs requires the cooperation of the patient; the route cannot be used when the patient is unconscious or uncooperative. Parenteral administration may also be required if the patient is unable to retain drugs taken orally (e.g., in emesis).

Factors Affecting Absorption of Drugs from the Gastrointestinal (GI) Tract

Physicochemical Properties of the Drug. As discussed in an earlier section, the nature of the gastrointestinal epithelial barrier consisting of tight (or occluded) intercellular junctions is such that drug absorption is mainly determined by lipophilicity. Thus, highly polar or ionized (charged) substances are usually poorly absorbed after oral administration. Pharmaceutical properties (such as particle size and dissolution characteristics of tablets versus suspensions) of a drug preparation also can be important in determining absorption characteristics after oral administration. Consequently, variability in commercial formulations can lead to inconsistencies in the rate and extent of absorption. Differences in bioavailability have been reported for a number of drugs, including digoxin, penicillin G, erythromycin, hydrochlorothiazide, phenobarbital, l-dopa, prednisone, and warfarin, with the result that examples of therapeutic inequivalence resulting from bioinequivalence between some commercial preparations of digoxin, dicoumarol, and l-dopa have been noted. Although efforts to standardize drug formulations have effectively eliminated most problems relating to differences in bioavailability, caution always should be exercised when changing preparations of drugs with a low margin of safety.

Drug Complexation in the GI Tract. Complex formation between orally administered drugs and dietary components or other concomitantly administered pharmacologic agents can markedly reduce the rate and extent of absorption. The decreased effectiveness of tetracycline antibiotics when ingested together with milk or dairy products is attributable to the formation of a stable calcium-tetracycline complex that is poorly absorbed. A similar metal chelation process also is responsible for the impairment in absorption of tetracyclines when they are administered in combination with antacids containing hydroxides of magnesium or aluminum. Interestingly, antacids have also been found to interfere with the absorption of the histamine antagonist, cimetidine, resulting in decreases of 40–50 per cent in peak plasma concentrations of this commonly prescribed anti-ulcer drug. If the antacid is taken one hour before or one hour after cimetidine, this clinically relevant interaction can be avoided. A final example of drug interactions resulting in decreased oral absorption involves the bile acid-binding resin cholestyramine, which is used in the management of hypercholesterolemia. This cholesterol-lowering agent is a positively charged ion-exchange resin, and can bind a variety of other substances, including anticoagulants, digitalis glycosides, phenobarbital, thyroxine, and chlorothiazide, thereby reducing their absorption from the gut. Again, such interactions can be minimized by giving the drug in question one hour before or four hours after the cholestyramine.

Drug Stability in the GI Tract. An important consideration when drugs are administered by the oral route is their stability to the extremes of pH encountered in the digestive tract. The improved oral absorption of penicillin V and amoxicillin, synthetic analogues of naturally occurring penicillin G, reflects their greater stability to gastric acidity as compared with the parent compound. Pharmacologic agents may also be susceptible to enzymatic degradation in the gut.

This normally precludes the oral administration of substances such as the polypeptide hormone insulin. Much research effort has been directed to the development of orally effective insulin preparations for use in the management of diabetic patients. One of the more interesting approaches currently being investigated involves encapsulation in a polymeric substance that, although resistant to the action of digestive enzymes in the stomach, contains azo linkages susceptible to cleavage by intestinal bacteria. The released insulin can, despite its size, cross the mucosal barrier of the intestinal wall

Table 2.2 Comparison of Routes of Administration

Route	Advantages	Limitations
Oral	convenient, relatively safe, economical	relatively slow onset of action, variety of factors can influence rate and extent of absorption
Intravenous (IV)	rapid onset of action, exact control over magnitude and duration of response, no preabsorptive inactivation, permits administration of large volume of fluid and of highly irritating drugs	increased risk of adverse reactions, self-medication impractical, need for asepsis, thrombophlebitis risk with repeated use, drug must be in a soluble form
Intramuscular (IM)/ Subcutaneous (SQ)	permits effective administration of drugs showing poor oral absorption, drugs may be given as repository preparation (eg., in oily vehicle) for sustained action	absorption may be delayed if circulatory status impaired, bioavailability may be incomplete due to precipitation or inactivation at the site of administration, pain following injection, release of creatine phosphokinase into circulation following IM injection
Sublingual	rapid onset of action, minimal "first pass" hepatic inactivation	mucosal ulceration with repeated use, highly irritant drugs precluded
Rectal	can be used in uncooperative or unconscious patients, can minimize gastric irritant effects of drugs, reduced "first pass" hepatic inactivation	absorption may be variable, irritant drugs precluded
Inhalation	rapid onset of action, magnitude and duration of response can be rigorously controlled (in case of inhalation anesthetics)	practically limited to gases or vaporizable liquids
Transdermal	convenient, less fluctuation in blood levels	drug must possess considerable lipid solubility, expense
Miscellaneous		
Intra-arterial	used to localize effects of highly toxic agents by reducing their systemic distribution	
Intrathecal/ Epidural:	used to produce surgical anaesthesia in the conscious patient	
Intraperitoneal:	convenient and versatile, but use virtually restricted to experimental setting (risk of adhesions, infection)	

and be effectively absorbed into the circulation.[1] Although initial experimental results have been encouraging, the therapeutic potential of such oral insulin preparations remains to be established. Enzymes derived from bacteria in the gut may also participate in the degradation of orally administered drugs prior to their absorption. The increase in plasma concentrations of digoxin noted in patients being treated concomitantly with certain antibiotics (e.g., erythromycin or tetracycline) points to gut bacterial involvement in the preabsorptive metabolism of this orally effective digitalis glycoside preparation.

Gastric Emptying. Gastric emptying determines the time required for orally administered drugs to reach the primary sites of absorption located in the small intestine. Therefore, factors influencing gastric emptying will exert predictable effects on rates of drug absorption. Gastric emptying is most rapid in the fasting state, so that drugs will be most rapidly absorbed when taken on an empty stomach. Mild exercise and cold meals are also associated with relatively rapid rates of gastric emptying. Conversely, hot meals and intense pain, emotion, or strenuous exercise will all delay gastric emptying and thereby decrease the rate of drug absorption from the gut.

"First Pass" Metabolism (or Presystemic Elimination). Substances absorbed from the GI tract are delivered directly to the liver via the portal circulation. Some drugs are readily extracted and extensively metabolized on their "**first pass**" through the liver, so that very small amounts of active drug reach the systemic circulation. One such agent is the beta-adrenoceptor antagonist propranolol, which has therapeutically useful antianginal and antihypertensive effects. Propranolol is effective when given orally, but must be administered at doses that are much greater than those required to produce therapeutic blood levels after parenteral administration. This approach of using high oral doses of drugs subject to "first pass" hepatic metabolism, which involves saturation of the relevant metabolizing enzymes in the liver, can be used for drugs not producing potentially toxic metabolites. Alternatively, drugs that would be subject to high presystemic elimination if administered orally can be given by a different route. Two examples are lidocaine injected intravenously for treatment of ventricular dysrhythmias and nitroglycerine used sublingually to terminate attacks of angina. Both of these routes of administration (see below) also have the advantage of ensuring rapid onset of drug action, which is highly desirable in the above clinical situations.

Pathologic Factors. The presence of gastric ulceration has been reported to slow gastric emptying and might, therefore, delay drug absorption. Patients with congestive heart failure may also show a decreased rate of drug absorption from the gut. This may be caused by a reduction in splanchnic blood flow resulting from the decrease in cardiac output and an associated vasoconstrictor response in the mesenteric circulation.

Intravenous (IV)

This route of drug administration has many important advantages. It is frequently chosen to obtain a prompt pharmacologic response, which can be achieved within one circulation time (15–20 seconds). Drugs that undergo rapid inactivation in the body can be given by IV infusion, which permits a direct control (by appropriate adjustment of the rate of infusion) over the magnitude and duration of the desired therapeutic effect. Because of the powerful buffering capacity of blood, the IV route can be used for highly irritating drugs such as thiopental, for which the extreme alkalinity precludes its administration by any other route. Lipophilicity and size restrictions obviously do not apply to drugs given IV, so that virtually any type of substance can be administered, provided that it is available as a soluble preparation. However, this may require the use of organic vehicles, some of which may not be entirely inert pharmacologically. Furthermore, injectable drug preparations are frequently less stable and more costly than those for nonintravenous use. Other disadvantages of this route include its limited suitability for self-medication, the need for asepsis, the potential of rapidly achieving **toxic** drug concentrations, the irretrievability of the injected drug and the problem of thrombophlebitis with chronic therapy.

Intramuscular (IM) and Subcutaneous (SQ)

These two routes are considered together because they have many characteristics in common. Deltoid or gluteal muscles are frequent sites of IM injection; the skin of the shoulder, forearm, or leg is often used for the SQ administration of drugs. Gentle massage at the site of injection can accelerate absorption by increasing the surface area of drug exposure. As discussed above in Diffusion Through Porous Lipoidal Barriers, substances injected IM or SQ gain access to the circulation by passage through discontinuities between endothelial cells of peripheral blood vessels. As a consequence, highly polar drugs that would be poorly absorbed from the GI tract with its tight intercellular junctions can be effectively administered by the SQ or IM routes. The molecular dimensions of most pharmacologic agents are such that size restrictions governing passage across the porous capillary network do not apply. In certain therapeutic situations, substances may be injected in the form of macromolecular complexes (e.g., protamine zinc insulin) or subcutaneously implantable pellets or timed-release polymers (e.g., certain hormone replacement preparations), so that absorption is determined by the gradual release of active drug that can then readily enter the circulation. A similar effect can be achieved by the injection of drug in an oily vehicle. Such "depot preparations" are useful when sustained blood levels of drug are required or when patient compliance with a critical therapeutic regimen is thought to be unreliable.

Tissue perfusion is a critical factor determining rates of drug absorption from IM or SQ sites. Blood flow considerations correctly predict the greater rate of drug absorption from IM than from SQ sites, and from deltoid as compared with gluteal muscle. The delayed onset of drug action after IM or SQ injection in patients with hypotension, congestive heart failure, or circulatory shock can also be rationalized on this basis. Experimental studies examining factors that influence the rate of absorption of SQ administered insulin have demonstrated a marked enhancement of absorption by increased environmental temperature (e.g., induced by exposure to a sauna) or exercise, and a decrease associated with smoking (presumably the result of peripheral vasoconstriction). These results further reinforce the major role of circulatory status in the process of drug absorption from SQ sites and have important practical implications in the management of insulin-dependent diabetic patients. Vasoconstrictors are commonly administered to delay the systemic absorption of local anesthetics used to produce infiltration blockade in dental procedures, thereby increasing the duration of anesthesia and reducing the risk of toxicities.

Although most drugs can be effectively absorbed after IM or SQ injection, these routes of administration have some inherent limitations. One of these relates to the incomplete absorption seen with certain pharmacologic agents. In some cases, this may be attributable to low drug solubility, resulting in the precipitation of the agent at the site of injection. Digoxin and phenytoin are two drugs that cannot be reliably administered by the IM route for this reason. Second, drugs may be subject to degradation by tissue enzymes. This has been well documented in the case of SQ administered insulin, which can undergo extensive proteolysis (up to 50 per cent of an administered dose) prior to absorption into the bloodstream in some diabetic patients. Another limitation is the discomfort associated with injection. Pain is usually caused by the distention of muscle, particularly after the injection of a large volume of fluid, or by stimulation of pain receptors that are particularly abundant in skin and SQ tissue. The risk of sciatic nerve damage after gluteal injections can be minimized by avoiding the upper-outer quadrant of the gluteal region. Finally, IM injections can cause the release of muscle creatine phosphokinase and thereby interfere with certain diagnostic procedures that rely on estimates of this enzyme activity in plasma.

Sublingual

The sublingual region provides a richly vascular absorptive surface from which drugs can be rapidly taken up into the circulation by the process of passive diffusion. Because absorption from this route is into the systemic venous system rather than directly into the portal circulation, presystemic elimination by hepatic metabolism is minimized. Promptness of action and minimization of first-pass inactivation form the basis of sublingual nitroglycerin use in angina pectoris, as mentioned previously. Other drugs for which the sublingual route has some therapeutic application include ergotamine (used in the treatment of migraine headaches) and certain testosterone preparations. Highly irritating drugs cannot be administered sublingually. Likewise, irritation and mucosal ulceration can limit chronic therapy that depends on this route of administration.

Rectal

Drugs administered in suppositories can produce not only local effects but also systemic therapeutic actions. Although the rectum has a rich vascular and lymphatic supply, the absence of villi and the limited surface area result in a rather slow (and erratic) rate of drug absorption. Blood draining the lower part of the rectum largely bypasses the liver, so that drugs showing a high "first pass" metabolism when given orally are more effectively absorbed when administered rectally. This route can be used to advantage when oral medication is impractical, as in unconscious patients, or those with severe gastrointestinal disturbances, in children, and in the administration of drugs with an unpleasant taste or smell. Again, absorption is favored by a high lipid solubility and highly irritating drugs are obviously contraindicated.

Inhalation

Volatile or vaporized substances can be rapidly absorbed through the pulmonary epithelium and mucous membranes of the respiratory tract into the systemic circulation. The inhalation route has important therapeutic applications, most notably in the area of general anesthesia, but may also provide a route of access for various environmental toxicants. In addition, the administration of drugs by inhalation can be an appropriate route when treating pulmonary disorders, such as bronchial asthma. Although absorption from the respiratory tract is determined mainly by lipid solubility, the abundance of pinocytotic vesicles suggests that the formation of transient fenestrae may also permit the passage of highly water-soluble molecules such as nicotine and various types of allergens. The abundant vascular supply of pulmonary tissue and the very close apposition of the single layered alveolar epithelial wall and capillary endothelial cells permit the highly efficient and rapid but nonselective absorption of substances exposed in adequate concentration to the respiratory tract by inhalation. Mucus secretion and ciliary movement in upper respiratory tract epithelial cells play an important role in protecting the respiratory tract against inhaled particulate material. Detrimental effects of drugs or environmental toxicants on these crucial defense processes are likely to have serious pathologic implications.

Topical

The outer epidermal layer of the skin is an effective lipoidal barrier that normally limits the systemic absorption of most topically applied pharmacologic agents. In contrast, the underlying dermis is freely permeable and richly supplied with lymph and blood capillaries, so that drugs applied to denuded, abraded, or otherwise damaged skin may be readily absorbed into the systemic circulation. However, absorption of molecules through intact skin, which is favored by high lipophilicity and enhanced by the presence of an oily vehicle, is a frequent cause of poisoning after accidental exposure (especially on a chronic basis) to foreign chemicals, one of the more common examples being organophosphate insecticide toxicity and even death in agricultural workers. Increasing use is now being made of percutaneous (or transdermal) drug absorption for therapeutic purposes, the major advantages being convenience of administration, protection from GI inactivation or "first pass" hepatic metabolism, and the maintenance of relatively stable drug levels in the blood. Thus, in the management of patients with angina pectoris, nitroglycerin can be given as an ointment spread on the chest or arms, with blood levels attained being proportional to the surface area covered. Alternatively, the drug can be administered in a gel-like matrix attached to an adhesive bandage. Such dermal patch preparations are available for a number of other drugs, including nicotine, the anti-motion-sickness agent scopolamine, the antihypertensive clonidine, and estrogens used in hormone replacement therapy.

Other examples of the topical administration of drugs include ophthalmic agents applied as "eye drops" that are absorbed from the conjunctival sac in the treatment of glaucoma, and decongestants applied as a spray to nasal mucous membranes.

Miscellaneous

Intra-arterial

Highly toxic substances such as antineoplastic agents may be administered intra-arterially to localize their action and reduce systemic distribution. Certain diagnostic substances are also sometimes given in this manner.

Intrathecal

Polar drugs that do not readily cross the blood-brain barrier can be injected directly into the subarachnoid space for the production of spinal anesthesia or the antibiotic treatment of acute CNS infections.

Intraperitoneal

Drugs injected intraperitoneally leave the peritoneal cavity through intercellular gaps in the mesenteric wall and surrounding capillaries, allowing the effective absorption of a wide variety of substances regardless of their polarity or lipophilic character. However, drugs are still subject to "first-pass" metabolic inactivation when administered in this manner. The intraperitoneal route, although widely used in the laboratory, is rarely employed clinically because of problems relating to the development of adhesions and the risk of infection.

Summary

Drugs absorbed from the GI tract after their oral administration are the most commonly prescribed of all pharmacologic agents. Delivery of drugs to their target organs in order to produce the desired therapeutic effects is influenced by a number of factors that affect the rate and extent of absorption from the gut (bioavailability) and by hepatic "first-pass" metabolism. Depending on the therapeutic circumstances and the chemical properties of the drug in question, other specialized routes of administration may be required to obtain an optimal onset of action and magnitude of the desired pharmacologic response. In some instances, enhanced specificity of drug action may be achieved by localized administration of the drug.

Distribution

After their entry into the circulation, drugs become subject to two important distributional processes—binding to plasma proteins and accumulation in tissues[r10] (Fig. 2.1.). Both of these binding processes proceed according to mass action principles and their reversal can therefore serve as a capacitor to sustain the pharmacologically active free (or unbound) component of drugs in the circulation as total plasma concentrations are progressively reduced by metabolism and excretion. As will be discussed in detail below, clinically relevant alterations in drug handling relating to pathologic conditions or the concomitant administration of other pharmacologic agents are, in some instances, attributable to effects at the level of drug distribution.[r11]

Binding to Plasma Proteins

The extent to which drugs are bound to circulatory proteins ranges from 15 per cent or less (e.g., acetamin-

Table 2.3 Comparison of Pharmacokinetic Parameters for Cardiac Glycosides

	Bound in Plasma (%)	Volume of Redistribution (L/kg)	Half Life (hr)	Major Mode of Elimination
digoxin	25	9.14	42	glomerular filtration
digitoxin	97	0.51	166	hepatic metabolism

ophen, acyclovir, gentamicin, metronidazole, metoprolol, and ranitidine) to greater than 95 per cent (e.g., diazepam, digitoxin, furosemide, tolbutamide, and warfarin). Protein binding has a profound effect on drug handling in the body. This can be readily seen from a comparison of two digitalis glycoside preparations, digoxin and digitoxin, which share common pharmacodynamic actions but differ markedly in their pharmacokinetic properties (Table 2.3).

The greater degree of binding to plasma proteins (97%) shown by digitoxin, the more nonpolar of the two molecules, underlines the importance of lipophilicity as a driving force favoring drug-protein association in general. Lipophilicity considerations also correctly predict that digitoxin is better absorbed from the gut after oral administration than is digoxin. This comparison also illustrates the effect of extensive protein binding to limit both drug distribution into tissues (resulting in a lower volume of distribution for digitoxin) and filtration at the kidney glomerulus, which is restricted to the free (unbound) component (Fig. 2.1). Consequently, the elimination of digoxin is critically influenced by renal functional status, and careful adjustment of drug dosage is required in patients with renal disease. In contrast, the longer plasma half-life of digitoxin is determined by hepatic metabolism and the disposition of this agent may be altered in the presence of hepatic dysfunction. Another aspect of plasma protein binding and drug elimination relates to hemodialysis and peritoneal dialysis, in which the rate of drug removal varies inversely with the extent of plasma protein binding. Addition of albumin (see next Section) to the dialyzing solution can accelerate the rate of drug removal by these procedures.

Drug-Albumin Interactions

Albumin is the most abundant protein in plasma and is normally present at a concentration of 4–5 grams/100 ml (or approximately 7×10^{-4}M). Although albumin can bind a wide variety of substances in proportion to their lipophilicity, the protein has a particularly high affinity for weakly acidic substances, which at physiologic pH are present predominantly in the anionic form. Electrostatic forces are therefore likely to be important in binding, with additional contributions from hydrogen bonding and hydrophobic interactions. Binding is usually reversible, with association and dissociation time-constants typically being in the millisecond range. Mass action kinetics apply, predicting saturability at high ligand concentrations and competition among structurally related substances for common sites of interaction.

There are three distinct classes of binding sites on the albumin molecule. Competitive displacement studies have been performed with warfarin, diazepam, and digitoxin as specific markers for each of these binding domains. Information so obtained has provided a useful framework within which to understand and predict drug-drug interactions attributable to alterations in binding to plasma albumin. Great caution must be exercised when extrapolating results obtained in studies of drug-albumin interactions *in vitro* (under conditions that are often distinctly unphysiologic) to the *in vivo* situation. Furthermore, although there are undoubtedly numerous instances of statistically significant alterations in free and albumin-bound components of individual agents during the course of multiple drug therapy, only a relatively small number of these interactions actually have clinical significance, cases in which the conditions shown in Table 2.4 must apply. The application of the criteria listed in this Table can be illustrated by considering two different types of adverse drug reactions, both of which involve interactions at the level of plasma albumin.

The first example, which concerns the development of neonatal kernicterus[2] after the administration of certain antibacterial sulfonamides, has been discussed previously in a different context (see page 43). Early in the neonatal period, the breakdown of fetal hemoglobin releases large amounts of bilirubin that cannot be efficiently metabolized by conjugation to a more water-soluble metabolite due to the immaturity of the hepatic enzyme, glucuronyl transferase (see page 55). Bilirubin is extensively bound to albumin and this interaction (involving "warfarin-type" binding sites) is critical in preventing excessive increases in plasma concentrations of free bilirubin that, given the incomplete formation of the neonatal blood-brain barrier (see page 43), can produce severe neurologic damage. The tenuous balance which thus exists can be upset by agents such as antimicrobial sulfonamides that compete with bilirubin for common binding

Table 2.4 Criteria Predictive of Clinically Relevant Drug Interactions at the Level of Plasma Albumin

(i) the drug is extensively bound to albumin (usually in excess of 90–95%). Under these conditions, a small decrease in binding produced by a competing ligand causes a proportionally large increase in the pharmacologically active (unbound) component of the displaced drug.
(ii) the increase in the plasma level of unbound drug cannot be readily dissipated. Such is the case when the displaced drug has a relatively long plasma half-life or when its elimination is decreased in the presence of the displacing ligand.
(iii) the displaced drug has a narrow margin of safety.

sites on the albumin molecule in proportion to their lipophilicity. Resulting increases in the concentration of free bilirubin are likely to persist in view of the limiting glucuronyl transferase activity in the neonatal liver and lead to the production of kernicterus due to the deposition of bilirubin in the brain. For this reason, sulfonamides (particularly highly lipophilic, long-acting agents) are not used in neonates or in pregnant women near term.

Another well-documented drug interaction involves the oral anticoagulant warfarin and the nonsteroidal anti-inflammatory drug phenylbutazone. Patients being treated concomitantly with conventional doses of these drugs were found to exhibit an unexpected intensification of the anticoagulant response. In part, this interaction has a pharmacodynamic basis relating to the combined mechanistically distinct actions of warfarin (inhibition of vitamin K-dependent clotting factor synthesis) and phenylbutazone (decreased platelet aggregatability as a result of cyclooxygenase inhibition), both leading independently to a prolongation of bleeding time. However, pharmacokinetic factors serve to worsen the already precarious situation when these substances are given concomitantly. Warfarin is highly bound to albumin (99 per cent), has a long plasma half-life (approximately 35 hr) and a narrow margin of safety—thereby fulfilling the three drug interaction criteria under consideration (Table 2.4). Phenylbutazone is able to compete with warfarin for common sites of binding to plasma albumin and for sites of metabolism in the liver. As a consequence, plasma concentrations of free warfarin show a sustained increase. This situation can result in serious haemorrhagic complications unless an appropriate adjustment in anticoagulant dosage is made.

Drug Binding by Other Plasma Proteins

Although interaction with albumin accounts for most of the plasma protein binding of neutral and particularly of acidic (anionic) drugs, association with other circulatory components, notably lipoproteins and α_1-acid glycoprotein, may be quantitatively more important in the case of basic (cationic) drugs. In addition to their well documented role in the transport of cholesterol, phospholipids, and triglycerides, plasma lipoproteins may also be involved in the binding of highly lipophilic and/or basic substances, such as quinidine, reserpine, propranolol, tricyclic antidepressants, and certain insecticides.

While relatively little detailed information is available concerning the pharmacokinetic implications of drug binding to plasma lipoproteins, considerably more is known about α_1-acid glycoprotein, sometimes referred to as "acute phase reactant protein".[r12] This terminology reflects the fact that plasma concentrations of this protein increase (as much as 4–5 fold) in response to a number of pathologic conditions, including infection, inflammation, cancer, and trauma. The resulting decrease in the unbound fraction of weakly basic drugs showing appreciable affinity for α_1-acid glycoprotein can result in a reduced therapeutic response to usual doses of these agents.[r13] In the absence of such disease-related elevations, the concentration of α_1-acid glycoprotein in plasma is only $1–3 \times 10^{-5}$ M, which is almost two orders of magnitude less than that of albumin. Fetal plasma levels of α_1-acid glycoprotein have been found to be lower than those in the maternal circulation. This, in combination with a lower affinity of fetal albumin for drugs, may lead to an enhanced susceptibility of the fetus to drugs present in the maternal circulation. Under usual circumstances, however, the binding capacity of α_1-acid glycoprotein is unlikely to be limiting despite its relatively low concentration in plasma, because therapeutically effective plasma concentrations of weakly basic drugs tend to be considerably lower than those of weakly acidic drugs. There is one documented situation in which the drug binding capacity of α_1-acid glycoprotein becomes limiting *in vitro,* and this forms the basis of what has been termed the "vacutainer effect." Stoppers of vacutainer blood collection tubes contain a plasticizer (tris-2-butoxyethyl phosphate) that can cause the displacement of drugs such as quinidine, propranolol, and lidocaine from binding sites on the α_1-acid glycoprotein molecule. The redistribution of unbound drug to red cells causes an artifactual lowering of the measured concentration of drug in plasma.

Disease-related Alterations in Drug Binding to Plasma Proteins

The effect of various pathologic processes on plasma concentrations of α_1-acid glycoprotein, as discussed in the previous section, illustrates one mechanism by which drug handling may be modified under pathologic conditions. Abnormalities in the content or composition of various plasma lipoprotein components are also likely to be associated with changes in the distributional characteristics of pharmacologic agents, but these have yet to be examined in detail. In contrast, disease-related alterations in drug disposition involving plasma albumin have been very extensively characterized. These will be considered under two general categories: (a) changes attributable to hypoalbuminemia; (b) those resulting from modifications in the binding characteristics of the albumin molecule.

Hypoalbuminemia. Chronically reduced levels of plasma albumin occur most commonly in association with liver disease, renal failure, nephrotic syndrome, protein-losing enteropathy, and severe burns. For drugs showing appreciable binding to albumin, an increase in the level of the free (unbound) component would, therefore, be anticipated. Based on the scheme shown in Figure 2.1, an intensified pharmacologic response and an increased rate of drug elimination are two possible consequences of such an increase. As might have been predicted in the former case, an increased incidence of adverse drug reactions has generally been noted in patients with hypoalbuminemia. However, the complex interplay of pharmocokinetic and pharmacodynamic factors influencing drug action in the various disease states involved precludes a rigorous interpretation of this important clinical observation. The extent to which drug elimination is enhanced in patients with hypoalbuminemia is largely determined by the nature of the underlying disease process as it affects the relevant systems responsible for the excretion or metabolism of the particular agent in question.

As an illustrative example, let us consider alterations in the disposition of phenytoin observed in patients with burn injury-related hypoalbuminemia.[r14] Clinically, it has been noted that burn victims being treated for epilepsy with conventional dosing regimens for phenytoin show an increased incidence of seizure activity in association with reduced total plasma concentrations of drug. Experiments in burned rats have indicated that the clearance of phenytoin was increased in these animals (relative to controls), although no change in its plasma half-life was apparent. This suggests that the decreased plasma concentrations of phenytoin in burn injury are primarily determined by an enhanced redistribution of unbound drug to extravascular tissues. Although this increased availability of unbound drug is related to the extent of hypoalbuminemia, alterations in the binding characteristics of the albumin molecule may also be involved, as discussed in the next section.

Altered Binding Capacity of Albumin. In diseases of renal or hepatic origin, the binding capacity of albumin for certain drugs may be substantially modified by the presence in plasma of endogenous substances that accumulate in proportion to the degree of uremia or hepatic dysfunction present. Consistent with the previously noted heterogeneity of binding sites on plasma albumin, the extent to which drug binding is affected in a given disease state depends on the particular agent in question. Thus, in patients with liver cirrhosis, diazepam binding is usually decreased, while that of warfarin is minimally affected. Although alterations in drug binding have also been observed in other hepatic diseases (such as acute viral hepatitis), these alterations do not necessarily parallel those in cirrhosis. Uremia, on the other hand, is associated with a reduction in albumin binding capacity that is generalized and that encompasses agents bound to the warfarin site (e.g., phenytoin, phenylbutazone, sulfonamides) as well as the diazepam and digitoxin binding domains. Drugs primarily associated with α_1-acid glycoprotein (e.g., propranolol and quinidine) do not appear to be affected under these conditions.

Practical Clinical Implications. The extent to which a reduction in plasma protein binding produces a corresponding increase in the elimination rate of a drug (with a resultant decrease in total blood level) during the course of chronic therapy is critically influenced by the metabolic characteristics of the particular agent in question. For drugs that are rapidly cleared by the liver (e.g., lidocaine, meperidine, morphine, propranolol), protein binding is not a rate-limiting factor in elimination; conversely, protein-binding is often rate-limiting in the case of drugs that are relatively poorly extracted by the liver (e.g., phenytoin, phenylbutazone, tolbutamide). For agents in this latter category, an increased level of unbound drug in plasma is likely to result in an enhanced rate of drug elimination, provided that the relevant disposition mechanisms are not adversely affected by the associated pathologic condition.

Pharmacokinetic considerations regarding the use of phenytoin in patients with uremia or hypoalbuminemia secondary to the nephrotic syndrome illustrate practical consequences of the foregoing principles.[r15] In both of the above conditions, the reduced binding of phenytoin to plasma albumin gives rise to an increase in the rate of drug elimination with an attendant decrease in its average total circulating concentration achieved during chronic therapy. The net result of this decrease in the total plasma concentration of drug and the proportional increase in the unbound fraction is such that the level of the pharmacologically active free component is in the normal therapeutic range. In this situation, adjustments of phenytoin dosage based on measurements of **total** blood concentration would have produced circulating levels of **free** drug well into the toxic range. The crucial point to be emphasized, then, is that when binding characteristics of albumin are modified, the relationship between total circulating levels of drug and the corresponding pharmacologic response may be altered strikingly.

Drug Accumulation in Tissues

The unbound fraction of drugs in plasma exists in a dynamic equilibrium involving binding to plasma proteins and uptake by extravascular tissues (Fig. 2.1).[r10] Two main factors that influence the latter process are tissue perfusion and drug lipophilicity. The pharmacologic properties of the ultra-short acting barbiturate thiopental provide a useful illustration of some fundamental aspects of drug uptake by tissues. When used for the induction of general anesthesia, thiopental is given as a single bolus injection (typically at a dose of 4 mg/kg) that produces effects that are almost immediate in onset and that last only a matter of minutes. The rapid onset of action is determined both by the abundant supply of blood to the brain and the high lipophilicity of thiopental, which facilitates uptake into brain tissue. The importance of lipophilicity is emphasized by the considerably longer time required to produce anaesthesia with pentobarbital, an analogue of thiopental in which replacement of the sulfur atom with oxygen leads to an approximately 70-fold reduction in lipid solubility. Termination of thiopental action parallels the rapid **redistribution** of drug from the brain to other highly perfused tissues such as muscle, with uptake into fat and other poorly perfused tissues occurring very much more slowly. If thiopental is administered as a continuous IV infusion (4 mg/kg/hr over several days) rather than as a single 4 mg/kg bolus injection, the time required for termination of drug action after the cessation of the infusion is greatly increased. Under these conditions, hepatic metabolism rather than redistribution becomes the rate-limiting step in the dissipation of the pharmacologic effect. This striking dose-dependent alteration in thiopental pharmacokinetics may result from saturation of tissue storage sites and possibly also of enzymes mediating its hepatic metabolism.

A number of important generalizations concerning drug distribution can be made on the basis of the foregoing example. The crucial role of tissue perfusion predicts that in pathologic conditions associated with appreciable circulatory impairment, standard doses of drugs that show large apparent volumes of distribution (denoting extensive tissue sequestration) may produce excessively elevated plasma concentrations as a result of decreased tissue uptake, thereby necessitating a reduction in dosage. Such is the case, for example, with the antiarrhythmic lidocaine in patients with congestive heart failure. The reduction in muscle mass typically accompanying aging is likely to have similar functional consequences, which might be exacerbated by age-related impairment in drug disposition processes. Particular caution must, therefore, be exercised when drugs that show extensive accumulation in muscle and a low margin of safety (e.g., digoxin) are administered to elderly patients (see Chapter 3).

Given the importance of lipophilicity in distributional processes, the proportion of an ionizable drug in the uncharged form at physiologic pH (as predicted by the Henderson-Hasselbalch equation) is a critical factor determining the rate and extent of its equilibration with tissues. As a consequence, weakly acidic substances that exist predominantly in the ionized form under physiologic conditions, are largely confined to the aqueous extracellular compartment. For weakly basic drugs, on the other hand, appreciable amounts of the nonionized form are likely to be present at physiologic pH. As a result, these compounds show marked tissue accumulation, as reflected in apparent volumes of distribution that are typically two or more orders of magnitude larger than those for weakly acidic drugs. Another aspect of ionization-dependent partitioning concerns the development of an unequal distribution of drugs across lipoidal barriers separating various intracellular structures or tissue compartments when there is a pH gradient. Weakly acidic drugs will accumulate in regions of higher pH while weak bases are concentrated in regions of lower pH. The principle involved is referred to as "diffusion trapping" (Fig. 2.2).

Consider the distribution of a weakly basic drug (pKa = 7.4) across mammary gland epithelium, assuming pH values of 7.4 and 6.4 for blood and milk, respectively. The nonionized component is assumed to equilibrate freely across the epithelial wall and its concentration in both fluid compartments will thus be the same. If this concentration is taken as [C], application of the Henderson-Hasselbalch equation indicates that the concentrations of the ionized form [CH^+] in the media of pH 7.4 and 6.4 will be C and 10 C, respectively. Thus, a greater amount of drug becomes trapped in the compartment where the pH allows a greater degree of ionization; the total amounts (i.e., nonionized + ionized forms) of drug in each of the two compartments are such that a 5.5-fold greater concentration is present in milk as compared with blood. The development of such concentration gradients is independent of any energy expenditure, unlike the situation in active transport.[r16] This particular example of pH-dependent drug partitioning has important practical implications in nursing mothers and possibly also in the consumption of dairy products from cattle raised on feed that contains antimicrobial agents. More generally, the accumulation of basic drugs in intracellular structures with low internal pH (e.g., lysosomes) or in acidotic tissues and the pronounced effects of changes in urinary pH on the renal excretion of drugs (to be discussed in a later section) can all be understood in terms of the "diffusion trapping" concept.

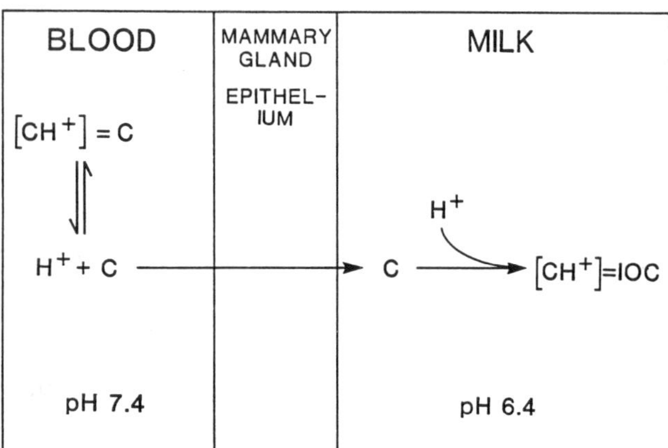

Figure 2.2 Example of diffusion trapping for a weakly basic drug ($CH^+ \rightleftharpoons C + H^+$) with a pKa of 7.4 that distributes across the mammary gland epithelium. After application of the Henderson-Hasselbalch equation, the concentration of the ionized form of the drug (CH^+) in blood will be equal to the uncharged form (C) because the pKa of 7.4 is equal to the pH of blood. For the milk compartment with a pH of 6.4, the concentration of the charged form (CH^+) will be equal to 10C. As a result of the "trapping" of drug due to the pH gradient, the total (C + CH^+) drug concentration in milk is 5.5 times the concentration in blood.

Finally, the potential saturability of tissue sites of drug accumulation, as suggested by the pharmacokinetic properties of thiopental when given as a continuous infusion, raises the possibility of drug interactions involving competition/displacement phenomena analogous to those previously described for plasma proteins. Such interactions at the level of tissues could, in principle, have more serious consequences, because displaced drugs would be redistributed back into the plasma, the volume of which is small in comparison with the extravascular tissue space. Digoxin and quinidine are two drugs that show extensive accumulation in tissues. When certain patients on chronic digoxin therapy are given quinidine (e.g., for the management of a digoxin-related cardiac rhythm disorder), serum digoxin concentrations may increase as much as 2–3-fold, with an attendant risk of cardiotoxicity.[r17] Although this finding was initially interpreted mainly in terms of competition for common sites of tissue uptake, it has since become clear that quinidine also exerts important effects on the absorption and elimination of digoxin. This interaction, which can be minimized by a reduction in digoxin dosage prior to the administration of quinidine, is another example of the pharmacokinetic complexities involved in drug-drug interactions.

Summary

The distribution of drugs is a critical factor in the therapeutic response to a specific pharmacologic agent. Distribution within the vascular compartment can be influenced by drug binding to plasma proteins, and is an important site of drug-drug interactions. In order to bind to or enter tissues to produce a cellular response, drugs usually must leave the vascular space. The redistribution of a drug can terminate its pharmacologic actions prior to metabolism and can influence its rate of elimination. Finally, there is a special and important situation involving the distribution of drugs into spaces or compartments in pregnancy, since drugs can cross the placenta by simple diffusion and thus have effects on the fetus (see Chapter 3).

Metabolism (Biotransformation)

The time-dependent characteristics of drug action are critically dependent on susceptibility to biotransformation *in vivo* (Fig. 2.1). The enzymatic processes involved affect pharmacologic activity both directly (by metabolic **inactivation** or, in some cases, **activation**) and indirectly by chemical modifications (typically involving increases in polarity) that favor **excretion** by increasing the water solubility of the drug. Lipophilicity generally increases substrate (drug) accessibility to sites of metabolism, particularly those in the liver. Enzyme systems responsible for the biotransformation of exogenous chemicals (or "xenobiotics") may also be important in the biosynthesis or degradation of certain endogenous substances.[r18] Thus, cytochrome P450-dependent hydroxylation reactions that figure prominently in the hepatic metabolism of drugs that contain aromatic ring structures (see below) are also involved in the biosynthesis of steroid hormones and bile acids. Furthermore, the pharmacologic actions of certain substances may reflect their ability to interact selectively with the metabolic pathways of endogenous compounds. This principle is illustrated by methyl dopa and captopril, two agents useful in the management of hypertension. Methyl dopa is converted to the central neurotransmitter α-methyl norepinephrine by enzymes that normally convert 3,4 dihydroxyphenylalanine (dopa) to norepinephrine. Captopril is an inhibitor of angiotensin converting enzyme (ACE), which is responsible for the conversion of the inactive angiotensin I to the active angiotensin II. Thus, the actions of both these drugs depend on enzyme systems involved in the metabolism of endogenous compounds.

Metabolism and Pharmacologic Activity

The chemical modification of drugs during the course of metabolism may result in complete or partial loss of pharmacologic activity. In addition there is an extensive list of drugs that produce **active metabolites**: sedatives (benzodiazepines and chloral hydrate), antidepressants (amitryptiline and imipramine), analgesics (acetanilid and codeine), β-adrenoceptor blockers (propranolol), and anti-inflammatory agents (phenylbutazone and prednisone). There may be therapeutically significant differences in metabolic disposition between drugs within the same pharmacologic category. Such is the case, for example, with the benzodiazepines. Some analogues (diazepam, chlordiazepoxide, and triazolam) form several active metabolites, whereas others, like clorazepate, undergo metabolic activation; some benzodiazepines (flurazepam and lorazepam) are directly converted to products devoid of pharmacologic activity. For drugs that produce significant quantitites of active metabolites, dose optimization based on plasma concentrations of parent drug becomes complicated, such that there may be an increased likelihood of toxicity due to the cumulative effects of these metabolites during chronic therapy.

Sites of Drug Metabolism

Enzymes capable of catalyzing reactions involved in the biotransformation of exogenous as well as endogenous molecules are widely distributed throughout the body. In the GI tract, drugs are subject to the action not only of digestive hydrolases but also of enzymes present in mucosal cells or arising from gut bacterial flora. Although the contribution of the latter to drug disposition is usually relatively minor, a reduction in drug-metabolizing gut flora after the administration of certain antibiotics may have clinical significance, particularly in the case of agents with a narrow margin of safety (e.g., digitalis glycosides). Other sites involved in the biotransformation of certain chemical substances include the lung (prostaglandins), plasma (the local anesthetic procaine and the neuromuscular blocker succinylcholine, both of which are metabolized by plasma pseudocholinesterase), and the placenta. In terms of over-all drug metabolism, however, the liver occupies a central role by virtue of the large number and diversity of chemical transformations that can occur in this tissue.

Hepatic Metabolism of Drugs

General Features

The quantitative and qualitative characteristics of hepatic metabolism for individual agents are critically dependent on the chemical properties of each drug. Circulating substances gain access to intracellular sites of metabolism in proportion to their lipophilicity, which favors diffusion into the hepatocyte and subsequent accumulation in the smooth endoplasmic reticulum (see below). In general, within a given homologous series of compounds, increasing lipid solubility is associated with a greater contribution of hepatic metabolism to elimination with a correspondingly lesser contribution of renal excretion. This principle has already been discussed in relation to the differing pharmacokinetic characteristics of digoxin and digitoxin (see page 49 and Table 2.3). A similar comparison can be made with pentobarbital and barbital, the former being approximately 40 times more lipophilic than the latter. The elimination of pentobarbital is largely determined by its hepatic metabolism; that of barbital is mainly dependent on renal excretion. This difference in metabolism readily explains the observation that, whereas the hypnotic effect of barbital is minimally altered in the presence of hepatic dysfunction, that of pentobarbital is considerably increased under these conditions. These findings would suggest that particular caution should be exercised when administering highly lipophilic drugs to patients with liver disease.

The rate and extent of drug metabolism by the liver is influenced by the chemical structural characteristics of the molecule in question. Some substances, despite extensive protein binding, are readily extracted by the liver and their rates of metabolism are critically dependent on hepatic blood flow. Such agents, which include propranolol, lidocaine, and meperidine, show high "first pass" effects after oral administration. In contrast, the rate of metabolism of other drugs is limited not by rate of delivery but by intrinsic hepatic clearance. Examples of such poorly extracted compounds include theophylline, phenytoin, tolbutamide, and certain benzodiazepines.

Reactions involved in the biotransformation of drugs by the liver can be divided into two distinct categories: **Phase I** (nonsynthetic) and **Phase II** (synthetic or conjugation) processes (Fig. 2.3).

Phase I Reactions. The nonsynthetic phase of drug metabolism, which typically involves simple **oxidation** or **reduction** reactions, is largely dependent on enzymes associated with the smooth endoplasmic reticulum (SER), a subcellular tubular network continuous with both the outer plasma membrane and the nuclear membrane. Fragmentation of SER due to the homogenization of the liver produces vesicles (termed "microsomes") that retain drug metabolizing activity. Such microsomal fractions, which can be isolated by high-speed ultracentrifugation of postmitochondrial supernatants from liver homogenates, have been extensively used in the elucidation of the chemical processes involved in drug biotransformation.

The term "Mixed Function Oxidase" (MFO) system is used to describe collectively the hepatic microsomal enzymatic components mediating Phase I metabolic reactions[r19] (Fig. 2.4). A characteristic feature of this system is the dual requirement for molecular oxygen and a reducing agent, principally NADPH, derived from the hexose monophosphate (HMP) shunt pathway of glucose metabolism. A key cofactor in the oxidative metabolism of both endogenous substances

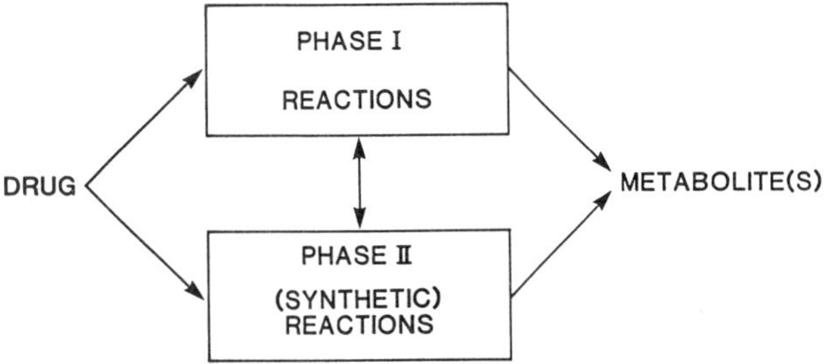

Figure 2.3 Drug metabolism, classified according to Phase I or Phase II (synthetic) reactions.

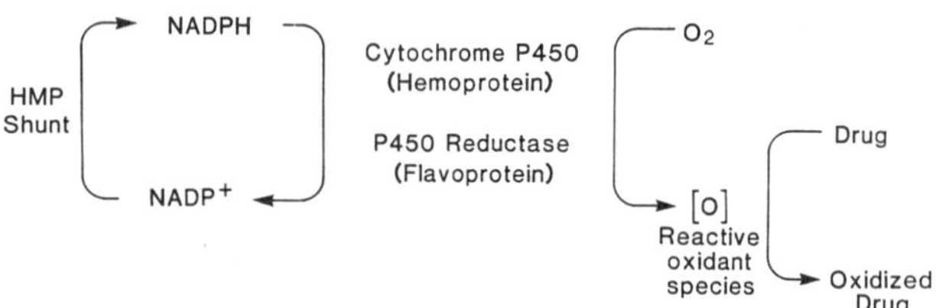

Figure 2.4 Mixed function oxidase (MFO) system. The hepatic MFO system is composed of two cofactors (NADPH and molecular oxygen) and two proteins (enzymes), a hemoprotein (cytochrome P450), and a flavoprotein (cytochrome P450 reductase). NADPH, derived from cellular metabolism via the hexose monophosphate (HMP) shunt pathway, is an electron donor; the reductase catalyzes the transfer of this electron to a cytochrome P450-drug complex which then reacts with molecular oxygen to form a reactive oxidizing species (cytochrome P450 is a terminal oxidase that produces "activated oxygen"), resulting in the formation of an oxidized substrate (drug).

(e.g., steroids) and exogenous drugs is the **cytochrome P450** complex, named for the absorption peak at 450 nm that appears when hepatic microsomal metabolism is inhibited by carbon monoxide. This group of hemoproteins may also play a role in certain biotransformation processes in adrenal cortex, kidney, and intestinal mucosa. A considerable degree of biochemical heterogeneity is present in cytochrome P450-dependent enzymes, and evidence has been found for the existence of multiple isoenzymes. The P450 enzymes that metabolize xenobiotics are part of a superfamily of heme-containing monooxygenases that include enzymes involved in the synthesis of steroids and bile acids.[r18,r20] Specific forms of P450 enzymes (e.g., P450 2A6 that catalyzes the 7-hydroxylation of coumarin) have been classified into families (designated by numbers; 1, 2, 3, 4, etc.) and subfamilies (letters; A, B, C, D) on the basis of amino acid sequence similarities from cDNA cloning studies. Thus far, 19 P450 isoenzymes have been identified in human tissues (liver, lung, intestine).[r18]

The NADPH-dependent redox cycling of cytochromes P450 involves an intermediary flavoprotein component that seems identical with **NADPH-cytochrome c reductase.** The passage of reducing equivalents through such coupled cofactor systems is associated with the generation of a reactive oxidizing species,[r19] likely a partially reduced form of molecular oxygen, that participates in the oxidative biotransformation of a wide range of molecules (see Fig. 2.4). Some typical Phase I reactions of pharmacologic relevance involving oxidations and reductions catalyzed by the hepatic MFO system are shown in Table 2.5.

A chemical property that is an important determinant of susceptibility to biotransformation in the liver is chirality. Marked differences in rates of metabolism of enantiomers have been reported for a number of drugs, including mephenytoin, metoprolol, warfarin, and propranolol. The fact that drugs are frequently administered as racemic mixtures can lead to pharmacokinetic complexities if, for example, one enantiomer can effectively inhibit the metabolism of the other. Furthermore, there may also be qualitative differences in the metabolic disposition of isomers. In the case of mephenytoin, the S(+) isomer is metabolized primarily by aromatic ring hydroxylation, but the R(–) compound is N-demethylated at a slower rate. Similarly, the R(+) isomer of warfarin is converted by reduction of the acetonyl side chain ketone function to a metabolite excreted by the kidney but S(⁻)–warfarin mainly undergoes aromatic ring hydroxylation with subsequent excretion in the bile. Finally, metabolic disposition

Table 2.5 Typical Phase I Metabolic Transformations Catalyzed by Hepatic Mixed Function Oxidase System

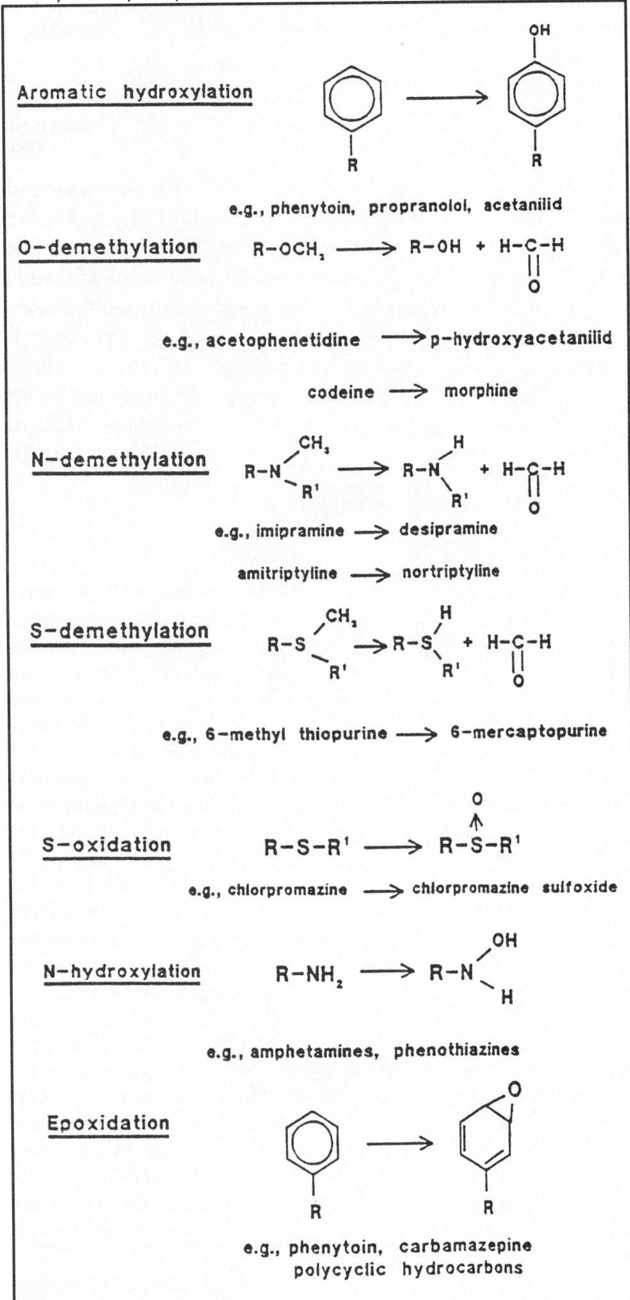

patterns for isomeric substances can show striking species differences. Thus, whereas aromatic ring hydroxylation of propranolol occurs more readily with the S(-) isomer in the dog, the R(+) enantiomer is preferentially metabolized in humans, accounting for the greater bioavailability of the S(-) compound that is responsible for the β-adrenoceptor blocking activity of the racemate.

Stereochemical factors, therefore, are critical determinants of drug biotransformation characteristics. This and the recognition that stereoselectivity can also extend to processes such as binding to plasma albumin, uptake by tissues, and renal excretion, not to mention interactions with pharmacodynamically relevant sites of drug action, have led to increasing concern regarding the use of racemic drug mixtures for either therapeutic or investigational purposes.

Phase II Reactions. The synthetic phase of drug metabolism is an energy-requiring process that involves the enzymatically catalyzed coupling of highly polar endogenous substances to the Phase I reaction product or, in some cases, the parent drug (Table 2.6). Phase II **conjugation reactions** are catalyzed by both microsomal and cytosolic enzymes. The formation of glucuronic acid conjugates is important in the biotransformation of both endogenous substances such as bilirubin and exogenous drugs.[r21] Hydroxyl groups are common sites of glucuronidation (see Fig. 2.5 for the Phase I oxidation of phenytoin, followed by Phase II conjugation). While N- and S-glucuronides have also been reported, they are somewhat less stable than O-glucuronides. It seems likely that functionally distinct glucuronyl transferases are responsible for the production of these various types of glucuronide derivatives. The glucuronidation of some drugs (e.g., morphine) can be direct, i.e. without the requirement of a preceding Phase I reaction. Conjugation with sulfate (derived from sulfur-containing amino acids), sometimes referred to as "ethereal sulfate" synthesis, is important in the metabolism of phenolic compounds such as estrone. Glycine conjugation is the major pathway in the biotransformation of agents like salicylates, leading to the formation of salicyluric acid, which accounts for approximately 80 per cent of the administered dose of aspirin (acetylsalicylic acid), after the esterase Phase I reaction (Fig. 2.6). Glucuronidation of the phenolic hydroxyl group also can occur to a limited extent, for example, after the deacetylation of acetylsalicylic acid.

Table 2.6 Hepatic Phase II (Synthetic) Reactions

Conjugation Reaction	Examples of Drug Substrates
1. Glucuronidation	acetaminophen, chloramphenicol, digitoxin, phenytoin, morphine, oxazepam, and lorazepam
2. Sulfate conjugation	acetaminophen, estrone
3. Glycine conjugation	salicylates
4. Acetylation	hydralazine, isoniazid, procainamide, sulfonamides
5. Glutathione conjugation	metabolites (arene oxides, epoxides, quinoids)

Figure 2.5 Phase I (mixed function oxidase) and Phase II (glucuronyl transferase) metabolic processes, as exemplified by phenytoin metabolism.

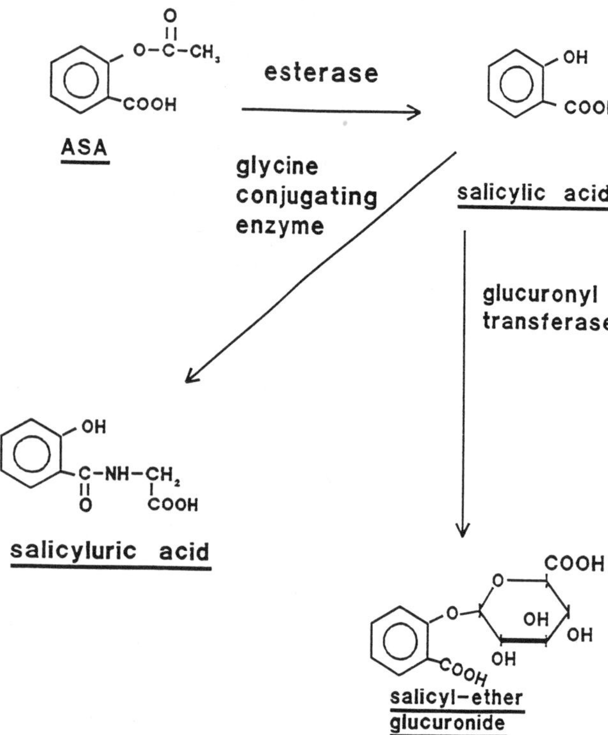

Figure 2.6 Metabolism of acetylsalicylic acid (ASA) by Phase I (esterase) and Phase II reactions (conjugation with glycine or glucuronide).

The polar salicyluric acid and glucuronide derivatives are readily excreted by the kidney. A critical feature of salicylate metabolism is the saturability of the glycine conjugation reaction at high plasma concentrations produced by doses of acetylsalicylic acid in excess of 600 mg. Under these conditions, a disproportionate increase in steady state plasma concentrations of drug relative to administered dose can occur, with a resulting risk of serious toxicity. Thus, aspirin can be seen as a prototype for drugs that exhibit dose-dependent pharmacokinetics. This important topic will be dealt with in more detail in a later section. Drugs with a primary amine constituent can be acetylated. For isoniazid, acetylation (Phase II reaction) precedes hydroxylation (Phase I reaction). The acetylator enzymes are subject to genetic polymorphism (see below).

Reactive Metabolites and Drug Toxicity

The metabolism of pharmacologic agents can, in some instances, lead to the formation of chemically reactive intermediates capable of covalent binding to functionally important cellular constituents.[r22] Among the possible adverse clinical consequences of such drug-related modifications of essential molecular structures are hepatocellular necrosis, aplastic anemia, teratogenesis, and carcinogenesis. In addition, the covalent attachment of a reactive drug product to biologic macromolecules can render it antigenic, resulting in subsequent immunologically-based disorders (e.g., drug-induced lupus).

A number of examples illustrating the generation of reactive species during the course of drug metabolism will now be considered. The first relates to the production of arene oxides (Fig. 2.7). These substances are reactive epoxide derivatives that can arise as intermediates during the metabolism of aromatic compounds by microsomal mixed function oxidases. Their formation can be demonstrated with an *in vitro* system in which changes in the viability of lymphocytes after incubation with drug precursor, NADPH, and a microsomal preparation are monitored. Lymphocytes contain en-

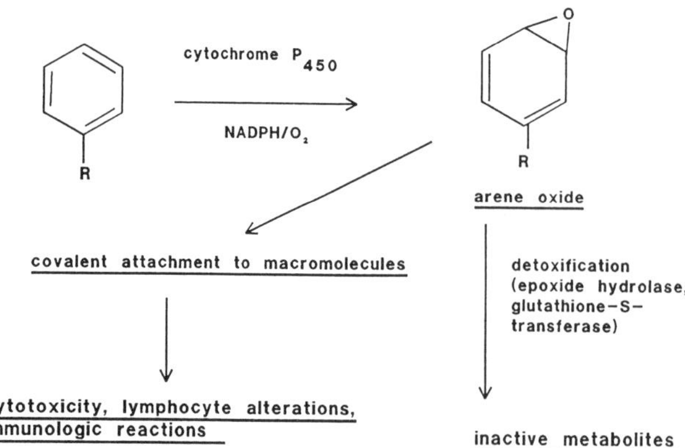

Figure 2.7 Production of toxic arene oxide intermediates by xenobiotic metabolism, and cellular detoxification mechanisms.

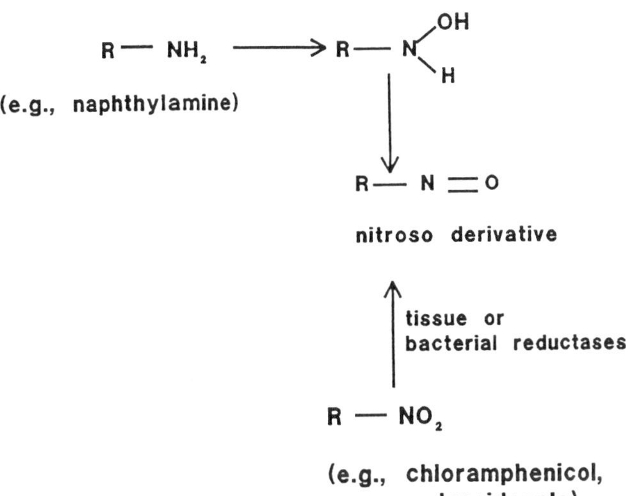

Figure 2.8 Formation of toxic nitroso derivatives as metabolic products of N-hydroxylation or nitro group reduction.

zymes (e.g., epoxide hydrolase and glutathione-S-transferase) capable of converting these potentially deleterious substances to nontoxic derivatives (Fig. 2.7). The extent of lymphocyte damage should, therefore, be a reflection both of reactive metabolite formation and the integrity of cellular defense mechanisms. Good correlations among *in vitro* lymphocyte injury, arene oxide production, and clinical toxicity have been shown for various compounds. Arene oxide formation has been implicated in certain manifestations of phenytoin toxicity, namely hepatotoxicity (a rather rare idiosyncratic reaction), birth defects, and gingival hyperplasia. With regard to phenytoin-induced hepatotoxicity, *in vitro* studies with lymphocytes from affected individuals have pointed to a defect in epoxide detoxification as the likely basis of the idiosyncracy. Furthermore, it has been suggested that the concomitant administration of two or more substances capable of being converted to arene oxide derivatives may, under certain conditions, give rise to cumulative toxic effects. A clinical report documenting the development of aplastic anemia in a patient given phenytoin and carbamazepine (both of which form arene oxide intermediates) would be consistent with this possibility.[3]

A second class of reactive metabolic intermediates that can be responsible for drug-induced toxicity are nitroso derivatives (Fig. 2.8). These can arise from unstable N-hydroxylated products of aromatic amine metabolism, from the reaction of amines with nitrates or nitrites, and from the action of tissue or bacterial reductases on nitro group-containing xenobiotics (e.g., chloramphenicol, metronidazole). Nitroso compounds have toxicologic significance in that they can produce mutagenic and carcinogenic effects *in vivo*. The identification of such activities has been facilitated by the introduction of the *in vitro* Ames test originally developed to detect mutagenicity but also used to screen potentially carcinogenic compounds. Briefly, this procedure utilizes a histidine-requiring strain of *Salmonella typhimurium* that has a mutation in the gene for phosphoribosyl adenosine triphosphate synthetase, an enzyme required for the production of histidine. The ability of this mutant strain to grow on a histidine-deficient medium can be restored by chemicals capable of inducing a reverse mutation at the level of the defective gene, thereby restoring its functional capacity. Since the expression of mutagenic or carcinogenic properties frequently requires prior metabolic activation (e.g., to nitroso or other chemically reactive derivatives), hepatic microsomal material is routinely incorporated into the test system. Although the Ames test provides a rapid and sensitive means of screening chemicals for mutagenic and carcinogenic activity, extrapolation of the results obtained to the situation in humans must be undertaken with great caution. In the case of metronidazole, for example, although carcinogenic and mutagenic activity has been demonstrated in rats and bacteria, respectively, and mutagenic material has been shown to be present in the urine of patients receiving the drug, studies to date have failed to provide definitive evidence for an increased incidence of carcinogenesis or mutagenesis in patients treated with this useful antimicrobial agent. Nonetheless, very close surveillance is obviously warranted for any therapeutic agent showing a positive response in the Ames test.

A final example illustrates a practical application of knowledge concerning the generation of reactive metabolites as it applies to the treatment of acute acetaminophen overdose. At usual doses of the drug, glucuronide and sulfate conjugation are the principal routes of metabolism for acetaminophen (Table 2.6). As plasma concentrations increase beyond the therapeutic range, these processes progressively become saturated, with a greater proportion of drug metabolism proceeding via the hepatic MFO system. In this pathway, acetaminophen is converted to a reactive quinone-like derivative by way of a semiquinone free radical intermediate (Fig. 2.9). Glutathione, a cysteine-containing tripeptide that acts as a general scavenger of reactive drug metabolites in the liver (Table 2.6) initially serves to detoxify the quinoid compound by converting it to a mercapturic acid derivative. As tissue glutathione concentrations are gradually depleted, irreversible modification of essential macromolecular components can occur, with resulting hepatocellular necrosis.

Recognition of the important roles of reactive metabolite generation and of glutathione scavenging in the setting of liver damage that may occur with acute acetaminophen overdose has led to the development of a rational therapeutic approach for acetaminophen poisoning.[r23] The approach involves the use of N-acetyl-cysteine

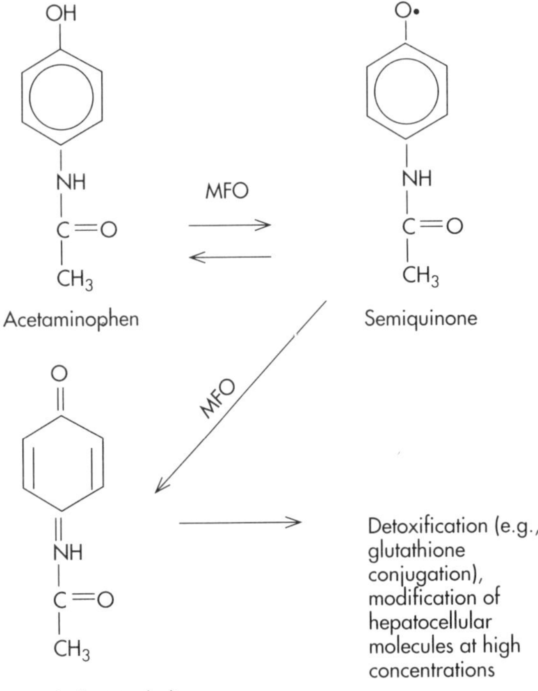

Figure 2.9 Metabolism of acetaminophen by mixed function oxidase (MFO) to produce a reactive quinoid-like intermediate that is toxic because depletion of tissue glutathione levels results in a reduced ability of the liver to detoxify the quinoid compound.

(NAC), which enters cells more readily than the free amino acid and acts either by direct scavenging of the reactive metabolic intermediate or by increasing the synthesis of glutathione. Early intervention (within 8–10 hours) after ingestion of acetaminophen is essential in order to derive appreciable benefit from NAC administration.

Factors that Influence Hepatic Metabolic Capacity

Enzyme Induction. Repeated exposure of the liver to certain lipophilic substances can cause an enhancement in tissue metabolic activity.[r24] Phenobarbital exemplifies one class of compound that, when administered chronically, produces a marked proliferation of the hepatic SER network and an increased production (via new protein synthesis = **induction**) of P450-type cytochromes (P450 2B1 and 2B2),[r25] cytochrome P450 reductase, and other enzymes involved in biotransformation processes.

The inducible forms of cytochromes P450 are distinguished by distinct molecular weights, substrate specificities, immunologic reactivities, and by distinct light-absorbing (spectral) characteristics. As a consequence of enzyme induction, the rate of hepatic metabolism of a wide variety of molecules (that may or may not include the inducer) is increased. In contrast, the stimulation of liver microsomal enzymes by polycyclic hydrocarbons affects the metabolism of a rather narrow range of substrates. The molecular mechanism responsible for P450 1A1 enzyme induction by polycyclic aromatic hydrocarbons (e.g., 3-methylcholanthrene and related compounds) has been established.[r26] The aromatic hydrocarbon enters the cell and binds to a cytosolic (Ah) receptor. The ligand-receptor complex then undergoes translocation to the nucleus where it interacts with specific DNA regulatory sequences in the 5′ flanking region of the CYP 1A1 gene, resulting in increased gene transcription and enhanced P450 1A1 (aryl hydrocarbon hydrolase) activity in the endoplasmic reticulum. This molecular mechanism for enzyme induction is the same as that previously described for the action of steroid hormones on intracellular nuclear receptors (see Chapter 1). Other substances known to be capable of inducing human P450 enzymes to varying degrees after chronic exposure include phenytoin, rifampicin, ethanol, insecticides, dietary substances, and cigarette smoke.[r20] Although effects on metabolic activities are gradually reversible when the inducer is discontinued, this process may be fairly protracted, depending on the particular agent and the cumulative dose involved. Thus, for example, the enzyme induction produced by the hydrocarbon components in tobacco smoke can persist for up to three months after cessation of smoking. Enzyme induction, although most prominent in the liver, can also occur to some extent in other tissues, such as lung, placenta, kidney, and skin. For example, the P450 1A1 isoenzyme is expressed in the lungs of cigarette smokers.[r18]

The induction of metabolic enzymes by pharmacologic agents or environmental substances has important functional implications. The enhanced hepatic metabolic activity produced by the anticonvulsant phenobarbital can increase the dosage requirements of concomitantly administered therapeutic agents for which the disposition is critically dependent on hepatic metabolism (e.g., the oral anticoagulant warfarin). Among the enzyme activities increased by repeated phenobarbital administration is glucuronyl transferase. The induction of this enzyme has been used effectively to lower serum bilirubin concentrations in patients with cholestasis and in infants with neonatal jaundice. Long-term management of epileptic patients with phenobarbital or phenytoin can be associated with the development of overt rickets or abnormalities in calcium metabolism as a result of an acceleration in the metabolism of vitamin D or its biologically active derivatives. Enhancement of metabolic enzyme activities by inducers can increase the likelihood and/or severity of drug-related toxicities caused by chemically reactive metabolic intermediates; such is the case for the previously discussed hepatocellular necrosis resulting from acute acetaminophen overdose. It has also been suggested that individual variations in metabolic activation by P450-related enzyme activities (that can be influenced by genetic factors, as described in the next section) may be important in determining the risk of adverse consequences in a given animal or human after exposure to potentially mutagenic or carcinogenic drugs or environmental chemicals. Conversely, the inducibility of detoxifying enzymes (such as glucuronyl transferase or glutathione-S-transferase) may provide a means by which organisms can respond adaptively to the potentially deleterious effects of exposure to environmental or therapeutic xenobiotics. Recently, Talalay and coworkers have screened vegetables for their ability to induce a Phase II enzyme, quinone reductase, in cultured hepatic cells that will detoxify carcinogens formed by a Phase I reaction.[4] A potent Phase II enzyme inducer was isolated from broccoli and characterized chemically.[5] Thus, dietary modifications that influence hepatic drug metabolizing enzymes may reduce the risk of cancer.

Genetic Factors. The sometimes widely divergent steady state concentrations of drugs administered at a fixed standard dose to an apparently homogeneous group of individuals point to an important influence of genetic factors on processes involved in drug disposition.[r27] Generally, this is a reflection of the polygenic control of drug metabolism. In certain instances, however, the distribution of such steady state plasma concentrations of drug in a representative population sample is polymodal (see Fig. 1.3, Chapter 1), indicating the presence of subgroups that can be distinguished on the basis of differences in drug handling. Studies of the biochemical determinants of such drug-related "polymorphism" comprise the field of **Pharmacogenetics.**

One illustration of such pharmacogenetic polymorphism is the existence of rapid and slow metabolizers by acetylation (Phase II reaction; Table 2.6) of the antituberculosis drug isoniazid, reflecting differences in the synthesis of liver acetyl transferase, a nonmicrosomal enzyme.[r28,r29] The "slow acetylator" phenotype is inherited as an autosomal recessive trait and shows a distribution that is highly race-dependent. Approximately half of the individuals in North American populations are slow acetylators. A considerably lower proportion of "slow acetylators" is found among those of Asian and Inuit descent, whereas a greater preponderance of "slow acetylators" is found in persons of northern European ancestry. With regard to clinical implications of acetylator status, slow metabolizers are more prone to develop peripheral neuropathies when given isoniazid, although this toxicity is readily preventable by the concomitant administration of pyridoxine. Acetylator status does not seem to be a useful predictor of isoniazid-induced hepatotoxicity; patient age is the critical factor. In the treatment of tuberculosis, rapid acetylators may show a diminished therapeutic response if isoniazid is administered on a once-weekly basis. Other drugs for which metabolism is similarly affected by acetylator phenotype include procainamide, hydralazine, and sulfasalazine. It is claimed that slow acetylators are at increased risk of developing hydralazine-induced systemic lupus erythematosus and require lower daily doses of sulfasalazine than do fast acetylators in order to maintain ulcerative colitis in remission. Finally, it has been suggested that the slow acetylator phenotype may be associated with a greater incidence of bladder cancer, especially in individuals exposed to high levels of arylamines. Thus, it can be seen that genetic polymorphism in terms of a Phase II metabolic pathway (acetylation) can have a direct bearing on the clinical toxicity of drugs.

The microsomal cytochrome P450-dependent oxidative metabolism of the antihypertensive debrisoquin (Phase I reaction; Table 2.5) has also been found to exhibit a bimodal distribution consisting of rapid and slow hydroxylators. The prevalence of the slow hydroxylator phenotype varies considerably among racial groups and is present in 3–10 per cent of Caucasians. The defect appears to involve faulty expression of cytochrome P450 2D6[r29,r30] and is inherited as an autosomal recessive trait. This oxidation polymorphism is also reflected in the disposition of numerous other agents, including tricyclic antidepressants, phenformin, dextromethorphan, and beta adrenoceptor blockers. In the latter category, the cardioselectivity of agents such as metoprolol is likely to be compromised seriously at the markedly elevated plasma concentrations expected in slow hydroxylators receiving standard doses of the drug.

Finally, studies of human lymphocyte cytochrome P450-dependent aryl hydrocarbon hydroxylase have indicated that genetic factors influence its susceptibility to induction. This may have important implications in determining individual susceptibilities to the mutagenic or carcinogenic effects of pharmacologic or environmental agents after their metabolic activation by cytochromes P450-associated systems.[r31] In summary, genetically determined alterations in Phase I or Phase II metabolic processes can have important clinical consequences in terms of individual susceptiblities to the deleterious effects of drugs or environmental components. Knowledge of the drug-metabolizing phenotype status of patients would have the following therapeutic benefits: (i) design of dosage regimens to minimize toxicities; (ii) avoidance of interactions with co-administered drugs that share the same metabolic pathway; and (iii) avoidance of potential environmental carcinogens.

Age- and Disease-related Considerations. Pathophysiologic factors associated with aging and disease processes are known to affect the biotransformation of drugs markedly.[r30,r32] Alterations in plasma albumin binding, liver blood flow, and in the intrinsic activity of metabolic enzymes can, individually or in combination, produce changes in drug disposition that may require adjustments to drug dosing regimens in order to prevent the occurrence of serious toxicities.

The increased sensitivity of the very young and the elderly to the adverse effects of drugs, particularly when doses are estimated solely on the basis of body size, has long been recognized (see Chapter 3). In the neonate, enzymes catalyzing microsomal oxidation and Phase II conjugation reactions (e.g., glucuronidation of morphine, bilirubin, and chloramphenicol) are incompletely developed and do not attain full adult functional capacity until several weeks after birth. A clinical condition in which the immaturity of glucuronyl transferase has been directly implicated is the "gray baby" syndrome, which has been reported after chloramphenicol use in newborn infants. Glucuronidation accounts for approximately 90 per cent of chloramphenicol metabolism in adults, so that its administration during the neonatal period can produce markedly elevated plasma concentrations that predispose to this potentially life-threatening cyanotic condition. The limiting activity of glucuronyl transferase in the neonate also contributes to the risk of kernicterus when free bilirubin levels are increased in plasma due to displacement from albumin binding sites, as discussed on page 49. The factors that predispose to kernicterus are summarized in Table 2.7.

Although the metabolism of numerous agents tends also to be compromised at the opposite extreme of the age spectrum, changes are not uniform with all agents and the multiplicity of interacting variables involved makes generalizations concerning aging-related dosage adjustments difficult.[r33,r34] One important factor that can alter drug metabolism with increased age is hepatic blood flow, which can be decreased by as much as 50 per cent in persons above the age of 65. Thus, in the elderly, drugs normally showing high hepatic clearance values indicative of blood flow-limited rates of metabolism (e.g., propranolol, lidocaine, meperidine), would be expected to show decreased clearance rates and an increased incidence of toxicity. Conversely, it has been reported that for a drug such as phenytoin, where metabolism is limited by binding to plasma proteins rather than by the rate of delivery via the hepatic portal system and the hepatic artery, metabolic clearance may actually be increased in patients over 65 years when compared with individuals 45 years of age. This increased clearance rate has been attributed to age-dependent reductions both in the concentration and in the binding capacity of albumin. The reduction in plasma binding results in an increased accessibility of circulating drug to hepatic metabolism. The biotransformation of phenytoin (Fig. 2.5) is also highly sensitive to changes in the activity of liver metabolic enzymes. Other poorly extracted substances that are similarly affected include theophylline, imipramine, meperidine, quinidine, tolbutamide, and antipyrine. The elimination half-life of antipyrine is frequently used experimentally as a convenient measure of hepatic metabolic capacity *in vivo*. Studies of alterations in rates of hepatic metabolism for a wide variety of pharmacologic agents as a function of increasing age have indicated that, whereas nonmicrosomal metabolism and Phase II conjugation processes are minimally affected, the activity of the microsomal MFO system decreases progressively with increasing age. Differences in the disposition of various benzodiazepine derivatives are illustrative in this regard. Analogues converted mainly to inactive derivatives by conjugation with glucuronic acid (e.g., lorazepam and oxazepam) exhibit rates of hepatic biotransformation that do not vary appreciably with age. For this reason, these relatively short-acting benzodiazepines are considered agents of choice to produce sedation in the geriatric population. In contrast, benzodiazepines that undergo Phase I microsomal oxidations with the formation of pharmacologically active metabolites (e.g., alprazolam, chlordiazepoxide, diazepam, and flurazepam) have plasma half-lives that

Table 2.7 Conditions that Predispose to the Development of Kernicterus in the Newborn

1. Increased production of bilirubin, resulting from breakdown of fetal haemoglobin.
2. Immaturity of hepatic glucuronyl transferase, resulting in impaired metabolic disposition of bilirubin.
3. Displacement of albumin-bound bilirubin by a drug (e.g., sulfonamide), leading to increased circulating levels of free bilirubin.
4. Incomplete formation of blood-brain barrier, allowing deposition of excess free (unbound) bilirubin in the brain.

are considerably increased in elderly individuals. Although these analogues are generally best avoided in elderly patients, diazepam is still sometimes used to obtain sedation prior to investigative or therapeutic procedures (such as endoscopy or dental extraction). In addition to the reduced rates of hepatic metabolism, lipophilic derivatives such as diazepam and chlordiazepoxide also exhibit age-related increases in their volumes of distribution. As a result, drug accumulation in plasma would be less than expected on the basis of the impairment in hepatic metabolism. In addition to these pharmacokinetic considerations, pharmacodynamic factors further complicate the issue. On the one hand, elderly patients tend to show an increased sensitivity to acutely administered sedative-hypnotics, while the long-term use of these agents can lead to the development of tolerance. Clearly, then, benzodiazepines should be administered with particular caution to elderly patients and dosage requirements should be determined individually on an empirical basis. It should be noted that the interplay of pharmacokinetic and pharmacodynamic factors, which is particularly complex in the case of benzodiazepine action in the geriatric population, is nonetheless a feature of therapeutic drug effects generally.

In contrast to the effects of kidney disease on drug elimination, which are reasonably straightforward to predict (see below), the effects of liver disease and other pathologic conditions on drug metabolism are complex and often unpredictable.[r35] Although drug elimination is frequently impaired in hepatic disorders, this is not invariably the case. The nature of the underlying disease process can influence the severity of alterations in drug disposition, these generally being less marked in acute viral hepatitis than in cirrhosis, for example. The distinction between readily-extracted and poorly-extracted drugs (with reference to relative rates of hepatic metabolism) is also an important functional consideration. Indeed, the same conceptual framework previously used to analyze the pharmacokinetic consequences of aging is directly relevant to the problem of disease-related changes. Although the present section will view this area from the pharmacokinetic perspective, alterations in drug sensitivity (i.e., pharmacodynamic considerations) also may be clinically relevant. This is particularly so in the case of centrally acting sedatives or analgesics for which the high potential for precipitating hepatic coma in patients with liver disease very likely involves an interplay of pharmacokinetic and pharmacodynamic factors.

The pharmacokinetic implications of compromised blood flow to the liver have already been discussed in connection with the effects of aging on drug disposition. Functionally significant reductions in hepatic blood flow under pathologic conditions (e.g., cirrhosis or congestive heart failure) can result from the formation of intra- or extrahepatic shunts. It has been estimated that in chronic liver disease, up to 50 per cent of portal flow may be shunted through mesenteric and splenic vascular beds. As a consequence, the elimination of readily extracted drugs is likely to be markedly impaired and their presystemic elimination ("first pass" effect) after oral administration decreased correspondingly. By way of illustration, the clearance of propranolol from the plasma (see page 71: Quantitative Pharmacokinetics) is typically reduced in cirrhotic patients from a normal value of 860 L/min (indicative of highly efficient, flow-limited hepatic metabolism) to approximately 580 L/min. Whereas the clearance of highly-extracted drugs is generally reduced in hepatic disease, changes in distributional characteristics and plasma half-lives are relatively variable, although the latter are frequently decreased.

Factors responsible for the reduction in drug binding capacity of plasma accompanying renal or liver dysfunction have already been discussed (see page 51). The metabolism of poorly extracted drugs is likely to be accelerated under these conditions, as has been shown to be the case with tolbutamide in patients with acute viral hepatitis, for example. However, the functional status of the system primarily involved in the process of drug disposition is critical in determining the extent to which elimination is altered. Furthermore, disease-related increases in drug biotransformation may occur independently of changes in plasma protein binding. This appears to be the case for the oxidative metabolism of agents such as phenytoin in patients with uremia. Conversely, the activity of hepatic drug metabolizing enzymes may be impaired to varying degrees in a number of pathologic states, including acute drug-induced or viral hepatitis, active or inactive liver cirrhosis, hemochromatosis, hepatocellular carcinoma, heavy metal poisoning, and porphyria.[r30] Microsomal cytochromes P450-linked enzyme systems seem most vulnerable to inactivation under these conditions, while nonmicrosomal enzymes involved in Phase II synthetic reactions are frequently spared;[r35] a similar pattern was noted previously with aging.[r34] Thus, with regard to benzodiazepine disposition in chronic liver disease, the elimination of analogues principally metabolized by glucuronidation (e.g., lorazepam and oxazepam) is largely unaffected, while the metabolism of derivatives undergoing extensive Phase I oxidative metabolism (e.g., diazepam and chlordiazepoxide) can be markedly impaired. Apart from such generalizations, however, disease-associated alterations in drug biotransformation are usually difficult to predict *a priori* and to quantify with conventional clinical indices of liver function, unlike the situation with impaired drug elimination in renal failure (see page 63).

Inhibition of Biotransformation by Pharmacologic Agents. The relatively broad range of specificities exhibited by enzymes that catalyze Phase I or Phase II metabolic processes allows for competition between pharmacologic agents at common sites of biotransformation.[r30] The simultaneous administration of such compounds, therefore, can lead to an impairment in the elimination of the more slowly metabolized drug, with potentiation of its pharmacologic effects. Individuals who metabolize a drug slowly because of pharmacogenetics (see section above) will be particularly susceptible to toxicities arising from competition. The consequences of such interactions will be most serious if the enzyme inhibited is solely (or primarily) responsible for drug inactivation, or if major metabolic pathways are readily saturable. Saturability of disposition mechanisms at doses in the upper therapeutic range is a characteristic feature of theophylline, dicumarol, and phenytoin, three drugs commonly implicated in clinically significant interactions involving inhibition of metabolism, as described below.

It has been reported that children show an intensified response to theophylline, characterized by unexpected nausea and vomitting, when treated concomitantly with erythromycin, a known inhibitor of drug metabolism. The potentiation of dicumarol action by cimetidine has also been attributed to an impairment of anticoagulant metabolism at the microsomal level. In contrast to this potentially serious drug interaction, the reduction in diazepam metabolism produced by cimetidine, although statistically significant, is not usually associated with clinical evidence of daytime fatigue or excessive sedation. The increase in plasma concentrations of the diazepam after cimetidine administration is likely to be gradual (given the long half-life of this benzodiazepine) and the development of tolerance could minimize any functional consequences. With regard to phenytoin, on the other hand, severe ataxia and drowsiness have been reported in patients that receive the drug in combination with dicumarol or chloramphenicol. Interestingly, these two agents are substrates for different metabolic pathways in liver, cytochromes P450-dependent oxidation in the case of dicumarol and glucuronidation for chloramphenicol. As noted previously (see Fig. 2.5), both of these systems figure prominently in the biotransformation of phenytoin. Given the wide variety of xenobiotics dependent on microsomal MFO-dependent metabolism for inactivation, it seems likely that competition at this level is functionally relevant in many instances of drug interactions. Although effects of competing substrates on metabolic systems in liver are usually reversible, irreversible inactivation of cytochromes P450 during the course of metabolism can occur with some agents (e.g., secobarbital, allobarbital). Competition for glucuronidation, which is likely the basis of the chloramphenicol/phenytoin interaction,[6] has also been implicated in the impaired metabolism of acetaminophen and lorazepam produced by probenecid,[7] a uricosuric agent better known for its effects on renal tubular secretory processes (see page 62).

The foregoing examples have generally focused on the potentially adverse consequences of reductions in drug metabolic capacity produced by various pharmacologic agents. However, the specific inhibition of enzymes involved in the biotransformation of endogenous or exogenous substances can be used to therapeutic advantage. Thus, anticholinesterases are used after surgery to reverse skeletal muscle relaxation produced by curare-like compounds, monoamine oxidase inhibitors can be effective in the treatment of depression, and inhibition of xanthine oxidase with allopurinol decreases excessive uric acid production in patients with hyperuricemia. The use of drugs that interfere with the activity of enzymes catalyzing the breakdown of naturally occurring substrates can also produce important changes in the disposition of other exogenously administered pharmacologic agents, as illustrated by the following two examples. The antineoplastic drug 6-mercaptopurine undergoes metabolism by xanthine oxidase, so that it must be used at substantially reduced dosage when allopurinol is given to prevent the complications of secondary hyperuricemia resulting from increased cell turnover and breakdown. In the treatment of Parkinson's disease, levodopa is combined with carbidopa, an inhibitor of aromatic L-amino acid decarboxylase, in order to reduce the breakdown of levodopa in peripheral tissues, thereby increasing its accessibility to nigrostriatal sites of action in the brain.

Summary

The metabolism or biotransformation of drugs has two important functions: (i) inactivation of some (but not all) drugs, thereby terminating their therapeutic effect (it must be remembered, however, that many drugs have metabolites that are pharmacologically active and that some drugs (pro-drugs) are activated by metabolism); and (ii) conversion of the drug to a more water-soluble compound in order to aid in the renal elimination of the drug from the body. The liver is the principal site of drug metabolism. A number of factors influence the rate and extent of the hepatic metabolism of drugs. For example, the administration of one drug can either increase (through enzyme induction) or decrease (by simple competition) the metabolism of a second drug. Various physiologic (genetics; development) and pathophysiologic (hepatic disease) situations also can affect the rates of drug metabolism. A detailed understanding of these factors is required in order that the therapeutic effectiveness of drugs can be optimized and the risk of adverse drug-drug interactions minimized. Finally, the "inactivation" of drugs by hepatic metabolism can, in fact, produce highly reactive metabolic intermediates that are themselves very toxic.

Excretion

Drugs and their Phase I or Phase II metabolites are most commonly excreted in the **urine** or in the **bile.** Biliary excretion is usually followed by fecal elimination in inverse proportion to lipid solubility, which also determines the degree of subsequent intestinal reabsorption. Conversely, lipophilicity favors the elimination of volatile agents (e.g., inhalational anesthetics, ethanol) via the lungs and the partitioning of drugs into body fluids such as sweat, saliva, tears, and milk. The accumulation of weakly basic substances in milk is also related to the pH gradient across mammary gland epithelium (Fig. 2.2). Drugs bound extensively to plasma proteins can partition into milk to varying degrees and, in the case of nursing mothers, possibly attain concentrations sufficient to exert pharmacologic actions in the child—two documented examples are warfarin and sulfisoxazole.

Renal Excretion

A number of drugs such as antibiotics are excreted in **unchanged active forms** by the kidney (Table 2.8). Consequently, the rate of renal elimination determines the duration of action for these agents. As presented previously, however, one of the functions of drug metabolism is to convert the drug to a more polar form that exhibits an **increased water-solubility,** so that elimination by the kidney can be increased. The kidneys, which are critically dependent on a high degree of tissue perfusion, receive approximately 20 per cent of the cardiac output; renal plasma flow is of the order

Table 2.8 Drugs Excreted by the Kidney Largely in the Unchanged, Pharmacologically Active Form

Antibiotics:	amikacin, cephalexin, ethambutol, flucytosine, gentamicin, kanamycin, spectinomycin, trimethoprim, vancomycin
Cardiovascular/ Renal:	acetazolamide, atenolol, digoxin, hydrochlorothiazide, isosorbide, dinitrate, nadolol, practolol
Miscellaneous:	barbital, hexamethonium, methotrexate, pyridostigmine

of 650 ml/min. A portion of this blood supply is diverted to the glomerular capillary network of the afferent arteriole, resulting in the production of plasma ultrafiltrate at a rate of 120–130 ml/min. The efferent arteriole arborizes to provide a richly vascular supply to renal tubules that carry out two types of active transport processes, namely, reabsorption of glomerular filtrate constituents (e.g., sodium, chloride, amino acids, glucose, uric acid, etc.) and the secretion of weakly acidic or basic molecules (both endogenous and exogenous) from the vascular compartment into the tubular lumen. The extent to which filtered and/or secreted substances are subsequently excreted in the urine increases in proportion to their polarity or degree of ionization, both of which limit their passive diffusion (reabsorption) through the lipoidal tubular wall.

The three key processes that determine the renal excretion of drugs, then, are: (1) **filtration** at the glomerulus; (2) active tubular **secretion** and (3) passive tubular **reabsorption** (Fig. 2.10). The contribution of each of these processes to drug excretion varies with the particular agent in question.[r36] Under normal conditions (i.e., in the absence of proteinuria), only the unbound component of drug in plasma is subject to glomerular filtration. Pathologic or pharmacologic factors leading to a reduction in drug association with plasma protein components (e.g., phenytoin and hypoalbuminemia; page 50) can, therefore, result in an increased rate of renal drug elimination. In contrast, protein binding is not rate-limiting for tubular secretion, given the highly efficient, ATP-energized active transport systems involved. By way of illustration, penicillin G shows appreciable binding to plasma albumin and yet is readily eliminated by the kidney at a rate that approximates renal plasma flow. This result indicates a rapid transfer of drug from blood to urine by active tubular transport.

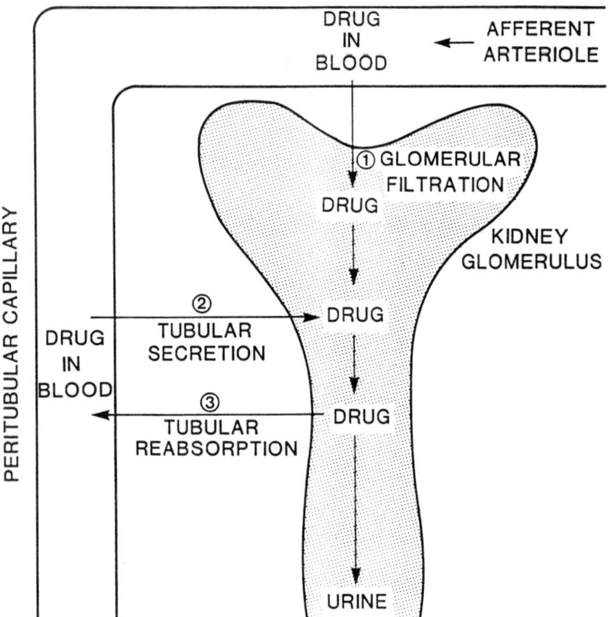

Figure 2.10 Kidney processes involved in the excretion of drugs: (1) glomerular filtration of free (nonprotein-bound) drug in the blood; (2) active secretion of drugs into the tubular urine; (3) passive reabsorption of drugs from the tubular urine back to the blood. Processes that reduce drug reabsorption (formation of water-soluble metabolites, alteration in tubular pH) will enhance drug excretion.

The secretion of anionic (weakly acidic) and (weakly basic) cationic substances is effected by two independent carrier-mediated systems located in the proximal segment of renal tubules. Although both systems are capable of bidirectional transport, secretion is usually favored. The accumulation of circulating anionic molecules by renal tubular cells utilizes carriers located in the plasma membrane and may be dependent on the transmembrane sodium gradient. Accumulated substances then move into the tubular lumen by passive or facilitated diffusion. Cation transport can occur at both basolateral and brush border membranes. The former may involve gated channels, while the latter operates as a carrier-mediated system. Transmembrane proton gradients generated by amiloride-sensitive Na^+/H^+ antiport activity appear to be important in the renal transport of cationic substances.

The structural requirements for renal tubular transport[r37] are rather broad, with overall charge being the major determinant. As a consequence, competition can occur among endogenous and exogenous weak acids or bases for transport by their respective carriers. Although little overlap occurs, there are a few instances in which a given compound may utilize both systems, two notable examples being cefalexin (β-lactam antimicrobial agent) and the antineoplastic drug cisplatinum.

Competition at the level of renal tubular transport carriers can result in therapeutically advantageous effects or, alternatively, can give rise to adverse drug interactions. In the former category, probenecid (which can be viewed as an inert organic acid) has been used to reduce the renal excretion of penicillin by reducing tubular **secretion,** thereby increasing the effectiveness of penicillin in the single-dose treatment of certain infectious disorders (Fig. 2.10). Besides blocking tubular secretion, probenecid can also interfere with the carrier-mediated **reabsorption** of uric acid in the proximal tubule, (Fig. 2.10), a property that determines the usefulness of probenecid in the management of patients with hyperuricemia. The renal excretion of uric acid is complex and consists of filtration at the glomerulus, the aforementioned reabsorptive phase followed by active tubular secretion. Interference by endogenous substances (e.g., lactic acid) or weakly acidic drugs (e.g., salicylates, numerous diuretics) at this final secretory phase can produce elevations in plasma uric acid concentrations sufficient to precipitate attacks of acute gout in predisposed individuals. In a similar fashion, salicylates and probenecid impair the renal excretion of methotrexate, while, at the weak base carrier, the tubular secretion of H_2–antihistamines such as cimetidine can be inhibited by a variety of agents, including quinidine, quinine, tolazoline, and procainamide.

Alterations in urinary pH (which may vary from 4.5–8.0) can be effectively used to enhance the elimination of ionizable drugs by minimizing the extent of passive reabsorption after glomerular filtration or tubular secretion. Urinary alkalinization can be of use in managing overdoses of weakly acidic drugs, such as salicylates. At usual therapeutic doses, salicylate (Fig. 2.6) is predominantly eliminated in the form of its polar glycine conjugate and hence is relatively unaffected by changes in urinary pH. At high doses, levels of free salicylate in the tubular fluid progressively increase, owing to saturation of the glycine conjugation pathway. Under these conditions, the administration of sodium bicarbonate to increase urinary pH can produce a marked (4–6 fold) increase in the rate of drug excretion due to an increase in the proportion of the drug as the ionized (anionic) species according to the Henderson-Hasselbalch equation for a weak acid with a pKa of 3, and the resulting decrease in passive reabsorption. Sodium bicarbonate is also sometimes included in the therapeutic regimen of patients with hyperuricemia who are receiving allopurinol or probenecid. The resulting increase in urinary pH favors the conversion of uric acid to its more soluble urate salt form, thereby both hastening its elimination and reducing the risk of uric acid precipitation, a process favored by low urinary pH. On the other hand, acidifying salts such as ammonium chloride generally enhance renal clearance of weakly basic drugs such as amphetamine, chloroquine, codeine, imipramine, and meperidine. Effects of urinary pH manipulation on the renal excretion of ionizable drugs vary considerably and are greatest for substances that are weakly acidic (pK values in the range of 3–6) or strongly basic (pKa values greater than 8). In contrast, strongly acidic and weakly basic drugs already exist almost entirely in their ionized states under physiologic conditions. Thus, the changes in urinary pH that result from the administration of acidifying or alkalinizing agents are unlikely to alter appreciably the proportions of charged and uncharged forms. Consequently, the rates of drug elimination of strong acids and weak bases will not be significantly affected by changes in urinary pH.

Given the paramount role of the kidney in drug elimination, changes in renal functional status can have profound pharmacologic implications.[r38] This is particularly important in the case of drugs with narrow margins of safety that are excreted with minimal prior metabolic biotransformation (Table 2.3). Two notable examples are aminoglycoside antimicrobials and digoxin. When administering agents such as these to patients with reduced renal function, it is essential to adjust drug dosages according to the severity of the impairment. This important problem will be considered in a later section (page 68) dealing with pharmacokinetic calculations. However, mention should be made at this point of one complexity concerning drugs for which elimination is decreased in patients with compromised kidney function. In such individuals, increases in the activity of alternative nonrenal pathways can, to varying extents, depending on the agent and pathologic condition involved, compensate for a reduction in renal excretion. As a result, the extent to which over-all rates of drug clearance from plasma are altered cannot always be inferred directly from the degree of renal functional impairment. For this reason, nomograms relating changes in drug elimination (usually expressed in terms of plasma half-life values) to creatinine clearance (a quantitative measure of renal functional status) have been constructed for many commonly used drugs, thereby providing a convenient means of adjusting dosing regimens to the needs of each individual patient.[r38] Creatinine clearances of 50–80 ml/min are typical of patients with relatively mild renal impairment; values in the range 10–50 ml/min denote moderate impairment; and clearances below 10 ml/min are indicative of severe kidney dysfunction.

Although reductions in dosage and/or increases in dosing intervals are required for many drugs when used in patients with clinically significant uremia, the following are exceptions to this generalization: phenytoin, warfarin, corticosteroids, tricyclic antidepressants, and most narcotic analgesics. Besides renal dysfunction, developmental factors also may be important in limiting drug elimination by the kidney. In premature and newborn infants, rates of glomerular filtration and renal tubular secretion are less than 50 per cent of the adult values; full maturity is not attained until six months to one year. This reduced functional capacity of renal excretion processes must be considered in the choice of drugs and dosing regimens to be used in the neonatal period. Renal function is also decreased significantly with age, even in the absence of kidney disease.

Additional details of the cellular processes involved in the excretion of drugs are described in Chapter 37 on General Principles of Renal Cellular Mechanisms of Drug Transport.

Biliary Excretion

Bile is produced by the liver at a rate of 0.5–1.0 L/day in the adult human and reaches the duodenum via the common bile duct. Circulating drugs and drug metabolites can accumulate in bile by passage across the hepatic parenchymal cell membrane followed by active secretion into the biliary tract. Their subsequent elimination in the feces is favored by high polarity, which minimizes the extent of passive reabsorption through the intestinal wall. For certain substances secreted largely unchanged into the bile or in the form of Phase II conjugates readily hydrolyzeable in the intestine, the reabsorption of the parent compound may be considerable. This process, referred to as "enterohepatic circulation," plays an important physiologic role in the conservation of bile acids and may delay the elimination of some pharmacologic agents (e.g., tetracyclines, morphine, digitoxin). Other drugs that show significant elimination in bile include streptomycin, quinine, colchicine, vinblastine, d-tubocurarine, and steroid hormones.

Chemicals are secreted into bile by mechanisms functionally analogous to those previously described for renal tubular transport. Independent carrier systems are utilized by anions, cations, and neutral substances (such as steroids). Within each group, relative rates of transport are determined by chemical structural characteristics, and competition between related molecules can occur. Drug elimination by this route is favored by metabolic alterations that produce an increase in polarity, with glucuronide conjugates being particularly susceptible to biliary secretion. Compounds with molecular weights below 300 daltons are not efficiently eliminated, probably because these are extensively reabsorbed during the passage of bile through small canaliculi. A number of endogenous substances (such as bilirubin and bile acids) and some exogenously administered pharmacologic agents are actively concentrated in bile and can attain concentrations that are 10–1000 times greater than those in plasma. As is the case for active transport systems in the kidney, binding to plasma proteins is not rate-limiting under these conditions.

Biliary secretory activity determines the elimination of sulfobromophthalein (BSP), a diagnostic agent used in the assessment of liver function. Normally, more than 90 per cent of this dye is cleared from the circulation 30 minutes after its IV administration as a 5 mg/kg test dose. Abnormally elevated blood concentrations can, therefore, provide useful information concerning the severity of hepatic functional impairment. Biliary secretion also has important diagnostic implications in the use of cholecystographic contrast media for the radiographic visualization of gall bladder and bile duct structures.

Summary

The kidney is the most important organ for the elimination of drugs and their metabolites. Drugs can be excreted unchanged by the kidney, so that rates of renal elimination can determine the duration of the pharmacologic response to a particular drug. Excretion of drugs by the kidney is determined by the net balance between glomerular filtration and active tubular secretion, and tubular reabsorption. A drug such as probenecid can block either of these tubular transport processes and thus influence the excretion of endogenous compounds or other drugs. Many drugs are metabolized to more water-soluble compounds in order to enhance their elimination by the kidney by reducing the extent of tubular reabsorption. Manipulation of urinary pH can accelerate the elimination of drugs that are weak acids or bases by increasing the proportion of the drug in the ionized form that will not be reabsorbed by passive diffusion. For a drug that is eliminated predominantly as the active (parent) compound by the kidney (Table 2.8), alterations in the function of the kidney due to disease can have a marked effect on the therapeutic action of the drug and on the incidence of toxic side-effects. Other routes of drug elimination include hepatic secretion into bile, exhalation of volatile agents by the lungs, and excretion via milk and sweat.

Quantitative Pharmacokinetics

As outlined in the Introductory section (2.1) of this chapter, the two fundamental pharmacokinetic parameters—apparent volume of distribution (Vd) and half-life ($t^{1/2}$)—provide a quantitative over-all description of the distributional and elimination phases, respectively, of drug disposition following drug administration. Standard Vd and $t^{1/2}$ values as well as other useful pharmacokinetic information (e.g., plasma protein binding, oral availability, clearance) are included in most comprehensive pharmacology textbooks, often in a separate Appendix section (cf. Goodman and Gilman, *The Pharmacological Basis of Therapeutics*). The multiplicity of pathophysiologic factors influencing drug handling by the body can lead to considerable variations in the magnitude of Vd or $t^{1/2}$. Clearly, these must be anticipated and taken into account in order that drug administration be individualized to the needs of each particular patient. The sections that follow will illustrate a rational approach to drug dosing protocols based on the fundamental pharmacokinetic principles discussed earlier in this chapter.

Apparent Volume of Distribution

The ratio of the administered dose of a drug divided by the resulting maximal concentration attained in plasma (usually estimated by extrapolation) is defined as the apparent volume of distribution (Vd) of the drug. Values can be expressed either in liters (assuming an "ideal" weight of 70 kg) or in L/kg, the latter allowing a more meaningful estimate of Vd based on actual body weights.

Example. The anticonvulsant drug valproic acid is administered at a dose of 500 mg to a patient weighing 55 kg. The extrapolated initial plasma concentration is found to be 70 μg/ml. What is the apparent volume of distribution of this drug?

Solution. In this, as in all pharmacokinetic calculations, it is essential to ensure uniformity of units. Plasma concentration units of μg/ml are equivalent to those expressed as mg/L:

$$\text{Vd} = \frac{\text{dose}}{\text{plasma concentration}} = \frac{500\ \text{mg}}{70\ \text{mg/L}} = 7.1\ \text{L}$$

In this patient, then, the Vd value for valproic acid would be 7.1 L/55 kg = 0.13 L/kg.

As a first approximation, Vd can be thought of as that **hypothetical volume** in which a given dose would have to distribute in order to produce the estimated peak concentration achieved in plasma. This makes the simplifying assumption of uniform distribution in a single homogeneous compartment that, in some instances, may correspond to (or approximate) a functional anatomic space in the body. In fact, chromophoric or isotopically-labeled reference compounds with well-defined distributional characteristics can be used to determine the volumes occupied by these compartments under normal or pathologic conditions. Substances such as the dye Evans blue (which binds with a high affinity to plasma proteins) or ^{131}I-albumin yield Vd values in man of about 3 L (or 4% body weight), which represents plasma volume. In the case of highly polar, low molecular weight substances, such as sodium thiosulfate or mannitol, the value of 14 L (or 20% of body weight) provides an estimate of extracellular water. Isotopic water (D_2O or T_2O) equilibrates with total body water as indicated by a Vd equal to 42 L (or 60% of body weight).

The foregoing reference values provide a framework within which to derive some insight into the considerably more complex distributional properties of therapeutic agents based on the magnitude of their Vd. A number of illustrative examples are presented in Table 2.9. Heparin, as may have been expected based on the high degree of binding to albumin, is largely confined to the plasma compartment, the primary site of its anticoagulant effect. However, warfarin, which also is extensively bound to plasma proteins, shows considerably greater extravascular distribution, consistent with its hepatic site of action. The Vd for acetylsalicylic acid is approximately equal to the volume of the extracellular water space. Very similar values are found for a variety of other weakly acidic substances, including ibuprofen, naproxen, probenecid, sulfisoxazole, and valproic acid, all of which are very much more highly bound to plasma proteins (>90%) than is acetylsalicylic acid (bound to the extent of only 50%). The Vd for ethanol is indicative of its well-known ability to traverse biologic membranes, thereby allowing it to equilibrate with aqueous compartments throughout the body. The very high "apparent" volumes of distribution for metoprolol and propranolol, which bear no obvious relation to the extent of plasma protein binding, are a characteristic feature of drugs that show marked uptake and accumulation by tissues. The resulting sharp decrease in measured plasma concentrations leads to an artifactual increase in the dose/plasma concentration ratio that defines Vd, yielding a value that obviously exceeds any "real" volume compartment within the body.

Table 2.9 Distributional Characteristics of Some Pharmacological Agents

Agent	Vd (L)*	Comments
heparin	4.1	extensively bound to albumin, distributed predominantly in plasma compartment.
wafarin	7.7	extensively bound to albumin, distribution consistent with its extravascular site of action.
acetylsalicylic acid	10.5	binding to plasma protein relatively low (50%), exists largely in ionized form at physiologic pH, distribution volume approximates that of extracellular water.
ethanol	38	negligible binding to plasma albumin, accessible to most aqueous compartments within the body.
metoprolol	294	minimal binding to plasma proteins (13%), extensive accumulation in tissues is reflected in high Vd value.
propranolol	273	despite a high degree of binding to plasma protein (93%), high affinity for tissues gives rise to a high Vd value.

*Values for apparent volume of distribution (Vd) are with reference to a standard 70-kg individual.

A number of important general conclusions can be drawn based on the type of information contained in Table 2.9.

(a) Weakly acidic substances typically have much smaller Vd values than weak bases. The more extensive distribution of weak bases likely reflects the greater proportion, at physiologic pH, of nonionized (permeant) to ionized (impermeant) forms as compared with weak acids, the latter existing almost completely in the ionized form at pH 7.4 (see page 41).

(b) For chemically-related substances, the magnitude of Vd does not correlate with the extent of binding to plasma proteins.

(c) The fact that molecules with a high affinity for plasma proteins can also show appreciable tissue accumulation underlines both the dynamic nature of the distribution process and the degree of oversimplification in the initial assumption that drug distribution involves a single homogeneous compartment. The use of multicompartmental analysis in pharmacokinetics will be dealt with on page 67.

(d) Although numerical Vd values provide useful quantitative information concerning drug distribution under various pathophysiologic conditions, the fact that they are derived solely from measurements in plasma is a serious drawback that generally precludes their interpretation in specific structural or functional terms. This becomes most apparent for agents whose calculated Vd exceeds by one or more orders of magnitude any real anatomic domain in the body.

(e) Despite the foregoing limitations, Vd values can serve to identify those agents most likely to be involved in drug-drug interactions relating to displacement from plasma proteins, namely, substances with a *low* Vd, and drugs that may require a reduction in dosage under conditions of severe circulatory impairment (e.g., lidocaine (Vd = 77 L) in patients with congestive heart failure), namely, compounds with a *high* Vd, indicating a propensity for accumulation in highly perfused tissues.

Kinetics of Drug Elimination

Mathematical analysis of the decrease in plasma levels of drugs with time after their administration by single bolus injection provides useful information concerning processes involved in their elimination. In the simplest case, the decline is monoexponential, indicating that drug distribution and elimination can be described in terms of a single (central) compartment (Fig. 2.11). Under these conditions, the rate at which

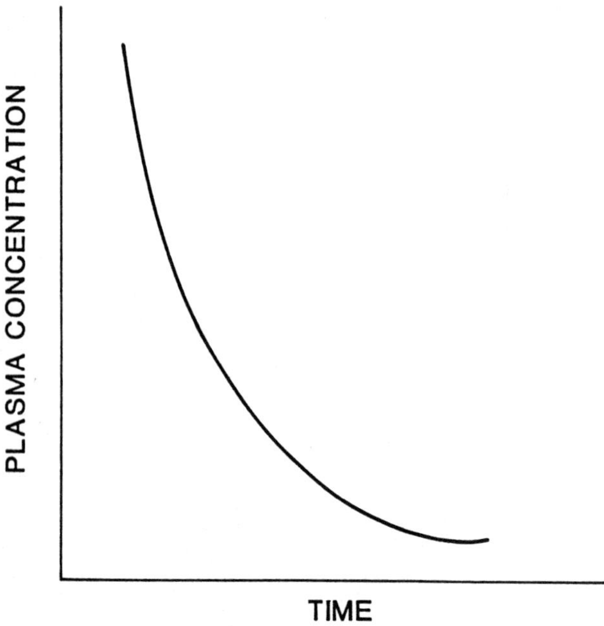

Figure 2.11 Monoexponential decrease in plasma concentrations of a drug after its IV administration.

drug concentration falls (as reflected in the steepness of the curve) progressively decreases in proportion to the amount of drug remaining. This is characteristic of a "first order" exponential decay process, which can be expressed mathematically as follows:

$$\text{Rate of decline in plasma drug concentration (C) with time (t)} = -\frac{dC}{dt} = kC \tag{1}$$

with k being the first order rate constant. The value of k, which has dimensions of reciprocal time (min^{-1}, hr^{-1}, etc.), denotes the constant fraction of remaining drug that is being eliminated per unit time. The differential equation (1) can be solved by separating the variables and integrating, applying the boundary condition that at t½ = O, C = Co, to give:

$$C = Co \, . \, e^{-kt} \tag{2}$$

This useful relationship enables the fraction of drug remaining (C/Co) or eliminated (1-C/Co) to be determined at any time t, given the value of k.

Example. A drug with an elimination rate constant (k) equal to 0.2 hr^{-1} is given as a rapid IV bolus injection. What fraction of the loading dose given will have been eliminated by 4 hours?

Solution. From Equation 2, the fraction of the administered dose remaining at any time t is given by e^{-kt}. Prior to calculation, it is *essential* to ascertain uniformity of the time units in k and t—in this case both are in hours, so that no conversion is required:

$$\text{fraction remaining} = e^{-(0.2/hr)(4\,hr)} = e^{-0.8} = 0.45$$

(*Note*: it is important to include the negative sign when determining the value of $e^{-0.8}$ from natural logarithm tables or using a calculator).

The fraction of drug eliminated is, therefore, 1.00 – 0.45 = 0.55. Thus, 55 percent of the loading dose will have been eliminated by four hours.

On a cautionary note, it should be reiterated that first order elimination is an **exponential** rather than a **linear** process. Thus, in the foregoing problem, it would be invalid to assume, on the basis of a k value = 0.2 hr^{-1} that after four hours 4 × 20%/hr = 80% of the drug would be eliminated.

In a related application, equation (2) can also be used to estimate the dosing interval that would be required to maintain plasma concentrations of a drug within a given range.

Example. A drug is to be administered as a loading dose followed by repeated maintenance doses such that plasma concentrations do not decrease by more than 20%. If the elimination rate constant of the drug is 0.150 hr^{-1}, what would be the maximal allowable dosing interval?

Solution. If plasma levels cannot decrease by more than 20 percent, the maximal dosing interval will be the time at which fractional residual drug concentration has decreased to 0.80. Thus, from Equation (2):

$$0.8 = e^{-k.t} = e^{-(0.150/hr)(t)}$$

taking natural logarithms and rearranging:

$$t = \frac{\ln 0.9}{-(0.150/hr)} = \frac{-0.223}{-0.150}\,hr = 1.5\,hr$$

The drug could, therefore, be given every 1.5 hr, and the relevant maintenance dose under these conditions would be 20 percent of the initial loading dose.

Rate constants characterizing first order drug elimination processes can be determined from semilogarithmic plots of plasma concentration versus time as follows. Equation (2) expressed in natural logarithmic form can be written:

$$\ln C = -k.t + \ln Co \tag{3}$$

This predicts that ln C will be a linear function of t, with a y intercept equal to ln Co (which can be used in the estimation of Vd) and a negative slope that provides a direct measure of the elimination rate constant k as shown in Figure 2.12 (upper tracing) for a drug given by the intravenous route. The lower curve illustrates the general pattern expected for the same drug when an absorption phase is present (as would be the case for oral, subcutaneous, or intramuscular routes of administration). Two salient features of this biphasic curve should be noted. First, absorption, like elimination, is typically a first order exponential process, so that plasma levels of drug (when plotted on a logarithmic scale) show a linear increase with time. Thus, the rate of absorption progressively decreases

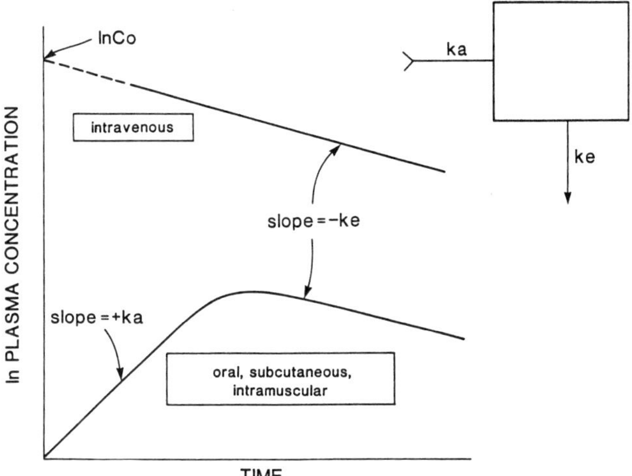

Figure 2.12 Time-dependent alterations in plasma concentrations of a drug (IV, oral, SQ, and IM administration) following single-compartment kinetics (for further details, see text).

as the concentration of drug at the site of uptake into the circulation falls. Secondly, the slope of the linear portion of the curve describing drug elimination is identical to that seen when the drug is injected IV, both being a measure of the elimination rate constant characteristic of the particular drug in question. Figure 2.12 also shows the conventional scheme used to depict the pharmacokinetic behavior of a drug distributed in a single homogeneous compartment, with k_a and k_e being rate constants for absorption and elimination phases, respectively.

For many drugs, the decrease in plasma levels with time after their intravenous administration cannot be accurately described by a monoexponential function.[8] A typical pattern is that illustrated in Figure 2.13, in which the elimination phase is preceded by a distributive component involving uptake of drug by peripheral tissues. In the simplest case, the pharmacokinetic data conform to a two-compartment open model. Drugs enter and are eliminated from a central compartment (1 in Fig. 2.13) that usually consists of blood and/or the extracellular fluid space of highly perfused organs (e.g., heart, kidneys and lungs). The peripheral compartment (2 in Fig. 2.13) can be comprised of muscle, skin, or body fat, all of these acting as potential reservoirs that drugs can enter or leave according to the law of mass action. Again, processes of absorption, distribution, and elimination are all assumed to exhibit first order kinetics, with rate constants of k_a, k_{12} or k_{21}, and k_a, respectively, as shown in Figure 2.13. The apparent distribution volume of the central compartment (V_1) is less than that of the peripheral compartment (V_2), the relative magnitude of each value being determined by blood flow and the physicochemical properties of the molecule in question. The concentrations of drug in the central (C_1) and peripheral (C_2) compartments will exhibit complex time– and dose–dependent variations that can be described by the following differential equations:

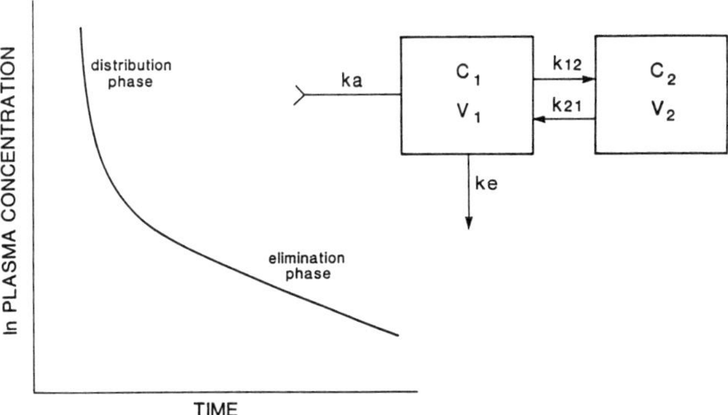

Figure 2.13 Time-dependent alterations in plasma concentration of a drug following two-compartment kinetics (for further details, see text).

$$\frac{dC_1}{dt} = -(k_{12} + k_e).C_1 + k_{21}.C_2 \quad (4)$$

$$\frac{dC_2}{dt} = -k_{21}.C_2 + k_{12}.C_1 \quad (5)$$

These equations can be solved using Laplace transforms with the boundary condition that initially C_1 = dose/V_1 and C_2 = O.

The variation in experimentally determined concentrations of drug in plasma (C_1) as a function of time can be expressed in the form:

$$C_1 = A.e^{-\alpha t} + B.e^{-\beta t} \quad (6)$$

A plot of ln C_1 *vs.* time will, therefore, give the biphasic pattern shown in Figure 2.13, with α and β being the slopes of the linear segments characterizing the distribution and elimination phases, respectively. Values for A and B can be estimated from the y intercepts of these two lines (i.e., by extrapolation of each to zero time). Standard pharmacokinetic equations (presented in Table 2.10) can then be used to evaluate each of the kinetic parameters that describe the two-compartment open model depicted in Figure 2.13. Table 2.11 shows the application of Equation (6) to describe the pharmacokinetics of chlordiazepoxide in terms of a 2-compartment open model. For several drugs (e.g., diazepam, digoxin, furosemide), a 3-compartment model, which includes two different peripheral com-

Table 2.10 Pharmacokinetic Parameters for a Two-Compartment Open Model System

Calculation of pharmacokinetic parameters using values of A, B, α, and β from the equation $C_1 = A.e^{-\alpha t} + B.e^{-\beta t}$ for a 2 compartment open model system (see Fig. 2.13).

$$k_e = \frac{A + B}{\frac{A}{\alpha} + \frac{B}{\beta}}$$

$$k_{21} = \frac{\alpha - \beta}{k_e} = \frac{A\beta + B\alpha}{A + B}$$

$$k_{12} = \frac{AB}{(A + B)^2} \cdot \frac{(\beta - \alpha)^2}{k_{21}}$$

$$V^1 = \frac{dose}{A + B} \qquad V_2 = V_1 \cdot \frac{k12}{k21}$$

At steady-state (when net transfer of drug from the peripheral to the central compartment equals zero):

$$(Vd)_{SS} = V_1 \left[1 + \frac{k12}{k21}\right]$$

Table 2.11 Calculation of Pharmacokinetic Parameters for Chlordiazepoxide

The use of Equation (6) to describe the pharmacokinetics of chloradiazepoxide in terms of a 2-compartment open model system (from Greenblatt and Koch-Weser, New Engl J Med 1975; *293*:702–705).

$C_1 = A.e^{-\alpha t} + B.e^{-\beta t}$
$= 3.18\ e^{-3.31\,t} + 1.02\ e^{-0.0575\,t}$
$\alpha = 3.31\ hr^{-1}$ $t½ = 0.2\ hr$
$\beta = 0.057\ hr^{-1}$ $t½ = 12\ hr$
$K_e = -225\ hr^{-1}$ $Vd = 23.3\ L$

partments (termed shallow and deep), provides a more accurate description of the observed pharmacokinetic properties. For most practical purposes, however, standard Vd and elimination rate constant (k_e) values (or clearance values that are the product of Vd and k_e) provide sufficient information for establishing optimal drug dosing regimens, as will be described throughout the remainder of this section.

Although pharmacokinetic calculations that involve drug elimination (e.g., estimation of maintenance doses) generally use k values, it is more conventional to describe first-order drug elimination in quantitative terms with reference to its plasma half-life (t½), i.e., the time required for drug concentrations to fall by 50 percent. Intuitively, an inverse relationship between respective k and t½ values is expected (i.e., a very high rate constant of elimination would predict a short plasma half-life and vice versa). This can readily be demonstrated by substituting t = t½ and C = ½Co in Equation (3) and rearranging algebraically to obtain:

$$t½ = \frac{\ln 2}{k} = \frac{0.693}{k} \qquad (7)$$

By way of illustration, if the elimination rate constant (k_e) of a drug is 0.5 day^{-1}, the corresponding t½ is $\frac{0.693}{0.5/day}$ = 1.4 days. Clearly, then, it cannot be concluded from a k_e equal to 0.5 per day that 50 per cent of the drug is eliminated in one day (i.e., that t½ = 1 day). This would only be so if the initial rate of elimination persisted; given that drug elimination is a first-order exponential process, the rate will gradually decrease in proportion to the amount of drug remaining.

As indicated earlier, drug dosing regimens are developed on the basis of pharmacokinetic information contained in Vd and t½ values. The following clinical example involving digoxin demonstrates the general approach used.

Example. Digoxin is to be administered to a 70-kg patient with normal renal function as a loading dose to achieve an initial (maximal) plasma level of 1.5 ng/ml followed by daily maintenance doses. The Vd and t½ of digoxin are 500 L and 1.6 days, respectively. What would be appropriate loading and daily maintenance doses for this patient?

Solution. Loading dose is given by the product of Vd and maximal plasma concentration. Uniformity of volume units can be simply achieved because ng/ml is equivalent to μg/L. Thus:

$$\text{loading} = 500\ L \times 1.5\ \mu g/L = 750\ \mu g\ (0.75\ mg)$$

This is a typical loading dose for digoxin that, given the narrow therapeutic index of this drug, would likely be administered in two or three divided doses.

The fraction of this loading dose remaining after one day is given by

$$e^{-kt} = e^{-(.693/1.6\ days)(1\ day)} = e^{-0.433} = 0.65$$

It therefore follows that the fractional elimination is 1.00 − 0.65 = 0.35, so that the daily maintenance dose of digoxin will be 0.35 × 0.75 mg = 0.25 mg.

In the foregoing example, the stated fact that the patient had normal renal function is significant, because it allowed the use of the "standard" value for t½ in the calculation. The rate of digoxin elimination is likely to be decreased in the presence of renal functional impairment. The pharmacokinetic consequences of a prolongation in digoxin t½ are explored in the following example.

Example. How should the dosing regimen for digoxin described in the previous example be modified in a patient with a reduction in kidney function sufficient to cause a twofold increase in the elimination half-life of digoxin (i.e., t½ is increased from 1.6 to 3.2 days)?

Solution. Loading dose. In the absence of any information indicating a change in Vd, the magnitude of the loading dose would remain the same. (*Note:* There is a common misconception that initial loading doses of drugs usually should be reduced if their elimination is impaired. This is not generally the case, unless there is an associated change in Vd).

Maintenance dose. Because drug-elimination is impaired, one would expect a reduction in maintenance dose under these conditions, which in fact is the case. The fraction of digoxin eliminated per day is now given by

$$1 - e^{-(.693/3.2\ days)(1\ day)} = 1 - e^{-0.216} = 0.20$$

Therefore, a doubling of the elimination t½ reduces the magnitude of the maintenance dose by approximately one-half.

Multiple Dose Drug Administration

Drugs used for chronic therapy are, as a general rule, administered at dosing intervals approximately equal to the elimination half-life of the agent in question. As a result, drug accumulates in the body and levels gradually increase until a steady state is reached such that the amount of drug eliminated in the dosing interval becomes equal to the dose administered.[9] The time required to achieve this steady state is strictly determined by the half-life of the drug and is approximately equal to five times the t½ value (this is frequently referred to as the **plateau rule**). These important general principles become readily apparent by considering the following situation.

A drug is to be given once every t½ at a constant dose D that produces an incremental increase in plasma drug concentration of 1.0 unit. For simplicity, we will assume the absorption of the drug is instantaneous. The expected variation in plasma levels is depicted in Figure 2.14. Initially, plasma concentration increases to 1.0, but declines to 0.5 after one half-life has elapsed. At this point, another dose D is administered, producing a total plasma concentration of 1.5, which will have decreased by half (to 0.75) by the next half-life. As this process is continued, it is apparent that peak plasma concentrations of drug gradually increase toward a maximal value of 2.0. The approach to this plateau is such that approximately 88, 94 and 97 per cent of this maximum has been attained by 3, 4 and 5 half-lives, respectively. Furthermore, as a steady state is approached, the amount of drug lost in each dosing interval progressively increases such that at steady state an exact balance between the amount of drug given and the amount eliminated has been established. This dose D of drug, if administered continually at the same dosing interval (equal to the t½ in this example), will maintain the steady state, and can therefore be referred to as the "maintenance dose." Alternatively, peak steady state plasma concentrations of drug could have been achieved immediately by giving a loading dose (equal to 2D in this case), followed by regular

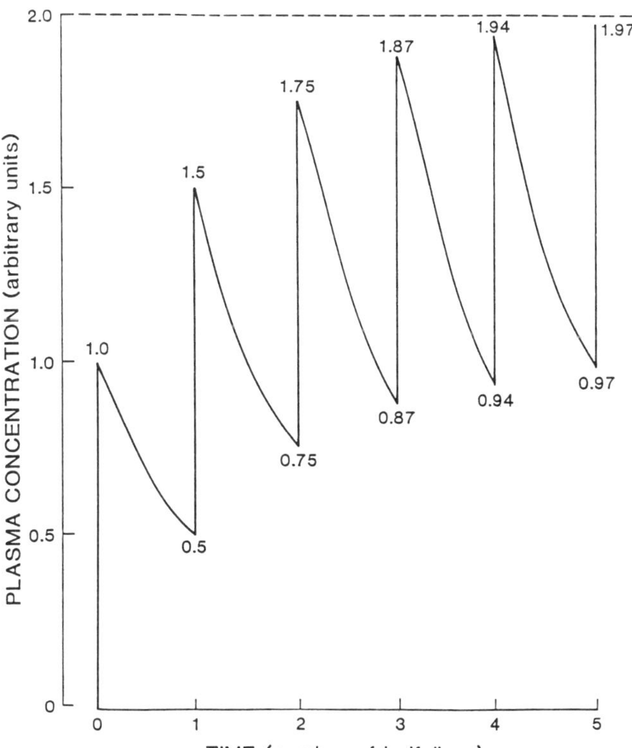

Figure 2.14 Drug accumulation following administration at intervals equal to the elimination half-life, showing the maximal and minimal drug concentration in plasma (arbitrary units).

maintenance doses of D every half-life. It must be emphasized, however, that the **same** steady state would be reached **in either case.**

A number of general pharmacokinetic principles important in chronic drug dosing regimens emerge from the foregoing example.

(a) When drugs are administered at regular dosing intervals approximately equal to their elimination half-lives, a steady state is reached wherein the amount of drug eliminated becomes equal to the amount administered; this being referred to as the "maintenance dose."

(b) The time required to achieve the steady state is determined by the elimination half-life of the drug, with greater than 90 per cent of peak plasma levels being attained after four half-lives.

Corollary. If the elimination half-life of a drug is increased in a particular clinical situation, the time required for peak plasma concentrations (and possibly dose-related drug toxicity) to develop will be correspondingly delayed.

(c) Whether a drug is given as a loading dose followed subsequently by regular maintenance doses or as repeated maintenance doses (without an initial loading dose), the *same* steady state is attained in either case.

Corollary. The choice between these alternative therapeutic approaches is influenced by a number of factors, including the half-life of the drug (loading doses are often used for drugs with very long half-lives), the margin of safety of the particular drug, and, most importantly, the urgency of the clinical situation.

(d) In any steady state resulting from repeated drug administration, plasma concentrations of drug exhibit time-dependent variations between predictable maximum and minimum values, with the extent of such fluctuations being inversely proportional to the duration of the dosing interval (e.g., a reduction in the dosing interval will lessen the degree of variation in plasma levels of drug).

Corollary. Optimization of drug dosing regimens consists of establishing conditions such that, at steady state, the peak plasma concentration of drug is below that likely to produce toxicity while the minimum plasma concentration of drug is above that required to produce the desired therapeutic effect.

Administration of Drugs by IV Infusion and the Concept of Drug Clearance

IV Infusion

Any chronic therapeutic regimen must ultimately entail some compromise between the avoidance of large fluctuations in plasma concentrations of drug and convenience of drug administration, with specific reference to the frequency of daily dosing. For practical purposes, the dosing interval, which is determined by the plasma half-life of the drug, usually should not be less than 5–6 hours. It may, therefore, be necessary to administer drugs with short plasma half-lives by continuous IV infusion. Among the more common examples of clinically useful drugs used in this manner are: lidocaine, sodium nitroprusside, and heparin.

When a drug is to be given as a constant IV infusion to achieve and maintain a particular steady state concentration in plasma (C_{ss}), it is administered at a rate equal to that which will characterize drug elimination at steady state. At any time, rate of drug elimination is given by the product of the elimination rate constant (k) and the amount of drug present (A). At steady state (ss), the rate of drug elimination is given by $k.A_{ss}$, which can also be written $k.Vd.C_{ss}$ (where Vd is the apparent distribution volume). Thus, the IV infusion rate required to produce a steady state drug concentration in plasma equal to C_{ss} can be estimated from the following relationship:

$$\text{infusion rate} = k.Vd.C_{ss} \qquad (8)$$

The time required for plasma concentration of a drug to approximate the steady state value (C_{ss}) is determined by its elimination half-life as predicted by the "plateau rule" (see page 69). This is illustrated graphically in Figure 2.15.

Example. An antibiotic is to be administered as an IV infusion to attain and maintain a plasma concentration of 4 μg/ml. Calculate the infusion rate required, given that this antibiotic has a Vd value of 125 L and an elimination half-life equal to 5 hr.

Solution. Using Equation (8), the infusion rate is given by:

$$\frac{0.693}{5\text{ hrs}} \times 125\text{ L} \times 4\text{ mg/L} = 69.3\text{ mg/hr (or 1.16 mg/min)}$$

Based on Figure 2.15, it can be estimated that after 5 hr (1 × t½) the concentration of antibiotic in the plasma will be 2 μg/ml (i.e., 50 per cent of maximum) and after 25 hr (5 × t½) a value of 3.88 μg/ml (i.e., 97 per cent of maximum) is expected.

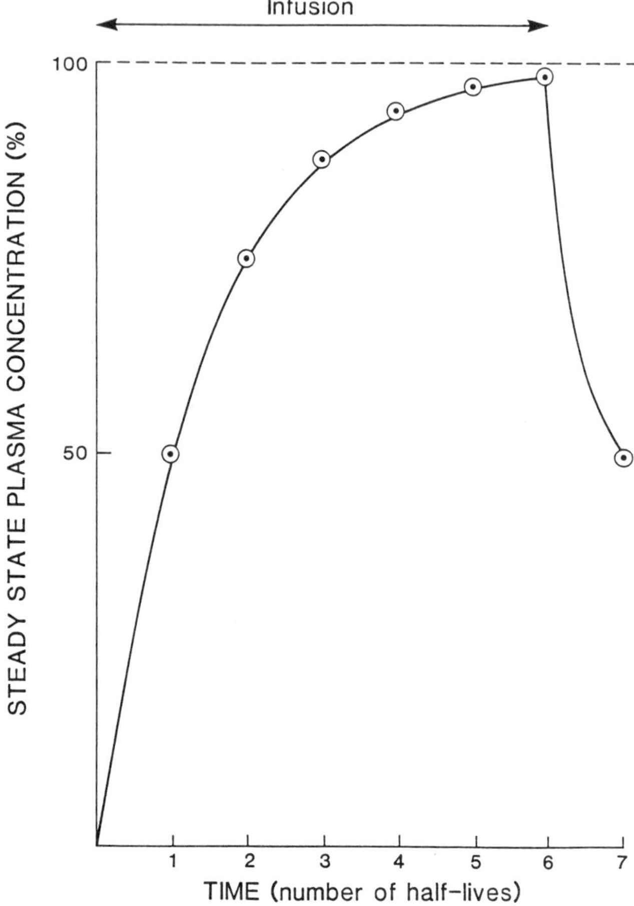

Figure 2.15 Increasing plasma concentrations of a drug during the course of IV infusion, according to multiples of the drug's half-life.

Drug Clearance

The **clearance (Cl)** of a drug can be defined in pharmacokinetic terms as the product of its elimination rate constant (k) and apparent volume of distribution (Vd):

$$Cl = k.Vd \qquad (9)$$

Clearance, therefore, has dimensions of volume/time and represents the **volume of plasma cleared of the drug per unit time.** Equations (8) and (9) may be combined to yield the following:

$$Cl = \text{infusion rate}/C_{ss} \qquad (10)$$

Clearance values can, therefore, be determined by studying the relationship between rates of IV infusion and resulting steady state plasma concentrations. Given that infusion rate is equal to the rate of excretion at steady state as stated above, Equation (10) can also be expressed as follows:

$$Cl = \frac{\text{amount excreted/time}}{C_{ss}} \qquad (11)$$

This forms the basis of the more conventional approach to estimating clearance, which for any substance is given by the ratio of the amount excreted in a fixed time interval (e.g., 24 hr) divided by its concentration in plasma.

The clearance concept has practical applications in the area of clinical pharmacokinetics. Clearance values can provide valuable insights into mechanisms involved in the elimination of exogenous or endogenous compounds. Thus, substances freely filtered at the glomerulus and minimally reabsorbed (e.g., creatinine, inulin) have clearance values that provide a measure of glomerular filtration rate (normally 120–130 ml/min). Alterations in creatinine clearance accompanying renal functional impairment provide a convenient means of assessing the severity of the underlying disease process and of monitoring its progress (see page 63). Substances eliminated by active renal tubular secretion with negligible postsecretory reabsorption (e.g., p-aminohippuric acid) show clearances that approximate renal plasma flow (600–650 ml/min). Many agents known to undergo probenecid-sensitive active tubular secretion (e.g., various penicillin derivatives, thiazide diuretics) typically have clearance values in the range of 300–400 ml/min, indicative of appreciable postsecretory passive reabsorption. Finally, drugs showing extensive "first pass" hepatic metabolism are characterized by high clearance values (usually in the range of 800–1200ml/min) that approach total hepatic plasma flow (1500 ml/min).

The clearance of drugs is usually expressed in terms of an over-all or total body clearance (Cl_T) value. This represents the summation of all processes involved in drug elimination, the two major components usually being renal (Cl_R) and hepatic (Cl_H) clearance. Thus, in general, one can write:

$$Cl_T = C_R + Cl_H \tag{12}$$

The relative contribution of each elimination process depends on the pharmacologic agent involved, with one or the other component frequently being dominant. However, minor pathways of drug disposition may assume greater importance under pathophysiologic conditions associated with impaired functioning of the primary pathway. For this reason, the extent to which the over-all clearance of a given drug subject to excretion by the kidney is decreased in a patient with renal disease need not be directly proportional to (or predictable from) the reduction in creatinine clearance. As indicated in a previous section (page 63), dosage adjustments in the presence of renal failure are most conveniently made using a nomogram that describes, in quantitative terms, the relationship between creatinine clearance and over-all elimination characteristics for the particular pharmacologic agent being used.

Alterations in Cl_T arising from the hepatic component (Cl_H) are usually referable to changes either in intrinsic metabolic capacity (which may be increased by enzyme inducers or reduced in certain forms of liver disease) or in hepatic blood flow. The extent to which either is likely to be involved can, to some degree, be predicted from the categorization of drugs as readily extracted or poorly extracted. The clearance of the former is likely to be markedly affected by changes in blood flow to the liver, while the disposition of agents in the latter group is more dependent on the intrinsic metabolic capacity of the liver (see page 60).

Estimation of Average Plasma Drug Concentrations Associated with Chronic Oral Dosing Regimens

As indicated in the section above, the repeated administration of a drug at a dosing interval comparable to its plasma half-life eventually produces a steady state in which plasma concentrations of drug vary in a regular, time-dependent manner between maximum and minimum values determined by the dose administered, the dosing interval, and the clearance value for the drug. A simple transformation of Equation (10) provides a useful formula for estimating average plasma concentrations of drug in any given chronic oral dosing regimen. From Equation (10) we have that:

$$C_{ss} = \frac{\text{infusion rate}}{Cl} = \frac{\text{dose}}{\text{time}} \cdot \frac{1}{Cl} \tag{13}$$

The corresponding relationship for the average plasma concentration (C_{av}) of a drug given at an "effective" dose of F.D (where F = fractional oral absorption and D is the administered dose) and a dosing interval of t is:

$$C_{av} = \frac{F.D}{\Delta t} \cdot \frac{1}{Cl} = \frac{F.D}{\Delta t.k.\ Vd} \tag{14}$$

Example. Metoprolol is being used orally to treat a 65-kg hypertensive patient who has been taking two 50-mg tablets per day, one at 8:00 AM and another at 8:00 PM. The optimal plasma level of metoprolol in the treatment of hypertension is reported to be 25 ng/ml.

Determine whether the average steady state plasma concentration of metoprolol expected from the foregoing regimen is in the optimal therapeutic range, given the following pharmacokinetic information for metoprolol: oral absorption 38 per cent, Vd 4.2 L/kg, and plasma half-life 3.2 hr.

Solution. From Equation (14) we have that:

$$C_{av} = \frac{0.38 \times 50 \text{ mg}}{12 \text{ hr} \times \frac{9.693}{3.2 \text{ hr}} \times \frac{4.2\text{L}}{\text{kg}} \times 65 \text{ kg}} = 0.027\text{mg/L} = 27 \text{ ng/ml}$$

Clearly, then, this oral dosing regimen does produce average plasma levels that are in the optimal therapeutic range. However, the fact that the dosing interval chosen is approximately four times greater than the half-life of the drug predicts that plasma concentrations of metoprolol will show large fluctuations about the average steady state value. Application of Equation (2) predicts that plasma concentrations of drug will decrease by more than 90 per cent during the 12-hr dosing interval. These fluctuations could be considerably reduced while still maintaining the same average plasma concentration by giving smaller doses of metoprolol more frequently.

Dose-Dependent (or Nonlinear) Pharmacokinetics

At therapeutic doses of most pharmacologic agents, rates of metabolism and elimination vary in direct proportion to the concentration of drug present at the relevant site(s) of biotransformation or elimination; that is, these processes exhibit first-order kinetics. Under these conditions, plasma half-life and clearance values are independent of drug dose. The potential saturability of enzymatic or carrier-mediated processes involved in drug disposition does, however, allow for the possibility of a transition to zero-order kinetics at sufficiently high doses (or plasma concentrations) of drug (Fig. 2.16). The occurrence of this phenomenon with a limited number of commonly used substances (including acetysalicylic acid, phenytoin, and ethanol) has important pharmacologic consequences.[10] Such compounds exhibit pharmacokinetic properties that are dose-related, and minor adjustments in dosage can lead to exaggerated pharmacologic responses and potentially serious toxicities[11–14].

With the transition from first order to zero order (saturation) kinetics, the relationship between administered dose and resulting plasma levels of drug deviates progressively from linearity and elimination half-life

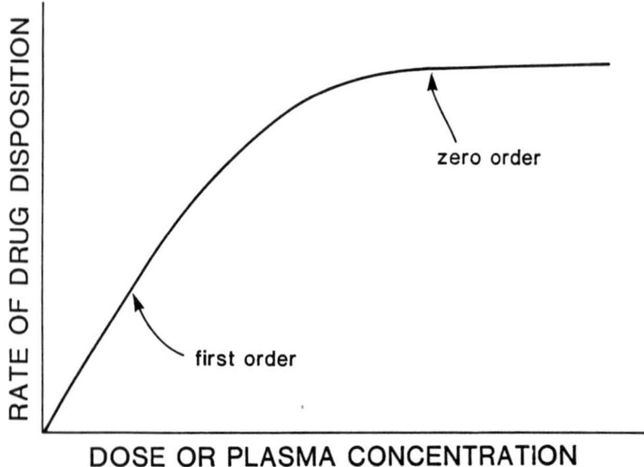

Figure 2.16 First-order and zero-order phases of drug disposition, according to the dose or plasma concentration.

becomes dose-dependent (Fig. 2.17). By way of illustration, consider the following example.

Example. A drug exhibits first order kinetics at doses between 5 and 40 mg, but zero-order (saturation) kinetics at doses in excess of 50 mg. The drug has a volume of distribution equal to 5 L, a first-order elimination half-life of 2 hr, and a maximal rate of elimination (at saturation) of 100 mg/hr.

(a) How long would it take for plasma concentrations to fall from 6 mg/L to 3 mg/L?

(b) How long would it take for plasma concentrations to fall from 200 mg/L to 100 mg/L?

Solution

(a) A plasma concentration of 6 mg/L would correspond to a dose of 6 mg/L × 5 L = 30 mg. Since this is still in the range where first-order kinetics apply, the elimination half-life value of 2 hr is applicable.

(b) At plasma concentrations of 200 and 100 mg/L, the total amounts of drug present (as estimated from the Vd value) are 1000 and 500 mg, respectively, both of which are well beyond the range where first-order kinetics apply.

Given that the zero-order rate of metabolism is 100 mg/hr, a 50 per cent reduction in plasma levels will now occur in five hours.

Let us now consider in some detail the implications of zero-order kinetics in the pharmacologic properties of acetylsalicylic acid, phenytoin, and ethanol. As discussed in an earlier section (page 55), the crucial step in salicylate disposition involves its conjugation with glycine to form salicyluric acid. The enzyme system involved undergoes saturation at doses of acetylsalicylic acid somewhat in excess of 600 mg. This accounts for the high incidence of salicylism in patients with rheumatoid arthritis being treated with acetylsalicylic acid at daily doses typically in the range of 4 to 6 grams.

Phenytoin has clinically useful anticonvulsant properties. However, optimization of drug treatment in epileptic patients is complicated by the unpredictability of the therapeutic effect and dose-related toxicities such as nystagmus and ataxia. Such variability in response is a characteristic feature of drugs showing elimination half-lives which vary with the dose administered. In the case of phenytoin, the transition from first-order to zero-order kinetics occurs at plasma concentrations between 10 and 20 μg/ml, which encompass the optimal therapeutic range for this drug. The saturable process in question is the Phase I Mixed Function Oxidase-mediated hydroxylation step in the hepatic metabolism of phenytoin (see Fig. 2.5).

As a final illustrative example, the rate of ethanol metabolism *in vivo* approaches a constant (maximal) value of 10 ml absolute ethanol/hr for virtually all plasma concentrations capable of exerting effects on the CNS. The biochemical basis of the predominantly zero-order disposition of ethanol relates to the kinetic properties of alcohol dehydrogenase. This enzyme, which catalyzes a rate-limiting step in ethanol metabolism, shows a half maximal rate *in vitro* at a substrate concentration of approximately 1 mM. By comparison, at an inebriating blood alcohol reading of 100 mg % (corresponding to an ethanol concentration of 20 mM) the enzyme would be essentially fully saturated. The progressive accumulation of unmetabolized ethanol resulting from its injudicious consumption produces the all too familiar deleterious effects characteristic of this most common substance of abuse. In addition to the foregoing examples of well characterized enzyme systems exhibiting zero-order kinetics, there is also evidence that suggests the possible involvement of readily saturable processes

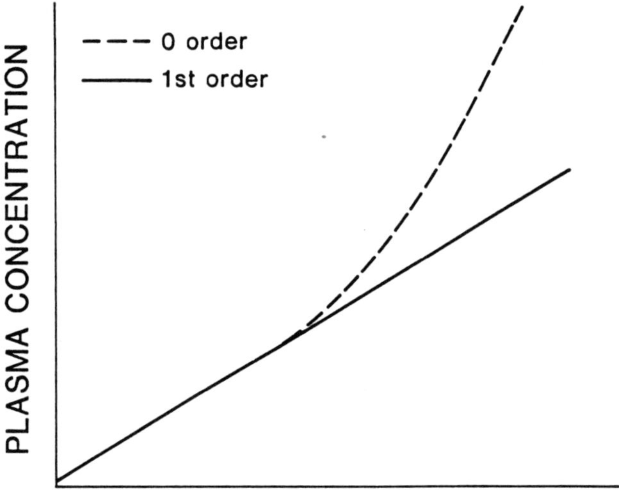

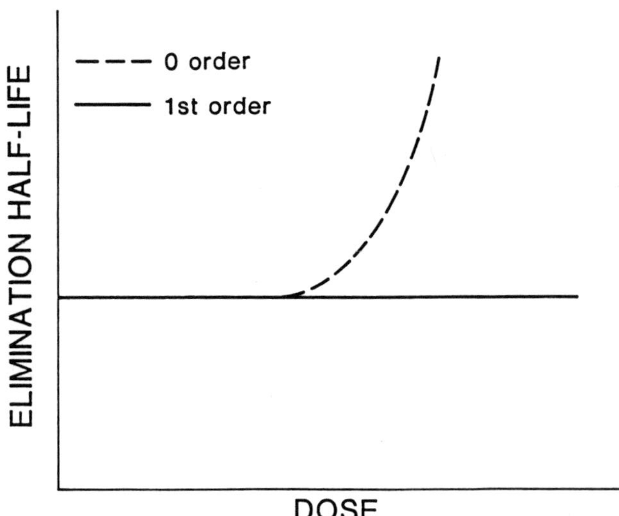

Figure 2.17 Variation in plasma concentration and elimination half-life as a function of drug dose, under zero-order or first-order kinetic conditions.

in the disposition of several other pharmacologic agents, including clonidine, dysopyramide, heparin, theophylline, and prednisolone. Dose-related alterations in pharmacokinetic properties should, therefore, be included with age, disease, and heredity as an important potential source of variability in clinical responses to drugs.

References

Research Reports

1. Saffran M, Kumar GS, Saviar C, Burnham JC, Williams F. A new approach to the oral administration of insulin and other peptide drugs. Science 1986;*233*:1081–1084.
2. Walker PC. Neonatal bilirubin toxicity. Clin Pharmacol 1987;*13*:26–50.
3. Gerson WT, Fine DG, Spielberg SP, Sensenbrenner LL. Anticonvulsant-induced aplastic anemia: increased susceptibility to toxic drug metabolites in vitro. Blood 1983;*61*:889–893.
4. Prochaska HJ, Santamaria AB, Talalay P. Rapid detection of inducers of enzymes that protect against carcinogens. Proc Natl Acad Sci USA 1992;*89*:2394–2398.
5. Zhang Y, Talalay P, Cho C-G, Posner GH. A major inducer of anticarcinogenic protective enzymes from broccoli: Isolation and elucidation of structure. Proc Natl Acad Sci USA 1992;*89*:2399–2403.
6. Rose JQ, Choi HK, Schentag JJ, Kinkel WR, Jusko WJ. Intoxication caused by interaction of chloramphenicol and phenytoin. J Am Med Assoc 1977;*237*:2630–2631.
7. Abernathy DR, Greenblatt DJ, Ameer B, Shader Rl. Probenecid impairment of acetaminophen and lorazepam clearance: direct inhibition of ether glucuronide formation. J Pharmacol Exp Ther 1985;*234*:345–349.
8. Gillespie WR. Noncompartmental versus compartmental modelling in clinical pharmacokinetics. Clin Pharmacokin 1991;*20*:253–262.
9. Bjornsson TD. The method of relative drug accumulation: A simple method for illustrating the effects of different drug dosing regimens and variability in drug elimination on time courses of drug concentrations. Clin Pharmacol Therap 1992;*51*:266–270.
10. Luden TM. Nonlinear pharmacokinetics: clinical implications. Clin Pharmacol 1991;*20*:447–462.
11. Levy G, Tsuchiya T. Salicylate accumulation kinetics in man. New Engl J Med 1972;*287*:430–432.
12. Lambie DG, Nanda RN, Johnson RH, Shakir RA. Therapeutic and pharmacokinetic effects of increasing phenytoin in chronic epileptics on multiple drug therapy. Lancet 1976;*2*:386–389.
13. Stanski DR, Mihm FG, Rosenthal MH, Kalman SM. Pharmacokinetics of high-dose thiopental used in cerebral resuscitation. Anesthesiology 1980;*53*:169–171.
14. Butts JD, Secrest B, Berger R. Nonlinear theophylline pharmacokinetics. Arch Int Med 1991;*151*:2073–2077.

Reviews

- r1. Aronson JK, Hardman M. Measuring plasma drug concentrations. Br Med J 1992;*305*:1078–1080.
- r2. Kwong TC. Free drug measurements: methodology and clinical significance. Clin Chim Acta 1985;151:193–216.
- r3. Lee EJD, Williams KM. Chirality: clinical pharmacokinetic and pharmacodynamic considerations. Clin Pharmacokin 1990;*18*:339–345.
- r4. Walle T, Walle UK. Pharmacokinetic parameters obtained with racemates. Trends Pharmacol Sci 1986;*7*:155–158.
- r5. Butterworth JF, Strichartz GR. Molecular mechanisms of local anesthesia: a review. Anesthesiology 1990;*72*:711–734.
- r6. Concepcion M, Covino BG. Rational use of local anesthetics. Drugs 1984;*27*:256–270.
- r7. Bradbury MWB The blood-brain barrier (transport across the cerebral endothelium). Circ Res 1985;*57*:213–222.
- r8. Neuwelt EA, Frenkel EP. Is there a therapeutic role for blood-brain barrier disruption? Ann Int Med 1980;*93*:137–139.
- r9. Joo F. New aspects to the function of the cerebral endothelium. Nature 1986;*321*:197–198.
- r10. Pacifici GM, Viani A. Methods of determining plasma and tissue binding of drugs. Pharmacokinetic consequences. Clin Pharmacokinet 1992;*23*:449–468.
- r11. McElnay JC, D'Arcy PF. Protein binding displacement interactions and their clinical importance. Drugs 1983;*25*:495–513.
- r12. Thompson D, Milford-Ward A, Whicher JT. The value of acute phase protein measurements in clinical practice. Ann Clin Biochem 1992;*29*:123–131.
- r13. Kremer JMH, Wilting J, Janssen LMH. Drug binding to human alpha-1-acid glycoprotein in health and disease. Pharmacol Rev 1988;*40*:1–47.
- r14. Bonate PL. Pathophysiology and pharmacokinetics following burn injury. Clin Pharmacokin 1990;*18*:118–130.
- r15. Levine M, Chang T. Therapeutic monitoring of phenytoin. Rationale and current status. Clin Pharmacokin 1990;*19*:341–358.
- r16. Atkinson HC, Begg EJ. Prediction of drug distribution into human milk from physicochemical characteristics. Clin Pharmacokin 1990;*18*:151–167.
- r17. Doherty JE. The digoxin-quinidine interaction. Ann Rev Med 1982;*33*:163–170.
- r18. Gonzalez FJ. Human cytochromes P450: problems and prospects. Trends Pharmacol Sci 1992;*13*:346–352.
- r19. Coon MJ, Ding X, Pernecky SJ, Vaz ADN. Cytochrome P450: progress and predictions. FASEB J 1992;*6*:669–673.
- r20. Guengerich FP. Characterization of human cytochrome P450 enzymes. FASEB J 1992;*6*:745–748.
- r21. Kromer HK, Klotz U. Glucuronidation of drugs. A re-evaluation of the pharmacological significance of the conjugates and modulating factors. Clin Pharmacokin 1992;*23*:292–310.
- r22. Gillette JR, Mitchell JR, Brodie BB. Biochemical mechanisms of drug toxicity. Ann Rev Pharmacol 1974;*14*:271–288.
- r23. Prescott LF, Critchley JAJH. The treatment of acetaminophen poisoning. Ann Rev Pharmacol Toxicol 1983;*23*:87–101.
- r24. Gelehrter TD. Enzyme induction. New Engl J Med 1976;*294*:522–526; 589–595; 646–651.
- r25. Waxman DJ, Azaroff L. Phenobarbital induction of cytochrome P-450 gene expression. Biochem J 1992;*281*:577–592.
- r26. Okey AB. Enzyme induction in the cytochrome P-450 system. Pharmac Ther 1990;*45*:241–298.
- r27. Wood AJJ, Zhou HH. Ethnic differences in drug disposition and responsiveness. Clin Pharmacokin 1991;*20*:350–373.
- r28. Clark DWJ. Genetically determined variability in acetylation and oxidation. Drugs 1985;*29*:342–375.

r29. Guttendorf RJ, Wedlund PJ. Genetic aspects of drug disposition and therapeutics. J Clin Pharmacol 1992;*32*:107–117.

r30. Murray M. P450 enzymes. Inhibition mechanisms, genetic regulation and effects of liver disease. Clin Pharmacokinet 1992;*23*:132–146.

r31. Gelboin HV. Carcinogens, drugs and cytochromes P450. New Engl J Med 1983;*309*:105–107.

r32. Durnos C, Lai C-M, Cusack BJ. Hepatic drug metabolism and aging. Clin Pharmacokin 1990;*19*:359–389.

r33. Birnbaum LS. Pharmacokinetic basis of age-related changes in sensitivity to toxicants. Ann Rev Pharmacol 1991;*31*:101–128.

r34. Tumer N, Scarpace PJ, Lowenthal DT. Geriatric pharmacology: Basic and clinical considerations. Ann Rev Pharmacol Toxicol 1992;*32*:271–302.

r35. McLean AJ, Morgan DJ. Clinical pharmacokinetics in patients with liver disease. Clin Pharmacokinet 1991;*21*:42–69.

r36. Somogyi A. New insights into the renal excretion of drugs. Trends Pharmacol Sci 1987;*8*:354–357.

r37. Neilson P, Rasmussen B. Relationship between molecular structure and excretion of drugs. Life Sci 1975;*17*:1495–1512.

r38. St. Peter WL, Redic-Kill KA, Halstenson CE. Clinical pharmacokinetics of antibiotics in patients with impaired renal function. Clin Pharmacokinet 1992;*22*:169–210.

General

Incardi JF, Willits NH. Setting confidence intervals for drug concentrations from pharmacokinetic parameters. Ann Pharmacother 1992;*26*:1070–1074.

Scheuplein RJ, Shoaf SE, Brown RN. Role of pharmacokinetics in safety evaluation and regulatory considerations. Ann Rev Pharmacol Toxicol 1990;*30*:197–218.

Banerjee PS, Robinson JR. Novel drug delivery systems: an overview of their impact on clinical pharmacokinetic studies. Clin Pharmacokin 1991;*20*:1–14.

Goldman P. Rate-controlled drug delivery. New Engl J Med 1982;*307*:286–290.

Greenblatt DJ, Koch-Weser J. Clinical Pharmacokinetics. New Engl J Med 1975;*293*:702–705;964–970.

Atkinson Jr. AJ, Kushner W. Clinical Pharmacokinetics. Ann Rev Pharmacol Toxicol 1979;*19*:105–127.

Norman J. One compartment kinetics. Br J Anaesthesia 1992;*69*:387–396.

Williams RL, Benet RL. Drug pharmacokinetics in cardiac and hepatic disease. New Engl J Med 1980;*20*:389–413.

Williams RL. Drug administration in hepatic disease. New Engl J Med 1983;*309*:1616–1622.

Reidenberg MM, Drayer DE. Drug therapy in renal failure. Ann Rev Pharmacol Toxicol 1980;*20*:45–54.

Brosen K. Recent developments in hepatic drug oxidation. Implications for clinical pharmacokinetics. Clin Pharmacokinet 1990;*18*:220–239.

CHAPTER 3

Drug Development, the Evaluation of New Drugs, and Principles of Therapeutics

Keith L. MacCannell
Henry J. Duff

Introduction

Consider the four words: drug, medicine, chemical, toxin. All words have dramatically different semantic connotations for the public; yet the general pharmacologist would recognize only those differences that are quantitative or relate to social usage. A **drug** is a chemical; it may or may not be used for medicinal purposes; when given in doses that are excessive for a given individual, it may become a toxic compound. Substances taken for their nutrient value are foods rather than drugs; yet vitamins, when taken to treat vitamin deficiencies or in large quantities become drugs, and may even be toxins (e.g., vitamins A and D). Moreover, some drugs, such as ethyl alcohol, clearly also have nutrient value. In addition to these interests of the general pharmacologist, the clinical pharmacologist and physician must be concerned with the therapeutic value of drugs in a clinical setting.

The goal of *clinical pharmacology* is to apply an understanding about drug mechanisms and toxicology gained from basic pharmacologic principles, such as those presented in Chapters 1 (pharmacodynamics) and 2 (pharmacokinetics), to the patient in a way that yields therapeutic benefit(s) without introducing toxicity. In the context of some interventions, such as the treatment of a bacterial infection with antibiotics, the principle of selective toxicity can be applied, capitalizing on the differences in cellular structure and/or function between the microbe and the human cell. Unfortunately, selective toxicity is never complete, and even relatively nontoxic antimicrobials, antihelminthics, etc., usually exact some toll on the human cell. It is the objective of this chapter to summarize briefly some of the principles used to discover new therapeutic drugs, to evaluate the efficacy and toxicity of such agents, and, where necessary, to regulate their use by law. For more extensive discussions of these topics, the reader is encouraged to consult texts dealing exclusively with clinical pharmacology.[r1–4]

Discovering New Drugs

Many drugs still in use today have been derived from herbal remedies or poisons (e.g., arrow poison) employed since antiquity by practitioners of "Folk Medicine." The precise chemical structures are now known of a large number of the active ingredients in such preparations found to be useful therapeutically (e.g., cinchona alkaloids, curare, ephedrine, reserpine, cardiac glycosides). In principle, the discovery of these drugs depended on: (i) knowledge of the clear-cut efficacy of a given herbal preparation for a specific indication; and (ii) a useful and reliable screening assay capable of identifying the "active principle" in such preparations, during the course of its chemical isolation and characterization. Many herbal preparations are still widely used today, both in North America and in the Far East. These mixtures of natural products potentially represent a major resource for the discovery of new drugs. However, for many herbal remedies, there may not be sufficient documentation of a clear-cut therapeutic benefit; and for some putative therapeutic effects (e.g., promoting longevity), a quantitative estimate of drug efficacy may prove problematic. Considering the number of alkaloids and other chemicals present in herbal preparations, and considering the difficulties of designing a suitable bioassay for the active principles, it is perhaps not surprising that the discovery and characterization of the active ingredient(s) present in these herbal remedies has proved to be a relatively low-yield process. Nonetheless, well-recognized herbal preparations have served as a source of a large proportion of the new drugs that were developed over the first half of the 20th century.

More recently, the rational development of new drugs, both in university laboratories and in industry, has taken on a new dimension, largely because of: (i) recent advances in the understanding of biochemistry, cell biology, pathophysiology, and molecular biology; (ii) the evolution of wide-ranging novel drug screening protocols that can efficiently identify "lead compounds" among a large number of widely divergent chemicals. In the past, traditional drug screens employed standardized animal bioassays to measure effects such as analgesia, anticonvulsive activity, anti-inflammatory activity, bronchodilation, etc. Based on such assays, new drugs have been developed by identifying "lead compounds" and by building on the structure-activity relationships observed for a series of synthetic compounds.

Often, the use of such widespread screens has led in unexpected serendipitous directions. For instance, sulfa drugs, initially studied for their antibacterial properties, were observed in screening assays to reduce blood sugar and to inhibit carbonic anhydrase. Based on these preliminary observations with the parent sulfa compounds, new chemical syntheses led ultimately to the development of oral hypoglycemic agents (sulfonylureas) and carbonic anhydrase inhibitor diuretics. Further work with the carbonic anhydrase inhibitors led ultimately to the synthesis of the benzothiodiazine diuretics and to the loop diuretic, furosemide.

In addition to the bioassay screens that monitor over-all organ function or animal behavior, more targeted procedures, employing receptor binding methods,[r5] enzyme inhibition assays, and specific electrophysiologic measurements (e.g., specific ion channel properties) are now in use for the selective screening of putative sources of new drugs or for the conduct of structure-activity studies.

As a complement to drug "screening protocols," the improved understanding of the molecular basis of many physiologic pathways and certain diseases has led to the design of specific agents targeted to selected receptors or enzymatic pathways. For instance, a knowledge of the renin-angiotensin-aldosterone system that regulates blood pressure has spawned the development of the angiotensin-converting enzyme inhibitors (e.g., captopril) that have proved so effective for the treatment of hypertension. Similarly, an understanding of the voltage-operated calcium channels in the plasma membrane of myocardial and smooth muscle tissue has led not only to the development of effective antiarrhythmic drugs, but also to the development of calcium channel blockers that are effective dilators of vascular smooth muscle (e.g., nifedipine) and that are therefore useful agents for the treatment of essential hypertension.

In a similar vein, the explosive growth in knowledge about drug receptors (see Chapter 1) now provides a basis for the rational design of receptor subtype-specific agents, such as the histamine (H_2)-receptor blockers (e.g., cimetidine) that have proved their usefulness in the context of peptic ulcer disease. A promising new area is the study of the three-dimensional structure of target proteins, allowing a definition of the topology of potential receptor sites and the design of new drugs to fit that receptor. It is fair to say that the process of rational drug design, based on basic cell biology and molecular biology, is as yet in its infancy.

Despite the above-mentioned developments in drug discovery, bringing a new safe and efficacious drug to the marketplace is still a laborious, time-consuming, and exceedingly expensive enterprise. A high proportion of potentially useful drugs, developed either within the pharmaceutical industry or via university-industry interactions, fall by the wayside, either because of an inadequate spectrum of activity or because of the discovery of unexpected toxicity (Table 3.1). Any agent that shows a promising pharmacologic profile (e.g., antiarrhythmic activity) must also be evaluated for acute and chronic toxicity, teratogenicity, mutagenicity, and carcinogenicity. In addition, much information must be developed concerning absorption, distribution, and clearance of these putative drugs. These considerations are reviewed in Chapter 2 (Pharmacokinetics).

Table 3.1 Toxic Responses to Drugs

*1. Dose-related (predictable) toxicity
2. Idiosyncratic (unpredictable) responses
3. Allergic reactions
4. Drug interactions (pharmacokinetic factors)
*5. Drug reactions (additive or synergistic pharmacodynamic effects)
6. Carcinogenicity
7. Specific tissue-toxicity (e.g., hepatotoxicity, lymphopenia)

*most common

In terms of absorption of the putative drug, attention frequently will focus on the possible presence of a "first pass effect," where liver metabolism may limit the plasma concentration of an orally-administered drug. In terms of metabolism, attention must be paid to whether the chemical acts as a "prodrug" that has to be converted to an active drug in the body; other active drugs may prove to have potentially toxic metabolites. In terms of drug distribution,[1] there is a need to delineate such factors as how disease states might modify the protein binding of the putative drug, and what drug-drug interactions might be anticipated. With respect to clearance, there again is concern about how the disease states for which the drug might be intended might modify the clearance of the drug, and about issues such as whether saturable metabolic clearance of the drug might result in a nonlinear increase in plasma concentration when the dose is increased. An example of an "established" drug where such is the case is phenytoin. Thus, at the point a drug is considered for clinical trial, a great deal is known about its structure, stability and appropriate formulation, its range of activities, its metabolism and toxicity in several animal species, and its efficacy in normal animals as well as in animal disease models. All of this information provides the essential basis for a clinical trial.

The Clinical Evaluation of New Drugs

The evaluation of a drug in the clinic represents a specialized version of a clinical trial done either to generate or to test a particular hypothesis. Generally, clinical drug trials are prospective studies designed to test a specific hypothesis (e.g., drug A is effective in condition A; or drug A is more efficacious than drug B in a targeted patient population. Retrospective studies, which may be used to generate but not to test hypotheses, may also be done in the context of evaluating drug actions, subsequent to the introduction of a drug in the general population (so-called "Phase IV" studies). For any study, preliminary considerations are essential in terms of establishing inclusion/exclusion criteria for the selection of an appropriate study group, identifying therapeutic end-points for assessing drug effects, establishing an appropriate sample size required to confirm efficacy, and developing suitable ethical criteria to protect patients and to establish end-points for terminating the trial. Clinical drug trials are subject to the same statistical considerations as are all clinical trials[r6,r7] in terms of defining the sample size required to avoid either "Type I" (declaring erroneously that an effect exists) or "Type II" (failing to identify a truly meaningful difference between treated and untreated groups) errors.

The clinical trial of drugs is usually considered in terms of four phases (Table 3.2). In Phase I, a new agent is administered for the first time to a restricted number of healthy, drug-free volunteers (usually young males) in a tightly controlled environment (e.g., a metabolic unit of a hospital) with appropriate equipment to monitor the drug's cardiovascular impact. The Phase I studies are designed to establish effective dose ranges, to monitor acute toxicity, to determine appropriate routes of administration, and to evaluate the pharmacokinetics (e.g., volume of distribution, clearance, half-life, etc.) and metabolism. Upon establishing safe and effective dose ranges in the Phase I study, investigators may proceed to "Phase II" studies that involve small numbers of patient volunteers (again, usually males) who have the disease for which the new drug is expected to be of value. Usually, patients with organ diseases are excluded from such studies and, as with the Phase I studies, patients are usually not permitted the concurrent administration of other drugs that might interfere with the interpretation of the drug effects. The Phase II studies are also performed in a hospital or clinic setting, usually under conditions where (i) both the subject and the investigator know when active drug is being given (open study) or (ii) only the investigator knows when the active drug is being administered (single blind). These studies may involve a comparison of different doses and different routes of administration, plus studies on the metabolism of the drug (pharmacokinetics) and can yield considerable information, both about the drug's potential therapeutic value in a disease state and about its poten-

Table 3.2 General Features of Clinical Drug Trials

Phase I:	Small numbers of normal male volunteers studied in a controlled setting (hospital metabolic unit)
Phase II:	Larger numbers of patient volunteers (usually male), selected for the disease under investigation, investigated in a hospital setting as an open or single-blind study.
Phase III:	Less stringent patient selection to include both male and female subjects with multiple diseases, investigated under outpatient conditions as a double-blind study with the investigative drug and either placebo or "standard treatment."
Phase IV:	Open studies (postmarketing surveillance).

tial toxicity. However, Phase II studies are far removed from clinical relevance because of the necessarily rigid selection of patients.

Phase III studies more closely approximate the world of clinical practice. Patient subjects may have more than one disease, and female subjects are usually included, although some assurance that the patient will not become pregnant is often sought. The Phase III study is commonly done under outpatient conditions. The main question being asked relates to the efficacy of the putative drug, usually in comparison with a placebo or a "standard treatment." For example, in clinical studies on drugs in peptic ulcer disease, it is considered unethical to offer the patient only a placebo; an active "standard drug," such as an antacid, must be used for comparison with the drug under investigation. The study is performed under double-blind conditions, where neither the subject nor the investigator knows which drug (new investigative drug, placebo, or standard treatment) is being dispensed. Many types of protocols have been devised for Phase III studies; most involve dose finding, "crossover" of active and standard or placebo preparations, and "washout" periods between the administration of the active drug and the administration of the control drug. In most instances the drugs are given orally. Many Phase III studies are done on a multicenter basis to generate sufficiently large numbers of patients for investigation, particularly when interest focusses on relatively uncommon illnesses. Multicenter Phase III trials introduce problems in terms of standardization of protocols, but they are efficient in identifying possible therapeutic benefits of a drug and in identifying unexpected toxicities, since these studies are usually many months in duration. Most drugs enter the marketplace on the basis of Phase III studies.

It should be emphasized that at the time a drug enters the market, notwithstanding the extensive investigations in Phases I to III, very little is known about its action in specific population groups, such as the young, the old, and those who are pregnant; and data obtained from the nonpregnant female population are also somewhat limited. Some of these data are developed during Phase IV studies. These are usually open studies initiated after the drug has been approved for general use, and intended to develop "field" information on efficacy and toxicity. Because of their uncontrolled nature and attendant difficulties with data collection, Phase IV studies are difficult to evaluate; they do, however, come closest to replicating the general clinical situation in which the putative drug will be used. It is probable that, in the future, pharmaceutical companies and government regulatory bodies will give greater attention to Phase IV studies.

General Principles of Therapeutics

Therapeutics may be defined as the rational application of pharmacologic principles to the treatment of diseases in patients. Those proficient in therapeutics will require:

(i) Skill in making a diagnosis, so that the correct pharmacologic intervention can be chosen (rarely, drugs may be used empirically to treat symptoms before the diagnosis is established)
(ii) Knowledge of the therapeutic interventions possible (pharmacologic and nonpharmacologic, such as changes in life-style, diet, etc.)
(iii) Knowledge of the pharmacokinetics of the drugs available (see Chapter 2)
(iv) Knowledge of how disease states (e.g., antecedent liver and kidney disease) may alter the dose of the drug required or the therapeutic response to the drug, together with an awareness of other drugs the patient may be receiving
(v) Knowledge of drug side-effects, including awareness of potential drug interactions
(vi) Awareness of risk/benefit ratios and the cost of the medication
(vii) Awareness of the importance of designing drug treatments to foster compliance

The choice of a specific drug is based on a detailed knowledge of both the patient and the principles of pharmacology. Frequently, more than one drug can be used effectively to treat a given condition; if all elements are considered, one drug may emerge as most appropriate for a given patient. In some instances, some "theoretical" considerations may be at odds with others, and clinicians will then have to use their expert judgment to optimize a therapeutic regimen. Compromises are often necessary. For example, a knowledge of kinetics (see Chapter 2 for quantitative pharmacokinetic considerations) may dictate that two separate drugs required for a therapeutic benefit be given on quite different dosage schedules or regimens because of differences in half-life. However, patient compliance in actually taking the two medications over such an irregular time-course may suffer because of the complexity of the dosing schedule. The wise clinician will thus usually settle for good compliance and accept suboptimal drug kinetics by giving both drugs on a convenient dosage schedule. Knowledge of pharmacokinetics may be crucial to limit toxicity in situations of drug overdoses.[r8] The following sections outline further considerations for the clinical use of drugs.

Application of Clinical Trial Principles to Routine Therapeutics

The principles of a clinical trial design can also be applied to routine patient care. These principles include: (i) the identification of a clear rationale for the use of that drug; (ii) the definition of a specific goal and a clear therapeutic end-point; (iii) reproducible and quantitative estimation of a desired end-point; (iv) individualization of drug selection, depending on the underlying disease process and specific characteristics of the patient (such as age); (v) adjusting the dose, beginning with the lowest dose possible, with gradual increments until the desired end-point is achieved (this may not be necessary in the case of inexpensive drugs that have a wide therapeutic index); and (vi) simplifying the drug regimen to avoid drug interactions and to promote compliance.

Route of Administration

The route of administration is dependent on the clinical situation. The advantages and limitations of the different routes of administration for drugs are presented in Chapter 2 (Table 2.2). Some drugs must be given parenterally, and parenteral use offers both advantages and disadvantages. It is possible to achieve therapeutic levels very rapidly; however, it is equally possible to achieve toxic concentrations. Many drugs absorbed from the intestine undergo a significant "first pass effect" in the liver, so that substantial metabolism occurs before the drug can enter the systemic circulation. This first pass effect is obviated by parenteral administration. Finally, drugs may be administered orally without moment-to-moment supervision. In contrast, skilled professionals must administer parenteral drugs, except in those cases where patients are specifically trained to administer their own parenteral medications (e.g., insulin). More recently, patients may control the rate of narcotic analgesic administration, but "fail-safe" computer-controlled pumps are required to prevent overdosage.

Drug Toxicities

Toxic responses to drugs may be dose-related (pattern predictable), idiosyncratic (pattern unusual and frequently unpredictable), allergic, or may be based on drug interactions involving pharmacokinetic factors (competition for protein binding, enzyme induction, enzyme inhibition; see Chapter 2 for general principles, Table 2.4). Clinically significant drug reactions that are a consequence of drug interactions are relatively uncommon. Most adverse drug reactions are due to additive or synergistic (pharmacodynamic) effects of drugs at the cellular level (e.g., CNS depressants), or to dose-related toxicity (Table 3.1).

Dose-related Toxicity

Most drugs have a wide safety ratio (therapeutic index), but most will poison an individual if enough is given. Patients will be poisoned at "usual" doses if the drug is normally metabolized by the liver and the patient has hepatic failure,[r9] or if the drug is excreted in active form by the kidney and the patient's renal function is compromised.[r10,r11]

Idiosyncratic Responses

It is likely that most "idiosyncratic" drug responses will not remain idiosyncratic. Many of these responses, such as drug-induced hemolysis, lupus-like syndromes, and prolonged apnea, can already be explained on the basis of genetic variability or pharmacogenetics. For example, as discussed in Chapter 2, the "slow acetylator" phenotype results in an increased risk of hydralazine-induced systemic lupus erythematosus.

Allergic Reactions

These involve antigen-antibody responses, with the drug combining with an endogenous protein to form a hapten that is antigenic. Examples include anaphylaxis, urticaria, contact dermatitis, drug-induced asthma, polyarteritis, drug fever, and serum sickness.

Drug Reactions and Multiple Drug Administration

Although not common clinically, drug reactions are usually preventable; thus, they merit an importance disproportionate to their frequency. About one-third of all prescribed drugs are mixtures of more than one chemical. Moreover, many patients self-medicate with "over-the-counter" preparations, which usually contain many different chemical entities. Finally, physicians frequently overprescribe, and patients may visit more than one physician; thus, it is not unusual for a patient to be receiving 10–15 separate prescriptions. Obviously, patients may be exposed to a multitude of different chemicals. Moreover, it is known that the incidence of adverse drug reactions rises exponentially (rather than linearly) with the number of drugs taken.

The Young and Old

Persons over the age of 65 account for about 11 percent of the North American population, yet they consume about 22 percent of all prescribed drugs and over-the-counter preparations. The chance of a person over 65 having an adverse drug reaction is about seven times that of one who is 25. A number of factors that determine drug pharmacokinetics are altered in the elderly.[r12] By way of example, body fat is about 10 per cent of body weight at age 20, but increases to 24 per cent at age 60; body water accounts for 25 per cent of weight at age 20, but decreases to 18 per cent at 60. In addition, metabolizing capability and renal clearance decrease with age (Chapter 2). Consequently, the effect of age on pharmacokinetic parameters (drug absorption, distribution, metabolism, and excretion) must be considered.[r12]

Drug Absorption

Gastric atrophy with achlorhydria may influence absorption of highly ionized drugs. Diminished intestinal blood flow may decrease drug absorption. These effects, however, are rarely important clinically. Absorption of drugs may be decreased, however, in "short-gut syndrome" or in situations where there is a shortened intestinal transit time; conversely absorption may be increased if there is intestinal stasis.

Drug Distribution

Serum albumin may decrease (hypoalbuminemia) with age, with resultant effects on protein binding of drugs. Some common drugs are known to show decreased protein binding as a function of age. These include warfarin, phenytoin, meperidine, tolbutamide, salicylate, phenylbutazone, and sulfadiazine. The decreased muscle mass in the elderly also influences the distribution of drugs that are subject to tissue binding. All these alterations in drug distribution will increase the effective plasma concentration of certain drugs, resulting in enhanced drug effects and perhaps toxicities.

Drug Metabolism

Between the ages of 25 and 65, cardiac output decreases 30–40 per cent, with corresponding changes in liver blood flow. As a result, the clearance of a drug such as propranolol that is blood flow-limited (Chapter 2) will be reduced, resulting in an increased risk of toxicity. Liver blood flow may also be further decreased in pathologic states associated with aging, such as heart failure. With aging, there may be a deterioration in hepatocyte function. As discussed in Chapter 2, Phase II conjugation reactions are minimally affected by age, but Phase I microsomal oxidation reactions are reduced in the elderly. As a result, the duration of action ($t^{1/2}$) of certain benzodiazepines that undergo microsomal oxidation in the liver to produce active metabolites (e.g., alprazolam) is increased. Therefore, these drugs should be avoided in the elderly; instead, consideration should be given to the use of other benzodiazepines (e.g., oxazepam) that are metabolized by glucuronidation.

Renal Excretion

Between ages 25 and 65, renal blood flow decreases by 40–50 percent. Renal blood flow and glomerular filtration rate may also deteriorate with heart failure so as to affect adversely the excretion of drugs.

In summary, the elderly may exhibit enhanced sensitivity to pharmacologic agents, largely because of pharmacokinetic alterations. In addition, sensitivity of receptors to drugs (e.g., benzodiazepines) also may change with age.[r12]

The aged individual encounters other problems that may influence the over-all drug response. Problems with respect to vision and cerebration, may influence drug *compliance*, as may poverty. An increased number of physician visits (the elderly account for 30 per cent of health care expenditures in North America) provide more opportunities for overprescribing. Drugs given to the elderly are apt to be those with narrow safety margins and with cardiovascular and CNS side-effects. Moreover, deteriorating organ function and altered homeostatic mechanisms may leave the elderly less tolerant of drug side-effects. For instance, an elderly man with prostatic hypertrophy does not tolerate drugs well that have an anticholinergic action; patients with reduced tone in the lower esophageal sphincter are prone to develop gastroesophageal reflux when exposed to smooth muscle relaxants; and elderly individuals are at increased risk of developing glaucoma.

At the other end of the age spectrum are the very young, who have been described as "therapeutic orphans." This designation acknowledges the fact that children are not "little adults," and that a pediatric data base of drug information, corresponding to the adult data base, is frequently absent.[2] This situation exists even though children are exposed to large numbers of drugs. The range of drugs given during uncomplicated labor is 0–14, and averages six. Within a few days of birth, the infant has been exposed, on average to 18.7 drugs (intrauterine and extrauterine). If the mother breast feeds, one adds, on an average, 7.7 drugs, for a total of 26.4! The accumulation of weakly basic drugs in milk due to the pH gradient across the mammary gland epithelium (diffusion trapping) was discussed in Chapter 2 (Fig. 2.2).

As in the geriatric patient, there are physiologic departures from the adult in the young that may influence drug kinetics. Body fat is scant in the premature; this may also be true of the normal newborn. Subcutaneous fat increases in early infancy, only to fall in the period between nine months and six years, and increase again from six years to puberty. During the period from one year to puberty, total body water maintains a reasonably constant relationship to body weight, but intracellular water increases and extracellular water decreases.

Absorption of drugs is not markedly different in the infant or child than in the adult. The distribution of many drugs, however, may be different. The so-called "blood-brain barrier" is less of a "barrier" in the newborn and the infant. There is also a decreased concentration of serum albumin and a decreased affinity of serum albumin for many drugs. These features explain why some drugs, such as sulfas, displace bilirubin from albumin, so that bilirubin may be deposited in the basal ganglia and cause kernicterus (Chapter 2, Table 2.7). The metabolism of many drugs is reduced in the newborn because of the immaturity of conjugating systems (glucuronidation) in the liver. Drug excretion may also be compromised. In the newborn and young infant, glomerular filtration is only one-third to one-half that of the adult. There is also immaturity in terms of tubular secretion and tubular reabsorption (Chapter 2).

None of these differences in the geriatric or pediatric age groups present major problems with respect to therapeutics, provided that the clinician is aware of them and is prepared to alter the drug selection or the dosage regimen accordingly.

Drugs and Pregnancy

Pregnancy can alter the pharmacokinetics and pharmacodynamic responses to many drugs. Specifically, pregnancy can alter absorption, distribution, clearance, and end-organ sensitivity to drugs.[3] Pregnancy increases body fat, thus altering tissue distribution and uptake of lipophilic drugs. Pregnancy increases cardiac output and liver and renal blood flow. Changes in blood flow to clearing organs can alter drug clearance, particularly drugs with a high extraction ratio (for details see Chapter 2). Metabolic clearance also can be altered by hormonal alteration in enzyme activity. Pregnancy can alter receptor density, and thus can alter end-organ sensitivity. Finally, the embryonic-placental unit provides an additional pharmacokinetic compartment that also can absorb, clear, and metabolize drugs.[4,5]

Drug transfer across the placenta to the embryo depends on the same factors presented in Chapter 2 for drug absorption and distribution (see Table 2.1 and Fig. 2.1): (i) lipid solubility; (ii) molecular size; and (iii) protein binding. Lipophilic drugs generally diffuse across the placenta wall. Examples of this type of drug are anesthetics. Drugs of a molecular size of 200–500 generally cross the placenta wall, whereas agents of greater than 1000 molecular weight cross poorly. Some drugs that are highly protein-bound or ionized do not cross the placenta.

The embryonic-placental unit also can actively clear drugs by metabolism (Chapter 2). The placenta is a very active metabolizing tissue. In addition, some of the blood from the placenta entering the fetal circulation enters the fetal liver; as a result, fetal drug metabolism can have clinical implications.[r13] First-pass hepatic metabolism in the fetus can have a potentially protective effect, except for those drugs that generate toxic active metabolites.[5]

Drugs may affect the embryo in a number of ways. Drugs can be teratogenic; they can alter the physiology and the growth of the fetus. The teratogenic potential of an agent depends on the timing of exposure to the drug, the duration and quantity of the exposure, and drug-specific characteristics. The greatest risk for teratogenesis is during the first trimester of pregnancy, although this may not be true for all drugs. Teratogenic effects may manifest immediately at birth (congenital defects), but adverse effects may not appear until adulthood. For example, diethylstilbestrol increases the risk of adenocarcinoma of the vagina at puberty. Drug-abuse also can affect fetal development. Consumption of alcohol and cocaine during pregnancy can have deleterious effects on the development of the CNS and can affect general growth characteristics and facial features, making the fetus an innocent bystander of recreational drug intoxication. This avoidable problem results in major intellectual and developmental impairments for those affected. The cost to society is enormous. Education is critically important to avoid these problems (see Chapter 21).

Drugs can be given to the mother in order to treat conditions in the embryo.[4] For example, corticosteroids have been used to stimulate fetal lung maturation in women with a history of premature labor.[6] Other examples of fetal drug treatment include the use of antiarrhythmic drugs to treat cardiac arrhythmias of the fetus.[7]

Drugs also can alter labor. The therapeutic agent oxytocin stimulates contraction of the uterus, but should be used only by trained personnel and under conditions where uterine and fetal activity are monitored. Anesthetics and opioids can slow labor; β2 adrenergic agonists have been used to inhibit labor.[5] Obviously, treatment with β2 adrenergic agonists affects the cardiovascular system of both fetus and mother, as well as causing many other systemic effects, including sodium retention. This adrenergic agent is contraindicated when cardiovascular disease exists in the mother or the fetus.

As mentioned above, drugs can be excreted into breast milk and may have adverse effects on the newborn. Sedatives may make the baby drowsy and may interfere with feeding. In addition, some drugs (such as diuretics) can decrease the amount of breast milk being produced by the mother.

Therapeutic Drug Monitoring

Technological advances have provided the opportunity to measure the concentrations of drug in blood and other body fluids. Clinically, therapeutic drug monitoring has both limitations and potential value.[3] One of its limitations relates to the wide variability in pharmacodynamic response to any given concentration of drug (see Chapter 1: Quantal dose-response curves, Fig. 1.3). Some individuals require concentrations of drugs higher than the upper limit of the "normal therapeutic range" in order to achieve efficacy. Some of these can be treated at such high doses without side-effects. Others develop adverse effects at concentrations below the lower limit of the normal therapeutic range. Given these major limitations, what is the clinical utility of therapeutic drug monitoring? The normal therapeutic range can be thought of as a measure of the probability of efficacy that can be achieved by increasing the dose of the medicine. For example, if a patient is taking a normal dose of any medicine, and if its concentration is relatively low (below the lower limit of the therapeutic range) in plasma, then the probability of additional efficacy being achieved by increasing the dose is substantial. In contrast, if the concentration of drug in plasma in this individual is at the top of the normal therapeutic range, the probability for achieving efficacy for that medicine by increasing the dose is relatively low because the probability of side-effects at such an increased dose is high.

The other legitimate indication for obtaining blood samples is to assess drug plasma levels when toxicity or drug interactions are suspected. In addition, some clinical pharmacokineticists obtain blood samples to provide data for computer simulations to individualize drug dosing for a patient. Given the substantial variance in pharmacodynamic response to a given drug concentration, a physiologic measure of the amount of the drug at the active site may be a better strategy to optimize drug dosing. Unfortunately, this is rarely possible. Even so, the use of therapeutic drug monitoring has value for decreasing the probability of toxicity when administering a number of drugs such as antibiotics psychotherapeutic agents, phenytoin, and, probably, digoxin.[r14]

Measures of drug concentration in biologic fluids have other research indications. Pharmacokinetic and pharmacodynamic data may provide information about the presence of active metabolites, pharmacogenetic differences, or other mechanistic information. Finally, therapeutic drug monitoring services offered by a team providing health care may provide a useful teaching resource for physicians and other health care workers, so as to optimize patient care.

The Prescribing and Regulation of Drugs

A drug prescription is an order, given verbally or in written form by a physician to a pharmacist, that offers instructions for the dispensing of a medication. Not all drugs require prescriptions; those that do not are referred to as "over-the-counter" medications (OTCs). In the past, OTCs were sometimes called "patent" drugs. The spectrum of drugs that require a prescription differs from country to country. National regulatory agencies establish lists of prescription drugs. In the US, the national regulatory agency is the Food and Drug Administration (FDA); in Canada, it is the Health Protection Branch (HPB). Such lists of prescription drugs are established on the basis of the toxicity and abuse potential of specific chemicals, balancing these considerations against efficacy. Drugs requiring a measure of control in terms of distribution are designated "prescription" drugs; that is to say, they cannot be dispensed without a prescription. Those not requiring such control are eligible for OTC status. OTC drugs are usually safe when taken in recommended doses, although efficacy is frequently questionable. Prescription drugs, on the other hand, while usually efficacious, have a potential for doing serious harm, even when administered at recommended doses. Narcotic drugs and, by extension, non-narcotic drugs that are often abused are usually covered by separate legislation that adds additional levels of difficulty in gaining access to the drug. In the US, prescription drugs are regulated by the Food, Drug, and Cosmetic Act and the Controlled Substances Act. In Canada, the corresponding acts are the Food and Drug Act and the Narcotic Control Act. These national lists may be expanded at a regional level (states, provinces, etc) to include drugs not covered on the national lists. In both the United States and Canada, local regulations are included in either state (USA) or provincial (Canada) pharmacy acts.

Prescription drugs are authorized for use in specific clinical situations. Thus, a drug may be authorized for use in peptic ulcer disease, but not in gastroesophageal reflux. Of course, once a drug is available, there is nothing to prevent usage for a nonapproved indication. There could, of course, be legal consequences if a patient came to harm because of a drug used in a nonapproved context. Newer drugs will almost certainly be listed in national or regional regulations. Some older drugs (e.g., digitalis glycosides) may not be regulated and theoretically may be nonprescription drugs. In fact, custom usually will dictate that the pharmacist will demand a prescription before dispensing such drugs.

The ways countries handle "problem" drugs differ. By way of example, heroin cannot be prescribed in the US. In Canada, it is a legal narcotic, included with other narcotics, under the Narcotic Control Act. In Canada, the term "controlled drugs" refers to drugs such as barbiturates and amphetamines. In the US "controlled drugs" refers to both narcotics and other drugs of potential abuse. In the US "controlled drugs" are subdivided into classes (C1 to C4).

C1: High abuse potential; little medical use; can't be prescribed; e.g. LSD.

C2: High abuse potential; significant medical use; prescriptions may be verbal, but must be confirmed in writing within 72 hours; e.g., morphine. In Canada, such drugs are under the Narcotic Control Act; written prescriptions are necessary.

C3: Some potential for abuse; verbal or written prescriptions are acceptable; e.g., glutethimide; mixtures of codeine and acetaminophen or acetylsalicylic acid

C4: Lower potential for abuse; e.g., diazepam.

C5: Low abuse potential; e.g., cough mixtures.

In the US and Canada, physicians and pharmacists are licensed at a state or provincial level. Thus, a prescription written by a licensed physician in one jurisdiction need not be honored in a contiguous state or province.

Therapeutic Decisions and Sources of Information on Drugs

There are a number of sources of information that assist therapeutic choices. Many hospitals issue a drug formulary on a regular basis. Formularies are restricted lists of drugs, selected by knowledgeable pharmacologists, physicians, and pharmacists, who collectively comprise an entity such as a Pharmacy and Therapeutics Committee. The physician usually can be confident that drugs of little value or whose risk or cost profile is unacceptable have been excluded from the formulary. Some hospital formularies are very restrictive, others much less so. In some jurisdictions, there are state or provincial formularies in addition to those of hospitals.

Newsletters, of which the best known is the "Medical Letter on Drugs and Therapeutics," provide an objective assessment of drugs. Because they are published on a regular basis, the reviews are always current. Many general medical journals such as the *New England Journal of Medicine* periodically review newer drugs or current management of given illnesses. "Drug Evaluations," published by the American Medical Association, is another reliable source of information on new drugs. Physicians will also find useful *"Facts and Comparisons"* and the *"Handbook to NonPrescription Drugs."*

Pharmacology textbooks are useful for basic information on drugs, but may be weak in the area of therapeutics; publishing can make delays some textbooks out-of-date at the time of publication because of new clinical data. "Free" publications and "free" meetings sponsored by pharmaceutical companies may or may not be reliable sources of information on drugs. Postgraduate course offered by continuing education departments usually provide reliable assessments of newer drugs.

Many countries have publications that are commonly used by physicians as references in drug therapy. In the US, the most popular is the *Physicians' Desk Reference (PDR)*; the corresponding publication in Canada is the Compendium of Pharmaceuticals and Specialties (CPS). Such publications are usually sponsored by pharmaceutical companies, and therefore may or may not be impartial with respect to the information offered on indications for use of a given product. These publications are usually based on "package inserts," and therefore provide useful information on pharmacology, dosage forms, known side-effects, and contraindications.

References

Research Reports

1. Pacifici GM, Viani A. Methods of determining plasma and tissue binding of drugs. Pharmacokinetic consequences. Clin Pharmacokinet 1992;*23*:449–468.
2. Gilman JT, Gal P. Pharmacokinetic and pharmacodynamic data collection in children and neonates. A quiet frontier. Clin Pharmacokinet 1992;*23*:1–9.
3. Knott C, Reynolds, F. Therapeutic drug monitoring in pregnancy-rationale and current status. Clin Pharmacokinet 1990;*6*:425–433.
4. Miller RK. Fetal drug therapy-principles and issues. Clin Obstet Gynecol 1991;*34*:241–250.

5. Rurak DW, Wright JM, Axelson JE. Drug disposition and effects in the fetus. J Dev Physiol 1991;*15*:33–44.

6. Roberts WE, Morrison JC. Pharmacologic induction of fetal lung maturity. Clin Obstet Gynecol 1991;*34*:319–327.

7. Pinsky WW, Rayburn WF, Evans MI. Pharmacologic therapy for fetal arrhythmias. Clin Obstet Gynecol 1991;*34*:304–309.

Reviews and Textbooks

r1. Grahame-Smith DG, Aronson JK. Oxford Textbook of Clinical Pharmacology and Drug Therapeutics, Second Edition. Oxford: Oxford University Press (1992).

r2. Spector R. The Scientific Basis of Clinical Pharmacology—Principles and Examples. Boston: Little, Brown (1986).

r3. Young LY, Koda-Kimble MA. Applied Therapeutics—The Clinical Use of Drugs Fourth Edition, Vancouver: Applied Therapeutics (1988).

r4. Evans WE, Schentag JJ, Jusko WJ. Applied Pharmacokinetics: Principles of Therapeutic Drug Monitoring Third Edition. Vancouver: Applied Therapeutics (1992).

r5. O'Brien RA. Receptor Binding in Drug Research. New York: Dekker (1986).

r6. Feinstein AR. Clinical Biostatistics. St. Louis: Mosby (1977).

r7. Friedman LM, Furberg, CD, Demets DL. Fundamentals of Clinical Trials. Boston: Wright (1981).

r8. Sue Y-J, Shannon M. Pharmacokinetics of drugs in overdose. Clin Pharmacokinet 1992;*23*:93–105.

r9. McLean AJ, Morgan DJ. Clinical pharmacokinetics in patients with liver disease. Clin Pharmacokinet 1991;*21*:42–69.

r10. Fillastre J-P, Singlas E. Pharmacokinetics of new drugs in patients with renal impairment (Part I). Clin Pharmacokinet 1991;*20*:293–310.

r11. St. Peter WL, Redic-Kill KA, Halstenson CE. Clinical pharmacokinetics of antibiotics in patients with impaired renal function. Clin Pharmacokinet 1992;*22*:169–210.

r12. Tumer N, Scarpace PJ, Lowenthal DT. Geriatric pharmacology: Basic and clinical considerations. Ann Rev Pharmacol Toxicol 1992;*32*:271–302.

r13. Krauer B, Dayer P. Fetal drug metabolism and its possible clinical implications. Clin Pharmacokinet 1991;*21*:70–80.

r14. Dobbs RJ, O'Neill CJA, Deshmukh AA, Nicholson PW, Dobbs SM. Serum concentration monitoring of cardiac glycosides. How helpful is it for adjusting dosage regimens? Clin Pharmacokinet 1991;*20*:175–193.

SECTION II

Peripheral Neuropharmacology

Section Editors:
S. Z. Langer
Robert R. Ruffolo, Jr.

CHAPTER 4

Chemical Neurotransmission: Peripheral Autonomic Nervous System

Robert R. Ruffolo, Jr.
Ullrich G. Trendelenburg
S. Z. Langer

Introduction

Neurohumoral transmission is now firmly established as the mechanism by which nerves interact with effector organs of the body. The basic premise behind neurohumoral transmission is that a nerve releases a chemical mediator, termed a neurotransmitter, that diffuses across a small, but defined area, the synaptic cleft, to interact with a suitable receptor on the effector organ, thereby evoking a response in the effector organ. The nerve terminal contains all the apparatus necessary for synthesis, storage, release, and subsequent inactivation of the neurotransmitter; cells of the effector organ contain, on their cell surface membranes, the receptors with which the neurotransmitter interacts and the enzymes necessary for degradation of the neurotransmitter. Intracellularly on the effector cells, the "signal transduction" mechanisms transmit information from the receptor to the "cellular machinery" that produces the end-organ response.

The release of the neurotransmitter by the nerve terminals on the peripheral nervous system is under the regulation of nerve impulses originating within the CNS. Nerves that have cell bodies in the CNS and that innervate the skeletal muscle are termed "somatic" nerves. In contrast, nerves that originate within the CNS and that innervate the visceral organs, such as the heart, blood vessels, GI tract, reproductive organs, and many others, are termed "autonomic" nerves. Almost all autonomic nerves have relay centers, called ganglia, that are outside the CNS; whereas neuronal connections for the somatic nervous system are entirely within the CNS. Furthermore, most somatic nerves that control motor function are myelinated and transmit impulses rapidly, but most autonomic nerves are nonmyelinated and conduct impulses relatively slowly. The function of peripheral autonomic nerves is to modulate the ongoing activity of the involuntary viscera by eliciting either excitatory or inhibitory responses.

Because peripheral autonomic nerves have ganglia outside the CNS, autonomic nerves are actually composed of two neurons, termed "preganglionic" and "postganglionic," named for their anatomic location relative to the ganglia. The preganglionic neuron has its cell body in the spinal cord or brain stem and is modulated by higher centers in the brain and by spinal reflexes. The axon originating from the cell body of the preganglionic neuron exits the spinal cord or brain stem from the cranial, thoracic, lumbar, or sacral regions, and forms a synaptic connection in the autonomic ganglia with the cell body of the postganglionic autonomic nerve fiber. The postganglionic neurons send their axons directly to the effector organs to complete the pathway of autonomic innervation to the peripheral involuntary viscera.

Divisions of the Peripheral Autonomic Nervous System

There are two major divisions of the peripheral autonomic nervous system: the sympathetic or adrenergic division; and the parasympathetic or cholinergic division. A number of anatomic and functional differences distinguish these two separate entities of the peripheral autonomic nervous system. An anatomic depiction of the sympathetic and parasympathetic divisions of the peripheral autonomic nervous system is presented in Figure 4.1, page 89.

Sympathetic Nervous System

Cell bodies for the preganglionic neuron of the sympathetic division of the autonomic nervous system originate in the intermediolateral cell column of the spinal cord at the thoracic and lumbar levels (T1 to L2 or L3). Relatively short preganglionic neurons exit the spinal cord at the thoracic and lumbar levels, giving rise to the term "thoracolumbar outflow," which describes the sympathetic division of the peripheral autonomic nervous system. These short preganglionic axons send projections to the sympathetic ganglia, which consist of two chains of 22 segmentally arranged ganglia located bilaterally with respect to the spinal cord outside the spinal vertebrae. Postganglionic neurons with their cell bodies located in these paravertebral sympathetic chain ganglia send relatively long postganglionic fibers to the effector organs innervated by the sympathetic nervous system. Although most preganglionic sympathetic neurons synapse in the paravertebral sympathetic ganglia, a few preganglionic sympathetic fibers pass through these vertebral ganglia without making synaptic connections and travel by way of the splanchnic nerves to the prevertebral ganglia in front of the vertebral column. These ganglia are situated in the pelvis and abdomen and are named the celiac, superior mesenteric, and inferior mesenteric (hypogastric) ganglia. They lie close to the organs they innervate, principally the urinary bladder and rectum. Acetylcholine mediates synaptic transmission between preganglionic and postganglionic nerve fibers in the sympathetic ganglia of adrenergic nerves. In contrast, norepinephrine, liberated by the long postganglionic sympathetic nerves, mediates the end-organ responses at the adrenergic neuroeffector junction—although there are a few exceptions, such as the sweat glands, where the neurotransmitter of the postganglionic sympathetic neuron is acetylcholine.

The adrenal medulla is a chromaffin tissue embryologically and anatomically homologous to the sympathetic ganglia in that it is derived from the neural crest. The adrenal medulla, unlike the postganglionic sympathetic nerve terminals, releases epinephrine (directly into the blood) as the primary catecholamine, although smaller quantities of norepinephrine are also released by the adrenal gland. The chromaffin cells of the adrenal medulla are innervated by typical preganglionic sympathetic nerve terminals, whose neurotransmitter is acetylcholine.

Parasympathetic Nervous System

The parasympathetic division of the autonomic nervous system differs markedly from the sympathetic division. Cell bodies giving rise to preganglionic parasympathetic nerves have their origins in the brain stem and spinal cord. They exit the brain stem and spinal cord at the cranial and sacral levels, giving rise to the term "craniosacral outflow" to describe the parasympathetic division of the autonomic nervous system. The cranial (tectobulbar) portion of the parasympathetic outflow innervates structures in the head, neck, thorax, and abdomen. These fibers travel in the oculomotor (III), facial (VII), glossopharyngeal (IX), and vagal (X) cranial nerves. The sacral (S2 to S4) division of the parasympathetic nervous system forms the pelvic nerve and innervates the remainder of the intestines and the pelvic viscera, including the bladder and reproductive organs. The preganglionic neurons of the parasympathetic division of the autonomic nervous system are extremely long, such that the parasympathetic ganglia are located in or near the effector organs. Thus, the postganglionic parasympathetic neurons are short. The neurotransmitter mediating synaptic transmission in the parasympathetic ganglia is acetylcholine. Acetylcholine is also liberated by postganglionic parasympathetic nerves innervating the effector organs.

Autonomic Regulation of Peripheral Involuntary Organs

Most organs of the body receive dual innervation from both the sympathetic and parasympathetic components of the autonomic nervous system. Although there are some exceptions, the parasympathetic and sympathetic neurons mediate opposing responses in the effector organ. Because of the balance in most organs between the sympathetic and parasympathetic divisions, blockade or inhibition of one system leads to exaggeration in the response mediated by the other. Some organs of the body, such as the vasculature and spleen, receive only one type of innervation, which, in these cases, is sympathetic.

In thoracolumbar sympathetic outflow, one preganglionic neuron may ramify and ultimately synapse with many postganglionic sympathetic neurons, leading to diffusion of sympathetic responses. In contrast, the craniosacral parasympathetic preganglionic neurons in general form only single synaptic connections with postganglionic parasympathetic neurons, giving rise to a more discrete and localized response—although Auerbach's plexus in the small intestine is a notable exception. This anatomic distinction between sympathetic and parasympathetic divisions of the autonomic nervous system has profound physiologic sig-

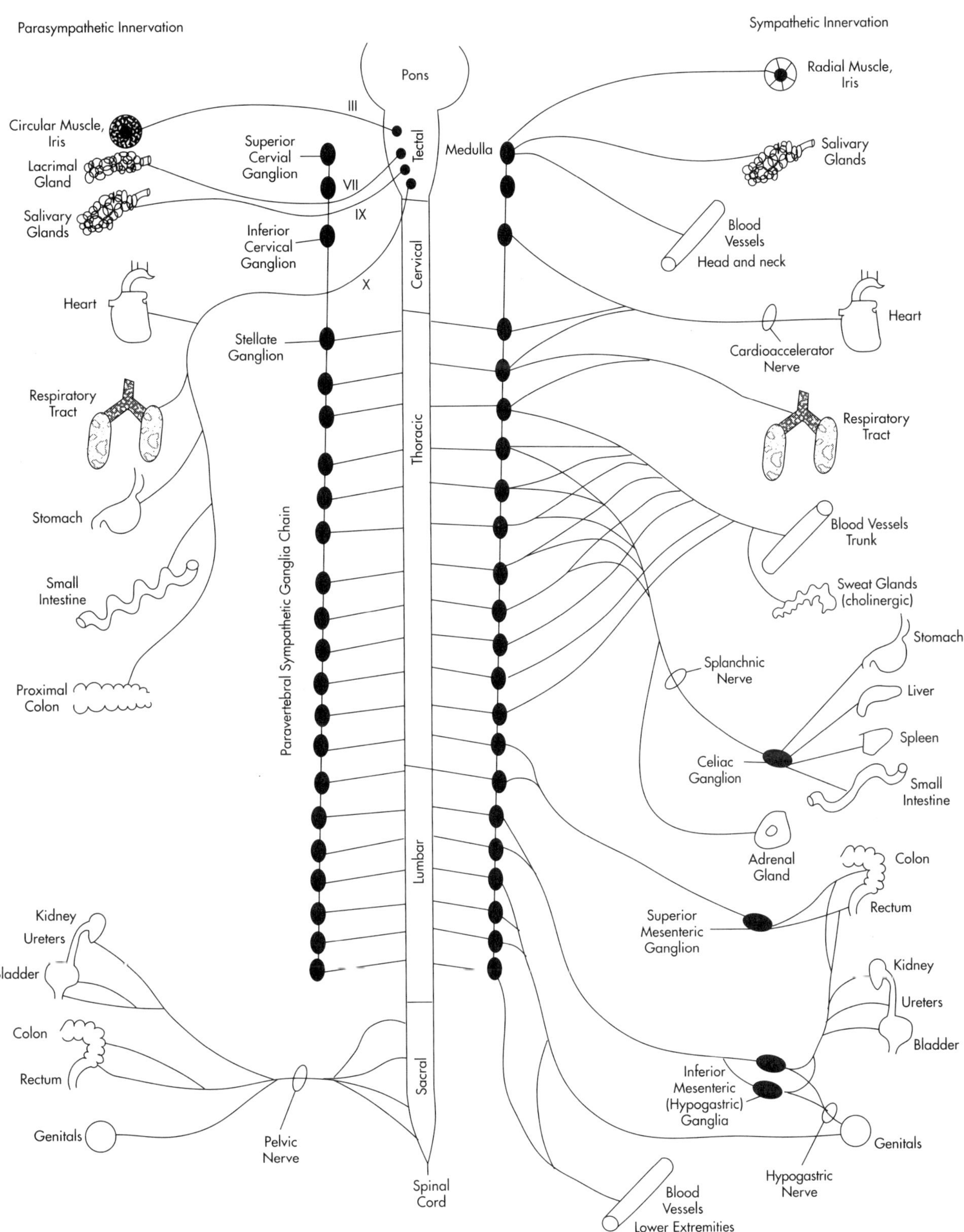

Figure 4.1 Schematic representation of the autonomic nervous system depicting the functional innervation of peripheral effector organs and the anatomic origin of peripheral autonomic nerves from the spinal cord. Although both paravertebral sympathetic ganglia chains are presented, the sympathetic innervation to the peripheral effector organs is shown only on the right part of the figure; parasympathetic innervation of peripheral effector organs is depicted on the left. The Roman Numerals on nerves originating in the tectal region of the brain stem refer to the cranial nerves that provide parasympathetic outflow to the effector organs of the head, neck and trunk.

nificance, because activation of sympathetic outflow, resulting from anger, fear, or stress, prepares the body for a ready state of activation: the "fight or flight" response. Thus, heart rate is accelerated, blood pressure is increased, perfusion to skeletal muscle is augmented through redirection of blood flow away from the skin and splanchnic region, blood glucose is elevated, bronchioles and pupils are dilated, and piloerection occurs. In contrast, because the cholinergic system is more discrete and localized, activation of parasympathetic outflow is associated with conservation of energy and maintenance of organ function during minimal activity. Activation of parasympathetic outflow produces a reduction in heart rate and blood pressure, activation of GI movements and emptying of the urinary bladder and rectum. Furthermore, glandular cells, such as lacrimal, salivary, and mucus cells, are activated; and smooth muscle of the bronchial tree is constricted. Based on these responses, it is clear that widespread activation of the parasympathetic nervous system would not be beneficial.

Although the parasympathetic nervous system is essential for life, the sympathetic nervous system is not, and animals completely deprived of it will survive, albeit with a lower level of efficiency. A decrease in sympathetic tone in the viscera occurs during times of stress, when activation of sympathetic outflow to other organs (e.g., heart and vasculature) is essential.

Neurohumoral Transmission in the Autonomic Nervous System

Transmission of information from preganglionic neurons to postganglionic neurons, or from postganglionic neurons to the effector organs, involves chemical transmission of nerve impulses for both the sympathetic and parasympathetic divisions of the autonomic nervous system. The sequence of events has been studied in great detail, and is illustrated for the sympathetic and parasympathetic ganglia, as well as for the postganglionic sympathetic and parasympathetic neurons, in Figure 4.2. Electrical impulses originating from within the CNS result in local depolarization of the neuronal membrane owing to the selective increase in the permeability of sodium ions that flow inwardly in the direction of their electrochemical gradient. Repolarization of the membrane follows immediately, resulting from the selective increase in permeability to potassium ions. These ionic flows are mediated by separate and distinct ion channels. The transmembrane ion fluxes that lead to ion currents produced in a local circuit result in the generation of an action potential propagated throughout the length of the axon. The arrival of the action potential at the preganglionic or postganglionic nerve terminal augments the quantal release of neurotransmitter stored in intracellular vesicles. The synthesis of the neurotransmitter occurs in the nerve terminal, where it is maintained in storage vesicles until a sufficient action potential stimulus is obtained.[1] The adrenergic storage vesicles in sympathetic nerve terminals and in adrenal chromaffin cells range in diameter from 400 to 1300A, whereas cholinergic storage vesicles in parasympathetic nerve terminals range in diameter from 200 to 400 A.

When sufficient action potential stimuli arrive, the release of neurotransmitter occurs through a calcium-dependent process known as exocytosis, in which the storage vesicle migrates to the nerve terminal membrane, fuses with the neuronal plasma membrane, and then opens to the extracellular space. This allows the contents of the storage vesicle, including the neurotransmitter, to be discharged into the synaptic cleft. The neurotransmitter diffuses across the synaptic cleft and interacts with a specific receptor located on either the cell body of the postganglionic neuron or on the effector cell. In both the sympathetic and parasympathetic ganglia, the neurotransmitter released by preganglionic neurons is acetylcholine, which activates postjunctional membrane receptors on the cell body of the postganglionic neuron, leading to an increase in ion permeability (and, therefore, ionic conductance) in the postganglionic neuron. This increase in permeability of ions ultimately results in the generation of action potentials that are propagated along the length of the postganglionic nerve. As at preganglionic nerve terminals, neurotransmitter is released when these action potentials reach the postganglionic sympathetic and parasympathetic nerve terminals. As indicated above, the neurotransmitter liberated by postganglionic sympathetic nerve terminals is norepinephrine, whereas the neurotransmitter in the postganglionic parasympathetic neuron is acetylcholine. The response mediated in the effector organ subsequent to the release of the neurotransmitter depends on the neurotransmitter, acetylcholine or norepinephrine, and, just as important, on the nature of the postjunctional receptor or receptor subtype present in the neuroeffector junction of the effector organ. These autonomic receptors are discussed in greater detail later in this chapter.

Following release of the neurotransmitter, the effect of the neurotransmitter must be rapidly terminated to avoid the loss of fine control provided by the autonomic nervous system and to prevent excessive activation of the postjunctional elements. Most cholinergic synapses and neuroeffector junctions contain a highly specialized enzyme, acetylcholinesterase, that rapidly hydrolyzes acetylcholine into two inactive products, acetic acid and choline, thereby terminating the effect of the neurotransmitter. Choline is then rapidly accumulated in the cholinergic nerve terminal by an active neuronal membrane pump in order to be reused for the synthesis of acetylcholine by the enzyme, choline acetyltransferase, which is present in the cytoplasm of the cholinergic nerves. Acetylcholine is then accumulated in the storage vessels of the cholinergic nerve terminal until required for release, thereby conserving the neurotransmitter.

At adrenergic neuroeffector junctions, the response to norepinephrine is not terminated by rapid

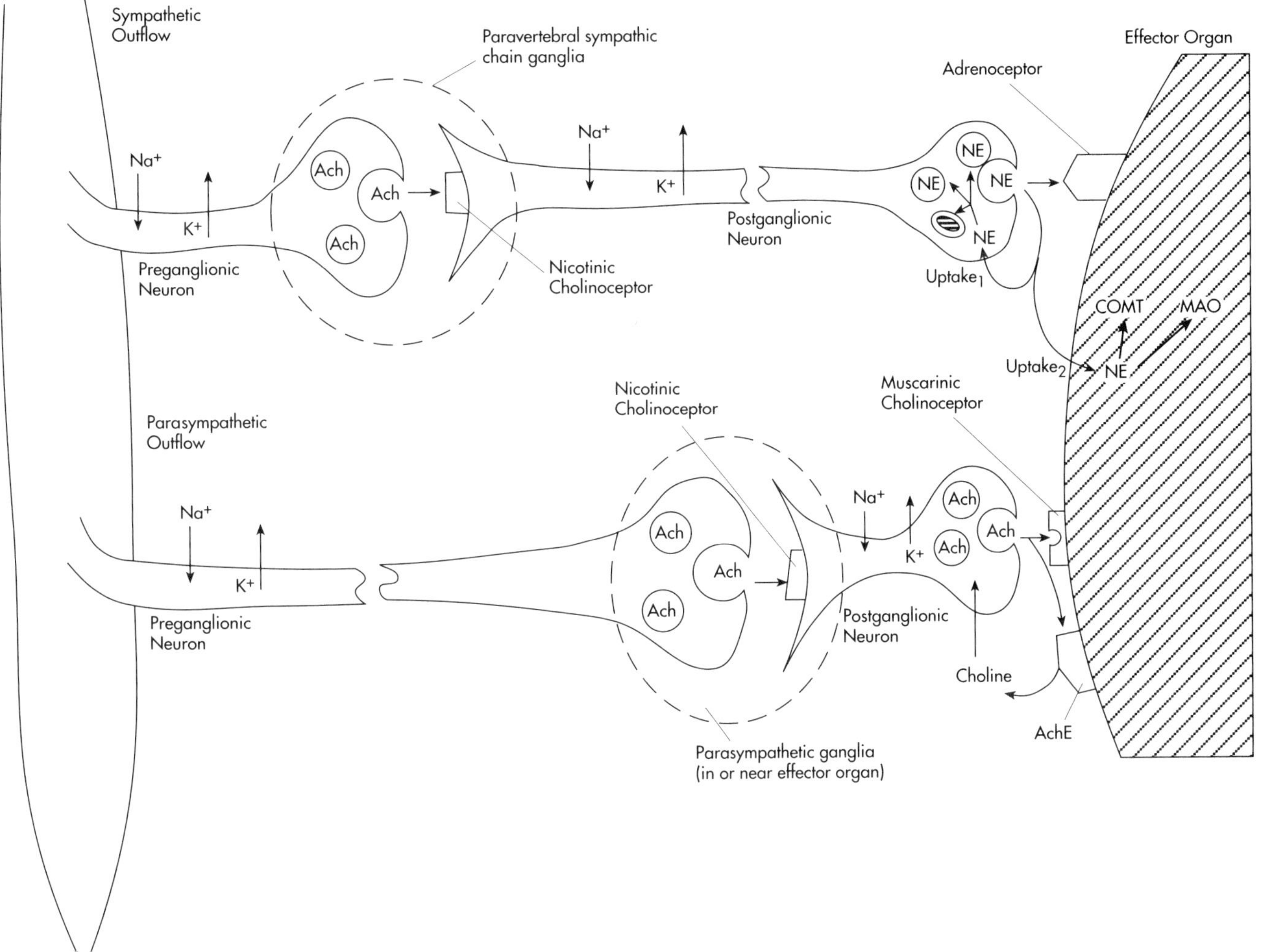

Figure 4.2 Schematic representation of neurohumoral transmission in the sympathetic and parasympathetic divisions of the peripheral autonomic nervous system. Short preganglionic neurons originate from the spinal cord and make synaptic connections in peripheral autonomic ganglia. The neurotransmitter liberated in both sympathetic and parasympathetic ganglia is acetylcholine (Ach), which is liberated through an exocytocic process upon the arrival of an action potential to the preganglionic nerve terminal. The electrochemical generation of these action potentials results from the influx of sodium ions (NA^+) and the efflux of potassium ions (K^+). Acetylcholine liberated from preganglionic neurons in both the sympathetic and parasympathetic ganglia diffuses across the synaptic cleft to interact with cholinoceptors on cell bodies of the postganglionic neuron. The interaction of acetylcholine with ganglionic cholinoceptors results in the generation and propagation of action potentials that elicit the release of neurotransmitter at the postganglionic nerve terminal. The neurotransmitter liberated from postganglionic sympathetic nerves is norepinephrine (NE), which diffuses across the neuroeffector junction to stimulate the adrenoceptors and elicit the end-organ response. Most of the liberated NE is taken back up into the sympathetic nerve terminal by $uptake_1$ and is either stored in the adrenergic storage vesicles or is metabolized by monoamine oxidase (MAO) in the mitochondria. A smaller amount of the liberated NE may diffuse away from the adrenoceptors and be transported by extraneuronal cells by $uptake_2$, after which it may be metabolized by the enzyme, catechol-O-methyl-transferase (COMT) and to a lesser extent monoamine oxidase (MAO). A similar process occurs in the postganglionic parasympathetic neuron, except that the neurotransmitter released is acetylcholine, which diffuses across the synaptic cleft and activates cholinoceptors on the effector organ. The liberated acetylcholine is rapidly metabolized by acetylcholinesterase (AchE) located in the extracellular space; the product, choline, is taken up into the parasympathetic nerve terminal and used to synthesize additional acetylcholine subsequently stored in the cholinergic storage vesicles.

enzymatic catabolism, but rather by a combination of neuronal reuptake of the neurotransmitter into the postganglionic sympathetic nerve terminal by an energy-dependent amine uptake pump, called $uptake_1$,[r2] and by simple diffusion away from the region of the receptors and subsequent accumulation by an extraneuronal uptake process[r3] often called $uptake_2$. Norepinephrine accumulated by sympathetic nerves by the $uptake_1$ pump may be: (1) oxidatively deaminated by the metabolic intracellular enzyme, monoamine oxidase, in the mitochondria of the sympathetic nerve terminal; or (2) sequestered in storage vessels for subsequent release. Norepinephrine diffusing away from the receptors to the extraneuronal site of $uptake_2$ may be further inactivated by O-methylation by the enzyme, catechol-O-methyltransferase. The metabolism of the catecholamines, norepinephrine and epinephrine, by the catabolic enzymes, monoamine oxidase and catechol-O-methyltransferase, results in many inactive degradation products found in tissues, blood, and urine. The scheme for the metabolic breakdown of the catecholamines has been well established and is depicted in Figure 4.3.

Biosynthesis of Neurotransmitters

Catecholamines

The pathway for the biosynthesis of the catecholamines, epinephrine and norepinephrine, is well established and is illustrated in Figure 4.4 (page 94). The basic precursor for the synthesis of all catecholamines is the amino acid, tyrosine. Tyrosine is first hydroxylated in the meta position by the enzyme, tyrosine hydroxylase, to form the catechol derivative, 3-4-dihydroxyphenylalanine. Tyrosine hydroxylase is the rate-limiting enzyme in the biosynthesis of all catecholamines, and this step takes place in the cytoplasm of the postganglionic sympathetic nerve terminal. Tyrosine hydroxylase is highly regulated, and its regulation is complex, involving both feedback inhibition by cycloplastmic norepinephrine and activation of the enzyme by cAMP-dependent protein kinase and possibly calcium-dependent protein kinases.

3-4-Dihydroxyphenylalanine (DOPA) is subsequently decarboxylated by the enzyme, L-aromatic amino acid decarboxylase, to form dopamine. This step also occurs in the cytoplasm. Dopamine is then actively accumulated by the storage vesicles in the sympathetic nerve terminals. After this transport process, dopamine is β-hydroxylated by the enzyme, dopamine-β-hydroxylase, which is inside the storage vesicle and on the storage vesicle membrane. The product of this enzymatic reaction is norepinephrine, which is retained within the storage vesicle in association with adenosine triphosphate (ATP) until an action potential arrives at the sympathetic nerve terminal. Dopamine-β-hydroxylase represents the terminal enzyme in the biosynthesis of catecholamines in the postganglionic sympathetic neuron. As such, adrenergic nerves release only norepinephrine as the neurotransmitter.

In contrast, however, norepinephrine and epinephrine coexist in the adrenal medulla. The synthesis of epinephrine in the adrenal occurs because of the presence of the enzyme, phenethanolamine-N-methyltransferase, which N-methylates norepinephrine (that has leaked from the varicosity) to form epinephrine in the cytoplasm.[r4] Cytoplasmic epinephrine is then accumulated by the storage granule in the chromaffin cell, where it is stored until released. In the human adult, epinephrine accounts for approximately 80% of the catecholamines in the adrenal medulla, norepinephrine making up the remainder.

Acetylcholine

The biosynthesis of acetylcholine in cholinergic neurons is achieved by the acetylation of the substrate, choline, by the enzyme, choline acetyltransferase, in association with acetyl coenzyme A, which serves as the donor for the acetyl group (Fig. 4.5, page 95). Choline is actively accumulated into the axoplasm of the neuron from extraneuronal sites by a high-affinity choline uptake process. The synthesis of acetylcholine from choline occurs in the axoplasm, with the product, acetylcholine, being actively accumulated by the storage vesicles in the cholinergic nerve terminal, which release the neurotransmitter upon the arrival of sufficient action potential stimuli.

Neurotransmitter Receptors in the Peripheral Autonomic Nervous System

It is not surprising that such distinct chemical entities as the neurotransmitters, acetylcholine and norepinephrine, would have different pharmacologic receptors mediating their end-organ responses. However, studies over the last century have shown that each neurotransmitter may interact with a variety of receptor types and subtypes as defined by pharmacologic methods. Because the end-organ response is as much a function of the receptor mediating the response as it is of the neurotransmitter that elicits the response, a detailed description of the adrenergic and cholinergic receptors mediating these end-organ responses is necessary. A diagram of the currently known adrenergic and cholinergic receptor subtypes is presented in Figure 4.6 (page

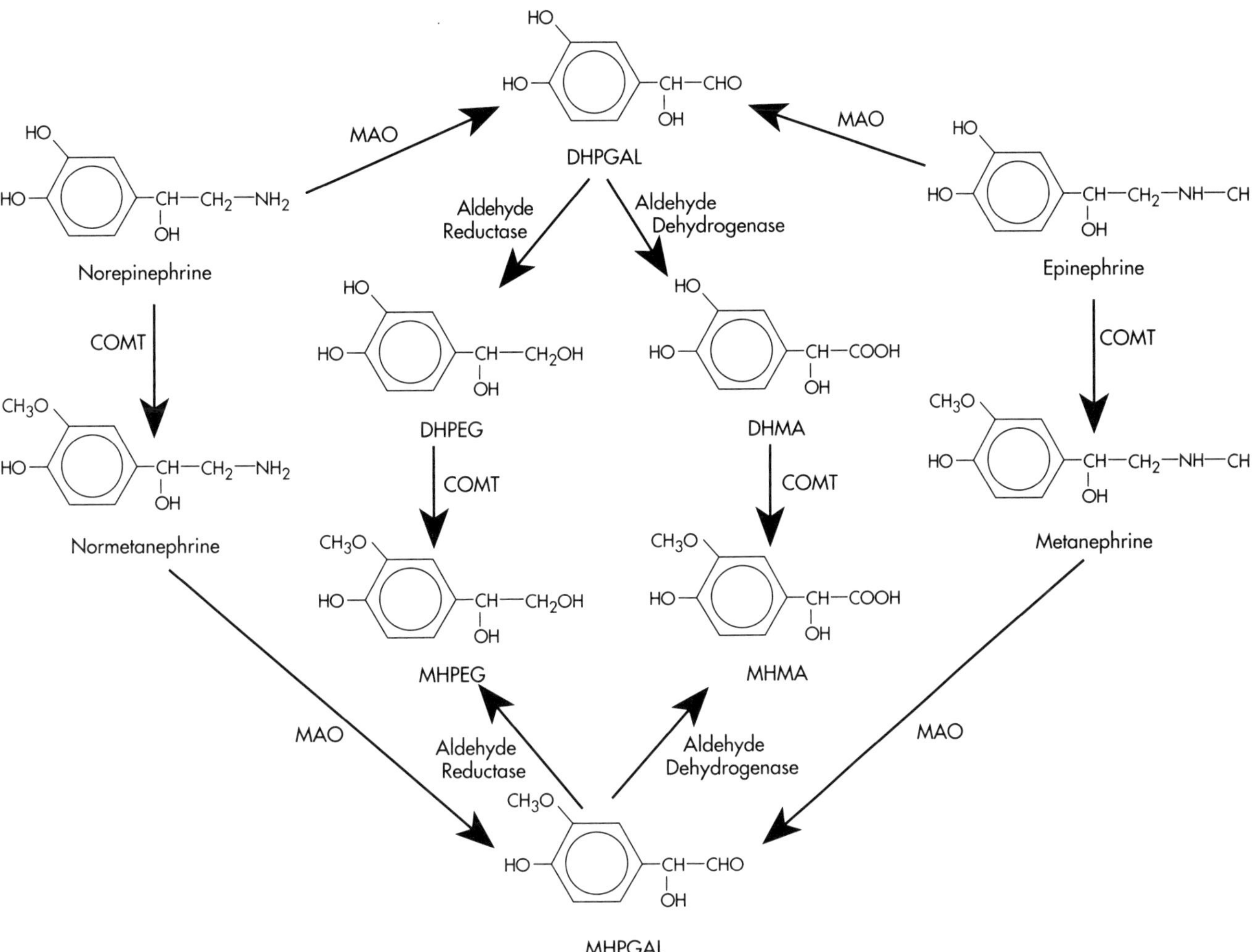

Figure 4.3 Metabolism of NE and epinephrine by monoamine oxidase (MAO) and catechol-O-methyltransferase (COMT). The abbreviations for the individual metabolites are as follows:

DHPGAL, 3,4-dihydroxyphenylglycol aldehyde; DHPEG, 3,4-dihydroxy- phenylethylene glycol; DHMA, 3,4-dihydroxylmandelic acid; MHPEG, 3-methoxy-4-hydroxphenylethylene glycol; MHMA, 3-methoxy-4-hydroxymandelic acid; MHPGAL, 3-methoxy-4-hydroxyphenylglycol aldehyde.

96), along with examples of agents that stimulate (agonists) or block (antagonists) these receptor subtypes.

Adrenergic Receptors (Adrenoceptors)

In the classic study of Ahlquist,[1] a series of sympathomimetic amines was investigated, providing the first evidence that the neurotransmitter, norepinephrine, and the adrenal catecholamine, epinephrine, could activate more than one type of adrenoceptor. For stimulation of smooth muscle in the vasculature, uterus, ureter, and dilator pupillae, and inhibition of intestinal smooth muscle, the following rank order of potency was obtained: epinephrine > norepinephrine > α-methylnorepinephrine > α-methylepinephrine > isoproterenol. In contrast, the rank order of potency for these same agonists for inhibition of vascular and uterine smooth muscle and for stimulation of the myocardium was: isoproterenol > epinephrine > α-methylepinephrine > α-methylnorepinephrine > norepinephrine. Based on these distinct potency orders, it was proposed that two types of adrenoceptors existed, termed α when the first order of potency was obtained, and β when the second was obtained. The existence of distinct α- and β-adrenoceptors was subsequently confirmed by the development of selective α- and β-adrenoceptor antagonists.

For many years, only two adrenoceptors were known to exist, the α and the β types just defined. Subsequent studies indicated that β-adrenoceptors did not belong to one homogeneous population, but rather

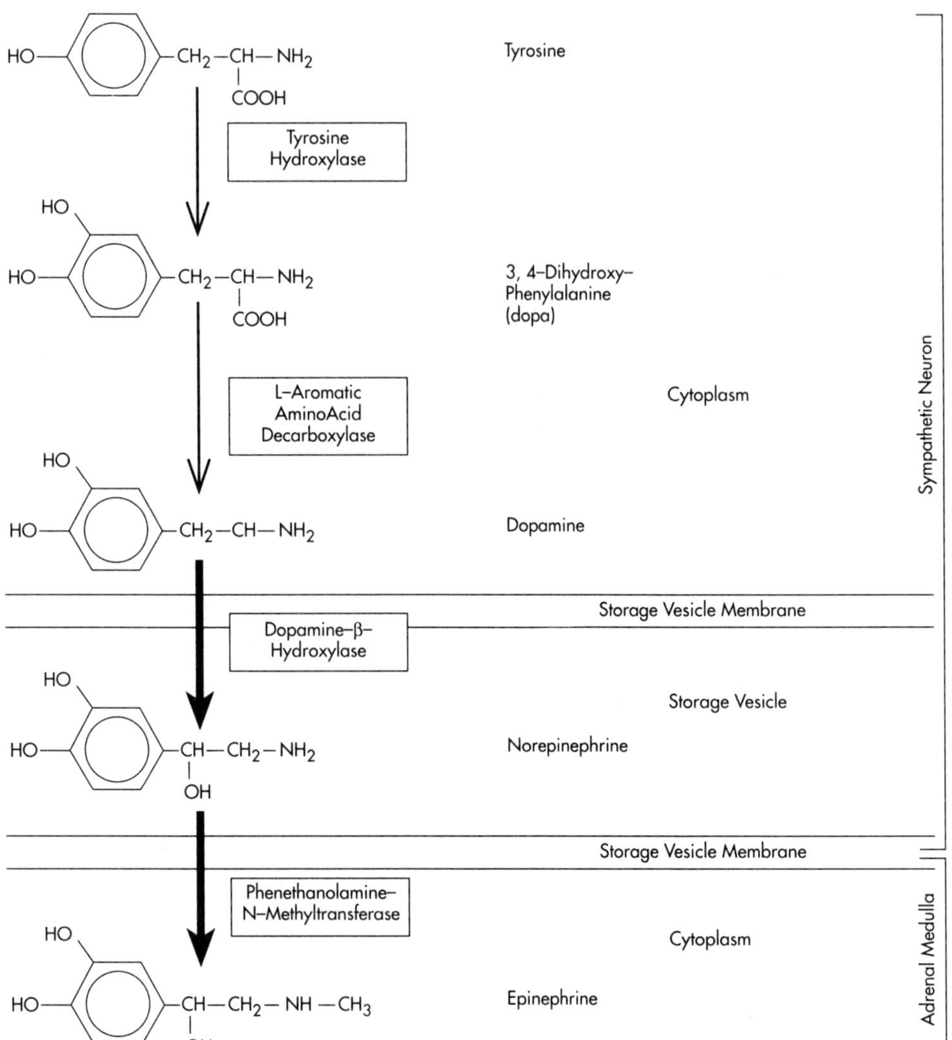

Figure 4.4 Steps in the enzymatic biosynthesis of the catecholamines, dopamine, NE, and epinephrine. The enzymes involved in each catalytic step are enclosed in boxes. The first three enzymatic steps occur in postganglionic sympathetic nerve terminals leading to the synthesis of NE, and all four enzymatic steps occur in the adrenal medulla, resulting in the synthesis of epinephrine.

could be subdivided further into the β_1- and β_2-subtypes.[2] Thus, β_1-adrenoceptors are characterized by the following rank order of potency: isoproterenol > epinephrine = norepinephrine. In contrast, β_2-adrenoceptors are characterized by the following order of potency: isoproterenol > epinephrine >> norepinephrine. The development of β-adrenoceptor antagonists with high selectivity for either the β_1- or β_2-adrenoceptors has confirmed this subclassification. Recently, a β_3-adrenoceptor has been identified that may play a role in fat cells to promote lipolysis.

In an analogous manner, recent studies have confirmed that α-adrenoceptors do not represent one homogeneous population, but may be further subdivided into at least two subtypes, α_1- and α_2-adrenoceptors.[3,4] α_1-Adrenoceptors are those showing high potency to selective agonists, such as methoxamine and phenylephrine and specific blockade by prazosin; α_2-adrenoceptors show high potency to specific agonists such as clonidine and α-methyl-norepinephrine and specific antagonism by yohimbine. Recent studies in which various adrenoceptors have been cloned confirmed the existence of three major families of adrenoceptors (i.e., α_1-, α_2-, and β), each of which may be further subdivided into two or more subtypes (Fig. 4.6, page 96), which represent separate and distinct molecular entities.[r5,r6,r7] Comparison of the amino acid sequences of the adrenoceptors shows a high degree of homology for those receptor subtypes within a given adrenoceptor family.[r8,r9] All of the adrenoceptors possess seven hydrophobic regions, suggesting that the amino acid chain traverses the membrane seven times, as depicted in Figure 4.7 (page 97) for the α_2-adrenoceptor of human kidney.[5]

Cholinergic Receptors (Cholinoceptors)

The neurotransmitter of the cholinergic nervous system is acetylcholine; as expected, differences in responses mediated by acetylcholine result from actual differences in cholinoceptors (Fig. 4.6). The actions of acetylcholine can be mimicked in certain organs by the alkaloid, muscarine, whereas in other organs the response to acetylcholine is mimicked by the alkaloid, nicotine. Thus, responses evoked by acetylcholine or by activation of the parasympathetic nervous system are described as being either "nicotinic" or "muscarinic," and have led to the subclassification of cholinoceptors as either nicotinic cholinoceptors or muscarinic cholinoceptors. The responses of most autonomic effector cells in peripheral visceral organs is typically muscarinic, whereas the response in parasympathetic and sympathetic ganglia, as well as responses of skeletal muscle, are nicotinic. The nicotinic receptors of autonomic ganglia and skeletal muscle are themselves not homogeneous, since they can be blocked by different antagonists. Thus, d-tubocurarine effectively blocks nicotinic responses in skeletal muscle, whereas hexamethonium is more effective in blocking nicotinic responses in autonomic ganglia—thereby confirming heterogeneity in nicotinic cholinoceptors. Molecular cloning studies have made the reasons for differing responses to nicotinic cholinoceptor agonists apparent. The nicotinic cholinoceptors of muscle contain α, β and, γ subunits, whereas the nicotinic cholinoceptor of ganglia contains only α and β subunits. The latter are also found in brain, and are referred to as neuronal nicotinic cholinoceptors. The heterogeneity of neuronal nicotinic cholinoceptors may be considerable. Currently five α-subunits and even multiple β-subunits are known.

Recently, it has been shown that muscarinic receptors also may be subdivided into at least two subtypes, termed M_1 and M_2, based on the pharmacologic specificities of certain agonists and antagonists. Atropine will block both M_1 and M_2 muscarinic cholinoceptors

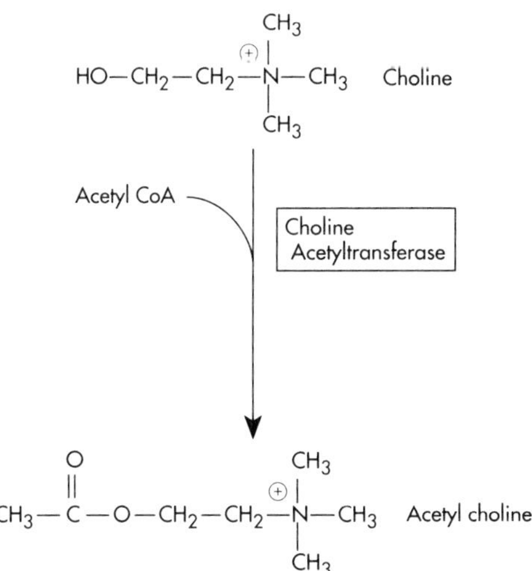

Figure 4.5 Enzymatic biosynthesis of acetylcholine which is catalyzed by the enzyme, choline acetyltransferase. The acetyl group is donated by the cofactor, acetyl coenzyme A.

with virtually the same potency. However, the drug, pirenzepine, has proved to be a selective antagonist of the M_1 subtype. In general, muscarinic cholinoceptors with the pharmacologic profile characteristic of the M_1 subtype are found to exist in the autonomic ganglia and in the CNS, whereas M_2 muscarinic receptors exist at neuroeffector junctions of organs innervated by the parasympathetic nervous system.

Molecular techniques currently are used to explore the heterogeneity of cholinoceptors and where they fit into the classification scheme being developed for receptors. The cholinoceptor population, like the adrenoceptor situation, is complex. For example, five different human genes have been identified that produce functional muscarinic cholinoceptors of the same family (M_1 through M_5), but with subtle structural and mechanistic differences.

Prejunctional Autoreceptors

In recent years, the functional significance of prejunctional autoreceptors has been established.[3,r10] Their distribution and function are illustrated schematically in Figure 4.8 (page 97). On most adrenergic and cholinergic nerve terminals, prejunctional α-adrenoceptors belonging to the α_2-subtype have been identified. Activation of these receptors by the released neurotransmitter, norepinephrine, or by exogenously administered α_2-adrenoceptor agonists, will decrease the release of norepinephrine.[6] This presynaptic inhibitory autoreceptor mechanism has been proposed to be involved in the normal regulation of neurotransmitter release as evidenced by the fact that blockade of this prejunctional α_2-adrenoceptor will lead to an enhanced overflow of the neurotransmitter, norepinephrine. There are also presynaptic α_2-adrenoceptors on most peripheral cholinergic nerve terminals; when these presynaptic α_2-adrenoceptors are activated, the release of acetylcholine is inhibited.[r11] These prejunctional α_2-adrenoceptors on cholinergic nerves may be activated by exogenously administered α_2-adrenoceptor agonists, and may also play a physiologic role in regulating the release of acetylcholine when activated by norepinephrine liberated from postganglionic sympathetic neurons that impinge on postganglionic cholinergic nerve terminals.

Presynaptic β-adrenoceptors belonging to the β_2-adrenoceptor subtype also have been identified on adrenergic nerve terminals. Activation of these receptors by β_2-adrenoceptor agonists, such as epinephrine, leads to facilitation of norepinephrine release, an effect opposite to that observed with presynaptic α_2-adrenoceptor activation. The physiologic role of the presynaptic β_2-adrenoceptor is not known.

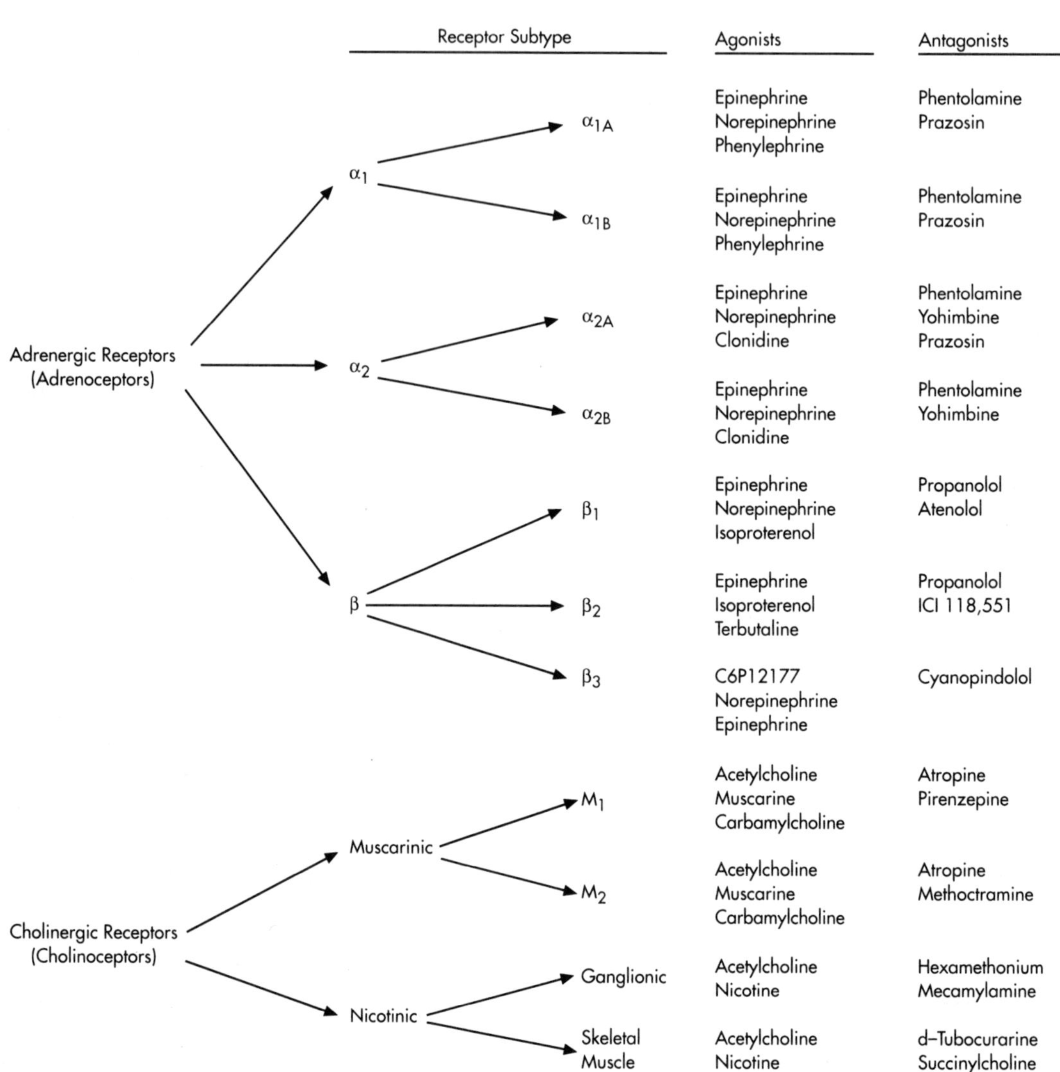

Figure 4.6 Division of the adrenoceptors and cholinergic receptors into individual receptor subtypes. Drugs that stimulate (agonists) or block (antagonists) each of the individual adrenergic and cholinergic receptor subtypes are listed.

It also has been proposed that there are presynaptic muscarinic cholinergic receptors on postganglionic parasympathetic neurons; when activated, these receptors mediate a decrease in the release of acetylcholine. There also may be prejunctional nicotinic cholinergic receptors on cholinergic nerve terminals that facilitate the release of acetylcholine.

Mechanisms of Signal Transduction Utilized by Autonomic Receptors

Until recent years, little was known about the intracellular molecular events set into motion when a cell-surface receptor was stimulated by a neurotransmitter. The mechanisms by which receptor activation is coupled to a cellular response are beginning to be understood for the peripheral autonomic receptors. These mechanisms of "signal transduction" appear to be different for many of the adrenoceptor and cholinoceptor subtypes, and may even differ for a given receptor subtype in different tissues. A brief summary of the recent developments in our understanding of the signal transduction processes utilized by autonomic receptors is given below.

β-Adrenoceptors

The mechanism by which activation of β_1- and β_2-adrenoceptors leads to the ultimate generation of a pharmacologic response is now beginning to be understood. Stimulation of β_1- and β_2-adrenoceptors leads to the activation of the membrane-bound enzyme, adenylate cyclase, which catalyzes conversion of adenosine triphosphate (ATP) to cyclic adenosine monophosphate (cAMP). The activation of adenylate cyclase by β_1- and β_2-adrenoceptors involves a third protein, which serves to couple the β-adrenoceptor subtypes to the catalytic enzyme. These recently identified coupling proteins, or guanine nucleotide regulatory proteins (G-proteins; G_s for stimulation and G_i for inhibition), are absolutely essential for receptor-mediated activation of adenylate cyclase.[7] The sequence of events is believed to be as follows:

(1) β-Adrenoceptor agonists bind to either β_1- and β_2-adrenoceptors.

(2) The resulting receptor-agonist complex will have high affinity for, and bind to, the G_s protein.[r12,8]

(3) Formation of the receptor-agonist-G_s protein complex facilitates the exchange of guanine disphosphate (GDP) for guanine triphosphate (GTP) on the G_s protein.

(4) The complex between the G_s protein and GTP dissociates from the receptor-agonist complex and interacts with the catalytic subunit of adenylate cyclase,[r9] thereby promoting the conversion of ATP to cyclic AMP (cAMP).

(5) cAMP then causes the activation of an intracellular protein, called cAMP-dependent protein kinase, which then can phosphorylate a variety of intracellular proteins, ultimately leading to a pharmacologic response.

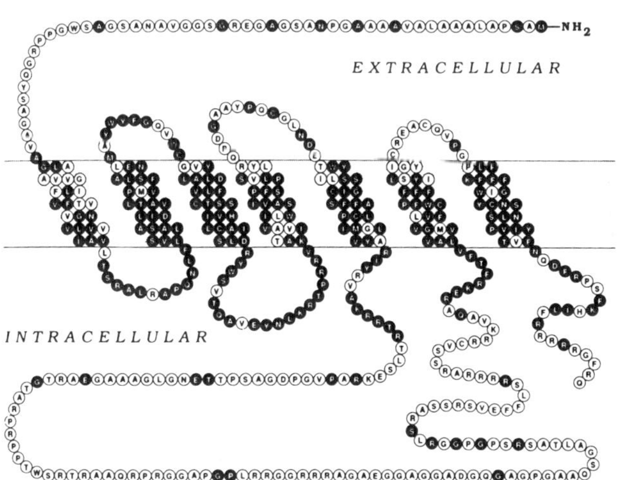

Figure 4.7 Primary structure of the human kidney α_2-adrenoceptor. The amino acid sequence is represented by the one letter code. The arrangement of the receptor structure within the membrane is based on a model of rhodopsin and is thought to represent a general model for other G protein-coupled receptors. The darkened residues represent identical amino acids between the human kidney and platelet α_2-adrenoceptors.

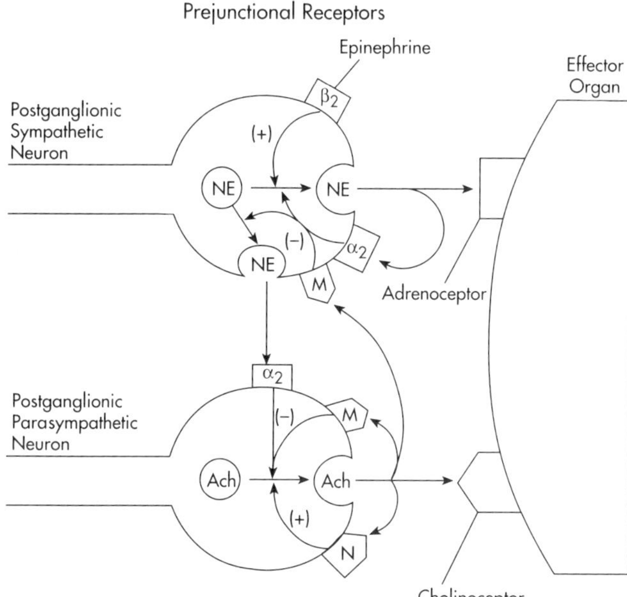

Figure 4.8 Schematic representation of the presynaptic autoreceptors that regulate neurotransmitter release in adrenergic and cholinergic neurons. Presynaptic α_2- and β_2-adrenoceptors exist on sympathetic nerve terminals and inhibit and facilitate, respectively, the release of the neurotransmitter, NE. Presynaptic muscarinic (M) and nicotinic (N) cholinergic receptors exist presynaptically on cholinergic neurons and inhibit and facilitate, respectively, the release of acetylcholine (Ach). Presynaptic α_2-adrenoceptors also exist on cholinergic neurons and inhibit acetylcholine release.

(6) Desensitization of β-adrenoceptors is mediated in part by phosphorylation of the receptor proteins.[r13] Multiple kinases recognize and modify the β-adrenoceptors. One group of kinases, termed β-*a*drenergic *r*eceptor *k*inases (BARK), has the unique property of only recognizing the agonist-occupied or "activated" form of the receptor.[r13] Phosphorylation of the receptor by BARK is localized to serine and threonine residues in the carboxy terminal tail. Two forms of BARK have been identified as separate gene products.[r14] BARK1 and BARK2 both modify the agonist-occupied form of the β-adrenoceptor, but BARK1 is twice as efficient. BARK-mediated phosphorylation by itself does not appear to alter the function of the β-adrenoceptor directly. The phosphorylated receptor binds a cytosolic factor, β-arrestin, that uncouples the receptor from G_s, thus attenuating signal transduction through adenylyl cyclase.[r14]

α_2-*Adrenoceptors*

In many systems, α_2-adrenoceptors are coupled to the inhibition of adenylate cyclase, with the net effect being the opposite of that observed for β_1- and β_2-adrenoceptor activation. Thus, α_2-adrenoceptors are coupled to adenylate cyclase in an inhibitory manner[10] through a guanine nucleotide regulatory protein termed G_i. When α_2-adrenoceptors are activated, the G_i protein ultimately will inhibit the catalytic activity of adenylate cyclase, thereby leading to a reduction in intracellular levels of cAMP, which decreases the activation of cAMP-dependent protein kinase.

Although the inhibition of adenylate cyclase by α_2-adrenoceptor activation occurs in many systems, it is important to note that α_2-adrenoceptors may also utilize other mechanisms of signal transduction in different systems. For example, in the human platelet, activation of α_2-adrenoceptors leads to stimulation of a sodium-hydrogen exchange system that produces an influx of sodium and an efflux of hydrogen ions. The net effect is intracellular alkalinization, which leads to an elevation in intracellular calcium levels. As calcium levels inside the cell rise, membrane-bound phospholipase A_2 becomes activated, which leads to the release of arachidonic acid from the cell membrane. The intracellular enzymes, cyclooxygenase and thromboxane synthetase, convert arachidonic acid to thromboxane A_2, which is released from the platelet and interacts with a specific membrane-bound thromboxane A_2 receptor to produce platelet aggregation.[11]

In blood vessels, yet a different mechanism for signal transduction is utilized by α_2-adrenoceptors, although the details have not been fully elucidated. It appears that the activation of α_2-adrenoceptors in blood vessels is associated with a G_i protein that in some as yet unidentified manner leads to activation of a membrane calcium channel, resulting in the influx of calcium from extracellular sites.[r15]

α_1-Adrenoceptors

α_1-Adrenoceptors produce their effects through increases in intracellular phosphatidylinositol turnover.[12] That is, activation of the α_1-adrenoceptor leads to stimulation of membrane-bound phospholipase C, the latter being coupled to the α_1-adrenoceptor by a guanine nucleotide regulatory protein termed G_p. The activation of phospholipase C results in the hydrolysis of phosphatidylinositol bisphosphate (PIP_2) to produce diacylglycerol (DAG) and inositol-1,4,5-trisphosphate (IP_3).[13,r16] Diacylglycerol has been shown to activate the enzyme, protein kinase C, which leads to phosphorylation of a variety of intracellular proteins. IP_3 can release intracellular calcium from stores in the endoplasmic reticulum. Thus, diacylglycerol and IP_3 can be considered as the intracellular messengers that lead to pharmacologic responses mediated by α_1-adrenoceptor activation.

Muscarinic Cholinoceptors

Muscarinic cholinoceptors also may utilize a signal transduction process similar to α_1-adrenoceptors, in that they produce their effects through increases in intracellular phosphatidylinositol turnover.[r17] Thus, activation of the muscarinic cholinoceptor leads to association with a guanine nucleotide regulatory protein (G_p) and the activation of phospholipase C. The subsequent generation of diacylglycerol and inositol trisphosphate from phosphatidylinositol bisphosphate following hydrolysis by phospholipase C ultimately mediates the muscarinic cholinergic effect. In some cells, activation of muscarinic cholinoceptors also leads to the inhibition of adenylate cyclase and a decrease in cAMP concentrations in a manner similar to that described for α_2-adrenoceptors.

Nicotinic Cholinoceptors

The details of signal transduction for nicotinic cholinergic responses have not yet been fully elucidated. Activation of the nicotinic cholinergic receptor does not require interaction with a guanine nucleotide regulatory protein. Rather, the nicotinic cholinoceptor itself forms an ion channel (selective for sodium), which, when activated by acetylcholine, undergoes a conformational change leading to a change in quaternary structure and opening of the ion channel.

Functional Responses Mediated by the Autonomic Nervous System

Many organs of the body receive both adrenergic and cholinergic innervation. Therefore, the responses in these organs represent a complex interplay between these two divisions of the autonomic nervous system. It is not uncommon for one type of innervation to predominate, such that an organ may be predominantly under the control of only one division of the autonomic nervous system, even though both components are present and can modulate any given response. Organs receiving dual innervation from the sympathetic and parasympathetic divisions of the autonomic nervous system include the heart, eye, bronchial tree, GI tract, urinary bladder, and reproductive organs. Some organs receive only a single type of innervation, which is generally that of the sympathetic nervous system. Thus, blood vessels, spleen, and piloerector muscle receive predominantly adrenergic innervation. As indicated earlier, the predominant cholinoceptor located postjunctionally on the visceral effector organs and mediating the response to acetylcholine is the muscarinic cholinoceptor of the M_2 subtype. In contrast, the α_1-, α_2- or β-adrenoceptor subtypes can mediate the adrenergic responses to nerve stimulation in the various visceral effector organs receiving adrenergic innervation. A detailed account of the adrenergic and cholinergic responses that occur in a number of important organs of the body is presented in Table 4.1. It is apparent from Table 4.1 that, in most instances, sympathetic and parasympathetic nerves mediate physiologically opposing effects. That is, if one system inhibits a certain function, the other system usually enhances that function. It is important to emphasize that the responses presented in Table 4.1 correspond to the responses mediated by stimulation of sympathetic or parasympathetic nerves; therefore, they represent responses mediated by the neurotransmitter interacting only with the innervated autonomic receptors located directly in the neuroeffector junction. However, autonomic receptors also are commonly found at sites away from the neuroeffector junction. These non-innervated receptors may be different from the receptors or receptor subtypes located directly in the neuroeffector junction. While these "extrajunctional" receptors are functional and may mediate responses to exogenously administered drugs, they probably play little or no physiologic role in the normal autonomic response mediated by sympathetic or parasympathetic nerves; therefore, they are not listed in Table 4.1.

Pharmacology of the Autonomic Nervous System

Detailed discussions of pharmacologic agents that alter the adrenergic and cholinergic divisions of the autonomic nervous system are presented in later chapters of this book. The present section presents a relatively brief overview of the targets of pharmacologic manipulation and intervention possible in the autonomic nervous system, and provides a few examples of drugs that interfere with processes involved in autonomic regulation.

Ganglionic Blockers

Drugs that block autonomic ganglia interfere with the chemical transmission of nerve impulses from preganglionic nerve terminals to the cell bodies of postganglionic neurons. Because the neurotransmitters (acetylcholine) and receptors (nicotinic cholinoceptors) are identical in autonomic ganglia of both sympathetic and parasympathetic nerves, ganglionic blockers seem to impede equally the neurohumoral transmission between pre- and postganglionic fibers of both divisions of the autonomic nervous system. The classic ganglionic blockers are hexamethonium and mecamylamine.

Although the ganglionic blockers inhibit equally ganglionic neurohumoral transmission in both the sympathetic and parasympathetic ganglia, the effects on end-organ response may nonetheless show a predominant adrenergic or cholinergic effect. The reason for this is that the degree of innervation by the adrenergic and cholinergic nervous system, and the extent of the adrenergic and cholinergic dominance in a given organ, may not be equivalent, as indicated in Table 4.1. Therefore, interruption of ganglionic transmission will have the over-all effect of selectively eliminating the component of the autonomic nervous system that generally dominates, leading to a response characteristic of the less dominant component. For example, the cholinergic system appears to dominate in the heart over the adrenergic component, and the administration of a ganglionic blocker will therefore have the greatest effect on the cholinergic component, giving rise to an apparent adrenergic end-organ effect (e.g., tachycardia). Thus, to predict the effect in a given organ mediated by interruption of ganglionic neurotransmission, one must consider the types of responses mediated by adrenergic and cholinergic nerves in that organ, as well as the dominance of one division of the autonomic nervous system over the other.

Drugs that Inhibit the Synthesis of Neurotransmitter

The rate-limiting step in the biosynthesis of norepinephrine and epinephrine involves the enzyme, tyrosine hydroxylase. α-Methyltyrosine blocks tyrosine hydroxylase, and thereby inhibits the conversion of tyrosine to 3,4-dihydroxyphenylalanine (see Fig. 4.4, page 94). The next step in the biosynthesis of the catecholamines is the conversion of 3,4-dihydroxyphenylalanine to dopamine by the enzyme, L-aromatic amino acid decarboxylase. This enzyme is inhibited by carbidopa and α-methyldopa, the latter also being a substrate for the decarboxylase, which converts it to α-methylnorepinephrine, a "false" transmitter that is also a potent and selective α_2-adrenoceptor agonist.

Dopamine synthesized in the cytoplasm is actively accumulated in the adrenergic storage vesicles by an active amine uptake pump in the vesicular membrane. After the transport of dopamine into the storage vesicle, the enzyme, dopamine-β-hydroxylase, which is associated with the storage vesicle membrane and also located within the varicosity, hydroxylates dopamine at the benzylic carbon atom. The natural neurotransmitter, norepinephrine, is formed, and is trapped within the adrenergic storage vesicle by low intravesicular pH, which protonates the neurotransmitter and prevents outward diffusion through the storage vesicle membrane. The norepinephrine trapped in the storage vesicle is associated with ATP to prevent excessive osmotic pressure inside the vesicles. Fusaric acid, a selective inhibitor of dopamine-β-hydroxylase, produces a significant reduction in norepinephrine levels and a concomitant increase in dopamine levels.

Table 4.1 Responses Elicited in Effector Organs by Stimulation of Sympathetic and Parasympathetic Nerves

Effector Organ	Adrenergic Response	Adrenoceptor Involved	Cholinergic Response	Dominant Response A or C*
Heart				
Rate of Contraction	Increase	β_1	Decrease	C
Force of Contraction	Increase	$\beta 1$	Decrease	C
Blood Vessels				
Arteries (most)	Vasoconstriction	α_1 (α_2)	—	A
Skeletal muscle	Vasodilator	β_1/β_2	—	A
Veins	Vasoconstriction	α_2 (α_1)	—	A
Bronchial Tree	Bronchodilation	$\beta 2$	Bronchoconstriction	C
Splenic Capsule	Contraction	α_1	—	A
Uterus	Contraction	α_1	Variable	A
Vas deferens	Contraction	α_1	—	A
Prostatic Capsule	Contraction	α_1	—	A
Gastrointestinal Tract	Relaxation	α_2	Contraction	C
Eye				
Radial Muscle, iris	Contraction (mydriasis)	α_1	—	A
Circular Muscle, iris	—		Contraction (miosis)	C
Ciliary Muscle	Relaxation	β	Contraction (Accommodation)	C
Kidney	Renin Secretion	β_1	—	A
Urinary Bladder				
Detrusor	Relaxation	β	Contraction	C
Trigone and Sphincter	Contraction	α_1	Relaxation	A,C
Ureter	Contraction	α_1	Relaxation	A
Insulin Release from Pancreas	Decrease	α_2	—	A
Fat Cells	Lipolysis	β_1 (β_3)	—	A
Liver glycogenolysis	Increase	α_1	—	A
Hair folicles smooth muscle	Contraction (piloerection)	α_1	—	A
Nasal Secretion	Decrease	α_1	Increase	C
Salivary Glands	Increased Secretion	α_1	Increase Secretion	C
Sweat Glands	Increase Secretion	α_1	Increase Secretion	C

*A, adrenergic, C, cholinergic

The synthetic step involving dopamine-β-hydroxylase is the terminal step in the biosynthesis of catecholamines in postganglionic sympathetic nerve terminals. Thus, high levels of norepinephrine are found in these neurons. However, in the adrenal medulla, there is an additional enzyme, phenethanolamine-N-methyltransferase, this catalyzes the N-methylation of norepinephrine to form epinephrine, the major catecholamine of the adrenal. Phenethanolamine-N-methyl-transferase can be inhibited by agents such as 2,3-dichloro-α-methylbenzylamine.

Reserpine, a rauwolfia alkaloid, can inhibit the synthesis of norepinephrine (and epinephrine in the adrenal gland), even though the drug does not inhibit any of the enzymes involved in the synthesis of the catecholamines. Reserpine is a potent inhibitor of the uptake process that occurs at the level of the storage vesicle, and thus it blocks the transport of dopamine into the varicosity. When uptake of dopamine into the varicosity is inhibited, the enzyme, dopamine-β-hydroxylase, cannot convert dopamine into norepinephrine. As a result of the continued leakage of norepinephrine from the storage vesicles, and the inability of the storage vesicles to replenish stores of norepinephrine through the β-hydroxylation of dopamine, norepinephrine levels in the nerve terminal are depleted by reserpine. Because leakage of norepinephrine from the storage vesicles is required for the synthesis of epinephrine by phenethylamine-N-methyl-transferase, epinephrine as well is depleted from the adrenal.

The synthesis of acetylcholine involves the one-step conversion of choline to acetylcholine by choline acetyltransferase conjunction with acetyl coenzyme A (Fig. 4.5). Although there are no potent and specific inhibitors of choline acetyltransferase, it is possible to inhibit the biosynthesis of acetylcholine indirectly through the use of hemicholinium, a synthetic compound that blocks the high affinity transport system that accumulates choline into the cholinergic nerve terminal. By reducing the stores of substrate, hemicholinium inhibits the synthesis of acetylcholine, resulting in depletion of acetylcholine from cholinergic neurons.

Drugs that Inhibit the Release of Neurotransmitter

The release of norepinephrine from postganglionic sympathetic nerve terminals involves an exocytotic process in which the storage vesicle membrane fuses with the neuronal membrane, allowing the storage vesicle to release its contents into the synaptic cleft. This process may be inhibited by such drugs as bretylium and guanethidine. Thus, bretylium and guanethidine also are known as adrenergic neuron blocking agents and can interfere with adrenergic neurotransmission.

The release of acetylcholine also occurs through exocytosis. Botulin toxin has been shown to prevent the release of acetylcholine from all types of cholinergic nerve fibers. Because the cholinergic nervous system is essential for survival, botulin toxin is lethal.

Drugs that Promote the Release of Neurotransmitter

It is possible to promote the release of norepinephrine from postganglionic sympathetic nerve terminals by two processes. One is activation of nicotinic ganglionic cholinoceptors by either nicotine or 1,1-dimethyl-4-phenylpiperazinium (DMPP), which will evoke the generation of action potentials in the cell body of the postganglionic neuron. These action potentials are propagated to the nerve terminal and activate the calcium-dependent exocytoxic release of norepinephrine from storage vesicles into the synaptic cleft.

It is possible to evoke the release of cytoplasmic stores of norepinephrine with the indirectly-acting sympathomimetic amines, such as tyramine, ephedrine, and amphetamine. These drugs enter the sympathetic nerve terminal by the $uptake_1$ pump and liberate norepinephrine into the synaptic cleft by a process that does not involve calcium or exocytosis.[r18]

Indirectly-acting sympathomimetic amines, e.g., tyramine, liberate, norepinephrine from postganglionic sympathetic nerve terminals, and the liberated neurotransmitter acts postjunctionally on the adrenoceptors to produce the end-organ response. The mechanism of action of the indirectly-acting sympathomimetic amines has been investigated in detail and is outlined below.

(1) Indirectly-acting sympathomimetic amines, such as tyramine, are transported into the postganglionic sympathetic nerve terminal by the active uptake process, $uptake_1$ (see above).

(2) This increases the number of $uptake_1$ transporters on the inside of the neuronal membrane, and therefore increases the availability of these transporters to carry norepinephrine in the reverse direction out of the nerve terminal because the $uptake_1$ transporters are bidirectional.

(3) Although cytoplasmic concentrations of norepinephrine are kept very low, owing to the high efficiency of the vesicular uptake process (and intraneuronal AMO), axoplasmic norepinephrine concentrations are typically too low to occupy the increased number of carriers made available on the inside of the cell membrane. However, because the indirectly-acting sympathomimetic amines also block the vesicular uptake pump, the uptake of norepinephrine (that has leaked from the storage vesicles) back into the storage vesicles is inhibited. Thus, there is a net leakage (without subsequent uptake) of norepinephrine from the storage vesicles, which ultimately increases cytoplasmic norepinephrine concentrations to the point where they can occupy the increased number of available carriers on the inside of the cell membrane for transport to the outside of the sympathetic nerve terminal. This results in the over-all net release of norepinephrine.

(4) Normally, approximately 90 percent of the liberated norepinephrine is immediately accumulated by the sympathetic nerve terminal via $uptake_1$, as described previously. However, because the indirectly-acting sympathomimetic amines are also substrates for $uptake_1$, they accordingly compete with the released norepinephrine for available carrier sites, and in that way significantly inhibit the reuptake of liberated norepinephrine.

(5) The net effect of a sympathomimetic amine is to increase the availability of carriers on the inside of the nerve terminal, to increase cytoplasmic concentrations of norepinephrine due to blockade of the vesicular uptake process, and to prevent the reuptake of norepinephrine following its release due to competitive inhibition of $uptake_1$. All these effects result in the excess liberation of norepinephrine caused by sympathomimetic amines.

The release of acetylcholine from postganglionic cholinergic nerve terminals also can be evoked by activation of ganglionic nicotinic cholinoceptors by nicotine or DMPP. As is the case for the release of norepinephrine, DMPP will elicit the generation of action potentials that ultimately produce the exotoxic release of acetylcholine. No known drugs will displace acetylcholine from neuronal stores and thereby indirectly elicit release of this neurotransmitter. Because acetylcholine is a positively charged quaternary ammonium compound, it cannot readily penetrate the neuronal membrane; therefore, the ability of cholinergic agents to promote the release of acetylcholine is limited.

Drugs that Interfere with the Storage of Neurotransmitter

Following its synthesis in the cytoplasm, norepinephrine is ultimately accumulated and maintained in the storage granules until subsequent release through exocytosis. There is an energy-dependent amine uptake pump at the level of the storage vesicle membrane that is involved in this accumulation.[r1] As discussed previously, reserpine can block the uptake of catecholamines into the storage vesicles, thereby decreasing the amount of norepinephrine synthesized (and stored) and available for release upon nerve stimulation. Reserpine eventually leads to complete depletion of catecholamines from postganglionic sympathetic nerve terminals through this mechanism.

At present, no known drugs can interfere with the accumulation of acetylcholine by the storage vesicles in the cholinergic nerve terminal. However, as indicated above, hemicholinium will lead to depletion of acetylcholine stores in cholinergic neurons by interfering with the accumulation of choline, the precursor for acetylcholine biosynthesis.

Drugs that Affect Neuronal Uptake

Following exocytotic release of norepinephrine from postganglionic sympathetic nerve terminals, most of the released catecholamine is actively taken up and accumulated into the sympathetic nerve terminal by an energy- and sodium-dependent neuronal uptake pump called uptake$_1$. Many drugs, such as cocaine and desipramine, are known to block this amine uptake pump, thereby increasing synaptic levels of norepinephrine and enhancing or facilitating adrenergic neurotransmission.

Acetylcholine is not taken up into cholinergic neurons after its release. However, as indicated above, there is a high-affinity uptake process for choline generated from enzymatic hydrolysis of acetylcholine by acetylcholinesterase, and this uptake process is inhibited by hemicholinium.

Drugs that Inhibit the Metabolism of Neurotransmitter

The two enzymes involved in the metabolism of the catecholamines are monoamine oxidase and catechol-O-methyltransferase. Monoamine oxidase can be inhibited by pargyline or tranylcypramine, and catechol-O-methyltransferase can be inhibited by other catechols, such as pyrogallol. Inhibition of monoamine oxidase and catechol-O-methyltransferase leads to higher levels of norepinephrine in peripheral tissues.

Acetylcholinesterase is the major enzyme involved in the hydrolysis of acetylcholine and in the termination of the cholinergic effect of the neurotransmitter. Acetylcholinesterase is inhibited by physostigmine, which serves to enhance the magnitude and duration of effects elicited by stimulation of cholinergic neurons.

Drugs that Block Autonomic Receptors

As indicated previously, there are four types of adrenoceptors, termed α_1, α_2, β_1, and β_2. The prototypic α-adrenoceptor blockers were such drugs as phenoxybenzamine, phentolamine, and tolazoline, which block both α_1-and α_2- adrenoceptors. Recently developed drugs such as prazosin have the capacity to block α_1-adrenoceptors selectively. It has also been shown that such compounds as yohimbine and idazoxan have the capacity to block α_2-adrenoceptors with relatively high selectivity.

The prototypic β-adrenoceptor blockers, such as propranolol, block both β_1- and β_2-adrenoceptors and show relatively little selectivity for either subtype. Recently, a number of selective-adrenoceptor blockers have been discovered. Betaxolol and atendolol are relatively selective β_1-adrenoceptor antagonists; butoxamine and ICI-118551 are known to be reasonably selective β_2-adrenoceptor antagonists.

Most effector organs of the autonomic nervous system contain muscarinic cholinoceptors, and these receptors are blocked in a competitive manner by atropine. Nicotinic cholinoceptors are of two types; those in skeletal muscle and those in autonomic ganglia. Nicotinic cholinoceptors in skeletal muscle are selectively antagonized by d-tubocurarine; ganglionic nicotinic cholinoceptors are selectively inhibited by hexamethonium or mecamylamine.

Drugs that Stimulate Autonomic Receptors

The neurotransmitter, norepinephrine, will activate α_1-, α_2-, and β_1-adrenoceptors, with relatively weak activity at β_2-adrenoceptors. Epinephrine, on the other hand, will activate all known adrenoceptor subtypes with similar potency. A several drugs have recently been discovered that will selectively activate each of the adrenoceptor subtypes. Phenylephrine is a potent and highly selective α_1-adrenoceptor agonist, and clonidine is a selective α_2-adrenoceptor agonist. Isoproterenol is equally effective at stimulating both β_1- and β_2-adrenoceptors. However, dobutamine has been proposed to be a selective β_1-adrenoceptor agonist, whereas terbutaline is a reasonably selective agonist of β_2-adrenoceptors.

The natural neurotransmitter, acetylcholine, will activate both muscarinic and nicotinic cholinergic receptors, as well as each of the individual subtypes of these cholinergic receptors. Muscarinic cholinoceptors may be selectively stimulated by the alkaloids muscarine and pilocarpine, or by synthetic agonists such as carbamylcholine. Nicotinic cholinoceptors may be selectively stimulated by nicotine, and stimulation of ganglionic nicotinic cholinoceptors can be achieved with DMPP.

References

Research Reports

1. Ahlquist RP. The study of the adrenotropic receptors. Am J Physiol 1948;*153*:586–600.
2. Lands AM, Arnold A, McAuliff JP, Luduena FP, Brown RG, Jr. Differentiation of receptor systems activated by a sympathomimetic amine. Nature 1967;*214*:597–598.
3. Langer SZ. Presynaptic regulation of catecholamine release. Biochem Pharmacol 1974;*23*:1793–1800.
4. Berthelsen S, Pettinger WA. A functional basis for classification α-adrenergic receptors. Life Sci 1977;*21*:595–606.
5. Regan JW, Kobika TS, Yang-Feng TL, Caron MG, Lefkowitz RJ, Kobika BK. Cloning and expression of a human kidney cDNA for an α_2-adrenergic receptor subtype. Proc Natl Acad Sci USA 1988;*85*:6301–6305.
6. Starke K, Endo T, Taube HD. Relative pre- and postsynaptic potencies of α-adrenoceptor agonists in the rabbit pulmonary artery. Naunyn-Schmiedeberg's Arch Pharmacol 1975;*291*:55–78.
7. Gilman AG. Guanine nucleotide-binding regulatory proteins and dual control of the adenylate cyclase. J Clin Invest 1984;*73*:1–4.
8. Cerione RA, Sibley DR, Codina J, Benovic JL, Winslow J, Neer J, Birnbaumer L, Caron MG, Lefkowitz RJ. Reconstitution of a hormone-sensitive adenylate cyclase system: The pure beta adrenergic receptor and guanine nucleotide regulatory protein confer hormone responsiveness on the resolved catalytic unit. J Biol Chem 1984;*239*:9979–9982.
9. Strader CD, Dixon RAF, Cheung AA, Candelore MR, Blake AD, Sigal IS. Mutations that uncouple the β-adrenergic receptor from G_s and increase agonist affinity. J Biol Chem 1987;*262*:16439–16443.
10. Clare KA, Scrutton MC, Thompson NT. Effects of α_2-adrenoceptor agonists and of related compounds on aggregation of, and on adenylate cyclase activity in human platelets. Br J Pharmacol 1984;*82*:467–476.
11. Sweatt JD, Johnson SL, Cragoe EJ, Limbird LE. Inhibition of Na^+/H^+ exchange block stimulus-provoked arachidonic acid release in human platelets. J Biol Chem 1985;*260*:12910–12918.
12. Cotecchia S, Leeb-Lundberg IMF, Hagen P-O, Lefkowitz RJ, Caron MG. Phorbol ester effects on α_1-adrenoceptor binding and phosphatidylinositol metabolism in cultured vascular smooth muscle cells. Life Sci 1985;*37*:2389–2398.
13. Fain JN, Garcia-Sainz JA. Role of phosphatidylinositol turnover in α_1- and of adenylate cyclase inhibition in α_2-effects of catecholamines. Life Sci 1980;*26*:1183–1194.

Reviews

r1. Euler US von. Synthesis, uptake and storage of catecholamines in adrenergic nerves. The effects of drugs. In Blaschko H, Muscholl E. Catecholamines. Handbook of Experimental Pharmacology, Vol. 33. Berlin: Springer-Varleg, (1972); pp 186–230.

r2. Iversen LL. The uptake and storage of noradrenaline in sympathetic nerves. London: Cambridge University Press, 1967.

r3. Trendelenburg U. A kinetic analysis of the extraneuronal uptake and metabolism of catecholamines. Rev Physiol Biochem Pharmacol 1980;*87*:33–115.

r4. Weiner N. Control of the biosynthesis of adrenal catecholamines by the adrenal medulla. In Blaschko H, Sayers G, Smith AD. Adrenal Gland, Vol. *6*, Section 7. Endocrinology. Handbook of Physiology, Washington D.C.: American Physiological Society, 1975; pp 357–366.

r5. Nichols AJ, Ruffolo RR Jr. α-Adrenoceptor subclassification. In: Ruffolo RR Jr. α-Adrenoceptors: Molecular Biology, Biochemistry and Pharmacology. Prog Basic Clin Pharmacol Basel: Karger, 1991; Vol. 8, pp 1–23.

r6. Bylund DB. Subtypes of α_1- and α_2-adrenergic receptors. FASEB 1992;*6*:832–839.

r7. Hieble JP, Ruffolo RR Jr. Subclassification of β-adrenoceptors. In: Ruffolo RR Jr. α-Adrenoceptors: Molecular Biology, Biochemistry and Pharmacology. Prog Basic Clin Pharmacol Basel: Karger vol 8, pp 1–25, 1991.

r8. Stadel JM. Molecular biology of α-adrenoceptors. In: Ruffolo RR Jr. α-Adrenoceptors: Molecular Biology, Biochemistry and Pharmacology, Prog Basic Clin Pharmacol Basel: Karger vol 8 pp 24–43, 1991.

r9. Stadel JM, Nakada MT. Molecular biology of β-adrenoceptors. In: Ruffolo RR Jr. β-Adrenoceptors: Molecular Biology, Biochemistry and Pharmacology, Prog Basic Clin Pharmacol Basel: Karger vol 7 pp 26–66, 1991.

r10. Langer SZ. Presynaptic regulation of the release of catecholamines. Pharmacol Rev 1981;*32*:337–362.

r11. Ruffolo RR Jr, Nichols AJ, Stadel JM, Hieble JP. Pharmacologic therapeutic applications of α_2-adrenoceptor subtypes. Ann Rev Pharmacol Toxicol 1993;*32*:243–279.

r12. Gilman AG. G-proteins: transducers of receptor-generated signals. Ann Rev Biochem 1987;*56*:615–650.

r13. Hausdorff WP, Caron MG, Lefkowitz RJ. Turning off the signal: desensitization of β-adrenergic receptor function. FASEB 1990;*4*:2881–2889.

r14. Palczewski K, Benovic JL. G-protein-coupled receptor kinases. TIBS 1991;*16*:387–391.

r15. Ruffolo RR Jr, Nichols AJ, Stadel JM, Hieble JP. Structure and function of α-adrenoceptors. Pharmacol Rev 1991;*43*:475–505.

r16. Putney JW Jr. Phosphoinositides and alpha-1 adrenergic receptors: In: Ruffolo RR Jr. The Alpha-1 Adrenergic Receptors. ed. Clifton, Humana Press, 1987; pp 189–208.

r17. Harden TK, Tanner LI, Martin MW, Nakahata N, Hughes AR, Hepler JR, Evans T, Masters SB, Brown JH. Characteristics of two biochemical responses to stimulation of muscarinic cholinergic receptors. Trends Pharmacol Sci 1986;*8*:14–18.

r18. Trendelenburg U. Factors influencing the concentration of catecholamines at the receptors. In Blaschko H, Muscholl E. Catecholamines, Handbook of Experimental Pharmacology, Vol. *33*, Berlin: Springer-Varleg, 1972; pp 726–761.

CHAPTER 5

J. Paul Hieble
Robert R. Ruffolo, Jr.

Pharmacology of Cholinergic Transmission

Introduction

Acetylcholine serves as a neurotransmitter at many sites within the peripheral and central nervous systems, and cholinergic neurotransmission is involved in the control of many physiologic processes. Moreover, the distribution of membrane receptors for acetylcholine is even more extensive than that of cholinergic synapses, since tissues not receiving cholinergic innervation (e.g., many blood vessels) retain functional cholinergic receptors. Thus, in addition to vascular smooth muscle acetylcholine receptors mediating vasoconstriction, vasodilator acetylcholine receptors are present on the vascular endothelium. In the latter case, acetylcholine acts via the release of a novel paracrine mediator, either nitric oxide or a nitric oxide precursor, from the endothelial cell.[r1]

The cholinergic system has served as a representative example for many novel pharmacologic observations, from the initial postulate by Dixon in 1907[r2] that a nerve can liberate a chemical neurotransmitter resembling a plant alkaloid (muscarine), through the experimental confirmation of chemical neurotransmission by Otto Loewi in the 1920s and the characterization of the mechanisms involved in the storage, release, and degradation of acetylcholine in the 1930–1960 era. More recently, the cholinergic receptor was the first neurotransmitter receptor protein to be purified to homogeneity, and the cholinergic receptors have provided early examples of the utility of radioligand binding assays to characterize the affinity of drugs for membrane receptors. Likewise, studies to characterize the second messengers responsible for transducing receptor action, as well as molecular cloning and expression techniques to identify receptor subtypes were pioneered in the cholinergic system.

Sites of Cholinergic Synapses

Cholinergic synapses are found at several sites, and the anatomy and pharmacology of the synapse depends on its location. Acetylcholine is the principal neurotransmitter at the neuromuscular junction. This specialized synapse between motor nerve and skeletal muscle is described in detail in Chapter 4. Acetylcholine is also the neurotransmitter for all preganglionic autonomic neurons, both sympathetic and parasympathetic divisions. Transmission of an impulse through the sympathetic ganglion can involve the activation of several dissimilar acetylcholine receptors (see below). Postganglionic parasympathetic neurons also release acetylcholine, although in many cases, peptide or purine cotransmitters may play an important physiologic role following stimulation of these nerves. In addition, some postganglionic sympathetic neurons, primarily those innervating the sweat glands, release acetylcholine as a neurotransmitter. Cholinergic receptors are also present at prejunctional sites, both on acetylcholine releasing neurons, and on norepinephrine-releasing, postganglionic sympathetic neurons.

Acetylcholine is also an important neurotransmitter in the CNS. Immunohistochemical studies using antibodies directed against choline acetyltransferase, the rate-limiting enzyme in acetylcholine biosynthesis, allow the localization of cholinergic cell bodies and axonal terminals within the brain[1,2,3]. Nevertheless, the specific location and synaptic distribution of all of the central cholinergic neurons are not yet conclusively established. As in the periphery, acetylcholine receptors are found at both pre- and postsynaptic sites. Presynaptic cholinergic receptors have been shown to control the release of several neurotransmitters, including dopamine, GABA, glutamate, and aspartate.

Subclassification of Cholinergic Receptors

As noted above, early in this century it was recognized that the alkaloid, muscarine, would mimic many of the responses of cholinergic nerve activation. As a consequence, a subset of cholinergic receptors was designated as "muscarinic." The other major class of cholinergic receptors are sensitive to another alkaloid, nicotine, and hence are designated as "nicotinic."

Muscarinic and nicotinic cholinergic receptor-mediated responses can be easily distinguished. Indeed, only acetylcholine itself and a few close structural analogues, such as methacholine and carbachol, can stimulate both muscarinic and nicotinic cholinergic receptors. Selective activation of muscarinic cholinergic receptors can be produced by a variety of agents, including muscarine, other alkaloids (e.g., pilocarpine and acecholine), substituted acetylcholine derivatives (e.g., bethanechol), as well as other synthetic molecules (areclidine, oxotremorine). Many potent and selective antagonists are available for the muscarinic receptor, the prototype being atropine. Nicotinic cholinergic receptors can be selectively activated by nicotine, other alkaloids (lobeline), and synthetic analogues (tetramethylammonium and dimethylphenylpiperazinium [DMPP]). Nicotinic (but not muscarinic) responses can be antagonized by bisquaternary amines, such as hexamethonium and pentolinium. The chemical structures of the various muscarinic and nicotonic cholinergic receptor agonists are presented in Figure 5.1.

Muscarinic Cholinergic Receptor Subtypes

In the past decade, it has become clear that muscarinic cholinergic receptors can be further subdivided. A comprehensive review of the history and current status of muscarinic cholinergic receptor subclassification is described by Hulme et al., 1990.[4] The impetus for this subclassification was provided by the observation that a novel antagonist, pirenzipine, can selectively antagonize certain muscarinic responses. Other antagonists that also block only some muscarinic responses, but with selectivity patterns different from pirenzipine, have been identified, and, based on their ability to block functional responses to muscarinic stimulation, it is now generally accepted that there are as many as five subtypes of the muscarinic receptor, designated M_1–M_5 (Fig. 5.2). The pharmacologic characteristics of M_1, M_2, and M_3 receptors are well established. M_1 receptors, having high sensitivity to pirenzipine, are located primarily at autonomic ganglia and in the CNS. M_2 receptors, which are selectively antagonized by AF-DX 116 or methoctramine, are located primarily in cardiac tissue, although they may also be present in the CNS. M_3 receptors, antagonized by hexahydrosiladifenidol, are located on smooth muscle and secretory glands. Earlier literature often refers to the M_2 and M_3 receptors as "cardiac" and "glandular" subtypes, respectively, of the M_2 receptor. Hexahydro-siladifenidol can differentiate M_3 from M_2 receptors, but does not show substantial selectivity between the M_3 and M_1 subtypes. Less is known about the M_4 receptor, but this subtype may mediate presynaptic inhibition of neurotransmitter release,[5] and is the predominant subtype in rabbit lung.[6] Inhibition of adenylate cyclase activity in rat striatum may also be mediated by the M_4 receptor.[7,8] The M_4 receptor is characterized by a high affinity for himbacine and an affinity for pirenzipine intermediate between that of the M_1 and M_2 subtypes.[9]

Subtype selective muscarinic cholinergic agonists have not been studied as extensively as have the antagonists, and fewer chemical tools are available. McN A-343 can produce selective activation of the M_1 subtype. Conversely, arecaidine propargyl ester stimulates M_2 and M_3, but not M_1 cholinergic receptors. By comparison of the relative potencies of bethanechol and McN A-343, M_2 and M_4 muscarinic-cholinergic receptors can be differentiated.[8] Some agonists can show functional selectivity, acting as partial agonists at M_1 receptors, and competitive antagonists in M_2 and M_3 muscarinic cholinergic receptor systems.[10] Characterization of the pharmacology of the muscarinic cholinergic receptor subtypes has been hindered by the lack of subtype selective agonists and the lack of antagonists having high affinity for only one subtype.

This functional subclassification of muscarinic cholinergic receptors is supported by radioligand binding assays that use nonselective ligands, such as [^{3}H]QNB (quinuclidyl benzoate) or [^{3}H] NMS (N-methylscopolamine) (Fig. 5.3), where pirenzipine and methoctramine are more potent inhibitors of binding to M_1 and M_2 sites, respectively. Consistent with functional studies, hexahydrosiladifenidol is a more potent inhibitor of [^{3}H]NMS binding to M_3 vis-a-vis M_2 cholinergic receptor sites.[9] [^{3}H] Pirenzipine and [^{3}H] AF-DX 116 have also been utilized to show that the number of cholinergic receptors labeled by each of these selective ligands is less than that labeled by a nonselective radioligand.[11]

Muscarinic receptor cloning experiments have identified five

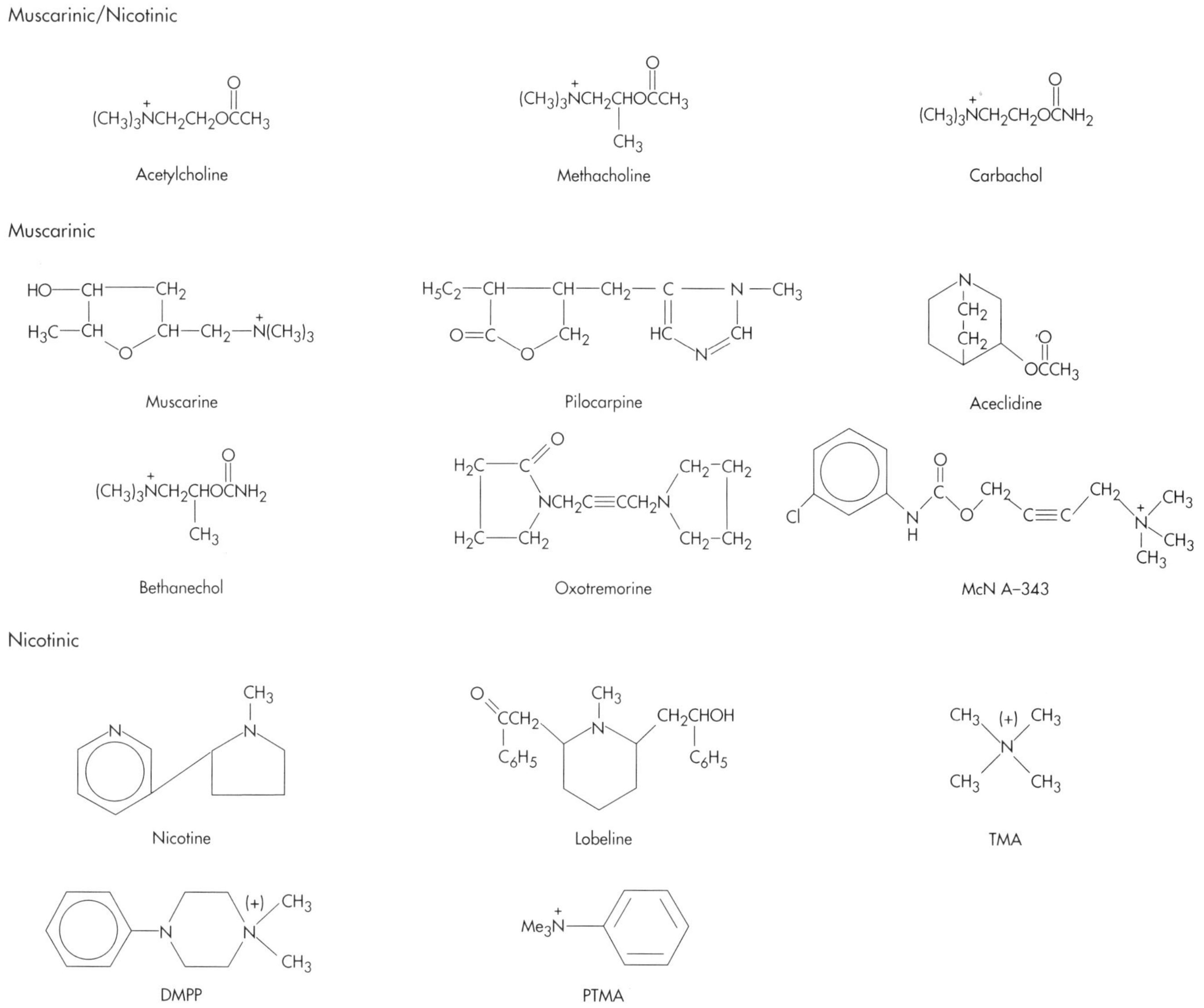

Muscarinic/Nicotinic

$(CH_3)_3\overset{+}{N}CH_2CH_2OCCH_3$ (C=O)
Acetylcholine

$(CH_3)_3\overset{+}{N}CH_2CHOCCH_3$ (C=O; CH_3 on CH)
Methacholine

$(CH_3)_3\overset{+}{N}CH_2CH_2OCNH_2$ (C=O)
Carbachol

Muscarinic

Muscarine

Pilocarpine

Aceclidine

$(CH_3)_3\overset{+}{N}CH_2CHOCNH_2$ (C=O; CH_3 on CH)
Bethanechol

Oxotremorine

McN A-343

Nicotinic

Nicotine

Lobeline

TMA

DMPP

PTMA

Figure 5.1 Cholinoceptor Agonists

proteins that, when expressed in tissue culture, have binding characteristics compatible with an endogeneous muscarinic receptor. Furthermore, expression of these muscarinic receptors confers functional biochemical responsiveness to muscarinic agonists in a cell line previously unresponsive. This response can be reflected either by a stimulation of phosphoinositide hydrolysis or by a stimulation (or inhibition) of adenylate cyclase. Although the nature of this response has been used to differentiate muscarinic cholinergic receptor subtypes, it appears that the particular second messenger system stimulated by receptor activation can depend on the cell line used to express the receptor protein. Like many neurotransmitter receptors, the cloned muscarinic cholinergic receptor proteins have amino acid sequences compatible with seven membrane spanning regions. A high degree of homology is observed in the transmembrane regions, with considerable diversity in both size and amino acid composition in the remaining portions of the molecule, particularly in the third intracellular loop, postulated to be the site of interaction between receptor and second messenger. This region shows greater amino acid identity within those subtypes postulated to mediate phosphotidyl inositol hydrolysis (M_1, M_3, and M_5) and within those mediating inhibition of adenylate cyclase (M_2 and M_4) than between these groups.[4]

When the ability of selective muscarinic cholinergic agents to inhibit the binding of $[^3H]$NMS to cloned muscarinic receptors is compared with their binding profile in homogenates of native tissues, it appears that three of the five expressed clones have pharmacologic profiles corresponding reasonably well with the M_1, M_2, and M_3. As noted above, the M_4 clone appears to have a functional counterpart in rabbit lung,[9] and may also correspond to the muscarinic cholinergic receptor mediating contraction in the guinea pig uterus.[12] Hybridization studies using probes prepared from the M_5 clone suggest this receptor to have a very limited distribution, with a low density detected only in a few discrete areas of the CNS.[13] The functional response, if any, to this muscarinic-cholinergic receptor subtype has not been characterized. It is possible that multiple muscarinic receptor subtypes participate in the response of an individual tissue to cholinergic stimulation of exogenous administration of a muscarinic cholinergic agonist.

Compound	Selectivity Profile
Pirenzipine	$M_1 > M_2 = M_3$
AF-DX 116	$M_2 > M_1 > M_3$
Methoctramine	$M_2 > M_1 > M_3$
Hexahydrosiladifendol	$M_3 \geq M_1 > M_2$
4-DAMP	$M_3 > M_1 > M_2$
Silahexocyclium	$M_3 = M_1 > M_2$

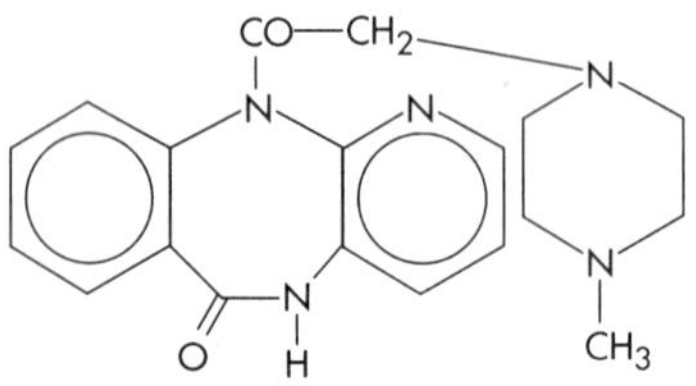

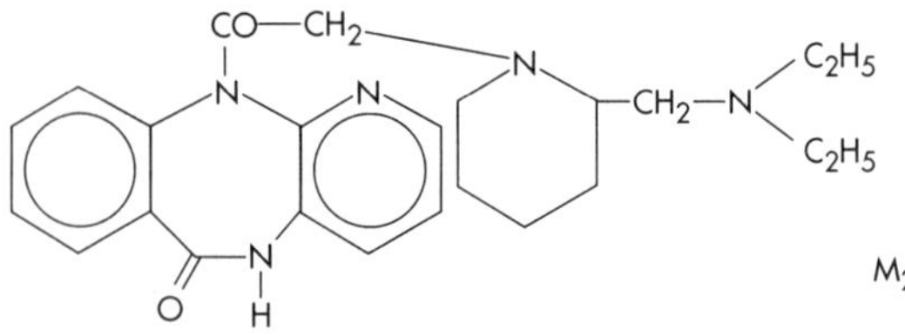

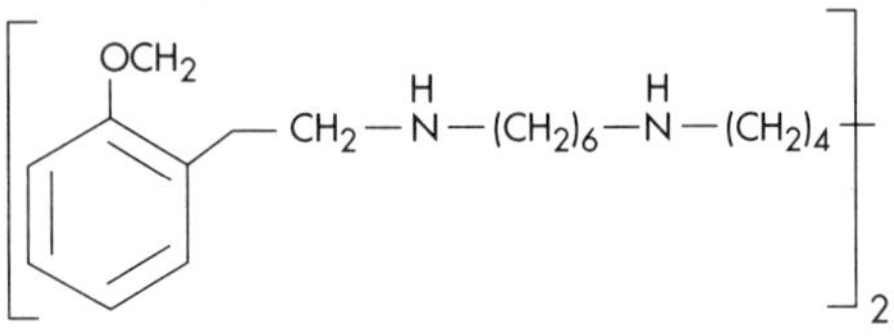

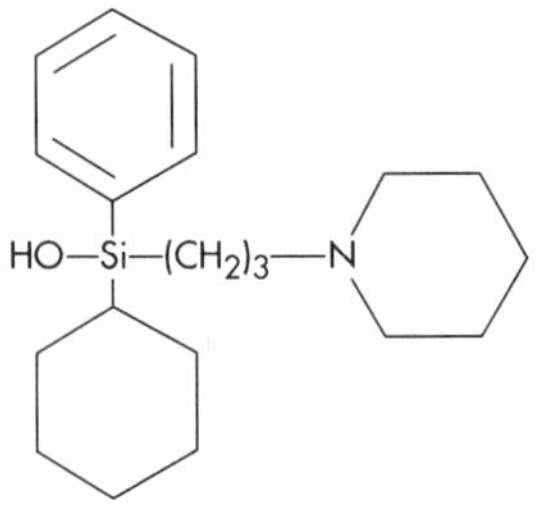

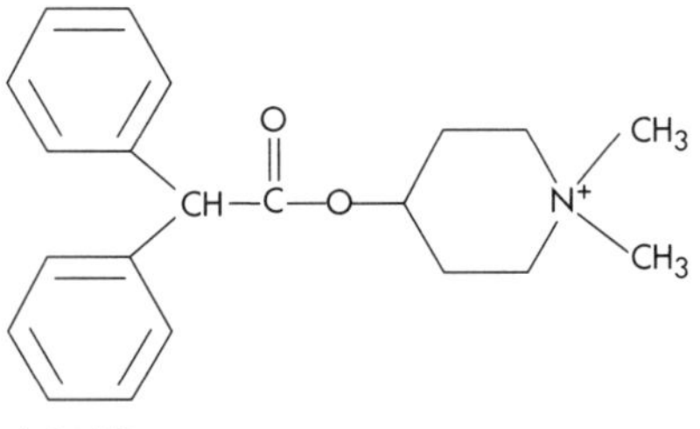

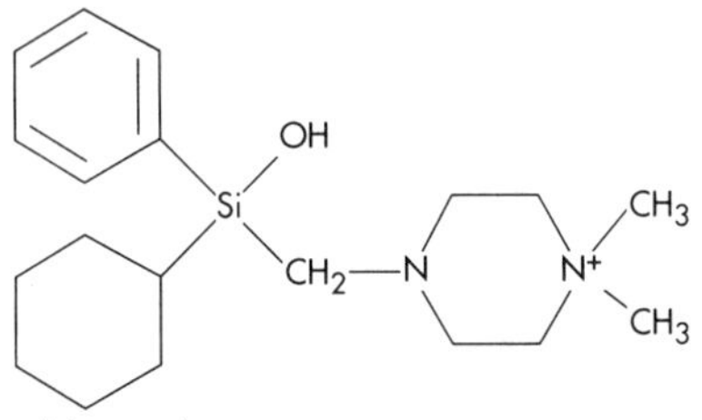

Figure 5.2 Subtype Selective Muscarinic Cholinergic Antagonists

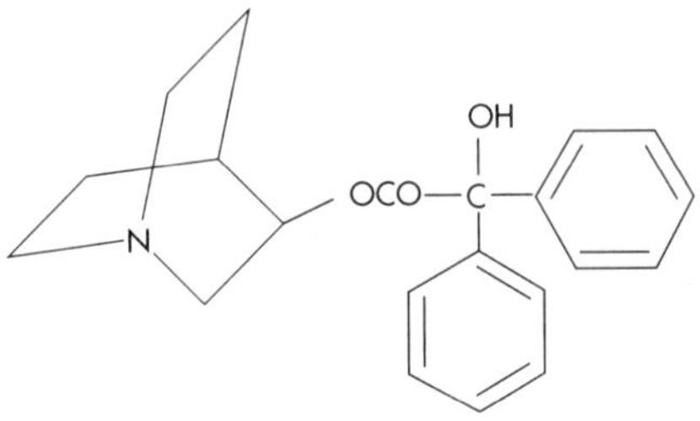

[^{3}H] QNB

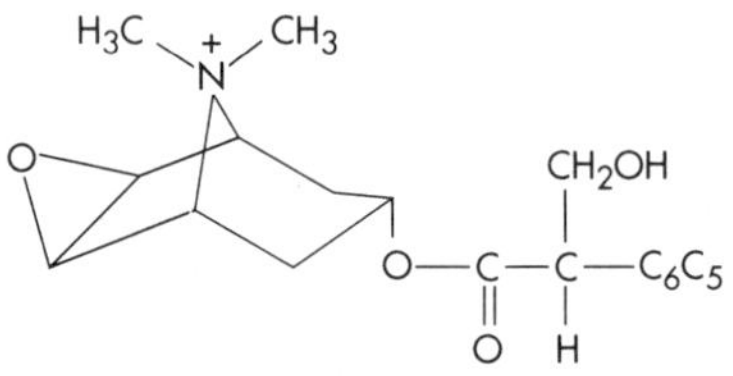

[^{3}H] NMS

Figure 5.3 Radioligands Utilized for Labeling Muscarinic Cholinergic Receptors

It was mentioned above that muscarinic cholinergic receptors can be either coupled to phosphatidyl inositol hydrolysis or inhibition of adenylate cyclase, and that the preferred second messenger depends on the receptor subtype.[14] Several other intracellular events can be induced by muscarinic cholinergic receptor activation, including calcium influx, phosphodiesterase activation, and increases in cyclic GMP,[15] although it is not clear whether these are independent events or whether one signal transduction system can secondarily activate others. It appears that an individual muscarinic receptor subtype can be coupled to multiple signal transduction mechanisms.[15]

Nicotinic Cholinergic Receptor Subtypes

It has long been known that there are two major classes of nicotinic acetylcholine receptors—those located at the neuromuscular junction (muscular) and those located at sympathetic ganglia and in the CNS (neuronal). This subdivision is based on both agonist and antagonist selectivity. The quaternary amines, DMPP and PTMA (phenyltrimethylammonium), activate neuronal and muscular-nicotinic cholinergic receptors, respectively. Furthermore, although both nicotinic cholinergic receptors are blocked by bisquarternary amines and related compounds (Fig. 5.4), the optimum distance between cationic centers differs substantially between muscular and neuronal receptors. Hexamethonium has little or no neuromuscular blocking activity, whereas the longer molecule, decamethonium, can depolarize and subsequently block the neuromuscular junction at concentrations having only minor effects at autonomic ganglia.

The pharmacology and structure of the skeletal muscle nicotinic cholinergic receptor has been studied extensively, aided by the availability of very similar receptors in high density in several marine organisms. This receptor is described in Chapters 1, 4, and 7. The neuronal nicotinic cholinergic receptor seems to have a similar structure, with multiple subunits surrounding a central ion channel. However, in contrast to the skeletal muscle receptor, the neuronal nicotinic cholinergic receptor is generally composed of only two different subunits. These subunits, each of which has four putative transmembrane spanning domains, are designated as α and β. The α subunit contains two adjacent cysteine molecules thought to be involved in acetylcholine binding. The configuration of the neuronal nicotinic receptor is not known with certainty. Although the assembled receptor must contain at least two of each subunit, the receptor could be either tetrameric (α_2, β_2) or pentameric ($\alpha_3\beta_2$).[r3] It is likely that at least some neuronal nicotinic cholinergic receptors contain two different α subunits.[16]

Most neuronal nicotinic cholinergic receptors are insensitive to α-bungarotoxin, a polypeptide component of a snake (*Bungarus multicinctus*) venom binding with extremely high affinity to the α-subunit of skeletal muscle nicotinic cholinergic receptors. Another component in the venom of this snake, neuronal bungarotoxin, will bind to neuronal nicotinic cholinergic receptors in autonomic ganglia and produce functional blockade of ganglionic transmission. However, at least some of the nicotinic receptors within the CNS have been shown to be insensitive to both α- and neuronal bungarotoxin.[r4] This possible heterogeneity in neuronal nicotinic cholinergic receptors is consistent with the identification of multiple forms of both the α and β subunits by receptor cloning and expression techniques. At the present time, seven distinct α subunits and four β subunits have been identified from mammalian or avian sources. Experimental recombination of these subunits can form receptors having characteristics similar to native neuronal nicotinic cholinergic receptors.[r4] It appears that nicotinic cholinergic receptors at peripheral autonomic ganglia have a different subunit composition compared with those in the CNS, and the particular α and β subunits comprising these receptors have been tentatively identified.[17,18] However, considerable additional research will be required to identify all of the physiologically significant nicotinic cholinergic receptors from the almost limitless number of receptors that can be assembled using various proportions of the subunits currently identified.

Although most neuronal nicotinic cholinergic receptors do not bind α-bungarotoxin, there are central binding sites for this toxin. The distribution of α-bungarotoxin binding sites and nicotine binding sites within the CNS is different,[19,r5,20] with the α-bungarotoxin sites being located predominantly extrasynaptically.[21] Recent evidence suggests that these sites may correspond to neuronal cholinergic receptors having characteristics similar to the nicotinic receptor at the neuromuscular junction, but differing in the primary amino acid sequence of each subunit.[22] Nicotinic cholinergic receptors sensitive to blockade by α-bungarotoxin have been identified in the chick optic lobe[23] and cerebellum,[24] consistent with the cloning of an α-subunit, designated as α_7, from avian brain having high affinity for this toxin. Reconstitution of cloned α_7 units in an amphibian oocyte membrane results in an ion channel that can be activated by nicotine and acetylcholine, and blocked by d-tubocurarine.[25] Using a fluorescence assay, nicotine was shown to induce an increase in intracellular calcium in chick ciliary ganglion neurons that could be blocked by low concentrations of α-bungarotoxin, showing that these sites can act as functional cholinergic receptors.[26] In some neuronal populations, these α-bungarotoxin sensitive receptors, whose function is still unknown, outnumber those nicotinic cholinergic receptors sensitive to neuronal bungarotoxin by five–tenfold,[27] although it is clear that cholinergic transmission is mediated by the latter group of receptors. Hence, it appears that there are at least three functional subclasses of the neuronal nicotinic cholinergic receptor, based on pharmacology, with further heterogeneity at the molecular level being likely.

Functional Role of Cholinergic Receptor Subtypes

Nicotinic Cholinergic Receptors

Neuromuscular Junction

Acetylcholine is the neurotransmitter at the specialized junction between the motor nerve and skeletal muscle. Synaptically released acetylcholine acts on nicotinic cholinergic receptors to initiate muscle contraction. This process has been studied extensively, and has been shown to result from an opening of the receptor-associated ion channel that initiates an action potential

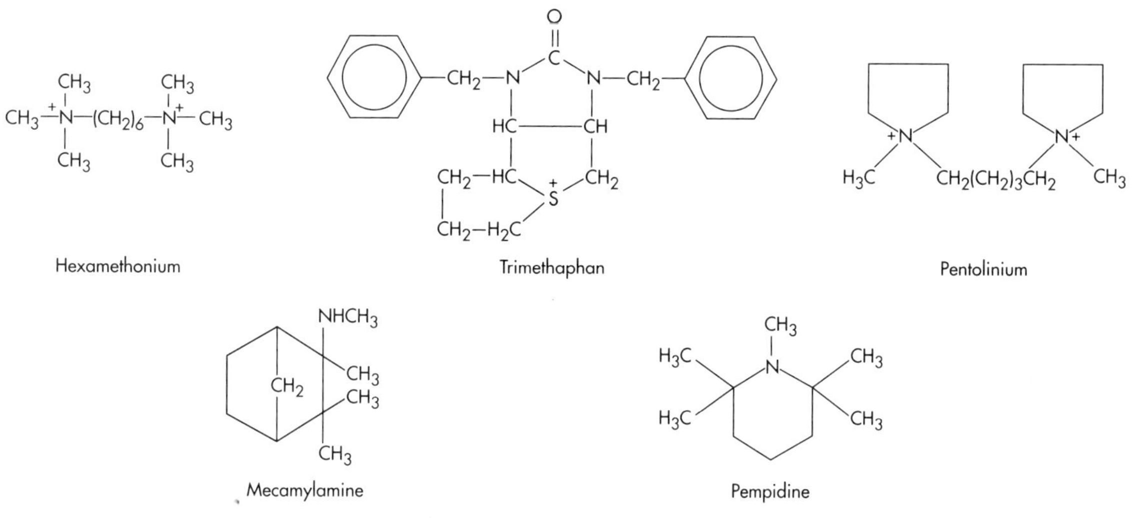

Hexamethonium

Trimethaphan

Pentolinium

Mecamylamine

Pempidine

Figure 5.4 Ganglionic Blocking Agents

in skeletal muscle cells. This process is described in more detail in Chapter 7.

Autonomic Ganglia

Acetylcholine is the principal neurotransmitter at both sympathetic and parasympathetic ganglia. Although the neuronally released acetylcholine activates both nicotinic and muscarinic cholinergic receptors, the initial rapid EPSP (excitatory postsynaptic potential) induced by activation of nicotinic cholinergic receptors on the cell bodies of postganglionic neurons is responsible for the chemical transmission of the neuronal action potential through the ganglion. A nicotinic cholinergic receptor antagonist, such as hexamethonium, is capable of completely abolishing ganglionic transmission. As in skeletal muscle, activation of the nicotinic cholinergic receptor initiates an action potential via the opening of an ion channel, which allows the rapid translocation of Na^+ ions into the neuron.

Central Nervous System

Although nicotinic cholinergic receptors are present at a variety of locations within the mammalian CNS, few neurons have been shown to produce a classic nicotinic cholinergic response to electrical stimulation or to the administration of exogenous acetylcholine. The classic example of a nicotinic response in a CNS neuron is the Renshaw cell, a spinal interneuron responsible for recurrent inhibition of spinal motor neurons. The fast and sharp increase in activity produced by cholinergic stimulation of the Renshaw cell is quite similar to peripheral nicotinic cholinergic responses. Other central neurons showing such responses are found in the lateral geniculate nucleus, medulla, thalamus, and supraoptic hypothalamic nucleus. However, in all of these neurons, even the Renshaw cell, a muscarinic response is often produced, and may predominate under some experimental conditions. Some neurons have been shown to exhibit an "intermediate" response to acetylcholine, sensitive to blockade by both muscarinic and nicotinic antagonists.

Presynaptic Nicotinic Cholinergic Receptors

Koelle[28,29] postulated that activation of presynaptic nicotinic cholinergic receptors could enhance the stimulation-evoked release of acetylcholine from preganglionic autonomic fibers and from motor nerve terminals. This positive feedback system appears to function in the intestinal myenteric plexus, but evidence in other peripheral autonomic neurons and at postganglionic cholinergic terminals is less conclusive, as are experiments in brain slice and synaptosomal preparations from various areas of the CNS.[r6] Perhaps some of the conflicting data result from the ability of presynaptic nicotinic receptor stimulation to either facilitate or depress ganglionic neurotransmission, depending on experimental conditions and the preparation studied.[r7] Nicotinic cholinergic receptor activation can also facilitate acetylcholine release at the neuromuscular junction, at least under some conditions. Agonist and antagonist sensitivity confirms that these prejunctional nicotinic cholinergic receptors have characteristics of neuronal, as opposed to skeletal muscle, nicotinic cholinergic receptors.

Nicotinic cholinergic receptors are present on postganglionic sympathetic nerve terminals, where their activation results in enhancement of stimulation-evoked release of norepinephrine. This prejunctional receptor has the characteristics commonly associated with nicotinic cholinergic receptors at other sites, (e.g., rapid onset of biologic response followed by a rapid desensitization). There is no convincing evidence for presynaptic nicotinic cholinergic receptors on central noradrenergic neurons. In contrast, presynaptic nicotinic cholinergic receptors appear to be present on striatal dopaminergic terminals, where their activation accelerates neurotransmitter release.

Muscarinic Cholinergic Receptors

Autonomic Ganglia

Although the primary impulse transmission through autonomic ganglia in mediated by nicotinic cholinergic receptors (see above), the muscarinic cholinergic receptor plays an important role in the modulation of this impulse transmission. Muscarinic receptor activation is responsible for the slow EPSP generated by iontophoretic application of acetylcholine to autonomic ganglia. This response appears to be mediated by M_1 receptors. Muscarinic cholinergic receptor activation also appears to contribute to the inhibitory postsynaptic potential (IPSP) observed upon recording from postganglionic cell bodies. This IPSP can be blocked both by muscarinic and α-adrenergic receptor antagonists, leading to the hypothesis that it is mediated by the activation of muscarinic-cholinergic receptors located on adrenergic interneurons which inhibit the postganglionic neuron. The muscarinic cholinergic receptor involved in this response has been shown to be of the M_2 subtype in certain ganglia.

Parasympathetic Effector Organs

Many organs receive parasympathetic innervation, including the heart, stomach, bladder, and secretory glands. Acetylcholine released from postganglionic parasympathetic neurons acts on muscarinic cholinergic receptors. In contrast to the nicotinic cholinergic receptor, which usually initiates an action potential when activated, muscarinic cholinergic receptor stimulation generally modulates ongoing mechanical and/or electrical activity of an effector organ. Activation of muscarinic cholinergic receptors may mediate an excitatory response, such as stimulation of smooth muscle contraction (GI system, bladder, uterus, respiratory tract), stimulation of glandular secretion (parietal cell, other secretory cells of the stomach, pancreas, salivary gland), contraction of specialized smooth muscles in the eye (sphincter of iris and ciliary muscle of the lens) or an inhibitory response (inhibition of the depolarization rate of the SA nodal pacemaker). Conduction through the AV node is also inhibited as a result of muscarinic cholinergic receptor activation. Muscarinic receptor activation also generally reduces tone of sphincters in the GI and urogenital systems. Parasympathetic vasodilator nerves innervate some blood vessels, including those of the brain, tongue, salivary glands, and penis. Although stimulation of muscarinic cholinergic receptors on vascular smooth muscle generally induces vasoconstriction, nerve-induced cholinergic vasoconstriction is not commonly observed in mammalian species (see Chapter 4).

The muscarinic cholinergic receptor mediating the effects of parasympathetic stimulation appears to be of either the M_2 (cardiac tissue) or M_3 (GI and bronchial smooth muscle and secretory glands) subtype. Based on the relatively low antagonist potency of AF-DX 116, the urinary bladder may also represent an M_3 response.[30] Although the functional contraction of smooth muscle induced by cholinergic receptor activation may be mediated primarily by the M_3 receptor, radioligand binding studies generally show the presence of both the M_2 and M_3 receptor subtypes in smooth muscle. Experiments in the isolated guinea pig uterus indicated that the pharmacology of carbachol-induced contraction differs from other smooth muscle preparations. The response in this tissue can be blocked both by preferential M_2 (AF-DX 116 and methoctramine) and M_3 (4-DAMP and silahexocyclium) antagonists. The correlation between antagonist potency values and ability to inhibit radioligand binding to rat striatum has led to the proposal that the guinea pig uterus represents an M_4-mediated functional response.[12]

Cholinergic Sympathetic Effector Organs

Although most postganglionic sympathetic nerves release norepinephrine, those innervating sweat glands and some specialized blood vessels release acetylcholine, which acts on muscarinic cholinergic receptors. Vasodilation in skeletal muscle can result from activation of sympathetic cholinergic fibers. Some sympathetic cholinergic neurons innervate the blood vessels of the skin, but appear not to play an important role in the regulation of cutaneous blood flow.

Blood Vessels and Endothelium

Although parasympathetic or cholinergic sympathetic nerves do not play a major role in the control of blood flow in vascular beds, most arteries possess muscarinic cholinergic receptors on both smooth muscle and vascular endothelium. At least in the CNS, combined histochemical/functional studies provide convincing evidence for nerve-induced vasoconstriction mediated by acetylcholine acting at muscarinic cholinergic receptors.[31] In isolated vessels with intact endothelium, and in the intact animal, activation of endothelial muscarinic receptors results in vasodilation. This effect has been shown to be mediated via the release of nitric oxide, either free or complexed with a carrier molecule, from the endothelial cell. If the endothelium is damaged, muscarinic stimulation results in vasoconstriction as a result of activation muscarinic cholinergic receptors on the vascular smooth muscle. Characterization of the muscarinic cholinergic receptors subtypes involved in these responses has yielded inconclusive results to date. Recent functional evidence shows the endothelial and smooth muscle receptors of rabbit aorta have M_3 and M_2 cholinergic receptor characteristics, respectively, although radioligand binding[32] and second messenger studies[33] in this tissue are not consistent with this assignment.

Central Nervous System

Muscarinic cholinergic receptors are widely distributed throughout the CNS. Radioligand binding studies suggest the presence of all known receptor subtypes, and molecular biologic probes show expression of all of the receptor proteins which have been cloned. As noted above, almost all central cholinergic neurotransmission involves muscarinic cholinergic receptor activation, even where a nicotinic-cholinergic response in present. Often, only the muscarinic component can be demonstrated. Muscarinic cholinergic receptor activation usually produces a slow depolarization of central neurons, although examples of hyperpolarization are known. It was initially proposed that the central muscarinic effect is a consequence of a decrease in potassium conductance. However, recent evidence with subtype selective agents suggests that M_2 receptor activation may increase potassium conductance, whereas the M_1 subtype is associated with a decrease in potassium permeability.[34] In most cases cholinergic neurotransmission within the CNS is inferred from the presence of enzymatic pathways for the synthesis and degradation of acetylcholine, and an uptake system for choline. The actual demonstration of central cholinergic synapses is impossible in most cases.

The central cholinergic system is concentrated in a diffuse tract ascending from the tegmentum through the mesencephalon to the cortex. In addition to the cortex, structures such as the cerebellum, septum, limbic system, and habenula receive cholinergic innervation from branches of this neuronal tract. This pathway is generally excitatory, although inhibitory cholinergic systems may also terminate in the cortex. A pharmacologically important pathway is present in the striatum, where dopaminergic neurons originating in the substantial nigra block the activity of cholinergic interneurons. As expected from the diversity of central cholinergic pathways, central cholinergic transmission is involved in a multitude of physiologic and pharmacologic responses. Some examples of the many effects which can be induced by general or localized central cholinergic stimulation include: the induction of seizures; the production REM (rapid eye movement) sleep; the enhancement of memory acquisition; the induction of catalepsy or stereotype; enhanced aggression; polydipsia; stimulation of hypothalamic somatostatin release; analgesia; and enhanced sexual activity. In many cases, muscarinic cholinergic receptor blockade will induce the opposite effect, suggesting that these effects are modulated by ongoing activity of cholinergic neurons, acting through muscarinic receptors.

Presynaptic Muscarinic Cholinergic Receptors

There is now substantial experimental evidence to suggest that the often conflicting data regarding the effect of muscarinic stimulation and blockade on neuromuscular transmission may be explained by the presence of both inhibitory and facilitory muscarinic cholinergic receptors on the motor nerve terminal.[r8] There is extensive evidence for prejunctional muscarinic cholinergic receptors acting to inhibit neurotransmitter release from peripheral cholinergic nerve terminals. Functional inhibition of transmission or acetylcholine release has been demonstrated from postganglionic innervation of the GI system, bronchi, bladder, and heart. In contrast, some preganglionic sympathetic nerves (e.g., those supplying the superior cervical ganglion and adrenal medulla) appear not to possess presynaptic muscarinic cholinergic receptors, although muscarinic stimulation can inhibit acetylcholine release from preganglionic myenteric neurons.

Inhibitory muscarinic autoreceptors (i.e., receptors modulating transmitter release from cholinergic nerve terminals) have been demonstrated in brain slice and synaptosomal preparations of cerebral cortex, hippocampus, striatum and brainstem. In vivo experiments measuring striatal acetylcholine release also support the presence of central muscarinic autoinhibition, although actions on cholinergic receptors located on the cell body cannot be discounted.

Stimulation of prejunctional muscarinic receptors on postganglionic sympathetic neurons can inhibit adrenergic neurotransmission (e.g., in isolated blood vessels). Within the CNS, presynaptic muscarinic cholinergic receptors have been identified on noncholinergic neurons on dopaminergic, excitatory amino acid (glutamate, aspartate), and GABAergic neurons.[35] In contrast to the other muscarinic cholinergic receptors, which inhibit neurotransmitter release, the presynaptic muscarinic receptor on striatal dopaminergic neurons results in a facilitation of dopamine release.[36] It appears that prejunctional and presynaptic muscarinic cholinergic receptors may be of the M_1, M_2, or M_3 subtype, and there appear to be significant species differences. As noted above, the M_4 subtype also may contribute to this action.

Drugs Interacting with Nicotinic Cholinergic Receptors

Nicotinic Receptor Agonists

Stimulation of nicotinic cholinergic receptors at the neuromuscular junction has therapeutic application in several myasthenic states characterized by pre- or postjunctional defects in cholinergic transmission. This is accomplished either by promoting the release of acetylcholine, with agents such as 4-aminopyridine, or by inhibition of the degradation of endogenously released acetylcholine with inhibitors of acetylcholinesterase. For a further description of the use of these agents, see Chapter 7.

Stimulation of ganglionic or CNS nicotinic cholinergic receptors has no known therapeutic application, although the systemic administration of nicotine (i.e., from inhaled tobacco products) has widespread pharmacologic actions. A small clinical trial has provided evidence suggesting that systemic administration of nicotine may have beneficial effects on memory and information processing deficits in patients with Alzheimer's disease.[37] Selective ganglionic stimulants (e.g., DMPP) are utilized as pharmacologic tools. Therapeutic doses of cholinergic receptor agonists having activity at the nicotinic receptor, (e.g., carbachol) do not produce effects attributable to stimulation of ganglionic nicotinic cholinergic receptors. Neuromuscular blockade with pancuronium can increase blood pressure, possibly as a result of blockade of cardiac muscarinic cholinergic receptors, with subsequent tachycardia and increased cardiac output.

Nicotinic Cholinergic Antagonists

Antagonists of the action of acetylcholine at nicotinic cholinergic receptors of the neuromuscular junction are used extensively as neuromuscular blocking agents during surgical procedures (see Chapter 13).

Blockade of ganglionic neurotransmission was one of the first approaches to the pharmacologic treatment of hypertension. Both the bis-quaternary agents (hexamethonium, pentolinium) as well as singly charged species (trimethaphan) and tertiary amines (mecamylamine, pempidine) have been employed for acute or chronic therapy. However, the cardiovascular effects of ganglionic blocking agents are complex, since transmission through both sympathetic and parasympathetic ganglia is blocked, and the net effect depends on the balance between sympathetic and parasympathetic tone prior to drug administration. Orthostatic hypotension is frequent and often severe. In addition to effects on vascular tone, ganglionic blocking agents inhibit propulsive activity of the GI system, which can result in erratic absorption of orally-administered agents. Micturition, penile erection, and ejaculation also are impaired. With the development of newer antihypertensive drugs with more selective action and fewer side-effects, there is no longer much use for ganglionic blocking agents in the chronic treatment of essential hypertension, or even in the acute management of hypertensive crisis. However, ganglionic blockade is still used in the initial control of blood pressure in acute dissecting aortic aneurysm, the acute relief of pulmonary edema associated with severe pulmonary hypertension, the acute control of autonomic hyperreflexia during surgical procedures on patients with upper spinal cord lesions, and in the induction of controlled hypotension during surgery. Intravenous administration of trimethaphan, or other short-acting ganglionic blockers, has been used for these indications.

Several early trials with hexamethonium showed beneficial effects in congestive heart failure, consistent with current hypotheses suggesting that excess sympathetic activity is detrimental in this condition.[38] However, chronic therapy with ganglionic blocking drugs is not practical, owing to the many side-effects caused by their nonselective action. Although acid secretion is also inhibited by ganglionic blocking agents, other approaches with lower side-effect liability are available for the treatment of gastric and duodenal ulcer.

Drugs Acting at Muscarinic Cholinergic Receptors

Stimulation of muscarinic cholinergic receptors has several important therapeutic applications. This effect can be achieved either via administration of exogenous muscarinic cholinergic agonists, or by inhibition of the degradation of endogenous acetylcholine with anticholinesterase agents.

Cholinesterase Inhibitors

The chemical structures of therapeutically useful cholinesterase inhibitors, and their biochemical mechanisms of action are presented in Chapter 7. In addition to their use in myasthenic states, these drugs can stimulate the smooth muscle of the urinary bladder or GI tract. This is sometimes required to relieve paralytic ileus and bladder atony following surgery. Neostigmine is the drug most commonly employed agent for these conditions. For example, SQ administration will generally restore intestinal peristaltic activity within 30 minutes and cause the return of spontaneous urination. Oral neostigmine is also effective for these indications, but the onset of therapeutic action is substantially slower. Short-acting cholinesterase inhibitors, such as edrophonium, can be used to terminate episodes of paroxysmal supraventricular tachycardia.

Topical administration of cholinesterase inhibitors is useful in reducing the elevated intraocular pressure associated with glaucoma. Although muscarinic cholinergic receptor stimulation will lower intraocular pressure in both narrow-angle and wide-angle glaucoma, the utility of cholinesterase inhibitors is limited primarily to chronic therapy of wide-angle glaucoma, since narrow-angle glaucoma usually requires a rapid reduction in intraocular pressure, which may be more easily attained by direct application of a muscarinic agonist (see below) and/or by the IV administration of agents capable of reducing intraocular pressure by other mechanisms (i.e., reducing aqueous humor secretion or inducing ocular dehydration).

Although there is no anatomic obstruction to aqueous humor outflow in wide-angle glaucoma, constriction of the sphincter and ciliary muscles increases tone and changes the alignment of the trabecular network so as to facilitate the outflow of aqueous humor into the canal of Schlemm.[39] Both short-acting, reversible, cholinesterase inhibitors, such as physostigmine or neostigmine, and long-acting agents, either reversible (demecarium) or irreversible (echothiophate, isoflurophate) have been used.

Significant potential for the production of side-effects exists for the topical cholinesterase inhibitors. These may be mechanism-based, such as impairment of accommodation and exacerbation of myopia as a result of actions on the ciliary muscle. Symptoms related to systemic cholinesterase inhibition also can result, especially with the irreversible inhibitors; systemic effects can involve any of the many organ systems under cholinergic control, including the cardiovascular (bradycardia), urinary (incontinence), exocrine glands (salivation, sweating), or GI (abdominal cramps, diarrhea) systems. In addition to mechanism-based side-effects, long-term treatment with topical cholinesterase inhibitors can be associated with the development of lens opacities and iris cysts. Ocular administration of long-acting cholinesterase inhibitors is also useful in cases of convergent strabismus resulting from alterations in accommodation.

Muscarinic Cholinergic Agonists

Direct-acting muscarinic agonists are used for several of the indications discussed above for the cholinesterase inhibitors. Some of the preparations available for clinical use in the US are shown in Table 5.1. Although potential selectivity of agonists for muscarinic cholinergic receptors has not been investigated extensively, oral and SQ administration of certain muscarinic agonists can result in apparent tissue selectivity. For example, carbachol and bethanechol can produce therapeutic actions on the smooth muscle of the urinary bladder and GI tract with no substantial effect on blood pressure. This is a consequence of the ability of baroreceptor reflexes to compensate for the vasodilation produced by activation of muscarinic cholinergic receptors on the vascular endothelium, provided that plasma levels of the agonist rise slowly. If the same drugs are administered IV, this apparent selectivity is lost. Methacholine has been used to produce vasodilation in peripheral vascular disease, both by systemic and local iontophoretic administration, and to terminate episodes of paroxysmal supraventricular tachycardia through its vagomimetic action. Other modes of therapy have proved superior in both indications, and methacholine is not in current clinical use.

Bethanechol, via the oral or SQ route, is useful for postsurgical stimulation of the GI tract or urinary bladder, as described above for the cholinesterase inhibitors. This agonist is also occasionally used to increase the tone of the lower esophageal sphincter to reduce reflux. Although carbachol has a similar clinical profile, it is not currently administered systemically, owing to its greater propensity to stimulate nicotinic cholinergic receptors. Since both GI and bladder smooth muscle is stimulated by bethanechol, it is difficult to stimulate one system without producing side-effects related to stimulation of the other (i.e., vomiting and abdominal cramps or urinary urgency). Other side-effects commonly associated with cholinergic agonists are sweating, salivation, stimulation of GI secretions, and bronchoconstriction, which can precipitate an asthma attack in susceptible subjects. Aerosol administration of methacholine can be used as a diagnostic test to detect asymptomatic individuals with enhanced airway responsiveness.

In view of the experimental evidence for a role of central muscarinic cholinergic receptors in memory acquisition and the observed deficits in cholinergic function observed in patients with Alzheimer's disease,[39] there has been extensive research directed toward drugs capable of enhancing central muscarinic receptor activation as an approach to this debilitating condition. Mechanistic approaches evaluated have included: acetylcholine precursors (e.g., choline); agents stimulating synaptic acetylcholine release (e.g., 4-aminopyridine analogues); and acetylcholinesterase inhibitors as well as directly-acting muscarinic agonists. Most muscarinic agonists do not cross the blood-brain barrier. However, a recent study using continuous intracerebroventricular administration of bethanechol via a surgically-inserted cannula has shown some evidence of a beneficial effect on symptoms and memory capability in Alzheimer's patients, although beneficial effects were observed only in a narrow dosage range.[40]

Ocular application of muscarinic cholinergic agonists is a common therapeutic approach to glaucoma (see rationale above for cholinesterase inhibitors). Pilocarpine is the agonist typically employed for this indication. This agonist, unlike those possessing a quaternary nitrogen atom (Fig. 5.1) is not fully protonated at physiologic pH and hence has better access to the interior of the eye. Combination of pilocarpine with other antiglaucoma drugs, such as epinephrine or β-adrenoceptor antagonists, can produce a synergistic effect. Ocular side-effects induced by pilocarpine (paralysis of accommodation, enhanced myopia) are similar to those observed with the cholinesterase inhibitors, although an increased incidence of lenticular opacities is not observed with pilocarpine, and systemic side-effects are uncommon. Carbachol is also employed for

Table 5.1 Clinical Parameters for Cholinergic Agonists

Name	Preparation	Approx Dose Freq & Route
Bethanechol	Injection 5mg/ml	2.5–5 mg, SQ
	Tablet 5–50 mg	10–50 mg, tid-qid
Carbachol	Opthalmic Solution 0.75–3%	2 drops, tid
Pilocarpine	Opthalmic Solution 0.25–10%	2 drops, tid-qid
	Ocular Insert .02–.04 mg/hr	1 insert per week

the treatment of glaucoma, and may be effective in patients resistant to pilocarpine. Systemic side-effects may be more common with carbachol than with pilocarpine. Either carbachol or acetylcholine are used in ophthalmic surgery when rapid induction of miosis is required.

Muscarinic Cholinergic Receptor Antagonists

Muscarinic cholinergic receptor antagonists, including the plant alkaloids, atropine and scopolamine, and many synthetic molecules of widely varied chemical structure (Fig. 5.5) have been used extensively both as pharmacologic tools and therapeutic agents for a wide variety of indications. Data on some of the particular drugs used clinically in the US are provided in Table 5.2. In its native form, atropine has been used for its medicinal and toxic effects for many centuries, and the anticholinergic activity of the purified alkaloid has been known for over 100 years. Since potent and selective muscarinic antagonists have long been available, and since many systems of the body are under parasympathetic control, muscarinic blockade has been utilized for a wide array of clinical indications. In the past, muscarinic antagonists were used as primary therapy for peptic ulcer, bronchial asthma, and Parkinson's disease. Although significant therapeutic benefit is observed in each of these conditions, the diversity of parasympathetic innervation leads to multiple side-effects of generalized muscarinic blockade. Therefore, as other pharmacologic approaches offering greater selectivity have been developed, these uses of muscarinic antagonists have declined. The muscarinic antagonists remain important drugs, however, and the availability of subtype selective antagonists may increase their therapeutic utility even further.

Cardiovascular actions of muscarinic cholinergic antagonists are usually utilized for acute therapy to blunt the effects of excessive vagal activity. Following myocardial infarction, atropine is often used to prevent excessive bradycardia and atrioventricular block. However, the dose must be titrated carefully, since atropine can often produce a paradoxical bradycardia at low doses, and tachycardia if the dose is too high. The bradycardic action of atropine in man is now known to be due to a slight selectivity of this antagonist for M_1 receptors, resulting, at low doses, in preferential blockade of inhibitory prejunctional M_1 receptors and a consequent enhancement of vagal acetylcholine release. As the dose of atropine is increased, muscarinic subtype selectivity is lost, and the net effect is tachycardia as a result of blockade of M_2 receptors in the sinoatrial node.[r10] Atropine is also effective in cases of bradycardia associated with a hyperactive carotid sinus reflex. It is possible that selective M_2 receptor antagonists, such as AF-DX 116, may eventually be used for these indications.

Muscarinic cholinergic antagonists will blunt vagally-induced gastric acid secretion and will reduce intestinal motility. Before the introduction of the histamine H_2 receptor antagonists, muscarinic blockade was widely used as anti-ulcer therapy. Side-effects due to blockade of other muscarinic receptors (dry mouth, mydriasis, failure of accommodation, tachycardia, urinary retention) were unavoidable with the nonselective antagonists employed clinically, especially since the gastric secretory response is relatively resistant to muscarinic receptor blockade. Effects on the CNS could be avoided by the use of quaternary compounds, such as methantheline and propantheline. These compounds were also purported to show fewer peripheral side-effects when used in anti-ulcer therapy, although some evidence of ganglionic and neuromuscular receptor block is often observed with propantheline (e.g., impotence or muscular weakness). The availability of M_1 selective antagonists, such as pirenzipine and its analogues, has stimulated renewed interest in muscarinic cholinergic antagonists as anti-ulcer agents, especially since the effects of M_1 muscarinic and H_2 histaminergic receptor blockade may be synergistic. Although muscarinic cholinergic antagonists are effective against symptoms of intestinal hypermotility and diarrhea induced by adrenergic neuronal blockers or by mild infectious conditions, they are not generally effective against more severe conditions induced by salmonella, ulcerative colitis, or regional enteritis.

Muscarinic cholinergic antagonists also have a long history of utility in respiratory disorders. These agents can block nerve-induced bronchoconstriction and inhibit secretion from the upper and lower respiratory tract. The symptomatic efficacy of "over-the-counter" cold remedies results largely from the antimuscarinic activity of the antihistamines present in these mixtures. Although the bronchodilator activity of muscarinic antagonists may at times be useful in bronchial asthma, the reduction in volume of bronchial secretion can result in viscous secretions that obstruct airflow and predispose to infection. Ipratropium, the N-isopropyl derivative of atropine, appears to have bronchodilator effects without affecting the volume or viscosity or bronchial secretions and is effective in relieving the bronchospasm associated with chronic obstructive pulmonary disease.

The ability of muscarinic antagonists to inhibit secretions from the respiratory tract makes these agents useful as adjuncts to general anesthesia, since manipulation of the airway increases secretion via an irritant action. Muscarinic blockade is also commonly used in combination with neostigmine to achieve selective stimulation of nicotinic receptors after administration of cholinesterase inhibitors to reverse the action of nondepolarizing neuromuscular blocking agents (see Chapters 7 and 13).

Cholinergic neurons play an important role in the control of motor function by the basal ganglia. In general, cholinergic and dopaminergic neurons oppose one another in this system. In Parkinson's disease, the degeneration of dopaminergic neurons results in a dominance of cholinergic activity. Central muscarinic blockade can restore the balance between dopaminergic and cholinergic tone. Prior to the availability of levodopa, muscarinic antagonists represented the only effective therapy for Parkinsonism. Although the efficacy of muscarinic cholinergic antagonists is less than levodopa, these drugs still have an important role in the treatment of Parkinsonism, being used in patients with mild disease, in those where levodopa or other dopaminergic agonists cannot be tolerated, and as a supplement to levodopa therapy to improve the degree of therapeutic benefit. The specific muscarinic antagonists used for this indication (Fig. 5.5) all cross the blood-brain barrier readily, and appear to produce side-effects associated with peripheral muscarinic blockade less frequently than do the naturally occurring alkaloids. Nevertheless, paralysis of accommodation, constipation, and urinary retention are commonly observed.

Although the ocular actions of muscarinic cholinergic antagonists have no therapeutic application, and often give rise to side-effects when muscarinic receptor blockade at other sites is desired, muscarinic cholinergic antagonists are commonly used to induce mydriasis and cycloplegia (paralysis of accommodation) during ocular examination and to allow effective therapy of certain ocular

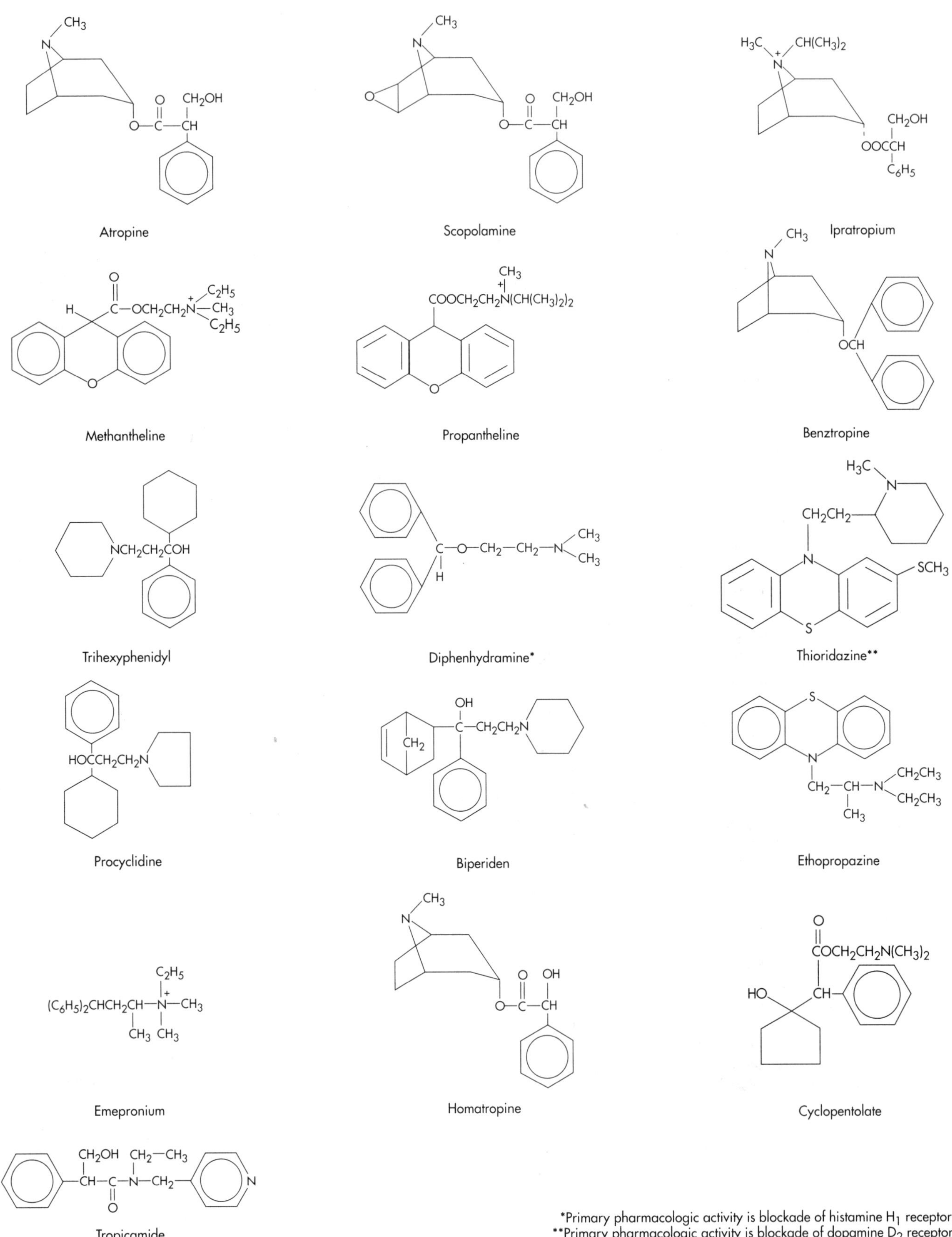

Figure 5.5 Examples of Therapeutically Useful Muscarinic Cholinergic Antagonists

Table 5.2 Clinical Parameters for Muscarinic Antagonists

Name	Approx Dose (mg) Freq & Route	Potency (Atropine = 1)
Atropine	*	1
(Hyoscyamine)	0.25–0.5 mg, IM, IV or SQ 0.125–0.25 mg, PO, hid	2
Scopolamine	0.5 mg delivered transdermally over 3-day period	1
Biperiden	2 mg, IM OR IV 2–4 mg, PO, qid	0.1–1[a]
Dicyclomine	20 mg, IM 20–40 mg, PO, qid	0.01–0.1[a]
Propantheline	7.5–15 mg, PO, tid-qid	
Mepenzolate	25–50 mg, PO, qid	
Benztropine	0.5–6 mg, IM or IV 1–2 mg, PO, bid-tid	0.5–1
Trihexyphenidyl	2–5 mg, PO, tid	0.1–1[a]
Procyclidine	2.5–5 mg, PO, tid	0.03–0.1
Ipratropium	36 μg, via inhalation, bid	1
Oxybutynin	5 mg, PO, bid-qid	0.3–1

*Although atropine (dl-hyoscyamine) is a component of many pharmaceutical preparations, it is not currently prescribed in the USA in a preparation containing only atropine as the active agent. The active enantiomer (l-hyoscyamine) is available in both oral and parenteral preparations.

[a]Shows moderate (10–50 fold) selectivity for M_1 versus M_2 muscarinic cholinergic receptors in functional isolated tissue (Lambrecht *et al.*, 1988) or radioligand binding (Lazareno et al., 1990) assays.

inflammations. Atropine or scopolamine is used to produce mydriasis and cycloplegia of prolonged duration, as is required in the treatment of inflammation, while shorter-acting agents, such as homatropine, cyclopentolate, and tropicamide, are used for diagnostic procedures. Alternative treatment with a muscarinic receptor agonist and antagonist can be useful in breaking adhesions between the iris and lens. Ocular or even systemic administration of a muscarinic cholinergic antagonist can precipitate an attack of narrow-angle glaucoma in susceptible individuals. Careful ophthalmologic examination should be performed before initiating intensive or prolonged mydriatic therapy, since complete and rapid reversal of mydriasis induced by atropine or scoploamine is nearly impossible.

Muscarinic receptor blockade is useful in the treatment of urinary incontinence associated with detrusor instability. The pharmacologic approach commonly used is to combine muscarinic receptor blockade with another pharmacologic action that also affects bladder smooth muscle, such as nonspecific spasmolytic activity (flavoxate, dicyclomine) or calcium channel blockade (terodiline) (Fig. 5.6). Muscarinic cholinergic antagonists having some nicotinic receptor antagonist activity, such as methantheline, propantheline or emepronium, may also offer a greater therapeutic to side-effect ratio. However, despite the additional pharmacologic actions of these agents, the effects on micturition appear to correlate with their antimuscarinic activity, at least in experimental animal models.[41]

In conclusion, it is clear that, although much recent progress has been made, many aspects of cholinergic neurotransmission are not yet completely understood. Whether the M_4 and M_5 receptor binding sites represent

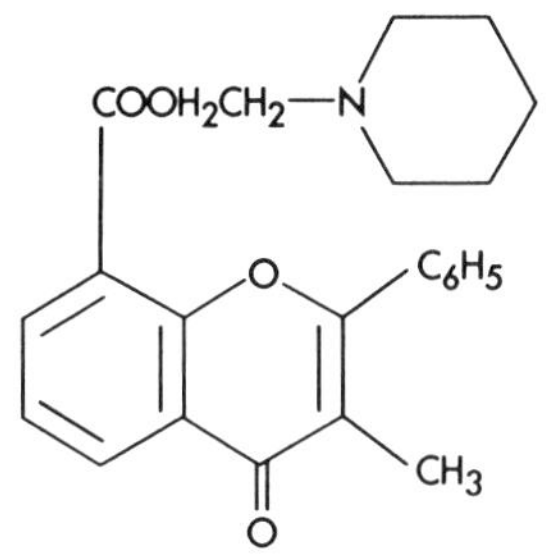

Flavoxate

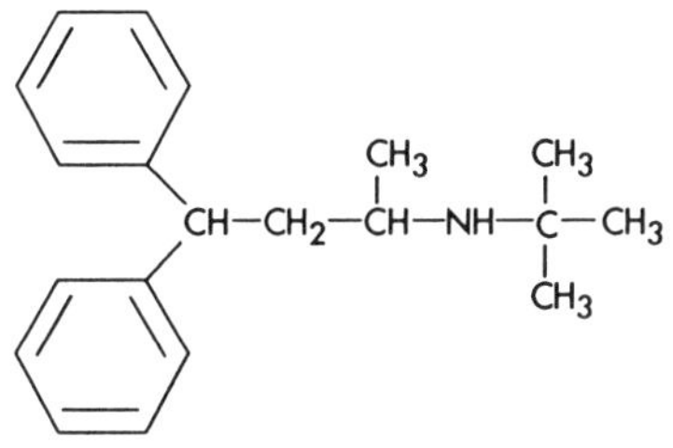

Terodiline

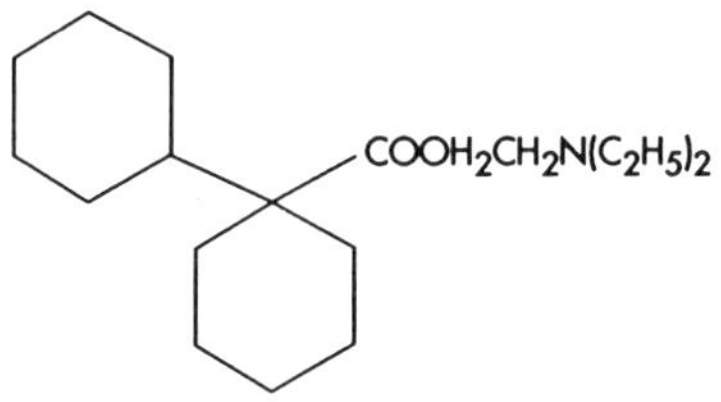

Dicylomine

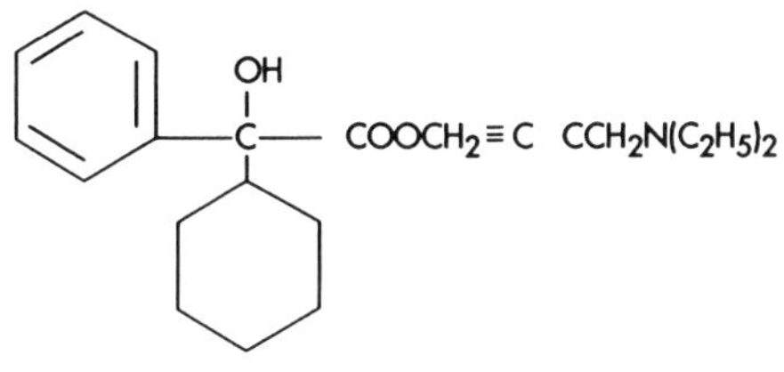

Oxybutinin

Figure 5.6 Muscarinic Antagonist/Antispasmodics

functional muscarinic cholinergic receptors is unknown, as is their role in physiologic regulation and as targets for drug action. Although most cholinergic receptor agonists and antagonists in current clinical use have little receptor subtype selectivity, they are important therapeutic tools. However, as more selective agents become available, more effective therapy, and perhaps even new therapeutic indications, are a likely consequence.

References

Research Report

1. Kimura H, McGeer PI, Peng JH, McGeer EG. The central cholinergic system studied by choline acetyltransferase immunohistochemistry in the cat. J Compar Neurol 1981;*200*:151–201.
2. Mesulam M-M, Mufson EJ, Wainer BH, Levey AI. Central cholinergic pathways in the rat: An overview based on an alternative nomenclature. Neurosci 1983;*4*:1185–1201.
3. Woolf NJ, Butcher LL. Cholinergic systems in the rat brain: III. Projections from the pontomesencephalic tegmentum to the thalamus, tectum, basal ganglia and basal forebrain. Brain Res Bull 1986;*16*:603–637.
4. Hulme EC, Birdsall NJM, Buckley NJ. Muscarinic receptor subtypes. Ann Rev Pharmacol Toxicol 1990;*30*:633–673.
5. Caulfield MP, Brown DA. Pharmacology of the putative M4 muscarinic receptor mediating Ca-current inhibition in neuroblastoma x glioma hybrid (NG 108-15) cells. Brit J Pharmacol 1991;*104*:39–44.
6. Dorje F, Levey AI, Brann MR. Immunological detection of muscarinic receptor subtype proteins (m1–m5) in rabbit peripheral tissues. Mol Pharmacol 1991;*40*:459–462.
7. Keen M, Nahorski SR. Muscarinic acetylcholine receptors linked to the inhibition of adenylate cyclase activity in membranes from the rat striatum and myocardium can be distinguished on the basis of agonist efficacy. Mol. Pharmacol. 1988;*34*:769–778.
8. McKinney M, Miller JH, Gibson VA, Nickelson L, Aksoy S. Interactions of agonists with M2 and M4 muscarinic receptor subtypes mediating cyclic AMP inhibition. Mol Pharmacol 1991;*40*:1014–1022.
9. Lazareno S, Buckley NJ, Roberts FF. Characterization of muscarinic M_4 binding sites in rabbit lung, chicken heart and NG108-15 cells. Mol Pharmacol 1990;*38*:805–815.
10. Freedman SB, Patel S, Harley EA, Iversen LL, Baker R, Showell GA, Saunders J, McKnight A, Newberry N, Scholey K, Hargreaves R. L-687,306: A functionally selective and potent muscarinic M_1 receptor agonist. Eur J Pharmacol 1992;*215*:135–136.
11. Roeske WR, Wang J-W, Gulya K, Yamamura HI. [^{3}H] AF-DX 116 labels a subset of muscarinic receptors. Trends Pharmacol (Suppl) 1988;*81*.
12. Dorje F, Friebe T, Tacke R, Mutschler E, Lambrecht G. Novel pharmacological profile of muscarinic receptors mediating contraction of the guinea pig uterus. Naunyn-Schmiedeberg's Arch Pharmacol 1990;*342*:284–289.
13. Weiner DA, Levey I, Brann MR. Expression of muscarinic acetylcholine and dopamine receptor mRNA's in rat basal ganglia. Proc Natl Acad Sci USA. 1990;*87*:7050–7054.
14. Lambert DG, Burford NT, Nahorski SR. Muscarinic receptor subtypes: inositol phosphates and intracellular calcium. Biochem Sci Trans 1992;*20*:130–135.
15. Parekh AB, Brading AF. The M_3 muscarinic receptor links to three different transduction mechanisms with different efficacies in circular muscle of guinea pig stomach. Br J Pharmacol 1992;*106*:639–643.
16. Conroy WG, Vernallis AB, Berg DK. The α5 gene product assembles with multiple acetylcholine receptor subunits to form distinctive receptor subtypes in brain. Neuron 1992;*9*:679–691.
17. Lukas RJ, Audhya T, Goldstein G, Lucero L. Interactions of the thymic polypeptide hormone thymopoietin with neuronal nicotinic α-bungarotoxin binding sites and with muscle-type but not ganglia-type nicotinic acetylcholine receptor ligand-gated ion channels. Mol Pharmacol 1990;*38*:887–894.
18. Whiting PJ, Schoepfer R, Conroy WG, Gore MJ, Keyser KT, Shimaski S, Esch F, Lindstrom JM. Expression of nicotinic acetylcholine receptor subtypes in brain and retina. Mol Brain Res 1991;*10*:61–70.
19. Clarke PBS, Schwartz RD, Paul SM, Pert CB, Pert A. Nicotinic binding in rat brain: Autoradiographic comparison of [^{3}H]-acetylcholine [^{3}H]-nicotine and [^{125}I] α-bungarotoxin. J Neurosci 1985;*5*:1307–1315.
20. Cimino M, Marini P, Fornasari D, Cattabeni F, Clementi F. Distribution of nicotinic receptors in cynomolgus monkey brain and ganglia: Localization of α_3 subunit mRNA, α-bungarotoxin and nicotine binding sites. Neurosci 1992;*51*:77–86.
21. Loring RH, Dahm LM, Zigmond RE. Localization of α-bungarotoxin binding sites in the ciliary ganglion of the embryonic chick: An autoradiographic study at the light and electron microscopic level. Neurosci 1985;*14*:645–660.
22. Joy AM, Siegel HN, Lukas RJ. Photoaffinity labeling of muscle-type nicotinic acetylcholine receptors and neuronal/nicotinic α-bungarotoxin binding sites with a derivative of α-bungarotoxin. Mol Brain Res 1993;*17*:95–100.
23. Gotti C, Esparis Ogando A, Hanke W, Schlue R, Moretti M, Clementi F. Purification and characterization of an α-bungarotoxin receptor that forms a functional nicotinic channel. Proc Nat Acad Sci USA. 1991;*88*:3258–3262.
24. Gotti C, Hanke W, Schlue W-R, Briscini L, Moretti M, Clementi F. A functional α-bungarotoxin receptor is present in chick cerebellum: Purification and characterization. Neuroscience 1992;*50*:117–127.
25. Bertrand D, Bertrand S, Ballivet M. Pharmacological properties of the homomeric α7 receptor. Neurosci Lett 1992;*146*:87–90.
26. Vijayaraghavan S, Pugh PC, Zhang Z, Rathouz MM, Berg DK. Nicotinic receptors that bind α-bungarotoxin on neurons raise intracellular free Ca^{2+}. Neuron 1992;*8*:353–362.
27. Halvorsen SW, Berg DK. Identification of a nicotinic acetylcholine receptor on neurons using an α-neurotoxin that blocks receptor function. J Neurosci 1986;*6*:3405–3412.
28. Koelle GB. A proposed dual neurohumoral role of acetylcholine: Its functions at the pre and post-synaptic sites. Nature 1961;*190*:208–211.
29. Koelle GB. A new general concept of the neurohumoral functions of acetylcholine and acetylcholinesterase. J Pharm Pharmacol 1962;*14*:65–90.
30. Del Tacca M, Danesi R, Blandizzi C, Bernardini MC. Differential affinities of AF-DX 116, atropine and pirenzipine for muscarinic receptors of guinea pig gastric fundus, atria and urinary bladder:

Might atropine distinguish among muscarinic receptor subtypes? Pharmacology 1990;*40*:241–249.

31. Miao FJ-P, Lee TJ-F. VIP-ergic and cholinergic innervations in internal carotid arteries of the cat and rat. J Cardiovasc Pharmacol 1991;*18*:369–378.
32. Manjeet S, Sim MK. Atropine and scopolamine-resistant subtypes of muscarinic receptors in the rabbit aorta. Eur J Pharmacol 1989;*174*:99–105.
33. Sim MK, Manjeet S. Properties of muscarinic receptors mediating second messenger responses in the rabbit aorta. Eur J Pharmacol 1990;*189*:399–404.
34. Egan TM, North RA. Acetylcholine hyperpolarized central neurones by acting on an M_2 muscarinic receptor. Nature 1986;*319*:405–407.
35. Sugita S, Uchimura N, Jiang ZG, North RA. Distinct muscarinic receptors inhibit release of γ-aminobutyric acid and excitatory amino acids in the mammalian brain. Proc Nat Acad Sci USA 1991;*88*:2608–2611.
36. Raiteri M, Marchi M, Paudice P. Presynaptic muscarinic receptors in the central nervous system. Ann NY Acad Sci 1990;*604*:113–129.
37. Sahakian B, Jones G, Levy R, Gray J, Warburton D. The effects of nicotine on attention, information processing and short-term memory in patients with dementia of the Alzheimer type. Brit J Psychiatr 1989;*154*:797–800.
38. Freis ED. Hexamethonium, a forgotten drug in relation to "new" concepts in the management of heart failure. Am Heart J 1989;*118*:426–427.
39. Francis PT, Palmer AM, Sims NR, Bowen DM, Davidson AN, Esiri MM, Neary D, Snowden, JS, Wilcock GK. Neurochemical studies of early-onset Alzheimer's disease. Engl J Med 1985;*313*:7–11.
40. Read SL, Frazee J, Shapira J, Smith C, Cummings JL, Tomiyasu U. Intracerbroventricular betanechol for Alzheimer's Disease. Arch Neurol 1990;*47*:1025–1030.
41. Noronha-Blob L, Lowe VC, Peterson JS, Hanson RC. The anticholinergic activity of agents indicated for urinary incontinence is an important property for effective control of bladder dysfunction. J Pharmacol Exp Ther 1989;*251*:586–593.
42. Connolly J, Boulter J, Heinemann SF. α4-2β2 and other nicotinic acetylcholine receptor subtypes as targets of psychoactive and addictive drugs. Br J Pharmacol 1992;*105*:657–666.
43. Jaiswal N, Lambrecht G, Mutschler E, Tacke R, Malik KU. Pharmacological characterization of the vascular muscarinic receptors mediating relaxation and contraction in rabbit aorta. J Pharmacol Exp Ther 1991;*258*:842–850.
44. Lambrecht G, Feifel R, Moser U, Aasen AJ, Waelbroeck M, Christophe J, Mutschler E. Stereochemistry of the enantiomers of trihexyphenidyl and its methiodide at muscarinic receptor subtypes. Eur J Pharmacol 1988;*155*:167–170.

Reviews

r1. Moncada S, Palmer RMJ, Higgs EA. Nitric oxide: Physiology, pathophysiology and pharmacology. Pharmacol Rev 1991;*43*:109–142.

r2. Dixon WE. On the mode of action of drugs. London: Med Mag 1907;*16*:454–457.

r3. Lindstrom J, Whiting P, Schoepfer R, Luther M, Das M. Structure of nicotinic acetylcholine receptors from muscle and neurons. In: Computer-assisted modeling of receptor-ligand interactions: Theoretical aspects and applications to drug design. New York: Liss (1989); pp 245–266.

r4. Deneris ES, Connolly J, Rogers SW, Duvoisin R. Pharmacological and functional diversity of neuronal nicotinic acetylcholine receptors. Trends Pharmacol Sci 1991;*12*:34–40.

r5. Clarke PBS. Mapping of brain nicotinic receptors by autoradiographic techniques and the effect of experimental lesions. Prog Brain Res 1989;*79*:65–71.

r6. Starke K, Gothert M, Kilbinger H. Modulation of neurotransmitter release by presynaptic autoreceptors. Physiol Rev 1989;*69*:864–989.

r7. Volle RL. Nicotinic ganglion-stimulating agents. Handbook of Experimental Pharmacology. 1980;*53*:281–312.

r8. Wessler I. Control of transmitter release from the motor nerve by presynaptic nicotinic and muscarinic autoreceptors. Trends Pharmacol Sci 1989;*10*:110–114.

r9. Hoskins HD, Kass M. Diagnosis and therapy of the glaucomas, 6th Ed. St Louis: Mosby, 1989.

r10. Pitschner HF, Schlepper M, Schulte B, Volz C, Palm D, Wellstein A. Selective antagonists reveal different functions of M cholinoceptor subtypes in humans. Trends Pharmacol Sci 1989; (Suppl) 92–96.

CHAPTER 6

J. Paul Hieble
Andrew J. Nichols
S. Z. Langer
Robert R. Ruffolo, Jr.

Pharmacology of the Sympathetic Nervous System

Introduction

Most involuntary (autonomic) control of physiologic activity within the body is regulated, at least in part, by the sympathetic nervous system. Several examples of important systems under sympathetic control include heart rate, vascular tone, GI motility, lipolytic activity of the adipocyte, and secretions from most exocrine glands. In some cases, such as in the control of heart rate, two branches of the autonomic nervous system, the sympathetic and parasympathetic, exert reciprocal control. Hence, activation of the sympathetic and parasympathetic nerves innervating the heart result in an increase or decrease in heart rate, respectively. In other cases, as in the control of vascular tone, the parasympathetic system does not play a significant role, and both vasoconstriction and vasodilation can be a consequence of sympathetic nerve stimulation. This occurs because the primary sympathetic neurotransmitter, norepinephrine (NE), can activate two distinct adrenoceptors, the α-adrenoceptor, which mediates vasoconstriction, and the β-adrenoceptor, which mediates vasodilation. The relative contribution of α- and β-adrenoceptors can vary substantially between different vascular beds.

The basic principles of chemical neurotransmission, and the anatomic organization of the sympathetic nervous system, are described in detail in Chapter 4. Briefly, the activation of neuronal cell bodies within the brain stem or spinal cord results in the activation of neurons with cell bodies in sympathetic ganglia, usually in a ganglion chain adjacent to the spinal cord. These neurons send postganglionic sympathetic fibers to the organs receiving sympathetic innervation. An action potential initiated in a postganglionic sympathetic neuron results in the release of NE from storage vesicles in varicosities in the distal region of the neuronal fiber arborization. The released neurotransmitter crosses the neuroeffector junction to activate adrenoceptors on the cell membrane of the innervated tissue. Neurotransmitter released into the neuroeffector junction will also activate prejunctional adrenoceptors on sympathetic nerve terminals, and activation of these prejunctional "autoreceptors" will modulate vesicular neurotransmitter release, thereby exerting feed back control on neurotransmitter release.

An important function of the sympathetic nervous system is the control of epinephrine secretion from the adrenal medulla, which can be considered as a specialized sympathetic ganglion. The action of epinephrine, a circulating hormone, can reinforce the action of neuronally released NE, inasmuch as both molecules can activate α- and β-adrenoceptors. However, since there are differences in the selectivity profile of epinephrine and NE at the adrenoceptor subtypes (see below), a specific organ system sometimes can be affected differently by localized sympathetic stimulation (i.e., primarily NE release) and generalized sympathoadrenal activation (i.e., both NE and epinephrine release).

Sympathetic Neurotransmitters

Nearly a century ago, it was known that adrenal extracts could mimic many of the physiologic effects of sympathetic nerve stimulation.[1,2] Experiments in the 1920s[3,4] established the release of an excitatory neurotransmitter from sympathetic nerves. Taken together, these two observations suggested that the catecholamine, epinephrine, may be a sympathetic neurotransmitter. However, there were sufficient differences, primarily relating to increased vasodilation with the epinephrine-containing extracts, to eliminate epinephrine as the only neurotransmitter. Because the concept of α- and β-adrenoceptors was not postulated until 1948, early attempts to identify the sympathetic neurotransmitter were impeded by the presence of both "excitatory" and "inhibitory" responses to sympathetic nerve stimulation. Synthetic drugs capable of reproducing the physiologic effects of sympathetic nerve stimulation were identified and designated as sympathomimetic amines. Some of these sympathomimetic amines could selectively produce excitatory or inhibitory effects. This observation was consistent with the commonly held belief that there were separate sympathetic neurotransmitters for excitation and inhibition. Although early experiments suggested that a primary amine, such as NE, might be the neurotransmitter, this was not conclusively established until 1946, when von Euler developed quantitative assay procedures of sufficient sensitivity to measure NE.

Although NE is the primary neurotransmitter at most sympathetic neuroeffector junctions, some postganglionic sympathetic neurons release acetylcholine as a neurotransmitter—principally those innervating the sweat glands. Furthermore, epinephrine is released from the adrenal gland as a neurohormone. Although epinephrine-releasing neurons are present in the CNS, peripheral sympathetic neurons do not synthesize epinephrine. However, sympathetic varicosities can accumulate and store circulating epinephrine, and it has been postulated that under some conditions epinephrine release after uptake from the peripheral circulation may have pathophysiologic consequences in the etiology of hypertension.[5]

Both NE and epinephrine are synthesized from dopamine by the enzyme, dopamine β-hydroxylase. Specific receptors for dopamine are found on most neuronal varicosities and on the postjunctional membrane at several neuroeffector junctions. Furthermore, substantial quantities of dopamine are present in the sympathetic varicosity; however, most of this accumulation of dopamine represents a precursor pool for NE synthesis. The high levels of dopamine found in postganglionic sympathetic neurons has led to the postulate of dopamine-releasing neurons in the periphery. Although dopaminergic neurotransmission plays a significant role in the CNS and dopaminergic interneurons may be present in sympathetic ganglia, a physiologic role of peripheral dopamine-releasing neurons has not been conclusively established.

Both NE and epinephrine can activate either α- or β-adrenoceptors. In many effector systems, such as blood vessels, adipocytes, the endocrine pancreas, and prejunctional control of NE release, α- and β-adrenoceptor activation results in opposing effects. For example, activation of α-adrenoceptors will contract vascular smooth muscle, whereas β-adrenoceptor activation induces relaxation. Since the affinity of epinephrine for most vascular β-adrenoceptors (i.e., β_2-adrenoceptors) is much higher than that of NE, with both agents having nearly equivalent affinity for α-adrenoceptors, the two catecholamines can produce substantially different effects on blood pressure when administered to animals or humans. Epinephrine has a greater tendency to decrease pressure, and any pressor effect observed after administration of epinephrine is converted to a depressor effect after α-adrenoceptor blockade, a phenomenon known as "epinephrine reversal". In other tissues, such as cardiac muscle, both α- and β-adrenoceptor activation will produce stimulatory effects, whereas in others, such as intestinal smooth muscle, both adrenoceptors cause inhibition of contractile activity.

It is now clear that most neuronal varicosities release more than one neurotransmitter in response to an axonal action potential. Both the primary neurotransmitter and cotransmitter(s) have specific receptors on the postjunctional membrane and/or on the axonal varicosity, and the activation of the receptors for the cotransmitters can modulate neuroeffector transmission. For example, adenosine triphosphate (ATP) is stored with NE in the adrenergic storage vesicles and is coreleased with NE upon stimulation. In some tissues, neuronally released ATP, acting on discrete purinergic receptors, makes a significant contribution to the functional response observed following sympathetic nerve stimulation. Indeed, neuronally released ATP is likely responsible for the α-adrenoceptor antagonist resistant electrophysiologic effects produced by field stimulation in certain blood vessels; these responses previously were postulated to result from activation of a different class of adrenoceptors, termed γ-adrenoceptors.[6]

In recent years, the role of neuropeptide Y (NPY) in sympathetic neurotransmission also has been recognized. This 36-amino acid peptide is also co-stored and co-released with NE in the adrenergic varicosity. NPY has multiple actions, including direct vasoconstriction in some blood vessels, potentiation of the α-adrenoceptor-mediated actions of exogenous and neuronally released NE, and modulation of NE release via activation of prejunctional NPY receptors.[7] In addition to its vesicular localization with NE, discrete NPY-containing vesicles are also found in many adrenergic varicosities. The contents of these vesicles are released upon high frequency nerve stimulation, suggesting that NPY may have an additional functional role under conditions of intense sympathetic activation.

Subclassification of Adrenoceptors

As noted above, it has long been recognized that both excitatory and inhibitory responses are produced by sympathetic nerve stimulation. It was also known that agents such as the ergot alkaloids were capable of blocking the vasoconstrictor action of sympathetic nerve stimulation, and could produce "epinephrine reversal".[8] However, most inhibitory responses to epinephrine or sympathetic nerve stimulation, as well as the stimulation of cardiac rate and force of contraction, were insensitive to blockade by the ergot alkaloids. In contrast to the qualitative division of sympathetic responses into excitatory and inhibitory, Ahlquist[9] used a semiquantitative approach to propose the existence of two adrenoceptor subtypes, based on different rank orders of potency of a series of structurally related natural and synthetic sympathomimetics evaluated in different tissues. Ahlquist designated these two subtypes of adrenoceptors as α and β. This mode of receptor subclassification was consistent with that based on antagonist sensitivity, with those responses designated by Ahlquist as "β" being insensitive to ergot alkaloids. The concurrent identification of the β-haloalkylamines as more selective α-adrenoceptor antagonists, relative to the ergot alkaloids, provided additional support for Ahlquist's proposal. Final proof came ten years later, with the description of dichloroisoproterenol, the first agent capable of antagonizing β-but not α-adrenoceptor-mediated responses.

α-Adrenoceptors

Soon after prejunctional α-adrenoceptors were identified in the early 1970s, it became apparent that pre- and postjunctional α-adrenoceptors had different pharmacologic characteristics.[10,11] Langer[11] suggested the designation of α_1- and α_2-adrenoceptors for postjunctional and prejunctional α-adrenoceptors, respectively. Studies on the interactions of agonists and antagonists with these α-adrenoceptors extended this subclassification scheme to a functional, as opposed to an anatomic basis.[12] Although most vascular contraction is mediated by α_1-adrenoceptors, certain vessels or vascular beds have postjunctional α_2-adrenoceptors that also mediate a contractile response. In addition to the prejunctional control of NE release from the neuronal varicosity, α_2-adrenoceptors mediate functions such as platelet aggregation and inhibition of insulin secretion. Potent and highly selective agonists and antagonists have now been identified for both α_1- and α_2-adrenoceptors. Several of these pharmacologic classes represent useful therapeutic agents (see below).

With the advent of new techniques for studying drug-receptor interactions, such as radioligand binding assays, the ability to isolate and purify receptor proteins, and the ability to determine the nucleotide sequence of genes encoding individual receptor subtypes, it has become clear that there are multiple subclasses of both α_1- and α_2-adrenoceptors.[r1,r2,13] Currently, molecular biology techniques have identified three distinct subtypes of both α_1- and α_2-adrenoceptors, whose pharmacologic characteristics correspond, in general, to the subtypes identified using radioligand binding techniques.[13] Furthermore, apparently independent of this subclassification scheme, α_1- and α_2-adrenoceptors can be pharmacologically subclassified based on the ability of certain antagonists to block the action of norepinephrine (or other agonists).[14,r2] The subclassification of α_1- and α_2-adrenoceptors offers additional opportunities for selective actions of drugs at a particular tissue. Although α-adrenoceptor subtype selectivity has not yet been utilized for the development of new drugs, the particular adrenoceptor subtypes present in many target tissues are now being identified with the goal of designing more effective therapeutic agents.

β-Adrenoceptors

In 1967, Lands and coworkers,[15] comparing rank orders of potency of agonists in a manner similar to that of Ahlquist, concluded that there were two subtypes of the β-adrenoceptor. The β_1-adrenoceptor, the dominant receptor found in heart and adipose tissue, was equally sensitive to NE and epinephrine, whereas the β_2-adrenoceptor, responsible for relaxation of vascular, uterine, and airway smooth muscle, was much less sensitive to NE vis-a-vis epinephrine. Selective agonists and antagonists of β_1- and β_2-adrenoceptors have been identified, and several of these drugs have been utilized extensively as therapeutic agents. Evidence has accumulated over the years for the existence of an "atypical" β-adrenoceptor that is insensitive to the commonly used antagonists. Selective agonists are now available for this receptor, now commonly known as the β_3-adrenoceptor. These agents may offer novel therapeutic opportunities through their action at β_3-adrenoceptors on the adipocyte or pancreatic islet cell. In contrast to the results observed for responses mediated by the β_2-adrenoceptor, NE is more potent than epinephrine in activating the β_3-adrenoceptor, which is responsible for stimulation of thermogenesis in brown adipose tissue and lipolysis in the white adipose tissue of some species.

Genes encoding the three β-adrenoceptors have been cloned and expressed; the pharmacologic characteristics of the purified receptors obtained in this manner corresponds well with those of the three β-adrenoceptor subtypes identified in native tissues. The molecular pharmacology of the β-adrenoceptors has been studied extensively. The β_2-adrenoceptor was the first adrenoceptor to be cloned, and analysis of the hydrophobicity of the 418 amino acids making up its sequence suggested a folded structure passing through the cell membrane seven times, with an extracellular amino terminus and intracellular carboxyl terminus.[16] This seven-transmembrane-domain structure has now been postulated for many neurotransmitter and hormone receptors and, although not yet confirmed by physical techniques, such as X-ray crystallography, appears to be consistent with the results obtained from techniques such as site-directed mutagenesis and the artificial assembly of chimeric receptors to study the mode of the interaction between the receptor and either agonists/antagonists or second messenger regulatory proteins (see below).

Signal Transduction Processes

α-*Adrenoceptors*

α_1- and α_2-Adrenoceptors utilize different signal transduction processes to translate receptor occupation by an agonist to a functional cellular response. α_1-Adrenoceptor activation increases intracellular calcium concentrations. The activation of α_2-adrenoceptors is consistently associated with inhibition of adenylate cyclase. However, this does not necessarily represent the mechanism for α_2-adrenoceptor signal transduction in all tissues. Both α_1-adrenoceptor-mediated calcium effects and α_2-adrenoceptor-mediated inhibition of adenylate cyclase involve a guanine nucleotide regulatory protein (G-protein) that binds guanine nucleotides and acts to convey the signal from the receptor to the catalytic unit responsible for calcium translocation or adenylate cyclase inhibition, respectively. Molecular biologic studies have clearly demonstrated that the G-protein interacts with the third intracellular loop of the α-adrenoceptor. Many distinct G-proteins have been identified, and subtle changes in amino acid sequence in the third intracellular loop of the α-adrenoceptors can influence both the efficiency of coupling between the receptor and G-protein as well as which G-protein interacts with the receptor.[r3] Interestingly, the third intracellular loop represents the region of least homology between the α-adrenoceptor subtypes. There is a high degree of structural divergence in this region, both in length and in amino acid sequence, between the many neurotransmitter receptors sharing the general seven transmembrane-spanning domain structure.

α_1-Adrenoceptor-mediated elevation in intracellular calcium concentration is often a result of calcium release from intracellular stores; it occurs through a G-protein-mediated activation of phospholipase C. This enzyme hydrolyzes phosphatidylinositol-4,5-bisphosphate to generate inositol-1,4,5-triphosphate, which acts, in turn, to release intracellular calcium stores from the sarcoplasmic reticulum, and diacylglycerol, which activates protein kinase C. However, other α_1-adrenoceptor mediated responses depend on the influx of extracellular calcium through voltage-gated calcium channels. There is often a correlation between the relative contribution of intracellular versus extracellular calcium and the intrinsic efficacy of an α_1-adrenoceptor agonist, with agonists of lower efficacy being more dependent on translocation of extracellular calcium to produce a response. It has been postulated that the α_1-adrenoceptor in vascular smooth muscle is linked to two G-proteins, one mediating phospholipase C activation, and another linked to a membrane calcium channel. In this model, occupation of the α_1-adrenoceptor by a full agonist results in activation of both G-proteins, while partial agonists can activate only the G-protein linked to the calcium channel.[18]

Activation of α_2-adrenoceptors results in the inhibition of adenylyl cyclase activity, mediated through an inhibitory G-protein (G_i).[19] In some tissues, inhibition of adenylyl cyclase appears to represent the true signal transduction mechanism (e.g., the functional inhibition of the action of vasopressin on the renal collecting duct). However, in other tissues, although adenylyl cyclase may be inhibited, another second messenger system, as yet unidentified, appears to mediate the functional response to receptor activation. In vascular smooth muscle, it is unlikely that adenylyl cyclase could be sufficiently activated under basal conditions for α_2-adrenoceptor mediated increases in blood pressure to result from inhibition of cyclase activity. Alternatively, the vascular postjunctional α_2-adrenoceptor appears to be linked to a calcium channel, allowing translocation of extracellular calcium to mediate the response to receptor activation.[r4] α_2-Adrenoceptors have been shown to activate other potential signal transduction mechanisms, including potassium channels, phospholipase A_2, and Na^+/H^+ exchange.

β-*Adrenoceptors*

All three β-adrenoceptor subtypes appear to be linked to adenylyl cyclase activation through a stimulatory G protein (G_s), with no evidence for subtype-related differences in receptor-cyclase interaction. The β-adrenoceptors have been the prototype for studies on the linkage between receptor, G-protein, and the catalytic subunits of adenylyl cyclase, and much is known regarding the molecular interactions between these three proteins.[r5] There is evidence to suggest that in certain tissues, such as cardiac muscle, there could be a direct coupling between G_s and a voltage-sensitive calcium channel.[20]

Functional Effects of Sympathetic Nerve Activation

The sympathetic nervous system, acting through α- and β-adrenoceptors, mediates effects on most of the body's organ systems. Additional effects can be produced by exogenous administration of α- and β-adrenoceptor agonists, since many adrenoceptors do not receive direct sympathetic innervation. This section will concentrate on the major effects mediated by sympathetic nerve stimulation, principally those demonstrated in human subjects and having physiologic, pathophysiologic, or therapeutic relevance. For a more detailed description of the functional effects mediated by α- and β-adrenoceptor activation, see reviews by Nichols and Ruffolo[r6] and Hieble and Ruffolo.[r7]

Control of Blood Pressure

The sympathetic nervous system plays an important role in the control of blood pressure, primarily through the modulation of vascular tone, although effects on cardiac rate and contractility (see below) also may contribute. As previously noted, sympathetic nerve stimulation can produce either vasoconstriction, mediated via α-adrenoceptors, or vasodilation, mediated via β-adrenoceptors. Most blood vessels receive sympathetic innervation, although the relative density of α- vis-a-vis β-adrenoceptors and the subtype distribution of both classes of adrenoceptors, can vary substantially between different vascular beds and between large and small vessels of a particular bed.

Most vasoconstrictor responses to sympathetic nerve activation are mediated via α_1-adrenoceptors. It is interesting to note that, although blood pressure can be increased in experimental animals via activation of both postjunctional α_1- and α_2-adrenoceptors, it is difficult to detect the presence of α_2-adrenoceptor-mediated contraction on most isolated arteries. There is evidence in isolated human arteries to suggest that vascular α_2-adrenoceptors may play a functional role only in smaller blood vessels. In contrast, postjunctional α_2-adrenoceptor-mediated vasoconstriction in response to both exogenous agonists and sympathetic nerve activation can readily be demonstrated in certain veins, such as the saphenous vein, from both humans and experimental animals.

Postjunctional α_2-adrenoceptors make an important contribution to the control of cutaneous blood flow. Activation of α_2-adrenoceptors in the cutaneous circulation is likely of clinical relevance in the etiology of Raynaud's disease, which is characterized by intense cutaneous vasoconstriction leading to pain and even loss of digits. Symptoms of Raynaud's disease are induced by cold and other conditions leading to sympathetic nerve activation. Studies in isolated blood vessels have demonstrated that lower temperatures potentiate α_2-adrenoceptor mediated vasoconstriction, while attenuating the response to α_1-adrenoceptor stimulation.[21]

Whereas α-adrenoceptor-mediated vasoconstriction is the net response to sympathetic stimulation in most vascular beds, β-adrenoceptor-mediated vasodilation is observed as the primary response in the coronary and skeletal muscle vasculature. Although in vitro studies demonstrate that β-adrenoceptors on coronary arteries are primarily of the β_1-subtype, most in vivo studies show a substantial or even predominant role of the β_2-adrenoceptor in the control of coronary vascular tone.[22]

Control of Heart Rate and Force of Myocardial Contraction

Sympathetic nerve stimulation to the heart increases both the rate and force of cardiac contraction. This response is mediated primarily via activation of β_1-adrenoceptors, both by NE released from nerve terminals and by epinephrine released from the adrenal medulla. β_2-Adrenoceptor activation can also increase cardiac rate and force of contraction, whereas α-adrenoceptor activation preferentially increases the force of contraction vis-a-vis rate. Cardiac β_2-adrenoceptors are present in human atrial and ventricular muscle, and may make a significant contribution to the cardiac stimulation produced by the sympathetic nervous system. Although an α_1-adrenoceptor-mediated increase in cardiac contractile force can be demonstrated in vitro, and myocardial α_1-adrenoceptors may play a functional role in the cardiac response to sympathetic nerve stimulation in certain pathologic states, as well as contribute to the inotropic selectivity of certain exogenous agonists,[23] they are rarely activated by an exogeneous α_1-adrenoreceptor agonist.

Control of Airway Resistance

The role of the sympathetic nervous system in the control of pulmonary resistance is not clearly established, although field stimulation of isolated tracheal strips can induce a β-adrenoceptor mediated relaxation. Although β_2-adrenoceptor agonists are commonly employed as bronchodilators in humans, in vitro studies suggest that both β_1- and β_2-adrenoceptors can induce relaxation of human pulmonary smooth muscle.[r8] There is no evidence for a physiologically significant role of the α-adrenoceptors in the control of pulmonary smooth muscle tone.

Control of Renal Electrolyte Balance

Activation of renal sympathetic nerves stimulates renin release from the juxtaglomerular apparatus. This action, at least in humans, appears to result from activation of the β_1-adrenoceptor. It appears that juxtaglomerular cells are under a constant adrenergic tone, since β-adrenoceptor antagonists inhibit basal renin release. Renal sympathetic nerves also influence tubular sodium and water reabsorption via actions on the proximal tubule, the ascending limb of the distal convoluted tubule, and the collecting duct. An increase in sympathetic nerve activity produces an α_1-adrenoceptor mediated antinatriuretic response in several species, although, in the rat following chronic α_1-adrenoceptor blockade, the α_2-adrenoceptor apparently can mediate the same response.[24] Likewise, in the rat, α_2-adrenoceptor stimulation can produce a functional antagonism of the action of vasopressin on the collecting duct, resulting in a water diuresis. This phenomenon, however, appears to be limited to the rat.[25]

Effects on Urogenital Structures

Activation of sympathetic nerves innervating the bladder results in a contraction of the bladder neck and proximal urethra, contributing to the ability of the bladder to retain urine. This response is mediated via α_1-adrenoceptors. In contrast, the bladder dome contains a low density of α-adrenoceptors, but will exhibit a β_2-adrenoceptor mediated relaxation. A physiologic role for these bladder β-adrenoceptors has not been established, but they may contribute to the ability of the bladder to relax in response to filling. In general, sympathetic stimulation mediates functions promoting urine storage, in contrast to parasympathetic stimulation, which mediates the micturition process.

The prostate gland receives a dense sympathetic innervation, which induces contraction via activation of α_1-adrenoceptors on the fibromuscular stromal tissue of the gland. The role of the sympathetic nervous system in the control of normal prostate function is not known; however, when the gland undergoes hypertrophy, the increased tone resulting from sympathetic activation can impose an additional "dynamic" component to the static obstruction of the urethra produced by the glandular enlargement, as occurs in benign prostatic hypertrophy. Radioligand binding studies in hypertrophic human prostate have detected the presence of both α_1- and α_2-adrenoceptors, but functional studies show the contractile response to be mediated only by α_1-adrenoceptors. Autoradiographic studies show the α_2-adrenoceptors in the human prostate to be localized primarily at the base of secretory acini, suggesting a potential role in the control of prostatic secretion.

Activation of sympathetic nerves to the penis results in contraction of the trabecular smooth muscle of the corpus cavernosum. Contraction of this muscle expels the blood responsible for maintenance of the erect state.[26] This effect is mediated via the α_1-adrenoceptor. Consequently, drugs blocking α_1-adrenoceptors are used to treat impotence.

Control of Lipolysis

There is reciprocal adrenergic regulation of lipid breakdown in the adipocyte, with lipolysis being activated by β-adrenoceptor stimulation and inhibited by activation of α-adrenoceptors. This regulation occurs both via sympathetic innervation of adipose tissue and hormonal control via adrenal epinephrine. The effects of β- and α-adrenoceptor activation are mediated through the activation and inhibition of adenylyl cyclase, respectively, which in turn controls the activity of hormone-sensitive-lipase.[r9]

Adipocyte β-adrenoceptors were initially classified as the β_1-subtype, based on potent activation by NE. However, the relative contribution of β_1- and the recently characterized β_3-adrenoceptors to the lipolytic response varies substantially between species. The receptor reserve for the β_3-adrenoceptor in human adipocytes may be lower than in rodents, inasmuch as selective β_3-adrenoceptor partial agonists produce a marked lipolytic response in rat adipose tissue, but are inactive on human adipocytes.[27]

Inhibition of lipolysis is mediated via the α_2-adrenoceptor. The relative density of β- and α_2-adrenoceptors appears to determine the nature of the response of a particular adipose tissue site to adrenoceptor activation, since NE and epinephrine can activate either β-adrenoceptors (to promote lipolysis), or α_2-adrenoceptors (to inhibit ongoing lipolytic activity). Under conditions of caloric restriction, α_2-adrenoceptor responsiveness may be enhanced, shifting the balance from lipolysis to an antilipolytic response, with a consequent decrease in lipid mobilization.[28] In isolated human adipose tissue, an α_2-adrenoceptor antagonist will potentiate the lipolytic effect of epinephrine.

The relative density of α_2- and β-adrenoceptors is dependent both on species and on anatomic site within a given species. Subcutaneous fat deposits contain a higher relative density of α_2-adrenoceptors than does internal adipose tissue. There are also sex differences, with females having a higher relative density of α_2-adrenoceptors in gluteal subcutaneous adipose tissue than males; this may relate to the resistance of these fat deposits to diet-induced lipolysis. In the rat, a specialized adipose tissue known as brown adipose tissue receives dense sympathetic innervation. Sympathetic stimulation of this brown adipose tissue induces a thermogenic response, mediated primarily via the β_3-adrenoceptor. Localized deposits of brown adipose tissue are not found in humans or other nonrodent species, although a thermogenic response may be produced in humans by β_3-adrenoceptor activation.

Control of Gastrointestinal Motility and Secretion

Activation of the sympathetic innervation of the intestine results in an inhibition of peristaltic activity and a reduction in tone. Reduction in tone is also produced in the stomach. This inhibitory effect is mediated by both α- and β-adrenoceptors. Both α_1- and α_2-adrenoceptors appear to be involved in this action. Activation of prejunctional α_2-adrenoceptors on parasympathetic nerve terminals also may play an important role in the inhibitory action of sympathetic nerve stimulation of GI motility by inhibiting acetylcholine release. α_2-Adrenoceptor activation also will cause inhibition of gastric acid secretion from the parietal cells of the stomach induced by parasympathetic nerve stimulation. This action results from prejunctional inhibition of acetylcholine release.

Although the intestinal β-adrenoceptor has been classified as the β_1-subtype, a component of the inhibitory effect of the sympathetic nervous system appears to be mediated by the β_3-adrenoceptor. The sympathetic nervous system also may control the balance between absorption and secretion in the ileum through activation of mucosal α_2-adrenoceptors. Stimulation of these receptors in isolated segments of ileum results in a decrease in ionic fluxes, consistent with the ability of α_2-adrenoceptor agonists to inhibit intestinal fluid secretion in both humans and experimental animals.

Control of Pancreatic Hormonal Secretion

The pancreatic islet cells receive a dense sympathetic innervation, and the sympathetic nervous system plays an important role in the control of the two hormones of the endocrine pancreas, insulin and glucagon. There is reciprocal adrenergic control of insulin secretion, with a β-adrenoceptor activation mediating stimulation and α-adrenoceptor activation mediating inhibition. The α-adrenoceptor-mediated effect generally predominates, since stimulation of sympathetic nerves, or infusion of epinephrine, produces a reduction in insulin secretion, whereas β-adrenoceptor-mediated stimulation of secretion is observed only following α-adrenoceptor blockade. The β-adrenoceptor stimulating insulin secretion appears to be of the β_2-subtype, and α-adrenoceptor mediated inhibition results from activation of an α_2-adrenoceptor. This α-adrenoceptor-mediated inhibition of insulin release appears to be operative under physiologic conditions, since an α_2-adrenoceptor antagonist will blunt the hyperglycemic response to oral glucose challenge. β-Adrenoceptor stimulation enhances glucagon secretion. This action results from facilitation of the stimulatory effects of the principal physiologic mediator, plasma amino acids. Hence, the dominant actions of sympathetic nerve stimulation on both insulin and glucagon secretion result in increases in plasma glucose.

Other Metabolic Actions

Sympathetic nerve stimulation results in an increased output of glucose from the liver into the circulation. This is a consequence of both enhanced breakdown of hepatic glycogen stores (glycogenolysis) and stimulation of de novo glucose synthesis (gluconeogenesis). In contrast to many of the adrenoceptor control mechanisms, both α- and β-adrenoceptor activation stimulate hepatic glucose output. In experimental animals, the relative roles of hepatic α- and β-adrenoceptors in the control of glucose output can be altered markedly by age and by the levels of several circulating hormones. α-Adrenoceptor-mediated stimulation of both glycogenolysis and gluconeogenesis appears to involve the α_1-adrenoceptor subtype. Stimulation of gluconeogenesis by α_1-adrenoceptor activation can occur by two independent pathways, one being sensitive to calcium, the other to insulin.

β-Adrenoceptor-mediated stimulation of glycogenolysis in the liver is produced via activation of glycogen phosphorylase. The receptor subtype responsible for this effect still has not been established. It has long been recognized that epinephrine-induced hyperglycemia is insensitive to blockade by propranolol and other β-adrenoceptor antagonists. This insensitivity is similar to that observed for responses now thought to be mediated by the β-adrenoceptor. However, the similar effect mediated by both α- and β-adrenoceptor activation, plus the redundancy of mechanisms controlling plasma glucose levels, makes the characterization of specific receptor subtypes responsible for this effect difficult.

Functional Role of Prejunctional Adrenoceptors

Several examples have been noted where the sympathetic nervous system can attenuate the responses mediated by the parasympathetic nervous system through activation of prejunctional α_2-adrenoceptors on parasympathetic nerves to inhibit the release of acetylcholine. Prejunctional α_2-adrenoceptors on sympathetic varicosities (autoreceptors) also are activated under physiologic conditions, since α_2-adrenoceptor antagonists elevate plasma catecholamine levels in both human subjects and in experimental animals. A functional role of the prejunctional β-adrenoceptor, which facilitates neurotransmitter release from sympathetic nerves, is less certain. Most available data suggest that this prejunctional β-adrenoceptor is of the β_2-subtype, which would be relatively insensitive to the NE released into the synaptic cleft by sympathetic nerves under normal conditions. Circulating epinephrine can be accumulated by sympathetic varicosities and subsequently coreleased with NE. Because epinephrine has higher affinity for the prejunctional β_2-adrenoceptor, neurotransmitter release may thereby be facilitated, and greater activation of postjunctional adrenoceptors produced. It has been postulated[5] that this process may contribute to essential hypertension, especially since plasma epinephrine levels are elevated in many hypertensive patients. Although studies testing this "epinephrine hypothesis" in human subjects have yielded controversial results, recent clinical studies have demonstrated that epinephrine can facilitate sympathetic vascular neurotransmission, suggesting that, at least in a particular subset of the hypertensive population, the activation of prejunctional β-adrenoceptors may contribute to the elevation of vascular resistance.[29]

Principal Therapeutic Indications

The functional effects mediated by the sympathetic nervous system result in many potential therapeutic opportunities for drugs inhibiting or enhancing sympathetic function. The primary mechanisms by which the functional effects of sympathoadrenal activity can be inhibited include: (1) decreased central activation of sympathetic outflow; (2) inhibition of ganglionic neurotransmission; (3) inhibition of NE synthesis, storage, or release; (4) adrenoceptor blockade. Although ganglionic blockers (e.g., hexamethonium, mecamylamine) and inhibitors of NE storage (e.g., reserpine) and release (e.g., guanethidine) have been used extensively in the past, and are still in limited use today, most current therapy and the development of new therapeutic agents is concentrated on receptor antagonists. Blockade of the action of a neurotransmitter at its receptor offers greater potential for selective action on a particular organ system, especially considering the rapidly developing capability for achieving receptor subtype selective blockade.

The functional effects of sympathoadrenal activity can be enhanced by: (1) inhibition of synaptic neurotransmitter reuptake; (2) liberation of NE from its storage vesicles; (3) stimulation of adrenoceptors by exogenous agonists. Norepinephrine uptake inhibitors (e.g., desipramine) are used clinically as antidepressants, based on their ability to enhance postsynaptic adrenoceptor activation in the CNS. Agents capable of releasing vesicular NE into the synaptic cleft (indirectly-acting sympathomimetic amines) are widely used, primarily in over-the-counter preparations as nasal decongestants. A variety of directly-acting sympathomimetic amines are used clinically, including the physiologic catecholamines, close structural analogues, and newly-developed agents having enhanced selectivity for a particular adrenoceptor subtype. The primary therapeutic indications for adrenoceptor agonists and antagonists are discussed below. Specific drugs for these indications are described in the following section.

Hypertension

Because the sympathetic nervous system plays an important role in the control of blood pressure, many therapeutic approaches involving modulation of sympathoadrenal activity have been employed in the treatment of hypertension (see Chapter 26). The first drugs capable of reducing blood pressure in humans were the ganglionic blockers. These reduced vascular sympathetic tone, but had many unacceptable side-effects, since parasympathetic neurotransmission was also blocked. Somewhat greater selectivity was achieved with the adrenergic neuronal blockers, such as guanethidine, which are still used in the treatment of severe hypertension. Current modes of antihypertensive therapy that act through inhibition of one or more components of sympathetic activity include α_1-adrenoceptor antagonists (e.g., prazosin), centrally-acting α_2-adrenoceptor agonists (e.g., clonidine), and β-adrenoceptor antagonists (e.g., propranolol).

The first α-adrenoceptor antagonists, such as phenoxybenzamine and phentolamine, which blocked both α_1- and α_2-adrenoceptors, were not generally effective as antihypertensive drugs. One potential explanation for the lack of efficacy is the blockade of the negative feedback loop involving the prejunctional α_2-adrenoceptor. As such, nonselective α-adrenoceptor antagonists increase plasma catecholamine levels, and the increased synaptic NE concentrations counteract the postjunctional α-adrenoceptor blockade produced by these drugs.

This hypothesis led to the design and testing of selective α_1-adrenoceptor antagonists, which do not interfere with the prejunctional α-adrenoceptor-mediated feedback control of NE release. This pharmacologic class has proved to be effective in the control of hypertension, presumably through blockade of the action of NE and epinephrine at postjunctional vascular α_1-adrenoceptors. It is possible that an action in the CNS also contributes, to inhibit sympathetic nerve firing rate because α_1-adrenoceptor antagonists do not produce reflex tachycardia to the same extent as do other arterial vasodilators, such as hydralazine. The primary side-effect of α_1-adrenoceptor antagonists is orthostatic hypotension, which is especially prevalent upon initiation of therapy ("first dose effect"). This often can be eliminated by dose-titration and by administering the first dose at bedtime.

Clonidine, a moderately selective α_2-adrenoceptor agonist, and α-methyldopa, which is converted to α-methyl-norepinephrine, the latter also being a selective α_2-adrenoceptor agonist, have been used as antihypertensive drugs for many years. Other α_2-adrenoceptor agonists, some having much greater selectivity than clonidine, have been introduced as antihypertensive agents. A large body of experimental evidence, both in animals and human subjects, supports the concept that clonidine and other α_2-adrenoceptor agonists lower blood pressure via activation of medullary α_2-adrenoceptors in the nuclei controlling sympathetic outflow to the periphery. Activation of medullary α_2-adrenoceptors results in an inhibition of vascular and cardiac sympathetic tone.

Several research groups currently postulate that clonidine produces its sympatholytic effect by acting on receptors, distinct from the α-adrenoceptor, in the brain stem that recognize the imidazoline moiety present in the molecule. The evidence in experimental animals for an antihypertensive action of locally administered clonidine on central "imidazoline" receptors, rather than α_2-adrenoceptors, appears convincing.[30] New antihypertensive drugs having greater selectivity for imidazoline receptors versus α_2-adrenoceptors are being introduced, with the goal of eliminating α_2-adrenoceptor-mediated sedation, the principal side-effect associated with this pharmacologic class. Nevertheless, the similar antihypertensive profile of the α_2-adrenoceptor agonists, some of which do not interact with the imidazoline receptor, would suggest that stimulation of central α_2-adrenoceptors is primarily responsible for their antihypertensive activity in humans.

Propranolol, the prototypic β-adrenoceptor antagonist, was initially evaluated in humans as an antianginal drug. It was soon observed that propranolol produced a clinically significant reduction in blood pressure in hypertensive patients. β-Adrenoceptor antagonists remain one of the most prescribed classes of antihypertensive drugs, and at least 100 different β-adrenoceptor antagonists have been evaluated in humans. Both nonselective β-adrenoceptor blockers, such as propranolol, which block both β_1- and β_2-adrenoceptors, as well as drugs having high selectivity for the β_1-adrenoceptors, are clinically effective.

Despite the extensive evaluation of β-adrenoceptor antagonists in hypertension, the mechanism for the blood pressure reduction is still not known. Some proposed mechanisms include: (1) reduction in cardiac output; (2) CNS effects to decrease sympathetic outflow; (3) reduction in renin secretion; (4) decreases in plasma volume; (5) resetting of baroreceptor threshold; (6) reduction in the vasopressor effects of stress-induced catecholamine release and decreased peripheral neurotransmitter release as a result of prejunctional β-adrenoceptor blockade. None of these individual mechanisms will explain the effects of all β-adrenoceptor antagonists on blood pressure, since the clinically effective drugs vary widely in β-adrenoceptor subtype selectivity, ability to enter the CNS, and the presence of additional actions, such as intrinsic sympathomimetic activity or membrane stabilization. It is likely that several of the putative mechanisms listed above contribute to the clinical antihypertensive actions of the β-adrenoceptor antagonists, with the contribution of each varying among the individual agents.[31] It is interesting to note that the onset of antihypertensive action requires days to weeks, although β-adrenoceptor blockade can be demonstrated within hours of initial drug administration.

Cardiac Arrhythmias

Activation of cardiac sympathetic nerves, or elevation of plasma catecholamines, can, at least under some circumstances, increase the likelihood of cardiac arrhythmia. Thus, adrenoceptor antagonists have been evaluated extensively as antiarrhythmic agents. Drugs used for this condition are also discussed in Chapter 25. Although α_1-adrenoceptor antagonists are highly effective in some animal models of ischemia/reperfusion-induced arrhythmias, and although α_1-adrenoceptor antagonists, such as abanoquil, which has apparent cardiac selectivity, are now being evaluated in humans,[32] most of the clinical experience has been with β-adrenoceptor antagonists.

β-Adrenoceptor antagonists are effective against a variety of cardiac arrhythmias. Most of their clinical efficacy results from blockade of the β-adrenoceptor-mediated effects of sympathetic nerve activation on the specialized conducting tissues, such as the sinoatrial and atrioventricular nodes. β-Adrenoceptor antagonists are most useful against supraventricular arrhythmias, where their ability to decrease heart rate can contribute to the therapeutic action. β-Adrenoceptor antagonists have been designated as class II antiarrhythmics in the Vaughan-Williams classification of antiarrhythmic drugs. Some, but not all, β-adrenoceptor antagonists have other potential mechanisms of antiarrhythmic action unrelated to β-adrenoceptor blockade, such as membrane-stabilizing activity or the ability to prolong action potential duration (Class III action).

Angina Pectoris, Myocardial Infarction, and Congestive Heart Failure

Sympathetic stimulation enhances cardiac work and increases myocardial oxygen requirements. In patients with exercise-induced angina pectoris, a flow-limiting coronary stenosis prevents increases in coronary blood flow in response to exercise, causing an imbalance between myocardial oxygen supply and demand (see Chapter 24). β-Adrenoceptor antagonists are effective as antianginal agents as a consequence of their ability to decrease stress-induced increases in heart rate and myocardial contractility. If the angina patient is also hypertensive, the blood pressure-lowering effect of the β-adrenoceptor antagonist will also help by lowering cardiac afterload and myocardial wall tension. β-Adrenoceptor antagonists with intrinsic sympathomimetic activity are also able to increase exercise tolerance in these patients. This is consistent with the ability of a partial agonist to produce β-adrenoceptor blockade in the presence of a high degree of sympathetic activation. The agonist-induced stimulation of myocardial β-adrenoceptors observed under resting conditions offsets the cardiac depression observed with pure competitive antagonists that lack intrinsic sympathomimetic activity, whereas the β-adrenoceptor blocking effects that occur during sympathetic activation account for the antianginal effect.

Several large studies have shown substantially reduced incidence of second myocardial infarction in patients treated with β-adrenoceptor antagonists following their initial infarct.[33] The mechanism by which this beneficial effect is produced is not completely understood, but is likely to involve the antiarrhythmic action of β-adrenoceptor blockers, as well as their ability to inhibit the formation of atherosclerotic plaque, which has been consistently demonstrated in animal models.[r9] Despite this ability to prevent a second infarction, a reduction in primary myocardial infarcts has not been observed consistently in patients on β-adrenoceptor antagonist therapy. Intravenous β-adrenoceptor blockade is utilized in acute myocardial infarction. Release of intracellular enzymes is reduced, suggesting a decrease in infarct size.

Because β-adrenoceptor activation leads to enhanced myocardial contractility, β-adrenoceptor agonists would appear to represent a useful therapeutic approach in congestive heart failure (CHF), where myocardial function is depressed. Many β-adrenoceptor agonists have been studied for this indication, and a large body of clinical data has been generated, but no sustained clinical benefit (e.g., reduction in mortality) has been shown. However, IV infusion of a β-adrenoceptor agonist is a useful approach for acute maintenance of cardiac function in patients with heart failure over a short (usually less than 72-hr) interval. Cardiac output is increased, and cardiac afterload may be reduced, in part by withdrawal of sympathetic tone to the vasculature and in part by direct arterial vasodilation. Continuous β-adrenoceptor activation eventually will lead to β-adrenoceptor down-regulation, and consequent tolerance to the inotropic effect. Several β-adrenoceptor partial agonists, including some having selectivity for β_1-adrenoceptors, have been examined in CHF. Although initial hemodynamic improvement often is obtained, chronic oral therapy generally has not shown sustained clinical benefit.

Although β-adrenoceptor antagonists traditionally have been contraindicated in CHF, there is some clinical evidence for their utility in this condition under some circumstances. Elevated catecholamine levels in heart failure may actually contribute to the observed pathology. The ability of a β-adrenoceptor antagonist to decrease heart rate will result in a decrease in myocardial oxygen consumption, and will improve coronary blood flow owing to the increased percentage of time the heart spends in diastole as a consequence of the reduction in heart rate. Several groups have demonstrated that β-adrenoceptor blockade results in improved hemodynamic function and improved exercise tolerance in heart failure patients.[r10,r11]

Asthma

β-Adrenoceptor stimulation represents an important therapeutic approach to the treatment of the bronchospasm associated with asthma (see Chapter 29). In many cases, only acute aerosol therapy is required in response to an initiating event, such as cold air or exercise. In more severe cases, therapy with β-adrenoceptor agonists by aerosol is often used in combination with systemic administration of another class of antiasthmatic drug, such as a methylxanthine or glucocorticoid.

Although the nonselective adrenoceptor agonist, epinephrine, is highly effective in the treatment of asthma via the aerosol route, selective β_2-adrenoceptor agonists are now used almost always. These selective agents also can be used for oral or parenteral therapy; however, upon systemic administration, the separation between bronchodilator and cardiac stimulant doses is substantially less than with aerosol administration. This may result from the presence of cardiac β_2-adrenoceptors. β-Adrenoceptor stimulation also can inhibit the secretion of endogenous bronchoconstrictors, such as histamine, from pulmonary mast cells. It has also been suggested that the ability of β-adrenoceptor agonists to decrease the leakage of large macromolecules from the vascular system into the airways may make an important contribution to the antiasthmatic effect of β_2-adrenoceptor agonists.

Any therapeutic use of a receptor agonist carries the inherent risk of receptor down-regulation or desensitization. β_2-Adrenoceptor down-regulation has been demonstrated in asthmatic patients on long-term β_2-adrenoceptor agonist therapy, and has been postulated to account at least in part for the increase in deaths from asthma that occurred concurrently with increasing use of aerosol β-adrenoceptor agonist therapy in the 1960s.[r12] Loss of therapeutic response to β-adrenoceptor agonist therapy should be treated not by increasing the dose of β-agonist, but rather by adding another antiasthmatic drug that acts through a nonadrenergic mechanism. The concurrent use of glucocorticoids with β-adrenoceptor agonist therapy is important in the treatment of severe asthma. Other pulmonary obstructive diseases such as emphysema and chronic bronchitis involve an irreversible lesion. Nevertheless, a reversible bronchospasm may be superimposed on the fixed occlusion, and β-adrenoceptor agonist therapy is often found to be beneficial.

Benign Prostatic Hypertrophy

Sympathetic nerve stimulation induces contraction of prostatic smooth muscle, thereby exacerbating the obstruction of the prostatic urethra by the enlarged prostate. Based on the studies of Caine et al.,[34] who showed that contraction of human prostate is mediated by α-adrenoceptors, α-adrenoceptor antagonists were evaluated clinically and found to produce significant symptomatic improvement. More recently, the contractile response in the prostate has been shown to result primarily from α_1-adrenoceptor activation, and several selective α_1-adrenoceptor antagonists, such as prazosin, are now marketed for this indication. Recently, α_1-adrenoceptors have been further subclassified, and current drug discovery efforts are now focusing on the possibility of selective blockade of prostatic versus vascular α_1-adrenoceptors, with the goal of producing more complete blockade of the effects of sympathetic activation on prostatic tone without producing the side-effects, such as orthostatic hypotension, that result from vascular sympatholytic action.

Drugs Interacting with Adrenoceptors

Catecholamine Neurotransmitters and Analogues

The administration of NE or epinephrine or their metabolic precursor dopamine has several clinical applications. These agents produce a relatively nonselective stimulation of most adrenoceptors. Dobutamine, an analogue of dopamine, has a unique combination spectrum of activities on the adrenoceptors, making it useful as a cardiac stimulant.

Norepinephrine

Intravenous infusion of NE (Fig. 6.1) may be used to maintain blood pressure in the acute circulatory shock through activation of vascular α-adrenoceptors. However, in many cases of shock, particularly in cardiogenic shock, the sympathetic nervous system is already maximally activated; and the additional vasoconstriction induced by exogenous NE may exacerbate organ ischemia (see Table 6.1)

Epinephrine

Epinephrine (Fig. 6.1) also may be administered IV to elevate blood pressure in cases of shock or spinal anesthesia. More common is SQ administration in severe allergic reactions. A component of this action results from α-adrenoceptor-mediated vasoconstriction to relieve edema, which is particularly useful when edema of the glottis impairs airway patency. β-Adrenoceptor-mediated inhibition of histamine and leukotriene release from mast cells also may contribute to the therapeutic effect. Although formerly used extensively as an aerosol bronchodilator, epinephrine now is limited to low-strength, over-the-counter preparations for the relief of mild intermittent bronchospasm. (see Table 6.1)

Epinephrine is the sympathomimetic drug of choice for IV treatment of cardiac arrest. α-Adrenoceptor-mediated vasoconstriction elevates blood pressure, and therapy improves coronary perfusion pressure and coronary blood flow and preserves cerebral blood flow during resuscitation. (See Table 6.1). Topical administration of epinephrine will shrink mucous mem-

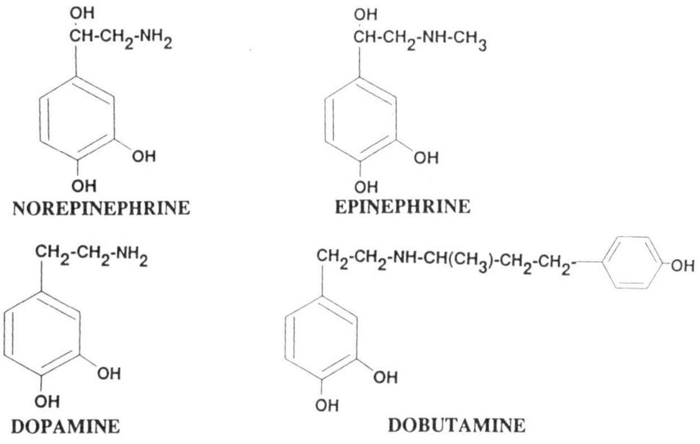

Figure 6.1 Catecholamine Neurotransmitters and Analogues

Table 6.1 Summary of Adrenergic Receptor Agonists

Drug	Route	Concentration	Dose	Onset	Duration of Response
Epinephrine					
Adrenalin	Parenteral	0.1–1 mg/ml	1–4 mg/min. infusion 1 mg for cardiac arrest	immediate	2–5 min
Primatene	Aerosol	7.0 mg/ml	0.2 mg/dose	1 min	5–10 min
Norepinephrine					
Levophed	Parenteral	1 mg/ml	2–12 mg/min. (IV)	immediate	1–2 min
Dopamine					
Intropin	Parenteral	40–160 mg/ml	1–5 mg/kg/min. (IV)	immediate	5–10 min
Dobutamine					
Dobutrex	Parenteral	12.5 mg/ml	1–15 mg/kg/min. (IV)	immediate	5–10 min
Phenylephrine					
Neosynephrine	Parenteral Nasal Spray	10 mg/ml 0.125–0.25%	0.1–0.5 mg (IV) 1–2 sprays q 3hr	immediate	5–10 min ¼–2 hr
Metaraminol					
Aramine	Parenteral	10 mg/ml	0.5–5 mg (IV)	1–2 min	10–30 min
Methoxamine					
Vasoxyl	Parenteral	20 mg/ml	3–5 mg (IV)	immediate	5–15 min
Phenylpropanolamine					
Dexatrim	Oral	Capsule 31.5–75 mg	20–25 mg q 4 hr	15–30 min	4–12 hr
Pseudoephedrine					
Novafed	Oral	tablets 30–120 mg suspension 15 mg/5 ml	60 mg q 4–6 hr	30 min	6 hr
Mephentermine					
Wyamine	Parenteral	15–30 mg/ml	30–45 mg initially (IV)	immediate	15–30 min
Ephedrine	Parenteral Oral	5–50 mg/ml 25–50 mg	5–10 mg (SQ, IM, IV) 25–50 mg	1–2 min 1–2 hr	15–30 min 3–4 hr

branes and limit hemorrhage. Simultaneous injection of epinephrine with local anesthetics constricts cutaneous blood vessels, which limits systemic absorption of the anesthetic and prolongs duration.

Dopamine

Dopamine (Fig. 6.1) can activate both α- and β-adrenoceptors. In addition, dopamine can inhibit sympathetic neuroeffector transmission and produce direct vasodilation in certain vascular beds that contain dopamine receptors. Dopamine is useful in the treatment of circulatory shock because of its actions on both β-adrenoceptors, which stimulate myocardial contractility, and α-adrenoceptors, which increase vascular tone. By control of infusion rates, β-adrenoceptor stimulation can be achieved with only minimal activation of α-adrenoceptors. Dopamine produces less stimulation of heart rate for a given degree of cardiac inotropic activity than many other β-adrenoceptor agonists. Dopamine receptor-mediated renal vasodilation (via the DA_1 receptor) and natriuresis also may contribute to the beneficial effects of dopamine in shock associated with oliguria. Acute IV dopamine can improve hemodynamics in severe CHF. This action results primarily from a β-adrenoceptor-mediated inotropic effect (See Table 6.1).

Dobutamine

Despite numerous references to its β_1-adrenoceptor subtype selectivity, dobutamine (Fig. 6.1) produces pharmacologically significant stimulation of β_1-, β_2- and α_1-adrenoceptors.[r13,33] Intravenous administration of dobutamine produces a relatively selective increase in myocardial contractility, with less effect on heart rate and blood pressure than other catecholamines. This clinical profile of dobutamine may result from the different pharmacologic profiles of the two enantiomers of dobutamine present in the racemic mixture used clinically. (+)-Dobutamine has selective agonist activity at β_1 and β_2-adrenoceptors, whereas the (−)-enantiomer has substantial α_1-adrenoceptor agonist activity. When the racemic mixture is administered, an α_1-adrenoceptor-mediated increase in vascular tone produced by the (−)-enantiomer opposes the β_2-adrenoceptor-mediated vasodilator activity of the (+)-enantiomer. Furthermore, an α_1-adrenoceptor-mediated inotropic activity of the (−)-enantiomer supplements the β_1-adrenoceptor-mediated inotropic and chronotropic activity of (+)-enantiomers, resulting in a preferential increase in cardiac force.[35] Dobutamine is useful in the short-term treatment of impaired cardiac contractility resulting from CHF, myocardial infarction, or cardiac surgery. In cases where infusion is continued for 24–72 hours, tolerance to the positive intropic activity often develops (see Table 6.1).

Indirectly-Acting Sympathomimetic Amines

Agents such as tyramine, which liberate endogenous NE from sympathetic varicosities to produce an indirect activation of post-junctional adrenoceptors, have been useful in the elucidation of the mechanisms involved in catecholamine synthesis, vesicular storage, exocytosis, and other aspects of chemical neurotransmission. In addition, several indirectly-acting sympathomimetic amines are used therapeutically, usually as a result of their ability to produce a relatively prolonged sympathomimetic effect following oral administration (see Table 6.1).

Ephedrine

Although acting primarily via an indirect mechanism, ephedrine (Fig. 6.2) has weak agonist activity at α- and β-adrenoceptors. Ephedrine is one of the active components of a plant extract used for centuries in Chinese herbal medicine. The primary uses of ephedrine are as a bronchodilator, acting through indirect stimulation of β-adrenoceptors, and for the treatment of urinary incontinence, resulting from indirect stimulation of α adrenoceptors on the bladder neck and vesicourethral sphincter. While available without other drug mixtures (Table 6.1), ephedrine is also commonly incorporated into oral bronchodilator preparations containing theophylline. Phenobarbital is also sometimes included to counteract the mild central stimulation produced by ephedrine. Ephedrine is also incorporated into nasal decongestant/antitussive preparations. Ephedrine has two asymmetric centers. Naturally-occurring ephedrine is the 1R,2S(−)-*erythro* form, which is most active pharmacologically.[36] The racemic (*erythro*) form is also used clinically, as is the (*threo*) isomer designated as "pseudoephedrine".[r14]

Pseudoephedrine

Pseudoephedrine (Fig. 6.2), one of the diastereomers of ephedrine, is, like ephedrine, an indirectly-acting sympathomimetic. It is available as tablets (see Table 6.1). Its primary use is as an oral or topical nasal decongestant. Pseudoephedrine also is incorporated into a wide variety of cold/cough preparations that contain a variety of ingredients.

Phenylpropanolamine

Phenylpropanolamine (Fig. 6.2), the des-hydroxy analogue of ephedrine, has pharmacologic actions similar to pseudoephedrine. It is incorporated into many cold/cough preparations for its nasal decongestant activity, and is the active ingredient in several over-the-counter appetite suppressants (see Table 6.1). Like ephedrine, phenylpropanolamine has two asymmetric centers. The form marketed as phenylpropanolamine is the racemic (*erythro*) form. The (*threo*) isomer, designated as norpseudoephedrine (Fig. 6.2), is not commonly used clinically.

α-Adrenoceptor Agonists

Several directly-acting α-adrenoceptor agonists having selectively for α-vis-a-vis β-adrenoceptors have been developed as therapeutic agents. Except for drugs used as topical vasoconstrictors in optical or nasal preparations (oxymetazoline, xylometazoline, tetrahydrozoline; Fig. 6.3), which activate both α_1- and α_2-adrenoceptors, most clinically useful α-adrenoceptor agonists are selective for either the α_1- or α_2-adrenoceptor subtype.

α_1-Adrenoceptor Agonists

Phenylephrine

Although phenylephrine (Fig. 6.3) is a close structural analogue of epinephrine, removal of the para-hydroxyl group from the aromatic ring results in a marked loss of agonist activity at α_2- and β-adrenoceptors, with only a slight reduction in potency at the α_1-adrenoceptor. Intravenous phenylephrine is used to maintain blood

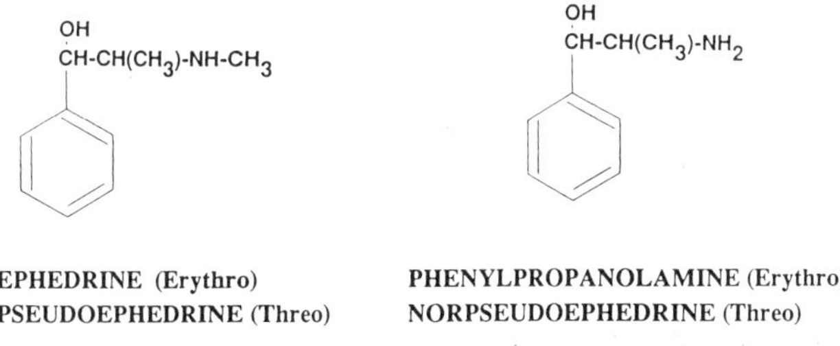

Figure 6.2 Indirectly Acting Sympathomimetics

NONSELECTIVE α-ADRENOCEPTOR AGONISTS

OXYMETAZOLINE XYLOMETAZOLINE TETRAHYDROZOLINE

α_1-ADRENOCEPTOR AGONISTS

PHENYLEPHRINE METARAMINOL METHOXAMINE

Figure 6.3 α-Adrenoceptor Agonists

pressure during general and spinal anesthesia. Since phenylephrine is a relatively poor substrate for both neuronal uptake and metabolic enzymes, the duration of action of an IV dose of phenylephrine is longer than that of epinephrine or NE. An additional advantage of phenylephrine as a vasopressor agent is the lack of β-adrenoceptor mediated cardiac stimulation. Intravenous administration of phenylephrine typically induces bradycardia as a result of reflex activation of the parasympathetic nervous system.

Phenylephrine also is used to prolong the action of spinal or regional anesthesia and as a local vasoconstrictor and mydriatic for ophthalmic surgery and diagnostic procedures. Phenylephrine is a component of many over-the-counter nasal decongestant preparations. Intravenous administration of phenylephrine and other vasopressor agents was formerly used to terminate episodes of paroxysmal supraventricular tachycardia, an effect that resulted from the ability of phenylephrine to produce reflex parasympathetic activation secondary to the increased blood pressure.

Metaraminol

Metaraminol (Fig. 6.3) is another close structural analogue of the catecholamine neurotransmitters, with a 3-hydroxyl group on the aromatic ring rather than the catechol moiety. Metaramimol can be accumulated by the adrenergic nerve varicosity, and hence can exert an indirect action from liberation of vesicular NE in addition to its direct action on the α-adrenoceptor. Metaraminol can be administered IV, IM, or SQ to maintain blood pressure during spinal anesthesia or to treat hypotension induced by drug reactions, surgery, or shock. Metaraminol, administered by either the systemic or intracavernosal route, is used to reverse priapism induced by a variety of causes, including the intracavernosal injection of α-adrenoceptor antagonists or other vasodilators. The pressor action of metaraminol is of longer duration than that induced by exogenous administration of the catecholamine neurotransmitters, since metaraminol is not a substrate for either monoamine oxidase or catechol-O-methyltransferase, the two enzymes responsible for degradation of endogenous catecholamines (see Table 6.1).

Methoxamine

Methoxamine (Fig. 6.3) does not have a phenolic hydroxyl group, but instead has methoxyl groups in the 2 and 5 positions. Nevertheless, methoxamine can produce direct activation of the α_1-adrenoceptor, and is a full agonist in most tissues. Methoxamine also is used primarily to support blood pressure during spinal and general anesthesia. Unlike the catecholamines and some other α-adrenoceptor agonists, methoxamine does not sensitize the heart to arrhythmias induced by general anesthetics, including cyclopropane (see Table 6.1).

α_2-Adrenoceptor Agonists

Clonidine

Clonidine (Fig. 6.4) was originally developed as a nasal decongestant; however, it was soon found that this compound lowered blood pressure and heart rate in both experimental animals and humans. Clonidine was a key pharmacologic tool in the identification of α-adrenoceptor subtypes in the early 1970s, since it was shown that this drug was significantly more potent as an agonist at prejunctional α-adrenoceptors (later designated as α_2-adrenoceptors) than at vascular postjunctional α-adrenoceptors (later designated as α_1-adrenoceptors). The ability of clonidine to lower blood pressure has been shown to result from activation of postjunctional α_2-adrenoceptors in medullary centers that control sympathetic outflow to the periphery. This action of clonidine results in decreased vascular and cardiac sympathetic tone, resulting in decreased blood pressure and heart rate, respectively. Although clonidine can activate peripheral prejunctional α_2-adrenoceptors on sympathetic varicosities to decrease NE release, this action does not contribute to its antihypertensive activity, since α_2-adrenoceptor agonists unable to penetrate the blood-brain barrier do not lower blood pressure.

CLONIDINE GUANABENZ GUANFACINE

RILMENIDINE MOXONIDINE α-METHYLDOPA (Pro-drug to α-Methylnorepinephrine)

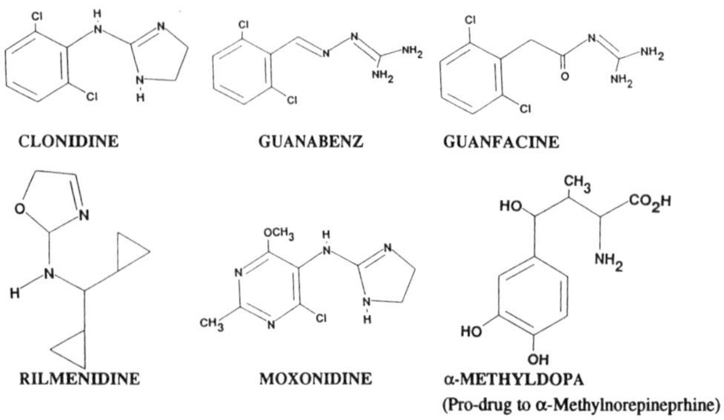

Figure 6.4 α_2-Adrenoceptor Agonists

As noted above, several studies in experimental animals, in which clonidine is administered directly into the medullary nuclei controlling sympathetic outflow, have shown that the reduction in sympathetic outflow results from the activation of imidazoline receptors, rather than α_2-adrenoceptors. The relevance of these findings to the mechanism by which orally administered clonidine lowers blood pressure in humans with essential hypertension has not yet been determined.

Clonidine is a clinically useful antihypertensive drug, either alone or in combination with a diuretic. This therapeutic action of Clonidine is discussed in Chapter 26, as are other drugs that are used to treat hypertension. The most troublesome and common side-effect is sedation, which also results from stimulation of central α_2-adrenoceptors, although these receptors are likely located presynaptically at a different site from those controlling sympathetic outflow. Dry mouth is also commonly observed, presumably resulting from stimulation of α_2-adrenoceptors controlling salivary gland secretion. Rebound increases in blood pressure, sometimes rising to levels higher than before therapy, may result if clonidine administration is terminated abruptly. Therefore, when one wants to transfer a patient to an antihypertensive drug that acts through another mechanism, clonidine doses should be lowered gradually. In addition to oral forms, clonidine is available in the form of transdermal patches that deliver drug at a constant rate for several days.

Besides its primary utility as an antihypertensive drug, clonidine also is useful for relief of symptoms in opiate withdrawal. This action results from stimulation of central α_2-adrenoceptors, which mimics the ability of opiates to inhibit the firing rate in the locus coeruleus. Clonidine is also useful in the treatment of attention deficit hyperactivity disorder in children.

Guanabenz

Guanabenz (Fig. 6.4) has some structural similarity to clonidine and a similar pharmacologic profile. As such, guanabenz is similar to clonidine as an antihypertensive, with sedation and dry mouth being the principal side-effects. Guanabenz does not activate imidazoline receptors; hence the similarity in the antihypertensive profiles of clonidine and guanabenz suggests that an α_2-adrenoceptor-mediated mechanism is involved in the action of both drugs.

Guanfacine

Guanfacine (Fig. 6.4) is structurally and pharmacologically similar to guanabenz, but has a longer plasma half-life and consequently a longer duration of antihypertensive action. Unlike clonidine and guanabenz, which are generally administered twice daily, guanfacine can be administered once daily. The longer duration of action of guanfacine also reduces the likelihood of a rebound increase in blood pressure when the drug is discontinued.

Rilmenidine

Rilmenidine (Fig. 6.4) is an oxazoline derivative that, like clonidine, can stimulate both α_2-adrenoceptors and imidazoline receptors. Rilmenidine is not yet available in all markets. Clinical trials indicate that rilmenidine may have less sedative liability than clonidine, which may result from a difference in the affinity ratio between imidazoline receptors and α_2-adrenoceptors, with rilmenidine having somewhat greater relative affinity for the imidazoline receptor.[37]

Moxonidine

Like rilmenidine, moxonidine (Fig. 6.4) has recently been introduced into some markets as an antihypertensive drug. It has been proposed to show less sedative liability than other α_2-adrenoceptor agonists as a consequence of its selectivity for imidazoline receptors; receptor affinity studies suggest that moxonidine has greater imidazoline receptor selectivity than does rilmenidine.[37]

α-Methyldopa

α-Methyldopa (Fig. 6.4) has been widely used as an antihypertensive drug, but such use is now declining. It is taken up into the CNS via a specific amino acid transporter, after which decarboxylation occurs from dopa decarboxylase and side-chain hydroxylation by dopamine β-hydroxylase to form α-methylnorepinephrine. α-Methylnorepinephrine has moderate selectivity for α_2-versus α_1-adrenoceptors, and the action of this catecholamine at brain stem α_2-adrenoceptors is postulated to account for the antihypertensive action of α-methyldopa. The clinical antihypertensive profile of α-methyldopa is similar to that of clonidine and other α_2-adrenoceptor agonists, with sedation common, especially upon initiation of therapy. α-Methyldopa also can induce a positive direct Coombs test, occasionally associated with hemolytic anemia. α-Methyldopa rarely may induce granulocytopenia or hepatic necrosis. The methyl ester of α-methyldopa is available for IV therapy when blood pressure must be lowered rapidly.

β-Adrenoceptor Agonists

Nonselective Agonists

Isoproterenol

Isoproterenol (N-isopropylnorepinephrine; Fig. 6.5) is the prototypic β-adrenoceptor agonist, producing stimulation of both β_1- and β_2-adrenoceptors, with little effect on the α-adrenoceptors. Isoproterenol is used IV for its cardiac stimulant effects in the treatment of heart block or cardiac arrest. Intravenous administration of isoproterenol also may be used to relieve bronchospasm during general anesthesia.

Isoproterenol also may be administered by aerosol in acute asthma or in bronchospasm associated with chronic obstructive pulmonary disease. When administered by aerosol, cardiac β-adrenoceptor stimulation usually is not produced at doses required to relieve bronchospasm.

β_1-Adrenoceptor Agonists

As noted above, several β-adrenoceptor partial agonists having some degree of selectivity for the β_1-adrenoceptor subtype have been evaluated in humans as cardiac stimulants, with no clear evidence for sustained therapeutic benefit. Xamoterol, considered to be a partial agonist at the β_1-adrenoceptor,[r15] may actually be more correctly represented as a β-adrenoceptor antagonist with intrinsic sympathomimetic activity at the

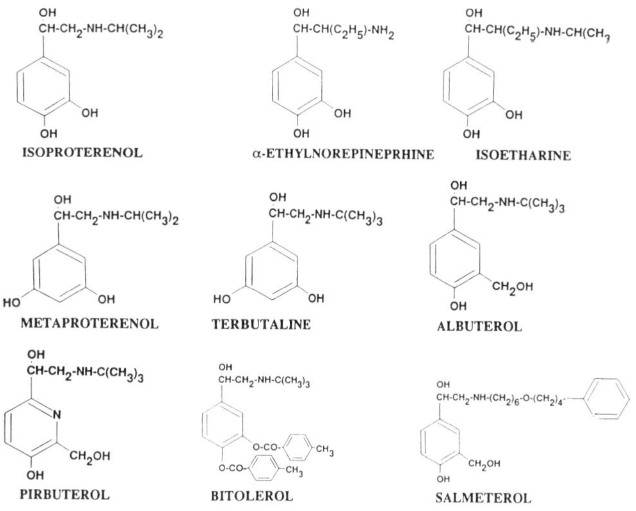

ISOPROTERENOL
α-ETHYLNOREPINEPRHINE
ISOETHARINE
METAPROTERENOL
TERBUTALINE
ALBUTEROL
PIRBUTEROL
BITOLEROL
SALMETEROL

Figure 6.5 β-Adrenoceptor Agonists

β_1-adrenoceptor. No other selective β_1-adrenoceptor agonists are currently available for clinical use.

β_2-*Adrenoceptor Agonists*

β_2-Adrenoceptor agonists represent the treatment of choice for the acute bronchospasm associated with asthma or other pulmonary obstructive diseases (see also Chapter 29). Drugs in this class include older agents, derived from epinephrine or isoproterenol, that have only moderate selectivity for β_2- versus β_1-adrenoceptors, as well as the more recently developed compounds with a higher degree of selectivity for β_2-adrenoceptor. Although few side-effects are observed upon aerosol administration, systemic administration is commonly associated with tremor (due to activation of β_2-adrenoceptors on skeletal muscle), nervousness, and excitability (presumably resulting from an action within the CNS), and cardiac stimulation (tachycardia and palpitations) resulting from activation of cardiac β-adrenoceptors.

Clinical trials have been performed with several of the β_2-adrenoceptor agonists in CHF, based on the premise that cardiac β_2-adrenoceptors may not be down-regulated in this disease.[38] However, β_2-adrenoceptor stimulation does not appear to result in any sustained symptomatic benefit to these patients.

α-Ethylnorepinephrine

The selectivity of α-ethylnorepinephrine (Fig. 6.5) has not been studied extensively; however, based on its clinical profile and chemical structure, the compound has a moderate degree of selectivity for β_2-adrenoceptors. α-Ethylnorepinephrine is administered SQ or IM for acute bronchospasm.

Isoetharine

Isoetharine (α-ethylisoproterenol; Fig. 6.5) has been demonstrated to have selective agonist activity at the β_2-adrenoceptor. Isoetharine is available in several preparations for aerosol administration as a bronchodilator.

Metaproterenol

Metaproterenol (Fig. 6.5), a structural isomer of isoproterenol differing in the position of the aromatic hydroxyl groups, has some selectivity for the β_2-adrenoceptor. Aerosol preparations of metaproterenol are available for acute treatment of bronchospasm. Unlike the catecholamines, metaproterenol has been shown to be effective as a bronchodilator when administered by the oral route, and both solid and liquid formulations are available.

Terbutaline

Terbutaline (Fig. 6.5), structurally similar to metaproterenol, but bearing a *tert*-butyl substituent on the nitrogen atom, may have slightly greater β_2-adrenoceptor selectivity than metaproterenol. Like metaproterenol, terbutaline is available in aerosol and oral preparations. Terbutaline is also available in a parenteral solution for SQ administration in acute bronchospasm.

Albuterol (Salbutamol)

Albuterol (Fig. 6.5) is probably the most widely used β_2-adrenoceptor agonist. It is structurally derived from *tert*-butylnorepinephrine by replacement of the *meta*-hydroxyl group by a hydroxymethyl substituent. Albuterol shows a higher degree of β_2-adrenoceptor selectivity than the catecholamine analogues or terbutaline. The compound is available in both aerosol and oral formulations.

Pirbuterol

Pirbuterol (Fig. 6.5) is structurally similar to albuterol, with a heterocyclic aromatic nucleus, and has a similar degree of selectivity for the β_2-adrenoceptor. Pirbuterol is available only as an aerosol.

Bitolterol

In contrast to the other β_2-adrenoceptor agonists described above, bitolterol (Fig. 6.5) is a pro-drug, where the aromatic hydroxyl groups of *tert*-butylnorepinephrine are esterified with 4-methylbenzoic acid. Since tertbutylnorepinephrine has only slight β_2-adrenoceptor selectivity, the selectivity of bitolterol results from selective ester hydrolysis to yield the active β-adrenoceptor agonist in the lung. Bitolterol is available only for aerosol administration.

Salmeterol

Salmeterol (Fig. 6.5) is the most recently introduced β_2-adrenoceptor agonist. This compound is an analogue of albuterol where the *tert*-butyl nitrogen substituent has been replaced by a long-chain aralkyl ether. As with albuterol, salmeterol has high β_2-adrenoceptor selectivity, but the large, lipophilic nitrogen substituent results in longer duration of action. Hence, in contrast to the other β_2-adrenoceptor agonists available for aerosol use, which must be administered every 4–6 hours, a single inhalation of salmeterol can exert a therapeutic effect for 12 hours.

β_3-*Adrenoceptor Agonists*

While not yet available for clinical use, several selective β_3-adrenoceptor agonists are being developed for treatment of Type II non-insulin dependent diabetes and as adjuncts to caloric restriction in obesity. The rationale for a β_3-adrenoceptor agonist in Type II diabetes is the ability of β_3-adrenoceptor stimulation to mimic the effect of exercise. Although humans do not have the localized brown adipose tissue deposits found in rodents, β_3-adrenoceptor stimulation does induce a thermogenic effect in human subjects. Furthermore, an increase in insulin sensitivity is observed. Currently available drugs are limited by side-effects, such as increased heart rate and muscle tremor. Whether these side-effects can be eliminated by improved β_3- versus β_2-adrenoceptor selectivity remains to be established.

α-Adrenoceptor Antagonists

Nonselective α-Adrenoceptor Antagonists

Several nonselective α-adrenoceptor antagonists are available clinically, but these compounds have limited therapeutic utility.

Phenoxybenzamine

Phenoxybenzamine (Fig. 6.5) is used occasionally for the long-term treatment of the hypertension associated with pheochromocytoma when surgical removal of the tumor is not possible or inadvisable. Phenoxybenzamine inhibits the vascular actions of the high levels of circulating catecholamines associated with pheochromocytoma. The irreversible α-adrenoceptor blockade produced by phenoxybenzamine may be desirable, since plasma catecholamine levels may rise to levels sufficient to overcome the effect of a competitive α-adrenoceptor antagonist. Phenoxybenzamine has been shown to be effective for the chronic treatment of benign prostatic hypertrophy, but its use for this indication has been limited by its carcinogenicity in rodent models. However, no evidence of human carcinogenicity has been observed with the drug. Phenoxybenzamine is available only in an oral preparation.

Phentolamine

Phentolamine (Fig. 6.6) is a competitive antagonist of α_1- and α_2-adrenoceptors. Unlike phenoxybenzamine, phentolamine has a short duration of action, and is administered IV during surgical removal of a pheochromocytoma to prevent hypertension due to catecholamines released into the circulation during manipulation of the tumor. Intravenous phentolamine also can be used to test whether hypertension is due to pheochromocytoma, since a profound reduction in blood pressure is produced immediately after administration if the elevated blood pressure is due to α-adrenoceptor stimulation. Oral preparations of phentolamine were formerly available, but the bioavailability of drug is poor and highly variable by this route.

Intracavernosal injection of smooth muscle relaxants is now a common treatment for impotence. Erection is produced by relaxation of the trabecular smooth muscle, allowing filling of the corpus cavernosum with blood. The most commonly employed regimen for this indication is combined administration of phentolamine with papaverine, a nonselective smooth muscle relaxant. Although the treatment generally results in a functional erection, repeated treatment is often associated with fibrosis and priapism, usually requiring reversal by intra-cavernosal injection of an α-adrenoceptor agonist.

Tolazoline

Tolazoline (Fig. 6.6), a relatively weak α-adrenoceptor antagonist with slight selectivity for α_2-adrenoceptors, is specifically indicated for persistent pulmonary hypertension in the newborn. Its mechanism of action in this condition has not been established, but α_2-adrenoceptor blockade in the pulmonary vasculature is likely, based on experimental studies in animals.

Selective α_1-Adrenoceptor Antagonists

Several highly selective α_1-adrenoceptor antagonists are available for the treatment of hypertension. Prazosin, the prototype of this pharmacologic class, as well as alfuzosin and indoramin, are currently approved for treatment of benign prostatic hypertrophy in certain markets. Clinical trials in benign prostatic hypertrophy are ongoing with several of the other α_1-adrenoceptor antagonists.

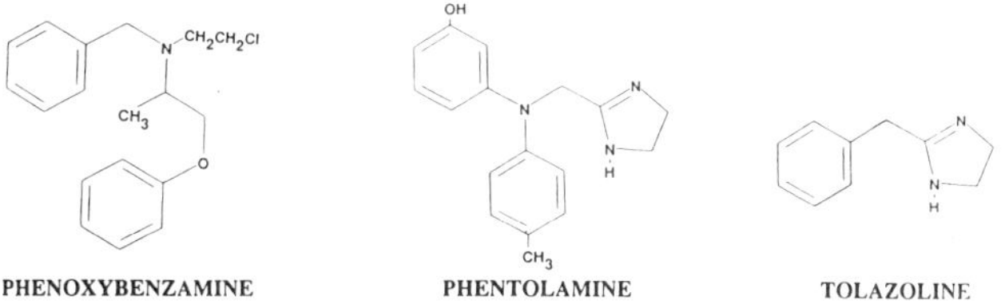

Figure 6.6 Nonselective α-Adrenoceptor Antagonists

PRAZOSIN TERAZOSIN DOXAZOSIN

ALFUZOSIN BUNAZOSIN TAMSULOSIN

INDORAMIN

Figure 6.7 Selective α_1-Adrenoceptor Antagonists

Several analogues of prazosin are available worldwide, including terazosin, doxazosin, alfuzosin, and bunazosin. The pharmacology of these drugs is remarkably similar, and the principal differences relate to duration of action, with the newer drugs, such as doxazosin and terazosin, requiring only once-daily dosing, in contrast to prazosin and alfuzosin, which must be administered two to three times daily.

α_1-Adrenoceptor antagonists are associated with a favorable effect on plasma lipoprotein profile, with a reduction in very low density lipoproteins and either no change or a slight increase in high density lipoprotein.[39] Although the effects of α_1-adrenoceptor blockade on atherosclerotic plaque formation in humans is not known, initial studies in experimental animals generally show an inhibition of diet-induced atherogenesis. α_1-Adrenoceptor blockade also may reverse the loss in insulin sensitivity associated with human essential hypertension.[39]

Prazosin

Prazosin (Fig. 6.7) was the first highly selective α_1-adrenoceptor antagonist to be identified and the first α-adrenoceptor antagonist to be highly effective as an antihypertensive drug (see Chapter 26). Although some other activities of prazosin can be demonstrated at high concentrations in vitro (e.g., phosphodiesterase inhibition), the effects of prazosin in intact animals or in humans can be attributed to α_1-adrenoceptor blockade. Prazosin produces a relatively selective arterial vasodilation. Prazosin is a useful antihypertensive drug, either as monotherapy, or in combination with other agents, such as diuretics. In contrast to other vasodilators, reflex tachycardia is not commonly observed with prazosin. Systolic blood pressure is reduced to a greater extent than diastolic, and orthostatic hypotension can be observed, especially upon initiation of therapy or when the dose is increased. This "first-dose phenomenon" can be minimized by initiating therapy with a low dose and by giving the initial dose immediately prior to retiring. In markets where prazosin is approved for benign prostatic hypertrophy, a prolonged dose titration is used, beginning therapy at subeffective doses to prevent orthostatic reactions.

Although initial treatment with prazosin produces a favorable hemodynamic profile in CHF patients, tolerance often develops. A long-term evaluation showed prazosin to have no effect on survival in heart failure patients, in contrast to the increased survival observed with a combination vasodilator regimen producing mixed arterial and venous dilation.[40]

Doxazosin

Doxazosin (Fig. 6.7), a close structural analogue of prazosin, has a similar pharmacologic profile and similar therapeutic utility. The longer half-life of doxazosin allows once-daily dosing, and may also contribute to a lower incidence of the first-dose phenomenon, although dose titration is used in an attempt to prevent severe orthostatic reactions.

Terazosin

Like doxazosin, terazosin (Fig. 6.7) is a longer-acting analogue of prazosin, having essentially an identical pharmacologic profile. Terazoxin is administered once-daily in the treatment of hypertension. Several chronic clinical trials of terazosin in benign prostatic hypertrophy have been reported, demonstrating sustained symptomatic benefit after dosing of up to 24 months.[41] As with other α_1-adrenoceptor antagonists, dose titration is used to limit orthostatic hypotension.

Indoramin

Although having selectivity for α_1- versus α_2-adrenoceptors, indoramin (Fig. 6.7) is structurally dissimilar from prazosin and its analogues. Indoramin is used for the treatment of both benign prostatic hypertrophy and hypertension. Orthostatic hypotension and the first-dose phenomenon are not commonly associated with indoramin, especially at the lower doses often found to be effective in benign prostatic hypertrophy. However, sedation is more commonly associated with indoramin than with other α_1-adrenoceptor antagonists.

α_2-Adrenoceptor Antagonists

Although studies in experimental animals and in humans have shown that the α_2-adrenoceptor plays an important role in a variety of pathophysiologic processes, selective α_2-adrenoceptor antagonists have not yet been introduced as therapeutic agents. In most markets, the only α_2-adrenoceptor antagonist approved for clinical use is yohimbine. In addition, α_2-adrenoceptor blockade may contribute to the antidepressant action of drugs such as mianserin, which also block NE and serotonin uptake into neuronal varicosities within the CNS. Selective α_2-adrenoceptor antagonists, such as idazoxan and its analogues, have been evaluated in human subjects as antidepressants; however, a drug acting only via α_2-adrenoceptor blockade has not yet been marketed for this indication. A potent and selective α_2-adrenoceptor antagonist, SL 84.0418, was evaluated clinically for the treatment of Type II diabetes, acting through its ability to block α_2-adrenoceptor-mediated inhibition of insulin secretion by the pancreatic islet cell.[42]

Yohimbine

Yohimbine (Fig. 6.8) has moderate selectivity for α_2- versus α_1-adrenoceptors; however, yohimbine also has pharmacologically significant antagonist activity at serotonin and dopamine receptors. The primary therapeutic use of yohimbine is in impotence. A modest improvement in sexual performance is observed in both psychogenic and organic impotence; the mechanism of this effect has not been established, but may involve blockade of the contractile effects of sympathetic activation on the trabecular smooth muscle of the penis, thereby facilitating erectile actions mediated through the parasympathetic nervous system.

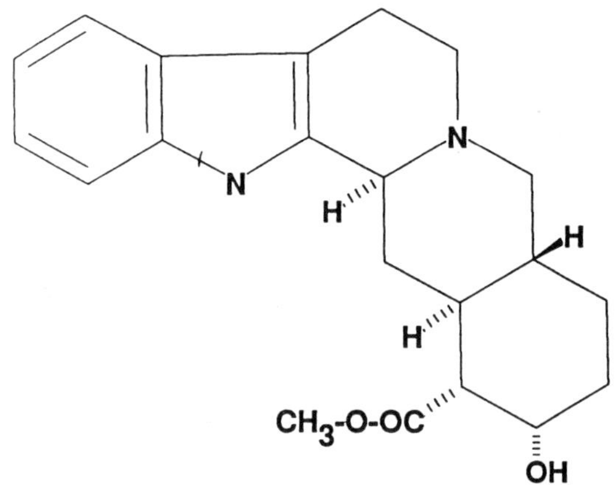

Figure 6.8 Yohimbine—an α_2-Adrenoreceptor Antagonist

β-Adrenoceptor Antagonists

β-Adrenoceptor antagonist are used extensively for the treatment of hypertension, angina pectoris, cardiac arrhythmias, and for the secondary prevention of myocardial infarction. Topical β-adrenoceptor blockade is used as a primary treatment for glaucoma. β-Adrenoceptor blockers are also used for migraine headaches, essential tremor, and performance anxiety. Many β-adrenoceptor antagonists are available for clinical use, including both nonselective and β_1-adrenoceptor selective compounds, some having partial agonist activity, often referred to as intrinsic sympathomimetic activity, and/or membrane stabilizing activity. All drugs bear structural similarity to one another, with an alkylaminoethanol side-chain attached to an aromatic nucleus, nearly always through an -O-CH_2- linkage. Pharmacologic properties and clinical profiles are influenced by changes in the nature of the aromatic ring system and its substituents. It is not practical to list all available drugs; therefore, the properties of representative examples will be described.

A phenomenon observed on long-term treatment with β-adrenoceptor antagonists is up-regulation of the β-adrenoceptor. Because of this up-regulation, caution is required when terminating therapy with this class of drug, since the β-adrenoceptor can remain up-regulated after antagonist is no longer present, and an exacerbation of the symptoms of angina or hypertension can be observed. β-Adrenoceptor antagonists with intrinsic sympathomimetic activity do not induce receptor up-regulation,[43] and may induce fewer clinical problems upon abrupt termination.

Nonselective β-Adrenoceptor Antagonists

Propranolol

There is extensive clinical experience with propranolol, which has been marketed for over 20 years. Propranolol (Fig. 6.9) is a potent antagonist at β_1- and β_2-adrenoceptors, with membrane stabilizing activity but no intrinsic sympathomimetic activity. Orally-administered propranolol is used in chronic hypertension, angina pectoris, cardiac arrhythmia, cardioprotection following a myocardial infarction, migraine, essential tremor, and hypertrophic subaortic stenosis. The therapeutic effectiveness is discussed in other chapters. The doses required vary widely between individual patients and different therapeutic indications. Dose titration often is required with propranolol and other β-adrenoceptor antagonists. An IV form is available for treatment of serious cardiac arrhythmias.

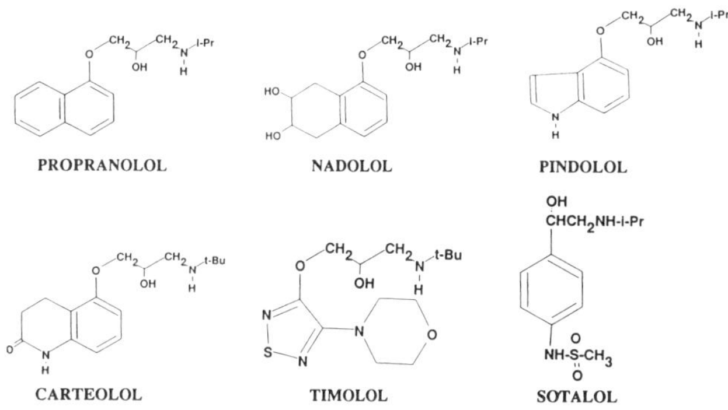

Chronic therapy with propranolol or other β-adrenoceptor antagonists should be tapered gradually if it is desired to change to alternate therapy, since exacerbation of angina pectoris and occasional myocardial infarction has occurred when therapy is terminated abruptly in angina patients. Propranolol is normally administered two to four times daily, but sustained-release preparations are available that allow once-daily dosing. In the treatment of hypertension, propranolol can be combined with other modes of therapy, including diuretics, vasodilators and α_1-adrenoceptor antagonists. Dosage forms combining propranolol and a diuretic are available.

PROPRANOLOL NADOLOL PINDOLOL

CARTEOLOL TIMOLOL SOTALOL

Figure 6.9 Nonselective α-Adrenoceptor Antagonists

Most side-effects of β-adrenoceptor antagonists can be attributed to an extension of their therapeutic actions (e.g., excessive bradycardia) or to blockade of β-adrenoceptors at other sites (e.g., bronchospasm due to blockade of pulmonary β-adrenoceptors, or impaired peripheral circulation due to blockade of vascular β-adrenoceptors). β-Adrenoceptor antagonists are contraindicated in asthmatic patients because of their ability to block β-adrenoceptor-mediated bronchodilation, which may be required to maintain pulmonary function in these individuals. Because bronchial β-adrenoceptors in humans are primarily of the β_2-adrenoceptor subtype, nonselective β-adrenoceptor antagonists have a greater tendency to induce bronchospasm than do selective β_1-adrenoceptor antagonists. Their ability to block the tachycardia resulting from sympathetic nerve activation can mask the warning signs of acute hypoglycemia and thyrotoxicosis. β-Adrenoceptor antagonists can also act within the CNS to produce a variety of side-effects, mainly expressed as depression, disorientation and lethargy, although hallucinations and vivid dreams can also occur. The relationship of these centrally-mediated effects to β-adrenoceptor blockade is not clearly established. Although β-adrenoceptor antagonists can produce effects considered unfavorable on plasma lipoproteins and triglycerides, animal studies have shown that β-adrenoceptor blockers reduce atherosclerosis induced either by diet or behavioral stress, and there are suggestions that the atherosclerotic process may also be favorably influenced in humans.[r9]

Nadolol

Nadolol (Fig. 6.9), like propranolol, is a nonselective β-adrenoceptor antagonist with no intrinsic sympathomimetic activity. However, nadolol has substantially less membrane-stabilizing activity than propranolol, perhaps as a consequence of its reduced lipophilicity. This reduced lipophilicity also may explain the low incidence of centrally-mediated side-effects associated with nadolol. In addition to withdrawing sympathetic tone, many β-adrenoceptor antagonists have a direct depressant effect on myocardial contractility resulting from local anesthetic activity. Nadolol has little direct depressant activity on the heart. Nadolol is used in hypertension and angina pectoris. A combination of nadolol and a thiazide diuretic is available. The drug is effective when given once daily.

Pindolol

Pindolol (Fig. 6.9) does not have membrane-stabilizing activity, but does possess a clinically significant degree of intrinsic sympathomimetic activity. This results in less bradycardia at rest with pindolol compared with other nonselective β-adrenoceptor antagonists. Cardiac output also is reduced to a lesser degree at rest. β-Adrenoceptor antagonists with intrinsic sympathomimetic activity do not produce the inhibition of renin secretion commonly associated with β-adrenoceptor blockade. There is some evidence to suggest that a component of the sympathomimetic action of pindolol results from activation of β_3-adrenoceptors.[44] As with other β-adrenoceptor antagonists, pindolol has been shown to be effective in the treatment of hypertension and angina, either as monotherapy or in combination with other antihypertensive agents. The drug is normally administered twice daily. Because of the intrinsic sympathomimetic activity, pindolol is less effective in preventing a second myocardial infarction than are other β-adrenoceptor blockers.

Carteolol

Carteolol (Fig. 6.9), which bears a structural resemblance to pindolol, also has intrinsic sympathomimetic activity without membrane stabilization. Carteolol is used as an antihypertensive, with a clinical profile similar to that of pindolol. Carteolol is normally administered once daily.

Timolol

Timolol (Fig. 6.9) is structurally distinct from most other β-adrenoceptor antagonists, with a heterocyclic thiadiazole nucleus replacing the substituted benzene or naphthalene nucleus commonly found in this pharmacologic class. Timolol does not have intrinsic sympathomimetic activity or membrane-stabilizing activity. Timolol is used for the treatment of hypertension, secondary prevention of myocardial infarction and prophylactic treatment for migraine headache. The drug is normally administered twice daily. A combination preparation with a thiazide diuretic is available for the treatment of hypertension. In addition to the oral preparations, solutions of timolol are available for the topical treatment of glaucoma. Ocular administration of this solution will rapidly reduce intraocular pressure, with significant effects often maintained for up to 24 hours. The drug normally is administered twice daily in the treatment of glaucoma. The lack of membrane-stabilizing activity is necessary in a β-adrenoceptor antagonist used topically in glaucoma, since it is important not to inhibit the blink reflex.

Sotalol

In contrast to most other β-adrenoceptor antagonists in clinical use, sotalol (Fig. 6.9) lacks the -O-CH_2-linkage between the aromatic ring and ethanolamine side-chain. As noted previously, sotalol is unique among the β-adrenoceptor antagonists in that it also possesses Class III antiarrhythmic activity as a result of its ability to prolong action potential duration. The combination of Class II (i.e., β-adrenoceptor blockade) and Class III (i.e., potassium channel blockade) antiarrhythmic activity makes sotalol especially useful in the prevention of ventricular tachycardia and fibrillation. Sotalol has no intrinsic sympathomimetic activity. Although it has Class III antiarrhythmic activity, sotalol does not have the membrane stabilizing activity classically associated with lipophilic β-adrenoceptor antagonists, such as propranolol. The Class III antiarrhythmic action is present in both enantiomers of sotalol, in contrast to the β-adrenoceptor antagonist activity, which, as with other molecules in this pharmacologic class, is found primarily in the S(–)-enantiomer. Hence, R(+)-sotalol acts as a relatively selective Class III antiarrhythmic agent without β-adrenoceptor antagonist activity, and has been evaluated clinically for use in situations where β-adrenoceptor blockade is undesirable.

Selective β_1-Adrenoceptor Antagonists

Metoprolol

Metoprolol (Fig. 6.10) is one of a series of phenoxypropanolamines bearing a substituent in the 4-position. While this 4-substituent decreases absolute potency as a β-adrenoceptor antagonist, these compounds have selectivity for the β_1- versus the β_2-adrenoceptor. Although selectivity for the β_1-adrenoceptor reduces the likelihood for the induction or exacerbation of bronchospasm, even the selective β_1-adrenoceptor antagonists should be used with extreme caution in patients with asthma and other bronchospastic diseases. None of the clinically available β-adrenoceptor antagonists has absolute selectivity for the β_1-adrenoceptor, and there is evidence that the β_1-adrenoceptor also may mediate a component of the bronchodilator response to adrenoceptor activation in humans. Metoprolol has no intrinsic sympathomimetic activity, and membrane-stabilizing activity is not observed at doses normally administered to block the β_1-adrenoceptor.

Metoprolol is used in hypertension, angina pectoris, and myocardial infarction (see Chapters 24, 25 and 26.) For chronic therapy, the drug usually is administered twice daily, although a sustained-release preparation is now available, allowing for once-daily administration. A combination preparation of metoprolol and a thiazide

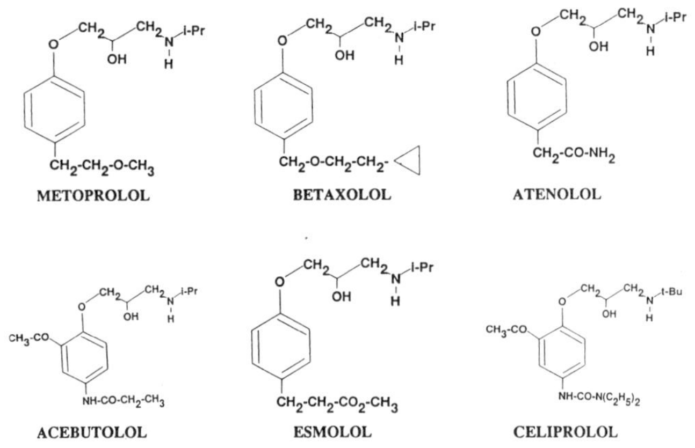

Figure 6.10 Selective β_1-Adrenoceptor Antagonists

diuretic is available for use in hypertension. An IV preparation is available for the acute treatment of myocardial infarction, where the drug may be administered as soon as hemodynamic parameters have stabilized in order to limit the ischemia-induced damage. This effect can be followed by chronic oral dosing to reduce the incidence of second infarction.

Betaxolol

Betaxolol (Fig. 6.10) is structurally similar to metoprolol, with an alkyl ether substituent in the 4-position. Betaxolol may have greater selectivity for the β_1-adrenoceptor than metoprolol, and has no intrinsic sympathomimetic activity or clinically significant membrane stabilizing activity. Betaxolol is available in an oral formulation for treatment of hypertension, where it is administered once daily, and as a topical solution for the treatment of glaucoma. The β-adrenoceptor subtype responsible for the ocular hypotensive action of β-adrenoceptor antagonists has not been conclusively established. At the high concentrations achieved in the eye following topical administration, both β_1- and β_2-adrenoceptors would likely be blocked, even by a selective β_1-adrenoceptor antagonist, such as betaxolol. A rationale for the use of a selective β_1-adrenoceptor antagonist as a topical antiglaucoma drug would be the reduced incidence of β_2-adrenoceptor-mediated side-effects (e.g., exacerbation of bronchospasm resulting from drug absorbed into the systemic circulation).

Atenolol

Like metoprolol and betaxolol, atenolol (Fig. 6.10) is a 4-substituted phenoxypropanolamine with moderate selectivity for the β_1-adrenoceptor, having no intrinsic sympathomimetic or membrane-stabilizing activity. The therapeutic indications are also similar, with atenolol being used chronically for the treatment of hypertension and angina pectoris, and acutely (IV) or chronically (oral) in CHF. Atenolol generally is administered once daily. A combination preparation of atenolol and a diuretic is available.

Esmolol

Like the other selective β_1-adrenoceptor antagonists described above, esmolol (Fig. 6.10) is a phenoxypropanolamine substituted on the 4-position of the phenyl ring. However, in the case of esmolol, the 4-substitutent contains an ester linkage susceptible to rapid hydrolysis by an esterase present in the erythrocyte cytosol. The carboxylic acid formed by this hydrolysis has low affinity for the β_1-adrenoceptor; hence, the duration of β-adrenoceptor blockade produced by an IV infusion of esmolol is short, with recovery within 10–20 minutes following termination of infusion. Esmolol is used for the acute IV treatment of supraventricular tachycardia occurring during or immediately following surgical procedures, or in other emergency situations.

Acebutolol

Acebutolol (Fig. 6.10) is a phenoxypropanolamine with substitutents in the 2- and 4- positions of the phenyl ring. The β_1-adrenoceptor selectivity of acebutolol is less than that of atenolol or metoprolol. Acebutolol has intrinsic sympathomimetic activity, but no clinically relevant membrane-stabilizing activity. Metabolic acetylation of the nitrogen atom of the 4-substituent results in an active metabolite of equal potency and even greater β_1-adrenoceptor selectivity than the parent molecule. Acebutolol is used for the chronic therapy of hypertension and cardiac arrhythmias. The drug is administered either once or twice daily.

Celiprolol

Celiprolol (Fig. 6.10), like acebutolol, is a 2,4-disubstituted phenoxypropanolamine with β_1-adrenoceptor selectivity and intrinsic sympathomimetic activity. Celiprolol appears to have a more prominent vasodilator component than do other β-adrenoceptor antagonists, which has been postulated to result from α-adrenoceptor blockade and/or intrinsic sympathomimetic activity, the latter being due to activation of β_2-adrenoceptors. However, evidence in experimental animals does not support either premise.[45] Interestingly, in contrast to other β-adrenoceptor antagonists, celiprolol may have a favorable effect on plasma lipoprotein profile.[46]

Selective β_2-Adrenoceptor Antagonists

No selective β_2-adrenoceptor antagonists are currently available for clinical use. The only compound of this class evaluated in humans is ICI 118,551 (Fig. 6.11). The results in hypertension were inconclusive, with only one of two studies showing efficacy. The compound showed efficacy comparable to propranolol in reducing essential tremor, a response presumed to result from β_2-adrenoceptor activation.[47]

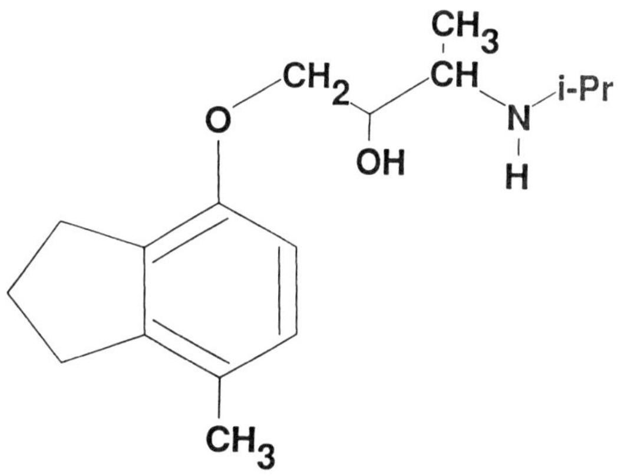

Figure 6.11 ICI 118,551—a β_2-Adrenoceptor Antagonist

Antagonists of α- and β-Adrenoceptors

Both α_1-adrenoceptor and β-adrenoceptor blockade lowers blood pressure in patients with hypertension, and agents of these classes can be combined as antihypertensive therapy. Single molecules have therefore been designed that block both α_1- and β-adrenoceptors. These molecules generally incorporate a complex aryl alkyl side chain conferring α_1-adrenoceptor antagonist activity on the nitrogen substituent of a phenoxypropanolamine or phenethylamine β-adrenoceptor antagonist.[r16] The potency ratio of β- and α_1-adrenoceptors ranges from 1 (amosulalol; Fig. 6.12) to 10 (carvedilol).

Labetolol

Labetolol (Fig. 6.12) is the only α/β-adrenoceptor antagonist widely available for clinical use. When ad-

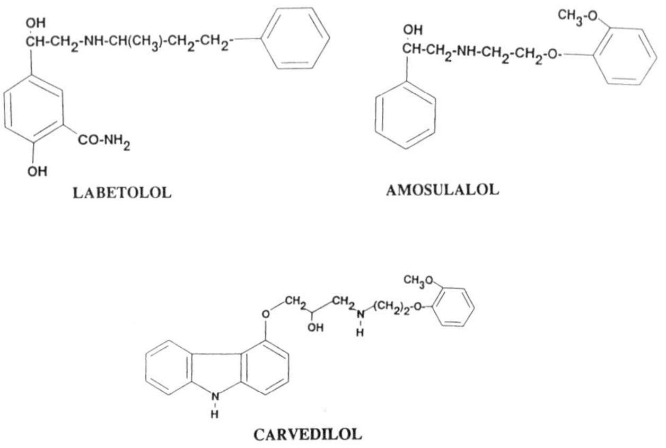

LABETOLOL

AMOSULALOL

CARVEDILOL

Figure 6.12 Mixed α-/β-Adrenoceptor Antagonists

ministered IV to human subjects, labetolol is approximately seven fold more potent as a β-adrenoceptor antagonist than as an α_1-adrenoceptor antagonist. Oral administration may result in a somewhat lower β-versus α-adrenoceptor potency ratio. Labetolol blocks β_1- and β_2-adrenoceptors with essentially equal potency, and has some intrinsic sympathomimetic activity. Interestingly, the sympathomimetic activity of labetolol may result from preferential activation of the β_2-adrenoceptor. Labetolol has two asymmetric centers, and is marketed as a mixture of four isomers (i.e., two pairs of diastereomers).[36] These isomers have been separated, and the R,R-isomer (dilevalol) has been reported to be more potent as a β-adrenoceptor antagonist, but with lower affinity for the α-adrenoceptor. Dilevalol was briefly marketed, but was withdrawn owing to liver toxicity. Labetolol is available for chronic oral use in the treatment of hypertension. A combination with a diuretic is also available. The drug is usually administered twice daily. An IV preparation is used for the acute treatment of hypertensive crisis (see Chapter 26 for other treatment details).

Carvedilol

Carvedilol (Fig. 6.12) has recently been introduced as an antihypertensive drug in some markets. It is a derivative of carazolol, with an aralkyl substituent on the nitrogen atom conferring α_1-adrenoceptor antagonist affinity. Carvedilol has one asymmetric center. As in all phenoxypropanolamines, β-adrenoceptor antagonist affinity is associated only with the S(−)-enantiomer; however, both enantiomers of carvedilol are equipotent as α_1-adrenoceptor antagonists. Carvedilol has equivalent affinity for β_1- and β_2-adrenoceptors, with approximately tenfold lower affinity for the α_1-adrenoceptor. Carvedilol has several other properties potentially useful for antihypertensive therapy, such as the ability to inhibit vascular proliferation[48] and the ability to inhibit LDL oxidation,[49] now thought to be a key step in the development of atherosclerotic plaque. The combination of vasodilation and β-adrenoceptor blockade may also make carvedilol useful in the treatment of CHF. Although β-adrenoceptor antagonists are traditionally contraindicated in heart failure, clinical studies show carvedilol to produce beneficial effects on exercise tolerance and quality of life in these patients. Extensive Phase III clinical studies with carvedilol are currently in progress to establish safety and efficacy in CHF.

Conclusions

The sympathetic nervous system acts on nearly all organ systems within the body, and controls many important physiologic functions. It is not surprising, therefore, that drugs modifying sympathetic function have many therapeutic applications.

Three important classes of antihypertensive drugs (α_2-adrenoceptor agonists, α_1-adrenoceptor antagonists and β-adrenoceptor antagonists) are effective by virtue of their ability to modulate sympathetic neurotransmission. β_2-Adrenoceptor agonists represent the primary mode of acute and chronic bronchodilator therapy for asthma and other bronchospastic diseases. Topical β-adrenoceptor antagonists are now the most common approach to chronic therapy of glaucoma. There is increasing interest in α-adrenoceptor antagonists in the treatment of benign prostatic hypertrophy. Several additional opportunities are currently being tested in patients, such as α_2-adrenoceptor blockade for noninsulin dependent diabetes, mixed α_1/β-adrenoceptor blockade for CHF, and β_3-adrenoceptor agonists for diabetes and obesity. The rapidly evolving ability to subclassify adrenoceptors is likely to allow the design of more selective, and consequently more effective, therapeutic agents.

References

Research Reports

1. Lewandosky M. Uber eine Wirkung des Nebennierenextractes auf das Auge. ZentBl Physiol 1898;*12*:599–600.
2. Langley JN. The difference of behavior of central and peripheral pilomotor nerve-cells. J Physiol (London) 1901;*27*:224–236.
3. Cannon WB, Uridil JE. Studies on the conditions of activity in endocrine glands. VIII. Some effects on the denervated heart of stimulating the nerves of the liver. Am J Physiol 1921;*58*:353–354.
4. Loewi O. Uber humorale Ubertragbarkeit der Herznervenwirkung. Pflugers Arch ges Physiol 1921;*214*:678–688.

5. Majewski H, Tung LH, Rand MJ. Adrenaline activation of prejunctional β-adrenoceptors and hypertension. J Cardiovasc Pharmacol 1982;*4*:99–106.

6. Sneddon P, Burnstock G. ATP as a co-transmitter in rat tail artery. Europ J Pharmacol 1984;*106*:149–152.

7. Edvinsson L, Hakanson R, Wahlestedt C, Uddman, R. Effects of neuropeptide Y on the cardiovascular system. Trends Pharmacol Sci 1987;*8*:231–235.

8. Dale HH. On some physiological action of ergot. J Physiol (London). 1906;*34*:163–206.

9. Ahlquist RP. A study of the adrenotropic receptors. Am J Physiol 1948;*153*:586–600.

10. Starke K, Montel H, Gayk W, Merker R. Comparison of the effects of clonidine on pre- and postsynaptic adrenoceptors in the rabbit pulmonary artery. Naunyn-Schmiedeberg's Arch Pharmacol 1974;*285*:133–150.

11. Langer SZ. Presynaptic regulation of catecholamine release. Brit J Pharmacol 1974;*60*:481–497.

12. Berthelsen S, Pettinger WA. A functional basis for the classification of α-adrenergic receptors. Life Sci 1977;*21*:595–606.

13. Bylund DB. Subtypes of α_1- and α_2-adrenergic receptors. FASEB 1992;*6*:832–839.

14. Muramatsu I, Ohmura T, Kigoshi S, Hashimoto S, Oshita M. Pharmacological subclassification of α_1-adrenoceptors in vascular smooth muscle. Brit J Pharmacol 1990;*99*:197–201.

15. Lands AM, Arnold A, McAuliff JP, Luduena FP, Brown TG. Differentiation of receptor systems activated by sympathomimetic amines. Nature 1967;*214*:597–598.

16. Dixon RAF, Kobilka BK, Strader DJ, Benovic JL, Dohlman HG, Frielle T, Bolanowski MA, Bennett GD, Rands E, Diehl RE, Mumford RA, Slater EE, Sigal IA, Caron MG, Lefkowitz RJ, Strader CD. Cloning of the gene and cDNA for mammalian β-adrenergic receptor and homology with rhodopsin. Nature 1986;*321*:75–79.

17. Powell CE, Slater IH. Blocking of inhibitory adrenergic receptors by a dichloro analogue of isoproterenol. J Pharmacol Exp Ther 1958;*122*:480–488.

18. Ruffolo RR Jr, Nichols AJ. The relationship of receptor reserve and agonist efficacy to the sensitivity of α-adrenoceptor mediated vasopressor responses to inhibition by calcium channel antagonists. Ann NY Acad Sci 1988;*522*:361–376.

19. Limbird LE. Receptors linked to inhibition of adenylate cyclase: Additional signaling mechanisms. FASEB 1988;*2*:2686–2695.

20. Yatani A, Codina J, Imoto Y, Reenes JP, Birnbaumer L, Brown AM. Direct regulation of mammalian cardiac calcium channels by a G-protein. Science 1987;*238*:1288–1312.

21. Flavahan NA, Lindblad LE, Verbeuren TJ, Shepherd JT, Vanhoutte PM. Cooling and α_1- and α_2-adrenergic responses in cutaneous veins: Role of receptor reserve. Am J Physiol 1985;*249*:H950–H955.

22. Vatner DE, Knight DR, Homcy CJ, Vatner SF, Young MA. Subtypes of β-adrenergic receptors in bovine coronary arteries. Circ Res 1986;*59*:463–473.

23. Ruffolo RR Jr, Morgan EL. Interaction of the novel inotropic agent, ASL-7022, with α- and β-adrenoceptors in the cardiovascular system of the pithed rat: Comparison with dobutamine and dopamine. J Pharmacol Exp Ther 1984;*229*:364–371.

24. Pettinger WA, Smyth DD, Umemura S. Renal α_2-adrenoceptors, their locations and effects on sodium excretion. J Cardiovasc Pharmacol 1985;*7* (Suppl 8): S24–S27.

25. Brooks DP, Edwards RM, DePalma PD, Frederickson TA, Hieble JP, Gellai M. The water diuretic effect of the alpha-2 adrenoceptor agonist, AGN 190851, is species dependent. J Pharmacol Exp Ther 1991;*259*:1277–1282.

26. Saenz de Tejada I, Kim N, Lagan I, Krane RJ, Goldstein I. Regulation of adrenergic activity in penile corpus cavernosum. J Urol 1989;*142*:1117–1121.

27. Langin D, Portillo MP, Saulnier-Blache J-S, Lafontan M. Coexistence of three β-adrenoceptor subtypes in white fat cells of various mammalian species. Europ J Pharmacol 1991;*199*:291–301.

28. Berlan M, Lafontan M. Evidence that epinephrine acts preferentially as an antilipolytic agent in abdominal subcutaneous fat cells: assessment by analysis of β- and α_2-adrenoceptor properties. Eur J Clin Invest 1985;*15*:341–348.

29. Floras JS. Epinephrine and the genesis of hypertension. Hypertension 1992;*19*:1–18.

30. Ernsberger P, Giuliano R, Willette RN, Reis DJ. Role of imidazole receptors in the vasodepressor response to clonidine analogs in the rostral ventrolateral medulla. J Pharmacol Exp Ther 1990;*253*:408–418.

31. Hansson L, Svensson A, Gudbransson T, Sivertsson R. Treatment of hypertension with β-blockers with and without intrinsic sympathomimetic activity. J Cardiovasc Pharmacol 1983;*5* (Suppl. 1): S26–S29.

32. Barin ES, Wong CK, Elstob JE, Davies DW, Nathan DW. An acute study of the electrophysiological and hemodynamic effects of intravenous UK 52,046, a novel alpha-1 adrenoceptor antagonist. Br J Clin Pharmacol 1990;*29*:359–362.

33. Frishman WH, Skolnick AE, Lazar EJ, Fein S. β-Adrenergic blockade and calcium channel blockade in myocardial infarction. Med Clin North Amer 1989;*73*:409–436.

34. Caine M, Raz S, Ziegler M. Adrenergic and cholinergic receptors in the human prostate, prostatic capsule and bladder neck. Br J Urol 1975;*47*:193–202.

35. Ruffolo RR Jr. The pharmacology of dobutamine. Am J Med Sci 1987;*294*:244–248.

36. Ruffolo RR Jr. Chirality in α- and β-adrenoceptor agonists and antagonists. Tetrahedron 1991;*47*:9953–9980.

37. Ernsberger P, Damon TH, Graff LM, Schafer SG, Christen MO. Moxonidine, a centrally acting antihypertensive agent, is a selective ligand for I_1-imidazoline sites. J Pharmacol Exp Ther 1993;*246*:172–182.

38. Bristow MR, Ginsburg R, Umans V, Fowler M, Minobe W, Rasmussen R, Zera P, Menlove R, Shah P, Jamieson S, Stinson EB. β_1- and β_2-adrenoceptor subpopulations in nonfailing and failing human ventricular myocardium: Coupling of both receptor subtypes to muscle contraction and selective β_1-receptor downregulation in heart failure. Circ Res 1986;*59*:297–309.

39. Suzuki M, Hirose J, Asakura Y, Sato A, Kageyama A, Harano Y, Omae T. Insulin insensitivity in nonobese, nondiabetic essential hypertension and its improvement by an α_1-blocker (bunazosin). Am J Hypertension. 1992;*5*:869–874.

40. Cohn JN, Archibald DG, Ziesche S, Franciosa JA, Harston WE, Tristani FE, Dunkman WB, Jacobs W, Francis GS, Flohr KH, Goldman S, Cobb FR, Shah PM, Saunders R, Fletcher RD, Loeb HS, Hughes VC, Baker B. Effect of vasodilator therapy on mortality in chronic congestive heart failure. N Engl J Med 1986;*314*:1547–1552.

41. Lepor H, Meretyk S, Knapp-Maloney G. The safety, efficacy and compliance of terazosin therapy for benign prostatic hyperplasia. J Urol 1992;*147*:1554–1557.

42. Angel I, Schoemaker H, Duval N, Oblin A, Sevrin M, Langer SZ. SL 84.018, a new alpha-2 antagonist with anti-hypergylcaemic properties. Europ J Pharmacol 1990;*183*:990–991.

43. Neve KA, Molinoff PB. Turnover of beta-1 and beta-2 adrenergic receptors after down-regulation or irreversible blockade. Mol Pharmacol 1986;*30*:104–111.

44. Kaumann AJ. Is there a third heart β-adrenoceptor? Trends Pharmacol Sci 1989;*10*:316–320.

45. Tung LH, Jackman G, Campbell B, Louis S, Iakovidis D, Louis WJ. Partial agonist activity of celiprolol. J Cardiovasc Pharmacol 1993;*21*:484–488.

46. Fogari R, Zoppi A, Pasotti C, Poletti L, Tettamanti F, Malamani G, Corradi L. Plasma lipids during chronic antihypertensive therapy with different β-blockers. J Cardiovasc Pharmacol 1989;*14* (Suppl. 7): S28–S32.

47. Teravainen H, Huttunen J, Larsen TA. Selective adrenergic beta-2 receptor blocking drug ICI 118,551 is effective in essential tremor. Acta Neurol Scand 1986;*74*:34–37.

48. Sung C-P, Arleth AJ, Ohlstein EH. Carvedilol inhibits vascular smooth muscle cell proliferation. J Cardiovasc Pharmacol 1993;*21*:221–227.

49. Yue T-L, McKenna PJ, Lysko PG, Ruffolo RR, Feuerstein GZ. Carvedilol, a new antihypertensive, prevents oxidation of human low density lipoprotein by macrophages and copper. Atherosclerosis 1992;*97*:209–216.

50. von Euler US. A specific sympathomimetic ergone in adrenergic nerve fibres (sympathin) and its relations to adrenaline and noradrenaline. Acta Physiol Scand 1946;*12*:73–97.

Reviews

r1. Ruffolo RR Jr, Nichols AJ, Stadel JM, Hieble JP. Structure and function of α-adrenoceptors. Pharmacol Rev 1991;*43*:475–505.

r2. Nichols AJ, Ruffolo RR. α-Adrenoceptor subclassification. In: Ruffolo RR Jr (ed). α-Adrenoceptors: Molecular biology, biochemistry and pharmacology. Prog Basic Clin Pharmacol Vol. 8 Basel: Karger, (1991); pp 1–23.

r3. Stadel JM, and Nakada MT. Molecular biology of β-Adrenoceptors. In: Ruffolo RR Jr (ed). β-Adrenoceptors: Molecular biology, biochemistry and pharmacology. Prog Basic Clin Pharmacol, Vol 7 Basel: Karger, (1991); pp 26–66.

r4. Nichols AJ. α-Adrenoceptor signal transduction mechanisms. In: Ruffolo RR Jr (ed). α-Adrenoceptors: Molecular biology, biochemistry and pharmacology. Prog Basic Clin Pharmacol Vol. 8 Basel: Karger, (1991); pp 44–74.

r5. Stadel JM. β-Adrenoceptor signal transduction. In: Ruffolo RR Jr (ed). β-Adrenoceptors: Molecular biology, biochemistry and pharmacology. Prog Basic Clin Pharmacol, Vol 7. Basel: Karger, (1991); pp 67–104.

r6. Nichols AJ, Ruffolo RR. Functions mediated by α-adrenoceptors. In: Ruffolo RR Jr (ed). α-Adrenoceptors: Molecular biology, biochemistry and pharmacology. Prog Basic Clin Pharmacol Vol. 8 Basel: Karger, (1991); pp 115–179.

r7. Hieble JP, Ruffolo RR Jr. Functions mediated by β-adrenoceptor activation. In: Ruffolo RR Jr (ed). β-Adrenoceptors: Molecular biology, biochemistry and pharmacology. Prog Basic Clin Pharmacol, Vol 7. Basel: Karger, (1991); pp 173–209.

r8. Hieble JP, Ruffolo RR Jr. Subclassification of β-adrenoceptors. In: Ruffolo RR Jr (ed). β-Adrenoceptors: Molecular biology, biochemistry and pharmacology. Prog Basic Clin Pharmacol, Vol 7. Basel: Karger, (1991); pp 1–25.

r9. Hieble JP, Ruffolo RR Jr. Effects of alpha and beta adrenoceptors on lipids and lipoproteins. In: Witiak DT, Newman HAI, Feller DR (eds) Antilipidemic drugs: Medicinal chemical and biochemical aspects. Pharmacochemistry Library, Vol 17. Amsterdam: Elsevier, (1991); pp 301–344.

r10. Packer M. Vasodilator and inotropic drugs for the treatment of chronic heart failure: Distinguishing hype from hope. J Amer Coll Cardiol 1988;*12*:1299–1317.

r11. Charlap S, Lichstein E, Frishman WH. β-Adrenergic blocking drugs in the treatment of congestive heart failure. Med Clin North Amer 1989;*73*:373–385.

r12. Conolly ME. Sympathomimetic amines, β-adrenoceptors and bronchial asthma. In: Trendelenburg U, Weiner N. (eds) Handbook of experimental pharmacology, Vol. 90 (II). Berlin: Springer-Verlag, (1989); pp 357–389.

r13. Malta E, McPherson GA, Raper C. Selective β_1-adrenoceptor agonists-fact or fiction? Trends Pharmacol Sci 1985;*6*:400–403.

r14. Patil PN, Miller and Trendelenburg U. Molecular geometry and adrenergic drug activity. Pharmacol Rev 1974;*2*:323–392.

r15. Hieble JP. Structure-activity relationships for activation and blockade of β-adrenoceptors. In: Ruffolo RR Jr (ed). β-Adrenoceptors: Molecular biology, biochemistry and pharmacology. Prog Basic Clin Pharmacol Vol 7 Basel: Karger, (1991); pp 105–172.

r16. Hieble JP, Ruffolo RR Jr. Imidazoline receptors: Historical perspective. Fund Clin Pharmacol 1992;*6* (Suppl. 1): 7s–13s.

r17. Kennedy C. Possible roles for purine nucleotides in perivascular neurotransmission. In: Burnstock G, Griffith SG. (eds) Nonadrenergic innervation of blood vessels. Boca Raton: CRC Press, (1988); pp 65–76.

r18. Minneman KP. α_1-Adrenergic receptor subtypes, inositol phosphates and sources of cell calcium. Pharmacol Rev 1988;*40*:87–119.

r19. Nickerson M. The pharmacology of adrenergic blockade. Pharmacol Rev 1949;*1*:27–101.

CHAPTER 7

Pharmacology of Neuromuscular Transmission

J. Paul Hieble
Robert R. Ruffolo, Jr.

Introduction

The anatomy of the neuromuscular junction, and the physiologic and pharmacologic aspects of neuromuscular transmission have been studied for over one hundred years. As a consequence, this process is now understood in great detail. The neuromuscular junction and the associated nicotinic cholinergic receptor has served as a prototype for the initial application of several new techniques, including selective staining techniques, freeze-fracture electron microscopy, receptor isolation and reconstitution, cloning of receptor proteins, and actual visualization of receptors via high resolution electron microscopy. These studies have been aided by the availability of tissue sources having high densities of receptor proteins, such as the electric organs of several marine species, and proteinaceous neurotoxins that have high affinity and selectivity for the nicotinic cholinergic receptor.

The neuromuscular junction has also served as a model system for study of chemical neurotransmission, the quantal release of neurotransmitter from neuronal varicosities to activate an ion channel, and the process of receptor desensitization. The mechanisms by which the neurotransmitter of the neuromuscular junction, acetylcholine, is synthesized, stored, released, and degraded have been investigated extensively, and drugs affecting these processes have been developed.

Studies on neuromuscular transmission also provide illustrations of the development of pharmacologic techniques and principles of drug discovery. Naturally-occurring alkaloids, such as curare, have been utilized for centuries as arrow poisons. Claude Bernard, in 1856, showed that curare acts to block neuromuscular transmission, representing one of the first examples of a pharmacologic study to determine the site of drug action. Once the utility of curare as an adjunct to anesthesia was recognized, many synthetic and semisynthetic analogues were investigated in both preclinical and clinical models in order to improve therapeutic utility and eliminate side-effects. As a consequence, neuromuscular blocking agents are now indispensable tools in modern anesthetic practice.

Anatomy and Physiology of the Neuromuscular Junction

Specialized synaptic connections between motor nerves and skeletal muscle are found in all species, from simple invertebrates to humans. A schematic representation of the vertebrate neuromuscular junction is shown in Figure 7.1. Most mammalian skeletal muscle fibers have a single neuromuscular junction, located near the center (focal innervation); the muscle spindles are examples of multiple neuromuscular junctions on a single fiber, positioned at regular intervals (distributed innervation).[r1]

The neuromuscular junction has multiple synaptic clefts, with active zones of the presynaptic membrane arranged in apposition with concentrated regions of nicotinic cholinergic receptors on a folded postjunctional membrane. The junctional folds result in a substantially greater area of postjunctional vis-a-vis prejunctional membrane, and serve to increase the efficiency of neurotransmission by increasing the access of acetylcholinesterase to the released acetylcho-

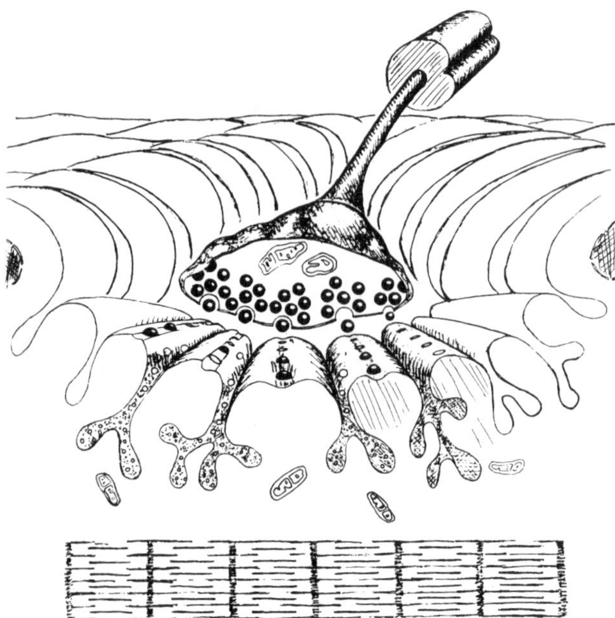

Figure 7.1 Schematic drawing depicting the chemical transmission of an impulse from a motor nerve to skeletal muscle. In the region of the neuromuscular junction, the motor nerve loses its myelin sheath; acetylcholine-containing vesicles are released into the synaptic cleft, where the neurotransmitter molecules can interact with nicotinic cholinergic receptors, concentrated in active zones on the region of muscle membrane in closest apposition with the nerve terminal. Acetylcholine diffusing away from the active zone into the junctional folds is more likely to be hydrolyzed by acetylcholinesterase. Acetylcholine-induced activation of the nicotinic receptors results in subsequent muscle contraction via interaction of the elements in the contractile protein array.

line once neurotransmitter diffuses away from the immediate vicinity of the synaptic cleft. This hypothesis is consistent with the presence of more extensive junctional folds in neuromuscular junctions of fast-twitch muscle fibers, compared with intermediate or slow-twitch fibers.[1]

Impulse transmission at the neuromuscular junction has been convincingly shown to result from quantal release of acetylcholine via vesicular exocytosis. Freeze-fracture electron microscopy, which can visualize the cytoplasmic face of the presynaptic membrane, can show sites of exocytosis at the active zone of the nerve terminal. Time course studies using extremely rapid freezing at defined intervals following nerve stimulation can actually identify vesicles in the process of exocytosis.[r2] The release process is calcium-dependent, and the particles shown by freeze-fracture studies to be present at the active zone of the presynaptic membrane may be voltage-dependent calcium channels.

Under resting conditions, sporadic release of acetylcholine maintains skeletal muscle tone. When the motor nerve is stimulated, the invading action potential results in a simultaneous exocytosis of several hundred vesicles. Each of these vesicles contains about 10,000 molecules of acetylcholine. Iontophoretic studies suggest that the amount of acetylcholine released in this manner by a single action potential is in the range of 10^{-17} moles (200,000–3,000,000 molecules).[r3] This acetylcholine activates the nicotinic cholinergic receptors on the postjunctional membrane (see following section) to produce an end-plate potential and open ionic channels to induce contraction of the muscle. Although this process generates an action potential in most skeletal muscles, neuromuscular transmission functions in a similar fashion in slow fibers where the end-plate potential propogates electrotonically. In most muscles, there is a substantial "safety factor," in that the amount of acetylcholine released is several fold greater than that required to initiate an action potential in the innervated muscle fiber.

In addition to the numerous acetylcholine vesicles, the neuronal terminal possesses a few giant synaptic vesicles, containing two to three times the amount of acetylcholine, as well as occasional dense-core vesicles. These dense-core vesicles have been thought to contain catecholamines, although recent studies[2] suggest that they may contain calcitonin gene related peptide. Synthetic enzymatic pathways for several neurotransmitters, including catecholamines, have been detected in the presynaptic terminal of the neuromuscular junction, although the contribution of neurotransmitters other than acetylcholine to neuromuscular transmission has not been established.

It is well known that transmission at the adrenergic neuroeffector junction can be modulated, both in vitro and in vivo, by a variety of neurotransmitter agonists acting at their respective prejunctional receptors. There is extensive evidence showing that nicotinic receptor agonists will induce repetitive antidromic firing in motor nerves. This action has been attributed to activation of prejunctional nicotinic receptors.[r4] Nevertheless, less is known concerning the role of prejunctional receptors in the modulation of transmitter release from motor vis-a-vis adrenergic nerve terminals.

Recent studies measuring the release of radiolabeled acetylcholine from the isolated phrenic nerve-diaphragm preparation in the rat have demonstrated that activation of prejunctional nicotinic cholinergic receptors can facilitate neuromuscular transmission. In addition, both inhibitory and facilitory muscarinic cholinergic receptors appear to be present in this preparation.[3] Whether these observations can be extended to other species and the extent of the functional contribution of positive or negative feedback regulation of acetylcholine release to neuromuscular transmission in the intact organism have yet to be established.

Several naturally occurring toxins can influence neuromuscular transmission. Of greatest clinical/ pathophysiologic relevance is the bacterial exotoxin, botulinum toxin, which acts prejunctionally to prevent quantal release of acetylcholine. Low doses of this toxin can block neuromuscular transmission, resulting in death by respiratory paralysis. Although the precise mechanism of action is not known, botulinum toxin is likely to inhibit the fusion of vesicles with the plasma membrane. The active component of black widow spider venom, α-latrotoxin, has the opposite effect, promoting exocytotic acetylcholine release, although the enhanced transmitter release produced by α-latrotoxin can eventually result in blockade of neuromuscular transmission as a result of depletion of acetylcholine stores.[2,4] β-Bungarotoxin, a component of krait venom, also produces blockade of neurotransmitter release from motor nerve terminals.[5] This action is thought to be a consequence of the phospholipase A_2 activity of β-bungarotoxin, perhaps by modification of the characteristics of the prejunctional plasma membrane. Alternatively, blockade of a specific calcium current may be involved.[6]

Another component of krait venom, α-bungarotoxin, acts at the postjunctional membrane and binds tightly to nicotinic cholinergic receptors. α-Bungarotoxin has been an invaluable tool in the isolation and characterization of nicotinic cholinergic receptors (see below). Histrionicotoxin, isolated from the skin of a Colombian frog, was used as an arrow poison. This toxin appears to bind to the nicotinic cholinergic receptor, thereby preventing passage of cations through the open channel[7] (see below). Local anesthetics appear to act in a similar fashion.

Molecular Characteristics of the Nicotinic Cholinergic Receptor

The characterization of the nicotinic cholinergic receptor on mammalian skeletal muscle has been greatly facilitated by the presence of a nearly identical receptor on the electrical organ of several species of fish. The most commonly studied are the electric eel (electrophorus) or marine ray (torpedo). The electric organs in these fish consist of stacks of flat cells over 1 cm in diameter. Cholinergic innervation is supplied to the ventral surface of each cell, with thousands of synapses per cell. Nerve stimulation results in ion fluxes, with consequent development of a large electrical charge. The electric organs are phylogenetically derived from skeletal muscle, and the anatomy of the cholinergic synapse and the physiology of synaptic transmission are remarkably similar to those at the mammalian neuromuscular junction. However, in contrast to mammalian skeletal muscle, which has a receptor density of less than 0.1 mg/kg of muscle, the electric organ of torpedo can contain over 100 mg of receptor protein per kg of organ. Since a large torpedo can carry over 2 kg of electrical organ, this ray represents a rich source of nicotinic cholinergic receptor. When the nicotinic cholinergic receptor was first isolated from mammalian sources, its morphologic characteristics were found to be identical to those isolated from the electrical organ, and a high degree of homology was found in the composition of the individual polypeptide chains comprising the receptor.

The nicotinic cholinergic receptor is composed of five subunits, oriented around a central transmembrane channel (Fig. 7.2).[8] In receptors of torpedo electrical organ, four similar but nonidentical polypeptides, designated α, β, γ, and δ, form the subunits, with two α-peptides being present. Each peptide is composed of approximately 500 amino acids. In mammalian skeletal muscle, the γ polypeptide is present in fetal skeletal muscle, but is replaced by an isoform, designated as ε, during maturation and consequent motor innervation.[9] The γ peptide sequence is retained in mature nicotinic cholinergic receptors spatially removed from the neuromuscular junction. A peripheral membrane protein (ν protein) is closely associated with the nicotinic receptor, and may serve to anchor the receptor at the postsynaptic site.[10]

As noted below, the subunit polypeptides have similar tertiary structure, but differ from one another substantially with respect to primary amino acid sequence. For example, in calf skeletal muscle, there is less than 40 percent homology between the α subunit and either the β, γ or δ subunit.[11] There is a greater degree of homology between γ, δ, and ε subunits (approximately 50%). The individual subunits are highly conserved within mammalian species (> 90% homology between human and calf) and substantial homology (55–80%, with the α-subunit being the most highly conserved) is retained between human and torpedo polypeptides.[12]

Hydrophilicity analysis suggests four membrane spanning domains for each subunit, with a fifth amphipathic sequence potentially forming an α-helix within the membrane, although controversy remains as to whether the peptide spans the membrane four or five times.[13] Despite the controversy regarding the conformation of each subunit,[14] electron microscopy has confirmed the pseudo-5-fold rotational symmetry of the intact receptor.[15] Both electron microscopy and electrophysiologic studies suggest a maximal density of 10,000 individual nicotinic cholinergic receptors per square micrometer on the postjunctional muscle membrane immediately opposed to the active sites of acetylcholine release.

Binding of acetylcholine molecules to the receptor triggers the opening of the central pore, allowing the passage of cations. Although the channel is likely to open only if two acetylcholine molecules are bound the receptor, one to each α-subunit,[16] there is a finite

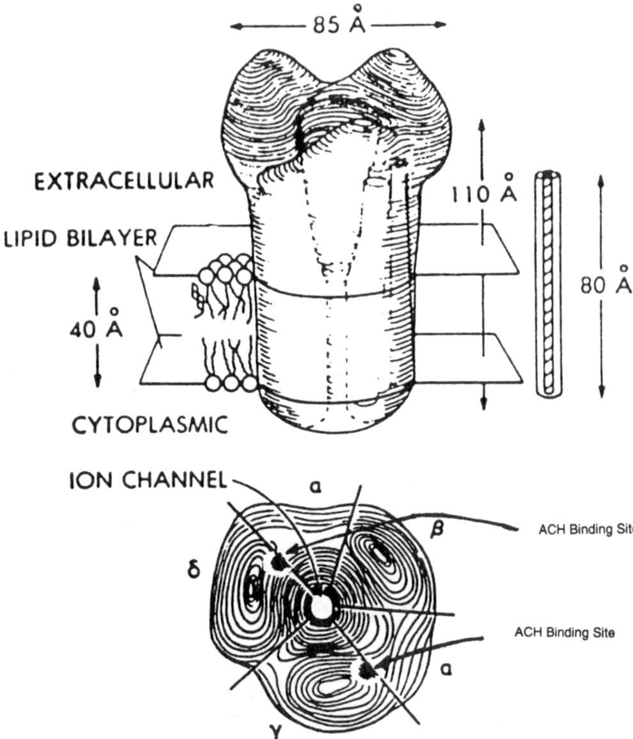

Figure 7.2 Three-dimensional model of nicotinic cholinergic receptor from *Torpedo californica*, showing the pentameric arrangement of the four distinct subunits. The specific assignment of subunit location around the central ion channel is tentative. The two binding sites for acetylcholine are thought to be located at the interfaces of the α-subunits with the λ and δ-subunit. Modified from McCarthy et al, The molecular neurobiology of the acetylcholine receptor. Am Rev Neurosci 1986;9:383–413.

probability of opening upon interaction of the receptor with one neurotransmitter molecule. The two binding sites in the intact receptor are not identical, perhaps as a consequence of differing degrees of glycosylation of the two α-subunits, or because of the asymmetry resulting from different subunits flanking the two α-subunits.[17] Although the binding of cholinergic receptor agonists or toxins is localized to the α-subunit, the adjacent subunits alter the receptor environment so as to enhance agonist affinity. The binding site has been localized to a specific region within the α-subunit polypeptide sequence (amino acids 185–196). A postulated model for the active site shows an interaction of the acetylcholine molecule with four amino acids.[18] Alteration of amino acid sequence in this region can have a dramatic effect on affinity of the receptor for nicotinic ligands and may explain species differences in receptor characteristics. For example, the nicotinic cholinergic receptors of snakes producing the neurotoxin, α-bungarotoxin, have amino acid differences in this key region, which result in loss of affinity for the toxin.[19]

Upon activation of the nicotinic cholinergic receptor, the channel has an open time of approximately one millisecond, although electrophysiologic studies of individual channels suggests that there may be brief intervals during which the pore is closed even though the agonist sites of the receptor remain occupied. This phenomenon is referred to as flickering or "Nachschlag." The open channel allows the passage of most positively charged species, including divalent cations, such as calcium, but is impermeable to anions. The primary ions traversing the channel under physiologic conditions are sodium and potassium. During the millisecond interval when the channel is open, approximately 10,000 sodium ions enter the skeletal muscle cell.

Prolonged contact of the nicotinic cholinergic receptor with agonists will induce receptor desensitization. This phenomenon, where the channel closes despite the continued presence of agonist at the active site, has been studied extensively but is still not completely understood. There is substantial evidence to suggest that there are two separate conformations of the desensitized receptor, and that the interaction of an agonist with the nicotinic cholinergic receptor may progress through the following stages:

Resting Receptor → Open Channel → Fast Onset Desensitized → Slow Onset Desensitized with the open channel and fast onset desensitized states being the most transient.[20] Receptor phosphorylation is thought to be involved in the desensitization process. The agonist binding sites responsible for induction of desensitization may be different from those responsible for channel opening, and it is possible that certain noncompetitive inhibitors of the nicotinic cholinergic receptor may act by stabilization of the fast onset desensitized state. The recovery from the desensitized state is quite slow (minutes), owing in part to greater affinity of desensitized vis-a-vis resting receptors. The isomerization constant between resting and desensitized nicotinic cholinergic receptors can vary considerably between species, with the torpedo receptor being significantly more susceptible to desensitization than that of human skeletal muscle. Based on studies of the frog neuromuscular junction, it appears that desensitization does not make an important contribution in vivo to neuromuscular transmission under physiologic conditions, because acetylcholine is rapidly degraded by acetylcholinesterase. However, desensitization of nicotinic cholinergic receptors can be readily observed in vivo when acetylcholinesterase is inhibited.

Disorders of Neuromuscular Transmission

Myasthenia Gravis

Myasthenia gravis, characterized by muscle weakness and abnormal fatigability upon exertion, has been studied clinically for over a century. Symptoms are variable, with only specific muscle groups (e.g., ocular muscles) affected in some patients, while other patients experience generalized muscle weakness. Furthermore, the severity of the disease can be highly variable within an individual patient. The observation of Patrick and Lindstrom[21] that rabbits develop myasthenic symptoms when immunized with purified electric eel nicotinic cholinergic receptor protein confirmed the hypothesis that myasthenia gravis results when antibodies are directed against the skeletal muscle nicotinic cholinergic receptor.

Although nearly all myasthenia gravis patients have circulating antibodies directed against the nicotonic cholinergic receptor, the nature of these antibodies is highly variable. The level of antibodies does not necessarily correlate with the severity of the disease. Although most antibodies are directed toward the α-subunit of the receptor, many patients also have antibodies directed against sites on the β and γ subunits. In most cases the antibodies do not interfere with the function of the nicotinic cholinergic receptor, but rather result in accelerated receptor degradation, causing a deficit in the number of postjunctional nicotinic cholinergic receptors.

The origin of the autoimmune response against the nicotinic cholinergic receptor remains controversial. The observation that myasthenic patients have a antibody profile similar to that observed in animals immunized with purified receptor proteins has been interpreted as evidence that the actual receptor serves as the immunogen in humans, rather than a cross reacting sequence in a foreign (e.g., viral or bacterial) protein. However, it is possible that most of the circulating antibodies in patients are the result of antigenic degradation products resulting from the accelerated catabolism of the nicotinic cholinergic receptor, and an infectious origin of myasthenia gravis cannot be excluded.[22] A subgroup of myasthenic patients have an associated thymoma, which has been postulated as a source of the antigen in this population.

Lambert-Eaton Myasthenic Syndrome

This condition is often associated with small cell carcinoma of the lung, although it can occur in patients with other malignancies, or without any tumor association. Onset of muscular contraction is delayed, with the proximal muscles of the lower extremities being most affected. In contrast to myasthenia gravis, Lambert-Eaton myasthenic syndrome results from a prejunctional deficit, such that the number of acetylcholine quanta released by a nerve impulse is reduced. Electron microscopy of the prejunctional membrane of neuromuscular junctions from affected patients suggest an alteration in the voltage-sensitive calcium channel,[23] consistent with electrophysiologic studies showing a reduced dependence of quantal acetylcholine release on external calcium concentration.[24]

Lambert-Eaton myasthenic syndrome is thought to have an autoimmune origin. Thus, the electrophysiologic and morphologic features of Lambert-Eaton myasthenic syndrome can be transferred from humans to experimental animals via injection of serum immunoglobulins. It is likely that in patients with malignant disease the myasthenic syndrome results from a tumor-associated antigen having similarity to the calcium channel of the motor nerve terminal. The antibodies generated by this antigen could interfere with calcium channel function via multiple mechanisms.[r5]

Congenital Myasthenic States

Several congenital myasthenic states have been characterized, and all are associated with muscular weakness. These can result from either prejunctional or postjunctional deficits, including alteration in acetylcholine mobilization, prolonged opening of the postjunctional ion channel, deficiency in acetylcholinesterase, or deficiency in the number of postjunctional nicotinic cholinergic receptors.[25]

Drugs Influencing Neuromuscular Transmission

Acetylcholinesterase Inhibitors

As noted above, the anatomy of the neuromuscular junction is designed to provide maximal exposure of the released acetylcholine to acetylcholinesterase, which hydrolyzes the neurotransmitter to its inactive precursor, choline, once it has diffused beyond the immediate region of the nicotinic cholinergic receptors. Rapid degradation of the neurotransmitter is required to prevent desensitization of the nicotinic cholinergic receptor. In view of the high density of acetyl-cholinesterase (2000–3000 molecules per square micrometer), the efficiency of the enzyme in hydrolyzing acetylcholine (30,000 molecules of acetylcholine hydrolyzed per minute per molecule of acetylcholinesterase), and the high concentration of acetylcholine released from the prejunctional nerve terminal, it is not surprising that inhibition of acetylcholinesterase has profound effects on neuromuscular transmission.

Acetylcholine has been shown to have a two-point attachment to the active site of the acetylcholinesterase molecule (Fig. 7.3). The positively charged quaternary nitrogen, binding electrostatically to a histidine residue, holds the neurotransmitter in a position placing the ester linkage in proximity to an activated serine residue capable of nucleophilic attack on the acyl carbon. Inhibitors of acetylcholinesterase bind to one or both of these sites. Representative agents are shown in Figure 7.4; typical doses and pharmacokinetic parameters of some of the agents commonly used clinically are shown in Table 7.1 . Physostigmine, a naturally-occurring alkaloid, has long been recognized as an inhibitor of acetylcholinesterase. The synthetic carbamate esters, neostigmine and pyridostigmine, incorporate the active moiety of the physostigmine molecule. Although carbamates containing a tertiary or quaternary nitrogen atom are of comparable potency as enzyme inhibitors, the quaternary agents are often more useful clinically because side-effects due to blockade of acetylcholinesterase within the CNS are eliminated. The carbamates bind to both sites of acetylcholinesterase, and are slowly hydrolyzed. The enzyme must then be reactivated by hydrolytic cleavage of the carbamoyl group from the esterase site.

Edrophonium attaches only to the cation binding site of acetylcholinesterase, thereby reversibly prevent-

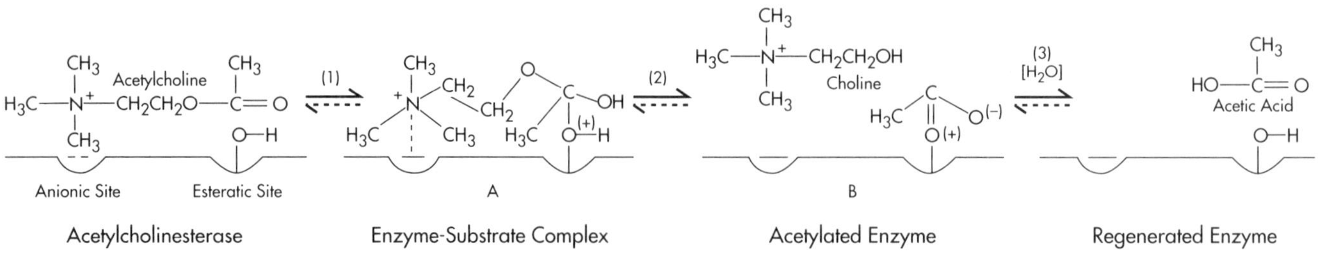

Figure 7.3 Mechanism of acetylchloline hydrolysis by acetylcholinesterase. The substrate combines with the enzyme by a bidentate electrostatic attraction between: (1) the quaternary nitrogen and an anionic site of the enzyme; and (2) the electrophilic carbon of the acetoxy group and a serine (residue 200) hydroxyl. This serine is made highly nucleophilic by an adjacent imidazole group. A tetrahedral complex is formed (step 1), followed by cleavage of the ester linkage (step 2). The acetylated enzyme then reacts with water to regenerate active enzyme.

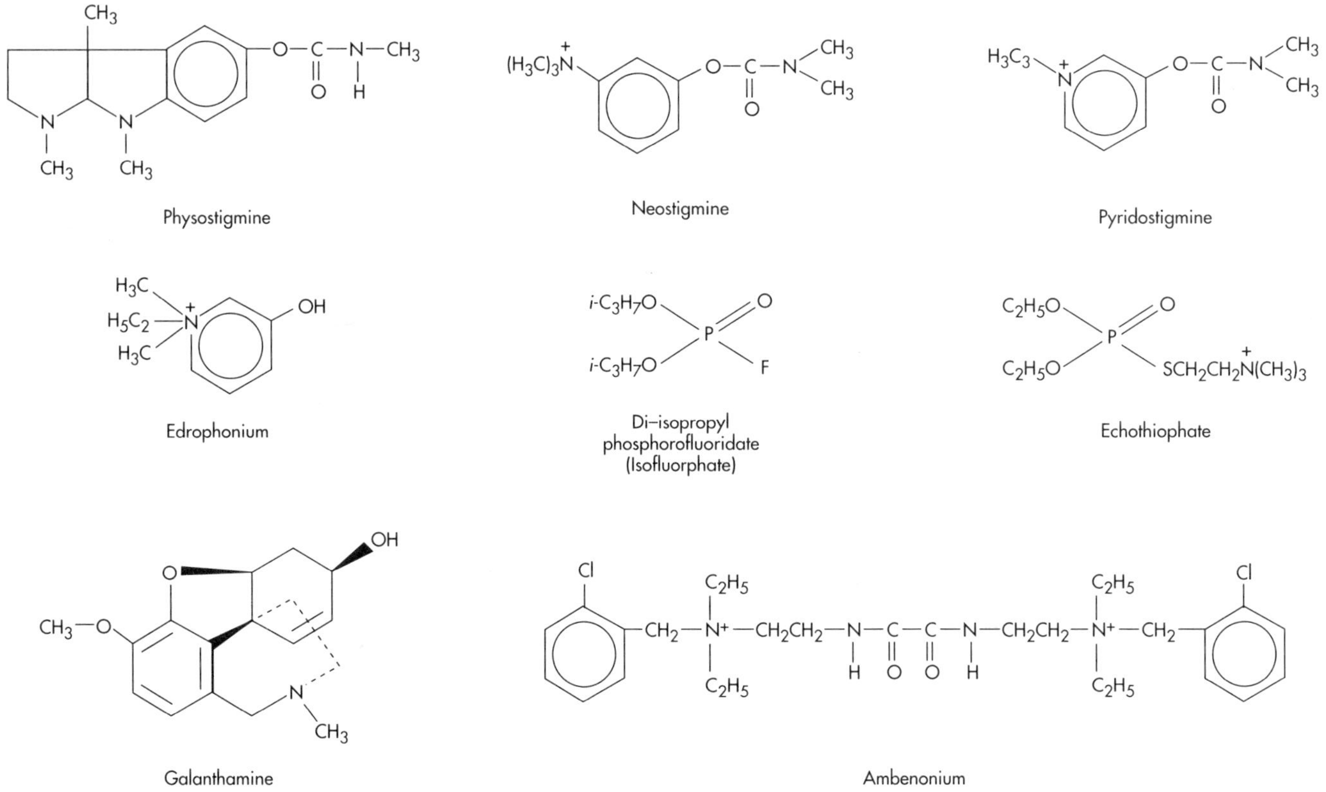

Figure 7.4 Inhibitors of Acetylcholinesterase

ing the binding of acetylcholine. This weak, one-point interaction between enzyme and inhibitor results in a short duration of action. A similar competitive inhibition is produced by simple quaternary ammonium compounds, such as tetraethylammonium salts. This principle has been used to develop agents, such as pralidoxine, capable of reactivating acetylcholinesterase following its "irreversible" inhibition by the organophorus derivatives described below.

In contrast, the organophosphorus derivatives, which also bind to only one of the acetylcholine binding sites, produce an irreversible inactivation of acetylcholinesterase. This results from the formation of an extremely stable covalent bond between the inhibitor and the esterase site. This bond is resistant to hydrolysis, and in many cases restoration of acetylcholinesterase activity requires the synthesis of new enzyme. Organophosphorus compounds can be applied topically in the treatment of glaucoma, and are utilized extensively as insecticides and chemical warfare agents, but are not used systemically in humans to influence neuromuscular transmission.

Table 7.1 Summary of Dosage and Pharmacokinetics of Cholinesterase Inhibitors

	Dosage			Pharmacokinetics			
Drug	**Route**	**Size**	**Dose**	**Peak**	**V_D**	**$t_{1/2}$**	**Clearance or Duration of Response**
Cholinesterase Inhibitors							
Edrophonium							
Tensilon	Parenteral	10 mg/ml	1–2 mg IV for myasthemia assessment				
			10–40 mg IV for antagonism of relaxants	1–2 min		Effects last 5–10 min	
Ambenonium							
Mytelase	Oral	10 mg tablet	5 mg tid or qid				Effects last 4–8 hr
Neostigmine	Oral	15-mg tablets	15 mg tid for myasthenia	1–2 hr			lasts 2–4 hr
Prostigmine	Parenteral	0.25–1 mg/ml	0.5–5 mg for antagonism of relaxants			52 min	
Physostigmine							
Antilirium	Parenteral	1 mg/ml	0.5–2 mg	immediate		15–40 min	lasts ½–5 hr
Pyridostigmine	Oral	60-mg tablets	60 mg tid initially	onset 40 min			Effect lasts 3–6 hr
Mestinon	Parenteral	5 mg/ml	10–20 mg	onset 5 min			lasts 2–3 hr

The alkaloid, galanthamine, and the oxalamide analogue, ambenonium, are examples of other chemical classes that have clinically useful acetylcholinesterase activity. Neither of these drugs are substrates for the enzyme, and they inhibit the enzyme primarily via a competitive action.

Therapeutic Applications

Although acetylcholinesterase inhibitors have several established therapeutic applications, and have been proposed for additional indications, discussion here will be limited to their utility in the treatment of myasthenic states and their use to reverse the effects of nondepolarizing neuromuscular blockade. Acetylcholinesterase inhibitors have been used extensively in the therapy of myasthenia gravis. Pyridostigmine is currently the drug of choice, owing to its relatively long duration of action and relatively low incidence of GI side-effects. The increase in acetylcholine concentration within the synaptic cleft partially compensates for the decreased postjunctional receptor density. The dose must be adjusted in response to changes in the severity of the disease. Because inhibition of acetylcholinesterase also increases acetylcholine concentrations at muscarinic cholinergic synapses of the autonomic nervous system, atropine or another muscarinic cholinergic receptor antagonist often must be employed to control the side-effects resulting from muscarinic cholinergic receptor overactivity, such as abdominal cramps, diarrhea, and salivation. In recent years, immunosuppressive therapy often has been used to supplement the use of acetylcholinesterase inhibitors in the treatment of myasthenic states, often allowing a reduction in dosage.

Acetylcholinesterase inhibitors are not generally effective in Lambert-Eaton myasthenic syndrome, and anticholinesterase inhibitor therapy is utilized in this condition only when other modes of therapy fail or are contraindicated.

When acetylcholinesterase is inhibited, stimulation of the nicotinic cholinergic receptor by acetylcholine can induce its desensitization, resulting in neuromuscular blockade. This is the mechanism by which the organophosphorus acetylcholinesterase inhibitors produce their toxic effects. Hence, in the myasthenic patient, the symptoms of overdosage with an acetylcholinesterase inhibitor often will resemble those of the untreated state or those of an insufficient dose. In order to assess whether muscle weakness results from under- or overdosage, the patient may be challenged with the short-acting acetylcholinesterase inhibitor, edrophonium. If the muscular weakness results from an insufficient degree of enzyme inhibition, edrophonium will produce a transient improvement in muscle strength. On the other hand, if the weakness results from excess nicotonic cholinergic receptor activation which produces desensitization, no improvement will be observed. Edrophonium can also be used in this manner to differentiate myasthenia gravis from other conditions that produce muscular weakness.

Acetylcholinesterase inhibitors are commonly utilized to antagonize the neuromuscular blockade produced by the nondepolarizing blocking agents (see below). This action is consistent with their ability to increase synaptic concentrations of acetylcholine, which will overcome the competitive blockade of the nicotinic cholinergic receptor. Inhibition of acetylcholinesterase will not attenuate, and often will exacerbate, neuromuscular blockade produced by depolarizing drugs. Reversal of surgical neuromuscular blockade is useful in order to allow the use of long-acting neuromuscular blocking agents to maintain muscular relaxation, and yet avoid long lasting respiratory depression following completion of the surgical procedure. Cholinesterase inhibitors commonly used for this purpose are neostigmine and edrophonium. Clinical evidence suggests that neostigmine is the more useful agent when reversal of profound neuromuscular blockade is required;[26] however, the efficacy of a cholinesterase inhibitor may depend on the particular neuromuscular blocker used.[27] The efficacy of edrophonium may be compromised by an additional action to inhibit opening time of the acetylcholine receptor coupled ion channel.[28]

Drugs Facilitating the Release of Acetylcholine

4-Aminopyridine (Pymadin)

4-Aminopyridine has been shown to facilitate the quantal release of acetylcholine from isolated nerve-muscle preparations in which neurotransmission has been partially impaired by a nondepolarizing blocker or by elevated magnesium ion.[r6] This action is thought to result from a prolongation of the neuronal action potential, resulting in a facilitation of the influx of extracellular calcium and the release of neurotransmitter. Electron microscopy shows that 4-aminopyridine increases the number of synaptic vesicles fused with the synaptic membrane.[29] Although 4-aminopyridine has been shown to be effective in both myasthenia gravis and Lambert-Eaton myasthenic syndrome, it produced frequent and severe side-effects, including grand mal seizures. A related agent, 3,4-diaminopyridine, has shown a good clinical response in Lambert-Eaton myasthenia, with only minor side-effects. 4-Aminopyridine is commonly used in some European countries to reverse nondepolarizing neuromuscular blockade.

Guanidine

Electrophysiologic studies have established that guanidine will potentiate calcium-dependent quantal acetylcholine release. Furthermore, this effect is maximal under conditions of low quantal release. This profile suggests that guanidine would be effective in Lambert-Eaton myasthenia. Although positive clinical results have indeed been obtained, several potentially fatal toxic effects, such as bone marrow depression and renal failure, severely limit use of the drug.

Neuromuscular Blocking Agents

Extensive research has been devoted to the identification of clinically useful neuromuscular blocking agents, primarily because these agents can produce skeletal muscle relaxation during surgical procedures. Most of these drugs contain two cationic sites, usually quaternary ammonium groups, linked by a spacing group (Fig. 7.6). This spacing group can range from a simple aliphatic chain, to a highly rigid steroidal ring system, or both ammonium groups and spacing link can be incorporated into a complex alkaloid. Neuromuscular blocking drugs can be divided into two classes, nondepolarizing agents, which produce competitive blockade of neuromuscular transmission without activation of the nicotinic cholinergic receptor, and the depolarizing agents, which produce an initial activation of the nicotinic cholinergic receptor, followed by blockade due to desensitization. Depolarizing agents have a highly flexible, generally unbranched chain linking the two cationic sites, whereas the nondepolarizing agents have a rigid or sterically hindered linkage. Increasing the rigidity of the link or dispersing the charge density of the cationic sites can convert the mechanism of a neuromuscular blocking agent from depolarizing to nondepolarizing. Owing to the side-effects associated with the depolarizing agents, most usage has centered on the nondepolarizing type, although succinylcholine, a depolarizing blocker, remains the drug of choice for producing the rapid and short-lasting neuromuscular blockade required for tracheal intubation.

Nondepolarizing Drugs

The first crude samples of the arrow poisons used by South American tribes arrived in Europe during the latter part of the 16th century. It was soon recognized that these substances caused death in animals through neuromuscular paralysis. Many years elapsed before the active alkaloids in these plant resins, generically termed "curare," were identified and isolated. It was eventually established that several groups of alkaloids, containing two tertiary or quaternary nitrogen atoms, were responsible for their neuromuscular blocking action. The first to be identified was d-tubocurarine, containing one tertiary and one quaternary amine group, produced by several species of *Strychnos* and *Chondrodendon*. *Strychnos toxifera* produces a different alkaloid, toxiferine, a bis quaternary amine, which is even more potent as a neuromuscular blocking agent. Many other alkaloids have been found to have neuromuscular blocking activity, and it is now recognized that almost all molecules containing a quaternary amine group can produce measurable blockade of neuromuscular transmission.

In 1857, Claude Bernard, using electrical stimulation of the sciatic nerve in a frog, localized the site of action of curare to skeletal muscle, as opposed to peripheral nerves or the CNS. Subsequent studies have localized its action to the neuromuscular junction, since curarized skeletal muscle is still responsive to direct electrical stimulation. Most of the mechanism of action studies involving nondepolarizing neuromuscular blockers have been performed using d-tubocurarine, although all of the nondepolarizing neuromuscular blockers (Table 7.2, Fig. 7.5) appear to interact with the neuromuscular junction in a similar fashion. Blockade of nerve-induced muscular contraction in an isolated preparation can be shown to result from three actions: (1) competitive blockade of the interaction between acetylcholine and the active site of the nicotinic cholinergic receptor; (2) impeding the passage of cations through open channels; and (3) impairment of quantal release of acetylcholine from the prejunctional nerve terminal, presumably via blockade of a facilitory prejunctional nicotinic cholinergic receptor. However, in the clinical use of nondepolarizing neuromuscular blocking agents, only competitive blockade of the nicotinic cholinergic receptor makes a significant contribution to the pharmacologic action. In some nicotinic cholinergic receptor preparations, d-tubocurarine can produce transient activation of the receptor; however, this has never been demonstrated in mammalian skeletal muscle, where this agent acts as a full competitive antagonist.

Therapeutic Utility

The first clinical use of d-tubocurarine was in the relief of spastic disorders. Although effective in some cases, its utility is limited by lack of oral absorption. The primary use of the neuromuscular blocking agents are as adjuncts to general anesthesia, in order to allow sufficient skeletal muscle relaxation to facilitate abdominal or orthopedic surgery. This use of neuromuscular blocking agents eliminates the need for higher concentrations of general anesthetics to produce skeletal muscle relaxation. As such, neuromuscular blocking agents reduce the incidence of cardiovascular depression and other side-effects associated with general anesthesia; they also speed the recovery from anesthesia. The first trial of d-tubocurarine as an adjunct to general anesthesia was reported in 1942; since that time many new neuromuscular blockers have been evaluated for this use and several have been introduced into clinical practice.

In both experimental animals and in humans, different skeletal muscles display different sensitivity to the neuromuscular blocking agents. When d-tubocurarine is administered IV to humans, small muscles of the head and neck are paralyzed first, as evidenced by difficulty in focusing, ptosis, and dysphagia. Muscles of the limbs are then paralyzed, as well as the intercostal muscles. The diaphragmatic control of respiration is last to be affected. Recovery occurs in the reverse order, with function being restored first to the diaphragm. Neuromuscular blocking agents have been studied extensively with respect to differential action on the various muscle groups, with the goal of identifying agents that can produce effective abdominal relaxation with little or no depression of respiration. While some agents, such as gallamine, do appear to spare the respiratory muscles to a greater degree than does d-tubocurarine, the magnitude of this selectivity is variable and of questionable clinical relevance. It should be noted that the neuromuscular blocking agents do not affect pain perception; supplementary analgesic agents must be utilized to relieve surgical pain if the general anesthesia employed does not produce sufficient analgesia.

The rate on onset and recovery from neuromuscular blockade by the nondepolarizing agents can be slow, and varies substantially between particular agents. It has been suggested that the primary determinant of recovery rate from nondepolarizing neuromus-

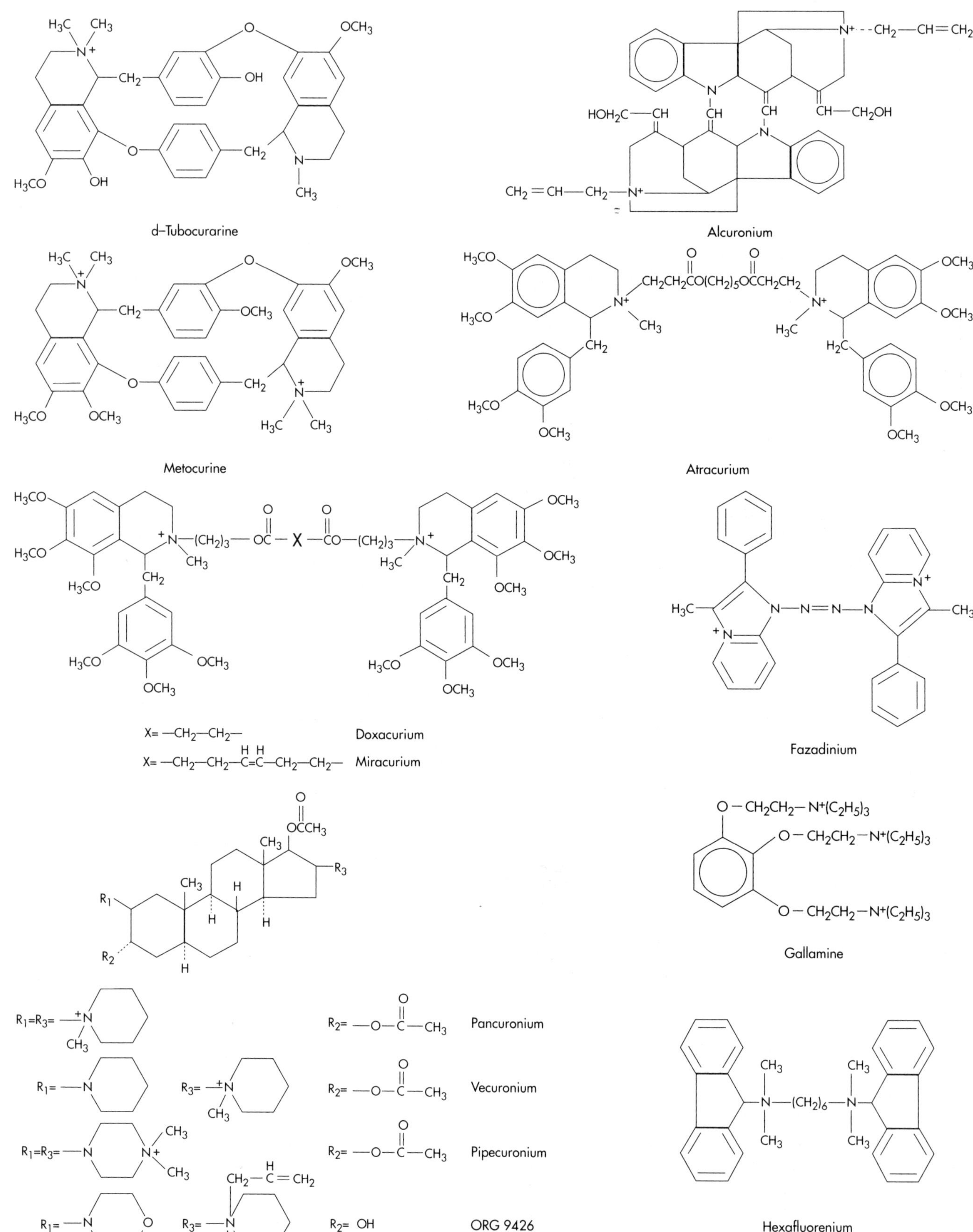

Figure 7.5 Nondepolarizing Neuromuscular Blocking Drugs

Table 7.2 Summary of Depolarizing and Nondepolarizing Muscle Relaxants

	Dosage			Pharmacokinetics			
Drug	**Route**	**Size**	**Dose**	**Peak**	**V_D**	**$t_{1/2}$**	**Clearance or Duration of Response**
Depolarizing Muscle Relaxant							
Succinylcholine							
Anectine	Parenteral	20–100 mg/ml	1 mg/kg IV 2–4 mg/kg IM	1 min			lasts up to 10 min
Nondepolarizing Relaxants							
Atracurium							
Tracrium	Parenteral	10 mg/ml	0.4–0.5 mg/kg	3–5 min	160 ml/kg	20 min	20–35 min
Doxacurium							
Nuromax	Parenteral	1 mg/ml	0.05 mg/kg	5 min	220 ml/kg	99 min	39–232 min
Gallamine							
Flaxedil	Parenteral	20 mg/ml	1 mg/kg	3 min			lasts 20–40 min
Metocurine							
Metubine	Parenteral	2 mg/ml	0.2–0.4 mg/ml		446 ml/kg	270 min	lasts 30–90 min
Mivacurium							
Mivacron	Parenteral	2 mg/ml	0.15 mg/kg	3 min			15–20 min
Pancuronium							
Pavulon	Parenteral	1–2 mg/ml	0.06–0.1 mg/kg	3 min	313 ml/kg	199 min	60 min
Tubocurarine							
Tubocucrarine	Parenteral	3 mg/ml	3–30 mg	2–5 min	425 ml/kg	173 min	30–45 min
Vecuronium							
Norcuron	Parenteral	10 or 20 mg/vial	0.08–0.1 mg/kg	3 min	120 ml/kg	30–80 min	20–30 min

cular blockade is the rate of drug-receptor dissociation.[30] Recent evidence supports the concept of a binding site for these drugs in the biophase surrounding the neuromuscular junction.[31]

While d-tubocurarine is still utilized clinically, this agent has several side-effects not associated with some of the newer drugs. d-Tubocurarine has the capability to induce histamine release from mast cells and basophilic leukocytes. This effect can be demonstrated in humans at neuromuscular blocking doses, and can result in bronchoconstriction, hypotension, and excessive salivation. In addition, although the ganglionic cholinergic nicotinic receptor is substantially less sensitive to blockade by d-tubocurarine compared with the nicotonic cholinergic receptor present at the neuromuscular junction, some ganglionic blockade is observed at clinically effective doses. The combination of ganglionic blockade and histamine release can produce marked hypotension if d-tubocurarine is injected rapidly.

d-Tubocurarine is not extensively metabolized, and is eliminated primarily in the urine. Hence, its duration of action is prolonged in patients with renal impairment. It is difficult to compare the rate of onset and recovery from neuromuscular blockade accurately in humans, since these parameters are dependent on several factors, such as the general anesthetic used and the relative dose of neuromuscular blocker given. However, d-tubocurarine appears to have an onset of action equivalent to that of the newer nondepolarizing drugs, but requires a somewhat longer period for complete recovery from neuromuscular blockade. If repeated doses are administered, recovery times for a given dose are prolonged. The interaction of d-tubocurarine with the nicotinic cholinergic receptor is stereoselective, since the l-enantiomer is 20–60-fold less potent than the naturally occurring d-enantiomer.

Metocurine is a derivative of d-tubocurarine in which both phenolic hydroxyl groups have been methylated, and both nitrogen atoms are quaternary. The pharmacologic properties of metocurine are similar to the parent, d-tubocurarine, except for a three-fold greater potency. Metocurine has less of a tendency to induce histamine release than d-tubocurarine. Absolute potency of metocurine as a ganglionic blocking agent is reduced, compared with d-tubocurarine, giving this agent a greater safety ratio with respect to this side-effect than d-tubocurarine, in view of its greater potency at the neuromuscular junction. This prediction is confirmed by a lack of prominent hemodynamic effect of therapeutic doses of metocurine. Another semisynthetic neuromuscular blocking agent, alcuronium (diallyl-bisnortoxiferine), is also approximately three-fold more potent than d-tubocurarine. Alcuronium does not appear to influence ganglionic neurotransmission at therapeutic doses.

Pancuronium has two quaternized piperidine nuclei joined by a steroid ring system. Pancuronium is a potent (ten-fold more potent than d-tubocurarine), long-lasting neuromuscular blocking agent, with no pharmacologically significant ganglionic blocking activity. In contrast to the hypotensive effect of d-tubocurarine, rapid injection of pancuronium can increase blood pressure, probably as a consequence of increased cardiac output. This hemodynamic action, and the commonly associated tachycardia, results from the ability of pancuronium to inhibit vagal activity. Like d-tubocurarine, multiple dosing with pancuronium is associated with an enhanced degree of neuromuscular blockade. Pancuronium is eliminated both by renal excretion and by hepatic hydroxylation. In contrast to other neuromuscular blockers, pancuronium produces potent inhibition of plasma cholinesterase. However, since its inhibitory activity at synaptic acetylcholinesterase is several orders of magnitude lower, and plasma cholinesterase has no known physiologic function (other than degradation of certain drugs such as procaine and succinylcholine), this activity probably is not important clinically.

Many derivatives of pancuronium have been evaluated clinically as neuromuscular blocking drugs.[r7] The most widely used of these analogs are vecuronium, in which only one piperidine nucleus is quaternized, and pipecuronium, in which the pyridine rings are replaced by quaternized piperazine rings. Vecuronium has a more rapid onset and shorter duration of action than pancuronium, while pipecuronium has comparable (slightly shorter duration) pharmacokinetics. Both analogues are at least as potent as pancuronium, with pipecuronium being significantly more potent in some assays. Neither vecuronium nor pipecuronium have the cardiovascular effects associated with pancuronium, consistent with their lack of vagolytic activity. Multiple dosing is associated with less enhancement of neuromuscular blocking activity, compared to pancuronium. A steroidal agent, ORG 9426, is currently undergoing clinical trials. This compound, although less potent, appears to have an even more rapid onset of action than vecuronium, with negligible cardiovascular side-effects.[32,33]

Several bis(benzylisoquinoline)esters have shown utility as nondepolarizing neuromuscular blocking drugs. This structural class includes atracurium, doxacurium, and mivacurium. Atracurium undergoes spontaneous, nonenzymatic degradation in the plasma, as a result of Hoffman elimination and ester hydrolysis. This suggests that the drug may be especially useful in patients with renal failure who are incapable of drug elimination via the kidney. Atracurium is three-fold more potent than d-tubocurarine, with a shorter duration of action than most of the commonly used nondepolarizing agents. Its short duration of action and rapid degradation allow administration as a continuous IV infusion for long surgical procedures. Some hypotension has been observed with the clinical use of atracurium, as well as evidence of histamine release. The potency of atracurium is enhanced in patients with low plasma potassium levels.[34]

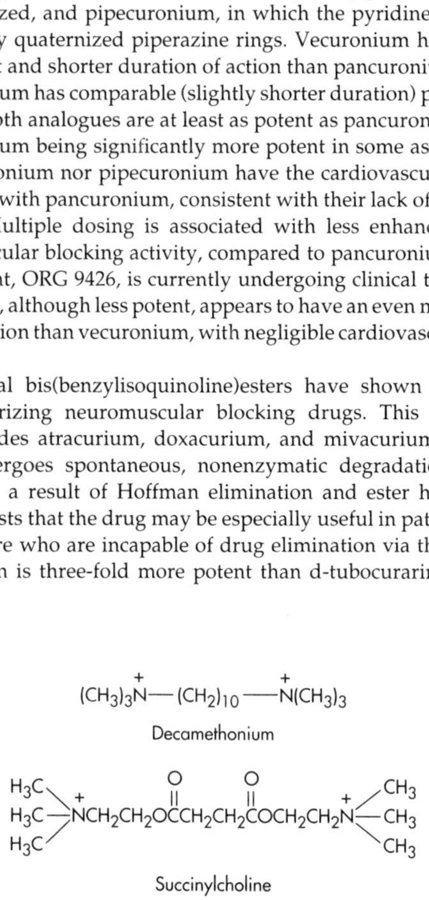

Mivacurium, another short-acting, rapid-onset agent, is readily hydrolyzed by plasma cholinesterase,[35] and, like atracurium, can be administered via continuous IV infusion. Prolonged neuromuscular block with mivacurium has been observed in patients with plasma cholinesterase deficiency.[36] Mivacurium is approximately ten-fold more potent than d-tubocurarine. In contrast to the other bis(benzylisoquinolines), doxacurium is relatively resistant to hydrolysis by plasma cholinesterase and therefore has a longer duration of action.[37] Doxacurium is one of the most potent neuromuscular blocking agents, being approximately 20-fold more potent than d-tubocurarine. In both experimental animals and in humans, doxacurium does not produce significant cardiovascular effects or induce histamine release. Its tendency to show intensified effects upon repeated administration is less than that of other long-acting neuromuscular blockers.

Gallamine, a simple tris-aminoethyl derivative of pyrogallic acid, is structurally distinct from the other nondepolarizing neuromuscular blocking agents. It is several-fold less potent than d-tubocurarine, with a slightly more rapid onset of action and shorter duration. Multiple dosing is associated with an accentuation of its neuromuscular blocking action. Like pancuronium, gallamine is often associated with tachycardia and hypertension. Gallamine is a potent vagolytic agent, probably acting as a competitive antagonist of cardiac muscarinic cholinergic receptors. When used in combination with halothane, gallamine occasionally can induce premature ventricular contractions or ventricular tachycardia. This may result from an indirect sympathomimetic action, which can be demonstrated in isolated myocardial preparations.

Another structurally novel neuromuscular blocking agent, fazadinium, is slightly less potent than d-tubocurarine, having a relatively rapid onset and long duration of action. Fazadinium is a potent vagolytic agent, which accounts for its tendency to increase heart rate and cardiac output. High concentrations can inhibit neuronal norepinephrine uptake. The rapid onset, in combination with long duration of action, make fazadinium useful in emergency surgery.

Depolarizing Agents

As noted above, in the presence of high concentrations of acetylcholinesterase inhibitors, the sustained presence of acetylcholine at the nicotinic cholinergic receptor will produce a sustained depolarization and consequent neuromuscular blockade due to nicotonic cholinergic receptor desensitization. This principle explains the ability of agents producing prolonged nicotinic cholinergic receptor activation to act as neuromuscular blocking agents (Fig. 7.6).

Although many additional actions have been postulated, it appears that the depolarizing agents act as simple agonists at the nicotinic cholinergic receptor,[r8,38] and muscle sensitivity is lost as a result of prolonged depolarization of the region surrounding the neuromuscular junction. This area of depolarization spreads

$(CH_3)_3\overset{+}{N}-(CH_2)_{10}-\overset{+}{N}(CH_3)_3$

Decamethonium

$(H_3C)_3\overset{+}{N}CH_2CH_2OC(=O)CH_2CH_2C(=O)OCH_2CH_2\overset{+}{N}(CH_3)_3$

Succinylcholine

Figure 7.6 Depolarizing Neuromuscular Blocking Drugs

as the presence of the agonist is maintained, and, in contrast to the nondepolarizing blockers, the sensitivity of this region of the muscle fiber to direct electrical stimulation is lost. Other actions of the depolarizing agents, such as their ability to produce blockade of the open ion channel, do not appear to make a substantial contribution to their clinical effects.

Neuromuscular blockade produced by depolarizing agents has different characteristics from that produced by nondepolarizing drugs, such as d-tubocurarine. Muscle fusiculation is commonly observed as a result of the initial depolarization of the postjunctional receptor. Acetylcholinesterase inhibition will enhance rather than reverse the neuromuscular blocking effects of the depolarizing antagonists. There are also differences between depolarizing and nondepolarizing agents with respect to species sensitivity, time sequence of muscle paralysis, and effects of changes in temperature.[r9]

A phenomenon known as "dual block" refers to change in character of the neuromuscular blockade produced by a depolarizing agent resembling that produced by nondepolarizing agents. This phenomenon can be explained by sufficient desensitization of the nicotinic cholinergic receptors produced by prolonged receptor activation, and the desensitization thereby allows a partial repolarization. This will cause some of the nicotinic cholinergic receptors to return to the resting state, although neuromuscular transmission is still impaired. Addition of an acetylcholinesterase inhibitor will now produce reversal of the blockade, since the high concentrations of neuronally-released acetylcholine will activate a greater percentage of the resting nicotinic receptors than those activated by the depolarizing blocker.[r8]

In contrast to the many nondepolarizing agents that have been used as neuromuscular blockers, only two depolarizing agents have been utilized clinically to a significant degree. One of these, decamethonium, is now primarily only of historical interest. Decamethonium (Fig. 7.6), can be considered the simplest neuromuscular blocker, with two quaternary ammonium groups linked by a simple alkyl chain. As noted above, most structural modifications to this alkyl chain result in agents that act by a nondepolarizing mechanism. Decamethonium produces neuromuscular blockade of moderate duration, does not interfere with ganglionic neurotransmission at clinical doses, and generally does not induce histamine release. Transient muscular fasciculations are observed prior to paralysis.

Succinylcholine also contains two quaternary ammonium groups linked by a ten-atom chain. However, unlike decamethonium, this chain contains two ester linkages susceptible to cleavage by plasma cholinesterase. This results in a short duration of neuromuscular blockade. A small percentage of the population has a genetic deficiency in the function of plasma cholinesterase. As such, succinylcholine produces neuromuscular blockade of longer duration in these individuals. The rapid onset of neuromuscular blockade and the rapid recovery following termination of infusion have made succinylcholine the preferred agent for procedures where neuromuscular relaxation of short duration is required, such as the insertion of an endotracheal tube. The short duration of succinylcholine also makes it the agent of choice for inducing neuromuscular blockade during electroshock procedures.

Succinylcholine can induce histamine release, although not to the extent observed with d-tubocurarine. Ganglionic blockade is not produced, although cardiovascular effects resulting from stimulation of parasympathetic or sympathetic ganglia occasionally are observed. Succinylcholine also may cause an increase in intraocular pressure. In contrast to the nondepolarizing agents, succinylcholine stimulates the efflux of potassium ions from skeletal muscle to a degree sufficient to induce transient hyperkalemia. This may be a result of the uncoordinated muscular activity occurring during the onset of neuromuscular blockade, and may be clinically significant in patients with congestive heart failure or pre-existing electrolyte imbalance. In conditions leading to muscle denervation, such as burns or neurologic injuries, hyperkalemia may be even more pronounced. This may result as a consequence of depolarization of a larger number of nicotinic cholinergic receptors, since these receptors spread over the entire muscle fiber following denervation. Muscular stimulation during onset of blockade by succinylcholine can result in soreness following recovery. This can be prevented by the use of a low dose of a nondepolarizing agent prior to induction of paralysis with succinylcholine;[39] hexafluorenium, a weak nondepolarizing blocker that also inhibits plasma cholinesterase, will both prevent muscular fasciculations and prolong the duration of action of succinylcholine. The administration of succinylcholine increases the sensitivity of patients to subsequently administered nondepolarizing neuromuscular blockers.[40] This is probably a consequence of nicotinic receptor depolarization, since a similar effect was produced by decamethonium.[41]

The problems resulting from muscle stimulation by depolarizing neuromuscular blockers have led to a search for a rapidly acting nondepolarizing agent with a short duration of action that could be substituted for succinylcholine. No agent meeting these criteria is yet available, although low-dose atracurium or vecuronium has been suggested as a useful alternative to succinylcholine in infants.[42]

References

Research Reports

1. Padykula HA, Gauthier GF. The ultrastructure of the neuromuscular junctions of mammalian red, white and intermediate skeletal fibers. J Cell Biol 1970;*46*:27–41.
2. Matteoli M, Haimann C, Torri-Tarelli F, Polak JM, Ceccarelli B, DeCamilli P. Differential effect of α-latrotoxin on exocytosis from small synaptic vesicles and from large dense-core vesicles containing calcitonin gene-related peptide at the frog neuromuscular junction. Proc Natl Acad Sci USA 1988;*85*:7366–7370.
3. Wessler I: Control of transmitter release from the motor nerve by presynaptic nicotinic and muscarinic autoreceptors. Trends Pharmacol Sci 1989;*10*:110–114.
4. Meldolesi J, Scheer H, Madeddu L, Wanke E. Mechanism of action of α-latrotoxin: The presynaptic stimulatory toxin of the black widow spider venom. Trends Pharmacol Sci 1986;*7*:151–155.
5. Harris JB. Phospholipases in snake venoms and their effects on nerve and muscle. Pharmacol Ther 1985;*31*:79–102.
6. Rowan EG, Pemberton KE, Harvey AL. On the blockade of acetylcholine release at mouse motor nerve terminals by β-bungarotoxin and crototoxin. Br J Pharmacol 1990;*100*:301–304.
7. Kato G, Changeaux JP. Studies on the effect of histrionicotoxin on the monocellular electroplax from Electrophorus electricus and on the binding of [^{3}H] acetylcholine to membrane fragments from Torpedo marmorata. Mol Pharmacol 1976;*12*:92–100.
8. Kistler J, Stroud RM, Klymkowsky MW, Lalancette RA, Fairclough RH. Structure and function of an acetylcholine receptor. Biophys J 1982;*37*:371–383.
9. Mishina M, Takai T, Imoto K, Noda M, Takahashi T, Numa S, Methfessel C, Sakmann B. Molecular distinction between fetal and adult forms of muscle acetylcholine receptor. Nature 1986;*321*:406–411.
10. Froehner SC, Luetje CW, Scotland PB, Patrick J. The postsynaptic 43K protein clusters of muscle nicotinic acetylcholine receptors in Xenopus oocytes. Neuron 1990;*5*:403–410.
11. Takai T, Noda M, Michima M, Shimizu S, Furutani Y, Kayano T, Ikeda T, Kubo T, Takahashi H, Takahashi T, Kuno M, Numa S. Cloning, sequencing and expression of cDNA for a novel subunit of acetylcholine receptor from calf muscle. Nature 1985;*315*:761–764.
12. Kubo T, Noda M, Takai T, Tanabe T, Kayano T, Shimizu S, Tanaka K, Takahashi H, Hirose T, Inayama S, Kikuno R, Miyata T, Numa S. Primary structure of δ-subunit precursor of calf muscle acetylcholine receptor deduced from cDNA sequence. Eur J Biochem 1985;*149*:5–13.
13. Leonard RJ, Labarca CG, Charnet P, Davidson N, Lester HA. Evidence that the M2 membrane-spanning region lines the ion channel pore of the nicotinic receptor. Science 1988;*242*:1578–1581.
14. Dwyer BP. Evidence for the extramembranous location of the putative amphipathic helix of acetylcholine receptor. Biochemistry 1988;*27*:5586–5592.
15. Giersig M, Kunath W, Pribilla I, Bandine G, Hucho F. Symmetry and dimensions of membrane bound nicotinic acetylcholine receptors from Torpedo californica electric tissue: Rapid rearrangement of two-dimensional ordered lattices. Membrane Biochem. 1989;*8*:81–93.
16. Neubig RR, Boyd ND, Cohen JB. Conformation of Torpedo acetylcholine receptor associated with ion transport and desensitization. Biochemistry 1982;*21*:3460–3467.
17. Pedersen SE, Cohen JB. d-Tubocurarine binding sites are located at α-γ and α-δ subunit interfaces of the nicotinic acetylcholine receptor. Proc Natl Acad Sci USA 1990;*87*:2785–2789.
18. Smythies JR, Kemp G. A possible structure for the nicotinic acetylcholine receptor. J Recep Res 1989;*9*:199–201.
19. Tzartos SJ, Remoundos MS. Fine localization of the major α-bungarotoxin binding site to residues α189–195 of the Torpedo acetylcholine receptor. J Biol Chem 1990;*265*:21462–21467.
20. Karlin A, Kao PN, DiPaola M. Molecular pharmacology of the nicotinic acetylcholine receptor. Trends Pharmacol Sci 1986;*7*:304–308.
21. Patrick J, Lindstrom JM. Autoimmune response to acetylcholine receptor. Science 1973;*180*:871–872.
22. Dieperink ME, Stafansson K. Molecular mimicry and microorganisms: A role in the pathogenesis of myasthenia gravis. Curr Topics Microbiol Immunol 1989;*145*:57–65.
23. Engel AG, Fukuoka T, Lang B, Newsom-Davis J, Vincent A, Wray D. Lambert-Eaton myasthenic syndrome IgG: Early morphologic effects and immunolocalization at the motor endplate. Ann NY Acad Sci 1987;*505*:333–345.
24. Kim YI. Lambert-Eaton myasthenic syndrome: Evidence for calcium channel blockade. Ann NY Acad Sci 1987;*505*:377–379.
25. Engel AG. Myasthenic syndromes. In: Engel AG, Banker BQ (Eds) Myology. New York: McGraw-Hill, (1986); pp 1955–1990.
26. Donati F, Smith CE, Bevan DR. Dose-response relationships for edrophonium and neostigmine as antagonists of moderate and profound atracurium blockade. Anesth Analg 1989;*68*:13–19.
27. Smith CE, Donati FR, Bevan, DR. Dose-response relationships for edrophonium and neostigmine as antagonists of atracurium and vecuronium neuromuscular blockade. Anesthesiology 1989;*71*:37–43.
28. Wachtel RE. Comparison of anticholinesterases and their effects on acetylcholine-activated ion channels. Anesthesiology 1990;*72*:496–503.
29. Heuser JE, Reese TS, Dennis MJ, Jan Y, Jan L, Evans L. Synaptic vesicle exocytosis captured by quick freezing and correlated with quantal transmitter release. J Cell Biol 1979;*81*:275–300.
30. Feldman SA, Tyrell MF. A new theory of the termination of action of the muscle relaxants. Proc Roy Soc Med 1970;*63*:692–694.
31. Feldman SA, Fauvel NJ, Hood JR. Recovery from pancuronium and vecuronium administered simultaneously in the isolated forearm and the effect on recovery following administration after cross-over of drugs. Anesth Analg 1993;*76*:92–95.
32. Quill TJ, Begin M, Glass PSA, Ginsberg B, Gorback MS. Clinical responses of ORG 9426 during isoflurane anesthesia. Anesth Analg 1991;*72*:203–206.
33. Woelfel SK, Brandom BW, Sarner JB, Cook DR, Cyran JA. Dose response of Org-9426 in children during nitrous oxide-halothane anesthesia. Anesth Analg 1991;*72*:S326.
34. Beemer GH, Bjorksten AR. Pharmacodynamics of atracurium in clinical practice: Effect of plasma potassium, patient demographics and concurrent medication. Anesth Analg 1993;*76*:1288–1295.
35. Savarese JJ, Ali HH, Basta SJ, Embree PB, Scott RPF, Sunder N, Weakly JN, Wastila WB, El-Sayad HA. The clinical neuromuscular pharmacology of Mivacurium Chloride. Anesthesiology 1988;*68*:723–732.

36. Petersen RS, Bailey PL, Kalameghan R, Ashwood ER. Prolonged neuromuscular block after mivacurium. Anesth Analg 1993;*76*:194–196.

37. Basta SJ, Savarese JJ, Ali HH, Embree PB, Schwartz AF, Rudd GD, Wastila WB. Clinical pharmacology of doxacurium chloride. Anesthesiology 1988;*69*:478–486.

38. Marshall CG, Ogden DC, Colquhoun D. The actions of suxamethonium (succinyldicholine) as an agonist and channel blocker at the nicotinic receptor of frog muscle. J Physiol (London) 1990;*428*:155–174.

39. Subhedar DV, Pashricha SK, Shibutani K. Does pre-curarization affect post-operative myalgia in cesarean section? Anesth Analg 1991;*72*:S283.

40. Donati F, Gill SS, Bevan DR, Ducharme J, Theoret Y, Varin F. The pharmacokinetics and pharmacodynamics of atracurium with and without previous exposure to suxamethonium. Brit J Anesth 1991;*66*:557–561.

41. Feldman S, Fauvel N. Potentiation and antagonism of vecuronium by decamethonium. Anesth Analg 1993;*76*:631–634.

42. McGregor D, Bires J, Lennon R. Intubation with low dose atracurium and vecuronium in infants and children. Anesth Analg 1991;*72*:S174.

Reviews

r1. Engel AG. The neuromuscular junction. In: Engel AG, Banker BQ (Eds) Myology, New York, McGraw-Hill, (1986); pp 209–253.

r2. Gershon MD, Schwarts JH, Kandel ER. Morphology of chemical synapses and patterns of interconnection. In: Kandel ER, Schwartz JH (Eds) Principles of neural science. New York: Elsevier/North-Holland, (1981); pp 91–105.

r3. McCarthy MP, Earnest JP, Young EF, Choe S, Stroud RM. The molecular biology of the acetylcholine receptor. Ann Rev Neurol 1986;*9*:383–414.

r4. Riker WF. Prejunctional effects of neuromuscular blocking and facilitatory drugs. In: Katz RK (ed.) Muscle relaxants. New York: American Elsevier, 1975; pp 60–102.

r5. Engel AG. Acquired autoimmune myasthenia gravis. In: Engel AG, Banker BQ (Eds) Myology. New York: McGraw-Hill, (1986); pp 1925–1954.

r6. Paskov DS, Agoston S, Bowman WC. 4-Aminopyridine hydrochloride (Pymadin). In: Kharkevich DA (ed) Handbook of Experimental Pharmacology, Vol. 79. Berlin: Springer-Verlag (1986); pp 679–718.

r7. Kharkecich DA, Shorr VA. Antimuscarinic and ganglion-blocking activity of neuromuscular blocking agents. In: Handbook of Experimental Pharmacology, Vol. 79. Berlin: Springer-Verlag, (1986); pp 191–224.

r8. Colquhoun D: On the principles of postsynaptic action of neuromuscular blocking agents. In: Kharkevich DA (ed) Handbook of Experimental Pharmacology, Vol. 79, Berlin: Springer-Verlag, (1986); pp 59–113.

r9. Zaimis E, Head S. Depolarizing neuromuscular blocking drugs. In: Zaimis E, (ed.) Neuromuscular junction. Berlin: Springer-Verlag, (1976); pp 365–420.

CHAPTER 8

Giora Z. Feuerstein
S. Z. Langer
Robert R. Ruffolo, Jr.

Adrenal Medulla

Introduction

The first demonstration of the possible physiologic role of the adrenal medulla was provided by Olivir and Schafer in 1895[1], who found that extracts of adrenal medulla injected IV evoked striking increases in arterial blood pressure. Subsequently, Abel and Crawford in 1897[2] isolated and purified the first active constituent of the gland and identified it as epinephrine. Shortly thereafter, adrenomedullary cells were described. Chromium stain was used and they came to be known as "chromaffin" cells. The similarity between pressor effects of adrenal extract and sympathetic nerve stimulation led Elliott in 1905[3] to propose that an epinephrine-like substance might be released from the sympathetic nerves. Subsequently, the role of epinephrine-like substances as neurohumoral mediators of sympathoadrenomedullary discharge in "fight or flight" responses was established by Cannon and Uridil in 1921.[4] The pressor epinephrine-like substance released from sympathetic nerves was identified as norepinephrine (NE) by von Euler in 1948.

Embryology

Chromaffin cells of the adrenal medulla arise from the neural crest and are formed in parallel with the peripheral sympathetic nervous system. In the fetus, at approximately seven weeks' gestation, neuroectodermal cells invade the adrenal cortex while undergoing differentiation from primitive sympathetic cells and pheochromoblasts to form chromaffin cells.[r1] Pheochromoblasts, which do not migrate, remain in close association with the developing sympathetic nervous system and form extra-adrenal chromaffin cells of paraganglia and chromaffin cell bodies. This extramedullary chromaffin tissue, located along the paravertebral sympathetic chain, may be the origin of extra-adrenal pheochromocytomas. Chromaffin and dense-core granules are found in the human fetus at approximately 12 to 16 weeks. At birth, the medulla is completely functional. The catecholamine-synthesizing enzymes appear early in fetal development of the medulla; however, the activities of the enzymes tyrosine hydroxylase and dopamine-β-hydroxylase are low at birth, but develop rapidly thereafter.[r1] In humans, the proportion of NE- to epinephrine-containing cells is higher in fetal and neonatal glands than in adult medullas.[r2]

Adrenal Circulation

The adrenal glands are situated on the upper poles of the kidneys. Adult adrenal medullas in humans weigh approximately 1 g. The gland receives its blood supply via three arteries: the superior adrenal artery, which is a branch of the inferior phrenic artery; the middle adrenal artery, which arises directly from the aorta; and the inferior adrenal artery, which branches off the renal artery. The adrenal medulla has both arterial and portal venous circulations. Cortical arteries form a plexus in the capsule and outer adrenal cortex from which blood flows inward to the sinusoids of the medulla. As a result, blood reaching the medulla contains high concentrations of the glucocorticoids that provide hormonal regulation for catecholamine synthesis (see below). The adrenal medulla is also supplied by a few direct medullary arterioles. In humans, and most other species, there is one large adrenal vein, which drains medullary blood either directly into the inferior vena cava or indirectly via the renal vein. Adrenomedullary blood flow is high, as is the case in other endocrine organs.

The functional unit of the adrenal medulla is the chromaffin cell, which is essentially a large sympathetic neuron. Its axon is lost, and the cell has become specialized to secrete its constituents directly into the bloodstream. Chromaffin cells are innervated by preganglionic cholinergic fibers that originate in the intermediolateral cell column between T3–L3 and pass through the sympathetic ganglia without synapsing.[r2] These fibers, carried in the splanchnic nerves, grow into the adrenal medulla at different periods of development, but in humans (and in rats) full innervation does not occur until after birth.[r2]

Histology

Chromaffin cells of the human adult adrenal medulla are of two types, producing either epinephrine or NE, with the majority (85%) producing epinephrine.[r2] Catecholamines are stored in dense-core granules similar to those present in postganglionic sympathetic neurons, and are osmiophilic, electron-dense, membrane-limited particles of 50–350 A.[r3] The composition of chromaffin granules has been studied extensively and found to consist of 21 percent catecholamines, 35 percent protein, 25 percent lipids, and 15 percent adenosine triphosphate (ATP). The human adrenal medulla contains 6 mg of catecholamines per gram of tissue. In addition to catecholamines and ATP, the major constituents of dense-core granules are chromogranin A, ascorbic acid, and peptides, such as enkephalins, β-endorphins, substance P, and neuropeptide Y.[r3] The chromaffin granule membrane contains a variety of proteins and enzymes, such as a proton pump ATP-ase, catecholamine carrier protein, nucleotide carrier protein, cytochrome b 561, actin, and dopamine-β-hydroxylase,[r3] which are all part of the complex system of catecholamine uptake, synthesis, storage, and release.

Biochemistry of Catecholamines

The primary hormone secreted by the adrenal medulla is epinephrine. The synthesis of epinephrine begins with the amino acid, tyrosine. Tyrosine is converted to 3,4-dihydroxyphenylalanine (dopa) by a cytosolic enzyme, tyrosine hydroxylase. The enzyme is present only in catecholamine-producing cells and requires molecular O_2, with tetrahydropteridine and NADPH as cofactors. This is the rate-limiting step, and, thus, alterations in tyrosine hydroxylase activity directly affect catecholamine synthesis. The activity of tyrosine hydroxylase is regulated through feedback inhibition by its end-product, dopa, and by dopamine and NE, all of which, when present in the cytosol, compete for the pteridine cofactor binding site on the enzyme.[5] Tyrosine hydroxylase in the adrenal medulla is subject to transsynaptic induction following depletion of catecholamines with reserpine.[6]

The next biosynthetic step is conversion of dopa to dopamine by aromatic L-amino acid decarboxylase, a pyridoxal-dependent enzyme. This enzyme is widely distributed and also acts on a variety of aromatic L-amino acids, including synthetic analogues (e.g., α-methyldopa) to produce "false transmitters".[5] After its formation, dopamine leaves the cytosol and is accumulated by the chromaffin granules, where it becomes oxidized to NE by a storage granule-limited enzyme, dopamine-β-hydroxylase. Accumulation of dopamine into the storage granules is accomplished by a stereoselective carrier (for norepinephrine/epinephrine), ATP- and Mg^{2+}-dependent, and saturable.[5] Hydroxylation by dopamine-β-hydroxylase requires O_2, with ascorbate and fumarate as cofactors.[5] Ascorbic acid acts as an electron donor for dopamine-β-hydroxylase, and in that process is converted to semihydroascorbate, which, in turn, is regenerated to ascorbate by a transfer of electrons via a membrane-bound cytochrome b 561. Dopamine-β-hydroxylase, like tyrosine hydroxylase, is found only in catecholamine-synthetizing cells, but is relatively substrate nonspecific, and can therefore β-hydroxylate many phenylethylamine derivatives.[5]

In epinephrine-producing cells, the NE produced in the dense-core granule leaks into the cytoplasm, where methylation to epinephrine by phenethanolamine-N-methyltransferase (PNMT: which transfers a methyl group from S-adenosyl-methionine to the nitrogen of NE) takes place. The presence of PNMT is limited to epinephrine-producing cells and is not substrate-specific.[5] The activity of adrenal PNMT is under continuous regulation by high concentrations of glucocorticoids present in the portal venous blood emanating from the adrenal cortex.[5] Thus, following hypophysectomy, PNMT activity markedly decreases, while replenishing physiologic levels of glucocorticoid restores both PNMT and epinephrine levels. Glucocorticoids may increase PNMT activity by preventing the degradation of the enzyme.[5] The regulatory role of glucocorticoids on epinephrine synthesis is also implied by the relatively selective localization of epinephrine to the outer (cortical) adrenal medulla, where glucocorticoid levels are at their maximum. Following its synthesis, epinephrine is accumulated by the dense-core granules, where it is trapped by low pH (i.e., intravesicular pH≈ 5) created by the proton pump until it is released.

In addition to the local hormonal control described above, the synthesis of epinephrine and NE also is regulated in adrenal medulla and in the sympathetic nerves by acute (minutes) and chronic (hours to days) neural mechanisms.[5,r4] It has been noted that nerve stimulation in vivo can release catecholamines from the adrenal medulla without producing changes in the catecholamine levels in the glands. This maintenance of catecholamine levels in the face of increased release results from a concomitant increase in catecholamine biosynthesis. Acutely, such regulation is provided via changes in the activity of tyrosine hydroxylase (without de novo synthesis) regulated by the free catecholamines in the cytosol. It has been postulated that nerve stimulation reduces the concentration of catecholamines in a small cytoplasmic pool (which is in equilibrium with the granular storage pool) and, therefore, releases tyrosine hydroxylase from end-product inhibition.[r3] In addition, acute splanchnic nerve stimulation leads to increased tyrosine hydroxylase activity by phosphorylation of the enzyme, which increases its affinity for substrate.[r3,r5] Prolonged stimulation (for more than 12 hours) involves tyrosine hydroxylase gene transcription and synthesis of additional enzyme molecules; this process is called "transsynaptic induction"[r3,r5] The induction of tyrosine hydroxylase increases the catecholamine-synthetizing capacity of chromaffin cells in response to chronically increased physiologic demand. The induction of dopamine-β-hydroxylase also occurs, but to a smaller degree.

Storage of Catecholamines in the Chromaffin Cell

The dense-core storage granules have an efficient system for the accumulation of epinephrine and NE from the cytoplasm and then concentrating these catecholamines 10,000-fold over levels found in the cytosol, yielding a concentration of 0.55 M.[r3,r5] Accumulation of dopamine for conversion to NE and of NE and epinephrine for storage in chromaffin granules is an active process requiring Mg^{2+} and ATP. The energy is supplied by a flow of protons down an electrochemical gradient. The proton gradient is produced by a transfer of protons from the outside to the inside of the granule during hydrolysis of ATP by the hydrogen-ATP-ase. The proton gradient responsible for catecholamine uptake lowers pH within the storage granule and thereby promotes internal trapping of protonated catecholamines in the granules.[r5] High osmotic concentrations of catecholamines would cause granule rapture if they were free in the solution. This is prevented by interaction of positively charged catecholamines with negatively charged ATP, which forms a reversible storage complex. Other substances are also involved in catecholamine storage, such as chromogranin A, an acidic granular protein.[r5]

The proton gradient from the inside to the outside of the storage granule also supplies energy for electron transport into the granules via a membrane-bound cytochrome b 561.[r3,r5] As noted earlier, the electrons are used in recharging of granular semidehydroascorbate to ascorbate, which is required for β-hydroxylation of catecholamines by dopamine-β-hydroxylase.

Release of Catecholamines by Exocytosis

Stimulation of the chromaffin cells mobilizes chromaffin granules and causes a discharge of their contents by exocytosis into the pericellular fluid by a process called "stimulus-secretion coupling".[r5] The physiologic stimulus for catecholamine release from the adrenomedullary chromaffin cells is acetylcholine liberated from the preganglionic sympathetic nerves. Acetylcholine then binds to nicotinic cholinoceptors on chromaffin cells and causes membrane depolarization by increasing its permeability to sodium ions.[r3,r5] As a result of these changes, the permeability of the chromaffin cell membrane to calcium increases, and calcium flows into the cell, elevating intracellular calcium concentration.[r3,r5] It is believed that the increase in cytosolic calcium is both necessary and sufficient to elicit secretion of catecholamines by exocytosis.

The mechanisms involved in the movement of the storage granules toward the inner cell membrane, and the fusion process between the granule and cell membrane,[r5] are not completely understood. This process of membrane fusion appears to involve Ca^{+2}-calmodulin binding to granular membrane and phosphorylation of certain proteins.[r5] In this process, a 47-kd protein, synexin, polymerizes and causes isolated chromaffin granules to aggregate with one another.[7] Synexin itself is regulated by calcium and an inhibitory protein, synhibin.[r5]

Control of Secretion

Adrenomedullary innervation classically has been regarded as purely cholinergic; however, studies suggest the existence of specific peripheral pathways for the differential release of epinephrine or NE, that are stimulated separately from specific brain sites. The preferential secretion of epinephrine (vis-a-vis NE) from the adrenal medulla also may be elicited by altering the pattern of nerve stimulation (bursting instead of continuous stimulation).[r4] Although nicotinic cholinoceptors are the primary receptors involved in catecholamine secretion, muscarinic cholinoceptors that inhibit catecholamine release also have been described.[r4] This dual receptor mechanism was proposed to provide a tonic inhibition of catecholamine secretion in the resting state and increased release during periods of stress. Stimulated release of catecholamines undergoes further modulation by adrenomedullary peptides, such as substance P and the enkephalins contained in the splanchnic nerves (see below).

In addition to neural stimuli, catecholamine secretion may be induced by humoral mechanisms. Neonatal adrenal medulla, which is not fully innervated, is particularly sensitive to this type of stimulation. Glucagon is a potent stimulus for delayed catecholamine secretion in response to hypoglycemia.[r3,r5]

Inactivation of Catecholamines Released from the Adrenal Medulla

Under basal conditions, plasma concentrations of epinephrine range between 20 and 50 pg/ml, and those

Table 8.1 Drugs Used for Adrenal Medullary Disorders

	Dosage			Pharmacokinetics			
Drug	Route	Size	Dose	Peak	V_D	$t_{1/2}$	Clearance or Duration of Response
Metyrosine							
Demser	Oral	250 mg	250 mg q.i.d.	1–3 hours		3–7 hours	lasts 3–4 days

of NE between 100 and 350 pg/ml.[5] While virtually all circulating epinephrine (systemic circulation) originates from the adrenal medulla, most plasma NE (in the resting state) is derived from peripheral sympathetic nerves. The half-lives of IV-administered catecholamines are estimated to be approximately 20 sec. The biologic effects of circulating catecholamines (see below) are terminated rapidly by uptake into the sympathetic nerve endings, followed by enzymatic degradation by monoamine oxidase (MAO), catechol-O-methyltransferase (COMT), and renal excretion.[5] Uptake into the postganglionic sympathetic nerves is a major inactivation route for NE, but plays a less important role with epinephrine. Neuronal uptake (uptake$_1$) is a chloride-and sodium-dependent, stereoselective [for (−)-enantiomers] and competitive process. There is a lower-affinity but high-capacity uptake system for epinephrine and NE in many extraneuronal tissues (i.e., extraneuronal uptake, or uptake$_2$) that also contributes to inactivation of circulating catecholamines, especially at high plasma concentrations.[5]

Catecholamines secreted from the adrenal medulla are, in large part, metabolized in the liver and excreted in the urine. Epinephrine is metabolized to metanephrine by liver COMT and further oxidized to 3-methoxy-4-hydroxymandelic acid and 3-methoxy-4-hydroxyphenylglycol by MAO found in the liver or neuronal tissues. The phenolic group of the catecholamines and their metabolites may be conjugated with sulfate (humans) or glucuronidate (rat) in the liver and in the gut. In the urine, 3.3 percent of epinephrine appears in the free form, 45 percent as 3-methoxy-4-hydroxymandelic acid, 7 percent as free metanephrine, 27 percent as conjugated metanephrine, and 6 percent as 3-methoxy-4-hydroxyphenylglycol.[5,r3] The synthetic pathways, storage, release and metabolic fate of catecholamines in the chromaffin cell are depicted schematically in Figure 8.1.

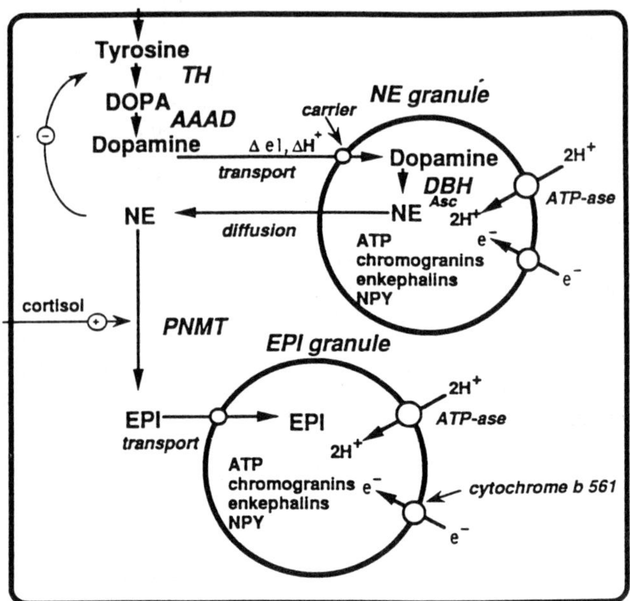

NOTE:
In NE-producing cells, only NE-containing granules are present;
in EPI-producing cells, NE diffuses into the cytosol for conversion to EPI which then re-enters into the same granule;
TH - tyrosine hydroxylase
AAAD - aromatic L-amino acid decarboxylase
DBH - dopamine-beta-hydroxylase
asc- ascorbatic acid
PNMT - phenylethanolamine-N-methyltransferase
Δ el, ΔH+ - electrical and proton grandients

Figure 8.1 Schematic Representation of the Synthesis and Storage of NE and Epinephrine in the Chromaffin Cell

Peptides of the Adrenal Medulla

The splanchnic nerves innervating the adrenal medulla contain peptides, such as substance P and enkephalins, in addition to acetylcholine.[r3] Substance P exerts an inhibitory action on nicotinic cholinoceptor-mediated secretion of catecholamines during resting conditions,[r3] but also prevents nicotinic cholinoceptor desensitization, thereby maintaining a prolonged secretory response at times of increased demand, as in stress situations.[r3] The opiate peptides, leu- and met-enkephalins, which are present in both preganglionic sympathetic nerves and in the chromaffin cells, are weak inhibitors of acetylcholine-induced release of catecholamines.[r3,r5] More potent inhibitory effects are mediated by other opiates, such as dynorphin$_{1-13}$ and metorphamide. At submicromolar concentrations, the enkephalins stimulate basal secretion of catecholamines, but the physiologic significance of this phenomenon is not known.[r3,r5] Met- and leu-enkephalins, and probably their precursors, are present in the chromaffin granules and are released during exocytosis together with epinephrine and NE. The release of opioids along with epinephrine and NE in stress situations may underlie the decreased perception of pain experienced during severe stress.[r3,r5]

In addition to the above adrenomedullary peptides, a 36-amino acid peptide, neuropeptide Y, is present in abundance in chromaffin cells of adrenal medulla of several mammalian species, including humans. In the adrenal medulla, neuropeptide Y is detected in the epinephrine-containing cells and to a lesser extent in the NE-containing cells, and in some cells neuropeptide Y is also co-localized with enkephalins.[8] The release of neuropeptide Y from the adrenal medulla occurs during splanchnic nerve stimulation,[9] but the only known pathophysiologic situation in which the adrenal medulla secretes large quantities of neuropeptide Y into the bloodstream is pheochromocytoma.[10] In the adrenal medulla, neuropeptide Y likely functions as a neuromodulator by inhibiting release of catecholamines induced by nicotinic cholinoceptor stimulation.[9] Furthermore, as a potent vasoconstrictor, neuropeptide Y also may amplify the vasoconstrictor responses of catecholamines,[11] and may be of potential importance in the local regulation of adrenomedullary blood flow.

Functions of Adrenomedullary Catecholamines

Adrenomedullary catecholamines are viewed as part of the hormonal response to stressful conditions. Their effects can be divided into cardiovascular, visceral, and metabolic.[r3,r5] Epinephrine produces α-adrenoceptor-mediated vasoconstrictor effects similar to those of NE but, additionally, at low concentrations, mediates vasodilation in vascular beds which possess β_2-adrenoceptors, such as skeletal muscle. At cardiac β_1-adrenoceptors, both catecholamines are equivalent in their ability to increase heart rate, the force of myocardial contraction, conduction velocity, and oxygen consumption, leading to an increase in cardiac output. Epinephrine also may dilate the coronary arteries directly by activation of β_2-adrenoceptors, and indirectly by increasing cardiac metabolism. Over-all, the systemic hemodynamic effects of epinephrine are characterized by reduced peripheral vascular resistance, lower diastolic blood pressure, increased systolic blood pressure, and, hence, a widened pulse pressure.

Epinephrine is more potent than NE at β_2-adrenoceptors, and is a powerful bronchodilator. Smooth muscle in the GI and urinary tracts is relaxed by epinephrine, whereas smooth muscle in the splenic capsule, erectores pili of the skin, and dilator pupilae of the iris is contracted by epinephrine.[r3,r5]

Most of the metabolic effects of catecholamines are mediated by β_2-adrenoceptors; therefore, epinephrine exerts stronger actions than NE.[r3,r5] Catecholamines have an over-all catabolic effect on stored fuels, carbohydrates, and lipids. One of the major metabolic functions of epinephrine is to mobilize substrates from the storage depots in liver, adipose tissue, and skeletal muscle, as is the case with glucagon.

The interaction of catecholamines with β_2-adrenoceptor results in the activation of adenylate cyclase, and thereby increases the formation of cyclic-AMP (cAMP), which activates cAMP-dependent protein kinase to increase the metabolism of glycogen.[r5] Epinephrine stimulates hepatic glycogenolysis by activating phosphorylase and, in addition, increases hepatic gluconeogenesis from lactate. Both of these processes lead to marked elevation of plasma glucose levels. α_1-Adrenoceptor stimulation by catecholamines also activates glycogenolysis, independently of cAMP[r3] The contribution of α- versus β-adrenoceptors varies in different species, and is regulated by such humoral factors, as steroids.[r3] Hepatic glucose output by epinephrine is further augmented by stimulation of glucagon and inhibition of insulin secretion.

In adipose tissue, epinephrine stimulates lypolysis by activating lipases that cleave triglycerides into glycerol and fatty acids, which are subsequently released into the bloodstream. This process involves activation of β_2- (and possibly β_3-) adrenoceptors, adenylate cyclase, and cAMP-dependent protein kinase, which in turn activates the lipase by phosphorylation. The lipolytic effect of catecholamines is potentiated by glucocorticoids, which are also secreted under the same stressful conditions. In skeletal muscle, epinephrine causes glycogenolysis solely by a β_2-adrenoceptor mechanism. Because muscles lack glucose-6-phosphatase, glycogen cannot be converted directly to glucose. As such, the glucose-6-phosphate is converted to lactate, which is then carried through the blood to the liver, where it is converted to glucose.[r3,r5]

The over-all metabolic effect of epinephrine, which is to increase the metabolic rate by breakdown of "fuel stores" (lipids, glycogen) and to enhance metabolism in peripheral tissues, leads to an increase in oxygen consumption and heat production.

Function of the Adrenal Medulla in Stress Situations

Hypoglycemia

Plasma levels of catecholamines are elevated in physiologic stress situations and in some pathophysiologic conditions. While sympathetic nerve activity plays a major role in maintaining resting blood pressure and minute-to-minute regulation of blood pressure (e.g., mediating postural changes), the adrenal medulla responds to emergency situations and metabolic stimuli.[5,r3,r5] When blood glucose falls below 95 mg/dl and, in particular, if it falls lower than 50 mg/dl, plasma epinephrine levels rise 10- to 50-fold, whereas the activity of the sympathetic nervous system is generally suppressed. The adrenomedullary response to hypoglycemia is mediated by specific neurogenic pathways originating in the glucose-sensitive areas in the CNS.

Exercise

Intense and prolonged exercise stimulates the secretion of adrenomedullary catecholamines, along with the over-all activation of the sympathetic nervous system.[5] The sympathoadrenomedullary system plays a critical role in adaptation to and survival in cold environments. The sympathetic nervous system plays a dominant role, but, when sympathetic function is impaired, the adrenal medulla can maintain adrenergic stimulation for survival in cold environments by providing the necessary metabolic and cardiovascular adaptations.

Circulatory Shock

The activity of the sympathoadrenomedullary system increases in certain pathophysiologic states, such circulatory shock, trauma, and hypoxia. In neonates, whose splanchnic innervation of the medulla is not yet mature, hypoxia increases the secretion of NE and epinephrine by a direct effect on the chromaffin cells.[r5]

In other pathophysiologic situations, responses of the sympathoadrenomedullary system are usually biphasic. The acute response is of adrenomedullary origin and the sympathetic nerve activity may even be decreased as in hypotensive hemorrhage or vasovagal syncope.[r3,r5] In more chronic situations, the secretion of adrenomedullary catecholamines gradually subsides, and sympathetic nerve activity increases. The adrenal medulla plays a pivotal role in survival from several forms of shock, in particular septic shock. Because the causal factor in all forms of circulatory shock is a progressive fall in cardiac output and systemic arterial blood pressure, the activation of cardiostimulatory and compensatory pressor mechanisms is important. In endotoxic shock, hypotension is associated with markedly reduced systemic vascular resistance, and adrenergic agonists are still used in therapy; however, their success is limited owing to progressively developing suppression of vascular adrenergic responsiveness.[12] In experimental, nonlethal models of endotoxic shock, adrenal demedullated animals show markedly impaired recovery,[11] and administration of epinephrine abolishes the fall in blood pressure.[11] Unfortunately, when marked elevation of circulating catecholamines persists for a prolonged period, severe restriction of organ blood flow occurs and leads to ischemia of visceral organs, which further complicates the shock state.

Pathology of the Chromaffin Cells

Pheochromocytoma

Chromaffin cells of adrenal medulla and the paraganglia can give rise to endocrine tumors, termed pheochromocytomas. Pheochromocytomas are rare, but, if not recognized and treated, may be fatal.[r3,r5] Pheochromocytomas are a rare cause of hypertension (<0.1% of hypertensive patients), but proper diagnosis and treatment can result in a complete cure. Most (90%) of the tumors are benign, but in some cases they may be a part of multiglandular neoplastic syndrome.[r5]

Pheochromocytomas have no markers to predict their hormonal activity and malignancy. Most secrete both epinephrine and NE, but NE usually is the predominant catecholamine. In rare cases, pheochromocytomas also liberate dopamine and dopa.[r3,r5] In contrast to normal chromaffin cells, secretion of catecholamines from pheochromocytomas is believed to be nonexocytotic. Interestingly, plasma neuropeptide Y levels are reported to increase several-fold,[10] and may contribute to systemic vasoconstriction.

The clinical presentation of pheochromocytoma can largely be predicted from the known physiologic and pharmacologic effects of the catecholamines. The hallmark of the disease is the occurrence of hypertensive "attacks" with or without sustained elevation of blood pressure in the intervening periods.[r3] Paroxysmal hypertension may be precipitated by pressure in the region of the tumor (operative manipulation), anxiety, or a variety of therapeutic or diagnostic agents (histamine, glucagon, tyramine, anesthesia). The attacks are abrupt and subside slowly; their clinical manifestations are due to the effects of excess circulating catecholamines and include headache, sweating, tachycardia with palpitations, pallor, severe anxiety, and fear of death. Other signs and symptoms are related to cardiovascular complications of catecholamine excess, leading to acute myocardial infarction, cardiomyopathy, dissecting aneurysm, cerebrovascular accidents, encephalophathy, ischemic enterocolitis, and shock.

Surgical removal of the pheochromocytoma is the only curative procedure. If the pheochromocytoma cannot be removed, prolonged treatment with α- and β-adrenoceptor antagonists can effectively control blood pressure for many years. Additionally, α-methyl-p-tyrosine (metyrosine), an inhibitor of tyrosine hydroxylase that blocks catecholamine synthesis, can be used in the management of chronic pheochromocytoma.[r3] Calcium channel blockers have recently been reported to suppress clinical symptoms of pheochromocytoma without reducing plasma catecholamine concentrations.

References

Research Reports

1. Oliver G, Schafer EA. The physiological effects of extracts on the suprarenal capsules. J Physiol (London) 1895;*18*:230–235.
2. Abel JJ, Crawford AC. On the blood pressure raising constituent of the suprarenal capsule. Bull Johns Hopkins Hos 1897;*8*:151–154.
3. Elliott TR. The action of adrenaline. J Physiol (London) 1905;*32*:401–404.
4. Cannon WB, Uridil JE. Studies on the conditions of activity in endocrine glands, VIII. Some effects of denervated heart of stimulating the nerves of the liver. Am J Physiol 1921;*58*:353–356.
5. Kopin IJ. Catecholamine metabolism (and the biochemical assessment of sympathetic activity). Clin Endocrinol Metab 1977;*6*:525–546.
6. Mueller RA, Otte U, Thoenen H. The role of adenosine cyclic 3′,5′-monophosphate in reserpine-initiated adrenal medullary tyrosine hydroxylase induction. Mol Pharmacol 1974;*10*:855–860.
7. Creutz CE, Pazoles CJ, Pollard HB. Identification and purification of an adrenomedullary protein (synexin) that causes calcium-dependent aggregation of isolated chromaffin granules. J Biol Chem 1978;*253*:2858–2863.
8. Allen JM, Adrian TE, Polak JM, Bloom SR. Neuropeptide Y (NPY) in the adrenal gland. J Autonomic Nerv System 1983;*9*:559–562.
9. Kataoka Y, Majane EA, Yang H-YT. Release of NPY-like immunoreactive material from primary cultures of chromaffin cells prepared from bovine adrenal medulla. Neuropharmacology 1985;*24*:693–695.
10. Corder R, Lowry, PJ, Emson PC, Gillard RC. Chromatographic characterisation of the circulating neuropeptide Y immunoreactivity from patients with pheochromocytoma. Regul Peptides 1985;*10*:91–95.
11. Evequoz D, Waeber B, Aubert JF, Fluckiger JP, Nussberger J, Brunner HR. Neuropeptide Y prevents the blood pressure fall induced by endotoxin in conscious rats with adrenal medullectomy. Circ Res 1988;*62*:25–30.
12. Parker MM, Parillo JE. Septic shock: hemodynamics and pathogenesis. JAMA 1983;*250*:3324–3327.

13. Von Euler US. A specific sympathomimetic ergone in adrenergic nerve fibers (sympathin) and its relations to adrenaline and noradrenaline. Acta Physiol Scand 1948;*12*:73–97.

Reviews

r1. Coupland RE. The development and fate of catecholamine secreting endocrine cells. In: Parvez H, Parvez S (eds) Biogenic amines in development, Amsterdam: Elsevier/North Holland, 1980, pp 3–28.

r2. Coupland RE. The chromaffin system. In: Blaschko H, Muscholl E (eds) Catecholamines, handbook of experimental pharmacology, Berlin: Springer-Verlag, 1972, vol. 33, pp 16–39.

r3. Landsberg L, Young JB. Catacholamines and the adrenal medulla. In: Wilson JD, Foster DW (eds) Williams Textbook of Endocrinology, 7th ed, Philadelphia: WB Saunders (1985); pp 891–965.

r4. Livett BG. The secretory process in the adrenal chromaffin cells. In: Cantin M (ed) Cell biology of the secretory process, Basel: Karger, 1984, pp 309–358.

r5. Tepperman J, Tepperman HM. Catecholamines. In: Metabolic and Endocrine Physiology, 5th ed Chicago, London: Year Book, (1987); pp 229–246.

CHAPTER 9

Autacoids in Peripheral Autonomic Functions

Giora Z. Feuerstein
Douglas W. P. Hay

Introduction

This chapter is devoted to a diverse group of biologically active substances normally produced by various cells and organs and traditionally excluded from the "hormone" class. They are generally short-lived (some, like thromboxane A_2 have a half-life of only a few seconds) and have little chance to survive effectively even one circulation time. Further, this class of compounds does not necessarily fit within the definition of "neurotransmitters," since many are not preformed, nor are they stored in secretory granules or vesicles (e.g., platelet activating factor, leukotrienes). Nevertheless, these biologically active substances are believed to be extremely important, each acting on the cell of origin (producer) itself, (hence the prefix-"autos") in a mode vital (hence "takos", or "remedial") to its own cell or to neighboring cells. This grouping is quite arbitrary for three reasons: (a) angiotensin II, which traditionally is lumped in this group, is believed to reflect more closely hormonal modes of action; (b) many peptides that are autacoid-like, e.g., gastrin, secretin, or lymphokines, usually are discussed as paracrine mediators, a term hard to differentiate from the classic autacoid realm of action; and (c) often, the autocrine/paracrine site of action is not the more important or critical one, as excessive production may overwhelm the metabolic/disposal barriers, leaving systemic, hormonel-like actions in effect and subject to pharmacologic intervention. Regardless of old semantics, this chapter will discuss the chemistry, biology, and pharmacology of eicosanoids and other lipid mediators, amines, peptides, and purines that are established mediators in physiologic and pathophysiologic processes and for which several therapeutic agents have been established.

Eicosanoids

Eicosanoids is a general term for various oxygenated products of arachidonic acid, including prostaglandins, thromboxanes, leukotrienes, lipoxins, epoxyeicosatrienoic acids, and others. Prostaglandins were the first substances studied, followed decades later by thromboxane, prostacyclin, and the leukotrienes. Lipoxins were discovered only recently, and their formation in vivo has not yet been demonstrated. The following sections will review the actions of the major products of arachidonic acid formation (prostaglandins, thromboxanes, and leukotrienes) on peripheral autonomic function.

Prostaglandins

Chemistry

The term "prostaglandin" was initially suggested for the lipid substance from seminal fluid that reduced blood pressure and produced contractile or relaxing effects on some nonvascular smooth muscle preparations, notably uterine tissue. The term prostaglandin was chosen because of the belief that the substance was produced by the prostate gland. Later investigations demonstrated that the predominant source was in fact the seminal vesicle. Currently, prostaglandins are considered to be one of the most ubiquitous biologic substances present in plants, prokaryotes, eukaryotes, and the animal kingdom, including humans.

Prostaglandins generally are of three types, referred to as the "one series," "two series," or "three series," to indicate the number of double bonds in their structure. All prostaglandins are synthesized from dihomo-δ-linoleic acid, arachidonic acid, or eicosapentaenoic acid, each of which is a 20-carbon fatty acid chain with 3, 4, or 5 double bonds, respectively. The free levels of prostaglandin precursors are generally extremely low, and, since prostaglandin products are not stored, levels often cannot be detected in organs or biologic fluids. Rather, prostaglandins are formed de novo when the precursor fatty acid is released from membrane phospholipids following specific stimuli associated with cell activation.

The most important phospholipases associated with prostaglandin synthesis are phospholipase A_2 and C. Phospholipase A_2 catalyzes the release of fatty acids from the C_2 position of the glycerol moiety. Phospholipase C catalyzes the release of the phosphate group from the phosphoglyceride, followed by the release of fatty acid from the 2 position of the glycerol moiety by diglyceride lipase. Activation of either phospholipase occurs after membrane stimulation (either receptor- or nonreceptor-mediated). Following the release of the appropriate fatty acid from the membrane phosphoglyceride stores, the fatty acid is cyclized and oxygenated by cyclooxygenase. This results in the formation of a prostaglandin endoperoxide, PGG_2. PGG_2 is reduced in a subsequent peroxidase reaction to the 15-hydroxy derivative, PGH_2. PGH_2 is the prostaglandin endoperoxide intermediate that subsequently can be converted to the prostaglandins (i.e., PGD_2, PGE_2, or $PGF_{2\alpha}$), prostacyclin (i.e., PGI_2), or thromboxane (Fig. 9.1).

At present, there is no generally accepted classification system for prostaglandin receptors. However, it has been advocated that the receptors can be divided into the following five groups: *DP*, *EP*, *FP*, *IP* and *TP* for which PGD_2, PGE_2, $PGF_{2\alpha}$, PGI_2 and TXA_2 are the most potent natural agonists, respectively.[1,r1] Furthermore, subtypes of EP receptors designated EP_1, EP_2, and EP_3 have been postulated; but there is conflicting evidence for the existence of these receptor subtypes.[r2] Although useful for characterizing eicosanoid responses, some controversy remains regarding this classification. One complicating factor, and an important consideration in receptor classification, is that individual eicosanoids interact to some degree with other eicosanoid receptor subtypes. Further, the prostanoid receptors are present in an array of cells. The confusion about classification of these receptors will be resolved with the cloning of all receptor subtypes.

Biology

The biologic effects of the prostaglandins defy simple description. There are substantial differences in biologic effects between the various prostaglandins, in addition to considerable organ and species differences. An important source of PGD_2 is mast cells, where it is released along with histamine and leukotrienes. PGD_2 is a potent bronchoconstrictor, but its vascular effects are more varied. In humans, infusion of PGD_2 produces a fall in arterial blood pressure, and additionally inhibits platelet aggregation. Inhibition of platelet aggregatory responses is mediated by a specific platelet receptor for PGD_2, and involves cAMP as the second messenger.[r2]

PGE_2 is widely formed in the body, including the brain, uterus, kidney, and the vessel wall. The primary sites of action of PGE_2 are on secretory cells and vascular smooth muscle. Like PGE_1, PGE_2 has an inhibitory effect on macrophages, granulocytes, and other inflammatory cells. In contrast to PGE_1, PGE_2 does not inhibit platelet aggregation. PGE_2 generally relaxes arterial vessels, but contracts venous vessels. PGE_2 relaxes or contracts airway smooth muscle, depending on the level of tone. PGE_2 also has an important role in inflammatory processes, including sensitization of pain receptors, inhibition of inflammatory cell function, and promotion of cytokine production. Finally, PGE_2, Like $PGF_{2\alpha}$, is important in the development of labor.

There are two stereoisomers of PGF; however, only the α isomers are biologically active. $PGF_{2\alpha}$ formation occurs throughout the body, by both an enzymatic and a nonenzymatic process. The predominant effects of $PGF_{2\alpha}$ are contraction of vascular, bronchial, and uterine smooth muscle. $PGF_{2\alpha}$ is an important uterine tone effector, and in subprimate species stimulates the regression of the corpus luteum. In humans, the clinical use of $PGF_{2\alpha}$ has been limited by undesirable side-effects; but in veterinary medicine it is used to induce abortion.

Certain prostaglandins have been reported to function as modulators of norepinephrine from sympathetic nerves. Evidence in support of the supposition for an inhibitory effect of PGE_1 and PGE_2 on catecholamine overflow has been shown in certain animal species and organ preparations, including the cat spleen, rabbit kidney, guinea pig vas deferens, and isolated perfused rabbit heart. Inhibition of prostaglandin synthesis by indomethacin, thereby removing the attenuating action of endogenously formed prostaglandins, indeed results in enhanced norepinephrine release, a finding consistent with the notion of a modulating effect of endogenously formed eicosanoids on norepinephrine release. However, other studies have challenged the original hypothesis of a prostaglandin-dependent mechanism for control of norepinephrine release. Thus, PGE_2 and PGI_2 did not decrease responses elicited by electrical stimulation of the isolated canine atrium, nor did they change plasma epinephrine or norepinephrine levels in spinal-cord-stimulated pithed rats.[r3] Finally, in intact anesthetized dogs, it was reported that neither PGE_2 nor PGI_2 influenced renal norepinephrine release. Therefore, the importance of the role of endogenous prostaglandins in modulating catecholamine release from sympathetic nerves has been seriously questioned. Moreover, the over-all effects of eicosanoids on adrenergic neurotransmitter release is considerably less than that achieved via modulation through the presynaptic α_2-adrenergic receptor.

Prostacyclin

Prostacyclin (PGI_2) was discovered by Vane and coworkers[4] in 1976 as the principal arachidonic acid metabolite of vascular tissue (Fig. 9.1). Studies exploring prostaglandin endoperoxide metabolism in a microsomal fraction of blood vessels revealed an unstable product that inhibited platelet aggregation and relaxed coronary vessels. This bicyclic substance, designated prostacyclin, is now termed PGI_2 to conform with commonly employed prostaglandin nomenclature.

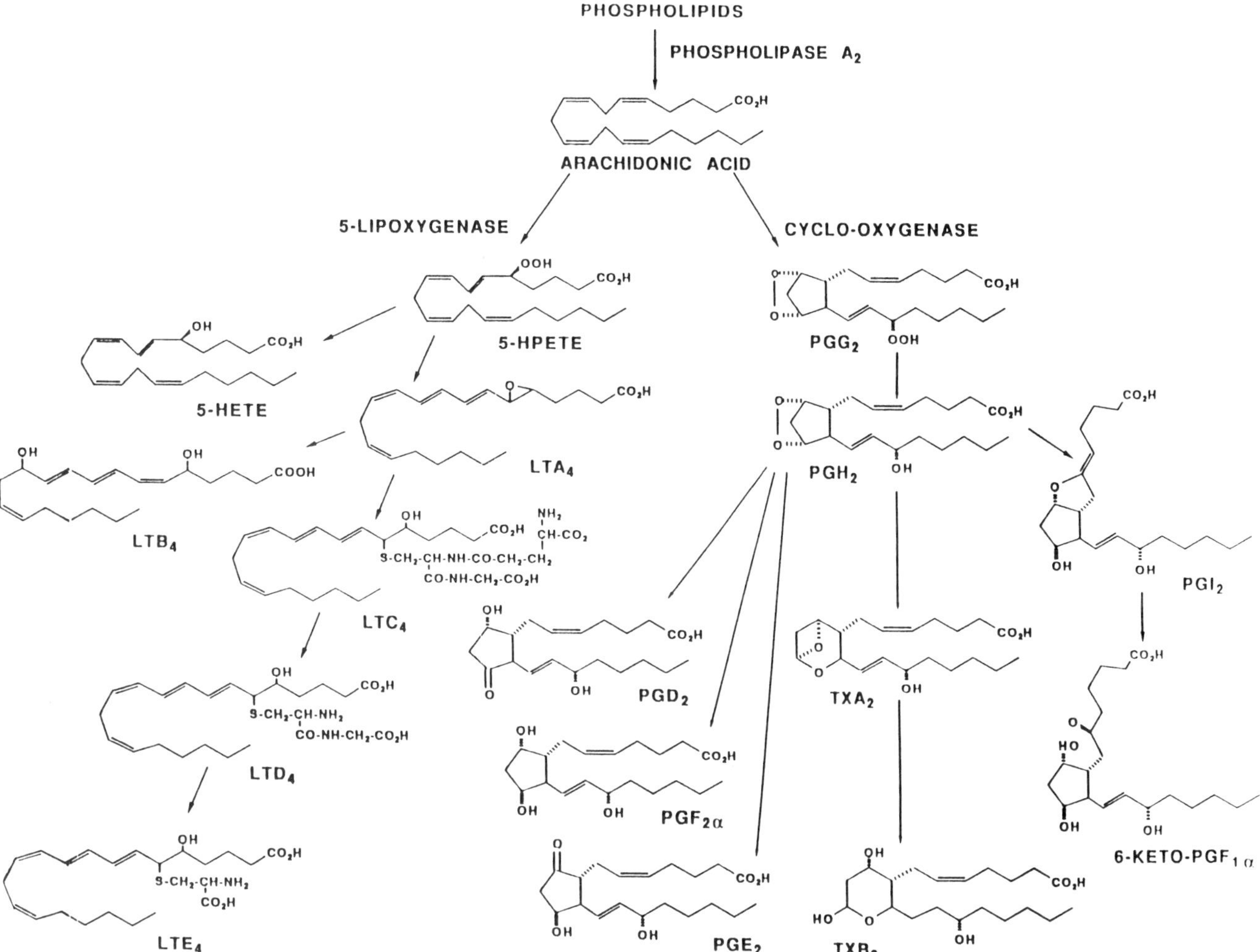

Figure 9.1 Pathways of arachidonic acid metabolism. Metabolism occurs primarily through either the cyclooxygenase of 5-lipoxygenase pathways. Abbreviations: PG: prostaglandin; TX: thromboxane; H(P)ETE: hydroxy(hydroxyperoxy) eicosatetrenoic acid; LT: leukotriene.

The formation of PGI_2 occurs through a pathway similar to that for the synthesis of the other prostaglandins. Prostacyclin synthase metabolizes the prostaglandin endoperoxides to PGI_2. In the vessel wall, Prostacyclin is present in the greatest amount at the intimal surface, progressively decreasing in activity toward the adventitial surface. Biologically, PGI_2 is a potent inhibitor of platelet aggregation,[5] and is approximately 10–30-fold more potent than PGE_1. Furthermore, PGI_2 disaggregates platelets in vitro and in vivo. PGI_2 relaxes most arterial preparations, including cat coronary, bovine coronary, human and baboon cerebral, and rabbit celiac and mesenteric vessels.

Generally, the major biologic effects of PGI_2, namely inhibition of platelet aggregation and vasodilation, are considered beneficial in many cardiovascular disorders, including myocardial infarction, circulatory shock, and peripheral vascular disease. Thus, inhibition of PGI_2 by cyclo-oxygenase inhibitors is not typically a specific therapeutic aim. A number of prostacyclin-mimetics have been characterized. Prostacyclin mimetics were developed in an attempt to produce an antithrombotic effect while avoiding or minimizing the hemodynamic side-effects. Although considerable effort has been expended in this area, a commonality of all PGI_2 mimetics is that they exhibit no substantially greater selectivity for platelets versus the vascular smooth muscle than PGI_2; hence, their side-effect profile (headache, nausea, vomiting, hypotension) appears similar to that of PGI_2.

Therapeutically, the antiaggregatory and vasodilatory actions of PGI_2 could be useful for the treatment of peripheral vascular disease and myocardial infarction, and for the reduction of platelet consumption in patients with extracorporeal circulation. This has stimulated interest in synthesizing PGI_2 analogues with greater chemical and biologic stability. Besides PGI_2, analogues that have been investigated include carbacyclin and iloprost.[5] PGI_2 and iloprost have already undergone investigations in small, limited clinical studies of myocardial infarction and peripheral vascular disease. Although in some cases the initial results were encouraging, significant cardiovascular side-effects occurred during IV administration. The narrow "therapeutic window" has generally hampered the widespread use of PGI_2 or similar analogues in larger, multicenter clinical studies. The hypotensive effects of PGI_2 and most other PGL_2 mimetics is likely to limit the broad clinical application of this otherwise useful class of drugs.

PGI_2 does not interfere with the physiologic nerve-stimulation-induced norepinephrine release or postjunctional adrenergic responses, but may in particular circumstances exert antiadrenergic actions. Following myocardial ischemia, catecholamines are released from sympathetic nerve terminals to the surrounding tissue,[6] a phenomenon considered to be associated with detrimental functions of the ischemic heart. PGI_2 attenuated this redistribution of catecholamines in the ischemic myocardium, and ultimately the containment of cardiac catecholamines within the adrenergic nerve endings.[6] Therefore, PGI_2 appears to be a potential therapeutic agent for treatment of myocardial ischemia. However, such potential has not been explored as yet in clinical situations.

At least 16 prostaglandin inhibitors (i.e., cyclo-oxygenase inhibitors) are available for use in humans. These include aspirin, ibuprofen, flurbiprofen, and naproxen, which are widely used as anti-inflammatory agents. These agents are discussed in detail in Chapter 74. They are generally associated with characteristic GI side-effects, including ulceration. However, a recently introduced compound, nabumetone, appears to have substantially fewer irritant effects in the GI tract.[r4] PGE_1, has been used as temporary therapy to maintain patency of the ductus arteriosus in neonates, and also for the treatment of severe forms of peripheral arterial occlusive disease. PGE_2, $PGI_{2\alpha}$, or more stable analogues previously were used to induce labor or in therapeutic abortions. However, because of undesirable side-effects, these agents are no longer favored for these indications.

Thromboxane

Chemistry

Thromboxanes are a unique class of cyclooxygenase products of arachidonic acid (Fig. 9.1), first isolated from platelets (i.e., thrombocytes, hence the prefix "thrombo"). The biologically active product is thromboxane A_2 (TXA_2), which is formed by the enzymatic conversion of the prostaglandin endoperoxide PGH_2. TXA_2 contains an extremely unstable acetal carbon susceptible to hydrolytic attack. Biosynthesis of TXA_2 from arachidonic acid requires prostaglandin endoperoxides and thromboxane synthase, which isomerizes PGH_2 to TXA_2. Formation of thromboxane A_2 is not limited to platelets,[7] as TXA_2 formation has been demonstrated in lung, umbilical artery, spleen, and brain. The half-life of TXA_2 in aqueous solution is less than 30 seconds at 37°C. The stable hydrolysis product, TXB_2, is the commonly measured metabolite of TXA_2, although TXB_2 can be further metabolized to other end-products, such as 2,3 dinor-TXB_2.

Biology

The major effects of TXA_2 are platelet aggregation, contraction of nonvascular (i.e., airway) and vascular smooth muscle, including arteries, veins, and lymphatic vessels, and enhanced membrane labilization and permeability.[r5] Because of these potent, and possibly deleterious effects, TXA_2 has been implicated in a number of thrombotic and cardiopulmonary disorders (see below). Consequently, intensive efforts to produce compounds to block the biologic activities of TXA_2 are being pursued.

Pharmacology

Several strategies are available for pharmacologic inhibition of TXA_2 formation and action. The least specific approach is inhibition of the cyclo-oxygenase enzyme. Included in this large group are the widely utilized anti-inflammatory drugs aspirin, indomethacin, and ibuprofen. The cyclo-oxygenase inhibitors are considered relatively nonspecific since, in addition to inhibiting a key enzymatic product necessary for the synthesis of thromboxanes A_2, they will also attenuate the formation of the potentially beneficial products of cyclooxygenase, such as PGE_2 and PGI_2. The development of thromboxane A_2 synthase inhibitors represents a more specific approach for inhibition of TXA_2 formation. Thromboxane synthase inhibitors inhibit the enzyme that converts the prostaglandin endoperoxides, PGG_2 and PGH_2, to TXA_2. Included within this class of drugs are dazoxiben, dazmegrel, CGS 13080, and others. However, thromboxane synthesis inhibition leads to the accumulation of the endoperoxide substrate PGH_2, which has affinity for the same receptor and has the same pharmacologic profile as TXA_2. This phenomenon may negate to some degree the effects of inhibition of TXA_2 formation.[r4,r5] Another specific approach involves the development of potent antagonists of the thromboxane A_2 receptor. Several potent compounds have been identified, including sulotroban, daltroban, SQ 29548, and GR 32191. These agents have been reported to antagonize the platelet proaggregatory and vasoconstrictor effects of TXA_2 or TXA_2-mimetics. Additionally, the TXA_2 receptor antagonists block the effects of the prostaglandin endoperoxides, such as PGH_2.[r4] Some compounds with combined TXA_2 receptor antagonism and thromboxane synthase inhibitory activity have been identified. From a theoretical standpoint, this class of compounds may have the best potential for therapeutic benefit in diseases in which TXA_2 has been implicated.[r4]

Increased circulating levels of TXB_2 (the stable metabolite of TXA_2, see Fig. 9.1) are found in a number of cardiovascular conditions where platelets are activated during transit, including atherosclerosis, unstable angina, myocardial infarction, septic shock, stroke, and diabetes mellitus. Additionally, increased urinary TXB_2 excretion has been considered an early prognostic indicator of renal transplant rejection. Despite Numerous reports that show a beneficial effect of thromboxane synthase inhibitors or thromboxane receptor antagonists in numerous animal models of disease, the limited clinical trials with thromboxane synthase inhibitors and thromboxane receptor antagonists have been disappointing. Accordingly, the clinical usefulness of these classes of compounds remains to be determined.

The interaction of TXA_2 with adrenergic nerve responses is of a complex nature. First, the contractile effects of TXA_2 on vascular smooth muscle would potentiate postjunctional adrenergic neurotransmitter responses. Second, there is increasing evidence that thromboxane A_2 increases exocytotic release of norepinephrine from adrenergic fibers. It was reported that the stable thromboxane mimetic, U46619, increased norepinephrine-release and consequently enhanced contractions of the isolated rabbit vas deferens. Under physiologic conditions, TXA_2 levels are extremely low; therefore, it is not suspected that humoral TXA_2 is an important physiologic modulator of adrenergic neurotransmitter release. Further studies will be required to characterize more precisely the effect of TXA_2 on neural function under more physiologic conditions, as well as during pathophysiologic events.

Leukotrienes

Chemistry

The leukotrienes (LTs) are a family of potent mediators consisting of the sulfidopeptidoleukotrienes (also known as the peptido-n-cysteinyl-leukotrienek), LTC_4, LTD_4, and LTE_4, and the chemoattractant, LTB_4. The leuotrienes are produced from the metabolism of membrane-derived arachidonic acid by the action of the 5-lipoxygenase enzyme that controls two steps in the synthetic pathway: first, there is 5-lipoxygenase-induced formation of an unstable intermediate 5-S-hydroperoxy-6,8-*trans*-11,14 *cis*-eicosatetraenoic acid (5-HPETE) and, second, 5-HPETE is either transformed subsequently by a hydroperoxidase to 5-hydroxyeicosatetraenoic acid (5-HETE) or converted by the catalytic activity of 5-lipoxygenase to another unstable intermediate, the allylic epoxide LTA_4 5S, 6S (5S, 6S-*trans*-oxido-7,9-*trans*-11,14-*cis*-ei cosatetraenoic acid. LTA_4 is then converted either enzymatically to LTB_4 (5S-12R-6,14-*cis*-8,10 *trans*-eicosatetraenoic acid) by LTB synthetase, or nonenzymatically to isomers of LTB_4. Additionally, LTA_4 is converted to LTC_4 (5-S-hydroxy-6-R-glutathionyl-7,9-*trans*-11,14-cis-eicosatetraenoic acid) by conjugation of LTA_4 with glutathione under the activity of glutathione-5-transferase. LTC_4 is then transformed by γ-glutamyltranspeptidase-induced reversal of a glutamic acid residue to yield LTD_4 (5S-hydroxy-6R-S-cysteinylglycyl-7,9-*trans*-11,14-eicosatetraenoic acid), which undergoes further metabolism by an aminopeptidase that removes the glycinyl residue to produce LTE_4 (5S-hydroxy-6R-S-cysteinyl-7,9-*trans*-11,14-*cis*- eicosatetraenoic acid. LTC_4, LTD_4, and LTE_4 comprise the active ingredients of what was previously referred to as "slow-reactive substance" of anaphylaxin (SRS-A).[8-10]

The mammalian 5-lipoxygenase has been cloned and its molecular mechanism characterized.[11,12] It is a Ca^{2+}- and ATP-dependent enzyme with a molecular weight of approximately 78 kDa. Recent studies isolated and identified an 18 kDa membrane protein, designated 5 (five)-lipoxygenase activating protein (FLAP) essential for activation of the 5-lipoxygenase enzyme and the production of the LTs.[r6,14]

Biology

There are several sources of the LTs, including a variety of inflammatory cells such as eosinophils, mast cells, basophils, macrophages, neutrophils, and monocytes. The qualitative and quantitative profile of release of the LTs depends on the cell type as well as the stimulus, which may include antigenic and nonantigenic provocation. The LTs exert a diverse array of biologic effects that are mediated following interaction with specific plasma membrane receptors. For example, the peptidoleukotrienes elicit contraction of a variety of smooth muscle preparations, increase mucous secretion, stimulate microvascular permeability, elicit pressor and depressor responses, produce excitation of Purkinje neurons and cause stimulation of prostaglandin release.[r7] The most notable feature of the biologic activity of LTB_4 is its prominent effects on leukocyte function, including stimulation of adhesion and enhanced neutrophil chemotaxis, aggregation, and degranulation. Other examples of the potent proinflammatory profile of LTB_4 are its ability to enhance vascular permeability and increase C3b expression.[r4,r8] Furthermore, elevated levels of the leukotrienes, especially LTB_4, have been detected in various animal models of inflammatory diseases, as well as in humans.[r9]

In human airways, unlike guinea pig airways and other tissues, contractions elicited by LTC_4, LTD_4, and LTE_4 appear to be mediated via an interaction with a homogeneous LT receptor population.[r10] Following activation, the LTD_4 receptor can interact with either pertussis toxin-sensitive or insensitive proteins, depending on the cell type. Receptor stimulation results in marked influences on Ca^{2+} mobilization and formation of second messengers, including a rapid, transient increase in intracellular Ca^{2+} from extracellular and intracellular sources, including translocation via receptor-operated Ca^{2+} channels, and activation of a phosphoinositide-specific phospholipase C and release of Ca^{2+} from the sarcoplasmic reticulum. The enhanced phosphoinositide turnover results in increases in the levels of the second messengers inositol phosphates, such as IP_3 and diacylglycerol, that activate protein kinase C.[13,r11] Phospholipase A_2 is also activated subsequently resulting in the formation and release of arachidonic acid and its potent biologically active metabolites.[r11,14]

The biologic effects of LTB_4 are mediated via two populations of specific receptors. For example, in human neutrophils, radioligand binding experiments have identified two separate, stereospecific populations of LTB_4 binding sites: a high-affinity site (K_D = 0.4nM) that mediates chemotaxis and chemokinesis and aggregation, and a low-affinity site (K_D = 61nM) responsible for degranulation.[16,21] Unlike peptidoleukotriene receptors, LTB_4 receptors utilize only a pertussis toxin-sensitive G protein.[r11] Largely as a result of their many, potent biologic effects, the LTs have been implicated in the pathogenesis of a variety of disorders. For example, LTB_4 has been proposed to play a significant role in psoriasis and other skin disorders, arthritis, and inflammatory bowel disease. In addition, levels of LTB_4, or its metabolite 20-OH-LTB_4, were elevated in several diseases, including asthma, cystic fibrosis, chronic bronchitis, gout, and rheumatoid arthritis. It was also been postulated that LTB_4 is involved in pain and immune response modulation by induction of T-lymphocyte supressor cells.[r9] The peptidoleukotrienes have been postulated to be involved in several cardiopulmonary disorders, including bronchitis, allergic rhinitis, endotoxemia or septic shock, adult respiratory distress, cystic fibrosis, myocardial ischemia, cardiac anaphylaxis, cerebral vasospasm, and ischemia.[r7,12] Asthma is the disease for which there is the most convincing evidence that the leukotrienes, particularly the peptidoleukotrienes, play a pivotal role,[r12,r9] and this area has been the focus of much of the work in the field of LT biology. Thus, the LTs mimic several of the cardinal features of asthma. For example, the peptidoleukotrienes are very potent bronchoconstrictor agonists in human airways in vitro and in vivo, having up to more than 1000-fold the potency of histamine or cholinergic agonists. They potently stimulate mucus secretion in human airways in vitro, and they increase microvascular permeability. Furthermore, increased LT levels are detected in the body fluids of asthmatics, and a correlation has been observed between the amounts of the LTs and the severity of the disease. In addition, LTs are released from human airways both in vitro and in vivo following antigen provocation.

Pharmacology

For the past decade or so the pharmaceutical industry has committed a considerable amount of resources to the development of drugs to control the deleterious actions of the LTs in various systems and diseases. Two strategies have been employed: (a) synthesis of potent and selective receptor antagonists for the peptidoleukotrienes on the one hand, and LTB_4 on the other; (b) synthesis of inhibitors of 5-lipoxygenase activity, either inhibitors of the enzyme itself or the FLAP. Several potent, selective, and stimulating diverse members of the different classes of compounds have been identified, primarily peptidoleukotriene receptor antagonists and 5-lipoxygenase and FLAP inhibitors; and many are in clinical trials. Research on LTB_4 receptor antagonists has lagged somewhat behind efforts directed toward the development of the other classes of compounds and, to date, there is no information on potent and selective LTB_4 receptor antagonists. The therapeutic focus with compounds that have entered clinical trials thus far has been asthma, with studies also performed in arthritis, inflammatory bowel disease, allergic rhinitis, and psoriasis.

The first peptidoleukotriene receptor antagonists identified was FPL-55712 in the early 1970s. Although widely and effectively utilized as an experimental tool, FPL-55712 has an inadequate profile (of potency, selectivity, and pharmacokinetic performance) to test clinically the pathophysiologic roles of the LTs. Subsequently, several much more potent and selective competitive receptor antagonists have been identified, and examples of these structurally diverse drugs have been involved in significant clinical trials, including ICI 204,219, MK-571, SK&F 104353, and ONO-1078. Several of the compounds demonstrate impressive in vitro and in vivo activity against LT-induced and also antigen-induced bronchoconstriction in animals.[r8,16] For example, IV administration of SK&F 104353 (in the presence of an antihistamine)[17] or oral administration of MK-571[18] inhibited antigen-induced bronchoconstriction in monkeys. Furthermore, several compounds, including SK&F 104353,[19] MK571,[18] and ONO-1078[19] inhibit antigen-induced constriction of isolated human bronchus.

Thus far, the data from clinical trials in asthma are interesting and encouraging, with preliminary reports of efficacy in this population. For example, several compounds have been demonstrated to inhibit antigen-induced bronchoconstriction (both early and late phases) and also exercise-induced asthma.[r13,20] In addition, inhibitory effects against cold air-, PAF-, or aspirin-induced bronchoconstriction, with improvement in baseline pulmonary function, has been noted.[r4] Thus, there is the realistic potential that, in the 1990s, the peptidoleukotriene receptor antagonist may represent the first new class of compounds for treatment of asthma for about a quarter of a century.

Some protective effects have been observed with peptidoleukotriene receptor antagonists in models of endotoxic shock.[20,r14] From a theoretical standpoint, 5-lipoxygenase inhibitors possess an exciting therapeutic potential in that they will inhibit the release of both the peptidoleukotrienes and LTB_4, and thus may exhibit greater efficacy in some diseases than selective peptidoleukotrienes or LTB_4 receptor antagonists.

Several different classes of compounds have been demonstrated to be 5-lipoxygenase inhibitors, and they have shown anti-inflammatory activity in in vivo animal models.[r4] For example, one group that has been extensively studied is the hydroxyureas, hydroxamic acid derivatives whose 5-lipoxygenase inhibitory activity is thought to be due to their iron-chelating capacity.[15] An example of this class of compound is A64077 (zileuton).[r15] A-64077 is currently the most advanced 5-lipoxygenase inhibitor in Phase III clinical trials for multiple indications, including asthma, inflammatory bowel disease, and arthritis. While zileuton is a potent 5-lipoxygenase inhibitor, it has a disappointing pharmacokinetic profile. BWA4C also is a potent inhibitor of 5-lipoxygenase with a relatively long duration of action, and has undergone clinical evaluation. Probably the most interesting of recent compounds are the methoxyalkyl thiazoles, such as ICI D2138, a novel class of potent and selective 5-lipoxygenase inhibitors that appear to act via a direct mechanism involving competitive inhibition of the enzyme rather than redox inhibition or iron chelation. This compound is in Phase II clinical trials for asthma.[r16] Additional compounds that inhibit LT production include MK-886[r17] and MK-0591.[r18] The drugs act, not by inhibiting the 5-lipoxygenase enzyme per se, but by interacting with the regulatory FLAP. MK-0591 is currently in Phase II trials for asthma.

Thus, preclinical and clinical researchers now have a powerful arsenal of potent and selective compounds with which to elucidate definitively the role of products of the 5-lipoxygenase pathway in various diseases. The potential and hope is that some of these compounds may become anti-inflammatory and antiasthma drugs in the not-too-distant future.

Lipoxins

Lipoxins are a group of trihydroxy fatty acids with a conjugated tetraene structure.[22] The lipoxins are metabolites of arachidonate via an interaction of 15- and 5-lipoxygenase pathways; alternatively, lipoxins can also be produced from 5,15-di-HPETE via a 12-lipoxygenase system.

Lipoxin A_4 (5S, 6R 15S-trihydroxy-7,9,13-*trans*-11-*cis*-eicosatetraenoic acid) and B_4 (5S, 14R, 15S-trihydroxy-6,10,12-*trans*-8-*cis*-eicosatetraenoic acid) are produced primarily by neuthrophils and eosinophils, and possibly by platelets when interacting with neutrophils. Lipoxin A_4 stimulates superoxide anion generation and granule secretion in neutrophils; chemotaxis, but not aggregation, also is elicited. Some lipoxins can affect vascular activity, eliciting vasoconstriction or vasorelaxation via an endothelium-dependent mechanism. Lipoxins A_4 and B inhibit natural killer cell cytotoxicity. Lipoxins A_4, A_5, and B_4, but not B_5, contract guinea pig lung parenchyma through a mechanism that involves the same receptor stimulated by the peptidoleukotrienes. The excessive release of lipoxins in patients with hypereosinophilia suggests their involvement in immune and allergic reactions. Lipoxin A was a more potent activator of protein kinase C than either diacylglycerol or arachidonic acid, suggesting a role as an intracellular modulator.[23] However, the precise role of lipoxins in normal physiology and in disease processes is unclear, and currently is under investigation.

Platelet Activating Factor

Chemistry

Platelet activating factor (PAF) is an ether-containing phospholipid originally isolated from IgE-stimulated basophils and ultimately identified primarily as 1-0-alkyl-2-acetyl-sn-glycerol-3-phosphocholine.[24] PAF is composed mainly of two different alkyl chain homologs, 1-0-hexadecyl and 1-0-octadecyl, but the existence of a variety of other species stresses the molecular heterogeneity of PAF molecules. PAF is produced by a variety of cell types, such as monocytes, endothelial cells, polymorphonuclear leukocytes, and platelets. PAF is produced via the "PAF cycle" (Fig. 9.2), a term describing the reactions that shuttle the transfer of acetate and arachidonic acid to lyso-PAF, the obligatory common intermediate in the formation and inactivation of PAF.[25] Lyso-PAF can be acetylated by either an acetyltransferase or by arachidonyl-transcylase. PAF is inactivated by acetylhydrolase, an enzyme present in tissues and blood.[25]

Biology

The effects of extracellular PAF are mediated by interaction of PAF with specific cell membrane receptors of high affinity, such as those found on platelets, neutrophils, monocytes, neurons, mesangial, and endothelial cells. PAF interacts with specific receptors that elicit multiple biochemical events, including activation of GTPase, increased Ca^{+2} influx, release of Ca^{+2} from intracellular stores, and activation of phospholipases. A central event in the transduction mechanism of PAF is activation of cytoplasmic protein kinase C and phosphorylation of critical cellular proteins.

The actions of PAF have been extensively studied in multiple organs and systems. Systemic administration of PAF in vivo consistently results in hypotension, reduction of cardiac output, pulmonary hypertension, and increased capillary permeability.[r19,26] In most species, PAF produces thrombocytopenia and leukopenia. Of primary importance are PAF effects on cardiac function, which include coronary constriction, myocardial depression, arrhythmias, and low cardiac output. The over-all actions of PAF on the cardiovascular system

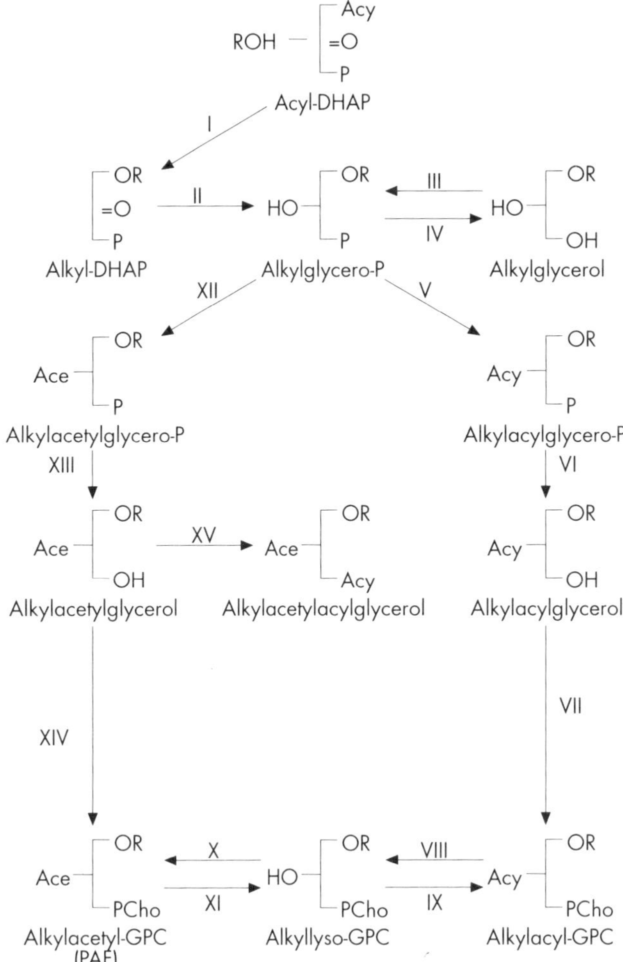

Figure 9.2 General pathways for the metabolism of the alkyl ether lipids and PAF. The Roman numerals refer to the following enzymes: (1) alkyl-DHAP synthase; (II) NADPH:alkyl-DHAP oxidoreductase; (III) ATP:1-alkyl-sn-glycerol-3-P phosphotransferase; (IV) 1-alkyl-2-lyso-sn-glycero-3-P phosphohydrolase; (V) acyl-CoA: 1-alkyl-2-lyso-sn-glycero-3-P acyltransferase; (VI) 1-alkyl-2-acyl-sn-glycero-3-P phosphydrolase; (VII) CDP-choline: 1-alkyl-2-acyl-sn-glycerol DTT-sensitive cholinephosphotransferase; (VIII) phospholipase A_2; (IX) phosphatidyl-choline: 1-alkyl-2-lyso-sn-glycero-3-phosphocholine polyenoic-specific transcyclase (CoA-independent); (X) acetyl-CoA: 1-alkyl-2-lyso-sn-glycero-3-phosphocholine acetyltransferase; (XI) 1-alkyl-s-acetyl-sn-glycero-3-phosphocholine acetylhydrolase; (XII) acetyl-CoA: 1-alkyl-2-lyso-sn-glycero-3-P acetyltransferase; (XIII) 1-alkyl-2-acetyl-sn-glycero-3-P phosphohydrolase; (XIV) CDP-choline: 1-alkyl-2-acetyl-sn-glycerol DTT-insensitive choline-phospho-transferase; (XV) acyl-CoA: 1-alkyl-2-acetyl-sn-glycerol acyl-transferase. Ace, acetyl; Acy, acyl; Cho, choline; GPC, sn-glycero-3-phosphocholine. This figure is reproduced with permission from F. Snyder.

lead to circulatory shock.[r14] However, PAF acts on virtually every organ. In the CNS, PAF affects cerebral blood flow and metabolism, and disrupts the blood-brain barrier.[35] In the bronchopulmonary system, PAF produces long-lasting airway inflammation and increased bronchial sensitivity to a variety of bronchoconstrictors (e.g., histamine, acetylcholine). PAF is also a potent pathogen in the GI tract, where it was shown to produce mucosal damage and hemorrhage.[27] PAF also may play a role in reproduction, because large quantities of PAF appear in human amniotic fluid during labor, and the myometrium contracts in response to similar high levels of PAF. Furthermore, evidence has been raised in support of PAF involvement in the process of nidation and implantation. The potential pulmonary origin of PAF present in amniotic fluid suggests a role for PAF in lung surfactant biosynthesis.

While numerous pharmacologic studies clearly support a role for PAF in tissue injury, information on PAF production in pathophysiologic states is sparse. Most notable are studies indicating PAF accumulation in various organs as well as in blood during endotoxic shock. Likewise, excessive PAF production was reported in rectal mucosa specimens taken from patients suffering from ulcerative colitis. However, at the present time, methodologic difficulties in PAF assay in biologic fluids call for caution in interpretation of plasma or tissue levels of PAF.

PAF receptors recently have been cloned, and their structure and function have been elucidated significantly. PAF receptors belong to the type with 7-transmembrane spanning regions that are linked to G-proteins. Activation of PAF receptors leads to elevation of $[Ca^{2+}]_i$ and IP_3, and, in some cells, activation of protein kinases and phospholipases.

Pharmacology

Potent and selective PAF-antagonists have provided more definite information on the role PAF may play in disease situations. For example, PAF antagonists prevent circulatory shock and mortality in several models of endotoxemia.[28] In animal models, PAF-antagonists also were shown to prevent such pathologic consequences of brain ischemia as edema, cerebral hypoperfusion, and neurologic deficits.[r20] PAF-antagonists also ameliorate allergic reactions and inflammatory processes.[r19]

Taken together, a plethora of evidence has accumulated to support an important role for PAF in a large range of disease processes. It is also apparent that the pathologic states that lead to PAF production are complex and involve multiple mediators that act in parallel or concert with PAF to initiate or propagate the pathologic process. Asthma is a perfect example, where PAF can reproduce some of the cardinal features of the disease—yet little can be achieved in animal models by treatment with PAF antagonists. While it is possible that the human disease may not be reflected in animal models, one should always keep in mind the multifactorial nature of chronic inflammatory disorders or acute tissue injury where blockade of one mediator may not be sufficient to modify the disease state.

Angiotensin

Chemistry

Angiotensin II, an octapeptide hormone, is a potent vasoconstrictor hormone of great importance in regulation of the cardiovascular system. The initiating mechanism for increasing circulating angiotensin II levels is found in the juxtaglomerular cells of the kidney, which secrete an aspartyl-protease enzyme, renin, into the blood in response to decreases in arterial blood pressure, a renal perfusion pressure, and plasma sodium, or to increased sympathetic nervous activity. Renin acts on angiotensinogen, a circulating α_2-globulin, that serves as a precursor for the decapeptide angiotensin I (Fig. 9.3). Angiotensinogen is continuously synthesized and released by the liver in such excess that this step is not a rate-limiting factor for angiotensin II production. A second enzyme present in the plasma and on endothelial cells throughout the cardiovascular system, angiotensin converting enzyme, rapidly converts angiotensin I to angiotensin II by proteolytic cleavage of the two terminal amino acids. Subsequently, angiotensin II is converted to the heptapeptide angiotensin III by aminopeptidase. In general, the order of the biologic activity is: angiotensin II ≥ angiotensin III >>> angiotensin I.

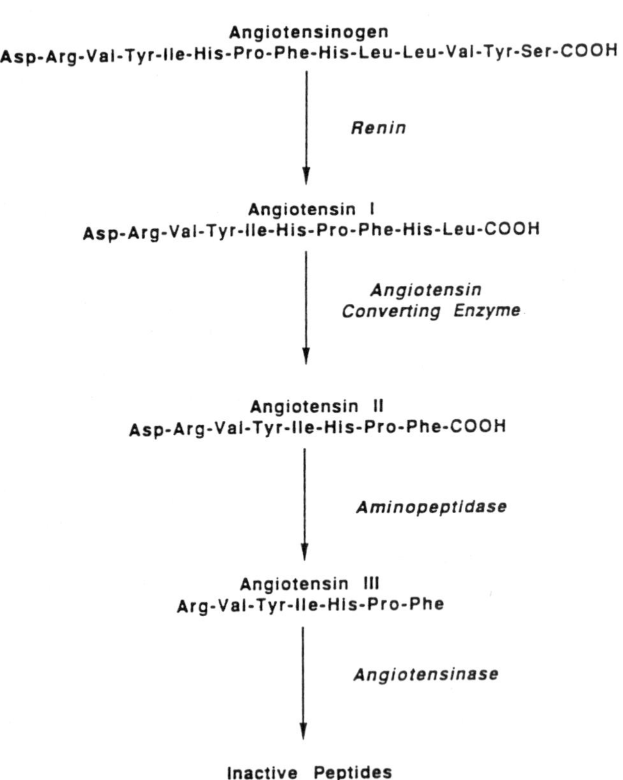

Figure 9.3 Synthesis and metabolism of angiotensin II. Angiotensin II is formed following sequential enzymatic cleavage of the precursor octapeptide, angiotensinogen.

Biology

The major biologic effects of angiotensin II are vasoconstriction, positive inotropic effects on the myocardium, vascular smooth muscle proliferation, stimulation of aldosterone release from the adrenal cortex, and stimulation of thirst. The predominant site of the vasoconstrictor effect of angiotensin II is on the arterioles; however, venoconstriction by angiotensin II has also been reported. In addition, angiotensin II promotes electrolyte and fluid resorption by the kidney, which results in a further decrease in electrolyte and fluid excretion by the kidney, and hence increased blood volume and elevated arterial pressure. Angiotensinogen and angiotensin I have limited pharmacologic activities, whereas angiotensin III maintains most of angiotensin II activities but is somewhat weaker than angiotensin II.[r21,r22]

The diverse responses to angiotensin II are mediated by angiotensin (AT) receptors coupled through G-proteins to effectors including phospholipase C and adenylyl cyclase. Most of the known actions of angiotensin II are mediated by stimulation of phosphoinositide hydrolysis and Ca^{+2} mobilization via a pertussis toxin-insensitive G-protein, which most likely is the Gq subtype. In some tissues, angiotensin II also inhibits adenylyl cyclase via a pertussis toxin-sensitive (Gi) protein, an action of unknown functional significance. Two binding sites for angiotensin receptors have been identified pharmacologically. The AT_1-receptors have high affinity to DuP53 (losartan) and SK&F 108566. The AT_2-binding site has high affinity to selective peptides (CGP42112A) and nonpeptide (PD123177) antagonists. Recently, the AT_1-receptor was cloned[29,r23] and proved to possess the seven transmembrane domain structure typical of G-protein-coupled receptors. Unlike the AT_1 receptor, the AT_2 receptor does not appear to be coupled to G-protein, nor is it sensitive to reduction by dithiothreitol as is AT_1. In addition, the AT_1 and AT_2 receptors have markedly different tissue distributions, providing further evidence for the distinct characteristics of these receptor subtypes. AT_1-receptors predominate in the vascular smooth muscle and the zona glomerulosa cells (aldosterone releasing); AT_2 receptors are abundant in the uterus, chromaffin cells, and several fetal tissues.

In addition to its potent vasoconstrictor effects, angiotensin II may potentiate the responses to norepinephrine released from sympathetic nerves by two distinct mechanisms. Angiotensin II may contribute to postjunctional sensitivity to NE in vascular tissue by a direct effect on smooth muscle. Second, angiotensin II may enhance the response to nerve stimulation by increasing the release of NE from nerve endings. Experimental evidence in support of such interaction between angiotensin II and the sympathetic system includes studies showing that depletion of endogenous catecholamines by pretreatment with reserpine or by acute sympathectomy attenuate the pressor responses to angiotensin II,[30] and that angiotensin II[31] increased the response to sympathetic stimulation. Direct evidence that angiotensin II enhances catecholamine release was provided by numerous studies demonstrating that angiotensin II increased overflow of NE following sympathetic nerve stimulation.[30,32] The potentiating effects of angiotensin II on NE release can be blocked with specific angiotensin II receptor antagonists, such as saralasin. Correspondingly, the facilitation of adrenergic neurotransmitter release by angiotensin I is blocked by an angiotensin converting enzyme inhibitor. Therefore, angiotensin II can act in a direct fashion to potentiate NE responses by increasing vascular tone, as well as indirectly, by increasing adrenergic responses by enhancing NE release.[30] The precise mechanism by which angiotensin II facilitates the release of NE during sympathetic nerve stimulation is still unknown.

In addition to the diverse peripheral actions of angiotensin II, this autacoid has significant effects in the brain, in part the result of potential synergy to its peripheral hypertensive, volume-expanding effects. Activation of angiotensin II receptors in the brain (both A_1 and A_2 are present) lead to increase in blood pressure, water intake,[33] stimulation of natriuresis, salt appetite, and secretion of vasopressin and adrenocorticotrophic hormone. These central actions of angiotensin II, except for natriuresis which is opposite to the peripheral action of angiotensin II, may support the overall pressor and volume-expanding actions of peripherally acting angiotensin II.[34] All these central actions of angiotensin II are mediated by the AT_1 receptor, the role of AT_2 receptors is still an enigma.

Pharmacology

Pharmacologic manipulation of angiotensin falls into three broad categories: (1) inhibition of angiotensin converting enzyme (ACE); (2) receptor antagonists; (3) renin inhibitors. The most widely used agents are the ACE inhibitors, such as captopril, enalapril, and lisinopril.[35–37] See chapter 26 for additional discussion of the use of these drugs. It is suspected that bradykinin formation following ACE inhibitors is associated with some complications, such as cough, angioedema, and hypotension.

A second means by which one can manipulate the effects of angiotensin II pharmacologically is through the use of specific receptor antagonists. The most widely studied angiotensin receptor antagonist is saralasin, which is a peptide analogue of angiotensin II with sarcosine in position 1 and alanine in position 8. Saralasin has been demonstrated to be useful for characterizing the role of angiotensin II in hypertension by blocking the effects of exogenously administered angiotensin II, lowering arterial blood pressure in hypertensive rats and to a certain extent in hypertensive patients. However, peptide angiotensin II receptor antagonists have not met with significant clinical success owing to the necessity of IV administration, short half-life, and partial agonist activity.[38,39] There has recently been renewed interest in developing angiotensin II receptor antagonists that theoretically would improve on the shortcomings of the earlier peptide compounds. Recently, research has led to the development of potent and specific nonpeptide angiotensin II receptor antagonists, two of which, losartan and SK&F 108566, are orally active.[40,r24] Losartan has already proved to be efficacious in lowering high blood pressure in hypertensive patients, but many nonpeptide angiotensin II antagonists are expected to become part of the armamentarium of antihypertensive drugs. The key potential advantage of angiotensin II antagonists over ACE inhibitors is their lack of interference with bradykinin metabolism; therefore, they are expected to be free of such side-effects as cough and the rare but potentially life-threatening complication, angioedema.[r25]

Angiotensin formation also can be manipulated by inhibiting the activity of renin.[41] Theoretically, renin inhibitors have greater specificity than the ACE inhibitors because the latter agents also modify bradykinin metabolism. However, better oral bioavailability is needed for this class of compounds to become a competitive therapeutic strategy in chronic hypertension. Further studies will be required to determine whether renin inhibitors offer any advantage over other classes of angiotensin II modifying agents.

While ACE inhibitors such as captopril and enalapril are routinely used to control mild to moderate blood pressure and occasionally severe hypertensive crises,[r25] they have also gained increasing acceptance in the treatment of patients with congestive heart failure. There is also the potential of utility in renal failure, but data are still inconclusive. Both captopril and enalapril are now established therapy in this disease, as they have proved to reduce morbidity and mortality.[41–43] In addition, the proliferative action of angiotensin II in vascular smooth muscle cells calls for trials with angiotensin II inhibitors (both converting enzyme and receptor antagonists) in combating arteriosclerosis and acute and chronic restenosis following such vascular manipulations as angioplasty or coronary by-pass surgery.

Kallikrein-Kinin System

Chemistry

Kinins are peptides formed in plasma or tissues through a cascade of protease actions on kininogens (substrates) (Fig. 9.4). Normally, kinins are found in extremely low ($<10^{-9}$M) concentrations in biologic fluids due to tight inhibitory regulation of natural kallikreins present in inactive form—the prekallikreins. Under special circumstances, such as exposure of blood to artificial surfaces or exposure to activated serine proteases (e.g., trypsin), prekallikreins are converted to kallikreins, which convert readily available substrate, a high molecular weight (HMW) kininogen, to the nonapeptide bradykinin (Fig. 9.4). Bradykinin, a highly potent peptide, has only a short half-life in the circulation owing to rapid conversion into inactive fragments by kininase II and/or kininase I, which are particularly abundant in endothelial cells of the lung and renal capillaries.[r26,r27,44]

Of special interest is the linkage between the activation of the kallikrein-kinin system and the coagulation system; both systems are activated by the same event—artificial surface activation of Hagemen Factor (HF, factor XII) to activated factor XII ($FXII_\alpha$), a serine protease capable of further activation of factor XI to FXI_α, and plasma prekallikrein to kallikrein.[45] Upon initiation, propagation of coagulation-kinin system activation is amplified further by the action of kallikrein on the inactive form of Factor XII to form Factor XII_α; thereby, amplification and acceleration of the cycle are set in motion. Additional support for a close association of coagulation and kinin formation is maintained by the permissive action of the circulating HMW-kininogen on Factor XIIα, activation of Factor XI, and plasma prekallikrein. However, the two systems are subject to different regulatory mechanisms that may allow continuous bradykinin generation while confining coagulation.[45]

Biology

Bradykinin has diverse biologic actions, including both relaxation and contraction of smooth muscles. Systemic administration of bradykinin consistently results in hypotension, believed to be the result of endothelium-dependent vasodilation.[44] However, capillary and venular endothelium as well as bronchial, GI, and urinary smooth muscle (bladder) contract in response to bradykinin. Unique to bradykinin is its unusual action on sensory nerve endings, which results in complex hemodynamic and neuroendocrine responses, such as vasopressin release. In addition to its sympathetic and parasympathetic effects, bradykinin stimulates sensory nerves to elicit algesia, an effect partly mediated through activation of phospholipase A_2, release of arachidonic acid, and production of prostaglandins of the E series. In addition, bradykinin has been shown to stimulate the production and release of several other endogenous autacoids, such as histamine and serotonin.

Bradykinin exerts its biologic actions by stimulating two types of receptors, termed B_1 and B_2. Interestingly, B_1 receptors are induced in situations of tissue injury such as inflammation or endotoxemia, but the role of B_1 receptors in mediating pathophysiologic reac-

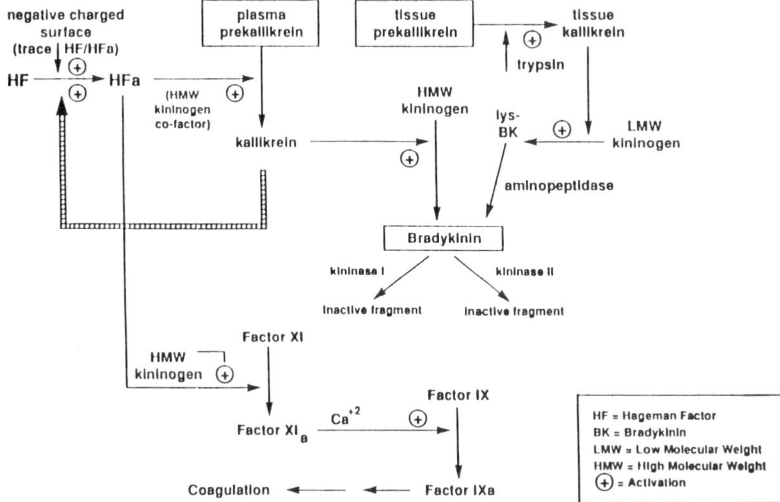

Figure 9.4 Co-activation of the kallikrein/kinin and the coagulation system. HF: Hageman factor; LMW: low molecular weight; HMW: high molecular weight; (+): activation; a: activated form of the zymogen; lys: lysine.

tions such as inflammation is still unknown. The primary receptor associated with the pathologic effects of bradykinin is the B_2 subtype, which elicits endothelial cell-derived relaxing factor(s) (EDRF)-mediated vasodilation, hypotension, microvascular permeability, and sensory nerve stimulation. A common metabolic response to activation of B_2 receptors in various organs is the release of arachidonic acid, which ultimately results in prostaglandin and prostacyclin production. The relationship of bradykinin to the eicosanoid cascade is believed to be of primary importance in such organs as the kidney, where bradykinin-induced renal blood flow redistribution is mediated by prostaglandins.[46] The kidney is an organ where all the components of kinin production and metabolism exist, with the distal nephron believed to be the primary source of urinary kinins. The renal kallikrein-kinin system has been associated with water and electrolyte metabolism in the distal nephron, yet the evidence in favor of such a physiologic role is incomplete. Furthermore, since the vasodilator and renal activities of bradykinin have been appreciated, efforts have been made to suggest a role for low kallikrein-kinin tone as a cause for hypertension.[r28] However, such evidence is only circumstantial, and indirect evidence is based on reduced kallikrein-kinin activity in experimental and clinical hypertension.

In summary, the kallikrein-kinin system is a carefully regulated system of yet unproved physiologic significance. Its activation is tightly coupled to systems involved in hemostasis and inflammation. Although specific analogues of agonistic and antagonistic activity have helped to discern subtypes of bradykinin receptors, such analogues have not yet been used therapeutically.

Histamine

Chemistry

Histamine is found in almost all tissues of the body. Its source is the amino acid histidine, which is acted upon by L-histidine decarboxylase to form histamine directly (Fig. 9.5). The predominant sources of histamine in the body are mast cells and to some degree the circulating blood basophils, in which histamine is stored in secretory granules. Histamine is released in response to many different chemical or physical stimuli. The most important stimulus for histamine release appears to be antigen bridging of IgE antibodies fixed on the cell surface membrane. However, other substances such as adenosine triphosphate, substance P, and complement by-products also induce mast cells to release histamine.[r29] Subsequent to mast cell activation by such stimuli, intracellular calcium increases consequent to influx of calcium into the cell and, ultimately, to the release of secretory granules containing histamine.

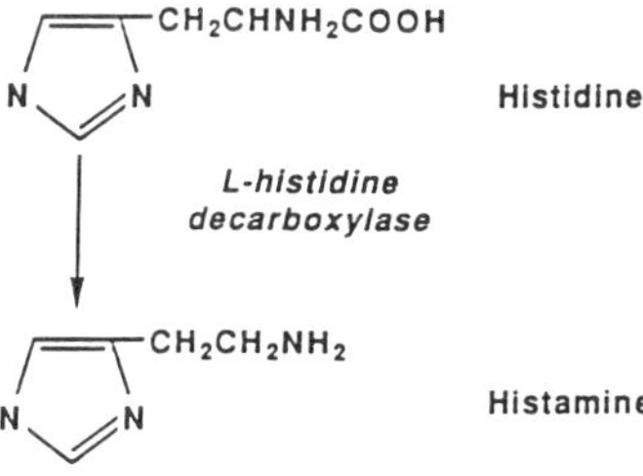

Figure 9.5 Formation of histamine occurs via transformation of the amino acid histidine, by the enzyme histidine decarboxylase.

Biology

Histamine is a potent vasodilator of arterioles; it also increases microvascular permeability. This latter effect allows leakage of plasma into the extravascular space, resulting in edema. Intradermal injection of histamine produces a classic reaction known as the "triple response".[r30] The triple response consists of an immediately developing red spot around the injection site due to microvascular dilation, a larger reddened area due to an axon-mediated vasodilatory reflex response, and finally the appearance of a wheal due to increased capillary permeability. Histamine phosphate (0.1 or 1.0 mg/ml base) is available for evaluating allergenic responses.

The role of histamine in the physiologic regulation of the cardiovascular system is unknown. In many pathologic conditions, arteriolar vasodilation and increased microvascular permeability result in a considerable loss of plasma to the extravascular space, leading to edema. Along with other substances, including the leukotrienes, histamine may contribute to anaphylactic shock. Anaphylaxis is a condition in which cardiac output and arterial blood pressure are severely compromised. It results primarily from an antigen-antibody reaction that occurs in a sensitized individual following the introduction of antigen into circulatory system. Darius et al.[48] have shown that the anaphylactic response in guinea pigs is the result of a complex interaction between platelet activating factor, leukotrienes, and histamine.

Pharmacology

Histamine acts on two types, of specific receptors designated as H_1 and H_2. Activation of the H_1 receptors produces bronchoconstriction, contraction of GI smooth muscle, and increased microvascular permeability. H_1 receptor responses can be blocked by specific receptor antagonists such as pyrilamine, diphenhydramine, and chlorpheniramine. Various types of antihistamines with H_1 antagonist properties are listed in Table 9.1. Such compounds are widely used in allergic reactions such as "hay fever" rhinitis. The presence of another histamine receptor subtype was suspected by the observation that H_1 blockers antagonized histamine-induced contractions of the guinea pig ileum, but were without effect on histamine-induced increases in gastric acid secretion. H_2 receptors increased gastric acid secretion), which is specifically blocked by H_2 receptor antagonists, such as burimamide, cimetidine, and ranitidine.[49,50] These H_2-antagonist drugs are discussed in Chapter 67. The hypotensive effect of histamine is mediated by both the H_1 and H_2 receptors, and is blocked only with a combination of H_1 and H_2 receptor antagonists. In smaller animal species, notably the rat and rabbit, histamine produces a vasoconstrictor response. In humans, histamine infusion produces flushing, headache, and hypotension.[51]

In the periphery, histamine has been reported to decrease the amount of NE released in response to sympathetic nerve stimulation. In the isolated dog saphenous vein, histamine decreased the release of labeled NE, as well as the contractile response to nerve stimulation. The regulation of NE release by prejunctional histaminergic receptors appears to be by activation of H_2-receptor, since the response is blocked by H_2-receptor antagonists.

Histamine does not cross the blood-brain barrier to any significant effect; therefore, CNS responses are generally not elicited following IV administration of histamine. Direct administration of histamine into the cerebral ventricles has been reported to elevate blood pressure, increase heart rate, elicit an emetic response, and alter body temperature. These central effects appear to be mediated by both H_1 and H_2 receptors, and suggest the existence of histaminergic involvement in brain regulation of these functions. Central effects consist of sedation and even hypnosis in patients using therapeutic doses of H_1-receptor antagonists that cross the blood-brain barrier. The mechanisms mediating the sedative effects of H_1-receptor blockers are unknown. There is no obvious correlation between the potency of H_1 blockers to antagonize histamine responses in the periphery and their tendency to produce sedation.[52]

Histamine does not appear to have a role as a major mediator in any significant cardiovascular disorders other than anaphylactic shock. Thus, there is no convincing evidence that histamine is involved in hypertension, myocardial infarction, stroke, or various forms of circulatory shock, such as hemorrhagic or septic shock. In anaphylactic shock, the precise role of histamine is not well-defined because of the involvement of other mediators, such as platelet activating factor and leukotrienes. It is thought that histamine-induced arteriolar vasodilation and increase in microvascular permeability contribute to decreased venous return and ultimately reduction in cardiac output during anaphylactic shock. Treatment of anaphylaxis is generally most successful if therapy can be initiated prior to onset of the anaphylactic reaction. Treatment generally includes synthetic glucocorticoids, such as dexamethasone, to prevent histamine release, or epinephrine, which functionally antagonizes histamine responses at the bronchopulmonary and cardiovascular systems. Histamine receptor antagonists (H_1) are utilized as adjunctive therapy.

Adenosine and Purine Nucleotides

Chemistry

The purine nucleotides and nucleosides are intercellular messengers. Adenosine is a metabolic product constantly produced in

Table 9.1 Histamine-1 Receptor Antagonists

Drug	Route	Dosage Form†	Dose	Duration of Response
Azatadine				
Optimine	oral	1 mg tablet	1–2 mg b.i.d.	12 hr
Brompheniramine	oral	2–5 mg/ml liquid	4–8 mg t.i.d.	
Dimetane		4–12 mg tablets		4–6 hr
Histaject	parenteral	10 mg/ml solution	5–10 mg q 6–12 hr	
Carbinoxamine	oral	4 mg/5 ml syrup	4 mg q.i.d.	6–10 hr
Cardec				
Chlorpheniramine	oral	2 mg/5 ml liquid	4 mg q.i.d.	4–6 hr
Chlortrimeton		2–12 mg tablets; injectable		
Clemastine	oral	0.67 mg/5 ml solution	1.34–2.68 mg	6–12 hr
Tavist		1.34–2.68 mg tablets	b.i.d. or t.i.d.	
Cyproheptadine	oral	2 mg/5 ml solution	4 mg t.i.d.	6–9 hr
Periactin		4 mg tablets		
Diphenhydramine	oral	12.5 mg/5 mt liquid	25–50 mg t.i.d.	4–6 hr
Benadryl		25–50 mg tablets		
Doxylamine	oral	25 mg tablet	25 mg at bedtime	4–6 hr
Unisom				
Methdilazine	oral	4 mg/5 ml liquid	8 mg b.i.d.-q.i.d.	6–12 hr
Tacaryl		8 mg tablet		
Promethazine	oral	6.25–25 mg/ml liquid	25 mg at bedtime or	4–12 hr
Phenergan		12.5–50 mg tablets	t.i.d. as required	
	parenteral	25–50 mg/ml solution	25–50 mg; i.m.	
Terfenadine	oral	60 mg tablet	60 mg b.i.d.	12 hr
Seldane				
Trimeprazine	oral	2.5 mg/5 ml liquid	2.5 mg q.i.d.	4–6 hr
Temaril		2.5–5 mg tablets		
Tripelenamine	oral	25 mg/5 ml liquid	25–50 mg q 4–6 hr	4–6 hr
PBZ		25–100 mg tablets		
Triprolidine	oral	1.25 mg/5 ml liquid	2.5 mg q 4–6 hr	4–6 hr
Actidi		2.5 mg tablets		

†Some of the drugs are available in over-the-counter preparations with and without multiple drugs.

every cell as part of the energy "supply and demand" situation. Intracellular 5′-nucleotidase dephosphorylates adenosine monophosphate (AMP) to yield adenosine, which is transported out of the cell by the symmetric nucleoside transporter (Fig. 9.6). Thus, in situations where depletion of the cell from energy sources such as ATP takes place (e.g., ischemia), accumulation of adenosine in the tissue is instantaneous. However, adenosine is also formed extracellularly from ATP released into the extracellular space during exocytotic processes, such as the extrusion of catecholamine storage vesicles containing ATP. The relative importance of these two pathways in vivo in adenosine metabolism is still unclear.

The primary pathways of adenosine metabolism are: (1) enzymatic phosphorylation to AMP by adenosine kinase; (2) conversion to inosine by the enzyme adenosine deaminase; and (3) rapid uptake into red blood cells and endothelium. Selective inhibitors of these enzymes are available: 5-iodolubericin for the kinase and erythrononyladenine for the adenosine deaminase. Inhibition of adenosine transport can be achieved by drugs such as dipyridamole, and together with 5′-nucleotidase inhibitors (α, β-methylene analogues of ADP), it was possible to demonstrate that intracellular originated ADP, and not extracellular hydrolysis of ATP released from cells, is the primary source of adenosine found in tissues.

Biology

The biologic actions of adenosine are well documented and extensively reviewed.[r31,r32] Most notably, adenosine produces bradycardia in many species, along with hypotension and coronary vasodilation (See Table 9.2). In general, the purines have a potent peripheral vasodilator effect in all vascular beds except the kidney, where they produce vasoconstriction. The mo-

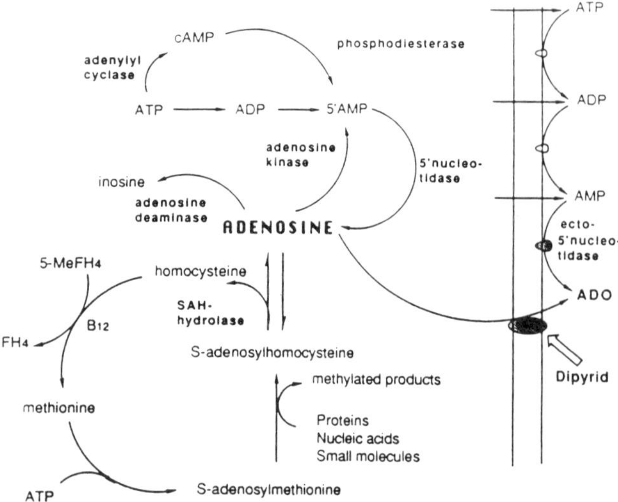

Figure 9.6 Synthesis and metabolism of adenosine. The figure demonstrates that adenosine exists intracellularly mainly in its phosphorylated forms at concentration below 1 μM. Most of basal adenosine production produced is derived from action of 5-adenosylhomocysteine transferase (SAH) which under circumstances of enhanced oxygen demand or reduced supply increased amounts of adenosine are formed by the action of 5′-nucleotidase. Adenosine then passes the cell membrane by facilitated diffusion and in the extracellular space is mainly inactivated via the nucleotide carrier sensitive to dipyridamole (Dipyrid). Subsequent deamination and phosphorylation at intra and extracellular sites keep adenosine (ADO) levels very low.

lecular mechanisms involved in the cellular actions of adenosine are still controversial. However, in in vitro cardiac preparations, adenosine was shown to shorten the atrial action potential duration and membrane hyperpolarization by activation of K^+ conductance. Such observation is supported by less direct studies in humans, which also emphasized the lack of adenosine effect on the ventricular system.[53] The regional electrophysiologic effects of adenosine and its antiarrhythmic properties are of major clinical interest for diagnosis and treatment of cardiac arrhythmias, where the atrioventricular node is involved. The generalized vasodilation achieved by continuous infusions of adenosine, in conjunction with its antiplatelet aggregation effect, led to therapeutic trials with adenosine infusion in hope of reducing pulmonary hypertension, and achieving improved cardiovascular outcome following cardiopulmonary bypass and controlled hypotension during neurosurgical procedures.[54]

Adenosine acts on two classes of receptors, A_1 and A_2, which are subclasses of the purinergic P_1 receptors. These receptors were recently cloned (see Chapter 12). There are two subclasses of A_{2x}—A_{2a} and A_{2b} receptors. The adenosine receptors are classified based on the actions of adenosine and adenosine analogues on adenylyl cyclase and recent cloning of these receptors. The A_1 subtype denotes those adenosine receptors that block the activity of adenylyl cyclase. Stimulation of the A_2 subtype activates this latter enzyme. However, this classification in many organs is unsatisfactory, owing to the difficulties in adequately correlating the functional and biochemical events associated with the actions of adenosine.

Both A_1 and A_2 receptors are widely distributed in peripheral organs and in the CNS. Therefore, agonists to any of the adenosine receptors could be expected to elicit multiple and diverse actions. For example, a long-acting A_1 receptor agonist would be of value in cardiac arrhythmias, yet could potentially compromise renal function owing to A_1 receptors' mediating reduction in glomerular filtration rate. On the other hand, a selective A_2 receptor agonist could provide vasodilation in the pulmonary and cardiac circulation, yet the strong sedative effect mediated by A_2 adenosine receptors in the CNS might confound the hemodynamic goals.

A_1 receptors have recently attracted attention for their role in modulation of excitatory amino acid (glutamate, aspartate) release during brain ischemia. Since adenosine action on A_1-receptors reduces release of glutamate, agonists for this receptor subtype may be of benefit in treating stroke, neurodegenerative disorders, or epileptic disorders, which were associated with uncontrolled release of such excitotoxic neurotransmitters as glutamate.[55] The case for adenosine's role in neuroprotection has been studied extensively, and several lines of evidence suggest a neuroprotective role for adenosine in ischemic brain damage. Adenosine as well as several adenosine agonist analogues (e.g., cyclohexyladenosine, 2-chloro-adenosine) have been reported to improve neuronal survival and functional outcome in animal models of stroke, whereas most studies utilizing adenosine antagonists (e.g., caffeine, dipropylcyclopeniaxanthine, theophylline) in such models resulted in exacerbated brain damage. Furthermore, modulation of adenosine metabolism by inhibiting adenosine transport with drugs such as nitrobenzylthioinosine or hydroxynitro-benzylthioguanosine, propentofylline, or inhibitional adenosine deaminase (pentostatin), also reduced brain damage in animal models of focal or global ischemia.[56]

Adenine nucleotides such as ATP or ADP also possess broad pharmacologic actions, including relaxation or contraction of many smooth muscles. ATP, acting via P_2 (purinergic) receptors (distinguished from adenosine-activated receptors) is believed to act as a nonadrenergic, noncholinergic transmitter in the autonomic nervous system.[57] ATP contracts smooth muscle in organs such as the urinary bladder or portal vein,

Table 9.2 Drugs Acting on Adenosine Receptors

Agonists	Route	Dosage Form	Dose	Onset
Adenosine				
Adenocard	parenteral	6 mg/2 ml	6 mg i.v.	immediate
Adenosine Phosphate	parenteral	25 mg/ml	25 mg i.m., b.i.d.	rapid

but relaxes smooth muscle of the aorta or taenia coli muscles. In blood vessels, ATP as a rule will cause relaxation by releasing the endothelium-derived relaxing factor (EDRF) and prostacyclin, while in exposed vascular smooth, muscle ATP elicits contractions.[r33] However, one should also keep in mind that in vivo released ATP and ADP will be rapidly dephosphorylated by ectonucleotidases present on the surface of the cell to yield adenosine, which is a general vasorelaxing agent.

In conclusion, the purine nucleoside adenosine and the related nucleotides ATP and ADP are ubiquitous and act through multiple subtypes of receptors present in virtually every organ and tissue. They are part of the fundamental energy metabolism of every cell, yet they appear to serve also as neurotransmitters/modulators and physiologic regulators in normal and pathologic states. Better understanding of the structure activity relationships of the purine receptor subtypes and the emergence of selective analogues of adenosine and ATP provide hope for developing tools for manipulation of subtype-specific purinergic receptors for clarifying the cellular functions associated with the purine nucleoside and adenosine receptors.

5-Hydroxytryptamine (Serotonin)

Chemistry

The chemical nature of 5-hydroxytryptamine (5-HT), a 3-(β-aminoethyl)-5-hydroxyindole, was elucidated in 1948. Its presence in serum, the "vasoconstrictor material of blood allowed to clot" (hence the name, serotonin), or histochemical evidence obtained from enterochromaffin cells of the GI mucosa (hence the name enteramine) had been known two decades earlier).

5-HT is a highly ubiquitous natural product found in plants, invertebrates, and vertebrates. In humans, 5-HT is found in many organs as well as blood, lymph, and CSF. While some 5-HT found in the diet is absorbed, it contributes virtually nothing to tissue levels (except platelets, where it is taken up from the circulation) owing to metabolism in the lungs and liver. 5-HT is synthesized de novo from the essential amino acid tryptophan, which is taken up into the cell and converted first to 5-hydroxytryptophan by the relatively selective and rate-limiting enzyme, tryptophan 5-hydroxylase. Conversion of 5-hydroxytryptophan to 5-HT is completed by the nonspecific L-aromatic amino acid decarboxylase (an enzyme also involved in catecholamine synthesis from L-DOPA). 5-HT is protected from further metabolism by uptake into storage granules, where it is bound to ATP. 5-HT is released by mechanisms common to neurotransmitters and hormones, i.e., receptor-mediated and Ca^{+2}-dependent release of the 5-HT storage granules.

Biology

The most studied functions of 5-HT in mammals, including humans, are those related to the CNS, where it is believed to act as a neurotransmitter. The serotoninergic neurons are clustered in a few discrete sites, in brain, with the Raphé nuclei in the mesenephalon a primary location for such serotonin-containing cells. These 5-HT neurons are involved in pain perception, behavior, and regulation of such autonomic functions as temperature, blood pressure, and respiration. An important function of the brain 5-HT system is in regulation of neuroendocrine functions such as ACTH, growth hormone, prolactin, and TSH release. However, the largest pool of 5-HT in the body is in the GI tract, where 5-HT is found in enterochromaffin cells. While the physiologic role of the 5-HT system in the gut is largely unknown, tumors arising from enterochromaffin cells (carcinoid tumors release large quantities of 5-HT) produce marked stimulation of the intestinal smooth muscle, leading to severe diarrhea and abdominal pain.

Pharmacology

The pharmacologic actions of 5-HT are extremely broad and have been studied in virtually every organ and tissue. In all cells, the actions of 5-HT are mediated by specific, high-affinity receptors. The 5-HT receptors are classified as 5-HT_1, 5-HT_2, and 5-HT_3, and, recently, evidence for 5-HT_4 receptors has been raised. 5-HT_2 and 5-HT_3 receptors are defined by selective antagonists; 5-HT_1 is defined by selective agonists and nonselective antagonists.[81] The 5-HT_1 binding sites have been further classified into four distinct subtypes, 5-HT_{1A}, 5-HT_{1B}, 5-HT_{1C}, and 5-HT_{1D}; and other binding sites are probably yet to be found.[85] The molecular biology of several 5-HT receptors has been elucidated (e.g., 5-HT_2, 5-HT_{1C}, 5-HT_{1A}), which indicate that they are part of the G-protein receptor superfamily and the family of ligand gated ion channels (5-HT_3) See chapter 12 for other details about serotonin receptors.[r34]

The functional dimensions of the 5-HT receptor

classification have been reviewed[59] and can be briefly summarized as follows: 5-HT_1 receptors mediate inhibition of neurotransmitter release, contraction or relaxation of smooth muscle, and release of EDRF. In the CNS, 5-HT_1 receptors mediate autonomic functions such as hypothermia, hyperphagia, analgesia, and diverse behavioral paradigms. The compound 5-carboxamidotryptamine is an agonist at the 5-HT_1 receptor; no highly selective antagonists are available for this receptor, but methiothepin and methysergide have significant affinity for 5-HT_1 receptors. Recently, a 5-HT_{1D} receptor agonist, sumatripan, has been developed for treatment of migraine, since 5-HT_{1D} receptors on cerebral blood vessels mediate vasoconstriction and, thereby, relieve the headache believed to result from profound vasodilation of cerebral blood vessels. Sumatripan is already a marketed antimigraine drug. Interestingly, 5-HT_{1D} agonists might act as antimigranotic agents via presynaptic inhibition of inflammatory mediated releases that elicit pain and vasomotion in the cerebral vessels[84] (see Chapter 27).

5-HT_2 receptors mediate primarily smooth muscle contraction, platelet-aggregation, and increased capillary permeability; in the CNS, they elicit aberrant behavioral responses, excitation, and neuroendocrine effects. The pharmacologic agents ketaserin and cyproheptadine are antagonists of the 5-HT_2 receptor, yet some overlap with other receptors has been noted. 5-HT_2 receptor antagonists have a limited use clinically to treat hypertension. Ketanserin is a prototype of these drugs, although part of its antihypertensive action involves blockade of α_1-adrenoceptors. Ritanserin is a more selective 5-HT_2 blocker; both drugs may enhance their vascular effect by counteracting platelet aggregation and 5-HT-induced amplification of catecholamine release. A potential therapeutic avenue for development of antihypertensive drugs is 5-HT_{1A} agonist activation of central 5-HT_{1A} receptors, since flesinoxan and 8-OH-DPAT lower blood pressure and heart rate.

The 5-HT_3 receptor mediates excitation of peripheral nerves (both afferent and efferent), gastric motility, emesis, and anxiogenic effects that may be associated with dopamine release. Selective antagonists of the 5-HT_3 receptor include MDL 72222, ondansetron, and ICS 205-930; 2 methyl-5-HT is an agonist of this receptor. 5-HT_3 receptor antagonists might be useful in migraine since the neurogenic pathway for migraine initiation might include 5-HT_3-receptor mediated axon reflex in the cranial vasculature, resulting in vasodilation.[r35] These potential avenues for new therapeutics based on selective 5-HT_3 receptor agonists/antagonists remain to be investigated.

While efforts to elucidate the diverse biologic actions mediated by 5-HT receptor subtypes is actively pursued for new therapeutic indications, other strategies have yielded highly efficacious drugs. Since increased levels of 5-HT in the brain have been associated with mood elevation, a strategy based on inhibition of endogenous 5-HT elimination via inhibition of 5-HT reuptake into tryptaminergic neurons, has yielded efficacious antidepressant drugs, such as fluoxetine and paroxetine (see Chapter 17). These 5-HT transport inhibitors have become the first line treatment for a variety of depressive illnesses in many countries; however, a side-effect, shared by the conventional tricyclic antidepressant, conversions to manic excitements, must still be closely monitored.

In summary, while 5-HT is one of the oldest autacoids known to pharmacologists, it is still one of the most actively investigated. The elucidation of the multiplicity of the receptors, their transduction mechanisms, and their regulation will, no doubt, result in yet more novel therapeutic agents.

Endothelium Dependent Relaxing Factor (EDRF)

The ability of acetylcholine to produce marked vasodilation in various vascular beds in vivo has been known for many years. Following early demonstrations in animals, numerous laboratories have shown that acetylcholine and other muscarinic agonists produce relaxation of isolated blood vessels precontracted by sympathetic nerve stimulation.[60,61] These phenomena were originally attributed to inhibition by the cholinergic agonists of preconjunctional sympathetic nerve and, hence, reduction in the adrenergic constrictor neurotransmitter.[62] These historical milestones, however, were not uniformly admired by all vascular experimentalists because, acetylcholine-induced contraction of helical aortic strips were frequently reported. It was only when Furchgott's laboratory replaced the spiral aortic strip, the traditional vascular preparation, with the more economical and easier to prepare aortic ring preparation that acetylcholine was found to relax this aortic preparation consistently. However, only systematic search to resolve the enigmatic difference between the spiral vs. ring aortic responses to acetylcholine led to the first recognition of the role of the endothelial cells in vascular tone regulation. In short, the spiral aortic preparation was shown to have severely impaired or absent endothelium (and, hence, responded with contraction), while the more preserved aortic ring, which carried an intact endothelial layer, showed relaxation. Removal of the endothelial layer from the ring preparation converted the relaxation back to constriction, whereas more careful handling of the spiral preparations, which preserved the endothelial layer, resulted in a preparation that, if precontracted by norepinephrine, showed complete relaxation to acetylcholine.[63] The obligatory role of endothelial cells in acetylcholine-induced relaxation was rapidly demonstrated, not only for the rabbit aortic preparation but for all other arteries in many animals (dog, cat, rat, guinea pig) and humans. It was also found that removal of the endothelial cells did not alter the sensitivity of such nonmuscarinic relaxing agents as glyceryl trinitrate, sodium azide, adenosine, adenylic acid (AMP), or isoproterenol, nor did endothelial denudation affect the sensitivity of the preparation to contracting agents. Further, endothelial dependent relaxation was rapidly recognized as a phenomenon that applies to many autacoids, including: ATP, ADP, Substance P, Choleystokinin, bradykinin, histamine, serotonin, thrombin, arachidonic acid, vasoactive intestinal peptide (VIP), vasopressin, mellitin, and calcitonin-gene-related peptide (CGRP). Furthermore, nonbiologically vasoactive chemicals like the Ca^{2+}-ionophore, A23187, also elicit endothelium-mediated relaxation of precontracted aortic rings.[r37]

An early hypothesis set to explain the obligatory role of the endothelium in the relaxation induced by various relaxing factors was that the relaxing agent, e.g., acetylcholine, acts on a receptor (muscarinic) on the endothelium to release a factor from the endothelium, which then relaxes the smooth muscle cells. This hypothesis was substantially supported by an elegant procedure called the "sandwich" mount, where aortic strips with or without intact endothelium were mounted in close proximity and in an orientation that allowed observation of the relaxation of the muscle strip (without endothelium), only when in close contact to an endothelium-intact, acetylcholine-stimulated strip.[64] Following this demonstration, many procedures were established to confirm that an endothelium-derived relaxing factor is produced and released in response to many known relaxing factors. Most popular procedures include the cascade perfusion and superfusion procedures.[65,r38]

The nature of the EDRF has been the subject of an intensive research effort in numerous laboratories. It was easy to demonstrate that EDRF was not cAMP, cGMP, adenosine, AMP, prostacyclin (PGI_2) or other eicosanoids. It was also clear from the very early stages that EDRF release can be blocked by such conditions as anoxia or by radical scavengers, and this led to the belief that EDRF might be a free radical. Parallel to this information, vascular researchers associated certain smooth muscle relaxants to an increase in cGMP.[r39] Likewise, it was observed that some EDRF producing agents (e.g., arachidonate hydroyperoxides) markedly stimulated guanylate cyclase.[66] Finally, it was noted that nitric oxide was a potent relaxing factor, acting via guanylate cyclase activation.[r39] It had been proposed that nitrovasodilators (e.g.) sodium nitroprusside, organic nitrates, azide, and inorganic nitrates) activate guanylate cyclase indirectly via nitric oxide released by chemical reaction.[r39] Thus, prior to the identification of nitric oxide as the primary EDRF, evidence pointed to the possibility that EDRF, like the nitrovasodilators, stimulates guanylate cyclase in smooth muscle cells. However, more definitive evidence on the nature of EDRF was obtained by Palmer et al.,[70] who identified nitric oxide (NO) as EDRF.

Biochemistry

The biosynthesis of EDRF/NO (Fig. 9.7) involves tetrahydrobiopterin, FAD, FMN, molecular oxygen (O_2), and the intermediary of N-OH-L-arginine.[r40] This general scheme applies to all cells studied so far, including endothelium, neurons, and macrophages. Several forms of nitric oxide synthase (NOS) already have been characterized biochemically and by molecular biology techniques; the NOS isozymes display cellular and biochemical diversities,[r40] are probably derived from three different NOS genes[71–76] of which at least one exhibits alternative splicing of the transcripts. The information now available classifies NOS as: (a) those dependent on exogenous Ca^{2+} and calmodulin (cNOS); (b) those independent of exogenous Ca^{2+} and calmodulin (iNOS). The cNOSs appear to be constitutive; iNOSs are inducible.

Biology

The biologic targets of NO are multiple and diverse. The cardinal mechanism of NO actions is believed to be activation of guanylate cyclase (Fig. 9.8), which, in smooth muscle cells, is associated with relaxation. However, NO can also activate an ADP-ribosyltransferase and interact with nerve proteins, such as hemoglobin and myoglobin. This latter effect is the basis of the old practice of using nitrates to cure meat. A prominent clinical use of macrophage-derived NO is its action on tumor cell DNA via inhibition of the rate-limiting enzyme, ribonucleotide reductase.[77] Another important target for NO is the oxygen radical O_2- (superoxide). Both of these oxygen reactive molecules interact in ways that depend on the chemical conditions. NO interaction with O_2- may lead to detoxification of either molecule or to generation to an extremely potent oxidant—peroxynitrite.[78] Furthermore, interactions of NO with sulfhydryls may result in S-nitrosothiols, which can serve to prolong the availability of bioactive NO. Also, S-nitrosylation can enhance catalytic function of some enzymes, such as plasminogen activators.

The biologic significance of NO function is under intense investigation. Since NO is a powerful cerebrovasodilator and is produced by neurons, it has been suggested that NO might be the long sought-for mediator that couples brain activity to cerebral blood flow.[92] This hypothesis is supported by recent data suggesting that NO plays a role in the maintenance of resting cerebral blood flow and in the cerebrovasodilation elicited by increased neural activity induced either by activation of selected neuronal pathways or by NMDA-receptor activation.

Data showing stimulation of NO production by the excitatory amino acid, glutamate, also have led to suggestions that NO may be involved in long-term potentiation,[79] a phenomenon associated with synaptic plasticity and with memory formation. Furthermore, since glutamate may be associated with neuronal death during ischemia/trauma or convulsive disorders, NO was also implicated in the neurotoxicity that follows ischemia. Recent studies support this possibility, demonstrating the salutary effect of NOS inhibitors in a mouse stroke model.[80] However, many more studies must be performed to clarify the issue.

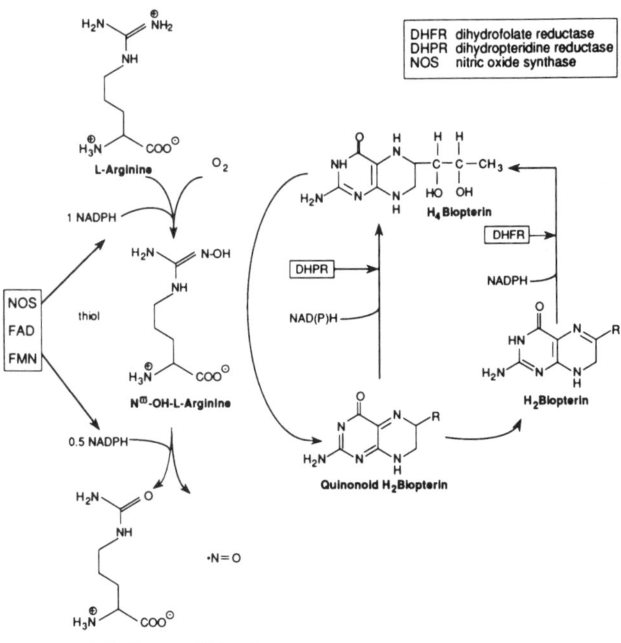

Figure 9.7 Biosynthesis of nitric oxide. A guanidino nitrogen of L-arginine undergoes a five-electron oxidation to yield the gaseous radical nitric oxide (• NO) via an N^{ω}-hydroxyl-L-arginine intermediate. NADPH donates two electrons for the formulation of this intermediate and one electron for its further oxidation. Both steps are catalyzed by the FAD- and FMN-containing enzyme, nitric oxide synthase (NOS). Molecular oxygen is incorporated both into the ureido group of product citrulline and into NO itself (see text). Tetrahydrobiopterin is also required; the amounts needed are substoichiometric with respect to NO generated, provided that tetrahydrobiopterin can be regenerated from its oxidized form, quinonoid dihydrobiopterin. Regeneration of tetrahydrobiopterin proceeds both through methotrexate-sensitive enzyme, dihydrofolate reductase and through the methotrexate-resistant enzyme, dihydropteridine reductase. Oxidative inactivation of NOS in cells lysates is retarded by inclusion of a thiol. Reprinted with permission from reference'40.

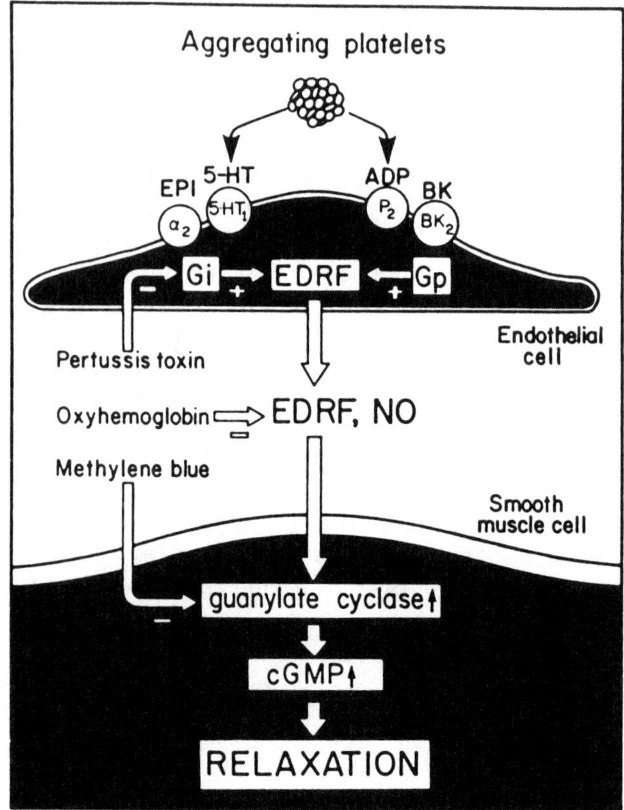

Figure 9.8 A representing scheme of EDRF/NO release and action from the endothelium. Stimuli such as epinephrine (EPI), serotonine (5HT) adenosine-diophosphate (ADP) or bradykinin (BK) act on their respective receptors which are coupled to a G-protein (Gi or Gp). EDRF/NO is released from the endothelium and diffuses into the muscle cell, activates guanylate cyclase, accumulation of cGMP and hence relaxation. The figure also depicts inhibitory actions by oxyhemoglobin (direct scavenging of NO) or methylene blue-and inhibitor of guanylate cyclase. Pertussis toxin is a known inhibitor of the Gi component of the G-protein system.

In addition to a potential role of NO in CNS function, it is also likely that it may act in the peripheral nervous system. cNOS reactive ganglia have been identified, and a NO-like substance is released by stimulation of nonadrenergic, noncholinergic neurons in the GI system.

The cardiovascular system has been most extensively studied for a potential physiologic role for NO. The original work on EDRF associated NO with endothelial and vascular function. Thus, NO was thought to figure in basal blood pressure regulation.[81,82] Further, the ability of NOS inhibitors to block the hypotension induced by cytokines or endotoxins suggested that NO may play a role in endotoxic shock[83] (see also Chapter 24).

In addition, NO has been shown to inhibit platelet

adhesion and aggregation, leukocyte adhesion to endothelium, and the synthesis and release of endothelin (a potent vasoconstrictor) and smooth muscle cell mitogen.[84] Furthermore, NO also directly inhibits smooth muscle cell proliferation.[85] Taken together, NO may be important in protecting blood vessels from inflammatory cell damage and thrombosis. In addition, scavenging NO by plasma lipoproteins and proteins may be associated with the generation of advanced glycosylated end-products (AGE) implicated in diabetic vasoculopathy and atherosclerosis. Impaired NO-mediated vasorelaxation in atherosclerotic vessels may contribute to accelerated thrombosis, spasm and myocardial (or cerebral) infarction.[86–88]

Pharmacology

At this time, no isozyme-selective NOS antagonists are available; therefore, it is still difficult to identify the role of each NOS isozyme in a particular cell or tissue function. The potential pharmacologic utility of NOS inhibitors is widely debated. Therapeutic effects can be achieved by NO delivery, as in ARDS patients,[89] where inhalation of NO may result in improved ventilation/perfusion ratios. NO's role in penile venous flow regulation suggests possible use of NO or NO agonists in some forms of impotence.[90] Also, the potent relaxing effect of NO in the coronary circulation may offer protection against coronary spasm and thrombosis.[91] Inhibitors of NO release may prove useful in cases of excessive production of NO. This latter goal may be difficult to achieve until we can direct such inhibitors to localized, isozyme-specific targets. The current trend of pharmacologic intervention in NO metabolism is based on substrate analogues, which may have beneficial effects in septic shock, cerebral ischemia (stroke), and migraine. A major chemical effort will be devoted to developing potent and isoform-selective NOS inhibitors, because significant toxicity has already been cited for some substrate analogs.

References

Research Reports

1. Kennedy I, Cleman RA, Humphrey PPA, Levy GP and Lumley P. Studies on the characterization of prostanoid receptors: a proposed classification. Prostaglandins 1982;*24*:667–668.
2. Gryglewski RJ, Bunting S, Moncada S, Flower RJ, Vane JR. Arterial walls are protected against deposition of platelet thrombi by a substance (prostaglandin X) which they make from prostaglandin endoperoxides. Prostaglandins 1976;*2*:685–713.
3. Schrör K, Ohlendorf R, Darius H. Beneficial effects of a new carbacyclin derivative, ZK 36374, in acute myocardial ischemia. J Pharmacol Exp Ther 1981;*719*:243–249.
4. Schrör K, Darius H, Addicks K, Koster R, Smith EF III. PGI_2 prevents ischemia-induced alterations in cardiac catecholamines without influencing nerve-stimulation-induced catecholamine release in non-ischemic conditions. J Cardiovasc Pharmacol 1982;*4*:741–749.
5. Needleman P, Minkes MS, Raz A. Thromboxanes: Selective biosynthesis and distinct biological properties. Science 1976;*193*:163–165.
6. Kellaway CH, Trethewie RE. The liberation of a slow reacting smooth muscle stimulating substance of anaphylaxis. Q J Exper Physiol 1940;*30*:121–145.
7. Murphy RC, Hammastrom S, Samuelsson B. Leukotriene C: A slow-reacting substance from murine mastocytoma cells. Proc Natl Acad Sci 1979;*76*:4275–4279.
8. Samuelsson B. Leukotrienes: Mediators of immediate hypersensitivity reactions and inflammation. Science 1983;*220*:568–575.
9. Dixon RAF, Jones RE, Diehl RE, Bennett CD, Kargman S, Rouzer CA. Cloning of the cDNA for human 5-lipoxygenase. Proc Natl Acad Sci USA 1988;*85*:416–420.
10. Rouzer CA, Rands E, Kargman S, Jones RE, Register RB, Dixon RAF. Characterization of cloned human leukocyte 5-lipoxygenase expressed in mammalian cells. J Biol Chem 1988;*263*:10135–101340.
11. Dixon RAF, Diehl RE, Opas E, Rands E, Vickers PJ, Evans JF, Gillard JW, Miller DK. Requirement of a 5-lipoxygenase-activating protein for leukotriene synthesis. Nature 1990;*343*:282–284.
12. Samuelsson B, Dahlén S-E, Lindgren JA, Rouzer CA, Serhan CN. Leukotrienes and lipoxins: Structures, biosynthesis, and biological effects. Science 1987;*237*:1171–1176.
13. Sarau H, Mong S, Foley H, Wu H, Crooke ST. Identification and characterization of leukotriene D_4 receptors and signal transduction processes in rat basophilic leukemia cells. J Biol Chem 1987;*262*:4034–4041.
14. Clark MA, Littlejohn D, Conway TH, Mong S, Steiner S, Crooke ST. Leukotriene D_4 treatment of bovine aortic endothelial cells and murine smooth muscle cells in culture results in an increase in phospholipase A_2 activity. J Biol Chem 1986;*261*:10713–10718.
15. Garland LG, Salmon JA. Hydroxamic acids and hydroxyureas as inhibitors of arachidonate 5-lipoxygenase. Drugs of the Future 1991;*16*:547–558.
16. Busse WW, Gaddy JN. The role of leukotriene antagonists and inhibitors in the treatment of airway disease. Am Rev Resp Dis 1991;*143*:S103–S107.
17. Osborn RR, Hay DWP, Wasserman MA, Torphy TJ. SK&F 104353, a selective leukotriene receptor antagonist inhibits leukotriene D_4- and antigen-induced bronchoconstriction in cynomolgus monkeys. Pulmon Pharm 1992;*5*:153–157.
18. Jones TR, Zamboni R, Belley M, et al. Pharmacology of L-660, 711 (MK-571): A novel potent and selective leukotriene D_4 receptor antagonist. Can J Physiol Pharmacol 1989;*67*:17–28.
19. Yamaguchi T, Kohrogi H, Honda I, et al. A novel leukotriene antagonist, ONO-1078, inhibits and reverses human bronchial contraction induced by leukotrienes C_4 and D_4 and antigen in vitro. Am Rev Respir Dis 1992;*146*:923–929.
20. Spector SL, Glass M, Minkwitz MC, ICI Asthma Trial Group. The effect of six weeks of therapy with oral doses of ICI 204,219 in asthmatics. Am Rev Resp Dis 1992;*145*:A16.
21. Smith EF III, Kinter LB, Jugas M, Wasserman MA, Eckardt RD, Newton JF. Beneficial effects of the peptidoleukotriene receptor

antagonist, SK&F 104353, on the responses to experimental endotoxemia in the conscious rat. Circ Shock 1988;*25*:21–31.

22. Serhan CN, Hamberg M, Samuelsson B. Lipoxins: Novel series of biologically active compounds formed from arachidonic acid in human leukocytes. Proc Natl Acad Sci 1984;*81*:5335–5339.
23. Stahl GL, Tsao P, Lefer AM, Ramphal JY, Nicolaou KC. Pharmacologic profile of lipoxins A5 and B5: new biologically active eicosanoids. Eur J Pharmacol 1989;*163*:55–60.
24. Benveniste J. Platelet activating factors: A new mediator of anaphylaxis from rabbit and human basophils. Nature 1974;*249*:581–584.
25. Snyder F. Biochemistry of platelet-activating factor: A unique class of biologically active phospholipids. Proc Soc Exper Biol Med 1988;*190*:125–135.
26. Siren A-L, Feuerstein G. Effect of platelet-activating factor and its antagonist, BN 52021, on cardiac function and regional blood flow in the conscious rat. Am J Physiol 1989;*257*:H25–H32.
27. Whittle JL, Horishita T, Ohya T, Leung FW, Guth PH. Microvascular actions of platelet-activating factor on rat gastric mucosa and submucosa. Am J Physiol 1986;*251*:G772–G778.
28. Rabinovici R, Yue T-L, Farhat M, Smith E. III, Esser K, Slivjak MJ, Feuerstein GZ. Platelet activing factor (PAF) and tumor necrosis factor-α (TNFα) interactions in endotoxic shock. Studies with BN 50739, a novel PAF antagonist. J Pharmacol Exper Ther 1990;*255*:256–263.
29. Murphy TJ, Alexander RW, Griendling KK, Runge MS, Bernstein KE. Isolation of a cDNA encoding the vascular type-1 angiotensin II receptor. Nature 1991;*351*:233–236.
30. Zimmerman BG. Actions of angiotensin on adrenergic nerve endings. Fed Proc 1978;*37*:199–202.
31. Benelli G, Della Bella D, Gandini A. Angiotensin and peripheral sympathetic nerve activity. Brit J Pharmacol 1964;*22*:211–219.
32. Starke K. Interaction of angiotensin and cocaine on the output of noradrenaline from isolated rabbit hearts. Naunyn-Schmiedeberg's Arch Pharmacol 1970;*265*:383–386.
33. Elfont RM, Fitzsimons JT. Renin dependence of captopril-induced drinking after ureteric ligation in the rat. J Physiol (Lond) 1983;*343*:17–30.
34. Steckelings UM, Pottari SP, Unger T.: Angiotensin receptor subtypes in the brain. TIPS 1992;*13*:365–368.
35. Cushman DW, Cheung HS, Sabo EF, Ondetti MA. Design of potent inhibitors of angiotensin-converting enzyme. Carboxyalkanoyl and mercaptoalkanoyl amino acids. Biochemistry 1977;*16*:5484–5491.
36. Sweet CS. Pharmacological properties of the converting enzyme inhibitor, enalapril maleate (MK-421). Fed Proc 1983;*42*:167–170.
37. Antonaccio MJ, Robin B, Horovitz ZP. Effects of captopril in animal models of hypertension. Clin Exper Hypertension 1980;*2*:613–637.
38. Anderson GH Jr, Streeten DHP, Dalakos TG. Pressor response to 1-Sar-8-Ala-angiotensin II (saralasin) in hypertensive subjects. Circ Res 1977;*40*:243–250.
39. Laragh JH, Case DB, Wallace JM, Keim H. Blockade of renin or angiotensin for understanding human hypertension: A comparison of propranolol, saralasin and converting enzyme blockade. Fed Proc 1977;*36*:1781–1787.
40. Edwards RM, Aiyar N, Ohlstein E, Weidley EF, Griffin E, Ezekiel M, Keenan RM, Ruffolo RR, Weinstock J. Pharmacological characterization of the nonpeptide angiotensin II receptor antagonist, SK&F 108566. J Pharmacol Exp 1 Ther 1991;*260*:175–181.
41. Haber E. Why renin inhibitors? Hypertension 1989;*7*(Suppl. 2):S81–S86.
42. Packer M, Lee MH, Yushak M, Medina N. Comparison of captopril and enalapril in patients with severe chronic heart failure. N Engl J Med 1986;*315*:847–853.
43. Sharpe DN, Murphy J, Coxon R, Hannan SF. Enalapril in patients with chronic heart failure. a placebo-controlled, randomized, double-blind study. Circulation 1984;*70*:271–278.
44. Regoli D. Neurohumoral regulation of precapillary vessels. The kallikrein-kinin system. J Cardiovasc Pharmacol 1984;62: 401–413.
45. Kaplan AP, Silverberg M. The coagulation-kinin pathway of human plasma. Blood 1987;*70*:1–15.
46. Terrango NA, Lonigro AJ, Malik KU, McGiff JC. The relationship of renal vasodilator action of bradykinin to the release of prostaglandin E-like substance. Experientia 1972;*28*:437–439.
47. Friedman MM, Kaliner M. The human lung mast cell and asthma. Am Rev Respir Dis 1987;*135*:1157–1164.
48. Darius H, Lefer DJ, Smith JB, Lefer AM. Role of platelet-activating factor-acether in mediating guinea pig anaphylaxis. Science 1986;*232*:58–60.
49. Black JM, Duncan WAM, Durant CJ, Ganellin CR, Parsons EM. Definition and antagonism of histamine H_2-receptors. Nature 1972;*236*:385–390.
50. Brimblecombe RW, Duncan WAM, Durant GJ, et al. Characterization and development of cimetidine as a histamine H_2-receptor antagonist. Gastroenterology 1978;*74*:339–347.
51. Kaliner M, Shelhamer JH, Ottesen EA. Effects of infused histamine: Correlation of plasma histamine levels and symptoms. J Allergy Clin Immunol 1982;*69*:283–289.
52. Carruthers SG, Shoeman DW, Hignite CE, Azarnoff DL. Correlation between plasma diphenhydramine level and sedative and antihistamine effects. Clin Pharmacol Ther 1978;*23*:375–382.
53. DiMarco JP, Lerman BB, Kabell G, Belardinelli L. Adenosine produces different effects on monophasic action potentials in human atrium and ventricule. J Am Coll Cardiol 1988;*11*:A227.
54. Clarke B, Coupe M. Adenosine: Cellular mechanisms, pathophysiological roles and clinical applications. Internat J Cardiol 1989;*23*:1–10.
55. Bowmer CJ, Yates MS. Therapeutic potential for new selective adenosine receptor ligands and metabolism inhibitors. TIPS 1989;*10*:340–342.
56. Rudolphi KA, Schubert P, Parkinson FE, Fredholm BB. Neuroprotective role of adenosine in cerebral ischemia. TIPS 1992;*13*:439–445.
57. Burnstock G: The changing face of autonomic neurotransmission. Acta Physiol Scand 1986;*126*:67–91.
58. Bradley PB, Engel G. Feniuk W, Fozard JR, Humphrey PPA, Middlemiss DN, Mylecharane EJ, Richardson BP, Soxena PR. Proposals for the classification and nomenclature of functional receptors for 5-hydroxytryptamine. Neuropharmacology 1986;*25*:563–576.
59. Mylecharane EJ. The classification of 5-hydroxytryptamine receptors. Clin Exp Pharmacol Physiol 1989;*16*:517–522.
60. Vanhoutte PM. Inhibition by acetylcholine of adrenergic neurotransmission in vascular smooth muscle. Circ Res 1974;*34*:317–326.
61. Steinsland OS, Furchgott RF, Kirpekar SM. Inhibition of adrenergic neurotransmission by parasympathetics in the rabbit ear artery. J Pharmacol Exp Ther 1973;*184*:346–356.

62. Loffelholz K, Muscholl E. A muscarinic inhibition of noradrenaline release evoked by postganglionic sympathetic nerve stimulation. Naunyn Schmiedebergs Arch Pharmacol 1969;*265*:1–15.

63. Furchgott RF, Zawadzki JV. The obligatory role of endothelial cells in the relaxation of arterial smooth muscle by acetylcholine. Nature 1980;*288*:373–376.

64. Furchgott RF. Role of endothelium in responses of vascular smooth muscle. Circ Res 1983;*53*:557–573.

65. Gryglawski PJ, Palmer RM, Moncada SA. Superoxide anion is involved in the breakdown of endothelium derived relaxing factor. Nature 1986;*320*:454–456.

66. Hidaka H, Asano T. Stimulation of platelet guanylate cyclase by unsaturated fatty acid peroxides. Proc Natl Acad Sci 1977;*74*:3657–3661.

67. Rapaport RM, Murad F. Agonist-induced endothelium dependent relaxation in rat thoracic aorta may be mediated through CGMP. Circ Res 1983;*52*:352–257.

68. Diamond J, Chu EB. Possible role for cyclic GMP in endothelium dependent relaxation of rabbit aorta by acetylcholine comparison with nitroglycerin. Res Comm Chem Pathol Pharmacol 1983;*41*:369–381.

69. Ignarro LJ, Harbison RG, Wood KS, Kadowitz PJ. Activation of purified soluble guanylate cyclase by endothelium -derived relaxing factor from intrapulmonary artery and vein: stimulation by acetylcholine bradykinin and arachidonic acid. J Pharmacol Exp Ther 1986;*237*:893–900.

70. Palmer RMJ, Ferrige AG, Moncada S. Nitric oxide release accounts for the biological activity of endothelium-derived relaxing factor. Nature 1987;*327*:524–526.

71. Bredt DS, Hwang PM, Glatt CE, Lowenstein C, Reed RR and Snyder SH. Cloned and expressed nitric oxide synthase structurally resembles cytochrome P-450 reductase. Nature (London) 1991;*351*:714–718.

72. Xie Q-w, Cho HJ, Calaycay J, Mumford RA, Swiderek KM, Lee TD, Ding A, Troso T, Nathan C. Cloning and characterization of inducible nitric oxide synthase from mouse macrophages. Science 1992;*256*:225–228.

73. Lyons CR, Orloff GJ and Cunningham JM. Molecular cloning and functional expression of an inducible nitric oxide synthase from a murine macrophage cell line. J Biol Chem 1992;*267*:6370–6374.

74. Lowenstein CJ, Glatt CS, Bredt DA and Snyder SH. Cloned and expressed nitric oxide synthase contrasts with brain enzyme. Proc Natl Acad Sci USA. 1992;89:6711–6715.

75. Lamas S, Marsden PA, Li GK, Tempst P, Michel T. Endothelial nitric oxide synthase: molecular cloning and characterization of a distinct constitutive enzyme isoform. Proc Natl Acad Sci USA 1992;*89*:6348–6352.

76. Janssens SP, Shimouchi A, Quertermous T, Bloch DB, Bloch KD. Cloning and expression of a cDNA encoding human endothelium-derived relaxing factor/nitric oxide synthase. J Biol Chem 1992;*267*:14519–14522.

77. Kwon NS, Stuehr DJ, Nathan CF. Inhibition of tumor cell ribonucleotide reductase by macrophage derived nitric oxide. J Exp Med 1991;*174*:761–768.

78. Beckman JS, Beckman TW, Chen J, Marshall PA, Freeman BA. Apparent hydroxyl radical production by peroxynitrite: Implication for endothelial injury from nitric oxide and superoxide. Proc Natl Acad Sci 1990;*87*:1620–1624.

79. Bohme GA, Bon C, Stutzman JM, Doble A, Blanchard JC. Possible involvement of nitric oxide in long term potentiation. Eur J Pharmacol 1991;*199*:379–381.

80. Nowicki JP, Duval D, Poignet H, Scatton B. Nitric oxide mediates neuronal death after focal cerebral ischemic in the mouse. Eur J Pharmacol 1991;*204*:339–340.

81. Aisaka K, Gross SS, Griffith OW, Levi R. N^G-methylarginine, an inhibitor of endothelium-derived nitric oxide synthesis, is a potent pressor agent in the guinea pig; does nitric oxide regulate blood pressure in vivo? Biochem Biophys Res Comm 1989;*160*:881–886.

82. Rees DD, Palmer RMJ, Moncada S. Role of endothelium derived nitric oxide in the regulation of blood pressure. Proc Natl Acad Sci 1989;*86*:3373–3378.

83. Kilbourn RG, Jurban A, Gross AS, Griffith OW, Levi R, Adams J, Lodato RF. Reversal of endotoxin-mediated shock by N^G-methyl-L-arginine, an inhibitor of nitric oxide synthesis. Biochem Biophys Res Comm 1991;*172*:1132–1138.

84. Boulanger C, Luscher TF. Release of endothelin from the porcine aorta. Inhibition of endothelium derived nitric oxide. J Clin Invest 1990;*85*:587–590.

85. Nakaki T, Nakayama M, Kato R. Inhibition by nitric oxide and nitric oxide producing vasodilators of DNA synthesis in vascular smooth muscle cells. Eur J Pharmacol 1990;*189*:347–353.

86. Bucala R, Tracey KJ, Cerami A. Advanced glycosylation endproducts quench nitric oxide and mediate defective endothelium-dependent vasodilation in experimental diabetes. J Clin Invest 1991;*87*:432–438.

87. Panza JA, Quyyumi AA, Brush JE Jr, Epstein SE. Abnormal endothelium-dependent vascular relaxation in patients with essential hypertension. N Engl J Med 1990;*323*:22–27.

88. Drexler H, Zeiher AM, Meinzer K, Just H. Correction of endothelial dysfunction in coronary microcirculation of hypercholesterolaemic patients with L-arginine. Lancet 1991;*338*:1546–1550.

89. Rossaint R, Falke KJ, Lopez F, Slama K, Pison U, ZapolWM. Inhaled nitric oxide for the adult respiratory distress syndrome. N Engl J Med 1993;*328*:399–405.

90. Rejfer J, Aronson WJ, Bush PA, Dorey FJ, Ignarro LJ. Nitric oxide as a mediator of relaxation of the corpus carvernosum in response to nonadrenergic, non-cholinergic neurotransmission. N Engl J Med 1992;*326*:90–96.

91. Mathies G, Sherman MP, Buckberg GD, Hayborn DM, Young HH, Ignarro LJ. Role of L-arginine-nitric oxide pathway in myocardial reoxygenation injury. Am J Physiol 1992;*262*:H616–H620.

92. Iadecola C. Regulation of the cerebral microcirculation during neural activity is nitric oxide the missing link? Trends Neurosci 1993;*16*:206–214.

Reviews

r1. Gardiner PJ. Classification of prostanoid receptors. In: Samuelsson B, Dahlén SE, Fritsch J, Hedqvist P, eds. Prostaglandin, thromboxane and leukotriene research. Vol. 20. New York: Raven Press, (1990); pp 110–118.

r2. Giles H, Leff P. The biology and pharmacology of PGD_2. Prostaglandins 1988;*35*:277–300.

r3. Feuerstein G, Kopin IJ. Effect of PGD_2, PGE_2, $PGE_{2\alpha}$ and PGI_2 on blood pressure, heart rate and plasma catecholamine responses to spinal cord stimulation in the rat. Prostaglandins 1981;*21*:189–206.

r4. Hay DWP, Griswold D. Inhibitors of fatty acid-derived mediators. In: Cunningham F (ed.) Handbook of immunology. Vol. 10. London: Academic Press, (1993); pp 117–179.

r5. Ogletree ML. Overview of physiological and pathophysiological effects of thromboxane A_2. Fed Proc 1987;*46*:133–138.

r6. Miller DK, Gillard JW, Vickerst PJ, Sadowski S, Léveillé C, Mancini JA, Charleson P, Dixon RAF, Ford-Hutchinson AW, Fortin R, Gauthier JY, Rodkey J, Rosen R, Rouzer C, Sigal IS, Strader CD, Evans JF. Identification and isolation of a membrane protein necessary for leukotriene production. Nature 1990;*343*:278–281.

r7. Feuerstein G. Autonomic pharmacology of leukotrienes. J Autonomic Pharmacol 1985;*5*:149–168.

r8. Hammarstrom S, Hua X-Y, Dahlén SE, Lindberg JM, Hedqvist P. Microcirculatory effects of leukotriene C4, D4 and E4 in the guinea pig. In: Lefer A, Gee MH, eds. Leukotrienes in cardiovascular and pulmonary function. New York: Alan Liss, Progress Clin Biol Res 1985;*59*:35–46.

r9. Ford-Hutchinson AW. Leukotriene B_4 in inflammation. Crit Rev Immunol 1990;*10*:1–12.

r10. Hay DWP, Muccitelli RM, Tucker SS, et al. Pharmacologic profile of SK&F 104353: A novel, potent and selective peptidoleukotriene receptor antagonist in guinea pig and human airways. J Pharmacol Exp Ther 1987;*243*:474–481.

r11. Crooke ST, Mattern M, Sarau HM, et al. The signal transduction system of the leukotriene D_4 receptor. TIPS 1989;*10*:103–107.

r12. Drazen JM, Austen KF. Leukotrienes and airway responses. Am Rev Respir Dis 1987;*136*:985–998.

r13. Nakagawa T, Mizushima Y, Ishii A, et al. Effect of a leukotriene antagonist on experimental and clinical bronchial asthma. In: Sameulsson B, ed. Advances in prostaglandin, thromboxane, and leukotriene Research. Vol. 21. New York: Raven Press, (1990); pp 465–468.

r14. Feuerstein G, Hallenbeck JM. Prostaglandins, leukotrienes and platelet activating factor in shock. Ann Rev Pharmacol Toxicol 1987;*27*:301–313.

r15. Bell RL, Young PR, Albert D, et al. The discovery and development of zileuton: an orally active 5-lipoxygenase inhibitor. Int J Immunopharmac 1992;*14*:505–510.

r16. McMillan RM, Walker ERH. Designing therapeutically effective 5-lipoxygenase inhibitors. TIPS 1992;*13*:323–330.

r17. Gillard, J, Ford-Hutchinson AW, Chan C, et al. L-663,536 (MK-886) (3-[1-(4-chlorobenzyl)-3-t-butyl-thio-5-isopropylindol-2-yl]-2, 2-dimethyl propanoic acid), a novel, orally active leukotriene biosynthesis inhibitor. Can J Physiol Pharmacol 1989;*67*:17–28.

r18. Brideau C, Chan C, Charleson S, et al. Pharmacology of MK-0591(3-[1-(4-chlorobenzyl)-3-(*t*-butylthio)-5-(quinol in-2-yl-methoxyl)-indol-2-yl]-2,2-dimethyl propanoic acid), a potent, orally active leukotriene biosynthesis inhibitor. Can J Physiol Pharmacol 1992;*70*:799–807.

r19. Braquet P, Touqui L, Shen TY, Vargaftig BB. Perspectives in platelet activating factor research. Pharmacol Rev 1987;*39*:97.

r20. Feuerstein G, Yue T-L. PAF as a putative mediator in cardiac and cerebrovascular diseases. In: Saito K, Hanahan DJ, (eds.) Platelet-activating factor and diseases. Tokyo: International Medical Publishers, (1989); pp 103–112.

r21. Regoli D, Park WK, Rioux F. Pharmacology of angiotensin. Pharmacol Rev 1974;*26*:69–123.

r22. Peach MJ. Renin-angiotensin system: biochemistry and mechanisms of action. Physiol Rev 1977;*57*:313–370.

r23. Sasaki K, Yamano Y, Bardan S, et al. Cloning and expression of a complementary DNA encoding a bovine adrenal angiotensin II type-1 receptor. Nature 1991;*351*:230–233.

r24. Timmermans PBMWM, Wong PC, Chiu AT, Heblin WF. Non-peptide angiotensin II receptor antagonists. TIPS 1991;*12*:55–66.

r25. Opie LH. Angiotensin converting enzyme inhibitors. New York: Wiley-Liss, 1992.

r26. Margolius HS. The kallikrein-kinin system and the kidney. Ann Rev Physiol 1984;*46*:309–326.

r27. Regoli D. Kinins. British Medical Bull 1987;*43*:270–284.

r28. Sharma JN. Interrelationship between the kallikrein-kinin system and hypertension. A review. Gen Pharmacol 1988;*19*:177–187.

r29. Metcalfe DD, Kaliner M, Donlon MA. The mast cell. CRC Crit Rev Immunol 1981;*3*:23–74.

r30. Lewis T. The blood vessels of the human skin and their responses. London: Shaw & Sons, Ltd. 1927.

r31. Williams M. Adenosine antagonists. Med Res Rev 1989;*9*:219–243.

r32. Williams M. Purine receptors in mammalian tissues: Pharmacological and functional significance. Ann Rev Pharmacol Toxicol 1987;*27*:315–345.

r33. Furchgott RF. The role of endothelium in the responses of vascular smooth muscle to drugs. Ann Rev Pharmacol Toxicol 1984;*24*:175–197.

r34. Hartig PR. Molecular biology of 5-HT receptors. TIPS 1989;*10*:64–69.

r35. Moskowitz MA. Neurogenic versus vascular mechanisms of sumitriptan and ergot alkaloids in migraine. TIPS 1992;*13*:307–311.

r36. van Heuven-Nolsen D. 5-HT receptor subtype-specific drugs and the cardiovascular system. TIPS 1988;*9*:423–425.

r37. Furchgott RF. Endothelium-dependent relaxation in systemic arteries. In: Vanhoutte PM, (ed.) Relaxing and contracting factors, New York: Humana Press, (1989); pp 1–26.

r38. Rubanyi GM, Vanhoutte PM. Modulation of the release of biological activity of endothelium-derived relaxing factor by oxygen-derived free radicals. In: Vanhoutte PM, (ed.) The endothelium, relaxing and contracting factors. New York: Humana Press (1988); pp 91–106.

r39. Murad F, Arnold WP, Mittal CK, Brauglier JM. Properties and regulation of guanylate cyclase and some proposed functions of cyclic GMP. Adv Cyclic Nucleotide Res 1979;*11*:175–204.

r40. Nathan C. Nitric oxide as a secretory product of mammalian cells. FASEB 1992;*6*:3051–3064.

CHAPTER 10

J. Paul Hieble
Robert R. Ruffolo, Jr.

Local Anesthetics

Introduction

Local anesthetics act by blocking the conduction of an action potential along a sensory nerve. This property can be used for the relief of pain or irritation, or to allow surgery or other procedures to be performed without induction of pain. Depending on the location of the nerve to be blocked, and consequently the anatomic region in which insensitivity to pain is desired, the local anesthetic may be administered via a variety of routes. Topical administration, infiltration, injection near a nerve fiber either peripherally or where it exits from the spinal cord, or localized IV administration are used. Several local anesthetics are useful upon systemic administration for the treatment of cardiac arrhythmias or, occasionally, as systemic analgesics. Although their antiarrhythmic effect is produced by the same mechanism as their local anesthetic effect, i.e., the blockade of membrane sodium channels to prevent the propagation of an action potential, the systemic application of these agents will not be discussed in this chapter, but in Chapter 25.

Historical Background

The local anesthetic properties of the extract of leaves of *Erythoxylon coca* were known to the Incas centuries ago, and this extract was used for pain relief in surgical procedures. Over 100 years ago, the active alkaloid, cocaine, was introduced as the first local anesthetic by Karl Koller. Sigmund Freud also played an important role in the discovery and use of cocaine as a local anesthetic.

Although cocaine was clinically effective as a local anesthetic, and still has some application, it had several liabilities, such as high toxicity, short duration of action, and thermal instability that prevented heat sterilization of its solutions. An effort was therefore devoted to the design of new molecules to overcome these limitations. In 1905, the synthesis of procaine was reported. Procaine retains several of the structural elements found in cocaine (see Table 10.1), and has a similar ability to block axonal conduction. However, procaine does not block neuronal catecholamine uptake, and lacks many of the CNS effects associated with cocaine. Many new agents have been tested in experimental models, and several have become effective clinical tools with advantages over procaine, which still remains a useful drug.

The mechanism by which cocaine, procaine, and other related compounds block neuronal action potentials and produce local anesthesia has been studied extensively and is now well understood, having been localized to an action on the voltage-gated neuronal sodium channel, interfering with depolarization induced by influx of extracellular sodium ions.[1] Nevertheless, the exact molecular interaction between anesthetic and sodium channel that induces the block is still not known.

Mechanism of Action

The initiation and propagation of an action potential along an axon depends on depolarization of the neuronal membrane. This depolarization is produced by the opening of specific channels that allow the movement of sodium from the extracellular space into the cell. The sodium channel is a complex transmembrane protein, which has been isolated in pure form and biochemically characterized.[2] A large body of experimental evidence has clearly demonstrated that local anesthetics prevent axonal conduction by functional blockade of these sodium channels.

Table 10.1 Local Anesthetic Preparations

Drug	Route	Concentration	Dose	Onset	Duration of Response
Bupivacaine HCl					
Marcaine	Parenteral	0.25–0.75%	depends on application	2–10 min	lasts 3–9 hr
Chloroprocaine HCl					
Nesacaine	Parenteral	1, 2, 3%	depends on application	6–12 min	lasts 1–1.5 hr
Lidocaine HCl					
Xylocaine	Parenteral	0.5–4%	depends on application	5–10 min	lasts 60 min
Mepivacaine HCl					
Carbocaine	Parenteral	1, 1.5, 2, 3%	depends on application	7–15 min	lasts 1.5–2 hr
Prilocaine HCl					
Citanest	Parenteral	4%	depends on application	2–4 min	lasts 2 hr
Procaine HCl					
Novocaine	Parenteral	1, 2, 10%	depends on application	2–5 min	lasts 2–3 hr
Propoxycaine HCl					
Ravocaine	Parenteral	0.4%	depends on application	2–5 min	lasts 3/4–1 hr
Tetracaine HCl					
Pontocaine	Parenteral	10% solution 20 mg powder	depends on application	15 min	lasts 1.5–3 hr
Etidocaine HCl					
Duranest	Parenteral	1%	depends on application	2–20 min	lasts 4–13 hr
Proparacaine HCl					
Alcaine	Intra-ocular	0.5%	1–5 drops	2–5 min	lasts 1.5–3 hr

Studies using isolated invertebrate axons have shown that the clinically used local anesthetics, most of which are tertiary amines, act at an intracellular site. Quaternary amine analogues of these drugs, which have a permanent charge, cannot readily cross the axonal membrane. Hence, they are not active when applied to the extracellular surface, but do produce blockade when administered intracellularly. Similar results recently have been obtained with isolated mammalian sodium channels incorporated into planar lipid bilayers.[3] This is consistent with the observation, made both clinically and in experimental models, that the speed of onset of impulse blockade produced by a tertiary amine depends on its ionization constant[4,r1] and is enhanced by raising the extracellular pH, which increases the percentage of molecules in the unionized state.

The sodium channel can exist in at least three states: resting (closed); active (open); and inactivated (closed). The difference between the resting and inactivated channel is that the resting state can be activated by depolarization, whereas the inactivated is in a desensitized state. Following the action potential and repolarization of the plasma membrane, there is a slow reversion of channels from the inactivated to resting states. During this reversion, the channel does not pass through the active state.

Local anesthetics appear to interact preferentially with the inactivated state of the sodium channel, interfering with its reversion to the resting state. Although the details of the interaction of local anesthetic molecules with the sodium channel are not completely understood, and some experimental controversies have not yet been resolved, there appear to be two modes of interaction of these molecules with the channel—one nonspecific and one that may be receptor-mediated.

Support for a specific, receptor-mediated action of the local anesthetics is based primarily on the observation of "use-dependent" blockade. If an isolated nerve fiber is repeatedly depolarized in the presence of a local anesthetic, the degree of impulse blockade can be substantially enhanced.[r2,5] This phenomenon appears to result from increased accessibility of the local anesthetic to its site of action during depolarization of the membrane and opening of the sodium channel. When sodium channels are converted to the inactive state subsequent to depolarization, their affinity for the local anesthetic is enhanced.

Since use-dependent blockade is more pronounced for relatively hydrophilic anesthetics, it has been postulated that the local anesthetic may actually traverse the sodium channel while open, and hence gain access to a binding site located near the cytoplasmic end of the channel.[r2] This internal binding site is distinct from that for the non-nitrogenous agents such as tetrodotoxin and saxitoxin, which produce potent and selective blockade of the sodium channel via interaction with a site near its external terminus. The local anesthetic does not appear to interact directly with the sodium ion, i.e., the anesthetic molecule does not actually "plug" the sodium channel.

In addition to the specific interaction, local anesthetics may interact with the sodium channel in a nonspecific fashion to block axonal conduction, apparently via passage of the lipophilic anesthetic molecules through the plasma membrane. This nonspecific mechanism may explain the local anesthetic action seen with molecules structurally unrelated to the tertiary amine agents, such as general anesthetics, aliphatic alcohols, and other molecules such as propranolol.

There is a substantial "safety factor" for action potential propagation, in that saltatory conduction normally produces a much greater nodal depolarization than that required to regenerate the action potential. Hence a substantial blockade of the sodium channel must be produced to block axonal transmission. Drugs that block 80 to 90 percent of the channels only reduce the amplitude of the compound action potential by 50 percent.[6] Consequently, any treatment that reduces the number of conducting sodium channels, or that decreases the passage of ions through the channel, will increase the apparent potency of a local anesthetic in producing impulse blockade.[7]

Early experiments suggested that small nerve fibers (C fibers), such as those conducting nociceptive impulses, were more sensitive to block by local anesthetics than larger fibers (A and B fibers). Clinical practice suggests that in many cases pain insensitivity can be produced without loss of motor function. It also has been suggested that the relative ability to produce sensory and motor blockade varies between different local anesthetics. The selectivity of bupivacaine for sensory responses has been used as a rationale for its use in obstetric procedures, since pain relief must be produced without loss of motor function. However, more recent data have shown that, when isolated nerve fibers are studied, the larger A fibers are actually more sensitive than B or C fibers.[8,9] The in vivo selectivity for C fibers often observed may be a consequence of easier accessibility of the anesthetic to these fibers under in vivo conditions, since the smaller fibers may be located closer to the surface of nerve bundles, and may have less extensive barriers (i.e., myelin sheath) through which the anesthetic must diffuse. Furthermore, because of increased accessibility, blockade of C fibers may have a more rapid onset, but when equilibrium blockade is attained, the block in all classes of fibers may be nearly equal.

Local anesthetics also can block the potassium channel, which would tend to oppose its primary effect on the sodium channel. In practice, however, potassium channel effects do not make a substantial contribution to the net potency of local anesthetics, since higher concentrations are required to block potassium vis-a-vis sodium channels, and the potassium conductance does not make a major contribution to the rising phase of the action potential.

Structure Activity Relationships

As noted above, the synthetic local anesthetics were designed to mimic the nerve blocking action of cocaine, while eliminating some of the undesirable side-effects. While many molecules will inhibit axonal conduction, we will consider here only those agents that have been shown to produce clinically useful local anesthesia.

Figure 10.1 shows the structures of a variety of local anesthetics. Most of these compounds have an aromatic group linked to a secondary or tertiary aliphatic amide via either an ester or an amide bond. The exceptions are agents such as benzocaine, which is an analogue of procaine lacking the amine moiety, and a few agents used as topical anesthetics in which the aromatic and amine groups are joined by an ether or ketone group. The preparations for commonly used local anesthetics are presented in Table 10.1.

In studies measuring action potential amplitude in isolated nerve fibers, procaine is approximately twofold weaker than cocaine. Although procaine is the least potent of the clinically used local anesthetics, absolute potency is not a major factor in determining the utility of a drug of this type, as long as effective anesthesia of sufficient duration can be produced without limiting toxicity. Although having an action similar to cocaine on the sodium channel, procaine does not block neuronal catecholamine uptake. An advantageous property of cocaine not found in procaine or other synthetic molecules is the ability to produce vasoconstriction, which tends to keep the anesthetic localized to its desired site of action. As a consequence, many of these agents are administered with a vasoconstrictor, such as epinephrine. Procaine also does not share the topical efficacy of cocaine. This may be a result of the rapid hydrolysis of procaine by pseudocholinesterase, since topical administration of procaine is effective if given in combination with physostigmine, an inhibitor of this enzyme.

It is difficult to compare the absolute potencies of the compounds in Table 10.1 as inhibitors of axonal conduction, since no single study comparing all agents in a particular experimental preparation has been performed. Data from different laboratories cannot be readily compared, since the absolute potency of an anesthetic molecule is highly dependent on the nerve fiber studied, the nature of the bathing solution (pH, ionic composition, temperature, etc.), and the accessibility of the anesthetic to the fiber.

Nevertheless, some general patterns relating local anesthetic potency to structure have become clear:

(1) Within a structural series, as lipophilicity is increased by adding carbon atoms on either the aromatic or aliphatic amine portions of the molecule, potency is enhanced. The potency of the piperidine analogues increases in the order

mepivacaine < ropivacaine < bupivacaine

Etidocaine, which bears additional alkyl substitution on both the amine nitrogen and the adjacent carbon, is fourfold more potent than lidocaine in reducing action potential amplitude in rabbit vagal/sciatic fibers.[8] The addition of the relatively lipophilic butyl group markedly enhances the potency of the ester-linked molecules, since tetracaine is more than tenfold more potent than procaine in most models, even though the steric bulk on the aliphatic amine group is reduced.

(2) Although the chemical nature of the link between aromatic group and aliphatic amine is not critical, increasing the distance between these moieties substantially reduces potency.[10] This may be

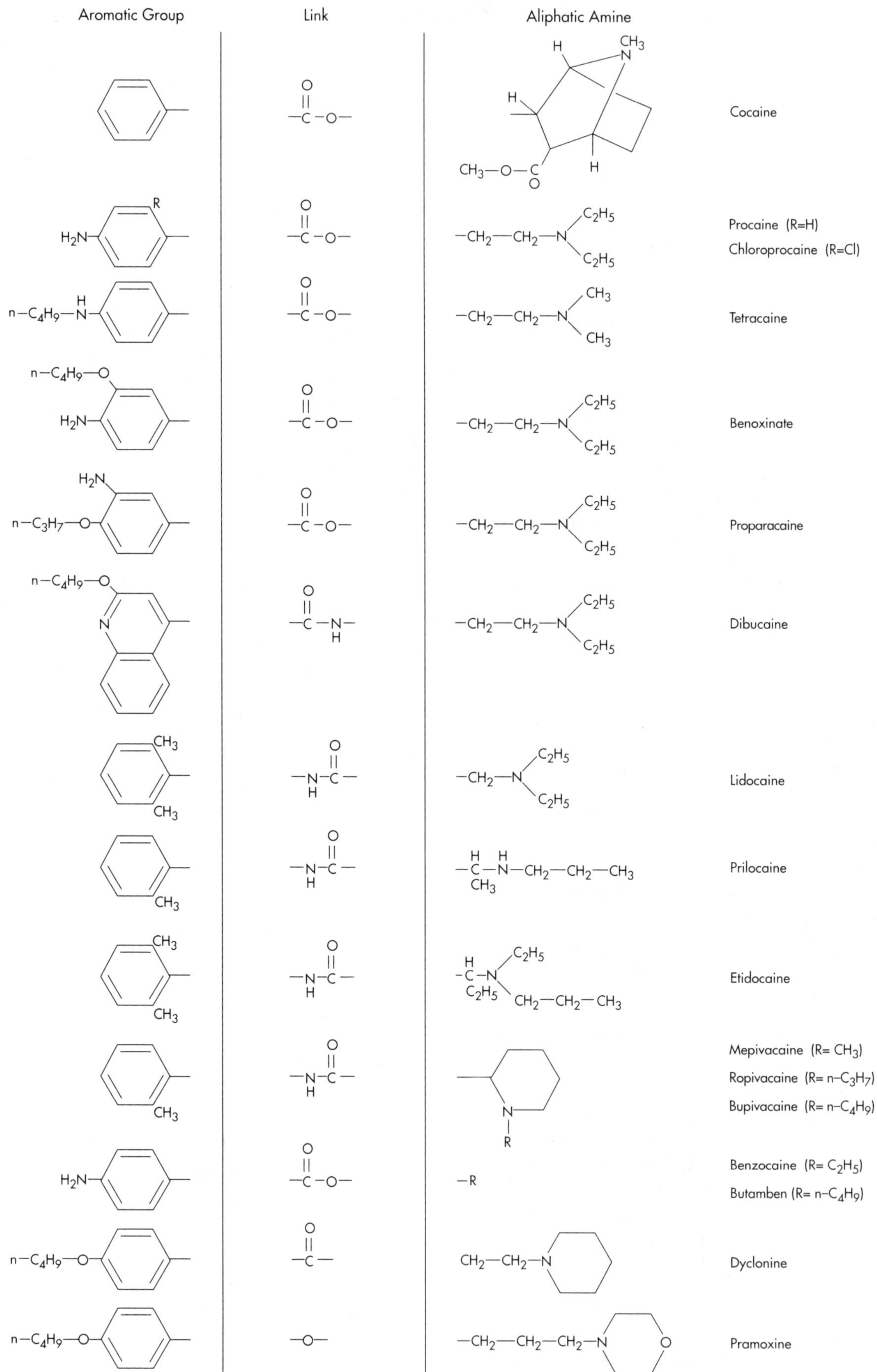

Figure 10.1 Structures of Clinically Used Local Anesthetics

a consequence of the increase in basicity of the amine nitrogen in these compounds.

(3) Although the aliphatic amine group is a key element in most local anesthetics, removal of this group does not necessarily influence potency, since benzocaine and procaine were essentially equipotent as inhibitors of action potential generation in isolated frog nerve fibers.[11] Nevertheless, the presence of the amine is required to provide sufficient aqueous solubility for utility as an injectable drug.

Stereoselectivity

One of the criteria for a drug-receptor interaction is a preferential interaction of one enantiomer of a drug containing an asymmetric center. Many of the local anesthetics have an asymmetric center, and some stereoselectivity has been observed with such molecules in isolated nerve preparations, especially under conditions favoring "use-dependent blockade" (see above).[12] The magnitude of the stereoselectivity is low, with enantiomeric potency differences being less than 5 in most cases. This is consistent with the postulate that these molecules can act by both a receptor-mediated and by a nonspecific mechanism. The (–) enantiomer of bupivacaine was found to produce a longer duration of analgesia in man,[13] but this may relate to stereoselective vasoconstriction by this enantiomer, causing selective retention at the site of action. Interestingly, ropivacaine, now undergoing clinical trials, is being studied as the S (–) enantiomer.[14]

Therapeutic Applications

Local anesthetics are used to produce loss of pain sensitivity in a specific region to allow a surgical procedure or other manipulation to be performed without general anesthesia. Use of local rather than general anesthesia often is advantageous with respect to safety and speed of recovery, and is required in surgical procedures that require interaction with the patient.

The anesthetic may be applied via several routes: (1) Topical; (2) infiltration; (3) regional nerve block; (4) spinal; and (5) localized IV injection. Although in theory many of the local anesthetics shown in Table 10.1 could be used by any of these routes, in practice certain local anesthetics are used for a specific application (see description of the individual agents below).

Although many different local anesthetics are available, there are no qualitative differences in their mechanism of action, and therapeutic ratios are generally similar, since their therapeutic action, and most side-effects, result from interference with sodium fluxes. Some specific side-effects associated with individual agents are noted later in this chapter. Apart from specialized applications, only a few different drugs of this class commonly are required in clinical practice.

Alteration of the chemical or physical nature of a local anesthetic can influence its clinical profile. Recent clinical evidence supports the premise (7) that alkalinization of solutions of tertiary amine local anesthetics will decease the time required for onset of action and will improve the degree of anesthesia produced.[16] Administration of a local anesthetic in combination with a lipid drug carrier can prolong its duration of action, and encapsulation into liposomes can both prolong duration of action and reduce systemic toxicity.

Topical Anesthesia

The topical application of local anesthetics to the skin can relieve pain and itching associated with toxic (e.g., poison ivy) or chronic dermatitis or from minor burns. Although absorption of these agents from intact skin is poor, they are more effective on inflamed or abraded skin, or on mucous membranes. A eutectic mixture of lidocaine and prilocaine can penetrate intact skin, and has been shown to be useful in preventing the pain associated with venous cannulation and ultrasonic destruction of kidney stones.

A mixture of tetracaine, epinephrine, and cocaine is commonly used for topical anesthesia in emergency treatment of wounds of the scalp and face.[r1] The degree of anesthesia produced by this mixture is comparable to that achieved with local infiltration of lidocaine although it is less useful for wounds of the trunk or extremity.[r1]

Topical anesthesia is useful for procedures involving the cornea or the nasal, oral, or urogenital mucous membranes. Since local anesthetics are efficiently absorbed into the systemic circulation via this route, caution must be exercised, and large quantities of anesthetic must be avoided. Absorption is especially rapid from the tracheobronchial tree. Tetracaine/epinephrine/cocaine mixtures are rapidly absorbed from mucous membranes or denuded or burned skin, and should not be allowed to come into contact with these surfaces.[r1]

Infiltration

Infiltration of a local anesthetic directly into the operative field is useful for minor procedures, such as those limited to the skin (suturing, insertion of cannulae). While there is no theoretical limit to the area which can be anesthetized, and deeper structures can also be affected, the total dose of anesthetic required rapidly increases with the size and depth of the area to be anesthetized, so that toxicity from systemically absorbed anesthetic represents the limiting factor.

In field block anesthesia, a technique bridging infiltration and nerve block, anesthesia is produced in an area larger than that directly in contact with the anesthetic, by SQ infiltration so as to block axonal transmission, and consequently produce anesthesia in an area distal to the injection site. Since the total dose of anesthetic is reduced by this technique, the potential for systemic toxicity is reduced.

As noted above, alkalinization of local anesthetic solutions can enhance the onset of action. Alkalinization also can reduce the pain associated with infiltration anesthesia, since most local anesthetics are marketed as relatively acidic solutions of their hydrochloride salts.[25]

Peripheral Nerve Block

Blockade of action potential generation in a major nerve bundle will produce anesthesia in the axon arborization distal to the block. For example, axillary block can anesthetize the entire arm. The amount of anesthetic required is inversely proportional to the proximity of the injection site to the nerve bundle. If the anesthetic can be delivered within the fascia surrounding the nerve, the anesthetic will be anatomically confined, and will produce a block of longer duration with less systemic absorption.

In contrast to infiltration or field block, nerve block techniques produce motor blockade in addition to analgesia. This is not normally a problem, although axillary block with long-lasting anesthetics such as bupivacaine can produce motor paralysis for up to 24 hours.

Direct infusion of local anesthetic into the femoral nerve sheath or intrapleural space has been employed for the relief of postsurgical pain. Anesthetic infusions can be continued for extended periods (24 hours or even longer).

Spinal Anesthesia

Introduction of local anesthetic directly into the subarachnoid space surrounding the spinal cord will block impulse flow in all sensory and motor nerves exiting from the cord. The injection site is usually between the third and fourth lumbar vertebra, below the termination of the cord itself. The area anesthetized will depend on the extent of cephalad travel of the anesthetic solution. The extent of travel will depend on: (1) the amount of anesthetic injected; (2) the direction of needle placement; (3) the density of the solution injected (hyperbaric and hypobaric solutions can be prepared by mixing the local anesthetic with 10% glucose or sterile distilled water, respectively); and (4) the position of the patient if a hyper- or hypobaric solution is utilized.

Since relatively small doses of anesthetic are administered and the clearance of drug from the subarachnoid space is slow, systemic effects of the anesthetic are not observed. However, since the preganglionic sympathetic fibers are blocked, a generalized sympatholytic effect is observed. The sympathetic fibers are more sensitive to the drug-induced block than the pain afferents, so that loss of sympathetic tone is observed in dermatomes corresponding to two spinal segments higher than the region where pain sensitivity is lost. On the other hand, since the motor axons are less sensitive to the local anesthetic action, motor blockade is observed only in areas corresponding to spinal segments up to two below the limit of anesthesia. For example, if surgical anesthesia is produced up to the level of the dermatome supplied by the first lumbar root, motor paralysis will be observed only in regions up to those supplied by the third lumbar root, but sympathetic tone will be lost up to the level supplied by the eleventh thoracic segment.

Epidural Anesthesia

In epidural anesthesia the local anesthetic is injected into the space surrounding the spinal cord (via caudal, lumbar, or occasionally thoracic injection), and the nerve fibers are blocked as they exit from the dural coating. Since the subarachnoid space is not entered, the potential side-effects (e.g., headache) related to loss of CSF are not observed. However, the anesthetic can diffuse through the dura and act on nerve roots and on the superficial layers of the spinal cord. Continuous epidural infusion can be used to relieve postoperative pain.

As in spinal anesthesia, the area of anesthesia is proportional to the amount of drug administered. The segmental difference between abolition of pain sensitivity and blockade of sympathetic tone is not observed, but the level of motor blockade is four to five segments below that of pain insensitivity.

Since the total dose of anesthetic administered into the epidural space is higher than that used for spinal anesthesia, and since the clearance into the systemic circulation is more rapid, blood levels sufficient to produce systemic effects can be observed following this mode of anesthesia.

The epidural administration of an opiate agonist will reduce the amount of local anesthetic required to produce analgesia. This combined therapy is commonly used during labor and delivery. Conversely, small amounts of epidural local anesthetic will reduce the dose of opiate agonist required to produce effective analgesia.

Epidural and general anesthesia can be combined, with the epidural administration of a local anesthetic continued during the recovery period from general anesthesia. A double-blind study in patients undergoing arterial reconstructive surgery has shown that the epidural administration of a local anesthetic-opiate agonist combination reduces postoperative complications and thrombosis in the arterial graft.

Regional IV Block

If the circulation to an extremity is isolated from the systemic circulation by means of a pneumatic tourniquet, local anesthetic may be administered IV to produce anesthesia of the limb. This technique is most often used for the arm. Prior to anesthetic administration, most of the blood is expressed from the extremity by means of a pressure bandage. When the tourniquet is released after completion of the surgical procedure, a substantial percentage of the administered anesthetic is released into the systemic circulation. However, peak blood levels are generally less than those observed following axillary nerve block or lumbar epidural block. Addition of low doses of fentanyl, an opiate receptor agonist, and pancuronium, a neuromuscular blocking agent, has been shown to improve the degree of regional anesthesia produced by IV lidocaine. The fentanyl may act to potentiate the lidocaine-induced conduction blockade via a mechanism independent of the opiate receptor, since these receptors are not present on peripheral nerve fibers.

Therapeutic Nerve Block

Nerve block is sometimes employed for the relief of intractable pain in a localized area. The relief of pain often persists for longer periods than would be predicted, based on the pharmacokinetics of the local anesthetic. Intrapleural administration of a local anesthetic has been used for the treatment of chronic arm pain associated with reflex sympathetic dystrophy. In some cases, neurotoxic agents such as phenol are used to produce permanent destruction of a sensory nerve.

Concurrent Use of Vasoconstrictor Agents

As noted above, cocaine will produce vasoconstriction upon local administration, at least in part as a consequence of its ability to block neuronal catecholamine uptake. This vasoconstriction reduces local blood flow, and consequently reduces the amount of drug removed from the application site into the systemic circulation. This principle has been applied to the synthetic local anesthetics, which usually do not produce vasoconstriction when administered alone, by administering these agents in combination with a vasoconstrictor agent. This technique increases the amount of local anesthetic that can be administered without producing systemic toxicity. Many preparations of local anesthetics contain a vasoconstrictor agent, and the combination of local anesthetic and vasoconstrictor can be used for all routes of local anesthesia. Vasoconstrictors should be avoided in terminal vascular beds, such as the fingers or toes.

Epinephrine is the most commonly used vasoconstrictor, but alpha-methyl norepinephrine is used in some preparations. Phenylephrine is advantageous for prolonging the action of topical anesthetics, since epinephrine is not well absorbed by this route. Vasopressin analogs are also occasionally utilized. Although used in the past, the combination of epinephrine and cocaine should be avoided, since cocaine can sensitize the heart to the arrhythmogenic effects of epinephrine.

Toxicity

Clinically used local anesthetics are toxic drugs, and their safe use depends on limiting their distribution to the desired site of action. Many toxic reactions to local anesthetics are due to inadvertent systemic administration, such as accidental IV dosing or premature release of the tourniquet during regional IV block. However, use of large amounts of local anesthetic via the appropriate route to produce regional block, especially in areas with a rich vascular supply, can result in toxic systemic concentrations.

Systemic toxicity from the injected local anesthetic is not a problem in spinal anesthesia; however, hypotension and cardiovascular depression associated with blockade of sympathetic outflow is commonly observed.

Toxic reactions to local anesthetics can be considered an extension of their therapeutic effect, i.e., their ability to block the membrane sodium channel. The most sensitive target usually is the CNS. Overdoses of any clinically used local anesthetic can produce central effects, with initial dizziness progressing to visual and auditory disturbances, twitching and tremors and eventual generalized convulsions. These effects appear to result from paralysis of inhibitory centers, primarily in the amygdala. Central nervous system depression, accompanied by respiratory depression or arrest, is seen only with massive systemic overdose. The potency of local anesthetics for induction of central stimulation is directly proportional to their therapeutic potency, with the exception of cocaine, which has distinct CNS effects as a result of its unique pharmacology. Although all agents can produce convulsions at high doses, initial sedation or even loss of consciousness is seen often with lidocaine and procaine, but not with mepivacaine, bupivacaine, or etidocaine.[r3] Treatment of convulsions induced by local anesthetic overdose involves assurance of a patent airway, assisted ventilation with oxygen, and administration of an ultrashort-acting barbiturate or a benzodiazepine if the convulsions persist.

Although local anesthetics can produce dramatic cardiovascular effects, the concentrations required are higher than those affecting the CNS. The predominant effect is a depression of cardiac impulse conduction, which leads to a fall in cardiac output and a fall in blood pressure. Although the initial effect of local anesthetics is to increase vascular resistance, particularly in the pulmonary bed, the cardiac effect usually predominates, and elevation of blood pressure is not observed. At very high doses, a direct vasorelaxant effect can contribute to profound hypotension and cardiovascular collapse. Hypotension and cardiovascular depression induced by local anesthetics is responsive to IV fluids and, when appropriate, vasopressor agents such as α-adrenoceptor agonists.

Although local anesthetics, particularly lidocaine, have clinically useful antiarrhythmic actions, bupivacaine overdose has been associated with the development of ventricular arrhythmias. Animal studies confirm the ability of bupivacaine, but not lidocaine, to induce ventricular fibrillation; and cardiac dysrhythmias can be observed with bupivacaine at nonconvulsant doses.

Although local anesthetics can depress neuromuscular transmission, this effect is not clinically relevant unless local anesthetics are used in combination with neuromuscular blocking agents, in which case prolongation of neuromuscular blockade can be observed. Since procaine and succinylcholine are both hydrolyzed by psuedocholinesterase, a clinically significant interaction can occur between these agents.

Local Tissue Toxicity

Local anesthetics do not produce any direct neurotoxic effect at the concentrations required to block axonal transmission. Skeletal muscle is more sensitive to the local irritant effects of these molecules. The more lipophilic agents are more irritating. Animal studies have shown that the ability of local anesthetics to produce skin irritation increases continuously with increasing lipophilicity, even beyond the point where peak anesthetic potency has been attained. Allergic reactions are rare with the amino-amides, although sensitization may occur to the aminobenzoic acid derivatives sometimes present as preservatives in commercial preparations of the amide anesthetics.[36]

Allergic Reactions

Allergic reactions are more commonly observed with the ester-linked anesthetics. This may be the result of hydrolysis of these agents to p-aminobenzoic acid, which is known to be a potential allergen. Proparacaine, in which the amino group is in the meta- rather than the para-position, does not exhibit cross-sensitization with the para-amino agents, such as procaine.

Persons suspected of having a genetic propensity toward malignant hyperpyrexia should not receive the amide-linked local anesthetics, since these agents are more likely to trigger a hyperthermic response.

Specific Properties of Individual Agents

This section lists some of the many local anesthetics in clinical use in various countries. Most agents are available in a variety of distinct preparations that vary in concentration of active drug, as well as the presence of vasoconstrictors and/or preservatives. Combinations containing two or more local anesthetics are also available in some markets. Specific local anesthetic preparations are presented in Table 10.1. As noted before, the structures of these local anesthetics are compared in Figure 10.1.

Cocaine

Cocaine is now used exclusively as a topical anesthetic, primarily in otolaryngeal and urogential procedures, and as a mixture with tetracaine and epinephrine in emergency treatment of wounds. Ophthalmic use is decreasing because of the tendency of cocaine to damage the corneal epithelium. When applied to the cornea, cocaine will produce mydriasis. In addition to systemic effects common to all local anesthetics, cocaine has other characteristic side-effects. Most prominent are its unique effects on the CNS, including the euphoria responsible for its high abuse potential. Higher doses can produce depression of brain function, leading eventually to respiratory arrest. The initial effect on the cardiovascular system is usually tachycardia and hypertension. A direct toxic action on the heart may induce rapid and lethal cardiac failure. Marked elevation in body temperature is also associated with cocaine overdose. This pyrexia may result from both a peripheral and central action. Since solutions of cocaine cannot be heat-sterilized, they usually are prepared immediately prior to use.

Procaine

Procaine is used for local anesthesia via infiltration, for producing peripheral nerve block, and for spinal anesthesia. It is not effective topically.

Chloroprocaine

Chloroprocaine is used for local anesthesia via infiltration and for producing either peripheral or epidural nerve block. A primary use of chloroprocaine is for labor and delivery, since the rapid hydrolysis of this molecule by pseudocholinesterase prevents toxic levels from accumulating in the fetal circulation. Chloroprocaine is also useful for procedures when rapid onset with short duration of action is desirable.

Tetracaine

Tetracaine is effective via all routes, including topical and spinal. It is generally used when long duration of anesthesia is desired.

Benzoxinate Hydrochloride

Benzoxinate hydrochloride is used as a topical anesthetic for ophthalmology.

Proparacaine

Proparacaine is used as a topical anesthetic for ophthalmology, when rapid onset with short duration of action is desirable.

Lidocaine

Lidocaine is the most commonly used of the amide-linked local anesthetics. It is used by all routes and is available in a wide variety of preparations, including topical solutions, oral sprays, viscous preparations (including gels and ointments), and many injectable preparations.

Lidocaine is also combined with dexamethasone in an injectable formulation for the relief of pain in joint inflammation.

Etidocaine

Etidocaine produces anesthesia of longer duration than its close analogue, lidocaine. It is administered via infiltration, or for peripheral or epidural nerve blocks. Etidocaine is not used for spinal anesthesia.

Prilocaine

Prilocaine has a time course similar to lidocaine. It is not currently used for nerve block or spinal anesthesia, owing to its tendency to induce methemoglobinemia, but is a component of a topical cream containing 5 percent of the eutectic (lowest melting point) mixture of prilocaine and lidocaine.

Mepivacaine

Mepivacaine has a time course similar to lidocaine, and is used for infiltration, peripheral nerve block, and epidural block.

Bupivacaine

Bupivacaine has a slower onset and longer duration of action than its close analogue, mepivacaine. Bupivacaine is used via infiltration, for peripheral and epidural nerve block, and for spinal anesthesia. Although widely used for obstetric anesthesia, studies in isolated placental tissue show that bupivacaine can readily gain access to the fetal circulation. The use of bupivacaine for regional IV block is not recommended, owing to its potential for systemic toxicity. The kinetic properties of its interaction with the sodium channel give bupivacaine a greater liability for depressing normal cardiac rhythm than local anesthetics having shorter durations of action. While useful in the treatment of postoperative pain, continuous intrapleural or epidural infusion of bupivacaine has been associated with convulsions in pediatric patients.

Ropivacaine

Ropivacaine is not yet available for clinical use, but experimental studies in both man and experimental animals show it to have properties similar to bupivacaine.[14] Animal studies suggest that ropivacaine has equivalent CNS toxicity to bupivacaine, but less tendency to induce ventricular arrhythmias.

Dibucaine

Dibucaine was formerly used for nerve block and spinal anesthesia, but now is available only in topical form.

Benzocaine, Butamben

Benzocaine is used only topically and is available in a variety of forms, such as a gel, solution, or aerosol. These preparations are used for anesthesia of mucous membranes and to suppress the gag reflex during endoscopy. It is also an ingredient in many multicomponent topical preparations for the relief of pain and irritation, including Cetacaine, a mixture of benzocaine, butamben, and tetracaine, available in spray, liquid, ointment, and gel forms for general pain relief when applied to mucous membranes.

Pramoxine

Pramoxine is the active ingredient in cream, lotion, and suppositories for the relief of the pain and irritation association with hemorrhoids. It is also available in a cream, lotion or ointment combined with hydrocortisone for pain relief in corticosteroid-sensitive dermatitis.

Dyclonine

Dyclonine is well absorbed from the skin and mucous membranes, and is used for topical anesthesia in otolaryngology and urology.

References

Research Reports

1. Butterworth JV, Strichartz GR. Molecular mechanisms of local anesthesia: A review. Anesthesiology 1992;*72*:711–734.
2. Wollner DA, Messner DJ, Catterall WA. Beta-2 subunits of sodium channels from vertebrate brain. J Biol Chem 1987;*262*:14709–14715.
3. Wang GK. Cocaine-induced closures of single batrachotoxin-activated Na^+ channels in planar lipid bilayers. J Gen Physiol 1988;*92*:747–765.
4. Covino BG. New developments in the field of local anesthetics and the scientific basis for their clinical use. Acta Anesth Scand 1982;*26*:242–249.
5. Raymond SA. Subblocking concentrations of local anesthetics: Effects on impulse generation and conduction in single myelinated sciatic nerve axons in frog. Anesth Analg 1992;*75*:906–921.
6. Hahin R, Strichartz GR. Effects of deuterium oxide on the rate and dissociation constants for saxitonin and tetrodotoxin action. J Gen Physiol 1981;*78*:113–139.
7. Wong K, Strichartz GR, Raymond SA. On the mechanisms of potentiation of local anesthetics by bicarbonate buffer: Drug structure-activity studies on isolated peripheral nerve. Anesth Analg 1993;*76*:131–143.
8. Gissen AJ, Covino BG, Gregus J. Differential sensitivities of mammalian nerve fibers to local anesthetic agents. Anesthesiology 1980;*53*:467–474.
9. Wildsmith JAW, Gissen AJ, Gregus J, Covino BG. Differential nerve blocking activity of amino-ester local anesthetics. Brit J Anesthesiol 1985;*57*:612–620.
10. Bokesch PM, Post C, Strichartz G. Structure-activity relationship of lidocaine homologs producing tonic and frequency-dependent impulse blockade in nerve. J Pharmacol Exp Ther 1986;*237*:773–781.
11. Belyaev VI. Comparative study of the effects of procaine, bencain, cocaine and anesthesin on electical activity of the node of Ranvier of single frog nerve fibers. Bull Exp Biol Med USSR 1973;*76*:1425–1427.
12. Yeh JZ. Blockade of sodium channels by stereoisomers of local anesthetics. Prog Anesthesiol 1980;2:35–44.

13. Aps C, Reynolds F. An intradermal study of the local anesthetic and vascular effects of the isomers of bupivacaine. Brit J Clin Pharmacol 1978;*6*:63–68.

14. Wood MB, Rubin AP. A comparison of epidural 1% ropivacaine and 0.75% bupivacaine for lower abdominal gynecologic surgery. Anesth Analg 1993;*76*:1274–1278.

15. Bezon, HT, Toleikis JR, Dixit P, Goodman I, Hill JA. Onset, intensity of blockade and somatosensory evoked potential changes of the lumbosacral dermatomes after epidural anesthesia with alkalinized lidocaine. Anesth Analg 1993;*76*:328–332.

16. Tetzlaff JE, Yoon HJ, Brems J, Secic M. Alkalinization of mepivacaine improves the quality of the interscalene brachial plexus block for shoulder surgery. Anesth Analg 1993;*76*:S432.

17. Langerman L, Grant GJ, Zakowski M, Golomb E, Ramanathan S, Turndork H. Prolongation of epidural anesthesia using a lipid drug carrier with procaine, lidocaine and tetracaine. Anesth Analg 1992;*75*:900–905.

18. Mashima T, Uchida I, Pak M, Shibata A, Nishimura S, Inagaki Y, Yoshiya I. Prolongation of canine epidural anesthesia by liposomal encapsulation of lidocaine. Anesth Analg 1992;*72*:827–834.

19. Boogaerts J, Declercq A, Lafont N, Benemeur H, Akodad EL, Dupont J-C, Legros FJ. Toxicity of bupivacaine encapsulated into liposomes and injected intravenously: Comparison with plain solutions. Anesth Analg 1993;*76*:553–555.

20. Soliman IE, Broadman LM, Hannallah RS, McGill WA. Comparison of the analgesic effects of EMLA (eutectic mixture of local anesthetics) to intradermal lidocaine infiltration prior to venous cannulation in unpremedicated children. Anesthesiology 1988;*68*:804–806.

21. Tiselius H-G Cutaneous anesthesia with lidocaine-prilocaine cream: A useful adjunct during shock wave lithotripsy with analgesic sedation. J Urol 1993;*149*:8–11.

22. Hegenbarth MA, Alteri MF, Hawk WH, Greene A, Ochsenschlager DW, O'Donnell R. Comparison of topical tetracaine, adrenaline and cocaine anesthesia with lidocaine infiltration for repair of lacerations in children. Ann Emerg Med 1990;*19*:63–67.

23. Tipton GA, DeWitt GW, Eisenstein SJ. Topical TAC (tetracaine, adrenaline, cocaine) solution for local anesthesia in children: Prescribing inconsistency and acute toxicity. South Med J 1989;*82*:1344–1346.

24. Bartfield JM, Gennis P, Barbara J. Buffered versus plain lidocaine as a local anesthetic for simple laceration repair. Ann Emerg Med 1990;*19*:1387–1390.

25. Cheney PR, Molzen G, Tandberg D. The effect of pH buffering on reducing the pain associated with subcutaneous infiltration of bupivacaine. Am J Emerg Med 1991;*9*:147–148.

26. Edwards ND, Wright EM. Continuous low-dose 3-in-1 nerve blockade for postoperative pain relief after total knee replacement. Anesth Analg 1992;*75*:265–267.

27. van Kleef JW, Logeman EA, Burm AGL, de Voogt JWH, Mooren RAG, van Kleef-Mannot IM. Continuous interpleural infusion of bupivacaine for postoperative analgesia after surgery with flank incisions: A double blind comparison with 0.25% and 0.5% solutions. Anesth Analg 1992;*75*:268–274.

28. Desparmet J, Meistelman C, Barre J, Saint-Maurice C. Continuous epidural infusion of bupivacine for postperative pain relief in children. Anesthesiology 1987;*67*:108–110.

29. Cohen S, Amar D, Pantuck CB, Pantuck EJ, Umanott M, Landa S. Epidural bupivacaine 0.015% reduces sufentanil requirements for labor analgesia. Anesth Analg 1993;*76*:S51.

30. Truman KJ, McCarthy RJ, March RJ, DeLaria GA, Patel RV, Ivankovich AD. Effects of epidural anesthesia on coagulation and outcome after major vascular surgery. Anesth Analg 1991;*73*:696–704.

31. Abdulla WY, Fadhi, NM. A new approach to intravenous regional anesthesia. Anesth Analg 1992;*75*:597–601.

32. Fields HL, Einson PC, Keigh BK, Gilbert RFT, Iversen LL. Multiple opiate receptor sites on primary afferent fibers. Nature 1980;*284*:351–353.

33. Reiestad F, McIlvaine WB, Kvalheim L, Stokke T, Pettersen B. Intrapleural analgesia in treatment of upper extremity reflex sympathetic dystrophy. Anesth Analg 1989;*69*:671–673.

34. Covino BG. Local anesthetic agents for peripheral nerve blocks. Reg Anaesth 1980;*3*:33–37.

35. Badgwell JM, Heavner JE, Turner D, Kao YJ, Smith DF. The toxic effects of bupivacaine are age dependent in young pigs. Anesth Analg 1989;*68*:S14.

36. Aberg G, Dhuner KG, Sydnes G. Studies on the duration of local anesthesia: Structure/activity relationships in a series of homologous local anesthetics. Acta pharmacol et toxicol. 1977;*41*:432–443.

37. Johnson RF, Johnson V, Herman N, Downing JW. Bupivacaine transfer across the human term placenta. Anesth Analg 1993;*76*:S168.

Reviews

r1. Norris RL. Local anesthetics. Emerg Med Clin N Amer 1992;*10*:707–718.

r2. Hille B. Ionic channels of excitable membranes. Sunderland, MA: Sinauer Associates, 1992.

r3. Covino BG. Toxicity and systematic effects of local anesthetic agents. In: Strichartz GR (ed.) Handbook of experimental pharmacology, Vol 81. Local anesthetics. Berlin: Springer-Verlag (1987); pp 187–212.

CHAPTER 11

Andrew J. Nichols
Robert R. Ruffolo, Jr.

Uterine Pharmacology

Basic Anatomy and Physiology of the Uterus

Anatomy

The uterus has three parts: the corpus (or main body); the cervix that connects the uterus to the vagina; and the isthmus that forms the narrowing between the corpus and the cervix. The outer serous layer consists of connective tissue that attaches the uterus to the body wall by the broad ligaments and round ligaments and to the ovaries by the ovarian ligaments. The thick middle layer of the corpus contains fibrous and elastic connective tissue and smooth muscle, known as the myometrium, arranged in layers that run in various directions. These layers give rise to the powerful expulsive actions during parturition and cause the mechanical compression of the uterine vasculature that prevents bleeding following detachment of the placenta during parturition. The cervix consists predominantly of collagenous and elastic tissue, with blood vessels and some smooth muscle fibers arranged in a predominantly circular fashion to form a sphincter. The inner layer of the uterus, the endometrium, consists of two layers, the superficial *stratum functionalis* and the inner *stratum basalis*, which contain glands, blood vessels, and lymphatics in loose connective tissue with a lining of epithelial cells. It is the *stratum functionalis* that undergoes cyclic changes of destruction and regeneration under the influence of the ovarian hormones, estradiol and progesterone, during the menstrual cycle. The cervical mucosa, which embryologically is a continuation of the endometrium, consists of a single layer of ciliated columnar epithelial cells. The secretory cervical glands extend from the surface of the mucosa to the underlying connective tissue.

Physiology

Myometrium

Uterine smooth muscle has a high degree of spontaneous electrical and contractile activity.[r1] Smooth muscle contraction is initiated by membrane potential spike activity produced by waves of spontaneous membrane depolarization triggered by pacemaker cells. The ionic basis of the pacemaker potential generation is uncertain, but most likely involves a slow depolarizing sodium current. Extracellular calcium enters the smooth muscle cells through voltage-operated calcium channels during the electrical spike activity. However, the amount of calcium that enters the myometrial cells is insufficient to cause contraction directly. Instead, this short burst of calcium entry triggers the release of much larger amounts of calcium from the sarcoplasmic reticulum,[1,r2] which in turn binds to calmodulin and activates myosin light-chain kinase to phosphorylate the light chains of myosin, allowing them to interact with actin to form the contractile actomyosin complex.[r3] The spread of electrical activity from cell to cell is facilitated by gap junctions, which are low resistance pathways that connect cells. These gap junctions and the frequency of pacemaker potential generation are regulated by ovarian hormones, with estrogens being excitatory and progestins being inhibitory. However, the number of gap junctions normally is very low until the onset of labor, at which time their number and size increase.[r4]

Estrogens also stimulate the synthesis of actin and myosin and hyperpolarize the myometrial plasma membrane from an electrically stable resting level of –35 mV to an electrically excitable level of –50 mV.[r5] In contrast, progestins stabilize the membrane potential near its resting level and do not induce the synthesis of contractile proteins.[r5] Since the force of uterine smooth muscle contraction is regulated by the frequency and duration of spike discharges, the degree of spread of electrical excitation between cells, and the levels of actin and myosin, spontaneous and stimulated uterine smooth muscle activity is enhanced by estrogens and inhibited by progestins. Thus, uterine smooth muscle activity increases at puberty and varies with the menstrual cycle. During pregnancy, the placenta produces large quantities of progesterone that act to reduce myometrial activity and reduce the sensitivity to oxytocin. However, the marked increase in estriol production and the decrease or leveling off of progesterone production by the placenta that occurs in the final weeks of pregnancy are believed to be partly responsible for the increase in spontaneous myometrial activity and increase in sensitivity to oxytocin that may be responsible for the initiation and progression of labor (see below).

Endometrium

The function of the endometrium is also controlled by ovarian hormones. The menstrual cycle starts with the onset of menstruation, in which the the superficial layer of the endometrium, the stratum functionalis, degenerates and is shed in response to a fall in the secretion of estradiol and progesterone. Following menstruation, the stratum functionalis regenerates in the proliferative phase in response to the slowly increasing levels of estrogen, with an increase in the number and height of the endometrial cells and number and length of the tubular endometrial glands.[r6] Moreover, there is a marked estrogen-induced increase in vascularity in the stratum functionalis.[r6] Toward the end of the proliferative phase, the preovulatory surge of estradiol induces an increase in endometrial proliferation. In addition, the activation of estrogen receptors in the endometrium increases the synthesis of progesterone receptors and thus renders the endometrium sensitive to the action of progesterone secreted from the *corpus luteum* following ovulation.[r6]

During the secretory or luteal phase, progesterone induces secretion from the glandular cells in the stratum functionalis and increases endometrial blood flow.[r6] The effects of progesterone are antagonized by estrogens, but progesterone receptor activation suppresses estrogen receptor synthesis and thus reduces the inhibitory effects of estrogens.[r6] At the end of the secretory phase, as the production of estradiol and progesterone fall, the glandular cells degenerate and secretion falls in the predecidual phase. The further fall in the production of estradiol and, in particular, progesterone below a certain level is the stimulus for menstruation. It is the fall in progesterone that is the stimulus for the onset of menstruation, since progesterone withdrawal in the presence of maintained estrogen levels induces menstruation, whereas estrogen withdrawal in the presence of progesterone levels does not.

The cervical endometrium contains many mucus-secreting cells, respond to the peak of estradiol at the end of the proliferative phase by producing a copious, watery, alkaline secretion rich in carbohydrate and protein. This mucus is believed to facilitate the passage of sperm through the uterus during the fertile period. In the postovulatory luteal phase, the progesterone causes the cervical mucus cells to produce a small quantity of viscous mucus.[r6]

Parturition

The precise mechanism by which parturition is initiated and maintained is unknown. There is much controversy regarding the importance of oxytocin as a mediator of parturition, since plasma levels of oxytocin do not change dramatically prior to onset of labor but have been observed to increase during its first phase.[2] However, there may be a complex interplay between estrogens, progesterone, oxytocin, and eicosanoids, in which oxytocin plays a central role in parturition without any changes in circulating levels. Figure 11-1 shows the likely sequence of events that lead to the onset of labor and delivery.[r7] The actions of oxytocin and eicosanoids are discussed below.

Drug Affecting Uterine Motility

Uterine-Stimulating (Oxytocic) Drugs

Oxytocin

Oxytocin is a nonapeptide synthesized in the supraoptic and paraventricular nuclei of the hypothalamus. Its structure oxytocin is similar to that of the antidiuretic hormone, vasopressin. However, it is only at very high concentrations that oxytocin interacts with vasopressin receptors to produce an antidiuretic response. At physiologic plasma concentrations, or at therapeutic doses, oxytocin interacts selectively with specific oxytocin receptors and has little or no antidiuretic activity. The effect of oxytocin on uterine smooth muscle depends on the hormonal status of the uterus. As described above, estrogens increase and progestins decrease the sensitivity of the myometrium to oxytocin, most likely by affecting both the electrical properties of the myometrial plasma membrane and the intracellular concentration of actin and myosin, and by changing the density of oxytocin receptors. For example, the density of myometrial oxytocin receptors increases gradually during pregnancy, with an abrupt further increase during early labor.[r7] At low concentrations, oxytocin increases spike discharge activity of the smooth muscle membrane by increasing the frequency, spike number, and amplitude of the spike discharges without affecting resting membrane potential. At higher concentrations, oxytocin also produces a sustained decrease in membrane potential. These electrophysiologic actions of oxytocin lead to an increase in both the frequency of spontaneous contractile activity and the force of contraction of uterine smooth muscle.[r1] The importance of extracellular calcium influx through voltage-operated calcium channels is highlighted by the high sensitivity of these responses to inhibition by calcium channel blockers.

Oxytocin is the drug of choice for the induction of labor when continuation of the pregnancy is considered to be more harmful to the mother and/or fetus than the possible effects of pharmacologic intervention. Toward the end of pregnancy the myometrium is highly sensitive to oxytocin (see above); therefore, only very low doses, given by increasing rates of infusion until the desired effect is produced, are required to induce labor. (See Table 11.1) for preparations available for this purpose. Thus, the likelihood of producing an antidiuretic response as a result of interaction with vasopressin receptors, during induction of labor is low. Uterine contractions produced by oxytocin at term are powerful and sustained, and may even lead to an increase in resting tone if higher doses are used. As a result, uterine activity should be carefully monitored during infusion of oxytocin so that the lowest possible infusion rate that will allow adequate progression of labor can be used. Moreover, oxytocin should not be used to augment labor in progress, albeit slowly, except in certain nulliparous patients in whom prolonged labor may be considered potentially dangerous to the mother and/or fetus. Another use of oxytocin is in the treatment of postpartum hemorrhage resulting from uterine atony. However, ergot alkaloids are more commonly used for this purpose (see below).

Eicosanoids

Eicosanoids (see Chapter 9) consist of the prostaglandins, prostacyclin, thromboxane A_2; and the leukotrienes. Prostaglandins were discovered when the ability of seminal fluid to contract smooth muscle was noted. They are lipid-derived (mainly from arachidonic acid), 20-carbon unsaturated carboxylic acids with a cyclopentane ring. The endometrium and decidua, the specialized endometrium of pregnancy, are rich in prostaglandin synthase activity. The first enzyme in the catabolic pathway of prostaglandins, NAD^+-dependent 15-hydroxyprostaglandin dehydrogenase (PGDH) is regulated by progesterone and thus decreases just prior to menstruation as progesterone levels fall.[3] As a result of the progesterone withdrawal-induced reduction in this catabolic enzyme, prostaglandin levels increase just before and during menstruation. It is believed that the hypercontractility and pain experienced in primary dysmenorrhea are produced by the higher levels of prostaglandins due to decreased catabolism in the degenerating endometrium. Prostaglandin production by the decidua, which is also rich in arachidonic acid, is markedly enhanced during labor,[4] possibly as a result of increased sensitivity to oxytocin resulting from an increase in decidual oxytocin receptor density.[r7]

Of the many naturally-occurring prostaglandins, PGE_2 and $PGF_{2\alpha}$ have the most pronounced activity on uterine motility. PGE_2 can interact with EP_3 receptors to produce uterine smooth muscle contraction[16] and with EP_2 receptors to produce uterine relaxation.[r13] On the other hand, $PGF_{2\alpha}$ interacts with both the EP_3 receptor and the FP receptor to produce smooth muscle contraction. $PGF_{2\alpha}$ produces uterine contractions in both the pregnant and nonpregnant state, whereas PGE_2 causes relaxation of the nonpregnant uterus and contraction of the pregnant uterus at low concentrations, but relaxation at high concentrations. The ability of high concentrations of PGE_2 to relax the pregnant uterus may be the result of an interaction with the prostacyclin IP receptor, which is known to exist in the uterus and to mediate relaxation, rather than with the EP_2 receptor.[r8]

As with oxytocin, the sensitivity of the myometrium to the contractile effects of PGE_2 and $PGF_{2\alpha}$ increases during pregnancy, although the magnitude of the increase in sensitivity is much less than that seen with oxytocin.[5] As a result, in the early stages of pregnancy, the uterus is more sensitive to $PGF_{2\alpha}$ than to oxytocin, but in the last month of pregnancy oxytocin is significantly more potent than $PGF_{2\alpha}$ or PGE_2 at inducing uterine contractions. These differences in increase in uterine sensitivity to oxytocin compared with the prostaglandins may be a consequence of the increased sensitivity to oxytocin that results from both steroid-induced changes in myometrial excitability and an increase in oxytocin receptor density, whereas the increase in sensitivity to prostaglandins results only from an increase in myometrial excitability, with no change in receptor density.

In addition to contractile actions on the myometrium, PGE_2 and $PGF_{2\alpha}$ also act on the cervix to produce ripening and dilation.[6] The mechanism by which this occurs is unknown, but may involve an effect on collagen metabolism in the cervix.

The major therapeutic use of prostaglandins is for induction of midtrimester abortion and to aid in expulsion of the fetus in the course of abortion by other methods, by causing contraction of the myometrium and softening of the cervix (see Table 11.1). Both PGE_2 and 15-methyl $PGF_{2\alpha}$ are used for these purposes. Another common use is promotion of ripening and dilation of the cervix by local instillation before induction of labor with oxytocin. Other uses include the treatment of postpartum hemorrhage resulting from uterine atony and softening of the cervix to aid in first trimester abortions by dilatation and evacuation.

Prostaglandins play an important role in the onset and progression of labor. Inhibition of the synthesis of prostaglandins with nonsteroidal antiinflammatory drugs (NSAIDs; i.e., cyclooxygenase inhibitors), such

Table 11.1 Summary of Drugs Affecting Uterine Tone

Drug	Route	Form	Dose	Peak	$t_{1/2}$	Duration of Response
Oxytocin						
Pitocin	parenteral	10 units/ml	0.5–1 milliunit/min initially to induce labor 20–40 milliunits/min postpartum	immediate	3–5 min	1 hr IV 1–3 hr IM
Syntocinon	nasal	40 units/ml	1 spray 3 min before nursing	3–5 min	3–10 min	1 hr–2 hr
Ergonovine	oral	0.2-mg tablet	0.2–0.4 mg po q 6–12 hr	30 min	0.5–2 hr	3 hr
Maleate						
Ergotrate	parenteral	0.2 mg/ml	0.2 mg IV q 2–4 hr	immediate	0.5–2 hr	45–2 hr
Methylergonovine	oral	0.2-mg tablet	0.2–0.4 mg po q 6–12 hr	30 min	0.5–2 hr	3 hr
Methergine	parenteral	0.2 mg/ml	0.2 mg IV q 2–4 hr	immediate	0.5–2 hr	45 min
ABORTAFACIENTS						
Dnoprostone						
Prostin-E_2	vaginal suppository	20 mg	20 mg 3 hr	20 min	very short in plasma	2–3 hr
Urea (40–50 %)	intraamniotic	40 g	80 g in 200 ml D_5W	4 hr	—	Up to a 24-hr infusion
Ureaphil	intraamniotic	20%	200 ml			
TOCOLYTICS						
Ritodrine	oral	10-mg tablet	10 mg q 2 hr initially up to 120 mg/day	30–60 min	10 hr	As required
Yutopar	parenteral	10–15 mg/ml	50–100 μg/min initially and gradually increased to no more than 350 μg/min	50 min	10 hr	
Terbutaline						
Brethine	oral	2.5–5 mg tablets	2.5 mg tid	2–3 hr		4–8 hr
Bricanyl	parenteral	1 mg/ml solution	0.25 mg q 4 hr, sq	30–60 min		

as aspirin, indomethacin, or ibuprofen, increases the length of gestation, prolongs spontaneous labor, and can interrupt premature labor.[7] The importance of the prostaglandins in parturition is presented in Figure 11.1, from which it can be seen that the effect of prostaglandins, produced primarily in the decidua, is to induce cervical ripening and dilatation, increase myometrial contractile sensitivity to oxytocin, and produce myometrial contraction. Thus, inhibition of prostaglandin production would be expected to inhibit parturition. However, the use of cyclooxygenase inhibitors for the prevention of labor is not without problems, and is not recommended. The ductus arteriosus in the fetus appears to remain patent in utero owing to the presence of vasodilator prostaglandins, such as prostacyclin (PGI_2). Inhibition of the synthesis of these prostaglandins by cyclooxygenase inhibitors may lead to premature closure of the ductus arteriosus. Although the use of cyclooxygenase inhibitors to delay premature labor is not recommended, they are effective in the treatment in uterine hypercontractility and cramping pain in primary dysmenorrhea, suggesting that prostaglandins released from the degenerating endometrium play a significant role in the uterine hypercontractility and pain sensitivity in this state.[8]

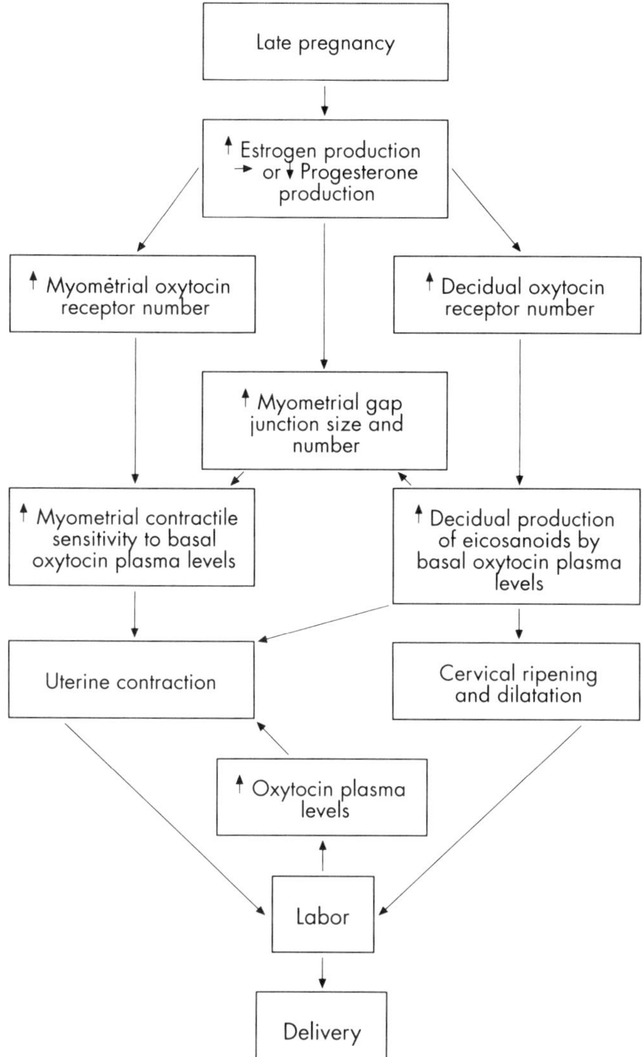

Figure 11.1 Schematic model of the interplay between steroid hormones, oxytocin, and eicosanoids in the initiation and progression of labor (modified from r7).

Ergot Alkaloids

The ergot alkaloids are derivatives of 6-methylergoline and comprise a class of compounds with a diversity of pharmacologic properties that include interactions with serotonin (5-HT) receptors, dopamine receptors, α-adrenoceptors, and uterine smooth muscle. Some ergot alkaloids are selective for only one of these actions (e.g., methysergide is a serotonin receptor antagonist), whereas others have varying degrees of activity at two or more of these sites (e.g., dihydroergotamine has actions at all four sites). The ability of ergot alkaloids to contract uterine smooth muscle results from their agonist activity at either 5-HT_2 receptors and/or α_1-adrenoceptors. Thus, the uterine contractile responses to both serotonin and ergonovine are blocked by the serotonin receptor antagonist, cyproheptadine, whereas the responses to norepinephrine and ergotamine are blocked by the α-adrenoceptor antagonist, phentolamine.[9,r9] The ergot alkaloids at low doses increase the force and frequency of uterine contraction followed by normal relaxation, whereas at high doses, the ergot alkaloids produce prolonged sustained contractions. Although the nonpregnant uterus is sensitive to ergot alkaloids, as is the case with other uterine contractile agents, the sensitivity of the uterus becomes increased during pregnancy.[r8]

Ergonovine and its derivative, methylergonovine, are the most commonly used ergot alkaloids (see Table 11.1). Because of their ability to produce a prolonged, sustained contraction of the uterus, particularly when uterine sensitivity is increased as pregnancy progresses, the ergot alkaloids are not used to induce labor. However, they are useful in treating the postpartum hemorrhage that results from uterine atony by producing a sustained uterine contraction that causes mechanical compression of the uterine vasculature and thereby prevents bleeding. In addition, when involution of the uterus following delivery is delayed because of uterine atony, ergonovine or methylergonovine can be used to initiate this process.

Uterine-Relaxing (Tocolytic) Drugs

β_2-Adrenoceptor Agonists

The myometrium contains β-adrenoceptors, which when activated produce relaxation of uterine smooth muscle by reducing the frequency and amplitude of spontaneous activity and by inhibiting the actively induced contractile responses to prostaglandins and oxytocin. β_2-Adrenoceptors mediate uterine relaxation. There is little or no evidence for relaxation induced by β_1-adrenoceptors, even though β_1-adrenoceptors exist in the uterus in significant numbers. Activation of myometrial β_2-adrenoceptors stimulates adenylate cyclase to increase intracellular cAMP concentrations, which promote the uptake of intracellular calcium by the sarcoplasmic reticulum and activate cAMP-dependent protein kinase. The activation of cAMP-dependent protein kinase leads to the phosphorylation of myosin light-chain kinase, leading to its inhibition.[10,r10,r2] The resulting reduction in intracellular calcium concentration and inhibition of myosin light-chain kinase produces smooth muscle relaxation in the uterus.

The pharmacologic properties of β_2-adrenoceptor agonists makes them suitable for use as tocolytic agents (see Table 11.1). The most commonly used β_2-adrenoceptor agonists for this purpose are ritodrine, fenoterol, albuterol, and terbutaline. The major use of tocolytic agents is to delay or prevent premature delivery when nonpharmacologic means are inadequate and when the risk of pharmacologic prolongation of gestation is less than that of premature delivery of an immature fetus.[r11] In addition, tocolytic agents used to slow labor temporarily or to stop it to allow other therapeutic procedures to be performed.

Calcium Channel Blockers

Calcium channel blockers can be divided into two major classes: inorganic (e.g., magnesium salts); and organic, (e.g., 1,4-dihydropyridines). Magnesium ions act as inorganic calcium channel blockers by entering, but not passing through, voltage-operated calcium channels; whereas 1,4-dihydropyridines reduce the probability of opening of voltage-operated calcium channels. Thus, magnesium salts and 1,4-dihydropyridines inhibit the entry of calcium into uterine smooth muscle cells that occurs during spike discharge activity. Because the calcium that produces uterine smooth muscle contraction is derived from the sarcoplasmic reticulum, and because this is regulated by the amount of calcium that enters the cell during the action potentials that constitute the spike discharges (see above), inhibition of extracellular calcium influx by both magnesium salts or 1,4-dihydropyridines results in relaxation of uterine smooth muscle. However, since the pacemaker potentials that give rise to the electrical activity and subsequent contractile response in uterine smooth muscle are not mediated by the voltage-operated calcium channels, calcium channel blockers reduce contractile amplitude but do not affect the frequency of uterine contractions.[11]

The most commonly used calcium channel blocker for tocolysis is magnesium sulfate. A dose higher than that used for the prevention of the seizures associated with eclampsia and severe preeclampsia is required to produce a tocolytic response. However, magnesium sulfate is effective in the treatment of preterm labor, and is associated with fewer side-effects than produced by β_2-adrenoceptor agonists.[12] The use of 1,4-dihydropyridines as tocolytic agents is still experimental, with nifedipine, nitrendipine, and nicardipine being the most commonly studied.

Drugs Affecting Endometrial Function

Steroids

Estrogens

One of the target organs for estrogens is the endometrial lining of the uterus. Other endocrine effects of estrogen are described in Chapter 46. Estrogens cause endometrial hyperplasia and are responsible for the growth of the stratum functionalis that occurs during the menstrual cycle (see above). Following withdrawal of the estrogenic stimulus, the stratum functionalis breaks down, and menstrual bleeding ensues. With threshold doses of estrogen, the stimulus may be sufficient to cause hyperplasia, but insufficient to maintain this response, leading to breakthrough bleeding even in the presence of continued estrogen administration. Because they can produce a hyperplastic response in the endometrium, long-term administration of estrogens to postmenopausal women is associated with a five- to 15-fold increase in the risk of developing endometrial carcinoma.[13] The magnitude of this effect depends on both the dose and duration of treatment. The risk of endometrial carcinoma declines following cessation of estrogen treatment, and is lower when the estrogen is given in low doses in a cyclic fashion or when combined with a progestin. The use of oral contraceptives in premenopausal women is not associated with an increase in endometrial carcinoma. Indeed, such use is associated with a decrease in the incidence of endometrial carcinoma.[14]

The major therapeutic use of estrogens is as oral contraceptives, either alone or in combination with a progestin. Short-term large doses of estrogens are also used as postcoital contraceptives, where their action is to change endometrial structure and function to a state that is inhospitable for implantation and to induce endometrial breakdown following the cessation of the short-term therapy. In addition, dysmenorrhea may be treated with estrogens by inhibiting ovulation. However, NSAIDs are more commonly used in this disorder (see above).

Progestins

Progesterone plays an important role in the control of endometrial function and leads to the development of a secretory endometrium. The abrupt withdrawal of progesterone at the end of the menstrual cycle is responsible for the breakdown of the stratum functionalis, with subsequent menstruation. Although estrogen treatment maintains endometrial integrity, and withdrawal can lead to menstruation, brief progesterone treatment and subsequent withdrawal in the presence of continued estrogen treatment will produce endometrial breakdown and menstruation. Interestingly, one of the genes whose transcription is increased by estrogen treatment is the gene that encodes for the progesterone receptor. Thus, estrogen treatment increases endometrial progesterone receptor density and primes the endometrium for the progesterone that is released from the corpus luteum following ovulation.

The major therapeutic use of progestins is the same as that of the estrogens, namely as oral contraceptives. Although the major mechanism by which oral contraceptives produce their effect is inhibition of release of gonadotropins, LH and FSH, which results in inhibition of follicular development and ovulation, other progestin effects on the endometrium may contribute the over-all contraceptive effect.[r12] Progestins lead to the production of a scant viscous secretion from the endocervical glands that gives rise to an inhospitable environment for the passage of sperm through the cervix into the uterus. Moreover, progestin therapy at sufficient doses over long periods leads to endometrial atrophy. In combination with the progestin-induced inhibition of ovulation, these other effects most likely contribute to the contraceptive efficacy of progestins.

Besides their use as oral contraceptives, progestins can be used in a variety of endometrial disorders.[r12] Dysfunctional uterine bleeding, characterized by prolonged hemorrhage, is most likely due to the continuous action of estrogen, which causes endometrial hyperplasia and angiogenesis, combined with an insufficient amount of progesterone such that the endometrium is incompletely sloughed off and is continually being stimulated by estrogen.[r12] Progestin therapy will cause complete sloughing of the endometrium, even in the presence of continued estrogen (see above); thus, following removal of the stratum functionalis, progestins will cause the severe bleeding to stop. To prevent a recurrence, cyclic progestin therapy may be used to raise the low levels during the secretory phase. A further use of progestins is in endometriosis, which is the development of extra-uterine masses of endometrial tissue. Without treatment, these masses undergo cyclic episodes of bleeding into the abdominal cavity, with subsequent inflammation and pain. Prolonged progestin treatment inhibits menstruation, and thus the concomitant intraabdominal bleeding, leading to atrophy and regression of the endometrial masses. In addition, progestins can be used in dysmenorrhea, either alone or in combination with an estrogen to inhibit ovulation and initiate prompt menstruation. However, as mentioned previously, NSAIDs are more commonly used for this purpose. Another much touted use of progestins has been the prevention of spontaneous abortion. However, in most patients there is little or no evidence of benefit, although in a small subset with a luteal phase defect and deficient secretion of progesterone, progestin treatment in the first trimester may provide benefit and prevent spontaneous abortion.

Antiprogestins

Competitive progesterone receptor antagonists (see Chapter 52) have been developed and studied for a variety of gynecologic and obstetric indications. The most commonly studied compound, and the only currently available antiprogestin, is mifepristone, also known as RU-486.[r12] This compound, a weak partial agonist at the progesterone receptor, like all partial agonists acts as an antagonist of the full agonist, progesterone. When given during the luteal phase of the menstrual cycle, when the endometrium is under the influence of progesterone, mifepristone will elicit a progesterone withdrawal response that induces the breakdown of the endometrium. Additionally, because progesterone is required for the maintenance of the endometrium during pregnancy, administration of mifepristone, usually in combination with prostaglandins, will induce abortion in early pregnancy. Mifepristone is also being studied for the induction of labor after intrauterine fetal death. Withdrawal of progesterone leads to cervical ripening, and mifepristone produces a cervical ripening that will aid its abortifacient actions.[15]

References

Research Reports

1. Huszar G, Roberts JM. Biochemistry and pharmacology of the myometrium and labor: Regulation at the cellular and molecular levels. Am J Obst Gynecol 1982;*142*:225–237.
2. Fuchs AR, Goeschen K, Husslein P, Rasmussen AB, Fuchs F. Oxytocin and the initiation of human parturition. III. Plasma concentrations of oxytocin and 13, 14-dihydro-15-keto-prostaglandin $F_{2\alpha}$ in spontaneous and oxytocin induced labor. Am J Obstet Gynecol 1983;*147*:497–502.
3. Casey ML, Hemsell DL, MacDonald PC, Johnston JM. NAD+-dependent 15-hydroxyprostaglandin dehydrogenase activity in human endometrium. Prostaglandins 1980;*19*:155–118.
4. Casey ML, MacDonald PC. Biomolecular processes in the initiation of parturition: Decidual activation. Clin Obstet Gynecol 1988;*31*:533–540.
5. Behrman HR, Anderson GG. Prostaglandins in reproduction. Arch Int Med 1974;*133*:77–84.
6. Brindley BA, Sokol RJ. Induction and augmentation of labor: Basis and methods for current practice. Obstet Gynecol Surv 1988;*43*:730–743.
7. Moise KJ, Huhta JC, Sharif DS, Ou CN, Kirshon B, Wasserstrum N, Cano L. Indomethacin in the treatment of premature labor N Engl J Med 1988;*319*:327–331.
8. Shapiro SS. Treatment of dysmenorrhea and premenstrual syndrome with nonsteroidal anti-inflammatory drugs. Drugs 1988;*36*:475–490.
9. Hashimoto H, Hayashi M, Nakahara Y, Niwaguchi T, Ishii H. Actions of D-lysergic acid diethylamide (LSD) and its derivatives on 5-hydroxytryptamine receptors in the isolated uterine smooth muscle of the rat. Eur J Pharmacol 1977;*45*:341–348.
10. Carsten ME, Miller JD. A new look at uterine muscle contraction. Am J Obstet Gynecol 1987;*157*:1303–1315.
11. Holbrook RH Jr, Lirette M, Katz M. Cardiovascular and tocolytic effects of nicardipine HCL in the pregnant rabbit: Comparison with ritodrine HCL. Obstet Gynecol 1987;*69*:83–87
12. Thiagarajah S, Harbert GM, Bourgeois FJ. Magnesium sulfate and ritodrine hydrochloride: Systemic and uterine hemodynamic effects. Am J Obstet Gynecol 1985;*153*:666–670.
13. Shapiro S, Kelly JP, Rosenberg L, Kaufman DW, Helmrich SP, Rosenhein NB, Lewis JL, Knapp RC, Stolley PD, Schottenfeld D. Risk of localized and widespread endometrial cancer in relation to recent and discontinued use of conjugated estrogens. N Engl J Med 1985;*313*:969–972.
14. Centers for Disease Control: Combination oral contraceptive use and the risk of endometrial cancer. JAMA 1987;*257*:796–800.
15. Baulieu EE. Contragestation and other clinical applications of RU 486, an antiprogesterone at the receptor. Science 1989;*245*:1351–1357.
16. Senior J, Marshjall K, Sangha R, Baxter GS, Clayton JK. In vitro characterization of prostanoid EP-receptors in the non-pregnant human myometrium. Br J Pharmacol 1991;*102*:747–753.

Reviews

r1. Kao CY. Electrophysiological properties of the uterine smooth muscle. In: Wynn, RM. Biology of the uterus. New York: Plenum Press, 1977, pp 423–496.

r2. van Breemen C, Saida K. Cellular mechanisms regulating [Ca^{2+}]i in smooth muscle. Ann Rev Physiol 1989;*51*:315–329.

r3. Hai CM, Murphy RA. Ca^{2+}, crossbridge phosphorylation, and contraction. Ann Rev Physiol 1989;*51*:285–298.

r4. Garfield RE. Structural and functional studies of the control of myometrial contractility and labor. In: McNellis D, Challis JRG, MacDonald PC, Nathanielsz P, Roberts J. Cellular and integrative mechanisms in the onset of labor. Ithaca: Perinatology Press, (1988); pp 55–78.

r5. Marshall JM. Vertebrate smooth muscle. In: Mountcastle VB. Medical physiology 14th ed. St Louis: CV Mosby, 1980, pp 120–148.

r6. Goodman HM. Reproduction. In: Mountcastle VB. Medical physiology, 14th ed. St Louis: CV Mosby, 1980, pp 1602–1637.

r7. Soloff MS, Fuchs AR, Fuchs F. Oxytocin receptors and the onset of parturition. In: Albrecht E, Research in perinatal medicine, Vol 4, Pepe GJ. Ithaca: Perinatology Press, (1985); pp 289–311.

r8. Rall TW. Drugs affecting uterine motility. In: Gilman AG, Rall TW, Nies AS, Taylor P. Goodman and Gilman's Pharmacological Basis of Therapeutics, 8th ed. New York: Pergamon Press, (1990); pp 933–953.

r9. Berde B, Stümer E. Introduction to the pharmacology of the ergot alkaloids and related compounds as a basis of their therapeutic applications. In: Berde B, Schild HO. Handbook of experimental pharmacology, Vol 49, Berlin: Springer-Verlag, (1978); pp 1–28.

r10. Kamm KE, Stull JT. Regulation of smooth muscle contractile elements by second messengers. Ann Rev Physiol 1989;*51*:299–313.

r11. Creasy RK, Resnik R. Maternal fetal medicine: Principles and practice. Philadelphia: WB Saunders, 1984.

r12. Murad F, Kuret JA. Estrogens and progestins. In: Gilman AG, Rall TW, Nies AS, Taylor P. Goodman and Gilman's Pharmacological Basis of Therapeutics, 8th ed, New York: Pergamon Press, (1990); pp 1384–1412.

r13. Halushka PV, Mais DE, Mayeux PR, Morinelli TA. Thromboxane, prostaglandin and leukotriene receptors. Ann Rev Pharmacol Toxicol 1989;*29*:213–219.

SECTION III

Central Neuropharmacology

Section Editor:
Fridolin Sulser

Associate Editor:
George Breese

CHAPTER 12

Relationship of Drugs Acting on the Central Nervous System to Neurotransmission

George R. Breese
Robert A. Mueller

Drugs that act to influence brain function have long been essential to medical practice. Because of the importance of brain to normal physiologic and psychologic function, the actions of centrally acting drugs are diverse. Drugs acting on the CNS can induce anesthesia, relieve pain and fever, prevent or modify seizures, induce sleep, reduce anxiety, and ameliorate symptoms of major mental illness. The positive aspects of centrally active drugs must be tempered by the fact that the functional consequences of these drugs can lead to abuse and physical or psychologic dependence, with many social implications that extend from the individual to national priorities of health care and law enforcement.

Scientists who study how drugs alter CNS function are known as neuropharmacologists, neuropsychopharmacologists, or simply neuroscientists. The ever-increasing knowledge of neural mechanisms and molecular processes that control brain function no doubt will have a synergistic effect on the over-all knowledge available concerning drug actions on brain. As distinct molecular actions of centrally-acting drugs are understood, our understanding of brain function will increase. Furthermore, drugs continue to be used as specific molecular probes to understand pathophysiologic mechanisms associated with central malfunctions in various central disorders.

The purpose of the present chapter is to provide a background on fundamental mechanisms responsible for neural transmission within the CNS in order to provide a basis for understanding the many mechanisms by which centrally acting drugs influence brain function. Included in this summary will be fundamental knowledge about central neurotransmitters, the receptor systems on which these endogenous compounds act, and the cellular components that allow the receptive cell to change its functions.

One aspect of drug action was the discovery that drugs have great specificity for sites, which are referred to as receptors. This term was originally coined to explain the action of drugs on biologic systems, because at that time there was little known about the biology of sites where drugs acted (see Chapter 1 for additional historical perspective). Regardless, the mathematical description of these receptive sites allowed predictions about dosage and potency. As will become apparent later, it was discovered subsequently that receptor sites had specificity for second messenger systems that provided a communication with other cellular events. While originally related to events postsynaptic to nerve terminals, concepts concerning receptors have no bounds in relation to neural structure. Receptors can be found on presynaptic terminals, postsynaptic membranes, intracellularly on organelles, and even on the nucleus. Recent work identifying the structures of proteins that make up receptors has led to the realization that receptors belong to large families of proteins that are modified to respond to specific neurotransmitters and whose structures predict second messenger responses. The activation of second messenger systems also can influence neural mechanisms that lead to formation of compounds that act on the nucleus to influence other cellular events or of chemicals that act on distinct neural systems by diffusing to other sites.

To understand the material in this chapter, the reader is assumed to be conversant with neurophysiology, neurochemistry, and neuroanatomy. The focus here will be the review of principles of biochemistry, physiology, and anatomy useful in explaining the sites and mechanisms of action of drugs effective in altering CNS function. The reader is referred to several excellent textbooks on neurophysiology, neurochemistry, and neuroanatomy to explain in more detail the concepts to be discussed.[r1–r6,1,2,3] Cells within the CNS are present in an almost infinite variety of form; their metabolism and the neurotransmitters within these neurons are just as diverse. A diagram applicable to many cells within CNS cells is provided to illustrate their general functional components (Fig. 12.1).

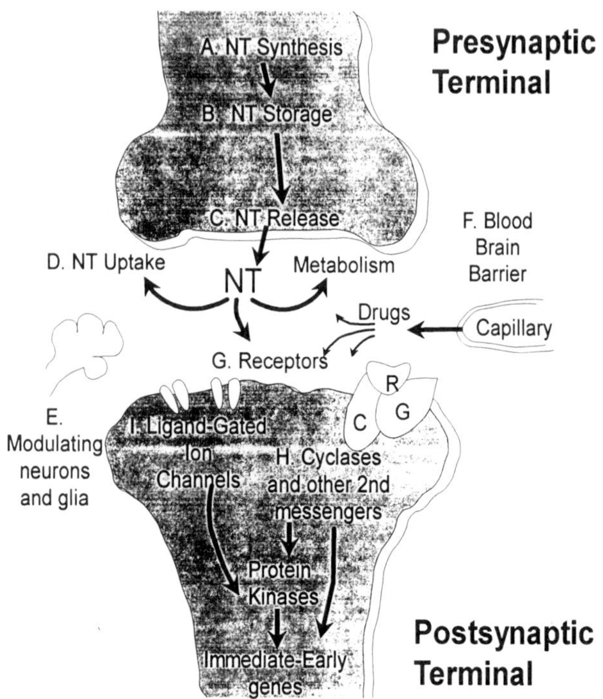

Figure 12.1 Example of drug interdiction of synaptic transmission in brain. As this diagram depicts, there are numerous mechanisms associated with pre and postsynaptic neurons that can be disturbed by drugs. As noted in the text, there are some drugs which are believed to affect neural membranes in nonspecific ways, but nonetheless, disturb synaptic function. Such drugs include local anesthetics, anesthetics, and ethanol. In spite of this belief, data are being collected that suggest greater specificity of these drugs than once believed. The best example to date is the specificity of ethanol to alter ligand-gated ion channel function.[8] **[Site A]** depicts the specific enzymes which are responsible for the synthesis of each neurotransmitter. There can be more than one neurotransmitter within a single neuron. **[Site B]** denotes the storage of neurotransmitters within vesicles. As noted in the text "False Transmitters" can be stored in these vesicles.[r12] These vesicles also contain specific uptake sites that can be affected by drugs. **[Site C]** illustrates the release of neurotransmitters. **[Site D]** is the site whereby neurotransmitter can be pumped back into the neuron after release to allow termination of the action of the neurotransmitter. Several drug classes have this capability. **[Site E]** illustrates the involvement of glia and modulatory neurons on function. Some drugs are believed to affect the synthesis of compounds elaborated from glia. **[Site F]** is the blood system that delivers the drug to brain. This delivery seems to depend on the physical-chemical properties of the drug. **[Site G]** depicts the receptive site for neurotransmitters on postsynaptic membranes that alter activity of this neuron. These receptive area are called receptors. Drugs which attach to this site without an agonist action can antagonize the action of the neurotransmitter. **[Site H]** indicates that the receptors are linked to second messenger systems like adenylate cyclase and phosphoinositol **[Site I]** illustrates a second kind of receptor that is linked to ion channels and are referred to as ligand-gated ion channels. Specific channels are depicted. As noted in Fig. 12.2, we also note that downstream mechanisms are operative that affect a variety of proteins involved in appropriate neural function (see p. 217).

Ionic Equilibrium

The neurons in the brain are different from most cells in the body in that they maintain one of the greatest negative resting membrane potentials, reflecting an enhanced cellular dedication of energy resources toward maintaining an excitable responsive state, which provides a vulnerable site at which drugs may act. Any drugs that alter cell threshold for depolarization, such as general or local anesthetics, usually produce dramatic effects in those cells with a high resting membrane potential. For this reason, the CNS and peripheral nervous system are depressed significantly by such drugs before function of other organ systems is altered. The major exception to this generalization is the heart, where specialized conducting (Purkinje) and ventricular cells also have a large membrane potential (see section on autonomic function and Chapters 23 and 25). Some compounds such as local anesthetics (e.g., lidocaine) are used both as antiarrhythmics in the heart and to produce regional or local anesthesia in nervous tissue because of their activity to inhibit sodium channel conductance (see Chapters 10 and 25). Other drugs such as phenytoin were initially used as anti-seizure medications, but have subsequently proved valuable in the management of cardiac dysrhythmias (depressing cardiac excitability). Some drugs thought of as cardiovascular drugs, such as digitalis glycosides, have a high incidence of CNS side-effects. Cardiac glycosides interfere primarily with cardiac sodium potassium ATPase linked to the sodium pump, thereby reducing resting membrane potential (less negative) and increasing the frequency of premature depolarization in the heart. In the CNS, similar alterations in membrane potential produce the central side-effects usually thought of as "toxic" events of the digitalis glycosides, since slightly higher doses are required. Similarly, Class I cardiac antiarrhythmics are potent sodium channel blockers; thus, side-effects often include CNS changes in function. Though drugs that are very potent inhibitors of sodium channels (e.g., local anesthetics, antiarrhythmics, and anti-seizure medications) are widely known and under constant development, drugs that interfere with potassium channels in these tissues have only recently appeared and have yet to gain clinical acceptance.

Perhaps the most widely utilized divalent ion channel susceptible to drug intervention is the calcium channel (see I in Fig. 12.1). Though calcium plays an important role in both CNS postsynaptic membrane function and in neurotransmitter secretion from presynaptic terminals, most calcium antagonist drugs used clinically are potent inhibitors of calcium translocation used in dysfunctions of the heart and vasculature. Such drugs produce few side-effects in the CNS, even though they may be of use in preventing calcium accumulation in neural cells after ischemic insults.[1] The reason for this selectivity is dependent on CNS calcium channels having different structural characteristics and, consequently, being less perturbed by these drugs.[2] It is becoming increasingly apparent that multiple receptor systems of different neurotransmitters in brain produce their responses by indirectly altering calcium channel activity (e.g., altering membrane potential or threshold), not by directly affecting the channel itself. Nevertheless, the increasing knowledge that voltage-sensitive calcium channels have differing protein structures provides considerable latitude for the development of drugs with specific effects on those calcium channel receptor subtypes in the CNS.[3] Recently, the glutamate receptor subtype acted on by N-methyl-d-aspartic acid (NMDA) has been cloned.[4] This receptor directly controls a calcium channel.[5]

The second major divalent ion, magnesium, has a much wider application in CNS disorders. Magnesium salts are very potent inhibitors of CNS excitability as well as of peripheral neuromuscular transmission. Thus, magnesium sulfate is still commonly used in conditions such as toxemia of pregnancy where seizures and hypertension are highly visible CNS manifestations. Besides the direct depressant effect of magnesium on cellular function with increasing extracellular concentrations, there also is evidence that an increase in intracellular magnesium may modulate or decrease the functional activity of any calcium channel pores that may have been opened in the course of normal function or in pathologic states, such as ischemia or hypoxia.[6] As ischemia develops in cells and ATP values decrease, ionized magnesium increases. Furthermore, magnesium may be an important endogenous calcium channel blocker. In this regard, magnesium can prevent the action of glutamate on NMDA receptors by modulating the function of this receptor, which has important actions to increase calcium flux in ischemia.[5,6]

Turning to the anions, which are differentially localized across the cell membrane as a result of normal membrane function, the most important pharmacologic target concerns drugs that change chloride ion flux across the membrane (see I in Fig. 12.1). The chloride pore or channel is closely linked to the normal endogenous transmitters gamma-aminobutyric acid (GABA) and glycine.[r3] The action of CNS depressant drug groups such as the benzodiazepines, barbiturates, central steroids, and ethanol are closely associated with receptor proteins forming the chloride channel specifically recognized by GABA ([7,8]; see Chapter 14 for more details about Drugs Acting on the GABA receptor). Opening of the chloride pore by GABA or administration of the synthetic compounds acting on this receptor produces a hyperpolarization of the membrane as chloride enters from the higher extracellular concentration, which in turn reduces further the membrane potential and the excitability of the cell. In contrast to the case of calcium, most of the drugs that alter chloride flux are active in the CNS. Only at higher doses do these drugs change chloride flux of peripheral cells, because these chloride channels are not responsive to GABA (see section on structure of receptors). Glycine receptors are also associated with chloride flux, resulting in an inhibition of cellular function,[9] but presently there are no useful therapeutic agents associated with glycine receptor function. However, strychnine, a convulsant, antagonizes the action of glycine, and alcohol is known to enhance some but not all responses to this neurotransmitter.[8] Another receptor that controls ion channels is the nicotinic cholinergic receptor (see Chapters 5 and 7). Within the CNS, the function of the nicotinic cholinergic receptor is complex and depends on different peptide components forming the receptor subtypes than used for the peripheral nicotinic receptor.

Neurotransmitter Synthesis and Metabolism

The normal synthesis of a neurotransmitter usually begins with the availability of a metabolic precursor (e.g., amino acids for catecholamines, acetate and choline for acetylcholine, etc.), but the enzymes required to produce neurotransmitters from these precursor molecules are limited to neuronal or, similarly, neuronal crest-derived tissues (e.g., adrenal medulla, chromaffin cells; see A and B, Fig. 12.1). Enzymes relevant to various neurotransmitters are listed in Table 12.1. There are now drugs that interfere with the synthesis of transmitters made in the terminal regions of the neuron (see Table 12.2). For example, the drug alpha-methyl tyrosine binds very strongly to the enzyme tyrosine hydroxylase, the first enzyme required to synthesize dopamine and norepinephrine. Since this drug is a poor substrate for this enzyme, it competes for tyrosine, resulting in a functional inhibition of catecholamine synthesis.[r7] Another drug interfering with neurotransmitter synthesis is p-chlorophenylalanine.[10] This drug binds to the enzyme tryptophan hydroxylase, which is specific for synthesis of the immediate precursor for serotonin[10] (Table 12.2).

For neurotransmission to be effective, the brain must possess mechanisms for terminating the presence of transmitter as well as for providing for its synthesis, secretion, and postsynaptic perception. Some neurotransmitters, such as norepinephrine, are effectively reaccumulated into the presynaptic cell via neurotransmitter transport proteins,[11] as discussed elsewhere for the peripheral nervous system (see Chapter 6). Perhaps no neuron is more efficient at this function than the norepinephrine-containing neurons within the CNS, where over 90 percent of released transmitter is believed to be reaccumulated into the presynaptic nerve terminal and can thus again participate in transmitter release (see D in Fig. 12.1). However, this uptake mechanism is also common to other monoamine-containing neurons, such as dopamine- and serotonin-containing fibers.[12,13] It can be expected that the structure of the various transporters for neurotransmitters and their precursor amino acids will be determined in the near future by molecular biologic approaches (see Table 12.2). Drugs that inhibit reuptake of monoamines, such as selected antidepressants, increase the local amount of transmitter (e.g., norepinephrine or serotonin) available for combining with receptor proteins on postsynaptic neurons (see Chapter 17). Subsequently, the increased availability of these neurotransmitters triggers postsynaptic receptors to down-regulate (i.e., decrease their number). This is one mechanism proposed to account for the therapeutic effect of this class of drugs (see Chapter 17). The specificity of these transporters led to the discovery of neurotoxins that could be used to cause destruction of specific monoamine-containing neurons.[r8]

Table 12.1 lists enzymes involved in the metabolism of various neurotransmitters. Metabolism of catecholamines is in large part via catechol-O-methylation by an enzyme called catechol-O-methyltransferase.[r9] In addition, released monoamines are metabolized via oxidative deamination by an enzyme monoamine oxidase (MAO). Inhibition of this enzyme by MAO inhibitors permits larger amounts of transmitter to remain in the extracelluar space for a longer time, thus initially magnifying the behavioral effects associated with stimulation of norepinephrine, serotonin, or dopamine, but later causing down-regulation of monoamine receptors (see Chapter 17). It is the actions of MAO inhibitors that are believed to be responsible for their ability to

Table 12.1 Brain Enzymes Associated with Neurotransmitter Metabolism

Neurotransmitter System	Synthesis Enzymes	Metabolism Enzymes
Norepinephine	Tyrosine hydroxylase DOPA decarboxylase Dopamine-β-hydroxylase	MAO[†] COMT[†]
Serotonin	Tryptophan hydroxylase 5-HTP Decarboxylase	MAO[†]
Dopamine	Tyrosine hydroxylase DOPA decarboxylase	MAO[†] COMT
Acetylcholine	Choline acetyltransferase	Choline esterases
Glycine	Serine hydroxymethylase	Glycine oxidase
GABA	Glutamic acid decarboxylase	GABA transaminase
Glutamate	Aspartate aminotransferase; Gutaminase; Ornithine-amino transferase*	Amino acid Acetyltransferase[+]
Neuropeptides	Synthesized from mRNA[#]	Peptidases

[†]MAO = Monoamine oxidase; COMT = catechol-o-methyl transferase.
[+]Uptake may be more important for termination than metabolism of glutamate.
*Specific enzyme responsible for glutamate synthesis has not been determined. Glutamate may come from the activity of all these enzymes.
[#]Generally neuropeptides are synthesized in a form that there are repeats within a pro-protein that can be "cut" to provide the neuropeptide. Detailed information on the general metabolism of such a protein has been described for pro-opiomelanocortin, proenkephalin, and prodynorphin.[73-75]

Table 12.2 Drugs Inhibiting Synthesis and Metabolism of Neurotransmitters

Neurotransmitter	Synthesis Inhibitor	Metabolism Inhibitor	Reuptake Inhibitor
Norepinephrine	α-methyltyrosine Decarboxylase inhibitor	MAO inhibitors U-14624†	Tricyclic ADs+ Nisoxetine, Cocaine
Dopamine	α-methyltyrosine Decarboxylase inhibitor	MAOI	GBR-12935 Cocaine WIN-35428
Serotonin	p-Chlorophenylalanine Decarboxylase inhibitor	MAO inhibitors	Fluoxetine Citalopram Paroxetine
Acetylcholine	Hemicholinium*	Cholinesterase inhibitors	Hemocholinium*
Glycine	—	—	Transporter Cloned#
γ-Aminobutyric acid (GABA)	Allylglycine	Amino-oxyacetic acid	Nipecotic Acid
Enkephalin	GEMSA**	Thiorphan	—

+Tricyclic ADs = tricyclic antidepressants.
*Inhibition of choline uptake by hemocholinium blocks acetylcholine synthesis.
#No drugs known that specifically antagonize transporter cloned (see reference[76]).
**GEMSA = quanidinoethylmercaptosuccinic acid (see reference[77]).
†U-14624 in a dopamine-β-hydroxylase inhibitor.

antagonize depressed states[r10] or ameliorate Parkinson's disease symptoms.[14] With cholinergic neurons, inhibition of destruction of acetylcholine by cholinesterase inhibitors may be therapeutic by increasing synaptic concentrations of acetylcholine for longer periods once presynaptic release occurs (e.g., myasthenia gravis, antagonism of competitive nondepolarizing neuromuscular blockade, and in Alzheimer's disease). Indeed, organophosphorus insecticides, which are irreversible cholinesterase inhibitors, can produce such a massive accumulation of acetylcholine that postsynaptic cells are overstimulated, impairing function and causing death by asphyxia if symptoms are not treated (see Chapter 5). Thus, drugs that affect termination of action of neurotransmitters can produce profound changes in CNS function. Table 12.2 provides examples of drugs that interfere with metabolism of selected neurotransmitters.

Altered Presynaptic Release of Neurotransmitters

The ability of presynaptic nerve impulses to alter the release of neurotransmitter stored in the presynaptic terminals is another point for pharmacologic manipulation (see B and C in Fig. 12.1). For example, a drug such as reserpine depletes the normal storage of monoamines in the dense-core vesicles of monoamine-containing neurons in brain by inhibiting uptake and retention of monoamines into these vesicles.[r11,15] Even though vesicles remain, they are not filled with transmitter, and this deficiency of a normal complement of neurotransmitter released per depolarization inhibits neurotransmission.

Some drugs can displace or release transmitter from presynaptic stores without depolarization of the nerve. Amphetamine, a central stimulant, may owe some of its CNS activation properties to its ability to release vesicular dopamine into the interstitial space by this mechanism.[16] Similarly, in patients given a monoamine oxidase inhibitor, dietary tyramine found in cheese and red wine can accumulate to very high levels and displace norepinephrine from the postganglionic sympathetic neurons. The released norepinephrine acts on adrenergic receptors of the heart (beta receptors) and vasculature (alpha receptors), and this may produce tachycardia and hypertension of dangerous proportions (see Chapter 17 for details).

Some drugs may act as "false transmitters" by utilizing the synthetic and storage capacity of one neuron to permit release of a false transmitter. For example, levodopa, a drug used to treat Parkinson's disease, can enter the presynaptic nerve terminals of serotonergic neurons of the basal ganglia after dopamine-containing neurons have been lost.[17] After decarboxylation of the levodopa to dopamine, the release onto dopamine receptors may restore the deficiency in motor function caused by the initial destruction of the dopamine-containing neurons in Parkinson's disease. Other drugs not normally present in the body, such as alpha-methyldopa, are similarly metabolized by decarboxylation to produce a "false neurotransmitter," alpha-methyl dopamine, which can in turn be metabolized to alpha-methyl norepinephrine.[r12] Release of these unnatural false neurotransmitters in the peripheral nervous system or CNS produces altered responses relative to a similar amount of the appropriate endogenous catecholamine. Thus, alpha-methyldopa by interfering with noradrenergic function has found a place in the clinical management of hypertension (see Chapter 26). Likewise, this specific drug by interfering with dopamine function can precipitate severe motor dysfunction in Parkinson's patients (see Chapter 18).

Receptors for the released transmitter found on presynaptic terminals of neurons have been referred to as autoreceptors.[r13,18] These presynaptic receptors provide a mechanism by which neurotransmitters alter the efficiency of their own release from intracellular stores. The presumed function of these receptors is to modulate or prevent the uncontrolled release of the neurotransmitter, since activation of these autoreceptors retards subsequent release of depolarization-induced transmitter. Many of these presynaptic autoreceptors for the released neurotransmitter have been found to be a receptor subtype similar to that found postsynaptically. For example, synthetic agonists for the alpha-2-noradrenergic receptors serve to inhibit both peripheral and central norepinephrine release.[r13] Such agents are effective at inhibiting release and can be used as antihypertensive drugs (e.g., clonidine). If these autoreceptors are blocked with a receptor antagonist, however, release of the neurotransmitter is enhanced. Such enhanced release of dopamine is observed when antischizophrenic drugs are administered, because these agents block the dopamine presynaptic autoreceptor.[19] Although decreased dopamine receptor activation postsynaptically in the cerebral cortex may explain the antischizophrenic potency of the drugs and some Parkinson-like symptoms, enhanced release of dopamine within basal ganglia areas may be responsible for the dyskinetic side-effects of this drug class. Recently, drugs have been found that inhibit release of glutamate, but a specific mechanism has not been attributed to this action.[22]

Table 12.3 Coexistence of Neurotransmitters in Neurons*

Neurotransmitter 1	Neurotransmitter 2
Serotonin	TRH, Substance P, GABA
Norepinephrine	Neuropeptide Y, Enkephalin, Vasopressin
Dopamine	Cholecystokinin, Neurotensin, GABA
Acetylcholine	Galanin, VIP, Substance P, GABA
GABA	Dynorphin, Substance P, Glycine
Glutamate	Substance P, Epinephrine

*This listing is not exhaustive. TRH, Thyrotropin-releasing hormone; VIP, vasoactive intestinal peptide. The cloning of the various peptides associated with the opioid receptors as well as other peptides has allowed their distribution to be determined in brain.[73-75] See references[21,22,r14,r15] for additional information in this area.

Corelease of Transmitters

It is now apparent that many neurons in brain contain not one but several different chemicals[r14-r16,21,22] that may alter postsynaptic cell activity, sometimes in different ways. This is illustrated by B and C in Fig. 12.1. For example, some norepinephrine-containing neurons contain a peptide that has a high content of the amino acid tyrosine (termed Y in amino acid shorthand); thus, the peptide was named "neuropeptide Y." This peptide is released with norepinephrine and produces postsynaptic cell effects much like those previously ascribed to alpha-noradrenergic receptors.[24] While the norepinephrine released will activate both alpha and beta-noradrenergic receptors, neuropeptide Y is also neurally active. Since the peptide is not reused (as is norepinephrine) by the presynaptic neuron, its relative effects will fade with repeated stimulation. In this regard, if alpha-noradrenergic antagonists are given via the blood, alpha-noradrenergic-like activity due to nerve stimulation will be prevented, but the action of neuropeptide Y will not be antagonized. Rather, the apparent degree of disruption of transmission will vary, depending on the local importance of neuropeptide Y in normal neurotransmission dynamics. With the knowledge that neurotransmitters are co-localized in brain it can be assumed that similar processes between peptides and classic neurotransmitters occur in brain, as has been demonstrated in the peripheral nerves; but little is known about the consequences of this co-localization. A summary of known neurotransmitters that co-localize in neurons in brain is presented in Table 12.3. As more is known about the function of neurotransmitters co-localized within the CNS, therapy of central disorders may be improved.

Membrane Receptor Mechanisms

Focus will now shift from a concern of drug activity on presynaptic membrane components and specific ion permeability changes to those functional sites found primarily on the postsynaptic membrane surface (see G in Fig. 12.1 and Fig. 12.2). These sites are referred to as postsynaptic receptors and in some cases can be observed by electron microscopy as well-defined anatomic structures. Furthermore, the proteins making up these receptors have a high affinity for endogenous neurotransmitters. Exogenous drug agonists and antagonists have been designed specifically to bypass the presynaptic innervation and combine with these receptors to alter their intended function. Based on the variable action of structural analogues of the endogenous transmitters, it was postulated that there were different receptors for the same transmitter. The first example related to this phenomenon was the discovery that acetylcholine acted in distinctly different ways in specific regions of the peripheral nervous system in the presence of certain receptor agonist and antagonist drugs (see Chapter 4). There were sites activated by nicotine that were referred to as nicotinic cholinergic receptors (see Chapters 4 and 5). In addition, there were sites with acetylcholine receptors that gave responses that resembled the action of the alkaloid muscarine, which led to these receptors being called muscarinic cholinergic receptors (see Chapters 4 and 5). This concept of multiple receptors for a given neurotransmitter has been fully confirmed in recent years for all known neurotransmitters, with the number of subtypes progressively increasing as our knowledge of specific receptor structure has increased.

Specific examples of the classification of receptor subtypes for selected classic neurotransmitters are listed in Tables 12.4 and 12.5. Initial classification of these neurotransmitters was based on pharmacologic results as well as the binding of radiolabeled ligands to these particular sites.[r18] Dozens of specific receptor proteins have now been sequenced, their genes cloned,[24–29] and expressed in model systems (e.g., transfected cells) that permit careful study of their properties and further classification of subtypes for each of the neurotransmit-

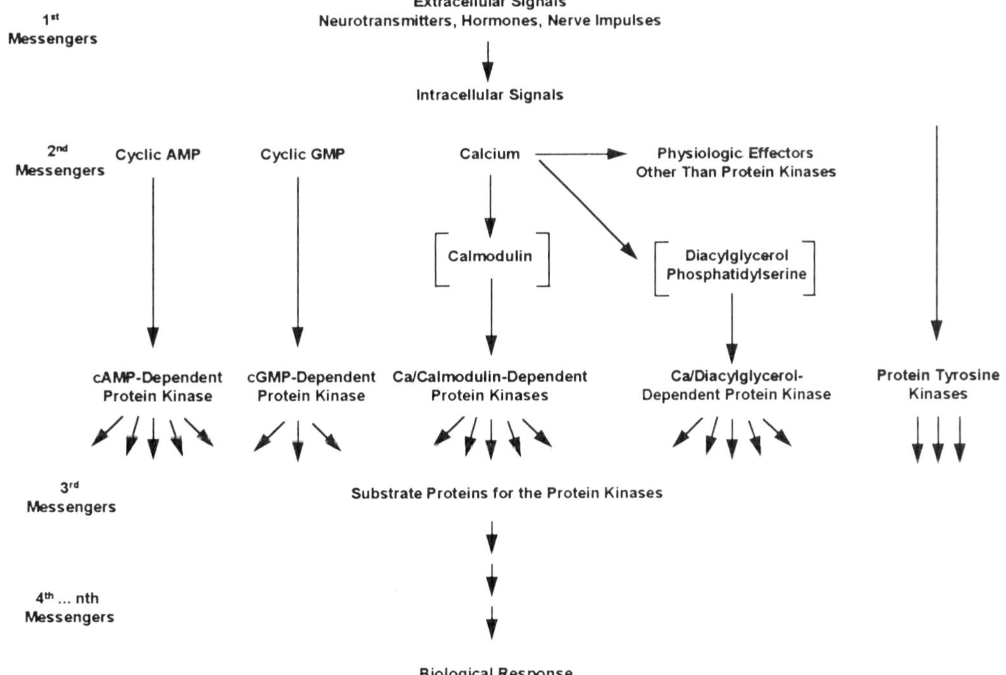

Figure 12.2 Scheme for various transduction pathways. Compounds that activate specific receptors on the cell surface cause changes in second messenger systems which include cyclic AMP, cyclic GMP and calcium. The cyclic nucleotides activate cAMP- and cGMP-dependent protein kinases. Calcium flux caused by neural translocation exerts its actions on calmodulin-dependent protein kinases which includes phosphorylase kinase, myosin kinase, calmodulin-dependent protein kinases I, II, and III. These protein kinases in turn affect the activity of other proteins which affect cellular function. In addition, there are tyrosine kinases in brain which have important actions. Calcium also acts to facilitate the formation of diacylglycerol which activates other protein kinases. Intense research is underway to understand the biological significance of each of the protein kinases for normal cellular function. Illustration adopted from Nestler and Greengard.[r28]

Table 12.4 Neurotransmitter Receptor Subtypes Associated with G-Proteins

Transmitter	Receptor Subtypes	Agonists	Antagonists
Norepinephrine	α1	Phenylephrine	Prazosin
	α2[#]	Clonidine	Yohimbine, Idazoxan
	β1	Isoproterenol	Practolol, Metoprolol
	β2	Isoproburenol Terbutaline	IPS 339
Dopamine	D_1[##]	SKF-38393	SCH-39166, SCH-23390
	D_2	Quinpirole	Sulpiride
	D_3	Quinpirole (NS); Trans-7-OH-PIPAT***	(+) Butaclamol
	D_4	Quinpirole (NS); CP-96501	Clozapine
Serotonin	$5HT_{1A}$	8-OH-DPAT	WB-4101, MDL-72832
	1B	RU-24969	Metergoline (NS)
	1C	—	Mianserin (NS); Mesulergine (NS)
	1D	5-methoxytryptamine	Metergoline (NS)
	$5\text{-}HT_2$	DOB	Ketanserin* (NS)
	Others[+]		
Acetylcholine	M1	MN-343	Pirenzepine
	M2	—	Methoctramine AFDX-116
	M3	—	Hexahydro-siladifendol
	M4	—	—
	M5	—	—
GABA	$GABA_B$	Baclophen	Phaclophen
Glutamate	Metabotropic	Quisqualate, ACPD** Ibotenate	—

NS = Not Specific ; [–] = compounds not known with this specificity.
[#]Known that two forms of receptor exist, an α2a agonist is guanfacine, while clonidine has greater but not absolute specificity for α2b. Rauwolscine appears to have greater action on α2b, whereas idazoxan blocks both α2 subtypes.
[##]A receptor referred to as D_5 receptor is a receptor with properties of a D_1 receptor (see references[79,80]).
*Has effects on α noradrenergic receptor.
[+]A variety of other serotonin receptor subtypes have now been cloned (see reference[39]).
**ACPD=aminocyclopentane- 1,3-dicarboxylate.
***Trans-7-OH-PIPAT-A = (R_1S) trans-7-hydroxy-2-(N-n-propyl-N-3'-iodo-2' propenyl) amino tetralin.[81]

ters. This latter process not only confirmed earlier predictions made from the pharmacologic and binding studies, but also revealed many closely related receptor subtypes not previously recognized.[r16] This list no doubt will grow as other neurotransmitter receptor related structures are defined. For example, the opioid receptor has recently been cloned—the first for this drug class of receptors, as have the adenosine receptors.[30–32] This no doubt will lead to the molecular characterization of other receptor subtypes known to exist for this group of receptors. The cannabinoid receptor has also been cloned and found to be widely localized in brain.[33,34] This seminal discovery then led to the discovery that an arachidonic acid derivative appears to be the endogenous ligand for this receptor.[34]

An additional group of specific cell surface receptors important to neural function are those that mediate the actions of neurotrophins.[r17] There appear to be two components for proper function of these receptors. The low affinity receptor is a glycoprotein that binds the known neurotrophins.[35,r17] In addition, there is a high-affinity binding site for these substances associated with a protein that has the tyrosine kinase (TRK) activity essential for proper function of the neurotrophin receptor.[36] It is now apparent that there is a family of these TRK proteins that relates to specific neurotrophins.[37] Since these receptors are expressed in developing as well as adult brain, it presumed that the neurotrophins are not only important to growth of neurons during ontogeny, but also play an important role in the maintenance of mature neurons.

Comparison of the receptor structures for various neurotransmitters show apparent homology.[38,39] This likely accounts for the fact that many drugs developed primarily for one receptor type may influence receptors of other types, particularly when administered at higher doses. A future challenge will be to apply this new knowledge about the structure of the recep-

Table 12.5 Receptors for the Superfamily of Ligand-gated Ion Channels

Neurotransmitter	Subunits*	Agonists	Antagonists
$GABA_A$	α1-6; β1-3 γ1-3; Delta	Muscimol Chlordiazepoxide Zolpidem	Bicuculline Picrotoxin Flumazenil
Glutamate Subtypes**			
Kainate	KA-1 & KA-2	AMPA	NBQX
Kainate-AMPA	GLUR 1–4	Kainate, AMPA	CNQX
AMPA	GLUR 5–7	—	MK-801,CGS-19755⁺
NMDA	NMDAR-1; NMDAR1a,b,c,d	NMDA	
Nicotinic Cholinergic	α2–7 β2–5	Nicotine	n-Bungarotoxin Mecamylamine
Glycine	α1–3 β	Glycine	Strychnine
$5\text{-}HT_3$	1 Clone	2-Methy-Serotonin 1-Phenyl-Biguanide	MDL-72222 ICS-205-903 LY-278584 GR-65630

*Evidence indicates that homology is found in the M II transmembrane for each subunit and that multiple subunits combine in a pentameric structure (see general reading for other details).
⁺NMDA receptor can be antagonized by drugs blocking a glycine and polyamine on this receptor complex.
**Other glutamate receptors include Delta-1 and Delta-2, the 8 variants for the NMDAR-1 subunit,[82,83] and the Flip and Flop variants for the GLUR-1-4 subunits.[84]

tors to the design of drugs with greater receptor specificity.

Receptors Linked to G Proteins

Careful analysis of the homology of neurotransmitter receptors suggests that there are two major classes: (a) G-protein-coupled receptors; (b) receptors associated with the superfamily of ligand gated-ion channels (see II and I in Fig. 12.1). One type of structural organization for receptors is a single protein that crosses the membrane seven times with a distinct extracellular amino-terminal domain. A third intracellular loop and/or the carboxyl-terminal peptide both permit coupling of the receptor via guanosine triphosphate (GTP) binding to "G-proteins" (see[31,32,38–40,r20,41–44]). These receptor proteins that are present as multimolecular complexes with G-proteins provide a means by which cellular metabolism, via GTP availability, influences the sensitivity of a neuron to the receptor agonist.[r19,r21,r22] The requirement for GTP for optimal receptor activity and the ability of the G-proteins to hydrolyze the terminal phosphate group in turn provide a mechanism by which receptors can be modulated by cell metabolic function. There are at least three major types of G-proteins in brain. One termed G_s produces a stimulation of the second messenger system (e.g., adenylate cyclase to produce cAMP from ATP); one termed G_i inhibits adenylate cyclase in the presence of GTP; and G_o, which stands for "other" GTP binding proteins that as yet have no clear link to specific receptors or catalytic cellular processes. Thus, G_s can be activated by agents such as beta-adrenergic receptor agonists (norepinephrine) once combined with their β-receptor protein. $Alpha_2$-adrenergic receptor agonists (e.g., clonidine) or muscarinic cholinergic receptor agonists (e.g., acetylcholine) in turn activate G_i and antagonize the effect of G_s activation on adenylate cyclase. Recently it has been discovered that glutamate can interact with G-proteins. This subtype of glutamate receptor is defined as a metabotropic glutamate receptor (see Table 12.4).

Drugs also can exert a part of their CNS stimulation effect by an ability to prevent the breakdown of cAMP, thus perturbing normal function dependent on adenylate cyclase activity. Aminophylline, a drug that antagonizes adenosine, can also inhibit phosphodiesterase, causing an accumulation of cAMP. Rolipram, another drug that inhibits phosphodiesterase breakdown of cAMP, is known to be an effective antidepressant.[45] Cyclic AMP has been shown to participate in subsequent intracellular signaling processes, such as activation of protein kinase A,[r23] or expression of immediate-early genes such as the proto-oncogenes (c-fos c-jun, etc.) in brain.[46] These immediate-early gene proteins can then activate AP-1 sites in the nucleus that in turn initiate mRNA synthesis. Alterations in transcription by these immediate-early genes can alter the proteins synthesized by the cell and may produce long-term changes in structure and neuronal function, such as habituation, changes in memory processes, or drug tolerance.[46] One must assume that cyclic GMP, which is formed by an action of nitric oxide on guanylate cyclase, has similar roles in intracellular signaling processes.[r27]

Another second messenger linked to receptors associated with G-protein mechanisms is the hydrolysis of phospholipids. In the early 1950s, it was discovered that inorganic phosphate could be incorporated into phosphatidyl inositol.[47] In the 1980s, the importance of this second messenger system to intracellular signaling in brain was established.[47,r24,r25] It is believed that the receptor activation allows hydrolysis of GTP with the appropriate binding of a G-protein linked to a phospholipase C. Activation of phospholipase C results in the release of inositol phosphate (IP_3) and diacylglycerol, both of which are compounds that result in the activation of protein kinases.[r25,r26] The IP_3 also produces mobilization of calcium, thus activating calmodulins. These calcium binding proteins can in turn phosphorylate other specific proteins.[r16,r23] The diacylglycerol proceeds through a different pathway to act on a protein kinase C.[r19] The biochemical mediators associated with the G-proteins and the subsequent involvement of protein kinases are depicted in Figures 12.2, 12.3, and Table 12.6.

Receptors Linked to Ion Channels

It is now recognized that there is structural homology among a distinct group of receptor proteins for a family of neurotransmitters associated with ion channels.[r1,7,8,48–51] These ligand-gated ion channels (see I in Fig. 12.1) are glycoproteins with considerable amino acid sequence homology in the transmembrane domains and are believed to form a pentameric complex from the subunits to form a functional receptor.[52] Because of the homology of these receptors, they form a superfamily of ligand-gated ion channels.[7,52,53] These transmembrane regions of the ligand-gated ion channels seem to function in mediating or modulating ion transport, whereas a large amino terminal extracellular chain may be important in determining the specificity of agonist binding for each specific neurotransmitter.[52] It has recently been recognized that some subunits for the ligand-gated ion channels have splice variants, increasing the diversity of this important family of receptors.[54–56] The intracellular loop portions of these proteins between the transmembrane domains or at the carboxyl end may also provide sites for drug action, although they usually are responsive to changes in cellular metabolism, including phosphorylation by various protein kinases.[r23,57,58] In fact, the make-up of these transmembrane proteins is very similar to those channel proteins that do not recognize extracellular neuronal transmitters or neural modulators, but are voltage-sensitive (e.g., the voltage-sensitive sodium channel). Table 12.5 lists the receptor-gated ion channels and includes selected drugs known to affect the function of these receptors.

Receptor Controls and Modulation

Receptors are not changeless segments of the cell membrane, but can be altered in response to changes in neurotransmitter traffic (or agonist/antagonist drug concentrations). Thus, the responsiveness of the receptors can be increased (up-regulated) by increasing the number of receptors or altering their affinity to the neurotransmitter as the concentration of neurotransmitter is decreased. Conversely, the responsiveness of receptors may be decreased (down-regulated) by opposite mechanisms when the amount of neurotransmitter is increased. Such alterations appear to serve to maintain synaptic transmission at a constant level. Some of these alterations may be critical in explaining the phenomenon of tolerance to drug action as well as side-effects produced by centrally acting drugs. From this perspective, the response to receptor occupation can be influenced by the recent history of receptor occupation. In a sense, this is an elementary memory capacity, and may play an important role in normal neuronal function and behavioral imprinting. This receptor modulation may take place at three different levels: (1) the affinity of the receptor for agonist; (2) the number of receptors; (3) spatial placement of the receptors in the postsynaptic cell relative to the site of presynaptic transmitter release. As outlined above, any change in coupling via second messengers (cAMP, cGMP, inositol phosphates, arachidonic acid, etc.) or subsequent messenger mechanisms (protein kinases A or C, phospholipase C, immediate-early genes, etc.) could accomplish the same result (see[r22,46]). The general process by which protein phosphorylation can alter biologic responses is illustrated in Figure 12.2. Specific examples of biologic systems affected by protein kinases (i.e., phosphorylated) are listed in Table 12.6.

The first type of receptor modification is a change in affinity for its natural transmitter or agonist (or antagonist) drug as a result of prior stimulation (or inhibition). A decrease in subsequent responses after a receptor combines with agonist has been termed desensitization.[59] In the desensitized state, there is some rapid change in secondary structure of the recep-

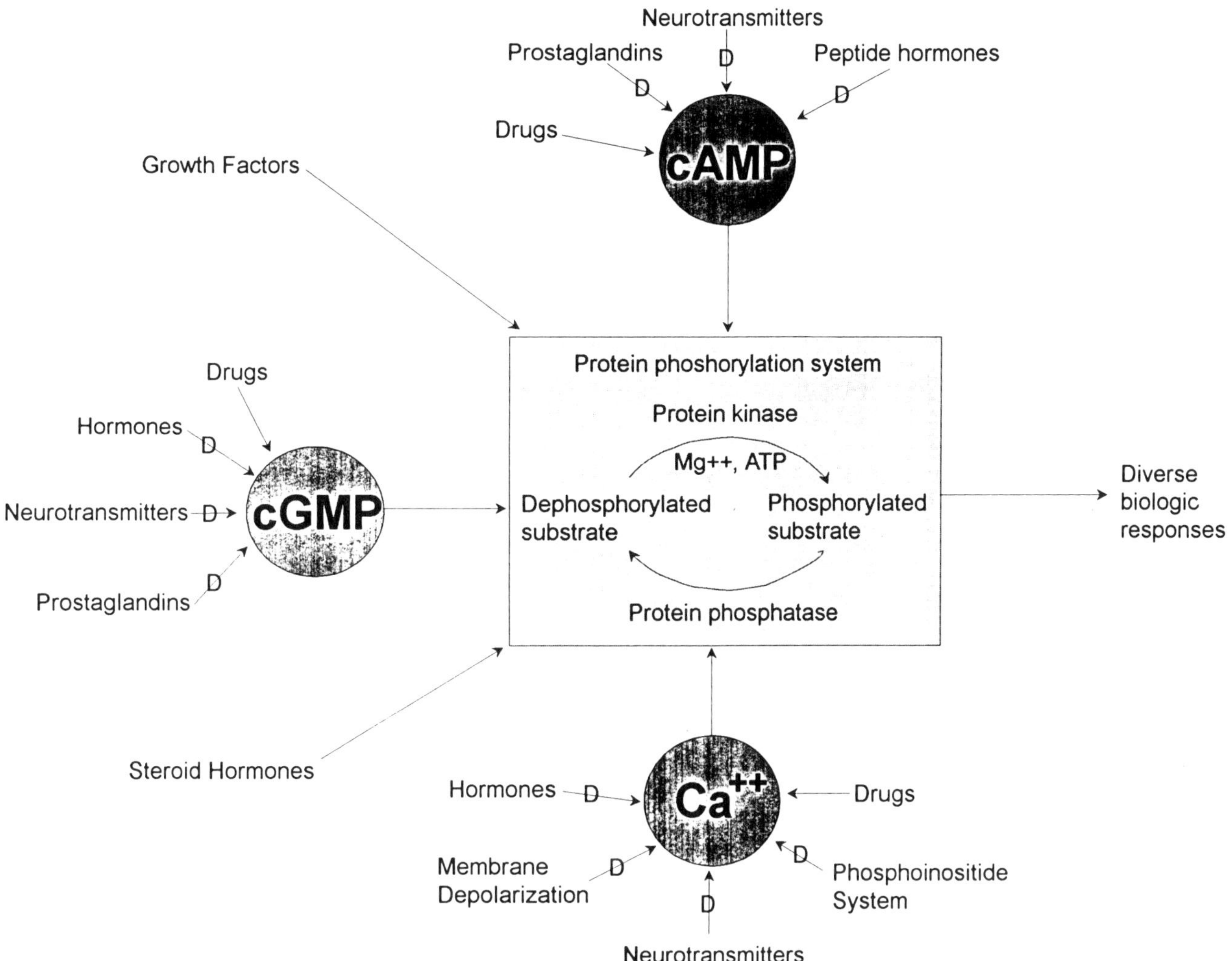

Figure 12.3 Expanded view of factors activating protein phosphorylation. It should be apparent from this diagram that phosphorylation is closely linked to the cyclic nucleotides and calcium metabolism. Only a few agents such as hormones and growth factors have a direct action on protein phosphorylation. The "D" over the various substances influencing the cyclic nucleotides or calcium flux represents additional sites where drugs can act to influence protein phosphorylation (Nestler and Greengard[r28]).

Table 12.6 Selected Examples of Substrate Proteins Regulated by Phosphorylation*

Enzymes Involved in Neurotransmitter Biosynthesis
Neurotransmitter Receptors
Ion Channels
Proteins Involved in the Regulation of Second Messengers
Protein Kinases
Protein Phosphatase Inhibitors
Cytoskeletal Proteins
Synaptic Vesicle Proteins
Transcription Factors
Proteins Involved in mRNA Translation

*List is intended to provide examples of classes of proteins found in brain that are affected by selected protein kinases. Adapted from O'Callaghn.[78]

tor that changes its affinity for subsequent agonist molecules. Although desensitization may be due to a decrease in affinity for agonist, there are exceptions, such as the nicotinic acetylcholine receptor, where the receptors increase affinity as desensitization occurs after exposure to acetylcholine.[60] In this latter change, the number of receptors more than compensates for the small increase in affinity. When agonists combine with receptor proteins, intracellular activation of protein kinase,[r23] as outlined above, may produce phosphorylation of the receptor itself or closely allied G-proteins, and thus secondary structure and responsiveness of the receptor may be altered. This type of desensitization also has been noted at NMDA and GABA receptors in brain.[57] Likewise, phosphorylation of β-adrenergic receptors has been proposed as one mechanism of desensitization.[r26,61]

The second means to alter receptor complex function is to change the number of receptor sites without altering their affinity.[59] Occasionally, 90 percent or more receptor sites or proteins may be lost as a result of continued excitation by a receptor agonist. This "down-regulation" is a slow process and occurs over a period of many hours. Thus, this process is generally far slower than the desensitization mechanisms discussed above. It has been proposed that one form of down-regulation of receptors is the loss of the receptor from the membrane in the postsynaptic cell membrane. Thus, agonists are physically not able to contact the receptor proteins that are wholly within the cytoplasm. Such a mechanism, referred to as internalization,[62,63] has been proposed for both muscarinic cholinergic as well as beta-adrenergic receptors. Internalization does not necessarily entail destruction of the receptor, since the receptor may, in fact, be able to be recycled back into the membrane. In some systems, changes in messenger RNA that encode the receptor proteins and permit protein synthesis can be altered after agonist or antagonist administration.[64] If such changes in synthetic template availability for protein synthesis are directly related to the rate of synthesis of receptors, this would eventually alter the number of receptors per unit membrane area, provided the receptor protein degradation rate remains constant.

The third mechanism of receptor modulation is brought about by changing the placement of receptors on the cell membrane. For instance, upon denervation of skeletal muscle and loss of acetylcholine availability, the nicotinic receptors migrate away from the motor end-plate region into other less specific areas of membrane function.[r27] Upon IV administration of a depolarizing muscle relaxant such as succinylcholine, a greatly magnified cellular loss of potassium may ensue upon activation of these more accessible receptors. This may prove lethal owing to high blood potassium concentrations that depress the heart. Although regional cellular localization of both ion channels and receptors in nerve cells has been reported, at the moment no similar pharmacologically relevant changes in CNS transmission are recognized that employ this mechanism. However, some evidence has appeared for redistribution of surface receptors as a result of lesions of CNS regions.

A final mechanism by which ligand-gated ion channel receptors alter receptor function is by changing the composition of the receptor proteins that make up the channel. For example, during ontogeny the proteins expressed for these ligand-gated channels differ from those expressed in adult brain.[65] Since these proteins dictate the channel characteristics and whether or not certain drugs influence these isoreceptors during development, this particular modification may have importance to our understanding of drug actions that differ between children and adults. Some data suggest that chronic drug treatment[67] or severe neural challenges (e.g., anoxia) may also alter the components forming the ligand-gated ion channels in adult brain. Thus, the expression of differing proteins for these receptors may be another approach by which this family of receptors adapts to various insults to CNS function. Neural function may also be affected by glia (see E in Figure 12.1), but little is known about this role of this interaction.

Transmembrane Non-Receptor-Dependent Intercellular Communications

In the peripheral nervous system, it has been recognized that the endothelial cells release a factor (EDRF) that results in the relaxation of the smooth muscle in blood vessels.[r27] Recently, this factor was identified as nitric oxide (NO).[68] Although there are at least three enzymes responsible for the formation of NO, one nitric oxide synthetase enzyme is localized in brain and accounts for the previous localization of NADPH diaphorase immunohistochemical staining.[69] NO synthetase has been found in a variety of brain structures, and recent evidence suggests that activation of some NMDA receptors increases the formation of NO.[70] NO seems to be a novel neurotransmitter, since it does not require vesicular storage, voltage-dependent release, or cell surface receptors. The function in the postsynaptic cell is changed because NO binds to the heme group of guanylyl cyclase, which activates it to increase cGMP concentrations.[71] There may be other volatile substances (e.g., CO) that also serve such a transneuronal function.[72] Many other compounds, such as arachidonic acid and the platelet activating factor, have been proposed to be involved in neuronal communication as well (see Chapter 9 for additional information).

Drug Delivery to the CNS

Any drug that produces changes in the CNS must first gain access to the extracellular space from the blood or CSF. At the extracellular site it must interact with pre- or postsynaptic receptors by augmenting or inhibiting the normal synaptic transmitter traffic (see F in Fig. 12.1). This extracellular milieu is affected both by the function of the neuronal and glial cells within the brain and by changes in permeability of the blood brain barrier that variably prevent (or permit) foreign compounds to enter the brain. Lipid-soluble, nonpolar compounds generally enter brain quickly and can profoundly alter CNS activity. This barrier is similarly responsible for the inability of polar drugs to penetrate the brain rapidly, thus limiting the development of CNS side-effects. If the blood brain barrier is temporarily rendered more permeable by pathologic processes in the brain (e.g., infection, high blood pressure), compounds normally devoid of CNS action may exert pronounced effects (e.g., penicillin may produce seizures).

The neurotransmitter content in the extracellular space is a function of both the rate of release of transmitter from neighboring presynaptic neurons and the rates of transmitter removal by reuptake into the presynaptic terminal, diffusion, or metabolism. Changes in the rate of presynaptic depolarization (or perhaps the number and different nearby presynaptic terminals that simultaneously release competing or similar-acting neurotransmitters) will determine the concentration of each transmitter available to activate the receptors on the postsynaptic cell. The response to drugs that mimic or antagonize the natural neurotransmitter will depend on the rate of release and dissipation of all endogenous presynaptic neurotransmitters. For example, if little endogenous transmitter is being released, an antagonist will not produce a marked effect; but an exogenous agonist may have an augmented response. Opposite results would be seen if endogenous transmitter release were elevated in the initial state. This basic view should be considered as the action of various centrally active drugs are studied. Similarly, if a neuron is sensitive to release of three different excitatory transmitters (e.g., glutamate, aspartate, and substance P), blockade of only one of these may be overridden by increased compensatory activity of the remaining two transmitters.

Functional Changes Follow CNS Drug Treatment

The foregoing discussion reviews the rich variety of mechanisms by which drugs may alter CNS synaptic activity. However, when drugs are given to patients, we must use much simpler monitors of their pharmacologic effects in the clinic. Obviously, specific changes in behavior and neurologic signs are readily assessed by physical and psychometric testing, as well as questionnaires. These tools for evaluating central drug action also help the therapist decide whether more or less drug is needed, or indeed if a different drug is required. The selection of the best drug for a specific patient is dictated not only by the patient's therapeutic response but also by the severity of side-effects (see Chapter 15). Besides simple observations, electroencephalography techniques can be used to permit titration of some anesthetics and narcotics in unconscious patients, and therapy is often monitored by close scrutiny of drug levels.

In addition to the therapeutic usefulness of medications, many drugs now serve as probes to "label" receptor populations in patients in an attempt to understand mechanisms of pathologic CNS function or to refine CNS disease diagnostic categories using MRI spectroscopy or PET scanning. While such technologic procedures are being investigated, little effort has yet been made to study brain function to monitor drug distribution and effectiveness in specific patients with these technologies. The recent elucidation of the heterogeneity of receptors in the brain and the unique structures for each receptor subtype holds out hope for the development of new, more specific therapeutic agents to affect CNS functions. Furthermore, potentially new probes for diagnosis of lesions in brain will become available as drugs acting on specific receptors and neurotransmitter uptake sites are delineated and their neuroanatomic locus is defined.

References

Literature

1. Jarvis RA, Triggle DJ. Drugs acting on calcium channels, In: Calcium antagonists; their function, pharmacology and clinical relevance. Boca Raton; CRC Press, 1991; pp 197–249.
2. Kennedy MB. Regulation of neuronal function by calcium. Trends Neurosci 1989;*12*:417–424.
3. Miller RJ. Voltage-sensitive Ca^{2+} channels. J Biol Chem 1992;*267*:1403–1406.
4. Nakanishi S. Molecular diversity of glutamate receptors and implications for brain function. Science 1992;*258*:597–603.
5. Aster P, Nowak L. Electrophysiological studies of NMDA receptors. Trends Neurosci 1987;*10*:284–288.
6. McDonald JW, Silverstein FS, Johnson MV. Magnesium reduces n-methyl-D-aspartate (NMDA)-mediated brain injury in prenatal rats. Neurosci Letters, 1990;*109*:234–238.
7. Schofield PR, Darlison MG, Fujita N, Burt DR, Stephenson FA, Rodriguez H, Rhee LM, Ramachandran J, Reale V, Glencourse TA, Seeburg PH, Barnard EA. Sequence and functional expression of the $GABA_A$ receptor shows ligand-gated receptor superfamily. Nature 1987;*328*:221–227.
8. Criswell HE, Simson PE, Duncan GE, McCown TJ, Herbert JS, Morrow AL, Breese GR. Molecular basis for regionally specific action of ethanol on $GABA_A$ receptors: Generalization to other ligand-gated ion channels. J Pharmacol Exp Ther 1993;*267*:522–537.
9. Betz H, Becker C-M. The mammalian glycine receptor: Biology and structure of a neuronal chloride channel protein. Neurochem Int 1988;*13*:137–146.
10. Koe KB, Weissman A. p-Chlorophenylalanine: A specific depletor of brain serotonin. J Pharmacol Exp Ther 1966;*154*:499–516.
11. Glowinski J, Axelrod J. Effect of drugs on the uptake, release, and metabolism of ^{3}H-norepinephrine in the rat brain. J Pharmacol Exp Ther 1965;*149*:43–49.

12. Hoffman BJ, Mezey E, Brownstein MJ. Cloning of a serotonin transporter affected by antidepressants. Science 1991;*254*:579–580.

13. Kilty JE, Lorang D, Amara SG. Cloning and expression of a cocaine-sensitive rat dopamine transporter. Science 1991;*254*:278–579.

14. LeWitt PA. Deprenyl's effect at slowing progression of parkinsonian disability: The data to study. Acta Neurol Scand 1991;*84*: suppl 136:79–86.

15. Henry JP, Scherman D. Radioligands of the vesicular monoamine transporter and their use as markers of monoamine storage vesicles Biochem Pharmaocl 1989;*38*:2395–2404.

16. Hollister AS, Breese GR, Cooper BR. Comparison of tyrosine hydroxylase and dopamine-β-hydroxylase inhibition with the effects of various 6-hydroxydopamine treatments and d-amphetamine-induced activity. Psychopharmacologica 1974;*36*:1–16.

17. Hollister AS, Breese GR, Mueller RA. Role of monoamine neural systems in L-dihydroxyphenylalanine stimulated activity. J Pharmacol Exp Ther 1979;*208*:37–43.

18. Langer SZ. Presynaptic regulation of catecholamine release. Biochem Pharmacol 1974;*23*:1793–1800.

19. Carlsson A. Dopamine autoreceptors. In: Almgren O, Carlsson A, Engel J. Chemical tools in catecholamine research, Vol. II. North Holland Publishing, 1975; pp 219–224.

20. Meldrum BS, Swan JH, Leach MJ, Millan MH, Gwinn R, Kadota K, Graham SH, Chen J, Simson RP. Reduction of glutamate release and protection against ischemic brain damage by BW 1003C87. Brain Res 1992;*593*:1–6.

21. Hökfelt T, Johansson O, Goldstein M. Chemical anatomy of brain. Science 1984;*225*:1326–1334.

22. Hökfelt T, Millhorn D, Serology K, Tsuruo Y, Ceccatelli S, Lindh B, Meister B, Melander T, Schalling M, Bartfai T, Terenius L. Coexistence of peptides with classical neurotransmitters. Experientia 1987;*43*:768–780.

23. Dale HH. the action of certain ethers and ethers of choline, and their relation to muscarinic. J Pharmacol Exp Ther 1974;*6*:147–190.

24. Weinshank RL, Zgombick JM, Macchi MJ, Branchek TA, Hartig PR. Human serotonin 1D receptor is encoded by a subfamily of two distinct genes: $5HT_{1D\alpha}$ and $5\text{-}HT_{1D\beta}$. Proc Natl Acad Sci USA 1992;*89*:3630–3634.

25. Regan JW, Kobilka TS, Yang-Feng TL, Caron MG, Lefkowitz RJ, Kobilka BK. Cloning and expression of a human kidney cDNA for an α_2-adrenergic receptor subtype. Proc Natl Acad Sci USA 1988;*85*:6301–6305.

26. Lovenberg TW, Erlander MG, Baron BM, Racke M, Slone AL, Siegel BW, Craft CM, Burns JE, Danielson PE, Sutcliffe G. Molecular cloning and functional expression of 5HTIE-like rat and human 5-hydroxytryptamine receptor genes. Proc Natl Acad Sci USA 1993;*90*:2184–2188.

27. Adham N, Kao H-T, Schechter LE, Bard J, Olsen M, Urquhart D, Durkin M, Hartig PR, Weinshank RL, Branchek TA. Cloning of another human serotonin receptor ($5\text{-}HT_{1F}$): A fifth $5\text{-}HT_1$ receptor subtype couple dot the inhibition of adenylate cyclase. Proc Natl Acad Sci USA 1993;*90*:408–412.

28. Albert PR, Zhou QY, Van Tol HHM, Bunzow JR, Civelli O. Cloning mRNA tissue distribution and functional expression of the rat $5\text{-}HT_{1A}$ receptor gene. J Biol Chem 1990;*265*:5825–5832.

29. Cotecchia S, Schwinn DA, Randall RR, Lefkowitz RJ, Caron MG, Kobilka BK. Molecular cloning and expression of the cDNA for the hamster α_1-adrenergic receptor. Proc Natl Acad Sci USA 1988;*85*:7159–7163.

30. Evans CJ, Keith DE, Morrison H, Magendzo K, Edwards RH. Cloning of a delta opioid receptor by functional expression. Science 1992;*258*:1952–1955.

31. Mahan LC, McVittie LD, Smyk-Randall RM, Nakata H, Monsma FJ Jr, Gerfen CR, Sibley DR. Cloning expression of an A_1 adenosine receptor from rat brain. Mol Pharmacol 1991;*40*:1–7.

32. Pierce KD, Furlong TJ, Selbie LA, Shine J. Molecular cloning and expression of an adenosine A2b receptor from human brain. Biochem Biophys Res Comm 1992;*187*:86–93.

33. Marsuda LA, Lolait SJ, Brownstein MJ, Young AC, Bonner TI. Structure of a cannabinoid receptor: Functional expression of the cloned cDNA. Nature 1990;*346*:561–563.

34. Devane WA, Hanus L, Breuer A, Pertwee RG, Stevenson LA, Griffin G, Gibson D, Mandelbaum A, Etinger A, Mechoulam R. Isolation and structure of a brain constituent that binds to the cannabinoid receptor. Science 1992;*258*:1946–1949.

35. Radeke MJ, Misko TP, Hsu C, Hersenberg LA, Shooter EM. Gene transfer and molecular cloning of the rat nerve growth factor receptor. Nature 1987;*325*:593–597.

36. Klein R, Jing SQ, Nanduri V, O'Rourke E, Barbacid M. The trk proto-oncogene encodes a receptor for nerve growth factor. Cell 1991;*65*:189–197.

37. Merlio J-P, Ernfors P, Jaber M, Persson H. Molecular cloning of rat trkC and distribution of cells expressing messenger RNAs for members of the trk family in the rat central nervous system. Neurosci 1992;*51*:513–532.

38. Lefkowitz RJ, Kobilka BK, Caron MK. The new biology of drug receptors. Biochem Pharmacol 1989;*38*:2941–2948.

39. Hartig PR. Molecular biology of 5-HT receptors. Trends Pharmacol 1989;*10*:64–69.

40. Venter JC, Fraser CM, Kerlavage AR, Buck MA. Molecular biology of adrenergic and muscarinic cholinergic receptors Biochem Pharmacol 1989;*38*:1197–1208.

41. Bunzow JR, Van Tol HHM, Grandy DK, Albert P, Salon J, Christie M, Machida CA, Neve KA, Civelli O. Cloning and expression of rat D2-dopamine receptor cDNA. Nature 1988;*336*:783–787.

42. Dearry A, Gingrich JA, Falardeau P, Fremeau RT, Bates MD, Caron MG. Molecular cloning and expression of the gene for a human D1 dopamine receptor. Nature 1990;*347*:72–76.

43. Civelli O, Bunzow JR, Grandy DK, Zhou Q-Y, Van Tol HHM. Molecular biology of the dopamine receptors. Eur J Pharmacol Mol Pharmacol 1991;*207*:277–286.

44. Mountjoy KG, Linda SR, Mortrud MT, Cone RD. The cloning of a family of genes that encode the melanocortin receptors. Science 1992;*257*:1248–1251.

45. Zeller E, Stief J-J, Pflug B, Sastre-y-Hernandez M. Results of a phase II study of the antidepressant effect of rolipram. Pharmacopsychiatr 1984;*17*:188–190.

46. Morgan JI, Curran T. Stimulus-transcription coupling in neurons: role of cellular immediate-early genes. Trends Neurosci 1989;*12*:459–462.

47. Fisher SK, Agranoff W. Receptor activation and inositol lipid hydrolysis in neural tissues. J Neurochem 1987;*48*:999–1017.

48. Deneris ES, Connolly J, Rogers SW, Duvoisin R. Pharmacological and functional diversity of neuronal nicotinic acetylcholine receptors. Trends Pharmacol Sci 1991;*12*:34–40.

49. Hollman M, O'Shea-Greenfield A, Rogers SW, Heinemann S. Cloning of functional expression of a member of the glutamate receptor family. Nature 1989;*342*:643–648.

50. Betz H. Glycine receptors: Heterogeneous and widespread in mammalian brain. Trends Pharmacol Sci 1991;*14*:458–461.

51. Sommer B, Keinanen K, Verdoorn TA, Wisden W, Burnashev N, Herb A, Kohler M, Takagi T, Sakmann B, Seeburg PH. Flip and flop: A cell-specific functional switch in glutamate-operated channels of the CNS. Science 1990;*249*:1580–1585.

52. Betz H. Ligand-gated ion channels in brain: The amino acid receptor superfamily. Neuron 1990;*5*:383–392.

53. Stroud RM, McCarthy MP, Shuster M. Nicotinic acetylcholine receptor superfamily of ligand-gated ion channels. Biochemistry 1990;*29*:11009–11023.

54. Kofuji P, Wang JB, Moss SJ, Huganir RL, Burt DR. Generation of two forms of the γ-aminobutyric $acid_A$ receptor γ2-subunit in mice by alternative splicing. J Neurochem 1991;*56*:713–715.

55. Sugihara H, Moriyoshi K, Ishii T, Masu M, Nakanishi S. Structures and properties of seven isoforms of the NMDA receptor generated by alternative splicing. Biochem Biophys Res Comm 1992;*185*:826–832.

56. Malosio M-L, Grenningloh G, Kuhse J, Schmieden V, Schmitt B, Prior P, Betz H. Alternative splicing generates two variants of the alpha-1 subunit of the inhibitory glycine receptor. J Biol Chem 1991;*266*:2048–2053.

57. Swope SL, Moss SJ, Blackstone CD, Huganir RL. Phosphorylation of ligand-gated ion channels: A possible mode of synaptic plasticity. FASEB 1992;*6*:2514–2523.

58. Betz H. Homology and analogy in transmembrane channel design: Lessons from synaptic membrane proteins. Biochemistry 1990;*29*:3593–3599.

59. Klein WL, Sullivan J, Skorup A, Aguilar JS. Plasticity of neuronal receptors. FASEB 1989;*3*:2132–2140.

60. Neubig RR, Boyd ND, Cohen JB. Confirmations of topedo acetycholine receptor associated with ion transport desensitization. Biochemistry 1982;*21*:3460–3467.

61. Lefkowtiz RJ, Hausdorff WP, Caron MG. Role of phosphorylation in desnsitization of the β-adrenoreceptors. Trends Pharmacol Sci 1990;*11*:190–194.

62. Chuang D-M, Costa E. Evidence for internalization of the recognition site of the β-adrenergic receptors during receptor subsensitivity induced by (-)-isoproterenol. Proc Natl Acad Sci USA 1979;*76*:3024–3028.

63. Hollenberg MD. Structure-activity relationship for transmembrane signaling: The receptor's turn. FASEB 1991;*5*:178–186.

64. Haddock JR, Malbon CC. Down-regulation of beta-adrenergic receptors: agonist-induced reduction in receptor mRNA. Proc Natl Acad Sci USA 1988;*185*:5021–5025.

65. Malosio M-L, Marqueze-Pouey B, Kuhse J, Betz H. Widespread expression of glycine receptor subunit mRNAs in the adult and developing rat brain. The EMBO J. (European Molecular Biology Organization) 1991;*10*:2401–2409.

66. Laurie DJ, Wisden W, Seeburg PH. The distribution of thirteen $GABA_A$ receptor subunit mRNAs in the rat brain. III. Embryonic and postnatal development. J Neurosci 1992;*12*:4151–4172.

67. Morrow AL, Herbert JS, Montpied P. Differential effects of chronic ethanol adminstration on $GABA_A$ receptor α1 and α6 subunit mRNA levels in rat cerebellum. Mol Cell Neurosci 1992;*3*:251–258.

68. Palmer RMJ, Ferrige AG, Moncada S. Nitric oxide release accounts for the biological activity of endothelium-derived relaxing factor. Nature 1987;*327*:524–526.

69. Dawson TM, Bredt DS, Fotutii M, Hwang PM, Snyder SH. Nitric oxide synthase and neuronal NADPH diaphorase are identical in brain and peripheral tissues. Proc Natl Acad Sci USA 1991;*88*:7797–7801.

70. Bredt DS, Snyder SH. Nitric oxide: A novel neuronal messenger. Neuron 1992;*8*:3–11.

71. Stamler JS, Singel DJ, Loscalzo J. Biochemistry of nitric oxide and its redox-activated forms. Science 1992;*258*:1898–1902.

72. Verma A, Hirsch DJ, Glatt CE, Ronnett GV, Snyder SH. Carbon monoxide: A putative neural messenger. Science 1993;*259*:381–384.

73. Howells RD, Kilpatrick DL, Bhatt R, Monahan JJ, Poonian M, Udenfriend S. Molecular cloning and sequence determination of rat preproenkephalin cDNA: Sensitive probe for studying transcriptional changes in rat tissues. Proc Natl Acad Sci USA 1984;*81*:7651–7655.

74. Yoshikawa K, Williams C, Sabol SL. Rat brain preproenkephalin mRNA. cDNA cloning, primary structure, and distribution in the central nervous systems. J Biol Chem 1984;*259*:14301–14398.

75. Civelli O, Douglass J, Goldstein A, Herbert E. Sequence and expression of the rat prodynorphin gene. Proc Natl Acad Sci USA 1985;*82*:4291–4295.

76. Smith KE, Borden LA, Hartig PR, Branchek T, Weinshank RL. Cloning and expression of a glycine transporter reveal colocalization with NMDA receptors. Neuron 1992;*8*:927–935.

77. Lynch DR, Strittmatter SM, Snyder SH. Enkephalin convertase localization by [3H]guanidinoethylmercaptosuccinic acid autoradiography: Selective association with enkephalin-containing neurons. Proc Natl Acad Sci USA 1984;*81*:6543–6547.

78. O'Callaghan JP. A potential role for altered protein phosphorylation in the mediation of developmental neurotoxicity. Neurotox 1994;*15*:27–38.

79. Grandy DK, Zhang Y, Bouvier C, Zhou Q, Johnson RA, Auen L, Buck K, Bunzow JR, Salon J, Cirelli O. Multiple D_5 dopamine receptor genes: a functional receptor and two pseudogenes. Proc Natl Acad Sci USA 1991;*88*:9175–9179.

80. Strange PG. New insights into dopamine receptors in the Central Nervous system. Neurochem Int 1993;*22*:233–236.

81. Kung M, Kung HF, Chumpradit S, Foulon C. In vitro binding of a novel dopamine D_3 receptor ligand: [^{125}I] trans 7-OH-PIPAT-A. Europ J Pharmacol 1993;*235*:165–166.

82. Hollmann M, Boulter J, Maron LB, Sullivan J, Pecht G, Heinemann S. Zinc potentiates agonist-induced currents at certain splice variants of the NMDA receptor. Neuron 1993;*10*:943–954.

83. Lugihara H, Moriyoshi K, Ishii T, Masu M, Nakanishi S. Structures and properties of seven isoforms of the NMDA receptor generated by alternative splicing. Biochem Biophys Res Comm 1992;*185*:826–832.

84. Sommer B, Keinänen K, Verdoorn TA, Wisden W, Burnashev N, Herb A, Köhler M, Takagi T, Sakmann B, Seeburg PH. Flip and Flop: A cell-specific functional switch in glutamate-operated channels of the CNS. Science 1990;*249*:1580–1585.

Reviews

r1. Siegel GJ, Agranoff BW, Albers RW, Molinoff PB. Basic Neurochemistry: Molecular cellular and medical aspects 5th ed. New York: Raven Press, 1994, pp 1–1080.

r2. Carpenter MB, Sutin J. Human neuroanatomy, 8th ed. Baltimore; Williams & Wilkins 1983, pp 1–872.

r3. Hille B. Ionic channels of excitable membranes, 2d ed. Sunderland, MA: Sinauer Associates, Inc, 1992, pp 1–607.

r4. Adams RD, Victor M. Principles of neurology, New York: McGraw Hill, 1989, pp 1–1286.

r5. Dowling JE. Neurones and networks—An introduction to neuroscience. Cambridge: Belknap, 1992, pp 1–447.

r6. Kandel ER, Schwartz JH, Jessell TM. Principles of neuroscience, 3d ed. Norwalk CT: Appleton & Lange, 1991, pp 1–1135.

r7. Spector S. Inhibitors of norepinephrine synthesis. Pharmacol Rev 1966;*18*:599–609.

r8. Breese GR. Chemical and immunochemical lesions by specific neurotoxic substances and antiserum. In Handbook of Psychopharmacology 1975;*1*:137–189.

r9. Guldberg HC, Marsden CA. Catechol-o-methyl transferase: Pharmacological aspects and physiological role. Pharmacol Rev 1975;*27*:137–206.

r10. Kopin IJ. Catecholamine metabolism: Basic aspects and clinical significance. Pharmacol Rev 1985;*37*:333–364.

r11. Stitzel RE. The biological fate of reserpine. Pharmacol Rev 1977;*28*:179–205.

r12. Kopin IJ. False adrenergic transmitters. Ann Rev Pharmacol 1968;*8*:377–394.

r13. Ruffolo RR, Nichols AJ, Stadel JM, Hieble JP. Structure and function of α-adrenoceptors. Pharmacol Rev 1991;*43*:475–505.

r14. Hökfelt T, Fuxe K, Pernow. Coexistence of neuronal messengers—a new principle in chemical transmission. In: Advances in Brain Research, Vol. 68. New York: Elsevier, 1968.

r15. Hökfelt T. Neuropeptides in perspective: The last ten years. Neuron 1991;*7*:867–879.

r16. Cooper JR, Bloom FE, Roth RH. Biochemical Basis of Neuropharmacolgy, 6th ed. New York: Oxford University Press, 1991, pp 1–450.

r17. Meakin SO, Shooter EM. The nerve growth factor family of receptors. TINS 1992;*15*:323–331.

r18. Yamamura HI, Enna SJ, Kuhar MJ. Methods in neurotransmitter receptor analysis. New York: Raven Press, 1990, pp 1–282.

r19. Birnbaumer L. Transduction of receptor signal into modulation of effector activity by G proteins: The first 20 years or so. . . . FASEB J. 1990;*4*:3068–3078.

r20. Huline EC, Birdsall NJM, Buckley NJ. Muscarinic receptor subtypes. Ann Rev Pharmacol Toxicol 1990;*30*:633–673.

r21. Freissmuth M, Casey PJ, Gilman AG. G-proteins control diverse pathways of transmembrane signaling. FASEB J. 1989;*3*:2125–2131.

r22. Hille B. G-Protein-coupled mechanisms and nervous signaling. Neuron 1992;*9*:187–195.

r23. Walaas SI, Greengard P. Protein phosphorylation and neuronal function. Pharmacol Rev 1991;*43*:299–349.

r24. Moncada S, Palmer RMJ, Higgs EA. Nitric oxide: Physiology, pathophysiology, and pharmacology. Pharmacol Rev 1991;*43*:109–142.

r25. Berridge MJ. Inositol trisphosphate and diacylglycerol: This interacting second messengers. Ann Rev Biochem 1987;*56*:159–193.

r26. Harden TK. Agonist-induced desensitization of the β-adrenergic receptor-linked adenylate cyclase. Pharmacol Rev 1983;*35*:5–32.

r27. Schuetze SM, Pole LN. Developmental regulation of nictonic acetylcholine receptors. Ann Rev Neurosci 1987;*10*:403–451.

r28. Nestler ET, Greengard P. Protein Phosphorylation and the regulation of neural function. In basic neurochemistry molecular cellular & medical aspects Siegel, Agranoff, Albers, Molinoff (Eds.) New York: Raven Press 1994, pp 449–474.

CHAPTER 13

Robert A. Mueller

General Anesthetic Drugs

Inhalational Anesthetics

In 1846, Morton demonstrated the effectiveness of diethyl ether for surgical anesthesia, marking the beginning of modern anesthesiology.[1] In subsequent years, numerous other compounds have been developed. Many of these generally small, simple molecules have been discarded because of flammability or explosive potential (diethyl ether, divinyl ether, cyclopropane, fluroxene, etc.), and some because of unacceptable coexisting toxicity (e.g., cardiac dysrhythmias and hepatitis with chloroform).[2] The chemical structures of volatile anesthetics are very diverse, and range from inert noble gases, such as xenon (Xe_2) to polyhalogenated ethers or hydrocarbons. Obviously, all currently used drugs produce a relatively predictable, totally reversible state of unresponsiveness to surgical procedures.

Anesthesia for surgical procedures in animals and humans attempts to produce reversible (1) analgesia, (2) amnesia, and (3) muscle relaxation. Initial studies attempted to produce all three of these modalities with a single volatile or gaseous drug. More recently, techniques of surgical anesthesia use specific drugs to achieve each of these three goals. Thus, a "balanced anesthetic technique" employing narcotic analgesics for analgesia and tranquilizers such as diazepam or midazolam for amnesia are combined with muscle relaxants.[3] The use of these drugs and, at the conclusion of anesthesia, their antagonists, increases the potential for drug interactions with other medications taken by the patient.

This chapter will focus mainly on drugs administered by inhalation. Although totally inert gases like nitrogen and xenon can produce CNS depression and anesthesia, only a few agents are of practical importance. Only properly trained anesthesiologists or certified registered nurse anesthetists commonly administer these potent drugs; however, all medical personnel should be familiar with their properties, since their patients will occasionally require anesthesia for surgical or diagnostic procedures.

History

Following the development of diethyl ether by Morton in 1842 there was a rapid appearance of two other anesthetics: chloroform was introduced by Simpson in 1847; nitrous oxide by Wells in 1844.[4] Before this time, surgical procedures were done without anesthesia, except for occasional resort to opiate preparations or alcohol. Thus, surgical procedures were necessarily short. It was still to be many years (some 40 years later) before local anesthetics provided practical, equivalent options to general anesthesia. In addition to the alleviation of pain, modern anesthesia drugs have now provided the surgeon with the luxury of more time to operate and the subsequent development of such adjunctive support and technical systems as cardiopulmonary bypass and microscopic surgery.

Modern halogenated anesthetics began with the introduction of fluroxene by Shukys in 1951.[5] The goal was to find new agents that were nonexplosive when mixed with oxygen in the patient's breathing circuit and also less toxic. Subsequently, halothane, methoxyflurane, enflurane, and isoflurane were developed. Other compounds were tried but not found acceptable because of enhanced frequency of cardiac dysrhythmias (trichloroethylene, halopropane, teflurane, etc.). In the search for new agents other characteristics besides reversibility and low incidence of side-effects also are important, such as chemical stability, especially in high pH environments as found in CO_2 absorbers on anesthetic machines, and freedom from the need of preservatives. In general, low solubility in blood and fat is desirable, since induction and emergence from anesthesia is then more rapid.[6] In addition, less of the drug is stored in body tissues; hence, less is available for possible metabolism or delayed "hang-over" in patients.

Chemistry and Occurrence

Several generalizations should be emphasized. To have drugs with a sufficiently high vapor pressure, all volatile anesthetic molecules are rather simple structures with low molecular weights. Nitrous oxide is a gas at ambient temperature and pressure and is supplied as a liquid in pressurized cylinders. All other agents are supplied as liquids at ambient pressures and require vaporization in an anesthetic machine to control inspired concentration accurately. Except for nitrous oxide, the presence of at least one hydrogen atom is required for anesthetic activity. Thus, carbon tetrachloride is not an anesthetic, but chloroform ($HCCL_3$) is. On the other hand, too many hydrogen atoms confer a capacity to oxidize; hence they produce chemicals that are flammable or explosive in air (e.g., cyclopropane, diethyl ether). As hydrogen atoms are replaced with halogen atoms, potency is increased (a lower inspired and cerebral partial pressure is required for anesthesia) and flammability is decreased; however, cardiac irritability and hepatic and renal damage become more likely.[7] The presence of an ether linkage produces a drug with potent analgesic properties even at sub-ED_{50} partial pressures, but the incidence of nausea and respiratory tract irritation (coughing, breath holding, and secretion production) is increased. There are many other low molecular weight hydrocarbons that are not useful as general inhalation anesthetics because of toxic side-effects, nonreversible depression, or low volatility.

Therapeutic Uses of General Anesthetic Drugs

Doses of most drugs covered in this book are expressed as an ED_{50}, or the weight of compound that produces the desired response in 50 percent of individuals at some interval after an arbitrary time of drug administration. Because of the tidal nature of ventilation, not all anesthetic gas-phase molecules inspired during inspiration are absorbed through the alveolar-capillary membrane. Thus, in order to compare the relative potencies of volatile drugs, we need to know not the percentage of anesthetic, but the percentage present (or partial pressure) in the brain. Once a patient is given a certain partial pressure of anesthetic to breathe, the partial pressure of anesthetic changes at different rates for different body membrane and fluid compartments. Moreover, when one wishes to compare different anesthetics, because of their different solubilities in blood and brain, all these rates of equilibration are different and specific for each drug. For these reasons, drugs can be compared as to potency only when all partial pressures are at equilibrium, and when the partial pressures of the anesthetic in the alveoli, blood, and brain are equal. Only under these conditions will the measurement of anesthetic partial pressure inspired equal the partial pressure in the brain. Alveolar partial pressure that, at equilibrium, blocks the reflex response of 50 percent of patients or animals to a standard skin incision is then determined and expressed (an ED_{50} value) but it is termed the "MAC" or Minimum Alveolar Concentration.[8] Thus, MAC concentration of an anesthetic is that which prevents movement in 50 percent of patients. It should be interpreted much like an ED_{50}, since one MAC dose would be satisfactory in only 50 percent of people. Obviously, inspired partial pressures 1 1/3–1 1/2 times MAC are required at equilibrium to produce good surgical conditions in *all* people.

The administration of these drugs in the practice of anesthesiology is dependent on a wide variety of dispensing equipment and monitoring devices. The anesthetic machine used for administration of the gas or vapor is designed to produce reliable concentrations of each drug in concentrations from 70 percent (N_2O) to 0.1 percent (volatile halogenated hydrocarbons) in air or oxygen, to recirculate exhaled respiratory gas to remove CO_2, and finally to scavenge and remove discarded exhaled anesthetic gas and vapor from the operating room area. The monitoring equipment that is an integral part of an anesthesia machine is designed to quantitate changes in those organ systems most dramatically altered by inhalation anesthetics and surgical manipulation. The measurement of the electrocardiogram, blood pressure monitors, inspired O_2 and anesthetic gas partial pressures, as well as exhaled CO_2 and anesthetic gas tensions, neuromuscular transmission, temperature, and blood oxygenation are now routine. In addition, computer-processed EEG now is used increasingly to monitor the CNS alterations produced by anesthetic uptake and removal, as well as subconscious neurologic responses of patients to surgical stimuli.

It should be emphasized that several inhalational agents often are used together. For example, one may be used to aid the uptake of the other (see second gas

Table 13.1 Chemical Structures of Seven Commonly Used Anesthetic Agents

Halogenated Ethers		
Nitrous Oxide	Enflurane	Sevoflurane
N_2O	HCF_2–0–CF_2–CHFCL	CF_3
Halothane	Isoflurane	H_2CF–O–CH
F Cl	HCF_2–0–CHCL–CF_3	CF_3
F–C–C–H	Methoxyflurane	Desflurane
F Br	H_3C–0–CF_2–$CHCL_2$	HCF_2–O–CHF–CF_3

effect, below) or to cancel out the side-effect of one drug with another. In addition, the patient often is given a minor or major tranquilizer and/or an opiate narcotic as premedication before arriving in the operating room or before induction of anesthesia.[9] Finally, during the anesthetic, if profound skeletal muscle paralysis is required for tracheal intubation or surgical manipulation, a specific muscle relaxant is selected to accentuate the paralysis due to the volatile drug. Obviously, over the course of an anesthetic a patient may receive 10 to 15 drugs to provide exactly the mixture of cardiovascular, respiratory, and metabolic alterations required for the surgical procedure and that patient's individual physiologic and pathologic processes.

Pharmacologic Effects and Mechanism of Action of General Anesthetic Drugs

The mechanism by which inhalation anesthetics produce unconsciousness is not completely understood. The partial pressures of anesthetic gases that produce anesthesia effect no important changes in cytoplasmic or mitochondrial function. Cell membrane function studies show that anesthetics increase the lateral mobility of such macromolecules as ion pores, cell surface proteins, etc., enmeshed in a sea of phospholipid molecules (Fig. 13.1).[10,11] Thus, the motion arrow may be increased in magnitude (*arrow x*), with the net

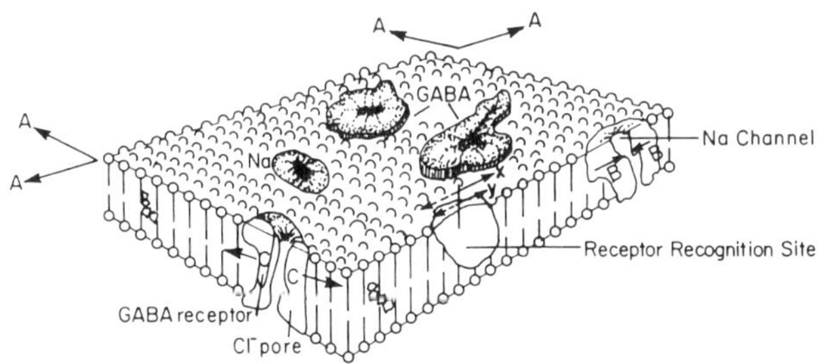

Figure 13.1 Membrane Effects of Inhalation Anesthetics. A stylized presentation of the external nerve cell membrane is used to represent sites of anesthetic action on (1) the GABA receptor-chloride channel complex, where anesthetic may open the Cl^- channel (C), thus hyperpolarizing the cell, (2) the Na^+ channel, where hydrophobic interactions with aromatic amino acids or clathrate formation (B) may increase impedance to ion flow, thus raising threshold potential, and (3) membrane proteins (e.g., Receptor Recognition Site) which has a normal lateral freedom of movement designated by vector arrow *y*, but may evidence enhanced lateral mobility (designated by vector arrow *x*) in the presence of inhalation anesthetics. This enhanced mobility may underlie the slight increase in membrane volume (0.6%) at anesthetic partial pressures, and also the compression of membrane channels (e.g., Na^+ channel, above) to render the cell less excitable.

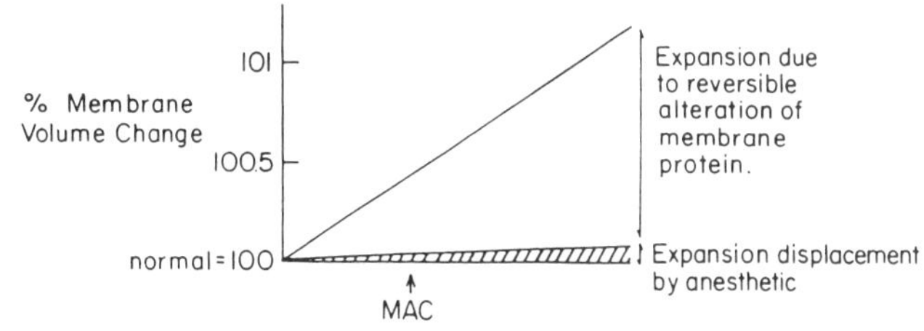

Figure 13.2 Membrane Volume Changes Produced by Anesthetics. Progressive addition of anesthetic molecules to a given membrane volume of synthetic membrane (e.g., phosphatidylcholine emulsion) from left to right, gradually increases (*cross hatched area*) the volume in that in vitro membrane, much like adding sugar to a cup of coffee. Addition of a similar range of partial pressure of anesthetic gases to a biologic membrane (*upper line*) such as erythrocyte ghosts or brain synaptosomes produces almost a 10X greater expansion of their membrane volume, perhaps as a result of unfolding of membrane proteins and enhanced lateral kinetic freedom of these protein molecules. At a partial pressure that produces anesthesia in 50% of subjects (*vertical arrow*), labeled "MAC" (the ED_{50} for the anesthetic), the biologic membrane has expanded by about 0.6%. Application of extremely high (100+) atmospheres of environmental pressures to the system sufficient to reduce the membrane volume to that present before anesthetic exposure will abolish the anesthetic effects on membranes, isolated nerves, or indeed whole animals.

result of an increase in membrane volume (*A*, Fig. 13.1). Coincident with this increase in kinetic activity and decreased mechanical organization, electrical conductivity across the membrane is reduced, producing a state of electrical quiescence.[12] Resting membrane potential and Na^+K^+-ATPase activity are unaltered. However, the ability of external or electrical impulses to produce a depolarization of the cell membrane is sharply reduced. Since anesthetic concentrations of these volatile drugs produce a small expansion of the membrane (about 0.06%) (Fig. 13.2), and extremely high environmental partial pressures (100 atmospheres) that reverse the anesthetic state,[13] compress biologic membranes to a similar degree, it has been proposed that the increase in cell membrane surface area may be a critical index of how anesthetics disrupt membrane excitability. It is also apparent that other non-neuronal cells of the body that also depend on an excitable cell membrane, such as that of the cardiovascular system, will also demonstrate changes in their apparent activity.[14] These changes are often responsible for the side-effects of anesthetics (cardiac depression, dysrhythmias).[15]

The cell membrane can be divided into two different general types of physical regions: *lipid* and *aqueous*. Since anesthetic potency is positively correlated with lipid solubility, Meyer[16] and Overton[17] proposed at the turn of the 20th century that the anesthetic effect was exerted by the molecules in the lipid regions, either in hydrophobic regions of cell membrane proteins or in the lipid bilayer milieu in which they reside. In an opposite interpretation, Pauling[18] and Miller[19] more recently noted that foreign molecules placed in an aqueous phase tend to stabilize the orientation of the water molecules to produce cagelike structures or clathrates. The stability of these iceberg-like structures is quantitated by measuring the hydrate dissociation pressure or pressures necessary to produce these structures. This pressure is high when the structures are unstable and low when they tend to form spontaneously. Thus, the presence of these cages or clathrates could function as impediments to ion translocation in the aqueous core of ion pores, thus rendering the membrane more resistant to excitation (see *B*, Na^+ channel, Fig. 13.1). In fact, very potent anesthetics such as halothane do have a low hydrate dissociation pressure, and low potency anesthetics such as nitrous oxide require a much higher pressure to promote the formation of clathrates.

Comparison of these two hypotheses by measuring the potency of a series of anesthetics revealed that *potency* actually correlates much better with their relative *lipid solubility* than with the reciprocal of their hydrate dissociation pressures.[20] In fact, the simple measurement of lipid solubility of a volatile drug permits one to predict fairly accurately the partial pressure required to produce anesthesia in humans or other animals.[21] Thus, (lipid solubility) $(1/ED_{50})$ = constant. In a more modern construct of this relationship (Seeman), it has been suggested that the free energy of absorption of the anesthetic, rather than simply the number of molecules of anesthetic per unit volume of lipid phase, probably predicts anesthetic potency even more accurately.[22] This free energy term allows for differences in polarity, molecular size, etc., to be considered. More recently, Brunner and Cheung have suggested that the hydrophobic region of the GABA-gated chloride pore is a more specific site of anesthetic disruption (see CC, Chloride pore, Fig. 13.1).[23] Opening of this pore (see *arrows*) permits the more ready translocation of chloride, thus hyperpolarizing the neuron as chloride ions move down their concentration gradient into the cell, making it less excitable.

It is apparent that the synaptic regions of neurons are more susceptible to disruption by anesthetics than are axonal membranes.[24] Perhaps for this reason, polysynaptic pain pathways in general are more sensitive to disruption by all anesthetics than are oligosynaptic (e.g., motor) pathways. Thus, a patient's muscle tone is well preserved even though analgesia is effective. Exactly how synaptic transmission is disturbed, i.e., pre- or postsynaptic sites of action, is not uniform for all anesthetics or all synapses that have been examined.

Krnjevic has recently reviewed the host of publications that have attempted to examine the effects of general anesthetics on classical specific neurotransmitters in brain.[84] Studies in isolated cortical mammalian brain suggest that excitatory neurotransmission is inhibited, whereas synaptic inhibition is enhanced. Whereas intracellular to extracellular K^+ current and extracellular to intracellular Na^+ currents are altered only at anesthetic dosages somewhat higher than those used to produce clinical anesthesia, a wide range of agonist and voltage-activated Ca currents in nerve cells are more sensitive to anesthetic perturbation. Such changes in Ca availability in the cytoplasm may in turn potentiate inhibitory postsynaptic potentials by lengthening the open time of gamma-aminobutyric acid linked Cl^- pores. Disruption of intracellular Ca availability of presynaptic terminals of excitatory synapses would similarly explain the inhibitory effects at these sites as well.

Although at the gross anatomic level early study with diethyl ether suggested that newer phylogenetic regions of brain (neocortex) were more susceptible to anesthetic depression than are the more primitive CNS areas (such as the pons-medulla), the introduction of newer halogenated anesthetics has revealed that the pattern of CNS regional sequential depression is quite specific for each drug (Fig. 13.3).[25] Thus, one recently developed anesthetic, enflurane, actually produces excitation of the electroencephalogram, a sensitive index of CNS function, at partial pressures that produce surgical anesthesia (Fig. 13.3). The development of seizures is probably due to widely different rates of regional CNS depression that relieve some areas of tonic inhibitory neuronal influences, consequently producing seizure-like discharges. Other drugs, such as halothane, produce a progressive quiescence of all CNS regions.[26]

Since cortical EEG signals in different patients are not reliable enough to use in gauging the depth of anesthesia, the effects of anesthetics on CNS-dependent functions such as reflexes, pupil diameter, etc., are used to identify the onset and depth of anesthesia.[27] Thus, changes in eyeball position and pupil configuration reflect changes in cranial nerves 3, 4, and 6 (midbrain) and altered balance

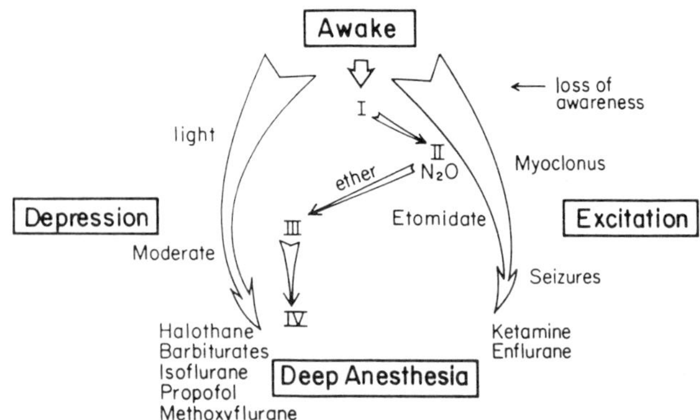

Figure 13.3 CNS Depression and Excitation by General Anesthetics. In proceeding from the awake to deep anesthetic states, the CNS can evidence largely progressive neuronal depression (left side of figure), excitatory changes (right side of figure) or a mixture of the two (center). Ether demonstrates a mixed pattern, with initial excitation followed by depression. Other anesthetics are placed on the figure in proportion to their tendency to promote depression or excitation of the CNS.

between sympathetic and parasympathetic influences on the eye. A decrease in blood pressure and respiratory activity suggest depression of the pons-medulla regions. A loss of muscle tone in the abdomen or extremities reflects depression of spinal cord reflexes. Since any one of the available anesthetics can produce the goals of anesthesia, the side-effects of inhalation anesthetics are often used as criteria for selecting the specific drug for a given patient (Table 13.2). Thus, the severe cardiac depression produced by halothane would make it a poor choice for someone in congestive heart failure, and the peripheral arteriolar vasodilating properties of isoflurane make it a useful choice to decrease aortic impedance and reduce oxygen demands on the heart. Similar variations in effect of anesthetics on respiration, CNS function, muscle relaxation, and metabolism are used to choose the most appropriate anesthetic for a specific patient (Table 13.2).

Undesirable Side-Effects of General Anesthetic Drugs at Therapeutic Doses (Table 13.2)

At higher concentrations—near those that produce loss of consciousness—all of the inhalation anesthetics depress non-neuronal cells of organs other than brain. The cardiovascular system demonstrates these depressant effects by a progressive decrease in cardiac output and peripheral vascular resistance. These changes are summarized in Figure 13.4. With halothane, the fall in cardiac output develops at low concentrations (see Fig.

Table 13.2 Side-Effects of General Anesthetic Drugs

Cardiovascular	**CHF_2-O-CF_2-C HFCl (Ethrane)**	**CHF_2-O-CHCl-CF_3 (Forane)**	**CF_3-CClBrH Halothane**	**Ketamine**	**N_2O**
Peripheral Vascular Resistance	↓↓	↓↓	–↓	↑	—
Heart Rate	↑ 33% @ 2.3%	↑ 25% @ 2%	↓↓	↑	
Blood Pressure	↓ @ higher doses –35% @2.3%	↓ @ higher doses –42% @ 2%	↓ ↓↓	↑	—
Sensitivity to Epinephrine Dysrhythmias	+1	+1	+3	—	—
Respiratory System					
Tidal Volume	↓	↓	↓	—	—
Respiratory Rate	—	—	↑	—	—
Changes in $PaCO_2$	↑↑	↑↑	↑	slight ↑	—
Irritate Airways	+1	+2	0	0	—
Bronchodilatation	+2	+1	+3	+2	—
Brain					
Excitatory EEG	+2	—	—	+4	—
Intracerebral Pressure	↑	↑	↑	↑	—
Neuromuscular Transmission					
Relaxation by Anesthetic Alone	+3	+3	0 (+ 1 in children)	–3	—
Potentiation of Muscle Relaxants & Paralysis	2 fold	2 fold	slight increase	—	—
Metabolism in Vivo	2–4%	1–2%	30%	All	—
Contraindications	Renal Impairment Seizure	? Induction	Hepatic Disease Recent Anesthesia (within 3 months) ↑ CSF Pr.	Hallucinations in 12% adults Visceral procedures Elevated intraocular pressure Hypertension Cardiac Disease	Loculated air pockets Bone marrow depression

— = no change
↑ = increase ↑↑ = marked increase
↓ = decrease ↓↓ = marked decrease

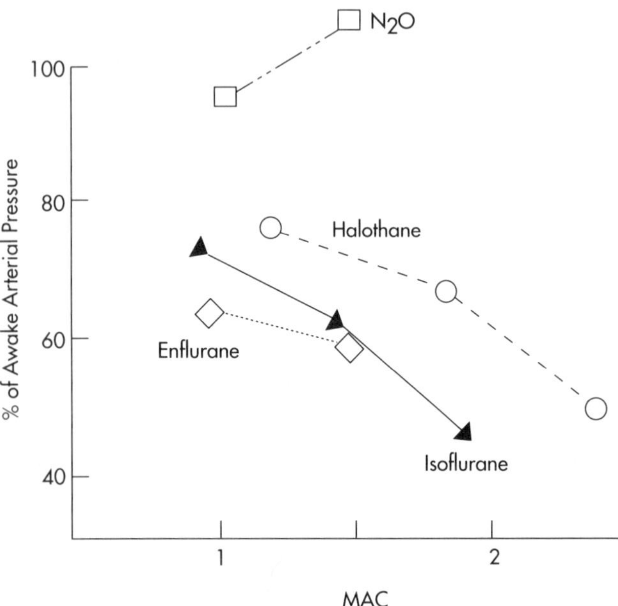

Figure 13.4 Isoflurane, halothane, and enflurane, but not nitrous oxide, decrease arterial blood pressure from preanesthetic value in a dose-related fashion (asterisks indicate a significant change). (Data from Winter et al., 1972, Calverley et al., 1978b, and Eger et al., 1970, Stevens et al., 1971. Reproduced with permission from Eger E. I. Isoflurane. BOC Inc. (1984); pp 38.

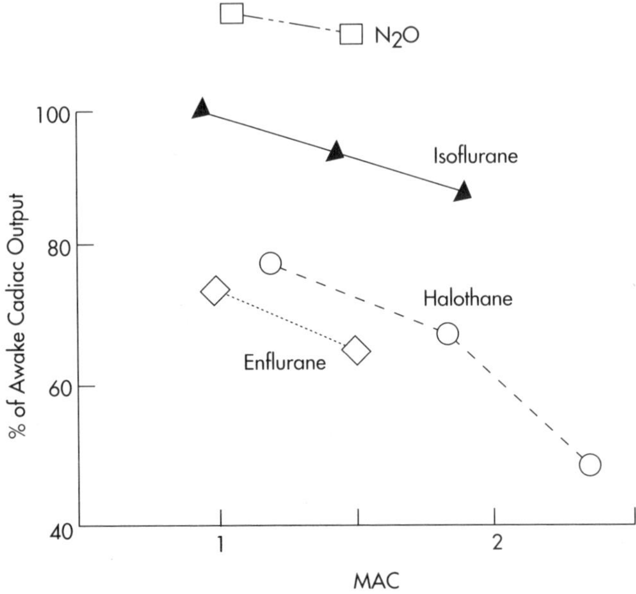

Figure 13.5 Neither isoflurane nor nitrous oxide depressed cardiac output below awake levels in volunteers. In contrast, both halothane and enflurane decreased output significantly (*asterisks*) and did so to a greater extent at deeper levels of anesthesia. The data are from Winter et al., 1972, Calverley et al., 1978b and Eger et al., 1970, Stevens et al., 1971. Reproduced with permission from Eger E.I. Isoflurane. BOC Inc. (1984); pp 35.

13.5) as a result of a decrease in heart rate and inotropic activity. This cardiac depression can be reversed by calcium,[28] which implies that the initial depression may be secondary to an interference in calcium availability for cardiac contractile activity via blockade of calcium channels.[29] Only at somewhat higher concentrations does the peripheral vascular resistance decline. Cerebral blood flow is increased by the halogentated drugs (see Fig. 13.6).[30] Many smooth muscles besides arteriolar muscle are relaxed by halothane. Thus, uterine tone and bronchial muscle activity are reduced (see Fig. 13.7).[31] Recent evidence suggests that this decline in smooth muscle contractility is secondary to an increase in cyclic AMP as a result of a nonreceptor-mediated increase in adenylate cyclase activity. Enflurane and isoflurane have similar effects on cardiovascular dynamics, except that the changes in peripheral resistance develop at lower concentrations than do the myocardial alterations.[32,33] Arrhythmias are more common with any of the halogenated hydrocarbons than in the awake state. Such changes are rarely seen with nitrous oxide, however, since only fractions of one MAC are used.

With the four commonly used hydrocarbon anesthetics, respiratory drive is progressively decreased with increasing anesthetic concentrations.[34,35,36,37] The

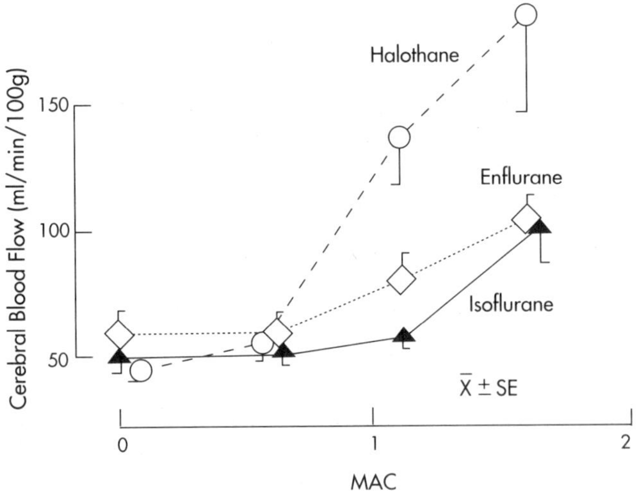

Figure 13.6 Cerebral blood flow was measured in volunteers at various levels of MAC for three anesthetic agents. The volunteers were paralyzed with d-tubocurarine and their $PaCO_2$ and systemic blood pressure were kept at normal levels. Flow increased at light levels of enflurane and halothane anesthesia, but did not increase at the same levels of isoflurane. All 3 agents increased flow at 1.6 MAC. Reproduced with permission from Eger E. I. Isoflurane. BOC Inc. (1984); p 66.

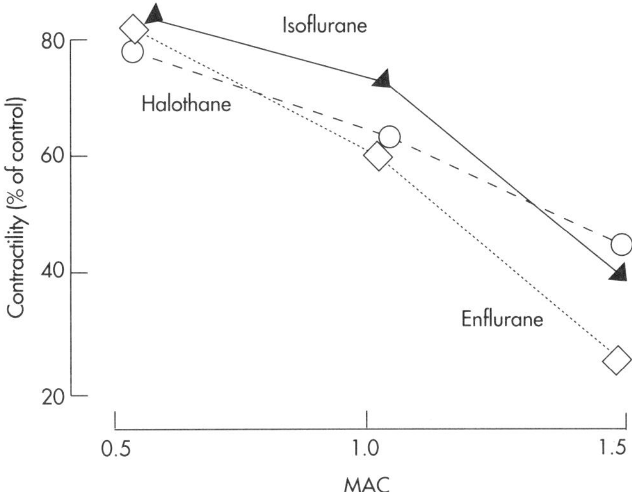

Figure 13.7 Isoflurane, enflurane and halothane equally depress in vitro contractions of human uterine muscle strips. Asterisks indicate a significant difference from control values. (Data from Munson and Embro 1977). Reproduced with permission from Eger E. I. Isoflurane. BOC Inc. (1984); p 95.

respiratory stimulant effects of hypoxia are the most sensitive to depression by inhalation anesthetics (see Fig. 13.8), but CO_2 sensitivity is also progressively but linearly reduced. The drugs all reduce bronchiolar muscle tone, thus helping to antagonize bronchospasm in the asthmatic patient. Many anesthesiologists still believe that halothane is the most potent agent in this regard. One of the great advantages of the volatile anesthetics is that they can be given safely to patients with very impaired renal or hepatic function, since pulmonary excretion terminates their action on the CNS. However, metabolism of the drug is important in understanding some toxic responses to these drugs. As shown in Table 13.3 most of the commonly used anesthetics are metabolized to some extent.[38,39,40]

During metabolism of halothane in laboratory animals with induced hepatic microsomal drug metabolizing capacity, the histologic appearance of a toxic inflammatory reaction or hepatitis develops in the liver.[41] Very rarely in humans (1/10,000 or less) a similar fulminating hepatitis develops several days after administration of halothane. The mechanism is probably secondary to the covalent attachment of reactive free radical metabolites of halothane to macromolecules in the liver cell, rendering them antigenic. When the patient is then challenged several weeks to months later, the amnestic release of antibodies toxic to the liver constituents from the immune system most probably produces the damage.[42] Some anesthesiologists now seek to avoid halothane unless specifically indicated (e.g., severe asthma). A similar reaction to enflurane has been described,[43] but isoflurane appears virtually free from this interaction.

Table 13.3 Properties of Inhalational Anesthetics

Drug	Oil/Gas Partition Coefficient	MAC(ED_{50}) % Atmospheric	Metabolism % of Absorbed Drug
Nitrous Oxide	1.36	101	0
Halothane	224	0.7	20
Enflurane	95	1.7	2–4
Isoflurane	98	1.15	1–2
Methoxyflurane	950	0.16	50

The use of methoxyflurane has been sharply reduced since it was established that as much as 50 percent of an absorbed dose may be metabolized to free fluoride ion.[44] This ion is a direct nephrotoxin, and if the inspired concentration was high enough or the anesthetic exposure sufficiently prolonged to permit sufficient methoxyflurane accumulation in lipid phases of the body, the levels of fluoride subsequently produced can easily reach toxic levels. Although both isoflurane and enflurane can also be metabolized to free fluoride ion, their low fat-solubility and hence rapid loss from the body through the lungs, keeps the amounts metabolized so small as to pose no danger, even to patients with impaired renal function.[45]

As a rule those anesthetics that contain an ether linkage are reasonably good skeletal muscle relaxants (enflurane, isoflurane), whereas nitrous oxide and halothane produce little relaxation in adults. Even with the ether derivatives, however, it is usually far safer to produce total muscle relaxation with drugs specifically intended for that purpose, rather than to use high doses of the inhalation drug, producing unneeded degrees of CNS or cardiovascular depression. The ether anesthetics do potentiate the effect of the nondepolarizing muscle relaxants by a factor of about two.[46] Thus, by producing unconsciousness with a halogenated ether, only about one-half of the usual dose of a muscle relaxant should be required. Little or no potentiation of muscle relaxants is visible with N_2O or halothane.[47]

Individual Drugs

Isoflurane (Forane)

(1-chloro-2,2,2-trifluoroethyl difluoromethyl ether—Table 13.1), shows moderate solubility in blood and lipid and provides a faster uptake and recovery from anesthesia than seen with more soluble agents such as halothane.[48] Its MAC for anesthesia is about 1.2 percent.

As shown in Figure 13.4, the blood pressure is progressively decreased as anesthetic concentrations are increased, largely as a result of reduced peripheral resistance. This reduction appears to be due in part to a calcium channel blocking activity in smooth muscle cells. Similar changes in cardiac cells are seen at higher doses. Cardiac output is reflexly sustained, largely by a faster heart rate (Fig. 13.5).[49] Since the chance of epinephrine-induced dysrhythmias is lower with this drug than with halothane, it is a preferred choice when epinephrine is to be used for surgical hemostasis.[50] Respiration is progressively decreased, whether CO_2 or hypoxic drive is assessed; thus, the patient frequently requires assisted ventilation even at low doses of the drug (Fig. 13.8). The drug's pungent odor is also quite irritating to the airways, making it a poor choice for mask-inhalation induction of anesthesia. However, the drug is a potent bronchodilator of bronchial smooth muscle, perhaps secondary to its nonspecific activation of adenylate cyclase and cAMP accumulation.[51] Thus, the drug is a useful alternative to halothane in anesthetizing patients with bronchospastic disease.

The CNS effects of isoflurane are essentially those of progressive depression without excitation, and an isoelectric EEG can be produced for protection from ischemic damage during elective circulatory arrest.[52] Cerebrovascular vasodilatation produced does increase intracranial pressure in a dose-dependent fashion, (Fig. 13.6), but is easily overcome by hyperventilation-induced hypocarbia.[53] The drug is a potent paretic agent of skeletal muscles by effects partly in the spinal cord (tonic reflex suppression) and partly at motor neuron end-plate regions. Similarly, it evidences an apparent enhancement of paralysis due to neuromuscular blocking drugs. The drug is sufficiently lipid insoluble that pulmonary excretion clears the drug before significant metabolism develops, probably accounting for the absence of hepatic and renal toxicity.

Enflurane (Ethrane)

(2-chloro-1,1,2-trifluoroethyl difluoromethyl ether) is a halogenated ether, and a chemical isomer of isoflurane (see Table 13.1 for structure).[54] Although introduced before isoflurane, its use has declined recently because of its CNS excitation properties and biotransformation.[55] The MAC for anesthesia is about 1.7 percent.

A dose-dependent loss of blood pressure is produced by this drug (Fig. 13.4), largely the result of its calcium channel blockade of smooth muscle cells of the arterioles. Consequently, a reflex tachycardia usually develops that tends to raise cardiac output but, unfortunately, cardiac inotropic activity is also reduced, probably again by interfering with calcium influx (Fig. 13.5). The summation of these changes is an impressive depression of cardiovascular stability at high doses (2 MAC). Fortunately, of all the halogenated hydrocarbons, enflurane appears to produce the least sensitization to epinephrine-induced dysrhythmias.[50]

Respiratory stimulation by either CO_2 or hypoxia is dramatically depressed (Fig. 13.8), often necessitating the use of mechanical ventilation.[35] When spontaneous ventilation is permitted, the tidal volume is decreased progressively with increasing doses, whereas respiratory rate is almost constant. The vapor is relatively nonirritating, but its bronchodilating capabilities are minimal relative to halothane or isoflurane.

Enflurane produces an EEG pattern reminiscent of idiopathic epilepsy, and peripheral tonic-clonic skeletal muscle activity is frequently noted at higher doses if the patient is not paralyzed by neuromuscular blocking drugs.[55] Hypocarbia enhances the chance of this excitatory phenomena just as it does the occurrence of idiopathic seizure discharge foci, so controlled mechanical ventilation should not be so vigorous as to decrease $PaCO_2$. There is an increase in cerebral blood flow if systemic blood pressure is maintained (Fig. 13.6). Since perfusion pressure is often reduced, as described above, changes in intracerebral pressure are inconsistent. Because of the variable effects on cerebral perfusion and neuronal excitation, the drug is perhaps best avoided in patients with seizures or head injury, although no studies have shown detrimental effects.

Although enflurane has low fat solubility and is rapidly excreted through ventilation, 5 percent may be dehalogenated, producing elevated blood fluoride levels. This metabolism may be enhanced by induction of some isoforms of hepatic microsomal cytochrome P450, specifically those responsive to barbiturates or isoniazid.[56] Although human studies have failed to show that even long anesthesia with high doses of this drug produce serum fluoride levels recognized as toxic, some isolated reports of impaired renal tubule urine concentrating activity at low fluoride levels have appeared. Moreover, since the toxic fluoride threshold concentration is not known for the various renal diseases, as a general rule the drug is perhaps best avoided in patients with recognized kidney disease. Only a few reports of hepatic damage have been attributed to this drug worldwide.[43] The neuromuscular actions of enflurane are about equivalent to those of isoflurane; like that drug, enflurane potentiates the apparent relaxation produced by specific nondepolarizing neuromuscular blocking drugs such as pancuronium.

Halothane (Fluothane)

(2-bromo-2-chloro-1,1,1-trifluoroethane) is a halogenated alkane (see Table 13.1). The drug is sensitive to decomposition by light, producing bromine, chlorine, and phosgene; thus, it is dispensed with a 0.01 percent mixture of thymol to antagonize decomposition. It is more lipid-soluble than the halogenated ethers isoflurane and enflurane; it thus has a lower MAC (0.75%).[8]

The blood pressure reduction (Fig. 13.4) produced by this drug is largely the result of cardiac depression (Fig. 13.5), where the cardiac calcium channels are very sensitive to depression. This dramatic depression usually is accompanied by an increase in ventricular filling pressures, reflecting the decreased inotropic state. Peripheral vascular resistance is sustained well until higher doses are reached. Cardiac rate is often unchanged or slightly decreased, and the refractory period of the AV node is prolonged.[57] This latter change, plus an increase in sensitivity of ventricular muscle to endogenous or injected catecholamines (epinephrine), provides a high incidence of junctional nodal rhythms and premature ventricular beats. In the presence of cardiac disease, where ventricular foci are more likely to depolarize, a variety of dysrhythmias can develop, including ventricular fibrillation. For this reason, the drug is avoided if epinephrine is to be used by the surgeon or if the patient presents with cardiovascular disease that may involve cardiac abnormalities.

Respiratory drive by CO_2 or hypoxia is very quickly abolished as anesthetic concentrations are increased (Fig. 13.8), often mandating mechanical ventilatory assistance.[36] The drug is nonirritating, has a sweet smell, and minimal stimulation of secretions, making it very useful for inhalational induction, especially in children. Moreover, it is perhaps the best tolerated bronchodilator of the inhalation anesthetic drugs currently available.

Neuromuscular paresis is very poorly achieved, except in children, where specific muscle relaxants may not be needed. Only a very slight apparent potentiation of the paralyzing effects of nondepolarizing relaxants is seen. Because of its appreciable lipid solubility, as much as 20 percent of absorbed agent may be retained long enough to permit metabolism during the postanesthesia days.[58] Because of the possibility of immunologic antigenicity of halothane metabolites, the drug should not be administered repeatedly within a six-month–one-year period after the last exposure (see above).

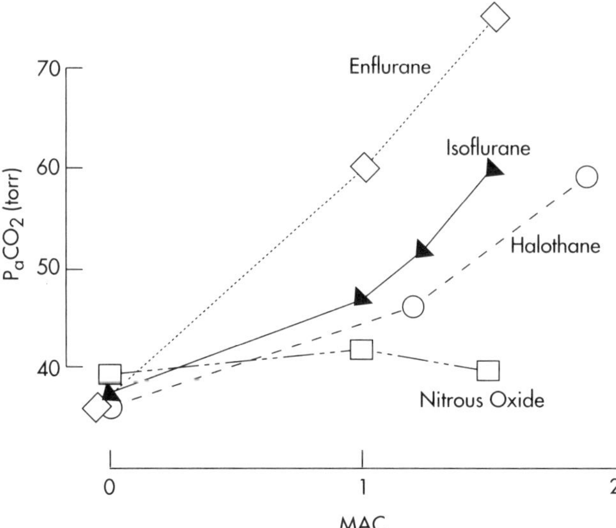

Figure 13.8 Healthy male volunteers were given one of four anesthetics in oxygen. Increasing levels of enflurane, isoflurane and halothane but not nitrous oxide increased $PaCO_2$. The order of their ability to depress respiratory function (highest to lowest) was as follows: enflurane (Calverley et al, 1978a), isoflurane (Cromwell et al, 1971), halothane (Bahlman et al, 1972) and nitrous oxide (Winter et al., 1972). Nitrous oxide was given in a pressure chamber at 1.1 and 1.55 atmospheres (total pressure in both cases was 1.9 atmospheres). Reproduced with permission from Eger E. I. Isoflurane. BOC Inc., (1984); p 24.

Methoxyflurane (Penthrane)

(2,2-dichloro-1,1-difluoro ethyl methyl ether) is a halogenated ether and the most soluble of all currently available volatile anesthetics, however, it has now been abandoned in most countries. Its MAC is about 0.16 percent, making it also the most potent general anesthetic.[59] Although the high lipid solubility would suggest a very slow rate of attainment of anesthetic equilibration, its potency permits as much as a ten fold excess over MAC to be given initially to aid delivery of molecules into the brain.

Cardiovascular depression is similar to that seen with halothane, with decreases in both cardiac and vascular smooth muscle contractility. Heart rate actually remains quite constant. The heart is sensitized to epinephrine, but less so than that seen with halothane. Respiratory drive from CO_2 and hypoxia are progressively decreased as a function of increasing dose. The nonirritating nature of the drug and its moderate bronchodilating capacity make it a good choice for patients with bronchospastic disease; however, its high lipid solubility makes gas induction noticeably slower. The EEG of the brain is progressively reduced in power, and cerebrovascular vasodilation and elevation of intracranial pressure may be seen.

Methoxyflurane is a potent muscle paretic, and the responses to specific nondepolarizing muscle relaxants are potentiated. Unfortunately, because of the drug's high lipid solubility, as much as 50 percent may be metabolized within a few weeks after anesthesia.[60] Although a large variety of metabolites are produced, the major one of clinical concern is inorganic fluoride. This toxic ion can produce a tubular lesion manifested as a high-output renal failure. Since the amount of fluoride produced depends on the dose of drug used and its duration of administration, attempts have been made to develop nomograms of dose and duration of anesthesia designed to preclude excess fluoride production. A limitation to 2–2 1/2 "MAC hours" = [(MAC Concentration) × (time of administration)] of anesthetic exposure, has been proposed. Unfortunately, a variety of inducers of hepatic microsomal P450 enzymes facilitate the production of fluoride. Other nephrotoxins (e.g., aminoglycosides) summate with fluoride to produce a damaging effect, making the choice of a "safe dose" or duration imprecise.[61] Because of the poor predictability of fluoride production, the use of methoxyflurane has almost ceased.

Sevoflurane

This fluorinated isopropyl ether is now licensed for clinical use and doubtless will be more widely used soon. It is more insoluble than other older halogenated ethers (with a blood/gas partition coefficient of 0.60), and its vapor pressure at room temperature should make it possible to use standard vaporizer technology for administration.[62] Soda lime to remove CO_2 from the breathing circuit of anesthetized patients is now widely used, and there is some evidence that sevoflurane may either be adsorbed to some components of soda lime, or that the alkaline environment together with the heat and moisture of the breathing circuit may foster some decomposition of sevoflurane.[63] Current efforts are directed toward elucidation of the magnitude of this problem, how soda lime might be altered, and the potential toxicity of the breakdown products.

The insoluble nature of sevoflurane should permit more rapid induction and emergence from anesthesia than is seen with older agents. MAC has been found in the range of 1.7–2.1 percent inspired concentration. The heart rate may be decreased, but no sensitization of the myocardium to catecholamines has been noted. Cardiovascular and respiratory changes are minor at inhaled concentrations up to 1 MAC, but progressive depression is noted at higher concentrations. Increasing concentrations of sevoflurane progressively depress the CNS, and the EEG may evidence burst suppression at high doses; dose-dependent cerebral vasodilatation may increase intracranial pressure.[64]

Sevoflurane does undergo some metabolism, but the minor nature of this probably reflects the low fat-solubility and rapid elimination of the drug from the body. Fluoride levels in the plasma are below the toxic level for renal impairment, similar to those produced from enflurane in man. Hepatic blood flow has been reported as increased, and some animal studies have shown that sevoflurane may cause hepatic damage. However, the magnitude and significance of this in humans is presently unknown.

Desflurane

Desflurane is a newer fluorinated methylethyl ether that has recently been released. It has the lowest blood/gas partition coefficient of any of the volatile anesthetics (0.42), but its boiling point of 23.5°C makes special dispensing equipment necessary.[65] As expected, the insolubility of this agent has made it possible to rapidly induce and terminate the anesthetic effect. The unpleasant ether odor of the molecule and the propensity to produce coughing and excitement in patients have made induction with desflurane less rapid than one might suppose, however. Elimination is so rapid that, less than three minutes after discontinuing 1 MAC concentrations of the drug (6%), volunteers were responding well. The drug does not bind or react with soda lime, and hepatic metabolism has not been described. Observed hemodynamic changes are largely a decrease in peripheral vascular resistance at higher doses and little change in the heart rate. Respiration is dose-dependently depressed with decreased minute ventilation and elevated $PaCO_2$ at doses of about 1 MAC.[66] The EEG shows dose-dependent changes, and burst suppression may be achieved. Cerebral blood flow is increased, and intracranial pressure may be minimally elevated. With increased emphasis on outpatient anesthesia and surgery, this agent should be used more widely.

Nitrous Oxide

(N_2O) Unlike the halogenated agents, which have a liquid phase at ambient temperature and pressure, nitrous oxide has a critical temperature slightly above room temperature; thus, it is considered a gas rather than a volatile liquid. It is supplied in compressed-gas cylinders under sufficient pressure (750 psi) to produce an appreciable liquid phase. The drug has a slightly sweet odor and a MAC value of 101 percent. This indicates that adequate anesthesia can be given with this agent alone only in a hyperbaric chamber. Therefore, the drug is often combined with IV narcotics, tranquilizers, or other volatile anesthetics to provide a part of the intended anesthetic effect. Since the patient normally breathes 20 percent oxygen (and ventilation/perfusion abnormalities produced by unconsciousness necessitate a higher FI O_2 (25–30%), 70–75 per cent N_2O are the highest concentrations that can safely be used clinically. The use of nitrous oxide as a mixture with other volatile drugs reflects the fact that when one combines several different drugs, the ED_{50} (or MACs) of the drugs will summate.[67] Thus, in order to produce 1.2–1.3 MAC of anesthesia (sufficient for most patient populations), one could use 1.3 MAC of halothane (about 1% inspired concentration), or 0.7 MAC of N_2O (70% inspired) plus 0.6 MAC of halothane (about 0.42 percent inspired concentration). Thus, the unwanted side-effects of higher doses of the potent volatile anesthetics (halothane in the above example) can be avoided. Nitrous oxide is the least soluble of the available inhalation drugs; thus, the onset and elimination of the drug are extremely rapid.

Because of the relatively low potency of this drug, cardiovascular, respiratory, CNS, and neuromuscular effects of the drug are minor.[68] Nitrous oxide, even at 0.7 MAC, can produce significant analgesia; yet patients are still conscious and responsive, though often somewhat disoriented. Patients will often remark about increased auditory acuity and mild euphoria or dysphoria. Prolonged exposure to the drug, as in abuse, produces megaloblastic changes in the bone marrow and CNS deterioration similar to that seen in vitamin B_{12} deficiency.[69] This is a result of oxidation of the biologically active cobalt^{+1} to inactive Co^{+2} in vitamin B_{12}, with a loss of the vitamin's cofactor potency and inhibition of methionine synthetase and folate cofactors required for DNA synthesis. Recently, concern has arisen that patients receiving other antimetabolites that interfere with cell replication (and folate-dependent DNA synthesis) or patients with depleted vitamin B_{12} as a result of pernicious anemia or multiple organ system failure in the ICU setting may be more sensitive to this untoward response. Fortunately, the administration of B_{12} or folinic acid at the conclusion of surgery counteracts any detrimental effects in any case.

The one major restriction to the use of N_2O is in patients who have an enclosed air pocket as part of their pathologic process (pneumothorax, distended loops of bowel, air in the subarachnoid space, etc.).[70] Although N_2O is an insoluble gas, it is much more soluble than nitrogen in blood. Thus, N_2O is transported to the capillaries lining the gas pocket and into the space faster than the nitrogen already there is removed into the circulation and excreted. The net result is that the pressure of gas (or its volume, if pressure is constant) increases, and the disruption produced by the gas pocket is enhanced (e.g., collapse of the lung, perforation of bowel, increased intracranial pressure). For these special situations N_2O is to be avoided. Since N_2O can be combined with many IV drugs as well as other volatile anesthetics, it is the most widely used general anesthetic.

Toxic Effects of Overdoses of General Anesthetics

Overdoses of anesthetic produce accentuated responses in the same organs affected at anesthetic concentrations. Thus, profound decreases in blood pressure and respiration as well as a prolonged unconscious state are the hallmarks of such misadventure. Fortunately, if the circulation is supported with cardiotonics and vasoconstrictors, and if ventilation with lower anesthetic concentrations is maintained, the toxic effects usually are reversible. Exceptions are those patients whose cardiovascular system cannot tolerate the decrease in blood pressure because of preexisting pathology. The reversibility of inhalation anesthetics by simply maintaining alveolar exchange is one of the major safety factors for this group of drugs. The competent anesthesiologist is forever varying the titration of anesthetic dose to match the severity of surgical stimulus, ever mindful of the patient's unique physiologic state. If this titration is carefully done, both overdosage and underanesthetization should be uncommon.

Principles of Uptake and Distribution of Volatile Anesthetics—Pharmacokinetics

The physical characteristics and biologic principles that determine uptake of volatile anesthetics into the body are of interest not only to anesthesiologists but also to other medical disciplines. Similar principles govern uptake of all volatile pollutants, and thus are also important in environmental health and toxicology. The major factors that affect uptake of a volatile drug from the atmosphere into the brain are outlined in Table 13-4.[71]

Each of these processes will now be discussed as it relates to the onset of anesthetic effect, i.e., the approach of the partial pressure in each successive compartment toward the partial pressure of inspired anesthetic.

Uptake into the Alveoli

It is intuitively apparent that the greater the inspired tension of an anesthetic, the more rapidly will its partial pressure increase in the alveoli. In addition, however, the absorption of some of the gas initially delivered to the alveolus, also makes possible the delivery of more gas to the absorptive surfaces of the lung from immediately adjacent nonrespiratory passageways. This increased delivery of gas has been termed the *Concentration Effect,* since the amount of such in-

Table 13.4 Factors that Determine the Rate of Increase in Anesthetic Partial Pressure in the Brain

1. Equilibration between inspired gas tension and alveolar tension.
   a. inspired concentration
   b. minute ventilation
2. Equilibration between alveolar tension and blood tension.
   a. solubility of gas in blood
   b. pulmonary blood flow
   c. [alveolar tension—arterial tension] Difference
3. Equilibration between the blood tension and brain tension.
   a. solubility of gas in brain
   b. cerebral blood flow
   c. [arterial tension—brain tension] Difference

creased delivery of drug is greater when the drug makes up a larger proportion (i.e., higher concentration) of the inhaled mixture.[72] In addition, when two volatile or gaseous drugs are present simultaneously in an inhaled mixture, the presence of one of them as a significant large proportion of the mixture will aid the delivery of the other, second gas to the alveolar absorptive surface as just described. This facilitatory effect of one drug on the delivery of the second has been termed the *Second Gas Effect*.[73] In addition, hyperventilation will aid the delivery of gas to the alveoli, but the speed of delivery to the brain is little affected because of low CO_2-induced cerebral vasoconstriction (see below).

Uptake of Drug Across Alveolar-Capillary Membrane

By definition, the more soluble a volatile drug is, the more molecules will enter the liquid or blood phase at a given partial pressure. Thus, for a more soluble drug, which has already achieved anesthetic partial pressure in the alveoli, more molecules must cross the membrane and enter the blood to produce an equivalent partial pressure than would be required if an insoluble drug were used. The clinical result of these considerations is that with soluble anesthetic drugs more time is required to transfer more molecules into the lipid phase of cells and equilibrate the blood with the inhaled anesthetic partial pressures.[6] Thus, with a more lipid-soluble drug, induction of the anesthetic state is delayed. Even though more soluble drugs are more potent at equilibrium (i.e., lower MAC), the achievement of equilibrium is more leisurely than with less potent, more insoluble agents.

The rate of pulmonary blood flow (or cardiac output) also governs the achievement of equilibrium between the partial pressure in the alveolus and that in blood leaving the lung. With even relatively insoluble drugs, the pulmonary blood partial pressure when it leaves the lung capillaries has not achieved equilibrium with the alveolar partial pressure. If the patient has an abnormally high cardiac output, the blood will leave the alveolus less saturated, and its partial pressure will be lower when it arrives at the brain, thus delaying induction of anesthesia. Conversely, patients in circulatory shock with low cardiac output will deliver to the brain blood that has had more time to equilibrate with alveolar partial pressures and that has not delivered anesthetic to non-CNS tissues. Thus, induction of anesthesia will be more rapid. This dependency on cardiac output is greatest for those anesthetics which are more soluble in blood and is less important with an insoluble drug, such as nitrous oxide. Moreover, increased blood flow to non-CNS tissues at high cardiac output states prevents those molecules from being delivered to the brain. Cerebral blood flow is autoregulated by the brain and, thus, with increased cardiac output, flow to the brain is virtually unaltered. In a patient with a high cardiac output, a lower percentage of the anesthetic absorbed into pulmonary capillary blood is actually directed to the brain, with the rest of the body acting as an inactive sink for anesthetic molecules.

Finally, it is obvious that the rate of uptake of anesthetic molecules will be most rapid at the start of anesthesia, when the number of anesthetic molecules in venous blood returning to the lungs is zero and the partial pressure of anesthetic in the alveolus is high. This rate will gradually decrease as uptake proceeds, and the net uptake will be zero at equilibrium.

Uptake of Anesthetic from the Blood into the Brain

The factors important for this process are very similar to those discussed above for the alveolus-to-blood transfer of drug. Thus, for more soluble drugs, transport of more molecules into the brain is required in order to reach the partial pressure present in blood. This achievement of partial pressure, like that of chemical reactions of gases, is the property that produces anesthesia. Thus, achieving a certain partial pressure produces anesthesia, not a certain number of molecules per unit volume. More lipid-insoluble drugs again approach equilibrium faster because fewer molecules must be delivered into brain before the partial pressure increases toward that in blood.

As brain blood flow increases, so does the rate of delivery of anesthetic molecules to brain. Brain blood flow is finely controlled by arterial carbon dioxide tension, as well as by local metabolic needs of the brain. Thus, a patient who hyperventilates due to anxiety at the start of an anesthetic administration will increase the delivery of anesthetic molecules to the alveoli, but this same hyperventilation will lower arterial carbon dioxide, thus decreasing cerebral blood flow and retarding entry of anesthetic molecules into brain. Thus, the net effect of hyperventilation on rate of loss of consciousness is really very small. The partial pressure difference between the brain and the arterial blood also determines the rate of delivery of anesthetic into the brain, and is again maximal at the start and progressively decreases with continued anesthetic administration.

When anesthetic administration is terminated and the patient is allowed to awaken, the same processes determine the rate of loss of anesthetic through the lungs. It is the rate of pulmonary excretion that determines the rate of recovery, not hepatic metabolism or renal excretion.

Intravenous Anesthetics

One of the major drawbacks to the use of IV drugs to produce unconsciousness and analgesia has been that their terminal half-lives are quite long (e.g., ketamine, droperidol). Thus, for short surgical procedures, or for those in which the intensity of surgical stimulation is highly variable from minute to minute, the administration of an IV drug sufficient to blunt the patient's response at the height of stimulation may be a gross overdosage a few minutes later, once the surgical stimulus is removed. At that point, unfortunately, the drug cannot be retrieved, and only time or antagonists of the drug's effects can be used to support the patient until the drug is redistributed from brain or metabolized. That consideration also points out the great utility of inhalation agents, i.e., not only can they be given to patients lacking a capacity to metabolize or renally excrete the drug or its metabolites, their concentration is also easily varied by enhancing pulmonary delivery or excretion as surgical stimulation or cessation may require.

Many of the drugs used in anesthesiology currently are discussed in other sections of this book. Short-acting, potent narcotics (fentanyl, sufentanyl, and alfentanil) are discussed in Chapter 20. The barbiturates used mainly in anesthesiology (thiopental, thiamylal and methohexital) are discussed in Chapter 14 on sedatives and hypnotics. Droperidol, a butyrophenone, is discussed in the section on antipsychotics (Chapter 16). Thus, only ketamine, etomidate, and isopropophenol will be discussed here.

Ketamine

This chemical relative of phencyclidine is regarded as a "dissociative anesthetic." Behaviorally, the individual seems grossly unresponsive to his or her environment (dissociated) with analgesic or cognitive testing assessments, yet not asleep.[74] From a neurophysiologic point of view, afferent impulses cannot produce efferent responses dependent on cortical function (Fig. 13.3). Diencephalic hypersynchronous or epileptiform electrical patterns are seen on the EEG, and the tone of the body muscles is increased rather than reduced as with most inhalation agents. It has been recognized since antiquity that a variable period of analgesia develops in patients with idiopathic epilepsy during the postictal period of many minutes after the seizure has ended. Presumably this ability of seizures to impair integrated neuronal responses (e.g., ketamine and enflurane) is responsible for their utility as anesthetics. Ketamine also has a significant local anesthetic potency, and is associated with hallucinations postoperatively in 12–15 percent of patients. This spectrum of pharmacologic effects is similar in many regards to that of cocaine.

Ketamine produces little cardiovascular depression, and, largely due to a brain stem mediated increase in CNS sympathetic efferent activity, an increase in heart rate, cardiac output, and peripheral resistance all contribute to the increase in blood pressure (Table 13.2).[75] This spectrum of effects has made the drug useful in the management of patients who require a resting sympathetic tone to maintain cerebral and cardiac perfusion, as seen in trauma victims. Obviously, patients with primary cardiac disease do not tolerate ketamine because of tachycardia with coincident elevated myocardial oxygen consumption and decreased diastolic perfusion interval. In fact, in patients already receiving beta-adrenergic receptor antagonists, ketamine will further depress myocardial performance. Fortunately, despite the indirect sympathetic activation and elevated circulating catecholamines produced, the drug is not dysrhythmogenic, possibly because of its local anesthetic or sodium channel-blocking capabilities (c.f., lidocaine).[76]

Respiratory drive due to CO_2 is transiently decreased for only a few seconds by high doses of ketamine, but with slow careful titration, only minimal respiratory depression usually accompanies analgesic doses of the drug. The sympathetic activation probably contributes to the bronchodilation observed with ketamine, and it is useful for rapid induction of anesthesia in individuals with bronchospastic disease.[77] Because of the generalized increase in muscle tone, the upper airway usually remains unobstructed. Unfortunately, the reflex laryngospasm produced by pharyngeal secretions or stimulation is also enhanced. The use of anticholinergic drugs (e.g., atropine and glycopyrrolate) prior to ketamine to prevent accumulation of secretions or the need for airway insertion is therefore important. Any attempt to suction the pharynx should be pursued only once all arrangements have been made to paralyze the patient and intubate the trachea should laryngospasm occur.

Ketamine increases cerebral blood flow and intracranial pressure, and should not be used when intracranial surgery is contemplated. Ketamine is an antagonist at excitatory N-methyl D aspartate receptors in brain,[78] and this action may explain a portion of its CNS effects. In addition, animal studies suggest that blockade of these receptors may protect CNS neurons from the glutamic acid-induced inflow of calcium produced by ischemic insults to brain. Studies of this effect are currently under way. The hallucinations are uncomfortable to most people, but sought by some, making ketamine a potential drug of abuse like its congener, phencyclidine.

Ketamine is cleared by redistribution initially, (t 1/2 = 11 min.), with subsequent hepatic metabolism providing a terminal t 1/2 of 2–3 hours. This latter, relatively long half-life makes it essential that patients be carefully watched in a special "recovery room" area for several hours after receiving ketamine or repeated small boluses of drug. The drug is supplied in multidose vials, and a usual IM dose is about 5–7 mg/kg; the initial IV dose should be 1–2 mg/kg, and should be followed by an infusion (25–50 μg/kg/min.). The drug is most widely used in short, superficial procedures, such as diagnostic tests, dressing changes, or for induction of anesthesia.

Ketamine is not a good drug if:

1. muscle relaxation is required but specific relaxants are to be avoided
2. the cardiovascular system would be detrimentally affected by increased sympathetic tone
3. the patient would be distressed by emergence hallucinations
4. the patient evidences increased intraocular or intracerebral pressure

Etomidate (Amidate) (R-(+)ethyl-1-(1-phenylethyl)-1H-imidazole-5 carboxylate)

Like ketamine, this imidazole derivative has a very high therapeutic index (unlike the barbiturates), and appears to depress CNS function by combination with the barbiturate recognition site linked to gamma aminobutyric acid (GABA) activated chloride pores (see Chapter 12).[79] Like the barbiturates, it provides no analgesia. The drug has a very short t 1/2 for redistribution (2–5 min.) and, thus, its effect is rapidly dissipated.

Though myoclonic activity is often noted in limb muscles, the drug is actually a potent anticonvulsant. Thus, the muscular activity (seen in 30% of patients) probably results from disinhibition of spinal reflex circuits by higher modulating cortical centers.[80]

Cardiovascular stability is very good with this drug, and it has been used with minimal changes in blood pressure. Respiratory activity is usually well maintained, but short periods of apnea may be seen with rapid IV administration.[81] Over half the patients given the drug as a peripheral IV bolus will complain of pain at the injection site.

Although the redistribution half-life is very short, much like the barbiturates, its terminal t 1/2 is about five hours, owing to hepatic metabolism. Thus, it should be used only for induction of anesthesia, not as an infusion or intermittent drug for long procedures. Prolonged infusion of the drug suppresses adrenal cortical hormone plasma levels by suppressing their synthesis in the adrenal cortex, as indicated by elevation of plasma ACTH levels.[82]

The induction dose is 0.2–0.6 mg/kg, and the drug is supplied in a concentration of 2 mg/ml.

Propofol (Diprivan) (2,6 Diisopropyl Phenol)

Because of its limited water solubility, propofol is formulated in a fat emulsion (10% soy bean oil, 1.2% egg phosphatide, 2.25% glycerol), which makes many patients (50%) complain of pain on injection. The drug is very lipid-soluble, is 97 percent bound to plasma protein (largely albumin), and has a volume of distribution of 6–7 l/kg. A dose of 1.5–2.5 mg/kg (70 μg/kg/min.) is used for the rapid induction of anesthesia, though infusion protocols also seem to be useful for longer procedures. There is usually a decrease in blood pressure due to a decrease in systemic vascular resistance.[83] The drug has a triphasic disappearance curve from plasma with redistribution t 1/2α of 2 min, t 1/2β of 30 min and a terminal t 1/2 of 4–5 hr, as a result of hepatic hydroxylation and conjugation.

Although cardiovascular stability is quite good, the baroreceptors may be reset, since the heart rate does not increase to the degree expected for a similar fall in blood pressure in the awake patient when blood pressure is reduced similarly with a vasodilator. Up to 40 percent of patients will evidence transient apnea for a few seconds, and 30 percent will demonstrate spontaneous involuntary movements or tremors with hypertonic limb muscle contractions. Reawakening is very rapid, and the drug is very useful in the outpatient anesthesia setting, since the incidence of nausea and vomiting is quite low.

Induction of anesthesia is usually produced with 1–2 mg/kg IV, and maintenance infusions often require 50 to 200 μg/kg/min.

References

Research Reports

1. Morton WTG. (1847) A memoir to the Academy of Science at Paris on a new use of sulfuric ether. Reprinted by Henry Schuman, New York, 1946.
2. Flourens MJP. (1847) Note touchant l'action de l'éther sur les centres nerveux. CR Acad Sci Pars *24*:340.
3. Hug CC Jr. New perspectives on anesthetic agents. Am J Surg 1988;*156*:406–415.
4. Keys TE. The history of surgical anesthesia. New York: Schuman (1945);14–20.
5. Krantz JC, Carr C, Lu G, Bell FK. The anesthetic action of trifluoroethyl vinyl ether. J Pharmacol Exp Therap 1953;*108*:488.
6. Eger EI II, Larson CP Jr. Anesthetic solubility in blood and tissues: values and significance. Brit J Anesth 1964;*36*:140–149.

7. Rudo FG, Krantz JC Jr. Anesthetic molecules. Brit J Anesth 1974;*46*:181–189.

8. Saidmen LJ, Eger EI II. Effect of nitrous oxide and of narcotic premedication on the alveolar concentration of halothane required for anesthesia. Anesthesiology 1964;*25*:302–306.

9. Munson ES, Saidman LJ, Eger E I II. Effect of nitrous oxide and morphine on the minimum anesthetic concentration of fluroxene. Anesthesiology 1965;*26*:134–139.

10. Ueda I, Hirakawa M, Arakawa K, Kamaya H. Do anesthetics fluidize membranes? Anesthesiology 1986;*64*:67–71.

11. Miller KW. The nature of the site of general anesthesia. Int Rev Neurobiol 1985;*27*:1–61.

12. Richards CD. Actions of general anesthetics on synaptic transmission in the CNS. Brit J Anesth 1983;*55*:201–207.

13. Johnson FH, Flagler EA. Hydrostatic pressure reversal of narcosis in tadpoles. Science 1950;*112*:91–92.

14. Atlee JL III. Perioperative Cardiac Dysrhythmias: Mechanisms, Recognition, Management. Chicago: Yearbook Medical Publishers (1985);156.

15. Brown BR Jr, Crout JR. A comparative study of five general anesthetics on myocardial contractility. Anesthesiology 1971;*34*:236–245.

16. Meyer H. Welche Eigenshaft der Anaesthetica bedingt ihre Narkotische Wirkung. Naunyns-Schmiedeberg's Arch Exp Pathol Pharmakol 1899;*42*:109–118.

17. Overton E. Studien uber die Narkose. zugleich ein Beitrag zur allgemeinen Pharmakologie. Jena: Gustav Fischer (1901).

18. Pauling L. A molecular theory of general anesthesia Science 1961;*134*:15–21.

19. Miller SL. A theory of gaseous anesthetics Proc Nat Acad Sci USA 1961:*47*:1515–1524.

20. Eger EI, Lundgren C, Miller SL, Stevens WC. Anesthetic potencies of sulfur hexafluroide carbon tetrafluoride, chloroform and ethrane in dogs. Anesthesiology 1969;*30*:129–135.

21. Saidman LJ, Eger EI II, Munson ES, Babad AA, Muallem M. Minimum alveolar concentration of methoxyflurane, halothane, ether and cyclopropane in man: correlation with theories of anesthesia. Anesthesiology 1967;*28*:994–1002.

22. Seeman P. The membrane action of anesthetics and tranquilizers Pharmacol. Rev 1972;*24*:583–656.

23. Cheng SC, Bruner EA. A hypothetical model on the mechanism of anesthesia. Med Hypothesia 1987;*23*:1–9.

24. Larrabee MG, Pasternak JM. Selective action of anesthetics on synapses and axons in mammalian sympathetic ganglia. J Neurophysiol 1952;*15*:91–114.

25. Winters WD, Ferrar-Allodo T, Guzman-Florez C, Alcarz M. The cataleptic state induced by ketamine: A review of the neuropharmacology of anesthesia. Neuropharmacology 1972;*11*:303–317.

26. Clark DL, Rosner BS. Neurophysiologic effects of general anesthetics. Anesthesiol 1973;*39*:564–81.

27. Guedel AE. Inhalation Anesthesia, 2d ed. New York: The Macmillan Co (1951).

28. Price HL. Calcium reverses myocardial depression caused by halothane. Anesthesiol 1974;*41*:576–579.

29. Lynch C, Vogel S, Sperelakis N. Halothane depression of myocardial slow action potentials. Anesthesiology 1981;*55*:360–368.

30. Wollman H, Alexander SC, Cohen PJ, Chase PE, Melman E, Behar MG. Cerebral circulation of man during halothane anesthesia. Anesthesiology 1964;*25*:180–184.

31. Hirshman CA, Edelstein G, Peetz S, Wayne R, Downes H. Mechanism of action of inhalational anesthesia on airways. Anesthesiology 1982;*56*:107–111.

32. Calverley RK, Smith NT, Prys-Roberts C, Eger EI, Jones CW. Cardiovascular effects of enflurane anesthesia during controlled ventilation in man. Anesth Analg 1978;*57*:617–628.

33. Eger EI II. Isoflurane (Forane) A compendium and reference. Madison, Wisconsin: Ohio Medical Products (1981).

34. Knill RL, Kievaszewicz HT, Dodgson BG, Clement JL. Chemical regulation during isoflurane sedation and anesthesia in humans. Can Anesth Soc J 1983;*30*:607–614.

35. Hirshman CA, McCullough RE, Cohen PJ, Weit JV. Depression of hypoxia ventilatory response by halothane, enflurane and isoflurane in dogs. Brit J Anesth 1977;*49*:957–963.

36. Knill RH, Gelb AW. Ventilatory responses to hypoxic and hypercarbia during halothane sedation and anesthesia in man. Anesthesiology 1978;*49*:244–251.

37. Holaday DA. Sevoflurane: an experimental anesthetic In: Brown (Ed). New pharmacologic vistas in anesthesia. Philadelphia: FA Davis Co (1983); pp 45–60.

38. Carpenter RL, Eger EI II, Johnson BH, Unadkat JD, Sheiner LB. The extent of metabolism of inhaled anesthetics in humans. Anesthesiology 1986;*65*:201–205.

39. Carpenter RL, Eger EI II, Johnson BH, Unadkat JD, Sheiner LB. Phamacokinetics of inhaled anesthetics in humans: measurements during and after the simultaneous administration of enflurane, halothane, isoflurane, methoxyflurane, and nitrous oxide. Anesth Analg 1986;*65*:575–582.

40. Cousins MJ, Mazze RI, Kosek JC, Hitt BA, Love FV. The etiology of methoxyflurane nephrotoxicity. J Pharmacol Exp Therap 1974;*190*:530–541.

41. Pohl LR, Gillette JR. Editorial. A perspective on halothane-induced hepatotoxicity. Anesth Analg 1982;*61*:809–811.

42. Vergani D, Mieli-Vergani G, Alberti A, Neuberger J, Eddlston ALWF, Davis M, Williams R. Antibodies to the surface of halothane-altered rabbit hepatocytes in patients with severe halothane associated hepatitis. N Engl J Med 1980;*303*:66–71.

43. Eger EI II, Schmuckler EA, Ferrel LD, Goldsmith CH, Johnson BA. Is enflurane hepatotoxic? Anesth Analg 1986;*65*:21–30.

44. Holaday DA, Rudofsky S, Treuhaft PS. The metabolic degradation of methoxyflurane in man. Anesthesiol 1970;*33*:579–593.

45. Bentley JB, Vaughan RW, Miller MS, Calkins JM, Gandolfi AJ. Serum inorganic fluoride levels in obese patients during and after enflurane anesthesia. Anesth Analg 1979;*58*:409–412.

46. Vitez TS, Miller RD, Eger EI II. An in vitro comparison of halothane and isoflurane potentiation of neuromuscular blockade. Anesthesiol 1974;*41*:53–56.

47. Ngai SH. Action of general anesthetics in producing muscle relaxation: Interaction of anesthetics with relaxants in muscle relaxants ed. Katz RL. Amsterdam Excerpta Medica (1975); pp 279–297.

48. Wade JG, Stevens WC, Isoflurane: an anesthetic for the eighties? Anesth Analg 1981;*60*:666–682.

49. Shimosato S, Carter JG, Kemmotsa O, Takakashi T. Cardiocirculatory effects of prolonged administration of isoflurane in normocarbic human volunteers Acta Anesth Scand 1982;*26*:27–30.

50. Johnston RR, Eger EI II, Wilson C. A comparative interaction of epinephrine with enflurane, isoflurane and halothane in man. Anesth Analg 1976;*55*:709–711.

51. Heneghan CPH, Bergman NA, Jordan C, Lehane JR, Cathey DM. Effect of isoflurane on bronchomotor tone Br J Anesth 1983;*55*:248P–249P.

52. Eger EI II, Stevens WC, Cromwell TH. The electroencephalogram in man anesthestized with forane. Anesthesiol 1971;*35*:504–508.

53. Adams RW, Cucchiara RF, Gronert GA, Messick JM, Michenfelder JD. Isoflurane and cerebrospinal fluid pressure in neurosurgical patient. Anesthesiology 1981;*54*:97–99.

54. Virtue RW, Lund LO, Phelps M Jr, Vogel JHK, Beckwith H, Heron M. Difluromethyl 1, 1, 2, trifluoro-2-chloroethyl ether as an anesthetic agent: results with dogs and a preliminary note on observations in man. Can Anesth Soc J 1966;*13*:233–241.

55. Lebowitz MH, Blitt CD, Dillon JB. Enflurane-induced central nervous system excitation and its relation to carbon dioxide tension. Anesth Analg 1972;*51*:355–363.

56. Mazze RI. Metabolism of the inhaled anesthetics: implications of enzyme induction. Brit J Anesth 1984;*56*:27S–41S.

57. Atlee JL III, Rusy BF. Halothane depression of AV conduction studied by electrograms of the bundle of His in dogs. Anesthesiol 1972;*36*:112–718.

58. Rehder K, Forbes J, Alter H, Hessler O, Stier A. Halothane biotransformation in man: a quantitative study. Anesthesiol 1967;*28*:711–715.

59. Walker JA, Eggers GWN, Allen CR. Cardiovascular effects of methoxyflurane anesthesia in man. Anesthesiol 1962;*23*:639–642.

60. Yoshimura N, Holaday DA, Fiserova-Bergerova V. Metabolism of methoxyflurane in man. Anesthesiol 1976;*44*:372–380.

61. Van Dyke RA. Metabolism of volatile anesthetics III. Induction of microsomal dechlorinating and ether-cleaving enzymes. J Pharmacol Exp Therap 1966;*154*:364–369.

62. Wallin RF, Regan BM, Napoli MD, Stern IJ. Seroflurane: a new inhalational anesthetic agent. Anesth Analg 1975;*54*:758–765.

63. Kudo M, Kudo T. Reaction products of seroflurane with components of soda lime under various conditions. Masui 1990;*39*:39–44.

64. Holaday DA, Smith FR. Clinical characteristics and biotransformation of seroflurane in healthy human volunteers. Anesthesiol 1981;*54*:100–106.

65. Jones RM, Cashman JN, Mant TGK. Clinical impressions and cardiorespiratory effects of a new fluorinated inhalational anesthetic. Desflurane (I-653) in volunteers. Br J Anesth 1990;*64*:11–15.

66. Jones RM, Cashman JN, Eger EI II, Damask MC. Kinetics and potency of desflurane (I-653) in volunteers. Anesth Analg 1990;*70*:3–7.

67. Quasha AL, Eger EI II, Ticker JH. Determination and applications of MAC Anesthesiology 1980;*53*:315–334.

68. Hill GE, English JE, Lunn, Stanley TH, Sentker CR, Loeser E, Liu WS, Kawamura R, Bidwai AV, Hodges M. Cardiovascular response to nitrous oxide during light, moderate and deep halothane anesthesia. Anesth Analg 1978;*57*:84–94.

69. Nunn JF, Chanarin I. Editorial Nitrous oxide and vitamine B_{12}. Brit J Anesth 1978;*50*:1089–1090.

70. Eger EI II, Saidman LJ. Hazards of nitrous oxide anesthesia in bowel obstruction and pneumothorax. Anesthesiol 1965;*26*:61–66.

71. Eger EI II, Anesthetic uptake and action. Baltimore: Williams and Wilkins (1974); pp 77–192.

72. Stoelting RK, Eger EI II. An additional explanation for the second gas effect: a concentrating effect. Anesthesiology 1969;*30*:273–277.

73. Epstein RM, Rackow H, Salanitre E, Wolf GL. Influence of the concentration effect on the uptake of anesthetic mixtures: the second gas effect. Anesthesiol 1964;*25*:364–371.

74. Corssen G, Domino EF. Dissociative anesthesia: further pharmacologic studies and first clinical experience with the phencyclidine derivative CI-581. Anesth Analg 1966;*45*:29–40.

75. Domino EF, Chodoff P, Corssen G. Pharmacological effects of CI-581, a new dissociative anesthetic in man. Clin Pharmacol Ther 1965;*6*:279–291.

76. Nedergaard OA. Cocaine-like effect of ketamine in vascular adrenergic neurons. Europ J Pharmacol 1973;*23*:153–161.

77. Corssen G, Guitierrez J, Reves JG, Huber FC. Ketamine in the anesthetic management of asthmatic patients. Anesth Analg 1972;*51*:588–596.

78. Anis NA, Berry SC, Burton NR, Lodge D. The disociative anesthetics, Ketamine and phencylidine, selectively reduces excitation of central mammalian neurones by N-methyl-aspartale. Br J Pharmacol 1983;*79*:565–575.

79. Morgan M, Lumley J, Whitwam J. Etomidate, a new water soluble nonbarbiturate intravenous induction agent. Lancet 1975; I 995–956.

80. Ghoneim MM, Uamada T, Etomidate: A clinical and electroencephalographic comparison with thiopental. Anesth Analg 1977;*56*:479–485.

81. Fragen RJ, Caldwell N, Brunner EA. Clinical use of etmidate for anesthesia induction: A preliminary report. Anesth Analg 1976;*55*:730–733.

82. Wagner RL, White PF, Kan PB, Rosenthal MH, Feldman D. Inhibition of adrenal steroidgenesis by the anesthetic etomidate. N Engl J Med 1984;*310*:1415–1421.

83. Prys-Roberts C, Davies JR, Calverley RK, Goodman NW. Hemodynamic effects of infusions of disopropylphenol (ICI 35868) during nitrous oxide anaesthesia in man. Brit J Anesth 1983;*55*:105–111.

84. Krnjevic K. Cellular and synaptic action of general anesthetics. Gen Pharmacol 1992;*23*:965–975.

Textbooks and Reviews

Albrecht RF, Miletich DJ. Speculations on the molecular nature of anesthesia. A reflective, thorough examination of theories of narcosis. Gen Pharmacol 1988;*19*:339–346.

Dale O, Brown BR Jr. Clinical Pharmacokinetics of the inhalational anesthetics. A useful reference for relating modern pharmacokinetic principles to anesthesiology applications. Clinical Pharmacokinetics 1987;*12*:145–167.

Eger EI II. Anesthetic Uptake and Action. A still up-to-date lucid description of basic science and clinical aspects important to understanding the pharmacokinetics of anesthetic drugs. Baltimore: Williams and Wilkins (1974); pp 77–96;113–145.

Wood M, Wood AJJ. Drugs and anesthesia: pharmacology for anesthesiologists, An in-depth discussion not only of anesthetic drugs, but also of their use with other adjuvant agents critical to the practice of anesthesiology. Baltimore: Williams and Wilkins (1982); 199–298.

Wrigley SR, James RM. New inhaled anesthetics. A concise review of newly released drugs of great promise. Current Opinion Anesthesiol 1991;*4*:534–538.

CHAPTER 14

Drugs Used for the Treatment of Anxiety and Sleep Disorders

James R. Martin
Willy E. Haefely

Chemotherapy of anxiety and sleep disorders has been sought since earliest times. Natural products have been used (opiates, ethanol, kawa pyrones) with some success. Bromides and chloral derivatives were very popular early in this century. However, with the discovery of barbiturates, the first synthetic organic compounds became available to counter many forms of central nervous system (CNS) overexcitability. Although still in use as injectable general anesthetics and as antiepileptics, barbiturates have largely been replaced as treatment for anxiety and sleep disorders—first, by propanediol carbamates (meprobamate) in the mid-1950s and later by benzodiazepines (BZs) since about 1960. At present, benzodiazepines dominate in the therapy of anxiety and sleep disorders.

History

The discovery of the BZs and their therapeutic profile, was serendipitous. The medicinal chemist Leo H. Sternbach, of Hoffmann-La Roche Inc. first synthesized a series of compounds based on the quinazoline 3-oxides, which had been the basis of his PhD thesis in Cracow, Poland, in the early 1930s. A ring system unknown at that time, a BZ, had been obtained. No biologic tests had been carried out with these novel compounds, but it was hoped that some useful activity might be discovered. Subsequently Lowell O. Randall discovered the pharmacologic profile of a compound, later named chlordiazepoxide, that included pronounced sedative, anticonvulsant, and muscle relaxant effects with excellent safety. Following clinical confirmation of the useful pharmacologic profile of chlordiazepoxide, this BZ compound was launched in 1960 under the trade name Librium for the treatment of psychosomatic disorders, anxiety, and related symptoms. It was followed in 1963 by a second BZ, diazepam (Valium). In rapid succession many other BZ derivatives appeared leading to the so-called "benzodiazepine boom" in the 1960s and 1970s. During this period, BZs were demonstrated to act through facilitation of synaptic transmission at the γ-aminobutyric acid (GABA) receptor.[1,2] Subsequently, specific receptors for this class of drugs were identified within the CNS in radioligand binding studies using tritiated diazepam.[3,4] The high correlation between the pharmacologic activity of BZs and radioligand binding affinity suggested that these binding sites represented the primary site of action, i.e. the benzodiazepine receptor (BZR). In early studies using tritiated diazepam as a radioligand, high-affinity binding sites were also found in various peripheral tissues, particularly in kidney, adrenal gland, and testis, but with a rank order of binding affinities for various ligands clearly different from that for brain (e.g., clonazepam binds only to the latter). These peripheral binding sites were inappropriately termed "peripheral BZRs" but are not part of the $GABA_A$ receptor channel complex as are BZRs, but rather are preferentially (or exclusively) located in the mitochondrial inner membrane. These mitochondrial BZRs should not be confused with the BZRs that are the topic of this chapter. A further important development occurred around 1980, with the discovery of a BZ derivative (flumazenil) that acts as a competitive antagonist at the BZR.[5] In addition, β-carbolines were identified as BZR ligands producing effects that were the exact mirror image of those produced by the classic BZs in therapeutic use with their known anxiolytic, hypnotic, muscle relaxant, and anticonvulsant properties.[6] The term "BZR inverse agonist" has been coined to describe the former compounds. Other non-BZs were subsequently found to act as BZR ligands; BZR agonists lacking the BZ structure have since been clinically introduced as hypnotics (zopiclone, a cyclopyrrolone, and zolpidem, an imidazopyridine) or anxiolytics (alpidem, an imidazopyridine). The isolation of the BZR led to the discovery that it is an integral part of the GABAergic system, acting as an allosteric modulatory site on the $GABA_A$ receptor channel complex. The first molecular cloning and sequencing of the cDNA encoding the subunits of the $GABA_A$ receptor channel complex was published by Schofield et al.[7] in 1987; since then, the structural complexity and polymorphism of this receptor channel has been progressively unraveled. The $GABA_A$ receptor channel contains, in addition to the BZR, other allosteric sites through which agents such as barbiturates, convulsants, ethanol, some general anesthetics, and steroids act. Very unexpectedly, BZs (e.g., diazepam, N-desmethyl-diazepam and several other derivatives) were recently found to be normally present (although in minute concentrations) in the brain and other organs of man and animals, as well as in several plant species.[8] These BZs are consumed with foodstuffs, but might also be synthesized by the intestinal flora. Interestingly, BZs have been reported to be present in increased concentrations in patients with acute liver dysfunction.[9]

This chapter focuses on the drug classes predominantly prescribed for the management of anxiety and sleep disorders. In classifying drugs, emphasis has been placed on the underlying mechanism of action rather than chemical structure, insofar as the mechanism has, in fact, been elucidated.

Drugs Acting Through the Benzodiazepine Receptor

This first section reviews the compounds exhibiting therapeutic effects through a specific interaction with a well-defined receptor protein, the so-called benzodiazepine receptor (BZR), with a focus on the prominent therapeutic effects obtained in anxiety and sleep disorders. However, BZR ligands exhibit a very broad sprectrum of clinically relevant activities that will also be discussed here. Initially, it was believed that affinity to the BZR was associated exclusively with a distinct chemical structure containing the benzodiazepine (BZ) ring system. This was proved incorrect and the BZR is now known also to interact with compounds belonging to other ("non-BZ") structural classes. Moreover, agents can interact with the BZR in different ways, producing quite different pharmacologic effects. The term "BZR ligands" encompasses all compounds that bind to BZR, irrespective of chemical structure or the pharmacologic activity resulting from this interaction. As will be described, BZR ligands can be classified on the basis of their pharmacologic profile (which is integrally related to the intrinsic efficacy) into agonists, antagonists, and inverse agonists.[10]

Chemistry

The basic BZ structure is illustrated in Figure 14.1; it consists of a benzene (ring A) fused to the seven-membered heterocycle diazepine with nitrogen atoms (ring B) in the 1 and 4 positions. Over 3000 derivatives of this structure have been synthesized and evaluated pharmacologically. The marketed BZs (see Fig. 14.2) are substituted in position 7 (chlorine, fluorine, bromine, nitro). The benzene ring can be replaced by another aromatic ring, e.g., thiophene. The nitrogen in position 1 carries an alkyl substituent (e.g., methyl) in most BZs. The carbon atom in position 2 carries a methyl-

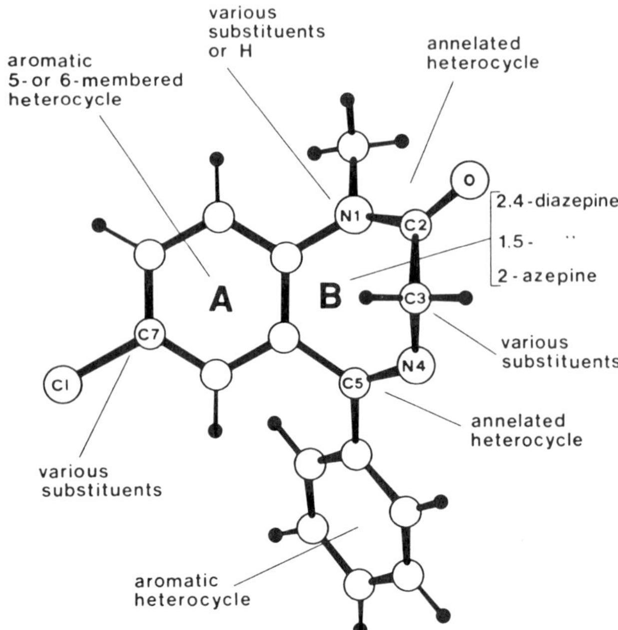

Figure 14.1 General Structure of the Benzodiazepine

amino group in chlordiazepoxide, but most frequently form a C = O function. The diazepine ring can be fused to a five-membered heteroaromatic cycle at positions 1 and 2 (triazol, imidazol). Clobazam is the only marketed example of a 1,5 benzodiazepine. A substituent on carbon 3 usually decreases activity, except for a hydroxyl group. The latter may be acylated to give an ester (oxazepam hemisuccinate) or form a carbamate (camazepam). A carboxyl group attached to carbon 3 allows water soluble salts to be obtained (clorazepate); however, the chemical stability of this compound is weak. Substituents in position 3 introduce a chirality center; only S-enantiomers interact with the BZR. Even in the absence of a 3-substituent, the diazepine ring exists in two energetically preferred boat forms (C_3 above or below the plane); the two conformations, however, easily interconvert. The nitrogen in position 4 is a N-oxide in chlordiazepoxide, but usually it is not oxidized. N_4 and C_5 usually are connected by a double bond. The diazepine ring may be 4,5-annelated (oxazolam, cloxazolam, ketazolam). These tetracyclic compounds are chemically very labile. Most BZs have a phenyl substituent in position 5, sometimes with a halogen in the ortho (2') position. The phenyl ring is replaced by a cyclohexenyl ring in tetrazepam or by a 2-pyridyl group in bromazepam and by a carbonyl function in the BZR antagonist flumazenil. A more extensive discussion of the structure-activity relationship (SAR) is available elsewhere.[11]

Diverse non-BZ structures have been found to exhibit high affinity to the BZR. The BZR agonist zopiclone belongs to the chemical class of cyclopyrrolones (Fig. 14.2), whereas BZR agonists zolpidem and alpidem are imidazopyridines (Fig. 14.2); these compounds are registered for the treatment of either sleep or anxiety disorders. The β-carbolines (e.g., 1,2,3,4-tetrahydro-β-carboline-3-carboxylic acid methyl and ethyl esters) are cyclic tryptophan derivatives that generated great interest as the first inverse agonists of the BZR. They were discovered during an attempt to identify putative endogenous ligands of the BZR. This chemical class also includes agonists, partial agonists, and antagonists at the BZR; none of these compounds has yet been approved for use, although clinical investigations have been carried out with several to date.

Pharmacology of BZR Agonists

Anxiolytic Activity

Many animal models have been developed in an attempt to predict the anxiolytic activity of novel compounds in humans.[12] Many of these paradigms evaluate animal behavior in a so-called "conflict" situation, i.e., a behavioral response is simultaneously under the influence of two opposing motivational states, such as approach and avoidance tendencies. Probably the best known model is the conditioned punishment conflict paradigm in which animals are trained to exhibit a certain response voluntarily (e.g., pressing a lever) in order to receive a reward (e.g., food for a hungry animal). Once the animals exhibit a constant rate of lever-press responding, then short periods are introduced (usually signaled by visual or acoustic signs) during which lever pressing is simultaneously rewarded by food and punished by mild electrical foot shock.[13] Animals exhibit a markedly reduced response rate during these conflict periods, which are also characterized by various overt signs of emotion. The characteristic effect of BZR full and partial agonists is the disinhibition of punished behavior (resulting in an increase in the rate of responding under punishment) at doses that fail to disrupt unpunished responding. Furthermore, these same active drugs produce an anxiolytic-like effect in the absence of actual punishment, i.e., when the rate of lever pressing is reduced by conditioned fear of punishment. The conflict task does not require conditioned behavioral responses: naive thirsty animals can be offered the opportunity to drink, with drinking punished via contact with an electrified spout.[14] Such punishment-suppressed drinking is disinhibited dose-dependently by BZR full and partial agonists. Exploratory activity can likewise be decreased by contingent punishment and released by treatment with known anxiolytics. Conflict models without punishment[15] are based on the presence of the natural opposing motivational states: on the one hand, the tendency to explore; on the other hand, fear of a novel environment (e.g., dark-light chamber task, elevated plus-maze, consumption of unfamiliar food or normal food in an unfamiliar environment, social interaction between animals unfamiliar with each other). While it is obvious to ascribe the behavioral disinhibitory effect of BZR agonism in these experimental situations to an anxiolytic-like action, their effect also can be interpreted as a general reduction of the influence of aversive factors or even to an impaired ability to withhold innate or conditioned responses. An antifrustration effect resulting from BZR agonism is suggested by the increase of responding maintained by response-contingent reward in the situation where the reward is reduced or omitted. Electrical stimulation of the periaqueductal gray area of the midbrain via chronically implanted electrodes in animals is aversive and elicits a number of emotional reactions; BZR agonists increase the aversive threshold. States of acute anxiety characterized by behavioral and physiologic symptoms (cardiovascular, endocrine) can be induced by chemicals known to be anxiogenic in man, e.g., convulsants such as pentylenetetrazol, inverse agonists at the BZR administered in subconvulsive doses, or even abrupt drug withdrawal after chronic treatment with high doses of sedatives. Ultrasonic distress cries by rat pups acutely separated from their mothers are decreased by BZR full and partial agonists.

The pharmacologic specificity of BZR full and partial agonists in the above paradigms is impressive, whereas antidepressants, analgesics, and antipsychotics are all relatively ineffective. However, it is possible that these animal models actually assess effects at the BZR *per se* rather than anxiolytic activity in general. Hence, it is controversial whether such tests are useful in identifying agents acting by mechanisms other than BZR agonism, but which might nonetheless be anxiolytic in humans.

Sedative and Hypnotic Effects

Sedation is a ambiguous term. It can indicate, on the one hand, the normalization of an abnormally elevated state of vigilance or arousal (speed and intensity of reaction to stimuli) that impairs normal function. On the other hand, it can mean a reduction from a normal to a subnormal level at which various brain functions of an individual are impaired. Sedative effects in animals usually are assessed by observing the spontaneous behavior (posture, locomotor, and social interaction), the reaction to various stimuli (e.g., the startle response), and performance in instrumental tests requiring continuous or timed-intermittent conditioned responding (e.g., continuous active avoidance). Reduction of vigilance also can be assessed by quantitative EEG monitoring. BZR agonists produce signs of sedation at doses that are higher than those eliciting anticonflict and anticonvulsant activity, although the dose ranges for these different effects can, nonetheless, overlap. For example, at low doses of BZR agonists, there is only an increase in the rate of punished responding (predictive of an anxiolytic effect), whereas at higher doses there is a concomitant reduction in the rate of unpunished responding (indicative of CNS depression). In diverse animal models the therapeutic index of BZR partial agonists has been found to be further improved beyond that of the full agonists.[16]

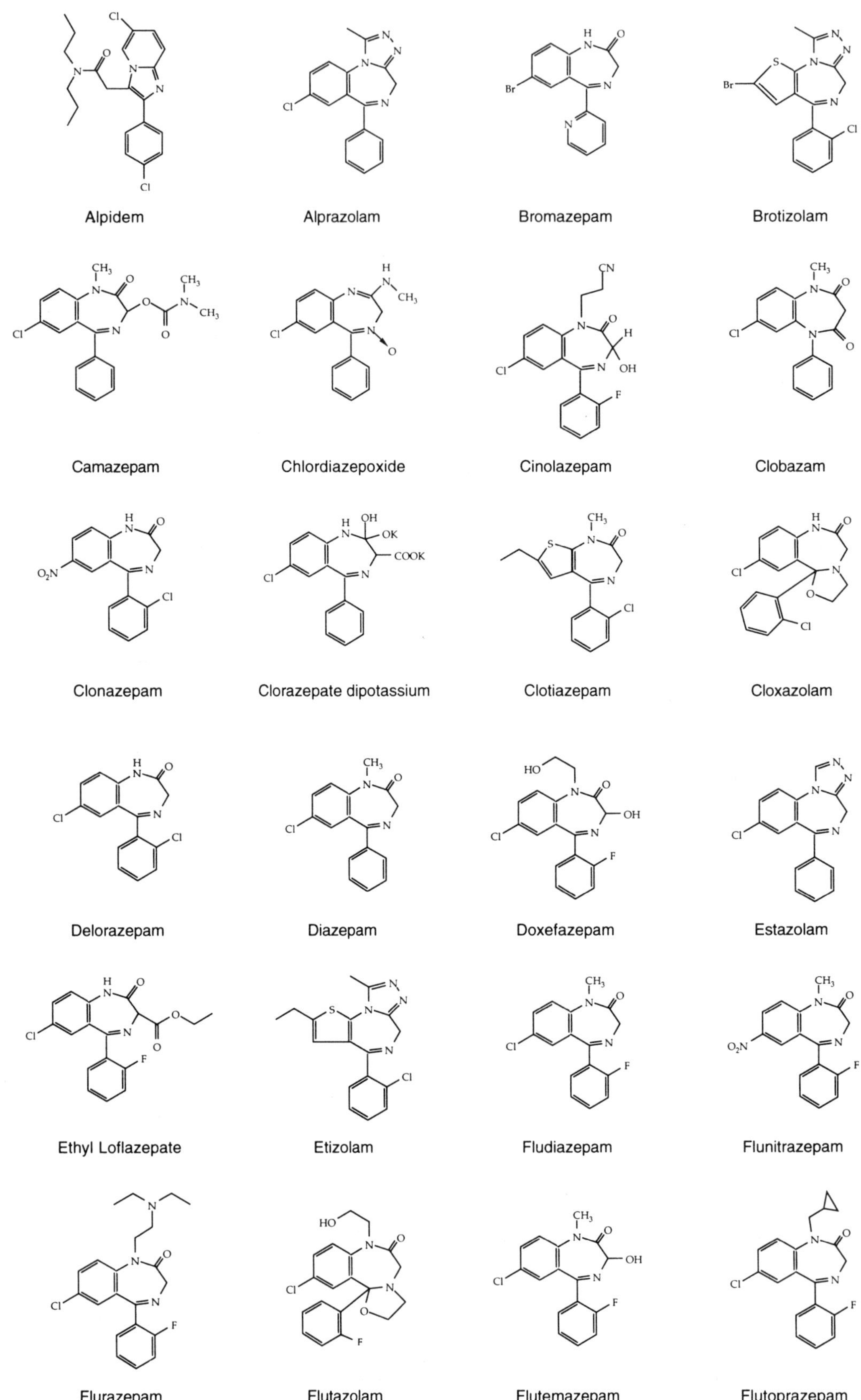

Figure 14.2 Chemical Structures of Marketed Benzodiazepine Receptor Agonists

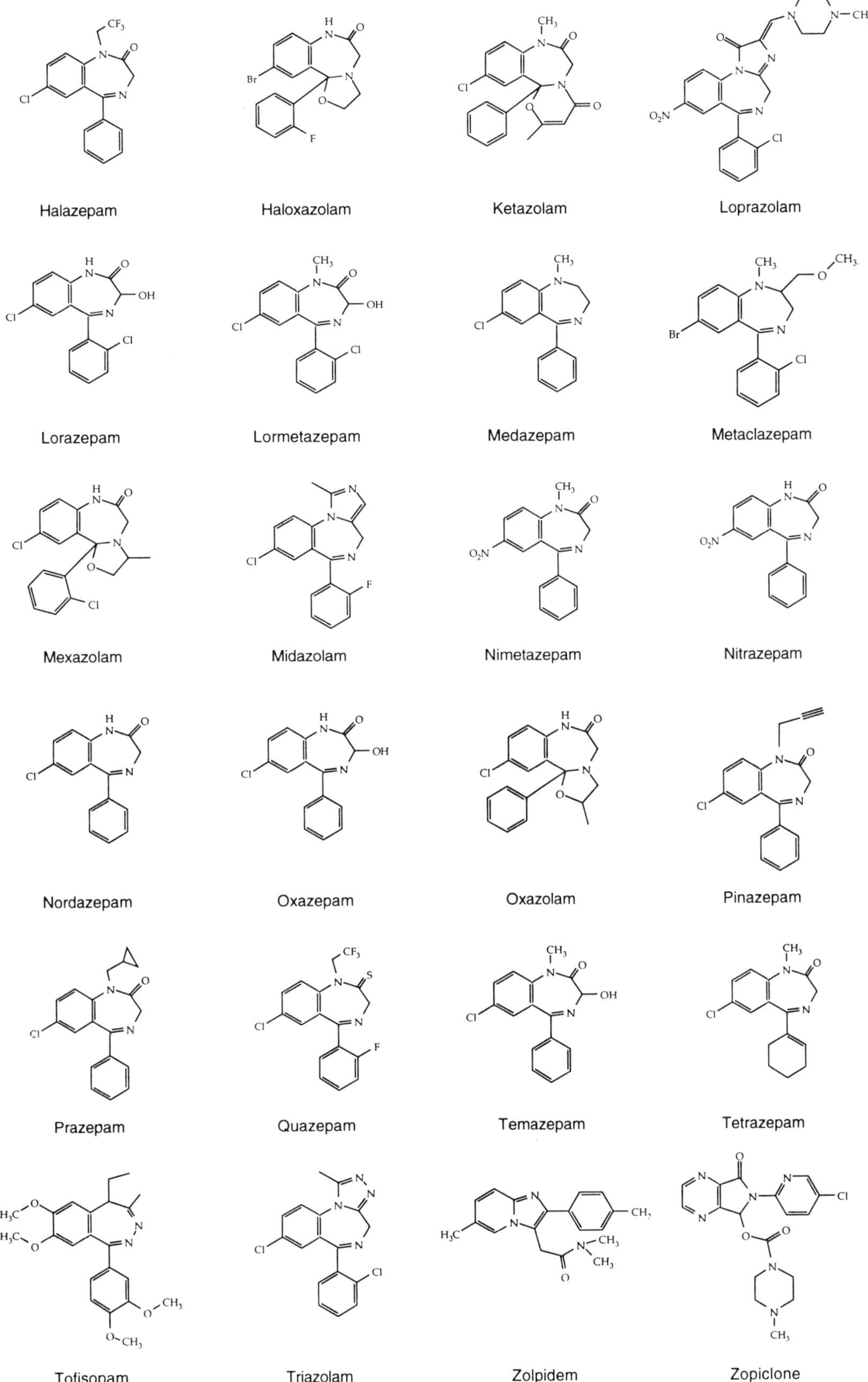

Halazepam
Haloxazolam
Ketazolam
Loprazolam
Lorazepam
Lormetazepam
Medazepam
Metaclazepam
Mexazolam
Midazolam
Nimetazepam
Nitrazepam
Nordazepam
Oxazepam
Oxazolam
Pinazepam
Prazepam
Quazepam
Temazepam
Tetrazepam
Tofisopam
Triazolam
Zolpidem
Zopiclone

Figure 14.2 *Continued*

The induction of anterograde amnesia, the inability to recall events that occurred while under the influence of the drug, is probably directly related to the occurrence of sedation. Anterograde amnesia produced by BZR full agonists is thought to be due mainly to impaired acquisition or early consolidation as a result of reduced vigilance.[17] This might be related to the observed blockade of long-term potentiation by such compounds. Full agonism at the BZR is apparently required to induce anterograde amnesia in animals, since various partial agonists failed to induce anterograde amnesia.[18]

The effect of BZR agonists on sleep in various species differs. Sleep assessed by electroencephalographic (EEG) methods in cats is drastically reduced, and wakefulness is increased over a wide dose range. In contrast, sleep in rabbits and rats is dose-dependently increased, with little alteration in sleep architecture. Unfortunately, there is very little information on the effect of BZR agonists in sleep-disturbed animals. BZR agonists given at relatively high doses have been found to affect the free-running, sleep-wakefulness rhythm in hamsters, with the direction and intensity of the change depending critically on the time of administration during the circadian cycle. It is a widely held but poorly documented view that to be effective in enhancing sleep it is necessary for the drug to reduce vigilance, i.e., that improved sleep is a direct consequence of sedation.

In the early days of BZR research, the taming effect of BZs (i.e., reduction of spontaneous and evoked aggression) received the most attention; however, subsequent studies clearly showed that BZR agonists lack specific antiaggressive properties.[19] They clearly reduce "anxious" or "defensive" aggression, but are relatively ineffective against various forms of innate or offensive aggressivity. In fact, these drugs sometimes can even induce aggressive behavior in some animal species under certain experimental conditions.

Anticonvulsant Activity

BZR agonists are among the most potent drugs known for use in preventing or abolishing seizures in animals induced acutely by chemicals administered systemically (e.g., pentylenetetrazol, bicuculline, picrotoxin, inhibitors of GABA biosynthesis, penicillin, local anesthetics, inhibitors of acetylcholinesterase) applied locally on the cortical surface or into the ventricular system (cardiac glycosides, the glutamate receptor stimulant NMDA), or applied chronically into the cortex (focal aluminum or cobalt epilepsy). They are also effective in protecting against hyperbaric seizures and seizures which develop after chronic intermittent electrical stimulation in the limbic system beginning at a subthreshold intensity (kindled seizures). Electroconvulsive seizures are also prevented by most (but not all) BZR agonists, although at doses considerably higher than those found to block chemically-induced seizures. Various genetic models of epilepsy (a petit mal-like phenotype in rats, seizures induced by acoustic stimulation in genetically-prone mouse strains, or myoclonic seizures induced by photic stimulation in genetically-prone baboons) respond to BZR agonists. Thus, BZR agonists are effective in all current animal epilepsy models predictive of efficacy in most forms of human epilepsy or convulsive states.[20] Consistent with their broad anticonvulsant activity, BZR agonists prevent or suppress epileptiform electric activity induced by various procedures (convulsants, change in ionic composition) in brain slices maintained in vitro, particularly hippocampal slices. They also reduce the neuronal afterdischarges induced in various brain regions by electrical stimulation. BZR agonists have been found to reduce epileptiform activities in foci, as well as to inhibit generalization. Partial agonists at the BZR have been less extensively studied, but are effective anticonvulsants in many test paradigms.[16]

Muscle Relaxant and Motor Incoordinating Action

Normal and increased skeletal muscle tone (spasticity, rigidity) of various forms is reduced by BZR agonists, e.g., after brain stem transection or ischemic lesion of the forebrain, monoamine depletion by reserpine, administration of spasmogens such as $GABA_A$ receptor blockers or glycine receptor blockers, as well as in certain genetic forms of spasticity. Transmission at the neuromuscular junction is not affected. The sites of the myorelaxant action of BZR agonists are clearly at both spinal and supraspinal levels. In the spinal cord, monosynaptic and particularly polysynaptic ventral root reflexes are dose-dependently depressed by BZR agonists; postsynaptic and, even more markedly, presynaptic inhibition (primarily afferent depolarization) of motoneurons is increased. Furthermore, BZR agonists reduce muscle tone and, in addition, impair supraspinal (in particular, cerebellar) control of motor coordination resulting in ataxia. However, under these conditions the maximal voluntary muscle force remains virtually unaffected.

Sensory Functions

No major changes in specific sensory perception are induced by BZR agonists at doses that do not reduce vigilance. Very subtle changes in visual perception have been observed in healthy volunteers. Most notably, these drugs when acting systemically do not induce antinociceptive (analgesic) effects except at doses producing severe sedation. In fact, they have even been found to reduce opiate analgesia. However, when applied directly into epidural or subarachnoid spaces (intrathecally) of the spinal cord, BZR agonists (e.g., midazolam) have been reported to produce pronounced analgesia.[21]

Respiratory and Cardiovascular Functions

At markedly sedating doses, BZR agonists dose-dependently depress respiration.[2] This effect results from a combination of muscle relaxation and the depressed sensitivity of the reticular formation to carbon dioxide. The respiratory depressant effect of other drugs (e.g., opiates) is increased by concomitant treatment with BZR agonists.

The effects of BZR agonists on the cardiovascular system are rather modest.[2] Heart rate may be increased moderately owing to preferential depression in the brain stem control of vagal activity. Arterial blood pressure is slightly reduced at high doses via a reduction of sympathetic outflow. Cardiovascular responses to various stimuli and emotional stress are very sensitive to BZR agonists. These drugs also moderately reduce blood pressure in various forms of experimental arterial hypertension. Antiarrhythmic effects have been described and are likely to result from a central reduction of vagal and sympathetic activities.

Effects on Central Monoamine Systems

In normal animals only very high doses of BZR agonists reduce the spontaneous electrical activity of identified neurons in nuclei of serotonergic (raphe nucleus), noradrenergic (locus coeruleus) and dopaminergic (substantia nigra) systems. Accordingly, the turnover of these amines is moderately decreased. The same is true for the cholinergic system. On the other hand, stress-induced activation of these monoaminergic neurons is robustly attenuated by BZR agonists.

Miscellaneous Effects

BZR agonists differ from most other CNS-active drugs by their virtual lack of direct activity in the periphery.[2] Thus, autonomic and endocrine functions are not affected directly. However, autonomic responses to emotional stress (cardiovascular, respiratory, GI, urogenital, hypothalamic-pituitary-adrenal cortical axis) can be attenuated by treatment with BZR agonists. BZR agonists produce hypothermia in animals maintained at a low ambient temperature; reduced locomotor activity and muscle tone, but also effects on central temperature control, are involved. Cerebral blood flow and oxygen consumption are reduced at high, markedly sedating doses of BZR agonists as a consequence of over-all reduced neuronal activity.

Therapeutic Uses of BZR Agonists

An overview of the main therapeutic uses of the marketed BZR agonists is provided in Table 14.1 (for a recent review of the literature see Ref. 22). Approximately 50 BZs and non-BZs acting as BZR agonists are now registered for clinical use (Table 14.2); therapeutic nuances of the individual compounds may differ (thereby providing the basis for differential patterns of approved, as well as actual, therapeutic use).

Anxiety

Anxiety is an emotion dominated by the perception or anticipation of danger for physical and/or psychic integrity, well-being, and self-esteem, or the fear of inability to cope with various problems or expectations. Anxiety, or fear, is a physiologic phenomenon that acts as a warning signal for a real or potential danger. Anxiety becomes pathologic when it occurs in the absence of any real danger or when the intensity of the emotion is exaggerated. Both physiologic and pathologic anxiety can be life-threatening when occurring in the face of pre-existing organic disorders and may create or perpetuate various physiologic dysfunctions. It is important to note that moderate and severe anxiety are very frequent and that psychiatrists come in contact with only a small proportion of anxious individuals, although true anxiety disorders are esti-

Table 14.1 Main Therapeutic Uses of BZR Agonists

Anxiety:
Generalized anxiety disorder
Phobic disorders
Panic disorder
Somatization disorder
Sleep Disorders
Vigilance Reduction
Seizures
Anesthesiology:
Premedication
Induction
Maintenance
Conscious Sedation
Muscle Relaxation
Acute Crisis Management
Dysthymia, Supportive Therapy of Depression

Table 14.2 Background Information on the Marketed BZR Ligands

Generic Name (Trade Names)	Dosage Forms	Main Therapeutic Areas (Representative Clinical Dosing Regimen)
Alpidem (INN, BAN, USAN) Ananxyl	tablet: 50 mg	tranquilizer oral: 50 mg given 3 times daily
Alprazolam (INN, BAN, JAN, USAN) Alplax, Alplax-Digest, Alprox, Apo-alpraz, Cassadan, Constan, Frontal, Medepolin, Mialin, Novo-Alprazol, Pazolam, Prazin, Prinox, Solanax, Talfil, Trankimazin, Tranquinal, Unilan, Valeans, Wideslow, Xanax, Xanor	tablet: 0.25, 0.5, 1, 2 mg	tranquilizer oral: 0.25–0.5 mg given 3 times daily, up to a maximal 4 mg/day
Bromazepam (INN, BAN, JAN, USAN) Atemperator, Bartul, Bromidem, Bromalex, Bromazanil, Bromazep, Brozam, Bromidem, Compendium, Creosedin, Deptran, Durazanil, Gasmol, Gityl, Lectopam, Lekotam, Lenitin, Lesotan, Lexantin, Lexatin, Lexaurin, Lexilium, Lexomil, Lexotan, Lexotanil, Lexpiride, Miopropan T, Neo-OPT, Neurozepam, Normoc, Nulastres, Octanyl, Pascalium, Seniran, Sipcar, Somalium, Sulpan, Ultramidol	capsule: 1.5, 3, 6, 12 mg drops tablet: 1.5, 2, 3, 5, 6, 12 mg	tranquilizer oral: 3–18 mg daily
Brotizolam (INN, BAN, JAN, USAN) Indormyl, Ladormin, Lendorm, Lendormin(e), Lindormin, Sintonal	tablet: 0.25, 0.5 mg	hypnotic oral: 0.125–0.25 mg at bedtime
Camazepam (INN) Albego, Limpidon, Nebolan, Panevril, Paxor	dragee: 10, 20 mg tablet: 20 mg	tranquilizer oral: 10 mg given 2–3 times daily
Chlordiazepoxide (INN, BAN, JAN, USAN) [Chlordiazepoxide Hydrochloride is BAN, JAN, USAN] Ansiacal, A-Poxide, Balance, Bent, Benzodiapin, Binomil, Brigen-G, Cebrum, Chemdipoxide, Chlorax, Chlordiazachel, Chlordiazepoxidum, Chlortran, Corax, C-Tran, Contol, Decacil, Diapax, Diazepina, Disarim, Eden-psich, Elenium, Elibrium, Endequil, Equibral, Gabil, Gene-Poxide, Helogaphen, Huberplex, I-Liberty, J-Liberty, Khlozepid, Klimax-S, Klipaks, Klopoxid, Labican, Lentotran, Liberans, Librelease, Libritabs, Librium, Librizan, Lipoxide, Lixin, Medilium, Mesural, Mitran, Multum, Murcil, Nack, Napoton, Neo Gnostoride, Normide, Novopoxide, Omnalio, Pantrop, Paxium, Peast C, Philicorium, Pneymic, Protensin, Psicofar, Psicosedin, Psicoterina, Radepur, Raysedan, Relaxedans, Relaxil, Reliberan, Relium, Reposal, Reposans, Retcol, Risachief, Risolid, Sakina, Sedans, Sereen, Seren, Serendyl, Servium, Silibrin, Sintesedan, SK-Lygen, Smail, Solium, Sonimen, Trilium, Sophiamin, Tabrium, Trakipearl, Tropium, Untensin, Viansin, Via-Quil, Zeisin, Zetran	capsule: 10, 25 mg dragee: 5, 10, 25 mg injectable formulation tablet: 5, 10, 25 mg capsule (HCl): 5, 10, 15, 25, 30 mg dragee (HCl): 5, 25 mg drops (HCl) injection formulation (HCl) tablet (HCl): 5, 10 mg	tranquilizer oral: 20–40 mg/day, up to a maximal of 100 mg/day; IV: dosage and administration varies according to indication
Cinolazepam (INN) Gerodorm	tablet: 40 mg	hypnotic oral: 40 mg at bedtime
Clobazam (INN, BAN, USAN) Castilium, Clarmyl, Clopax, Frisin, Frisium, Karidium, Noiafren, Odipam, Pixie, Sederlona, Sentil, Sulotil, Urbadan, Urbanil, Urbanol, Urbanyl	capsule: 5, 10 mg tablet: 10, 20 mg	tranquilizer, antiepileptic oral: 20–30 mg given as divided daily dose

continued

Table 14.2 *Continued*

Generic Name (Trade Names)	Dosage Forms	Main Therapeutic Areas (Representative Clinical Dosing Regimen)
Clonazepam (INN, BAN, JAN, USAN) Antelepsin, Clonazepamum, Clonex, Iktorivil, Klonopin, Landsen, Ravatril, Ravotril, Rivatril, Rivoril, Rivotril	drops injectable formulation tablet: 0.25, 0.5, 1, 2 mg	antiepileptic oral: 1–2 mg given 3–4 times daily; IV: dosage and administration varies according to indication
Clotiazepam (INN, JAN) Clozan, Distensan, Rize(n), Tienor, Trecalmo, Veratran	drops tablet: 5, 10, 20 mg	tranquilizer oral: 10–30 mg as divided daily dose
Cloxazolam (INN, JAN) Akton, Betavel, Cloxam, Elum, Enadel, Lubalix, Olcadil, Sepazon, Tolestan	capsule: 1, 2 mg tablet: 1, 2 mg	tranquilizer oral: 1–4 mg given 3 times daily
Delorazepam (INN) Briatum, Cipaxil, EN	drops injectable formulation tablet: 0.5, 1, 2 mg	tranquilizer oral: 3–6 mg as divided daily dose; IV: dosage and administration varies according to indication
Diazepam (INN, BAN, JAN, USAN) Aliseum, Alupram, Amiprol, Anksiyolin, Antenex, Ansiolin, Ansium, Anxium-5, Anzepam, Apaurin, Apollonset, Apozepam, Armonil, Assival, Atarviton, Atenex, Atensine, Atilen, Audium, Avex, Bensedin, Best, Betapam, Bialzepam, Bortalium, Calmpose, Canazepam, Cercine, Ceregulart, Condition, Cuadel, Cyclopam, Depocalm, Deprestop, Desconet, Diaceplex, Dialag, Dialar forte, Diapam, Diatran, Diazem, Diazemuls, Diazep, Diaz, Diazem, Diazepan, Diazidem, Dienpax, Dipam, Dipezona, Dizam, Domalium, Doval, Drenian, D-Tran, Dualid, Ducene, Duksen, Duradiazepam, E-Pam, Epanalium, Eridan, Erital, Euphorin-A, Eurosan, Evacalm, Faustan, Gewacalm, Gradual, Gubex, Hexalid, Hipofagin, Horizon, Inibex, Klarium, Lamra, Lembrol, Levium, Liberetas, Lizan, Lorinon, Mandro-Zep, Metamidol, Melil, Gobanal, Meval, Morostan, Neo-Calme, Neosorex, Nervium, Neurolytril, Noan, Notense, Novazam, Novodipam, Paceum, Pacipam, Pacitran, Pax, Paxate, Paxel, Plidan, Pro-Pam, Prantal, Psychopax, Q-Pam, Quetinil, Quievita, Relanium, Relivan, Renborin, Reval, Rival, Saromet, Scriptopam, Sedapam, Sedaril, Seduxen, Serenack, Serenamin(e), Serenzin, Servizepam, Setonil, Sico Relax, Solis, Somasedan, Sonacon, Spasmomen Somatico, Stedon, Stesolid, Stesolin, Stress-Pam, Tensium, Tensopam, Tepa Zepan, Timazepam, Tranimul, Tranquase, Tranquirit, Tranco-Puren, Tranquo-Tablinen, Umbrium, Unisedil, Usempax, Valaxona, ValCaps, Valibrin, Valiquid, Valiltran, Valium, Valoi, Valpinax, Valrelease, Vatran, Vazepam, Vicalma, Vival, Vivol, Zepam	capsule: 2, 3, 5, 6, 10, 15 mg slow release capsule: 15 mg dragee: 2, 5 mg drops injectable formulation sirup suppository: 2, 5, 10 mg tablet: 2, 2.2, 5, 10, 25 mg	tranquilizer, anticonvulsant, sedative oral: 2–10 mg given 3 times daily; IV: dosage and administration varies according to indication

continued

Table 14.2 *Continued*

Generic Name (Trade Names)	Dosage Forms	Main Therapeutic Areas (Representative Clinical Dosing Regimen)
Dipotassium Clorazepate (INN) [Clorazepate Dipotassium is JAN, USAN; Clorazepate Monopotassium is USAN] Anxidin, Audilex, Azene, Belseren, Clorazepatum, Covengar, Darkene, Dikalii Clorazepas, Dipot, Dorken, Enadine, Gen-Xene, Hypnodorm, Hypnor, Justum, Medipax, Mendon, Moderan, Modiur, Nansius, Noctran, Noriel, Novo-Clopate, Primum, Sedex, Silece, Softramal, Somnubene, Tencilan, Tranex, Transene, Tranxen(e), Tranxene-SD, Tranxilen, Tranxilen(e), Tranxilium, Tranxilium digest, Tranxilium Pediatrico, Uni-Tranxene, Valsera, Vegestabil, Vulbegal	capsule: 3.75, 5, 7.5, 10, 15, 20 mg drops injectable formulation sachet: 2.5 mg tablet: 3.75, 7.5, 11.25, 15, 20, 22.5, 50 mg	tranquilizer oral: 5–30 mg as divided daily dose; IV: dosage and administration varies according to indication
Doxefazepam (INN) Doxans	capsule: 10, 20 mg	hypnotic oral: 10–20 mg at bedtime
Estazolam (INN, JAN, USAN) Domnamid, Esilgan, Eurodin, Kainever, Noctal, Nuctalon, ProSom, Somnatrol, Tasedan	tablet: 1, 2 mg	hypnotic oral: 1–2 mg at bedtime
Ethyl Loflazepate (INN, JAN) Meilax, Victan	tablet: 2 mg	tranquilizer oral: 1–3 mg/day
Etizolam (INN, JAN) Arophalm, Capsafe, Demunatto, Depas, Dezolam, Eticalm, Etisedan, Guperies, Medipeace, Nonnerv, Palgin, Pasaden, Sedekopan, Sylazepam	capsule: 0.25 mg drops tablet: 0.1, 0.5, 1 mg	tranquilizer oral: 1–3 mg once daily at bedtime
Fludiazepam (INN, JAN) Elipsan, Elspan, Erispan, Landsen	granule tablet: 0.25 mg	tranquilizer oral: 0.25 mg given 3 times daily
Flumazenil (INN, BAN, USAN) Anexate, Lanexat, Romazicon	available only as injectable formulation	benzodiazepine antagonist parenteral: for reversal of benzodiazepine effects, e.g. 0.2 mg IV is given over 15 sec waiting 45 sec before further 0.2 mg doses repeated at 1 min intervals up to maximally 1 mg (higher titration for treating suspected benzodiazepine overdose)
Flunitrazepam (INN, BAN, JAN, USAN) Darkene, Flumipam, Flunipam, Flunitrax, Flunitrazepamum, Hipnosedon, Hypnodorm, Hypnor, Ilman, Libelius, Metopram, Narcozep, Noriel, Primun, Rohipnol, Rohypnol, Roipnal, Sedex, Somnubene, Valsera	drops injectable formulation tablet: 0.5m 1, 2 mg	hypnotic, anesthetic oral: 0.5–2 mg at bedtime; IV: dosage and administration varies according to indication
Flurazepam (INN, BAN, JAN) [Flurazepam Hydrochloride is USAN] Benozil, Dalmadorm, Dalmane, Dalmate, Dalmene, Domodor, Dormador, Dormodor, Durapam, Felison, Felmane, Flunox, Fluzepam, Fordrim, Insumin, Linzac, Lunipax, Midorm A.R., Morfex, Natam, Niotal, Novoflupam, Remdue, Somlan, Somnol, Som-Pam, Staurodorm, Staurodorm Neu, Valdorm	capsule: 10, 15, 27, 30 mg tablet: 15, 30 mg	hypnotic oral: 15–30 mg at bedtime

continued

Table 14.2 *Continued*

Generic Name (Trade Names)	Dosage Forms	Main Therapeutic Areas (Representative Clinical Dosing Regimen)
Flutazolam (INN, JAN) Coreminal	granule tablet: 4 mg	tranquilizer oral: 4 mg given 3 times daily
Flutemazepam (INN) Somnal	capsule: 2, 5 mg drops	hypnotic oral: 2–5 mg at bedtime
Flutoprazepam (INN, JAN) Restas	tablet: 2 mg	tranquilizer oral: 2–4 mg once daily
Halazepam (INN, BAN, USAN) Alapryl, Pacinone, Paxipam	tablet: 20, 40, 120 mg	tranquilizer oral: 20–40 mg given 3 times daily
Haloxazolam (INN, JAN) Somelin	granule tablet: 5, 10 mg	hypnotic oral: 5–10 mg at bedtime
Ketazolam (INN, BAN, USAN) Anseren, Ansieten, Anxon, Contamex, Larpaz, Loftran, Marcen, Parcil, Sedotime, Solatran, Unakalm	capsule: 15, 30, 45 mg tablet: 30 mg	tranquilizer oral: 15–60 mg as divided daily dose or as a single dose at bedtime
Loprazolam (INN, BAN), also as mesylate salt Avlane, Briantum, Dormonoct, Havlane, Somnovit, Sonin	tablet: 1, 2 mg	hypnotic oral: 1–2 mg at bedtime
Lorazepam (INN, BAN, JAN, USAN), also as pivalat derivative [lorazepam pivalat also named pivazepam] Albium, Almazine, Alzapam, Ansilor, Apo-Lorazepam, Aplacasse, Aripax, Ativan, Bonatranquan, Bonton, Control, Donix, Dorm, Duralozam, Efasedan, Emoten, Emotion, Emotical, Emotival, Grosanevron, Idalprem, Kalmalin, Larpose, Laubeel, Lorabenz, Lorafim, Loram, Lorans, Lorasolid, Loratensil, Loraus, Lorax, Loraz, Lorazepan, Lorenin, Loridem, Lorinax, Lorivan, Lorsedal, Lorsilan, Merlit, Mesmerin, Modium, Nervistop L, NIC, Nifalin, Noan-Gap, Novhepar, Novolorazem, Orfidal, Placidia, Placinoral, Pro Dorm, Proneurit, Psicopax, Punktyl, Quait, Sebor, Securit, Sedacalm, Sedarkey, Sedatival, Sedazin, Sedicepan, Sedizepan, Serenase, Sidenar, Somagerol, Tavor, Temesta, Thymal, Titus, Tolid, Trapax, Tran-quil, Trankilium, Tranquipam, Trapax, Trisedan, Wypax	slow release capsule: 2 mg dragee: 1, 2 mg drops injectable formulation tablet: 0.5, 1, 2, 2.5, 5 mg	tranquilizer, sedative oral, sublingual: 2–7.5 mg as divided daily dose; IV: dosage and administration varies according to indication
Lormetazepam (INN, BAN, JAN, USAN) Dilamet, Ergocalm, Evamyl, Lembrol, Loramet, Loretam, Minias, Noctamid(e), Pronoctan, Sedobrina, Stilaze	capsule: 0.5, 1, 2 mg drops injectable forumlation tablet: 0.5m 1, 2mg	hypnotic oral: 1–2 mg at bedtime; IV: dosage and administration varies according to indication
Medazepam (INN, BAN, JAN) [Medazepam Hydrochloride is USAN] Ansilan, Ansius, Anxitol, Azepamid, Becamedic, Benson, Camarines, Debrum, Diepin, Elbrus, Enobrin, Esmail, Glorium, Kobazepam Nichiiko, Lasazsepam, Lerisum, Medaurin, Medazepol, Megasedan, Metazepam Takeshim, Metonas, Mezepan, Narsis, Navizil, Nivelton, Nobraksin, Nobral, Nobritol, Nobrium, Pamnase, Pazital, Psiquium, Randum, Raporan, Resmit, Rudotel, Sedepam, Serenium, Siman, Siozepam, Stratium, Templane, Tranko Buskas, Tranquilax, Vegatar	capsule: 2, 5, 7.5, 10, 25 mg dragee: 5, 10, 25 mg drops tablet: 5, 10 mg	tranquilizer oral: 15–30 mg as divided daily dose

continued

Table 14.2 *Continued*

Generic Name (Trade Names)	Dosage Forms	Main Therapeutic Areas (Representative Clinical Dosing Regimen)
Metaclazepam (INN), also as hydrochloride salt Talis	drops tablet: 5, 10 mg	tranquilizer oral: 5–30 mg as divided daily dose
Mexazolam (INN, JAN) Melex	drops tablet: 0.5, 1 mg	tranquilizer oral: 0.5–1 mg given 3 times daily
Midazolam (INN, BAN, JAN) [Midazolam Hydrochloride and Midazolam Maleate are USANs] Doricum, Dormicum, Dormonid, Flormidal, Hypnovel, Sorenor, Versed	injectable formulation tablet: 7.5, 15 mg	hypnotic, anesthetic oral: 7.5–15 mg at bedtime; IV: dosage and administration varies according to indication
Nimetazepam (INN, JAN) Elimin, Erimin, Hypnon, Malmin	tablet: 3, 5 mg	hypnotic oral: 3–5 mg at bedtime
Nitrazepam (INN, BAN, JAN, USAN) Alodorm, Apodorm, Arem, Atempol, Benzalin, Calsmin, Cerson, Dormo-Puren, Dumolid, Eatan N, Eunoctin, Gerson, Grandaxin, Hipnax, Hipsal, Hirusukamin, Huberplex, Hypnotin, Ibrovek, Imadorm, Imeson, Insomin, Ipersed, Ipnozem, Lagazepam, Lyladorm, Megadon, Mitidin, Mogadan, Mogadon, Nelbon, Nelmat, Nemnamine, Neuchlonic, Nipam, Nirepam, Nitradorm, Nitrados, Nitrazepan Prodes, Nitrazepol, Nitrenpax, Noctem, Noctene, Novanox, Numdon, Ormodon, Pacisyn, Paxadorm, Paxisyn, Pelson, Persopir, Prosonno, Quill, Radedorm, Relact, Relax, Remnos, Seriel, Sindepres, Somitran, Somnased, Somnibel, Somnipar, Somnite, Sonebon, Sonnolin, Surem, Trazenin, Tri, Unisomnia	capsule: 5 mg drops tablet: 2.5, 5, 10 mg	hypnotic oral: 5–10 mg at bedtime
Nordazepam (INN) [also named desmethyldiazepam] Calmday, Demadar, Lomax, Madar, Nordaz, Praxadium, Sopax, Stilny, Tranxilium N, Vegesan	dragee: 2.5, 5, 10 mg drops tablet: 2.5, 5, 7.5, 15 mg	tranquilizer oral: 5–15 mg as divided daily dose
Oxazepam (INN, BAN, JAN, USAN) Adumbaran, Adumbran, Alepam, Alopam, Anchonat, Anxiolit, Aplakil, Apo-Oxazepam, Aslapax, Azutranquil, Benzotran, Blomsilan, Chemodiazine, Constantonin, Droxacepam, Durazepam, Enidrel, Expidet, Gnostorid, Iranil, Isodin, Januar, Limbial, Mepizin, Murelax, Neo Fargen, Nesontil, Neurofren, Noctazepam, Novoxapam, Nulans, Oksazepam, Opamox, Oxa, Oxabenz, Oxadin, Oxaline, Oxanid, Oxa-Puren, Oxepam, Oxazepamum Pharbita, Oxepam, Oxpam, Pankreoflat Sedant, Pausafren-T, Polidasa, Praxiten, Propax, Psicopax, Psiquiwas, Purata, Quen, Quilibrex, Redipax, Serax, Sedokin, Senepax, Serax, Serenal, Serenid D, Serepax, Seresta, Serpax, Sigacalm, Sobile, Sobril, Tazepam, Tranquo Buscopan, Uskan, Vaben, Wakazepam, Zapex, Zaxopam	capsule: 10, 15, 20, 30 mg dragee: 20 mg drops tablet: 10, 15, 20, 25, 30, 50 mg	tranquilizer oral: 15–60 mg as divided daily dose
Oxazolam (INN, JAN) Convertal, Hializan, Nebusn, Oxazolam, Ozonelum, Pelusarl, Quiadon, Serenal, Serumate, Toccala, Tranquit, Solaquionate	capsule: 10 mg granule tablet: 5, 10, 20 mg	tranquilizer, anesthetic oral: 30–60 mg as divided daily dose (1–2 mg/kg before anesthesia)

continued

Table 14.2 *Continued*

Generic Name (Trade Names)	Dosage Forms	Main Therapeutic Areas (Representative Clinical Dosing Regimen)
Pinazepam (INN) Domar, Duna	capsule: 2.5, 5, 10 mg	tranquilizer oral: 10–20 mg as divided daily dose
Prazepam (INN, BAN, JAN, USAN) Centrac, Centrax, Demetrin, Equipaz, Lysanxia, Mono-Demeterin, Prazene, Reapam, Sedapran, Trepidan, Verstran	capsule: 5, 10, 20 mg drops tablet: 10, 20, 40 mg	tranquilizer oral: 10–60 mg as divided daily dose
Quazepam (INN, BAN, USAN) Doral, Dormalin, Dorme, Dormyl, Hipnodane, Oniria, Prosedar, Quazium, Quiedorm, Selepam, Temodal	tablet: 7.5, 15, 30 mg	hypnotic oral: 7.5–15 mg at bedtime
Temazepam (INN, BAN, USAN) Cerepax, Euhypnos, Lenal, Levanxene, Levanxol, Mabertin, Maeva, Normison, Planum, Razepam, Redupax, Remestan, Reposium, Restoril, Signopam, Temaz, Temaze, Temazep, Temazepamum, Tenox, Texapam, Tonirem	capsule: 2, 5, 10, 15, 20, 30 mg elixir tablet: 5, 10, 20 mg	tranquilizer oral:10–30 mg at bedtime
Tetrazepam (INN) Clinoxan, Musaril, Myolastan	tablet: 50 mg	central muscle relaxant oral: 75 mg as divided daily dose
Tofisopam (INN, JAN) Grandaxin(e), Seriel	tablet: 50 mg	tranquilizer oral: 150–300 mg as divided daily dose
Triazolam (INN, BAN, JAN, USAN) Asasion, Dumozolam, Halcion, Halrack, Insomnium, Lightcall, Novidorm, Novodorm, Novo-Triolam, Nuctane, Nu-triazo, Onirium, Paruleon, Rilamir, Somniton, Songar, Trialam, Triasan, Triazoral, Trim	capsule: 0.25 mg dragee: 0.2 mg tablet: 0.125, 0.25, 1 mg	hypnotic oral: 0.125–0.25 mg at bedtime
Zolpidem (INN, BAN) [Zolpidem Tartrate is USAN] Ambien, Bikalm, Ivadal, Lorex, Niotal, Stilnoct, Stilnox	dragee: 10 mg tablet: 10 mg	hypnotic oral: 10–20 mg at bedtime
Zopiclone (INN, BAN, JAN) Amoban, Amovane, Cronus, Datolan, Imovance, Imovane, Limovan, Sopivan, Ximovan, Zimovane	dragee: 7.5 mg tablet: 7.5 mg	hypnotic oral: 7.5 mg at bedtime

Note: The clinical information contained in the above table is a compilation from numerous sources; it is very extensive but, especially in view of the difficulties in obtaining information at an international level, definitely not exhaustive. Further, the information provided on therapeutic doses (for which adequate differentiation is not made for the various salts, derivatives, and free base) and usage is intended for general comparative purposes and should not serve as the basis of any medical decisions with respect to individual patients. This is all the more the case in view of international differences in diagnostic and clinical practices, as well as precautions required for special patient populations which could not be adequately taken into account in such a general review. Combination preparations are excluded. Abbreviations: INN = International Nonproprietary Name; BAN = British Approved Name; JAN = Japanese Accepted Name; USAN = United States Adopted Name

mated to have a prevalence within the general population of between about 4 and 8 percent. An extensive review of the diagnosis, epidemiology, pathophysiology and management of anxiety disorders is provided elsewhere.[23,24]

BZs acting as full BZR agonists (e.g., alprazolam, lorazepam, diazepam, bromazepam) provide the predominant drug therapy of anxiety disorders. Recently, the non-BZ alpidem, which also acts at the BZR, was registered for this indication in France (but has subsequently been withdrawn from the market owing to the occurrence of hepatic side-effects). The most frequent use of BZs as anxiolytics is in situational anxiety in emergency medicine (severe injuries, cardiac infarction), in the hospital setting (before operations and stressful diagnostic interventions), and in acute stressful psychic situations, as well as severe physical illness. The immediate relief provided by BZR agonists in treating anxiety disorders is well documented. Although the efficacy of these drugs appears to be maintained over a long period, a series of issues arise when treatment is administered for more than several weeks (see below). As with all medical interventions, the balance between benefit and risk has to be evaluated (and periodically re-evaluated if treatment continues) on an individual basis. Alternative or concomitant treatments sometimes may be indicated for phobic or panic disorders, e.g., psychotherapy, behavioral therapy, or antidepressants. There is no convincing evidence to indicate that concomitant BZ treatment interferes with behavioral therapy.[25]

Sleep Disorders

The inability to initiate and/or maintain sleep (insomnia) is estimated to affect about one-third of the general population (with prevalence in women and the elderly even higher). Hypnotics continue to be commonly used, with some individuals taking them for relatively long periods. BZs acting as full BZR agonists are among the predominantly used drugs for treating sleep disorders (e.g., triazolam, flunitrazepam, temazepam, flurazepam); however, recently non-BZs that also act as BZR full agonists (zolpidem, zopiclone) have been added to the therapeutic armamentarium. Such BZR full agonists are the drugs of choice in this indication based on a superior therapeutic index.[26] Nonetheless, barbiturates, glutethimide, methyprylon, and chloral derivatives continue to maintain a place in the treatment of sleep disorders,[27] as have miscellaneous other compounds not further considered here, e.g., bromides, *L*-tryptophan, sulfonal, ethchlorvynol, ethinamate, triclofos, and chlomethiazole, as well as antidepressants, antihistamines, and phenothiazines.[28] A traditional view holds that any sedative agent will also induce or improve sleep at higher ("hypnotic") doses. This is not true. Insomniacs do not require drugs that make them sleepy or tired, but rather drugs that facilitate the onset of sleep from a normal level of vigilance and that maintain this sleep for an appropriate duration at a normal depth. BZR agonists in appropriate doses do exactly this. Latency to sleep and awakenings are reduced (to average values in good sleepers), latency to sleep after awakening during the normal sleep period is reduced, total sleep duration is normalized, and awakening at the end of sleep is easy and followed by normal vigilance. Doses to achieve this goal have to be adapted to the individual's sensitivity to centrally active drugs and to the severity of the insomnia. The effect of BZR agonists on sleep structure is well known from sleep laboratory studies in healthy volunteers. These drugs tend to increase the non-REM (rapid eye movement) sleep phases 2 and 3 at the expense of phase 4 and to prolong the latency to REM sleep and to reduce REM sleep at higher doses. It is, unfortunately, difficult to translate these findings to disturbed sleepers. The use of ultra-short acting BZR agonists to induce sleep with the apparent potential for induction of bizarre behavior and daytime withdrawal hyperactivity versus longer-acting BZR agonists with possible daytime sedation and motor impairment has remained a controversial issue.[29] Sleep disorders are very frequently a consequence of anxious apprehension and often the fear of a further sleepless night acts to maintain a vicious circle. This is another reason to use the lowest necessary anxiolytic dose (which will produce only minimal sedation).

Sedation

The term sedation is, unfortunately, used to indicate both the normalization of pathologically increased vigilance as well as the reduction of vigilance to a level below normal, whether as a therapeutic goal or, alternatively, as an undesired side-effect. Sedation is therapeutically indicated when vigilance is pathologically exaggerated to an extent that it disturbs well-being and performance. Such situations may occur acutely for various endogenous and exogenous reasons or even chronically, e.g., under continuous stressful living situations. Behavioral overexcitation may be overt, observed as agitation, or it may be masked, occurring as extreme inner tension. Of course, overexcitation generally accompanies anxiety; therefore, sedation concomitant to anxiolysis is, in fact, a desired drug effect in treating severe anxiety. BZR agonists are commonly used as sedatives.

BZR agonists have multiple uses in anesthesiology: as anxiolytics given beginning days or weeks prior to the diagnostic or surgical intervention; as hypnotics administered before, during, and after hospitalization; as premedication immediately before the intervention in order to induce anxiolysis, reduce sensory input and metabolic rate, minimize autonomic activation and, in general, facilitate the induction of anesthesia; and postoperatively to reduce agitation and promote sleep.[30] BZR agonists (e.g., midazolam, lorazepam, diazepam) are ideally suited for conscious sedation (i.e., a marked reduction of vigilance without complete loss of consciousness and with maintained ability to cooperate and communicate, amnesia for aversive events occurring within this state and robust anxiolysis), which is used increasingly for all kinds of endoscopies and in combination with analgesics to achieve tolerance of mechanical ventilation via an endotracheal tube when assisted respiration is required. Conscious sedation may be indicated for a relatively short time or may have to be maintained over days to even weeks. The ability of BZR full agonists to induce anterograde amnesia is valued in anesthetic practice. BZR agonists with the appropriate pharmacokinetic properties have to be chosen; for IV anesthesia the formulation becomes especially important (e.g., to avoid local reactions). It must be kept in mind that BZR agonists are not analgesic; therefore, analgesics must be given concomitantly if control of pain is required. Complete surgical anesthesia in the traditional sense (unconsciousness, loss of reflexes, analgesia) must not be the goal with a BZR agonist alone. The advantage of these drugs in maintenance (or balanced) anesthesia is their property to potentiate the effects of general anesthetics and, thus, the possibility of using smaller doses of the latter. The safety of BZR agonists in anesthesia has been increased further by the availability of a specific antagonist, flumazenil.[31] Sedation can be terminated, interrupted, or attenuated at any time with flumazenil. Use of BZR agonists in anesthesiology is very convenient because of their excellent tolerability, lack of unpleasant subjective effects, and, hence, good patient acceptance.

Anticonvulsant Activity

The potent and broad anticonvulsant activity of BZR agonists lends itself to many therapeutic applications, including petit mal and status epilepticus.[32] Diazepam, clonazepam, clobazam, and nitrazepam are therapeutically administered as antiepileptics. They are indicated in all acute convulsive states of any cause. Intravenous administration is then the most appropriate route but intrarectal instillation may be more convenient in children. The dose has to be adjusted to the therapeutic outcome. Severe sedation is inevitable but acceptable in these critical situations.

Epilepsy has a prevalence in the general population of approximately 1 percent and represents a chronic disorder characterized by recurrent seizures. Epilepsies represent a plethora of syndromes involving different seizure types, causes, and electroencephalographic characteristics. Drug therapy has remained the primary treatment modality, with surgical interventions carried out cautiously even in drug-refractory patients. For chronic treatment of epilepsies, BZR agonists are not the first choice (in spite of a much better tolerability than other antiepileptics), except for certain forms of epilepsy in children. The main reason for this restricted use is, on the one hand, the development of tolerance (resulting in so-called "therapeutic escape") in a considerable proportion of patients and, on the other hand, the potential pharmacologic side-effects (oversedation with impairment of cognitive functions). However, as adjunct therapy in patients refractory to monotherapy with other drugs, BZR agonists are very useful. No generally accepted rule for the optimal combination exists, empirical trials are necessary (also see Chapter 19).

Muscle Relaxation

The muscle relaxant activity of BZR agonists is much less suited for therapy than their other actions. A satisfactory muscle relaxant effect is obtained in many cases of acute or chronic increase of muscle tone; however, the doses required most often produce a degree of sedation that disrupts normal function. This is also true of barbiturates, with the additional problem of a narrow therapeutic index. Since there are no drugs with superior and more specific central muscle relaxant activity than BZR agonists, therapeutic use involving very careful dose titration may benefit many patients.

Psychosomatic Disorders

Owing to their effect on the central regulation of autonomic functions, BZR agonists are indicated in cardiovascular, respiratory, GI, and urogenital disorders for which no organic cause can be found in the affected organs, and where psychogenic factors cannot be eliminated by other treatments or procedures.

Mechanism of Action of BZR Agonists

The available BZR agonists produce their therapeutic effects by a single, highly specific molecular mechanism. The molecular target of these drugs is an elementary part of a major neurotransmitter system whose function in the CNS is more easily understood than that of most other neurotransmitter systems. Among CNS-active drugs, BZR agonists belong, therefore, to those whose actions are the currently best understood from the molecular level to the level of behavior. Since the target is the $GABA_A$ receptor, a brief description of the GABAergic system is needed.[33–35]

The GABAergic System

Since BZRs are an integral part of most, or all, of the $GABA_A$ receptors, a basic understanding of the effects of BZR ligands requires knowledge of the GABAergic system. Neurons using GABA as a neurotransmitter are among the most abundant neurons in the CNS. About a third of all synapses in the brain are believed to be GABAergic. GABAergic neurons occur mostly as local neurons or interneurons present in all areas of the CNS involved in the local modulation of neuron activity and, to a lesser extent, as projecting or principal neurons (e.g., cerebellar Purkinje cells, striatonigral, striatothalamic, and nigrothalamic pathways). GABA receptor blockers induce a general in-

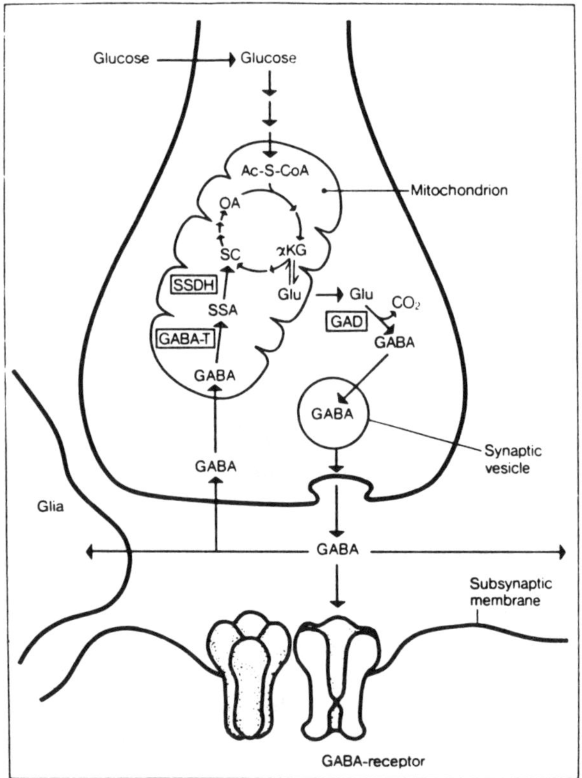

Figure 14.3 Schematic diagram of a GABAergic synapse. In a mitochondrion of the GABAergic nerve terminal glutamate is formed in the Krebs cycle. GAD = glutamic acid decarboxylase. GABA-T = GABA transaminase. SSA = succinic acid semialdehyde. SSDH = succinic semialdehyde dehydrogenase. A γ subunit is required for BZR-ligand binding.

crease in neuronal activity throughout the brain, leading dose-dependently to enhanced alertness, anxiety, muscular spasms, seizures, and even to death. GABAergic neurons synthesize GABA from the ubiquitous product of cell metabolism, glutamic acid, with the help of the enzyme glutamic acid decarboxylase (GAD) (Fig. 14.3). This enzyme is blocked by several agents, e.g., hydrazines. Using antibodies against GAD and GABA itself, GABAergic neurons can be identified in tissue slices. GABA is stored in synaptic vesicles and released upon arrival of an action potential at nerve endings. GABA released into the synaptic cleft is taken up by a specific transporter in GABAergic neurons and by a different one in glia cells. There are experimental compounds that block one or the other transporter. In the synapse, GABA interacts with receptors in the subsynaptic membrane of target neurons and, to a lesser extent, in the membrane of the presynaptic GABAergic neuron itself (GABA autoreceptor). Two classes of GABA receptors are known: the ionotropic $GABA_A$ and the metabotropic $GABA_B$ receptors. They differ by their structure, function, specific agonists and antagonists, and by their regulation through allosteric modulatory sites. The structure of $GABA_B$ receptor is not yet known. It probably belongs to a family of G-protein-coupled receptors. Its activation increases K^+ conductance, depresses a Ca^{2+} channel, and inhibits adenylylcyclase activity. The $GABA_B$ receptor is thought to be present on terminals of GABAergic neurons (as an autoreceptor) and on somadendritic and terminal membranes of GABA-responsive neurons. A late slow inhibitory postsynaptic current (IPSC) in hippocampal pyramidal neurons elicited by activation of GABAergic interneurons is mediated by $GABA_B$ receptors coupled to a K^+ channel. $GABA_B$ receptors also appear to be localized on nerve terminals of non-GABAergic neurons (e.g. noradrenergic neurons) that inhibit the release of various neurotransmitters. Although of apparently less over-all pharmacologic importance than $GABA_A$ receptors, the $GABA_B$ receptor is, nonetheless, of interest in view of the central muscle relaxant baclofen, a selective $GABA_B$ receptor agonist. There are experimental antagonists of the $GABA_B$ receptor also that have been reported to increase vigilance and improve cognitive functions. The BZR is tightly physically coupled to the $GABA_A$ receptor, but not to the $GABA_B$ receptor.

The $GABA_A$ receptor is one of the best-studied neurotransmitter receptors. Isolation of the $GABA_A$ receptor was facilitated by the fact that it copurifies with the BZR, for which excellent photoaffinity ligands were discovered around 1980. Molecular cloning and sequencing revealed that the $GABA_A$ receptor belongs to a superfamily of ligand-gated receptor channels, of which the nicotinic cholinoceptor is the best known and to which the inhibitory glycine and the excitatory glutamate receptors also belong. The $GABA_A$ receptor is probably a pentameric complex (Fig. 14.4) of noncovalently linked glycoprotein subunits pseudosymmetrically arranged to form a central transmembrane pore (channel). At least three different subunit types appear to be required for a fully functional receptor channel, as suggested by experiments using ectopically expressed subunit cRNAs in the *Xenopus* oocyte or mammalian cell lines. The subunits are called α (alpha), β (beta), γ (gamma), δ (delta) and ρ (rho). All subunits have a very similar structural plan and transmembrane topology. They are proteins of about 400 amino acids. Four approximately 20-amino acid long sequences are likely to traverse the lipid double layer of the cell membrane in the form of α-helices. The large extracellular N-terminal part contains a small loop stabilized by a disulphide bridge and contains potential glycosylation sites. Close to the transmembrane-spanning regions are positively charged amino acids. The intracellular part is formed mainly by the sequence between transmembrane segments 3 and 4. Transmembrane segment

II appears to form the inner wall of the channel pore and stabilize the complex in the membrane. The different subunit types show moderate structural homology; in particular, the transmembrane segments are highly homologous. A high polymorphism of the subunits has been discovered.[36] Six isoforms have been identified for the α-subunit, four for the β-subunit, three for the γ-subunit, one for the δ-subunit, and two for the ρ-subunit. Subunit isoforms are encoded by separate genes, but variability may be further increased by alternative splicing as shown so far for the β4 and the γ2-subunit. These splice variants give further diversity to these receptors. The functional roles of this polymorphism for the physiologic functions of the various combinational receptor assemblies and for pharmacologic interactions are not yet known with certainty. However, the α1β2γ2 subunit complex, which is regionally localized within the brain, is the receptor complex to which zolpidem binds[37] and it has been found that coexpression of the γ2 subunit with a selected α and β subunits yields $GABA_A$ receptors exhibiting high affinity binding to BZR ligands.[38]

The $GABA_A$ channel carries a number of other ligand binding sites apart from the GABA binding site (Fig. 14.4). These sites are allosteric modulatory sites, through which ligands can modulate the affinity of the GABA binding site or the conformational transition leading to channel opening. The $GABA_A$ receptor contains several binding sites on its surface that allow its function to be altered by small molecules. Most important, there are binding sites (probably two) for GABA, most likely on β-subunits. Compounds that bind to this site are isosteric or homotopic ligands. In addition, there are many binding sites that are structurally different and located at some distance from the GABA binding site. Compounds binding to these sites are called "allosteric" or "heterotopic" ligands. Most of the binding sites influence each other, i.e., binding of a ligand to another site. Most relevant for therapy is the allosteric interaction between the GABA binding site and the BZR receptor site.

The $GABA_A$ receptor functions as follows. When two molecules of GABA are bound to their specific binding sites on the extracellular domains, the subunits undergo a slight conformational change and the opening of the pore, which is selectively permeable for anions, in particular chloride ions (Fig. 14.4). As a consequence, the Cl^- conductance (g_{Cl^-}) of the membrane increases, and Cl^- ions can flow into or out of the neuron, depending on the concentration gradient between the extracellular space and the cytoplasm and on the actual membrane potential. Most frequently, $GABA_A$ receptor-mediated chloride conductance results in the influx of Cl^- and the hyperpolarization of the neuron; yet in some cells there is a Cl^- efflux and depolarization. The increased Cl^- conductance and the changes in membrane potential counteract the excitatory effect of the cation influx that underlies postsynaptic excitatory currents and the action potential, and hence are the physicochemical basis of the synaptic inhibitory action of GABA.

The operation of GABAergic neurons as inhibitory modules in neuronal circuits is shown schematically in Figure 14.5. Recurrent inhibition is particularly instructive as it shows that an excitatory principal output neuron excites a nearby GABAergic interneuron whenever it fires an action potential. The GABAergic interneuron responds with a burst of action potentials and releases GABA on the principal neuron, thereby depressing its excitability to all excitatory inputs for a short period. In this way, the maximal firing rate of a principal excitatory neuron is reduced. Blockade of $GABA_A$ receptors increases the responsiveness of neurons to even weak excitatory inputs and results in burst firing in response to strong inputs. Recurrent inhibition is a vital mechanism for the normal function of numerous neuron types, e.g., the pyramidal cells in the cortex and the hippocampus.

The Benzodiazepine Receptor

The BZR is an integral binding site on the $GABA_A$-receptor complex, located at some distance from the GABA binding site and mediating allosteric modulation. Allosteric modulation has been studied intensively with enzymes: allosteric enzyme modulators bind to a site different from the active catalytic site and alter the function of this site in a positive or negative direction. Applied to the $GABA_A$ receptor, allosteric modulation is the process whereby the allosteric modulator induces a conformational change of its binding protein; this change is transmitted intramolecularly to the GABA binding site (which alters its affinity for GABA) and/or to the other elements of the complex (that facilitate or depress the conformational transition of the channel induced by GABA, i.e., the channel gating). The BZR was identified by its high affinity for ^3H-labeled diazepam (later many other ligands were used). In tissue homogenates or membrane preparations typical specific saturation binding can be obtained with radioligands, and inhibition of this radioligand binding is used as the simplest test to assess the affinity of a compound for the BZR. Using autoradiographic techniques, the wide, but uneven, distribution of BZR in the CNS and other tissues can be visualized. The BZR antagonist flumazenil can easily be labeled with a short-lived positron emitting nuclide (e.g., ^{11}C) and, due to its very low nonspecific binding, can be used in PET (positron emission tomography) scanning to visualize BZR in the living human brain.

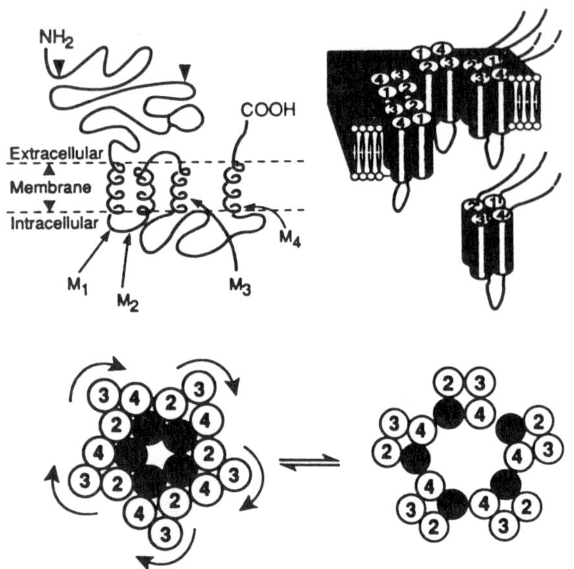

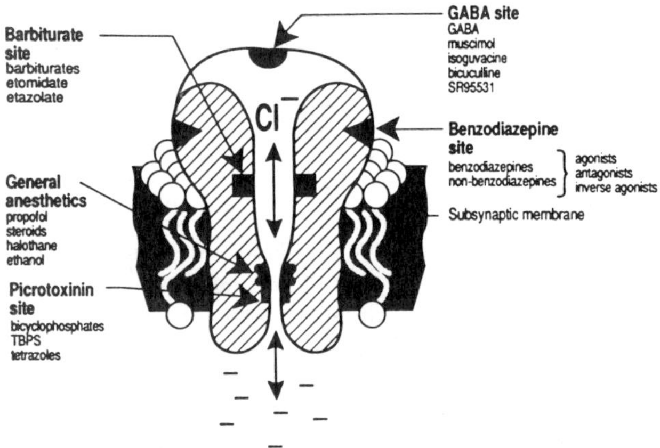

Figure 14.4 Schematic diagram of the GABA$_A$ receptor channel. (A) *Top left*: schematic drawing of a GABA receptor subunit with 4 membrane-spanning α-helical stretches (M_1 to M_4), the N-terminal extracellular position containing potential N-glycosylation sites (*arrowheads*), a disulfide stabilized loop, a larger cytosolic component consisting of the loop between M_3 and M_4 and containing (in some subunits) putative phosphorylation sites. *Top right*: assembly of 5 subunits (only the membrane spanning regions are shown as cylinders) in the lipid bilayer. *Bottom*: possible assembly of the transmembrane region of the 5 subunits in the closed state (*left*) and open state (*right*). (B) Transverse section through the GABA$_A$ receptor channel with the various currently known binding sites (their location is purely hypothetical).

The interaction of ligands with the BZR is unique. The BZR can exert both positive and negative modulation, depending on the ligand. Ligands with positive allosteric modulatory activity are the BZR agonists. They seem to increase the affinity of the GABA binding

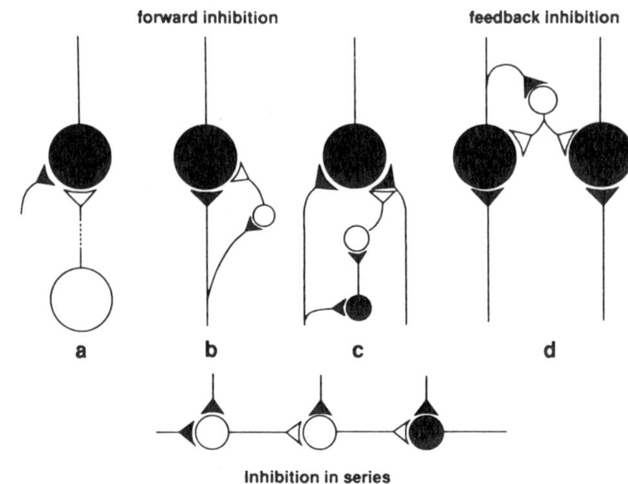

Figure 14.5 Typical synaptic connections of GABAergic neurons (indicated by empty symbols). Excitatory neurons are indicated by shaded symbols. Postsynaptic inhibition is represented by **a** (projecting GABAergic neuron impinging on an excitatory principal neuron, **b** (forward inhibition mediated via local inhibitory GABAergic neuron, and **d** (feedback of recurrent inhibition). Presynaptic inhibition is represented by **c**. GABAergic neurons arranged in a series are illustrated at the bottom.

site for its ligand. This makes the GABA$_A$ receptor more sensitive to the neurotransmitter (and other agonists). By plotting the log concentration of GABA on the abscissa against the chloride conductance induced (e.g., in a neuron in culture) on the ordinate, a characteristic sigmoid dose-response curve is obtained. *BZR agonists* shift this curve dose-dependently to the left without increasing the maximum. The maximal shift obtainable with agonists is about threefold. Another class of ligands (β-carbolines, BZs, and other chemical classes) produce a rightward shift, i.e., they depress the function of the GABA$_A$ receptor channel; they are called *inverse agonists*. Note that these agents do not act at the GABA binding site itself as, for example, the competitive GABA antagonist bicuculline does. However, the over-all effects on CNS function are similar for "isosteric" GABA antagonists and "allosteric" inverse agonists of the BZR. Yet other BZR ligands, of which flumazenil is representative, bind to the allosteric site without producing any appreciable alteration of the GABA gating function. However, these agents block selectively and competitively the action of BZR agonists and inverse agonists. Accordingly, they are called *BZR antagonists*. The ability of ligands to allosterically modulate the GABA$_A$ receptor function reflects this intrinsic efficacy, which is given the theoretical value +1 for agonists, −1 for inverse agonists, and 0 for pure antagonists. As is the case for other receptors, ligands of the BZR exist whose intrinsic efficacies are between those of agonists and antagonists or between inverse agonists and antagonists. These partial agonists and partial inverse agonists produce a less pronounced maximal shift of the GABA dose-response curve than do the full agonists and full inverse agonists. Several partial agonists of the BZR have been under clinical investigation because, based on preclinical results, they should offer several considerable advantages over the full agonists by maintaining the full therapeutic efficacy of the latter for indications like anxiety and sleep disorders, but with markedly reduced amnesia, sedation, ethanol potentiation, motor impairment, tolerance, physical dependence, and abuse liability.[16,18]

From the Molecular to the Neuronal Level

Knowing the functions and operation of GABAergic neurons and considering the basic effect of BZR agonists on the GABA dose-response curve, it becomes possible to make predictions in general terms about how these drugs will affect neuronal activity.[10] However, BZR agonists do not bind to all $GABA_A$ receptors in view of the fact that the actions of this drug class depend on the given $GABA_A$ receptor having the appropriate subunit components. Effective BZ agonists enhance the effect of GABAergic synaptic transmission. However, the extent of this potentiation will greatly differ at the various GABAergic synapses. At those synapses at which no GABA is being released at a certain point in time, BZR agonists will produce no effect. This will also be the case at synapses where the GABA concentration is high enough to saturate $GABA_A$ receptors (because the maximal effect of GABA is not enhanced). This is in contrast to the barbiturates, for example, which not only facilitate the effect of GABA but also open the chloride channel, even in the absence of GABA. BZR agonists will enhance transmission at those GABAergic synapses where the GABA concentration is suprathreshold for an effect but too low to produce the maximal effect. The effect of BZR agonists on neuronal activity will depend not only on the level of tonic or phasic GABAergic input to this neuron, but also on the level of excitatory input. The facilitated GABAergic influence will have either a minor or no effect on the activity of a neuron that receives only a weak or no excitatory input, but will markedly affect the discharge of neurons under a strong excitatory input. The effect of BZR agonists on the global CNS activity is not an even decrease of neuronal firing throughout the system for the reasons just given. Moreover, even though many neurons probably receive a GABAergic synaptic input, the neuronal network complicates the situation considerably. GABAergic neurons are arranged in series in some regions; therefore, the drugs may in fact produce disinhibition of the target neurons of the last GABAergic neuron in the series. GABAergic neurons innervate other neurons representing all neurotransmitter phenotypes, but to differing degrees. Target neurons may themselves produce an inhibitory effect through another transmitter, e.g., dopamine neurons (Fig. 14.6). The maximal over-all effect of BZR agonists is also restricted for another reason: taking the recurrent inhibitory circuit as an illustration, it is evident that with increasing efficiency of GABAergic feedback inhibition on the principal neuron the latter will produce less activation of the GABAergic interneuron, thus avoiding its own complete inhibition. In spite of this complexity, it is reasonable to explain the anxiolytic effect of BZR agonists by this preferential inhibition of neurons in the limbic system that are critical for the generation of the emotion of anxiety and its accompanying symptoms. The anticonvulsant action resides on the depression of the paroxysmal activity of pacemaker neurons and the reduced excitability of follower cells. The other effects of BZR agonists can logically be ascribed to similar influences on other neurons and neuronal systems. Correlating effective doses for the various effects and fractional receptor occupancy in the brain reveals that anxiolytic and anticonvulsant effects are obtained at a small fractional receptor occupancy, while severe sedation and muscle relaxation require a high to near total receptor occupancy.[16]

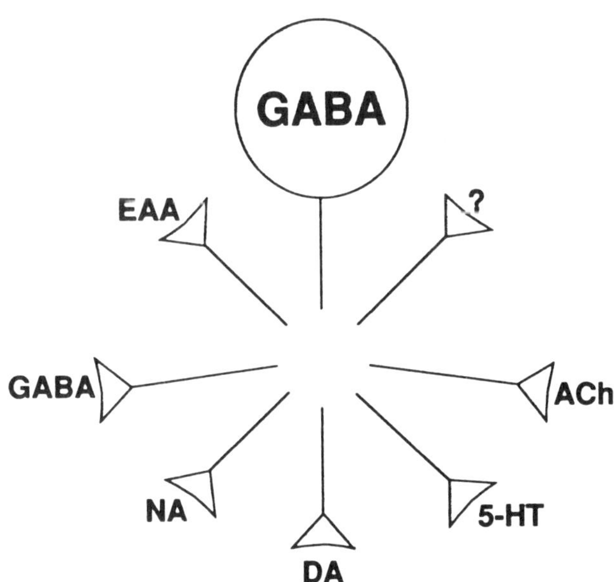

Figure 14.6 Primary target neurons of GABAergic neurons. These innervate neurons using excitatory neurotransmitter amino acids (EAA), GABA, noradrenaline (NA), dopamine (DA), serotonin (5-HT), acetylcholine (ACh) or possibly other neurotransmitters.

Other Possible Mechanisms of Action of BZR Ligands

Essentially no drug is absolutely specific for one biologic target. Nevertheless, as previously noted, most BZR ligands are remarkably selective for their receptor (recognition site) binding on the $GABA_A$ receptor. Some of the BZR ligands inhibit the cellular uptake of adenosine; the relevance of this for their pharmacologic and therapeutic profile is as yet unclear. At very high doses (e.g., those that can be achieved after IV injections to interrupt status epilepticus), some even have a depressant effect on voltage-dependent channels for Na^+ and Ca^{2+} ions.[39]

Some BZR ligands were found to bind to sites on neuronal and non-neuronal cells that are not part of the $GABA_A$ receptor channel.[40] These sites have been called "peripheral BZR" because they were initially found in peripheral tissues. Relative affinities of various BZR ligands for these sites are totally different from those at the allosteric site on $GABA_A$ receptor channels. Thus, although diazepam exhibits similar binding affinity for both the BZRs and the so-called "peripheral site," clonazepam and flumazenil bind only to the former. Furthermore, such "peripheral sites" are also located on glial cells in brain (which permits the monitoring of gliosis through the use of a high-affinity ligand of this binding site). Not suprisingly, the "peripheral site" is structurally totally different from the BZR, with the former sites located mainly on the mitochondrial membrane. These mitochondrial BZRs, as they are sometimes named, seem to be involved in the transport of cytosolic cholesterol into the mitochondrial inner membrane. It has been hypothesized that the mitochondrial BZR is a complex containing a steroid carrier, a voltage-dependent anion channel, and an adenosine nucleotide carrier that is involved in steroidogenesis and mitochondrial respiration. It has also been suggested that the peptide diazepam-binding-inhibitor (DBI) and its processing products regulate the mitochondrial BZR. A possible pharmacologic role of these mitochondrial BZRs at therapeutic doses of the BZR ligands that also exhibit high affinity binding to the mitochondrial BZRs has yet to be established.

Undesirable Side-Effects of BZR Agonists at Therapeutic Doses and Interaction With Other Drugs

Although undesirable side-effects can largely be avoided by optimizing dosage of BZR agonists for the individual patient, doses required for severe cases of anxiety and epilepsies as well as for reducing pathologic muscle tone frequently depress vigilance to a level that disturbs intellectual function and reduces attention and precision for various skills (operation of machines, car driving). The individual sensitivity to this oversedation varies greatly. Hangover with the use of BZR agonists in sleep disorders is the easily avoidable effect of overdosing or of the choice of a drug with an inappropriate duration of action. Muscle relaxation may result in blurred speech and disturbed gait, especially in elderly patients. Behavioral disinhibition (uncontrolled eloquence, aggressive behavior, bouts of eating and drinking) may occur at higher doses and even at normal doses in individuals having minimal experience with centrally active drugs. Such bouts of overactivity and amnesia for these periods can occur with all agonists with a very rapid onset of action that are taken as hypnotics. Criminal acts have on occasion been claimed to have been performed in such drug-induced states of disinhibition. There are few reported allergies to BZR agonists. Respiratory depression and apnea can occur from IV administration of BZR agonists (especially in bronchitic patients).

Problems can occur due to long-lasting exposure to BZR agonists. One such is the development of tolerance to a therapeutic effect. Loss of antiepileptic efficacy occurs in a fair proportion of patients (manifested as escape phenomena). In contrast, little loss of the sleep-improving effect of BZR agonists has been found in insomniacs with prolonged treatment[41] and, futhermore, anxiolytic efficacy has been demonstrated for a few BZR agonists in clinical trials lasting for two to six months.[42] Physical dependence manifested as drug discontinuation symptoms following abrupt withdrawal is a function of duration of drug exposure, dose, duration of action of the drug, and the personality of patients.[43] Drug discontinuation symptoms may be indicative of the recurrence of the original disorder (anxiety, insomnia, seizures) or, alternatively, true withdrawal. The mechanisms of tolerance and physical dependence are in principle identical (adaptation to the primary action of the drugs), although the neuronal systems involved may not all be the same. Basically, a reduced efficiency of the $GABA_A$ receptor channel develops that may involve the number and/or affinity of BZR and, more likely, a loss of the gating function of the $GABA_A$ receptor channel (possibly due to receptor phosphorylation). It should be recalled that this receptor shows a pronounced tendency to desensitize even in the absence of allosteric modulators. Consistent with this view is the fact that withdrawal symptoms are the mirror image of the primary action of BZR agonists and are simulated by blockade of $GABA_A$ receptors. Persistence of the original neuropsychiatric disorders during drug abstinence and physical dependence may lead to subsequent chronic drug use and abuse. However, the primary addictive property of BZR agonists is very weak and has been ascribed to BZR agonists almost exclusively by alcoholics and abusers of other drugs. This population, therefore, represents a group with a particularly high risk of abuse and dependence for BZR agonists. The controversy about the relative dependence liability of short- versus long-lasting BZR agonists probably reflects the fact that short-acting compounds are less prone to induce dependence; however, once dependence has developed, withdrawal reactions are more pronounced. A recent international survey of the views of numerous expert psychiatrists concluded that the qualitative differences among the marketed BZR agonists in abuse liability are minimal, with the development of physical dependence at therapeutic doses not considered to be a major clinical problem in view of its ready management by the treating physician.[44] Chronic personality changes and cognitive impairments have been reported in long-term users of

BZR agonists. These observations are rare and probably are more related to pretreatment personality disturbances than to primary drug effects.

Pharmacokinetic and pharmacodynamic factors may lead to interactions of BZR agonists with other drugs. Aspirin competes with protein binding of BZs and can enhance the pharmacologic effect of the latter. The histamine type 2 receptor antagonists cimetidine and ranitidine inhibit the metabolism of some BZs. The non-BZ zolpidem lacks this interaction. An additive or supra-additive pharmacodynamic interaction between BZR agonists and other agents with CNS depressant activity (barbiturates, general anesthetics, antipsychotics, antidepressants, opioids) is not surprising. The interaction with ethanol is complex, depending on both the dose of ethanol and that of the BZR agonist. Nevertheless, the possibility of a potentiating interaction has always to be considered. Stimulant drugs, e.g., caffeine, reduce all or some of the effects of BZR agonists. Although BZs do not generally excessively stimulate hepatic microsomal oxidizing systems,[45] the metabolism of BZs may nonetheless be affected by drugs that do so.

Toxic Effects of Overdoses of BZR Agonists

BZR agonists are remarkably free of organ toxicity.[45] Symptoms of overdosing, therefore, reflect exaggerated pharmacologic effects. The highest doses of BZR agonists that can be administered are not fatal in healthy subjects, unless taken in combination with other agents (e.g., ethanol). In overdose, the loss of consciousness can reach deep stages of coma, but is not dangerous by itself. However, depression of respiration in overdose can be a problem in those individuals with otherwise compromised respiratory function. Cardiovascular effects are rarely life-threatening. Death can occur in a cold environment owing to impaired temperature regulation. Treatment of overdose should concentrate on support of vital functions. The specific BZR antagonist flumazenil produces rapid reversal of intoxication with BZ and non-BZ compounds exerting their undesirable effects via the BZR. However, mixed overdoses involving BZR agonists and other agents are generally dominated by the effects of the latter. Flumazenil is capable of fully abolishing the effects of the BZR agonist, thus reducing the intoxication to those adverse effects induced by the other agents. A potential complication that has to be kept in mind when using flumazenil is that the BZR agonist involved in the overdose might in fact counteract some dangerous effects of another intoxicant (e.g., the convulsant effect of overdose with tricyclic antidepressants), which treatment with a BZR antagonist could then unmask.

Pharmacokinetics of the BZR Agonists

The pharmacokinetics of BZs and active metabolites are complex,[46] but differences in the pharmacokinetic profile of BZs often are presumed to provide a reasonable basis for clinical selection. BZs and the other available non-BZ agonists of the BZR are weak organic bases and largely undissociated at physiologic pH. Their water solubility is over-all rather poor except for some salts (oxazepam hemisuccinate, clorazepate dipotassium salt, midazolam hydrochloride, chlordiazepoxide hydrochloride, flurazepam hydrochloride). The lipid-water partition coefficient at physiologic pH varies enormously, from about 50 to 10,000. Absorption is mostly complete, although the rate of absorption can be slow (oxazepam) or very rapid (diazepam, triazolam, midazolam). Food can slow absorption without reducing its extent. Clorazepate is hydrolyzed and decarboxylated to desmethyldiazepam in the acid gastric content and absorbed as such. Binding to plasma albumin is high for many BZs; they share the same binding site as tryptophan and aspirin, and competition therefore occurs. A relevant liver first-pass effect is observed only with flumazenil. Owing to their high liposolubility BZs show a large tissue distribution (volume of distribution). For many BZs, tissue distribution rather than elimination half-life is the primary determinant of the duration of therapeutic action (e.g., flunitrazepam). Passage of the blood-brain barrier appears to be rapid. BZs and their metabolites also can cross the placenta to accumulate in fetal circulation. Elimination of BZs occurs mainly by metabolism on liver microsomes and subsequent renal excretion of water soluble metabolites. Terminal elimination half-time does not correlate with pharmacodynamic activity for most BZs because of the particularly complex metabolism, formation of active metabolites, and extensive distribution processes. There are pronounced variations in pharmacokinetic parameters among individuals; such factors as age, liver disease, smoking, and concomitant use of other drugs can exert a potentially important influence. Classification of these drugs according to $t_{1/2}\ \beta$ of the parent compound is, therefore, more often misleading than helpful; for example no simple relationship has been observed between clinical response, such as anxiolysis, and plasma concentration.[47,48]

BZs are biotransformed by various pathways.[49,50] N_1-alkyl compounds are oxidatively dealkylated to N-desalkyl derivatives (diazepam, flurazepam, prazepam) that exhibit pharmacologic activity. Chlordiazepoxide is N-demethylated in position 2 and then deaminated. Hydroxylation of C_3 and the phenylsubstituent in position 4′ leads to compounds that can be conjugated (glucuronides). The imidazo ring in midazolam and the triazolo ring in triazolam are hydroxylated in the α-position. 7-Nitro-substituted derivatives are reduced to the 7-amino compounds and further acetylated. Flumazenil undergoes rapid hydrolysis of the ester to the inactive free acid. While the formation of primary metabolites occurs virtually exclusively in the liver, conjugated secondary metabolites also can be formed extrahepatically. The biotransformation of BZs via oxidation can be reduced by hepatic disease; BZs that undergo only conjugation (e.g., oxazepam) are not affected. BZs in therapeutic doses do not induce microsomal enzymes to any appreciable degree.

BZR Antagonist Flumazenil

Flumazenil (Anexate, Lanexat, Romazicon) is a specific BZR antagonist.[51] It is an imidazobenzodiazepine, with a carbonyl substituent at C_5 instead of the more common aromatic ring and an ester function on the imidazo ring (structure shown in Fig. 14.7; also see Table 14.2). Flumazenil has a high affinity for the BZR, but does not bind to the "peripheral" mitochondrial binding site. It lacks any pharmacologically relevant binding affinity to other neurotransmitter receptors. The intrinsic efficacy of flumazenil at the BZR is extremely weak. More for theoretical reasons, it is interesting to note that flumazenil can reduce interictal epileptic activity, as well as having some anticonvulsant action in humans.[52,53] Such findings could be the result of intrinsic agonistic activity or, alternatively, of the blockade of an endogenous substance that has proconvulsive properties (e.g., a BZ inverse agonist). Flumazenil blocks all the effects of BZR agonists and inverse agonists that are mediated by the BZR. The doses required to prevent or abolish the various effects vary. Effects of agonists requiring high functional receptor occupancy (muscle relaxation, sedation) are antagonized with smaller doses of flumazenil than those effects occurring at low fractional receptor occupancy (anticonvulsant and anxiolytic effects). This leads to the situation that flumazenil more easily reverses (i.e., a lower dose is required) those effects induced by high doses of BZR agonists but requires a much higher dose of flumazenil to antagonize the low-dose effects of BZR agonists. Flumazenil is well and rapidly absorbed from the GI tract; however, a marked liver first-pass effect results in a low bioavailability. Metabolism to the free acid is also rapid after IV administration ($t\frac{1}{2}\ \beta < 1$ hour).

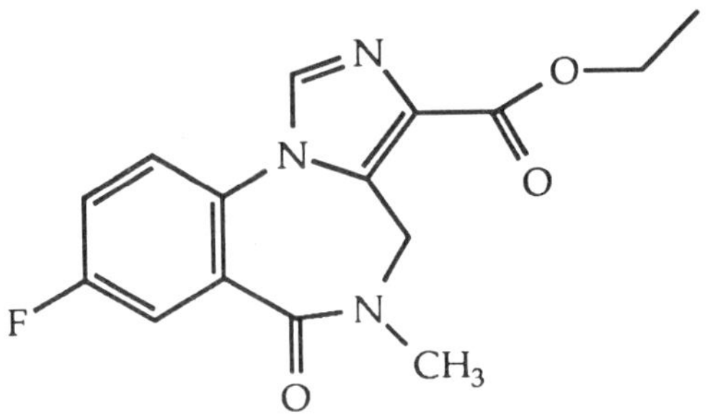

Figure 14.7 Chemical Structure of the BZR Antagonist Flumazenil

Intravenous flumazenil is used as a specific antidote of known or suspected (suicidal, accidental, and iatrogenic) mono-overdose with BZR agonists.[31] The antagonist is slowly injected IV in repeated doses of 0.5 mg until the required vigilance state is achieved. A too rapid awakening should not be induced in order to avoid possible subjective feelings of anxiety, sweating, and shivering. It must always be kept in mind that the patient might be a potential chronic user of BZR agonists and that, therefore, complete antagonism might precipitate a withdrawal syndrome. The precipitation of convulsions is extremely rare in treating mono-overdose, probably because of the modest anticonvulsant activity of flumazenil.

Shortening of postoperational unconsciousness after anesthesias involving a BZR agonist, if considered necessary, can easily be achieved using titrated IV doses of flumazenil.[54] It is imperative that the effect of neuromuscular blockers has disappeared before administering flumazenil. Conscious sedation performed over a long period in the intensive care unit may make it advisable to reduce sedation intermittently in order to be able to assess CNS function and to communicate with the patient. As flumazenil has a short duration of action, resedation may occur when high doses of BZR agonists had been given. Repeated IV injections of flumazenil can be given if required. Should the reversal by flumazenil be complete and stressful for the patient, a short-acting BZR agonist can be administered. A careful test using flumazenil may be helpful for diagnostic purposes in unexplained states of drowsiness. Flumazenil labeled with a positron-emitting radionuclide (e.g., ^{11}C) is used in PET scanning studies to investigate both the kinetics of BZR ligands and to assess their fractional receptor occupancy in the intact brain, as well as to study BZR alterations underlying CNS disease. The radiotracer iomazenil is an analogue of flumazenil labeled with ^{123}iodine, which permits the visualization of cerebral BZR density using single photon emission tomography (SPECT), thus further expanding diagnostic possibilities. Flumazenil has been reported to ameliorate the comatose state of some patients with hepatic encephalopathy,[55] possibly owing to an antagonism of natural BZs or other putative BZR agonists formed or increased in hepatic failure.[9]

Other Anxiolytics, Sedatives, and Hypnotics

Barbiturates, Primidone, Meprobamate, Methaqualone, Glutethimide, and Methyprylon

Chemistry

Barbituric acid is the condensation product of malonic acid and urea; centrally active barbiturates are obtained by double substitution at the position 5 (e.g., an ethyl and a phenyl group to yield phenobarbital). Thiobarbiturates (condensation of malonic acid and thiourea) represent another related series of compounds. Primidone is the 2-deoxy analog of phenobarbital. Only meprobamate of the propandiole class and methaqualone of the quinazoline class have achieved some clinical importance; piperidindiones such as glutethimide and methyprylon represent attempts to obtain barbiturate effects from another structural class. Some selected chemical structures are provided in Figure 14.8.

Pharmacology

Barbiturates and the other compounds listed above produce CNS depression that ranges in a steep dose-dependent manner from mild sedation and hypnosis to general anesthesia to coma and death. Barbiturates generally exhibit anticonvulsant effects; however, some analogues are, in fact, convulsant,[56] but the latter will not be considered here. Barbiturates disinhibit behavior suppressed by punishment, emotional conditioning, and frustration in animal models (considered predictive of anxiolytic activity in humans). However, compared to BZR agonists, the effects of barbiturates in these models are modest. Furthermore, there is only a narrow dose range in which such selective disinhibitory effects of barbiturates can be obtained without general behavioral depression. This poor separation of anxiolytic and sedative effects is consistent with clinical experience with barbiturates. Barbiturates have been shown to be effective against all kinds of experimentally induced epileptiform activities in animal models (electrically or chemically induced, genetic models). At nonsedative doses only some barbiturates are effective as anticonvulsants (e.g., phenobarbital), whereas at anesthetic doses all clinically used barbiturates inhibit convulsions. With respect to psychosedative and ataxic effects, barbiturates do not qualitatively differ from BZR agonists; however, the former are characterized by a much steeper dose-related increase in the magnitude of sedation than the latter. In contrast to BZR agonists, it is possible to obtain a state of general anesthesia with most barbiturates. This is characterized by total unconsciousness, loss of most autonomic reflexes, as well as somatic responses to somatic stimuli, but with maintenance of respiratory and cardiovascular functions. However, a small dose increment can result in irreversible coma and loss of vital functions.

BARBITURATES AND PRIMIDONE

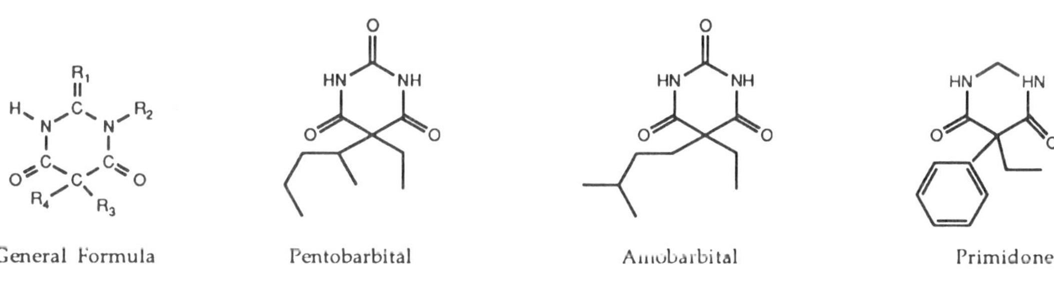

PIPERIDINDIONES QUINAZOLINE PROPANDIOLE

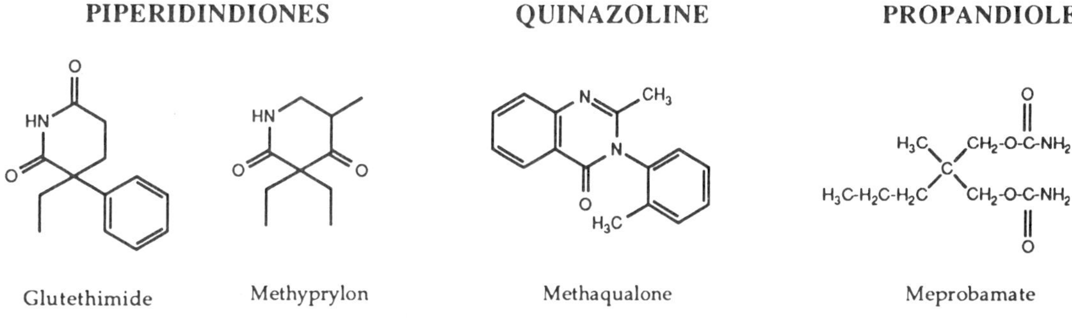

Figure 14.8 Structures of Some Commonly Prescribed Barbiturates, Primidone, Meprobamate, Methaqualone, Glutethimide, and Methyprylon

With BZR agonists it is difficult or impossible to obtain complete unconsciousness with a loss of somatic response to painful stimuli. Anterograde amnesia occurs under barbiturate treatment. Meprobamate exhibits a pharmacologic profile similar to BZR agonists except for a generally lower potency, as well as a much poorer therapeutic index. The lack of available results for methaqualone make comparisons to other compounds impossible. Similarly, piperidindiones have not been well studied; available results suggest a similarity in pharmacologic profile to the barbiturates.

Therapeutic Uses

An overview of the main therapeutic uses and background information on the marketed barbiturates, primidone, meprobamate, methaqualone, glutethimide, and methyprylon is provided in Table 14.3. As an alternative to BZs in treating various anxiety disorders, meprobamate and barbiturates are still used occasionally despite their narrower therapeutic index and higher dependence/abuse potential.[57] Secobarbital, pentobarbital, and amobarbital continue to be commonly prescribed as hypnotics. Glutethimide, methyprylon, and methaqualone are now generally considered to offer a rather similar profile to barbiturate sedative-hypnotics. Barbiturates are still used in anesthesiology for induction, maintenance, and conscious sedation. Phenobarbital has been used as an anticonvulsant since the beginning of the 20th century; primidone, which is metabolized to phenobarbital, and diverse barbiturates are also currently used in the management of epilepsy. Duration of action is one major factor in therapeutic use with, for example, the very short-acting sodium thiopental often chosen for IV anesthesia, short-to-intermediate acting secobarbital, pentobarbital, and amobarbital as hypnotics, and long-acting barbiturates like phenobarbital, metharbital, methylphenobarbital, and primidone for management of convulsions and as antiepileptics.

Mechanism of Action

Other allosteric modulatory sites of the $GABA_A$ receptor complex than the BZR mediate the effects of barbiturates, neurosteroids, and other related agents, with resulting pharmacologic effects different in part from those of BZR ligands. These are only poorly characterized, and to date none has been demonstrated to mediate bidirectional modulation like the BZR. By acting on their allosteric modulatory sites barbiturates and neurosteroids not only increase apparent potency of GABA but also increase the maximum effect of GABA and can even open the $GABA_A$ receptor channel in the absence of GABA. Thus, at low doses barbiturates have been shown to enhance GABAergic neurotransmission via positive allosteric modulation of the $GABA_A$ receptor, producing an even greater shift to the left of the dose-response curve for GABA than BZR agonists, with some barbiturates doing so even in the absence of GABA.[58] This may be the result of massive allosteric induction of the open configuration of the $GABA_A$ receptor. It has been demonstrated that the potentiating action of barbiturates results from an increase in the relative frequency of occurrence of long versus short bursts of channel opening and prolongation of the open state.[59] The allosteric modulatory site at which barbiturates act is different from the BZR, even acting at $GABA_A$ receptors lacking the γ-subunit required for the modulatory effect of BZR ligands.[60] The mechanism of action of the barbiturates is quite complex. At the electrophysiologic level, barbiturates prolong GABA-mediated presynaptic and postsynaptic inhibition and, at sufficiently high doses, mimic GABA effects at the subsynaptic membranes.[61] In the latter case, the effects of barbiturates involve the direct alteration of the chloride channel (in contrast to the modulatory effect of BZR ligands) within the GABAergic receptor complex. Specific sites on $GABA_A$ receptors have not been identified for barbiturates. Accumulation of barbiturates, which are lipophilic, within the cell membranes may be, at least in part, responsible for their actions. Barbiturates depress synaptic excitation at the same or higher doses than those required for prolongation of synaptic inhibition. The mechanism by which barbiturates enhance GABAergic transmission, and at high doses mimic the effect of GABA on chloride conductance, is most likely to occur on the postsynaptic membrane and to involve the coupling process between GABA receptors and chloride channels or alteration of the kinetics of the chloride channel. The mechanism of action of meprobamate does not appear to involve the enhancement of GABAergic transmission (whereas, methaqualone may do so). Little is known about the mechanism of action of glutethimide and methyprylon.

Undesirable Side-Effects

The acute toxicity of barbiturates is characterized by a pronounced central and peripheral nervous system depression combined with the impairment of function of most peripheral tissues (e.g., cardiovascular system) resulting from a generalized blockade of both active and passive membrane processes, as well as the activity of many enzymes, although no specific organ toxicity is known.[45] Adverse effects that are most common include confusion, drowsiness, hangover, skin rash, and nausea. Overdose symptoms range from profound sleep to coma characterized by marked respiratory depression and even ultimately death (in children, irritability and hyperactivity are commonly observed).

Table 14.3 Background Information on Marketed Barbiturates and Other Selected Anxiolytics and Sedative-Hypnotics

Generic Name (Trade Names)	Chemical Structure (R1 to R4 Refer to Substitutions on General Structure Shown in Fig. 14.8)	Main Therapeutic Areas (Dosage Forms and Regimen)
Allobarbital (INN, USAN) [also named Diallylbarbituric acid] Diadol, Dial, Katarin, Sediomed	R1 = O R2 = H R3 = allyl R4 = allyl	sedative-hypnotic
Amobarbital (INN, JAN, USAN), also as sodium salt and hydroquinine derivative [Amylobarbitone is BAN; Amobarbital Sodium is JAN, USAN] Altinal, Amosedil, Amsal, Amsebarb, Amycal, Amydorm, Amylbarb sodium, Amylobeta, Amytal (-Sodium), Barbamyl, Dorlotin, Dorminal, Dormytal, Estimal, Etamyl, Eunoctal, Isoamitil Sedante, Isobec, Isomytal, Isonal, Mudeka, Mylodorm Sustrels, Neur-Amyl, Novamobarb, Placidel, Robarb, Sednotic, Stadadorm, Talamo, Transital	R1 = O R2 = H R3 = isopentyl R4 = ethyl	sedative-hypnotic, anticonvulsant, preanesthetic [c, drg, e, inj, p, s, t] 50–300 mg po divided daily dose as sedative; 65–200 mg po at bedtime as hypnotic; 65–200 mg IV as anticonvulsant
Aprobarbital (INN), also as sodium salt Alurate, Isonal, Numal	R1 = O R2 = H R3 = isopropyl R4 = allyl	sedative-hypnotic [dr, drg, e, t] 40 mg po given 3 times daily as sedative; 40–200 mg po at bedtime as hypnotic
Barbexaclone (INN) Maliasin (combination of barbexaclone and phenobarbital)	[salt of levopropylhexedrin and phenobarbital]	antiepileptic [drg, t] 200–400 mg po in divided daily dose
Barbital (INN, JAN), **Barbital Sodium (sodium salt; INN)** [Barbitone and Barbitone Sodium are BANs] Barbimetten, Barbitalum, Diemal DAK, Dormileno, Hypnox, Nervo-OPT mono, Veroletten, Veronal	R1 = O R2 = H R3 = ethyl R4 = ethyl	sedative-hypnotic [drg, t] 100 mg po 1–3 times daily as sedative; 250–500 mg po at bedtime as hypnotic
Brallobarbital (INN), also as calcium salt Ucedorm	R1 = O R2 = H R3 = allyl R4 = 2-bromo-2-propenyl	sedative-hypnotic [t]
Butalbital (INN, USAN) [also named Allylbarbituric acid] Sandoptal, (also many combination products with acetaminophen, caffeine, aspirin, and/or codeine)	R1 = O R2 = H R3 = isobutyl R4 = allyl	sedative-hypnotic [t]
Butallylonal, also as sodium salt Pernocton, Sonbutal, Tempidorm	R1 = O R2 = H R3 = 1-methylpropyl R4 = 2-bromo-2-propenyl	sedative-hypnotic
Butobarbital [Butobarbitone is BAN; also named Butethal] Butobarbital Dipharma, Butobarbitalum, Butynoct, Etoval, Hypnasmine, Longanoct, Neonal, Sonabarb, Sonéryl, Supponéryl	R1 = O R2 = H R3 = ethyl R4 = butyl	sedative-hypnotic [s, t] 100–200 mg po as divided daily dose

continued

Table 14.3 *Continued*

Generic Name (Trade Names)	Chemical Structure (R1 to R4 Refer to Substitutions on General Structure Shown in Fig. 14.8)	Main Therapeutic Areas (Dosage Forms and Regimen)
Crotarbital Doladamon, Kalypnon	R1 = O R2 = H R3 = (E)-2-butenyl R4 = ethyl	sedative-hypnotic
Cyclobarbital (INN), also as calcium salt [Cyclobarbitone is BAN] Amnosed, Cyclobarbiton-Calcium, Cyclodorm, Cykldorm, Dormiphen, Fabadorm, Fanodormo Calcico, Irifan, Namuron, Palinum, Panodorm (-Calcium), Phanodorn (-Calcium), Phanotal (-Calcium), Pronox, Somnupan C, Union-nox	R1 = O R2 = H R3 = ethyl R4 = 1-cyclohexenyl	sedative-hypnotic [t] 100–400 mg po at bedtime as hypnotic
Cyclopentobarbital, also as sodium salt [also named Cyclopentylallybarbituric acid] Cyclopal (-Sodium)	R1 = O R2 = H R3 = allyl R4 = 2-cyclopentenyl	sedative-hypnotic 100–200 mg po at bedtime as hypnotic
5,5-Dipropylbarbituric acid Expectal	R1 = O R2 = H R3 = n-propyl R4 = n-propyl	sedative-hypnotic
Heptabarb (INN) [Heptabarbitone is BAN; also named Heptabarbital] Eudan, Medapan, Medomin, Medomine	R1 = O R2 = H R3 = ethyl R4 = 1-cycloheptenyl	sedative-hypnotic [t] 50 mg po single dose as sedative; 200–400 mg po at bedtime as hypnotic
Hexethal, also as sodium salt Hebaral, Ortal	R1 = O R2 = H R3 = ethyl R4 = n-hexyl	
Hexobarbital (INN, JAN), also as sodium salt [Hexobarbitone is BAN] Citopan, Cyclopan, Evipal (-Sodium), Evipan Natrium, Hexanastab, Narcosanum, Noctivane, Privénal, Sleepwell, Sodium Narcosate, Sombucaps, Sombulex, Tobinal, Toleran	R1 = O R2 = methyl R3 = methyl R4 = 1-cyclohexenyl	intravenous anesthetic, sedative-hypnotic [inj, t] 250 mg po 1–3 times daily as sedative; 250–500 mg po at bedtime as hypnotic
Metharbital (INN, JAN, USAN) [Metharbitone is BAN] Gemonil, Gemonit	R1 = O R2 = methyl R3 = ethyl R4 = ethyl	anticonvulsant [t] 100 mg po 1–3 times daily
Methitural (INN), also as sodium salt Neraval	R1 = S R2 = H R3 = 2-(methylthio)ethyl R4 = 1-methylbutyl	sedative-hypnotic
Methohexital (INN, USAN), also as sodium salt [Methohexitone is BAN; Methohexital Sodium is USAN] Brevimytal Natrium, Brevital (-Sodium), Brietal (-Sodium)	R1 = O R2 = methyl R3 = allyl R4 = 1-methyl-2-pentynyl	general anesthetic [inj, p] individualized dosage

continued

Table 14.3 *Continued*

Generic Name (Trade Names)	Chemical Structure (R1 to R4 Refer to Substitutions on General Structure Shown in Fig. 14.8)	Main Therapeutic Areas (Dosage Forms and Regimen)
Methylphenobarbital (INN) [Methylphenobarbitone is BAN; Mephobarbital is USAN, JAN] Mebaral, Menta-Bal, Mephytaletten, Phemiton, Prominal, Prominalette	R1 = O R2 = methyl R3 = ethyl R4 = phenyl	antiepileptic, sedative-hypnotic [t] 30–100 mg po 3–4 times daily as sedative; 200 mg po at bedtime as hypnotic; 300–600 mg po as divided daily dose as antiepileptic
Pentobarbital (INN, USAN), also sodium and calcium salts [Pentobarbitone is BAN; Pentobarbital Calcium is JAN; Pentobarbital Sodium is USAN] Barbopent, Butylone, Embutal, Hypnol, Insom Rapido, Isoamytal, Isobarb, Iturate, Mebumal DAK, Medinox Mono, Napental, Narcoren, Nembutal (-Sodium), Neodorm, Norkotral, Norkotral N, Nova-Rectal, Novopentobarb, Palapent, Pembule, Penbar, Penbon, Pentab, Pental, Pentanca, Pentogen, Pentone, Pentosol, Praecicalm, Prodormol, Repocal, Schlaffen, Sedanox, Sombutol, Somnopentyl, Somnotol, Sonistan, Sopental, Tamp-R-Tel Pentobarbital Sodium	R1 = O R2 = H R3 = ethyl R4 = 1-methylbutyl	sedative-hypnotic, anticonsulvant, preanesthetic [c, e, inj, p, s, t] 20 mg po 3–4 times daily as sedative; 100–200 mg po at bedtime as hypnotic; 100 mg po preoperative; 100 mg or more IV as anticonvulsant
Phenobarbital (INN, JAN, USAN), Phenobarbital Sodium (sodium salt; INN, JAN, USAN), also as calcium salt, cathine and diethylamine derivatives [Phenobarbitone is BAN] Adonal, Agrypnal, Ancalixir, Aparoxal, Aphenylbarbit, Austrominal, Barbellen, Barbilettae, Barbiphenyl, Barbita, Bialminal, Calminal, Comizial, Epanal Cinq, Ensobarb, Epidorm, Epsylone, Eskabarb Span, Fenemal, Fenilcal, Fenosed, Gardénal (-Sodium), Gardénale, Hypnaletten, Hypnolone, Hysteps, Kotabarb, Lepinal, Lepinaletten, Lethyl, Lumcalcio, Lumidrops, Luminal (-Sodium), Luminale, Luminaletas, Luminalette, Luminaletten, Luminalettes, Luminalum, Mediphen, Nervolitan S, Nova-Pheno, PEBA, Phenaemal, Phenaemaletten, Phenobal, Phenobarbiton, Phenobarbyl, Phenoturic, Sedabar, Sedadrops, Seda-Tablinen, Sevenal, Sevenaletta, Solfoton, Solu-Barb, Tamp-R-Tel Phenobarbital Sodium, Teolaxin, Tridezibarbitur, Valocordin N, Vegetamin, Versomnal, Zentramin	R1 = O R2 = H R3 = phenyl R4 = ethyl	sedative-hypnotic, antiepileptic, preanesthetic [c, dr, drg, e, inj, p, s, t] 15–30 mg po 2–4 times daily as sedative; 100–300 mg po at bedtime as hypnotic; 60–250 mg po divided daily dose as antiepileptic
Probarbital Sodium (sodium salt; INN) Ipral Sodium	R1 = O R2 = H R3 = ethyl R4 = isopropyl	sedative-hypnotic
Propallylonal [also named Ibomal] Noctal	R1 = O R2 = H R3 = 2-bromo-2-propenyl R4 = isopropyl	sedative-hypnotic 100–400 mg po at bedtime as hypnotic
Proxibarbal (INN) Axeen, Centralgol, Ipronal, Vasalgin	R1 = O R2 = H R3 = allyl R4 = 2-hydroxypropyl	sedative-hypnotic, antimigraine [c, drg, t] 100–200 mg po 3 times daily *continued*

Table 14.3 *Continued*

Generic Name (Trade Names)	Chemical Structure (R1 to R4 Refer to Substitutions on General Structure Shown in Fig. 14.8)	Main Therapeutic Areas (Dosage Forms and Regimen)
Secbutabarbital Sodium (sodium salt; INN), also as free base [Secbutobarbitone is BAN; Butabarbital, Butabarbital Sodium are USAÑs] BBS, Barbased, Bubartal, Busodium, Buta-Barb, Butabarpal, Butalan, Butamid, Butapro, Buticaps, Butisol (-Sodium), Da-Sed, Day-Barb, Mebutal, Merisyl, Neo-Barb, Quiebar, Renbu, Sarisol	R1 = O R2 = H R3 = ethyl R4 = 1-methylpropyl	sedative-hypnotic, preanesthetic [c, e, t] 15–30 mg po 3–4 times daily as sedative; 50–100 mg po at bedtime as hypnotic; 50–100 mg po preoperative
Secobarbital (INN, USAN), also as sodium salt [Quinalbarbitone sodium is BAN; Secobarbital Sodium is JAN, USAN] Dormatylan, Dormona, Evronal, Imménoctal, Immenox, Novosecobarb, Proquinal, Quinbar, S.C.B. Tal, Sebar, Secaps, Secogen, Seconal (-Sodium), Seral, Tamp-R-Tel Secobarbital Sodium	R1 = O R2 = H R3 = allyl R4 = 1-methylbutyl	sedative-hypnotic, preanesthetic, anticonvulsant [c, e, inj, p, s, t] 30–50 mg po 3–4 times daily as sedative; 50–200 mg po at bedtime as hypnotic; 5.5 mg/kg body weight IV repeated every 3–4 hours as needed as anticonvulsant
Talbutal (INN, USAN) Losate, Lotusate, Lutawin	R1 = O R2 = H R3 = allyl R4 = 1-methylpropyl	sedative-hypnotic [c,t] 15–40 mg po 2–3 times daily as sedative; 120 mg po at bedtime as hypnotic
Thiamylal Sodium (sodium salt; JAN, USAN), Thiamylal (USAN) Anestatal, Surital (-Sodium), Thiamylal, Thioseconal	R1 = S R2 = H R3 = allyl R4 = 1-methylbutyl	general anesthetic [inj] individualized dosage
Thiopental Sodium (sodium salt; INN, JAN, USAN) [Thiopentone Sodium is BAN] Farmotal, Hypnostan, Intraval Sodium, Leopental, Nesdonal, Pentothal (-Sodium), Sandothal, Thio-Barbityral, Thionembutal, Tiobarbital, Tiopental, Trapanal	R1 = S R2 = H R3 = ethyl R4 = 1-methylbutyl	general anesthetic, anticonvulsant [inj, p, s] individualized dosage
Vinbarbital (INN), also as sodium salt [Vinbarbitone is BAN] Delvinal, Diminal	R1 = O R2 = H R3 = ethyl R4 = 1-methyl-1-butenyl	sedative-hypnotic [s, t] 25–50 mg po 4 times daily as sedative; 100–200 mg po at bedtime as hypnotic
Vinylbital (INN) [Vinylbitone is BAN] Bykonox, Optanox, Speda, Suppoptanox	R1 = O R2 = H R3 = ethenyl R4 = 1-methylbutyl	sedative-hypnotic [s, t] 100–200 mg po at bedtime as hypnotic

continued

Table 14.3 *Continued*

Generic Name (Trade Names)	Dosage Forms	Main Therapeutic Areas (Dosage Forms and Regimen)
Buspirone (INN, BAN) [Buspirone hydrochloride is USAN] Ansial, Ansiced, Axoren, Bespar, Buspar, Buspimen, Buspinol, Buspisal, Buspon, Censpar, Lucelan, Narol, Nopiron, Travin	capsules: 5, 10 mg tablets: 5, 10 mg	tranquilizer 15–30 mg po individed daily dose
Chloral Hydrate (BAN, JAN, USAN), derivatives available Ansopal, Aquachloral, Chloradorm, Chloralate, Chloraldurat, Chloralix, Chloralixir, Cohidrate, Dormel, Elix-nocte, Escre, Eudorm, Hipnogal, H.S. Need, Kessodorate, Lanchloral, Médianox, Nervifene, Notec, Novochlorhydrate, Oradrate, Rectules, Somnifral, Somnos, Somnox, Sondrate, Suppojuvent	capsules: 250, 500 mg drops elixir siriup suppository: 250, 500, 648, 1296 mg tablets: 250, 500, 850 mg	sedative-hypnotic 250 mg po 3 times daily as sedative; 0.25–1.5 gram po at bedtime as hypnotic
Glutethimide (INN, BAN, USAN) Alfimid, Doriden, Doriglute Tabs, Dorimide, Elrodorm, Glimid, Rigenox, Rolathimide	capsules tablets: 250, 500 mg	sedative-hypnotic 250–500 mg po at bedtime as hypnotic
Meprobamate (INN, BAN, JAN, USAN) Acabmate, Amepromat, Andaxin, Ansietan, Ansiowas, Arcoban, Artolon, Ayeramate, Carb-A-Med, Cirponyl, Coprobate, Cyrpon, Dapaz, Dormabrol, Dormilfo M, Dystoid, Ecuanil, Epikur, Equanil, Equatrate, Exphobin N, Gene-Bamate, Kesso-Bamate, Lan-Dol, Mar-Bate, Meprotil, Meriprobate, Microbamat, Midixin, Milonorm, Miltaun, Miltown, Misedant, M.P. Transtabs, My-Trans, Neo-Tran, Nervonus, Neuramate, Novamato, Novomepro, Oasil, Pax, Paxin, Pensive, Perequil, Pertranquil, Praol, Prequil, Probamato, Probamyl, Probasan, Probate, Procalmadiol, Quaname, Quanil, Quietidon, Relaksin, Relax-Tablet, Reposo Mono, Restenil, Robamate, Sedabamate, Sedanyl, Selene, Setran, Sintown, SK-Bamate, Sonya, Sopanil, Sowell, Stensolo, Stersolo, Tamate, Trankilin, Tranmep, Tranquilin, Urbilat, Visano N, Wescomep	capsules: 200, 400 mg dragees injection ampoules tablets: 200, 250, 400, 600 mg	sedative-hypnotic, tranquilizer 200–400 mg po 3–4 times daily as tranquilizer; 800 mg po at bedtime as hypnotic
Methaqualone (INN, BAN, USAN), also as hydrochloride salt Bon-Sonnil, Cateudyl, Citexal, Dormigoa, Dormir, Dormised, Dormogen, Dormutil, Holodorm, Hyptor, Melsed, Melsedin, Melsomin, Mequalone, Mequelon, Mequin, Methadorm, Methasedil, Mollinox, Motolon, Mozambin, Nobadorm, Normi-Nox, Normorest, Noxybel, Oblioser, Optimil, Optinoxan, Pallidan, Parest, Parmilene, Paxidorm, Pexaqualone, Pro-Dorm, Revonal, Riporest, Rouqualone, Sedalone, Sleepinal, Somberol, Somnafac, Somnium, Somnomed, Somnotropon, Sovelin, Soverin, Sovinal, Spasmipront, Tiqualone, Toraflon, Torinal, Tualone, Tuazol, Tuazolona	tablets: 200, 250 mg	sedative-hypnotic 100–200 mg po daily
Methyprylon (INN, USAN) [Methyprylone is BAN] Noludar, Nolurate	capsules: 300 mg tablets: 50, 200 mg	sedative-hypnotic 50–100 mg po 3–4 times daily as sedative; 200–400 mg po at bedtime as hypnotic

continued

Table 14.3 *Continued*

Generic Name (Trade Names)	Dosage Forms	Main Therapeutic Areas (Dosage Forms and Regimen)
Primidone (INN, BAN, JAN, USAN) Apo-Primidone, Cyral, Granmid, Hexamidin, Lepsiral, Liskantin, Majsolin, Mizodin, Myidone, Myepsin, Mylepsine, Mylepsinum, Mysedon, Mysoline, Primoline, Prysoline, Resimatil, Sertan	sirup tablets: 50, 125, 250 mg	antiepileptic titration up to 1.5 grams po per day

Note: The clinical information contained in the above table is a compilation from numerous sources; it is very extensive but especially in view of the difficulties in obtaining information at an international level, it is definitely not exhaustive. Furthermore, the information provided on therapeutic doses (for which adequate differentiation is not made for the various salts, derivatives, and free base) and usage is intended for general comparative purposes and should not serve as the basis of any medical decisions with respect to individual patients. This is all the more the case in view of international differences in diagnostic and clinical practices, as well as precautions required for special patient populations which could not be adequately taken into account in such a general review. Combination preparations are excluded. Abbreviations: INN = International Nonproprietary Name; BAN = British Approved Name; JAN = Japanese Accepted Name; USAN = United States Adopted Name; po = oral; IV = intravenous; c = capsule; dg = dragee; dp = drops; e = elixir; inj = injection form; p = powder; s = suppository; t = tablet.

Barbiturate effects are potentiated by ethanol. The direct actions of barbiturates on peripheral tissues occur only at anesthetic doses and are most likely due to a depression of sodium and calcium fluxes involved in excitation, excitation-contraction, and excitation-secretion coupling. Less information is available concerning the toxicology of meprobamate, methaqualone, and the piperidindiones glutethimide and methyprylon. The adverse effects of these compounds are generally similar to those of the barbiturates. For meprobamate, the acute lethal dose is quite high. Methaqualone overdose involves epileptiform effects, which differentiates it clearly from BZR agonists and barbiturates. Acute toxic effects of the piperidindiones seems similar to barbiturates (except for the marked anticholinergic effects of glutethimide). Organ-specific toxic effects have not been clearly established for meprobamate, methaqualone, glutethimide, or methyprylon.

Barbiturates and primidone are known to induce rapid tolerance when given in large doses. Drowsiness is a frequent complaint at the start of treatment, but usually subsides within a few weeks. Such tolerance, in the case of some barbiturates, results predominantly from the alteration of drug disposition due to induction of microsomal enzymes involved in the metabolism of the inducing agent and/or from reduced absorption, altered tissue distribution, or increased renal excretion. The stimulation of hepatic microsomal oxidizing systems by barbiturates (especially phenobarbital) can result in the loss of therapeutic effects of concomitantly administered drugs when these are inactivated by cytochrome P450. The potential reduction of serum concentrations of antiepileptics such as phenytoin, carbamazepine, valproic acid, and clonazepam by phenobarbital treatment illustrates the clinical importance of such drug interactions.[62] Chronic barbiturate administration can alter vitamin D metabolism. Glutethimide, methyprylon, and methaqualone appear to stimulate hepatic microsomal oxidizing systems. Pharmacodynamic factors also may play a role in tolerance development to barbiturates and primidone. Acute tolerance has been described following a single administration. Cross-tolerance between barbiturates and other compounds occurs (e.g., to the sedative effect of BZR agonists or ethanol). Repeated administration of barbiturates also results in the development of physical dependence. Withdrawal signs in animals include hypermotility, muscle rigidity, altered sleep-wakefulness cycle, spontaneous seizures, and increased seizure susceptibility to exogenous stimuli; in humans withdrawal is typical of sedative/hypnotics, including BZR agonists and meprobamate. Barbiturates exhibit robust reinforcing effects in animals and have a high abuse potential in humans. The clear liability of meprobamate, methaqualone, glutethimide, and methyprylon to produce tolerance, physical dependence, and abuse is known from the clinical setting.[63]

Azapirones

Buspirone (structure shown in Fig 14.9, also see Table 14.3) has recently been approved for the symptomatic management of generalized anxiety disorder in many countries and is of special interest in view of the fact that this azaspirodecanedione derivative does not exert its actions via modulation of the $GABA_A$ receptor complex. The pharmacologic profile and therapeutic effects of buspirone have recently been reviewed in great detail.[64] This compound is structurally unrelated to the benzodiazepines, barbiturates, or the other anxiolytics and sedative/hypnotics discussed above. It has been hypothesized that the anxiolytic effects of buspirone are due to its demonstrated activity as a partial agonist at the 5-HT (5-hydroxytryptamine or serotonin) receptor of the 1A subtype, although it has also been speculated that there is some similarity of the profile of buspirone to that of dopamine receptor antagonists (note that neuroleptics are sometimes used to treat anxiety disorders), which possibly could contribute to its therapeutic activity. The pharmacologic profile of buspirone in both animals and in humans certainly differs substantially from that of the BZR agonists in that the former lacks anticonvulsant, muscle relaxant, and hypnotic effects and is less sedative, produces less psychomotor impairment in conjunction with ethanol consumption, has no reported liability to induce tolerance or physical dependence, and has a much lower abuse liability in view of its potential to induce dysphoria.[65] At most, only minimal anterograde amnesia has been observed after buspirone.[66] Not surprisingly, buspirone does not exhibit cross-tolerance with BZR agonists or barbiturates and, therefore, would not be useful in treating their withdrawal symptoms (furthermore, it is not anticonvulsant). Given in a divided daily dose of about 15 to 30 mg, buspirone is well tolerated. The most common adverse effects reported are headache, dizziness, nervousness, lightheadedness, excitement, and nausea. The lag time of a week or more before anxiolysis is achieved with buspirone makes it inappropriate for use when immediate anxiolysis is needed, and some studies indicate that buspirone may be less effective than BZR agonists in treating severe anxiety or patients with prior treatment experience with BZR agonists. In a single study, buspirone aggravated akathisia and dyskinesia in a small group of schizophrenics.[67] Buspirone is eliminated predominantly by hepatic metabolism and renal excretion (thus, use in patients with severe hepatic or renal impairment is not recommended); the hydroxylated metabolites of buspirone are not believed to contribute appreciably to its therapeutic activity.[68] Furthermore, buspirone is well absorbed, but due to extensive first-pass metabolism the systemic availability is only about 4% and is relatively rapidly eliminated in healthy subjects, with mean half-life values across several studies ranging from 2–11 hours. Buspirone is very highly protein-bound. With gradually increased clinical experience using this novel anxiolytic compound, the appropriate place for buspirone within the medical armamentarium will become more clearly defined.

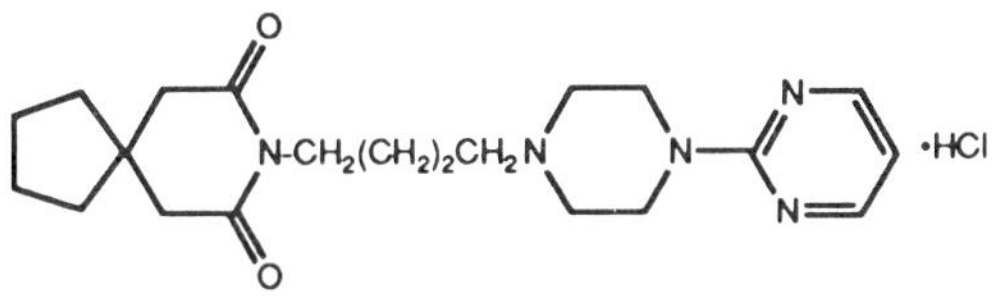

Figure 14.9 Structure of Buspirone (Hydrochloride Salt)

Conclusions

This chapter provides a description of the pharmacology of BZR agonists, barbiturates, meprobamate, as well as other miscellaneous agents currently used in the management of anxiety and/or sleep disorders. In view of their predominance in the clinical setting, the BZR agonists have received the greatest emphasis here. The profile and mechanism of action of the novel anxiolytic buspirone is quite different, requiring a separate consideration. The spectrum of somatic and behavioral effects of the BZR agonists and those of barbiturates are quite similar and occur rapidly; direct actions on peripheral tissues are virtually lacking. BZR agonists differ in potency, therapeutic index, and in the steepness of dose relation to the magnitude of CNS depression from the barbiturates, meprobamate, methaqualone, glutethimide, and methyprylon; the advantageous therapeutic index of the BZR agonists has been the basis of their widespread and now almost complete substitution for the other drugs over the past several decades. Prominent effects observed in animals treated with these compounds include the disinhibition of behaviors suppressed by either fear, punishment, or frustration and, additionally, the attenuation of arousal, vigilance, and attention. Furthermore, generally these drugs exhibit a broad spectrum of anticonvulsant effects, and decrease skeletal muscle tone and autonomic response to emotional stimuli. Only barbiturates are able to induce a full surgical anesthetic state. These different groups of compounds all produce tolerance and physical dependence and possess reinforcing properties that render them liable to abuse; however, BZR agonists again exhibit an advantageous profile relative to the barbiturates and other agents. BZR agonists, barbiturates, meprobamate, methaqualone, glutethimide, and methyprylon have no known organ-specific toxicity, with side-effects typically the result of exaggerated pharmacologic activity in overdose and lethal potential in monotherapy restricted almost exclusively to the barbiturates.

The considerable similarity in the pharmacologic profiles of BZR agonists and barbiturates can be attributed to their underlying mechanisms of action, i.e., modulation of GABAergic synaptic transmission through activation of two different allosteric modulation sites of the $GABA_A$ receptor/chloride channel in neuronal membranes. The $GABA_A$ receptor channel is involved, or capable of influencing, virtually all somatic and mental functions. Limited information is available concerning the mechanism of action of meprobamate, methaqualone, glutethimide, and methyprylon. The BZR recognizes ligands of both benzodiazepine structure (e.g., diazepam), as well as nonbenzodiazepine structures (e.g., zopiclone, zolpidem). BZRs mediate both the facilitation and inhibition of GABA-mediated chloride channel gating—effects that in turn can be blocked by BZR ligands lacking intrinsic modulatory activity (e.g., flumazenil). The classic benzodiazepine tranquilizers, anticonvulsants, muscle relaxants, and hypnotics have been demonstrated to be BZR full agonists which act via positive allosteric modulation of GABA-mediated chloride channel gating. Full inverse agonists exhibit a pharmacologic profile characterized by diametrically opposite effects (i.e., anxiogenic, convulsant, muscle spasticity inducing, arousing). There is evidence for a structural polymorphism of $GABA_A$ receptors, but in the absence of knowledge of the composition and stoichiometry of the native receptor(s) pharmacologic significance is difficult to judge (except possibly for the type 1 BZR). Furthermore, it has been speculated that in view of the observed heterogeneity of binding of diverse BZR ligands that different $GABA_A$ subunit combinations may confer diverse pharmacological possibilities.[69] Partial agonism within the context of different receptor reserves in various neuronal populations provides an alternative explanation of such heterogeneity of binding. The question of whether there is an endogenous substance that acts on the BZR under physiologic or pathologic conditions remains to be answered. What emerges quite clearly is that enhancement of GABAergic transmission is very effective in stabilizing the abnormal activity of neurons underlying symptoms of anxiety, regardless of whether the result of a deficit in the GABAergic or other neurotransmitter systems, probably because the fine-tuning possible with allosteric modulation of receptor function proves less disruptive to homeostasis of multiple, interacting neuronal systems. Barbiturates act predominantly by enhancing GABAergic transmission via a molecular mechanism different from that underlying the actions of BZR agonists. The receptors for barbiturates are poorly characterized, and there is evidence that barbiturates may interact directly with the GABA-regulated chloride channel. Unlike BZR agonists, barbiturates given in intermediate-to-high doses depress excitatory synaptic transmission, as well as various membrane and enzyme activities. No specific antagonist for barbiturates has been identified. In view of the existence of several allosteric modulatory sites located on the $GABA_A$ receptor complex, it would also be possible to focus drug discovery efforts on finding novel ligands of those sites possibly possessing therapeutic advantages.

In marked contrast to anxiolytics acting via BZR agonism (which exhibit anticonvulsant, muscle relaxant, and sedative/hypnotic effects), the azaspirodecanedione, buspirone, presents only anxiolytic activity. It has been hypothesized that the mechanism of action of buspirone involves partial agonism at the $5\text{-}HT_{1A}$ receptor. Advantages of buspirone include less sedation, less psychomotor impairment in conjunction with ethanol consumption, reduced physical dependence, and a much lower abuse liability than for BZR full agonists. However, the long latency in onset of anxiolytic activity is a pronounced difference to classic BZ tranquilizers, which act rapidly. In addition, there are possible problems in treatment compliance for buspirone and questions about efficacy in patients previously treated with BZR agonists or exhibiting severe anxiety. Buspirone is not only a valuable addition to the medical armamentarium whose place is gradually becoming more clearly defined, but also very important from the theoretical standpoint insofar as it is the first anxiolytic to meet the rigorous clinical efficacy and safety standards of modern times that does not act via modulation of GABAergic transmission.

The future for improved anxiolytics and hypnotics can be described as considerably brighter than at any time in recent decades. In view of the major advances achieved in the management of anxiety and sleep disorders in recent years it is clear, nonetheless, that improvements in symptomatic therapy will take place in increasingly smaller increments. The therapeutic efficacy of BZR agonists in general anxiety disorder, as well as in stress-induced and situational anxiety, is uncontested; and their potential benefits in panic and phobic disorders are judged more positively. Although proper medical use (dose and treatment duration, tapering off) can considerably reduce their undesirable effects (sedation, ethanol potentiation, physical dependence), the potential advantages offered by the BZR partial agonist approach would represent an important advance by maintaining full therapeutic efficacy while further minimizing such undesirable effects. Clinical investigations in anxiety and sleep disorders with such BZR partial agonists as bretazenil, imidazenil, divaplon, saripidem, and abecarnil should provide the basis for such an evaluation. The possibility of the existence of receptor subtypes with differential involvement in neuronal populations responsible for anxiolytic effects versus undesired effects in humans remains an intriguing approach that may yield an improved therapeutic index for novel anxiolytics and hypnotics. The clinical introduction of buspirone has paved the way to considering mechanisms other than those based on $GABA_A$ receptor function as a means to achieving anxiolytic activity; a number of related compounds acting as $5\text{-}HT_{1A}$ receptor partial agonists are currently in various stages of clinical development for this indication. Furthermore, exploratory approaches focusing on cholecystokinin receptor antagonism, $5\text{-}HT_2$ receptor antagonism, $5\text{-}HT_3$ receptor antagonism, neuropeptide Y_1 agonism, neurosteroids, and N-methyl-D-aspartate receptor antagonism as the basis of anxiolysis are actively being followed. Finally, increasing attention has been given to the clinical investigation of various marketed antidepressants (tricyclics, monoamine-oxidase inhibitors) in panic disorder with agoraphobia and/or social phobias. In conclusion, there is good reason to believe that, in view of the current high level of research interest in addressing the problems faced in the management of anxiety and sleep disorders, novel agents offering advantages over current therapy may soon become available.

Acknowledgements

The valuable contributions of many scientific colleagues are gratefully acknowledged, in particular, the critical evaluation of this manuscript by Prof. H. Möhler and Drs. W. Hunkeler and U. Widmer. Drs. J. Altenburger and J. Favre are thanked for assistance in conducting literature searches and Ms. J. Lindecker for her skillful preparation of the manuscript.

In Memoriam

Professor Willy E. Haefely died of a heart attack on April 19, 1993, while skiing in the Swiss Alps. Willy Haefely was an outstanding neuropsychopharmacologist whose broad scientific expertise and creativity in addressing the major issues of CNS pharmacology and moreover, his accessibility and irresistible enthusiasm as both teacher and research collaborator make him an enduring inspiration to all his colleagues.

References

Research Reports

1. Costa E, Guidotti A, Mao CC. Evidence for the involvement of GABA in the action of benzodiazepines: Studies on rat cerebellum. Adv Biochem Psychopharmacol 1975;*14*:113–130.
2. Haefely W, Pieri L, Polc P, Schaffner R. General pharmacology and neuropharmacology of benzodiazepine derivatives. In: Hoffmeister F, Stille G. Handbook of experimental pharmacology, vol. 55/II Berlin: Springer-Verlag, 1981; pp 9–262.
3. Möhler H, Okada T. Benzodiazepine receptor: Demonstration in the central nervous system. Science 1977;*198*:849–851.
4. Squires RF, Braestrup C. Benzodiazepine receptors in rat brain. Nature 1977;*266*:732–734.
5. Hunkeler W, Möhler H, Pieri L, Polc P, Bonetti EP, Cumin R, Schaffner R, Haefely W. Selective antagonists of benzodiazepines. Nature 1981;*290*:514–516.
6. Braestrup C, Schmiechen R, Neef G, Nielsen M, Petersen EN. Interaction of convulsive ligands with benzodiazepine receptors. Science 1982;*216*:1241–1243.
7. Schofield PR, Darlison MG, Fujita N, Burt DR, Stephenson FA, Rodriguez H, Rhee LM, Ramachandran J, Reale V, Glencose TA, Seeburg PH, Barnard EA. Sequence and functional expression of the $GABA_A$ receptor shows a ligand-gated receptor superfamily. Nature 1987;*328*:221–227.
8. Wildmann J, Möhler H, Vetter W, Ranalder U, Schmidt K, Maurer R. Diazepam and N-desmethyldiazepam are found in rat brain and adrenal and may be of plant origin. Neural Transm 1987;*70*:383–398.
9. Basile AS, Hughes RD, Harrison PM, Murata Y, Pannell L, Jones EA, Williams R, Solonick P. Elevated brain concentrations of 1,4-benzodiazepines in fulminant hepatic failure. N Engl J Med 1991;*325*:473–478.
10. Haefely WE. The $GABA_A$-benzodiazepine receptor: biology and pharmacology. In: Brown GD, Roth M, Noyer R. Handbook of Anxiety, Vol. 3: The Neurobiology of Anxiety (eds), 1990; Amsterdam: Elsevier, pp 165–188.
11. Haefely W, Kyburz E, Gerecke M, Möhler H. Recent advances in the molecular pharmacology of benzodiazepine receptors and in the structure-activity relationships of their agonists and antagonists. In: Testa B. Advances in Drug Research, vol. 14, 1985; London: Academic Press, pp 165–322.
12. Green S, Hodges H. Animal models of anxiety. In: Willner P. Behavioural models in psychopharmacology 1991; Cambridge: Cambridge University Press, pp 21–49.
13. Geller I, Seifter J. The effects of meprobamate, barbiturates, d-amphetamine and promazine on experimentally induced conflict in the rat. Psychopharmacologia 1960;*1*:482–492.
14. Vogel JR, Beer B, Clody DE. A simple and reliable procedure for testing anti-anxiety agents. Psychopharmacologia 1971;*21*:1–7.
15. Lister RG. Ethologically-based animal models of anxiety disorders. Pharmacol Ther 1990;*46*:321–340.
16. Haefely W, Martin JR, Schoch P. Novel anxiolytics that act as partial agonists at benzodiazepine receptors. Trends Pharmacol Sci 1990;*11*:452–456.
17. King DJ. Benzodiazepines, amnesia and sedation: Theoretical and clinical issues and controversies. Human Psychopharmacol 1992;*7*:79–87.
18. Martin JR, Schoch P, Jenck F, Moreau J-L, Haefely WE. Pharmacological characterization of benzodiazepine receptor ligands with intrinsic efficacies ranging from high to zero. Psychopharmacology 1993;*111*:415–422.
19. Miczek KA. The psychopharmacology of aggression. In: Iversen LL, Iversen SD, Synder SH. Handbook of psychopharmacology, vol. 19, New directions in behavioral pharmacology. 1987; New York: Plenum Press, pp 183–328.
20. Rogawski MA, Porter RJ. Antiepileptic drugs: Pharmacological mechanisms and clinical efficacy with consideration of promising developmental stage compounds. Pharmacol Rev 1990;*42*:223–286.

21. Goodchild CS, Noble J. The effects of intrathecal midazolam on sympathetic nervous system reflexes in man—a pilot study. Br J Clin Pharmacol 1987;*23*:279–285.

22. Hollister LE, Müller-Oerlinghausen B, Rickels K, Shader RI. Clinical uses of benzodiazepines. Clin Psychopharmacol 1993;*13:(Suppl 1)*, 1S–169S.

23. Dommisse CS, Hayes PE. Current concepts in clinical therapeutics: Anxiety disorders, part 2. Clin Pharmacy 1987;*6*:196–215.

24. Hayes PE, Dommisse CS. Current concepts in clinical therapeutics: Anxiety disorders, part 1. Clin Pharmacy 1987;*6*:140–147.

25. Wardle J. Behavioural therapy and benzodiazepines: allies or antagonists? Br J Psychiatry 1990;*156*:163–168.

26. Oswald I. Benzodiazepines and sleep. In: Trimble MR. Benzodiazepines divided, 1983; Chichester: Wiley pp 261–276.

27. Mendelsen WB. Human sleep: Research and clinical care. 1987; New York: Plenum, pp 1–436.

28. Sneader W. Hypnotics. Drug News Persp 1993;*6*:182–186.

29. Laverty R. Hypnotics and sedatives. In: Dukes MNG. Meyler's Side Effects of Drugs, 12th edition, 1992; Amsterdam: Elsevier, pp 93–104.

30. O'Boyle CA. Benzodiazepine-induced amnesia and anaesthetic practice: A review. In: Hindmarch I, Ott H. Benzodiazepine receptor ligands, memory and information processing. 1988; Berlin: Springer-Verlag, pp 146–165.

31. Brogden RN, Goa KL. Flumazenil: A reappraisal of its pharmacological properties and therapeutic efficacy as a benzodiazepine antagonist. Drugs 1991;*42*:1061–1089.

32. Ling W, Wesson DR. Seizure disorders. In: Smith DE, Wesson DR. The benzodiazepines: Current standards for medical practice. 1985; Hingham, MA, MTP Press, pp 149–157.

33. Möhler H, Benke D, Rhyner T, Sigel E. Molecular pharmacology of $GABA_A$-receptors. In: Schousboe A, Diemer NH, Kofod H. Drug research related to neuroactive amino Acids, Alfred Benzon symposium 32. 1992; Copenhagen: Munksgaard, 1992, pp 87–102.

34. Olson RW, Tobin AJ. Molecular biology of $GABA_A$ receptors. FASEB J 1990;*4*:1469–1480.

35. Seeburg PH, Wisden W, Verdoorn TA, Pritchett DB, Werner P, Herb A, Lueddens H, Sprengel R, Sakmann B. The $GABA_A$ receptor family: Molecular and functional diversity. Cold Spring Harb Symp Quant Biol 1990;*55*:29–40.

36. Lueddens H, Wisden W. Function and pharmacology of multiple $GABA_A$ receptor subunits. Trends Pharmacol Sci 1991;*12*:49–51.

37. Criswell HE, Simson PE, Duncan GE, McCown TJ, Herbert JS, Morrow AL, Breese GR. Molecular basis for regionally specific action of ethanol on γ-aminobutyric $acid_A$ receptors: Generalization to other ligand-gated ion channels. J Pharmacol Exper Therap 1993;*267*:522–537.

38. Pritchett DB, Sontheimer H, Shivers BC, Ymer S, Kettenmann H, Schofield PR, Seeburg PH. Importance of a novel $GABA_A$ receptor subunit for benzodiazepine pharmacology. Nature 1989;*338*:582–585.

39. Polc P. Electrophysiology of benzodiazepine receptor ligands: Multiple mechanisms and sites of action. Prog Neurobiol 1988;*31*:349–423.

40. Giesen-Crouse E. Peripheral Benzodiazepine Receptors. 1993; London: Academic Press. pp 1–281.

41. Kales A, Kales JD, Bixler EO, Scharf MB. Effectiveness of hypnotic drugs with prolonged use: Flurazepam and pentobarbital. Clin Pharmacol Therap 1975;*18*:356–363.

42. Rickels K, Case WG, Dowing RW, Winokur A. Long-term diazepam therapy and clinical outcome. JAMA 1983;*250*:767–771.

43. Woods JH, Katz JL, Winger G. Benzodiazepines: Use, abuse, and consequences. Pharmacol Rev 1992;*44*:151–347.

44. Balter MB, Ban TA, Uhlenhuth EH. International study of expert judgment on therapeutic use of benzodiazepines and other psychotherapeutic medications: I. Current concerns. Human Psychopharmacol 1993;*8*:253–261.

45. Hines LR. Toxicology and side-effects of anxiolytics. In: Hoffmeister F, Stille G. Handbook of experimental pharmacology, vol. 55/II 1981; Berlin: Springer-Verlag, pp 359–393.

46. Guentert TW. Pharmacokinetics of benzodiazepines and of their metabolites. Prog Drug Metabol 1984;*8*:241–386.

47. Lader M. Correlation of plasma concentrations of benzodiazepines with clinical effects. In: Priest RG, Pletscher A, Ward J. Sleep Research 1979; Lancaster, England: MTP Press, pp 99–108.

48. Norman TR, Burrows GD. Plasma concentrations of benzodiazepines—A review of clinical findings and implications. Prog Neuro-Psychopharmacology Biological Psychiatry 1984;*8*:115–126.

49. Garzone PD, Kroboth PD. Pharmacokinetics of the newer benzodiazepines. Clin Pharmacokinet 1989;*16*:337–364.

50. Jochemsen R, Breimer DD. Pharmacokinetics of benzodiazepines: Metabolic pathways and plasma level profiles. Curr Med Res Opin 1984;*8*:60–79.

51. Geller E, Thomson D. Proceedings of the international symposium on flumazenil—The first benzodiazepine antagonist. Eur J Anaesthesiol 1988;*Supplement 2*:1–332.

52. Scollo-Lavizzari G. The clinical anticonvulsant effects of flumazenil, a benzodiazepine antagonist. Eur J Anaesthesiol 1988;*5 (Supplement 2)*:129–138.

53. Sharief MK, Sander JWAS, Shorvon SD. The effect of oral flumazenil on interictal epileptic activity: Results of a double-blind, placebo-controlled study. Epilepsy Res 1993;*15*:53–60.

54. Thomson D. Midazolam and flumazenil—The agonist-antagonist concept for sedation and anaesthesia. Acta Anaesthesiol Scand 1990;*34 (Supplement 92)*:1–109.

55. Jones EA, Basile AS, Mullen KD, Gammal SH. Flumazenil: Potential implications for hepatic encephalopathy. Pharmacol Therap 1990;*45*:331–343.

56. Andrews PR, Jones GP, Poulton DB. Convulsant, anticonvulsant and anaesthetic barbiturates: In vivo activities of oxo- and thiobarbiturates related to pentobarbitone. Eur J Pharmacol 1982;*79*:61–65.

57. Koch-Weser J, Greenblatt DJ. The archaic barbiturate hypnotics. N Engl J Med 1974;*291*:790–791.

58. Haefely W, Polc P. Physiology of GABA enhancement by benzodiazepines and barbiturates. In: Olsen RW, Venter JC. Benzodiazepine/GABA receptors and chloride channels: Structural and functional properties. 1986; New York: Alan R. Liss, pp 97–133.

59. Macdonald RL, Rogers CJ, Twyman RE. Barbiturate regulation of kinetic properties of the $GABA_A$ receptor channel of mouse spinal neurones in culture. J Physiol 1989;*417*:483–500.

60. Pritchett DB, Sontheimer H, Gorman CM, Kettenmann H, Seeburg PH, Schofield PR. Transient expression shows ligand gating and allosteric potentiation of $GABA_A$ receptor subunits. Science 1988;*242*:1306–1307.

61. Haefely WE. GABA and the anticonvulsant action of benzodiazepines and barbiturates. Brain Res Bull 1980;*5 (Supplement 2)*:873–878.

62. Engel J. Seizures and epilepsy 1989; Philadelphia: FA Davis, pp 1–536.

63. Leutner V. Schlaf, Schlafstörungen, Schlafmittel. 1993; Stuttgart: Wissenschaftliche Verlagsgesellschaft, pp 1–224.

64. Tunnicliff G, Eison AS, Taylor DP. Buspirone: Mechanisms and clinical aspects. 1991; San Diego: Academic Press, pp 1–335.

65. Goa KL, Ward A. Buspirone: A preliminary review of its pharmacological properties and therapeutic efficacy as an anxiolytic. Drugs 1986;*32*:114–129.

66. Unrug-Neervoort A, van Luijtelaar G, Coenen A. Cognition and vigilance: Differential effects of diazepam and buspirone on memory and psychomotor performance. Neuropsychobiology 1992;*26*:146–150.

67. Brody D, Adler LA, Kim T et al. Effects of buspirone in seven schizophrenic subjects. J Clin Psychopharmacol 1990;*10*:68–69.

68. Gammans RE, Mayol RF, Labudde JA. Metabolism and disposition of buspirone. Am J Med 1986;*80 (Supplement 3B)*:41–51.

69. Doble A, Martin IL. Multiple benzodiazepine receptors: No reason for anxiety. Trends Pharmacol Sci 1992;*13*:76–81.

Reviews

r1. Balter MB, Manheimer DI, Mellinger GD, Uhlenhuth EH. A cross-national comparison of anti-anxiety/sedative drug use. Curr Med Res Opin 1984;*8 (Suppl. 4)*:5–20.

r2. Freedman DX. Benzodiazepines: Therapeutic, biological and psychosocial issues. J Psychiatr Res 1990;*24 (Suppl. 2)*:169–174.

r3. Friedel B, Staak M. Benzodiazepines and driving. Rev Contemp Pharmacotherap 1992;*3*:415–474.

r4. Ghoneim MM, Mewaldt SP. Benzodiazepines and human memory: A review. Anesthesiology 1990;*72*:926–938.

r5. Greenblatt DJ, Shader RI. Benzodiazepines in clinical practice. 1974; New York: Raven Press.

r6. Hindmarch I, Beaumont G, Brandon S, Leonard BE. Benzodiazepines: Current Concepts. 1990; New York: John Wiley.

r7. Lyons JS, Larson DB, Hromco J. Clinical and economic evaluation of benzodiazepines. PharmacoEconomics 1992;*2*:397–407.

r8. Marks J. Techniques of benzodiazepine withdrawal in clinical practice: A consensus workshop report. Med Toxicol 1988;*3*:324–333.

r9. Roy-Byrne PP, Cowley DS. Benzodiazepines in clinical practice: Risks and benefits. 1991; Washington: American Psychiatric Press.

r10. Senay EC. Drug abuse and public health: A global perspective. Drug Safety 1991;*6 (Suppl. 1)*:1–65.

r11. Shader RI, Greenblatt DJ. Use of benzodiazepines in anxiety disorders. N Engl J Med 1993;*328*:1398–1405.

r12. Smith DE, Wesson DR. The benzodiazepines: Current standards for medical practice. 1985; Lancaster, England: MTP Press Ltd.

r13. Woods JH, Katz JL, Winger G. Use and abuse of benzodiazepines: Issues relevant to prescribing. JAMA 1988;*260*:3476–3480.

CHAPTER 15

General Principles of Drug Therapy in Psychiatric Disorders

Richard C. Shelton
Peter T. Loosen
Michael H. Ebert

It is possible to lose sight of the significant contribution that psychopharmacology has made to the practice of psychiatry. Prior to 1949, psychiatrists were limited to using either psychotherapy or crude somatic treatments (including insulin-induced hypoglycemia or other convulsive therapies) or to therapies not specific to the diseases being treated (including barbiturates and bromides). This situation was changed dramatically by the successive introduction of lithium salts, the antipsychotic chlorpromazine, the monoamine oxidase inhibitor antidepressant iproniazid, the tricyclic antidepressant imipramine, and the benzodiazepine chlordiazepoxide. These drugs revolutionized both treatment and research in major mental illnesses. Biologic psychiatry research thus experienced a renaissance, recalling earlier decades in this century when it was in the forefront. It has been said that 90 percent of all knowledge about mental illness has been accumulated in the past 30 years; this can be attributed in a significant degree to psychopharmacology.

Psychotropic drugs traditionally have been classified according to their therapeutic action, e.g., antipsychotics, antidepressants, and antianxiety drugs. Although this nosology is heuristically useful in clinical practice, it appears to be arbitrary and limited. Some of the drugs have different therapeutic actions but are similar in chemical structure (e.g., compare imipramine [chapter 17], chlorpromazine [chapter 16], carbamazepine [chapter 19], and chlorpheniramine [chapter 9]). In addition, drugs can be used for more than one therapeutic indication (e.g., carbamazepine for seizures, depression, and bipolar disorder, and imipramine for depression, panic disorder, and enuresis). Caution is needed to avoid rigid views of drugs that limit therapeutic versatility.

The physician-patient relationship is critical in the discussion of the use of psychopharmacologic agents. Many concerns were raised by mental health professionals when drugs were first introduced into clinical practice. There was worry that drugs would interfere with the delicate therapeutic relationship and that drugs could be used to manipulate or control patients. Today, most psychiatrists skillfully and successfully blend psychopharmacologic and psychosocial approaches, and the dichotomy appears increasingly semantic. In fact, there is evidence that psychotherapy and psychopharmacology may act synergistically, at least in the treatment of major depression[1] and schizophrenia.[2] Medications are powerful tools in the management of psychiatric disorders and function as important components of the comprehensive approach to psychiatric disorders.

Diagnostic Nosology

At this point, psychiatric disorders are syndromes largely without known discrete biologic substrates. In practice there is often significant diagnostic overlap between disorders. The common necessity of using indirect behavioral data and short-term, cross-sectional observation contributes to this problem. It is not surprising, then, that diagnostic systems have proliferated and that there is confusion in nomenclature. Attempts to improve diagnostic uniformity include the World Health Organization International Classification of Diseases (ICD) and the American Psychiatric Association Diagnostic and Statistical Manual of Mental Disorders (third, revised edition [DSM-IIIR]).[3] The ICD is a collection of diagnostic terms, not a diagnostic system per se. The DSM-IIIR, on the other hand, has derived from a conscious attempt to develop an empirically derived, nontheoretical approach to diagnostic classification. The current version, though remaining controversial, is widely used as the standard of psychiatric diagnosis in the US.

In clinical practice, there is no substitute for a careful diagnostic evaluation. This should include longitudinal data as well as information from various sources, especially families. Special attention should be given to the use of alcohol and other drugs of abuse. Diagnoses should be periodically re-evaluated, especially in patients who have not responded well to standard therapies.

Pharmacokinetics and Pharmacodynamics

Most drugs used to treat psychiatric disorders are highly lipophilic and interact with receptors or uptake sites of catecholamines, indolamines, acetylcholine, and histamine. Most of these drugs (except lithium salts) are variations based on a cyclic amine nucleus. This nucleus facilitates efficient binding to receptors and explains most beneficial and adverse effects (Table 15.1). Understanding the binding properties and other chemical actions of the drugs is useful to the clinician in predicting these effects. Other important determinants of the therapeutic actions of drugs are such pharmacokinetic principles as absorption, distribution, biotransformation, and elimination.[r1,r2]

Administration and Absorption

There are various potential routes of administration of drugs, IV, oral, sublingual, subcutaneous, IM, intrathecal, intraperitoneal, aerosol (i.e., pulmonary), cutaneous, and rectal. Of these, only two, oral and IM, are widely used in psychiatry. Access to the CNS requires that the drug pass through cell membranes, and depends on relative lipid solubility. Most psychotropic drugs are fairly rapidly and completely absorbed from oral and IM sites and cross the blood-brain barrier, since they are highly lipid-soluble (i.e., have a high partition coefficient). Some notable exceptions to this rule will be discussed elsewhere in this volume. Since psychotropic drugs generally are weak bases, the low pH of the stomach will delay absorption by converting a higher percentage of the drug into the less soluble ionized form. In addition, the stomach has relatively little surface area compared to the small intestine, and many drugs have enteric coatings that prevent release into the stomach. Gastric emptying into the small bowel with its higher pH allows for more complete absorption of the nonionized species. Anything that delays gastric emptying, such as the presence of food or the use of drugs that slow GI motility, will delay absorption. Since the drugs are absorbed relatively slowly, and since there is significant "first-pass metabolism" (i.e., extensive metabolism in the liver after absorption but before distribution) for most psychotropics, oral administration affords a greater margin of safety than parenteral.

Intramuscular administration, on the other hand, delivers the drug to the bloodstream (and hence the CNS) in a more rapid and predictable pattern in most circumstances. Most drugs are rapidly absorbed from the extra-cellular fluid (ECF) into the capillaries. Further, they reach the CNS without having been extensively metabolized by the liver. Parenteral administration provides more predictable delivery of drug than does oral because it avoids the variability inherent in GI absorption and hepatic metabolism. This affords a quick onset of action and higher plasma levels, but is also associated with a greater degree of adverse reactions. Intramuscular administration is usually reserved for emergency circumstances where a rapid onset of action is mandatory. The one significant exception to this is the use of long-acting depot forms of antipsychotics. Drugs like fluphenazine and haloperidol are available in oil bases for IM use. This produces slow absorption and a prolonged duration of action. This is discussed in the chapter on antipsychotic agents (see chapter 16).

Distribution

After absorption, the lipophilic psychotropic drugs are rapidly distributed and largely bound to such plasma proteins as $alpha_1$ acid glycoproteins. Only a relatively small percentage of the drug is therefore available in the free (i.e., unbound) fraction. It is this free fraction, however, that is pharmacologically active. Since a drug may be 80 to 90 percent protein-bound, displacement of even a small fraction, either by competition with other drugs or a reduction of the amount of plasma protein, will have large effects on its availability to brain. This is of practical importance in considering the effects of drugs in the elderly and medically ill, as discussed below.

Table 15.1 The Relationship Between Mechanism of Action and Both Beneficial and Adverse Effects of Psychotropic Drugs (Adapted in part from Richelson, 1987[25])[a]

Mechanism of Action	Therapeutic Effect	Adverse Effect
Acetylcholine (muscarinic) blockade	None[b]	Dry mouth, blurred vision, tachycardia, reduced GI motility (constipation, ileus), exacerbation of narrow angle glaucoma, urinary retention, confusion, delirium.
Alpha 1 adrenergic blockade	None[b]	Orthostatic hypotension, reflex, tachycardia, dizziness, syncope.
Benzodiazepine agonism	Antianxiety Anticonvulsant	Drowsiness, lethargy, sedation, exacerbation of depression, ataxia, impairment of visuomotor coordination, augmentation of CNS depressants, paradoxical excitement, tolerance and dependency.
Dopamine (D_2) blockade	Antipsychotic	Extrapyramidal effects (dystonia, rigidity, pill-rolling tremor, shuffling gait, etc.), blunted affect, apathy, neuroleptic malignant syndrome, elevation of prolactin (gynecomastia, galactorrhea).
Dopamine reuptake blockade	None[b]	Exacerbation of psychosis, insomnia, anxiety, tremor.
Histamine 1	Antihistamine	Drowsiness, lethargy, weight gain, blockade augmentation of CNS depressants.
Monoamine oxidase inhibition	Antidepressant Antiparkinsonian (Deprenyl)	Pressor effect (hypertensive crisis), crisis, inhibition of metabolism of other drugs (e.g., meperidine), insomnia, myoclonus, tremor, anxiety, nervousness, headache exacerbation of psychosis.
Norepinephrine reuptake inhibition	Antidepressant	Anxiety, tremor, insomnia, nervousness, tachycardia.
Serotonin reuptake inhibition	Antidepressant	Anxiety, headache, insomnia, nervousness nausea, vomiting, diarrhea, myoclonus, weight loss.

[a]For a more complete discussion of the beneficial and adverse effects of each drug class refer to the appropriate chapter heading.
[b]No therapeutic indication with psychotropic drugs.

Drugs are distributed to receptor sites throughout the body, which accounts for their peripheral side-effects. In addition, distribution of lipophilic drugs in body fat will tend to reduce the amount of drug available in the blood by increasing the apparent volume of distribution. These sites serve as reservoirs of drug in the body. Increased body fat will, therefore, reduce the bioavailability of a given dose of drug. Distribution of drugs to the CNS is limited by the blood-brain barrier. This barrier consists of tight gap junctions between the endothelial cells of the capillaries of the CNS. Polar compounds are prevented from distributing in the ECF of the brain and spinal cord. Lipophilic drugs, on the other hand, can rapidly pass through the endothelial cell membrane by passive diffusion. This accounts for both accumulation and elimination of drug in the CNS.

Biotransformation

As a drug is being distributed via the circulation it passes through the liver. Essentially all psychoactive agents except lithium are metabolized by the liver, via the microsomal enzymes. These drugs undergo one or more metabolic steps prior to inactivation, usually through formation of water-soluble glucuronides that can be eliminated via the kidney. This metabolic action is particularly important for drugs administered orally since they are absorbed in the stomach and small intestine and are distributed first to the liver via the portal circulation. A large percentage (> 80%) of the drug may be metabolized before the drug enters the general circulation.

The amount of time required to metabolize and eliminate one-half of a given dose of drug from the system is referred to as the half-life of elimination ($T_{1/2e}$). Most drugs metabolized by the liver, however, have one or more active metabolites, each with its own $T_{1/2e}$. Therefore the biologic half-life of action of a drug depends on the metabolism and elimination of the parent compound and all its active metabolites. Alterations in hepatic metabolism can have significant effects on the relative activity of a given drug.

Elimination

Once the drug is in a hydrophilic form it can be eliminated from the body by excretion in the renal glomeruli. Reductions in renal function usually do not have a significant effect on the bioactivity of most drugs, since the glucuronidated drug is inactive. An exception to this is lithium. Lithium is not metabolized in the liver, and elimination is predominantly via filtration in the kidney. Renal impairment results in accumulation of lithium, with resulting toxicity. Other forms of elimination, such as through the bile, sweat, and respiratory tract, are generally of limited significance for most psychoactive agents.

Drug-Drug Interactions

Interactions between drugs can be either antagonistic or synergistic. Each step in drug action, from absorption to elimination, can be a potential site for drug interactions. Absorption of drugs can be slowed by reduction in GI motility, for example, and this commonly occurs with muscarinic cholinergic antagonists. Distribution can be affected by drug-drug interactions. Drugs can compete for plasma protein binding sites and mutually increase the relative free fraction of drug. Adding a drug to an established regimen can increase the pharmacologic effect, while discontinuing a drug may significantly reduce the relative effect by lowering the free fraction of the remaining drug as it is absorbed by the plasma proteins.

Bioavailability is also affected by the effects of drugs on metabolism. Some drugs, such as phenothiazines and tricyclic antidepressants, compete for the same metabolic enzymes in the liver. Co-administration will result in a mutual increase in available drug through reduction in metabolism. On the other hand, some drugs can increase the metabolic capacity by enzyme induction. This is important, for example, for carbamazepine and the barbiturates. Such agents will reduce the plasma levels of other drugs by induction of metabolism in the cytochrome P450 system. Such interactional effects on metabolism are important factors to consider if drugs are to be given together.

Drugs can also interact synergistically or antagonistically at effector sites in target organs. The dopamine D_2 receptor blocking action of antipsychotics will antagonize the beneficial effects of L-dopa in Parkinson's disease (see chapter 18). The tricyclic antidepressants will oppose the effect of antihypertensives such as guanethidine that require presynaptic uptake (see chapter 17). It is important to know the basic pharmacologic effects of drugs to prevent these interactions.

Plasma Level Monitoring

One important application of clinical pharmacokinetics is plasma level monitoring of drugs. Many psychotropics, including the tricyclic antidepressants and the antipsychotics, exhibit wide inter-individual variation in metabolism, producing widely varying plasma levels. All drugs have dose-response relationships, but only a relatively few have established effective plasma level ranges. The most extreme case is that of lithium, where plasma monitoring of all patients is a part of accepted clinical practice. The benzodiazepines and buspirone fall on the other end of a spectrum with no plasma monitoring commonly used. Antidepressants and antipsychotics fall in between. Therapeutic ranges have been worked out for several tricyclics, but not for other antidepressants.[4,5] Similarly, though a number of studies of antipsychotic plasma level-response relationships have been published, the clinical utility remains obscure.[6–9] A number of factors can come into play to determine whether or not a clear relationship can be established between plasma level and response. A slightly modified version of the list of requirements of May and Van Putten[10] would include:

1. A sensitive and reliable drug assay.
2. An adequate number of patients in the study to provide the statistical power to establish the effect.
3. Careful diagnostic selection of patients to ensure a homogeneous and treatment-responsive group.
4. The use of fixed dosages to ensure that plasma levels remain independent of clinical improvement.
5. The use of randomized double-blind conditions when more than one dosage level is used.
6. An adequate length of treatment.
7. Avoidance of other treatments that may obscure drug-therapy effects.
8. Age-and sex-matching the samples.
9. Preventing contamination from prior drug therapies by allowing the longest "washout period" ethically feasible.
10. Avoiding over-reliance on coefficients of correlation between "steady-state" blood levels and determinants of clinical outcome, either of which can be confounded by a variety of factors.
11. The use of appropriate statistical analysis.[9]
12. Avoiding a high level of placebo response in the sample that will "dilute" the relationship between level and response.
13. Consideration of the presence of one or more active metabolites that may obscure plasma level-response relationships for the parent compound.
14. Avoidance of the incorrect use of collection tubes that alter the plasma level determination.
15. Assuring patient compliance, particularly for steady-state studies.[11] From this list it seems clear that establishing plasma level-response relationships can be daunting.

When plasma levels are both available and clinically useful, when should they be used? In a review of the tricyclic plasma level monitoring, Preskorn, et al.[5] state that monitoring is now the "standard of care" for all patients being treated with tricyclics. The authors give five reasons why plasma monitoring may be used. These seem applicable to all drugs in which plasma levels are currently available:

1. *As a means of assessing compliance.* This is an important use of plasma level monitoring but can cause problems with the therapeutic alliance if not approached carefully with the patient.

Patients should always be informed that this is one reason for obtaining a plasma level so that they will not be "surprised" later with the information.

2. *As a means of maximizing response.* Marginal plasma levels may result in an incomplete response, particularly when subsequent induction of hepatic metabolism may lower the levels. When the response is incomplete or when relapse occurs in patients who are being treated, plasma levels can be useful. It is particularly important to assess plasma levels when a patient has not responded to a presumably adequate trial.
3. *As a means of avoiding toxicity.* Certain patients (e.g., the elderly, those who are medically ill, and slow metabolizers) may be particularly sensitive to the toxic effects of drugs. Plasma levels can aid in maximizing response while avoiding unnecessary toxicity. In particular, when toxic effects are uncertainly related to the drug (such as with a drug-induced delirium), the plasma level can assist in the determination. In addition, if higher than usual doses are used, testing the plasma level can help avoid reaching toxic levels.
4. *As a means of minimizing cost.* Noncompliance or low concentrations will clearly delay the onset of action of drugs and this may increase the length of hospital stay and produce longer-term compliance problems that may increase morbidity and mortality and reduce productivity. Further, high plasma levels (particularly in slow metabolizers) can produce toxicity, resulting in complications in treatment, avoidable hospitalizations (or prolongation of hospital care), and death. Thus, plasma level monitoring can reduce overall health care expenditures.
5. *As a means of avoiding medical-legal problems.* Unusual toxic events, such as the accumulation of plasma levels in slow metabolizers can result in untoward reactions that may lead to malpractice litigation. Avoiding malpractice should not, in and of itself, be a reason for obtaining plasma levels. The important consideration should be quality medical practice, the "standard of care." Plasma levels of lithium are now required to meet the standard, and for tricyclics this is increasingly so. Reliance on laboratory testing at the expense of careful patient monitoring, however, also is not acceptable.

To this list we would add:

6. *As a means of assessing potential drug-drug interactions.* Concomitant use of other drugs (such as carbamazepine in patients treated with antipsychotics, antidepressants, or benzodiazepines) may adversely affect plasma levels and produce either toxicity or loss of effect. Plasma levels are often mandatory in evaluating such interactions.

Special Populations

Children and adolescents present a special set of problems for the clinician.[r3] Children usually have a highly efficient cytochrome system and a high relative percentage of hepatic mass, producing a greater fraction of elimination on first pass through the liver of most psychotropics. Since these drugs are highly metabolized in all populations, even a minor increase in relative metabolism produces a substantial reduction in the available drug. There is a lower percentage of body fat relative to adults, decreasing the apparent volume of distribution. Children are usually physically healthy, and are on few or no competing drugs. Dosage adjustments also have to be made for a slow but virtually constant increase in weight. Taken together, this pharmacokinetic profile indicates that the average child will require a higher dose on a mg/kg basis than an adult. Very rapid titration to high doses should not be undertaken, however. Careful dosage adjustment still should be performed to minimize side-effects. Adolescents, on the other hand, resemble young adults in their pharmacokinetics. Percentage of body fat approaches adult levels by early to mid-adolescence, and there is a corresponding reduction in relative hepatic activity. Therefore, adolescents usually will require doses at near the adult levels. Plasma level monitoring, when available, is often helpful to optimize treatment.[12]

The choice of psychopharmacologic management of children is often difficult. First, sometimes drug management is necessary, as in an acute psychosis. Here it is advantageous to help the patient and family to view the mental problem as a brain disorder that can be treated much like diabetes or other physical conditions. On the other hand, the long-term consequences of pharmacologic management, both physical and psychologic, are at times unclear. Second, there is evidence that children may not respond as well to some psychopharmacologic agents (such as antidepressants), even at adequate plasma levels.[13] Third, diagnostic nosology is less precise in childhood conditions, and environmental factors (such as disturbed families) have a greater impact on children.[14] Considerable progress has been made, however, with the introduction of standard diagnostic systems such as the Research Diagnostic Criteria and the DSM-III-R.[15] However, children are not likely to have an optimal response to pharmacologic management when they are maintained in an abusive or otherwise highly stressful environment. Fourth, children and adolescents may be less sensitive to the effects of psychotropics in general. Drug treatment for children and adolescents should be undertaken only when necessary and as a component of a comprehensive treatment plan.

Pregnancy is another difficult situation for the psychopharmacologist because of the potential for birth defects related to drug treatment. Of the commonly used psychotropics, only lithium has been established to be clearly teratogenic, but benzodiazepines and such anticonvulsants as carbamazepine have been strongly implicated in the literature. Other drugs have also been implicated. The first trimester of pregnancy is the most vulnerable period for birth defects. In addition, if drugs are used they should be withdrawn at least two weeks before delivery in order to eliminate the drug from the newborn. This will help prevent such untoward reactions as excessive sedation or withdrawal in the newborn.

The first step in the management of drugs in pregnancy always should be reproductive counseling. All women of reproductive potential (i.e., who are not one year postmenopause or have not been surgically sterilized) should be counseled to avoid pregnancy or to inform the physician before becoming pregnant. Generally, all drugs should be treated as potential teratogens and eliminated if possible. Judicious pharmacologic treatment may be required despite the teratogenic risk, however, when severe mental symptoms are present and not amenable to psychotherapeutic management. This is often the case with manic, psychotic, or severely depressed women, though the latter group may be treated with electroconvulsive therapy as an alternative. A risk-benefit analysis for both the mother and unborn child should be undertaken when psychotropics are used in this situation. The informed consent procedure should be modified to apprise the patient and family of the potential for birth defects.

The risk to nursing infants when the mother is using psychopharmacologic agents is unclear. It is useful to avoid using any pharmacologic agents when nursing since many drugs are secreted into breast milk. In reality, the amount actually excreted is small, but the absolute short- and long-term risks are unknown. This, coupled with the availability of acceptable milk substitutes, makes the avoidance of psychotropics in nursing mothers prudent.

Geriatric psychopharmacology is becoming increasingly important as the population ages.[r4,r5] This group of patients presents its own set of special problems. First, older persons are usually on a number of medications, and the potential for drug-drug interactions is very high. Second, effective management requires thorough understanding of the pharmacokinetics of the elderly:

1. GI motility can be slowed by age, disease (e.g., diabetes), or drugs, including antacids, milk of magnesia, or anticholinergics. These can delay and reduce the peak serum levels achieved after an oral dose.
2. After absorption, drugs with high hepatic clearance may show a reduction in "first-pass" metabolism, especially when cardiac output is reduced. This effect is magnified by the reduction in cytochrome-dependent metabolism (particularly demethylation and hydroxylation) induced by both age and the presence of competing drugs. The effect is a prolonged $T_{1/2e}$ of parent drug and any active metabolites, causing accumulation. In addition, the activity of monoamine oxidase (MAO) is reduced. This enzyme is involved in the metabolism of the catecholamines and indolamines. Reduced MAO activity will increase the effects of drugs, such as antidepressants, that augment the availability of the monoamines.
3. The relative percentage of body fat increases with aging. This expands the apparent volume of distribution, and thereby reduces drug plasma levels.
4. Availability of plasma proteins, including albumin and $alpha_1$ acid glycoproteins, is reduced with age, increasing the free fraction and therefore the bioavailability of protein-bound drugs. This is especially important for drugs that are highly protein-bound.
5. Renal clearance of drugs is reduced in the elderly through declines in blood flow (and attendant glomerular filtration rate) and tubular excretion. This is particularly important for lithium treatment, where serum levels depend mainly on renal excretion. On the whole, although some effects of aging, e.g., an increase in the apparent volume of distribution, act to reduce the availability of drug at the effector site, the over-all pharmacokinetic effect of aging is to increase the available drug in the average patient.[16,17]

Age also can produce changes in the pharmacodynamics of drugs. A loss of neurons in the CNS occurs with aging, especially those neurons containing acetylcholine and dopamine. With this loss comes an increase in sensitivity of receptors. Clinically, this can manifest itself as an increased sensitivity to (for example) agents that block dopamine and muscarinic acetylcholine receptors, with associated cognitive impairment and extrapyramidal reactions at low doses. In addition, there is a particular sensitivity to sedative agents, including benzodiazepines, which puts elderly patients at increased risk for daytime drowsiness, confusion, ataxia, reduced motor coordination, and falls. The latter can be particularly troublesome because of the potential for fractures, especially of the hip. Clearly, this increased sensitivity to drugs, coupled with the fact that elderly patients are likely to be on multiple medications, makes drug management particularly difficult. As a rule of thumb, the elderly are more sensitive to the effects of drugs, and lower doses should be used than in younger adults.

Medically ill patients also require special consideration in clinical psychopharmacology. Many diseases produce psychiatric symptoms or can exacerbate underlying psychiatric illnesses; the same can be true of drugs used to treat medical conditions. Persons with chronic diseases, e.g., cancer patients, may experience depletion in body fat and plasma proteins, increasing the drug's access to the CNS and its potential for toxicity. Patients with reduced cardiac output will also have lower first-pass metabolism, as seen in elderly patients. Finally, persons with hepatic disease will show altered metabolism, prolonging the $T_{1/2e}$ and increasing the serum level. The commonest cause of adverse reactions in the medically ill, however, is drug-drug interactions. Such factors must be considered whenever a patient presents for psychiatric treatment. A complete medical history and physical examination are necessary components of the thorough psychiatric evaluation.

Principles of Psychopharmacologic Management[r6]

The establishment and maintenance of a *therapeutic alliance* are important steps to maximize compliance and outcome.[18] *Compliance* is critical in patient management because drugs don't work if they are not taken. Many factors interact to determine compliance. The quality of the relationship with the physician is not the least of these. This is particularly important since psychotropics often produce side-effects, but their beneficial effects may be delayed. Establishing a positive therapeutic relationship in which the treatment is viewed as a cooperative venture between patient and physician will help. In such a situation, the patient can see him/herself as the vital link in effective management. In addition, factors like limiting the number of medications prescribed, giving the medication as infrequently during the day as possible, and using an informed family monitor are likely to increase compliance.

Pharmacologic treatment must be seen as one of several potential means to achieve symptom relief. Drugs are obviously not required for everyone presenting with psychologic distress. Further, they should be used as a component of a more comprehensive biopsychosocial treatment plan that should addresses issues like psychosocial stress, family problems, work and living situation, and other related factors in addition to symptom reduction. Although psychopharmacologic drugs are used by all physicians, the biopsychsocial integration usually remains in the realm of the psychiatrist.

Among the suggested elements of successful psychopharmacologic treatment are the following:

1. Establish rapport with the patient, family, and significant others.
2. Perform a comprehensive medical, psychologic, and social assessment.
3. Choose appropriate psychosocial and pharmacologic interventions *after* an adequate risk-benefit analysis has been performed.
4. Inform the patient about the rationale for each element of treatment (including psychotherapy) and obtain informed consent after all reasonable risks, benefits, and alternative treatments have been reviewed.
5. Follow the guidelines of the "therapeutic trial," i.e., use dosages within the therapeutic range, allow the drug enough time to be beneficial (which may take up to six weeks for tricyclics), document treatment response, and avoid polypharmacy if possible, prescribing the minimum effective dosage and duration required to achieve the therapeutic goals.
6. Manage adverse reactions and other problems in treatment such as lack of compliance.
7. Periodically reassess the goals and treatments, making suitable adjustments if necessary. Terminate treatment when the targeted treatment goals have been achieved or if no beneficial effect can be documented.

Lack of adequate treatment response with psychopharmacologic agents is a relatively common phenomenon in clinical practice. Effective management of this problem is required. Managing treatment failure begins before initiation of treatment by careful informed consent, including telling the patient about side-effects, the likelihood of responding, and the latency of onset of action. Subsequently, the physician must ensure that adequate plasma levels and duration of treatment are achieved. Noncompliance is an important issue, and can be evaluated by testing plasma levels as noted above. In face of an acceptable drug treatment trial without the expected outcome, specific steps should be undertaken. The diagnosis should be carefully re-evaluated, and the patient should be reassessed for suicidal potential. The treatment plan should be reviewed with the patient with appropriate rationale. This may involve changing the medication or the use of augmenting agents. The review should always have the intent of instilling realistic hope in the patient. Finally, consultation with a colleague should be considered.

Side-effects are often an unavoidable element in pharmacologic management. When comparative beneficial effects are equal between agents, however, the side-effect profiles should be used to select the preferred medication. Our first goal should be to minimize side-effects. However, in some situations side-effects may be exploited. For example, sedating agents (such as certain antidepressants or antipsychotics) may be chosen when patients are experiencing either agitation or insomnia. Therefore, it is important for the physician to have a thorough understanding of both the beneficial actions and the side-effects of drugs.

Psychopharmacology and the Law[r7,r8]

In the US, as well as in many other countries, all physicians, including psychiatrists, have had to pay increasing attention to the legal aspects of practice.[19] Informed consent, for example, will play an expanding role in clinical practice. The concept of informed consent is not new to medicine. Written informed consent prior to elective surgery has been the standard in the US for many years, and it is now the standard of care in all clinical medicine. Failure to obtain informed consent can result in a successful lawsuit when an untoward event occurs, even when standard practice has been followed.

Informed consent has three main elements: information; voluntariness; and competence. The first (and in many ways most important) aspect is *information*. Enough information should be delivered to allow the patient to make a rational decision. Potential benefits, relevant risks, and alternative treatments should be explained, including the risk of taking no action. In addition, the patient needs to be informed of the risk of no treatment. This should be done in a clear and coherent manner, avoiding technical language, and using terms that the patient can readily understand. It is virtually impossible to inform patients of every side-effect ever reported with a drug. Informing the patient of the relatively common (i.e., ≥1% occurrence) adverse effects may overcome the dilemma, except in cases where the side-effect may be serious or life threatening (such as agranulocytosis with carbamazepine), or when the patient's knowledge is required in order to avoid a problem (such as the hypertensive crisis with monoamine oxidase inhibitors). Written materials may be used in the informed consent process. They should be used as supplement to the discussion, not as a substitute. Such materials often are available from the US Food and Drug Administration, from pharmaceutical companies, and in standard references. Practitioners are encouraged to develop their own hand-outs for patients to carry with them.

These materials can include information that is particular to the population that the physician faces in his/her own practice.

The second element of informed consent is *voluntariness*. Patients must be as free as possible from outside influence in making their decision. The purpose of the informed consent discussion is not to coerce the patient into compliance, but to allow an informed decision. This must concede the possibility that the informed patient may disagree with the physician, even when this is clearly not in his/her own best interest. Though closely linked to competence, these issues are not identical. In order for the consent procedure to be truly voluntary, there must be no negative consequences for refusal alone.

The final element of informed consent is *competence*. This principle states that the person to whom the treatment is being proposed should be of adequate mental capacity to make an informed decision. Roth et al.[20] have proposed a five-step evaluation of competency, based on whether.

1. The patient evidences a choice;
2. That choice is a reasonable one;
3. The choice is based on rational reasons;
4. The patient can understand the information vital to the decision-making process; and
5. The patient actually understands the process.

Persons who may be incompetent include those who are delirious, demented, or psychotic. Children and some adolescents, depending on local statutes or precedent, cannot make a legally competent decision. Competence must be evaluated for both informed refusal or acceptance of treatment. If the patient is incompetent, a guardian is required for all but emergency treatment.

In most states in the US, emergency treatment can be given against the objections of the individual, or when the person cannot otherwise give consent (as in delirium or coma), in order to save the person's life or when such treatment is clearly in his/her best interest. Closely linked to this standard is the commitment process. Commitment is usually governed by statute in each state. In general, involuntary hospitalization is allowed if the person has a mental illness, is a danger to himself or others, or is clearly incapable of caring for himself, and hospitalization is the least restrictive alternative to treatment.

Tardive dyskinesia (TD) also poses a particular problem in informed consent. Usually, the consent is obtained before treatment commences. This may not be practical when a patient is acutely psychotic. In addition, many patients may not agree to treatment in the face of the potential for TD if they do not experience the benefit of treatment. Since there is negligible risk for TD within the first three months, it is possible, when required, to postpone informing the patient of the risk for TD for up to that period. This does not obviate the need for information about other risks and side-effects. The best rule of thumb is to inform the patient about the risk as soon as possible.[21]

The last element of the informed consent process is documentation. Some have advocated a written informed consent process, especially for antipsychotic drugs. Written consent should never be used, however, as a substitute for verbally informing the patient. It is adequate to use the written record as documentation of the process, as long as the various elements are included.

Nonapproved Uses of Drugs

The US FDA determines what drugs can be marketed in the US. Drugs must be certified as "safe and effective" in the treatment of a specific disorder before they can be used. Nonetheless, the FDA does not certify all possible uses of a drug. Therefore, the practitioner can use drugs for nonapproved indications within reason.[22,23] If a drug has been used for a particular indication in the research literature, it usually can be used for that indication without difficulty. Whenever this happens, the clinician should inform the patient that the use of the drug has not been approved by the FDA. In addition, the practitioner can use a drug outside the approved dosage ranges as long as there is a clear, documented therapeutic rationale for doing so. Again, informing the patient is mandatory. Consultation with another clinician, especially one with special training in pharmacology, can be helpful to both the patient and physician in such circumstances.[24]

Psychopharmacology remains an exciting and ever-changing field. The recent release of the selective serotonin reuptake inhibitor antidepressants is an example of the dramatic shifts in available agents. Future research will focus on medications effective on both cell surface receptors and intracellular sites of action, both pre- and postsynaptically. These and related findings will broaden the range of effective drugs while reducing adverse events.

References

Research Reports

1. Rounsaville BJ, Klerman GL, Weissman MM. Do psychotherapy and pharmacotherapy for depression conflict? Empirical evidence from a clinical trial. Arch Gen Psychiatr 1981;*38*:24–29.
2. Sarti P, Cournos F. Medication and psychotherapy in the treatment of chronic schizophrenia. Psychiatric Clin N Amer 1990;*13*:215–228.
3. American Psychiatric Association. Diagnostic and Statistical Manual of Mental Disorders, 3d ed, revised. Washington: American Psychiatric Association Press, 1987.
4. American Psychiatric Association, Task force on the use of laboratory tests in psychiatry: Tricyclic antidepressants-blood level measurements and clinical outcome. Am J Psychiatr 1985;*142*:155–162.
5. Preskorn SH, Dorey RC, Jerkovich GS. Therapeutic drug monitoring of tricyclic antidepressants. Clin Chem 1988;*34*:822–828.
6. Shvartsburd A, Sajadi C, Morton V, Mirabi M, Gordon J, Smith RC. Blood levels of haloperidol and thioridazine during maintenance neuroleptic treatment of schizophrenic outpatients. J Clin Psychopharmacol 1984;*4*:194–198.
7. Mavroidis ML, Garver DL, Kanter DR, Hirschowitz J. Plasma haloperidol levels and clinical response: Confounding variables. Psychopharmacol Bull 1985;*21*:62–65.
8. Shostak M, Perel JM, Stiller RL, Wyman W, Curran S. Plasma haloperidol and clinical response: A role for reduced haloperidol in antipsychotic activity? J Clin Psychopharmacol 1987;*7*:394–400.

9. Midha KK, Hawes EM, Hubbard JW, Korchinski E, McKay G. The search for correlations between neuroleptic plasma levels and clinical outcome: A critical review. In: Melzer HY (ed), Psychopharmacology, the third generation of progress, New York: Raven, (1987), pp 1341–1352.
10. May PRA, Van Putten T. Plasma levels of chlorpromazine in schizophrenia. Arch Gen Psychiatry 1979;*35*:1081–1087.
11. Potter WZ, Linnoila M. Tricyclic antidepressant concentrations: Clinical and research implications. In: Post RM, Ballenger JC (eds), Neurobiology of mood disorders, Baltimore: Williams & Wilkins (1984), pp 698–709.
12. Rave E, Wilson JT. In: Gibaldi M, Prescott L (eds) Handbook of clinical pharmacokinetics, New York: Adis Health Science Press, (1983), pp 142–168.
13. Puig-Antich J, Ryan JD, Rabinovich H. In: Weiner JM (ed) Diagnosis and psychopharmacology of childhood and adolescent disorders, New York: John Wiley, (1985), pp 149–178.
14. Simeon JG. Pediatric psychopharmacology. Can J Psychiatr 1989;*34*:115–122.
15. Ambrosini PJ. Pharmacotherapy in child and adolescent major depressive disorder. In: Meltzer HY (ed) Psychopharmacology: The Third Generation of Progress, Raven, New York, 1987, pp 1247–1254.
16. Salzman C. Basic principles of psychiatric drug prescription in the elderly. Hosp Comm Psychiatry 1981;*33*:133–136.
17. Salzman C. A primer on geriatric psychopharmacology. Am J Psychiatr 1982;*139*:67–74.
18. Gutheil TG, Havens LL. The therapeutic alliance: Contemporary meanings and confusions. Int Rev Pscyhoanal 1979;*6*:467–481.
19. Gutheil TG, Appelbaum PS. Clinical handbook of psychiatry and the law. New York: McGraw-Hill (1982), pp 304–371.
20. Roth LH, Meisel A, Lidz CW. Tests of competency to consent to treatment. Am J Psychiatr 1977;*134*:279–284.
21. Mills MJ, Norquist GS, Shelton RC, Gelenberg AJ, VanPutten T. Consent and liability with neuroleptics: The problem of tardive dyskinesia. International Journal of Law and Psychiatry 1986;*8*:243–252.
22. Use of approved drugs for unlabeled indications. FDA Drug Bull, April 1982.
23. The FDA does not approve uses of drugs (editorial). JAMA 1984;*252*:1054–1055.
24. Schatzberg AF, Cole JO. Manual of clinical psychopharmacology, Washington: American Psychiatric Press (1986), pp 4–9.
25. Richelson E. Pharmacology of antidepressants. Psychopathology 1987;*20*(suppl 1):1–12.

Reviews

r1. Gibaldi M. Biopharmaceutics and clinical pharmacokinetics, 4th ed. Philadelphia: Lea & Febiger, 1991.
r2. Shargel L, Yu ABC. Applied biopharmaceutics and applied pharmacokinetics, 3d ed. Norwalk: Appleton & Lange, 1993.
r3. Green WH. Child and adolescent clinical psychopharmacology. Baltimore: Williams & Wilkins, 1991.
r4. Jenike MA. Geriatric psychiatry and psychopharmacology. Baltimore: Williams & Wilkins, 1989.
r5. Salzman C. Clinical geriatric psychopharmacology, 2d ed. Baltimore: Williams & Wilkins, 1992.
r6. Schatzberg AF, Cole JO. Manual of clinical psychopharmacology. Washington: American Psychiatric Association Press, 1991.
r7. Applebaum PS, Gutheil TG. Clinical handbook of psychiatry and the law, 2d ed. Baltimore: Williams & Wilkins, 1991.
r8. Gutheil TG (ed). Decision-making in psychiatry and the law. Baltimore: Williams & Wilkins, 1991.

CHAPTER 16

Paul A. J. Janssen
Frans H. L. Awouters

Antipsychotic Agents

Psychoses are mental disorders in which changes in brain structure can frequently be detected, but in which associated changes in brain function remain largely unpredictable.[1] These disorders involve the human faculties of thought, judgment, and emotion, and are presented in manifestations of profound disruption between common events and corresponding inner experiences. Descriptive psychiatry has long employed various patterns in psychotic phenomena. Spectrum and intensity of symptoms are the major bases used to distinguish between the many diagnostic groups of functional psychoses.[r1,r2] Current thinking on the biologic basis of psychoses focuses on rather subtle disturbances in central neurotransmission, which may have a hereditary background. Schizophrenia and manic depressive psychoses are the most typical indications for antipsychotic treatment. A manic episode is associated with symptoms of inflated self-esteem or grandiosity, decreased need for sleep, pressure of speech, flight of ideas, distractibility, increased involvement in goal-directed and pleasurable activities, and psychomotor agitation. Episodes begin suddenly, escalate rapidly, and last from a few days to months. They are briefer and terminate more abruptly than do major depressive episodes.

In an acute phase of schizophrenia, delusions, hallucinations, loosening of associations, catatonic behavior, incoherence in thought and speech, and flat affect are prominent. Psychosocial functioning is markedly below the earlier level, but may recover slowly. In acute exarcerbations of schizophrenia, "positive" symptoms (delusions, hallucinations, thought disorder, excitement) prevail over "negative" symptoms (social withdrawal, flat affect, apathy, impoverished thought). Medicinal tradition (rauwolfia alkaloids), the clinical discovery of the first synthetic antipsychotic (chlorpromazine), and pharmacologic antagonism of psychostimulants (haloperidol) have greatly contributed to the creation and expansion of the class of neuroleptic drugs. A variety of compounds are currently used in the treatment of psychosis. They have been shown to induce a regression of core symptoms in disorders such as schizophrenia and mania and, by maintenance treatment, to protect patients with schizophrenia from relapse. With antipsychotic treatment, positive symptoms usually regress to a larger extent than negative symptoms. At the same time, common practice reveals restrictions in their use. Some restrictions are mainly practical, such as patients' compliance and management of side-effects. Others are more fundamental, including absence of response in some patients and a residue of mainly negative symptoms after control of the more florid symptoms. Although it is of great interest to illustrate how current thinking on central neurotransmission is trying to correct the restrictions of the available neuroleptics, the emphasis in this chapter will be on what has been achieved: a distillate from pharmacologic and clinical experience.

Historical Perspective of Antipsychotic Drug Action to Dopaminergic Mechanisms

Chemotherapy of psychoses was virtually nonexistent before the discovery of chlorpromazine. Chemically, chlorpromazine was developed from antihistamines of the promethazine type, and it was first tested clinically in anesthesia to potentiate the narcotic activity of meperidine. Chlorpromazine produced a state of quietness and indifference, which suggested further studies of possible uses in psychiatry. The specific antipsychotic activity of chlorpromazine in acute psychosis was first described in 1952.[2] In the ensuing years, this activity was confirmed, and therapy was extended to chronic schizophrenia. These clinical observations led to the introduction of the term "neuroleptic" activity, which in its original definition indicates the improvement of psychotic symptoms in association with some neurologic and neurovegetative effects.[3] For several years, neuroleptic activity was considered to be an exclusive property of a few phenothiazine derivatives closely related to chlorpromazine and of the rauwolfia alkaloid, reserpine.

When the pharmacologic actions of chlorpromazine were first described, the relationship to clinical antipsychotic activity was not clear. A further experimental development followed in 1958 with the synthesis of haloperidol, the archetype of the butyrophenone series of neuroleptics,[4] which eliminated certain of the actions of chlorpromazine. Chemically, this butyrophenone resulted from progressive modifications of meperidine-like analgesics, unrelated to phenothiazines. Pharmacologically, the new compounds showed gradually more neuroleptic and less analgesic activity until full specificity was reached with haloperidol. The predicted antipsychotic activity of haloperidol was soon confirmed in the clinic. The introduction of haloperidol greatly stimulated the exploration of newly synthesized molecules for neuroleptic activity, resulting in the availability of more than 100 compounds that have received detailed study. Such availability of drugs has facilitated the discussion of similarities and differences between neuroleptics.

Pharmacologic methods first established that neuroleptics inhibited abnormal behavior induced by amphetamine or apomorphine. Meanwhile, developments in neuroscience showed the presence of dopamine as a normal constituent of the brain with a potential neurotransmitter function. Subsequently, the behavioral stimulation induced by amphetamine and apomorphine was found to be either the result of increased release of dopamine from the nerve terminals (amphetamine) or of a direct stimulation of dopamine receptors (apomorphine).[5] Interference of chlorpromazine or haloperidol with the central dopaminergic system in animals also was suggested from the observation that there was a pronounced increase in dopamine metabolites.[6] Based on such data, neuroleptics were proposed to act by blocking dopamine receptors in brain.[r3]

Dopaminergic Mechanisms

With the view that antipsychotic drugs are antagonists at dopamine receptors, mechanisms associated with dopaminergic function will be described briefly. Figure 16.1 illustrates schematically the pathways that use dopamine as a neurotransmitter. The cell bodies of the dopaminergic neurons are concentrated in the ventral tegmental area (VTA; A8, A10) and in the substantia nigra pars compacta (SN; A9). Axonal projections run from the SN mainly to the striatum, in which the caudate nucleus and the globus pallidus receive heavy dopaminergic input. This latter projection is referred to as the nigrostriatal pathway. The VTA cell bodies also send projections that reach "mesolimbic" and cortical areas in the forebrain.

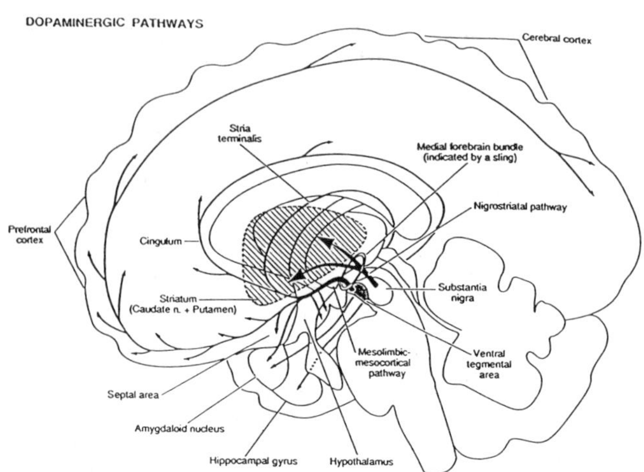

Figure 16.1 Main Dopaminergic Pathways in the Human Brain

Receptors important to dopaminergic function are localized neuroanatomically both pre- and postsynaptically (see Chapters 1 & 12). In addition, another site associated with dopamine function is responsible for dopamine uptake into the presynaptic site after release. This carrier protein has been cloned and is believed to be a major site of action of d-amphetamine and cocaine.[r4] Presynaptic receptors (or autoreceptors) are defined as dopamine sensitive receptors located on the releasing neuronal terminal. The consequence of activating this receptor is a decrease of further release of dopamine even at constant stimulation frequency (see also Chapters 1 & 12). Apomorphine at low doses, which can decrease locomotor activity in animals, is thought to act on these presynaptic autoreceptors.[7] However, as the dose of apomorphine is increased, postsynaptic dopamine receptors are activated, resulting in an increase in locomotor activity and increased agitation. It is proposed that exogenous agonists acting on this autoreceptor could conceivably decrease transmitter release and reduce dopaminergic stimulation; the functional consequence is thought to be the same as that observed after progressive blockade of postsynaptic dopaminergic receptors. However, more selective autoreceptor agonists are required to test this latter concept. Blockade of these presynaptic dopamine receptors is involved in the increase in dopamine metabolites observed after antipsychotic administration, but feedback pathways activated by the blockade of postsynaptic receptors appear to be more important.[r5]

Microanatomically classical postsynaptic receptors are membrane components of the neuron that receives the impact of the released neurotransmitter. The dopamine receptors in brain belong to the group of proteins that cross the cell membrane seven times (seven transmembrane domains) and are functionally linked to intracellular G-proteins[8] (see Chapters 1 & 12). Two types of dopamine receptors, D_1 and D_2, were first recognized by differences in this functional link. Activation of D_1-receptors increases adenylyl cyclase activity and thus accelerates the formation of cAMP. Activation of D_2-receptors indirectly decreases adenylyl cyclase activity. Antipsychotic activity of the known effective drugs is now recognized to correlate with affinity to D_2-receptors, but not with affinity to D_1-receptors.[r6] Pharmacologically the specific D_1-receptor antagonist SCH-23390 differs from the D_2-antagonists mainly by the lack of antiemetic and prolactin-releasing activity. Antipsychotic effects may be found to be based on anti-D_1-activity when clinically acceptable antagonists become available.[r7]

The direct demonstration of the common site of action of neuroleptics was made in 1975. It was found that the striatal membrane sites labeled with radioactive haloperidol correspond to specific dopamine receptors.[9,10] These dopamine receptors are presently known as D_2-receptors, and they are abundant in postsynaptic membranes of brain structures with dopaminergic terminals, such as the striatum. These receptors bind the endogenous neurotransmitter, dopamine, at micromolar concentrations, whereas binding of potent neuroleptics occurs at nanomolar concentrations. Blockade of the receptors in vivo has functional consequences such as decreased dopaminergic neurotransmission, increased dopamine turnover and formation of dopamine metabolites, increased prolactin secretion, and enhanced release of striatal acetylcholine. Following prolonged administration, there is a modest increase in receptor number, which is associated with the development of D_2-receptor supersensitivity. Benzamide neuroleptics, such as sulpiride and remoxipride, act selectively on dopamine D_2-receptors. Despite lack of action on D_1-receptors, remoxipride is reported to be an effective antipsychotic at daily doses around 400 mg, inducing relatively few extrapyramidal symptoms (EPS).[11]

These findings have generated the view that inhibition of the dopaminergic neurotransmission by blockade of D_2-receptors is the only requirement for effective treatment of schizophrenia-like psychoses. Pharmacology could then be reduced to screening for selective, high affinity binding to a membrane preparation of these receptors. Brain biology, however, offers many other opportunities for optimalization of antipsychotic drugs. It has frequently been suggested that the antipsychotic effect of D_2-receptor antagonists is due to occupation of the receptors in mesolimbic and cortical areas and the EPS-liability to occupation off striatal D_2-receptors. "Mesolimbic" selectivity is hence predicted to limit side-effects. The concept has been tested in animals, and soon after administration many antipsychotics have a tendency to greater occupation of the "mesolimbic" than the striatal receptors. In patients, however, common therapeutic doses of antipsychotic drugs from all chemical classes induce 65–85 percent occupancy of the putamen D_2-receptors.[12] Another topic is the cooperativity between D_1- and D_2-receptors and their precise cellular localization and function. D_1-dopamine receptors are also widely expressed in the brain in regions virtually devoid of D_2-receptors, and may have roles different from the postsynaptic modulation of motor functions.[13]

Molecular biology studies have now described additional clones for dopaminergic receptors,[r8,8,14] which include the major D_1- and D_2-receptors, splice variants of the D_2-receptors, and the newly cloned D_3-, D_4-, and D_5-receptors. The D_3- and D_4-receptors have great homology with the D_2, whereas the D_5-receptor has homology with the D_1-receptor. Pharmacologically, the D_1/D_2 classification persists until the consequences of specific interaction with the new receptor subtypes have been elaborated more completely.

There is, therefore, exciting research going on to affect central dopaminergic neurotransmission by means other than dopamine D_2-receptor occupation. For completeness, two additional historical approaches are briefly mentioned, because they once were believed to yield appropriate solutions to decreased dopaminergic overactivity. The biosynthesis of dopamine by inhibition of the key enzyme tyrosine hydroxylase was an early target. Analogues of tyrosine, like α-methyltyrosine, possess the required activity, but nonspecific inhibition of the synthesis of all catecholamines precludes therapeutic use. The mechanism of action of reserpine is also based on reduction of the neuronal dopamine content. Again the depletion is not very selective, and peripheral norepinephrine stores are affected to a large extent. Hypotension but also depression frequently accompany the use of reserpine.

The chemical diversity of the presently known antipsychotics, and especially compounds classified as "miscellaneous," give further impetus to the study of more appropriate drugs for treating schizophrenia. After all, psychosis and in particular schizophrenia, is not likely a disease caused by a single, well-defined mechanism. Therefore, optimal treatment may require the use of medications having distinct and differing mechanisms.

Serotonergic Function

As will be noted later in this chapter, many antipsychotic drugs also affect the function of the serotonin system. Pathways for serotonin-containing neurons are presented in Figure 16.2. The diffuse distribution of serotonergic neurons suggest a widespread influence

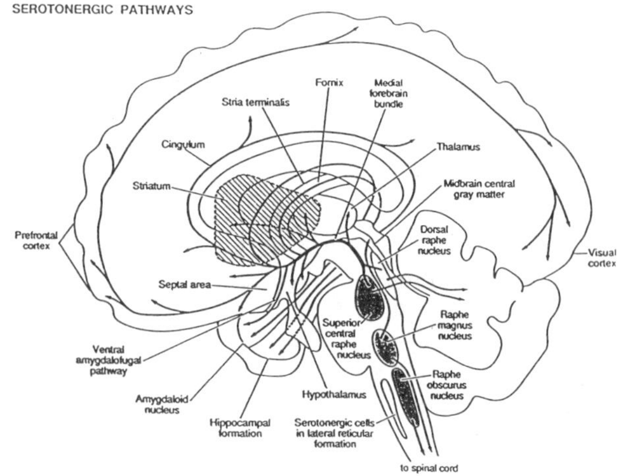

Figure 16.2 Main Serotonergic Pathways in the Human Brain

on many regions of the CNS. The synaptic connections to many serotonergic receptors seem to lack the specialization relevant to other types of synaptic transmission. Pharmacologically, it is now known that there are many serotonergic receptor subtypes. These are discussed in the introductory chapter to the section on drugs affecting the CNS. As will be noted, antipsychotic drugs affect primarily serotonin-S_2 receptors. These receptors are found in many brain regions.[r9] In order to have some view of the physiologic consequences of blocking these receptors, selective serotonin S_2-antagonism has been studied intensively with ritanserin, a potent antagonist. Doses of ritanserin around 10 mg increase the time spent in slow wave sleep, and reduce symptoms of depression and anxiety. In comedication with neuroleptics, the negative symptoms of schizophrenia show greater improvement, and some Parkinson-like motor disturbances and the EPS induced by antipsychotic drugs decrease.[r10] Therefore, new antipsychotics like risperidone and ocaperidone have been selected as clinically effective drugs on the basis of very potent S_2-antagonism associated with potent or equivalent D_2-antagonism. With clozapine, the serotonin S_2-antagonism is also more prominent than the D_2-antagonism.[r11,r12] Other activities of clozapine appear in Table 16.1. Known actions of clozapine occur in a narrow range of doses or concentrations affecting a variety of receptors including α_1, D_1, D_2, D_3, D_4, H_1, 5-HT_{1c}, 5-HT_2-(S_2)-receptors as well as muscarinic receptors. Therefore, no other antipsychotic deserves as much the label of "nonspecific" as clozapine. The high incidence of many side-effects other than EPS has long prompted the search for a new less toxic clozapine-like drug, but, because of a multitude of receptor interactions with unknown consequences, the properties of clozapine appear to be a confusing starting point for this goal.

Meanwhile, there is an area in which receptor binding, pharmacologic activity, and clinical experience are in close agreement, which is the fact that drugs of this class act on D_2-receptors. However, despite common dopamine D_2-antagonism, the available neuroleptics differ markedly in relation to interference with other neurotransmitters, including serotonin, norepinephrine, histamine, and acetylcholine. The resulting pharmacologic profiles to be described make up an important experimental basis to guide the clinical use of individual antipsychotics.[r12] Before going to these latter data, the varied chemistry of drugs making up the groups classified as neuroleptics or antipsychotics is discussed.

Chemistry

Medicinal research has made available approximately 100 neuroleptics for which at least some clinical data are available. They belong to more than ten different chemical classes and are discussed here on the basis of structure (Figures 16.3–16.6) and pharmacologic activity in the apomorphine test in rats, which measures central dopamine antagonism.[r12]

Class 1, *the reserpine-like compounds* (Fig. 16.3), contains all aryl-annulated quinolizine derivatives. It includes reserpine, which is in fact not a dopamine antagonist (Table 16.1) but a monoamine depleting agent, and butaclamol, which is used mainly as a tool in receptor binding studies.

Class 2, the largest group of compounds, are *phenothiazines*, which are subdivided into promazines, perazines, phenazines, and piperidinophenothiazines (Fig. 16.4, A-D) according to the chemistry of the side-chain. Chlorpromazine, known as a rather sedating antihistamine when its clinical exploration began, is a moderately potent apomorphine antagonist (ED_{50} = 0.26 mg/kg). The potency of the phenothiazines is highly dependent on substitution in carbon 2 of the phenothiazine nucleus: –H < –Cl < –CF3. Triflupromazine (Fig. 16.4, A), trifluperazine (Fig. 16.4, B), and fluphenazine (Fig. 16.4, C) are about equipotent (ED_{50}s of 0.074, 0.037, and 0.056 mg/kg, respectively); therefore, the different side-chains do not produce major shifts in pharmacologic activity. The prototype of the piperidino-phenothiazines, thioridazine (Figure 16.4, D), is a weak apomorphine antagonist (ED_{50} = 4.10 mg/kg), in comparison with other members of the same class. Duoperone is a combination of two interesting pharmacophores for neuroleptics, but activity against apomorphine remains low.

Class 3 drugs include the thioxanthenes (Figure 16.5, 3), which resemble phenothiazines both chemically and pharmacologically (chlorprothixene vs. chlorpromazine; flupenthixol vs. fluphenazine). The introduction of an extra fluoro substitution in pifluthixol results in very high activity as an antagonist of apomorphine (ED_{50} = 0.0071 mg/kg).

Class 4 drugs include the butyrophenones, a completely different chemical series of neuroleptics, of which haloperidol is the prototype (ED_{50} = 0.019 mg/kg; Fig. 16.5, 4). Generally, the butyrophenones are potent neuroleptics.[4] An interesting exception is pipamperone, which is a weak apomorphine antagonist (ED_{50} = 3.1), but more potent as a serotonin antagonist. Serotonin antagonism is also a component of the action of spiperone, which is widely used to label dopamine D_2-as well as serotonin S_2-receptors.

Class 5 compounds include the diphenylbutylamines (Fig. 16.5, 5), with pimozide as the archetype; these drugs are potent apomorphine antagonists. All act longer than the corresponding butyrophe-

1. Reserpine related structures

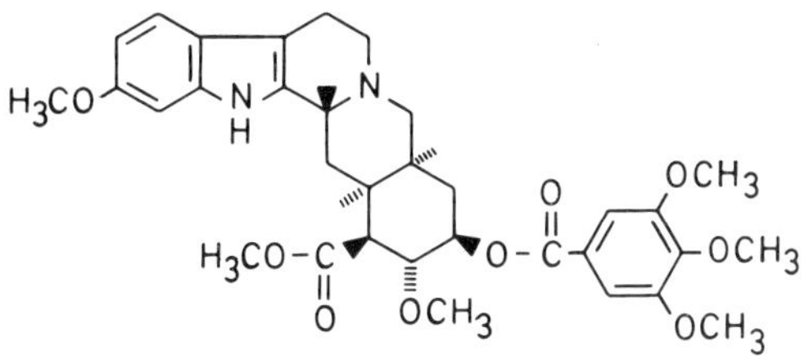

Reserpine (>20)[1]

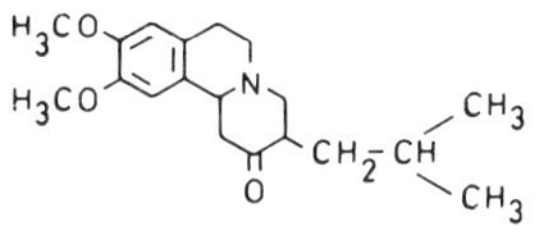

Tetrabenazine (5.4)

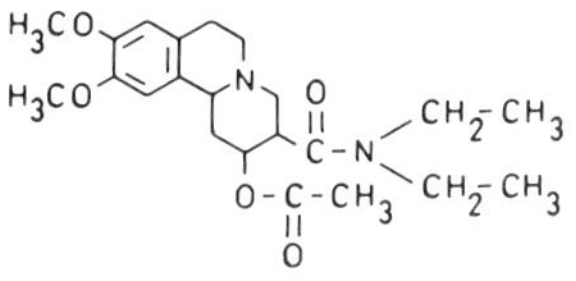

Benzquinamide (3.1)

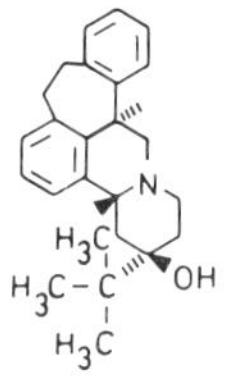

Butaclamol (0.098)

Figure 16.3 Chemical Structures of Antipsychotics. 1. Reserpine-related Compounds.

nones. The highly lipophilic character of these compounds favors a more gradual occupation of the dopamine receptors.

Class 6 compounds (Fig. 16.6, 6) include various tricyclic derivatives with a central 7-membered ring to which methylpiperazine is linked. The activity of this group is widely scattered, containing among the weakest (clozapine, 6.20 mg/kg) and the most potent (clorotepine, 0.043 mg/kg) of the apomorphine antagonists.

Class 7 compounds include the aminoalkylbenzamides, open-chain alkylamines of the metoclopramide type, pyrrolidines of the sulpiride type, and piperidines of the clebopride type (Figure 16.6, 7). Potencies as apomorphine antagonists vary widely within this class. Sulpiride (ED_{50} = 21.4 mg/kg) is considerably less potent than the recent benzamide, remoxipride (ED_{50} = 0.17 mg/kg) and than metoclopramide (ED_{50} = 0.76 mg/kg), which is used mainly for GI applications.

The aminoethylindoles of Class 8 (Fig. 16.6, 8) are markedly less potent than the phenoxyalkylamines of Class 9 (Fig. 16.6, 9)

Finally Group 10 drugs (Fig. 16.6, 10) includes miscellaneous structures, of which risperidone offers the best perspectives for an antipsychotic of a new type.[15]

The Pharmacologic Basis of Neuroleptic Effects

The activity of neuroleptics in relation to therapeutic usefulness, side-effects, and toxic effects will be discussed mainly on the basis of in vivo pharmacologic data obtained in a series of tests that have been described repeatedly.[r12,16] Nevertheless, there are many other tests that have provided relevant pharmacologic information on neuroleptics (e.g., procedures based on turning behavior, increased prolactin secretion, 5-hydroxytryptophan-induced head twitches, in vivo neurotransmitter release and its metabolism, to name some). For the present survey, data are provided from procedures in which hundreds of compounds have been studied in the same way. The precise meaning of the activity in each of these pharmacologic tests has generally been confirmed by independent measurements, in different biologic systems. Therefore, the information obtained in these tests provides a concise summary of the general pharmacology of these drugs.

Pharmacologic Profiles Obtained in Rats

As noted above, a series of tests are performed in rats to obtain the pharmacologic profile of an antipsychotic. These include the apomorphine test, the tryptamine test, the norepinephrine test, the antihistaminic test, the anticholinergic test, and general assessment of motor function. In the apomorphine test,[r12] the IV dose of 1.25 mg/kg of apomorphine to rats induces intense agitation (mainly continuous upper body movements) and stereotyped gnawing, licking, and sniffing. Maximal intensity (score 3 on a scale from 0 to 3) of this abnormal behavior lasts about 40 min (when scoring behavior every 5 min, score 3 is present 7 to 9 times). In animals pretreated with neuroleptics there is a dose-dependent decrease of high-intensity scores. ED_{50}-values reflect a significant decrease of the frequency of these behaviors in half of the test animals. ED_{50}-values for apomorphine antagonism by antipsychotic drugs correlate well with in vitro dopamine D_2-receptor binding. However, affinity for D_2-receptors is not essential, since the experimental D_1-antagonist SCH 23390 is also a potent apomorphine antagonist. For the antipsychotics discussed in this chapter, it is assumed that apomorphine antagonism results primarily from in vivo D_2-receptor occupation, with the possible exception of some thioxanthene neuroleptics. Furthermore, blockade of central α_1-,5-HT_2- or H_1-receptors in itself does not affect apomorphine behavior. Blockade of muscarinic cholinergic recep-

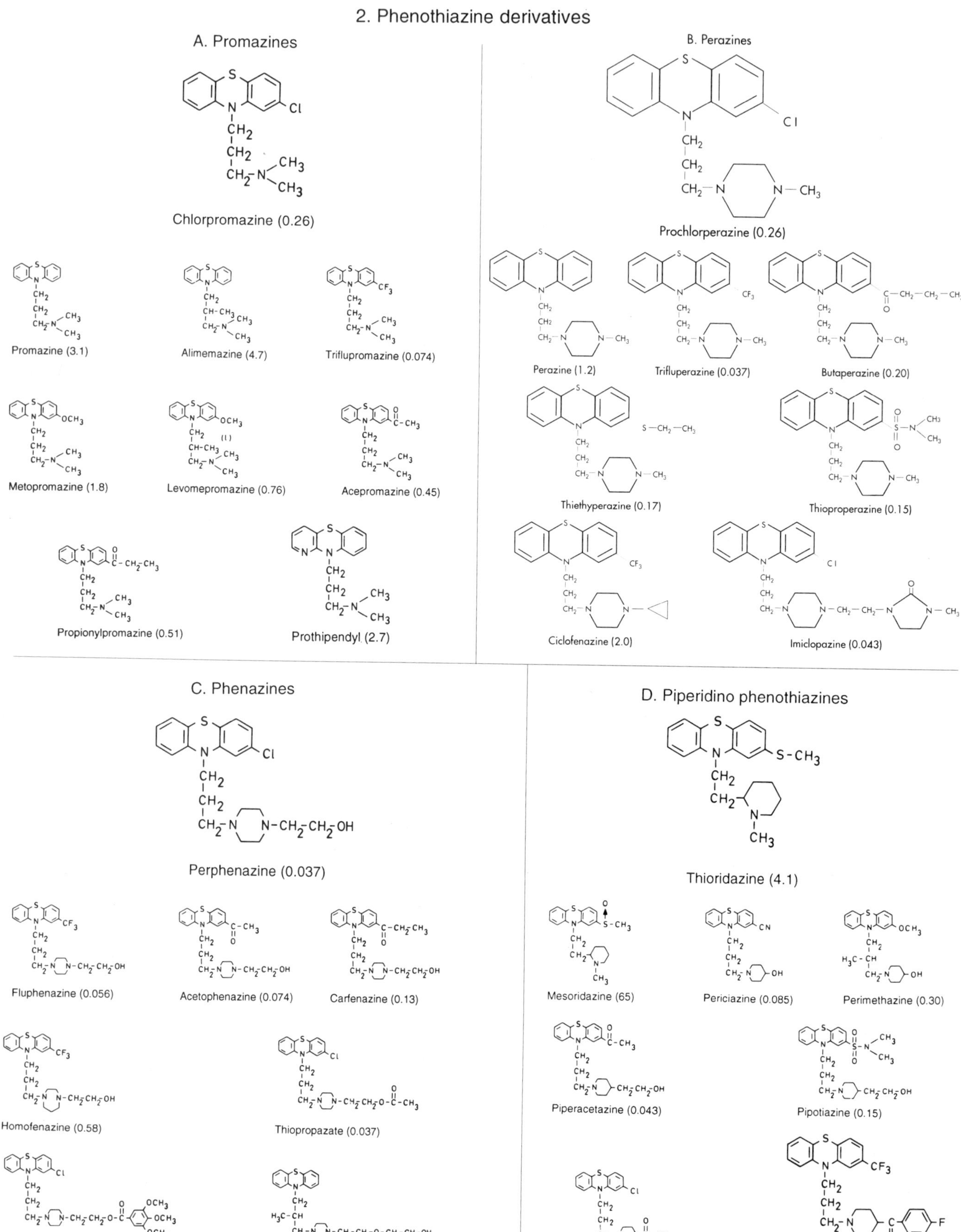

Figure 16.4 Chemical Structures of Antipsychotics. 2. Phenothiazine Derivatives: *A*. Promazines, *B*. Perazines, *C*. Phenazines, *D*. Piperidines

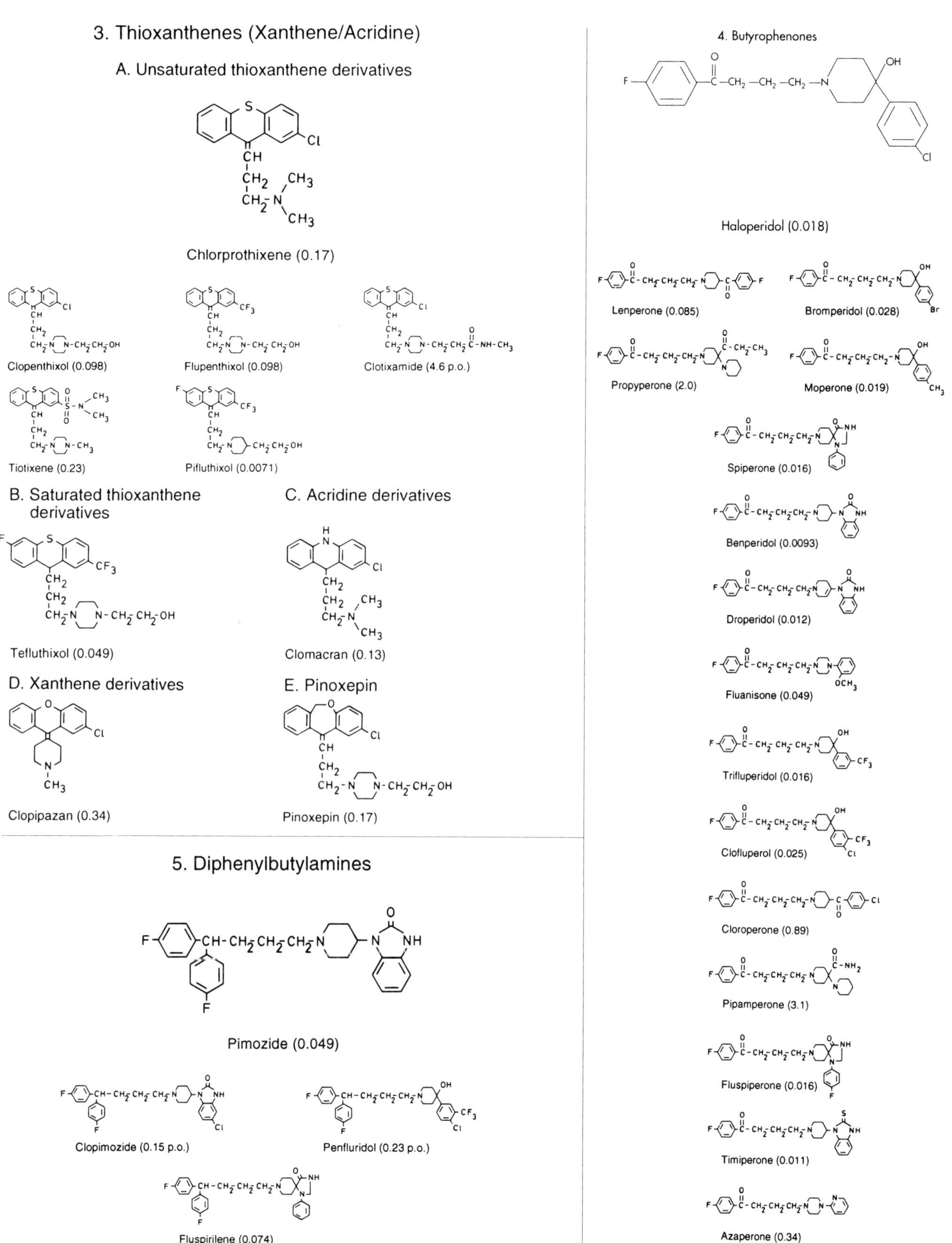

Figure 16.5 Chemical Structures of Antipsychotics. 3. Thioxanthenes and Related Compounds. 4. Butyrophenones. 5. Diphenylbutylamines

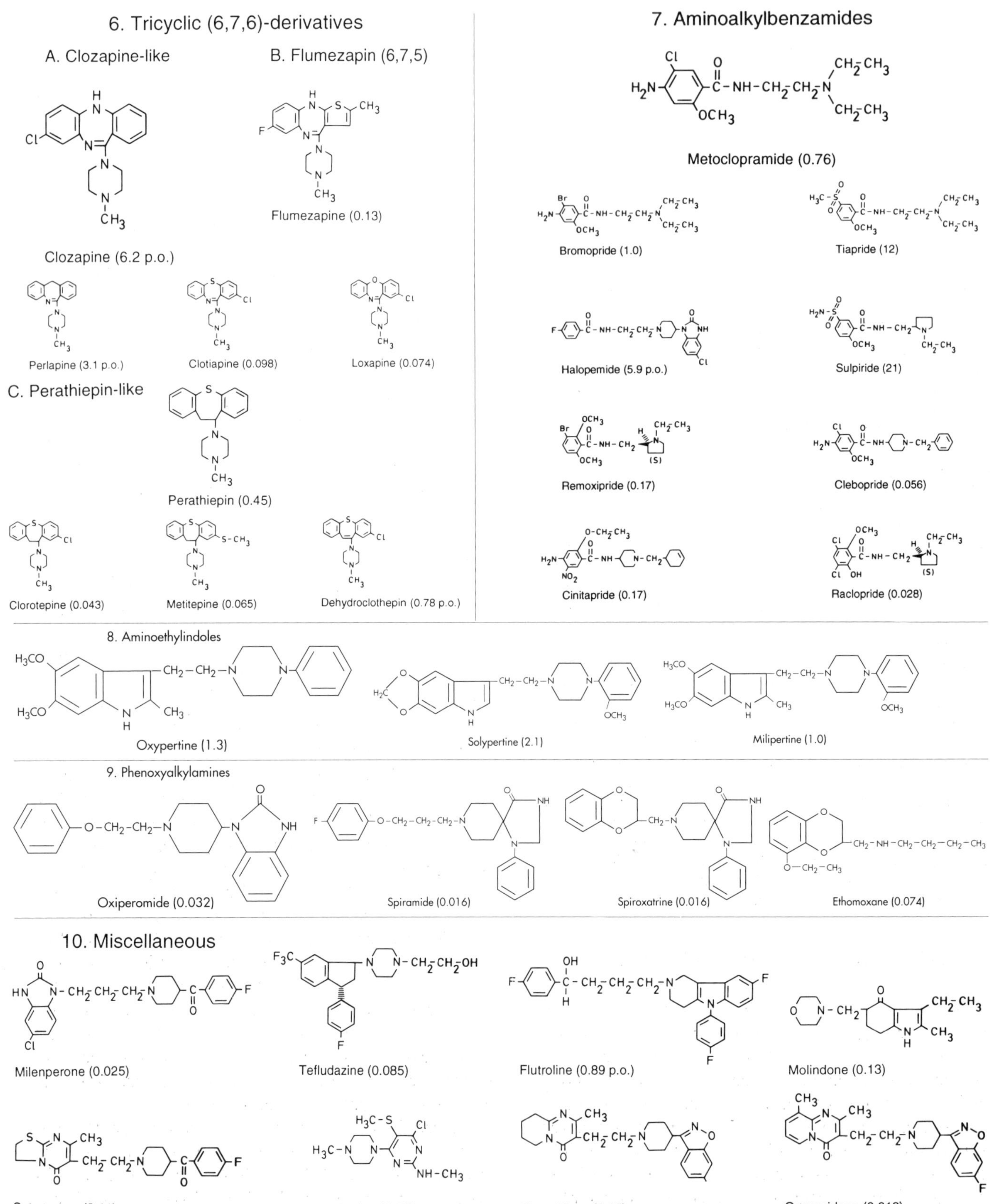

Figure 16.6 Chemical Structures of Antipsychotics. 6. Tricyclic (6,7,6)-derivatives. 7. Aminoalkylbenzamides. 8. Aminoethylindoles. 9. Phenoxyalkylamines. 10. Miscellaneous Structures.

tors, which potentiates apomorphine behavior, can be supplanted completely by concomitant D_2-blockade.

In the tryptamine test, the IV dose of 40 mg/kg of trypamine induces bilateral seizures of the forepaws and causes body tremors of high intensity during 1–2 min. This behavior has been shown to result from central serotonergic overstimulation and reaches the intensity score of 3 in virtually all untreated rats. Tryptamine antagonism is reflected in the dose-dependent occurrence of scores lower than 3, which primarily reflect a reduction of the forepaw seizures. ED_{50}-values obtained in this test correlate well with binding to 5-HT_2-receptors. Central serotonin 5-HT_2 antagonism varies widely in antipsychotics, but, when sufficiently potent, has recently been found to be important for the improvement of negative symptoms and a lower EPS-liability.[17]

In the norepinephrine test, the IV dose of 1.25 mg/kg of norepinephrine induces lethal hypertension. Survival for more than 15 min reflects peripheral α_1-adrenergic blockade of the test compounds. ED_{50} values correlate with α_1-receptor affinity and with clinical effects such as orthostatic hypotension and reflex tachycardia, a greater tendency for sedation, and reduction of psychomotor agitation early in the treatment.

In the compound 48/80 lethality test, 0.5 mg/kg of compound 48/80 IV releases histamine and serotonin and induces anaphylactic shock within about 30 min. Protection from the lethal shock, (i.e., survival at 4 hr), is obtained with all histamine H_1-antagonists, which block vascular H_1-receptors and prevent the hypovolemia caused by the released histamine. In rats, serotonin is released from mast cells by compound 48/80, along with histamine, and also contributes to the shock syndrome. It is likely, therefore, that potent 5-HT_2 antagonists, such as risperidone, are active in this test by blocking 5-HT_2- rather than H_1-receptors. This histamine H_1-antagonism of neuroleptics reflects their ability to cause sedation.

In the physostigmine test, pupil diameter is measured just before the IV injection of 1.0 mg/kg of physostigmine. Both mydriasis (pupil diameters exceeding 0.8 mm) and protection from physostigmine death (survival at 2 hr) are observed with drugs that have anticholinergic activity and cross the blood-brain barrier. Relatively high doses of various sedating agents may protect from the central cholinergic excess produced by physostigmine, without inducing mydriasis. Compounds with anticholinergic activity at central muscarinic receptors show fewer parkinson-like side-effects and clinically are associated with blurred vision and dry mucosa.

Catalepsy and palpebral ptosis are evaluated hourly over 8 hr after drug administration, mainly to confirm the neuroleptic (catalepsy, central dopamine D_2-antagonism) and associated actions (palpebral ptosis, favored by α_1-adrenergic blockade) of the drug.

Conclusions From the Pharmacologic Tests

Apomorphine antagonism is believed to reflect dopamine D_2-antagonism. Similarly, inhibition of tryptamine effects (serotonin-S_2), norepinephrine mortality (α_1-adrenoceptor blockade), compound 48/80 lethal shock (histamine-H_1), and physostigmine lethality (central muscarinic blockade) reflect interference of the antipsychotic drug with other specific neurotransmitters. For all these tests, there is a highly significant correlation between the active doses of neuroleptics and the binding affinity to the corresponding receptors in vitro measured with radioligands ($n = 20 - 30$ neuroleptics; rank correlation coefficients > 0.7; $p < 0.01$).[r3] Two tests, induction of catalepsy and palpebral ptosis, measure direct behavioral effects of the compounds.

Table 16.1 summarizes the data obtained with 19 representative antipsychotics in order of decreasing potency as apomorphine antagonists. All ED_{50} values refer to inhibition of apomorphine-induced agitation, since ED_{50}s based on sniffing and licking are not significantly different.[r12] There is about a thousandfold difference between the most potent of the list, spiperone, and the weakest, sulpiride. The order of activity on apomorphine-induced agitation is generally in agreement with in vitro affinity for dopamine D_2-receptors (column 1) and with clinical potency. The result of a single SQ administration, however, is dictated not only by differences in receptor affinity, but by many other factors, such as the rate of crossing biologic barriers. As an example, sulpiride is a very weak apomorphine antagonist in rats because of poor brain penetration, but a potent antiemetic in dogs (ED_{50} about 0.1 mg/kg for this peripheral activity). The results of several other tests in rats are in close agreement with apomorphine antagonism: antagonism of amphetamine-induced agitation, cocaine antagonism,[16] inhibition of intracranial self-stimulation and other conditioned reactions, and the induction of catalepsy. All these tests appear to reflect central dopamine D_2-antagonism (or a combination of D_2 - D_1-antagonism). For induction of catalepsy, the active doses are about four to 30 times higher than the ED_{50}-values for apomorphine antagonism, but there is no difference between potent and weak neuroleptics with respect to the ability to induce catalepsy in rats.

Major differences between the antipsychotic compounds arise in tests related to other neurotransmitters (Table 16.1). Tryptamine antagonism (serotonin S_2) is the dominant basic activity of risperidone, and is also more pronounced than dopamine antagonism for pipamperone and clozapine. Tryptamine and apomorphine antagonism are equivalent for levomepromazine. Tryptamine antagonism is relatively less marked ($^{++++}$) for spiperone, flupenthixol, chlorprothixene, chlorpromazine, and thioridazine. It is still weaker ($^{+++}$) for perphenazine and fluphenazine. Finally, haloperidol, bromperidol, trifluoperazine, and sulpiride are very weak ($^{++}$), and raclopride and remoxipride are extremely weak ($^{+}$) tryptamine antagonists. Pimozide is devoid of tryptamine antagonism.

Norepinephrine (NE) antagonism of the 16 compounds compared is most pronounced with thioridazine, and is a significant activity component of eight other neuroleptics of the list. Histamine (H_1) antagonism, measured as protection from compound 48/80-lethality, is the dominant basic activity of levomepromazine. It is pronounced with clozapine and

Table 16.1 Pharmacologic Activity Profiles of 19 Representative Neuroleptics in Rats

	APO ant. ED50 mg/kg D_2	D_2 rec. Affinity K_i, nM	Relative potency of indicated activities			
			TRY ant. S_2	NE ant. α_1	48/80 ant. H_1	PHY ant. AcCh
Spiperone	0.016	0.16	++++	0	0	0
Ocaperidone	0.018	0.75	+++++	+++	+	0
Haloperidol	0.019	1.6	++	0	0	0
Bromperidol	0.028	—	++	0	0	0
Raclopride	0.028	—	+	0	0	0
Perphenazine	0.037	3.0	+++	+	+++	0
Trifluoperazine	0.037	3.9	++	0	0	0
Pimozide	0.049	1.2	0	0	+	0
Fluphenazine	0.056	6.2	+++	++	++	0
Flupenthixol	0.098	—	++++	+++	+++	0
Risperidone	0.15	3.0	+++++++	+++++	++++	0
Chlorprotixene	0.17	11	++++	++++	+++	+
Remoxipride	0.17	(240)	+	0	0	0
Chlorpromazine	0.26	18	++++	++++	++++	+
Levomepromazine	0.76	—	+++++	++++	+++++++	++
Pipamperone	3.1	124	++++++	++++	+++++	0
Thioridazine	4.1	16	++++	++++++	+++++	+++
Clozapine	6.2	156	++++++	++++	++++++	+++++
Sulpiride	21	31	++	0	++++	0

D_2-receptor affinity: all values using ^{3}H-haloperidol as ligand[r3] except one for remoxipride (^{3}H-raclopride).
Abbreviations: APO, apomorphine; ant., antagonism; TRY, tryptamine; NE, norepinephrine; 48/80, compound 48/80; PHY, physostigmine.
All symbols derive from calculated ratios (ED_{50} in indicated test/ED_{50} in the apomorphine test). When both ED_{50}s are equivalent, i.e., ratio between 0.50 and 2.00, the symbol +++++ is used. Activity in other tests can be greater (++++++) or markedly greater (+++++++). Activity in the other tests can be lower: slightly (++++ up to 6 times), moderately (+++ up to 18 times), markedly (++ up to 54 times), very markedly (+ up to 150 times) or not measurable (0:>150).

equivalent to dopamine antagonism for pipamperone and thioridazine. For six other neuroleptics of the list, histamine antagonism is moderate to potent. Few neuroleptics protect rats from physostigmine (PHY)-induced lethality, which measures central antimuscarinic activity. In this regard, the most potent is clozapine, followed by thioridazine, levomepromazine, chlorprothixene, and chlorpromazine.

Although there is a pronounced tendency for the more potent neuroleptics to be the most specific dopamine antagonists, the data of Table 16.1 indicate that each compound has its individual pharmacologic activity profile. Between pimozide, which is virtually devoid of non-dopamine-related activities, and clozapine, which represents the profile of a completely nonspecific neuroleptic, virtually all combinations of activity can be found among the known neuroleptics.[12] Differences in pharmacologic profile have clinical relevance with respect to the potential effects and side-effects of the administered neuroleptic. Central dopamine D_2-antagonism, as measured in the apomorphine test, is considered to be the basis of the marked effect of neuroleptics on the positive symptoms of schizophrenia (delusions, hallucinations, thought disorder). At the same time this central activity is also the basis for neurologic side-effects, particularly the EPS.

The importance of central serotonin S_2-antagonism, as measured in the tryptamine test, for neuroleptics with this action has been much clarified by the development of ritanserin, a potent and selective serotonin S_2-antagonist.[r10,11,18] Up to high doses, the administration of ritanserin does not induce characteristic behavioral changes. In contrast, anxiety-like behavior such as reduced exploration of a novel environment, is disinhibited. In animals, as well as in humans, the time spent in slow wave sleep is markedly increased, and it is possible that the clinical thymosthenic properties of ritanserin in neurotic depressed and anxious patients (i.e., decreased fatigue, improved mood, relief of anxiety) are linked to the improved quality of sleep produced by this drug. In schizophrenic patients, ritanserin was studied as an additional therapy to their established neuroleptic medication. With this combination therapy, the clinical global impression improved mainly by a reduction of negative symptoms and a decrease of the extrapyramidal symptoms.[19] From the clinical experience gained with ritanserin, central serotonin S_2-antagonism, if sufficiently expressed, appears to bring about two corrections to the therapeutic spectrum of classic dopamine antagonism: a major improvement of negative symptoms (i.e., related to social withdrawal, anxiety, depression, anergy); and therapeutic effectiveness in the virtual absence of EPS.[r10] The recently selected benzisoxazole derivative, risperidone, appears to possess the required pharmacologic profile[16] to reach these therapeutic objectives. The value of serotonin S_2-antagonism is sustained by receptor classification studies of antipsychotics[20] and by functional interaction studies between the dopaminergic and serotonergic neurotransmission.[21–23]

Norepinephrine antagonism has been shown to correlate with α_1-adrenoceptor binding. Although it has been proposed that this interaction with the neurotransmitter norepinephrine may contribute to the therapeutic effects of antipsychotic drugs, it is generally accepted that it is the basis of autonomic side-effects of this drug class. The risk for (orthostatic) hypotension and tachycardia is directly linked to blockade of cardiovascular α_1-adrenoceptors. Sedation may also be favored by neuroleptics with high affinity to α_1-adrenoceptors. In a clinical trial, psychotic symptoms were not affected by treatment with the potent, specific antagonist prazosin.[24] Histamine H_1-antagonism is another activity component favoring sedation. Neuroleptics by definition act centrally, and a potent association with histamine H_1-antagonism will cause the common somnolence of classic antihistamines. The side-effects associated with histamine and norepinephrine antagonism tend to disappear with chronic administration of neuroleptics.

Finally, central antimuscarinic activity can be an important component of the pharmacologic profile of a neuroleptic. It is often presented as a therapeutic advantage by providing an automatic protection against the EPS of dopaminergic over-blockade. Centrally-acting anticholinergics, however, also can induce, at "therapeutic" doses, confusion, memory impairment, and psychotic reactions. As a rule, therefore, the antipsychotic effects of neuroleptics have to be pursued in the absence of an anticholinergic drug, because neuroleptic overdose may go unobserved in the presence of anticholinergic medication (i.e., mask the EPS). As discussed further later in this chapter, the appearance of EPS marks the patients' tolerance to dopaminergic inhibition. Therefore, many patients would be exposed to unnecessarily high doses of antipsychotics when this signal for excess dosing is deliberately obscured by anticholinergic medication.

Although neuroleptics are generally considered to be relatively nontoxic, safety margins evaluated on the basis of activity and acute toxicity in rats increase with increasing potency.[r12] Compounds that are active in the apomorphine test in rats at doses between 0.01 and 0.1 mg/kg may be nonlethal up to 20,000 times the effective dose, whereas this factor may be as low as 30 with neuroleptics active at doses of $\geq$ 1.0 mg/kg. Clinically, therefore, when high doses of a neuroleptic are required, the choice of a potent neuroleptic is evident.

Pharmacologic Data Obtained in Dogs and Relation to Pharmacokinetics

In dogs, the pharmacologic activities of neuroleptics include antagonism of apomorphine-induced emesis and inhibition of learned behavior in the shuttle box as a prototype of conditioned reactions.[r12] As part of the selection process of useful drugs, especially antiemetics and neuroleptics, these specific tests greatly facilitate their quantitative evaluation. Apomorphine antagonism in dogs measures the pronounced emetic response to the SQ dose of 0.31 mg/kg of apomorphine. Dose-dependent protection from emesis is obtained with all dopamine D_2-antagonists. The ED_{50} at peak effectiveness can be markedly lower than the ED_{50} for apomorphine antagonism in rats (a typical example is domperidone) or be of the same order (a typical example is haloperidol). This difference in potency is more related to brain penetration than to species differences. This test has particular advantages for time-activity relationships and functional oral bioavailability.

The clinical correlate of apomorphine antagonism in dogs is the antiemetic and antinauseant activity of the antipsychotics. In the shuttle box test in dogs, the central activity of antipsychotics is measured on the basis of failure to perform learned behavior. The activity of antipsychotics in this test is slightly to markedly lower than activity in the apomorphine antagonism test. This latter test also correlates well with inhibition of D_2-receptor binding exhibited by neuroleptics.

In Table 16.2, results obtained with eight antipsychotics in the dog tests are combined with estimated parameters from human pharmacokinetic studies. Risperidone and fluphenazine are equipotent antiemetics, followed by four other potent compounds. Chlorpromazine and thioridazine are markedly less active in this test. Following oral administration, thioridazine, risperidone, pimozide, and haloperidol are nearly as active as by SQ injection, and the same four compounds are active from 12 to 20 hr. Haloperidol and chlorpromazine, when compared to the remaining compounds, inhibit learned behavior in the shuttle box test at doses closer to their antiemetic dose. For other compounds, the results in dogs are suggestive of their use as an antiemetic at low doses with little risk of EPS, and their use as antipsychotics in the higher dose range. With the peripherally acting dopamine D_2-antagonist domperidone, the risk of EPS is virtually nil.

Apomorphine emesis in dogs has been of great value to detect the very long acting drugs, fluspirilene and penfluridol, which protect from emesis as long as seven days, and in the evaluation of esterified depot preparations, some of which may act up to one month. In the human data, the estimated oral bioavailability is lowest for the compounds with low oral activity in dogs. There is moderate agreement between duration of action in dogs and terminal elimination half life in the human studies, probably because their action at the receptor level is, in general, poorly related to elimination rate. The distribution volume is highest for the most lipophilic compound,

Table 16.2 Antagonism of Apomorphine Emesis in Dogs. Estimation of Antiemetic Dose, Oral Activity, and Duration of Action, in Relation to Human Pharmacokinetics.

	Apomorphine Emesis in Dogs			
Compound	**Lowest ED_{50} mg/kg sq**	**Relative Oral Activity %**	**Approximate Duration of Action, hr**	**Relative Central Activity (Shuttle Box, sq)**
Risperidone	0.0057	80	20	++
Fluphenazine	0.0060	8	12	+
Pimozide	0.011	70	20	++
Haloperidol	0.015	60	12	+++
Perphenazine	0.015	5	8	++
Flupenthixol	0.020	3	8	++
Chlorpromazine	0.54	10	8	+++
Thioridazine	2.0	≥100	20	++
	Human Pharmacokinetics[1]			
Compound	**Estimated Oral Bioavailability %**	**Elimination Half-life $t_{1/2\beta}$h**	**Distribution Volume l/kg**	**Active Metabolites**
Risperidone	≥80	24	1.5	+
Fluphenazine	≤10	16	—	+
Pimozide	90	50	30	0
Haloperidol	60	20	18	0
Perphenazine	15	9	20	+
Flupenthixol	55	26	14	+
Chlorpromazine	30	30	21	++
Thioridazine	80	30	4	+

[1]r21 and various other sources.

pimozide, and lowest for risperidone. For chlorpromazine, the contribution of active metabolites to over-all clinical effect is marked, whereas this contribution is absent for pimozide and haloperidol.

The Clinical Study of Antipsychotics

From the vast body of clinical studies in schizophrenia accumulated since 1952, a general consensus arises: *antipsychotics are effective drugs*. In double-blind studies lasting four to eight weeks, 50 to 80 percent of the treated patients showed marked improvement, i.e., about three times more than the percentage of patients improving with placebo. In the maintenance therapy of schizophrenia, the relapse rate of patients treated with antipsychotics is several times lower than that of placebo-treated patients.[r13] Efficacy in mania or in acute psychotic reactions is at least as great as in schizophrenia. In several other indications (e.g., delusional disorders, borderline psychoses, neurologic conditions), the clinical study is less comprehensive, often limited to particular neuroleptics or cases, but also positive in terms of the remarkable improvement of the related patients. Over-all, antipsychotics are among the most effective drugs used in psychiatry and reach the level of efficacy common for accepted medications in other fields of medicine.

Furthermore, the available drugs, with their prominent dopamine antagonism and inherent neurologic effects, appear to act in a way that is appropriate for psychosis. Unlike purely sedating drugs, all of which may reduce psychomotor agitation, they decrease the intensity of virtually *all* psychotic symptoms, although not necessarily to the same extent and with the same time course.[r14] Negative symptoms, related to withdrawal and flat affect, ultimately may persist to a much more striking degree than delusions, hallucinations, and thought disorder. There is a dose-related incidence of extrapyramidal side-effects. At fixed, high doses of potent antipsychotics, the incidence and intensity of EPS are frequently judged to be excessively high. In other studies, however, the same drugs are used at individually adapted doses below the neuroleptic threshold and yet produce the expected antipsychotic effect. For most patients adequate clinical improvement does not appear to depend on doses with disturbing side-effects. Some of the more potent antipsychotics can be used IM for rapid neuroleptization.[r15] The advantages of rapid control of psychosis must be weighed against the fact that in many patients thought disorder and other symptoms may require weeks of treatment to be resolved.

There are relatively few double-blind comparative clinical trials that show a significant difference in global improvement between different antipsychotics. It is, therefore, generally assumed that all available antipsychotics have a level of effectiveness similar to that of the archetype, chlorpromazine. This assumption is reflected in the concept of "chlorpromazine-equivalence": all drugs are considered essentially equal on the condition of using equipotent doses. Treatment of schizophrenia with common clinical doses of different neuroleptics, in fact, produces a similar level of striatal D_2-receptor occupation of about 75 percent in patients. In daily practice, an antipsychotic is rarely selected at random, because the known differences in pharmacologic spectrum and in pharmacokinetics lead to differential prescriptions according to the severity of the condition, the characteristics of the patient, his or her sensitivity to various potential side-effects, and the requirements of rapid and complete recovery with the lowest possible dose.

The Clinical Concept of Antipsychotic Action

The preceding portion of this chapter summarized the conclusions drawn from controlled clinical trials with antipsychotics set up to define the level of therapeutic benefit that can be reached. In daily psychiatric practice, the results of the use of antipsychotics should be superior. All limitations inherent to a study protocol can be avoided. In daily practice, a treatment trial with a moderate dose of a familiar drug should be the rule. Nevertheless, the most appropriate antipsychotic can be selected for the needs of an individual patient, and dosage can be chosen based on previous history, physical condition, age, and clinical evolution. Additional measures, including psychotherapy, family education, and social steps, may consolidate the results of pharmacotherapy. The most disturbing side-effects can be avoided by using the most appropriate drugs and dosages.

As noted earlier, antipsychotic drugs are D_2-receptor antagonists and inhibit dopaminergic neurotransmission in direct relation to the dose. The relationships of the dopaminergic system to mental disease is likely complex, in view of the marked heterogeneity of schizophrenia and of the large number of other psychoses that respond to antipsychotics. Nevertheless, there is a good agreement between the concept of dopaminergic equilibrium and therapeutic effectiveness. In psychotic exacerbations, in mania, and acute schizophrenia, relatively high doses of antipsychotics are indicated. In disorders with minimal involvement of psychosis, treatment is started with a low dose that may be increased slowly according to tolerance and therapeutic response. The clinical observation that patients with mania and schizophrenia tolerate much higher doses of antipsychotics than normal volunteers reflects the hyperactive dopaminergic condition and justifies neuroleptic treatment as long as the dose does not induce an hypodopaminergic state, which can be recognized by the appearance of parkinsonism. However, there are other markers for excessive doses, such as subjective dysphoric reactions.[25] When these signs appear, the logical step is a timely reduction of the dose. It has been repeatedly shown, also recently,[26] that most patients with schizophrenia attain a good clinical response with doses of antipsychotic drugs not inducing distinct EPS. The neuroleptic threshold for EPS can be artificially raised by concomitant treatment with an anticholinergic. However, this second therapeutic agent has its own side-effect profile and in fact conceals the effects of a neuroleptic overdose. Overdose may lead to other toxic effects, such as tardive dyskinesia, especially when combined with a drug that masks the neurologic signs of the antipsychotic.

Practical Use of Antipsychotics

When, on the basis of clinical evidence and history, the decision is taken to treat a patient with an antipsychotic, practical details of the administration have to be considered. Experience has shown that the therapeutic needs of patients vary greatly.[r16] Guidelines for practical use may still appear confusing because of the wide range of applications, the large chemical and pharmacologic differences between the available antipsychotics, and the wide therapeutic dose ranges. In the different applications of antipsychotic drugs, certain patterns of current use can be recognized. Potent neuroleptics (haloperidol equivalents from 1 to about 10 in Table 16.4) are used about twice as often as the less potent neuroleptics in treating schizophrenia and mania. In major depression with psychotic features, personality disorder, or substance abuse, the potent neuroleptics are used much less frequently.[r17] Indications for antipsychotics are briefly reviewed in Table 16.3.

Selection of a Drug

Pharmacologic and pharmacokinetic considerations favor the specific, potent antipsychotics with

Table 16.3 Use of Antipsychotics in Medicine

—History and diagnosis of the patient should establish the presence of symptoms known to be responsive to pharmacotherapy.

—Antipsychotics reduce symptom intensity. In complex disease, such as schizophrenia, a wide range of symptoms is usually seen to improve, but in individual patients the extent of improvement can vary among various symptoms.

—Optimal therapy (drug, dosage, route, frequency of administration) varies with the individual patient and his evolution, more than in any other therapeutic field.

1. Schizophrenia
   —Acute episodes (relapses are usually treated with oral or IM preparations (choice of IM preparations is limited to potent, specific neuroleptics); symptom improvement includes excitement, assaultiveness (calming effect); negativity, uncooperation (change in mood); thought disorder, hallucinations, delusions (core symptoms of schizophrenia).
   —Maintenance therapy is preferably carried out with long-acting IM depot preparations, at initial dosage corresponding to the prior dose which stabilized the patient; almost always the dosage can be further reduced by at least 50% in periodic adaptations every 3–6 months.
2. Paranoia
   —Refers to paranoid, but also schizoid and schizotypal personality disorder. Suspiciousness, distrust, easy anger, many associated features may respond to low doses of antipsychotics.
3. Mania
   —Recurring episodes of the disturbed affective state respond more rapidly to antipsychotics than to lithium.
4. Schizophreniform psychosis and other acute psychotic syndromes
   —Acutely psychotic patients (with symptoms as agitation, destructiveness, hostility, assaultive behavior, pressurized speech, incoherency, delusions, hallucinations) are given low dose IM injection —(e.g., haloperidol 0.5–2.0 mg) in first instance to allow a more complete examination and define the psychosis (schizophreniform? due to drugs, amphetamine, LSD? linked to alcohol? chronic brain syndrome?). Subsequent short-term neuroleptic medication is frequently sufficient to allow other appropriate therapeutic steps.
5. Borderline psychosis
   —Less rigorously diagnosed psychiatric disorders (with fluctuating symptoms of anger, anxiety, anhedonia, self-destructive behavior, inconsistent social relations, etc.) frequently respond to low-dose treatment.
6. Agitation in the elderly
   —In the elderly patient symptoms of restlessness, assaultiveness, violence, aggression may require medication. The effectiveness of neuroleptics is well documented and is seldom matched by other pharmacotherapy. Low doses are used because of the greater sensitivity of the elderly for cardiovascular side-effects related to α_1-adrenergic blockade and to EPS related to D_2-receptor blockade.
7. Infantile autism
   —Low doses, particularly of haloperidol (0.5–4 mg daily) are known to decrease stereotypes, hyperactivity and negativism, and to facilite learning. After prolonged neuroleptic treatment, abnormal involuntary movements may occur; these disappear spontaneously but slowly (≥2 weeks) when treatment is stopped.
8. Combination therapies
   —In several conditions neuroleptics are used as an adjunct to drugs, which are primarily indicated. In depression with some positive psychotic features (delusions, aggressiveness, irritability) short-term addition of a neuroleptic to the antidepressant; in severe chronic pain, especially cancer pain, addition to an analgesic; in a manic episode addition to lithium are examples of current combination therapies. Appropriate doses of neuroleptics do not aggravate the side-effect liability of the primary therapy.
9. Emesis
   —Dopamine-mediated stimulation of the chemoemetic trigger zone and gastric motor reflexes is inhibited by neuroleptics. Several phenothiazines, the butyrophenones droperidol and haloperidol, and the benzamide metoclopramide are widely used as antiemetics. The peripherally acting dopamine antagonist domperidone is an antiemetic devoid of the side-effects of neuroleptics, except for prolactin release. All can be used in the management of nausea and vomiting in cancer chemotherapy, although there is no completely effective single agent for all circumstances at doses that are relatively free of side-effects.
10. Neurolepantalgesia
   —The origin and development of the phenothiazine neuroleptics owes much to studies in the operating theatre, particularly as potentiators of analgesia. A combination fentanyl-droperidol, either in a fixed proportion or administered separately at a selected time and dose, is a well-known preparation for neuroleptanalgesia.
11. Neurologic conditions
   —Symptoms of various neurologic conditions often rapidly respond to some neuroleptics: Gilles de la Tourette's syndrome (haloperidol, pimozide; up to high doses); Huntington's chorea; chorea in general (the movement disorder responds to various neuroleptics at moderate doses); movements in hemiballismus, torticollis, persistent hiccups.
12. General medical uses
   —For suddenly occurring episodes of brain disorder with agitation and other symptoms, e.g., in hospitalized patients low doses of neuroleptics should be considered.

Table 16.4 Available Preparations of Antipsychotic Drugs and Usual Doses[1]

Antipsychotic (Common Trade Name)	HAL eq.[2]	INJ Forms[3]	Typical Oral Daily Doses[4], mg Start/ Target	Common Range	Extreme Range
Haloperidol (Haldol)	1	P/D	5	1–20	0.25–100
Fluphenazine (Prolixin)	1	P/D	5	2.5–10	0.5–30
Pimozide (Orap)	1	—	4	1–10	—
Bromperidol (Impromen)	1	D	6	2–12	—
Risperidone (Risperdal)	1	—	(6)	(2–10)	1–16
Droperidol (Inapsine)	2	P	(5 inj)	5–20	—
Tiotixene (Navane)	3	P	15	2–30	—
Trifluoperazine (Stelazine)	3	P	15	4–40	—
Perphenazine (Trilafon)	6	P/D	24	4–64	—
Thiopropazate (Dartal)	6	—	30	15–100	—
Molindone (Moban)	8	—	75	20–225	15–400
Loxapine (Loxitane)	10	P	20/80	15–250	—
Periciazine (Neulactil)	12	P	30	10–300	—
Prochlorperazine (Compazine)	12	P	50	20–150	—
Acetophenazine (Tindal)	15	—	100	40–400	—
Triflupromazine (Vesprin)	(25)	P	(40 inj)	(20–80 inj)	—
Chlorprotixene (Taractan)	40	P	200	50–600	—
Remoxipride (Roxiam)	40	—	200	80–600	—
Mesoridazine (Serentil)	50	P	150/300	30–400	—
Clozapine (Clozaril)	60	—	50/300	100–600	100–900
Thioridazine (Mellaril)	80	—	150/400	20–700	—
Chlorpromazine (Thorazine)	100	P	50/500	25–800	25–2,400
Promazine (Sparine)	150	P	50/500	25–1,000	—
Sulpiride (Dogmatil)	150	P	600	200–2,400	—

[1]Main sources: Physicians Desk Reference, 1990; Martindale, The Extra Pharmacopoeia, 29th Ed., 1989; recent clinical comparative trials.
[2]Approximate oral dose, equivalent to 1 mg haloperidol.
[3]Antipsychotics available for injection (generally IM only) as the Parent drug (P) or as a Depot preparation (D, commonly as the decanoate ester in sesame oil, see Table 16.5).
[4]Individual optimal doses vary greatly (see text). For many antipsychotics the target dose (a typical dose for an adult with moderate psychosis) can be administered from the beginning of treatment (usually divided over 2 to 4 daily administrations); for others it is recommended to reach the target dose slowly, by gradual increases, in order to reduce acute side-effects; very low or very high extreme doses occasionally have been found to be useful.

good oral bioavailability. Clinically, spectrum and intensity of symptoms, desirability of initial sedation, differences in potential side-effects, in- or out-patient conditions, and other factors may vary sufficiently to consider several options from haloperidol-like to thioridazine-like antipsychotics.[r18] In several clinical indications, the selection of particular drugs is imperative. For intense acute psychotic reactions, injectable preparations of potent antipsychotics with minimal cardiovascular or other autonomic effects are available. The same compounds are preferable for other short-term or high-dose applications. If sedation is required, benzodiazepines are the most reliable agents. If high-dose treatment of schizophrenia during the first four to six weeks is therapeutically ineffective or not tolerated, switching to a different antipsychotic for a second, third, . . . treatment period may lead to improvement. Patients not responding to several antipsychotics may still benefit from clozapine treatment. The possibility of antipsychotic activity with clozapine in the virtual absence of EPS has long been used to some extent in Europe. Following clinical studies in nonresponders to classic neuroleptics,[27] clozapine is available in the US for refractory patients, subjected to a weekly control of the WBC count to detect early signs of potentially fatal agranulocytosis. Although acute schizophrenic patients give a global rating of their neuroleptic treatment that is predominantly positive,[28] in the event of open rejection a change in neuroleptic may reduce the risk of noncompliance.

For borderline psychosis, elderly patients, and general medical indications, low doses of potent antipsychotics are considered the most adequate and safe. In monodelusional disorders and in the predominantly negative schizophrenic syndrome, pimozide has distinct effectiveness. The injectable diphenylbutylpiperidine, fluspirilene, in low-dose therapy has marked activity in minor tranquilizer indications. In "tic" disturbances (including Gilles de la Tourette disease and Huntington's chorea), haloperidol, pimozide, fluphenazine, and penfluridol are effective drugs.

Selection of a Dose

The following scale (0.25–400 mg) gives the approximate useful daily dose range of haloperidol in various conditions. The scale suggests that, for a patient with acute mania or schizophrenia presenting with moderately intense symptoms, a dose of 5 to 10 mg of haloperidol may be a good initial dose.

Common dose range in elderly patients and nonpsychotic disorders — Dose requirement for rapid control of florid symptoms

—0.25mg ——— 2 ——— 5 ——— 10 ——— 40... 100... 400 mg

Common maintenance antipsychotic dose range — Acutely nontoxic doses tested in emergencies

Similar scales can be drawn for other antipsychotics and clinical experience is summarized in Table 16.4. The antipsychotics are listed in approximate order of oral dose requirement for maintenance therapy of schizophrenia. The conversion of a 1-mg dose of haloperidol to the mg-equivalent of another antipsychotic should be applied with caution, since there is no proof of linear pharmacokinetics of the drugs over the full common dose range, and the marked differences in pharmacologic profiles do not sustain equivalent clinical effects. Target doses are most representative for the average oral dose required to maintain optimal symptom reduction in chronic schizophrenia. They do not apply to antiemetic or other general medical uses of antipsychotics.

Readjustment of the Dose

It is not uncommon that patients starting on a 10 mg dose will be adjusted within two weeks to doses ranging from 1 to 30 mg daily. Despite all efforts to use parameters, such as plasma levels of the antipsychotic or of increased prolactin, there is no substitute for careful clinical observation (symptom intensity and side-effects) in the decision to decrease or increase dose. Patients with mania, when showing improvement, are immediate candidates for dose reduction, in anticipation of the risk of dopaminergic blockade. Thus, short-term treatment is the rule in these patients. Patients with schizophrenia are generally treated with larger doses, usually for six weeks to three months, until a maximal level of improvement is reached. Usually this level can be maintained by rather gradual dose reduction to 20–50 percent of the highest dose, in order to establish the lowest effective dose. When there is no exacerbation of symptoms, long-term prevention of relapses is the next objective.

Maintenance Treatment

In schizophrenia, the use of the long-acting ester preparations of antipsychotics has several advantages. Moderate doses of the preparations providing the lowest initial plasma level after IM injection and the most stable levels over the next weeks are preferable [Table 16.5].[r19] There is no consensus at the present time how long such treatment has to be continued. In well-stabilized patients after several years of treatment, it is reasonable to check the requirement for antipsychotics by at least a further reduction in dose. Maintenance therapy in patients with manic-depressive illness is more controversial, although frequently applied in rapid cycling disease and when manic relapses occur despite adequate lithium levels.

Adverse Effects: Occurrence, Prevention, Management

After nearly 40 years of clinical use of antipsychotics, the emphasis is even more on the prevention of side-effects. For example, moderate, individually adapted doses limit the incidence of disturbing EPS. Early recognition of treatment failures and avoidance of coadministration of anticholinergics with antipsychotics eliminate in large part many other difficulties associated with antipsychotic treatment. In Table 16.6, side-effects of antipsychotics are described in three groups. The first group includes the *extrapyramidal side-effects* (EPS), which are typical for antipsychotics. The second group of side-effects involves non-EPS side-effects related to common activity components of the known antipsychotics. The third group includes general side-effects. The symptoms associated with EPS are dose-dependent and are observed with all antipsychotics at common clinical doses, but with variable incidence and severity. The lowest incidence, about 4 percent, is observed with clozapine, and it increases up to several times with the more specific, potent antipsychotics. Two known factors have a major impact on the incidence of EPS. One is related to the pharmacologic profile. Antimuscarinic and antiserotonin activity decrease the relative risk of EPS. The other is related to practical use. Dose increment is usually slower, and the upper limit is lower, with the less specific and weak antipsychotics, leading to more gradual and less extreme D_2-receptor occupation. More conservative use of potent antipsychotics in sensitive subjects can prevent part of the EPS observed in clinical studies at fixed doses.

Expectations from Antipsychotic Treatment

Treatment of schizophrenia-related, florid psychosis is a major application of antipsychotics. Diagnosis rests on a multiplicity of symptoms, mainly reflecting cognitive dysfunction and on their persistence in time.[r20] Current antipsychotic treatment of patients with schizophrenia is started and continued for four to six weeks with vigorous dosing (e.g., 5–20 mg halo-

Table 16.5 Characteristics of Some Depot Antipsychotics

Preparation Dose	Common Dose Range (mg)	Intervals (Weeks)	Plasma Level (ng/ml)	Half-life (Days)	Ratio First IM Dose/ Last Oral
Fluphenazine decanoate in sesame oil	12.5–100	1–4	0.5–3.0	8	1.6
Flupenthixol decanoate in viscoleo	10–50	2–4	0.5–2.0	15	5
Haloperidol decanoate in sesame oil	25–400	4	3.0–10	20	15
Perphenazine enanthate in sesame oil	50–200	1–4	2.0–10	4	2
Bromperidol decanoate in sesame oil	25–400	4	1.0–8.0	25	15
Fluspirilene in aqueous suspension	1–15	1–2	0.5–4.0	8	—

Fluphenazine esters were the first preparations available for IM use. Solutions of the decanoate in sesame oil are injected at intervals of 1 to 4 weeks to provide a usual dose between 12.5 and 100 mg. The conversion from oral to IM therapy is based on an empirical factor of 1.6 for one week's duration of action, which indicates that the bioavailability of IM fluphenazine is considerably larger than that of oral fluphenazine.
Monthly injections providing the most stable plasma levels are the common use for haloperidol and bromperidol decanoate, which are esters of tertiary alcohols and hence the most slowly hydrolyzing.
The relationship between plasma level and dose is rather good for IM depot preparations; for doses of haloperidol decanoate between 20 and 400 mg the correlation coefficient reached 0.86.

peridol equivalents), that is adapted to clinical response if clearly insufficient or not tolerated. However, higher dosages for many patients give no additional benefit.[29] Apparent effectiveness (greater calmness, less assaultiveness . . .) is first seen as a reduction of psychomotor agitation, which is a preliminary step to a change in other "core" symptoms.

True antipsychotic effects are obtained in the course of weeks of treatment, in which signs of hallucinations, delusions, and thought disorder may regress. Insight by the patients into their condition is the critical goal and requires other therapeutic steps, such as psychotherapy and social rehabilitation. Frequently, the effect of appropriate doses of antipsychotics on negative and positive symptoms is sufficiently large to avoid long-term hospitalization. When the expected remission does not start within six weeks and there are no disturbing side-effects, higher doses can be used for a limited time, even though the proportion of responders decreases with increasing doses. Maintenance treatment at a dose lower than the acutely effective dose will markedly reduce relapse rate. Every relapse further complicates the outcome of the patient.

Pharmacokinetics and Metabolism

As can be expected from the chemical heterogeneity of neuroleptics, the metabolic and pharmacokinetic behavior of these compounds is not uniform. Some neuroleptics appear to be better candidates for therapeutic monitoring than others. The ability to monitor pharmacokinetic parameters of a given neuroleptic has in part a technical basis. High pressure liquid chromatography generally provides the best separation of parent drug, isomers, and metabolites; however, this approach may not always provide needed sensitivity. Radioimmunoassays are usually very sensitive, but specificity of the assay depends on the antiserum batch. For example, chemically related molecules, such as haloperidol and reduced haloperidol, may be measured together in one case and separately in another. The gas chromatographic/mass spectrometer approach is specific and sensitive, but the costs are high for such an instrument, and specially trained professionals are required for the assays and for maintaining the equipment. For practical drug monitoring, the radio-receptor assay may have advantages, because it measures in the plasma sample the total binding activity of the drug and active metabolites to dopamine D_2-receptors. Some data from human pharmacokinetic studies of the antipsychotic drugs are presented in Table 16.2

The potential of plasma concentrations for therapeutic monitoring is illustrated in two recent studies. In a study with perphenazine, 228 patients were treated for at least five weeks.[30] Plasma levels were then determined to give three groups of patients: one within the therapeutic range of 2 to 3 nM (established on the basis of previous

Table 16.6 Side-Effects of Antipsychotics

1. Extrapyramidal side-effects	
Parkinsonism	Parkinson-like symptoms include general slowness of movement down to akinesia; rigidity; unsteadiness; tremor. The intensity and time of occurrence (days to several weeks) are dose-related. Reduction of the dose and anticholinergics reverse the symptoms.
Dystonia	Irregular spasms of facial, neck, and trunk muscle and sustained abnormal postures. They can occur early in the treatment and respond to anticholinergics.
Akathisia	Is experienced by the patient as an irresistible urge to move within minutes from any sitting, lying, or standing position. The purposeless motor activity can be misdiagnosed as related to psychotic agitation, but discrimination is possible. Akathisia is subjectively very distressing and responds satisfactorily to dose reduction and possibly to anticholinergics and propranolol.
Tardive dyskinesia	Oro-facio-lingual daytime movements, which may be associated with larger movements of trunk and extremities. They can be induced by long-term (months–years) treatment with antipsychotics, but identical dyskinesia is a feature of chronic psychosis by itself. Dose adjustment to the real needs of the patient is a general measure to prevent or slowly reverse the iatrogenic part of dyskinesia.
Neuroleptic malignant syndrome	Hyperthermia associated with other symptoms such as rigidity, tachycardia, hypertension, stupor, and leukocytosis. The syndrome is rare, unpredictable, and only superficially resembles malignant hyperthermia in surgery. Antipsychotic treatment should be stopped and maximal supportive care instituted. Other measures have not been shown to hasten recovery or prevent the often fatal outcome.
2. Profile-linked side-effects	
α_1-blockade	First-dose effects of antipsychotics with prominent α_1-adrenergic blocking activity include tachycardia, hypotension (as a result of vasodilation), dizziness, nausea, and fainting. Tolerance to these effects usually allows gradual dose increase.
H_1-blockade	Somnolence, sedation.
Muscarinic blockade	Dry mouth, blurred vision, urinary retention, bowel obstruction, and possibly central effects (positive symptoms of psychosis, memory impairment).
D_2-blockade	Increased prolactin secretion, as a result of blockade of peripheral pituitary D_2-receptors, is observed with low doses of antipsychotics. Prolonged hyperprolactinemia favors breast enlargement and galactorrhea. The relation between prolactin response and diagnostic systems used to define schizophrenia remains complex.
Related to D_1, D_3, D_4, 5-HT_{1B}, 5-HT_{1C}, 5-HT_3, α_2, σ-sites, etc	Most of these receptor interactions have not yet been studied sufficiently at the clinical level to define the related side-effects.
3. General side-effects	
Allergic reactions	Hypersensitivity develops more frequently with phenothiazines than with most other chemical classes of antipsychotics. Retinitis pigmentosa can occur with excessive doses of thioridazine.
Agranulocytosis	Decrease in circulating white blood cells has been reported for many antipsychotics. Stringent, weekly control to avoid lethal infection is required for clozapine only.
General toxicity Sialorrhea convulsions	Liver dysfunction and other general disturbances of body function are primarily a function of total daily dose. Absolute doses exceeding 1000 mg daily rapidly increase the risk of general toxicity symptoms. Clozapine is prone to signs of this type.
Teratogenicity	There is no substantial evidence of teratogenicity from human surveys, but cautious use (such as avoiding prescription for antiemetic effects) during pregnancy is recommended because very high doses in animals induce malformations.
Interactions	A well-known, valuable interaction is potentiation of analgesia in anesthesia generally without increasing recovery time. The suspected toxic interaction between neuroleptics and lithium is toxicity of the components, frequently that of a (too) high lithium dose.

experience); one above; and one below this range. The group within the "therapeutic range" achieved the best clinical response (86%) with the lowest level of EPS (9%). For the patients of the group with good clinical response but associated with EPS, a dose reduction ultimately resulted for 24 out of 41 patients in the three objectives: therapeutic plasma range; good clinical response; no EPS. In the last group, 17 of the 38 patients eligible for dose increase achieved the same goals.

In the second study, 33 schizophrenic patients were treated with haloperidol and rapidly adjusted to a point at which slight hypokinesia–rigidity (neuroleptic threshold) first appeared on clinical examination.[26] The mean daily dose at that point was 4.2 ± 2.4 mg. Plasma levels ranged from 1 to 12 ng/ml, with a mean of 4.9 ± 2.9. At least moderate therapeutic improvement was reached in 67 percent of the patients within three weeks of treatment at neuroleptic threshold doses. The correlation, however, between plasma levels and oral dose was rather low (r = 0.37).

In accordance with a wide range of therapeutically adapted individual doses, it is not to be expected that narrow therapeutic plasma level ranges have to be respected for optimal antipsychotic treatment. Individual variability, phase of treatment, age differences, and perhaps other conditions will challenge the concept. A recent double-blind study in 176 acutely exacerbated patients confirms this. Only minor differences in clinical responses were noted among three plasma levels of haloperidol: low (≤ 13 ng/ml); medium or high (> 24 ng/ml).[31] However, in an individual patient, regular determination of plasma levels may be important in clinical evaluation and the follow-up of compliance.

Summary

In 40 years, more than 100 antipsychotic agents have been prepared and studied, mainly in comparison to the first phenothiazine, chlorpromazine (1952) and the first butyrophenone, haloperidol (1958). The single common action of the antipsychotics is a central dopamine D_2-antagonism. In rats, this is expressed as inhibition of behavior elicited by dopaminergic stimuli, such as amphetamine and apomorphine. In human PET scan studies, striatal D_2-receptor occupation of up to 85 percent is found at therapeutic doses in schizophrenia. Major differences between the compounds reside in potency, relative ease to cross barriers such as the blood-brain barrier, duration of action, and profile of activities associated with dopamine antagonism. Potent and specific dopamine D_2-antagonists are preferred in the most typical applications of mania, schizophrenia, and paranoia. The target dose for optimal control of psychosis is generally reached readily in the absence of side-effects, except EPS. Severe EPS, resulting from excessive D_2-receptor blockade, call for dose reduction. New antipsychotics with reduced risk of EPS are studied partly on the basis of the pharmacologic profile of clozapine, partly on the basis of advances in the functional organization of the dopaminergic system. At the present time, prominent central serotonin S_2-antagonism, associated with D_2-antagonism, as is found in risperidone, appears to provide the broadest antipsychotic effectiveness with low EPS risks.

References

Research Reports

1. D'Amato T, Rochet T, Dalery J, Laurent A, Chauchat J-H, Terra J-L, Marie-Cardine M. Relationship between symptoms rated with the positive and negative syndrome scale and brain measures in schizophrenia. Psychiatr Res 1992;*44*:55–62.
2. Delay J, Deniker P, Harl JM. Utilisation en thérapeutique psychiatrique d'une phénothiazine d'action centrale élective (4560 RP). Ann Med Psychol 1952;*110*:112–116.
3. Delay J, Deniker P. Méthodes chimiothérapeutiques en psychiatrie. Paris: Masson, 1961.
4. Janssen PAJ, Niemegeers CJE, Schellekens KHL. Is it possible to predict the clinical effects of neuroleptic drugs (major tranquillizers) from animal data? Part I: "Neuroleptic activity spectra" for rats. Arzneimittelforschung 1965;*15*:104–117.
5. Ernst AM. Mode of action of apomorphine and dexamphetamine in gnawing compulsion in the rat. Psychopharmacologia 1967;*10*:316–323.
6. Carlsson A, Lindqvist M. Effect of chlorpromazine or haloperidol on formation of 3-methoxytyramine and normetanephrine in mouse brain. Acta Pharmacol Toxicol 1963;*20*:140–144.
7. Skirboll LR, Grace AA, Bunney BS. Dopamine auto- and postsynaptic receptors: electrophysiological evidence for differential sensitivity to dopamine agonists. Science 1979;*206*:80–82.
8. Sibley DR, Monsma FJ. Molecular biology of dopamine receptors. TIPS 1992;*13*:61–69.
9. Burt DR, Enna SJ, Creese I, Snyder SH. Dopamine receptor binding in the corpus striatum of mammalian brain. Proc Natl Acad Sci (USA) 1975;*72*:4655–4659.
10. Seeman P, Chau-Wong M, Tedesco J, Wong K. Brain receptors for antipsychotic drugs and dopamine: direct binding assays. Proc Natl Acad Sci (USA) 1975;*72*:4376–4380.
11. Lewander T, Westerbergh S-E, Morrison D. Clinical profile of remoxipride—a combined analysis of a comparative double-blind multicentre trial programme. Acta Psychiatr Scand 1990;*82* (Suppl. 358):92–98.
12. Farde L, Wiesel FA, Halldin C, Sedvall G. Central D_2-dopamine receptor occupancy in schizophrenic patients treated with antipsychotic drugs. Arch Gen Psychiatr 1988;*45*:71–76.
13. Fremeau RT, Duncan GE, Fornaretto MG, Dearry A, Gingrich JA, Breese GR, Caron MG. Localization of D_1 dopamine receptor mRNA in brain supports a role in cognitive, affective and neuroendocrine aspects of dopaminergic neurotransmission. Proc Natl Acad Sci USA 1991;*88*:3772–3776.
14. Niznik HB, Van Tol HHM. Dopamine receptor genes: new tools for molecular psychiatry. J Psychiatr Neurosci 1992;*17*:158–180.
15. Chouinard G, Jones B, Remington G, Bloom D, Addington D, Mac Ewan GW, Labelle A, Beauclair L, Arnott W. A Canadian multicenter placebo-controlled study of fixed doses of risperidone and haloperidol in the treatment of chronic schizophrenic patients. J Clin Psychopharmacol 1993;*13*:25–40.
16. Janssen PAJ, Niemegeers CJE, Awouters F, Schellekens KHL, Megens AAHP, Meert TP. Pharmacology of risperidone (R 64

766), a new antipsychotic with serotonin-S_2 and dopamine-D_2 antagonistic properties. J Pharmacol Exp Ther 1988;*244*:685–693.

17. Janssen PAJ. The development of new antipsychotic drugs: towards a new strategy in the management of chronic psychosis. J Drug Ther Res 1987;*12*:324–328.
18. Bersani G, Pozzi F, Marini S, Grispini A, Pasini A, Ciani N. 5-HT_2-receptor antagonism in dysthymic disorder: a double-blind placebo-controlled study with ritanserin. Acta Psychiatr Scand 1991;*83*:244–248.
19. Gelders Y, Vanden Bussche G, Reyntjens A, Janssen P. Serotonin-S_2 receptor blockers in the treatment of chronic schizophrenia. Clin Neuropharmacol 1986;*9*:325–327.
20. Meltzer HY, Matsubara S, Lee J-C. Classification of typical and atypical antipsychotic drugs on the basis of dopamine D_1, D_2 and serotonin$_2$ pK_i values. J Pharmacol Exp Ther 1989;*251*:238–246.
21. Awouters F, Niemegeers CJE, Megens AAHP, Janssen PAJ. Functional interaction between serotonin-S_2 and dopamine-D_2 neurotransmission as revealed by selective antagonism of hyper-reactivity to tryptamine and apomorphine. J Pharmacol Exp Ther 1990;*254*:945–951.
22. Saller CF, Szupryna MJ, Salama AI. 5-HT_2 receptor blockade by ICI 169,369 and other 5-HT_2 antagonists modulates the effects of D-2 dopamine receptor blockade. J Pharmacol Exp Ther 1990;*253*:62–70.
23. Iqbal N, Asnis GM, Wetzler S, Kay SR, Van Praag HM. The role of serotonin in schizophrenia. New findings. Schizophr Res 1991;*5*:181–182.
24. Hommer DW, Zahn TP, Dickar D, Van Kammer DP. Prazosin, a specific alpha-1-noradrenergic receptor antagonist, has no effect on symptoms but increases autonomic arousal in schizophrenic patients. Psychiatr Res. 1984;*11*:193–204.
25. Van Putten T, May PRA. Subjective response as a prediction of outcome in pharmacotherapy. Arch Gen Psychiatr 1978;*35*:477–480.
26. McEvoy JP, Stiller RL, Farr R. Plasma haloperidol levels drawn at neuroleptic threshold doses: a pilot study. J Clin Psychopharmacol 1986;*6*:133–138.
27. Kane J, Honigfeld G, Singer J, Meltzer H. Clozapine for the treatment-resistant schizophrenic: a double-blind comparison versus chlorpromazine/benztropine. Arch Gen Psychiatr 1988;*45*:789–796.
28. Windgassen K. Treatment with neuroleptics: the patient's perspective. Acta Psychiatr Scand 1992;*86*:405–410.
29. Rifkin A, Doddi S, Karajgi B, Borenstein M, Wachspress M. Dosage of haloperidol for schizophrenia. Arch Gen Psychiatr 1991;*48*:166–170.
30. Bolvig Hansen L, Larsen N-E. Therapeutic advantages of monitoring plasma concentrations of perphenazine in clinical practice. Psychopharmacology 1985;*87*:16–19.
31. Volavka J, Cooper T, Czobor P, Bitter I, Meisner M, Laska E, Gastanaga P, Krakowski M, Chou JC-Y, Crowner M, Dovyon R. Haloperidol blood levels and clinical effects. Arch Gen Psychiatr 1992;*49*:354–361.

Reviews and Textbook Chapters

r1. American Psychiatric Association. Diagnostic and statistical manual of mental disorders (4th ed). Washington DC: DSM-III-R 1987.

r2. World Health Organization. Mental disorders: glossary and guide to their classification in accordance with the ninth revision of the international classification of diseases. Geneva: WHO, 1978.

r3. Leysen JE, Niemegeers CJE. Neuroleptics. In: Handbook of neurochemistry, Vol. 9. New York: Plenum, 1985;331–361.

r4. Uhl GR, Hartig PR. Transporter explosion: update on uptake. TIPS 1992;*13*:421–425.

r5. Bannon MJ, Freeman AS, Chiodo LA, Bunney BS, Roth RH. The electrophysiological and biochemical pharmacology of the mesolimbic and mesocortical dopamine neurons. In: Iversen LL, Iversen SD, Snyder SH (Eds.) Handbook of psychopharmacology, Vol 19. New York: Plenum 1987;329–374.

r6. Seeman P. Brain dopamine receptors. Pharmacol Rev 1980;*32*:229–313.

r7. Waddington JL. Minireview. Therapeutic potential of selective D_1-dopamine receptor agonists and antagonists in psychiatry and neurology. Gen Pharmacol 1988;*19*:55–60.

r8. O'Dowd BF. Structures of dopamine receptors. J Neurochem 1993;*60*:804–816.

r9. Jacobs BL, Azmitia EC. Structure and function of the brain serotonin system. Physiol Rev 1992;*72*:165–229.

r10. Niemegeers CJE, Awouters F. Current status and perspectives of pharmacotherapeutic research related to schizophrenic psychoses. In: Schizophrenia and youth. Heidelberg: Springer-Verlag (1991):169–181.

r11. Meltzer HY. Clinical studies on the mechanism of action of clozapine: the dopamine-serotonin hypothesis of schizophrenia. Psychopharmacology 1989;*99*:S18–S27.

r12. Niemegeers CJE, Janssen PAJ. Minireview. A systematic study of the pharmacological activities of dopamine antagonists. Life Sci 1979;*24*:2201–2216.

r13. Davis JM, Andriukaitis S. The natural course of schizophrenia and effective maintenance drug treatment. J Clin Psychopharmacol 1986;6(Suppl.):2S–10.

r14. Cole JD. Phenothiazine treatment in acute schizophrenia. Arch Gen Psychiatr 1964;*10*:246–261.

r15. Ayd FJ. Guidelines for using intramuscular haloperidol for rapid neuroleptization. In: Haloperidol Update 1958–1980. Baltimore: Ayd Medical Communications, (1980); pp 53–65.

r16. Settle EC, Ayd FJ.: Haloperidol: a quarter century of experience. J Clin Psychiatr 1983;*44*:440–448.

r17. Baldessarini RJ, Katz B, Cotton P. Dissimilar dosing with high-potency and low-potency neuroleptics. Am J Psychiatr 1984;*141*:748–752.

r18. Martin RL. Practical therapeutics. Outpatient management of schizophrenia. Am Fam Physician 1991;*43*:921–933.

r19. Marder SR, Hubbard JW, Van Putten T, Midha KK. Review. Pharmacokinetics of long-acting injectable neuroleptic drugs: clinical implications. Psychopharmacology 1989;*98*:433–439.

r20. Andreasen NC. Schizophrenia: diagnosis and assessment. In: Psychopharmacology, the Third Generation of Progress. New York: Raven Press (1987); pp 1087–1094.

r21. Senon JL. Pharmacocinétique des neuroleptiques. Encéphale 1990;*16*:99–109.

CHAPTER 17

Drugs Used for the Treatment of Affective Disorders

Elaine Sanders-Bush
Fridolin Sulser

The affective disorders—bipolar and unipolar depression, mania, obsessive-compulsive, panic, and anxiety disorders—are human diseases exclusively. Therefore, it is not surprising that the prototypes of clinically effective drugs for the treatment of these disorders have been discovered in humans. Only after observations in the clinic were various animal models of depression introduced to screen for potential new therapeutic agents. Animal models of depression include pharmacologic (reserpine reversal; amphetamine potentiation); biochemical (blockade of amine uptake; receptor binding studies); and behavioral (learned helplessness, behavioral despair, olfactory bulbectomy; separation models) tests. Not surprisingly, these models have led to the proliferation of a large number of drugs with a similar pharmacologic profile, with none displaying more efficacy than the original prototypes. Indeed, this approach may have precluded the discovery of novel and more efficacious drugs for the treatment of affective disorders.

Currently available drugs for the treatment of depression include monoamine oxidase (MAO) inhibitors, the classic tricyclic antidepressants, selective and/or specific serotonin (5HT) uptake inhibitors, selective inhibitors of norepinephrine (NE) uptake, and a number of newer antidepressants collectively known as "second generation" or "atypical" antidepressants. Drugs for the treatment of mania include lithium salts and the anticonvulsant carbamazepine. Drugs to treat anxiety disorders are covered in Chapter 15. A discussion of the pharmacology of drugs used in affective disorders follows.

Monoamine Oxidase (MAO) Inhibitors

Monoamine oxidase (MAO) is a FAD-containing enzyme that catalyzes the oxidative deamination of monoamines thought to serve as neurotransmitters, including epinephrine, norepinephrine, dopamine, 5HT, and histamine. Localized in the outer membrane of mitochondria of nerve terminals, postsynaptic cells, and glia, MAO is involved in the metabolism and inactivation of synaptically released neurotransmitters and is responsible for the inactivation of intraneuronal unbound amines, formed by local synthesis or reuptake from the synaptic cleft. MAO produces an aldehyde intermediate product that is rapidly converted to an alcohol via the action of aldehyde reductase or to the corresponding carboxylic acid via aldehyde dehydrogenase (Fig. 17.1).The proportions of these products vary from tissue to tissue, depending on the relative presence of the reductase and dehydrogenase enzymes. The products are physiologically inactive; hence, MAO serves to limit the action of monoamine neurotransmitters. Other monoamines that may be formed endogenously (octopamine and tryptamine) or that may be obtained in the diet (tyramine) are also MAO substrates.

MAO exists in two isozyme forms, A and B, differentiated by their substrate specificity and inhibitor selectivity. For example, MAO-A preferentially oxidizes epinephrine, norepinephrine (NE), and 5HT and is selectively inhibited by clorgyline. MAO-B prefers phenylethylamine and benzylamine as substrates and is preferentially inhibited by deprenyl. Dopamine, tyra-

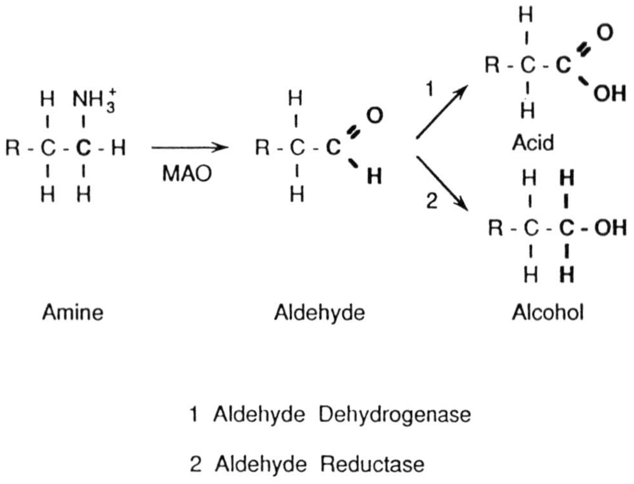

Amine → (MAO) → Aldehyde → (1) Acid; (2) Alcohol

1 Aldehyde Dehydrogenase

2 Aldehyde Reductase

Figure 17.1 General Scheme of Oxidative Deamination of Biogenic Amines

mine, and tryptamine are metabolized equally well by both forms. Recent cloning confirms that MAO A and B are close relatives, but coded by separate genes.[1] MAO activity is widely distributed in both neuronal and nonneuronal tissue, with most tissues, including brain and liver, containing both isozymes. The A form predominates in sympathetic neurons and intestine, while platelets contain only the B form. Less than 10 percent of total MAO in brain is localized intraneuronally.

MAO inhibitors available for clinical use in the US irreversibly inhibit both MAO-A and MAO-B forms. Several new drugs have been developed that are reversible, selective inhibitors of MAO-A. This new generation of MAO inhibitors is generally safer because of their reversibility and shorter duration of action.

History

Iproniazid, a hydrazine derivative, was the first MAO inhibitor used for treatment of endogenous depression. In the early 1950s, iproniazid was developed for and used in the treatment of tuberculosis. Its mood-elevating effect was recognized in tuberculosis patients, leading to the evaluation and discovery of antidepressant activity in patients with unipolar depression. In subsequent years, other hydrazine and nonhydrazine inhibitors were developed and used for the treatment of depression.

Today, MAO inhibitors are usually confined to patients resistant to the tricyclic antidepressants. The clinical decline of the MAO inhibitors was due primarily to their interaction with the pressor amine tyramine. Ingestion of foods rich in tyramine can precipitate a severe, life-threatening hypertensive crisis in patients maintained on MAO inhibitors.

A new class of drugs that selectively and reversibly block MAO-A was developed. These reversible MAO inhibitors appear to have comparable therapeutic actions, and are likely to be a valuable addition. Drug effects are more readily controlled, side-effects are fewer, and the toxic interactions with tyramine and other pressor agents appear to be less severe. Promising new reversible MAO-A inhibitors with therapeutic activity comparable to that of the older generation of MAO inhibitors include moclobemide and brofaromine (Fig. 17.2).

Chemistry

The irreversible MAO inhibitors can be subdivided into two categories: hydrazine and nonhydrazine derivatives. Included in the nonhydrazine group are a class of inhibitors with an acetylenic (2-propynylamine) group that includes drugs selective for MAO-A and MAO-B. Representative structures are shown in Figure 17.2.

Pharmacologic and Biochemical Effects of MAO Inhibitors

MAO inhibitors elevate the levels of amine neurotransmitters and reduce the levels of the corresponding deaminated metabolites; e.g., they increase NE and lower 3-methoxy-4-hydroxymandelic acid (VMA) and 3-methoxy-4-hydroxyphenylglycol (MHPG) or they increase 5HT and reduce 5-hydroxyindole acetic acid (5HIAA). Trace monoamines, such as tryptamine and octopamine, are also increased after MAO inhibition.

Even though intraneuronal levels of amines increase after MAO inhibition, this does not necessarily translate into elevated levels at the physiologically relevant amine receptor sites. There is, however, experimental evidence in laboratory animals that the extracellular levels of NE and 5HT are elevated, exposing

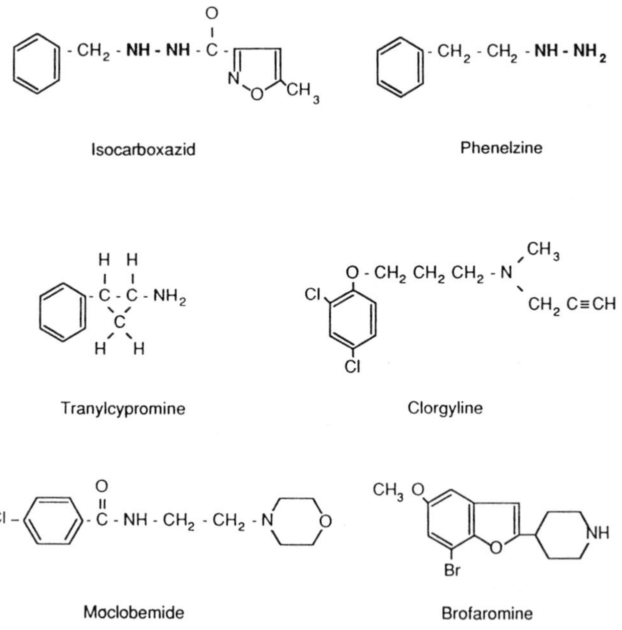

Isocarboxazid   Phenelzine

Tranylcypromine   Clorgyline

Moclobemide   Brofaromine

Figure 17.2 Chemical Structures of Representative MAO Inhibitors

synaptic receptors to higher levels of these neurotransmitters. Neurons adapt to this perturbation and attempt to maintain homeostasis. These adaptations after chronic MAO inhibition occur both presynaptically and postsynaptically. Presynaptically, the synthesis and turnover of monoamines decrease, while postsynaptically the density of receptors is reduced and receptor sensitivity is attenuated. These adaptive processes blunt but do not entirely offset the enhanced neurotransmission elicited by MAO inhibitors.

Two pharmacologic actions of the MAO inhibitors are important therapeutically: mood elevation and lowering of blood pressure. Unlike the tricyclic antidepressants, some MAO inhibitors produce hyperactivity in laboratory animals. In addition to alleviating the symptoms of depression, the administration of an MAO inhibitor can produce CNS stimulation in depressed patients and in normal individuals. In addition, some MAO inhibitors lower blood pressure. Since not all MAO inhibitors cause hypotension, a different mechanism may mediate these effects. Several mechanisms have been proposed, including blockade of adrenergic neurons, ganglionic blockade, and accumulation of octopamine, a false neurotransmitter. Only the latter would result directly from MAO inhibition. MAO inhibitors also have antianginal effects that may be secondary to the lowering of systemic blood pressure.

MAO inhibitors possess a variety of pharmacologic effects in addition to MAO inhibition, including inhibition of amine uptake and receptor blockade. These effects are not shared by all MAO inhibitors, but instead reflect the intrinsic properties of a particular drug class and are unrelated to MAO inhibition. Some MAO inhibitors, particularly the hydrazines, interfere with other enzyme systems, including diamine oxidase, cholinesterase, amino acid decarboxylase, and hepatic drug metabolizing enzymes. Hydrazines are chemically reactive and may interact with physiologically important substances. For example, hydrazines and vitamin B_6 (pyridoxine) can interact to form hydrazones, which could lead to vitamin B_6 deficiency.

Therapeutic Uses of MAO Inhibitors

The principal therapeutic indication for MAO inhibitors is endogenous unipolar depression. Compounds available and their doses are presented in Table 17.1. Other less prominent indications include panic disorders, bulimia, and post-traumatic reactions. Clinical studies suggest that 80 percent or more inhibition of MAO is required for an antidepressant effect. MAO inhibitors generally are used as a second line of assault, only after the tricyclic antidepressant drugs fail. The selective MAO-B inhibitor deprenyl (selegiline) is of some value for the treatment of parkinsonism (enhancement of the therapeutic efficacy of levodopa; see Chapter 18).

Table 17.1 Available Preparations of MAO Inhibitors and Usual Doses

Generic Name	Trade Name	Dosage Form*/mg	Daily Doses mg/d
Isocarboxazid	Marplan	(T) 10	10–30
Phenelzine	Nardil	(T) 15	60–90
Tranylcypromine	Parnate	(T) 10	30–60
Moclobemide	Aurorix	(T) 100–150	300–600

*T = Tablet

Mechanism of Therapeutic Action of MAO Inhibitors

Because inhibition of MAO has a more rapid onset than the therapeutic response, it is generally thought that delayed, adaptive processes may be important in mediating the therapeutic effects of this class of drugs in the treatment of depression and other CNS disorders. Like the tricyclic antidepressants, MAO inhibitors produce a delayed down-regulation of beta-adrenoceptors in brain and this finding has contributed to the revised catecholamine hypothesis of depression (discussed in more detail later). Chronic administration of MAO inhibitors to rats also elicits a delayed down-regulation of $5HT_1$ and $5HT_2$ receptors in brain. In addition, the behavioral and electrophysiologic effects of 5HT agonists are attenuated by chronic MAO inhibition, presumably mediated by down-regulation of receptors. The role of adaptive changes in 5HT systems in antidepressant action is the subject of ongoing investigations.

Undesirable Side-Effects of MAO Inhibitors at Therapeutic Doses and Interaction with Other Drugs

Numerous side-effects and adverse reactions occur in patients treated with MAO inhibitors. These can include insomnia, irritability, motor restlessness, tremor, agitation, and seizures. Orthostatic hypotension occurs and may require a reduction of dose or complete withdrawal. MAO inhibitors have been reported to precipitate a psychotic episode in patients with a history of schizophrenia, to initiate hypomania, and to convert a retarded depression into an agitated or anxious depression. Liver toxicity was more common with the early hydrazine MAO inhibitors than with currently used drugs that inhibit MAO.

The most important drug-drug interaction of MAO inhibitors is with tyramine, a naturally occurring monoamine. The tyramine concentration is especially high in aged cheeses, wines, and pickled products. A severe, life-threatening hypertensive crisis is precipitated in patients treated with MAO inhibitors who ingest large amounts of foods rich in tyramine. This interaction is frequently referred to as the "cheese effect." The MAO inhibitors prevent the inactivation of tyramine by hepatic MAO and potentiate its pressor effects. Moreover, MAO inhibition potentiates the effects of catecholamines released by tyramine. The symptoms of a "cheese attack" consist of severe occipital headache, with sudden onset of other symptoms including vomiting, hyperpyrexia, chest pain, muscle twitches, and restlessness. Symptoms usually disappear in a few hours, but in some cases fatal intracranial bleeding has occurred. Because of the severity of these attacks, patients taking MAO inhibitors should be cautioned to refrain from eating foods rich in tyramine. If a hypertensive crisis develops, the MAO inhibitor should be withdrawn immediately; however, because of the irreversible action of all but the newer drugs, several weeks must elapse before it is safe to consume tyramine-containing foods. Risks of life-threatening "cheese reactions" is thought to be reduced during treatment with the reversible MAO-A inhibitors. A toxic interaction may also occur if sympathomimetic amines or amphetamine-like drugs are administered to patients on irreversible MAO inhibitors. The mechanism involves a potentiation of the drug itself as well as the catecholamines released by these drugs (see Chapter 22 on Central Stimulants).

Care should be taken if MAO inhibitors are combined with tricyclic antidepressants. Early evaluations of such drug combinations carried alarming reports of severe toxic interactions, although more recently this combination has been used safely. MAO inhibitors interfere with the metabolism of barbiturates, aminopyrine, acetanilide, cocaine, and meperidine, thus potentiating and prolonging the action of these drugs.

Toxic Effects of Overdoses of MAO Inhibitors

Acute overdose with MAO inhibitors precipitates a number of central abnormalities, including agitation, hallucinations, hyperpyrexia, hyperreflexia, and convulsions. Abnormal blood pressure, either high or low, is a common toxic sign. Gastric lavage and maintenance of cardiopulmonary function may be required. Conservative treatment to maintain body temperature, blood pressure, and electrolyte balance is often successful.

Pharmacokinetics

All available MAO inhibitors are rapidly absorbed after oral administration. The onset of action of the hydrazines may be delayed, perhaps because they are converted to active products by enzymatic cleavage. N-acetylation is a major route of metabolism of hydrazines, such as phenelzine and isoniazid. Phenelzine-treated patients can have markedly different rates of acetylation. Some, but not all, studies of the metabolism of hydrazines suggest that patients exhibiting fast or slow acetylation of these drugs may differ in therapeutic response and toxic reactions. Isocarboxazid is metabolized by cleavage to benzylhydrazine, with ultimate secretion in the urine as hippuric acid, the glycine conjugate of benzoic acid. Hippuric acid is also a major urinary metabolite of tranylcypromine, formed by oxidative cleavage of the side-chain to benzoic acid and subsequent conjugation with glycine. Since all currently prescribed MAO inhibitors irreversibly inhibit MAO, recovery of MAO activity may take several weeks after cessation of treatment. The duration of action is determined by enzyme regeneration of MAO, rather than drug inactivation.

Tricyclic Antidepressants

The classic tricyclic antidepressants are either tertiary or secondary amines of structurally related chemicals with a three-ring core. The secondary amines can be formed in vivo by oxidative N-demethylation of the corresponding tertiary amines (e.g., desipramine is derived from imipramine, and nortriptyline from amitriptyline).

The tricyclic antidepressants are the most widely prescribed drugs for the treatment of major depression, particularly endogenous depression. Some of the tricyclic antidepressants are also successfully employed for the treatment of panic and obsessive compulsive disorders, and tricyclics such as chlorimipramine are reported to be effective in the treatment of chronic pain.

History

The synthesis of iminodibenzyl, which provided the starting material for substituted derivatives including imipramine, occurred 90 years ago. The discovery by Delay and Deniker[2] in France of the unusual therapeutic value of the phenothiazine derivative, chlorpromazine, for the treatment of schizophrenic patients, revived interest in clinical evaluations of the structurally related iminodibenzyl-derivatives that had previously been shown to exert antihistaminic, analgesic, anticholinergic, and sedative properties.[3] It was during the clinical evaluation for potential antipsychotic activity that the unexpected therapeutic value of imipramine in endogenous depression was discovered.[4] Synthesis of new tricyclic antidepressants followed quickly with structural modifications of either the ring system or the aliphatic side chain (Fig. 17.3). By and large, such structural modifications led to the introduction of drugs with pharmacologic and therapeutic profiles similar to those of imipramine. None of the newer tricyclic antidepressants turned out to be more efficacious than imipramine, and, contrary to some earlier claims, their onset of therapeutic action is not faster.

Studies of the mechanism of action of tricyclic antidepressants have significantly advanced our understanding of presynaptic aminergic function and of adaptive regulation of receptor-mediated events involved in signal transduction. Moreover, the more mechanistically oriented studies have contributed to the formulation of simple but heuristic hypotheses on the pathophysiology of affective disorders, e.g., the catecholamine (norepinephrine) and the indolealkylamine (serotonin) hypotheses of affective disorders.[6] Historically, studies on the mode of action of tricyclic antidepressants and other psychopharmacologic agents have decisively contributed to the emergence of biologic psychiatry as a medical discipline.

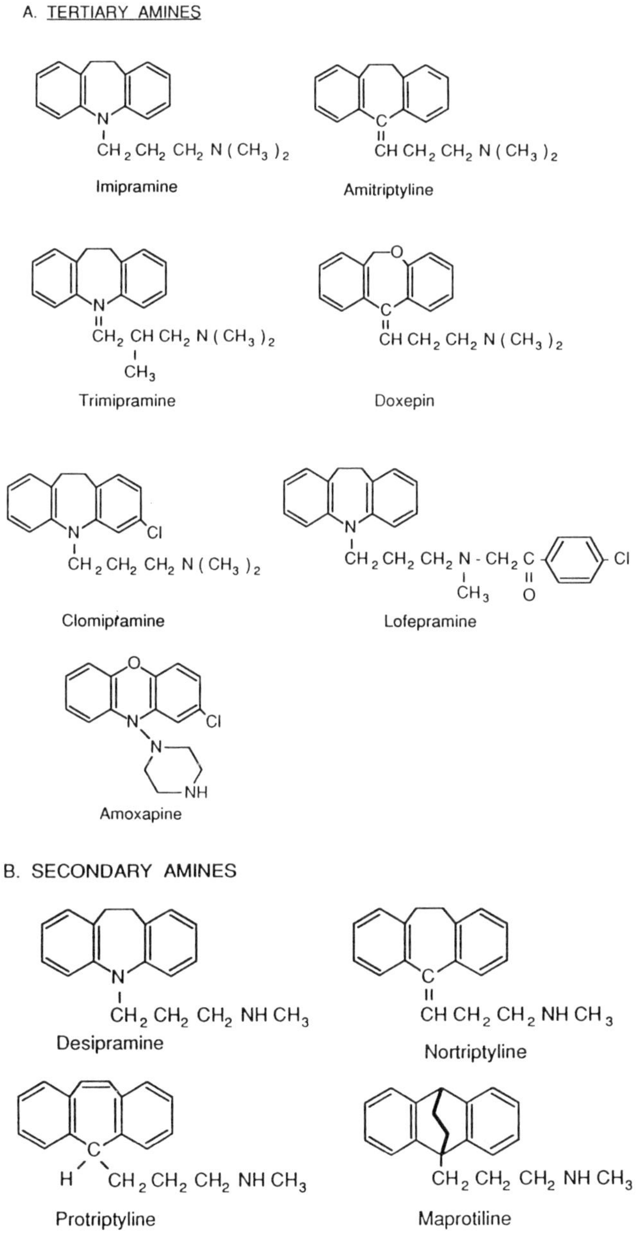

A. TERTIARY AMINES

$CH_2CH_2CH_2N(CH_3)_2$ Imipramine

$CHCH_2CH_2N(CH_3)_2$ Amitriptyline

$CH_2CHCH_2N(CH_3)_2$ (CH_3) Trimipramine

$CHCH_2CH_2N(CH_3)_2$ Doxepin

$CH_2CH_2CH_2N(CH_3)_2$ Clomipramine

$CH_2CH_2CH_2N(CH_3)$-$CH_2C(=O)$-C_6H_4-Cl Lofepramine

Amoxapine

B. SECONDARY AMINES

$CH_2CH_2CH_2NHCH_3$ Desipramine

$CHCH_2CH_2NHCH_3$ Nortriptyline

$CH_2CH_2CH_2NHCH_3$ Protriptyline

$CH_2CH_2CH_2NHCH_3$ Maprotiline

Figure 17.3 Chemical Structures of Tricyclic Antidepressants

Chemistry

Imipramine, the prototype of tricyclic antidepressants, was developed through structural modification of the phenothiazine nucleus in promazine, i.e., by replacement of the sulfur with an ethylene group. Although inspection of the structures of the tricyclic antidepressants at first glance shows similarities with the phenothiazines, there are subtle differences that must be responsible for the remarkable differences in therapeutic activity. In the phenothiazine ring system, the S-atom enables the conjugation of the benzene rings to extend over the bridge, whereas the ethylene group in the middle ring of imipramine acts as a barrier to conjugation. Moreover, promazine is a symmetrical molecule, whereas imipramine is asymmetrical, the two benzene rings being twisted against each other.[5]

The chemical structures of currently available tricyclic antidepressants are shown in Figure 17.3. They are either tertiary or secondary amines of iminodibenzyl (imipramine, desipramine, trimipramine), dibenzocycloheptadiene (amitriptyline, nortriptyline), dibenzocycloheptatriene (protriptyline), dibenzothiepin (prothiadene, northiadene), or dibenzoxepine (doxepin, desmethyldoxepin) derivatives. Two additional tricyclics with slightly different chemical structures are maprotiline, which contains an additional ethylene bridge across the middle six-carbon ring, and amoxapine, a dibenzoxazepine derivative, with mixed antidepressant and antipsychotic properties. Halogen substitution in the 3-position of imipramine led to the introduction of clomipramine.

Pharmacological and Biochemical Effects

In normal animals, most tricyclic antidepressants share anticholinergic, antihistaminic, sympatholytic, and sedative properties with the structurally related phenothiazine derivatives. These effects occur rapidly and can easily explain many of the side-effects of tricyclic antidepressants, such as dry mouth, blurred vision, cardiotoxicity (see below), and sedation; but they probably have little relevance to the delayed therapeutic action. Like the phenothiazines, tricyclic antidepressants potentiate the action of barbiturates and alcohol and reduce the arousal reaction to sensory stimuli.

Although many behavioral and biochemical tests are currently used to screen for potential antidepressant drugs, historically, the reserpine-like "model depression" has been useful for distinguishing qualitatively between antipsychotic and antidepressant drugs. Both tricyclic antidepressants and MAO inhibitors antagonize the reserpine-like syndrome to varying degrees. While antagonism of peripheral autonomic symptoms elicited by reserpine is not specific to antidepressants, evaluation of gross behavioral changes (sedation, decreased locomotor activity) has been a more discriminating test for antidepressant action. Antagonism of reserpine-induced behavioral changes by tricyclics depends on the synaptic availability of NE as the drugs fail to antagonize behavioral manifestations of reserpine in animals with selective depletion of brain catecholamines.[6] The reserpine-induced "model depression" in animals may have clinical relevance, since reserpine occasionally precipitates severe depressive reactions in humans.[7] Tricyclic antidepressants, MAO inhibitors, and electroconvulsive treatment (ECT) also alleviate the behavioral depression in rats exposed to uncontrollable shock[8] and severe stress. Since the stress-induced behavioral depression accompanying these behavioral challenges may be mediated by an increase in noradrenergic activity in the locus coeruleus, these findings are compatible with the suggested mode of action of antidepressant treatments (see later).

Although it has been shown that tricyclic antidepressants can inhibit MAO-B in vitro, there is no convincing evidence that drugs of this class exert their therapeutic action by blocking MAO in vivo. However, the classic tricyclic antidepressants increase the synaptic availability of catecholamines and of 5HT by blocking neuronal reuptake, thereby prolonging their physiologic action at corresponding receptor sites. Thus, MAO inhibitors and tricyclic antidepressants accomplish a similar effect—increased synaptic availability of NE or 5HT—but by two different mechanisms. The tricyclic antidepressants act as competitive inhibitors of the high affinity uptake of NE and 5HT. Generally, tertiary amines of tricyclic antidepressants are more potent in blocking the reuptake of 5HT, while secondary amines are more potent inhibitors of the reuptake of NE. Readers interested in detailed structure-activity relationships and stereochemical considerations are referred to Maxwell and White.[r2] Blockade of amine uptake can explain many of the acute pharmacologic effects of this class of drugs, e.g., the potentiation of exogenously administered or endogenously released NE and, in part, the antagonism of the reserpine-like syndrome. The different potencies of tertiary and secondary amines of tricyclic antidepressants as inhibitors of the uptake of biogenic amines are reflected in the effect of these drugs on the firing rate of noradrenergic and serotonergic neurons, respectively. Thus, secondary amines (preferential blockers of NE reuptake) markedly depress the spontaneous activity of noradrenergic locus coeruleus neurons, whereas the corresponding tertiary amines exert little or no effect. Alternatively, tertiary amines (preferential blockers of 5HT reuptake) decrease the firing rate of serotonergic raphe neurons, while secondary amines exert minimal or no effect in equivalent doses. Following administration, tertiary amines of tricyclic antidepressants are converted by oxidative N-demethylation to the corresponding secondary amines (see Pharmacokinetics below). Consequently, any of the multitude of factors that are known either to stimulate or to impair hepatic drug metabolism will alter both the pharmacologic and the toxic profile of a given tricyclic antidepressant by affecting the relative amounts of the parent compound and its active metabolites. Recently, more selective uptake inhibitors have been made available for clinical use, e.g., maprotiline and oxaprotiline (selective NE uptake inhibitors) and fluvoxamine, sertraline, citalopram, and fluoxetine (selective 5HT uptake inhibitors). Fluoxetine is of particular interest because its N-demethylated metabolite—unlike the secondary amines generated from tertiary amines of the classical tricyclic antidepressants—does not alter either potency or selectivity for inhibiting 5HT uptake.

Although inhibition of reuptake of NE and/or 5HT by tricyclic antidepressants occurs rapidly, other effects occur only following prolonged treatment. These delayed pharmacologic effects appear to be more relevant to the slow onset of the therapeutic action of tricyclic antidepressants. They include adaptive changes at presynaptic sites, i.e., a decrease in the activity of tyrosine hydroxylase in brain areas with noradrenergic projections (e.g., locus coeruleus and hippocampus), which may explain the decreased rate of turnover of NE following chronic administration of tricyclic antidepressants. One of the most consistent findings after chronic administration of tricyclic and other antidepressants, and also following ECT, is a delayed desensitization of the NE receptor-coupled adenylate cyclase in brain, accompanied in most cases by a down-regulation of the number of beta adrenoceptors.[9] In most brain regions, this reduction in beta adrenoceptor density is primarily the result of a reduction in $beta_1$ adrenoceptors.[10] The reduction in beta adrenoceptor density is confined to the receptor population displaying high agonist affinity, i.e., those receptors linked via nucleotide regulatory proteins (G-proteins) to adenylate cyclase. The molecular basis of the substantial and exclusive loss of central beta adrenoceptors with high agonist affinity is still unknown. The findings that chronic but not short-term exposure of human fibroblasts to therapeutic doses of some antidepressants leads to changes in the cellular phospholipid pattern[11] are of interest, as changes in phospholipid patterns have been implicated in changes of membrane-embedded neurotransmitter receptors.[12] Chronic administration of many tricyclic antidepressants, MAO inhibitors, and atypical antidepressants (e.g., mianserin) also causes a reduction in the density of cortical $5HT_2$ receptors linked to phosphatidylinositol turnover,[r3] while selective serotonin uptake inhibitors may act at a postreceptor site to blunt $5HT_2$ transmission.[13] The possible relationship between these changes and those in the beta adrenoceptor/adenylate cyclase signal cascade is an area of great scientific interest. Electrophysiologic studies show that in rats other 5HT receptor subtypes, including cell body and terminal autoreceptors and $5HT_{1A}$ receptors in hippocampus, are regulated by antidepressant treatments leading to enhanced 5HT neurotransmission.[r7] The recent observation that there is a time-dependent adaptation of monoamine receptors within various brain regions may be relevant to the delayed therapeutic activity of these drugs.[14,15]

Numerous studies have shown that the high affinity binding of [^{3}H]-imipramine is potently inhibited by tricyclic antidepressants in both brain and platelets and that this binding often is reduced in animals and humans following chronic treatment with some antidepressants.[16,r4] Since [^{3}H]-imipramine labels a high-affinity site associated with the 5HT transporter, the regulation of these sites by tricyclic antidepressants may be physiologically relevant. Whether these sites will turn out to be useful biologic markers for depression remains to be seen. The recent cloning of the 5HT transporter opens up new possibilities for exploring this protein in humans.[17,18] Changes in alpha$_2$ adrenoceptor number and benzodiazepine and GABA-B receptors after chronic administration of tricyclic and other antidepressants have been reported, but these changes have been rather inconsistent. Finally, it has been a consistent finding that tricyclic antidepressants antagonize NMDA responses, but any relationship this action may have to the therapeutic action of these drugs has yet to be established.

Therapeutic Uses

Tricyclic antidepressants are the most widely used drugs for the treatment of endogenous unipolar depression and bipolar depression diseases characterized by extreme sadness, despair, and anhedonia. The first clinical observations by Kuhn[4] that tricyclics are effective in severe endogenous depression but of little or no value in reactive and neurotic depressions have been revalidated repeatedly. Generally, if anxiety and restlessness are predominant, the use of tertiary amines with more sedative properties (e.g., amitriptyline, imipramine) may be preferred. In more retarded depressions, the less sedative secondary amines (desipramine, nortriptyline) may be more beneficial. Although "noradrenergic" vs. "serotonergic" depressions have been hypothesized, the onset of action and the efficacy of the various tricyclics with a predominantly noradrenergic vs. a predominantly serotonergic profile are not different. The over-all improvement rate with tricyclic antidepressants is not dramatic, generally ranging around 65 to 70 percent vs. 20 to 30 percent for placebo.

More recently, some tricyclic antidepressants have been successfully used to treat panic and obsessive-compulsive disorders and agoraphobia.[19] In these conditions, tricyclics often work in much lower doses than those used for the treatment of depressive disorders. There is considerable overlap in the therapeutic spectrum of tricyclic antidepressants and benzodiazepines (see Chapter 15). However, unlike the benzodiazepines, the tricyclic compounds lack the potential to cause dependency and addiction. Other indications for treatment with tricyclic antidepressants are listed in Table 17.2 Imipramine seems to be particularly effective for the treatment of enuresis in children in a dose of 25–75 mg/kg/d given one hour or more before bedtime.[r8] Clinical studies also indicate that chlorimipramine is particularly effective in obsessive-compulsive disorders.[19] Finally, chronic pain syndromes (e.g., lower back pain) may respond favorably to tricyclic antidepressants. See Table 17.3 for preparations and doses of the tricyclic antidepressants.

Amoxapine shares many of the pharmacologic properties of tricyclic antidepressants and the structurally related phenothiazines, including anticholinergic, sedative, and 5HT- and NE-uptake blocking actions. In addition, the drug exerts D_2-dopamine receptor blocking properties, and thus can produce extrapyramidal side-effects and tardive dyskinesia. Its indication should be restricted to psychotic depressions.

Since insomnia is often a major symptom of depression, and since many tricyclic antidepressants have sedative properties, it is convenient to give part of the daily dose at bedtime to counteract insomnia and to minimize the sedative effects during the daytime. The usual daily dose is 50 to 100 mg/d, reaching 150 mg/d by the end of the first week of treatment. The usual maximum therapeutic doses are in the range of 250–300 mg (see Table 17.3). It is advisable to continue the treatment after remission with lower doses of the particular tricyclic antidepressant for several months to prevent or reduce the frequency of relapses. In general, elderly depressed patients seem to require lower dosages of tricyclics because they metabolize the drugs more slowly.

It is important to realize that the onset of therapeutic activity of the tricyclic antidepressants is rather slow, and two to three weeks of treatment usually are required for clinical improvement. Some patients fail to respond to any tricyclic antidepressant, despite adequate doses, adequate blood levels, and adequate duration of treatment (therapy-resistant depression). The suffering of these patients is often immense, and the risk of suicide is pre-eminent. In such cases, lithium carbonate may be combined with either a tricyclic antidepressant or an MAO inhibitor, particularly in patients with bipolar illness where a rapid conversion of a therapy-resistant to a therapy-responsive depression frequently has been observed.[20] Also, switching to an atypical antidepressant or to an MAO inhibitor may be beneficial. The combination of a tricyclic antidepressant with an MAO inhibitor has been used successfully for tricyclic-resistant patients, though such a combination may be toxic (see earlier discussion) and is not approved by the US Food and Drug Administration. Finally, if all chemotherapy has failed, electroconvulsive therapy (ECT) should be considered, as it may produce full remissions. Also, there is some evidence that patients resistant to tricyclic compounds prior to ECT may respond favorably after ECT therapy. Importantly, supportive psychotherapy remains an essential supplement in the "total" therapy for depression.

Mechanism of Therapeutic Action

In the absence of a clear understanding of the pathophysiology of affective disorders, it is difficult to

Table 17.2 Therapeutic Uses of Tricyclic Antidepressants

A. *Well-established indications:*
- Acute major depression
- Prevention of relapse of major, nonbipolar depression for at least one year
- Secondary depression in psychiatric, neurologic, or medical disorders, especially given melancholic features
- Panic disorder
- Obsessive-compulsive disorders (especially chlorimipramine).
- Enuresis (particularly imipramine)
- Attention deficit disorder with hyperactivity in children
- "Pseudodementia" with depression in the elderly
- Bulimia

B. *Less well-established indications:*
- Peripheral diabetic neuropathy symptoms
- Chronic pain
- Narcolepsy
- Migraine syndrome
- Sleep apnea
- School phobia and other separation anxiety disorders of children
- Peptic ulcer disease
- Some behavioral disorders marked by aggression and agitation in the mentally retarded or brain damaged
- Substance abuse

conclude with certainty which one of the many pharmacologic effects and biochemical actions elicited by tricyclic antidepressants is clinically most relevant. Biogenic amine hypotheses of affective disorders—the catecholamine hypothesis and the indolealkylamine hypothesis—have clearly dominated the field during the last 25 years. These hypotheses were initially "deficiency hypotheses," implying a lack of catecholamines[21] or indolealkylamines [5HT][22,23] as being responsible for the depressive mood. Consequently, tricyclic antidepressants were hypothesized to correct the deficiency by blockade of the high-affinity uptake of either NE or 5HT or both, thereby alleviating the depressive mood. Based on these concepts, a large number of drugs that block either 5HT or NE reuptake, some with greater specificity for one or the other amine, have been developed by the pharmaceutical industry. By and large, such drugs are therapeutically effective. Does this mean that blockade of the reuptake of 5HT and/or NE is responsible for or is a prerequisite for therapeutic activity? Certainly not. There are marked differences in relative potencies and in selectivity of tricyclic antidepressants with regard to blockade of amine uptake; but, clinically, the various tricyclics are about equally effective. Also, inhibition by tricyclic antidepressants of NE and/or 5HT uptake occurs rapidly within minutes after the administration of the drugs, while the therapeutic action is delayed, generally requiring treatment for several weeks. Moreover, L-DOPA and amphetamine, both of which increase the availability of NE and dopamine, elicit poor or no therapeutic responses. Moreover, a number of antidepressant drugs that do not block the neuronal uptake of either NE or 5HT (e.g., iprindole, mianserin, clenbuterol, rolipram) exert clinical antidepressant efficacy comparable to that of the uptake blockers.

In the mid-1970s, the research emphasis on the mode of action of tricyclic antidepressants (and antidepressants in general) shifted from acute presynaptic to delayed postsynaptic receptor mediated events.[r1] The delayed deamplification of the NE beta adrenoceptor-coupled adenylate cyclase system—in most cases linked to a down-regulation of beta adrenoceptors—is a common feature of most if not all clinically effective antidepressant treatments, including tricyclic antidepressants, MAO inhibitors, atypical antidepressants, and ECT. Adaptive responses occurring at alpha$_2$ adrenoceptors and at 5HT$_2$ receptors linked to phosphatidylinositol hydrolysis or at subtypes of 5HT$_1$ receptors may also contribute to the therapeutic profile of antidepressants. While the decrease in the beta adrenoceptor-linked adenylate cyclase system following chronic treatment appears to be quite specific for clinically effective antidepressants,[24] the reduction in the density of 5HT$_2$ receptors is not restricted to drugs with antidepressant properties, and ECT, the most efficacious antidepressant treatment, upregulates both the density and function of 5HT$_2$ receptors.

Considerable evidence suggests that the beta adrenoceptor-coupled adenylate cyclase system in neuronal tissue is involved in the modulation of the sensitivity of other receptor systems. Heteroreceptor regulation is widespread, and the interdependence of NE and 5HT in the synaptic pharmacology of antidepressants is of particular interest. For example, the development of supersensitivity to 5HT, evidenced electrophysiologically or behaviorally after chronic administration of tricyclic antidepressants, is prevented by denervation of noradrenergic neurons.[25] Although implications for the etiology of affective disorders are premature at this time, the delayed adaptive changes in the noradrenergic and serotonergic cascades of signal transduction after chronic treatment with clinically effective antidepressants are presumed to represent the therapeutically most relevant biochemical actions. The findings that the beta adrenoceptor antagonist propranolol is not only devoid of antidepressant activity but can precipitate depressive reactions do not, contrary to suggestions in the literature, refute this notion. Propranolol also blocks 5HT receptors and, on repeated administration, increases the density of beta adrenoceptors and, like reserpine, amplifies the beta adrenoceptor-mediated NE signal transduction. For a more complete discussion of the monoamine hypotheses of affective disorders, the interested reader is referred to a review.[r1]

Undesirable Side-Effects at Therapeutic Doses and Interaction with Other Drugs

In comparison with MAO inhibitors, the tricyclic antidepressants are relatively safe drugs, although they are by no means devoid of side-effects. Generally, the side-effects represent an extension of the drug's pharmacologic action and, consequently, occur more frequently at higher doses. Since all antidepressants are equally effective therapeutically, the side-effect profile may determine the choice of drug.

The most frequent side-effects of the tricyclics are due to their anticholinergic properties, resulting in dry mouth, blurred vision, constipation, and urinary retention. Confusion and delirious behavior have been observed during treatment with tricyclic antidepressants—particularly in elderly patients—which may reflect anticholinergic intoxication. Desipramine seems to have fewer anticholinergic side-effects than do other tricyclics; and lofepramine, which is metabolized to desipramine, is also reported to have a low incidence of dry mouth and other anticholinergic side-effects. In general, the "second generation" antidepressants, mianserin, and the selective 5HT uptake inhibitors (fluoxetine, fluvoxamine) are less likely to cause disturbing anticholinergic side-effects and may thus be preferred in elderly patients or in patients with glaucoma or prostate disorders. Many tricyclic antidepressants cause mild sedation, probably as a consequence of central histamine H_1-receptor blockade (protriptyline is an exception and elicits CNS stimulation). Tricyclic antidepressants have been reported to trigger a switch from depression to hypomania in patients with bipolar illness, and latent schizophrenias may become overt. Seizures during treatment with therapeutic doses of tricyclic antidepressants have occurred, although the incidence is low.

The classic tricyclics can exert cardiovascular side-effects at therapeutic doses, including orthostatic hypotension (the most common cardiovascular complication), tachycardia, and a number of changes in cardiac conduction (flattened or inverted T-waves, prolonged PR and QRS intervals). Though severe cardiotoxicity including arrhythmias, bundle branch, and complete heart blocks are observed only after large overdoses or in elderly patients, the use of tricyclic antidepressants in patients with known cardiac disease should nevertheless be carefully considered.

Other side-effects occasionally seen at therapeutic doses of tricyclics include impaired erectile or orgasmic sexual function, amenorrhea, galactorrhea, and excessive weight gain. The latter is one of the major reasons for noncompliance. Interestingly, the selective 5HT uptake-inhibitor fluoxetine frequently induces weight loss. Occasionally, tricyclic antidepressants have been reported to cause cholestatic jaundice, rash, agranulocytosis, and bone marrow depression. Over-all, however, severe toxic effects at therapeutic doses of tricyclics are low, occurring in 5 to 10 percent of patients treated.[r8]

Tricyclic antidepressants inhibit liver microsomal enzymes and thus may potentiate and prolong the action of many other drugs (e.g., amphetamine, propranolol, phenobarbital) and potentiate the CNS depression caused by alcohol and antihistamines. Moreover, tricyclics are contraindicated in patients whose hypertension is controlled with guanethidine-like drugs (guanethidine, bethanidine). Because tricyclics block the neuronal uptake of hydrophilic amines including guanethidine, the therapeutic activity of guanethidine can be nullified by coadministration of a tricyclic antidepressant. Since withdrawal symptoms (mostly mild GI symptoms) have been reported occasionally after abrupt discontinuation of tricyclic antidepressants, gradual withdrawal, particularly after large doses, is recommended.

Toxic Effects of Overdoses and Mechanisms Responsible for These Effects

Overdosage with tricyclic antidepressants may cause severe and life-threatening symptoms. The physician must keep in mind that overdosage (in excess of 2 grams) with tricyclics may provide a means for successful suicide. The toxic effects after overdosage are essentially an extension of the anticholinergic effects and include severe central excitation and seizures, myocardiotoxicity, and cardiorespiratory arrest. The risk of seizures seems to be somewhat higher with high dosages of the newer drugs, such as maprotiline and nomifensin (the latter has since been removed from the market). Gastric lavage may be helpful. The symptoms of severe anticholinergic activity (sinus tachycardia, arrhythmias) are treated with IM or IV injections of neostigmine methylsulfate. Seizures respond to IV-administered benzodiazepines (e.g., diazepam). According to Pinder,[26] antidepressant overdosage is the most common life-threatening drug ingestion worldwide. Since acute doses in excess of 2 grams can be fatal, the dispensing of more than 1 gram of imipramine or the equivalent of another tricyclic to depressed patients should be avoided.

Fatal complications (hyperpyrexia, hypertensive crises, convulsions) have been reported after the combination of tricyclic antidepressants with MAO inhibitors. However, such combined treatment may be efficacious in refractory depressions, and its danger may have been greatly exaggerated.

Pharmacokinetics

Tricyclic antidepressants are rapidly and completely absorbed from the GI tract. The tricyclics are very lipophilic compounds and highly bound to plasma proteins (more than 90 percent) and to tissues. This makes it difficult to remove these drugs by hemodialysis in case of overdosage. A significant portion of an oral dose is metabolized during the first pass through the liver. The principal routes of metabolism by liver microsomal enzymes (Fig. 17.4) are:[r5] (1) oxidative N-demethylation leading to secondary and primary amines; (2) hydroxylation in 2-position of the ethylene bridge with subsequent glucuronide formation and urinary excretion; (3) N-oxidation and oxidative side chain dealkylation. The N-demethylated metabolites generally have a longer biologic half-life than the corresponding tertiary amines, accumulate in tissues including brain, and are pharmacologically and therapeutically active.

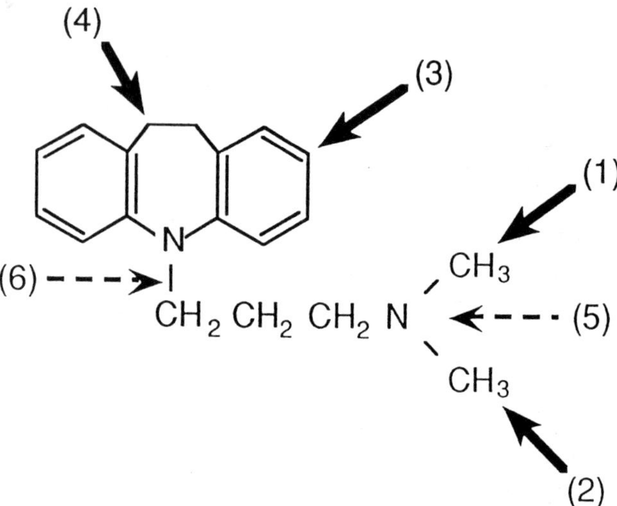

Figure 17.4 Principal routes of metabolism of tricyclic antidepressants: The metabolically vulnerable parts of the Imipramine Molecule.

(1) N-demethylation to secondary (−1 CH_3 group).

(2) and primary amines (−2 methyl groups).

(3) Aromatic hydroxylation followed by glucuronic acid conjugation.

(4) Aliphatic hydroxylation followed by glucuronic acid conjugation.

(5) N-Oxidative side-chain dealkylation.

(Adapted from Bickel, 1980).

Though N-demethylation and aliphatic and aromatic hydroxylation represent the major metabolic pathways, the relative contribution of each varies from species to species. For example, after the administration of imipramine, the N-demethylated secondary amine desipramine accumulates in tissues of rats and humans, but not in those of rabbits and mice. In the latter two species, hydroxylation followed by conjugation is the major metabolic pathway. While imipramine is hydroxylated in position 2 of the aromatic ring forming phenolic metabolites, amitriptyline is hydroxylated at the ethylene bridge forming alcoholic metabolites. The 2-hydroxy metabolites of imipramine and desipramine and the 10-hydroxy metabolite of amitriptyline and nortriptyline are biologically active; however, a significant contribution to the central action of the parent drugs is questionable. Because of the differences between tertiary and secondary amines in modifying central noradrenergic and serotonergic neuronal activity (see above), any of the multitude of factors known to influence hepatic microsomal enzyme activity will influence the ratio of the tertiary to the secondary amines and thus modify the pharmacologic profile and perhaps the therapeutic activity of a particular drug.

In humans, the genetically most heterogeneous species, the biologic half-lives of tricyclic antidepressants and their metabolites, particularly the N-demethylated secondary amine metabolites, are relatively long and vary considerably. Steady-state plasma levels after a fixed dose of desipramine vary between 8–280 ng/ml,[27] indicating that dose alone is not a reliable indicator of the amount of drug available at presumptive active sites. However, blood levels obtained after a fixed dose are relatively stable characteristics of individual patients, probably reflecting genetic control. Measurements of steady-state plasma levels provide a more rational guide for predicting individual dosage requirements. Generally, plasma steady-state levels (after 1 to 2 weeks of treatment) below 50 ng/ml are likely to be therapeutically ineffective, while levels above 500 ng/ml are likely to be associated with toxic effects.[r8] The biologic half-life of tricyclic antidepressants and hence the incidence of toxicity increase in the elderly. Therefore, it is prudent to monitor blood levels of the tricyclic antidepressant to assure appropriate drug concentrations. Because of the long half-life of tricyclics (up to 126 hours for protriptyline) and their accumulation in tissues, one cannot assume a patient to be drug free (much less drug-effect free) even weeks after discontinuation of treatment.

Table 17.3 Available Preparations of Tricyclic Antidepressants and Usual Doses

Generic Name	Trade Name	Dosage Forms* mg	Daily Doses mg/d
Tertiary Amines			
Imipramine	Tofranil, Presamine	(T) 10, 25, 50 (A) 25/2 ml	150–300
Amitriptyline	Elavil, Endep, Laroxyl	(T) 10, 25, 50, 75, 100 (A) 10/ml	150–300
Doxepin	Sinequan, Adapin, Curetin	(C) 10, 25, 50, 75, 100, 150	75–200
Trimipramine	Surmontil	(C) 25, 50, 100	75–250
Lofepramine	Gamonil	(T) 35, 70	140–210
Clomipramine	Anafranil	(T) 10, 25 (A) 25/2 ml	50–150
Secondary Amines			
Desipramine	Norpramin, Pertofrane	(T) 25, 50, 75, 100 (C) 25,50	150–250
Nortriptyline	Aventyl, Pamelor	(C) 10, 25	75–150
Protriptyline	Vivactyl	(T) 5, 10	15–60
Maprotiline	Ludiomil	(T) 25, 50, 75 (A) 25/5 ml	100–150
Amoxapine	Ascendin	(T) 50, 100, 150	200–300

*T = Tablet
C = Capsule
A = Ampule
d = day

"Second Generation" or "Atypical" Antidepressants

The term "second generation" antidepressants has been assigned to a number of new drugs, many of which share pharmacologic properties with those of tricyclic antidepressants but are structurally different. They include the selective 5HT-uptake inhibitors fluoxetine, sertraline, and fluvoxamine; the tetracyclic compound mianserin; the triazolopyridine derivative trazodone; the chlorpropiophenone bupropion; and the cyclohexanol derivative venlafaxine (Figure 17.5). Many of these newer drugs have expanded the range of clinical options for the treatment of depression but mostly in terms of potential unwarranted side-effects, particularly a reduction in anticholinergic properties. However, these newer drugs are by no means free of side-effects. Trazodone produces considerable sedation, and has caused sustained penile erections (priapism) necessitating surgery in some cases. Bupropion exerts some stimulant properties and has triggered seizures in a small number of patients (0.4%). The former is probably the consequence of increased dopaminergic activity. Major complaints following selective

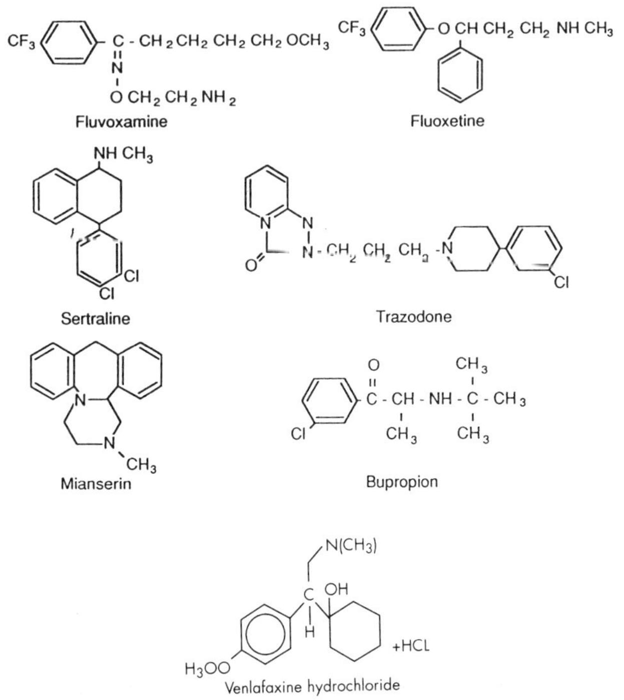

Figure 17.5 Chemical Structures of "Second Generation" or "Atypical" Antidepressants

5HT-uptake inhibitors and after venlafaxine are nausea, nervousness, and insomnia. Fluoxetine in particular has been associated with unusual toxic reactions, such as violent behavior and increased suicide attempts.[28] However, it has to be realized that all depressed patients are at increased risk for suicide as they begin to emerge from their severe depressed states, and there seems to be no evidence that fluoxetine triggers suicidal ideation over and above rates that may be associated with depression and other antidepressants.[29] Venlafaxine inhibits both the uptake of NE and 5HT without blocking muscarinic cholinegic, H_1-histaminergic or α_1-adrenergic receptors.[30] Its profile is thus clearly different from the classic tricyclic antidepressants. Doses used for these agents are presented in Table 17.4.

Advertising claims to the contrary, none of these newer drugs appears to provide significant advantage over the traditional tricyclic antidepressants in clinical efficacy, speed of onset of therapeutic action, or in the range of affective disorders responsive to drug treatment. It remains to be seen whether the clinical impression of a more favorable therapeutic ratio of these newer agents will survive the test of time.

"Second Generation" Antidepressants Undergoing Clinical Evaluation

A number of experimental drugs with interesting pharmacologic properties are currently undergoing clinical trials. These drugs include the β_2 adrenoceptor antagonists salbutamol and clenbuterol, the cyclic AMP phosphodiesterase inhibitor rolipram, S-adenosyl-L-methionine, the triazolobenzodiazepine alprazolam, levoprotiline, and the partial $5HT_{1A}$ agonist gepirone. A definite answer regarding clinical efficacy is still outstanding, but these putative antidepressants are of pharmacologic and theoretical interest. For example, clenbuterol down-regulates predominantly the β_2 adrenoceptor population, while rolipram desensitizes the beta adrenoceptor-coupled adenylate cyclase by a mechanism operating beyond the receptor. Though the pharmacologic action of S-adenosyl-methionine is unknown, this methyl donor may cause changes in the composition of methylated phospholipids in the membrane, thereby influencing signal transduction through membranes. Alprazolam has been claimed to exert antidepressant activity, particularly in patients whose depression is associated with anxiety. Since anxiety is a core symptom of many depressive disorders, the beneficial effect of alprazolam in anxious depressive patients is not surprising. Levoprotiline is the (–)-enantiomer of oxaprotiline and does not affect NE reuptake or beta adrenoceptor function; it has thus been of great theoretical interest. Although early clinical trials have suggested possible therapeutic activity of levoprotiline, more extensive placebo-controlled, double-blind studies failed to substantiate unequivocal efficacy.[31]

Since an enhancement of serotonergic function by classic tricyclic antidepressants is presumed to be involved in the therapeutic action, results from controlled clinical studies with the partial $5HT_{1A}$ agonist gepirone and congeners are eagerly awaited.

Table 17.4 Available Preparations of "Second Generation" Antidepressants and Usual Doses

Generic Name	Trade Name	Dosage forms* mg	Daily doses mg/d
Fluvoxamine	Fevarin	(T) 50	100–200
Fluoxetine	Prozac	(C) 20	20–80
Sertraline	Zoloft	(T) 50, 100	50–200
Other New Antidepressants			
Mianserin	Tolvin	(T) 10, 30	30–120
Trazodone	Desyrel	(2) 50, 100	150–600
Bupropion	Wellbutrin	(T) 75, 100	100–300
Venlafaxine	Effexor	(T) 25, 37.5, 50, 100	75–225

*T = Tablet
C = Capsule

Lithium Salts and Carbamazepine

History

The therapeutic benefit of lithium carbonate in mania was discovered four decades ago by the Australian physician, J. F. Cade. Prior to that, lithium chloride had been used as a salt substitute, but severe toxic reactions and even deaths occurred, probably due to the now-recognized potentiating action of sodium depletion on lithium toxicity. In early medicine, salts of lithium were used for the treatment of gout.

Chemistry

Lithium, the lightest known metal, belongs to the class of alkali metals that includes sodium and potassium. It is found in trace amounts in the body, but has no known physiologic role. Lithium is easily quantitated by flame photometry and atomic absorption spectroscopy.

Pharmacologic and Biochemical Effects

At therapeutic concentrations, lithium does not elicit CNS depression, excitation, or euphoria. Instead, the ion tends to stabilize mood, preventing the marked mood swings that are a hallmark of manic-depressive illness.

Lithium has a myriad of effects on cellular transport mechanisms, second messenger pathways, and neurotransmitter dynamics. Of the two major neurotransmitters (5HT and NE) implicated in the pathogenesis of affective disorders, 5HT has been most extensively investigated. Lithium alters both presynaptic and postsynaptic function of 5HT neurons.[32] In experimental animals, lithium increases the high-affinity uptake of tryptophan and increases the synthesis of 5HT. Lithium also enhances 5HT release and potentiates $5HT_1$ receptor-mediated behaviors, but it attenuates

$5HT_2$ receptor-mediated responses. It is not known whether these effects are primary or secondary, but it is clear that the initial, net effect of lithium is to enhance central 5HT function. Whether this effect on 5HT function changes with long-term administration has not been resolved. Evidence suggests that $5HT_2$ receptor desensitization is elicited after long-term administration of lithium, and 5HT receptor regulation after prolonged lithium administration remains an area of active research. Furthermore, the effects of lithium on 5HT function in humans are not well documented, although most clinical studies suggest enhanced central 5HT function.

The actions of lithium on noradrenergic neurons generally are to decrease noradrenergic transmission. Although lithium enhances NE turnover initially, turnover is decreased after long-term administration. Lithium also has been shown to decrease NE release and, within the clinically relevant therapeutic range, to inhibit basal and beta adrenoceptor-dependent adenylate cyclase, perhaps by interfering with the activity of G-proteins.

At therapeutic concentrations, lithium markedly alters phosphatidylinositol turnover. Phosphatidylinositol turnover mediates signal transduction at many central receptors, including $5HT_2$, $alpha_1$ noradrenergic, muscarinic cholinergic, and glutamate receptors. Lithium blocks a number of steps in the phosphatidylinositol pathway; the most sensitive site is the phosphatase that converts inositol-monophosphates to inositol.[33] Inositol recycling is the major mechanism for resynthesis of phosphoinositides, so lithium administration would theoretically attenuate neurotransmission at the receptors coupled to the phosphatidylinositol pathway.

Therapeutic Uses

Lithium is the drug of choice for the treatment of acute mania and for prophylactic treatment of recurrent bipolar manic-depressive illness. In acute mania, treatment with lithium leads to improvement in 60–100 percent of patients. Lithium is disease-specific and, unlike the phenothiazines that cause a "drugged state," lithium specifically reduces manic symptoms without sedation. In patients with bipolar manic-depressive illness, lithium decreases the recurrence of manic-depressive episodes and also lessens the duration and severity of episodes that do occur. The value of lithium in the treatment of unipolar endogenous depression is less well-established. Some accumulating evidence shows that lithium is beneficial in treatment-resistant depressed patients when combined with tricyclic antidepressants or MAO inhibitors.

Lithium has a narrow therapeutic window. Plasma levels ranging from 0.6 to 1 mEq/L are therapeutically effective (see Table 17.5). At higher plasma levels, the incidence of side-effects increases, with severe toxicity occurring at levels of 2 mEq/L or higher. Care should be taken at the initiation of treatment, including monitoring of blood levels, first daily and then periodically throughout the course of treatment.

Mechanism of Therapeutic Action

The mechanism of the therapeutic action of lithium is not known. Because it is an ion that substitutes for sodium, lithium can have multiple effects on cells; furthermore, its interaction with the inositol lipid signaling cascade could have widespread effects, since receptors for a large number of neurotransmitters are coupled to this pathway. Even so, the scientific community currently favors a primary role for 5HT in mediating the antidepressant effects and the potentiative interactions of lithium and tricyclic antidepressants, while other systems in addition to or instead of 5HT may mediate the antimanic effects of lithium.

Undesirable Side-Effects

At therapeutic plasma levels (0.6–1.0 mEq/L), the side effects of lithium are generally mild and include nausea, muscular weakness, fatigue, and fine tremors of hands. Polydipsia and polyuria also may occur. Hypothyroidism is the most common endocrinologic consequence of chronic lithium treatment. Diffuse benign goiters develop infrequently. All of these symptoms are reversible on discontinuation of treatment. If serum levels rise to 2 mEq/L or greater, more severe toxic signs including ataxia, slurred speech, drowsiness, and confusion may occur. The toxicity of lithium is increased by factors that deplete the body of sodium. Restriction of dietary sodium, e.g., salt-free diets, dramatically increases the renal reabsorption of lithium and can lead to severe toxicity. Similarly, diuretics that lead to sodium loss may augment lithium toxicity.

Toxic Effects of Overdoses

Symptoms following severe acute overdoses include vomiting, diarrhea, cardiac arrhythmias, seizures, and other neurologic abnormalities, which can progress to coma and death. Treatment of acute lithium poisoning is primarily supportive. Since the kidney is the important route of elimination of lithium, increasing the renal clearance of lithium by dialysis or infusion of saline may be beneficial.

Pharmacokinetics

Lithium is readily absorbed, with peak plasma levels 2–4 hours after a single oral dose of lithium carbonate. Lithium distributes rapidly to liver and kidney, and more slowly to muscle, brain, and bone. Lithium enters cells via sodium channels. Once inside, it is extruded by the active cation pump at about one-tenth the rate of sodium. Consequently, lithium accumulates within the cell, which may explain why the levels of lithium in red blood cells show a stronger correlation with brain levels than do the levels in serum. The thyroid gland concentrates lithium to concentrations that are two to five times higher than the serum concentration.

Elimination is predominantly via the kidneys. Lithium is reabsorbed in the proximal tubule with sodium and water. Restriction of dietary sodium can lead to the accumulation of lithium and severe toxicity; conversely, the addition of salt to the diet increases the excretion of lithium.

Carbamazepine

Carbamazepine (Fig. 17.6) was first introduced in the 1960s as an antiepileptic drug for treatment of partial or focal seizures. When it was recognized that mood improved, carbamazepine was evaluated in depression and mania. It is the latter, mania, where carbamazepine has proved most beneficial. Carbamazepine is now the alternative treatment for acute mania if lithium is unsuccessful or poorly tolerated.[r6] Carbamazepine may also have value as an alternative in bipolar manic-depressive illness and, if added to tricyclic antidepressants, may be of value in patients with therapy-resistant unipolar depression.[34]

The usual route of administration is oral. Absorption is complete, with peak plasma levels occurring 2.5–8 hours after dosing (see Table 17.5). The plasma half-life varies from 30–50 hours and is shortened after chronic administration because carbamazepine induces drug metabolizing enzymes, including the enzymes responsible for its own metabolism. Unlike the neuroleptics that are sometimes used for mania, carbamazepine has no sedative properties. Side-effects include nausea, dizziness, ataxia, and visual disturbances, which occur soon after dosing and disappear rapidly. Hypersensitive reactions with rash are infrequent and are slow in onset. The most serious toxicity involves the bone marrow; aplastic anemia occurs but with low incidence. Carbamazepine is a potent enzyme inducer and may lower levels of other drugs, including other anticonvulsants, steroids, theophylline, warfarin, and haloperidol. Carbamazepine affects catecholamines, 5HT, and adenosine systems.[27] However, its mode of action is not known.

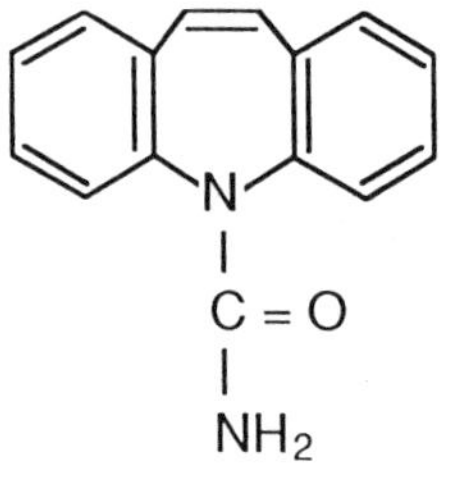

Figure 17.6 Chemical Structure of Carbamazepine

Table 17.5 Available Preparations of Lithium Salts and of Carbamazepine and Usual Doses

Generic Name	Trade Name	Dosage Forms* mg	Daily Doses mg/day
Lithium Carbonate	Eskalith, Lithane, etc.	300 (T,C)	900–1200[a]
Carbamazepine	Tegretol	2 00 (T)	400–800

[a]Dosage must be individualized to a desirable serum level of 0.6–1.2 mEq/L.
*T = Tablet
C = Capsule

References

Research Reports

1. Bach ANJ, Lan NG, Johnson DL, Ahell, CW, Bembenek ME, Kwau SW, Seeberg PH, Shih JC. cDNA cloning of human monoamine oxidase A and B: molecular basis of differences in enzymatic properties. Proc Nat Acad Sci USA 1988;*85*:4934–4938.
2. Delay J, Deniker P, Harl JM, Grasset A. Traitement d'états confusionnels par le chlorate de diméthyl aminopropyl-N-chlorophenothiazine (4500 RP). Ann Med Psychol 1952;*110*:398–403.
3. Schindler W, Häfliger F. Über Derivate des Iminodibenzyls. Helv Chim Acta 1954;*37*:472–480.
4. Kuhn R. The treatment of depressive states with G 22355 (imipramine hydrochloride). Am J Psychiatry 1958;*115*:459–464.
5. Häfliger F. Chemistry of Tofranil. Can Psychiat Assoc J 1959; *4* (Special Suppl.) 69–74.
6. Sulser F, Bickel MH, Brodie BB. The action of desmethylimipramine in counteracting sedation and cholinergic effects of reserpine-like drugs. J Pharmacol Exp Ther 1964;*144*:321–330.
7. Müller JC, Pryor WW, Gibbons JE, Orgain ES. Depression and anxiety occurring during Rauwolfia therapy. J Am Med Assoc 1955;*159*:836–839.
8. Simson PE, Weiss JM. Altered activity of the locus coeruleus in an animal model of depression. Neuro-psychopharmacol 1988;*1*:287–295.
9. Vetulani J, Sulser F. Action of various antidepressant treatment reduces reactivity of noradrenergic cyclic AMP generating system in limbic forebrain. Nature 1975;*257*:495–496.

10. Ordway GA, Gambarana C, Frazer A. Quantitative autoradiography of central beta adrenoceptor subtypes: Comparison of the effects of chronic treatment with desipramine or centrally administered *d*-isoproterenol. J Pharmacol Exp Ther 1988;*247*:379–389.

11. Fauster R, Honegger U, Wiesmann U. Inhibition of phospholipid degradation and changes of the phospholipid pattern by desipramine in cultured human fibroblasts. Biochem Pharmacol 1983;*32*:1737–1744.

12. Mallorga P, Tallman JF, Henneberry RC, Hirata F, Strittmatter WT, Axelrod J. Mepacrine blocks the β-adrenergic agonist induced desensitization in astrocytoma cells. Proc Natl Acad Sci USA 1980;*77*:1341–1345.

13. Sanders-Bush E, Breeding M, Knoth K, Tsutsumi M. Setraline-induced densensitization of the serotonin 5HT-2 receptor transmembrane signaling system. Psychopharmacology 1989;*99*:64–69.

14. Duncan GE, Paul IA, Powell KR, Fassberg SB, Stumpf WE, Breese GR. J Pharmacol Exp Ther 1989;*248*:470–477.

15. Ordway GA, Gambarana C, Tejani-Butt SM, Areso P, Hauptmann W, Frazer A. Preferential reduction of binding of ^{125}I-Iodopindolol to beta$_1$ adrenoceptors in the amygdala of rat after antidepressant treatments. J Pharmacol Exp Ther 1991;*257*:681–690.

16. Cortés R, Soriano E, Pazos A, Probst A, Palacios JM. Autoradiography of antidepressant binding sites in the human brain: Localization using [^{3}H]-imipramine and [^{3}H]-paroxetine. Neuroscience 1988;*27*:473–496.

17. Blakely RD, Berson HE, Fremeau RT Jr, Caron MG, Peek MM, Prince HK, Bradley CC. Cloning and expression of a functional serotonin transporter from rat brain. Nature 1991;*354*:66–70.

18. Hoffman BJ, Mezey E, Brownstein MJ. Cloning of a serotonin transporter affected by antidepressants. Science 1991;*254*:579–80.

19. Insel GR, Zohar T, Benkelfat CH, Murphy DL. Serotonin in obsessions, compulsions, and the control of aggressive impulses. NY Acad Sci 1990;*600*:574–586.

20. deMontigny C, Greenberg F, Mayer A, Deschenes JP. Lithium induces rapid relief of depression in tricyclic antidepressant drug non-responders. Br J Psychiatr 1981;*138*:252–256.

21. Schildkraut JJ. The catecholamine hypothesis of affective disorders: A review of supporting evidence. Am J Psychiatr 1965;*122*:509–522.

22. Coppen A, Wood K. 5-Hydroxytryptamine in the pathogenesis of affective disorders. Adv Biochem Psychopharmacol 1982;*34*:249–258.

23. Coppen A, Prange AJ, Whybrow PC, Noguera R. Abnormalities of indoleamines in affective disorders. Arch Gen Psychiatr 1972;*26*:474–478.

24. Sellinger MD, Mendels J, Frazer A. The effect of psychoactive drugs on beta adrenergic receptor binding sites in rat brain. Neuropharmacology 1980;*19*:447–454.

25. Gravel P, DeMontigny C. Noradrenergic denervation prevents sensitization of rat forebrain neurons to serotonin by tricyclic antidepressant treatment. Synapse 1987;*1*:233–239.

26. Pinder RM. The benefits and risks of antidepressant drugs. Human Psychopharmacol 1988;*3*:73–86.

27. Hammer W, Sjöqvist F. Plasma levels of monomethylated tricyclic antidepressants during treatment with imipramine-like compounds. Life Sci 1967;*6*:1895–1903.

28. Teicher MH, Glod C, Cole JO. Emergence of intense suicidal preoccupation during fluoxetine treatment. Am J Psychiatr 1990;*147*:207–210.

29. Consensus statement by the ACNP; suicidal behavior and psychotropic drug medication. Neuropsychopharmacology 1993;*8*:177–183.

30. Muth EA, Haskins JT, Moyer JA, Husbands GE, Nielsen ST, Sigg EB. Antidepressant biochemical profile of the novel bicyclic compound Wy-45030, an ethyl cyclo-hexanol derivative. Biochem Pharmacol 1986;*35*:4493–4497.

31. Katz RJ, Lott M, Landaw P, Waldmeier P. A clinical test of noradrenergic involvement in the therapeutic mode of action of an experimental antidepressant. Biol Psychiatry 1993;*33*:261–266.

32. Price LH, Charney DS, Delgado P, Heninger GR. Lithium and serotonin function: implications for the serotonin hypothesis of depression. Psychopharmacology 1990;*100*:3–12.

33. Nahorski SR, Ragon CI, Challiss RAJ. Lithium and the phosphoinositide cycle: an example of uncompetitive inhibition and its pharmacological consequences. TIPS 1991;*12*:297–303.

34. DelaFuente TM, Mendlewicz J. Carbamazepine addition in tricyclic antidepressant resistant unipolar depression. Biol Psychiatr 1992;*32*:369–374.

Reviews, monographs, textbooks

r1. Pryor JC, Sulser F. Evolution of the monoamine hypotheses of depression. In Horton RW, Katona C (Eds.) Biological aspects of affective disorders; London: Academic Press, (1990); pp 77–94.

r2. Maxwell RA, White HL. Tricyclic and monoamine oxidase inhibitor antidepressants: Structure–activity relationships. In Iverson LL, Iverson SD, Snyder SH (Eds). Handbook of Psychopharmacology, Volume 14. New York: Plenum Press (1978); pp 83–155.

r3. Frazer A, Offord SJ, Lucki I. (1988). Regulation of serotonin receptors and responsiveness in the brain. In Sanders-Bush E Ed. The serotonin receptors. Clifton, New Jersey: The Humana Press (1988); pp 319–362.

r4. Langer SZ, Galzin AM, Lee CR, Shoemaker H. Antidepressant-binding sites in brain and platelets. In: Antidepressants and receptor function; Ciba Foundation Symposium 123. Chichester, Sussex: John Wiley (1986); pp 3–17.

r5. Bickel, MH. Metabolism of antidepressants. In Hoffmeister F, Stille G (Eds.) Psychotropic Agents, Part I. Berlin: Springer-Verlag, (1980); pp 551–572.

r6. Post RM. Mechanisms of action of carbamazepine and related anticonvulsants in affective illness. In Meltzer HY (Ed). Psychopharmacology: The third generation of progress. New York: Raven Press (1987); pp 567–576.

r7. deMontigny C, Blier P, Chaput Y. Electrophysiological investigation of the effects of antidepressant treatments on serotonin receptors. In Paoletti R, Vanhoutte PM, Brunello N, Maggi FM. Serotonin: from cell biology to pharmacology and therapeutics. (Eds) Dordrecht: Kluver Academic Publishers (1990); pp 499–504.

r8. Baldessarini RJ. Chemotherapy in psychiatry—principles and practice. Cambridge MA: Harvard University Press (1985).

r9. Akiskal HS. (1985). A proposed clinical approach to chronic and "resistant depressions: Evaluation and treatment. J Clin Psychiatr 1985;*46*:32–36.

r10. Davis JM, Freedman DJ, Lindsey RD. A review of the new antidepressant medications. In Davis JM, Maas JW. The Affective Disorders. (Eds) Washington DC: American Psychiatric Press (1983); pp 1–29.

r11. Sulser F. Serotonin-norepinephrine interactions in the brain: Implications for the pharmacology and pathophysiology of affective disorders. J Clin Psychiatr 1987;*48*:12–18.

r12. Sulser F, Sanders-Bush E. The serotonin-norepinephrine link hypothesis of affective disorders: Receptor-receptor interactions in brain. In Ehrlich YH, Lenox RH, Kornecki E, Berry WO. Molecular basis of neuronal responsiveness, (Eds) New York: Plenum Press (1987); pp 439–502.

r13. Youdim MBH, Da Prada M, Amrein R. (Eds) The Cheese effect and new reversible MAO-A inhibitors. J Neural Transm Supplement 26 1988; 136 pages.

r14. Elphick M. Clinical issues in the use of carbamazepine in psychiatry: A review. Psychological Medicine 1989;*19*:591–604.

r15. Schöpf J. Treatment of depression resistant to tricyclic antidepressants, related drugs or MAO-inhibitors by lithium addition: Review of the literature. Pharmacopsychiatr 1989;*22*:174–182.

r16. Refractory Depression. In Amsterdam JD, (ed) Adv Neuropsychol Psychopharmacol Volume 2. New York: Raven Press (1991).

r17. Horton RW, Katona CLE. Biological affects of affective disorders. London: Academic Press, 1991.

r18. Sulser F. Mode of action of antidepressants: From traditional biochemical to molecular neuropsychopharmacology. In Leonard B, Spencer P. Antidepressants. London: CNS Publishers (1990); pp 23–35.

r19. Hyman StE, Nestler EJ. The molecular foundations of psychiatry. Washington, DC: American Psychiatric Press, (1993).

CHAPTER 18

Drug Treatment of Movement Disorders

R. Stanley Burns
J. Martin Rabey

Movement Disorders

Movement disorders are a subgroup of neurological disorders that are operationally defined based on the characteristics of the abnormal movements. The basic types of abnormal movements represent qualitative changes in motor function and behavior and can be produced by a variety of different diseases (Table 18.1). Movement disorders reflect disturbances in extrapyramidal motor function and are a prominent manifestation of diseases affecting the basal ganglia. Although our knowledge of the pathophysiology of the diseases that produce movement disorders is limited, many types of abnormal movements can be symptomatically controlled by the use of drugs. The mechanisms of action of drugs used to treat movement disorders are closely related to the physiological mechanism underlying the abnormal movements.

Basic Types of Movement Disorders

Parkinsonism: The motor syndrome of parkinsonism is specifically attributable to a loss of dopaminergic activity in the striatum. Its cardinal features are bradykinesia, rigidity, resting tremor, flexed posture, and impaired balance. The hallmark of parkinsonism is bradykinesia. The syndrome of parkinsonism can be produced by a number of disorders other than Parkinson's disease. Diseases that produce degeneration of the dopamine neurons in the substantia nigra compacta (SNc) or damage the nigrostriatal dopamine pathway can result in parkinsonism.

Dystonia: Dystonia is a motor syndrome dominated by involuntary, sustained muscle contraction frequently causing twisting and repetitive movements or abnormal postures.[1] A descriptive approach based on the concept of dystonia as a syndrome with emphasis on the body distribution of the abnormal movements has been useful in guiding diagnosis and treatment. The most common forms of dystonia are spasmodic torticollis, oromandibular dystonia, writer's cramp, spasmodic dysphonia, generalized dystonia, and blepharospasm. The physiological mechanism that produces dystonia is unknown. Several different classes of drugs alter dystonia, suggesting that the underlying mechanism is complex and no single dominant factor is involved.

Tremor: Tremor is defined as involuntary, rhythmic oscillations involving any part of the body.[2] The basic types of tremor are rest tremor, action and postural tremor, exaggerated physiological tremor, and tremors associated with cerebellar disease.[r1] Rest tremor occurs when voluntary muscle activity is absent and the limb is fully supported. It is almost always associated with other features of parkinsonism. Action tremor occurs on voluntary muscle activity. It is commonly associated with a postural tremor that occurs on maintenance of a posture. Action and postural tremor are prominent features of the disorder known as essential tremor. There are a number of variants of these basic tremor types as well as rarer forms of tremors.

Chorea: Chorea is made up of rapid, jerky, purposeless movements that appear to be random in their location and timing and

Table 18.1 Basic Types of Movement Disorder

Parkinsonism
Dystonia
Chorea
Tremor
Myoclonus
Motor tics
Motor restlessness
Hypertonicity
Muscle spasms
Ataxia

occur both at rest and during voluntary movements. A variety of different disease processes can lead to the development of chorea.

Myoclonus: Myocolonus is comprised of very rapid, brief, shock-like, jerky movements that occur spontaneously or in response to sensory stimuli or voluntary motor activity. The basic types of myoclonus include cortical, subcortical, and spinal myoclonus.[r2] They differ in the sites of origin of the abnormal discharges that produce the movements. Myoclonus can be produced by a wide variety of different disease processes occurring at different levels in the central nervous system. A hyperexcitability of neurons is thought to be the common mechanism of myoclonus.

Motor Tics: Tics are simple or complex, jerky or rapid, stereotyped movements that most often affect the face and head and are associated with an inner obsession and are voluntarily suppressible. Chronic motor tics accompanied by vocal tics are seen in Gilles de la Tourette syndrome.[r3]

Motor Restlessness: The distinguishing features of disorders of motor restlessness are the presence of a subjective component and the fact that the associated movements, like voluntary movements, are comprised of normal elements. Akathisia is a state of generalized motor restlessness manifesting as ceaseless movements of the limbs and changes in body position associated with a state of inner tension. It is most often a side effect of treatment with neuroleptic drugs, but can also occur in disorders such as Parkinson's disease and postencephalitic parkinsonism. Tardive akathisia represents a delayed response to the use of neuroleptic drugs and responds differently to drugs than the more typical forms of akathisia. In restless leg syndrome, there is a peculiar sensation in the lower legs which is associated with the need to consciously move the legs or walk.

Hypertonicity: Disorders of muscle tone are frequently associated with movement disorders and can affect voluntary movement when present in isolation. Rigidity represents a general increase in muscle tone that is typically present in both limb and axial muscles. It is one component of the motor syndrome of parkinsonism. Spasticity is a velocity-dependent increase in muscle tone associated with hyperreflexia and other features of the upper motor neuron syndrome.[r4] In pure spasticity, walking and leg movements have a stiff quality. In addition to rigidity and spasticity, the component of increased muscle tone in dystonia and the rigid state in neuroleptic malignant syndrome might also be considered to be forms of hypertonicity.

Muscle Spasms: Disorders producing muscle spasms are a heterogeneous group of disorders. This category includes common disorders such as hemifacial spasm, dystonic spasms, and extensor and flexor spasms related to spasticity as well as rare conditions such as stiff-man syndrome[r5] and progressive muscle spasm syndrome.[3]

Ataxia: Ataxia refers to incoordination of the movements of the limbs or of the gait. The physiological mechanisms involved in the coordination of movement are complex and involve the cerebellum and its circuits.

The Basal Ganglia and The Extrapyramidal Motor System

The extrapyramidal motor system is a clinically based concept referring to the basal ganglia and their circuitry.[r6] The basal ganglia are now considered to include the caudate nucleus, putamen, globus pallidus, subthalamic nucleus, and substantia nigra.[r7] Other structures that are part of the basal ganglia circuitry and play an important role in extrapyramidal motor function are the premotor cortex, primary motor cortex, and thalamus. The somatotopic organization of function is preserved within the basal ganglia and its circuits (Fig. 18.1).

There have been important recent contributions to our knowledge of the circuitry of the basal ganglia.[4] Interest has centered on the role in motor function of the nuclear complex comprised of the putamen, the internal (GPi) and external (GPe) segments of the globus pallidus, the subthalamic nucleus (STN) and the SNc. Widespread cortical inputs to the striatum influence the activity of the motor cortex via this complex. The single input nucleus of this complex is the putamen. The single output nucleus is the GPi. The key to an understanding of the function of this nuclear complex is knowledge of the two parallel pathways that connect the putamen to the GPi and the modulating role of the SNc.

The input to the putamen from the cortex involves glutamatergic neurons and has been shown to be excitatory in nature. The putamen in turn projects to the GPi via two pathways, the so-called "direct" and "indirect"

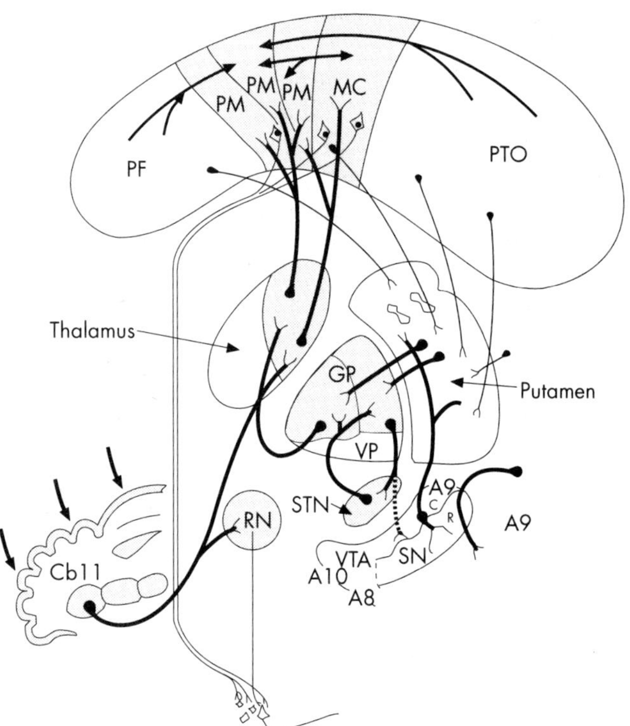

Figure 18.1 Schematic of extrapyramidal motor system. Pallido-thalamo-cortical and cerebello-thalamo-cortical pathways in heavy lines. Also shown in heavy lines are inputs to globus pallidus from the striatum and the putamen and the pallido-subthalamo-pallidal loop. MC, motor cortex; PM, premotor cortex; PF, prefrontal cortex; PTO, parieto-temporo-occipital association cortex; GP, globus pallidus; SN, substantia nigra; A9, dopaminergic cells comprising substantia nigra compacta; STN, subthalamic nucleus.[r104]

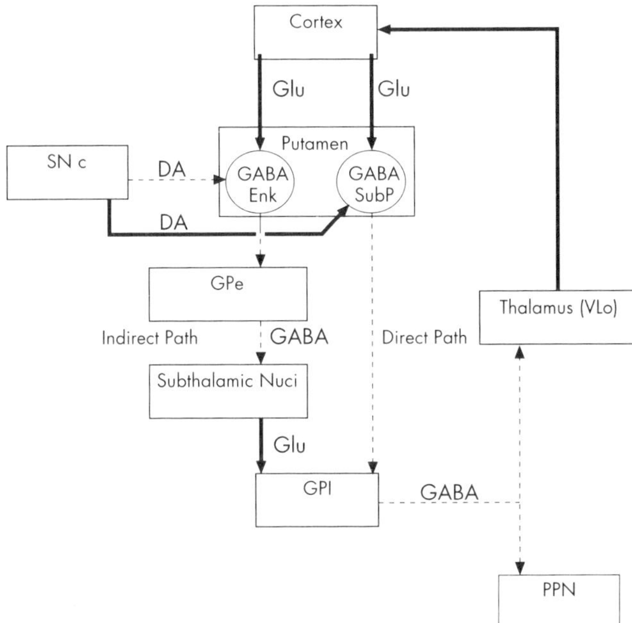

Figure 18.2 Schematic of "direct" and "indirect" pathways. Solid lines indicate excitatory pathways and dashed lines indicate inhibitory pathways. Glu, glutamate; GABA, γ-aminobutyric acid; Enk, enkephalin; SubP, substance P; SNc, substantia nigra compacta; GPe, external division of globus pallidus; GPi, internal division of globus pallidus; PPN, pedunculopontine nucleus; VLo, pars oralis of ventrolateral thalamus.[r105]

pathways.[4] This concept is illustrated in Figure 18.2. The "direct" pathway from the putamen to the GPi involves both GABA and substance P neurons and is thought to be primarily inhibitory in nature. The "indirect" pathway is more complex and involves two other nuclei, the GPe and STN. The primary projection from the putamen to the GPe via GABA and enkephalin neurons and the secondary projection from the GPe to the STN via GABA neurons are both inhibitory pathways. The tertiary projection from the STN to the GPi is excitatory and involves glutamatergic neurons. The output from this nuclear complex to the motor cortex occurs via inhibitory GABA neurons that project from the GPi to the thalamus and excitatory neurons in the thalamus that project to the motor cortex. The dopaminergic neurons of the SNc project to the putamen leading to excitation of striatal neurons of origin of the "direct" pathway and inhibition of neurons of the "indirect" pathway and, thus, modulate activity in both pathways.

The basal ganglia is one of the most chemically complex regions of the brain.[r8] Chemical transmission in extrinsic and intrinsic projections and of interneurons of these nuclei involve several different neurotransmitter and neuromodulator systems and multiple subtypes of receptors. The principal neurotransmitter systems involved include: glutamatergic projections from the cortex to the striatum; dopaminergic projections from the SNc to the striatum; cholinergic striatal interneurons; GABAergic projections from the striatum to the GPi and GPe; glutamatergic projections from the STN to the GPi; and, GABAergic projections from the GPi to the thalamus. The basal ganglia and its connections comprise a complex network of neurotransmitter-specific pathways with functional localization.

Because cerebellar disorders produce abnormalities of movement and tone in the absence of weakness, the cerebellum and its connections are considered to be closely related to the extrapyramidal motor system.[r6]

Changes in muscle tone are associated with abnormalities of movement. An example of this is the effect of pure spasticity on voluntary movements. The pyramidal tract and associated descending motor pathways and spinal circuits play an important role in the production of spasticity.

Muscle spasms and other forms of overactivity of muscle can also alter voluntary movement and posture. These disorders involve the basic mechanisms of neuromuscular transmission and muscle fiber contraction.

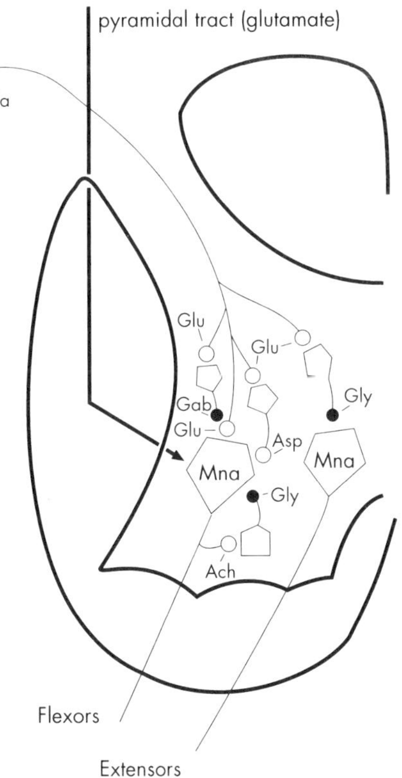

Figure 18.3 Spinal pathways and circuits involved in spasticity. αMn, alpha motor neuron; ACh, acetylcholine; Gly, glycine; Glu, glutamate; GABA, γ-aminobutyric acid; ASP, aspartate.[r68]

Pharmacology of Drugs Used to Treat Movement Disorders

L-Dihydroxyphenylalanine (L-DOPA, Levodopa)

History: In 1960, Ehringer and Hornykiewicz discovered that dopamine levels in the striatum, substantia nigra and globus pallidus were low in Parkinson's disease.[216] In 1962, Birkmeyer and Hornykiewicz reported that 50–150 mg of L-DOPA administrated intravenously produced a decrease in akinesia in patients with Parkinson's disease.[217,218] The effects were maximal at 2–3 hr and lasted up to 24 hr. MAO inhibitors intensified the effects and dopamine, D-DOPA and 5-HTP did not produce these effects. In the same year, Barbeau and his colleagues reported that small oral doses of L-DOPA temporarily decreased rigidity and, when combined with MAO inhibitors, reduced akinesia.[r77] In 1967, Cotzias reported that 3–16 gm of oral DL-DOPA given over long periods of time could produce a marked and persistent improvement in the symptoms and signs of Parkinson's disease.[219]

Chemistry: L-DOPA, (-)-3(3,4-dihydroxyphenyl)-L-alanine, the naturally occurring form of DOPA, exists as a zwitterion at physiological pH. It is readily soluble in dilute hydrochloric acid, but has limited solubility in water (1.65 mg/ml).[r9] In the presence of moisture, L-DOPA is oxidized by oxygen in the air to form a dark brown product.

Pharmacological effects: The amino acid L-DOPA is the biological precursor of dopamine and other catecholamines. L-DOPA exerts its effects only after being metabolized to dopamine. Dopamine is a neurotransmitter and an intermediate in the biosynthesis of norepinephrine and epinephrine. The enzyme aromatic L-amino acid decarboxylase (AADC), which is present in various peripheral organs and the brain, represents the biological receptor for L-DOPA. L-DOPA must enter catecholamine-containing neurons in the brain and be decarboxylated to dopamine to exert its central actions.

In the normal state, dopamine in the brain is synthesized within the neuron from tyrosine, which originates in blood. The metabolism of tyrosine to L-DOPA by the cytosolic enzyme tyrosine hydroxylase (TH) is the rate-limiting step in the synthesis of dopamine. L-DOPA synthesized from tyrosine is rapidly metabolized within the cytoplasm to dopamine by the enzyme AADC. In pathological states with reduced TH activity, the rate of synthesis of L-DOPA is low. When exogenous L-DOPA is administered, blood becomes the source of L-DOPA for catecholamine neurons in the brain. L-DOPA, like tyrosine, is transported across the brain capillary endothelial cell and nerve cell membrane by the L-system, a carrier-mediated transport system for neutral amino acids with branched or ringed side chains.[r10] L-DOPA entering cells containing AADC is thought to be metabolized nonselectively to dopamine. AADC is found almost exclusively within catecholaminergic and serotonergic neurons in the brain.[5,6] The highest levels of activity of AADC are found in the caudate nucleus and putamen.[7,8] In experimental animals, the systemic administration of L-DOPA leads to a dose-dependent increase in brain dopamine levels and an increase in the activity of dopamine at D1 and D2 receptors in the striatum.[9,10] Whether dopamine synthesized from extracellular L-DOPA within serotonergic nerve terminals in the striatum plays a role in the motor effects of L-DOPA is uncertain.[11,12,r11]

The absorption of L-DOPA across the wall of the gastrointestinal tract is restricted to the upper small intestine and occurs via the L-transport system.[13,14,15] Absorption is relatively rapid with peak plasma levels occurring 1–3 hr after ingestion.[14,16,17] The occurrence of multiple peaks in plasma suggests that gastrointestinal function influences absorption. AADC activity is high in the mucosa of the gastrointestinal tract including the stomach, which accounts for the extensive first pass metabolism of L-DOPA after oral administration.[18,19,20] L-DOPA is not absorbed from the stomach. A delay in gastric emptying can lead to metabolism of L-DOPA by AADC within the stomach reducing its bioavailability. The action of dopamine on local receptors can further slow emptying. The capacity of the mucosal L-transport system is high and normally occurring concentrations of amino acids in the intestine probably do not saturate it.[13]

Based on studies in the mouse, L-DOPA is widely distributed and accumulates in the pancreas, salivary glands, gut, liver, kidneys, and skin after intraperitoneal administration.[21] Only about 0.1% of the dose is found in the form of DOPA or dopamine in the brain. The entry of L-DOPA into the brain can be competitively inhibited by high blood concentrations of other natural substrates of the L-transport system including phenylalanine, tyrosine, tryptophan, leucine, isoleucine, methionine, valine, and histadine.[22] The apparent Km value of L-DOPA resulting from competition from other amino acids is determined by the equation $Km(aa) = Km\ (1 + [AAi]/Km)$, where [AAi] is the concentration of an competing amino acid (i) and Km is the absolute Km for L-DOPA.[23] The reversal of the clinical effects of an intravenous infusion of L-DOPA by the administration of a large dose of phenylalanine presumably occurs by this mechanism.[24] There is a substantial uptake of L-DOPA into muscle tissue, which is deficient in AADC and COMT.[25]

Up to 90% of an oral dose of L-DOPA is metabolized prior to reaching the systemic circulation.[26–30] This takes place mainly in the gastrointestinal tract with the liver contributing little to the presystemic metabolism of L-DOPA. After intavenous administration, decarboxylation of L-DOPA by AADC accounts for about 70% of its elimination.[30] It is metabolized primarily by AADC in the gastrointestinal wall, although this enzyme is present in liver, kidney, and other tissues and the transport of L-DOPA across cell membranes of these tissues is relatively unrestricted.[18,r12] AADC is also contained within sympathetic noradrenergic neurons and chromaffin cells of the adrenal gland, but this represents only a small fraction of the total.

Decarboxylation of L-DOPA in peripheral tissues results in the formation of dopamine, which is further metabolized to 3,4-dihydroxyphenylacetic acid (DOPAC) and homovanillic acid (HVA). Other pathways of metabolism include 3-*O*-methylation, oxidative deamination, and transamination.[32,33,r13] The major urinary metabolites of L-DOPA in humans are HVA, DOPAC, and vanillyl-lactic acid, the end product of 3-*O*-methylation.[29,34–36,r13] Less than 1% of an oral dose of L-DOPA is found unchanged in urine and up to 5% is excreted as dopamine. Only a small fraction is excreted as vanilmandelic acid, a metabolite of norepinephrine.[37,38] The major pathway for the metabolism of extracellular L-DOPA in the brain is decarboxylation by AADC. AADC in the brain is localized to nerve cells and found almost exclusively within catecholaminergic and serotonergic neurons. The degree to which extracellular L-DOPA is metabolized by COMT contained within glial cells and other neurons is unknown. Dopamine formed from extracellular L-DOPA is further metabolized by MAO and COMT to DOPAC, 3-methoxytyramine and HVA. In humans, the end product of the metabolism of L-DOPA in the brain is HVA.

The distribution half-life of L-DOPA in humans is about 5–10 min.[39–42,r14] Its plasma elimination half-life is estimated to be 0.6–0.9 hr.[15,29,42,43] In the presence of inhibitors of AADC, the plasma half-life is increased to 1.3–2.2 hr.[41] The oral administration of 250 mg of L-DOPA results in peak plasma levels in the range of 1 to 4 μg/ml. The plasma half-life of the metabolite 3-*O*-methyl-DOPA is about 15–17 hr.[44,r15]

Preparations of L-DOPA: L-DOPA (levodopa) is available alone (Dopar, Laradopa), in a fixed combination with carbidopa at a weight ratio (carbidopa to levodopa) of 1:10 (Sinemet 10/100, Sinemet 25/250) or 1:4 (Sinemet 25/100) and in combination with benserazide at a ratio of 1:4 (Madopar 62.5, Madopar 125, Madopar 250). Symptomatic treatment of Parkinson's disease with L-DOPA alone requires a dose in the range of 1.6–6 g per day.[r17] When used in combination with a peripheral decarboxylase inhibitor, the required daily dose of L-DOPA is in the range of 200–2000 mg (see Table 18.3).

Oral preparations of L-DOPA that release the drug at a slow rate have been developed.[r18] (see Table 18.3) Sinemet CR (Sinemet 25/100 CR, Sinemet 50/200 CR) is a slow-eroding polymer matrix containing carbidopa and L-DOPA, which releases its contents into the stomach over 2–2.5 hr and prolongs the absorption of L-DOPA.[48] Peak levels of L-DOPA occur at 1.6 hr.[49] The bioavailability of Sinemet CR is 20–30% less than standard Sinemet preparations.[r18] Madopar HBS remains in the stomach and forms a mucous body that floats on the gastric contents and slowly releases L-DOPA and benserazide over 6–8 hr.[50] Peak L-DOPA levels occur at about 2–4 hr after ingestion of Madopar HBS.[r18] Its bioavailability is 40–50% less than the standard forms of Madopar.[r18]

Incompatibilities: Co-administration of iron preparations containing the ferrous ion can lead to oxidation of up to 50% of a dose of L-DOPA prior to its absorption.[51] Anticholinergic drugs, which delay gastric emptying, can decrease the bioavailability and slow the absorption of L-DOPA.[52,53] Pyridoxine (vitamin B6) when transformed to pyridoxal phosphate increases the activity of peripheral AADC and limits the therapeutic effects of L-DOPA when given alone.[r13,r15] In the presence of a peripheral decarboxylase inhibitor, pyridoxine does not interfere with the effects of L-DOPA.[r19] The antihypertensive agent alpha-methyldopa enters the brain and can act as a weak inhibitor of AADC potentially reducing the rate of decarboxylation of L-DOPA to dopamine in the brain.[54] Reserpine reduces the vesicular storage of dopamine in neurons and might interfere with the therapeutic effects L-DOPA. Phenothiazines, butyrophenones, and other dopamine antagonists can completely block the therapeutic effects of L-DOPA. MAO A inhibitors when used concurrently with L-DOPA can produce hypertension.[r20]

Therapeutic Use in Parkinson's Disease: L-DOPA is the most effective and widely used drug in the treatment of Parkinson's disease. An estimated 85% of patients respond to L-DOPA with about 15% of patients showing no improvement.[76,220] L-DOPA acts on all of the motor signs and symptoms of Parkinson's disease[217,219,221–223] but not all of the features improve to the same degree.[76,220,224] L-DOPA is more effective in reducing bradykinesia and rigidity than in suppressing resting tremor. Complex motor functions like writing, speech and swallowing show the least improvement. It is questionable whether balance improves to any extent. Bradyphrenia can also improve in response to L-DOPA. L-DOPA therapy greatly improves longevity and general state of health in patients with Parkinson's disease.[r17]

The effects of L-DOPA are dependent on the stage of the disease.[224] Bradykinesia and tremor, which respond well to L-DOPA, are prominent features of the early stages of the disease. Dysarthria, dysphagia, and balance impairment, which respond poorly, are features of the later stages of the disease. Certain aspects of the motor response to L-DOPA change with progression of the underlying disease. The duration of the motor effects becomes shorter and shorter and the dose which produces chorea becomes progressively smaller.[225] These changes appear to be related to the severity of the underlying disease rather than chronic exposure to L-DOPA since they can occur within weeks of beginning L-DOPA therapy.[226,227]

Atypical parkinsonism: L-DOPA is also highly effective in the postencephalitic, MPTP-induced, and reserpine-induced forms of parkinsonism and neuroleptic persistent parkinsonism. In other disorders producing parkinsonism, such as progressive supranuclear palsy and multiple system atrophy, its effectiveness is limited. It does not reverse acute neuroleptic-induced parkinsonism.

Other: In addition to Parkinson's disease, treatment with oral L-DOPA produces a improvement in the symptoms of DOPA-responsive dystonia and restless leg syndrome. In addition to its motor effects, L-DOPA is effective in suppressing the sensory or subjective component of restless leg syndrome and the leg pain associated with the "off" state in Parkinson's disease.

Treatment Problems with L-DOPA

Clinical fluctuations: The duration of the response to oral L-DOPA becomes progressively shorter (from 4–8 hr to <2 hr) as the disease advances leading to predictable wearing off of the effects prior to the next dose and to fluctuations in motor function during the day, referred to as clinical or motor fluctuations.[228,229] The onset (15 min to 1 hr) and termination (1–3 hr) of the effects become more abrupt also. In contrast to simple wearing off, on–off reactions are abrupt and extreme switches between mobility and akinesia occurring over 5–10 minutes or less.[230,r78] Although seemingly random, the timing of the off periods has been shown to be related to the ingestion of L-DOPA.[42,r78] On–off reactions may be associated with alterations in mood or the ability to concentrate or with the occurrence of pain or anxiety during the off state. More than 50% of patients (10% per year) with Parkinson's disease develop clinical fluctuations after 2–5 years of chronic L-DOPA therapy.[228,230–232] An estimated 15% of patients develop on-off reactions after 6 years of treatment with L-DOPA.[230]

Clinical fluctuations appear to be related to alterations in the level of dopamine available to act in the striatum. In rats with unilateral 6-OHDA lesions of the nigrostriatal dopamine pathway, peak striatal dopamine concentrations on the lesioned side are lower and fall more rapidly after L-DOPA than on the control side.[233] In patients with on–off reactions, injections of apomorphine and lisuride can rapidly reverse akinesia suggesting that postsynaptic receptor mechanisms remain intact during the off periods.[42,234,235] The loss of the storage capacity of synaptic vesicles due to continual degeneration of dopamine terminals in the striatum has been proposed as the mechanism responsible for clinical fluctuations.[236] Other proposed mechanisms include a desensitization or depolarization block of dopamine receptors,[232,r79] an inhibitory effect of L-DOPA,[237] a reduction in striatal AADC activity by end-product inhibition[238,r78] and axonal sprouting of surviving dopamine neurons with loss of synchronization of function.[r17]

The relationship between the plasma levels of L-DOPA and its motor effects in Parkinson's disease is complex and changes during the course of the illness.[229] In patients with mild disease who have a stable response to oral L-DOPA, no direct relationship between the plasma concentration and therapeutic effects is found. In patients with advanced Parkinson's disease who exhibit clinical fluctuations, the motor effects are closely related to the plasma levels of L-DOPA. It has now been demonstrated in several studies that patients with clinical fluctuations on oral L-DOPA show a stable response during a constant-rate intravenous infusion of L-DOPA producing steady-state levels above 1–2 μg/ml.[24,239,240] Thus, in patients with advanced disease, the plasma kinetics of L-DOPA become a major factor influencing dopaminergic activity in the brain.

Altering the dosage schedule by giving smaller, more frequent doses is the simplest approach to reducing the variation in blood levels of L-DOPA. Slow or continuous release formulations of L-DOPA (Sinemet-CR, Madopar HBS) have proved to be moderately effective in reducing fluctuations.[241,r80,r81] Continuous intravenous infusions of L-DOPA are impractical because of the low solubility and poor stability of L-DOPA in aqueous solutions at physiological pH. The delivery of L-DOPA by constant rate infusions into the duodenum via a jejuenostomy tube is limited by the problems with large volume infusion pumps and the need for surgery.[242] The use of COMT inhibitors in combination with peripheral decarboxylase inhibitors has the potential to significantly reduce clinical fluctuations.[243] In some cases, MAO-B inhibitors can prolong the effects of L-DOPA and reduce fluctuations. Combined therapy with synthetic dopamine agonists which have a longer duration of action can provide a moderate antiparkinson effect during the wearing off phase. The use of subcutaneous infusions of apomorphine or lisuride is effective but limited by the frequent development of psychosis and the occurrence of nodules and abscesses at the infusion site.

Because plasma levels of L-DOPA are less variable over time with Sinemet CR than after standard Sinemet. The use of Sinemet CR reduces the required frequency of the doses and the number of daily off periods.[r18] These slow release preparations of L-DOPA are useful for patients with simple wearing off, nocturnal akinesia or off dystonia occurring on awakening in the morning. They are usually not helpful in patients with complicated fluctuations or on–off reactions. The use of a slow release preparations can produce prolonged periods of dyskinesia in patients who are sensitive to L-DOPA. When used at bedtime, they can produce an increase in vivid dreams or hallucinations or nocturnal dyskinesia. A greater delay to onset is consistent with a slower rate of absorption and a longer time to reach peak concentrations.

Loss of efficacy: The need for a higher dose of L-DOPA to maintain the same degree of symptomatic improvement in Parkinson's disease is a measure of loss of efficacy. After the initial dose of L-DOPA is optimized, efficacy usually declines requiring an increase in the dose of L-DOPA within 6–24 months. Over the course of the illness, L-DOPA can continue to be effective in reversing bradykinesia and rigidity for more than 10–20 years. Even in patients with severe akinesia during their off periods, the maximal effect of L-DOPA can be striking. The development of dysarthria, dysphagia and postural instability in the later stages of the disease, features which are less responsive to L-DOPA, might add to the impression that the efficacy of L-DOPA has declined.[224] The observed loss of the efficacy of L-DOPA is thought to be due to the more extensive degenerative changes in presynaptic and postsynaptic structures and nondopaminergic neurons with progression of the underlying disease.[224,r17]

Side Effects: The acute side effects of L-DOPA are related to high circulating levels of dopamine formed from L-DOPA in peripheral tissues. Anorexia, nausea, and vomiting are thought to be due to the action of dopamine on receptors in the region of the area postrema and chemoreceptor trigger zone in the brainstem.[r21] Cardiovascular side effects of L-DOPA include postural hypotension. A peripheral mechanism involving dopamine and baroreceptor reflexes and a central mechanism involving cardiovascular regulatory centers and resting blood pressure have been proposed.[55–58,r12] Symptomatic and persistent problems with orthostatic hypotension in response to L-DOPA are seen in multiple system atrophy with autonomic impairment (Shy–Drager syndrome). Dopamine formed from L-DOPA also stimulates cardiac β-adrenergic receptors and can produce cardiac arrhythmias.[r12] This most commonly takes the form of asymptomatic ventricular irritability with extra systoles. Increased urinary frequency at night might be related to the effects of L-DOPA on glomerular filtration, renal plasma flow and Na+ excretion.[r15] Other side effects include pupillary dilation and a brownish discoloration of urine, saliva and vaginal secretions.[r13] L-DOPA can also induce myoclonus.

Patients with postencephalitic parkinsonism develop more unusual side effects of L-DOPA including oculogyric crises, motor tics, and behavioral changes. Theoretically, there is a risk that L-DOPA generates superoxide radicals or other metabolic products that are harmful in Parkinson's disease and other degenerative diseases.[60–62] Increased growth of malignant melanomas has also been reported.[63]

Dyskinesia: A major side effect of chronic L-DOPA treatment in Parkinson's disease is dyskinesia. Patients with Parkinson's disease frequently develop choreoathetotic movements in response to L-DOPA, which are referred to as dyskinesia. It generally appears simultaneously with onset of the antiparkinson effect and is maximal at the time of peak plasma levels of L-DOPA. Dyskinesia frequently begins and is greatest in intensity on the side first affected by Parkinson's disease.[r17] It usually affects the limbs and the neck more than the face, tongue, jaw, and trunk.[r17] Dyskinesia is often mild at first but increases in severity and becomes more widespread in its distribution with time.[r17] As the disease progresses, smaller and smaller doses of L-DOPA induce dyskinetic movements.[244,r23] They may progress to the point of interfering with speech, the use of the arms and walking and producing severe disability. The presence of dyskinesia is correlated with the duration of Parkinson's disease.[r17] It is generally more marked in patients who develop the disease before the age of 50 years.[r22]

The development of striatal dopamine receptor supersensitivity secondary to degeneration of substantia nigra dopamine neurons has been proposed as the mechanism underlying dyskinesia in response to L-DOPA.[245–247,r17] Dyskinesia can also be induced by apomorphine, a D1 and D2 receptor agonist, a finding which is consistent with a dopaminergic mechanism.[248] Bromocriptine, a selective D2 agonist, rarely if ever induces dyskinesia suggesting that activity at the D1 receptor is important in the production of dyskinesia.[r22]

The intensity of dyskinesia is related to the size of the individual dose of L-DOPA and the resultant plasma levels of L-DOPA.[249] The use of smaller doses of L-DOPA given more frequently can reduce dyskinesia. If dyskinesia is severe, the dose of L-DOPA may be limited to 50 mg or less and require an interval of 90 min or less. The addition of a dopamine agonist and secondary reduction of the dose of L-DOPA can also reduce dyskinesia. The concurrent use of MAO-B inhibitors and anticholinergics can increase dyskinesia by indirect mechanisms.[168,250,r19] It is not known if it is damaging to the brain to maintain a mild to moderate dyskinetic state.

Psychosis: Psychosis is a side effect of chronic treatment with L-DOPA in advanced Parkinson's disease. The mechanism of psychosis is thought to be dopamine receptor supersensitivity in the limbic regions of the brain. Vivid dreams occur initially and progress to visual hallucinations at night and later to daytime hallucinations with a loss of insight. This is frequently associated with a paranoid state. In the past, L-DOPA treatment was withdrawn with the attendant risks of aspiration, deep vein thrombosis or injury due to falling. The treatment approach has changed with the availability of clozapine, a novel antipsychotic agent that is devoid of extrapyramidal side effects.[r82] Clozapine suppresses the psychotic symptoms and does not interfere with the antiparkinson effects of L-DOPA. A dose of clozapine in the range of 6.25–100 mg per day is effective.

Peripheral Decarboxylase Inhibitors

Carbidopa, Benserazide

Pharmacological Effects: Carbidopa, (-)-L-*a*-hydrazino-3,4-dihydroxy-*a*-methylbenzene proprionic acid, and benserazide, (+–)-DL-seryl-2-(2,3,4-trihydroxybenzyl) hydrazine, are reversible inhibitors of AADC[64,65] in peripheral tissues and blood. Structures of the peripheral AADC inhibitors are shown in Fig. 18.4. They inhibit AADC contained within capillary endothelial cells of the cerebral vessels,[66] the so-called enzymatic blood-brain barrier, but do not enter the brain and, therefore, are devoid of central activity. When used in combination with L-DOPA, their major effect is on the presystemic metabolism of L-DOPA to dopamine in the gut. Inhibitors of AADC, which are restricted by the blood-brain barrier to tissues outside the central nervous system, are referred to as extracerebral or peripheral decarboxylase inhibitors.

In humans, 40–70% of an oral dose of carbidopa is absorbed with peak concentrations occurring at 0.5–5 hr after administration.[67,68] In the case of benserazide, 66–74% of an oral dose is absorbed with peak concentrations occurring within 1 hr.[69] Carbidopa and benserazide are concentrated in the kidneys, lungs, small intestine, and liver with lower concentrations found in the heart.[r15] These compounds do not enter the brain to any significant extent.[69,r25] In the rat, carbidopa crosses into the placenta and appears in breast milk.[r15] The plasma half-life of carbidopa is about 2 hr.[r15] The half-life of benserazide in plasma is less than 2 hr.[r15]

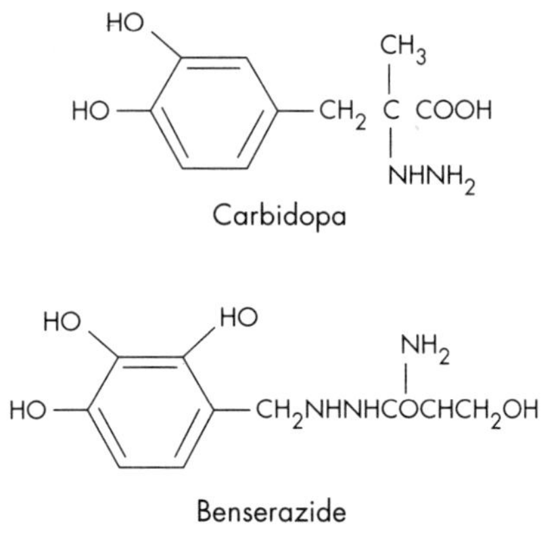

The co-administration of a peripheral decarboxylase inhibitor with oral L-DOPA increases the bioavailability of L-DOPA and the plasma concentrations of L-DOPA (2–10 fold).[70–74] In the presence of a peripheral decarboxylase inhibitor, 3-*O*-methylation of L-DOPA by COMT becomes the major pathway of metabolism of L-DOPA.[32,33] Because of the presence of alternate metabolic pathways, the change in the plasma half-life of L-DOPA produced by peripheral decarboxylase inhibitors (from 0.6–0.9 hr to 1.3–2.2 hr) is limited. The chronic administration of carbidopa leads to a 3-fold increase in plasma AADC activity in humans.[75]

Therapeutic Use: Peripheral decarboxylase inhibitors reduce the oral dose of L-DOPA that is required in Parkinson's disease and alleviate most of the acute side effects of L-DOPA. The average daily dose of L-DOPA needed to reverse the symptoms of Parkinson's disease, when administered alone, is 3.5–4.5 g (range 0.5–12 g/day).[76,r17] Combined treatment with a peripheral decarboxylase inhibitor reduces this dose by about 75% to 800 mg (range 300–1200 mg).[r17] Carbidopa and benserazide inhibit the metabolism of L-DOPA to dopamine by AADC in peripheral tissues and thus prevent high circulating levels of dopamine and the associated side effects of nausea and vomiting, orthostatic hypotension, cardiac arrhythmias, and pupillary dilation. These compounds do not influence side effects of L-DOPA, which are due to its central actions such as dyskinesia.

L-DOPA is routinely administered in combination with carbidopa or benserazide. Carbidopa is available in a fixed combination with L-DOPA at a weight ratio of 1:10 or 1:4. The combination of benserazide and L-DOPA is available in a ratio of 1:4. Patients with Parkinson's disease typically receive a total of 30–150 mg of carbidopa per day. It has been estimated that a minimum of 75 mg per day of carbidopa is required to produce adequate inhibition of peripheral decarboxylase activity.[73,77,78]

The use of peripheral decaboxylase inhibitors prevents the gastrointestinal side effects of L-DOPA in most patients. In patients with persistent gastrointestinal intolerance to combination preparations of L-DOPA and peripheral decarboxylase inhibitors, pretreatment with domperidone can control these side effects. Mild postural hypotension secondary to L-DOPA is relatively common but generally asymptomatic. Peripheral decaboxylase inhibitors influence only the peripheral

HO
HO — [benzene ring] — CH_2 — C(CH_3)($NHNH_2$) — COOH

Carbidopa

HO HO
HO — [benzene ring] — $CH_2NHNHCOCH(NH_2)CH_2OH$

Benserazide

Figure 18.4 Structure of Peripheral AADC Inhibitors

component of the underlying mechanism. Symptomatic postural hypotension is treated with elastic stockings or 9-*a*-fludrocortisone and an increase in sodium intake.[r17,r22,r23] Supplemental doses of carbidopa or propranolol have been used to limit the cardiac effects of L-DOPA.[59,r12,r24] The optimum daily dose of carbidopa appears to vary between individuals with some patients requiring more than 200 mg of carbidopa per day to control the gastrointestinal side effects of L-DOPA.[79] Carbidopa (Lodosyn 25 mg) is available to be used as a supplement to the fixed combination in patients requiring a higher dose (see Table 18.3).

Catechol-O-Methyltransferase (COMT) Inhibitors

Tolcapone, Entacapone

Biochemical effects: Tolcapone, 3,4-dihydroxy-4′-methyl-5-nitrobenzophenone, and entacapone, *N,N*-diethyl-2-cyano-3-(3, 4-dihydroxy-5-nitrophenyl) acrylamide, are selective and reversible, competitive inhibitors of COMT.[80,81] The structures of these compounds are found in Figure 18.5.

Therapeutic Use: The elimination rate and half-life of L-DOPA become important in advanced Parkinson's disease because of the close relationship between the plasma kinetics of oral L-DOPA and fluctuations in motor function. In the presence of a peripheral decarboxylase inhibitor, 3-*O*-methylation of L-DOPA by COMT becomes the major pathway for the metabolism of L-DOPA. This shift to an alternate route of metabolism limits the effect of peripheral decarboxylase inhibitors on the rate of elimination of L-DOPA.

Tolcapone and entacapone are nontoxic, potent inhibitors of COMT, which have been developed to be used in combination with peripheral decarboxylase inhibitors to further reduce the peripheral metabolism of exogenous L-DOPA. These agents substantially decrease the plasma clearance rate and increase the plasma half-life of L-DOPA.[82,83] Unlike AADC inhibitors, the central activity of COMT inhibitors does not interfere with the mechanism of action of L-DOPA. To the contrary, central inhibition of COMT might augment the effects of L-DOPA by inhibiting the metabolism of extracellular L-DOPA or the catabolism of dopamine.

HO, HO, CO, CH_3, NO_2

Tolcapone

HO, HO, CHCNCON, C_2H_5, C_2H_5, NO_2

Entacapone

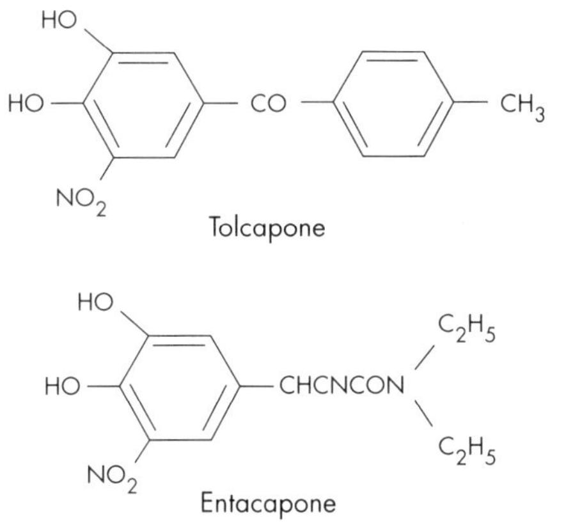

Figure 18.5 Structure of COMT Inhibitors

Monoamine Oxidase (MAO) Inhibitors

Deprenyl (Selegiline)

Pharmacological effects: Deprenyl, (−)-deprenyl, R(−)-*N,a*-dimethyl-*N*-(2-prop-2-inyl)-phenethylamine hydrochloride, is a selective,[84,85,r26,r27] "suicide" inhibitor of MAO type B (MAO-B).[r28,r29] Its structure is shown in Figure 18.6. It is metabolized by MAO-B to form a product which binds irreversibly to the covalently bound flavin moiety of MAO.[86] Because deprenyl is selective for MAO-B, it inhibits the oxidation of dopamine and phenylethylamine (PEA) but not that of serotonin or norepinephrine.[87,r30] In humans, a dose of 10 mg/day produces complete inhibition of platelet MAO,[95] which is exclusively of the B type, and about 90% inhibition of brain MAO-B.[97,98] No substantial change in MAO-A activity is found in postmortem brain in patients with Parkinson's disease treated with deprenyl.[93] An increase in the concentration of PEA in brain[93] and increased urinary excretion of PEA can be demonstrated in man after deprenyl.[99]

Dopamine is metabolized by MAO to DOPAC. MAO is localized within the cell to the mitochondria. There is evidence that catecholaminergic neurons contain MAO type A (MAO-A) and that serotonergic neurons and glial cells contain MAO-B[89]. Although the affinity of MAO-B for dopamine is greater than that of MAO-A, dopamine is a substrate for both forms of MAO. In humans, dopamine in the brain is metabolized predominantly by MAO-B.[90,91]

In animals, deprenyl produces an increase in the level of dopamine in the brain[r31] and prolongs the contralateral rotation produced by L-DOPA in the unilateral 6-OHDA lesioned rat.[92] Deprenyl is thought to inhibit the catabolism of dopamine and prolong the activity of dopamine at the receptor.[r31] Other actions

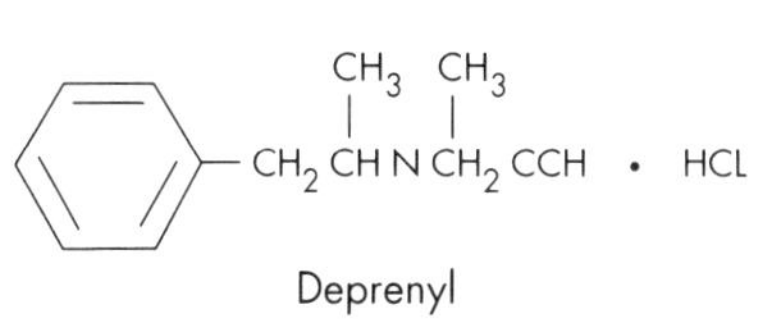

CH_3 CH_3, CH_2 CH N CH_2 CCH · HCL

Deprenyl

Figure 18.6 Structure of Deprenyl

of deprenyl include inhibition of the presynaptic uptake of dopamine.[87] In humans, deprenyl is converted to methamphetamine and smaller amounts of amphetamine as well as desmethyl-deprenyl.[88] The metabolites are thought to be the L-isomers of these compounds.[88,r28,r29] Formation of these amphetamine metabolites[93,94] and the inhibition of the catabolism of PEA[95] adds further to the enhancement of dopaminergic activity. Amphetamines are known to enhance dopaminergic transmission[93,94] and PEA has been shown to have indirect dopaminergic activity.[96]

Therapeutic Uses: Deprenyl is used both as a neuroprotective agent and an adjunct to L-DOPA therapy in the treatment of Parkinson's disease. Clinical studies have shown that deprenyl prolongs the effects of L-DOPA[112] and improves clinical fluctuations in patients with Parkinson's disease who are treated with L-DOPA.[110,281,282] Deprenyl has also been shown to have a dose-sparing effect allowing a 20% reduction in the dose of L-DOPA.[110,282] Based on the DATATOP study, a dose of 10 mg/day is used for protective therapy.[107] Some patients are given 5 mg/day because of side effects at higher doses. The dose of deprenyl used for adjunct therapy in Parkinson's disease is in the range of 5–20 mg/day. Inhibition of MAO-A is thought to become clinically significant at doses above 40 mg/day.[99,113,114]

Oxidative damage has been proposed as one component in the complex disease process leading to the degeneration of dopaminergic neurons in Parkinson's disease.[100] Interest has centered on the potential role of the enzyme MAO in this process. MAO catalyzes the oxidation of dopamine and in the process generates hydrogen peroxide and, in turn, leads to the formation of oxygen free radicals that can induce lipid peroxidation and damage a wide variety of cellular components.[100,101,r32] There is thought to be a specific regional vulnerability of dopamine neurons in the SNc in Parkinson's disease because autooxidation of dopamine produces highly reactive quinones, iron found in increased concentrations in the substantia nigra[r33] promotes hydrogen peroxide formation, and glutathionine peroxidase, superoxide dismutase, catalase and glutathione which protect against such damage are deficient.[100–105]

Birkmayer, in an uncontrolled retrospective study, reported that deprenyl might prolong life expectancy in Parkinson's patients.[106] This report and the finding that inhibitors of MAO-B prevented MPTP-induced parkinsonism in primates, led to clinical studies of the neuroprotective properties of deprenyl in Parkinson's disease. It was hypothesized that deprenyl would decrease the rate of degeneration of dopamine neurons in the SNc in Parkinson's disease by decreasing hydrogen peroxide formation and subsequent damage by oxygen free radicals.[107] Two studies in patients with early Parkinson's disease showed that deprenyl prolonged the time to reach a level of disability requiring treatment with L-DOPA by about 10 to 11 months.[107,108] This finding was interpreted as evidence that deprenyl has a protective effect in Parkinson's disease. The interpretation as a protective effect became controversial because it was discovered that deprenyl can produce a symptomatic effect in Parkinson's disease.[107] To establish the neuroprotective effect of deprenyl in Parkinson's disease will ultimately require demonstration that the rate of degeneration of remaining dopamine neurons is reduced by treatment with deprenyl.[109]

Various actions of deprenyl have been proposed as the mechanism of its symptomatic effect.[109] The inhibition of MAO-B by deprenyl reduces the catabolism of dopamine and increases the concentration and activity of dopamine in the brain. MAO-B inhibition leads to the accumulation of PEA, which increases the activity of dopamine by an indirect mechanism.[96] The metabolites of deprenyl include L-methamphetamine and L-amphetamine, which enhance the release and block the reuptake of dopamine. An increase in dopamine activity in the brain by one or more of these mechanisms might account for the symptomatic effect of deprenyl.

Deprenyl is also used as an adjunct to L-DOPA therapy.[110] The substitution of amphetamine for deprenyl in patients with Parkinson's disease treated with L-DOPA produces worsening suggesting that the effects of deprenyl are not due to its amphetamine metabolites.[111] Deprenyl does not alter the peripheral kinetics or metabolism of L-DOPA.[112]

Side Effects: The side effects of deprenyl in the dose range of 10–50 mg/day include nausea, dryness of mouth, dizziness, headache, insomnia, and confusion.[99,113,114] Deprenyl can also lead to the reactivation of peptic ulcer disease. In patients with Parkinson's disease, deprenyl intensifies the side effects of L-DOPA including nausea, orthostatic hypotension, dyskinesia, and psychosis. Acute and chronic treatment with deprenyl is devoid of the cheese effect.[95,115] Deprenyl does not inhibit the oxidation of tyramine[116] and it does not cause hypertension when administered concurrently with tyramine or L-DOPA.[105] Co-administration of meperidine and deprenyl can lead to the development of delirium and marked muscle rigidity.[117]

Dopamine Agonists

Bromocriptine, Pergolide, Lisuride

Chemistry: The ergot derivatives, bromocriptine mesylate, 2-bromo-2β-isopropyl-5*a*-isobutyl-ergopeptine methanesulfonate, lisuride hydrogen maleate, 1,1 diethyl-3-(9,10-didehydro-6-methyl-8*a*-ergolinyl) urea and pergolide mesylate, (8β)-8-[(methylthio)methyl]-6-propylergoline methanesulfonate, are the principal dopamine agonists used in the treatment of Parkinson's disease. Lisuride hydrogen maleate is soluble in water or saline up to a concentration of 1 mg/ml.[r34]

The dopaminergic ergots compounds fall into two groups, the ergopeptines and the ergolines. The ergopeptines, like bromocriptine, consist of the naturally occurring D-lysergic acid linked to a tricyclic peptide moiety by a peptide bond. The simpler ergolines, which include lisuride and pergolide, contain the unsubstituted tetracyclic structure of lysergic acid. Buried in the ergoline nucleus, which is common to both groups, is the structure of dopamine and serotonin. Small changes in the substituents can increase one dopaminergic effect and decrease another.

Pharmacological effects: Bromocriptine is the prototype of ergot derivatives with marked central dopaminergic activity. It is a potent agonist at D2 receptors in the striatum and produces contralateral turning in the 6-OHDA lesioned rat.[118–121,r35,r36,r37] This effect is inhibited by pretreatment with *a*-methyl-para-tyrosine, an inhibitor of TH, indicating that its motor effects are dependent on the presence of some endogenous dopamine.[118,119,r36,r37] Bromocriptine, lisuride, and pergolide all possess potent agonist properties at the D2 receptor but they have diverse actions at D1 receptor sites. Lisuride is a partial agonist/antagonist at the D1 receptor[r34] whereas pergolide is a partial agonist[122–124,r38]

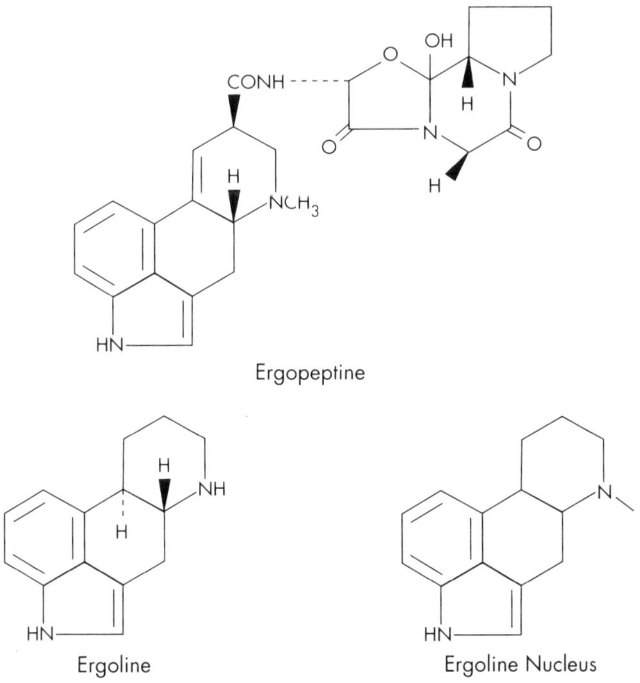

Figure 18.7 Structure of Two Classes of Ergot Compounds

Table 18.2 Activity of Agonists at Dopamine Receptors*

Agonist	D1	D2
L-DOPA (Dopamine)	*Agonist*	*Agonist*
Apomorphine	*Agonist*	*Agonist*
Pergolide	*Partial agonist*	*Agonist*
Bromocriptine	*Weak partial agonist*	*Agonist*
Lisuride	*Partial agonist/ antagonist*	*Agonist*

*D1 and D2 refer to dopamine receptor subtypes.

and bromocriptine is weak partial agonist (Table 18.2).[119] There is evidence that lisuride and pergolide at low doses preferentially act on presynaptic dopamine receptors, or autoreceptors, and inhibit dopamine turnover.[r34,r39] The clinical effects of bromocriptine, lisuride and pergolide in Parkinson's disease are thought to be related to their activity at D2 dopamine receptors in the striatum.[r34,r39] The activity of the dopaminergic ergot compounds on different subtypes of dopamine receptors is more selective than that of dopamine. Lisuride also has a high affinity for serotonin receptors where its effects are complex.[r34] The highest levels of lisuride in the brain are found in the caudate nucleus, putamen, parts of the thalamus and lamina IV of cortex.[125]

Lisuride is completely absorbed[126,127] and more than 55% of an oral dose of pergolide is absorbed in man.[128] Studies in primates have shown that only 37% of an oral dose of bromocriptine is absorbed.[r40] Six percent of the absorbed dose of bromocriptine reaches the systemic circulation unchanged.[129,r37] The bioavailability of oral lisuride in man is only 10–22%.[126,127] Ninety-four to 98% of a dose of bromocriptine is excreted in the bile and feces with 2–6% excreted in urine.[129,r37] Sixty percent of a dose of lisuride is excreted in the urine with 40% excreted in the feces.[r40] In the case of pergolide, 55% of the dose is excreted in urine and 40% in the feces.[128]

The major sites of metabolism of the ergolines include the 1-methyl, the 6-methyl, and the 8-substituent and the aromatic ring. Ergopeptines undergo biotransformation almost exclusively in the proline fragment of the peptide moiety.[r41] Although many of the metabolites of bromocriptine have not been identified, they do not appear to be active.[129] None of the metabolites of lisuride account for more than 10% of the total metabolites and it is doubtful that any of them have a significant clinical effect.[r34,r42]

Ninety to 96% of bromocriptine,[r37] 70% of lisuride[r43] and 95–96% of pergolide[128] present in blood are bound to plasma proteins. Peak plasma levels of bromocriptine and lisuride after oral administration occur at about 1–3 hr[r37,r43] and 0.5–2 hr,[127] respectively. The plasma half-lives of bromocriptine and lisuride are 3 and about 2 hr, respectively.[129,130,r43] The plasma clearance rates of bromocriptine (900 ml/min)[r37] and lisuride (740–800 ml/min)[126,127,131] approach the rate of hepatic blood flow. The volume of distribution of lisuride in man has been calculated to be 2.3–2.4 L/kg.[r34]

Bromocriptine

Therapeutic Use: Bromocriptine was the first ergot derivative to be studied for the treatment of Parkinson's disease.[r83] It has been shown to be effective and to alleviate all the major motor features of the disease.[251–253,r84,r85] Bromocriptine is used either as monotherapy or as an adjunct to L-DOPA therapy.[r86,r87] Monotherapy is usually effective only for the first 1–2 years in patients with early, mild disease or in patients with slowly progressive disease. In most patients, concurrent treatment with L-DOPA is required for optimum results. Low doses of bromocriptine combined with L-DOPA are useful in patients with mild to moderate Parkinson's disease. High doses in combination with L-DOPA are required in patients with more advanced disease. Indications for its use include a loss of efficacy of L-DOPA or the development of clinical fluctuations or dyskinesia. The reduction in dyskinesia is probably due to the downward adjustment in the dose of L-DOPA. Using bromocriptine as the sole therapy for Parkinson's disease for the purpose of preventing the development of clinical fluctuations and dyskinesia is controversial.

The usual oral dose of bromocriptine when used as monotherapy is 40–80 mg per day.[r13,r86,r87] An occasional patient requires a dose of greater than 100 mg per day. A low dose of 5–25 mg per day is employed when bromocriptine is used as an adjunct to L-DOPA therapy.[254,r88] Because some patients develop symptomatic hypotension in response to the first dose, a test dose of 1.25 mg is given prior to starting therapy.[r13] A starting dose of 2.5 mg per day is followed by titration of the dose with an increase of 2.5 mg every 3 days until a therapeutic effect or side effect occurs. The systemic availability of dopaminergic ergot compounds depends on the drug metabolizing enzyme activity of the liver that may vary greatly between individuals. This may explain the large individual variation in plasma drug levels and wide therapeutic dosage range of these compounds.[255,r40,r89] In addition to Parkinson's disease, dopaminergic ergot compounds have been used in the treatment of dystonia and neuroleptic malignant syndrome (Table 18.4, page 341 and Table 18.10, page 349).

Side Effects: The acute side effects of bromocriptine include nausea, vomiting, and postural hypotension.[r13,r43] These effects are related to its dopamine agonist activity and can be controlled by a reduction in the dose. An occasional patient experiences severe hypotension after the first dose. The chronic side effects of bromocriptine include hallucinations, paranoia, confusion, dyskinesia, erythromelalgia, fibrotic reactions, and digital vasospasm. Psychotic symptoms are more frequent and severe with bromocriptine than with L-DOPA. Erythromelalgia is manifest as a burning discomfort of the feet and ankles associated with edema and tenderness. The lower extremities are found to be erythematous and warm to the touch. This condition resolves rapidly when the drug is stopped.[r13] Bromocriptine, like methysergide, can produce fibrotic reactions.[132,133] Retroperitoneal fibrosis can be manifest as back pain (hydronephrosis), urinary frequency or deep vein thrombosis. Pulmonary fibrosis can produce a feeling of breathlessness. Such fibrotic reactions represent serious but reversible effects of the drug. More uncommon side effects include elevation of serum transaminase levels, nasal congestion, headache, diplopia, sedation, cardiac arrhythmias, symptoms of angina, and gastrointestinal hemorrhage.[r13]

Lisuride

Therapeutic Uses: Lisuride is effective in Parkinson's disease when used as monotherapy or in combination with L-DOPA. Like bromocriptine, it improves all of the features of the disease and produces an optimum response when used with L-DOPA. The addition of lisuride to L-DOPA therapy can reduce clinical fluctuations and allow a decrease in the L-DOPA dose of 20–50% with improvement in dyskinesia. Oral lisuride is used in a dosage range of 0.4–5 mg per day. The average dosage used in combination with L-DOPA is in the range of 0.6–1.6 mg per day.[r34,r42]

Lisuride is the only dopamine agonist available that can be administered parenterally. The water solubility of lisuride as the hydrogen maleate and its intrinsic potency and lipid solubility make it suitable for administration by the intravenous or subcutaneous routes.[256,257] Single intravenous bolus doses have been used as acute treatment for severe akinesia (0.025–0.15 mg)[r34] or a test of responsiveness to dopamine agonists (0.025–0.2 mg).[r90] They produce dose-dependent effects with an onset of about 10 min and a duration of up to 3–4 hr. Doses in the range of 0.2 mg produce dyskinesia. Lisuride has also been administered chronically as a constant-rate intravenous infusion (0.3–1.0 mg/hr)[258] or as a continuous subcutaneous infusion (1–2 mg/day)[259,260] to treat clinical fluctuations. Lisuride infusions can improve fluctuations and dyskinesia and improve functional capacity. Domperidone is used to block the acute side effects of lisuride. The develop-

Table 18.3 Preparations and Doses of Drugs Used to Treat Parkinson's Disease

Generic Name	Trade Name	Dosage Forms mg	Daily Doses
Carbidopa/Levodopa	Sinement, etc. Sinemet CR (slow release)	10/100 (T) 25/100 (T) 25/250 (T) 25/100 CR (T) 50/200 CR (T)	30/300–150/1500
Benserazide/Levodopa	Madopar	62.5 (12.5/50 (T) 125 (25/100) (T) 250 (50/200) (T) HBS (25/100) (T)	75/300–200/800
Carbidopa	Lodosyn	25 (T)	75–200
Bromocriptine	Parlodel, etc.	2.5 (T) 5 (C)	10–60
Pergolide	Permax	0.05 (T) 0.25 (T) 1 (T)	1–6
Amantadine	Symmetrel, etc.	100 (C) 50 mg/5 ml (Syrup)	100–300
Trihexyphenydil	Artane, etc.	2 (T) 5 (T) 5 (C) (Slow release) 2 mg/5 ml (Elixir)	2–15
Benztropine	Cogentin, etc.	0.5 (T) 1 (T) 2 (T)	1–6
Procyclidine	Kemadrin, etc.	2 (T) 5 (T)	5–20
Biperiden	Akineton, etc.	2 (T)	2–8
Ethopropazine	*Parsitane, etc	10 (T) 50 (T) 100 (T)	50–200
L-Deprenyl	Eldepryl, etc.	5 (T)	5–10
Damperidone	*Motilium, etc.	10 (T)	30–80

*Available in Canada and Europe

ment of psychosis and local tissue reactions are frequent side effects. The water solubility of lisuride as the hydrogen maleate and its intrinsic potency make it suitable for administration by the intravenous or subcutaneous route.

Side Effects: The side effects of lisuride are similar to those of bromocriptine.[r34,r42] Nausea, vomiting, and postural hypotension can be prevented or diminished by pretreatment with domperidone or sulpiride.[134,135] Tolerance to these effects usually develops within 8–12 weeks. Headache and sedation are of central origin and are not affected by dopamine antagonists. The development of psychosis is frequent after continuous treatment with lisuride infusions for several months.[136] Subcutaneous infusion of lisuride produces granulomas at the site of the infusion.[134,135]

Pergolide

Therapeutic Use: Like the other dopaminergic ergot derivatives, pergolide is effective in the treatment of Parkinson's disease when used as monotherapy or in combination with L-DOPA.[r39,r91] The addition of pergolide can allow a reduction in the dosage of L-DOPA of up to 30–50%. Chronic treatment with pergolide has been shown to be effective in Parkinson's disease for up to 5 years.[r39] Some patients have responded to pergolide after failing to respond to bromocriptine. Monotherapy with pergolide is advised in patients who cannot tolerate L-DOPA. Its use as monotherapy for the purpose of preventing the late complications associated with L-DOPA therapy is controversial. The effective dose of pergolide ranges from 1–15 mg per day.[r39,r91] When pergolide is combined with L-DOPA, doses of up to 6 mg per day are used. As a general rule, the effect of 0.25 mg of pergolide is considered to be equivalent to that of 2.5 mg of bromocriptine (1:10 ratio). After first determining the effects of a single test dose of 0.05–0.125 mg, the dose is slowly titrated to produce the desired motor response or until side effects occur.

Side Effects: The side effects of pergolide are similar to those of the other ergot compounds.[r34,r39] Postural hypotension can occur with the first dose of pergolide and be absent thereafter. The concern regarding the occurrence of cardiac arrhythmias appears to have been unwarranted since patients with cardiac disease tolerate pergolide without major problems.[r44] As a general rule, the dose should not exceed 3.0 mg per day in patients with known heart disease. The abrupt withdrawal of pergolide can precipitate worsening of parkinsonism and increased hallucinations and confusion.[137,r39]

Apomorphine

Chemistry : The alkaloid apomorphine, (R)-5,6,6*a*,7-tetrahydro-6-methyl- 4*H*-dibenzo[de,g]quinoline-10,11-diol, is a synthetic opiate obtained by treating morphine with concentrated HCl or by heating morphine with ZnCl[r45]. Apomorphine hydrochloride is soluble in water at 20 mg/ml.[r45]

Pharmacological effects: Apomorphine is an agonist at both D1 and D2 dopamine receptors.[138,r46] At low doses, it preferentially acts on presynaptic autoreceptors and inhibits dopamine turnover.[139,140] Apomorphine undergoes extensive first-pass metabolism. Its plasma half-life is about 30 min.[141]

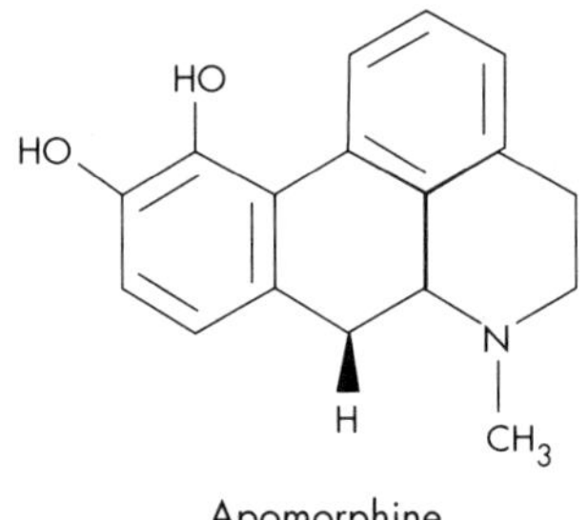

Figure 18.8 Structure of Apomorphine

Therapeutic Use: The effects of apomorphine on the symptoms of Parkinson's disease are attributed to its activity at dopamine receptors since they are blocked by pretreatment with haloperidol.[142] Apomorphine was the first dopamine agonist to be employed in the treatment of Parkinson's disease.[261,r92] Before its dopamine agonist properties were known, apomorphine was given to patients with Parkinson's disease because it reduced decerebrate rigidity in animals.[r92] Oral doses of 160–600 mg per day were found to be effective in early studies.[143,262] The use of oral apomorphine was limited by the occurrence of nausea and vomiting and the impairment of renal function.[262] Parenteral administration avoids the problem of extensive first pass metabolism and substantially reduces the required dose. Doses as small as 0.5–2 mg administered subcutaneously can produce symptomatic improvement.[248,263] Apomorphine has agonist properties at both D1 and D2 receptors.[r46] It improves akinesia, rigidity and tremor and the degree of its effect is similar to that of L-DOPA.[r19]

Apomorphine hydrochloride is water soluble. It has been administered by the intravenous, subcutaneous,[145,146,264–266,267] sublingual,[268,269] intranasal,[270] and rectal routes.[271] Apomorphine given by intravenous or subcutaneous injection (0.5–10 mg) is used as "rescue therapy" for the acute treatment of akinesia in patients on chronic L-DOPA therapy.[145] The effects occur after 5–15 min, reach a maximum after 30 min and last for 60–120 min.[272,r22] The response to apomorphine is considered to be a predictor of responsiveness to other dopaminergic agonists. Apomorphine is also used by continuous subcutaneous infusion (up to 12 mg/hr; 12–24 hr/day) for the treatment of patients who develop severe clinical fluctuations on oral L-DOPA.[146,257,266] Tachyphylaxis or loss of efficacy has not been observed. Renal failure has not reported after chronic subcutaneous administration.

Side Effects: Apomorphine is potent in producing nausea and vomiting. These side effects can be blocked by pretreatment with domperidone. Tolerance to these side effects develops after several weeks. Chronic oral administration of high doses of apomorphine is associated with renal damage and azotemia.[143] Continuous subcutaneous infusions of apomorphine frequently lead to the development of subcutaneous nodules, cutaneous necrosis and other dermatological complications.[144–146] Chronic therapy with apomorphine in Parkinson's disease is frequently associated with the development of dyskinesia and psychosis.[147–149]

Dopamine Antagonists

Haloperidol, Pimozide

Modes of therapeutic action: Haloperidol and pimozide are the most frequently used dopamine antagonists in the treatment of movement disorders. Dopamine antagonists are used in the treatment of chorea, hemiballismus, motor tics and dystonia (Table 18.9, page 348). Other details about the general pharmacology of this drug class is presented in Chapter 18.

Presynaptic Dopamine Depleters

Tetrabenazine

Pharmacological effects: Tetrabenazine, 1,3,4,6,7, 11b-Hexahydro-9, 10-dimethoxy-3-(2-methylpropyl)-2H-benzo[*a*]quinolizin-2-one methanesulfonate, like reserpine, acts on neurons to deplete synaptic vesicles of dopamine and other monamines[150] (see Fig. 18.9). It causes the release of dopamine from synaptic vesicles and blocks its uptake into the vesicles.[150] Tetrabenazine produces a decrease in the content and activity of dopamine, norepinephrine and serotonin in the brain. It also acts to block postsynaptic dopamine receptors.[151] The central activity of tetrabenazine relative to its peripheral activity is greater than that of reserpine.[150]

Therapeutic Use: Tetrabenazine has been found to be useful in the treatment of chorea,[152–154] tardive dyskinesia,[155] hemiballismus and, to a more limited extent, in dystonia[153,156,r47,r48] (Table 18.3). Tetrabenzaine is used in doses of 50–150 mg/day.[r48]

Side Effects: The side effects of tetrabenazine are similar to those of reserpine but it has fewer peripheral side effects and is less likely to cause orthostatic hypotension.[10] The major side effects are sedation, parkinsonism, akathisia, depression, and orthostatic hypotension. Other side effects include hypersalivation, insomnia, anxiety, headache and impotence.[156,r15,r47,r48] Tetrabenzazine has not been associated with the development of tardive movement disorders.

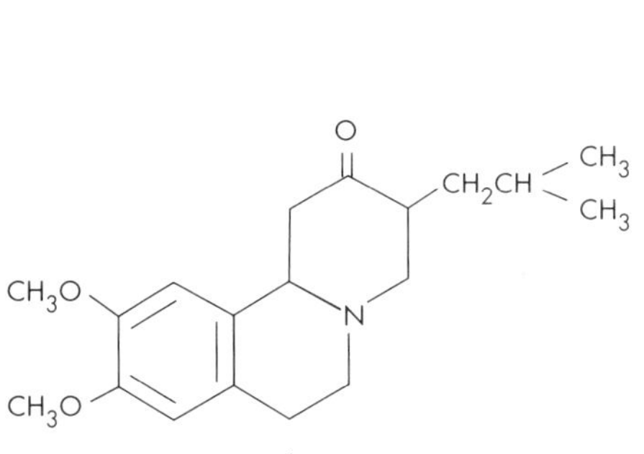

Tetrabenazine

Figure 18.9 Structure of Tetrabenazine

Anticholinergic Drugs

Trihexyphenidyl, Benztropine, Others

History: Atropine and scopolamine, naturally occurring alkaloids with anticholinergic properties, were the first effective therapeutic to be used in the treatment of parkinsonism.[r49,r50,r51] Synthetic, centrally active anticholinergic drugs with fewer peripheral side effects were developed and eventually replaced the use of the belladonna alkaloids.

Chemistry: The prototypic synthetic centrally acting anticholinergic agents are trihexyphenidyl hydrochloride (Artane), *a*-cyclohexyl-*a*-phenyl-l-piperidine-propanol hydrochloride, and benztropine mesylate, 3-(diphenylmethoxy)-8-methyl-8-azabicyclo [3,2,1] octane methanesulfonate. Trihexyphenidyl hydrochloride is soluble in water at 10 mg/ml.[r52] Structures of these drugs are presented in Figure 18.10. Benztropine mesylate is also soluble in water. Other commonly used anticholinergic agents are procyclidine hydrochloride, biperiden hydrochloride and ethopropazine.

Pharmacological effects: The synthetic anticholinergic agents block muscarinic receptors in the peripheral and central nervous system but are thought to act more selectively on central cholinergic receptors. These compounds have a greater affinity for the low-affinity M1 site than the high-affinity M2 site for pirenzepine although the relative selectivity of the different compounds for the muscarinic receptor subtypes varies.[157] Trihexyphenidyl is the prototype of this group. There

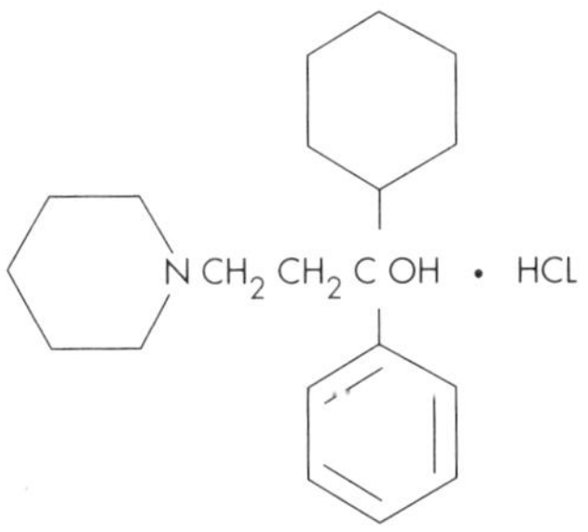

Trihexyphenidyl Hydrochloride

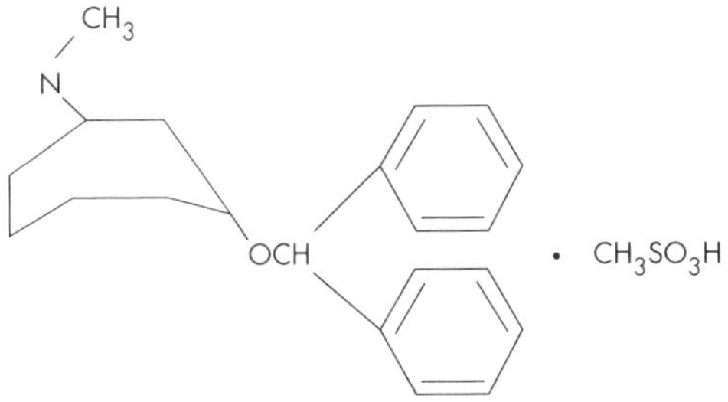

Benztropine Mesylate

Figure 18.10 Structure of Prototypic Anticholinergic Drugs

is evidence that many of these compound inhibit the active reuptake of dopamine.[158,159] Benztropine is a potent dopamine reuptake blocker. Ethopropazine is a phenothiazine with significant anticholinergic activity.

Peak serum levels of trihexyphenidyl occur 1.3 hr after an oral dose.[160] The half-life of trihexyphenidyl in normal subjects was found to be 1.7 hr.[161] The half-life of trihexyphenidyl in dystonic patients on chronic, high-dose therapy was 3.7 hr.[160] Preparations and daily doses are presented in Table 18.3, page 337. Other details about the pharmacology of the anticholinergic drugs are found in Chapter 5.

Therapeutic Use: Nigrostriatal dopamine neurons exert a tonic inhibitory effect on striatal cholinergic interneurons.[r53] Anticholinergic drugs are thought to improve parkinsonism by decreasing the activity of disinhibited striatal cholinergic interneurons.[r54] Physostigmine, a centrally active acetylcholinesterase (AChE) inhibitor, worsens parkinsonism while edrophonium, an AChE inhibitor and quaternary compound that does not enter the brain, is without effect.[162] The effect of physostigmine can be blocked by anticholinergic drugs with central activity like benztropine.

Anticholinergic drugs are effective in the treatment of Parkinson's disease. They are generally more effective in reducing tremor and rigidity than bradykinesia and can produce mild to moderate improvement.[273,r93] Treatment with these agents is considered in patients with early, mild disease or tremor-predominant Parkinson's disease. They are considered the treatment of choice for neuroleptic-induced parkinsonism and are used prophylactically to prevent its occurrence.[r94] Anticholinergic drugs provide a secondary benefit in the form of reduction of sialorrhea and urinary frequency. The abrupt discontinuation of anticholinergic drugs can produce marked symptomatic worsening.[274] Acetylcholine receptor hypersensitivity has been proposed as the mechanism underlying rebound withdrawal worsening.[275]

The muscarinic rather than the nicotinic properties of anticholinergic drugs are thought to be responsible for their antiparkinson effects. Atropine has an antiparkinson effect but has no effect on nicotine-induced tremor in animals.[163] Nicotine administered intravenously actually reduces rather than increases resting tremor in Parkinson's disease.[163] Since the postulated site of action of anticholinergic drugs is distal to the presynaptic dopamine neuron, they might be effective in other forms of parkinsonism even in the absence of a response to L-DOPA.[164,r54]

In addition to their use in various forms of parkinsonism, anticholinergic drugs are used in the treatment of dystonia and certain forms of akathisia (see Table 18.10, page 349). The activity of anticholinergic drugs on the striatum is also thought to be responsible for their antidystonia effects.[r55]

Side Effects: The peripheral side effects of the synthetic anticholinergic drugs include dry mouth, blurred vision, constipation, and urinary retention.[r55,r56] Mydriasis and loss of accommodation produce the symptom of blurred vision. Their use is contraindicated in patients with narrow angle glaucoma[165] or prostatic hypertrophy. Pyridostigmine bromide, a peripherally active AChE inhibitor, can be used at a dose of 30–60 mg four times per day to antagonize the peripheral side effects.[r55]

The central side effects of these agents include memory impairment, confusion, delirium, and hallucinations. The sensitivity of adults to the central side effects is thought to be due to age-related changes in cholinergic systems in the brain.[166] If severe, the central side effects can be treated with parenteral physostigmine at a dose of 2–4 mg.[r56] Centrally active anticholinergic drugs can produce worsening of chorea, classic tardive dyskinesia (orofacial dyskinesia) and L-DOPA-induced dyskinesia.[167,168,r57]

Other Treatments for Movement Disorders

Serotonergic Agents

L-5-Hydroxytryptophan (L-5HTP)

Chemistry: L-5-Hydroxytryptophan (L-5-HTP), (-)-L-*a*-hydrozino-*a*-methyl-β-(3, 4-dihydroxybenzene) propanoic acid monohydrate, is a naturally occurring aromatic amino acid. It is soluble in water at 10 mg/ml (5°C) and stable in aqueous solutions at low pH.[r58]

Pharmacological effects: The amino acid L-5-HTP is the biological precursor of serotonin. Exogenous L-5-HTP is transported across the brain capillary endothelial cell and nerve cell membranes by the L-transport system and converted to serotonin by AADC. L-5-HTP is thought to be decarboxylated to serotonin in catecholaminergic neurons as well as serotonergic neurons in the brain. Brain levels of serotonin and 5-HIAA are elevated in postmortem brain after the administration of L-5-HTP in humans.[169] Plasma levels of serotonin and 5-HIAA, the serotonin content of platelets and the 24 hr urinary excretion of 5-HIAA are increased during treatment with L-5-HTP.[r59]

L-5-HTP is absorbed from the upper small intestine via the L-transport system. When administered with carbidopa, 47–84% of an oral dose of L-5-HTP is absorbed.[r59] Other amino acid substrates for the L-system competitively inhibit the transport of L-5-HTP at the intestinal wall and brain capillary sites.[r60] Peak plasma

Table 18.4 Effectiveness of Different Classes of Drugs in Movement Disorders

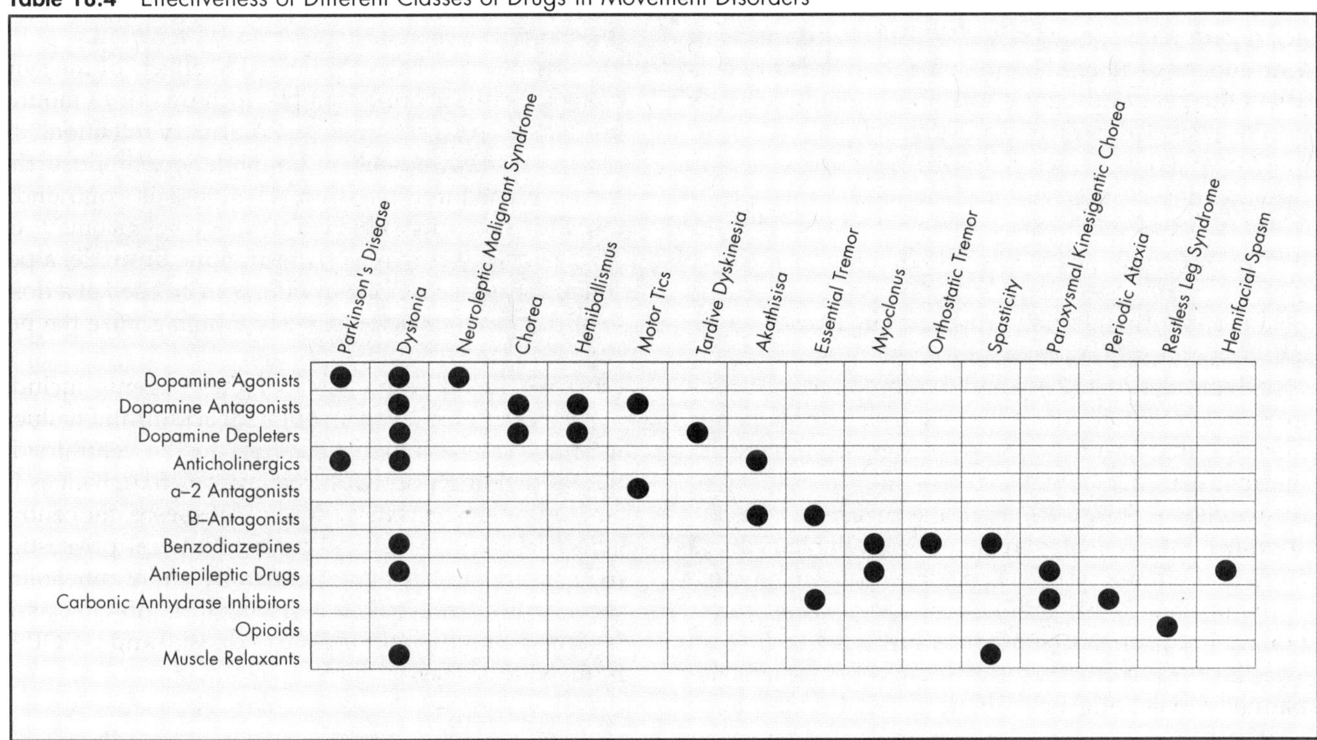

	Parkinson's Disease	Dystonia	Neuroleptic Malignant Syndrome	Chorea	Hemiballismus	Motor Tics	Tardive Dyskinesia	Akathisisa	Essential Tremor	Myoclonus	Orthostatic Tremor	Spasticity	Paroxysmal Kinesigenic Chorea	Periodic Ataxia	Restless Leg Syndrome	Hemifacial Spasm
Dopamine Agonists	●	●	●													
Dopamine Antagonists		●		●	●	●										
Dopamine Depleters		●		●	●		●									
Anticholinergics	●	●						●								
α-2 Antagonists						●										
B-Antagonists								●	●							
Benzodiazepines		●								●	●	●				
Antiepileptic Drugs		●								●			●			●
Carbonic Anhydrase Inhibitors									●				●	●		
Opioids															●	
Muscle Relaxants		●										●				

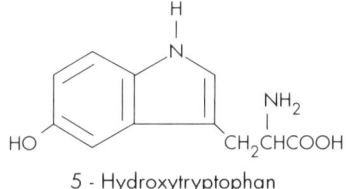

Figure 18.11 Structure of 5-Hydroxytryptophan

concentrations are reached about 1–3 hr after an oral dose of L-5-HTP.[r59] In the presence of carbidopa, the plasma half-life of L-5-HTP is 2–7 hr.[r59] The CSF levels are proportional to the plasma levels with an average CSF:plasma ratio of 0.24.[r59]

The major pathway for the metabolism of L-5-HTP in peripheral tissues is decarboxylation by AADC to serotonin. The co-administration of carbidopa produces a 5–15-fold increase in the plasma levels of 5-HTP and a corresponding decrease in the levels of 5-HIAA, the major metabolite of serotonin.[r59] Treatment with carbidopa permits the use of a smaller dose of L-5-HTP and reduces the side effects due to high peripheral levels of serotinin.

Therapeutic Use: L-5-HTP has usefulness in treating myoclonus.[170,301] The effective dose of L-5-HTP is usually in the range of 1000–2000 mg per day.[r22,r59,r61] Carbidopa is coadministered with L-5-HTP in a dose of 100 to 300 mg per day to prevent or reduce the acute side effects of L-5-HTP.[r22,r61]

Side Effects: The major acute side effects of L-5-HTP are diarrhea, anorexia, nausea, and vomiting.[170,r59,r60] Diarrhea responds to treatment with diphenoxylate hydrochloride 2.5 mg four times per day.[r61] Prochlorperazine 5–10 mg or trimethobenzamide 250 mg four times a day can be used to control anorexia and nausea.[r61] These agents can usually be stopped after several weeks. Other reported side effects include mydriasis, lightheadedness, abdominal pain, blurring of vision, bradycardia, sleepiness.[r59,r61] Central side effects in the form of mental changes include euphoria, hypomania, restlessness, anxiety, insomnia, aggressiveness, and agitation.[r59] An acute overdose can produce respiratory difficulties and hypotension.[r59] A sclerodermalike skin reaction has been reported.[r59] L-5-HTP is known to reduce plasma cholesterol levels by about 20%.[r61]

Adrenergic Agents

Propranaolol, Clonidine

Therapeutic Use in Movement Disorders: Propranolol and clonidine are the most frequently used adrenergic agents for the treatment of movement disorders. Propranolol is used in the treatment of essential tremor and akathisia. Clonidine is used in the treatment of Tourette syndrome (Table 18.9, page 348). For details about the pharmacology of these drugs and their side effects, consult Chapters 6 and 26.

Glutamatergic Agents

Amantadine

History: Amantadine was first developed as an antiviral agent.[171] It inhibits the replication of strains of influenza A virus.[171,172] and has prophylactic value in individuals who have had contact with an active case. Its antiparkinson properties were discovered by chance.[173]

Chemistry: Amantadine, 1-adamantanamine, is the 1-amino derivative of adamantane. Adamantane has a 10 carbon symmetrical tricyclic structure. Amantadine hydrochloride is water soluble (at 1:20).[r62] Memantine is the *N*-ethyl analog of amantadine.

Pharmacological effects: Amantadine has indirect dopamine agonist properties. It increases the presynaptic synthesis and release of dopamine[174,175] and inhibits dopamine reuptake.[176] There is some evidence that amantadine has direct effects on postsynaptic dopamine receptors[177,178,r63] and alters the affinity of postsynaptic dopamine receptors.[r64] Some of its clinical effects suggest that it has anticholinergic properties but anticholinergic activity has not been demonstrated. It has now been shown that amantadine is an antagonist at the *N*-methyl-D-aspartate (NMDA) subtype of glutamate receptor.[179] In postmortem human frontal cortex, amantadine and memantine bind to the MK-801 binding site of the NMDA receptor.[180] Of the 1-amino-adamantanes tested, memantine exhibits the highest affinity for the MK-801 receptor site in human brain tissue.

Amantadine is rapidly and relatively completely absorbed after oral administration[181,r65] with peak plasma concentrations occurring at about 1–4 hr.[182] About 90% of an oral dose is excreted in the urine as unchanged drug.[182,183,r65] The renal clearance rate of amantadine appears to be greater than that of creatinine suggesting secretion of the drug by renal tubular cells.[183] Amantadine accumulates when renal function is impaired.[r43] The plasma half-life of amantadine is 16 hr.[181] Its plasma clearance rate is 0.3 L/kg·hr.[181] About 67% of the drug present in blood is bound to plasma proteins.[184] An oral dose of 200 mg results in peak plasma concentrations of 0.3–0.6 μg/ml.[r65] The half-life of amantadine is increased in patients with renal impairment[r65] and in the elderly.[r66]

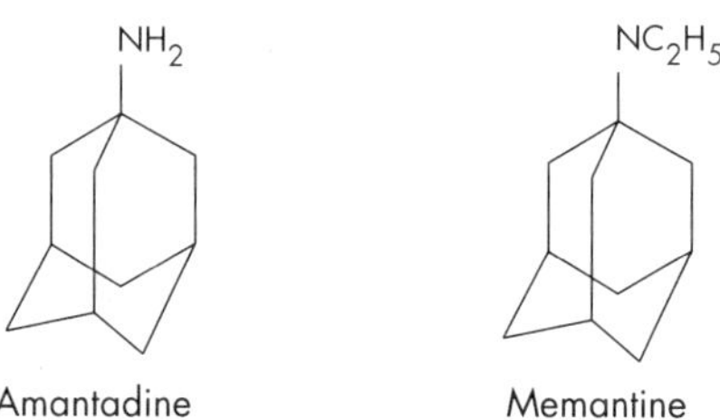

Figure 18.12 Structure of the 1-Amino-Adamantanes

The mechanism of action of amantadine in Parkinson's disease is unclear. Its effects have been assumed to be due to its capacity to increase presynaptic synthesis and release of dopamine and to inhibit dopamine reuptake. It is now thought that amantadine might act by blocking glutamate receptors in the brain. Studies in experimental animals suggest that overactivity of the subthalamic nucleus (STN) is involved in the mechanism underlying the motor syndrome of parkinsonism. It is known that the pathways to and from the STN utilize the excitatory amino acid L-glutamate as their neurotransmitter. The injection of glutamate antagonists into the internal segment of the globus pallidus, a target region for glutamatergic neurons from the STN, reverses the motor signs of parkinsonism in monkeys.[185] NBQX, a selective antagonist of the AMPA (alpha-amino-3-hydroxy-5-methyl-4 isoxazole propionate) subtype of the glutamate receptor, has antiparkinson effects and potentiates the actions of L-DOPA in the MPTP-treated monkey.[186]

Therapeutic Use: Amantadine is effective in reducing bradykinesia, rigidity and tremor in Parkinson's disease.[276–278,r66] The efficacy of amantadine is less than that of L-DOPA.[279,280] About two-thirds of patients respond with an estimated 15–25% improvement.[r54] The effects of amantadine are additive or synergistic with those of L-DOPA or anticholinergic agents. Chronic therapy with amantadine can produce sustained benefits.[r54] The loss of efficacy seen in some patients might be due to progression of the underlying disease. A rebound withdrawal worsening can occur on abrupt discontinuation of amantadine. The usual dose of amantadine is 200–300 mg per day.

Side Effects: Livedo reticularis associated with ankle edema is a relatively common side effect of amantadine.[187,188] It is thought to result from the local release of catecholamines and changes in the permeability of blood vessels in the skin.[189,190] Other peripheral side effects include dry mouth, constipation and urinary retention. The central side effects of amantadine include anxiety, restlessness, depression, dizziness, confusion, hallucinations, and paranoia.[191,192] Amantadine can also produce myoclonus. The acute side effects and psychiatric symptoms usually resolve within 36–72 hr.[r54] Drug levels in the range of 1–5 μg/ml are associated with central nervous system toxicity.[r65] In general, the use of amantadine in patients with renal impairment should be avoided. The combination of hydrochlorothiazide and triamterine reduces the excretion rate of amantadine.[193] Guidelines are available for the use of amantadine in patients with renal failure.[194]

Benzodiazepines

Clonazepam, Diazepam

Therapeutic Use in Movement Disorders: Clonazepam and diazepam are the most frequently used benzodiazepines in the treatment of movement disorders. Clonazepam is used in the treatment of myoclonus, dystonia and orthostatic tremor. Diazepam is used for the treatment of dystonia and spasticity (Table 18.4, page 341 and Table 18.10, page 349). For detailed pharmacology and side effects consult Chapter 14.

Antiepileptic Agents

Carbamazepine, Valproic Acid, Phenytoin, Acetazolamide

Modes of therapeutic action: Carbamazepine, valproic acid, phenytoin and acetazolamide are drugs with antiepileptic properties drugs which are used in the treatment of movement disorders (Table 18.4). Carbamazepine and phenytoin are used in the treatment of paroxysmal kinesigenic forms of chorea and dystonia. Valproic acid is used in the treatment of myoclonus. Acetazolamide, a carbonic anhydrase inhibitor, is used in the treatment of paroxysmal chorea and dystonia, and periodic ataxia. Methazolamide, an analog of acetazolamide, is effective in some cases of essential tremor.[195] For details about the pharmacology and side effects of these drugs see Chapter 19.

Opioids

Propoxyphene, Codeine

Therapeutic Use in Movement Disorders: Propoxyphene and codeine have been used in the treatment of restless leg syndrome (Table 18.4, page 341). See Chapter 20 for additional information about the pharmacology of these drugs.

Muscle Relaxants

Dantrolene, Diazepam, Baclofen, Tizanidine

Therapeutic Use: Dantrolene, diazepam, baclofen and tizanidine are muscle relaxants used for the treatment of spasticity (Table 18.4, page 341). Dantrolene acts directly on the muscle to reduce calcium release to the sarcoplasmic reticulum and alter actin and myosin interaction and decrease muscle contraction force.[196,197] Diazepam appears to enhance presynaptic GABAergic inhibition.[r67] Baclofen, which has antispasticity properties, is thought to reduce the release of the neurotransmitters aspartate and glutamate and decreases excitatory input to alpha motor neurons.[198] Tizanidine is potent in reducing spasticity.[199] It acts at the α-2 adrenergic receptor and probably at GABA and glycine receptors. It is postulated that tizanidine enhances both presynaptic and reciprocal spinal inhibitory mechanisms.[r68]

Botulinum Toxin Type A

Chemistry: Botulinum toxin is produced by certain strains of the bacterium Clostridium botulinum. There are seven serotypes (A, B, C1, D, E, F, G) that differ in their antigenicity, molecular weight, amino acid content, electrophoretic mobility, species specificity, and pharmacological effects. Human disease is associated with types A, B, E, and F.[200] Botulinum toxin is synthesized as a single chain protein of about 150 kDa. It undergoes post-translational proteolytic processing or "activation" to form a dichain protein with a light (L) chain (50 kDa) and heavy (H) chain linked by a disulfide (S–S) bond.[201,r69] The toxin is associated with one or more proteins which are thought to protect it from inactivation or enhance its absorption. Type A is associated with the protein hemagglutinin forming a toxic complex with a molecular weight of about 500 kDa.[r70] Botulinum toxin on a weight basis is the most potent toxin known. The lethal dose in humans is estimated to be less than 50 μg by the oral route and less than 1 pg per kg given parenterally. Botulinum toxin is inactivated by high temperature (212 °C × 10 min) or alkaline pH conditions.

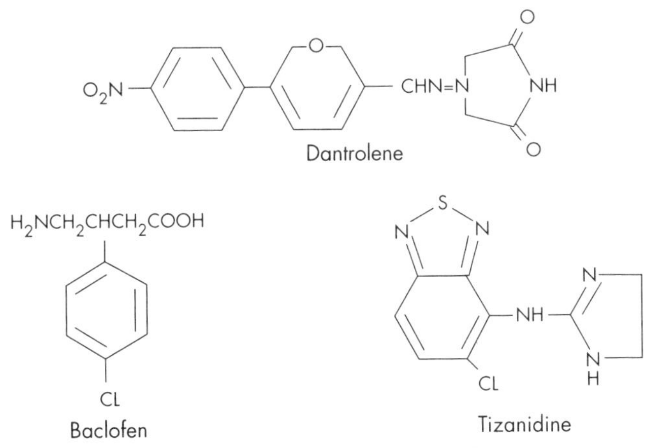

Figure 18.13 Structure of Compounds with Muscle Relaxant Properties

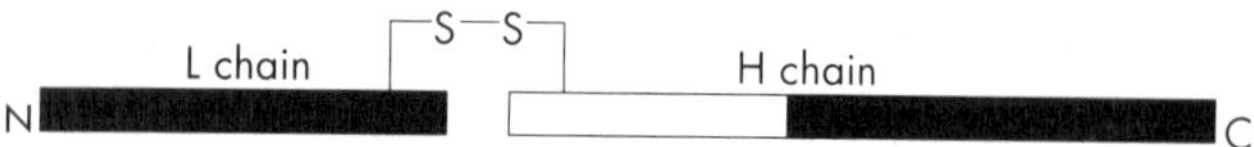

Figure 18.14 Structure of botulinum toxin L, light chain; H, heavy chain; S–S, disulphide bond; N, N–terminal; C, C-terminal.

Pharmacological effects: Botulinum toxin acts selectively on cholinergic synapses to block the release of ACh. Its effects are greater at the neuromuscular junction than at autonomic cholinergic synapses. The mechanism of action involves three steps: binding of the toxin to the nerve terminal, internalization by endocytosis and internal activity of the toxin.[202,203,r71] The H chain is responsible for the binding of the toxin to the nerve terminal, which is saturable and highly selective with high- and low-affinity sites. The toxin is internalized via a receptor-mediated, endocytotic-lysosomal vesicle pathway. The H chain is also responsible for the translocation of the L chain across the endosomal membrane into the cytosol. It is the L-chain which is responsible for the toxic activity.

Botulinum toxin blocks Ca^{2+} mediated release of ACh.[r72,r73,r74] It does this by interfering with the merging of the synaptic vesicle with the plasmalemma. The intracellular receptor for the toxin is thought to be a membranous or cytoskeletal site. Botulinum toxins affect several steps in the ACh releasing process. Serotypes B, D, and F affect a step beyond the influx of Ca^{2+}, which is involved in the synchronization of quantal ACh release. Type B has protease activity and cleaves synaptobrevin-2 which alters recognition of the binding protein on the plasma membrane and impairs vesicle fusion.

Unlike axotomy, botulinum toxin does not cause degeneration of the neuromuscular junction. Terminal motor axons are still capable of conducting impulses. The entry and intraneuronal levels of C^{2+} are unchanged. ACh synthesis and storage is also unchanged. The muscle still responds to applied ACh. Spontaneous miniature end plate potentials are still present but markedly reduced in frequency. Axonal sprouting of the preterminal axons occurs in the region of the neuromuscular junction. There is an increase in extrajunctional ACh receptors.

Therapeutic Use: An aqueous solution containing the botulinum toxin A (Botox), albumin and sodium chloride is injected intramuscularly into selected muscles to produce local neuromuscular blockade. One mouse unit is equal to the amount of toxin that produces a 50% death rate in 18–20 g female Swiss–Webster mice.[204] A concentration of 25–100 mouse units per 1 ml is commonly used. The dose of toxin injected varies according to the site and muscle injected. To optimize the effect, an attempt is made to inject the toxin near the motor end plate region and into the center of the muscle and to inject at multiple sites in each muscle. In experimental animals, it has been shown that the toxin spreads with a diffusion diameter of 4.5 cm (1.8 in) and that muscle facia does not act as a barrier.[205] Intramuscular botulinum toxin produces weakness and atrophy of the injected muscle and adjacent muscles. The effects are first apparent 24–72 hr (1 to >30 days) after injection, maximal by 2–4 weeks and persist for 2–4 months (1–9 months).

The spectrum of clinical applications of local intramuscular botulinum toxin injections is listed in Table 18.5.[r75] In general, botulinum toxin is used in the treatment of focal overactivity of skeletal muscle in any part of the body. The most frequent uses of botulinum toxin are for cervical dystonia, blepharospasm, and hemifacial spasm. Its use has been expanded to the treatment of spasticity and tremor.

Side Effects and Toxicity: the LD50 of botulinum toxin in the monkey is about 40 mouse units per kg given parenterally.[206] Based on this finding, it is estimated that a dose of 3000 mouse units or greater given intramuscularly could be lethal in a 70 kg human. Intramuscular botulinum toxin can produce excessive weakness or unintended involvement of adjacent muscles. Antitoxin cannot inactivate the toxin once it enters the nerve terminal. Agents to antagonize the effects of botulinum toxin are currently under study. Repeated injections of botulinum toxin can lead to pathological

Table 18.5 Clinical Applications of Intramuscular Botulinum Toxin

Dystonia:	*Blepharospasm*
	Cervical dystonia
	Spasmodic dysphonia
	Oromandibular dystonia
	Focal hand dystonia
	Limb dystonia
Muscle Spasms:	*Hemifacial spasm*
	Facial synkinesis
	Masticatory spasms
Spasticity:	*Multiple sclerosis*
	Cerebral Palsy
	Head injury
	Paraplegia
	Stroke
Tremor:	*Dystonic tremor*
	Essential tremor
	Vocal tremor
	Palatal tremor (myoclonus)
Other:	*Bruxism*

changes in the muscle including fibrosis, atrophy, axon sprouting and motor end plate abnormalities.[207,208] Systemic effects have been found including single fiber EMG changes (jitter) in distal muscles and minor changes in cardiac reflexes.[209] Treatment with botulinum toxin is contraindicated in patients with myasthenia gravis or Eaton-Lambert syndrome or those receiving aminoglycosides.

A small number of patients develop antibodies to botulinum toxin type A and no longer respond to treatment.[210] Clinical indicators of antibody formation are a loss of benefit and lack of muscle atrophy. The presence of antibodies can be tested using an in vivo mouse neutralization assay.[211] In an effort to prevent the development of antibody formation, high doses and short intervals between injections are avoided.

Neurotrophic Factors

GM-1 Ganglioside, Glial Derived Neurotrophic Factor (GDNF)

Therapeutic Use: Neurotrophic factors or drugs that modulate them might prove to be useful for the treatment of Parkinson's disease and other degenerative diseases of the basal ganglia. GM-1 ganglioside, a glycosphingolipid, may protect against or assist in repair of nervous system injury. There is evidence that GM-1 ganglioside has a neuroprotective action on experimental parkinsonism in primates.[212] It has also been shown that GM-1 ganglioside injected subcutaneously is well tolerated and may have a positive effect on Parkinson's disease.[213] Gangliosides may act by themselves or by modulating a neurotrophic factor. Glial-derived-neurotrophic factor (GDNF) is a compound capable of promoting axonal sprouting in adult dopaminergic neurons.[214] The gene for GDNF has been identified and human cell lines have been established to produce this factor. Clinical application of these compounds is still limited by the problem of delivery of the compounds to the brain.

General Principles of Movement Disorder Treatment

Drugs are used in a number of different ways in both the diagnosis and treatment of basal ganglia diseases (Table 18.6). Most drugs are administered as symptomatic therapy to reduce the intensity and frequency of the abnormal movements. In some disorders, the drug response is highly characteristic of the disease and critical to the diagnosis. In other disorders, drugs have been used to provoke abnormal movements to support the diagnosis. Drugs are also used as preventative agents to prevent toxic injury to the brain or as neuroprotective agents to protect the nervous system from further damage by the disease process. A more recent approach is the use of drugs to promote regeneration or recovery of function in degenerative diseases.

Different types of movement disorders generally respond to different classes of drugs (Table 18.7). The mechanisms of action of drugs used are closely related to the physiological mechanisms underlying the abnormal movements. Movement disorders occur in the context of brain disease and the pathophysiology of the disease also determines the response to drugs. Different diseases of the basal ganglia involve different pathways and transmitter systems and their pharmacological response properties differ. The optimum use of drugs for the symptomatic treatment of movement disorders requires an understanding of their effects on extrapyramidal motor function and a knowledge of the pharmacological response properties of basal ganglia diseases.

Drugs that modify extrapyramidal motor function generally act by altering neurotransmitter concentrations or interacting selectively with their receptors in the brain. Dopaminergic agents that act on the nigrostriatal dopamine system or other components of circuits involving this pathway provide the best example. The treatment of hypertonicity and muscle spasms and the use of botulinum toxin have extended the target sites of interest to transmitter systems within the spinal cord and peripheral sites such as the neuromuscular junction and muscle spindles. Exceptions to this gen-

Table 18.6 Different Uses of Drugs in Basal Ganglia Diseases*

Purpose	Examples
Symptomatic therapy:	L-DOPA in Parkinson's disease Dopamine antagonists in Huntington's disease
Protective therapy:	Copper chelators in Wilson's disease Deprenyl in Parkinson's disease
Regenerative therapy:	GM1 gangliosides in Parkinson's disease
Diagnostic response:	L-DOPA in DOPA-responsive dystonia Acetazolamide in periodic ataxia
Provocative testing:	L-DOPA in presymptomatic Huntington's disease

*See table 18.4 for other information.

Table 18.7 Drug Response Profile of Various Movement Disorders

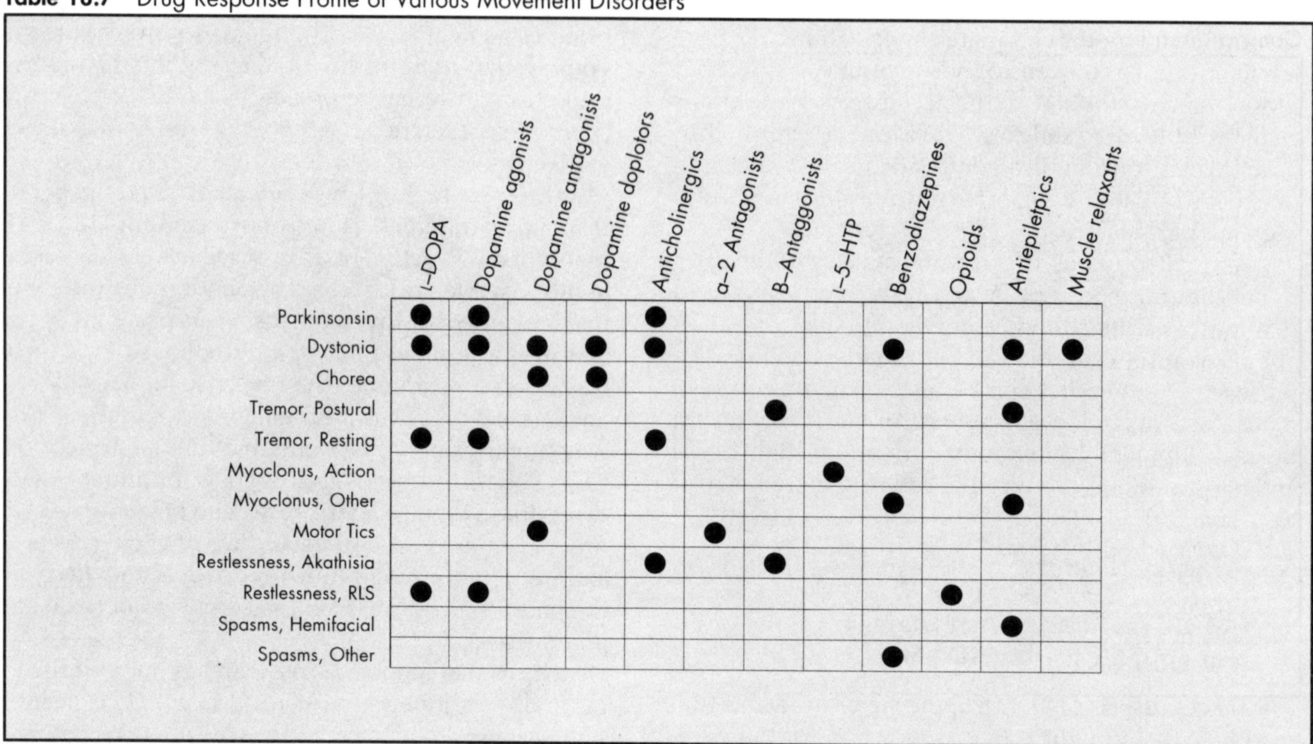

	L-DOPA	Dopamine agonists	Dopamine antagonists	Dopamine doplotors	Anticholinergics	a-2 Antagonists	B-Antaggonists	L-5-HTP	Benzodiazepines	Opioids	Antiepiletpics	Muscle relaxants
Parkinsonsin	●	●			●							
Dystonia	●	●	●	●	●				●		●	●
Chorea			●	●								
Tremor, Postural							●				●	
Tremor, Resting	●	●			●							
Myoclonus, Action								●				
Myoclonus, Other									●		●	
Motor Tics			●			●						
Restlessness, Akathisia					●		●					
Restlessness, RLS	●	●								●		
Spasms, Hemifacial											●	
Spasms, Other									●			

eral mechanism are antiepileptic agents and certain muscle relaxants which act at the level of the cell membrane.

Drugs with selective activity on neurotransmitters are effective because certain neurotransmitter-specific pathways play a major role in extrapyramidal motor function. The effectiveness of L-DOPA in Parkinson's disease reflects the dominant role of the nigrostriatal dopamine system in the motor syndrome of parkinsonism. Functional localization within basal ganglia circuits constituted by diverse neurotransmitter pathways extends the sites at which drugs can be designed to act. The use of anticholinergic drugs to block the output of striatal interneurons receiving input from the nigrostriatal dopamine neurons is an example. The proposed use of glutamate antagonists to block the output of the STN and alter the balance between activity in the "indirect" and "direct" pathways and, ultimately, the output of the GPi, is a more complex example.

The development of drugs that act at different steps in the synthesis, storage, or catabolism of dopamine or are selectively active at different subtypes of dopamine receptors is based on the important role of dopamine in basal ganglia function. In addition to its role in parkinsonism, dopamine plays a major role in the mechanism of chorea, ballismus, restless leg syndrome and some forms of dystonia and a more limited role in many other movement disorders. Dopaminergic drugs used to treat movement disorders now include L-DOPA, dopaminergic agonists, peripheral AADC inhibitors, MAO-B inhibitors, COMT inhibitors, presynaptic dopamine depleters and dopamine antagonists. Other drugs which act indirectly to modify the effects of dopamine on striatal output include anticholinergic agents and the proposed glutamate antagonists.

The pattern of abnormal movements that develops during the course of the illness and the profile of pharmacological responses are highly characteristic of an individual disease. Both properties reflect the complex and subtle effects of the disease process on neuronal circuits and chemical transmission in the brain. The changing response to L-DOPA during the course of Parkinson's disease exemplifies the subtle relationship between drug effects and brain disease. The variability in the effects of a specific drug on a particular movement disorder is a measure of the differences between disease states producing the same type of abnormal movement. In diseases of the basal ganglia that produce a mixture of different types of abnormal movements, e.g., Huntington's disease, the drug response can be complex with suppression of some types of movements and aggravation of others.

Basal ganglia disorders vary in the degree of improvement that occurs in response to drug therapy (Table 18.8). In general, drug-induced forms, e.g., neuroleptic-induced acute dystonic reactions, are highly responsive to drug therapy. This reflects the selectivity

Table 18.8 Drug Responsiveness of Various Basal Ganglia Diseases

Highly Responsive
Neuroleptic-induced, acute dystonic reactions
Paroxysmal kinesigenic choreoathetosis/dystonia
Paroxysmal hypnogenic dystonia
Hereditary periodic ataxia
DOPA-responsive dystonia
Postanoxic action myoclonus
Neuroleptic 'persistent' parkinsonism
Parkinson's disease
Restless leg syndrome
Poorly Responsive
Striatonigral degeneration
Blepharospasm
Spasmodic dysphonia
Oromandibular dystonia
Palatal tremor (myoclonus)
Writer's cramp
Rubral tremor
Cerebellar tremor

of the drugs that cause these disorders and the absence of underlying damage to the brain. Some paroxysmal or periodic forms of movement disorders, e.g., paroxysmal kinesigenic choreoathetosis, are also well controlled with drug therapy. In these cases, the underlying abnormality is probably a disturbance in membrane function and, again, connectivity and chemical transmission in the brain are basically intact. Certain forms of myoclonus, e.g., cortical and reticular reflex myoclonus, represent another example of a functional change in the membrane or local circuits which are highly responsive to drug therapy. In some diseases, e.g., DOPA-responsive dystonia and acetazolamide-sensitive periodic ataxia, the dramatic response to a specific drug is a defining characteristic of the disease. In these cases, a close association between the mechanism of the drug and the disease state is indicated by the degree of response to the drug.

Other types of movement disorders respond poorly to drugs (Table 18.8). In some cases, e.g., striatonigral degeneration, the disease damages cell populations or neurotransmitter systems critical to the mechanisms of action of the drugs used to treat the abnormal movements. In general, movement disorders affecting laryngeal, orofacial, lingual, jaw, and hand muscles, which are involved in highly complex motor functions, are resistant to drug therapy. Degenerative and destructive lesions of the cerebellum or its connections lead to changes in motor function which are complex in their mechanism and generally not modifiable with drugs.

The temporal aspect of the disease can affect drug response and influence drug therapy (Table 18.9). Progressive disorders like Parkinson's disease require repeated adjustments of medications over time to optimize motor function. In diseases like progressive supranuclear palsy, the response to drug treatment seen early in the course of the illness is lost with progression of the disease. Some diseases like essential tremor progress very slowly over several years and drug response and dosage requirement appear relatively stable. Disorders such as postencephalitic parkinsonism are relatively static and may not require any major changes in drug therapy over a several year period. Paroxysmal and periodic disorders can also be considered to be static disorders. Other diseases like Sydenham's chorea are essentially self-limited and the abnormal movements improve over time and eventually resolve. In these diseases, the decision of when to discontinue drug therapy is based on a knowledge of the course of illness and the drug response properties of the disease. Concepts concerning drug treatments for each of the movement disorders is detailed below.

Parkinson's Disease

As noted earlier in this chapter, Parkinson's disease is a progressive neurological disease caused by a degeneration of dopaminergic neurons in the SNc resulting in a marked loss of dopamine in their terminal projection region, the striatum.[215,r76] In a pathological state like parkinsonism with reduced TH activity, the rate of synthesis of dopamine in the brain is low. If the rate of synthesis of dopamine in the striatum falls below the physiological threshold of 20% of normal, the motor signs of parkinsonism appear.[45] In Parkinson's disease, TH activity in the striatum is reduced to 5–20% of normal.[r16] The administration of tyrosine does not produce symptomatic improvement presumably because the low level of TH limits the rate of synthesis of dopamine from tyrosine.[r16] Although the activity of AADC in the striatum in Parkinson's disease is reduced to 5–15% of normal,[9,46] the residual capacity of the enzyme appears to be sufficient, since postmortem studies show that striatal levels of dopamine and HVA are increased after L-DOPA treatment.[46,47] Treatment with L-DOPA also increases the lumbar cerebrospinal fluid level of HVA. In the late stages of the disease, the levels of AADC might be insufficient to convert exogenous L-DOPA to dopamine. It has been suggested that under these conditions, dopamine might be formed from L-DOPA within serotonergic nerve terminals in the striatum.

Atypical parkinsonism: Other forms of parkinsonism vary in their response to drugs. Highly treatable forms

Table 18.9 Temporal Aspects of Drug Response and Basal Ganglia Diseases

Pattern	Examples
Progressive disorders:	Development of dyskinesia and fluctuations in response to L-DOPA in *Parkinson's Disease*
	Loss of efficacy in response to L-DOPA in *Progressive Supranuclear Palsy*
Static disorders:	Stable response to L-DOPA in *Postencephalitic Parkinsonism*
Paroxysmal disorders:	Stable control with antiepileptic drugs in *Paroxysmal Kinesigenic Choreoathetosis*
	Stable control with antiepileptic drugs in *Paroxysmal Hypnogenic Dystonia*
Periodic disorders:	Stable control with acetazolamide in *Hereditary Periodic Ataxia*
Self-limited disorders:	Chorea resolves and no further therapy is required in *Syndenham's Chorea*
	Neuroleptic drugs are restarted and slowly withdrawn in *Withdrawal Emergent Chorea*
	Ballismus resolves and no further therapy is required in *Hemiballismus*
	Need for L-DOPA diminishes over weeks or months in *Neuroleptic Persistent Parkinsonism*

include postencephalitic parkinsonism, neuroleptic persistent parkinsonism, reserpine-induced parkinsonism and MPTP-induced parkinsonism. A more limited response is seen in progressive supranuclear palsy, multiple system atrophy, the rigid form of Huntington's disease, corticobasal ganglionic degeneration and other diseases. The drugs which are effective in the treatment of Parkinson's disease and its atypical forms are listed in Table 18.3, page 337. Their pharmacology has been described earlier in this chapter.

Other disorders which produced parkinsonism vary in their response to drugs. Highly treatable forms include Parkinson's disease, postencephalitic parkinsonism, neuroleptic persistent parkinsonism, reserpine-induced parkinsonism and MPTP-induced parkinsonism. A more limited response is seen in progressive supranuclear palsy, multiple system atrophy, the rigid form of Huntington's disease, corticobasal ganglionic degeneration and other diseases.

Parkinsonism induced by dopaminergic antagonists which persists after the drug is stopped can appropriately be called neuroleptic persistent parkinsonism. Two-thirds of patients recover over a period of several weeks.[283] However, it can last as long as 20 months and recovery can be followed after a few years by the development of Parkinson's disease. In some cases, the response to L-DOPA is essentially complete and the daily dosage requirement decreases over several months until treatment is no longer required. Parkinsonism lasting for a prolonged period after limited exposure to neuroleptic drugs is thought to indicate the presence of subclinical Parkinson's disease.[284]

Dystonia

In general, dystonia is only moderately treatable. The number of different agents which can influence dystonia is large and the ability to predict which agents will be effective and the degree of response in individual cases is limited. Exceptions to this general property of dystonia are a small number of highly treatable forms of dystonia which respond dramatically to specific agents. They include neuroleptic-induced acute dystonic reactions, DOPA-responsive dystonia, paroxysmal kinesigenic dystonia and paroxysmal hypnogenic dystonia. The existence of these forms of dystonia and their pharmacological properties suggest that the mechanism of dystonia involves cholinergic and dopaminergic neurotransmitter systems and conduction in specific motor circuits. See Table 18.10 for various drugs and their doses for treating dystonia.

Anticholinergic Sensitive Dystonia: High dose anticholinergic therapy is the most frequently used treatment of dystonia in its various forms.[285,286,r55] A greater percentage of patients improve in response to anticholinergic drugs than with any other class of drugs. An estimated 50% of children and 40% of adults with dystonia obtain moderate or greater benefit from anticholinergic drugs. Two forms of dystonia that respond well are dystonia secondary to perinatal injury and tardive dystonia.[287] About 40% of patients with tardive dystonia benefit from treatment with anticholinergic drugs.[288] Patients with DOPA-responsive dystonia can respond to low dosages of anticholinergic drugs.[r95] These drugs are highly effective in reversing neuroleptic-induced acute dystonia reactions.[289–291] A dose of 2 mg of benztropine mesylate given intramuscularly or 50 mg of diphenhydramine, an antihistamine with anticholinergic properties, given intravenously is recommended for acute dystonic reactions.[r55]

DOPA-Responsive Dystonia: DOPA-responsive dystonia is a form of childhood-onset dystonia that predominantly affects gait and balance and responds dramatically to treatment with L-DOPA.[r96] Patients with

Table 18.10 Doses of Drugs Used to Treat Other Movement Disorders

Type of Disorder	Generic Name	Trade Name	Daily Doses (mg)
Dystonia	Trihexyphenidyl	Artane	6–60
	Clonazepam	Klonopin	1–10
	Baclofen	Lioresal	30–120
	Tetrabenazine	Nitoman	25–150
	Pimozide	Orap	4–12
	Carbamazepine	Tegratol	600–1200
	Bromocriptine	Parlodel	10–60
Chorea	Haloperidol (or Pimozide)	Haldol	1–8
	Tetrabenazine	Nitoman	25–150
Tremor, postural	Propranolol	Inderal	80–240
	Primidone	Mysoline	50–250
	Acetazolamide	Diamox	500–1000
Myoclonus, action	5-Hydroxytrypophan	L-5-HTP	1000–2000
Myoclonus, other	Clonazepam	Klonopin	1–10
	Valproic acid	Depakote	500–2000
Motor tics	Pimozide (or haloperidol)	Orap	2–8
	Clonidine	Catapres	0.1–0.8
Akathisia, typical	Benztropine	Cogentin	1–4
	Propranalol	Inderal	30–120
Akathisia, tardive	Tetrabenazine	Nitoman	25–150
	Pimozide	Orap	2–8
Restless leg syndrome	L-DOPA	Sinemet (or Sinemet CR)	25/100–250/1000
	Bromocriptine	Parlodel	5–25
	Propoxyphene	Darvon	100–400
Spasticity	Baclofen	Lioresal	30–120
	Dantrolene	Dantrium	100–300
	Diazepam	Valium	30–50
	Tizanidine	Sirdalud	6–12

DOPA-responsive dystonia can show improvement as early as after the first or second dose and with doses as low as 50–100 mg.[r96] The marked and immediate improvement and the absence of peak-dose dyskinesia and clinical fluctuations with chronic L-DOPA treatment are characteristic of this disorder. In DOPA-responsive dystonia, there is evidence of a decrease in dopamine synthesis and a marked decrease in striatal dopamine content[292] in the presence of a normal number of substantia nigra neurons and a normal striatal 6[^{18}F] L-DOPA uptake.[293] The exceptional response to L-DOPA in DOPA-responsive dystonia is probably related to the structural integrity of dopamine neurons in this disorder.

Paroxysmal Hypnogenic Dystonia: Paroxysmal hypnogenic dystonia is characterized by painful, dystonic spasms lasting less than a minute which awaken the patient from sleep and occur several times a night or during daytime naps.[294] Mesial frontal lobe seizures are suspected to be the cause of these dystonic spasms. Treatment with carbamazepine, which has antiepileptic properties, is effective in controlling the spasms.[295]

Tremor

The basic types of tremor respond differentially to drugs suggesting that their underlying mechanisms differ (see Table 18.10). Dopaminergic agonists and anticholinergic agents with central activity are effective in suppressing rest tremor. This effect can be dramatic and in some cases results in complete control of the tremor. β-Adrenergic antagonists are effective in reducing action tremor, postural tremor and exaggerated physiological tremor. They are thought to act at peripheral β-2 receptors present on extrafusal muscle fibers of muscle spindles.[296] Although two-thirds of patients with essential tremor respond to β-adrenergic antagonists, the effect is unpredictable in individual patients. Many of the drugs which provoke or exacerbate physiological and pathological forms of tremor also act on central cholinergic or dopaminergic systems or on peripheral adrenergic systems.

Tremors associated with cerebellar disease are generally unresponsive to drug therapy. This could reflect the degree or extent of damage or the functional organization of neurotransmitter pathways within the cerebellum and its circuits.

Chorea

In general, chorea is highly treatable. The number of agents which suppress chorea is relatively small and their effects are predictable (see Table 18.10). The degree of response is relatively nonspecific with regard to the nature of the underlying disease. The direction of the change in chorea is specific to the type of drug. Dopaminergic antagonists and presynaptic dopamine depleters reduce or abolish chorea whereas anticholinergic agents intensify chorea. These effects suggest that the mechanism which produces chorea involves dopaminergic pathways and the dopaminergic-cholinergic balance of activity in the striatum. The pattern of effects is the inverse of that found in parkinsonism and suggests that chorea is produced by a relative increase in dopaminergic activity in the striatum. Paroxysmal kinesigenic choreoathetosis appears to be fundamentally different from other forms of chorea based on its pharmacological response properties.

Huntington's Disease: Huntington's disease is an autosomal dominant disorder characterized by widespread degenerative changes of the basal ganglia and other brain regions and the development of prominent chorea and dementia.[r97] Other types of movement disorders also occur in this disease including dystonia, bradykinesia and cerebellar dysfunction. Chorea which dominates during the early stages can be replaced by dystonia and bradykinesia late in the disease. The most prominent pathological changes are atrophy of the caudate nucleus and putamen with selective loss of intrinsic spiny neurons which utilize GABA/metenkephalin or GABA/substance P as transmitters. The early loss of GABA/met-enkephalin neurons projecting to the GPe, a component of the 'indirect' pathway, with a decrease in the inhibitory output of the GPi to the thalamus and disinhibition of the thalamocortical pathway has been proposed as the mechanism producing chorea.[297,r98] Treatment with dopaminergic antagonists by decreasing the activity within the 'direct' pathway might restore the balance and suppress chorea.

Hemiballismus: Ballismus refers to rapid, large amplitude, proximal movements of the limbs which have a rotational component giving them a flinging quality or making them resemble throwing movements. It is associated with lesions of the subthalamic nucleus or its afferent or efferent connections with the globus pallidus.[298,299] It is thought that an interruption of subthalamopallidal pathways or of the pallido-thalamic inhibitory pathway is responsible for hemiballismus. Lesions of the "indirect" pathway leading to a relative overactivity of the "direct" pathway might explain the effectiveness of dopaminergic antagonists and presynaptic dopamine depleters in hemiballismus.

Paroxysmal kinesigenic choreoathetosis: Paroxysmal kinesigenic choreoathetosis (PKC) is characterized by brief attacks starting in childhood of choreiform or dystonic movements precipitated by voluntary movements such as rapidly arising from a chair or starting to walk.[r99] The attacks typically last less than 5 minutes and can occur up to 100 times per day. Phenytoin and other antiepileptic drugs are effective in controlling the attacks. PKC is thought to represent a form of seizure disorder involving the basal ganglia.

Myoclonus

Highly treatable forms of myoclonus include postanoxic action myoclonus, cortical myoclonus and reticular reflex myoclonus, a subtype of subcortical myoclonus. Action myoclonus is associated with a low cerebrospinal fluid level of 5-hydroxyindolacetic acid (5-HIAA),[300] the major metabolite of serotinin in brain, and a dramatic response to treatment with L-5-hydroxytryptophan (5-HTP), the precursor of serotonin.[170,301] These findings suggest that serotonergic systems play a role in the mechanism of this form of myoclonus. Benzodiazepines, in particular clonazepam, and valproic acid are effective in other forms of myoclonus. It is thought that GABAergic mediated inhibition might be responsible for the actions of these drugs.

Action myoclonus: L-5-HTP has been shown to be effective in the treatment of postanoxic action myoclonus.[170,301] The reduction in myoclonus is thought to be due to the enhancement of serotonin synthesis in the brain. There are a limited number of reports of improvement in patients with other forms of myoclonus. L-5-HTP has not been demonstrated to have therapeutic effects in other types of abnormal movements. Other drugs available to treat myoclonus are listed in Table 18.10.

Motor Tics

Dopaminergic antagonists[100] and presynaptic dopamine depleters are effective in tic disorders suggesting that dopaminergic systems are involved in the mechanism of tics. There is evidence that clonidine, an α-2 adrenergic agonist, reduces tics suggesting possible involvement of noradrenergic mechanisms.[302]

Motor Restlessness

The pharmacological response profiles of akathisia and restless leg syndrome are relatively distinct compared to other movement disorders.

Akathisia: Dopaminergic antagonists and presynaptic dopamine depleters can elicit typical forms of akathisia and anticholinergic agents, β-adrenergic antagonists and opioids can partially suppress them.[303,304] These effects suggests that dopaminergic, cholinergic, noradrenergic and opioid systems are involved in the mechanism of akathisia. In contrast, tardive akathisia can be completely suppressed by dopaminergic antagonists and β-adrenergic antagonists are ineffective. Anticholinergic agents can produce worsening of tardive akathisia. Although the neurotransmitter systems and circuits involved in tardive akathisia and the more typical forms of akathisia are probably the same, the balance of activity between the components appears to differ. The partial extent of the response to drug treatment also suggests a complex underlying mechanism with no single dominant factor (see Table 18.10).

Restless Leg Syndrome: Restless leg syndrome responds dramatically to treatment with L-DOPA and opioid agonists indicating participation of dopaminergic and opioid systems in the underlying mechanism[305,306] (see Table 18.10).

Hypertonicity

Doses of drugs to treat hypertonicity are listed in Table 18.10. Disorders in this category are discussed individually below.

Rigidity: The pharmacological properties of rigidity are similar to those of the bradykinesia component of parkinsonism. Dopaminergic agonists and anticholinergic drugs are effective in reducing rigidity. The response to dopaminergic agonists is predictable and the effect can be almost complete in its extent. There is frequently a dissociation in the response of bradykinesia and rigidity and that of rest tremor to these agents. This indicates that differences exist in the underlying mechanisms of the various components of parkinsonism. An understanding of these differences is important in improving the treatment of the tremor- and bradykinesia-predominant forms of Parkinson's disease.

Although rigidity does not appear to impair movement directly, it is associated with a chronic, aching pain in the proximal limbs and lower back and makes assisting patients with parkinsonism more difficult. For these reasons, drug therapy directed at reducing rigidity is useful.

Spasticity: The advances in drug therapy of spasticity have paralleled an understanding of the mechanism of spasticity. Spasticity appears to result from decreased activity in spinal inhibitory pathways and increased excitability of flexor reflex interneurons and to involve both GABAergic and glycinergic inhibitory pathways.[r101] In spasticity, alpha motor neurons and interneurons involved in flexor reflexes are in a hyperexcitable state and presynaptic inhibition of 1A terminals and reciprocal inhibition is reduced. In general, drugs used to treat spasticity have greater effects on polysynaptic reflexes than on monosynaptic ones. Drugs which are effective in reducing spasticity have multiple and complex actions involving GABAergic, glutamatergic, glycinergic and adrenergic transmission and the basic contractile mechanism of muscle fibers.

Spasticity is of interest in the context of movement disorders because it alters movement and responds to drug therapy. Treatment of spasticity can result in functional improvement in patients with relatively preserved extensor muscle strength in the legs. Patients who depend on extensor spasticity in the legs for support while standing can become worse if aggressively treated for spasticity.

Neuroleptic Malignant Syndrome: Neuroleptic malignant syndrome is characterized by muscle rigidity, extreme hyperthermia, autonomic instability, a decreased level of consciousness, leukocytosis and an elevated CPK level.[r102] It is a potentially fatal side effect of neuroleptic drugs but can also be caused by treatment with presynaptic dopamine depleters or the withdrawal of dopamine agonists. The rigidity of the skeletal muscles can lead to dyspnea, dysphagia and rhabdomyolysis. Blockade of dopamine receptors in the striatum, hypothalamus and spinal cord has been proposed as the underlying mechanism. Treatment with the dopaminergic agonists L-DOPA, bromocriptine and lisuride and the muscle relaxant dantrolene has been suggested.

Stiff-Man syndrome: Stiff-man syndrome is a progressive disorder characterized by the insidious development of stiffness of the lower back, neck and proximal limbs associated with painful spasms triggered by movement or various stimuli.[r5] Lumbar lordosis, a slow, stiff-legged gait and falling forward in response to spasms are characteristic of this disorder. Electromyography shows continuous motor unit activity in both agonist and antagonist muscles that is reduced by diazepam. It is thought to be an autoimmune disorder with antibodies directed against glutamic acid decarboxylase (GAD) which result in a decrease in GABA synthesis and activity within the central nervous system. Anti-

GAD antibodies are found in serum and cerebrospinal fluid (CSF). Diazepam and clonazepam in high doses are effective in the treatment of the stiffness and spasms.

Muscle Spasms

Hemifacial spasm is characterized by clonic jerks or twitches of facial muscles innervated by the seventh cranial nerve. Alterations in the facial nerve nucleus leading to ephaptic transmission between the nerve fibers or ectopic excitation of nerve fibers have been proposed as possible mechanisms.[307–309] The kindling phenomenon has been used to explain the hyperactivity of motor neurons found in this disorder. Carbamazepine, which has antiepileptic properties, is the most effective drug in the treatment of hemifacial spasm.

Ataxia

In general, ataxia does not improve with drug therapy. However, there are a few diseases which produce ataxia where treatment with specific agents can reverse the ataxia or prevent or arrest progression of the neurological symptoms. These include hereditary periodic ataxia, acquired and hereditary disorders with vitamin E deficiency and ataxia, and cholestanolosis.

Ataxia associated with vitamin E deficiency: Vitamin E deficiency can be associated with the development of spinocerebellar degeneration and ataxia.[r103] Diseases which affect the bile salt concentration in the small intestine or its absorptive surface can lead to fat malabsorption and vitamin E deficiency. In abetalipoproteinemia and pure vitamin E deficiency, both autosomal recessive disorders, treatment with vitamin E can prevent or arrest the progression of the neurological dysfunction.[310] The pathophysiological mechanism by which a deficiency of vitamin E produces ataxia is unknown.

Cholestanolosis: Cholestanolosis, or cerebrotendinous xanthomatosis, is an autosomal recessive disorder characterized by ataxia and tendon xanthomata. Treatment with chenodeoxycholic acid is reported to improve neurological function in cholestanolosis.[311]

Hereditary Periodic Ataxia: Periodic ataxia is a rare autosomal dominant disorder characterized by attacks of limb and gait ataxia associated with nystagmus, dysarthria and intention tremor. The attacks can be completely controlled by treatment with the carbonic anhydrase inhibitor acetazolamide.[312] The physiological mechanism of ataxia in this disorder is unknown.

References

Research Reports

1. AD HOC COMMITTEE (1984) Ad Hoc Committee of the Dystonia Medical Research Foundation met in February 1984. Its members included Drs. A. Barbeau, D.B. Calne, S. Fahn, C.D. Marsden, J. Menkes and G.F. Wooten.
2. Findley LJ, Gresty MA. Tremor. Br J Hosp Med 1981;*26*:16–32.
3. Satoyoshi E. A syndrome of progressive muscle spasms, alopecia, and diarrhea. Neurolgy 1978;*28*:458–461.
4. Alexander GE, Crutcher MD. Functional architecture of basal ganglia circutis: neural substrates of parallel processing. Trends Neurosci *13*:266–271.
5. Lovenberg W, Weissbach H, Udenfriend S. Aromatic L-amino acid decarboxylase. J Biol Chem 1962;*237*:89–93.
6. Lloyd KG, Hornydiewicz O. Occurrence and distribution of aromatic L-amino acid (L-DOPA) decarboxylase in the human brain. J Neurochem 1972;*19*:1549–1559.
7. Sourkes TL. Dopa decarboxylase: substrates, coenzyme, inhibitors. Pharmacol Rev 1966;*18*:53–60.
8. Lloyd KG, Hornykiewicz O. Parkinson's disease: activity of L-dopa decarboxylase in discrete brain regions. Science 1970;*170*:1212–1213.
9. Everett GM, Borcherding JW. L-Dopa: effect on concentrations of dopamine, norepinephrine and serotonin in brains of mice. Science 1970;*168*:849–850.
10. Langelier P, Roberge AG, Boucher R, Poirier LJ. Effects of chronically administered L-dopa in normal and lesioned cats. J Pharmacol Exp Ther 1973;*187*:15–26.
11. Ng LKY, Chase TN, Colburn RW, and Kopin IJ. L-dopa in parkinsonism: a possible mechanism of action. Neurology 1972;*22*:688–696.
12. Melamed E, Hefte F, Liebman J, Schlosberg AJ, Wurtman RJ. Serotoninergic neurones are not involved in action of L-dopa in Parkinson's disease. Nature 1980;*283*:772–774.
13. Wade DN, Mearrick PT, Morris JL. Active transport of L-dopa in the intestine. Nature 1973;*242*:463–465.
14. Morris JGL, Parsons RL, Trounce JR, Groves MJ. Plasma dopa concentrations after different preparations of levodopa in normal subjects. Brit J Clin Pharmacol 1976;*3*:983–990.
15. Sasahara L, Nitanai T, Habara T et al. Dosage form design for improvement of bioavailability of levodopa V: absorption and metabolism of levodopa in intestinal segments of dogs. J Pharm Sci 1981;*70*:1157–1160.
16. Hare TA, Beasley BL, Chambers RA, Boehme DH, Vogel WH. Dopa and aminoacid levels in plasma and cerebrospinal fluid of patients with Parkinsons disease before and during treatment with L-Dopa. Clinica Chimica Acta 1973;*45*:274–280.
17. Imai K, Sugiura M, Tamura Z, Hirayama K, Narabayashi H. The plasma levels of DOPA and catecholamines after oral administration of L-DOPA. Chem Pharm Bull 1971:*19*:439–440.
18. Rivera-Calimlin L, Morgan JP, Dujovne DA, Bianchine JR, Lsagna L. L-3,4-dihydroxyphenylalanine metabolism by the gut in vitro. Biochem Pharmacol 1971;*20*:3051–3057.
19. Mearrick PT, Graham GG, Wade DN. The role of the liver in the clearance of L-dopa from plasma. J. Pharmacokin Biopharm 1975;*3*:13–23.
20. Cotler S, Holazo A, Boxenbaum HG, Kaplan SA. Influence of route of administration on physiological availability of levodopa in dogs. J Pharm Sci 1976;*65*:822–827.
21. Wurtman RJ, Chow C, Rose CM. The fate of ^{14}C-dihydroxyphenylalanine (^{14}C-dopa) in the whole mouse. J Pharmacol Exp Ther 1970;*174*:351–356.

22. Eriksson R, Granerus A, Linde A, Carlsson A. 'On-off' phenomenon in Parkinson's disease: relationship between dopa and other large neutral amino-acids in plasma. Neurology 1988;*38*:1245–1248.

23. Knudsen GM, Pettigrew KD, Patlak CS, Hertz MM, Paulson OB. Asymmetrical transport of amino acids across the blood-brain barrier in humans. J. Cereb Blood Flow and Metab 1990;*10*:698–706.

24. Nutt JG, Woodward WR, Hammerstad JP, Carter JH, Anderson JL. The 'on-off' phenomenon in Parkinson's disease: relation to levodopa absorption and transport. N Engl J Med 1984;*310*:484–488.

25. Ordonez LA, Arbrus M, Borson S, Goodman MN, Ruderman NB, Wurtman RJ, Skeletal muscle: reservoir for exogenous L-Dopa. J Pharmacol Exp Ther 1974;*190*:187–191.

26. Andersson I, Granerus A, Jagenburg R, Svanborg A. Intestinal decarboxylation of orally administered 1-dopa. Acta Med Scand 1975;*198*:415–420.

27. Sasahara K, Nitanai T, Habara T, Morioka T, Nakajima E. Dosage form design for improvement of bioavailability of levodopa IV: possible causes of low bioavailability of oral levodopa in dogs. J Pharm Sci 1981;*70*:730–733.

28. Coutinho DB, Spiegel HE, Kaplan SA et al. Kinetics of absorption and excretion of levodopa in dogs. J Pharm Sci 1971;*60*:1014–1019.

29. Granerus AK, Jagenburg R, Svanborg A. Intestinal decarboxylation of L-dopa in relation to dose requirement in Parkinson's disease. Naunyn Schmiedeberg's Arch Pharmacol 1973;*280*:429–439.

30. Sasahara K, Nitanai T, Habara T, Moroiki T, Nakajima E. Dosage form design for improvement of bioavailability of levodopa II: bioavailability of marketed levodopa preparations in dogs and Parkinsonian patients. J Pharm Sci 1980;*69*:261–265.

31. Goodall MC, Alton H. Metabolism of 3,4-dihydroxyphenylalanine (L-DOPA) in human subjects. Biochem Pharmac 1972;*21*:2401–2408.

32. Sandler M, Johnson RD, Ruthven CRJ, Reid JL, Calne DB. Tranamination is a major pathway of L-dopa metabolism following peripheral decarboxylase inhibition. Nature 1974;*247*:364–366.

33. Bronaugh RL, Wenger GR, Garver DL, Rutledge CO. Effect of carbidopa on the metabolism of L-dopa in the pigtail monkey. Biochem Pharmacol 1976;*25*:1679–1681.

34. Calne DB, Karoum F, Ruthven DRJ, Sandler M. The metabolism of orally administered L-DOPA in Parkinsonism. Br J Pharmacol 1969;*37*:57–68.

35. Peaston MJT, Bianchine JR. Metabolic studies and clinical observations during L-dopa treatment of Parkinson's disease. Br Med J 1970;*1*:400–403.

36. Imai K, Sugiura M, Kubo H et al. Studies on the metabolism and excretion of L-3-,4-dihydroxyphenylalanine (L-DOPA) in human beings by gas chromatography. Chem Pharm Bull 1972;*20*:759–764.

37. Morgan JP, Bianchine JR, Spiegel HE, Rivera-Calimlim L, Hersey RM. Metabolism of levodopa in patients with Parkinson's disease. Arch Neurol 1971;*25*:39–44.

38. Cotzias GC. Parkinsonism and dopa. J Chronic Dis 1969;*22*:279–301.

39. Fabbrini G, Juncos J, Mouradian M, Serrati C, Chase T. Levodopa pharmacokinetic mechanisms and motor fluctuations in Parkinson's disease. Amm Neurol 1987;*21*:370–376.

40. Gancher S, Nutt J, Woodward W. Peripheral pharmacokinetics of levodopa in untreated, stable and fluctuating patients. Neurology 1987;*37*:940–944.

41. Nutt JG, Woodward W, Anderson J. The effect of carbidopa on the pharmacokinetics of intravenously administered levodopa: the mechanism of action in the treatment of Parkinsonism. Ann Neurol 1985;*18*:537–543.

42. Hardie RJ, Lees AJ and Stern GM. On-off fluctuations in Parkinson's disease: a clinical and neuropharmacological study. Brain 1984;*107*:487–506.

43. Hardie RJ, Malcolm S, Lees AJ et al. The pharmacokinetics of oral and intravenous levodopa in patients with Parkinson's disease who exhibit on-off fluctuations. Br J Clin Pharmacol 1986;*22*:429–436.

44. Cedarbaum J, Hoey M, McDowell F. A double-blind crossover comparison of Sinemet CR4 and standard Sinemet 25/100 in patients with Parkinson's disease and fluctuating motor performance. J Neurol Neurosurg Psych 1989;*52*:207–212.

45. Bernheimer H, Birkmayer W, Hornykiewicz O, Jellinger K, Seitelbergger FF. Brain dopamine and the syndromes of Parkinson and Huntington. J Neurol Sci 1973;*20*:415–455.

46. Lloyd KG, Davidson L, Hornykiewicz O. The neurochemistry of Parkinson's disease: effect of L-DOPA therapy. J Pharmacol Exp Ther 1975;*195*:453–464.

47. Rinne UK, Sonninen V. Brain catecholamines and their metabolites in Parkinsonian patients. Arch Neurol 1973;*28*:107–110.

48. Dempski R, Scholtz E, Oberholtzer E, Yeh K. Pharmaceutical design and development of a Sinemet controlled release formulation. Neurology 1989;*39*(supp):.

49. Cedarbaum JM, Kutt H, McDowell F. A pharmacokinetic and pharmacodynamic comparison of Sinemet CR (50/200) and standard Sinemet (25/100). Neurology 1989;*39*(supp):).

50. Erni W, Held K. The hydrodynamically balanced system: a novel principle of controlled drug release. Eur Neurol 1987;(supp):21–27.

51. Campbell NRC, Hasinof B. Ferrous sulfate reduces levodopa bioavailability: chelation as a possible mechanism. Clin Pharmacol Ther 1989;*45*:220–225.

52. Messiha FS, Morgan JP. Imipramine-mediated effects on levodopa metabolism in man. Biochem Pharmacol 1974;*23*:1503–1507.

53. Fermaglich J, O'Doherthy S. Effect of gastric morility on levodopa. Dis Nerv Syst 1972;*33*:624–625.

54. Sweet RD, Lee JE, McDowell FH. Methyldopa as an adjunct to levodopa treatment of Parkinson's disease. Clin Pharmacol Ther 1972;*13*:23–27.

55. Henning M, Rubenson A. J Pharm Pharmacol 1970;*22*:241.

56. Reid JL, Calne DB, George CF, Vakil SD et al. Plasma concentration of levodopa in Parkinsonism before and after inhibition of peeipheral decarboxylase Neurol Sci 1972;*17*:45–51.

57. Dhasmana KM, Spilker BA. Brit J Pharmacol 1973;*47*:437.

58. Calne DB, Reid JL, Vokel SD, George CF, Rao S. Effect of carbidopa and L-DOPA on blood pressure in man. Adv Neurol 1973;*2*:149–160.

59. Parks LC, Watanabe AM, Kopin IJ. Prevention or reversal of levodopa induced cardiac arrhythmias by decarboxylase inhibition. Lancet 1970;*2*:1014–1015.

60. Graham DG, Tiffany SM, Bell WR, Gutnecht WF. Auto-oxidation versus covalent binding of quinones as the mechanism of toxicity of dopamine, 6-hydroxydopamine and related com-

pounds toward c1300 neuroblastoma cells in vitro. Mol Pharmacol 1978;*14*:644–653.

61. Dexter DT, Carter C, Agid F et al. Lipid peroxidation as a cause of nigral cell death in Parkinson's disease. Lancet 1986;*2*:639–640.

62. Sandler M. The dopa effect: possible significance of transamination and tetrahydroisoquinolone formation. Adv Neurol 1973;*2*:255–264.

63. Lieberman AN, Shupack JL. Levodopa and melanoma. Neurology 1974;*24*:340–343.

64. Heubert ND, Palfreyman MG, Haegele KD. A comparison of the effects of reversible and irreversible inhibitors of aromatic L-amino acid decarboxylase on the half-life and other pharmacokinetic parameters of oral L-3,4-dihydroxyphenylalanine. Drug Metab 1983;*11*:195–200.

65. Baldessarini RJ, and Greiner E. Inhibition of catechol-O-methyl transferase by catechols and polyphenols. Biochem Pharmacol 1973;*22*:247–256.

66. Burkard WP, Gey KF, Pletscher A. Inhibition of decarboxylase of araomatic amino acids by 2,3,4-trihydroxybenzylhydrazine and its seryl derivative. Arch Biochem Biophysics 1964;*107*:187–196.

67. Vickers S, Stuart EK, Bianchine JR, Hucker HB, Haffe ME, Rhodes RF, Vandenheuval WJA. Metabolism of carbidopa [L-(-)-2-hydrazino-3, 4-dihydroxy-a-methylhydrocinnamic acid monohydrated], an aromatic amino acid decarboxylase inhibitor, in the rat, dog, rhesus monkey and man. Drug Metab Distrib 1974;*2*:9–22.

68. Vickers S, Stuart EK, Hucker HB and Vandenheuval WJA. Further studies on the metabolism of carbidopa (-)-L-a-hydrazino-3, 4-dihydroxy-b-methylbenzenepropanoic acid monohydrate, in the human, rhesus monkey, dog and rat. J Med Chem 1975;*18*:134–138.

69. Schwartz ED, Jordan JC, Ziegler WH. Pharmacokinetics of the decarboxylase inhibitor benserazide in man: its tissue distribution in the rat. Eur J Clin Pharmacol 1974;*7*:39–45.

70. Bartholini G, Pletscher A. Cerebral accumulation and metabolism of C^{14}-DOPA after selective inhibition of peripheral decarboxylase. J Pharmcol Exp Ther 1968;*161*:14–20.

71. Tissot R, Bartholini G, Pletscher A. Drug-induced changes of extracerebral dopa metabolism in man. Arch Neurol 1969;*20*:187–190.

72. Dunner DL, Brodie KH, Goodwin FK. Plasma DOPA response to levodopa administration in man: effects of a peripheral decarboxylase inhibitor. Clin Pharmacol Exp Ther 1971;*12*:212–217.

73. Kuruma I, Bartholini G, Tissot R, Pletscher A. Comparative investigation of inhibitors of extracerebral dopa decarboxylase in man and rats. J Pharm Pharmacol 1972;*24*:289–294.

74. Messiha FS, Hsu TH, Bianchine JR. Effects of peripheral aromatic L-amino acids decarboxylase inhibitor on L-($2^{14}C$)-dopa metabolism in man. Biochem Pharmacol 1972;*21*:2144–2147.

75. Boomsma F, Meerwaldt JD, Veld AJ, et al. Induction of aromatic-l-amino acid decarboxylase by decarboxylase inhibitors in idiopathic parkinsonism. Ann Neuro 1989;*25*:624–628.

76. McDowell FH, Lee JE, Swift T, Sweet RD, Ogsbury JS. Kessler JR. Treatment of Parkinson's disease with L-dihydroxyphenylalanine (levodopa). Ann Int Med 1970;*72*:29–35.

77. Hoehn M. Increased dosage of carbidopa in patients with Parkinson's disease receiving low doses of levodopa. Arch Neurol 1980;*37*:146–149.

78. Bianchine JR, Messina FS, Hsu TH. Peripheral aromatic l-amino acids decarboxylase inhibitor in parkinsonism II: effect on metabolism of ^{14}C-DOPA. Clin Pharmacol Ther 1972;*13*:584–594.

79. Calne DB. Brit Med J 1971;*3*:693.

80. Zurcher G, Keller HH, Kettler R, Borgulya J, Bonetti EP, Eigenmann R, Da Prada M. Ro 40-7592, a novel, very potent and orally active inhibitor of catechol-O-methyltransferase: a pharmacological study in rats. Adv Neurol 1990;*53*:497–503.

81. Mannisto PT, Kaakkola S, Nissinen E, Linden I-B, Pohto P. Properties of novel effective and highly selective inhibitors of catechol-O-methyltransferase. Life Sci 1988;*43*:1465–1471.

82. Dingemanse J, Schmitt M, Fotteler B, Gieschke R, Zurcher GG, Timm U, Nielsen T, Goggin T. A single ascending oral dose study of tolerability, safety, pharmacodynamics and pharmacokinetics of Ro 40-7592 in young healthy male volunteers.

83. Keranen T, Gordin A, Harjola V-P, et al. The effects of catechol-O-methyltransferase inhibition by entacapone on the pharmacokinetics and metabolism of levodopa in healthy volunteers. Clin Neuropharm 1993;*16*:145–156.

84. Birkmayer W, Riedener P, Ambrozi L, Youdin MBH: Implications of combined treatment with Madapar and L-deprenyl in Parkinson's disease. Lancet 1977;*2*:439–440.

85. Yahr MD. Levodopa. Ann Int Med 1975;*83*:677–682.

86. Youdim MBH. The active centres of monoamine oxidase types 'A' and 'B' binding with (^{14}C)-Clorgyline and (^{14}C)-Deprenyl. J Neural Transm 1978;*43*:199–208.

87. Knoll J. (–) Deprenyl-the MAO inhibitor without the 'cheeseeffect'. Trends Neurosci 1979;*2*:11–13.

88. Reynolds GP, Elsworth JD, Blau K, Sandler M, Lees AJ, Stern GM. Deprenyl is metabolised to metamphetamine and amphetamine in man. Brit J Clin Pharmacol 1978;*6*:542–544.

89. Westlund KN, Denney RM, Kochersperger LM, Rose RM, Abell CW. Distinct monoamine oxidase A and B populations in primate brain. Science 1985;*230*:181–183.

90. Glover V, Elsworth JD, Sandler M. Dopamine oxidation and its inhibition by (-)-deprenyl in man. J Neural Trans 1980;*16* (supp):163–172.

91. Glover V, Sandler M, Owen F, Riley GJ. Dopamine is a monoamine oxidase B substrate in man. Nature 1977;*265*:80–81.

92. Heikkila RE, Cabbat FS, Manzino L, Duvoisin RC. Potentiation by deprenil of l-dopa induced circling in nigral-lesioned rats. Pharmacol Biochem Behav 1981;*15*:75–79.

93. Reynolds GP, Riederer P, Sandler M, et al. Amphetamine and 2-Phenylethylamine in post-mortem Parkinsonian brain after (–) deprenyl administration. J Neural Transm 1978;*43*:271–277.

94. Reynolds CP, Riederer P, Sandler M. 2-Phenylethylamine and amphetamine in human brain: effects of L-deprenyl in Parkinson's disease. Biochem Soc Trans 1979;*7*:143–145.

95. Elsworth JD, Glover V, Reynolds GP, Sandler M, Lees AJ, Phuapradit P, Shaw KM, Stern GM, Kumar P. Deprenyl administration in man: a selective monoamine oxidase B inhibitor without the 'cheese effect'. Psychopharmacology 1978;*57*:33–38.

96. Jackson DM. 2-Phenylethylamine and locomotor activity in mice. Arzneim-Forsch 1975;*25*:622–626.

97. Riederer P, Youdim MBH. Monamine oxidase activity and monoamine metabolism in brains of parkinsonian patients treated with 1-deprenyl. J Neurochem 1986;*46*:1359–1365.

98. Reynolds GP, Riederer P. Assessment of MAO inhibitors using postmortem brain tissue: biochemical and therapeutic implications. Mod Prob Pharmacopsych 1983;*19*:255–259.

99. Liebowitz MR, Karoum F, Quitkan FM, Davies SO, Schwaetz D, Levitt M, Linnoila M, Biochemical effects of L-deprenyl in atypical depressives. Biol Psych 1985;558–565.

100. Spina MB, Cohen G. Dopamine turnover and glutathione oxidation: implications for Parkinson's disease. Proc Natl Acad Sci 1989;*86*:1398–1400.

101. Cohen G. The pathobiology of Parkinson's disease: biochemical aspects of dopamine neuron senescence. J Neural Trans 1983;*19*(supp):89–103.

102. Robinson DS. Changes in monoamine oxidase and monoamines with human development and aging. Fed Proc 1975;*34*:103–107.

103. Ambani LM, Van Woert WH, Murphy S. Brain peroxidase and catalase in Parkinson's disease. Arch Neurol 1975;*32*:114–118.

104. Perry TL, Godin DV, Hansen S. Parkinson's disease: A disorder due to nigral glutathione deficiency? Neuroscience Letters 1982;*33*:305–310.

105. Kish SJ, Morito C, Hornykiewicz O. Glutathione peroxidase activity in Parkinson's disease brain. Neurosci Lett 1985;*58*:343–346.

106. Birkmayer W, Knoll J, Riederer P, Youdim MBH, Hars V, Marton J. Increased life expectancy resulting from the addition of L-deprenyl to Madopar treatment in Parkinson's disease. J Neural Trans 1985;*64*:113–127.

107. Datatop Study. Effect of Deprenyl on the progression of disability in early Parkinson's disease. N Engl J Med 1989;*321*:1364–1371.

108. Tetrud JW, Langston JW. The effect of deprenyl (selegiline) on the natural history of Parkinson's disease. Science 1987;*245*:519–522.

109. Olanow CW, Calne D. Does selegiline monotherapy in Parkinson's disease act by symptomatic or protective mechanisms? Neurology 1991;*42*(supp):13–26.

110. Golbe LI. Deprenyl as symptomatic therapy in Parkinson's disease. Clin Neuropharm 1988;*11*:387–400.

111. Stern GM, Lees AJ, Hardie R, Sandler M. Clinical and pharmacological aspects of (–) deprenyl treatment in Parkinson's disease. Mod Probl Pharmacopsychiat 1983;*19*:215–219.

112. Cedarbaum J, Clark M, Silvestri M, Harts A, Kutt H. Deprenyl, levodopa pharmacokinetics and modification of response fluctuations in Parkinson's disease. 1989.

113. Mann JJ, Frances A, Kaplan RD, Kocsis J, Peselow ED, Gershan S. The relative efficacy of L-deprenyl, a selective monoamine oxidase type B inhibitor. J Clin Psychopharmacol 1982;2:54–57.

114. Mandlewicz J, Youdim MBH. L-deprenil, a selective monoamine oxidase type B inhibitor, in the treatment of depression: a double blind evaluation. Brit J Psych 1983;*142*:508–511.

115. Knoll J, Vizi ES, Somogyi G. A phenylisopropylmethyl-propinylamine (E-250), tyraminantagonist hatasa. MTA V Oszt Kozl 1967;*18*:33–37.

116. Youdim MBH, Finberg JPM. Monoamine oxidase B inhibition and the "cheese effect". J Neuro Transm 1987;*25*(supp):27–33.

117. Zornberg GL. Severe adversive interaction between pethidine and selegiline. Lancet 1991;*337*:246.

118. Markstein R, Herrling PL. The effect of bromocriptine on rat striatal adenylate cyclase and rat brain monoamine metabolism. J Neurochem 1978;*31*:1163–1172.

119. Markstein R. Neurochemical effects of some ergot derivatives: a basis for their antiparkinson actions. J Neural Transm 1981;*51*:39–59.

120. Schwartz R, Fuxe K, Agnati LF. Effect of bromocriptine on ^{3}H-spiroperidol binding sites in rat striatum—evidence for actions of dopamine receptors not linked to adenylate cyclase. Life Sci 1978;*23*:465–470.

121. Fuxe K, Agnati LF, Kohler C. Characterization of normal and supersensitive dopamine receptors: effects of ergot drugs and neuropeptides. J Neural Transm 1981;*51*:3–37.

122. Lees AJ, Stern GM. Pergolide and lisuride for levodopa-induced oscillations. Lancet 1981;*2*:577.

123. Goldstein M, Lieberman A, Lew JY, Asano T, Rosenfeld MR, Makman MH. Interaction of pergolide with central dopaminergic receptors. Proc Natl Acad Sci USA 1980;*77*:3725–3728.

124. Horowski R. Differences in the dopaminergic effects of the ergot derivatives bromocriptine, lisuride and D-LSD as compared with apomorphine. Eur J Pharmacol 1978;*51*:157–166.

125. Strumpf WE, Detmer WM, Sar M, Horowski R, Dorow R. Autoradiographic studies with [^{3}H] dopamine, and [^{3}H] domperidone in pituitary and brain. In Macleod RM, Thorner MO, Scapagnini U (Eds). Prolactin, basic and clinical correlates. Padova: Liviana (1985); pp 27–35.

126. Humpel M, Nieuweboer B, Hasan SH, Wendt H. Radioimmunoassay of plasma lisuride in man following intravenous and oral administration of lisuride hydrogen maleate: effects on plasma prolactin level. Eur J Clin Pharmacol 1981;*20*:47–51.

127. Humpel M. Pharmacokinetics of lisuride in animals species and humans. In Calne DB, Horowski R, McDonald RJ, Wuttke W (Eds). Lisuride and other dipamnine agonists. New York: Raven (1983); pp 141–152.

128. Rubin A, Lemberger L, Dhahir P and Crabtree RE. Paper presented at World Conference on Clinical Pharmacology and Therapeutics, London, August 1980.

129. Aellig WH, Neuesch E. Comparative pharmacokinetic investigations with tritium-labelled ergot alkaloids after oral and intravenous administration in man. Int J Clin Pharmacol 1977, *15*:106–112.

130. Krause W, Nieuweboer B, Ruggieri ST, Stocchi F, Suchy I. Pharmacokinetics of lisuride after subcutaneous infusion. J Neural Trans 1988;*27* (supp):71–74.

131. Humpel M, Toda T, Oshino N, Pommerenke G. Eur J Metab Pharmacokin 1981.

132. Bowler JV, Ormerod IE, Legg NJ. Retroperitoneal fibrosis and bromocriptine. Lancet 1986;*ii*:466.

133. Wiggins J, Skinner C. Bromocriptine induced pleuropulmonary fibrosis. Thorax 1986;*41*:328–330.

134. Dorow R, Brietkopf M, Graf K-J, Horowski R. Neuroendocrine effects of lisuride and its 9,10-dihydrogenated analog in healthy volunteers. In Calne DB, Horowski, R, McDonald RJ, Wuttke W (Eds). Lisuride and other dopamine agonists. New York: Raven Press (1983); pp 161–174.

135. Cangi F, Fanciullacci M, Pietrini U, Boccuni M, Sicuteri F. Emergence of pain and extrapain phenomena from dopaminomimetics in migraine. In Pfaffenrath V, Lindborg PO, Sjaastads O (Eds). Updating in Headache Heidelberg: Springer (1985); pp 276–280.

136. Critchley P, Perez F, Quinn M. Coleman R, Parkes D, Marsden CD. Psychosis and the lisuride pump. Lancet 1986;*2*:349.

137. Tanner CM, Chhablani R, Goetz CG, Klawans HL. Pergolide mesylate: Lack of cardiac toxicity in patients with cardiac disease. Neurology 1985;*35*:918–921.

138. Tsang D, Lal S. Canad J Physiol Pharmacol 1977;*55*:1263–1269.

139. Davidson M, Kendler KS, Mohs RC, Hollander E, Ryan T, Davis KL. Effect of apomorphine infusion on plasma homovanillic acid in normal subjects. J Psychiat Res 1986;*20*:131–135.

140. Springer J, Hannigan JH, Isaacson RL. Changes in dopamine and DOPAC following systemic administration of apomorphine and 3,4-dihydroxyphenylamino-2-imidazoline (DPI) in rats. Brain Res 1981;*220*:226–230.

141. Nutt JG, Hammerstad JP, Gancher ST. Therapy: dopamine agonists. In Nutt JG, Hammerstad JP and Gancher ST (Eds). Parkinson's disease. 100 Maxims in neurology, vol. 2 St Louis; Mosby Year Book (1992); pp 93–101.

142. Corsini FU, Del Zompo M, Cianchetti C, Mangoni A, Gessa GL. Psychopharmacologia 1976;*47*:169–173.

143. Cotzias GC, Papavasiliou PS, Tolosa ES, Mendez JS, Bell-Midura M. Treatment of Parkinson's disease with apomorphines: possible role of growth hormone. N Engl J Med 1976;*294*:567–572.

144. Pollak P, Champay AS, Gaio JM, et al. Administration souscutanee d'apomorphine dans les fluctuations motrices de la maladie de Parkinson. Rev Neurol 1990;*116–122*.

145. Stibe CM, Kempster PA, Lees AJ, Stern GM. Subcutaneous apomorphine in Parkinsonian on-off fluctuations. Lancet 1988;*1*:403–406.

146. Stibe CM, Lees AJ, Stern G. Subcutaneous infusion of apomorphine and lisuride in the treatment of parkinsonian on-off fluctuations. Lancet 1987;*1*:871.

147. Ruggieri S, Stocchi F, Carta A, et al. Side-effects of subcutaneous apomorphine in Parkinson's disease. Lancet 1989;*1*:566.

148. Gaucher ST, Nutt JG, Woodward WR. Tolerance to antiparkinsonian effects of apomorphine. Neurology 1991;*41*(supp):211.

149. Poewe W, Luef G, Kleedorfer B, Wagner M, et al. Side-effects of subcutaneous apomorphine in Parkinson's disease. Lancet 1989;*1*:1084–1085.

150. Pletscher A, Brosi A, Gey KF. Benzoquinoliaine derivatives: a new class of monoamine decreasing drugs with psychotropic action. Int Rev Neurobiol 1962;*4*:275–306.

151. Login IS, Cronin MJ, MacLeod RM. Tetrabenazine has properties of a dopamine receptor antagonist. Ann Neurol 1982;*12*:257–262.

152. Dalby MA. Effect of tetrabenazine in extrapyramidal movement disorders. Brit Med J 1969;*2*:422–423.

153. Swash M, Roberts AH, Zakko H, Heathfield KWG. Treatment of involuntary movement disorders with tetrabenazine. J Neurol Neurosurg Psych 1972;*35*:186–191.

154. McLellan DI, Chalmers RJ, Johnson RH. A double blind trial of tetrabenazine, thiopropazate and placebo in patients with chorea. Lancet 1974;*1*:104–107.

155. Kazamatsuri H, Chien C-P, Cole JO. Long term treatment of tardive dyskinesia with haloperidol and tetrabenazine. Am J Psych 1973;*1304*:479–483.

156. Jankovic J. Treatment of hyperkinetic movement disorders with tetrabenazine: a double-blind cross-over study. Ann Neurol 1982;*11*:41–47.

157. Burke RE. The relative selectivity of anticholinergic drugs for the M_1 and M_2 muscarinic receptor subtypes. Movement Dis 1986;*1*:135–144.

158. Coyle JT, Snyder SH. Antiparkinsonian drugs: Inhibition of dopamine uptake in the corpus striatum as a possible mechanism of action. Science 1969;*166*:899–901.

159. Farnebo L, Fuxe K, Hamberger B, Ljungdahl H. Effect of some antiparkinsonian drugs on catecholamine neurons. J Pharm Pharmacol 1970;*22*:733–737.

160. Burke RE, Fahn S. Pharmacokinetics of trihexyphenidyl after short-term and long-term administration to dystonic patients. Ann Neurol 1985;*18*:35–40.

161. Burke RE, Fahn S. Pharmacokinetics of trihexyphenidyl after acute and chronic administration. Ann Neurol 1982;*12*:94.

162. Duvoisin RC. Cholinergic-anticholinergic antagonism in parkinsonism. Arch Neurol 1967;*17*:124–136.

163. Marshall J, Schnieden H. Effects of adrenaline, noradrenaline, atropine and nicotine on some types of human tremor. J. Neurol Neurosung Psychiatry 1966;*29*:214–218.

164. Jankovic J. Parkinsonism-plus syndromes. Movement Disord 1989;*4*:5–s95–s119.

165. Friedman Z, Neumann E. Benzhexol-induced blindness in Parkinson's disease. Br Med J 1972;*1*:605.

166. Burke RE, Fahn S. Serum trihexyphenidyl levels in the treatment of torsion dystonia. Neurology 1985;*35*:1066–1069.

167. Fahn S, David E. Oral-facial-lingual dyskinesia due to anticholinergic medication. Trans Am Neurol Assoc 1972;*97*:277–299.

168. Birket-Smith E. Abnormal involuntary movements in relation to anticholinergics and levodopa therapy. Acta Neurol Scand 1975;*52*:158–160.

169. Van Woert MH, Rosenbaum D, Chung E. Biochemistry and therapeutics of postanoxic myoclonus. Adv Neurol 1986;*43*:171–182.

170. Van Woert MH, Rosenbaum D. L-5-Hydroxytryptophan therapy in myoclonus. Advances in Neurology 1979;*26*:107–115.

171. Davies WL, Grunert RR, Haff RF et al. Antiviral activity of l-adamantanamine (amantadine). Science 1964;*144*:862–863.

172. Skehel JJ, Hay AJ, Armstrong JA. On the mechanism of inhibition of influenza virus replication by amantadine hydrochloride. 1978;*38*:97–110.

173. Schwab RS, England AC, Poskanzer DC, Young RR. Amantadine in the treatment of Parkinson's disease. JAMA 1969;*208*:1168–1170.

174. Stromberg V, Svensson TH. Further studies on the mode of action of amantadine. Acta Pharmacologica et Toxicologica 1971;*30*:161–171.

175. Scatton B, Cheramy A, Besson MJ, Glowinski J. Europ J Pharmacol 1970;*13*:131.

176. Von Voigtlander PF, Moore KE. Dopamine: release from the brain 'in vivo' by amantadine. Science 1971;*174*:408–410.

177. Stone TW. Responses of neurons in the cerebral cortex and caudate nucleus to amantadine, amphetamine and dopamine. Br J Pharmacol 1976;*1*:101–110.

178. Pycock C, Milson JA, Tarsy D et al. The effects of blocking catecholamine uptake on amphetamine-induced circling behaviour in mice with unilateral destruction of striatal dopaminergic nerve terminals. J Pharm Pharmacol 1976;*28*:530–532.

179. Kornhuber J, Bormann J, Retz W, Hubers M. Rieder P. Memantine displaces [3H]MK-801 at therapeutic concentrations in post-mortem human frontal cortex. Cur J Pharmacol 1989;*166*:589–590.

180. Kornhuber J, Bormann J, Hubers M, Rusche K, Reiderer P. Effects of the 1-amino-adamantanes at the MKL-801 binding site of the NMDA receptor gated ion channel: a human postmortem brain study. Eur J Pharmacol 1991;*206*:297–300.

181. Aoki FY, Siter DS. Clinical pharmacokinetics of amantadine hydrochloride. Clin Pharmacokin 1988;*14*:35–51.

182. Bleidner WE, Harmon JB, Hewes WE, Lynes TE, Hermann EC. Absorption, distribution and excretion of amantadine hydrochloride. J Pharmacol Exp Ther 1965;*150*:484–490.

183. Horadam VW, Sharp JG, Smilack JD, McAnalley BH, Garriott JC, Stephens MK, Prati RC, Braer DC. Pharmacokinetics of amantadine hydrochloride in subjects with normal and impaired renal function. Ann Intern Med 1981;*94*:454–458.

184. Liu P, Cheng PJ, Ing TS, Daugirdas JT, Jeevanandhan R, Soung LS, Galinis S. In vitro binding of amantadine to plasma proteins. Clin Neuropharmacol 1984;*7*:149–151.

185. Bergman H, Wichman T, DeLong MR. Reversal of experimental parkinsonism by lesions of the subthalamic nucleus. Science 1990;*249*:1436–1438.

186. Kockgether T, Turski L, Honore T, Zhang Z, Gash DM, Kurlan R, Greenamyre JT. The AMPA receptor antagonist NBQX has antiparkinsonian effects in monoamine-depleted rats and MPTP-treated monkeys. Ann Neurol 1991;*30*:717–723.

187. Shealey CN, Weeith JB, Mercier D. Livedo reticularis in patients with parkinsonism receiving amantadine. JAMA 1970;*212*:1522–1523.

188. Parkes JD, Curzon G, Knott PJ, Tatersall R, Baxter RCH, Knill-Jones RP, Marsden CD, Vollum D. Treatment of Parkinson's disease with amantadine and levodopa. Lancet 1971;*1*:1083–1086.

189. Parkes JD, Baxter RC, Galbraith A, Marsden CD, Rees JE. Amantadine treatment in Parkinson's disease. Adv Neurol 1973;*3*:105–114.

190. Pearce LA, Waterbury LD, and Green HD. Amantadine hydrochloride: alteration in peripheral circulation. Neurology 1974;*24*:46–48.

191. Harper RW, Knothe BU. Coloured lilliputian hallucinations with amantadine. Med J Aust 1973;*1*:444.

192. Postma JU, Van Tilburg W. Visual hallucinations and delerium during treatment with amantadine (Symmetrel). J Am Geriatr Soc 1975;*23*:212–215.

193. Wilson Tw, Rajput AH. Amantadine-dyazide interaction. Can Med Assoc J 1983;*129*:974–975.

194. Ing TS, Daugirdas JT, Soung LS, Klawasns HL, Mahurkar SD, Hayashi JA, Geis WP, Hano JE. Toxic effects of amantadine in patients with renal failure. Can Med Assoc J 1979;*120*.695–698.

195. Meunter MD, Daube JR, Miller PM. Treatment of essential tremor with methazolamide. Mayo Clin Proc 1991;*66*:991–997.

196. Van Winkle WB. Calcium release from skeletal muscle sacroplasmic reticulum: site of action of drantolene sodium? Science 1976;*193*:1130–1131.

197. Desmedt JE, Hainaat K. Dantrolene and A23187 ionophore: specific action on calcium channels revealed by the acquoricn method. Biochm Pharmacol 1979;*28*:957–964.

198. Bowery NG, Hill DR, Hudson AL. Baclofen decreases neurotransmitter release in the mammalian CNS by an action at a novel GABA receptor. Nature 1980;*283*:92–94.

199. Newman PM, Nogues M, Newmain PK, Weightman D, Hodgson P. Tizanidine in the treatment of spasticity. Eur J Clin Pharmacol 1982;*23*:31–35.

200. Simpson LL. Kinetic studies on the interaction between botulinum toxin type A and the cholinergic neuromuscular junction. J Pharmacol Exp Ther 1980;*212*:16–21.

201. DasGupta BR. Dekieva ML. Botulinum neurotoxin type A: sequence of amino acids at the N-terminus and around the nicking site. Biochimie 1990;*72*:661–664.

202. Bandyoipadhyay S, Clark AW, Das Gupta BR, Sathyamoorthy V. Role of the heavy and light chains of botulinum neurotoxin in neuromuscular paralysis. J Biol Chem 1987;*262*:2660–2663.

203. Black JD, Dolly JO. Interaction of 125-I-labeled botulinum neurotoxins with nerve terminals. II. Autoradiographic evidence for its uptake into motor nerves by acceptor-medicated endocytosis. J Cell Biol 1986;*103*:521–534.

204. Sellin LC. The action of botulinum toxin at the neuromuscular junction. Med Biol 1981;*59*:11–20.

205. Borodic GE, Joseph M, Fay L, Cozzolino D, Ferrante RJ. Botulinum A toxin for the treatment of spasmodic torticollis: dysphaggia and regional toxin spread. Head Neck 1990;*12*:392–398.

206. Scott AB, Suzuki D. Systemic toxicity of botulinum toxin by intramuscular injection in the monkey. Movement Dis 1988;*3*:33–35.

207. Harris CP, Alderson K, Nebeker J, Hols JB, Anderson RL. Histology of human obicularis muscle treated with botulinum toxin. Arch Ophthalmol 1991;*109*:393–395.

208. Borodic GE, Ferrante R. Histological effects of repeated botulinum toxin over many years in human obicularis oculi muscle. J Clin Neuro-Ophthalmol 1992;*12*:121–127.

209. Lange DJ, Rubin M, Greene PE, et al. Distant effects of locally injected botulinum toxin: a double blind study of single fiber EMG changes. Muscle Nerve 1991;*14*:672–675.

210. Greene P, Fahn S. Development of antibodies to botulinum toxin type A in patients with torticollis treated with injections of botulinum toxin type A.

211. Hatheway CG, Snyder JD, Seals JE, Edell TA, Lewis GE. Antitoxin levels in toulism patients treated with trivalent equine botulism antitoxin to toxin types A, B, and E. J Infect Dis 1984;*150*:407–412.

212. Schneider JS, Pope A, Simpson K, Taggart J, Smith MG, DiStefano L. Recovery from experimental parkinsonism in primates with GM1 ganglioside treatment. Science 1992;*256*:843–846.

213. Schneider JS, Rothblat DS, Roeltgen DP. GM1 ganglioside (Sygen) in Parkinson's disease: safety and efficacy. Neurology 1994;*44*:258.

214. Lin LF, Doherty DH, Lile JD, Bektesh S, Collins F. GDNF: a glial cell line-derived neurotrophic factor for midbrain dopaminergic neurons. Science 1993;*260*:1130–1132.

215. Burns RS, LeWitt PA, Ebert MH, Pakkenberg H, Kopin IJ. The clinical syndrome of striatal dopamine deficiency: parkinsonism induced by 1-methyl-4-phenyl-1,2,3,6-tetrahydropyridine (MPTP). N Eng J Med 1985;*312*:1418–1421.

216. Ehringer H and Hornykiewicz O. Verteilung von noradrenalin und dopamin (3-hydroxytrptamin) in gehirn des menschen und ihr verhalten bei erkrankungen des extrapyramidalen systems. 1960;*38*:1236–1239.

217. Birkmayer W and Hornykiewicz o. Der L-dioxyphenylalanin (L-dopa)—effekt bei der Parkinson-akinese. Wiener Klinische Wochenschrift 1961;*73*:787–788.

218. Birkmayer W, Hornykiewicz O. The L-DOPA effect in Parkinson's syndrome in man. Arch Psychiatr Nervenkr 1962;*203*:560–574.

219. Cotzias GC, Van Woert MH, Schiffer LM. Aromatic amino acids and modification of parkinsonism. N Engl J Med 1967;*276*:374–379.

220. Yahr MD, Duvoisin RC, Schear MJ, Barrett RE, Hoehn MM. Treatment of parkinsonism with levodopa. Arch Neurol 1969;*21*:343–354.

221. Barbeau A. Excerpta Med Int Congr Ser 1961;*38*:152.

222. Yahr MD, Duvoisin RC, Hoehn MM, Schear MJ, and Barrett RE. Trans Amer Neurol Ass 1968;*93*:56.

223. Calne DB, Spiers ASD, Stern GM, Laurence DR, Armitage P. Lancet 1969;*2*:973.

224. Bonnet AM, Loria Y, Saint-Hilaire MH, Lhermitte F, Agid Y. Does long-term aggravation of Parkinson's disease result from nondopaminergic lesions? Neurology 1987;*37*:1539–1542.

225. Marsden CD, Parkes JD. "On-off" effects in patients with Parkinson's disease on chronic levodopa therapy. Lancet 1976;*1*:292–296.

226. Cotzias GC, Papavasiliou PS, Gellene R. Modification of parkinsonism-chronic treatment with L-dopa. N Engl J med 1969;*280*:337–345.

227. Langston JW, Ballard P. Parkinsonism induced by 1-methyl-4-phenyl-1,2,3,6-tetrahydropyridine (MPTP): implications for treatment and the pathogenesis of Parkinson's disease. Can J Neurol Sci 1984;*11*:160–165.

228. Marsden CD, Parkes JD. Success and problems of long-term levodopa therapy in Parkinson's disease. Lancet 1977;*1*:345–349.

229. Meunter MD, Tyce Gm, L-dopa therapy of Parkinson's disease: plasma L-dopa concentrations, therapeutic response, and side effects. Mayo Clin Proc 1971;*46*:231–239.

230. Shaw KM, Lees AJ, Stern GM. The impact of treatment with levodopa on Parkinson's disease. Q J Med 1980;*49*:283–293.

231. Fahn S. 'On-off' phenomenon with levodopa therapy in parkinsonism. Neurology 1974:*34*:431–441.

232. Barbeau A, Roy M. Ten-year results of treatment with levodopa plus benserazide in Parkinson's disease. In: Rose FC, Capildeo R (Eds). Research progress in Parkinson's disease. London: Pitman Medical (1981): pp 241–247.

233. Spencer SE, Wooten GF. Altered pharmacokinetics of L-dopa metabolism in rat striatum deprived of dopaminergic innervation. Neurology 1984;*34*:1105–1108.

234. Duby SE, Cotzias GC, Papavasiliou PS, Lawrence WH. Injected apomorphine and orally administered levodopa in parkinsonism. Arch Neurol 1972;*27*:474–480.

235. Yahr MD, Clough CG, Bergmann KJ. Cholinergic and dopaminergic mechanisms in Parkinson's disease after long-term levodopa administration. Lancet 1982;*2*:709–710.

236. Marsden CD and Jenner P. L-DOPA's action in Parkinson's disease-reply to Hefti and Melamed. Trends Neurol Sci 1980;*4*:148–150.

237. Nutt JG, Gancher ST, Woodward WR. Does an inhibitory action of levodopa contribute to motor fluctuations? Neurology 1988;*38*:1553–1557.

238. Melamed E. Initiation of levodopa therapy in Parkinsonian patients should be delayed until the advanced stages of the disease. Arch Neurol 1986;*43*:402–405.

239. Shoulson I, Glaubiger GA, Chase TN. On-off response-clinical and biochemical correlations during oral and intravenous levodopa administration in parkinsonian patients. Neurology 1975;*25*:1144–1148.

240. Quinn N, Parkes JD, Marsden CD. Control of on-off phenomenon by continuous intravenous infusion of levodopa. Neurology 1984;*34*:1131–1136.

241. Cedarbaum JM. The promise and limitation of controlled release oral levodopa administration. Clin Neuropharm 1989;*12*:147–166.

242. Sage JI, Trooskin S, Sonsalla PK et al. Long-term duodenal infusion of levodopa for motor fluctuations in Parkinsonism. Ann Neurol 1988;*24*:87–88.

243. Mannisto PT, Kaakkola S. Rationale for selective COMT inhibitors as adjuncts in drug treatment of Parkinson's disease. Pharm Tox 1990;*66*:317–323.

244 Barbeau A. Long-term side-effects of levodopa. Lancet 1971;*1*:395–.

245. Klawans HL, Goetz C, Nausieda PA, Weiner WJ. Levodopa-induced dopamine receptor hypersensitivity. Ann Neurol 1977;*2*:125–129.

246. Creese I, Burt D, Snyder S. Dopamine receptor binding enhancement accompanies lesion-induced behavioral supersensitivity. Science 1977;*197*:596–598.

247. Lee R, Seeman P, Rahput A, Farlay I, Hornykiewicz O. Receptor basis for dopaminergic supersensitivity in Parkinson's disease. Nature 1978;*278*:59–61.

248. Cotzias GC, Papavasiliou PS, Fehling C, Kaufman B, Mena I. Simularities between neurological effects of L-dopa and apomorphine. New Egl J Med 1970;*282*:31–33.

249. Nutt JG, Woodward WR. Levodopa pharmacokinetics and pharmacodynamics in fluctuating parkinsonian patients. Neurology 1986;*36*:739–744.

250. Tarsy D, Leopold N, Sax D. Physostigmine in choreiform movement disorders. Neurology 1974;*24*:28–34.

251. Calne DB, Williams AC, Neophytides A, Plotkin C, Nutt JG, Teychenne PF. Long-term treatment of parkinsonism with bromocriptine. Lancet 1978;*1*:735–738.

252. Debono AG, Donaldson I, Marsden CD and Parkes JD. Lancet 1975;*2*:987–988.

253. Lieberman A, Zolfaghar IM, Boal D, Hassouri H, Vogel B, Battista A, Fuxe K. Goldstein M. The antiparkinson efficacy of bromocriptine. Neurology 1976;*26*:405–409.

254. Teychenne PF, Bergsrud D, Racy A. Bromocriptine: low dose therapy in parkinsonism. Neurology 1982;*32*:577–583.

255. Burns RS, Gopinathan G, Humpel M, Dorow R, Calne DB. Disposition of oral lisuride in Parkinson's disease. Clin Pharmacol Ther 1984;*35*:548–556.

256. Dorow R, Graf K-J, Nieuweboer B, Horrowski R. Intravenous lisuride: a new tool for testing responsiveness to dopaminergic agonists and neuroendocrine function. Acta Endocrinol 1980;*94* (supp):9.

257. Obeso JA, Luquin M.r, Martinez-Lage JM. Lisuride infusion pump. A device for the treatment of motor fluctuations in Parkinson's disease. Lancet 1986;*1*:467–470.

258. Obeso JA, Luquin MR, Martinez-Lage JM. Intravenous lisuride corrects oscillations of motor performance in Parkinson's disease. Ann Neurol 1986;*19*:31–35.

259. Horowski R, Marsden CD, Obeso JA. Continuous dopaminergic stimulation: state of the art and outlook. J Neural Transm 1988;*27* (supp):249–253.

260. Agnoli A, Stocchi F, Carta A, Antonini A, Bragoni M, Ruggierei SA. Continuous dopaminergic stimulation in the management of complicated Parkinson's disease. Mt Sinai J Med 1988;*55*:62–66.

261. Struppler A, v. Uexhuell T. Untersuchungen ueber die wirkungsweise des apomorphins auf den parkinson tremor. Ztschr Klin Med 1951;*76*:251–253.

262. Cotzias GC, Lawrence WH, Papavasiliou PS, Duby SE, Ginos JZ, Mena I. Apomorphine and parkinsonism. Trans Amer Neurol Assoc 1972;*97*:156–159.

263. Braham J, Sarova-Pinhas I, Goldhammer Y. Brit Med J 1970;*2*:768.

264. Obeso JA, Grandas F, Vaamonde J, Luquin MR, Martinez-Lage JM. Apomorphine infusion for motor fluctuations in Parkinson's disease. Lancet 1987;*1*:1376–1377.

265. Pollak P, Champay AS, Hommel M, Perret JE, Benabid AL TI. Subcutaneous apomorphine in Parkinson's disease: therapeutic efficacy of apomorphine combined with an extracerebral inhibitor of dopamine receptors in Parkinson's disease. J Neurol Neurosurg Psych 1989;*52*:544.

266. Frankel JP, Lees AJ, Kempster PA, Stern GM. Subcutaneous apomorphine in the treatment of Parkinson's disease. J Neurol Neurosurg Psych 1990;*55*:96–101.

267. Chaudh KR, Critchley P. Abbott RJ, et al. Subcutaneous apomorphine for on-off oscillations in Parkinson's disease. Lancet 1989;*2*:1260.

268. Lees AJ, Montastruc JL, Turjanske N et al. Sublingual apomorphine and Parkinson's disease. J of Neurology, Neurosurgery and Psychiatry 1990;*52*:1439.

269. Gancher ST, Nutt JG, Woodward WR. Sublingual apomorphine in Parkinsons disease. Movement Dis 1990;*5*(supp):53.

270. Kapoor R, Turjanske N, Frankel J, et al. Intranasal apomorphine: a new treatment in Parkinson's disease. J Neurol Neurosurg Psych 1990;*53*:1015.

271. Hughes AJ, Bishop S, Lees AJ, et al. Rectal apomorphine in Parkinson's disease. Lancet 1991;*337*:118.

272. Barker R, Duncan J, Lees A. Subcutaneous apomorphine as a diagnostic test for dopaminergic responsiveness in parkinsonian syndromes. Lancet 1989;*1*:675.

273. Parkes JD, Baxter RC, Marsden CD, Ree JE. Comparative trial of benzhexol, amantadine and levodopa in the treatment of Parkinson's disease. J Neurol Neurosurg Psych 1974;*37*:422–425.

274. Hughes RC, Polgar JG, Weightman D, Walton JN. Levodopa in parkinsonism: the effects of withdrawal of anticholinergic drugs. Br Med J 1971;*2*:487–491.

275. Ruberg M, Ploska A, Javoy-Agid F, Agid Y. Muscarinic binding and choline acetyltransferase activity in parkinsonian subjects with reference to dementia. Brain Res 1982;*232*:129–139.

276. Dallos V, Heathfield K, Stone P, Allen FAD. Use of amantadine in Parkinson's disease. Results of a double-blind trial. Br Med J 1970;*4*:24–26.

277. Fahn S, Isgreen WP. Long-term evaluation of amantadine and levodopa combination in Parkinsonism by double-blind crossover analysis. Neurology 1975;*25*:695–700.

278. Butzer JF, Silver DE, Sahs AL. Amantadine in Parkinson's disease. A double-blind, placebo-controlled, crossover study with long-term follow-up. Neurology 1974;*25*:603–606.

279. Parkes JD, Zikha KJ, Calver DM, Knill-Jones RP. Controlled trial of amantadine hydrochleride in Parkinson's disease. Lancet 1970;*1*:259–262.

280. Mawdsley C, Williams IR, Pullar IA, Davidson DL, Kinloch NE. Treatment of parkinsonism by amantadine and levodopa. Clin Pharmacol Ther 1972;*13*:575–583.

281. Stern GM, Lees AJ, Hardie RJ, Sandler M. Clinical and pharmacological problems of deprenyl (selegiline) treatment in Parkinson's disease. Acta Neurol Scand 1983;95 (supp):113–116.

282. Lees AJ, Shaw KM, Kohout LJ, Stern FM, Elsworth JD, Sandler M, and Youdim MBH. Deprenyl in Parkinson's disease. Lancet 1977;*2*:791–796.

283. Klawans HL, Bergen D, Bruyn GW. Prolonged drug-induced parkinsonism. Contemp Neurol 1973;*35*:368–377.

284. Rajput AH, Rozdilsky B, Hornykiewicz O, Shannak K, Lee T, Seeman P. Reversible drug-induced parkinsonism: clinicopatholigic study of two cases. Arch Neurol 1982;*39*:644–646.

285. Greene P, Shale H, Fahn S. Analysis of open-label trials in torsion dystonia using high dosages of anticholinergics and other drugs. Movement Dis 1988;*3*:46–60.

286. Fahn S. High dosage anticholinergic therapy in dystonia. Neurology 1983;*33*:1255–1261.

287. Burke RE, Fahn S, Jankovic J, Marsden CD, Lang AE, Gollomp S, Ilson J. Tardive dystonia: Late-onset and persistent dystonia caused by antipsychotic drugs. Neurology 1982;*32*:1335–1346.

288. Kang UJ, Burke RE, Fahn S. Natural history and treatment of tardive dystonia. Movement Dis 1986;*1*:193–208.

289. Paulson G. Procyclidine for dystonia caused by phenothiazine derivatives. Dis Nerv Syst 1960;*21*:447–448.

290. Waugh WH, Metts JC. Severe extrapyramidal motor activity induced by prochloprperzine. N Engl J Med 1960;*262*:353–354.

291. Smith MJ, MIller MM. Severe extrapyramidal reaction to perphenazine treated with diphenhydramine. N Engl J Med 1961;*264*:396–397.

292. Zhong XH, Rajput AH, Hornykiewicz O, Kish SJ. Striatal dopamine, tyrosine hydroxylase and dopamine transporter are markedly reduced in a patient with dopa responsive dystonia. Soc Neurosci Abstr 1992;*18*:1247.

293. Sawle GV, Leenders KL, Brooks DJ, et al. Dopa-responsive dystonia: [^{18}F]dopa positron emission tomography. Ann Neurol 1991;*30*:24–30.

294. Lugaresi E, Cirignotta F. Hypnogenic paroxysmal dystonia. Epileptic seizure or a new syndrome? Sleep. 1981;*4*:129–138.

295. Lee BI, Lesser RP, Pippenger CE. et al. Familial paroxysmal hypnogenic dystonia. Neurology 1985;*35*:1357–1360.

296. Young RR, Growdon JH, Shahani BT. Beta-adrenergic mechanisms in action tremor. N Eng J Med 1975;*293*:950–953.

297. Reiner A, Albin RL, Anderson KD, D'Amato CJ, Penney JB, Young AB. Differential loss of striatal projection neurons in Huntington's disease. Proc Natl Acad Sci 1988;*78*:233–238.

298. Martin JP. Hemichorea (hemiballismus) without lesion in the corpus Lusyii. Brain 1957;*80*:1–10.

299. Mitchell IJ, Jackson A, Sambrook MA, et al. Common neurological mechanism in experimental chorea and hemiballismus in the monkey. Evidence from 2-deoxyglucose autoradiography. Brain Res 1985;*339*:346–350.

300. Guilleminault C, Tharp BR, Cousin D. HVA and 5-HIAA CSF measurements and 5-HTP trials in some patients with involuntary movements. J Neurol Sci 1973;*18*:435–441.

301. Lhermitte F, Peterfalvi M, Marteau R, Gazengel J, Serdara M. Analyse pharmacologique d'un cas de myoclonus d'intention et d'action postanoxique. Rev Neurol 1971;*124*:21–31.

302. Cohen DJ, Detlor J, Young JG, Shaywitz BA. Clondine ameliorates Gilles de la Tourette's syndrome. Arch Gen Psychiat 1980;*37*:1350–1357.

303. Lipinski JF, Zubenko GS, Barreira P, Cohen BN. Propanolol in the treatment of neuroleptic-induced akathisia. Lancet 1983;*2*:685–686.

304. Walters A, Hening W, Chokroverty S, Fahn S. Opioid responsiveness in patients with neuroleptic-induced akathisia. Movement Dis 1986;*1*:119–127.

305. Akpinar S. Restless legs syndrome treatment with dopaminergic drugs. Clin Neuropharmacol 1987;*10*:69–79.

306. Walters A, Henning W, Cote L, Fahn S. Dominantly inherited restless legs with myoclonus and periodic movements in sleep: a syndrome related to the endogenous opiates? Adv Neurol 1986;*43*:309–319.

307. Nielsen VK. Pathophysiology of hemifacial spasm. I. Ephaptic transmission and ectopic excitation. Neurology 1984;*34*:418–426.

308. Nielsen VK. Pathophysiology of hemifacial spasm: II. Lateral spread of the supraorbital nerve reflex. Neurology 1984;*34*:427–431.

309. Moller AR, Janetta PJ. Hemifacial spasm: results of electrophysiologic recording during microvascular decompression operations. Neurology 1985;*35*:969–974.

310. Muller DPR, Lloyd JK, Wolff OH. Vitamin E and neurological function. Lancet 1983;*1*:225–228.

311. Berginer VM, Salen G, Shefer S. Long-term treatment of cerebrotendinous xanthomatosis with chenodeoxycholic acid. N Engl J Med 1984;*311*:1649–1651.

312. Griggs RC, Moxley RT, Lafrance RA, McQuillen J. Hereditary paroxysmal ataxia: response to acetazolamide. Neurology 1978;*28*:1259–1264.

Reviews

r1. Marsden CD. Origins of normal and pathological tremor. In Findley LJ, Capildeo (Eds). Movement Disorders: Tremor New York: Oxford University Press (1984); pp 15–26.

r2. Marsden CD. Hallet M, Fahn S. The nosology and pathophysiology of myoclonus. In Marsden CD, Fahn S (Eds): Movement Disorders London: Butterworths (1981); pp 196–248.

r3. Shapiro AK, Shapiro ES, Bruun RD, Sweet RD. Gilles del la Tourette Syndrome New York: Raven Press (1978).

r4. Lance JW. Symposium synopsis. In Feldman RG, Young RR, Koella WP (Eds.). Disordered motor control Chicago: Year Book (1980); pp 485–494.

r5. McEvoy KM. Stiff-man syndrome. Semin Neurol 1991;*11*:197–204.

r6. Anthoney TR. Neuroanatomy and the Neurologic Exam Ann Arbor:CRC Press (1994); pp 233–238.

r7. Anthoney TR. Neuroanatomy and the Neurologic Exam Ann Arbor:CRC Press (1994); pp 106–109.

r8. Graybiel AM, Ragsdale CW. Biochemical anatomy of the striatum. In Emson PC (Ed). Chemical Neuroanatomy New York: Raven Press (1983); pp 427–504.

r9. The Merck Index Rahway, NJ: Merck & Co., Inc. (1976); pp 715.

r10. Christensen HN. Recognition sites for material transport and information transfer. In Bonner F, Kleinzeller A (Eds). Current Topics in Membranes and Transport New York: Academic Press (1975); pp 227–258.

r11. Hornykiewicz O. The mechanisms of action of L-DOPA in Parkinson's disease. Life Sci 1975;*15*:1249–1259.

r12. Nutt JG, Hammerstad JP, Gancher ST. Therapy: levodopa in early stages of parkinsonism. In Nutt JG, Hammerstad JP, and Gancher ST (Eds). Parkinson's disease, 100 Maxims in Neurology, vol 2 St Louis; Mosby Year Book (1992); pp 63–70.

r13. Calne DB. Parkinsonism. In Calne DB (Ed). London: Blackwell Scientific Publications (1980); pp 235–255.

r14. Nutt JG. Pharmacokinetics of levodopa. In Killer WC (Ed). Handbook of Parkinson's disease New York; Marcel Dekker (1987); pp 339–356.

r15. Eadie MJ, Tyrer JH. Disorders of motor function, II: involuntary movement disorders. In Eadie MJ, Tyrer JH (Eds.). Neurological Clinical Pharmacology Sydney:ADIS Press (1980): pp 81–152.

r16. Hornykiewicz 74, b6 c8
Hornykiewicz O. The mechanisms of action of L-DOPA in Parkinson's disease. Life Sci 1974;1249–1259.

r17. Klawans HL, Weiner WJ. Parkinsonism. In Klawans HH Weiner (Eds). Textbook of clinical neuropharmacology New York: Raven Press (1981); pp 1–35.

r18. Cedarbaum JM. The promise and limitations of controlled-release oral levodopa administration. Clin Neuropharmacol 1989;*12*:147–166.

r19. Klawans HL. The pharmacology of extrapyramidal movement disorders. Basel: S Karger (1973).

r20. Sjoqvist F. Psychotropic drugs, vol 2: interaction between monoamine oxidase (MAO) inhibitors and other substances. Proc Royal Soc Med 1965;*58*:967–978.

r21. Dobbing J. Blood brain barrier. Physiol Rev 1961;*41*:131–188.

r22. Morris FGL. Involuntary movement disorders. In Eadie MJ (Ed). Drug Therapy in Neurology London: Churchill Livingstone (1992): pp 247–309.

r23. Kutt H, McDowell F. Extrapyramidal syndromes. In Kutt H, McDowell F (Eds). Clinical Neuropharmacology New York: Churchill Livingstone (1979); pp 54–75.

r24. Yahr MD. Abnormal involuntary movements induced by dopa: clinical aspects. In Barbeau A, McDowell F (Eds). L-DOPA and parkinsonism Philadelphia: F.A. Davis (1970); pp 101–108.

r25. Porter CC. Inhibitors of aromatic amino acid decarboxylase—their biochemistry. Adv Neurol 1973;*2*:37–58.

r26. Knoll J. Deprenyl (selegiline): the history of its development and pharmacological action. Acta Neurol Scand 1983 (supp);*95*:57–80.

r27. Knoll J. Analysis of the pharmacological effects of selective monoamine oxidase inhibitors. In Wolstenholme GEW, Knight J (Eds). Monoamine Oxidase and its inhibition Amsterdam:Elsevier (1976); pp 135–155.

r28. Singer TP, VonKorff RW, Murphy DL (Eds). Monoamine oxidase: structure, function, and altered functions New York: Academic Press (1979).

r29. Sandler M, Stern GM. Deprenyl in Parkinson disease. In Marsden CD, Fahn S (Eds). Neurology 2: movement disorders London: Butterworths (1982): pp 166–173.

r30. Youdim MBH, Finberg JPM. In Grahame-Smith DG (Ed). Psychopharmacology 1 Amsterdam: Excerpta Medica (1982); pp 38–70.

r31. Snyder SH, D'Amato RJ. MPTP: a neurotoxin relevant to the pathophysiology of Parkinson's disease. Neurology 1986;*36*:50–258.

r32. Cohen G. Oxidative stress in the nervous system. In Sies H (Ed). Oxidative Stress London: Academic Press (1985): pp 383–402.

r33. Olanow CW. Oxidation reactions in Parkinson's disease. Neurology 1990;*40*(suppl):32–37.

r34. Gopinathan G, Horowski R, Suchy I. Lisuride pharmacology and treatment of parkinson's disease. In Calne DB (Ed). Drugs for the treatment of Parkinson's disease, Handbook of Experimental Pharmacology, vol 88 Berlin: Springer-Verlag (1989); pp 471–513.

r35. Reavill C, Jenner P, Marsden CD. Pharmacological and biochemical aspects of the mechanism of action of bromocriptine. Res Clin Forums 1981;*3*:7–17.

r36. Goldstein M, Lew JY, Makamura S. Dopaminephilic properties of ergot alkaloids. Fed Proc 1978;*37*:2202–2205.

r37. Schran HF, Bhuta SI, Schwarz HJ, and Thorner MO. The pharmacokinetics of bromocriptine in man. In Goldstein M, Calne DB, Lieberman A, Thorner MO (Eds.). Ergot compounds and brain function: neuroendocrine and neuropsychiatric aspects New York: Raven Press (1980); pp 125–139.

r38. Reavill C, Jenner P. Marsden CD. Puzzles of the mechanism of action of bromocriptine. In Gessa EL, Corsini FU (Eds). Basic pharmacology, vol 1. Apomorphine and other dopaminomimetics New York: Raven (1981); pp 229–239.

r39. Sage JI, Duvoisin RC. Pergolide in Parkinson's Disease. In Koller WC, Paulson G (Ed). Therapy of Parkinson's disease New York: Marcel Dekker (1990); pp 311–323.

r40. Burns RS, Calne DB. Treatment of Parkinsonism with artificial dopaminomimetics: pharmacokinetic consideration. In Corsini FU, Gessa GL (Eds). Apomorphine and other dopaminomimetics, vol 2 New York: Raven Press (1981): pp 93–106.

r41. Eckert H, Kiechel JR, Rosenthaler J, Schmidt R, Schreier E. Biopharmaceutical aspects. Analytical methods, pharmacokinetics, metabolism and bioavailability. In Bede B, Schild HO (Eds). Ergot alkaloids and related compounds, Handbook of experimental pharmacology, vol 49 Berlin: Springer-Verlag (1978); pp 719–803.

r42. Horowski R, Obeso JA. Lisuride: a direct dopamine agonist in the treatment of Parkinson's disease. In Koller WC, Paulson G (Ed). Therapy of Parkinson's disease New York: Marcel Dekker (1990); pp 269–309.

r43. Bianchine JR. Drugs for Parkinson's disease, spasticity, and acute muscle spasms. In Gilman AG, Goodman LS, Rall TW, Murad F (Eds). The pharmacological basis of therapeutics New York: Macmillan (1985); pp 473–490.

r44. Goetz CG, Tammer CM, Glantz RH, Klawans HL. Pergolide in Parkinson'ss disease. Arch Neurol 1983;*40*:785–787.

r45. The Merck Index Rahway, NJ: Merck & Co., Inc. (1976); pp 101.

r46. Seeman P, Grigoriadis DE. Dopamine receptors in brain and periphery. J Neurochem 1987;*1*:1–25.

r47. Asher SW, Aminoff MJ. Tetrabenazine and movement disorders. Neurology 1981;*31*:1051–1054.

r48. Lang AE, Marsden CD. Alphamethylparatyrosine and tetrabenazine in movement disorders. Clin Neuropharm 1982;*5*:375–387.

r49. Ordenstein L. Sur la paralysie agitante et la sclerose en plaque generalise Paris: Martinet (1867).

r50. Charcot JM. Clinical lectures on diseases of the nervous system, vol I, 2nd edition, translated by Sigerson G. Philadelphia, Henry C. Lea (1879).

r51. Erb W. Paralysis agitans (Parkinson's disease). In Church A (Ed). Diseases of the nervous system. New York: Appleton (1909); pp 801–898.

r52. The Merck Index. Rahway, NJ: Merck & Co., Inc. (1976); pp 1243.

r53. Bunney BS. The electrophysiological pharmacology of midbrain dopaminergic systems. In Horn AS, Korf J, Westernick BHC (Eds). The neurobiology of dopamine London: Academic Press (1979); pp 417–452.

r54. Lang AE, Blair RDG. Anticholinergic drugs and amantadine in the treatment of Parkinson's disease. In Calne DB (Ed). Drugs for the treatment of Parkinson's disease Berlin: Springer-Verlag (1989); pp 307–323.

r55. Fahn S, Burke R, Stern Y. Antimuscarinic drugs in the treatment of movement disorders. Prog Brain Res 1990; *84*:389–397.

r56. Calne DB. Therapeutics in neurology, 2nd edition Oxford: Blackwell Scientific Publications (1980).

r57. Fahn S. The tardive dyskinesias. In Matthews WB, Blaser GH (Eds). Recent advances in clinical neurology, vol 4 Edinburgh: Churchill Livingstone (1984); pp 229–260.

r58. The Merck Index. Rahway, NJ: Merck & Co., Inc. (1976); pp 645.

r59. Summary of information pertinent to the safety and possible usefulness of the investigational drug combination L-5HTP-Carbidopa. Copiague, NY: Bolar Pharmaceutical Co., Inc.

r60. Fuller RW. Biochemical pharmacology of the serotonin system. Adv Neurol 1986;*43*:469–480.

r61. Calne DB. Myoclonus. In Calne DB. Therapeutics in neurology. 2nd edition London: Blackwell Scientific Publications (1980); pp 274–278.

r62. The Merck Index. Rahway, NJ: Merck & Co., Inc. (1976); pp 50.

r63. Randrup A, Mogilnicka E. Spectrum of pharmacological actions on brain dopamine. Indications for development of new psychoactive drugs. Discussion of amantadines as examples of new drugs with special actions on dopamine systems. Pol J Pharmacol Pharm 1976;*28*:551–556.

r64. Allen RM. Role of amantadine in the management of neuroleptic induced extrapyramidal syndromes: overview and pharmacology. Clin Neuropharmacol 1983;*6* (supp):s64–s73.

r65. Sande MA and Mandell GL. Antifungal and antiviral agents. In Gilman AG, Goodman LS, Rall TW, Murad F (Eds). The pharmacological basis of therapeutics New York: Macmillan (1985); pp 1219–1239.

r66. Birdwood GFB, Gilder SSB, Wink CAS (Eds). Parkinson's disease, a new approach to treatment London: Academic Press (1971).

r67. Costa E, Cuidotti A. Molecular mechanisms in the receptor action of benzodiazepines. Ann Rev Pharmacol Toxicol 1979;*19*:531–545.

r68. Delwaide PJ. Electrophysiological analysis of the mode of action of muscle relaxants in spasticity. Ann Neurol 1985;*17*:90–95.

r69. Hambleton, P. Clostridium botulinum toxins: a general review of involvement in disease, structure, mode of action and preparation for clinical use. J of Neurology 1993;*239*(1):16–20.

r70. Blum K, Manzo L. Neurotoxicology New York: Marcel Dekker Inc (1985).

r71. Simpson LL. Molecular pharmacology of botulinum toxin and tetanus toxin. Ann Rev Pharmacol Toxicol 1986;*26*:427–453.

r72. Simpson LL. The origin, structure, and pharmacological activity of botulinum toxin. Pharmacol Rev 1981;*33*:155–188.

r73. Simpson LL. Botulinum neurotoxins and tetanus toxin San Diego: Academic Press (1989).

r74. Simpson LL. The actions of clostridial toxins on storage and release of neurotransmitters. In: Harvey A (Ed). Natural and synthetic neurotoxins San Diego: Academic Press (1993); pp 278–317.

r75. Brin MF. Clinical usefulness of botulinum toxin. Workshop #450, Annual Meeting of the American Academy of Neurology, New York, May 1, 1993.

r76. B12 C15 Hornykiewicz 66
Hornykiewicz O. Dopamine (3-hydroxytyramine) and brain function. Pharmacol Rev 1966;*18*:925–962.

r77. Barbeau A. The pathogenesis of Parkinson's disease. Can Med Assoc J 1962;*87*:802–807.

r78. Hardie RJ, Levodopa-related motor fluctuations. In Stern G (Ed). Parkinson's Disease Baltimore: The Johns Hopkins University Press (1990): pp 559–596.

r79. Mouradian MM, Juncos JL, Fabbrini G, Schlegel J, Bartko J, Chase T. Motor fluctuations in Parkinson's disease: central pathophysiological mechanisms, Part II, Ann Neurol 1988;*24*:372–378.

r80. Marsden CD, Rinne UK, Koella WP, Dubuis R (Eds). Madopar HBS. International workshop on the 'on-off' phenomenon in Parkinson's disease: new possibilities for its management. Europ Neurol 1987;*27*(supp):1–142.

r81. Duvoisin RC (Ed). New strategies in dopaminergic therapy of Parkinson's disease: the use of a controlled-release formulations. Neurology 1989;*39* (supp 2): 1–106.

r82. Baldessarini RJ, Rankenburgg FR. Clozapine, a novel antipsychotic agent. NEJM 1991;*325*:746–754.

r83. Calne DB, Teychenne PF, Claveria LE, Eastman R, Greenacre JK, Petric A. Bromocriptine in parkinsonism. Br Med J 1974;*4*:442–444.

r84. Fahn S, Cote LH, Snider SR, Barrett RE, Isgreen Wp. In Fuxe K, Calne DB (Eds). Dopaminergic ergot derivatives and motor function Oxford: Pergamon Press (1979): pp 303–312.

r85. Rinne UK, Marttila R, Sonninen V. Relationship between brain dopamine turnover and the therapeutic response to bromocriptine. In Fuxe K and Calne DB (Eds). Dopaminergic ergot derivatives and motor function Oxford: Pergamon Press (1979): pp 319–324.

r86. Lieberman AN, Goldstein M. Bromocriptine in Parkinson's disease. Pharmacol Rev 1985;*37*:217–227.

r87. Lieberman A. Bromocriptine in Parkinson's disease. In Koller WC, Paulson G (Eds). Therapy of Parkinson's disease New York: Marcel Dekker (1990); pp 255–267.

r88. Lieberman AN, Goldstein M. Update on bromocriptine in Parkinson's disease. In Calne DB (Ed). Drugs for the treatment of Parkinson's disease Berlin: Springer-Verlag (1989); pp 443–458.

r89. Burns RS, Calne DB. Disposition of dopaminergic ergot compounds following oral administration. In Calne DB, Horowski R, McDonald RJ, Wuttke W (Eds). Lisuride and other dopamine agonists New York: Raven Press (1983): pp 153–160.

r90. Quinn N, Marsden CD, Schachter M. Thompson C, Lang AE, Parkes JD. Intravenous lisuride in extrapyramidal disorders. In Calne DB, Horowski R, McDonald RJ, Wuttke W (Eds) Lisuride and other dopamine agonists. New York: Raven (1983); 383–393.

r91. Markam CH, Diamond SG. Pergolide in the treatment of Parkinson's disease. In Calne (Ed). Drugs for the treatment of Parkinson's disease, Handbook of Experimental Pharmacology, vol 88 Berlin: Springer-Verlag (1989); pp 459–470.

r92. Schwab RS, Amador LV, Leevin JY. Apomorphine in Parkinson's disease. Trans Am Neurol Assoc 1951; *76*:251–253.

r93. Marsden CD. Advances in the management of Parkinson's disease. Scott Med J 1976;*21*:139–148.

r94. Simpson GM, May PRA. Schizophrenia: somatic treatment. In Kaplan HI, Sadock BJ (Eds). Comprehensive textbook of psychiatry, 4th edition Baltimore: Williams & Wilkins (1985); pp 713–724.

r95. Fahn S, Marsden CD. The treatment of dystonia. In Marsden CD, Fahn S (Eds). Movement disorders, vol 2 London: Butterworths (1987); pp 359–382.

r96. Nygaard TG. Idiopathic dystonia-parkinsonism. In Stern MB, Koller WC (Eds). Parkinsonian syndromes New York: Marcel Dekker (1993); pp 451–466.

r97. Harper PS (Ed). Huntington's disease Philadelphia: W.B. Saunders Company Ltd. (1991).

r98. Albin RL, Young AB, Penney JB. The functional anatomy of basal ganglia disorders. Trends Neurosci 1989;*12*:366–375.

r99. Buruma OJS, Roos RAC. Paroxysmal choreoathetosis. In Vinken PR, Bruyn GW, Klawans HL (Eds). Handbook of Clinical Neurology, vol 49 Amsterdam: Elsevier (1986); pp 349–367.

r100. Shapiro AK, Shapiro E, Sweet RD. Treatment of tics and Tourette syndrome. In Barbeau A (Ed). Disorders of movement Lancaster, England: MTP Press (1981); pp 105–132.

r101. Delwaide PJ. Medical treatment of spasticity. J Drugtherapy Res 1987;*12*:1–5.

r102. Guze BH, Baxter LR. Neuroleptic malignant syndrome. NEJM 1985;*313*:163–166.

r103. Harding AE. Clinical features and classification of inherited ataxias. Adv Neurol 1993;*61*:1–14.

r104. Graybiel A. Neurochemically specified subsystems in the basal ganglia. In Functions of the basal ganglia. Ciba Foundation symposium 107. London: Pitman (1984); pp 114–149.

r105. Hallet M. Neurophysiologic aspects of basal ganglia disorders. In Jankovic J (Ed.) Movement Disorders, Course #240, Annual Meeting of the American Academy of Neurology, Washington, DC, May 2, 1994.

r106. DasGupta BR. Structures of botulinum neurotoxin, its functional domains, and perspectives on the crystalline type A toxin. In Jankovic J, Hallet M (Eds). Therapy with botulinum toxin. New York: Marcel Dekker, Inc.; pp 15–39.

r107. Lebeda FJ, Hack DC, Gentry MK. Theoretical analyses of the functional regions of the heavy chain of botulinum neurotoxin. In Jankovic J, Hallet M (Eds). Therapy with botulinum toxin. New York: Marcel Dekker, Inc.; pp 51–61.

CHAPTER 19

Epilepsy and Antiepileptic Drugs

G. Kenneth Lloyd
Gail Gillenwater

Epilepsy is one of the most common neurologic disorders, affecting about 1 percent of the population, second only to stroke.[r1] Today, the prognosis for seizure control is excellent in most patients. Comprehensive Epilepsy Centers, supported by the National Institutes of Health, provide research, direct services, and education to improve the quality of life of patients and their families. Over the past two decades, substantial progress has been made in understanding the causes of epilepsy. Novel treatment strategies including epilepsy surgery are being developed. Several new antiepileptic drugs recently have been approved by the FDA, and numerous others are under investigation worldwide.

Epilepsy is a *chronic neurologic condition* characterized by recurrent spontaneous seizures not caused by active cerebral disease. Seizures are sudden, involuntary, time-limited alterations in behavior associated with excessive discharges of cerebral neurons. Epileptic disorders can be *primary* or *secondary*. Primary disorders are presumed to result from a genetic disturbance; secondary disorders are presumed to result from a brain injury, such as penetrating head trauma or cerebral infarction. Seizures associated with sleep deprivation, abrupt withdrawal of alcohol or sedative drugs, fever, or use of convulsive drugs are not reflective of a chronic epileptic disorder.

Classification of Epileptic Seizures

Epileptic seizures can be characterized by specific EEG patterns and behavioral events during the seizures. The classification of seizures is of clinical relevance since many antiepileptic drugs are effective only in certain seizure types and are contraindicated for others. The most widely used classification system is the International Classification of Epileptic Seizures (ICES) introduced in 1981 by the International League Against Epilepsy[1] (see Table 19.1).

According to the ICES system, seizures are classified as either *partial* or *generalized*. Partial seizures originate in one cerebral hemisphere; generalized seizures originate in both. When partial seizures evolve to generalized seizures, they are referred to as *secondarily generalized seizures*.

Partial seizures are classified further into *simple* and *complex* seizures. Simple partial seizures occur with no loss of consciousness. These are further classified according to whether there are motor, sensory, autonomic, or psychic symptoms. Simple partial seizures that occur before the progression to a loss of consciousness are referred to as *auras*. Complex partial seizures may either begin as simple partial seizures or begin with a loss of consciousness.

Generalized seizures are either *convulsive* or *nonconvulsive*. Convulsive seizures include tonic-clonic, clonic, and tonic seizures. Nonconvulsive seizures include absence, myoclonic, and atonic seizures. Most generalized seizures are presumed to be an inherited disorder and are frequently referred to as *primary generalized seizures*.

Tonic-clonic seizures are the most common type of convulsive seizure. Usually the seizures begin suddenly with an abrupt loss of consciousness. Tonic con-

Table 19.1 The International Classification of Epileptic Seizures (Simplified)*

Seizure Type	Seizure Subgroup
I. Partial seizures (focal, local seizures)	A. Simple partial seizures (consciousness not impaired) 1. With motor symptoms 2. With somatosensory symptoms or special sensory symptoms 3. With autonomic symptoms 4. With psychic symptoms B. Complex partial seizures (with impairment of consciousness) 1. Beginning as simple partial and progressing to impairment of consciousness 2. With impairment of consciousness at onset C. Partial seizures evolving to secondarily generalized seizures (these may be generalized, tonic-clonic, tonic, or clonic) 1. Simple partial seizures evolving to generalized seizures 2. Complex partial seizures evolving to generalized seizures 3. Simple partial seizures evolving to complex partial seizures evolving to generalized seizures.
II. Generalized seizures (convulsive or nonconvulsive)	A. Absence 1. Absence seizures 2. Atypical absence seizures B. Myoclonic seizures C. Clonic seizures D. Tonic seizures E. Tonic-clonic seizures F. Atonic seizures
III. Unclassified epileptic seizures	

*Simplified from: Commission on Classification and Terminology of the International League Against Epilepsy.[1]

tractions occur with arms and legs extended. After 10 to 20 seconds the tonic phase ends, the clonic phase begins, and tonic rigidity is interrupted by brief intermittent muscle relaxation. During this type of seizure, heart rate and blood pressure increase and glandular hypersecretion and prolonged apnea occur. The seizure duration ranges from seconds to a few minutes. As consciousness is regained, incontinence often occurs, and headache and fatigue are frequent. Patients may fall into a deep sleep and then awaken disoriented and confused with no memory of the seizure.

Absence seizures are characterized by sudden onset and sudden offset. The seizures are brief and rarely last longer than 10 seconds. Generally they are characterized by lapses of consciousness, complete cessation of all ongoing activities, and a brief motionless stare. To an onlooker, the seizure resembles daydreaming. Absence seizures are associated with a characteristic 3-Hz spike-and-wave discharge on the EEG. Atypical absence seizures have a slower, less sharp onset and recovery than absence seizures, and the alteration in consciousness may not be complete.

Myoclonic seizures consist of sudden, brief, shock-like muscle contractions. Myoclonic seizures can occur in other neurologic conditions as well as in epilepsy. Myoclonic seizures are not associated with loss of consciousness. However, myoclonic seizures may progress to tonic-clonic seizures.

Atonic seizures consist of sudden loss of tone in postural muscles. In the severe form, the patient collapses to the floor. Atonic seizures are associated with impaired consciousness. Frequent falls often result in injury to the patient. Atonic seizures also are referred to as *drop attacks* or *astatic* seizures.

Although the ICES classification is useful in diagnosing seizures, the terminology is different from that previously used to describe seizures and currently used by many clinicians. The ICES term tonic-clonic designates a "grand mal" seizure; absence designates a "petit mal" seizure; complex partial designates a "psychomotor," "temporal lobe," or "limbic" seizure, and simple partial designates a "focal" or "Jacksonian" seizure.

Management of the Patient with Epilepsy

Diagnosis of Epilepsy

Epilepsy must be correctly diagnosed before appropriate treatment can be initiated. Also, a diagnosis of epilepsy has major implications for the patient and the patient's family and should be made only after a complete evaluation of the patient.

Obtain a Complete History. The most critical aspect in diagnosing epilepsy is a detailed seizure history from the patient and from someone who has observed the seizures, including a careful description of events preceding, during, and following the seizures. Any precipitating factors such as excessive fatigue, consumption of alcohol or drugs, photosensitivity, etc., should be identified. The history should indicate whether the patient was responsive during the seizure. The frequency and duration of seizures should be specified. Most epileptic seizures are brief, and seizures lasting for more than a few minutes usually are not epileptic. The age of onset is important because many causes of epilepsy are age-related. It is important to obtain a complete list of all previously used antiepileptic drugs, the treatment regimen, plasma concentration, duration of treatment, effectiveness in reducing seizures, adverse events associated with the drug, and reasons for discontinuation if the drug was withdrawn. It is also important to obtain a complete medical history from the patient. If other family members have experienced epileptic disorders, this may be helpful in determining whether the patient has a hereditary disorder.

Perform a Physical Examination. A general physical examination should be performed to identify specific diseases or disorders that might be the cause of the seizures. A neurologic examination should be performed, and results may aid in differentiating partial (focal) seizures from generalized seizures.

Perform Laboratory Tests. Clinical laboratory tests such as blood chemistry and hematologic testing can provide information about underlying disease states, especially liver and renal function. They also provide a baseline measure for evaluating abnormalities in clinical laboratory tests associated with initiation of or changes to existing antiepileptic drug therapy. Lumbar punctures are seldom indicated in the routine evaluation for epilepsy, unless an infection of the CNS is suspected. The electroencephalograph (EEG) is important for diagnosing the patient with newly identified seizures. Specific epileptiform discharges can help localize seizures and aid in the classification of seizures. In patients with partial seizures, a localized abnormality usually is detectable; in patients with primary generalized seizures, EEG abnormalities usually are bilateral. In some cases, the EEG findings are negative or inconclusive. Specialized diagnostic tests such as computerized tomography (CT) or magnetic resonance imaging (MRI) usually are conducted on new patients to demonstrate brain lesions. Despite the additional cost, MRI usually is preferable to CT. In some patients, seizures are difficult to diagnose or control, and intensive monitoring involving simultaneous videotaping and recording of the EEG may be indicated.

Treatment of Epilepsy

Once a diagnosis of epilepsy is made, medical treatment should be initiated. The goals of therapy should be to reduce seizures and preserve the patient's quality of life. If a specific cause of seizures is found, such as a brain tumor, treatment may consist of removing the cause. However, most frequently a treatable cause cannot be determined, and the patient will require antiepileptic drugs to control the seizures. Because some seizures respond only to specific classes of antiepileptic drugs and because some antiepileptic drugs can exacerbate specific types of seizures, it is important that the seizures be identified correctly before antiepileptic drugs are prescribed. Generally, about half of the patients will have their seizures satisfactorily controlled with antiepileptic drugs; the remaining half will be divided into patients having occasional seizures and patients who have uncontrolled seizures and/or unacceptable adverse effects from antiepileptic medications.

Monotherapy vs. Polytherapy

An important issue when developing treatment strategy is whether to prescribe only one antiepileptic drug (monotherapy) or more than one (polytherapy). Current practice advocates monotherapy whenever possible. When one antiepileptic drug fails, its replacement by a second is recommended. Monotherapy has several advantages over polytherapy. Adverse effects are more manageable since it is difficult to evaluate the role of more than one drug in producing a specific reaction. A further important advantage is that compliance is improved when patients have fewer drugs to take; also, monotherapy avoids some of the unpredictable adverse effects associated with drug-drug interactions. The initial antiepileptic drug should be chosen based on its efficacy for the patient's type of seizures. If the seizures are frequent, a loading dose sometimes is administered. If seizures are not controlled, the dosage should be slowly increased until seizures are controlled or unacceptable adverse effects occur. Generally, dosages should only be changed after five drug elimination half-lives have passed. If the drug fails after an adequate course of therapy, a second drug should be added and the first drug tapered very slowly to avoid seizure recurrence. Polytherapy usually is not recommended unless three antiepileptic drugs have failed to control seizures with acceptable adverse effects when administered as monotherapy.

Selection of Antiepileptic Drugs

Currently in the US, the most common antiepileptic drugs for treating partial seizures with and without secondary generalization are carbamazepine, phenytoin, and valproate. Two new drugs were recently approved as treatment for partial seizures. Gabapentin was approved as adjunctive therapy. While Felbamate was approved as monotherapy and adjunctive therapy, its use was recently suspended (see page 385). Also, approval of lamotrigine as adjunctive therapy is expected soon. Clinical experience will determine the optimal uses of these new drugs. The most common drugs for treating primary generalized seizures are valproate, ethosuximide (absence only), and phenytoin. Carbamazepine has been used successfully in treating some patients with tonic-clonic seizures, but may worsen absence, myoclonic, or atonic seizures. Phenobarbital is widely used as an alternative drug for treating partial and generalized seizures. Diazepam is the standard drug for treating status epilepticus.

It is noteworthy that common usage of antiepileptic drugs in the US is not totally consistent with the indications approved by the FDA. This is especially true for valproate, which is a standard treatment for partial and generalized seizures but approved as monotherapy only for simple and complex absence seizures and as adjunctive therapy for multiple seizure types that include absence seizures.

Single Seizures

There is a controversy regarding whether to initiate antiepileptic drug therapy in a patient who has a single, unprovoked seizure. Because of the impact of a diagnosis of epilepsy, it is often not in the patient's best interest to give antiepileptic medication following a single seizure. However, if clinical and laboratory evaluations indicate focal symptoms, the seizure could be predictive of a chronic epilepsy disorder and treatment is often indicated. There is a reasonable probability that seizures will recur. In any case, there is always risk of a second seizure. The advantages and disadvantages of treating a single seizure must be weighed and decided for each patient.

Psychogenic Seizures

Nonepileptic, seizure-like episodes of psychogenic origin can be mistaken for epileptic seizures and inappropriately treated with antiepileptic drugs. Often, if a psychogenic seizure is observed, it can be identified by behaviors that are not typical of epileptic seizures. Patients with epileptic seizures may have concurrent psychogenic seizures, and it is often difficult to differentiate between them. Psychogenic seizures also have been termed *pseudoseizures.*

Status Epilepticus

Status epilepticus occurs when seizures are continuous or occur so frequently that there is no recovery between attacks for more than 30 minutes. The seizure may be partial or generalized (e.g., tonic-clonic or absence). The longer an episode continues, the more likely it will result in permanent neuronal damage. Both the clinical and EEG convulsive states should be terminated as soon as possible. Untreated or ineffectively treated status epilepticus can be fatal.

Psychosocial Considerations

Epilepsy has significant psychologic, social, and financial implications. Patients and their families can greatly benefit from a treatment strategy that takes into consideration the nonmedical aspects of epilepsy. Educational information gives patients and their families an understanding of how epilepsy will impact their lives. It also can provide ways to deal with the physical consequences of epilepsy, the adverse effects of drug therapy, and the psychologic aspects of epilepsy, including feelings of guilt, shame, and inadequacy. By providing psychosocial support and assisting the patient and the patient's family in taking advantage of community resources, the goal of enhancing the quality of life can be obtained. The disabling potential of epilepsy can be greatly reduced by knowledgeable and understanding friends, family, and co-workers.

Mechanism of Action of Antiepileptic Drugs

Most of the presently used antiepileptic drugs and their forbears were discovered by screening without a rationale as to mechanism of action. Anticonvulsant activity and clinical efficacy, together with an acceptable safety profile, were (and still are) sufficient to present a compound for marketing authorization. The mechanisms of action of the classic antiepileptics were discovered many years after these compounds entered clinical use.

The strategy for the discovery of antiepileptic drugs began to change in the late 1970s, when different synaptic mechanisms were shown to play a fundamental role in seizure generation, propagation, and suppression. The GABA (γ-aminobutyric acid) hypothesis of epilepsy and antiepileptic drug action stimulated drug research and discovery.[r2,r3] As a result, two novel compounds have reached the European market (progabide and vigabatrin) and several others are in clinical trials.[r4,r5,r6,r7] Several classic antiepileptic drugs exhibit GABAergic mechanisms (e.g., barbiturates, benzodiazepines, valproate). Rational drug design based on an identified mechanism of action has become the standard for embarking on a new antiepileptic drug discovery program.

Seizures and subsequent epilepsy result from a

regional imbalance of inhibitory and excitatory neuronal inputs and from alterations in neuronal membrane stability and permeability. The resultant hyperexcitability of specific neurons and circuits produces a series of synchronous neuronal discharges with typical EEG patterns, convulsions, and behavioral abnormalities reflective of the neuronal circuitry involved. The rationale for a new antiepileptic drug discovery program generally addresses this imbalance of excitation/inhibition, hyperexcitability, and synchronous discharges.

There are basically three hypotheses for the fundamentals of antiepileptic drug action: enhanced inhibition, decreased excitation; and increased neuronal membrane stability. This translates into specific molecular (e.g., receptor, ion channel, enzyme) subtypes as the most frequent targets for antiepileptic drug action. The neurotransmitter-based mechanisms are outlined in Table 19.2. An excess of any of these mechanisms leads to a lack of therapeutic specificity and unacceptable side-effects.

Enhancement of Inhibitory Synaptic Activity. $GABA_A$ synapses are the most prevalent inhibitory synapses in the cerebrum. Those thought to be most relevant to epilepsy are distributed in the hippocampus, amygdala, thalamus, deep forebrain nuclei, and many cortical areas.[r8,r9,r10] There is substantial evidence that GABAergic transmission is diminished in epileptic foci.[r9,r11,2] It is also clear that not all $GABA_A$ synapses are directly relevant to epilepsy.

The $GABA_A$ receptor complex is a multimeric structure composed of combinations of different molecular subunits (α, β, γ, ∂, epsilon) and several functional sites that modulate a chloride ion channel in the neuronal membrane. These functional sites include the $GABA_A$ receptor itself and various allosteric recognition sites (e.g., benzodiazepine, barbiturate, neurosteroid) and sites within the chloride ion channel.[3] Sufficient inhibition of any of these sites will produce convulsions. Conversely, enhancement of the function of the $GABA_A$ receptor complex has an anticonvulsant effect, which is translated into an antiepileptic action in man.[r7,r12,r13] Enhancing the function of specific sites within the $GABA_A$ receptor complex, or by increasing the availability of synaptic GABA, has proved to be a most successful approach (see Table 19.2). Other inhibitory neurotransmitter synapses may also be relevant to seizure generation and control. These include the strychnine-sensitive glycine receptors in the brainstem and dopamine receptors relevant to photosensitive epilepsy.

Diminution of Excitatory Synaptic Activity. The preponderance of fast excitatory neurotransmission is mediated by the amino acid glutamate; in many instances aspartate appears to subserve the same role. Although the physiology and pharmacology of the different types of glutamate receptors have not been exploited as potential targets for antiepileptic drug action to the same extent as $GABA_A$ synapses, this is presently a very competitive field. At least two types of glutamate receptor-gated ion channel complexes have relevance to seizure generation and control, the N-methyl-d-aspartate (NMDA) receptors and the AMPA/kainate receptors, named after their prototypic agonists. Overactivation of either of these receptor types will produce convulsions, although the seizure characteristics and pharmacology differ markedly. The metabotropic glutamate receptors do not directly mediate excitability, and likely play a more subtle role in epilepsy via regulation of intracellular events including calcium storage, negative cyclic AMP regulation, and phosphoinositide metabolism. Preliminary evidence suggests that glutamate levels are increased in some epileptic patients,[4] and the new antiepileptic drug lamotrigine has been shown to decrease glutamate release.[5]

NMDA receptors modulate a specific calcium channel, and excess activity of these receptors is associated with convulsions and, if sufficiently severe, neuronal death. Antagonism of either the glutamate recognition site or any of the allosteric sites within the NMDA receptor complex is an effective anticonvulsant mechanism. Unfortunately, to date, the anticonvulsant compounds that interfere with the function of the NMDA receptor complex have had an unacceptable safety profile, which includes psychotomimetic (PCP-like) activity, neuropathologic changes (in animals), and impairment of cognitive function.[r16,r17] It is very possible that compounds highly selective for specific subtypes of NMDA receptors will prove to be useful antiepileptics.

Investigations of AMPA/kainate receptor antagonists, or compounds active at the metabotropic glutamate receptor are too preliminary to assess for an antiepileptic potential. However, it is probable that several interesting compounds will evolve from this line of drug discovery.

Control of Neuronal Membrane Excitability and Ionic Permeability. A major determinant of neuronal membrane excitability is the functional state of voltage-dependent calcium, potassium, and sodium channels. Of these, the calcium channels are presently receiving considerable attention following the observations that: the paroxysmal depolarizing shift associated with burst firing is mediated by the activation of calcium channels; excessive calcium entry leads to neuronal death; and certain anti-absence drugs appear to block a T-type calcium channel in the rat thalamus.[r14,9,10] Other than flunarizine, the calcium blockers presently used for various cardiovascular indications do not seem to have antiepileptic potential; most either do not penetrate the blood-brain barrier sufficiently, or do not have the desired calcium channel subtype selectivity.

Modulation of neuronal sodium channels decreases cellular excitability and diminishes the axonal propagation of nerve impulses. This is a clinically useful mechanism and has been demonstrated to be integral to the activity of major antiepileptic drugs such as carbamazepine and phenytoin.[r14,r15,11]

Animal Models in the Discovery of New Antiepileptic Drugs. Screening compounds in rodents against convulsions induced by different stimuli is the classic route for the discovery of new antiepileptic drugs. Discoveries in molecular biology have provided highly specific tools for mechanism-based rational drug design at a stage prior to *in vivo* testing. Thus, cloned subtypes of human (or rat when the human is not available) receptors expressed either transiently or in stable cell lines can be used as initial targets for antiepileptic drug screening. Based on either cell biology or electrophysiology, functional techniques have been developed for different neuronal calcium channels, subtypes of NMDA receptors and recombinant $GABA_A$ receptors. As these techniques progress and the physiologic combinations of subunits become known, recombinant technology will be an important step in screening for new antiepileptic drugs.

Even with the advancement of *in vitro* screening

Table 19.2 Neurotransmitter-Based Mechanisms of Action for the Rational Design of Antiepileptic Drugs

Synaptic Activity	Molecular Target: Activity	Subtype(s)	Seizure Indication	Example of Antiepileptic Drug
Inhibitory: GABA	$GABA_A$ receptor complex: GABA mimetics	Agonist site	Not absence	Progabide[r4]
		Benzodiazepine site	Status epilepticus	Clonazepam[r7,r14]
		Barbiturate site	Partial and generalized tonic-clonic, clonic, tonic, status epilepticus	Phenobarbital[r7,r14]
		Neurosteroid site	?	Epalons in preclinical[6,7]
		Chloride ion channel	?	None as yet; barbiturates?
	GABA transporter: GABA uptake inhibitor	Neuronal and glial	?	Tiagabine in clinical trials[r6,r7]
	GABA transaminase: inhibitor	?	Refractory partial epilepsy	Vigabatrin[r5]
Inhibitory: Dopamine	Receptor agonist	D_1–D_5 identified	Photosensitive seizures	Apomorphine as experimental drug in clinical trials[8]
Inhibitory: Taurine	Receptor agonist	?	?	Taltrimide in clinical trials[r6,r7]
Inhibitory: Glycine	Receptor mimetic	Strychnine sensitive	?	Milacemide?[r6,r7]
Excitatory: Glutamate	NMDA receptor complex: antagonist	Agonist site	?	Remacemide in clinical trials[r6]
		Calcium channel	?	None known; potential psychotomimetic effects
		Glycine site	?	None known
	AMPA/kainate receptor: antagonist	Multiple subtypes $GluR_1$–$GluR_4$	?	None known
	Metabotropic: antagonist	Multiple subtypes $mGluR_1$–$mGluR_6$	?	None known
	Glutamate release	?	Partial seizures	Lamotrigine[r7,5]
Excitatory: Acetylcholine	Neuronal nicotinic: antagonist or partial agonist	Multiple subunits	?	None known
Excitatory: Norepinephrine	Alpha noradrenergic receptors	Multiple subtypes	?	None known
Membrane stabilization: voltage dependent ion channels	Calcium channels: antagonist	Multiple subtypes and subunits: T-type	Absence	Ethosuximide[9]
	Potassium channels: block	Multiple subtypes	?	None known
	Sodium channels: antagonist	Multiple subtypes	Partial and generalized tonic-clonic seizures	Carbamazepine, phenytoin[r7,r15]

based on recombinant receptors and ion channels, animal models will continue to play key roles in the discovery of new antiepileptic drugs. A wide variety of such animal models exist: chemically-induced convulsions, either rationally (decreased inhibition, increased excitation) or empirically based; convulsive states that are genetic in origin (photosensitive baboons, sound-sensitive mice, Wistar rats with spontaneous "absence" seizures); and those that are electrogenic in origin (amygdala kindling, transorbital or transauricular electroshock). A list of the most common primary screening models and some of the more relevant secondary models is given in Table 19.3.

Traditionally, it was perceived that activity in the electroshock model indicated potential efficacy against partial seizures and generalized tonic and/or clonic seizures, whereas antipentylenetetrazol activity was predictive for anti-absence drugs. However, it is becoming clear with the development of new compounds that drugs effective against complex partial seizures may be inactive in the electroshock test.[r6] More complex models such as the amygdala kindling model appear to be more indicative of clinical efficacy against different partial seizures. When screening for an antiepileptic potential, it is the profile of anticonvulsant activity which is important, rather than the activity in any particular animal model.

Antiepileptic Drugs Commercially Available in the United States

Major Antiepileptic Drugs

Phenytoin

Phenytoin is a diphenyl substituted hydantoin. (Fig. 19.1). It is one of the most widely used antiepileptic drugs, even though it has been available for more than 50 years. Phenytoin is useful in treating both complex partial and generalized epileptic seizures.

Chemistry. Phenytoin (Figure 19.1; 5,5-diphenyl-2,4-imidazolidinedione) is related to the barbiturates in structure, but has a five-membered ring. A 5-phenyl or other aromatic substituent appears to be necessary for anticonvulsant activity. Alkyl substituents at position 5 result in a molecule with sedative properties. Other hydantoins used in epilepsy include ethotoin and mephytoin (see below).

History. Phenytoin was first synthesized in 1908 by Blitz. The anticonvulsive properties of phenytoin were discovered in 1938 by Merritt and Putnam[12] during a screening program that used electroshock-induced seizures in laboratory animals to test the anticonvulsive effects of potential antiepileptic drugs. Phenytoin was selected for clinical trials because it had substantial anticonvulsant effects and minimal sedative properties. Phenytoin was the first antiepilep-

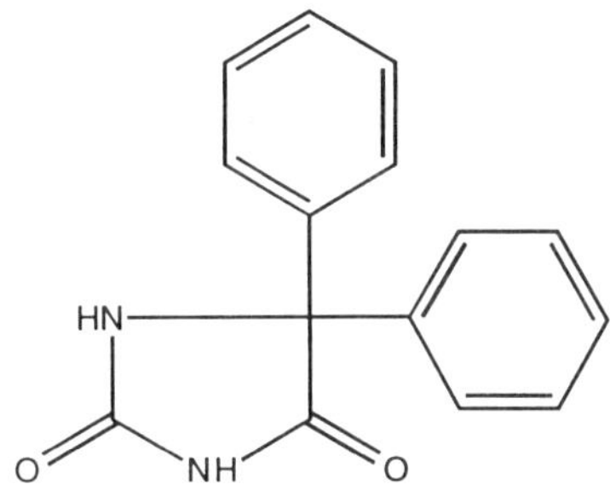

HN
NH
O
O
PHENYTOIN

Figure 19.1 Structure of Phenytoin

Table 19.3 Commonly Used Models for Antiepileptic Drug Discovery[r6,r18]

Convulsant Stimulus	Species	Seizure Type	Clinical Correlate
Primary screening models			
Maximal electroshock (transauricular, transorbital)	Mice, rats	Tonic	Simple or complex partial; tonic and/or clonic primary generalized
Pentylenetetrazol	Mice, rats	Generalized clonic and tonic seizures	Absence; myoclonic
Sound	DBA/2J mice	Wild running; clonic/tonic	Absence
Decreased $GABA_A$ function (bicuculline, isoniazid)	Mice, rats	Clonic, tonic/clonic	Partial seizures; tonic and/or clonic primary generalized
Secondary Screening Models			
Amygdala kindling	Rat	After-discharge threshold; seizure severity	Partial seizures with secondary generalization
Spontaneous spike-wave discharge	Wistar rat strain	EEG spike-wave discharge; "absences"	Partial seizures; absence seizures
Intermittent photic stimulation	Papio papio	EEG spiking; myoclonic jerks	Photosensitive epilepsy

tic drug without significant sedation at therapeutic doses. Diverse mechanisms have been proposed to account for the antiepileptic action of phenytoin. The most convincing is that the compound shares a similar mechanism of action with carbamazepine, blocking neuronal sodium channels by binding to the inactivated state of the channel.[r7,r.14,r15,11,13,14] This reverses the paroxysmal depolarization shift observed in epileptic foci.

Therapeutic Uses and Limitations.[r19,r20,15,16] Phenytoin is indicated in adults and children for the control of generalized tonic-clonic and complex partial seizures and for the prevention and treatment of seizures occurring during or following neurosurgery. Phenytoin is ineffective in treating absence seizures. Some patients develop hypersensitivity reactions resulting in discontinuation of phenytoin. The risk of birth defects in infants of mothers treated with phenytoin is not clearly established, but is probably twice normal. The "fetal hydantoin syndrome" that includes mild-to-moderate growth and mental retardation, microcephaly, craniofacial abnormalities, and nail and digital hypoplasia has been reported in infants born to mothers treated with phenytoin. However, similar syndromes have been reported after use of other antiepileptic drugs, such as phenobarbital, carbamazepine, and valproic acid. Because seizures pose a risk to the mother and developing fetus, most patients should continue treatment with antiepileptic drugs during pregnancy. Abrupt withdrawal of phenytoin in epileptic patients may precipitate status epilepticus.

Effects of the Drug Responsible for Its Therapeutic Usefulness.[r2,r7,r14] In animal models, phenytoin has been shown to modify the pattern of maximal electroshock seizures in a manner similar to other antiepileptic drugs that are effective against generalized tonic-clonic seizures. Phenytoin blocks the spread of seizure activity. In contrast to the barbiturates, phenytoin does not elevate the seizure threshold to electroshock or to convulsant drugs such as pentylenetetrazol, picrotoxin, or strychnine.

Phenytoin has a stabilizing effect on neuronal membranes that may be associated with interference with ionic currents, primarily sodium and calcium. In excitable tissues, phenytoin blocks sodium channels, which normalizes the paroxysmal depolarizing shift observed in epileptic foci. Phenytoin also limits membrane permeability to calcium, leading to decreased intracellular calcium concentration.

Undesirable Effects.[16,17,18] The adverse effects of phenytoin depend on the dosage, route of administration, and duration of therapy. The most common adverse effects are associated with the CNS. These effects usually are dose related and include nystagmus, ataxia, slurred speech, decreased coordination, and mental confusion. It is still debated whether cognitive impairment occurs at therapeutic doses. In rare instances, patients treated with phenytoin experience nausea and vomiting, which can be minimized by taking the drug at mealtimes. At high plasma levels a paradoxical exacerbation of seizures may occur. When phenytoin is administered IV at a rapid rate, cardiovascular toxicity and respiratory depression may occur.

Hypersensitivity reactions can be seen in susceptible patients within four weeks of starting treatment. A rash is the most common sign and can be accompanied by fever, lymphadenopathy, eosinophilia, and hepatitis. Rarely, more serious forms of dermatitis such as exfoliative dermatitis, lupus erythematosus, or Stevens-Johnson syndrome are associated with this therapy.

Cosmetic adverse effects unrelated to dose have been reported in some patients treated with phenytoin. Gingival hyperplasia can develop in both adults and children. Many investigators have found that this effect can be prevented or controlled by routine dental procedures. Hirsutism may occur, but is rarely severe enough to require withdrawal of phenytoin. Facial coarsening, manifested as broadening of the lips and nose, has been reported but is extremely rare and occurs only after many years of treatment.

Following chronic treatment with phenytoin, a small number of patients may develop uncommon adverse effects including hematologic reactions (e.g., megaloblastic anemia that responds to folic acid therapy), endocrine effects (e.g., decreased serum protein-bound iodine in euthyroid patients or hyperglycemia), immunologic effects (e.g., decrease in serum immunoglobulin A), peripheral nervous system effects (e.g., sensory peripheral polyneuropathy), and skeletal effects (e.g., osteomalacia manifested by hypocalcemia).

Drug Interactions.[r21,r22,16,19] Phenytoin is highly bound to plasma proteins and is metabolized by the hepatic microsomal oxidase system. Consequently, most interactions between phenytoin and other drugs are pharmacokinetic interactions and are associated with altered plasma protein binding, inhibition of metabolism or induction of metabolism. Certain antacids may interfere with the absorption of phenytoin from the GI tract, but their effect probably is of limited importance. Drugs that displace phenytoin from plasma protein binding sites generally result in a decrease in the optimal plasma concentration as the free phenytoin fraction rises and metabolism and clearance increase. Intoxication can occur with drugs such as valproic acid, which also inhibit phenytoin metabolism.

Because the metabolism of phenytoin is saturable, a small degree of inhibition can lead to a large increase in phenytoin concentration. On the other hand, stimulation of phenytoin metabolism and a fall in plasma levels is relatively unusual. Interactions of phenytoin with phenobarbital or benzodiazepines are usually clinically insignificant. Treatment with phenytoin can lead to accelerated turnover or a variety of drugs. Table 19.4 provides a list of substances that may have an effect on phenytoin serum levels and also drugs that are affected by concurrent treatment with phenytoin.

Overdosage.[r19,r20,16,17] Initial signs of overdosage are associated with the CNS and include nystagmus, ataxia, dysarthria, lethargy, and mental changes. Other signs include tremor, hyperreflexia, slurred speech, nausea, and vomiting. The patient may become comatose and hypotensive. Death may result from respiratory and circulatory depression. The estimated lethal dose in adults is 2 to 5 grams and is unknown in children. There is no known antidote, and treatment includes maintaining the respiratory and circulatory systems with appropriate supportive measures. Where appropriate, emesis or gastric lavage may be tried and hemodialysis can be considered.

Pharmacokinetics.[r19,16,20,21] Phenytoin is absorbed slowly and incompletely after oral and IM administration; peak plasma levels occur three to 12 hours after

Table 19.4 Drug Interactions Involving Phenytoin

Phenytoin on Plasma Levels of Other Drugs			Other Drugs on Phenytoin Plasma Levels	
Increase	**Decrease**	**Increase or Decrease**	**Increase**	**Decrease**
acute alcohol intake	carbamazepine	phenobarbital	carbamazepine	corticosteroids
amiodarone	reserpine	sodium valproate		coumarin
chloramphenicol	sucralfate	valproic acid		anticoagulants
chlordiazepoxide	molindone hydrochloride			digitoxin
diazepam	chronic alcohol intake			doxycycline
dicumarol				estrogens
disulfiram				felbamate
estrogens				furosemide
felbamate				lamotrigine
H_2-antagonists				oral contraceptives
halothane				quinidine
isoniazid				rifampin
methylphenidate				theophylline
phenothiazines				vigabatrin
phenylbutazone				vitamin D
salicylates				
succinimides				
sulfonamides				
tolbutamide				
trazodone				

a single oral dose. Phenytoin is about 90 percent bound by plasma proteins. Approximately 95 percent of phenytoin is excreted as metabolites, with less than 5 percent excreted unchanged in urine. The half-life after oral administration ranges from seven to 42 hours, with a mean of 22 hours; the half-life after IV administration is 10 to 15 hours. The major route of metabolism is by hepatic microsomal enzymes to inactive metabolites. At lower dosages, phenytoin follows first-order kinetics. However, at higher doses, when the hepatic system is near saturation, phenytoin follows zero-order kinetics. Thus, at higher plasma concentrations, a very small increase in dosage can result in a very large increase in plasma concentrations, resulting in intoxication. Because phenytoin is metabolized by hepatic enzymes, phenytoin levels are influenced by concomitant medication and by factors such as pregnancy, age, and liver and renal disease.

Available Preparations and Usual Doses.[16] Phenytoin is available in a variety of dosage forms including 30- and 100-mg extended release capsules, 50-mg tablets, solutions containing 500 mg/mL for parenteral injection, and suspensions for oral administration. Capsules containing a combination of phenytoin and phenobarbital also are available. The usual starting adult dosage for phenytoin is 100 mg three times a day, with the dosage adjusted to suit individual requirements up to 600 mg/day. Once-a-day dosing may be appropriate for some individuals. The pediatric dosage is 4 to 8 mg/kg/day. The therapeutic range of phenytoin plasma levels is 10 to 20 µg/ml. When changing formulations, dosage adjustments and plasma level monitoring may be necessary. A loading dose may be administered to adults. In treating adults with status epilepticus, a loading dose of 10 to 15 mg/kg should be administered slowly IV (less than 50 mg/min) and followed by maintenance doses.

Carbamazepine

Carbamazepine is a tricyclic compound of the iminostilbene family. It is closely related to the tricyclic antidepressants, and was derived from a series of imipramine analogues. The medical indications for use in the US for carbamazepine include certain types of epileptic seizures (partial seizures, and primary and secondary generalized tonic, clonic, and tonic/clonic) and trigeminal neuralgia.[22] It may have some use in other neurologic disorders and in manic-depressive disorder. Carbamazepine also has antidiuretic effects.

Chemistry. Carbamazepine (Figure 19.2, 5H-dibenz[b,f]azepine-5-carboxamide) is a neutral lipophilic compound virtually insoluble in water but readily soluble in organic solvents. It has a molecular weight of 236.26. The three-dimensional structure has considerable overlap with other tricyclic compounds such as chlorpromazine, imipramine, maprotyline, phenobarbital, phensuximide, clonazepam, and phenytoin.[23] Within the iminostilbene family, the carbamyl group is essential for good anticonvulsant activity.[24]

History. An anticonvulsant potential of iminostilbene-like compounds has been known and exploited since the 1890s. Carbamazepine was first synthesized at Geigy in the mid-1950s and clinical trials in epilepsy started late in the same decade. It was introduced in Europe as an antiepileptic in 1963 and in the US in 1974. Carbamazepine was the first antiepileptic drug that had efficacy in all seizure types except for absence seizures.[23]

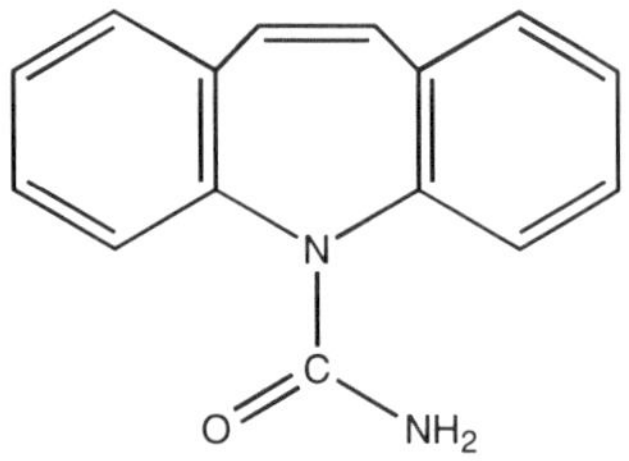

CARBAMAZEPINE

Figure 19.2 Structure of Carbamazepine

It is presently thought that the molecular basis of the antiepileptic activity of carbamazepine is inhibition of voltage-dependent sodium channels by preferentially binding to the inactivated state of the sodium channel.[11,13,14] This results in a decreased cell excitability and a reduction in sustained repetitive bursting of action potentials in response to repetitive stimulation. In epileptic foci this translates as a reversal of the paroxysmal depolarizing shift. This inhibition of voltage-dependent sodium channels occurs at therapeutic carbamazepine concentrations. Carbamazepine also has an effect on the type-3 ("peripheral") benzodiazepine receptor, adenosine receptors, and alpha-2 noradrenergic receptors.[r23] It does not exhibit activity at excitatory amino acid receptors or at $GABA_A$ receptors.

Therapeutic Uses and Limitations.[22,23] Carbamazepine is the drug of choice for the monotherapy of newly diagnosed partial seizures with or without secondary generalization in both children and adults. It is also the antiepileptic drug of choice for benign focal epilepsies of children. Carbamazepine is considered as a first-line therapy for any uncontrolled patient with partial seizures and secondary generalized tonic, clonic, or tonic-clonic seizures. Generalized tonic-clonic seizures are generally thought to be the seizures most responsive to carbamazepine therapy. Once seizure control and stable carbamazepine blood levels are attained, an attempt may be made to wean the patients off other antiepileptic drugs. Carbamazepine is not a drug of choice for the control of absence seizures, which may actually be enhanced or activated by this drug in some patients.[25]

Carbamazepine should not be used in patients with a history of bone marrow depression or with a sensitivity to structurally-related tricyclic compounds (e.g., imipramine). The use of volatile anesthetic agents should be avoided for patients receiving carbamazepine. Patients with increased intraocular pressure should be carefully monitored during carbamazepine therapy. Aplastic anemia and agranulocytosis have been associated with the use of carbamazepine. A patient receiving carbamazepine who exhibits low or decreased leukocyte or platelet counts should be monitored closely. Discontinuation of carbamazepine should be contemplated upon evidence of bone marrow depression.

Upon initiation of carbamazepine therapy, especially in a polytherapy situation, renal, hepatic, and complete hematologic parameters need to be monitored in addition to establishing stable therapeutic blood levels of carbamazepine.

In pregnant women, carbamazepine monotherapy is recommended. Polytherapy, especially the combination with phenobarbital and valproate, seems to be associated with an enhanced risk of teratology.[22,26] Epidemiologic data suggest an association between carbamazepine use in pregnancy and congenital malformations, including spina bifida.[r24,15]

Effects of the Drug Responsible for Its Therapeutic Usefulness. The clinical and preclinical anticonvulsant profile of carbamazepine is similar to that of phenytoin, although carbamazepine is more active in the amygdala kindling, pentylenetetrazole and electroshock seizure models. Both compounds have a similar blocking action on sodium channels, resulting in a preferential inhibition of high frequency discharges at concentrations that do not alter physiologic synaptic activity.[r14,11,13] The activation of noradrenergic neurons in the locus coeruleus by carbamazepine may be integral to its anticonvulsant activity as clonidine and norepinephrine depletion antagonize the action of the compound.[27]

Undesirable Effects.[r24,22,23] The undesirable effects of carbamazepine observed at therapeutic doses fall into two general categories: (1) rare and life-threatening; (2) relatively common, reversible, and generally tolerable. Between 30 and 50 percent of patients receiving carbamazepine experience undesirable effects; about 10 percent of patients discontinue the drug, most commonly for exanthema. The epoxide metabolite of carbamazepine has intrinsic toxicity, and carbamazepine toxicity is associated with enhanced levels of this metabolite. The frequency and severity of undesirable effects is enhanced in the elderly and during polytherapy.

Serious life-threatening effects are rare and generally occur with a frequency of one to five per million patient years. These are mainly aplastic anemia, Stevens-Johnson syndrome, and toxic epidermal necrolysis. These events usually are observed in the first three months of therapy and are associated with a mortality rate of 33 to 50 percent. The incidence of aplastic anemia and agranulocytosis is about 11 times greater than in the general population. Other serious adverse events are for the most part hematologic (leukopenia, thrombocytopenia purpura) or dermatologic (systemic lupus erythematosus), often the result of a drug-sensitivity reaction, possibly due to activation and proliferation of a subset of T-lymphocytes. Also reported are jaundice of either cholestatic or hepatic origin, which occasionally progresses to hepatitis; oliguria with hypertension, left ventricular failure, thrombophlebitis and cardiovascular collapse; lymphadenopathy and myocarditis.

The commonly observed undesirable effects can be minimized by initiating carbamazepine therapy at low doses with a slow increase to maintenance levels. CNS effects most frequently observed are diplopia, blurred vision, drowsiness, dizziness, ataxia, and dyskinesia. The incidence of altered cognitive function is lower than for phenobarbital, phenytoin, or primidone. Gastrointestinal adverse events include nausea, vomiting, and diarrhea. A decrease in white blood cell count is frequent as is splenomegaly or hepatomegaly with an increase in liver enzymes. Long-term administration of carbamazepine may result in lowered thyroxine levels and a clinically evident goiter.

Drug Interactions.[r21,22,23] Drug interactions involving carbamazepine are frequent, varied and often with therapeutic significance (see Table 19.5). Carbamazepine is a very effective inducer of hepatic mixed function drug metabolizing enzymes. Carbamazepine increases phenytoin levels (with a risk of phenytoin toxicity) and phenytoin enhances carbamazepine metabolism to the epoxide, which may result in toxic carbamazepine-epoxide levels together with low carbamazepine concentrations. It is recommended that blood levels of all three compounds be monitored for the first month upon initiation of combination therapy. Co-administration of carbamazepine and lithium may produce undesirable effects, even when the blood levels of both substances remain within therapeutic limits. These are mainly CNS events, which include cerebellar signs, coarse tremor, hyperreflexia, drowsiness, confusion, and weakness. The antidiuretic effect of carbamazepine is enhanced by valproate and phenobarbital, which can result in hyponatremia, hypocalcaemia, and hypochloremia. It should be noted that when carbamazepine therapy is withdrawn there will be a readjustment of the blood levels whose steady state was affected by carbamazepine, and that monitoring of the blood levels of the relevant compound may be appropriate.

Overdosage.[22,23,28] The outcome of acute overdoses of carbamazepine are related to the blood concentrations attained. Of 300 overdoses, nine fatalities were recorded, usually in combination with other drugs or alcohol. The lethal single dose of carbamazepine seems to be at least 60 grams for an adult. The formation of carbamazepine epoxide as a toxic metabolite is an important aspect of carbamazepine overdose. Carbamazepine plasma levels of 11 to 15 µg/ml are associated with drowsiness and ataxia; levels of 15 to 25 µg/ml give rise to hallucinations, combativeness, and choreiform movements; levels in excess of 25 µg/ml are associated with coma and seizures, which may lead to death. Treatment involves symptomatic therapy together with elimination of the drug and its toxic metabolite via gastric lavage together with peritoneal or hemodialysis. The seizures can be treated with benzodiazepines.

Pharmacokinetics.[22,23,29,30] Salient features of carbamazepine pharmacokinetics are: time-dependency due to autoinduction of hepatic metabolism; the 10,11-epoxide has intrinsic anticonvulsant activity and toxicity; lipophilicity which results in slow absorption but rapid distribution and penetration into the brain. Brain levels approximate plasma levels and CSF concentrations equate with plasma free drug levels. The lipophilicity is also relevant to the treatment of toxic overdoses as adipose tissue acts as a carbamazepine reservoir.

The time of maximum plasma levels after administration is relatively long, varying from four to eight hours, may be up to 24 hours for very high doses. Although the absorption is delayed, it is essentially complete. Carbamazepine is about 75 percent bound to plasma proteins. The plasma half-life is about 35 hours for the initial dose, which decreases to 10 to 20 hours once autoinduction is complete. When coadministered with phenytoin or phenobarbital the half-life of carbamazepine is from nine to ten hours.

Therapeutic blood concentrations of carbamazepine range from 6 to 12 µg/ml. There is not a simple concentration-effect relationship. CNS adverse effects are observed at blood levels > 8.5 µg/ml. Carbamazepine epoxide levels may reach 50 percent of the parent compound, especially when polytherapy includes phenobarbital or phenytoin. The epoxide is metabolized to the 10,11 diol, which is further metabolized and excreted as glucuronides. Another metabolite, 9-hydroxymethylcarbamylacridone also is formed. Very small amounts of carbamazepine or its epoxide are excreted in the urine. Free carbamazepine is excreted in breast milk, tears, and saliva.

Different pathologic conditions are known to alter the pharmacokinetics of carbamazepine. Mild liver dis-

Table 19.5 Drug Interactions Involving Carbamazepine

Carbamazepine on Plasma Levels of Other Drugs		Other Drugs on Carbamazepine Plasma Levels	
Decrease	**Increase**	**Decrease**	**Increase**
clobazam	phenytoin	phenytoin	erythromycin
clonazepam	lithium	primidone	isoniazid
primidone	imipramine	phenobarbital	meconazole
phenobarbital		felbamate	verapamil
valproate		cisplatin	diltiazem
ethosuximide			viloxazine
haloperidol			cimetidine
oral contraceptives			
theophylline			
cyclosporin			
doxycycline			

ease is associated with a decrease in plasma protein binding, whereas severe hepatic disease can result in carbamazepine intoxication. Malabsorption, especially of proteins, decreases the bioavailability of carbamazepine. Renal disease apparently has little effect on carbamazepine pharmacokinetics.

Available Preparations and Usual Doses.[22,23] Carbamazepine is available in the US as 100-mg chewable tablets, 200-mg tablets, and a suspension of 20 mg/ml. In Europe, a slow-release formulation has recently been introduced. Dosing may be commenced either at 200 mg bid in adults (100 mg bid in children) in 100-mg increments every 12 hours followed by increases of 100 mg/day at weekly intervals or, in a more conservative manner, at 50 mg/day increased by 50 mg/day every second day. Maintenance doses in adults range from 600 to 1200 mg/day (administered in three doses).

Valproic Acid/Divalproex Sodium (Valproate)

Valproate is a branched-chain fatty acid which has use exclusively as an antiepileptic agent. It is indicated as monotherapy and adjunctive therapy in the treatment of simple and complex absence seizures. It is also indicated for use as an adjunct in patients with multiple seizure types which include absence seizures. Valproate has been studied for use in other CNS indications including bipolar depressive disorders and trigeminal neuralgia.

Chemistry. The structure of valproic acid (dipropylacetic acid or 2-propylpentenoic acid) is shown in Figure 19.3. Valproic acid is an organic solvent and is highly soluble in water and polarized organic solvents. At physiologic pH, valproic acid is predominantly in the ionized form (pKa = 4.56). Divalproex sodium is the sodium salt of valproic acid and has the same pharmacologic and clinical spectrum as the free acid. Divalproex sodium is a stable coordination complex of valproic acid and sodium valproate in a 1:1 ratio. Both valproic acid and divalproex sodium dissociate to the valproate ion in the GI tract. These drugs share the same clinical profile as valproic acid and are commonly referred to as valproate.

History and Mechanism of Action. Valproate was first synthesized by Burton in 1882 as an organic solvent. The anticonvulsant activity was discovered in the early 1960s during its use as a vehicle for testing potential anticonvulsants. Valproate was first used clinically in 1967 in France and was approved for use in the US in 1978.[r25,r26] Diverse proposals have been advanced as to the mechanism of the antiepileptic action of valproate, many of them involving the inhibitory neurotransmitter GABA.[r2,r7] It was originally proposed that valproate exerts its clinical effect by enhancing CNS GABA levels subsequent to inhibition of the catabolic enzyme GABA-transaminase. This was questioned, since the degree of enzyme inhibition associated with therapeutic concentrations of valproate probably is too low to account fully for the antiepileptic effect. Other hypotheses invoking a GABAergic component include inhibition of succinic semialdehyde dehydrogenase (the step subsequent to GABA transaminase activity) and the activation of GABA synthesis and release. More recently it has been demonstrated that valproate inhibits voltage-dependent sodium channels as well as T-type calcium channels in afferent neurons[r14] (but not the ethosuximide-sensitive calcium channels in the thalamus).[9] It is highly probable that the clinical activity of valproate is the sum of several convergent mechanisms including both enhanced GABAergic inhibition and decreased transmembrane current flow.

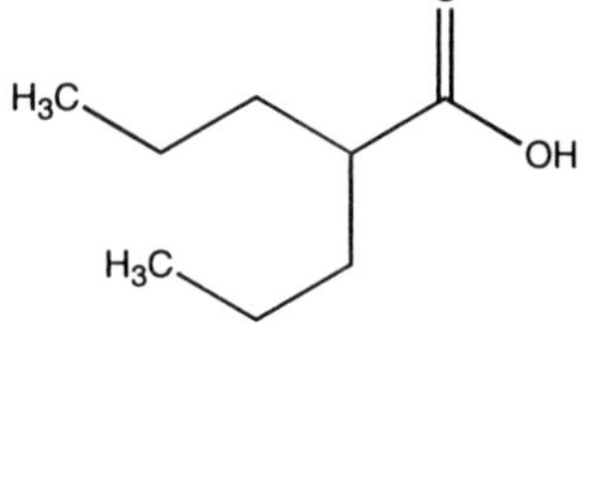

H_3C O OH H_3C

VALPROIC ACID

Figure 19.3 Structure of Valproic Acid

Therapeutic Uses and Limitations.[r25,r26,15,31,32,33] In the US valproate is indicated for use as monotherapy and add-on therapy in the treatment of simple and complex absence seizures. It is also indicated for use as an adjunct therapy when absence seizures are an aspect of multiple seizure types. Valproate use is growing as a broader-spectrum antiepileptic for other types of primary generalized seizures, including tonic-clonic seizures, myoclonus, Lennox-Gastaut syndrome, and West's syndrome.

The major limitations to the use of valproate are the potential for fatal hepatotoxicity and a teratogenic potential. A history of hepatitis or jaundice is a relative contraindication of valproate therapy; valproate is contraindicated in patients with hepatic disease or significant hepatic dysfunction. Liver function tests should be performed prior to initiation of therapy and at frequent intervals thereafter, especially during the first six months of therapy, when the incidents usually occur. The incidence of hepatotoxicity decreases markedly with age. Patients receiving valproate may develop clotting abnormalities, including thrombocytopenia, platelet aggregation, and low fibrinogen levels. Prior to surgery patients receiving valproate should be monitored for platelet count and coagulation. Children under two years have a considerably increased risk for fatal hepatotoxicity. Those on multiple anticonvulsants, those with congenital metabolic disorders, those with severe seizures accompanied by mental retardation, and those with organic brain dysfunction are at special risk. Valproate products should be used with extreme caution and as monotherapy in these patients. Valproate may have teratogenic effects when administered during pregnancy. The incidence of neural tube defects may be increased by the administration of valproate in the first trimester of pregnancy, and other congenital anomalies have been reported.

Effects of the Drug Responsible for Its Therapeutic Usefulness.[r2,r7,r26,34] Valproate exhibits activity in models for both generalized and focal seizures. Valproate increases CNS GABA levels both in animals and in the CSF of epileptic patients receiving the drug. As valproate prevents seizure spread, seizure generation, and high frequency sustained repetitive firing, it appears that the compound acts at several steps in the generation of spike and wave formation. It is possible that 2-en-valproic acid, a metabolite with a long half-life, contributes to the *in vivo* activity of valproate.

Undesirable Effects.[r25,r26,31,32,33] In addition to the limitations described above, valproate is associated with a number of undesirable effects, most of which are not serious. Gastrointestinal effects are common, often transient, and include nausea, vomiting and dyspepsia (reduced by enteric coating), and weight gain. CNS effects are infrequent and include hand tremor, ataxia, and sedation. Other common side-effects are rash, hair loss, and ankle edema. Rarer, more serious reactions include an acute pancreatitis that is potentially fatal, carnitine deficiency, and idiosyncratic reactions such as neutropenia and bone marrow suppression. Thrombocytopenia and inhibition of platelet aggregation already have been mentioned.

Drug Interactions.[r21,r22,35] Valproate is an inhibitor of hepatic oxidative metabolism. Valproate increases the plasma concentrations of phenobarbital, ethosuximide, carbamazepine, and carbamazepine epoxide. This latter effect may result in carbamazepine toxicity. Valproate both inhibits the metabolism of phenytoin and displaces it from plasma protein binding. Other antiepileptic drugs have an effect on valproate pharmacokinetics. Phenytoin, phenobarbital, primidone and carbamazepine all increase the clearance and lower plasma concentrations of valproate. Thus, higher doses of valproate may be appropriate in polytherapy as compared with monotherapy. The combination of valproate and clonazepam may rarely result in absence status epilepticus. Aspirin inhibits valproate metabolism, and salicylic acid displaces valproate from its protein binding sites. The former increases total blood levels and the latter increases free plasma concentrations of valproate.

Overdosage. Overdosing with valproate can have a fatal outcome. Overdosage is associated with somnolence, deep coma, and heart block. It has been reported that naloxone reverses the central depressant effects of valproate. However this should be used with caution owing to the possible reversal of the antiepileptic effect of valproate by naloxone.

Pharmacokinetics.[r25,r26,31,32,36,37] The different formulations of valproate are rapidly and completely absorbed after oral administration. Maximal plasma concentrations are reached one to four hours postdosing, and can be altered by administration with meals or by formulation. Valproate is normally 90 percent protein-bound; however, this is saturable at blood concentrations of 80 μg/ml. The plasma half-life of valproate is about 15 hours in monotherapy and decreases to seven to nine hours in patients receiving polytherapy. The therapeutic window for valproate plasma concentrations is in the range of 30 to 150 μg/ml; however, there is a lack of correlation between plasma concentrations and the antiepileptic or toxic effect. There is equilibration of valproate between blood and brain. Valproate is almost completely metabolized, mainly by glucuronidation as well as by mitochondrial oxidation. There are at least five metabolic routes of valproate metabolism in man. Two active metabolites are formed, one of which accumulates in brain and plasma (2-propyl-2-pentanoic acid), whereas 2-propyl-4-pentanoic acid does not.

Available Preparations and Usual Doses.[31,32] Valproic acid is available in the US as 250-mg capsules and as a syrup of 250 mg/5 ml. The initial daily dose is usually 15 mg/kg. This is increased weekly by 5 to 10 mg/kg/day to a maximum dose of 60 mg/kg/day. When the daily dose is greater than 250 mg, it is administered bid or tid. The onset of efficacy may take several weeks to appear. Divalproex sodium is available as 125-mg, 250-mg, and 500-mg tablets with or without enteric coating. Divalproex sodium is administered to the same dose schedule as valproate. BID administration is usual for patients on monotherapy, whereas divalproex is administered tid to patients receiving polytherapy. Divalproex sodium is also formulated as sprinklets for children, which is a particulate formulation that can be mixed with food. A slower absorption results from admixture with food.

Benzodiazepines

The benzodiazepines are used primarily in clinical medicine for anxiety disorders and insomnia; however, most have anticonvulsant properties. Diazepam, clorazepate, and clonazepam are approved for the treatment of epilepsy in the US. Benzodiazepines being investigated as antiepileptic drugs include lorazepam (approved in the US for other uses), clobazam, and nitrazepam, which are approved as antiepileptic drugs in many countries outside the US. Most benzodiazepines have a 1,4 configuration; however, clobazam, a newer benzodiazepine, has a 1,5 configuration.

Chemistry. The structures of the benzodiazepines are shown in Figure 19.4. The CNS potency of benzodiazepines is correlated with their affinity for the benzodiazepine recognition site within the $GABA_A$ receptor complex. Potency is enhanced by a chloride or nitro group at the 7 position or a methyl group on the N at position 1.[r27]

History.[r27] The first benzodiazepines were synthesized by Sternbach in Poland in the 1930s but were not exploited until the 1950s at Hoffman-La Roche. Chlordiazepoxide, which was the first benzodiazepine to be used clinically, was synthesized in 1933 and introduced in 1960 as an anxiolytic agent. The first use of a benzodiazepine as an antiepileptic drug occurred in 1965, when diazepam was used to treat status epilepticus.

Benzodiazepines act at a specific set of recognition sites within the $GABA_A$ receptor-chloride ion complex. These act as allosteric modulators of the $GABA_A$ agonist site, with the anticonvulsant benzodiazepines increasing the affinity of the GABA recognition site. Benzodiazepines appear to increase the opening frequency of the $GABA_A$-receptor gated chloride ion channels without changing channel conductance. See chapter 14 on benzodiazepines used for other CNS disorders for extensive discussion of mechanisms.

Therapeutic Uses and Limitations. Benzodiazepines are used in the management of epilepsy either as a treatment for status epilepticus or as a treatment for partial and generalized seizures. Most benzodiazepines are not suitable for chronic treatment because

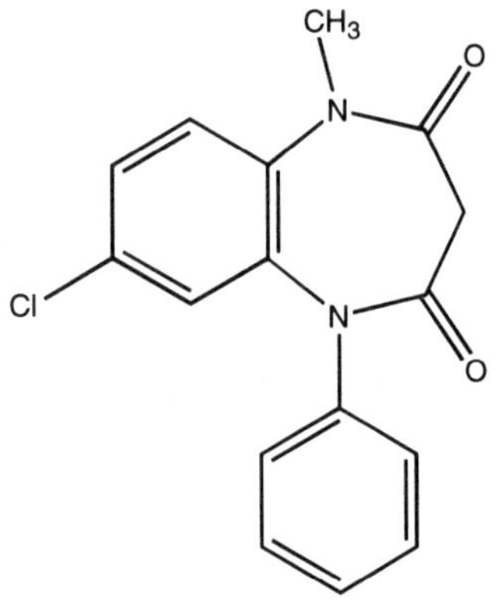

CLOBAZAM

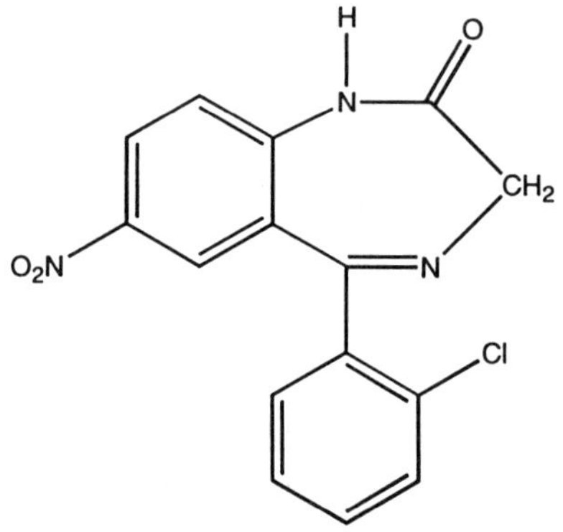

CLONAZEPAM

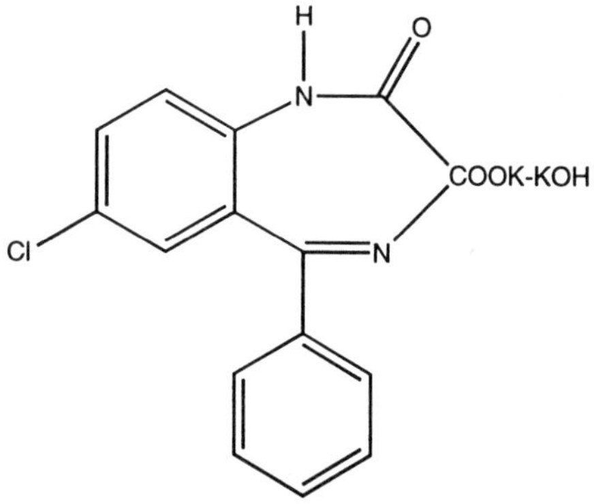

CLORAZEPATE

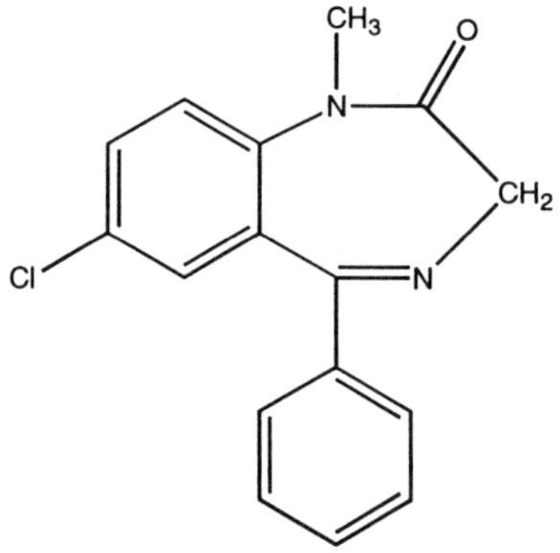

DIAZEPAM

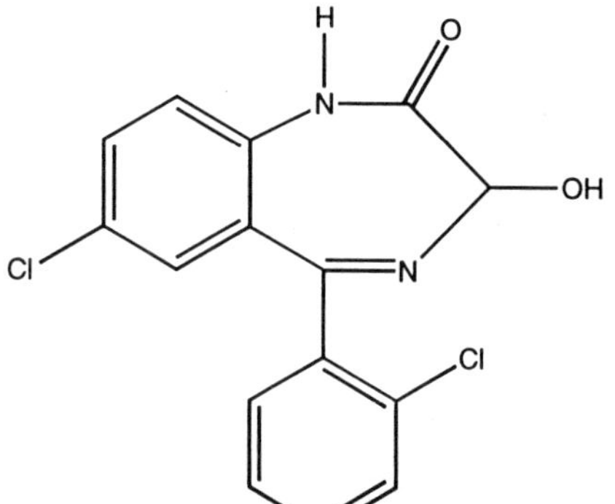

LORAZEPAM

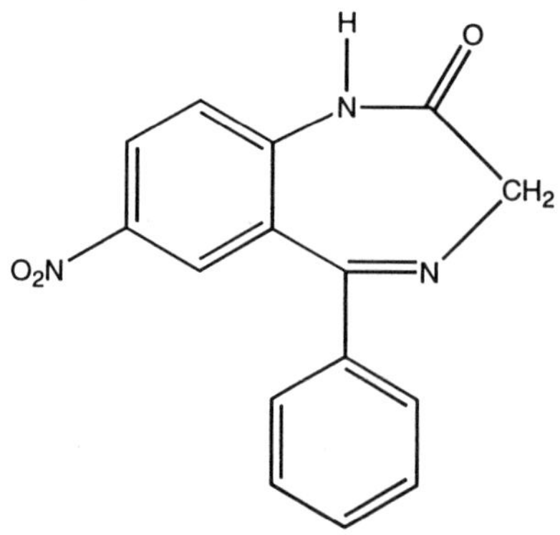

NITRAZEPAM

Figure 19.4 Benzodiazepine Structures

tolerance develops to the clinical effectiveness. Only clorazepate has been shown to have continued therapeutic activity in long-term studies.[38] Also, dependence, both physical and psychologic, develops in many patients treated with this class of drugs. Abrupt discontinuation of benzodiazepines results in such withdrawal phenomena as anxiety, agitation, restlessness, insomnia, and tension, which usually are delayed several days because of the long half-life of most of these drugs or their active metabolites. Abrupt discontinuation of benzodiazepines may be associated with a temporary increase in the frequency or severity of seizures.

The effects of individual benzodiazepines in pregnancy have not been studied adequately to determine the risk of fetal abnormalities. An increased risk of congenital malformations has been associated with the use of minor tranquilizers[39], including diazepam, and the use of other anticonvulsant drugs. Because seizures pose a risk to the mother and developing embryo, most patients should continue treatment with antiepileptic drugs during pregnancy. Women taking benzodiazepines should not breast feed their infants. Benzodiazepines are contraindicated in all patients with acute narrow angle glaucoma and also in patients with open angle glaucoma unless they are receiving appropriate therapy.

Status Epilepticus.[r28,r29,39,40] Injectable diazepam is the drug of choice for the treatment of status epilepticus. Although seizures may be brought under control promptly, many patients experience a return to seizure activity, and it may be necessary for the drug to be readministered. However, diazepam is not recommended for maintenance. Once seizures are brought under control, other antiepileptic drugs should be initiated for long-term control.

Lorazepam is available in the US as an IV preparation, and there have been reports of success with this drug in treating status epilepticus. The advantage of lorazepam is that, when administered IV, it has a longer duration of action than diazepam, allowing up to 12 hours of coverage before maintenance therapy is to be initiated. In a small percentage of patients, IV administration of diazepam and/or lorazepam can lead to respiratory depression, apnea, or hypotension.

Chronic Treatment of Partial and Generalized Seizures.[r30,r31,38,41] In the US, clorazepate and clonazepam are approved for the chronic treatment of epileptic seizures. Clorazepate is indicated as adjunctive therapy in the management of partial seizures. As previously mentioned, clorazepate differs from other benzodiazepines in that it is effective during prolonged treatment. Clonazepam is effective as monotherapy or as adjunctive therapy in treating patients with Lennox-Gastaut syndrome, akinetic seizures, and myoclonic seizures. However, tolerance to the antiepileptic effects of clonazepam develop within three months in about 30 percent of patients.

Two benzodiazepines that are investigational and not approved in the US are clobazepam and nitrazepam. *Clobazam* has been reported to be useful as adjunctive therapy in treating refractory partial and generalized seizures. However, long-term use of this drug is limited by tolerance that develops in many patients within three months of starting treatment. Nitrazepam has been used primarily to treat infantile spasms, although it also is useful in the management of myoclonic seizures and Lennox-Gastaut syndrome. Long-term use is limited by the development of tolerance to its antiepileptic effects.

Effects of the Drug Responsible for Its Therapeutic Usefulness.[r27] Benzodiazepines are effective in preventing pentylenetetrazol- and maximal electroshock-induced seizures in experimental models of epilepsy. The clinical effects of the benzodiazepines are considered to be due to the potentiation of the inhibitory neurotransmitter GABA by increasing the frequency of openings of the $GABA_A$-receptor coupled chloride ion channel and increasing the affinity of the $GABA_A$ receptor for GABA. Although both the barbiturates and the benzodiazepines potentiate inhibition mediated by GABAergic transmission, they act by different mechanisms which explains the different anticonvulsant profiles of these classes of drugs.

Undesirable Effects.[r30] All benzodiazepines produce CNS depression, and sedation is their most common adverse effect. At the initiation of treatment with these drugs, drowsiness, ataxia, and dizziness may occur. These effects frequently decrease with continued therapy or with a dose adjustment. Behavior problems have been noted in approximately 25 percent of patients treated with clonazepam. Children and elderly patients taking benzodiazepines may experience alterations in cognitive function and emotional state. Benzodiazepines are controlled substances in the US and have a potential for dependence or abuse.

Drug Interactions. The most prominent drug interactions are pharmacodynamic and occur when benzodiazepines are administered concurrently with other drugs acting on the CNS. Because benzodiazepines have a CNS depressant effect, patients should be advised against concurrent use of alcohol and other CNS-depressants during benzodiazepine therapy. Also, the actions of the benzodiazepines may be potentiated by narcotics, barbiturates, nonbarbiturate hypnotics, anti-anxiety agents, phenothiazines, monoamine oxidase inhibitors, tricyclic antidepressants, or other antidepressants. In contrast, pharmacokinetic interactions with other antiepileptic drugs are infrequent. Benzodiazepines are not potent enzyme inducers, nor do they strongly affect plasma protein binding of other drugs.

Overdosage. Symptoms of benzodiazepine overdosage are similar to those produced by other CNS depressants and include somnolence, confusion, and coma. Overdosage by benzodiazepines alone is not associated with a fatal outcome. Treatment includes monitoring of vital signs, general supportive measures and immediate gastric lavage. Intravenous fluid should be administered and an adequate airway maintained. Hypotension, though rarely reported, may occur with large overdoses and usually can be controlled with levarterenol or metaraminol. Dialysis is of no known value. Administration of flumenazil,[42] a benzodiazepine antagonist, rapidly reverses all the actions of benzodiazepines, including both the undesirable and antiepileptic effects.

Pharmacokinetics.[r27,r32] Generally, the benzodiazepines are rapidly and completely absorbed with peak plasma concentrations reached within a few hours. The benzodiazepines are very lipophilic and rapidly penetrate the brain. Plasma protein binding is high. Benzodiazepines are metabolized primarily in the liver and excreted in the urine. The pharmacokinetics of the benzodiazepines discussed in this chapter are shown in Table 19.6.

Available Preparations and Usual Doses. The available preparations of the benzodiazepines approved in the United States are described in this section.

Clonazepam[41] is available as 0.5-, 1- and 2-mg tablets. In adults, the initial dose should not exceed 1.5 mg/day in three divided doses. Dosage may be increased by 0.5 to 1 mg every three days up to a maximum daily dose of 20 mg. In infants and children (up to 10 years of age or 30 kg of body weight), the dose should be between 0.1 and 0.3 mg/kg/day but not exceeding 0.5 mg/kg/day given as two or three divided doses. Dosage may be increased by 0.25 to 0.5 mg every three days up to a maintenance dose of 0.1 to 0.2 mg/kg of body weight.

Clorazepate[38] is available as 3.75-, 7.5-, and 15-mg tablets and in 11.25- and 22.5-mg sustained release tablets. In adults or children over 12 years of age, the maximum initial dose is 22.5 mg/day in three divided doses. Dosage may be increased by no more than 7.5 mg every week and should not exceed 90 mg/day. In children 9–12 years of age, the maximum initial dose is 15 mg/day in two divided doses. Dosage may be increased by no more than 7.5 mg/week and should not exceed 60 mg/day. Owing to limited clinical experience, clorazepate is not indicated for children under nine years.

Diazepam[39] is available as 2-, 5-, and 10-mg tablets, in 2-ml ampules, and in 10-ml vials of sterile 5-mg/ml solution for injection. For status epilepticus, diazepam is administered IV. In adults, the usual dosage is 5 to 10 mg administered at a rate of 5 mg/min or less and may be repeated if necessary at 10-to 15-minute intervals, up to a maximum dose of 30 mg. In children five years of age or older, the dose is 1 mg every 2 to 5 minutes up to a maximum of 10 mg. If necessary, therapy for adults and older children may be repeated 2 to 4 hours later, with consideration being given to residual active metabolites. In infants over 30 days of age and children under five years, the dose is 0.2 to 0.5 mg administered slowly every 2 to 5 minutes up to a maximum of 5 mg.

Phenobarbital

Phenobarbital is a derivative of phenylbarbituric acid, which has found diverse medical uses. A related drug, mephobarbital, is also marketed as an antiepileptic agent and is metabolized to phenobarbital. Mephobarbital was available as an antiepileptic until 1990, when the manufacturer ceased marketing this compound. The most prevalent medical uses of these barbiturates include treatment of epilepsy and nonepileptic convulsions, use as sedative/hypnotics, and use in anesthesia and reduction of cerebral edema. The use of barbiturates for most CNS indications has declined with the introduction of benzodiazepines, as the barbiturates have a lower therapeutic index, a greater abuse potential and more numerous drug interactions than do the benzodiazepines. Barbiturates are also used for the treatment of kernicterus and hyperbilirubinemia in the neonate.

Chemistry.[43] Phenobarbital (Fig. 19.5, 5-ethyl, 5-phenylbarbitaric acid) is an archiral molecule which was first patented in 1911. The molecular weight is 234.24. Barbituric acid derivatives are poorly soluble in water but dissolve readily in nonpolar solvents. The sodium salts form alkaline solutions, which are often unstable. The maximum anticonvulsant activity of barbituric acid derivatives occurs with a phenyl substituent at the 5-position. However, the 5,5 diphenyl substituted compound has less anticonvulsant activity than phenobarbital. The parent compound, barbituric acid, is without anticonvulsant or sedative activity. Very large substituents at the 5-position are convulsant. The pKa of phenobarbital is 7.3. Thus, the tissue/plasma distribution is dependent on plasma pH, and an alkaline urine enhances the renal clearance of phenobarbital.

History. Barbituric acid was first synthesized in 1864, which led to the discovery of barbital, the first synthetic sedative/hypnotic drug. Phenobarbital was the first effective organic antiepileptic substance to be discovered, synthesized by Hauptmann at Bayer (German patent in 1911, US patent in 1912). Its clinical use as an antiepileptic began in 1912, and thus it is the oldest AED in use at present.

Table 19.6 Pharmacokinetic Parameters of Benzodiazepines

	Time to Peak Plasma Level after Oral Administration (hr)	Elimination Half-Life (hr)	Protein Binding (%)	Active Metabolite
Diazepam	1–2	20–60	>90	Nordiazepam ($T_{1/2}$:30–90 hr)
Clorazepate	1	30–90 (Nordiazepam)	99% (Nordiazepam)	Nordiazepam
Clonazepam	1–2	24–48	86	None
Lorazepam	2	12 (po) 16 (im,iv)	85	None
Clobazam	1–4	18	90	Norclobazam ($T_{1/2}$:42 hr, weakly active)
Nitrazepam	1	24–31	86	None

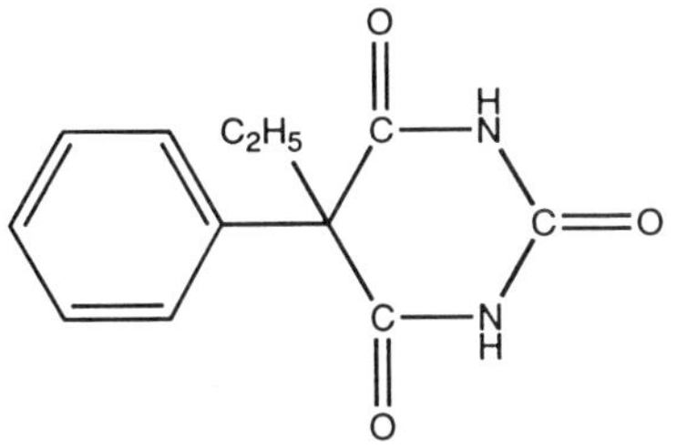

PHENOBARBITAL

Figure 19.5 Structure of Phenobarbital

It was not until the late 1970s that animal studies demonstrated that $GABA_A$ receptor-gated chloride ion channels are the target for the CNS activities of the barbiturates. The anticonvulsant activity appears to be related to a potentiation of physiologic $GABA_A$ receptor activation, whereas the hypnotic effects result from a direct action of the compound on the $GABA_A$ chloride ion channel receptor complex. The molecular recognition site of phenobarbital appears to be at the α and β subunits of the $GABA_A$ receptor complex. This produces an increased duration of chloride channel open time without altering conductance or opening frequency. At supratherapeutic doses, phenobarbital decreases the synaptic response to glutamate and decreases neurotransmitter release via a selective block of voltage-dependent N-type calcium channels.[r2,r14,44,45]

Therapeutic Uses and Limitations.[r33,r34,r35,15,46,47] Phenobarbital is generally not considered as a first-line treatment except in neonatal seizures. Phenobarbital is used for the control of generalized tonic, tonic-clonic, and partial seizures of all age groups. The long duration of action of phenobarbital makes its use possible in the maintenance control of status epilepticus. The use of phenobarbital (and other antiepileptic drugs) for the prophylaxis and treatment of febrile seizures has become controversial. As oral administration of phenobarbital takes two days to achieve therapeutic blood levels (stable levels after two to three weeks), the use of phenobarbital for the treatment of febrile seizures should be considered only if treatment is to last at least several days. Phenobarbital is the initial antiepileptic drug used for the treatment of neonatal seizures, either epileptic or nonepileptic in origin. An initial loading dose is administered IV, followed by oral maintenance dosing. Phenobarbital is also used for the control of seizures resulting from alcohol and drug withdrawal, although benzodiazepines are more commonly used for these conditions (see Chapter 21).

The limitations to the use of phenobarbital depend on the seizures and the patient population treated. In adults, sedation is the major dose-limiting factor, although on long-term administration, impaired perceptual motor performance, impaired memory, and depression occur with some regularity. Induction of hepatic microsomal drug metabolizing enzymes with subsequent effects on antiepileptic drug levels plays an important role. During the treatment of status epilepticus, the limitations to the use of phenobarbital are respiratory depression, hypotension, and sedation. The limitations to the use of phenobarbital in children are due mainly to the behavioral effects of the drug, which are principally sedation and hyperactivity. These may occur in 40 percent or more of treated children and are more frequent in patients with a predisposition to behavioral abnormalities. In neonates, the limiting factors to phenobarbital use are cardiovascular (bradycardia resulting in reduced perfusion) and a potential deleterious effect on brain growth and development (as shown in rats). The indications and use of mephobarbital are the same as those for phenobarbital, with no evident advantage.

Effects of the Drug Responsible for Its Therapeutic Usefulness.[r2,r7,r14,44,45] Phenobarbital decreases neuronal firing and raises the convulsant threshold as a result of enhanced inhibitory neurotransmission (potentiation of $GABA_A$ synaptic activity, see above). Phenobarbital is active at nonsedative doses in a wide variety of seizure models, including pentylenetetrazol, bicucculine, and electroshock, although in some models the anticonvulsant activity is seen only at doses that are clearly sedative. Phenobarbital blocks both seizure activity and seizure spread, actions that probably are highly relevant to its clinical effectiveness.

The combined actions of phenobarbital on potentiating $GABA_A$-mediated inhibitory neurotransmission and decreasing the activity of excitatory glutamatergic synapses provide an explanation for the relatively wide spectrum of activity of phenobarbital in animal models and in severe seizures in the clinic (generalized seizures, status epilepticus).

Undesirable Effects.[r33,r34,15,46,47,48] Undesirable effects depend on the age of the patient population considered. In neonates, the risk of bradycardia and resultant poor perfusion (due to lack of compensatory mechanisms) is present. In children and infants, the most frequent (up to 40% of patients) undesirable effects are behavioral and cognitive in nature, including hyperactivity, aggression, insomnia, and somnolence. As noted earlier, the occurrence is greater in children with a predisposition to behavioral abnormalities. In infants, an 8- to 12-month follow-up study demonstrated a significant negative relation between plasma phenobarbital levels and performance on memory tasks. It has also been reported the phenobarbital is associated with a failure to maintain the normal age-related progression in IQ scores. It should be noted, however, that cognitive improvement has also been demonstrated in epileptic children treated with phenobarbital.

In adults, sedation is the foremost undesirable effect of therapeutic doses of phenobarbital and frequently diminishes with continued therapy. Behavioral/cognitive effects also occur at therapeutic doses in adults, of which depression is the most severe. This has been reported in up to 40 percent of patients and may not spontaneously remit upon cessation of phenobarbital. Some memory impairment in adults has also been noted.

The antiepileptic barbiturates are relatively free of toxicity as compared to other antiepileptic drugs. There is a very low incidence of hematologic effects and a low incidence of idiosyncratic, dysmorphic, motor, or GI side-effects. An allergic reaction (morbilliform or scarlatiniform rash) to phenobarbital is observed sufficiently often to advise patients of its probability. Other reactions to phenobarbital include hepatitis, bone marrow depression, and a systemic lupus erythematosus-like reaction. Chronic use of phenobarbital may result in megaloblastic anemia due to low folic acid levels; this condition responds to folate administration. The osteomalacia that may appear responds to high doses of vitamin D.

The fetal syndrome observed involves hypoprothrombinemia, which leads to bleeding and possibly hemorrhage in the newborn period. This is treatable with vitamin K and prevented by including vitamin K in the mother's diet during the final trimester of pregnancy. The reproductive toxicology potential of phenobarbital is generally thought to be less than that for phenytoin or valproic acid. In animals, phenobarbital is only mildly teratogenic, and relatively high doses are needed to induce malformations such as cleft palate or urogenital and cardiac defects. The combination of phenobarbital and phenytoin is associated with a higher rate of malformations than either compound alone.

Drug Interactions.[r21,r22,r33,46,49] Phenobarbital is well known as an inducer of hepatic and extrahepatic metabolic enzymes, notably the hepatic microsomal drug metabolizing enzymes. This alters plasma concentrations of many concomitantly administered medications. A phenobarbital-induced increased clearance has been reported for at least 25 compounds, including other antiepileptic drugs, oral contraceptives, beta blockers, digitoxin, and anticoagulants. Conversely, several drugs are known to increase plasma phenobarbital levels, and the interaction with valproic acid can result in barbiturate-induced coma. Phenobarbital levels should be measured in patients with impaired hepatic or renal function.

Overdosage.[46] Overdoses of phenobarbital result in ataxia and nystagmus and eventual loss of consciousness. Death can result from respiratory depression. The onset of symptoms may be delayed for several hours due to slow absorption.

Pharmacokinetics.[r34,46,50,51] The pharmacokinetics of phenobarbital are age-dependent. Neonates have low plasma protein building, erratic absorption due to slow gastric emptying and achlorhydria, low hepatic drug metabolizing enzyme activity and a low rate of renal excretion. The plasma clearance in neonates is very variable with a reported range of 40 to 200 hours. Infants and children, as compared to adults, have a higher rate of gastric emptying, peristalsis, and gastric blood flow, resulting in rapid absorption. The clearance is relatively rapid (40–75 hours) as compared to adults (60–140 hours). Thus, steady state levels take three to four weeks to attain, and single daily dosage is sufficient and appropriate. These data suggest that the mean dosage will decrease with age, which is supported by statistical studies. However, owing to the large variability and overlap between ages, this cannot be used to predict attainment of therapeutic blood levels. In adults, oral bioavailability is essentially complete.

Therapeutic plasma levels of phenobarbital range from 10 to 40 μg/ml. Plasma protein binding is 40 to 60 percent in adults but very low in neonates (up to day 7 postpartum). Few undesirable effects occur at plasma levels lower than 30 μg/ml, whereas marked secondary effects are noted in nontolerant subjects when plasma levels attain 60 μg/ml. Plasma levels greater than 30 to 40 μg/ml should be maintained only if this is essential for treatment and are well tolerated. The major route of metabolism of phenobarbital is via hepatic microsomal enzymes, resulting in inactive metabolites and conjugates which are then excreted in the urine. Less than 25 percent of a dose is eliminated as the parent compound via pH-dependent renal excretion. The kinetics of phenobarbital are altered during pregnancy, often necessitating a modification of the dosage. Late in the first trimester, plasma concentrations decrease due to an increased volume of distribution and an increased hepatic and renal clearance. The plasma clearance decreases following childbirth.

Available Preparations and Usual Doses.[46] Phenobarbital is available for use in epilepsy as an injectable (IV, IM) solution (phenobarbital sodium 30 mg/ml, 60 mg/ml, 65 mg/ml, and 130 mg/ml). It is also available as an elixir at a strength of 20 mg/5 ml and in tablet strength of 15 mg, 30 mg, 60 mg, and 100 mg. No single manufacturer provides all formulations. The compound is available in a wide range of generic forms.

Normal antiepileptic dosages vary as to the age of the patient. In neonates, a loading dose of 10–20 mg/kg IV is suggested with a maintenance dose of 3–4 mg/kg. Children are usually started at 3–6 mg/kg/day and the dosage adjusted as needed. The normal maintenance dose is 1–4 mg/kg/day. In adults a starting dose of 30–60 mg is common for 3–4 days. The usual maintenance dose is 1–5 mg/kg/day (60–240 mg/day). Phenobarbital can be administered once or twice daily.

Primidone

Primidone is a deoxybarbiturate used exclusively for the treatment of partial and generalized seizures, except for absence seizures.

Chemistry. The structure of primidone (5-ethyldihydro-5-phenyl-4,6(1H,-5H)-pyrimidinedione;5-desoxyphenobarbital) is shown in Figure 19.6. Although, from a strict chemical perspective, primidone is not a derivative of barbituric acid (lacking one of the three carbonyl groups), it is closely related to phenobarbital. The molecular weight of primidone is 218. An important metabolite of primidone is phenobarbital and much of the therapeutic activity of primidone can be attributed to this metabolite.

History. Primidone was patented and first introduced into the therapy of epilepsy in 1952.[52,53] It has been used steadily since then. One of the most important aspects of primidone is its metabolism, with two active metabolites identified. Phenylethylmalonamide was immediately identified, but it was not until 1956 that phenobarbital was identified as a metabolite of primidone.[54]

The mechanism of action of primidone is complex and related to its metabolism. Primidone itself has intrinsic anticonvulsant activity, as is shown by its rapid onset of action (before the appearance of phenobarbital) and activity when metabolism to phenobarbital is blocked by inhibition of the metabolizing enzymes.[55,56] The molecular mechanism of action of the intrinsic anticonvulsant activity of primi-

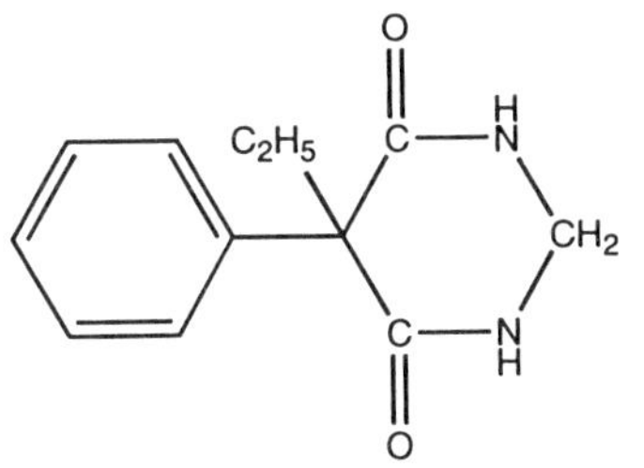

PRIMIDONE

Figure 19.6 Structure of Primidone

done is not clear. The portion of activity due to metabolism to phenobarbital is related to a potentiation of GABAergic synaptic activity (see section on phenobarbital).

Therapeutic Uses and Limitations.[r35,15,57,58] Primidone is not a first-line medication for any type of seizure or form of epilepsy because of the risk of serious neurologic adverse events. Primidone is used for all types of epilepsy except absence seizures; the main use is for generalized tonic-clonic seizures, simple and complex partial seizures, and juvenile myoclonic epilepsy, after the preferred antiepileptic drugs have been shown to be insufficient. If possible, primidone should be used as monotherapy or combined with an antiepileptic that does not induce drug-metabolizing enzymes. In spite of this advice, primidone generally is used in combination with phenytoin or carbamazepine. The efficacy of primidone is considered to be equivalent to that of phenobarbital, but may be associated with more side-effects. Withdrawal of primidone should be undertaken with caution as this may exacerbate seizures.

Primidone is contraindicated in patients with porphyria and in patients with a hypersensitivity to phenobarbital. The limitations to primidone use include an acute toxic reaction of mainly CNS origin, which is severe but usually transient. This is decreased in patients who previously have been treated with phenobarbital.

Neonatal hemorrhage may occur in the newborns of primidone-treated patients, and serious idiosyncratic reactions have been reported in patients, usually cutaneous (rash) or hematologic in origin. There is no specific teratogenic profile reported with primidone; cases of microcephaly, ventriculoseptal defects, and poor somatic development have been reported.

Effects of the Drug Responsible for Its Therapeutic Usefulness.[r35,52,55,56] As stated above, primidone exerts antiepileptic activity both by an intrinsic activity as well as metabolism to active compounds, phenyl ethyl malonamide (PEMA) and phenobarbital. The intrinsic activity of primidone is short-lasting and may account for the acute effects of primidone, including the acute toxic reaction. In animal models, PEMA has been demonstrated to exert a rather weak anticonvulsant activity and it is unlikely that this metabolite makes a major contribution to the clinical activity of primidone. However, PEMA has been shown to potentiate the anticonvulsant activity of phenobarbital. It is considered that phenobarbital contributes significantly to, and may largely explain, the therapeutic activity of repeated doses of primidone. The anticonvulsant profile of primidone in animal models parallels that of phenobarbital, but has considerably lower potency.

Undesirable Effects.[r35,57,58] The undesirable effects of primidone are related to primidone plus PEMA plus phenobarbital. The acute toxic syndrome that can occur in patients never previously treated with primidone may be severe but is transient. This consists of CNS (sedation, dizziness, diplopia, vertigo, ataxia, nystagmus) and GI (nausea, vomiting) symptoms. This acute toxic reaction is believed to be related to primidone itself. An acute psychotic reaction has also been reported. Serious side-effects which occur on continued treatment are probably related to phenobarbital and include rash, osteomalacia, hematologic effects (leukopenia, thrombocytopenia, systemic lupus erythematosus, megaloblastic anemia), and lymphadenopathy. A neonatal syndrome (hemorrhage) has been observed with primidone.

Drug Interactions.[r21,r22,56,57,59] Drugs that induce drug-metabolizing enzymes will increase the metabolism of primidone and result in lower blood levels of the parent compound and higher levels of phenobarbital. In this case, lower doses of primidone are needed to maintain steady-state phenobarbital levels and therapeutic activity. Phenytoin seems to accelerate primidone metabolism the greatest amount. Carbamazepine has been reported to both increase and reduce the metabolism of primidone, although an enhanced conversion is the usual observation. Nicotinamide and isoniazid block the metabolism of primidone. Acetazolamide reduces its oral absorption.

Overdosage.[r35,57,59] Primidone overdose (serum primidone levels > 90 μg/ml) results in CNS depression, flaccidity, somnolence, and lethargy. Symptoms correlate with plasma concentrations of the parent compound, rather than the metabolites. Crystallization is a consistent sign of overdose. Primidone is relatively safe, and greater than ten times the daily dose has been taken without permanent effect. Overdose is treated with gastric lavage and supportive measures.

Pharmacokinetics.[56,57,60,61] Primidone is rapidly and almost completely absorbed after oral administration. Peak plasma concentrations occur about three hours post-administration in adults and four to six hours in children. The half-life for patients on primidone monotherapy is 10 to 15 hours; this is reduced to six to eight hours when primidone is co-administered with other antiepileptics. In newborns the half-life of primidone is reported to be 8 to 80 hours owing to a slow rate of biotransformation. Primidone is a hepatic enzyme inducer and is metabolized to two active compounds, PEMA (which has much weaker activity than primidone or phenobarbital in animal models) and phenobarbital. The half-life of PEMA is about 16 hours, and this compound accumulates on long-term therapy. Significant amounts of PEMA appear soon after primidone administration, whereas phenobarbital levels are measurable about 24 hours following the first dose of primidone. Approximately 40 percent of the primidone dose is excreted as unchanged compound in the urine, the remainder excreted as PEMA, phenobarbital, and other metabolites.

Primidone and PEMA exhibit only a small degree of plasma protein binding (10–30%), whereas phenobarbital is 50 percent plasma protein-bound. Brain primidone concentrations are lower than plasma concentrations. There are marked individual differences in the plasma ratios of primidone, PEMA, and phenobarbital. Normally about 25 percent of the primidone dose is converted to phenobarbital. Steady state plasma concentrations (per 1 mg/day primidone) are: primidone = 1 μg/ml; PEMA = 1–2 μg/ml and phenobarbital = 2 μg/ml. Monotherapy dosage of 20 mg/kg/day produces steady-state phenobarbital levels of 30 μg/ml after two to three weeks. A high primidone:phenobarbital ratio is an indication of poor compliance due to the low accumulation of phenobarbital. Plasma primidone levels greater than 10 μg/ml are associated with significant toxic effects, but there is not a significant relationship between plasma levels and therapeutic effect.

Available Preparations and Usual Doses.[57] Primidone is available as 50- and 250-mg tablets and as a 250 mg/5 ml oral suspension. The usual daily dose is from 750 to 1500 mg in adults and 10 to 25 mg/kg for children less than eight years of age. The therapeutic plasma concentration range is 5–12 μg/ml. Therapy usually commences at low doses (62.5 or 125 mg at bedtime) owing to the high incidence of transient but severe neurologic and gastric effects. It may take three weeks to reach maintenance doses, which can be given once daily or bid. If blood levels are used to adjust the dosage, phenobarbital levels are more appropriate than primidone levels.

Ethosuximide

Ethosuximide is the most active of a group of antiepileptic compounds having in common the succinimide nucleus. Ethosuximide is indicated for use in childhood absence epilepsy. Other related compounds are phensuximide for absence therapy, which shows lower efficacy than the other succinimides; methsuximide as add-on therapy for partial complex seizures. Epilepsy is the only indication for the use of the succinimides in the US.

Chemistry. The structure for ethosuximide (2-ethyl-2-methylsuccinimide) is shown in Figure 19.7. Substitution at the 2-C position greatly influences activity in different animal models. Phenyl substitution exhibits anti-maximal electroshock activity, whereas alkyl substitution results in anti-pentylenetetrazol effects. The occurrence of a methyl group at the 5-N position enhances anti-pentylenetetrazol activity (and also sedative effects). The combined substitutions of methyl at 5-N and phenyl and alkyl at 2-C produces both anti-electroshock and anti-pentylenetetrazol effects. Of these compounds ethosuximide is the most active and phensuximide (N-methyl-2-phenyl-succinimide) is the least effective.[62] The succinimides are nonpolar water-soluble compounds that do not accumulate in fat deposits.

History. Phensuximide, the first of the antiepileptic succinimides, was to be introduced by Zimmerman in 1951. Methsuximide was introduced in 1956; the first clinical trials for ethosuximide were reported in 1958. The mechanism(s) of action of the succinimides are still under study. It is probable that more than one mechanism enters into play, given the different selectivities for the electroshock and pentylenetetrazol models. The following mechanisms have been proposed: altered neurotransmitter release; control of calcium entry into nerve terminals; modulation of sodium, potassium, or chloride conductance. The specific anti-absence effect of ethosuxilmide has been proposed to be due to blocking specific low-threshold voltage-dependent calcium channels in the intralaminar nucleus of the thalamus, which will disrupt the synchronous spike-wave discharge pattern controlled by intrathalamic and thalamocortical circuits.[r7,r14,9]

Therapeutic Uses and Limitations.[63,64,65] Ethosuximide is indicated for the control of absence epilepsy, especially for children and adolescents, and may be used in monotherapy. Some authors consider ethosuximide to be specifically indicated for the control of childhood absence epilepsy. It is the drug of choice in infants. As ethosuximide exhibits very few drug interactions, it can be combined with other antiepileptic drugs when other seizure types are present together with absence. Ethosuximide is not effective in generalized tonic-clonic seizures or in partial seizures. There are relatively few limitations to the use of ethosuximide. The drug is contraindicated in patients with a history of hypersensitivity to succinimides. In patients with mixed types of epilepsy ethosuximide monotherapy may increase the frequency of tonic-clonic seizures in some patients.

Ethosuximide has been reported to be associated with abnormal renal and hepatic function and thus should be administered with utmost caution to patients with known kidney or liver disease. Periodic blood counts should be measured as ethosuximide has been reported to be associated with blood dyscrasias, some with a fatal outcome. Indications of an infection (e.g., fever, sore throat) indicate a consideration of performing blood counts. The possibility of ethosuximide-in-

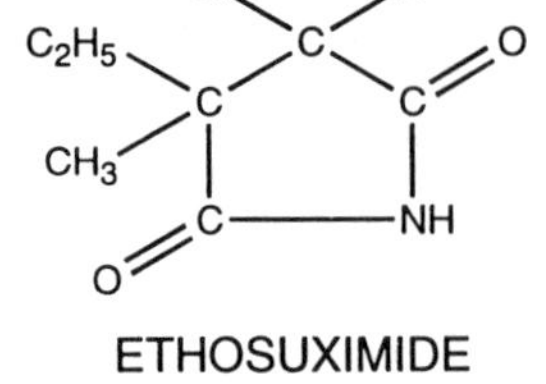

ETHOSUXIMIDE

Figure 19.7 Structure of Ethosuximide

duced systemic lupus erythematosus should be remembered. There are no specific fetal malformations reported with the use of ethosuximide and the compound has been shown to have a very limited teratology in rodents.

Effects of the Drug Responsible for Its Therapeutic Usefulness. Ethosuximide desynchronizes the 3 Hz spike-wave discharges that occur in absence patients and are thought to reflect an abnormal synchronization involving intrathalamic and thalamocortical circuits. This action of ethosuximide is apparently via the depression of inhibitory pathways.

Undesirable Effects.[63,64,65] Dose-related undesirable effects mainly involve the GI tract and CNS. The compound is associated with diarrhea, epigastric and abdominal pain, nausea, vomiting, and anorexia. CNS effects include agitation, psychosis, night terrors, drowsiness, lethargy, euphoria, dizziness, headache, hiccough, and parkinsonian symptoms. In the case of a previous psychiatric history, multiple behavioral effects may occur, including aggression, anxiety, and restlessness. Rarely, paranoid psychosis, increased libido, and exacerbated depression with suicidal intentions have been reported. Ethosuximide treatment has been associated with photophobia as well as myopia. Vaginal bleeding and microscopic hematuria have been exhibited during ethosuximide therapy. The idiosyncratic events which have been reported for ethosuximide include hematologic events, such as eosinophilia, leukopenia (which may be transient but has led to fatal bone-marrow depression), thrombocytopenia, aplastic anemia, and agranulocytosis. Dermatologic reactions have been reported:urticaria; Steven-Johnson syndrome; systemic lupus erythematosus; erythremia multiforme; hirsutism.

Drug Interactions.[r21,r22,63] Ethosuximide does not induce or inhibit hepatic drug metabolizing enzymes. Carbamazepine has been observed to decrease blood ethosuximide concentrations and valproic acid to both increase and decrease them. Ethosuximide may increase plasma levels of phenytoin.

Overdosage.[63,64] Acute overdoses are associated with nausea and vomiting. CNS depression may occur, leading to coma with respiratory depression. No relationship between plasma levels and ethosuximide toxicity has been demonstrated. Treatment is symptomatic, with emesis (unless contraindicated), gastric lavage, and activated charcoal.

Pharmacokinetics.[63,66,67] After oral administration, ethosuximide is rapidly and almost completely (90–95%) absorbed. Maximal blood concentrations are reached in three to seven hours. The plasma half-life is 20 to 60 hours in adults and approximately 30 hours in children. There is very little plasma protein binding and at steady state there is equilibration between plasma and CSF. Steady state concentrations are attained in four to six days in children and more than six days in adults. The therapeutic range at steady state is 40 to 100 μg/ml for the control of absence seizures. Ethosuximide is excreted as 25 percent unchanged compound in the urine. Forty per cent of the drug is metabolized to the inactive hydroxyethyl metabolite, which is excreted either unchanged or as the glucuronide.

Available Preparations and Usual Doses.[63] Ethosuximide is supplied as 250-mg capsules and as a flavored syrup of 250 mg/5 ml. The latter should be protected from high temperatures (>86 degrees F or 30 degrees C), freezing, and light. Ethosuximide is administered by the oral route. For patients between three and six years old, the usual initial dose is one capsule or one teaspoonful (250 mg) per day. Patients six years or older usually start at 500 mg per day (2 capsules or 2 teaspoons). Dosage should be increased by small increments, and the final dose needs to be determined according to the patient's response. Dosage may be increased by 250 mg/day every four to seven days. The optimal dose for most children is about 20 mg/kg/day. Doses should not exceed 1.5 grams per day unless administered under strict medical supervision.

Trimethadione

Trimethadione is a member of the oxazolidenedione family. Trimethadione is used exclusively as an antiepileptic agent for the treatment of absence, myoclonic, and akinetic seizures in patients who have an insufficient response to other antiepileptic drugs.

Chemistry. Three oxazolidendiones are effective antiepileptics, trimethadione (Fig. 19.8, 3,5,5-trimethyl-2,4-oxazolidenedione), its active metabolite dimethadione, and paramethadione. A 5-alkyl substitution is essential for anti-pentylenetetrazol activity in animal models and for selective anti-absence actions in man.[r36]

History. Trimethadione was introduced by Lennox in 1945 as the first selective agent for the treatment of absence (petit mal) seizures. Trimethadione was the drug of choice for absence seizures for almost 15 years until the availability of ethosuximide (1958) followed by valproic acid and clonazepam.[r36] Trimethadione and some other agents for the treatment of absence seizures appear to exert their antiepileptic action by the blockade of a subset of voltage dependent low threshold T-type calcium channels located in the thalamic relay nuclei.[r7,r14,9] Other antiepileptics do not appear to exert their primary activity at such channels. Trimethadione has also been reported to block calcium channels in the hippocampus.

Therapeutic Uses and Limitations.[r36,68,69] Trimethadione is indicated only for the control of absence seizures in patients who are poorly controlled by other therapy. Close medical supervision is recommended; prior to commencing therapy with trimethadione, a complete blood count, urinalysis, and biochemistry profile should be performed owing to the occurrence of severe (at times fatal) hematologic reactions.

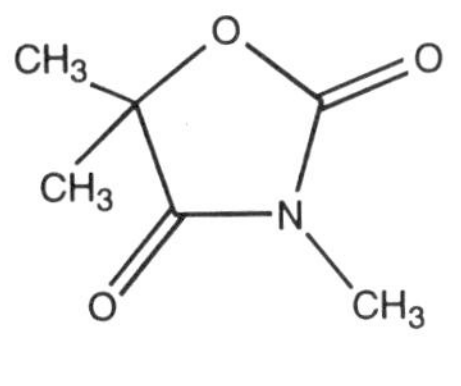

TRIMETHADIONE

Figure 19.8 Structure of Trimethadione

Trimethadione has been established to be teratogenic in humans, with a high rate of stillbirths and major abnormalities in the surviving newborn. Cardiac defects are highly prevalent, and a fetal trimethadione syndrome (facial anomalies, congenital heart disease, and mental retardation) is recognized. In animals, trimethadione is highly embryotoxic and teratogenic in several species.

Effects of the Drug Responsible for Its Therapeutic Usefulness. Trimethadione exhibits a marked selectivity for protecting rodents from pentylenetetrazol-induced seizures, being much more active than phenytoin. This is likely related to the blockade of calcium channels in the hippocampus and thalamus.

Undesirable Effects.[r36,68,69] The most common adverse effects are sedation, to which tolerance develops, and hemeralopia, for which dark glasses can be worn. Agitation and psychosis may occur and may respond to a reduction in dose. Less frequent and more severe adverse (may be fatal) effects include: blood dyscrasias, such as neutropenia, aplastic anemia, agranulocytosis, pancytopenia; skin conditions—rashes, exfoliate dermatitis, lupus erythematosus; hepatitis; nephritis; mysathenia gravis; and aggravation of primary generalized seizures. This drug also has been demonstrated, as noted above, to be teratogenic.

Drug Interactions.[68,70] The metabolism of trimethadione is induced by phenobarbital and inhibited by cimetidine.

Overdosage.[r36,68,69] Acute overdoses of trimethadione result in drowsiness, ataxia, dizziness, visual disturbances and nausea. Coma may be induced by huge overdoses. Treatment of overdose is by gastric evacuation (emesis, lavage) and supportive measures. Following recovery, the patient should be assessed for blood count, and hepatic and renal function.

Pharmacokinetics.[r36,68,71,72] Trimethadione is rapidly and completely absorbed after oral administration, with maximum plasma levels at 0.5 to two hours. It is N-demethylated by liver microsomal enzymes to dimethadione, which accounts for most of the antiepileptic activity of trimethadione. Dimethadione is excreted unchanged in the urine. The plasma half-life of dimethadione is six to 13 days, as compared to 16 hours for the parent trimethadione. Concurrent hepatic disease decreases the metabolism of trimethadione. Several weeks' therapy are needed to attain steady-state levels of dimethadione. Combined steady state levels need to be in excess of 700 μg/ml in order to attain effective seizure control. Dimethadione levels (12 μg/ml per 1 mg/kg/day administered) are about 20-fold those of trimethadione (0.6 μg/ml per 1 mg/kg daily dose).

Available Preparations and Usual Doses.[68] Trimethadione is available as 300-mg capsules, 150-mg chewable tablets, and as a flavored oral solution of 40 mg/ml. The final daily dose is 30–50 mg/kg/day for adults and 20–60 mg/kg/day for children, as a single dose. It is advised to start young children (less than 6 years) at 150 mg bid, increasing to 300 mg tid as necessary. Older children should start at 300 mg bid and increase to 600 mg tid, as seizure control demands. Once steady state is attained then once-daily dosing should be sufficient.

Recently Approved Drugs

Gabapentin

Gabapentin is one of the new anticonvulsants approved by the US FDA in the early 1990s (approved Dec. 30, 1993). Gabapentin is a cyclic GABA analogue, and its only approved medical use is as an antiepileptic.

Chemistry. Gabapentin (Fig. 19.9, 1-(aminomethyl)-cyclohexaneacetic acid) is an amino acid designed as a GABA agonist or prodrug with greater liposolubility and thus greater penetration into the brain than GABA itself. The compound enters the brain, but there is no evidence that it exerts an action as a GABA agonist or mimetic. Gabapentin is water soluble and has a molecular weight of 171.

History.[r6,r7,r14,r22,73,74,75] Gabapentin was discovered and developed in Europe in the 1970s by Goedecke. As stated above, it was designed to act as a liposoluble GABA-mimetic or prodrug. However, extensive studies have failed to demonstrate an action on GABA receptors (either $GABA_A$ or $GABA_B$), GABA uptake or GABA metabolism. A GABAergic mechanism is not completely excluded, as gabapentin enhances GABA synthesis and turnover in select brain areas.

Therapeutic Uses and Limitations.[r7,73,76] The indications for gabapentin in the US are as adjunctive therapy in the treatment of refractory partial seizures in adults. As the use of this compound grows, it is possible that other indications will be added. The data available at present indicate that gabapentin is well tolerated. Insufficient data are available to be able to predict accurately the limitations to its therapeutic use. However, gabapentin may exacerbate absence seizures in some patients. Caution in renally-impaired patients may be indicated, as excretion of unchanged compound via the urine is the major route of elimination. There is a report of acute onset of renal failure in a renally-impaired patient.

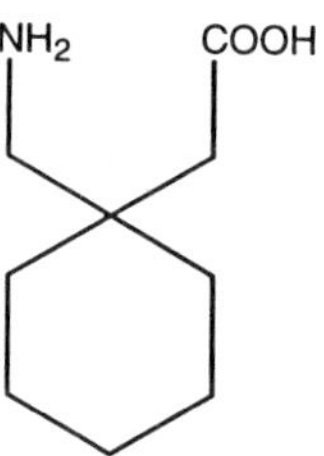

Figure 19.9 Structure of GABApentin

Effects of the Drug Responsible for Its Therapeutic Usefulness.[r7,r14,73,74,76] The molecular basis for the anticonvulsant and antiepileptic activities of gabapentin are unknown. In animal models, gabapentin exerts a marked anticonvulsant activity. This includes activity against seizures in genetic models, and against electroshock-induced convulsions, bicuculline-induced convulsions, strychnine-induced seizures, and convulsions induced by NMDA. Gabapentin exhibits a weaker activity against pentylenetetrazole (clonic seizures) and the photosensitive baboon (papio papio). In contrast, gabapentin does not block the seizures resulting from electrical kindling. In the spontaneous spike-wave discharge model for absence epilepsy in Wistar rats, gabapentin worsened the EEG phenomena. This may be related to similar events seen in some patients with absence seizures (see below).

Gabapentin does not exert an activity at the strychnine-sensitive glycine receptor, at neuronal voltage-dependent calcium channels, nor at the recognition site or ion channel associated with the NMDA subtype of glutamate receptors. An action at the glycine site within the NMDA/glutamate receptor complex has not been excluded. An interesting aspect is that gabapentin binds to a specific recognition site in the rat brain; however, the identity and function of this site remains to be determined.

Undesirable Effects.[r7,73,76] The undesirable effects observed are mainly of CNS origin and for the most part are those observed frequently with antiepileptic drugs. These are somnolence, fatigue, dizziness and ataxia. In many instances, tolerance develops rapidly to these effects. Additionally, weight gain has been observed as has depression. Very little has been published on the toxicity of gabapentin. The compound is not genotoxic; however, in the two-year carcinogenicity study in the male rat, an increased incidence of acinar cell carcinomas of the pancreas was observed at the high dose. This was not observed in the females, nor was it observed in the mouse carcinogenicity studies. The implications and relevance of this finding to humans is unknown.

It is possible that a small subgroup of patients respond to gabapentin with an exacerbation of seizures. The demographics of this population are not clear.

Drug Interactions.[73,76] To date, there is an absence of interactions between gabapentin and other antiepileptic drugs (carbamazepine, phenobarbital, phenytoin, valproate) or oral contraceptives.

Overdosage.[76] In five cases of overdose with gabapentin there were no fatalities and recovery was uneventful. The symptoms observed included drowsiness, diplopia, dizziness, and diarrhea.

Pharmacokinetics.[76,77] In humans, gabapentin has a plasma terminal elimination half-life of five to six hours. This is consistent with tid administration. The bioavailability was determined to be 59 percent, with maximal plasma concentrations occurring between two and three hours. There was not any apparent effect of food on bioavailability, but this may be decreased by antacids. The major route of elimination is via renal excretion of the unchanged compound (80–100% of administered dose). In humans, gabapentin is not metabolized and does not induce hepatic mixed-function drug metabolizing enzymes. The compound does not bind to plasma proteins.

Available Preparations and Usual Doses.[76] Gabapentin is available in the US in tablets of 100 mg, 300 mg, and 400 mg. The starting dose is 900 mg/day, and the recommended dose range is 900–1800 mg/day. It appears that a rapid titration is possible (3 days).

Felbamate

Felbamate is a dicarbamate structurally related to meprobamate, an anxiolytic. The indications for the use of felbamate are as monotherapy and adjunctive therapy in partial seizures with and without generalization in adults with epilepsy and as adjunctive therapy in the treatment of partial and generalized seizures associated with the Lennox-Gastaut syndrome in children. Although structurally related to meprobamate, felbamate appears to have a low incidence of sedation. After being approved, the FDA and Carter-Wallace (the manufacturer of felbamate) recommended that the use of felbamate be limited to patients with severe epilepsy for whom the benefits outweigh the risks. The restricted use of felbamate is due to the occurrence of several cases of aplastic anemia and acute liver failure in the first year of approval in the US.[78]

Chemistry. Felbamate (Fig. 19.10, 2-phenyl-1,3-propanediol dicarbamate) is an achiral structural analogue of the anxiolytic meprobamate Felbamate has greatly reduced sedative and myorelaxant effects as compared to meprobamate, and from animal studies appears to be without the addictive potential associated with the latter compound. Felbamate is a crystalline powder with a white to off-white color and a characteristic odor. It is only very slightly soluble in water, slightly soluble in ethanol, and highly soluble in dimethyl sulfoxide and other organic solvents. Felbamate (pure substance) is stable at room temperature for at least one year and is stable in acid conditions for at least four hours; it is less stable in basic conditions. Formulations of felbamate (tablets, suspension) may be less stable

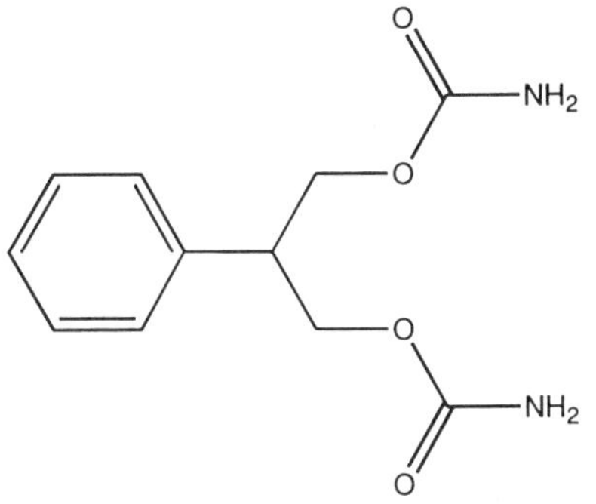

O
NH_2
O
O
NH_2
O
FELBAMATE

Figure 19.10 Structure of Felbamate

than the pure substance. Owing to the synthetic route used, it is possible that felbamate could contain small amounts of two known animal carcinogens, urethane and methyl carbamate. Maximum possible levels of these compounds in felbamate are much below (<1/5000) those causing cancer in rodents. No tumors were observed during the felbamate lifetime carcinogenicity studies.[79,80]

History. Felbamate was discovered by Carter-Wallace during the screening and study of meprobamate analogues. The compound was approved for marketing as an antiepileptic drug by the US FDA during the third quarter of 1993. This was the first anti-seizure medication to receive FDA approval for monotherapy since 1978 (clorazepate was approved in 1981 for use as an adjunctive therapy). The development of felbamate has been succinct and limited to the US; it consists of five well-controlled double-blind trials in partial onset epilepsy with or without generalization and one well-controlled double-blind trial in Lennox-Gastaut syndrome. The trial with felbamate is the first instance of a well-controlled study to demonstrate efficacy in Lennox-Gastaut syndrome.[79,80,81,82,83,84,85] Nonetheless, as noted above, it has been recommended that the use of felbamate be limited to patients with severe epilepsy.

Therapeutic Uses and Limitations.[79,80,85] Felbamate is indicated for use in epilepsy as monotherapy and adjunctive therapy in the treatment of partial seizures with or without generalization in adults and as adjunctive therapy in the treatment of partial and generalized seizures associated with the Lennox-Gastaut syndrome in children.

In renally or hepatically impaired patients the effects of felbamate have not been systematically evaluated. However, several cases of acute liver failure (some fatal) have been reported. No studies exist of pregnant women. Felbamate is detected in human milk, and in rats felbamate was associated with a decrease in pup weight and an increase in pup mortality during lactation. No systematic studies in geriatric patients have been performed, and it is not known whether this patient group responds differently from younger subjects. Dosing for the elderly patient should be cautious. The oral administration of felbamate was not associated with any carcinogenic, teratogenic, reproductive, or mutagenic effects in toxicologic studies. In rats there was a decrease in pup weight and an increase in pup mortality during lactation. Although the data available submitted in the felbamate NDA strongly suggested that the toxicology and clinical safety of felbamate would be satisfactory[79,80,88] several fatal cases of liver failure and aplastic anemia have been reported. Prior to treatment, liver function tests should be obtained and during treatment weekly blood tests should be performed to monitor liver function. If liver problems are found, patients should be withdrawn from the drug. Patients with preexisting liver disease should not be treated with felbamate.

Effects of the Drug Responsible for Its Therapeutic Usefulness.[79,86] The mechanism of action of felbamate is still to be determined; however, the spectrum of its anticonvulsant activity in laboratory models is suggestive of both a reduction in seizure spread and an elevation in seizure threshold. Felbamate exhibits a anticonvulsant profile in rodents different from that of the classic antiepileptic drugs. The most potent activity is demonstrated against electroshock-induced convulsions and seizures induced by the intracerebral injection of glutamate or the glutamate agonist NMDA. The antiepileptic effects of felbamate appear to be due to an intrinsic activity as the metabolites tested exhibit weaker anticonvulsant effects than the parent compound.

In terms of a cellular mechanism of action, felbamate apparently does not enhance the function of the $GABA_A$-chloride ion channel receptor complex, nor does it act within the calcium channel of the NMDA subtype of excitatory amino acid receptors. However, felbamate does exert an effect at the glycine modulatory site within the NMDA receptor. It is very possible that an interaction with noradrenergic synapses is relevant to the mechanism of action of felbamate as decreased noradrenergic transmission (inhibition of synthesis or antagonism of $alpha_1$ receptors) diminishes the anticonvulsant effect of felbamate. Conversely increasing the synaptic concentration of norepinephrine enhances the anticonvulsant activity of felbamate.[79,86,87]

Undesirable Effects.[78,79,80,85] Felbamate has been administered to a limited number of adults and children under the artificial conditions of clinical pharmacology and clinical trials, usually in severely refractory patients. Given these circumstances it was impossible to predict what would eventually emerge as the adverse effect profile of felbamate after extensive patient exposure and well-conducted postmarketing surveillance. The emerging profile has resulted in the FDA recommending that felbamate be limited to patients with severe epilepsy. During the combined clinical trials in adults, felbamate was associated with several generally mild-to-moderate undesirable effects. These were more frequent when felbamate was administered as adjunctive therapy than as monotherapy. A similar profile of undesirable effects was reported for adults and children.

The most commonly observed undesirable effects were GI (nausea, vomiting, dyspepsia, weight loss, constipation, abdominal pain), diplopia and abnormal vision, rhinitis, CNS (headache, fatigue, somnolence, insomnia, dizziness, ataxia, and abnormal gait), rash, and upper respiratory tract infection. Elevated SGPT levels were observed in 5 percent of adult patients receiving the high dose (3600 mg/day) of felbamate as monotherapy. The incidence of severe adverse events was very low in this limited patient population, and those reported (< 0.1% incidence) were mainly associated with hypersensitivity: photosensitive allergic reaction; agranulocytosis; Stevens-Johnson Syndrome. However, since becoming commercially available, felbamate has been associated with several fatal cases of aplastic anemia and acute liver failure.

No studies on the addictive or abuse potential of felbamate have been performed in humans. In rats receiving a high daily dose of felbamate, there was no weight loss when the drug was withdrawn one day per week over a five-week treatment period.

Drug Interactions.[79,80,85] Felbamate therapy frequently necessitates a dosage reduction of concomitantly administered antiepileptic drugs owing to clinically significant pharmacokinetic interactions.

Felbamate (3600 mg/day) increases phenytoin plasma steady state concentrations, necessitating a reduction in the phenytoin dosage by 20 to 40 percent. Valproate clearance is decreased by felbamate resulting in an increase in valproate steady state concentrations in a dose-related manner; plasma protein binding of valproate is not altered. Plasma carbamazepine concentrations are reduced by felbamate, with a concomitant increase in the levels of carbamazepine-epoxide and other metabolites. Both carbamazepine and phenytoin increase felbamate clearance, resulting in a 40 to 50 percent lowering of felbamate steady state trough concentrations. Valproate administration apparently does not alter felbamate plasma steady state levels. Antacids are reported to be without effect on the absorption of felbamate.

Overdosage.[79,80] A limited number of felbamate overdoses have been reported (5400 to 7200 mg/day for six to 51 days). No serious adverse experiences were described. The only adverse events noted upon the acute ingestion of 12000 mg of felbamate was mild gastric distress and a heart rate of 100 beats/minute.

Pharmacokinetics.[79,80,85] In man, felbamate appears to be well absorbed, with maximum plasma levels at 2–6 hours; it has a small volume of distribution, a relatively long half-life (16–19 hours), is not extensively metabolized, and is excreted mainly via the renal route. The pharmacokinetic parameters of the tablet and suspension are similar. There is no effect of food on the absorption of the tablets. Plasma concentrations are all proportional to the dose administered. The terminal half-life is similar following single or multiple doses. The dosing schedule (tid or qid) is not consistent with the half-life; this is in order to enhance the tolerance to the undesirable GI effects.

Felbamate does not bind extensively to plasma proteins. Binding ranges from 22 to 25 percent, mostly to albumin, and is independent of felbamate plasma concentrations. Unchanged felbamate represents 40 to 50 percent of urinary excretion. Metabolites include p-OH-phenylfelbamate, 2-OH felbamate, and monocarbamate felbamate derivatives.

Available Preparations and Usual Doses.[80] Felbamate is available as 400-mg and 600-mg tablets and as a suspension of 600 mg/5 ml. Felbamate is stored at room temperature. *In adults,* felbamate has not been extensively studied as initial monotherapy. For adults, the manufacturer recommends initiation with 1200 mg/day divided in three or four doses. Previously untreated patients should be titrated under close clinical supervision, with dosage increases of 600 mg every two weeks to a dose of 2400 mg/day based on clinical response. A daily dose of 3600 mg may be attained if indicated. In patients receiving other antiepileptic drugs, felbamate should be started at 1200 mg/day. If felbamate is intended as add-on therapy to existing antiepileptics, the dosage of the concomitant antiepileptics should be reduced by 20 percent (or greater if needed to minimize side-effects) to control the plasma concentrations of valproate, phenytoin, and carbamazepine and its metabolites. The felbamate dosage is increased by 1200 mg/day at weekly intervals to a maximum dose of 3600 mg/day. If the goal is conversion to felbamate monotherapy, felbamate should be started at 1200 mg/day in three or four divided doses; the other antiepileptics should be decreased by one-third at the start of felbamate. At week 2, the felbamate dosage should be increased to 2400 mg/day and the other antiepileptics reduced by up to one-third of the original dosage. At week 3, felbamate may be increased up to 3600 mg/day and the dosage of the concomitant antiepileptics reduced as indicated by the clinical situation. As with other antiepileptic drugs, felbamate should not be discontinued abruptly owing to the possibility of increased seizures. *In children with Lennox-Gastaut syndrome (2–14 years old),* felbamate is administered as add-on therapy, commencing with 15 mg/kg/day in three or four divided doses. Concomitant antiepileptics should be reduced by 20 percent or more if needed to minimize side-effects. Dosage increases of felbamate in increments of 15 mg/kg/day may occur at weekly intervals to a maximum of 45 mg/kg/day or 3600 mg/day.

Infrequently Used Antiepileptic Drugs

Several of the antiepileptic drugs still available for use in the US, as listed in the Physician's Desk Reference are used infrequently. These drugs are listed in Table 19.7.

Antiepileptic Drugs Not Commercially Available in the United States

Of the antiepileptic drugs not yet approved for the US market, lamotrigine, vigabatrin, and zonisamide appear the most likely to be available soon. They are discussed in some detail below. Others that either are marketed elsewhere or are in clinical trials and appear to be some distance from US approval are also listed in Table 19.8.

Oxcarbazepine

Oxcarbazepine is a prodrug that is rapidly and extensively metabolized to a monohydroxide derivative, 10-hydroxycarbazepine, that is responsible for the drug's therapeutic effects.[97] Oxcarbazepine has been reported to effectively treat partial and generalized tonic-clonic seizures. It is marketed in Europe, Mexico, and South America, and is under investigation in the US.

Chemistry. Oxcarbazepine (10,11-dihydro-10-oxo-carbamazepine) is a ketohomologue of carbamazepine. The chemical structure is shown in Figure 19.11.

History.[98] Oxcarbazepine was developed by Ciba-Geigy to avoid the epoxide metabolite of carbamazepine, which has been associated with many of the untoward effects of carbamazepine. Oxcarbazepine shares the sodium-channel blocking action of carbazepine, and additionally exhibits an antagonism of neuronal potassium channels.

Therapeutic Uses and Limitations.[r40,99,100] Clinical studies have indicated that the over-all efficacy of oxcarbazepine in reducing seizure frequency in epileptic patients is essentially equivalent to that of carbamazepine, with the dosage of oxcarbazepine being approxi-

Table 19.7 Antiepileptic Drugs with Relatively Infrequent Usage

Drug	Chemical Class	Indication	Comments
Mephobarbital[89]	Barbiturate	Tonic-clonic Absence	Prodrug for phenobarbital Controlled substance Induces hepatic drug-metabolizing enzymes Withdrawal symptoms include status epilepticus Fetal abnormalities Sedative, hypnotic
Pentobarbital[90]	Barbiturate	Emergency control of status epilepticus and other acute convulsions	Available as injectable solution Anticonvulsant only at anesthetic doses Controlled substance Synergistic with other CNS depressants
Mephenytoin[91]	Hydantoin	Refractory patients with tonic-clonic, focal, Jacksonian and complex partial seizures	Close medical supervision necessary. Serious adverse reactions include blood dyscrasias, fatal dermatologic reactions, CNS effects, hepatitis and nephrosis.
Ethotoin[92]	Hydantoin	Tonic-clonic Complex partial	Possible neonatal coagulation defect Isolated cases of lymphadenopathy and systemic lupus erythematosus
Paramethadione[93]	Oxazalidenedione	Refractory absence seizures	Fetal malformations Severe adverse events include exfoliative dermatitis, hepatitis, fatal nephrosis, myasthenia gravis-like syndrome
Methsuximide[94]	Succinimide	Refractory absence seizures	Severe adverse events include blood dyscrasias, systemic lupus erythematosus, neurologic and psychiatric abnormalities Extreme caution in patients with hepatic or renal disease.
Phensuximide[95]	Succinimide	Absence seizures	As monotherapy may increase frequency of clonic-tonic seizures. Severe adverse events include blood dyscrasias, systemic lupus erythematosus Extreme caution in patients with hepatic or renal disease
Phenacemide[96]	Substituted acetyl-urea	Severe refractory complex partial epilepsy	Potentially fatal effects include hepatoxicity, aplastic anemia Severe adverse events include personality changes (suicide attempts and psychosis) and allergic reactions. Birth defects have been reported.

mately 50 percent higher than that of carbamazepine. However, oxcarbazepine has been reported to be better tolerated than carbamazepine. Hyponatremia is an adverse effect that occurs more frequently at clinically relevant doses of oxcarbazepine than carbamazepine. The decrease in serum sodium levels appears to be related linearly to the oxcarbazepine dose and 10-hydroxycarbazepine serum concentrations. Although patients generally are asymptomatic, this effect is a concern in the elderly and patients treated with high doses of oxcarbazepine.

Effects of the Drug Responsible for Its Therapeutic Usefulness.[98] Like carbamazepine, the mechanism of action of 10-hydroxycarbazepine appears to occur by blockade of voltage-sensitive sodium channels. Additionally, 10-hydroxycarbazepine also appears to block potassium channels, which is not an action of carbamazepine. In standard animal seizure models, oxcarbazepine and 10-hydroxycarbazepine have anticonvulsant activity similar to that of carbamazepine.

Undesirable Effects.[r32,r40] The most frequently reported adverse effects of oxcarbazepine are similar to those of carbamazepine and

Table 19.8 Selected Antiepileptic Drugs Not Commercially Available in the United States

Drug	Indication	Clinical Phase	Animal Models	Mechanism of Action	Comments
Flunarizine[r6,r7]	Refractory epilepsy	Marketed (Europe)	MES ++ PTZ 0	Calcium channel blocker	—
Clobazam[r6,r7]	Refractory partial and generalized seizures	Marketed (Europe)	MES ++ PTZ ++	GABA potentiation	Tolerance may develop
Lamotrigine†	Refractory partial seizures	Registration (US)	MES + PTZ 0	Reduced glutamate release	Very few drug interactions
Oxcarbazepine†	Partial seizures	Marketed (Europe)	MES ++ PTZ ++	Sodium channel blockade	Prodrug for 10-OH carbazepine
Piracetam[r37]	Progressive myoclonic epilepsy	Marketed (UK)	MES 0 PTZ 0	Unknown	Low toxicity
Progabide[r4]	All types except absence	Marketed (France, Italy)	MES ++ PTZ ++	GABA agonist	Potential liver toxicity
Vigabatrin†	Partial seizures	Marketd (Europe)	MES 0 PTZ +	Increased GABA levels	Very few drug interactions
Zonisamide†	Partial seizures	Marketed (Japan) (Phase III US)	MES + PTZ 0	Sodium channel	—
5-hydroxy-tryptophan[r38]	Progressive myoclonic epilepsy	Orphan drug status	—	Serotonin precursor	—
Tiagabine[r6,r7]	Refractory epilepsy	Phase III	MES +/− PTZ +	GABA uptake inhibitor	Transient memory impairment
Topiramate[r6,r7]	Refractory partial epilepsy	Phase III	MES ++ PTZ 0	GABA (?)	Very few drug interactions
Remacemide[r6,r7]	GTCS; CPS	Phase II	MES ++ PTZ 0	NMDA antagonist (?)	
Taltrimide[r6,r7]	Primary generalized	Phase II	MES + PTZ +	Taurine agonist	—
ACTH[r39]	Infantile spasms; West syndrome	Marketed	—	—	—

Abbreviations: MES = Maximal electroshock (mice), PTZ = Pentylene tetrazole convulsions (mice), ++ = Marked effect, + = Moderate effect and 0 = No effect, † = See text for references.

include sedation, headache, dizziness, and ataxia. However, serious adverse effects requiring discontinuation occur more frequently in patients treated with carbamazepine. Oxcarbazepine is considerably less likely to cause skin reactions at the onset of treatment. Also, approximately 75 percent of patients with skin reactions to carbamazepine tolerate oxcarbazepine, allowing substitution in most of these patients.

Drug Interactions.[101,102] Compared to carbamazepine, oxcarbazepine is less likely to be associated with pharmacokinetic drug interactions. Oxcarbazepine is only moderately bound to plasma proteins, so drug interactions at this level are unlikely. Because oxidative enzymes play a minor role in the metabolism of oxcarbazepine, the metabolism of other antiepileptic drugs is not induced by oxcarbazepine. Consequently, the substitution of oxcarbazepine for carbamazepine may result in an increase in serum concentrations of other concurrent antiepileptic drugs. However, oxcarbazepine does induce a subgroup of cytochrome P-450 enzymes responsible for the metabolism of some oral contraceptives. Thus, estrogen levels may be decreased in women taking ethinylestradiol, resulting in possible break-through bleeding and loss of contraceptive protection.

Overdosage. No data are available to date on the effects of oxcarbazepine overdosage.

Pharmacokinetics.[r7,r40,97] Oxcarbazepine is quickly and almost completely absorbed. There is a linear cor-

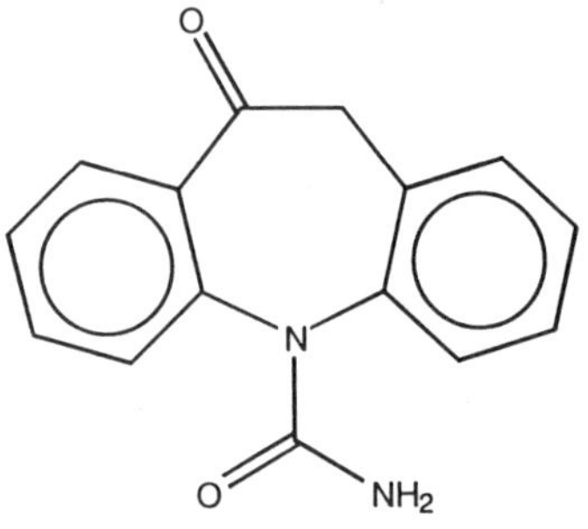

Figure 19.11 Structure of Oxcarbazepine

relation between the dosage of oxcarbazepine and plasma drug and metabolite concentrations. Both oxcarbazepine and 10-hydroxycarbazepine are widely distributed in the body. The 10-hydroxycarbazepine metabolite is approximately 40 percent bound to plasma proteins. Peak serum concentrations are reached in three to eight hours, and steady state levels are achieved in about three days. The elimination half-life of 10-hydroxycarbazepine is about eight to ten hours, and elimination kinetics are not affected by repeated administration of oxcarbazepine. The primary route of elimination of 10-hydroxycarbazepine is a glucuronide conjugate excreted in the urine.

Unlike carbamazepine, which is metabolized by hepatic microsomal enzymes, oxcarbazepine is catalyzed primarily by reductase enzymes, which are not subject to induction. The different metabolic profile of oxcarbazepine gives it several potential advantages compared with carbamazepine. First, oxcarbazepine causes less induction of hepatic microsomal enzymes, resulting in less difficulty in adjusting dosages when used concurrently with other antiepileptic drugs and in a lower potential for drug-drug interactions. Second, oxcarbazepine does not appear to induce its own metabolism; thus, steady state plasma levels can be quickly achieved. Third, by avoiding the production of carbamazepine epoxide, serious adverse events such as allergic skin reactions may occur less frequently.

Available Preparations and Usual Doses.[103] The recommended dosage of oxcarbazepine in adult patients with epilepsy is 600–1200 mg/day in three divided doses. Oxcarbazepine has been well tolerated in patients at dosages of 3000–4000 mg/day. When oxcarbazepine is substituted for carbamazepine, the dosage of oxcarbazepine is approximately 1.5 times the dosage of carbamazepine. At the initiation of treatment with oxcarbazepine the dose should be increased slowly to decrease the probability of skin reactions. Serum concentrations of concurrently administered antiepileptic drugs should be monitored when oxcarbazepine is substituted for an inducing agent and the doses of associated drugs should be reduced to avoid possible toxicity.

Lamotrigine

Lamotrigine has been shown to have clinical efficacy as adjunctive therapy in the treatment of adult epileptic patients with partial seizures. It was initially approved for marketing in Ireland in 1990, and has subsequently been approved for marketing in an additional 23 countries including the UK and Germany. In the US, the drug is under review by the FDA and marketing approval is expected as this book goes to press.

Chemistry. Lamotrigine (Fig. 19.12, 6-(2,3-dichlorophenyl)-1,2,4-triazine-3,5-diamine) is a triazine derivative structurally related to antifolate drugs. It is chemically unrelated to currently marketed antiepileptic compounds.

History. Lamotrigine was synthesized in the early 1970s at Burroughs-Wellcome as part of a screening program for compounds with antifolate activity. Lamotrigine has only very weak antifolate activity; a more plausible mechanism of action is a somewhat selective reduction in synaptic glutamate release. Lamotrigine has anticonvulsant activity in several animal models of epilepsy and has been successfully used as adjunctive therapy in controlled clinical trials.[5,104]

Therapeutic Uses and Limitations.[r41,105,106,107,108] The clinical efficacy of lamotrigine has been established as adjunctive therapy in adult epileptic patients with refractory partial seizures, both with and without secondary generalization. Results from uncontrolled studies have suggested that lamotrigine may also be effective in treating patients with atypical absence, juvenile myoclonic epilepsy, and Lennox-Gastaut syndrome.

Treatment with lamotrigine is limited by the presence of rash in approximately 3 percent of patients. Rash and other adverse events may increase when lamotrigine is added to valproate, and the efficacy of lamotrigine may be reduced in the presence of enzyme-inducing drugs such as carbamazepine and phenytoin.

Effects of the Drug Responsible for Its Therapeutic Usefulness.[5,104,109] The proposed mechanism of action of lamotrigine is a reduction of glutamate release

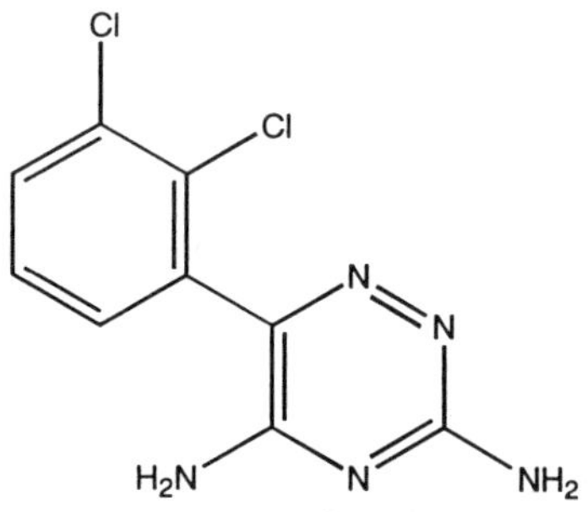

Figure 19.12 Structure of Lamotrigine

subsequent to blockade of voltage-sensitive sodium channels. This drug does not have activity at the NMDA receptor. Lamotrigine has broad spectrum anticonvulsant effects in experimental animal models of epilepsy.

Undesirable Effects.[r41,105,106,107,108] Lamotrigine is generally well tolerated. In controlled clinical trials, the most frequently reported adverse events were associated with the nervous system or GI system and included dizziness, headache, diplopia, ataxia, nausea, blurred vision, somnolence, and rash. The most common cause of discontinuation of treatment with lamotrigine was rash, which was generally maculopapular and resolved after lamotrigine was discontinued.

Drug Interactions.[r22,r41,107,110] Lamotrigine can be administered concurrently with most other drugs without altering their pharmacokinetic profiles. Lamotrigine lacks enzyme-inducing actions and thus does not seem to affect the metabolism of most drugs. Lamotrigine does not interfere with the efficacy of oral contraceptive agents. No significant changes occur in plasma concentrations of carbamazepine, phenytoin, phenobarbital, or valproic acid. However, lamotrigine may increase plasma levels of the active epoxide metabolite of carbamazepine, resulting in adverse effects associated with the CNS.

Conversely, because lamotrigine is metabolized by glucuronidation, treatment with many other antiepileptic drugs alters lamotrigine pharmacokinetics. The half-life of lamotrigine is decreased to approximately 15 hours when the drug is administered with enzyme-inducing drugs, such as carbamazepine, phenytoin, or phenobarbital. However, when lamotrigine is administered with valproate, the half-life is increased to approximately 60 hours. When lamotrigine is administered with both enzyme-inducing antiepileptic drugs and valproate, the opposing effects on lamotrigine elimination appear to counteract each other and the half-life is about 30 hours, similar to that found when lamotrigine is administered alone.

Overdosage.[r41] One patient overdosed in a suicide attempt by taking 30 tablets of 100-mg lamotrigine. The patient experienced ataxia, vomiting, and nystagmus, which disappeared within two days. There were no persistent adverse effects.

Pharmacokinetics.[r41,110] Lamotrigine is almost completely absorbed, and peak plasma concentrations are reached in approximately one to three hours. The absorption of lamotrigine is not affected by the presence of food. Plasma protein binding of lamotrigine is about 55 percent. The elimination of lamotrigine occurs primarily by hepatic metabolism and about 70 percent of a single dose is recovered in the urine, primarily as a glucuronide conjugate. The half-life in healthy subjects is approximately 25 hours and ranges from 14 to 50 hours. At doses up to 500 mg/day lamotrigine follows first-order linear kinetics. The pharmacokinetic parameters are similar for single- and multiple-dose administration but are significantly altered in the presence of enzyme-inducing drugs and valproate (See section on Drug Interactions).

Available Preparations and Usual Doses.[r41] The dosage of lamotrigine depends on existing therapy. In the presence of enzyme-inducing antiepileptic drugs, the recommended dosage is about 300 to 500 mg/day. When lamotrigine is administered in the presence of both valproate and enzyme-inducing drugs (e.g., phenytoin), the recommended dose is about 150 mg/day. The drug is usually administered twice daily.

Vigabatrin

Vigabatrin is a structural derivative of the inhibitory amino acid neurotransmitter GABA, and is a suicide inhibitor of the GABA metabolizing enzyme γ-aminobutyrate-α-ketoglutaric acid aminotransferase (GABA transaminase). The therapeutic indication to date is as an antiepileptic drug for the control of complex partial seizures with or without generalization. Vigabatrin also has beneficial effects in some childhood epilepsies. Vigabatrin has been reported to have some effects in the control of tardive dyskinesia and in spasticity due to spinal cord lesions or multiple sclerosis.

Chemistry. Vigabatrin (Fig. 19.13, R,S-gamma-vinylGABA) is a racemate of which the (+) isomer is the active form. This is a member of a series of compounds designed to be suicide inhibitors of the GABA-metabolizing enzyme GABA-transaminase, and thus increase brain GABA levels and enhance GABAergic transmission. Whereas some of the compounds in this series also inhibited GABA synthesis (e.g., gamma-acetylenic GABA) vigabatrin appears to be devoid of this property.[r5]

History.[r5,r6,r7,111,112] Vigabatrin has been developed by Merrell-Dow. The inhibition of GABA-transaminase by vigabatrin was first published in 1977, and its anticonvulsant properties in 1978. Antiepileptic activity in double-blind trials was demonstrated in 1984, followed by studies in several different seizures types. The results indicate that complex partial seizures with or without generalization are the most responsive to vigabatrin, whereas an exacerbation of absence and myoclonic seizures may occur. Vigabatrin is the result of a rational drug design aimed at enhancing brain GABA levels subsequent to an irreversible inhibition of the GABA metabolizing enzyme GABA-transaminase. Vigabatrin acts as a substrate for this enzyme, the reaction producing an intermediate which binds covalently to the active site of GABA transaminase. As this inhibition is irreversible, new enzyme molecules must be synthesized to overcome the action of vigabatrin.

Therapeutic Uses and Limitations.[r5,r6,r7] Vigabatrin has been studied mainly as add-on therapy in refractory patients. In these refractory patients vigabatrin has exhibited a marked activity, both in terms of seizure reduction and in enhancement of the quality of life.

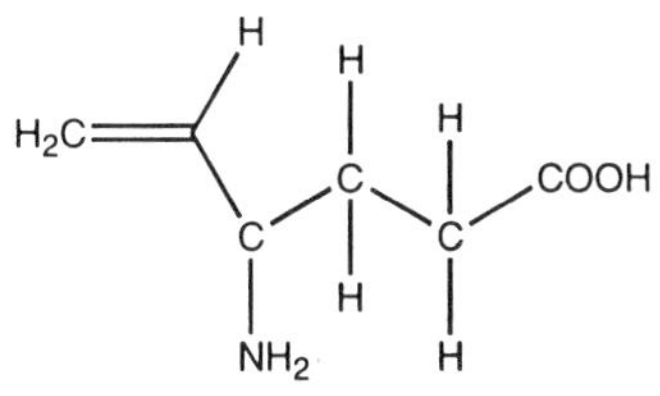

$H_2C{=}CH{-}CH(NH_2){-}CH_2{-}CH_2{-}COOH$

VIGABATRIN

Figure 19.13 Structure of Vigabatrin

The greatest efficacy in adults has been attained in complex partial seizures with or without generalization. Effectiveness in children has been demonstrated for cryptogenic partial epilepsy and symptomatic infantile spasm. Vigabatrin may aggravate absence or myoclonic seizures. As the compound has recently been marketed in Europe, information on a broader population of epileptic patients should soon be available.

Vigabatrin should not be used during pregnancy (a low incidence of cleft palate was reported in studies in the rabbit). Care should be exercised in patients with a previous history of psychiatric illness or mental retardation. Vigabatrin should be used with caution in patients with compromised renal function; in such cases a reduction in dosage may be necessary. The induction of intramyelinic edema demonstrated in non-primate animal studies does not seem to be translated to man.

Effects of the Drug Responsible for Its Therapeutic Usefulness.[r5,r6,r7,111,112] Vigabatrin increases synaptic GABA levels in the brain by irreversible inhibition of GABA metabolism at the level of GABA-transaminase. The inhibition of GABA transaminase is rapid (within minutes) and long lasting (several days), recovery depending on the synthesis of new enzyme. Unlike some structurally related compounds, vigabatrin does not inhibit glutamic acid decarboxylase, the enzyme accounting for the neuronal synthesis of GABA. However, GABA synthesis is reduced in animals after several days of repeated administration of high doses of vigabatrin.

Vigabatrin exhibits anticonvulsant activity in a wide variety of animal models; however, it was without beneficial effect in a rat model of absence epilepsy. In a genetic murine model of epilepsy, it has been demonstrated that the anticonvulsant activity of vigabatrin is highly correlated with the enhancement of brain GABA levels. In humans, brain GABA levels are increased as evidenced by CSF levels of GABA and homocarnisine (a dipeptide of GABA and histidine). The effect of vigabatrin on brain GABA metabolism seems to be responsible for its antiepileptic activity as no other relevant effects of the compound have been described.

Undesirable Effects.[r5] The information available on the adverse effects of vigabatrin must be considered as preliminary in nature as it is obtained from use as add-on therapy in a limited (in number) restricted (to refractory) group of epileptic patients. As the drug is used in the general epileptic population a much more accurate profile will be obtained.

To date most adverse events seem to be of CNS origin and usually are mild and transitory. These include sedation, fatigue, headache, confusion and memory impairment, ataxia, diplopia, and insomnia. Transient psychiatric adverse events may occur; rarely, a clinically evident psychosis or aggression has been reported, especially in patients with a previous history of psychiatric illness, behavioral disturbances, or mental retardation. From the limited autopsy material available from patients who had received vigabatrin, it appears that the intramyelinic edema reported in non-primate animal studies is not reproduced in man. Experience in children is even more limited. CNS events are the most common, and include agitation, insomnia, and behavioral changes.

Drug Interactions.[r5,r22] Vigabatrin appears to be without any clinically significant interactions with most of the commonly used antiepileptic drugs, with the exception of phenytoin, for which plasma concentrations may be decreased up to 30 percent. This may necessitate adjustment of the phenytoin dosage.

Overdosage.[r5] Overdoses of up to 30 g of vigabatrin have been without sequelae. Supportive therapy is indicated.

Pharmacokinetics.[r5] Vigabatrin is available as the racemate in which the therapeutic activity resides in the S(+) isomer. The two isomers have somewhat different pharmacokinetic properties but there is not any interference between the two, nor is there any chiral interconversion. There is no apparent food effect and vigabatrin appears to be almost completely absorbed. Tmax occurs about one hour after administration of a 1.5 g dose. CSF concentrations of vigabatrin are much lower than plasma levels. The plasma half-life is about six to eight hours, but this does not reflect the duration of action of the compound. Vigabatrin does not exhibit plasma protein binding. The pharmacokinetics of vigabatrin appear to be similar in adults and children, although in the latter bioavailability may be lower.

Vigabatrin is excreted in the urine mainly as the unchanged compound without undergoing hepatic metabolism. No metabolites have been identified in man. Excretion is impaired when creatinine clearance is < 60 ml/min; dosage adjustment may be necessary owing to toxicity.

Available Preparations and Usual Doses.[r5] At the time of writing, vigabatrin is not available for prescription in the US, but is marketed in several European countries (England, France, Italy, Sweden). Vigabatrin exists as 500-mg tablets. The usual daily dose in adults is 2 g per day and may be increased to 4 g per day if necessary (increments of 0.5–1 g/day per week). In young children (3–9 years) the usual dose of vigabatrin is 1 g/day and in older children 2 g/day. Vigabatrin is administered either as a single daily dose or bid. As for all antiepileptic drugs, withdrawal of vigabatrin should be done gradually.

Zonisamide

Zonisamide is a sulfonamide derivative of the 1,2-benzisoxazole series. The principal use of zonisamide is in epileptic patients with partial seizures. At time of press, zonisamide is marketed only in Japan, with clinical trials ongoing in Europe and the US.

Chemistry. Zonisamide (Fig. 19.14, 1,2-benzosoxazole-3-methanesulphonamide) does not have an asymmetric carbon atom. Halogenation at the 5-position enhances anticonvulsant activity but also increases neurotoxicity. Substitution of the sulfamoyl group decreases activity.

History.[r7,r42,113] Zonisamide was discovered by Uno and collaborators in the mid-1970s at the Dainippon Pharmaceutical Company during screening of a series of benzisoxazole derivatives. The compound has undergone clinical testing in Japan (where it is currently marketed), Europe, and the US. The molecular mechanism of action is not yet defined. It has been proposed that zonisamide acts at a novel site within the $GABA_A$-chloride ion channel complex; however, GABA responses are not altered by the compound. Another possible site of action is at T-type calcium channels or neuronal voltage-dependent sodium channels. Apparently zonisamide does not act at glutamate receptors or on carbonic anhydrase activity.

Therapeutic Uses and Limitations.[r7,r42,114] Zonisamide is useful in the treatment of partial seizures, either simple or complex, and also secondary generalized seizures and compound seizures. It is used in Japan for adults and children as either monotherapy or as add-on therapy to other antiepileptic drugs. It has a profile similar to that of carbamazepine and phenytoin, but at this time no long-term, double-blind trials versus phenytoin, carbamazepine, or valproate have been published.

The limitations to zonisamide usage are related to the toxicity resulting from concomitant therapy with other antiepileptic drugs. Before zonisamide add-on therapy is initiated, as well as after therapy has commenced, the following should be evaluated: blood chemistry; urinalysis; neuropsychologic profile; memory; learning.

Effects of the Drug Responsible for Its Therapeutic Usefulness.[r42,115,116,117] Zonisamide has a profile of anticonvulsant activity in animal models very similar to that of phenytoin or carbamazepine, with activity in the maximal electroshock and kindling models. In addition, zonisamide is active in cortical focus models and is more active against the tonic phase than the clonic phase of the different models. Zonisamide blocks the sustained repetitive firing of depolarized spinal cord neurons in culture. These activities suggest that zonisamide suppresses the focus as well as blocking seizure propagation.

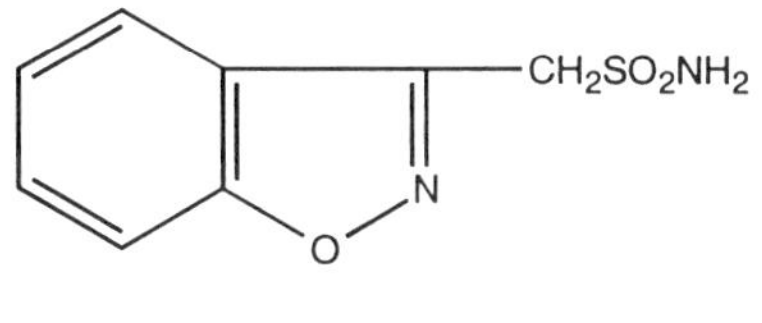

$CH_2SO_2NH_2$

N

O

ZONISAMIDE

Figure 19.14 Structure of Zonisamide

Undesirable Effects.[r42,r43,114,118] The common adverse effects of zonisamide monotherapy include an adverse effect on cognition, weight loss, drowsiness, and parasthesia. Drowsiness can occur at plasma concentrations > 30 μg/ml, and adverse events are common at plasma levels > 40 μg/ml.

When zonisamide is administered as adjunctive therapy to other antiepileptic drugs, adverse effects are relatively frequent and may limit zonisamide therapy. CNS events are the most frequent and commonly include drowsiness, verbal and nonverbal memory impairment, ataxia, nystagmus, diplopia, tremors, psychosis, and dysarthria. Educational and occupational performances may be impaired. Non-CNS events include GI problems, nephrolithiasis (which has a lower reported rate in Japan than elsewhere), and allergic reactions such as dermatitis, Stevens-Johnson syndrome, and leukopenia.

Drug Interactions.[r42] Zonisamide exhibits multiple interactions with other drugs. Many other antiepileptic drugs increase the clearance of zonisamide, with phenytoin having a greater effect than carbamazepine. Conversely zonisamide decreases the clearance rate of other antiepileptic drugs, with carbamazepine being the most sensitive. The plasma protein binding of zonisamide is not altered by phenobarbital or phenytoin.

Overdosage. A single case of zonisamide overdose together with clonazepam in a suicide attempt has been reported without a fatal outcome.[119]

Pharmacokinetics.[r42,120] In studies performed in the US, zonisamide exhibits nonlinear first-order pharmacokinetics, with a decreased clearance and greater than expected trough plasma levels with increasing dose. In Japanese studies, the pharmacokinetics were demonstrated to be of a linear nature. Zonisamide has virtually complete absorption in animal studies and very good oral bioavailability was demonstrated in human volunteers.

Zonisamide is approximately 50 percent bound to plasma proteins and is concentrated in erythrocytes (up to nine-fold). Therapeutic plasma levels are 20 to 40 μg/ml, with adverse events occurring at > 30 μg/ml. The terminal plasma half-life is 50 to 68 hours in monotherapy and 27 to 36 hours in polytherapy. Maximum plasma concentrations occur 2.4 to 3.6 hours postdose.

The major metabolic route of zonisamide is via ring cleavage and metabolism to the glucuronide. Acetylation also occurs. Urinary excretion of zonisamide plus metabolites is the major route of excretion but accounts for less than half the dose administered. In rodents, zonisamide is also excreted via the bile.

Available Preparations and Usual Doses.[r42] In Japan, zonisamide is available as 100-mg tablets and a 20% powder. Starting doses in adults are recommended as 100 to 200 mg/day (in one, two or three doses), increasing to 200 to 400 mg/day over two weeks. The maximum recommended doses are 12.5 mg/kg/day. In children starting doses are 2 to 4 mg/kg/day, increasing to 4 to 8 mg/kg/day.

References

Research Reports

1. Commission on Classification and Terminology of the International League Against Epilepsy (1981). Proposal for revised clinical and electroencephalographic classification of epileptic seizures. Epilepsia **22**, 489–501.
2. Savic I, Roland P, Sedvall G, Persson A, Pauli S, Widen L. (1988). In-vivo demonstration of reduced benzodiazepine receptor binding in human epileptic foci. Lancet **1**, 863–866.
3. DeLorey TM, Olsen RW. (1992). γ-Aminobutyric $acid_A$ receptor structure and function. J. Biol. Chem. **267**, 16747–16750.
4. During MJ, Spencer DD. (1993). Extracellular hippocampal glutamate and spontaneous seizure in the conscious human brain. Lancet **341**, 1607–1610.
5. Leach MJ, Marden CM, Miller AA. (1986). Pharmacological studies on lamotrigine, a novel potential antiepileptic drug: II. Neurochemical studies on the mechanism of action. Epilepsia **27**, 490–497.
6. Anonymous (1994). CCD-3045. Pharmaprojects **15A** (May), 1435.
7. Lan NC, Gee KW, Bolger MB, Chen JS. (1991). Differential responses of expressed recombinant human γ-aminobutyric $acid_A$ receptors to neurosteroids. J. Neurochem. **57**, 1818–1821.
8. Quesney LF, Reader T. (1984). Role of cortical catecholamine depletion in the genesis of epileptic photosensitivity. In: Neurotransmitters, Seizures, and Epilepsy II; RG Fariello et al., eds., Raven Press, New York, 11–20.
9. Coulter DA, Huguenard JR, Prince DA. (1989). Specific petit mal anticonvulsants reduce calcium currents in thalamic neurons. Neurosci. Lett. **98**, 74–78.
10. Sugaya E, Sugaya A. (1991). Cellular physiology of epileptogenic phenomena and its application to therapy against intractable epilepsy. Comp. Biochem. Physiol. **98C**, 249–270.
11. Schwarz DJ, Grigat G. (1989). Phenytoin and carbamazepine: potential-and frequency-dependent block of Na currents in mammalian myelinated nerve fibers. Epilepsia **30**, 286–294.
12. Merritt HH, Putnam TJ. (1938). Sodium diphenyl hydantoinate in the treatment of convulsive disorders. JAMA **111**, 1068–1073.
13. Wakamori M, Kaneda M, Oyama Y, Akaike N. (1989). Effects of chlordiazepoxide, chlorpromazine, diazepam, diphenylhydantoin, flunitrazepam and haloperidol on the voltage-dependent sodium current of isolated mammalian brain neurons. Brain Res. **494**, 374–378.
14. Tomaselli G, Marban E, Yellen G. (1989). Sodium channels from human brain RNA expressed in *Xenopus* oocytes: basic electrophysiologic characteristics and their modifications by diphenylhydantoin. J. Clin. Invest. **83**, 1724–1732.
15. Dansky LV, Finnell RH. (1991). Parental epilepsy, anticonvulsant drugs, and reproductive outcome: epidemiologic and experimental findings spanning three decades; 2: Human studies. Reprod. Toxicol., 301–335.
16. Parke-Davis (1994). Dilantin® prescription drug labeling. In: Physicians' Desk Reference; DW Sifton, ed., Medical Economics Data Production Company, Montvale, NJ, 1730–1735.
17. Dam M. (1982). Phenytoin: Toxicity. In: Antiepileptic Drugs; DM Woodbury, JK Penry and CE Pippenger, eds., Raven Press, New York, 247–256.
18. Pisciotta AV. (1982). Phenytoin: Hematological toxicity. In: Antiepileptic Drugs; DM Woodbury, JK Penry and CE Pippenger, eds., Raven Press, New York, 257–268.
19. Kutt H. (1982). Phenytoin: Interactions with other drugs. In: Antiepileptic Drugs; DM Woodbury, JK Penry and CE Pippenger, eds., Raven Press, New York, 227–240.
20. Woodbury DM. (1982). Phenytoin: Absorption, distribution, and excretion. In: Antiepileptic Drugs; DM Woodbury, JK Penry and CE Pippenger, eds., Raven Press, New York, 191–207.
21. Chang T, Glazko AJ. (1982). Phenytoin: Biotransformation. In: Antiepileptic Drugs; DM Woodbury, JK Penry and CE Pippenger, eds., Raven Press, New York, 209–226.
22. Basel Pharmaceuticals, Ciba-Geigy Corporation (1994). Tegretol® prescription drug labeling. In: Physicians' Desk Reference; DW Sifton, ed., Medical Economics Data Production Company, Montvale, NJ, 585–587.
23. Sillanpää M. (1993). Carbamazepine. In: The Treatment of Epilepsy: Principles and Practices; E Wyllie, ed., Lea & Febiger, Philadelphia, 867–887.
24. Schindler W, Hälliger F. (1954). Über derivate de iminostilbenzyls. Helv. Chim. Acta. **37**, 472–483.
25. Snead OC, Hosey LC. (1985). Exacerbation of seizures in children by carbamazepine. N. Engl. J. Med. **313**, 916–921.
26. Lindhout D, Höppener RJEA, Meinardi H. (1984). Teratogenicity of antiepileptic drug combinations with special emphasis on epoxidation (of carbamazepine). Epilepsia. **25**, 77–83.
27. Quattrone A, Samanin R. (1977). Decreased anticonvulsant activity of carbamazepine in 6-hydroxydopamine-treated rats. Eur. J. Pharmacol. **41**, 333–336.
28. Weaver DF, Camfield P, Fraser A. (1988). Massive carbamazepine overdose: clinical and pharmacologic observations. Neurology **38**, 755–759.
29. Morselli PL, Bossi L. (1982). Carbamazepine: Absorption, distribution, and excretion. In: Antiepileptic Drugs; DM Woodbury, JK Penry and CE Pippenger, eds., Raven Press, New York, 465–482.
30. Faigle JW, Feldmann KF. (1982). Carbamazepine: Biotransformation. In: Antiepileptic Drugs; DM Woodbury, JK Penry and CE Pippenger, eds., Raven Press, New York, 483–495.
31. Abbott Laboratories (1994). Depakene® prescription drug labeling. In: Physicians' Desk Reference; DW Sifton, ed., Medical Economics Data Production Company, Montvale, NJ, 411–413.
32. Abbott Laboratories (1994). Depakote® prescription drug labeling. In: Physicians' Desk Reference; DW Sifton, ed., Medical Economics Data Production Company, Montvale, NJ, 413–415.
33. Jeavons PM. (1982). Valproate: Toxicity. In: Antiepileptic Drugs; DM Woodbury, JK Penry and CE Pippenger, eds., Raven Press, New York, 601–610.
34. Löscher W, Nau H, Marescaux C, Vergnes M. (1984). Comparative evaluation of anticonvulsant and toxic potencies of valproic acid and 2-en-valproic acid in different models of epilepsy. Eur. J. Pharmacol. **99**, 211–218.
35. Mattson RH. (1982). Valproate: Interactions with other drugs. In: Antiepileptic Drugs; DM Woodbury, JK Penry and CE Pippenger, eds., Raven Press, New York, 579–589.
36. Levy RH, Lai AA. (1982). Valproate: Absorption, distribution, and excretion. In: Antiepileptic Drugs; DM Woodbury, JK Penry and CE Pippenger, eds., Raven Press, New York, 555–565.

37. Schobben F, van der Kleijn E. (1982). Valproate: Biotransformation. In: Antiepileptic Drugs; DM Woodbury, JK Penry and CE Pippenger, eds., Raven Press, New York, 567–578.

38. Abbott Laboratories (1994). Tranxene® prescription drug labeling. In: Physicians' Desk Reference; DW Sifton, ed., Medical Economics Data Production Company, Montvale, NJ, 452–454.

39. Roche Products (1994). Valium® prescription drug labeling. In: Physicians' Desk Reference; DW Sifton, ed., Medical Economics Data Production Company, Montvale, NJ, 1967–1969.

40. Wyeth-Ayerst Laboratories (1994). Ativan® prescription drug labeling. In: Physicians' Desk Reference; DW Sifton, ed., Medical Economics Data Production Company, Montvale, NJ, 2514–2517.

41. Roche Laboratories (1994). Klonopin® prescription drug labeling. In: Physicians' Desk Reference; DW Sifton, ed., Medical Economics Data Production Company, Montvale, NJ, 1935–1936.

42. Roche Laboratories (1994). Romazicon™ prescription drug labeling. In: Physicians' Desk Reference; DW Sifton, ed., Medical Economics Data Production Company, Montvale, NJ, 1949–1952.

43. Johannessen SI. (1982). Phenobarbital: Chemistry and methods of determination. In: Antiepileptic Drugs; DM Woodbury, JK Penry and CE Pippenger, eds., Raven Press, New York, 297–307.

44. Barker JL, Gratz E, Owen DG, Study RE. (1984). Pharmacological effects of clinically important drugs on the excitability of cultured mouse spinal neurons. In: Actions and Interactions of GABA and Benzodiazepines; NG Bowery, ed., Raven Press, New York, 203–216.

45. Verdoorn TA, Draguhn A, Ymer S, Seeburg PH, Sakmann B. (1990). Functional properties of recombinant rat $GABA_A$ receptors depend upon subunit composition. Neuron **4**, 919–928.

46. Lilly Research Laboratories (1994). Phenobarbital. In: Physicians' Desk Reference; DW Sifton, ed., Medical Economics Data Production Company, Montvale, NJ, 1255–1257.

47. Hooper WD, Eadie MJ. (1992). Mephobarbital. In: The Medical Treatment of Epilepsy; SR Resor Jr, H Kutt, eds., Marcel Dekker, Inc, New York, 363–369.

48. Mattson RH, Cramer JA. (1982). Phenobarbital: Toxicity. In: Antiepileptic Drugs; DM Woodbury, JK Penry and CE Pippenger, eds., Raven Press, New York, 351–363.

49. Kutt H, Paris Kutt H. (1982) Phenobarbital: Interactions with other drugs. In: Antiepileptic Drugs; DM Woodbury, JK Penry and CE Pippenger, eds., Raven Press, New York, 329–340.

50. Maynert EW. (1982). Phenobarbital: Absorption, distribution, and excretion. In: Antiepileptic Drugs; DM Woodbury, JK Penry and CE Pippenger, eds., Raven Press, New York, 309–317.

51. Maynert EW. (1982). Phenobarbital: Biotransformation. In: Antiepileptic Drugs; DM Woodbury, JK Penry and CE Pippenger, eds., Raven Press, New York, 319–327.

52. Bogue JY, Carrington HC. (1953). The evaluation of "mysoline"—a new anticonvulsant drug. Br. J. Pharmacol. **8**, 230–236.

53. Handley R, Stewart ASR. (1952). Mysoline: a new drug in the treatment of epilepsy. Lancet **1**, 742–744.

54. Butler TC, Waddell WJ. (1956). Metabolic conversion of primidone (Mysoline) to phenobarbital. Proc. Soc. Exp. Biol. Med. **93**, 544–546.

55. Baumel IP, Gallagher BB, Mattson RH. (1972). Phenylethylmalonamide (PEMA). An important metabolite of primidone. Arch. Neurol. **27**, 34–41.

56. Fincham RW, Schottelius DD. (1982). Primidone: Relation of plasma concentration to seizure control. In: Antiepileptic Drugs; DM Woodbury, JK Penry and CE Pippenger, eds., Raven Press, New York, 429–440.

57. Wyeth-Ayerst Laboratories (1994). Mysoline® prescription drug labeling. In: Physicians' Desk Reference; DW Sifton, ed., Medical Economics Data Production Company, Montvale, NJ, 2560–2561.

58. Leppik IE, Cloyd JC. (1982). Primidone: Toxicity. In: Antiepileptic Drugs; DM Woodbury, JK Penry and CE Pippenger, eds., Raven Press, New York, 441–447.

59. Fincham RW, Schottelius DD. (1982). Primidone: Interactions with other drugs. In: Antiepileptic Drugs; DM Woodbury, JK Penry and CE Pippenger, eds., Raven Press, New York, 421–427.

60. Schottelius DD. (1982). Primidone: Absorption, distribution, and excretion. In: Antiepileptic Drugs; DM Woodbury, JK Penry and CE Pippenger, eds., Raven Press, New York, 405–413.

61. Schottelius DD. (1982). Primidone: Biotransformation. In: Antiepileptic Drugs; DM Woodbury, JK Penry and CE Pippenger, Raven Press, New York, 415–420.

62. Chen G, Weston JK, Bratton AC. (1963). Anticonvulsant activity and toxicity of phensuximide, methsuximide and ethosuximide. Epilepsia **4**, 66–76.

63. Parke-Davis (1994). Zarontin® prescription drug labeling. In: Physicians' Desk Reference; DW Sifton ed., Medical Economics Data Production Company, Montvale, NJ, 1773–1774.

64. Dreifuss FE. (1982). Ethosuximide: Toxicity. In: Antiepileptic Drugs; DM Woodbury, JK Penry and CE Pippenger, eds., Raven Press, New York, 647–653.

65. Sherwin AL. (1993). Ethosuximide. In: The Treatment of Epilepsy: Principles and Practices; E Wyllie, ed., Lea & Febiger, Philadelphia, 923–929.

66. Glazko AJ, Chang T. (1982). Ethosuximide: Absorption, distribution, and excretion. In: Antiepileptic Drugs; DM Woodbury, JK Penry and CE Pippenger, eds., Raven Press, New York, 623–629.

67. Chang T, Glazko AJ. (1982). Ethosuximide: Biotransformation. In: Antiepileptic Drugs; DM Woodbury, JK Penry and CE Pippenger, eds., Raven Press, New York, 631–635.

68. Abbott Laboratories (1994). Tridione® prescription drug labeling. In: Physicians' Desk Reference; DW Sifton, ed., Medical Economics Data Production Company, Montvale, NJ, 454.

69. Booker HE. (1982). Trimethadione: Toxicity. In: Antiepileptic Drugs; DM Woodbury, JK Penry and CE Pippenger, eds., Raven Press, New York, 701–703.

70. Withrow CD. (1982) Trimethadione: Interactions with other drugs. In: Antiepileptic Drugs; DM Woodbury, JK Penry and CE Pippenger, eds., Raven Press, New York, 693–695.

71. Withrow CD. (1982). Trimethadione: Absorption, distribution, and excretion. In: Antiepileptic Drugs; DM Woodbury, JK Penry and CE Pippenger, eds., Raven Press, New York, 681–687.

72. Withrow CD. (1982). Trimethadione: Biotransformation. In: Antiepileptic Drugs; DM Woodbury, JK Penry and CE Pippenger, eds., Raven Press, New York, 689–692.

73. Chadwick D. (1994). Gabapentin. Lancet **343**, 89–91.

74. Taylor CP, Vartanian MG, Yuen PW, Bigge C, Suman-Chauhar N, Hill DR. (1993). Potent and stereo-specific anticonvulsant activity of 3-isobutyl GABA relates to in vitro binding at a novel site labeled by tritiated gabapentin. Epilepsy Res. **14**, 11–15.

75. Loscher W, Honack D, Taylor CP. (1991). Gabapentin increases amino-oxyacetic acid-induced GABA accumulation in several regions of rat brain. Neurosci. Lett. **128**, 150–154.

76. Parke-Davis (1994). Neurontin® prescription drug labeling. Parke-Davis, Div. of Warner-Lambert Co., Morris Plains, NJ.

77. Vollmer K-O, von Hodenberg A, Kölle EU. (1986). Pharmacokinetics and metabolism of gabapentin in rat, dog and man. Arzneim.-Forsch./Drug Res. **36(I)**, 830–839.

78. Food and Drug Administation. (September 27, 1994). Felbatol Update. FDA Talk Paper.

79. Anonymous (1993). Felbatol™: review and evaluation of clinical data. In: Carter-Wallace NDA No. 20-189.

80. Wallace Laboratories, Carter-Wallace, Inc. (1994). Felbatol™ prescription drug labeling. In: Physicians' Desk Reference; DW Sifton, ed., Medical Economics Data Production Company, Montvale, NJ, 2473–2476.

81. Sachdeo R, Kramer LD, Rosenberg A, Sachdeo S. (1992). Felbamate monotherapy: controlled trial in patients with partial onset seizures. Ann. Neurol. **32**, 386–392.

82. Jensen PK. (1993). Felbamate in the treatment of refractory partial-onset seizures. Epilepsia **34** (Suppl. 7), S25–S29.

83. Ritter et al. (1993). Efficacy of felbamate in childhood epileptic encephalopathy (Lennox-Gastaut syndrome). N. Engl. J. Med. **328**, 29–33.

84. Dodson WE. (1993). Felbamate in the treatment of Lennox-Gastaut syndrome: results of a 12-month open-label study following a randomized clinical trial. Epilepsia **34** (Suppl. 7), S18–S24.

85. Leppik IE, Kupferberg HJ. (1992). Felbamate. The Medical Treatment of Epilepsy; SR Resor Jr, H Kutt, eds., Marcel Dekker, Inc., 655–660.

86. White HS, Wolf HH, Swinyard EA, Skeen GA, Sofia RD. (1992). A neuropharmacological evaluation of felbamate as a novel anticonvulsant. Epilepsia **33**, 564–572.

87. McCabe RT, Wasterlain CG, Kucharczyk N, Sofia RD, Vogel JR. (1993). Evidence for anticonvulsant and neuroprotectant action of felbamate mediated by strychnine-insensitive glycine receptors. J. Pharmacol. Exp. Ther. **264**, 1248–1252.

88. Schmidt D. (1993). Felbamate: successful development of a new compound for the treatment of epilepsy. Epilepsia **34** (Suppl. 7), S30–S33.

89. Sanofi Winthrop Pharmaceuticals (1994). Mebaral® prescription drug labeling. In: Physicians' Desk Reference; DW Sifton, ed., Medical Economics Data Production Company, Montvale, NJ, 2107–2108.

90. Abbott Laboratories (1994). Nembutal® Sodium Solution prescription drug labeling. In: Physicians' Desk Reference; DW Sifton, ed., Medical Economics Data Production Company, Montvale, NJ, 433–435.

91. Sandoz (1994). Mesantoin® prescription drug labeling. In: Physicians' Desk Reference; DW Sifton, ed., Medical Economics Data Production Company, Montvale, NJ, 2059–2060.

92. Abbott Laboratories (1994). Peganone® prescription drug labeling. In: Physicians' Desk Reference; DW Sifton, ed., Medical Economics Data Production Company, Montvale, NJ, 448–449.

93. Abbott Laboratories (1994). Paradione® prescription drug labeling. In: Physicians' Desk Reference; DW Sifton, ed., Medical Economics Data Production Company, Montvale, NJ, 445–446.

94. Parke-Davis (1994). Celontin® Kapseals® prescription drug labeling. In: Physicians' Desk Reference; DW Sifton, ed., Medical Economics Data Production Company, Montvale, NJ, 1721.

95. Parke-Davis (1994). Milontin® prescription drug labeling. In: Physicians' Desk Reference; DW Sifton, ed., Medical Economics Data Production Company, Montvale, NJ, 1757.

96. Abbott Laboratories (1994). Phenurone® prescription drug labeling. In: Physicians' Desk Reference; DW Sifton, ed., Medical Economics Data Production Company, Montvale, NJ, 449.

97. Lloyd P, Flesch G, Dieterle W. (1994). Clinical pharmacology and pharmacokinetics of oxcarbazepine. Epilepsia **35** (Suppl. 3), S10–S13.

98. McLean MJ, Schmutz M, Wamil AW, Olpe H-R, Portet C, Feldmann KF. (1994). Oxcarbazepine: mechanisms of action. Epilepsia **35** (Suppl. 3), S5–S9.

99. Leppik IE. (1994). Antiepileptic drugs in development: prospects for the near future. Epilepsia **35** (Suppl. 4), S29–S40.

100. Gram L. (1994). Clinical experience with oxcarbazepine. Epilepsia **35** (Suppl. 3), S21–S22.

101. Baruzzi A, Albani F, Riva R. (1994). Oxcarbazepine: pharmacokinetic interactions and their clinical relevance. Epilepsia **35** (Suppl. 3), S14–S19.

102. Jensen PK, Saano V, Haring P, Svenstrup B, Menge GP. (1992). Possible interaction between oxcarbazepine and an oral contraceptive. Epilepsia **33**, 1149–1152.

103. Dam M. (1994). Practical aspects of oxcarbazepine treatment. Epilepsia **35** (Suppl. 3), S23–S25.

104. Leach MJ, Baxter MG, Critchley MAE. (1991). Neurochemical and behavioral aspects of lamotrigine. Epilepsia **32** (Suppl. 2), S4–S8.

105. Richens A, Yuen AWC. (1991). Overview of the clinical efficacy of lamotrigine. Epilepsia **32** (Suppl. 2), S13–S16.

106. Hamilton MJ, Cohen AF, Yuen AWC, Harkin N, Land G, Weatherley BC, Peck AW. (1993). Carbamazepine and lamotrigine in healthy volunteers: relevance to early tolerance and clinical trial dosage. Epilepsia **34**, 166–173.

107. Brodie MJ. (1992). Lamotrigine. Lancet **339**, 1397–1400.

108. Betts T, Goodwin G, Withers RM, Yuen AWC. (1991). Human safety of lamotrigine. Epilepsia **32** (Suppl. 2), S17–S21.

109. Lang DG, Wang CM, Cooper BR. (1993). Lamotrigine, phenytoin and carbamazepine interactions on the sodium current present in N4TG1 mouse neuroblastoma cells. J. Pharmacol. Exp. Ther. **266**, 829–835.

110. Peck AW. (1991). Clinical pharmacology of lamotrigine. Epilepsia **32** (Suppl. 2), S9–S12.

111. Hammond EJ, Wilder BJ. (1985). Gamma-vinyl GABA. Gen. Pharmac. **16**, 441–447.

112. Schechter PJ, Hanke NFJ, Grove J, Huebert N, Sjoerdsma A. (1984). Biochemical and clinical effects of γ-vinyl GABA in patients with epilepsy. Neurology **34**, 182–186.

113. Uno H, Kurokawa M, Masuda Y, Nishimura H. (1979). Studies on 3-substituted 1,2-benzisoxazole derivatives. 6. syntheses of 3-(sulfamoylmethyl)-1,2-benzisoxazole derivatives and their anticonvulsant activities. J. Med. Chem. **22**, 180–183.

114. Yagi K, Seino M. (1992). Methodological requirements for clinical trials in refractory epilepsies—our experience with zonisamide. Prog. Neuropsycho-pharmacol. Biol. Psychiatry **16**, 79–85.

115. Ito T, Hori M, Masuda Y, Yoshida K, Shimizu M. (1980). 3-sulfamoylmethyl-1,2-benzisoxazole, a new type of anticonvul-

sant drug: electro-encephalographic profile. Arzneim.-Forsch./ Drug Res. **30**, 603–609.

116. Wada Y, Hasegawa H, Okuda H, Yamaguchi N. (1990). Anticonvulsant activity of zonisamide and phenytoin on seizure activity of the feline visual cortex. Brain Dev. **12**, 206–210.

117. Rock DM, McDonald RL, Taylor CP. (1989). Blockade of sustained repetitive action potentials in cultured spinal cord neurons by zonisamide (AD-801, CI 912), a novel anticonvulsant. Epilepsy Res. **3**, 138–143.

118. Leppik IE, Willmore LJ, Homan RW, Fromm G, Dommen KJ, et al. (1993). Efficacy and safety of zonisamide: results of a multicenter study. Epilepsy Res. **14**, 165–173.

119. Naito H, Itoh N, Matsui N, Eguchi T. (1988). Monitoring plasma concentrations of zonisamide and clonazepam in an epileptic attempting suicide by an overdose of the drugs. Curr. Ther. Res. **43**, 463–467.

120. Ito T, Yamaguchi T, Miyizaki H, Sekine Y, Shimizu M, et al. (1982). Pharmacokinetic studies of AD-810, a new antiepileptic compound. Arzneim.-Forsch./Drug Res. **32**, 1581–1586.

Textbooks and Review Articles

r1. Porter RJ. (1993). Classification of epileptic seizures and epileptic syndromes. In: A Textbook of Epilepsy; J Laidlaw, A Richens and D Chadwick, eds., Churchill Livingstone, Edinburgh, 1–22.

r2. Morselli PL, Lloyd KG. (1985). Mechanism of action of antiepileptic drugs. In: The Epilepsies; RJ Porter, PL Morselli, eds., Butterworth & Co. Ltd., London, 40–81.

r3. Meldrum B. (1981). GABA-agonists as anti-epileptic agents. In: GABA and Benzodiazepine Receptors; E Costa, et al., eds., Raven Press, New York, 207–217.

r4. Morselli PL, Bartholini G, Lloyd KG. (1986). Progabide. In: New Anticonvulsant Drugs; BS Meldrum, RJ Porter, eds., John Libbey & Co, Ltd., London, 237–253.

r5. Grant SM, Heel RC. (1991). Vigabatrin: a review of its pharmacodynamic and pharmacokinetic properties, and therapeutic potential in epilepsy and disorders of motor control. Drugs **41**, 889–926.

r6. Löscher W, Schmidt D. (1993). Central & peripheral nervous system: new drugs for the treatment of epilepsy. Curr. Opin. Invest. Drugs **2**, 1067–1095.

r7. Rogawski MA, Porter RJ. (1990). Antiepileptic drugs: pharmacological mechanisms and clinical efficacy with consideration of promising developmental stage compounds. Pharmacol. Rev. **42**, 223–286.

r8. McNamara JO. (1986). Kindling model of epilepsy. In: Advances in Neurology, Vol. 44; AV Delgado-Escueta, AA Ward Jr, DM Woodbury and RJ Porter, eds., Raven Press, New York, 303–318.

r9. Ribak CE. (1986). Contemporary methods in neurocytology and their application to the study of epilepsy. In: Advances in Neurology, Vol. 44; AV Delgado-Escueta, AA Ward Jr, DM Woodbury and RJ Porter, eds., Raven Press, New York, 739–764.

r10. Babb TL, Pretorius JK. (1993). Pathologic substrates of epilepsy. In: The Treatment of Epilepsy: Principles and Practice; E Wyllie, ed., Lea & Febiger, Philadelphia, 55–70.

r11. Lloyd KG, Bossi L, Morselli PL, Munari C, Rougier M, Loiseau H. (1986). Alterations of GABA-mediated synaptic transmission in human epilepsy. In: Advances in Neurology, Vol. 44; AV Delgado-Escueta, AA Ward Jr, DM Woodbury and RJ Porter, eds., Raven Press, New York, 1033–1044.

r12. Lloyd KG, Zivkovic B, Scatton B, Bartholini G. (1984). Evidence for functional roles of GABA pathways in the mammalian brain. In: Actions and Interactions of GABA and Benzodiazepines; NG Bowery, ed., Raven Press, New York, 59–79.

r13. Meldrum B, Braestrup C. (1984). GABA and the anticonvulsant action of benzodiazepines and related drugs. In: Actions and Interactions of GABA and Benzodiazepines; NG Bowery, ed., Raven Press, New York, 133–153.

r14. Macdonald RL, Kelly KM. (1993). Antiepileptic drug mechanisms of action. Epilepsia **34** (Suppl. 5), S1–S8.

r15. Catteral WA. (1987). Common modes of drug action on Na^+ channels: local anesthetics, antiarrhythmics and anticonvulsants. TIPS **8**, 57–65.

r16. Rogawski MA. (1992). The NMDA receptor, NMDA antagonists and epilepsy therapy: a status report. Drugs **44**, 279–292.

r17. Meldrum BS. (1992). Excitatory amino acids in epilepsy and potential novel therapies. Epilepsy Res. **12**, 189–196.

r18. Fisher RS. (1989). Animal models of the epilepsies. Brain Res. Rev. **14**, 245–278.

r19. Wilder BJ, McLean JR, Uthman BM. (1993). Phenytoin. In: The Treatment of Epilepsy: Principles and Practices; E Wyllie, ed., Lea & Febiger, Philadelphia, 887–897.

r20. Leppik IE. (1992). Phenytoin. In: The Medical Treatment of Epilepsy; SR Resor Jr, H Kutt, eds., Marcel Dekker, Inc., New York, 279–289.

r21. Pisani F, Perucca E, Di Perri R. (1990). Clinically relevant antiepileptic drug interactions. J. Int. Med. Res. **18**, 1–15.

r22. Brodie MJ. (1992). Drug interactions in epilepsy. Epilepsia **33** (Suppl. 1), S13–S22.

r23. Post RM. (1988). Time course of clinical effects of carbamazepine: implications for mechanisms of action. J. Clin. Psychiatry **49** (Suppl.), 35–48.

r24. Schmidt D, Rohrer E. (1992). Carbamazepine. In: The Medical Treatment of Epilepsy; SR Resor Jr, H Kutt, eds., Marcel Dekker, Inc., New York, 293–303.

r25. Dean JC, Penry JK. (1992). Valproate. In: The Medical Treatment of Epilepsy; SR Resor Jr, H Kutt, eds., Marcel Dekker, Inc., New York, 265–275.

r26. Dean JC. (1993). Valproate. In: The Treatment of Epilepsy: Principles and Practices; E Wyllie, ed., Lea & Febiger, Philadelphia, 915–921.

r27. Homan RW, Rosenberg HC. (1993). Benzodiazepines. In: The Treatment of Epilepsy: Principles and Practice; E Wyllie, ed., Lea & Febiger, Philadelphia, 932–949.

r28. Kutt H. (1992). Diazepam. In: The Medical Treatment of Epilepsy; SR Resor Jr, H Kutt, eds., Marcel Dekker, Inc., New York, 341–343.

r29. Kutt H, Resor Jr SR. (1992). Lorazepam. In: The Medical Treatment of Epilepsy; SR Resor Jr, and H Kutt, eds., Marcel Dekker, Inc., New York, 353–355.

r30. Larbisseau AL. (1992). Clonazepam and nitrazepam. In: The Medical Treatment of Epilepsy; SR Resor Jr, and H Kutt, eds., Marcel Dekker, Inc., New York, 329–337.

r31. Trimble MR. (1992). Clobazam. In: The Medical Treatment of Epilepsy; SR Resor Jr, H Kutt, eds., Marcel Dekker, Inc., New York, 319–327.

r32. Richens A, Perucca E. (1993). Clinical pharmacology and medical treatment. In: A Textbook of Epilepsy; J Laidlaw, A Richens and D Chadwick, eds., Churchill Livingstone, Edinburgh, 495–559.

r33. Gallagher BB. (1992). Phenobarbital. In: The Medical Treatment of Epilepsy; SR Resor Jr, H Kutt, eds., Marcel Dekker, Inc., New York, 357–361.

r34. Painter MJ, Gaus LM. (1993). Phenobarbital. In: The Treatment of Epilepsy: Principles and Practices; E Wyllie, ed., Lea & Febiger, Philadelphia, 900–907.

r35. Bourgeois BFD. (1993). Primidone. In: The Treatment of Epilepsy: Principles and Practices; E Wyllie, ed., Lea & Febiger, Philadelphia, 909–913.

r36. Uthman BM, Wilder BJ. (1993). Less commonly used antiepileptic drugs. In: The Treatment of Epilepsy: Principles and Practices; E Wyllie, ed., Lea & Febiger, Philadelphia, 959–973.

r37. Shafer SQ. (1992). Piracetam. In: The Medical Treatment of Epilepsy; SR Resor Jr, H Kutt, eds., Marcel Dekker, Inc., New York, 489–490.

r38. Van Woert MH, Chung E. (1992). L-5-Hydroxytryptophan. In: The Medical Treatment of Epilepsy; SR Resor Jr, H Kutt, eds., Marcel Dekker, Inc., New York, 485–487.

r39. Snead III OC. (1993). Adrenocorticotropic Hormone (ACTH). In: The Treatment of Epilepsy: Principles and Practices; E Wyllie, ed., Lea & Febiger, Philadelphia, 950–953.

r40. Grant SM, Faulds D. (1992). Oxcarbazepine: a review of its pharmacology and therapeutic potential in epilepsy, trigeminal neuralgia and affective disorders. Drugs **43**, 873–888.

r41. Goa KL, Ross SR, Chrisp P. (1993). Lamotrigine: a review of its pharmacological properties and clinical efficacy in epilepsy. Drugs **46**, 152–176.

r42. Peters DH, Sorkin EM. (1993). Zonisamide: a review of its pharmacodynamic and pharmacokinetic properties, and therapeutic potential in epilepsy. Drugs **45**, 760–787.

r43. Henry TR, Sackellares JC. (1992). Zonisamide. In: The Medical Treatment of Epilepsy; SR Resor Jr, H Kutt, eds., Marcel Dekker, Inc., New York, 423–427.

CHAPTER 20

Andrew P. Smith
Nancy M. Lee
Horace H. Loh

Opioid Analgesics and Antagonists

The opioids are a highly diverse group of drugs, including plant-derived alkaloids, a number of synthetic compounds, and a large group of peptides found in the mammalian brain. They have a broad range of physiologic effects, but are used primarily because of their ability to induce analgesia (relief of pain) and euphoria (a feeling of intense pleasure). Their analgetic properties have made opioids the drugs of choice for alleviating the intense pain and/or anxiety associated with such conditions as heart attack and traumatic injuries, for postsurgical anesthesia, and to ease the chronic pain of patients suffering from cancer and other terminal illnesses. The euphoria or "high" induced by opioids, on the other hand, has resulted in extensive recreational use.[r1]

Another characteristic and often problematical feature of most opioids becomes apparent during their chronic administration. Repeated use generally leads to tolerance, a state in which increasing doses of drug are needed to achieve a given effect, and to physical dependence, in which regular administration of drug is required to prevent painful withdrawal symptoms. Tolerance limits the clinical usefulness of opioids in long-term pain management, because it progressively blunts their analgetic effectiveness. Physical dependence, together with a less measurable psychologic dependence, makes these drugs highly addictive.

The first opioids, including **morphine, codeine,** and **papaverine,** were isolated and characterized from the juice (Greek, οποχ) of the opium poppy, and for many years most known opioids were such plant-derived substances, or their chemically synthesized congeners. In the mid-1970s, however, our understanding of opioids underwent a profound transformation, with the discovery of peptides in mammalian brain with opioid-like properties. The existence of such endogenous opioids had actually been predicted much earlier, since other classes of drugs had been shown to be closely related structurally to endogenous substances.

Subsequent work has provided strong evidence that the endogenous opioid peptides play important roles in the brain in pain regulation and other functions. Like other biologic messengers, they mediate their effects by interacting with specific receptors, which are located on the surface of certain cells in the CNS. Exogenous alkaloids such as morphine interact with the same receptors as the endogenous opioids.

Because of this recent work, opioids can be now regarded in the same way that has become conventional with most other drugs—that is, as substances that mimic natural biologic messengers in the body. In this chapter, we shall take that approach. After a brief discussion of the history of these drugs, we will examine the endogenous opioids and the receptors through which they are thought to act. Subsequently, we will consider the pharmacologic effects and clinical uses of the exogenous opioids.

History

As is the case with other substances having powerful subjective effects, the use of opioids goes very far back in history; indeed, they may be the oldest psychoactive substances known to humanity. Apparently opium juice was used as a general sedative or sleep-promoting treatment by the ancient Babylonians as early as 4000 BC, and was well known subsequently to both the Greeks and the Romans. It was later introduced into China by merchants from the Middle East. It became popular in Europe during the Renaissance. Morphine, the major opioid drug present in opium, and still the one most commonly used clinically today, was isolated in the beginning of the 19th century.

Throughout this period, opium was viewed as a highly beneficial medicine. One of the earliest warnings against its addictive liabilities was raised by the Chinese emperor Tao Kuang, who banned opium smoking. However, after victory by the British in the subsequent Opium Wars, the drug continued to be imported into China. In America, thousands of soldiers developed serious opioid habits during the Civil War, when the drug, readily administered through the newly-invented hypodermic syringe, was commonly used during treatment of battle injuries.

Nevertheless, opioid addiction was not recognized as a serious problem in the US until the beginning of the 20th century. By this time, the use of opioids had been greatly enhanced by the general availability of pure preparations of morphine, and by the widespread availability of syringes. The Narcotic Act of 1914 outlawed the general use of morphine. Though its clinical use as an analgesic was still permitted, it became illegal for physicians to use morphine to maintain or reduce the habit of addicts.

Since this time, the use/abuse of opioids among the general population has occurred in cycles. Use of heroin, now the most widely-abused opioid, reached a peak in the US, estimated at three quarters of a million, in the early 1970s. The abuse of opioids has declined somewhat since that period, stabilizing at about 500,000 users. Abuse of other opioids, primarily meperidine and morphine, also occurs among doctors, nurses, and other professionals who have direct access to these drugs.

Chemistry

Opioid Alkaloid Agonists and Antagonists

Morphine is the major alkaloid component of opium, and its properties make it typical of this group of substances. Its structure and those of some commonly-used derivatives are shown in Figure 20.1A. The three-ring motif is known as the phenanthrene nucleus; it is found in other natural and synthetic opioids with analgetic activity, including heroin, codeine, and levorphanol. All of them possess a structure basically similar to morphine, differing only in the nature of the groups found at the 3 and 6 positions and on the nitrogen. Most exhibit the same range of pharmacologic effects as morphine, though at widely different potencies.

Since the turn of the century, chemists have synthesized a large number of compounds structurally related to morphine. The goal of these studies—to develop an opioid compound capable of inducing analgesia without the side-effects and addictive liability of morphine—was not realized; but this work did provide an enormous amount of information about the structural requirements for opioid activity. These studies indicated that opioid receptors have distinct sites that interact with specific groups at the 3 and 6 positions of the phenanthrene complex, and with the nitrogen. Other portions of the molecule apparently are not critical for opioid activity. This conclusion has been reinforced by the synthesis of compounds that are not closely related to morphine structurally, yet which have many of its properties, including the ability to induce analgesia. Examples include **methadone, meperidine,** and **propoxyphene,** which contain a 2-ring nucleus (Fig. 20.1B). These compounds, despite their limited structural resemblance to morphine, contain substituents that can interact with critical portions of the opioid binding site.

Some compounds, however, bind to opioid receptors but do not induce analgesia or other effects of opioids. In fact, when given with morphine or other active opioids, they *inhibit* analgesia and other opioid effects. These substances, known as **opioid antagonists,** include synthetic alkaloids such as **naloxone** and **naltrexone** (Fig. 20.1C). The structure of these drugs differs from that of morphine and other agonists primarily in that they possess relatively bulky substituents on the pyridine nitrogen. It is believed that these bulky N-substituents prevent normal interaction of the compound with an appropriate site on the receptor responsible for the effects of opioids. Therefore, while the antagonist can bind to the receptor, it cannot trigger the subsequent biochemical processes necessary to mediate the effects of opioids; it can, however, prevent the action of endogenously released or exogenously administered opioids.

Some opioids have both agonistic and antagonistic effects. As will be discussed in more detail below, several different opioid receptor types are present in brain, and are thought to mediate somewhat different pharmacologic effects. Mixed agonist-antagonists, such as **pentazocine** and **nalorphine** (Fig. 20.1D), act at more than one of these receptors. Finally, several other opioids, known as partial agonists, can have both agonist and antagonist effects for a different reason. Though they induce analgesia, they do not achieve the full analgetic effect seen with morphine and related opioid agonists. Thus, when given in conjunction with the latter, they compete with morphine, reducing its effects to some degree. **Buprenorphine** is one such partial agonist (Fig. 20.1E).

Endogenous Opioid Peptides

Like the opioid alkaloids, the endogenous opioid peptides are extremely diverse, and include both natural and synthetic substances. They can be grouped into three major classes: β-endorphin and related peptides; the enkephalins; and dynorphin and related peptides (Fig. 20.1F; Tables 20.1 and 20.2). Members of each class derive from a genetically distinct, larger precursor molecule: β-endorphin from pro-opiomelanocortin (POMC); the enkephalins from pro-enkephalin A; and dynorphin from pro-enkephalin B (pro-dynorphin).[1,2,r2] All are distributed fairly widely throughout the CNS (Table 20.1).

Although the endogenous opioid peptides vary greatly in length, all share a common sequence at their amino-terminus, consisting of the amino acids tyrosine-glycine-glycine-phenylalanine-methionine (or leucine). As shown in Fig. 20.1F, the conformation of this sequence bears a resemblance to the active portion of opioid alkaloids. Thus the opioid peptides and the opioid alkaloids, though chemically very different molecules, apparently present a somewhat similar conformation to their receptors. Since the N-terminal sequence of all opioid peptides is the same, it is apparently differences in the length and amino acid sequence of the C-terminal portions of these peptides that determine their selectivity for different types of opioid receptors (see Fig. 20.1F). This has led to the proposal that some of the longer opioid peptides, such as β-endorphin and dynorphin, interact with additional sites besides those that interact with morphine and other alkaloids.[3]

Opioid peptides are produced from their respective precursors by a series of steps in which the large precursor molecule is broken down into smaller peptides by specific enzymes. Most of these enzymes cleave the bonds between adjacent basic amino acids, arginine and lysine; thus, by identifying where in the precursor sequence these basic amino acid pairs are located, investigators have been able to predict the sequences of smaller opioid peptides that should be formed by proteolytic cleavage. A large number of these peptides can be produced from each of the three major precursor peptides, and many of these smaller peptides have now been isolated and to some extent characterized. Each smaller opioid peptide may have a distinct pattern of selectivity for particular types of opioid receptors. Thus,

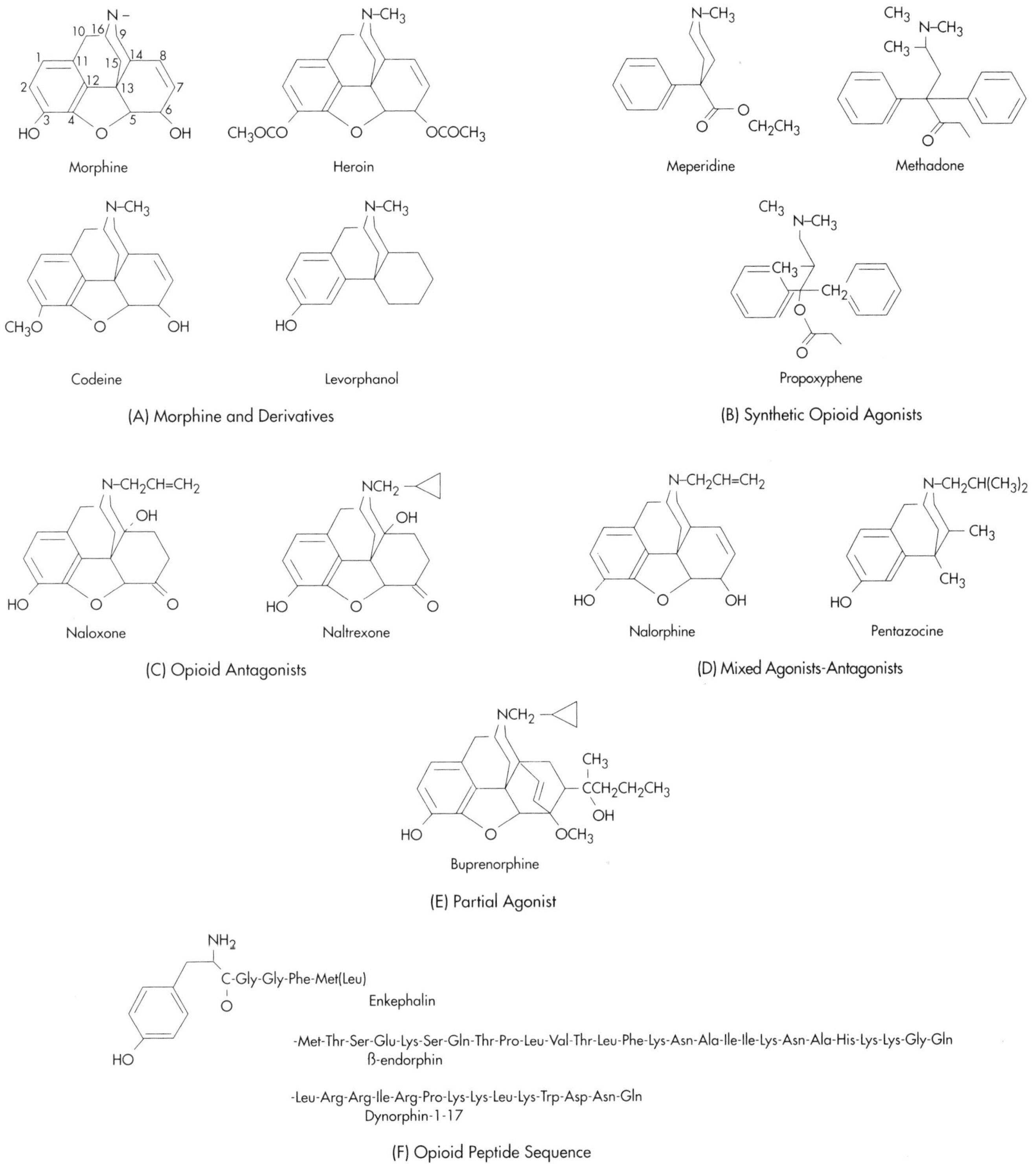

Figure 20.1 Chemical Structures of Various Opioids. See text for other details.

differential processing is probably an important regulatory mechanism by which the cell can determine the specificity of its opioid messengers. Even when different regions of the CNS contain the same concentration of opioid peptide precursors, they may vary widely with respect to the type and concentration of smaller opioid peptides because of differences in their content of processing enzymes.[4,5]

Endogenous Alkaloids

Although most endogenous opioids are peptides, several laboratories recently have reported the detection of opioid alkaloids in some mammalian systems. Morphine and codeine have been identified in rat brain and in bovine hypothalamus and adrenal;

Table 20.1 Opioid Peptide Classes

Precursor	Typical Members	CNS Localization
Pro-opiomelanocortin	β-endorphin	Primarily pituitary, hypothalamus, stria terminalis, amygdala, thalamic periventricular nucleus, periaqueductal gray, pons
Pro-enkephalin A	Leucine and methionine enkephalin	Throughout CNS, with highest concentrations in amygdala, globus pallidus, hypothalamus, thalamus, pons, spinal cord
Pro-enkephalin B	Dynorphin A(1-17)	Throughout most of CNS, with highest concentrations in hippocampus, hypothalamus, substantia nigra, spinal cord

Table 20.2 Classes, Ligands, and CNS Distribution of Multiple Opioid Receptors

Receptor Type	Representative Agonists	Endogenous Agonists	CNS Localization
Mu (μ)	D-ala^2-N-met^4-enkephalin-gly-ol (DAMGO)	β-endorphin	Throughout brain and spinal cord, with highest concentrations in amygdala, nucleus accumbens, thalamus, interpeduncular nucleus, superior and inferior colliculi, nucleus tractus solitarus
Delta (δ)	D-Pen^{2,5}-enkephalin (DPDPE)	leucine and methionine enkephalin, β-endorphin	Primarily telencephalon
Kappa (κ)	U-50,488H	Dynorphin A (1–17)	Throughout brain and spinal cord, with highest concentrations in preoptic area, hypothalamus, nucleus tractus solitarus

morphine has also been detected in toad skin.[6,7] In addition, an enzyme that catalyzes a critical step in the synthesis of morphine in the opium poppy has been detected in rat liver.[8] Since no endogenous opioid peptide with high selectivity for mμ opioid receptors has been reported, it has been proposed that morphine is the endogenous ligand for this type of receptor. However, the physiologic significance of endogenous morphine has not yet been established.

Pharmacologic Effects of Opioids

Though their signal property and most important clinical action is analgesia, opioids have a broad range of effects in the body, both within and outside the CNS (summarized in Table 20.3). In the descriptions that follow, we will consider primarily the actions of morphine, which to some extent are typical of most opioids. However, other opioids do differ significantly in some of their nonanalgetic effects, and this may make them preferable to morphine under certain conditions.

Analgesia and Other Subjective Effects

The opioids have a wide range of effects in the body, but the most important is the relief of pain (see Table 20.4). A dose of 5–10 mg of morphine per 70 kg body weight, given subcutaneously (SQ) or intramuscularly (IM) to a nontolerant individual (no previous exposure to the drug) induces a general analgesia beginning within 15–20 min, and lasting for several hours. Analgesia (or more accurately, since analgesia refers to a subjective state, antinociception) is also observed in other mammals, as determined by their resistance to thermal stimuli such as heat applied to the

Table 20.3 Principal Pharmacologic Effects of Morphine

Analgesia
Respiratory Depression
Motor Effects
Constipation
Hypothermia
Vasodilation
Hormonal Effects
Immunomodulation
Feeding Behavior
Response to Trauma
Suppress Cough Reflex

Table 20.4 Clinical Parameters for Morphine and Other Opioid Analgesics

Class & Generic Name	Proprietary Name	Approx. Dose (mg) & route	Oral: Parenteral	Duration of Action Onset (min)	Peak (min)	$T_{1/2}$ (hr)	Potency (morphine=1)
(A) Morphine and Derivatives							
Morphine	—	8–20 IM	1:3	60	60–90	3	1
Heroin[1]	—	5–10 IM	1:25	20–30	30–45	3	1.5
Codeine[2]	—	30–60 PO	1:1.5	30	45–60	3	0.08
Levorphanol	Levo-Dromoran	2–3 IM	1:2–1:1	20–60	60–120	12–16	5
(B) Synthetic Opioid Agonists							
Methadone	Dolophine	2.5–10 IM	1:2	30–60	30–120	15	0.8
Meperidine	Demerol	60–80 IM	1:3	40–60	60–120	2.5	0.125
Propoxyphene[2]	Darvon	100 PO	—[3]	40–60	90–180	6–12	0.06
(D) Mixed Agonist—Antagonist							
Pentazocine	Talwin	25–100 PO	1:4	40–60	60–180	2	0.06
(E) Partial Agonist							
Buprenorphine	Buprenex[4]	0.2–0.6 IM	1:0.75	60–120	120–240	3.5	25–50
(F) Opioid Anaesthetics[5]							
Fentanyl	Sublimaze	0.2 IV	—	rapid	20–30	3.7	50
Sufentanil	Sufenta	0.5 IV	—[1]	v. rapid	mins	2.5	600–700
Alfentanil	Rapifen	0.5 IV	—[1]	rapid	5–10	1.6	16.5

[1]Not used in U.S.
[2]Codeine and propoxyphene are usually supplied in combination with acetaminophen or aspirin. This combination produces an analgesic potency greater than the sum of the two alone.
[3]IV administration of propoxyphene produces irritation and damage to veins.
[4]Also administered subligually (Temgesic).
[5]Administered IV alone or in combination with a neuroleptic agent to produce anesthesia.

tail or the feet. This resistance can be quantitated, for example, by measuring the time taken for the animal to withdraw from the noxious stimulus, and in this manner constitutes a standard laboratory assay for opioids.

In humans, morphine and other commonly-used opioids may have other subjective effects as well. Morphine often induces euphoria, a state of profound pleasure, which is its chief attraction for recreational drug users. However, in many individuals, particularly those taking the drug for the first time, morphine may have unpleasant effects, inducing dysphoria, nausea, vomiting, changes in mood, and a general disorientation or confusion. These effects are frequently also prominent with mixed agonists-antagonists such as nalorphine or pentazocine. However, compared with other drugs that may also induce some analgesia at sufficient doses (such as ether, alcohol, barbiturates, and nitrous oxide), morphine at analgetic doses interferes relatively little with other mental functions, or with consciousness itself.

Morphine also has sedative effects, and apparently was used for this purpose by the ancients. It may induce drowsiness and sleep, but of a different, more pleasant nature than that of general depressants. Opioids generally decrease aggression, as well as such other fundamental drives as feeding, drinking, and sex.

The opioid peptide β-endorphin is also a potent analgesic, but the natural enkephalins, leucine- and methionine-enkephalin, have little or no analgetic activity, even when injected directly into the brains of experimental animals. Most investigators believe the lack of analgetic potency of enkephalins is due at least in part to the presence of enzymes in the blood and the brain that rapidly degrade these peptides. In support of this, several enkephalin analogues have been synthesized that resist degradation and show analgetic potency.

The opioid peptide dynorphin also does not exhibit analgetic activity when injected into the brain, though it does in the spinal cord. In this case, enzymatic degradation does not appear to account for the lack of analgesia, for dynorphin has other effects when injected into the brain. It modulates the analgesia produced by other opioids such as morphine, inhibiting it in previously untreated animals, yet potentiating it in morphine-tolerant animals.[9] Dynorphin has also been shown to suppress withdrawal symptoms in morphine-dependent monkeys and in human heroin addicts, suggesting that it might be a useful tool in treating opioid addiction.[10] Finally, some early studies reported that β-endorphin could induce a psychosis-like state in human patients, suggesting that certain forms of mental illness might involve alterations in the level or distribution of endogenous opioid peptides.[11] High doses of this peptide also induce unusual behavior in laboratory animals.

Respiration

An important clinical limitation of morphine and other opioids is their ability to depress respiration; both respiratory rate and the volume are affected. Respiration is highly sensitive to morphine, with significant depression detectable even at doses where no analgesia is apparent. Hence, this effect often limits the use of opioids as analgetics, and is the usual direct cause of death by an overdose of opioids. In addition, since morphine crosses the placenta and can depress fetal respiration, it should not be used during labor or in other obstetric procedures.

Morphine is thought to exert its depressant effects on respiration by acting directly on centers in the brain stem that regulate breathing. These centers are responsive to hydrogen ions and to carbon dioxide in the blood, increasing respiration when the concentrations of these metabolites rise. Morphine decreases the responsiveness of these brain stem centers to these physiologic signals, hence inhibiting respiration. It also depresses the activity of other centers in the pons and the medulla that regulate the rhythmicity of breathing. Other opioid alkaloids also depress respiration to about the same degree as morphine at doses that have comparable analgetic effects. Thus, they offer no particular clinical advantage or disadvantage with respect to this side-effect. The opioid peptide β-endorphin also depresses respiration; dynorphin has no effect on respiration by itself, but it increases the respiratory depression induced by morphine when coadministered with this latter opioid.

Motor Effects

Opioids may have a number of effects on central motor control, but as these are usually observed only at relatively high doses, they are generally not regarded as a clinical limitation. Indeed, patients on morphine can usually perform motor tasks without difficulty. At sufficiently high doses, morphine can induce muscular rigidity in humans, and in animals has been observed to cause circling motions and stereotyped behavior patterns. The receptors responsible for these actions are thought to be distinct from those mediating analgesia, and exist in the substantia nigra and in the striatum. However, morphine and β-endorphin at high doses can also induce catalepsy in laboratory animals; in this case they seem to act through the hypothalamus. Opioids may also affect motor behavior by action at the spinal cord level. Generally, morphine stimulates monosynaptic reflexes while inhibiting those mediated by several neurons.

Gastrointestinal (GI) Motility

Morphine and other opioids have a number of effects on the GI tract, which taken together, result in spasmogenicity and constipation. Hence these drugs are useful as antidiarrheals, particularly as they have a significant effect at doses less than those necessary to induce analgesia. A general decrease in motility and increase in tone occurs throughout the stomach and the small and large intestine. Propulsive contractions are decreased in both the large and small intestine; gastric secretions are reduced. The effects of opioids on the GI tract are to a large extent locally mediated, for these effects are observed in experimental animals in which innervation to the intestine has been transected. However, a central effect on intestinal motility has been observed in experiments in which morphine is injected directly into the brain, with the effect being blocked by injections of an opioid antagonist.

Morphine and other opioids also inhibit electrically-induced contractions in the isolated guinea pig ileum, an effect that is used as another important pharmacologic assay for these drugs. A section of the ileum is removed from the animal, placed in a physiologic bathing medium, and set up so that electrical current can be applied to the tissue and the strength of its contractions measured. When added to the bathing medium, morphine and other opioid agonists inhibit these contractions in a dose-dependent fashion, and this effect is blocked by antagonists such as naloxone. Tolerance to this action is also observed. When the ileum is exposed to opioid continuously over a period of time, the ability of the drug to inhibit electrical contractions is gradually reduced.[12]

Temperature Control

Administration of morphine or other opioid agonists results in hypothermia. Opioids are thought to act directly on temperature control areas in the hypothalamus to produce this change. β-endorphin has a similar effect, but dynorphin has little effect on body temperature when given alone. When given together with morphine to animals, however, it enhances the morphine-induced hypothermia.[13]

Cardiovascular Effects

Morphine and other opioids have little effect on blood pressure and heart beat. However, they do have dilatory effects on peripheral veins that can result in orthostatic or postural hypotension. Constriction of these vessels in the musculature is normally an important mechanism by which the cardiovascular system responds to sudden changes in gravity, as occurs when a patient stands up from a prone position. Therefore, opioids should be used with caution in patients suffering from low blood pressure, as in the case of shock. In addition, morphine may release histamine, reducing venous return by this mechanism and through inhibition of centrally-mediated adrenergic tone. Furthermore, blood pressure may be lowered in patients suffering from acute opioid intoxication, as an indirect result of respiratory depression and subsequent hypoxia. As discussed earlier, respiratory depression is highly sensitive to morphine, so its indirect effect on blood pressure may be significant even at subanalgetic doses.

Hormonal Effects

Morphine and other opioids have effects on a wide variety of hormones. While many of these effects depend on the opioid used and the schedule of administration, morphine generally increases circulating levels of antidiuretic hormone (ADH), prolactin (PRL), growth hormone, and somatotropin; it decreases levels of luteinizing hormone (LH), corticotropin, and pituitary gonadotropin.[14,15,16] Since tolerance develops only incompletely at best to many of these effects, chronic opioid users may exhibit significant hormonal imbalances, especially in sex hormones. For example, male opioid addicts have been observed to have decreased sex drive; menstruation may be suppressed in females.

With the discovery of the endogenous opioid peptides, the connection between opioids and hormones has become clearer. For example, pro-opiomelanocortin (POMC), the precursor for β-endorphin, also contains the adrenocorticotropic hormone (ACTH) sequence. Hence, it might be expected that processes that regulate the levels of ACTH would also affect levels of β-endorphin, and this has been observed experimentally in some tissues, under certain conditions. Endogenous opioids, in their putative roles as neurotransmitters or neuromodulators, may also directly affect the activity of cells in the pituitary and other tissues that release hormones.

Immunomodulation[r3]

A large body of evidence indicates that morphine and other opioids can have major effects on the functioning of the immune system. Over 20 years ago, it was shown that opioid abusers frequently have increased incidences of various infectious diseases and alterations in such immune parameters as complement levels and the number and proliferative response of T-cells.[17,18,19,20] However, such effects could obviously be indirect, the result of sharing of needles, poor diet, and other factors. More recently, direct effects of opioids on the immune system have been demonstrated in animals and in isolated human cell cultures.[21] Both morphine and endogenous opioids such as β-endorphin alter the proliferative response of T-cells, a major weapon of the body in fighting foreign cells and substances.[22,23,24] They also may alter the activity of natural killer (NK) cells, which nonspecifically attack invading cells and viruses.[25,26] Opioids have also been reported to alter the circulating levels of lymphokines,[27] chemical growth factors that play a critical role in the maturation and proliferation of many types of immune cells. A recent study found that opioids could also suppress proliferation of bone marrow cells, which are the progenitors of all mature immune cells.[28]

How opioids achieve these effects on the immune system is not known, but opioid receptors and opioid peptides have also been detected in several kinds of immune cells. Many of the in vivo and in vitro effects of opioids on the immune system are not prevented by naloxone, indicating that the drugs do not act through conventionally defined opioid receptors. Furthermore, different laboratories have reported both increases and decreases of many immune functions in response to opioids. Regardless of how opioid effects on the immune system are mediated, they must be regarded as a major side-effect of opioid use.

Feeding Behavior

Considerable interest in the involvement of opioids in feeding behavior has arisen in recent years.[29] Several laboratories have reported that either acute or chronic administration of opioid agonists stimulates food intake in experimental animals, whereas antagonists such as naloxone have the opposite effect. Both mu and kappa agonists, and possibly delta agonists, can alter feeding behavior.[30,31] Opioid agonists may also alter dietary patterns. Generally speaking, agonists result in a greater increase in intake of fats than of carbohydrates. Some studies have also shown changes in the levels of opioid receptors in the brain as a result of fasting or other dietary manipulations. These studies suggest that endogenous opioid peptides are involved in feeding behavior, and raise the possibility that opioid antagonists might be used to help control weight in humans. However, it is not yet clear whether opioids have a direct effect on feeding behavior by regulating brain centers involved in the sensation of hunger, or whether their effects on food intake are mediated indirectly, through other kinds of behavior.

Response to Stress or Trauma

Much evidence has implicated endogenous opioid systems in the body's response to stress.[32,33] Levels of these peptides are altered in specific regions of the brain and spinal cord of laboratory animals by acute or chronic stress. Several studies have also shown that both morphine and endogenous opioids have anticonvulsant activity. Opioids have also been implicated in the response to brain injury. Several laboratories have reported that in both humans and experimental animals morphine exacerbates the effects of stroke, whereas antagonists such as naloxone can prolong survival and in some cases improve neurologic deficits.[34,35] Dynorphin has also been reported to prolong post-stroke survival in animals.[36] These opioids do not result in significant repair of damaged tissue, but may facilitate the process by which uninjured portions of the brain take over functions of injured ones. To date, these promising findings have not been applied clinically.

Centrally-Mediated Reflexes

Morphine and most other opioids suppress the cough reflex. Unlike most other actions of opioids, this effect is not stereospecific; thus D-racemic forms such as dextromethorphan, which lack the analgetic activity and other effects of opioids, can be used as safe, effective antitussive agents.

Morphine and other opioids stimulate brain stem centers that result indirectly in nausea and vomiting, which are the commonest unpleasant side-effects of these drugs in the initial user. However, morphine can also inhibit the vomiting center directly. Opioid agonists also produce pupillary contraction, or miosis, by action on the nucleus of the third cranial nerve. This is an important diagnostic indicator of opioid use in patients who cannot or will not provide this information. It is especially useful in that tolerance does not develop to this effect of opioid agonists. Thus, miosis is present in both chronic and acute users of opioids.

Therapeutic Uses and Limitations of Opioids

The primary use of opioids is to relieve intense pain, both physical and psychologic. They are most commonly administered to patients suffering from heart attacks, shock, and serious traumatic injuries, and may also be used to relieve postoperative pain and to alleviate both physical pain and anxiety in individuals with terminal illnesses, such as cancer. They are used, to a lesser extent, for treating relatively minor problems, including coughing and diarrhea. While all opioid agonists have these effects, different opioids may be preferred in specific situations. For example, codeine and meperidine are relatively more effective orally than morphine. In addition, codeine is much weaker than most other opioid agonists, and thus may be useful in controlling relatively minor forms of pain with less risk of inducing dependence. Meperidine is less spasmogenic than morphine, and so has fewer severe effects on the digestive organs.

Whenever opioid use is indicated, the physician should be aware of the addictive potential of these drugs. Patients given opioids to relieve relatively temporary pain generally do not develop a significant dependence on the drug; however, when opioids are given repeatedly over a period of several weeks, some tolerance and physical dependence is inevitable, and psychologic dependence also may emerge. With tolerance, the patient requires increasingly larger doses to achieve a given degree of analgesia, and in some extreme cases, the full analgetic effect may be lost, even at very high doses. Such patients are also physically dependent on the opioid, in that regular administration of the drug is necessary to prevent withdrawal symptoms. These chronic effects of opioids should not be a consideration with the terminally ill, as the use of these drugs is generally the only alternative to a life of unremitting pain. For those whose pain is not permanent, however, the situation is not as clear-cut, and the physician's choice is more difficult. The conventional attitude, born of a deep fear of inducing addiction, is to avoid prescribing opioids except in the most extreme cases, and then only at low doses that may be insufficient to relieve pain completely. While addiction may be avoided, the patient may pay a very high price in pain and discomfort.

A newer school of thought holds that physicians should not hesitate to prescribe these drugs in whatever doses are necessary to relieve pain. This approach is based on evidence that individuals who take opioids to relieve physical pain, rather than for their euphoric effects, rarely develop a serious addiction.[37] These studies also suggest that when the patients themselves are allowed to control their drug dosage, through self-administration, they avoid much of the anxiety that would otherwise arise as the effects of the most recent dose wear off. It is probably safe to say that undermedication, rather than overmedication, is currently a greater problem with opioids. However, it should always be kept in mind that any medical patient who has a prior significant abuse problem with some drug—and studies suggest these people comprise 10–20 percent of the population—is very likely to develop an abuse problem if administered opioids over a prolonged period. Alternative methods of alleviating pain, involving not only newer types of drugs, but nonchemical approaches such as electrical stimulation of discrete areas in the brain or spinal cord, may eventually make this a moot issue. For the present, however, both physician and patient should be aware of the benefits and risks of opioids. In many cases, a satisfactory degree of pain relief can be achieved by using a relatively weak and less addicting opioid, such as codeine, or by using a low dose of a stronger opioid such as morphine in conjunction with caffeine, which enhances the analgetic effect of opioid agonists.

Other limitations of opioids may arise in specific cases. As discussed previously, respiratory depression occurs with very low doses of opioids, and this may be an important consideration in treating patients who have diseases, such as emphysema or asthma, that make breathing difficult. In the case of asthma, other opioid effects may also aggravate the condition, including cough suppression and histamine release. Morphine is sometimes contraindicated for patients with head injury, as this may aggravate the respiratory depression. Subsequent elevation of carbon dioxide in the blood increases cerebral blood flow and thus intracranial pressure. The respiratory depressive effects of morphine seem to be more acute on fetuses, and thus this drug should be used only with great caution to alleviate the pain of childbirth.

As discussed earlier, opioids lower blood pressure, and must be used with caution in treating patients in shock or with significant blood loss. Morphine and many other opioids may also aggravate liver disease, as they are metabolized primarily in this organ and may overburden it.

Opioids may interact with several other classes of drugs, particularly with antidepressants and antipsychotics. These drugs generally enhance the depressive and/or sedative effects of opioids, and in some cases their analgetic effects as well. Contrary to this general conclusion, some phenothiazines reduce the analgetic effect of morphine. Monoamine oxidase (MAO) inhibitors in combination with meperidine may result in excitation, delirium, convulsions, and severe respiratory depression. Caffeine and amphetamine have the well-documented effect of greatly enhancing opioid analgesia. Coadministration of such drugs with opioids can reduce the amount of opioid needed to alleviate pain.

Mechanisms of Action of Opioids

The most important action of morphine and other opioids, analgesia, is thought to be mediated through a series of descending pathways from brain centers to the spinal cord (Fig. 20.2). The end-effect of this system is to inhibit the electrical activity of neurons in the dorsal horn of the spinal cord that transmit pain impulses from peripheral receptors—on the body's surface or from internal organs—to the brain. According to a recent hypothesis, opioids act initially in the periaqueductal gray (PAG) region of the brain; PAG neurons, in turn, project to and activate medullary centers, particularly the nucleus raphe magnus (NRM).[38] Axons from NRM neurons descend in a tract in the dorsal horn of the spinal cord, making inhibitory contact at each segmental level with the pain-transmitting dorsal horn neurons (Fig. 20.2).

This hypothesis has been supported by several lines of evidence. Injection of opioids such as morphine directly into the PAG induces analgesia, as does electrical stimulation of either the PAG or the NRM. Electrical stimulation of these supraspinal centers is, in fact, a promising means of alleviating pain in some patients. Transection of the descending projections from the NRM blocks opioid analgesia, presumably by removing the inhibitory influence of these projections on incoming pain impulses from the periphery. Finally, opioid receptors and endogenous opioid peptides are present in the PAG and also in the spinal cord. In agreement with the latter finding, opioids can induce analgesia not only via the PAG, but also by direct injection into the spinal cord.[39]

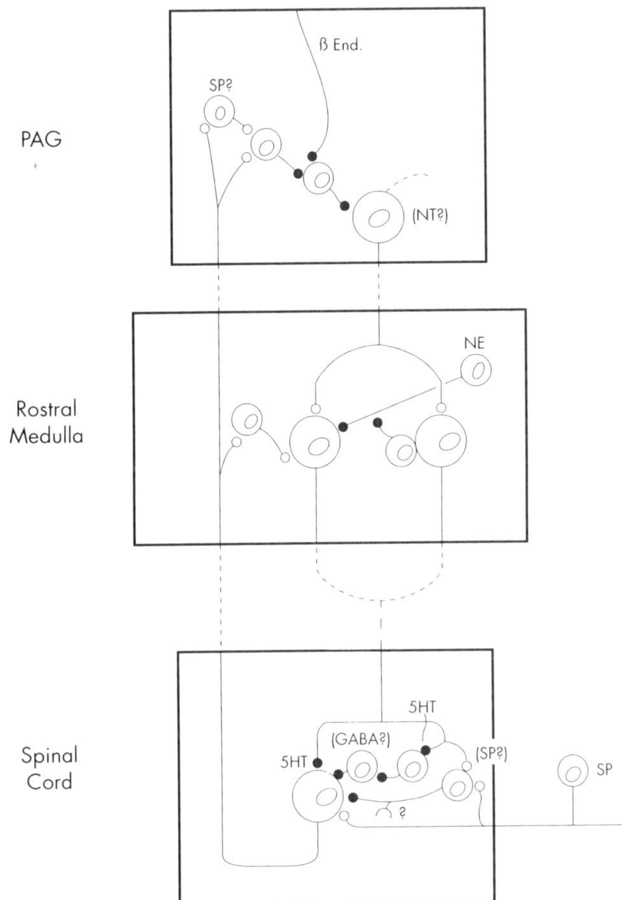

Figure 20.2 Spinal and supraspinal components of proposed opioid pain modulation system (from ref. 7). The system consists of 3 interacting levels, the periaqueductal gray (PAG), rostral medulla, and dorsal horn of the spinal cord. Participating neurons are indicated schematically as a large soma with a single process ending in a presynaptic terminal. Shaded somae indicate the presence of an endogenous opioid peptide, while unfilled somae contain a nonopioid neurotransmitter. Excitatory and inhibitory presynaptic terminals are indicated by clear and solid knobs, respectively. βEnd, β-endorphin; SP, substance P; NT, neurotensin; NE, norepinephrine; 5HT, serotonin; GABA, γ-aminobutyric acid.

Opioid Receptors[r4,r5]

As with other drugs, the initial action of opioids is binding to specific receptor molecules present in certain cells. Opioid receptors were first identified in mammalian brain in the early 1970s, when it was shown that radioactive opioids bound specifically to subcellular fractions of brain.[40,41,42] This binding satisfied many of the criteria conventionally used to identify opioids in pharmacologic assays. The binding was stereospecific, with only the L-forms of opioids interacting with the receptor; and it could be blocked by naloxone. In addition, there was a good correlation between binding potency and analgetic potency, with the most potent opioid analgetics generally showing the highest affinity for receptors.

Multiple Opioid Receptors[r6]

Although all opioid agonists share certain physiologic effects, most notably analgesia, significant differences in the effects of these drugs also have been observed. For example, ketocyclazocine and related drugs lack the euphoria-inducing properties of morphine, producing sedation instead. These latter drugs also cannot prevent withdrawal symptoms in morphine-dependent animals, though they do induce both analgesia and tolerance by themselves. Another opioid, the synthetic compound SKF-10047, induces dysphoria and hallucinations. Such observations, demonstrating different actions of opioids, originally led to the postulation of multiple opioid receptors—receptors that differ in their specificity for different opioids and for the pharmacologic effects that they mediate. The original classification included mu (μ) receptors, selective for morphine; kappa (κ), selective for ketocyclazocine; and sigma (σ), selective for the synthetic compound SKF-10047.[43] However, subsequent work has indicated that σ receptors are not conventional opioid receptors. They interact with numerous nonopioid compounds, and the effects of either these compounds or opioids on σ receptors are not blocked by low doses of naloxone.

Another class of opioid receptors, delta (δ), was discovered during studies of an isolated tissue preparation, the mouse vas deferens.[44] The isolated vas deferens contracts in response to electrical stimulation, and opioid agonists inhibit these contractions; as with analgesia and other in vivo effects of opioids, opioid inhibition of these contractions occurs in a dose-dependent fashion, and the inhibition is reversed by antagonists such as naloxone. However, enkephalins were shown to have much greater potency, relative to alkaloid opioids, than is the case for their whole animal in vivo effects. These data led to the proposal that the deferens contains a distinct receptor, δ, specific for enkephalins.

None of the alkaloid opioids nor the natural endogenous peptides is completely specific for a particular receptor type. For example, morphine has some affinity for δ receptors, and the natural enkephalins interact with μ receptors. Recently, however, investigators have synthesized new opioids that have a fairly high degree of selectivity for a particular opioid receptor type.[45] These compounds have been useful in further characterization of these receptor types, and some may prove to be useful clinically.[46] Subsequent work has indicated that δ receptors, like μ and κ receptors, are present in ammalian brain. Still other opioid receptor types have been postulated,[47,48] and recent work has made it clear that μ, δ, and κ opioid receptors are themselves heterogeneous, consisting of two or more receptor subtypes.[49,50,51] However, the three major types of opioid receptors differ substantially in their regional distribution[2] (Table 20.2). Mu opioid receptors have the widest CNS distribution, followed by κ receptors, then δ receptors.

Different opioid receptor types are also found in certain isolated tissue systems with opioid sensitivity. As mentioned above, the pharmacologic selectivity of the mouse vas deferens constituted a main line of evidence for the existence of δ receptors. Opioids also inhibit electrically-induced contractions in the isolated guinea pig ileum; this tissue contains primarily μ and κ receptors. Still another isolated system, consisting of cultured cells formed by fusing neuronal and glial tumor cells, contains exclusively δ opioid receptors.[52] Some of the phamacologic properties of these isolated systems will be discussed below.

The physiologic significance of the different opioid receptor types is not well understood. It is known that μ opioid receptors mediate analgesia, and some evidence suggests that, in brain, they are primarily responsible for this effect. This receptor subtype is found in substantial concentrations in areas involved in opioid analgesia, such as the periaqueductal gray (PAG), and μ-selective opioids appear to be the most potent in inducing analgesia.[53,54,55] While both δ agonists and κ agonists can induce analgesia, understanding the role of their specific receptors in this process is complicated by the fact that most of these agonists can also interact to some extent with μ receptors. In addition, there is evidence that μ and δ receptors may in some cases be physically associated, so that ligands binding to one type of receptor influence activity of the other type.[56] However, opioids also can induce analgesia by acting in the spinal cord, in the dorsal horn where sensory neuron cell bodies are located. All three opioid receptor types are found in the dorsal horn, and there is good evidence that κ as well as μ receptors can mediate analgesia here.

Elucidation of the exact relationship of different opioid receptor types to each other presumably will require knowledge of their structure, obtained, as has been the case with many other cell surface receptors, from purification and cDNA cloning. Purification of opioid receptors has been exceptionally difficult for several reasons, including not only their multiplicity but their sensitivity to detergents commonly used to solubilize receptors. Recently, however, two independent laboratories have reported cloning of the cDNA for the opioid receptor present in NG108-15 cells,[57,58] a neuroblastoma x glioma hybrid. These cells contain exclusively δ opioid receptors, and expression of the cDNA yielded receptors with δ selectivity and the ability to inhibit adenylate cyclase, another feature of receptors in these cells (see below). Moreover, the predicted amino acid sequence of the receptor indicated it is a member of a superfamily of proteins that interact with GTP-binding proteins, and this is also consistent with what is known about opioid receptors in these cells (see below). It will now be possible to determine whether other opioid receptor types have a similar structure, as well as to search for still other types, not identified pharmacologically but with distinct structural differences.

Second Messengers

The binding of a drug molecule to its receptor is only the first step in its physiologic action. Receptors are thought to mediate their pharmacologic effects by interacting with other cellular molecules, known as second messenger systems. In this way, a chain of metabolic events, often quite complex, is triggered in the cell (see Chapters 1 & 12). One of the best known of these second messengers is cyclic AMP, which is synthesized by the enzyme adenylate cyclase. Cyclic AMP may modify the action of other enzymes in the cell, and is particularly intimately involved in the phosphorylation of proteins. A large class of neurotransmitter receptors, including those for α- and β-adrenergic ligands, muscarinic cholinergic ligands, and some serotonergic ligands, has been shown to be coupled closely to adenylate cyclase. This coupling is mediated by a guanosine triphosphate (GTP)-binding protein, or G-protein;[59] see Fig. 20.3). Different G-proteins may have stimulatory or inhibitory effects on adenylate cyclase. Adenylate cyclase has been shown to be associated with δ-type opioid receptors in NG108-15 neuroblastoma x glioma hybrid cells,[60] and in mammalian striatum.[61,62] Opioid receptors in both these systems are coupled to adenylate cyclase through an inhibitory G-protein; thus, opioid agonists induce a decrease in intracellular cyclic AMP levels. More recently, it has been reported that μ and κ opioid receptors inhibit adenylate cyclase in brain and spinal cord, respectively.[63,64,65]

Other studies have shown that μ, δ and κ receptors may be associated with ion channels, which control the influx of cations into the cell.[66] Mu agonists have been shown to increase K^+ conductance in the locus coeruleus and the guinea pig myenteric system, and δ agonists have a similar effect in the latter.[67] Kappa agonists, in contrast, reduce Ca^+ influx in dorsal root ganglion cells as well as in the myenteric plexus.[68] In either case, the end-result is a reduction of transmitter release, and hence a blockade of synaptic transmission. It is not clear whether these effects of opioids are also mediated through G-proteins, but this seems likely, as opioid receptors appear to be coupled to G-proteins throughout the brain.[69,70]

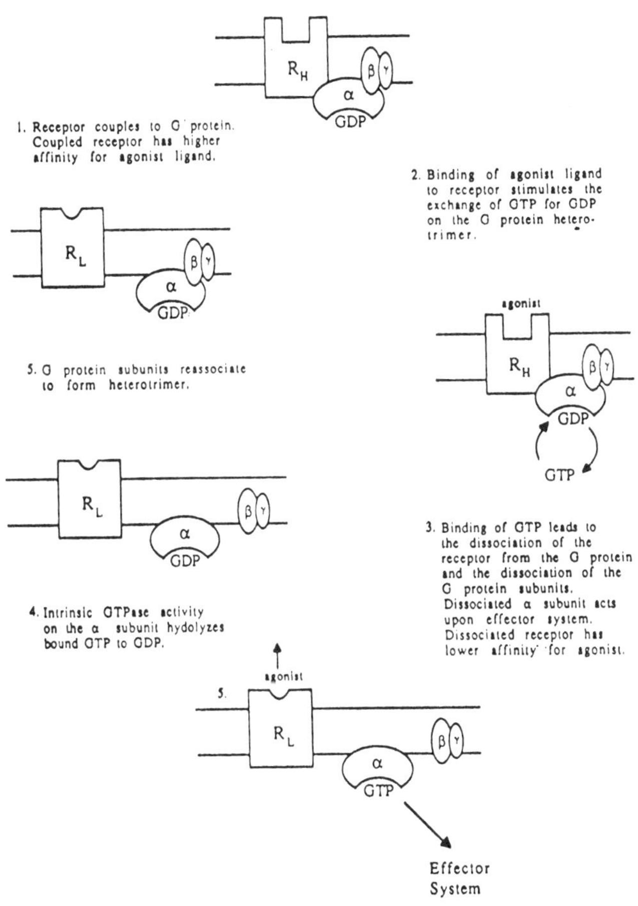

Figure 20.3 Coupling of membrane receptors to G-proteins. The binding of agonist to its receptor is promoted when the latter is in its high-affinity state (RH), as a result of association with a G-protein (1). Following agonist binding, GTP is exchanged for GDP on the α subunit of the G-protein (2), resulting in a dissociation of the α subunit (3). This subunit then affects some intracellular process, such as inhibition of adenylate cyclase. Hydrolysis of the bound GTP results in reassociation of α with the other two subunits (4,5), so that coupling with receptor can reoccur.

Undesirable and Toxic Effects

In addition to addiction, which will be discussed in a later section, the most serious liability of opioids is respiratory depression. In severe cases, resulting from an overdose of drug, this effect may be lethal. In addition to respiratory depression, symptoms of opioid overdose may include deep sleep, sometimes a coma; cold, clammy skin; muscular flaccidity; and pupillary miosis. Of these symptoms, the coma and pinpoint pupils, together with very low breathing rate, are usually sufficient to establish diagnosis of overdose, though naloxone-induced reversal or withdrawal is the definitive test.

Treatment for opioid overdose includes reestablishing respiration and administration of an opioid antagonist, generally naloxone. Since antagonists frequently have a shorter duration of action than agonists, their use should be continued until it is certain that the toxic effects of the agonist have been completely reversed, and do not reemerge. Naloxone has little, if any, physiologic effect on the nondependent organism; so if the patient is known not to have had prior exposure to opioids there is no danger of administering too much antagonist. However, in a person dependent on heroin, morphine, or another opioid, naloxone can provoke a severe withdrawal syndrome, such that its administration must be carried out with great caution.

At lower doses, where there is no threat to life, morphine and other opioids may have other, less serious side-effects, including nausea, vomiting, and difficulty in concentration. These effects are generally most prominent in first-time users, and not in patients who receive the drug chronically to alleviate the pain of a terminal illness. Generally, these effects are also not a problem with patients receiving opioid for surgery, as mental clarity is obviously not necessary at this time.

Opioid Tolerance, Dependence, and Addiction

When an opioid drug is administered repeatedly over an extended period, tolerance and physical dependence generally develop, becoming manifest clinically after about three weeks. **Tolerance** is a state in which progressively larger doses of the drug are required to achieve a particular effect. Such tolerance occurs to some opioid effects (e.g., analgesia and respiratory depression) to a greater degree than to others (e.g., pupillary miosis and constipation). Physical dependence, usually associated with tolerance, is characterized by the need to continue taking the opioid to avoid withdrawal symptoms.

Opioid addiction has a less precise definition, but refers to a compulsive need to take the drug. **Addiction** generally includes physical dependence, but may also have a psychologic component. That is, the individual takes the opioid not only to suppress withdrawal symptoms, but to satisfy a craving. This craving may be a more serious and deep-rooted aspect of addiction, in the sense that it can persist even after withdrawal from physical dependence, frequently leading to a renewed period of drug-seeking (see Chapter 21).

Characteristics of Tolerance and Physical Dependence

Though tolerance is generally associated with opioid use occurring over a period of at least several weeks, it can actually be observed after administration of a single dose to experimental animals. If the animal continues to receive opioids, a very high degree of tolerance may be attained—the effective dose of morphine may be increased as much as 100-fold. Indeed, patients taking opioids to relieve the pain of terminal illness sometimes become so tolerant to the analgetic effects that they no longer are able to obtain complete analgesia from any dose of opioid, no matter how high.

Tolerance to one opioid is generally associated with tolerance to other opioids, a phenomenon known as **cross-tolerance.** Consequently, an animal or human patient tolerant to morphine is also tolerant to other alkaloids, such as heroin or methadone, and to opioid peptides such as β-endorphin. The subject is also cross-dependent on these substances, and any of the other opioids can suppress the withdrawal symptoms resulting from morphine abstinence. However, there is no cross-tolerance or cross-dependence between mu opioids (e.g., morphine) and the kappa opioids (e.g., ketocyclazocine).

When an opioid-tolerant animal ceases to take opioid, or is given an antagonist such as naloxone, it undergoes a characteristic withdrawal syndrome. In humans, this is associated initially with sweating, abdominal cramps, aches and stiffness in all the limbs, and increasing anxiety. These symptoms, in the case of withdrawal from morphine, reach their peak intensity several days after the last dose, and gradually subside over a period of a week or more. Somewhat similar symptoms are observed in the case of withdrawal from other opioids, but the time course may be different. For example, withdrawal from methadone is considerably slower than that from morphine, but generally less intense.

Cellular and Biochemical Bases of Opioid Tolerance and Physical Dependence

Although tolerance and physical dependence have been intensively studied in laboratory animals for several decades, little is yet known about the cellular and biochemical processes underlying them. One of the most popular theories has been that tolerance results from a change in the number or affinity of opioid receptors, so that the animal is less responsive to a given dose of drug. With the identification of opioid receptors in the brain, it became possible for the first time to test this hypothesis. However, studies from many laboratories have been unable to confirm the existence of such changes in a manner consistent with tolerance/dependence development.[71]

Nevertheless, chronic opioid treatment does affect opioid receptors in certain systems, including, under certain conditions, mammalian brain. For example, incubation of NG108-15 cells with opioid agonist initially results in opioid receptor uncoupling from G-proteins, and a reduction in affinity for agonist. Subsequently, the receptors undergo down-regulation, that is, loss of number on the cell surface.[72] Opioid receptor down-regulation has also been observed following chronic opioid agonist treatment of hippocampal slices,[73] neonatal rats,[74] and chronic treatment of adult animals with selective μ and δ opioid agonists.[75,76] These findings, together with other work documenting opioid receptor up-regulation in brains of animals chronically treated with opioid antagonists,[77] establish that opioid receptors are in a dynamic state, sensitive to concentrations of endogenous as well as exogenous ligands. Thus, alterations in these receptors may play some role in tolerance/dependence that has not yet been elucidated.

Chronic opioid agonist treatment can also alter the concentrations of certain G-proteins in both brain[64,78] and spinal cord,[79] suggesting another possible mechanism of tolerance/dependence. However, G-proteins generally exist in much higher concentrations than their corresponding receptors, so it is not clear that even a large reduction in this concentration could affect signal transduction. Another problem with this idea is that G-proteins are believed to be shared extensively among different receptors, so that any alteration in signal transduction that did occur would probably affect several different receptors. This is not consistent with the specific nature of opioid tolerance/dependence, which alters the sensitivity of only these drugs.

Other theories of opioid tolerance have suggested a change in brain levels of some substance that antagonizes the action of opioids. For example, several small endogenous peptides have been detected in the brain that do not bind to opioid receptors, but which can antagonize the analgetic effects of opioids.[80] Accordingly, it has been proposed that opioid tolerance results from an increase in the levels of these peptides. Antagonism of this kind would presumably be directed not against opioid receptors directly, but against opioid-mediated effects, such as second messenger systems. Other researchers have studied the effects of chronic opioids on such second messenger systems as adenylate cyclase in brain and in simpler nervous system preparations. Opioid tolerance could also conceivably result from a change in the levels of opioid peptides in the brain. In vivo, opioid receptors are presumably activated by endogenous opioids, and a change in the levels of these opioids might be expected to alter the response to exogenously administered opioid. To date, however, no such changes in tolerant animals have been observed, although changes in the levels of POMC, the β-endorphin precursor, have been reported.

Characteristics and Treatment of Opioid Addiction

The euphoric effects of morphine and other opioids, coupled with their ability to induce tolerance and physical dependence, make them readily subject to abuse. As with other drug abusers, the number of opioid abusers in the U.S. fluctuates over time, but is now estimated at about 500,000. This figure has been quite stable for the past decade, after a peak of about 750,000 occurred about 20 years ago. The great majority of opioid addicts take heroin, which is readily bought in the street subculture; but opioid abuse is also a significant problem among doctors, nurses, and other health care professionals with access to these drugs. In the latter case, morphine or meperidine is usually the drug of choice. As discussed earlier, some individuals may become dependent on opioids as a result of being administered them during medical treatment, although this appears to be quite rare.

While a small proportion of opioid users take the drug purely for its euphoric effects, and are apparently able to avoid becoming physically dependent on the drug, the great majority of those who take opioids for any length of time probably do so because of underlying psychologic problems. Thus, opioid addiction is generally a symptom of a deeper central pathology that needs to be confronted and treated. This constitutes the most cogent argument for encouraging the addict to seek treatment for his or her problem (see Chapter 21).

In addition to the purely pharmacologic problems associated with opioid addiction, there is a cultural one. Because opioids are illegal, except under prescribed medical circumstances, they are relatively expensive when acquired outside of a medical context. In order to support his or her habit, the addict may be forced to turn to crime, including dealing the drug to others. Heroin abuse is also a major risk factor in contracting Acquired Immunodeficiency Syndrome (AIDS) through the sharing of contaminated needles. It has been the experience of most health professionals who attempt to treat addicts that they must have a genuine desire to end the habit if they are to be helped. Regardless of how destructive the drug habit may appear to others, attempts to force the addict to accept treatment are generally futile. Unfortunately, it is only when the addict has hit bottom in life—running out of money, friends, and perhaps everything else—that he or she is likely to be interested in treatment. At that time, those still close to the addict can play a major role in introducing him or her to a treatment program.

There are two major kinds of treatment available to opioid addicts in the U.S. The most widely used approach has been methadone maintenance. The addict is given a daily dose of 40–100 mg. methadone, which induces tolerance to this drug and, in effect, weans the addict off whatever other opioid was being taken previously. Although methadone has most of the effects of other opioids, including euphoria and addictive liability, its relatively great oral potency allows it to be administered in a single daily dose, so that the addict's intake can be strictly controlled. It has freed many thousands of addicts from dependence on the street culture to support the habit, making them more accessible to therapy that may help them eliminate their habit entirely. Nevertheless, as long as the addict is dependent on methadone, the addiction, and the fundamental problems underlying it, cannot be fully resolved. Furthermore, while methadone withdrawal is less intense than that from most other opioids, it is also much longer, and is considered by many addicts to be more difficult. Consequently, complete withdrawal from opioids in the addicted patient is an increasingly attractive, if very difficult, option.

Opioid withdrawal is best carried out in a hospital setting, where not only may the patient's access to drug be strictly monitored and controlled, but where other medications may be administered if necessary. The support of friends, family, and experienced health care professionals is also extremely important. While it is often stated that opioid withdrawal is usually not life-threatening, this is true only in the direct sense that the withdrawal process will not cause a fatal breakdown of any of the body's essential processes. The fact is that the withdrawing addict usually experiences enormous pain, both physical and psychologic, and the possibility of a suicide attempt should never be discounted. Because withdrawal is such an intense and agonizing experience, medication throughout the peak period as well as during the time after this critical period is extremely important. In some programs, a relatively small dose of methadone (10–20 mg.) is given for the first few days, which suppresses withdrawal symptoms to some extent. When this latter treatment is discontinued, the withdrawal symptoms are somewhat less intense than would be the case with abrupt withdrawal. Another increasingly popular drug that seems to help considerably is clonidine, an a_2-adrenergic antagonist. While clonidine does not suppress withdrawal symptoms directly, it alleviates their intensity, and relieves much of the fear and anxiety associated with removal of opioid. Abrupt withdrawal takes 7–10 days before symptoms subside. This process may be accelerated by administration of an antagonist such as naloxone during the later stages. In the earlier stages in particular, the patient is likely to be in enormous pain, experiencing such symptoms as nausea, sweating, abdominal cramps, and stiffness in the joints to the point of near-immobility. Thus, both medical and psychologic support are critical during this period.

While complete physical withdrawal represents an enormous step forward in the addict's life, it is only one step. The physical dependence on the drug is gone, but there is still a strong psychologic dependence for drug abuse. The addict may experience craving for the drug and may also feel a profound malaise or meaninglessness with the elimination of what has been for so long a major focus and ritual in his or her life. As a recovering addict once pointed out, withdrawal is much like an operation, in which a vital organ has been removed from the body. Even after the initial pain and shock of the operation itself subsides, an extensive period of adjustment is required, in order to learn to live without something that for so long has been an intimate part of one's body. To get past this latter stage may take several months, and even then the recovering addict will still have to confront the psychologic problems that led to the addiction in the first place. It is for this reason that the rate of relapse among recovering addicts is so high, and that addicts themselves say there is no real cure for their condition. It has been said that there are no ex-addicts, only recovering ones, and that the recovery process goes on for the remainder of one's life.

The recovery period is best undertaken with the aid of a support group. One of the fastest growing of these groups is Narcotics Anonymous (NA), an international organization that has chapters and regular meetings in all large American cities as well as in many foreign countries. NA is modeled after Alcoholics Anonymous, and in particular, is based on the 12-Step Program. In the groups, which are essentially leaderless, the recovering addicts are encouraged to confront their problem by discussing it openly, to take responsibility for their lives, and to make amends to those who may have suffered as a result of the addiction. NA, like AA, also encourages the recovering addict to seek spiritual guidance, though in a nondenominational sense.

Is Addiction a Disease?

Support groups of recovering addicts, like NA, promote the view that addiction to opioids and other substances is a *disease,* in the sense that it results from a biologic problem that may be medically treatable—in the future if not today—but over which the addict him- or herself has only limited control. This view is relatively new and highly significant in our history; it challenges the long-time belief that drug abuse represents criminal behavior that should be severely punished. The newer attitude implies that education and medical treatment, not fines or jail sentences, should be the major weapons in combating drug abuse. Nevertheless, the "addiction as disease" concept has been criticized by some both within and outside the medical profession on the grounds that it seems to remove all blame from the addict, encouraging him or her not to take any responsibility for the condition.

To what degree an addict can exercise free will is extremely difficult, pitting long-established legal and cultural mores against emerging new medical views. On the one hand, our country has a long tradition of holding adult individuals responsible for all their actions; our entire legal system depends on this belief, no matter how accurate it may actually be, in order to function effectively. On the other hand, the factors that lead people to take drugs such as opioids are extremely complex, and no one can really say to what extent someone may have felt compelled to begin abusing them. Moreover, anyone who has either been addicted to drugs such as the opioids, or who has worked with someone who has, knows that once in the grip of the addiction it is almost impossible for the addict to break out of it without assistance.

In light of this conflict, the most effective strategy may be to regard the addiction as a disease, but require the addict to be held responsible for seeking treatment. Just as someone with a clearly physical problem, such as high blood pressure or diabetes, is expected to seek treatment for that problem, so the addict may be held responsible for seeking treatment for the addiction. If the addict is willing to admit he or she has a problem, and to seek regular help for that problem, then regarding addiction as a disease over which the addict has little direct control encourages, rather than discourages, individual responsibility for treatment.

In addition to being practically constructive for

treatment strategies, the assumption that addiction is a disease can be vital to strategies for medical research. While physical withdrawal, followed by a group-supported recovery process, represents the best hope for opioid addicts today, there has been a long-time presumption that further pharmacologic advances will lead to more effective treatment of the addiction process. If, as many researchers believe, the tendency to take opioids, in at least some individuals, results from a metabolic defect in the brain, then it may be alleviated pharmacologically, much as the symptoms of diabetes can be alleviated by taking insulin. Furthermore, if the defect has a genetic basis, it might some day be cured by genetic counseling, if not by genetic engineering.

Pharmacokinetics

Opioids are most commonly administered either by IM injection, or orally in the form of tablets. Occasionally, to treat severe, acute pain, they are administered IV, and this is also the route preferred by most opioid users/abusers. Opioids also may enter the body via the lungs, as in the smoking of opium. Regardless of the route of administration, the drug rapidly enters the bloodstream. About one-third of the morphine present in the blood becomes protein-bound. The free portion, being highly lipophilic, can cross the capillary wall, and rapidly accumulates in organs such as the kidney, liver, lungs, spleen, and, of course, the brain. However, although the major sites of action of opioids are in the brain, only about 2 percent of systemically administered morphine finds its way to this site, owing to the difficulty opioids have in crossing the blood-brain barrier. More lipophilic opioids, such as heroin and methadone, accumulate in the brain in somewhat larger quantities than do other substances in this class.

Because they are rapidly metabolized, most opioids have a duration of action not exceeding 4–5 hours. Metabolism occurs primarily in the liver, and only traces of an opioid remain in the body by 24 hours after administration. The drug is first conjugated with glucuronic acid, with the conjugated product then excreted in the urine. If taken orally, most opioids are also metabolized to a significant extent before absorption into the bloodstream, which accounts for their significantly lower oral potency. Exceptions to this rule, such as codeine, are thought to contain structural features that make them resistant to such metabolism.

Available Preparations and Usual Doses

Morphine has traditionally been available in the form of both crude opium powder, containing 10 percent morphine, and as the pure base or salt. However, morphine salts (hydrochloride or sulfate) are now used almost exclusively, often as preparations predissolved in sterile saline. These preparations are customarily administered IM to patients, with a dose of 10 mg/70 kg sufficient to control most types of pain (see Table 20.4). Morphine is occasionally given IV when quicker action is needed to control pain in medical emergencies, such as severe cardiac pain. Under these conditions, morphine is approximately as potent as when given IM or SQ. On the other hand, morphine given orally is only about one-tenth as potent per mg as that given IM or SQ.

Of the other most commonly-used opioids, methadone, meperidine (Demerol), oxycodone (Percodan), and propoxyphene (Darvon) are available both as tablets and as sterile solutions. While all these opioids share the general properties of morphine, some possess particular properties that may make them advantageous in specific treatment situations. For example, meperidine is less spasmogenic than morphine, such that its effects on the biliary tract are less severe. Meperidine is also relatively more potent than morphine when taken orally. Methadone, as discussed earlier, also has high oral efficiency, and is commonly used to treat heroin addicts. Codeine is available in oral tablets as sulfate or phosphate salts in varying doses, up to 60 mg. Codeine is much less potent than morphine, but is relatively much more effective orally. Since its addictive liability is considerably less than that of morphine, it is useful for controlling relatively moderate forms of pain.

Less commonly-used opioids available include levorphanol (Levo-Dromoran), fentanyl (Sublimaze), pentazocine (Talwin), butorphanol (Stadol), nalbuphine (Nubain), and buprenorphine (Temgesic). Several of these drugs, including pentazocine, nalbuphine and buprenorphine, were developed as candidate nonaddictive analgesics, and have been used with varying degrees of success to treat opioid addicts. Buprenorphine is currently considered the most promising in this regard, and patients receiving the drug regularly do not experience withdrawal upon naloxone administration. However, withdrawal symptoms do occur when the drug is discontinued.

Summary

The opioids are a highly diverse group of drugs, including plant-derived alkaloids, a number of synthetic compounds, and a large group of peptides found in the mammalian brain. They have a broad range of physiologic effects, but are used primarily because of their ability to induce analgesia (relief of pain) and euphoria (a feeling of intense pleasure). Their analgetic properties have made opioids the drugs of choice for post-surgical anesthesia and to alleviate the chronic pain of patients suffering from cancer and other terminal illnesses. The euphoria or "high" induced by opioids, on the other hand, has resulted in extensive recreational use and abuse.

Opioids achieve their analgetic and other physiologic effects by interacting with specific receptors present in the brain and, in some cases, the spinal cord. Several different types of opioid receptors have been identified, which differ in their specificity for different classes of opioid ligands. The mu (μ) type, selective for morphine and other alkaloids, is thought to mediate analgesia in the brain.

In addition to analgesia, opioids have a number

of other physiologic effects, including respiratory depression, inhibition of GI motility, hypothermia, alterations in the circulating levels of several hormones, alteration of several immune system parameters, alteration of feeding behavior, modulation of the response to stress, and effects on certain centrally-mediated reflexes. Of these, respiratory depression is the most serious undesired side-effect of opioids, and is the usual cause of death by overdose.

The major liability of opioids, in addition to respiratory depression, is their addictive potential. Continued use of most opioids leads to tolerance, a state in which increasing doses of drug are needed to achieve the same analgetic effect, and dependence, in which regular administration of drug is required to prevent withdrawal symptoms. Opioid dependence has conventionally been treated by methadone maintenance, which does not cure the addiction, but substitutes controlled administration of methadone for the abused drug. Newer treatment programs emphasize complete withdrawal from opioid, followed by extensive therapy.

References

Research Reports

1. Hollt V. Multiple endogenous opioid peptides. Trends in Neurosci 1983;*6*:24–26
2. Mansour A, Khachaturian H, Lewis ME, Akil H, Watson SJ. Anatomy of CNS opioid receptors. Trends in Neurosci 1988;*11*:308–314.
3. Schwyzer R. Molecular mechanism of opioid receptor selection. Biochem 1986;*25*:6335–6342.
4. Young E, Bronstein D, Akil H. Proopiomelanocortin biosynthesis, processing and secretion: Functional implications. In Herz A (ed). Handbook of Experimental Pharmacology. Opioids I Berlin: Springer-Verlag (1993); 393–421.
5. Fricker LD. Opioid Peptide Processing Enzymes. In Herz A (ed). Handbook of Experimental Pharmacology Berlin: Springer-Verlag (1993); 529–545.
6. Spector S, Kantrowitz JD, Oka K. Presence of endogenous morphine in toad skin. Prog Clin Biol Res 1985;*192*:329–332.
7. Donnerer J, Cardinale G, Coffey J, Lisek CA, Jardine I, Spector S. Chemical characterization and regulation of endogenous morphine and codeine in the rat. J Pharmacol Exper Ther 1987;*242*:583–587.
8. Weitz CJ, Faull KF, Goldstein A. Synthesis of the skeleton of the morphine molecule by mammalian liver. Nature 1987;*330*:674–677.
9. Friedman HJ, Jen MF, Chang JK, Lee NM, Loh HH. Dynorphin: a possible modulatory peptide on morphine or beta-endorphin analgesia in mouse. Eur J Pharmacol 1981;*69*:351–360.
10. Wen HL, HO WKK. Suppression of withdrawal symptoms by dynorphin in heroin addicts. Eur J Pharmacol 1982;*82*:183–186.
11. Lehmann H, Nair NP, Kline NS. β-Endorphin and naloxone in psychiatric patients: Clinical and biological effects. Am J Psychiat 1979;*136*:762–766.
12. Hammond MD, Schneider C, Collier HOJ. Induction of opiate tolerance in guinea pig ileum and its modification by drugs. In Kosterlitz HW (ed.) Opiates and Endogenous Opioid Peptides Amsterdam: Elsevier/North Holland (1976); pp 169–176.
13. Lee NM, Smith AP Possible regulatory function of dynorphin and its clinical implications. Trends Pharm Sci 1984;*55*:108–110.
14. Holaday JW, Gilbeau PM, Smith CG, Pennington LL. Multiple opioid receptors in the regulation of neuroendocrine responses in the conscious monkey. In Delitala G, Motta M, Serio M. (Eds.) Opioid Modulation of Endocrine Function New York: Raven (1984); pp 21–32.
15. Koenig JI, Krulich L. Differential role of multiple opioid receptors in the regulation and secretion of prolactin and growth hormone in rats. In Delitala G, Motta M, Serio M. (Eds.) Opioid Modulation of Endocrine Function New York: Raven (1984); pp 89–98.
16. Gilbeau PM, Almirez RG, Holaday JW, Smith CG. Opioid effects on plasma concentrations of luteinizing hormone and prolactin in the adult male rhesus monkey. J Clin Endocrinol Metab 1985;*60*:299–305.
17. Wetli CV, Noto TA, Fernandez CA. Immunologic abnormalities in heroin addiction. South Med J 1974;*67*:193–197.
18. Louria DB. Infectious complications of non-alcoholic drug abuse Ann Rev Med 1974;*25*:219–231.
19. McDonough RJ *et al.* Alteration of T and null lymphocyte frequencies in the peripheral blood of human opiate addicts: In vivo evidence for for opiate receptor sites on T lymphocytes. J Immunol 1980;*125*:2539.
20. Brown SL, Van Epps DE. Suppression of T lymphocyte chemotactic factor production by the opioid peptides β-endorphin and met-enkephalin. J Immunol 1985;*134*:3384–3390.
21. Sibinga NES, Goldstein A. Opioid peptides and opioid receptors in cells of the immune system. Ann Rev Immunol 1988;*6*:219–249.
22. Gilman SC, Schwartz JM, Milner RJ, Bloom FE, Feldman JD. β-endorphin enhances lymphocyte proliferative responses. Proc Nat Acad Sci USA 1982;*79*:4226–4230.
23. Puppo F, Corsini G, Mangini P, Bottaro L, Barreca T. Influence of β-Endorphin on phytohemagglutinin-induced lymphocyte proliferation and on the expression of mononuclear cells surface antigens in vitro. Immunopharmacol 1985;*10*:119–125.
24. Kusnecov AW, Husband AJ, King MG, Pang G, Smith R. In vivo effects of beta-endorphin on lymphocyte proliferation and interleukin 2 production. Brain Behav Immun 1987;*1*:88–97.
25. Kay N, Allen J, Morley JE. Endorphins stimulate normal human peripheral blood lymphocyte natural killer activity. Life Sci 1984;*35*:53.
26. Mandler RN, Biddison WE, Mandler R, Serrate SA. β-Endorphin augments the cytolytic activity and interferon production of natural killer cells. J Immunol 1986;*136*:934–939.
27. Bessler H, Sztein MB, Serrate SA. Beta-endorphin modulation of IL-1-induced IL-2 production. Immunopharmacol 1990;*19*:5–14.
28. Roy S, Ramakrishnan S, Loh HH, Lee NM. Chronic morphine treatment selectively suppresses macrophage colony formation in bone marrow. Eur J Pharmacol 1991;*195*:359–363.
29. Morley JE, Levine AS, Gosnell BA, Billington CJ. Which opioid receptor mechanism modulates feeding? Appetite 1984;*5*:61–81.
30. Morley JE, Levin AS. Involvement of dynorphin and the k opioid receptor in feeding. Peptides 1983;*4*:797–800.

31. Gosnell BA, Morley JE, Levine AS. Opioid-induced feeding: localization of sensitive brain sites. Brain Res 1986;*369*:177–184.

32. Holaday JW, Loh HH. Endorphin-opiate interaction with neuroendocrine systems. Adv Biochem Psychopharmacol 1979;*20*:227–258.

33. Smith AP, Lee NM. Pharmacology of dynorphin. Ann Rev Pharmacol Toxicol 1988;*28*:123–140.

34. Jabaily J, Davis JN. Naloxone partially reverses neurologic deficits in some but not all stroke patients. Neurology 1982;*32*:A197.

35. Hosobuchi Y, Baskin DS, Woo SK. Reversal of induced ischemic neurologic deficits in gerbils by the opiate antagonist naloxone. Science 1982;*215*:69–71.

36. Baskin DS, Kuroda H, Hosobuchi Y, Lee NM. Treatment of stroke with opiate antagonists—effects of exogenous antagonists and dynorphin 1–13. Neuropeptides 1985;*5*:307–310.

37. Melzack R. The tragedy of needless pain. Sci Amer 1990;*262*:27–33.

38. Basbaum AI, Fields HL. Endogenous pain control systems: brainstem spinal pathways and endorphin circuitry. Ann Rev Neurosci 1984;*7*:309–338.

39. Yaksh TL, Rudy TA. Narcotic analgetic CNS sites and mechanisms of action as revealed by intracerebroventricular injection techniques. Pain 1978;*4*:299–359.

40. Pert CB, Snyder SH. Opiate receptor: its demonstration in nervous tissue. Science 1973;*179*:1011–1014.

41. Simon EJ, Hiller JM, Edelman J. Stereospecific binding of the potent narcotic analgesic [3H] etorphine to rat brain homogenate. Proc Nat Acad Sci USA 1973;*70*:1947–1949.

42. Terenius L. Stereospecific interaction between narcotic analgesics and a synaptic plasma membrane fraction of rat cerebral cortex. Act Pharmacol (Kbh) 1973;*32*:317–320.

43. Martin WR, Eades CG, Thompson JA, Huppler RE, Gilbert PE. The effects of morphine and nalorphine-like drugs in the nondependent and morphine-dependent chronic spinal dog. J Pharmacol Exp Ther 1976;*197*:517–532.

44. Lord JAH, Waterfield AA, Hughes J, Kosterlitz HW Endogenous opioid peptides: multiple agonists and receptors. Nature 1977;*267*:495–499.

45. Chang KJ. Opioid receptors: multiplicity and sequelae of ligand-receptor interactions. In Conn M. (ed.) The Receptors. New York: Academic Press (1984); pp 1–81.

46. Schiller PW. Development of receptor-selective opioid peptide analogs as pharmacologic tools and as potential drugs. In Herz A (ed) Handbook of Experimental Pharmacology Berlin: Springer-Verlag (1993); pp 681–710.

47. Schulz R, Wuster M, Herz A. Pharmacological characterization of the epsilon-opiate receptor. J Pharmacol exp Ther 1981;*216*:604–606.

48. Grevel JT, Sadee W. An opiate binding site in the rat brain is highly selective for 4,5-epoxymorphinans. Science 1983;*221*:1198–1201.

49. Nishimura SC, Recht LD, Pasternak GW. Biochemical characterization of high-affinity ^{3}H-opioid binding. Further evidence for Mμ_1 Sites. Mol Pharmacol 1984;*25*:29–37.

50. Loew G, Keys C, Luke B. Polgar W, Toll L. Structure-activity relationships of morphiceptin analogs: receptor binding and molecular determinants of mu-affinity and selectivity. Mol Pharmacol 1986;*29*:546–553.

51. Iyengar S, Kim HS, Wood PL. Effects of kappa opiate agonists on neurochemical and neuroendocrine indices: evidence for kappa receptor subtypes. J Pharmacol exp Ther 1986;*238*:429–436.

52. Chang KJ, Cuatrecasas P. Multiple opiate receptors: enkephalins and morphine bind to receptors of different specificity. J Biol Chem 1979;*254*:2610–2618.

53. Vaught JL, Rothman RB, Westfall TC. μ and δ-receptors, their role in analgesia and in the differential effects of opioid peptides on analgesia. Life sci 1982;*30*:1443–1455.

54. Fang F, Fields H, Lee NM. Action at the mu receptor is sufficient to explain analgesic action of opiates. J Pharmacol exp Ther 1986;*238*:1039–1044.

55. Fedynyshyn JP, Lee NM. Mu-type opioid receptors in rat periaqueductal gray-enriched P_2 membrane are coupled to guanine nucleotide binding proteins. Brain Res 1989;*476*:102–109.

56. Rothman RB, Westfall TC. Allosteric coupling between morphine and enkephalin receptors in vitro. Mol Pharmacol 1982;*21*:548–557.

57. Evans CJ, Keith DE Jr, Morrison H, Magendzo K, Edwards RH. Cloning of a delta opioid receptor by functional expression. Science 1992;*258*:1952–1955.

58. Kieffer BL, Befort K, Gaveriaux-Ruff C, Hirth CG. The δ-opioid receptor: isolation of a cDNA by expression cloning and pharmacological characterization. Proc Natl Acad Sci USA 1992;*89*:12048–12052.

59. Rodbell M. The role of hormone receptors and GTP regulatory proteins in membrane transduction. Nature 1980;*284*:17–22.

60. Sharma S, Nirenberg M, Klee W. Morphine receptors are regulators of adenylate cyclase activity. Proc Natl Acad Sci USA 1975;*72*:590–594.

61. Law PY, Wu J, Koehler JE, Loh HH. Demonstration and characterization of opiate inhibition of the striatal adenylate cyclase. J Neurochem 1981;*36*:1834–1846.

62. Cooper DMF, Londos C, Gill DL, Rodbell M. Opiate receptor-mediated inhibition of adenylate cyclase in rat striatal plasma membranes. J Neurochem 1982;*38*:1164–1167.

63. Schoffelmeer AN, Rice KC, Heijna MH, Hogenboom F, Mulder AH. Fentanyl isothiocyanate reveals the existence of physically associated mu- and delta-opioid receptors mediating inhibition of adenylate cyclase in rat neostriatum. Eur J Pharmacol 1988;*149*:179–182.

64. Nestler RJ, Erdos JJ, Terwilliger R, Duman RS, Tallman JF. Regulation of G proteins by chronic morphine in the rat locus coeruleus. Brain Res 1989;*476*:230–239.

65. Attali B, Saya D, Nah SY, Vogel Z. Kappa opiate agonists inhibit Ca^{++} influx in rat spinal cord-dorsal root ganglion cocultures. Involvement of a GTP-binding protein. J Biol Chem 1989;*264*:347–353.

66. Childers SR. Opioid receptor-coupled second messenger systems. In Herz A (Ed). Handbook of Experimental Pharmacology Berlin: Springer-Verlag (1993); pp 189–216.

67. North RA, Williams JT, Surprenant A, Christie MJ. Mu and delta receptors belong to a family of receptors that are coupled to potassium channels. Proc Natl Acad Sci USA 1987;*84*:5487–5491.

68. North R, Williams JT. Opiate activation of potassium conductance inhibitory calcium action potentials in rat locus coeruleus neurons. Brit J Pharmacol 1983;*80*:225–228.

69. Blume AJ, Lichtchstein D, Boone G. Coupling of opiate receptors to adenylate cyclase: requirements for Na^+ and GTP. Proc Nat Acad Sci 1979;*76*:5626–5630.

70. Abood ME, Law PY, Loh HH. Pertussis toxin treatment modifies opiate action in the rat brain striatum. Biochem Biophys Res Comm 1985;*127*:477–483.

71. Smith AP, Law PY, Loh HH. Role of opioid receptors in narcotic tolerance/dependence. In Pasternak GW (Ed). The Opioid Receptors New York: Academic Press (1988); pp 441–485.

72. Law PY, Griffin MT, Loh HH. Mechanisms of multiple cellular adaptation processes in clonal cell lines during chronic opiate treatment. In Sharp CW (ed). Mechanisms of Tolerance and Dependence NIDA Research Monograph (Washington DC: US Government Printing Office) (1984); pp 119–135.

73. Dingledine R, Valentino RJ, Bostock E, King ME, Chang K-J. Downregulation of delta but not mu opioid receptors in the hippocampal slice associated with loss of physiological response. Life Sci 1983;*33*:Suppl I, 333–336.

74. Tempel A, Habas J, Paredes W, Barr GA. Morphine-induced downregulation of mu-opioid receptors in neonatal rat brain. Brain Res 1988;*469*:129–133.

75. Tao PL, Chang L-R, Law PY, Loh HH. Decrease in δ-opioid receptor density in rat brain after chronic [D-Ala^2, D-Leu^5]enkephalin treatment. Brain Res 1988;*462*:313–320.

76. Tao PL, Lee HY, Chang LR, Loh HH. Decrease in mu-opioid receptor binding capacity in rat brain after chronic PL017 treatment. Brain Res 1990;*526*:270–275.

77. Zukin RS, Tempel A, Gardner EL. Opiate receptor upregulation and functional supersensitivity. In Sharp CW (Ed). Mechanisms of Tolerance and Dependence (Washington DC: US Government Printing Office) (1984); pp 146–161.

78. Cox BM. Opioid receptor-G protein interactions: acute and chronic effects of opioids. In Herz A (Ed). Handbook of Experimental Pharmacology Berlin: Springer-Verlag (1993); pp 145–188.

79. Attali B, Vogel Z. Long-term opiate exposure leads to reduction of the alpha$_i$-1 subunit of GTP-binding proteins. J Neurochem 1989;*53*:1636–1639.

80. Yang H-YT, Fratta W, Majane EA, Costa E. Isolation, sequencing, synthesis and pharmacological characterization of two brain neuropeptides that modulate the action of morphine. Proc Nat Acad Sci USA 1985;*82*:7757–7761.

Reviews

r1. Levinthal CF. Messengers of paradise: opiates and the brain. New York: Anchor. (1988) A brief history of opioid use and opioid research.

r2. .Li CH. Chemistry of beta-endorphin Adv Biochem Psychopharmacol 1979;*20*:145–163.
A summary of pioneering studies into the chemistry and structure of β-endorphin and related opioid peptides.

r3. Sibinga NES, Goldstein A. Opioid peptides and opioid receptors in cells of the immune system. Ann Rev Immunol 1988;*6*:219–249.
The most comprehensive and critical summary of studies demonstrating a link between endogenous opioids and the immune system.

r4. Loh HH, Smith AP. Molecular characterization of opioid receptors. Ann Rev Pharmacol Toxicol 1990;*30*:123–147.
A summary of current knowledge of the molecular structure of opioid receptors.

r5. Snyder SH. Brainstorming. The science and politics of opiate research. Cambridge MA: Harvard University Press (1989).
A colorful history of the discovery and characterization of opioid receptors, by one of the leading researchers in the field.

r6. Mansour A, Khachaturian H, Lewis ME, Schafer MK, Watson SJ. Anatomy of the CNS opioid systems. Trends Neurosci 1985;*8*:111–119.
Summary of studies localizing opioid receptors and opioid peptides in the brain, with maps included.

CHAPTER 21

Peter R. Martin
David M. Lovinger
George R. Breese

Alcohol and Other Abused Substances

The use of psychoactive substances is inexorably intertwined in the socioeconomic fabric of most cultures. Accordingly, psychoactive substance use, abuse, and dependence have widespread interest in our society,[r1–r3] and considerable attention has been paid to this subject in art, music, literature, and the social sciences.[r13,r16,r62,r67] Furthermore, owing to the protean clinical manifestations of psychoactive substance use disorders, the clinician must consider these disorders in the differential diagnosis of a myriad of medical illnesses.[r1,1,2,68,110,109] In particular, it is recognized that psychoactive substance use can contribute to and/or result from various forms of psychopathology.[r4,r5,2,3]

Psychosocial factors, which tend to be similar for diverse pharmacologic agents, are probably of greater importance in the pathogenesis of psychoactive substance use disorders and in the maintenance of pathologic drug use than is the unique psychopharmacologic profile of a given drug.[r6] Therefore, generic social and behavioral strategies provide the theoretical underpinnings for currently accepted approaches to long-term management of patients suffering from psychoactive substance use disorders.[r6–r11,4,5] Although there is considerable interest in pharmacologic treatment of patients with psychoactive substance use disorders,[6–7] these must be viewed, for the present, as adjunctive and experimental.

For the psychopharmacologist, an understanding of psychoactive substance use disorders can serve to elucidate fundamental brain mechanisms underlying mood, thought, perception, and cognition, all of which may be modified by the use of psychoactive agents. Further, understanding of the pharmacologic characteristics of psychoactive substances of abuse is vital for appropriate management of intoxication, withdrawal, and the medical complications associated with drug abuse.

This chapter will define for each of the drugs of abuse discussed the pattern of pathologic drug use, syndromes of intoxication, the pharmacologic mechanisms that influence drug-seeking behavior, adaptive changes in the nervous system resulting from drug use, the generic features of the drug dependence syndrome, and the medical complications associated with these compounds. Nonetheless, primary emphasis in this chapter will be on the pharmacology of the major psychoactive substances of abuse. Particular attention is directed to substances used predominantly for other than medical reasons (Table 21.1). Following this will be a section that deals in more detail about the pathogenesis of drug abuse in general and the clinical course of psychoactive substance use disorders.

Terminology Associated with Drug Abuse

Terminology used in relation to psychoactive substance use disorders historically has been plagued by imprecision, lack of consensus, and regular revisions punctuated by heated debate.[9] Much of the controversy has resulted from the differing needs of the constituent groups who must deal with psychoactive substance use at very different levels of analysis (e.g., societal or government regulation, basic research, clinical diagno-

Table 21.1 Classification of Psychoactive Substances with Liability for Abuse

Class	Common Examples
CNS Depressants	alcohol, benzodiazepines (diazepam, chlordiazepoxide, alprazolam), barbiturates, nonbarbiturate hypnosedatives (ethchlorvynol, glutethimide, chloral hydrate, methaqualone)
Psychostimulants	amphetamine and related compounds, cocaine, methylphenidate
Opioids	heroin, morphine, methadone, codeine, hydromorphone, oxycodone, meperidine, pentazocine
Tobacco	nicotine, cigarettes and other types of tobacco products
Cannabinoids	marijuana, hashish, delta-9-tetrahydrocannabinol (THC)
Psychedelics or hallucinogens	lysergic acid diethylamide (LSD), psilocybin, dimethyltryptamine, mescaline
Arylcyclohexylamines	phencyclidine, ketamine
Caffeine	coffee, tea, soft drinks
Hydrocarbon inhalants	aliphatic, aromatic, and halogenated hydrocarbons (gasoline, glue, paint, paint thinners, spray paints, and other volatile compounds)
Other	anesthetic gases (nitrous oxide, ether), vasodilators (amyl or butyl nitrate)

sis, psychopharmacologic therapy as well as other treatment approaches). Therefore, it is necessary to define terms used in this chapter that are commonly used to describe the effects of drugs of abuse and the consequences of chronic exposure to such drugs.

Intoxication refers to the subjective effects of a drug perceived by the individual as well as the changes in a user's behavior observed by others. *Tolerance* refers to greater amounts of a drug being required to produce the same physiologic, subjective, or behavioral change after repeated exposure than would be required when the agent was first administered. *Dependence* refers to the neuroadaptive physiologic changes that occur after repeated exposure to a drug as well as the clinical syndrome characterized by *drug-seeking behavior* and other psychosocial consequences. One sign of dependence is the occurrence of a withdrawal syndrome following cessation of prolonged drug use. The emergence of a withdrawal syndrome upon drug discontinuance is referred to as *physical dependence,* whereas the craving for a drug has been referred to as *psychosocial (psychologic) dependence.* The term *drug-seeking behavior* is largely self-explanatory in that it describes characteristics that develop in individuals who regularly use an abused substance. These patterns will differ depending on the drug involved and the time the individual has been using the drug. The notation *dependence syndrome* has come to represent the elements of psychologic dependence, including drug-seeking and psychosocial consequences of drug use.[9] However, it is currently recognized that removal of the drug in a dependent individual can also result in a *protracted abstinence syndrome.*[10] It is probably because of this protracted withdrawal syndrome that there is an increased relapse risk during the six-month period after discontinuance of the abused substance.

Tolerance to a psychopharmacologic agent is usefully conceptualized in terms of: 1. *dispositional (pharmacokinetic or metabolic) tolerance* due to increased capacity for clearance of the drug by metabolizing enzymes in the liver which results in decreased concentrations of the drug at the site of pharmacologic action; 2. *functional (pharmacodynamic) tolerance* due to neuronal adaptation resulting in reduced response from the same molar drug concentrations at the site of action in the nervous system; and 3. *behavioral (learned) tolerance* due to behavioral accommodation to drug effects through learning acquired while the organism was in the intoxicated "state" or in the environment in which intoxication occurred. Tolerance is an adaptive physiologic response of the intact organism which opposes the pharmacologic effects of the drug with its mechanistic underpinnings residing in molecular changes at the cellular level and in the interactions of the organ systems of the body. Tolerance may not develop equivalently to all pharmacologic actions of a given drug nor within all organ systems of the body. Nonetheless, after repeated exposure to CNS stimulants, *reverse tolerance,* or a *greater* pharmacologic effect, also may be observed. Acquired tolerance should be distinguished from: 1. *initial tolerance* or sensitivity to a given drug on first administration; 2. *acute tolerance,* which develops over the course of a single exposure to the drug. Differences in the population in initial and/or acute tolerance to a given drug are innate characteristics of the CNS that may influence individual vulnerability to development of psychoactive substance use disorders.[r1,r2]

Dependence can only be defined indirectly in terms of: 1. the presence of tolerance or the emergence of a withdrawal (abstinence) syndrome (immediate) upon drug discontinuation or the administration of a specific antagonist (also referred to as physical dependence); 2. the "craving" experienced (protracted withdrawal) or drug-seeking behavior manifested as a result of conditioned stimuli (psychologic dependence).[10–13] Accordingly, the term neuroadaptation has been coined to refer (in the broadest sense) to the neuronal changes and consequent clinical signs and symptoms encompassing the biologic substrata of tolerance and "physical" (as opposed to "psychologic") dependence that occur as a result of repeated drug administration. Physical dependence usually develops in concert with tolerance; it is still controversial whether or not they are simply different manifestations of the same neuronal changes.[14,15] The reacquisition of both tolerance and physical dependence are accelerated following repeated cycles of drug administration and withdrawal,[12,16] suggesting certain similarities between these phenomena and learning and memory.[17-20]

The withdrawal syndrome is believed to involve a reversal of an "abnormal" homeostatic state in the presence of the drug to the normal state. Behavioral signs of the withdrawal syndrome are often opposite to the acute effects of the abused drug. For example, withdrawal following use of CNS depressants usually involves neuronal hyperexcitability, whereas withdrawal from stimulants involves depression and lethargy. The severity of withdrawal is related to the cumulative dose (dosage and duration of administration).[r12,21-23] In addition to these drug-specific manifestations for most drugs of abuse, the withdrawal syndrome also involves homeostatic responses to the reversal of the neuroadaptive changes that have occurred as a result of long-term drug administration with significant activation of the autonomic nervous system.[24-26]

Brief History of Psychoactive Substance Use

Since earliest times, members of almost every society known to man have used psychoactive substances indigenous to their region for widely-accepted medical, religious, or recreational purposes. Archeological studies of the early Sumerian city-states of the late fourth millennium BC, one of the oldest literate civilizations in the world, have provided the earliest chemical evidence for beer.[27] Opium was used for medicinal purposes by Roman and Greek physicians, and the drug was widely available in Egypt, Persia, and India prior to the Christian era.[r3] The source of opium was the poppy plant, *Papaver sominferum*. Throughout history, the plant material derived from *Cannabis sativa* has been reported to have clinical utility for the treatment of pain, convulsions, glaucoma, muscle spasticity, bronchial asthma, nausea, and vomiting.[28] The history of caffeine use is inseparable from that of coffee, tea, and various other caffeine-containing beverages that have been used since before recorded time throughout the world. In the 16th century, smoking of tobacco (*Nicotiana tabacum*) leaves, a source of nicotine, was introduced into European culture by the Spanish explorers of the New World, where smoking tobacco had been a common practice among native Americans. Subsequently, this habit spread throughout other continents.

The native Indians of South America have chewed the leaves of the shrub *Erythroxylon coca*, from which the stimulant cocaine is derived, for at least 2000 years, as evidenced by ancient statues with puffed out cheeks (presumably representing a wad of coca in the mouth).[r13] Cocaine (*Erythroxylon coca*) has not been the only stimulant used in history. The history of the use of stimulant compounds in Chinese folk medicine from the Ephedra plant extends for more than 5000 years. The substance extracted from this plant was ephedrine, a sympathomimetic derivative. The history of this drug is described by Chen and Schmidt.[r14] Subsequent analogues of ephedrine, such as amphetamine, methamphetamine, and their derivatives, were made synthetically and possessed strong CNS stimulant actions.[r15] Amphetamine use increased dramatically in the US with the introduction of medicinal forms such as Benzedrine in the 1930s. Widespread use of these stimulants developed in the West in the 20th century. A steady increase in amphetamine abuse persisted up to the late 1960s, with steadily increasing prescribed use of amphetamine for a variety of medical purposes. During the past century, pharmaceutical science has led to the de novo syntheses of a wide range of CNS depressants and stimulants, hallucinogens, and dissociative anesthetics as well as modifications of various existing psychoactive compounds that have been abused.

Prevalence of Drug Use

Dramatically shifting attitudes toward the use of psychoactive substances over the past 200 years have resulted in cycles of widespread drug use followed by periods of prohibition.[r16,28] However, not until the late 1960s were the techniques of epidemiology applied to the study of drug abuse to document the magnitude of this problem.[29] Cross-sectional and longitudinal surveys conducted by various government agencies at fixed intervals since that time have allowed us to monitor changes in the attitudes of the population, the prevalence of different types of drug use, health consequences and estimated costs to society, and treatment outcome. Epidemiologic surveys in the US have documented epidemics of marijuana abuse in the 1960s, heroin in the 1970s, and cocaine in the 1980s, with a background of an upward trend in the usage of all drugs and alcohol during the 1970s, followed by a downward trend in the 1980s.[29,r17] Although more Americans use alcohol than any other drug (see below), younger individuals tend to combine alcohol with multiple other drugs, whereas older cohorts (age ≥ 35) predominantly use alcohol alone. National data have consistently shown that both use and abuse/dependence of alcohol and drugs are most prevalent among the young (age 18–34), with the highest rates observed for younger men. Cross-sectional epidemiologic studies provide clinicians with valuable knowledge concerning the prevalence of drug-related problems and, hence, the likelihood that these may be encountered in the patient population they serve.[r18] Longitudinal population studies of cohorts of drug users are particularly informative with respect to understanding antecedents of psychoactive substance use disorders, dose-response relationships for consequences of use, and determinants of effective treatment and outcome variables.

The lifetime prevalence rate of a substance (except nicotine or caffeine) use disorder (16.7 per 100 persons 18 years and older) was higher than that for any other mental illness.[r4,3] Alcohol abuse or dependence was present (during their lifetime) in 13.5 percent and other drug abuse/dependence in 6.1 percent of the population. In the one sample in this study in which cigarette smoking was surveyed, the reported lifetime prevalence was 36.0 percent.[30] Lifetime prevalence rates for abuse/dependence on other psychoactive substances were: marijuana (4.3%), amphetamines (1.7%), barbiturates and other depressants (1.2%), opiates (0.7%), hallucinogens (0.3%), and cocaine (0.2%).[3,r4] The odds of having a mental disorder were 2.7 times greater if one also had alcohol and/or other drug abuse/dependence (excluding nicotine or caffeine) in comparison with no drug use disorder. Drug use disorders occurred at higher rates in individuals suffering from alcohol abuse/dependence (21.5%) than in those who were not (3.7%) Also, alcohol use disorders were more prevalent among those who met criteria for drug abuse/dependence (47.3%) than among those who did not (11.3%). In a recent survey, more males (73%) than females (64%) used alcohol. The rates of use for males versus females for use of cigarettes (35% vs 30%), marijuana (12% vs 8%), psychostimulants (6% vs 3%), and depressants (2% vs 2%) were overall only slightly in favor of males.

Diagnostic Considerations of Dysfunctional Use of Psychoactive Substances

The descriptors ("excessive use," "abuse," "misuse," "addiction") employed to convey the magnitude, context, and consequences of psychoactive drug use pose difficult value judgments.[9] The general conceptual formulations on which medical diagnoses are made need to stand on firmer ground. The focus for development of meaningful diagnostic criteria that are generalizable across cultures has been to define maladaptive patterns of use in terms of consequences that are (presumably) less influenced by value judgments. Implicit in the term "maladaptive" is the emphasis on behavioral, rather than purely medical complications of use, or physiologic effects of the drug. This conceptual advance has its theoretical base in the biopsychosocial model of health care.[5] This approach is readily amenable to preventing abuse and has important implications for treatment strategies.[r18] This perspective is quite different from the traditional medical model of considering drug use merely a bad "habit" until organ damage is diagnosable, or the social model according to which even use sufficient to cause physical complications is not considered an illness.[9,r19] In summary, the diagnostic focus has shifted from the drug per se to encompass the interactions of drug, individual, society and medical consequences.[31–34] This concept is expanded at the end of this chapter in the section referred to as Etiological, Diagnostic, and Legal factors.

Physicians are most likely to encounter patients with psychoactive substance use disorders when they present for treatment of a complicating or associated physical or emotional illness.[1–3] Medical and psychiatric complications of drug use are attributable to: 1. acute and chronic *direct* pharmacologic actions of the substance (e.g. overdose, organ toxicity, and metabolic consequences); 2. *indirect* effects of drug administration on life-style (e.g., use of other than the primary drug of abuse, including tobacco, inappropriate use of prescribed medications such as analgesics or anxiolytics, lack of compliance with the medical regimen for coexistent illnesses, malnutrition, trauma, infection, and neglect). Treatment of severe medical complications clearly takes precedence if the illness is life-threatening or incapacitating. However, unless the underlying substance use disorder and emotional concomitants are recognized and addressed, initial treatment efforts may be for naught. Psychiatric syndromes that may be a complication of substance abuse are presented in Table 21.2.

Table 21.2 Psychiatric Syndromes that May Accompany Substance Use Disorders*

Psychiatric Syndrome	Psychoactive Drugs Causing Complications
Delirium	depressants (I/W), stimulants (I), opioids (I), cannabinoids (I), hallucinogens (I), arylcyclohexylamines (I), inhalants (I)
Dementia	depressants (P), inhalants (P)
Amnestic disorder	depressants (P)
Psychotic disorder	depressants (I/W), stimulants (I), opioids (I), cannabinoids (I), hallucinogens (I/P), arylcyclohexylamines (I), inhalants (I)
Mood disorder	depressants (I/W), stimulants (I/W), opioids (I), hallucinogens (I), arylcyclohexylamines (I), inhalants (I)
Anxiety disorder	depressants (I/W), stimulants (I), caffeine (I), cannabinoids (I), hallucinogens (I), arylcyclohexylamines (I), inhalants (I)
Sexual dysfunction	depressants (I), stimulants (I), opioids (I)
Sleep disorder	depressants (I/W), stimulants (I/W), opioids (I/W), caffeine (I)

*This table is adapted from DMS-IV of the American Psychiatric Association. (I) denotes that the disorder has its onset during intoxication. (W) denotes that disorder occurs during withdrawal. (I/W) denotes that syndrome can occur during intoxication or withdrawal.
(P) denotes that the disturbance persists long after the acute effects of intoxication or withdrawal.

Conceptualization of psychoactive substance use disorders in terms of the biopsychosocial model, rather than simply the physiologic consequences of chronic drug use, has led to recognition of the central role of conditioning and learning in drug dependence.[20,35,r20] The value of the behavioral perspective is that it provides a framework for understanding the entire spectrum of psychoactive substance use, from its initiation to its progression to compulsive drug use, as well as the acquisition of tolerance and physical dependence.[r20,r21] Psychopharmacologic processes that initiate, maintain, and regulate drug-seeking behavior are: 1. positive reinforcing and discriminative effects of drugs;[r21] 2. environmental (conditioning) stimuli associated with drug effects (which facilitate drug-seeking);[20,35] and 3. aversive effects of drugs (which extinguish drug-seeking), all of which are modulated by social,[r6,r8] environmental,[r7] psychopathologic,[r4,r5] and genetic factors,[r1,r2] including the previous behavioral and pharmacologic history of the individual (Fig. 21.1). Behavioral factors that influence psychoactive drug use are amenable to detailed analysis utilizing drug self-administration models in laboratory animals, whereas the underlying neural mechanisms can be explored by studying the neuropharmacology and neuroanatomy of the brain systems that mediate reward.[r20–r22]

The concept of a *dependence syndrome* also is an important advance in our thinking about psychoactive

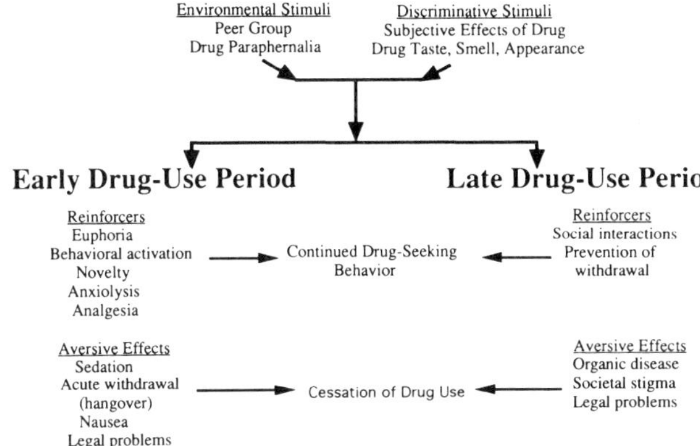

Factors that Modulate Drug Use at All Stages: Socioeconomic status; genetic predisposition to drug abuse; success or failure in career/family; social and cultural milieu; psychologic stress, health; financial and legal problems.

Figure 21.1 Factors Contributing to Drug-Seeking Behavior

substance use disorders because it frames, for the first time, the interactions among the pharmacologic actions of the drug, individual psychopathology, and the effects of the environment in a clinically meaningful construct that is *generalizable* to all drugs of abuse.[9,36,37] This concept is derived from the clinical observation that patients may have maladaptive behavior as a result of drug use. Neuroadaptation is not necessarily dysfunctional if there is no desire to continue the use of the drug.[9] For example, driving while drunk may have devastating consequences, particularly in the sporadically drinking young driver; the postsurgical patient who has been receiving morphine for pain relief clearly exhibits neuroadaptation (tolerance), but is not likely to develop the dependence syndrome. Fundamental to the concept of the dependence syndrome is the central role of *drug-seeking behavior* (priority of drug-seeking over other behaviors) in the maintenance of dysfunctional drug use. In this syndromatic diagnostic approach, the dualism inherent in the use of the terms "psychologic" and "physical" dependence is avoided.

Specific psychiatric diagnoses such as major depressive disorder, bipolar disorder, schizophrenia, anxiety disorders, and antisocial personality disorder have been associated with psychoactive substance use disorders, leading to theories of common pathogenesis.[r4] Furthermore, this association suggests that the clinician should have a high index of suspicion for diagnosing psychoactive substance use disorders when dealing with certain clinical populations,[2,3] and be circumspect about prescribing to such patients medications that have dependence liability (see text below).

It may be exceedingly difficult to determine whether psychopathology in a given individual who has a psychoactive substance use disorder is a consequence of drug use or is due to an additional psychiatric diagnosis. It is apparent from Table 21.2 how broad is the overlap between substance-induced and other mental disorders. Diverse psychiatric signs and symptoms, including those of delirium, psychotic, mood, and anxiety disorders, sexual dysfunction, and sleep disorders can have their onset during intoxication or withdrawal, and dementia and amnesic disorder (and even flashbacks from hallucinogen use) may persist long after the acute effects of intoxication and withdrawal. Accordingly, it is helpful to determine, preferably by longitudinal observation, or by history, the timing of the onset of psychopathology with respect to the initiation of drug use and whether it is present when drug use has ceased, recognizing that the duration of abstinence can be a determining variable. Pharmacotherapy of a complicating psychiatric disorder is currently considered appropriate only if it is independent (a primary disorder), but not if it is a consequence (a secondary disorder), of a psychoactive substance use disorder.[6,7] It is important to underline that the distinction between whether a complicating psychiatric disorder is primary or secondary to substance dependence is not easily made, particularly if both disorders started early in life or if they are historically closely intertwined.[2] Nevertheless, the use of medications with dependence liability (e.g., benzodiazepines, methylphenidate, barbiturates, anticholinergics) for the treatment of a secondary coexisting psychiatric disorder or failing to address the primary disorder (substance dependence) may be detrimental to the patient.

Alcohol and Other CNS Depressants

The CNS depressants include ethanol, available for consumption in brewed or distilled alcoholic beverages, and various pharmaceutical agents prescribed for treatment of insomnia, anxiety, and, less frequently, for control of seizure disorders or as muscle relaxants (Table 21.1). Alcoholic beverages are readily available at affordable cost with minimal legal restrictions. Accordingly, there is widespread use of alcohol in diverse recreational and work-related circumstances. Although each new wave of synthetic CNS depressants has been marketed initially with claims of pharmacologic novelty—particularly, a lack of dependence liability and, hence, minimal risk of abuse—strikingly similar problems (shared with alcoholic beverages) have emerged as they have become more widely available. To date, no CNS depressant has been developed that is free of abuse liability and the potential for withdrawal symptoms upon drug discontinuation. Benzodiazepines are currently (as barbiturates were previously) among the most widely prescribed drugs in the world, ranking in the top 50 most commonly prescribed drugs since the late 1960s. The following material will define the pharmacology of ethanol in more detail than the other CNS depressant drugs because the pharmacology of these latter drugs is described in detail in Chapter 14. Particular attention will be given to the dependence liability of this general drug class.

Alcohol

A quotation attributed to Sir William Osler, "Alcohol does not make people do things better, it makes them less ashamed of doing them badly," superbly summarizes the human behavioral pharmacology of this CNS depressant. Because there are so few legitimate medical uses of systemically administered ethanol, the misuse of this agent is not the result of patient abuse of a drug prescribed for medical reasons. Rather, this is a substance readily available to the public in the form of beer, wine, and purified alcoholic mixtures. Ethanol abuse stands as the most prevalent drug abuse problem in the US (see page 419).

Pharmacologic Effects of Ethanol

Ethyl alcohol (ethanol, alcohol) (Fig. 21.2) is used primarily for its effects on the CNS. Alcohol produces a slowing of the brain wave rhythm. Apparent CNS stimulation and euphoria caused by ethanol that occurs early during intoxication results from depression of inhibitory control mechanisms. Following alcohol intake, aspects of discrimination, memory, and insight are reduced. There can be impulsive speech as inhibition is lost. The reaction to ethanol will depend in part on the personality of the individual, whether the person is tolerant to the amount of ethanol ingested, and the environment. Dulling of performance that depends upon training and previous experience and expectation occurs after moderate doses of ethanol. Higher blood ethanol concentrations cause loss of motor coordination. Traumatic injuries sustained while under the influence of elevated blood alcohol concentrations are probably the most common public health problems associated with ethanol abuse.[38] Heavy drinkers, who often have blood alcohol concentrations that impair judgment and motor skills, are particularly at risk for alcohol-related traumatic injury and death. The combination of ethanol with other CNS depressants greatly increases the risk associated with its use and is the most common clinical presentation for severe drug overdoses. Still higher concentrations of ethanol depress midbrain functions and interfere with spinal reflexes and temperature regulation. Finally, neurons in the medullary centers controlling cardiorespiratory functions are depressed by extremely high doses of ethanol, with predicted consequences. Ethanol can have anticonvulsant properties with acute administration, but hyperexcitability occurs upon withdrawal from chronic alcohol exposure and puts epileptic individuals in jeopardy of seizures (see Medical Complications). Cardiovascular measures do not change significantly following moderate amounts of alcohol. However, cutaneous vessels are dilated, producing a flushed feeling.

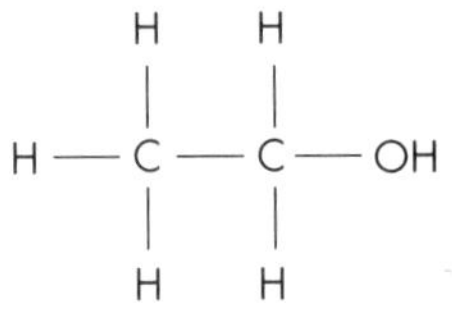

```
     H   H
     |   |
H —  C — C — OH
     |   |
     H   H
```

Figure 21.2 Structure of Ethanol (Alcohol)

Pharmacokinetic Considerations

Absorption and Distribution

The rate-limiting step in systemic absorption of ethanol is gastric emptying, because the absorption of alcohol is much faster and more extensive from the small intestine than from the stomach. The rate of rise of the blood alcohol concentration is more rapid and the peak is higher when alcohol is taken on an empty stomach. Food, particularly fatty foods, delay gastric emptying and slow absorption of alcohol, especially from drinks with low volume and high alcohol concentration. The rate of absorption from carbonated beverages is greater than from noncarbonated ones, also probably because of an increased rate of gastric emptying. Alcohol distributes in total body water which is about 55 percent of body weight for women and 68 percent for men.

The plasma (and saliva) concentration is about 1.15 times that in whole blood. The physicochemical basis for use of the breathalyzer which allows accurate determinations of blood alcohol concentrations is that the partition coefficient between blood and air is about 2000 to 1.

The dose-response curve of ethanol has been studied in depth under varied circumstances (Table 21.3). The sensitivity to alcohol intoxication among the population as a whole varies widely. For example, at a blood ethanol concentrations of 50, 100–150, and 200 mg/100 ml, it is estimated that approximately 10 percent, 64 percent, and almost all of the general population would appear overtly intoxicated. On the other hand, at 300 mg/100 ml some alcoholics may appear only mildly intoxicated, even though their psychomotor performance and judgment are significantly impaired. According to the Council of Scientific Affairs of the American Medical Association, blood alcohol concentrations of 60, 100, and 150 mg/100 ml increase the relative probability of causing an automobile accident two-, six-, and 25-fold, respectively. Legal limits of blood ethanol concentration for automobile drivers are 100 mg/100 ml (the term in common use

Table 21.3 Relationship of Drinks Consumed and Blood Ethanol Concentration to CNS Functions

Whiskey (Ounces) Beer (Drinks)	Blood Ethanol (mg/100 ml)	Impaired Function
0.5	15	Vision
1–1.5	30–40	Fine muscle coordination
2–3	80	Reaction time
4	100	Judgment

is 0.10) for most of the US, 80 mg/100 ml for most countries in Western Europe, and between 0 and 50 mg/100 ml for Scandinavian and Eastern European countries.

Metabolism and Elimination

Elimination of ethanol is 90 to 98 percent by oxidation, largely via alcohol dehydrogenase and aldehyde-dehydrogenase.[22] Thus, elimination of ethanol from the body depends upon near-total metabolism.[r23,r24] Above blood alcohol concentrations of about 9 mg/100 ml, elimination is by zero order kinetics (actually, Michaelis-Menten kinetics). As a rule of thumb, the mean rate of ethanol elimination is about 100 mg/kg/hr or about 15 mg/100 ml/hr (for a 70-kg person this corresponds to 8–10 ml/hr). So, it takes about 1.5 hours to metabolize the alcohol in 1 ounce of 100-proof whiskey or in 12 ounces of beer. The liver is the main site of systemic ethanol metabolism. Blockade of acetaldehyde dehydrogenase with an enzyme inhibitor to prevent metabolism of acetaldehyde formed from ethanol has been one approach for treating alcohol abuse (see disulfiram in section on Treatments).

Recently, orally administered ethanol was shown to undergo significant presystemic oxidation by alcohol dehydrogenase in gastric mucosa. Moreover, ethanol was found to have greater oral bioavailability in women (approximately 90%) than in men (approximately 75%). The difference was associated with lower gastric alcohol dehydrogenase activity in women than in men.[39] Ordinarily, only a small amount of alcohol is oxidized by the hepatic microsomal mixed function oxidase system. However, at high blood alcohol levels or during long-term consumption of alcohol, this system may be a more important pathway of metabolism. A nonoxidative enzyme system found in several organs converts ethanol to ethyl esters of fatty acids. It has been suggested that these products contribute to nonhepatic organ damage.[40]

Drug Interactions

There is a broad range of pharmacokinetic and pharmacodynamic interactions between alcohol and prescribed medications which can result in either increased or decreased drug effect. Although alcohol can alter absorption of certain drugs (e.g., increase the absorption of diazepam), the demonstrated basis for the majority of pharmacokinetic ethanol-drug interactions involves the alcohol dehydrogenase pathway and liver microsomes.[41,69] Alcohol is metabolized predominantly by alcohol dehydrogenase, whereas the microsomal mixed function oxidase system is responsible for the biotransformation of a large number of drugs. Microsomal drug metabolism is inhibited in the presence of high concentrations of ethanol, in part through competition for a common microsomal detoxification process. Therefore, when ethanol and prescribed drugs are taken together, the drug's effect may be augumented (e.g., phenytoin, warfarin) or the alcohol effect may be prolonged (e.g., chloral hydrate, chlorpromazine, cimetidine). Microsomal induction after long-term alcohol consumption contributes to accelerated ethanol metabolism only at high blood ethanol concentrations. Increased drug metabolism and activation of xenobiotics (e.g., carcinogens) due to microsomal induction persist after cessation of long-term alcohol consumption, potentially resulting in lower than therapeutic blood levels (e.g., barbiturates, phenytoin, isoniazid, meprobamate, and warfarin) or increased production of toxic metabolites (e.g., acetaminophen). Common mechanisms for pharmacodynamic drug-ethanol interactions include increased drug effect due to additive CNS depression (e.g., antihistamines, other CNS depressants, antipsychotics, and antidepressants) or diminished drug effect due to the presence of cross-tolerance to other CNS depressants. The major medical concern of ethanol interactions with other CNS depressants is a severe depression of the CNS that leads to respiratory arrest because of a pharmacodynamic interaction.

Proposed Mechanisms of Ethanol Action in the CNS

For many years, the most popular theory of the pharmacologic action of alcohol has been that it associates with hydrophobic areas of neuronal membranes and makes the membranes more fluid, thus increasing the mobility of membrane components and altering functions of membrane proteins.[15,r24] For example, while acute alcohol fluidizes cell membranes, chronic alcohol exposure results in alterations in the lipid composition that render synaptic membranes more "rigid."[42] Consequently, unlike many other CNS-active drugs (e.g., opiates, benzodiazepine, etc.), alcohol has been thought not to interact directly with specific receptors. However, it has been shown in vitro that ethanol, in concentrations that occur after consuming one to three drinks (5–50 mM), selectively activates GABA-stimulated chloride channels,[43] inhibits NMDA-activated ion currents,[44] and potentiates 5-HT_3-activated ion currents.[45] Similarly, ethanol has been demonstrated to have such actions on these receptors as well as on glycine and nicotinic cholinergic receptors in vivo in intact animals.[46,47] These findings led to the conclusion that ethanol has the capability of influencing all ligand-gated ion channels.[47–49] It is unknown whether these effects of ethanol mediated by receptors linked to ion channels are caused by its direct actions on the proteins involved or by alteration of lipid-protein microenvironments.

Another recent finding important to ethanol's action in brain is that it affects responses induced by agonists interacting with ligand-gated ion channels at some but not all neurons.[47,50] For GABA, Criswell et al.[47] proposed that a specific receptor subtype associated

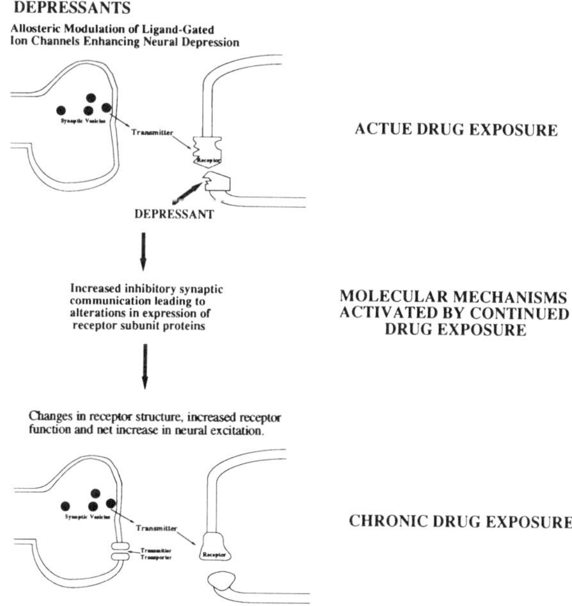

Figure 21.3 Neuroadaptive changes in $GABA_A$ and other ligand-gated ion channels after acute and chronic treatment with ethanol and other CNS depressants.

with zolpidem binding accounted for the enhancement of GABA by ethanol on the majority of neurons and the selectivity of ethanol within selected brain regions. It is proposed that this selectivity of ethanol for a specific $GABA_A$ receptor subtype will generalize to specific receptor subtypes for the other ligand-gated ion channels, because ethanol has been demonstrated to affect responses to agonists for these channels on only a subset of neurons.[47,50]

The $GABA_A$ receptor binds the major inhibitory neurotransmitter in brain and is also the target for the pharmacologic actions of both barbiturates and benzodiazepines. Depressant agents acting at this receptor may alter acute ethanol intoxication and changes in $GABA_A$ receptor characteristics when coadministered with ethanol, and may contribute to tolerance and dependence associated with chronic ethanol ingestion. On the other hand, the NMDA-receptor binds the major excitatory neurotransmitter (glutamate) in the brain, activation of which allows calcium to enter neurons and act as a secondary messenger. Activation of the NMDA-receptor has been implicated in synaptic plasticity, kindling, learning, and excitotoxicity.[51] Up-regulation of NMDA-receptors and down-regulation of $GABA_A$ receptors following chronic alcohol intake may contribute to alcohol withdrawal seizures.[52] Finally, antagonists of the 5-HT_3 receptor, which is activated by serotonin and potentiated by ethanol, block subjective recognition of intoxication, reduce alcohol intake, and inhibit ethanol-stimulated dopamine release in the nucleus accumbens.[53–55] Although low doses of ethanol stimulate locomotor activity and produce marked increases in extracellular dopamine levels in the nucleus accumbens of the rat,[56] there is considerable evidence for dopamine-independent ethanol reward, particularly via the $GABA_A$ receptor complex which plays a significant role in modulating endogenous stress levels in the organism.[r25] The recent observation[47] that ethanol enhances the excitatory action of nicotine on nicotinic receptors may be a contributing factor in acute stimulant effects related to ethanol.

Work performed in parallel to that on ligand-gated ion channels, relevant to the action of ethanol on the CNS, is that ethanol affects at least some receptors linked to phospholipase C (PLC) and also affects protein kinase C (PKC).[57,58] PLC is an enzyme that causes hydrolysis of phosphoinosital phosphate resulting in a change in calcium levels.[r26] PKC is capable of phosphorylating specific proteins, including the ligand-gated ion channels.[r27] Future work should determine whether only those receptor subtypes, with phosphorylation sites affected by PKC or linked to PLC, are sensitive to ethanol.

Sources of Alcoholic Beverages

Alcoholic beverages contain between 3 to 50 percent (or ml per 100 ml) of ethanol, and the typical "drink" has approximately 15 g of ethanol. For example, the ethanol content of beer, wine, "fortified" wines (port, sherry), and whiskey (80–100 proof) are 3–5, 10–12, 18–20, and 40–50 percent, respectively. The "proof" of alcohol is twice the percentage by volume (i.e., 45% = 90 proof, etc.). The density of ethanol is about 0.8, so 100 ml of 100-proof whiskey contains about 40 grams.

Alcohol, USP is 95 percent ethanol. Absolute alcohol is 100 percent, but takes up water rapidly when exposed to air, diluting itself to 95 percent. "Rubbing alcohol" is 70 percent ethanol (denatured), which is more bactericidal than higher concentrations of ethanol. "Denatured alcohol" is ethanol used in many household and industrial products and contains small amounts of any of a number of agents to discourage its consumption (e.g., pyridine, castor oil, acetone, sucrose octa-acetate, amyl alcohol, gasoline, benzene).

Alcohol Dependence Syndrome

There is considerable support for the view that ethanol has a reinforcing component to its pharmacology.[r25,r28] The longitudinal course of chronic self-administration of alcohol (alcohol dependence) is probably the most studied of all psychoactive substance use disorders[31–33,r2,r29] and can be used as a paradigm for understanding the development of psychoactive substance use disorders in general (see sections for each agent). Elements of this paradigm include: 1. Predisposing factors (biologic, psychologic, social); 2. psychopharmacologic effects of the drug; 3. tolerance, dependence (physical, or psychologic) and withdrawal; 4. brain damage and other medical complications. These elements are highly interrelated and can influence each other, as suggested in Figure 21.1. Alcohol abuse in family members disrupts family life and affects development of children within that family. It is not surprising that there are higher rates than normal of alcohol dependence as well as other forms of psychopathology among children of alcoholics.

It is well recognized that there are large differences among groups of alcoholic patients. The challenge has been to identify characteristics of these patients that would allow classification of individuals into more homogeneous subgroups that are useful predictors of etiology, longitudinal course, and response to different treatment modalities. One heuristically useful classification system is based predominantly on the age of alcohol dependence onset. Type 1 is after age 25; Type 2 is before age 25. Alcohol-related problems and personality traits tend to differ between these two types. In general, Type 2 patients tend to be more recalcitrant to treatment and to have a greater genetic loading. Environmental background for Type 2 patients seems to be relatively less important than it is for Type 1 alcoholics.[31]

Comorbidity of Mental Disorders with Alcohol Dependence

As noted earlier in this chapter, it is important to consider whether evidence of an underlying major psychiatric condition is present in any patient believed to be alcohol-dependent,[2,3,59,r4] since an underlying mental disorder may be a component of the alcohol dependence syndrome (see Table 21.2). If a mental disorder is discovered, the appropriate pharmacologic and psychotherapeutic interventions should be instituted.

Nonetheless, other treatments that deal with the alcohol dependence syndrome also should be undertaken.[r7]

Inheritance and Gender in Alcohol Dependence

Several studies have been undertaken to determine if a genetic component is a contributing factor in alcoholism.[60–62] Twin and adoption studies have allowed partialling out of the relative contributions of genetic and environmental factors in alcohol dependence. The concordance rate for severe alcoholism is substantially higher in monozygotic (0.70) than dizygotic (0.33) twins, whereas concordance rates are no different for less severe forms of alcohol abuse (0.8 for both monozygotic and dizygotic twins). Adoption studies show that men with alcoholic biologic parents have an increased likelihood of developing alcoholism regardless of whether they are raised in an alcoholic environment. In general, the severity of parental alcoholism tends to influence the prevalence of alcoholism in adopted-out sons (most severe alcoholics have the highest rate of alcoholism in offspring). These studies suggest that the role of environment in the development of alcoholism may vary with the severity (or type) of alcohol dependence inherited. Although the above studies suggest that genetic factors are important contributors to the development of alcohol dependence, the mechanisms involved that result in alcoholism remain to be elucidated. This is an exciting area of research, but there are no current hypotheses that have real clinical applicability. Examples suggesting a genetic contribution include differences in subjective intoxication, ethanol metabolism, and brain (EEG) evoked potentials between children who have and those who do not have a biologic parent with alcoholism.[63–65]

Women and Alcohol Dependence

There are definite differences between the sexes in the presentation and longitudinal course of alcoholism. It is particularly important to understand alcoholism in females because of the adverse effects of drinking on the developing fetus and the disruptive effects of alcohol dependence on the maternal/child relationship, both of which can perpetuate the transmission of alcoholism from one generation to the next (via nongenetic means). Females tend to have lower rates of alcohol dependence (although these rates are rapidly rising) relative to males, but women have a greater likelihood of a genetic contribution. However, this is offset by lower rates of alcohol consumption by females in the general population. Even though females start drinking later than males, they tend to develop more serious complications at about the same age as males. For example, women are more at risk for alcohol-induced liver disease than are men.[1]

Tolerance, Dependence and Withdrawal

Tolerance

Extended use of alcohol results in metabolic as well as functional tolerance. Owing to adaptation of alcohol dehydrogenase, alcoholics ingesting large amounts of alcohol have an increased capacity to metabolize ethanol (i.e., metabolic tolerance). Consequently, higher levels of alcohol are necessary to produce a deficit in motor and other functions in alcoholics than in normals. Accompanying this metabolic tolerance is a central neuroadaptation to the actions of ethanol. This type of tolerance to ethanol is shared with most other CNS depressants including the barbiturates and benzodiazepines, but not the opioids. Tolerance may not develop at the same rate to all actions of alcohol. For example, there is no marked attenuation of the effect of repeated ethanol use on respiratory function in dependent individuals. Therefore, with a severe overdose of ethanol superimposed on chronic consumption, respiratory arrest can occur. The neuroadaptive changes that accompany chronic ethanol exposure are illustrated in Fig. 21.3.

Alcohol Dependence and Withdrawal

Maintenance of high doses of ethanol produces a functional state of dependence. In alcohol-dependent individuals, removal of ethanol results in symptoms associated primarily with a sensitization of the CNS to sensory input. This syndrome is characterized by anxiety, apprehension, restlessness, irritability, and insomnia with clinically apparent tremor and hyperreflexia. Moderately severe cases progress to signs of autonomic hyperactivity with tachycardia, hypertension, diaphoresis, hyperthermia, and muscle fasciculations. Often patients experience anorexia and nausea and vomiting with subsequent dehydration and electrolyte disturbances. Sleep is markedly disturbed and nightmares are often described. Eventually, the most severe cases may develop delirium (agitation, disorientation, fluctuating levels of consciousness, visual and auditory hallucinations and intense autonomic arousal). In older literature, this syndrome was referred to as "delirium tremens" or "rum fits." During withdrawal, generalized tonic-clonic seizures may occur in those patients who have undergone repeated withdrawals over years.[16] Typically, seizures will occur between 12 to 48 hours after the last drink, and delirium tremens begins at between 48 to 72 hours. Ballenger and Post[16] proposed that the appearance of seizure activity in alcoholic patients is due to a kindling process caused by repeated withdrawal. This view is supported by other clinical[66] as well as preclinical studies.[67] The treatment of choice for acute withdrawal from ethanol is a long-acting benzodiazepine (see Treatment), but all CNS depressants will suppress withdrawal symptoms. The acute withdrawal syndrome observed in the dependent individual usually subsides within three to seven days if untreated. Regardless, brain dysfunction may persist for weeks to months in severe cases of withdrawal.[r29]

Medical Complications of Alcohol Abuse

The medical complications of chronic alcoholism derive from the pharmacologic effects of ethanol, the changes in intermediary metabolism resulting from its biotransformation to acetaldehyde in the liver, and the toxic effects of this metabolite in various tissues of the body.[68,69] Alcoholics are likely to have a shorter life span than nonalcoholics owing to such medical complications associated with chronic ethanol exposure.[68]

Consequences of Ethanol Metabolism: Liver Disease Associated With Alcohol Abuse

The hepatic oxidation of ethanol causes the consumption of NAD because this proceeds faster than the reoxidation of NADH; as a result there is an increase in the NADH/NAD ratio (e.g., the metabolism of 100 gm of ethanol—about six strong drinks—requires about 2 moles of NAD). Ethanol metabolism leads to conversion of pyruvate to lactate and to the formation of acetoacetate, acetone, and betahydroxybutyrate. These agents can interfere with renal tubular secretion of uric acid, causing modest increases in blood urate, thus exacerbating gout. Heavy drinking after a period of not eating can cause severe, even fatal hypoglycemia. This is the result of the combination of low hepatic glycogen stores and inhibition by ethanol of gluconeogenesis.

The pathologic conditions that constitute alcoholic liver injury are fatty liver, alcoholic cirrhosis, and alcoholic hepatitis. The possible mechanisms for alcohol induction of these conditions are related primarily to its effects on metabolism and a background of malnutrition in the alcohol dependent individual.[41,69] Alcoholic fatty liver is the most common consequence of chronic alcohol abuse and is completely reversible with abstinence and proper nutrition. The pathogenesis of fatty liver is related to the reduction of hepatic lipid oxidation by ethanol. Fatty liver can be caused by even single doses of ethanol. Fatty acids are released from fat by ethanol, and their conversion to hepatic triglycerides is promoted by the increased NADH/NAD ratio. Chronic fatty liver, probably with the help of nutritional deficiencies, progresses to alcoholic hepatitis and finally to cirrhosis. Acetaldehyde can be hepatotoxic, and ethanol can induce an isozyme of cytochrome P-450 that converts some chemicals to hepatotoxic metabolites.[69]

Alcohol is the major cause of cirrhosis in developed nations. Alcoholic cirrhosis is the second most common cause of death in the 24- to 44-year-old age group in large urban areas and the third most common in the 45 to 64 group. Deaths from cirrhosis are highly correlated with the availability of alcohol in the population and the duration and amount of consumption (e.g., epidemiologic studies have shown that rates of cirrhosis were significantly reduced during Prohibition).

Acute symptomatic alcohol hepatitis results in death (20%), chronic symptomatic disease (40%), or recovery of asymptomatic state (40%). It is not understood with certainty why certain individuals with alcoholic hepatitis develop cirrhosis, whereas in others the liver recovers. However, it is recognized that multiple factors may contribute to these differences [e.g., ethanol dose (duration of drinking), host (gender, genetics, immunity), and environment (diet, toxins)]. However, the ability of the patient to maintain abstinence remains the major determinant of the clinical outcome of alcoholic hepatitis. For example, 80 percent of abstinent individuals recover or improve following acute alcoholic hepatitis, and 20 percent develop cirrhosis; whereas, of those who continue drinking, 50 to 80 percent develop cirrhosis and 30 to 50 percent have continued alcoholic hepatitis. Survival after the diagnosis of alcoholic cirrhosis (5 years) with abstinence is 63 percent, whereas it is 40.5 percent with continued drinking.

The presence of cirrhosis in an alcoholic patient is an important consideration in the pharmacotherapy of any concomitant illness because the pharmacokinetics of many drugs are altered by cirrhosis and the consequent diminished hepatocellular functions. Complications of cirrhosis that can complicate pharmacotherapy include portal hypertension (GI bleeding, portosystemic encephalopathy, hypersplenism), salt and water retention (ascites/edema, functional renal failure), hepatoma, coagulopathy, defective immune function, defective leukocyte function, glucose intolerance (diabetic-like), hemosiderosis (increased GI iron absorption), peptic ulcer, gall stones, and renal tubular acidosis.

Certain ethanol-related compounds that are metabolized by alcohol dehydrogenase, methanol and isopropyl alcohol, are important for toxicologic reasons. Alcoholics sometimes substitute these alcohols for ethanol when "spirits" are not available to them. Methanol is a less potent CNS depressant than is ethanol, but it is much more toxic owing to its metabolism to formaldehyde and formic acid. The formic acid formed from methanol causes a profound systemic acidosis, and one or both metabolites cause retinal damage and permanent blindness. Death has resulted from drinking as little as 60 ml of methanol and blindness from 4 ml. Treatment of methanol poisoning includes correcting the acidosis, for example with bicarbonate, and inhibiting the metabolism of methanol with ethanol.

Isopropyl alcohol is a more potent CNS depressant than is ethanol, but has such a bad taste that it is not often used by alcoholics when they cannot get ethanol. Isopropyl alcohol is commonly used as an agent to clean skin areas (i.e., substitute for rubbing alcohol). Those who are in coma because of drinking isopropyl alcohol have acetonemia, acetone odor on the breath, and thus may be confused with ketoacidotic diabetics. They are not, however, acidotic or glycosuric.

Cardiovascular Disease

Heavy alcohol consumption increases cardiovascular and coronary heart disease mortality/morbidity due to direct toxicity of ethanol and/or its metabolites and indirectly through hyperlipidemia, vitamin or protein deficiencies, hypertension, and effects on calcium/mineral metabolism and thrombosis/fibrinolysis.[69] Chronic ethanol alters kidney function,[70] which also can contribute to cardiovascular disease. Possible protective effects of moderate alcohol consumption include decreased coronary heart disease,[71] which may be offset by the increased associated cancer and stroke mortality with chronic excessive amounts of ethanol. Finally, ethanol consumption increases HDL_3, but not HDL_2, which is associated with decreased arteriosclerotic heart disease.[72] Methodological issues (ex-drinkers, behavior and life-style variables) complicate interpretation of these epidemiologic studies of the possible protective effects of moderate alcohol consumption.

Endocrine Effects

The diuresis associated with drinking alcoholic beverages is caused primarily by inhibition of ADH release from the posterior pituitary.[73] The volume of water ingested is only a minor factor. Oxytocin release also is inhibited by ethanol, and uterine contractions are inhibited. Alcohol also increases the release of ACTH and glucocorticoids[74] and catecholamines.[75] The synthesis of testosterone is inhibited, and its hepatic metabolism is increased.[76] Consequently, male alcoholics often have signs of hypogonadism and feminization.

Gastrointestinal Effects

Ethanol stimulates the secretion of gastric and pancreatic juices. This effect on gastric juices and the direct irritant action of concentrated solutions of ethanol help explain why one of every three heavy drinkers suffers from chronic gastritis.[68] In high doses, vomiting may occur independently of any local irritation. Alcohol abuse is associated with acute and chronic pancreatitis and esophagitis. Heavy users of alcoholic beverages have an increased incidence of carcinoma of the pharynx, larynx, and esophagus.

Malnutrition

Malnutrition is common among alcohol-dependent patients and is manifested by weight loss or obesity, impaired protein synthesis, altered amino acid metabolism, immune-incompetence, mineral and electrolyte imbalance, and vitamin deficiencies.[r30] The following vitamin deficiencies have been observed in alcoholic patients: thiamine (30–80%); folic acid (6–80%); pyridoxine (50%); nicotinic acid (35%); ascorbic acid; and vitamins A and D. The possible mechanisms for thiamine deficiency in chronic alcoholism are inadequate intake, decreased activation of thiamine to thiamine pyrophosphate, reduced hepatic storage, inhibition of intestinal transport, and impairment of absorption due to ethanol-related nutritional deficiency states.[77]

Central Nervous System Brain Disease

Neuropsychologic studies indicate that intellectual impairment probably is the earliest complication of chronic alcoholism.[78–80] Early evidence indicated that this impairment is related to neuropathology,[81] a conclusion backed by recent magnetic reasonance imaging results of alcohol-dependent patients[r31,r32] and basic research on chronic alcohol administration.[82] Factors that contribute to neurotoxicity and brain damage associated with alcohol dependence[83,84] include alcohol pattern of use/abuse and duration of abstinence and secondary effects of life-style such as nutrition, head trauma, hepatic dysfunction, anoxia, and concomitant abuse of other drugs. The most common neuropathologic findings in the chronic alcoholic patient include cerebellar degeneration (40%), Wernicke-Korsakoff syndrome (13%), and reduced brain weight/volume (mechanism unknown).[85] Alcoholic organic mental disorders are usefully conceptualized as two clinically and neuropathologically differentiable syndromes of impairment: 1. alcohol amnesic disorder (commonly called Wernicke-Korsakoff syndrome); 2. alcoholic dementia.[85] It is well established that thiamine deficiency in the chronic alcoholic patient may cause the Wernicke-Korsakoff syndrome,[r33] but the relative contribution of thiamine deficiency and alcohol neurotoxicity in alcoholic dementia is still controversial. Of patients with Wernicke's encephalopathy (an acute neuropsychiatric syndrome characterized by ataxia, confusion, and abnormalities of eye movement), 80 to 90 percent develop Korsakoff's psychosis (a chronic syndrome characterized by subtle behavioral abnormalities and disproportionate impairment of memory over other cognitive functions). Over one year, approximately 20 percent of patients with Korsakoff's psychosis make a complete recovery, 20 percent recover incompletely, and 60 percent have long-lasting deficits requiring institutionalization. Thus, the treatment of chronic organic mental disorders associated with alcoholism must involve abstinence and improved nutrition, if any advantage is to be gained.

Fetal Alcohol Effects

Alcohol exposure of the fetus during gestation results in a continuum of effects that are related to the dose, intensity, individual factors (in fetus or mother), and timing of exposure, including spontaneous abortions, growth retardation, stillbirths, neonatal behavioral effects, and impaired neonatal status (decreased APGAR scores).[r34] For the most severe cases of ethanol exposure, malformations, retarded developmental milestones, decreased IQ, and perinatal mortality occur. Exposure to alcohol during the first trimester can result in major morphologic abnormalities. There is an increased risk of spontaneous abortion if alcohol exposure occurs during the second trimester. Decreased fetal growth characterizes exposure during the third trimester.

The most severe fetal alcohol effects have been termed the fetal alcohol syndrome (FES).[86] This syndrome is characterized by prenatal or postnatal growth retardation in weight, height, and/or head circumference; altered morphogenesis, especially a characteristic facial dysmorphology; and CNS involvement with mental retardation. The facial features in fetal alcohol syndrome include microcephaly, short palpebral fissures, flat midface, indistinct philtrum, thin upper lip, micrognathia, short nose, minor ear anomalies, low nasa bridge, and epicanthal folds. Manifestations of CNS dysfunction include irritability in infancy, altered muscle tone (especially hypotonia in infancy), poor motor coordination, hyperactivity in childhood, mental retardation, with the severity of the dysmorphogenesis tending to be correlated with IQ. However, it is becoming increasing apparent that dysmorphogenesis in some affected individuals can be minimal, even though individuals show severe behavioral abnormalities once they have reached puberty.[87]

Acute and Protracted Treatment of Alcohol Dependence

Acute Withdrawal Treatment

Owing to the prevalence of alcohol use, it is not unexpected that the most common drug management problem that the physician will see pertains to alcohol abuse/dependence. Initial management of the alcohol-dependent patient involves diagnosis, and if necessary treatment of those patients who manifest the alcohol withdrawal syndrome.[23] Withdrawal from a CNS depressant like ethanol results in hyperexcitability.[88] Anxiety is often a prominent symptom of withdrawal. It has been proposed that CRF and/or a benzodiazepine inverse agonist in brain released during withdrawal contribute to this anxiety observed during acute abstinence from chronic self-administration of large doses of ethanol.[89,90] Treatment objectives are relief of symptoms, prevention or treatment of complications (e.g., seizures, arrhythmias, delirium), and preparation for postwithdrawal rehabilitations.[23] *The treatment of choice for the acute alcohol withdrawal syndrome is 60 mg of the long-acting benzodiazepine, diazepam.*[91,92] Prior to any extended treatment, a careful clinical evaluation needs to be conducted with emphasis on the complications of alcohol dependence including trauma, malnutrition/CNS dysfunction, fluid-electrolyte disturbances/hypoglycemia, infections, gastritis, pancreatitis, liver disease, cardiopulmonary disease, history of seizures/delirium, and use of other drugs of abuse.[23]

Treatment of Alcohol Dependence

Disulfiram. Disulfiram (Antabuse), a drug that inhibits aldehyde dehydrogenase, has been used to diminish ethanol abuse. Its effects in the drinker are largely if not entirely, due to accumulation of acetaldehyde. Taken alone, disulfiram causes little or no effect (although it does inhibit dopamine-beta-hydroxylase). When given with alcohol, it causes intense flushing of the face and neck, tachycardia, hypotension, nausea, and vomiting. Death in individuals who have taken ethanol when treated with disulfiram has occurred. Therefore, its use in treating alcoholism must be combined with psychosocial treatment modalities. Patients taking disulfiram may experience reactions similar to those with ethanol after exposure to other organic solvents.[93] Disulfiram inhibits other drug-metabolizing enzymes and increases the elimination half-life of several drugs, including phenytoin, warfarin, thiopental, and caffeine. The success rate of disulfiram versus placebo showed disulfiram to have minimal effectiveness (see details in outcome). Calcium carbimide, which is available in Canada and other countries but not in the US, acts similarly to disulfiram to inhibit aldehyde dehydrogenase, and is said by some to be less toxic than disulfiram.[94]

Experimental Treatments. At the present time no ideal pharmacologic agent has been approved by the FDA for use in treating chronic alcoholism. Nonetheless, recent data have provided reason to be optimistic. For example, based on animal research,[r35] naltrexone, an opioid antagonist, has undergone a few successful clinical trials for treating alcoholism.[95] It was concluded that this treatment was safe and effective for reducing alcohol relapse.[95] Additionally, there are positive reports that drugs that block serotonin re-uptake may be useful in preventing relapse in alcoholics.[96] It is too early to tell whether these drugs will be found to be effective in treating all alcohol dependence, but it appears that basic studies are providing important clues about how this disease state may be treated with pharmacologic agents.

Psychosocial Strategies. Psychosocial strategies have been among the best approaches for reducing drinking in susceptible individuals (i.e., alcoholics). The most noted organization for supporting alcoholics is Alcoholics Anonymous (AA).

Whereas detoxification (treatment of withdrawal) varies for individual agents due to pharmacologic considerations, long-term management is more similar than different for the different substances of abuse. The degree of outside social support and stability in the patient's environment is the major determinant of whether in- or outpatient treatment is indicated. Both forms of treatment include psychotherapies (social or milieu, insight-oriented, behavioral, individual, and group in various combinations) with introduction and encouragement to participate in 12-step self-support groups such as AA. Aftercare (i.e., care following the treatment program) is equivalently (if not more) important than the initial treatment program itself. Individuals with disorganized family situations and/or no outside supports may benefit from halfway houses. Development of pharmacologic strategies for treatment of psychoactive substance use disorders is an exciting new field of research, but at this stage its clinical utility remains to be demonstrated. Pharmacotherapy of concomitant psychiatric disorders requires careful diagnosis and avoidance of the misuse of pharmacotherapy to treat a disorder that is a consequence of the psychoactive substance use disorder. Treatment is given additional attention later in the chapter where the general basis of a psychosocial approach is suggested as a model to treat all types of drug abuse.

Outcomes of Diagnosed Alcohol Dependent Patients

The five- to seven-year outcome for 1289 diagnosed alcoholics treated during a two-year period (between 1973–1975) showed that only 1.6 per cent of the subjects showed stable moderate drinking at follow-up, 15 per cent were totally abstinent, and 4.6 per cent were mostly abstinent with occasional drinking. The only predictors of moderate drinking found were female sex and less severe alcoholism. The evolution to stable moderate drinking appears to be a rare outcome among alcoholics treated at medical or psychiatric facilities.[97] Accordingly, it seems reasonable that the goals of long-term treatment should focus on abstinence.

At present, psychotherapeutic and social strategies are the cornerstone of treatment; however, there is some excitement concerning psychopharmacologic strategies. The most widely used pharmacologic strategy for reduction of alcohol consumption in patients has involved aversive agents such as alcohol-sensitizing drugs (disulfiram and calcium carbamide) and emetics (apomorphine, emetine).[94] The efficacy of disulfiram has been very carefully evaluated in a VA Cooperative Study of 605 men who received concomitant counseling bimonthly for one year.[98] Total abstinence, time to first drink, employment, or social stability were not significantly different among patients who received disulfiram 250 mg or 1 mg (double blind) or placebo. However, the reported drinking days among nonabstinent patients were as follows: 250 mg (49.0 ± 8.4), 1 mg (75.4 ± 11.9), no disulfiram (86.5 ± 13.6), suggesting a subtle benefit of disulfiram. Therefore, one must weigh the relative benefits of disulfiram treatment, which are not impressive based on the VA Cooperative Study, versus the risks which are significant (e.g., unknown optimal dose/schedule, unknown therapeutic margin, several contraindications [liver disease, pregnancy, heart disease, etc.], substantial/diverse toxicity [CNS, liver, etc.], drug interactions, and the toxicity/reinforcing effects of acetaldehyde).

Better understanding of the neurobiologic mechanisms regulating alcohol consumption is expected to lead to development of medications that can reduce the urge to drink.[r25] Drugs that have been used in the treatment of primary alcoholism include antidepressants (zimelidine, citalopram, serotonin precursors), lithium, dopaminergic agents (apormophine, bromocriptine, amantadine, L-DOPA), vitamins, β-blockers, carbamazepine, and hydroxyzine. As noted above, naltrexone can also be added to this list.[95] Drugs that have been used in the treatment of alcoholism secondary to a psychiatric disorder predominantly address the underlying psychopathology. Medications for the pharmacologic treatment of alcoholism should have the predictable effect of attenuating ethanol intake in the target population without having positive reinforcing effects (low abuse/dependence potential). Furthermore, such medications should have no deleterious interactions with alcohol, should be administrable by the oral route and be long-acting and well tolerated in order to facilitate compliance. Finally, they should have a wide therapeutic margin (minimal overdose potential) with no serious drug-related toxicity, especially in organs damaged by alcohol.

Benzodiazepines and Sedative-Hypnotics

Benzodiazepines are often prescribed for management of patients with anxiety and insomnia. Other drugs in the general category of sedative and hypnotics, such as the barbiturates, are not used to the degree they once were. The material here will focus on the abuse of these agents since the pharmacology of the benzodiazepines, barbiturates, and other CNS depressants has been described in Chapter 14.

Pharmacology

CNS depressant intoxication proceeds in stages that depend on dose and time following administration. Euphoric feelings are often reported during the initial stage of intoxication and typically are the expressed reason for drug self-administration. Mild impairment of motor skills and slowing of reaction time can be seen, followed by sedation, decreased motor coordination, impaired judgment, memory and other cognitive deficits, and diminished psychomotor activity as drug concentration increases in the brain. At very high concentrations most CNS depressants can induce general anesthesia, although it is difficult to obtain surgical depth anesthesia with benzodiazepines. (See Chapter 14 for other details.)

Mechanism of Action

Benzodiazepines and barbiturates have classic sedative/hypnotic actions which correlate well with their ability to modulate GABA-induced Cl-fluxes, as discussed in Chapter 14. These drugs produce a release of punished responding in conflict situations, which correlates well with their ability to act as anxiolytics. The anxiolytic/tension-reducing property of CNS depressants may be a major component of their reinforcing actions and abuse potential.[r22,r36] GABA function in some limbic and extrapyramidal regions such as the amygdala, ventral forebrain, olfactory tubercle, and globus pallidus could influence drug reward. $GABA_A$ receptor antagonists block their anticonflict (antianxiety) effects and $GABA_A$ receptor agonists potentiate these effects.

Abuse of Benzodiazepines and Barbiturates

Continued use of depressant drugs results in tolerance, and larger doses are needed in order to achieve symptomatic relief. If the physician does not provide education and carefully monitor prescribing, the patient may eventually administer larger doses of these medications, with attendant side-effects including mood disorders, cognitive dysfunction, social difficulties, impaired work performance, and traumatic injury due to falls or vehicular accidents. In order to maintain symptomatic relief in the face of tighter controls by the prescribing physician, the patient may combine alcohol, other prescribed medications or illicit drugs (e.g., marijuana, opiates) with the prescribed dose of these CNS depressants, seek other physicians to provide further prescriptions, or even engage in illegal activities such as forging prescriptions. Cessation of drug use leads to undesirable, even potentially harmful withdrawal symptoms. Occasionally, fulminant withdrawal may occur in patients who discontinue CNS depressant use due to illness or other unforeseen circumstances such as hospitalization.

Tolerance, Dependence and Withdrawal

Tolerance and Dependence

Adaptive neuronal changes to the continued presence of benzodiazepines or barbiturates involves a decrease in inhibitory functions of the CNS. The behavioral consequences are well characterized and include the development of tolerance and dependence, which usually proceed in parallel (see Chapter 14). The development of tolerance and dependence to these CNS depressants can occur after only a few days of repeated ingestion, and, as with all drugs, is determined by dose and frequency of use.[r12] For example, a dose of drug that initially caused sedation may in time be insufficient to cause sleep or reduce anxiety, necessitating higher doses to attain these therapeutic goals. The acute and adaptive changes that follow alcohol and other CNS depressants are illustrated in Figure 21.3, page 423.

Tolerance may not develop at the same rate to all actions of a CNS depressant. For example, whereas sedation usually diminishes after the first few days of treatment with most benzodiazepines, anxiolytic effects may persist for months without need to increase the dose. Euphoric effects may not be as predictable, and this can cause rapid increases in dose if the drug is being self-administered for this purpose. In general, for all CNS depressants there is no marked elevation of the lethal dose with repeated use, and respiratory depression may be superimposed on chronic consumption with a severe acute overdose.

Withdrawal

Cessation of benzodiazepine and barbiturate intake following prolonged use is associated with a syndrome of neuronal hyperexcitability with increased peripheral sympathetic and adrenocortical activity.[88] Among the CNS depressants, the most severe and potentially dangerous withdrawal syndrome results from short-acting barbiturates and nonbarbiturate hypnosedatives, followed by alcohol, and then benzodiazepines. The onset, amplitude, and duration of the withdrawal syndrome in a given class of CNS depressants are determined by the rate of elimination of the drug and metabolites from the body.[99,r12] For example, among the barbiturates, nonbarbiturate hypnosedatives, and benzodiazepines, withdrawal usually begins within 12 hours and is most severe for rapidly eliminated compounds (e.g., amobarbital, methyprylon, and triazolam). For slowly metabolized compounds (e.g., phenobarbital, diazepam, or clonazepam), the syndrome may be delayed for several days after drug discontinuation.

Like ethanol withdrawal, the withdrawal syndrome for these other CNS depressants is characterized initially by anxiety, apprehension, restlessness, irritability, and insomnia with clinically apparent tremor and hyperreflexia. Signs of autonomic hyperactivity are seen in moderately severe cases of withdrawal (e.g., tachycardia, hypertension, diaphoresis, hyperthermia). Patients often experience anorexia, nausea, or vomiting, with subsequent dehydration and electrolyte disturbances. Eventually the most severe cases may develop delirium (agitation, disorientation, fluctuating level of consciousness, visual and auditory hallucinations, and intense autonomic arousal). Paroxysmal EEG discharges may proceed to generalized tonic-clonic seizure activity. Cross-tolerance and cross-dependence among alcohol and other CNS depressants occur, as would be expected of drugs that share cellular and molecular mechanisms of action.

The general pharmacologic approach to treat withdrawal from chronic abuse of all CNS depressants is to administer an appropriate drug which has a longer elimination half-life than the drug from which the patient is being withdrawn, once obvious clinical signs of withdrawal are apparent.[99,100] *For the CNS depressants other than alcohol (barbiturates, benzodiazepines and other sedative-hypnotics), the slowly-eliminated barbiturate phenobarbital is the treatment of choice for withdrawal symptoms.*[99,100] The typical patient who manifests moderately severe signs of withdrawal from barbiturates, nonbarbiturate hypnosedatives, or benzodiazepines may need 900 to 1500 mg of phenobarbital.[99,100] Doses of phenobarbital for withdrawal from these CNS depressants are administered until the patient manifests signs of mild intoxication.[99,100] It is important to recognize that phenobarbital and all drugs currently used for the treatment of CNS depressant withdrawal have dependence liability. Accordingly, a major challenge for pharmacologists is to develop agents that can ease CNS depressant withdrawal with little liability for abuse and dependence.

Treatment of Depressant Dependence

Acute Treatment of Overdose

Any patient who enters an emergency room setting comatose from an overdose of a CNS depressant could be dependent on any of the CNS depressants, including alcohol. Therefore, such individuals could experience withdrawal when brain levels of the depressant are reduced below a critical level. Obviously, this possibility can be a complicating factor in the treatment of patients overdosed with this drug class. If a patient is overdosed on a benzodiazepine, IV flumazenil is a specific antidote (see Chapter 14). However, the physician must be cautious; if the patient is dependent on a benzodiazepine and the antagonism by flumazenil of benzodiazepine receptors is complete, withdrawal symptoms may emerge in a dependent individual. Overdose of CNS depressants other than the benzodiazepines is treated symptomatically to avoid respiratory arrest and to facilitate the excretion of the compound, as no specific antagonists exist for these other CNS depressants.

Protracted Treatment

The strategy to treat CNS depressant dependence is generally like that described for alcohol earlier in this chapter. However, there are no aversive drugs to prevent recurrence nor is any specific agent presently available to treat CNS depressant dependence. It would seem reasonable to test whether naltrexone and drugs that block serotonin uptake (which have promise for treating ethanol dependence) would be effective in reducing CNS depressant relapse. As with the treatment of alcoholics, the long-range strategy is to keep the patient abstinent from these CNS depressants. This involves treating any psychopathology, altering the environment to reduce conditioning-related relapse and providing psychotherapeutic and psychosocial support.

Psychostimulants: Cocaine and Amphetamines

Cocaine is an alkaloid derived from the shrub *Erythroxylon coca*, a plant indigenous to South America, where its leaves have long been chewed for their stimulating effect. Cocaine was isolated in 1860; after 1884, it became the first effective local anesthetic, the only purpose for which it is still used in medicine (see Chapter 10 and History earlier in this chapter). Until 1914, when cocaine was placed under the same laws as morphine and heroin and was legally classified as a narcotic, the drug was used "therapeutically" in a variety of ways.

Amphetamine has been used clinically as a nasal decongestant, analeptic, antidepressant, an adjunct to dieting, and for treatment of hyperactive children—among other things (see Chapter 22). Use of amphetamine has permeated many socioeconomic strata of society, with amphetamine abuse being fashionable among the poor, working, and middle classes at different times, primarily because of its availability and low cost. In some western societies, amphetamine is second only in prevalence to marijuana among abused drugs.

Widespread manufacture of amphetamine by pharmaceutical companies contributed to the availability and low cost of this drug.[r11] The low cost of amphetamines also has, in turn, fueled their widespread distribution as a cheaper, longer lasting alternative to cocaine and other stimulants. More recently, illegal manufacture of methamphetamine derivatives has burgeoned, especially within countercultures. In the mid- to late 1980s, a new crystallized, smokable form of methamphetamine appeared that became known by the street name "ice." It was believed to have originated in East Asia and was first introduced to the US in California. The high potency and extremely long-lasting effects of "ice" appear to have increased the abuse liability of the drug and may have contributed to individuals switching from "crack" cocaine to "ice" abuse.

Pharmacology[r11,r37,21]

The structure of cocaine is described in Chapter 10. Amphetamine is a racemic β-phenyl isopropylamine (d and l isomers; see Chapter 22). The d-isomer is several times more potent than the l isomer with respect to its CNS actions. The main clinically relevant pharmacologic effect of the central stimulants related to cocaine and amphetamine is the blockade of reuptake of catecholamine neurotransmitters, noreprinephrine, and dopamine.[r22,r37] Thus, many of the peripheral and CNS effects of amphetamine and cocaine are similar. The consequences of noradrenergic reuptake blockade are primarily peripheral and include tachycardia, hypertension, vasoconstriction, mydraisis, and diaphoresis. Other details of the actions of norepinephrine on peripheral functions when released by amphetamine can be found in Chapters 4 and 6.

Dopamine reuptake blockade resulting from central stimulant administration results in prominent effects on the CNS function (see Chapter 22). These include enhanced intracranial self-stimulation, euphoria, anorexia, stereotypes, and hyperactivity. It is these central dopaminergic effects that are believed to be responsible for the cocaine "high" as well as the strong reinforcing properties of the drug. The fact that cocaine effects are relatively short-lasting contributes to the high rate of intake, which, in turn, probably increases tolerance, dependence and abuse liability. Studies in animal models show that animals will self-administer cocaine preferentially over food, leading to emaciation and death (in contradistinction to other highly reinforcing agents such as opiates). Amphetamine is also a strongly reinforcing drug in animal models, and dopamine is implicated in amphetamine reward as well as that of cocaine. Amphetamine will substitute for cocaine in drug discrimination paradigms, but discrimination between the two drugs can be achieved only with extensive training. Thus, while the subjective state produced by the two drugs is similar, there are subtle differences that may alter abuse liability. Although cocaine is clearly a highly efficacious positive reinforcer, environmental manipulations such as punishment, increasing the amount of behavior required to obtain the drug, or offering alternative reinforcers are effective in decreasing self-administration.[r22] As described in Chapter 10, cocaine also has direct vasoconstriction action on blood vessels and is a local anesthetic. These properties, associated with its use as a local anesthetic, also make it more dangerous because of the potential for seizures and cardiac arrest when administered systemically (see Medical Complications of Abuse).

Routes of Administration and Absorption

Methods of use of the central stimulants include inhalation (snorting), subcutaneous or IV injection, and freebasing (smoking). Inhalation is the most common and least dangerous method, but does not provide the ecstatic sensation of smoking or injection. These latter routes of administration allow rapid access of the drug to the brain, thereby increasing its reinforcing effect as well as its toxicity.[21,r11]

Mechanism of CNS Action

It is widely accepted at the present time that the pharmacologic effects of cocaine and the amphetamines on the CNS are related to the ability of these drugs to enhance the action of released dopamine.[101,r22] The reinforcing action of d-amphetamine to increase brain stimulation reward was demonstrated to be due to the action of these drugs on dopaminergic neurons, not to the release of norepinephrine,[102] a view now widely accepted. The mechanism by which these drugs act is to antagonize the reuptake of dopamine by binding to a reuptake site on presynaptic neurons. This reuptake site has been cloned recently.[103–105] Thus, dopamine seems to be the major neurotransmitter involved in the positive reinforcement of central stimulants.[r22]

Our understanding of the neuroanatomic basis of dopaminergic involvement in stimulant reinforcement is also being clarified.[r22,r37] The cell bodies of the mesocorticolimbic dopamine system, anatomically an anterior component of the reticular formation, originate in the ventral tegmental area (VTA) and project to the forebrain, largely to the nucleus acumbens, olfactory tubercle, frontal cortex, amygdala, and septal area. Destruction of these dopaminergic fibers diminishes motor responses to environmental stimuli or produces a syndrome of perseveration with reduced distraction to irrelevant information including decreased behavioral flexibility, spontaneity, and reversal of previously learned habits. Likewise, experimental lesions of the nucleus accumbens and the VTA extinguish cocaine and amphetamine self-administration.[r22,r37] In vivo microdialysis studies confirm that dopamine release is increased in the nucleus accumbens during IV self-administration of cocaine.[r22]

Stimulant Abuse

The typical pattern of abuse begins with introduction to the drug in pill (amphetamine) or powder (cocaine) form as a way to increase energy or by prescription for mood elevation or diet control. Because of their "energizing" effect, stimulants are often used by workers on the job. As with most drugs that produce intense euphoria, the user seeks to reproduce the initial high experienced upon first exposure and ingests amphetamine or cocaine more frequently and at higher doses.[106] Eventually, addiction ensues and the route of administration may change to smoking or IV intake.[r11,106,107]

A sense of profound well-being and optimism appears to pervade the individual intoxicated with stimulants (cocaine, amphetamines methylphenidate; Table 21.1). The most striking pharmacologic characteristic of cocaine and amphetamine are their tremendous reinforcing effects.[r11,r21,r22] Stimulants produce profound euphoric feelings coupled with behavioral activation and signs of increased sympathetic nervous system activity.[r11] Locomotor activity increases profoundly in laboratory animals following treatment with these central stimulants.[101] Human users appear to be more energetic after stimulant administration. A major difference between the two stimulants is that the initial euphoric effect of cocaine appears to be more pronounced than that of amphetamine, while amphetamine intoxication far outlasts that of cocaine.

The differences in intensity of the initial euphoric effects by amphetamine and cocaine may relate to the preferred route of administration for these drugs. For example, drugs that are smoked or inhaled have more rapid access to the brain than do those ingested orally. However, the cocaine "high" is relatively short-lived. Mood elevation begins to dissipate within 10s to minutes after cocaine administration, and an acute depression may follow. Amphetamine intoxication is of much longer duration. Mood elevation and increased activity can persist for hours, especially following ingestion of methampetamine. This prolonged high is almost always followed by a period of listlessness, drowsiness, and depressed mood. Long periods of sleep may follow intoxication induced by high drug doses. Appetite suppression occurs during stimulant intoxication and lasts for hours after amphetamine ingestion. This effect often results in significant weight loss in patients who abuse stimulants.

Cocaine is almost always used with another psychoactive substance, most commonly alcohol. In this regard, alcohol may be a "gateway" drug for cocaine use, as it accentuates the "high" obtained from cocaine, but alleviates some of the adverse effects ("wired" feelings). There may well be common predisposing factors (genetic, environmental, and psychological) that lead to the abuse of both agents.

Tolerance, Dependence and Withdrawal

Tolerance

The most significant feature of tolerance to stimulant drugs is that the desirable effects of the drug become less pronounced while the undesirable and even lethal effects increase. In addition, effects that initially seemed desirable, such as increased sociability, change to less desirable effects, such as paranoia and socially unacceptable behavior.[r11]

As with amphetamine, acute tolerance develops to the subjective effects of cocaine, and this can play a major role in dose escalation and subsequent toxicity. On the other hand, it is possible that sensitization[r39] plays a role in stimulant-induced panic attacks, paranoia, seizures, and lethality. Repeated use of stimulants results in loss of the euphoric, anorexic drug effects and the cognitive coherence that marks initial intoxication. Enhanced activity and talkativeness continue, but begin to take ever more bizarre forms such as incoherent speech and stereotypic movements. Mood changes also persist. While initial use results in euphoria, continued use leads to cyclic emotional highs and lows. Unwanted perceptual changes such as hallucinations and delusions of persecution may appear.[107] Prolonged stimulant use can lead to a psychotic state characterized by paranoia, hallucinations (both auditory and visual), and delusions. Violent acts are not uncommon in long-time stimulant users.

Dependence

Stimulant dependence is characterized by marked craving for the drug and its euphoric and energizing effects as well as a need to prevent the emotional and energetic low experienced after cessation of the drug's effect. In the case of cocaine, the desire for euphoric feelings predominates during the early period of chronic use, but is diminished as use persists. Amphetamine intoxication can be followed by pronounced physical and psychologic depression even after the first use. Thus, dependence even in the early stages of stimulant use is characterized by a desire to recapture the euphoria and energy of the "high". Furthermore, there is an accompanying need to alleviate the lethargy and depression taking place after this major effect of the stimulants dissipates. Once significant tolerance has taken place, larger doses are used to regain the effects previously observed. In the absence of the drug, craving occurs. Dackis and Gold[108] have suggested a dopamine depletion hypothesis to account for the dependence syndrome that accompanies prolonged stimulant abuse. Robinson and Berridge[r39] have suggested that the craving for stimulants is due to receptor sensitization. These views are illustrated in Figure 21.4.

Withdrawal

In humans, discontinuation of cocaine after repeated administration can lead to dysphoria (a so-called "crash") and cocaine craving.[r11] During withdrawal patients are anxious and restless. Hypersomnolence, dysphoria, anergia, and general depression also occur. As a result, the typical cycle of cocaine use consists of periods of binging, followed by the crash (9 hours to 4 days), followed by a period of

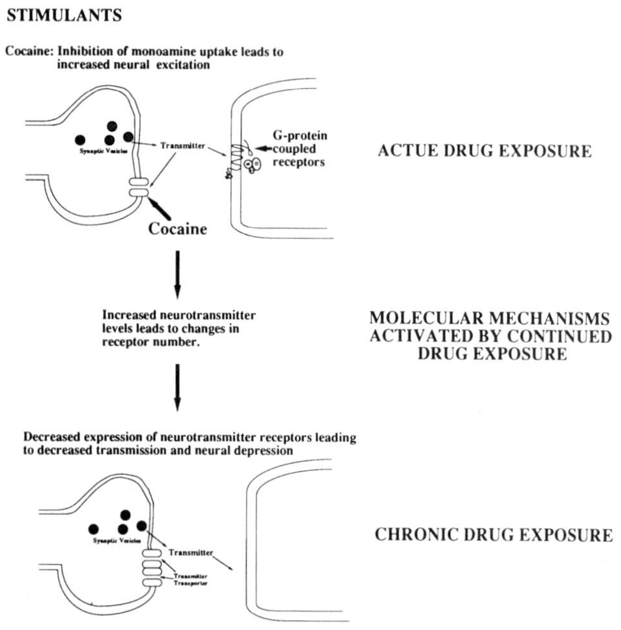

STIMULANTS

Cocaine: Inhibition of monoamine uptake leads to increased neural excitation

Transmitter G-protein coupled receptors ACTUE DRUG EXPOSURE

Cocaine

Increased neurotransmitter levels leads to changes in receptor number.

MOLECULAR MECHANISMS ACTIVATED BY CONTINUED DRUG EXPOSURE

Decreased expression of neurotransmitter receptors leading to decreased transmission and neural depression

Transmitter CHRONIC DRUG EXPOSURE

Figure 21.4 Neuroadaptive changes in dopaminergic function after acute and chronic treatment with cocaine. Amphetamine and other central stimulants are presumed to have a similar action.

withdrawal (1 to 10 weeks) during which relapse is very common.[107]

Cessation of chronic amphetamine use also leads to anxiety, depression, and irritability. These symptoms are accompanied by reports of listless feelings and a profound increase in appetite. Later these symptoms subside and are followed by prolonged sleep and drowsiness. Suicidal ideation may accompany this depressed state. These symptoms last for at least several days after withdrawal and may persist for months after cessation of amphetamine use in some individuals.

Two significant neurochemical changes occur following cessation of chronic stimulant use. Depletion of dopamine is thought to result from constant blockade of uptake systems exceeding the ability of neurons to synthesize new transmitter.[108,r39] This action likely contributes to the dysphoria and anhedonia reported during withdrawal since normal dopamine release, and hence normal neural reward pathways, are disrupted. The second significant change is an increase in dopamine receptor number. This receptor change appears to be a secondary consequence of dopamine depletion or a reduced release. Receptors are "up-regulated" to enhance the efficiency of transmission. The increase in receptor number probably contributes to "sensitization" to any dopamine released, as discussed above.[r37] This receptor supersensitivity may also underlie stereotypic movements observed in chronic amphetamine abusers.

Medical Complications of Stimulant Abuse

It is a moot point whether there are small changes in rates of cocaine use over the last five to ten years because medical complications of cocaine use (which tend to follow estimates of use in a population with a lag of a few years) are still very high, as indicated by both nonfatal events and deaths reported by the Drug Abuse Warning Network of the National Institute of Drug Abuse. Excessively high doses of stimulants can elicit paranoia, hallucinations, stereotypic behaviors, convulsions, stroke, or even death.[109] In addition, the effects of cocaine on cardiac function can elicit arrythmias and death.[r40] Physical complaints that have been reported in cocaine abusers include sleep problems, chronic fatigue, severe headaches, nasal sores and bleeding, chronic cough and sore throat, nausea, vomiting, and seizures or loss of consciousness. Cardiovascular complications of cocaine abuse include angina pectoris, myocardial infarction, syncope, sudden arrhythmic death, aortic dissection, stroke, and pulmonary edema. Neurologic complications of cocaine abuse include seizures, cerebrovascular accidents, cerebrovasculitis, hyperpyrexia and rhabdomyolysis, headaches, dystonias, and loss of consciousness. Psychologic symptoms include depression, anxiety, irritability, apathy, paranoia, difficulty concentrating, memory problems, sexual disinterest, and panic attacks.

Psychiatric complications of cocaine abuse include acute organic mental disorders (intoxication, withdrawal, delirium, delusional disorder) possibly chronic organic mental syndrome(s), schizophreniform psychosis, affective disorders, anxiety disorders, and sexual dysfunction. Affective disorder is a particularly important complicating factor in management of cocaine dependence that differentially affects the genders.[110a] Females who are cocaine-dependent have higher rates of major depression (primary), leading to the concept that drug use is a form of "self-medication." Men with cocaine dependence have higher rates of antisocial personality disorder. Mechanisms for neuropsychiatric complications include cerebrovascular vasoconstriction, neurotransmitter depletion, and reduced limbic seizure threshold resulting from repeated subconvulsant stimulation. Adverse social and other effects include dealing cocaine to support their habit, stealing from work, family or friends, arrest for dealing or possession, automobile accidents, loss of job, loss of spouse, and severe financial debt. Females who become pregnant during chronic stimulant use deliver "crack" babies.[r41] The impact of these infants on health and social care has not been fully realized at this time. Additionally, individuals who share needles to administer cocaine IV are at risk for HIV infection and AIDs (see Opiate Abuse).[110]

Treatment of Stimulant Overdose and Dependence

The major problem with stimulant abuse is overdose. Treatment of amphetamine intoxication involves acidification of the urine by administering ammonium chloride, which also has a mild diuretic action. One of the antipyschotics such as chlorpromazine is administered to diminish the CNS symptoms. An α-adrenergic blocker usually is administered to reduce hypertension.

The treatment of cocaine overdose is much more complex than that for amphetamines. The major consideration is to prevent convulsions, respiratory failure, and cardiac arrest. Artificial respiration may be necessary. Chlorpromazine is useful for reducing CNS excitation as well as the cardiovascular effects due to its mild α-adrenergic blocking activity. If seizures occur, they are treated symptomatically. If the serious consequences are minimized, prognosis is favorable because cocaine is rapidly metabolized.

Efforts to treat chronic CNS stimulant dependence require proper support. Only if the patient can maintain abstinence beyond the withdrawal period can extinction and ultimate abstinence follow. Therefore, treatment should address the conditions that lead to relapse, i.e., reducing the effects of conditioned cues that trigger craving (such as persons with whom—or situations in which—the individual has used cocaine and the availability of cocaine in one's neighborhood). Adjunctive pharmacologic treatments that hold promise for treating the stimulant dependent syndrome include tricyclic antidepressants or the anticonvulsant carbamazepine.[21,111] The principles for dealing with this aspect of drug abuse treatment is discussed later in this Chapter.

Opioids

The present discussion will focus entirely on the issue of abuse of this class of drugs. The pharmacology of the opioids has been described in detail in Chapter 20. Opiates are considered to be highly addictive, and individuals often will persist in using these drugs for years. For example, heroin and its predecessor morphine are widely abused in Asia, Europe, and the Americas. Periods of discontinuation and relapse are frequent among opiate addicts, with relapse often occurring years after cessation of drug use. Former users commonly report remembering positive experiences with the drugs even after long periods of abstinence.[r42,r43]

Pharmacology

Opium has been used for centuries; its active ingredients are the opioid alkaloids. The structures of opioids are found in Chapter 20. Effects of opioids can be attributed to their action on opiate receptors. Because of their action on peripheral opiate receptors, opioids have been used for the treatment of diarrhea, but better agents are now available that do not have the abuse liability of this drug class. Central effects of opioids in both animals and humans are biphasic, with behavioral activation at low doses and sedation at higher doses. The major pharmacologic action of opioids is analgesia. These drugs also depress respiration, produce miosis, and can induce sleep. Death from opioid overdose is invariably from respiratory arrest.

The receptor subtypes for opiates are detailed in Chapter 20. The mu-opioid receptor subtype appears to be important for the reinforcing actions of opiates. Delta-opioid receptors appear to have an important role in the opioid motor stimulation that is dopamine-dependent. Endogenous opioid peptides that act on opiate receptors are distributed throughout the brain and form three major functional systems defined by their precursor molecules: β-endorphin from pro-opiomelanocortin; enkaphalins from proenkephalin; and dynorphin from prodynorphin.[r44] Modulation of nociceptive response to painful stimuli and stressors, reward, and homeostatic adaptive functions such as food, water, and temperature regulation are associated with these endogenous substances. Therefore, opioid administration would be expected to mimic the same physiologic functions controlled by these endogenous substances,[112] particularly those that act on mu-opiate receptors.

In laboratory animals, opiate drugs can serve as rewarding stimuli and also facilitate brain-stimulation reward. Furthermore, morphine-like opiates can lower the electric current threshold for intracranial electrical self-stimulation, indicating an ability of the opiate to facilitate the central reward mechanism itself. Thus, opiates act as powerful reinforcing agents.[r22,r45] Sterotypic movements are also elicited in laboratory animals and likely involve opiate actions on brain motor systems. Rats will self-administer opioid peptides into the VTA and nucleus accumbens. Intra-VTA morphine lowers the electric current threshold for intracranial electrical self-stimulation, induces conditioned place preference, and supports self-administration through microcannulae or micropipettes implanted into the VTA. After self-administration behavior has been extinguished, it can be reinstated by administration of morphine into VTA, but not into the nucleus accumbens. Intra-VTA morphine administration also reinstates cocaine self-administration. These results specifically implicate the dopaminergic projections from the VTA to the nucleus accumbens in the rewarding actions of opiates and may explain why cocaine, which also acts at this site, is coadministered with opioids.[r22,r37,r40,r45] Opiates, like other substances of abuse, can increase dopamine release in the nucleus accumbens as measured by in vivo microdialysis in awake, freely moving animals, but the reinforcing effect of opiates in the nucleus accumbens can be independent of dopamine release. Therefore, the reinforcing actions of opiates may involve both a dopamine-dependent (VTA) and a dopamine-independent (nucleus accumbens) mechanism. Like the central stimulants, these results suggest that neural elements in the region of the nucleus accumbens are responsible for the reinforcing properties of opiates.[r45] Other regions supporting rewarding effects for opioids are the hippocampus and hypothalamus.

Finally, chronic morphine treatment of rats has been shown to increase G proteins, cyclic AMP-dependent protein kinase, and the phosphorylation of a number of proteins.[113] It is likely that alteration of several of these mechanisms may occur during neuroadaptation, but it is not yet clear whether there is one final common pathway, perhaps akin to the alterations that occur at the molecular level during learning and memory, that all psychoactive substance of abuse may share.[19,20] Keys to molecular changes during neuroadaptation have clear implications in the pharmacotherapy of dependence and withdrawal of opiates and other substances abused.

Opiate Abuse[r42]

Throughout the 20th century a proportion of the population has been addicted to opiates. This "subculture" of opiate users has grown in proportion in the latter half of the century. Heroin, a potent opiate, has largely replaced morphine among illicit users in most countries. A large group of patients abuse opiates prescribed for treatment of chronic pain. Finally, a small number regularly use opium, particularly in Asian countries.

Heroin and morphine usually are injected IV, and this is the overwhelmingly preferred route of administration among opiate addicts. IV administration of an opioid produces a change described by dependent individuals as a "rush." This feeling, which lasts less than a minute, appears to be the basis of abuse of opioids. When suitable vessels become unavailable, subcutaneous administration or "skin-popping" sometimes is substituted. A small number of users inhale refined opiates. This route of administration is most popular among relatively inexperienced users. Unrefined opium usually is smoked from a water pipe. Administration or ingestion of heroin or morphine induces a profound euphoric state that is maximal minutes after ingestion. This is associated with analgesia and is followed by the onset of a "dreamlike" state characterized by decreased responsiveness to the environment. The analgesic and sedative effects of opiates usually persist for hours and thus outlast the intense euphoria. The less efficacious opiates usually produce milder euphoria with some analgesia and sedation.

Heroin addiction is associated with particular patterns of behavior that are worthy of mention. Addicts often engage in criminal behavior (petty theft, burglary) or prostitution to obtain money for drug purchases. Heroin addiction thus has a large impact on society via secondary unlawful consequences in addition to the effects of the drug itself. Dependence also represents a major public health problem because it contributes to the spread of communicable diseases. IV heroin users are susceptible to a variety of infections, which they spread to others via sharing of hypodermic paraphernalia. Most notable among these diseases transmitted is AIDS by HIV infection. AIDS is extremely widespread among heroin addicts. Likewise many venereal diseases also can be spread by unprotected sexual activity in this patient group.[110]

Other opiates carry abuse liability. These include the prescription drug pentazocine, often used in conjunction with anticholinergics and antihistaminics (see section of psychedelics), and codeine, which is a component of several nonprescription medications. These opiates sometimes are used by heroin addicts when heroin is unavailable, but are also used by others seeking their narcotic effects.

Tolerance, Dependence and Withdrawal

As morphine and methadone are relatively selective agonists for mu-opioid receptors, these receptors may be regarded as the primary sites involved in the acquisition, maintenance, and relapse of opiate addiction. This cyclic process for opiate dependence has been described.[10,r42]

Tolerance

A characteristic feature of opioids is the tolerance that develops from repeated use. However, tolerance does not develop to all actions of the opioids. Increases in the amount of drug necessary to achieve euphoric and analgesic effects are the main symptoms of tolerance. The depressant effects on respiration and physical activity also dissipate with repeated use. In contrast, psychomotor stimulation appears to increase during early phases of chronic use. This latter behavioral sensitization to opiates may coincide with an increased perception of the desirable or reinforcing effects of the drug. Eventually, tolerance develops even to the reinforcing and psychomotor drug effects and increasing drug doses are self-administered.[r42] Tolerance does not develop to the action on the eye (miosis) or to the constipating effect of the opioids with repeated use.

Dependence and Withdrawal

The dependence on opioids is characterized by a withdrawal syndrome. Hyperalgesia, GI cramps, joint and muscle aches, yawning, and sweating accompany acute withdrawal in dependent opioid users. Following acute symptoms in dependent individuals, a characteristic syndrome of depressed mood and dysphoria occurs. The withdrawal symptoms depend on the opioid used, the duration, and the dose. Following the period of depression, excessive autonomic output (dilated pupils, anorexia, etc.) nausea, elevated blood pressure, diarrhea, and gooseflesh are common. These symptoms usually abate over a period of 4 to 7 days. The degree of physical dependence does not predict the intensity of craving. Neither does detoxification and recovery from physical dependence prevent relapse into addiction. The motivational (affective) properties of withdrawal are independent of the intensity and pattern of the physical symptoms of withdrawal.[r42]

Medical Complications of Opioid Abuse

The medical complications associated with opioid use are described in detail in Chapter 20 and are related directly to the pharmacologic properties of this drug class. Except for overdose, opioid compounds are relatively safe. The major medical problem is treating the craving of the dependent individuals. Another indirect medical complication related to sharing of needles is the contraction of the HIV virus and AIDS,[110] as noted earlier.

Treatment of the Opioid Dependence Syndrome

As with other drugs of abuse discussed, one major problem area encountered in individuals abusing opiates is drug overdose. Any individual entering an emergency room who is comatose with reduced respiration and constricted pupils should be considered as a case of opioid overdose. Attention must be given to correcting the respiratory depression. This is dealt with by administering naloxone, an opioid antagonist. However, care must be taken to prevent precipitation of withdrawal in such patients if they are dependent on opioids. Also, owing to the short halflife of naloxone, patients aroused may serendipitously slip into a coma as the action of the naloxone wears off.

Once it is determined that a patient has dependence to an opiate, one course of action is to administer methadone (which itself has considerable dependence liability) in increasingly lower doses until the individual is abstinent. Alternately, clonidine, which suppresses many symptoms of withdrawal, can be administered.[114] This latter approach is an advantage because its use is without risk of cross-dependence with opioids. Following this medical course, the individual usually is associated with support groups that attempt to maintain abstinence. As with all drugs of abuse, it is important that life-style and environment change because of condition.[115] Another approach for treatment of opioid dependence is methadone maintenance to prevent the psychosocial problems associated with the opiate dependence.[r46] (See Chapter 20 p. 401, for the structure of methadone.) This would seem a particularly important approach for dependent individuals with a history of relapse, given the current AIDS epidemic. Other pharmacotherapeutic strategies to prevent relapse include the use of naltrexone and buprenorphine (see Chapter 20).

Marijuana: Cannabinoids

Marijuana is the common name for the plant *Cannabis sativa*. Other names for the plant or its products include hemp, hashish, chasra, bhang, and daga. On the street, marijuana is referred to as "grass," "pot," and "reefer." The use of marijuana has been documented to have occurred for centuries (see historical background). Highest concentrations of the psychoactive cannoabinoids are found in the flowering tops of both male and female plants. Most commonly the plant is cut, dried, chopped and then incorporated into cigarettes. Marijuana is often the first illicit drug tried by individuals. The likelihood of using other drugs increases with the extent of marijuana use in all age groups. The epidemiology of marijuana use, therefore, can be viewed as a predictor of drug-related problems in a given population.

Pharmacology

The pharmacology and neurobiology of THC have been reviewed in detail.[r47–r50] The primary psychoactive constituent of marijuana is (-)-delta-9-tetrahydrocannabinol (THC), although the hemp plant synthesizes at least 400 chemicals.[r49] Its structure is presented in Figure 21.5. Studies have clearly documented the action of THC on brain, but for many years the underlying mechanism responsible for these central changes was unknown. This situation has now changed. The newly isolated cannibinoid receptor provides the basis for the actions of THC.[116] Actions on this receptor are responsible for the reduction of spontaneous activity, catalepsy, antinoception, and hypothermia caused by THC, as well as the "high" associated with its administration.[r50] There is dilation of conjunctival blood vessels, and tachycardia occurs after marijuana or THC administration. Blood pressure remains relatively unchanged unless high doses are used, in which case orthostatic hypotension ensues. Although increased appetite frequently is attributed to marijuana, appetite has not been consistently enhanced in controlled studies, and increased food intake is not observed in intoxicated animals.

THC acts as an agonist at the cannabinoid receptor. This receptor is extremely abundant in the brain, especially in cerebral cortex, as demonstrated by radioligand binding[117] and localization of the mRNA for the

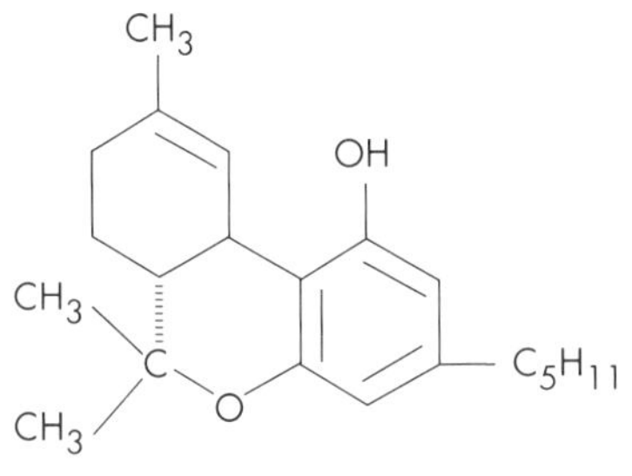

CH_3 OH CH_3 C O C_5H_{11} CH_3

Figure 21.5 Structure of Δ9-Tetrahydrocannabinol

receptor protein.[118] The pharmacologic profile of agonist action suggests that virtually all intoxicating cannabinoids act as agonists at this receptor, and that their potencies for receptor activation closely parallel their potency for producing intoxication in laboratory animals. However, upon chronic administration of THC, no change in cannabinoid receptor number has been observed, indicating that tolerance is not associated with a change in receptor number.

The THC receptor is related to G-protein transduction linked to inhibition of adenylate cylcase.[119,r47] This receptor has not been shown to be linked to other receptors that inhibit adenylyl cyclase. However, the physiologic consequences of this inhibitory effect on adenylate cyclase are not well understood. It has been observed that cannabinoid receptor activation will inhibit voltage-gated calcium channels and activate voltage-gated potassium channels.[120] Inhibition of excitatory synaptic transmission in the hippocampus by cannabinoids may be another consequence of receptor activation.[121] Much additional work is needed to establish the mechanism by which activation of this abundant receptor leads to changes in CNS functions.

It is noteworthy that an endogenous chemical has been shown to possess activity at the cannabinoid receptor.[122] Thus, the possibility that endogenous cannabinoid-like agents contribute to neural function and behavior is worthy of serious consideration. A "peripheral" cannabis receptor also has recently been described that is closely related in structure to the brain form, but with potentially important differences.[123] It has been postulated that activation of this receptor is responsible for the immunosuppressant actions of cannabinoids. These recent discoveries are certain to stimulate new research to define the physiologic role of cannabinoid receptors in brain and peripheral function.

Absorption, Distribution and Metabolism[r49]

The amount of active material that reaches the bloodstream is highly dependent on the smoking technique, the cannabinoid content of the sample, and the amount altered by pyrolysis during smoking. Plasma levels are attained within approximately 10 minutes, and subjective effects begin 20 to 30 minutes later, seldom lasting beyond 2 hours.[124,r49] In vivo, THC is converted rapidly into a centrally active metabolite, 11-hydroxy-9-THC. While most of the other 60 cannabinoids present in the plant are either inactive or only weakly active, they have the potential of interacting with THC to either increase or decrease its potency. Hundreds of additional compounds are produced by pyrolysis when marijuana is smoked, which may contribute either to acute effects or to its long-term toxicity. The half-life of THC in plasma is relatively short,[r49] apparently due to a redistribution to fatty tissues. This redistribution of THC likely accounts for the long period before THC and its metabolites are cleared from the body. The metabolites of THC are excreted in the urine and feces.[r49]

Marijuana Abuse[r51]

Marijuana use has been falling in young adults, but use rates in females are nearly as high as those in males.[29] This suggests the possibility that the sex-related differences described for alcoholism (see above) may be changing in the current generation of substance abusers. The subjective effects of marijuana vary somewhat from individual to individual, determined in part by highly variable pharmacokinetic variables, dose, route of administration, setting, experience and expectation, and individual vulnerability to certain psychotoxic effects. Typically, intoxication is characterized by an initial period of "high" that has been described as a sense of well-being and happiness. Euphoria frequently is followed by a period of drowsiness or sedation. Perception of time is altered, along with distortions in both hearing and vision. The subjective effects include dissociation of ideas. Illusions and hallucinations occur infrequently.

Impaired functioning in a variety of cognitive and performance tasks, including impaired memory, altered time sense, and decrements in tasks such as reaction time, concept formation, learning, perception, motor coordination, attention, and signal detection occur. At doses equivalent to one or two cigarettes, processes involved in driving and flying are impaired. This impairment persists for four to eight hours, long after the user perceives the subjective effects of the drug. The impairment produced by alcohol is additive to that induced by marijuana. Tolerant individuals may perform somewhat better on the above measures when given marijuana. At higher doses, acute panic reactions or mild paranoia have been observed due to the alterations in perception produced by the drug. With extremely high doses, an acute toxic psychosis accompanied by depersonalization and loss of insight has been reported. This latter response seems to affect only extremely heavy users.

Tolerance, Dependence and Withdrawal

Tolerance

Tolerance appears to develop mainly following frequent usage of high doses of the drug.[r11,r50] The drug effects to which tolerance develops include most of the acute actions of THC. Tolerance to THC appears to reflect mostly pharmacodynamic rather than pharmacokinetic changes.[r50] Tolerance has been well documented for actions of THC in animals.[r48]

Dependence[r11,r50,r51]

Chronic users of marijuana report craving for the drug. It is unclear if this represents a specific desire to experience the psychologic effects of the drug or to maintain a pattern of behavior that has become habitual to the user.[r48] Some evidence of a dependence syndrome in humans has been reported, mostly from anecdotal reports of symptoms observed upon drug withdrawal. Some drug effects, mild withdrawal symptoms, and craving may persist for months. This is probably the result of the fact that the drug is only slowly removed from fatty tissues and thus is slowly released to the rest of the body long after cessation.

The evidence for dependence from studies of animal models is scant. Animals will not self-administer THC, and THC does not readily substitute for other drugs of abuse.[r48,r50] In all, THC does not appear to have marked abuse or dependence liability in animals, perhaps suggesting some physical or psychologic interaction unique to humans that increases abuse potential.

Withdrawal[r11,r50,r51]

There is no pronounced, well-characterized withdrawal syndrome associated with cessation after prolonged THC use. However, symptoms including irritability, restlessness, insomnia, anorexia, and mild nausea have been reported in humans upon withdrawal. These changes were accompanied by weight loss, slight fever, and hand tremor. However, few analogous changes have been noted in animal models of THC withdrawal.

Medical Complications[r51]

An "amotivational syndrome" frequently has been described in the literature; however, well-controlled clinical studies have failed to provide strong evidence that an amotivational syndrome is a direct consequence of marijuana use. Nonetheless, chronic marijuana users have been noted to exhibit apathy, dullness, and impairment of judgment, concentration, and memory, as well as loss of interest in personal appearance and pursuit of conventional goals.[125] There has been some evidence of alterations in the reproductive system, immune system, and respiratory function with chronic use of marijuana.[126,r51]

Nicotine and Tobacco

Tobacco is widely abused by individuals ranging in age from teens to senior citizens.[29] The most prevalent form of tobacco use is cigarette smoking. Cigar and pipe smokers account for a much smaller percentage of abusers. Tobacco is also administered via the "smokeless" route (snuff). This involves placing tobacco leaf or powder adjacent to the gums, which slowly releases tobacco juice into the microvasculature of the mouth allowing the absorption of nicotine—the major pharmacologic agent in tobacco.

Pharmacology

Nicotine acts on nicotinic receptors for acetylcholine in autonomic ganglia and brain to produce its pharmacologic actions (see Chapter 4, 5). Nicotine is a highly selective agonist at these receptors. Activation of these receptors throughout the peripheral nervous system and musculature is the likely source of the autonomic activating effects of the drug. The CNS action of nicotine results in a pleasant feeling and a reduction in appetite.[r11] Nicotine produces dependence in animal models as well as in humans. Conditioned place preference behavior is supported by the drug, and rodents will self-administer nicotine. However, the ability of nicotine to support self-administration is less than that of drugs of abuse with marked euphoric effects, such as the central stimulants and opiates. Thus, activation of nicotinic receptors in the CNS is believed to play a role in nicotine dependence. Nicotine is unusual among drugs of abuse in that it is highly dependence-producing without strong euphoric, sedative, or anxiolytic actions.

Several subtypes of central nicotinic cholinergic receptors have been identified using ligand binding assays.[127,128] More recently, the structures of specific subunits making up central nicotinic receptors have been identified using molecular biologic techniques.[129,r52] The variable localization of these subunits for nicotinic receptors in brain reinforces the view that there are differing nicotinic cholinergic receptors in brain with distinct neuroanatomic locations. Nonetheless, the physiologic role of these CNS nicotinic cholinergic receptors in various behaviors is not as clear as their function in the periphery. Definition of the involvement of specific nicotinic cholinergic receptors in the rewarding action of nicotine that leads to dependence ultimately should provide clues for treating the dependence caused by chronic tobacco exposure.

Tobacco Abuse

Tobacco use in North America has declined over the last 20 years, due mostly to information about the health hazards of use provided in large part by government sources.[r53] Despite these efforts, people still use tobacco on a daily basis. Thus, tobacco (nicotine) abuse remains a substantial public health problem, not only in the US,[29] but throughout the world. This ingredient is believed to be responsible for the psychoactive actions and dependence properties of tobacco. When tar and nicotine levels of cigarettes are varied, user reports of strength and satisfaction depend on nicotine content.[r11] This idea has received support from animal studies indicating abuse liability of nicotine as well as the observation that nicotine gum or dermal applications can substitute for tobacco use in individuals.

Tolerance, Dependence and Withdrawal

Tolerance

It has been well established in animals and humans that tolerance can develop to selected actions of nicotine, in particular the dizziness and nauseous feeling. However, others may go through periods of mini "withdrawals" before continuing the use of tobacco. Irrespective of tolerance to some effects of nicotine, the chronic smoker exhibits an acute change in cardiovascular function (i.e., increased heart rate and blood pressure) suggesting that tolerance to this action of nicotine is minimal.

Dependence

Long-term smokers often express a "need" or craving for tobacco after abstinence that suggests a dependence on the drug. Other signs of dependence include an inability to discontinue drug use even with a strong desire to do so. In the most serious cases, tobacco use continues in spite of the development of serious tobacco-related diseases, such as emphysema, cardiovascular disease, and lung cancer, even though tobacco inhalation increases the severity of these disease states (see Medical Complications). It is this resolute continuation of an obviously dangerous habit that constitutes the most dramatic, if not the most convincing, evidence for tobacco dependence in humans.

Withdrawal

Most tobacco users experience withdrawal due to a "cold turkey" sudden cessation of use. If removed from a nicotine source, the irritability, anxiety, restlessness, headaches, lack of concentration and sleep disturbances persist for several days to weeks. The psychologic dependence may take several months before it subsides. Subjective reports of strong craving for tobacco are common among individuals during the early stages of withdrawal. Some evidence of craving can persist for years after cessation of tobacco use, indicating that psychologic dependence remains long after intake has been halted and dependence broken.

Medical Complications Associated With Tobacco

Since the use of tobacco is a major medical problem for society,[29] it would be desirable that it be eliminated. While smoking and other uses of tobacco have decreased in the last decade, approximately 36 percent of the population continues to use this substance. The major medical complications include cardiovascular diseases, particularly coronary heart disease.[130] Pulmonary diseases such as emphysema are associated with smoking.[131] Further, the symptoms associated with peripheral vascular disease are worsened by chronic tobacco use. The pulmonary complications of smoking appear to be particularly severe in individuals who work in situations associated with dust (coal miners, fiber industry, and weaving industries). A final area of concern is the high incidence of lung cancer among smokers.[132,133] Additionally, mothers who smoke have children with reduced birth weight.

Treatment of Nicotine Dependence

The obvious solution for preventing the undesirable chronic consequences of tobacco (nicotine) intake is to have individuals cease their use of this substance. However, even though individuals wish to stop, it often is difficult if not impossible (see Dependence and Withdrawal). Some individuals undergoing withdrawal from smoking tobacco (nicotine) respond to clonidine.[26] Another strategy for treating individuals with dependence on tobacco is the administration of nicotine to alleviate craving.[134] The FDA has approved nicotine-containing gum and a dermal patch. Over time the concentration in these delivery systems is reduced in the patch and fewer gum pieces are used until dependence on nicotine is eliminated. This latter approach is said to have some success in treating individuals who are resistant to other approaches. It has the advantage of removing behavioral cues associated with smoking fewer and fewer cigarettes. Presumably, the course of the patch or gum treatments is sufficiently limited in scope that any detrimental effects of the nicotine administration are minimal. Since administration of nicotine via oral or dermal routes decreases craving, this provides strong evidence that nicotine is the chemical agent sought following withdrawal from tobacco. Increased food intake often occurs during prolonged withdrawal, and significant weight gain can be an undesirable consequence of cessation of nicotine intake.

Other Drugs of Abuse

Beyond the drugs previously reviewed, there are only a few other substances abused. Because the use of these substances is only a minor component of the over-all problem of drug abuse, we have included them under a single heading. They will be discussed individually below, but to a lesser degree then the other drugs of abuse reviewed.

Psychedelic and Hallucinogenic Drugs

Several pharmacologic classes of compounds, which can be referred to as psychedelic, have hallucinogenic or psychotomimetic properties.[r11] The prototype hallucinogenic drug is lysergic acid diethylamide (LSD). Natives of the Americas were using psychedelics at the time Spanish were exploring Mexico and the southwest US. These drugs included peyote (mescaline) and mushrooms (psilocybin & psilocin).[r54] In 1943, Hoffman discovered the remarkable hallucinogenic effects of lysergic diethylamide (LSD). The description of this event was recorded by Hoffman.[r55] Additional drugs having this general property include belladonna alkaloids such as scopolamine, traditional plant derivatives such as mescaline, and the amphetamine "designer drugs." The structure of these drugs are presented in Fig. 21.6. The structure activity relationship of psychotomimetic drugs has been reviewed.[r56] Hallucinogenic drug usage was quite prevalent during the late 1960s and early 1970s. A sharp decrease in usage occurred thereafter, but levels of use remained steady and significant over the next two decades (see section on Prevalence).

Pharmacology[r11,r56,r57]

The feature that characterizes this drug group is their ability to include altered perception and thoughts.[r57] In particular, sensory

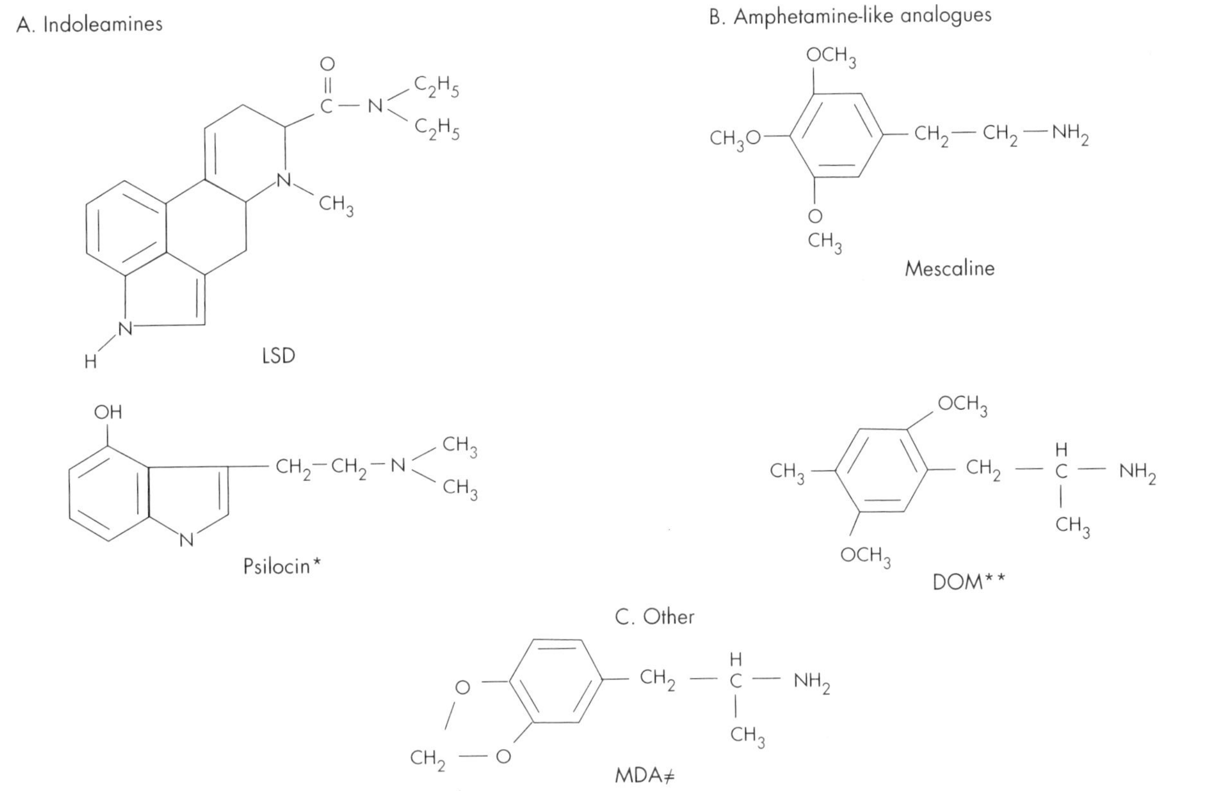

A. Indoleamines

LSD

Psilocin*

B. Amphetamine-like analogues

Mescaline

DOM**

C. Other

MDA≠

Figure 21.6 Structures of Selected Psychedelic Drugs
LSD = Lysergic Acid Diethylamide; DOM = 2,5-Dimethoxy-4-methyl Amphetamine; MDA = 3,4-methylenedioxy amphetamine
* DMT (Dimethyltryptamine) does not have the -OH group.
** DMA (Dimethoxyamphetamine) does not have the CH_3 on the phenyl ring.
≠ MMDA (5-methoxy-3,4 methylenedioxy amphetamine) differs from MDA by the presence of a ring-OCH_3

perceptions seem to be affected by these agents, but there is an inability of the individual to control the inputs. One group of drugs is related to indoalkylamnes and includes LSD, psilocybin, psilocin, dimethyltryptamine (DMT), and diethyltryptamine (DET). The other group, derivatives of phenylethylamine, includes mescaline, 2,5-dimethoxy-4-methyl amphetamine (DOM, STP), 3,4-methoxy-3,4 methyl-dioxy-amphetamine (MMDA), 3,4-methylenedioxy amphetamine (MDA), and 3,4-methylendioxy methamphetamine (MDMA, "ecstasy").[r57]

There is no common site of action for all psychedelic/hallucinogenic drugs. However, the widely used indoleamine and phenylalkylamine hallucinogens are serotonin receptor agonists. The activation of phosphatidylinositol hydrolysis that follows activation of these receptors by this group of drugs generally increases excitability of individual neurons in the cortex, limbic system, and certain brain stem regions. It is believed that this action mimics overstimulation of serotonergic systems involved in the processing of sensory information, leading to distortions of perception. These drugs also may interfere with the brain's endogenous system for selective attention such that information that normally is not consciously perceived becomes more salient. The receptor systems acted upon by other psychedelics are less well defined.

While patterns of intoxication vary widely among the individual hallucinogenic drugs, certain common features can be observed for drugs with similar pharmacologic actions.[r56,r57] Drugs such as phenylethylamines (e.g., mescaline) and indoleamines (e.g., lysergic acid diethylamide-25, LSD) produce giddiness, alterations in perception, behavioral activation, and visual hallucinations. Hallucinations vary in intensity from simple changes in perception of light patterns to mistaken identification of objects or movement patterns of objects. Beliefs in a bond with other users that have been called "depersonalization" also may occur. Both euphoria and dysphoria (the "bad-trip") may result from ingestion of the same hallucinogen. These opposite affective states are sometimes seen in the same individual at different times following drug ingestion. Interestingly, no clear evidence of cognitive or memory impairment is observed during or after intoxication.

Ingestion of methoxyamphetamine (phenylisopropylamines) psychedelics leads to a heightened response to sensory stimulation, particularly tactile sensations. Thus, MDMA is referred to as "ecstasy" because it produces pleasurable enhancement of such sensations. These compounds also have mood elevating effects similar to other amphetamines. Outright hallucinations are rarely induced by these drugs, but some users report perceptual changes. Physical symptoms of intoxication include bruxism, sweating, nausea, ataxia, and dizziness.

Phenylisopropylamines appear to act via inhibition of catecholamine and indoleamine neurotransmitter uptake. These drugs may themselves be transported into serotonergic neurons. It is not yet clear how these pharmacologic effects induce intoxication. However, increased catecholamine levels probably contribute to the energizing effects of the drugs, while increased concentrations of serotonin may activate the same receptors that are affected by other hallucinogens. This class of psychedelics *has* toxic effects on serotonergic neurons at high doses.[r135] Similarly, the toxic compound MPTP was an unwanted contaminant of batches of illicitly manufactured 1-methyl-4-phenyl-propionoxy piperidine (MPPP), a "designer heroin." MPTP is toxic to dopaminergic neurons and induces an irreversible parkinsonian condition.[136]

Anticholinergics with intoxicating and hallucinogenic actions are muscarinic receptor antagonists.[r11] Anticholinergics are used by a relatively small percentage of the population. Anticholinergics, such as the belladonna alkaloids atropine, scopolamine, and antihistamines, such as tripelennamine, produce euphoria, social stimulation, sedation, and induction of a "dreamlike" state. Hallucinations can be induced by high doses and often are accompanied by paranoia and disorientation. Doses taken for intoxication are often below those which produce marked hallucinations and drowsiness, and probably are used for mood elevation. Several subtypes of muscarinic receptors are found in the brain. These receptors can both excite and inhibit the activity of neurons. They have strong connections with higher brain regions such as the cerebral cortex. These antagonists are nonselective in their ability to block muscarinic receptors, and thus it is not clear if one class of muscarinic cholinergic receptor contributes more to the hallucinogenic actions than any other. One intriguing possibility is that interactions between brain cholinergic and serotonergic systems are involved in the hallucinogenic effects of anticholinergics.

Abuse of Psychedelic Drugs[r57]

Recent years have witnessed an upsurge in psychedelic drug use among teenage and college age youths. In particular, "designer drugs" have become more prevalent. Psychotomimetic drugs commonly are taken by individuals seeking some form of mental escape or an experience of alternative modes of thinking or emotion. Drug use in American society has generally been heaviest among those aged 14 to 30, becoming less prevalent among older adults. In addition, certain Native American and other aboriginal peoples continue to use hallucinogenic plant derivatives as a part of traditional mystic ceremonies. However, this accounts for only a small proportion of the total drug use in North American society. Psychedelic drugs are nonaddictive or induce only a mild dependence syndrome. Thus, repeated, regular usage, such as that seen in alcoholics and heroin addicts, is comparatively rare. In general, use is episodic.

Drugs with anticholinergic action have been used as antiparkinsonian medication and as an adjunct to antipsychotic treatment to prevent extrapyramidal side-effects. There is significant abuse liability among patients using the drugs for these purposes. In the "street," antihistamines that possess anticholinergic activity have been used in conjunction with mild opiates to produce a profound euphoria. This combination, known as "Ts and Blues" or "Juice and Beans," has undergone periodic episodes of abuse and is sometimes used to substitute for heroin when availability is low. The constituents of these drug cocktails are now available only through prescription, which may reduce the incidence of abuse.

Tolerance, Dependence and Withdrawal[r11]

The intoxicating effects of LSD and related psychedelics are lost within days of continued use. This rapid tolerance is matched by an equally rapid return of the effects of a subsequent dose after a few days of abstinence. Cross-tolerance develops between LSD and other indoleamines, but not the phenylethylamine-related psychedelics. Tolerance after prolonged use of anticholinergic drugs has been reported. It is most often the social stimulation and euphoria that are reduced after repeated drug usage. Higher and more toxic doses are then taken to achieve the same desired effects.

Dependence. Dependence on most psychedelic drugs is rare. Frequent users do not report craving. Psychedelics are not self-administered by laboratory animals. The phenylisopropylamines have greater liability for dependence, presumably due to their amphetamine-like effects. However, reports of addiction to these drugs are infrequent. Animals will self-administer MDMA-like drugs. Patients taking anticholinergics for medication sometimes exhibit craving and signs of dependence. This may take the form of resistance to decreased medication or requests for increases in prescription dose.

Withdrawal. Withdrawal after prolonged anticholinergic use is characterized by signs of increased parasympathetic and central cholinergic function. The symptoms include enhanced perspiration, tachycardia, anxiety, depression, motor agitation, and hallucinations. The other compounds in general do not appear to display such symptoms of dependence.

Medical Complications

The medical consequences associated with the use of psychedelic drugs can relate to both acute and chronic effects. Acutely, sympathomimetic effects (e.g., hypertension) are seen with the administration of these drugs particularly those with phenylisopropylamine structures.[r11,r57] Intoxication after ingestion of anticholinergic drugs is accompanied by signs of autonomic blockade, such as photophobia and blurred vision (which results from dilation of pupils), increased intracular pressure, dry mouth, dryness and warming of the skin, constipation, bronchodilation, tachycardia, urinary retention, and decreased capacity for penile erection. Anticholinergics also induce a profound amnesia and hallucinations resulting from blockade of central cholinergic systems important for learning and memory. Other complications of psychedelic drugs can include panic and euphoria. In some individuals, psychedelics can precipitate seizures and psychopathology, including depression, paranoid behavior, or prolonged psychotic episodes. These effects associated with psychedelics are treated symptomatically.

The psychedelics can have significant long-term effects. One of these is referred to as "flash back," which is a recurrence of the drug consequence after even years of abstinence from the drug. The mechanism of this effect is unknown but is commonly precipitated by anxiety and fatigue. This may persist for several years after exposure to LSD. High doses of MDMA and MDA have been demonstrated to cause selective damage to serotinergic nerve terminals.[135] Since the amount producing this change in animals is as little as two times that used for the psychedelic actions, this effect could be a serious consequence if the usual dose of this group of compounds is raised. Animal studies suggest that, even though some recovery of serotonin-containing neurons occurs, the recovery of these neurons is not complete.

Arylcyclohexylamines

The commonly used arylcyclohexylamines are the "dissociative" anesthetics, ketamine and phencyclidine (PCP). These compounds originally were developed as clinical anesthetics, and ketamine is still used, particularly in veterinary medicine. Abuse patterns and illicit use of these compounds are widely variable and somewhat inconsistent in pattern.[r58] PCP, commonly known by the street moniker "angel-dust," has undergone intense periods of high usage in inner cities and suburbs; the most recent period being the mid-to late 80s. PCP is used alone and in conjunction with other drugs, most notably alcohol and marijuana.

Pharmacology[r11,r57–r60]

As noted above, this class of drugs is referred to as dissociative anesthetics (see Chapter 13 for details about ketamine). The behavioral pharmacology of PCP has been reviewed.[r59] The arylcyclohexylamines are antagonists of the N-methyl-D-aspartate (NMDA) type glutamate receptor, an ion channel.[137,r11] NMDA receptor binding associated with these drugs is widely distributed in forebrain.[138] Early reports of human tests of the newer compounds blocking NMDA receptors indicate that they produce undesirable effects much like ketamine.[139] Thus, NMDA receptor blockade is a good candidate mechanism for the intoxication profile of arylcyclohexylamines. Transmission involving this receptor mediates facets of learning and memory, perception of pain and other sensations, cardiovascular control, development of the brain, and quite likely other facets of higher cognitive function.

While PCP inhibits NMDA receptor function, PCP also has an appreciably high affinity for the sigma type opiate receptor in addition to its actions on the NMDA receptor.[140] However, the physiologic role of this receptor is not well defined, and thus it is unclear how PCP actions on the receptor contribute to intoxication.[r60] Arylcyclohexylamines also block catecholamine uptake. This action may underlie the increase in extracellular dopamine concentration observed after administration to laboratory animals or application to brain slice preparations. This latter neuropharmacologic action might contribute to the abuse potential of the drug (see section on Central Stimulants).

Abuse

Ketamine is abused less frequently than PCP and generally is not available on the street.[r57,r58] Abuse by professional medical workers is a distinct liability among those with regular access to the drug. Long-term use of PCP is uncommon, presumably due to the many problems encountered by users. These include incidences of paranoid hallucinations, self-abuse, and negative encounters with legal authorities, which seem to be more common among PCP users than among other drug abusers. The "RED DANES" acronym describes the physical and behavioral symptoms of PCP intoxication.[r11] This refers to the *R*ed skin, *E*nlarged pupils and *D*elusions as well as the *D*issociations, *A*mnesia, *N*ystagmus, *E*xcitement, and dry *S*kin of the user. The most prominent neural effects of arylcyclohexylamine intoxication are alterations in motor function, cognition, and mood. A "psychotomimetic" state somewhat akin to schizophrenia is seen in many users.[r11] Low doses of the drugs primarily impact on cognitive function. Impairment of judgment and complex reasoning are affected, and evidence of delusions and hallucinations may be present as well. In addition to visual hallucinations, ketamine and PCP also induce auditory and even tactile hallucinations, especially at high doses.

Medical Complications

Symptoms of mild to moderate intoxication may include agitation, anxiety, catalepsy, diaphoresis, irritability, excitement, fever, hyperreflexia, hypersalivation, myoclonus, rigidity, and stereotyped movement.[r11] Stereotyped movements are prominent in laboratory animals in the first stages of PCP or ketamine intoxication. Higher doses can induce cardiac arrythmias, hypertension, hyporeflexia, and paranoia. Caretakers may see violent and irrational behaviors. Overdose can induce convulsions and catatonia and can be lethal. Treatment of overdose is symptomatic. Antipsychotic medications are used to treat psychosis.

Amnesia is often observed following arylcyclohexylamine abuse such that users will not remember events taking place during intoxication.[r11] This cognitive impairment and a profound dysphoria, including nightmares, are often reported by patients given ketamine as an injectable anesthetic. These undesirable consequences minimize the clinical use of these agents. The arylcyclohexylamines are also analgesic, presumably owing to actions at the level of the spinal cord and brain stem. This may account for the unusual tolerance for pain and bodily injury sometimes reported among PCP users. The combination of violent behavior and analgesia among users has added to the perception of the "crazed" PCP user. These compounds also have anesthetic actions and induce a hypnotic state after administration of high doses. However, the anesthesia is "dissociative" in that the recipient often feels a separation from the environment. These compounds are not potent muscle relaxants. Indeed, bizarre, stereotyped movements are observed during sedation and anesthesia. Treatment of intoxication requires reduced sensory stimulation and may require sedation with a benzodiazepine or neuroleptics.

Volatile Inhalants

The drugs in this category are varied, as noted in Table 21.1. These include volatile compounds, which are aliphatic, aromatic, and halogenated hydrocarbons. Other compounds included in this discussion will be nitrous oxide (an anesthetic and amyl nitrite (a vasodilator). Users tend to be in the preteen to teen years. Mixtures containing these compounds are often available for purchase.

Pharmacology

The cellular and molecular bases of inhalant intoxication are not well understood. It has been postulated that nitrous oxide has effects on membrane fluidity, as proposed for a number of general anesthetic agents. There is no clear theoretical basis for understanding the CNS actions of the various types of hydrocarbons. However, given the recent results obtained on ethanol, actions on ion channels and neurotransmitter receptors should be explored. These compounds in the hydrocarbon group can have severe toxicological effects with chronic use.[r61]

Abuse

Paint thinner and other highly volatile compounds are used as solvents and are contained in glues and some aerosol products. These compounds are inhaled to produce the desired intoxicant effect.[r61] Individuals will buy these volatile compounds on a daily basis for "binges" of intoxication. Amyl nitrate or "poppers" also have undergone periods of heavy use. This compound is inhaled from sealed vials or capsules and has been used during sexual intercourse to enhance arousal. The last period of enhanced use, during the late 1970s and early 1980s, saw prevalent use among young adults. Inhalant ingestion leads to an intense but short-lived euphoric state. The intoxicated state generally lasts no more than two to five minutes. Amyl nitrate intoxication may be over within 30 seconds. In the case of toluene and related solvents, this feeling is accompanied by dizziness and temporary cognitive impairment. High doses can lead to loss of consciousness.

Nitrous oxide is also inhaled to produce euphoric sensations. This gas is usually dispensed from pressurized cylinders or canisters. Nitrous oxide is used as a short-lasting general anesthetic, particularly for dental operations, and thus cylinders are available commercially. Nitrous oxide induced euphoria is characterized by ready elicitation of laughter (hence the term "laughing gas"). Use is sporadic and generally observed among teens and young adults, with the occasional incidence of an abusing dentist.

Medical Complications

The type of medical complication will depend in part on the type of inhalant. The long-term consequences of organic-based solvents would be the acute and chronic toxic manifestations of such agents. The major concern with this group is the neuropathies that result in dementia.[r4,7] However, cardiac arrhythmia, pulmonary edema, and renal and liver dysfunction can follow the administration of these compounds.[141,142,r61] Nitrous oxide may be lethal if used in an enclosed environment where extended atmospheric contamination may lead to asphyxiation. It is reported that chronic use of amyl nitrite can suppress the immune system.[143]

Etiologic, Diagnostic, and Legal Factors of Substance Abuse Disorders

Etiologic Factors

It is unlikely that a single causal factor exists that can explain why, in the face of widespread availability of alcohol and drugs, some individuals develop a psychoactive substance use disorder and others do not. It no doubt is due to psychoactive substance use disorders being complex and multifaceted and to the circumstances that lead to drug use differing among individuals (i.e., possible genetic predisposition). Equally difficult to understand is why in certain cases psychoactive substance use disorders continue inexorably to death, whereas, in others, drug use can be decreased or arrested. Therefore, it is widely accepted that psychoactive substance use disorders are most usefully conceptualized in terms of multiple simultaneous variables interacting over time.[32,33,r63] This concept is embodied in Figures 21.1 and 21.7. The typical longitudinal course of psychoactive substance use disorders begins by exposure of a vulnerable individual to a given psychopharmacologic agent within a sociocultural context, progresses to dependence, characterized by compulsive drug use, and eventually results in the development of social, neuropsychiatric, and medical complications (Fig. 21.7).

The fact that not all individuals who self-administer psychoactive agents during given developmental stages or life circumstances progress to repeated problematic use has led to the search for factors that determine individual vulnerability. Biologic factors that may contribute to the development of psychoactive substance use disorders include interindividual differences in: 1. susceptibility to acute psychopharmacologic effects of a given drug; 2. metabolism of the drug; 3. cellular adaptation within the CNS to chronic exposure to the drug; 4. predisposing personality characteristics (sensation seeking or antisocial traits); 5. susceptibility to medical and neuropsychiatric complications of chronic drug self-administration; and 6. possibly a genetic predisposition.[31–34,r2,r63]

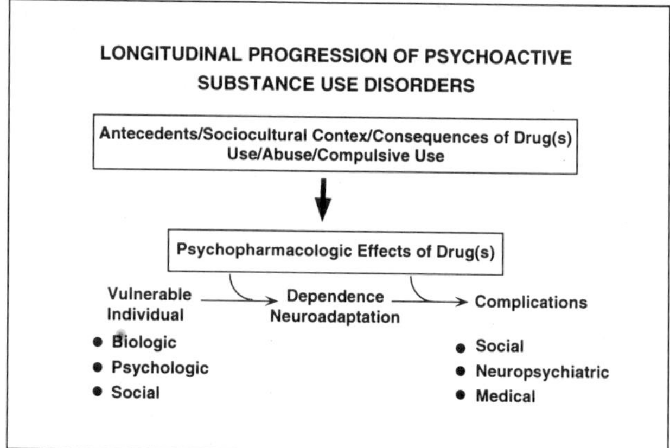

Figure 21.7 Longitudinal Course of Psychoactive Substance Use Disorders

Although psychologic factors, such as the presence of comorbid psychopathology (e.g., depression, anxiety, attention deficit disorder, psychosis), medical illnesses (e.g., chronic pain, essential tremor), severe stress (crime, battle, sexual, economic), or post-traumatic effects have received considerable attention as possible causes for "self-medication", susceptibility to these psychologic stressors may also represent a shared etiology with psychoactive substance use disorders. Finally, social factors, such as peer group attitudes toward, and shared expectations of the benefits of drug use, the availability of competing reinforcers in the form of educational, recreational, and occupational alternatives to substance use, and the availability of the drug during particular developmental stages also contribute to the initiation of drug use and progression of psychoactive substance use disorders.

The fact that individuals often use more than one drug simultaneously, or give a history of having used different drugs sequentially during their lifetime, has led to the emphasis on the similarities rather than the differences among psychoactive substances of abuse with respect to the ontogeny of drug use behaviors.[r5,r7,r20,r43] The concept of "gateway drug" implies that legal, readily available substances (tobacco, alcohol) are normally first used by youngsters, and illicit drugs (marijuana, heroin, and cocaine) tend to be used at a later stage in the development of psychoactive substance use disorders. A direct corollary of this hypothesis is that prevention aimed at "softer" drugs may eventually reduce the abuse of more "serious" drugs as an individual matures. This orderly progression can be disturbed in certain sociocultural contexts, such as inner cities where crack cocaine is often made available to preadolescents. Furthermore, the stepwise acquisition of different drugs based on availability over time suggests common mechanisms of susceptibility among all drugs. This allows generalization to diagnostic criteria and treatment strategies for all drugs abused.

If a drug is repeatedly administered under given circumstances (situation, time, place), environmental stimuli can become associated with effects of the drug by means of classic (Pavlovian) conditioning processes.[144,145] Subsequently, the circumstances under which the drug was administered (without actual presentation of the drug) includes certain environmental (conditioned) stimuli that can modify drug-seeking behavior, subjective state, or psychophysiologic responses (conditioned reinforcement). For example, patients who have been abstinent from IV heroin for many years can experience a desire to use heroin when they return to the location where they previously used, or view a film that portrays others who are injecting drugs IV. The importance of conditioned stimuli in the response to drugs is also readily demonstrated in laboratory animals by the greater tolerance present when a drug is tested in an environment where it was previously administered rather than in a distinctly different environment.[144,145]

The tempo of progression and severity of drug abuse can differ considerably based on various characteristics of the agent(s) involved, including availability (cost, purity, etc.), route of administration, physical-chemical properties, and psychopharmacologic actions. For example, the duration of time between initial exposure to alcohol and the development of compulsive use is months to years,[r29] compared to weeks to months for cocaine.[106] Similarly, serious complications related to drinking typically occur 10 to 15 years after initial exposure to alcohol, whereas for cocaine, the time to develop the complications associated with cocaine use may be less than one to two years. The behavioral mechanisms that mediate the positive reinforcing effects of drugs are positive effects on mood (euphoria), alleviation of negative affective states (anxiety, depression), functional enhancement (improved psychomotor or cognitive performance), and alleviation of withdrawal. Furthermore, drug effects (aversive, positive reinforcing, discriminative, and conditioned) are modulated by variables such as social context, genetic factors, behavioral history, including the presence of psychopathology (e.g., anxiety, depression, or thought disorders), and previous exposure to psychoactive drugs (e.g., expectancy) (Figs. 21.1, 21.7).

Patients are unlikely to present to physicians complaining of having difficulty with their use of psychoactive substances. Rather, they present for treatment of the complications of psychoactive substance use. Such patients also are unlikely to offer that they use psychoactive agents or admit to problematic drug use. Most likely, patients deny that they, in fact, have a drug problem when questioned. The nonspecificity and wide variety of symptoms that accompany psychoactive substance abuse, as well as the unreliable report of patients, makes the diagnosis of these disorders difficult. Therefore, the physician must approach patients who present with signs and symptoms consistent with a psychoactive substance use disorder with a high index of suspicion. Only if the physician is open to making the diagnosis will it be appropriately made. Recognition may be particularly difficult if the patient also suffers from a comorbid condition (both medical and psychiatric) that can complicate and influence the course of psychoactive substance use disorders. Post-withdrawal rehabilitation constitutes a complement of interventions organized within a treatment program including individual and group psychotherapy, family therapy, and self-help groups. Currently, there is considerable interest in developing pharmacologic adjuncts to these treatment programs to reduce the likelihood that a patient will use drugs.

Diagnostic Criteria

What constitutes "inappropriate" or "excessive" self-administration of psychoactive substances—and, hence, a "disorder"—has varied throughout history and in different cultures (see History). The etiology of psychoactive substance use disorders has been conceptualized in terms of biologic, psychologic, and social theories as well as theories that attempt integration of these perspectives.[r62] The milestones in development of psychoactive substance use disorders are strikingly similar, as evidenced by the use of common diagnostic criteria across drugs of different pharmacologic classes and as depicted in Figures 21.1 and 21.7.

The specific criteria for diagnosis of psychoactive substance use disorders presented by the American Psychiatric Association (Diagnostic and Statistical Manual of Mental Disorders [DSM] and the World Health Organization (International Classification of Diseases [ICD])[r65,r66] both draw heavily on the concepts of the dependence syndrome. In general, three clusters of symptoms, of which a given number need to be part of the clinical presentation, are required for the diagnosis of psychoactive substance dependence: 1. loss of control (the substance is taken in larger amounts or over a longer period than intended, or there are unsuccessful efforts to reduce use); 2. salience to the behavioral repertoire (a great deal of time is spent in substance-related activities at the expense of important social, occupational, or recreational activities, which are reduced or given up, or there is continued substance use despite knowledge of having a persistent or recurrent physical or psychologic problem likely to have been caused or exacerbated by the substance); and 3. neuroadaptation (the presence of tolerance or withdrawal). Dependence syndromes are specified in DSM-IV for the following substances: alcohol; amphetamine (or related substance); cannabis; cocaine; hallucinogen; inhalant; nicotine; opioid; phencyclidine (or related substance); sedative/hypnotic/anxiolytic; polysubstance; and other (e.g., anabolic steroids, nitrite inhalants, nitrous oxide, and various over-the-counter and prescription drugs that do not readily fall into the above categories).[r65]

The distinction between substance abuse and dependence in the DSM classification system has been particularly controversial, and, hence, inconsistent. For example, in DSM-III-R,[r66] the criteria for dependence were considerably broadened compared with DSM-III such that an individual could be diagnosed as substance-dependent without ever having exhibited tolerance or withdrawal. As a result, substance abuse became a residual category in DSM-III-R,[r66] only applied to individuals who manifested a "maladaptive pattern of psychoactive substance use" who did not meet criteria for substance dependence. In contrast, in DSM-IV,[r65] a greater emphasis is given to the presence of neuroadaptation in that dependence can be subtyped according to whether or not there is "physiologic dependence" (tolerance or withdrawal). Furthermore, certain descriptive terms have been added to distinguish among different clinical courses of the dependence syndrome to better characterize individual patients. For example, a dependent patient may be in remission, which in turn, may be early or sustained, full or partial, and on agonist therapy or in a controlled environment. Even with the redefinition of psychoactive substance dependence in DSM-IV, it remains to be determined whether the abuse category is actually more meaningfully defined (individuals experiencing "clinically significant impairment or distress" in life functioning as a result of substance use but who have never had the full dependence syndrome) than it was in DSM-III-R.[r66] This is not surprising if one views substance use disorders in terms of continuities rather than categories (see above). Nevertheless, it would be important to develop diagnostic criteria that identify the substantial minority of individuals with a history of psychoactive substance abuse who do not progress to dependence in the future, despite continuing substance use and associated problems.

As mentioned, integration via a multiaxial classification system of the physical, psychologic, and social domains of each patient's clinical presentation has been an important feature of the DSM diagnostic system. However, no multiaxial classification approach is fully satisfactory in describing the effects on the dependence syndrome of complex drug use patterns (more than one drug via different routes of administration), disabilities resulting from drug use, or the existence of different clinical syndromes in terms of diverse personality and cultural presentations.

Medical and Legal Considerations of Substance Abuse

As noted above from historical and clinical perspectives, the rehabilitation of individuals suffering from psychoactive substance use disorders falls either within the realm of medicine or the criminal justice system.[r67] But this dichotomy is not as clear-cut as it may initially seem, because the social control mechanisms used for prevention (medical) or deterrence (legal) of drug use-related behaviors are interrelated in the minds of most members of society. In addition, there are distinct inconsistencies and tensions between the medical and legal systems, as evidenced by the lack of a straightforward relationship between a drug's pharmacologic properties and effects on health and whether it is considered licit or illicit within criminal law.[r68] For example, drugs such as alcohol and nicotine (as smoked in tobacco), which carry the greatest health and safety risks in our society, are not currently illegal. In fact, for all drugs that present society with problems today, ongoing controversy concerning how or whether they should be controlled is the topic of intense discussion. For example, it is being recommended by several review agencies such as FDA that the content of nicotine in cigarettes be controlled. Ever-changing drug laws document, perhaps most succinctly, the history of society's struggles to control dysfunctional drug use.[r16,r64,r67,r68] These laws reflect cyclical changes in attitudes, including permissiveness, criminal prohibition, enforcement, nonenforcement, noncriminal regulation, and cultural acceptance, toward so-called nonpredatory behaviors (offenses that involve voluntary participation with no perceived direct victim), to which psychoactive drug use per se belongs.[r67]

The focus of intensive legal suppression at different times during the 20th century has had its impetus from the moral pressure of temperance ideology rather than a concern for health (e.g., alcohol, heroin, cannabis, and cocaine.[r67]) However, drinking did continue during Prohibition, because the laws were largely unenforceable and widely broken as a result of corruption and violence perpetrated by thriving criminal organizations that maintained a steady supply of alcoholic beverages for illegal distribution. Prohibition was repealed (in spite of demonstrated health benefits) when it was recognized that this form of legal control had severe limitations with respect to a substance such as alcohol for which demand was so widespread. Criminalization of opiates by the Harrison Act of 1914 resulted in a decrease in the socioeconomic status of opiate addicts and a particularly damaging lifestyle,[r67,r68] characterized by predatory crime and self-neglect, which includes malnutrition, severe psychopathology, and infectious diseases. Nonetheless, it is clear that well-controlled opiate use is probably less physically dangerous than several psychoactive agents not legally sanctioned. The ensuing highly negative stereotype of the addict and the relatively low prevalence of opiate use in the population have facilitated continued criminal controls. However, allowing medical prescription of heroin for addicts (United Kingdom) and methadone maintenance (United States) do represent acceptable alternatives to categorical sanctions based predominantly on moral disapproval, especially in light of the recognized spread of HIV with IV drug use.

The large increase in use of cannabis during the 1960s and 1970s by a significant proportion of a generation (rather than the disenfranchised few) led to a mismatch between the perceived risks and benefits of strict adherence to legal control of the "marijuana problem." Specifically, it became apparent that there were considerable social costs (felt to this day) to criminalization of millions of mainly young users of a drug with few demonstrable adverse effects on health. Further, legal controls were mostly ineffective (when compared to nonlegal influences) in reducing the prevalence and consequences of cannabis use.[r67] Eventually, concerns about cocaine eclipsed those related to marijuana, and the role of marijuana as a "gateway" to other illicit drugs (especially cocaine) received most attention.

In the late 1970s, cocaine use by sniffing was considered a harmless diversion of the economic elite.[21] By the 1980s, alarm over the devastating consequences of cocaine use was being fueled by the falling price and increased availability of street cocaine ("crack") and enormous media coverage of the deaths of promising young athletes, the economic drain on the health care system of cocaine-related psychiatric and medical emergencies, the AIDS epidemic, "cocaine babies," and lurid accounts of inner city violence and police corruption juxtaposed on immensely wealthy and powerful drug lords who seemed immune to governmental controls. Some contend that current reductions of cocaine use are not attributable to legal controls, whereas others see the change representing a shift in public attitudes away from drug use, which throughout history have followed periods of relative permissiveness.[21,r16] The fluidity of these trends, well documented by epidemiologic studies, likely represents attitudinal changes over time which tend to influence our definitions of these disorders.

It is difficult to understand the apparent paradox of why certain psychoactive drugs with aversive effects can nonetheless maintain drug-seeking behavior and have dependence liability. Aversive effects of drugs counteract the tendency toward self-administration and may limit drug use if they result in dose-dependent toxicity. For example, initial exposure to nicotine in the form of cigarettes often results in distressing symptoms, such as coughing, nausea, and lightheadedness, which may terminate smoking. Similarly, severe gastritis in the chronic alcoholic patient may result in attempts to cut down drinking or limit continued alcohol ingestion. It is now recognized that the stimulus properties of most drugs of abuse, a major determinant of drug-seeking behavior, are complex and multifaceted. Specifically, their pharmacologic profiles include both positive reinforcing and aversive components and their effects are readily modified by associated environmental stimuli and interindividual differences among drug users. (Fig. 21.1).

The approach to the treatment of individuals who suffer from dysfunctional psychoactive substance use is determined by the widely-held attributions within society of where responsibility for causation of the problem—and for its solution—lies, rather than an understanding of etiology.[r19,r67,4] In simplified terms, such attributions can lead to a broad range of responses, the most extreme forms of which include viewing the addict as either a patient or a criminal, and hence, as moral or immoral, innocent or guilty, and victim or perpetrator.[r67] If physicians are to interact effectively with national and international organizations for legal consultation, disability assessments, and development of health care legislation (as they are called to do on a regular basis), these issues cannot be ignored. Emphasis should be on the similarities rather than the differences (as had been the case in the past) among psychoactive substances of abuse, such as common neurochemical mechanisms of drug-seeking behavior and underlying psychopathology. Future directions in research are likely to involve understanding issues of comorbid psychiatric conditions, the development of psychopharmacologic treatments, and the combined use of pharmacotherapy and psychotherapy in the management of the substance use disorder.

Acknowledgment: This effort was supported in part by the National Institute on Alcohol Abuse and Alcoholism (AA08492, AA07515 and AA-09122).

References

Research Reports

1. Van Thiel DH. (1991) Gender differences in the susceptibility and severity of alcohol-induced liver disease. *Alcohol Alcoholism, Suppl. 1.*, pp 9–18.
2. Deykin EY, Buka SL, Zeena TH. (1992) Depressive illness among chemically dependent adolescents. *Am. J. Psychiatry* 149:1341–1347.
3. Regier DA, Kramer ME, Rae DS. (1990) Comorbidity of mental disorders with alcohol and other drug abuse: Results from the Epidemiologic Catchment Area study. *JAMA* 264:2511.
4. Brickman P, Rabinowitz VC, Karuza J, Coates D, Cohn E, Kidder L. (1982) Models of helping and coping. *Am. Psychol.* 37:368–385.

5. Engel GL. (1977) The need for a new medical model: a challenge for biomedicine. *Science* 196:129–136.

6. Meyer, RE. (1989) Prospects for a rational pharmacotherapy of alcoholism. *J. Clin. Psychiatry* 50:403–412.

7. Meyer RE. (1992) New pharmacotherapies for cocaine dependence . . . revisited. *Arch. Gen. Psychiatry* 49:900–904.

8. Yamaguchi K, Kandel DB. (1984) Patterns of drug use from adolescence to young adulthood: III. Predictors of progression. *Am. J. Public Health* 74:673–681.

9. Edwards G, Arif A, Hodgson R. (1981) Nomenclature and classification of drug- and alcohol-related problems: a WHO memorandum. *Bull. WHO* 59:225–242.

10. Martin WR, Jasinski DR. (1969) Physiological parameters of morphine dependence in man-tolerance, early dependence, protracted abstinence. *Psychiat. Res* 7:9–17.

11. Childress AR, McLellan AT, O'Brien CP. (1986) Abstinent opiate abusers exhibit conditioned craving, conditioned withdrawal and reductions in both through extinction. *Br. J. Addict.* 81:655–660.

12. Isbell H, Fraser HF, Wikler A, Belleville RE, Eisenman AJ. (1955) An experimental study of the etiology of "rum fits" and delirium tremens. *Q. J. Stud. Alcohol* 16:1–33.

13. Ludwig A, Stark LH. (1974) Alcohol craving: subjective and situational aspects. *Q. J. Stud. Alcohol* 35:899–905.

14. Ritzmann RF, Tabakoff B. (1976) Dissociation of alcohol tolerance and dependence. *Nature* 263:418–420.

15. Koob, GF, Bloom FE. (1988) Cellular and molecular mechanisms of drug dependence. *Science* 242:715–723.

16. Ballenger JC, Post RM. (1978) Kindling as a model for alcohol withdrawal syndromes. *Brit. J. Psychiatry* 133:1–14.

17. Hoffman PL, Ritzmann RF, Walter R, Tabakoff B. (1978) Arginine vasopressin maintains ethanol tolerance. *Nature* 276:614–616.

18. Petrides M, Alivisatos B, Evans AC, Meyer E. (1993) Dissociation of human mid-dorsolateral from posterior dorsolateral frontal cortex in memory processing. *Proc. Natl. Acad. Sci. U.S.A.* 90:873–877.

19. Kandel ER. (1989) Genes, nerve cells, and the remembrance of things past. *J. Neuropsychiat. Clin. Neurosci.* 1:103–125.

20. Kalant H. (1985) Tolerance, learning, and neurochemical adaptation. Can. J. Physiol. Pharmacol. 63:1485–1494.

21. Gawin FH, Ellinwood EH Jr. (1988) Cocaine and other stimulants. *N. Engl. J. Med.* 318:1173–1182.

22. Benowitz N.L. (1988) Pharmacologic aspects of cigarette smoking and nicotine addiction. *N. Engl. J. Med.* 319:1318–1330.

23. Sellers EM, Kalant H. (1976) Alcohol intoxication and withdrawal. *N. Engl. J. Med.* 294:757–762.

24. Martin PR, Ebert MH, Gordon EK, Weingartner H, Kopin IJ. (1984) Catecholamine metabolism during clonidine withdrawal. *Psychopharmacology* 84:58–63.

25. Walinder J, Balldin J, Bokstrom K, Karlsson I, Lundstrom B, Svensson, TH. (1981) Clonidine suppression of the alcohol withdrawal syndrome. *Drug Alcohol Depend.* 8:345–348.

26. Glassman AH, Jackson WK, Walsh T, Roose SP, Rosenfeld B. (1984) Cigarette craving, smoking withdrawal, and clonidine. *Science* 226:864–866.

27. Michel RH, McGovern PE, Badler VR. (1992) Chemical evidence for ancient beer. *Nature* 360:24.

28. Musto DF. (1991) Opium, cocaine and marijuana in American history. *Sci. Am.* 265:40–47.

29. Kozel NJ, Adams EH. (1986) Epidemiology of drug abuse: an overview. *Science* 234:970–974.

30. Robins LN, Helzer JE, Weissman MM. (1984) Lifetime prevalence of specific psychiatric disorders in three sites. *Arch. Gen. Psychiatry* 41:949–958.

31. Cloninger CR. (1987) Neurogenetic adaptive mechanisms in alcoholism. *Science* 236:410–416.

32. Kissin B. (1979) Biological investigations in alcohol research. *J. Stud. Alcohol* 8:146–181.

33. Tarter RE, Alterman AI, Edwards KL. (1985) Vulnerability to alcoholism in men: A behavior-genetic perspective. *J. Stud. Alcohol.* 46:319–356.

34. Crabbe JC, Belknap JK, Buck KJ. (1994) Genetic animal models of alcohol and drug abuse. *Science* 264:1715–1723.

35. Wikler A. (1977) The search for the psyche in drug dependence. *J. Nerv. Ment. Dis.* 165:29–40.

36. Kosten TR, Rounsaville BJ, Babor TF, Spitzer RL, Williams JBW. (1987) Substance use disorders in DSM-III-R: evidence for the dependence syndrome across different psychoactive substances. *Brit. J. Psychiatry* 151:834–843.

37. Schuckit M, Helzer J, Crowley T, Nathan P, Woody G, Davis W. (1991) DSM-IV in progress. Substance use disorders. *Hosp. Commun. Psychiatry* 42:471–473.

38. Brewer RD, Morris PD, Cole TB, Watkins S, Patetta MJ, Popkin C. (1994) The risk of dying in alcohol-related automobile crashes among habitual drunk drivers. *N. Engl. J. Med.* 331:513–517.

39. Frezza M, di-Padova C, Pozzato G, Terpin M, Baraona E, Lieber CS. (1990) High blood alcohol levels in women. The role of decreased gastric alcohol dehydrogenase activity and first-pass metabolism. *N. Engl. J. Med.* 322:95–99.

40. Laposata EA, Lange LG. (1986) Presence of nonoxidative ethanol metabolism in human organs commonly damaged by ethanol abuse. *Science* 231:497–99.

41. Lieber CS. (1991) Biochemical mechanisms of alcohol-induced hepatic injury. *Alcohol Alcoholism Suppl. 2,* 283–290.

42. Chin JH, Goldstein DB. (1977) Drug tolerance in biomembranes: a spin label study of the effects of ethanol. *Science* 196:684–685.

43. Harris RA, Allan AM. (1989) Alcohol intoxication, ion channels and genetics. *FASEB J.* 3.1689–1695.

44. Lovinger DM, White G, Weight FF. (1989) Ethanol inhibits NMDA-activiated ion current in hippocampal neurons. *Science* 243:1721–1724.

45. Lovinger DM, White G. (1991) Ethanol potentiation of 5-hydroxytryptamine$_3$ receptor-mediated ion current in neuroblastoma cells and isolated adult mammalian neurons. *Mol. Pharmacol.* 40:263–270.

46. Simson PE, Criswell HE, Breese GR. (1991) Ethanol potentiates GABA-mediated inhibition in the inferior colliculus: Evidence for local ethanol/GABA interactions. *J. Pharmacol. Exp. Ther. 259*:1288–1293.

47. Criswell HE, Simson PE, Duncan GE, McCown TJ, Herbert JS, Morrow AL, Breese GR. (1993) Molecular basis for regionally specific action of ethanol on GABA$_A$ receptors: Generalization to other ligand-gated ion channels. *J. Pharmacol. Exp. Ther.* 267:522–537.

48. Breese GR, Morrow AL, Simson PE, Criswell HE, McCown TJ, Duncan GE, Keir WJ. (1993) The neuroanatomical specificity

of ethanol action on ligand-gated ion channels: A hypothesis. *Alcohol Alcoholism, Suppl.* 2, pp 309–313.

49. Sanna E, Harris RA. (1993) Recent developments in alcoholism: neuronal ion channels. Recent Dev. Alcohol. 11:169–186.
50. Simson PE, Criswell HE, Breese GR. (1993) Inhibition of NMDA-evoked electrophysiological activity by ethanol in selected brain regions: evidence for ethanol-sensitive and ethanol-insensitive NMDA-Evoked responses. *Brain Res.* 607:9–16.
51. Muller D, Joly M, Lynch G. (1988) Contribution of quisqualate and NMDA receptors to the induction and expression of LTP. *Science* 242:1694–1975.
52. Gulya K, Grant KA, Valverius P, Hoffman PL, Tabakoff B. (1991) Brain regional specificity and time course of changes in the NMDA receptor-ionophore complex during ethanol withdrawal. *Brain Res.* 547:129–134.
53. Knapp DJ, Pohorecky LA. (1992) Zacolpride, a 5-HT3 receptor antagonist, reduces voluntary ethanol consumption in rats. *Pharmacol. Biochem. Behav.* 41:847–850.
54. Fadda F, Garau B, Marchie F, Colombo G, Gessa GL. (1991) MDL 72222, a selective 5-HT3 receptor antagonist, suppresses voluntary ethanol consumption in alcohol-preferring rats. *Alcohol-Alcoholism* 26:107–110.
55. Grant KA, Barrett JE. (1991) Blockade of the discriminative stimulus effects with 5-HT3 receptor antagonists. *Psychopharmacol. Berl.* 104:451–456.
56. Imperato A, DiChiara G. (1986) Preferential stimulation of dopamine release in the nucleus accumbens of freely moving rats by ethanol. *J. Pharmacol. Exp. Ther.* 239:219–228.
57. Allison JH, Cicero TJ. (1980) Alcohol acutely depresses myo-inositol 1-phosphate levels in the male rat cerebral cortex. *J. Pharmacol. Exp. Ther.* 213:24.
58. Wafford KA, Whiting PJ. (1992) Ethanol potentiation of $GABA_A$ receptors requires phosphorylation of the alternatively spliced variant of the gamma-2 subunit. *FEBS Lett.* 313:113–117.
59. Ross HE, Glaser FB, Germanson T. (1988) The prevalence of psychiatric disorders in patients with alcohol and other drug problems. *Arch. Gen. Psychiatry* 45:1023–1031.
60. Kaprio J, Viken R, Koskenvuo M, Romanov K, Rose RJ. (1992) Consistency and change in patterns of social drinking: a 6 year follow-up of the Finnish Twin Cohort. *Alcohol Clin. Exp. Res.* 16:234–240.
61. Cloninger CR, Bohman M, Sigvardsson S, von Knorring AL. (1981) Inheritance of alcohol abuse: Cross-fostering analysis of adopted men. *Arch. Gen. Psychiat.* 38:861–868.
62. Prescott CA, Hewitt JK, Truett KR, Heath AC, Neale MC, Eaves LJ. (1994) Genetic and environmental influences on lifetime alcohol-related problems in a volunteer sample of older twins. *J. Stud. Alcohol.* 55:184–202.
63. Schuckit MA. (1985) Ethanol-induced changes in body sway in men at high alcoholism risk. Arch. Gen. Psychiat. 42:375–379.
64. Schuckit MA. (1980) Biological markers: Metabolism and acute reactions to alcohol in sons of alcoholics. *Pharmacol. Biochem. Behav. 13: (Suppl. 1)*:9–16.
65. Porjesz B, Begleiter H. (1991) Neurophysiological factors in individuals at risk for alcoholism. *Recent Dev. Alcohol.* 9:53–67.
66. Brown ME, Anton RF, Malcolm R, Ballenger JC. (1988) Alcohol detoxification and withdrawal seizures: Clinical support for a kindling hypothesis. *Biol. Psychiat.* 23:507–514.
67. McCown TJ, Breese GR. (1990) Multiple withdrawals from chronic ethanol "kindles" inferior collicular seizure activity: evidence for kindling of seizures associated with alcoholism. *Alcoholism: Clin & Exp. Res. 14*:394–399.
68. Eckardt MJ, Harford TC, Kaelber CT, Parker ES, Rosenthal LS, Ryback RS, Salmoiraghi GC, Vanderveen E, Warren KR. (1981) Health hazards associated with alcohol consumption. *JAMA* 246:648–666.
69. Lieber CS. (1988) Biochemical and molecular basis of alcohol-induced injury to liver and other tissues. *N. Engl. J. Med.*, 319:1639–1650.
70. De Marchi S, Cecchin E, Basile A, Bertotti A, Nardini R, Bartoli E. (1993) Renal tubular dysfunction in chronic alcohol abuse-effects of abstinence. *N. Engl. Med.* 329:1927–1934.
71. Gaziano JM, Buring JE, Breslow JL, Goldhaber SZ, Rosner B, VanDenburgh M, Willett W, Hennekens CH. (1993) Moderate alcohol intake, increased levels of high-density lipoprotein and its subfractions, and decreased risk of myocardial infarction. *N. Engl. J. Med.* 329:1829–1834.
72. Sillanaukee P, Koivula T, Jokela H, Myllyharju H, Seppa K. (1993) Relationship of alcohol consumption to changes in HDL-subfractions. *Eur. J. Clin. Invest.* 23:486–491.
73. Murray MM. (1932) The diuretic action of alcohol and its relation to pituitrin. *J. Physiol. (London)* 76:379–386.
74. Adinoff B, Martin PR, Bone GHA, Eckardt MJ, Roehrich L, George DT, Moss HB, Eskay R, Linnoila M, Gold PW. (1990) Hypothalamic-pituitary-adrenal axis functioning and cerebrospinal fluid CRH and ACTH in alcoholics following recent and long-term abstinence. *Arch. Gen. Psychiatry* 47:325–330.
75. Cryer PE, Haymond MW, Santiago JV, Shah SD. (1976) Norepinephrine and epinephrine release and adrenergic mediation of smoking associated hemodynamic and metabolic events. *N. Engl. J. Med.* 295:573–577.
76. Castilla GA, Santolaria-Fernandez FJ, Gonzalez-Reimers CE, Satista-Lopez N, Gonzalez-Garcia C, Jorge-Hernandez JA, Hernandez-Nieto L. (1987) Alcohol-induced hypogonadism: reversal after ethanol withdrawal. *Drug Alcohol. Depend.* 20:255–260.
77. Hoyumpa AM. (1986) Mechanisms of vitamin deficiencies in alcoholism. *Alcohol Clin. Exp. Res.* 10:573–581.
78. Tuck RR, Jackson M. (1991) Social, neurological and cognitive disorders in alcoholics. *Med. J. Aust.* 155:255–259.
79. Lee K, Moller I, Hardt F, Haubek A, Jensen E. (1979) Alcohol-induced brain damage and liver damage in young males. *Lancet* 2:(8146)759–761.
80. Eckardt MJ, Rawlings RR, Graubard BI, Faden V, Martin PR, Gottschalk LA. (1988) Neuropsychological performance and treatment outcome in male alcoholics. *Alcohol Clin. Exp. Res.* 12:88–93.
81. Lynch MJG. (1960) Brain lesions in chronic alcoholism. *Arch. Pathol.* 69:342–353.
82. Lovinger DM. (1993) Excitotoxicity and alcohol-related brain damage. *Alcohol. Clin. Exp. Res.* 17:19–27.
83. Torvick A. (1987) Brain lesions in alcoholics: neuropathological observations. *Acta. Med. Scand.* 717:47–54.
84. Charness ME. (1993) Brain lesions in alcoholics. *Alcohol Clin. Exp. Res.* 17:2–11.
85. Martin PR, Adinoff B, Weingartner H, Mukherjee AB, Eckardt MJ. (1986) Alcoholic organic brain disease:nosology and pathophysiologic mechanisms. *Prog. Neuro-Psychopharmacol. Biol. Psychiat.* 10:147–164.

86. Streissguth AP, Landesman-Dwyer G, Martin DC, Smith DW. (1980) Teratogenic effects of alcohol in humans and animals. *Science* 209:353–361.

87. Streissguth AP. (1993) Fetal alcohol syndrome in older patients. *Alcohol Alcoholism*, Suppl 2. pp 209–212.

88. Glue P, Nutt D. (1990) Overexcitement and disinhibition: dynamic neurotransmitter interactions in alcohol withdrawal. *Brit. J. Psychiatry* 157:491–499.

89. Baldwin HA, Rassnick S, Rivier J, Koob GF, Britton KT. (1991) CRF antagonist reverses the "anxiogenic" response to ethanol withdrawal in the rat. *Psychopharmacol.* 103:227–232.

90. Criswell HE, Breese GR. (1993) Similar effects of ethanol and flumazenil on acquisition of a shuttle-box avoidance response during withdrawal from chronic ethanol treatment. *Brit. J. Pharmacol.* 110:753–761.

91. Devenyi P, Harrison ML. (1985) Prevention of alcohol withdrawal seizures with oral diazepam loading. *Can. Med. Assoc. J.* 132:798–800.

92. Sellers EM, Naranjo CA, Harrison M, Devenyi P, Roach C, Sykora K. (1983) Diazepam loading: simplified treatment of alcohol withdrawal. *Clin. Pharmacol. Ther.* 34:822–826.

93. Scott GE, Little FW. (1985) Disulfiram reaction to organic solvents other than ethanol. *New Engl. J. Med.* 312:790.

94. Sellers EM, Naranjo CA, Peachey JE. (1981) Drugs to decrease alcohol consumption. *N. Engl. J. Med.* 305:1255–1262.

95. Volpicelli JR, Alterman AI, Hayashida M, O'Brien CP. (1992) Naltrexone in the treatment of alcohol dependence. *Arch. Gen. Psychiat.* 49:876–880.

96. Naranjo CA, Poulos CX, Bremner KE, Lanctot KL. (1992) Citalopram decreases desirability, liking, and consumption of alcohol in alcohol-dependent drinkers. *Clin. Pharmacol. Therm.* 51:729–739.

97. Helzer JE, Robins LN, Taylor JR, Carey K, Miller RH, Combs-Orme T, Farmer A. (1985) The extent of long-term moderate drinking among alcoholics discharged from medical and psychiatric treatment facilities. *New Eng. J. Med.* 312:1678–1682.

98. Fuller RK, Branchey L, Brightwell DR, Derman RM, Emrick CD, Iber FL, James KE, Lacoursiere RB, Lee KK, Lowenstam I, Manny I, Neiderhiser D, Nocks S, Shaw JJ. (1986) Disulfiram treatment of alcoholism: a Veterans Administration cooperative study. *JAMA* 256:1449–1455.

99. Martin PR, Kapur BM, Whiteside EA, Sellers EM. (1979) Intravenous phenobarbital therapy in barbiturate and other hypnosedative withdrawal reactions: A kinetic approach. *Clin. Pharmacol. Ther.* 26:256–264.

100. Robinson GM, Sellers EM, Janecek E. (1981) Barbiturate and hypnosedative withdrawal by a multiple oral phenobarbital loading dose technique. *Clin. Pharmacol. Ther.* 30:71–76.

101. Hollister AS, Breese GR, Cooper BR. (1974) Comparison of tyrosine hydroxylase and dopamine-beta-hydroxylase inhibition with the effects of various 6-hydroxydopamine treatments on d-amphetamine induced motor activity. *Psychopharmacologia 36*:1–16.

102. Cooper BR, Konkol RJ, Breese GR. (1978) Effects of catecholamine depleting drugs and d-amphetamine on self-stimulation of the substantia nigra and locus coeruleus. *J. Pharmacol Exp. Ther. 204*:592–605.

103. Shimada S, Kitayama S, Lin C-L, Patel A, Nanthakumar E, Gregor P, Kuhar M, Uhl G. (1991) Cloning and expression of a cocaine-sensitive dopamine transporter complementary DNA. *Science* 25:576–578.

104. Kilty JE, Lorange D, Amara SG. (1991) Cloning and expression of a cocaine-sensitive rat dopamine transporter. *Science* 254:578–579.

105. Usdin TB, Mezey E, Chen C, Brownstein MJ, Hoffman BJ. (1991) Cloning of the cocaine-sensitive bovine dopamine transporter. *Proc. Natl., Acad. Sci. USA.* 88:11168–11171.

106. Gorelick DA. (1992) Progression of dependence in male cocaine addicts. *Am. J. Drug Alcohol Abuse* 18:13–19.

107. Gawin FH, Kleber HD. (1986) Abstinence symptomatotolgy and psychiatric diagnosis in cocaine abusers. *Arch. Gen. Psychiatry.* 43:107–113.

108. Dackis CA, Gold MS. (1985) New concepts in cocaine addiction: the dopamine depletion hypothesis. *Neurosci. Biobehav. Rev.* 9:469–477.

109. Levine SR, Brust JCM, Futrell N, Ho KL, Blake D, Millikan CH, Brass, LM, Fayad P, Schultz LR, Selwa JF, Welch KMA. (1990) Cerebrovascular complications of the use of "crack" forms of alkaloidal cocaine. *N. Engl. J. Med.* 323:699–704.

110. Haverkos HW. (1991) Infectious diseases and drug abuse: Prevention and treatment in the drug abuse treatment system. *J. Subst. Abuse Treat.* 8:269–275.

110a. Griffin ML, Weiss RD, Mirin SM, Lange U. (1989) A comparison of male and female cocaine abusers. *Arch. Gen. Psychiat.* 48:122–128.

111. Halikas JA, Crosby RD, Carlson GA, Crea F, Graves NM, Bowers LD. (1991) Cocaine reduction in unmotivated crack users using carbamazepine versus placebo in short-term, double blind crossover design. *Clin. Pharmacol. Ther.* 50:81–95.

112. Raynor K, Kong H, Chen Y, Yasuda K, Yu L, Bell GI, Reisine T. (1994) Pharmacological characterization of the cloned kappa-, delta-, and mu-opioid receptors. *Mol. Pharmacol.* 45:330–334.

113. Guitart X, Nestler EJ. (1989) Identification of morphine- and cyclic AMP-regulated phosphoproteins (MARPP's) in the locus coeruleus and other regions of rat brain: regulation by acute and chronic morphine. *J. Neurosci.* 9:4371–4387.

114. Gold MS, Redmond DE, Kleber HD. (1978) Clonidine in opiate withdrawal. *Lancet* 1:929–930.

115. Childress AR, McLellan AT, O'Brien CP. (1986) Abstinent opiate abusers exhibit conditioned craving, conditioned withdrawal and reductions in both through extinction. *Brit. J. Addict.* 81:655–660.

116. Matsuda LA, Lolait SJ, Brownstein MJ, Young AC, Bonner TI. (1990) Structure of a cannabinoid receptor and functional expression of the cloned cDNA. *Nature* 346:561–564.

117. Herkenham M, Lynn AB, Little MD, Johnson MR, Melvin LS, DeCosta BR, Rice KC. (1990) Cannabinoid receptor localization in brain. *Proc. Natl. Acad. Sci. USA* 87:1932–1936.

118. Matsuda LA, Bonner TI, Lolait SJ. (1993) Localization of cannabinoid receptor mRNA in rat brain. *J. Comp. Neurol.* 327:535–550.

119. Howlett AC, Qualy JM, Khachaturian LL. (1986) Involvement of Gi in the inhibition of adenylate cyclase by cannabinomimetic drugs. *Mol. Pharmacol.* 29:307–313.

120. Mackie K, Hille B. (1992) Cannabinoids inhibit N-type calcium channels in neuroblastoma-glioma cells. *Proc. Natl. Acad. Sci. USA* 89:3825–3829.

121. Heyser CJ, Hampson RE, Deadwyler SA. (1993) Effects of delta-9-tetrahydrocannabinol on delayed match to sample performance in rats: alterations in short-term memory associated with

changes in task specific firing of hippocampal cells. *J. Pharmacol. Exp. Ther.* 264:294–307.

122. Devane WA, Hanuš L, Breuer A, Pertwee RG, Stevenson LA, Griffin G, Gibons D, Mandelbaum A, Etinger A, Mechoulam R. (1992) Isolation and structure of a brain constituent that binds to the cannabinoid receptor. *Science* 258:1946–1949.

123. Lynn AB, Herkenham M. (1994) Localization of cannabinoid receptors and nonsaturable high-density cannabinoid binding sites in peripheral tissues of the rat: implications for receptor-mediated immune modulation by cannabinoids. *J. Pharmacol. Exp. Ther.* 268:1612–1623.

124. Johansson E, Agurell S, Holister LE, Halldin MM. (1988) Prolonged apparent half-life of tetrahydrocannabinol in plasma of chronic marijuana users. *J. Pharm. Pharmacol.* 40:374–375.

125. Thomas H. (1993) Psychiatric symptoms incannabis users. *Brit. J. Psychiatry* 163:141–149.

126. Wu, T-C, Tashkin DP, Djahed B, Rose JE. (1988) Pulmonary hazards of smoking marijuana as compared to tobacco. *N. Engl. J. Med.* 318:347–351.

127. Clarke PBS, Schwartz RD, Paul SM, Pert CB. (1985) Nicotinic binding in rat brain: Autoradiographic comparison of [^{3}H]acetylcholine, [^{3}H]nicotine, and [^{125}]-α-bungarotoxin. *J. Neurosci.* 5:1307–1315.

128. Schulz DW, Loring RH, Aizenman E, Zigmond RE. (1991) Autoradiographic location of putative nicotinic receptors in the rat brain using ^{125}I-neuronal bungarotoxin. *J. Neurosci.* 11:287–297.

129. Sequela P, Wadiche J, Dineley-Miller K, Dani JA, Patrick JW. (1993) Molecular cloning, functional properties, and distribution of rat brain α7: A nicotinic cation channel highly permeable to calcium. *J. Neurosci.* 13:596–604.

130. McCall MR, van-den-Berg JJ, Kuypers FA, Tribble DL, Krauss RM, Knoff LJ, Forte TM. (1994) Modification of LCAT activity and HDL structure. New links between cigarette smoke and coronary heart disease risk. *Arterioscler Thromb.* 14:248–253.

131. Vial WC. (1986) Cigarette smoking and lung disease. *Am. J. Med. Sci.* 291:130–142.

132. Newcomb PA, Carbone PP. (1992) The health consequences of smoking. Cancer. *Med. Clin. North. Am.* 76:305–331.

133. Hecht SS, Carmella SG, Murphy SE, Akerkar S, Brunnemann KD, Hoffmann D. (1993) A tobacco-specific lung carcinogen in the urine of men exposed cigarette smoke. *N. Engl. J. Med.* 329:1543–1546.

134. Levin ED, Westman EC, Stein RM, Carnahan E. Sanchez M, Herman S, Behm FM, Rose JE. (1994) Nicotine skin patch treatment increases abstinence, decreases withdrawal symptoms, and attenuates rewarding effects of smoke. *J. Clin. Psychopharmacol.* 14:41–49.

135. O'Hearn E, Battaglia G, DeSouza EB, Kuhar MJ, Molliver ME. (1988) Methylenedioxyamphetamine (MDA) and methylenedioxymethamphetamine (MDMA) cause selective ablation of serotonergic axon terminals in forebrain: Immunocytochemical evidence for neurotoxicity. *J. Neurosci.* 8:2788–2803.

136. Langston JW, Ballard P, Tetrud JW, Irwin I. (1983) Chronic parkinsonism in humans due to a product of meperidine-analog synthesis. *Science* 219:979–980.

137. Anis NA, Berry SC, Burton NR, Lodge D. (1983) The dissociative anesthetics, ketamine and phencylidine, selective by reduced excitation of central mammalian neurones by N-methyl-aspartate. *Br. J. Pharmacol.* 79:565–575.

138. Sakurai SY, Penney JB, Young AB. (1993) Regionally distinct N-methyl-D-Aspartate receptors distinguished by quantitative autoradiography of [^{3}H]MK-801 binding in rat brain. *J Neurochem.* 60:1344–1353.

139. Sveinbjornsdottir S, Sander JWAS, Upton D, Thompson PJ, Patsalos PN, Hirt D, Emre M, Lowe D, Duncan JS. (1993) The excitatory amino acid antagonist D-CPP-ene (SDZ EAA-494) in patients with epilepsy. *Epilepsy Res.* 16:165–174.

140. Mendelsohn LG, Kalra V, Johnson BG, Kerchner GA. Sigma opioid receptor: Characterization and co-identity with the phencyclidine receptor. *J. Pharmacol. Exp. Ther.* 233:597–602, 1985.

141. Rosenberg HC, Kleinschmidt-DeMasters BK, Davis KA, Dreisbach JN, Hornes JT, and Filley CM. (1988) Toluene abuse causes diffuse central nervous system white matter changes. *Ann. Neurol.* 23:611–614.

142. McIntyre AS, Long RG. (1992) Fatal fulminant hepatic failure in a solvent abuser. *Postgrad. Med. J.* 68:29–30.

143. Dax EM, Nagel JE, Lange WR, Adler WH, Jaffe JH. (1988) Effects of nitrites on the immune system of humans. *Natl. Inst. Drug Abuse Res. Monogr. Ser.* 83:75–80.

144. Le AD, Poulos CX, Cappell H. (1979) Conditioned tolerance to the hypothermic effects of ethyl alcohol. *Science* 206:1109–1110.

145. Siegel S. (1976) Morphine analgesic tolerance: situation specificity supports pavolovian conditioning model. *Science* 193:323–325.

Reviews

r1. Crabbe JC, Belknap JK. (1992) Genetic approaches to drug dependence. *Trends Pharmacol. Sci.* 13:212–219.

r2. Schuckit MA. (1991) A longitudinal study of children of alcoholics. In Galanter M (ed.), *Recent Developments in Alcoholism, Volume 9,* Plenum Press, New York. pp 5–19.

r3. Kolb L. (1962) *Drug Addiction: A Medical Problem,* Charles C Thomas, Springfield, Illinois.

r4. Regier DA, Farmer ME, Goodwin FK. (1992) Comorbidity of mental and substance abuse disorders. In Michels R, Cooper AM, Guze SB, Judd LL, Klerman GL, Solnit AJ, Stunkard AJ, Wilner PJ (eds.), *Psychiatry, Volume 3,* J.B. Lippincott Company, Philadelphia. pp 1–23.

r5. Meyer RE. (1986) *Psychopathology and Addictive Disorders,* The Guilford Press, New York, NY.

r6. Johnson BD, Muffler J. (1992) Sociocultural aspects of drug use and abuse in the 1990s. In Lowinson JH, Ruiz P, Millman RB, Langrod JG (eds), *Substance Abuse: A Comprehensive Textbook,* Williams and Wilkins, Baltimore, MD. pp 118–137.

r7. Prochaska JO, DiClemente CC. (1986) Toward a comprehensive model of change. In Miller WE, Heather N (eds.), *Treating Addictive Behaviors,* Plenum Press, New York, NY. pp 3–27.

r8. Marlatt GA, Gordon JR. (1980) Determinants of relapse: Implications of the maintenance of behavior change. In Davidson PO, Davidson SM (eds.), *Behavioral Medicine: Changing Health Lifestyles,* Brunner/Mazel, New York, NY. pp 410–452.

r9. Brehm NM, Khantzian EJ. (1992) A psychodynamic perspective. In Lowinson JH, Ruiz P, Millman RB, Langrod JG (eds.), *Substance Abuse: A Comprehensive Textbook,* Williams and Wilkins, Baltimore, MD. pp 106–117.

r10. Lowinson JH, Ruiz P. (1981) *Substance Abuse: Clinical Problems and Perspectives,* Williams and Wilkins, Baltimore, MD.

r11. Giannini AJ, Slaby AE. (1989) *Drugs of Abuse*, Medical Economics Books, Oradell, NJ.

r12. Kalant H, LeBlanc AE, Gibbins RJ. (1971) Tolerance to and dependence on some non-opiate psychotropic drugs. *Pharmacol. Rev.* 2:135–191.

r13. Grinspoon L, Bakalar JB. (1985) *Cocaine: A Drug and its Social Evolution*, Basic Books, Inc., New York.

r14. Chen KK, Schmidt CF. (1930) Ephedrine and related substances. *Medicine* 9:1–117.

r15. Haley TJ. Desoxyphedrine—a review of the literature. *J. Am. Pharm. Ass.* (Scientific Edition) (1947) 36:161–169.

r16. Musto DF. (1992) Historical perspectives on alcohol and drug abuse. In Lowinson JH, Ruiz P, Millman RB, Langrod JG (eds.), *Substance Abuse: A Comprehensive Textbook*, Williams and Wilkins, Baltimore, MD. pp 2–14.

r17. Kandel DB. (1992) Epidemiology of drug use and abuse. In Michels R, Cooper AM, Guze SB, Judd LL, Klerman GL, Solnit AJ, Stunkard AJ, Wilner PJ (eds.), *Psychiatry, Volume 3*, J.B. Lippincott Company, Philadelphia, PA. pp 1–30.

r18. *Prevention and Treatment of Alcohol Problems: Research Opportunities*, National Academy Press, Washington, DC. 1989.

r19. Fingarette H. (1988) *Heavy Drinking: the Myth of Alcoholism as a Disease*, University of California Press, Berkeley.

r20. Stolerman I. (1992) Drugs abuse: behavioral principles, methods and terms. *Trends in Pharmacol. Sci.* 13:170–176.

r21. Bozarth MA. (1987) *Methods of Assessing the Reinforcing Properties of Abused Drugs*, Springer-Verlag, New York, NY.

r22. Koob GF. (1992) Drugs of abuse: anatomy, pharmacology and function of reward pathways. *Trends Pharmacol. Sci.* 13:177–184.

r23. Agarwal DP, Goedde HW. (1992) Pharmacogenetics of alcohol metabolism and alcoholism. *Pharmacogenetics* 2:48–62.

r24. Goldstein DB. (1983). *Pharmacology of alcohol*. New York: Oxford University Press.

r25. Samson HH, Harris RA. (1992) Neurobiology of alcohol abuse. *Trends Pharmacol. Sci.* 13:206–211.

r26. Wolfe LS, Horrocks LA. (1994) Eicosanoids. In: Siegel GJ, Agranoff BW, Albers RW, Molinoff PB (eds), *Basic Neurochemistry (Fifth Edition)* Raven Press, New York, NY, pp 475–490.

r27. Nestler EJ, Greengard P. (1994) Protein phosphorylation and the regulation of neuronal function. In: Siegel GJ, Agranoff BW, Albers RW, Molinoff PB (eds), *Basic Neurochemistry (Fifth Edition)* Raven Press, New York, NY, pp 449–474.

r28. Meisch RA. (1977) Ethanol self-administration: infrahuman studies. In Thompson T, Dews PB (eds.), *Advances in Behavioral Pharmacology, Volume 1*, Academic Press, New York, N.Y. pp 36–84.

r29. Pokorny AD, Kanas TE. (1980) Stages in the development of alcoholism. In Fann WE, Karacan I, Pokorny AD, Williams RL (eds.), *Phenomenology and Treatment of Alcoholism*, Spectrum Publications, Inc., New York. pp 45–68.

r30. Watson RR, Watzl B. (1992) *Nutrition and Alcohol*. CRC Press, Ann Arbor, MI.

r31. Pfefferbaum A, Lim KO, Rosenbloom M. (1992) Structural imaging of the brain in chronic alcoholism. In Zakhari S, Witt E (eds), *Imaging in Alcohol Research—Research Monograph—21*. U.S. NIAAA DHHS publication (ADM) 92-1890, Rockville, MD pp 99–120.

r32. Jernigan TL, Butters N, Cermak LS. (1992) Studies of brain structure in chronic alcoholism using magnetic resonance imaging. In Zakhari S, Witt E (eds), *Imaging in Alcohol Research—Research Monograph—21*. U.S. NIAAA, DHHS publication (ADM) 92-1890, Rockville, MD pp 121–133.

r33. Victor M, Adamson RD, Collins GH. (1989) *The Wernicke-Korsakoff Syndrome* 2nd ed., F.A. Davis Co, Philadelphia.

r34. Streissguth AP, LaDue RA. (1987) Fetal alcohol: teratogenic causes of developmental disabilities. *Monogr. Am. Assoc. Ment. Defic.* 8:1–32.

r35. Reid LD, Delconte JD, Nichols ML, Bilsky EJ, Hubbell CL. (1991) Tests of opioid deficiency hypotheses of alcoholism. *Alcohol Journal*. 8:247–257.

r36. Woods JH, Katz JL, Winger G. (1987) Abuse liability of benzodiazepines. *Pharmacol. Rev.* 39:251–419.

r37. Woolverton WL, Johnson KM. (1992) Neurobiology of cocaine abuse. *Trends Pharmacol. Sci.* 13:193–200.

r38. Byck R. (1987) Cocaine use and research: three histories. In Fisher S, Raskin A, Uhlenhuth EH (eds.), *Cocaine: Clinical and Biobehavioral Aspects*, Oxford University Press, Inc., New York, NY. pp 3–20.

r39. Robinson TE, Berridge KC. (1993) The neural basis of drug craving: an incentive-sensitization theory of addiction. *Brain Res. Rev.* 18:247–291.

r40. Benowitz NL. (1992) How toxic is cocaine? *Ciba Found Symp.* 166:125–143; discussion 143–148.

r41. Gonzalez NM, Campbell H. (1994) Cocaine babies: does prenatal exposure to cocaine affect development. *J. Am. Acad. Child Adoles. Psychiat.* 33:16–23, 1994.

r42. Jaffe JH. (1992) Opiates: clinical aspects. In Lowinson JH, Ruiz P, Millman RB, Langrod JG (eds.), *Substance Abuse: A Comprehensive Textbook*, Williams and Wilkins, Baltimore. pp 186–194.

r43. O'Brien CP, Childress AR, McLellan AT, Ehrman R. (1992) A learning model of addiction. In O'Brien CP, Jaffe JH (eds.), *Addictive States*, Raven Press, New York. pp 157–177.

r44. Simon EJ. Opioid receptors and endogenous opioid peptides. *Med. Res. Rev.* 11:357–374, 1991.

r45. DiChiara G, North RA. (1992) Neurobiology of opiate abuse. *Trends Pharmacol. Sci.* 13:185–193.

r46. Lowinson JH, Marion IJ, Joseph H, Dole VP. (1992) Methadone maintenance. In Lowinson JH, Ruiz P, Millman RB, Langrod JG (eds.), *Substance abuse: a comprehensive textbook*, Williams and Wilkins, Baltimore, MD. pp 550–561.

r47. Martin B. (1986) Cellular Effects of cannabinoids. *Pharmacol. Rev.* 38:45–74.

r48. Dewey WL. (1986) Cannabinoid pharmacology. *Pharmacol. Rev.* 38:151–178.

r49. Agurell S, Halldin M, Lindgren J-E, Ohlsson A, Widman M, Gillespie H, Hollister L. (1986) Pharmacokinetics and metabolism of Δ^1- tetrahydrocannabinol and other cannabinoids with emphasis on man. *Pharmacol. Rev.* 38:21–43.

r50. Abood ME, Martin BR. (1992) Neurobiology of marijuana abuse. *Trends Pharm. Sci.* 13:201–206.

r51. Hollister LE. (1986) Health aspects of cannabis. *Pharmacol. Rev.* 38:1–20.

r52. Deneris ES, Connolly J, Rogers SW, Duvoisin R. (1991) Pharmacological and functional diversity of neuronal nicotinic acetylcholine receptors. *Trends in Pharmacol. Rev.* 121:34–40.

r53. Ravenholt RT. (1985) Tobacco's impact on the Twentieth Century: US Mortality patterns. *Am. J. Rev. Med.* 1:4–16.

r54. Schultes RE. (1978) Plants and plant constituents as mind-altering agents throughout history. *Handbook of Psychopharmacology* (eds. Iversen LL, Iversen SD, Snyder SH) Vol. 11: pp 219–241.

r55. Hoffman A. (1963) *Readings in Pharmacology* (eds. Holmstedt B, Liljestrand J). pp 209–213 The MacMillan Company, New York.

r56. Shulgin AT. (1978) Psychotomimetic drugs: structure-activity relationships. *Handbook of Psychopharmacology* (eds. Iversen LL, Iversen SD, Snyder, SH) Vol. 11: pp 243–333.

r57. Hollister LE. (1978) Psychotomimetic drugs in man. *Handbook of Psychopharmacology* (eds. Iversen LL, Iversen SD, Snyder SH) Vol. 11: pp 389–424.

r58. Crider R. (1986) Phencyclidine: changing abuse patterns. *In Phencyclidine:* an Update (Clouet DH, ed)., pp. 163–173. Natl. Inst. on Drug Abuse Research Monogran 64. DHHS publication (ADM) 86–1443.

r59. Balster RL. (1987) The behavioral pharmacology of phencyclidine. In *Psychopharmacology: the Third Generation of Progress* (Meltzer HY, ed.). pp 1573–1579. Raven Press, New York.

r60. Johnson KM. (1987) Neurochemistry and neurophysiology of phencyclidine. *In Psychopharmacology: the Third Generation of Progress* (Meltzer HY, ed.) pp 1581–1588. Raven Press, New York.

r61. Blum K. (1984) Solvent and aerosol inhalants ("glue sniffing") in Handbook of Abusable Drugs, Gardner Press, NY pp 211–236.

r62. Chaudron CD, Wilkinson DA. (1988) *Theories on Alcoholism,* Addiction Research Foundation, Toronto, Canada.

r63. Schuckit MA, Smith TL, Anthenelli R, Irwin M. (1993) Clinical course of alcoholism in 639 male inpatients. Am. J. Psychiatry 150:786–792.

r64. Black D. (1989) *Sociological Justice,* Oxford University Press, New York, NY.

r65. Diagnostic and Statistical Manual of Mental Disorders (Fourth Edition) (1993), American Psychiatric Association, Washington, D.C.

r66. *Diagnostic and Statistical Manual of Mental Disorders* (*Third Edition—Revised*), (1987) American Psychiatric Association, Washington, D.C.

r67. Erickson PG. (1992) The law in addictions: principles, practicalities and prospects. In Erickson PG, Kalant H (eds.), *Windows on Science,* Addiction Research Foundation, Toronto, Canada. pp 125–160.

r68. Inciardi JA, Chambers C. (1974) *Drugs and the Criminal Justice System,* Sage, Beverly Hills, CA.

CHAPTER 22

Aaron J. Janowsky
Richard L. Hauger

CNS Stimulants

Central nervous stimulants include drugs with a wide variety of chemical structures, pharmacologic activity, and clinical uses. Although many of these drugs have been (ab)used for decades or even centuries, their mechanisms of action as stimulants are not completely understood. Recent studies involving the use of amphetamine and the other stimulants in treating a variety of neuropsychiatric disorders indicate that lack of response to a particular medication may not predict the response to another drug in the same class. The drugs described below are currently available by prescription and, for the most part, are administered for their systemic or central nervous system (CNS) effects. Drugs available by prescription for topical or local effects but abused *via* systemic administration are included in the chapter on drug abuse.

Amphetamine and Related Compounds

The noncatecholamine amphetamine, a β-phenylisopropylamine, possesses strong central psychostimulant actions and indirect sympathomimetic activity in the periphery.[r1–r7] A number of amphetamine analogues, including methamphetamine, methylphenidate, fenfluramine, diethylpropion, phentermine, and phendimetrazine, share some effects and are discussed below. As a general neurochemical mechanism of action, amphetamine stimulates the release of dopamine and norepinephrine from a newly-synthesized cytoplasmic pool of monoamines that is reserpine-insensitive.[1,2,r1–r8] The CNS stimulant actions of amphetamine in humans include psychomotor activation, anorexia, diminished sleep and fatigue, hypodypsia, respiratory stimulation, hyperthermia, and the induction of a euphoric mood.[3–5,r6,r9–r11] In preclinical studies, amphetamine has been found to increase spontaneous and operant locomotor behavior; at high doses, it increases continuous stereotypy in laboratory animals.[6,7,r6,r7,r9]. Among its peripheral effects, amphetamine activates the sympathetic nervous system, but with a delayed onset.[5,r2,r6] Amphetamine also has a delayed effect on blood pressure, but a longer duration of action compared with the effects of a single equipressor dose of norepinephrine.[5,r2,r6] Direct sympathomimetic drugs activate sympathetic effector cells by binding to postsynaptic catecholamine receptors. However, amphetamine's peripheral stimulation of the sympathetic nervous system depends on the release of norepinephrine from presynaptic stores, followed by an indirect activation of alpha- and beta-adrenergic receptors.[1,2,r1–r6,r8] Hypertension secondary to vasoconstriction, bronchodilation, mydriasis, and contraction of the urinary bladder sphincter are among the peripheral autonomic effects of amphetamine.[r2,r6] Chronic administration of amphetamine decreases the newly-synthesized cytoplasmic stores of norepinephrine, resulting in the tachyphylaxis typical for indirectly acting sympathomimetic agents.[2,6,7,r6,r9] Amphetamine and related compounds are "positively reinforcing" drugs based on their ability to promote repetitive self-administration by laboratory animals, sometimes at a lethal dose, and to cause drug addiction to humans.[6,7,r6,r7,r9–r11] The administration of high doses of amphetamine in humans can cause a toxic paranoid psychosis.[r9,r12] In the past, the principal medical uses of amphetamine have been for weight reduction in obesity, for narcolepsy and refractory depression, and inattention-deficit disorder with hyperactivity (ADDH) in children.[r13–r16] The euphoriant and psychostimulant properties of amphetamine, however, create a substantial risk for drug abuse and addiction.[7,16,r10] These adverse effects usually outweigh the therapeutic benefits of amphetamine, limiting its use in clinical medicine.

History

Eight years before the discovery of the pressor activity of suprarenal extracts (later to be named "epinephrine" by Abel in 1899), Edeleanu first synthesized amphetamine in 1887 as part of his research studies on aliphatic amines.[r16–r17] In the same year, Nagai isolated ephedrine from Ephedra plants, which were used as a source of the Chinese herbal drug Ma Huang. Schmidt synthesized methamphetamine in 1914. Alles also reported the synthesis of amphetamine in 1927 during his search for sympathomimetics that could be substituted for ephedrine in the treatment of asthma. Piness and associates first demonstrated the long-acting pressor activity of amphetamine in 1930. Since these investigators gave both oral and subcutaneous doses of 50 mg amphetamine to their human subjects, psychostimulant responses must have occurred.

Three years later, Alles demonstrated other pharmacologic effects of amphetamine, including bronchodilation and respiratory stimulation. Amphetamine was also found in 1933 to act as an analeptic, causing reversal of barbiturate anesthesia. However, amphetamine's CNS psychostimulant properties were not appreciated until 1933—46 years after it was first synthesized. It may not have been appreciated that amphetamine was a psychostimulant, because the first pharmacologic characterization of amphetamine (in 1910 by Barger and Dale) was performed in anesthetized animals, which probably blocked stimulant responses. In 1935, Prinzmetal and Bloomberg first treated narcolepsy with amphetamine. The following year an oral form of amphetamine was available by prescription. In 1938, Hauschild demonstrated the psychostimulant activity of methamphetamine in laboratory animals.[r13,r14,r16,r17] Hauschild also self-administered 5 mg methamphetamine (which he called Per-Vatin) and noted that its effects on behavior were similar to those of amphetamine.

With the recognition of its psychostimulant effects, amphetamine quickly became a drug of abuse. The euphoriant, fatigue-reducing, and insomnia-producing properties of amphetamine were clearly described in 1930 when nasal amphetamine inhalers were used in Germany: "Patients treated in the afternoon were noted to be refreshed, have a sense of well being and competence and, for the most part, could not sleep that night." Between 1936 and the beginning of World War II, amphetamine was used to treat many different medical patients besides narcoleptics. These included individuals with alcoholic stupor and acute alcohol intoxication; barbiturate and morphine overdoses; myasthenia gravis; postencephalitic parkinsonism; hypotensive conditions; nasal congestion; obesity; enuresis; migraine; asthma; vomiting during pregnancy; sea sickness; carotid sinus syndrome; and gastrointestinal spasms. Amphetamine was also administered to psychiatric patients with organic psychoses, "dementia praecox" (schizophrenia), and manic-depressive psychosis.[r13,r14,r16,r17] In 1938, the first report appeared indicating that amphetamine was a psychotomimetic. The previous year, Guttman and Sargeant had recognized amphetamine's potential for addiction. Nevertheless, amphetamine continued to be used indiscriminately as a possible therapeutic agent. In fact, many physicians doubted that amphetamine was addictive because there were no withdrawal symptoms as occurred with classic addiction syndromes such as opiate withdrawal. Stimulant "craving" *per se* was not appreciated as a sign of psychologic dependence.

Methylphenidate's synthesis was described in 1944, and reports describing drug-induced stereoptyped behavior in animals appeared about ten years later, although it was noted that methylphenidate was less potent than amphetamine. Clinical trials involving the treatment of various neuropsychiatric disorders, including depression, followed shortly thereafter, and in the drug was marketed as a "mood elevator.[r13,r14,r16,r17] During World War II, amphetamine stimulants were distributed to German soldiers to induce aggressiveness and belligerence. In wartime Japan, amphetamine was used to reduce fatigue and increase productivity in soldiers and civilians. In 1947, the classic study of Monroe and Drell revealed that 25% of inmates in military prisons used amphetamine, documenting four who became psychotic after using 15 to 670 mg amphetamine every 2 to 4 hours.[8] An epidemic of IV methamphetamine abuse occurred in Japan after World War II, when the large wartime supplies became available. It is noteworthy that amphetamine abuse is associated with a paranoid "schizophreniform psychosis" in Western psychiatric literature,[r10,r12] while the Japanese literature noted the presence of both schizophrenic and affective symptoms in amphetamine users. In the 1960s, amphetamine abuse ("speed freaks") became widespread in the US and other western countries, especially Sweden. In addition, reports of methylphenidate-induced dependence and psychosis also appeared in the literature at this time. It is interesting that episodes of stimulant abuse tend to be discrete, while opiate addiction is more persistent than episodic.[7,r10,r16] In addition, very high amphetamine abuse is found in the US and Japan, and relatively low rates are found in Europe.[7,r10,r16] It is possible that psychosocial aspects of life in the US and Japan contribute to the preferential use of psychostimulants.

Chemistry

The chemical structure of amphetamine is depicted in Figure 22.1. D-Amphetamine is the prototype for indirect sympathomimetics. Many other stimulant drugs such as methamphetamine, methylphenidate, phenmetrazine, pipradrol, ephedrine, and nomifensine have a structure consisting of a benzene ring and an ethylamine side-chain (i.e., beta-phenylethylamine), and cause psychomotor stimulation and anorexia.[1–3,r1–r4,r18] Beginning with the classic structure-activity studies of Barger and Dale, it has been recognized that chemical substitutions on the aromatic ring, the alpha- and beta-carbon atoms, and the terminal amino group modify the sympathomimetic activity of this beta-phenethylamine compound.[r6,r18] First, there are two stereoisomers of amphetamine owing to the asymmetry of the side-chain alpha-carbon. The D-form of amphetamine, created by dextrorotatory substitution on the alpha-carbon, possesses a significantly greater behavioral stimulant effect (*e.g.*, the d-isomer has two- to tenfold more potent central psychostimulatory activity, as compared to the L-isomer, based on the behavioral or neuropharmacologic parameter) in comparison to L-amphetamine. Ephedrine, amphetamine, and methamphetamine cross the blood-brain barrier more readily because their aromatic nuclei are unsubstituted or have an alkyl group.[r1,r18] The greater lipophilic nature increases their stimulant activity in the CNS.[r1,r2,r6,r18] In general, the separation of the benzene ring from the side-chain amino group by two carbon atoms is essential for significant sympathomimetic activity.[r16,r18]

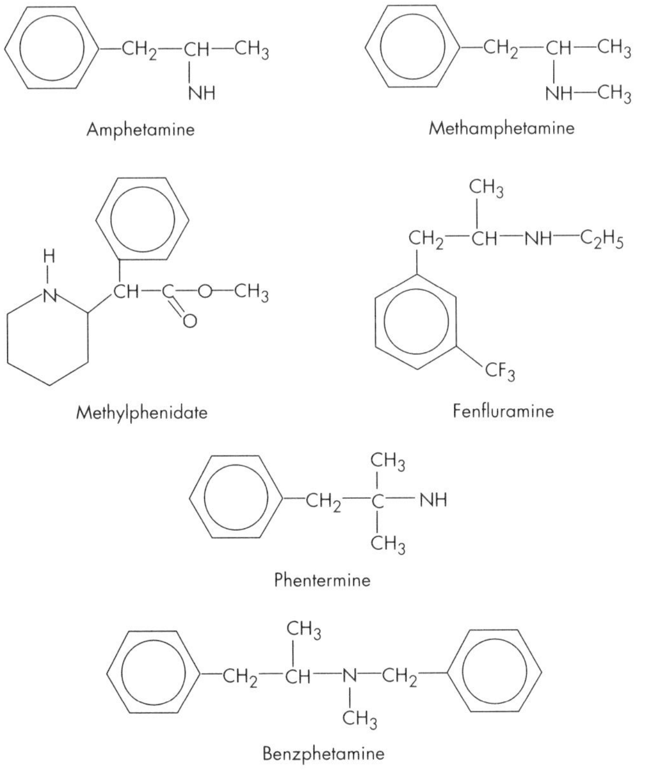

Amphetamine

Methamphetamine

Methylphenidate

Fenfluramine

Phentermine

Benzphetamine

Figure 22.1

Benzene Ring

The anorectic action can be dissociated from the CNS stimulant effects of amphetamine derivatives. For example, fenfluramine is formed by a trifluoromethyl substitution at the meta position of the aromatic benzene ring (Fig. 22.1). Fenfluramine and its N-dealkylated derivative, norfenfluramine, retain potent anorectic activity while losing CNS psychostimulant properties.[r2,r3,r6,r18] In fact, fenfluramine is actually a behavioral depressant. Replacement of the benzene ring with an aliphatic chain (triaminoheptane, methylhexaneamine), a saturated ring (cyclopentamine, propylhexedrine), or a different unsaturated ring (naphozaline) does not affect alpha- or beta-receptor psychostimulant activity.[r6,r18] The potent alpha-receptor stimulant naphozaline is a behavioral depressant like fenfluramine, which also has a substituted benzene ring.

Alpha-Carbon

Phenylethylamine drugs are largely inactivated by intraneuronal monoamine oxidase (MAO) but not catechol-O-methyltransferase (COMT).[r1,r6,r18,r19] The presence of an alpha-carbon atom substitution to form the noncatecholamines ephedrine or amphetamine changes the duration of action of the phenylethylamine from minutes to hours.[r6,r18,r19] The slow inactivation of amphetamine derivatives due to the alpha-methyl group is important for the ability of these drugs to release norepinephrine from presynaptic storage sites.

Beta-Carbon

Polar substituents (*e.g.*, -OH group) on the beta-carbon atom make the drug less lipophilic, diminishing its entry into the CNS.[r6,18,r19] Therefore, ephedrine, which has a -OH substituent on the beta-carbon, has low psychostimulant activity but increased activity as both a direct and an indirect alpha- and beta-receptor agonist. The stimulant phenylpropanolamine, which also has a -OH group in the beta carbon position, is the major ingredient in a large number of over-the-counter agents, including nasal decongestants and diet pills.

Ethylamine Side-Chain

The length of the ethylamine side-chain is also an important determinant of psychostimulant potency in the CNS. Stimulant activity of the amphetamine derivatives is decreased by shortening or lengthening this side-chain.[r2,r6,r18] Psychostimulant potency is also diminished if a group larger than a methyl substitution is placed on the primary nitrogen. The potent psychostimulants methylphenidate and pipradrol were synthesized by making the amino alkyl side-chain into a piperidine ring structure. In contrast to amphetamine steroisomers, only the L-form of pripradrol possesses stimulant activity. Methylphenidate, which has two assymetric centers, exists as diastereomers (i.e., isomers that are not mirror images), with the *threo* form of the drug possessing the stimulant properties, and the *erythro* form of the drug being inactive.[r6,r18] The cardiovascular and anorectic effects of methylphenidate and related ritalinic acid ester compounds are generally less pronounced, as compared with the effects of amphetamine and other phenethylamines, although the pharmacologic effects of these drugs are similar.

Therapeutic Uses and Limitations

Up until 30 years ago, amphetamine and its derivatives often were used to treat depression. However, amphetamine is not an effective antidepressant for long-term maintenance treatment of depressed patients because of its addictive potential, its ability to produce agitation and dysphoria, and an exacerbation of the somatic, neurovegetative symptoms associated with depression (e.g., insomnia, anorexia, sexual dysfunction, impaired cognition, anergy, anhedonia).[r10–r14] Typically, chronic administration of amphetamine results in a progressive reduction in its euphoriant effects owing to the development of tolerance.[6,7,r7] The loss of the mood-elevating action of amphetamine leaves only its dysphoric effect on mood to be experienced by the patient. It is interesting to note the increased incidence of psychostimulant abuse in psychiatric patients suffering from bipolar affective disorder (*e.g.*, manic-depressive illness).[r19] Many bipolar patients may self-adminster stimulants in order to induce hypomanic mood and the cognitive and behavioral changes they desire. The high degree of amphetamine and cocaine abuse in bipolar patients also may result from a genetic abnormality in mood regulation common to both disorders. The co-morbid presence of psychostimulant abuse in bipolar affective disorder is also associated with a poor treatment response, prolonged periods of affective illness, and suicide—further emphasizing that amphetamine is not an effective treatment for mood disorders.[r19]

Amphetamines also were prescribed in an effort to decrease fatigue and enhance mental attention and performance. They were administered to elderly patients with cognitive impairment and apathy.[r13,r14,r16] However, amphetamine administration to these patients produces tolerance, dysphoria, agitation, and other adverse effects, resulting in no therapeutic benefits, as described above.

Recent reviews of the literature indicate that, based on careful studies of the effects of psychostimulants, including amphetamine, their use in treating neuropsychiatric disorders may be limited. The current Physicians' Desk Reference (PDR) indicates the following uses for dextroamphetamine sulfate (dexedrine): (1) narcolepsy; (2) attention deficit disorder with hyperactivity (ADDH); and (3) obesity.

Narcolepsy

Dextroamphetamine treatment can reduce the episodes of uncontrollable sleepiness in narcolepsy.[r13,r14,r16] However, tricyclic antidepressants such as imipramine and chlorimipramine appear to be more effective in treating the cataleptic attacks that often are part of the narcoleptic syndrome.[r20]

Attention Deficit Disorder with Hyperactivity

Many research studies have demonstrated that amphetamine significantly reduces ADDH symptoms, improves behavior in school, and increases the child's ability to acquire study skills and to learn more effectively.[r13–r15] These clinical effects of dextroamphetamine have been observed with daily oral doses ranging between 2.5 to 40 mg and, in some studies have correlated with circulating levels of plasma amphetamine.

Morbid Obesity

The anorectic effect of amphetamine is dose-dependent.[3,r6,r11] Fenfluramine also suppresses appetite. Amphetamine may cause anorexia by its interaction at neuronal sites in the lateral hypothalamus or other appetite regulatory centers in the brain.[r6,r8,r11] There also may be peripheral sites mediating amphetamine's anorexic effect.[r8,r11] However, the anorectic effect of amphetamines only occurs for one to two weeks and is followed by the development of tolerance. Thus, the use of amphetamine for the treatment of obesity is questionable.

Methylphenidate has been used with some success in the treatment of a number of neuropsychiatric disorders, including depression in medically ill and (or) stroke patients, except those with delirium. The antidepressant effect of methylphenidate administration was, in these cases, apparent within 48 hours of drug administration, suggesting that the etiology of the ("secondary") depression, and the mechanism of the drug are different from the mechanisms involved in the effects of typical antidepressants, and that the underlying cause of the depression in these patients differed from that of primary depression. Methylphenidate also has been used successfully as an adjunct to narcotic analgesic treatment of pain in patients with advanced cancer and for the primary sensory symptoms that accompany Parkinson's disease. The effects of the drug in the latter example disappeared when patients were also treated with beta and (or) serotonin receptor blockers, suggesting that the drug's mechanism of action, in these specific cases, involved noradrenergic and serotonergic neurotransmitter systems.

For the most part, however, current use of methylphenidate is limited to the treatment of narcolepsy or behavioral problems including ADDH.[r15] With regard to the latter, methylphenidate has been used to treat similar behavioral problems in patients with fragile X syndrome and children who were also taking antiseizure medication (see Undesirable Effects, below). Methylphenidate also has been used to treat craving associated with cocaine abuse in adult patients with ADDH, but other cocaine abusers treated with methylphenidate experienced an increase in craving for cocaine.

Mechanisms of Action

A prevailing mechanism of psychostimulants is the inhibition of the presynaptic uptake of dopamine and norepinephrine. Behavioral stimulants also strongly promote the synaptic release of dopamine. Amphetamine psychostimulants are potent releasers of dopamine from the reserpine-insensitive cytoplasmic pool of dopamine, which is dependent on replenishment by newly formed amine. In contrast, the non-amphetamine class of stimulants such as methylphenidate, cocaine, and nomifensine, can be distinguished from amphetamine on the basis that these latter stimulants promote the release of dopamine from the granular, reserpine-sensitive storage pool of vesicular dopamine. Amphetamine is a more potent stimulator of the release of dopamine than of norepinephrine. In addition to their stimulatory effect on catecholamine release, amphetamines also block the reuptake and metabolism by monoamine oxidase of dopamine and norepinephrine. At higher doses, amphetamine inhibits norepinephrine reuptake to a greater extent than dopamine reuptake.

Recent radioligand binding studies have demonstrated the direct action of psychostimulants at the dopamine transporter located on presynaptic neurons. [^{3}H]-Threo-(±)-methylphenidate (ritalin), [^{3}H]-cocaine, and [^{3}H]-nomifensine are preferentially bound to presynaptic sites on catechol and indole amine nerve terminals.[r8] The interaction of motor stimulant drugs at methylphenidate binding sites in the corpus striatum appears to mediate psychostimulant action at the dopamine transport complex in striatal nerve terminals. All the other psychostimulants (e.g., cocaine, nomifensine) appear to define a similar site related to the striatal dopamine transport system which, at least in part, mediates the central action of non-amphetamine psychostimulants.

Although the amphetamine binding site in the striatum does not appear to have a presynaptic location, binding of amphetamine stimulants to the presynaptic dopamine carrier site may be an important initial event in the psychostimulant effects of amphetamine. This hypothesis is supported by the observations that methylphenidate inhibits in vitro amphetamine-induced dopamine release and in vivo amphetamine-stimulated behaviors. Other stimulants such as phencyclidine also may interact at presynaptic dopamine transport sites. Recently, the DNA for the human dopamine transporter of the CNS has been cloned, and other stimulants appear to bind to this site, but may have different effects on transporter function (see mazindol, below).

Therefore, this recent work on the labeling of the dopamine transport complex with tritiated ritalin, cocaine, mazindol, and nomifensine, and the classic studies of psychostimulant mechanisms have demonstrated that stimulants act on presynaptic monoamine neurons in the CNS. However, although these psychostimulants do not directly interact with postsynaptic receptors, stimulant drugs can mimic catecholamines at their postsynaptic receptor sites via their stimulation of biogenic amine release and inhibition of neuronal reuptake and neurotransmitter inactivation. These presynaptic effects subsequently can produce regulatory changes in postsynaptic monoamine receptor sites. In addition to these indirect effects of stimulants on postsynaptic catecholamine neurons, recent studies have identified postsynaptic binding sites in the CNS for [^{3}H]-(+)-amphetamine and [^{3}H]-mazindol, which may represent an intrasynaptosomal sequestration site essential for the neurochemical action of amphetamines on monoamine release.

These neuropharmacologic mechanisms do not fully explain amphetamine's efficacy in such neuropsychiatric disorders as ADDH. For example, methylphenidate is a more potent inhibitor of in vitro presynaptic reuptake of dopamine and norepinephrine. However, methylphenidate is clearly not as effective in treating ADDH. This discrepancy may relate to the ability of amphetamine to stimulate in vivo greater release of catecholamines.

Methylphenidate when used for the treatment of ADDH causes a decrease in behavioral problems in children, including aggression, noncompliance, and negative verbalizations, and an increase in positive peer interactions. When used for the treatment of narcolepsy, methylphenidate causes an increase in maintenance of wakefulness and sleep latency.

The etiology for these specific behaviors is not clear; thus, methylphenidate's known neurochemical actions are invoked as reflections of the pathophysiology. As mentioned above, methylphenidate and related compounds appear to bind to sites on the presynaptic dopamine, norepinephrine, and serotonin transport complexes and to block the reuptake of the respective neurotransmitter. The relative potency of ritalinic acid ester analogues at blocking the specific binding of [^{3}H]-threo-(±)-methylphenidate to brain membrane preparations correlates with their motor stimulant properties, and radioligand binding correlates with the degree of intact dopaminergic innervation. Thus, the disposition of dopamine, and perhaps norepinephrine, may be involved in the etiology of the disorders, and the blockage of the dopamine and (or) norepinephrine uptake complex may be the neurochemical mechanism of action for methylphenidate. This contrasts with a neurochemical effect of amphetamine, which blocks neurotransmitter transport, and is also a substrate for the transporter.

Undesirable Effects at Therapeutic Doses and Interactions with Other Drugs

Amphetamine at therapeutic doses can acutely increase systolic and diastolic pressure and produce a reflex slowing of the heart rate. This cardiovascular effect could be detrimental in patients with significant cardiac disease, arrhythmias, and hypertension. Amphetamine also can produce hyperthermia, EEG desynchronization, insomnia, psychomotor agitation, dysphoria, and confusion. Of most concern is its potential to cause tolerance and physical dependence when amphetamine is given chronically at higher doses. Abrupt withdrawal from amphetamine after chronic administration can cause an anhedonic state or depression with excessive fatigue (as compared to agitated depression).

When amphetamine is administered to children, anorexia and insomnia can occur. Although children may also experience a slowing of stature growth, there has been no documented permanent impairment of growth. It is interesting that the therapeutic effect of amphetamine in ADDH patients has a rapid onset, and children with this condition treated with amphetamine do not appear to develop tolerance. Children with ADDH can experience a dysphoric mood on amphetamine, but do not seem to develop physical dependence. The addition of amphetamine or other psychostimulants to a monoamine oxidase inhibitor antidepressant regimen should be avoided, as it could cause a hypertensive crisis and death.

Methylphenidate causes euphoria, and its therapeutic use has been limited because of its abuse potential (e.g., the development of tolerance and dependence). In addition, ritalinc acid esters are anorectic agents and have cardiovascular effects that are dose-dependent. These latter effects, however, are minimal in comparison to the effects of amphetamine and related compounds. One of the most notable undesirable effects of methylphenidate administration in children with ADDH is a slowing in growth rate. Retrospective studies indicate that this slowing is reversible; the height of adults who had been treated with methylphenidate as children does not differ from normal values. The stimulant effects of methylphenidate preclude its use in patients with anxiety or insomnia.

Most of the undesirable effects of methylphenidate may involve the drug-induced increase in the synaptic availability of neurotransmitter that results from the inhibition of catechol- and (or) indole-amine uptake. Toxic effects of overdose are similar to those described for amphetamine.

Toxic Effects of Overdoses

When 60 mg or more of amphetamine is consumed as a single dose or within a few hours in nontolerant individuals, an acute intoxication syndrome occurs. Symptoms include agitation, mood lability, confusion, headache, periods of sweating and chills, and vomiting. Blood pressure can be increased and cardiac arrhythmias can occur when a high amphetamine dose has been ingested. Severe intoxication results in hyperpyrexia, seizures, and hallucinations, especially visual and tactile. These toxic effects of amphetamine are mediated by its indirect sympathomimetic actions, which alter brain excitability, thermoregulation, and sympathetic function as discussed earlier.

Chronic psychostimulant abusers who have developed tolerance can ingest orally or inject IV 1000 mg or more per day of dextroamphetamine or methamphetamine during a binge without developing these toxic symptoms. Preclinical studies in laboratory animals have demonstrated neuronal damage during chronic administration of psychostimulants. Serotonergic neurons in the CNS seem to be the most vulnerable to stimulant-induced neurotoxicity. Ring-substituted amphetamines such as 3,4-methylenedioxyamphetamine (MDA) and 3,4-methylenedioxymethamphetamine (MDMA, "ecstasy") are the most potent neurotoxins in these animal models. It is uncertain whether chronic amphetamine abuse is neurotoxic in humans. Since the neurotoxic doses in animal studies ranges from 10 to 100 mg/kg, the higher doses may not be reached in amphetamine-abusing human addicts (see Chapter 21).

One other important toxic effect of amphetamines is psychosis. Although patients who have a past history of psychosis or a genetic or other predispositon are most vulnerable, normal volunteers with no previous psychiatric history have developed a paranoid delusional psychosis when given large doses of amphetamine. Amphetamine psychosis generally occur when doses of 100 mg or more daily are taken for a prolonged period (weeks to months).

Pharmacokinetics

The therapeutic route of administration is oral. Amphetamine addicts often resort to IV injection. Oral administration (0.45 mg/kg) results in rapid absorption with peak plasma concentrations (60 to 70 ng/ml) being reached with three to four hours.[r21] The elimination half-life is approximately seven to 12 hours.[5] Circulating levels of plasma amphetamine in the range of 10 to 20 ng/ml may be therapeutic. The metabolism of amphetamine involves its oxidation and hepatic conjugation. Amphetamine is converted to p-hydroxyamphetamine via an aromatic hydroxylation reaction. This is followed by a deamination, producing benzoic acid and its conjugates. The primary route of elimination is renal excretion.

The two available forms of methylphenidate, though readily absorbed, have slightly different pharmacokinetic properties. The SR (sustained release) tablet is absorbed more slowly, and the time to peak plasma rate in children varies from about five hours for the SR form to about two hours for the other tablets. The plasma half-life is one to two hours. The drug is metabolized by deesterification and the resulting ritalinic acid is excreted in the urine.

Pemoline

Pemoline has a unique chemical structure (Fig. 22.2) that includes a heterocyclic ring system incorporating a substituted side-chain of amphetamine.

Therapeutic Uses of Pemoline

This drug is used for the treatment of ADDH, and appears to be at least as effective as other medications for treating this disorder.[9] Pemoline also is useful for the treatment of narcolepsy, with dose ranges similar to those used for ADDH.

Mechanism of Therapeutic Action of Pemoline

Early studies involving non-human primates suggest that pemoline is not self-administered and will not substitute for cocaine, methylphenidate, or amphetamine when access to those drugs is removed from animals that self-administer cocaine. Thus, the potential for abuse of pemoline may be lower than that of other stimulants.

The clinical effects of pemoline resemble those of methylphenidate, and the sympathomimetic effects are minimal. In animal studies, pemoline appears to share some pharmacologic effects with methylphenidate; when administered at reasonable doses, it does not deplete monoamines, compared with the more neurotoxic effects of amphetamine and methamphetamine.[10] At higher doses there is a perturbation of some biogenic amine and metabolite levels. Thus, the neurochemical mechanisms underlying the effects of pemoline are not at all clear.

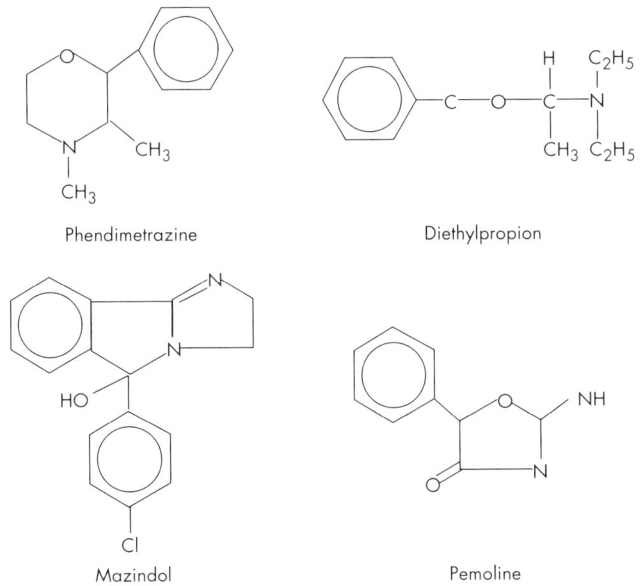

Figure 22.2

Pharmacokinetics

Time of onset for the therapeutic effects of pemoline are rapid (2 hours) and may require three to four weeks to reach a maximal effect. However, liver damage associated with use of pemoline prevents its use as a drug of first-choice (see below).

Oral preparations of pemoline are rapidly absorbed, with peak serum concentrations occurring at two to three hours. The half-life reportedly varies from about seven to 12 hours, and steady-state levels are reached in about three days. The drug is metabolized in the liver, and liver dysfunction has been reported in some children.[11] Thus, liver function (aminotransferase) values should be determined before treatment and periodically afterward. Pemoline should not be administered to patients with impaired liver function. Administration of pemoline for up to three weeks does not appear to alter its pharmacodynamics.[12]

Available Preparations and Usual Doses (Table 22.2)

Pemoline (Cylert) is available in 18.75-, 37.5-, and 75-mg tablets, and as a 37.5-mg chewable tablet. The optimal dose in ADDH appears to be 37 to 75 mg per day, with side effects (insomnia) dissipating over the first three days of treatment.[13] In all cases, initiation of treatment should begin with a minimal dose, and the patient should be titrated to the desired (behavioral) effect.

Mazindol

Recent preclinical studies of mazindol (Sanorex) have resulted in the re-examination and potential increase in clinical use of this relatively weak psychostimulant, which shares a number of neurochemical effects with amphetamine and related compounds. It is a substituted imidazoisoindole and is structurally dissimilar to other stimulants (Fig. 22.2).

Table 22.1 Available Preparations of Amphetamine Derivatives and Usual Doses

Generic Name	Trade Name	Dosage Forms* mg	Daily Doses mg/day
Amphetamine	Obetrol Dexedrine	(T) 10,20 (C) 5,10,15 (T) 5	2.4–40
Methamphetamine	Desoxyn	(T) 5,10,15	10–15
Methylphenidate	Ritalin Ritalin SR	(T) 5,10,20 (T) 20	20–30 20–30
Benzphetamine	Didrex	(T) 25,50	25–150
Fenfluramine	Pondimin	(T) 20	60–120
Diethylpropion	Tenuate Tenuate Dospan	(T) 25 (T) 75	75
Phentermine	Ionamine Adipex-P	(C) 15,30 (T,C) 37.5	15–30
Phendimetrazine	Prelu-2 Bontril Slow Release Plegine Bontril PDM	(C) 105 (T) 35	105 70–105

*(T) Tablet; (C) Capsule

Table 22.2 Available Preparations of Other Stimulants and Usual Doses

Generic Name	Trade Name	Dosage Forms* mg	Daily Doses mg/day
Pemoline	Cylert	(T) 18.75,37.5,75 (T) 37.5	56–75
Mazindol	Sanorex	(T) 1,2	1–3

*(T) Tablet; (C) Capsule

Therapeutic Uses of Mazindol

Mazindol has been used to treat a number of neuropsychiatric and/or medical disorders, including obesity[14] and narcolepsy.[15] Some studies have indicated that mazindol may be more efficacious than other drugs in producing weight loss, and tolerance to the anorectic effect is minimal compared with tolerance observed with other medications.[16] Craving associated with cocaine dependence is also attenuated by mazindol, and the maximal effect requires up to seven days of treatment.[17] Preclinical studies involving monkeys tend to support these findings.[18] Based on reports that mazindol decreases growth hormone release and so may be beneficial for retarding the development of Duchenne dystrophy, a series of clinical trials were executed. The results of those studies were equivocal at best, and most suggested that the drug was of limited usefulness and, in many cases, resulted in effects that were not well tolerated by the patients.[19]

Mechanism of Therapeutic Action

Studies to uncover the mechanisms and effects involved in mazindol's anorexogenic activity indicate that mazindol inhibits gastric emptying,[20] and gastric acid secretion.[14] Radiolabeled mazindol binds to a site in the lateral hypothalamus, and displacement of the radioligand by drugs in vivo correlates well with their potencies as anorectic agents and with their potencies at inhibiting uptake of serotonin via the presynaptic serotonin transporter.[21] Thus, it appears that mazindol binds to an "anorexogenic" site that may involve regulation of serotonin concentrations in the synapse.

Like other stimulants and abused substances, such as cocaine (see Chapter 21), mazindol blocks the reuptake of dopamine by the presynaptic dopamine transporter.[22] However, the drug appears to have unique effects on transporter-mediated release of dopamine via the human transporter expressed in mammalian cell lines.[23] Thus, while abused substances including cocaine or amphetamine and amphetamine analogues either have no effect on dopamine release or stimulate release (respectively), mazindol actually inhibits basal dopamine release through the human dopamine transporter. This effect of mazindol, i.e., blocking both uptake and release of dopamine, could be involved in its effects at attenuating the craving associated with cocaine abuse.

Perhaps of greatest importance are the reports that indicate that many stimulants including mazindol are self-administered by animals, but that mazindol may be relatively unique because of its low potential for abuse by humans.[4]

Undesirable Effects of Mazindol

The effects of mazindol are similar to those of other stimulants, and include tolerance to the stimulant effect of the drug.

Methylxanthines

The methylated xanthines, caffeine, theophylline, and theobromine, are the most widely used psychoactive substances in the world. Descriptions of their extraction from vegetable matter and of their use were described centuries ago, and they are included in a number of beverages, including coffee, tea, cocoa products, chocolate, prescription, and over-the-counter medications. All three methylxanthines are CNS stimulants that elevate mood and increase alertness. These agents have neurochemical mechanisms of action and therapeutic uses that clearly differ from those of amphetamine and related compounds. Since theophylline is available by prescription, much of the discussion of methylxanthines, below, concerns this drug.

History

It is likely that ancient humans discovered the effects of tea, and extracted appropriate plants for their "medicinal" value.[r22,r23] One of the first descriptions of the benefits of tea, which contains caffeine as the predominant methylxanthine and also contains theophylline and theobromine, dates back to the year 2737 B.C., when the Emperor Shen Nung of China is reported to have accidentally discovered the benefits and potential medicinal value of tea (from *Camellia Sinensis*). Descriptions from China around 350 A.D. describe the cultivation of plants and the use of tea in commerce. Tea as a recreational beverage was described 50 to 100 years later. The introduction of tea to western culture occurred in 1610, when Dutch traders brought it to Europe from China and Japan. In 1657 it was introduced in England and eventually became the national beverage.

Coffee arabica plants are indigenous to Ethiopia, and were introduced into Yemen on the Arabian peninsula in the fifteenth century. Europeans delivered *Coffee arabica* to their South American colonies late in the seventeenth century, and cultivation of plants in Brazil began early in the eighteenth century.

Cocoa and chocolate, which contain predominantly theobromine and a small amount of caffeine, are derived from the cocao tree of the western hemisphere. Columbus introduced cocao beans into Europe in 1502, but it took almost 200 years before drinking cocoa became commonplace in England.

Caffeine was first isolated from green coffee beans in Germany in 1820, and subsequently was isolated from mat and kola nuts. The complete synthesis of caffeine was reported by Fischer and Ach in 1895. Theobromine was first isolated from cocoa beans in 1842, and was methylated to form caffeine in 1861, thus proving that caffeine was a trimethylxanthine and that theobromine was a dimethylxanthine. In 1888 theophylline was isolated from tea leaves and identified as a dimethylxanthine.

Chemistry

Caffeine, theophylline, and theobromine are methylated analogues of xanthine. All are derived from a core purine ring structure (Fig. 22.3). Purine is also the parent compound for nucleic acids, including adenosine, and this fact is important for understanding the pharmacologic mechanisms of methylxanthine actions (see below). Caffeine is a trimethylxanthine, and theophylline and theobromine are dimethylxanthine derivatives. Structure-activity studies related to the behavioral effects of these drugs suggest that theobromine is an extremely weak CNS stimulant, while theophylline is probably the most potent methylxanthine stimulant.

Mechanisms of Drug Action

The pharmacologic mechanisms of action for the methylxanthines are not well understood. Evidence

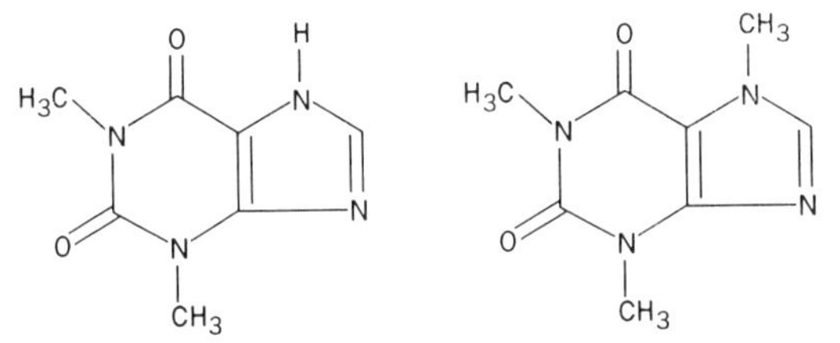

Theophylline

Caffeine

Figure 22.3

gathered over many decades suggested that the methylxanthines inhibit phosphodiesterase, the enzyme that metabolizes cyclic adenosine monophosphate (cAMP), causing an accumulation of cyclic nucleotide. Concentrations required for this biochemical effect, however, are much higher than the therapeutic circulating plasma concentrations of caffeine or theophylline.

More recent evidence suggests that the therapeutic effect of the methylxanthines involves blockade of adenosine receptors, some of which have been characterized at the molecular and physiologic levels. Structure-activity relationships for methylxanthines at some of these receptors have been described.

Therapeutic Uses and Limitations

Caffeine and theophylline, especially aminophylline (theophylline ethylene diamine, the soluble salt), but not theobromine, are currently included in a number of prescription and nonprescription medications, including aspirin and nonaspirin analgesics. The main prescription use for theophylline, however, is as a smooth muscle relaxant for the treatment of bronchial asthma and for tension or muscle contraction headaches. In addition, theophylline and caffeine are under active investigation for use in the treatment of apnea in preterm infants, and for prevention of sudden infant death (sleep apnea) in full-term infants.[24]

Undesirable Effects at Therapeutic Doses and Interactions with Other Drugs

Even though methylxanthines are widely used, they have a number of side-effects at therapeutic doses. Theophylline alone and in combination with other agents will cause irritation of the stomach and nausea resulting in vomiting. Thus, medications containing theophylline should be taken after meals if possible. Some coated capsules that bypass the stomach are available. As with other drugs that have cardiovascular effects, palpitation, headaches, and dizziness may occur at therapeutic doses. In addition, theopylline at therapeutic doses can cause insomnia, diarrhea, and palpitation.

Pharmacokinetics

The half-life of theophylline is affected by coadministration of many agents, or by pre-existing pathology. Thus, impaired liver function, or impaired cardiac function will increase elimination time. Cigarette smoking, on the other hand, will increase elimination time.[25] Drugs that increase theophylline levels include but are not limited to cimetidine, erythromycin, lithium carbonate, and oral contraceptives. Phenytoin and rifampin, however, decrease theophylline serum levels.

Toxic Effects of Overdose

Theophylline toxicity occurs at serum levels over 20 μg/ml. The CNS-stimulating effects of the methylxanthines, as well as interindividual variations in response to a particular dose are the primary concerns that limit their use. Restlessness, insomnia, tachycardia, ventricular arrhythmias, vomiting, seizures, delirium, and death can result from overdose. Activated charcoal is effective in cases of oral medication overdose. Treatment of seizures with diazepam—or general anesthesia in severe cases—may be required.

Available Preparations and Usual Doses

Theophylline is available by prescription in tablet, capsule, and liquid form. There are currently over a dozen preparations that contain theophylline as one of many major components, and nearly as many preparations that contain theophylline as the sole pharmacotherapy.

Acknowledgements

The work described in this review article was done as part of our employment with the federal government and is therefore in the public domain. All descriptions of the clinical and pharmacologic effects of drugs and of drug pharmacokinetics have been previously published in research articles or review articles. The authors gratefully acknowledge the helpful suggestions of Drs. Kim A. Neve and S. Paul Berger and the assistance of Anna Evenson in the preparation of this manuscript.

References

Research Reports

1. Glowinski J, Axelrod J. Effect of drugs on the uptake, release, and metabolism of ^{3}H-norepinephrine in brain. J Pharmacol Exp Ther 1965;*149*:43–49.
2. McMillen BA, German DC, Shore PA. Functional and pharmacological significance of brain dopamine and norepinephrine storage pools. Neuropharmacology 1980;*29*:3045–3050.
3. Cox RH Jr, Maickel RP. Comparison of anorexogenic and behavioral potency of phenylethylamines. J Pharmacol Exp Ther 1972;*181*:1–9.
4. Chait LD, Uhlenhuth EH, Johanson CE. Reinforcing and subjective effects of several anorectics in normal human volunteers. J Pharmacol Exp Ther 1987;*242*:777–783.

5. Angrist B, Corwin J, Bartlik B, Cooper T. Early phamacokinetics and clinical effects of oral d-amphetamine in normal subjects. Biol Psych 1987;*22*:1357–1368.

6. Segal DS, Weinberger SB, Cahill J, McCunney SJ. Multiple daily amphetamine administration: Behavioral and neurochemical alterations. Science 1980;*207*:904–907.

7. Koob GF, Bloom FE. Cellular and molecular mechanisms of drug dependence. Science 1988;*242*:715–723.

8. Monroe RR, Drell HZ. Oral use of stimulants obtained from inhalors. JAMA 1947;*135*:909–915.

9. Pelham WE Jr, Greenslade KE, Vodde-Hamilton M, Murphy DA, Greenstein JJ, Gnagy EM, Guthrie KJ, Hoover, MD, Dahl, RE. Relative efficacy of long-acting stimulants on children with attention deficit-hyperactivity disorder: A comparison of standard methylphenidate, sustained release methylphenidate, sustained release dextroamphetamine, and pemoline. Pediatrics 1990;*86*:226–237.

10. Zaczek R, Battaglia G, Contrera JF, Culp S, De Souza EB. Methylphenidate and pemoline do not cause depletion of rat brain monoamine markers similar to that observed with methamphetamine. Toxical Appl Pharmacol 1989;*100*:227–233.

11. Pratt DS, Dubois RS. Hepatotoxicity due to pemoline (Cylert): A report of two cases. J. Pediatr Gastroenterol Nutr 1990;*10*:239–241.

12. Sallee FR, Stiller RL, Perel JM. Pharmacodynamics of pemoline in attention deficit disorder with hyperactivity. J Am Acad Child Adolesc Psychiatry 1992;*31*:244–251.

13. Swanson JM, Lerner M, Cantwell D. Blood levels and tolerance to stimulants in ADDH children. Clin Neuropharmacol 1986;*9*:(suppl.4)523–525.

14. Inoue S, Egawa M, Satoh S, Saito M, Suzuki H, Kumahara Y, Abe M, Kumagai A, Goto Y, Shizume K. Clinical and basic aspects of an anorexiant, mazindol, as an antiobesity agent in Japan. Am J Clin Nutr 1992;*55* (Supp 1):199S–202S.

15. Alvarez B, Dahlitz M, Grimshaw J, Parkes, JD. Mazindol in long-term treatment of narcolepsy. Lancet 1991;*337*:1293–1294.

16. Murphy, JE, Donald JF, Molla AL, Crowder D. A comparison of mazindol (Teronac) with diethylpropion in the treatment of exogenous obesity. J Int Med Res 1975;*3*:202–206.

17. Berger P, Gawin F, Kosten TR. Treatment of cocaine abuse with mazindol. Lancet 1989;*1*:283.

18. Kleven MS, Woolverton WL. Effects of three monoamine uptake inhibitors on behavior maintained by cocaine or food presentation in rhesus monkeys. Drug Alcohol Depend 1993;*31*:149–158.

19. Griggs RC, Moxley RT, Mendell R, Fenichel GM, Brooke MH, Miller PJ, Mandel S, Florence J, Schierbecker J, Kaiser, KK. Randomized, double-blind trial of mazindol in Duchenne dystrophy. Muscle Nerve 1990;*13*:1169–1173.

20. Jonderko K, Kucio C. Extra-anorectic actions of mazindol. Isr J Med Sci 1989;*25*:20–24.

21. Angel I, Taranger MA, Claustre Y, Scatton B, Langer SZ. Anorectic activities of serotonin uptake inhibitors: correlation with their potencies at inhibiting serotonin uptake *in vivo* and ^{3}H-mazindol binding *in vitro*. Life Sci. 1988;*43*:651–658.

22. Javitch AJ, Blaustein RO, Snyder SH. [^{3}H]-Mazindol binding associated with neuronal dopamine and norepinephrine uptake sites. Mol Pharmacol 1984;*26*:35–44.

23. Eshleman AJ, Henningsen RA, Neve KA, Janowsky A. Dopamine transport *via* the human transporter. Mol Pharmacol 1994;*45*:312–316.

24. Peliowski A, Finer NN. A blinded, randomized, placebo-controlled trial to compare theophylline and doxapram for the treatment of apnea of prematurity. J. Pediatr 1990;*116*:648–653.

25. Crowley, JJ, Cusak, BJ, Jue SG, Koup JR, Park BK, Vestal RE. Aging and drug interactions. II. Effect of phenytoin and smoking on the oxidation of theophylline and cortisol in healthy men. J. Pharmacol Exp Ther 1988;*245*:513–523.

Reviews, Monographs and Textbooks

r1. Axelrod, J. Amphetamine: Metabolism, physiological disposition, and its effects on catecholamine storage. In: Costa E, Garrattini S. Amphetamines and Related Compounds. New York: Raven Press, (1979), pp 207–216.

r2. Biel JH, Bopp BA. Amphetamines: Structure-activity relationships. In: Iversen LL, Snyder SH. Handbook of Psychopharmacology, Vol. 11. New York: Plenum Press (1979), pp 1–39.

r3. Bizzi A, Bonaccoorsi A, Jespersen S, Jori A, Garattini S. Pharmacological studies on amphetamine and fenfluramine. In: Costa E, Garattini S. Amphetamines and Related Compounds. New York: Raven Press, (1970), pp 577–595.

r4. Carlson A. (1970): Amphetamine and brain catecholamines. In: Costa E, Garratini S. Amphetamines and Related Compounds, New York: Raven Press, (1970), pp 289–300.

r5. Kuczenski R. Biochemical actions of amphetamines and other stimulants. In: Creese I. Stimulants: Neurochemical, Behavioral, and Clinical Perspectives. New York: Raven Press, (1983); pp 31–61.

r6. Moore KE. Amphetamines: Biochemical and behavioral actions in animals. In: Iversen LL, Snyder SH. Handbook of Psychopharmacology, Vol. 11. New York: Plenum Press (1979), pp 41–98.

r7. Robbins TW, Sahakian BJ. Behavioral effects of psychomotor stimulant drugs: clinical and neuropsychological implications. In: Creese I. Stimulants: Neurochemical, Behavioral, and Clinical Perspectives. New York: Raven Press, (1983), pp 301–338.

r8. Hauger RI, Angel I, Janowsky A, Berger P, Hulihan-Giblin B. Brain recognition sites for methylphenidate and the amphetamines: Their relationship to the dopamine transport complex, glucoreceptors, and serotonergic neurotransmission in the central nervous system. In: Deutsch SI, Weizman A. Application of Basic Neuroscience to Child Psychiatry, New York: Plenum (1990), pp 77–100.

r9. Robinson TE, Becker JB. Enduring changes in brain and behavior produced by chronic amphetamine administration: A review and evaluation of animal models of amphetamine psychosis. Brain Res Rev 1986;*11*:157–198.

r10. Schuckit MA. Drug and Alcohol Abuse. New York: Plenum (1989).

r11. Silverston T. Appetite suppressants. Drugs 1992;*43*:820–836.

r12. Segal DS, Schuckit MA. Animal models of stimulant induced psychosis. In: Creese, I. Stimulants: Neurochemical, Behavioral, and Clinical Perspectives. New York: Raven Press, (1983); pp 131–167.

r13. Chiarello RJ, Cole JO. The use of psychostimulants in general psychiatry. Arch Gen Psychiat 1987;*44*:286–295.

r14. Warneke L. Psychostimulants in Psychiatry. Can J Psychiatry 1990;*35*:3–10.

r15. Swanson JM, Cantwell D, Lerner M, McBurnett K, Hanna G. Effects of stimulant medication on learning in children with ADHD. J Learning Disabilities *24*:219–230.

r16. Angrist B, Sudilovsky A. Central nervous system stimulants: Historical aspects and clinical effects. In: Iversen L, Iversen SD, Snyder SH. Handbook of Psychopharmacology, Vol. 11. New York: Plenum Press (1978), pp 99–153.

r17. Caldwell J. Amphetamine and related stimulants: Some introductory remarks: In: Caldwell, J. Amphetamines and Related Stimulants: Chemical, Biological, Clinical, and Sociological Aspects. Boca Raton FL, CRC Press (1980); pp 2–11.

r18. Weiner N. Norepinephrine, epinephrine, and the sympathomimetic amines. In: Gilman AG, Goodman LS, Gilman A. The Pharmacological Basis of Therapeutics, 6th ed. New York: Macmillan (1980); pp 138–175.

r19. Goodwin FK, Jamison KR. Alcohol and drug abuse in manic depressive illness. In: Goodwin FK, Jamison KR. Manic-Depressive Illness, New York: Oxford University Press (1990); pp 210–226.

r20. Baldessarini RJ. Chemotherapy in Psychiatry. Cambridge: Harvard University Press (1985).

r21. Vree TB, Henderson PT. Pharmacokinetics of amphetamines: In vivo and in vitro studies of factors governing their elimination. In: Caldwell J Amphetamines and Related Stimulants: Chemical, Biological Clinical, and Sociological Aspects. Boca Raton, FL, CRC Press (1980); pp 49–68.

r22. Barone JJ, Roberts H. Human consumption of caffeine. In: Dews, PB. Caffeine. New York: Springer-Verlag (1984); pp 59–73.

r23. Spiller GA. Overview of the methylxanthine beverages and food and their effect on health. Progress in Clinical and Biological Research 158: 1984; 1–7.

SECTION IV

Cardiovascular and Pulmonary Pharmacology

Editor:
Théophile Godfraind

Associate Editors:
C. Advenier
A. Kaba Sengele

CHAPTER 23

Agents Used in the Management of Heart Failure

Théophile Godfraind

This chapter deals with several classes of drugs used to treat cardiac failure. As discussed below, cardiac failure is an evolving process. Heart failure has been classified into four degrees by the New York Heart Association, with worldwide acceptance. The choice of drugs depends on the severity of the disease; ambulatory patients should not receive the same treatment as patients with acute cardiac failure in intensive care units. As heart failure involves both the heart and the peripheral vessels, treatment of the disease is selective. Agents most commonly used for outpatients belong to differing pharmacologic groups: beta-adrenoceptor agonists; inhibitors of phosphodiesterase; angiotensin-converting enzyme (ACE) inhibitors; diuretics; and cardiac glycosides. In addition, potent vasodilators are used in intensive care units to decrease afterload; they will not be examined in this chapter. Diuretics (discussed in another chapter) are effective in eliminating edema, one of the symptoms of heart failure. Although attempts have been made to improve the prognosis of ischemia-evoked cardiac failure with second-generation calcium antagonists, this interesting approach is still experimental.[r20,r28,r32] There also have been trials with β-blockers, a practice not recommended for outpatients.[r3,r13]

As an introduction to this section, the pathophysiology of heart failure will be examined in order to rationalize the choice of the various agents.

Pathophysiologic Aspects of Heart Failure

Heart failure is a complex pathophysiologic situation that can be caused by various diseases and also by drug intoxications.[r14,r15] Heart failure involves several compensatory mechanisms, and this led to the introduction of successive models describing its pathophysiology. Those models consider the disease from a cardiorenal point of view, from a cardiocirculatory point of view, and from a neurohormonal point of view. In its final stage, cardiac failure is characterized by all three disorders—cardiorenal, cardiocirculatory, and neurohormonal.[r9,r11,r16,r25,r29]

In heart failure, cardiac output and O_2 delivery are inadequate to sustain the aerobic metabolism of working tissues. As a reflex response to systemic blood flow reduction, the sympathetic nervous and renin-angiotensin-aldosterone systems are activated. These two pressor systems promote an arteriolar vasoconstriction that preserves central aortic pressure and thereby ensures the perfusion of the heart and brain. This acute neuroendocrine response evokes an increase in peripheral resistance that serves to redistribute blood flow away from less vital organs (for example, renal, splanchnic and cutaneous). These tissues receive less than their usual fraction of cardiac output in order to ensure perfusion to the heart and brain; however, as a compensatory mechanism, they

Table 23.1 Agents Increasing Cardiac Output

Receptors Involved in Direct Action	Main Responses	
α	inotropic effect, vasoconstriction	
β_1	inotropic effect, tachycardia	
β_2	vasodilatation, some inotropic effect	
D_1	vasodilatation, natriuresis	
D_2	bradycardia vasodilatation (presynaptic inhibition of norepinephrine release)	
Digitalis	bradycardia, inotropic effect (peripheral resistance?)	
PDE III	PDE III is a phosphodiesterase subtype which shows high affinity for cAMP and is not stimulated by calmodulin, whereas PDE I and PDE II have no cAMP/cGMP specificity	
AGENTS		
β adrenoceptor agonists		
Isoprenaline	$\beta_1 > \beta_2$	(tachycardia)
Pirbuterol	$\beta_2 > \beta_1$	
Salbutamol	$\beta_2 > \beta_1$	
Dobutamine	$\beta_1 > \beta_2 > \alpha$	
β_1 adrenoceptor partial agonists		
Xamoterol	β_1 stabilization	
Dopaminergic agonists		
Lèvodopa	$D_1 + D_2 + \beta_1 + \beta_2$	(CNS)
Dopexamine	$D_1 + \beta_2$	
Ibopamine	$D_1 + D_2$, $\beta_2 > \beta_1$	
PDE III selective inhibitors:	+ inotropic effect, vasodilators	
Amrinome		
Milrinome		
Epoxinome		
Piroxinome		
PDE III inhibitors + contractile proteins sensitizers		
Sulmazole		
Isomazole		
Digitalis receptors and Na Channels		
Cardiac glycosides		
Experimental compounds:		
OPC-8212, DPI-201.106		
Anthopleurin - A		

extract more O_2 to satisfy their aerobic requirements.

Increased resting levels of plasma norepinephrine (NE) have been reported in patients with severe cardiac failure. During exercise, increased release of NE has been observed. It is essential to accentuate the reflex vasoconstriction, mainly if hypotension has to be prevented when there is vasodilation in working skeletal muscle.

Angiotensin II, through its action on vascular smooth muscle, kidney, and adrenal, promotes vasoconstriction and enhances aldosterone secretion and the reabsorption of salt and water by the kidney. In very severe heart failure, intense functional tubular reabsorption of sodium and water inhibits the kidney's ability to excrete free water. The resultant hyponatremia is often accompanied by peripheral edema and ascites. This hypo-osmolality may be accentuated by the increased secretion of antidiuretic hormone. Finally, decline of hepatic perfusion leads to a reduced metabolic degradation of various endogenous circulating factors such as aldosterone.

An increase in cardiac filling pressure is a major determinant of the release of atrial natriuretic peptides (ANP) from the heart, a release that may be enhanced by activation of the sympathetic nervous system. The venous blood content of ANP is related to the dilatation of the atria. These peptides exert potent direct vasodilator action by virtue of their ability to increase intracellular cyclic GMP. ANP may be considered as functional antagonists of angiotensin II.

Humoral changes occurring during heart failure are not completely understood; indeed, humoral factors other than those discussed here also change in heart failure.

In addition, to these humoral-mediated reflexes,

there are compensatory mechanisms occurring in the heart as well as tissue alterations promoted by the underlying disease.[r32] A disease process involving the coronary arteries, such as atherosclerosis or hypertension, ultimately will affect cardiac contractility. Moderate chamber dilatation may sustain cardiac pump function by utilizing the length-dependent property of muscle (Frank-Starling mechanism), but this beneficial effect is lost when chamber dimensions are excessively increased and oxygen consumption exceeds supply. Another cardiac compensatory mechanism is cardiac muscle hypertrophy, as reflected by increased thickness of the myocardium. This may improve pump function, but this process is also limited by the extent to which coronary blood supply may be adequate. An increase in the collagen fibers in hypertrophied hearts has also been reported in systemic hypertension, and may entrap muscle and reduce the efficiency of the contractile response.[10,11] An increase in the diastolic wall stress in ventricles leads to the induction of specific proto-oncogenes of Class 3 (c-fos and c-myc) that trigger synthesis of myofibrillar proteins. In addition, there is evidence that proto-oncogenes of Classes 1 and 2 are induced, which may play a role in cardiac and vascular growth.[r10,11] The major growth factors so far identified, angiotensin II, platelet-derived growth factor, and endothelin, also are potent vasoconstrictors. Furthermore, endothelin at subthreshold concentrations enhances a vasoconstriction evoked by catecholamines that is sensitive to blockade by calcium antagonists.[6] In addition, proto-oncogenes of Class 2 encode growth factor receptors and thereby increase the reactivity of the cardiovascular system to several neurohormones. Metabolic factors promoted by anoxia and by ischemia also may greatly affect the ability of the muscle to contract and to respond to drugs.

Such metabolic alterations may be caused by cardiovascular diseases, as well as by therapeutic drugs with cardiac toxicity profiles, e.g., inhalational anesthetics, ethanol, antidepressants, antineoplastic drugs, anthracycline antibiotics, cyclophosphamide, 5-fluorouracil, or overaggressive use of drugs used to treat heart failure, e.g., antihypertensive vasodilators and sympathomimetics. Cardiac cellular injury is characterized by alterations in electrical properties, alterations in contractility, and cell death. The first two factors are easy to demonstrate and may be reversible. They are also some of the signs of drug-induced cardiotoxicity. There are three main mechanisms of cardionecrosis: ischemia (reduction of blood flow), anoxia (reduction of oxygen supply), and direct toxic actions on the heart. The rate at which cardionecrosis occurs and its extension are influenced by a number of factors, including the duration and degree of vascular alteration, the dosage of a drug directly responsible for the severity of ischemia or hypoxia, the age and sex, the hormonal, nutritional, and metabolic status of the tissue, and the coexistence of other disease processes. A striking and important characteristic of ischemia and, to a lesser extent of hypoxia, is its macroscopic and microscopic heterogeneity. Varying conditions of work load and tissue perfusion may create a transient or patchy ischemia. In the latter instance, islands of severely ischemic tissue may be interspersed with, or lie adjacent to, areas of normal tissue. This is well illustrated by the multifocal distribution of the cardionecrotic areas resulting from the injection of large doses of catecholamines in rats.

Immediately after the onset of ischemia (within a few seconds) there is a decline of contractile activity (Fig. 23.1). This decline occurs at a time when excitability remains essentially normal. During these first few seconds in anoxia tissue or in severely ischemic tissue, available oxygen dissolved in the cytoplasm will be utilized and anerobic conditions will develop within the cell. Associated with this will be a major reduction or even a complete abolition of oxidative metabolism, electron transport, and mitochondrial ATP production and only the much less efficient anerobic pathways of metabolism remain for the production of ATP. Re-

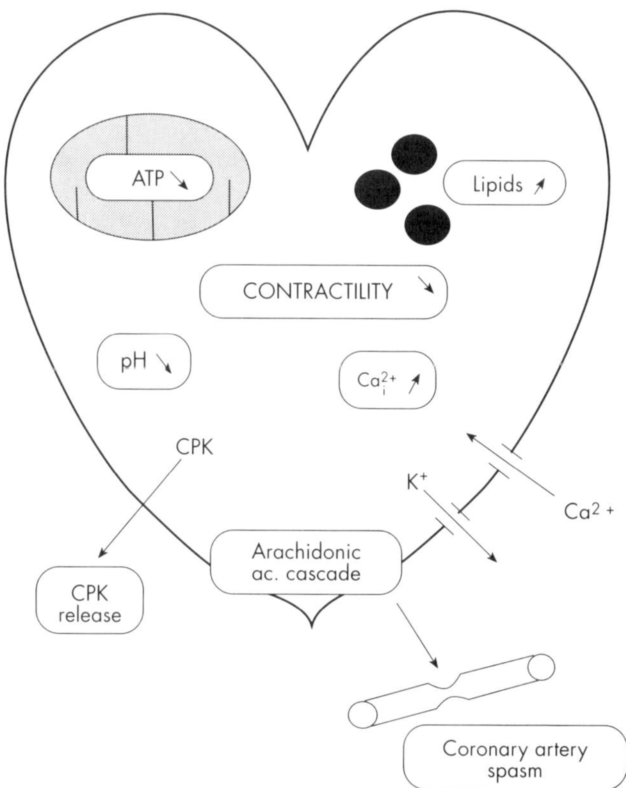

Figure 23.1 Schematic representation of the main alterations evoked by ischemia in cardiac tissue.

duced mitochondrial metabolism will result in a rapid reduction in the flux through the β-oxidation pathway for fatty acids. Despite the reduction of fatty acid utilization, uptake may not be diminished; as a result of these two factors, fatty acid acylCoA derivatives may accumulate during ischemia. This accumulation may be exacerbated by cyclic-AMP-mediated lipolysis of endogenous triglycerides, which, itself, may be triggered by the early ischemia-induced release of catecholamines. The stimulation of anerobic glycolysis (the Pasteur effect) represents an attempt to maintain, through nonoxidative mechanisms of substrate-level phosphorylation, the declining myocardial ATP content. The stimulation of glycolysis in the face of reduced mitochondrial activity leads to the accumulation of glycolytic intermediates such as reduced nicotinamide adenine dinucleotide phosphate (NADPH). In an attempt to regenerate declining and limited reserves of NAD for continued glycolytic activity, pyruvate is reduced to lactate, which accumulates and leaks from the cells.

An early feature of myocardial ischemia is the accumulation in the cytoplasm of protons and the progressive development of intracellular acidosis. In addition to their inhibitory effect on glycolytic activity and their possible role in early contractile failure, protons may contribute to the development of later stages of ischemic damage.

The progressive evolution of ischemia is associated with the loss of intracellular constituents to the extracellular space and ultimately to the circulating blood. This may be divided into three relatively distinct phases of loss: ions; metabolites; and macromolecules. The loss of potassium reflects opening K channels and deficit of the ion pumps and is associated with some electrical disturbances. The loss of the metabolites, as of adenine nucleotide precursors, has an extreme importance for the lack of restoration of cell function when the aggregation factor declines. The loss of macromolecules reflects the alteration of membrane integrity. Macromolecules such as CPK may be detected in the blood as indicators of the lesion and of its size. However, only large lesions can be recognized.

The alteration of the membrane is associated with the activation of phospholipases leading to a stimulation of the arachidonic acid cascade with the formation of potent vasoconstrictor products. Release of endothelin from endothelium has been reported to occur in anoxic conditions. This peptide is one of the most powerful vasoconstrictors. Furthermore, at very low concentrations, it potentiates the action of vasoconstrictors acting by opening of calcium channels. In cardiac failure, both heart and vessels are involved in the pathologic process.

Another factor responsible for reduction of cardiac contractility is the denovo production of NO by cardiomyocytes as a result of the induction of the inducible NO synthase following the pathologic release of various cytokines.[1]

Pharmacologic Principles in the Management of Heart Failure

The main therapeutic objective in the treatment of heart failure is the reduction of mortality. Unfortunately, this has been shown objectively only for angiotensin converting enzyme (ACE) inhibitors and nitrodilators. Thus, many drugs that effectively enhance performance acutely, such as β_1 stimulants and digitalis glycosides, unequivocally enhance patient performance and reduce symptoms, but do not significantly prolong life expectancy. The benefits are achieved by actions on the neuroendocrine response, by global hemodynamics, and by a prevention of the progression of myocardial disease.

The neuroendocrine response responsible for sodium retention may be managed with diuretics and ACE inhibitors. The improvement of hemodynamics may be achieved by drugs with actions on the contractility of the heart and (or) on the tone of the resistance vessels.

The management of the progress of the myocardial disease is still a hope with new calcium antagonists endowed with vascular selectivity, but ACE inhibitors prolong survival by reducing ventricular hypertrophy.

As far as the myocardium is concerned, we have seen above that energy starvation is a common situation in heart failure. Therefore, energy demand can be reduced by decreasing wall tension in the ventricles as a result of reduced afterload (aortic pressure or ventricular filling pressures). These goals may be achieved by arterio- and venovasodilators, respectively. The use of inotropic agents acting primarily on the myocardium is not satisfactory when used alone, because any increase in contractile or rate performance must be balanced by enhanced delivery of oxygen and substrates to the heart, which usually are already limited. Thus, if afterload is too high, an increase in cardiac contractility will increase metabolic expenditure with only a small benefit in cardiac output. Therefore, pharmacologic interventions to stimulate the heart will restore hemodynamics in a more optimal way only after the afterload has been decreased. Single agents that act both to stimulate the heart and reduce aortic pressure are also available and are termed "inodilators."

Pharmacologic Agents

Angiotensin-Converting Enzyme (ACE) Inhibitors

We have seen above that the neuroendocrine response in heart failure is characterized by activation of the renin-angiotensin system. ACE inhibitors will blunt this activation by blocking the transformation of angiotensin-1 into angiotensin-2. Several inhibitors are now available; the classic ones are captopril, lisinopril, enalapril, and enalaprilat, the deesterified product of enalapril.[r33]

There is increasing experimental evidence that the therapeutic effect of ACE inhibitors is related to inhibition of tissue ACEs, especially in blood vessels and not only to inhibition in the circulation. ACEs not only transform angiotensin-1 to angiotensin-2, but also degrade the smooth muscle relaxant peptide bradykinin. Therefore, through an effect on the metabolism of those two peptides, ACE inhibitors decrease peripheral resistance. This results in a decrease in afterload and thus an increase in cardiac output to improve tissue perfusion. In addition, since angiotensin-2 stimulates aldosterone secretion, there is a decreased activity of this hormone responsible for sodium retention and edema production.

When administered to patients with congestive heart failure (NYHA class III–IV), ACE inhibitors decrease right atrial, pulmonary arterial and pulmonary capillary wedge pressures and systemic arterial pressure, thus permitting an increase in cardiac output.

ACE inhibitors are active not only in acute treatment, but also after long-term treatment. This results in symptomatic improvement and an increase in exercise tolerance. The detailed pharmacology of these drugs is discussed in Chapter 26.

Adverse Effects

The major side-effect is hypotension, which may be increased by hyponatremia resulting from diuretic therapy and restriction of sodium intake. Another potential side-effect is the development of hyperkalemia. ACE inhibitors also cause a dose-related disturbance in taste and increase the frequency of coughing by an unknown mechanism.

β-Adrenoceptor Agonists and Inhibitors of Phosphodiesterase

The chemistry of those agents is examined in another section. Their chemical structures are illustrated in Figure 23.2.

Ahlquist classified tissue adrenoceptors as α and β on the basis of the relative potency of various chemical analogues of catecholamines. Later, it was suggested that at least two major subtypes of β-adrenoceptors, the β_1 and the β_2, can be distinguished according to a variety of pharmacologic criteria. Both β_1- and β_2-adrenoceptors stimulate the membrane-bound enzyme adenylate cyclase; this action leads to the intracellular accumulation of adenosine 3′–5′-cyclic phosphate (cAMP). The intracellular concentration of cAMP is also dependent on the activity of specific phosphodiesterases. It is known that phosphodiesterase inhibitors mimic β-adrenoceptor stimulation and evoke a potentiation of β agonists through an increase in cAMP levels.

Figure 23.3 summarizes how an increase in cAMP could allow changes in cardiac contractility through the phosphorylation of three main intracellular systems. The contraction of cardiac muscle is due to the interaction between actin and myosin following the increase of $[Ca^{2+}]_i$. The stimulatory effect of calcium is mediated by its binding to a system of regulatory proteins present with actin in the thin filament. This system is represented by the tropomyosin-troponin complex. The cardiac troponin complex is a substrate for cAMP-dependent protein kinases. Phosphorylation of cardiac troponin I has been demonstrated both in vitro and in vivo. The phosphorylation of troponin I is associated with a decrease in the calcium sensitivity of actomyosin interaction as determined by measurements of actomyosin-ATPase activity, isometric force measurement, and immediate stiffness. This desensitization favors relaxation by reducing the proportion of cardiac troponin bound to calcium at any level of $[Ca^{2+}]_i$.

Calcium uptake into the sarcoplasmic reticulum is effected by an ATP-dependent calcium pump. Hydrolysis of ATP is coupled to formation of a high-energy phosphorylated intermediate with pump protein in which calcium is bound to a high-affinity binding site. One specific sarcoplasmic reticulum (SR) site of phosphorylation by cAMP-dependent protein kinases is a 22,000 dalton protein called phospholamban, which, when phosphorylated, appears to enhance the Ca^{2+}-ATPase activity and the Ca^{2+} uptake by isolated cardiac SR. This mechanism could be responsible for an enhanced rate of diastolic relaxation.

Voltage clamp studies of Ca^{2+} current have provided the evidence that Ca^{2+} current is increased in response to catecholamines by rapidly increasing the number of Ca^{2+} channels in the membrane. It has been shown by patch clamp analysis that cAMP-dependent calcium channel phosphorylation increases the conductance of the channel responsible for calcium entry and thus increases the force of contraction.

Relaxation of smooth muscle contraction by cAMP has been postulated to involve stimulation of Ca pumps. cAMP-dependent protein kinase increases Ca accumulation into the sarcoplasmic reticulum of skinned arterial smooth muscle. Studies on subcellular fractions have yielded contradictory results, some investigators reporting that cAMP stimulated microsomal Ca uptake, while others were unable to find any stimulatory effect. In cardiac sarcoplasmic reticulum, there is an important cAMP-dependency of Ca transport.

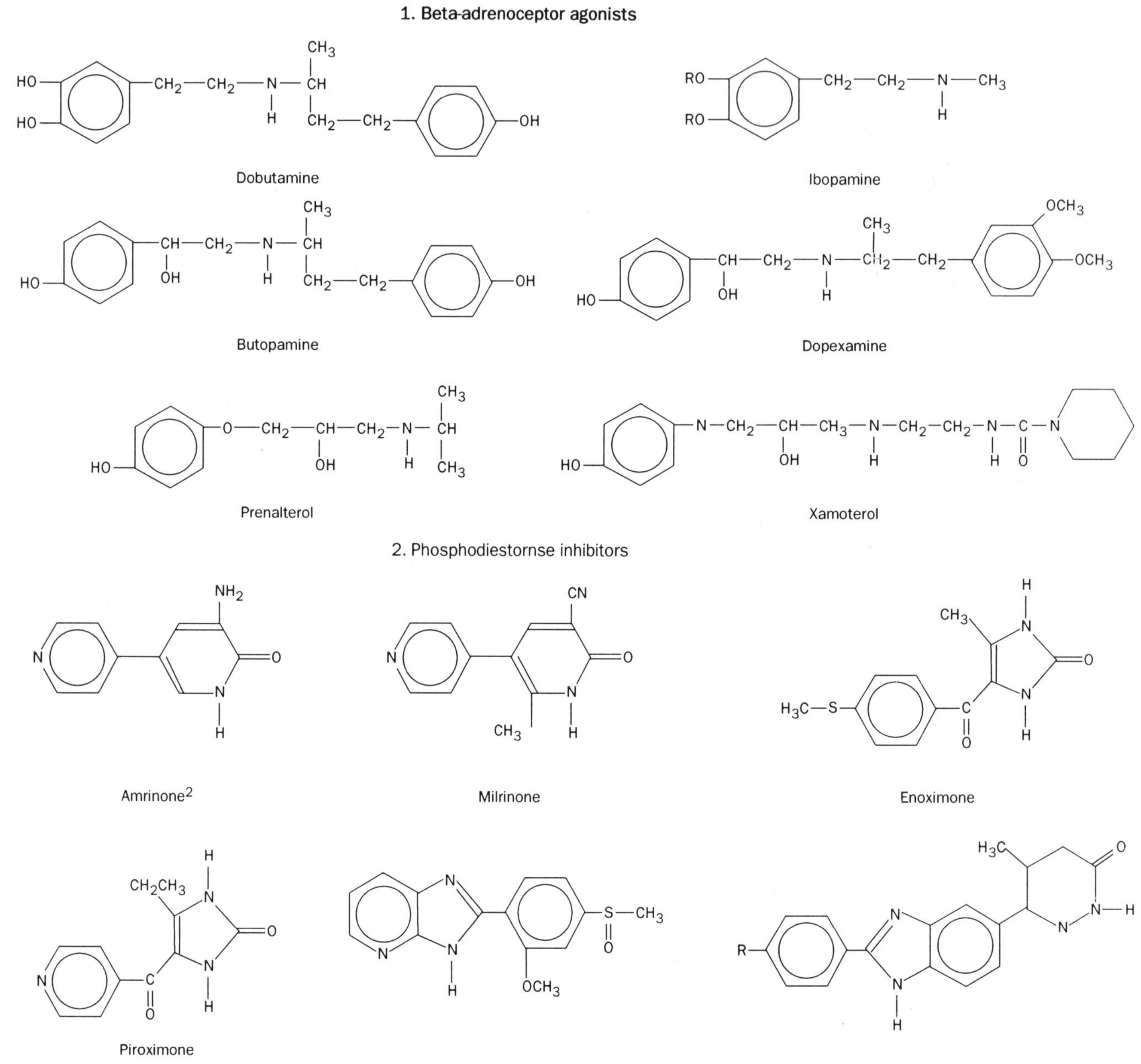

1. Beta-adrenoceptor agonists

Dobutamine

Ibopamine

Butopamine

Dopexamine

Prenalterol

Xamoterol

2. Phosphodiestornse inhibitors

Amrinone[2]

Milrinone

Enoximone

Piroximone

Figure 23.2 Structure of Beta receptor agonists and of Phosphodiesterase (type III) inhibitors.

Smooth muscle behaves differently from cardiac muscle, since there is some evidence that cAMP-dependent phosphorylation of calcium channels could exert an opposite effect in cardiac and smooth muscle where phosphorylation could close (and not open) membrane Ca^{2+} channels.

Recently, evidence has been put forward suggesting a prominent role for cGMP in relaxation of vascular smooth muscle. This role appears well-established in the action of nitrocompounds and in endothelium-dependent relaxation by acetylcholine.

It therefore appears that there is agreement between observations on cellular action and general hemodynamic actions of catecholamines since β_1-adrenoceptor stimulation increases heart contractility and β_2-adrenoceptor stimulation causes skeletal muscular vasodilatation. Therapeutic interest is not only focused on β_1 and β_2 agonists such as dobutamine and salbutamol, respectively, but also on the adrenergic agonists dopamine and epinine and on partial β_1-adrenoceptor agonists (xamoterol, which has not fulfilled appropriate criterias).

Recent findings on β-adrenoceptors are based not only on studies of the response of isolated organs but

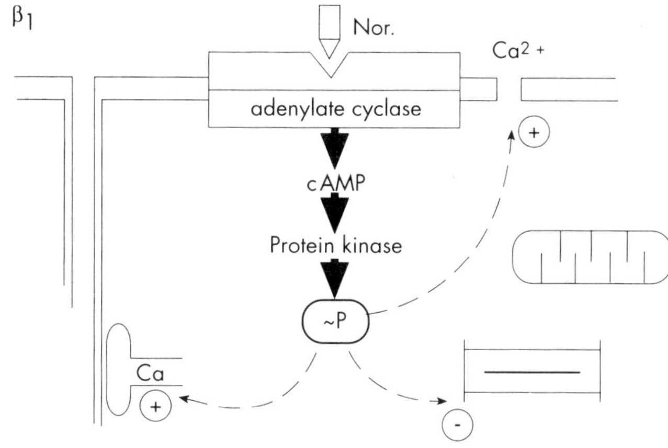

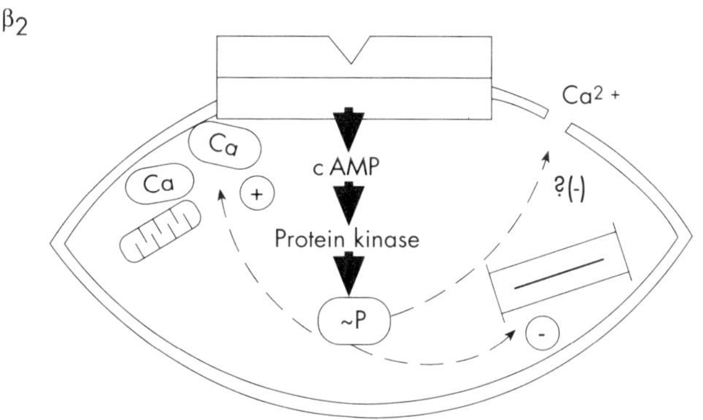

Figure 23.3 Schematic representation of the intracellular action of cAMP in cardiac muscle after stimulation of β_1-adrenoceptors and in smooth muscle after stimulation of β_2-adrenoceptors.

also on ligand binding studies, which have shown that the human heart, like a number of tissues, contains both β_1- and β_2-receptors. Ligand studies also have related to reduction of receptors density the observation that long-term treatment with β-adrenergic agonists evokes a loss of responsiveness to NE of both the cardiac contractile response and the increase in cAMP levels. This decrease in responsiveness has been found in every species examined as well as in human patients.

Chronic heart failure patients have increased circulating endogenous catecholamines and decreased numbers of cardiac β-receptors.[r4] Although many feel that the reduced number of receptors is a compensation for the elevated NE in plasma, others have suggested that in some cases of cardiomyopathy the decrease in receptors is primary. If this latter view is correct, the use of β_1 antagonists, such as propranolol, should increase the number of β-receptors and alleviate symptoms.[r3]

There have been enthusiasts for β-adrenoceptor blockade in idiopathic dilated cardiomyopathy, with apparent improvement in both symptoms and survival. An intermediate approach between β_1 blockade and β_1 stimulation has been the development of β_1-adrenoceptor partial agonists such as xamoterol that stabilize β_1-adrenoceptor activity at about half maximum, thereby avoiding the adverse hemodynamic consequences of inadequate or excessive endogenous stimulation. In preliminary studies, this drug seems to have improved both systolic and diastolic left ventricular function, at rest and during stress, without increasing myocardial oxygen consumption, but confirmatory trials are not available.

The administration of dopamine results in substantial improvement in the performance of a failing heart. Its beneficial hemodynamic action has been attributed not only to a potent positive inotropic effect mediated by action of the β_1-adrenoceptors, but also to its agonist activity at the level of vascular dopamine receptors.[r6,r7] In addition, dopamine increases the release of NE from presynaptic membranes. Activation of the dopamine receptors leading to an increase in renal blood flow has been advocated to be the major factor responsible for the important increase in diuresis observed after administration of dopamine whereas dobutamine increases femoral flow without changing renal flow. Dopamine prodrugs such as levodopa and ibopamine are active orally and could allow a more comfortable therapy than possible with parenteral adrenoceptor agonists.

Ibopamine is a prodrug that releases epinine as the active compound. Ibopamine has been shown to possess inotropic activity after oral administration and to increase cardiac output without affecting heart rate in humans. Animal studies have shown that epinine increases myocardial contractility by a β_1-adrenoceptor mediated effect. In view of the absence of a positive chronotropic effect of ibopamine in humans, it may be anticipated that the action of epinine is not simply a β_1 effect that is associated with a marked tachycardia. In humans, the receptors involved in the inotropic effect of epinine are not identical to those involved in the inotropic effect of dopamine.[r19]

As already pointed out, inhibition of phosphodiesterase leading to increase in cellular cAMP levels may mimic the activation of β-adrenoceptors in the cardiovascular system. Much of our information on those agents is based on studies with methylxanthines, which affect cardiac and smooth muscle as well as other systems. Three possible mechanisms of action have been considered for the cardiac effect of the methylxanthines: (1) the increase in cAMP levels due to their effects on phosphodiesterases; (2) a direct action on cellular calcium control, namely by the release of calcium from sarcoplasmic reticulum; (3) their ability to block adenosine receptors, counteracting negative inotropic influences of locally released cardiac adenosine.[r8,r9,r11]

The cardioactive bipyridines, amrinone and milrinone and the cardioactive benzimidazoles (see below) have a complex mode of action in which phosphodiesterase inhibition could likely contribute.

Among inhibitors of phosphodiesterases that increase the cAMP content of the cell and thereby evoke a positive inotropic effect and a decrease in vascular tone, some have in addition an effect on the Ca^{2+} sensitivity of the contractile proteins. This property has initially been illustrated with sulmazole (AR-L 115).

It has been shown that this agent increases active tension development and unloads shortening velocity of chemically skinned heart muscle preparations at submaximal activating levels of free Ca^{2+}. The calcium concentration-effect curve is displaced to the left when the myofibrillar ATPase is used as an index of calcium effect. Similarly, calcium binding to myofibrillar protein is also increased. These experimental data indicate that sulmazole increases the affinity of myofibrillar troponin C for calcium. Therefore, the action of sulmazole is to increase cAMP leading to an increase in $[Ca^{2+}]_i$ (see above) and to enhanced sensitivity of the myofilament for calcium. Owing to its toxicity, sulmazole has not reached large clinical trials. There are several other experimental compounds in this group, including imobendan, which shows stereoselectivity for its Ca^{2+}-sensitizing effect. Indeed, in chemically skinned heart muscle the force developed by the preparation at pCa 6.75 is enhanced by L-imobendan more than by D-imobendan. This action may be responsible for the difference in inotropic action of the two isomers. It remains to be demonstrated that phosphodiesterase inhibitors (selective for PDE III) with or without Ca sensitizing action may be useful for the long-term management of heart failure.

Adverse Effects

In therapy, desensitization is a strong limitation for the long-term utilization of β-adrenoceptor agonists. In acute conditions, their use may nevertheless be beneficial. However, while β_1-adrenoceptor stimulation increases heart rate and contractility, it may provoke or worsen myocardial ischemia by increasing oxygen requirements and may also precipitate tachyarrhythmia. On the other hand, β_2-adrenoceptor stimulation causes coronary and skeletal muscular vasodilatation, thereby increasing flow. But it may further increase myocardial oxygen requirements by direct inotropic and chronotropic effects. Moreover, the renin-angiotensin cascade is activated via β_2-adrenoceptors and thus hyperglycemia, hypokalemia, and lactic acidosis may ensue. To reduce these unwanted effects while retaining the hemodynamic benefits, several different therapeutic approaches to β_1-adrenoceptor manipulation in heart failure have been devised. Most attempt to separate inotropic and chronotropic effects or attempt to use partial agonists. The separation of inotropic and chronotropic effects has been claimed for a number of adrenergic agents, including dopamine, dobutamine, and the partial agonists prenalterol and xamoterol. In general, this separation of effects seems more evident in intact animals than in isolated preparations, suggesting that enhanced cardiac stroke volume is secondary to increased venous return via reduced venous capacitance (an α-receptor effect) rather than direct myocyte β-receptor activation.

Phosphodiesterase inhibitors evoke several adverse effects. Treatment with oral amrinone causes thrombocytopenia in about 20 percent of patients. Other adverse effects are GI symptoms such as nausea, vomiting, and abdominal pain and abnormal liver function. It has been reported that withdrawal of the drug was required in about 34 percent of patients. Milrinone, a derivative of amrinone, does not produce thrombocytopenia and the side-effects appear to be better tolerated. The other agents of this group may be considered as still in the experimental stage. Adverse reactions have not yet been reported with ibopamine.

Cardiac Glycosides

Cardiac glycosides are still utilized because they are inotropic drugs that can be given by the oral route for long-term treatment. Their long-term efficacy has been questioned, but this is not a very new problem. Hemodynamic studies during management of acute cardiac failure have shown that cardiac glycosides increase cardiac output and decrease peripheral resistance, and thus they remain widely used.

Digitalis is a challenge for both basic and clinical research. It is surprising that it has been used for so many centuries and that no modern substitute has yet emerged, such as for opiates.[r1,r2,r10,r12,r17,r18,r22,r23,r26,r27,r30,r31,3]

History

Cardiac glycosides are the active principles of various plants (foxglove). The common medical language is to name "digitalis" the purified principles, which may cause some confusion because digitalis is a botanical term. Extracts of foxglove were introduced into therapy two centuries ago by Withering, who wrote a most remarkable book, "An Account of the Foxglove," published in 1785. In this book, Withering insisted on the importance of using a low dose in order to avoid toxicity. In January 1785, Erasmus Darwin also published, in the Medical Transactions of the Royal College of Physicians, a case-report on the use of digitalis. Digitoxin was the first cardiac glycoside crystallized by J. F. Nativelle in 1871.

Chemistry

Cardiac glycosides are made up of a steroid nucleus (the genin), one or more C-3 glycosidically linked sugar moieties, and at C-17 a five-membered unsaturated lactone ring, in the case of plant derived cardenolides. Bufadienolides are chemically similar compounds that contain a six-membered lactone ring in C-17 and are found in toad skin (Fig. 23.4).

The most commonly used cardiac glycoside is digoxin. Digitoxin is less used, β-methyldigoxin is a semisynthetic derivative of digoxin. Ouabain is a rapidly acting glycoside used in research studies. The various cardiac glycosides differ mainly by their bioavailability and their pharmacokinetics.

Binding

The binding of cardiac glycosides to their receptors, the Na^+, K^+-ATPases of the cell membrane, has been studied using intact tissues or microsomal preparations. Although earlier studies reported the existence of only one class of binding sites, recent studies support the concept of the heterogeneity of cardiac glycoside binding sites. In guinea pig atria, a high-affinity, low-capacity binding of ouabain has been identified in the nanomolar range and a low-affinity high-capacity binding can be identified in a concentration range two or three orders of magnitude higher. The high affinity binding sites represent 5 to 10 percent of the total number of sites. At first glance, this figure might appear to be very low, but it corresponds to about 10^4 molecules bound per cardiac cell when high-affinity sites are saturated. Similar observations have been carried out in rat heart, where the proportion of high-affinity sites is higher.

There are several experimental arguments suggesting that high- and low-affinity binding sites are related to two Na^+, K^+-ATPase isozymes and that the high-affinity receptors are associated with Na-H exchangers and the low-affinity ones with Na-Ca exchangers. The amino acid sequence and the spatial organization of several Na^+, K^+-ATPase isozymes have been reported.

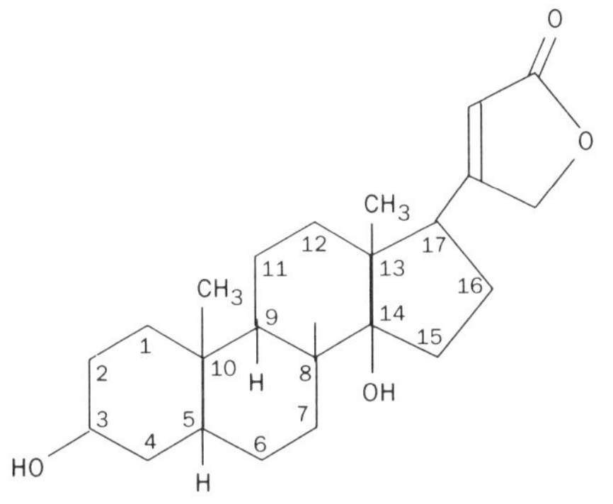

Digitox

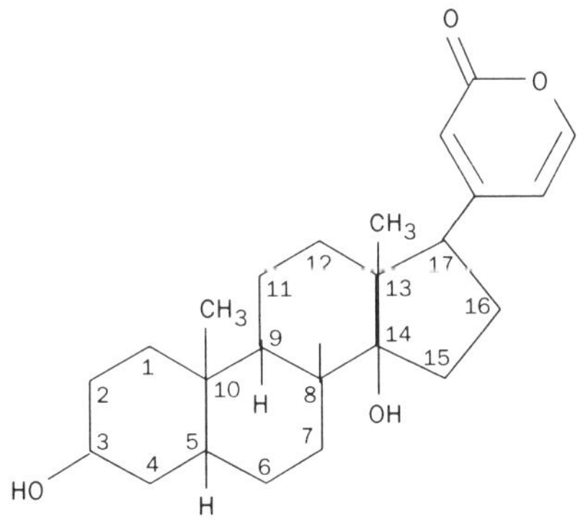

Bufalin

	R_3	R_{14}	R_{12}	R_{16}
Digitoxigenin	OH	OH	H	H
Gitoxigenin	OH	OH	H	OH
Gitaloxigenin	OH	OH	H	OCHO
Digoxigenin	OH	OH	OH	H
Diginatigenin	OH	OH	OH	OH

Figure 23.4 Planar structure of the main genins of the digitals family compared to bufalin.

Pharmacologic Action

The contractility of cardiac muscle is largely controlled by intracellular Ca_I^{++} concentrations, which can be increased by: (1) increasing extracellular calcium; (2) opening voltage sensitive calcium channels; and (3) by increasing the exchange of intracellular Na_I^+ for extracellular calcium.

A decrease in the activity of the sodium pump elevates Na_I^+ since less sodium is extruded to the cell exterior per unit time. Increased intracellular Na^+ activity stimulates Na-Ca exchange, leading to increased intracellular activator Ca^{2+}, and enhanced contractility, as previously outlined. However, detailed analysis has shown that it is necessary to distinguish two concentration ranges in the inotropic effect of cardiac glycosides: a low- and a high-dose effect, and that the inotropic effect of ouabain is likely the result of two mechanisms. One, observed at high concentrations, is related to inhibition of low affinity Na^+, K^+ pumps and most likely to toxicity. The other, observed at low concentrations, may be considered as the therapeutic action resulting from interaction of ouabain with high-affinity Na^+, K^+-ATPases.

Pharmacologic Action

The use of digitalis for the treatment of congestive heart failure (CHF) has declined following the introduction of oral diuretic therapy. However, more recently, it has been recognized that long-term digitalis therapy improves left ventricular function in heart failure. Digitalis should be considered as a mild inotropic agent. Another and important indication of digitalis is atrial fibrillation or flutter, in which digitalis is used to produce a partial A–V block, thus slowing the rate of ventricular contraction enough to permit adequate ventricular filling.

The actions of digitalis are divided into cardiac and extracardiac ones; another classification considers direct effects on the target organ and indirect ones related to the neurovegetative system (Table 23.2). Among the cardiac actions, the most obvious is the positive inotropic effect. In normal subjects, this effect is accompanied by an increase in peripheral resistance that does not allow an increase in cardiac output. However, in patients with heart failure, the peripheral resistance is already elevated as a result of enhanced sympathetic nervous system tone, and digitalis treatment decreases peripheral resistance by reflexly decreasing sympathetic activity as cardiac output improves. The positive inotropic effect is associated with a negative chronotropic effect, part of which is related to an increase in vagal tone, also responsible for the GI effects characterized by nausea and vomiting, the most common adverse effects of this treatment.

Other common side-effects are disturbances of cardiac rhythm, which may be avoided by a careful dose titration controlled by blood level monitoring. Special care must be taken when using digoxin in patients with renal failure and in older patients with reduced renal clearance. This is due to the fact that digoxin is mainly eliminated by the kidney, unlike digitoxin, which is mainly eliminated by hepatic metabolism and biliary excretion.

Another factor responsible for intoxications is related to the simultaneous use of digitalis and diuretics responsible for K-loss. There is competition between cardiac glycosides and KCl at the level of low-affinity Na^+, K^+-ATPase sites. A decrease in extracellular KCl concentration increases the inhibition of the low-affinity Na^+, K^+-ATPase and thereby the incidence of digitalis-induced toxicity.

Toxicity may also be caused during initiation of therapy. Indeed, the efficacy of digitalis is related to maintenance of a steady-state in blood level (about 1 ng/ml for digoxin). In order to avoid delays due to the relatively long half-life of orally active cardiac glycosides, a loading dose is commonly used, known as "digitalization."

Table 23.2 Cardiac Actions of Digitalis

Effect	Atria	A - V node	Ventricles
Direct	↑contractility ↑refractory period ↓conduction ↑automaticity	↑refractory period ↓conduction	↑contractility ↓refractory period ↑automaticity
Indirect (vague)	↓refractory period ↑conduction	↑refractory period ↓conduction	no effect
ECG	P wave changes	↑PR internal	↓QT interval T and ST segment depressed
Overdose Response	tachycardia, fibrillation or flutter	A - V block	Ventricular Excitability fibrillation

Calcium Antagonists

These drugs are also discussed in Chapter 5, 25 and 26 since calcium antagonists (discovered in the laboratories of Fleckenstein and of Godfraind) were first introduced to treat hypertension and coronary disease.[r32,r20,r21,r25,3,5,6,10,12,13,14] Because cardiac infarction and heart failure are complications of the above diseases, the question has been raised whether calcium antagonist therapy should not be discontinued in these life-threatening situations. The first generation of calcium antagonists—such agents as nifedipine, diltiazem and verapamil—were negative inotropic agents. Nevertheless, in large clinical trials, it appeared that subgroups of patients showed benefit from this therapy. The actual trend is to test the new generation of calcium antagonists in ischemic left ventricular dysfunction.[7,9] The term "left ventricular dysfunction" is all-embracing, and covers a spectrum of myocardial ischemic dysfunction including postinfarct dysfunction, reperfusion stunning, and hibernation. Ischemic dysfunction also includes overt systolic heart failure, accompanied by diastolic abnormalities.

Postischemic myocardial stunning is due to at least two mechanisms: cytosolic calcium overload and formation of free radicals. The first can be alleviated by calcium antagonists, given at the time of reperfusion in the rat heart. In the dog heart, verapamil, given post-reperfusion, also can lessen stunning. These benefits, relating to the use of calcium antagonists relatively early in the course of stunning, do not mean that these agents can benefit established post-cardioplegic myocardial failure in patients.

It is of interest that calcium antagonist treatment has been associated with benefits against other aspects of ischemic dysfunction, including hibernation and post-infarct left ventricular diastolic dysfunction.

Thus, morbidity (e.g., progression toward CHF and angina pectoris) and mortality remain high despite treatment with ACE inhibitors. Hence, the new generation of dihydropyridine calcium antagonists may represent an improvement. Their afterload-reducing action, coupled with powerful coronary vasodilatation, might delay the progression of ischemic left ventricular dysfunction. In addition, the improved pharmacokinetic profile of these drugs, without wide variations in peak and trough plasma levels, may avoid triggering a neurohormonal reflex. Therefore, multicenter trials have been designed to test the action of calcium antagonists on cardiac performance after acute myocardial infarction.

The Defiant-I study was a multicenter, multinational, double-blind, randomized study of the effects of the new calcium antagonist nisoldipine on left ventricular size and function after acute myocardial infarction. Randomization to placebo or to long-acting nisoldipine coat-core (20 mg once daily) was performed in 135 eligible patients with mild to moderate systolic left ventricular dysfunction (left ventricular ejection fraction of 50% or less) 20 days (range 7–35) after infarction; serial clinical, echocardiographic, and Doppler cardiographic measurements were taken during a four-week follow-up period. At the end of the follow-up period, exercise capacity was determined by bicycle ergometry.

Nisoldipine improved indices of diastolic left ventricular function. No change was seen in systolic and diastolic left ventricular volume or left ventricular ejection fraction. Exercise capacity was greater in patients receiving nisoldipine.

The observed changes in diastolic left ventricular function during nisoldipine therapy may reflect an anti-ischemic effect of the drug or may be due to an improvement in myocardial relaxation. The Defiant-II study, presently in progress, will examine the effect of higher doses of nisoldipine on left ventricular function and on exercise performance after acute myocardial infarction, with a longer (six-month) follow-up period. Studies are also in progress with amlodipine and other calcium antagonists which could allow complete neurohumoral control when potent vasoconstrictor forces such as endothelin-1 remain activated.

References

Research Reports

1. Balligand JL, Kelly RA, Marsden PA, Smith TW, Michel T. Control of cardiac muscle cell function by an endogenous nitric oxide signalling system. Proc Natl Acad Sci USA 1993;*90*:347–351.
2. Beuckelmann DJ, Nabauer M, Erdmann E. Intracellular calcium handling in isolated ventricular myocytes from patients with terminal heart failure. Circulation 1992;*85*:1046–1055.
3. Bolognesi R, Tsialtas D, Manca C. Digitalis and heart failure: Does digitalis really produce beneficial effects through positive inotropic action? Card Drugs Ther 1992;*6*:459–464.
4. Cowley AJ, Wynne RD, Swami A, Birkhead J, Skene A, Hampton, JR. A comparison of the effects of captopril and flosequinan in patients with severe heart failure. Card Drugs Ther 1992;*6*:465–470.
5. Die Cas L. Acute and chronic effects of the dihydropyridine calcium antagonist nisoldipine on the resting and exercise hemodynamics, neurohumoral parameters and functional capacity of the patients with chronic heart failure. Card Drugs Ther 1993;*7*:103–110.
6. Finet M, Godfraind T, Khoury G. The positive inotropic action of a nifedipine analogue, Bay K 8644, in guinea-pig and rat isolated cardiac preparations. Br J Pharmacol 1985;*86*:27–32.
7. Godfraind T, Egleme C, Finet M, Jaumin P. The actions of nifedipine and nisoldipine on the contractile activity of human coronary arteries and human cardiac tissue in vitro. Pharmacol Toxicol 1987;*61*:79–84.
8. Godfraind T, Mennig D, Morel N, Morelin N, Wibo M. Effect of endothelin-1 on calcium channel gating by agonists in vascular smooth muscle. J Cardiovasc Pharmacol 1989;*13* (Suppl 5):S112–S117.
9. Godfraind T, Salomone S, Dessy C, Verherlst B, Dion R, Schoevaerts JC. Selectivity scale of calcium antagonists in the human cardiovascular system (based on in vitro studies). J Cardiovasc Pharmacol 1992;*20* (Suppl 5):S34–S41.
10. Jalil JE, Doering CW, Janicki JS, Pick R, Shroff SG, Weber KT. Fibrillar collagen and myocardial stiffness in the intact hypertrophied rat left ventricle. Circ Res, 1989;*64*:1041–1050.
11. Nadal-Ginard B, Mahdavi V. Molecular basis of cardiac performance: Plasticity of the myocardium generated through protein isoform switches. J. Clin. Invest 1989;*84*:1693–1700.
12. Takahashi T, Allen PD, Lacro RV, Marks AR, Dennis AR, Schoen FJ, Grossman W, Marsh JD, Izumo S. Expression of dihydropyridine receptor (Ca^{2+} channel) and calsequestrin genes in the myocardium of patients with end-stage heart failure. J Clin Invest 1992;*90*:927–935.
13. Wagner JA, Sax FL, Weisman, HF. Calcium-antagonist receptors in the atrial tissue of patients with hypertrophic cardiomyopathy. N Engl J Med 1989;*320*:755–761.
14. Wibo M, Bravo G, Godfraind T, Porterfield J, McIntosh C, Weisfeldt ML, Snyder SH, Epstein SE. Postnatal maturation of excitation-contraction coupling in rat ventricle in relation to the subcellular localization and surface density of 1,4-dihydropyridine and ryanodine receptors. Cir Res 1991;*68*:662–673.

Reviews

r1. Akera T, Brody TM. The role of Na^+ K^+-ATPase in the inotropic action of digitalis. Pharmacol Rev 1978;*29*:187–220.

r2. Arnold SB, Byrd RC, Meister W, Melanon K, Cheitlin MD, Bristow D, Parmley WW, Chatterjee K. Long-term digitalis therapy improves left ventricular function in heart failure. N Engl J Med 1980;*30325*, 1443–1448.

r3. Bristow MR. Pathophysiologic and pharmacologic rationales for clinical management of chronic heart failure with beta-blocking agents. Am J Cardiol 1993;*71*:1C-22C.

r4. Brodde OE. β_1- and β_2-Adrenoceptors in the human heart: properties, function, and alterations in chronic heart failure. Pharmacol Rev 1991;*43*:203–242.

r5. Captopril-Digoxin Multicenter Research Group: Comparative effects of therapy with captopril and digoxin in patients with mild to moderate heart failure. Heart Failure Ther 1988;*259*:4, 539–544.

r6. Cohn, JN, Franciosa JA. Vascular therapy of cardiac failure. N Engl J Med 1977;*297*:27–31; 254–258.

r7. Cohn JN. Future directions in vasodilator therapy for heart failure. Am Heart J 1991;*121*:969–974.

r8. Colucci WS, Wright RF, Brauwald E. New positive inotropic agents in the treatment of congestive heart failure. N Engl J Med 1986;*314*:3290–3299; 349–358.

r9. DiBianco R, Shabetai R, Kostuk W, Moran J, Schlant RC, Wright R. A comparison of oral milrinone, digoxin, and their combination in the treatment of patients with chronic heart failure. N Engl J Med 1989;*320*:11, 677–683.

r10. Erdmann E et al. Cardiac Glycosides 1785–1985. Steinkopff Verlag Darmstadt, Springer Verlag New York (1985).

r11. Farah AE, Alousi AA, Schwarz RP. Positive inotropic agents. Ann Rev Pharmacol Toxicol 1984;*24*:275–328.

r12. Fleg JL, Gottlieb SH, Lakatta EG. Is digoxin really important in treatment of compensated heart failure? A placebo-controlled crossover study in patients with sinus rhythm. Am J Med 1982;*73*:244–250.

r13. Fowler MB. Controlled trials with beta blockers in heart failure: Metoprolol as the prototype. Am J Cardiol 1993;*71*:45C-53C.

r14. Francis GS, Cohn JN. Heart failure: mechanisms of cardiac and vascular dysfunction and the rationale for pharmacologic intervention. FASEB J 1990;*4*:3068–3075.

r15. Frohlich ED, Apstein C, Chobanian AV, Devereux RB, Dustan HP, Dzau V, Faudd-Tarazi F, Horan MJ, Marcus M, Massie B. The heart in hypertension. N Engl J Med 1992;*327*:998–1008.

r16. Gillis RA, Quest JA. The role of the nervous system in the cardiovascular effects of digitalis. Pharmacol. Rev 1980;*31*:19–97.

r17. Godfraind T. Cardiac glycoside receptors in the heart. Biochem Pharmacol 1975;*24*:823–827.

r18. Godfraind T. Withering: 200 years is not enough. Trends Pharmacol Sci 1985;*6*:360–363.

r19. Godfraind T. Comparative pharmacology of cardiac and vascular tissues in heart failure. J Cardiovasc Pharmacol 1989;*14*:(Suppl. 8); S1–S20.

r20. Godfraind T. The cardioselectivity of calcium antagonists. Cardiovasc Drugs Ther. In press, 1994.

r21. Godfraind T, Miller R, Wibo M. Calcium antagonism and calcium entry blockers. Pharmacol Rev 1986;*38*:321–416.

r22a. Greef K. Cardiac glycosides. Part I: Experimental pharmacology. 1981; Berlin: Springer-Verlag.

r22b. Greef, K. Cardiac glycosides. Part II: Pharmacokinetics and clinical pharmacology 1981; Berlin: Springer-Verlag.

r23. Marcus FI. The use of digitalis for the treatment of congestive heart failure: a tale of its decline and resurrection. Cardivasc Drugs Ther 1989;*3*:473–476.

r24. Min Ae Lee, Böhm MS, Paul M, Ganten D. Tissue renin-angiotensin systems. Their role in cardiovascular disease. Circ 1993; Suppl IV, *87*:5, 7–13.

r25. Morgan JP. Abnormal intracellular modulation of calcium as a major cause of cardiac contractile dysfunction. N Engl J Med 1991;*325*:625–632.

r26. Murray RG, Tweddel AC, Martin W, Pearson D, Hutton I, Lawne TDV. Evaluation of digitalis in cardiac failure. Br Med J 1982;*284*:1526–1528.

r27. Noble D. Mechanism of action of therapeutic levels of cardiac glycosides. Cardiovasc Res 1980;*14*:495–514.

r28. Opie LH. Clinical Use of Calcium Channel Antagonists Drugs, 2d ed. Boston: Kluwer Academic Publishers (1990).

r29. Packer M. How should physicians view heart failure? The philosophical and physiological evolution of three conceptual models of the disease. Am J Cardiol 1993;*71*:3C–11C.

r30. Schwartz A, Lindenmayer GE, Allen JC. The sodium-potassium adenosine triphosphatase: Pharmacological, physiological and biochemical aspects. Pharmacol Rev 1975;*27*:1–134.

r31. Smith, TW, Butler VP, Haber E, Fozzard H, Marcus FI, Bremner F, Schulman IC, Phillips A. Treatment of life-threatening digitalis intoxication with Fab fragments of digoxin-specific antibodies. N Engl J Med 1982;*307*:1357–1362.

r32. Spedding M, Paoletti R. Classification of calcium channels and the sites of action of drugs modifying channel function. Pharmacol Rev 1992;*44*:363–376.

r33. Thind GS. Angiotensin converting enzyme inhibitors: Comparative structure, pharmacokinetics and pharmacodynamics. Card Drugs Ther 1990;*4*:199–206.

CHAPTER 24

P. A. Calle
M. G. Bogaert

Anti-ischemic Drugs

This chapter deals primarily with several classes of drugs used in the prevention and treatment of angina pectoris attacks: organic nitrates; β-adrenergic blocking agents; calcium antagonists; and some substances belonging to other pharmacologic groups.[r1,r2,r3] There is also much interest in the use of the same drugs for other ischemic cardiac disease states, such as silent ischemia and myocardial infarction. In these conditions, however, other agents are also used, e.g., acetylsalicylic acid and other platelet anti-aggregating agents, thrombolytic substances, heparin, and oral anticoagulants, angiotensin-converting enzyme (ACE) inhibitors, hypolipidemic drugs, and antiarrhythmics;[r1,r2,r3,r4] these drugs are extensively dealt with in other chapters of this book.

As introduction to this chapter, the different ischemic syndromes will be described briefly, with a schematic outline of the appropriate medical treatment (Table 24.1). Discussions of the role in these syndromes of coronary graft surgery[1] and the various technologies in interventional cardiology such as percutaneous transluminal coronary angioplasty[2] are beyond the scope of this chapter.

Table 24.1 Drug Treatment of Ischemic Heart Disease

— Stable angina pectoris
Acute attack: sublingual nitrates (and oral nifedipine)
Maintenance treatment: nitrates, β-blockers, calcium antagonists, various drugs (molsidomine, amiodarone, acetylsalicylic acid)

— Unstable angina
Nitrates, β-blockers, calcium antagonists, heparin, acetylsalicylic acid

— Silent ischemia
Nitrates, β-blockers, calcium antagonists, acetylsalicylic acid

— Acute phase of myocardial infarction
Thrombolytic agents, acetylsalicylic acid, anti-arrhythmic agents, β-blockers, heparin and oral anticoagulants

— Secondary prophylaxis after myocardial infarction
β-blockers, acetylsalicylic acid, ACE-inhibitors? oral anticoagulants, hypolipidemic drugs

— Primary prevention of ischemic heart disease
Hypolipidemic agents? acetylsalicylic acid? antihypertensive treatment?

Clinical Syndromes and Therapeutic Considerations

Angina pectoris attacks result from a disequilibrium between oxygen requirement and oxygen supply of the myocardium. These attacks are usually the consequence of organic narrowing of the coronary arteries and often occur during physical exercise or stress, when an increased heart rate leads to increased oxygen demand. Attacks can also occur at rest, however, and this has drawn attention to the role of coronary spasm in anginal attacks, even in those that are exercise-induced.[r5,r6]

Treatment of the acute anginal attack consists of sublingual administration of nitrates. Sublingual nitrates can also be used prophylactically, shortly before an expected attack, e.g., pre-exercise.[r1,r3]

Maintenance treatment in the patient with angina pectoris consists of administration of organic nitrates, β-blockers, calcium antagonists, or sometimes other agents such as molsidomine or amiodarone. The choice between different drugs often will be made on the basis of individual patient characteristics and the side-effects and contraindications of specific agents.[r1,r3,r7] In some patients, drugs from different classes have to be combined in order to reach a satisfactory reduction of the attacks, although results from some studies suggest that most patients treated with multiple drugs probably do not experience greater symptomatic or prognostic benefits, but may suffer more adverse effects.[r7,r8,r9,3,4,5,6]

It is not known whether anti-ischemic drug treatment influences the prognosis of the angina pectoris patient with the exception of β-blockers in selected patients after myocardial infarction.[r10] On the other hand, administration of acetylsalicylic acid[7] or ACE-inhibitors,[r11] drugs that have no effect on the ischemic threshold, has recently been shown to improve outcome in patients with stable ischemic heart disease.

In patients with *unstable angina,* intensive drug treatment is given for relief of symptoms, but more so for avoiding progression toward infarction; nitrates, β-blockers, calcium antagonists, and/or heparin are administered, and antiaggregating agents such as acetylsalicylic acid are also commonly used. Most of these substances have shown beneficial effects, but there is a need for controlled studies about what drug(s) should be given to a particular patient.[r2,8,9,10,11,12]

In recent years, *silent ischemia* episodes—i.e., electrocardiographic signs suggestive of ischemia, but without pain—have been recognized to occur frequently, mainly by 24-hour EKG monitoring and exercise testing. Such painless episodes of ST-T depression can be found in most patients with ischemic heart disease, whether or not painful attacks also occur. Patients with unstable angina who also show frequent silent ischemic episodes are considered to be of higher risk for myocardial infarction and sudden death; similarly, silent ischemia outside unstable angina is known to be of prognostic significance.[r12,r13] On the other hand, it has not yet been shown clearly that treatment aimed at eliminating all silent ischemic episodes (nitrates, β-blockers, calcium antagonists) has a beneficial effect on prognosis, either in unstable angina or in other circumstances.[r12,r14,13]

Patients with *acute myocardial infarction* are, whenever possible, treated with thrombolytic agents[r4,r15,r16] and, nowadays, according to the results of the ISIS-II study,[14] also with acetylsalicylic acid. Antiarrhythmic agents (e.g., lidocaine) are indicated only in the presence of life-threatening arrhythmias.[r4,r17] Treatment with β-blockers, first IV and then orally, has been shown to reduce early mortality and/or reinfarction, regardless of whether thrombolytics are given.[r4,r16,r18,r19,15] Treatment during the acute phase with heparin—but without thrombolytics—followed by oral anticoagulants, has been shown to reduce mortality and reinfarction-rate, the risk of mural thrombosis with peripheral embolism, and the risk of peripheral venous thrombosis with acute pulmonary embolism.[r4] The influence of heparin on mortality in patients treated with thrombolytics is under investigation; similarly, the discussion on the optimal way to administer heparin is still going on.[r4,r16]

Magnesium sulfate has been suggested to reduce early mortality;[r20] the first reports about the ongoing ISIS 4-trial tend to weaken this point of view. Other drugs still under investigation for this indication are nitrates, molsidomine, and ACE inhibitors. The available data provide some evidence for a beneficial effect of IV nitrates,[r21] but not of IV ACE-inhibitors[16] in the acute situation. Neither oral nitrates nor oral ACE-inhibitors seem to be beneficial, according to the first reports about the ISIS-4 trial. Routine use of calcium antagonists is of no use and may even be deleterious,[r22,r23] with the possible exception of diltiazem in patients with non-Q wave infarction.[17]

In *secondary prophylaxis after myocardial infarction,* β-blocking agents undoubtedly reduce mortality in the first years.[r24,r25] The role of calcium antagonists is less clear, and only diltiazem and verapamil may be beneficial.[r22,r23] Indeed, diltiazem given in patients without heart failure has been shown to reduce cardiac mortality and nonfatal reinfarction,[18] and in DAVIT-II[r23,19] a favorable trend on mortality and reinfarction was observed with verapamil. Acetylsalicylic acid has been used more and more in secondary prophylaxis, as a beneficial effect has been inferred from meta-analysis of trials with rather limited numbers of patients.[r26] Secondary prophylaxis with oral anticoagulants is frequently used in some countries, as some studies have yielded positive results.[r27] The value of hypolipidemic substances in secondary prophylaxis is still under investigation.[r28] Antiarrhythmic drugs, especially Class I antiarrhythmic drugs, should not be used, except for symptomatic or life-threatening arrhythmias. An exception may be amiodarone. Indeed, prophylactic use of this class III-antiarrhythmic agent has been shown to be beneficial in some small studies; large, multicenter studies are ongoing.[r29,r30] In recent studies in patients with heart failure—overt or silent—mainly due to ischemic heart disease, ACE-inhibitors have been shown to improve survival.[r11]

Primary prevention of ischemic heart disease has attracted much interest lately. Dietary and general hygienic measures (mainly cessation of smoking) are thought to be of use, but definite proof has been difficult to come by. For hypolipidemic agents the results of population trials in primary prevention have not yet been convincing.[r31] Two large trials with acetylsalicylic acid in primary prevention have yielded conflicting results.[r32] Trials of the effect of long-term antihypertensive treatment on progression of ischemic heart disease in patients with mild hypertension also yielded disappointing results.[r33]

Pharmacologic Agents

Organic Nitrates

Organic nitrates have been used in cardiovascular diseases for more than 100 years, first in patients with angina pectoris and now also in patients with congestive heart failure.

Chemistry

The organic nitrates most used are nitroglycerin (glyceryl trinitrate), isosorbide 5-mononitrate, isosorbide dinitrate, and pentaerythritol tetranitrate. Their structural formulas are given in Figure 24.1. The vascular activity of the organic nitrates correlates quite well with their liposolubility: the metabolites, whose structures are also shown in Figure 24.1, are less liposoluble but also less potent.

History

Amyl nitrite was first used in angina pectoris in 1867. It lowered blood pressure, and blood pressure-lowering due to blood-letting had been observed to have a beneficial effect on nocturnal angina. In 1879, nitroglycerin was proposed for the treatment of angina pectoris, because its effect on the peripheral pulse was similar to that of amyl nitrite. In the 1940s, the organic nitrates isosorbide dinitrate and pentaerythritol tetranitrate were synthezised. In the 1970s, the nitrated metabolites of the above-mentioned drugs were tested for vascular activity; of these, isosorbide-5-mononitrate was marketed as a drug.

Whereas originally the emphasis was put on the peripheral vasodilation induced by nitrates, gradually the notion of coronary vasodilation was introduced, and was thought to be the main mechanism of the antianginal effect of these substances. In the last 20 years, however, the effect of the nitrates on the peripheral circulation, mainly on venous capacitance or preload, was rediscovered and again emphasized as an important mechanism of the antianginal effect. This led to the more recent use of nitrates in congestive heart failure.[r34,r35]

For many years it was thought that nitrates were effective only via the sublingual route. In the last 15 to 20 years, however, the value of oral administration for maintenance therapy has become clear, while the sublingual route remains the mainstay for prevention and treatment of the acute attack.[r1,r3] Intravenous infusion of nitroglycerin isosorbide and of isosorbide dinitrate has been introduced for treatment of unstable angina[r2,20,21] and myocardial infarction.[r21,r34] Nitroglycerin has been applied transdermally for many years in the hope of obtaining a prolonged and sustained effect; this culminated in the development of transdermal controlled release systems that allow maintenance of rather stable plasma concentrations of nitro-

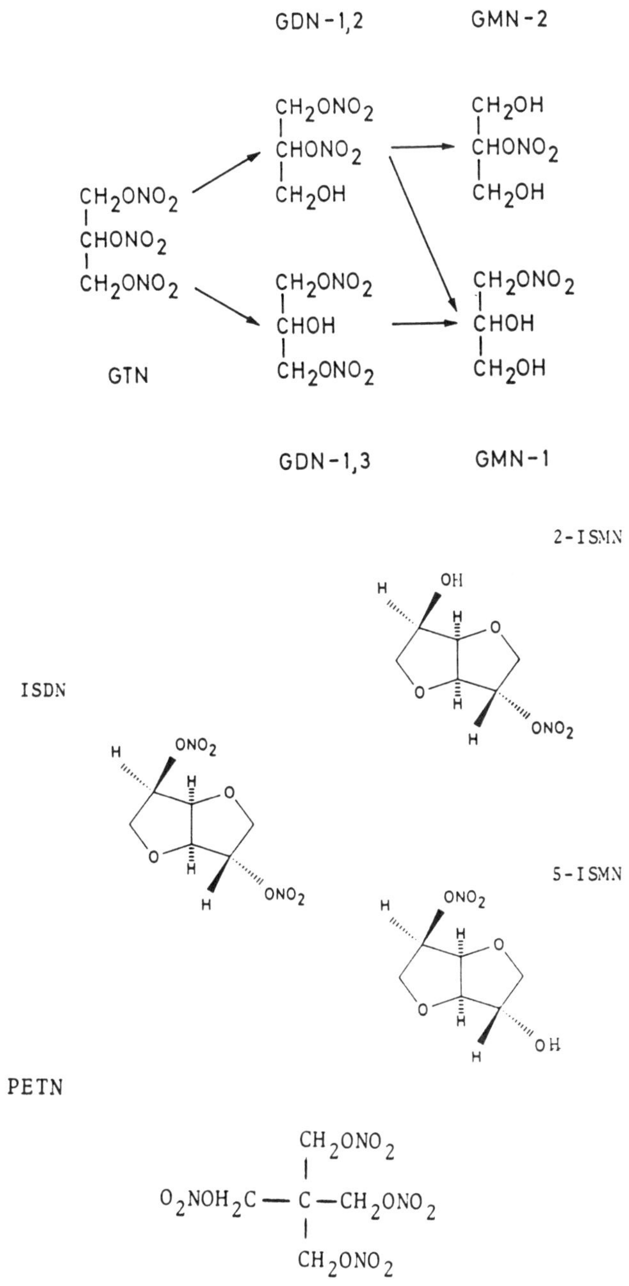

Figure 24.1 Structural formulas of the organic nitrates and their metabolites.

GTN : glyceryl trinitrate; GDN-1,2 : glyceryl-1,2-dinitrate; GDN-1,3 : glyceryl-1,3-dinitrate; GMN-2 : glyceryl-2-mononitrate; GMN-1 : glyceryl-1-mononitrate.

ISDN : isosorbide dinitrate; 2-ISMN : isosorbide-2-mononitrate; 5-ISMN : isosorbide-5-mononitrate.

PETN : pentaerythritol tetranitrate

glycerin and of its nitrated metabolites with one daily renewal of the plaster.[r34,r35]

The main object of current research in the nitrate field is the attenuation of the effects of these substances with their chronic use and how to prevent it.[r35,r36,r37]

Therapeutic Uses and Limitations

Organic nitrates are also used in congestive heart failure (see Chapter 23); only their use in ischemic heart disease will be discussed here.

Nitroglycerin and isosorbide dinitrate are administered sublingually to stop an anginal attack or to prevent an expected anginal attack, e.g., by administration immediately before an effort or before sexual intercourse. After sublingual administration of isosorbide dinitrate, the onset of action is probably somewhat slower and the duration of the protective effect longer than for nitroglycerin. Sublingual administration of a nitrate in chest pain can be helpful in differentiating angina from myocardial infarction. Nitrates could be harmful, mainly on sublingual administration, in patients suffering from hypertrophic obstructive cardiomyopathy. Likewise, aggravation of the already compromised diastolic filling may occur in patients with cardiac tamponade or constrictive pericarditis.[r34]

Attention has been drawn to new formulations of nitroglycerin: sprays and a buccal delivery formulation. However, whether administered sublingually by spray or in the old-fashioned tablet, nitroglycerin is found to be similarly effective in timing and extent of hemodynamic response.[22] A buccal delivery formulation of nitroglycerin showed an effect comparable to that of sublingual tablets in the treatment of acute anginal attacks, but a more prolonged duration of the effect.[23]

In the maintenance therapy of angina pectoris, the different organic nitrates are given orally, often together with β-blockers and/or calcium antagonists. Slow-release preparations of these oral forms are used in the hope of prolonging the therapeutic effect.[r1,r3,r34] Nitroglycerin ointment can also be used: although absorption of nitrates from these preparations is unpredictable, several studies have shown their efficacy in angina pectoris.[24] Nowadays, transdermal controlled delivery systems are often used,[r1,r3,r35,25,26] although some doubt remains concerning their usefulness.[27,28]

The attempts to maintain stable plasma concentrations through application of a transdermal system, by use of slow-release oral formulations, or by very frequent oral dosing, lead in many patients to rapid attenuation of the therapeutic effects, probably within hours[r35,r36,r37] (see below). Therefore, nitrate-free intervals are recommended, by giving the oral nitrate only in the morning and at noon (not in the evening), or by removing the nitroglycerin plaster approximately eight hours out of 24.[25,26] It probably is not possible to have a protective effect 24 hours out of 24.[r35,r36,r37]

Organic nitrates are also used in unstable angina: here the IV route is often preferred.[r2,r34,20,21] Intravenous nitrates have been shown to reduce mortality after myocardial infarction, probably by lessening pulmonary congestion or preload in patients with left ventricle failure.[r21] Obviously, IV doses have to be titrated under careful hemodynamic monitoring. At present, orally-given nitrates are under investigation in the acute and subacute phase of myocardial infarction.

All organic nitrates probably have the same therapeutic value in maintenance therapy, but the doses needed differ, owing to differences in potency and pharmacokinetics.

Effects and Mechanisms

The hemodynamic effects, the clinical efficacy, and the side-effects of nitrates are probably all related to their vasodilatory effect, although other mechanisms of action—such as antiaggregating effects[r38]—have been postulated.[r34,r35]

The cellular mechanism for the vasodilation is not entirely understood. Increased prostacyclin production by nitrates is probably not of major importance. Evidence is accumulating that vasodilation is linked to stimulation of guanylate cyclase in the vascular smooth muscle cells, with production of cyclic guanosine monophosphate, which then leads to lowered intracellular free calcium concentration and relaxation of contractile proteins (Fig. 24.2). The guanylate cyclase activation is thought to result from the formation of nitric oxide, which is now recognized as one of the endothelial relaxing factors that modulate arteriolar tone. Conversion of the nitrate into nitric oxide involves reaction with sulfhydryl groups; tolerance, i.e., a decreased response of the vascular smooth muscle cells toward nitrates, is thought to be partly due to depletion of free sulfhydryl groups.[r35,r36,r37]

Relaxation of the vascular smooth muscle cells leads to dilation of the coronary arteries, with increased oxygen supply to the myocardium. The coronary dilation probably does not lead to a coronary steal effect, i.e., shunting of blood away from the ischemic areas;

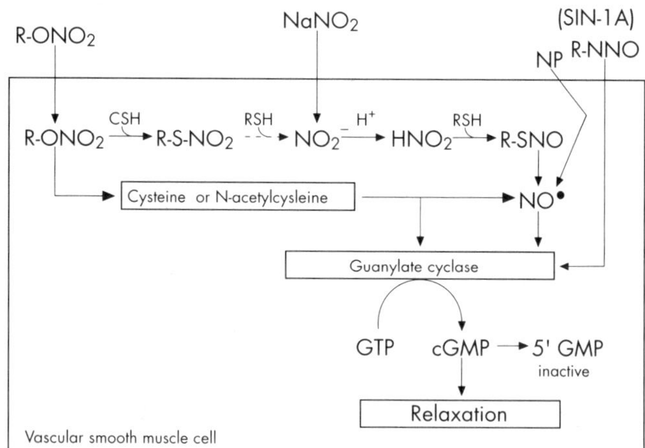

Figure 24.2 Possible steps leading to stimulation of the guanylate cyclase activity by nitrates (R-ONO2).

NP : nitroprusside, SIN-1A : active metabolite of molsidomine; GTP : guanosine trisphosphate; cGMP : 3′ 5′-cyclic guanosine monophosphate (from Romanin and Kukovetz, with permission, J. Mol. Cell. Cardiol., vol. 20, 389–396, 1988, figure 5).

in fact nitrates seem to redistribute blood flow preferentially toward the zones with the highest oxygen requirements ("inverted steal"). There is also dilation of peripheral vessels, i.e., the resistance vessels, with decreased afterload, but mainly dilation of venous capacitance vessels, with decreased preload; the decreased myocardial wall tension will lead to decreased oxygen requirements. The relative importance of these two mechanisms (increased oxygen supply versus decreased oxygen requirement) probably differs from patient to patient, depending on preexisting hemodynamic conditions.[r35]

The mechanism of action and the hemodynamic effects are probably similar for all organic nitrates, although there are differences in vasodilator potency, e.g., between the parent drugs and their nitrated metabolites. Pharmacokinetic differences can, however, alter the onset and the duration of the effect, although one should not assume that maintenance of nitrate concentrations equals maintainance of hemodynamic effects. As with other vasodilators, the speed of onset of the effect will influence the reflex responses of the organism and the eventual results.[r35]

Undesirable Effects and Interactions

Hypotension, even syncope, can occur due to peripheral vasodilation, with coronary hypoperfusion and reflex tachycardia;[r34] oxygen supply may decrease and oxygen requirements may increase. Individual sensitivity toward this hypotensive effect is variable, and patients should be advised to start with a small dose and, if possible, not to take a sublingual nitrate while standing. Hypotension also can occur with other routes of administration, mainly with IV administration. Special attention should be paid to patients with right ventricle infarction; as a rule, nitrates are contraindicated in these patients because of the danger of too excessive preload reduction of the right ventricle, resulting in a reduced cardiac output. Abrupt interruption of IV administration in patients with unstable angina at rest has been shown to induce rebound myocardial ischemia.[29] Similarly, some data suggest that a withdrawal phenomenon may occur after removal of dermal nitroglycerin patches, and controlled-release preparations.[30]

The side-effect that is most annoying for most patients is headache, a throbbing headache (e.g., immediately after taking a sublingual nitrate) and a longer lasting, dull constant headache with photophobia and sometimes nausea. Individual susceptibility to the nitrate headache is variable. Patients should be warned of this side-effect and should be told that the headache usually wears off with chronic intake of the drug, and that the disappearance of the headache does not necessarily mean that the therapeutic efficacy has decreased.[r34] If hypotension or headache poses a problem, it is worth trying lower doses, which subsequently may be increased gradually.

Although glaucoma is traditionally stated as a contraindication for use of nitrates, increased intraocular pressure probably is not a real problem. Occasionally edema of the legs can be seen, as with other vasodilators.

The undesirable effects of organic nitrates probably are correlated with the intensity of the vasodilator effect, and there is therefore no essential difference between the side-effects encountered with the different organic nitrates. With transdermal nitrate preparations, contact dermatitis can be seen.

An important problem with nitrates is the attenuation of their effects with chronic administration,[r35,r36,r37] a problem often somewhat inaccurately referred to as "nitrate tolerance" (see below). Workers in explosives industries knew well that their headaches occurred mainly on Monday morning and disappeared with continuous contact with the nitrates as the week went on. Headache on initial medical use of nitrates also wears off and disappears in many patients. The hemodynamic effects and the therapeutic efficacy also tend to decrease with continuous treatment, although it should not be assumed that disappearance of the headache equals disappearance of the therapeutic benefit, but exact quantitation of the attenuation of the nitrate effects is difficult. The attenuation has been found to be mainly pronounced with higher doses and short dosing intervals; uninterrupted application of nitroglycerin transdermal patches, which leads to sustained plasma concentrations of the nitrate, is accompanied by a rapid decrease of the effect, as well in angina pectoris as in cardiac failure. The same holds true for oral administration of sustained release formulations[31] and, probably to a lesser extent, also for IV administration.

The attenuation of the effects of nitrates with chronic use is probably due to more than one factor: on the one hand counterregulation, i.e., activation of hormones and baroreflex adaptation of the organism, as seen with all substances that influence the cardiovascular system; and on the other hand true tolerance, i.e., a decreased response of the vascular smooth muscle toward a given concentration of the nitrate. Vascular tolerance has been explained, within the framework of the suggested biochemical mechanism of vasodilation, as depletion of the sulfhydryl groups necessary for the formation of nitric oxide from nitrates (Fig. 24.2).[r35,r36,r37] Whether administration of sulfhydryl groups, e.g., with N-acetylcysteine[32] or the ACE-inhibitor captopril can reverse or prevent tolerance, is still a matter of debate. Similarly, studies on the blockade of the neurohumorally-mediated rebound vasoconstriction with, e.g., ACE-inhibitors gave equivocal results.[33]

There is cross-tolerance between the different organic nitrates, and probably also cross-attenuation of the therapeutic effects of these products.[r37] The sublingual administration of nitroglycerin or isosorbide dinitrate for the acute attack seems, however, still to be efficacious, even in patients who have been taking maintenance nitrate therapy for a long time.[25]

Clinically relevant pharmacokinetic interactions with nitrates have not been described. From a pharmacodynamic point of view one should be aware of the possibility that nitrates could interact with other cardiovascular drugs and, as such, lead to exaggerated hypotension, e.g., when treating patients with unstable angina simultaneously with nitrates, β-blockers, and calcium antagonists at high doses.

Resistance to heparin has been described in patients receiving IV nitroglycerin.[34,35]

Pharmacokinetics

After oral administration, nitroglycerin undergoes extensive hepatic first-pass extraction, and bioavailability is low and erratic. In contrast with what was thought formerly, nitroglycerin is efficacious after oral administration, possibly through formation of active metabolites, which are indeed present in plasma. After sublingual administration (tablets, liquids, spray) bioavailability of nitroglycerin is moderate. Transdermal absorption from traditional dermal preparations, and more recently from controlled release systems, has been well demonstrated.

Nitroglycerin is rapidly broken down to glyceryl dinitrates and glyceryl mononitrates (Fig. 24.1) that are less potent as vasodilators. This biotransformation takes place in the liver, but also elsewhere in the organism (blood, vascular wall). The half-life of disappearance of nitroglycerin from the plasma is of the order of a few minutes. The pharmacokinetics of nitroglycerin are still incompletely understood, and the usual pharmacokinetic models cannot be applied, probably because of the extremely rapid biotransformation of the substance and because of the role of extrahepatic elimination sites.[r39,r40]

Isosorbide dinitrate also undergoes hepatic first-pass extraction after oral administration, but to a lesser extent than nitroglycerin. It is transformed in the liver to the less potent metabolites isosorbide-2-mononitrate and isosorbide-5-mononitrate (Fig. 24.1), and its half-life of disappearance from plasma is probably of the order of 30 minutes. The pharmacokinetics of isosorbide-5-mononitrate and isosorbide-2-mononitrate have been studied extensively. They are rapidly and completely absorbed and there is no first-pass extraction; the half-life is about two hours for the 2-mononitrate and five hours for the 5-mononitrate. They are further biotransformed in the liver.[r40]

Pentaerythritol tetranitrate has been studied less than the other nitrates; there is also an important first-pass extraction and breakdown to partially denitrated substances with varying vasodilator potency.

After administration of glyceryl trinitrate, isosorbide dinitrate or pentaerythritol tetranitrate, plasma concentrations of the respective metabolites are often much higher than those of the parent products and they last longer. It is not known to what extent these metabolites contribute to the effects when the parent product has been given.[r40]

For many years, attempts have been made to obtain sustained concentrations of the nitrates in plasma in the hope of prolonging their therapeutic effect: this has led to development of oral slow-release nitrate preparations,[r1,r3] of a buccal delivery formulation that combines a rapid onset of action and protracted plasma levels,[23,36] and of transdermal controlled-release nitroglycerin systems.[r3] There is, however, no direct relationship between the plasma concentrations of the nitrates and the intensity and duration of their effect.[r41] This is due, at least in part, to the decreased effectiveness with continuous contact with the substances, as discussed above, but perhaps also to the presence of the vasoactive metabolites. Moreover, it could be that the effects are related to concentrations in the vascular smooth muscle cells and not to those in plasma. Attempts to define a "therapeutic plasma concentration range" for the nitrates have therefore not been successful.

The pharmacokinetics of the different organic nitrates have been studied extensively in disease states such as renal failure and cirrhosis; moreover, the kinetics of nitroglycerin are influenced by posture, exercise, etc.[r41,37] However, the clinical relevance of the concentration changes encountered in such situations is probably minor, and dose alterations are not necessary.

Available Preparations and Usual Doses

Nitroglycerin. *Sublingual*: tablets, chewable tablets, oral spray, usually 300 to 600 μg; start with a low dose and increase if necessary. Nitroglycerin tablets should be kept in an appropriate container to avoid loss of activity.

Oral: usually as slow-release preparations, containing several milligrams of the substance to be taken several times a day, to a total daily dose of 5 to 10 mg.

Buccal tablet (not yet available world-wide): to be placed in the buccal pouch between the upper teeth and the inner lip. Doses up to 10 mg every 4 to 6 hours may be needed, e.g., in unstable angina.

Transdermal: ointment, 20 mg or more per application, several times daily, or controlled delivery systems releasing 5, 10, 20 mg/24 hr. Doses to be adapted in consideration of efficacy and side-effects.

Intravenous: doses in the order of 0.6 to 12 mg/hr, to adapt to hemodynamic responses and side-effects.

Nitroglycerin in solution can be adsorbed to the surface of containers, to tubing etc., mainly to polyvinyl, less to glass or high-density polyethylene material. Use of high flow rates and presaturation can minimize the adsorption.[r34] When high doses (and volumes) are infused, the alcohol[38] or propylene glycol[39] content of some IV preparations may lead to toxicity.

Isosorbide Dinitrate. *Sublingual*: tablets or chewable tablets, usually 2.5 to 5 mg.

Oral: 5 to 20 mg 3 to 4 times daily; slow release preparations 2 to 3 times daily.

Intravenous: 2 to 10 mg/hr, to be adapted. Adsorption of isosorbide dinitrate to containers and tubing is less a problem than for nitroglycerin.

Isosorbide-5-Mononitrate. *Oral*: 20 to 40 mg 3 times daily.

Pentaerythrytol Tetranitrate. *Oral*: 20 to 40 mg 3 to 4 times daily.

Note. As mentioned before, attenuation of the effects with chronic administration probably occurs much more easily when plasma concentrations are kept constant. Therefore, it is better to introduce a nitrate-free period, e.g., by giving the oral preparations only in the morning and at noon, not at night-time, or by applying the nitroglycerin patch only 16 hours out of 24. The optimal length of this nitrate-free interval and the doses to be used are still to be determined.[r37]

Summary

Organic nitrates have been used in the treatment of angina pectoris for more than 100 years, and have now also been introduced in the treatment of congestive heart failure. For treatment or short-term prophylaxis of the acute attack, the sublingual administration

Nitro Dilator Summary Table

	Dosage			Pharmacokinetics		
Drug	**Route**	**Size**	**Dose**	**Peak**	$t_{1/2}$	**Cl or Duration of Response**
Nitroglycerin						
Nitrogard	Oral tablet Transmucosal	1, 2.3 mg	1 tablet initially	acts in 2–3 min.	1–4 min.	lasts 3–5 hours
Nitrostat	Oral tablet sublingual	0.15, 0.3, 0.4, 0.6 mg	1 tablet may repeat in 5 minutes	acts in 2 min.		lasts 30 minutes
Nitrolingual	Oral Spray	0.4 mg/dose	1–2 sprays			
NitroBid	Oral Capsule	2.5, 6.5, 9,13 mg	1 capsule initially			
Nitrostat	Parenteral	0.5, 0.8, 5 mg/ml		immediately	1–4 min.	
NitroDur	Topical Ointment	0.1, 0.2, 0.3, 0.4, 0.6 mg/hr	5μg/minute	acts in 30 min.		lasts 3 hours
Pentaerythritol Tetranitrate						
Peritrate	Oral tablet	10, 20, 40 mg	10–20 mg tid or qid	onset in 20 min.	10 min.	lasts 20–60 min.
Isosorbide						
Dinitrate	Oral tablets	5, 10, 20, 30, 40 mg	10–20 mg tid	onset 1 hour		lasts 5–6 hours
Isordil	Oral sublingual tablets	2.5, 5, 10 mg	2.5–10 mg	onset in 3 min.		lasts 2 hours
Erythrityl Tetranitrate						
Carditate	Oral tablet	10 mg	5–10 mg	acts in 5 min.		lasts 3 hours

of nitroglycerin or isosorbide dinitrate is still preferred. In maintenance treatment with oral preparations, nitrate-free intervals should be introduced in order to avoid the decrease of the effects seen when giving the substances with short intervals or as slow-release formulations. Full protection throughout the 24 hour-day is not possible with nitrates. Transdermal controlled release formulations are a technologic success, but here again the decrease of the effect with time does not allow their uninterrupted use. Intravenous nitrates are of interest in acute situations, such as unstable angina.

Beta-Adrenergic Blocking Agents

The β-blockers are described extensively elsewhere in this book. (see Chapters 25, 26) Their use in ischemic heart disease is discussed here.

History

Sir James Black, Nobel Prize winner in 1988, postulated that some substances with β-adrenergic antagonist properties that had been described in the literature could be of interest in the treatment of cardiac disease states where orthosympathetic stimulation is deleterious, such as angina pectoris. Due to Sir James' recommendation, the ICI company in the 1960s developed a series of β-blockers. The first clinical trials with these compounds proved Black's prediction to be correct. Since then, β-blockers have been extensively used in the maintenance therapy of angina pectoris[r1,r2,r3,r7,r8] and, of course, of other cardiovascular diseases.[r33] About 10 years ago, the value of β-blockers in the secondary prevention of myocardial infarction was proved in several trials.[r24,r25] β-blockers have also been given with some success in the acute phase of myocardial infarction,[r18] but their precise role in that situation is not clear.[r19]

Therapeutic Uses and Limitations

The therapeutic uses of β-blockers in ischemic heart disease can be defined as follows.

In *angina pectoris,* β-adrenergic blockers are used

as maintenance therapy of attacks elicited by exercise or emotion.[r1,r3] In angina at rest and in unstable angina, where a spastic component is thought to be present, β-blockers are, from a theoretical point of view, less appropriate, although they are often being used with success.[r2] In this respect, the ultra-short acting β-blocker esmolol should be mentioned. Indeed, because of its short half-life (9 min), esmolol can be titrated rapidly and safely in unstable angina.[40,41]

β-blockers are also used in patients with silent ischemia, where they reduce the number of ischemic episodes, even those not preceded by tachycardia.[r12,r13,r14,13] Comparative studies between antianginal drug classes show no clear-cut results, but β-blockers tend to be better than calcium-antagonists.[42] Beta-blockers also significantly attenuate the morning peak in ischemic activity—overt and silent—ascribed to the circadian variation in sympathetic tone,[43,44] whereas calcium antagonists do not.[44]

In all these situations, β-blockers are often used together with other drugs, such as nitrates and calcium antagonists, although reports on combined therapy reveal conflicting results.[r7,r8,r9,3,4,5,6,43]

In the *acute phase of myocardial infarction,* IV administration of cardioselective β-blockers has been shown to lead to a reduction of early mortality.[r18] With the success of the thrombolytic agents and of acetylsalicylic acid in the acute phase,[r4,r15,r16,14] the role of β-blockers during that period is not fully clarified; most authors, however, recommend the combination of β-blockers and thrombolytics.[r4,r19,15]

In *secondary prevention of myocardial infarction* many studies on large numbers of patients have been carried out. From the meta-analysis of these trials one can conclude that long-term treatment with β-blockers after myocardial infarction decreases mortality and/or the risk of cardiac death and/or reinfarction and/or sudden death by about one-fourth,[r24,r25,45,46,47,48,49] and this for at least three to six years.[r42,47,48] Furthermore, during the period following the withdrawal of the trial preparation in a chronic postinfarction metoprolol trial, mortality tended to be higher in those previously treated with metoprolol than in those previously treated with placebo.[50] Whether the β-blocker is well tolerated by the patient is obviously also a factor in deciding how long to continue the treatment. From these studies it is not possible to define exactly which patients will benefit and which will not. It is best to use a β-blocker for which a beneficial effect has been proved clearly in one of these studies: timolol,[47] propranolol,[45,46] metoprolol,[48] sotalol.[49] For the subgroup of patients with non-Q-wave infarction, however, the precise role of β-blockers in secondary prevention is not clear.[r43,51]

β-adrenergic blockers should be used only with utmost care in patients at risk for cardiac failure, atrioventricular block, and bronchospasm. In such patients it is often better to use other drugs, e.g., calcium antagonists.[r1,r3] Another option may be to titrate esmolol carefully, since clinical deterioration by β-blockade can be expected to be easily reversible by stopping the administration after this ultra-short acting β-blocker.[40,41]

Effects and Mechanism

The most important mechanism for the beneficial effect of β-blockers in angina pectoris is certainly the reduction of oxygen consumption: this reduction is brought about by a decrease of heart rate, of myocardial contractility, and of ventricular systolic pressure; the accompanying increase in intraventricular volume and myocardial tension, however, tends to counteract partially the reduction in oxygen requirement.[r1,r2,r3,r7] Whether other properties, such as the anti-aggregating effect or redistribution of coronary flow, are important is not known. The mechanism of the protective effect during the acute phase of acute myocardial infarction and in secondary prophylaxis also is likewise not clear: factors such as decreased orthosympathetic tone, reduction of infarct size, and anti-arrhythmic effect could be important.[52]

Ancillary properties such as partial β-agonism and β_2-agonism, resulting in vaso- and bronchodilatory properties probably do not have a major impact on the efficacy of these drugs in ischemic heart disease.[53] There have, however, been suggestions that substances with partial agonism are less suitable in secondary prophylaxis after myocardial infarction;[r24,r25,54] furthermore, this property could be deleterious in patients who develop angina pectoris at very low heart rate increases. Whether the metabolic effects of the β-blockers[r44] (see below) influence the evolution of ischemic heart disease during long-term treatment, e.g., of angina pectoris or in secondary prophylaxis, is not known, as well-controlled long-term studies are not available.

Undesirable Effects and Interactions

The undesirable effects of these substances are described in detail elsewhere, but some points particularly relevant in patients with ischemic heart disease are taken up here. Congestive heart failure can be precipitated or worsened, although some recent studies suggest a beneficial effect of small doses of β-blockers in selected subgroups with heart failure.[55,56] In patients with bronchospasm, β-blockers should be avoided in situations where alternatives, e.g., calcium antagonists, are available.[r1,r3] The feeling of fatigue and lack of drive are often major handicaps, mainly in active patients without symptoms, as in secondary prophylaxis after myocardial infarction.[r3,r24]

Lipid changes (increased triglycerides and decreased HDL-cholesterol) are seen mainly with nonselective agents without partial agonism, less with cardioselective agents, and even less with agents with partial agonism.[r44] It is not known what the impact of these "atherogenic" changes is on prognosis. Nevertheless, the metabolic changes induced have been cited as possible reasons why, in long-term trials of β-blockers in patients with mild hypertension, ischemic heart disease was not favorably influenced, although global prognosis was improved, mainly through a decrease of the incidence of stroke.[r33]

After abrupt stopping of chronic β-blocker therapy in patients with severe ischemic heart disease and/or hypertension, rebound phenomena with worsening of angina, ventricular arrhythmias, and sudden death have been observed.[r3,57] Although the extent of this problem is not known, β-blocker therapy should, when possible, be stopped gradually, e.g., by reducing the dose to 50 percent and then to 25 percent over several days.

Pharmacodynamic drug interactions between β-adrenergic blocking agents and calcium antagonists should be mentioned here, as substances of these two classes are often combined in patients with ischemic heart disease. One should be aware of the possibility of excessive bradycardia, blood pressure fall, and cardiodepression with such a combination. Calcium antagonists with an important cardiac depressant or heart rate-lowering effect, such as verapamil and diltiazem, carry a higher risk for untoward interaction with β-blockers than do calcium antagonists with higher vascular selectivity, such as the dihydropyridines.[r7,r8,r45] One should never give a calcium antagonist IV when the patient is taking a β-blocker, and vice versa, unless continuous monitoring and possibilities for direct intervention and resuscitation are available.[r45] Pretreatment with IV calcium chloride could perhaps attenuate this interaction.

Pharmacokinetic interactions with β-blockers are possible. As β-blockers decrease cardiac output and splanchnic blood flow, they can alter the presystemic (first pass) and the postsystemic hepatic elimination of drugs with a high hepatic extraction, such as lidocaine and the calcium antagonists. In fact, many β-blockers are high-extraction substances and as such can alter their own hepatic elimination.

Available Preparations and Usual Doses

Beta-blockers are usually given orally but some of them are also available for IV use, e.g., in arrhythmias or in the acute phase of myocardial infarction.

The doses used in angina pectoris are those leading to inhibition of exercise or stress-induced tachycardia; the daily dose and rhythm of administration will depend on the agent used, but also on patient characteristics. The degree of β-blockade cannot be judged solely from the heart rate at rest: dose adaptation should be done preferentially on the basis of exercise testing, but only on condition that this procedure is not dangerous for the patient concerned.[r3] Slow-release preparations can be used to limit the need for frequent administration.

The optimal dosage of β-blockers for secondary prevention after myocardial infarction is not clear. Indeed, in most studies a fixed dosage was administered. Consequently, one can only state that for the whole group 10 mg timolol b.i.d. (5 mg b.i.d. for the first two days),[47] 60–80 mg propranolol t.i.d. (according to blood propranolol levels, and after gradually increasing the dosage),[45,46] 100 mg metoprolol b.i.d. (50 mg t.i.d. for the first three days)[48] or sotalol (320 mg once daily)[49] offer some benefit. Whether higher or lower doses offer more protection, e.g., in some subgroups, is unknown.

Summary

Beta-blockers are used in the maintenance treatment of angina pectoris and silent ischemia and in unstable angina. In the latter patients and in patients where a spastic component is important, care should be taken because in some individuals β-blockers could be deleterious. The choice of a particular β-blocker, or of a β-blocker instead of a calcium antagonist, will depend on the characteristics of the individual patient.

Beta-blockers are used with success in the secondary prophylaxis of myocardial infarction. In the acute phase of myocardial infarction, monotherapy with β-blockers also has been shown to be beneficial; their role in the thrombolytic era is, however, not clear.

Calcium Entry Blockers

Calcium-entry blockers (or calcium antagonists) are used in the treatment of different disease states, mainly of the cardiovascular system. The calcium antagonists used in ischemic heart disease belong to WHO classes 1 to 3[r46] i.e., drugs selective for slow Ca^{++}-classes: the phenylethylamines (verapamil), the benzothiazepines (diltiazem), and the dihydropyridines (nifedipine, nisoldipine, isradipine). Recently, bepridil, a combined sodium-calcium channel blocker belonging to the group of drugs not selective for slow Ca^{++} channels, was introduced.[58,59] These drugs are discussed more completely in Chapters 23, 25 and 28. Only aspects of importance to their use in angina pectoris will be reviewed here.

History

In the 1960s calcium antagonists were used in Prinzmetal angina. When coronary spasm was discovered as being important in many other patients with ischemic heart disease, calcium antagonists were also used in these situations. Nowadays, these agents have also proved to be useful in exercise-induced angina.

Therapeutic Uses and Limitations

In *angina pectoris* the calcium antagonists are frequently used in maintenance treatment of both exercise-induced attacks and rest attacks.[r1,r3,r7,60,61,62,63,64,65] The choice between β-blockers and calcium antagonists will often be based on possible contraindications and/or expected or observed side-effects. Well-controlled studies, especially long-term studies, comparing the therapeutic effects of calcium antagonists and β-blockers are scarce, and generally show little differences.[r7,3,5,65] Factors in favor of β-blockers, however, are the retrospective observations that patients treated with a β-blocker may have a better outcome if myocardial infarction occurs,[66,67] and the finding that nifedipine and probably also the other dihydropyridines may increase the frequency of ischemic periods in patients with stable angina pectoris and good collateral flow, probably because of a coronary steal phenomenon.[68] In some patients β-blockers and/or calcium antagonists and/or nitrates are combined, although conclusive trials showing improved efficacy or fewer side-effects for the same efficacy are scarce.[r7,r8,r9,3,4,5,6] There seems to be little or no difference in efficacy between calcium antagonists in the treatment of stable angina pectoris,[60,61,63,64,65] although it cannot be excluded that for a particular patient one calcium antagonist could be better than another[59,61,62] and that some patients may benefit from a combination of calcium antagonists from different classes.[61,64]

Nifedipine can be used for treatment of acute angina attacks (after biting the capsule, the liquid should be swallowed), but it seems to have no advantage over the sublingual nitrates.

Calcium antagonists are also used in patients with *silent ischemia.* Their definite place, like that of other agents, is still not clear, although most data suggest that calcium antagonists, especially nifedipine and probably also the other dihydropyridines, are less effective than β-blockers.[r12,r13,r14,13,42,44,68]

In *unstable angina,* in view of the role of coronary spasm, the calcium antagonists seem at first sight the agents of choice.[r2,r6,9,10,69] The results obtained with these agents, however, have been variable, and in some studies a deleterious effect, i.e., more frequent progression toward myocardial infarction, was seen.[r22,8] The difference in outcome seen in different studies may be due to the choice of the agent, because for different calcium antagonists the balance between cardiac depression and peripheral vasodilation is different. One should keep in mind, however, that patient selection in these studies was not uniform, and no comparative trial of different calcium antagonists was carried out in this situation. Moreover, the response to calcium antagonists in unstable angina is probably to a large extent dependent on individual patient characteristics, e.g., the degree of coronary spasm. It is therefore likely that in a given patient a calcium antagonist of one class could be beneficial, but one of another class deleterious. Unfortunately, definition of these patient characteristics and prediction of the outcome with a particular agent are not possible at this moment.

The role of calcium antagonists, especially dihydropyridines, in the *acute and chronic phases of myocardial infarction* is probably limited.[r16,r22,r23,70,71] With diltiazem started 24–72 hr after myocardial infarction, reduction of cardiac events was seen in patients with non-Q-wave infarction.[17] In patients without left ventricular dysfunction, chronic diltiazem treatment may reduce cardiac mortality and reinfarction, but in the same study an increase of cardiac events was seen in patients with left ventricular dysfunction.[18] Similarly, verapamil started several days after myocardial infarction may prevent death and reinfarction,[19] especially in patients without impaired cardiac function.[72] Consequently, as in unstable angina, it could be that only a subpopulation within myocardial infarction patients benefits from calcium antagonist therapy, and that there are differences between calcium antagonist classes.

Effects and Mechanisms

The cellular mechanism of calcium-entry blockade is discussed in Chapter 23. Both (1) vascular effects (coronary dilation, increase in venous capacitance with decreased preload, and decrease of the arterial resistance with decreased afterload) and (2) cardiac effects (depression of myocardial contractility and heart rate) are important determinants of the beneficial effect in ischemic heart disease.[r3,r7,r9,r45]

The relative contribution of these factors will depend on the properties of the calcium antagonist used and on the characteristics of the patient. The dihydropyridines present more vascular selectivity (i.e., less cardiac depression for the same degree of peripheral vasodilation) than verapamil. Newer dihydropyridine molecules with more vascular selectivity than nifedipine have been developed. It is not clear, however, whether such pharmacologic differences are relevant to clinical efficacy (and to side-effect incidence).[73]

The clinical relevance of the antiatherosclerotic properties of calcium entry blockers is unclear. In two studies dihydropyridines were found to have no effect on advanced coronary atherosclerosis. They may, however, slow down the progression of minimal lesions or suppress the appearance of new lesions.[74,75]

Undesirable Effects and Interactions

These are discussed in detail elsewhere. In patients with ischemic heart disease, particular attention should be paid to the peripheral vasodilation, which may lead to a fall in systemic blood pressure, coronary hypoperfusion, and reflex tachycardia. These effects are more important for dihydropyridines and have been suggested as possible explanations for unfavorable effects of calcium antagonists seen in some studies.[r16] Paradoxical angina, i.e., increased frequency and severity of anginal attacks, probably due to coronary hypoperfusion and reflex tachycardia, has been described mainly with nifedipine.[68] Whether paradoxical angina also occurs with other dihydropyridines is unclear, mainly because clinical experience with the other agents is less extensive.

Calcium antagonists have been shown not to interfere with lipid and carbohydrate metabolism, and this could be important in the long-term treatment of patients with ischemic heart disease, although there is no proof for the clinical relevance thereof.

Interactions of calcium antagonists with β-blockers have been discussed in the section on β-blockers.

Available Preparations and Usual Doses

For treatment of ischemic heart disease, the calcium antagonists are routinely given via the oral route. The doses for nifedipine are 10 to 20 mg three times daily; for nicardipine 20 to 30 mg three times daily; for verapamil 40 to 120 mg three times daily; for diltiazem 60 mg three times daily; for bepridil 100–400 mg daily; the doses have to be adapted according to efficacy and side-effects.

For some calcium antagonists, slow release preparations are available that allow twice-or once-daily dosing; for nifedipine, in one study an improvement in anti-ischemic efficacy was found with a slow-release GI therapy system (acronym: GITS).[r47]

In angina attacks nifedipine solution can be swallowed, e.g., after biting the capsule, although no advantage above nitrates is to be expected.

Diltiazem also can be administered IV with a bolus of 0.15 to 0.25 mg/kg over 2 min followed by 10 to 20 mg/hr.

Summary

Calcium antagonists are used in many cardiovascular diseases. In ischemic heart disease they are useful mainly in angina pectoris, perhaps also in silent ischemia. They have a limited role in unstable angina. There seems to be no major role for calcium antagonists in the acute phase of myocardial infarction or in the secondary prophylaxis after acute myocardial infarction, except perhaps for diltiazem after non-Q-wave infarction.

Various Substances

Besides nitrates, β-blockers, and calcium antagonists, some other substances are also used as antiischemic agents. For *dipyridamole,* besides its antiaggregating properties, an antianginal efficacy has been claimed, but a clear-cut benefit has not been shown[r48] and the possibility of coronary steal has been suggested.

Amiodarone, which is described in detail with the antiarrhythmic agents, has definite antianginal properties. However, in view of its side-effects, its use is limited to patients with angina pectoris not responding to the usual antianginal drugs, and is not widely accepted. Its prophylactic use after infarction is under study.[r29]

Molsidomine is converted in the organism to the vasoactive metabolite sin-1A, which, as nitroglycerine, activates guanylate cyclase and leads to dilation of vascular smooth muscle (Fig. 24.2). Its hemodynamic effects and, probably, also its efficacy and side-effects are rather similar to those of the nitrates. In view of the direct effect of molsidomine on guanylate cyclase, without involvement of sulfhydryl groups, there is much interest in the possibility that tolerance would not occur with this substance.[76,77] Some data suggest more inhibition of platelet inhibition with molsidomine than with nitrates.[78]

References

Research Reports

1. Rogers WJ, Coggin CJ, Gersh BJ, Fisher LD, Myers WO, Oberman A, Sheffield LT for the CASS investigators. Ten-year follow-up of quality of life in patients randomized to receive medical therapy or coronary artery bypass graft surgery. Circulation 1990;*82*:1647–1658.
2. Baim DS. Angioplasty as a treatment for coronary artery disease. N Engl J Med 1992;*326*:56–58.
3. Findlay IN, MacLeod K, Ford M, Gillen G, Elliott AT, Dargie HJ. Treatment of angina pectoris with nifedipine and atenolol: efficacy and effect on cardiac function. Brit Heart J 1986;*55*:240–245.
4. El-Tamimi H, Davies GJ, Kaski J-C, Vejar M, Galassi AR, Maseri A. Effects of diltiazem alone or with isosorbide dinitrate or with atenolol both acutely and chronically for stable angina pectoris. Am J Cardiol 1989;*64*:717–724.
5. Hill JA, Gonzalez JI, Kolb R, Pepine CJ. Effects of atenolol alone, nifedipine alone and their combination on ambulant myocardial ischemia. Am J Cardiol 1991;*67*:671–675.
6. Akhras F, Jackson G. Efficacy of nifedipine and isosorbide mononitrate in combination with atenolol in stable angina. Lancet 1991;*338*:1036–1039.
7. Juul-Möller S, Edvardsson N, Jahnmatz B, Rosén A, Sorensen S, Ömblus R for the Swedish Angina Pectoris Aspirin Trial (SAPAT) Group. Double-blind trial of aspirin in primary prevention of myocardial infarction in patients with stable chronic angina pectoris. Lancet 1992;*340*:1421–1425.
8. Holland Interuniversity Nifedipine/Metoprolol Trial (HINT) Research Group. Early treatment of unstable angina in the coronary care unit: a randomised, double blind, placebo controlled comparison of recurrent ischaemia in patients treated with nifedipine or metoprolol or both. Brit Heart J 1986;*56*:400–413.
9. André-Fouet X, Usdin JP, Gayet Ch, Wilner C, Thizy JF, Viallet M, Apoil E, Vernant P, Pont M. Comparison of short-term efficacy of diltiazem and propranolol in unstable angina at rest. A randomized trial in 70 patients. Eur Heart J 1983;*4*:691–698.

10. Colombo G, Zucchella G, Planca E, Grieco A. Intravenous diltiazem in the treatment of unstable angina : a study of efficacy and tolerance. Clin Ther 1987;*9*:536–547.

11. Théroux P, Ouimet H, McCans J, Latour J-G, Joly P, Lévy G, Pelletier ED, Juneau M, Stasiak J, DeGujise P, Pelletier GB, Rinzler D, Waters DD. Aspirin, heparin, or both to treat acute unstable angina. N Engl J Med 1988;*319*:1105–1111.

12. Lewis HD, Davis JW, Archibald DG, Steinke WE, Smitherman TC, Doherty JE, Schnaper HW, LeWinter MM, Linares E, Pouget JM, Sabharwal SC, Chesler E, DeMots H. Protective effects of aspirin against acute myocardial infarction and death in men with unstable angina. N Engl J Med 1983;*309*:396–403.

13. Koehn DK, Glasser SP. The impact of antianginal drug therapy on asymptomatic myocardial ischemia. J Clin Pharmacol 1989;*29*:722–727.

14. ISIS-2 (Second International Study of Infarct Survival) collaborative group. Randomised trial of intravenous streptokinase, oral aspirin, both, or neither among 17,187 cases of suspected acute myocardial infarction : ISIS-2. Lancet 1988;*ii*:349–360.

15. TIMI Study Group. Comparison of invasive and conservative strategies after treatment with intravenous tissue plasminogen activator in acute myocardial infarction. N Engl J Med 1989;*320*:618–627.

16. Swedberg K, Held P, Kjekshus J, Rasmussen K, Rydén L, Wedel H. on behalf of the CONSENSUS II Study Group. Effects of the early administration of enalapril on mortality in patients with acute myocardial infarction. N Engl J Med 1992;*327*:678–684.

17. Gibson RS, Boden WE, Théroux P, Strauss HD, Pratt CM, Gheorghiade M, Capone RJ, Crawford MH, Schlant RC, Kleiger RE, Young PM, Schechtman K, Perryman MB, Roberts R and the Diltiazem Reinfarction Study Group. Diltiazem and reinfarction in patients with non-Q-wave myocardial infarction. N Engl J Med 1986;*315*:423–429.

18. The Multicenter Diltiazem Postinfarction Trial Research Group. The effect of diltiazem on mortality and reinfarction after myocardial infarction. N Engl J Med 1988;*319*:385–392.

19. The Danish Study Group on Verapamil in Myocardial Infarction. Effect of verapamil on mortality and major events after acute myocardial infarction (The Danish Verapamil Infarction Trial II - DAVIT II). Am J Cardiol 1990;*66*:779–785.

20. Conti CR. Use of nitrates in unstable angina pectoris. Am J Cardiol 1987;*60*:31H–34H.

21. Kaplan K, Davison R, Parker M, Przybylek J, Teagarden JR, Lesch M. Intravenous nitroglycerin for the treatment of angina at rest unresponsive to standard nitrate therapy. Am J Cardiol 1983;*51*:694–698.

22. Laslett LJ, Baker L. Sublingual nitroglycerin administered by spray versus tablet: comparative timing of hemodynamic effects. Cardiology 1990;*77*:303–310.

23. Bray CL, Jain S, Faragher EB, Myers A, Myers P, MacIntyre P, Rae A, Goldman M, Alcorn M. A comparison of buccal nitroglycerin and sublingual nitroglycerin in the prophylaxis and treatment of exertional (situation-provoked) angina pectoris. Eur Heart J 1991;*12*(Suppl A):16–20.

24. Reichek N, Goldstein RE, Redwood DR, Epstein SE. Sustained effects of nitroglycerin ointment in patients with angina pectoris. Circulation 1974;*50*:348–352.

25. de Milliano PA, Koster RW, Bär FW, Janssen J, de Cock C, Schelling A, van de Bos A. Long-term efficacy of continuous and intermittent use of transdermal nitroglycerin in stable angina pectoris. Am J Cardiol 1991;*68*:857–862.

26. Gumbrielle T, Freedman SB, Fogarty L, Ogasawara S, Sobb P, Kelly DT. Efficacy, safety and duration of nitrate-free interval to prevent tolerance to transdermal nitroglycerin in effort angina. Eur Heart J 1992;*13*:671–678.

27. Bassan M. The day-long antianginal effectiveness of nitroglycerin patches. A double-blind study using dose-titration. Chest 1991;*99*:1120–1125.

28. Waters DD, Juneau M, Gossard D, Choquette G, Brien M. Limited usefulness of intermittent nitroglycerin patches in stable angina. JACC 1989;*13*:421–425.

29. Figueras J, Lidon R, Cortadellas J. Rebound myocardial ischaemia following abrupt interruption of intravenous nitroglycerin infusion in patients with unstable angina at rest. Eur Heart J 1991;*12*:405–411.

30. Rehnqvist N, Olsson G, Engvall J, Rosenqvist U, Nyberg G, Aberg A, Ulvenstam G, Uusitalo A, Keyriläinen O, Reinikainen P, Härkönen R, Nilsson B. Abrupt withdrawal of isosorbide-5-mononitrate in Durules[R] (Imdur[R]) after long term treatment in patients with stable angina pectoris. Eur Heart J 1988;*9*:1339–1347.

31. Bassan MM. The daylong pattern of the antianginal effect of long-term three times daily administered isosorbide dinitrate. JACC 1990;*16*:936–940.

32. Boesgaard S, Aldershvile J, Enghusen Poulsen H. Preventive administration of intravenous N-acetylcysteine and development of tolerance to isosorbide dinitrate in patients with angina pectoris. Circulation 1992;*85*:143–149.

33. Katz RJ, Levy WS, Buff L, Wasserman AG. Prevention of nitrate tolerance with angiotensin converting enzyme inhibitors. Circulation 1991;*83*:1271–1277.

34. Becker RC, Corrao JM, Bovill EG, Gore JM, Baker SP, Miller ML, Lucas FV, Alpert JA. Intravenous nitroglycerin-induced heparin resistance : a qualitative antithrombin III abnormality. Am Heart J 1990;*119*:1254–1261.

35. Habbab MA, Haft JI. Heparin resistance induced by intravenous nitroglycerin. Arch Intern Med 1987;*147*:857–860.

36. Dellborg M, Gustafsson G, Swedberg K. Buccal versus intravenous nitroglycerin in unstable angina pectoris. Eur J Clin Pharmacol 1991;*41*:5–9.

37. Lefebvre RA, Bogaert MG, Teirlynck O, Sioufi A, Dubois JP. Influence of exercise on nitroglycerin plasma concentrations after transdermal application. Brit J Clin Pharmacol 1990;*30*:292–296.

38. Shook TL, Kirshenbaum JM, Hundley RF, Shorey JM, Lamas GA. Ethanol intoxication complicating intravenous nitroglycerin therapy. Ann Intern Med 1984;*101*:498–499.

39. Demey H, Daelemans R, De Broe ME, Bossaert L. Propyleneglycol intoxication due to intravenous nitroglycerin. Lancet 1984;*I*:1360.

40. Hohnloser SH, Meinertz T, Klingenheben T, Sydow B, Just H, for the European Esmolol Study Group. Usefulness of esmolol in unstable angina pectoris. Am J Cardiol 1991;*67*:1319–1323.

41. Barth C, Ojile M, Pearson AC, Labovitz AJ. Ultra short-acting intravenous β-adrenergic blockade as add-on therapy in acute unstable angina. Am Heart J 1991;*121*:782–788.

42. Stone PH, Gibson RS, Glasser SP, DeWood MA, Parker JD, Kawanishi DT, Crawford MH, Messineo FC, Shook TL, Raby K, Curtis DG, Hoop RS, Young PM, Braunwald E, ASIS Study Group. Comparison of propranolol, diltiazem, and nifedipine in the treatment of ambulatory ischemia in patients with stable angina. Circulation 1990;*82*:1962–1972.

43. Egstrup K. Attenuation of circadian variation by combined antianginal therapy with suppression of morning and evening increases in transient myocardial ischemia. Am Heart J 1991;*122*:648–655.

44. Mulcahy D, Keegan J, Cunningham D, Quyyumi A, Crean P, Park A, Wright C, Fox K. Circadian variation of total ischaemic burden and its alteration with anti-anginal agents. Lancet 1988;*ii*:755–759.

45. Beta-blocker Heart Attack Trial Research Group. A randomized trial of propranolol in patients with acute myocardial infarction. I. Mortality results. JAMA 1982;*247*:1707–1714.

46. Beta-blocker Heart Attack Trial Research Group. A randomized trial of propranolol in patients with acute myocardial infarction. II. Morbidity results. JAMA 1983;*250*:2814–2819.

47. Pedersen TR for the Norwegian Multicenter Study Group. Six-year follow-up of the Norwegian Multicenter Study on timolol after acute myocardial infarction. N Engl J Med 1985;*313*:1055–1058.

48. Olsson G, Rehnqvist N, Sjögren A, Erhardt L, Lundman T. Long-term treatment with metoprolol after myocardial infarction: effect on 3 year mortality and morbidity. JACC 1985;*5*:1428–1437.

49. Julian DG, Prescott RJ, Jackson FS, Szekely P. Controlled trial of sotalol for one year after myocardial infarction. Lancet 1982;*i*:1142–1147.

50. Olsson G, Odén A, Johansson L, Sjögren A, Rehnqvist N. Prognosis after withdrawal of chronic postinfarction metoprolol treatment : a 2–7 year follow-up. Eur Heart J 1988;*9*:365–372.

51. Yusuf S, Wittes J, Probstfield J. Evaluating effects of treatment in subgroups of patients within a clinical trial: the case of non-Q-wave myocardial infarction and beta blockers. Am J Cardiol 1990;*66*:220–222.

52. ISIS-1 Collaborative Group. Mechanisms for the early mortality reduction produced by beta-blockade started early in acute myocardial infarction : ISIS-1. Lancet 1988;*i*:921–923.

53. Frishman WH, Heiman M, Soberman J, Greenberg S, Eff J for the Celiprolol International Angina Study Group. Comparison of celiprolol and propranolol in stable angina pectoris. Am J Cardiol 1991;*67*:665–670.

54. Boissel J-P, Leizorovicz A, Picolet H, Peyrieux J-C for the APSI Investigators. Secondary prevention after high-risk acute myocardial infarction with low-dose acebutolol. Am J Cardiol 1990;*66*:251–260.

55. Waagstein F, Caidahl K, Wallentin I, Bergh C-H, Hjalmarson A. Long-term β-blockade in congestive cardiomyopathy: effects of short- and long-term metoprolol treatment followed by withdrawal and readministration of metoprolol. Circulation 1989;*80*:551–563.

56. Swedberg K, Hjalmarson A, Waagstein F, Wallentin I. Beneficial effects of long-term β-blockade in congestive cardiomyopathy. Brit Heart J 1980;*44*:117–133.

57. Psaty BM, Koepsell TD, Wagner EH, LoGerfo JP, Inui TS. The relative risk of incident coronary heart disease associated with recently stopping the use of β-blockers. JAMA 1990;*263*:1653–1657.

58. B.I.S. Research Group. Controlled clinical trial of bepridil, propranolol and placebo in the treatment of exercise induced angina pectoris. Fund Clin Pharmacol 1989;*3*:597–611.

59. Singh BN for the Bepridil Collaborative Study Group. Comparative efficacy and safety of bepridil and diltiazem in chronic stable angina pectoris refractory to diltiazem. Am J Cardiol 1991;*68*:306–312.

60. Ardissino D, Savonitto S, Mussini A, Zanini P, Rolla A, Barberis P, Sardina M, Specchia G. Felodipine (once daily) versus nifedipine (four times daily) for Prinzmetal's angina pectoris. Am J Cardiol 1991;*68*:1587–1592.

61. De Caprio L, Acanfora D, Odierna L, DiPalma A, Romaniello C, Rengo C, Giordano A, Rengo F. Acute effects of nifedipine, diltiazem and their combination in patients with chronic stable angina : a double-blind, randomized, cross-over, placebo-controlled study. Eur Heart J 1993;*14*:416–420.

62. Subramanian VB, Bowles MJ, Khurmi NS, Davies AB, Raftery EB. Rationale for the choice of calcium antagonists in chronic stable angina. Am J Cardiol 1982;*50*:1173–1179.

63. Crean PA, Waters DD, Lam J, Chaitman BR. Comparative antianginal effects of nisoldipine and nifedipine in patients with chronic stable angina. Am Heart J 1987;*113*:261–265.

64. Pucci PD, Pollavini G, Zerauscheck M, Fazzini P. Acute effects on exercise tolerance of felodipine and diltiazem, alone and in combination, in stable effort angina. Eur Heart J 1991;*12*:55–59.

65. Chaitman BR, Wagniart P, Pasternac A, Brevers G, Scholl J-M, Lam J, Methe M, Ferguson RJ, Bourassa MG. Improved exercise tolerance after propranolol, diltiazem or nifedipine in angina pectoris : comparison at 1, 3 and 8 hours and correlation with plasma drug concentration. Am J Cardiol 1984;*53*:1–9.

66. Nidorf SM, Parsons RW, Thompson PL, Jamrozik KD, Hobbs MST. Reduced risk of death at 28 days in patients taking a β-blocker before admission to hospital with myocardial infarction. BMJ 1990;*300*:71–74.

67. Ellis SG, Muller DW, Topol EJ. Possible survival benefit from concomitant beta- but not calcium-antagonist therapy during reperfusion for acute myocardial infarction. Am J Cardiol 1990;*66*:125–128.

68. Egstrup K, Andersen PE. Transient myocardial ischemia during nifedipine therapy in stable angina pectoris, and its relation to coronary collateral flow and comparison with metoprolol. Am J Cardiol 1993;*71*:177–183.

69. Mehta J, Pepine CJ, Day M, Guerrero JR, Contl CR. Short-term efficacy of oral verapamil in rest angina. A double-blind placebo-controlled trial in CCU patients. Am J Med 1981;*71*:977–982.

70. Wilcox RG, Hampton JR, Banks DC, Birkhead JS, Brooksby IAB, Burns-Cox CJ, Hayes MJ, Joy MD, Malcolm AD, Mather HG, Rowley JM. Trial of early nifedipine in acute myocardial infarction: the Trent study. BMJ 1986;*293*:1204–1208.

71. The Danish Study Group on Verapamil in Myocardial Infarction. Verapamil in acute myocardial infarction. Eur Heart J 1984;*5*:516–528.

72. Jespersen CM and the Danish Study Group on Verapamil in Myocardial Infarction. The effect of verapamil on major events in patients with impaired cardiac function recovering from acute myocardial infarction. Eur Heart J 1993;*14*:540–545.

73. Currie P, Saltissi S. Isradipine therapy in chronic stable angina pectoris—comparison with nifedipine. Eur Heart J 1991;*12*:807–812.

74. Lichtlen PR, Hugenholtz PG, Rafflenbeul W, Hecker H, Jost S, Deckers JW on behalf of the INTACT Group investigators. Retardation of angiographic progression of coronary artery disease by nifedipine. Lancet 1990;*335*:1109–1113.

75. Waters D, Lespérance J, Francetich M, Causey D, Théroux P, Chiang Y-K, Hudon G, Lemarbre L, Reitman M, Joyal M, Gosselin G, Dyrda I, Macer J, Havel RJ. A controlled clinical trial to assess the effect of a calcium channel blocker on the progression of coronary atherosclerosis. Circulation 1990;*82*:1940–1953.

76. Wagner F, Gohlke-Bärwolf C, Trenk D, Jähnchen E, Roskamm H. Differences in the antiischaemic effects of molsidomine and isosorbide dinitrate (ISDN) during acute and short-term administration in stable angina pectoris. Eur Heart J 1991;*12*:994–999.

77. Dalla-Volta S, Scorzelli L, Razzolini R. Evaluation of the chronic antianginal effect of molsidomine. Am Heart J 1985;*109*:682–684.

78. Drummer C, Valta-Seufzer U, Karrenbrock B, Heim J-M, Gerzer R. Comparison of anti-platelet properties of molsidomine, isosorbide-5-mononitrate and placebo in healthy volunteers. Eur Heart J 1991;*12*:541–549.

Reviews

r1. Thadani U. Medical therapy of stable angina pectoris. Cardiology Clinics 1991;*9*:73–87.

r2. Gottlieb SO, Flaherty JT. Medical therapy of unstable angina pectoris. Cardiology Clinics 1991;*9*:89–98.

r3. Shub C. Stable angina pectoris: 3. Medical treatment. Mayo Clin Proc 1990;*65*:256–273.

r4. American College of Cardiology/American Heart Association Task Force on Assessment of Diagnostic and Therapeutic Cardiovascular Procedures. ACC/AHA guidelines for the early management of patients with acute myocardial infarction. Circulation 1990;*82*:664–707.

r5. Fuster V, Badimon L, Badimon JJ, Chesebro JH. The pathogenesis of coronary artery disease and the acute coronary syndromes (I+II). N Engl J Med 1992;*326*:242–250, 310–318.

r6. Selwyn AP, Yeung AC, Ryan TJ, Raby K, Barry J, Ganz P. Pathophysiology of ischemia in patients with coronary artery disease. Progr Cardiovasc Dis 1992;*35*:27–39.

r7. Challenor VF, Waller DG, George CF. Beta-adrenoceptor antagonists plus nifedipine in the treatment of chronic stable angina pectoris. Cardiovasc Drugs Therap 1989;*3*:275–285.

r8. Packer M. Combinated beta-adrenergic and calcium-entry blockade in angina pectoris. N Engl J Med 1989;*320*:709–718.

r9. Lessem JN, Singh BN. Calcium channel antagonism and beta blockade in combination—a therapeutic alternative in cardiovascular disorders. A review. Cardiovasc Drugs Ther 1989;*3*:355–373.

r10. Hilton TC, Chaitman BR. The prognosis in stable and unstable angina. Cardiology Clinics 1991;*9*:27–38.

r11. Cohn JN. The prevention of heart failure. A new agenda. N Engl J Med 1992;*327*:725–727.

r12. Epstein SE, Quyyumi AA, Bonow RO. Myocardial ischemia—silent or symptomatic. N Engl J Med 1988;*318*:1038–1043.

r13. Bertolet BD, Hill JA, Pepine CJ. Treatment strategies for daily life silent myocardial ischemia : a correlation with potential pathogenic mechanisms. Progr Cardiovasc Dis 1992;*35*:97–118.

r14. Gottlieb SO. Asymptomatic or silent myocardial ischemia in angina pectoris: pathophysiology and clinical implications. Cardiology Clinics 1991;*9*:49–61.

r15. Rapaport E. Thrombolytic agents in acute myocardial infarction. N Engl J Med 1989;*320*:861–864.

r16. Yusuf S, Sleight P, Held P, McMahon S. Routine medical management of acute myocardial infarction. Lessons from overviews of recent randomized controlled trials. Circulation 1990;*82*(Supp II): 117–134.

r17. Nattel S, Arenal A. Antiarrhythmic prophylaxis after acute myocardial infarction. Drugs 1993;*45*:9–14.

r18. Sleight P. Early intravenous β-adrenoceptor blockade for victims of heart attack. TIPS 1988;*9*:52–54.

r19. Sobolski JC. What data support our current thrombolytic management of patients with acute myocardial infarction? Progr Cardiovasc Dis 1992;*34*:367–378.

r20. Shechter M, Kaplinsky E, Rabinowitz B. The rationale of magnesium supplementation in acute myocardial infarction. A review of the literature. Arch Intern Med 1992;*152*:2189–2196.

r21. Yusuf S, Collins R, MacMahon S, Peto R. Effect of intravenous nitrates on mortality in acute myocardial infarction: an overview of the randomised trials. Lancet 1988;*i*:1088–1092.

r22. Held PH, Yusuf S, Furberg CD. Calcium channel blockers in acute myocardial infarction and unstable angina: an overview. BMJ 1989;*299*:1187–1192.

r23. Yusuf S, Held P, Furberg C. Update of effects of calcium antagonists in myocardial infarction or angina in light of the second Danish Verapamil Infarction Trial (DAVIT-II) and other recent studies. Am J Cardiol 1991;*67*:1295–1297.

r24. Yusuf S, Peto R, Lewis J, Collins R, Sleight P. Beta blockade during and after myocardial infarction: an overview of the randomized trials. Progr Cardiovasc Dis 1985;*27*:335–371.

r25. Baber NS, Lewis JA. Confidence in results of beta-blocker post-infarction trials. BMJ 1982;*284*:1749–1750.

r26. Antiplatelet Trialists' Collaboration. Secondary prevention of vascular disease by prolonged antiplatelet treatment. BMJ 1988;*296*:320–331.

r27. Jafri SM, Gheorghiade M, Goldstein S. Oral anticoagulation for secondary prevention after myocardial infarction with special reference to the Warfarin Re-Infarction Study. Progr Cardiovasc Dis 1992;*34*:317–324.

r28. Rossouw JE, Lewis B, Rifkind BM. The value of lowering cholesterol after myocardial infarction. N Engl J Med 1990;*323*:1112–1119.

r29. Cowan JC, Coulshed DS, Zaman AG. Antiarrhythmic therapy and survival following myocardial infarction. J Cardiovasc Pharmacol 1991;*18*(Suppl 2):92–98.

r30. Gheorghiade M, Goldstein S. Arrhythmia suppression in post-myocardial infarction patients with special notation to Cardiac Arrhythmia Suppression Trial. Progr Cardiovasc Dis 1991;*33*:213–218.

r31. Editorial. Primary prevention of ischaemic heart disease with lipid-lowering drugs. Lancet 1988;*i*:333–334.

r32. De Gaetano G. Primary prevention of vascular disease by aspirin. Lancet 1988;*i*:1093–1094.

r33. Collins R, Peto R, MacMahon S, Hebert P, Fiebach NH, Eberlein KA, Godwin J, Qizilbash N, Taylor JO, Hennekens CH. Blood pressure, stroke, and coronary heart disease. Part 2, short-term reductions in blood pressure: overview of randomised drug trials in their epidemiological context. Lancet 1990;*335*:827–838.

r34. Corwin S, Reiffel JA. Nitrate therapy for angina pectoris. Arch Intern Med 1985;*145*:538–543.

r35. Flaherty JT. Nitrate tolerance: a review of the evidence. Drugs 1989;*37*:523–550.

r36. Abrams J. Clinical aspects of nitrate tolerance. Eur Heart J 1991;*12*(Suppl E):42–52.

r37. Elkayam U. Tolerance to organic nitrates: evidence, mechanisms, clinical relevance, and strategies for prevention. Ann Intern Med 1991;*114*:667–677.

r38. Stamler JS, Loscalzo J. The antiplatelet effects of organic nitrates and related nitroso compounds in vitro and in vivo and their relevance to cardiovascular disorders. JACC 1991;*18*:1529–1536.

r39. Bogaert MG. Clinical pharmacokinetics of glyceryl trinitrate following the use of systemic and topical preparations. Clin Pharmacokin 1987;*12*:1–11.

r40. Fung H-L. Pharmacokinetics and pharmacodynamics of organic nitrates. Am J Cardiol 1987;*60*:4H–9H.

r41. Bogaert M. Introductory remarks about clinically relevant pharmacokinetic properties of organic nitrates. Z Kardiol 1990;*79*(Suppl 3):47–49.

r42. Goldman L, Sia STB, Cook EF, Rutherford JD, Weinstein MC. Costs and effectiveness of routine therapy with long-term beta-adrenergic antagonists after acute myocardial infarction. N Engl J Med 1988;*319*:152–157.

r43. Boden WE. Management of non-Q-wave myocardial infarction: role of diltiazem versus β-blocker therapy. J Cardiovasc Pharmacol 1990;*16*(Suppl 6):55–60.

r44. Roberts WC. Recent studies on the effects of beta blockers on blood lipid levels. Am Heart J 1989;*117*:709–714.

r45. McTavish D, Sorkin EM. Verapamil. An updated review of its pharmacodynamic and pharmacokinetic properties, and therapeutic use in hypertension. Drugs 1989;*38*:19–76.

r46. Vanhoutte PM. The Expert Committee of the World Health Organization on classification of calcium antagonists: the viewpoint of the raporteur. Am J Cardiol 1987;*59*:3A–8A.

r47. Editorial. Nifedipine: a new life with GITS? Lancet 1992;*340*;1507–1508.

r48. Sacks HS, Ancona-Berk VA, Berrier J, Nagalingam R, Chalmers TC. Dipyridamole in the treatment of angina pectoris: a meta-analysis. Clin Pharmacol Ther 1988;*43*:610–615.

CHAPTER 25

B. A. Dupuis
M. M. Adamantidis

Antiarrhythmic Drugs

The treatment of cardiac arrhythmias requires both an accurate diagnosis and, as far as possible, knowledge of the factors triggering or favoring rhythm disturbances. If antiarrhythmic therapy is needed, its rationale should be established at once, and the selection of drug should be based on physiopathologic, pharmacologic, and pharmacokinetic data. In all cases, knowledge of the therapeutic and adverse effects, potential drug interactions, and possible correlations between plasma concentrations and observed effects is necessary to monitor carefully the course of therapy.

The understanding of physiopathologic mechanisms involved in abnormalities of cardiac rhythm and the mechanism of action of antiarrhythmic drugs results mostly from recent investigations about the electrophysiologic modifications of membrane electrical activity in cardiac cells.

Cardiac Electrophysiology

Transmembrane Ion Transport

Like other excitable cells, cardiac cells maintain a large ionic gradient across their surface membrane by the action of ion pumps, exchangers, and intermittent selective permeabilities.

Sarcolemmal Pumps

Sarcolemmal pumps transport ions actively across the cell membrane against concentration gradients (Fig. 25.1). These proteins utilize energy stored in the cell. The best known pump is the sodium pump that transports Na out and K into the cell by deriving energy from the hydrolysis of ATP. This catalytic function is dependent on magnesium ions. Most evidence points to a coupling ratio of 3 Na to 2 K transported for every ATP molecule hydrolyzed: one positive charge is

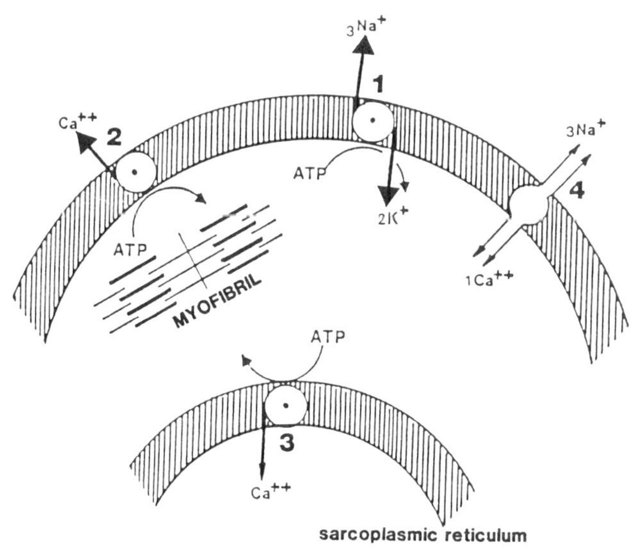

Figure 25.1 Active transport of ions across the membranes.

lost intracellularly at each exchange. This pump is thus electrogenic, leading to a "pump current" and it participates in the membrane polarization. Similarly ATP-dependent Ca pumps are located in the sarcolemma and especially the sarcoplasmic reticulum membrane, where they play an essential role in the relaxation process.

Na–Ca Exchange

A Na–Ca exchange system has been demonstrated to extrude Ca ions and permit Na ions to enter the cell or, conversely, to extrude Na ions and permit Ca ions to enter the cell, the direction being governed by the Na gradient. This exchange is not symmetric, with the stoichiometry of the exchange process at 3 Na/1 Ca, and it is thus electrogenic.

Selective Permeabilities

In cardiac cells, ions flow selectively and passively across the membrane according to two modes (Fig. 25.2):

(1) Constant permeabilities. These lead to leak currents (mainly K ions leak out of cells) independent of physiologic stimuli.

(2) Intermittent permeabilities. These are characteristic of excitable membranes that can suddenly change in response to a single chemical or electrical stimulus with a high degree of amplification that modifies the electrical properties of the membrane, leading to transmembrane ionic fluxes and ionic currents.

Resting Membrane Potential

At rest, the membrane potential (Er) in nonautomatic cells (atrial cells, myocardial cells, and Purkinje fibers) is determined predominantly by the passive permeability of K ions across the cell membrane and lies near –90 mV (Fig. 25.3). In the nodal cells, the maximum diastolic membrane potential never becomes more negative than –60 mV and lies normally between –30 and –40mV.

Action Potential

Stimulation of the cardiac cell membrane initiates membrane potential changes secondary to alterations of ionic fluxes that have a characteristic time course called the "action potential" (Fig. 25.4).[r1] For convenience, in normal nonautomatic cells, the action potential has been subdivided into five phases as follows: (i) Phase 0 is the initial, rapid membrane depolarization or upstroke that raises the membrane potential from –90 mV to +35 mV. Between 0 and +35 mV, the intracellular potential is positive with respect to the extracellular potential. The most positive value is called "overshoot." The maximal rate of rise of depolarization is usually chosen as an important characteristic of action potential. It depends on the membrane potential and

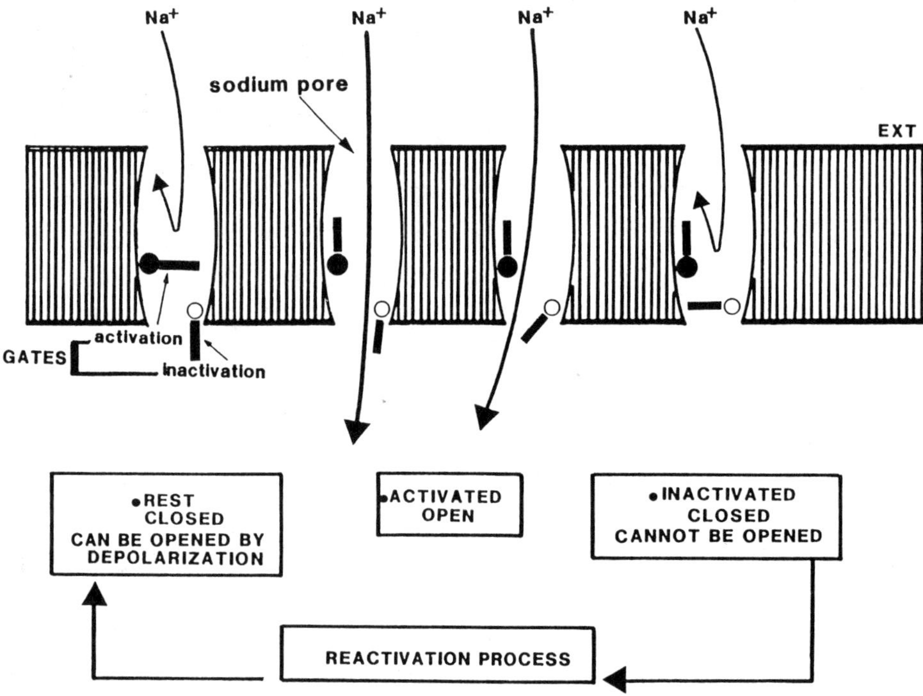

Figure 25.2 Schematic mechanisms of the voltage-operated sodium channel.

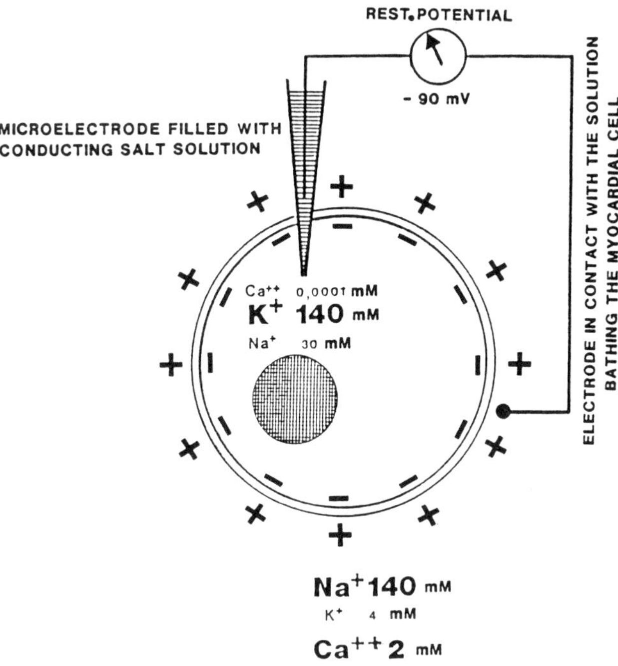

Figure 25.3 In excitable tissues, the potential difference maintained across the cell membrane in the absence of stimulation is called "resting potential" (about -90mV in Purkinje cells and cardiac contractile fibers).

governs the conduction velocity of the cardiac impulse.[1] (ii) Phase 1 consists of initial and rapid repolarization. (iii) Phase 2 is the "plateau" or prolonged depolarization, the most diagnostic feature of the action potential of cardiac cells. (iv) Phase 3 is the terminal repolarization that brings the membrane potential back to the resting level. (v) Phase 4 covers the period of diastole.

In automatic cells, the diastolic potential or Phase 4 is unstable, showing gradual loss of negativity until it reaches threshold potential at which an impulse is initiated. This slow diastolic depolarization is a normal property of cardiac cells in the sinus node, the atrioventricular node, and the His-Purkinje system. The rate of impulse initiation due to automaticity of cells in the sinus node is sufficiently high that other potentially automatic cells are excited by propagated impulses before they can spontaneously depolarize to their threshold potential. The sinus node is therefore referred to as the dominant pacemaker. The steeper the diastolic depolarization and/or the closer the threshold potential, the higher is the pacemaker rate. The adrenergic system can increase the rate of automaticity by increasing the diastolic depolarization rate, whereas the cholinergic system causes hyperpolarization, moving the membrane potential away from the threshold potential and thus decreasing the rate of automaticity.

The ionic channels are made up of protein complexes located in the sarcolemma, and include multiple substructures that support their selectivity and kinetics. They possess two fundamental properties: permeability and excitability.[r2,2,r3] The channels can exist in three primary states: rested (R), activated (A), and inactivated (I). The transition between these states is governed by the membrane potential. Antiarrhythmic agents interact with these three states with characteristic association and dissociation rate constants, the association of the drug with ionic channels leading to the blockade of activation processes.

The transmembrane ionic movements lead to the depolarizing inward currents and repolarizing outward currents given in Table 25.1 (the multiple K conductances are not described in detail).

Refractory Periods

Refractoriness has been defined in many different ways, but the term is now used to refer to the duration

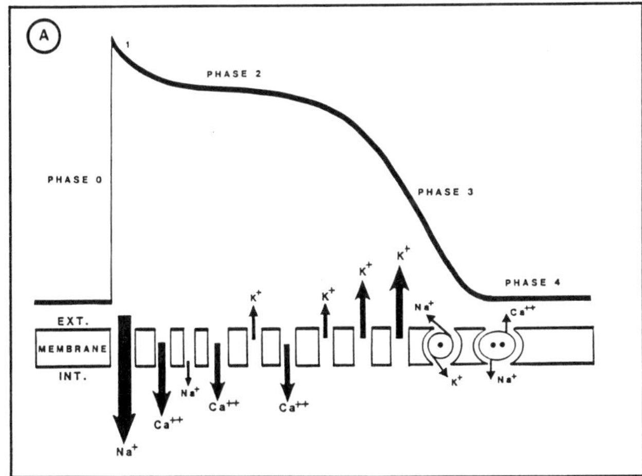

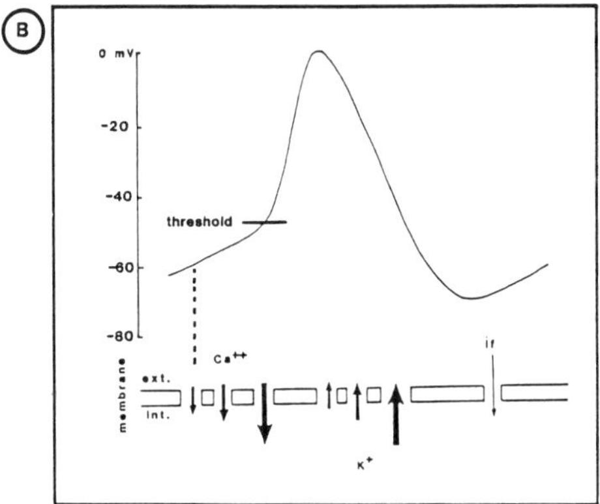

Figure 25.4 Ionic movements underlying the action potential:
A. In Purkinje and contractile fibers.
B. In nodal cells.

Table 25.1 Major Ionic Currents and the Cardiac Action Potential

Current	Ion	Phase of Action Potential	Direction of Current Flow	Role
I_{Na}	Na^+	0	Inward	• Depolarizes cell
I_{Ca}	Ca^{++}	1, 2	Inward	• Triggers the release of internal calcium • Contributes to plateau
I_{to}	K^+	1	Outward	• Early repolarization
I_k	K^+	2, 3	Outward	• Repolarizes fibers
I_{K1}	K^+	0, 1, 2, 3, 4	Outward	• Repolarizes fibers
I_f	Na^+	4	Inward	• Promotes spontaneous depolarization

of the effective refractory period (ERP), which is the minimal interval between two propagated responses.[r1] In most cardiac cells, the ERP depends on the state of either fast Na channels (His-Purkinje fibers, atrial and ventricular contractile cells) or slow Ca channels (sinus node, A-V node). Excitability depends on the number of fully reactivated channels. In fast Na-dependent cells, the ERP is closely related to the action potential duration because recovery from inactivation of the Na channel closely parallels repolarization. In slow Ca-dependent cells, opening, closing, and reactivation are markedly time-dependent; refractoriness can outlast full repolarization, and ERP is much longer than the duration of the action potential.

Intracardiac Conduction

In the heart, the ability of cell-to-cell propagation of influx results from the low electrical resistance between the connecting structures (intercalary disks, gap junctions). The heart pump function needs the sequential activation of cardiac chambers allowed by an adequate coordination of contractile fibers. This sequence is performed through specialized fibers (Fig. 25.5) that have lost the property to contract and have modified their capacity to conduct impulses (Table 25.2).

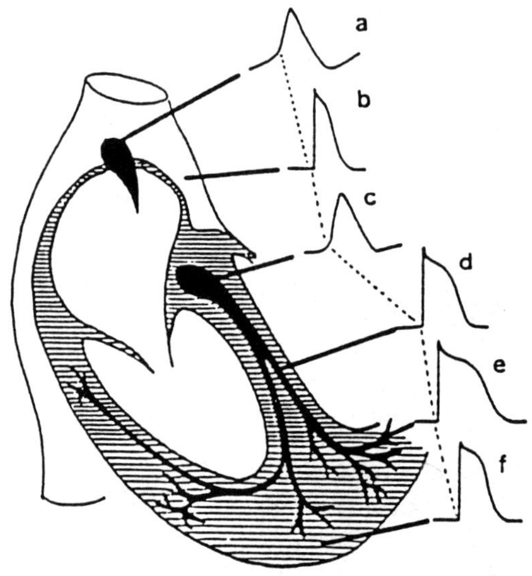

Figure 25.5 Action potentials in (a) sinus node; (b) atrial myocardium; (c) atrioventricular node; (d) proximal Purkinje fiber; (e) terminal Purkinje fiber; (f) ventricular myocardium.

Table 25.2 Conduction Velocity and Automatism in Diverse Cardiac Tissues

	Conduction Velocity meters/seconds	Firing Rate/min
Sinus Node		70
Atrium	1–1.2	
A-V Node	0.02–0.05	40–50
His-Purkinje Fibers	2–4	25–40
Ventricle	0.5–1	

The Relationship Between Cardiac Period and Action Potential Duration

The action potential duration is regulated by the cardiac period. This relation is based on the gating kinetics of the time-dependent repolarizing currents (mainly I_K). Because of the slow kinetics of deactivation of these K channels, a premature action potential will find them in partially opened state, therefore accelerating the repolarization process. Conversely, the prolonged cardiac period give these K channels the possibility to close fully; therefore their opening needs a longer time, delaying repolarization.

The interrelation between the cardiac period and the action potential duration subsequently exerts an influence on the effective refractory period (Table 25.3), and can explain the phenomenon of "aberrant conduction" and the variable severity of premature extrasystole during bradycardia.

Table 25.3 Effect of Antiarrhythmic Agents on Conduction Times and Effective Refractory Periods

			Effective Refractory Period				
Agent	**AH**	**HV**	**Atrium**	**AV Node**	**His Purkinje**	**Ventricle**	**Accessory Pathway**
Quinidine	0/↓	↑	↑	0/↓	↑	↑	↑
Procainamide	↑	↑	↑	0/↓	↑	↑	↑
Disopyramide	0/↑	↑	↑	0/↓	↑	↑	↑
Lidocaine	0/↑	0/↑	0	0	0/↓	0/↓	0/↓
Propafenone	↑	↑	↑	↑	↑	↑	0/↑
Encainide	↑	↑	0	↑	0	0	↑
Propranolol	↑	0	0	↑	0	0	0
Amiodarone	↑	0	↑	↑	↑	↑	↑
Verapamil	↑	0	0	↑	0	0	0/↓
Digitalis	↑	0	0/↓	↑	0/↓	0/↓	↓

↑: Lengthening
↓: Shortening
0: No significant change
AH: Interval between atrial electrogram and His deflection
HV: Interval between His deflection and ventricular electrogram

The Relationship Between the Action Potential and Electrocardiogram

The electrocardiogram (EKG) is the consequence of unitary electrical activities (Fig. 25.6). At the ventricular level, the rate of cellular depolarization determines the width of the ventriculogram, and the duration of phases 1, 2, and 3 is responsible for the QT duration.

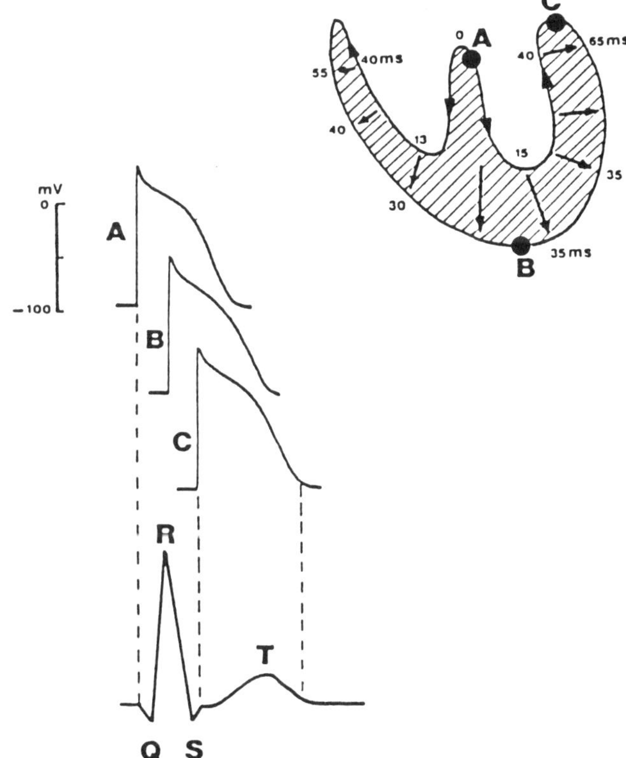

Figure 25.6 Action potential-electrocardiogram relationship.
A. First depolarized ventricular cell.
B. Apex cell.
C. Last depolarized ventricular cell.
The ventriculogram (QRS) begins with the phase 0 of the first action potential and ends with the phase 0 of the last action potential. The repolarization phase (QT) begins with the phase 0 of the first action potential and ends when the last depolarized cell has completed its repolarization.

Mechanisms Responsible for Cardiac Arrhythmias

An arrhythmia is an abnormality of the rate, site of origin of the cardiac impulse, or a disturbance in conduction that leads to alterations in the sequence of activation of the atria and ventricles. Arrhythmias may arise due to abnormal impulse generation, abnormal conduction, or both.[3]

Altered Normal Automaticity

It should be recalled that a few types of cardiac cells develop normal automaticity (sinus node, A-V node, His-Purkinje system) that can be altered by autonomic activity. At the sinus node level, increased vagal activity can slow and even stop sinus node pacemakers by increasing potassium conductance. The sympathetic system exerts opposite effects by accelerating the rate of Phase 4 depolarization (pacemaker current). Impulse initiation by the subsidiary pacemakers may arise when there is slowing or impairment of the dominant pacemaker. Augmented automaticity in the His-

Purkinje system is a common cause of arrhythmias (Fig. 25.7).

Abnormal Impulse Generation

The numerous mechanisms involved in abnormal impulse generation may be categorized as either abnormal automaticity or triggered activity.

Abnormal Automaticity. This term is used to refer to spontaneous diastolic depolarization that occurs at a low (depolarized) level of membrane potential in a cell that normally has a high (well-polarized) level of membrane potential during diastole. Thus Purkinje fibers, atrial, and ventricular cells can show spontaneous diastolic depolarization (Fig. 25.8) and repetitive firing when the membrane potential is brought to about −60 mV (or less negative values).[4,r4] The ionic mechanisms are still not fully understood, but alterations in potassium and/or calcium conductances are probably involved.

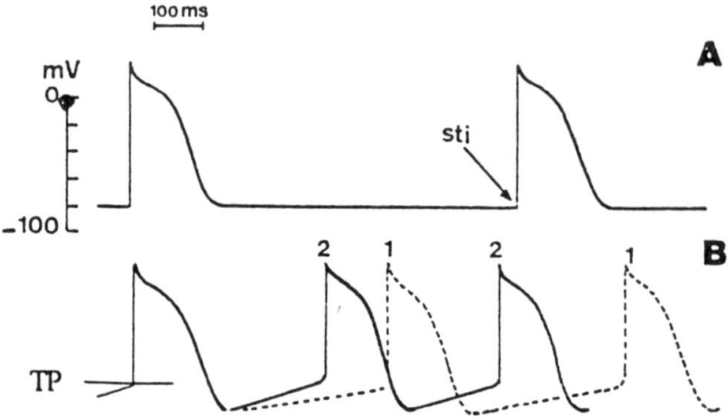

Figure 25.8 Abnormal automaticity.

A. Quiescent cell. The diastolic membrane potential is stable. Depolarization requires external stimulus. (sti)

B. Occurrence of spontaneous diastolic depolarization. (1) Once the thresold potential (TP) is reached, cell depolarizes. (2) Increasing the slope of diastolic depolarization leads to increase the rate of discharge.

Triggered Activity. This is the generation of impulses arising from afterdepolarizations that attain a threshold potential.[r5]

Early afterdepolarizations are depolarizing afterpotentials that begin prior to the completion of repolarization, thus delaying or interrupting the normal repolarization process (Fig. 25.9). Early afterdepolarizations can attain a threshold potential and induce a second upstroke, which propagates into cardiac muscle and thus begins a burst of triggered activity. They are caused by a reduction in net outward current that can result either from an actual reduction in outward currents (I_K and I_{K1}) or from an actual increase in inward currents (slowly inactivated I_{Na}, I_{Ca} slow) or from both. They are hypothesized as one of the mechanisms responsible for polymorphous ventricular tachyarrhythmias (so-called "Torsade de Pointes") during antiarrhythmic treatment with quinidine, sotalol, or N-acetylprocainamide.

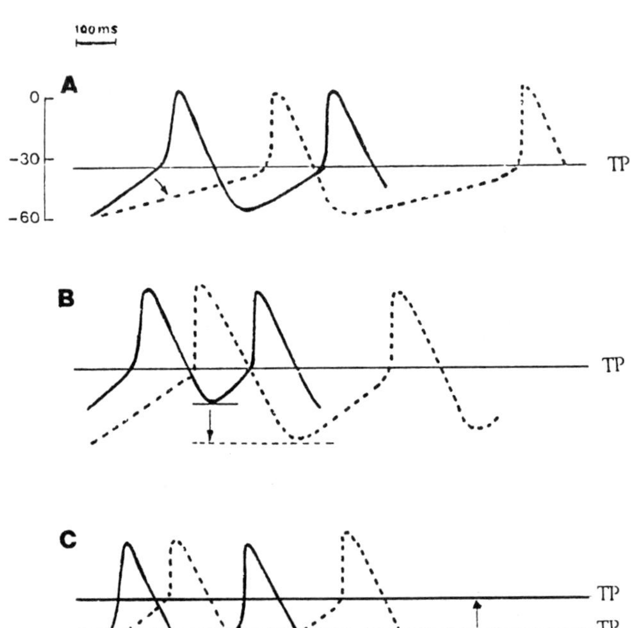

Figure 25.7 Altered normal automaticity: slowing in the rate of discharge of the sinus node.

A. By a decrease in the slope of the diastolic depolarization.

B. By hyperpolarization of the maximal diastolic potential (primary mechanism for vagal bradycardia).

C. By an increase in the threshold potential (TP).

Delayed afterdepolarizations are depolarizing afterpotentials that begin after full repolarization. A delayed afterdepolarization that reaches threshold potential gives rise to another action potential and may initiate sustained rhythmic activity (e.g., ventricular tachycardia).[r5]

The delayed afterdepolarization is not self-initiated but is dependent on a prior action potential. Its amplitude and coupling interval are linked with the driving rate: the amplitude increases at shorter cycle lengths, whereas the coupling interval decreases, these features favoring the occurrence of triggered activity (Fig. 25.10). Delayed afterdepolarizations are linked with the transient inward current,[5,r5] which is carried mainly by Na ions and suggested as deriving from either a Na-Ca exchange current or a nonselective cation current. They are accompanied by an aftercontraction. They are seen in cells exposed to digitalis, cate-

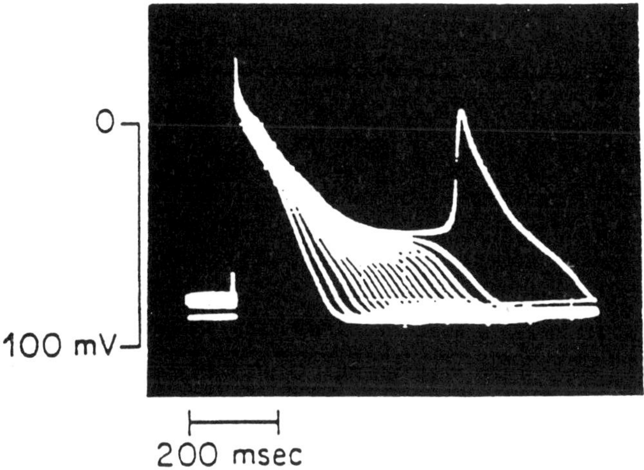

Figure 25.9 Typical example of an early afterdepolarization induced in a canine cardiac Purkinje fiber exposed to Tyrode's solution containing 2.7 mM K and 1 μM quinidine. The fiber was initially driven at a cycle length of 1000 ms (shortest action potential), then at cycle lengths prgoressively increased to 8000 ms. The action potential duration increased gradually until an early afterdepolarization gave rise to a second (nondriven) upstroke (from Fig. 9, Roden and Hoffman, 1985 ref in r5).

cholamines, increased extracellular calcium, myocardial infarction, or ischemia—all of these situations leading to intracellular calcium overload.

Although triggered activities cannot be self-initiated, they can be self-sustained. They can be initiated by a single premature stimulus and may also be terminated by a single premature stimulus. The same characteristics are found in reentrant arrhythmias and make it difficult to assign a mechanism for a given clinical tachyarrhythmia.

Abnormal Impulse Conduction

Focal Reexcitation. Altered extracellular conditions (acidosis, elevated extracellular K concentration, decreased pO_2) may induce heterogeneous action potential duration and lead to different levels of excitability in neighboring cells. Some depolarized cells can act like a stimulus and reexcite the cells recovering from a refractory period and initiate an extrasystolic beat. Myocardial ischemia, which shortens action potential duration, is a typical example of a situation that allows focal reexcitation. Taking into account the relation between membrane potential and rate of depolarization, conduction disturbances will be observed.

Decremental Conduction. Because the conduction velocity is critically dependent on the membrane potential at the time of activation, incompleted reactivation of Na channels results in slowing of conduction velocity. This is observed in ischemic areas because of increased intracellular Na and Ca concentrations and decreased intracellular K concentration that cause partial depolarization in the resting potential and slow Na channel reactivation.

Nevertheless, decremental conduction is a physiologic property of the atrioventricular junction in which the low conduction velocity is attributed to: (i) the slow depolarizing rate; and (ii) the high electrical resistance due to fewer gap junctions and the small diameter of the cells.

After decrementally slowing, the conduction velocity can recover to normal values when the impulses reach healthy areas with well-polarized cells. Ultimately, the decremental conduction may lead to a reduction of the action potential to such an extent that the membrane response cannot successfully propagate.[6] These conduction blocks can occur in different regions of the heart (sinus node, A-V node, His-Purkinje system, contractile myocardium) and play an essential role in the development of reentrant pathways.

Reentrant Arrhythmias. The reentry mechanism is usually involved in the occurrence of premature

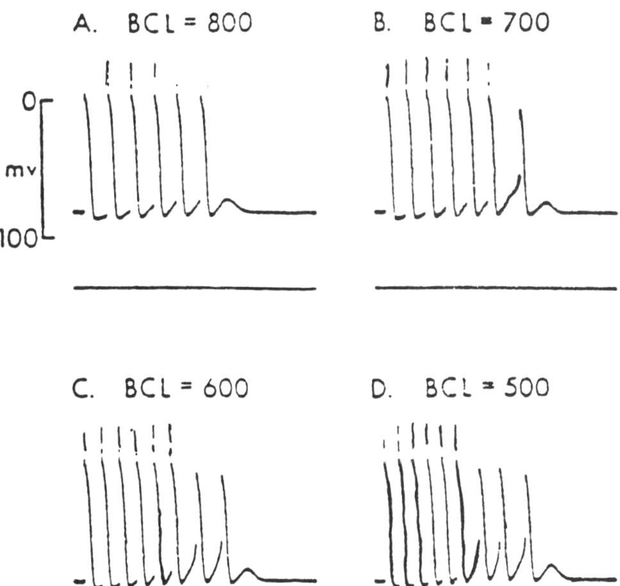

Figure 25.10 Example of delayed afterdepolarizations and triggered activity induced in a canine cardiac Purkinje fiber by exposure to acetylstrophantidin. Decreasing from 800 to 500 ms the basic cycle length (BCL) of stimulation led to a subthreshold delayed afterdepolarization (A) then to a single (B), two (C) and three (D) nondriven action potentials arising after termination of pacing from a delayed afterdepolarization that attains its threshold potential. In each case, the last nondriven action potential was followed by a subthreshold delayed afterdepolarization. Note the absence of Phase 4 depolarization during quiescence. (From Fig. 6, Ferrier et al., 1973 ref in r5.)

beats and ventricular tachycardia.[r6] For reentry to be initiated, both unidirectional block of conduction and slow conduction must occur (Fig. 25.11). Furthermore, an anatomic and functional barrier must exist and form a circuit, the pathlength of the circuit being greater than the wavelength of the cardiac impulse. In that case the impulse will continue to find excitable myocardial cells as the depolarizing wavefront progresses. Arrhythmias that result from such circus movements are self-sustained, but are not self-initiated. They can be initiated by a single premature stimulus and terminated by a single premature stimulus.[7]

Antiarrhythmic Therapy

Besides the antiarrhythmic drugs, interventions that are aimed to minimize and even suppress factors and drugs that act through the autonomic nervous system also must be considered (Table 25.4). For example, in cardiac failure, cardiotonic or vasodilator drugs can exert beneficial effects by improving hemodynamic conditions and therefore suppressing the existing arrhythmias. Acceleration of the cardiac rhythm by external pacing is the most suitable treatment for the ventricular tachycardia "Torsade de Pointes." Modification of the potassium pool can by itself either suppress arrhythmias or influence the efficacy of antiarrhythmic drugs. For some arrhythmias, surgical procedures can be useful (e.g., resection of an abnormal pathway, such as a ventricular aneurysm).

Last but not least, in a notable percentage of patients (about 10%), the discontinuation of antiarrhythmic drugs can be enough to suppress the rhythm disorder. This possibility must be kept in mind.

Some mechanisms that contribute to arrhythmogenesis appear to be intimately related to autonomic

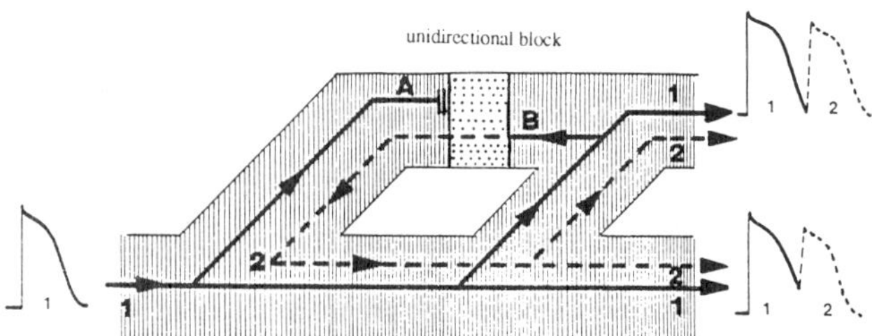

Figure 25.11 In the A direction, the front of depolarization cannot propagate into the area of unidirectional block. A few milliseconds later, a retrograde response can successfully pass through in the B direction. In such conditions of associated unidirectional block and slowed conduction, a single action potential (1) entering the circuit leads to a double response (1 + 2). Dashed line = reentry pathway.

Table 25.4 Medical Management of Dysrhythmias

A - Drugs or interventions aimed to minimize or suppress factors favoring rhythm disturbances
- O_2
- Potassium and magnesium salts
- Pacing
- Surgery
- Withdrawal of antiarrhythmic agent.
- —

B - Drugs acting via the autonomic nervous system
- Atropine
- Beta-blockers
- Bata-agonists
- Digitalis
- —

C - Drugs acting (mainly) through alteration of the transmembrane currents
- Quinidine
- Lidocaïne
- Amiodarone
- Verapamil
- —

neural influences. This explains the efficacy of drugs that act through either the cholinergic or the adrenergic systems.

Drugs Influencing the Cholinergic System

Digitalis

Despite the appearance of new antiarrhythmic drugs, digitalis is still widely used in the treatment of some supraventricular rhythm disturbances: atrial fibrillation and other supraventricular tachyarrhythmias. Because most of the latter are due to junctional reentry mechanisms digitalis can improve the relation between effective refractory period and orthograde conduction. A detrimental fast ventricular response rate can be decreased by both the direct and indirect (vagal) slowing of conduction at the AV node. Therefore digitalis can stop the ventricular conveyance of the arrhythmia and hinder its recurrence.[8,9,10]

Adenosine

Through its effect of activating or opening the GTP binding protein that controls potassium conductance, G_K, adenosine allows recovery of many supraventricular tachycardias to sinus rhythm (up to one minute) in the majority of reciprocal paroxysmal tachycardias (Bouveret syndrome) with or without accessory pathways. Reentry is interrupted through the transitory hyperpolarization block of conduction in the AV node, thus allowing the resumption of sinus rhythm.

Adenosine is administered IV at a dose of 5–10 mg in adult humans.

Disopyramide

The anticholinergic effect of this class IA antiarrhythmic drug will be beneficial whenever either exaggerated vagal tone is involved in the genesis of arrhythmia or its own electrophysiologic effects have to be counterbalanced: slowed sinus rate, aggravating effect of sinus rate slowing, lengthening of the AV conduction time.

Drugs Influencing the Adrenergic System

Beta-Blocking Drugs

In the heart, these agents counteract competitively the effects of catecholamines on beta-1 receptors. Catecholamines enhance the slope of slow diastolic depolarization in Purkinje fibers, thus increasing the rate of discharge of normal and latent pacemakers, leading to emergence of ectopic foci. In ischemia-induced arrhythmias, the beta-blocking drugs may act through either their specific or indirect effects (see Chapter 6).

Amiodarone

Amiodarone exerts noncompetitive antiadrenergic (alpha and beta) effects[11] and reduces norepinephrine release from presynaptic nerve endings.[12] The effect is observed rapidly, even before the electrophysiologic effects (lengthening in action potential duration and refractory periods) develop.

Antiarrhythmic Drugs

Substances that directly alter the electrophysiologic properties of cardiac cells are termed antiarrhythmic drugs.

Many classification have been proposed, but the most widely accepted is that established by Vaughan-Williams (Table 25.5).[13] One limitation of this classification is that it relies on effects produced in vitro on fragments of cardiac tissues. Therefore, it is supported by the electrophysiologic effects of the tested drug and does not take into account either the drugs' other effects, particularly those on the autonomic nervous system, or the possible influence of metabolites.

Table 25.5 Classification of Antiarrhythmic Drugs

Class	Mechanism of Action	Drugs
I	Sodium Channel Blockade	
	A. Moderate phase 0 depression Prolonged repolarization	*quinidine* procainamide disopyramide
	B. Minimal phase 0 depression Shortened repolarization	*lidocaine* phenytoin tocainide mexiletine
	C. Marked phase 0 depression Little effect on repolarization	*encainide* flecainide propafenone moricizine
II	Beta adrenergic blockade	beta-blockers
III	Prolonged repolarization	*amiodarone* sotalol bretylium
IV	Calcium channel blockade	*verapamil* diltiazem

Theory of Modulated Receptor

The theory of modulated receptors proposes that a drug interacts with its receptor (ionic channel) in a time- and voltage-dependent fashion.[r7] The conformation of membrane proteins is different, depending on the membrane potential. Furthermore there may be transient conformational states characteristic for negative-to-positive and positive-to-negative transitions. The modulated receptor theory suggests that each of these states may have proper affinities for specific drugs and that occupation of a receptor by a drug leads to modifications in protein behavior. Therefore, a drug can be bound to each state of a given channel (rested, activated, inactivated), and the drug-associated channels are assumed not to conduct ions and to have their voltage dependence of inactivation shifted to more negative potentials (Fig. 25.12).[r8]

Thus, a concentration of drug that exerts a minimal effect in a quiescent fiber at normal resting potential could block a significant fraction of channels during one action potential. During repeated action potentials, the number of drug-associated channels increases, the channels accumulate in the inactivated state, and ionic current decreases until a steady state is attained. This phenomenon is called use-dependent block, as opposed to the tonic (not use-dependent) block observed through interaction with channels in a rested state. If the kinetics of association and dissociation of the drug are both relatively rapid, the use-dependent block will reach a steady state in a few action potentials. On the other hand, if dissociation is slow, the use-dependent block may develop fully over many action potentials during which the fraction of inactivated channels continues to increase, thus leading to incremental block.

Therefore a drug can have little effect at one membrane potential and heart rate and, at the same concentration, a markedly greater effect at another potential and heart rate.[r7] This has been demonstrated for sodium, calcium,[r7] and potassium[14] blocking drugs.

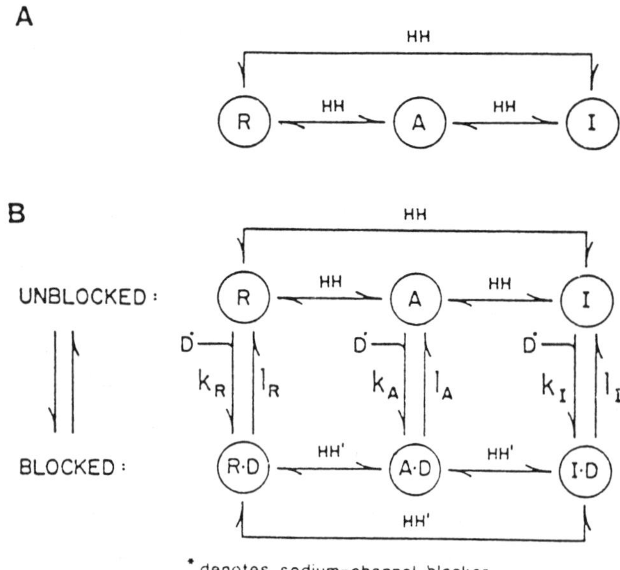

Figure 25.12 Schematic diagram of the modulated receptor hypothesis.

A: A kinetic scheme for sodium channels under drug-free conditions. There are three primary states: rested (R), the predominant state at normal diastolic potential; activated (A), the predominant state during the action potential upstroke; and inactivated (I), the predominant state during the action potential plateau and at low diastolic potentials. Transitions between the three states are assumed to obey Hodgkin-Huxley (HH)-kinetics.

B: Possible channel states in the presence of drug. Drug molecules (D) can associate or dissociate with channels in resting, activated, or inactivated states. Drug-associated channels (R-D, A-D, and I-D) do not conduct ions (are blocked) and behave as if they are at a less negative transmembrane potential; that is, their Hodgkin-Huxley kinetic parameters (HH') are shifted to more negative values. (From Fig 30-2, Clarkson and Hondeghem[r8])

General Warnings

The dosage of antiarrhythmic agents must be individualized on the basis of: (i) the patient's pre-existing cardiac status (automaticity, conduction, and contractility); (ii) the antiarrhythmic response and development of tolerance, both of which are generally dose-related. Most of these agents depress excitability. Consequently, pacemaker reprogramming may be required in patients with permanently implanted devices.

Encainide and flecainide were included in the National Heart Lung and Blood Institute's Cardiac Arrhythmia Suppression Trial (CAST)[15,16,r9,17,18] a long-term multicenter, randomized, double-blind study in asymptomatic patients with life-threatening arrhythmias who had had a myocardial infarction more than six days but less than two years previously. An excess of deaths due to arrhythmias and deaths due to shock after acute recurrent myocardial infarction was seen in patients treated with these drugs compared with a carefully matched placebo-treated group.

The applicability of these results to other populations (e.g., those without recent infarction) is uncertain; however, at present it is prudent to consider the risks of Class IC agents, coupled with the lack of any evidence of improved survival, as generally unacceptable in patients who have no life-threatening ventricular arrhythmias—even if the patients are experiencing unpleasant, but not life-threatening, symptoms or signs.

It is now well-established that potentially malignant ventricular arrhythmias are independent predictors of mortality. But it is not known whether reducing potentially malignant ventricular arrhythmias significantly reduces mortality. Although small-scale trials have been conducted with antiarrhythmic drugs, no definitive studies have been undertaken in an attempt to answer this important question.

Beta-blockers form the only class of drugs (Class II) that have consistently demonstrated the potential to reduce total mortality and, specifically, sudden death rates in patients after myocardial infarction. However, beta-blockers have many effects other than antiarrhythmic actions that may be related to their cardioprotective effects.

Class I Antiarrhythmic Drugs

Quinidine

History

Quinidine is the dextrostereoisomer of quinine. It was first described in 1848 by Van Heyningen, then prepared and given its present name by Pasteur in 1853. Wenckebach (1914) reported the antiarrhythmic effects of quinine alkaloids, and Frey (1918) found quinidine the most effective.

Cellular Electrophysiologic Effects

Quinidine is the prototype of Class IA antiarrhythmic agents.

(1) Resting membrane potential. In normal cardiac cells, therapeutic concentrations of quinidine do not affect the resting potential, whereas in depolarized (e.g., ischemic) cells, low levels of quinidine induce depolarization and can even lead to inexcitability. In sinus and AV nodal cells and in His-Purkinje cells that develop normal automaticity, quinidine decreases the slope of Phase 4 depolarization and slows down the firing rate.

(2) Phase 0 depolarization. Quinidine decreases the maximal upstroke velocity (Vmax) in atrial, ventricular, and Purkinje cells, and shifts the curve Vmax-

Table 25.6 Clinical Parameters for Antiarrhythmic Drugs

Class and Generic Name	Trade Name	Approx. Dose (mg) and Route	Bioavailability	Hepatic First-Pass	Binding to Plasma Proteins	Plasma Concentration ug/ml	Elimination Half-Life hr	Metabolism Route	Metabolites (+) Genetic Variations	Plasma Clearance ml/min
IA										
Quinidine	Duraquin Quinaglut Dura-Tabs Quinalan Cardioquin Quinidex	600–1200 mg/d po	70–90%	+(20%)	80–90%	2–5	4–10	Hepatic	3-OH quinidine 2′-oxo-quinidinone active (unknown)	210 ml/min
Procainamide	Pronestyl Procan	100–1000 mg IV/d 1–4 g/d po	80–90%	0	15%	4–10	3	Hepatic renal	N-acetyl procainamide active Desethyl procainamide Desethyl-N-acetyl-procainamide (+)	600 ml/min
Disopyramide	Norpace Rythmodan	400–800 mg/d po	60–90%	+	25–40%	1.7–6	5–8	Hepatic (50%)	Mono-N-dealkyl disopyramide active (0)	200 ml/min
IB										
Lidocaine	Xylocaine	100 mg IV 300 mg IM	70%	+	35–80%	1.5–4	< 2 h	Hepatic	Glycine-xylidine mono-ethylglycylxylidine active	750 ml/min
Mexiletine	Mexitil	250 mg IV 600–800 mg po	90%	± O	60%	0.75–2	10 h	Hepatic	inactive	200 ml/min
Phenytoin	Dilantin		90%		90%	10–15	16–24 h –40 h	Hepatic	Hydroxylated inactive	25 ml/min
Tocainide	Tonocard	1200–1800 mg/d po	98%	0	50%	4–10	12–15 h	Hepatic	inactive	130 ml/min
IC										
Encainide	Enkaid	75–200 mg/d po	30% 80% (depending on genetic phenotype)	+	70–80%	0.03 (E) 0.10 (ODE) 0.11 (MODE)	1–2 h 8–11 h (depending on genetic phenotype)	Hepatic	O-demethylencainide (ODE) 3-methoxy-O-demethyl-encainide (MODE) more active than encainide (+)	200 ml/min
Flecainide	Tambocor	100–400 mg/d po 1.5–5 mg/d IV	90%	0	40%	0.2–1	0.24–14 h	Hepatic renal	dealkylated little active	500 ml/min
Propafenone	Rythmol	50–100 mg IV 300–900 mg/d po	3–50%		90%	0.5–3	2–32 h	Hepatic	active (+)	1000 ml/min
Moricizine	Ethmozine	600–900 mg/d po	35%	+	95%	0.2–1.2	2–4 h	Hepatic	active and inactive	
III										
Amiodarone	Cordarone	Loading doses 800–1600 mg/d po than 600–800 mg/d and 400 mg/d for maintenance	22–86%	variable	95%	1–4	14–20 hr (single dose) 13–63 d (prolonged treatment)	Hepatic	N-mono-desethyl amiodarone active (unknown)	100–700 ml/min
Sotalol	Under development Sotalex in Europe	0.2–0.5 mg/kg IV 160–400 mg/d po	near 100%	0	5–10%	0.5–4	7 Hr (healthy) 7–42 hr (renal failure)	Absent	—	150 ml/min
Bretylium	Bretylol	10 mg/kg/d IV		0	10%	0.5–1.5	13 hr	Renal	—	420 ml/min
IV										
Verapamil	Isoptin Calan Verelan	5–10 mg IV 120–480 mg/d po	10–20%	+	90%	0.1–0.4	5 hr	Hepatic and renal	N-demethyl verapamil (unknown)	500–1500 ml/min

Em to more negative values of Em. This effect is dose-, frequency-, and use-dependent, while the time-dependent changes are most marked at low (less negative) values of Em. This suggests that quinidine effects on sodium channels are more marked on activated sodium channels than on inactivated or resting ones, leading to the depression of premature beats.[19] The quinidine-induced decrease in Vmax results in a slowing in intracardiac conduction and a decrease in cell excitability.

(3) Action potential duration and refractoriness. Quinidine causes a significant increase in action potential durations of atrial, His-Purkinje, and ventricular cells. This lengthening affects mainly final repolarization since the plateau phase is shortened. The Purkinje cells located proximal to contractile fibers ("gate system" of Myerburg) undergo a shortening in duration that contributes to a decrease of the inhomogeneity in repolarization.[14,20]

The effective refractory period (ERP) increases much more than would be expected from the changes in the action potential duration (APD), therefore leading to an increase in the ERP/APD ratio.

Electrophysiologic Effects in Humans

(1) Sinus function. Minor changes are induced by quinidine on normal sinus function. An increase in sinus rate may be observed after IV administration of quinidine by reflexly increasing sympathetic activity (consecutive to both vasodilator and negative inotropic effects of quinidine) or cholinergic blockade (still under discussion). In sinus dysfunction, quinidine is usually contraindicated, although recent studies do not report any significant change in such patients.[21]

(2) Refractory periods. Quinidine increases the duration of refractory periods in atrial, ventricular, and His-Purkinje cells.

(3) Conduction. Both atrial and intraventricular conduction velocities are slowed by quinidine. At the atrioventricular junction, its effects may be different: actually, in more than 50 percent of patients, quinidine causes an *increase* in conduction velocity (as estimated by AH interval shortening) and a shortening in effective refractory period. These effects are explained mainly by the drug's anticholinergic properties. Thus, the net atrioventricular transmission is facilitated, and acceleration in ventricular rate has been reported in cases of atrial tachyarrhythmias. This is never observed in transplanted hearts deprived of autonomic influence.

Electrocardiographic Effects

At therapeutic concentrations in man, quinidine causes a moderate increase in the QRS duration[22] without modifying significantly the PR interval. Prolongation of repolarization is observed: the QTc interval is lengthened, along with flattening of the T wave.

Hemodynamic Effects

Quinidine decreases myocardial contractility in a dose- and frequency-dependent manner. This adverse effect on ventricular function can be striking in patients who have preexisting ventricular failure. Blood pressure is moderately lowered by quinidine. This response is probably due to both local anesthetic and alpha-adrenergic blocking effects.

Pharmacokinetics

When administered orally, quinidine absorption depends on the pharmaceutical form. Bioavailability ranges from 70 to 90 percent. The first-pass hepatic metabolism of quinidine (20%) explains rather large individual variations in plasma concentrations. About 80–90 percent of quinidine is bound to plasma proteins. The peak concentration in plasma is reached within two hours for quinidine tablets. The apparent volume of distribution is 210 L (2–3 L/kg). The elimination half-life is about six hours (from 4 to 10 hr).

Quinidine is largely metabolized by the liver and excreted in the urine. Most urinary metabolites are hydroxylated. About 20 percent of quinidine is excreted unchanged by the renal route. Quinidine is both filtered at the glomerulus and secreted by the proximal renal tubule. Passive back-diffusion of the unchanged molecule occurs in the distal nephron. The plasma clearance is 210 ml/min. The two major metabolites, 3-hydroxy quinidine and 2′-oxo quinidinone, contribute to over-all quinidine effects.[23] In case of hepatic or renal insufficiency or in cardiac failure,[24] quinidine distribution, protein binding, and renal excretion are altered, and dosage should be reduced by 20 to 50 percent.

Untoward Effects

(1) Cardiotoxicity. The cardiac toxicity of quinidine includes atrioventricular and intraventricular block, ventricular tachyarrhythmias, and depression of myocardial contractility.[25] The dosage must be individualized.

Quinidine syncope and/or sudden arrhythmic death are uncommon, but major complications of quinidine therapy are due to ventricular tachyarrhythmias. The role of an atypical polymorphous ventricular tachycardia called "Torsade de Pointes" has been underlined.[26] This particular arrhythmia is associated with bradycardia, heterogeneous lengthening in repolarization, and slowing in conduction. The treatment of this life-threatening arrhythmia requires discontinuation of therapy, ventricular pacing, and correction of ionic disturbances.

(2) Extracardiac adverse reactions. (a) Gastrointestinal: nausea, vomiting and diarrhea.

(b) Hypersensitivity reactions: drug fever, skin rashes, thrombocytopenia, hemolytic anemia, and agranulocytosis. A lupus-like syndrome attributed to quinidine has been reported but is still controversial.

(c) Cinchonism: dizziness, tinnitus, loss of hearing, blurred vision, diplopia, headache.

(d) Musculoskeletal: exacerbation of myasthenia.

Therapeutic Uses

Quinidine continues to play an important role in the acute and chronic treatment of supraventricular and ventricular arrhythmias. Quinidine is useful as chronic oral therapy to prevent recurrences of atrial fibrillation and flutter after DC cardioversion and ventricular tachycardia.

Contraindications

Hypersensitivity reactions have to be detected with a test dose. In addition, quinidine is prohibited in cases of sick sinus syndrome and sinus node dysfunction, intraventricular conduction defect, myasthenia, digitalis intoxication, overt congestive heart failure (CHF), and hypokalemia.

Precautions for Use

Constant vigilance is required in managing every patient suffering first-degree AV block, sinus bradycardia, arterial hypotension, mild CHF, association with digitalis, or renal and/or hepatic insufficiency.

Drug Interactions

Quinidine increases the plasma concentrations of digoxin. The mechanism of this reaction has not been completely elucidated. Drugs that induce microsomal enzyme activity may significantly modify quinidine bioavailability.

Dosage

Quinidine dosage ranges from 600–1200 mg/d and must be individually adjusted, both for conversion and maintenance.

Procainamide

History

Procainamide was discovered in 1951 as a result of a systematic study of derivatives of procaine that exert antiarrhythmic and antifibrillatory effects similar to those of quinidine.

Cardiac Electrophysiologic Effects

The direct effects of procainamide on the electrical activity of myocardial cells are very similar to those produced by quinidine and other Class IA antiarrhythmic drugs.[27] In humans, procainamide causes depression in sinus activity (this direct negative chronotropic effect may be counteracted in part by the anticholinergic action of procainamide), and the lengthening in duration of the atrial, ventricular and His-Purkinje refractory periods.[28]

Hemodynamic Effects

Procainamide exerts negative inotropic effects and has vasodilating properties that can lead to systemic hypotension.[29]

Pharmacokinetics

Procainamide is nearly completely absorbed after oral administration and does not undergo first-pass hepatic elimination. Thus, its bioavailability ranges from 80–90 percent. Procainamide is weakly bound to plasma proteins. The peak concentration in plasma is reached within one hour. The apparent volume of distribution is about 120–150 L. The half-life is brief (3 hr).

Procainamide is eliminated by hepatic metabolism and renal excretion. The major metabolic pathway is N-acetylation.[30] In slow acetylators, the plasma half-life is prolonged.[31] Fifty percent of a dose of procainamide is eliminated unchanged in the urine. The plasma clearance is 600 ml/min. Metabolites are desethyl-procainamide, N-acetylprocainamide (NAPA), and desethyl-N-acetylprocainamide. NAPA contributes to the antiarrhythmic (and proarrhythmic) effects of procainamide, and its elimination half-life is more prolonged.[28] The concentration in plasma needed for antiarrhythmic effects ranges from 4–10 µg/ml, and side-effects (e.g., systemic lupus erythematosus-like syndrome) are more often observed in slow-acetylators. In renal insufficiency, the elimination half-life of procainamide is prolonged. Because NAPA is almost entirely eliminated by renal excretion, procainamide and NAPA can accumulate to excessive levels in plasma. Congestive heart failure does not affect the elimination half-life of procainamide.

Untoward Effects

Except for hypersensitivity reactions, the incidence of adverse effects is related to plasma concentrations. Moreover rapid IV infusion can decrease myocardial performance and can cause hypotension and conduction disturbances. Lengthening of QT interval and "Torsade de Pointes" have been reported.[32]

The hypersensitivity reaction is the most common adverse effect: skin rashes, pruritus, and agranulocytosis have been reported. A systemic lupus erythematosus-like syndrome has been described: arthralgia, fever, myalgia, and even hemorrhagic pericardial effusion with tamponade. Antinuclear antibodies reach high levels. It is not yet clear whether patients who acetylate procainamide slowly have an increased risk of developing this syndrome because they synthetized little NAPA or have prolonged half-life of the parent compound.[33]

Procainamide may cause GI (nausea, vomiting, diarrhea) and neuropsychiatric (giddiness, hallucination, mental disorders) symptoms.

Therapeutic Uses

Procainamide is generally employed to treat ventricular arrhythmias (premature beats and paroxysmal tachycardia) and, less often than quinidine and disopyramide, to prevent recurrences of atrial flutter and atrial fibrillation. Procainamide is also effective in treating the Wolff-Parkinson-White syndrome.

Contraindications

The drug is contraindicated in patients with a hypersensitivity reaction to paraaminobenzoyl group, atrioventricular block (second and third degree), bundle branch block, severe CHF, myasthenia, or severe renal insufficiency.

Precautions for Use

During IV administration, hemodynamics must be monitored in all patients, particularly if they suffer from: first degree of atrioventricular block; renal or hepatic insufficiency; atrial flutter and atrial fibrillation; or mild CHF.

Dosage

When given by the IV route patients should receive 100 mg over 5 minutes, repeated every 5 minutes up to 1 g total dose. By the oral route, 1 to 4 g daily can be given, at intervals of 6 or (better) 4 hours.

Disopyramide

Electrophysiologic and Cardiovascular Effects

In vitro, disopyramide exerts typical Class IA electrophysiologic effects (cf. quinidine).[r10,r11,34] In addition to Class IA antiarrhythmic effects, disopyramide has cholinergic blocking properties, thus inducing an increase in sinus rate and shortening the sinus recovery time. Disopyramide should be used with caution in patients suffering from sinus node dysfunction. Refractory periods are minimally changed or weakly increased at atrial and ventricular levels, whereas in the His-Purkinje system and in accessory pathways, refractory periods are lengthened.[35,36]

Disopyramide does not depress the conduction velocity in the atrium. Its effects on the AH interval are variable (lengthening through direct effects, shortening by anticholinergic effects). Conduction velocity is slowed down in the His-Purkinje system and accessory pathways. The heart rate may slightly increase. Usually the PR interval and QRS are modified only if they have previously been lengthened. Lower dosage or discontinuation is indicated if the QRS duration widens more than 25 percent. Disopyramide increases the QT interval dose-dependently.

At therapeutic concentrations, disopyramide decreases myocardial performance[37] and should be avoided in CHF.[38]

Pharmacokinetics

An oral dose of disopyramide is rapidly and nearly totally absorbed. Bioavailability ranges from 60 to 90 percent, perhaps due to a first-pass hepatic metabolism. The peak concentration is reached in plasma within 30–120 minutes. The apparent volume of distribution is about 100 L. The elimination half-life ranges from five to eight hours, and little (25–40%) is bound to plasma proteins.[39]

Only 20 to 30 percent of a dose of disopyramide is metabolized as the mono-N-dealkylated metabolite and eliminated in the stools. The rest of the dose is excreted unchanged in the urine. The mono-N-dealkylated derivative exerts a less potent antiarrhythmic but more marked anticholinergic action in addition to its weak positive inotropic effects.[40]

The usual therapeutic concentration ranges from 1.7–4 μg/ml, with 7 μg/ml considered toxic.

Drug Interactions

In patients receiving lidocaine therapy, disopyramide gives rise to a 25 percent increase in the unbound form of lidocaine. Similarly, administration of quinidine causes an increase in disopyramide level and concomitantly a decrease in plasma concentration of quinidine.

Untoward Effects

The anticholinergic action of disopyramide causes a dry mouth, pharynx, nose, and eye, with blurred vision, urinary hesitancy and retention as well as constipation.[41] Hypoglycemia has been reported. Disopyramide can induce or worsen CHF, and can cause a decrease in atrioventricular conduction with QRS widening.[42] Particularly in patients with pre-existing conduction disturbances, disopyramide can impair atrioventricular and intraventricular conduction.

Hypotension may occur in patients who have cardiomyopathy or CHF. Prolongation of the QT interval is not infrequent and if the increase is beyond 25 percent, the change should be considered as toxic and arrhythmogenic.

Therapeutic Uses

Disopyramide is used for the suppression or prevention of atrial and ventricular premature beats, complex ventricular arrhythmias, and for maintenance and management of atrial flutter and atrial fibrillation. Its efficacy is not influenced by digitalis. Furthermore, recent studies have shown that disopyramide may be effective in acute myocardial infarction for reducing arrhythmias resistant to lidocaine.

Contraindications

Disopyramide is contraindicated in patients with: cardiogenic shock; preexisting second- or third-degree atrioventricular block; CHF; prolonged repolarization (long QT syndrome); glaucoma; urinary retention; or myasthenia gravis.

Precautions for Use

Great care should be exercised when prescribing the drug for patients with CHF due to rhythm disturbances, first degree atrioventricular block, and those in atrial flutter or atrial fibrillation. These latter patients should be treated with digitalis before administering disopyramide in order to avoid the disopyramide-induced heart rate acceleration.

Also patients with sinus rhythm disorders, bundle branch block, cardiomyopathies, renal and hepatic insufficiency, and those who are already consuming other class 1 antiarrhythmic drugs or have potassium imbalance should be carefully watched.

Dosage

Oral administration: the usual total daily dose is 400–800 mg divided into three or four doses.

Lidocaine

Electrophysiologic and Hemodynamic Effects

Lidocaine is the prototype of Class 1B antiarrhythmic agents. Therapeutic concentrations of lidocaine have no effect on the action potential and firing rate of the sinus node. At higher doses, the slope of Phase 4 depolarization is decreased.[43] Like other Class 1B antiarrhythmic drugs, lidocaine moderately depresses the maximal rate of rise of Phase 0 depolarization (Vmax),[43,44,45] and the kinetics of Na channel reactivation are slowed down. Lidocaine causes a net decrease in action potential duration,[20] and the effective refractory period is shortened in the intraventricular conducting system. This shortening is more marked as the action potential duration becomes longer. Lidocaine can counteract automaticity in depolarized, stretched Purkinje fibers and delayed afterdepolarizations caused by digitalis.[46] This could result from an increase in I_{K1} and/or from a decrease in inward Na current.

Some cases of sinus node arrest have been reported, and care must be taken in the presence of sinoatrial conduction disturbances.[r12] Refractory periods are slightly shortened in the atrial and ventricular muscle, whereas in terminal Purkinje fibers that normally have the longest refractory period, lidocaine effects are more prominent. At therapeutic concentrations, lidocaine increases the conduction velocity in the junction Purkinje fiber-contractile ventricular cell and may accelerate the conduction in accessory pathways. At higher concentrations, lidocaine depresses the conduction in all cardiac tissues.[47,48]

At usual doses, lidocaine causes quite negligible changes in the EKG. At toxic levels, lidocaine induces a decrease in contractility and blood pressure, both of which may develop at low doses, especially with pre-existing congestive heart failure.

Pharmacokinetics

After oral administration, lidocaine is well-absorbed; its bioavailability, however, is low because of extensive first-pass hepatic metabolism (about 70%) with only one-third of the drug reaching the general circulation. Thus only IM and IV routes are usually employed. About 60 percent of lidocaine in plasma is bound to proteins, but there are large interindividual variations (35 to 80 percent),[48] and they may explain why in some patients untoward effects occur in the presence of a therapeutic level of drug.[49] The peak concentration in plasma is reached within two minutes after IV injection and 15 to 20 minutes when the IM route is used. The apparent volume of distribution ranges from 90 to 120 L. The elimination half-life is short (1.5–2 hr). Hepatic insufficiency and reduced perfusion of the liver as a result of heart failure lengthen the elimination half-life of lidocaine and require dosage reduction.[50]

Lidocaine is mostly metabolized in the liver, and only 10 percent is excreted unchanged in the urine. The clearance of lidocaine is 750 ml/min. The two main metabolites are glycine xylidine and monoethylglycylxylidine, the latter having antiarrhythmic activity, while the former has almost none.[51] The range of effective concentrations is large: 1.5 to 6 μg/ml; the toxicity threshold is about 9 μg/ml.

Drug Interactions

Enhanced microsomal enzyme activity may accelerate the metabolism of lidocaine. The beta-blockers, particularly propranolol, can decrease hepatic blood flow and cause a subsequent increase in plasma concentrations of lidocaine. Similar effects are reported with other negative inotropic agents (cf. disopyramide).

Untoward Effects

The main adverse effects are on the CNS: paresthesias; muscle tremor; convulsions; disorientation; blurred vision; and hypersensitivity reactions. After rapid injection of high dosages or in severely compromised heart function, lidocaine may cause heart failure, hypotension, bradycardia, sinus arrest, and respiratory depression.

Therapeutic Uses

Intravenously administered, lidocaine is specifically indicated in the acute management of ventricular arrhythmias, such as those occurring with acute myocardial infarction,[52] or during cardiac manipulation, as in cardiac surgery. In addition, lidocaine is effective in the treatment of digitalis-induced arrhythmias.

Contraindications

The drug is contraindicated in patients who have hypersensitivity to local anesthetics of the amide type, Wolff-Parkinson-White syndrome (because of the facilitating effect on conduction velocity in accessory pathways), and severe degrees of sinoatrial, atrioventricular, or intraventricular block in the absence of an artificial pacemaker.

Precautions for Use

Great care should be used when giving the drug to patients with CHF, conduction disturbances, bradycardia, or hepatic insufficiency.

Dosage

An initial single direct IV injection (bolus) of 50–100 mg should be followed by infusion of 4 mg/min for the following two hours, then 3 mg/min for four hours, and finally 2 mg/min for the next 18 following hours in order to achieve a constant plasma level.

Intramuscular injection (in deltoid muscle) of 300 mg can be followed by IV infusion one to two hours later to maintain plasma concentrations.

Mexiletine

Electrophysiologic and Hemodynamic Effects

Mexiletine is a Class 1B antiarrhythmic agent and exerts electrophysiologic effects similar to those of lidocaine: dose-dependent slowing in the maximal rate of rise of Phase 0 depolarization and shortening of the action potential duration and effective refractory period.[53]

In patients with sinus dysfunction, mexiletine may cause bradycardia and sinus node arrest. Although mexiletine shortens the effective refractory period, this effect is minimal in normal nodal and contractile tissues and more noticeable in the His-Purkinje system. In patients with impaired or abnormal A-V nodal and ventricular conduction, mexiletine may reduce conduction velocities.[54]

Mexiletine has little effect on the EKG.[55] In patients with pre-existing abnormalities, it may cause bradycardia, lengthening of the PR interval and QRS widening. At therapeutic doses, a negative inotropic effect may occur in ischemic myocardium.

Pharmacokinetics

Mexiletine is readily absorbed after oral administration (70%), with a systemic bioavailability of about 90 percent.[56] About 60 percent of mexiletine in plasma is bound to albumin, and the peak concentration in plasma is reached between two and four hours after oral administration. The apparent volume of distribution is about 500 L and the elimination half-life is approximately 10 hours. The clearance of mexiletine is 200 ml/min.

The drug is eliminated after hepatic metabolism as inactive metabolites. Less than 10 percent of a dose is found unchanged in the urine. Hepatic or renal insufficiency and reduced perfusion of the liver lengthen the elimination half-life and require reduction of dosage.

The therapeutic concentrations in plasma range from 0.75 to 2 μg/ml. At 4 μg/kg untoward effects occur.[57,58]

Untoward Effects

Gastrointestinal symptoms are the most frequent side-effects. Cardiotoxicity and adverse effects on the CNS are also observed.

Therapeutic Uses

Like lidocaine, mexiletine is indicated in the treatment of ventricular arrhythmias when an oral medication is desired.[58,59]

Dosage

By the IV route: 250 mg should be given within 15 min, with 250 mg during the following hour and then 1 mg/min for each following hour.

Oral dosage is 200 mg every six to eight hours.

Phenytoin

Electrophysiologic and Hemodynamic Effects

Phenytoin is a Class 1B antiarrhythmic agent[60] that causes modest depression in automaticity. At therapeutic concentrations of phenytoin, the maximal rate of rise of Phase 0 depolarization is not modified, but it is slowed at higher concentrations. Some authors have reported hyperpolarizing effects of phenytoin with a concomitant increase in Vmax leading to positive dromotropic effects; however, these effects may be determined by experimental conditions and are still controversial.

As with other Class 1B antiarrhythmic agents, phenytoin shortens the action potential duration and effective refractory period. The electrophysiologic effects of phenytoin are more marked in ischemic than in normal cells.[61] A slight sinus tachycardia may be observed, due to the adrenergic reflex triggered by phenytoin-induced vasodilatation. Refractory periods are unchanged in atrial, nodal, and contractile tissues and are decreased in the His-Purkinje system. Phenytoin slightly increases conduction velocity in the His-Purkinje system, and, in rare cases, in the atrioventricular node. Like lidocaine, phenytoin has little effect on the EKG. However, a recent report has shown a lengthening in repolarization (QTc) after two years' treatment with phenytoin.[62] At low concentrations, a slight vasodilation may occur. At higher doses, hypotension and negative inotropic effects are observed.[63]

Pharmacokinetics

Phenytoin is slowly absorbed, with a bioavailability of 90 percent. About 90 percent of phenytoin in plasma is bound to albumin, and the peak concentration in plasma is reached between 6 and 12 hours after oral administration. The apparent volume of distribution ranges from 35 to 55 L, with an elimination half-life directly proportional to dosage (as a consequence of the saturation of hepatic hydroxylation): it ranges from 16 to 24 hr for a single dose, and can reach 40 hr during prolonged therapy. The plasma clearance of phenytoin is 2.5 ml/min. Hepatic insufficiency prolongs the elimination half-life.[64]

Because phenytoin is hydroxylated in the liver by an enzyme system that is saturable, small incremental doses may produce very substantial increases in serum levels, when the doses are in the upper range. Moreover, large interindividual variations exist (limited vs. extensive metabolizers). Most of the drug is excreted in the bile as inactive metabolites, which are then reabsorbed from the intestinal tract and excreted in the urine.

The therapeutic concentrations in plasma range from 10–15 μg/ml. Beyond 20 μg/ml, toxic signs occur.

Drug Interactions

There are many drugs that may increase or decrease phenytoin levels or may be affected by phenytoin (phenylbutazone, tranquilizers, dicoumarol, chloramphenicol, tolbutamide, phenothiazines, cimetidine, carbamazepine).

Untoward Effects

The most prominent adverse reactions of phenytoin are in the CNS (diplopia, speaking disorders, mental aberration) and particularly cerebellar signs (vertigo, nystagmus, ataxia). In addition, digestive (nausea, vomiting) hematologic symptoms (anemia, leukopenia, thrombocytopenia) and gingival hyperplasia are observed; some cases of teratogenic effects have been reported.

Therapeutic Uses

In cardiology, phenytoin is mainly used to treat ventricular arrhythmias associated with digitalis toxicity because phenytoin does not depress (and even improves) conduction velocity in heart. Phenytoin is poorly effective in the treatment of supraventricular arrhythmias.[r13] Phenytoin has been proposed in ventricular arrhythmias due to delayed repolarization.[65]

Dosage

The usual dose is 3.5 to 5 mg/kg body weight administered by slow IV injection at a uniform rate of not more than 50 mg/min; this dose may be repeated once if necessary.

Tocainide

Electrophysiologic and Hemodynamic Effects

Tocainide belongs to Class 1B antiarrhythmic drugs[r14] and exerts effects similar to those of lidocaine. Tocainide slightly decreases (or depresses) sinus automatism. Increases[66] or decreases[67] in atrial refractory periods have been reported, whereas in nodal tissue and the intracardiac conducting system the refractory periods are shortened. Only the AH interval is moderately lengthened. The effects of tocainide on electrocardiographic intervals are identical to those of other Class IB antiarrhythmic drugs—namely, nothing highly significant. Tocainide does not significantly influence hemodynamic variables; after slow IV administration (7.5 to 11 mg/kg), hemodynamic parameters remain almost unchanged.

Pharmacokinetics

Tocainide is completely absorbed after oral administration, and bioavailability is nearly 100 percent.[r14] There is no first-pass hepatic elimination, and about 50 percent is bound to proteins in plasma. The peak concentration in plasma is reached within 1 hour, and the apparent volume of distribution ranges from 70 to 150 L, with a clearance in plasma of 130 ml/min. The elimination half-life in plasma is 12–15 hr, with 60 percent of a dose metabolized by the liver and the remainder excreted unchanged in the urine. The major metabolites do not participate in antiarrhythmic action. Therapeutic concentrations range from 4–10 μg/ml.

Untoward Effects

Gastrointestinal symptoms (anorexia, nausea, vomiting, abdominal pain, constipation) are frequent but transient side-effects occurring at the initiation of therapy and lead to discontinuation in less than 10 percent of patients. Headache, vertigo, muscle tremor, blurred vision, and anxiety have also been observed.

Therapeutic Uses

Tocainide, like lidocaine, is used for the treatment of ventricular arrhythmias. Responsiveness to IV lidocaine is quite predictive of a response to oral therapy with tocainide.[68,69]

Dosage

The recommended initial dosage is 400 mg every 8 hours. The usual adult daily dosage is between 1200 and 1800 mg/day in three divided doses.

Encainide

Electrophysiologic and Hemodynamic Effects

Encainide is the prototype of Class 1C antiarrhythmic drugs.[70] It decreases the maximal rate of rise of Phase 0 depolarization (Vmax) of Purkinje fibers and ventricular muscle in a frequency-dependent manner without modifying resting membrane potential.[71] In normal cells, encainide slightly shortens the action potential duration, but does not alter the effective refractory periods; like other Class 1 agents, encainide prolongs the effective refractory period of ischemic and/or depolarized cells.

Intravenous administration of encainide (0.5–0.9 mg/kg) produces no change in sinus rate or in corrected sinus recovery time or in nodal and atrial refractory periods. On the contrary, conduction velocity is slowed through the His-Purkinje system and ventricular muscle; thus, A-H interval is markedly increased (+30%).[72] As predicted by the above electrophysiologic effects, encainide dose-dependently alters the EKG by significantly prolonging the PR and QRS intervals. The QTc interval is prolonged to a lesser degree. This prolongation is solely a result of the prolongation of the ventriculogram, as shown by the absence of prolongation of the JT interval. Encainide does not modify myocardial performance, and only slighly depresses myocardial contractility in subjects with severe cardiac insufficiency.

Pharmacokinetics

The absorption of encainide after oral administration is nearly complete, with peak plasma levels present 30 to 90 minutes after dosing.

There are two major genetically determined patterns of encainide metabolism. In over 90 percent of patients, the drug is rapidly and extensively metabolized, with an elimination half-life of 1–2 hr.[73] These patients convert encainide to two active metabolites: O-desmethyl-encainide (ODE) and 3-methoxy-O-demethylencainide (MODE), that are more active (on a per mg basis) than encainide itself. These metabolites are eliminated more slowly than encainide, with half-lives of 3–4 hr for ODE and 6–12 hr for MODE.[74]

In less than 10 percent of patients, metabolism of encainide is slower, and the estimated encainide elimination half-life is 6–11 hr.[75] Despite the differences in pharmacogenetic phenotype, all patients require three to five days of dosing to achieve a steady-state plasma level. Encainide and ODE are bound to a moderate extent to plasma proteins, while the binding of MODE is somewhat greater (92%).

Untoward Effects

As with all antiarrhythmics of this class, aggravation of a pre-existing disorder of cardiac rhythm or provocation of a different type of arrhythmia is possible.[76] The risk of proarrhythmic events is particularly marked in patients with histories of ventricular fibrillation or sustained ventricular tachycardia and altered myocardial function. The occurrence of such an event is independent of sex, age, and the basic electrocardiogram or the electrocardiogram during treatment by encainide.

QRS widening is regularly observed and linked to the plasma concentrations. An increase of more than 50 percent should suggest a decrease in dosage. The slowing in intraventricular conduction velocity is responsible for the worsening of pre-existing ventricular tachyarrhythmias.

The noncardiac adverse effects of encainide are infrequent and neurologic in nature (dizziness, headache, visual blurring, paresthesia, muscle cramps) but do not necessitate discontinuation of therapy.

Therapeutic Uses

The results of a long-term randomized study in patients with asymptomatic non-life-threatening ventricular arrhythmias,[15,16,r9,17,18] who had a myocardial infarction more than six days, but less than two years previously, has resulted in restricted use to the treatment of only life-threatening ventricular arrhythmias, in particular sustained ventricular tachycardia, in patients who are intolerant of, or unresponsive to, other antiarrhythmic agents.

Contraindications

This drug should not be used in patients with second or third degree atrioventricular block (in the absence of a pacemaker), or in complete left bundle-branch block or bifascicular block in the absence of previous exploration of the bundle of His.

Dosage

It is recommended that treatment with encainide be initiated in a hospital setting with facilities for cardiac rhythm monitoring after a full-assessment of cardiac function. The recommended initial dosing schedule for adults is 25 mg three times daily at 8-hr intervals. After a period of three to five days the dose may be increased to 100 mg/d, then to 150 mg/d.

Dosages of more than 200 mg/d or a too-rapid dose escalation should be avoided. Each single dose should not exceed 75 mg.

Flecainide

Electrophysiologic and Hemodynamic Effects

Flecainide is a Class IC antiarrhythmic agent; it exerts effects on cellular activity quite similar to those of encainide.[77] Moreover, flecainide delays repolarization, indicating a possible additional Class III-type property.

Flecainide does not affect normal sinus function, but in patients with intrinsic sinus node disease the corrected sinus recovery time may increase.[78] Flecainide produces a dose-related decrease in intracardiac conduction in all part of the heart, with the greatest effect on the His-Purkinje system. A significant increase in refractory period is observed only in the ventricle.[79] Flecainide produces alterations in the EKG quite similar to those described with encainide: concentration-related increases in PR, QRS, and to a lesser extent QT intervals.

In animals and isolated myocardium, a negative inotropic effect of flecainide has been demonstrated. Decreases in ejection fraction, consistent with a negative inotropic effect, have been observed after the single administration of 200 to 250 mg of the drug in man; both increases and decreases in ejection fraction have been encountered during multidose therapy in patients at usual therapeutic doses.[80]

In humans, flecainide has a negative inotropic effect and may cause or worsen CHF, particularly in patients with cardiomyopathy, pre-existing severe heart failure, or low ejection fractions. Congestive heart failure develops rarely in patients who have no previous history of congestive heart failure.

Pharmacokinetics

After oral administration absorption is nearly complete, and flecainide does not undergo presystemic elimination. The elimination half-life depends on the route of administration: biphasic after a single IV dose (0.24–14 hr), but the half-life in plasma is about 14 hr after oral administration.[r15] The clearance is 500 ml/min, and the apparent volume of distribution is 7.9 L/kg. Approximately 60 percent of flecainide is metabolized by the liver, producing two main metabolites (one active but only one-fifth as potent).

Untoward Effects

The most frequent cardiac side-effects are new or exacerbated ventricular arrhythmia,[81] and new or worsened congestive heart failure.[82] The most frequent extracardiac side-effects are vertigo, blurred vision, tremor, nausea, headache, and asthenia.

Therapeutic Uses

Flecainide is indicated in the treatment of life-threatening ventricular arrhythmias, Wolff-Parkinson White syndrome, and supraventricular arrhythmias in patients without impaired left ventricular function.[15,16,r9,17,18]

Contraindications

This drug should not be used in patients with cardiogenic shock, second- or third-degree atrioventricular block (in the absence of a pacemaker), or in complete left bundle branch block or bifascicular block in the absence of previous exploration of the bundle of His.

Dosage

It is recommended that treatment with flecainide be initiated in a hospital setting with facilities for cardiac rhythm monitoring and after a full assessment of cardiac function.

Flecainide is administered orally 100–200 mg twice daily. In patients with left ventricular function impairment or with renal failure, the initial dose is reduced from 100–50 mg twice daily. In all patients, doses should be increased slowly at intervals of no less than four days and in increments of 50 mg twice daily.

With IV administration, the daily dose is 1.5 to 5 mg/kg, given initially at 1 to 2 mg/kg and injected slowly (over at least a 5-minute period).

Propafenone

Electrophysiologic and Hemodynamic Effects

Propafenone is a Class IC antiarrhythmic drug with its major effect the slowing of the rate of depolarization.[84] Propafenone does not modify the duration of the action potential, but at high concentrations and like the other Class I drugs, propafenone induces a decrease in the slow calcium current. Its chemical structure is similar to that of beta-blockers, and a beta-blocking effect of propafenone (competitive antagonism) has been established in experimental and clinical studies.[85]

Propafenone induces a slowing in sinus rate, but the corrected sinus recovery time is not modified.[86] Refractory periods are lengthened in atrial, ventricular, and His-Purkinje fibers. The sinoatrial, atrial, and intraventricular conduction velocities are slightly slowed by propafenone, which therefore increases moderately the A-H and H-V intervals (10 and 18% respectively). The conduction is also depressed in accessory pathways.[87]

The PR interval and the QRS duration are lengthened by propafenone in a plasma concentration-dependent manner. The time for repolarization tends to increase, but this effect is less marked with propafenone than with quinidine. Propafenone exerts a moderate negative inotropic effect, which is observed only after IV administration.[88] A decrease in blood pressure has been reported in some cases.

Pharmacokinetics

Bioavailability is between 3 and 50 percent (first-pass effect), and the peak concentration in plasma is reached within two to four hours, with a variable elimination half-life ranging from two to 32 hours. Propafenone shows genetic polymorphism of its metabolic fate.[89] In extensive metabolizers plasma levels of active metabolites are high and pharmacokinetics are nonlinear because of metabolic saturation.[90,91] Propafenone is highly metabolized in the liver, and less than 5 percent of an administered dose is excreted as such in the urine. The clearance is 1 L/min, and the volume of distribution 2–4 L/kg. The plasma concentration range is from 0.5–3 μg/ml.[92]

Untoward Effects

Less than 20 percent of patients exhibit side-effects, but these do not require the discontinuation of treatment. The most frequent propafenone-induced adverse effects are GI (nausea, vomiting, anorexia, and, rarely, cholestatic icterus), neurologic (dizziness, tremor, headache, blurred vision), or cardiac (bradycardia, conduction disturbances, or depression of myocardial contractile force).

Therapeutic Use, Contraindications, Precautions for Use

Propafenone is administered by both the venous and oral routes. Its therapeutic use, contraindications, and precautions for use are the same as the prototype class IC agent, encainide. Propafenone is also effective in the treatment of the Wolff-Parkinson-White syndrome.

Dosage

The initial IV dose is: 1–2 mg/kg; the oral dose is: 300 to 900 mg/day in three divided doses.

Moricizine

Electrophysiologic and Hemodynamic Effects

The predominant cellular electrophysiologic effect of moricizine (a phenothiazine derivative) is a frequency-dependent inhibition of the fast sodium current in cardiac tissue with a slow onset and a slow offset kinetics.[r16] Therefore, moricizine reduces the upstroke velocity of Phase 0 of the action potential and produces a relative prolongation of the effective refractory period, but has minimal effects on action potential amplitude, maximum diastolic potential, and normal automaticity. Although moricizine does not readily conform exactly to Vaughan-Williams' classification, "moricizine has all the attributes of a Class 1C antiarrhythmic agent".[93]

In some cases, moricizine may increase sinus node automaticity (anticholinergic effect) and depress sinoatrial conduction (attributed to its membrane stabilizing properties).[94] Moricizine lengthens the A-V and H-V intervals, and widens the QRS complex, but has little effect on the ERP, JT, or QTc intervals.[95,96] In patients with supraventricular tachycardia associated with Wolff-Parkinson-White syndrome, moricizine increased antero- and retrograde accessory pathway refractoriness.

Moricizine produces no measurable changes in myocardial performance at rest or during exercise. This suggests that moricizine possesses relatively weak cardiodepressant activity.[r16]

Pharmacokinetics

Moricizine is rapidly and almost completely absorbed from the GI tract and is subject to extensive first-pass hepatic metabolism.[97] Its bioavailability is about 35 percent with oral doses of 300–500 mg, and the peak plasma concentration is reached within two hours. Moricizine is highly bound (95%) to plasma proteins, with a volume of distribution is 8.3–11.1 L/kg.

Moricizine undergoes extensive hepatic biotransformation, and less than 1 percent of the parent drug is excreted unchanged in the urine and faeces following oral administration. Nine metabolites have been identified in humans, but it is unclear whether any exerts antiarrhythmic activity. The plasma elimination half-life after a single oral dose is 2–4 hr, reaching 9 hr on chronic oral administration.

Untoward Effects

Proarrhythmic responses to therapeutic doses of moricizine have been described, but are less problematic than with encainide or flecainide.[76] In patients with pre-existing severely depressed left ventricular function, the incidence of moricizine-induced aggravation of congestive heart failure is low (<1%).[98]

The predominant noncardiac adverse effects involve the GI tract (nausea, abdominal discomfort) and CNS (dizziness, headache, perioral paresthesia).[99] The over-all incidence of adverse effects ranges from 0 to 33 percent of patients.

Therapeutic Uses

Moricizine is effective in treating nonmalignant ventricular arrhythmias by suppressing single and repetitive forms of premature ventricular complexes. Moricizine was significantly less effective in patients with spontaneous sustained ventricular tachycardia and/or ventricular fibrillation than in those with unsustained ventricular tachycardia.

After discontinuation of the study of flecainide and encainide as a result of highly significant excess mortality, only the moricizine-arm of the AST trial was continued.[15,16,r9,17,18] Recently, an intermediate analysis established that deleterious effects of moricizine (excess mortality) also occurred, and the trial has been suspended. Despite the lack of precise data, moricizine must be considered as a proarrhythmic agent.

Contraindications

The presence of a previous history of coronary artery disease, severe CHF, myocardial infarction, myocarditis, pacemaker insertion and conduction abnormalities may increase the risk of a proarrhythmogenic effect of moricizine. Caution is required in patients with renal or hepatic dysfunction.

Dosage

It is recommended that treatment with moricizine be initiated in a hospital setting with facilities for cardiac rhythm monitoring after a full assessment of cardiac function. The initial oral dose is 600 mg/d administered on a thrice-daily regimen. This may be increased to a maximum of 900 mg/d.

Class II Antiarrhythmic Drugs

Propranolol and other beta-blockers constitute the Class II antiarrhythmic agents.[r17] The pharmacology of these drugs is discussed in another chapter (see Chapter 6); only their use in the treatment of arrhythmias is considered here.

Beta-Adrenergic Activity and Arrhythmias

Beta-adrenergic receptor stimulation increases during the acute phase of myocardial infarction,[r18] ischemic episodes, and CHF due both to local ischemia-induced norepinephrine release from sympathetic nerve terminals and an excessive increase in compensatory sympathetic tone. All the cardiac structures are innervated by the adrenergic system, whereas the cholinergic system affects only the sinus node, atria, and atrioventricular junction.

In the healthy heart, stimulation of beta-adrenergic receptors gives rise to: (i) an enhancement of automaticity (increased slope of slow diastolic depolarization (Phase 4)) leading to faster firing rates of latent pacemakers; (ii) an increase in conduction velocity, especially at the atrioventricular junction; (iii) a decrease in effective refractory periods. An excessive adrenergic stimulation results in clinically significant arrhythmias in many cardiomyopathies. Although the involved mechanisms are still insufficiently understood, several consequences may be outlined:

The stimulated cardiac activity leads to an increase in the consumption of O_2 and other substrates. The imbalance between myocardial supply and demand in coronary disease is aggravated, and the already abnormal electrogenesis becomes further depressed (less negative membrane potential, with subsequent slowing in Vmax, and abnormal recovery from inexcitability).

The shortening in effective refractory periods (and duration of action potential) may be nonhomogeneous in adjacent cell areas (at the margin of the ischemic area) and because of heterogeneity in excitability, responsiveness, and conduction, circuits of reentry around the ischemic zone or scar may develop. The long QT syndrome is also related to abnormalities in adrenergic function.

In infarcted or ischemic areas, cells such as Purkinje fibers are particularly sensitive to catecholamines and can become spontaneously active even in the presence of normal sympathetic tone. When they are partially depolarized due to ischemia (i.e., when the resting membrane potentials range from −55 to −40 mV), the generated action potentials are due only to calcium ion translocation and are called "slow responses" (Phase 0 depolarization then depends on the calcium inward current).

Hyperactivity of the adrenergic nervous system is also encountered in digitalis intoxication due to the CNS effects of the glycosides. In hyperthyroidism the apparent hyperactivity is probably the result of summation of the abilities of norepinephrine and thyroid hormones to elevate cyclic AMP, the second messenger of β receptor occupation.

Cellular Electrophysiologic Effects

In isolated cardiac preparations deprived of adrenergic influence, acute administration of therapeutic concentrations of beta-blockers (except sotalol) does not induce any significant effects on electrical activity. At 50- or 100-fold higher concentrations, several beta-blockers (such as propranolol and alprenolol) exert additional Class I effects (quinidine-like effect, "membrane-stabilizing" activity). However, such effects are not involved in their antiarrhythmic properties since: (i) their dextroisomers (inactive on β receptors) possess similar quinidine-like activity but low antiarrhythmic effects;[100] (ii) the antiarrhythmic effect is evident at dosages where quinidine-like activity is nearly insignificant; (iii) several beta-blockers are devoid of membrane stabilizing property but manifest antiarrhythmic effects.

During prolonged administration, the beta-blockers lengthen the duration of action potentials and effective refractory periods in animals and in humans.[101,102] This effect may be beneficial only if the lengthening is homogeneous throughout the myocardium or if it reduces heterogeneous repolarizations (long QT syndrome).

Electrophysiologic Effects in Humans

The observed effects are quite similar with all beta-blocking drugs—namely a decrease in sinus rate and recovery time, an increase in A-H interval, atrial and AV node effective refractory periods, and in AV node functional refractory period. The conduction velocity in the His-Purkinje system and in ventricular myocardium is not modified by beta-blockers.[103,104,105] Whether a beta-blocker possesses partial agonist activity seems of minor importance in the determination of the electrophysiologic effects, since equipotent effects are obtained with pindolol (which exhibits marked partial agonist activity) and propranolol (which is devoid of such activity). Similarly the relative selectivity for beta-1 or beta-2 receptors does not influence the antiarrhythmic effects.[106,107]

Therapeutic Uses

Beta-blocking drugs are effective and widely used in the treatment of various arrhythmias:[r19]

(1) When adrenergic activity increases to an abnormally high level or if patients do not tolerate normal adrenergic activity: e.g., sinus tachycardia; tachyarrhythmias; hyperthyroidism; pheochromocytoma, atrial or ventricular arrhythmias related to stress, myocardial infarction, and mitral valve prolapse; supraventricular and ventricular arrhythmias linked with digitalis intoxication.

(2) In decreasing ventricular response rate secondary to atrial fibrillation, atrial flutter, supraventricular tachycardia, and tachycardia following nodal reentry.

(3) In long QT syndrome.

Dosage

Dosages must be adapted to each patient or situation. Beta-blocking drugs are usually administered at the same doses used in coronary disease (see Chapter 24). Under conditions of high sympathetic tone, the beta-blocking drugs with intrinsic sympathetic activity have to be avoided because of the possibility of a further increase in heart rate or lowering of ventricular fibrillation threshold.

The property of "membrane stabilizing activity" is manifest only at very high dosage (e.g., propranolol at dosages of 640 mg/d) and does not contribute to the clinical effects of beta-blocking drugs.

Class III Antiarrhythmic Drugs

As explained above, most currently used Class I drugs may not adequately protect against sudden cardiac death from ventricular tachycardia and fibrillation.[15,16,r9,17,18] Such results provide further rationale for continued search for alternative drug therapy to prevent or reduce the likelihood of ventricular fibrillation. Recently, much attention has been focused on Class III antiarrhythmic drugs as the most promising candidates for antifibrillatory activity.[r20]

Class III antiarrhythmic agents are defined as antiarrhythmic drugs that act primarily by prolonging the action potential duration.[108] The cardiac membrane needs to repolarize to a certain negative voltage before a response to a stimulus can be obtained.[109] Therefore, interventions that prolong the action potential duration are likely to lengthen cardiac refractoriness. In pacemaker (normal or abnormal) tissues, lengthening the action potential duration will delay attaining the maximal diastolic potential and result in delay of the onset of the next spontaneous diastolic depolarization. Thus the cycle length of the tachycardia will be prolonged. In nonpacemaker tissue, the increase in the action potential duration and in the voltage-dependent refractoriness will slow the tachycardia (regardless of its mechanism). In addition, experimental and clinical data suggest that antiarrhythmic agents that lengthen cardiac repolarization are not negatively inotropic and may even exert a weak positive inotropic action.[110]

Class III effects merely require: (i) a relative reduction in outward currents; (ii) an increase in inward currents. Furthermore, the latter does not necessarily imply an increase of peak inward current since, for example, slowing of inactivation of the sodium or the calcium current resulting in more inward current toward the end of the action potential could also lengthen the action potential duration. The interaction with the time-dependent outward current (I_K) of antiarrhythmic agents that exert multiple mechanisms of action (Class I, Class II or Class IV) has been demonstrated to be modulated by time and voltage.[14] The block of potassium channels exhibits reverse use dependence:[108] the block increases during diastole and declines during the plateau, resulting in less block with increasing use, contrasting with the use-dependent block of sodium channels that develops primarily during depolarization and declines during diastole.

Therefore, Class III effects lead to lengthening of the action potential duration and refractoriness at slow heart rates. As the heart rate increases, these desired effects decline. Furthermore, the drug effect may become excessive, resulting in repolarization disturbances. At times, these can be so severe that they lead to Torsade de Pointes.[r20,111,112]

An "ideal" Class III agent needs to do little or nothing at normal heart rates, but should increase refractoriness steeply as the heart rate accelerates.[r21] To date, the only agent that sustains its Class III effect during tachycardia is amiodarone (see below).

There are now a growing number of pharmacologic agents that might exert their major antiarrhythmic actions by selectively lengthening repolarization. These can be classified by their mechanism of Class III activity: (i) activation of inward current; (ii) block of outward currents.

Activation of Inward Current

DPI 201-106, an activator of the fast Na current, has been reported to produce Class III effects primarily at slow heart rates,[113] but its usefulness as an antiarrhythmic agent seems unlikely, and safety needs require further investigations.

Ibutilide, a compound under clinical development, is a substituted methane sulfonamide derivative that has been shown to be effective against atrial and ventricular arrhythmias in dogs[114] and atrial arrhythmias in humans.[115] Ibutilide was recently reported to prolong action potential duration in guinea pig ventricular cells through activation of a slow inward sodium current that would play an important role in the plateau region of the ventricular action potential and that would be a new target for Class III activity without altering potassium currents.[116] Studies of the pharmacokinetic and pharmacodynamic effects of ibutilide are incomplete. Ibutilide induces QT interval prolongation correlated with plasma concentrations[117] but does not alter other parameters (blood pressure, heart rate, QRS duration or PR interval).[118]

Ipazilide exerts Class III antiarrhythmic effects through binding to a specific site associated with cardiac sodium channels (a site identified as "site 2 neurotoxin-batrachotoxin-B"), but causes minimal changes in contractility.[119]

Block of Outward Currents

The development of Class III antiarrhythmic drugs is mostly focused on the block of outward repolarizing current usually considered a primary target for Class III action. The number of potassium channels reported in cardiac tissue is large, but three major currents can be distinguished: I_{to}, a major repolarizing current early during the action potential; I_K, an important repolarizing current during the late portion of the plateau and fast repolarization phase; I_{K1} a prominent potassium current during final repolarization and diastole.

Tedisamil appears to inhibit selectively the transient outward potassium current I_{to} and prolong the action potential duration.[120] However its Class III effect would be expected to be much less in the ventricle, where Ito is of lesser importance than in atrial tissue.

A number of new Class III agents have been found to be selective for one type of the delayed rectifier potassium current I_K, namely the fast, inwardly rectifying component. Among these drugs are ambasilide (LU-47110),[121] sematilide that exerts Class III effects in vitro[122] as well in patients with arrhythmias,[123] almokalant,[124,125,126] and MS-551.[127]

The structurally related variant of the Class III antiarrhythmic d-sotalol, E-4031, has been found to exert its effects at much lower concentrations than sotalol,[125] to enhance contractility,[128] and to suppress sustained ventricular tachycardia in experimental models of sudden cardiac death.[129]

Dofetilide (UK 68, 798) is the most extensively studied new Class III agent. It is a recently synthesized bis (arylalkyl) amine[130] that exhibits potent and selective Class III antiarrhythmic effects. In animal studies dofetilide selectively inhibits the rapid component of the time-dependent outward potassium current I_K, and therefore increases the action potential duration and effective refractory period without affecting the sodium and calcium currents.[131] As would expected of any agent that prolongs action potential duration in the sinus node, dofetilide expresses a negative chronotropic potency that is not mediated by beta-receptors but is entirely accounted for by the increase in sinoatrial action potential duration.[132]

Studies in dogs showed that dofetilide prolongs the effective refractory period and the QT interval in a dose-dependent manner, elevates ventricular fibrillation threshold, facilitates conversion of electrically-induced ventricular fibrillation to sinus rhythm, does not influence conduction within the His-Purkinje system or within the myocardium, does not impair cardiac contractility, and reduces dispersion in repolarization.[133]

In humans, dofetilide causes dose-dependent effects on myocardial repolarization, as evidenced by prolongation of the QTc interval. This is reflected in significant prolongation in the effective and functional refractory periods throughout the myocardium. No effects on sinus node function, conduction parameters or cardiac contractility have been detected in any of the clinical studies performed in healthy volunteers or in patients with angina pectoris.[134,135]

In healthy volunters[134] dofetilide is well absorbed, with a bioavailability of 99%. The peak plasma concentration is reached about 2–5 hr after oral administration, and elimination half-like is 2–5 hr. Approximately 50 percent of the dose appears unchanged in the urine; the other 50 percent is metabolized in the liver to inactive metabolites. After IV administration, a clearance of 4.7 ml/min/kg and a volume of distribution of 3.6 L/kg were found. No interactions with digoxin, propranolol, and warfarin were detected. In patients with ischemic heart disease, pharmacokinetic parameters were very similar to those described in normal healthy volunteers.[135]

Dofetilide has generally been well tolerated. Side-effects have been reported occasionally (headache, sinus tachycardia, muscle cramps), but were usually mild and transient. One case of proarrythmia has been reported: a short self-terminating run of polymorphic ventricular tachyarrhythmia occurred in association with an excessive prolongation of the QT interval that was already prolonged at entry into the study.

Amiodarone

Amiodarone was first introduced in 1967 in Belgium and France as an antianginal agent.[r22]

Electrophysiologic and Hemodynamic Effects

In sinus node cells, amiodarone prolongs the duration of the action potential and lowers the slope of diastolic depolarization, producing a bradycardia that is resistant to atropine. Amiodarone does not alter resting membrane potential and action potential amplitude in cardiac (atrial and ventricular) muscle or conducting tissue, but does decrease moderately the maximal rate of rise of Phase 0 depolarization.

The most prominent effect of amiodarone is to prolong the duration of the action potential and the effective refractory period. These effects are more marked if the action potential is initially abnormally short before administration of the drug. Thus, amiodarone also tends to decrease or even abolish physiologic disparities in duration as well (Purkinje-ventricle junction). Amiodarone increases the diastolic excitability threshold and noncompetitively antagonizes alpha and beta adrenergic effects.[136,137] In addition, amiodarone exerts both Class I antiarrhythmic effects by blocking inactivated Na channels[138] and Class III antiarrhythmic effects by blocking K channels.[139]

Amiodarone slows the sinus rhythm and lengthens the sinus node recovery time through its direct and indirect effects.[140] Refractory periods are prolonged in the atria, atrioventricular node, ventricular contractile, normal conducting tissues, and in abnormal accessory pathways.[141] Amiodarone depresses conduction, leading to significant increases in sinoatrial and atrioventricular conduction times. Amiodarone reduces the heart rate, lengthens the P-R interval and, through its effects of prolonging repolarization, increases the Q-T interval, flattens the T wave, and may produce U-waves and changes in T-wave contour.[r23]

Amiodarone exerts vasodilating effects through a significant reduction in peripheral arterial resistance, particularly of the coronary arteries. Long-term oral treatment with amiodarone does not appear to have clinically significant hemodynamic effects.[142] Intravenous administration of 10 mg/kg amiodarone results in only a minimal negative inotropic effect; use of this drug rarely necessitates discontinuation of therapy due to CHF.[143]

Pharmacokinetics

The pharmacokinetic properties of amiodarone are well documented. Nevertheless, some aspects are complex and still poorly characterized for many reasons: the circulating levels are low, the kinetics are nonlinear, and the number of metabolites are numerous (15 metabolites have been identified, among them the N-monodesethyl derivative, which possesses some antiarrhythmic activity), and, finally, the cardiac tissue concentrations are unknown.

Oral absorption is low (40–50%),[r24,144] and a first-pass hepatic metabolism cannot be ruled out. The plasma protein binding is high; levels of around 95 percent have been reported.[r23] The peak plasma concentration after single oral administration is reached after 4–7 hr, and a steady state is achieved after three to five weeks of oral therapy.[r25] The elimination half-life in plasma differs from one study to another, but averages 14–20 hr for amiodarone and about 80 hr for its major metabolite. During prolonged administration the elimination half-life is between 13 and 63 days (about 40, on average) for amiodarone and 65 days for N-monodesethyl amiodarone. The therapeutic plasma concentrations range from 1 to 4 μg/ml, but large interindividual variations have been observed.

The most prominent feature in amiodarone pharmacokinetics is the strong tissue binding (largely in adipose and muscular tissues); complete elimination of amiodarone and N-monodesethyl amiodarone from the body could take four to six months or longer following termination of long-term treatment.[145] Amiodarone is partially deiodized, and the resulting iodide is either excreted in the urine or fixed in the thyroid gland.

Untoward Effects

Adverse reactions have been very common in virtually every series of patients treated with relatively large doses of drug (40 mg/d and above), occurring in about three-fourths of all patients and causing discontinuation in 7–18 percent.[146,147] The most serious reactions are pulmonary toxicity, exacerbation of arrhythmias, and hypo- or hyperthyroidism.[148] Recently, pulmonary fibrosis after large doses of amiodarone has been reported and thought to be due to structural alterations in membrane lipids.[149,150,151]

"Torsade de Pointes" may occur, and the number of case reports is increasing since this side-effect was first linked with amiodarone therapy.[152,153] Its occurrence is explained through the effects of amiodarone to prolong repolarization concomitantly with slowed conduction and a decreased heart rate. Pronounced sinus bradycardia may be observed if there are pre-existing alterations in sinus node function, and conduction delays may precipitate complete atrioventricular block.

One of the most frequent untoward effects of amiodarone is thyroid dysfunction. Amiodarone interfers with the peripheral conversion of T_4 to T_3, leading to formation of inactive "reverse" T_3 (rT_3) in a dose-dependent manner.[151,154,155,163,164] Hyperthyroidism and, most often, hypothyroid symptoms have been reported. Patients with pre-existing goiter or hyperthyroid conditions are more prone to these toxic effects. Hyperthyroid treatment needs inexplicably high dosages of antithyroid drugs. Hypothyroidism may be corrected by thyroxine if necessary. Before beginning amiodarone, assessment of thyroid function should be performed in all patients, even if it cannot give quite predictive results concerning the risk of side-effects.

The most common side-effect of amiodarone is asymptomatic corneal microdeposits of the drug or one of its metabolites.[147] These microdeposits consist of lipofuscin granules located in the intermediate and basal cells of the cornea. Usually they do not interfere with vision, but occasionally some patients experience halo vision, discomfort, or smarting. The deposition appears to be dose-related and reversible on discontinuation of therapy.

Amiodarone causes photosensitivity and skin discolorations that are likewise due to lipofuscin microdeposits, which give bluish-gray pigmentation of skin. These effects are not dose-related and occur with treatment of more than 20 weeks.[147,151] Malaise and fatigue, tremor, abnormal involuntary movements, lack of coordination, abnormal gait, ataxia, dizziness, and paresthesias represent neurologic side-effects.[147,160] Thrombophlebitis has been observed at the injection site. During IV administration, hypotension, nausea, and vomiting have been reported, but these effects are not very troublesome and quickly disappear.

Therapeutic Uses

Because of its life-threatening side-effects, amiodarone is indicated only for treatment of supraventricular and ventricular arrhythmias that are life-threatening or refractory to other currently available antiarrhythmic agents.

Contraindications

The drug should not be prescribed for patients with sinus bradycardia, abnormalities in sinoatrial and atrioventricular conduction, abnormal trifascicular conduction, cardiogenic shock, severe hypotension, abnormal thyroid or pre-existing thyroid disease, or pregnancy (thyroid risk for the fetus).

Drug Interactions

Amiodarone may interfere with other drugs that are bound with plasma proteins, leading to elevated plasma levels of these drugs, particularly digitalis, heparin, vitamin K antagonists, and many Class I antiarrhythmics (including quinidine, procainamide and flecainide), some beta-blockers (e.g., propranolol), and calcium channel blockers (e.g., diltiazem and verapamil).[156]

Dosage

Loading doses of 800–1600 mg/d are required for one to three weeks until the initial therapeutic response occurs. Upon starting amiodarone therapy, an attempt should be made to discontinue prior antiarrhythmic drugs gradually. When adequate arrhythmia control has been achieved, or if side-effects become prominent, the amiodarone dose should be reduced to 600–800 mg/d for one month and then to the maintenance dose, usually 400 mg/d.

Sotalol

In addition to its adrenergic beta-blocking effect, sotalol (MJ 1999) possesses Class III antiarrhythmic properties.

Electrophysiologic and Hemodynamic Effects

Sotalol increases the duration of the action potential in a concentration-dependent fashion with a concomitant lengthening in the effective and the absolute refractory period.[157] Sotalol does not change Vmax except when concentrations were 100 μM or greater.[158]

The dextroisomer of the drug has been found essentially devoid of beta-blocking properties but prolongs the refractory period identically to the levo isomer. This was reported in both experimental[158] and clinical studies.[159] Thus, d-sotalol is now under clinical development and exerts similar electrophysiologic and antiarrhythmic effects to the racemic drug.[160]

The property of lengthening cardiac action potential duration has been attributed to a substantial reduction in the delayed rectifier current I_K associated with a small decrease in the inward rectifier current I_{K1}.

Intravenous d-sotalol lengthens the effective refractory period in the atria, atrioventricular node, and ventricle, and increases the intranodal conduction time. It significantly prolongs the sinus node recovery time, the QT interval, the PR and the A-H but not the H-V intervals, but it has little effect on His-Purkinje conduction.[161]

Hemodynamic studies following IV administration of sotalol have reported a reduction in heart rate, cardiac index, and stroke work index without changing stroke volume index or increasing left ventricular end-diastolic pressure.[162] However sotalol is a weaker cardiac depressant than other β-adrenergic blockers. It appears that the property of lengthening of the action potential duration tends to augment contractility, which offsets, at least in part, the depressant effect of beta-blockade on the myocardium. The absence of beta-blocking activity in the dextro isomer d-sotalol would reduce the negative inotropic effect that may exacerbate cardiac failure.

Pharmacokinetics

The bioavailability of orally administered sotalol approaches 100 percent with negligible first-pass hepatic metabolism. Sotalol is little protein-bound (5–10%) and over 75 percent is excreted unchanged in the urine. Excretion of the drug tends to be reduced in patients with renal failure, but the kinetics are unaffected by changes in hepatic function. Elimination half-life is about 7 hr in healthy volunteers, and may reach 42 hr in renal insufficiency. Biotransformation is negligible with no active metabolites.[r26,163] There is a nearly linear relationship between the plasma concentration of the drug and the prolongation of the QT interval.

Untoward Effects

The adverse reactions due to sotalol may be attributed to its beta-blocking action (bradycardia, hypotension, conduction disturbances in AV node) and its propensity to lengthen the QT interval of the EKG. Although the incidence of side-effects with sotalol is comparable to that of other beta-blockers, the incidence of heart failure aggravation appears to be lower.[161]

Worsening of arrhythmias and Torsade de pointes have been associated with the prolongation of the QT interval.[164] Torsade de pointes has occurred in cases of overdosage in the presence of hypokalemia, severe bradycardia[165] or in situations of high plasma concentrations (e.g., renal failure). When the disorders develop, sotalol therapy should be withdrawn, potassium and magnesium infusion begun and ventricular pacing instituted or, if impossible, isoproterenol infusion given.

Therapeutic Use

Because of its Class III antiarrhythmic action combined with its beta-blocking properties, sotalol is indicated in the control of supraventricular and ventricular tachyarrhythmias. Sotalol has been shown to convert atrial flutter or fibrillation and paroxysmal supraventricular tachycardias[166] to sinus rhythm, even in the Wolff-Parkinson White syndrome[167] (by its effect on the bypass tract). However, the major interest in sotalol is in the control of ventricular arrhythmias, particularly in the reduction of the frequency of premature ventricular contractions,[168] in the prevention of life-threatening ventricular arrhythmias, and in patients with inducible ventricular tachycardia by programmed electrical stimulation.

Contraindications

The drug should not be given to patients with non-compensated heart failure, bradycardia of less than 50 beats/min, greater than first degree atrioventricular block, bronchial asthma, or in association with monoamine oxidase inhibitors, verapamil, cardiac depressant drugs, or other drugs that prolong repolarization.

Dosage

With slow IV administration, doses of sotalol between 0.2 and 1.5 mg/kg are given in patients with normal as well as depressed ejection fractions.

The oral sotalol dosage is 160 mg once daily or 80 mg twice daily. This dose may be increased to a maximum of 480 mg daily. In patients with reduced renal function, a careful dosage adjustment is necessary.

Bretylium

Bretylium tosylate was introduced as an antihypertensive agent in the 1950s; in 1978, it was approved as an antiarrhythmic agent in the US in emergency situations when other antiarrhythmic drugs prove ineffective.

Electrophysiologic and Hemodynamic Effects

Bretylium tosylate interferes markedly with the autonomic nervous system by entering the adrenergic nerve terminals. Its action is biphasic, first inducing then inhibiting norepinephrine release.

In automatic cells (S-A node, His-Purkinje system) low concentrations of bretylium increase the firing rate. In atrial cells and in the intraventricular conducting system, it accelerates the rate of rise of Phase 0 depolarization and decreases the duration of the action potential. The diastolic electrical current threshold is lowered.[169] These effects are probably caused by the release of catecholamines and are abolished by pretreatment with reserpine or propranolol. They may be involved in the improvement of electrical activity and in the increased conductivity in partially depolarized cells. Higher concentrations of bretylium tosylate elevate the ventricular fibrillation threshold, lengthen the duration of the action potential and the effective refractory period in Purkinje fibers, and lower the slope of diastolic depolarization in automatic cells.[170,171] These actions do not depend only on the adrenergic neuron blocking effect of bretylium, since other blockers (such as guanethidine) do not elevate the ventricular fibrillation threshold.[172] Direct membrane effects are likely implied through its quaternary amine function.

A transient sinus tachycardia during the first few minutes after administration is usually followed by a slight bradycardia. Refractory periods are lengthened in the His-Purkinje system and in ventricular myocardium. Only in ischemic zones does bretylium increase conduction velocity. An initial increase in heart rate, cardiac output, and systemic pressure is followed after two hours by a decrease in total peripheral resistance.

The intense postural hypotension caused by bretylium restricts its use to patients confined to bed. On the other hand, even high concentrations of bretylium tosylate do not depress the myocardial contractility that may increase as a result of catecholamine release.

Pharmacokinetics

Oral absorption is less than 40 percent, with no first-pass hepatic metabolism and only a weak binding to proteins.[173] After IM doses, the peak concentration in plasma is reached within 30 minutes. The average half-time elimination is about 13 hours, with large interindividual variations.

Bretylium is eliminated almost entirely by renal excretion and is found unchanged in the urine. The effective concentrations range between 0.5–1.5 μg/ml. Renal insufficiency markedly lengthens the elimination half-life of bretylium tosylate and requires reduction in dosage.

Untoward Effects

The main adverse effects are related to arterial pressure: a transient initial hypertension with tachycardia is followed by hypotension that frequently necessitates discontinuation of therapy. Parotid pain has also been reported.

Therapeutic Uses

Currently bretylium tosylate is recommended only for life-threatening ventricular arrhythmias that fail to respond to other antiarrhythmic drugs. Suppression of ventricular fibrillation without countershock has been reported, but is unusual.

Contraindications

The drug should not be given to patients with hypotension, severe CHF, or digitalis-induced arrhythmias.

Precautions for Use

The use of bretylium tosylate should be limited to intensive care units. Patients treated with bretylium are highly sensitive to adrenergic drugs. Renal insufficiency requires reduction of drug dosage.

Dosage

Only IV use is possible (10 mg/kg/day) diluted in 500-ml glucose solution. In extreme emergencies, a dose of 5 mg/kg of the undiluted solution can be slowly injected IV.

Class IV Antiarrhythmic Drugs: Calcium Antagonists

Calcium antagonist drugs[r27,r28] are currently used as antianginal agents. They specifically block the voltage-operated calcium channels of the L-type. The blocking action of verapamil and diltiazem occurs in cardiac and vascular smooth cells at quite similar concentrations.[174,r29] In contrast, therapeutic levels of the 1-4 dihydropyridines exert their blocking effects almost exclusively on the smooth muscle cells of the vasculature. Therefore, the 1-4 dihydropyridines are not indicated as antiarrhythmic agents. At the cardiac level, the effects of verapamil and diltiazem alter all slow Ca channel-dependent mechanisms: the plateau phase of the cardiac action potential, nodal (SA and AV nodes) cells, partially depolarized atrial and ventricular cells, and excitation-contraction coupling in contractile cells. Consequently, they reduce the plateau of the action potential and induce bradycardia and slowing in atrioventricular conduction, depression and suppression of abnormal rhythms initiated in depolarized cells, and exert a negative inotropic effect.

Verapamil and diltiazem have been demonstrated to depress the fast Na current concomitantly with the Ca current, and therefore also exert some Class I antiarrhythmic effects. The involvement of Ca ions as coupling ions in a great number of physiologic processes leads to a variety of effects, mainly hemodynamic: a decrease in arterial blood pressure, vasodilating effects, and activation of the baroreflex.

The calcium antagonists are poorly effective in the treatment of ventricular arrhythmias. In myocardial ischemia, their beneficial effects may be related both to the improvement of local conditions (decrease in cardiac work, delayed intracellular Ca overload, increase in oxygen and substrate supply, and improvement in conduction through ischemic areas) and to their direct electrophysiologic effects.

Verapamil

Electrophysiologic and Hemodynamic Effects

Verapamil depresses sinus automatism and lengthens sinus recovery time, but does not modify the refractory periods in the atria, ventricles, and conducting system. In contrast, verapamil strongly lengthens, dose-dependently, the refractory period in the atrioventricular node and slows down the conduction velocity, thus leading to an increase in the A-H interval.[r30] As with other Ca antagonists, verapamil depresses cardiac contractility and lowers systemic vascular resistance and arterial blood pressure.[r31] These effects are obvious with IV administration in patients with pre-existing left ventricular function impairment.[175]

Pharmacokinetics

Verapamil is 90 percent absorbed from the GI tract, however, its bioavailability is only 10 to 20 percent, indicating extensive first-pass metabolism in the liver[176] and explaining large interindividual variations in plasma levels with similar doses of drug.[177] Verapamil is highly bound to plasma proteins (about 90%). The peak concentration in plasma is reached within about 30 minutes, the apparent volume of distribution is 450 L, and the elimination half-life averages five hours.[177,178] Verapamil is metabolized in the liver with its major metabolite (norverapamil) produced by N-demethylation. This metabolite is biologically active, but a less potent vasodilator than the parent drug.

In liver insufficiency the elimination half-life may be increased fourfold.[179] Verapamil and its main metabolite norverapamil are also excreted in the urine, thus, impaired renal function causes an increase in duration and intensity of drug effects. Congestive heart failure leads to similar modifications of pharmacokinetics because of the decreased hepatic blood flow.

Drug Interactions

Chronic administration of verapamil produces a significant increase in serum digoxin concentration. Moreover, verapamil and digitalis may act synergistically on the sinus and atrioventricular nodes and lead to increased atrioventricular block.

Untoward Effects

Side-effects are rather infrequent if careful attention is paid to both drug indications and cautions for use.[r32] The majority of adverse effects reported in the literature are cardiovascular: hypotension (2.9%), peripheral edema (1.7%), third degree A-V block (0.8%), bradycardia (less than 50 beats/minute: 1.1%), and worsening of CHF or pulmonary edema (0.9%). Central nervous system adverse effects due to verapamil are headache (1.8%), weakness (1.1%), and vertigo (3.6%). Gastrointestinal side-effects are constipation (6.3%) and nausea (1.6%).

Therapeutic Uses

Intravenous verapamil is a preferred drug for treating paroxysmal supraventricular tachycardia, since conversion to sinus rhythm has been reported in about 90 percent of cases.[r28] Oral verapamil is often used as an adjunct to digitalis to slow the ventricular response rate in atrial fibrillation and atrial flutter.

Although verapamil has significant effects on ventricular arrhythmias, it does not play a major role in their treatment because alternatives are available. In addition, its efficacy in the treatment of ventricular arrhythmias is less marked, particularly when they are not due to ischemia.[180,181,182,183]

Contraindications

The drug is contraindicated in patients with severe left ventricular dysfunction, hypotension (i.e., systolic pressure less than 80 mm Hg), atrial flutter or atrial fibrillation and an accessory pathway, e.g., Wolff-Parkinson-White syndrome, cardiogenic shock, sick sinus syndrome, or if second- or third-degree atrioventricular block is present, except in patients with an artificial ventricular pacemaker.

Precautions for Use

Combined use with beta-blocking drugs may result in additive negative effects on cardiac contractility, atrioventricular conduction, and heart rate (careful monitoring is mandatory). Great care must be used when using this drug in patients with first degree atrioventricular block, obstructive cardiomyopathy, hypotension, hepatic and renal impairment, and digoxin consumption.

Administration with other antihypertensive drugs may cause hypotension, and disopyramide should not be administered during the preceding 48 hours and following 24 hours of verapamil treatment.

Verapamil in association with quinidine may result in significant hypotension.

Usual Dosages

Intravenous route: Slow infusion of 5–10 mg in intensive care units, possibly repeated once after 15 minutes; then 15 mg slowly for the following 8 hr. Oral dosage may be given 2 hr before the end of the infusion.

Oral route: 40 to 120 mg every 6–8 hr.

References

Research Reports

1. Weidmann S. The effect of the cardiac membrane potential on the rapid availability of the sodium system. J Physiol (Lond) 1955;*127*:213–224.
2. Beeler GW, Reuter H. Reconstruction of the action potential of ventricular myocardial fibers. J Physiol (Lond) 1977;*268*:127–210.
3. Hoffman BF, Rosen MR. Cellular mechanisms for cardiac arrhythmias. Circ Res 1981;*49*:69–83.
4. Gadsby D, Cranefield PF. Two levels of resting potential in cardiac Purkinje fibers. J Gen Physiol 1977;*70*:725–746.
5. Lederer WS, Tsien RW. Transient inward current underlying arrhythmogenic effects of cardiac steroids in Purkinje fibers. J Physiol (Lond) 1976;*263*:73–100.
6. Cranefield PF, Klein HO, Hoffman BF. Conduction of the cardiac impulse. I–Delay block and one-way block in the depressed Purkinje fibers. Circ Res 1971;*28*:199–219.
7. Wit AL. Cranefield PF. Reentrant excitation as a cause of cardiac arrhythmias. Am J Physiol 1978;*235*:H1–H17.
8. Dhingra RC, Amat-Y-Leon F, Wyndham C, Wu D, Denes P, Rosen KM. The electrophysiological effects of ouabain on sinus node and atrium in man. J Clin Invest 1975;*56*:555–562.
9. Goodman DJ, Rossen RM, Cannom DS, Rider AK, Harrison DC. Effects of digoxin on atrioventricular conduction. Circulation 1975;*51*:251–256.
10. Bissett JK, de Soyza NDB, Kane JJ, McConnell JR, Doherty JE. Effect of digitalis on human ventricular refractoriness. Cardiovasc Res 1978;*12*:288–293.
11. Charlier R. A new antagonist of adrenergic excitation not producing competitive receptor blockade. Br J Pharmacol 1970;*39*:668–674.
12. Bacq ZM, Blackeley AG. The effects of amiodarone, an alpha and beta receptor antagonist, on adrenergic transmission in the cat spleen. Biochem Pharmacol 1976;*25*:1195–1199.
13. Vaughan-Williams EM. A classification of antiarrhythmic actions reassessed after a decade of new drugs. J Clin Pharmacol 1984;*24*:129–147.
14. Roden DM, Bennett PB, Snyders DJ, Balser JR, Hondeghem LM. Quinidine delays IK activation in guinea-pig ventricular myocytes. Circ Res 1988;*62*:1055–1058.
15. The CAPS Investigators. The Cardiac Arrhythmia Pilot Study. Am J Cardiol 1986;*57*:91–95.
16. The Cardiac Arrhythmia Suppression Trial Investigators. Preliminary report: effects of encainide and flecainide on mortality in a randomized trial of arrhythmia suppression after myocardial infarction. N Engl J Med 1989;*321*:406–412.
17. Echt D, Liebson P, Brent-Mitchell L et al. and the CAST Investigators. The Cardiac Arrhythmia Suppression Trial: Mortality and morbidity in patients receiving encainide, flecainide and placebo. N Engl J Med 1991;*324*:781–788.
18. Akiyama T, Pawitan Y, Gremberg M, Kuoc S, Reynolds-Haerthle R and the CAST investigators. Increased risk of death and cardiac arrest from encainide and flecainide in patients after non-q-wave acute myocardial infarction in the cardiac arrhythmia suppression trial. Am J Cardiol 1991;*68*:1551–1555.
19. Hondeghem LM, Matsubara T. Quinidine blocks cardiac sodium channels during opening and slow inactivation in guinea-pig papillary muscle. Br J Pharmacol 1988;*93*:311–318.
20. Colatsky TJ. Mechanism of action of lidocaine and quinidine on action potential duration in rabbit cardiac Purkinje fibres. An effect on steady-state sodium current? Circ Res 1982;*50*:17–27.
21. Vera Z, Licht J, Klein R, Harris F, McMillin D, Mason DT. Effect of acute procainamide and subacute quinidine administration on sinus node function in sick sinus syndrome. Clin Res 1978;*26*:98A.
22. Nademanee K, Stevenson WG, Weiss JN, Frame VB, Antimisiaris MG, Suithichaiyakul T, Pruitt CM. Frequency-dependent effects of quinidine on the ventricular action potential and QRS duration in humans. Circulation 1990;*81*:790–796.
23. Holford NHG, Coates PE, Guentert TW, Riegelman S, Sheiner LB. The effect of quinidine and its metabolites on the electrocardiogram and systolic time intervals: concentration effect relationships. Br J Clin Pharmacol 1981;*11*:187–195.
24. Drayer DE, Hughes M, Lorenzo B, and Reidenberg MM. Prevalence of high (3S)-3-hydroxyquinidine/quinidine ratios in serum and clearance of quinidine in cardiac patients with age. Clin Pharmacol Ther 1980;*27*:72–75.
25. Josephson ME, Seides SF, Batsford WP et al. The electrophysiological effects of intracellular quinidine on the atrioventricular conducting system in man. Am Heart J 1974;*87*:55–64.
26. Bauman JL, Bauernfeind RA, Hoff JV, Strasberg B, Swiryn S, Rosen KM et al. Torsade de pointes due to quinidine: observations in 31 patients. Am Heart J 1984;*107*:425–430.
27. Arnsdorf MF, Bigger JT. The effects of procaine amide on components of excitability in long mammalian cardiac Purkinje fibers. Circ Res 1976;*38*:115–122.
28. Woosley RL, Roden DM, Reele SB, Smith RF, Wilkinson GR, Oates JA. Comparative clinical pharmacology of procainamide and N-acetylprocainamide (acecainide). Circulation 1979;*60*:84–89.
29. Giardina EGV, Heissenbuttel RH, Bigger JT. Intermittent intravenous procainamide to treat ventricular arrhythmias: correlations of plasma concentration with effect on arrhythmias, electrocardiogram and blood pressure. Ann Intern Med 1973;*78*:183–193.
30. Giardina EGV, Dreyfuss J, Bigger JT et al. Metabolism of procainamide in normal and cardiac subjects. Clin Pharmacol Ther 1976;*19*:339–351.
31. Reidenberg MM, Drayer DE, Levy M et al. Polymorphic acetylation of procainamide in man. Clin Pharmacol Ther 1975;*17*:722–730.
32. Chow MJ, Piergies AA, Bowsher DJ, Murphy JJ, Kushner W, Ruo TI, Asada A, Talano JV, Atkinson AJ Jr. Torsade de pointes induced by N-acetylprocainamide. J Am Coll Cardiol 1984;*4*:621–624.
33. Woosley RC, Drayer DE, Reidenberg MM, Nies AS, Carr K, Oates JA. Effect of acetylator phenotype on the rate at which procainamide induces antinuclear antibodies and the lupus syndrome. N Engl J Med 1978;*298*:1157–1159.
34. Danilo P, Hordof AM, Rosen MR. Effect of disopyramide on electrophysiological properties of canine cardiac Purkinje fibers. J Pharmacol Exp Ther 1977;*201*:701–710.

35. Bergfeldt L, Schenck-Gustafsson K, Dahlqvist R. Comparative class 1 electrophysiologic and anticholinergic effects of disopyramide and its main metabolite (mono-N-dealkylated disopyramide) in healthy humans. Cardiovasc Drugs Ther 1992;*6*:529–537.

36. Spurrell RAJ. The effects of disopyramide on the human heart: an electrophysiological study. J Int Med Res 1976;*4*(suppl1): 31–36.

37. Kotter V, Linderer T, Schroder R. Effects of disopyramide on systemic and coronary hemodynamics and myocardial metabolism in patients with coronary disease. Am J Cardiol 1980;*46*:469–475.

38. Podrid PJ, Schoeneberger A, Lown B. Congestive heart failure caused by oral disopyramide. N Engl J Med 1980;*302*:614–616.

39. Meffin PJ, Robert EW, Winkle RA, Harapat SR, Peters FA, Harrison DC. The role of concentration-dependent plasma protein binding in disopyramide disposition. Clin Exp Pharmacol Physiol 1976;*6*:657–658.

40. Chiang WT, Von Bahr C, Calissendorff B, Dahlqvist R, Emilsson H, Magnusson A, Schenk-Gustafsson K. Kinetics and dynamics of disopyramide and its dealkylated metabolite in healthy subjects. Clin Pharmacol Ther 1985;*38*:37–44.

41. Bauman JL, Gallastegui J, Strasberg B, Swiryn S, Hoff J, Welch WJ, Bauerfeind RA. Long-term therapy with disopyramide phosphate: side effects and effectiveness. Am Heart J 1986;*III*:654–660.

42. Nicholson WJ, Martin CE, Gracey JG, Knoch HR. Disopyramide-induced ventricular fibrillation. Am J Cardiol 1979;*43*:1053–1055.

43. Brennan FJ, Cranefield PF, Wit AL. Effects of lidocaine on slow response and depressed fast response action potentials of canine cardiac Purkinje fibers. J Pharmacol Exp Ther 1978;*204*:312–324.

44. Rosen MR, Hoffman BF, Wit AL. Electrophysiology and pharmacology of cardiac arrhythmias. V Cardiac antiarrhythmic effects of lidocaine. Am Heart J 1975;*89*:526–536.

45. Grant AO, Dietz MA, Gilliam FR, Starmer CF, Durham NC. Blockade of cardiac sodium channels by lidocaine: single channel analysis. Circ Res 1989;*65*:1247–1262.

46. Rosen MR, Danilo P. Effects of tetrodotoxin, lidocaine, verapamil and AHR-2666 on ouabain-induced delayed afterdepolarizations in canine Purkinje fibers. Circ Res 1980;*46*:117–124.

47. Arnsdorf MF, Bigger JT Jr. Effects of lidocaine hydrochloride on membrane conductance in mammalian cardiac Purkinje fibers. J Clin Invest 1972;*51*:2252–2263.

48. Benowitz ML, Meister W. Clinical pharmacokinetics of lignocaine. Clin Pharmacokinetics 1978;*3*:177–201.

49. Pieper JA, Wyman MG, Goldreyer BN, Cannom DS, Slaughter RL, Lalka D. Lidocaine toxicity: Effects of total versus free lidocaine concentrations. Circulation 1980;*62*:181–186.

50. Thomson PD, Melmon HL, Richardson JA, Cohn K, Steinbrunn W, Cudihee R, Rowland M. Lignocaine pharmacokinetics in advanced heart failure, liver disease and renal failure in humans. Ann Inter Med 1973;*78*:499–508.

51. Di Fazio CA. Metabolism of local anesthetics in the fetus, newborn and adult. Brit J Anaesth 1979;*S1*:suppl:29–34.

52. De Silva RA, Hennekens CH, Lown B, Cascells W. Lignocaine prophylaxis in acute myocardial infarction: an evaluation of randomised trials. Lancet 1981;*2*:855–858.

53. Yamaguchi I, Singh B, Mandel W. Electrophysiological action of mexiletine on isolated rabbit atria and canine ventricular muscle and Purkinje fiber. Cardiovasc Res 1979;*13*:288–296.

54. Roos JC, Paalman ACA, Dunning AR. Electrophysiological effects of mexiletine in man. Br Heart J 1976;*38*:1262–1271.

55. Chew CYC, Collett J, Singh BN. Mexiletine: a review of its pharmacological properties and therapeutic efficacy in arrhythmias. Drugs 1979;*17*:161–181.

56. Woosley RL, Wang T, Stone W, Siddoway L, Thompson K, Duff HJ, Cerskus I, Roden D. Pharmacology, electrophysiology and pharmacokinetics of mexiletine. Am Heart J 1984;*107*:1058–1065.

57. Mehta J. Conti CR. Mexiletine, a new antiarrhythmic agent for treatment of premature ventricular complexes. Am J Cardiol 1983;*49*:455–460.

58. Franck MJ, Watkins LO, Prisant M, Smith MS, Russel SL, Abdulla AM, Manwaring RL. Mexiletine versus quinidine as first-line antiarrhythmic therapy: results from consecutive trials. J Clin Pharmacol 1991;*31*:222–228.

59. Jewitt D, Jackson G, McCormish M. Comparative antiarrhythmic efficacy of mexiletine, procainamide and tolamolol in patients with symptomatic ventricular arrhythmias. Postgrad Med J 1977;*53*:Suppl 1:158–172.

60. Rosen MR, Danilo P Jr, Alonso MB, Pippenger CE. Effects of therapeutic concentrations of diphenylhydantoin on transmembrane potentials of normal and depressed Purkinje fibers. J Pharmacol Exp Ther 1976;*197*:594–604.

61. El-Sherif N, Lazzara R. Reentrant ventricular arrhythmias in the late myocardial infarction period. Mechanism of action of diphenylhydantoin. Circulation 1978;*57*:465–473.

62. Ishida K, Uchida A, Yabuki S, Seki K. Effect of long-term sodium diphenylhydantoin on QT and U (TU) wave. Acta Neurol Scand 1980;*62* Suppl.79:119.

63. Mixter CG, Moran JM, Austen WG. Cardiac and peripheral vascular effects of diphenylhydantoin sodium. Am J Cardiol 1966;*17*:332–339.

64. Richens A. Clinical pharmacokinetics of phenytoin. Clin Pharmacokinet 1979;*4*:153–169.

65. Lovell RRH. Phenytoin after recovery from myocardial infarction. Lancet 1971;*2*:1055–1058.

66. Danilo P. Tocainide. Am Heart J 1979;*97*:259–262.

67. Zipes DP, Troup PJ. New antiarrhythmic agents. Amiodarone, aprindine, disopyramide, ethmozin, mexiletine, tocainide, verapamil. Am J Cardiol 1978;*41*:1005–1024.

68. Maloney JD, Nissen RG, McColgan JM. Open clinical studies at a referral center: chronic maintenance of tocainide therapy in patients with recurrent sustained ventricular tachycardia refractory to conventional antiarrhythmic agents. Am Heart J 1980;*100*:1023–1030.

69. Young MD, Hadizian Z, Horn HR, Johnson JL, Vassalo HG. Treatment of ventricular arrhythmias with oral tocainide. Am Heart J 1980;*100*:1041–1045.

70. Woosley RL, Wood AJJ, Roden DM. Encainide. N Engl J Med 1988;*318*:1107–1115.

71. Carmeliet E. Electrophysiological effects of encainide on isolated cardiac muscle and Purkinje fibers and the Langendorff-perfused guinea-pig heart. Eur J Pharmacol 1980;*61*:247–262.

72. Sami M, Mason JW, Peters F, Harrison DC. Electrophysiologic effects of encainide, a newly developed antiarrhythmic. Am J Cardiol 1979;*44*:526–532.

73. Wang T, Roden DM, Wolfenden HT, Woosley RL, Wood AJJ, Wilkinson GR. Influence of genetic polymorphism on the metabolism and disposition of encainide in man. J Pharmacol Exp Ther 1984;*228*:605–611.

74. Anderson JL, Stewart JR, Johnson TA, Lutz JR, Pitt B. Encainide therapy of malignant arrhythmias: concentration of parent drug and metabolites. Clin Res 1982;*30*:3–8.

75. Woosley RL, Roden DM, Dai G, Wang T, Altenbern D, Oates J, Wilkinson GR. Co-inheritance of the polymorphic metabolism of encainide and debrisoquin. Clin Pharmacol Ther 1986;*39*:282–287.

76. Podrid PJ, Lambert S, Graboys TB, Blatt CM, Lown B. Aggravation of arrhythmia by antiarrhythmic drugs. Incidence and predictors. Am J Cardiol 1987;*59*:38E–44E.

77. Borchard U, Boisten N. Effects of flecainide on action potentials and alternating current-induced arrhythmias in mammalian myocardium. J Cardiovasc Pharmacol 1982;*4*:205–212.

78. Vik-Mo H, Ohm OJ, Lund-Johonsen P. Electrophysiologic effects of flecainide acetate in patients with sinus nodal dysfunction. Am J Cardiol 1982;*50*:1090–1094.

79. Estes NA 3d, Garan H, Ruskin J. Electrophysiological properties of flecainide acetate. Am J Cardiol 1984;*53*:26B–29B.

80. Legrand V, Vandormael M, Collignon P, Kulbertus HE. Hemodynamic effects of a new antiarrhythmic agent flecainide R 818 in coronary heart disease. Am J Cardiol 1983;*51*:422–426.

81. Nathan AW, Hellestrand KJ, Bexton RS, Spurrell RAJ, Camm AJ. The proarrhythmic effects of flecainide. Drugs 1985;*29*(Suppl 4):45–53.

82. Josephson MA, Ikeda N, Singh BN. Effects of flecainide on ventricular function: clinical and experimental correlation. Am J Cardiol 1984;*53*:95B–100B.

83. Gentzkow GD, Sullivan JY. Extracardiac adverse effects of flecainide. Am J Cardiol 1984;*53*:101B–105B.

84. Kohlhardt M, Seifert C. Inhibition of Vmax of action potential by propafenone and its voltage-time and pH-dependance in mammalian ventricular myocardium. Naunyn-Schmied Arch Pharmacol 1980;*315*:55–62.

85. Dukes ID, Vaughan-Williams EM. The multiple modes of action of propafenone Eur Heart J 1984;*5*:115–125.

86. Waleffe A, Mary-Rabine L, De Rijbel R, Soyeur D, Legrand V, et al. Electrophysiological effects of propafenone studied with programmed electrical stimulation of the heart in patients with recurrent paroxysmal supraventricular tachycardia. Eur Heart J 1981;*2*:345–352.

87. Clementy J, Falquier JP, Danis C, Roudaut R, Bricaud H. Etude des propriétés électrophysiologiques de la propafénone intraveineuse. Méd Hyg (Genève) 1980;*38*:4277–4281.

88. Shen EN, Sung RJ, Morady F, Schwartz AB, Scheinman MM, DiCarlo L, Shapiro W. Electrophysiological and haemodynamic effects of intravenous propafenone in patients with recurrent ventricular tachycardia. J Am Coll Cardiol 1984;*3*:1291–1297.

89. Siddoway LA, Thompson KA, McAllister CB, Wang T, Wilkinson GR, Roden DM, Woosley RL. Polymorphism of propafenone metabolism and disposition in man: clinical and pharmacokinetic consequences. Circulation 1987;*75*:785–791.

90. Kates RE, Yee YG, Winckle RA. Metabolic cumulation during chronic propafenone dosing in arrhythmia. Clin Pharmacol Ther 1985;*37*:610–614.

91. Giani P, Landolina M, Giudici V, Bianchini C, Ferrario G, Marchi S, Riva E, Latini R. Pharmacokinetics and pharmacodynamics of propafenone during acute and chronic administration. Eur J Clin Pharmacol 1988;*34*:187–194.

92. Keller K, Meyer-Estorf G, Beck OA, Hochrein H. Correlation between serum concentration and pharmacological effect on atrioventricular conduction time of the antiarrhythmic drug propafenone. Eur J Clin Pharmacol 1978;*13*:17–20.

93. Vaughan-Williams EM. Classification of the antiarrhythmic action of moricizine. J Clin Pharmacol 1991;*31*:216–221.

94. Chazov EI, Shugushev KK, Rosenshtraukh LV. Ethmozin I. Effects of intravenous drug administration on paroxysmal supraventricular tachycardia in the ventricular preexcitation syndrome. Am Heart J 1984;*108*:475–482.

95. Chazov EI, Rosenshtaukh LV, Shugushev KK. Ethmozin. II. Effects of intravenous drug administration on atrioventricular nodal reentrant tachycardia. Am Heart J 1984;*108*:483–489.

96. Bigger JT. Cardiac electrophysiologic effects of moricizine hydrochloride. Am J Cardiol 1990;*65*:15D–20D.

97. Woosley RL, Morganroth J, Fogoros RN, McNahon G, Humphries JO, Mason DL, Williams RL. Pharmacokinetics of moricizine HCl. Am J Cardiol 1987;*60*:35F–39F.

98. Podrid PJ, Bean SL. Antiarrhythmic drug therapy for congestive heart failure with focus on moricizine. Am J Cardiol 1990;*65*:56D–64D.

99. Kennedy HL. Noncardiac adverse effects and organ toxicity of moricizine during short- and long-term studies. Am J Cardiol 1990;*65*:47D–50D.

100. Jewitt DE, Singh BN. The role of beta-adrenergic blockade in myocardial infarction. Prog Cardiovasc Dis 1974;*16*:421–438.

101. Vaughan-Williams EM, Raine AEG, Cabrera AA. The effect of prolonged beta-adrenoceptor blockade on heart weight and cardiac intracellular potentials in rabbit. Cardiovasc Res 1975;*9*:579–592.

102. Edvardsson N, Olsson SB. Effects of acute and chronic beta-receptor blockade on ventricular repolarization in man. Eur Heart J 1980;*1*:335–343.

103. Seides SF, Josephson ME, Batsford WP, Weisfogel GM, Lau SH, Damato AN. The electrophysiology of propranolol in man. Am Heart J 1974;*88*:733–741.

104. Robinson C, Birkhead J, Crook B, Jennings K, Jewitt D. Clinical electrophysiological effects of atenolol. A new cardioselective beta-blocking agent. Br Heart J 1978;*40*:14–21.

105. Rizzon P, Di Biase M, Chiddo A, Mastrangelo D, Sorgente L. Electrophysiological properties of intravenous metoprolol in man. Br Heart J 1978;*40*:650–655.

106. Ward DE, Camm AJ, Spurrell RA. The acute cardiac electrophysiological effects of intravenous sotalol hydrochloride. Clin Cardiol 1979;*2*:185–191.

107. Di Biase M, Brindicci G, Rizzon P. Effects of pindolol on impulse formation and conduction in man. J Electrocardiol 1977;*10*:45–50.

108. Hondeghem LM, Snyders DJ. Class III antiarrhythmic agents have a lot of potential but a long way to go. Reduced effectiveness and dangers of reverse use dependence. Circulation 1990;*81*:686–690.

109. Weidmann S. Effects of calcium ions and local anesthetics on electrical properties of Purkinje fibers. J Physiol (Lond) 1955;*129*:568–582.

110. Platou ES, Refsum H, Hotvedt R. Class III antiarrhythmic activity linked with positive inotropy: electrophysiological and he-

modynamic effects of the sea anemone polypeptide ATXII in the dog heart in situ. J Cardiovasc Pharmacol 1986;*8*:459–465.

111. Roden DM, Hoffman BF. Action potential prolongation and induction of abnormal automaticity by low quinidine concentration in canine Purkinje fibers: relationship to potassium and cycle length. Circ Res 1985;*56*:857–67.

112. El-Sherif N, Bekheit SS, Henkin R. Quinidine-induced long QT interval and Torsade de pointes: role of bradycardia-dependent early afterdepolarization. J Am Coll Cardiol 1989;*14*:252–257.

113. Mortensen E, Tande PM, Klow NE, Platou ES, Refsum H. Positive inotropy linked with class III antiarrhythmic action: electrophysiological effects of the cardiotonic agent DP1 201–106 in the dog heart in vivo. Cardiovasc Res 1990;*24*:911–917.

114. Buchanan LV, Kabell G, Turcotte UM, Brunden MN, Gibson JK. Effects of ibutilide on spontaneous and induced ventricular arrhythmias in 24-hour-canine myocardial infarction. A comparative study with sotalol and encainide. J Cardiol Pharmacol 1992;*19*:256–263.

115. DiMarco JP. Cardioversion of atrial flutter by intravenous ibutilide. A new class III antiarrhythmic agent. J Am Coll Cardiol 1991;*17*:2324A.

116. Lee KS. Ibutilide, a new compound with potent class III antiarrhythmic activity, activates a slow inward Na^+ current in guinea-pig ventricular cells. J Pharmacol Exp Ther 1992;*262*:99–108.

117. Jungbluth GL. Della Colletta AA. Vanderlugt JT. Evaluation of the pharmacokinetics and pharmacodynamics of ibutilide fumarate and its enantiomer in healthy male volunteers. Pharm Res 1991;*8*:S249.

118. Vanderlugt JT, Gaylor SK, Wakefiels LK, Jungbluth GL, Walters RR, Kabell GG. Effects of ibutilide fumarate, a new class III antiarrhythmic agent in man. Clin Pharmacol Ther 1991;*49*:188.

119. Hill RJ, Grant AM, Dessingue OC, Harris AL, Ezrin AM. Ipazilide, a new antiarrhythmic drug: inhibition of 3H-batrachotoxin binding to cardiac sodium channels and effects on papillary muscle contractility. Br J Pharmacol 1991;*104*:Suppl, 187P.

120. Dukes ID, Morad M. Tesidamil inactivates transient outward K^+ current in rat ventricular myocytes. Am J Physiol 1984;*247*:H1746–H1749.

121. Takanaka C, Sarma JSM, Singh BN. Electrophysiologic effects of ambasilide (LU-47110) a new class III antiarrhythmic agent, on isolated canine rabbit cardiac muscle. J Cardiovasc Pharm 1992;*19*:290–301.

122. Lumma WC Jr, Wohl RA, Dovey DD, Argentieri TM, De Vito RJ, Gomez RP, Jain VK, Marisca AJ, Morgan TK, Reiser HJ, Sullivan ME, Wiggins J, Wong SS. Rational design of 4-[(methyl-(sulfonyl)amino] benzamides as class III antiarrhythmic agents. J Med Chem 1987;*30*:755–758.

123. Wong W, Pavlou HN, Birgersdotter UM, Hilleman DE, Mohiuddin SM. Roden DM. Pharmacology of the class III antiarrhythmic agent sematilide in patients with arrhythmias. Am J Cardiol 1992;*69*:206–212.

124. Carlsson L, Abrahamson C, Almgren O, Lundberg C, Duber G. Prolonged action potential duration and positive inotropy induced by the novel class III antiarrhythmic agent H234/09 (almokalant) in isolated human ventricular muscle. J Cardiovasc Pharmacol 1991;*18*:882–887.

125. Wettwer E, Groundke M, Ravens U. Differential effects of the new class III antiarrhythmic agents almokalant, E-4301 and D-sotalol, and of quinidine, on delayed rectifier currents in guinea pig ventricular myocytes. Cardiovasc Res 1992;*26*:1145–1152.

126. Wiesfeld ACP, Crijns HJGM, Tobe JJM, Almgren O, Bergstrand RH, Aberg J. Electropharmacologic effects on pharmackinetics of almokalant, a new class III antiarrhythmic, in patients with healed or healing myocardial infarcts and complex ventricular arrhythmias. Am J Cardiol 1992;*70*:990–996.

127. Nakaya H, Tohse N, Takeda Y, Kanno M. Effects of MS-551, a new class III antiarrhythmic drug on action potential and membrane currents in rabbit ventricular mycocytes. Br J Pharmacol 1993;*109*:157–163.

128. Wettwer E, Scholtysik G, Schaad A, Himmel H, Ravens U. Effects of the new class III antiarrhythmic drug E-4031 on myocardial contractility and electrophysiological parameters. J Cardiovasc Pharm 1991;*17*:480–487.

129. Chi L, Mu D, Lucchesi BR. Electrophysiology and antiarryhythmic actions of E-4031 in the experimental animal model of sudden coronary death. J Cardiovasc Pharmacol 1991;*18*:137–143.

130. Cross PE, Arrowsmith JE, Thomas GN, Gwilt M, Burges RA, Higgins AJ. Selective class III antiarrhythmic agents. I Bis(arylalkyl)amines. J Med Chem 1990;*33*:1151–1155.

131. Gwilt M, Arrowsmith JE, Blackburn KJ, Burges RA, Cross PE, Dalrymple HW, Higgins AJ. UK-68,798: a novel potent and highly selective class III antiarrhythmic agent which blocks potassium channels in cardiac cells. J Pharmacol Exp Ther 1991;*256*:318–324.

132. Tande PM, Bjornstad H, Yang T, Refsum T. Rate-dependent class III antiarrhythmic action, negative chronotropy and positive inotropy of a novel IK blocking drug UK-68,798: potent in guinea-pig but no effect in rat myocardium. J Cardiovasc Pharmacol 1990;*16*:401–410.

133. Rasmussen HS, Allen MJ, Blackburn KJ, Butrous GS, Dalrymple HW. Dofetilide, a novel class III antiarrhythmic agent. J Cardiovasc Pharmacol 1992;*20* (Suppl 2) S96–S105.

134. Sedgwick M, Rasmussen HS, Walker D, Cobbe SM. Pharmacokinetic and pharmacodynamic effects of UK-68,798, a new potential class III antiarrhythmic drug. Br J Clin Pharmacol 1991;*31*:S15–S19.

135. Sedgwick M, Rasmussen HS, Cobbe SM. Clinical and electrophysiologic effects of intravenous dofetilide UK (68,798) a new class III antiarrhythmic drug in patients with angina pectoris. Am J Cardiol 1992;*69*:513–517.

136. Singh BN, Vaughan-Williams EM. The effect of amiodarone, a new antianginal drug, on cardiac muscle. Br J Pharmacol 1970;*39*:657–667.

137. Goupil N, Lenfant J. The effects of amiodarone on the sinus node activity of the rabbit heart. Eur J Pharmacol 1976;*39*:23–31.

138. Follmer CH, Aomine M, Yeh JZ, Singer DH. Amiodarone-induced block of sodium current in isolated cardiac cells. J Pharmacol Exp Ther 1987;*243*:187–194.

139. Takanata C, Singh BN. Barium-induced nondriven action potentials as a model of triggered potentials from early afterdepolarizations: significance of slow channel activity and differing effects of quinidine and amiodarone. J Am Coll Cardiol 1990;*15*:213–221.

140. Touboul P, Atallah G, Gressard A, Kirkorian G. Effects of amiodarone on sinus node in man. Br Heart J 1979;*42*:573–578.

141. Wellens HJJ, Lie KI, Bar FW, Wesdorp JC, Dohmen HJ, Duren DR, Durrer D. Effect of amiodarone in the Wolff-Parkinson-White syndrome. Am J Cardiol 1976;*38*:89–194.

142. Sheldon RS, Mitchell LB, Duff HJ, Wyse DG, Manyari DE. Right and left ventricular function during chronic amiodarone therapy. Am J Cardiol 1988;*62*:736–740.

143. Rosenbaum MB, Chiale PA, Halpern MS, Nau GJ, Przybylski J, Levi RJ, L'Azzari JO, Elizari MV. Clinical efficacy of amiodarone as an antiarrhythmic agent. Am J Cardiol 1976;*38*:934–944.

144. Pfeifer A, Vidon N, Bovet M, Rongier M, Bernier JJ, et al. Intestinal absorption of amiodarone in man. J Clin Pharm 1990;*30*:615–620.

145. Poirier JM, Escoubet B, Jaillon P, Coumel Ph, Richard MO, et al. Amiodarone pharmacokinetics in coronary patients: differences between acute and one-month chronic dosing. Eur J Drug Metab Pharmacokinet 1988;*13*:67–72.

146. Murphy JAM, Fitzsimons BM, Meute MA, Wilkinson WC, Luck JC, Wiley SW. Amiodarone: a postmarketing evaluation of monitoring for drug-induced toxicity. Drug Int Clin Pharm 1990;*24*:1001–1006.

147. Wilson JS, Podrid PJ. Side effects of amiodarone. Am Heart J 1991;*121*:158–171.

148. Lubbe WF, Mercer CJ. Amiodarone: its side effects, adverse reactions and dosage schedules. N Z Med J 1982;*95*:502–504.

149. Morena J, Vidal R, Morell F, Ruiz J, Bernardo L, Laporte JR. Pulmonary fibrosis and amiodarone. Brit Med J 1982;*285*:895.

150. Kennedy JI. Clinical aspects of amiodarone pulmonary toxicity. Clin Chest Med 1990;*11*:119–129.

151. Counihan PJ, McKenna WJ. Risk-benefit assessment of amiodarone in the treatment of cardiac arrhythmias. Drug Safety 1990;*5*:286–304.

152. McComb JM, Logan KR, Khan MM, Geddes JS, Adgey AAJ. Amiodarone-induced ventricular fibrillation. Eur J Cardiol 1980;*11*:381–385.

153. Selarovski S, Lewin RF, Kracoff O, Strasberg B, Arditti A, Admon J. Amiodarone-induced polymorphous ventricular tachycardia. Am Heart J 1983;*105*:6–12.

154. Nademanee K, Melmed S, Hendrickson JA, Reed AW, Hershman JM, Singh BN. Role of serum T "and reverse T" in monitoring antiarrhythmic efficacy and toxicity of amiodarone in resistant arrhythmias. Am J Cardiol 1981;*47*:482–486.

155. Kennedy RL, Griffiths H, Gray TA. Amiodarone and the thyroid. Clin Chem 1989;*35*:1881–1887.

156. Lesko LJ. Pharmacokinetic drug interactions with amiodarone. Clin Pharmacokinet 1989;*17*:130–140.

157. Singh BN, Vaughan-Williams EM. A third class of antiarrhythmic action: effects on atrial and ventricular intracellular potentials and other pharmacological actions on cardiac muscle of MS 1999 and AH 3676. Br J Pharmacol 1970;*39*:675–689.

158. Carmeliet E. Electrophysiologic and voltage clamp analysis of effects of sotalol on isolated cardiac muscle and Purkinje fibers. J Pharmacol Exp Ther 1985;*232*:817–825.

159. Johnston GD, Finch MB, McNeill JA, Shanks RG. A comparison of the cardiovascular effects of (+) sotalol and (±) sotalol following intravenous administration in normal volunteers. Br J Clin Pharm 1985;*20*:507–510.

160. Brachmann J, Beyer T, Schmitt C, Schoels W, Montero M, Hilbel T. Electrophysiologic and antiarrhythmic effects of D-sotalol. J Cardiovasc Pharmacol 1992;*20*:Suppl 2:591–595.

161. Nademanee K, Feld G, Hendrickson JA, Singh PN, Singh BN. Electrophysiologic and antiarrhythmic effects of sotalol in patients with life-threatening ventricular tachyarrhythmias. Circulation 1985;*72*:555–563.

162. Yusuf S, Peto R, Lewis J, Collius R, Sleight P. Beta-blockade during and after myocardial infarction: an overview of the randomized trials. Prog Cardiovasc Dis 1985;*27*:335–371.

163. Meier J. Pharmacokinetic comparison of pindolol with other beta-adrenoceptor blocking agents. Am Heart J 1982;*104*:364–373.

164. Neuvonen PJ, Elonen E, Vuorenmaa T, Laakso M. Prolonged QT interval and ventricular to tachyarrhythmias: common features of sotalol intoxication. Eur J Clin Pharm 1981;*20*:85–89.

165. Mc Kibbin JK, Pocock WA, Barlow JB, Scottmillon RN, Obel JWP. Sotalol, hypokalemia, syncope and torsade de pointes. Br Heart J 1984;*51*:157–162.

166. Teo KK, Harte M, Hogan JH. Sotalol infusion in the treatement of supraventricular tachyarrhythmias. Chest 1985;*87*:113–118.

167. Bennett D. Acute prolongation of myocardial refractoriness by sotalol. Br Heart J 1982;*47*:521–526.

168. Anderson JL, Askins JC, Gilbert EM, Miller RH, Keefe DL, Somberg JC, Freeman RA, Haft LR, Mason JW, Lessem JN. Multicenter trial of sotalol for suppression of frequent complex ventricular arrhythimas: a double blind, randomized, placebo-controlled evaluation of two doses. J Am Coll Cardiol 1986;*8*:752–762.

169. Wang CM, Maxwell RA. The electrophysiologic effects of bretylium on isolated cardiac tissue of normal and immunosympathectomized rats. Pharmacologist 1974;*16*:267–273.

170. Bigger JT Jr, Jaffee CC. The effect of bretylium tosylate on the electrophysiologic properties of ventricular muscle and Purkinje fibers. Am J Cardiol 1971;*27*:82–92.

171. Cardinal R, Sasyniuk BJ. Electrophysiological effects of bretylium tosylate on subendocardial Purkinje fibers from infarcted canine hearts. J Pharmacol Exp Ther 1978;*203*:159–174.

172. Kniffen FJ, Lomas TE, Counsell RE, Lucchesi BR. The antiarrhythmic and antifibrillatory actions of bretylium. J Pharmacol Exp Ther 1975;*92*:120–128.

173. Anderson JL, Paterson E, Wagner JG, Johnson TA, Lucchesi BR, Pitt B. Clinical pharmacokinetics of intravenous and oral bretylium tosylate in survivors of ventricular tachycardia or fibrillation: clinical application of a new assay for bretylium. J Cardiovasc Pharmacol 1981;*3*:485–499.

174. Singh BN, Vaughan-Williams EM. A fourth class of antiarrhythmic action? Effect of verapamil on ouabain toxicity, on atrial and ventricular intracellular potentials and other features of cardiac function. Cardiovasc Res 1972;*6*:109–119.

175. Agabih-Rosei E, Muiesan ML, Romanelli G, Beschi M, Castellano M, Muiesan G. Reversal of cardiac hypertrophy by long-term treatment with calcium antagonists in hypertensive patients. J Cardiovasc Pharm 1988;*12*(Suppl 6):S75–S78.

176. Woodcock BG, Hopf R, Kaltenbach M. Verapamil and norverapamil plasma concentrations during long-term therapy in patients with hypertrophic obstructive cardiomyopathy. J Cardiovasc Pharm 1980;*2*:17–23.

177. Mc Allister RG, Kirsten EB. The pharmacology of verapamil. IV Kinetics and dynamic effects after single intravenous and oral doses. Clin Pharm Therap 1982;*31*:418–426.

178. Haman SR, Blouin RA, Mc Allister RG. Clinical pharmacokinetics of verapamil. Clin Pharmakinet. 1984;*9*:21–41.

179. Finucci GF, Padrini R, Piovan D, Melica E, Merkel C, et al. Verapamil pharmacokinetics and liver functions in patients with cirrhosis. Int J Clin Pharm Res 1988;*VII*:123–126.

180. Rinkenberger RL, Prystowski EW, Heger JJ. Effect of intravenous and chronic oral verapamil administration in patients with supraventricular tachyarrhythmias. Circulation 1980;*62*:996–1010.

181. El-Sherif N, Lazzava R. Re-entrant ventricular arrhythmias in the late myocardial infarction period. Effect of verapamil and D600 and the role of "slow channel." Circulation 1979;*60*:605–615.

182. Elharrar V, Gaum WE, Zipes DP. Effect of drugs on conduction delay and the incidence of ventricular arrhythmias induced by acute coronary occlusion in dogs. Am J Cardiol 1977;*39*:544–549.

183. Danish study group on verapamil in myocardial infarction. Effects of verapamil on mortality and major events after acute myocardial infarction (The Danish Verapamil Infarction Trial II - DAVIT II) Am J Cardiol 1990;*66*:779–785.

Reviews and Books

r1. Katz AM. The cardiac action potential. In Physiology of the heart, 2nd Ed. New York: Raven Press, (1992); 438–472.

r2. Hille B. Ionic channels in nerve membranes. Prog Biophys Molec Biol 1970;*21*:1–11.

r3. Hille B. Gating in sodium channel nerve. Annu Rev Physiol 1976;*38*:139–152.

r4. Cranefield PF. The conduction of the cardiac impulse. In: The slow response and cardiac arrhythmias. Mount Kisko, New York: Futura, 1975.

r5. Cranefield PF, Aronson RS. Cardiac arrhythmias: the role of triggered activity and other mechanisms. Mount Kisko, New York: Futura, 1988.

r6. Moe GK. Evidence for reentry as a mechanism for cardiac arrhythmias. Rev Physiol Biochem Pharmacol 1975;*72*:56–66.

r7. Hondeghem LM, Katzung BG. Antiarrhythmic agents: The modulated receptor mechanism of action of sodium and calcium channel-blocking drugs. Ann Rev Pharmacol Toxicol 1984;*24*:387–423.

r8. Clarkson CW, Hondeghem LM. Effects of antiarrhythmic drugs on conduction and automaticity. In Rupp H (ed.): The regulation of heart function. Basic concepts and clinical applications. New York: Thieme, (1986); pp 407–420.

r9. A Symposium: The Cardiac Arrhythmia Suppression Trials: Does it alter our concept of and approaches to ventricular arrhythmias? Am J Cardiol 1990;*65*:1B–42B.

r10. Broogden RN, Todd PA. Disopyramide—A reappraisal of its pharmacodynamic pharmacokinetic properties and therapeutic use in cardiac arrhythmias. Drugs 1987;*34*:151–187.

r11. Anderson JL, Harrison DC, Meffin PJ, Winkle RA. Antiarrhythmic drugs: clinical pharmacology and therapeutic uses. Drugs 1978;*15*:271–309.

r12. Bigger JT Jr, Reiffel SA. Sick sinus syndrome. Ann Rev Med 1979;*30*:91–118.

r13. Atkinson AJ Jr, Davidson R. Diphenylhydantoin as an antiarrhythmic drug. Ann Rev Med 1974;*25*:99–105.

r14. Roden DM, Woosley RL. Drug therapy: Tocainide. N Engl J Med 1986;*315*:41–45.

r15. Roden DM, Woosley RL. Drug therapy: Flecainide. N Engl J Med 1986;*315*:36–41.

r16. Fitton A, Buckley MM-T. Moricizine. A review of its pharmacological properties, and therapeutic efficacy in cardiac arrhythmias. Drugs 1990;*40*:138–167.

r17. Ijzerman AT, Sondjin W. The antiarrhythmic properties of β-adrenoceptor antagonists. TIPS 1989;*10*:31–36.

r18. Brachman J, Schömig A. Adrenergic system and ventricular arrhythmias in myocardial infarction. Berlin, Heidelberg, New York: Springer Verlag (1989).

r19. Singh BN. When is a drug therapy warranted to prevent sudden cardiac death. Drugs 1991;*41*:Suppl 2:24–46.

r20. Singh BN, Sarna JSM, Zhong ZH, Tanaca C. Controlling cardiac arrhythmias by lengthening repolarization: rationale for experimental finding and clinical considerations. In Hashiba K, Moss AJ, Schwartz PJ, Eds QT prolongation and ventricular arrhythmias, New York: New York Academy of Science, (1992); pp 187–209.

r21. Hondeghem LM. Development of class III antiarrhythmic agents. J Cardiovasc Pharmacol 1992;*20*(Supplb2):S17–S22.

r22. Gill J, Heel RC, Fitton A. Amiodarone. An overview of its pharmacological properties, and review of its therapeutic use in cardiac arrhythmias. Drugs 1992;*43*:69–110.

r23. Singh BN, Venkatesh N, Nademanee K, Josephson MA, Kannan R. The historical development, cellular electrophysiology and pharmacology of amiodarone. Prog Cardiovasc Dis 1989;*31*:249–280.

r24. Nattel S, Talajic M. Recent advances in understanding the pharmacology of amiodarone. Drugs 1988;*36*:121–131.

r25. Rotmensch H, Belhasse B. Amiodarone in the management of cardiac arrhythmias: current concepts. Med Clinics North Am 1988;*72*:321–357.

r26. Sundquist H. Basic review and comparison of beta-blocker pharmacokinetics. Curr Ther Res 1980;*28*:388–448.

r27. Nayler WG. Calcium antagonists. London: Academic Press 1988.

r28. Singh BN, Nademanee K, Baky SH. Calcium antagonists: clinical use in the treatment of arrhythmias. Drugs 1983;*25*:125–153.

r29. Fleckenstein A. Calcium antagonism in heart and smooth muscle. Experimental facts and therapeutic prospects. New York: Wiley, 1983.

r30. Mitchell LB, Schroeder JS, Mason JW. Comparative clinical electrophysiologic effects of diltiazem, verapamil and nifedipine: a review. Am J Cardiol 1982;*49*:629–635.

r31. Stone PH, Antman EM, Muller JE, Braunwald E. Calcium channel blocking agents in the treatement of cardiovascular disorders. Part II. Hemodynamic effects and clinical applications. Am Int Med 1980;*93*:886–904.

r32. Lewis JG. Adverse reactions to calcium antagonists. Drugs 1983;*25*:196–222.

CHAPTER 26

Antihypertensive Drugs

Philippe Lechat

Although the negative implications of extreme elevated blood pressure have been noted for over a hundred years, only in the last several decades has it been appreciated that even mild elevations in systemic pressure may have negative prognostic implications. Initial attempts to reduce hypertension were nonpharmacologic and included surgical sympathectomy as well as dietary manipulations (low sodium or rice diets). Even today nonpharmacologic interventions are the first line of attack in managing hypertension, with reduced body weight, cessation of smoking, relaxation therapy, and increased exercise as initial weapons. When these avenues cannot restore blood pressure to a normal range, then a cornucopia of drugs is reviewed for the best medical intervention for each specific patient.

Blood pressure is the result of many dynamic regulatory mechanisms, but the ones most useful as a framework for discussion of pharmacotherapeutic principles are diagrammed in Figure 26.11. In this framework, the kidney occupies the top-central, dominant point of importance because it modulates changes in blood volume directly. The two primary modulators of renal effects on circulating blood volume are the renin-angiotensin-sodium system (left side of figure) and the autonomic sympathoadrenal nervous system (right side). Actions of these two systems control changes in renal manipulation of circulating blood volume as well as the capacitance of the arterial (and venous) vascular tree. This capacitance and the volume inside that space ultimately determine the blood pressure. More important, when one of these two systems is impaired as a result of antihypertensive therapy, the compensatory increase in activity of the other one will often be responsible either for failure of therapy or for the type and severity of side-effects.

As the drugs in this section are reviewed, repeated instances of this principle will be discussed. As an initial example, the use of a vasodilator such as hydralazine to reduce arteriolar resistance would seem the most direct way to cure hypertension, a disease whose hallmark is increased peripheral vascular resistance. During therapy, however, increased activity of the sympathetic nervous system will produce a tachycardia due to increased baroreceptor firing and increased sympathetic activity. Dependent edema is also frequent after hydralazine, owing to a compensatory increase in renin secretion because of diminished renal blood flow (again a result of the reduced blood pressure) and increased sympathetic outflow via the baroreceptor activation mentioned above.

When a diuretic is used as initial therapy compensatory sympathetic activation often follows; conversely, sympatholytics (reserpine) lead to subsequent sodium and water retention. Because of these somewhat parallel compensating systems, the best avenue for patients with moderate or severe hypertension is to interdict both systems simultaneously. By similar reasoning, if one sympatholytic is not effective in restoring normal blood pressure, addition of another similar type of drug, i.e., another sympatholytic, usually will not achieve the target reduced blood pressure; it may only increase side-effect symptoms. Similar observations accrue to adding a second diuretic when the first has been unsuccessful. For these reasons many patients may be best managed by a mixture of antihypertensive drugs that act at different sites in the panoply of mechanisms that control blood pressure. Figure 26.11 also denotes the several primary points at which drug therapy is now possible.

Calcium Antagonists

Antagonism of calcium entry into smooth muscle cells has become established in the management of essential hypertension. Calcium overload represents one major factor of stiffness of large arteries as well as vasoconstriction of arterioles. Furthermore, calcium ions could play a role as a factor influencing the progression of atherosclerosis and coronary sclerosis. The calcium antagonists (calcium entry blockers) decrease calcium in the arterial wall, as demonstrated by the pioneer work of Godfraind and of Fleckenstein.[r1,r2] They also represent a group of antihypertensive drugs that preserve regional blood flow.

The group of calcium antagonists includes a long list of substances with rather different pharmacologic characteristics. Only a few of these drugs have been used in the treatment of hypertension (see Table 26.1): Verapamil (a phenylalkylamine), diltiazem (a benzothiazepine), and some dihydropyridine derivates such as nifedipine, nicardipine, nitrendipine, amlodipine, and felodipine. Although, all behave as selective competitors of calcium ion transport into cells, they have different binding locations on calcium channels and tissue-specific variable affinities for these binding sites. Less specific calcium antagonist drugs such as piperazine derivates, bepridil or perhexilline, have not been used as antihypertensive drugs, and will not be discussed in this chapter.

Chemistry

Verapamil

(5 - [N - (3,4 - Dimethoxyphenethyl, - N -methylamino] - 2 - (3,4 - dimethoxyphenyl) - 2 -isopropylvaleronitrite hydrochloride (Fig. 26.1).

This substance is a derivate of papaverine, a naturally occurring alkaloid. It contains an aryl cycle with a lateral chain and an asymmetric carbon. The L- compound is inactive; the D-verapamil is the active drug.

Diltiazem

This molecule is a benzothiazepine derivative, and was developped in the early 1970s. It is the d-cis isomer of 3-acetoxy-2, 3-dihydro-5-[2-(dimethylamino) ethyl]-2-(p-methoxyphenyl)-1, 5-benzothiazepin-4 (5H) - one hydrochloride. It is a weak base with a pKa of 7.7.

Dihydropyridine Derivates

All substances in this group are phenyl dihydropyridine derivatives. They all have high affinity for the identical receptor binding site on calcium channels. Most of the compounds have asymmetric carbons, and affinities of stereoisomers for binding sites may differ greatly. Amlodipine, for instance, has been found to inhibit calcium-induced contractions of potassium-depolarized rat aorta with approximately twice the potency of nifedipine but with a much slower onset of effect for amlodipine.[1]

The potency of dihydropyridine derivates is enhanced with membrane depolarization,[2] and this property participates in both the selectivity and intensity of vascular sensitivity among different compounds.

Anti-Hypertensive Properties of Calcium Entry Blockers

Although the action of calcium antagonists in hypertension may be attributed to their effect on resistance vessels, calcium channel blockade inhibits excitation contraction coupling in cardiac muscle as well as in vascular smooth muscle. This induces a direct relaxant effect on vascular smooth muscle that is responsible for the antihypertensive effects. The specific result depends on the type of calcium antagonist and on the patient's pathologic condition.

In normal subjects, calcium antagonists do not greatly modify blood pressure unless high doses are used. A 10 to 15 percent decrease in mean blood pressure is obtained after oral administration of 20 mg of nifedipine, 160 mg of verapamil, or 120 mg of diltiazem. Hypertensive patients with mild and moderate hypertension, however, appear to be much more sensitive to calcium antagonists.[r2,r3,r4] Using regional arterial infusions, it has been demonstrated that verapamil produces a greater increase in forearm blood flow in hypertensive patients than in normotensive subjects.[3] Smooth muscle relaxation of large arteries by calcium antagonists improves arterial compliance,[4] which prevents deterioration of elastic properties of large arteries.

Hemodynamic and Reflex Responses

All calcium antagonists reduce blood pressure by vasodilatation while maintaining blood flow to organs such as the kidney, brain, myocardium, and skeletal muscles. With dihydropyridine derivatives, the fall in blood pressure is associated with an immediate reflex tachycardia of approximately 10 beats/min. Cardiac index and plasma norepinephrine concentrations increase while calculated systemic resistance decreases suggesting reflexly mediated sympathoneural activation due to arterial vasodilatation.

After chronic treatment, blood pressure is further

Table 26.1 Calcium Antagonists: Available Preparations and Dosage for Antihypertensive Treatments

	Presentation and Dosage	Antihypertensive Dose/Day
Verapamil	Tablets = 40 mg (not indicated for hypertension) Capsule = 120 mg Slow release capsule = 240 mg	120–340 mg 240–360 mg
Diltiazem	Tablets = 60 mg (not indicated for hypertension) Slow release tablet = 300 mg	300 mg
Nifedipine	Capsule = 10 mg (sublingual route for hypertensive crisis) Slow release tablet = 20 mg	20–40 mg
Nicardipine	Tablets = 10, 20 mg	20–40 mg
Nitrendipine	Tablets = 20 mg Slow release tablet = 50 mg	50–100 mg
Amlodipine	5 mg tablets	5–10 mg
Felodipine	5 mg Slow release : 5 mg	5–10 mg
Lacidipine	2, 4 mg tablets	2 and 8 mg
Isradipine	2.5, 5 mg tablets (Slow release)	5 mg

reduced, while heart rate, cardiac index, and plasma norepinephrine concentrations return to pretreatment values. The further decrease of blood pressure seems to be mediated by a return toward control values of acutely increased sympathetic activity. These findings suggest a resetting of arterial baroreflexes in responders.[5] However, baroreflex sensitivity was found unchanged after nifedipine therapy.[6] With high doses, however, neurohormonal activation induced with dihydropyridines may persist during chronic treatment.[7] In contrast, owing to a direct cardiac depressant effect, heart rate is slightly reduced by verapamil and diltiazem, though cardiac output remains unchanged.

Exercise Hemodynamics

Blood pressure is decreased during exercise without any decrease in cardiac output. The fall in blood

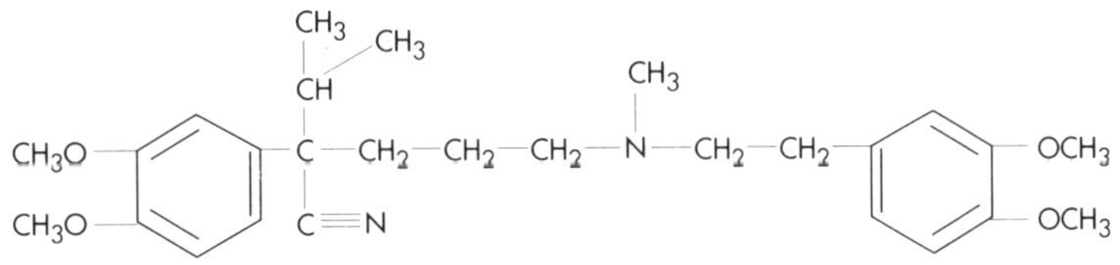

Verapamil

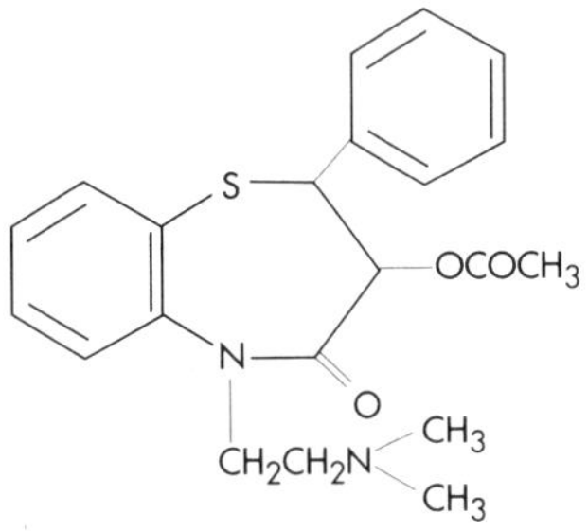

Diltiazem

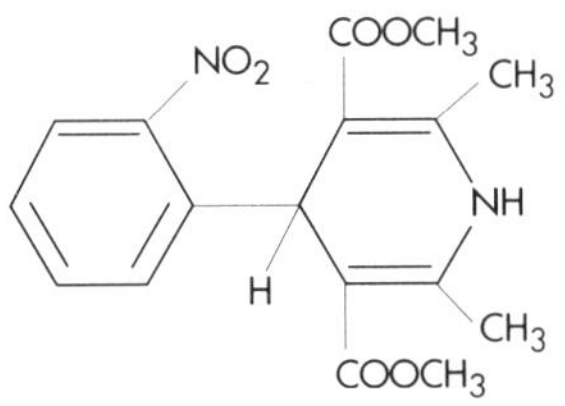

Nifedipine

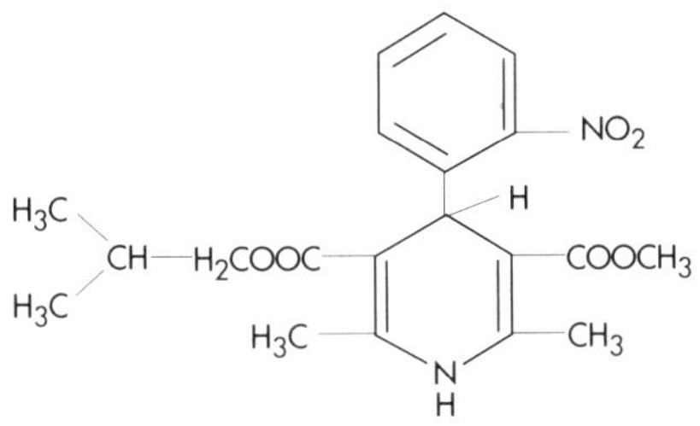

Nisoldipine

Figure 26.1 Calcium Antagonists

pressure is related to a reduction in total peripheral resistance.[8] Long-term studies have shown that blood pressure control during exercise is excellent with nifedipine. Other dihydropyridines show a similar pattern of effects on exercise performance (nifedipine, nisoldipine, nitrendipine, amlodipine).

Renal Effects

Most studies have shown that the vasodilatation and fall in blood pressure are associated with maintenance of renal blood flow. In vitro, calcium entry blockers alter the response of the isolated rat kidney to vasoconstrictor agents. In the presence of norepinephrine, calcium antagonists markedly enhance glomerular filtration rate but produce only a modest improvement in renal perfusion. This preferential augmentation of glomerular filtration rate may be attributable to a selective vasodilatation of preglomerular vessels. Clinical implications remain to be evaluated, but calcium antagonists might exert beneficial effects in clinical settings characterized by impaired renal hemodynamics.[9]

Acute administration of calcium antagonists enhances natriuresis.[10] This could result from direct inhibition of distal tubular sodium reabsorption. The relation of such an acute natriuretic response to the antihypertensive action of calcium antagonists, however, needs to be further investigated. Such effects on renal sodium handling might be as important for the long term antihypertensive effect as is the vasodilator effect per se.

Regression of Left Ventricular Hypertrophy

Left ventricular hypertrophy represents an adaptative response to pressure overload in hypertension. It might in itself become an independent aggravating factor of coronary artery disease complications.[11] Reversal of cardiac hypertrophy is one of the goals of antihypertensive therapy and has been obtained with different calcium entry blockers. For example, after a six-month period of therapy with nifedipine (10 mg/d) or verapamil (240 mg/d) a reduction of left ventricular mass was obtained from 234 ± 54 to 190 ± 71 ($p < 0,05$) and from 207 g ± 48 to 182 g ± 57 (g/m2), respectively, in hypertensive patients without alteration of left ventricular performance.[12]

In another study, the long-term effects (5 years) of antihypertensive therapy on echocardiographically proven left ventricular hypertrophy were studied in 117 previously untreated patients.[13] Five treatments were compared: gallopamil (100 mg), metoprolol (200 mg), acebutolol (200 mg) + nifédipine, and atenolol (50 mg) + enalapril (10 mg). For the entire population there was a significant (24.5%) decrease in left ventricular mass index after one year, which increased to 44 percent after five years of treatment. In 82 percent of the patients, almost complete regression of hypertrophy was achieved. However, the time course of regression of hypertrophy differed between groups, despite similar blood pressure reduction.

It has been suggested that angiotensin II and cardiac catecholamines could play important roles in modifying the influence of various drugs on regression of cardiac hypertrophy and that they possibly exert their effect by influencing cardiac protein synthesis and collagen content, which was reduced by nifedipine treatment.[14]

Therapeutic Use of Calcium Antagonists in Hypertension

Verapamil, diltiazem, and nifedipine (and many other related compounds; see Table 26.1) may be used in monotherapy in mild and moderate hypertension.[r5–r9] The maximal daily dose for verapamil is around 320 mg, for nifedipine 80 mg, and for diltiazem 300 mg. Slow-release tablets of such substances allow twice or even single administration per day.

Patients with contraindications to other antihypertensive agents such as beta blockers or diuretics may be potential candidates for the calcium entry blockers. These drugs seem to be a good alternative in patients with hypertension and peripheral vascular disorders. In the elderly, some authors found that the response rate was better than in younger hypertensives. This was not confirmed in some other centers; however, it is generally accepted that elderly patients are good candidates for the calcium entry blockers.

Result of Trials with Calcium Antagonists in Hypertension. Comparison with Other Anti-Hypertensive Treatments

The first trial with verapamil in hypertension was published by Lewis et al. in 1978.[15] More extensive studies with calcium antagonists have been initiated by Bülher et al.[r6] They administrated verapamil in increasing doses from 120 bid up to 240 mg tid (mean: 427 mg/day), and observed that systolic blood pressure decreased from 171 ± 16 to 152 ± 14 mm Hg and that diastolic blood pressure decreased from 108 ± 6 to 93 ± 9 mm Hg. Target blood pressure was reached in 25 of 43 patients. In their study the blood pressure decrease with verapamil was related to three specific pretreatment values: age of the patients (the older the patients, the larger the blood pressure decrease), and pretreatment renin level (inverse correlation). However, no such correlation was found between magnitude of response and age in other studies. The efficacy of antihypertensive action of verapamil persists after one year of treatment. The magnitude of the blood pressure decreasing effect of verapamil compared with beta-blocking agents is currently under study in a large multicenter European study (EMIHL study). Verapamil in a slow-release preparation (240–480 mg/day) is being compared with metoprolol 100–200 mg/day.

With nitrendipine, different studies showed that the antihypertensive effectiveness is similar to that of diuretics and beta-blockers. During long term (one year) nitrendipine treatment in mild to moderate hypertension, the blood pressure reduction is well sustained in "short-term" nitrendipine responders. In patients with severe hypertension, nitrendipine has a potent antihypertensive effect in combination with beta-blockers and/or diuretics. In mild-moderate hypertension, a single daily dose (10–40 mg) may be sufficient, whereas two daily doses (20–80 mg/day) seem necessary in severe hypertension.

At least four parallel placebo-controlled studies have investigated the antihypertensive effects of nicardipine. Even at 10 mg three times daily, the decrease was significantly greater than that achieved with placebo, and the reduction increased in proportion to the dosage. Serious side-effects were rare.

Combination Therapy with Other Antihypertensive Drugs

In many hypertensive patients it may be necessary to combine antihypertensive drugs. When a diuretic is given in combination with the calcium antagonist, a further decrease in systolic as well as in diastolic blood pressure can be observed. Combination of calcium antagonists with beta-blockers is of special interest. Several controlled studies have shown that such a combination is remarkably potent and better tolerated than a combination between beta-blocking drugs and hydralazine.

Undesirable Effects

The side-effects of calcium antagonists result mainly from an exaggeration of the intended vasodilatation. Episodes of flushing or headache may occur when treatment is started. There is, however, a tendency for these reactions to disappear after some time. The most disturbing side-effect is ankle edema. This has been reported in about 1–5 percent of the patients during long-term treatment with nifedipine, less often with diltiazem or verapamil.

Verapamil and diltiazem may cause sinus bradycardia and AV conduction delay. This can be potentiated when these drugs are administrated with beta-blocking substances, digitalis, or amiodarone, and especially when sinus dysfunction or first degree AV block are present before treatment. With verapamil, constipation has been reported in up to 25 percent of the patients.

Toxic Effects or Overdose

Toxic doses of verapamil and diltiazem may cause excessive sinus bradycardia and third degree AV block. This appears as a direct consequence of excessive calcium channel blockade at the sinus and atrio-ventricular nodes, which are "slow calcium current" dependent cells. Treatment of such events may include isoproterenol infusion, calcium chloride, and/or electrostimulation.

Pharmacokinetics and Relations Between Therapeutic Efficacy and Plasma Concentrations

We shall review below characteristics of the three classic calcium antagonists. See Table 26.1 for dosage forms, Table 26.2 reports pharmacokinetic data for the most recent ones.

Verapamil. The disposition of verapamil in healthy subjects following IV or oral administration showed a biexponential decline, with an initial rapid phase with a half-life of 18 to 31 minutes followed by a slower phase with a half-life of 161 to 442 minutes. The liver extracts approximately 80 percent of this drug after oral dosing, and systemic clearance approaches hepatic blood flow. Conditions that significantly alter liver blood flow, therefore, result in altered clearance and elimination half-time.

During long term oral verapamil therapy, the half-life approximately doubles (within one week after beginning therapy). This appears to be a consequence of reduction in liver blood flow related to the effect of verapamil as a nonselective vasodilator. After initial IV or oral doses both the hemodynamic and electrophysiologic effects of verapamil appear to be directly related to its concentration in plasma. During long-term oral verapamil administration, however, plasma drug concentrations vary by more than tenfold in hypertensive patients given the same total daily dose and in whom similar intensities of drug effects are seen. This wide variation in plasma drug levels may derive in part from a stereoselective presystemic hepatic extraction. In neither patients with angina nor those with hypertension can a distinct therapeutic plasma level range be defined.

Dihydropyridines. After oral dosing the bioavailability of nifedipine is about 45 percent, and the drug is metabolized in the liver to inactive products. Its elimination half-life is about four hours after oral doses with the capsule formulation. The tablet formulation has the properties of a sustained release product and induces more sustained plasma drug levels. In slow release form, nifedipine has a half-life of 10–12 hours with a similar bioavailability. Plasma concentrations of nifedipine in patients receiving the drug for long-term hypertension control were two- to threefold higher than those seen with similar doses given initially. In normotensive subjects there appears to be a linear correlation between hemodynamic effects and drug plasma levels. In hypertensive patients, plasma drug levels associated with therapeutic efficacy are considerably higher than those producing hypotensive effects after initial doses in normal subjects. In all cases, a great interindividual variability has been observed concerning plasma levels after a given dose of nifedipine. After intake of a tablet of slow-release nifedipine, blood levels can vary by eightfold. The same interindividual variability concerning pharmacokinetic parameters has been found with other dihydropyridines.

Among the dihydropyridines, amlodipine possesses a particular pharmacokinetic profile.[16] It has a long elimination half-life of 35–50 hours. It is slowly absorbed, its absolute bioavailability is high, and it is extensively metabolized in the liver. The long half-life is associated with a prolonged (<24hr) duration of pharmacodynamic action. Felodipine and lacidipine also have a prolonged duration of action over 24 hours with once-daily administration.

Diltiazem. After oral doses bioavailability is approximately 45 percent. The drug is metabolized in the

Table 26.2 Pharmacokinetic Data

	Intestinal Resorption (%)	Apparent Elimination Half-life (hr)	Plasma Protein Binding (%)	Metabolism and Elimination
Verapamil	>90	3–7; with slow-release form, 11	90	First-pass effect ++: bioavailability = 25 to 35% Intense hepatic metabolism Several metabolites; some are active. Renal elimination metabolites
Diltiazem	90	4–8	80–85	First-pass effect ++ Bioavailability = 35%. Intense hepatic metabolism Several metabolites
Nifedipine	95	3; 10–12 (with slow-release form)	90–95	First-pass effect ++ Bioavailability = 70% 80% to 90% eliminated by urinary tract under metabolite forms
Nicardipine	>95	3–4	95	Bioavailability = 15 to 40% Intense hepatic metabolism
Nitrendipine	>95	8–23	98	Bioavailability = 5 to 40% First-pass effect
Amlodipine	63 (bioavailability)	35	98	Extensive hepatic metabolism inactive metabolites
Felodipine	15 (bioavailability)	15–22 (depend on formulation)	99	Extensive hepatic metabolism inactive metabolites
Lacidipine	2 to 9 (bioavailability)	1.9	>95	Hepatic metabolism
Isradipine	95 (bioavailability = 17)	8	>95	Hepatic metabolism

liver to deacetylated and inactive forms. Elimination half-life after initial dose ranges from three to seven hours. After repeated oral dosing, bioavailability of diltiazem increases from 38–90 percent after the sixteenth dose, suggesting saturation of hepatic elimination mechanisms.

In patients given single IV or oral doses of diltiazem, systolic blood pressure and systemic vascular resistance decreased in relation to the diltiazem levels in plasma, with vasodilating effects seen only at drug concentrations above 100 µg/ml. In conclusion, with the different calcium entry blockers, pharmacokinetic parameters show a great interindividual variability, and there appears to be substantial variation from single to long-term administration.

Because of the poor correlation of plasma levels with the antihypertensive response, measurements of drug concentrations in plasma for these agents should serve primarily to identify noncompliance in patients with abnormal mechanisms of drug handling, not therapeutic/toxic differentials.

Angiotensin-Converting Enzyme Inhibitors

Angiotensin-converting enzyme (ACE) inhibitors represent a major advance in the treatment of hypertension. The first orally active ACE inhibitor to be marketed was captopril. More recently, several other compounds have been developed: enalapril; lisinopril; perindopril; ramipril; quinapril; etc.

All these drugs inhibit the cleavage of inactive angiotensin I to angiotensin II, which is a powerful vasoconstrictor that stimulates the secretion of aldosterone and antidiuretic hormone, promotes thirst, and stimulates the sympathetic nervous system, while inhibiting vagal tone. Several aspects of this range of actions can become deranged in a number of forms of hypertension. ACE inhibitors are known to inhibit other peptidases as well, including the conversion of the vasodilator autacoid, bradykinin, to inactive metabolites. Several controlled trials have shown that ACE inhibitors have antihypertensive effects in essential hypertension comparable to those seen with thiazide diuretics and with beta-blockers when used as sole therapy.[r10–r14]

Chemical Structure (Fig. 26.2)

- Captopril = 1 - [(25) - 3 mercapto - 2 -methylpropionyl/1 - L - proline
- Enalapril = N - [(8) - 1 - (ethoxy - carbonyl) - 3 - phenylpropyl] - L - ala - L -proline
- Enalaprilic acid: active metabolite of enalapril
- Lisinopril: Lysine analog of enalaprilic acid.

The captopril molecule contains a sulfhydryl group, which appears necessary for its action but is also responsible for some adverse effects. More recently developed substances, such as enalapril, lisinopril, ramipril, quinapril, perindopril, etc. are devoid of such a moiety and its toxic effects. Some compounds are only prodrugs, and a metabolite is their active substance: enalaprilic acid is formed from enalapril, quinalaprilic acid from quinapril. Captopril and lisinopril are directly active.

Structure–Activity Relationship

Captopril and alacepril bind to the enzyme by means of a sulfhydryl group, but the other ACE Inhibitors do not. They have in common a 2 - methylpropanolol - L - proline moiety, a group of critical importance in blocking the active site of the angiotensin-converting enzyme.

Binding of converting enzyme to its substrates or inhibitors includes:

- Binding of the terminal carboxyl group to a positively charged location on the enzyme
- Binding of the carboxylamide - C - N - to the enzyme by a hydrogen link

The terminal proline ring (or lysine group of Angiotensin) favors the binding to the enzyme.

Mechanism of Antihypertensive Action of ACE Inhibitors

Within the circulation, renin reacts with angiotensinogen, resulting in production of the inactive decapeptide, angiotensin I. Subsequently, angiotensin I is transformed into angiotensin II by the action of converting enzyme by removal of two amino acid residues. Inhibition of converting enzyme suppresses the synthesis of angiotensin II and thus its vasoconstrictor effects and stimulatory action on aldosterone production. It also prevents the degradation of bradykinin. The antihypertensive effect of ACE inhibitors may depend on all three of these actions. In hypertensive subjects, acute or chronic administration of ACE inhibitors induces hemodynamic effects that are qualitatively identical to those observed in normal subjects. In essential hypertension, levels of angiotensin II are often within a range having a direct immediate effect on arterial pressure. Thus, one would expect an initial fall in arterial pressure with ACE inhibitors in proportion to the circulating level of angiotensin II. This is indeed the case. Sustained ACE inhibition, however, produces an additional fall in arterial pressure over 3–4 weeks of treatment beyond the initial response. With long-term therapy, the relationship between the blood pressure fall and the fall in angiotensin II is less robust.

In addition, converting enzyme inhibitors show antihypertensive effects when the plasma renin activity is normal or low—even in anephric patients where the renal source of renin is eliminated. The ACE inhibitors also act on other systems such as the kallikrein-kinin system and the prostaglandin system. Inhibition of the converting enzyme inhibits degradation of bradykinin, which is a powerful vasodilating agent that stimulates release of some vasodilating prostaglandins, such as PGE2 and prostacyclin. Investigation of systems such as bradykinin that interfere with local regulation of vascular tone is difficult, and their precise role in the antihypertensive action of ACE inhibitors has not been determined. Indomethacin, however, a drug that inhibits PGE synthesis, partly inhibits the antihypertensive effects of captopril, enalapril, and perindopril.[17] In addition, angiotensin may stimulate vascular smooth muscle cell growth by inducing the expression of growth regulatory genes, thereby modulating the long-term regulation of vascular resistance by influencing changes in vascular structure.

It has been suggested that the circulating renin-angiotensin system is primarily involved with the short-term regulation of cardiovascular function, whereas a tissue-localized renin-angiotensin system may be more important in the chronic long-term influence of vascular tone and structure (e.g., hypertrophy).[18] However, if renin can be present at tissue levels, it originates from the plasma compartment by diffusion. Forty-eight hours after bilateral nephrectomy, no more renin activity can be detected in any tissue nor in plasma. The angiotensin-converting enzyme is exposed to the plasma, since it is linked to the endoluminal face of the endothelium membrane and part of it can be released into the plasma. Angiotensin II can then only be synthesized in plasma by the converting enzyme. Angiotensin II, however, can diffuse into the tissue and act at the tissue level. The relevance of a

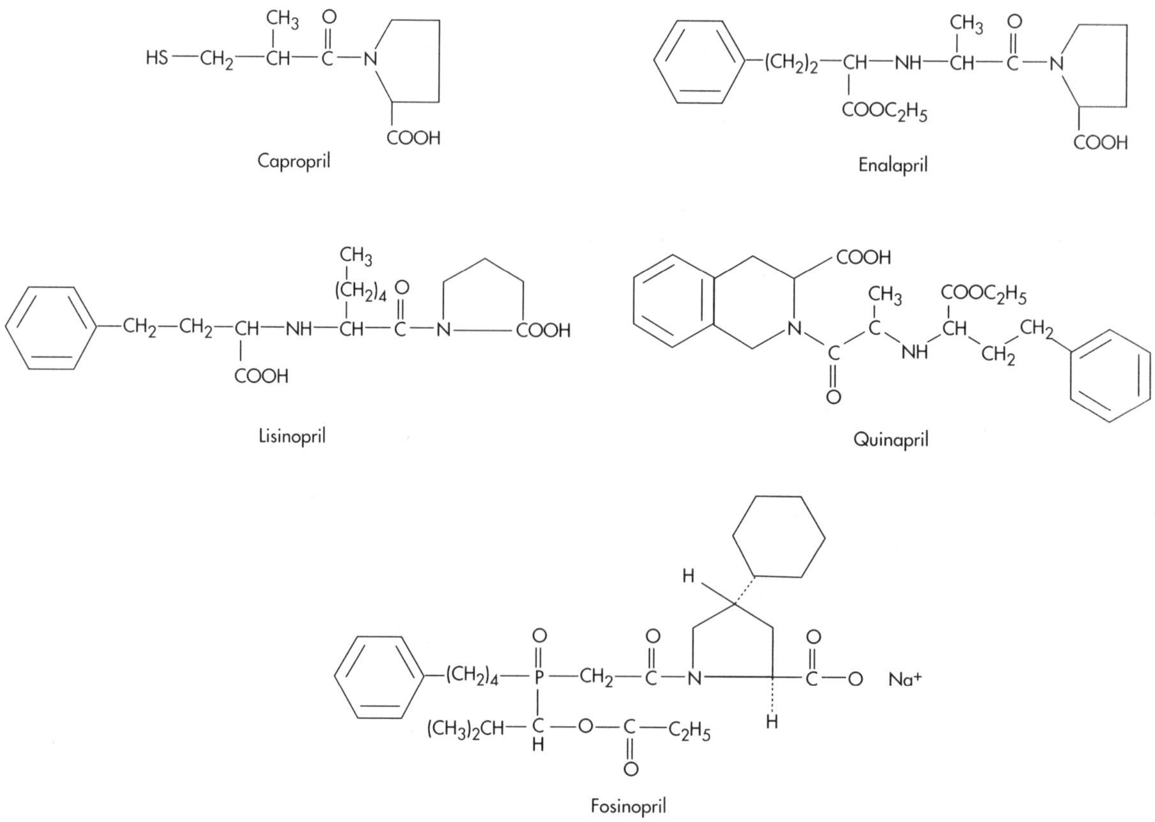

Figure 26.2 ACE Inhibitors

functional duality of a plasma renin angiotensin system and a tissue system seems very unlikely. Much of the controversy about the separate or identical nature of these enzyme activities has arisen from the difficulties and nonspecificity of angiotensin II detection and determination of concentration.[19]

Antihypertensive Efficacy

Efficacy and Hemodynamic Effects

ACE inhibitors have been as effective as other antihypertensive agents (35–70% of patients respond with diastolic blood pressure below 90 mmHg) when used as monotherapy. Initially these drugs were reserved for treating patients with severe, resistant hypertension or with renal vascular hypertension. They have been progressively recommended for more widespread use equal to beta-blockers and diuretics as first-step treatment of mild to moderate essential hypertension. This is a consequence of the recognition of the appropriate dose of an ACE inhibitor and the absence of adverse metabolic effects. When sodium depletion induced by diet or the administration of diuretics is combined with these inhibitors, blood pressure normalization can be achieved in more than 90 percent of patients. In general, the fall in blood pressure induced by ACE Inhibitors has ranged from 15 to 25 percent, affecting both diastolic and systolic blood pressure. The hemodynamic effect of ACE inhibitors is induced via a systemic vasodilation without substantial change in cardiac output. Blood flow to vital organs is not decreased and may be increased despite the reduction in perfusion pressure. Local and reflex mechanisms involved in cardiovascular regulation are not impaired and may even be improved by ACE inhibitors.[20] Baroreceptor control of blood pressure, which is altered in hypertension, can be reset and its sensitivity improved by ACE inhibition.[21] In addition, the presynaptic stimulation of angiotensin II on norepinephrine release from sympathetic nerve terminals is suppressed by ACE inhibition. These two actions explain why the hypotension induced by this class of drugs is not associated with tachycardia or an increase in sympathetic stimulation that might counteract the therapeutic effect. It also explains why during ACE inhibitor treatment no alteration in blood pressure homeostasis is observed during exercise or orthostasis.[21]

When the drug is given once daily, the control of blood pressure to a normal level over an entire 24 hours generally is not obtained with captopril, which has a short half-life of only 1–2 hours. Enalapril, with a longer half-life, can reduce blood pressure during 24 hours, but such a result is not constantly achieved with one daily administration. With longer acting drugs, such as lisinopril, quinapril or perindopril, however, 24-hour blood pressure control is more regularly achieved. Comparison of antihypertensive efficacy of different ACE inhibitors has yielded equivalent results.[22,23]

This antihypertensive effect is obtained with few side-effects, even in elderly hypertensive patients. In a multicenter tolerance study of 418 elderly hypertensive patients treated with captopril for at least 12 months, blood pressure was reduced from 193/105 ± 30/16 to 159/88 ± 25/12 mmHg.[24] Few side-effects were observed, and renal function remained undisturbed in most of the patients; even those with elevated serum creatinine level upon entry into the study did not reduce their renal function further over the 12-month treatment period. Similar results have been obtained with other ACE inhibitors.

Patients with renovascular hypertension respond usually with a marked blood pressure drop to ACE inhibition. However, since renal perfusion pressure behind the stenosis may become very low and, because ACE inhibition, will lower angiotensin II availability to maintain postglomerular resistance, the stenotic kidney not infrequently reduces glomerular filtration rate further or stops filtration. For this reason, long-term treatment of renovascular hypertension by ACE inhibition is probably not advisable unless alternative therapy, primarily correction of the stenosis, is not available or is impossible.

As a general rule, ACE inhibitors have an equivalent efficacy to beta-blockings drugs, diuretics, or calcium antagonists. Like calcium antagonists,[25] they increase arterial compliance of the great vessels. This effect should be beneficial, especially for the heart, since great vessel compliance represents one of the components of left ventricle impedance. One would then expect for a same antihypertensive effect a greater reduction of left ventricular hypertrophy with drugs that increase great vessel compliance. This is partly true when vasodilators are compared. Regression of left ventricular hypertrophy is obtained with ACE inhibitors and calcium antagonists, but not with hydralazines and minoxidil. However, an equivalent regression of ventricular hypertrophy can be obtained by drugs that do not modify arterial compliance, such as beta-blocking drugs devoid of partial agonist activity. Inconstant results have been found with diuretics that also do not modify arterial compliance.

Particular effectiveness of ACE inhibitors can be expected on left ventricular hypertrophy, since angiotensin II and possibly aldosterone stimulate protein synthesis. Indeed, the HYCAR study recently demonstrated that low doses of ramipril (1.25 mg and 5 mg) can induce a significant reduction, compared with placebo, in hypertensive patients with left ventricular hypertrophy. In this study, all patients received a baseline antihypertensive treatment with furosemide (20 mg daily).

As far as the long-term complications of hypertension are concerned, the large trials in hypertension have enrolled patients receiving beta-blocking drugs and/or diuretics. These trials have demonstrated a reduction of incidence of stroke and heart failure. Such long-term trials with ACE inhibitors have not yet been performed.

ACE inhibitors have been used effectively in combination with other agents, particularly diuretics and calcium antagonists. In general, adding thiazide diuretics normalizes blood pressure in an additional 20 to 25 per cent of patients. ACE inhibitors used in combinations with nonspecific vasodilators (hydralazine) or beta-blockers appear less efficient than with calcium-channel blockers or diuretics.

Treatment of Special Groups

Several studies have reported that black patients respond less well to ACE inhibitors than do white patients. In elderly patients, ACE inhibitors and diuretics are similarly efficacious. In diabetic patients with hypertension and renal deterioration, ACE inhibitors are of particular interest. Indeed, renal dysfunction in diabetics could be the result of increased intraglomerular pressure mainly due to an increase in intrarenal levels of angiotensin II. Several studies have suggested that the administration of captopril to diabetic patients with renal dysfunction reduces the rate of deterioration of the kidney.[26] In a double-blind placebo-controlled trial in 20 normotensive diabetics, microalbuminuria decreased in the enalapril-treated group after six months but increased in the placebo group. These studies suggest a beneficial effect of ACE inhibitors on the renal dysfunction of diabetic patients—even those who are normotensive.

Undesirable Effects

ACE inhibitors are well-tolerated drugs and interfere with the quality of life of patients to a lesser extent than do other antihypertensive agents.[27]

Some side-effects are common to all ACE inhibitors:

Hypotension can be exaggerated by administration of diuretics, low salt intake, and high levels of renin. This can be reduced by lowering the dose.

Functional renal insufficiency can occur in patients with bilateral renal artery stenosis or stenosis on a solitary kidney. This is a consequence of suppression of the compensatory vasoconstrictor effect of angiotensin on the glomerular efferent arterioles that maintain glomerular filtration.

Furosemide

Hydrochlorothiazide

Xipamide

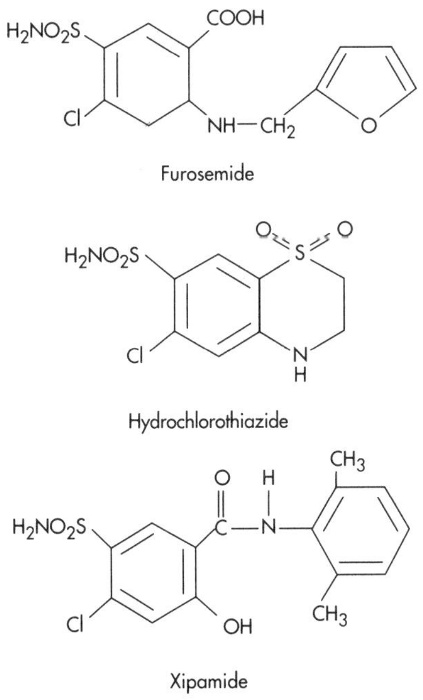

Figure 26.3 Diuretics

Hyperkalemia also can occur, particularly if sodium intake is restricted, or when potassium-sparing diuretics or nonsteroidal anti-inflammatory agents are given along with ACE inhibitors.

Coughing can occur in 1–5 percent of patients secondary to the effects of ACE inhibitors on bradykinin or prostaglandin production, and subsequent pulmonary inflammatory response.

Angioedema is a very rare side effect (0.1%). It may be secondary to a change in bradykinin metabolism. Almost invariably, when it occurs, it is within the first month of therapy, sometimes after the first dose; it is more frequent with the longer-acting converting enzyme inhibitors (enalapril, lisinopril) than with captopril. Early warning signs (localized edema and respiratory stridor) must be recognized to minimize its lethal potential (respiratory arrest by airway obstruction).

Some undesirable effects have been observed only with captopril (neutropenia, nephrotic syndrome, skin rash, and taste disturbance). These seem to be a consequence of the sulfhydryl moiety of the compound. Most patients with neutropenia and agranulocytosis under captopril therapy had renal insufficiency or an immune disorder or had been given high doses.

Pharmacokinetics

Duration of Action (Table 26.3)

Some of the ACE inhibitors are prodrugs (enalapril, quinapril, ramipril) and have to be converted (de-esterification) by the liver into an active compound. The active forms of the drugs reach a peak level in the serum later when it must first be metabolized (2–4 hours, compared with 1–2 hours). The elimination half-life varies with the different compounds; however, a short half-life may be associated with a longer action when affinity for the angiotensin-converting enzyme is high (e.g., ramipril or quinapril). The primary route of elimination of these drugs is the kidney. Therefore, patients with impaired renal function require a reduction of dosage.

Diuretics

Introduction

Diuretics have become a mainstay of antihypertensive therapy. Numerous studies have shown that 50 to 60 percent of patients with mild hypertension (diastolic blood pressure between 90 and 104 mmHg) respond favorably to a diuretic alone. The basic pharmacology to thise compounds[r15–r18] is discussed in Chapter 38; this discussion will focus on clinical antihypertensive applications.

Loop diuretics and thiazide diuretics (and related compounds) are widely used. Apart from these, xipamine is neither simply a thiazide nor a loop diuretic; indapamine and cicletanine (for structures see Fig. 26.3) are both diuretics but have antihypertensive activity separate from their diuretic properties. As antihypertensive drugs, thiazide and related compounds

Table 26.3 ACE Inhibitors: Pharmacokinetics

	Oral Resorption (%)	Protein Binding (%)	Elimination Half-life (hr)	Metabolism	Presentation (tablets) (mg)	Usual Antihypertensive Dose (mg/d)
Captopril	>25	30	1.7	Partly metabolized	25–50	50
Enalapril	60	≤80 (enalaprilat)	11 (enalaprilat)	Partly converted to enalaprilat; both eliminated by the urinary tract	5–20	20
Lisinopril	25	0	41	Nonmetabolized	5–20	20
Perindopril	70	<30	25	Perindopril = active inactive metabolites	4	4
Quinapril	60	97	11; 3 for quinalaprilat	3 inactive metabolites + quinaprilat = active	5 20	20–40
Fornopril Monopril	36	>95	12	fornoprilat = active	10 20	10–80 max
Benazepril	≥37	95	0, 6, 22 for benazeprilat	benazaprilat = active	5, 10, 20, 40	5 to 80 initially max
Ramipril	60	73	13 to 17	remiprilat = active	5, 10, 25, 2.5	2.5

have been used preferentially. When there is significant potassium loss, they can be combined with aldosterone antagonists or potassium-sparing diuretics. The more potent loop diuretics are used mainly in severe hypertension, especially that associated with renal failure. They are, however, quite effective in moderate hypertension as well.

Mechanism of Antihypertensive Action of Diuretics

The diuretics, especially thiazides and related compounds, have become a mainstay of antihypertensive therapy. Sodium and water depletion appear to provide a basis for the antihypertensive effect of these substances. At the beginning of treatment a decrease in extracellular fluid and plasma volumes, cardiac output, and total exchangeable sodium occur. This decrease is associated with a compensatory increase in systemic resistance. The reduction in blood volume makes maintenance of the blood pressure highly dependent on vascular tone, particularly that of capacitance vessels. After several months of diuretic administration, plasma volume, total body sodium and water, and cardiac output progressively return almost to pretreatment walues, while systemic resistance then decreases. This last effect appears to be enough to account for the persistent antihypertensive effect.[r19,r20] The hypotensive effect of diuretics unrelated chemically to the thiazides has led to the suggestion that the ultimate mechanism of the persistent reduction in peripheral vascular resistance may involve local altered sodium metabolism or a compensation for it. Irrespective of the ultimate machanism, it appears that the diuretic thiazides relax peripheral arteriolar smooth muscle. At this arteriolar level, spironolactones tend to increase extracellular potassium, which favors sodium and calcium extrusion from the smooth muscle cell. Such a reduction of sodium content of cells in the vascular wall induces a vasorelaxant effect. In elderly subjects, this reduction of total peripheral resistance represents the major hemodynamic effect of thiazide therapy, and there seems to be little over-all change in cardiac output or plasma volume.[28-30] There is, however, a spectrum of hemodynamic responses, with some patients (young to middle-aged hypertensive subjects) exhibiting a sustained decline in plasma volume and cardiac output.[31]

R_1—CHOH—CH_2—NH—R_2

Chemical Structure

R_1		R_2
1-naphthyl—O—CH_2—	Propranolol	—CH(CH_3)$_2$
4-indolyl—O—CH_2—	Pindolol	—CH(CH_3)$_2$
H_3C—SO_2—HN—C_6H_4—	Sotalol	—CH(CH_3)$_2$
H_3C_3—CO—HN—C_6H_3(CO—CH_3)—O—CH_2—	Acebutolol	—CH(CH_3)$_2$
H_2N—CO—CH_2—C_6H_4—O—CH_2—	Atenolol	—CH(CH_3)$_2$
H_3C—O—CH_2—CH_2—C_6H_4—O—CH_2—	Metoprolol	—CH(CH_3)$_2$
(CH_3)$_2$CH—O—CH_2—CH_2—O—CH_2—C_6H_4—????—	Bisoprolol	—CH(CH_3)$_2$

Figure 26.4 Beta Adrenoceptor Antagonists

Antihypertensive Efficacy

General Use

Diuretics are widely used as antihypertensive agents. Many studies have shown that 50 to 60 percent of patients with mild hypertension (diastolic pressure between 90 and 104 mmHg) respond to a diuretic alone. The drugs are easy to titrate and generally well tolerated. In the VA Cooperative Study,[32,33] the mean systolic blood pressure was reduced by 17.5 mmHg in the diuretic group (hydrochlorothiazide 50–200 mg/

d), compared with 8.3 mmHg in the propranolol group, 66.5 percent of patients being controlled with diuretic, 52.8 percent with propranolol. Somes studies have shown that hydrochlorothiazide may be even more effective at reducing blood pressure in certain subgroups of patients than are beta-blockers, ACE inhibitors, or calcium antagonists. If monotherapy with one of these substances does not achieve normotensive blood pressure levels, the addition af a diuretic greatly improves the outcome.

Addition of a low-sodium diet does not improve the antihypertensive effects of diuretics. Moreover, this association enhances the risk of onset of hypokalemia by increasing the magnitude of secondary hyperaldosteronism. Usually thiazides and related compounds do not induce a significant potassium depletion in hypertensive patients with a normal diet. Combining the use of these diuretics with potassium-sparing diuretics is not systematically necessary.

Among diuretics given for antihypertensive treatment, thiazides are the most extensively used compounds (for pharmacokinetic parameters, refer to Table 26.4). The great potency and rapid onset of loop action diuretics (for pharmacokinetic parameters, see Table 26.5) does not provide any advantage for chronic daily treatment of hypertension (without renal insufficiency). Prevention of diuretic-induced side-effects is mainly secured by using the lowest effective dose regimen. Potassium-sparing diuretics (for pharmacokintec parameters, see Table 26.6) should be given to patients when they are vulnerable to hypokaliema, especially those with a history of cardiac dysrhythmias, those receiving digitalis, or those with certain abnormal EKG findings.

In hypertensive patients, potassium-sparing diuretics should be reserved for those who have developed hypokalemia from thiazide therapy.

Among substances with diuretic properties, two nonthiazide drugs are currently used: xipamide and cicletanine. Xipamide is neither a thiazide nor a loop diuretic. It is one of various substituted derivatives of 4-chlorosalicylic acid. The major site of the diuretic action of xipamide is in the distal tubule. Its antihypertensive action is comparable to that of thiazide diuretics. Cicletanine was synthetized in 1984. Its chemical structure is characterized by a fluropyridine group. The mechanism by which cicletanine lowers blood pressure has not been established. It could act on vascular smooth muscle by increasing prostacyclin synthesis and by interaction either directly with cytosolic calcium pools or indirectly through various agents capable of mobilizing intracellular calcium. With higher doses, cicletanine induces a saluretic effect. Both actions account for the antihypertensive properties of the drug. Several controlled studies have demonstrated the antihypertensive effects of cicletanine. It appears to be well tolerated with few side-effects.

Result of Large Scale Clinical Trials

All large scale trials have shown stroke benefit as a result of the blood pressure reduction, whereas coronary heart disease benefit has not been convincingly demonstrated in any of the trials. Some

Table 26.4 Benzothiadiazides and Thiazide-like Diuretics

Agent	Range of Optimally Effective Oral Anti-pertensive Diuretic Dose in man (mg/day)	Duration of Action (hr)	Intestinal Resorption (%)	Plasma Protein Binding (%)	Elimination Half-life (hr)	Renal Elimination
Hydrochlorothiazide	25–100	12	60–80	40	6–15	70% of the drug excreted in urine within 48 hr; 95% unchanged
Hydroflumethiazide	50–100	12	50	80	17	
Bendroflumethiazide	2–5	24	95	95	3	30% of the drug excreted in urine
Polythiazide	4–8	30	>80	80	26	20% excreted in urine
Chlorthalidone	25–100	72	65	75	40–50	Elimination by both biliary and urinary tract; 90% in unchanged form
Indapamide	2.5	12–24	>95	79	18	60%
Tienilic acid	125–250	12–24	80	95	6	80% of the administered dose is excreted in urine within 24 hr

Table 26.5 Loop Diuretics

	Chemical Structure	Range of Effective Oral Diuretic Dose (mg)	Intestinal Resorption (%)	Plasma Protein Binding (%)	Elimination Half-life (min)	Renal Elimination
Furosemide	4 chloro-N-furfuryl-5-sulphamoyl-thianilic acid-4-chloro-2-furfuryl amino-5-sulfamoyl-benzoic acid	20–500	65	99	90	Largely unchanged + glucuronide and free amine metabolite
Bumetanide	3-butylamino-4-phenoxy-5-sulfa-moylbenzoic acid	0.5–5	>95	>95	90	50% unchanged
Ethacrynic acid	2,3-dichloro-4-(2-ethylacryloyl) phenoxyacetic acid	50	95	90	50	2/3 excreted in unchanged form and conjugates with sulfydryl compounds

Table 26.6 Aldosterone Antagonists and Potassium-sparing Diuretics

	Range of Effective Oral Diuretic Dose (mg)	Intestinal Resorption (%)	Plasma Protein Binding (%)	Elimination Half-life (hr)	Renal Elimination
Spironolactone	50 to 100	>90	90–98		Elimination of metabolites
Canrenone	50 to 200	>90	>90	20	15% eliminated unchanged
Triamterene	100 to 300	variable	67		Elimination of triamterene and metabolites
Amiloride	5 to 20	15–26		10	> 60% unchanged

have thought that the adverse metabolic effect of thiazide diuretics, which form the basis of the antihypertensive regimen in most of the trials, may have diminished the cardiac benefit that would have been expected from the degree of blood pressure reduction.

The Veterans Administration double blind 58-week trial compared the efficacy of hydrochlorothiazide (HCTZ) with propranolol in controlling mild hypertension.[32,33] It was found that propranolol reduced diastolic blood pressures to < 90 mmHg in 53 percent of the patients, whereas 66 percent were controlled on HCTZ ($p < 0.03$). In three trials (IPPPSH, HAPPHY, and MRC),[34–36] the effects of thiazide and beta-blocking agents were compared. No significant differences in stroke were found between thiazide and beta-blocker treated subjects in the IPPPSH and HAPPHY studies. In the MRC trial, the thiazide (bendrofluazide) conferred stroke benefit greater than that attributable to its blood pressure lowering effect, whereas the stroke benefit associated with the beta-blocker was entirely explained by its effects on blood pressure. In the MRC trial (see also beta-blocking drugs, Chapter 6) the diuretic (bendrofluazide) reduced stroke rates and all cardiovascular events, but not coronary events.

In hypertensive patients aged 60 and older, the EWPHE trial (European Working Party on Hypertension in the Elderly) evaluated the effects of a thiazide-triamterene combination versus placebo.[37] At the end of 4.7 years, there was a significant reduction (38%) in total cardiovascular mortality. Cardiac mortality alone was reduced by 47 percent, and the death rate from myocardial infarction was significantly reduced by 60 percent. The results of this study support the conclusion that elderly patients with diastolic hypertension benefit from antihypertensive therapy.

In another study, the Australian national blood pressure trial, 3427 subjects with mild to moderate hypertension receiving either a diuretic drug (chlorothiazide) or a placebo were included.[38] There was a 68 percent reduction in cardiovascular mortality in the diuretic group compared with the placebo group and a 25 percent reduction in nonfatal cardiovascular events in the actively treated group. The MRC (multiple risk factor intervention trial) found that a subgroup of hypertensive men with EKG abnormalitics at rest receiving hydrochlorothiazide were at increased risk of cardiovascular mortality. There is controversy about the statistical significance of this result. It suggests that diuretic-induced hypokalemia may have placed patients who have electrocardiographic abnormalities at rest at risk for acute arrhythmias.

In the HAPPHY trial, an identical antihypertensive effect was obtained in both diuretics and metoprolol groups; after a follow-up of ten years, mortality was, however, lower in the metoprolol group with a smaller rate of sudden death. The pooled incidences of fatal and nonfatal coronary heart disease (CHD), i.e., the first CHD event of sudden death of fatal myocardial infarction (MI) or definite acute MI or definite silent MI, are as follows: the first CHD event was fatal in 25 percent of cases (29 vs 54 cases in the diuretic group), was an acute MI in 38 percent (44 vs 54 cases), and was a silent MI in 36 percent (38 vs 55 % cases), a total of 111 cases in the metoprolol group and 144 cases in the diuretic group ($p < 0.001$).

Among the arguments given to explain the decreased efficacy of diuretics to reduce coronary events in the hypertensive patients is the fact that diuretic drugs tend to increase blood lipid levels, do not improve compliance of large arteries, and do not reduce left ventricular hypertrophy, which represents an independent cardiovascular risk factor.[39] This effect on hypertrophy was not confirmed by most recent trials in which diuretics proved to be most effective on regression of left ventricular hypertrophy compared to other antihypertensive drugs.

Use of Diuretics in Renal Disease

In patients with renal disease, the decreased population of intact nephrons may be in part responsible for the diuretic resistance. Accumulated endogenous organic acids in uremia compete with the diuretics for transport into the urine by the tubular organic anion pathway, and the loop diuretics depend on this transport for their access into the urine. Both of these factors may be involved in resistance to the loop diuretic effects. In addition, at the beginning of treatment, the diuretic-induced hypovolemia induces a decrease in glomerular filtration. This can further decrease renal function in case of renal failure tolerance and side-effects. Most frequent undesirable effects responsible for treatment withdrawal with thiazide diuretics in the MRC trial were gout and sexual impotence (12.8/1000 patient years in men). Other less frequent side-effects were impaired glucose tolerance, nausea, dizziness, skin disorders, and lethargy.

Metabolic Disturbances

Serum lipids and thiazides. Diuretics may increase cholesterol and triglyceride levels, but these return to pretreatment levels after long-term therapy.

Glucose tolerance. Thiazides and related compounds reduce glucose tolerance, but induce very small glycemic variations in nondiabetic patients.

Uric acid. All diuretics, except tielinic acid, reduce uric acid renal elimination and enhance uricemia. This can induce acute gouty arthritis in patients suffering from gout.

Calcium ion. Unlike loop diuretics, thiazide diuretics decrease the renal excretion of calcium by failing to block its reabsorption in the distal nephron. The excretion of magnesium, in contrast, is enhanced by the thiazides. This effect on calcium renal excretion recently has been associated with a lower incidence of hip fracture in elderly patients on thiazide diuretics.

Toxic Effects or Overdoses

The only relevant toxic effects of overdose of diuretics are encountered with the powerful loop diuretics. Excessive administration of loop diuretics without an increase in water intake can lead to extracellular fluid depletion, dehydratation, and hypotension. Use of very high doses of furosemide, especially in an attempt to convert established oliguric acute tubular necrosis to the nonoliguric form, may induce an irreversible ototoxicity.

Beta-Adrenoceptor Antagonists

Large scale trials have demonstrated the efficacy of beta-blocking agents as antihypertensive drugs. They can indeed reduce cardiovascular mortality and morbidity. The expectation that beta-blockers might also exert a primary preventive action on ischemic heart disease in patients with hypertension, however, has not been substantiated by any of the trials. Please see Chapter 6 for a complete discussion of the basic pharmacology of these drugs. Only their use in hypertension will be discussed here.

Mechanism of Antihypertensive Effect of Beta Adrenoceptor Antagonists

General Concept

Although beta-blocking drugs have been used for many years in the treatment of hypertension, their mode of action is still a matter of debate. The difference between the many beta-adrenergic blocking agents (see Fig. 26.6 for structures) do not result in clinically significant different antihypertensive action (see Table 26.7 for comparative pharmacodynamic and pharmacokinetic properties). Their action may be effected, in part, through reduction in cardiac output, reduction in plasma renin activity, effects on the CNS and peripheral effects on presynaptic beta receptors.

If cardiac output indeed initially decreases after beta-blocker administration, however, it progressively returns to normal values while blood pressure remains lowered. After an oral dose of 80 mg of propranolol, cardiac output returns to normal values after four hours in hypertensive patients. In the study of Van der Meiracker et al., acebutolol, atenolol, pindolol, and propranolol were compared. Although renin activity was suppressed to 60–70 percent in all treatment groups, the changes in renin or pretreatment values of renin levels were not correlated with the fall in blood pressure.[40] Despite similar hypertensive effects of the four drugs, the changes in flow and resistance underlying the fall in blood pressure differed considerably. With pindolol, the fall in blood pressure was associated with a fall in vascular resistance (26%), whereas with propranolol it was predominantly associated with a fall in cardiac output (11%). No significant changes in

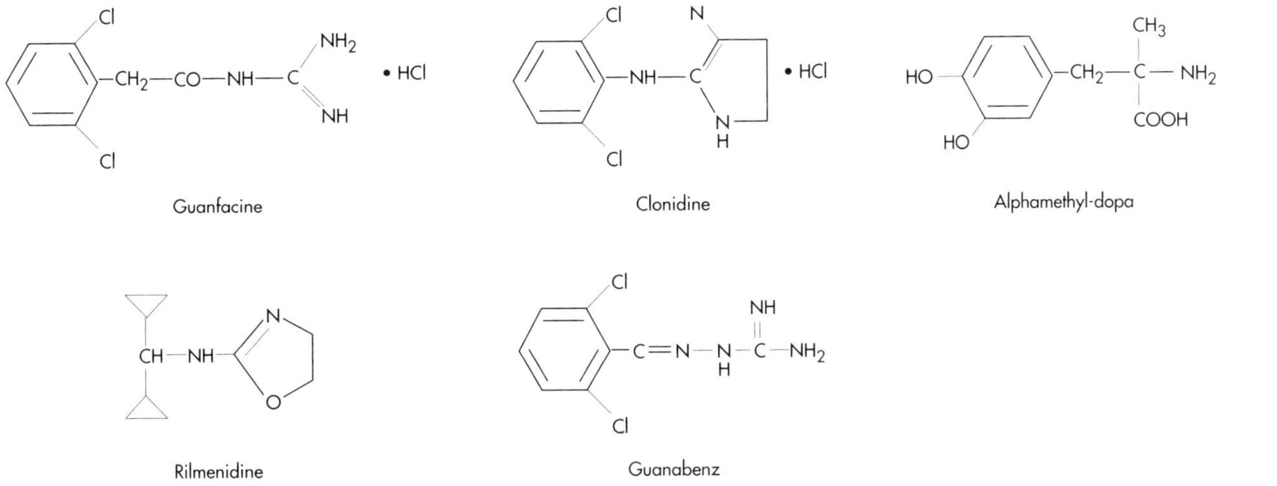

Guanfacine

Clonidine

Alphamethyl-dopa

Rilmenidine

Guanabenz

Figure 26.5 Centrally Acting Anti-hypertensive Drugs

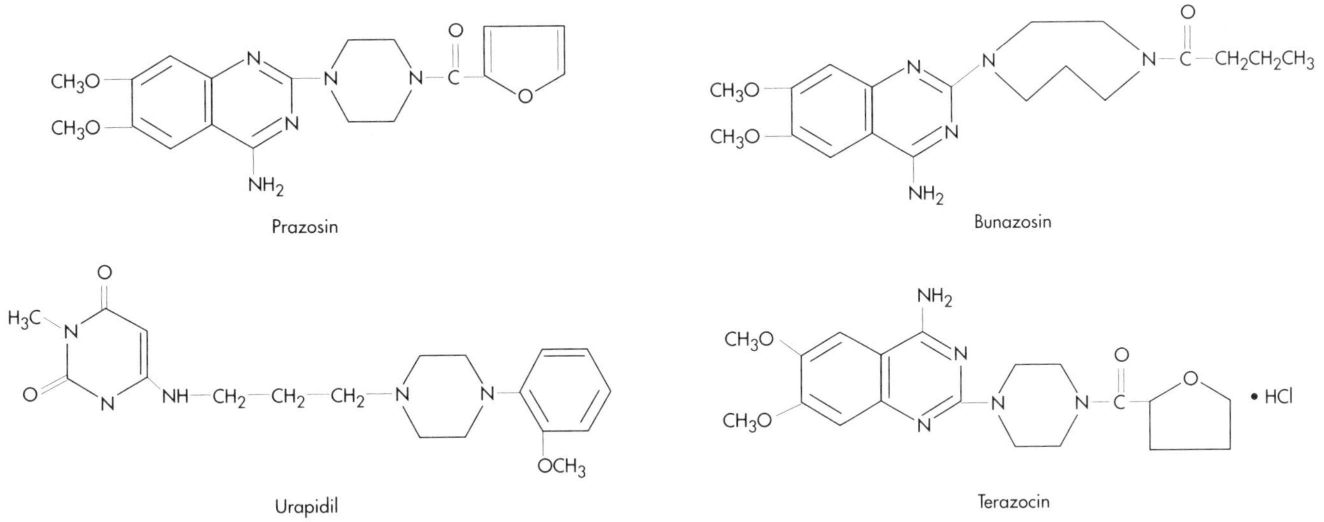

Prazosin

Bunazosin

Urapidil

Terazocin

Figure 26.6 Alpha Adrenergic Blocking Agents

vascular resistance or cardiac output occurred with atenolol or acebutolol.

Stimulation of presynaptic beta adrenoceptors leads to an increase in norepinephrine release from sympathetic nerves. Blockade of these receptors could lead to an antihypertensive effect through a reduction of norepinephrine release. Although exaggerated activity of the sympathetic nervous system has often been considered to be a major factor for inducing and/or maintaining high blood pressure levels in essential hypertension, a clear increase in the concentration of plasma norepinephrine in essential hypertension has not been demonstrated.[41,42] Such an increase is found more often in young hypertensive patients, however. As proposed by Bühler, a beta- and alpha-adrenoceptor response adaptation characterizes the sympathetic nervous system contribution in essential hypertension.[43] In an early phase of hypertensive disease and in younger patients, mainly increased beta-adrenoceptor-mediated functions prevail. In a later phase and in older patients in whom beta adrenoceptor-mediated functions are blunted, increased alpha adrenoceptor-mediated and calcium influx-dependent vasconstriction predominates.

In some studies, patients with hypertension showed a hyperreactivity to pressor responses, in particular those that involved vasoconstriction mediated by sympathetic activity and adrenoceptors. At postsynaptic sites in the vascular bed of the human forearm in hypertensives, drugs that are alpha-adrenoceptor agonists tend to produce a more pronounced vasoconstriction than in normotensive subjects. In the study of Lenders et al., however, an increased cardiovascular sensitivity to exogenous norepinephrine was not found in hypertensive patients compared with control patients when differences in metabolic clearance of norepinephrine were taken into account.[44]

Though neither the slightly elevated sympathetic tone nor the inconstant increased reactivity to noradrenaline could alone be responsible for the blood pressure elevation both factors together appear to form an important determinant of the level of arterial blood pressure.

Selectivity (Table 26.7)

Beta-blocking agents can preferentially bind to beta receptors of either the β1 or the β2 type. There are theoretical grounds for believing that cardioselective drugs (β1) might be better antihypertensive agents than nonselective ones. Indeed, beta 2 blocking activity prevents the vascular relaxation induced by beta 2 stimulation. In practice, however, it is not possible to demonstrate differences in efficacy with chronic maintenance therapy with the two types of antagonists at equipotent doses in hypertensive patients. In many cases, cardioselective agents might be of interest in patients with peripheral vascular disease or Raynaud's phenomenon. Vascular sparing could also be important in situations when increased epinephrine secretion occurs. In the presence of a nonselective drug, a marked diastolic response may result. This can occur during insulin-induced hypoglycemia in diabetics, during mental stress, cigarette smoking, and coffee drinking.

Partial Agonist Activity (Table 26.7)

Some beta-adrenoceptor antagonists partly stimulate beta receptors while occupying them (i.e., a partial agonist activity). Such an agonist activity remains much less than that produced by a full agonist such as isoproterenol. Available drugs that possess this property are pindolol, oxprenolol, alprenolol, acebutolol, and bopindolol. Pindolol has the most potent partial agonist activity, which is a preferential beta 2 activity. The result of administering these drugs depends on the degree of activation of the sympathetic nervous system at the time. Under resting conditions, when sympathetic activity is low, they cause less cardiac slowing than drugs without agonist activity. At high rates of sympathetic activity, beta blockade is the predominant effect. Under conditions of submaximal exercise, oxprenolol and pindolol are only slightly less effective than propranolol in inhibiting exercise tachycardia. The antihypertensive efficacy of these drugs with partial agonist activity may be less effective.

Mixed Properties

Some beta-blocking agents also antagonize catecholamine effects at the alpha-receptor level (labetalol, dilevalol, carvedilol). Dilevalol is one of the four isomers of labetalol. Its alpha-blocking activity is weaker than that of labetalol. Moreover, dilevalol has a strong β 2-partial agonist activity. One possible advantage of dilevalol compared with labetalol includes the ability to reduce peripheral resistance without postural hypotension.

Nebivolol, a highly selective beta 1 adrenoceptor antagonist, has vasodilating properties unrelated to beta 2 stimulation or alpha blockade. Sotalol has antiarrhythmic properties of beta-blocking drugs (Class II antiarrhythmic drugs) as well as of Class III antiarrhythmics.

Antihypertensive Efficacy

Although it is a common belief that all antihypertensive agents are equally effective in reducing blood pressure, there are, however, some differences. In black patients, monotherapy with beta-blockers or ACE inhibitors has been shown to be less effective than diuretics. After age 60, the percentage of responders to monotherapy beta-blockers (see Table 26.8) seems to be less than with calcium antagonists.

The decrease in blood pressure after administering an ACE inhibitor or a calcium antagonist appears to be equivalent to that of a beta-blocker, although some studies indicate that the percentage of responders to beta-blockers may be slightly greater.

Combination Therapy Efficacy

Data from many centers indicate that if monotherapy with a beta-blocker (or ACE inhibitor or calcium antagonist) does not achieve normotensive blood pressure, the addition of a diuretic greatly improves the outcome. In one study, when hydrochlorothiazide was added to the nonresponder's regimen of either diltiazem (120–360 mg/d) or propranolol (160–480 mg/d), 50 percent of those in the diltiazem group and 60 percent of the propranolol group became normotensive. Combination of beta-blockers with an ACE

Table 26.7 Beta Adrenoceptor Blocking Agents Properties

Drug	Cardio-selectivity	Partial Agonist Activity	Membrane Stabilizing Activity	Bioavailability (%)	Elimination Half-life (hr)	Liposolubility Lipophilic : L Hydrophylic : H
Propranolol	–	–	+	30	2–5	L
Oxprenolol	–	+	+	40	1–4	L
Timolol	–	–	–	55	2–5	L
Metoprolol	+	–	+	95	3–4	L
Acebutolol	+	+	+	50	3–4	H
Pindolol	–	+	–	85	2–5	L
Nadolol	–	–	–	16–25	17–22	H
Bisoprolol	+	–	–	88	10	H
Sotalol	–	–	–	>90	7–18	H
Atenolol	+	–	–	50	6–9	H
Labetolol	–	–	+	90+	2.5–8	L

Table 26.8 Large Scale Trials with Beta-Blockers as First-Step Therapy in One Group

	Schedule	Patients	Result		
Medical Research Council Trial (MRC)	5,5 years follow up Three groups: Placebo, propranolol, bendrofluazide	35–64 years of age 17,000 patients	**Morbidity Reduction**		
				Diuretic (%)	**Propranolol (%)**
			Stroke	67	24
			Coronary events	–2	13
			All cardiovascular events	20	18
International primary prospective prevention study in hypertension (IPPPSH)	3–5 yr follow-up Two Groups: Oxprenolol (+ diuretics if necessary), Placebo (+ diuretics if necessary)	40–64 years of age 6357 patients	**Incidence of Stroke and Cardiac Events (rate/1000 patient year)**		
				Non-Beta-Blocker	**Oxprenolol**
			Stroke	3.6	3.5
			Cardiac event	8.4	7.6
			Myocardial infarction	5.7	4.7
Heart attack primary prevention in hypertension (HAPPHY)	Average follow-up = 3.7 yr Two Groups: Diuretics, Beta-blockers: Atenolol, Metoprolol (MAPHY)	40–64 years of age 6569 patients	**Incidence of Stroke and Cardiac Events (rate/1000 patient year)**		
				Diuretic	**Beta Blockade**
			Stroke	3.35	2.58
			Cardiac events	9.48	10.62

inhibitor may, however, not always add to the effectiveness of the single agent.

Results of Large-Scale Trials with Beta Adrenoceptor Antagonists in Hypertension

The goal of antihypertensive therapy is focused on prevention of its complications. Dramatic benefit was initially demonstrated for pharmacotherapy of patients with severe hypertension (see Table 26.8). With moderate hypertension, the effects of antihypertensive treatment on cerebrovascular and coronary heart disease end-points reported in large-scale national trials have differed (MRC, IPPSH, HAPPHY; see Table 26.8). All trials have shown stroke benefit, with a reduction of incidence of 40 percent by diuretics or beta blockade treatment.[45–47] Prevention of coronary heart disease, however, has not been convincingly demonstrated in any of the trials. These large-scale trials have shown that normalization of blood pressure is not consistently obtained with diuretics or beta blockade used as monotherapy. A 5-mmHg reduction of diastolic blood pressure is, however, associated with a 24 percent reduction of cardiac risk and with a 43 percent reduction of stroke risk. Propranolol was the beta-blocking agent studied in MRC trial, oxprenolol in the IPPSH trial, atenolol in the HAPPHY trial and metoprolol in the MAPHY trial.

In the MRC trial, stroke rate and the incidence of all cardiovascular events were significantly reduced for patients actively treated either by diuretics or propranolol compared with placebo. However, neither treatment could reduce coronary events in men or women who smoked: such a finding was found in the IPPSH but not in the HAPPHY trial. In both trials, beta-blocking agents and diuretics provided equal benefit. In the MAPHY trial (extension of the HAPPHY trial), the pooled incidence of fatal and nonfatal coronary heart disease events were significantly lower in the metoprolol group compared with placebo.[48]

Some explanations have been proposed for the absence of better results with beta-blocking drugs on morbidity and mortality from myocardial infarction. Most likely, antihypertensive treatment with beta-blockade treatment does not correct all the coronary risk factors, especially the lipid profile. However, in the MRC trial, although there was a statistically significant elevation of cholesterol by treatment, the effect was very small and could not have explained the lack of benefit on coronary events. It is, however, fair to say that there is still controversy about the precise extent and duration of blood lipid disturbances after long-term treatment with beta-blockers. In a recent meta analysis of trials on hypertension, reduction of stroke incidence was 42 ± 6 percent, compared with 14 ± 5 percent for coronary events in 14 controlled trials.[49,50]

Undesirable Effects

Most of the clinical trials have concluded that beta-blockers are generally well tolerated, with subjective side-effects occurring in only 10 percent of patients. Most frequently reported are: sleep disturbances; cold extremities; headache; depressed mood; tiredness; sex problems.

Undesirable cardiac effects can be excessive sinus bradycardia or AV block. Patient factors that foster such events include latent sinus node dysfunction or AV dysfunction, and associated treatments such as digitalis, diltiazem, or verapamil. Some cases of heart failure decompensation have been observed with high doses of beta-adrenoceptor antagonists in compensated hypertensive heart failure. When they are progressively administrated with relatively low dosage, however, beta-blocking agents do provide long-term benefit in heart failure patients. However, this remains to be demonstrated conclusively.

Beta-adrenoceptor antagonists may increase plasma triglyceride concentrations, decrease high density lipoproteins, and increase low density lipoproteins. Cardioselective substances may have a lesser effect but the difference appears to be very small. However, these induced blood lipid modifications returned to normal values after long-term treatment with beta-blocking drugs.

It has recently been suggested that the beta-blocker-induced changes in both triglycerides and cholesterol are the result of inhibition of lipoprotein lipase by predominantly alpha adrenergic stimulation. In any case, the clinical relevance of such blood lipid modifications remains to be demonstrated.

Pharmacokinetics

As a general rule, liphophilic beta adrenergic substances are extensively metabolized and have a short elimination half-life (1 to 4 hours) (see Table 26.7). On the contrary, water-soluble substances are eliminated unchanged by the kidney and have longer half-lives (6 to 22 hours). For lipophilic substances, first-pass hepatic metabolism is a biologically variable phenomenon and induces large interindividual differences in plasma concentrations. These drugs may be involved in interactions with drugs that affect microsomal enzyme activity. In addition, they gain access to the CNS and can produce more central side-effects. In contrast, water-soluble beta-adrenoceptor antagonists, such as atenolol, nadolol, or sotalol, are less well absorbed but are not metabolized in the liver. They also exhibit less interpatient variability in plasma concentrations.

Centrally Acting Antihypertensive Drugs

The brain exerts broad control over the circulation. In particular, the medulla and hypothalmus appear to exert a tonic outflow of sympathetic activity to the heart and blood vessels, the absence or decrease of which can result in dramatic reductions in heart rate and blood pressure. Several drugs whose primary action is located in the CNS can be used as antihypertensive drugs, e.g., clonidine, methyldopa, guanabenz, guanfacine, and rilmenidine. The important role of the sympathetic nervous system in the development of high blood pressure in animals has been emphasized by several authors. In human hypertension, however, the role of the sympathetic nervous system in hypertensive disease is more difficult to demonstrate.[51]

Mechanism of Action

All these substances depress sympathetic tone by an action on CNS receptors (alpha adrenergic or imidazoline receptors). Their chemical structures are shown in Figure 26.5. Drugs such as clonidine, rilmenidine, and guanfacine, could mimic an endogenous substance, or "endazoline" according to Bousquet;[52] but, if so, the endogenous receptor ligand has not yet been characterized. All these substances are alpha-adrenergic agonists, and part of their antihypertensive action could be related to stimulation of presynaptic alpha-adrenergic receptors on peripheral sympathetic nerve terminals. Such stimulation decreases the efficiency of norepinephrine release in response to nerve depolarization.

When given IV as a bolus, clonidine induces a dramatic initial increase in blood pressure that is followed immediately by a progressively marked fall in blood pressure. The initial increase in blood pressure is probably mediated by the direct postsynaptic stimulation of peripheral vascular alpha-adrenergic receptors. This is followed by a decrease in heart rate and cardiac output without change in total peripheral resistance. Clonidine has little or no effect on either renal blood flow or glomerular filtration rate, but reduces renal vascular resistance, a pattern similar to that observed with methyldopa.

Centrally acting antihypertensive drugs reduce both renin levels and renin release in animals and hypertensive patients. The contribution of this centrally mediated decrease in renin levels to the antihypertensive action is unclear. Although some of the bradycardia caused by these substances is a result of the reduction of sympathetic nerve activity, clonidine also decreases heart rate by activating brain vagal centers. In addition, clonidine is able to potentiate the baroreceptor response resulting from an increase in systemic blood pressure. Most recent developments suggest that the antihypertensive action of imidazoline compounds could result mainly from stimulation of specific receptors in the medulla, but that most side-effects, like sedation, could result from central stimulation of alpha-adrenergic receptors.

The pharmacokinetic information on drugs of this class is presented in Table 26.9.

Table 26.9 Pharmacokinetics of Centrally-Acting Antihypertension Drugs

	Oral Bioavailability (%)	Plasma Protein Binding (%)	Metabolism	Elimination Half-life (hr)	Urinary Elimination of Unchanged Drug (%)	Usual Antihypertensive Dose (mg)
Clonidine	75	30	30 to 40% metabolization Unactive metabolites	20–24	30–40	0.150–0.600
Alphamethyl dopa	8–62	30	Hepatic metabolization : methyl-dopa-mono-O-sulfate (partly active)	1.7	60	500 to 3g
Guanfacine	100	20–30 (60% bound to erythrocytes)	No first-pass effect Major metabolite : 3-hydroxy derivative	17	30	1–3
Rilmenidine	100	10	No first-pass effect	7	66–68	0.5–2
Guanobenz	70–80	90	Extensive first-pass metabolism	4–21	1	4 bid.

Antihypertensive Efficacy

Clonidine

When given as a sole agent to patients with mild essential hypertension, clonidine lowers pressure to normal levels in approximately 50 to 60 percent of patients. Approximately a 25/15 mmHg (systolic/diastolic) drop in blood pressure is obtained and might be expected in mild or moderate hypertension when clonidine is given alone in a maximally effective and tolerated dose. When combined with diuretics such as chlorthalidone, a 20–25 percent decline in both systolic and diastolic pressure is usually obtained.

Alphamethyldopa

Methyldopa has been shown to reduce blood pressure approximately 20/13 mmHg (systolic/diatolic) in mild hypertension and approximately 38/22 mmHg in moderate or severe hypertension (with a mean maximal daily doses of 3.8 g). Tolerance (actually a pseudotolerance) frequently develops, however, after several weeks of methyldopa due to an expanded plasma volume. For this reason, alphamethyldopa generally has been used in association with diuretics. Good results have been reported with such a combination in severe hypertension. In one study in hypertensives with pretreatment blood pressures averaging 190/130 mmHg, administration of both drugs resulted in post-treatment mean blood pressures of 159/104.[53] The usual daily dose of alphamethyldopa ranges between 750 mg and 1.5 g daily. In severe hypertension, mean daily doses must be much higher, up to 4 g/day.

Guanfacine

Guanfacine, like clonidine, exerts its antihypertensive action primarily by its effect on total peripheral resistance. Reflex tachycardia is not observed, and heart rate is decreased after guanfacine administration. One mg/day appears to be an effective monotherapy in hypertensive patients and is obtained without frequent side-effects (only 3%) and without metabolic disturbances.[54] Doses of guanfacine at 2–3 mg/day are not more effective than the 1 mg/day dose, but are associated with more side-effects. Compared with clonidine as a step 2 therapy of mild to moderate hypertension, guanfacine was equally efficacious.[54] Fifty-five percent of patients with guanfacine and 59 percent with clonidine achieved good diastolic reduction to pressures below 90 mmHg. Abrupt withdrawal of clonidine produced a rapid increase in diastolic and, especially, systolic blood pressure, whereas guanfacine withdrawal produced more gradual increases.[56]

Rilmenidine

Rilmenidine differs greatly from clonidine with respect to sedative activity, which could not be demonstrated even for high doses in animal models. In one multicentric study on patients with mild to moderate hypertension, blood pressure was normalized in 61

Table 26.10 Summary Table: Other Antihypertensive Drugs

Drug	Dosage			Pharmacokinetics			Cl or Duration of Response
	Route	Size	Dose	Peak	V_D	$t_{1/2}$	
K Channel Activators							
Diazoxide Hyperstat	Parenteral	15 mg/ml	1–3 mg/Kg over 5–15 min initially	immediate		21–45 hr	Effect lasts 3–72 hr
Minoxidil Loniten	Oral	2.5–10 mg tablets	5 mg qid initially	1 hr		4.2 hr	lasts 2–5 d
Adrenergic Neurone Blockers							
Guanadrel Hylorel	Oral	10, 25 mg tablets	5 mg bid initially	1.5–2 hr		10–12 hr	effect lasts 4–14 hr
Guanethidine Ismelin	Oral	10, 25 mg tablets	10 mg qid initially	1–3 weeks		5 d	effect lasts 1–3 weeks
Vasodilators							
Hydralazine	Oral	10, 25, 50, 100 mg tablets	10 mg qid	2 hr		8 hr	
Apressoline	Parenteral	20 mg/ml	10–20 mg IV 10–50 mg IM	5–10 min			lasts 2–6 hr lasts 2–6 hr
Adrenergic Transmitter Depletors							
Reserpine	Oral	0.1–0.25 mg	0.1 mg	2 hr		13 d	4–10 hr
Rauwolfin Serpentina	Oral	50, 100 mg	50 mg	2 hr		13 d	4–10 hr
Deserpidine	Oral	0.25 mg	0.25 mg	2 hr		13 d	4–10 hr
Ganglonic Blockers							
Mecamylamine Inversine	Oral	2.5 mg tablet	2.5 mg qid × 2 d	3–5 hr		lasts 6–12 hr	
Trimethaphan camsylate Arfonad	Parenteral	50 mg/ml	0.5–1 mg/min	immediate			lasts minutes
α_1Adrenergic Antagonists							
Prazocin Minipress	Oral	1,2,5 mg capsults	1 mg bid or tid	2–3 hr		2–4 hr	lasts under 24 hr
Terazocin Hytrin	Oral	1,2,5 mg tablets	1 mg qid initially	1–2 hr	17–30 L	12 hr	lasts 2–3 d

percent of the patients taking rilmenidine (1mg/day) as opposed to 23 percent of those taking placebo.[55] With 1 mg/day, no significant difference in the incidence of either dry-mouth or daytime drowsiness could be found between rilmenidine and placebo. Increasing the dose to 2 mg/day tended to increase the incidence of dry-mouth. Compared with clonidine, 1 mg rilmenidine appears to provide an equivalent antihypertensive action to 0.15 mg clonidine.[56]

Undesirable Effects

Undesirable effects are relatively frequent with clonidine and alphamethyldopa. Rilmenidine appears to be better tolerated.

Clonidine

About 7 percent of patients must discontinue the drug because of persistence of side-effects. The most common reactions associated with clonidine therapy are dry mouth and drowsiness. They tend to disappear in two to four weeks of treatment. Other reactions: GI disturbances, weight gain, vivid dreams or nightmares, insomnia, anxiety, mental depression, urinary retention, and impotence.

Alphamethyldopa

Most frequent undesirable effects with alphamethyldopa are sedation (28%), dizziness (15%), dry-mouth (9%), headache (9%). Occasionally (0.5 to 5%): diarrhea, sleep disturbances, nasal congestion, depression, and impotence.

On discontinuation of therapy with clonidine, a rebound effect can be observed. A great deal has been written about the existence of such a syndrome. In many of the published cases, concomitant therapy or recent cessation of beta-blockade therapy may have exacerbated the clinical result; also, most of these patients had prior severe hypertension. Only rarely was an overshoot of blood pressure noted; usually the pressure simply returned to the pretreatment level. A positive direct Coombs test, with or without production of hemolytic anemia can be found in 20 percent of patients treated with alphamethyldopa. Hemolytic anemia occurs much less frequently, with an incidence of 0.1–0.2 percent. Sixty percent of these hemolytic anemias occur within 18 months of initiation of therapy. Hepatic derangement occurs in approximately 3 percent of patients taking alphamethydopa. Most reports of the more severely affected patients describe a viral hepatitis-type picture that occurs approximately eight weeks after exposure to the drug, but is reversible.

Guanfacine

With guanfacine, dry mouth, tiredness, and sedation are the most commonly reported side-effects. After drug withdrawal, symptoms of increased sympathetic activity within 24 to 72 hours occurred in 2 percent of patients. Compared with clonidine, guanfacine withdrawal produced more gradual increases in blood pressure. In one study, somnolence was less frequently observed with guanfacine (21%) than with clonidine (35%).

Rilmenidine

This compound provides an antihypertensive effect equivalent to clonidine but with fewer undesirable effects such as sedation and somnolence. Fewer patients are withdrawn from treatment with rilmenidine compared with clonidine. In one multicentric trial, at equihypotensive doses, rilmenidine induced two to three times less dry mouth, daytime drowsiness, and constipation than clonidine, and with a weaker intensity.

Alpha-Adrenergic Blocking Drugs

The basic pharmacologic description is presented in Chapter 6; only points of interest for clinical management of chronic hypertension will be discussed here.

Prazosin

Prazosin was the first available selective alpha 1-adrenergic blocking drug and was introduced in 1976 for hypertension therapy. A number of other compounds with a similar mechanism have since been synthesized and marketed, such as urapidil and doxazosin (see Fig. 26.6 for chemical structures).

Mechanism of Action

Presynaptic alpha adrenoceptors that inhibit norepinephrine release with postganglionic sympathetic nerve depolarization are almost exclusively of the alpha 2 subtype, whereas both alpha 1 and alpha 2-adrenoceptors occur in comparable numbers at the postsynaptic sites on the effector cells (e.g., smooth muscle). The postsynaptic alpha 2-adrenoceptors appear not to be innervated; in other words, their location is extrasynaptic, and they react to circulating catecholamines rather than to norepinephrine released from presynaptic nerve endings. Prazosin, doxazosin, and trimazosin are selective alpha 1-antagonists. These drugs preserve prejunctional alpha 2-receptor function and prevent an unmodulated disproportionate increase in norepinephrine release with sympathetic activation. Heart rate and renin release will then increase less than with other older nonselective alpha blocking agents (e.g., phenoxybenzamine, phentolamine).

Antihypertensive Effect

There is a close relationship between alpha-blocking activity and decrease in peripheral vascular resistance of prazosin and its hypotensive effect. Its antihypertensive efficacy has been clearly documented in a number of therapeutic trials.[57] The percentage of patients classified in various trials as "responders" has ranged from 50 to 70 percent. Although the antihypertensive effects of prazosin, when used alone, may be modest, they are comparable to those of diuretics and alphamethyldopa. The antihypertensive efficacy of prazosin, when used as a single agent, may be limited by fluid retention and an increase in plasma volume in some patients.[58] Addition of a diuretic in these cases results in an additive antihypertensive effect and increases the incidence of clinical response.

Therapy with prazosin is generally initiated with an initial dose of 1 mg at bedtime and then continued at 1 mg two or three times daily. The prominent orthostatic hypotension seen initially is generally not sustained after two or three days of continuous treatment. The reduction in blood pressure observed after several days of continuous treatment is well sustained. Because of the balanced reduction in both capacitance and resistance vessel tone, right atrial pressure decreases slightly or remains unchanged. Prazosin does not produce adverse metabolic effects. Indeed, its use may be associated with potentially favorable effects on blood lipids.

Undesirable Effects

Side-effects with prazosin are not frequent. The most prominent is postural dizziness, which usually is transient but has been reported in up to 38 percent of patients. Initial marked hypotension with syncope may occur. This can usually be avoided by initiating therapy with low doses (1 mg) and with a bedtime dose. The incidence of syncopal episodes is approximately 1 percent in patients given an initial dose of 2 mg or greater. Nasal congestion, depression, edema, constipation, impotence, and skin rash have occasionally been observed.

Pharmakokinetic Data

Prazosin has a markedly variable biovailability of about 60 percent and is extensively metabolized (97%) by the liver via O-dealkylation and glucuronide formation. Prazosin is 97 percent albumin-bound and the elimination half-life is 3–4 h. In the presence of liver disease, one would expect to have a prolonged antihypertensive action, but doses need not be reduced in renal failure.

Other Alpha Blocking Agents

Prazosin Analogues. Doxazosin, trimazosin, and bunazosin. A number of prazosin analogues have been developed that, in preliminary trials, showed promise as antihypertensive agents.[59] These quinazoline derivatives also selectively block alpha 1 adrenergic receptors, and trimazosin may possess additional antihypertensive properties. Bunazosin is also a quinazoline derivative and, in addition, appears to have calcium antagonistic action on experimental preparations.

Indoramin. Indoramin possesses an indol structure with a piperidine chain. It is relatively selective for alpha 1-adrenergic receptors. It also possesses antihistamine and antiserotonin properties. At the CNS level, these actions can explain the somnolence induced by this compound. It has a prophylactic action against migraine.

Terazosin. This drug is a very close analogue of prazosin; it exerts its antihypertensive effect by blocking postsynaptic α adrenergic receptors, with a subsequent decrease in peripheral vascular resistance. Some reports suggest that preload as well as afterload on the heart are both reduced. No adverse effects on blood lipid profiles have been noted. The drug is more completely absorbed (90%) after oral administration, but is over 85 percent metabolized in the liver. The higher water solubility relative to prazosin produces a larger elimination half-time and a dependence on renal excretion, as well as less frequent dose repetition. Almost half the hypertensive patients begun on terazosin as monotherapy required the addition of a duirectic to achieve a normal blood pressure. Adverse effects include weight gain (fluid retention), dizziness (10%) and asthenia (7%). As weith all α antagonists, the first dose must be low, and the patient should be warned of syncope due to postural hypotension. After several days, the dose should be slowly increased if blood pressure has not yet reached target values. If control is not reached with doses of 20 mg/d, a second antihypertensive drug (usually a diuretic or ACEI) should be added.

Urapidil. Urapidil is a phenyl piperazine derivative (see Fig. 26.6). Its antihypertensive effects are the result of reduction of peripheral vascular resistance. The drug has no significant effect on the heart rate. Experimental studies in animals have shown that urapidil lowers sympathetic tone by a central action and selectively inhibits vascular postsynaptic alpha-adrenoceptors. Urapidil is well absorbed orally. Its absolute bioavailability in man is 56%.

In hypertensive patients, clinical trials of up to two years have demonstrated the efficacy and tolerance of monotherapy with urapidil sustained-release capsules in primary and secondary hypertension. The absence of drug-specific side-effects and the relatively low rate of adverse reactions and the simple dose regimen suggest that urapidil sustained-release capsules may become available for the treatment of hypertension.[59]

Hydralazine

Hydralazine was introduced in 1959 as an antihypertensive agent and was often administered alone or in combination with a ganglionic-blocking agent. Although it provided oral treatment for essential hypertension, it caused frequent discomfort and side-effects. Because of development of other major antihypertensive drugs, hydralazine is now less widely used.

Chemical Structure

Hydralazine is a phthalazine derivate (see Fig. 26.7). A number of other compounds appear to have very similar hemodynamic effects, such as minoxidil.

Mechanism of Hypotensive Action

The hypotensive action of hydralazine is entirely due to the relaxation of arterial smooth muscle, which results in a reduction of peripheral resistance. Resistance decreases less in skin and muscle than in other vascular beds, such as cerebral, renal, splanchnic, and coronary beds. Since the venous side of the circulation is relatively unaffected by hydralazine and compensatory cardiovascular reflexes reamin unaltered by the drug, blood pressure is reduced equally in both the supine and erect positions.

The antihypertensive potency of hydralazine is limited by a reflex increase in sympathetic outflow. The sympathetically mediated increase in tachycardia and cardiac output can reduce the antihypertensive effect of the vasodilator by as much as 75 percent. In addition, sodium and water retention occur due to renin-angiotensin-aldosterone compensatory activity. Thus, hydralazine is seldom used as sole therapy in hypertension, but rather in association with a beta-blocker and/or a diuretic.[60,61] Glomerular filtration, renal tubular function, and urine volume are not consistently affected, but hydralazine usually increases plasma renin activity. The over-all compensated hyperdynamic state of the circulation induced by hydralazine may accentuate specific inadequacies. Indeed, hydralazine can cause anginal pain in those with coronary insufficiency, owing to the decrease in coronary perfusion pressure and compensatory tachycardia.

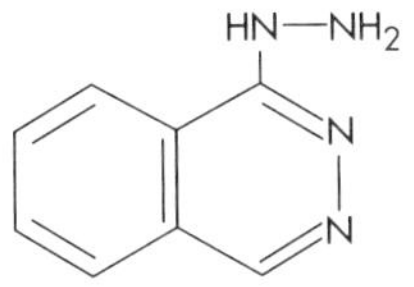

HN—NH_2

Hydralazine
(chemical structure)

Figure 26.7 Hydralazine

Antihypertensive Efficacy and Use

The therapeutic usefulness of oral hydralazine is as an adjunct to other drugs. It induces a dose-related response, with mean reductions in blood pressure in the range of 14/8 mmHg (systolic/diastolic with doses of 120 mg per day). Therapy with hydralazine is now limited to doses under 200 to 300 mg per day. Hydralazine is usually added to a diuretic when the latter fails to reduce the pressure adequately. Several studies showed that the thiazide-hydralazine regimen produced a mean decrease in blood pressure of 12/11 mmHg in mild and moderate hypertension.[61] The most effective use of hydralazine has been as "triple therapy" with thiazide, propranolol, and hydralazine. Hydralazine corrects the arteriolar vasoconstriction, propranolol blocks the reflex increase in heart rate and the increase in renin release, and the thiazide diuretic compensates for the tendency of the hydralazine hypotensive effect to retain sodium and increase the extracellular fluid compartment. Addition of hydralazine to propranolol and hydrochlorothiazide further decreases the blood pressure by an average of 22 mmHg.

Hydralazine, IV, has been used in hypertensive crises. The dose, frequency of administration, and therapeutic effectiveness are variable, however. Other drugs including diazoxide, nitroprusside, and sublingual calcium antagonists are faster-acting and are generally preferred for this use.

Undesirable Effects

Hydralazine produces a high incidence of untoward reactions. The Boston Collaborative Surveillance Program found hydralazine produced an 18.5 percent rate of adverse reactions in hospitalized patients. Most adverse reactions to oral hydralazine when used alone are of an acute nature: headache; nausea; tachycardia; postural hypotension; and palpitations are the most frequent adverse reactions. Occasionally observed: diarrhea, constipation, anxiety, nightmares, sleep disturbance, and angina pectoris. In some patients a delayed hydralazine toxicity, lupus-like syndrome may develop. It occurrence seems to be related to:

1. Duration of exposure. The incidence increases with time of exposure, with an average of 12 months needed to develop this syndrome.
2. Slow hepatic acetylation phenotype (about 50% of the population). Almost all toxic reactions occur in individuals who are genetically slow acetylators of hydralazine. Such patients should be limited to doses of 200 mg daily.

3. An average maximal dose over 400 mg daily. The reported cases of toxicity involving dosages over 400 mg daily represent 67 percent of cases.

Pharmacokinetics

Hydralazine is quickly and almost totally absorbed from the GI tract. Hydralazine is metabolized in the gut and the liver with an important first-pass effect. Bioavailibility is only 22 to 55 percent. A bimodal distribution of plasma concentration occurs after ingestion of hydralazine. This is related to partition of population between two phenotypes: slow and fast acetylators. The drug is widely distributed, and is concentrated in the walls of arterial muscle. Hydralazine is 85 percent bound to albumin, and the plasma half-life is two to four hours. The antihypertensive action, however, is much longer than the plasma half-life, with hydralazine persisting within arterial wall muscle long after being cleared from the blood.

Recommended Doses

Oral dosages are given initially four times daily, although twice a day doses also appear to be effective. A common regimen is to start with 10 mg 4 times daily for the first two days, then increase to 25 mg 4 times for the first week. For the second and subsequent weeks, increase dosage to 50 mg 4 times daily or 100 mg twice a day. Maximal dose is usually 300 mg a day. The usual maintenance dose is 100–200 mg orally per day.[62]

Sympatholytic Drugs

Guanethidine (Fig. 26.8)

Guanethidine, a guanine derivative, is an adrenergic neuronal blocking agent introduced in 1959. Its basic pharmacology and structure are covered in Chapter 6. Its use as an antihypertensive agent has greatly declined. The major antihypertensive effect of guanethidine is inhibition of responses to sympathetic adrenergic nerve activation due to reduced release of norepinephrine. Chronic administration of guanethidine produces a supersensitivity of effector cells very similar to that due to sympathetic postganglionic denervation, the earliest surgical therapy of hypertension.

Hemodynamic Effects

Guanethidine induces a reduction of both arteriolar and venous tone, leading to a fall in blood pressure. Since venous return and compensatory adrenergic reflexes are impaired by the drug, orthostatic hypotension occurs, and heart rate, myocardial contractility, and cardiac output are reduced. Under resting conditions, the distribution of blood flow is not greatly affected, although the hepatosplanchnic and renal beds may receive a smaller percentage of the cardiac output after guanethidine. During chronic administration, the cardiac output may return toward the initial level as a result of sodium and water retention and increased blood volume.

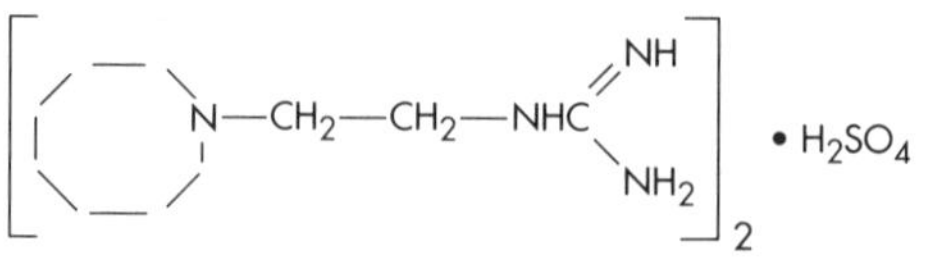

$$\left[(CH_2)_7N{-}CH_2{-}CH_2{-}NHC(=NH)NH_2 \right]_2 \cdot H_2SO_4$$

Guanethidine (chemical structure)

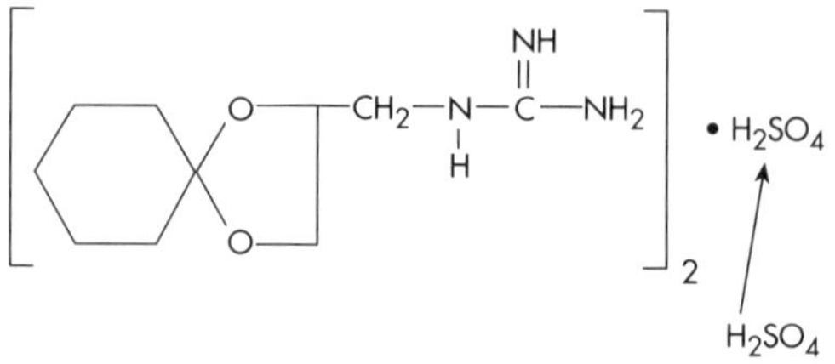

$$\left[C_6H_{10}(O{-}CH_2{-})O \;\; {-}CH_2{-}NH{-}C(=NH){-}NH_2 \right]_2 \cdot H_2SO_4$$

H_2SO_4

Guanadrel

Figure 26.8 Guanethidine

Antihypertensive Action

Guanethidine in combination with a diuretic is effective in lowering blood pressure in patients with moderate or severe hypertension. Guanethidine is effective in treating ambulatory patients but is more appropriately used in treating hospitalized patients with malignant or accelerated severe hypertension. Side-effects related to sympathetic ablation have limited its use as a common antihypertensive drug. Combined with a diuretic, gaunethidine reduces supine blood pressure of 21/17 mmHg and 35/23 mmHg in the erect position. The addition of a diuretic affords the opportunity to decrease the maintenance dose of guanethidine and simultaneously reduce side-effects.

Adverse Reactions

The most important adverse reaction is postural hypotension, which may be associated with symptoms of cerebral and myocardial ischemia. In contrast to the ganglionic blocking agents, guanethidine per se does not produce impotence. However association with diuretic drugs can induce it. Muscular weakness and fatigue, ejaculatory impairment, diarrhea, headache, edema, and weight gain may occur. Adverse effects can appear or progress for many days or even weeks after an increase in dosage, and may not subside for several days after cessation of therapy.

Drug Interactions

Because guanethidine is dependent on uptake into sympathetic nerve endings to be effective, it is subject to interactions with many other drugs that also act at the same site of uptake. The tricyclic antidepressants prevent the action of guanethidine by not allowing it to enter the neuron. Sensitization by guanethidine to some sympathomimetics found in "cold remedies" (e.g., ephedrine) can result in hypertensive crises. Conversely, dietary drugs such as tyramine (e.g., wine, cheese) will have little or no effect since they require uptake in order to have any action at all.

Pharmacokinetics

Gastrointestinal resorption of guanethidine can vary from 3 to about 30 percent. Differences in absorption account for only part of the wide variation of the dose required for a satisfactory antihypertensive effect. After oral administration, the plasma level and rate of excretion of unchanged drug suggest that guanethidine is absorbed continuously over a period of at least 12 hours. There is some degree of first-pass metabolism by the liver. However, a significant amount of drug is metabolized by the liver. Elimination half-life is about five days. Approximately half the drug is excreted unchanged in the urine. Metabolites have no antihypertensive activity.

Formulation

Tablets: 10 and 25 mg.
Antihypertensive dose: Onset of treatment, 10 mg.
Increase the dose by increments of 10 mg weekly.
Average daily dose: 25–50 mg per day (once a day).

Guanadrel

Guanadrel is another guanidine-containing adrenergic neuron blocking agent (Fig. 26.8). Its bioavailability is higher than that of guanethidine (85%), and its elimination half-life much shorter (10 hours). Thus guanadrel must be given twice daily to produce a sustained effect. Guanadrel has been shown to be as effective and as potent as guanethidine. Both drugs caused a statistically significant reduction in blood pressure when compared to placebo, with no significant difference between the two drugs. However, its duration of action is considerably shorter than that of guanethidine, in the order of 6 to 8 hours. Adverse effects are similar with both drugs, with the exception of a lower incidence of diarrhea with guanadrel.

Guanadrel sulfate is available in 10- and 25-mg tablets for oral administration. The usual initial dose is 10 mg/day; maintenance doses range from 20 to 75 mg/day. Concomitant use of a diuretic potentiates the antihypertensive effect and helps reduce side-effects.

Ganglionic Blockers

These drugs were discussed with the drugs that affect the peripheral autonomic nervous system in Chapter 4. *Mecamylamine* is an orally active drug that blocks postsynaptic nicotinic ganglionic transmission in both the sympathetic and parasympathetic autonomic nervous system divisions. Though very potent and always able to reduce the blood pressure to target values, the ablation of baroreceptor reflexes produces marked postural hypotension and other adverse effects similar to the adrenergic neuron blockers above. In addition, however, the blockade of the parasympathetic division tends to add additional incapacitating side-effects, such as bladder atony, constipation, inability to focus vision, photophobia (dilated pupils), dry mouth, and a decreased ability to sweat. At high doses it can produce a curare-like neuromuscular transmission blockade. Because of the severity of side-effects the drug is used only in the management of severe hypertension.

Trimethaphan Camsylate

The drug is similar to mecamylamine in its mechanism of action and side-effects, but since it is only available as a parenteral solution for IV use, the postural triggering of hypotensive episodes is less likely when the patient is confined to bed. Tachyphylaxis does develop to this drug, but not to mecamylamine. Unlike mecamylamine, trimethaphan is metabolized by plasma pseudocholinesterase, which accounts for its very short (minutes) plasma half-life. The drug is used mainly in the management of severe hypertension or to produce deliberate hypotension during surgical procedures. Its advantage over diazoxide or nitroprusside in the latter application is that it is less likely to provoke a compensatory tachycardia. As noted above, however, its interruption of parasympathetic functions makes neurologic assessment of the unconscious patient more difficult. In addition, some patients demonstrate a histamine-release when given this drug, which, although helpful to lower the blood pressure, may make ventilation and oxygenation suboptimal.

Rauwolfia Alkaloids

These drugs are discussed in more detail in Chapter 6, but their use in hypertension will be discussed here. Since most research studies have used only one alkaloid, reserpine, the discussion will focus on that compound, but similar statements could be made for deserpidine, another purified alkaloid, or the dried powdered, whole-plant root. The reduced peripheral vascular resistance is thought to be secondary to the alkaloid depletion of norepinephrine neurotransmitter in postganglionic neurons, although an additional action to lower blood pressure by an effect in the CNS is still a possibility. Since the noradrenergic transmitter stores are reduced, but not absent, postural hypotension is not a common problem. The unantagonized effects of parasympathetic activity may be quite prominent, with bradycardia, diarrhea, nasal congestion, gastric acid oversecretion, and miosis in evidence. Edema fluid may accumulate unless a diuretic is added to the drug therapy. The easy penetration of the alkaloids into brain, where serotonin neurotransmitter stores are sharply reduced, may be responsible for the lassitude, and even depression some patients manifest. Combinations of this drug with other CNS depressants may produce states of deep coma. Parkinson symptoms are occasionally observed, probably as a result of reduced brain dopamine availability. Patients treated with L-DOPA for Parkinson's disease may lose the beneficial response. The lipid-soluble nature of the drugs is responsible for the long terminal half-life (weeks) and persistence of primary and side-effects for many weeks once the drug is stopped.

These drugs are used for more moderate to severe forms of hypertension when first-line drugs and their combinations have been ineffective. When used with a diuretic, blood pressure may be controlled with a minimum of side-effects. If vasopressors are used in a patient receiving reserpine or related alkaloids, the effects of direct-acting α agonists (e.g., neosynephrine) and β agonists (isoproterenol) may be accentuated, owing to up-regulation of postsynaptic receptors.

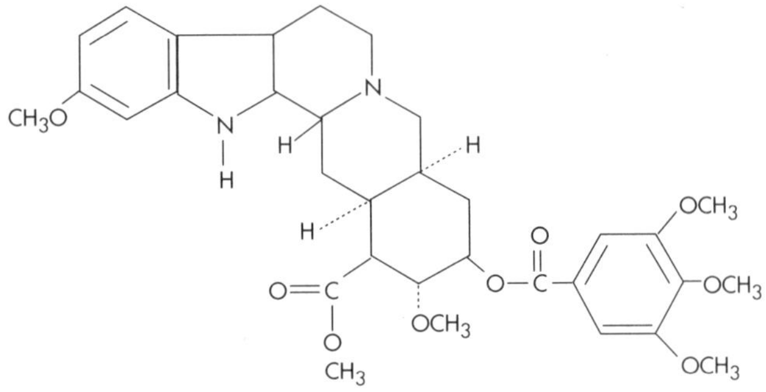

Reserpine

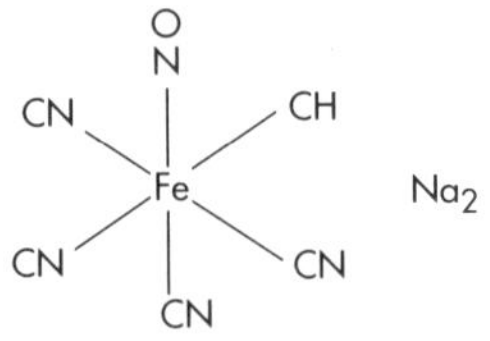

Nitroprisside

Figure 26.10

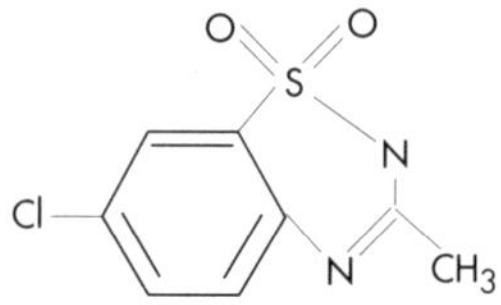

Diazoxide

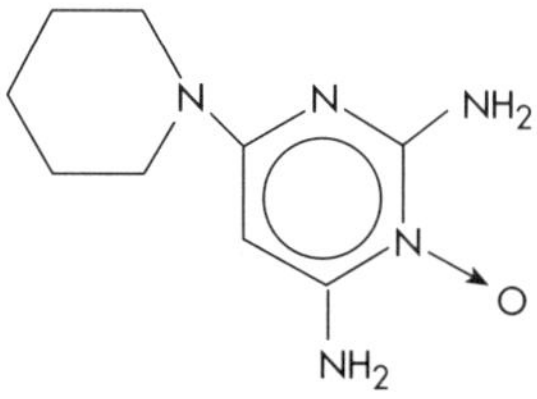

Minoxidil

Ganglionic Blockers

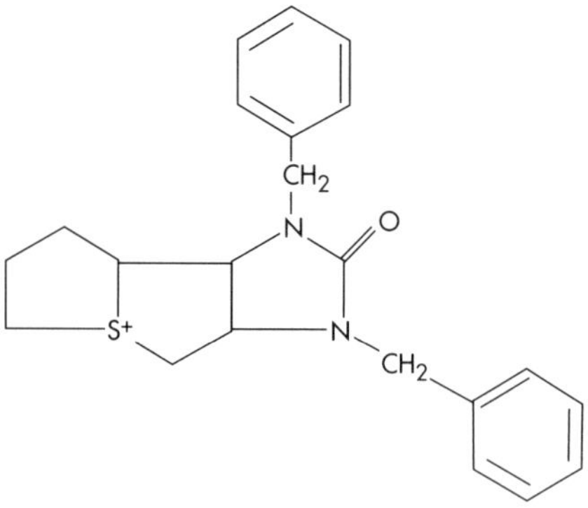

Trimethaphan Camuylate

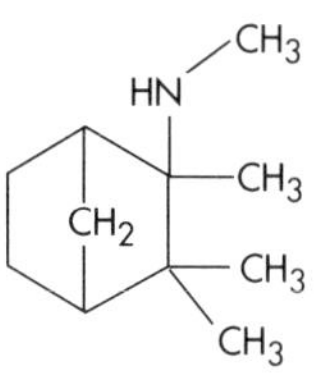

Mecamylamine

Figure 26.9 Potassium Channel Activators

Potassium Channel Activators

Mechanism of Antihypertensive Action

A series of vasodilators induce their vasodilatory properties through opening of potassium channnels.[63] This results in hyperpolarization of the cell membrane, which reduces calcium entry through calcium channels. In smooth muscle cells, the resulting decrease of

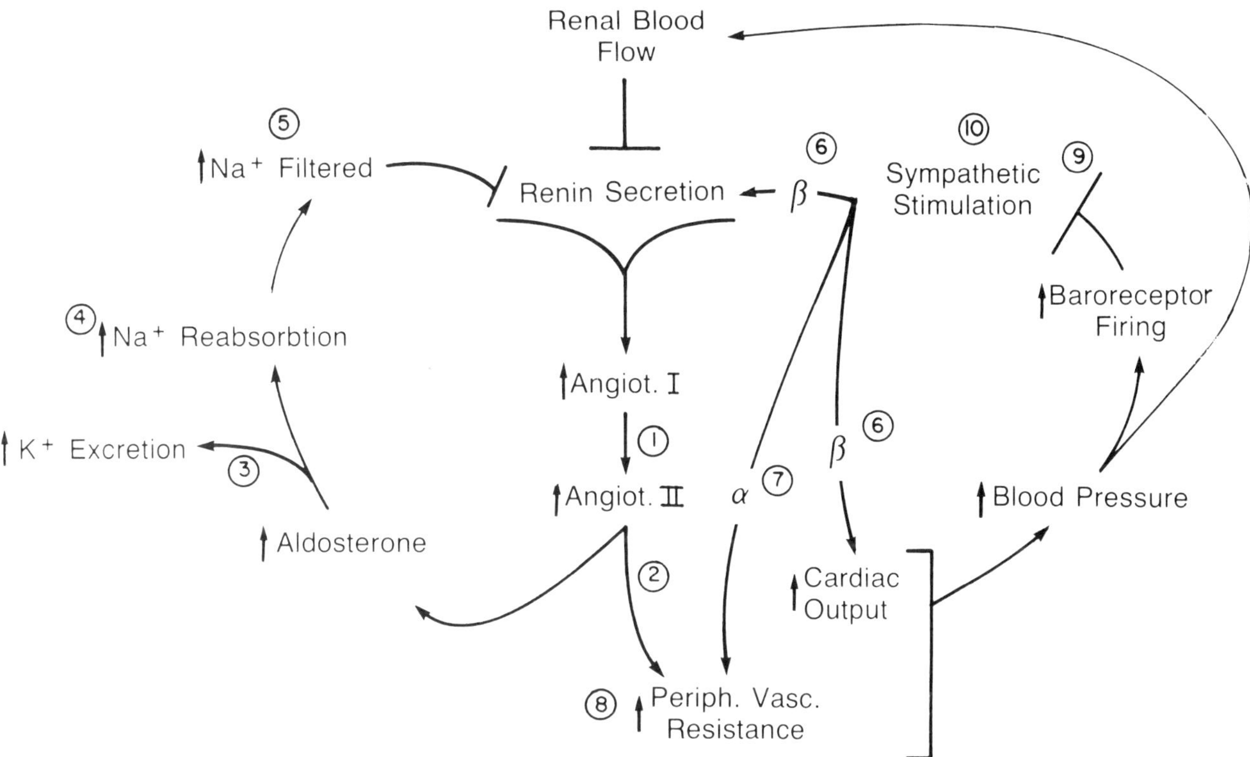

Figure 26.11 Systems that Modulate Blood Pressure. An arrow pointing to a word or phase indicates that the preceding factor increases or stimulates activity; conversely a perpendicular line implies an inhibition or decrease in activity. Each circled number designates a point at which pharmacotherapy is available, as noted below.

1. Angiotensin converting enzyme inhibitors
2. Angiotensin receptor antagonists (experimental)
3. Aldosterone antagonists
4. Diuretics
5. Experimental only
6. Beta receptor antagonists
7. Alpha receptor antagonists
8. Direct vasodilators
9. Alpha$_2$ receptor agonists in CNS
10. Noradrenergic neuron blockers, ganglionic blockers, and reserpine

intracellular calcium produces relaxation, particularly in blood vessels. Such a vasorelaxant effect has been used for antihypertensive purposes.

Three such substances have been marketed for years (diazoxide, minoxidil, and pinacidil). Their antihypertensive effect is uniquely related to a dose-dependent reduction of vascular resistances, and induces stimulation of compensatory mechanisms such as sympathetic and renin-angiotensin stimulations. The reflex tachycardia can be blunted by pretreatment with beta adrenergic blockade.

Experimental data show that these substances do not prevent development of genetic hypertension in spontaneous hypertensive rats, without any effect on cardiac hypertrophy.

Antihypertensive Efficacy and Therapeutic Use

Diazoxide is available only for IV administration, and its use is restricted to emergency treatment of severe hypertensive crisis. Opening of ATP-dependent potassium channels at the pancreatic levels with the same range of concentrations induces a marked elevation of glucose blood levels due to decreased insulin release.

Cromakalim shows modest antihypertensive activity. Use of higher doses is limited by tachycardia and headaches.[64]

Antihypertensive efficacy of pinacidil (12.5–75 mg bid) appears higher than that of placebo or prazosin.[65] Better results are obtained with combinations of pincacidil with diuretics.[66] However, adverse effects remain frequent (tachycardia, headache, edema). These appear to be dose-dependent. Minoxidil has been available for a long time; its use in hypertension has been limited by specific side-effects such as hypertrichosis, in addition to baro-reflex and renin-angiotensin system stimulation. Other potassium channel activators are currently under evaluation. Some of them, such as nicorandil, possess also properties of nitrate vasodilator compounds.

In conclusion, development of potassium channel activators in hypertension appears greatly limited by their adverse effects, especially baro-reflex and renin-angiotensin system stimulation.

Nitroprusside

Although sodium nitroprusside is not used for its direct action against cardiac ischemia, it is nevertheless used to reduce aortic impedence (or afterload) and thus can reduce the cardiac metabolic demands for coronary perfusion. Its major medical indication is in acute management of severe hypertension, and thus it will be discussed in this chapter along with antihypertensive drugs, even though it is a nitrovasodilator.

Chemistry

This nitrovasodilator is stable only when stored as a dry solid. When the compound is dissolved in 5 percent dextrose for infusion it must be protected from light to prevent decomposition The brown-red tint of freshly made solutions will change to blue as decomposition proceeds, with conversion of Fe^{+2} to Fe^{+3}. Fresh drug must be used every 24 hours.

When used for therapy of hypertensive states or to produce deliberate hypotension during surgical procedures (to decrease blood loss), the primary response is a decrease in peripheral vascular resistance, with slightly less fall in venous tone. These responses are the result of release of NO and its diffusion into the smooth muscle cell, where it activates guanylate cyclase. The increase in cGMP in the cell produces a relaxation in the smooth muscle cell by as yet unclear mechanisms probably related to a decrease in intracellular Ca^{+2} ion activity. Activation of the baroreceptors by the reduced systemic blood pressure increases a sympathetic outflow to the heart, and an impressive compensatory tachycardia may be seen. This, together with the decrease in vascular resistance, usually increases the cardiac output markedly. The hypotensive effect dissipates within minutes of cessation of infusion because of the very short half-time (a few minutes). Reaction with sulfhydryl groups in proteins and red blood cell membranes rapidly decomposes the drug to cyanide ion, which is subsequently converted to thiocyanate in the liver and kidney by rhodanese. Prolonged use of nitroprusside may permit cyanide ion concentrations normally in blood to increase to toxic levels. The inclusion of 0.5 g $Na_2S_2O_3$ in each infusion of nitroprusside (50 mg) supplies enough of the co-substrate to convert the released cyanide to the relatively inactive thiocyanate, precluding the development of cyanide intoxication evidenced by acidosis and increase in venous oxygen tension. Because of the need for parenteral administration of this extremely potent agent, the patient should be started on a longer acting, more manageable (noninfusion) medication as soon as possible. Small amounts of hemoglobin are converted to cyanomethemoglobin as the cyanide radical is released. The thiocyanate ion itself is weakly neurotoxic and a thyroid suppressant (inhibits iodine uptake and organification) at high doses. Such high blood levels are most common in patients with renal insufficiency who have a reduced capacity to excrete thiocyanate ions. The much more common signs of acute overdose of nitroprusside are the result of inadequate perfusion of organ systems (cerebral, cardiac, renal, hepatic) after too-abrupt, large, or long lasting a reduction of blood pressure. This is especially dangerous with patients who already have fixed vascular stenoses in the arterial supply to these organs.

References

Research Reports

1. Burges RA, Gardiner DG, Gwilt M, Higgins AJ, Blackburn KJ, Campbell SF, Cross PE, Stubbs JK. Calcium channel blocking properties of amlodipine in vascular smooth muscle and cardiac muscle in vitro: evidence for voltage modulation of vascular dihydropyridine receptors. J Cardiovasc Pharmacol 1987;*9*:110–119.
2. Godfraind T, Salomone S. Functional interaction of lacidipine with calcium channels in vascular smooth muscle. J Cardiovasc Pharmacol 1991;*18*(Suppl. 11):S1–S6.
3. Hulthen UL, Bolli P, Amann FW, Kiowski W, Bulher FR. Enhanced vasodilatation in essential hypertension by calcium channel blockade with verapamil. Hypertension 1982;*4*:II-26–II-31.
4. Simon AC, Safar ME, Levenson JA, Borthier JE, Benetos A. Action of vasodilating drugs on small and large arteries of hypertensive patients. J Cardiovasc Pharmacol 1983;*5*:626.
5. Kiowski W, Bolli P, Erne P, Hulthen VL, Buhler FR. Mechanisms of action of calcium antagonists in hypertension. J Cardiovasc Pharmacol 1987;*10*:523–527.
6. Kiowski W, Erne P, Bertel O, HUlthen UL, Ritz R, Buhler FR. Unchanged baroreflex sensitivity during acute and chronic antihypertensive therapy with nifedipine. J Hypertens 1983;*1*(suppl. 2):365–367.
7. Leenen FHH, Holliwell DL. Antihypertensive effect of felodipine assciated with persistent sympathetic activation and minimal regression of left ventricular hypertrophy. Am J Cardiol 1992;*69*:639–645.
8. Pool PE, Seagren SC, Salel AF, Skalland ML. Effects of diltiazem on serum lipids, exercise performance and blood pressure: randomized, double-blind, placebo-controlled evaluation for systemic hypertension. Am J Cardiol 1985;*56*:86H–91H.
9. Loutzenhiser RD, EpsteinM. Renal hemodynamic effects of calcium antagonists. J Cardiovasc Pharmacol 1988;*12*(Suppl. 6):548–552.
10. Ritz E, Schmid M, Ji-Zhen G, Mann J. Salt and action of calcium antagonists J Cardiovasc Pharmacol 1988;*12*(Suppl6):553–556.
11. Messerli FM, Ketelhut R. Left ventricular hypertrophy: an independent risk factor. J Cardiovasc Pharmacol 1991;*17*(Suppl. 4):S59–S67.
12. Agabiti-Rossi E, Muiesan ML, Ramasielli G, Beshi M, Castellano M, Muiesan G. Reversal of cardiac hypertrophy by long term treatment with calcium antagonists in hypertensive patients. J Cardiovasc Pharmacol 1988;*12*(Suppl. 6):575–578.

13. Franz IW, Ketelhut R, Behr U, Tonnesmann U. Long term studies on regression of left ventricular hypertrophy. J Cardiovasc Pharmacol 1991;*17*(Suppl. 2):S87–S93.

14. Motz W, Strauer BE. Left ventricular function and collagen content after regression of hypertensive hypertrophy. J Hypertens 1989;*13*:43–50.

15. Lewis GRJ, Morley KD, Lewis, Bones PJ. The treatment of hypertension with verapamil. NZ Med J 1978;*87*:351–354.

16. Stopher DA, Beresford AP, Macrae PV, Humphrey MJ. The metabolism and pharmacokinetics of amlodipine in humans and animals. J Cardiovasc Pharmacol 1988;*12*(Suppl. 7):355–359.

17. Abdel-Hag B, Magagna A, Favilla S, Salvetti A. Hemodynamic and humoral interactions between perindopril and indomethacin in essential hypertensive subjects. J Cardiovasc Pharmacol 1991;*18*(Suppl. 7):S33–S36.

18. Dzau VJ. Short long term determiants of cardiovascular function and therapy contributions of circulating and tissue renin-angiotensin systems. J Cardiovasc Pharmacol 1989;*14*(Suppl. 4):S1–S5.

19. Corvol P, Clauser E, Beeber B. Circulating and tissular renin-angiotensin systems. J Cardiovasc Pharmacol 1989;*14*(Suppl. 4).

20. Paulson OB, Walderman G, Anderson AR. Role of angiotensin in autoregulation of cerebral blood flow. Circulation 1988;*77*(Suppl. I):I55–I58.

21. Mancia G, Parati G, Pomidossi G, Grassi G, Bertinieri G, Buccino N, Ferrari A, Greggorini L, Rupoli L, Zanchetti A. Modification of arterial baroreflexes in essential hypertension. Am J Cardiol 1982;*49*:1415–1419.

22. Vlasses PH, Conner DP, Rotmensch HA, Fruncillo RJ, Danzeisen JR, Shepley KJ, Ferguson RK. Double blind comparison of captopril and enalapril in mild to moderate hypertension. J Am Coll Cardiol 1986;*7*:651–660.

23. Thind GS, Jonhson A, Bhatnagar D, Henkel TW. A parallel study of enalapril and captopril and 1 year of experience with enalapril treatment in moderate to severe essential hypertension. Am Heart J 1985;*109*:852–858.

24. Jenkins AC, Knill JR, Dresbinsky GR. Captopril in the treatment of the elderly hypertensive patient. Arch Int Med 1985;*145*:2029–2031.

25. Safar M, Bouthier JA, Laurent SM, Simon AC. Captopril and common carotid blood flow in patients with essential hypertension a review. Postgrad Med J 1986;*62*(Suppl. 1):31–33.

26. Taguma Y, Kitamote Y, Futaki G, Ueda H, Monma H, Ishizaki M, Takahashi H, Sekino H, Sasaki Y. Effect of captopril on heavy proteinuria in azotemic diabetics. N Engl J Med 1985;*313*:1617–1620.

27. Croog SH, Levine S, Testa MA, Brown B, Bulpitt CJ, Jenkins CD, Klerman GL, Williams GH. The effects of antihypertensive therapy on the quality of life. N Engl J Med 1986;*314*:1657–1664.

28. Varden S, Mookherjee S, Warner R, Smulyan H. Sytolic hypertension in the elderly: hemodynamic response to longterm thiazide diuretic therapy and its side effects. JAMA 1983;*250*:2807–2813.

29. Cranston WI, Juel-Jensen BE, Semmence AM, Handfield-Jones RPC, Forbes JA, Muctch LMM. Effects of oral diuretics on raised arterial pressure. Lancet 1963;*2*:966–970.

30. Varden S, Dunsky MH, Hill NE, Mehrotra KG, Mookherjee S, Smulyan H, Warner RA. Effect of one year of thiazide therapy on plasma volume, renin, aldosterone, lipids and urinary metanephrines in systolic hypertension of elderly patients. Am J Med 1987;*60*:388–390.

31. Yan Brummelen P, Man in't Veld A, Scholodamp MADH. Hemodynamic changes during long-term thiazide treatment of essential hypertension in responders and nonresponders. Clin Pharmacol Ther 1980;*27*:328–336.

32. Veterans Administration Cooperative Study Group on Antihypertensive agents. Comparison of propranolol and hydrochlorothiazide for the initial treatment of hypertension. I. Results of short-term titration. JAMA 1982;*248*:1996–2003.

33. Veterans Administration Cooperative Study Group Comparison of propranolol and hydrochlorothiazide for the initial treatment of hypertension. II. Results of long term therapy. JAMA 1982;*248*:2004–2011.

34. The IPPPSH Collaborative Group Cardiovascular risk and factors in a randomized trial of treatment based on the beta blocker oxprenolol: the international prospective primary prevention study in hypertension (IPPPSH). J Hypertens 1985;*3*:379–392.

35. The Heart Attack Primary Prevention in Hypertension Trial Research Group. Beta-blockers versus diuretics in hypertensive men: main results from the HAPPHY trial. J Hypertension 1987;*5*:561–572.

36. Multiple Risk Factor Intervention Trial Research Group. Baseline rest electrocardiographic abnormalities, antihypertensive treatment and mortality in the multiple risk factor administration intervention trial. Am J Cardiol 1985;*55*:1–15.

37. European Working Party on High Blood Pressure in the Elderly (EWPHE). Amery A, Birkenhger W, Brixko P, Bulpitt C, Clement D, Deruyttere M, De Schaepdryver A, Dollery C, Fagard R, Forette F. Mortality and morbidity results from the European Working Party on High Blood Pressure in the Elderly Trial. Lancet 1985;*1*:1349–1354.

38. Australian National Blood Pressure Study Management Committee. The Australian therapeutic trial in mild hypertension. Lancet 1980;*i*:1261–1267.

39. Wikstrand J, Warnold I, Olsson G, Tuomilehto J, Elmfeldt D, Berglund G. On behalf of the advisory committee primary prevention with metoprolol in patients with hypertension: mortality results from the MAPPHY study. JAMA 1988;*259*:1976–1982.

40. Meiracker AH, Man in't Veld AJ, Boosma F, Fischer DJ, Molinoff PB, Schalekam MA. Hemodynamic and beta-adrenergic receptor adaptations during long term beta adrenoceptor blockade. Circulation 1989;*80*:903–914.

41. Philipp TH. Sympathetic nervous activity in essential hypertension: activity and reactivity. J Cardiovasc Pharmacol 1987;*10*(Suppl. 4):S31–S35.

42. Philip T, Disthler A, Hecking E. Reactivity to tyramine and norepinephrine, plasma dopamine beta-hydroxylase activity and norepinephrine excretion in hypertensive patients with normal and with low plasma renin concentration. In. Frontiers of Internal Medicine. Basel: Karger (1975); pp 86–90.

43. Bühler FR, Kiowski W, Bolli p, Müller FB, Jones RC. The beta and alpha adrenoceptor response adaptation in hypertension development. J Cardiovasc Pharmacol 1987;*10*(Suppl. 4):S76–S80.

44. Lenders JWM, De Boo TH, Lemmens WAJ, Willemson JJ, Thein T. Am J Cardiol 1989;*63*:1231–1234.

45. Medical Research Council Working Party. MRC trial of treatment of mild hypertension. Principal results. Br Med J 1985;*291*:97–104.

46. The IPPPSH Collaborative Group. Cardiovascular risk and factors in a randomized trial of treatment based on the beta blocker oxprenolol: the international prospective primary prevention study in hypertension (IPPPSH). J Hypertens 1985;*3*:379–392.

47. The Heart Attack Primary Prevention in Hypertension Trial Research Group. Beta-blockers versus diuretics in hypertensive men: main results from the HAPPHY trial. J Hypertens 1987;*5*:561–572.

48. Wikstrand J, Warnold I, Olsson G, Tuomilehto J, Elmfeldt D, Berglund G. On behalf of the advisory committee primary prevention with metoprolol in patients with hypertension: mortality results from the MAPPHY study. JAMA 1988;*259*:1976–1982.

49. Mac Mahon SW, Peto R, Cutler J, Collins R, Sorlie P, Neaton J, Abbot R, Godwin J, Dyer A, Stamler J. Blood pressure, stroke, and coronary heart disease: part I. prolonged differences in blood pressure: prospective observiational studies corrected for the regression dilution bias. Lancet 1990;*335*:765–774.

50. Collins R, Peto R, Mac Mahon SW, Herbert P, Fiebach NH, Eberlein KA, Godwin J, Qizilbash N, Taylor JO, Hennekens CH. Blood pressure, stroke and coronary heart disease. Part 2. Short term reductions in blood pressure: overview of randomised drug trials in their epidemiological context. Lancet 1990;*335*:827–838.

51. Leonetti G. Centrally acting antihypertensive agents. J Cardiovasc Pharmacol 1988;*12*(Suppl. 8):S68–S73.

52. Bousquet P, Feldman J, Schwartz J. Central cardiovascular effects of alpha adrenergic drugs; differences between catecholamines and imidazolines. J Pharmacol Exp Ther 1984;*230*:2.

53. Horwitz D, Pettinger WA. Effects of methyldopa in fifty hypertensive patients. Clin Pharmacol Ther 1967;*8*(2):224.

54. Wilson MF, Haring O, Lewin A, Bedsole G, Stepansky W, Fillington J, Hall D, Roginsky M, MacMahon FG, Jagger P. Comparison of guanfacine versus clonidine for efficacy, safety and occurrence of withdrawal syndrome in step-2 treatment of mild to moderate essential hypertension. Am J Cardiol 1986;*57*:43E–49E.

55. Osterman G, Brisgand B, Schmitt J, Fillastre JP. Efficacy and acceptability of rilmenidine for mild to moderate systemic hypertension. Am J Cardiol 1988;*61*:76D–80D.

56. Fillastre JP, Letac B, Galinier F, Le Bihan G, Schwartz J. A multicenter double blind comparative study of rilmenidine and clonidine in 333 hypertensive patients. Am J Cardiol 1988;*61*:81D–85D.

57. Lund-Johansen P. Hemodynamic changes at rest and during exercise in long term prazosin therapy of essential hypertension. In: Cotton DWK, (ed.) Prazosin. Evaluation of a New Antihypertensive agent. Amsterdam: Excerpta Medica (1974); pp 43–53.

58. Koshy MC, Mickley D, Bourgoignie J, Blaufox MD. Physiologic evaluation of a new antihypertensive agent: prazosin hydrochloride. Circulation 1977;*55*:533–537.

59. Schoetensack W, Bruckschen EG, Zech K. Urapidil. In: Scriabine A (ed), New drugs annual: cardiovascular drugs, New York: Raven 1983.

60. Zacest R, Gilmore E, Kocher Weser J. Treatment of essential hypertension with combined vasodilatation and beta adrenergic blockade. N Engl J Med 1972;*286*:617.

61. Veterans Administration Multi-Clinic Cooperative Study on antihypertensive agents. Double blind controlled study of antihypertensive agents. III chlorothiazide alone and in combination with other agents; preliminary results. Arch Intern Med 1962;*110*:230.

62. McMahon FG. Management of essential hypertension. Mount Kisco, New York: Futuran, 1978.

63. Cook NS. The pharmacology of potassium channels and their therapeutic potential. TIPS 1988;*9*:21–28.

64. Vandenburg MJ, Woodard SMA, Stewart-Long P, Tasker T, Pilgrim AJ, Dews IM, Fairhurst G. Potassium channel activators: antihypertensive activity and adverse effect profile of BRL 34915. J Hypertens 1987;*5*:S193–S195.

65. Sterndorff B, Johansen P. Comparative trial of pinacidil versus prazosin in mild to moderate arterial hypertension. Drugs 1988;*12*:102–109.

66. Goldberg MR, Offen WW. Pinacidil with and without hydrochlorothiazide: dose response relationships from results of 4 × 3 factorial design study. Drugs 1988;*36*(Suppl. 7):83–92.

Reviews

r1. Godfraind T, Miller R and Wibo M. Calcium antagonism and calcium entry blockade. Pharmacological reviews, 1986;*38*:321–416.

r2. Fleckenstein A, Frey M, Leder O. Prevention by calcium antagonists of arterial calcinosis. In: Fleckenstein A, Hashimoto K, Hermann M, Schawartz A, Seipel L (eds.) New calcium antagonists. Recent developments and prospects. Stuttgart, & New York: G. Fischer (1983); pp 15–31.

r3. Moser M. Calcium entry blockers in the treatment of hypertension. A review and report of comparative studies with diltiazem. Am J Cardiol 1987;*59*:115A–121A.

r4. Halperin AK, Cubeddu LX. The role of calcium channel blockers in the treatment of hypertension. Am Heart J 1986;*111*:363–382.

r5. Chaffman M, Brogden RN. Diltiazem. A review of its pharmacological properties and therapeutic efficacy. Drugs 1985;*29*:387–454.

r6. Bühler FR, Hulthen LU, Kiowski W, Müller FB, Bolli P. The place of the calcium antagonist verapamil in antihypertensive therapy. J Cardiovasc Pharmacol 1982;*4*(Suppl. 3):S350–S357.

r7. Reinfrank J, Eckardt A, Halin KJ. Long term efficacy and safety of verapamil s.1. in hypertension. American Society of Hypertension Second Annual Meeting. New York, 1987 (poster).

r8. Hulten VL, Katzamn PL. Review of long term trials with nitrendipine. J Cardiovasc Pharmacol 1988;*12*(Suppl. 4):S11–S15.

r9. Agre K. An overview of the safety and efficacy of nicardipine in clinical trials. Am J Cardiol 1987;*59*:31J–35J.

r10. Jenkins AC, Dreslinski DPGR, Tadros SS, Groel JT, Faud R, Herczeg SA. Captopril in hypertension: seven years later. J Cardiovasc Pharmacol 1985;*7*(Suppl. 1):S96–S101.

r11. Dollery CT. Safety and efficacy of enalapril. Summing-up the evidence. J Hypertens 1983;*1*(Suppl. 1):155–157.

r12. 1989 Guidelines for the management of mild hypertension: memorandum from a WHO/ISH Meeting. J Hypertens 1989;*7*:698–693.

r13. Lund-Johansen P, Omvik P. Long term hemodynamic effects of enalapril (alone and in combination with hydrochlorothiazide) at rest and during exercise in essential hypertension. J Hypertens 1984;*2*(Suppl. 2):49–56.

r14. Thurston H, Desche P. Assessment of antihypertensive efficacy of perindopril: results of double blind multicenter studies versus reference drugs. J Cardiovasc Pharmacol 1991;*18*(Suppl. 7):S45–S49.

r15. Burg MB. Tubular chloride transport and the mode of action of some diuretics. Kidney Int 1976;*9*:189–197.

r16. Imai M. Effect of bumetanide and furosemide on the thick ascending limb of Henle's loop of rabbits and rats perfused in vitro. Eur J Pharmacol 1977;*41*:409–407.

r17. Schlatter E, Gregar R, Weidtke C. Effect of high ceiling diuretics on active salt transport in the cortical thick ascending limb of Henle's loop of rabbit kidney. Pflugers Arch 1983;*396*:210–217.

r18. Roberts CJC, Homeida M, Roberts F. Effects of piretanide, bumetanide and furosemide on electrolyte and urate excretion in normal subjects. Br J Clin Pharmacol 1978;*6*:129–133.

r19. Dikshit D, Wyden J, Forrester JS, Chatterjee K, Prakash R, Swann HJC. Renal and extrarenal hemodynamic effects of furosemide in congestive heart failure after acute myocardial infarction. N Engl J Med 1973;*228*:1087–1090.

r20. Conway J, Palmero H. The vascular effect of the thiazide diuretics. Arch Int Med 1963;*111*:203–207.

CHAPTER 27

Jean-Louis Montastruc
Olivier Rascol
Jean-Michel Senard

Vascular Disorders

Cerebral Circulation

Stroke and Acute Vascular Disturbances

Stroke remains the third leading cause of death in the US and Europe and one of the most important causes of definitive disability. The term "stroke" encompasses a wide variety of pathophysiologic processes that end in a focal deficit that persists for more than 24 hours. This chapter will review the therapeutic approach to transient ischemic attacks (TIAs) and subarachnoid hemorrhage.[1] Since no specific drugs are now available for intracerebral hemorrhage and cerebral infarction, these conditions will not be discussed.[r7]

Transient ischemic attacks (TIAs) are episodes of temporary *focal neurologic deficit that begin abruptly and resolve within 24 hours* without residual neurologic defect. A TIA must be treated; epidemiologic studies indicate that it may be a harbinger of stroke. When TIAs are due to cardiac embolic events, the underlying cardiopathy must be treated. Most the TIAs, however, are related to local thromboembolic mechanisms.

Anticoagulant therapy has not been shown to be of any benefit with respect to mortality.[2] It is of interest to note that all the nonrandomized studies report a decreased incidence of stroke in patients with TIA treated with anticoagulants, whereas all randomized studies failed to show any significant improvement. In fact, effective anticoagulation is associated with increased risk of hemorrhage, including intracerebral bleeding.

Antiplatelet drugs alter both platelet adhesiveness and aggregation in vitro. The most studied drugs in the preventive treatment of TIAs are aspirin, sulfinpyrazone, and dipyridamole. Although conflicting results have been reported, the general agreement is in favor of aspirin, which appears to reduce the risk of subsequent thromboembolic stroke significantly. Early studies used high daily dosages (1 g), whereas it now seems likely that lower doses could be as effective with fewer side-effects. Neither dipyridamole nor sulfinpyrazone shows increased benefit over aspirin alone, and no clear synergism between these agents has been demonstrated. Recent large controlled studies have demonstrated that ticlopidine also may be useful.[3]

The *calcium channel blocker,* nimodipine, was introduced for the treatment of subarachnoid hemorrhage.

Table 27.1 Some "Cerebroactive" and "Vasodilator" Agents

Bamethan	Naftidrofuryl
Bencyclane	Nicergoline
Bethahistine	Nicotinic acid derivatives
Cyclandelate	Nylidrin
Cinnarizine	Pentoxifylline
Citicoline	Papaverine
Dihydroergocristine	Piracetam
Dihydroergotoxine	Piribedil
Ebunamonine	Raubasine
Flunarizine	Suloctidil
Ginko-biloba extracts	Vincamine
Isoxsuprine	

Table 27.2 Summary Table

Drug	Dosage: Route	Dosage: Size	Dosage: Dosage Protocol	Pharmacokinetics: Peak	Pharmacokinetics: V_D	Pharmacokinetics: $t_{1/2}$	Pharmacokinetics: Cl or Duration of Response
Cerebral Vasodilators							
Nimodipine Nimotop	Oral Capsule	30 mg	20–90 mg q4hr	1 hour	0.94–2.3 l/kg	2–9 hours	0.5–1.2 l/kg/hr
Antimigraine Drugs							
Ergotamine	Oral Tablets Rectal Supp.	1–2 mg 2 mg	1–2 mg q30min till effective	1/2–3 hours		21 hours	
Dihydroergotamine DHE 45	Parenteral	1 mg/ml	1 mg qhr till response or 3 mg total dose given				
Methysergide Sansert	Oral Tablet	2 mg	4–8 mg/d in divided doses			10 hours	
Sumatriptan Imitex	Parenteral s.q.	6 mg	6 mg s.q. initially may repeat once after 1 hour if no response	1/3–1 hour		2 hours	
Peripheral Vasodilators							
Papaverine	Oral Tablets	300 mg	75–300 mg qid				
Pavabid	Oral Capsules	150 mg					
Genabid	Parenteral	30 mg/ml					
Pentoxifylline Trental	Tablets	400	400 mg tid	1 hour		1.6 hours	
Antivertigo Agent							
Scopolamine	Topical	0.5 mg/inch²/72 hours	1 patch 4 hours before challenge	1 hour			72 hours duration of effect
Other Vasodilators							
Cyclandelate							
Cyclospasmol	Oral Capsule	200, 400 mg	1.2–1.6 g/d in 3 or 4 divided doses				
Dipyridamole							
Persantine	Oral Tablets	25, 50, 75 mg	75–100 mg q.i.d.	3/4–3 hour onset		10–12 hours	
Isoxsuprine							
Vasodilan	Oral Tablet	10, 20 mg	10–20 mg q.i.d.	1 hour		1.25 hours	lasts 3 hours
Nylidrin							
Arlidin	Oral Tablet	6, 12, mg	3–12 mg q.i.d.	30 minutes			lasts 2 hours
Tolazoline							
Priscoline	Parenteral	25 mg/ml	10–50 mg q.i.d.	30–60 mg post IM		1.5–4 hours	

Nimodipine is a dihydropyridine derivative with a more selective effect on cerebral vessels than the other drugs in this group (especially nifedipine). It penetrates well into the brain and preferentially increases CBF in hypoperfused areas. It produces less systemic hypotension and cardiac effects than do the other calcium channel antagonists. Nimodipine is rapidly absorbed from the GI tract (Cmax: 30–60 min) with a low bioavailability (8 to 10%) due to a marked hepatic first-pass effect. It is mostly transported by plasma proteins (98%), and it is metabolized by the liver to inactive metabolites. Its plasma half-life is very short (60–120 min). Owing to variations in its hepatic first-pass effect, plasma levels of nimodipine are variable and largely unpredictable. Like the other dihydropyridines, nimodipine can induce cutaneous rashes, vasodilation of the face, GI pain, and arterial hypotension. Nimodipine must be used cautiously when given with other antihypertensive or calcium channel blocking drugs because of increased risks of hypotension and cardiac arrhythmias. Its action appears to be more pronounced when it is administered early after bleeding. Oral nimodipine is recommended for the preventive treatment of ischemic complications elicited by arterial vasospasm after subarachnoid hemorrhage. More recently, IV nimodipine has been introduced for acute treatment of such ischemic complications; however, its use by the IV route is limited by its high cost and the lack of definitive controlled trials.[r1]

Antimigraine Drugs

Pathophysiology of Migraine

The precise mechanism of migraine headache remains obscure. The oldest theories involved vascular disturbances in extracranial territories due to platelet dysfunction and serotonin (5HT) release leading to a first phase of vasoconstriction followed by vasodilation. Now it is believed that the migraine process starts from neurons in the brain and then proceeds to dilate the blood vessels, leading to pain.[4] Whatever the exact mechanism, the treatment of migraine headache includes drugs: (1) for the attack; (2) for prophylactic treatment. Evaluation of new antimigraine drugs appears to be very difficult because of the large variability of inconsistent symptoms and the large placebo effect in these patients.[r10]

Antiemetics (Metoclopramide or Domperidone). These drugs are widely used for the treatment of nausea or vomiting associated with migraine attack. They act through blockade of dopamine D2 receptors and accelerate both gastric emptying and absorption of orally administered analgesics. Metoclopramide also displays high affinity for 5HT3 receptors, which may participate in expression of symptoms.

Analgesics. Most of the nonsteroidal antiinflammatory drugs (aspirin, acetaminophen, ibuprofen, naproxen, or diclofenac) have been shown to be active in the treatment of attacks.

Ergotamine Tartrate. This ergot derivative exerts agonist activity for 5HT1-like receptors and behaves as an antagonist on both 5HT2 and alpha-adrenergic receptors. Its poor bioavailability (60%) can be increased by simultaneous administration of caffeine. Its delay of action is long (Tmax: 120 min) and plasma half-life is 21 hours, leading to accumulation in cases of frequent intake. It is excreted mainly in the bile after hepatic metabolism. The association of ergotamine with macrolide antibiotics can lead to ergotism (a syndrome of intense vasospasm, often with ischemia) since these antimicrobial agents are potent enzymatic inhibitors of the metabolism of ergotamine. The other side-effects of ergotamine, explained by activation of 5HT3 receptors located on the chemoreceptor trigger-zone of the brain-stem, are mainly digestive (nausea, vomiting). Rectal administration of ergotamine can be used in vomiting. Owing to its potent vasoconstrictor effect, it must not be used in patients with angina pectoris, arterial hypertension, Raynaud's disease, or pregnancy.

Sumatriptan. Recently, a new drug has been approved by the FDA for migraine therapy and appears to be extremely effective in managing migraine headaches.[2] Sumatriptan is not an analgesic but is an agonist at $5HT_1$ receptors on the cerebral vascular smooth muscles, provoking a contractile response. Presumably the vasoconstriction of these dilated edematous vessels decreases the pain due to vasodilatation of intracranial vessels. The large conducting blood vessels are decreased in size, yet intracerebral blood flow is not altered. There is also evidence that $5HT_1$ receptors on sensory dendrites of the 5th cranial nerve that supply the large vessels at the base of the brain are the real locus of drug action. At this site, the decreased dendritic release of calcitonin gene-related peptide (CGRP) may be important in resolving the enhanced edema formation and pain perception.[3]

Dihydroergotamine. This drug is also effective for management of attacks; however, since it is also particularly susceptible to first-pass metabolism in the liver, it must be administered by nasal spray or a parenteral route for the treatment of attacks. Pharmacodynamic and pharmacokinetic parameters are similar to those of ergotamine.

Prophylactic Drugs

The poor understanding of the pathogenesis of migraine explains both the wide range of drugs proposed for preventive treatment and the controversial results of clinical trials. Thus, several pharmacologic classes of drugs have been used.

Beta-Adrenoceptor Antagonists. Their usefulness in the prophylaxis of migraine was first demonstrated for propranolol and secondly extended to nadolol, atenolol, metroprolol, and timolol. Only beta-adrenoceptor antagonists devoid of intrinsic sympathomimetic activity are effective. The other properties (cardioselectivity, liposolubility, or membrane anesthetic effect) do not appear to be important variables. Thus, the exact mechanism of action still remains unknown, but does not appear to involve an interaction with beta-adrenoceptors since d-propranolol, devoid of any effect on beta-adrenoceptors, is also effective. Recent studies have suggested that the antimigraine efficacy can be explained by an interaction with 5HT1 receptors.

Antiserotonergic Drugs. The discovery of changes in plasma 5HT levels and 5HT release from platelets during migraine attacks led to the introduction of antiserotonergic drugs for migraine prophylaxis. Most of them are 5HT2 antagonists but most also have other properties of possible relevance for migraine treatment.

Methysergide: This ergot derivative has a high affinity for brain 5HT2 receptors but is also a 5HT1C agonist. It is the most active drug in migraine prophylaxis. Methysergide blocks 5HT induced-platelet aggregation and histamine release from mast cells; it also decreases the release of prostaglandin and kinins. After oral administration, its bioavailability is 100 percent. Tmax is obtained after 1 hour, and its plasma half-life is 10 hours, mainly through demethylation by liver. Side-effects are frequent and do not allow the use of methysergide as the first preventive treatment of migraine. Drowsiness, vertigo, nausea, vomiting, and weight gain are linked to interactions with 5HT receptors. The structure of methysergide (i.e., an ergot derivative) explains the possible occurrence of distal paresthesias, intermittent claudication, or angina pectoris secondary to vasospasm. Its most severe side-effect is retroperitoneal, pericardial, or pleural fibrosis, which can occur after long-term treatment. A one-month drug holiday every six months may prevent this complication. Biologic evaluation of renal function and regular radiologic investigations of the urinary tract must be performed. Regression may be complete after drug withdrawal.

Pizotifene: this tricyclic derivative has a mechanism of action similar to that of methysergide. Its enteric absorption is 80 percent with the Tmax obtained after five hours; plasma half-life is 20 hours. Pizotifene is strongly bound to proteins (91%). Like methysergide, pizotifene can induce drowsiness, nausea, or weight gain. It also possesses anticholinergic properties, and its use must be avoided in patients with glaucoma or prostatic hypertrophy. Its clinical efficacy is well-documented, and it is often used as a reference treatment in clinical pharmacologic studies of new antimigraine drugs.

Tricyclic Antidepressants. Amitriptyline has been shown to be effective for migraine prophylaxis. This effect, distinct from the antidepressant one, is thought to be linked to 5HT2 antagonist properties and inhibition of 5HT uptake. Its use can be limited by the side-effects resulting from anticholinergic properties or sedation. Curiously, other tricyclic drugs (clomipramine, desipramine) have not been found to be clearly effective.

Oxetorone. This antiserotonergic and antihistaminic compound also has sympatholytic properties. After oral administration, Tmax is obtained in 4 hours, with a plasma half-life of 24 hours. More than 95 percent is metabolized and eliminated by the liver. The side-effects of oxetorone are those of other antiserotonergic drugs (gastric disturbances, sedation).

Calcium Channel Blockers. Several calcium channel blockers have recently been studied in migraine. The rationale for their introduction seems incompatible with current views on the pathophysiology of migraine. It has been suggested that these drugs could inhibit the intracellular penetration of calcium observed during cerebral hypoxia.

Most of the studies carried out with the dihydropyridines were not conclusive. Recent studies with nimodipine, a drug with high selectivity for cerebral vessels, failed to demonstrate its antimigraine efficacy. Flunarizine (a diphenylalkylamine calcium channel blocker) may be effective because of its affinity for 5HT2 and D2 receptors, not its ability to block calcium channels. After oral administration, 80 percent of the drug reaches the systemic circulation, and Tmax is obtained after 2.4 hours. More than 90 percent of flunarizine binds to plasma alpha and beta globulins. Elimination is mainly due to intensive hepatic metabolism leading to hydroxylated or dealkylated derivatives. Its half-life is very long (19 days), and flunarizine is highly lipophilic. Side-effects of flunarizine are extrapyramidal syndromes (parkinsonism, tardive dyskinesia), depression, and amenorrhea or galactorrhea. Other adverse effects (sedation, weight gain) are explained by its H1 and 5HT antagonist properties.

Other Prophylactic Drugs for Migraine. Antiplatelet drugs were proposed to correct increased platelet aggregation and to prevent 5HT release observed in the early stages of a migraine attack. These drugs also inhibit synthesis of thromboxane A2 and prostaglandins. Aspirin has been shown to be effective, but its long-term use may be limited by its side-effects. The usefulness of dipyridamole or nonsteroidal antiinflammatory drugs remains controversial.

Lithium salts. Controlled studies have shown the usefulness of lithium salts for preventing migraine attack. This action is thought to be linked to inhibition of 5HT or norepinephrine release.

Alpha-adrenergic drugs: Use of these drugs also lacks any rationale in view of the present concept of migraine pathophysiology. Both $alpha_1$-adrenergic antagonists and $alpha_2$-adrenergic agonists have been proposed. Among the alpha blocking drugs, indoramine is the only drug marketed for migraine; prazosin is not. The pharmacology of indoramine is quite complex: apart from its $alpha_1$-adrenergic antagonist properties, it also behaves as an antagonist of 5HT, dopaminergic, and H1 histamine receptors. It is rapidly absorbed from the intestinal tract, with a bioavailability ranging from 8 to 75 percent because of variable hepatic first-pass effects. Its plasma half-life is four hours. After hepatic metabolism, indoramine is eliminated by the liver and kidney. Skin rashes, sedation, xerostomia, and priapism have been reported as side-effects. Indoramine also exerts antihypertensive actions and must be cautiously combined with other antihypertensive drugs. Some (but not all) studies have demonstrated the efficacy of the alpha 2-agonist clonidine (used at low doses) in the prophylaxis of migraine. However, it is not being used in clinical practice for this indication.

Peripheral Circulation

Drugs for Intermittent Claudication

The prevalence of intermittent claudication is about 10 percent in patients over 65 years. It is now well accepted that careful hygienodietetic care improves the natural history of claudication. When examining the efficacy of drugs widely prescribed for intermittent claudication, a divergence between medical practice and close analysis of pharmacologic trials appears. The latter indicate that drug therapy for intermittent claudication is of scant value. Misleading interpretation of the conclusions of atrial may be due to inconsistent patient characterization, small sample size, short duration of treatment, bad study design (open studies, lack of evaluation of placebo effect), inappropriate use of statistical methods, comparison of new drug trials with an agent without demonstrated efficacy, and inconsistent methods of assessing patient status. Thus, most of the 30 different drugs tested in intermittent claudication do not fulfill sufficient criteria for clinical efficacy. According to the pathophysiologic mechanisms of intermittent claudication (decrease in peripheral blood flow in ischemic areas secondary to vascular obstruction), several kinds of drugs have been proposed.[r11]

Vasodilators

These drugs with heterogeneous pharmacologic profiles are supposed to increase peripheral blood flow in ischemic areas. Despite their wide use, there is no clear evidence of their efficacy. Moreover, vasodilators decrease arterial blood pressure, increasing vascular dilatation in normal areas. As discussed for CBF (in Chapter 28), these two effects can induce a paradoxical negative effect in the ischemic regions (steal phenomenon) as the arterial pressure falls with generalized vasodilatation and flow past a fixed partial occlusion is reduced.

The Musculotropic Vasodilators. These drugs act through nonspecific mechanisms, inducing a direct relaxation of smooth muscle.

Papaverine and derivatives (ethaverine, eupaverine, dioxyline) inhibit cyclic nucleotide phosphodiesterase leading to cyclic AMP accumulation and vasodilatation. Although a vasodilator effect can be clearly demonstrated in normal subjects or in patients after acute treatment, no clear beneficial effect was demonstrated after long-term use in patients. Moreover, these drugs can induce side-effects such as flushes, arterial hypotension, tachycardia, and cardiac arrhythmias. The vascular actions of cyclandelate are similar to those of papaverine, although their characterization is incomplete.

Nicotinic acid and derivatives are potent skin vasodilators; however, only high doses are known to increase blood flow in the extremities. Such doses are associated with side-effects: flushes; nausea and vomiting; abdominal pain; and diarrhea.

Other drugs: Vincamine derivatives; cinapazide; and cietiedil have been proposed.

Calcium Channel Blockers. Cellular injuries induced by anoxia lead to excessive intracellular accumulation of calcium and cell death. Limitation of the toxic effects of calcium and inhibition of an hypothesized spastic component are the two theoretical reasons for the use of these drugs in intermittent claudication. However, results from controlled studies have been controversial.

Drugs Acting on Rheologic Factors

Pentoxifylline has been included in more studies than any other drug for intermittent claudication. The clinical response is thought to be the result of both an improvement in erythrocyte flexibility and a decrease in plasma fibrinogen, thus resulting in decreased blood viscosity. The exact mechanism of action of this methylxanthine derivative remains poorly defined and its definitive clinical efficacy unproved.

Isovolemic hemodilution by macromolecules (e.g., dextran, hespan, pentastarch, etc.) has seemed effective in acute trials, but usefulness in long-term use remains undemonstrated.

Antithrombotics

The efficacy of antiplatelet drugs (ticlodipine, dipyridamole) remains controversial. Anticoagulants are not useful.

Drugs for Raynaud's Syndrome

The original concept of Raynaud was based on the existence of an increased sympathetic tone. The pathophysiology of Raynaud's syndrome remains unclear however, and several mechanisms appear to be involved: vascular abnormalities (medial hyperplasia, increased alpha/beta adrenoceptor ratio); low perfusion pressure; elevated blood viscosity; and/or immunologic disturbances. This uncertain pathophysiology explains the lack of etiologic treatment. From the many drugs proposed for symptomatic treatment, only a few have been evaluated in humans using adequate methods. Moreover, controlled studies in Raynaud's syndrome appear to be difficult because of the importance of the placebo effect and the influence of environmental factors.

Alpha-Adrenoceptor Antagonists and Sympatholytic Drugs

These drugs might prevent the attack through a decrease in sympathetic vasoconstrictor tone. The efficacy of prazosin is the best documented, although its clinical usefulness is limited by side-effects (10%). Other alpha-adrenoceptor antagonists have been proposed: phenoxybenzamine; phentolamine; and indoramine or ergot derivatives (nicergoline, ifenprodil, dihydroergocryptine). However, they have been studied mainly in open, uncontrolled studies. The sympatholytic drugs, reserpine (used by oral or intra-arterial routes) and guanethidine, have been claimed to be of interest in severe cases.

Calcium Channel Blockers

These structurally heterogeneous agents induce vasodilation by inhibition of calcium entry in the vascular smooth cells. Several drugs (especially diltiazem and nifedipine) have been found to be of interest in controlled studies decreasing both the frequency of attacks the cold exposure-induced side-effects.

Other Drugs

5 HT2 antagonists (ketanserin) and prostaglandin PGI_2 agonists are potential drugs that act as vasodilatators and inhibitors of platelet activation. Local application of trinitrine remains uncomfortable and of unimpressive efficacy. Papaverine and sodium nitroprusside must be administrated IV and remain of little interest. Chronic treatment with buflomedil, oxpentifyline, naftidrofuryl or cinepazide was proposed as preventive treatment. However, the value of such therapy remains to be demonstrated.

Finally, prophylactic measures may also be effective, such as protection from cold and avoidance of provocative agents (ergot compounds, beta-blocking agents). Pharmacologic treatment has been proposed for severe symptoms; the calcium channel blockers are the most effective and best tolerated drugs.

Other Vasodilators

A variety of compounds have been developed in the hope of beneficially restoring blood flow to ischemic tissues. All of these agents are of marginal efficacy because the vasculature of ischemic tissues usually is already fully vasodilated as a result of local autoregulatory mechanisms. Thus, since the pathologic vasculature is already maximally vasodilated, the vascular beds that have unused vasodilation potential (the non-ischemic parts of the body) will constitute most of the decrease in peripheral vascular resistance response to any vasodilator. The effect of these changes, of necessity in the body as a whole, result in a decrease in arterial blood pressure. Since the ischemic tissue is already fully dilated before the vasodilator is given, blood flow to the tissue is dependent on arterial perfusion pressure. Thus, paradoxically, the vasodilating drug may, in fact, worsen the ischemic state of the tissues at maximum risk.

The defense of the use of these vasodilators is that perhaps increasing flow via collateral vessels by their dilatation may permit greater numbers of cells to survive. The indication for use of any of these drugs is thus more a function of belief of the prescriber rather than therapeutic fact established via experimental trials.

Cyclandelate

The drug dilates vascular and some nonvascular smooth muscles. It has been used for claudication, Raynaud's phenomenon, and ischemic cerebrovascular disease. Side-effects are largely those of vasodilation, with flushing, headache, dizziness, and palpitations from the compensatory tachycardia. The drug should be avoided in glaucoma patients, and may prolong the bleeding time.

Dipyridamole

This drug antagonizes the uptake of adenosine into endothelial and other cells, thus magnifying the vasodilator effect of endogenously released adenosine in response to local hypoxia. Platelet aggregation also may be antagonized since adenosine inhibits a variety of mechanisms that enhance platelet aggregation. Platelet survival has been reported as prolonged by dipyridamol in patients on cardiopulmonary bypass perfusion or in patients with valvular heart disease. The drug has also been used to aid anticoagulation in patients with prosthetic cardiac valves when given together with coumarin anticoagulants. The drug has been shown useful in angina in some studies, but has been reported to precipitate angina in occasional patients, probably due to systemic hypotension and compensatory tachycardia.

Isoxsuprine

This direct smooth muscle relaxant alters contractility in both vascular and uterine tissue. It has been used much as cyclandelate (see above), and side-effects are similar.

Nylidrin

This is a structural homologue of isoxsuprine, and its uses and side-effects are similar.

Tolazoline

This drug is a chemical relative of the α antagonist phentolamine, but the decrease in peripheral resistance is probably more the result of a direct smooth muscle relaxation than α receptor blockade. In addition, the drug stimulates intestinal motility and gastric acid secretion. The decrease in pulmonary arterial pressures initially made it a drug of choice for persistent pulmonary hypertension in the newborn, but it does not enjoy great favor in this application now, since its effects are slight and antagonized in the presence of acidosis. Concurrent ethanol consumption may produce a dysphoric reaction like that seen after disulfiram administration.

Drugs for Vertigo

Pathophysiology

Today, the symptom of vertigo is not considered to have a vascular etiology. Indeed, if one excludes the out-of-date physiopathologic hypotheses and empirical data, very few objective links remain between vertigo and vascular disease. Only 50 percent of the true vestibular syndromes can be clearly diagnosed as Meniere's disease, benign positional paroxysmal vertigo, acoustic neuroma, etc. The diagnosis of the other 50 percent is generally limited to "peripheral" or "central" vertigo; in these cases, according to habit, experience, and lack of better explanations, the physician will frequently come to the conclusion that a vascular mechanism is responsible for the lesion, especially if the patient is old and presents with vascular risk factors or arterial lesions. These are not objective direct proofs, however, and many "vascular" vertigos probably result from problems other than circulatory ones. In fact, very few vestibular syndromes—namely, true vertebrobasilar insufficiency (diagnosed according to a very strict neurologic definition and not fanciful arguments such as "old age," cervical arthrosis, abnormal doppler data, etc.) and the occlusion of the internal cochlear artery—can be related with reasonable enough arguments to a vascular etiology. Other cases generally refer to the old erroneous idea of chronic vascular insufficiency, which should be abandoned in vestibular pathology as it has been in the case of "cerebrovascular insufficiency" or "cerebrosclerosis." Moreover, according to a hypothetical notion of vasculovestibular insufficiency, the object of treatments that tend to dilate the small vessels of the inner ear should also be criticized: in the ear, there is very little, if any, collateral circulation; maximal vasodilatation has then probably already been achieved in cases of circulatory insufficiency and before any drug has been prescribed. In fact, since vasodilators influence all systemic peripheral vessels, the question of a possible steal syndrome must again be raised, actually compromising local perfusion. Finally, at the central level, nothing has ever been demonstrated about any benefit on vertigo obtained from vasodilating the brainstem vessels.

Apart from this "vascular" aspect of vertigo, many limits persist in the approach of vestibular pharmacology.[r12] Experimentally, the aim of an antivertiginous drug still remains unclear. Should it "depress" the vestibular system? If so, it is supposed to reduce the symptoms by decreasing the imbalance between the lesion and the intact peripheral vestibular afferences. However, in this way it also probably impairs another important phenomenon: "vestibular compensation." This term defines the spontaneous rearrangement of the CNS that allows the symptoms to disappear after a vestibular lesion. Its normal achievement requires that the nervous system should be informed of the erroneous signal secondary to the vestibular lesion. Vestibular suppression reduces this information, and by this means can delay or avoid normal compensation.

Very little is known about the neurotransmitters of the vestibular systems. This ignorance represents an important check on vestibular pharmacologic research and new drug development. There are also several clinical pharmacologic inadequacies in terms of vestibular pharmacology: major methodologic limits or imperfections still impair correct assessment of drug effects on vertigo. Motion sickness is often confused with pathologic vestibular syndromes; defined types of vertigos are mixed in the trials; judgment criteria are frequently erroneous, assessing electronystagmographic data (sometimes in healthy volunteers) instead of clinical evaluation of vertigo (e.g., diazepam reduces rotational nystagmus in the monkey but has no effect on the recovery of patients from vestibular lesions). Placebo-controlled and long-term studies are very rare, whereas in this disorder the placebo effect is huge and spontaneous evolution is capricious. Thus, many, if not all, antivertiginous effects of drugs used in man have been studied according to methods open to criticism.

Drug Management

At the moment, any antivertigo drug must be seen as symptomatic treatment. There is therefore no reason, except for marketing purposes, to advise one compound or another preferentially in any type of vertigo, especially the "vascular" ones.

Anticholinergic Drugs. Anatomic, electrophysiologic, and pharmacologic data support the evidence that acetylcholine is the neurotransmitter of the afferent vestibular nerve. In animals, anticholinergics exert vestibulodepressant effects and induce overcompensation. In humans, the antimuscarinic properties of belladonna alkaloids were the first ones successfully used in motion sickness. They are more effective if prophylactically prescribed. By extension, several antimuscarinic drugs are also believed to have antivertigo efficacy, but this fact is not well documented in humans. Anticholinergics are used via oral or parenteral routes; recently, transdermal presentation of scopolamine has become more and more popular, since it is supposed to reduce the incidence of the systemic side-effects that markedly impede the usefulness of anticholinergics. Nevertheless, the occurrence of peripheral (dry mouth, constipation, urinary retention, impaired accomodation) or central (amnesic or confusional syndromes) antimuscarinic side-effects still may develop.

Antihistamine Drugs. In animals, H1 histamine receptors are present in the vestibular nuclei. H1 antihistaminic drugs induce vestibular depression. A decrease of alertness also reduces vestibular nystagmus responses, and somnolence represents one of the main central side-effects of the antihistamine drugs. It is therefore possible to relate part of the depressive effect of these drugs to a reduction of vigilance. Histamine antagonists also possess anticholinergic properties, and could explain some vestibular effects of histamine antagonists and several of their side-effects. H1 antagonists (mostly belonging to the piperazine derivatives family) are the more widely used antimotion sickness drugs. Their use in the treatment of vertigo is empirical, and an antiemetic effect is probably beneficial.

Among antihistamines, two piperazine derivatives, namely cinnarizine and flunarizine are now promoted for their concomitant calcium channel blocking properties. Flunarizine is marketed in France as an antivertiginous drug. It seems devoid of anticholinergic properties but its antihistaminic effects are perhaps sufficient to explain an antivertiginous effect (especially since very little is known about any putative role of calcium in the vestibular system). Besides various pharmacologic properties (antimigrainous, antiepileptic . . . "justifying" a surprisingly large number of various therapeutic indications in different European countries), flunarizine produces vasodilator and vestibulosuppressive effects and promotes vestibular compensation. This profile appears attractive for an antivertiginous drug. However, not enough well-conducted clinical trials have studied the antivertiginous properties of flunarizine in man. The potential interest in this drug for such an indication requires additional methodologically satisfying trials, since, beside somnolence and weight gain, severe central neurologic side-effects (extrapyramidal and depressive syndromes) have been reported.

Histamine Agonists. Histamine-like drugs such as betahistine (beta 2 pyridylalkylamine) are also used widely in the treatment of vertigo. They act as relatively pure H1 agonists. This fact seems rather paradoxical if one remembers the vestibular properties of the H1 antagonists. Betahistine is largely used in Meniere's disease, but its alleged mechanism, i.e., its ability to increase microvascular perfusion of the inner ear, is questionable. Reports of therapeutic value of the drugs have not been totally convincing because of methodologic criticisms. Few side-effects have been reported, mainly of a digestive nature.

Amphetamines. Although no clear catecholaminergic innervation has been demonstrated in the vestibular system, sympathomimetics are widely used in the prevention of motion sickness. In animal models, amphetamines accelerate vestibular compensation. Amphetamines appear to potentiate the antivertiginous activity of antimuscarinic drugs, and are frequently associated with them.

Antidopamine Drugs. Neuroleptics are used in vestibular pathology because of their antiemetic property (blockade of dopaminergic receptors in the area postrema), which reduces the GI symptoms of vestibular dysfunction.

Acetyl D, L-Leucine. The mechanism of action of this drug is still unknown, though it has been used as an antivertiginous drug in France since 1957. Contrasting with the empirical reputation of a very potent antivertiginous effect of the drug, no real clinical trial has been performed to try to demonstrate this property. This compound can be given IV, which is a useful route during the acute stage of vertigo frequently associated with vomiting.

Other Drugs. Tetrahydrocannabinol is used to treat vomiting during cancer therapy; its efficacy as an antivertiginous drug has not been demonstrated, however. This is also true for several vasodilators or psychotropic drugs. Benzodiazepines can be useful in the treatment of motion sickness, probably because of their anxiolytic effect; their possible effect on the vestibular function is controversial. Diuretic and osmotic drugs are proposed in Meniere's disease, with the theoretical purpose to induce a rebalance in the inner ear fluids.

Finally, it must be emphasized that several marketed preparations combine two different pharmacologic agents, for example, amphetamine with an anticholinergic or antihistaminic. One should be careful not to give the same patient drugs with opposed properties (antihistamine and histamine) or cumulative side-effects (e.g., two anticholinergic drugs). New compounds that seek mainly to promote vestibular compensation, such as ACTH analogues, may represent future pharmacologic possibilities.

References

Research Reports

1. Buzzi MG, Moskowitz MA, Peroutka SJ, Byun B. Further characterization of the putative 5-HT receptor which mediates blockade of neurogenic plasma extravasation in rat dura mater. Brit J Pharmacol 1991;*103*:1421–1428.
2. The Subcutaneous Sumatriptan International Study Group. New Eng J Med 1991;*325*:316–321.
3. Ferrari MD, Saxena PR. Clinical and experimental effects of sumatriptan in humans. Trends in Pharmacol Sci 1993;*14*:129–132.

Reviews

r1. Spagnoli A, Tognoni G, Darmansjah I, Laporte JR, Urhovac B, Tuacher DF, Warlow CP. A multinational comparison of drug treatment in patients with cerebrovascular disease. Eur Neurol 1985;*24*:4–12.

r2. Scheinberg P. Controversies in the management of cerebral vascular disease. Neurology 1988;*38*:1609–1616.

r3. Walkowitz OM, Tinklenberg JR, Weingartner H. A psychopharmacological perspective of cognitive functions. 1. Theoretical overview and methodological considerations. 2. Specific pharmacologic agents. Neuropsychobiology 1985;*14*:88–155.

r4. Zee DS. Perspectives on the pharmacotherapy of vertigo. Arch Otolaryngol 1985;*111*:609–612.

r5. Cameron HA, Waller PC, Ransay LE. Drug treatment of intermittent claudication: a critical analysis of the methods and findings of published clinical trials, 1965–1988. Br J Clin Pharmacol 1988;*26*:569–576.

r6. Peatfield R. Drugs and the treatment of migraine. Trends Pharmacol Sci 1988;*9*:141–145.

r7. Silva CA. Prophylaxis and treatment of stroke; The state of the art. Drugs 1993;*45*:329–337.

r8. Jonas S. Anticoagulant therapy in cerebrovascular disease: review and metaanalysis. Stroke 1988;*19*:1043–1048.

r9. Spagnoli A, Tognoni G. Cerebroactive drugs. Clinical pharmacology and therapeutic role in cerebrovascular disorders. Drugs 1983;*26*:44–69.

r10. Tfelt-Hanse P, Olesen J. Methodological aspects of drug trials in migraine. Neuroepidemiology 1985;*4*:204–226.

r11. Verstraete M. Current therapy for intermittent claudication. Drugs 1982;*24*:240–248.

r12. Norris CH. Drugs affecting the inner ear. A review of their clinical efficacy, mechanisms of action, toxicity and place in therapy. Drugs 1988;*36*:754–772.

CHAPTER 28

Ralph A. Kelly
Elliott M. Antman
Thomas W. Smith

Monitoring of Cardiovascular and Pulmonary Drugs

Introduction

Techniques of therapeutic drug monitoring have undergone an evolution since the 1940s, when a good correlation first was established between blood levels of anti-anginal chemotherapeutic agents and clinical outcome.[1] The notion that monitoring blood levels of drugs, particularly those with low toxic/therapeutic ratios, could help prevent the development of toxicity and ensure efficacy made sense and became widely accepted. Subsequently, the deployment in the developed world of techniques sufficiently sensitive and reliable for routine monitoring of a variety of therapeutic agents in the 1960s and 1970s provided clinicians with easy access to drug level data. Indeed, the rapid acceptance of drug monitoring as an integral and often indispensable tool of modern therapeutics was due, in part, to the widespread availability of drug analysis techniques. In the 1990s, however, the appropriateness of routine blood level testing for many drugs is being questioned, driven in part by the growing need to justify the cost of any health-related technology, but largely because of careful analyses based on 40 years of experience of the assumptions that underlie therapeutic drug monitoring.

There remain two broad indications that are not in dispute for obtaining blood levels of drugs. Most clinical pharmacologists would obtain levels of a potentially toxic drug early in the course of therapy in order to individualize dosage because of the large number of pharmacokinetic variables from patient to patient that can influence the maintenance dosage regimen. This allows the clinician to screen easily and inexpensively for patients who have marked abnormalities in bioavailability and, importantly, genetic alterations in drug clearance rates, as well as for checking patient compliance. The second well-established use of drug monitoring is during the development of new pharmaceuticals by industry, when a new drug's pharmacokinetic profile is first defined, and during the large-scale clinical trials that attempt to define rigorously the relationship of drug levels with clinical outcome. At present, however, these two indications account for only a small percentage of the total number of drug assays performed.

Spector et al.[2] and others[3,4] have summarized this reassessment by clinical pharmacologists of the utility of routine therapeutic drug monitoring. In Table 28.1, Spector and colleagues outline the seven components of what they term the "target concentration strategy;" that is, the application of pharmacokinetic principles to manage patients with potentially toxic drugs. Most of the criteria are self-evident and do not require elaboration; for example, the concept that therapeutic efficacy and toxicity are related to dose, or that dosage may vary importantly from patient to patient in order to establish a target blood level. However, for most drugs for which drug monitoring is now routine—even deemed essential for proper management of patients—there is not a close and highly predictable correlation between blood levels and either efficacy or toxicity. There are many reasons for this, including factors that change the ratio of free, unbound drug in blood to total blood levels (the parameter that is usually measured in most drug assays, and discussed in more detail below); changes in the underlying disease state that alter tissue responsiveness to pharmacologic agents; age; and drug interactions. Most important, however, is the fact that clinical trials of sufficient

Table 28.1 The Target Concentration Strategy

Analytic
• An appropriate drug assay is available.
Pharmacokinetic
• Documented, significant interindividual variability in drug absorption, distribution, and clearance exists.
• Adequate pharmacokinetic data concerning the drug are available.
Pharmacologic
• Pharmacologic effect is predictably related to plasma drug concentration.
• A narrow "therapeutic window" between blood levels that result in clinical efficacy and blood levels that induce toxicity.
• Tolerance to the drug effect does not develop rapidly despite maintenance of blood levels.
Clinical
• Clinical studies are available that define the therapeutic and toxic range for plasma levels of the drug.

size and statistical power to generate widely applicable and useful guidelines for therapeutic drug monitoring and to identify subgroups of patients who are unusually sensitive or resistant to a given drug have, in most instances, simply not been done.

Thus, a fundamental assumption underlying the target concentration strategy—that there is a good correlation between appropriately obtained drug levels and efficacy or toxicity—is often invalid, even for agents for which blood monitoring has become routine, such as prevention of ototoxicity or renal toxicity with aminoglycoside antibiotics.[5,6] However, even if there were valid criteria for a range that reliably bracketed therapeutic and toxic levels for a drug, the clinician must always rely on his or her own assessment of the patient's response, regardless of the result obtained from clinical chemistry. Fortunately, in cardiovascular pharmacology, endpoints other than a pre-established therapeutic range of blood level are used routinely for many drugs, such as a fall in blood pressure or in heart rate with β blockers, or the extent of a natriuretic response with a diuretic. Most clinicians carefully titrate doses of these and other drugs to the patient's clinical response and symptoms, and would find the availability of drug testing for these agents to be of little if any use. Moreover, when a prescribed drug carries the risk of serious toxicity and/or when it becomes difficult to define the presence or absence of a therapeutic response, the availability of routine therapeutic drug monitoring may instill a false sense of security.

Free and Total Drug Level Monitoring

An important limitation of therapeutic drug monitoring not immediately obvious to nonpharmacologists is the fact that most drug assays measure total (free + protein bound) drug levels in plasma. Although the pharmacologically relevant concentration for many, but not all, drugs in cardiovascular therapeutics is the concentration of free drug—that is, the concentration available to interact with target receptors and enzymes as well as clearance mechanisms—the ratio of free to total drug usually does not change and is assumed to be constant. However, there are exceptions, the main causes of which are listed in Table 28.2.

The principal drug binding proteins in plasma are albumin and α-1 acid glycoprotein and, to a lesser extent, lipoproteins and immunoglobulins. Only α-1 acid glycoprotein levels (also referred to as orosomucoid) often change rapidly enough in response to physiologic stress to induce clinically relevant shifts in the ratio of free to total plasma levels of a drug. The best documented example of this is the rise in α-1 acid glycoprotein (an "acute phase reactant") following myocardial infarction. This results in enhanced plasma protein binding of lidocaine and disopyramide and a decline in free drug levels and therapeutic effectiveness, despite the fact that routinely available (i.e., total) plasma lidocaine and disopyramide levels would be unchanged.[7]

Regardless of the amount of drug binding proteins present in plasma, the binding interaction per se is typically of relatively low affinity and nonselective, and therefore subject to interference by many compounds with somewhat similar chemical structures. This is a common cause of "drug interactions" and is often unpredictable. Endogenous compounds, such as plasma nonesterified fatty acids, are also known to displace drugs from plasma protein binding sites. Nevertheless, the frequency and importance of this phenomenon is unknown in large part because most drug assays measure the total rather than the free concentration of drug in plasma. Thus, the sudden and unexplained reappearance of ventricular ectopy during constant infusion of an antiarrhythmic or the insidious development of toxicity with blood levels well within the "therapeutic range" should make the clinician sus-

Table 28.2 Factors that Alter the Expected Ratio of Free to Total Drug Levels in Plasma

1. Changes in plasma levels of principal drug-binding proteins
2. Displacement of drug from plasma protein binding sites by:
a) exogenous factors (e.g., other drugs)
b) endogenous factors
3. Large patient-to-patient variability in plasma protein binding of a given drug
4. Saturation of plasma protein binding within the standard dosing range (i.e., nonlinear binding)

pect the possibility of a change in the ratio of free to total drug in plasma.

Although unusual, in the case of certain drugs the ratio of free to total drug in plasma can differ markedly from patient to patient, making the relevance of a broad therapeutic range based on assays that measure total plasma levels questionable. Although a large interpatient variability in both the therapeutic and toxic response to quinidine has long been known, the wide variation in protein binding and, hence, free levels in plasma of this drug has only recently been appreciated.[8,9]

Protein binding may not be linear within the same patient for some drugs that saturate the number of protein binding sites, resulting in rapid increases in the ratio of free to total drug levels above a certain dosing level. Fortunately, this is uncommon. The classic example in cardiovascular therapeutics is that of disopyramide, where saturation of protein binding may occur well within the standard therapeutic dosing range.

Despite the obvious advantages of being able to quantitate free, pharmacologically active drug levels rather than total drug in plasma, the assay systems necessary to separate free from bound drug are not widely available, and the number of drugs for which determination of free drug level would be important is relatively small. Even if free drug levels were widely available, it would still be necessary to undertake large-scale clinical trials in order to define a meaningful therapeutic range for a given population of patients.

Specific Classes of Drugs

β-Adrenergic Blockers

The use of β-adrenergic blockers overlaps several major categories of cardiovascular therapeutics, including anti-anginal, antihypertensive, and antiarrhythmic therapy as well as numerous miscellaneous indications, and therefore will be discussed as a class here. Therapeutic monitoring of β blocker drug levels is not often indicated because physiologic endpoints (e.g., resting heart rate, heart rate response with exercise, or blood pressure) can usually be used to titrate dosage. In large part because of the common practice of titrating β blocker dosage to clinical response, there are few reliable data correlating blood levels with the degree of clinically relevant β-adrenergic receptor blockade.

Assays

Although all β-adrenergic antagonists have some chemical structural similarity, they often differ greatly in polarity, which necessitates an extraction technique tailored to each drug. Most β-adrenergic blockers in current clinical use, with the exception of esmolol,[10] are quite stable in biologic samples. Liquid chromatographic techniques with either UV or fluorescence detection have now replaced gas chromatography as the preferred method for detecting most β blockers in biologic samples. Radioimmunoassays are not routinely available, in part because of the difficulty in obtaining selective antibodies to many drugs in this class, but largely owing to the absence of any commercial source of antisera as a result of low demand for large scale assays of these drugs.

Drug Monitoring

Aside from pharmacokinetic analyses, there are few indications for measuring the plasma level of a β blocker: (1) checking compliance; (2) therapeutic failure despite seemingly adequate dosing; (3) evidence of toxicity despite reduced dosing. Apart from the first of these indications, it may simply be more efficient to switch to another category of cardiovascular drugs to achieve the desired therapeutic objective rather than attempt to monitor drug levels. The dosage range that has been suggested for propranolol, the only drug of this class for which there are substantial blood level data, is from 500–1000 ng/ml, with the treatment of angina often requiring lower blood levels and the treatment of hypertension with β blockade alone sometimes requiring much higher levels.[11–14]

Antiarrhythmic Drugs

The antiarrhythmic agents as a class have a relatively narrow therapeutic/toxic ratio; the "toxic" concentration exceeds the "effective" level only by two- to three-fold in many cases. The powerful ability of antiarrhythmic drugs to modify various currents (sodium, calcium, potassium) that flow across the cardiac sarcolemma at various points during the action potential is believed to be the basis for suppression of cardiac dysrhythmias. Experienced clinicians have learned to view these actions of antiarrhythmic compounds as a poisoning of the electrophysiologic state of cardiac cells with, it is hoped, a therapeutic effect on the cardiac rhythm disturbance. Unfortunately, because of the limited therapeutic "window" for these drugs, profound depressant effects on the myocardium can occur, resulting in bradycardia and hemodynamic compromise. In addition, the underlying electrophysiologic substrate may be altered in an adverse manner by antiarrhythmic drugs so that the tendency toward arrhythmias is actually increased rather than decreased; this is referred to as *proarrhythmia* and is especially important when dealing with ventricular arrhythmias.[15] Proposed definitions of proarrhythmia are shown in Table 28.3.

Techniques of Monitoring of Antiarrhythmic Drug Action

Common errors in the clinical use of antiarrhythmic drugs include:

1. Inappropriate decision to begin antiarrhythmic therapy. The risk/benefit ratio does not favor treatment of "benign" ventricular arrhythmias (e.g., isolated ventricular premature depolarizations in persons with normal function) and in many cases, does not favor treatment of "potentially malignant" ventricular arrhythmias (e.g.,

Table 28.3 A Definition of Primary Proarrhythmia for Ventricular Arrhythmias*

I. The new onset of:
   1. Ventricular premature complexes >5 hr
   2. Nonsustained ventricular tachycardia
   3. Sustained ventricular tachycardia
   4. Torsades de pointes (polymorphic ventricular tachycardia)
   5. Ventricular flutter/fibrillation

II. Change in the frequency of a previously documented ventricular arrhythmia:
   1. Increases in the frequency of ventricular premature complexes (VPCs):
      If the mean VPC/hr at baseline is from 10 to 50, a 10-fold increase is required for proarrhythmia.
      If the mean VPC/hr at baseline is from 51 to 100, a 5-fold increase is required for proarrhythmia.
      If the mean VPC/hr at baseline is from 101 to 300, a 4-fold increase is required for proarrhythmia.
      If the mean VPC/hr at baseline is >300, a 3-fold increase is required for proarrhythmia.
   2. A ≥10-fold increase in the mean hourly frequency of nonsustained ventricular tachycardia beats.

III. A significantly more difficult cardioversion or termination of ventricular tachycardia or ventricular flutter/fibrillation, as defined by the investigator.

IV. Occurrence of sudden cardiac death (defined as an unexpected, nontraumatic, non-self-inflicted fatality within 1 hour of the onset of the terminal event) or unexplained syncope.

*None of these events will be considered proarrhythmic if they: occur only within 72 hr after myocardial infarction; occur only after the patient has received the same daily dosage of active drug for ≥30 consecutive days; cannot be demonstrated on subsequent electrocardiographic monitoring when the patient is receiving the same daily dose (except for sustained ventricular tachycardia); can be clearly related to such other factors as hypokalemia and stopping medication.

asymptomatic nonsustained ventricular tachycardia in patients with moderately depressed ventricular function).

2. Inappropriate dosing of drug due to one or more of the following: improper dosing interval, inadequate time allowed to achieve steady state at a given dose level before moving to a higher dose, and failure to account for hepatic or renal failure and drug interactions.

3. Failure to interpret correctly serum concentrations of antiarrhythmic drugs.

In order to avoid these pitfalls, four broad areas of therapeutic monitoring of antiarrhythmic drug action are of value, as follows.

12-Lead EKG Monitoring. Inhibition of sinus node automaticity leads to sinus bradycardia. This is seen most prominently with β-adrenoceptor blockers, but may also be observed with the membrane-active antiarrhythmic agents (Classes IA, IB, and IC), certain Class III drugs such as amiodarone, and the Class IV drug (calcium antagonist) verapamil. Since the Class IA drugs (quinidine, procainamide, and disopyramide) inhibit the inward movement of sodium ions during the upstroke of the action potential and also inhibit the delayed outward rectifier current carried by potassium ions, their use is associated with a slowing of conduction velocity in the myocardium and prolongation of the effective refractory period of myocardial tissue. On the 12-lead EKG, this translates into widening of the QRS and prolongation of the QT interval. No formal studies have been performed to provide precise guidelines for "toxic" degrees of QRS widening and QT prolongation, but many authorities advocate caution once these measurements exceed 25 percent of baseline.

Serum Level Determinations. Although serum (or plasma) levels of antiarrhythmic drugs can be a valuable clinical aid, it is essential that the results be interpreted appropriately. While tables of "therapeutic levels" of antiarrhythmic drugs for prophylaxis against arrhythmias are available (Table 28.4), it should be understood that these are guidelines derived for the most part from population studies and that the precise serum level "therapeutic" for an individual patient may be outside the published range. Indications for monitoring serum levels of antiarrhythmic drugs include: determination of the drug concentration required to suppress an arrhythmia in a specific patient (often not needed clinically) and evaluation of apparent drug failure (e.g., "drug-resistant" arrhythmia); assessment of possible symptoms of drug toxicity (may also need to measure concentration of metabolites); assessment of the effects of alterations in the patient's physiologic state (e.g., congestive heart failure) and drug interactions; and investigation of possible noncompliance or drug abuse.

When the results of a serum level of an antiarrhythmic drug are reported from the laboratory, one should first determine whether it is in the usual therapeutic range. If it is, and the patient is doing well clinically, nothing further is required. If the level is in the usual therapeutic range but the patient appears toxic, a problem with decreased protein binding leading to a normal total drug level (but an increase in the concentration of free, non-protein-bound drug) should be considered. Should the value be outside the therapeutic range, it is important to confirm that the specimen was drawn at an appropriate interval after drug dosing (preferably a trough level immediately prior to the next dose). If the patient does not exhibit clinical signs of toxicity from the drug, in many cases the patient can be observed to be safe despite an isolated laboratory result. However, if toxicity is present clinically and/or the arrhythmia is not well controlled, the appropriate response would be to evaluate the dosage schedule and search for possible drug interactions and conditions that alter drug clearance.

Noninvasive EKG Monitoring Techniques. In this approach, antiarrhythmic drugs are chosen on the basis of the results of ambulatory EKG recordings ("Holter" monitoring). For patients with infrequent, troublesome paroxysms of arrhythmia, transtelephonic transmissions of the EKG are frequently utilized. Although somewhat less reproducible, exercise testing protocols are occasionally employed to determine whether arrhythmias are adequately suppressed during exertion. Because of spontaneous variation in the frequency of cardiac arrhythmias, the use of these noninvasive techniques is seriously compromised in the absence of adequate determinations of the frequency of arrhythmias in the baseline, drug-free state. For example, a patient may be incorrectly classified as a drug responder when the apparent decrease in arrhythmia on a 24-hour Holter monitor is nothing more than random variation in arrhythmia frequency. As a rough guide, when comparing a 24-hour baseline ambulatory EKG recording with one on an antiarrhythmic drug, there should be a minimum of a 75 percent reduction in total ventricular premature depolarizations, 90 percent reduction in ventricular couplets, and virtual elimination of ventricular tachycardia before one can conclude that a clinically significant antiarrhythmic effect has been ob-

Table 28.4

Drug	Proposed Therapeutic Range (μg/ml)	Comment
Quinidine	2–6	Numerous preparations are available but vary significantly in the amount of quinidine base contained in the tablet. When converting from dosing with quinidine sulfate to another preparation, there may be a drop in serum quinidine levels if the new regimen is not equivalent to the original dose of quinidine base.
Procainamide	3–8	An active metabolite, N-acetylprocainamide (NAPA), is formed in varying amounts depending on genetically determined acetylator phenotype. Slow acetylators generally have a serum procainamide concentration that is greater than NAPA and are more at risk for the lupus-like side effects associated with this drug. NAPA has Class III electrophysiologic action and is under investigation as an independent antiarrhythmic drug. The therapeutic concentration of NAPA is less well studied but has been proposed to be approximately 10–20 μg/ml. Sustained release preparations of the parent compound are in clinical use, but have a reduced bioavailability compared to regular formulations of the drug.
Disopyramide	2–5	Concentrations above 7 μg/ml are associated with a considerable risk of toxicity, most commonly due to the anticholinergic action of the drug. Individuals with a prior history of congestive heart failure may be predisposed to a recurrence of ventricular decompensation despite drug concentrations in the therapeutic range.
Lidocaine	1–5	Prolonged infusion of the drug (e.g., >24 hr) and/or co-administration of cimetidine and β-adrenoceptor blockers are associated with a decreased hepatic clearance of the parent compound and toxic levels begin to accumulate rapidly. Side-effects such as slurred speech and ataxia are seen initially and later convulsions as lidocaine levels approach 10 μg/ml.
Tocainide	5–12	Maximum 1-1.5 hr post-dose. Protein Binding = 10–50%. Multiple nonactive metabolites formed; the R-enantiomer is cleared more rapidly and is 3 times as potent as S-enantiomer. Measurement of serum levels (as total R + S enantiomers) probably not useful due to large interpatient variability in rates of clearance of R and S enantiomers.
Mexiletine	1–2	Maximum 1–3 hr post-dose. Protein Binding = 70%. Induction of hepatic enzymes by phenobarbital, primidone, rifampin, or phenytoin shorten elimination by up to 50%. Co-administration of INH, chloramphenicol, dicumarol, disulfiram, methylphenidate decrease hepatic clearance. Multiple nonactive metabolites formed; the R-enantiomer is cleared more rapidly and is probably more potent. Measurement of serum levels (as total R + S enantiomers) probably not useful due to large interpatient variability in rates of clearance of R and S enantiomers.
Flecainide	0.2–1.0 (>1.0 μg/ml increases risk of proarrhythmia)	Maximum 3–4 hr post-dose. Protein binding = 40%.
Encainide	Not Helpful	In over 90% of patients, 2 active metabolites of encainide: ODE and MODE are formed with an elimination half-life of 1–2 hr. These are more active than the parent compound and excreted more slowly with a half-life of 3–4 hr for ODE and 6–12 hr for MODE. 10% of patients metabolize encainide poorly (elimination half-life of 6–11 hr) and form a relatively inactive metabolite (NDE) in small amounts. Metabolizer phenotype correlates with ability to metabolize debrisoquin (and possibly dextromethorphan). Measurement of serum levels not helpful since the relative contribution of electrophysiologic effects of parent compound and metabolites is difficult to assess in an individual patient. ODE accumulates during long-term treatment and is primarily responsible for drug effect in extensive metabolizers.

continued

Table 28.4 *Continued*

<table>
<tr><th>Drug</th><th>Proposed Therapeutic Range (μg/ml)</th><th>Comment</th></tr>
<tr><td>Propafenone</td><td>Not Helpful</td><td>There are 2 genetically determined patterns of propafenone metabolism. In over 90% of cases, the drug is rapidly and extensively metabolized into 2 active metabolites: 5-hydroxy-propafenone and N-depropylpropafenone with a half-life of 2–10 hr. This pathway is easily saturated and as the dose increases, the serum levels rise in a nonlinear fashion. In less than 10% of cases (and in any patient concurrently receiving quinidine), the metabolism of propafenone is slower because the 5-hydroxy metabolite is not formed. The half-life of elimination in "slow" metabolizers is 10–32 hr. There are significant differences in plasma concentrations of propafenone in fast and slow metabolizers with the latter achieving levels 1.5–2.0 times those of the fast metabolizers. However, the recommended dosing regimen is the same in slow and fast metabolizers because the difference in levels lessens as the dose increases and the 5-hydroxy metabolite is active. Measurement of serum levels is probably not helpful, but the usual therapeutic range of propafenone is 1.2–1.5 μg/ml.</td></tr>
<tr><td>Amiodarone</td><td>1.5–2.5</td><td>The drug undergoes predominantly hepatic metabolism to a weakly active metabolite; desethylamiodarone (DEA). Serum levels should only be measured in a steady state which may take several weeks to establish when initiating dosing or making a change in maintenance dose. Amiodarone is avidly protein bound.</td></tr>
<tr><td>Moricizine (Ethmozine)</td><td>(see comments)</td><td>There is extensive first-pass hepatic metabolism and <0.1% of the dose ultimately is excreted unchanged in the urine. There are at least 26 metabolites (as is common for phenothiazine-like compounds). Two of these metabolites demonstrate some antiarrhythmic activity (moricizine sulfoxide and phenothiazine-2-carbonic acid ethyl ester sulfoxide). It has also been found that moricizine exhibits AUTO INDUCTION OF METABOLISM. With chronic dosing, serum levels of the parent compound may DECREASE. There is a linear dose relationship in the usual therapeutic range. Serum levels are not clinically useful when treating patients with moricizine.</td></tr>
<tr><td>Sotalol</td><td>(see comments)</td><td>Serum levels are maximum 2.5–4 hours post dose, blood levels not useful clinically, and protein binding is negligible. Sotalol is predominantly excreted via the kidney. Correct the dosing interval as follows:<table><tr><th>Creat Clearance (ml/min)</th><th>Dosing interval (hours)</th></tr><tr><td>>60</td><td>12</td></tr><tr><td>30–60</td><td>24</td></tr><tr><td>10–30</td><td>36–48</td></tr><tr><td><10</td><td>Dose should be individualized</td></tr></table></td></tr>
<tr><td colspan="3">Sotalol has both β-adrenoceptor blocking and cardiac action potential duration prolongation properties (Class II and Class III actions, respectively). The current preparation is a racemic mixture of d- and 1-sotalol. Both isomers have similar Class III actions while the 1-isomer is responsible for virtually all the β-blocking action. Sotalol is non-cardioselective and does not have partial agonist or membrane stabilizing activity. Maximal β blockade occurs at doses between 320–640 mg/day. Sotalol is roughly 1/3 as potent on a weight basis as propranolol as a β blocker.</td></tr>
</table>

served. In order to improve the chance of truly observing a beneficial treatment effect, it is preferable to obtain several recordings in the baseline state (e.g., 48 hours) and again with each antiarrhythmic drug tested.

Invasive Electrophysiologic Testing. This approach attempts to provoke the arrhythmia of interest under controlled circumstances in a cardiac catheterization laboratory. Multiple catheter electrodes are inserted into the heart and programmed electrical stimulation is performed. For example, critically timed atrial premature stimuli are used to provoke circus movement tachycardia in patients with the Wolff-Parkinson-White syndrome, or critically timed ventricular premature stimuli during ventricular pacing are used to provoke ventricular tachycardia or ventricular fibrillation in patients with a history of sudden cardiac near death. Because of the high likelihood of provoking an arrhythmia and the possibility of hemodynamic compromise, facilities for defibrillation must be routinely available during such testing. After the baseline study, during which the ease of provocation of the arrhythmia is noted along with its precise mechanism, one or more follow-up studies are performed with the patient in a steady state on the antiarrhythmic agent being evaluated. This "electropharmacologic" approach has been shown to be predictive of the long-term therapeutic efficacy of antiarrhythmic drug regimens for patients with reliably induced circus movement tachycardias (e.g., re-entrant supraventricular arrhythmias) and quite helpful in patients with a history of out-of-hospital ventricular tachycardia or fibrillation.

Clinical Perspective on Usefulness of Therapeutic Drug Monitoring of Antiarrhythmic Drugs

Despite advances in cardiovascular pharmacotherapeutics over the last several decades and refinements in the monitoring techniques described above, the prescription of a specific antiarrhythmic drug for an individual patient remains an inexact science. Even in the presence of an apparently positive response to a drug (as judged by the noninvasive and/or invasive techniques) and in the absence of abnormal EKG findings or serum concentrations of the drug, failures of antiarrhythmic therapy continue to occur commonly. These may take the form of recurrence of arrhythmia and/or the development of intolerable drug-related side-effects. It is disturbing to the clinician when adverse outcomes such as recurrent sudden cardiac death cannot be prevented despite a seemingly effective drug regimen. However, it is a particularly devastating result when drug treatment of an asymptomatic or minimally symptomatic individual is associated with increased mortality. This last point has been emphasized in several recent publications on both ventricular and supraventricular arrhythmias. Meta-analyses of the results of randomized control trials of lidocaine prophylaxis against primary ventricular fibrillation in patients with acute myocardial infarction have shown a reduction in the incidence of ventricular fibrillation, but at the cost of a tendency toward higher mortality in the drug treatment group as compared with the control group.[16] The Cardiac Arrhythmia Suppression Trial (CAST) reported a higher mortality rate in postinfarction patients randomized to receive encainide or flecainide (versus their matched placebos), despite the documented efficacy of these drugs in suppressing the frequency of ventricular arrhythmias as described in the noninvasive monitoring section above.[17,18] CAST II reported similar findings with moricizine (ethmozine).[19] No clues to an adverse electrophysiologic event developing were apparent on the 12-lead EKG of the patients who died. Finally, a meta-analysis of the randomized control trials of quinidine for suppression of recurrences of atrial fibrillation revealed a tendency toward increased mortality in the quinidine-treated group, despite a greater chance of maintaining sinus rhythm following cardioversion.[20,21]

These observations indicate a need for respecting the potentially harmful effects of antiarrhythmic drugs and for healthy skepticism concerning the results of therapeutic drug monitoring of such compounds. There is a clear need for improvement in the specificity of drug evaluation techniques. Many investigators have begun to explore nonpharmacologic options such as ablation, implantable devices (e.g., automatic implantable cardioverter defibrillator), and antitachycardia surgery as alternatives to drug treatment in symptomatic patients.

Adenosine is an endogenous nucleoside that, when administered in pharmacologic doses, has important electrophysiologic effects.[22] These include: a decrease in Ca influx via the slow inward channel; an increase in K conductance via K channels; and antiadrenergic effects.

Adenosine is indicated for treatment of paroxysmal supraventricular tachycardia (PSVT) and may be helpful in cases of atrial flutter or wide-complex tachycardia by exposing the atrial mechanism during AV block.[23-25] The drug should be given as a rapid 6-mg IV bolus. This should be repeated as a rapid 12-mg IV bolus if no response is seen in 1–2 minutes. Side-effects include: flushing; hypotension; palpitation; dyspnea; and chest pain. Because of the rapid metabolism of adenosine to the electrophysiologically inactive metabolite, inosine, and rapid uptake of adenosine intracellularly, measurement of adenosine blood levels is not clinically useful.

Digitalis Glycosides

The narrow margin between therapeutic and toxic doses of digitalis results in a high incidence of toxicity. This problem has stimulated the development of several methods for determining circulating cardiac glycoside concentrations. Measurements of serum or plasma concentration have clinical utility, but inappropriate use or interpretation of these laboratory values can limit their usefulness and potentially can lead to suboptimal decisions in patient management unless such data are properly interpreted in the clinical context.

Rationale

Evidence indicates that a useful relationship exists between serum levels of cardiac glycosides and their pharmacologic effect. First, both therapeutic and toxic effects are known to be dose-related phenomena. Since it is clear from numerous studies that serum digitalis levels rise with increasing dosage, correlation between serum level and clinical state (at least in the statistical sense) would be expected. In the case of digoxin, experimental and clinical studies have shown a relatively constant ratio of serum to myocardial or other tissue concentrations, provided adequate equilibration between the vascular and peripheral compartments has taken place.[26] In addition, the cardiac glycoside binding site of the putative digitalis receptor NaK-ATPase faces the outer cell surface, providing a basis for the translation of serum level to myocardial effect. Despite these considerations, many variables—in particular, the type and severity of existing heart disease—interact to determine the individual patient's response to a given serum cardiac glycoside concentration.

Studies Correlating Serum Digitalis Levels with Clinical State

Results of 41 separate studies designed to define the relationship between serum cardiac glycoside concentration and clinical effect are now available and are summarized in Reference 26. Data from over 1300 patients demonstrated that the mean serum digoxin level in patients judged to be receiving a therapeutically appropriate dose is about 1.4 ng/ml (1.8 nmole/L), while mean levels in patients with clinically overt toxicity (usually defined on the basis of characteristic cardiac rhythm disturbances) are usually two- to threefold higher. Although this difference is statistically significant in nearly all these reports, overlap of serum digoxin levels between groups of patients with and without evidence of toxicity is the rule, not the exception.

Data from 12 series involving patients receiving digitoxin are also summarized in Reference 26. Values are about tenfold higher than analogous serum digoxin concentrations because of serum protein binding of digitoxin. As in the case of digoxin, mean values for groups of patients considered to be receiving optimal therapeutic doses are significantly less than mean values for patients with symptoms and signs of toxicity, but appreciable overlap occurs between the two groups.

Use of serum digoxin measurement is reportedly associated with a lower incidence of digoxin intoxication in clinical practice.[27] For the clinician dealing with an individual patient, however, it is clear that no specific serum level can be chosen to define the separation between toxic and nontoxic states.[28,29]

Establishment of an accurate diagnosis of digitalis toxicity is often difficult, since virtually any abnormality of cardiac impulse formation or conduction that can result from digitalis excess can be caused by intrinsic heart disease as well, even in patients without a history of having taken digitalis. For these reasons, serum glycoside concentration values should be taken into account, along with all clinical data, before one can arrive at appropriate management decisions.

It is also difficult to correlate therapeutic cardiac glycoside effects with serum levels in humans. The correlation between serum digoxin concentration and slowing of previously rapid ventricular rates in patients with atrial fibrillation is rough at best. As might be expected, this correlation is not seen in patients with relatively slow ventricular responses when not receiving digitalis, and the wide variation in serum levels needed to maintain control of the ventricular response to atrial fibrillation and atrial flutter is well recognized. Ventricular rate and clinical symptoms serve as appropriate guides to dosage under these circumstances.

In patients with congestive heart failure and normal sinus rhythm, an even more difficult problem exists. Studies in experimental animals support the conclusion that increasing the dose of acutely administered cardiac glycoside will increase its inotropic effects, the limits of which are imposed by the emergence of overt rhythm disturbances.[30] More recent findings, however, suggest that this conclusion may need to be modified in the context of clinical cardiac glycoside use. Available studies suggest that, with regard to digoxin's inotropic response, a point of diminishing returns is reached at serum digoxin levels of 1 to 2 ng/ml.[31–33] Since the risk of digitalis-toxic arrhythmias clearly increases at serum concentrations beyond this range, the risk/benefit ratio appears to be optimal in the range of 1 to 2 ng/ml.

It must be emphasized, however, that available data on this important issue are quite limited, particularly regarding patients with advanced heart failure. Still needed are further studies in which the patient populations are stratified based on etiology, severity, and pathophysiologic manifestations of heart failure. In a recent prospective analysis of the prevalence of digoxin toxicity in almost 1000 patients with congestive heart failure, 56 percent of whom were receiving maintenance digoxin therapy, only four patients (0.8%) could be classified as definitely digoxin toxic, while another 16 were classified as possibly digoxin toxic (4.0%).[34] These authors also included a retrospective analysis of over 200 patients admitted to a large urban teaching hospital over eight years in the mid1980s with a diagnosis of digoxin toxicity. They concluded that in most patients there was little evidence to support a diagnosis of digoxin drug toxicity, and that the mortality rate in documented digoxin toxicity in patients receiving maintenance doses of the drug (as opposed to accidental or suicidal overdoses) was less than 5%, and possibly as low as 1 percent.[34]

Relatively limited data are available correlating noncardiac symptoms of toxicity with serum digitalis levels. Doering et al.[35] carried out an extensive study of 1148 patients and found considerable overlap among serum digoxin levels in patients with and without extracardiac symptoms of toxicity, even though the mean digoxin levels of the two groups differed significantly.

Eraker and Sasse[36] developed a Bayesian approach to using serum digoxin levels in clinical decision making. The relation between the estimated risk of toxicity in the patient population at risk and the predictive value of the serum digoxin concentration was established and was used to analyze the importance of the degree of elevation of the serum digoxin level. With a knowledge of a patient's serum level, the probability of toxicity can be made to cross the threshold probability for treatment for toxicity for an intermediate range of pretest risk. This interesting study formalized the approach we have long advocated in the use of serum digoxin concentration data, i.e., that the values be used in the over-all clinical context in formulating clinical decisions.

Clinical Use of Serum Cardiac Glycoside Concentrations

Assessment of timing and magnitude of digoxin doses, renal function, and body mass will permit a first approximation of the total body stores of the drug. When a patient on digoxin develops fatigue, visual changes, anorexia, nausea, vomiting, or cardiac rhythm abnormalities, a toxic response should be suspected, and knowledge of the digoxin level is likely to be useful. Since metabolic abnormalities, including hypokalemia, hypomagnesemia, hypercalcemia, and severe acid-base imbalance, predispose a patient to digitalis toxicity, a digoxin level within the usual "therapeutic" range should not be considered to exclude toxicity under such circumstances. Table 28.5 lists additional variables.

Underlying heart disease is an important variable in determining the individual patient's sensitivity to digitalis. Myocardial ischemia, myocardial infarction, and advanced cardiomyopathy may increase sensitivity to digitalis glycosides, and a digoxin level in the usual "therapeutic" range does not exclude digoxin toxicity in the presence of symptoms or signs consistent with digitalis excess. Hypothyroidism and pulmonary disease are also associated with an increased incidence of digoxin toxicity at any given serum digoxin concentration. Conversely, when there are contraindications to the use of other classes of drugs such as adenosine or β blockers, and in the absence of clinical symptoms or signs of digoxin toxicity, a digoxin level in the range of 2–3 ng/ml should not invariably dictate the withholding of digoxin when such levels are required to control the ventricular response to a supraventricular tachyarrhythmia.

Table 28.5 Causes of Altered Responsiveness to Cardiac Glycosides

- Digitalis Resistance
  - Apparent
    - Tablets not taken as prescribed
    - Inadequate bioavailability of tablets
    - Inadequate intestinal absorption
    - Increased metabolic degradation (e.g., by gut flora)
  - True end-organ resistance
    - Infancy
    - With respect to control of ventricular response in the presence of atrial fibrillation or atrial flutter
      - a. Fever
      - b. Elevated sympathetic tone from all causes, including uncontrolled congestive heart failure
      - c. Hyperthyroidism
- Digitalis Sensitivity
  - Apparent
    - Unsuspected use of digitalis
    - Change from poorly absorbed tablets to well-absorbed tablets
    - Decreased renal excretion
- Drug-drug interactions (e.g., quinidine)
  - True end-organ sensitivity to toxic effects
    - Advanced myocardial disease
    - Active myocardial disease
    - Active myocardial ischemia
    - Electrolyte imbalance (especially hypokalemia)
    - Acid-base imbalance
    - Concomitant drug administration (e.g., catecholamines)
    - Hypothyroidism
    - Hypoxemia (especially in setting of acute respiratory failure)
    - Altered autonomic tone (e.g., vagotonic states)

From Ref. 26, with permission.

A frequent clinical problem is failure to achieve an adequate therapeutic response in a patient receiving a conventional dose of digoxin. The clinician must decide whether the dose is inadequate (for example, because of noncompliance with the prescribed regimen or because of impaired absorption) or whether there are reasons why the patient may be resistant to usual doses and serum levels of digoxin (for example, occult thyrotoxicosis or mitral stenosis). In a compliant patient with a low serum digoxin concentration despite usually adequate dosage, the digoxin level may be a clue to other disorders or drug interactions. Hyperthyroidism tends to cause relatively low serum digoxin levels, in addition to true resistance to control of the ventricular response to supraventricular tachyarrhythmias. Malabsorption syndromes and preparations of digoxin with poor bioavailability will result in low serum digoxin values and clinical underdigitalization. Certain drugs, including cholestyramine, colestipol, kaolinpectin, and certain antacids, will bind digoxin in the gut and result in clinical and laboratory evidence of subtherapeutic digitalization.

Finally, skepticism is warranted when a laboratory result conflicts with clinical judgment. An isolated value should never be used as the sole criterion for determination of a drug's toxicity or efficacy.

Perhexiline Maleate

Perhexiline maleate is one of the few drugs in cardiovascular therapeutics for which routine drug monitoring is essential. Although introduced in Europe over 20 years ago with well-documented efficacy in the therapy of angina pectoris, the drug quickly developed a reputation for unacceptable toxicity.[37–39] Perhexiline was subsequently withdrawn from several markets and has never been marketed in the US owing to infrequent, but initially unpredictable and serious hepatic and neurologic toxicity. Following the development of straightforward and reliable methods for quantitating blood levels of perhexiline,[40,41] it became clear that the metabolism of the drug was highly variable and that the toxicity correlated best with perhexiline drug levels rather than dose or duration of therapy.[42,43]

Assay

In the first decade after the introduction of perhexiline as an anti-anginal agent, effective therapeutic monitoring was hampered by the lack of appropriate instrumentation and by the relative insensitivity of standard gas chromatographic techniques. The introduction of a liquid chromatographic method that incorporated a fluorescent derivitization step brought the limit of detection to 10 ng/ml.[40] Perhexiline is quite stable in biologic samples.

Therapeutic Drug Monitoring

Perhexiline provides an excellent example of a drug with a narrow therapeutic-to-toxic ratio, for which blood levels are essential not only during the initiation of therapy in order to exclude the small percentage of patients who are "poor metabolizers" of this drug, but also following initiation of a maintenance dose in order to detect those patients who exceed the threshold of saturable hepatic metabolism. Perhexiline undergoes classic "Phase I" oxidative metabolism in the liver by an isoform of the cytochrome P450 family of enzymes. The specific P450 isozyme responsible for perhexiline metabolism is now known to be a member of the type II, class D family, denoted $P450_{db1}$.[44,45] The subscript "db1" refers to "debrisoquine type 1" after the now rarely used sympatholytic antihypertensive drug that, in low doses, serves as a useful agent with which to determine hydroxylator phenotype in man. This enzyme is also responsible for the initial metabolism of many other drugs, including the newer type 1C antiarrhythmics (encainide, flecainide, propafenone) and some β blockers (timolol, metoprololol, propranolol). The slow hydroxylator phenotype is transmitted as an autosomal recessive trait with a prevalence of 5–10 percent among Caucasians, and is presumably due to the inheritance of two mutant alleles for the $P450_{dbl}$ gene, recently localized to chromosome 22.[46]

Although in theory a patient's genotype can now be established by identifying characteristic restriction fragment length polymorphism (RFLPs) on Southern analysis of genomic DNA, or his or her functional phenotype established by giving a test dose of debrisoquine, most clinical pharmacologists or cardiologists will not have access to the necessary instrumentation or expertise. Repetitive measurements of blood levels are necessary during the first week of therapy to identify those patients who are slow metabolizers. However, routine monitoring of plasma levels during chronic therapy is also necessary, for a significant percentage of patients will demonstrate saturable metabolism even after weeks or months on a stable dose. Horowitz et al.[43] studied prospectively a large number of ambulatory patients treated with perhexiline and documented that efficacy could be maintained with a minimum of toxicity when dosage was adjusted to keep plasma levels within a range of 150–600 ng/ml. Similarly, Cole et al., in a recent prospective randomized, doubly-blinded crossover trial, also confirmed anti-anginal efficacy and an absence of serious side effects in 17 patients with blood levels maintained within this range.[47] Horowitz et al.[43] determined that blood levels above 1000 ng/ml were associated with an unacceptably high incidence of toxicity.

Theophylline

Theophylline use—as with perhexiline maleate and a handful of other drugs routinely used in cardiovascular and pulmonary medicine—requires periodic monitoring of blood levels in order to assure both safety and efficacy. This is due to the fact that drug metabolism can be influenced by a number of factors, including increasing age, concurrently administered drugs, smoking history, etc. Although still widely and appropriately used in the therapy of chronic asthma in adults and in the elderly, theophylline is slowly being supplemented, at least as a first-line agent, by newer, more selective and long-acting sympathomimetics[48] and other classes of drugs, including anti-inflammatory agents.[49–53] The recent controversy surrounding the potential link between continuous use of inhaled β agonists and increased morbidity and mortality due to asthma[52,54–57] suggests that theophylline and related congeners will remain important in the therapy of asthma throughout the 1990s.

The role of theophylline in the treatment of chronic asthma in children has been questioned following reports of cognitive deficits in young patients on theophylline,[58,59] although more recent studies do not support any important effects of theophylline preparations on either behavior or cognitive processing.[60–62] As a consequence, clinicians may become less familiar with the prescription of theophylline products, including the recognition of side-effects and the anticipation of common drug interactions. In a commentary on the safety and efficacy of theophylline in the context of several highly publicized reports of severe theophylline intoxication in children, Hendeles, Weinberger and colleagues noted that ". . . the most common source of excessive serum concentrations and severe toxic effects in children has been patient, parent, or physician errors in dosing or in judgment".[63] This emphasizes all the more the importance of therapeutic drug monitoring for this agent.[63–67]

Assays

HPLC techniques have now completely supplemented the older spectrophotometric methods that did not require separation of theophylline from other blood components. This is due to the much superior selectivity of these newer, widely available chromatographic techniques. Despite the growing popularity of simpler methods that can be purchased in a kit format or that can be modified easily to measure other drugs (such as the enzyme immunoassay and immunochromatographic assay techniques), HPLC is still used by reference laboratories because of its specificity. The enzyme immunochromatographic method (e.g., Acculevel, Syntex) is one of the most popular as it measures theophylline concentration with acceptable reproducibility in whole blood with a minimum of necessary equipment, does not require specialized analytical chemistry skills, and therefore can be done outside a clinical chemistry laboratory. Although it lacks the specificity of HPLC-based methods, and cannot be rapidly converted to allow measurement of other drugs in blood, it is quite acceptable for use in facilities that lack clinical laboratories. The dissemination of this technology on a wide scale for therapeutic drug monitoring is probably justified in the case of theophylline, unlike most other commonly used cardiovascular drugs, as discussed above.

Therapeutic Drug Monitoring

Theophylline is rapidly and completely absorbed when given as a liquid or as a standard, nonsustained released formulation, and is metabolized primarily in the liver (90%) with only about 10 percent of ingested drug undergoing clearance unchanged in the kidney. The drug is metabolized into four major metabolites by the liver, which are subsequently cleared by the kidney, and liver metabolism is by a cytochrome P450 isoform enzyme.[64–67] Distinct differences in theophylline metabolism based on inheritance of specific cytochrome P450 isoform alleles has not been as well documented as in the case of debrisoquine or perhexiline, although some important individual differences in theophylline clearance based on this factor almost certainly do exist. Dosage adjustments during the rapid growth that accompanies puberty in children must also be considered.[68] More important, however, are concomitant illnesses and drug interactions that affect theophylline metabolism. Tobacco and marijuana smoking substantially increase the clearance rate of theophylline in any age group, and cessation of smoking only gradually results in a return to a more "normal" clearance rate. Similarly, phenytoin and phenobarbital increase theophylline clearance. Interestingly, a febrile illness alone may often reduce theophylline clearance, irrespective of concurrently administered drugs, although a number of drugs do interfere with theophylline metabolism (e.g., erythromycin, cimetidine (but not ranitidine)) while others have an unpredictable effects on theophylline clearance (e.g., corticosteroids and oral contraceptives). An extensive list of drug interactions is given in Reference 63 and in Chapter 32 of Reference 64. Importantly, theophylline metabolism changes dramatically with age, and is diminished in both the neonate and elderly, while clearance may be markedly enhanced in childhood compared to the adult. Finally, blood levels of theophylline can change with the formulation of sustained-release preparations, due to variation in absorption. Most of the older sustained-release formulations were affected by concurrent food intake, which delays final absorption and may diminish bioavailability. The application of new technologies for sustained-release preparations may mitigate these marked differences in the rates of absorption and bioavailability in older sustained-release tablets and capsules.

Therapeutic and toxic blood levels for theophylline are well established. The commonly accepted therapeutic range is 10–20 mg/L, and potentially severe side-effects occur commonly at drug levels of 30 mg/L and above, but they may occur at lower levels as well. Although serum theophylline levels can be used to predict unbound levels of theophylline in serum reliably in most patients, theophylline levels in mixed, stimulated saliva may be preferred in patients in whom the serum protein concentration may vary, as in cystic fibrosis, since they have been shown to reflect directly the concentration of unbound drug in serum.[65] Saturation of hepatic metabolism or of protein binding within the therapeutic range is rarely a problem, although congestive heart failure or concurrent hepatic disease, as well as drug interactions, can limit metabolism. Thus, the narrow toxic-therapeutic ratio and the difficulty in predicting blood levels due to variable absorption of the sustained-release preparations, numerous drug interactions, and other factors that affect hepatic metabolism, make routine monitoring of theophylline levels mandatory.[64,67,69] Recent reviews of the management of asthma have largely reaffirmed the value of theophylline preparations, in part because of new information supporting alternative mechanisms for the efficacy of theophylline in addition to bronchodilation[52,53] and in addition recommending that the serum concentrations for most patients be at the lower end of the accepted therapeutic range (i.e., <15 μg/ml).[51,52] In order to increase the margin of safety in pediatric patients, an algorithm that targets this lower serum theophylline concentration range is given in the commentary by Hendeles et al.[63]

Clinical Experience in the Reversal of Digitalis Toxicity with Specific Fab Fragments

Advanced digitalis toxicity has a potentially fatal outcome. The risk is particularly high in patients with advanced cardiac disease or following large doses given or taken by accident or with suicidal intent. Consequences of severe digitalis toxicity include hyperkalemia, atrioventricular block, and a variety of supraventricular and ventricular tachyarrhythmias. The extensive tissue distribution of digoxin and digitoxin limit the ability to treat toxic symptoms of these drugs successfully by hemodialysis or hemoperfusion methods, which are generally too slow in removing digoxin from tissue receptor sites to allow prompt reversal of life-threatening toxicity. Standard therapy for digitalis-induced conduction disturbances causing bradyarrhythmias consists of atropine or temporary pacing; ectopic tachyarrhythmias are conventionally treated with potassium repletion and lidocaine, with phenytoin as a potentially useful backup.[29]

Antibodies from exogenous sources have been used in diphtheria and tetanus and more recently in the management of organ transplant rejection. In 1967, Butler and Chen described digoxin-specific antibodies obtained from rabbits challenged with a conjugate prepared by chemically coupling digoxin as a hapten to a carrier protein.[70] These were found to have high affinity and specificity,[71] permitting their use in radioimmunoassay procedures for digoxin or digitoxin.[72,73] Recognizing the potential for therapeutic application, techniques were developed to immunize animals with a digoxin-protein conjugate and to cleave the resulting intact digoxin-specific IgG molecule into its Fab and Fc fragments, followed by isolation and purification of the digoxin-specific Fab fragments by affinity chromatography.[74] Initial clinical use in the setting of severe digoxin toxicity was reported in 1976.[75] Additional experiences demonstrating dramatic reversal of advanced toxicity led to a multicenter clinical trial of the safety and efficacy of digoxin-specific Fab fragments for the treatment of potentially life-threatening digitalis toxicity.[76]

A total of 21 medical centers, geographically distributed throughout the US, were provided with supplies of Fab fragments prepared by Burroughs Wellcome UK. To obtain information on the pharmacokinetics and antigenicity of the purified polyclonal sheep Fab fragments.

Following informed consent and hypersensitivity screening, Fab fragments were given IV over periods varying from 15 minutes to 2 hours. A dose of Fab equivalent on a molar basis to the amount of digoxin or digitoxin in the patient's body was infused through a sterile 0.22 μm membrane filter.

Clinical responses to Fab treatment are summarized in Figure 28.1 for 150 patients treated in the initial multicenter trial. Details of the patient population are found in Reference 76.

Manifestations of digitalis toxicity included second- or third-degree AV block in 53 percent of patients, ventricular tachycardia in 46 percent, ventricular fibrillation in 33 percent, asystole in 11

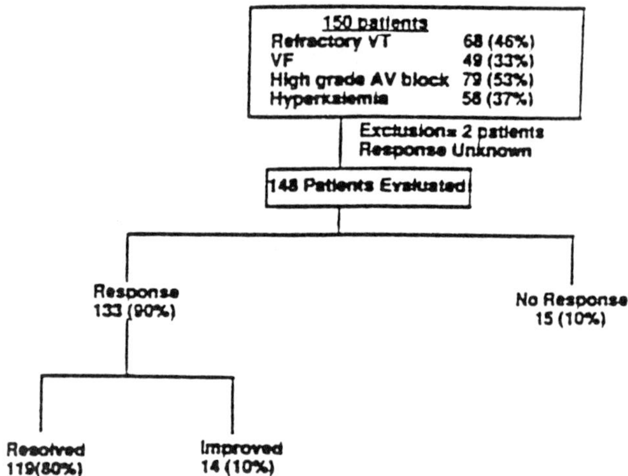

Figure 28.1 Clinical response to Fab fragment treatment in 150 patients with potentially life-threatening digitalis intoxication. VT, ventricular tachycardia; VF, ventricular fibrillation; AV, atrioventricular. From Antman EM, Wenger TL, Butler VP Jr, Haber E, Smith TW. Treatment of 150 cases of life-threatening digitalis intoxication with digoxin-specific Fab antibody fragments: Final report of a multi-center study. Circulation 1990; *81*:1742–1744, with permission.

percent, and hyperkalemia in 37 percent (Fig. 28.1). Serum digoxin concentrations of patients treated had a median value of 8.0 ng/ml; the median serum digitoxin level was 156 ng/ml. Doses of digoxin-specific Fab fragments given covered a wide range with a median of 200 mg. The highest dose administered was 40 vials, or 1600 mg.

As summarized in Figure 28.1, 80 percent of the patients treated with Fab showed resolution of all signs and symptoms of digitalis intoxication; 10 percent showed improvement; and 10 percent showed no response. All five patients treated for digitoxin toxicity had complete responses. Among the 80 patients for whom such data were available, the mean time to initial therapeutic response was 19 minutes from the termination of the Fab infusion. Mean time to full response was 88 minutes. Thus, most patients who responded favorably showed appreciable improvement by one hour after completion of Fab infusion, and a complete response by four hours. Among those patients who showed a partial response or no response, most were moribund when treated or were probably not suffering from digitalis toxicity.

In terms of laboratory evidence of Fab fragment response, as expected, falls in serum potassium concentration were commonly observed (from 5.0 meq-/l to 4.1 meq-/l). We view this as a direct consequence of the reversal of NaK-ATPase inhibition with restoration of the normal distribution of potassium ions across cell membranes throughout the body.

Data from the 150 patients were analyzed with particular attention to adverse events that could have been related to Fab administration. Thirty-two such events were identified. Fourteen of these 32 patients suffered adverse events possibly or probably caused by Fab administration. Hypokalemia with relatively rapid progression occurred in six patients (4%); four patients (3%) appeared to develop increased severity of congestive heart failure, thought possibly to be related to loss of inotropic support from digoxin. There were two instances of mild hypotension, one of nausea, and a neonate less than one day old developed transient apnea during the infusion of Fab fragments. Renal function, as judged by serum creatinine measurements, tended to be stable or improved following Fab therapy; there was no case in which impaired renal function could be clearly ascribed to Fab treatment.

In postmarketing surveillance experience, 717 adult treatments at 493 hospitals were reported, in addition to treatment of 28 children.[77] Follow-up forms were available for 75 percent of the 676 adults who survived beyond the time of completion of the initial form. More than 60 percent of patients were more than 70 years old; the median age for female patients was 75, for males 72 years.

In contrast to the experience in the initial multicenter trial, a vast majority of patients in the postmarketing surveillance study (94%) were proved to have underlying cardiovascular disease. About one-third had severe renal functional impairment, and another 43 percent mild to moderate impairment. Seventy-one per cent of patients receiving Fab had been on maintenance digoxin therapy using conventional doses. Of these, 40 percent had severe impairment of renal function. About 17 percent of instances of toxicity treated with Fab fragments resulted from single drug overdoses. Of these, only 7 percent had severe renal impairment. Manifestations of toxicity tended to be less severe than was the case in the initial multicenter clinical trial. Doses of Fab administered tended to be less in the postmarketing surveillance experience. The median dose was 120 mg and the most frequently administered dose was 80 mg (2 vials).

Data from the postmarketing surveillance study indicated that 50 percent of patients had complete reversal of toxicity, 24 percent had partial reversal, and 12 percent had no response to treatment. The response was reported as uncertain, or was not reported, for 14 percent of the patients treated. Treating physicians judged that 89 patients failed to respond to treatment under circumstances in which the residual abnormalities in 14 patients were still believed, in retrospect, to be due to digitalis toxicity. An independent cardiologist reviewed all these cases and concluded that four of 14 represented possible instances of treatment failure. The failure of response in the remaining 10 percent either could not be evaluated or was judged to be related to a questionable diagnosis of digoxin intoxication, and inadequate administered dose of Fab, or a moribund clinical state prior to Fab treatment.

Fifty-two patients were judged to have had adverse events possibly or probably related to Fab administration. These events could be categorized into four groups, including allergic responses; possible recrudescent digoxin toxicity; problems associated with digoxin readministration following Fab treatment; and other events.

The experience with the use of digoxin-specific antibodies in pediatric patients is more limited, in part because of the infrequent incidence of digitalis toxicity in these patients. For example, in a retrospective analysis of clinical outcome in only 41 well-documented cases of digoxin poisoning over a 10-year period in three academic pediatric medical centers, no patient had life-threatening arrhythmias and none died.[79] Recently, we reported our experience in 29 children (median age 1.5 years; range 1 day–18 years) treated with digoxin-specific Fab fragments for complications due to both chronic and acute digoxin intoxication.[80] Sixteen patients had underlying heart disease, and most had serum digoxin levels above 5.0 ng/ml. Although 27 of the 29 patients responded to the administration of digoxin-specific antibodies with a resolution of signs and symptoms of digoxin intoxication, most within three hour of administration, the mortality rate remained high (24%). Most of these deaths were due to complications unrelated to digoxin toxicity. There were no documented allergic reactions and only two clear adverse effects following administration of digoxin-specific Fab fragments: an exacerbation of underlying heart failure due to the abrupt withdrawal of the digoxin effect; and transient hypokalemia that resolved with supplemental potassium. The mortality rate noted in this trial is similar to those we reported in adults,[76] and reflects the influence of other, incapacitating medical problems. Nevertheless, this therapy appears to be safe and effective in the treatment of digoxin intoxication in children.

Taken together, the results of the multicenter trials[76,79] and the postmarketing surveillance study[77] provide evidence that purified Fab fragments with high affinity and specificity for digoxin rapidly and safely reverse advanced digitalis toxicity in patients with acute or chronic drug exposure.

The relative paucity of adverse clinical responses has led us to recommend the use of digoxin-specific Fab fragments under less dire circumstances than was the case during our early experience, when the risk of toxicity of the Fab fragments themselves had not been extensively assessed. However, the potential immunogenicity of the ovine Fab formulation, and its relatively high cost, argue against the routine use of this agent in the diagnosis of suspected digoxin toxicity. Clinically important side-effects related to treatment such as worsening of heart failure, increased ventricular rate of patients with atrial fibrillation, or clinically important hypokalemia have been observed in less than 10 percent of patients treated, and allergic phenomena occurred in less than 1 percent. Given the sometimes precipitous course of digitalis intoxication following large ingestions, we favor the early use of appropriate doses of Fab fragments as soon as reliable evidence of a large-scale ingestion resulting in overt cardiac toxicity is available.

References

Research Reports

1. Marshall EK. Experimental basis of chemotherapy in the treatment of bacterial infections. Bull NY Acad Med 1940;*16*:722–731.
2. Spector R, Park GD, Johnson GF, Vesell ES. Therapeutic drug monitoring. Clin Pharmacol Ther 1988;*43*:345–353.
3. Vozeh S. Cost-effectiveness of therapeutic drug monitoring. Clin Pharmacokin 1987;*13*:131–140.
4. Brodie MJ, Feely J. Practical clinical pharmacology. Therapeutic drug monitoring and clinical trials. Br Med J 1988;*296*:1110–1114.
5. Williams PJ, Hull JH, Sarubbi FA, Rogers JF, Wargin WA. Factors associated with nephrotoxicity and clinical outcomes in patients receiving amikacin. J Clin Pharmacol 1986;*26*:79–86.
6. Arroyo JC, Milligan WL, Davis J, Mitchell D. Impact of aminoglycoside serum assays on clinical decisions and renal toxicity. South Med J 1986;*79*:272–276.
7. David BM, Whitford EG, Ilett KF. Disopyramide binding to alpha$_1$-acid glycoprotein: Sequential effects following acute myocardial infarction. Clin Exp Pharmacol Physiol 1982;*9*:478.
8. Kates RE. Therapeutic monitoring of antiarrhythmic drugs. Therap Drug Monit 1980;*2*:119–126.
9. Woo E, Greenblatt DJ. Pharmacokinetic and clinical implications of quinidine-protein binding. J Pharmaceut Sci 1979;*68*:466–469.
10. Sum CY, Yacobi A, Kartzinel R, Stampfli H, Davis CS, Lai C-M. Kinetics of esmolol, an ultra-short-acting beta blocker, and of its major metabolite. Clin Pharmacol Ther 1983;*34*:427.
11. Naggar CZ, Alexander S. Propranolol treatment of VPC's. Engl J Med 1976;*294*:903–904.
12. Woosley RL, Kornhauser D, Smith RS, Reele S, Higgins SB, Nies AS, Shand DG, Oates JA. Suppression of chronic ventricular arrhythmias with propranolol. Circulation 1979;*60*:819–827.
13. Chidsey C, Pine M, Favrot L, Smith S, Leonetti G, Morselli P, Zanchetti A. The use of drug concentration measurements in studies of the therapeutic response to propranolol. Postgrad Med 1976;*52* (Suppl 4):26–32.
14. Pine M, Favrot L, Smith S, McDonald K, Chidsey CA. Correlation of plasma propranolol concentration with therapeutic response in patients with angina pectoris. Circulation 1975;*52*:886–893.
15. Morganroth J. Risk factors for the development of proarrhythmic events. Am J Cardiol 1987;*59*:32E–37E.
16. MacMahon S, Collins R, Peto R, Koster RW, Yusuf S. Effects of prophylactic lidocaine in suspected acute myocardial infarction. An overview of results from the randomized, controlled trials. J Am Med Assoc 1988;*260*:1910–1916.
17. Cardiac Arrhythmia Suppression Trial (CAST) Investigators. Preliminary Report: Effect of encainide and flecainide on mortality in a randomized trial of arrhythmia suppression after myocardial infarction. N Engl J Med 1989;*321*:406–412.
18. Echt DS, Liebson PR, Mitchell B et al. Mortality and morbidity in patients receiving encainide, flecainide, or placebo. The Cardiac Arrhythmia Suppression Trial. N Engl J Med 1991;*324*:781–788.
19. Greene HL, Roden DM, Katz RJ, Woosley RL, Salerno DM, Henthorn RW. The cardiac arrhythmia suppression trial: first CAST . . . then CAST II. JACC 1992;*19*:894–898.
20. Reimold SC, Berlin JA, Chalmers TC, Antman EM. Assessment of the efficacy and safety of antiarrhythmic therapy for chronic atrial fibrillation: Observations on the role of trial design and implications of drug-related mortality. Am Heart J 1992;*124*:924–932.
21. Coplen SE, Antman EM, Berlin JA, Jewitt P, Chalmers TC. Efficacy and safety of quinidine therapy for maintenance of sinus rhythm after cardioversion. A meta-analysis of randomized control trials. Circulation 1990;*82*:1106–1116.
22. Lerman BB, Belardinelli L. Cardiac electrophysiology of adenosine. Basic and clinical concepts. Circulation 1991;*83*:1499–1509.
23. DiMarco JP, Sellers TD, Berne RM, West GA, Belardinelli L. Adenosine: electrophysiologic effects and therapeutic use for terminating paroxysmal supraventricular tachycardia. Circulation 1983;*69*:1254–1263.
24. Rankin AC, Oldroyd KG, Chang E, Rae AP, Cobbe SM. Value and limitations of adenosine in the diagnosis and treatment of narrow and broad complex tachycardias. Br Heart J 1989;*62*:195–203.
25. Camm AJ, Garratt CJ. Adenosine and supraventricular tachycardia. N Engl J Med 1991;*325*:1621–1629.
26. Smith TW. Serum and plasma cardiac glycoside concentrations: clinical use and misuse. In Smith TW (ed). Digitalis glycoside. Orlando: Grune & Stratton Orlando. (1986); pp 153–167.
27. Duhme DW, Greenblatt DJ, and Koch-Weser J. Reduction of digoxin toxicity associated with measurement of serum levels. Ann Intern Med 1974;*80*:516–519.
28. Kelly RA, Smith TW. Use and misuse of digitalis blood levels. Heart Dis Stroke 1992;*1*:117–122.
29. Kelly RA, Smith TW. Recognition and management of digitalis toxicity. Am J Cardiol 1992;*69*:1080–1190.
30. Williams JR Jr, Klocke FJ, Braunwald E. Studies on digitalis. XIII. A comparison of the effects of potassium on the inotropic and arrhythmia-producing actions of ouabain. J Clin Invest 1965;*45*:346–352.
31. Lewis RP. Clinical use of digoxin levels. Am Heart J. (Still in Press).
32. Botker HE, Toft P, Klitgaard NA, Simonsen EE. Influence of physical exercise on serum digoxin concentration and heart rate in patients with atrial fibrillation. Br Heart J 1991;*65*:337–341.

33. Kolibash AJ Jr, Lewis RP, Bourne DW, Kramer WG, Reuning RH. Extension of the serum digoxin concentration-response relationship to patient management. J Clin Pharmacol 1989;*20*:300–306.

34. Mahdyoon H, Battilana G, Rosman H, Goldstein S, Gheorghiade M. The evolving pattern of digoxin intoxication: Observations at a large urban hospital from 1980 to 1988. Am Heart J 1990;*120*:1189–1194.

35. Doering W, Konig E, Sturm W. Digitalis intoxication: Specificity and significance of cardiac and extracardiac symptoms. I. Patients with digitalis-induced arrhythmias. Z Kardiol 1977;*66*:121.

36. Eraker SA, Sasse L. The serum digoxin test and digoxin toxicity: A Bayesian approach to decision making. Circulation 1981;*64*:409–420.

37. Chamberlain DA. The medical treatment of angina pectoris. Br Heart J 1987;*58*:547–551.

38. Wallace DC. Perhexiline maleate in the treatment of angina pectoris. Med J Aust 1978;*2*:466–495.

39. Vaughn Williams E. Antiarrhythmic action and the puzzle of perhexiline. Academic Press, London, 1980.

40. Horowitz JD, Morris PM, Drummer OH, Goble AJ, Louis WJ. High performance liquid chromatographic assay of perhexiline maleate in plasma. J Pharmac Sci 1981;*70*:320–322.

41. Pilcher J, Cooper JDH, Turnell DC, Matenga J, Paul R, Lockhart JDF. Investigations of long-term treatment with perhexiline maleate using therapeutic monitoring and electromyography. Ther Drug Monit 1985;*7*:54–60.

42. Horowitz JD, Morris PM, Drummer O, Goble AJ, Louis WJ. Saturable metabolism of perhexiline maleate: Correlations with long term toxicity. Am J Cardiol 1981;47:399.

43. Horowitz JD, Sia STB, MacDonald PS, Goble AJ, Louis WJ. Perhexiline maleate treatment for severe angina pectoris—correlations with pharmacokinetics. Int J Cardiol 1986;13:219–229.

44. Nebert DW, Gonzalez FJ. P450 genes and evolutionary genetics. Hosp Prac, March 15, 1987, pp 63–74.

45. Gonzalez FJ, Skoda RC, Kimura S, Umeno M, Zanger UM, Nebert DW, Gelboin HV, Hardwick JP, Meyer UA. Characterization of the common genetic defect in humans deficient in debrisoquine metabolism. Nature 1988;331:442–446.

46. Gonzalez FJ, Vilbois F, Hardwick JP, McBride OW, Nebert DW, Gelboin HV, Meyer UA. Human debrisoquine 4-hydroxylase (P45011D1): cDNA and deduced amino acid sequence and assignment of the CYP2D locus to chromosome 22. Genomics 1988;*2*:174–179.

47. Cole PL, Beamer AD, McGowan N, Cantillon CO, Benfell K, Kelly, RA, Hartley LH, Smith TW, and Antman EM. Efficacy and safety of perhexiline maleate in refractory angina: A double-blind, placebo-controlled clinical trial of a novel antianginal agent. Circulation 1990;*81*:1260–1270.

48. Pearlman DS, Chervinsky P, LaForce C, Seltzer JM, Southern DL, Kemp JP, Dockhorn RJ, Grossman J, Liddle RF, Yancey SW, Cocchetto DM, Alexander WJ, and van As, A. A comparison of salmeterol with albuterol in the treatment of mild-to-moderate asthma. N Engl J Med 1992;*327*:1420–1425.

49. Wrenn K, Slovis CM, Murphy F, and Greenberg RS. Aminophylline therapy for acute bronchospastic disease in the emergency room. Ann Intern Med 1991;*115*:241–247.

50. McFadden ER Jr. Methylxanthines in the treatment of asthma: The rise, the fall, and the possible rise again. Ann Intern med 1991;*115*:323–324.

51. Poe RH, Utell MJ. Theophylline in asthma and COPD: Changing perspectives and controversies. Geriatrics 1991;*46*:55–65.

52. Tattersfield AE. Bronchodilators: New developments. Br Med Bull 1992;*48*:190–204.

53. Barnes PJ. New therapeutic approaches. Br Med Bull 1991;*48*:231–247.

54. Spitzer WO, Suissa S, Ernst P, Horwitz RI, Habbick B, Cockcroft D, Boivin J-F, McNutt M, Buist AS, Rebuck AS. The use of β-agonists and the risk of death and near death from asthma. N Engl J Med 1992;*326*:501–506.

55. Burrows B, Lebowitz MD. The β-agonist dilemma. N Engl J Med 1992;*326*:560–561.

56. Grainger J, Woodman K, Pearce N, Crane J, Burgess C, Keane A, Beasley R. Prescribed fenoterol and death from asthma in New Zealand, 1981–7: a further case-control study. Thorax 1991;*46*:105–111.

57. Sears MR, Rea HH, Beaglehole R, Jackson R. Asthma mortality in New Zealand: a two year national study. NZ. Med J 1985;*98*:271–275.

58. Furukawa CT, DuHamel TR, Weimer L, Shapiro GG, Pierson WE et al. Cognitive and behavioral findings in children taking theophylline. J Allergy Clin Immunol 1988;*81*:83–88.

59. Rachelefsky GS, Wo J, Adelson J, Mickey MR, Spector SL, Katz RM, Siegel SC, Rohr AS. Behavior abnormalities and poor school performance due to oral theophylline use. Pediatrics 1986;*78*:1133–1138.

60. Schlieper A, Alcock D, Beaudry, P, Feldman W, Leikin L. Effect of therapeutic plasma concentrations of theophylline on behavior, cognitive processing, and affect in children with asthma. J Pediatr 1991;*118*:449–455.

61. Bender B, Milgrom H. Theophylline-induced behavior change in children. An objective evaluation of parents' perceptions. JAMA 1992;*1267*:2621–2624.

62. Lindgren S, Lokshin B, Stromquist A, Weinberger M, Nassif E, McCubbin M, Frasher R. Does asthma or treatment with theophylline limit children's academic performance? N Engl J Med 1992;*327*:926–930.

63. Hendeles L, Weinberger M, Szefler S, Ellis E. Safety and efficacy of theophylline in children with asthma. J Pediatr 1992;*120*:177–183.

64. Hendeles L, Massanari M, Weinberger M. In Evans WE, Schentag JJ, Jusko WJ, Harrison H. (eds). Applied Pharmacokinetics, principles of therapeutic drug monitoring, Second Edition. Spokane WA. Applied Therapeutics, 1986; pp 1105–1188.

65. Blanchard J, Harvey S, Morgan WJ. Relationship between serum and saliva theophylline levels in patients with cystic fibrosis. Therap Drug Monit 1992;*14*:48–54.

66. Hendeles L, Weinberger M. Theophylline. A "State of Art" Review. Pharmacotherapy 1983;*3*:2–44.

67. Bierman CW, Williams PV. Therapeutic monitoring of theophylline rationale and current status. Clin Pharmacokinet 1989;*17*:377–384.

68. Cary J, Hein K, Dell R. Theophylline disposition in adolescents with asthma. Therap Drug Monit 1991;*13*:309–313.

69. Bierman CW, Pierson WE, Shapiro GG, Furukawa CT. Is a uniform round-the-clock theophylline blood level necessary for optimal asthma therapy in the adolescent patient. Am J Med 1988;*85*:17–20.

70. Butler VP Jr, Chen JP. Digoxin-specific antibodies. Proc Natl Acad Sci USA 1967;*57*:71–78.

71. Smith TW, Butler VP Jr, Haber E. Characterization of antibodies of high affinity and specificity for the digitalis glycoside digoxin. Biochemistry 1970;*9*:331–337.

72. Smith TW, Butler VP Jr, Haber E. Determination of therapeutic and toxic serum digoxin concentrations by radioimmunoassay. N Engl J Med 1969;*281*:1212–1216.

73. Smith TW. Radioimmunoassay for serum digitoxin concentration: Methodology and clinical experience. J Pharmacol Exp Ther 1970;*175*:352–360.

74. Curd J, Smith TW, Jaton J-C, Haber E. The isolation of digoxin-specific antibody and its use in reversing the effects of digoxin. Proc Natl Acad Sci USA 1971;*68*:2401–2406.

75. Smith TW, Haber E, Yeatman L, Butler VP Jr. Reversal of advanced digoxin intoxication with Fab fragments of digoxin-specific antibodies. N Engl J Med 1976;*294*:797–800.

76. Antman EM, Wenger TL, Butler VP Jr, Haber E, Smith TW. Treatment of 150 cases of life-threatening digitalis intoxication with digoxin-specific Fab antibody fragments: Final report of a multi-center study. Circulation 1990;*81*:1744–1752.

77. Hickey AR, Wenger TL, Carpenter VP, Tilson HH, Hlatky MA, Furberg CD, Kirkpatrick CH, Strauss HC, Smith TW. Antibody therapy in the management of digitalis intoxication: Safety and efficacy results of an observational surveillance study. J Am Coll Cardiol 1991;*17*:590–598.

78. Kirkpatrick CH. The digibind study advisory panel. Allergic histories and reactions of patients treated with digoxin immune Fab (ovine) antibody. Am J Emer Med 1991;*9*:7–10.

79. Lewander WJ, Gaudreault P, Einhorn A, Henretig FM, Lacouture PG, Lovejoy FH Jr. Acute pediatric digoxin ingestion: a ten-year experience. Am J Dis Child 1986;*140*:770–773.

80. Woolf AD, Wenger T, Smith TW, Lovejoy FH Jr. The use of digoxin-specific Fab fragments for severe digitalis intoxication in children. N Engl J Med 1992;*326*:1739–1744.

81. Fowler RS, Rathi L, Keith JD. Accidental digitalis intoxication in children. J Pediatr 1964;*64*:188–200.

82. Smith TW, Lloyd BL, Spicer N, Haber E. Immunogenicity and kinetics of distribution and elimination of sheep digoxin-specific IgG and Fab fragments in the rabbit and baboon. Clin Exp Immunol 1979;*36*:384–396.

83. Lloyd BL, Smith TW. Contrasting rates of reversal of digoxin toxicity by digoxin-specific IgG and Fab fragments. Circulation 1978;*58*:280–283.

CHAPTER 29

Peter J. Barnes
Robert A. Mueller

Bronchodilators

Bronchodilator drugs have an antibronchoconstrictor effect, which may be demonstrated directly in vitro by a relaxant effect on precontracted airways.[r1,r2] Bronchodilators cause immediate reversal of airway constriction in vivo, and this is believed to be due to an effect on airway smooth muscle, although additional pharmacologic effects on other airway cells (such as reduced microvascular leakage and reduced release of bronchoconstrictor mediators from inflammatory cells) may contribute to the reduction in airway narrowing. The only classes of bronchodilator in current clinical use are beta-adrenoceptor agonists, methylxanthines, and anticholinergic drugs. Drugs such as disodium cromoglycate, which prevent bronchoconstriction, have no bronchodilator action and are ineffective once bronchoconstriction has occurred. Corticosteroids, while gradually improving airway obstruction, have no direct effect on airway smooth muscle and therefore are not considered to be bronchodilators.

Beta-Adrenoceptor Agonists

Epinephrine has been used in the treatment of asthma since the beginning of the 20th century. Dessicated adrenal gland was originally given to asthmatic patients in the belief that it would reduce the swelling of the bronchial mucosa in the same way that it produces blanching of the skin. Epinephrine stimulates both alpha- and beta-adrenoceptors and, because its bronchodilator effect is mediated by beta-receptors, selective beta-agonists were developed. Isoproterenol, which has only beta-agonist activity, evolved in the 1940s. Isoproterenol is a nonselective beta-agonist that stimulates β_1 and β_2 receptors with equal efficacy. Because bronchodilation is mediated by β_2 receptors alone, selective β_2 agonists, such as salbutamol and terbutaline, were introduced in the 1960s. The goals of reducing the incidence of β_1 activation of the heart with subsequent tachcardia or dysrhythmia has been partially achieved, but at high doses, some residual β_1 receptor stimulation is seen with all β_2 selective agonists.

Chemistry

The development of β_2 agonists was a logical development of substitutions in the catecholamine structure.[r3] The catechol ring consists of hydroxyl groups in the 3 and 4 positions of the benzene ring (Fig. 29.1). Norepinephrine differs from epinephrine only in the presence of a methyl group in the terminal amine group, which therefore indicates that addition of alkyl groups to the amine position confers beta-receptor selectivity. Epinephrine still possesses α and β receptor agonist potency, whereas the substitution of an isopropyl group for the methyl group results in loss of all α activity (e.g., isoproterenol). Further substitution of the terminal amine with even larger alkyl groups resulted in β_2 receptor selectivity (as in salbutamol and terbutaline) with reduced β_1 agonist activity.

Endogenous catecholamines are rapidly removed from the synaptic region by two active uptake processes (Fig. 29.2)[r4] (see also Chapter 6).

1. *Uptake*$_1$ is localized to sympathetic nerve terminals, and norepinephrine is rapidly returned to storage vesicles from the extracellular space.

2. *Uptake*$_2$ facilitates uptake into non-neural tissue, such as smooth muscle cells, where enzymatic degradation occurs by catechol O-methyl transferase (COMT). Isoproterenol is not a substrate for uptake$_1$, but is avidly taken up by uptake$_2$, whereas noncatecholamine beta-agonists are not substrates for either transport process. Catecholamines are rapidly metabolized by the enzyme COMT, which methylates in the 3-hydroxyl position, thereby destroying agonist activity, and along with uptake$_1$ accounts for the short duration of action of naturally occurring catecholamines. Modification of the catechol ring to remove the catechol configuration, as in salbutamol and terbutaline, prevents degradation by COMT and therefore

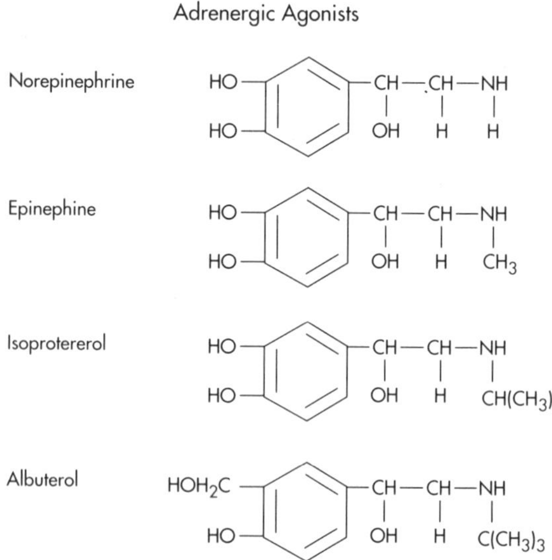

Figure 29.1 Structure of Adrenergic Agonists

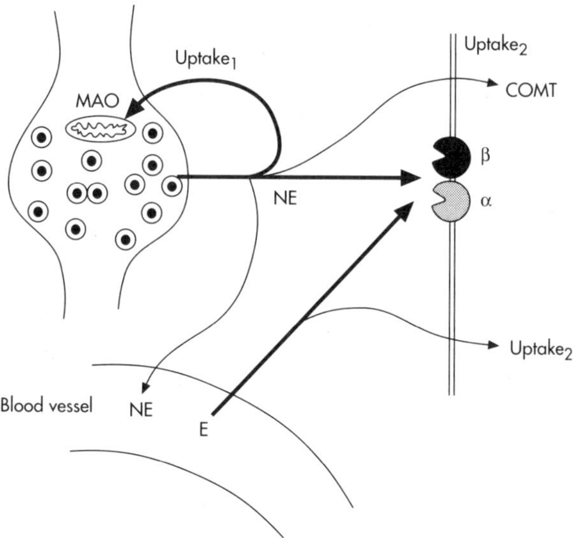

Figure 29.2 Uptake of catecholamines. Norepinephrine (NE) released from sympathetic nerves is taken up by neuronal uptake 1 and, to a lesser extent, by uptake 2 in tissues, whereas epinephrine (E) is taken up mainly by uptake 2.

prolongs their effects. The amine portion of the catecholamine nucleus is also metabolized to inactive compounds via side-chain cleavage by the enzyme monoamine oxidase (MAO) in sympathetic nerve terminals, liver, gastrointestinal, and many other tissues. Compounds such as ephedrine, which lack both the catechol and monamine structures, can be active after oral administration and aid in bronchodilation, whereas compounds with a catechol or monoamine group are inactive when given orally because of gut and hepatic metabolism.

Many β_2 selective agonists have now been introduced; while there may be differences in potency, there are no clinically significant differences in relative β_2/β_1 selectivity. Inhaled β_2 selective drugs in current clinical use have a similar duration of action, longer than endogenous catecholamines such as epinephrine, because of resistance to metabolism outlined above. Recently, β_2 selective drugs such as salmeterol and formeterol, which have a much longer duration of effect, have been introduced.

Mode of Action

Beta-agonists produce bronchodilation by directly stimulating beta-receptors in airway smooth muscle, which leads to relaxation. This can be demonstrated in vitro by the relaxant effect of isoproterenol on human bronchi and lung strips,[1] and in vitro by a rapid decrease in airway resistance. Beta-receptors have been demonstrated in airway smooth muscle by direct receptor binding techniques and autoradiographic studies and indicate that beta-receptors are localized to smooth muscle of all airways from trachea to terminal bronchioles.[2] The molecular mechanisms by which beta-agonists induce relaxation of airway smooth muscle have been extensively investigated. The β_2 receptor protein binds the alpha subunit of a binding protein (Gs), which in the presence of GTP increases the catalytic activity of adenylyl enclase. This enzyme subsequently increases intracellular cyclic adenosine 3′,5′ monophosphate (cAMP), leading to activation of cAMP-dependent protein kinase A and causing relaxation by several mechanisms: (1) lowering of free intracellular calcium ion concentration by active removal of free calcium ions from the cell and into intracellular membrane stores; (2) inhibition of myosin phosphorylation (Fig. 29.3); and (3) opening calcium-activated potassium channels, thus hyperpolarizing the cell membrane. Beta-agonists act as functional antagonists and reverse bronchoconstriction irrespective of the contractile agent, and this is a useful property, since many bronchoconstrictor stimuli are likely to be operative in asthma.

Beta-agonists may have additional effects on airways, and beta-receptors are localized to several different airway cells.[5]

1. Beta-agonists have potent effects in preventing mediator release from isolated human lung mast cells in vitro[5] and in vivo.[6]

2. Beta-agonists also may reduce microvascular leakage and thus the development of bronchial mucosa edema after exposure to mediators such as histamine.[7]

3. Beta-agonists increase mucus secretion from submucosal glands and ion transport across airway epithelium, and these effects may enhance mucociliary clearance, therefore reversing the defect on clearance found in asthma. Beta-agonists may also release a putative relaxant factor from epithelial cells.

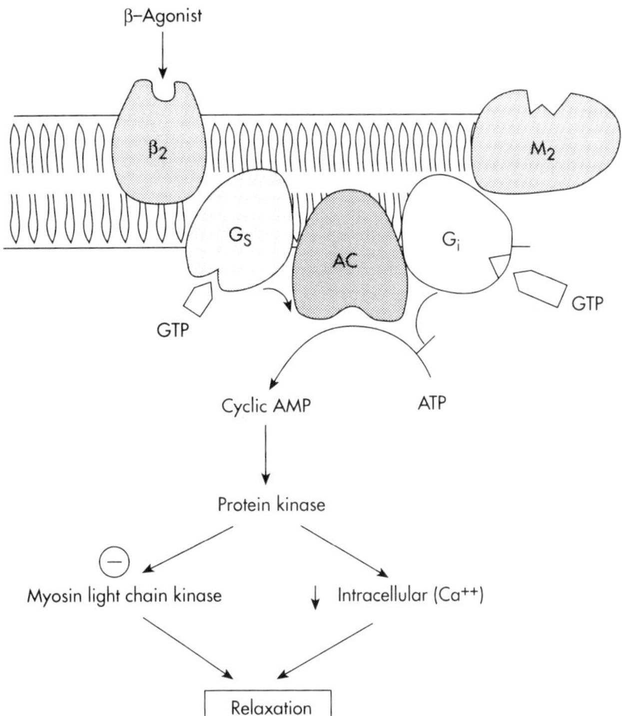

Figure 29.3 Molecular mechanisms of beta-adrenoceptor agonist action in airway smooth muscle cell. Stimulation of a β-receptor (β) activates adenylate cyclase (AC) via a guanine-nucleotide regulatory protein (G). Muscarine receptors (M) have the opposite effect on AC.

4. Beta-agonists reduce neurotransmission in cholinergic nerves by an action at prejunctional $β_2$ receptors to inhibit acetylcholine relase.[8]

Although these additional effects of beta-agonists may be relevant to the prophylactic use of these drugs against various challenges, their rapid bronchodilator action can probably be attributed to a direct effect on airway smooth muscle.

Choice of Drug

Epinephrine

Epinephrine is still the drug of choice for treatment of acute anaphylaxis, where a combination of alpha- and beta-adrenergic properties is desirable, but the agent is now no longer the first choice for treating asthma. The disadvantages of epinephrine are its lack of $β_2$ selectivity, resulting in $β_1$ receptor-mediated cardiac stimulation, and its short duration of action because of rapid metabolism and removal by the uptake and metabolic mechanisms discussed above. Its alpha-agonist effects could be an advantage in reducing microvascular leakage in airways (by a vasoconstrictor effect on bronchial arterioles).[9] Nebulized epinephrine offers no advantage over albuterol, at least in acute severe asthma.[10] There is no convincing evidence that epinephrine causes bronchoconstriction via activation of alpha-receptors on airway smooth muscle.

Isoproterenol

Isoproterenol is a nonselective beta-agonist and therefore is more likely to have cardiac side-effects. Pharmacologically it behaves as a full agonist, whereas $β_2$ selective drugs are partial agonists. Comparison of dose-response curves to isoproterenol with those of salbutamol, however, shows no greater bronchodilating effect with isoproterenol.[11] Isoproterenol has a relatively short bronchodilator effect (less than 2hr because of metabolism by COMT), although its onset is very rapid (peak effect 5 min). Orciprenaline is also nonselective, but is resistant to enzymatic degradation and so has a longer duration of action.

$β_2$ Selective Agonists

Several $β_2$ selective agonists are now available (Fig. 29.4). These drugs are as effective as nonselective agonists in their bronchodilator action, since airway effects are mediated only by $β_2$ receptors. However, they are less likely to produce cardiac stimulation than isoprenaline because $β_1$ receptors are stimulated relatively less. With the exception of rimiterol (which retains the catechol ring structure and is therefore susceptible to COMT), they have a longer duration of action because they are resistant to uptake and enzymatic degradation by COMT and MAO. There is little to choose between the various $β_2$ agonists currently available; all are usable by inhalation and orally, have a similar duration of action (usually 3–4 hr, but less in severe asthma) and similar side-effects. Differences in $β_2$ selectivity have been claimed but are not clinically important.

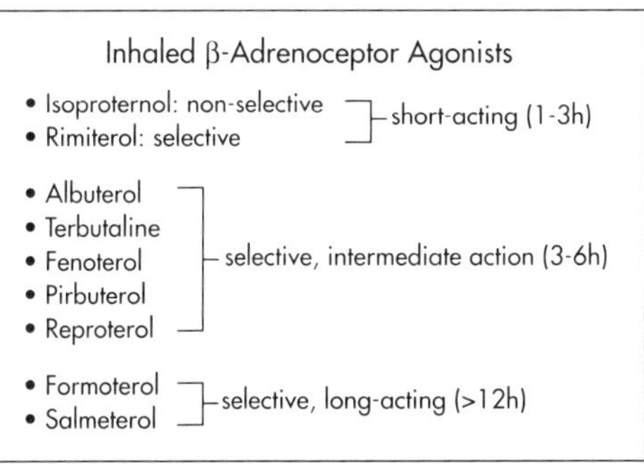

Figure 29.4 Inhaled B-Agonists

Drugs in clinical use worldwide include albuterol, terbutaline, fenoterol, pirbuterol, bitolterol, and reproterol.

Longer-acting β_2 agonists that are effective by inhalation are now available for clinical use in some countries. Formoterol and salmeterol have a bronchodilator effect of over 12 hr and are therefore suitable for twice-daily dosing.[12]

Mode of Administration

1. Inhalation

Inhalation is the method of choice for routine treatment; since side-effects are less likely, the therapeutic benefit may be greater, and the effect is more rapid in onset. Furthermore, beta-agonists may be more effective by inhalation; thus, inhaled albuterol can prevent exercise-induced asthma, whereas an oral dose with similar bronchodilator effect, cannot.[13] This may indicate that the inhaled drug may reach surface cells (e.g., mast cells) inaccessible to the orally administered drug. Beta-agonists are normally given by a metered dose inhaler (MDI), which is convenient and easy to use, provided proper instruction is given. For patients who are unable to use the MDI correctly, dry powder formulations using spacers to assure drug delivery at the most efficacious point in inspiration often work much better.

2. Oral

Oral administration of beta-agonists provides no advantage over the inhaled route and is more likely to be associated with side-effects. Sustained-release preparations are usually less effective than theophylline, but may be useful in treating nocturnal asthma in some patients.

3. Parenteral

Intravenous administration is associated with more frequent side-effects; for acute asthma it has not been shown to have any significant benefit over a nebulized beta-agonist.[14] Subcutaneous infusion of a beta-agonist has proved useful in some asthmatic patients, with "brittle" asthma characterized by sudden and unpredictable episodes of bronchospasm.[15]

Side-Effects

Unwanted effects are dose-related and are due to stimulation of extrapulmonary beta-receptors. Side-effects are unusual with inhaled therapy, but more common with oral or IV administration.

1. Muscle Tremor

Muscle tremor is due to stimulation of β_2 receptors in skeletal muscle, and is the commonest side-effect. It may be more troublesome in elderly patients.

2. Cardiovascular

Tachycardia and palpitations are due both to reflex cardiac stimulation secondary to peripheral vasodilation, and from direct stimulation of atrial β_2 receptors. The human heart is unusual in having a relatively high proportion of β_2 receptors, and stimulation of myocardial β_1 receptors as the doses of β_2 agonist are increased probably also occurs. These side-effects tend to disappear with continued use of the drug, reflecting the development of tolerance.

3. Metabolic

Metabolic effects (increase in plasma free fatty acid, insulin, glucose, pyruvate, and lactate) are usually seen only after large systemic doses. Hypokalemia is a potentially more serious side-effect.[16] This is due to β_2 receptor stimulation of potassium entry into skeletal muscle, which is not secondary to a rise in insulin secretion,[17] but is due to increased potassium transport into both liver and muscle cells. Hypokalemia, as well as hypomagnesemia, may have serious consequences in the presence of hypoxia and hypercarbia as in acute asthma, when there may be a predisposition to cardiac dysrhythmias. In practice, however, significant arrhythmias after nebulized β_2 agonists have been reported only infrequently in acute asthma.

4. Hypoxemia

Beta-agonists may increase ventilation-perfusion mismatching by causing pulmonary vasodilation in blood vessels previously constricted by hypoxia, resulting in the shunting of blood to poorly ventilated areas and a fall in arterial oxygen tension. Although in practice the effect of beta-agonists on PaO_2 is usually very small (5 mm Hg fall), occasionally in severe chronic airways obstruction it is large, although it may be prevented by increasing the inspired oxygen tension.[18]

Safety

Because of a possible relationship between adrenergic drug therapy and the rise in asthma deaths in the United Kingdom during the early 1960s, doubts were cast on the safety of beta-agonists. This causal relationship was never proved, and might be explained equally well by the concomitant reduction in corticosteroid usage and delay in seeking medical attention with the introduction of isoproterenol as an effective bronchodilator.[r7] More recently, these doubts have been revived, and the use of high doses of beta-agonists given by nebulizers at home has been linked to the increase in asthma deaths in New Zealand.[19] However, there is no convincing evidence that beta-agonists contribute to asthma deaths, which can usually as well be ascribed to underestimation and undertreatment of the disease.[20]

There is some concern about the use of beta-agonists alone without concomitant anti-inflammatory therapy, since beta-agonists (at least, those currently available to clinical use) do not seem to suppress the chronic inflammatory process in asthmatic airways.[9]

Tolerance

Continuous treatment with an agonist often leads to tolerance or subsensitivity, which may be due to down-regulation of the receptor. For this reason there have been many studies of bronchial beta-receptor function after prolonged therapy with beta-agonists. Tolerance of nonairway beta-receptor responses, such as tremor and cardiovascular and metabolic responses, is readily induced in normal and asthmatic subjects. But whether tolerance of airway beta-receptors occurs is debatable. Tolerance of human airway smooth muscle to beta-agonists in vitro has been demonstrated, although the concentration of agonists necessary is high and the degree of desensitization is variable. Animal studies suggest than pulmonary beta-receptors may be more resistant to desensitization than beta-receptors elsewhere. In normal subjects, tolerance has been demonstrated in some studies after high-dose inhaled albuterol, but not in others. Similarly, in asthmatic subjects, tolerance has been found in some studies but not in others. However, even when tolerance has been demonstrated, the effect is very small and probably clinically insignificant; the more readily demonstrable tolerance of extrapulmonary effects has the benefit that side-effects tend to disappear with continued use. The reason for the relative resistance of airway beta-receptors to desensitization remains uncertain, but perhaps reflects the fact that, in asthmatic airways, beta-receptors may always be "down-regulated" as a result of the chronic inflammatory process. It has been noted that whereas normal individuals show no change in airway resistance when given a β antagonist (e.g., propranolol), asthmatic individuals do show a decrease in airway conductivity, suggesting that there is little or no sympathetic tone or innervation of normal airways, and that this develops only with disease, such as asthma.

Experimental studies have shown that corticosteroids prevent the development of tolerance to β agonists in airway smooth muscle, and prevent or reverse the fall in pulmonary beta-receptor density. Similarly, IV hydrocortisone reverses the tolerance of airway beta-receptors in normal subjects. Thus, any tendency for tolerance to develop with high-dose inhaled beta-agonists should be prevented by concomitant administration of corticosteroids.

Clinical Use

Beta-agonists are the most widely used and effective bronchodilators in the treatment of asthma.[r2] When inhaled from metered dose aerosols they are convenient, easy to use, rapid in onset, and without significant side-effects. In addition to their acute bronchodilator effect, they are effective in protecting against various challenges, such as exercise, cold air, and allergens. They are the bronchodilators of choice in treating acute severe asthma, when the nebulized route of administration is as effective as IV use.[14] The inhaled route of administration is preferable to the oral route because side-effects are fewer, and it may be more effective. Beta-agonists are commonly used on a regular basis, but it may be preferable to give them as required by symptoms, since increased usage would then indicate the probable need for more anti-infammatory therapy as well.

Anticholinergics

Datura plants, which contain the cholinergic muscarinic antagonist strammonium, were smoked for relief of asthma two centuries ago. Atropine, a related naturally occurring compound, was also introduced for treating asthma; but, because these compounds gave side-effects, particularly drying of secretions,and CNS depression, less lipid soluble quaternary compounds, such as atropine methylnitrate and ipratropium bromide, which do not cross the blood-brain barrier were introduced. These ionized compounds are topically active but are not significantly absorbed from the respiratory tract. Ipratropium has now been in clinical use in Europe for several years.

Mode of Action

Anticholinergics are specific antagonists of muscarinic receptors and, in therapeutic use, have no other significant pharmacologic effects. There are now at least five different muscarinic receptors, but it is the M_2 and M_3 receptors that seem of most functional relevance in the lung. The bronchoconstrictor response to cholinergic agonists is mediated by M_3 receptors, but M_2 receptors also may be involved via inhibition of adenylyl cyclase.[59] In animals and normal humans there is a small degree of resting cholinergic bronchomotor tone that is probably due to tonic vagal nerve impulses that release acetylcholine in the vicinity of airway smooth muscle, since in both normal and asthmatic individuals it can be blocked by anticholinergic drugs.[r10] There is considerable evidence that cholinergic pathways may play an important role in regulating acute bronchomotor responses in animals, and there are a wide variety of mechanical, chemical and immunologic stimuli capable of eliciting reflex bronchconstriction via vagal pathways (Fig. 29.5). This suggested that cholinergic mechanisms might underly bronchial hyperresponsiveness and acute bronchoconstrictor responses in asthma, with the implication that anticholinergic drugs would be effective bronchodilators in asthma. An enhanced bronchoconstrictor response to acelylcholine was noted in asthmatic subjects over two decades ago.[21] Shah et al have reported that provocative tests to increase endogenous parasympathetic activity to the heart (deep breathing, Valsalva manuuver, and carotid massage) showed augmentation of airway resistance.[22] Many controlled studies have now been performed.[r11,r12] In general, while these drugs may afford protection against acute challenge by sulfur dioxide, inert dusts, cold air, and emotional factors, they are less effective against antigen challenge, exercise, and fog. This is not surprising, as anticholinergic drugs will only inhibit reflex cholinergic bronchoconstriction and would not be expected to have a significant blocking effect on the direct effects of inflammatory mediators, such as histamine and leukotrienes, on bronchial smooth muscle. Furthermore, cholinergic antagonists probably have little or no effect on mast cells and microvascular leakiness, and probably have less effect on the smallest caliber airways.

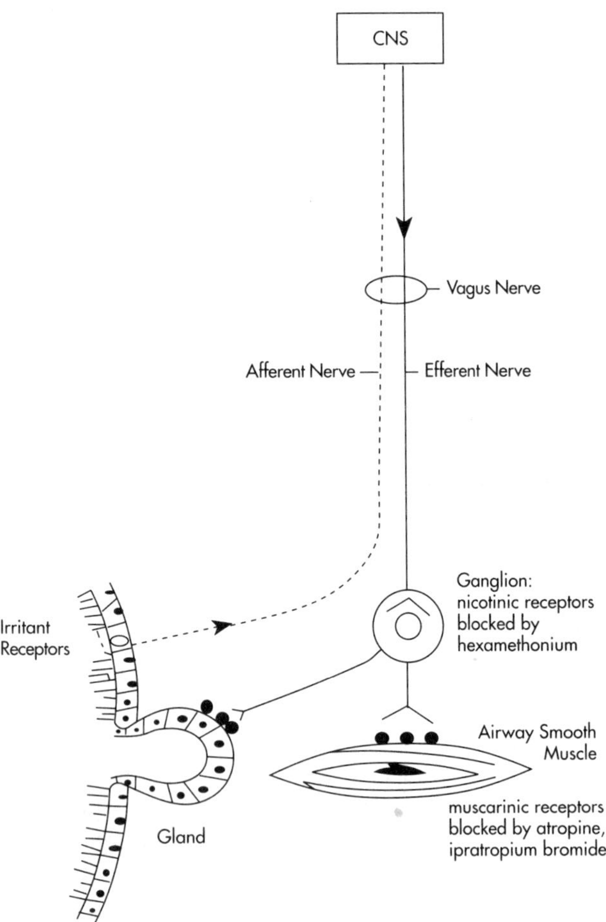

Figure 29.5 Cholinergic neural pathways. Acetylcholine released from postgaglionic pathways acts on muscarinic receptors on airway smoth muscle and glands and is blocked by antagonists such as atropine or ipratropium bromide. Cholinergic pathways may be activated reflexly in asthma from stimulation of sensory receptors in the airways.

Clinical Use

Asthma

In asthmatic subjects anticholinergic drugs usually are less effective as bronchodilators than are beta-agonists, and offer less efficient protection against various bronchial challenges, although their duration of action is significantly longer.[r11–r13] These drugs may be more effective in older patients with asthma.[23] Nebulized anticholinergic drugs are effective in acute severe asthma,[24,25] although they are less effective than beta-agonists in this situation. Nevertheless, in the acute and chronic treatment of asthma, anticholinergic drugs may have an additive effect with beta-agonists and should therefore be considered when control of asthma is not adequate with beta-agonists, particularly if there are problems with theophylline. The onset of bronchodilation with anticholinergic drugs is slower than with beta-agonists, reaching a peak only one hour after inhalation, but persists for over six hours, longer than the duration of most β_2 agonists.

Chronic Bronchitis

In chronic obstructive pulmonary disease (COPD), anticholinergic drugs may be as effective as, or even superior to, beta-agonists.[26] Their relatively greater effect in chronic obstructive airways disease than in asthma may be explained by an inhibitory effect on vagal tone that, while not necessarily being increased in COPD, may be the only reversible element of airway obstruction exaggerated by geometric factors in a narrowed airway (Fig. 29.6).

Side-Effects

Inhaled anticholinergic drugs are usually well tolerated, and there is no evidence for any decline in responsiveness with continued use. On stopping inhaled anticholinergics a small rebound increase in responsiveness has been described,[27] but the clinical relevance of this is uncertain. Atropine has side-effects that are dose-related and are due to cholinergic antagonism in other systems that may lead to dryness of the mouth, blurred vision, and urinary retention. Side-effects after ipratropium are far less common because there is less systemic absorption.[r13]

Because cholinergic agonists stimulate mucus secretion there have been several studies of mucus secretion with anticholinergic drugs, since there has been concern that these drugs may reduce secretion and lead to more viscous mucus. Atropine reduces mucociliary clearance in normal subjects and in patients with asthma and chronic bronchitis,[28] but the quaternary derivative, ipratropium bromide, even in high doses, has no detectable effect in either normal subjects or in patients with airway disease.[29] A significant unwanted effect is the unpleasant bitter taste of inhaled ipratropium, which may contribute to poor compliance with this drug. There are several reports of paradoxical bronchoconstriction with ipratropium bromide, particularly when given by nebulizer. This is largely explained by the hypotonicity of the nebulizer solution and by antibacterial additives, such as benzylkonium chloride. Nebulizer solutions free of such additives do not cause bronchoconstriction.[30] Alternatively, it is possible that bronchoconstriction is due to blockade of prejunctional M_2 receptors on cholinergic nerves that normally inhibit acetylcholine release.[31]

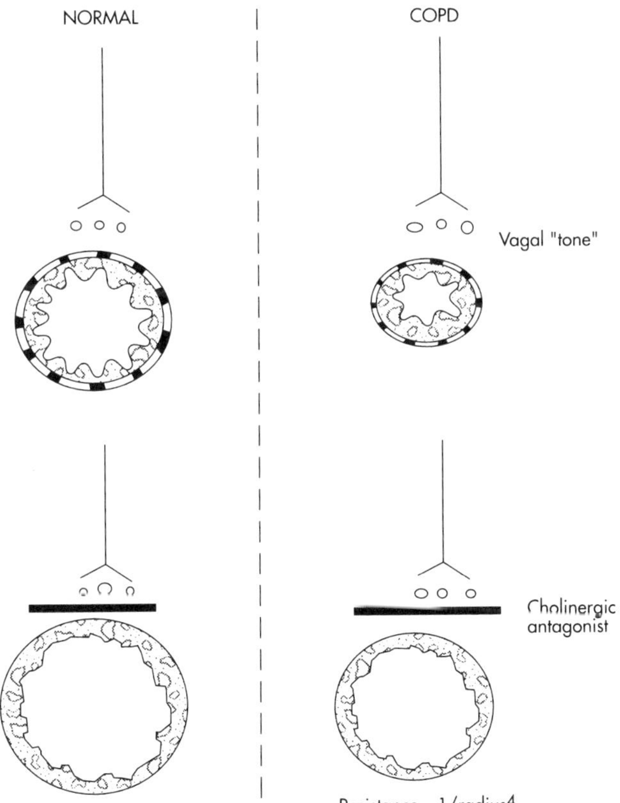

Figure 29.6 Anticholinergics may be particulary useful in chronic obstructive pulmonary disease (COPD) in which vagal cholinergic tone is the only reversible element in airway obstruction. The effect of anticholinergics is exaggerated by the fact that there is structural narrowing of the airways in COPD, and so inhibition of normal vagal tone has a relatively greater bronchodilator effect than in normal individuals.

Methylxanthines

The bronchodilator effect of strong coffee was described by Dr. Hyde Salter during the 19th centry, and methylxanthines such as theophylline, which are related to caffeine, have been used in the treatment of asthma since 1930. Indeed, theophylline is the most widely used antiasthma therapy worldwide. Theophylline has become a more useful therapy now that blood levels can readily be determined and reliable slow-relase preparations are available. However, the frequency of side-effects and the relative low efficacy of theophylline have led to reduced usage in many countries, since beta-agonists are far more effective as bronchodilators and inhaled steroids have a much greater anti-inflammatory effect.

Chemistry

Theophylline is a methylxanthine similar in structure to the common dietary xanthines, caffeine and theobromine (Fig. 29.8). Several substituted derivatives have been synthesized, but none has any advantage over theophylline, apart from the 3-propyl derivative, enprofylline, which is more potent as a bronchodilator and may have fewer toxic effects. Many salts of theophylline have also been marketed, the most common being aminophylline, which is the ethylenediamine salt used to increase solubility at neutral pH. Other salts, such as choline theophyllinate, do not have any advantage; others, such as acepifylline, are virtually inactive.[r14]

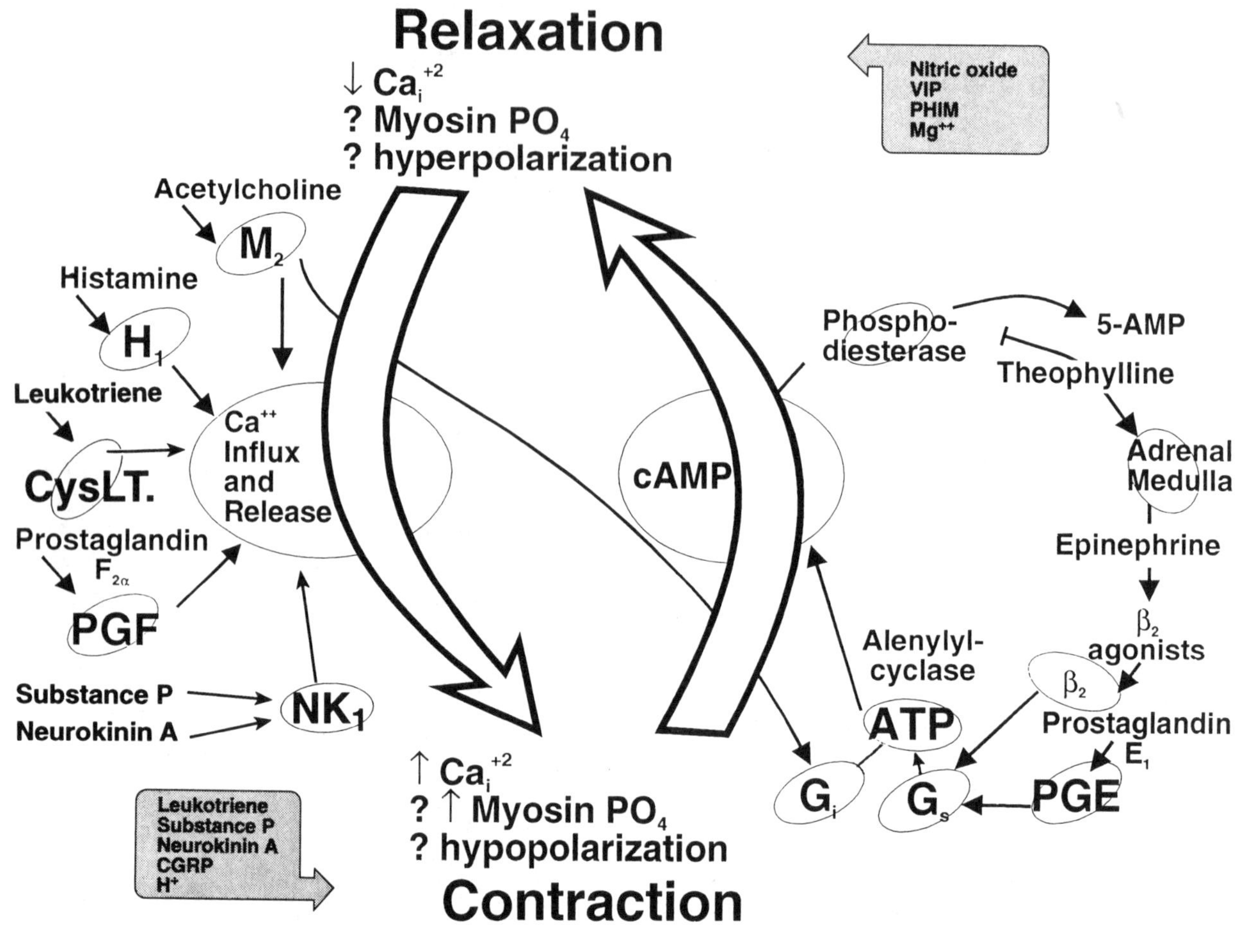

Figure 29.7 Factors that alter bronchomotor tone:
Ca_i = intracellular calcium ion activity
→ = stimulation
⊥ = inhibition or antagonism
G_i = GTP binding protein that inhibits adenylyl cyclase
G_s = GTP binding protein that stimulates adenylyl cyclase
5-AMP = Adenosine 5′ monophosphate
cAMP = 3′5′ cyclic adenosine monophosphate
ATP = adenosine 5′ triphosphate
VIP = vasoactive intestinal peptide
PHI/M = peptide histidine - isoleucine/methionine
CGRP = calcitonin gene related peptide
Shaded boxes = neural or nonneural autocoids locally synthesized or released in the vicinity of bronchiolar muscle.

Mode of Action

Although theophylline has been in clinical use for more than 50 years, its mode of action is still uncertain. Several modes have been proposed.[r15]

1. Phosphodiesterase Inhibition

It is still widely held that the bronchodilator effect of theophylline is due to inhibition of the Type III or IV phosphodiesterase (PDE), which breaks down cyclic AMP in smooth muscle cells, thereby leading to an increase in intracellular cyclic AMP concentrations.[59] However, the degree of inhibition of this enzyme is only trivial at therapeutically relevant concentrations of theophylline, and there is no evidence that airway smooth muscle cells concentrate theophylline to achieve higher intracellular than circulating concentrations. Other drugs that have a greater inhibitory effect on PDE, such as dipyridamole and papaverine, have no bronchodilator effect. Furthermore, inhibition of PDE should lead to synergistic interaction with beta-agonists, but this has not been convincingly demonstrated

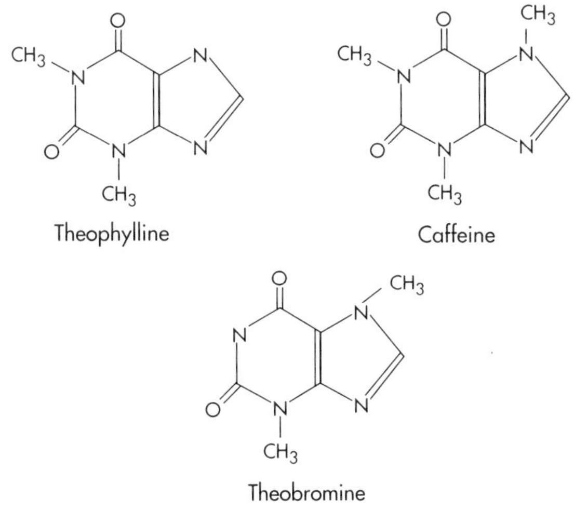

Theophylline

Caffeine

Theobromine

Figure 29.8

in vivo. Several isozymes of PDE have now been identified, and inhibitors of specific isoenzymes relevant to airway smooth muscle are now in clinical trials.[r18,33,59]

2. Adenosine Receptor Antagonism

Theophylline is a potent inhibitor of adenosine receptors at therapeutic concentrations, suggesting that this could be the basis for its bronchodilator effects.[34] Although adenosine has little effect on human airway smooth muscle in vitro, it causes bronchoconstriction in asthmatic subjects when given by inhalation.[35] This bronchoconstriction is prevented by therapeutic concentrations of theophylline.[36] However, this only confirms that theophylline is capable of antagonizing the effects of adenosine at therapeutic concentrations. Enprofylline, which is more potent than theophylline as a bronchodilator,[37] has no significant inhibitory effect on adenosine receptors, suggesting that adenosine antagonism is an unlikely explanation for the bronchodilator effect of theophylline. Adenosine antagonism may account for some of the side-effects of theophylline, however, such as CNS stimulation, cardiac arrhythmias and diuresis.[38]

3. Endogenous Catecholamine Release

Theophylline increases the secretion of epinephrine from the adrenal medulla, although the increase in plasma concentration is small and may be insufficient to account for any significant bronchodilator effect;[39] the tachycardia observed with high doses of theophylline is correlated with increased plasma catecholamine concentrations.

4. Prostaglandin Inhibition

Theophylline antagonizes the effect of some prostaglandins on vascular smooth muscle in vitro, but there is no evidence that these effects are seen at therapeutic concentrations or are relevant to airway effects.

5. Calcium Influx

There is some evidence that theophylline may interfere with calcium mobilization in airway smooth muscle.[40] Theophylline has no effect on entry of calcium ions via voltage-dependent channels, but it has been suggested that it may influence calcium entry via receptor-operated channels, release from intracellular stores, or have some effect on phosphatidylinositol turnover. Studies in airway smooth muscle have shown no effects of theophylline on receptor-operated calcium channels or on phosphatidylinositol turnover, however.[41]

6. Unknown Mechanisms

Despite extensive study, it has been difficult to elucidate a single molecular mechanism for the bronchodilating or other antiasthma actions of theophylline. It is possible that its beneficial effect in asthma is related to its action on other cells (such as platelets, neutrophils or macrophages) in addition to airway smooth muscle. It may be relevant that theophylline is ineffective when given by inhalation,[42] but is effective when a critical plasma concentration is reached. This may indicate that it is having important effects on cells other than those in the airway.

Actions of Theophylline

The primary effect of theophylline is assumed to be relaxation of airway smooth muscle, and in vitro studies have shown that it is equally effective in large or small airways.[43] However, theophylline is a rather weak bronchodilator at therapeutically relevant concentrations, suggesting that some other target cell may be more relevant. Theophylline inhibits mast cell mediator release, increases mucociliary clearance, and prevents the development of microvascular leakiness; therefore, it may be considered "anti-inflammatory".[r16] Theophylline has inhibitory actions on T-lymphocytes that may be relevant to the control of chronic airway inflammation, but has no effect on eosinophil degranulation at clinically relevant concentrations.[44]

In addition, aminophylline apparently increases the contractility of the fatigued diaphragm in humans,[45] although whether this is relevant clinically in respiratory failure is uncertain.

Pharmacokinetics

There is a close relationship between improvement in airway function and serum theophylline concentration. Below 10 mg/L, therapeutic effects are small; above 25 mg/L additional benefits are outweighed by side-effects; thus, the therapeutic range is usually taken as 10–20 mg/L.[1] The dose of theophylline required to give these therapeutic concentrations varies between subjects, largely because of differences in clearance. In addition, there may be differences in bronchodilator response to theophylline and, with acute bronchoconstriction, higher concentrations may be required to produce bronchodilation.[46]

Theophylline is rapidly and completely absorbed, but there are large interindividual variations in clearance, due to differences in hepatic metabolism. Theophylline is metabolized in the liver by the cytochrome P450/P448 microsomal enzyme system, and a large number of factors may influence hepatic metabolism[r14] (Table 29.1). Increased clearance is seen in children (1–16 years), and in cigarette and marijuana smokers, with concurrent administration of phenytoin and phenobarbital, so that higher doses may be required. Reduced clearance is found in liver disease, pneumonia, heart failure, and with drugs such as erythromycin, allopurinol, and cimetidine (but not ranitidine) that interfere with cytochrome P450. Thus, if a patient on maintenance theophylline requires a course of erythromycin, the dose of theophylline should be reduced. Viral infections and vaccination may also reduce clearance. Because of these variations in clearance, individualization of theophylline dosage is required; and plasma concentrations should be measured four hours after dosing with slow-release preparations when steady-state has been achieved. There is no significant circadian variation in theophylline metabolism,[47] although there may be delayed absorption at night, which may relate to the supine posture.[48]

Routes of Administration

Intravenous

IV aminophylline has been used for many years in the treatment of acute severe asthma. The recommended dose is now 6 mg/kg given IV over 20–30 minutes, followed by a maintenance dose of 0.5 mg/kg/hr. If the patient is already taking theophylline, or there are any factors that decrease clearance, these doses should be halved and the plasma level checked more frequently.

Table 29.1 Factors That Affect Theophylline Clearance

Increased clearance	Decreased clearance
Enzyme induction by rifampicin phenobarbitone ethanol	Enzyme inhibition by cimetidine erythormycin allupurinol
Smoking tobacco marijuana	Congrestive cardiac failure Liver disease
High-protein, low-carbohydrate diet	Pneumonia
Barbequed meat	Viral infection and vaccination
Childhood	High carbohydrate diet Old age

Oral

Plain theophylline tablets or elixir, which are rapidly absorbed, give wide fluctuations in plasma levels and are not recommended. Several effective sustained-release preparations are now available; these are absorbed at a constant rate and provide steady plasma concentrations over a 24-hour period.[r17] Although there are differences between preparations, these are minor and of no clinical significance. Both slow-release aminophylline and theophylline are available and are equally effective (although the ethylenediamine component of aminophylline has very occasionally been implicated in allergic reactions). For continuous treatment, twice daily therapy (approximately 8 mg/kg twice daily) is needed, although some preparations are designed for once-daily administration. For nocturnal asthma a single dose of slow-release theophylline at night is often effective.[49,50] Once optimal doses have been determined, plasma concentrations usually remain stable, provided no factors that alter clearance change.

Other theophylline salts, such as choline theophyllinate, have no advantgages; some derivatives, such as acepiphylline, diprophylline, and proxophylline, are less effective. Compound tablets that contain adrenergic agonists and sedatives in addition to theophylline should be avoided.

Other Routes

Aminophylline may be given as a suppository, but rectal absorption is unreliable and proctitis may occur, so this route is best avoided. Inhalation of theophylline is irritant and ineffective.[41] Intramuscular injections of theophylline are very painful and should never be given.

Side-Effects

Unwanted effects of theophylline are usually related to plasma concentration and tend to occur when plasma levels exceed 200mg/L. However, some patients develop side-effects even at low concentrations. To some extent side effects may be reduced by gradually increasing the dose until therapeutic concentrations are achieved. The commonest side-effects are headache, nausea and vomiting, abdominal discomfort, and restlessness. There may also be increased acid secretion and diuresis. At high concentrations, convulsions and cardiac arrthymias may occur. Some of the side-effects (central stimulation, gastric secretion, diuresis, and arrythmias) may be due to adenosine receptor antagonism and may therefore be avoided by using drugs such as enprofylline, which has no significant adenosine antagonism at bronchodilator doses.[37] There has recently been concern that theophylline, even at therapeutic concentrations, may lead to behavioral disturbance and learning difficulties in school children,[51] although it is difficult to design adequate controls for such studies.

Clinical Use

In patients with acute asthma iv aminophylline is less effective than nebulized beta-agonists,[52] and should therefore be reserved for patients who fail to respond to beta-agonists. Theophylline has little or no effect on bronchomotor tone in normal airways,[53] but reverses bronchoconstriction in asthmatic patients,[r14] although it is less effective than inhaled beta-agonists and is more likely to have unwanted effects. There is good evidence that theophylline and beta-agonists have additive effects, even if true synergy is not seen,[54]

Table 29.2 Summary Table

Drug	Dosage			Pharmacokinetics			
	Route	Size	Dose	Peak	V_D	$t_{1/2}$	Cl or Duration of Response
Aminophylline (Aminophyllin)	oral tablets	100+200 mg	3 mg/lg q 6–8 hr	1–2 hr	0.45 l/kg	3–13 hrs	0.65 ml/kg/hr
	oral extended release	225 mg		5 hour			
	parenteral	25 mg/m	load maintenance = 5 mg/kg hr				
	rectal suppositories	250 + 500 mg					
Dyphylline (Lufyllin)	Oral Tablets	200 mg					2 hours
	Parenteral	250 mg/ml					
Albuterol	oral-inhalation aerosol	90 µg/ inhalation	2 inhalations q 4–6 hours	2–5 min		2–7 hours	
(Salbutamol) (Proventil) (Ventolin)	Oral Tablets	2+4 mg					
	Oral Inhalation powder	200 µg/ inhalation					
Bitolterol (Tornalate)	Oral Inhalation aerosol	370 µg/ spray	2 inhalation q8hr	1 hour		3 hour	
Ephedrine	Oral Capsule	25+50 mg	25–50 mg q 3–4 hours	19–60 min.		6 hours	effect persists 2–4 hours
	Parenteral	5,25,50 mg/ml		immediate		6 hours	effect persists 1 hour
Epinephrine (Bronkaid)	Parenteral	1 mg/ml	0.1–0.5 mg sq	20 min			
(Primatene)	Oral aerosal	10 mg/ml	200 µg/spray				
Isoethorine	Oral Nebulization	0.062–1%	340 µg/spray	5–15 min			
Isoprotererol (Isuprel)	Oral	0.25% aerosol	120–262 µg/ inhalation	immediate			persists 1 hr
Metaproterenol		10 mg tablet or/5 ml solution	20 mg qid	1 hour			persists 1–3 hours
(Alupent)	Oral	0.65 mg/ aerosol spray	2–3 spray/ q 4 hours	immediate			
Terbutaline	Oral	2.55 mg tablets	qid	2–3 hours			lasts 4–8 hours
(Brethine)		200 µg/ aerosol spray	400 ug 4–6 x/ day	1–2 hours			last 2–4 hours
Ipratropium (Atrovent)	Oral	18 µmg/ inhalation aerosol	2 inhalation qid	1–2 hours		2 hours	last 3–4 hours

and there is evidence that theophylline may provide an additional bronchodilator effect even when maximally effective doses of beta-agonist have been given.[55] This means that, if adequate bronchodilation is not achieved by beta-agonist alone, theophylline may be added to the maintenance therapy with benefit. Theophylline is useful for nocturnal asthma, since slow-release preparations are able to provide therapeutic concentrations overnight and are more effective than slow-release beta-agonists. Although theophylline is less effective than a beta-agonist and corticosteroids, a minority of asthmatic patients appear to derive unexpected benefit, and even patients on oral steroids may show a deterioration in lung function when theophylline is withdrawn.[56]

Theophylline also may benefit patients with COPD, increasing exercise tolerance,[57] although without any improvement in spirometry tests unless combined with an inhaled beta-agonist. However, theophylline may reduce trapped gas volume, suggesting an effect on peripheral airways,[58] and this may explain why some patients obtain considerable symptomatic improvement.

New Bronchodilators

Although several new bronchodilators are under development (potassium channel openers, selective PDE inhibitors, etc), it is unlikely that they will have any major advantages over inhaled β_2 agonists.[r19]

Acknowledgement

We thank Madeleine Wray and Linda McKeel for preparing this manuscript.

References

Research Reports

1. Zaagsma J, van derHeijden RJCM, van der Schaar MWG, Blank CMC. Comparison of functional beta-adrenoceptor heterogeneity in central and peripheral airway smooth muscle of guinea pig and man. J Recept Res 1983;*3*:89–106.
2. Carstairs JR, Nimmo AJ, Barnes PJ. Autoradiographic visualization of beta-adrenoceptor subtypes in human lung. Am Rev Respir Dis 1985;*132*:541–547.
3. Torphy TJ, Freese WB, Rinard GA, Brunton LL, Mayer SE. Cyclic nucleotide-dependent protein kinases in airway smooth muscle. J Biol Chem 1982;*257*:11609–11616.
4. Silver PJ, Stull JT. Phosphorylation of myosin light chain kinase and phosphorylase in tracheal smooth muscle in response to KCL and carbachol. Mol Pharmacol 1984;*25*:267–274.
5. Church MK, Hiroi J. Inhibition of IgE-dependent histamine release from human dispersed lung mast cells by anti-allergic drugs and salbutamol. Br J Pharmacol 1987;*90*:421–249.
6. Howarth PH, Durham SR, Lee TH, Kay AB, Church MK, Holgate ST. Influence of albuterol, cromolyn sodium and ipratropium bromide on the airway and circulating mediator responses to allergen bronchial provocation in asthma. Am Rev Respir Dis 1985;*132*:986–992.
7. Erjefalt I, Persson OGA. Anti-asthma drugs attenuate inflammatory leakage into airway lumen. Acta Physiol Scand 1986;*128*:653–655.
8. Rhoden KJ, Meldrum LA, Barnes PJ. Inhibition of cholinergic neurotranmission in human airways by beta2-adrenoceptors. J Appl Physiol 1988;*65*:700–705.
9. Boschetto P, Roberts NM, Rogers DF, Barnes PJ. Effect of anti-asthma drugs on microvascular leakage in guinea-pig airways. Am Rev Respir Dis 1989;*139*:416–421.
10. Coupe MO, Guly U, Brown E, Barnes PJ. Nebulised adrenaline in acute severe asthma: comparison with salbutamol. Eur J Respir Dis 1987;*71*:227–232.
11. Barnes PJ, Pride NB. Dose-response curves to inhaled beta-adrenoceptor agonists in normal and asthmatic subjects. Br J Clin Pharmacol 1983;*15*:677–682.
12. Ullman A, Svedmyr N. Salmeterol, a new long acting inhaled β_2-adrenoceptor agonist: comparison with salbutamol in adult asthmatic patients. Thorax 1988;*43*:674–678.
13. Anderson SD, Seale JP, Rozea P, Bandler L, Theobald G, Lindsay DA. Inhaled and oral salbutanol in exercise-induced asthma. Am Rev Respir Dis 1976;*114*:493–498.
14. Williams S, Winner SJ, Clark TJH. Comparison of inhaled and intravenous terbutaline in acute severe asthma. Thorax 1981;*36*:629–631.
15. O'Driscoll BRC, Ruffles SP, Ayres JG, Cochrane GM. Long term treatment of severe asthma with subcutaneous terbutaline. Br J Dis Chest 1988;*82*:360–367.
16. Haalboom JRE, Deenstra A, Struyvenberg A. Hypokalaemia induced by inhalation of fenoterol. Lancet 1985;*1*:1125–1127.
17. Schnack C, Podolsky A, Watzke H, Schernthaner G, Burghuber OC. Effects of somatostatin and oral potassium administration on terbutaline-induced hypokalemia. Am Rev Respir Dis 1989;*139*:176–180.
18. Maguire WG, Nair S. Ventilation and perfusion effects of inhaled alpha and beta agonists in asthma patients. Chest 1978;*73*(Suppl):983–985.
19. Wilson JD, Sutherland DC, Thomas AC. Has the change to beta agonists combined with oral theophylline increased cases of fatal asthma? Lancet 1981;*1*:1235–1237.
20. Benatar SR. Fatal asthma. N Eng J Med 1986;*314*:423–429.
21. Makino S, Ouellette JJ, Reed CE, Fisher C. Correlation between increased bronchial response to acetylcholine and diminished metabolic and eosinopenic responses to epinephrine in asthma J Allergy 1970;*46*:178–179.
22. Shah PKD, Lakhotia M, Mehta S, Join SK, Gupta GL. Clinical dysautonomia in patients with bronchial asthma. Chest 1990;*98*:1408–1413.
23. Ullah MI, Newman GB, Saunders KB. Influence of age on response to ipratropium and salbutamol in asthma. Thorax 1981;*36*:523–529.
24. Ward MJ, Fentem PH, Roderick Smith WH, Daview D. Ipratropium bromide in acute asthma. Br Med J 1981;*282*:590–600.
25. Rebuck AS, Chapman KR, Abboud R, Pare PD, Kreisman H, Walkove N, Vickerson P. Nebulized anticholinergic and sympa-

thomimetic treatment of asthma and chronic obstructive airways disease in the emergency room. Am J Med 1987;*82*:59–64.

26. Gross NJ, Skorodin MS. Role of the parasympathetic system in airway obstruction due to emphysema. N Engl J Med 1984;*311*:321–325.
27. Newcomb R, Tashkin DP, Hu KK, Conolly ME, Lee E, Dauphinee B. Rebound hyperresponsiveness to muscarininc stimulation after chronic therapy with an inhaled muscarinic antagonist. Am Rev Respir Dis 1985;*132*:12–15.
28. Yeates DB, Aspin N, Levison H, Jones MT, Bryan AC. Mucociliary tracheal transport rates in man. J Appl Physiol 1975;*39*:487–495.
29. Pavia D, Bateman JRM, Sheahan NF, Clark SW. Effect of ipratropium bromide on mucociliary clearance and pulmonary function in reversible airways obstruction. Thorax 1979;*34*:501–507.
30. Rafferty P, Beasley R, Holgate ST. Comparison of the efficacy of preservative free ipratropium bromide and Atrovent nebuliser solution. Thorax 1988;*43*:446–450.
31. Barnes PJ. Muscarinic receptor subtypes: implications for lung disease. Thorax 1989;*44*:161–167.
32. Fredholm BB, Persson OGA. Xanthine derivatives as adenosine receptor antagonists. Eur J Pharmacol 1982;*81*:673–676.
33. Handslip PDJ, Dart AM, Davies BH. Intravenous salbutamol and aminophylline in asthma: a search for synergy. Thorax 1981;*36*:741–744.
34. Cushley MJ, Tattersfield AE, Holgate ST. Inhaled adenosine and guanosine on airway resistance in normal and asthmatic subjects. Br J Clin Pharmacol 1983;*15*:161–165.
35. Cushley MJ, Tattersfield AE, Holgate ST. Adenosine-induced bronchoconstriction in asthma: antagonism by inhaled theophylline. Am Rev Respir Dis 1984;*129*:380–384.
36. Persson OGA. Development of safer xanthine drugs for the treatment of obstructive airways disease. J Allergy Clin Immunol 1986;*78*:817–824.
37. Higbee MD, Kumar M, Galant SP. Stimulation of endogenous catecholamine release by theophylline: a proposed additional mechanism for theophylline effects. J Allergy Clin Immunol 1982;*70*:377–382.
38. Kolbeck RC, Speir WA, Carrier GO, Bransome ED. Apparent irrelevance of cyclic nucleotides to the relaxation of tracheal smooth muscle induced by theophylline. Lung 1979;*156*:173–183.
39. Grandordy B, Cuss FM, Barnes PJ. The effect of anti-asthma drugs on phosphatidylinositol turnover in airway smooth muscle. Life Sci 1987;*41*:1661–1667.
40. Cushley MJ, Holgate ST. Bronchodilator actions of xanthine derivatives administered by inhalation in asthma. Thorax 1985;*40*:176–179.
41. Finney MJB, Karlsson J-A, Persson OGA. Effects of bronchoconstrictors and bronchodilators on a novel human small airway preparation. Br J Pharmacol 1985;*85*:29–36.
42. Yukawa T, Kroegel C, Dent G, Chanez P, Ukena D, Barnes PJ. Effect of theophylline and adenosine on eosinophil function. Am Rev Respir Dis 1989;*140*:327–333.
43. Dutoit JI, Salome CM, Woolcock AJ. Inhaled corticosteroids reduce the severity of bronchial hyperresponsiveness in asthma, but oral theophylline does not. Am Rev Respir Dis 1987;*136*:1174–1178.
44. Aubier M, De Troyer A, Sampson M, Macklem PT, Roussos C. Aminophylline improves diaphragmatic contractility. N Engl J Med 1981;*305*:249–252.
45. Vozeh S, Kewitz G, Perruchoud A, et al. Theophylline serum concentration and therapeutic effect in severe acute bronchial obstruction: the optimal use of intravenously administered aminophylline. Am Rev Respir Dis 1982;*125*:181–184.
46. Taylor DR, Duffin D, Kinney CD, McDevitt DG. Investigation of diurnal changes in the disposition of theophylline. Br J Clin Pharmacol 1983;*16*:413–416.
47. Warren JB, Cuss F, Barnes PJ. Posture and theophylline kinetics. Br J Clin Pharmacol 1985;*19*:707–709.
48. Barnes PJ, Greening AP, Neville L, Timmers J, Poole GW. Single dose slow-release aminophylline at night prevents nocturnal asthma. Lancet 1982;*1*:299–301.
49. Neuenkirchen H, Wilkens JH, Cellerich M, Sybrecht GW. Nocturnal asthma and sustained release theophylline. Eur J Respir Dis 1985;*66*:196–204.
50. Rachelefsky GS, Wo J, Adelson J, Mickey MR, Spector SL, Katz RM, Siegel SC, Rahr AS. Behavior abnormalities and poor school performance due to oral theophylline use. Pediatrics 1986;*78*:1133–1138.
51. Rossing TH, Fanta CH, Goldstein DH, Snapper JR, McFadden ER. Emergency therapy of asthma: comparison of acute effects of parenteral and inhaled sympathomimetic and infused aminophylline. Am Rev Respir Dis 1980;*122*:365–371.
52. Estenne M, Yernault J, De Troyer A. Effects of parenteral aminophylline on lung mechanics in normal humans. Am Rev Respir Dis 1980;*121*:967–971.
53. Shenfield GM. Combination bronchodilator therapy. Drugs 1982;*24*:414–439.
54. Barclay J, Whiting B, Meredith PA. Addis GJ. Theophylline-salbutamol interactions: bronchodilator response to salbutamol at maximally effective plasma theophylline concentrations. Br J Clin Pharmacol 1981;*11*:203–208.
55. Brenner, Mo, Bgrkowitz NM, Strunk RC. Need for theophylline in severe steroid-requiring asthmatics. Clin Allergy 1988;*18*:143–150.
56. Taylor DR, Buick B, Kinney C, Lowry RC, McDevitt DG. The efficacy of orally administered theophylline, inhaled salbutamol, and a combination of the two as chronic therapy in the management of chronic bronchitis with reversible air-flow obstruction. Am Rev Respir Dis 1985;*131*:747–751.
57. Chrystyn H, Mulley BA, Peake MD. Dose response relation to oral theophylline in severe chronic obstructive airways disease. Br Med J 1988;*297*:1506–1510.
58. Tomkinson A, Karlsson JA, and Raeburn D. Comparison of the effects of selective inhibition of phosphodiesterase Types III and IV in airway smooth muscle with differing β adrenoceptor types. Br J Pharmacol 1993;*108*:57–61.

Reviews

r1. Barnes RJ. Asthma therapy: basic mechanisms. Eur J Respir Dis 1986;*68*(Suppl 144):217–265.

r2. Barnes RJ. Airway pharmacology. In: Murray JF, Nadel JA, (eds): Textbook of Respiratory Medicine (2nd Edition). Philadelphia: WB Saunders, press. 1988; pp 249–268.

r3. McFadden ER. Beta 2 receptor agonists—metabolism and pharmacology. J Allergy Clin Immunol 1981;*68*:91–96.

r4. Iversen LL. Role of transmitter uptake mechanisms in synaptic neurotransmission. Br J Pharmacol 1971;*41*:571–591.

r5. Nelson HS. Adrenergic therapy of bronchial asthma. J Allergy Clin Immunol 1986;*77*:771–785.

r6. Newhouse MT, Dolovich MB. Control of asthma by aerosols. N Engl J Med 1986;*315*:870–874.

r7. Barnes PJ, Chung KF. Questions about inhaled β_2 agonists in asthma. Trends in Pharmacol. Sci. 1993;*13*:200–203.

r8. Barnes RJ. New Approach to the treatment of asthma. N Engl J Med 1989;*321*:1517–1527.

r9. Barnes PJ. Muscarinic receptor subtypes in airways. Life Sci. 1993;*52*:521–528.

r10. Barnes PJ. State of art. Neural control of human airways in health and disease. Am Rev Respir Dis 1986;*134*:1289–1314.

r11. Gross NJ, Skorodin MS. Anticholinergic antimuscarinic bronchodilators. Am Rev Respir Dis 1984;*129*:856–870.

r12. Mann JS, George CF. Anticholinergic drugs in the treatment of airways disease. Br J Dis Chest 1985;*79*:209–228.

r13. Gross NJ. Ipratropium bromide. N Engl J Med 1988;*319*:486–494.

r14. Weinburger M. The pharmacology and therapeutic use of theophylline. Allergy Clin Immunol 1984;*73*:525–540.

r15. Barnes PJ. Mode of action of theophylline: a multiplicity of actions. Int Congr Symposia Series. 1988;*126*:39–45.

r16. Weinberger M, Hendeles L. Slow-release theophylline. Rationale and basis for product selection. N Engl J Med 1983;*308*:760–764.

r17. Persson OGA. Overview of effects of theophylline. J Allergy Clin Immunol 1986;*78*:780–787.

r18. Torphy TJ, Urdem BJ. Phosphodiesterase inhibitors: New Opportunities for the treatment of asthma. Thorax 1991;*46*:512–523.

r19. Barnes PJ. New drugs for asthma. Eur Resp J 1992;*5*:1126–1136.

r20. Torphy TJ. Selective inhibitors of phosphodiesterase as bronchodilators. In Barnes PJ, (ed) New Drugs for Asthma. London: IBC Publications 1989; pp 199.

CHAPTER 30

Anti-Inflammatory Management of Bronchospastic Disease

Peter J. Barnes
Robert A. Mueller

Corticosteroids

Corticosteroids were introduced for the treatment of asthma shortly after their discovery in the 1950s, and they remain the most effective therapy available for asthma. However, side-effects and fear of adverse effects have limited their use, and there has therefore been considerable research into discovering new or related agents that retain the beneficial action on airways, without unwanted effects. The introduction of inhaled steroids has been a major advance in the treatment of chronic asthma. Now asthma is viewed as a chronic inflammatory disease, and inhaled steroids may even be considered as first-line therapy.[r1]

Chemistry

The adrenal cortex secretes cortisol (hydrocortisone); by experimental modification of its structure, it was possible to develop derivatives such as prednisolone and dexamethasone that exhibited enhanced corticosteroid effects, but with reduced mineralcorticoid activity (see Chapter 44). Those derivatives with potent glucocorticoid actions were effective in asthma when given systemically, but had no antiasthmatic activity when given by inhalation.[r2] Further substitution in the 17α ester position resulted in steroids with high topical activity (such as beclomethasone dipropionate (BDP), betamethasone, and budesonide), which were potent on the skin and were later found to have significant antiasthma effects when given by inhalation.

The antiasthma potency of an inhaled steroid is approximately proportional to its anti-inflammatory potency, measured by a skin blanching test. Thus, budesonide is approximately twice as potent as BDP and 1000 times more potent than prednisolone.[r9] More recent studies have shown that to achieve maximal effects only a short exposure time to a steroid may be necessary, although the effects of the steroid may be slow in onset.[r3] This implies that, if topical steroids could be metabolized locally, the full local effect may be obtained but the incidence of systemic side-effects should be reduced, which would allow higher inhaled doses to be administered. Such local metabolism occurs to some extent with both budesonide and BDP, but further improvements may be possible.

Mode of Action

1. Steroid Receptors

Most steroid effects are mediated by interaction with specfic receptors, but, at concentrations higher than those used therapeutically, nonspecfic effects due to insertion into the cell membrane may be seen. Steroids enter target cells and combine with specific receptors within the cytoplasm (Fig. 30.1). These receptors are specific to certain classes of steroids (such as corticosteroids, androgens, estrogens) but each class is similar in all tissues. The steroid-receptor complex is transported to the nucleus, where it initiates (or represses) DNA transcription of specific messenger RNAs. This altered protein synthesis eventually brings about the steroid effect. This sequence of events may take some time and explains why the onset of steroid effects is usually several hours. However, corticosteroids can have more rapid effects on calcium ion flux and vascular permeability, which may be independent of protein synthesis.

2. Lipocortin

Corticosteroids inhibit the release of arachidonic acid metabolites from lung and macrophages by the

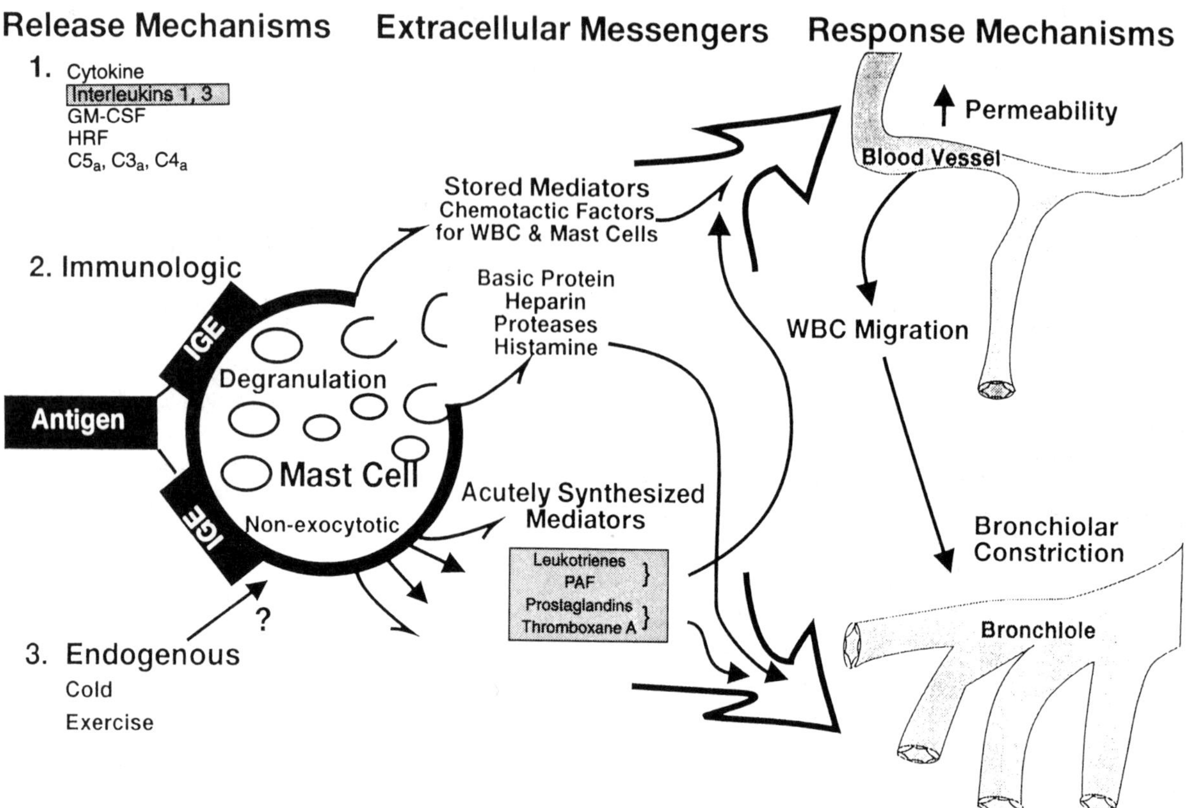

Figure 30.1 Initiation of inflammatory responses in the bronchial environment. On the left side of the figure are the three major types of mechanisms that can trigger a pulmonary airway inflammatory reaction by activating mast cells (left of center). Degranulation and/or nonexocytotic release of stored or rapidly synthesized mediators from the activated mast cells can produce bronchiolar constriction directly (lower right) or amplify the inflammatory response by increasing the permeability of the pulmonary capillaries and further white blood cell invasion (upper right).

GM-CSF = Granulocyte macrophage colony simulating factor
HRF = Histamine releasing factor
$C5_a$,$C3_a$,$C4_a$ = components of the complement cascade
IGE = Immunoglobulins of the E type
PAF = Platelet activating factor
Shaded areas = components whose synthesis or activity is thought to be inhibited by glucocorticoid administration.

production of a protein called macrocortin, which is thought to be an inhibitor of phospholipase A_2 in the cell membrane.[r4,2] Steroids similarly inhibit release of arachidonic acid from membrane phospholipids in neutrophils, and an inhibitory protein called lipomodulin has been isolated.[3] Purification and characterization studies indicate that macrocortin and lipomodulin are probably identical, so that they are now referred to as lipocortin. This 37kD protein has now been cloned and expressed. This provides a unitary hypothesis for the mode of action of steroids through inhibition of phospholipase A_2 (and thus the formation of prostaglandins, leukotrienes, and platelet activating factor) (Fig. 30.2). Steroids may also inhibit other phospholipases such as phospholipase C. It is now thought unlikely that lipocortin can account for all the effects of steroids. Although the rapid effects of steroids could not be mediated by synthesis of lipocortin, there is evidence that this protein may be stored in the cell. Inhibition of phospholipase A_2 may account for inhibition of neutrophil and macrophage chemotaxis, lymphocyte mitogenesis, and inflammatory mediator secretion; but is unlikely to account for all the actions of steroids (see Fig. 30.2). It is likely that steroids induce the synthesis of several regulatory proteins through multiple steroid-sensitive genes.

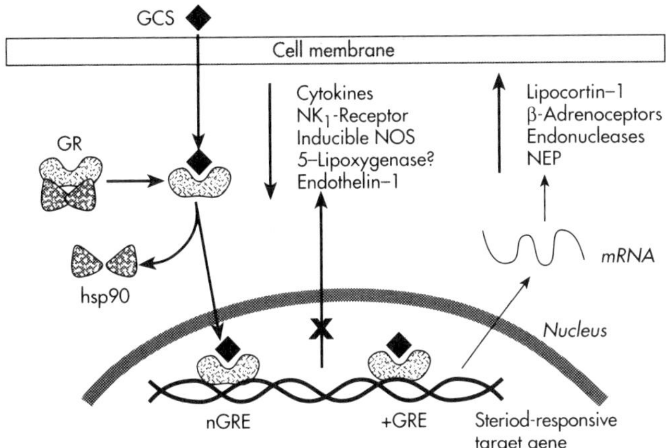

Figure 30.2 Possible mode of action of corticosteroids. Steroids bind to a cytosolic receptor that induces the transcription of a messenger RNA that codes for lipocortin and presumably other proteins (yet to be identified). Lipocortin inhibits phospholipase A_2 (PLA2), which is involved in the formation of lipid mediators such as prostaglandins (PG), leukotrines (LT) and platelet activating factor (PAF). GCS = Glucocorticosteroid; GR = Glucocorticoid Receptor; hsp 90 = Heat Shock Protein of 90 kDa molecular weight; GRE = Glucocorticoid Response Element, nGRE = negative Glucorticoid Response Element, NK_1 Receptor = $Neurokinin_1$ Receptor activation, NOS = Nitric Oxide Synthetase

Anti-Inflammatory Effects

The mechanism of action of corticosteroids in asthma is still poorly understood, but is most likely to be related to their anti-inflammatory properties.[r5–r8] There is increasing evidence that asthma and bronchial hyperresponsiveness are due to an inflammatory process in the airways and that several components of this inflammatory response might be inhibited by steroids.

Steroids potently inhibit the accumulation of neutrophils,[4] probably by inhibiting the production of chemotactic factors in tissues[5] (Fig. 30.2). They inhibit secretion by human pulmonary macrophages of leukotrienes and prostaglandins,[6] but have no direct action on human lung mast cells.[7] They also cause eosinopenia and inhibit degranulation and adherence of eosinophils.[8] In addition, they induce a fall in circulating T-lymphocytes and may lead to the formation of an IgE-binding suppressive factor.[9] Steroids also inhibit the formation of several cytokines, including interleukin-1, interleukin 2, interleukin-5, tumor necrosis factor α, and granulocyte-macrophage colony stimulating factor.[10] (See Fig. 30.2)

Steroids prevent and reverse the increase in vascular permeability due to inflammatory mediators and may therefore lead to resolution of airway edema.[11,12]

Effect on Airway Function

Steroids have no direct effect on airway smooth muscle, and improvement in lung function is presumably due to an effect on the chronic airway inflammation and bronchial reactivity.[r8] In a single dose, inhaled steroids have no effect on the early response to allergen (reflecting their lack of effect on mast cells), but do inhibit the late response (which may be due to an effect on macrophages and eosinophils); they also inhibit the increase in bronchial reactivity. Inhaled steroids also reduce bronchial hyperreactivity, but this effect may require several weeks or months and presumably reflects the slow healing of the damaged inflamed airway.[r9] Steroids have no immediate effect on the early bronchoconstrictor response to allergen or exercise but, if they are taken over several weeks, there is a reduction even in the acute constrictor responses.[13] This could be due to reduced bronchial responsiveness or to a reduction in mast cell numbers in airway tissue (which has been demonstrated in the nasal mucosa after topical steroids).[14]

Effect on Beta-Receptors

Steroids increase beta-adrenergic responsiveness, but whether this is relevant to their effect in asthma is uncertain. Steroids potentiate the effects of beta-agonists on bronchial smooth muscle and prevent and reverse beta-receptor tachyphylaxis in airways in vitro.[15] In vivo steroids similarly reverse tolerance to beta-agonists in dogs[16] and normal humans.[17] Steroids increase the density of beta-receptors in rat lung membranes,[18] increase the proportion of receptors in the high-affinity binding state in human leukocytes, and reverse and prevent the fall in leukocyte beta-receptor density after beta-agonists in normal and asthmatic subjects.[19] Steroids increase the synthesis of beta-receptor proteins at the mRNA transcription level.[20] This action of steroids of beta-receptor expression is unlikely to contribute to their anti-asthma effect, but may be clinically important in preventing the development of beta-receptor tolerance when high doses of nebulized beta-angonists are used.

Pharmacokinetics

Prednisolone is readily and consistently absorbed after oral administration with little interindividual variation. Enteric coatings to reduce the incidence of dyspepsia delay absorption but not the total amount of drug absorbed. Prednisolone is metabolized in the liver; drugs such as rifampicin, phenobarbital, or phenytoin, which induce hepatic enzymes, lower the plasma half-life of prednisolone.[21] The plasma half-life is 2–3hr, although its biologic half-life is approximately 24hr, so that it is suitable for daily dosing. There is no evidence that previous exposure to steroids changes their subsequent metabolism. Prednisolone is approximately 92 percent protein-bound, the majority to a specific protein, transcortin, and the remainder to albumin; it is the unbound fraction that is biologically active.

Some patients, usually with severe asthma, apparently fail to respond to corticosteroids. "Steroid-resistant" asthma is not due to impaired absorption or metabolism of steroids, but may be associated with a defect in responsiveness of certain cells to steroids.[22]

Routes of Administration

Oral

Prednisolone or prednisone are the most commonly used steroids, prednisolone being preferred, since prednisone is converted to prednisolone in the liver. Clinical improvement with oral steroids may take several days and the maximal beneficial effect is usually achieved with 30 mg prednisolone daily, although a few patients may need 60 mg daily to achieve control of symptoms. The usual maintenance dose is in the order of 10mg/day.

Oral steroids should be given in a single dose in the morning, since this coincides with the normal diurnal increase in plasma cortisol; there is therefore less adrenal suppression than when given in divided doses or at night. Furthermore, the amount of steroids bound to transcortin is less during the day, resulting in higher free concentrations, and this might contribute to the greater functional effect.[23] Alternate day treatment has advantages, since there is less adrenal suppression and other side-effects with similar control of asthma, although some patient's control is not optimal on this regime.

Intravenous

Parenteral steroids are indicated in acute exacerbations of asthma. Hydrocortisone is the steroid of choice as it has the most rapid onset (5–6 hr after administration),[24] being more rapid than prednisolone (8 hr). The dose required is still uncertain, but it is common to give hydrocortisone 4 mg/kg initially followed by a maintenance dose of 3 mg/kg/6 hr. These doses are based on the argument that it is necessary to maintain "stress" levels of plasma.[25]

Inhaled

Inhaled topical steroids (Table 30.1) have been a great advance in the management of chronic asthma as it may thus be possible to control symptoms without adrenal suppression or side-effects and still allow a reduction in the dose of oral maintenance steroids[r2,r7] (Table 30.2). The high topical activity of inhaled steroids means that only small doses are required, and any swallowed drug is immediately metabolized by the liver. Only when much larger doses are inhaled is sufficient steroid absorbed to cause adrenal suppression. Most patients get a maximal response at a dose of 400 μg budesonide/BDP per day, but some patients may benefit from higher doses (up to 1500 μg/day), and high-dose inhalers have therefore been introduced.[r2] Traditionally, steroid inhalers have been used four times daily, but twice-daily administration is usually as effective and compliance is better.[26]

Table 30.1 Inhaled Corticosteroids

- Beclomethasone
- Budesonide
- Triamcinoione
- Flunisolide
- Fluticasone

Table 30.2 Inhaled Steroid Preparations

	Dose	Frequency	Metab	$t_{1/2}$
Beclomethasone Dipropionate Beclovent Vanceril	42 μg/ spray	2 sprays tid/qid	high hepatic first-pass effect	15 hr
Triamcinolone Acetonide Azmacort	100 μg/ spray	2 sprays tid or qid		
Flunisolide Aerobid	250 μg/ spray	2 sprays bid		$t_{1/2}$ = 1–2 hr

Side-Effects

Steroids inhibit ACTH and cortisol secretion by a negative feedback effect on the pituitary gland. This suppression is dependent on dose, and usually occurs only when a dose of prednisolone greater than 7.5–10 mg daily is used. Significant suppression after short courses of steroid therapy usually is not a problem, but prolonged suppression may occur after several months or years. Steroid doses after prolonged oral therapy must therefore be reduced slowly. Symptoms of "steroid withdrawal syndrome" include lassitude, muscuoskeletal pains, and occasionally fever.

Side-effects of long-term corticosteroid therapy are well described and include fluid retention, increased appetitie, weight gain, osteoporosis, capillary fragility, hypertension, peptic ulceration, diabetes, cataracts, and psychoses. The frequency of side-effects increases with age. Occasionally adverse reactions (such as anaphylaxis) to IV hydrocortisone have been described, particularly in aspirin-sensitive asthmatics.

Side-effects of inhaled steroids are few.[r9] The most common problem is oropharyngeal candidiasis (which may occur in 5% of patients). Hoarseness and weakness of the voice (dysphonia) occasionally may occur and may be due to atrophy of the vocal cords. The incidence of these side-effects may be related to the local concentrations of steroid deposited and may be reduced by the use of various spacing devices that reduce oropharyngeal deposition.[27] There is no evidence for atrophy of the lining of the airway or of an increase in lung infections after inhaled steroids.

Clinical Use

Acute Asthma

Hydrocortisone is given IV in acute asthma. While the value of corticosteroids in acute severe asthma has been questioned, others have found that they speed the resolution of attacks.[r6] There is no apparent advantage in giving very high doses of IV steroids (such as methylprednisolone 1g). Intravenous steroids are indicated in acute asthma if lung function is less than 30 percent predicted and if the patient shows no significant improvement with nebulized beta-agonists. Intravenous therapy is usually given until a satisfactory response is obtained; then oral prednisolone may be substituted. Oral prednisolone has an effect similar to that of IV hydrocortisone and is easier to administer.[28] Inhaled steroids have no proved effect in acute ashtma.

Chronic Asthma

Corticosteroids are indicated if asthma is not adequately controlled with bronchodilators alone, although, increasingly, inhaled steroids are advocated as first-line therapy for chronic asthma.[r1] Inhaled steroids are the treatment of choice, and oral steroids are reserved for patients who cannot be controlled on other therapy, the dose being titrated to the lowest that provides acceptable control of symptoms. For any patient taking regular oral steroids, objective evidence of steroid responsiveness should be obtained before maintenance therapy is instituted.[29] Short courses of oral steroids (such as 30 mg prednisolone daily for 1–2 weeks) are indicated for exacerbations of asthma.

Inhaled steroids should be used twice daily, which improves compliance. If a dose of more than 500 μg daily is used, a spacer device should be considered, as this reduces the risk of orpharyngeal side-effects. Inhaled steroids also may be used in children, but disodium cromoglycate is the initial preferred anti-inflammatory treatment. In children, the dose should be kept under 500 μg daily, if possible, to reduce the risk of inhibitory effects on growth.[r7] Chronic bronchitis patients occasionally respond to steroids, and these patients may be undiagnosed asthmatics. Steroids have no objective benefit on airway function in patients with chronic bronchitis, although they may often produce subjective benefit because of their euphoric effect.

Because of the apparent benefit of the use of nedocromil,[30,31] an anti-inflammatory drug (see Chapter 31), other drugs developed for anti-inflammatory potency in other diseases by virtue of their immunomodulating activity have also been explored in asthmatics with some reports of benefits. Parenteral or oral gold compounds (see Chapter 74) have a weak, steroid-sparing effect,[32] but the many side-effects (dermatitis, thrombocytopenia, proteinuria) have deterred wide use. Nierop et al. have examined the effect of the oral gold compound auranofin on asthma symptoms, pulmonary function tests, and oral prednisone requirements.[33] In 32 patients with steroid-dependent asthma, a randomized, double-blind, placebo-controlled study found that 3 mg of auranofin twice daily permitted a greater reduction in steroid dosage and reduction in symptoms over a 26-week period of study than could be achieved in the control group, Dermatologic side-effects of auronofin were more frequent than in the treated group, however. In this study it was unclear whether the difference in steroid requirements was due simply to a delayed clearence of the remaining steroid dosages, however. There may be an effect of this compound separate from inhibition of steroid metabolism, since Honma et al. have reported that a similar dose of auranofin inhibited the hyper-responsiveness to inhaled methacholine of patients with moderate to severe asthma.[44] Methotrexate, a folate antimetabolite (see Chapter 58), has also been shown to reduce steroid requirements (as in musculoskeletal inflammatory diseases), but also has side-effects of hepatitis, pancytopenia, and frequent GI complaints.[35] Other studies in severe, steroid-dependent asthma patients have failed to confirm a beneficial effect of methotrexate (up to 30 mg/wk total) on airway reactivity or symptom scores.

Other compounds that interdict the effectiveness of inflammation-provoking mediators (Fig. 30.1) have also received increased attention in asthma management. Antagonists of platelet activating factor have now been found to be of benefit in asthma therapy,[36] but members of this class are still not approved for medical use.[36] Leukotriene antagonists are still under evaluation and show promise.[37] Few clinical studies of human airway responses to leukotriene receptor antagonists are available, but in one such study in patients with at least a 20 percent decrease in FEV_1, during exercise, an inhaled leukotriene inhibitor, SKF 104353, was as effective as cromolyn sodium in preventing the decrease in FEV_1.[38] This suggests that leukotrienes may play a role in the pathogenesis of some types of asthma.

References

Research Reports

1. Johanssen S-A, Andersson K-E, Brattsand R, Gruvstad E, Hedner P. Topical and systemic glucocorticoid potencies of budesonide, beclomethasone diproprionate and prednisolone in man. Eur J Respir Dis 1982;*63*:74–82.
2. Blackwell GJ, Carnuccio R, Di Rosa M, Flower RJ, Parente L, Persico P. Macrocortin: a polypeptide causing the anti-phospholipase effect of glucocorticoids. Nature 1981;*287*:147–149.
3. Hirata F, Axelrod J. Phospholipid methylation and biological signal transmission. Science 1980;*209*:1082–1090.
4. Mischler JM. The effects of corticosteroids on mobilization and function of neutrophils. Experimental Haematol (Suppl 5.) 1977; p 15.
5. Tsurufuji S, Kurihara A, Ojima F. Mechanisms of antiinflammatory actions of dexamethasone: blockade by hydrocortisone mesylate and actinomycin D of the inhibitory effect of dexamethasone on leukocyte infiltration in inflammatory sites. J Pharmacol Exp Ther 1984;*229*:237–243.
6. Fuller RW, Kelsey CR, Cole PJ, Dollery CT, MacDermot J. Dexamethasone inhibits the production of thromboxane B2 and leukotriene B4 by human alveolar and peritoneal macrophages in culture. Clin Sci 1984;*67*:653–656.
7. Schleimer RP, Schulman ES, MacGlashan DW, Peters SP, Adams GK, Lichtenstein LM, Adkinson NP. Effects of dexamethasone on mediator release from human lung fragments and purified human lung mast cells. J Clin Invest 1983;*71*:1830–1835.
8. Altman LC, Hill JS, Hairfield WM, Mularkey MF. The effects of corticosteroids on eosinophil chemotaxis and adherance. J Clin Invest 1981;*67*:28–36.
9. Yodoi J, Hirtshima M, Ishizaka K. Lymphocytes bearing Fc receptors for IgE. VI. Suppressive effects of clucocorticoids on the

expression of Fc, receptors and glycosylation of IgE-binding factors. J Immunol 1981;*127*:471–476.

10. Snyder DS, Unanue ER. Corticosteroids inhibit murine Ia expression and IL2 production. J Immunol 1982;*129*:1803–1805.

11. Erjefalt I, Persson OGA. Anti-asthma drugs attenuate inflammatory leakage into airway lumen. Acta Physiol Scand 1986;*128*:653–655.

12. Boschetto P, Rogers DF, Barnes PJ. Corticosteroid inhibition of airway microvascular leakage. Thorax 1989;*44*:358P.

14. Gomez E, Clague JE, Gatland D, Davies RJ. Effect of topical corticosteroids on seasonally induced increases in nasal mast cells. Br Med J 1988;*296*:1572–1573.

15. Davis C, Conolly ME. Tachyphylaxis to B-adrenoceptor agonists in human bronchial smooth muscle: studies in vitro. Br J Clin Pharmacol 1980;*10*:417–423.

16. Stephan WC, Chick TW, Avner BP, Jenne JW. Tachyphylaxis to inhaled isoproterenol and the effect of methylprednisolone in dogs. J Allergy Clin Immunol 1980;*65*:105–109.

17. Holgate ST, Baldwin CJ, Tattersfield AE. Beta-adrenergic agonist resistance in normal human airways. Lancet 1977;*2*:375–377.

18. Mano K, Akbarzadeh A, Townley RG. Effect of hydrocortisone on beta-adrenergic receptors in lung membranes. Life Sciences 1979;*25*:1925–1930.

19. Davis AO, Lefkowitz RJ. In vitro desensitization of beta-adrenergic receptors in human neutrophils. Attenuation by corticosteroids. J Clin Ivest 1983;*71*:565–571.

20. Collins S, Caron MG, Lefkowitz RJ. β2-Adrenergic receptors in hamster smooth muscle cells are transcriptionally regulated by glucocorticosteroids. J Biol Chem 1988;*263*:9067–9070.

21. Gambertoglio JG, Amend WJC, Benet LZ. Pharmakokinetics and bioavailability of prednisone and prednisolone in healthy volunteers and patients: a review. J Pharmacokin Biopharm 1980;*8*:1–52.

22. Carmichael J, Paterson K, Diaz P, Crompton GK, Kay AB, Grant IWB. Corticosteroid resistance in chronic asthma. Br Med J 1981;*282*:1419–1422.

23. Reinberg A, Halberg F, Falliers CJ. Circadian timing of methylprednisolone effects in asthmatic boys. Chronobiologica 1974;*1*:333–337.

24. Ellul-Micallef R, Fenech FF. Intravenous prednisolone in chronic bronchial asthma. Thorax 1975;*30*:312–315.

25. Collins JV, Clarke TJH, Brown D, Townsend J. The use of corticosteroids in the treatment of acute asthma. Q J Med 1975;*44*:259–273.

26. Meltzer EO, Kemp JP, Welch MJ, Orgel HA. Effect of dosing schedule on efficacy of beclomethasone diproprionate aerosol in chronic asthma. Am Rev Respir Dis 1985;*131*:732–736.

27. Toogood JH, Baskerville J, Jennings B, Lefcoe NM, Johansson S-A. Use of spacers to facilitate inhaled corticosteroid treatment of asthma. Am Rev Respir Dis 1984;*129*:723–729.

28. Harrison BDW, Hart GJ, Ali NJ, Stokes TC, Vaughan DA, Robinson AA. Need for intravenous hydrocortisone in addition to oral prednisolone in patients admitted to hospital with severe asthma without ventilatory failure. Lancet 1986;*2*:181–184.

29. Ricci M, Scano G. The aetiology of bronchial asthma and critical assessment of therapy. Europ Resp J 1991;*4*:1148–1151.

30. O'Byrne PM, Cook D. Is nedocromil sodium effective treatment for asthma? Eur Respir J 1993;*6*:5–6.

31. Edwards AM, Stevens MT. The clinical efficacy of inhaled nedocromil sodium (Tilade) in the treatment of asthma. Eur Respir J 1993;*6*:35–41.

32. Bernstein PI, Bernstein IL, Bodenheimer SS, Pietrusko RG. An open study of auranofin in the treatment of asthma. J Allergy Clin 1988;*81*:6.

33. Nierop G, Gizel NP, Bel EH, Zwinderman AH, Di, Kman JH. Auranofin in the treatment of steroid dependent asthma: a double blind study. Thorax 1992;*47*:349–354.

34. Honma M, Tamura G, Taniguchi Y, Taskishima T. The effect of an oral gold compound auronafin, on bronchial responsiveness to inhaled methacholine in well-controlled bronchial asthma. Arerogi 1991;*40*:1470–1476.

35. Mullarkey MF, Blumenstein BA, Andrade WP, Bailey GA, Olason I, Wetzel CE. Methotrexate in the treatment of steroid dependent asthma: A doubleblind cross-over study. N Engl J Med 1988;*318*:603.

36. Page CP. The role of platelet activity factor in asthma. J Allergy Clin Immunol 1988;*81*:145.

37. Robuschiem RE, Fuccella LM, Vida E, Barnale R, Rossi M, Gambaro G, Spagxotto S, Bianco S. Prevention of exercise-induced bronchoconstriction by a new leukotriene antagonist (Skasnd F. 104353). A doubleblind study versus disodium cromoglycate and placebo. Am Rev Respir Dis 1992;*145*:1285–1288.

Acknowledgement

We thank Madeleine Wray and Linda McKeel for preparing this manuscript.

Reviews

r1. Barnes PJ. Anti-inflammatory therapy for asthma Ann Rev Med 1993;*44*:229–249.

r2. Toogood JH, Jennings B, Baskerville JC. Aerosol corticosteroids. In Weiss EB, Segal MS, Stein M (eds): Bronchial asthma: mechanisms and therapeutics. Boston; Little, Brown. (1985); pp 698–713.

r3. Brattsand R. Glucocorticosteroids for inhalation. In Barnes PJ (ed): New drugs for asthma. London: IBC Publications. (1989); pp 117–130.

r4. Flower RJ. Lipocortin and the mechanism of action of the glucocorticosteroids. Br J Pharmacol 1988;*94*:987–1015.

r5. Morris HG. Mechanisms of action and therapeutic role of corticosteroids in asthma. J Allergy Clin Immunol 1985;*75*:1–14.

r6. Ellul Micalef R. Glucocorticosteroids In Barnes PJ, Rodger IW, Thomson NC (eds): Asthma: Basic mechanisms and clinical management (2nd ed.). London: Academic Press. (1992); pp 613–658.

r7. Konig P. Inhaled corticosteroids-their present and future role in the management of asthma. J Allergy Clin Immunol 1988;*82*:297–306.

r8. Barnes PJ. Effect of corticosteroids on airway hyperresponsiveness. Am Rev Respir Dis 1990;*141*:S70–76.

r9. Barnes PJ, Pedersen S. Efficacy and safety of inhaled steroids in asthma therapy. Ann Rev Resp Dis 1993, *148*:51–76.

r10. Dahl R, Venge P, Fredens K. Eosinophils. In: Barnes PJ, Rodger IW, Thomson NC (eds): Asthma: basic mechanisms and clinical management. London: Academic Press (1988); pp 115–129.

r11. Fleisch JH, Cloud ML, Marshall WS. A brief review of the preclinical and clinical studies with LY 171883. Ann NY Acad Sci 1988;*524*:356.

CHAPTER 31

Cromolyn Sodium and Related Drugs

C. Advenier

Introduction

Cromolyn sodium or, more precisely, disodium cromoglycate (DSCG), was discovered in the 1960s and was welcomed as a new approach to the treatment of asthma and some allergic diseases, since it was shown to exert a preventive effect on asthmatic attacks while being devoid of bronchodilator activity. DSCG acts on the immediate symptoms of asthma but also on delayed reactions and, in some cases, on bronchial hyperreactivity. Inhibition of mast cell degranulation is still thought to be one of its principal modes of action, but other theories have been put forward to explain all its clinical effects, since other substances that inhibit only mast cell degranulation do not possess all the properties of cromolyn sodium.

Nedocromil sodium has recently been introduced into the world market. On the other hand, it has been shown that several bronchodilators, such as theophylline and beta$_2$-adrenergic agonists, are also capable of inhibiting mast cell degranulation. These substances, however, differ from DSCG and nedocromil sodium in that they are without effect on delayed hypersensitivity reactions or bronchial hyperreactivity. The only drugs that exert a potent activity on both of these two phenomena are corticosteroids.

Drugs

Prominent among the compounds that exert a specific antiallergic and/or anti-inflammatory effect by inhibiting the degranulation of mast cells and/or the activity of other immunocompetent cells are (Fig. 31.1): (1) Disodium cromoglycate (DSCG), the sodium salt of 1,3-*bis*(2-carboxychromom-5-yloxy)-2-hydroxypropane. The first compound of this kind studied, DSCG is a white, hygroscopic, crystalline powder soluble in water and insoluble in alcohol, which explains why little or none is absorbed in the digestive tract. (2) Nedocromil sodium, the disodium salt of pyranoquinoline dicarboxylic acid.

Other compounds are also capable of exerting some of the effects of DSCG, notably mast cell stabilization, but they possess other pharmacologic properties that classify them within other categories of drugs. These are: (1) bronchodilators, such as isoproterenol, selective beta$_2$-adrenergic stimulants and theophylline; (2) histamine H1-receptor antagonists (antihistamines H_1), including ketotifen, terfenadine, loratadine, mequitazine, and promethazine.

A stabilizing effect on mast cells is also exerted by some other compounds, such as nonsteroidal anti-inflammatory agents and calcium antagonists, but only in extremely high and nontherapeutic doses or concentrations.

Finally, it has recently been shown that cyclosporine or FK 506 can partially inhibit the IgE-dependent release of histamine from human lung mast cells and basophils.[r1]

Therapeutic Uses and Limitations

Bronchopulmonary Pathology

The effects of DSCG and nedocromil sodium on allergen-induced asthma have been well demonstrated. Each of these drugs given before an antigen challenge has clearly been shown to block the occurrence of both the immediate bronchoconstrictive response and the more severe late onset or delayed response.[r2,r3;1] It will be recalled that inhalation challenge with an antigen results in immediate bronchoconstric-

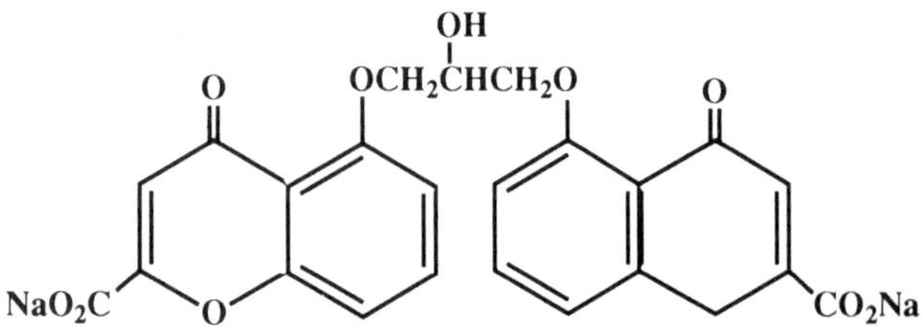

Sodium cromoglycate

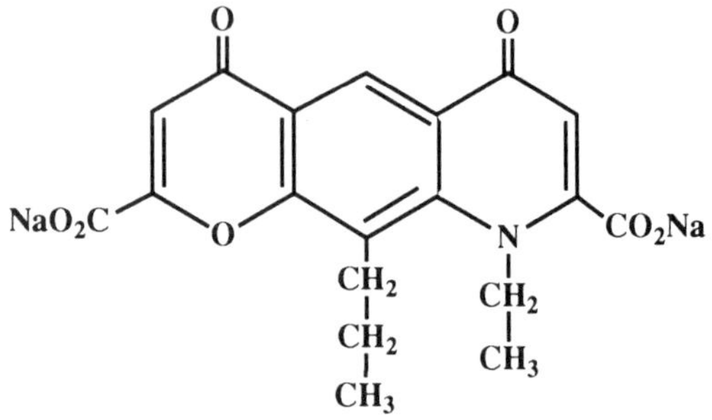

Nedocromil sodium

Figure 31.1

tion, but many asthmatics will undergo a second bronchoconstrictive response four to 12 hours after the first one, this being known as "late" or "delayed" asthmatic reaction. The early response can rapidly be reversed by beta$_2$-adrenoceptor agonists, whereas the late reaction responds poorly to these agents, is prolonged and more severe; corticosteroids are ineffective on the immediate response, but they inhibit the late response. Symptoms in asthmatic patients more closely resemble the late than the immediate response to antigens, which emphasizes the importance of the late asthmatic reaction. As regards pathophysiology, and roughly speaking, the immediate reaction is frequently associated with mast cell degranulation and with the production of mediators and their immediate effects. The late reaction is associated with cell mobilization and the resulting inflammatory phenomena. However, not all allergic patients are protected by DSCG. This might be due to the drug being less active or even inactive against antigen-antibody reactions that do not involve IgEs.

DSCG and nedocromil sodium are equally active on bronchoconstrictive responses induced by SO_2 and cold air. They also exert a protective effect against exposure to several types of industrial agents, including toluene diisocyanate, western red cedar, and colophony. Conflicting results have been reported about the immediate protective effect of DSCG against the nonspecific constricting agents methacholine and histamine.

Finally, DSCG reduces the bronchial hyperreactivity observed in asthma patients. Airway hyperreactivity is a characteristic feature of bronchial asthma, and the degree of bronchial responsiveness, as measured by methacholine, histamine, or allergen bronchoconstrictor response, has been shown to correlate with the occurrence and severity of asthma, with diurnal fluctuations in peak flow rate, with the amount of medication needed to control symptoms, and with airway responses to allergens.

However, the action of DSCG and nedocromil sodium on bronchial hyperreactivity has been demonstrated with treatments lasting more than two weeks, in allergic asthma in the pollen season, and when bronchial hyperreactivity is revealed by challenge tests performed with antigens or histamine. The reported decrease of response to acetylcholine remains questionable.

Nasal Allergy

Numerous nasal challenge tests and clinical trials have shown that DSCG also exerts a protective effect on the nasal mucosa, so that allergic seasonal rhinitis ("hay fever") is a good indication for the drug. The action of DSCG in other types of rhinitis is not so clear.

Eye Allergy

Cromolyn sodium has been used in the treatment of allergic conjunctivitis and vernal conjunctivitis. This treatment has the advantage of reducing the need for systemic or topical corticosteroid therapy.

Effects and Actions of Cromolyn and Nedocromil Sodium

The principal action of cromolyn sodium and nedocromil sodium in immunoallergic reactions is to inhibit the release of mediators stored in mast cells or basophils and the concomitant synthesis of other autocoids, including histamine, leukotrienes, PGD_2, eosinophil-chemotactic factor (ECFA), neutrophil chemotactic factors (NCFA), cytokines (including interleukin-1,3,4,5, and 6), tumor necrosis factor-α (TNF-α), proteases, and heparin.[r1,r2] This mechanism of action is, however, a matter of debate. In addition, these drugs reduce the activity of other cells involved in immunoallergic and inflammatory reactions. They also seem to be capable of inhibiting nerve impulse conduction in the nonadrenergic-noncholinergic (NANC) system of the vagus nerve.

It has been suggested that, together with mast cell degranulation, the accumulation of neutrophils and eosinophils or inflammatory cells contributes to airway narrowing and obstruction through mediator release, increased vascular permeability, mucosal edema, mucus secretion, and epithelial damage. Epithelial damage in turn may lead to bronchial hyperreactivity through the exposure of afferent nerve endings, producing vagally- or axonal reflex-mediated bronchoconstriction.

DSCG and nedocromil sodium, therefore, prevent the occurrence of the pathologic manifestations generated by allergic reactions in the bronchial, nasal, and ocular mucosa, which contain numerous mast cells and inflammatory cells.

DSCG has only weak effects on the intestinal mucosa and on skin, despite their high content of mast cells. This weak activity may in fact be due to pharmacokinetic factors (reduced tissue penetration and short half-life) or to a difference in the nature of mast cells or allergic processes.

Experimental Basis for the Action of Cromolyn and Nedocromil Sodium

Mast Cell Stabilization

The inhibitory effect of DSCG on mast cell degranulation was first demonstrated on rat peritoneal mast cells degranulated by reaginic antibodies (IgE) or by chemical substances (48/80, dextran, phosphatidylserine). It was demonstrated later on human basophils. As regards the human lung, DSCG acts preferentially on mast cells obtained by alveolar lavage,[2] these cells being regarded as most representative of mast cells in the lung lumen that come in contact with allergens.

The action of nedocromil sodium on rat mast cells is similar to that of DSCG, but the new compound is considerably more potent than DSCG on human mast cells obtained by bronchoalveolar lavage or dispersion of lung fragments.[r3]

The interest of this effect, however, is a matter of debate, because albuteral, for example, is 1000 times more effective than cromolyn sodium in this respect and a lot of compounds have been produced by various pharmaceutical companies, that were in some cases considerably more potent than cromolyn sodium as mast cell stabilizers in animal models but inefficient in man.

Effect on Other Inflammatory Cells

DSCG and nedocromil sodium have been shown to induce significant inhibition of fMLP-induced enhancement in both complement and IgG rosettes and in leukocyte cytotoxicity. In other in vitro studies DSCG was found to inhibit activation and chemotaxis to zymozan-activated serum of neutrophils.[3] Nedocromil sodium inhibits IgE-mediated activation of monocytes and platelets in rats and in man, and it prevents the abnormal response to aspirin of platelets derived from aspirin-sensitive patients.[4]

In asthmatics DSCG inhibits the enhanced neutrophil and monocyte activation that occurs during exercise challenge or fog-induced bronchospasm,[5] while nedocromil sodium inhibits the release of leukotriene B_4 and 5-hydroxyeicosatetraenoic acid by alveolar macrophages from asthmatic patients, as well as the complement-dependent release of eosinophil granule proteins.[6] It has potent activities on mediator release from and cytotoxic functions of eosinophils and neutrophils.[7]

Neuropharmacologic Effects

During bronchospasm, DSCG and nedocromil sodium can, to some extent, inhibit the parasympathetic reflex component or the occurrence of an axonal or NANC system reflex resulting in the release of bronchoconstrictor or proinflammatory peptides.[5,8] Thus, in dogs, DSCG inhibits the bronchospasm induced by capsaicin, a substance that induced the release of substance P and other bronchoconstrictor neuropeptides from NANC nerve endings. In some patients DSCG may reduce, at least partially, the intensity of the bronchospasm induced by inhalation of methacholine chloride, histamine, SO_2, or cold and dry air. Nedocromil sodium exerts a similar effect, but in addition it inhibits in dogs the cough induced by citric acid and in humans the bronchoconstriction induced by bradykinin, which is a potent stimulant of the sensitive bronchial nerve endings.

Effect on Smooth Muscle

Neither DSCG nor nedocromil sodium has a direct antagonistic activity toward the bronchoconstrictor or vasomotor effects of the various mediators released or generated in allergic reactions.

Mechanism of Action

Several theories have been put forward to explain the mechanism of action of DSCG. This drug has been claimed to inhibit: (i) cyclic nucleotide phosphodiesterase; (ii) Ca^{++} movements (it must be noted in this respect that organic antagonists of Ca^{++} movements, e.g., nifedipine, also can inhibit mast cell degranulation, but do so only in very high, supratherapeutic doses; (iii) anaphylatoxins C_{3a} and C_{5a} release; (iv) activation of protein C kinase (this applies only to nedocromil sodium); and (v) neuropeptide release. However, none of these theories, taken separately, seems to account for all the activities of DSCG.

Undesirable Effects

The undesirable effects of disodium cromoglycate are infrequent and usually mild and transient. They seldom require withdrawal of the drug. During inhalation, some patients may develop bronchospasm due to the product's being in powder form. In such cases it may be useful to inhale a puff of $beta_2$-adrenergic stimulant before inhaling DSCG.

The other side-effects of DSCG include irritation of the pharynx and larynx, bitter taste, and papular, erythematous, or urticarial rashes. These immediately regress after treatment is discontinued. A few cases of lung eosinophilia have been reported. Myositis and GI disorders occasionally have been noted. All these side-effects are rare, and as a rule sodium cromoglycate is very well tolerated. The side-effects most frequently associated with nedocromil are distinctive taste, headache, nausea, vomiting, and dizziness. They are usually mild and transient.

Pharmacokinetics

DSCG, being extremely water-soluble, is not absorbed in the digestive tract. When administered by inhalation, the drug is usually presented as a powder bound to inactive particles of lactose; for this reason it only partly penetrates the bronchopulmonary system. Part of it remains in the mouth, and a fraction of the amount that has succeeded in entering the lung is taken by bronchial secretions down to the digestive tract, so that the quasitotality of the dose taken is excreted in the feces.

A pharmacokinetic study performed by Fuller and Collier[9] in four healthy volunteers showed that when DSCG was administered IV its plasma half-life was 0.37 hr, its volume of distribution 0.2 $1 \cdot kg^{-1}$ and its plasma clearance 0.35 $1 \cdot h^{-1} \cdot kg^{-1}$. When DSCG was inhaled as a powder the plasma half-life of the fraction absorbed was longer (1.5hr) owing to slow absorption, and this may account for the relatively long duration of action of the drug.[10]

A study by Brown et al.[11] suggested that the amount of DSCG absorbed in the tracheobronchial tree is lower in asthmatics than in normal subjects, despite considerable inter- and intraindividual variations in both groups.

As regards nedocromil, when this drug is administered by inhalation in doses of 4 mg, its terminal half-life is equivalent to the absorption half-life at 2.3 hr, with absorption from the lung being rather limited. Bioavailability is 6 to 9 percent after inhalation, 2.5 percent of this being contributed by GI absorption. Nedocromil sodium is not metabolized, and there is no evidence of accumulation. After IV administration, the plasma clearance of nedocromil sodium is rapid at 0.61 $1 \cdot h^{-1} \cdot kg^{-1}$ via excretion in urine and bile. The pharmacokinetic profile of nedocromil sodium in patients with reversible obstructive airway disease is similar to that observed in healthy volunteers.

Available Preparations and Usual Doses

Cromolyn Sodium

Bronchopulmonary Use

There are three pharmaceutical forms of inhaled DSCG. Whatever the form utilized, it is important that the airways are patent for maximal drug delivery. There is a correlation between the degree of airway patency and the amount of cromolyn reaching the lungs.

Capsules for Inhalation. (Intal, Lomudal, 20-mg capsules for inhalation with a spinhaler) The spinhaler was developed to overcome coordination problems in aerosol therapy. It is a small open plastic tube containing a plastic propeller-like rotor that revolves at high speed when air is inhaled through the device. Twenty mg powdered cromolyn mixed with 20 mg lactose contained in a standard gelatin capsule is inserted into a cup in the propeller. Two perforations are made in the capsule by vertically sliding the sleeve down once, which activates a simple piercing mechanism. When air is inhaled through the mouthpiece, the turbo-vibratory action of the propeller causes the powdered drug to be dispersed into the inspired air through perforations in the capsule wall. The airstream inside the spinhaler and the action of the propeller cause agglomerates of drug and lactose to break up, with the resultant fine particles of cromolyn sodium passing with the inspired air into the respiratory tract. The remaining larger lactose particles are retained in the mouth and upper airway.

The spinhaler delivery system can be utilized by any patient over 4 years of age. Being a breath-actived system, it requires little coordination, and no spacer devices are necessary. The starting dose is usually one 20-mg capsule four times daily. When symptoms are in control, usually after 1–2 months of therapy, the dosage can be decreased to three times a day and then twice daily.

Nebulizer Solution. (Intal, Lomudal, 1 per cent solution for inhalation, 2-ml ampules containing 20 mg) Administered as a nebulizer solution, cromolyn sodium has proved to be especially useful for children under 4, patients who are unable to tolerate the powder formulation because of extremely hyperreactive airways, and patients with more severe disease who benefit from the bronchodilator/cromolyn mixture.

The usual dose is 4 ampules per day. Each nebulization lasts from 8 to 10 minutes.

Metered Dose Aerosol. Each metered spray of 1 mg delivers approximately 800 μg of cromolyn sodium. The recommended dose is two inhalations or 1.6 mg four times daily at regular intervals.

Intranasal Use

(Nasalcrom, Rynacrom, Lomusol, 2% solutions for intranasal use; Rynacrom cartridges each containing DSCG 10 mg and lactose 10 mg). The intranasal solution (Lomusol) seems to be preferable in most cases to the intranasal powder. The frequency of administration

Table 31.1 Clinical Parameters for Cromolyn Sodium and Nedocromil Sodium

Class and Generic Name	Proprietary Name	Approx Dose (mg) & route	Duration of Action		
			Onset (min)	Peak (min)	$T_{1/2}$ (hr)
Cromolyn sodium	Intal®	40–80 mg (inhalation)	15	60	15
Nedocromil sodium	Tilade®	8 mg (inhalation)	15	60	15

Table 31.2 Available Preparations of Cromolyn Sodium and of Nedocromil Sodium and Usual Doses

Generic Name	Trade Name	Dosage Forms* mg	Daily Doses
Cromolyn sodium	Intal®	Inhaler 1 mg/metered inhalation	2 or 10 mg 4 times daily
Sodium cromoglycate		5 mg/metered inhalation	20 mg 4 times daily (aerosol)
Disodium cromoglycate		10 mg/ml in ampules of 2 ml	20 mg 4 times daily
		Spincaps, 20 mg	
	Nalcrom®	Capsules 100 mg	200 mg 4 times daily
	Gastrocrom®		
	Opticrom®	Eyedrops 2% or 4%	4 times daily
	Nasalcrom®	Nasal solution 40 mg/ml	4 times daily
Nedocromil sodium	Tilade®	Inhaler 2 mg/metered inhalation	4 mg twice daily

Table 31.3 Summary Table

Sodium Cromoglycate and Nedocromil Sodium

- Given prophylactically these drugs prevent both immediate and late phase of asthma in many but not all patients.
- According to the international consensus on management of chronic asthma, cromolyn sodium and nedocromil sodium are recommanded in asthma of mild to moderate severity (steps 1 and 2).
- The mechanism of action uncertain: depression of axon reflex release of neuropeptides; inhibition of PAF interaction with platelets; inhibition of eosinophils migration; mast cell stabilization.
- Given by inhalation or local route.
- Unwanted effects are minor—respiratory tract irritation and (rarely) hypersensitivity.

varies according to the importance of the nasal discharge which interferes with the impregnation of the mucosa by the drug.

Applications of disodium cromoglycate onto the nasal mucosa are well tolerated by the majority of patients. In some patients, transient irritation may occur when the powder or the solution come in contact with the nasal mucosa.

Ophthalmic Use

(Opticrom, Opticron, 2% eye drops with benzalconium chloride 0.01%). One drop in each eye four times a day.

Other Proprietary Names. DSCG: Alercrom, Colimune, Cromo-asma, Freval, Lomudal, Lomyren, Nasmil, Nebulasma.

Nedocromil Sodium: Tilade

Inhaler, 2 mg/metered inhalation.

It is given by inhalation in the prophylactic treatment of asthma in usual doses of 4 mg twice daily, increased to 4 mg four times daily where necessary.

References

Research Reports

1. Aalbers R, Kauffman HF, Groen H, Koëter GH, De Monchy JGR. The effect of nedocromil sodium on the early and late reaction and allergen-induced bronchial hyperresponsiveness. J Allergy Clin Immunol 1991;*87*:993–1001.
2. Church MK, Young KD. The characteristics of inhibition of histamine release from human lung fragments by sodium cromoglycate, salbutamol and chlorpromazine Br J Pharmacol 1983;*78*:671–679.
3. Kay AB, Walsh GM, Moqbel R, MacDonald AJ, Nagakura T, Carroll MP, Richarderson HB. Disodium cromoglycate inhibits activation of human inflammatory cells in vitro. J Allergy Clin Immunol 1987;*80*:1–8.
4. Thorel T, Joseph M, Tonnel AB, Capron A. In vitro modulation by nedocromil sodium of IgE-mediated activation of mononuclear phagocytes and platelets from rats and man. Revista Espanola Allergol Immunologica 1987;2:78.
5. Moscato G, Rampulla C, Dellagianca A, Zanotti E, Candura S. Effect of salbutamol and inhaled sodium cromoglycate on the airway and neutrophil chemotactic activity in "fog" induced bronchospasm. J Allergy Clin Immunol 1988;*82*:382–388.
6. Godard P, Chavis C, Daures JP, Crastes de Paulet A, Michel FB, Daman M. Leucotriene B_4 and 5-HETE release by alveolar

macrophages in asthmatic patients: inhibition by nedocromil sodium. Am Rev Respir Dis 1987;*135*:A318.

7. Moqbel R, Cromwell O, Walsh GM, Wardlaw AJJ, Kurlak L, Kay AB. Effects of nedocromil sodium (Tilade®) on the activation of human eosinophils and neutrophils and the release of histamine from mast cells. Allergy 1988;*43*:268–276.
8. Verleden GM, Belvisi MG, Stretton CD, Barnes PJ. Nedocromil sodium modulates nonadrenergic, noncholinergic bronchoconstrictor nerves in guinea pig airways in vitro. Am Rev Resp Dis 1991;*143*:114–118.
9. Fuller RW, Collier JG. The pharmacokinetic assessment of sodium cromoglycate. J Pharm Pharmacol 1983;*35*:289–292.
10. Neale MG, Brown K, Hoddler RW, Auty RM. The pharmacokinetics of sodium cromoglycate in man after intravenous and inhalation administration. Br J Clin Pharmacol 1986;*22*:373–382.
11. Brown LA, Neale KMG, Auty RM, Hodder RW, Snashall P. The pharmacokinetics of sodium cromoglycate. In GW Kert, MA Ganderton (Eds): Proceedings of the eleventh international congress of allergology and clinical immunology, London, October 1982, Edited by London: Macmillan, 1983, pp 513–516.

Reviews

r1. Galli SJ. New concepts about the mast cell. New Engl J Med 1993;*328*:257–265.
Special focus on mast cells and cytokines.

r2. Murphy S. Cromolyn sodium. In Jenne JW, Murphy S Eds., Drug therapy for asthma. New York, Basel: Marcel Dekker, (1987); pp 669–717.

r3. Gonzalez JP, Brogden RN. Nedocromil sodium. A preliminary review of its pharmadodynamic and pharmacokinetic properties and therapeutic efficacy in the treatment of reversible obstructive airways disease. Drugs 1987;*34*:560–577.

r4. Kaliner M. Asthma and mast cell activation. J Allergy Clin Immunol 1989;*83*:510–520.

r5. Barnes PJ, Baraniuk JN, Belvesi MG. Neuropeptides in the respiratory tract. Am Rev Resp Dis 1991;*144*:1187–98 (Part I); 1391–1399 (Part II).

r6. Edwards AM, Stevens MT. The clinical efficacy of inhaled nedocromil sodium (Tilade) in the treatment of asthma. Eur Resp J 1993;*6*:35–41.
Overview meta-analysis of the effects of nedocromil sodium in 4723 patients.

r7. Bienenstock J. An update on mast cell heterogeneity. J Allergy Clin Immunol 1998;*81*:763–769.

CHAPTER 32

C. Advenier
P. Sadoul

Respiratory Stimulants

The use of respiratory stimulants, notably in the treatment of acute respiratory failure, has been fiercely debated. While the earliest analeptic drugs (lobeline, nikethamide, etamivan, prethcamide, dimefline) have rightly been discarded owing to their toxicity, notably on the CNS, modern respiratory stimulants have been the object of renewed interest and are being used in some anesthesia and intensive care units. Their long-term administration in patients with hypoxemia has occasionally proved useful, but this is not an approved use in the United States.

Classification and Chemistry—History

Respiratory stimulants may be divided into five groups. The chemical structures of the principal members of this category of drugs are shown on Figure 32.1.

Acidifiers

The only representative of this group is acetazolamide.

Older Analeptic Drugs

This group comprises several compounds (nikethamide or coramine, etamivan, prethcamide, dimefline) with respiratory stimulant properties. They have been abandoned owing to their side-effects, particularly their convulsant effect.

Nonspecific Respiratory Stimulants

This group contains a variety of compounds with a respiratory stimulant effect that is often impressive but never isolated. Typical examples are camphor and its derivatives, amphetamine, ephedrine, protriptyline (a tricyclic antidepressant), xanthines (theophylline and caffeine), and various hormones (e.g., progesterone) or antihormones (e.g., antialdosterone).

Specific Morphine Antagonists

Nalorphine, naloxone, naltrexone are of use only if respiration is depressed by narcotics.

Selective Respiratory Stimulants of the Carotid Chemoreceptors

Compounds in this group have little or no neuropsychic activity since they act selectively or exclusively on the carotid chemoreceptors. They are: doxapram, a pyrolidinone derivative in use since 1965; and almitrine dimesilate, a piperazine derivative not yet available in all countries.

Therapeutic Uses and Limitations

Acute Respiratory Failure (ARF)

Apart from naloxone, which is used in the treatment of morphine poisoning, the only respiratory stimulants given in severe ARF caused by major sedatives are doxapram and almitrine dimesilate. An IV infusion of doxapram or almitrine in doses of 1 to 2 mg/kg/

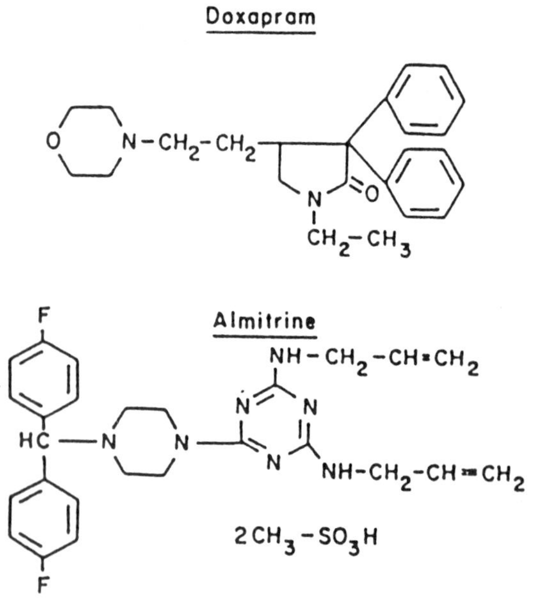

Doxapram

Almitrine

$2 CH_3-SO_3H$

Figure 32.1 Chemical Structure of Doxapram and Almitrine

hr or a single and slow IV injection may be a useful stimulant once the airways have been cleared of obstruction and the patient is no longer paralyzed. Both drugs are useful as a therapeutic test of the mechanism of respiratory failure prior to mechanical ventilation. In no case should the drugs be used instead of mechanical ventilation, and for this reason the respiratory stimulants are seldom indicated in anesthesia and intensive care. A well-conducted anesthetic should preclude postoperative hypoventilation.

Acute respiratory failure in patients with chronic obstructive lung disease often results in a marked increase of PCO_2 and a deep fall of PO_2. The use of analeptic drugs in such patients is severely condemned by some authors who argue that ventilatory fatigue is a frequent cause of ARF and that, based on occlusion pressure measurements, the respiratory center is already strongly stimulated in these patients. However, occlusion pressure is only one index of the complex ventilatory disorder that results in severe respiratory failure in chronic obstructive lung disease, and it is difficult to simplify a complex situation. An IV infusion of doxapram or almitrine (1–2 mg/kg/hr) over one to three hours occasionally avoids intubation and ventilatory support, but is rarely used. Infusions can be repeated two or three times in 24 hours.

Close supervision of the patient during the use of analeptic drugs is mandatory. If ventilatory frequency, signs of struggle, and ventilatory failure set in, one should have recourse to mechanical ventilation.

In respiratory disorders of the newborn, low-dose doxapram (0.05 mg/kg) and theophylline or the more classic caffeine are preferred.

Chronic Respiratory Failure

The chronic use of respiratory stimulants acting on the carotid chemoreceptors has occasionally been advocated in chronic bronchopulmonary diseases with associated hypoxemia, but is not widely practiced. Long-term treatment with almitrine dimesilate in doses of 50–100 mg per day may improve blood gas values (i.e., increase PaO_2 and decrease $PaCO_2$) in patients with chronic obstructive lung disease. However, in some patients PaO_2 may be considerably increased, whereas $PaCO_2$ remains virtually unchanged; this pattern suggests an improvement in the ventilation/perfusion ratio rather than a respiratory stimulant effect proper.[1] Indeed, improvement of blood and air distribution has been observed in patients receiving almitrine while being kept under constant ventilation; in other patients, both the hypoxemia and the hypercapnia are corrected in the same proportions.[2–4]

Absolute and Relative Contraindications

Respiratory stimulants are obviously contraindicated when arterial blood gases are within normal limits and when severe mechanical ventilatory disturbances are present. This is the case with asthma, some cases of COPD, or restrictive pulmonary syndromes. The refractory hypoxemia that characterizes the acute respiratory distress syndrome in adults is certainly not amenable to respiratory stimulants, and the same applies to asphyxia caused by myopathies, paralysis, or fatigue of the thoracic muscles and diaphragm.

Mechanism of Action

Acidifiers

Acidifiers, e.g., acetazolamide, stimulate ventilation by producing metabolic acidosis.

Older Analeptic Drugs

These drugs stimulate respiration by acting on the medulla oblongata as one aspect of their generalized stimulation of the CNS. They significantly increase cerebral oxygen consumption and therefore have a narrow margin of safety. The nausea, vomiting, and, above all, the convulsions they provoke preclude their administration in high doses, although only high doses are effective in alveolar hypoventilation.

Table 32.1 Clinical Parameters and Available Preparations for Doxapram and Almitrine

Class and Generic Name	Proprietary Name	Approx Dose (MG) & Route	Dosage Forms
Doxapram	Dopram* Doxapril*	0.5–1.5 mg/kg, IV	IV infusion: 2 mg/ml, in glucose IV infusion Injection: 20 mg/ml in ampules of 5 ml or 20 ml
Almitrine	Vectarion*	0.5–3 mg/kg/24h, IV 50–100 mg, po	Ampules: 15 mg/5 ml Tablets: 50 mg

*not available in all countries

Stimulants of the Carotid Chemoreceptors

Doxapram acts partly by stimulating the carotid chemoreceptors. Intravenous infusion in doses of 400 mg over two to four hours to patients with chronic hypercapnia lowers $PaCO_2$ by 10 mmHg on average. This action is prolonged for about two to four hours after the infusion is completed. It must be noted that pulmonary arterial hypertension has been reported in chronic hypercapnic and hypoxemic patients after an infusion of 200 mg. The respiratory stimulant effects of that drug are not always suppressed by oxygen therapy.

Almitrine dimesilate acts selectively on the carotid chemoreceptors. A significant increase of PaO_2 has been observed with doses that did not modify ventilation or $PaCO_2$. In dogs, doses as low as 10 μg/kg may increase PaO_2 by 10 mmHg. This increase of PO_2 without change in $PaCO_2$ has been found in patients under artificial ventilation or in hypercapnic chronic bronchitis patients. Measurements performed with gases of different solubilities suggest that this improvement is due to a decrease of blood flow in areas with low ventilation/perfusion ratio; these findings seem to be confirmed by radionuclide studies.[1,2,5] The mechanism responsible for this enhanced ventilation/perfusion matching, however, is unknown.

Undesirable and Toxic Effects of Stimulants of the Carotid Chemoreceptors

Doxapram

Side-effects are rare when this drug is given IV in doses of 400 mg over two to four hours, but are frequently observed with doses of 3 mg/kg/hr. They consist of tremor, sweating, agitation, and vertigo; moderate arterial hypertension is less frequent. Pulmonary arterial hypertension has been observed in chronic hypercapnic and hypoxemic patients after an infusion of 200 mg. Nausea and vomiting are exceptional. Pruritus and, more often, perspiration have been recorded. Shivers and tremor have been reported, but not seizures. However, doxapram is contraindicated in epilepsy or other convulsive disorders and in hypertension. In case of obstruction or severe pulmonary restriction, the drug may cause respiratory impairment due to its ventilatory effects.

Almitrine Dimesilate

In patients with severe airway obstruction or restriction due to parenchymal defect (kyphoscoliosis, pachypleuritis, etc.), ventilatory stimulation by almitrine produces a respiratory impairment that is more or less distinctly perceived by the patient, associated with anxiety and sometimes excitation. Seizures have never been reported, but with very high doses given to patients with mechanically normal thoraco-diaphragmatic musculature, ventilatory alkalosis with vertigo, tetany, and other symptoms may develop. In hypoxemic and hypercapnic patients, hemodynamic studies have shown that as the hypoxemia is corrected, pulmonary arterial pressure and vascular resistance are increased, often associated with a decrease of right ventricular end-diastolic pressure. There have been reports of peripheral neuropathy in patients taking almitrine dimesilate.[6–12] In contrast to perhexiline neuropathy, almitrine neuropathy is not related to slow oxidation of the compound with regard to the particular P-450 iso-enzyme (CYP2D6) involved in dextromethorphan and debrisoquine metabolism.[13]

Pharmacokinetics

Doxapram has a half-life of three to four hours, and bioavailability after oral administration is 60 percent. Most of it is degraded in the liver by an oxidative process.

Almitrine dimesilate is primarily excreted by the liver, and its elimination in the bile creates an enterohepatic cycle. The half-life of this drug is 31 ± 12 hours; it is prolonged up to 60 hours in patients with liver disease, but is little modified in patients with renal impairment.

Available Preparations and Usual Doses

Doxapram (Dopram, Doxapril)

Injection: doxapram hydrochloride 20 mg/ml in ampules of 5 ml. *Intravenous infusion:* doxapram hydrochloride 2 mg/ml (UK).

Doxapram hydrochloride has a short duration of action. It is used in the treatment of respiratory depression following anesthesia, usually in a dose of 0.5 to 1.5 mg/kg IV. This dose may be repeated at hourly intervals. It may also be given by IV infusion, initially administered at a rate of 2–5 mg/min and then reduced, according to the patient's response, to 1–3 mg/min. The recommended maximum total dosage is 4 mg/kg.

Doxapram may be infused at a rate of 1.5 to 4.0 mg per minute in the treatment of ARF.

Almitrine Dimesilate (Vectarion) (Not Available in All Countries)

Almitrine dimesilate is given orally as a respiratory stimulant in conditions such as chronic obstructive pulmonary disorders. Usual doses range from 50 to 100 mg daily, and treatment may be intermittent. Higher doses (0.5 to 3 mg/kg/24 hr) are given by IV perfusion in ARF or in respiratory depression following anesthesia.[8]

Table 32.2 Summary Table

- Respiratory stimulants or analeptics have been proposed for the management of severe respiratory failure responsible for hypoxemia with or without hypercapnia.
- The first drugs used (nikethamide, dimefline) produced multiple side-effects, including seizures.
- Currently used stimulants acting predominantly on the chemoreceptors of the carotid bodies (doxapram and almitrine) are well tolerated and effective. In addition to increasing ventilation, almitrine often improves the ventilation-to-perfusion ratio. Excessive use may still produce CNS excitation and seizures, however. Peripheral neuropathies have been reported with almitrine.
- Respiratory stimulants are indicated only in cases of arterial hypoxemia with or without hypercapnia. Their effect should always be monitored by clinical evaluations and arterial blood gas analysis. Contraindications include bronchial obstruction and major parenchymal restriction. The drugs should never be used without the immediate availability of mechanical ventilatory support and IV access for CNS sedation if seizures develop.

References

Research Reports

1. Castaing Y, Manier G, Guenard H. Improvement in ventilation-perfusion relationships by almitrine in patients with chronic obstructive pulmonary disease during mechanical ventilation. Am Rev Resp Dis 1986;*134*:910–916.
2. Connaughton JJ, Douglas NJ, Morgan AD, Shapiro CM, Critchley JA, Pauly N, Flenley DC. Almitrine improves oxygenation when both awake and asleep in patients with hypoxia and carbon dioxide retention caused by chronic bronchitis and emphysema. Am Rev Resp Dis 1985;*132*:206–210.
3. Dull WL, Polu JM, Sadoul P. The pulmonary haemodynamic effects of almitrine infusion in men with chronic hypercapnia. Clin Science 1983;*64*:25–31.
4. Powles ACP, Tuxen DV, Mahood CB, Pugsley SO, Campbell EJ. The effect of intravenously administered almitrine, a peripheral chemoreceptor agonist, on patients with chronic air-flow obstruction. Am Rev Resp Dis 1983;*127*:284–289.
5. Prost JF, Desche P, Jardin F, Margairaz J. Comparison of the effects of intravenous almitrine and positive end-expiratory pressure on pulmonary gas exchange in adult respiratory distress syndrome. Eur Resp J 1991;*4*:683–687
6. Chedru F, Nodzenski R, Dunand JF, Amarenco G, Ghnassia R, Ciaudo-Lacroix C, Said G. Peripheral neuropathy during treatment with almitrine. Br Med J. 1985;*290*:896.
7. Gherardi R, Louarn F, Benvenuti C, Perrier M, Lejonc JL, Schaeffer A, Dejos JD. Peripheral neuropathy in patients treated with almitrine dismesilate. Lancet 1985;*i*:1247–1249.
8. Blondel M, Arnott G, Defoort S, Bouchez B, Persuy P, Masingue M, Hache JC, Krivosic I. Onze cas de neuropathie à l'almitrine, dont un cas avec neuropathie optique. Rev Neurol (Paris) 1986;*8/9*:683–688.
9. Bouche P, Leger JM, Lacomblez L, Chaunu MP, Ratinahirana H, Brunet P, Haun JJ, Cathala HP, Laplane D. Peripheral neuropathy during treatment with almitrine bismesylate: report of 28 cases. Muscle & Nerve (Suppl.) 1986;*9*:122.
10. Gérard M, Léger P, Couturier JC, Robert D. Ten cases of peripheral neuropathy during microsomal cythrome P-450 involved in the 4-hydroxylation of debrisoquine, a prototype for genetic variation in oxidative drug metabolism. Biochem 1986;*23*:2787–2795.
11. Gherardi R, Baudrimont M, Gray F, Louarn F. Almitrine neuropathy. A nerve Biopsy study of 8 cases. Acta Neuropath (Berl.) 1987;*73*:20–28.
12. Watanabe S, Kanner RE, Cutillo AG, Menlove RL, Bachand RJ, Szalkowski MB, Renzetti AD. Long-term effect of almitrine bismesylate in patients with hypoxemic chronic obstructive pulmonary disease. Am Rev Resp Dis 1989;*140*:1269–1273.
13. Belec L, Larrey D, De Cremoux H, Tinel M, Louarn F, Pessayre D, Gherardi R. Extensive oxidative metabolism of dextromethorphan in patients with almitrine neuropathy. Br J Clin Pharmaol 1989;*27*:387–390.

Review

r1. Wang SC, Ward JW. Analeptics. In: Widdicombe JG. Respiratory Pharmacology. (1982); Oxford, Pergamon Press, pp 85–127.

CHAPTER 33

D. W. Empey

Antitussive Drugs

Cough is a protective reflex that rapidly ejects foreign material and sputum from the larger airways.[r1] The mucociliary escalator achieves the same result much more slowly for smaller particles and normal amounts of mucus within the smaller airways. Antitussive agents relieve or prevent cough. Expectorants aid the production of sputum; mucolytics reduce the viscosity of sputum and are discussed in Chapter 34. The cough reflex has three conceptual components: (1) The afferent perception and conduction to the CNS, probably via the vagus nerves. Cough is initiated by a peripheral stimulus to a "cough receptor," probably the fine nerve endings seen between the mucosal cells lining the pharynx, larynx, and the larger airways. (2) A central integrative area where the peripheral stimuli are combined with other behavioral inputs (e.g., voluntary suppression of the cough, inhibition if food is in the pharynx, etc.) This area is located in the dorsal medulla, near the solitary tract nuclei and dorsal expiratory neurons and can be examined in animal research preparations. (3) The efferent limb of the reflex arc is largely the somatic innervation of the larynx and thoracoabdominal skeletal muscles.

A typical cough stimulus, such as breathing in some dust, initiates a quick inspiration, followed by closure of the glottis and then rapid contraction of the expiratory muscles. The subsequent sudden opening of the glottis a fraction of a second later produces an explosive release of air that can propel sputum at 80 km/hr up to four to five meters beyond the mouth. Numerous standardized stimuli have been used in humans as stimulants of the cough reflex, such as hypotonic saline, paraldehyde, and citric acid aerosols. Application of endogenous compounds to the airway mucosa has also been found to trigger a cough reflex in experimental animals. Histamine or bronchoconstrictors of any type (bradykinin, prostaglandins) also have been examined. Obviously, particulate matter whether aspirated into the lung, parenchymal secretions, or inflammatory exudate are also potent cough stimulants. Dry air per se or a change from nose-to mouth-breathing can raise airway surface fluid osmolarity by almost 30 percent, thus triggering an increase in cough frequency or severity.

Pharmacologic Strategies for Inhibiting Cough

The management of a patient with cough should begin with an attempt to discover the cause. Usually it is in the larynx or the peripheral airways. Primary lung infections should be treated with drugs to which the offending orginsms are sensitive. A search for pharyngeal, esophageal, thyroid, and laryngeal neoplasms or infections always should be made, with chronic obstructive lung disease and asthma more frequent identifiable causes. Winter dry air may be provocative and effectively treated with humidification.

If primary attack on the pathogenic mechanisms is not possible, then the much more frequent purely symptomatic management becomes important. The great majority of such therapy is directed at interfering with the peripheral afferent input.

Interruption of Afferent Pathways

Demulcent agents such as honey and lemon may have a protective and soothing effect on the pharyngeal wall, but they do little to affect stimuli in the lung. Local anesthetics, such as nebulized lidocaine, are effective when used to suppress cough during fiberoptic bronchoscopy under mild sedation. A longer-term effect has been claimed in some cases of chronic nonspecific cough, but this is not an approved indication.[1] The local anesthetic activity in cough drops (menthol) is a common approach to block afferent pathways.

Bronchodilators may be effective antitussives in asthmatics and those patients with bronchial hyperreactivity. By inhibiting bronchoconstriction they reduce the distortion of the airways that can stimulate cough receptors.[2] Cough is a common presenting symptom in asthmatic children, and the bronchodilators can, together with anti-inflammatory asthma prophylactics, be very effective in this age group.[3] Both cholinerigic muscarinic antagonists (e.g., ipratropium) and beta$_2$ agonists (e.g., albuterol) have been shown to have antitussive activity. The use of antihistamines to decrease nasal secretions may be helpful in patients where postnasal drip may be the source of the irritation focus. The use of histamine type 2 antagonists (metaclopromide) to enhance gastric emptying may be helpful for patients where gastroesophageal reflux is responsible.

Centrally Acting Drugs

Most antitussives work centrally on the cough center, where opiates and opiate derivatives are the most effective agents. Those drugs that have relatively more antitussive action and relatively less euphoric, addictive, sedative, and constipating effects are to be preferred.

Codeine is probably the most widely used cough suppressant and is often employed as the standard by which other antitussives are judged. Pholcodine is an opiate used in Europe with cough suppressant but no analgesic properties, but it is not yet available in most countries. Potent opiates such as methadone and morphine are likely to be more effective as antitussives but carry a greater risk of adverse effects. In general, the antitussive dose is below the dose needed for analgesia. Other agents have not been convincingly shown to be superior to codeine in terms of antitussive activity. Though these agents are usually thought to act only in the brain on mμ and kappa opiate receptors,[4,5] part of their effectiveness may rely on their activity on peripheral afferent nerve terminals as well.[6]

Side-Effect Profile

Most antitussives are generalized CNS depressants and not specific for the cough center. Thus, they carry the potential for sedation, respiratory depression, and other central effects. Respiratory depression is unlikely to be a problem if codeine or pholcodine are used in standard antitussive doses, provided the patient is not already at risk. There is, however, a very real danger in overdose. Should this occur, it may be reversed with the opiate antagonist naloxone. Repeated dosing may be necessary because naloxone often has a shorter duration of action than the opiate. Other effects such as dizziness, sedation, nausea, and constipation may occur after antitussive doses of opiates and such nonopiate drugs as isoaniline. Diphenhydramine and other antihistamines are used as antitussives, but a marked tendency to produce drowsiness limits their usefulness to short-term treatment only. Patients should be warned of the possibility of sedation and the dangers of driving or operating machinery if affected. Nausea is unlikely to occur if standard doses are used, but constipation may be a problem. Tolerance to this effect does not develop.

Dextromethorphan is the methyl ester of the dextroisomer of the opiate levorphanol and lacks analgesic properties or addictive liability. It is said to have a specific effect on cough almost equal to that of codeine but to lack the tendency of other opiates to produce the unwanted effects outlined above. Despite this generalization, it is still known to cause drowsiness, dizziness, and GI upsets in susceptible patients or on overdosage. This drug is now recognized as a weak glutamic acid antagonist (NMDA type) and is undergoing trials to assess its efficacy in prevention of ischemic traumatic brain damage.

If the benefits of treatment outweigh the problems of constipation and other side-effects there is little to choose between antitussives on the basis of their side-effect potential. Codeine or pholcodine should be suitable for most patients. Dextromethorphan may be the safest choice, even if there is a special risk of respiratory depression. For this reason the drug is now available in over-the-counter preparations.

Effector Acting Drugs

Only skeletal muscle relaxants of the entire body musculature can abolish cough by this mechanism; thus, they are rarely used except for management of patients on mechanical ventilators.

Evaluation of Antitussives

There is no reliable model of cough that can be used in animal experiments, and induced cough in normal human volunteers does not exactly mimic that produced by lung diseases. Some drug classes, such as the angiotensin converting enzyme (ACE) inhibitors may increase the frequency of coughing, however.[5]

The inhalation of irritant substances (by animals or humans) will produce cough, and the frequency and intensity can be recorded. Unfortunately, tolerance develops, and this can confuse the interpretation of any drug effects.[6] In addition, efficacy in animal models does not guarrantee effectiveness in man, and studies with cough-provoking stimuli in volunteers with normal airways do not assure effectiveness of cough antagonists or suppressants in patients with disease-related coughs.

Studies of cough in patients with spontaneous cough due to lung disease are most relevant, but the variability both between and within patients is extremely high and the technical aspects of quantifying and analyzing such studies are complex. Also, there are wide discrepancies between subjective and objective benefits and side-effects.

The Place of Antitussives in Clinical Practice

Before deciding to prescribe an antitussive the physician must be clear about the diagnosis underlying the symptom. In cases where sputum (particularly infected sputum) is being produced, it may be very undesirable to administer antitussives. A case of acute bronchitis could become a case of pneumonia if this were done. The correct approach is usually to give treatment specific to the cause and use cough suppressants only as an adjunct or in cases such as terminal disease where the cough is a distressing aspect of the problem.

Causes of Cough

MINOR	Viral infections
	Postnasal drip
	Psychogenic
	Allergy
SERIOUS	Asthma
	Bronchitis
	Tuberculosis
	Lung cancer
	Heart failure
	Pneumonia
	Foreign body

When to Treat Cough

When cough is unproductive and, particularly, if it disturbs sleep or causes syncope, it may be wise to suppress it.[7] The complications of uncontrolled unproductive cough include: rib fractures; pneumothorax; rupture of subconjunctival veins; urinary incontinence; rupture of surgical wounds; and syncope.[r2] All of these provide good reasons for intervention.

Choosing an Antitussive

A report of the WHO Scientific Group stated that "the resources available for controlled clinical studies of antitussive agents are insufficient".[r3] Since an antitussive effect demonstrated in the laboratory is not always predictive of an effect in clinical practice, the choice of agent should be based on the efficacy and acceptability of the preparation for each individual patient. It is difficult to sort through the large number of antitussive preparations on the market, but a logical approach can be formulated from simple considerations of drug and patient factors.

Abuse Potential

Opiate antitussives are euphoriant and may produce dependence. Dextromethorphan is an exception; large doses have caused bizarre behavior, but the drug appears to produce little or no physical dependence.[r3]

Ancillary Constituents of the Preparation

Many antitussives are formulated as mixtures containing decongestants or expectorants, and the possible adverse effects of these should be borne in mind. The British National Formulary states that "there is no place for compound preparations in the treatment of respiratory diseases," and it is difficult to rationalize the use of a mixture of opposing actions such as an expectorant and an antitussive. In spite of this, such preparations are on sale in many countries of the world, including the US.

Drug Interactions

Some of the opiate and antihistamine compounds are sedative as well and can have additive effects with other CNS depressants.

Sugar Content

Many cough mixtures contain sugar, and this should be remembered when prescribing for children, whose teeth may be damaged, and for diabetics.

Age

Greater end-organ sensitivity to the pharmacologic effects of drugs coupled with reduced elimination capabilities place the very old or the very young at increased risk from adverse drug reactions. This generalization applies to many drugs, and antitussive agents are no exception. Careful evaluation of the need for treatment is required, with therapy initiated only if the anticipated benefits clinically outweigh the potential risk of adverse drug reactions in these susceptible groups.

Children

Most coughs in children are caused by viral infections that are often self-limiting, or by asthma, which is best treated with specific therapy and not with antitussive agents that will be ineffective anyhow. In the rare situation of a dry unproductive cough that is very irritating or dangerous, a pediatric sugar-free preparation of codeine, pholcodine, or dextromethorphan is likely to be a safe choice. Cough suppressants should not be used in children under the age of two years.[3]

Aging

Elderly patients may be particularly susceptible to the central and sedative effects of antitussive agents. It should be remembered that cough suppression may be positively harmful in those at risk of developing chest infections or in patients with chronic obstructive airways disease. Antitussive-induced constipation may be an additional problem, especially in the sedentary elderly person.

The Use of Antitussives in Pregnancy and Lactation

Administration of any drug to a pregnant woman is always a risk. In every case a careful assessment is needed to determine whether the benefit to the mother of pharmacologic intervention outweighs the risk to mother and fetus. The teratogenic potential of a drug is the major determinant of its safety during the first trimester of pregnancy. Unfortunately, for most drugs, this cannot be assessed with any degree of certainty. The results of animal experiments have a limited application owing to wide interspecies differences and the difficulty of proving cause and effect. Retrospective and prospective studies in humans are hampered by difficulties in study design.

Throughout pregnancy there are important differences between drug disposition in the mother and fetus. This is particularly relevant if the drug is given shortly before delivery. Drug elimination in the neonate may be reduced owing to immature metabolic and excretory capabilities. This may result in drug accumulation with enhanced and prolonged pharmacologic effects.

There are few data on the risk/benefit ratio of antitussives during pregnancy and the manufacturers of the preparation should be consulted for up-to-date information in individual cases. It is likely that indiscriminate use of codeine and other opiates carries some

Summary Table

	Dosage			Pharmacokinetics			
Drug	Route	Size	Dose	Peak	V_D	$t_{1/2}$	Clearance or Duration of Response
Dextromethorphan	Oral Lozenge	5 mg					
	Oral Solution	3.5 mg/5 ml					
	Oral Tablets	10–15 mg 10–20 mg	q 4 hours	30 minutes			lasts 3–6 hours
Codeine	Oral Solution	8.4 mg/5 ml					
	Oral Tablet	30–60 mg	10–20 mg q 4–6 hrs	1–2 hours			lasts 4 hours

risk to the fetus. Use of codeine during the first trimester has been associated with musculoskeletal defects such as dislocated hip and cleft mouth and palate, and with inguinal hernias and cardiac and circulatory system defects. Alimentary system defects are linked with codeine use during the second trimester.

Use of codeine and other opiates during labor may result in neonatal respiratory depression. Neonatal codeine withdrawal has been described in two infants of nonaddicted mothers who took codeine cough preparations during the last two weeks of pregnancy. In general, it is best to avoid these drugs during pregnancy.[8]

References

Research Reports

1. Howard P. Lignocaine aerosol spray for relief of intractable cough. Br J Dis Chest 1977;*71*:19–23.
2. Corrao, WM, Braman SS, Irwin RS. Chronic cough as the sole presenting manifestation of bronchial asthma. N Engl Med 1979;*300*:633–637.
3. Phelan PD, Pearce G. Cough mixtures in children. Curr Ther October 1986, 55–59.
4. Kamei J, Tanihara H, Kasuya Y. Modulation of μ-mediated antitussive activity in rats by a δ agonist. Eur J Pharamacol 1992;*203*:153.
5. Kamei J, Tanihara H, Kasuya Y. 1992, Modulation of K-mediated antitussive activity in rats by a δ agonist. Res Commun Pathol Pharmacol 1992;*76*:375.
6. Adcock JJ. Peripheral opiod receptors and the cough reflex. Resp Med 1991;*85*:43–46.
7. Karlberg BE. Cough and inhibition of the renin-angiotensin system. J Hypertension 1993;*11*:Suppl 3 S49–S52.
8. Empey DW, Laitinen LA, Young GA, Bye C, Hughes DTD. Comparison of the antitussive effect of codeine, dextromethorphan and noscapine. Eur J Clin Pharm 1979;*16*:393–397.
9. Empey DW. Cough production and suppression. Eur J Resp Dis 1980;*61*:Suppl 111, 16–17.
10. Gogan MP, Ritson EB. Dimyril abuse in the East Midlands. Br J Addict 1970;*65*:63–66.

Reviews

r1. Irwin RS, Rosen MJ, Braman SS. Cough. A comprehensive review. Arch. Intern. Med. 1977;*37*:1186–1191.

r2. Banner AS. Cough: Physiology evaluation and treatment. Lung 1986;*164*:79–92.

r3. WHO Technical Report No 495. Geneva, 1972.

CHAPTER 34

Alain Lurie
Martine Mestiri
Georges Strauch
Jean Marsac

Drugs Acting on Mucociliary Transport and Surface Tension

Drugs Acting on Mucociliary Transport

Mucus and particles are transported toward the oropharynx. Mucociliary transport can be efficient only if ciliary beats are coordinated (metachronism) and if cilia and mucus cooperate. This requires not only good functioning of the cilia but also the presence of mucus with adequate rheologic properties.[r1,r2] Since mucociliary transport is often abnormal in bronchial diseases, drugs have been devised to facilitate the clearance of the bronchial secretions and inhaled particles normally effected by the cilia-mucus system (Fig. 34.1).

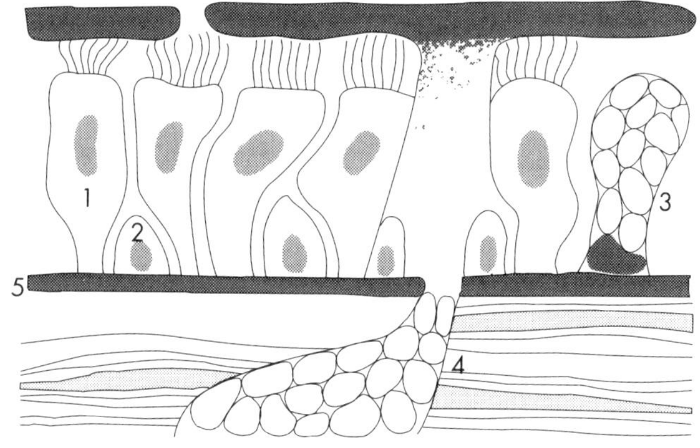

Figure 34.1 Bronchial Mucosa: (1) ciliated cell; (2) basal cell; (3) goblet cell, (4) submucous gland," (5) basal membrane.

Chemistry

Drugs that improve the mucociliary transport system are bronchodilators and expectorants. Bronchodilators will be described in another chapter of this book. Expectorants belong to a wide variety of physicochemical families. They are cysteine derivatives with either a free or blocked thiol group, alkaloids, piperazine, terpene, or phenol derivatives, and proteolytic enzymes of plant or pancreatic origin (Table 34.1 and Fig. 34.3).

Pharmacologic Effects

The pharmacologic effects of agents that influence mucociliary transport are listed in Table 34.1.

Anesthetics

When administered in high doses, lidocaine reduces mucociliary transport in vitro; in the doses usually given in vivo, it has no influence on the frequency

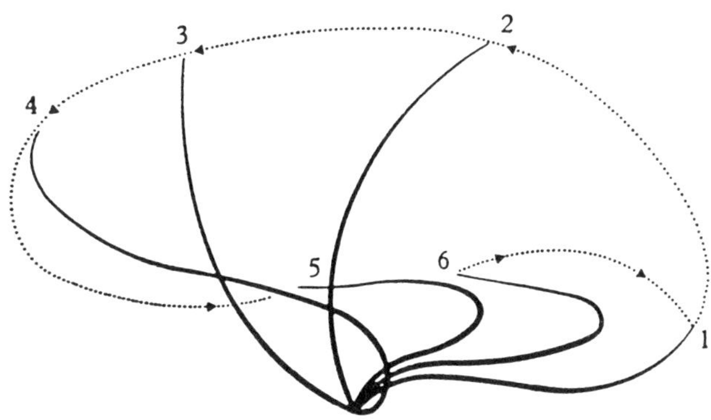

Figure 34.2 Ciliary Movement

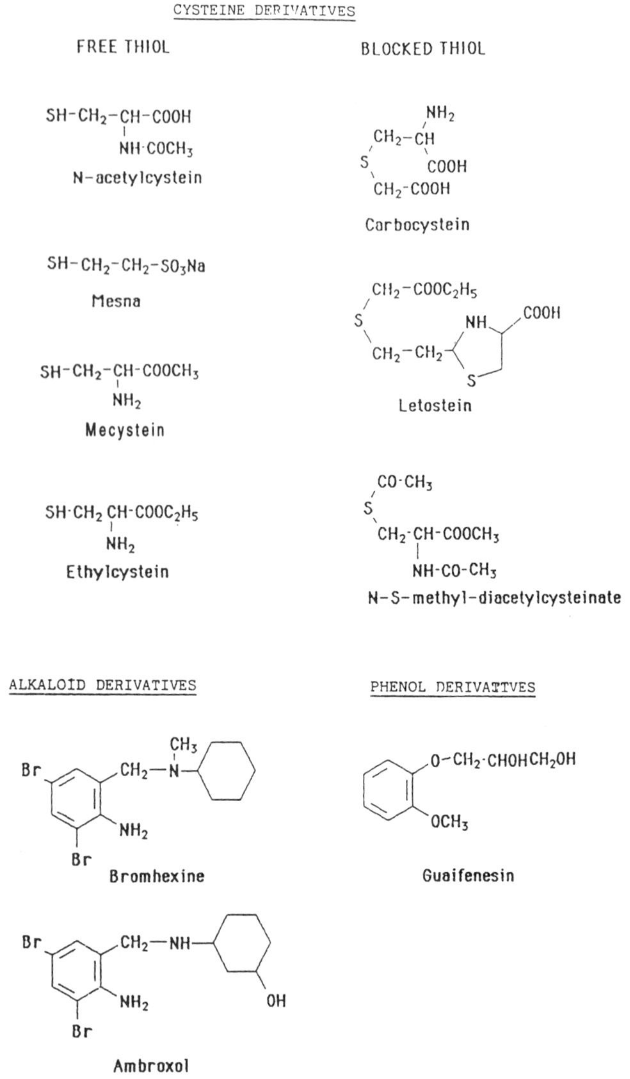

CYSTEINE DERIVATIVES

FREE THIOL

$SH-CH_2-CH(NHCOCH_3)-COOH$
N-acetylcystein

$SH-CH_2-CH_2-SO_3Na$
Mesna

$SH-CH_2-CH(NH_2)-COOCH_3$
Mecystein

$SH-CH_2-CH(NH_2)-COOC_2H_5$
Ethylcystein

BLOCKED THIOL

Carbocystein

Letostein

N-S-methyl-diacetylcysteinate

ALKALOID DERIVATIVES

Bromhexine

Ambroxol

PHENOL DERIVATIVES

Guaifenesin

Figure 34.3 Chemical Formulas of Expectorants (cysteine, alkaloid and phenol derivatives)

Table 34.1 Pharmacologic Activity of Compounds Acting on Mucociliary Transport

Compounds Tested	Effect on Mucociliary Transport
General anesthetics	Slowing down
Local anesthetics	No effect or slowing down
Synthetic parasympatholytics	No effect
Parasympathomimetics	Acceleration
Sympathomimetics	Acceleration
Theophylline	Acceleration
Expectorants	Controlled clinical trials needed

of ciliary beats. Other local anesthetics (procaine, chlorprocaine, cocaine, tetracaine, dibucaine) have been studied; they vary widely in their effects on mucociliary transport.[1,2]

Parasympatholytics

When inhaled in therapeutic doses, synthetic atropine-like compounds, such as ipratropium bromide, do not slow mucociliary transport in humans.[3]

Parasympathomimetics

Parasympathomimetic agents are potent stimulants of ciliary activity, bronchial secretion, and mucociliary transport.[4] Subcutaneous injections of pilocarpine stimulate submucosal gland and goblet cell secretion and accelerate mucociliary transport in man. However, parasympathomimetic drugs produce bronchonconstriction and cannot be used in the treatment of bronchial disease.

Sympathomimetics

In normal subjects, a 0.25 mg SQ injection of terbutaline, a sympathomimetic drug, produces a 50 percent increase in bronchial clearance.[5] Sympathomimetic drugs also increase mucociliary transport in patients with asthma, chronic bronchitis, and cystic fibosis. However, even after a 100 percent increase, bronchial clearance would remain very low in patients with bronchial obstruction when compared with the clearance measured in healthy subjects. Sympathomimetic drugs increase the frequency of ciliary beats and modify the characteristics of bronchial secretions.

Theophylline

Theophylline increases the frequency of ciliary beats and the production of mucus in vitro, and it accelerates mucociliary transport both in vitro and in vivo.[6]

Expectorants

It seems preferable to speak of expectorants rather than mucolytics (characterized by their ability to reduce the viscosity and elasticity of bronchial secretions in vitro) or mucoregulators, which are terms often used to designate this therapeutic class of drugs. Expectorants are defined as drugs whose objective is the removal of bronchial secretions (Table 34.2). In healthy subjects, although coughing has been found to enhance mucus clearance, the removal of bronchial secretions is mainly due to mucociliary transport.[7] In patients, this removal is effected by coughing and mucociliary transport.[8] Thus, expectorants should be evaluated on both of these aspects of bronchial secretion removal. Any other properties of expectorants are indirect and must be considered as such.

Assessment of Expectorants[r3]

Clinical Assessment. Symptoms of bronchial obstruction and ease of expectoration cannot be related specifically to qualitative or quantitative abnormalities of bronchial secretion, as the diseases concerned are accompanied not only by hypersecretion, but also by edema, bronchospasm, and obstructive scars that reduce the bronchial lumen.

Patients with chronic bronchial disease often produce larger amounts of secretion than usual, and a further increase due to the use of secretory stimulants may reduce mucus clearance. It is inaccurate to claim that bronchial secretions with greater fluidity are more easily transported; effective transport requires well-defined degrees of viscosity and elasticity. The amount of sputum expectorated depends on mucociliary transport, but also on the production of bronchial secretions. Therefore, an increase in the amount of sputum may be due both to improved transport and enhanced production. Therefore, measuring the amount of sputum collected is not a good method by which to evaluate the efficacy of expectorants.

By aiding the removal of bronchial secretions, expectorants will ease the act of coughing, but there are no appropriate objective methods for evaluating this. Cough frequency and severity are assessed, but expectorants are not antitussive agents (whose methodology of assessment is completely different from that of expectorants). The reduction of cough in patients with bronchial hypersecretion treated by expectorants may be considered as a consequence of their possible effect on the removal of bronchial secretions. Therefore, the reduction of cough is not a criterion of assessment of expectorants.[9] Nevertheless, the committee in charge of the "National Mucolytic Study" recognized that "both anecdotal reports and controlled studies provide data to support the improvement in symptoms such as the frequency and/or severity of cough, chest discomfort, difficulty in raising sputum, and subjective global evaluations of over-all pulmonary status in response to mucoevacuant therapy".[10] This position was taken because of "the difficulty associated with demonstrating effectiveness by objective criteria, the lack of definitive clinical data, and uncertainty about the patients who are likely to benefit from this therapeutic modality".[10]

The assessment of quality-of-life can be considered as a means to evaluate the usefulness of a drug for a patient. An attempt to evaluate the effect of expectorants on well-being has recently been performed in the "National Mucolytic Study",[10] but this assessment was an evaluation of comfort and ease of expectoration, not of quality-of-life of patients.

Lung Function Tests. The efficacy of expectorants is frequently evaluated by measuring lung function (airway resistance, peak expiratory flow rate, blood gases, etc.), but the relevance of these criteria has been questioned.[11,12] The effect of expectorants on lung function cannot be assessed without taking into account

Table 34.2 Classification of Expectorants

Class of Expectorant	Mechanism of Action	Examples
Mucolytics		
Compounds with free thiol group	Dostroy disulfide bonds of proteins and glycoproteins	N-acetylcysteine Ethylcysteine Mercaptoethane sodium sulfonate (Mesna) Mecysteine
Proteolytic enzymes	Hydrolyze peptide bonds of proteins or glycoproteins	Trypsine, chymotrypsine
Deoxyribonuclease	Destroys deoxyribonucleic acid fibers	Deoxyribonuclease
Mucoregulators	Alter the secretory activity of the bronchila mucosa	Bromhexine Ambroxol (bromhexine metabolite)
	Activate sialomucin synthesis	Carbocysteine
"Hydrating" Agents	Correct water and electrolyte disorders in secretions	Sodium chloride Sodium bicarbonate Water
Tensio-Active Agents	Make secretions less adhesive	Tyloxapol
Other Compounds	Modify fibrillate structures (?)	Eprazinone

whether these drugs are administered alone or combined with other treatments (physiotherapy, bronchodilator drugs, etc.). However, this effect can, to some extent, be estimated indirectly through lung function tests, provided there are no drug interactions. In any case, the modifications detected by such tests are small, and they seldom correlated with more direct evaluation methods, such as measurement of mucociliary clearance.[11] In addition, lung function tests are useful for evaluating the possible respiratory side-effects of expectorants.

Tracheobronchial Studies. Tracheobronchial studies have been extensively reviewed in the literature.[13–15] Their use for the study of the effect of drugs on bronchial secretion removal by mucociliary transport and cough is a useful pharmacologic approach, but they cannot replace therapeutic trials. Mucociliary function can be studied either directly, by measuring mucociliary transport, or indirectly, by measuring the mucociliary clearance that reflects this transport. Mucociliary transport is measured by the speed at which mucus travels over the tracheobronchial epithelium.[15] Mucociliary clearance is measured by detecting the radioactivity of inhaled particles outside the chest.[15] A number of factors that may influence the measurement of mucociliary clearance have been evaluated: site of deposition of tracer aerosol (size of the particle, pattern of inhalation, airway calibre); lung size; mucus-cilia interaction; mucosal surface damage; cough, exercise, disease, and drugs[13,14] (Table 34.2). Radionuclide techniques assess the efficacy of cough on the removal of bronchial secretions in patients as well as in healthy subjects.[7,8]

In Vitro and Ex Vivo Studies. Such studies are used in attempts at understanding the pathologic changes observed in mucociliary function and the mechanisms of action of the drugs investigated. They do not directly evaluate the changes that occur in vivo in the removal of bronchial secretions, and therefore the clinical efficacy of the expectorant tested. To study bronchial secretions is to study one of the components of mucociliary transport.

Chemical studies of secretions describe the relative importance of their various fractions (water, glycoproteins, etc.), which determine their rheologic properties such as viscosity, elasticity, spinability. The viscosity and elasticity of bronchial fluids often are analyzed in terms of viscoelasticity modulus, i.e., the ratio of the strain applied to the resulting elastic deformation. Mucociliary transport on frog palate provides information on the functional quality of bronchial secretions, but not on the mucociliary transport as a whole. Measurements are performed on freshly excised frog palate placed in a conditioned, water-saturated chamber kept at a temperature of 30°C.[16]

Other Properties of Expectorants. Some other properties of expectorants have been mentioned. These are indirect properties and must be evaluated as such. It has been reported that expectorants facilitate the diffusion of antibiotics in bronchial secretions, but the clinical significance of variations in local concentrations of antibiotic under the influence of expectorants remains to be determined. The antioxidant properties of expectorants should also be evaluated, but this is beyond the scope of this chapter.

Pharmacologic and Therapeutic Effects

Mucolytics include reducing agents, proteolytic enzymes, and deoxyribonuclease. Reducing agents act on cohesion linkage by destroying disulfide bonds, thereby disuniting the fibrillated structures. They possess a free thiol group, and the best known of them is N-acetylcysteine. In several studies N-acetylcysteine was found to reduce the elasticity and viscosity of secretions, but it did not reduce their amount and did not improve the patients' respiratory function.[17,18] Whenever a functional improvement was observed, it could be ascribed to the concomitant use of a bronchodilatator.[17] There is no evidence that use of N-acetylcysteine is superior to saline instillation or adequate humidification alone.

Proteolytic enzymes, such as trypsin or chymotrypsin, hydrolyze the peptide bonds of glycoproteins; deoxyribonuclease hydrolyzes the DNA fibers present in purulent secretions. In vitro, these enzymes significantly reduce viscidity and elasticity but, unfortunately, their in vivo activity is far from being similar to that observed in vitro. Chymotrypsin, trysin, and desoxyribonuclease are not approved for inhalation therapy in the US. Water, hypertonic saline, and potassium iodide have also been used to increase sputum fluidity.[19,20]

Mucoregulators activate in vivo the synthesis of sialomucin and/or surfactant. S-carboxymethylcysteine is a compound with a blocked thiol group. When studied in vitro on the dog tracheal mucosa it had no effect on the rheologic properties of mucus or on mucociliary transport.[21] It acts by activating sialyl transferase. In patients with chronic bronchitis, a significant diminution of sputum viscidity has been observed after nine days of treatment with this compound combined with an antibiotic. In the same category of patients, S-carboxymethylcysteine has been claimed to exert a mucoregulatory activity by increasing mucus viscidity and elasticity that were initially too low (rheologically nonfunctional secretions).[22] Not all authors, however, have found an increase in the amount of secretion and a reduction of viscidity after short or prolonged treatment with this drug: mucociliary clearance remains unmodified.[23] Bromhexine is derived from *Adhatoda vasica* (Acanthacae). In an uncontrolled study, bromhexine has been reported to increase mucociliary clearance in patients with chronic bronchitis (48 mg/d for 14 days).[24] Ambroxol is a bromhexine metabolite.

Undesirable Effects and Interactions

N-acetylcysteine is contraindicated in patients with advanced chronic bronchitis, since fluidifying a mucus that already has low viscidity and elasticity can only hinder and delay its transport. The drug is also unsuitable for patients with peptic ulcer; moreover, it may induce bronchial obstruction when inhaled as an aerosol. Side-effects such as gastric pain, cutaneous erythema, and hypothyroidism have been observed after treatment with potassium iodide;[25,26] it inactivates some antibiotics (penicillins, cephalosporins) and may inhibit the ciliary activity. The use of proteolytic enzymes is limited by a risk of sensitization. When inhaled, these drugs may be responsible for inflammation of the bronchial mucosa, bronchial obstruction, or anaphylactic shock. Oral administration is useless because these enzymes are destroyed by digestive enzymes. Mucoregulators may produce GI disorders. Inhaled agents active against surface tension, such as tyloxapol, may induce bronchial obstruction.

Pharmacokinetics

After oral administration, the plasma levels of N-acetylcysteine reach their peak in two to three hours and remain high after 24 hours; most of the active substance is bound to plasma proteins. Proteolytic enzymes are best absorbed by the sublingual route; their distribution and excretion are imperfectly understood. After oral administration of carbocysteine, peak plasma levels are obtained in two hours; the half-life of the drug is three hours, and it is excreted chiefly in the urine. The plasma levels of letosteine show a peak at three hours; much of the compound is taken up by the lungs, and excretion is mainly through the kidneys. After an oral dose of bromhexine, peak plasma levels are observed at three hours; the half-life of the drug is 24 hours, and it is excreted chiefly in the urine. Eprazinone shows a peak plasma level one hour after oral administration, and its half-life is six hours.

Available Preparations and Usual Doses

The principal presentations and usual therapeutic doses of expectorants are shown in Table 34.3.

Summary and Conclusion

The principal drugs acting on mucociliary transport are bronchodilators and expectorants. Among bronchodilators, beta-sympathomimetics and theophylline accelerate mucociliary transport, while synthetic atropine-like compounds have no effect on it. Expectorants include mucolytics, mucoregulators, "hydrating" agents, and surface tension-reducing agents. The effectiveness of these drugs and their usefulness to the patients need to be proved by controlled clinical trials. So far, the clinical assessment of their activity has been subjective, imprecise, and indirect. Mucociliary clearance, which reflects mucociliary transport, can be determined by inhalation of a radio-labeled aerosol, but its measurement cannot replace therapeutic trials. Respiratory tests do not directly measure the effects of expectorants but only their possible indirect effects. The changes observed are often minor and seldom correlate with the results of other methods of evaluation. In vitro and ex-vivo studies of bronchial secretions (chemical composition, rheologic properties, mucociliary transport as seen on the frog's palate) cannot predict in vivo changes in bronchial drainage produced by cough or mucociliary transport.

Drugs that Alter Surface Tension

"Surfactant" has long been recognized as an essential component of the aveolar walls of the lung, since

Table 34.3 Clinical Use of the Main Expectorants

Chemical Family	Chemical name	Route of administration	Daily doses
Free SH Group	N-acetylcysteine	Inhaler	0.5 to 2 g/24 hr
		Instillation	0.2 to 0.4 g diluted at 50 % in normal saline 1 to 4 hourly
		Oral	200 mg 3 times a day
	Mercaptoethane sodium sulfonate	Inhaler, instillation	600 mg 1 to 4 times a day, diluted in normal saline
	Ethylcysteine	Oral	300 mg 2 to 3 times a day
	Mecysteine	Inhaler	5 ml ampules (250 mg): 250 mg 2 to 6 times a day
		Oral	200 mg twice a day
Blocked SH Group	Carbocysteine	Oral	750 mg 2 to 3 times a day
	Letosteine	Oral	50 mg 3 times a day
Alkaloid Derivatives	Bromhexine	Inhaler	100 ml solution=200 mg (2 ml, 2 to 4 times a day)
		Injection	2 ml ampule (4 mg), 4 mg, 2 to 4 times a day
		Oral	4 to 8 mg 3 times a day
	Ambroxol	Oral	30 or 90 mg per day
Piperazine Derivatives	Eprazinone	Oral	50 mg 3 to 6 times a day
		Rectal	100 mg 2 to 3 times a day
Phenol Derivatives	Guaifenesine	Oral	400 mg 4 times a day

it keeps the surface tension at the water/air interface in the lung at low values. This property prevents alveoli with decreased diameters from collapsing as gases are expelled from the lung in expiration. The loss of surfactant has been proposed as a primary cause of neonatal (and perhaps other) respiratory distress syndromes (RDS). There are now preparations of beef "surfactant"[r4] (beractant in the US); (Surfactant-TA) and porcine surfactant (Curosurf) in Japan and Europe. Beractant contains phospholipids (25 mg/ml), triglycerides (0.5–1.75 mg/ml), and free fatty acids (1.4–3.5 mg/ml) derived from minces of beef lungs by shaking with cofosceril palmitate, palmitic acid, and tripalmatin. Two low molecular weight hydrophobic "surfactant associated proteins (SP-B and SP-C) contribute to the protein content (1 mg/ml) of this extract. Fortunately, antibovine antibody production has not yet been reported. These preparations are under investigation for even wider use in managing patients with pulmonary problems. Such extracts contain a widely divergent number of chemical entities, which might be a disadvantage, except that there is still some debate as to the most important surface tension lowering chemical. Thus, at least a wide variety of possible alternatives is received by the patient.

An alternative approach has been to treat patients with the chemical components that comprise the largest fraction of organic molecules. Since phosphatidylcholine and phosphatidylglycerol are the most common molecular entities, synthetic dipalmitoylphosphatidylcholine has been developed, utilizing cetyl alcohol to aid in spreading the phospholipid on the alveolar surfaces (Colfosceril-Exosurf). For tracheal administration the mixture is dispersed in a NaCl, $CaCl_2$ mixture using a detergent, tyloxapol, to aid by saponification. The drug is currently indicated for prophylaxis of RDS in infants under 1350 g, and in heavier infants with pulmonary immaturity, as well as for treatment of infants with RDS.[27] The use of the drug in adults with RDS appears promising, but is not yet an approved indication in the US. In infants the mortality of RDS has been reduced by this therapy,[1] but there is a chance of intrapulmonary hemorrhage, especially in patients whose ductus arteriosus has not yet closed. In addition, instillation of the dispersed material into the small conducting airways where it must go also often produces transient, but occasionally severe hypoxia (10%). The improved chest compliance after administration may produce dangerous hyperoxia and hypocarbia unless mechanical ventilatory parameters are decreased appropriately. Obstruction of the endotracheal tube with secretions, hypotension, and apnea are also common events during treatment. There are no direct comparative studies of the synthetic preparations with the bovine lung extracts.[28]

Available Preparations:

Exosurf, 5 ml/kg every 12 hr., via a special endotracheal tube adapter.

Beractant, 4 ml/kg every 6 hr., via endotracheal tube adapter.

References

Research Reports

1. Landa JF, Hirsch JA, LeBeaux MI. Effects of topical and general anesthetic agents on tracheal mucous velocity of sheep. J Appl Physiol 1975;*38*:946–948.
2. Patrick G, Stirling C. Measurement of mucociliary clearance from the trachea of conscious and anesthetized rat. J A Appl Physiol 1977;*42*:451–455.
3. Pavia D, Bateman M, Sheahan NF, Clarke SW. Effect of ipatropium bromide on mucociliary clearance and pulmonary function in reversible airways obstruction. Thorax 1979;*34*:501–507.
4. Sturgess J, Reid L. An organ culture study of the effects of drugs on the secretory activity of the human bronchial submucosal glands. Clin Sci 1972;*43*:533–543.
5. Foster WM, Bergofsky EH, Bohning DE, Lippman M, Albert RE. Effect of adrenergic agents and their mode of action on mucociliary clearance in man. J Appl Physiol 1976;*41*:146–152.
6. Sutton PP; Pavia D; Bateman JRM, Clarke SW. The effect of oral aminophylline on lung mucociliary clearance in man. Chest 1981;*80*:889–892.
7. Bennett WD, Foster WM, Chapman WF. Cough enhanced mucus clearance in the normal lung. J Appl Physiol 1990;*69*:1670–1675.
8. Pavia D, Agnew JE, Clarke SW. Cough and mucociliary clearance. Clin Respir Physiol 1987;*23*:41S–45S.
9. Irwin RS, Curley FJ, Pratter MR. The effects of drugs on cough. Eur J Respir Dls 1987;*71*:173–181.
10. Petty TL. The national mucolytic study. Results of a randomized, double blind, placebo-controlled study of iodinated glycerol on chronic obstructive bronchitis. Chest 1990;*97*:75–83.
11. Demets M. Assessment of airway secretions by pulmonary function tests. Eur J Respir Dis 1987;*71*:330–333.
12. Medici TC, Shang H, Grosgurin P, Berg P, Achermann R, Wehrli R. No demonstrable effect of sobrerol as an expectorant in patients with stable chronic bronchial diseases. Bull Eur Physiopathol Respir 1985;*21*:477–483.
13. Pavia D. Lung mucociliary clearance. In Clarke SW, Pavia D (Eds): Aerosols and the lung: clinical and experimental aspects. London: Butterworths (1984);*275*:127–155.
14. Yeates DB, Gerrity TR, Garrard CS. Characteristics of tracheobronchial deposition and clearance in man. Ann Occup Hyg 1982;*26*:245–257.
15. Pavia D, Sutton PP, Agnew JE, Lopez-Vidriero MT, Newman SP, Clarke SW. Measurement of bronchial mucociliary clearance. Eur J Respir Dis 1983;*64*:Suppl 127, 41–56.
16. Puchelle E, Tournier JM, Petit A, Zahm JM, Lauque D, Vidailhet M, Sadoul P. The frog palate for studying mucus transport velocity and mucociliary frequency. Eur J Respir Dis 1983;*64*:Suppl 128, 293–303.
17. Kory RC, Hirsch SR, Giraldo J. Nebulisation of N-acetyl cysteine combined with a bronchodilatator in patients with chronic bronchitis, a controlled study. Dis Chest 1968;*54*:504–509.

18. Multi Center Study Group. Long-term oral acetyl cysteine in chronic bronchitis: a double blind controlled study. Eur J Respir Dis 1980;*61*:(Suppl) 93–95.

19. Marriott C, Richards JG. The effects of storage and potassium iodide, urea, N-acetyl cysteine and trixon X-100 on the viscosity of bronchial mucus. Br J Dis Chest 1974;*68*:171–182.

20. Lieberman J, Kurnick MB. The induction of proteolysis in purulent sputum by iodides. J Clin Invest 1964;*43*:1892–1897.

21. Martin R, Mitchell L, Marriot C. The effect of mucolytic agents on the rheologic air transport properties of canine tracheal mucus. Am Rev Respir Dis 1980;*121*:495–499.

22. Puchelle E, Aug F, Polu JM. Effect of mucoregulator S-carboxymethyl-cysteine in patients with chronic bronchitis. Eur J Clin Pharmacol 1978;*14*:177–184.

23. Thomson ML, Pavia D, Jones JL, Mc Quinston TAC. No demonstrable effect of S-carboxymethyl cysteine on clearance of secretion from the human lung. Thorax 1975;*30*:669–673.

24. Thomson ML, Pavia P, Gregg I, Stark VE. The effect of bromhexine on mucociliary clearance from the human lung in chronic bronchitis. Scand J Respir Dis (Suppl) 1974;*90*:75–79.

25. Bernstein LI, Austenmore RW. Iatrogenic bronchospasm occurring during clinical trials of a new mucolytic agent, acetyl cysteine. Dis Chest 1964;*46*:469–472.

26. Bernecker G. Potassium iodide in bronchial asthma. Br Med J 1969;*4*:236–240.

27. Reynolds MS, Wallander KA. Use of surfactant in the prevention and treatment of neonatal respiratory distress syndrome. Clin Pharm 1989;*8*:559–576.

28. Soll RF, Lucey, JF. Surfactant replacement Therapy. Pediatr Rev 1991;*12*:261–267.

Reviews

r1. Brain JD, Proctor DF, Reid, LM. Respiratory defense mechanisms, part I & II. In Lenfant. C. Lung biology in health and desease. New York & Basel: Ed: Dekker, (1977).

r2. Phipps RJ. The airway mucociliary system. Int rev physiol 1981;*23*:213–260.

r3. Lurie A, Mestiri M, Huchon G, Marsac, J, Lockhart, A, Strauch G. Methods for clinical assessment of expectorants: a critical review. Int J Clin Pharm Res 1992;*12*:47–52.

r4. Jobe AH. Pulmonary surfactant therapy. N Engl J Med 1993;*328*:861–868.

SECTION V

Renal Pharmacology

Editor:
William O. Berndt

CHAPTER 35

Introduction to Renal Pharmacology

William O. Berndt

Introduction

The modern practice of the health professions, especially medicine, requires a thorough knowledge of drugs that alter fluid and electrolyte balance, whatever their mechanisms of action. However, drugs and chemicals that affect the kidney directly are most important. Many of the drugs that act on the kidney to reduce salt and water reabsorption are used extensively because they have actions beyond those specifically related to renal function. Nonetheless, their effects on renal function occur, whatever the intended use.

To understand drug effects on renal function, health practitioners must have a working knowledge of how the kidney performs. Without such information, an understanding of drug actions, mechanisms, etc., is extremely difficult if not impossible. Of course, not all aspects of renal function are relevant to drug effects on the kidney, but a knowledge of those renal activities that underlie drug effects is critical.

Not all drugs or potential drugs affect salt and water excretion uniformly. Some drugs alter salt reabsorption more than that of water; other drugs dramatically affect water movement more than that of sodium chloride. Most drugs that change sodium reabsorption also alter potassium movement across the renal tubular cells. Hence, drug effects on the kidney can be complex, but almost always are predictable if one's understanding of renal function is adequate.

Unfortunately, several drugs have effects on the kidney that are neither desirable nor intended. Many of these actions go beyond simple alterations of fluid and electrolyte balance. Having a knowledge of these adverse renal effects will help the practice of modern medicine tremendously. Many drugs have acute detrimental effects on renal function. Indeed, some extremely valuable therapeutic agents are of limited usefulness because of nephrotoxicity. Others produce more chronic effects.

Finally, it must be appreciated that the kidney serves an important function with respect to the elimination of many drugs and chemicals. The mechanisms that underlie these processes have revealed much about renal function. In addition, much has been learned about the mechanisms by which drug or chemical interactions occur. An understanding of renal excretory mechanisms for drugs and chemicals will facilitate an appreciation of drug toxicities and interactions.

In summary, this section has been developed to provide the reader with an essential knowledge of renal function as it underlies drug or chemical effects on the kidney. In addition, emphasis has been placed on the mechanisms by which the kidney eliminates drugs and thereby often terminates drug action.

Of course, drug effects on the kidney also have been emphasized since this knowledge provides a direct basis for therapeutics. Desirable and often predictable drug actions are presented along with those that are undesirable and often unpredictable. Except for one chapter, the focus is on drug effects and drug handling by the kidneys. The therapeutic value of fluid and electrolyte replacement is covered elsewhere in this book.

CHAPTER 36

Fluid and Electrolyte Balance

Peter A. Friedman

The kidneys normally maintain the volume and composition of the extracellular fluid (ECF) compartment within narrow limits. Retention of sodium may result from reductions of the glomerular filtration rate (GFR), as in acute glomerulonephritis. However, the pathologic accumulation of sodium leading to edema more commonly results from the same underlying mechanisms that are responsible for the physiologic conservation of salt in states of ECF volume contraction. These mechanisms are activated by reductions of actual plasma volume, as in hemorrhage, or by reductions of effective plasma volume, as in hypoalbuminemia or cardiac failure. In these latter instances, the kidneys can be viewed as attempting, although inappropriately, to restore a functionally adequate vascular volume.

Diuretics are drugs that have the pharmacologic property of increasing the renal excretion of salt and water, thereby producing a net negative sodium balance. Such an augmentation of urinary salt and water excretion, which is generally referred to as diuresis, results from direct inhibition by diuretic drugs of sodium absorption by renal tubules. The effectiveness of any particular diuretic will be determined largely by the nephron site where tubular sodium absorption is blocked, the quantity of salt delivered to that site, compensatory increases of salt absorption at nephron locations distal to the site of drug action, or to physiologic compensations in renal sodium conservation. In the first part of this chapter, a summary of the contribution of the integrated action of the kidney on ECF volume and osmotic homeostasis is presented; in the second part, the functions of individual nephron segments are discussed.

Body Fluid Compartments and Composition

Water is the most abundant component of the body and constitutes about 60 percent of body weight. In individuals with greater than average amounts of adipose tissue, water comprises a smaller percentage of body weight. Total body water is partitioned into several distinct compartments. The ECF compartment represents about one-third of the total body water, or 20 percent of body weight. The two major components of ECF are plasma (5% of body weight) and interstitial fluid plus lymph (15% of body weight). Transcellular fluids such as cerebrospinal fluid (CSF) and saliva account for 1.5% of body weight. The remainder of the body water is intracellular fluid (ICF), which represents two-thirds of body weight. The composition of ICF varies between tissues and its volume can be estimated only indirectly. The relative contribution of these different compartments to body weight is shown in Table 36.1.

The major electrolytes in plasma and interstitial fluids are Na^+, Cl^-, and HCO_3^-. Two characteristics of plasma electrolyte concentrations are especially noteworthy. First, because protein and lipids occupy some 7% of the plasma, the concentration of dissolved ions in plasma water exceeds that in plasma. Increases of plasma lipids further exaggerate the difference of elec-

Table 36.1 Selected Normal Values for Adults

Parameter	Value
GFR	125 ml/min, 180 L/d
Total body water	60% of body weight
Intracellular water	40% of body weight
Extracellular water (total)	20% of body weight
Extracellular water (plasma)	4% of body weight
Extracellular water (interstitial fluid)	16% of body weight

trolyte concentrations between plasma and plasma water. Second, although Na^+, K^+, Cl^-, and HCO^-_3 are, to a first approximation, completely dissociated (i.e., ionized) at plasma concentrations, this is not true for Ca^{2+} or Mg^{2+}. In the case of Ca^{2+}, 50–55 percent of the total serum calcium (see Table 36.2) is ionized. Moreover, 40% of calcium is bound to plasma proteins, and an additional 5–10% is complexed to anions such as phosphate and citrate. In the case of Mg^{2+}, 55% of the total plasma magnesium is ionized, 30 per cent is bound to plasma proteins, and 15% is complexed with anions.[r1]

Regulation of Extracellular Fluid Volume

As noted above and summarized in Table 36.2, about 60 percent of the body weight is water and one-third of that volume is contained in the ECF compartment. Sodium salts, mainly NaCl, constitute the bulk of the osmotically active solute in ECF. By virtue of the relatively high water permeability of cell membranes, changes in osmolality within a fluid compartment result in rapid equilibration of water between intracellular and extracellular compartments. The volume of ECF is determined primarily by the total amount of osmotically active solutes (and, therefore, of sodium salts), present in the ECF. Hence, simply stated, ECF volume is defended by alterations of renal NaCl conservation. Both intrarenal and extrarenal processes participate in regulating renal salt absorption.

Intrarenal regulation of salt absorption involves the macula densa (MD, Fig. 36.1), a component of the juxtaglomerular apparatus. In response to changes in the composition and rate of fluid flow emerging from the loop of Henle, renin is released into the circulation where it acts on angiotensin I to form the potent vasoconstrictor angiotensin II (AII). AII has dual actions on the kidneys, both of which amplify sodium conservation. First, AII decreases renal plasma flow (RPF) and GFR. However, preferential vasoconstriction of the efferent arteriole produces a greater fall of RPF than of GFR, thereby resulting in an increase of the renal filtration fraction (RPF/GFR). Increases of the filtration fraction, in turn, promote enhanced reabsorption of sodium by proximal tubules. Second, AII stimulates secretion of the mineralocorticoid aldosterone by the adrenal cortex. As discussed later, aldosterone enhances the reabsorption of sodium primarily by collecting duct principal cells, but also by increasing NaCl

Table 36.2 Electrolyte Composition of Extracellular Fluids

Ion	Plasma	Plasma Water	Interstitial fluid
	mEq/L		
Cations			
Na^+	141	152	144
K^+	4	4	4
Ca^{2+}	5	5	
Mg^{2+}	2	2	
Total cations	152	163	>148
Anions			
Cl^-	104	112	118
HCO_3^-	27	29	31
$HPO_4^{=}$	2	2	
$SO_4^{=}$	1	1	
Organic acids	3	3	
Protein	15	16	
Total anions	152	163	>149

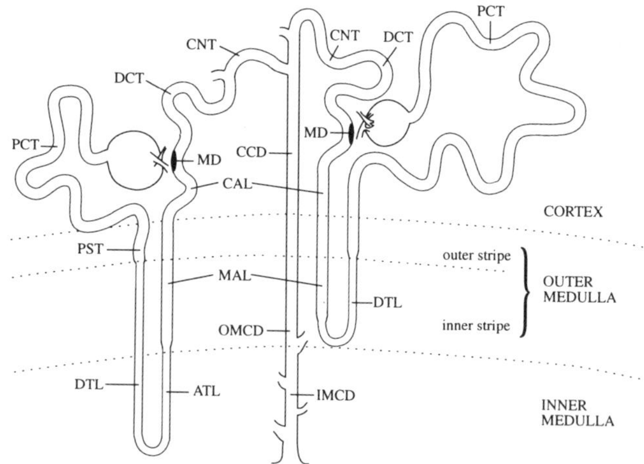

Figure 36.1 Schematic representation of human nephron. Glomeruli are located exclusively in the cortex. A long-looped juxtamedullary nephron is depicted on the left and a short-looped cortical nephron on the right. Abbreviations: PCT = proximal convoluted tubule; PST = proximal straight tubule; DTL = descending thin limb (of Henle's loop); ATL = ascending thin limb; MAL = medullary thick ascending limb; CAL = cortical thick ascending limb; MD = macula densa; DCT = distal convoluted tubule; CNT = connecting tubule; CCD = cortical collecting duct; OMCD = outer medullary collecting duct; and, IMCD = inner medullary collecting duct.

transport in thick ascending limbs. Under the influence of aldosterone, sodium wasting becomes negligibly small.

Extrarenal regulation of sodium absorption involves the coordinated activity of high and low pressure baroreceptors, neural pathways, and hormonal activity. High-pressure baroreceptors are located in the carotid sinus and aortic arch; low pressure baroreceptors are in the pulmonary vasculature and cardiac atria. These receptors influence renal sodium conservation both directly and indirectly. Direct effects involve increased renal sympathetic activity, resulting in elevation of the renal filtration fraction, and, indirectly, through their action on cardiovascular and circulatory reflexes.

An additional factor involved in the regulation of ECF volume is atrial natriuretic peptide (ANP). This hormone is produced in the atria and released in response to volume-induced stretch.[1] ANP acts on the kidney by vasodilating glomerular afferent and efferent arterioles, leading to an increase in GFR and, hence, in the filtered load of NaCl. ANP also acts directly on terminal nephron segments to reduce sodium reabsorption. Lastly, ANP inhibits renin release from the macula densa (see Fig. 36.1), aldosterone secretion by the adrenal cortex, and vasopressin release from the posterior pituitary. Taken together, these actions of ANP collectively serve to attenuate the effects of the renin-angiotensin-aldosterone axis on sodium conservation and of vasopressin on water reabsorption.

Regulation of Extracellular Fluid Tonicity

Although ECF volume is governed by mechanisms that regulate the amount of solute, principally NaCl, reabsorbed by the kidney, extracellular solute concentrations are determined by the volume of water excreted by the kidneys. Renal water excretion is regulated by vasopressin (antidiuretic hormone, ADH) in response to increases in plasma osmolality or to decreases of effective extracellular volume.[r2] Vasopressin is a polypeptide that is synthesized in the hypothalamus and stored in and released into the circulation from nerve terminals in the posterior pituitary. The release of vasopressin is highly sensitive to even small changes in plasma osmolality. Increases in plasma osmolality of as little as 1 percent provoke vasopressin release. In contrast, relatively large decreases (~10%) of effective plasma volume are necessary to trigger the release of vasopressin. However, in contrast to the *linear* increases in plasma vasopressin with increases in plasma osmolality, decreases in plasma volume elicit *exponential* elevations in plasma vasopressin. Irrespective of the stimulus to vasopressin release, water reabsorption is enhanced, leading to restoration of extracellular osmolality and inhibition of hormone release. Surgical stress may also induce vasopressin release and may cause water retention and hyponatremia.

Summary of Nephron Function

The functional unit of the kidney is the nephron. In humans, each kidney contains about one million nephrons. Each nephron consists of two parts, a glomerulus and a tubule. The glomerulus is a specialized vascular capillary bed, the surrounding capsule of which is continuous with the renal tubule. Renal tubules are formed from a cylindrical array of epithelial cells. The epithelial cells comprising the tubules are structurally and functionally polarized, thereby permitting net vectorial solute and solvent movement. Apical plasma membranes form the luminal (or mucosal) surface, whereas basolateral plasma membranes face the serosal peritubular interstitial space. Adjacent cells are connected at their apical membranes by tight junctions. Variations in tight junctional permeability between different nephron segments influence, and may dominate, the over-all permeability characteristics of individual nephrons. Some 25 different epithelial cell types, distributed largely into discrete nephron segments, confer much of the distinguishing features of sodium transport. Since the kidney exhibits a number of distinct mechanisms of sodium reabsorption, their transport properties should condition the choice of an appropriate diuretic. For this reason it is useful to review the mechanisms of NaCl reabsorption in the kidney. Two renal processes contribute to the formation and composition of the urine: glomerular filtration and tubular transport, either reabsorptive or secretory.

The first step in the formation of urine involves the separation at the glomerulus of an essentially protein-free ultrafiltrate from plasma. The glomerulus is composed of an outer glomerular capsule, the glomerular capillary tuft, and the basement membrane. To reach the lumen of the proximal tubule, fluid must cross the capillary endothelium, the basement membrane, and the epithelial cell layer of Bowman's capsule. The limiting barrier to the passage of solutes from Bowman's space into the lumen of the proximal tubule appears to involve endothelial, mesangial, and visceral layer epithelial cells, as well as the glomerular basement membrane.[3]

The forces regulating the filtration of fluid at the glomerulus are the same as those governing filtration in other capillary beds. Thus, the rate of glomerular filtration (GFR, ml/min, or L/day; see Table 36.1) is the product of the intrinsic ultrafiltration coefficient of the glomerulus (K_f), and the net sum of the forces favoring and opposing filtration:

$$GFR = K_f(\Delta P - \Pi_{GC})$$

where ΔP is the net hydrostatic pressure favoring ultrafiltration, and Π_{GC} is the average oncotic pressure in the glomerular capillary impeding ultrafiltration. As in other capillary networks, K_f itself is the product of the intrinsic capillary permeability and the surface area available for filtration. Although net filtration pressure is similar in glomerular capillaries as in other capillary beds, the magnitude of filtration is greater in glomerular capillaries. This increased filtration appears to result from the greater filtration surface area in glomerular capillaries.[r3]

Although diuretics do not directly alter GFR, two aspects of glomerular function affecting or affected by diuretics need to be considered. First, since all diuretics, except spironolactone, exert their inhibitory action from the apical membrane surface, they must be present at sufficiently high concentrations in the tubular fluid at their nephron site of action to inhibit sodium transport. However, many drugs, including diuretics, are extensively bound to plasma proteins[5] and therefore are filtered only to a limited extent at the glomerulus. For highly protein-bound agents, such as the loop diuretics furosemide and bumetanide, entry into the luminal fluid is accomplished primarily by tubular secretion in proximal tubules.[r4] Diuretics less extensively bound to plasma proteins, such as amiloride, reach the luminal fluid through a combination of glomerular filtration and tubular secretion. Second, many nondiuretic drugs are vasodilators that reduce renal plasma flow and hence, GFR. Under conditions of reduced ECF volume, regardless of its origin, the amount of sodium reaching the nephron site at which an administered diuretic acts may be so reduced that, operationally, there is nothing to inhibit. In other words, the failure of a diuretic to induce or to continue to effect a significant diuresis may result not from a loss of sensitivity to the diuretic per se, but from the lack of delivery of sufficient sodium to the nephron site at which the administered diuretic acts.[r5]

Proximal Tubule Solute and Water Absorption

The process of modification of the tubular fluid leading to the formation of the final urine begins in the proximal tubules (see Fig. 36.1). The composition of the tubular fluid is continuously modified along the length of the nephron by transepithelial transport of both solutes and water. Transepithelial solute transport may proceed, uniquely or simultaneously, in absorptive (lumen to blood) or in secretory (blood to lumen) directions. For most solutes, transport occurs, at least to some degree, in both directions, although not necessarily in the same nephron segment. Over-all movement in one direction generally exceeds that in the opposite direction, if present. The dominant direction of movement is referred to as the direction of net transport, i.e., net reabsorption or net secretion. Furthermore, movement of solute across the tubule epithelium may occur through cells and between cells.

In proximal tubules, sodium absorption is mediated by several different transport mechanisms. Importantly, solute absorption in proximal tubules proceeds isosmotically, i.e., the luminal fluid remains at the same total osmotic solute concentration as that in peritubular capillaries. Some 65–70 per cent of salt and water filtered at the glomerulus is reabsorbed along the length of the proximal nephron. Several different cellular processes contribute to NaCl absorption in proximal tubules. These include: sodium-coupled absorption of glucose, amino acids, phosphate, and, perhaps, chloride; sodium/proton (Na^+/H^+) exchange; chloride/formate ($Cl^-/HCOO^-$) and electrogenic sodium reabsorption, i.e., electrically conductive movement of sodium driven by combined electrical and chemical gradients.[r6]

Although it is accepted that NaCl absorption in proximal nephrons proceeds isosmotically, i.e., luminal fluid is virtually isosmotic to that in the peritubular space, it is now recognized that tubular fluid becomes slightly hypotonic with respect to plasma, thereby producing an osmotic gradient for the diffusion of water.[2,3] The importance of these observations is that they provide an explanation for the development of driving forces to account for fluid absorption in proximal tubules. The high osmotic water permeability of the proximal nephron assures that the luminal fluid remains near isotonic. The functional corollary of this high water permeability is that the presence in the luminal fluid of nonabsorbable or poorly permeable solutes will retard fluid absorption by proximal tubules. This effect provides the basis for the action of osmotic diuretics. In the presence of a nonabsorbable solute, proximal sodium absorption continues until a limiting transepithelial gradient is reached. However, as a result of the high water permeability and the presence of the nonabsorbable solute, fluid leaks back into the lumen at a rate sufficient to keep the contents isosmotic. The continued absorption of sodium, but now without concomitant fluid absorption, dissociates the normally near-isosmotic reabsorptive process, and may lead to hypernatremia.[r7]

An additional driving force for water absorption by proximal nephrons is due to differences in the anion composition of luminal and peritubular fluids.[4,5] This difference arises from the preferential absorption of bicarbonate in the first part of proximal convoluted tubules and leads to the development of high luminal chloride concentrations in the latter portion of proximal convoluted tubules.[6] The transepithelial gradient for chloride, in turn, serves as a driving force for solute and water absorption in the late proximal tubule.[7]

The secretion of protons (H^+) into the lumen of proximal tubules in exchange for sodium (Na^+/H^+ exchange, Fig. 36.2) results in the titration of filtered bicarbonate to carbonic acid (H_2CO_3) that, in turn, is dehydrated to CO_2 and H_2O. The CO_2 generated in this process diffuses into proximal tubule cells, where it combines with water and, in the presence of cytoplasmic carbonic anhydrase, forms carbonic acid. The carbonic acid, in turn, is ionized to bicarbonate (HCO_3^-) and hydrogen ions. The bicarbonate formed in the cytoplasm leaves the cell across basolateral membranes. This latter process may be mediated by one or more electrogenic mechanisms involving electrogenic sodium bicarbonate cotransport[7] (not shown in Fig. 36.2). Clearly, bicarbonate absorption mediated by such processes has several important implications. For instance, no "new" bicarbonate is formed by these cyclic processes; second, bicarbonate absorption is coupled thermodynamically to sodium.

Proximal Organic Ion Transport

The proximal nephron is also the site of organic anion and cation transport. Transport of organic ions proceeds in both secretory and absorptive (or reabsorptive) directions. Separate pathways are responsible for the transport of organic anions and for organic cations. Secretory and absorptive transport are mediated by specific proteins found in basolateral and apical plasma membranes, respectively. These transporters represent not only the means of reabsorption of endogenous solutes, such as urate, but also of the secretory movement of many organic anions, including all diuretic drugs except mannitol and spironolactone.

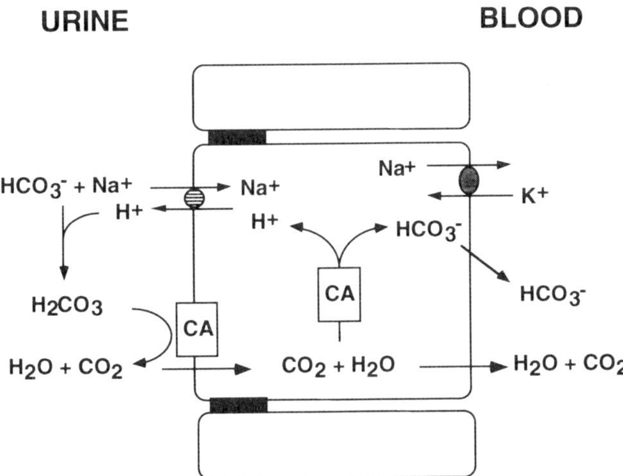

Figure 36.2 Mechanisms of proximal tubular fluid acidification and bicarbonate reabsorption. CA = carbonic anhydrase.

The secretory movement of weak organic electrolytes in proximal tubules is mediated by a two-step process involving carrier-mediated uptake into the cell across basolateral cell membranes, followed by facilitated diffusion across luminal (apical) cell membranes into the tubular fluid. Uptake across basolateral plasma membranes and accumulation above electrochemical equilibrium in the cytoplasm is an energy-dependent process. Diffusion of the anion from the cell into the luminal fluid is driven by the favorable chemical gradient from cell to lumen, together with the intracellular electronegativity.[r6]

Binding of weak organic acids to the basolateral membrane transporter can be competitively inhibited by other weak organic anions, but not by cations. This is a therapeutically important consideration since lactic acid and other anionic solutes that are products of intermediary metabolism may accumulate in plasma during renal failure. The elevated concentrations of these weak organic anions may competitively inhibit the tubular secretion of diuretics, thereby diminishing or even preventing their diuretic effect,[8] which depends on their antecedent secretion into the luminal fluid. Thus, it should be pointed out that the effect of diuretics acting in thick ascending limbs, distal convoluted tubules, or in collecting ducts may by blunted by reductions in the secretion of these compounds by proximal tubules. Raising the dose of the diuretic under these circumstances may overcome the inhibition and permit entry of sufficient amounts of the drug into the tubular fluid to restore its diuretic effect.

Calcium and Phosphate

Sixty per cent of the calcium filtered at the glomerulus is reabsorbed by proximal tubules. When sampled from accessible parts of proximal tubules, the ratio of calcium in the tubular fluid to that in glomerular filtrate ($[TF/GF]_{Ca^{2+}}$), i.e., in Bowman's space fluid, is greater than unity. This ratio stays constant along the length of proximal tubules, even following physiologic or experimental interventions that increase or decrease over-all renal calcium conservation. The basis for the elevated $[TF/GF]_{Ca^{2+}}$ and its constancy is uncertain. Irrespective of its origin, the increased luminal calcium concentration serves as a driving force for passive calcium reabsorption in the first (S1) portion of proximal convoluted tubules, where the permeability to calcium is high.

Calcium reabsorption closely parallels that of sodium by proximal convoluted tubules. These observations have led to the view that, in this nephron segment, the bulk of calcium absorption results from passive transport processes coupled, directly or indirectly, to active sodium transport. The remaining portion of calcium absorption, some 20 percent of total proximal tubule calcium absorption, is due to primary active transport of calcium. Finally, although the cellular mechanisms responsible for mediating apical membrane uptake of the active component of calcium absorption are not known, both Na^+/Ca^{2+} exchange and a Ca^{2+}-ATPase may participate in mediating basolateral efflux.[r8,9]

In contrast to proximal convoluted tubules, in the straight portion of proximal nephrons (S2, proximal straight tubule (PST), pars recta; Fig. 36.1), as much as 75 percent of transepithelial calcium absorption may be ascribed to active transport processes.[r8,10]

Calcium absorption by the S2 portion of proximal straight tubules is temperature-sensitive, but is not impaired by ouabain, suggesting that calcium efflux across basolateral membranes is not dependent on primary active sodium extrusion. These observations suggest that the Ca^{2+}-ATPase is the principal means of cellular calcium efflux, and that Na^+/Ca^{2+} exchange plays a negligible role in the efflux process in proximal straight tubules.

Proximal tubules are also the major site of phosphate reabsorption. Sixty to 70% of the filtered phosphate is reabsorbed by the end of the proximal tubule.[19] In the first part of the proximal tubule the rate of phosphate reabsorption exceeds the rate of fluid reabsorption. This relation holds until the phosphate concentration in the tubules declines by more than 30 percent below the plasma level. At this point, the rate of phosphate reabsorption parallels fluid reabsorption, and the tubular phosphate concentration stays relatively constant.

Although under experimental conditions a small component of distal and post-distal tubule phosphate reabsorption can be shown, this contribution to overall renal phosphate economy is minimal. Hence, for practical purposes, an increase in the excretion of phosphate following administration of a diuretic serves as a functional index that the drug inhibited, directly or indirectly, proximal tubule solute and fluid reabsorption. Similar considerations apply to the reabsorption and excretion of glucose and bicarbonate. That is, their appearance in voided urine following administration of a diuretic serves as a functional index that proximal tubule solute and water absorption were inhibited.

Descending Thin Limbs of Henle's Loop

The absorption of water continues in descending thin limbs of Henle's loop (DTL; Fig. 36.1). Descending thin limbs are characterized by low permeability to NaCl and urea, and a high permeability to water. This high water permeability, in the presence of a hypertonic medullary interstitium, provides the driving force for passive fluid absorption. Thus, unlike fluid absorption in proximal convoluted tubules, which is an isosmotic process, water movement in descending thin limbs proceeds without significant solute absorption. Hence, at the bend of the loop of Henle, the tubular fluid becomes hypertonic to plasma.[r10] Indeed, by virtue of the high water permeability of this nephron segment, the osmotic concentration of the tubular fluid at the bend of Henle's loop approximates that in the surrounding interstitium (2000 mOsm/kg H_2O).[r11] Except for osmotic diuretics, the descending thin limb does not represent a primary site of diuretic action. In the case of osmotic diuretics such as mannitol, the presence of nonabsorbable solute in the lumen of thin descending limbs limits net diffusional fluid exit.

Solute Absorption in Ascending Thin Limbs of Henle's Loop

The permeability properties of ascending thin limbs of Henle's loop (ATL, Fig. 36.1) are essentially opposite those of descending thin limbs. In ascending thin limbs, the tubule epithelium is impermeable to water but rather permeable to NaCl.[r12] Thus, NaCl reaching thin ascending limbs readily diffuses down its concentration gradient from tubular fluid into the interstitium. This process contributes to medullary interstitial osmolality and, in turn, supplies the thermodynamic driving force for the abstraction of water, in the presence of vasopressin, from collecting tubules. However, the ascending thin limb itself is not a site of diuretic action.

An additional aspect of solute movement in ascending thin limbs involves the contribution of urea to urinary concentrating ability by enhancing the passive diffusion of NaCl out of ATLs, as discussed above. Critical to this operation are the discrete and spatially separated permeabilities to water, sodium and to urea in descending thin and ascending thin limbs and in cortical and medullary collecting tubules.[11] The recycling of urea in the medulla causes urea to accumulate to high concentrations in the medullary interstitium, where it osmotically abstracts water from DTLs. This process, in turn, increases the NaCl concentration in the tubule fluid, since DTLs are poorly permeable to sodium. The stage is then set for sodium to diffuse out of the permeable ATL into the medullary interstitium. The fact that medullary interstitial osmolality is formed from the sum of salt and urea, instead of NaCl alone, permits this coupling and amplification effect to occur.

Solute Absorption in Thick Ascending Limbs of Henle's Loop

About 10–15% of the NaCl filtered at the glomerulus is normally reabsorbed by thick ascending limbs of Henle's loop (Fig. 36.1). Since thick ascending limbs represent the site at which one class of widely employed diuretics (so-called "loop diuretics," or "high-ceiling" diuretics) exerts its natriuretic effect, the physiologic properties and mechanism of sodium absorption in this nephron structure are discussed in some detail.

Thick ascending limbs consist of two anatomically and functionally distinct parts: the medullary thick ascending limb (MAL, Fig. 36.1), also referred to as the "medullary diluting site," and the cortical thick ascending limb (CAL, Fig. 36.1) or "cortical diluting site." These functional descriptions reflect the fact that, during maximal hydration, i.e., in the absence of vasopressin, urinary dilution begins in medullary and continues in cortical thick ascending limbs.

Both the permeability properties and the mechanism of sodium absorption are unique to this nephron segment. Thick ascending limbs of Henle's loop have hybrid permeabilities to water and sodium. Specifically, these nephron segments are negligibly permeable to water but exhibit very high rates of active sodium absorption.[12] Because thick ascending limbs are virtually water impermeable, salt absorption serves both to dilute the urine and to supply the energy for countercurrent multiplication.

Thick ascending limbs are not accessible to study through ordinary micropuncture techniques. Hence, our present understanding of the transport processes in this nephron site is derived from studies of isolated segments microperfused in vitro. Based on such investigations, it is generally accepted that NaCl absorption, in both medullary and cortical portions of thick ascending limbs, proceeds largely, if not entirely, by a secondary active transport process ultimately dependent on the activity of Na^+/K^+-ATPase in basolateral membranes (Fig. 36.3). Entry of chloride across apical membranes into cells is mediated by an electroneutral 1Na:1K:2Cl cotransport mechanism. This carrier-mediated process is driven by the chemical gradients for both Na^+ and Cl^-.[r13,r14] The movement of Na^+ into the cell provides the energy to drive K^+ absorption. Although the energy-dependent uptake of K^+ may seem to be thermodynamically dissipative and an inefficient use of the cotransporter, it can be shown that it contributes to over-all conservation of ATP. In fact, the recycling of K^+ across apical plasma membranes permits the electrical charge associated with the secretory flux of K^+ into the lumen to drive the absorptive transport of an equivalent amount of Na^+ through the Na^+-selective tight junctions. In this way, for every $3Na^+$ actively extruded by the basolateral Na^+/K^+-ATPase, an added $2Na^+$ are absorbed in parallel through the paracellular (or intercellular) pathway.[r13] Electroneutrality is maintained by the accompanying absorption of chloride. No significant net transport of K^+ occurs.

An additional mechanism is present in the cortical thick ascending limbs that may contribute to NaCl absorption. In some species, about 50 per cent of total NaCl absorption appears to be mediated by parallel

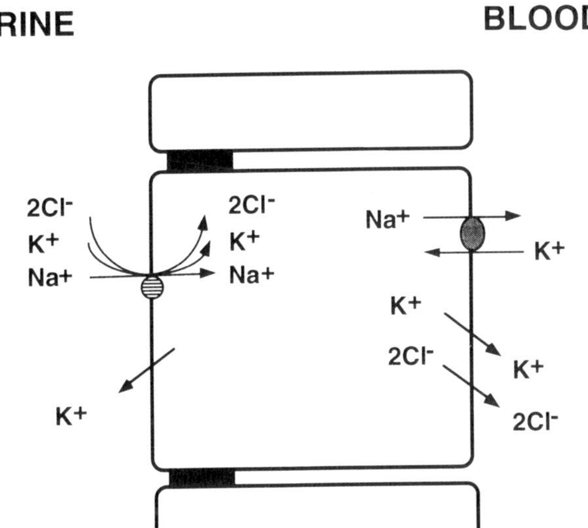

Figure 36.3 Cellular mechanism of NaCl absorption by thick ascending limb cells. Apical Na:K:2Cl cotransport is the target for the inhibitory action of loop diuretics such as furosemide, bumetanide, and piretanide.

Na^+/H^+ and Cl^-/HCO_3^- exchange.[13] This bicarbonate-dependent sodium transport is stimulated by carbonic anhydrase, an enzyme present in CALs of the mouse, the rat, and humans,[14] which supplies both H^+ and HCO_3^- to the respective countertransport exchangers.

Exit of chloride across basolateral membranes of MAL and CAL cells is passive and proceeds primarily through chloride-conductive channels.[r13] An electroneutral KCl exit process may also contribute to cellular chloride exit.[15] The asymmetric electrical properties of apical (primarily K^+ conductive) and basolateral (primarily Cl^- conductive) membranes results in the generation of a lumen-positive transepithelial voltage. The magnitude of this voltage correlates directly with the rate of net NaCl absorption. The greater the rate of NaCl absorption, the greater the magnitude of the transepithelial voltage that develops.[12] The electropositive transepithelial voltage, together with the cation-selective shunt pathway, permits the electrically conductive transport of 40–50 per cent of net sodium movement through the tight junction-paracellular route[16] (see above). The paracellular pathway in thick ascending limbs may also mediate, at least in part, the reabsorptive transport of K^+ and ammonium (NH_4^+). The basal, i.e., hormone-independent, passive absorption of the divalent cations Ca^{2+} and Mg^{2+} may also be mediated by the paracellular pathway in thick ascending limbs.[9] Thus, the rate of sodium absorption determines the amplitude of the transepithelial voltage that, in turn, establishes the magnitude of the passive absorption of permeable charged species through the paracellular pathway. Decreases in NaCl transport, secondary to the action of diuretics such as furosemide reduce the transepithelial voltage and, hence, the driving force for passive, paracellular absorption. Thus, reductions in NaCl absorption secondary to diuretic therapy, which result in significant urinary loss of calcium and magnesium, may be partly ascribed to this mechanism.

Besides the paracellular pathway, NH_4^+ absorption may also proceed through a cellular route. Transcellular absorption of NH_4^+ is mediated by the 1Na:1K:2Cl cotransporter, which accepts NH_4^+ on the potassium site of the cotransport protein.[17] Ammonium absorption by thick limbs may play an important role both in ammonium accumulation by the renal medullary interstitium and ammonium excretion by terminal nephron segments, as well as in base recovery by the kidney.[r15]

Both hormonal and nonhormonal factors regulate NaCl absorption by thick ascending limbs. The antidiuretic hormone vasopressin, acting through V_2 receptors, increases the rate of NaCl absorption in medullary, but not cortical, segments in murine species. It is unclear whether the human thick limb has V_2 receptors or if it responds to this hormone. In those species that are responsive to the hormone, vasopressin enhances countercurrent multiplication.[16] Prostaglandins of the E-series (e.g., PGE_2) competitively inhibit vasopressin-dependent NaCl absorption in response species,[18] but also reduces NaCl absorption in the vasopressin-insensitive rabbit thick limbs.[19,20]

The primary nonhormonal factor regulating NaCl absorption in thick ascending limbs is the rate of salt delivery to this nephron segment. NaCl absorption, which again proceeds in the absence of water absorption, leads to a reduction in the concentration of NaCl in tubular urine. The magnitude of this reduction depends on the pump-leak characteristics of the medullary and cortical segments.[21] In other words, active NaCl absorption and passive paracellular backleak establish a limiting NaCl concentration in tubular urine. As the load of NaCl to thick limbs is increased, the site within the thick limb at which this equilibrium is achieved is advanced toward the distal convoluted tubule, which increases the absolute magnitude of NaCl absorption. At very high delivery rates, a limiting NaCl concentration may not be reached. In this circumstance, backleak is minimized and the absolute rate of NaCl absorption is further increased. Thus, the more NaCl reaching the thick ascending limbs, the more that is absorbed. The greater NaCl absorption at this nephron site, the greater will be urinary dilution (free-water production, see below) in the absence of vasopressin, or the greater the magnitude of urinary concentration during hydropenia.

The elaboration of dilute urine is defined as a positive free-water clearance. The concept of "free-water" was introduced to provide an index of the relative magnitude of urinary concentrating or diluting capacity. According to this formulation, the rate of urine flow (V, ml/min) can be divided conceptually into two components; the first contains all the osmotically active solutes and the second consists of solute-free water. The rate of urine excretion is the sum of the osmolar clearance (C_{osm}, ml/min) and the free-water clearance (C_{H_2O}, ml/min):

$$V = C_{osm} + C_{H_2O}.$$

Since the rate of urine excretion and the osmolar clearance can both be measured, the clearance of free-water may be calculated. A positive free-water clearance indicates that the urine is dilute with respect to plasma (i.e., V > Cosm) and a negative free-water clearance, denoted, $T^c_{H_2O}$ indicates that the urine is more concentrated than plasma (i.e., $C_{osm} > V$). These concepts are also of some utility in assessing both the nephron site and mechanism of diuretic action. As noted above, free-water clearance is a reflection of delivery of NaCl to thick ascending limbs. Hence, in a hydrated individual, an increase of C_{H_2O} following administration of a diuretic reveals that the drug inhibited NaCl absorption at a nephron site prior to the thick ascending limb. Diuretics that decrease C_{H_2O} inhibit the reabsorption of NaCl in thick ascending limbs, or at more distal nephron sites.

NaCl absorption by cortical thick limbs alone does not lead to solute enrichment of the medullary interstitium, and hence, does not contribute to the abstraction of water from collecting ducts in the presence of vasopressin. This distinction permits the use of the clearance of positive or negative free-water to identify the site within the thick limb of a diuretic effect. Thus, a drug that impairs urinary dilution (i.e., decreases C_{H_2O}) during hydration and diminishes urinary concentrating capacity (reduces $T^c_{H_2O}$) during hydropenia must inhibit NaCl absorption in both cortical and medullary thick ascending limbs. On the other hand, decreases of C_{H_2O} in the absence of reductions in $T^c_{H_2O}$ result from the selective inhibition of salt reabsorption in cortical diluting sites, which include cortical thick limbs and distal convoluted tubules.

Distal Convoluted Tubules

The distal tubule consists of three distinct structural and functional elements. Considerable species heterogeneity attends the structural organization of this nephron segment, which was classically called the distal tubule. The distal convoluted tubule (DCT, Fig. 36.1) is now recognized as having a single cell type, known as the distal tubule convoluted cell. The connecting tubule, or intermediate portion, is composed of two cell types, the connecting tubule cell and the intercalated cell. Finally, the initial collecting duct (or late distal tubule), like the cortical collecting tubule, is formed from intercalated and principal cells. Transport functions of the distal convoluted tubule, connecting tubule, and initial collecting duct are discussed together in this section.

Sodium

The mechanism responsible for NaCl absorption in distal convoluted tubules (DCT, Fig. 36.1) is now generally thought to involve electroneutral NaCl cotransport, which does not require or transport potassium.[22,23] Although distal convoluted tubules bear some resemblance to cortical thick ascending limbs, the rate of net sodium absorption in thick limbs is about half that of distal convoluted tubules.[r12] The fact that the concentration of sodium reaching the early distal tubule is lower than that in peritubular capillary blood, together with the fact that the lumen is electronegative with respect to extracellular fluid, indicates that net sodium absorption in distal convoluted tubules proceeds against its transepithelial electrochemical gradient and therefore involves active transport.

Apical sodium entry in distal convoluted tubules had previously been ascribed to an electrically conductive pathway that was thought to shunt a parallel potassium conductance in this membrane. However, alterations in luminal sodium concentration do not produce appreciable changes of the transepithelial voltage.[24] These results suggest that apical membrane sodium conductance is slight, and that sodium ions cross this plasma membrane coupled to the transport of another species in an electroneutral fashion. Intracellular chloride activity of distal convoluted tubule cells is above its electrochemical equilibrium level.[22] Given the magnitude of the apical membrane voltage, it is likely that chloride entry into distal convoluted tubule cells is active. Thus, the entry of sodium is likely to be thermodynamically coupled to chloride through an apical membrane cotransport process.[25]

Sodium absorption in distal convoluted tubules, like that in the thick ascending limb of Henle's loop (see above), is load-dependent. As delivery of sodium to distal tubules increases, proportional augmentation of the rate of sodium absorption occurs. Even following tenfold increases in the delivery of sodium to distal convoluted tubules, the fractional reabsorption of sodium is maintained constant at 80%. The maintenance of a constant fractional sodium reabsorption reflects the large reserve reabsorptive capacity of distal convoluted tubules. This feature of sodium transport in distal convoluted tubules may be achieved by recruiting additional transport sites at more distal locations. In other words, as delivery to distal convoluted tubules is increased, the axial site at which the tubular sodium concentration reaches its equilibrium value is moved further along the distal tubule. Moreover, under all circumstances studied, this reserve capacity is not exceeded. This takes on particular importance in explaining the basis for the failure of diuretics acting in proximal tubules to reduce total renal salt reabsorption as much as they may block it in the proximal tubules.

Potassium

The magnitude and direction of potassium transport in distal tubule segments depends on internal and external potassium balance, mineralocorticoid and adrenergic status, the rate of tubular fluid flow, and the concentrations of sodium and, perhaps, of chloride and calcium delivered to distal nephrons. On low-potassium diets, net potassium absorption occurs along the length of the accessible superficial distal tubule. Conversely, high-potassium (or low-sodium) diets promote net potassium secretion. Most evidence now suggests that potassium secretion is a function of connecting and cortical collecting tubules; little net potassium transport occurs in distal convoluted tubules. Many diuretics provoke significant potassium wasting.[r5] Such losses of potassium result from a combination of increased tubular flow through the terminal portions of distal tubules, compensatory elevated levels of aldosterone leading to distal nephron potassium secretion, and from the increased delivery of sodium to the distal nephron, again resulting in enhanced potassium secretion.

Calcium and Magnesium

In nondiuretic animals, some 8–11 percent of filtered calcium and 5–10 percent of filtered magnesium is reabsorbed by distal tubules. Under a wide variety of circumstances the kidney exhibits close parallelism between net reabsorption of sodium and calcium. However, pathophysiologic conditions, such as metabolic acidosis or adrenocortical insufficiency, or pharmacologic intervention with thiazide diuretics or amiloride disrupts the normal relations between sodium and calcium handling. In each of these circumstances, the dissociation occurs in distal convoluted tubules.[9] The hypocalciuric action of thiazides or of amiloride is confined to the distal convoluted tubule. It should be noted that these agents have little or no effect on magnesium excretion.

Water

Water permeability of the distal tubule is low and dependent on the state of hydration. Moreover, unlike the connecting tubule, the distal convoluted tubule is not influenced by vasopressin.[26]

Protons/Bicarbonate

Filtered bicarbonate that escapes reabsorption by proximal tubules is recovered by initial collecting ducts (late distal tubules) and cortical collecting tubules. Both hydrogen ion secretion and bicarbonate absorption are mediated by intercalated cells in these segments. Thus, both distal tubules, as well as the more terminal collecting ducts, are involved in the regulation of acid-base balance. Distal acidification is modified by several factors, including the delivery of sodium, chloride, and bicarbonate, and by the mineralocorticoid status.[r17] Increases in the delivery of the sodium and its accompanying anion, on the one hand, and aldosterone on the other, stimulate distal acidification. Secondary hyperaldosteronism—that is, increases in circulating aldosterone consequent to the loss of sodium induced by diuretics—contributes to metabolic alkalosis attending the use of loop or thiazide-type agents. This effect is due to the exaggeration of H^+ secretion induced by the diuretic. Similarly, diuretics acting at more proximal nephron sites augment the delivery of sodium to initial collecting ducts and, hence, increase renal hydrogen ion loss and thereby contribute to the metabolic alkalosis induced by these agents.

Collecting Tubules

The final regulation of sodium reabsorption and potassium secretion proceeds in cortical and medullary collecting ducts (CCT, MCD; Fig. 36.1). As indicated previously, these segments are composed of principal and intercalated cells. Sodium absorption and potassium secretion proceed through principal cells, whereas intercalated cells are responsible for H^+ secretion and HCO_3^- absorption.

Collecting tubules reabsorb 5–7% of the filtered sodium. In these nephron segments, sodium absorption and potassium secretion are mediated by active transport processes dependent on the activity of Na^+/K^+-ATPase located in basolateral membranes of principal cells. This sodium-potassium exchange pump not only maintains the intracellular sodium activity lower and the potassium activity higher than in blood, it also renders the cell electronegative with respect to both blood and tubular urine. In this way a favorable gradient is created for apical sodium entry. Influx of sodium from the tubular urine into the cell is mediated by

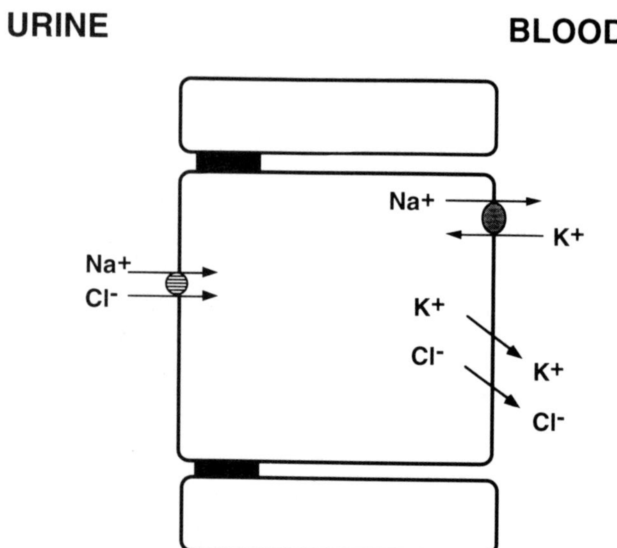

Figure 36.4 Cellular mechanism of NaCl absorption by distal convoluted tubule cells. Thiazide diuretics act from apical membranes to inhibit NaCl absorption.

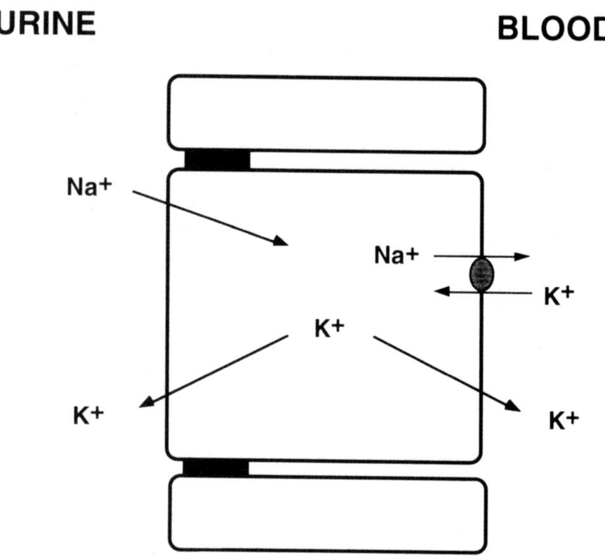

Figure 36.5 Cellular mechanism for Na^+ absorption and K^+ secretion by collecting duct principal cells. Sodium enters the cell through a sodium-selective channel that is inhibited by the potassium-sparing diuretics amiloride and triamterene. The driving force for K^+ secretion is determined by the magnitude of antecedent Na^+ entry.

selective ion channels that span the apical membrane (Fig. 36.5). Apical cell membranes also contain a channel that is selective for potassium, which represents the route for potassium secretion from the cell into the urine. Potassium is actively taken up into the cell from the peritubular fluid by the Na^+/K^+-ATPase and diffuses passively into the urine. High intracellular potassium activity favors, whereas the negative intracellular voltage retards, potassium movement from cell to tubular fluid.

Although sodium absorption from, and potassium secretion into, the urine occurs through separate channels in apical membranes of principal cells, these processes are generally operationally linked.

Studies in which single cells of the in vitro perfused rabbit cortical collecting tubule were impaled with voltage-sensing microelectrodes have established that sodium absorption modifies potassium secretion in two ways.[27,28] First, sodium entry into cells across apical plasma membranes alters the electrochemical gradient, favoring potassium secretion. As the rate of sodium transport through apical membrane sodium channels increases, the voltage across the membrane depolarizes (and the transepithelial voltage becomes more lumen-negative), thereby enhancing the driving force for potassium secretion into the urine. Conversely, reductions in apical sodium entry decrease conductive potassium secretion. Second, the activity of the basolateral membrane Na^+/K^+-ATPase, and hence, the rate of active potassium uptake from the peritubular space into cells, is dependent on the cytoplasmic sodium concentration. Hence, increases in sodium absorption enhance, whereas decreases in sodium absorption diminish, basolateral potassium uptake (and thus, secretion) by initial collecting tubules and cortical collecting ducts.

The two principal modulators of the magnitude of sodium absorption and potassium secretion by collecting tubules are the load of sodium delivered to this nephron site and the plasma mineralocorticoid level. Clearly, the sodium load delivered to these nephron segments may be altered by pathologic processes, as well as by diuretics acting in more proximal nephron segments. Both the transepithelial electrical conductance and the passive sodium permeability of cortical collecting tubules are quite low.[r12] Thus, sodium absorption in initial collecting tubules and cortical collecting tubules may lead to the development of steep transtubular concentration gradients for sodium that, in turn, diminish sodium entry into cells, thereby limiting further sodium absorption. As the load of sodium presented to these nephron segments is raised by increasing the sodium concentration or the tubule urine flow rate at the beginning of the initial collecting tubule, the point at which the limiting gradient for sodium is achieved moves further downstream in the nephron and the absolute amount of sodium absorbed is increased. This is the same type of load- (or flow-) dependent behavior of sodium transport described above for thick ascending limbs and distal convoluted tubules. Clearly, potassium secretion is altered in a pari-passu fashion with changes in sodium absorption.

The ability of mineralocorticoid hormones to enhance sodium absorption and potassium secretion in collecting tubules is well-established.[r18] This physiologic adaptation is accompanied by morphologic and biochemical changes in basolateral membranes. Increases of basolateral membrane area,[29] high-affinity aldosterone receptors, and in the activities of Na^+/K^+-ATPase and citrate synthetase[30] in initial collecting tubule and in cortical collecting tubules are consistent with a predominant effect of mineralocorticoid hormones on ion transport in these nephron segments. Within the first day of mineralocorticoid administration the sodium conductance of apical membranes increases.[31] This early primary increase of apical sodium permeability is sufficient to explain the enhancement in both sodium absorption and potassium secretion by this nephron segment following mineralocorticoid treatment.[32] Increases in the potassium permeability of apical membranes and in Na^+/K^+-ATPase activity in basolateral membranes occur later. These delayed effects further enhance both sodium absorption and potassium secretion.

Water

The collecting ducts, including the initial collecting ducts, absorb water in the presence of vasopressin, which increases the hydraulic permeability of these nephron segments. The mechanism by which vasopressin increases water permeability involves activation of basolateral membrane V_2 receptors, leading to the formation of cyclic AMP that, in turn, activates protein kinase A.[51] These events lead to the fusion of cytoplasmic, membrane-bound particles, thought to contain water channels, with apical cell membranes.[r19]

References

Research Reports

1. Volpe M. The physiological role of atrial natriuretic factor. Cardioscience 1992;*3*:217–225.
2. Green R, Giebisch G. Luminal hypotonicity: a driving force for fluid absorption from the proximal tubule. Am J Physiol 1984;*246*:F167–F174.
3. Green R, Giebisch G, Unwin R, Weinstein AM. Coupled water transport by rat proximal tubule. Am J Physiol 1991;*261*:F1046–F1054.
4. Barratt LJ, Rector FC, Jr., Kokko JP, Seldin DW. Factors governing the transepithelial potential difference across the proximal tubule of the rat kidney. J Clin Invest 1974;*53*:454–464.
5. Schafer JA, Patlak CS, Andreoli TE. Fluid absorption and active and passive ion flows in the rabbit superficial pars recta. Am J Physiol 1977;*233*:F154–F167.
6. Neumann KH, Rector FC, Jr. Mechanism of NaCl and water reabsorption in the proximal convoluted tubule of rat kidney.

Role of chloride concentration gradients. J Clin Invest 1976;*58*:1110–1118.

7. Rector FC, Jr. Sodium, bicarbonate, and chloride absorption by the proximal tubule. Am J Physiol 1983;*244*:F461–F471.
8. Rose HJ, Pruitt AW, Dayton PG, McNay JL. Relationship of urinary furosemide excretion rate to natriuretic effect in experimental azotemia. J Pharmacol Exp Ther 1976;*199*:490–497.
9. Friedman PA, Gesek FA. Calcium transport in renal epithelial cells. Am J Physiol 1993;*264*:F181–F198.
10. Rouse D, Ny RCK, Suki WN. Calcium transport in the pars recta and thin descending limb of Henle of rabbit perfused in vitro. J Clin Invest 1980;*65*:37–42.
11. Knepper MA, Star RA. The vasopressin-regulated urea transporter in renal inner medullary collecting duct. Am J Physiol 1990;*259*:F393–F401.
12. Hebert SC, Culpepper RM, Andreoli TE. NaCl transport in mouse medullary thick ascending limbs. I. Functional nephron heterogeneity and ADH-stimulated NaCl cotransport. Am J Physiol 1981;*241*:F412–F431.
13. Friedman PA, Andreoli TE. CO_2-stimulated NaCl absorption in the mouse renal cortical thick ascending limb of Henle. Evidence for synchronous Na^+/H^+ and Cl^-/HCO_3^- exchange in apical plasma membranes. J Gen Physiol 1982;*80*:683–711.
14. Dobyan DC, Magill LS, Friedman PA, Hebert SC, Bulger RE. Carbonic anhydrase histochemistry in rabbit and mouse kidneys. Anatomical Record 1982;*204*:185–197.
15. Greger R, Schlatter E. Properties of the basolateral membrane of the cortical thick ascending limb of Henle's loop of rabbit kidney. A model for secondary active chloride transport. Pflugers Arch Eur J Physiol 1983;*396*:325–334.
16. Hebert SC, Andreoli TE. Control of NaCl transport in the thick ascending limb. Am J Physiol 1984;*246*:F745–F756.
17. Kikeri D, Sun A, Zeidel ML, Hebert SC. Cell membranes impermeable to NH_3. Nature 1989;*339*:478–480.
18. Culpepper RM, Andreoli TE. Interactions among prostaglandin E_2, antidiuretic hormone, and cyclic adenosine monophosphate in modulating Cl^- absorption in single mouse medullary thick ascending limbs of Henle. J Clin Invest 1983;*71*:1588–1601.
19. Stokes JB. Effect of prostaglandin E_2 on chloride transport across the rabbit thick ascending limb of Henle. Selective inhibition of the medullary portion. J Clin Invest 1979;*64*:495–502.
20. Frazier LW, Yorio T. Eicosanoids: Their function in renal epithelia ion transport. Proc Soc Exp Biol Med 1992;*201*:229–243.
21. Burg MB. Thick ascending limb of Henle's loop. Kidney Int 1982;*22*:454–464.
22. Gesek FA, Friedman PA. Mechanism of calcium transport stimulated by chlorothiazide in mouse distal convoluted tubule cells. J Clin Invest 1992;*90*:279–288.
23. Ellison DH, Velázquez H, Wright FS. Thiazide-sensitive sodium chloride cotransport in early distal tubule. Am J Physiol 1987;*253*:F546–F554.
24. Hayslett JP, Boulpaep EL, Giebisch G. Factors influencing transepithelial potential difference in mammalian distal tubule. Am J Physiol 1978;*234*:F182–F191.
25. Velázquez H, Wright FS, Good DW. Luminal influences on potassium secretion: chloride replacement with sulfate. Am J Physiol 1982;*242*:F46–F55.
26. Costanzo LS, Windhager EE. Effects of PTH, ADH, and cyclic AMP on distal tubular Ca and Na reabsorption. Am J Physiol 1980;*239*:F478–F485.
27. Koeppen BM, Biagi BA, Giebisch G. Intracellular microelectrode characterization of the rabbit cortical collecting duct. Am J Physiol 1983;*244*:F35–F47.
28. O'Neil RG, Sansom S. Electrophysiological properties of cellular and paracellular conductive pathways of the rabbit cortical collecting duct. J Membrane Biol 1984;*82*:281–295.
29. Kaissling B, LeHir M. Distal tubular segments of the rabbit kidney after adaptation to altered Na- and K-intake. I. Structural changes. Cell Tissue Res 1982;*224*:469–492.
30. Marver D. Evidence for corticosteroid action along the nephron. Am J Physiol 1984;*246*:F111–F123.
31. Sansom S, O'Neil RG. Mineralocorticoid regulation of apical cell membrane Na and K transport of the cortical collecting duct. Am J Physiol 1985;*248*:F858–F868.
32. O'Neil RG, Hayhurst RA. Sodium-dependent modulation of the renal Na-K-ATPase: influence of mineralocorticoids on the cortical collecting duct. J Membrane Biol 1985;*85*:169–179.
33. Hébert RL, Jacobson HR, Breyer MD. Triple signal transduction model for the mechanism of PGE_2 actions in rabbit cortical collecting duct. Prostagl Leukotr Essen Fatty Acids 1991;*42*:143–148.

Reviews

r1. Walser M. Divalent cations: physicochemical state in glomerular filtrate and urine and renal excretion. In: Orloff J, Berliner RW (Eds.) Handbook of physiology, section 8: Renal physiology. Washington, D.C.: American Physiological Society, (1973); pp 555–586.

r2. Kriz W, Kaissling B. Structural organization of the mammalian kidney. In: Seldin DW, Giebisch G (Eds.) The kidney. Physiology and pathophysiology. New York: Raven Press, (1985); pp 265–306.

r3. Maddox DA, Brenner BM. Glomerular ultrafiltration. In: Brenner BM, Rector FC, Jr. (Eds.) The kidney. Philadelphia: WB Saunders, (1991); pp 205–244.

r4. Friedman PA. Biochemistry and pharmacology of diuretics. Seminars Nephrol 1988;*8*:198–212.

r5. Friedman PA, Hebert SC. Mechanisms of action of diuretics. In: Brenner BM, Stein JH (Eds.) Body Fluid Homeostasis. New York: Churchill Livingstone, (1987); pp 377–407.

r6. Aronson PS. The renal proximal tubule: A model for diversity of anion exchangers and stilbene-sensitive anion transporters. Ann Rev Physiol 1989;*51*:419–441.

r7. Rose BD. Clinical physiology of acid-base and electrolyte disorders. New York: McGraw-Hill, (1989); pp 1–853.

r8. Bourdeau JE. Renal handling of calcium. In: Brenner BM, Stein JH, eds. Divalent ion homeostasis. New York: Churchill Livingstone, (1983); pp 1–31.

r9. Suki WN, Rouse D. Renal transport of calcium, magnesium, and phosphorous. In: Brenner BM, Rector FC, Jr. (Eds.) The kidney. Philadelphia: WB Saunders, (1991); pp 380–423.

r10. Jamison RL, Kriz W. Urinary concentrating mechanism. New York: Oxford University Press, (1982); pp 3–332.

r11. Knepper MA, Rector FC, Jr. Urinary concentration and dilution. In: Brenner BM, Rector FC, Jr. (Eds.) The kidney. Philadelphia: WB Saunders (1991); pp 445–482.

r12. Sands JM, Kokko JP, Jacobson HR. Intrarenal heterogeneity: vascular and tubular. In: Seldin DW, Giebisch G (Eds.) The kidney: physiology and pathophysiology. New York: Raven Press, (1992); pp 1087–1155.

r13. Greger R. Ion transport mechanisms in thick ascending limb of Henle's loop of mammalian nephron. Physiol Rev 1985;*65*:760–797.

r14. Haas M. Properties and diversity of (Na-K-Cl) cotransporters. Ann Rev Physiol 1989;*51*:443–457.

r15. Knepper MA, Packer R, Good DW. Ammonium transport in the kidney. Physiol Rev 1989;*69*:179–249.

r16. Knepper MA. NH_4^+ transport in the kidney. Kidney Int 1991;*40* (Suppl.) *33*:S95–S102.

r17. Alpern RJ, Stone DK, Rector FC, Jr. Renal acidification mechanisms. In: Brenner BM, Rector FC, Jr. (Eds.) The kidney. Philadelphia: WB Saunders (1991); pp 318–379.

r18. Stanton BA, Giebisch GH. Renal potassium transport. In: Windhager EE, (ed.) Handbook of physiology. Section 8: Renal physiology. New York: Oxford University Press, (1992); pp 813–874.

r19. Wade JB. Role of membrane fusion in hormonal regulation of epithelial transport. Ann Rev Physiol 1986;*48*:213–223.

r20. Jamison RL, Maffly RH. The urinary concentrating mechanism. New Engl J Med 1988;*295*:1059–1067.

r21. Giebisch G, Koeppen BM. Transport of sodium and potassium across the epithelium of the distal nephron. In: Puschett JB, Greenberg A (Eds.) Diuretics II: Chemistry, pharmacology, and clinical applications. Elsevier Sciences Publishing (1987); pp 121–130.

r22. Knepper MA, Packer R, Good DW. Ammonium transport in the kidney. Physiol Rev 1989;*69*:179–249.

r23. Haas M. Properties and diversity of (Na-K-Cl) cotransporters. Ann Rev Physiol 1989;*51*:443–457.

r24. Bronner F. Renal calcium transport: mechanisms and regulation—an overview. Am J Physiol 1989;*257*:F707–F711.

r25. Maack T. Receptors of atrial natriuretic factor. Ann Rev Physiol 1992;*54*:11–27.

r26. Duchatelle P, Ohara A, Ling BN, et al. Regulation of renal epithelial sodium channels. Mol Cell Biochem 1992;*114*:27–34.

r27. Greger R, Lohrmann E, Schlatter E. Action of diuretics at the cellular level. Clin Nephrol 1992;*38* Suppl. 1:S64–S68.

CHAPTER 37

General Principles and Renal Cellular Mechanisms of Drug Transport

Peter D. Holohan

Maintenance of the body's internal homeostatic environment is one of the kidney's main functions. Homeostasis is achieved by the integration of multiple physiologic mechanisms, one of which is the capacity of the proximal tubule to secrete exogenous (xenobiotic) and endogenous (metabolic end-products) chemical coumpounds. Apparently, two secretory systems are present: one for organic anions; the other for organic cations. Each system displays broad specificity for the substrates it transports; moreover, each system can be subdivided into several components having overlapping specificities. The topic is how drugs (i.e., xenobiotics mostly) are secreted by the kidney.

Secretion of these organic compounds is an active process and represents the performance of work by the kidney. The capacity to produce work is a consequence of the polarized nature of the proximal tubule, which provides the mechanism by which metabolism is energetically coupled to transport. Secretion is a manifestation of transcellular movement and represents transport in series: uptake from the blood across the basolateral membrane and exit into the tubular fluid across the brush border membrane. Transepithelial transport is achieved by the asymmetric distribution between the basolateral and brush border membranes of integral membrane proteins, termed transporters, that facilitate the movement of drugs. These transporters, in turn, are coupled energetically to ion gradients generated across the plasma membranes at the expense of metabolism. The integration of the individual transporters into the physiologic capacity of the individual cell provides the functional unit; organization of the individual cells into a transporting epithelial layer provides the functional tissue.

Functional Organization of the Proximal Tubule

Anatomically the proximal tubule can be divided into at least three segments: S_1, the first part of the convoluted tubule just after the glomerulus; S_2, the last part of the convoluted tubule and the beginning portion of the straight; and S_3, the proximal straight tubule or pars recta. Functionally, the proximal tubule operates as a sheet of cells separating fluid compartments of different chemical composition; it thereby prevents equilibration of these compartments. The cell layer consists of individual cuboidal or columnar cells from 5 to 20 μm in diameter and 5 to 10 μm in height, resting on a basement membrane. The layer functions as a continuous sheet because the cells are held together by four types of intercellular junctions: one, tight junctions (zonula occuludens) usually found near the apical surface; two, belt desmosomes, which form a continuous band around each cell near the apical surface just below the tight junctions; three, spot desmosomes, which hold adjacent cells together; and four, gap junctions, which permit communication between adjacent cells.

The apical cell surface is increased fortyfold by the presence of as many as 1000 microvilli ("brush border") per cell. The basolateral surface is also increased by cellular indentations, and, in actuality, the brush border and basolateral membrane surface areas are approximately equal.[1] This organization of individual cells into a cohesive monolayer produces not only biochemically and physiologically distinct brush border and basolateral membrane domains, but also a unique cytoplasmic and cytoskeletal organization. It is clear that the establishment and maintenance of the cell's functional polarity is dependent on an intact polarized cytoskeleton. Disease states or drugs that disaggregate the cytoskeleton will consequently disrupt secretion.[2,3] The maintenance of this polarized organization depends on the targeting of proteins and lipids to specific membrane domains by as yet poorly-described mechanisms.[4] The lipid composition of the two membranes differs. The brush border membrane is high in cholesterol and sphingomyelin but low in phosphatidylcholine and phosphatidylinositol; the basolateral membrane has the opposite composition. Furthermore, the physical chemical properties of the two membranes are different: the brush border membrane has high electrical resistance but low fluidity; the basolateral membrane has physical chemical properties that are roughly the inverse.

The protein composition of the two membranes is different. Enzymes localized to either the basolateral or to the brush border membrane are listed in Table 37.1. Hormone receptors are in the basolateral membrane predominately, but not exclusively. Until recently it was assumed that these receptors were only in the basolateral membrane; however, it has now been shown that both the basolateral and brush border membranes contain a receptor for angiotensin II, and that the two receptors appear to be nearly identical in binding properties and physiologic responses. The physiologic advantage of having a receptor for a hormone at both faces of the cell remains an unclear but intriguing problem.

The feature of interest here is the asymmetric distribution of transport proteins, and several are listed in Table 37.1. This anatomic distribution of transporters and channels to selected membrane surfaces provides for the distribution and maintenance of ECF compartments of different chemical composition. The movement of solutes across the epithelial layer is accounted for by active and passive transport processes.

Two potential routes are available for movement across the monolayer: the cellular and paracellular pathways. Each represents transport in series across two barriers. The paracellular pathway is through tight junctions and lateral intracellular spaces. The cellular pathway is uptake across one plasma membrane, movement through the cytoplasm, and exit across the membrane on the opposite face of the cell. Secretion is via the cellular pathway exclusively, and is from blood to tubular fluid.

Table 37.1 Plasma Membrane Localization of Enzymes and Transporters

basolateral	brush border
Na^+, K-ATPase	H-ATPase
CA^{+2}-ATPase	P-glycoprotein
Adenylyl cyclase	hydrolytic enzyme
hormone receptors	-sucrase -maltase
glucose uniporter	alkaline phosphatase
Na^+-dicarboxylic cotransporter	Na^+ gradient-dependent glucose cotransporter
Na^+ gradient-dependent amino acid cotransporters	Na^+ gradient-dependent amino acid cotransporters
Na^+/HCO_3^- cotransporter Cl^-/HCO_3^- exchanger	Na^+/H^+ exchanger

Principles of Membrane Transport[r1,2]

Molecules traverse biologic membranes by mediated or nonmediated pathways. Mediated transport is achieved by a specific interaction between a solute molecule and a membrane component, giving the characteristics of specificity and saturation. Nonmediated transport is the simple diffusion of a solute molecule through the lipid bilayer, showing little specificity and no apparent saturation. It is generally held that mediated transport is reserved mainly, but not exlusively, to hydrophilic molecules, while nonmediated transport is the pathway for hydrophobic ones. Conceivably, both pathways contribute significantly to the renal disposition of drugs.

Nonmediated Transport[r2]

Diffusion is the process by which solute molecules move from a region of higher concentration to one of lower. It is quantitatively described by Fick's first law:

$$J_x = -D\, dc/_{dx} \qquad \text{(B-1)}$$

in which J_x is the flux of solute, x is a distance along the pathway, $dc/_{dx}$ is the change in concentration of the solute as it moves down its concentration gradient, and D is a constant of proportionality termed the diffusion coefficient. D has the dimensions of cm^2/sec., and its value increases in dilute solutions. Unfortunately this straightforward description is of little value for studying membrane transport because what is measured is the diffusion of the solute in a lipid matrix. Generally, D is an unknown under these conditions.

A more useful description can be derived by making certain assumptions and rearranging the Fick equation to the following:

$$J_x = PA[(x)_H - (x)_L] \tag{B-2}$$

in which J_x is the flux of solute perpendicular to the plane of the membrane, A is the area of membrane in cm^2, $(X)_H$ and $(X)_L$ are the solute concentrations, moles/cm^3, on the high and low sides, and P is the permeability coefficient with the dimensions of cm/sec. The permeability coefficient (P) has the dimensions of velocity (cm/sec) and is a measure of the ease with which a solute molecule crosses the membrane.

Nonmediated transport can be considered as a random-walk phenomenon. As solute molecules jump from one position to another, molecules will hit the membrane and whether or not the solute molecule penetrates the membrane will depend upon its size and chemical structure. Obviously, the side exposed to the greater concentration will experience the greater number of hits, and consequently a net flux will occur until equilibrium is reached, i.e., when the fluxes in opposite directions are equal. Thus, nonmediated transport depends not only on the concentration gradient of the solute across the membrane, but also requires that the solute dissolve in the membrane. The permeability coefficient measures the ease with which the solute enters the lipid phase of the membrane. As a generalization, smaller molecules are more permeable than larger ones; nonpolar molecules more permeable than polar. Yet, the actual situation is somewhat more complex.

The permeability coefficients for various solutes, measured in human red blood cells, differ by several orders of magnitude: for example, from 3.7×10^{-3} cm/sec for methanol to 6.7×10^{-9} cm/sec for erythritol. Moreover, the permeability coefficient for the same solute is different in different membranes; the value for methanol is 4.7×10^{-7} cm/sec in dog red blood cells.[r2] Obviously, the chemical composition of the membrane is a key parameter that determines the ease with which the solute dissolves in the lipid bilayer. The solubility of a solute in a lipid membrane is a measure of the balance between the solute-H_2O interactions occurring in the aqueous phase and the solute-lipid interactions occurring in the membrane. Solute-H_2O interactions are dominated by hydrogen bonds. Solute-lipid interactions are dominated by hydrophobic bonding resulting from structural changes in the lipid milieu, and reflect the chemical composition of the drug and the lipid make-up of the membrane. Consequently, the relative solubility of a solute is established by determining its partition coefficient: that is, the ratio of its concentration in an oil phase over its concentration in an aqueous phase, a dimensionless parameter. This proves to be valuable, since the permeability coefficient (see Equation B-2) can thus be defined in terms of its partition coefficient:

$$P = \frac{K\, D_{mem}}{\lambda} \tag{B-3}$$

in which K is the partition coefficient of the solute, D_{mem} is its diffusion coefficient within the membrane, and λ is the thickness of the hydrocarbon region of the membrane. Rewriting equation B-2:

$$J_x = \frac{K\, D_{mem}\, A\, [(x)_H - (x)_L]}{\lambda} \tag{B-4}$$

nonmediated transport is readily understandable: it is linearly related to the concentration gradient and to the partition coefficient of the solute. The value of the latter is influenced by the chemical structure of the solute and the chemical composition of the hydrocarbon layer of the membrane; since "like" dissolves "like", hydrophobic compounds penetrate faster than polar compounds and chemically similar compounds have similar permeabilities. Moreover, this description provides an empirical approach for predicting permeabilities. It has been found empirically that drugs with partition coefficients greater than 3 tend to enter cells by nonmediated transport. Any drug containing a substituent group that increases the lipid solubility of the compound (e.g., halogens, methylene, phenyl) would increase the partition coefficient, thereby increasing the permeability coefficient. On the other hand, any substituent that decreases lipid solubility (e.g., polar groups) would be expected to decrease the capacity of the drug to penetrate the cell membrane.

Another empirical finding is that smaller molecules cross biologic membranes at a significantly faster rate than larger ones. The reason for this behavior is not intuitively obvious. Rearranging equation B-3:

$$D_{men} = \frac{P\lambda}{K} \tag{B-5}$$

and recalling that D_{men} is the diffusion coefficient within the membrane, the observation must mean that D_{men} is large for smaller solutes and small for the larger solutes. A similar phenomenon is found in polymers where the polymer molecules cannot flow around the solute molecule. An explanation is: In biologic membranes, the phospholipids are anchored at the membrane-water interface and cannot flow past the solute—thus, smaller solutes diffuse more slowly than predicted.

Nonmediated transport, then, is a major pathway by which hydrophobic drugs passively enter a cell. There are two complicating factors, however. One is the presence of an unstirred water layer surrounding the cell; the other is the presence of a pH gradient across the cell membrane. The first can diminish the uptake of a drug; the second can enhance the drug accumulation. An unstirred water layer is, in essence, a hydrophilic barrier to the penetration of a highly lipid-soluble compound. This explains why some hydrophobic drugs with large partition coefficients are nonetheless poorly absorbed. Therefore, if nonmediated transport is the major pathway for drug uptake by a cell, the drug must have some water-soluble as well as lipid-soluble properties before it can enter the cell.

The other factor is the presence of a pH gradient across the membrane: it can have a profound effect on the final distribution of a solute, if the solute is a weak acid.

For a carboxylic group:

$$\underset{\text{(acid)}}{RCOOH} \rightleftharpoons H^+ + \underset{\text{(conjugate base)}}{R\text{-}COO^-} \tag{B-6}$$

The relative concentrations of the acid and its conjugate base depend on the pH of the medium and the pKa of the acid, as given by the Henderson-Hasselbalch equation:

$$pH = pk_a + \log \frac{[\text{conjugate base}]}{[\text{acid}]} \tag{B-7}$$

The partition coefficient would be expected to be greater for the noncharged species since it is less polar. Therefore, the permeability coefficient of the noncharged species can be significantly faster than that of the charged species. If, in addition, there is a pH gradient across the membrane, the noncharged species will reequilibrate in accordance with equation B-7. The significance of this is that at equilibrium the total number of charged plus uncharged molecules on both sides of the membrane must be equal, but the concentration of either species can be significantly different across the membrane, depending on the pKa value of the dissociable group.

For a solute containing an amino group:

$$\underset{\text{(acid)}}{RNH_3^+} \rightleftharpoons H^+ + \underset{\text{(conjugate base)}}{RNH_2} \tag{B-8}$$

and the same principles apply; consequently, the final disposition of the drug depends not only on the chemical composition of the solute and the lipid composition of the membrane, but also on the presence of dissociable groups.

Mediated Transport

Historically, it was found that many low molecular weight, water-soluble solute molecules penetrated cells more rapidly than could be accounted for by simple diffusion. It was concluded, correctly, that there must be something in the plasma membrane that facilitated solute movement—hence the term "facilitated diffusion." The next step in the development of membrane transport theory was the carrier concept: a membrane-bound entity binds the solutes on one side of the membrane; the complex diffuses across the membrane; and the solute molecule is released at the opposite side. The "carrier" model accurately describes the mechanism of action of some ionophores and remains a useful conceptual explanation of the established observation that mediated transport shows the properties of saturation and specificity.

Transport phenomena are often described from a thermodynamic viewpoint: they are either active or passive. Passive transport describes the process of the net flux of solute from a region of higher to one of lower electrochemical potential. At equilibrium, the rate of influx must equal the rate of efflux. Active transport describes the movement of a substrate against its electrochemical gradient. Since endergonic reactions do not occur spontaneously, active transport implies that the movement of the substrate against its electrochemical gradient is coupled to an exergonic reaction. The important point is that understanding the nature of the coupling reactions provides insight into the mechanisms by which cells can perform work.

A good deal is known about transport processes; conceptually, the transporters are likened to enzymes and the solute molecules to substrates. Consequently, throughout the remainder of this discussion, the term "substrate" will be used exclusively, instead of "solute", since this notation reinforces the concept of specificity. The membrane entity that binds the substrate is termed a transporter and is an integral membrane protein that spans the membrane several times, thereby providing a pocket within the membrane for substrate binding. The analogy to an enzymatic reaction can be extended to rate of flux, which can be described by simple Michaelis-Menten kinetics:

$$J = \frac{J_{max}\,[S]}{K_m + [S]} \qquad \text{(B-9)}$$

in which J is the flux, J_{max} is a limiting flux, and K_m is a measure of the affinity of the substrate. The rate is not necessarily proportional to the concentration gradient of the substrate, but to the concentration of the substrate:transporter complex. A useful conceptual model for describing transport is that after the substrate binds, the binding site reorients, substrate is released on the opposite face of the membrane, and the binding site reorients back to its starting position, either loaded with a different substrate or unloaded. The key feature is that the binding site alternately faces one side of the membrane and then the other. Presumably, the actual distance translocated by the binding site is only a small fraction of the entire width of the membrane (about 30_{nm}). This presumption is consistent with the observation that transport proteins undergo only minor conformational changes on substrate binding. While this conceptual model is useful, the fact remains that the molecular mechanisms underlying the transport reaction are largely unknown, and, furthermore, it is uncertain whether the transporter functions as a monomer or an oligomer; the issue is whether the translocation pathway is formed within the transporter molecule itself or within subunits.

The determination of whether a transport reaction is active or passive is a simple matter. The influx of substrate(s) into a cell is described thermodynamically by the change in free energy as given by the following:

$$\Delta G = \frac{RT \ln [S]_i + ZF\Delta\Psi}{[S]_o} \qquad \text{(B-10)}$$

Where: ΔG is the Gibbs free energy change and is a measure of work that can be performed by the system; R is the gas constant; T is the temperature in degrees Kelvin; $[S]_i$ and $[S]_o$ are the substrate concentrations inside and outside the cell; F is Faraday's constant; Z is the charge on the substrate; and $\Delta\Psi$ is the membrane potential measured as $\Delta\Psi = \Psi_i - \Psi_o$. If ΔG is positive, the transport reaction, as written, is energetically unfavorable and must be coupled to some source of energy to proceed; if ΔG is negative, the reaction proceeds, as written, in an energetically favorable fashion.

However, describing transport processes on the basis of the thermodynamic status of the substrate has led to many ambiguities. Therefore, the classification advanced by Mitchell that emphasizes the molecular nature of the reaction will be followed: transport reactions are categorized as either primary or secondary active.[r1]

Primary-Active Transport[r1]

Transport processes are placed in this category if the translocation of the substrate across the membrane is directly and obligatorily linked to the formation and rupture of a covalent bond. While several different types of chemical reactions have been identified, the hydrolysis of ATP is the reaction most frequently encountered. Members of this group include the Na^+, K^+-ATPase, the Ca^{2+}-ATPase, and the H^+-ATPases. They represent ion-motive ATPases and frequently are referred to as ion "pumps." The ATPases are subdivided into: F-type, e.g., the mitochondrial ATP synthase; V-type, e.g., the vacuolar and plasma membrane H^+-

ATPase; and P-type, e.g., Na^+, K^+-ATPase and Ca^+-ATPase where a phosphorylated intermediate is formed during the reaction cycle. It was thought that ATPases were not involved directly in the movement of drugs, but rather were responsible for the generation of ion gradients (e.g., Na^+ and/or H^+) to which the flux of drugs were coupled. Recent developments indicate, however, that the current description of secretion may have to be modified to include primary-active transport pathways. It is now recognized that the brush border membrane of the proximal tubule of the kidney possesses a P-glycoprotein that is a member of a superfamily of transporters found throughout phylogeny.[5] The P-glycoprotein functions as an ATP-dependent efflux pump. Its putative role in drug secretion will be addressed subsequently.

Secondary-Active Transport[r1]

This classification describes transport reactions in which the translocation step is not directly linked to covalent bond formation. The transporters are termed "porters" and can be subdivided depending on whether the translocation of one substrate is obligatorily coupled to the translocation of another.

Uniporters. Members of this group simply allow the substrate to respond to its electrochemical gradient until equilibrium is reached. They are passive processes and are incapable of work. Net flux occurs only if a chemical or an electrochemical gradient exists. An example is glucose uptake by red blood cells, liver, and muscle, where there is a concentration gradient of glucose from blood to cell.[6,7]

Conversely, the proximal tubule reabsorbs glucose by a mechanism that will be described subsequently; hence, a gradient exists for glucose from the cell to the blood. The basolateral membrane contains a uniporter for glucose that catalyzes the transport from cell to blood.[8] The glucose uniporters are members of a family of transport proteins whose anatomic disposition and kinetic properties correspond to the metabolic needs of their tissue localization.[9] Charged substrates are translocated by uniporters and therefore a uniport mechanism mediates transport in response to a membrane potential. For example, a cationic substrate accumulates intracellularly in response to an inside negative membrane potential. From a thermodynamic viewpoint, this is active transport, and fits the historical criterion that a metabolic poison would block transport; the membrane would become depolarized. However, since the translocation step is not linked to the movement of another substrate or to covalent bond formation, transport reactions fitting this description are termed "uniporters."

Exchange or Antiport. Transport reactions in this category describe the movement of one substrate to the countermovement of another. The final distribution of one substrate is dependent on the electrochemical gradient of the driver substrate and the stoichiometry of the coupling reaction. The substrate farthest from its electrochemical equilibrium is termed the "driver" substrate and the other the "driven" substrate.

Cotransport or Symport. Transport reactions in which the movement of one substrate is coupled to the movement of another in the same direction. As described with antiport mechanisms, the final disposition depends on the electrochemical potential of the "driver" substrate. Generally, the driver substrates are ions (Na^+, H^+) whose electrochemical gradients are generated by primary-active transporters, e.g., ATPases. For example, glucose is reabsorbed from the fluid of the proximal tubule by a Na^+:glucose cotransporter.[10] As a Na^+ enters the cell down its electrochemical gradient it carries glucose with it. The extent of glucose accumulation depends on the dimension of the electrochemical gradient for Na^+ and the stoichiometric coupling of the transport reaction. The size of the Na^+ gradient (out to in) depends on the activity of the Na^+, K^+ ATPase that is localized to the basolateral membrane.

Drug Secretion

The renal excretion of a chemical substance is the net result of glomerular filtration, reabsorption, and secretion. The disentanglement of these mechanisms, however, encompassed one of the most controversial periods in the history of science. The second half of the nineteenth century witnessed a long, sometimes acrimonious debate between proponents of the theory of filtration, as the explanation of excretion, and proponents of the theory of secretion. Those favoring filtration accused their opponents of necessarily invoking vitalism. The notion that solutes could be extracted selectively from the blood appeared to them purposeful and vitalistic because the discrimination of solutes by membrane transport systems was not merely unknown, it was incomprehensible as well. To them, the physical mechanistic theory, on the other hand, was intellectually satisfying. Ironically, however, renal physiology began with the concept of secretion. William Bowman proposed, in 1842, that water secreted by the glomerular capillaries washed out solutes secreted by the distal tubules. Two years later, Carl Ludwig introduced the concept of plasma ultrafiltration; the stage for the debate was set. The issue was finally resolved in 1923, when Marshall and Vickers firmly established the concept of secretion. They showed that 70 per cent of an injected dye, phenolsulfonphtalein, appeared in the urine during one circulation through the kidney, a value far in excess of any that could be accounted for by filtration alone. The intervening years have seen an evolution toward our present understanding.

Classification

Secretory systems can be divided into two broad categories: one for organic anions; and another for organic cations, with evidence for the existence of subsystems for each. (The issue of subsystems will be addressed subsequently.) The evidence overwhelmingly supports the view that the two systems are separate and distinct. Identification has rested primarily on the use of inhibitors. In fact, certain inhibitors have achieved the status of "indicator ions." For the organic anion system, the indicator ion is probenecid. If the secretion of a substance under study is inhibited by probenecid, the conclusion reached is that that substance is secreted by the organic anion system. As far as the organic cation system is concerned, no single inhibitor has achieved the same universal status. Mepiperphenidol accomplishes that end for in vitro experiments, but it cannot be used in vivo because of its potent cardiovascular side-effects. More recently, the histamine H_2 receptor antagonist, cimetidine, has been advocated as a clinically useful indicator ion of organic cation secretion. This lack of a generally accepted "indicator" has hampered development of a comprehensive description of organic cation secretion. Inhibition by both probenecid and an organic cation, e.g., cimetidine, is rarely seen; consequently, a clear-cut pattern of inhibition is the basis for concluding that the two systems are separate. Furthermore, the two systems can be distinguished anatomically.[r4] Species differences exist, not only in the anatomic disposition of the transport systems to different localizations within the proximal tubule, but also in the efficacy of particular drugs secreted by the different species.[r5,7] The general description presented does not elaborate on these complications.

Organic Anions

A bewildering variety of organic anions are secreted.[11–14] Generally, p-aminohippurate (PAH) is used as the prototypical organic anion and inhibition by probenecid as the defining condition. As will be discussed, secretion represents transport in series: entry across the basolateral membrane and exit across the brush border membrane. It is assumed that any drug that is a substrate for the transporter on one face of the cell is a substrate for the transporter on the opposite face as well, although this assumption has not been exhaustively confirmed. The list of substrates includes: glycine conjugates; amino acid conjugates; glucuronides; sulfates; benzoate derivatives; acetate and propionate derivatives; heterocyclic carboxylates; sulfonamides; sulfates; amino acid derivatives; heterocyclic compounds; and some miscellaneous compounds, including prostaglandins and cAMP. A list of drugs secreted by this system is given in Table 37.2. There have been several attempts at defining structure–activity relationships. It should be no surprise that none has ever been completely successful. Nonetheless, a tentative model has emerged: the substrate has an obligatory hydrophobic core and one or two electronegative groups capable of electrostatic or dipole interaction with matching positively charged groups on the transporter. The positive charges on the binding site are separated by a distance of 7.5 A.

Table 37.2 Drugs Secreted by the Organic Anion System

Acetazolamide	Penicillin G
Bumetanide	Phenylbutazone
Cephalothin	Probenecid
Chlorothiazide	Saccharin
Ethacrynic acid	Salicylate
Furosemide	Sulfisoxazole
Indomethacin	Sulfinpyrazone

Organic Cations

As with the anion system, a diverse group of chemically unrelated compounds are secreted.[15, 16] A representative list of some secreted cationic drugs is given in Table 37.3. Despite their variety of chemical structure, all contain a nitrogen atom and are positively charged at physiologic pH. Beyond these facts, the only other parameter for substrate specificity seems to be hydrophobicity: the greater the permeability coefficient for a drug, the higher its affinity.

Transepithelial Transport[r4–8]

Organic anions and organic cations are concentrated from the blood into the tubular fluid against their electrochemical gradients. Secretion is an active process: it requires the input of energy to move the system away from equilibrium. The question is how does the kidney perform work isothermally? At the expense of ATP hydrolysis, the Na^+, K^+-ATPase (a primary-active transporter) generates and maintains a Na^+ gradient across the plasma membrane (140mM out, 10–20 mM in). The consequence of this reaction in the cell is maintained at a state of disequilibrium, and the energy in the Na^+

Table 37.3 Drugs Secreted by the Organic Cation System

Amiloride	Mecamylamine
Amprolium	Mepiperphenidol
Atropine	Neostigmine
Cimetidine	Norepinephrine
Cisplatin	Paraquat
Creatinine	Procainamide
Dihydromorphine	Quinidine
Dopamine	Quinine
Epinephrine	Ranitidine
Hexamethonium	Thiamine
Histamine	Tolazoline
Isoproterenol	

gradient is used to create a gradient of other ions. Secretion of drugs (i.e., the movement of drugs against unfavorable electrochemical gradients) is achieved by coupling the movement of the drug to the co- or countermovement of another ion down energetically favorable pathways. The currently accepted models explaining secretion have been arrived at by a variety of experimental techniques. Each has its own advantages and disadvantages. Unfortunately, exhaustive studies quantifying the kinetic parameters of many drugs transported in a single species as determined by several techniques have not been conducted. Consequently, the models to be presented here are a general description.

Organic Anions

The prototypical organic anion is p-aminohippurate (PAH). A model describing the transepithelial movement of PAH is shown in Figure 37.1. PAH is concentrated intracellularly, from the blood side, at least 40 fold. This represents active transport and therefore, there must be an energy input. A mechanism of PAH uptake across the basolateral membrane has been proposed: PAH enters in exchange for ∝KG (Fig. 37.1, reaction 1); via a secondary-active exchanger (or antiporter).[17,18]

[Primary-active transport, as described above, is a mechanism that couples the translocation of solute directly to the hydrolysis of ATP; secondary-active transport is any mechanism that couples the translocation of one solute to that of another without the direct involvement of ATP hydrolysis.] The ∝KG gradient (in to out) is generated either by Na+ gradient-dependent dicarboxylic acid co-transporters (i.e., secondary-active) located at either face of the cell (Fig. 37.1, reaction 2) or by metabolism (Fig. 37.1, reaction 3), via the ∝KG/malate shuttle. The ∝KG/malate shuttle plays an important role in delivering reducing equivalents to the electron transport chain. The most important pathway for the coupling of ∝KG to PAH influx may, in fact, be reaction 3, since it is well extablished that PAH uptake across the basolateral membrane is intimately coupled to aerobic metabolism. As indicated, the kidney also has the capacity to take up αKG from the blood or tubular fluid by Na^+ gradient-dependent mechanisms. The ultimate driving force for PAH accumulation is the energy in the Na^+ gradient that was created at the expense of ATP hydrolysis (Fig. 37.1, reaction 4). Since the monovalent anion,

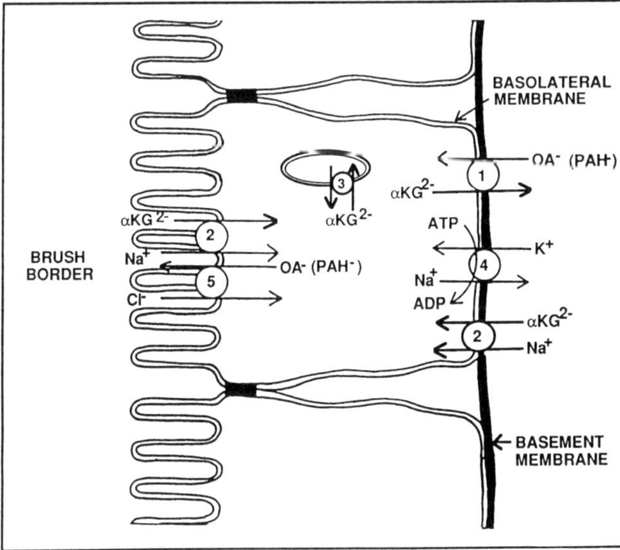

Figure 37.1 Model for Transepithelial Transport of Organic Anions

PAH, is taken-up in exchange for the divalent anion, ∝KG, the reaction is electrogenic; there is a net movement of charge. Consequently there are two driving forces: the Na^+ gradient and an electrical coupling reaction.

The importance of the electrical component is revealed by considering the thermodynamics of the reaction. The amount of energy available to do useful work is given by the Gibbs free-energy change (ΔG). The free energy change for the influx of PAH coupled to the efflux of ∝KG down its electrochemical gradients is given by:

$$\Delta G = -m_{\propto KG}\,\Delta G_{\propto KG} + m_{PAH}\,\Delta G_{PAH} \qquad \text{(C-1)}$$

where $m_{\propto KG}$ is moles of αKG transported and m_{PAH} moles PAH transported, per reaction cycle. $\Delta G_{\propto Kg}$ is the electrochemical potential of ∝KG, and ΔG_{PAH} is the electrochemical potential of PAH. At equilibrium ΔG = 0 (by definition), and rearrangement gives:

$$m_{PAH}\Delta G_{PAH} = m_{\propto kg}\Delta G_{\propto kg} \qquad \text{(C-2)}$$

$\frac{m_{PAH}}{m_{\propto kg}}$ = (n)stoichiometry or coupling ratio for the reaction

Consequently,

$$n\Delta G_{PAH} = \Delta G_{\propto kg} \qquad \text{(C-3)}$$

the electrochemical potential for PAH is:

$$\Delta G_{PAH} = \frac{RTln[PAH]_i + ZF\Delta\Psi}{[PAH]_o}$$

- the subscripts (i and o) refer to in and out respectively,

and Z, F, and ΔΨ are as described above.

A similar expression can be written for ∝KG with the exception Z = −2.

Thus, at equilibrium:

$$\frac{n(RTln[PAH]_i + ZF\Delta\Psi)}{[PAH]_o} = \frac{RTln[\propto KG]_i + ZF\Delta\Psi}{[\propto KG]_o} \qquad \text{(C-4)}$$

simplified to:

$$\frac{[PAH]_i}{[PAH]_o} = \frac{[\propto KG]_i^{\,n}e^{n\text{-}2\,F\Delta\Psi}}{[\propto KG]_o} \qquad \text{(C-5)}$$

Analysis of equation C-5 shows that, physiologically, there are two driving forces for the accumulation of PAH: a chemical force and an electrical force. The plasma concentration of ∝KG is approximately 50 μM and while its intracellular concentration is uncertain, it is at least 250μM. Putting these values into equation C-5 provides an appreciation of the coupling mechanisms. PAH could accumulate fourfold by the chemical gradient of αKG alone, but the electrical term provides a dramatic influence, and increases the energy available for concentrative transport by more than tenfold. Thus, with a coupling ratio of 1, and a fourfold $[\propto kg]_i/[\propto kg]_o$ ratio, PAH can be accumulated more than 40-fold! The physiologic advantage of electrical coupling is clear by considering the case where two moles PAH are moved for one mole ∝KG (i.e., an n of 2). The advantage of the electrical component is lost.

PAH exits the cell in exchange for another anion, either Cl^- or HCO_3^- in some species,[19] e.g., dog, or by a uniport mechanism in others,[20] e.g., rabbit. The physiologic advantages of the various efflux pathways is unclear. It may be that in those species where urate is reabsorbed, e.g., dog, PAH and urate ride on the same exchanger in the brush border membrane. Where urate is excreted, e.g., rabbit, PAH and urate efflux pathways are separate.[r8] The uniport mechanism means that the univalent anion PAH will distribute itself across the brush border membrane in accordance with the Nernst equation; for a (−)60 mV membrane potential, PAH would be concentrated in the tubular fluid tenfold. Thus, transepithelial transport (i.e., secretion) is achieved by the coordinated activity of secondary-active transporters at both plasma membranes, of the ∝KG/malate anion exchanger of the mitochondrion, of the Na^+ gradient-dependent dicarboxylic cotransporters, of the Na^+, K^+-ATPase, and ultimately, of the metabolic status of the cell. The capacity of the proximal tubule to secrete organic anions is dependent on the integrated physiologic capacity of the constituent renal cells.

Organic Cations

The prototypical organic cation to be used for this discussion is N^1-methylnicotinamide (NMN). Presumably, all cationic drugs are handled in a similar fashion. It is concentrated intracellularly from the blood by a uniport mechanism (Fig. 37.2, reaction 1). That is, the cationic substrate is driven (or "pulled") into the cell by the membrane potential and, in accordance with the above definitions, NMN uptake across the basolateral membrane is a secondary-active transport process. The membrane potential is maintained by the activity of the Na^+/K^+-ATPase. Any chemical reagent that inhibits metabolism or the Na^+, K^+-ATPase will block the uptake of NMN.

The extent to which NMN can be accumulated is given by:

$$\Delta G = \frac{RT \ln [NMN]_i + ZF\Delta\Psi}{[NMN]_o}$$

Solving this equation for the equilibrium conditions, shows that there is sufficient energy in a –70mV membrane potential to accumulate NMN 14-fold. Whether organic cations are accumulated to any extent greater than this value remains controversial.[21,22] If they are, some mechanism other than a uniport transport has to be involved. This issue awaits clarification.

The exit of NMN from the cell across the brush border membrane into the tubular fluid is accompanied by the movement of a H^+ into the cell[23] (Fig. 37.2, reaction 2). Since NMN is accumulated in the tubular fluid, this represents an active transport process. The energy is provided in the H^+ gradient (out to in) and NMN/H^+ exchange represents secondary-active transport. The pH gradient (tubular fluid acidic) is maintained by the activity of the Na^+/H^+ exchanger (Fig. 37.2, reaction 3); the Na^+ gradient is maintained by the Na^+/K^+-ATPase (Fig. 37.2, reaction 4). Thus, the active transport of NMN into the tubular fluid is achieved by the functional coupling of two secondary-active transporters (Fig. 37.2, reactions 2 and 3).

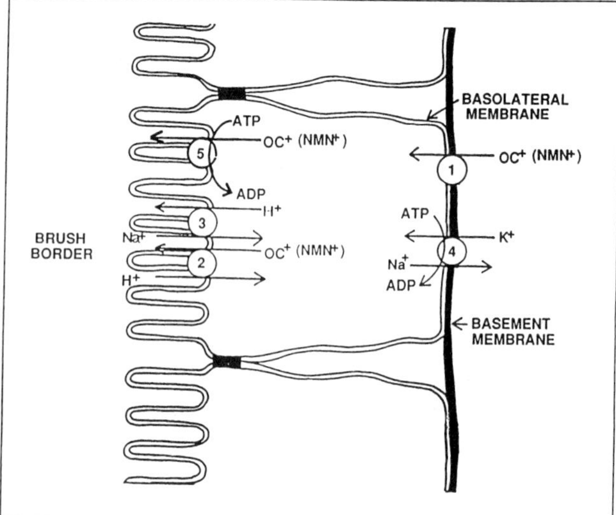

Figure 37.2 Model for the Transepithelial Transport of Organic Cations

The extent to which NMN can be accumulated is given by the thermodynamic relationship, as derived above:

$$\frac{[NMN]_o}{[NMN]_i} = \frac{[H^+]_o}{[H^+]_i}^{n \cdot e^{n-1\,F\Delta\Psi}}$$

The NMN/H^+ exchange reaction is electroneutral, that is, n = 1. Thus, for a tenfold proton gradient, NMN could be accumulated tenfold. (In actuality, the pH gradient across the brush border membrane is something less than tenfold.) At first glance, it might seem that the system would be more efficient if n > 2. However, the cost-effectiveness would be lost because the cell would have to expend more energy to expel the additional H^+. Hence, the transepithelial transport of organic cations is achieved by the coordinated activity of the uniporter, of the NMN/H^+ exchanger of the Na+/H^+ exchanger, of the Na^+, K^+-ATPase, and ultimately, of course, of the metabolic status of the cell. Drugs that are considered substrates compete with the prototypical (or indicator) substrate for transport.[24-26]

Summary

The secretion of ionic drugs is achieved by the polarized distribution between the basolateral and brush border membrane of secondary-active transporters specific for either class. Organic anions are probably taken up from the blood by an electrogenic anion exchange mechanism and exit by electroneutral anion exchange. Organic cations are taken up by a voltage-dependent uniport mechanism and exit by an electroneutral H^+ exchange mechanism. Transepithelial transport is achieved by the organic ions being "pushed" at both faces of the renal cell.

Other Pathways

The currently accepted models of drug secretion may have to be modified to include other pathways. It has been shown that the brush border (or apical) membrane contains a P-glycoprotein,[27] and ATP-dependent efflux pump, i.e., a primary-coupled transporter with broad substrate specificity (Fig. 37.2, reaction 5). The substrates for the P-glycoprotein are mostly, but not exclusively, cations.[28] While it is not clear what is the P-glycoprotein's over-all contribution to drug secretion, it is probably that neutral molecules, e.g., digoxin, are secreted by the P-glycoprotein.[29] Yet organic cations such as quinidine and verapamil are substrates for the P-glycoprotein also. Consequently, it seems likely that the well-established clinical entity of quinidine affecting the renal secretion of digoxin may be due to competition for transport via the P-glycoprotein. A still further complicating factor arises from the possibility that the organic cation/H^+ exchanger (Fig. 37.2, reaction 2) and the P-glycoprotein (Fig. 37.2, reaction 5) may have common substrates. Thus, it appears that there are two efflux pathways for organic cations across the brush border membrane of the proximal tubule: one, via primary-active transport; two, via secondary-active transport. The physiologic advantage of this transport redundancy is unclear, yet it is likely that the potential for competition among the various substrates for transport out of the cell is the site of deleterious drug–drug interactions.

Nonmediated Transport

There is no evidence that drugs move from blood to tubular fluid paracellularly. It is conceivable, however, that cationic drugs (but not anionic) could be accumulated in the tubular fluid by nonmediated transport and ion trapping. The transepithelial flux is determined largely by the permeability coefficient (P) (see Equation B-2) of both membranes. The contribution of nonmediated transport could be significant for hydrophobic, cationic drugs in particular. At physiologic pH, a sizeable portion of these molecules could be in a noncharged form, that is the more lipid-permeable form; but, when these molecules diffuse into the acidic tubular fluid, they become charged and trapped, i.e., ion-trapping. Conversely, the transepithelial movement of organic anions from blood to tubular fluid is not favored by nonmediated transport and ion-trapping. (They have low pK_a values.) Conversely, the phenomenon of ion-trapping favors the reabsorption of hydrophobic anionic drugs.

References

Research Reports

1. Welling LW, Welling DJ. Surface areas of brush border and lateral cell walls in the rabbit proximal nephron. Kidney Int 1975;*8*:343–348.
2. Molitoris BA, Chan LK, Shapiro JI, Conger JD, Falk SA. Loss of epithelial polarity: A novel hypothesis for reduced proximal tubule Na^+ transport following ischemic injury. J Membr Biol 1989;*107*:119–127.
3. Molitoris BA, Nelson WJ. Alterations in the establishment and maintenance of epithelial cell polarity as a basis for disease processes. J Clin Invest 1990;*85*:3–9.
4. Rodriguez-Boulan E, Powell SK. Polarity of epithelial and neuronal cells. Ann Rev Cell Biol 1992;*8*:395–427.
5. Higgins CF. ABC transporters: From microorganisms to man. Ann Rev Cell Biol 1992;*8*:67–113.
6. Baly DL, Horyle R. The biology and biochemistry of the glucose transporter. Biochim Biophys Acta 1988;*947*:571–590.
7. Mueckler M, Caruso C, Baldwin S, Panico A, Blench I, Morris HR, Allard WJ, Lienhard GE, Lodish HF. Sequence and tissue distribution of a human glucose transporter. Science 1985;*229*:941–945.
8. Fukumoto H, Seino S, Imura H., Seino Y, Eddy RL, Fukushima Y, Byers MG, Shows TB, Bell GI. Sequence, tissue distribution, and chromosomal localization of a mRNA encoding a human glucose transporter-like protein. Proc Natl Acad Sci USA 1988;*85*:5434–5438.
9. Elsas LJ, Longo N. Glucose transporters. Ann Rev Med 1992;*43*:377–393.
10. Turner RJ, Moran A. Stoichiometric studies of the renal outer cortical brush border membrane D-glucose transporter. J Membr Biol 1982;*67*:73–80.
11. Ullrich KJ, Rumrich G, Fritzsch G. Contraluminal paraaminohippurate transport in the proximal tubule of the rat kidney. I. Kinetics, influence of cations, anions and capillary preperfusion. Pflugers Arch 1987;*409*:229–235.
12. Ullrich KJ, Rumrich G, Fritzsch G, Klöss S. Contraluminal paraminohippurate (PAH) transport in the proximal tubule of the rat kidney. II. Specificity: Aliphatic dicarboxylic acids. Pflugers Arch 1987;*408*:38–45.
13. Ullrich KJ, Rumrich G, Klöss S. Contraluminal para-aminohippurate transport in the proximal tubule of the rat kidney. Pflugers Arch 1987;*409*:547–554.
14. Ullrich KJ, Rumrich G, Klöss S. Contraluminal para-aminohippurate (PAH) transport in the proximal tubule of the rat kidney: IV. Specificity: mono- and polysubstituted benzene analogs. Pflugers Arch 1988;*413*:134–146.
15. Ullrich KJ, Papauassiliou F, David C, Rumrich G, Fritzsch G. Contraluminal transport of organic cations in the proximal tubule of the rat kidney: I. Kinetics of N^1-methylnicotinamide and tetraethyl-ammonium; influence of K^+, HCO_3^-. pH; inhibition by aliphatic primary-, secondary-, tertiary amines, mono- and bisquaternary compounds. Pflugers Arch 1991;*419*:84–92.
16. Ullrich KJ, Rumrich G, Neiteler K, Fritzsch G. Contraluminal transport of organic cations in the proximal tubule of the rat kidney. II. Specificity: anilines phenylalkylamines (catecholamines), hetercyclic compounds (pyridines, quinolines, acridines). Pflugers Arch 1992;*420*:29–38.
17. Pritchard JB. Coupled transport of p-aminohippurate by rat basolateral membrane vesicles. Am J Physiol 1988;*255*:F597–F604.
18. Burckhardt G, Ullrich KJ. Organic anion transport across the contraluminal membrane-dependence on sodium. Kidney Int 1989;*36*:370–377.
19. Steffens TG, Holohan PD, Ross CR. Operational modes of the organic anion exchanger in canine renal brush-border membrane vesicles. Am J Physiol 1989;*256*:F596–F609.
20. Martinez F, Manganel M, Montrose-Rafizadeh C, Werner D, Roch-Ramel F. Transport of urate and p-aminohippurate in rabbit renal brush-border membranes. Am J Physiol 1990;*258*:F1145–F1153.
21. Sokol PP, McKinney TD. Mechanism of organic cation transport in rabbit renal basolateral membrane vesicles. Am J Physiol 1990;*258*:F1599–F1607.
22. Brändle E, Greven J. Transport of cimetidine across the basolateral membrane of rabbit kidney proximal tubules: Characterization of transport mechanisms. J Pharmacol Exp Ther 1991;*258*:1038–1045.
23. Holohan, PD, Ross, CR. Mechanisms of organic cation transport in kidney plasma membrane vesicles: 2. ΔpH studies. J Pharmacol Exp Ther 1981;*216*:294–298.
24. Sokol PP, Huiatt KR, Holohan PD, Ross CR. Gentamicin and verapamil compete for a common transport mechanism in renal brush border membrane vesicles. J Pharmacol Exp Ther 1989;*251*:937–942.
25. Sokol PP, Gates SB. Effect of endogenous and exogenous polyamines on organic cation transport in rabbit renal plasma membrane vesicles. J Pharmacol Exp Ther 1990;*255*:52–58.
26. Bendayan R, Sellers EM, Silverman M. Inhibition kinetics of cationic drugs on N^1-methylnicotinamide uptake by brush border membrane vesicles from dog kidney cortex. Can J Physiol Pharmacol 1990;*68*:467–475.
27. Croop JM, Rymond M, Haber D, DeVault A, Arceci RJ, Gros P, Hausman DE. The three mouse multidrug resistance (mdr) genes are expressed in a tissue-specific manner in normal mouse tissues. Mol Cell Biol 1989;*9*:1346–1350.
28. Ford JM, Hait WN. Pharmacology of drugs that alter multidrug resistance in cancer. Pharmacol Rev 1990;*42*:155–199.
29. Tanigawara Y, Okamura N, Hirai M, Yasuhara M, Veda K, Kioka N, Komano T, Hori R. Transport of digoxin by human P-glycoprotein expressed in a porcine kidney epithelial cell line (LLC-Pk_1). J Pharmacol Exp Ther 1992;*263*:840–845.
30. Rebbeor JF, Holohan PD. The physiological function of a normally expressed kidney P-glycoprotein. J Pharmacol Exp Ther *in press*.

Reviews

Suggested texts for an introduction to and for a clear understanding of the subject of membrane transport are the following:

r1. Harold FM. The vital force: A study of bioenergetics. New York, Freeman 1986.
This is a beautifully written, clear, concise, yet thorough description of the subject. The scope of the subject and the definitions of the phenomena studied are clearly presented. The importance of considering membrane transport phenomena within the integrated physiological capacity of the cell is presented forcefully.

r2. Stein, WD. Transport and diffusion across cell membranes. New York: Academic Press, 1986.
This is a more rigorous mathematical description of the subject. The description of diffusion is excellent and is highly recommended.

There are many excellent reviews on the renal secretory systems, the anatomical organization of the kidney, integrated physiological capacity of the kidney with its transport functions, and the experimental methods used to arrive at our present understanding. The following are recommended highly:

r3. Ross CR, Holohan PD. Transport of organic anions and cations in isolated renal plasma membrane vesicles. Ann Rev Pharmacol Toxicol 1983;23:65–85.

r4. Weiner IM. Organic acids, bases and uric acid. In Seldin DW, Giebisch G, (eds) The kidney: Physiology and pathophysiology. New York: Raven Press (1985); pp 1703–1724.

r5. Grantham JJ, Chonko AM. Renal handling of organic anions and cations; metabolism and excretion of uric acid. In Brenner GM, Rector FC (eds.) The kidney WB Saunders, (1986); Chap. 17, pp 663–700.

r6. Pritchard JB, Miller DS. Comparative insights into the mechanisms of renal organic anion and cation secretion. Am J Physiol 1991;*261*:R1329–1340.

r7. Brater DC, Sokol PP, Hall SD, McKenney TD. Renal elimination of drugs: Methods and determinants. In Seldin DW, Giebisch G (Eds) The Kidney: Physiology and pathophysiology, 2nd edition New York: Raven Press, 1992; Vol 3, pp 3597–3628.

CHAPTER 38

D. Craig Brater

Diuretics

Though all diuretics are used to increase renal excretion of sodium and water, they differ considerably in chemical derivation, efficacy, sites of action, and mechanism of effects (Table 38.1). The choice of a diuretic clinically is dictated by the objective of therapy and the pathophysiology of the patient's disease. For example, patients with renal insufficiency require loop diuretics because they do not respond to other agents to a clinically relevant degree. Patients with cirrhosis are noted for having secondary hyperaldosteronism as a cause of sodium retention; thus, diuretic treatment in such patients is initiated with an inhibitor of aldosterone, spironolactone. Effective use of diuretics, then, requires knowledge of the pharmacology of each diuretic agent coupled with an understanding of the pathophysiology of the patient's disease.

Diuretics are used in many clinical conditions (Table 38.2), the most common being the edematous disorders and hypertension. Other uses include the treatment of hypercalcemia with loop diuretics, the treatment of diabetes insipidus or hypercalciuria with thiazide diuretics, the treatment of glaucoma with carbonic anhydrase inhibitors, and the treatment of cerebral edema with osmotic agents.

When used for treating edematous disorders and hypertension, the fundamental objective of therapy is to cause a negative sodium balance; in other words, to cause excretion of sodium in excess of sodium intake. Doing so results in decreased vascular volume, which stimulates movement of sodium and water from the interstitium into the vascular space, thereby "mobilizing" edema. This effect in hypertensive patients who do not have edema results in a diminished vascular volume and consequent decrease in blood pressure. It should be apparent that attainment of a negative sodium balance can be prevented by too much sodium intake, and effective use of diuretics requires counseling patients to limit their intake of salt.

In patients with edematous disorders, it is important to assess clinically whether the patient has an expanded or contracted vascular volume. The former group may need—and can tolerate—a vigorous diuresis. In the latter, overly aggressive diuresis can exceed the rate at which interstitial edematous fluid can refill the vascular volume, with the risk of a vascular space sufficiently contracted to result in hypotension. Thus, in patients with normal or contracted vascular volumes, as typically occurs in nephrotic syndrome or cirrhosis, diuresis should be induced in a slow and controlled fashion, leading one to choose diuretics with less efficacy, such as the thiazides. On the other hand, patients with expanded volumes, such as those with congestive heart failure (CHF), are often treated with loop diuretics to cause a rapid and extensive diuresis. These examples stress the importance of linking pathophysiology to pharmacology to derive a more rational therapeutic strategy.

Chemistry and History

Carbonic Anhydrase Inhibitors

The structures of clinically used diuretics are presented in Figure 38.1. The carbonic anhydrase inhibitor, acetazolamide (Fig. 38.1,

Table 38.1 Characteristics of Diuretics

Type	Site of Action	Chemical Class	Relative Efficacy
Carbonic Anhydrase Inhibitors Acetazolamide	Proximal Tubule	Sulfonamide Derivative	2
Osmotic Agents Mannitol	Proximal Tubule and Thick Ascending Limb of Henie	Sugar	6
Loop Diuretics Bumetanide, Furosemide Ethacrynic Acid, Torsemide	Thick Ascending Limb of Henle; Na^+-K^+-2CL^-	Carboxylic Acid Sulfonamide Derivatives	10–15
Thiazide Diuretics Bendroflumethiazide, Benzthiazide, Chlorothiazide, Chlorthalidone, Cyclothiazide, Hydrochlorothiazide, Hydroflumethiazide, Indapamide, Methyclothiazide, Metolazone, Polythiazide, Quinethazone, Trichlormethiazide	Distal Tubule; Electroneutral NaCl Reabsorption	Sulfonamide Derivatives	4
Potassium-Retaining Diuretics Amiloride, Spironolactone, Triamterene	Distal Tubule and Collecting Duct; Na^+, K^+ Exchange	Pyrazinolyl-Guanidine, 17-Spirolactone, and Pteridine, respectively	1

Table 38.2 Therapeutic Uses of Diuretic Agents

Type	Uses	
	Diuretic	"Non Diuretic"
Carbonic Anhydrase Inhibitors	With Loop Diuretics in Patients With Diuretic Resistance	Glaucoma, Metabolic Alkalosis, Altitude Sickness
Osmotic Agents	Acute Renal Failure	Cerebral Edema
Loop Diuretics	Edematous Disorders, Acute Renal Failure, Hypertension in Patients with Cl_{CR}* < 40 ml/min or in those with Extensive Fluid Retention	Hypercalcemia, Hyponatremia, Renal Tubular Acidosis
Thiazide Diuretics	Edematous Disorders	Hypertension, Hypercalciuria, Diabetes Insipidus
Potassium-Retaining Diuretics	Edematous Disorders (Particularly Primary or Secondary Hyperaldosteronism; e.g., cirrhosis)	Potassium and/or Magnesium Loss

*CL_{CR} = Creatinine Clearance

Panel A) is a derivative of sulfonamide antibiotics. Its development was stimulated by the observation that the antibiotic, sulfanilamide, caused a diuresis but with metabolic acidosis as a side-effect. Further study showed that sulfanilamide inhibited carbonic anhydrase. Modification of the structure of the antibiotic yielded acetazolamide as a drug with more desirable diuretic features. Its inhibition of carbonic anhydrase explained not only its mechanism of action but also helped define the role of carbonic anhydrase in the kidney. This historical precedent is typical of the field of diuretics, in which pharmacology has been linked inextricably to fundamental discoveries in renal physiology.

Osmotic Diuretics

Mannitol is a sugar that remains within the vascular space and is freely filtered at the glomerulus (Fig. 38.1, Panel B). The osmotic effect while in the vasculature causes influx of interstitial and intracellular water into the vascular space, expanding blood volume and decreasing serum sodium concentrations. If there is any limitation to renal elimination of mannitol (as in patients with renal insufficiency) this effect can cause CHF. After being filtered at the glomerulus, mannitol creates an osmotic force throughout the length of the renal tubule that blunts reabsorption of sodium and water. This

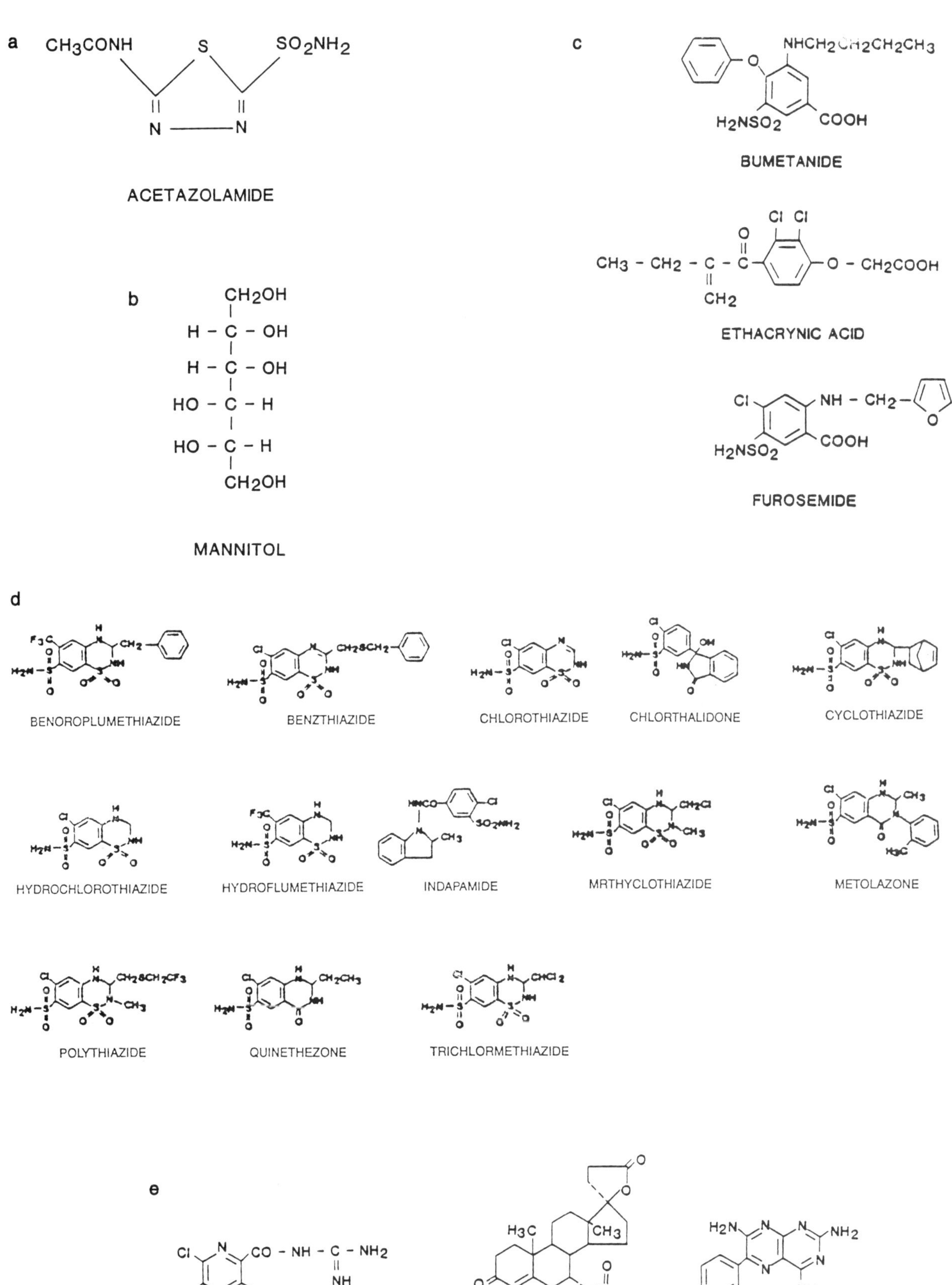

Figure 38.1 Structures of Diuretic Agents

same effect occurs with other sugars and causes the volume depletion seen in patients with uncontrolled diabetes mellitus in whom renal excretion of glucose results in osmotic diuresis.

Loop Diuretics

The first consistently effective diuretics had their site of effect at the thick ascending limb of the loop of Henle. These organic mercurials are no longer marketed because better agents have been developed that have more consistent efficacy and less toxicity.

Ethacrynic acid and furosemide were developed independently and virtually simultaneously (Fig. 38.1, Panel C). Development of ethacrynic acid focused on notions from the era of mercurial diuretics that inhibition of sulfhydryl groups in the kidney would cause a diuresis. Screening for such compounds led to the discovery of this agent. At the same time in Germany, screening of compounds for diuretic activity resulted in a group of active sulfamoylanthranilic acids that were substituted on the amine group of the aromatic ring. Of this group, furosemide was developed, followed by bumetanide (Figure 38.1, Panel C), azosemide, piretanide, and torsemide. Other structurally different agents with sites of action at the loop of Henle have been studied, but none have been marketed. These loop diuretics represented a major breakthrough. The magnitude of their effect made them useful in patients who did not respond to other drugs, including those with severe renal insufficiency, severe heart failure, etc. In addition, an extensive literature in renal physiology is focused on use of these drugs as probes to elucidate fundamental physiologic and pathophysiologic processes in the kidney.

Thiazide Diuretics

The discovery of acetazolamide led to the notion that compounds could be discovered that would result in a NaCl diuresis as opposed to the $NaHCO_3$ diuresis caused by carbonic anhydrase inhibitors. Such an effect was deemed to be beneficial because this type of drug might have greater effects but would also avoid the undesirable metabolic acidosis that attended carbonic anhydrase inhibition. Numerous chemical modifications of the sulfa nucleus were explored. One derivative resulted in ring closure that conferred the desired pharmacologic effect. This constituted the somewhat serendipitous discovery of chlorothiazide. Additional thiazides were then developed (Fig. 38.1, Panel D). They have different pharmacokinetic features, but all have the same magnitude of effect. Thus, these drugs are now selected clinically based primarily on their duration of effect (see below) and relative cost rather than distinguishing pharmacologic characteristics.

Other modifications of the sulfa nucleus resulted in quinethazone, metolazone, and chlorthalidone, which have pharmacologic effects identical to the classic thiazides but represent different chemical categories (Fig. 38.1, Panel D). Because their pharmacologic features are identical, these drugs are grouped with thiazides.

Like loop diuretics and carbonic anhydrase inhibitors, thiazides have played major roles in both therapeutics and in renal physiology. In fact, their use as probes of renal epithelial function has recently resulted in the discovery of a pathway of electroneutral NaCl reabsorption in the distal tubule, the site of action of these diuretics.

Potassium-Retaining Diuretics

Physiologic studies identified the role of aldosterone in stimulating reabsorption of Na^+ in the distal tubule and collecting duct in exchange for K^+ and H^+. Derivatives of the steroid nucleus of spirolactone were found to be active in animals with intact adrenals and inactive in those with adrenalectomy. Thus, it was presumed that the activity of these agents was by blocking aldosterone. As methods for studying steroid receptors and effects became available, these compounds were shown to block the receptor for aldosterone competitively. From this series of compounds, spironolactone (Fig. 38.1, Panel E) was developed clinically.

Triamterene (Fig. 38.1, Panel E) was discovered from studies of the biologic activity of pteridines, some of which were shown to have renal effects. Chemical modification of xanthopterin, a pigment in butterfly wings, resulted in the discovery and development of triamterene. Amiloride (Fig. 38.1, Panel E) is chemically similar to triamterene, in essence representing an open ring version of the pteridines. Like many of the other diuretics, it has been an extremely useful physiologic probe, since it specifically blocks Na^+ entry from the lumen of the distal tubule. In vitro it and its derivatives have also been used to block the Na^+/H^+ antiporter specifically, but this effect requires such high concentrations that this pharmacologic effect is probably not relevant to its clinical utility.

Pharmacology

General

All diuretics except spironolactone must reach the lumen of the renal tubule to achieve their effect.[1–3] Their primary routes of access and subsequent sites of effect are presented in Table 38.3. These discrete sites of action along the nephron account for the additive effects that occur with combinations of diuretics. Identification of these sites, together with an understanding of the physiology of nephron function at the sites, allows prediction of the various effects that are caused by the different diuretics.

Both the organic acid and organic base secretory sites for diuretics and other xenobiotics are in the proximal tubule.[1–3] Each of these is subject to competition. Thus, other organic acids (such as probenecid) can compete for transport of acidic diuretics, and other organic bases (e.g., trimethoprim) can compete for secretion of amiloride and triamterene. Such competition can limit the amounts of these diuretics that reach the lumen, diminishing response.

The amount of diuretic reaching its intraluminal site of action is reflected in its excretion rate in the voided urine. This quantity can be related to the amount of sodium excretion, as illustrated for loop and thiazide diuretics in Figure 38.2.[4] This relationship is a typical pharmacologic S-shaped (sigmoidal) curve. The greater efficacy of the loop compared to thiazide diuretics is shown. The major importance of these relationships is that an upper plateau occurs, above which no greater response will occur even if additional drug reaches the site of action. This upper plateau allows definition of the maximal doses of these diuretics that should be administered, as presented for loop diuretics in Table 38.4.

Table 38.3 Routes of Access to and Sites of Action of Diuretics

Diuretic	Route of Access	Site of Action
Carbonic Anhydrase Inhibitors	Organic Acid Secretion	Proximal Tubule
Osmotic Diuretics	Glomerular Filtration	Proximal Tubule and Thick Ascending Limb of the Loop of Henle
Loop Diuretics	Organic Acid Secretion	Thick Ascending Limb of the Loop of Henle
Thiazide Diuretics	Organic Acid Secretion	Proximal Tubule (Clinically Negligible) and Distal Tubule
Potassium-Retaining Diuretics		
Amiloride	Organic Base Secretion	Distal Tubule & Collecting Duct
Spironolactone	Peritubular Circulation	Distal Tubule & Collecting Duct
Triamterene	Organic Base Secretion	Distal Tubule & Collecting Duct

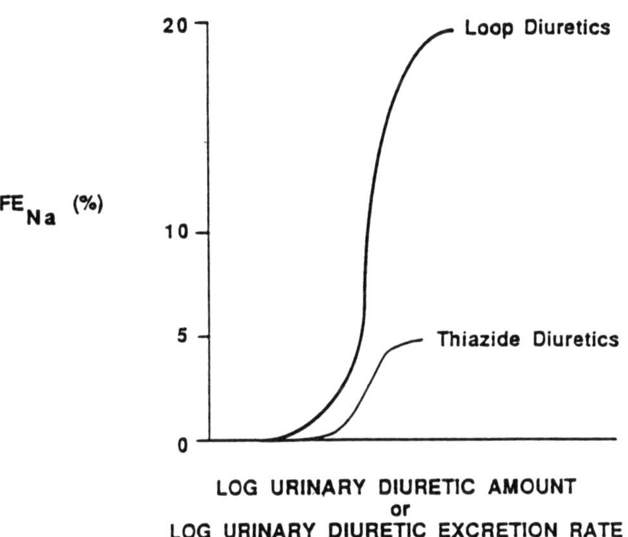

Figure 38.2 Relationship Between Urinary Excretion of Loop and Thiazide Diuretics and Excretion of Sodium

Carbonic Anhydrase Inhibitors

Efficacy

By catalyzing the hydration of bicarbonate at the proximal tubule, carbonic anhydrase facilitates the reabsorption of virtually all the bicarbonate filtered at the glomerulus (Fig. 38.3).[5] Sodium accompanies this anion to maintain electroneutrality. When the enzyme is inhibited, $NaHCO_3$ is lost in the urine, accompanied by water. This loss of base inevitably leads to a metabolic acidosis.

Much but not all of the sodium rejected from the proximal tubule is reabsorbed at the thick ascending limb of the loop of Henle. This reclamation diminishes the over-all efficacy of proximally acting diuretics. The increased delivery of sodium to the distal nephron and collecting duct results in increased exchange for potassium. Additionally, the luminal bicarbonate creates a negative charge that facilitates potassium secretion. The net result is that bicarbonate is excreted not only as $NaHCO_3$ but also as $KHCO_3$; carbonic anhydrase inhibitors thereby cause potassium depletion.

Table 38.4 Maximum (Ceiling) Doses of Loop Diuretics

	Dose (mg)				
	Furosemide		Bumetanide	Ethacrynic Acid	Torsemide
Clinical Condition	IV	PO	IV & PO	IV & PO	IV & PO
Renal Insufficiency					
$20 < Cl_{CR}^* < 50$	80	160	2	100	50–100
$Cl_{CR} < 20$	200	400	8–10	250	100–200
Nephrotic Syndrome	120	240	4	150	120**
Cirrhosis	40	80	1	50	20
Congestive Heart Failure	120	240	4	150	50–1

*Cl_{CR} = Creatinine Clearance; ** estimated

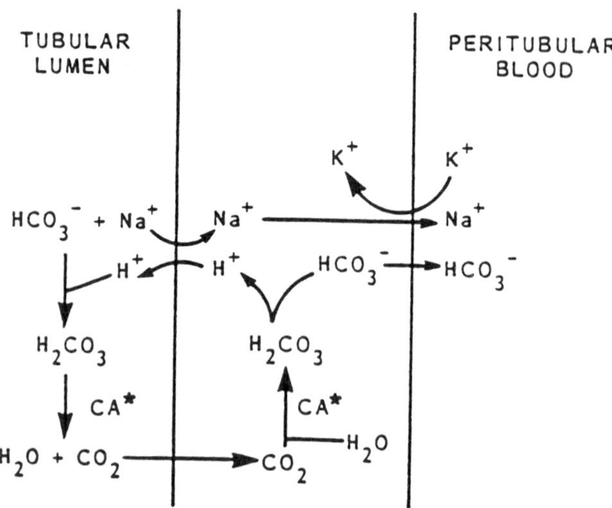

Figure 38.3 Mechanism of Effect of Carbonic Anhydrase on $NaHCO_3$ Reabsorption

Toxicity

The major toxicity of diuretics is in general an extension of their pharmacology. Thus, for carbonic anhydrase inhibitors, metabolic acidosis, and potassium depletion are the primary concerns. In addition, acetazolamide, particularly in large doses, can cause CNS side-effects, including light-headedness, paresthesias (particularly circumoral), weakness, and difficulty cerebrating. The mechanism(s) of these effects are unknown.

Pharmacokinetics (Table 38.5)

Because acetazolamide is now infrequently used and because it was developed before attention was paid to pharmacokinetics, little is known about its disposition. Its half-life of about 13 hours means that twice-a-day dosing is sufficient and that steady-state concentrations would be attained after two days of therapy.[6] Presumably, the renal elimination of acetazolamide is compromised in patients with renal insufficiency.

Therapeutic Uses (Table 38.2)

Acetazolamide is now used only rarely as a diuretic. It has been supplanted by better agents with fewer adverse effects. Since 60 percent or more of filtered sodium is reabsorbed in the proximal tubule, which is the site of action of acetazolamide, one might speculate that the drug would cause more sodium excretion than any other diuretic. However, only a fraction of proximal tubular sodium reabsorption is as $NaHCO_3$ and thereby linked to carbonic anhydrase; furthermore, much of the sodium rejected from the proximal tubule under the influence of acetazolamide is reabsorbed at more distal nephron sites, particularly the thick ascending limb of the loop of Henle. The net effect is that acetazolamide is a relatively weak diuretic (see Table 38.1 for relative efficacy compared with other diuretics).

The major use of acetazolamide as a diuretic is in the few patients with severe edematous disorders who are poorly responsive or refractory to large doses of potent loop diuretics.[7] Some of these patients, particularly those with heart failure, have increased proximal tubular reabsorption of sodium. Thus, the loop diuretic is limited in its efficacy because less sodium is being delivered to the loop. Coadministration of acetazolamide in this setting occasionally can cause a clinically important diuresis when such was unobtainable before.

Since carbonic anhydrase is also important for intraocular fluid formation, inhibitors of this enzyme are effective in decreasing intraocular pressure and are, therefore, used to treat glaucoma. Acetazolamide itself is now little used for this purpose, since derivatives of acetazolamide, such as methazolamide, were developed that have ample effects on ocular carbonic anhydrase but little systemic effect. As such, benefit is retained, but the diuresis and metabolic acidosis that inevitably occur with acetazolamide are decreased. Thus, acetazolamide itself is now mainly of historical interest.

The systemic metabolic acidosis caused by acetazolamide is used occasionally to correct metabolic alkalosis. The usual patient is one with severe chronic obstructive pulmonary disease in whom treatment with other diuretics resulted in Na^+, Cl^+, and K^+ loss, causing a severe metabolic alkalosis. If sufficiently severe, the alkalosis per se results in hypoventilation in order to raise blood CO_2 concentrations to correct systemic pH. This hypoventilation, however, can cause further hypoxemia in such patients. Correcting the alkalosis with short-term use of acetazolamide can improve oxygenation.

Acetazolamide has been proved effective in treatment of and prophylaxis against altitude sickness.[8] The mechanism of this effect is not known.

Osmotic Diuretics

Efficacy

Mannitol is freely filtered at the glomerulus. Since it is not reabsorbed in the nephron, it remains in the

Table 38.5 Diuretic Pharmacokinetics*

	Bio-availability (%)	Clearance (ml/min/kg)	Vd (L/kg)	Half-Life (hr)	Comments
Carbonic Anhydrase Inhibitor					
Acetazolamide				13	
Osmotic Agent					
Mannitol	N.A.	7	0.5	1	T1/2 in ESRD = 36 hrs
Loop Diuretics					
Bumetanide	80–90	2–3.5	0.15	0.3–1.5	T1/2 Unchanged in ESRD
Ethacrynic Acid					Kinetics Presumed Similar to Furosemide
Furosemide	40–60	1.5–3	0.15	0.3–3.4	T1/2 Prolonged in ESRD
Torsemide	80–100			3–4	T1/2 Unchanged in ESRD
Thiazide Diuretics					
Bendroflumethiazide	90	4.3	1–1.5	2.5–5	Duration of Action: 18–24 hr
Benzthiazide	100			10	Duration of Action: 12–18 hr
Chlorthalidone	65			24–55	Duration of Action: 24–72 hr
Chlorothiazide	30–50	4.3	1	15–25	Duration of Action: 6–12 hr
Clopamide				8–12	Duration of Action: 18–24 hr
Cyclothiazide					Duration of Action: 18–24 hr
Hydrochlorothiazide	65–75	4.6	2.5	3–10	Duration of Action: 6–12 hr
Hydroflumethiazide	75	6.4	5	6–10	Duration of Action: 18–24 hr
Indapamide	90		1.6	6–15	Duration of Action: 24–36 hr
Methyclothiazide					Duration of Action: 24–48 hr
Metolazone					Duration of Action: 12–24 hr
Polythiazide				25	Duration of Action: 24–48 hr
Quinethazone					Duration of Action: 12–24 hr
Trichlormethiazide		3.4		1–4	Duration of Action: 24 hr
Potassium-Retaining Diuretics					
Amiloride				17–26	T1/2 in ESRD = 100 hr
Spironolactone				1.5	T1/2 of Active Metabolites = 15 hr
Triamterene	83(55)	14(0.7)	3.0(0.14)	3(3)	Parentheses Denote Active Metabolite; T1/2 in ESRD = 10 hr

*Abbreviations: V_d = Volume of Distribution; T1/2 = Half-life; ESRD = Endstage Renal Disease

tubule lumen, where it exerts an osmotic effect, thereby impairing the ability of the proximal tubule and thick ascending limb to reabsorb sodium.[9,10] The reabsorptive pumps in these nephron segments have a limited ability to counteract the osmotic gradient caused by the intraluminal mannitol.

Though the proximal effect of mannitol causes some excretion of bicarbonate, the effect at the loop of Henle predominates, so that sodium is mainly excreted, along with chloride. In addition, the increased delivery of Na^+ to distal sites allows increased exchange for K^+ so that osmotic agents also cause enhanced potassium excretion. This effect accounts for the potassium deficits commonly encountered in patients with uncontrolled diabetes mellitus and a glucose-mediated osmotic diuresis.

Toxicity

The adverse effects of mannitol are a predictable consequence of its pharmacology. Thus, volume depletion and potassium loss are the risks in patients with adequate renal function. Patients with compromised renal function are at risk of volume expansion—risks of sufficient magnitude to limit, if not preclude, the use of mannitol in them.[11]

Pharmacokinetics (Table 38.5)

Mannitol is eliminated quickly, with a half-life in patients with normal renal function of about one hour. Thus, its effects begin quickly but also dissipate quickly. For this reason, it is often administered as a continuous IV infusion. Mannitol elimination is markedly impaired in patients with renal insufficiency (half-life = 36 hr).[12] Retention of this agent in such patients can be dangerous.[11]

Therapeutic Uses (Table 38.2)

Osmotic diuretics represent another group that has been used less since the advent of highly effective loop diuretics. The most common setting of osmotic diuresis, in fact, is disease-related rather than therapeutic; namely, that caused by the renal glucose excretion that occurs in uncontrolled diabetes mellitus.

Generation of a diuresis before virtually any renal insult (e.g., hypotension, aminoglycoside antibiotics, contrast agents, cis-platinum, etc.) has been shown to be protective of renal function in animal models. Mannitol is used by some as prophylaxis in patients likely to suffer ischemic insults to the kidney (as in some types of surgery), and at one time it enjoyed widespread use prior to chemotherapy with cis-platinum. There is little, if any, evidence to demonstrate that an osmotic diuresis is better than simply administering sufficient parenteral saline to cause a brisk diuresis. In fact, if an osmotic agent causes volume depletion, it could actually worsen the insult. In addition, recent data in animals suggest that a truly protective effect is best gained by decreasing renal metabolic demands by blocking Na^+ reabsorptive pump activity at the thick ascending limb.[13–15] Such an effect can be accomplished with loop but not osmotic diuretics. Over-all, rather than using osmotic agents for prophylaxis against renal injury, it is better to assure adequate volume status in the patient.

Mannitol also has been used in patients with acute renal failure in attempts to "open up" the kidney. There is no good evidence that this strategy is effective, and assuring adequate volume status in the patient is probably the best treatment. This latter strategy is reinforced by the fact that if mannitol is administered to a patient with acute renal failure, and the patient's renal function remains suppressed, the mannitol remains in the vascular space, where its osmotic effect expands blood volume and risks precipitating heart failure.[11] It seems, then, that mannitol should be used only rarely as a diuretic.

On the other hand, the osmotic effect of mannitol is highly effective in treating cerebral edema and has been used appropriately in neurosurgical procedures and head trauma. This use is inevitably associated with a pronounced osmotic diuresis that, in this setting, is an unwanted effect. Scrupulous attention must therefore be paid to the patient's volume status to make certain that too much volume depletion does not occur. Saline is usually given to the patient, titrating the volume loss.

Loop Diuretics

Efficacy

Loop diuretics inhibit the Na^+-K^+-$2CL^-$ reabsorptive pump at the thick ascending limb of the loop of Henle, causing a diuresis of NaCl and KCl. At this nephron site, 20 to 30 percent of filtered sodium is reabsorbed. Since loop diuretics can cause excretion of about 20 percent of filtered sodium, it is apparent that these agents can block virtually all reabsorption by this segment of the nephron. In doing so, the segment becomes metabolically quiescent, accounting for the protective effect of loop diuretics against ischemic insults.[13–15] The loop of Henle normally borders on hypoxemia: metabolic O_2 demands are great, while O_2 saturation is relatively low in this deep region of the kidney. Thus, the loop is uniquely susceptible to ischemic insults. By minimizing O_2 demands, loop diuretics can be protective. Unfortunately, most clinical ischemic insults are recognized only after the fact—beyond a point of rescue with loop diuretics.

Since a major component of calcium reabsorption occurs parallel to that of sodium at the thick ascending limb, loop diuretics will enhance calcium excretion sufficiently to be a useful therapeutic adjunct in patients with hypercalcemia. However, their use should be reserved until the volume depletion associated with hypercalcemia is corrected with infusions of saline.

The thick ascending limb is also important for urinary concentrating ability. Formation of a concentrated urine requires not only antidiuretic hormone (ADH), which permits reabsorption of water across the collecting duct, but also a hypertonic medullary interstitium to serve as the osmotic driving force for water reabsorption. In turn, the hypertonicity of the renal medullary interstitium is maintained by solute reabsorption at the thick ascending limb. Thus, loop diuretics decrease the driving force for water reabsorption, thereby preventing generation of a concentrated urine.[16]

Loop diuretics also have a short-lasting venodilating effect when administered IV.[17] This effect explains the immediate improvement that often occurs in patients with acute pulmonary edema, before any diuresis has occurred. The venodilation results in decreased cardiac preload, a fall in pulmonary artery wedge pressure, and symptomatic relief. Subsequently, the diuresis that ensues shrinks vascular volume, which also diminishes preload and results in more long-term benefit.

Toxicity

Most toxicity from loop diuretics is attributable to their effectiveness. The vigorous diuresis they can cause may result in volume depletion and/or potassium deficits. In addition, loop diuretics can cause both auditory and vestibular toxicity.[18,19] This is usually associated with high doses, particularly in patients with renal insufficiency and those receiving other ototoxic compounds, such as aminoglycoside antibiotics. This effect is reversible. Its mechanism is not well understood, but is associated with loss of cochlear hair cells. Most clinicians feel that the risk of ototoxicity is greatest with ethacrynic acid, which accounts for its infrequent use compared with other loop diuretics.

Allergic interstitial nephritis also occurs with chronic use of loop diuretics. This diagnosis should be entertained in historically stable patients whose renal function begins to deteriorate. If the diagnosis is made and the patient still needs a loop diuretic, ethacrynic acid is the best alternative, since it differs structurally, whereas the chemical structures of other loop diuretics are similar.

Pharmacokinetics (Table 38.5)

All loop diuretics are avidly bound to serum albumin (< 95% bound) and enter the urine by being actively secreted at the proximal tubule.[2,3] The high protein binding accounts for the small distribution volumes of these drugs, which are for the most part restricted to the vascular space. The short half-lives of these agents means their duration of action is brief.[20–27] Thus, they cause an intense, short-lived diuresis. When given IV, response occurs within minutes and is complete within two to three hours. When administered by mouth, peak response occurs within 30 to 90 minutes and is complete within another two to three hours. Because of their short duration of action, these drugs must be administered several times a day. Torsemide, a new loop diuretic has a longer half-life and duration of action.[27] It may be possible to administer it less frequently.

The bioavailabilities of these drugs differ, that for bumetanide and torsemide being essentially complete (≥80%), whereas that for furosemide is about 50 percent. Therefore, when switching a patient from IV to oral bumetanide or torsemide, dosing is the same; in contrast, the oral dose of furosemide needs to be twice the IV dose.

In patients with renal disease, less total drug appears in the urine. This accounts for the larger doses that are needed. In addition, with furosemide, entry into the urine is prolonged, so that the duration of response is longer than in patients with normal renal function.[28] For bumetanide and torsemide, the half-life and duration of response are unchanged in patients with renal disease. The mechanism for this difference is preservation of nonrenal pathways of bumetanide and torsemide elimination so that over-all clearance and half-life are not affected appreciably.[28]

Therapeutic Uses (Table 38.2)

Loop diuretics are the most effective diuretics currently available. For this reason and because they often succeed when other diuretics do not, they are also called "high-ceiling" diuretics. Their site of action is the thick ascending limb of the loop of Henle, which normally reabsorbs 20 to 30 percent of filtered sodium. The loop diuretics can block virtually all reabsorption at this site; this, coupled with the relatively small amounts of sodium that can be claimed at more distal nephron sites, allows these agents to cause excretion of up to 20 percent of the sodium filtered at the glomerulus. These drugs therefore cause a vigorous diuresis and should not be used when other, less active diuretics suffice.

Many patients, particularly those with severe heart failure, severe cirrhosis, nephrotic syndrome, and renal insufficiency, require loop diuretics to control edema. If creatinine clearance is less than about 40 ml/min, other diuretics, as single agents, are unlikely to be clinically effective, and loop diuretics will almost always be required. Patients may require large doses of these drugs, but their efficacy demands that small doses be tried first, followed by upward titration according to clinical response. Thus, 40 mg of furosemide or the equivalent dose of another agent is given first. If inadequate, the dose can be sequentially doubled until there is a response or a maximum dose is reached. The maximum single dose that should be tried differs for different clinical conditions (Table 38.3). The ceiling doses described in Table 38.4 are derived from studies in these diseases, showing that nothing is to be gained and that toxicity may occur if larger doses are used.[28]

Once an effective dose is found, the frequency of administration is determined individually and depends on the sodium excretion needed relative to the effectiveness of the drug and the amount of sodium restriction the patient will accept. For example, if the goal is to cause a net loss of 200 mEq of sodium and each dose of diuretic causes 100 mEq to be excreted, twice-daily dosing would be sufficient if the patient ingested no sodium. If the patient ingests 200 mEq of sodium, then dosing four times a day will be necessary. Unfortunately, noncompliance to sodium restriction is exceedingly common, mandating more frequent dosing of these diuretics than would otherwise be necessary.

Lastly, it should be emphasized that response to

loop diuretics is highly variable among patients, and most have less response than do healthy subjects. The mechanisms for this variable and blunted response are not understood. Clinically, one must tailor therapy with these drugs based on individual patient response.

As mentioned previously with osmotic diuretics, in animal models loop diuretics are effective in preventing renal damage from a number of different insults.[13–15] Again, there is little or no clinical evidence to support efficacy over and above adequate hydration. Large doses of loop diuretics have been tried in patients with acute renal failure (e.g., one or more grams of furosemide) with no evidence for a salutary effect.

Loop diuretics also are used to treat hypertension. Several studies demonstrate greater efficacy of thiazides compared to furosemide in mild hypertension, owing to their ability to decrease peripheral vascular resistance as well as produce diuresis.[29,30] On the other hand, low doses of torsemide have proved to be an effective antihypertensive with minimal or no diuretic effect.

Other renal effects of loop diuretics are used in treating hypercalcemia, hyponatremia, and occasionally renal tubular acidosis. The major site of calcium reabsorption is the thick ascending limb of the loop of Henle. Thus, by inhibiting solute reabsorption at this segment of the nephron, loop diuretics increase calcium excretion and are effective adjunctive therapy of hypercalcemia. Most patients with hypercalcemia are volume-depleted, so the first step of therapy is volume replacement with saline. The saline diuresis in and of itself will increase calcium excretion and is sufficient in most patients. If additional therapy is needed, loop diuretics plus replacement of fluid losses to maintain blood volume can be helpful.

Loop diuretics cause excretion of water in excess of sodium. As such, if patients who are hyponatremic have loop diuretic-induced volume losses replaced with iso- or hypertonic saline, there will be a net gain of sodium relative to water, causing the serum sodium concentration to increase.[31] This strategy is currently used only rarely, particularly since too-rapid correction of hyponatremia can be deleterious.

In some patients with distal renal tubular acidosis who are unable to maintain an adequate systemic pH with conventional therapy, loop diuretics will allow excretion of an acid urine and facilitate correction of the metabolic acidosis.

Thiazide Diuretics

Efficacy

Thiazide diuretics block electroneutral NaCl reabsorption at the distal convoluted tubule, connecting tubule, and early collecting duct.[32] These segments are usually collectively referred to as the "distal tubule." Additionally, in sufficient concentrations, all thiazides have inhibitory activity toward carbonic anhydrase, but, in usual doses, any effect at the proximal tubule is negligible.[33] Thiazides cause a NaCl diuresis, and the enhanced distal delivery of Na^+ facilitates potassium secretion, so these drugs can cause potassium depletion. Because the distal tubule reabsorbs only about 5 percent of filtered sodium, the maximal effect of thiazides is much less than that of loop diuretics. However, these drugs are still sufficient in most patients with mild edematous disorders unless they have concomitant renal dysfunction. In such cases, limited filtered sodium and diminished access of thiazides into the tubular lumen compromise efficacy sufficient to require loop diuretics.

The thiazide diuretics have a very shallow dose-response curve (Fig. 38.2). This means that there is little difference between the lowest dose having any effect and the dose having maximal effects. Thus, the starting dose of a thiazide is 12.5 mg of hydrochlorothiazide, or the equivalent of another agent, while the maximal dose is 50 mg. Higher doses result in no greater benefit but increase risks, particularly of potassium depletion and altered glucose and lipoprotein homeostasis.[34,35]

Toxicity

As with other diuretics, much of the toxicity from thiazides is predictable, based on the renal pharmacology of these agents. Thus, the same mechanism that causes decreased urinary calcium excretion causes increased serum calcium concentrations that can mimic hyperparathyroidism. Similarly, impairment in urinary dilution prevents patients who drink large volumes of hypotonic fluids from excreting them. Thus, free water is retained and hyponatremia can occur. In fact, thiazide diuretics are the most common drug-induced cause of hyponatremia.

The mild volume depletion caused by thiazide diuretics results in increased proximal tubular reabsorption with chronic therapy; thus, thiazide administration can affect other cations. The major component of lithium reabsorption occurs at the proximal tubule. Chronic treatment with thiazides increases lithium reabsorption, decreasing its renal excretion and causing accumulation to potentially toxic concentrations.[36] As a consequence, patients concomitantly treated with these drugs should be given lower doses of lithium, and dosing should be guided by measured serum concentrations of lithium.

Thiazide diuretics also cause other adverse effects, the mechanisms of which are poorly understood. They disrupt glucose homeostasis. This usually occurs clinically in a patient with borderline blood glucose control, who, with institution of thiazides, becomes sufficiently hyperglycemic to require oral sulfonylurea hypoglycemic agents. Alternatively, a patient well maintained on oral hypoglycemic agents may deteriorate after administration of thiazides and need insulin. Some have argued that this adverse effect is linked to potassium depletion and can thereby be prevented by maintaining potassium homeostasis. There seems to be little support for this hypothesis.

Pharmacokinetics (Table 38.5)

The disposition of some of the thiazide diuretics has been defined in detail, while that of others has been little studied.[37–41] Extensive clinical experience with this group of drugs has demonstrated their pharmacologic equivalence. Thus, the maximal response to all is the same, and all have shallow dose-response curves (Fig. 38.2). Since their potencies differ, different amounts are needed to achieve the same effect.

The major distinguishing features among these drugs are cost and duration of action. Costs vary among pharmacies, and patients should be given the option of receiving the thiazide that is least expensive for them. In addition to cost, the duration of effect is occasionally a factor in deciding which of these drugs to use. Importantly, duration of effect and elimination half-life are not always linked, and thiazides with short half-lives often have longer durations of action (Table 38.5). The reasons for this discrepancy are unclear. Thiazides are usually grouped according to short (6–12 hr), medium (12–24 hr) and long (>24 hr) durations of effect. It is best to use the short and medium drugs; those with longer duration of effect usually cause more potassium loss.

Therapeutic Uses (Table 38.2)

Thiazide diuretics are the initial choice for most patients with edematous disorders if renal function is not impaired, although not all patients will respond to them. If possible, a therapeutic trial of thiazides should be attempted before utilizing the more efficacious loop diuretics.

The greatest use of thiazide diuretics has been as antihypertensive agents. Initial doses of a thiazide are associated with diuresis-induced decreases in blood volume and a consequent blood pressure lowering effect. This decrease in blood volume, however, triggers homeostatic reflexes such as activating the plasma renin-angiotensin-aldosterone and sympathetic nervous systems, which cause renal sodium retention and restoration of blood volume. The antihypertensive effect, however, is maintained because chronic use of these agents results in diminished peripheral vascular resistance. This effect to lower vascular resistance, the mechanism of which is unknown, has made thiazide diuretics a mainstay of antihypertensive therapy.[42] They are not only effective as single agents in patients with mild hypertension, but also in multiple drug therapy of patients with more severe disease. They are particularly useful for blunting the sodium retention that occurs with vasodilators.

The homeostatic reflexes that restore blood volume when thiazides are used to treat hypertension can be helpful in treating hypercalciuria and diabetes insipidus. Some patients with nephrolithiasis have idiopathically increased urinary calcium excretion. Increased reabsorption of solute, including calcium, proximal to sites at which the thiazides act, plus increased distal reabsorption result in diminished calcium excretion and amelioration of renal stone formation.[44] This effect will also cause slight increases in serum calcium concentration. Thus, while loop diuretics can be used to lower serum calcium, thiazide diuretics can increase it. Importantly, these effects are predictable based on the pharmacology of the drugs and the physiology of calcium homeostasis.

The increased proximal solute reabsorption associated with chronic thiazide use is also accompanied by increased water reabsorption. In addition, the distal site at which thiazides act is also responsible for generating a dilute urine. As a consequence, thiazide diuretics impair the ability to dilute the urine maximally. Patients with central diabetes insipidus are plagued by a maximally dilute urine, which can result in urine volumes of up to 20 L/day. Use of thiazides in such patients can often diminish urinary output to half its pretreatment value, an effect sufficient to improve the quality of these patients' lives. Thus, a diuretic agent in this setting is actually used to diminish urinary volume, a seemingly paradoxical effect that makes sense once knowledge of the site of action and pharmacology of the drug is coupled with the pathophysiology of diabetes insipidus.

Potassium-Retaining Diuretics

Efficacy

In the distal nephron and collecting duct, sodium undergoes exchange with K^+ and H^+. This process depends on luminal entry into the cell of Na^+, a pathway blocked by amiloride and triamterene. Exchange of sodium for K^+ and H^+ is also stimulated by aldosterone. There are receptors for aldosterone in the cytoplasm of cells in this part of the nephron. Their interaction with aldosterone results in translocation of the hormone-receptor complex to the nucleus of the cell, where protein synthesis, presumably of Na^+ pumps, is stimulated. This entire sequence of events can be blocked by spironolactone, which blocks the receptor for aldosterone.

Thus, there are two different mechanisms by which this class of drugs blocks Na^+ reabsorption. That for amiloride and triamterene is independent of aldosterone, while that for spironolactone requires the presence of mineralocorticoid.[45,46] This latter mechanism of action is the rationale for specifically using spironolactone in patients with primary or secondary hyperaldosteronism. It should be apparent that the dose of spironolactone needed will depend on the endogenous level of mineralocorticoid in each individual patient. Thus, each patient must undergo titration until an effective dose is reached. Since the mechanism of action involves blockade of protein synthesis, the duration of effect of spironolactone is one or more days, and plateau effects are not reached until after three or four days of therapy. Therefore, in titrating patients, doses should not be increased more frequently than every three or four days.

The actions of amiloride and triamterene stand in contrast to spironolactone. They are effective in the absence of mineralocorticoid and additionally are shorter-acting, making dosage adjustments possible on a daily basis if necessary. These agents are preferable to spironolactone when a potassium-retaining diuretic is needed in a patient without mineralocorticoid excess.

Since only a small amount of sodium is reabsorbed at the site of action of these agents, they are not sufficiently effective to be of benefit in most patients (excluding mineralocorticoid excess). Their use, then, is to correct potassium and/or magnesium deficiency. The mechanism by which these drugs diminish magnesium excretion has not been fully elucidated.

Toxicity

Use of potassium-retaining diuretics predictably entails a risk of hyperkalemia, which can be life-threatening. Studies in large numbers of patients show this effect occurs in about 5 percent of patients treated prophylactically. Because hyperkalemia has a potentially lethal effect and because hypokalemia is both uncommon and relatively benign, prophylactic use of these drugs cannot be justified.

Other settings increase the risk of hyperkalemia with these agents. Coadministration of potassium supplements is obvious. Angiotensin converting enzyme inhibitors also can cause hyperkalemia and their combination with potassium-retaining diuretics is likely additive. Lastly, patients with renal insufficiency have diminished ability to eliminate potassium; these diuretics are particularly risky in such patients and should be avoided.

Blockade of H^+ exchange for Na^+ by these drugs causes a mild form of renal tubular acidosis called Type IV. Patients may have an acid urine, but they are unable to acidify maximally. They characteristically demonstrate a hyperchloremic metabolic acidosis with hyperkalemia. Patients with mild renal insufficiency or with diabetes mellitus may be particularly susceptible.

Other adverse effects of potassium-retaining diuretics are not extensions of their pharmacologic effects. Rarely, the metabolite of triamterene can precipitate in concentrated urine and serve as a nidus for stone formation. High doses of spironolactone have antiandrogenic effects and can cause gynecomastia. This occurs only rarely at conventional doses.

Pharmacokinetics (Table 38.5)

Triamterene has a short half-life and duration of effect. Thus, it needs to be dosed multiple times per day.[47] Triamterene itself is not active, and it must be converted to its active metabolite by the liver. This process can be impaired in patients with liver disease, making this drug ineffective in such patients.[48] Other drugs in this group should be selected for patients with liver disease. Triamterene, as well as amiloride and spironolactone, should be avoided in patients with renal insufficiency because of the increased risk of hyperkalemia.[49]

Though spironolactone has a short half-life, it appears that activity resides mainly in several metabolites with half-lives of about 15 hour.[50] In addition, the duration of effect is even longer (several days). Spironolactone exerts its effects through interference with protein synthesis. Because of this, peak effects do not occur until three or four days of dosing, if not longer.

Amiloride has a long half-life but the duration of effect is actually less than that of spironolactone since it parallels the kinetic half-life.[51] In patients with liver disease in whom an alternative to spironolactone is sought, amiloride is preferred over triamterene since it does not require metabolic activation. Amiloride can be administered twice a day, and steady state effects occur in two days.

Therapeutic Uses (Table 38.2)

Potassium-retaining diuretics are most frequently used in combination preparations with thiazide diuretics. The rationale for these preparations is that the thiazide component causes renal potassium and magnesium losses, whereas the potassium-retaining agents have the opposite effect. Hence, the combination is presumed to have a neutral effect on potassium and magnesium excretion while maintaining the effects needed to lower blood pressure. This rationale for combination products is, however, flawed.[52,53] First, only about 5 percent of patients receiving thiazide diuretics alone become potassium-depleted. Thus, the remaining 95 percent of patients do not need therapy with potassium-retaining diuretics. Second, potassium-retaining diuretics entail a risk of hyperkalemia, which may be more threatening than potassium depletion. This fact again argues against prophylactic use. Third, patients with a legitimate need for potassium-retaining diuretics often require amounts not available in fixed combination preparations. Thus, when used, these drugs should be individually titrated.

The most rational approach for use of these drugs to maintain potassium and magnesium homeostasis is to restrict them to patients who have become hypokalemic or hypomagnesemic. In these patients, potassium-retaining diuretics appear to be more effective at attaining and maintaining homeostasis of these cations than is exogenous replacement with supplements.

Although potassium-retaining diuretics are occasionally used in edematous disorders and in hypertension, their weak diuretic effects are insufficient to make them useful as single agents. In patients with excess aldosterone, the specific receptor antagonist, spironolactone, is the drug of choice. Such patients include those with mineralocorticoid tumors or adrenal hyperplasia (primary) or those with renal artery stenosis and cirrhosis (secondary). Its use requires titration to an individual dose sufficient to block endogenous levels of aldosterone for each patient.

Overall, then, spironolactone is best used in patients with excessive mineralocorticoid effects. The most common clinical setting is the patient with cirrhosis and fluid retention. Spironolactone, amiloride, or triamterene can be used in those who cannot maintain potassium or magnesium homeostasis. The long duration of action of spironolactone makes it more difficult to use in this setting, and the other two agents should be used as individual agents rather than in fixed combination with thiazides.

Combinations of Diuretics

The use of potassium-retaining diuretics combined with other diuretics that cause potassium and magnesium losses was discussed above.

Other diuretic combinations are used to obtain additive or even synergistic effects in patients who respond poorly to single agents. Such patients usually have severe disease, e.g., end-stage heart failure, severe renal insufficiency, severe cirrhosis with persistent ascites, etc. They have received maximal doses of loop diuretics, yet sodium excretion is inadequate. By blocking additional sites in the nephron, a greater response can many times be achieved.[54–47]

The most useful combination of agents for this purpose is that of a loop plus a thiazide diuretic. Response to a loop diuretic alone can be blunted considerably by increased reabsorption of sodium at sites distal to the thick ascending limb. In fact, chronic dosing of a loop diuretic causes hypertrophy of distal tubule cells with an enhanced capacity to reabsorb sodium.[58–60] Blocking reclamation of sodium at these distal sites with thiazide diuretics often increases response to a clinically important degree, and can occasionally result in a pronounced diuresis in patients with minimal or no response to a loop diuretic alone. Patients should be monitored carefully for volume and potassium status when such combinations are used.

Some patients, particularly those with severe heart failure, have increased proximal tubular reabsorption of sodium, which blunts response to more distally acting agents. Addition of an agent with proximal effects such as acetazolamide can be an helpful adjunct to therapy in some patients. It is best to try combinations of thiazides and loop diuretics first and reserve addition of acetazolamide for those still unresponsive patients. Fortunately, such patients are encountered only rarely.

Preparations and Doses

Preparations and doses of diuretics are presented in Table 38.6.

Summary

Diuretics are effective for edematous disorders and hypertension, and, for the most part, adverse effects are an extension of their pharmacology. All except spironolactone must reach the urine before sodium reabsorption is inhibited. Mannitol gains access by filtration at the glomerulus; acetazolamide, loop diuretics, and thiazides are actively secreted by the organic acid transport pump. Amiloride and triamterene are similarly secreted, but by the organic base pump.

Diuretics encompass a range of efficacy, with loop diuretics being the most effective and potassium-retaining diuretics the least. Loop diuretics can cause excretion of about 20 percent of filtered sodium, and they retain their effectiveness in all but the most severe disease states.

Acetazolamide inhibits carbonic anhydrase and blocks sodium reabsorption at the proximal tubule. It

Table 38.6 Diuretic Preparations and Doses

	Formulation	Available Doses (mg)	Clinical Doses (mg/d)
Carbonic Anhydrase Inhibitor Acetazolamide	Tablet	125, 250	250–1000
	Sustained Release	500	
	Injection	500	
Osmotic Diuretic			
Mannitol	Injection	5–25%	50–200 g/d
Loop Diuretics			
Bumetanide	Tablet	0.5, 1, 2	0.5–10 (See Table 38.4)
	Injection	0.5, 1, 2.5	
Ethacrynic Acid	Tablet	25, 50	50–400 (See Table 38.4)
	Injection	50	
Furosemide	Tablet	20, 40, 80	20–400 (See Table 38.4)
	Solution	10/ml, 40/5 ml	
	Injection	20, 40, 50, 60, 80, 100, 120	
Torsemide	Not yet available		
Thiazide Diuretics			
Bendroflumethiazide	Tablet	5, 10	5–20
Benzthiazide	Tablet	50	50–200
Chlorthalidone	Tablet	25, 50, 100	50–200
Chlorothiazide	Tablet	250, 500	500–2000
	Suspension	250/5 ml	
	Injection	500	
Cyclothiazide	Tablet	2	1–2
Hydrochlorothiazide	Tablet	25, 50, 100	25–200
	Solution	50/5 ml, 100/ml	
Hydroflumethiazide	Tablet	50	25–200
Indapamide	Tablet	2.5	2.5–5
Methyclothiazide	Tablet	2.5, 5	2.5–10
Metolazone	Tablet	0.5, 2.5, 5, 10	2.5–20
Polythiazide	Tablet	1, 2, 4	1–4
Quinethazone	Tablet	50	50–100
Trichlormethiazide	Tablet	2, 4	1–4
Potassium-Retaining Diuretics			
Amiloride	Tablet	5	5–20
Spironolactone	Tablet	25, 50, 100	50–400
Triamterene	Capsule	50, 100	100–300

causes a $NaHCO_3$ diuresis. Mannitol inhibits sodium reabsorption in the proximal tubule and also in the thick ascending limb, causing a NaCl diuresis. Loop diuretics block the Na^+ K^+ $2Cl^-$ reabsorptive pump at the thick ascending limb, causing a NaCl diuresis and impairing the ability to concentrate the urine. Thiazide diuretics inhibit electroneutral NaCl reabsorption in the distal tubule, causing a NaCl diuresis and impairing the ability to dilute the urine. These and all diuretics affecting more proximal sites cause K^+ loss concomitant with that of Na^+. In contrast, the more distally acting, potassium-retaining diuretics cause K^+ accumulation. Of these diuretics, amiloride and triamterene are independent of aldosterone, whereas spironolactone is a competitive antagonist of this mineralocorticoid.

Most patients are initially treated with thiazide diuretics because they are effective, moderately potent, and inexpensive. Members of this class of drugs differ only in cost and duration of action. They have shallow dose-response curves, so little dose titration is needed. Patients with renal insufficiency and those not responding to thiazide diuretics are treated with loop diuretics, beginning with small doses and titrating upward according to individual patient needs. Lack of response to ceiling doses of loop diuretics requires combining these and thiazide diuretics. Mannitol is used less as a diuretic per se but as a systemic osmotic agent to treat cerebral edema. Spironolactone is used primarily in patients with liver disease to reverse the secondary hyperaldosteronism associated with this disorder. Amiloride and triamterene are used for patients who become potassium-depleted from other, more proximally acting diuretics.

Knowledge of the pharmacology of diuretics coupled with the physiology of the nephron allows rational and predictable use of this useful group of agents.

References

Research Reports

1. Odlind B. Renal tubular secretion and effects of the alkaline diuretics amiloride, tizolemide (Hoe 740) and 2-aminomethyl-4-(1,1-dimethylethyl)-6-Iodophenol hydrochloride (MK-447). Arch Pharmacol 1981;*317*:357–363.
2. Odlind B. Relationship between tubular secretion of furosemide and its saluretic effect. J Pharmacol Exp Ther 1979;*208*:515–521.
3. Odlind B, Beermann B. Renal tubular secretion and effects of furosemide. Clin Pharmacol Ther 1980;*27*:784–790.
4. Chennavasin P, Seiwell R, Brater DC, Liang WMM. Pharmacodynamic analysis of the furosemide-probenecid interaction in man. Kidney Int 1979;*16*:187–195.
5. Rector FC. Sodium, bicarbonate, and chloride absorption by the proximal tubule. Am J Physiol 1983;*244*:F461–471.
6. Wallace SM, Shah VP, Riegelman S. GLC analysis of acetazolamide in blood, plasma, and saliva following oral administration to normal subjects. J Pharm Sci 1977;*66*:527–530.
7. Maren TH. Carbonic anhydrase inhibition. IX. Augmentation of the renal effect of meralluride by acetazolamide. J Pharmacol Exp Ther 1958;*123*:311–315.
8. Milledge JS. Acute mountain sickness. Thorax 1983;*38*:641–645.
9. Gennari FJ, Kassirer JP. Osmotic diuresis. N Engl J Med 1974;*291*:714–719.
10. Warren SE, Blantz RC. Mannitol. Arch Intern Med 1981;*141*:493–497.
11. Borges HF, Hocks J, Kjellstrand CM. Mannitol intoxication in patients with renal failure. Arch Intern Med 1982;*142*:63–66.
12. Cloyd JC, Snyder BD, Cleeremans B, Bundlie SR. Mannitol pharmacokinetics and serum osmolality in dogs and humans. J Pharmacol Exp Ther 1986;*236*:301–306.
13. Brezis M, Rosen S, Silva P, Epstein FH. Selective vulnerability of the medullary thick ascending limb to anoxia in the isolated perfused rat kidney. J Clin Invest 1984;*73*:182–190.
14. Brezis M, Rosen S, Spokes K, Silva P, Epstein FH. Transport-dependent anoxia cell injury in the isolated perfused rat kidney. Am J Pathol 1984;*116*:327–341.
15. Hays SR. Ischemic acute renal failure. Am J Med Sci 1992;*304*:93–108.
16. Goldberg M, McCurdy DK, Foltz EL, Bluemle LW. Effects of ethacrynic acid (a new saluretic agent) on renal diluting and concentrating mechanisms: Evidence for site of action in the loop of Henle. J Clin Invest 1964;*43*:201–216.
17. Dikshit K, Vyden JK, Forrester JS, Chatterjee K, Prakash R, Swan HJC. Renal and extrarenal hemodynamic effects of furosemide in congestive heart failure after acute myocardial infarction. N Engl J Med 1973;*208*:1087–1090.
18. Cooperman LB, Rubin IL. Toxicity of ethacrynic acid and furosemide. Am Heart J 1973;*85*:831–834.
19. Gallagher KL, Jones JK. Furosemide-induced ototoxicity. Ann Intern Med 1979;*91*:744–745.
20. Beermann B, Dalen E, Lindstrom B: Elimination of furosemide in healthy subjects and in those with renal failure. Clin Pharmacol Ther 1977;*22*:70–78.
21. Brater DC, Chennavasin P, Day B, Burdette A, Anderson S: Bumetanide and furosemide. Clin Pharmacol Ther 1983;*34*:207–213.
22. Cannon PJ, Heinemann HO, Stason WB, Laragh JH: Ethacrynic acid: Effectiveness and mode of diuretic action in man. Circulation 1965;*31*:5–18.
23. Cook JA, Smith DE, Cornish LA, Tankanow RM, Nicklas JM, Hyneck ML: Kinetics, dynamics, and bioavailability of bumetanide in healthy subjects and patients with congestive heart failure. Clin Pharmacol Ther 1988;*44*:487–500.
24. Hammarlund-Udenaes M, Benet LZ: Furosemide pharmacokinetics and pharmacodynamics in health and disease—an update. J Pharmacokinet Biopharm 1989;*17*:1–46.
25. Kim KE, Onesti G, Moyer JH, Swartz C: Ethacrynic acid and furosemide: Diuretic and hemodynamic effects and clinical uses. Am J Cardiol 1971;*27*:407–415.
26. Marcantonio LA, Auld WHR, Skellern GG, Howes CA, Murdoch WR, Purohit R: The pharmacokinetics and pharmacodynamics of bumetanide in normal subjects. J Pharmacokinet Biopharm 1982;*10*:393–409.
27. Brater DC, Leinfelder J, Anderson SA. Clinical pharmacology of torasemide, a new loop diuretic. Clin Pharmacol Ther 1987;*42*:187–192.
28. Voelker JR, Brown-Cartwright D, Anderson S, Leinfelder J, Sica DA, Kokko JP, Brater DC. Comparison of loop diuretics in patients with chronic renal insufficiency: Mechanism of difference in response. Kidney Int 1987;*32*:572–578.
29. Araoye MA, Chang MY, Khatri IM, Freis ED. Furosemide compared with hydrochlorothiazide: Long-term treatment of hypertension. JAMA 1978;*240*:1863–1866.
30. Holland OB, Gomez-Sanchez, CE, Kuhnert L, Poindexter C, Pak CYC. Antihypertensive comparison of furosemide with hydrochlorothiazide for black patients. Arch Intern Med 1979;*139*:1015–1021.
31. Schrier RW, Lehman D, Zacherle B, Earley LE. Effect of furosemide on free water excretion in edematous patients with hyponatremia. Kidney Int 1973;*3*:30–34.
32. Stokes JB: Electroneutral NaCI transport in the distal tubule. Kidney Int 1989;*36*:427–433.
33. Kunau RT, Weller DR, Webb HL: Clarification of the site of action of chlorothiazide in rat nephron. J Clin Invest 1975;*56*:401–407.
34. McVeigh G, Galloway D, Johnston D. The case for low dose diuretics in hypertension: Comparison of low and conventional doses of cyclopenthiazide. Br Med J 1988;*297*:95–98.
35. Carlsen JE, Kober L, Torp-Pederson C, Johansen P. Relation between dose of bendrofluazide, antihypertensive effect, and adverse biochemical effects. Br Med J 1990;*300*:975–978.
36. Jefferson JW, Kalin NH. Serum lithium levels and long-term diuretic use. JAMA 1979;*241*:1134–1136.
37. Beermann B, Groschinsky-Grind M: Pharmacokinetics of hydrochlorothiazide in patients with congestive heart failure. Br J Clin Pharmacol 1979;*7*:579–583.
38. Beermann B, Groschinsky-Grind M, Lindstrom B, Wikland B: Pharmacokinetics of bendroflumethiazide in hypertensive patients. Eur J Clin Pharmacol 1978;*13*:119–124.

39. Fleuren HLJ, Wissen CV, van Rossum JM: Dose-dependent urinary excretion of chlorthalidone. Clin Pharmacol Ther 1979;*25*:806–812.

40. Hobbs DC, Twomey TM: Kinetics of polythiazide. Clin Pharmacol Ther 1978;*23*:241–246.

41. Sketris IS, Skoutakis VA, Acchiardo SR, Meyer MC: The pharmacokinetics of trichlormethiazide in hypertensive patients with normal and compromised renal function. Eur J Clin Pharmacol 1981;*20*:453–457.

42. Welling PG. Pharmacokinetics of the thiazide diuretics. Biopharm Drug Disp 1986;*7*:501–535.

43. de Carvalho JGR, Dunn FG, Lohmöller G, Frohlich ED. Hemodynamic correlates of prolonged thiazide therapy: Comparison of responders and nonresponders. Clin Pharmacol Ther 1977;*22*:875–880.

44. Breslau N, Moses AM, Weiner IM. The role of volume contraction in the hypocalciuric action of chlorothiazide. Kidney Int 1976;*10*:164–170.

45. Frelin C, Vigne P, Barbry P, Lazdunski M: Molecular properties of amiloride action and of its Na^+ transporting targets. Kidney Int 1987;*32*:785–793.

46. Ochs HR, Greenblatt DJ, Bodem G, Smith TW: Spironolactone. Am Heart J 1978;*96*:389–400.

47. Gilfrich HJ, Kremer G, Mohrke W, Mutschler E, Volger KD: Pharmacokinetics of triamterene after i.v. administration to man: Determination of bioavailability. Eur J Clin Pharmacol 1983;*25*:237–241.

48. Villeneuve JP, Rocheleau F, Raymond G: Triamterene kinetics and dynamics in cirrhosis. Clin Pharmacol Ther 1984;*35*:831–837.

49. Knauf H, Mohrke W, Mutschler E: Delayed elimination of triamterene and its active metabolite in chronic renal failure. Eur J Clin Pharmacol 1983;*24*:453–456.

50. Gardiner P, Schrode K, Quinlan D, Martin B, Boreham DR, Rogers MS, Stubbs K, Smith M, Karim A: Spironolactone metabolism: Steady-state serum levels of the sulfur-containing metabolites. J Clin Pharmacol 1989;*29*:342–347.

51. Spahn H, Reuter K, Mutschler E, Gerok W, Knauf H: Pharmacokinetics of amiloride in renal and hepatic diseases. Eur J Clin Pharmacol 1987;*33*:493–498.

52. Tannen RL. Diuretic-induced hypokalemia. Kidney Int 1985;*28*:988–1000.

53. Kassirer JP, Harrington JT. Diuretics and potassium metabolism: A reassessment of the need, effectiveness and safety of potassium therapy. Kidney Int 1977;*11*:505–515.

54. Epstein M, Lepp BA, Hoffman DS, Levinson R: Potentiation of furosemide by metolazone in refractory edema. Curr Ther Res 1977;*21*:656–667.

55. Ram CVS, Reichgott MJ: Treatment of loop-diuretic resistant edema by the addition of metolazone. Curr Ther Res 1977;*22*:686–691.

56. Sigurd B, Olesen KH, Wennevold A: The supra-additive natriuretic effect addition of bendroflumethiazide and bumetanide in congestive heart failure. Am Heart J 1975;*89*:163–170.

57. Wollam GL, Tarazi RC, Bravo EL, Dustan HP: Diuretic potency of combined hydrochlorothiazide and furosemide therapy in patients with azotemia. Am J Med 1982;*72*:929–938.

58. Ellison DH, Velazquez H, Wright FS: Adaptation of the distal convoluted tubule of the rat. J Clin Invest 1989;*83*:113–126.

59. Kaissling B, Stanton BA: Adaptation of distal tubule and collecting duct to increased sodium delivery. I. Ultrastructure. Am J Physiol 1988;*255*:F1256–1268.

60. Stanton BA, Kaissling B: Adaptation of distal tubule and collecting duct to increased Na delivery. II. Na^+ and K^+ transport. Am J Physiol 1988;*255*:F1269–1275.

Reviews

r1. Beermann B, Groschinsky-Grind M. Clinical pharmacokinetics of diuretics. Clin Pharmacokinet 1980;*5*:221–245.
This review is a detailed assessment and compilation of pharmacokinetic data for all diuretics.

r2. Brater DC. Clinical pharmacology of loop diuretics. Drugs 1991;*41*(Suppl 3):14–22.
This review discusses the pathophysiology of resistance to loop diuretics and how to overcome it.

r3. Frazier HS, Yager H. The clinical use of diuretics. N Engl J Med 1973;*288*:246–249 and 455–457.
This is a comprehensive review of the pharmacology and clinical pharmacology of diuretics.

r4. Martinez-Maldonado M, Eknoyan G, Suki WN. Diuretics in nonedematous states. Physiological basis for the clinical use. Arch Intern Med 1973;*131*:797–808.
This review describes use of diuretics for nondiuretic indications, such as for disorders of calcium homeostasis and diabetes insipidus. The efficacy of diuretics in these settings is explained based on the pharmacology of the drugs and renal physiology.

r5. Seely JF, Dirks JH. Site of action of diuretic drugs. Kidney Int 1977;*11*:1–8.
This review discusses the sites and mechanisms of action of diuretics.

r6. Shear L, Ching S, Gabuzda GJ. Compartmentalization of ascites and edema in patients with hepatic cirrhosis. N Engl J Med 1970;*282*:1391–1396.
This classic study defines rates at which fluid can be mobilized in patients. It therefore provides guidelines as to aggressiveness of diuretic therapy.

r7. Tucker RM, Vandenberg CJ, Knox FG. Diuretics: Role of sodium balance. Mayo Clin Proc 1980;*55*:261–266.
This review discusses the importance of sodium balance relative to efficacy of diuretics and in turn, the need to modify the intake of sodium by patients.

r8. Rose BD. Diuretics. Kidney Int 1991;*39*:336–352.
This paper is a physiologically-based review of the clinical use of diuretics.

r9. Martinez-Maldonado M, Cordova HR. Cellular and molecular aspects of the renal effects of diuretic agents. Kidney Int 1990;*38*:632–641.
A recent, detailed review of the mechanisms of diuretic action.

r10. Gines P, Arroyo V, Rodes J. Pharmacotherapy of ascites associated with cirrhosis. Drugs 1992;*43*:316–332.
A comprehensive review of the treatment of ascites.

CHAPTER 39

Antidiuretic Hormones, Synthetic Analogues, and Related Drugs

Larry A. Walker

Antidiuretic hormone (ADH) is the peptide hormone of the posterior pituitary that serves to promote renal water conservation. In most mammals, including humans, the antidiuretic hormone is 8-arginine vasopressin (AVP). This hormone also has significant pressor activity, as its name implies, and has been used for that purpose; but such use is rarely justified. The principal use of ADH and antidiuretic analogues in medicine is for replacement therapy in disorders in which there is a deficient synthesis or release of the endogenous hormone, i.e., in hypothalamic diabetes insipidus. They are also used for diagnostic purposes in distinguishing between certain types of polyuric disorders. An analogue (desmopressin) is used under some conditions in von Willebrand's disease and some types of hemophilia to increase the levels of coagulation factors.

Table 39.1

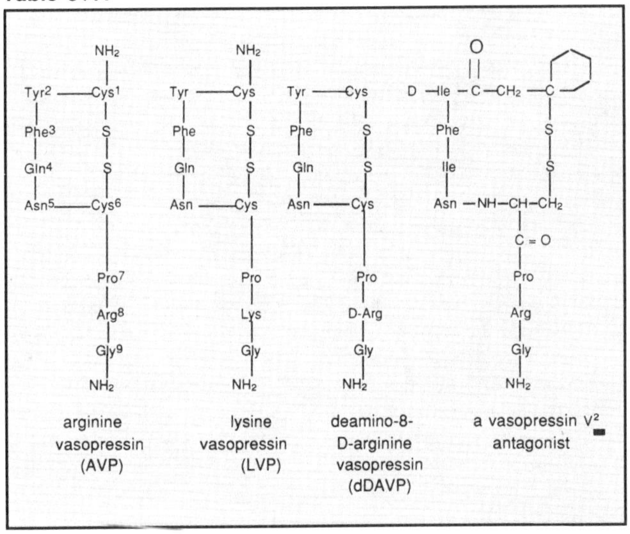

NH_2	NH_2		O ‖
Tyr^2 — Cys^1	Tyr — Cys	Tyr — Cys	D — Ile — C — CH_2 — C
Phe^3 S	Phe S	Phe S	Phe S
Gln^4 S	Gln S	Gln S	Ile S
Asn^5 — Cys^6	Asn — Cys	Asn — Cys	Asn — NH — CH — CH_2
			C = O
Pro^7	Pro	Pro	Pro
Arg^8	Lys	D-Arg	Arg
Gly^9	Gly	Gly	Gly
NH_2	NH_2	NH_2	NH_2
arginine vasopressin (AVP)	lysine vasopressin (LVP)	deamino-8-D-arginine vasopressin (dDAVP)	a vasopressin V^2 antagonist

Chemistry

AVP was chemically characterized and synthesized by Vincent duVigneaud and colleagues in the early 1950s.[1] Structurally, it is a nonapeptide in which the cysteine residues of positions 1 and 6 are linked by a disulfide bridge (thus forming a single amino acid, cystine). This linkage forms a cyclic moiety, with the amino acids in positions 7–9 extended from this ring (Table 39.1). Lysine vasopressin (LVP) is the peptide found in swine, and differs from AVP only in the substitution of lysine for arginine in position 8. Oxytocin also belongs to this family of peptides, differing from AVP in the substitution of isoleucine for phenylalanine at position 3 and leucine for arginine at position 8. Oxytocin shares antidiuretic and pressor activities with AVP, but is much less potent (approximately 1/100). LVP is only slightly less potent than AVP as regards antidiuretic action (depending on the species used for testing), and it retains substantial pressor activity. Scores of analogues of these hormones have been synthesized and evaluated for antidiuretic, vasopressor, and oxytocic activities. The structure-activity relationships are complex, but, in general, a basic amino acid (Arg or Lys) in position 8 is required for antidiuretic potency. An intact ring system has been shown to be essential for optimum biologic actions of the peptide. Changing the configuration of the amino acid at position 8 from the naturally occurring L-form to the D-form results in a drastic reduction in pressor activity, but retains antidiuretic potency. Deamination of the cysteine at position 1 yields a peptide that is resistant to degradation by peptidases; it also appears to confer some specificity of antidiuretic action. The combination of the latter two structural changes by Zaoral and coworkers in 1967 yielded 1-deamino-8-D-arginine vasopressin (desmopressin), a peptide with a long duration of action, excellent antidiuretic potency, and markedly reduced pressor activity.[2] This compound has proved to be therapeutically useful for treatment of hypothalamic diabetes insipidus. Substitution of amino acids with lipophilic side-chains (e.g., valine) at position 4 also generally results in decreased pressor activity and enhanced antidiuretic potency.[3]

As might be expected from the disassociation of antidiuretic and pressor activities, it has been demonstrated that there are at least two distinct subtypes of vasopressin receptors: V_1, found in vascular smooth muscle, liver, and several other tissues; and V_2, in renal tubular epithelium and perhaps in other cell types. The kidney also contains V_1 receptors, but their function remains obscure.

History

While pressor and uterotonic activities were described in extracts of the posterior pituitary gland as early as 1895, it was several years later that antidiuretic effects were uncovered. In 1913, it was demonstrated that posterior pituitary extracts could be used to treat diabetes insipidus. Although the identity of the antidiuretic principle was not established until the 1950s, many investigators studied the synthesis and release of the hormone. It had been generally regarded that ADH was synthesized in the cells of the posterior pituitary. However, it was demonstrated in the 1930s that experimental production of a permanent diabetes insipidus in animals could be accomplished by bilateral hypothalamic lesions that resulted in degeneration of the posterior pituitary. These studies, along with the work of anatomists, provided the basis for the hypothesis that the antidiuretic principle was actually synthesized in the hypothalamus and transported in neurosecretory granules to the posterior pituitary (see historical review by Share).

In 1937, Gilman and Goodman first demonstrated that dehydration or injections of hypertonic saline increased the excretion of antidiuretic activity in the urine of rats.[4] Chambers and coworkers suggested in 1945 that changes in osmotic pressure of the ECF rather than any specific solute determined the release of ADH from the pituitary.[5] Verney's classic experiments, reported in 1947,[6] demonstrated that intracarotid injection of hypertonic solutions in conscious dogs produced an antidiuresis that was comparable to that produced by injection of posterior pituitary extract. Verney suggested that since the intracarotid injections were much more effective than similar injections into the peripheral circulation, the osmotically sensitive cells were located in the brain.

After several decades of intense study, duVigneaud and colleagues were successful in isolating and purifying the antidiuretic and oxytocic principles of the neurohypophysis sufficiently to allow elucidation of the structures, which they then confirmed by total synthesis.[1] This was a landmark accomplishment because it demonstrated for the first time that relatively large biologically active peptides could be synthesized. It also provided the groundwork for subsequent investigations of structure-activity relationships, culminating in the first widely useful synthetic hormone analogue (desmopressin).

Biosynthesis and Release of ADH

The anatomic relationship between the hypothalamus and the neurohypophysis (posterior pituitary) is depicted schematically in Figure 39.1. Cell bodies located in the supraoptic nuclei (above the optic chiasm) and paraventricular nuclei (just lateral to the anterior third ventricle) send axonal projections along the hypothalamo-neurohypophysial tract. These axons terminate on capillary networks in the neurohypophysis. AVP and oxytocin are synthesized in the cell bodies of the supraoptic and paraventricular nuclei. Each peptide is synthesized as part of a large prohormone of approximately 20,000 Daltons. The precursor of AVP consists of a glycopeptide, a large binding protein termed neurophysin, and AVP. The prohormone is packaged into neurosecretory granules in the perikarya of the hypothalamic nuclei, then transported along axons of the hypothalamo-neurohypophysial tract. During transport, the components are cleaved by enzymatic action, and AVP (or oxytocin) is stored bound to its respective neurophysin in secretory granules in the nerve terminals of the neurohypophysis. The peptide and neurophysin are released simultaneously into the circulation in response to neuronal firing, which originates with stimulation of the cell bodies in the hypothalamus. Oxytocin and AVP are contained in two separate populations of vesicles in different neurons, and their release is controlled by different stimuli.

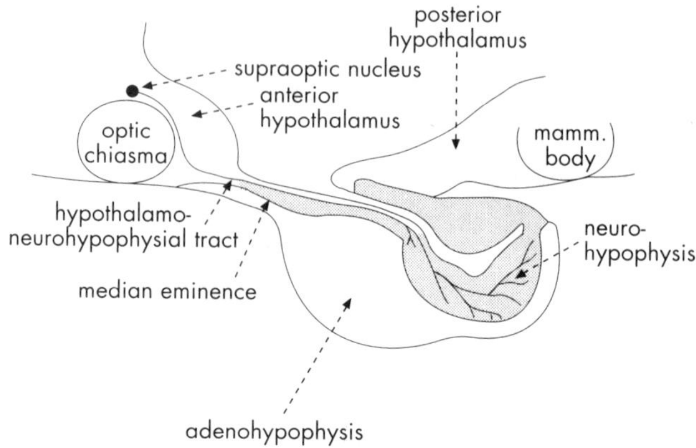

Figure 39.1 Schematic diagram of the hypothalamo-neurohypophysial system showing the axonal projections from the supraoptic nuclei to nerve terminals in the neurohypophysis. Mamm. body = mammillary body

The secretion of ADH is primarily under the control of sensory cells termed "osmoreceptors" in the vicinity of the AVP-synthesizing cell bodies of the supraoptic nuclei. These receptors are stimulated by elevated tonicity (i.e., osmolality) of the surrounding ECF, causing shrinkage of the receptor cell and resulting in activation of the adjacent neurons to release ADH from the nerve terminals in the neurohypophysis. It is conceived that above a certain "osmotic threshold," plasma AVP levels are increased in proportion to the osmolality of plasma[7] (Fig. 39.2). This system is ex-

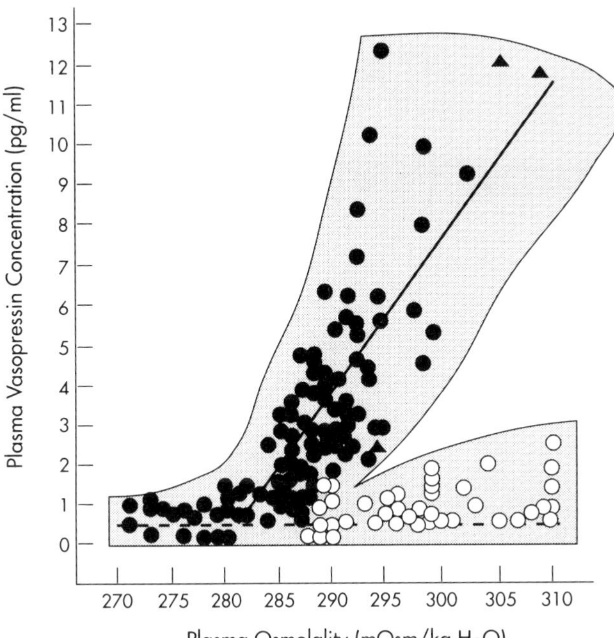

Figure 39.2 The relationship between plasma osmolality and plasma ADH concentration. Above a certain osmotic threshold, plasma levels increase in normal subjects (closed circles). Open circles depict a series of patients with hypothalamic diabetes insipidus who cannot synthesize or release ADH in appropriate amounts. Closed triangles represent patients who have been diagnosed with nephrogenic diabetes insipidus. These patients can release ADH, but the renal response is impaired, and therefore plasma osmolality tends to be elevated, along with levels of ADH. Reproduced from Reference 7, with copyright permission of the American Society of Clinical Investigation.

tremely sensitive in healthy individuals, and a rise in plasma osmolality of as little as 2 per cent can cause a detectable increase in AVP release.

Other stimuli can also affect the release of vasopressin. Volume and pressure-sensitive receptors in the circulation appear to exert a tonic inhibitory influence on secretion of the peptide. There is good evidence that baroreceptors in the carotid sinus and aortic arch, and especially in the left atrium and pulmonary veins,[8] are unloaded by decreases in blood pressure or blood volume, resulting in a decrease in their firing rate and, ultimately, in withdrawal of the tonic inhibition so that ADH release is enhanced. This control system is less sensitive than the osmoreceptor system, but may be critical in conditions of hypovolemia (e.g., during hemorrhage).

Other factors that may enhance ADH release include nausea, hypoglycemia, hypoxia, pain, cold, physical exercise, fever, and some drugs or hormones. In some of these cases, it is unclear whether the effect is direct or mediated by another control system, e.g. changes in blood pressure or distribution of blood volume.

Renal Effects of ADH

The therapeutic utility of ADH and analogues is based primarily on their actions in the kidney to promote conservation of water. In addition to its role in excretion of waste products and maintaining balance of electrolytes and metabolic substrates, the kidney is responsible for regulation of the tonicity of body fluids. Concentration or dilution of ECF is accomplished by the excretion or retention, respectively, of water in excess of solute. The kidney's ability to excrete either hypotonic or hypertonic urine is largely controlled by ADH. An understanding of the renal actions of this hormone will require a comprehension of the principal features of salt and water reabsorption along the nephron. These have been reviewed in Chapter 36 of this section, and are only highlighted here in order to characterize the action of ADH.

In all portions of the mammalian nephron, the movement of water is passive, driven by the active transport of solutes. It was a difficult problem for renal physiologists to conceive of a system that could form hyperosmotic urine in the absence of active water reabsorption. In 1942, two Swiss physical chemists (Kuhn and Ryffel) proposed the countercurrent mechanism for urinary concentration.[9] According to their scheme, the capacity for formation of hypertonic urine was attributable to: (a) the "hairpin" arrangement of the loops of Henle, with tubular fluid moving in opposite directions ("countercurrent") in the two limbs; (b) differential permeability characteristics of the two limbs; and (c) the ability to generate osmotic gradients between the two limbs by separating solute from water reabsorption in the ascending limbs of Henle. This architecture allows small transverse osmotic gradients between the limbs of the loop to be "multiplied" into large longitudinal gradients at the bend. The principal features of this model were verified and expanded by other investigators. The reader is referred to the brief descriptions by Valtin[10] and by Pitts[11] of the operation of the countercurrent system. Roy, Layton, and Jamison[12] have provided a detailed review. A schematic of the renal countercurrent system is presented in Figure 39.3a.

It is helpful to consider first the condition of water diuresis (absence of ADH). Approximately two-thirds of the glomerular filtrate is reabsorbed in an essentially isosmotic fashion by the proximal tubule. As tubular fluid traverses the descending limb of Henle's loop, water is abstracted osmotically into the surrounding interstitial spaces (the hypertonicity of the medullary interstitium is maintained by active transport of sodium and chloride out of the thick ascending limbs and by the sequestration of urea in the inner medulla). Tubular fluid is thus progressively concentrated until it reaches the bend of Henle's loop, where there are marked changes in the permeability and transport characteristics of the nephron. The ascending limb is relatively impermeable to water, while sodium and chloride are reabsorbed by active (thick ascending limb) and perhaps by passive (thin ascending limb) mechanisms. In this fashion, osmolality of tubular fluid is reduced as it ascends toward the cortex. At the beginning of the distal tubule, the fluid is distinctly hypotonic (approximately 100 mOsm/kg H_2O). In the absence of ADH, the distal tubule and collecting duct remain essentially impermeable to water, while small amounts of solute continue to be reabsorbed, so that the urine is maximally dilute, (about 50–75 mOsm/kg H_2O). Under these conditions, 10–12 percent of the filtered water may be excreted.

If in this setting one administers exogenous ADH or stimulates release of the hormone from the pituitary, several changes are effected along the nephron that allow for enhanced reabsorption of water and excretion of hypertonic urine (see Fig. 39.3b):

(1) the membranes of the late distal tubule and the entire collecting duct system have a greatly increased permeability to water, allowing osmotic equilibration of collecting duct fluid with the surrounding interstitium;

(2) the membranes of the terminal portion of the collecting duct are rendered more permeable to urea, allowing (at least in the early stages of antidiuresis) increased deposition of urea in the medullary interstitium;

(3) medullary blood flow is reduced, minimizing the "washout" of medullary solutes from the interstitial space;

(4) reabsorption of sodium and chloride out of the thick ascending limb into the medullary interstitium is enhanced.

These changes result in an enhanced osmotic gradient in the interstitium from cortex to papilla (increasing the driving force for water reabsorption) and also in osmotic equilibration of the collecting duct fluid with the hypertonic interstitial spaces. It is uncertain whether in humans the third and fourth mechanisms play a role, but experimental evidence in animals indicates that all of these effects are integrated to achieve optimum efficiency of the renal concentrating system. The combination of elevated interstitial osmolality and the enhanced water permeability of the distal portion

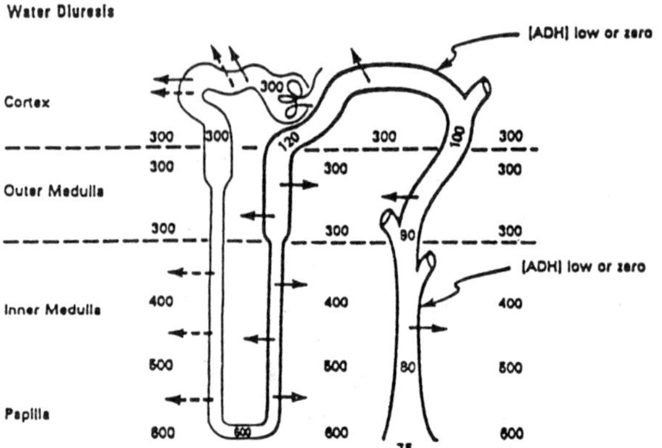

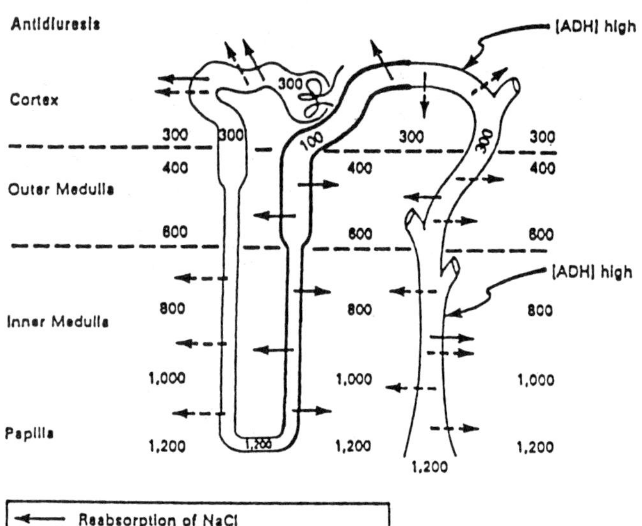

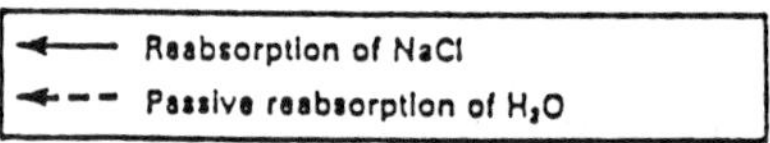

Figure 39.3 Operation of the renal countercurrent system in a normal human. Heavy boundaries indicate very low permeability to water. The numbers refer to osmolality (mOsm/kg H_2O) of either intratubular or interstitial fluid. Solid arrows denote reabsorption of NaCl, which is active except in the thin ascending limbs of Henle, where it may be largely passive; arrows with dashed line denote passive reabsorption of water. A. During water diuresis. B. During antidiuresis. Some important changes from (or 'compared to') water diuresis are (1) the lower interstitial osmolality in the medulla and papilla; (2) the virtual absence of ADH; and hence (3) the lack of osmotic equilibration between fluid in the collecting duct and the surrounding interstitium. Adapted from Reference 10, with permission of Little, Brown & Company.

of the nephron allows the reabsorption of water to be maximized. The highest urinary osmolality attainable in humans is approximately 1200 mOsm/Kg water, but other species, especially rodents, can achieve much higher concentrations.

Cellular Action of ADH

As mentioned above, ADH activates at least two distinct subtypes of receptors. V_1 receptors in many tissues are coupled to hydrolysis of phosphatidylinositol, giving rise to inositol trisphosphate (IP_3) and diacylglycerol (DAG). IP_3, in turn, elevates levels of intracellular calcium. It is by this mechanism that ADH elicits contraction of vascular smooth muscle, and analogous events can occur in the collecting duct, though perhaps only at high concentrations of ADH.[13,14] However, it is now well established that the ADH-elicited increase in water permeability of the distal nephron involves the adenylate cyclase–cyclic AMP system (Fig. 39.4) The hormone binds to and activates V_2 receptors on the peritubular side of the cells of the late distal tubule and collecting duct. The receptor stimulation is translated to activation of the enzyme adenylate cyclase, which catalyzes the conversion of adenosine triphosphate to cyclic AMP. As in other receptor-adenylate cyclase systems, the activation is mediated by a receptor-coupled G-protein, which interacts with the catalytic site.[14a] Cyclic AMP activates specific protein kinases that initiate a series of events that are not completely defined, but result in an increase in the permeability of the luminal membrane to water. The permeability change appears to involve actin microfilaments of the epithelial cells, since under some conditions disruptors of their integrity impair the response.[15] Microfilaments may be instrumental in the insertion of protein particle aggregates into the luminal membrane or in the rearrangement of aggregates within the membrane.[16] These aggregates are contained in cytoplasmic membranous structures that fuse with the apical cell membrane upon stimulation of the cell by ADH. The proteins appear to contain channels that actually allow the passage of water molecules, but exclude solutes. When ADH is withdrawn, these particle aggregates disappear from the membrane.[16,17]

The role of calcium in the cellular events leading to increased water permeability is incompletely understood. However, a persistent increase in intracellular calcium appears to exert an inhibitory effect on the adenylate cyclase response to ADH, and it increases

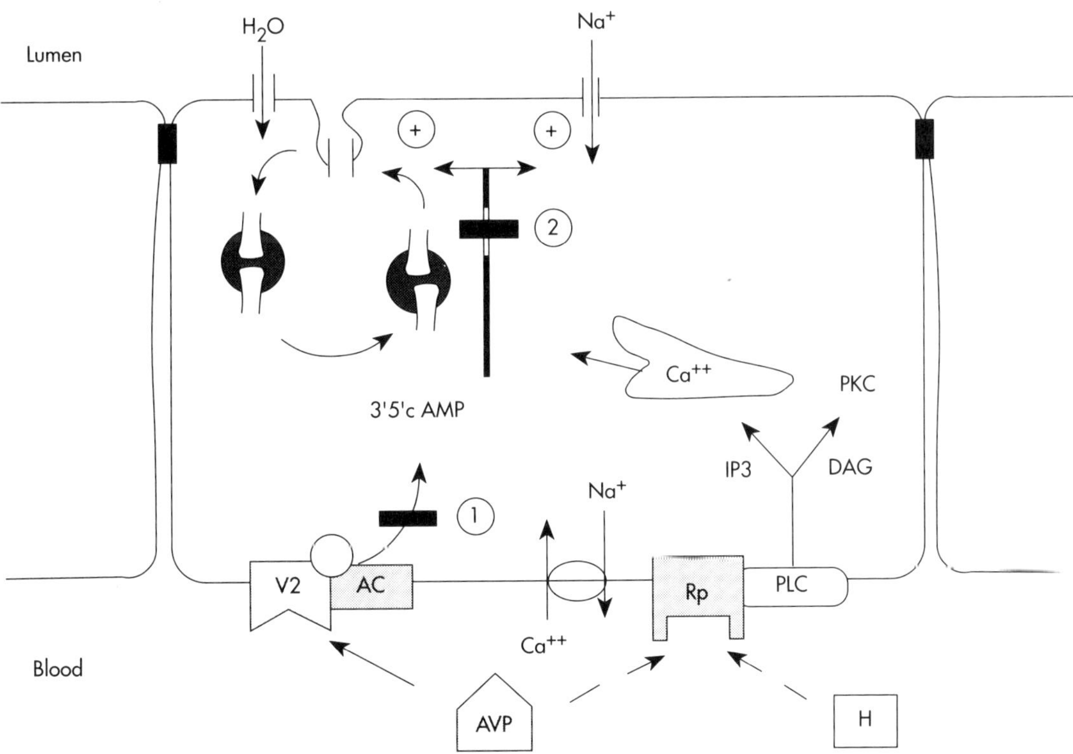

Figure 39.4 Schematic of the principal features of the water permeability response to ADH in a collecting duct cell. The principal mechanism involved is the adenylate cyclase system, which is activated by stimulation of V_2 receptors. The sequence of events between protein kinase activation and the fusion of vesicles containing protein particle aggregates is unclear, but appears to involve microfilamentous elements of the cell. Site 1 depicts effect of agents that inhibit at pre-cAMP level. Site 2 depicts inhibition at post-cAMP level. Vasopressin (AVP) and cAMP also stimulate sodium transport. Basolateral sodium-calcium exchange influences intracellular calcium concentration and sodium transport. AC, adenylate cyclase; DAG, diacylglycerol; H, hormone; IP_3, inositol trisphosphate; PKC, protein kinase C; PLC, phospholipase C; Rp, PLC-coupled receptor; V2, V_2 receptor. Adapted from Reference 14, with permission from the American Journal of Physiology.

breakdown of cyclic AMP by activation of phosphodiesterase;[18] in addition, activation of protein kinase C results in diminution of the effect of cyclic AMP on the hydro-osmotic response.[14] These mechanisms may serve to dampen the maximal effects of AVP or to hasten reversal of the response.

Disorders of Water Metabolism

Diabetes Insipidus

The term "diabetes insipidus" refers to a syndrome in which the patient passes large quantities of very dilute urine. The polyuria of diabetes insipidus is a water diuresis (relatively free of solute) that may result from one of three basic conditions: (1) a complete or partial defect in the synthesis or release of ADH from the hypothalamo-neurohypophysial system (hypothalamic diabetes insipidus); (2) a renal defect in which the response to circulating ADH is impaired (nephrogenic diabetes insipidus); or (3) chronic, excessive ingestion of fluid (primary polydipsia).

Hypothalamic (central) diabetes insipidus may result from several causes. A small fraction of patients have a hereditary disorder in which the synthetic mechanism for the hormone is absent or deficient. Other causes include trauma from accident or surgery, neoplasms, sarcoid or other granulomatous infiltration, and numerous other less common disorders. In addition, some drugs may cause a suppression of ADH release (see below). Since in hypothalamic diabetes insipidus the renal response to the hormone is intact, replacement with ADH or an analogue is the logical therapy. Because of its ease of administration and the relative absence of adverse effects, desmopressin (administered by nasal solution) is the preferred form of therapy in patients who can utilize this route.

As might be expected, in nephrogenic diabetes insipidus, exogenous ADH and analogues are ineffective because of the refractoriness of the kidney to the action of the hormone. This disorder can be hereditary, but it is most commonly encountered as a result of lithium therapy; it can also be caused by some other drugs.

Primary Polydipsia

Primary polydipsia is mentioned here because it is often difficult to distinguish this disorder from partial hypothalamic diabetes insipidus, yet the treatments for these two disorders are very different. Primary polydipsia is often of psychologic origin, and therefore is referred to as "psychogenic polydipsia" or "compulsive water drinking." In these patients, water restriction is the treatment required, and this often necessitates psychiatric evaluation and therapy. Clearly, treatment with vasopressin is contraindicated and could have deleterious results.

Inappropriate ADH Secretion

Inappropriate ADH Secretion (SIADH) is caused by excessive release of ADH, either from the pituitary or from ectopic malignancies (e.g., in bronchogenic carcinoma). Many different types of pulmonary and CNS disorders, as well as various carcinomas, have been associated with SIADH.[19] Chronically elevated levels of the hormone result in failure to dilute the urine maximally and, therefore, in hypoosmotic expansion of the ECF volume. The volume expansion is thought to lead, transiently, to excessive renal excretion of sodium and progressive hyponatremia, perhaps via elevation of levels of atrial natriuretic peptide.[20] The most serious sequelae of this disorder result from the hyponatremia and include neuropsychiatric disturbances, lethargy, disorientation, seizures, and coma.

Therapeutic Uses and Limitations

Diagnosis of Polyuric Disorders

Because of the differential response to ADH in patients with hypothalamic diabetes insipidus compared to the nephrogenic form, administration of AVP or desmopressin is often used diagnostically to distinguish between these two disorders. Following a period of fluid restriction (or infusion of hypertonic saline), patients with subnormal urine concentration receive a test dose of the antidiuretic agent. Patients with hypothalamic diabetes insipidus will respond with a prompt increase in urine osmolality; those with nephrogenic diabetes insipidus show little or no response to the hormone. For details of this test and possible pitfalls, the reader is referred elsewhere.[21,22]

Hypothalamic Diabetes Insipidus

The primary therapeutic use of antidiuretic peptides is in replacement therapy in complete and partial forms of central diabetes insipidus. Aqueous solutions of AVP for injection are available, but are unsuitable for long-term therapy because of short duration of action. For many years, vasopressin tannate in oil was the preferred form of therapy. It is given by IM injection, usually every two or three days. Desmopressin, administered intranasally, is now the drug of choice. In most patients, two doses daily will provide adequate control of polyuria, though the dose required is highly variable and must be individualized.

Nocturnal Enuresis

Desmopressin nasal spray, because of convenience of administration and long duration of action, has found utility in the management of nocturnal enuresis. In many cases, a bedtime dose reduces urine flow sufficiently that the condition can be controlled. Some patients may require adjunctive therapy.

Bleeding Disorders

ADH and desmopressin have both been discovered to have a beneficial action in patients with hemophilia A and in mild to moderate von Willebrand's disease (Type I), a related bleeding disorder.[23] Desmopressin is indicated for therapy in these patients who are about to undergo dental or surgical procedures or in those that need treatment for acute mild bleeding episodes. For this application, desmopressin is administered IV. The peptides are believed to exert their beneficial effects by increasing the circulating levels of clotting Factor VIII and perhaps other coagulation factors. Patients who are severely deficient in this factor (less than 5% of normal) and cannot respond with an increase in plasma levels receive no beneficial effect. Several recent reports also indicate beneficial hemostatic effects in patients with various platelet dysfunctions.[24]

Adverse Effects

As might be expected from their antidiuretic activity, ADH and anologues may produce water intoxication during chronic administration, particularly with excessive fluid intake. Consequences are similar to findings in the clinical syndrome of SIADH and include failure to dilute urine maximally, volume expansion, and hyponatremia. The hyponatremic patient may develop a number of CNS disturbances that can finally result in seizures, coma, and death. It should be noted that infants or elderly patients may be particularly susceptible to this complication.[25] Early signs of drowsiness, lethargy or disorientation should be recognized and therapy discontinued. It is recommended that the regimen of antidiuretic therapy be adjusted so that the patient experiences some polyuria and thirst intermittently, allowing excretion of any excess water that has been retained.[26]

The constrictor actions of AVP (and other analogues with pressor activity) may cause abdominal or uterine cramping, bronchoconstriction, and various cardiovascular sequelae, including headache and facial pallor. A more serious adverse reaction is possible coronary artery constriction. In patients with vascular disease, especially with coronary artery involvement, extreme caution should be exercised, particularly with IV administration, as anginal pain and even myocardial infarction may be precipitated. Desmopressin, due to its reduced activity at V_1 receptors, is largely free of adverse vasoconstrictor effects, but in rare instances headache, abdominal pain, flushing and sweating have occurred at high doses. LVP has the potential to cause vascular complications similar to AVP, but, since it is administered only by the intranasal route, the likelihood of serious problems is greatly reduced. Some adverse effects are peculiar to the route of administration of the drug. Both LVP and desmopressin, when given intranasally, can cause localized symptoms of rhinorrhea, nasal congestion, irritation, and pruritus. Administration of vasopressin tannate in oil (a repository formulation of the hormone for slow release) may result in sterile abcesses at the injection site.

Pharmacokinetics

Naturally occurring vasopressin, like most peptides, is poorly available on oral administration since digestive enzymes rapidly hydrolyze certain of the peptide linkages. AVP is therefore administered by the IM, SQ, or IV routes. LVP and desmopressin have been successfully administered by the intranasal route. Because of its long duration of action and relatively low incidence of adverse effects, desmopressin is particularly effective by this route, although its bioavailability is variable and averages only 10 percent compared with an IV dose.[26]

Following absorption (or release into the circulation), AVP and LVP are distributed throughout the extracellular compartment. They are rapidly cleared, with a half-life of 10–20 minutes. AVP is not bound to plasma proteins to any appreciable extent, and is metabolically cleared primarily in the liver and kidney. A small fraction of circulating AVP (< 20%) is excreted intact in the urine. Inactivation appears to occur by the action of various aminopeptidases, particularly those cleaving the 1,2 linkage. This metabolic reaction is retarded in peptides lacking the terminal amino group at 1-cysteine, as in desmopressin. Because of this feature, desmopressin persists in the circulation with a half-life of 70–90 minutes. The peptide also appears to be slowly absorbed across the nasal mucosa, resulting in an especially prolonged duration of action when administered by this route.[26]

AVP and its analogues are generally measured by radioimmunoassay.[27] Although measurement of the peptide is generally not necessary in the clinical setting, it often can be helpful in diagnosing polyuric disorders.

Available Preparations and Doses

For many years the preparations of neurohypophysial hormones that were available came from natural sources. For this reason, preparations varied in purity and had to be standardized by bioassay against a reference standard. In the US the standard is the USP Posterior Pituitary reference standard. For USP purposes, the vasopressin content of a preparation is expressed in terms of vasopressor activity in the rat. The reference standard contains approximately 0.5 Unit of vasopressor activity per mg of powder. By comparison, pure synthetic arginine vasopressin has a potency of approximately 400 Units per mg.

Vasopressin injection (Pitressin) is a sterile aqueous solution of synthetic vasopressin containing 20 pressor Units per ml. It is recommended for SQ or IM injection.

Vasopressin tannate (Pitressin Tannate in Oil) is a suspension of water insoluble vasopressin tannate in peanut oil. The suspension contains 5 pressor Units per ml. This preparation is utilized for IM administration only. For the treatment of hypothalamic diabetes insipidus, 0.3 to 1.0 ml is injected IM. The duration of action is usually two to four days.

Lypressin (Diapid) is a preparation of synthetic lysine vasopressin for use as a nasal spray. It contains 0.185 mg per ml and an activity of 50 pressor Units per ml. The only indication for use of lypressin nasal spray is for the control of the symptoms of diabetes insipidus. For this purpose the usual dose is one or two sprays (2–4 USP units) four times daily.

Desmopressin acetate injection (DDAVP or Stimate) is an aqueous solution of desmopressin acetate that contains 4 μg/ml. This preparation is used in the management of diabetes insipidus in cases where the intranasal route is unsuitable. It is usually administered SQ or IV at 2–4 μg daily in two divided doses. Desmopressin injection is also used in the management on acute bleeding disorders of patients with hemophilia or von Willebrand's disease, or prophylactically in these patients prior to dental or surgical procedures. The recommended dose is 0.3 μg/kg body weight, diluted in 50 ml of physiologic saline and infused over 15–30 minutes. This is generally recommended 30 minutes prior to any scheduled surgical or dental procedures.

Desmopressin acetate nasal solution (DDAVP) contains 100 μg/ml of desmopressin acetate in 2.5-ml bottles. These are supplied with a nasal catheter calibrated for administration of the solution. Dosage must be individualized, but ranges from 0.1 to 0.4 ml daily, usually in two divided doses.

Desmopressin acetate nasal spray (DDAVP) contains 100 μg/ml of desmopressin acetate in a 5 ml bottle with spray pump. Actuation of the pump supplies a metered dose of 10 μg of desmopressin. Dosage is 10–40 μg/day in one or two doses.

Drugs Affecting the Secretion or Action of ADH

Alteration of ADH Secretion

A large number of drugs and hormones have been shown to modulate ADH release. Nicotine, isoproterenol, vincristine, vinblastine, cyclophosphamide, colchicine, and morphine (depending on dose) have all been shown to stimulate secretion under certain conditions. These actions may be direct effects of the drugs on the osmoreceptor or neurosecretory system, or may be mediated by decreases in blood pressure or blood volume (or its distribution) or perhaps via other pathways. Some drugs that enhance ADH release have been used therapeutically in cases of partial central diabetes insipidus, i.e., where ADH is synthesized but its release is inadequate. Clofibrate and carbamazepine are agents that appear to enhance the release of endogenous AVP, but adverse effects make their use rarely advisable. Chlorpropamide, one of the sulfonylurea class of hypoglycemic agents, appears to be beneficial in partial diabetes insipidus, both by increasing the release of ADH and by augmenting the renal response to the hormone.[28] Although this drug has been used fairly extensively, the treatment of choice in AVP-responsive diabetes insipidus is desmopressin.

Among the drugs that inhibit the secretion of ADH, ethanol is perhaps the best known. Opiate agonists or partial agonists, including some opioid peptides, also have been shown to suppress release of ADH, seemingly elevating the "threshold" for osmotic stimulation.[29] Several recent studies suggest that opioids that stimulate the kappa receptor subtype are potent inhibitors of ADH secretion.[30] Phenytoin has been implicated as an inhibitor of the secretion of the peptide, and has been successfully used to suppress ADH levels in patients with the syndrome of inappropriate ADH secretion. Glucocorticoids also exert an inhibitory effect on release of ADH. This appears to be most readily demonstrated in states of glucocorticoid deficiency, where water excretion is impaired by elevated levels of ADH. The mechanism is unknown, but may relate to improvement of the compromised cardiac function in glucocorticoid-deficient states.

Modification of the Renal Response

Several pharmacologic agents have been shown to impair the ability of the kidney to concentrate urine. Lithium salts are used in therapy of manic-depressive disorders. A commonly observed adverse effect is nephrogenic diabetes insipidus.[31] This effect of lithium is thought to be mediated by inhibition of the stimulation of adenylate cyclase by ADH. This defect can be quite severe, with urine volumes of greater than 15 L per day; in most patients the condition is reversible. Gentamicin, cisplatin, and amphotericin B are drugs often associated with nephrotoxicity in clinical use. These agents usually cause increased serum creatinine or blood urea nitrogen due to impairment of glomerular filtration rate. However, all of them can also induce renal concentrating defects that are vasopressin-resistant. A compound of special interest is the antibiotic drug demeclocycline, which has also been shown to inhibit ADH-sensitive adenylate cyclase and therefore cause defects in urinary concentration. This agent has found some therapeutic utility because of its ability to inhibit the action of AVP. Demeclocycline is now the preferred treatment in SIADH because it can reliably induce hyporesponsiveness to the high circulating levels of AVP,[19] but development of effective antagonists for V_2 receptors may provide a new therapeutic approach (see below).

There are some pharmacologic agents that also potentiate the response to AVP. The nonsteroidal anti-inflammatory drugs (NSAIDs), of which indomethacin is a prototype, appear to potentiate the effects of AVP on water reabsorption, at least under some conditions. Prostaglandins synthesized in the kidney normally serve to antagonize the response to AVP.[32] The NSAIDs are potent inhibitors of the biosynthesis of prostaglandins, and therefore reduce this antagonism and allow an enhanced renal response. It is of interest that chlorpropamide, an oral hypoglycemic agent known for several years to enhance the renal response to ADH, also is an effective inhibitor of prostaglandin biosynthesis.[33] Chlorpropamide and the NSAIDs have been used successfully in therapy of nephrogenic diabetes insipidus.

Another class of drugs also potentiates the effects of ADH in vivo, although by a somewhat indirect mechanism. The thiazide diuretics, paradoxically, are useful in nephrogenic diabetes insipidus, where they reduce urine flow rather than increase it. This response is thought to be due to the sodium depletion that occurs with the diuretics, leading to enhanced reabsorption of sodium and water in the proximal tubule. This allows a smaller volume to be delivered to the later portions of the nephron, and therefore limits the load of water that must be reabsorbed by ADH-dependent mechanisms. The effect of these drugs on the kidney is fairly modest, and patients with severe nephrogenic diabetes insipidus often do not concentrate their urine very effectively, even with adjunctive therapy with other drugs. However, even a small improvement in urinary concentration (e.g., from 100–300 mOsm/kg water) provides a dramatic benefit to the patient in that urine flow may be reduced from 12 to 4 L per day.

AVP Receptor Antagonists

Beginning in the early 1960s, scores of peptide analogues of vasopressin were synthesized and evaluated for antagonistic activity in vasopressor or antidiuretic assays. Although some compounds were developed with moderate antivasopressor action, it was not until 1981 that effective antagonists of the antidiuretic action of vasopressin in vivo were developed.[34] Several of these compounds have a good selectivity for V_2 over V_1 receptors,[35] and thus may provide useful pharmacologic tools for characterizing ADH receptor populations and for studying the physiology and pathophysiology of ADH action. There is considerable structural diversity among these agents, but all have in common the lack of the N-terminal amino group at the cysteine residue in position 1, and substitution of a cyclopentamethylene group on the β - carbon of this same cysteine (see Table 39.1). Several of the more potent and selective agents have D- or L-aliphatic amino acids (leucine, isoleucine, or valine) substituted at positions 2 and/or 4.[34] From a clinical standpoint, however, the peptide antagonists have proved a disappointment. Although in vitro and animal studies indicated competitive antagonism of V_2 receptors, all compounds tested in man have unexpectedly shown agonist activity. The recent discovery of nonpeptide

Table 39.2 Available Preparations of Antidiuretic Hormone and Analogues

Non Propietary Name	Description	Trade Name	Preparation	Primary Usage	Dose/Route/Interval
Vasopressin (argipressin)	8-arginine vasopressin	Pitressin	20 U/ml Inj.	Central diabetes insipidus[a]	5–10 U i.m. or s.c. at 4 hr. intervals
Lypressin	8-lysine vasopressin	Diapid	50 U/ml nasal spray	Central diabetes insipidus[a]	2–4 U (1–2 sprays) each nostril 4 times daily
Desmopressin acetate	1-deamino-8-D-arginine-vasopressin acetate	DDAVP Stimate	4-μg/ml Inj.	Central diabetes insipidus	2–4 μg i.v. or s.c. daily in two divided doses
				bleeding disorders[b] in surgical or trauma patients	0.3 /μg/kg by i.v. infusion over 15–30 min.[c]
Desmopressin Acetate	1-deamino-8-D-arginine-vasopressin acetate	DDAVP	0.1 mg/ml nasal solution or spray	Central diabetes insipidus	10–40 μg/day in one or two doses
Terlipressin	triglycyl-lysine-vasopressin (inactive prodrug)	Glypressin	1 mg Inj., with diluent	bleeding esophageal varices, uterine hemorrhage	1–2 mg i.v. every 4–6 hrs.
Ornipressin	8-ornithine-vasopressin	Por-8	5 U/ml Inj.	Hemorrhage during surgery	1–20 U by i.v. or local infusion

a) Preferred maintenance drug is DDAVP.
b) Only certain types of disorders respond to vasopressin analogs. See text for details.
c) For preoperative use, infuse 30 min. prior to surgery.

OPC-21268

OPC-31260

Figure 39.5 Chemical structures of OPC-31260, [5-dimethylamino 1-{4-(2-methylbenzoylamino) benzoyl}-2,3,4,5-tetrahydro-1 H-benzazepine], a V_2 antagonist and OPC-21268, 1-{1-[4-(3-acetylaminopropoxy) benzoyl]-4-piperidyl}-3,4-dihydro-2 (IH)-quinolinone, a V_1 antagonist.

antagonists of V_1[36] and V_2[37] receptors offer new hope for development of orally active therapeutic agents for various pathophysiologic states involving ADH (Fig. 39.5). Of particular interest is OPC-31260, now in clinical trials, which will be indicated for treatment of SIADH. This agent displays potent V_2 receptor antagonism in vitro and excellent water diuretic activity when administered by the oral route. In preclinical and clinical studies, no agonist activity has been observed with this nonpeptide antagonist.

Summary

Antidiuretic hormone is a peptide hormone that serves to promote antidiuresis in the kidney. Arginine vasopressin, which is the form found in most mammals, is released from the posterior pituitary in response to an elevated tonicity of extracellular fluid. The hormone exerts its action in the kidney by increasing the permeability of the distal portions of the nephron to water. This increase in permeability allows enhanced reabsorption of water that is returned to the circulation and thereby dilutes body fluids, inhibiting ADH release. Under some conditions the biosynthesis and/or release of AVP from the pituitary is deficient, leading to an inability to adequately concentrate the urine, an elevation in urine flow, and dehydration. This disorder is referred to as hypothalamic diabetes insipidus, and it remains the primary indication for the use of ADH and its antidiuretic analogues. Desmopressin is a synthetic analogue of AVP that has a remarkably prolonged duration of action, good antidiuretic potency, and reduced pressor activity compared with vasopressin. Desmopressin is absorbed across the nasal mucosa, and intranasal administration of this peptide is the preferred mode of therapy for maintenance of patients with hypothalamic diabetes insipidus.

References

Research Reports

1. du Vigneaud V, Gish DT, Katsoyannis PG. A synthetic preparation with biological properties associated with arginine vasopressin. J Am Chem Soc 1954;*76*:4751–4751.
2. Zaoral M, Kole J, Sorm F. Amino acids and peptides. LXXI Synthesis of 1-deamino-8-D-aminobutyrine vasopressin, 1-deamino-8-D-lysine vasopressin and 1-deamino-8-D-arginine vasopressin. Coll Czech Chem Commun 1967;*32*:1250–1257.
3. Manning M, Sawyer WH. Development of selective agonists and antagonists of vasopressin and oxytocin. In Schrier RW. (Ed.): Vasopressin, New York: Raven Press, 1985; pp 131–144.
4. Gilman A, Goodman L. The secretory response of the posterior pituitary to the need for water conservation. J Physiol 1937;*90*:113–124.
5. Chambers GH, Melville EV, Hare et al. Regulation of the release of pituitrin by changes in the osmotic pressure of the plasma. Am J Physiol 1945;*144*:311–320.
6. Verney EB. The antidiuretic hormone and factors which determine its release. Proc Royal Soc London (Biol) 1947;*135*:25–106.
7. Robertson GL, Mahr EA, Athar S, et al. Development and clinical application of a new method for the radioimmunoassay of arginine vasopressin in human plasma. J Clin Invest 1973;*52*:2340–2352.
8. Henry JP, Gauer OH, Reeves JL. Evidence of the atrial location of receptors influencing urine flow. Circ Res 1956;*4*:85–90.
9. Kuhn W, Ryffel K. Herstellung konzentrierter Lusungen aus verdunnten durch blosse Membranwirkung: Ein Modellversuch zur Funktion der Niere. Z Physiol Chem 1942;*276*:145–178.
10. Valtin H. Renal function: Mechanisms preserving fluid and solute balance in health, 2d ed. Boston: Little, Brown 1983; pp 161–194.
11. Pitts RF. Physiology of the kidney and body fluids, 3d ed. Chicago; Yearbook Medical Publishers, (1974); pp 124–132.
12. Roy DR, Layton HE, Jamison RL. Countercurrent system and its regulation. In Seldin DW, Giebisch G (Eds) The kidney: Physiology and pathophysiology, 2d ed., Vol. 2. New York: Raven Press (1992); pp 1649–1692.
13. Star RA, Hiroshi N, Balaban R. et al. Calcium and cyclic adenosine monophosphate as second messengers for vasopressin in the rat inner medullary collecting duct. J Clin Invest 1988;*81*:1879–1888.
14. Breyer MD. Regulation of water and salt transport in collecting duct through calcium-dependent signaling mechanisms. Am J Physiol 1991;*260* (Renal Fluid Electrolyte Physiol. 29): F1–F11.

14a. Skorecki KL, Ausiello DA. Vasopressin receptor-adenylate cyclase interactions: A model for cAMP metabolism in the kidney. In Cowley AW Jr, Liard JF, Ausiello DA. (eds.): Vasopressin. New York: Raven Press, 1988; p 55.

15. Pearl M, Taylor A. Actin filaments and vasopressin-stimulated water flow in toad urinary bladder. Am J Physiol 1983;*245* (Cell Physiol. 20): C28–C35.

16. Verkman AS. Mechanisms and regulation of water permeability in renal epithelia. Am J Physiol 1989;*257* (Cell Physiol. 26): C837–C850.

17. Harris HW Jr, Handler JS. The role of membrane turnover in the water permeability response to antidiuretic hormone. J Membrane Biol 1988;*103*:207–216.

18. Jackson BA. Modulation of vasopressin-sensitive cyclic AMP levels by calcium in papillary collecting tubules. Mol Cell Endocrinol 1988;*57*:199–204.

19. Zerbe R, Stropes L, Robertson G. Vasopressin function in the syndrome of inappropriate antidiuresis. Ann Rev Med 1980;*31*:315–327.

20. Cogan E, Debieve M, Pepersack T, et al. Natriuresis and atrial natriuretic factor secretion during inappropriate antidiuresis. Am J Med 1988;*84*:409–418.

21. Miller M, Dalakes T, Moses AM, et al. Recognition of partial defects in antidiuretic hormone secretion. Ann Intern Med 1970;*73*:721–729.

22. Dashe AM, Cramm RE, Crist CA, et al. A water deprivation test for the differential diagnosis of polyuria. JAMA 1963;*185*:699–703.

23. de la Fuente B, Kasper CK, Rickles FR, et al. Response of patients with mild and moderate Hemophilia A and von Willebrand's disease to treatment with desmopressin. Ann Intern Med 1985;*103*:6–14.

24. DiMichele DM, Hathaway WE. Use of DDAVP in inherited and acquired platelet dysfunction. Am J Hematol 1990;*33*:39–45.

25. Shepherd LL, Hutchinson RJ, Worden EK, et al. Hyponatremia and seizures after intravenous administration of desmopressin acetate for surgical hemostasis. J Pediatrics 1989;*114*:470.

26. Richardson DW, Robinson AG. Desmopressin. Ann Intern Med 1985;*103*:228–239.

27. Robertson GL, Mahr EA, Athar S, et al. Development and application of a new method for the radioimmunoassay of arginine vasopressin in human plasma. J Clin Invest 1973;*52*:2340–2352.

28. Moses AM, Numann P, Miller M. Mechanism of chlorpropamide induced antidiuresis in man: Evidence for release of ADH and enhancement of peripheral action. Metabolism 1973;*22*:59–66.

29. Kamoi K, Robertson GL. Opiates and vasopressin secretion. In Schrier RW. Vasopressin. New York: Raven Press, (1985); pp 259–264.

30. Peters GR, Ward NJ, Antal EG, et al. Diuretic actions in man of a selective kappa opioid agonist: U-62066E. J Pharmacol Exp Ther 1987;*240*:128–131.

31. Cox M, Singer I. Lithium and water metabolism. Am J Med 1975;*59*:153–157.

32. Anderson RJ, Berl T, McDonald KM, et al. Evidence for an in vivo antagonism between vasopressin and prostaglandins in the mammalian kidney. J Clin Invest 1975;*56*:420–426.

33. Zusman RM, Keiser HR, Handler JS. Inhibition of vasopressin-stimulated prostaglandin E biosynthesis by chlorpropamide in the toad urinary bladder. J Clin Invest 1977;*60*:1348–1353.

34. Sawyer WH, Manning M. The development of vasopressin antagonists. Fed Proc 1984;*43*:87–90.

35. Kinter LB, Huffman WF, Stassen FL. Antagonists of the antidiuretic activity of vasopressin. Am J Physiol 1988;*254* (Renal Fluid Electrolyte Physiol. 23): F165–F177.

36. Yamamura Y, Ogawa H, Chihara T, et al. OPC-21268, an orally effective, nonpeptide vasopressin V_1 receptor antagonist. Science 1991;*252*:572–574.

37. Yamamura Y, Ogawa H, Yamashita H, et al. Characterization of a novel aquaretic agent, OPC-31260, as an orally effective, nonpeptide vasopressin V_2 receptor antagonist. Br J Pharmacol 1992;*105*:787–791.

Reviews

r1. Brownstein MJ. Biosynthesis of vasopressin and oxytocin. Ann Rev Physiol 1983;*45*:129–135.
A concise summary of the characterization and intracellular processing of the prohormones of AVP and oxytocin.

r2. Cowley AW, Liard J-F, Ausiello DA (eds.): Vasopressin: Cellular and integrative functions. New York: Raven Press, 1988.
A collection of papers on topics of current interest in vasopressin research, including chemistry, release, pathophysiology, cardiovascular actions, and cellular mechanisms.

r3. Robertson GL. Regulation of vasopressin secretion. In Seldin DW, Giebisch G. The Kidney: Physiology and Pathophysiology, 2d ed. New York: Raven Press, 1992; pp 1595–1614.
A detailed review of physiologic mechanisms controlling ADH release and their interrelationships, as well as pharmacologic agents that affect these processes.

r4. Valtin H. Renal Function: Mechanisms Preserving Fluid and Solute Balance in Health, 2d ed. Boston: Little, Brown 1983.
An excellent basic textbook in renal physiology, designed for medical students, including a very readable discussion of the countercurrent system.

r5. Pitts RF. Physiology of the Kidney and Body Fluids, 3d ed. Chicago: Year Book, 1974.
A classic basic textbook in renal physiology.

r6. Richardson DW, Robinson AG. Desmopressin. Ann Int Med 1985;*103*:228–239.
A useful review of the pharmacology and clinical uses of desmopressin, thoroughly referenced.

r7. Roy DR, Layton HE, Jamison RL. Countercurrent mechanism and its regulation. In Seldin DW, Giebisch G. The Kidney: Physiology and Pathophysiology, New York: Raven Press, 1992; pp 1694–1692.
A thorough and comprehensive treatment of the renal countercurrent system and its operation in urinary concentration and dilution.

r8. Sawyer WH, Manning M. The development of vasopressin antagonists. Fed Proc 1984;*43*:87–90.
A brief review of principal advances in the development of peptide antagonists to the cardiovascular and diuretic effects of ADH.

r9. Robertson GL, Berl T. Pathophysiology of water metabolism. In Brenner BM, Rector FC Jr. The Kidney (4th ed), Philadelphia: WB Saunders 1991; pp 677–736.
A detailed review of clinical and experimental pathophysiology of water imbalance, including diabetes insipidus and the syndrome of inappropriate ADH secretion.

r10. Hayes RM. Cell biology of vasopressin. In Brenner BM, Rector FC Jr. The Kidney (4th ed), Philadelphia: WB Saunders 1991; pp 424–444.
An excellent summary of current understanding of cellular responses to hormones, with detailed treatment of vasopressin.

r11. Share L. Vasopressin and regulation of water homeostasis and cardiovascular function. In McCann SM. Endocrinology: People and Ideas. American Physiological Society, 1988; pp 1–21.
An historical review of vasopressin discovery, characterization, and elucidation of function.

CHAPTER 40

Drug-Induced Kidney Disease

William O. Berndt
Mary E. Davis

Drug-induced renal disease accounts for a substantial portion of disease of the tubules. For some agents, such as the glycoside antibiotics, a resulting bout of acute renal failure can add days to a patient's hospitalization and additional costs that run into thousands of dollars.

Renal Exposure to Nephrotoxic Drugs

The kidneys are, in a sense, designed to be exposed to all types of chemicals, including endogenous hormones, factors, or other proteins, diet constituents, and nephrotoxic agents. To perform their functions of maintaining electrolyte homeostasis and eliminating waste products, the kidneys must process large volumes of blood. The kidneys receive approximately 20 percent of cardiac output, making them among the best perfused organs in the body, but also exposing them heavily to any toxic agent present in the blood. Of that 650 ml/min of blood, approximately one-fifth is filtered at the glomerulus and enters the lumen of the tubule. This means that the renal tubule is exposed to chemicals from both the plasma and tubular urine, if the compounds are present in plasma in free solution (not completely bound to proteins).

The transport systems in the proximal tubule actively move drugs that are organic anions or cations, into the cell; concentrations in the cell can reach up to tenfold that in the plasma that bathes the cell, increasing the likelihood of toxicity for drugs with intracellular actions. The cytochrome P450 mono-oxygenase system is localized predominantly in the cells in this region of the kidney, and this likely contributes to the regional selectivity of drugs that require bioactivation to reactive intermediates to become toxic.

All along the tubule, large volumes of water are reabsorbed. If the drug is not reabsorbed with water, the drug concentration will increase along the nephron, potentially contributing to toxic effects in more distal elements, such as the papillary necrosis induced by acetaminophen.

Finally, the kidney is subject to feedback control systems that serve to keep function optimal. The first, autoregulation of renal blood flow, maintains adequate perfusion of the kidneys in spite of perturbations of systemic vascular resistance and blood pressure that otherwise would drastically decrease renal blood flow. The second, glomerular-tubular feedback, serves to prevent massive fluid loss during episodes of impaired renal function by decreasing filtration at the glomeruli of tubules that are damaged and therefore not able to reabsorb the massive fluid load normally presented to the nephron tubule. These control mechanisms themselves are sites for drug action or toxicity.

Disease may increase the susceptibility of the kidneys to drug toxicity. This can occur even with diseases that do not involve the kidneys if cardiovascular function or water and electrolyte balance are altered. As do many organs, the kidneys have a reserve capacity that may be overwhelmed by ongoing disease processes; thus, renal toxicity may be seen in sick patients that would not be seen in otherwise healthy patients receiving the same drug treatment. That is, the drug may cause the same decrement of renal function in both groups, but only those with pre-existing deficits would lose sufficient renal function for signs of renal failure to be detectable. Similarly, renal function declines with age and so elderly patients, with less reserve capacity, would be expected to be more susceptible to drug-induced renal toxicity. Disease states can increase susceptibility to renal damage without direct renal involvement. For example, severe diarrhea or vomiting or ascites can result in a contraction of fluid volume and derangement of electrolyte balance that will decrease renal function without causing damage, but the kidneys will not be able to handle the additional insult presented by the drug.

Schemes for classifying acute renal failure are based on anatomy and on the mechanism of damage. Anatomically based schemes have the advantage of not requiring that the disease process be understood, but therefore also impart less information about the cause of the disease. Conversely, drugs, chemicals, and other agents that cause damage to the proximal tubule, for example, have similar signs and symptoms and treatments, and thus are diagnostically useful. The mechanisms of drug-induced renal failure can be broadly classified as allergic or cytotoxic. Cytotoxic reactions can be further subdivided according to where the damage occurs: prerenal; renal; or postrenal. Prerenal events alter renal hemodynamics and produce an ischemic-type damage. This occurs with the NSAIDs and possibly with cyclosporine A. Renal events include effects within the kidney or nephron, e.g., the tubular toxicity of such agents as the aminoglycosides, cisplatin, radiocontrast agents, and the NSAIDs. These include both chronic toxicity and the rare incidents of nephrotoxicity from acute overdose. Postrenal failure refers to actions that block the movement of urine out of the tubule and ultimately out of the body. Drugs that cause postrenal failure precipitate in the tubule, e.g., methotrexate, or increase the appearance of other agents that can precipitate, e.g., uric acid (suprofen, contrast agents) and oxalate (contrast agents).

Nonsteroidal Anti-Inflammatory and Analgesic Drugs

The nonsteroidal anti-inflammatory drugs (NSAIDs) are among the most widely used drugs. They are used for pain, dysmenorrhea, inflammation, and fever, and in connective tissue, rheumatologic, and autoimmune diseases. Several syndromes of renal toxicity are caused by the NSAIDs. Acute renal insufficiency, allergic interstitial nephritis, nephrotic syndrome, and hyperkalemia have resulted from therapy with several of the agents, and there are reports of acute tubular necrosis in cases of acetaminophen overdose.

Acute renal insufficiency has occurred with members of all classes of NSAIDs (fenoprofen, naproxen, ibuprofen, indomethacin, sulindac, tolmetin, zomepirac, mefenamic acid, ketoprofen, and piroxicam), and is due to inhibition of prostaglandin synthesis. Acute renal insufficiency or failure generally occurs in those whose renal function depends on the vasodilatory influences of the prostaglandins (Fig. 40.1). The NSAIDs inhibit prostaglandin synthesis and thus remove vasodilatory influences.[1] Acute renal failure results from the decreased blood flow, and is therefore termed "hemodynamically mediated renal failure." Acute renal insufficiency or failure is an extension of NSAID therapeutic effects. Dependence on prostaglandin synthesis occurs with decreased effective plasma volume or preexisting renal disorders. Examples of conditions that sensitize the kidneys to NSAID-induced hemodynamically mediated acute renal failure are outlined in Table 40.1. However, small reductions of GFR or renal plasma flow occur in healthy humans,[2] and acute overdose of ibuprofen has been reported to cause acute renal failure in a patient with no predisposing factors.[3]

Prostaglandins also decrease water reabsorption, by shifting blood from the cortical to medullary areas, decreasing the concentrating gradient, inhibiting both chloride transport in the ascending limb of the loop of Henle and the action of ADH in the collecting duct, and altering the Starling forces to decrease movement of water from the tubule into the interstitium. NSAIDs eliminate these effects of prostaglandins and thus increase water reabsorption. The reduction of renal blood flow and increased sodium reabsorption in the proximal tu-

Table 40.1 Factors Enhancing NSAID Nephrotoxicity

Decreased plasma volume
Blood loss
Diuretic use
Vomiting
Ascites
Alcoholic cirrhosis
Congestive heart failure
Atherosclerotic coronary vascular disease
Diabetes mellitus
Decreased renal function
Advanced age
Glomerulonephritis
Interstitial nephritis
Lupus nephritis
Hydronephrosis
Ureteral obstruction
Bartter's syndrome
Renovascular hypertension

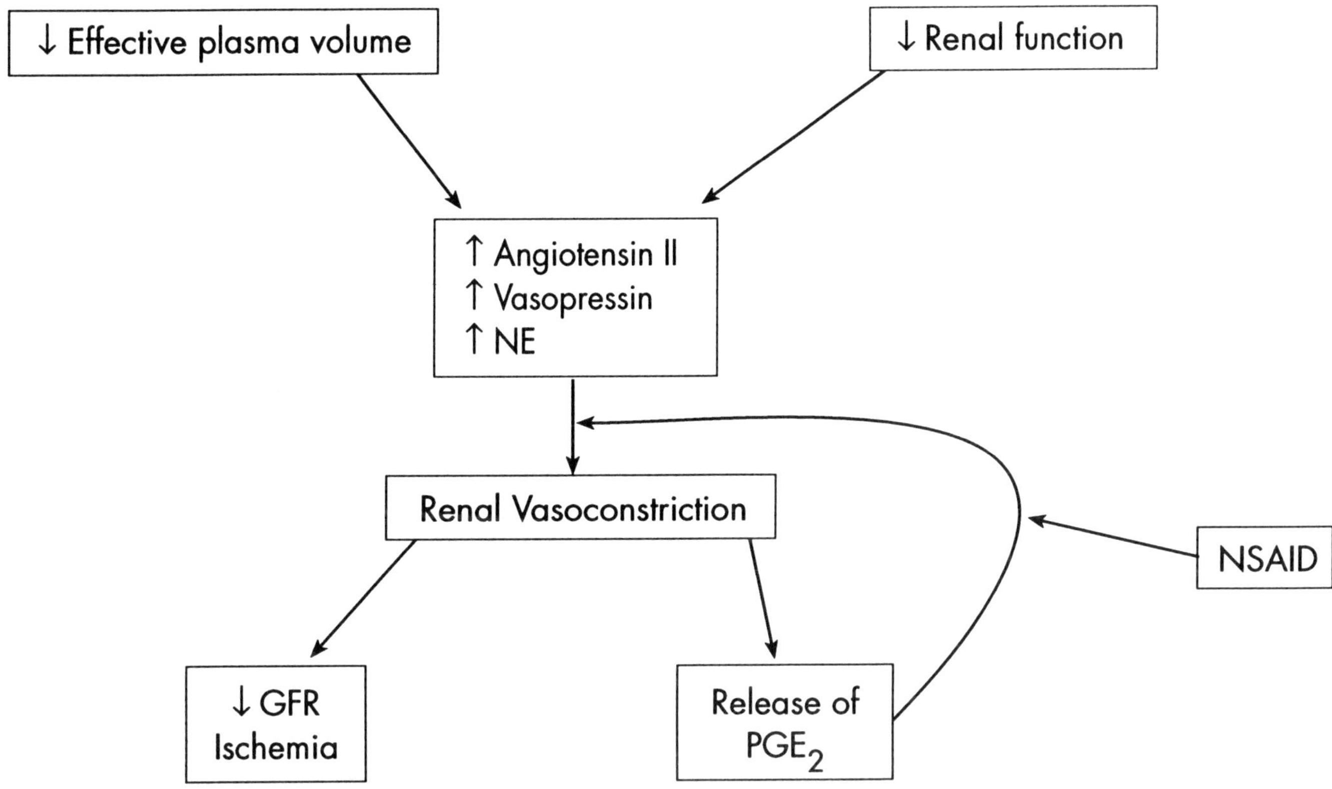

Figure 40.1 NSAID's inhibit synthesis of vasodilatory prostaglandins, allowing vasoconstrictor influences to be unopposed.

bule cause sodium retention in up to one-fourth of arthritis patients taking aspirin, ibuprofen, or fenoprofen.

NSAID-induced hemodynamic acute renal failure is characterized by decreased urine output, occasional oliguria, and weight gain; rapid rise of BUN and serum creatinine soon after therapy begins; and sodium retention and hyperkalemia. Biopsy often discloses acute tubular necrosis and interstitial nephritis with no glomerular involvement.

Risk factors for NSAID-induced hemodynamic renal failure are those conditions that sensitize the kidneys to NSAIDs (Table 40.1) and include situations of decreased plasma volume, renal disease or decreased renal function, hydronephrosis, ureteral obstruction, Bartter's syndrome, and renovascular hypertension. NSAIDs should be used cautiously, if at all, in these patients.

Overdose of acetaminophen has resulted in nephrotoxicity. In three cases reported[4,5] liver failure was prevented by treatment with N-acetylcysteine. Signs of nephrotoxicity appeared the second day after poisoning, and kidney function was impaired for up to a week. Urine volume was normal to increased, with proteinuria and hematuria. BUN and serum creatinine were increased.

Interstitial nephropathy after NSAIDs is relatively rare. It is more common in older patients and takes several months to develop. It is characterized by proteinuria in the nephrotic range and edema secondary to loss of plasma proteins. The presenting complaint is often edema or oliguria. Biopsy specimens show marked interstitial inflammatory changes and minimal change glomerulopathy, with fusion of epithelial foot processes. NSAID-induced interstitial nephropathy is believed to be a cell-mediated allergic reaction. The inhibition of prostaglandin synthesis, however, may prevent the body from fighting the disease, thus allowing the disease process to proceed relatively unimpeded. Furthermore, the NSAIDs inhibit cyclo-oxygenase, which could allow arachidonic acid metabolism to be shifted to the leukotriene pathway, increasing the synthesis of products that mediate inflammatory reactions.

Analgesic nephropathy occurs with long-term use or abuse of analgesics, usually mixtures including aspirin, phenacetin or acetaminophen, and caffeine, but also with salicylates, meclofenamate, ibuprofen, and phenylbutazone. Women are more frequently affected, and the incidence is higher in Australia and Switzerland and, within the US, in the southeastern states. The disease coexists with peptic ulceration, hypertension, anemia, atherosclerosis, and psychiatric instability. Patients generally deny use or abuse of analgesics, and relatives may provide more reliable information on the quantity of analgesic purchased weekly. BUN and serum creatinine are increased; renal tubular acidosis and inability to concentrate urine occur. Necrosis of the papilla is the classic sign of analgesic nephropathy; acute interstitial nephritis is also found in biopsy specimens. The toxicity is believed to be due to accumulation of toxic metabolites within the papilla, overwhelming cellular defense mechanisms. Dehydration allows higher papillary concentrations to be reached, and this is one factor in the higher incidence in hot climates. Deranged hemodynamics also may contribute.

Sulindac has been observed to be less nephrotoxic than other NSAIDs. Sulindac is a prodrug; the active metabolite, sulindac sulfide, is formed in the liver and oxidized in the kidney to the inactive sulfone. It was felt that oxidation in the kidney spared the kidney of toxic effects. Further studies have shown that sulindac decreases clearance of inulin (GFR) and PAH (*p*-aminohippurate, effective RBF) in a way similar to other NSAIDs when doses were equieffective for cyclo-oxygenase inhibition.

Suprofen occasionally causes uric acid nephropathy. Suprofen is uricosuric, and individuals who are volume-depleted are at risk for developing uric acid crystals within the tubules. The symptoms are bilateral flank pain, abdominal pain, constipation, polyuria, polydipsia, and elevation of BUN and serum creatinine. The urine is free of glucose, protein, and ketone bodies. The flank pain and renal effects resolve within one to two weeks after the drug is stopped.

Antibiotics

Aminoglycosides

Nephrotoxicity from antibiotic use is a major cause of acute renal failure, accounting for 5 to 30 percent of all cases. The aminoglycosides, particularly gentamicin, are well known for their nephrotoxicity; other nephrotoxic antibiotics include some cephalosporins. Gentamicin frequently causes frank renal damage, and subclinical damage occurs in a large portion of those treated with the drug. In one study of gentamicin use in the Philadelphia area, 7.3 percent of patients developed nephrotoxicity; the treatment for kidney dysfunction cost an average of $2501 per case, or $183 averaged for all patients treated with aminoglycosides.[6]

Gentamicin is the prototype of aminoglycoside antibiotics. It is used for gram-negative infections. Gentamicin is a cation, and the positive charge contributes to toxicity by allowing the drug to bind to anionic groups of membrane phospholipids.

Gentamicin is distributed throughout the ECF volume, and it is not appreciably protein-bound or metabolized. The clearance of gentamicin is the same as that for creatinine and inulin. Excretion is renal, and the drug will accumulate within the kidney and be elevated in plasma if the dose is not adjusted for inadequate renal function, including deficits of renal function brought about by treatment with gentamicin.

Nephrotoxicity generally becomes apparent after several days to weeks of gentamicin treatment. There is pronounced proteinuria, and β-$_2$-microglobulinuria. GFR is decreased in some patients in the first few days after even low doses of gentamicin.[7] On the second day after gentamicin, the GFR in the more affected group was substantially less than in the less responsive group (75 vs 114 ml/min); such differences would allow more gentamicin to accumulate in patients who did develop nephrotoxicity.

Tissue damage after gentamicin is characterized by the appearance within proximal tubule cells of concentric membranous structures called myeloid bodies. Gentamicin binds to the brush border membranes; the gentamicin-membrane complexes are taken up into the cells and accumulate in lysosomes. The presence of gentamicin prevents further processing, either by degradation of the membrane or by fusion of lysosomes during normal processing of the organelles; instead, the lysosomes develop into myeloid bodies, which have whorls of membrane material concentrated within them.[8] In a review of biopsy slides taken for diagnosis of glomerular disease,[9] 19 specimens were found to have myeloid bodies; of these, 15 had received gentamicin within six weeks of the study. Of the four not related to gentamicin treatment, one patient had been taking chloroquine, which may act similarly to gentamicin to stimulate myeloid body formation. Two of the others had much less conspicuous myeloid bodies. In the same study, 90 of the samples had no myeloid bodies, and the patient charts showed no history of gentamicin. However, myeloid body formation is not useful for diagnosing or predicting acute renal failure, as most patients develop myeloid bodies but do not develop renal failure. While myeloid bodies are a major site of gentamicin storage within the kidney, the role of myeloid bodies in the acute tubular necrosis that occurs is not clear.

Studies with isolated mitochondria have shown that gentamicin enhances production of hydrogen peroxide in mitochondria—and therefore, it seems likely, of hydroxyl radical.[10] Pretreatment of rats with hydroxyl radical scavengers protects against gentamicin-induced acute renal failure. Antioxidants were not effective, so the lipid peroxidation that occurs is a sign, rather than cause, of toxicity.

Calcium supplements have been shown to protect experimental animals against gentamicin toxicity, possibly by stimulating synthesis of anionic lipids for gentamicin to bind to, and decreasing the amount of drug available to sites that cause nephrotoxicity.[11,12]

Risk factors for gentamicin nephrotoxicity are listed in Table 40.2. Gentamicin nephrotoxicity is more likely in patients with preexisting deficits of either renal function or ability to eliminate gentamicin by excretion in urine. Thus, the elderly, critically ill, and patients who are volume-depleted or dehydrated are most at risk. Concomitant treatment with other nephrotoxic drugs increases the risk. Gentamicin in combination with cephalosporins may be beneficial therapeutically; however, the combination increases the risk of nephrotoxicity. Correlation studies have suggested that high-trough concentrations in blood, total dose, liver disease, and being female contribute to risk of kidney damage during gentamicin therapy.[13]

The likelihood of gentamicin nephrotoxicity can be decreased by correcting those factors that can be manipulated, such as dehydration or concurrent treatment with other nephrotoxic drugs or cyclo-oxygenase inhibitors. Plasma concentrations should be monitored, as a slowly rising through indicates that the dose is greater than the patient can eliminate. Toxicity is less if gentamicin is administered as a large bolus, rather than a slow infusion, as the high initial concentration saturates the uptake mechanism, and so rela-

Table 40.2 Factors Enhancing Gentamicin Nephrotoxicity

High total dose
Pre-existing renal disease
Liver disease
Being female
Advanced age
Critically ill
Volume depletion or dehydration
Hypocalcemia
Diuretic therapy
Metabolic acidosis
Cyclo-oxygenase inhibitors
Other nephrotoxic drugs

tively less of the dose is accumulated in the kidney. Bolus administration should be considered if therapeutic effectiveness will not be impaired. Dialysis can be used to remove (or administer) gentamicin.

Cephalosporin Antibiotics

The cephalosporins are active against most gram-positive cocci and many gram-negative bacilli, yet have little host toxicity. Therefore their use is increasing. Cephalosporins differ in degree of nephrotoxicity; cephaloridine is the most toxic, particularly if high doses are administered. Cephalothin, cephalexin, and cefamandole have all been reported to cause kidney damage, either after high doses or in patients with compromised renal function.

Cephaloridine toxicity is characterized by progressive azotemia and oliguria. There is tubular necrosis, with sloughing of the brush border and cast formation. Toxicity correlates with the renal cortical concentration of cephaloridine. Cephaloridine is accumulated actively in cells of the proximal tubules by the organic anion transport system; once in the cell, it tends to remain there. Cephaloridine is a zwitterion; it also has a positive charge, and therefore requires transport to leave the relatively electronegative intracellular fluid. Cephaloridine is a substrate for the organic cation transport system; however, only small amounts are transported out of cells.[14] Probenecid blockade of anion transport decreases cephaloridine nephrotoxicity.

Mitochondrial dysfunction and lipid peroxidation occur early in cephaloridine nephrotoxicity, and both have been considered as mechanisms of toxicity.[15] While there is much evidence that lipid peroxidation occurs after administration of cephaloridine, antioxidants did not protect against toxicity. Similarly, evidence for mitochondrial damage and impaired gluconeogenesis have been found in the initial stages of toxicity, but there are not sufficient data to conclude that either factor is responsible for the toxicity, and not an effect of the damage.

Cephaloridine nephrotoxicity is more likely with high doses (above 4–6 g/day) or if the dose is not adjusted for pre-existing renal function deficits. Older patients are more susceptible, as are those receiving other nephrotoxic agents or diuretics.

Cyclosporine A

Cyclosporine A is an eleven amino acid cyclic polypeptide synthesized by the fungus *Tolypocladium inflatum.* It is an an immunosuppressant with selective action against T-lymphocytes involved in the rejection process. Because of this selectivity, resistance to infectious agents is not compromised, and patients experience fewer and less severe episodes of infection with cyclosporine than with other broad acting immunosuppressive agents. Cyclosporine is more effective in preventing rejection than other immunosuppressants and use of cyclosporine has greatly improved the success of kidney, liver, heart, and bone marrow transplants. More recently, cyclosporine has been used in autoimmune disease.

Nephrotoxicity is the major, dose-limiting toxicity of cyclosporine.[16,17] In the initial period of cyclosporine therapy high doses were used, and both acute and chronic kidney damage were seen. The acute nephrotoxicity led to development of less toxic treatment protocols; nevertheless, nephrotoxicity appearing after weeks or months of treatment does occur in a significant number of patients.

Diminished kidney function or acute renal failure in the first weeks after transplant may occur from the effects of surgery on renal hemodynamics (especially in liver and kidney transplant patients), rejection of the kidney allograft, or cyclosporine nephrotoxicity. Differential diagnosis is difficult because decreases of GFR and effective renal plasma flow and increases of BUN and serum creatinine are signs of kidney failure common to all three factors. Intrarenal pressure increases in acute rejection, but not in nephrotoxicity or chronic rejection. Analysis of fine-needle aspirates for cells and cyclosporine deposits may be helpful.[18] Cyclosporine toxicity is likely if the trough concentration of cyclosporine in whole blood is greater than 800 ng/ml and unlikely if the concentration is less than 300 ng/ml. Whole blood measurements are used most frequently because red blood cells sequester plasma cyclosporine by a time-and temperature-dependent process.[19]

Chronic cyclosporine toxicity generally occurs after six months or more of therapy. There is persistent elevation of serum creatinine, often hypertension, but rarely proteinuria. Biopsy reveals mild to moderate and nonspecific glomerular lesions, arteriolopathy, interstitial fibrosis, and tubular atrophy. In one series, ischemic damage to the glomeruli preceded tubular atrophy; the pathology did not correlate with the reductions in GFR.[20] In a liver transplant series, mean serum creatinines had doubled after one year on cyclosporine; all patients had impaired renal perfusion after just two months on cyclosporine (trough levels between 200 and 800 ng/ml blood, generally between 300 and 400 ng/ml); and 66 percent of the 56 patients had become hypertensive. Kidney biopsies taken from eight patients on cyclosporine for one and one-half to four years showed little evidence of arteriole damage, whereas ischemic damage to the glomeruli and some tubular damage (insufficient to account for the glomerular damage) did occur.[21] Clearance of inulin, creatinine, and PAH are decreased, as is the ability to dilute urine in response to a water load. Sodium excretion may be normal, decreased, or increased. Decreased sodium excretion possibly may contribute to hypertension. Concurrent therapy with steroids also is implicated, because of mineralocorticoid effects. Hypertension occurs in all types of cyclosporine therapy.[r1] Stimulation of the renin-angiotensin-aldosterone system has been postulated to cause the hypertension; however, evidence is equivocal. More recently, cyclosporine therapy-associated hypertension has been related to sodium and volume retention.

Cyclosporine is metabolized, and some of the metabolites are measured by commercial radioimmunoassay (RIA). While RIA is the common method for analyzing cyclosporine in blood, the test gives values are higher than those by high pressure liquid chromatography, which is specific for cyclosporine. Toxicity correlates well with the RIA values for cyclosporine, suggesting that the metabolites also recognized by the RIA antibody are toxic to the kidney cells.[19] The role of metabolism in cyclosporine toxicity is not clear. It is possible that reactive metabolites are either formed in the kidney or accumulate there, contributing to the early acute renal failure of cyclosporine. In rats, phenobarbital induction of hepatic mixed function oxidase activity decreases plasma concentrations of cyclosporine (measured by HPLC techniques specific for cyclosporine) and acute tubular damage. Phenobarbital induction did improve survival of transplanted rats, compared to those receiving cyclosporine without phenobarbital induction, but did not improve the rate of survival or diminish the severity of histopathologic signs of chronic toxicity. These results suggest that metabolites of cyclosporine are involved in acute toxicity, but not in chronic toxicity, and therefore that the mechanisms are different in the two phases of toxicity.[22]

Vascular and hemodynamic effects of cyclosporine often are credited for playing a crucial role in the delayed, chronic toxicity, and the role of various endogenous mediators has been extensively examined. In cardiac transplant patients plasma renin activity increases after cyclosporine administration if the drug is given early after transplant—but not if cyclosporine therapy is delayed until four days after transplant. Cyclosporine administration causes increases of plasma renin activity in the first half-hour after its administration, and the increase of renal vascular resistance may increase susceptibility to ischemia and prevent transplanted kidneys from functioning.[23] Cyclosporine interferes with the release of endothelial derived relaxing factor from aorta.[24] Infusion of atrial natriuretic peptide improves renal plasma flow and glomerular filtration in renal transplant patients on cyclosporine.[25] Cyclosporine causes cultured endothelial cells to release endothelin, a potent vasoconstrictor,[26] and plasma endothlin is increased in patients on cyclosporine.[27] In experimental studies, pretreatment with an endothelin receptor antagonist prevented acute cyclosporine toxicity.[28] Calcium is involved in endothelin signal transduction. The ability of calcium antagonists to prevent or ameliorate cyclosporine toxicity[29,30] is consistent with a role for endothelin. Altering the balance of arachidonic acid metabolites, from vasodilation to vasoconstriction, also may play a role in cyclosporine nephrotoxicity. NSAIDs have been reported to augment the deterioration of filtration.[31] This interaction was attributed to decreasing the synthesis of vasodilatory prostaglandins, thus leaving vasoconstrictory influences unopposed.

Strategies for minimizing toxicity center on decreasing exposure of kidneys to cyclosporine. Maintaining trough blood concentrations below 250 ng/ml is recommended initially, tapering off to 80–200 ng/ml for the long-term phase.[19] In one series, 82 percent of acute rejection episodes had cyclosporine trough blood concentrations below 125 ng/ml. For renal allografts it may be beneficial to use conventional immunosuppression until the graft is functioning and then switch to cyclosporine. The cyclosporine dose should be lower in the perioperative period because excretion of cyclosporine is impaired by surgery. Frequent monitoring of blood trough levels is crucial for successful management of these patients. Cyclosporine is generally administered orally, in spite of erratic absorption, because of rare anaphylactic reactions upon IV administration.

AntiCancer Drugs

Renal toxicity, either acute or chronic, is a common occurrence in chemotherapy of cancer, and is the dose-limiting toxicity for some of these agents.[32,r2]

Cisplatin [cis-diamminedichloroplatinum II] is used to treat solid tumors, including tumors of the head and neck, urinary bladder, and cervix; and it is standard treatment for testicular and ovarian cancers. Nephrotoxicity was predicted from preclinical toxicology studies and was confirmed in early clinical studies to be dose-limiting. Recent efforts have focused on decreasing nephrotoxicity while maintaining therapeutic efficacy. Different approaches include modifying the dosing schedule and vehicle, coadministration of protective agents, and synthesizing non-nephrotoxic congeners of cisplatin.

Cisplatin exists in equilibrium between the chlorinated, nonionized species in high-chloride media, and dechlorinated, hydrated, ionized species in the low-chloride intracellular environment. The hydrated species is formed within cells and inhibits DNA synthesis. Cisplatin appears to be actively secreted into the tubular urine. The clearance of cisplatin exceeds that of inulin, and uptake of cisplatin by renal tissue can be blocked by drugs that are transported by the base transport system. In experimental animals given cisplatin, platinum is found in the kidneys, especially in the P3 segment of the proximal tubule.[33] Cisplatin generates superoxide anion and peroxide radicals. Superoxide dismutase can protect against toxicity, and quenching of superoxide toxicity may be part of mannitol's protection against cisplatin toxicity. Other radical scavenging agents are being tested for protection against nephrotoxicity. Cisplatin may be metabolized in kidney cells, as platinum in cells is not mutagenic but urinary platinum is mutagenic.

Signs of cisplatin nephrotoxicity are increases of blood urea nitrogen and plasma creatinine, and decreases of creatinine clearance. They generally occur within two to seven days of starting therapy. Tissue damage is seen as cortical swelling, congestion in the medulla, acute tubular necrosis with disruption of the brush border microvilli, and segmental necrosis in proximal and distal tubules. In electron micrographs, mitochondria are swollen and vacuolated and show signs of degeneration, the endoplasmic reticulum is dilated, and there are convolutions of the nuclear membrane. Proteinuria and casts of cellular debris are reported. Excretion of β-2-microglobulin and N-acetyl-β-D-glucosaminidase within 24 hour after cisplatin treatment have been reported as indicative of acute tubular damage, but neither is predictive for long-term renal damage.

Decreases of both GFR and effective renal plasma flow have been reported for humans as well as experimental animals. Indeed, a common criterion for nephrotoxicity in patients receiving cisplatin is a rise of plasma creatinine concentration, either above a fixed value or an allowable increase (i.e., 1 mg/dl) over pretreatment values. The role of hemodynamic factors for initiating the toxicity is the subject of debate. Studies of treatments with angiotensin converting enzyme inhibition and calcium channel blockade have both supported and refuted the hypothesis that hemodynamic factors are important for cisplatin toxicity. Tubular damage, expressed as excretion of lactate dehydrogenase (LDH) or γ-glutamyltranspeptidase (γ-GTP) in urine, was not prevented, but was reversible. A role for hemodynamic factors in the elaboration of cisplatin nephrotoxicity is not surprising, since hydration during therapy is also protective. Patients receiving cisplatin have elevated plasma and urinary endothelin,[34] consistent with the experimental observation that increases in renal vascular resistance occur early in cisplatin nephrotoxicity.[35] Administration of ANF or the ANF analogue A68828 is beneficial in established experimental cisplatin nephrotoxicity.[36]

Phase I and early Phase II studies with cisplatin showed therapeutic efficacy with substantial, and dose-limiting kidney toxicity. Subsequent studies focused on minimizing toxicity while maintaining therapeutic efficacy. Administering the same total dose divided over five days yielded less nephrotoxicity (and nausea and vomiting) without compromising antitumor activity. Initially the dose used was 100 mg/M^2; more recently, however, total doses of up to 250 mg/M^2 have been administered by infusion without nephrotoxicity. Vigorous hydration with half-normal saline (sometimes with dextrose) ranging from 1 to 6 L/d is protective. Hydration is sometimes combined with diuretics (either furosemide or mannitol) to insure adequate urine flow and is believed by some to be superior. Increasing the urine volume would effectively dilute the concentration of cisplatin in the kidney, and this would be expected to limit toxicity. High concentrations of chloride ion in hypertonic saline decrease formation of the hydrated species that can cross cell membranes and do damage to renal cells, yet the antitumor effectiveness of cisplatin is not impaired by hypertonic saline. Hypertonic saline does not change the pharmacokinetics of cisplatin, but the chloruresis does result in an increased urine volume. In a trial using the combination of methotrexate, 5-fluorouracil and cisplatin, however, hypertonic saline administration did not improve on adequate hydration with mannitol.

Other attempts to ameliorate cisplatin nephrotoxicity are based on the assumption that cisplatin toxicity is related to the platinum and its ability to bind to sulfhydryl groups, in analogy to the acute renal failure produced by heavy metals such as mercury. Administration of glutathione (an endogenous tripeptide with a free sulfhydryl group) prior to cisplatin protected against both transient nephrotoxicity and myelosuppression. The amelioration of nephrotoxicity was not better than that achieved with hydration, and higher doses were not used because of concern for antitumor efficacy.[37] The monoisopropyl ester of glutathione is also protective.[38] Thiosulfate provides short-term protection against cisplatin nephrotoxicity.[39] The sulfhydryl compound, WR-2721 (S-2-(3-aminoproplylamino)ethyl phosphorothioric acid), is protective against damage from radiation treatment and alkylating agents, and was tested for protection against cisplatin toxicity. There was transient nephrotoxicity at cisplatin doses ranging from 120 mg/M^2 to 150 mg/M^2, and the degree of protection was inversely related to the dose of cisplatin administered. Antitumor activity was not impaired, with objective responses to chemotherapy seen in 58 percent of all patients.[40] It is likely that the tumor cells were not able to accumulate WR-2721. In screening studies of sulfur-containing compounds, dimethyl sulfoxide, biotin, and sulfathiazole were found to protect against nephrotoxicity and did not impair anti-tumor effectiveness.[41,42] Probenecid blocks platinum accumulation in kidneys and protects against nephrotoxicity, again without impairing antitumor effectiveness.[43] Human trials confirmed the renal protection; as expected, ototoxicity and myelosuppression were not similarly protected.[44]

Carboplatin is a cisplatin analogue with cyclobutane groups substituted for the chlorine ligands. Carboplatin has less nephrotoxicity and emetic effects, but has myelosuppressive activity similar to cisplatin. Carboplatin is eliminated by the kidneys, and pre-existing kidney damage can allow carboplatin to accumulate to toxic concentrations.[39] The excretion of alanine aminopeptidase, N-acetyl-β-glucosaminidase, and total protein were greater after cisplatin therapy than after either carboplatin plus 5-fluorouracil or iproplatin (another cisplatin analogue). With carboplatin therapy, nephrotoxicity is seen at doses of 800 to 1600 mg/M^2, as a 25 to 50 percent reduction of GFR.[45]

Iproplatin [dichlorobis (isopropylamine) dihydroxyplatinum] is a cisplatin analogue that is not cross-resistant to cisplatin and has antitumor activity in cell lines comparable to that of cisplatin. Although adverse effects have been reported (myelosuppression, diarrhea, vomiting, and weight and hair loss), no nephrotoxicity was observed.[39]

Ifosfamide [(2-(bis-(2-chloroethyl)-amino-tetrahydro-2H-1,3,2-oxazaphosphorine-2-oxide] and cyclophosphamide are oxazophosphorine compounds that are metabolized in vivo to alkylating agents. The difference between cyclophosphamide and ifosfamide is the location of the second chloroethyl group: on the ring nitrogen for ifosfamide; on the amino nitrogen for cyclophosphamide. Both agents undergo hydroxylation of the carbon in position 4, followed by spontaneous formation of acrolein and a nitrogen mustard; for both, the primary dose-limiting toxicity is cystitis (both micro-and macrohemoglobinuria are seen). This toxicity is due to formation of acrolein within the kidney and bladder and can be prevented by administration of mesna (2-mercapto-ethane sulfonate sodium).[46] In contrast, the renal effects of cyclophosphamide and ifosfamide are quite different.

Cyclophosphamide causes a short-lived (less than one day) impairment of water excretion, manifested as decreased urine flow, high urine osmolality, hyponatremia, and weight gain.[r3] There is no proteinuria or impairment of creatinine clearance. The decreased urine flow occurs simultaneously with appearance of cyclophosphamide metabolites in urine, and is not related to stimulation of vasopressin release. Patients undergoing high-dose cyclophosphamide treatment are hydrated with saline before and during treatment. Hydration is necessary to decrease the incidence of hemorrhagic cystitis and to prevent hyperkalemia. The latter may occur if intracellular potassium is released by rapid tumor lysis. Hydration is needed to prevent formation of stone from uric acid and xanthine products.

Ifosfamide causes nephrotoxicity[r4] similar to adult Fanconi syndrome. Without mesna treatment, ifosfamide causes polyuria, glucosuria, proteinuria, and phosphaturia. Creatinine clearance decreases over several days and then recovers, whereas ability to concentrate urine (in response to dehydration or administered vasopressin) does not recover. Mesna treatment that prevents hemorrhagic cystitis is not adequate to prevent renal injury. In pediatric patients, tubular toxicity, measured as excretion of alanine aminopeptidase, N-acetyl-β-glucosaminidase, and protein, was seen in all patients after a five-day course of treatment with ifosfamide and mesna. The renal toxicity was reversible (enzymuria and proteinuria generally recovered), and none of the patients had elevations of serum creatinine of more than 0.1 mg/dl above pretreatment values three weeks after the treatment course. Ifosfamide is excreted in urine unchanged, and patients who have had cisplatin treatment with enzymuria indicative of nephrotoxicity have increased neuro- and hepatotoxicity.

Nitrosourea compounds used in cancer chemotherapy are streptozocin (formerly designated as streptozotocin), carmustine (BCNU), lomustine (CCNU) and semustine (methylCCNU). Renal toxicity occurs with carmustine, lomustine, and semustine only after high total doses, and then months to years after the last treatment course.[47] In contrast, streptozocin toxicity occurs after initial treatment.

Streptozocin is effective against pancreatic islet cell carcinoma, causing measurable decreases in tumor size as well as reductions of insulin secretion. It has the advantage of not being toxic to the hematopoietic system. Renal toxicity is the dose-limiting side-effect, and occurs in 30 to 60 percent of patients (in the first Phase I trial, all 18 patients developed renal tubular disease). The symptoms are those of adult Fanconi syndrome: proteinuria; glucosuria; phosphaturia; decreased creatinine clearance; elevated BUN and serum creatinine; and hypophosphatemia and osteomalacia. The toxicity usually is reversible, but becomes more severe and sometimes irreversible with continued treatment or high doses. Damage to proximal convoluted tubules, collecting duct, tubular atrophy, and interstitial inflammatory infiltrates and glomerular tufting have been seen. Between 10 and 20 percent of the dose is excreted in the urine as streptozocin. Urinary excretion of the drug is greatest in the first hour after administration, and it is likely that the presence of the parent compound in urine is crucial for toxicity. Unfortunately, therapeutic regimens to decrease nephrotoxicity have not been developed for streptozocin as they have been for other agents.

With the other nitrosoureas, nephrotoxicity is delayed after treatment and generally is not apparent until the cumulative dose exceeds 1.4 g/m^2; since few patients have survived long enough to reach that high a cumulative dose, nephrotoxicity is not seen commonly. The toxicity is seen as increased serum creatinine and urea nitrogen and decreased clearances of creatinine, inulin, and *p*-aminohippurate. The kidneys appear small. The failure is often, but not always, progressive, and patients may require dialysis. Ten per cent of patients in an early trial with carmustine experienced increases of BUN that could not be explained by other disease factors; in a study of nitrosourea nephrotoxicity, four patients who had received high doses of carmustine had chronic renal disease similar to that seen after semustine.

Radiocontrast Agents

Acute renal failure or insufficiency after radiologic examinations using contrast agents is not common; nevertheless, it is a significant cause of hospital-acquired renal insufficiency. In the past it was chiefly associated with IV doses of contrast agents for urography; more recently, procedures for computerized tomography and digital angiography use the highest doses of contrast agents. Acute renal failure is rare after cholecystographic agents and with the new nonionic contrast agents (iohexol, iopamidol, iopromide).

Contrast media-induced renal damage can be classified as either mild, nonoliguric dysfunction, or severe, oliguric renal failure. For both, the initial signs of renal impairment occur between 24 to 48 hours after the examination. Typically there is a diuresis of the osmotic load in the first hours after administration of the contrast agents. In mild renal dysfunction, peak increases of serum creatinine occur between three and five days, and patients recover within 10 to 14 days. In contrast, patients who develop severe renal failure become oliguric 24 to 48 hours after the examination and remain so for two to five days, the oliguria usually ending with spontaneous diuresis. In these patients, the peak increase of serum creatinine occurs between five and ten days, and recovery occurs between two and three weeks. Some of these patients require dialysis to correct azotemia and water and electrolyte imbalances. Biopsies from patients who did not develop renal insufficiency had vacuolization of the cytoplasm of epithelial cells and patchy tubule cell necrosis, with no involvement of the glomeruli or distal structures. Patients with renal failure had frank proximal tubular necrosis and atrophy and interstitial edema. The pattern of damage is similar to that of other tubular toxicants.

The histopathology observed in patients who did not develop renal failure is similar to the osmotic nephrosis that occurs after administration of hypertonic solutions. Hypertonic solutions and contrast agents initially increase blood flow to the kidneys; this delivers a large load of hyperosmolar fluid to the tubule, which decreases water reabsorption and, by increasing hydrostatic pressure within the kidney, decreases glomerular filtration. Vasoconstriction, perhaps mediated by activation of the renin-angiotensin system, contributes to decreases of GFR. Hypertonic iothalamate increases renal vascular resistance when added to the isolated perfused kidney preparation.[48] A role for tubular obstruction also has been suggested. Contrast agents are able to bind to and precipitate proteins, forming casts that can obstruct the tubule. Thus, the presence of abnormal amounts of protein in urine, as occurs in multiple myeloma and other diseases, increases the likelihood of cast formation. The concentrations of uric acid and oxalate in urine are increased by the contrast agent, and crystals of either may contribute to tubular obstruction. In oliguric renal failure the fractional excretion of sodium is low,

Table 40.3 Factors Enhancing Contrast Agent Nephrotoxicity

Dehydration
Diabetes mellitus
Multiple myeloma
Advanced age
Diuretic therapy
Renal insufficiency
Hyperuricemia
Radiocontrast within 24 hr
Proteinuria
Large dose
Hepatic disease

consistent with tubular obstruction. Contrast agents may also be cytotoxic, interfering with basic metabolic processes within the cells. Calcium antagonists can prevent or ameliorate contrast agent-induced nephrotoxicity.[49]

The risk of contrast agent-induced acute renal failure is greatly increased by pre-existing renal insufficiency and diabetes mellitus. In various studies, the percentage of patients responding with renal failure (most often assessed as an increase of serum creatinine, but occasionally by decreased creatinine clearance) increased with decreased glomerular filtration. In some, but not all, studies, patients with diabetes mellitus have had an even greater response. Other risk factors are given in Table 40.3. It is important that dehydration be avoided, even though it may improve contrast, and that high doses be avoided. Three days should be allowed between examinations, as some patients will have subclinical damage; if renal failure occurs, there should be complete recovery before repeat administration of a contrast agent.

References

Reading List

Brenner BM, Lazarus JM (Eds). Acute renal failure. New York: Churchill Livingstone, 1988.

Bibliography

1. Toto RD. The role of prostaglandins in NSAID induced renal dysfunction. J Rheumatol 1991;*18* Suppl 28:22–25.
2. Toto RD, Anderson SA, Brown-Cartwright D, Kokko JP, Brater DC. Effects of acute and chronic dosing of NSAIDs in patients with renal insufficiency. Kid Int 1986;*30*:760–768.
3. Perazella MA, Buller GK. Can ibuprofen cause acute renal failure in a normal individual? A case of acute overdose. Am J Kidney Dis 1991;*18*:600–602.
4. Kher K, Makker S. Acute renal failure due to acetaminophen ingestion without concurrent hepatotoxicity. Am J Med 1987;*82*:1280–1281.
5. Davenport A, Finn R. Paracetamol (acetaminophen) poisoning resulting in acute renal failure without hepatic coma. Nephron 1989;*50*:55–56.
6. Eisenberg JM, Koffer H, Glick RA, Connell ML, Loss LE, Talbot GH, Shusterman NH, Strom BL. What is the cost of nephrotoxicity associated with aminoglycosides? Ann Intern Med 1987;*107*:900–909.
7. Trollfors B, Alestig K, Krantz I, Norrby R. Quantitative nephrotoxicity of gentamicin in nontoxic doses. J Infect Dis 1980;*141*:306–309.
8. Giurgea-Marion L, Toubeau G, Laurent G, Heuson-Stiennon JA, Tulkens PM. Impairment of lysosomepinocytic vesicle fusion in rat kidney proximal tubules after treatment with gentamicin at low doses. Toxicol Appl Pharmacol 1986;*86*:271–285.
9. Houghton DC, Campbell-Boswell MV, Bennett WM, Porter GA, Brooks RE. Myeloid bodies in the renal tubules of humans: relationship to gentamicin therapy. Clin Nephrol 1978;*10*:140–145.
10. Walker PD, Shah SV. Evidence suggesting a role for hydroxyl radical in gentamicin-induced acute renal failure in rats. J Clin Invest 1988;*81*:334–341.
11. Elliott WC, Patchin DS, Jones DB. Effect of parathyroid hormone activity on gentamicin nephrotoxicity. J Lab Clin Med 1987;*109*:48–54.
12. Ernest S. Model of gentamicin-induced nephrotoxicity and its amelioration by calcium and thyroxine. Medical Hypotheses 1989;*30*:195–202.
13. Smith CR, Moore RD, Lietman PS. Studies of risk factors for aminoglycoside nephrotoxicity. Am J Kidney Dis 1986;*8*:308–313.
14. Williams PD, Hitchcook MJM, Hottendorf GH. Effect of cephalosporins on organic ion transport in renal membrane vesicles from rat and rabbit kidney cortex. Res Commun Chem Pathol Pharmacol 1985;*47*:357–371.
15. Goldstein RS, Smith PF, Tarloff JB, Contardi L, Rush GF, Hook JB. Biochemical mechanisms of cephaloridine nephrotoxicity. Life Sci 1988;*42*:1809–1816.
16. Kahan BD. Cyclosporine nephrotoxicity: Pathogenesis, prophylaxis, therapy, and prognosis. Am J Kidney Dis 1986;*8*:323–331.
17. Myers BD, Ross J, Newton L, Luetscher J, Perlroth M. Cyclosporine-associated chronic nephropathy. N Engl J Med 1984;*311*:699–705.
18. Salaman JR. Diagnosis of cyclosporine nephrotoxicity. Mt Sinai J Med 1987;*54*:457–459.
19. Moyer TP, Post GR, Sterioff S, Anderson CF. Cyclosporine nephrotoxicity is minimized by adjusting drug dosage on the basis of drug concentration in blood. Mayo Clinic Proc 1988;*63*:241–247.
20. Dische FE, Neuberger J, Keating J, Parsons V, Calne RY, Williams R. Kidney pathology in liver allograft recipients after long-term treatment with cyclosporin A. Lab Invest 1988;*58*:395–402.
21. Wheatley HC, Datzman M, Williams JW, Miles DE, Hatch FE. Long-term effects of cyclosporine on renal function in liver transplant recipients. Transplantation 1987;*43*:641–647.
22. Duncan JI, Heys SD, Thomson AW, Simpson JG, Whiting PH. Influence of the hepatic drug-metabolizing enzyme-inducer phenobarbitone on cyclosporine nephrotoxicity and hepatotoxicity in renal-allografted rats. Transplantation 1988;*45*:693–697.
23. Schuler S, Thomas D, Hetzer R. Cyclosporine A-related nephrotoxicity after cardiac transplantation: The role of plasma renin activity. Transplant Proc 1987;*19*:3998–4001.
24. Balligand JL, Godfraind T. Endothelium-derived relaxing factor and muscle-derived relaxing factor in rat aorta: Action of

cyclosporine A. J Cardiovasc Pharmacol 1991;*17* Suppl 3:S213–S221.

25. Lang CC, Henderson IS, Mactier R, Stewart WK, Struthers AD. Atrial natriuretic factor improves renal function and lowers systolic blood pressure in renal allograft recipients treated with cyclosporin A. J Hypertens 1992;*10*:483–488.

26. Bunchman TE, Brookshire CA. Cyclosporine-induced synthesis of endothelin by cultured human endothelial cells. J Clin Invest 1991;*88*:310–314.

27. Deray G, Carayon A, Le Hoang P. Increased endothelin level after cyclosporine therapy. Ann Intern Med 1991;*114*:809.

28. Fogo A, Hellings SE, Inagami T, Kon V. Endothelin receptor antagonism is protective in in vivo acute cyclosporine toxicity. Kidney Int 1992;*42*:770–774.

29. Morales JM, Andres A, Rodriguez Paternina E, Alcazar JM, Montoyo C, Rodicio JL. Calcium antagonist therapy prevents chronic cyclosporine nephrotoxicity after renal transplantation: A prospective study. Transplant Proc 1992;*24*:89–91.

30. Rooth P, Dawidson I, Diller K, Taljedal IB. Protection against cyclosporine-induced impairment of renal microcirculation by verapamil in mice. Transplantation 1988;*45*:433–437.

31. Erman A, Chen-Gal B, Rosenfeld J. The role of eicosanoids in cyclosporine nephrotoxicity in the rat. Biochem Pharmacol 1989;*38*:2153–2157.

32. Ries F, Klastersky J. Nephrotoxicity induced by cancer chemotherapy with special emphasis on cisplatin toxicity. Am J Kidney Dis 1986;*5*:368–379.

33. Safirstein R, Winston J, Goldstein M, Moel D, Dikman S, Guttenplan J. Cisplatin nephrotoxicity. Am J Kidney Dis 1986;*8*:356–367.

34. Ohta K, Hirata Y, Shichiri M, Ichioka M, Kubota T, Marumo F. Cisplatin-induced urinary endothelin excretion. JAMA 1991;*265*:1391–1392.

35. Winston JA, Safirstein R. Reduced renal blood flow in early cisplatin-induced acute renal failure in the rat. Am J Physiol (Renal, Fluid Electrolyte Physiol) 1985;*249*:F490–F496.

36. Pollock DM, Holst M, Opgenorth TJ. Effect of the ANF analog A68828 in cisplatin-induced acute renal failure. J Pharmacol Exp Ther 1991;*257*:1179–1183.

37. Oriana S, Bohm S, Spatti G, Zunio F, Di Re F. A preliminary clinical experience with reduced glutathione as protector against cisplatin-toxicity. Tumori 1987;*73*:337–340.

38. Anderson ME, Naganuma A, Meister A. Protection against cisplatin toxicity by administration of glutathione ester. FASEB Journal 1990;*4*:3251–3255.

39. Fuks JZ, Wadler S, Wiernik PH. Phase I and II agents in cancer therapy: two cisplatin analogues and high-dose cisplatin in hypertonic saline or with thiosulfate protection. J Clin Pharmacol 1987;*27*:357–365.

40. Glover D, Glick JH, Weiler C, Fox K, Turrisi A, Kligerman MM. Phase I/II trials of WR-2721 and cis-platinum. Int J Radiat Oncol Biol Phys 1986;*12*:1509–1512.

41. Jones MM, Basinger MA, Holscher MA. Control of the nephrotoxicity of cisplatin by clinically used sulfur-containing compounds. Fund Appl Toxicol 1992;*18*:181–188.

42. Jones MM, Basinger MA, Field L, Holscher MA. Coadministration of dimethyl sulfoxide reduces cisplatin nephrotoxicity. Anticancer Res 1991;*11*:1939–1942.

43. Ross DA, Gale GR. Reduction of the renal toxicity of cis-dichlorodiammineplatinum(II) by probenecid. Cancer Treatment Reports 1979;*63*:781–787.

44. Jacobs C, Kaubisch S, Halsey J, Lum BL, Gosland M, Coleman CN, Sikic BI. The use of probenecid as a chemoprotector against cisplatin nephrotoxicity. Cancer 1991;*67*:1518–1524.

45. Gore ME, Calvert AH, Smith LE. High dose carboplatin in the treatment of lung cancer and mesothioloma: a phase I dose escalation study. Eur J Cancer Clin Oncol 1987;*23*:1391–1397.

46. Brock N, Stekar J, Pohl J, Neimeyer U, Scheffler G. Acrolein, the causative factor of urotoxic side-effects of cyclophosphamide, ifosfamide, trofosfamide and sufosfamide. Arzneimittel-Forschung Drug Research 1973;*29*:659–663.

47. Weiss RB, Posada JG, Kramer RA, Boyd MR. Nephrotoxicity of semustine. Cancer Treatment Reports 1983;*67*:1105–1112.

48. Haylor JL, El Sayed AA, El Nahas AM, Morcos SK. The effect of sodium iothalamate on the vascular resistance of the isolated perfused rat kidney. Br J Radiol 1991;*64*:50–54.

49. Neumayer H-H, Junge W, Kufner A, Wenning A. Prevention of radiocontrast-media-induced nephrotoxicity by the calcium channel blocker nitrendipine: A prospective randomised clinical trial. Nephrol Dial Transplant 1989;*4*:1030–1036.

50. Mann JFE, Goerig M, Brune K, Luft FC. Ibuprofen as an over-the-counter drug: Is there a risk for renal injury. Clin Nephrol 1993;*39*:1–6.

Reviews

r1. Weidle PJ, Vlasses PH. Systemic hypertension associated with cyclosporine: A review. Drug Intell Clin Pharm 1988;*22*:443–451.

r2. Weiss RB, Poster DS. The renal toxicity of cancer chemotherapeutic agents. Cancer Treat Rev 1982;*9*:37–56.

r3. DeFronzo RA, Colvin OM, Braine H, Robertson GL, Davis PJ. Cyclophosphamide and the kidney. Cancer 1974;*33*:483–491.

r4. Brade WP, Herdrich K, Varini M. Ifosfamide-pharmacology, safety and therapeutic potential. Cancer Treat Rev 1985;*12*:1–47.

SECTION VI

Pharmacology of Hormones and Reproduction

Editor:
Paul L. Munson

Associate Editors:
Ranjit Roy Chaudhury
Irving M. Spitz

CHAPTER 41

Insulin, Glucagon, and Oral Hypoglycemic Agents in the Treatment of Diabetes Mellitus

Ethan A. H. Sims
Jorge Calles-Escandon

Insulin, a polypeptide produced and secreted by the beta cells of the pancreatic islets of Langerhans, is an essential hormone for normal growth, development, and metabolism. Insulin is especially important for the metabolism of carbohydrates, but is equally essential for metabolism of protein and fat. Glucagon is another hormone of the islets of Langerhans; it is produced by the alpha cells. In contrast to the hypoglycemic effect of insulin, glucagon increases plasma glucose, mainly by increasing hepatic glucose production.

Diabetes mellitus encompasses a group of serious disorders caused mainly either by a primary deficiency of insulin or by resistance to the actions of insulin combined with a relative deficiency of insulin. The sole therapeutic use of insulin is for the treatment of patients with diabetes in whom there is absolute deficiency of insulin or in whom relative deficiency cannot be corrected by measures to reduce insulin resistance or to increase the secretion of insulin. The principal therapeutic use of glucagon is acutely to correct serious insulin-reduced hypoglycemia in patients with diabetes.

The oral hypoglycemic agents are used in the treatment of diabetes that is associated with insulin resistance and cannot be managed by nonpharmacologic means. Two main types are in general use. The sulfonylureas act mainly by increasing insulin secretion by the pancreatic islets and may reduce insulin resistance directly or indirectly by reducing the effects of elevated glucose and free fatty acids. The biguanides are antihyperglycemic and increase the receptor and postreceptor actions within tissues targeted by insulin. They do not increase insulin secretion.

There can be no simple rules for the treatment of a condition as heterogeneous as diabetes, and for which treatment must vary so greatly according to the subtypes, stages of development, and associated complications.

Insulin

Insulin, the peptide hormone secreted by the beta-cells, was at first solely derived from animal pancreases, but is now also obtainable in human form by recombinant DNA technology.

Chemistry and Biosynthesis

Insulin is derived from preproinsulin. As depicted in Figure 41.1, the DNA-controlling synthesis of preproinsulin is located in chromosome 11 (short arm). Preproinsulin includes a "signal sequence" of 23 amino acids that is cleaved during the transport from its site of synthesis to the secretory granule, yielding proinsulin as a product that is packed into secretory granules. This is the immediate precursor of secreted insulin and includes the A and B chains and the connecting 31-residue C-peptide in a single polypeptide chain (Fig. 41.2). Once within the granule, proinsulin is cleaved to yield insulin and the C-peptide fragment. The A-chain of the insulin is composed of 21 amino acids and the B-chain of 30 amino acids; they are linked by disulfide bonds between cysteine residues. Both insulin and C-peptide are secreted into the portal vein on an equimolar basis. Their catabolic routes differ, however, in that almost 50 percent of the insulin is removed by the liver on the first pass, while C-

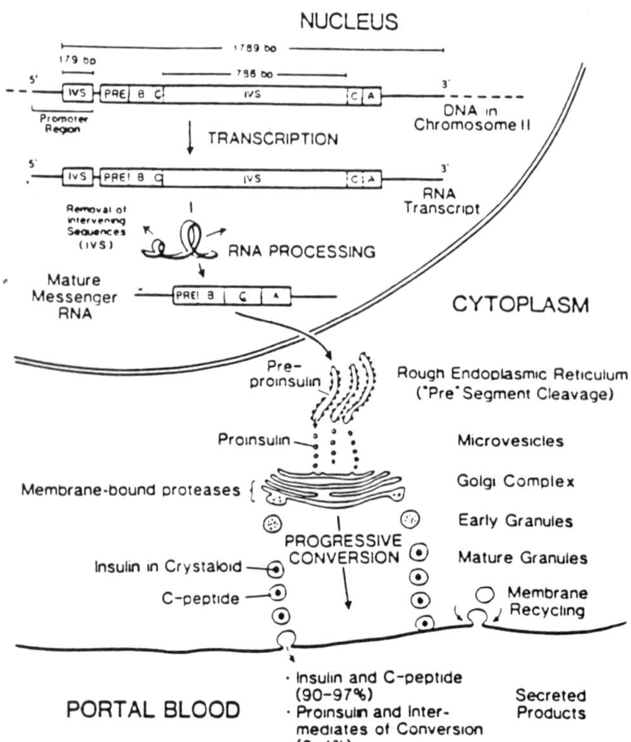

Figure 41.1 The biosynthesis of insulin in the pancreatic beta cell. IVS denotes intervening segment or intron; Pre, prepeptide segment or "signal peptide"; B, C, and A are peptide segments of the proinsulin; and bp, base pairs. The C-peptide is cosecreted with insulin. (From Robbins, DC, Tager HS, Rubenstein AH. New Eng J Med 1984; *310*:1165–75, with permission.)

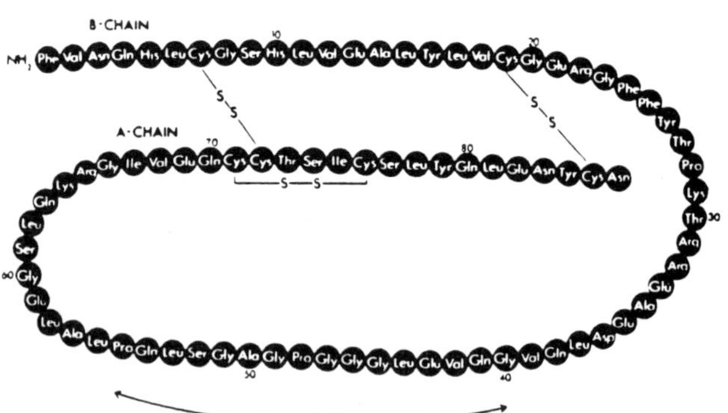

Figure 41.2. The Structure of proinsulin and its cleavage to insulin. The connecting C-peptide is freed when two basic amino acids are removed from the ends of its chair when it is cosecreted with insulin. Since it is not removed from the circulation on its passage through the liver, it serves as an index of insulin secretion. See text for structural differences in the A chain between animal and human insulins. (From Steiner DR Diabetes, vol 26. 1976. Copyright 1976 by the American Diabetes Assn. Reprinted with permission).

peptide is not extracted. In the presence of zinc, both proinsulin and endogenous and exogenous insulins form stable hexamers. The insulin derived from porcine pancreas differs in structure from the human only in having an alanine rather than threonine in the terminal amino acid in position 30 of the B chain. Beef insulin differs in the 8 and 10 positions of the A-chain in having alanine and valine in place of threonine and isoleucine. Fish insulins may be an alternative for those with immune reactions to human insulin.

The **Insulin unit** is based on the hypoglycemic effect in fasted rabbits. The potency of a specific insulin solution in units/ml is determined by bioassay in comparison with the USP or International (WHO) standard, which is a mixture of purified bovine and porcine insulins and contains 24 units/mg. Pure human insulin contains 25–30 units/mg.

Radioimmunoassay methods are available for measurement of plasma insulin, proinsulin, and C-peptide.

Insulin-like Growth Factors (IGF) are a closely related group of peptides, of which two, IGF-I and IGF-II, have been sequenced.[r1] They are homologous to proinsulin and are produced in many tissues. Originally termed somatomedins, they apparently mediate the mitogenic action of growth hormone and have some actions in common with insulin. Their receptors are related to that for insulin, and each has at least low affinity for its counterpart.

The Discovery of Insulin[r2]

The involvement of the pancreas in diabetes mellitus was demonstrated 100 years ago in Germany by Minkowski and von Mering in a series of definitive experiments in dogs.[r3] Langerhans discovered the insulin-producing islets named after him, but he confused them with lymph glands, and it was not until 1901 that Opie at Johns Hopkins suggested that the islets were the source of insulin. Early attempts at isolation of insulin failed, since the proteoloytic enzymes of the crude pancreatic extracts destroyed the peptide. In 1920, Banting, a young surgeon back from World War I, read an article in a surgical journal that sparked his imagination. It described a patient with atrophy of the pancreas from a ductal stone, who nonetheless suffered no damage to the pancreatic islets. During the summer of 1920, he and a medical student, Charles Best, at the University of Toronto obtained permission from the eminent Professor Macleod to attempt isolation of the pancreatic "hypoglycaemic factor" after ligation of the duct. J. B. Collip, a skillful biochemist from Alberta, joined the team and simplified the procedure by precipitating the crude extracts of ordinary pancreas with alcohol, which inactivates the degrading enzymes, and prepared the insulin that was first used to treat a person with diabetes. Insulin was crystallized by John Jacob Abel in 1926, and the amino acid sequence of bovine insulin was established by F. Sanger in 1960. Its three-dimensional structure was delineated by Hodgkin and coworkers in 1971. Production of human insulin by cloning of recombinant DNA in E. coli was accomplished by B. H. Frank and R. E. Chance in 1983.

Certain regions of both chains have been conserved over the past 500 million years of evolution and are common to insulins of insects, fish, and philosophers.[r4]

The Regulation of Secretion and Mechanism of Action of Insulin

The insulin-producing beta cells constitute 60 per cent of the pancreatic islets. Alpha-cells producing glucagon, delta-cells producing somatostatin, and F-cells producing pancreatic polypeptide are in close juxtaposition and are interconnected by gap junctions serving as low-resistance pathways that permit paracrine communication. However, it is not only the juxtaposition that allows this communication and coordination. The microvascular pattern of the islet is such that insulin flowing from the beta cells to the periphery exerts restraint on glucagon secretion by the alpha cells. As a result, inappropriate glucagon secretion occurs when beta cells are inhibited or destroyed.

Glucose serves as the major stimulus for insulin release and as the only promotor of its synthesis via translation of mRNA. Amino acids, particularly arginine and lysine, as well as free fatty acids and ketones, potentiate the effect of glucose in stimulating insulin secretion.[r5,1] Intravenous injection of glucose gives a peak release of insulin within 1–2 minutes (first phase), followed by a more sustained secretion (second phase). During a third phase, insulin concentration decreases, even though hyperglycemia persists. Diminution of the first-phase release is a characteristic of the early stages of the development of both main types of diabetes. When the first phase is blocked experimentally, disposal of glucose by nonoxidative routes is impaired, as is the increase in metabolic rate normally associated with a meal.[2] Basal insulin secretion is pulsatile, and early in the development of subtypes of diabetes involving insulin deficiency both the first phase secretion and the pulsatile quality are diminished or lost.[3]

The Regulation of Insulin Secretion and Its Metabolism

How glucose leads to release of insulin from the beta cell is not yet entirely clear, since its effect is both increased and decreased by many factors not yet fully understood.[r5] Glucokinase, a key enzyme of glucose metabolism in beta cells and in hepatocytes, has been proposed as a key regulator of insulin secretion.[r6,r7] Glocuse is readily transported into the beta cell or liver by GLUT-2 at a rate that reflects the extracellular concentration. There are genetic abnormalities in this enzyme in one kindred of the so-called maturity-onset diabetes of youth that explains the defective insulin secretion and mild hyperglycemia.[4] Following the activation of the kinase it is believed that glucose metabolism induces activation of membrane phospholipases, rapid turnover of phosphoinositides, and accumulation of inositol triphosphate (IP_3), arachidonic acid, and diacylglycerol. The first two mediators mobilize Ca^{++} stored in the endoplasmic reticulum, increasing intracellular Ca^{++} and activating calmodulin-dependent protein kinases. There is recent evidence that cyclic ADP-ribose generated in islets from glucose stimulation may be the predominant second messenger for mobilization of calcium and insulin release.[5] These phosphorylated proteins in the cytoskeleton lead to the extrusion of the secretory granules, which contain the C-peptide and the insulin, as well as amylin. Diacylglycerol activates protein kinase C, which may have a larger role in second- than first-phase insulin release. The metabolic products of glucose, particularly glucose-6-phosphate, may be the inhibiting signals, triggering sequestration of Ca^{++}. Amino acids in a pure protein meal stimulate insulin release, but less strongly than a meal of carbohydrate. In this condition, stimulation of glucagon secretion counteracts the hypoglycemic effect of the secreted insulin.

The CNS and the autonomic nervous system exert control over mechanisms involving carbohydrate metabolism in the liver, pancreas, and adrenal gland.[r8,r9] Alpha-receptor stimulation by epinephrine or norepinephrine in response to various stresses inhibits insulin secretion, whereas beta-2-receptor stimulation, as by isoproterenol, stimulates insulin release, possibly via cyclic AMP, as a second messenger. Vagal stimulation increases the release of insulin, and this effect can be blocked by atropine. Cholecystokinin also stimulates insulin secretion in the presence of adequate glucose. This and the vagal effect may be mediated by acetylcholine, with associated changes in flux of Ca^{++} and of K^+.

It is noteworthy that the hypothalamic center for autonomic control of insulin secretion is located near the centers related to hunger and satiety, and also that there are hepatic sensors for glucose in the liver, which serve an afferent limb to the CNS.[r8] Changes in the secretion of insulin in response to feast or famine directly affect these centers of the brain and affect intake of food. Conversely, the sight of appetizing food can stimulate an increase in insulin secretion, and this in turn can lower blood glucose and increase appetite.[r10]

A host of GI phenomena alert the pancreas to ingestion of food via release of enteric hormones and stimulate or inhibit insulin release via the entero-insular axis. The major stimulants are the glucose-dependent insulinotropic polypeptide from the small bowel and the newly-defined glucagon-like insulinotropic peptide, GLIP. Their action may explain why oral glucose gives a greater insulin response than does IV glucose. A new and possibly important player on this crowded field of neuropeptides is gelanin, which is widely distributed in the nervous system and acts directly at the pancreatic beta-cells to inhibit glucose-stimulated release of insulin, and may mediate adrenergic and stress-related inhibition of insulin secretion.[r11]

Islet amyloid polypeptide (IAPP or AMYLIN) has stimulated much interest as a possible modifier of insulin action in predominantly insulin-resistant diabetes.[r12,r13] It was isolated in 1976 from the pancreatic islet deposits of amyloid, which are prominent in this type of diabetes in humans. It is cosecreted with insulin, and in rats physiologic concentrations of synthetic human amylin inhibit glycogenolysis and gluconeogenesis and reduce glucose oxidation via the hexose monophosphate shunt.[6] Clamp studies involving infusion of amylin to yield probably superphysiologic concentrations indicate increased insulin resistance in rats,[7] and in dogs.[8] This could serve as a moderator of insulin secretion and action. However, production in healthy volunteers of plasma concentrations believed to be physiologic failed to show any acute effect on IV glucose tolerance.[9]

Many counter-regulatory hormones also have important effects on insulin secretion. GIP, CCK, and GLP-1, VIP, and acetylcholine in response to feeding stimulate insulin release. Stress-induced increase of epinephrine, norepinephrine, and galanin act directly on the pancreas to inhibit insulin secretion. Growth hormone increases peripheral insulin resistance and indirectly causes oversecretion of insulin. The physiologic insulin resistance of pregnancy is produced by the increase in placental lactogen and in the sex hormones progesterone and estrogen, along with free cortisol in the serum.

The Metabolic Fate of Endogenous Insulin[r14]

Half of the insulin in the portal blood is extracted on the first pass through the liver. It circulates in the blood stream as a monomer with a half-life of approximately 5–8 minutes in persons with normal glucose tolerance or uncomplicated diabetes. About 30 per cent is cleared from the blood by the kidney, and the remainder by bowel, muscle, and adipose tissue following binding to its cellular receptor. Only 3–4 per cent of the beta-cell secretion is in the form of uncleaved proinsulin, but because of a half-life six times longer than insulin, it may account for up to 30 percent of insulin immunoreactivity in the serum. On a molar basis, however, it exerts only about 8 per cent of the biologic action of insulin. When the pancreatic islets are stimulated by hyperglycemia and nearing exhaustion, or during other states of metabolic imbalance such as hypokalemia, they secrete a higher proportion of proinsulin.[r5] Surprisingly, it appears that the C-peptide cleaved from proinsulin is apparently not inert, since on short-term infusion it stimulates glucose utilization and also tends to correct the increased glomerular filtration rate of patients deficient in insulin and C-peptide.[10] Since the C-peptide cosecreted with insulin is minimally cleared by the liver, its concentration in plasma provides a useful index of insulin secretion. The ratio of C-peptide to fasting or stimulated glucose in the plasma serves as an indication of insulin resistance or deficiency.[r15]

The Effects and Mechanisms of Action of Insulin

The main physiologic effects of insulin are: (1) increased entry of glucose into insulin-sensitive cells such as myocytes, hepatocytes, and adipocytes; (2) decreased output of glucose as a result of increase in glycogen synthesis in liver by stimulation of glycogen synthase, and decrease in glycogenolysis and gluconeogenesis. Additional actions are increasing entry of amino acids into cells, promoting lipogenesis, and inhibiting proteolysis and lipolysis. Thus, anabolism, growth, and storage of metabolic fuels are all favored by its actions.

Clarification of the molecular mechanisms and messengers involved in the multiple actions of insulin are beginning to provide exciting opportunities for understanding and classification and for intervention in the two main types of diabetes.[r16,r17,r18]

The successive stages of insulin action and its functions are outlined in Figure 41.3. They include relatively rapid stimulation of glucose transport, and the less rapid effects on enzymes affecting carbohydrates and maintenance of extra- and intracellular ion gradients, the activity of lipoprotein lipase, and lipid and apolipoprotein metabolism.[r19] As pointed out recently,[r20] we tend to emphasize the sweet carbohydrate aspects of insulin action at the expense of its effect on lipids.

The long-term effects of insulin seen hours after its administration are dependent on nuclear messenger RNA synthesis and lead to protein and glycogen synthesis and cell growth. For a cell to respond to insulin, it must have the insulin receptor on its surface. The receptor is a dimer derived from a proreceptor and has extracellular, intramembranous, and intracellular domains. After insulin binds to the extracellular alpha unit, the protein tyrosine kinase, which is an intracellular extension of the beta unit, is activated by autophosphorylation.

The activated protein tyrosine kinase is essential for insulin action.[r16] An important role of the tyrosine kinase is activation of other enzymes that make available the more recently defined mediators of insulin action. These mediators are apparently derived from a unique phosphatidyl-inositol glycan bound to the surface of the cell membrane by a glycophospholipid anchor. Glucose transport into the cell is very rapidly increased in the presence of insulin. This is brought about by the translocation of glucose transporters from an intracellular compartment to the plasma membrane, and/or increased activity of the transporters. Here they facilitate diffusion of glucose via tubular passages into the cell by a mechanism not utilizing energy from ATP or ion transport. In obese subjects with predominantly insulin-resistant diabetes, a number of defects have been described in muscle, including activity of the receptor tyrosine kinase kinase[11,12,13] and reduced glycogen synthase,[14] and in adipocytes, as well as reduced insulin binding.[r21] Even partial weight-loss and increased physical activity may restore these toward or to normal.[14]

Clinical Effects of Deficiency of Insulin

The acute effects of insulin deficiency are summarized under diabetic ketoacidosis later in this chapter. Chronic insulin deficiency and the resulting hyperglycemia are strongly associated with the complications of diabetes. These include neuropathy, retinopathy, and nephropathy, among others. Two main mechanisms are contributory:

(1) Hyperglycemia leads to nonenzymatic glycosylation of cellular and extracellular proteins, including collagen, with alteration of their structure and function. Formation of the advanced glycosylation and products (AGE) is irreversible.[r22] This may thicken the basement membranes and contribute to development of nephropathy and neuropathy. Measurement of the percentage of glycosylation of either hemoglobin (HgbA1c) or the more readily measured total glycated serum protein (commonly referred to as "fructosamine") gives an index of the degree of control of hyperglycemia over the previous 8–12 weeks for the former and 2–3 weeks for the latter, and provides a useful incentive for improving regulation of the diabetes.

(2) Another mechanism involves the accumulation within cells of osmotically-active polyols, alcohols that are formed from the reduction by the enzyme aldose reductase of the carbonyl groups of aldoses, particularly glucose, or of ketones.

The Classification of Diabetes as a Basis of Treatment

In the ideal world, therapy of diabetes mellitus would be related to the mechanisms underlying the particular type of diabetes. In 1979 in the US, the National Diabetes Data Group published a landmark classification,[15] which continues to be used worldwide. The basic laboratory criteria are listed in Table 41.1, and the clinical criteria in Table 41.2. In clinical work and in much of research, assignment to a classification is based on clinical features alone. The NDDG group, however, specifically urged that additional data be collected on clinical patients and research subjects and that, as knowledge of diabetes developed further, the classification should be amended and revised. Since knowledge of the subtypes of diabetes has increased markedly over the past decade, we will use in this chapter an approach to diabetes that emphasizes the mechanisms and also the clinical stages as a basis for appropriate therapy.[r23]

Figure 41.4 shows diagrams of the two main etiologic groups that need to be considered in choosing pharmacologic and other therapy appropriate to sub-

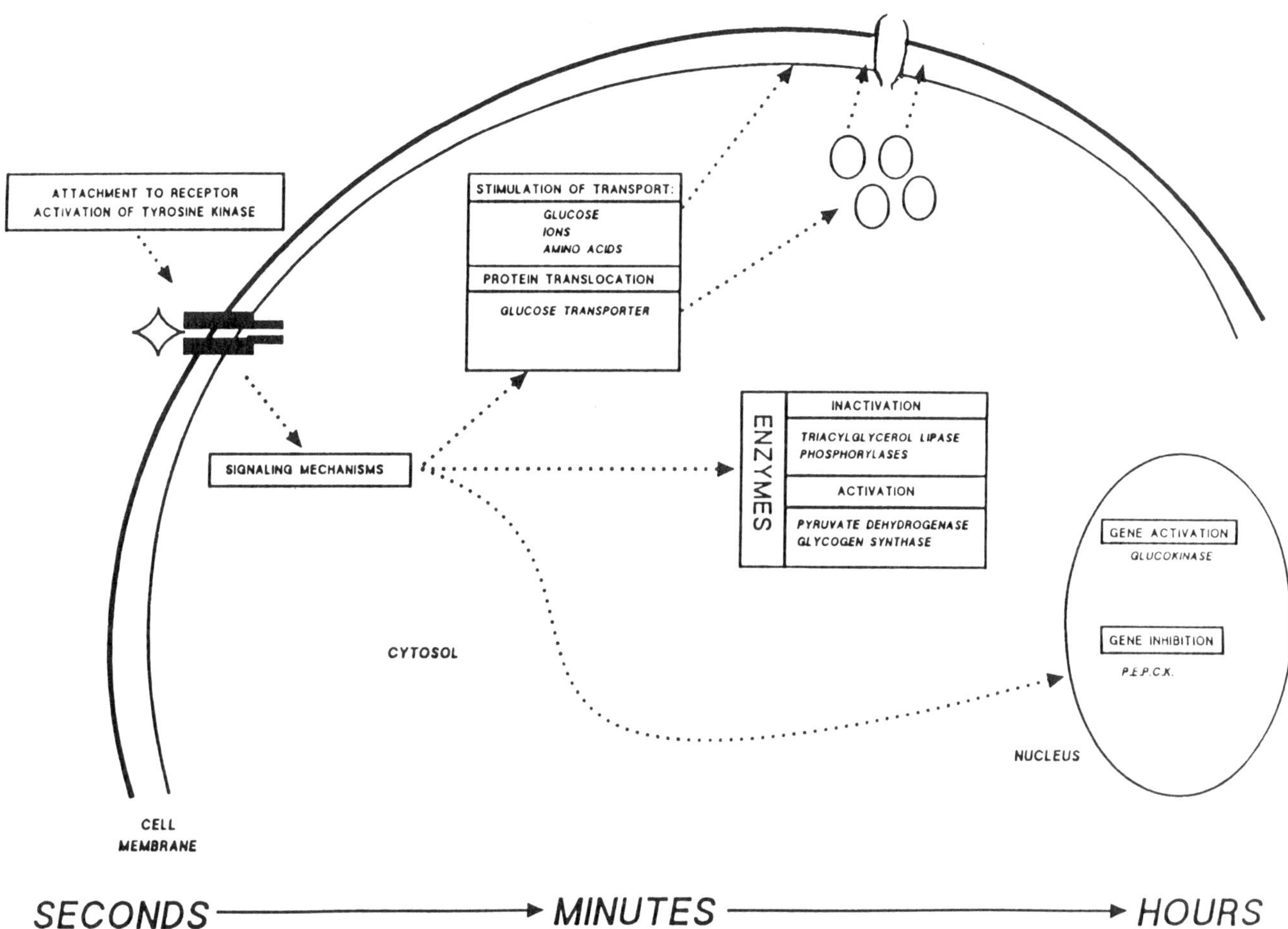

Figure 41.3 The Receptor, Cytoplasmic, and Nuclear Actions of Insulin and their Approximate Time Course

types of diabetes. The division is made initially between those subtypes in which (1) the disorder involves or leads ultimately to predominantly insulin deficiency (lower section), which includes autoimmune and pancreatic disease, and in which beta cell mass is ultimately decreased; and (2) those in which the primary disorder is predominantly insulin resistance (upper section), and in which there is a block in one or more of the stages of insulin action. Patients in the latter category are a heterogeneous group that com-

Table 41.1 Diagnostic Criteria for Diabetes and Impaired Glucose Tolerance of the 1979 National Diabetes Data Group

	Plasma glucose mg/100 ml (× 18 = mM/1)				
Class	**Fasting**		**Mid Test**		**2 hour test**
Normal	<115 (<6.4)	and	<200 (<11.1)	and	<140 (<7.8)
Impaired Glucose Tolerance	<140 (<7.8)	and	≥200(11.1)	and	140–199 (7.8–11.1)
Diabetes	≥140 (≥7.8)	or	≥200 (11.1)	and	≥200 (≥11.1)
Nondiagnostic	all other combinations of the three.				

A standard 75-gm oral glucose tolerance test with venous sampling is used.

In a subsequent revision by the World Health Organization (WHO), the mid-test criteria were deleted and the normal fasting value was increased to <140 (7.8) with the 2-hr test <140 (7.8). A fasting value of ≥140 (7.8), preferably repeated, is considered diagnostic of "diabetes".

Table 41.2 The NDDG and WHO Classification of Diabetes Mellitus and Allied Categories

A. Diagnostic Classes	**Usual Clinical Criteria**
Diabetes Mellitus (DM)	See Table 41.1
Insulin-dependent (IDDM) (IDDM-Type I)	Requires insulin to prevent ketosis Usually but not necessarily at early age with abrupt onset
Non-Insulin-Dependent (NIDDM-Type IIA & B)	Insulin not required to prevent ketosis Not secondary to other diseases 60–90 percent are obese (Subtype IIB)
Malnutrition-Related Tropical (MRDM)	Includes severe malnutrition, pancreatic calcification
Other Types	Associated with pancreatic disease, hormonal etiology, drug or chemical, abnormal insulin or receptor, genetic syndromes, and miscellaneous.

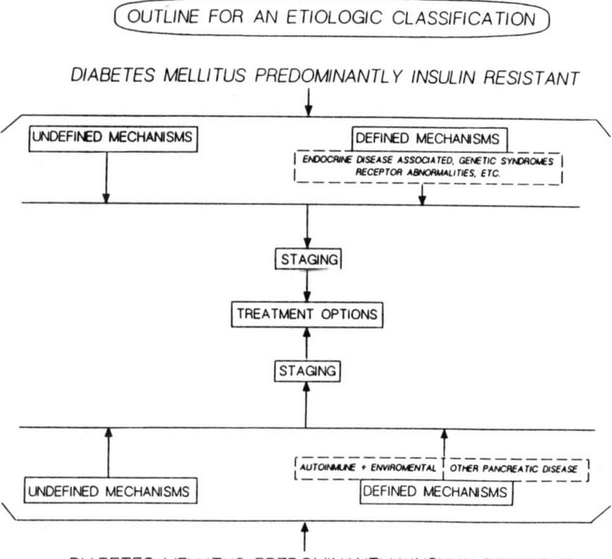

Figure 41.4 A basis for selection of therapy appropriate for the various types and stages of diabetes. See text and Figures 42.4 and 42.5 for staging and treatment options. (Modified with permission from Diabetes Care[13].)

prises about 85 per cent of those with diabetes. Approximately 80 per cent are obese, and often have the metabolically more important central abdominal visceral distribution of fat, which may occur with or without frank obesity or increase in body mass index.[r24,r25] It is this group that is most apt to respond to nonpharmacologic measures. Needless to say, regardless of the type of diabetes, all patients have at least relative insulin deficiency or they would not be diabetic. Hyperglycemia itself contributes both to decreased responsiveness of the beta cell to glucose and to increased insulin resistance from down-regulation of receptors.[r16] In uncontrolled primary insulin deficiency, hyperglycemia itself leads to increased insulin resistance.[r26]

The above two categories correspond roughly to the phenotypic division of the National Diabetes Data Group (NDDG)[15] into insulin-dependent diabetes (IDDM), Type I, and non-insulin-dependent (NIDDM), Type II.[15] The distinction between these two groups based on supposed requirement for insulin has recently become more blurred, since it is now apparent that 10–25 percent of patients with features considered typical of NIDDM actually have slowly developing autoimmune diabetes.[r23,16] Such patients may become candidates for preventive measures, and they must also be carefully watched as they develop the need for treatment with insulin. Measure of antibodies against the 64,000 M_r islet cell antigen, recently identified as glutamic acid decarboxylase (anti-GAD), is proving to be a valuable means of identifying and classifying such patients.[17,18,19,20] The assay is technically more feasible than the previous assays of islet cell antibodies, and remains positive longer in affected individuals.

The Stages of Diabetes and Options for Treatment

There is increasing emphasis on recognizing the various stages through which a patient with a particular underlying mechanism may pass. These are related to the changing amounts of insulin secretion, beta cell destruction, and insulin resistance, which are important in selecting appropriate therapy.[27] We suggest as a guide the following somewhat arbitrary divisions into the stages with the options for treatment, as diagrammed in Figure 41.5A and B.[r23]

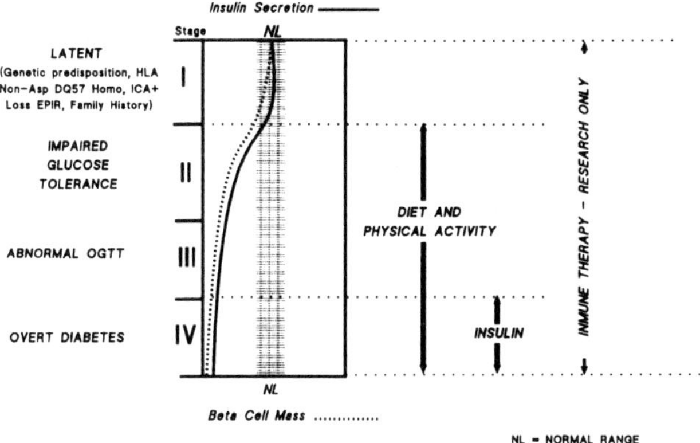

Figure 41.5A Stages of *predominantly insulin deficient* types of diabetes and their relation to therapeutic options. The evolution of the disorder is diagrammed in relation to the surviving beta cell mass (......) and to the insulin secretory capacity (——).

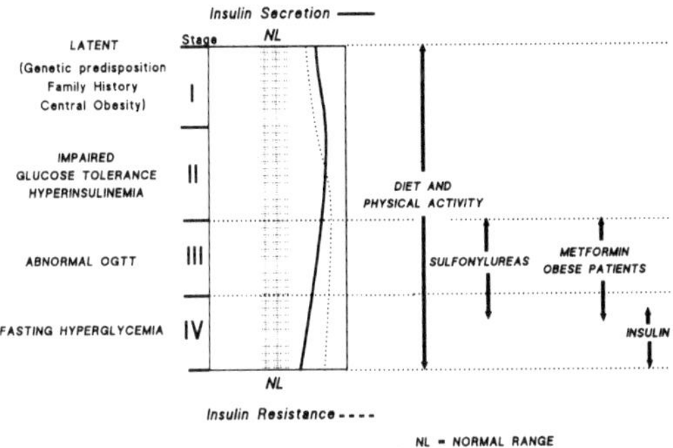

Figure 41.5B Stages of *predominantly insulin resistant* types of Diabetes and their relation to therapeutic options. The interplay of insulin resistance in indicated by (—) and insulin secretory capacity by (–). The double arrows indicate potential reversibility. (Modified with permission from Sims and Calles[13].)

The Stages of Predominantly Insulin-Deficient Diabetes

Figure 41.5A shows the diminishing insulin secretory capacity as beta cells are gradually destroyed by islet-cell antibodies in association with viral infection or other pancreatic disease.[r23] With poor control, hyperglycemia and hyperlipidemia insulin resistance develops secondarily (not diagrammed).

Stage I corresponds to potential abnormality of glucuse tolerance suggested by the above findings associated with insulin deficiency.

In Stage II, often asymptomatic, there is progression to impaired glucose tolerance by the 1979 NDDG criteria (Table 41.2). These first two stages provide the greatest opportunity for preventive measures.

In Stage III there is progression to abnormal glucose tolerance. The patient may still be asymptomatic or may have nonspecific symptoms, such as episodes of reactive hypoglycemia or lack of well-being.

In Stage IV there is "classic" overt insulin-dependent diabetes, with feasting hyperglycemia, glycosuria, and susceptibility to diabetic ketoacidosis and minimal stimulated or fasting plasma C-peptide. Immune intervention even for this stage is being evaluated in some research centers. Treatment with insulin is obligatory.

The Stages of Predominantly Insulin-Resistant Diabetes

Figure 42.5B shows the variable interplay between the response of insulin secretion and the degree of insulin resistance seen in this group of disorders. Specific defects in insulin action produce the various subtypes.[r23]

Stages I and II correspond to potential abnormality of glucose tolerance and impaired glucose tolerance. Nonpharmacologic preventive measures of dietary restriction and exercise are most effective in these first two stages.[21]

In Stage III, glucose tolerance is abnormal by NDDG criteria, and insulin resistance predominates. Tolerance often can be restored, at least temporarily, by caloric restriction and increased physical activity without recourse to drug treatment.

Early Stage IV includes progression of glucose intolerance to overt diabetes. Response to oral hypoglycemic agents may be satisfactory, while caloric restriction and exercise continue to be essential.

In Late Stage IV there is increase in fasting glucose, reflecting persistent and excessive hepatic glucose production, a major metabolic defect in this group of patients. Often this is not corrected by oral hypoglycemic agents (see below) alone, and addition of a single dose of evening insulin may be an alternative to total replacement with insulin. Approximately 50–60 per cent of patients with long-standing NIDDM by NDDG criteria, which we now know may include up to 10–25 percent of patients with slowly evolving autoimmune diabetes, ultimately progress to marked, although not necessarily total insulin deficiency.[r23] They are characterized by hyperglycemia and hyperlipidemia, but develop ketonemia only under severe stress. At this stage insulin treatment is usually necessary for satisfactory control of the hyperglycemia.

Use of Insulin in the Treatment of Diabetes

Historical Perspective

Before supplemental insulin became available, the dietary approach to management of diabetes was emphasized. As early as 1876, the English physician Rollo reported the treatment of a corpulent, young army captain, who was induced to follow a stringent regimen of caloric restriction, who achieved a remission of what must have been predominantly insulin-resistant diabetes, and who was able to return to his military career. Frederick Allen in the US was an advocate in the early 1900s of strict caloric and carbohydrate restriction for diabetes, since this was the only therapy then available. Children with insulin-dependent diabetes were virtually starved, and often died from wasting away. In January 1922, a 12-year-old boy in the terminal stages of a starvation regimen in Toronto was successfully treated with Dr. Collip's crude extract of insulin. Other dramatic successes followed. However, after an initial period when insulin was regarded as a cure, it gradually was realized that complete normalization of blood glucose and prevention of long-term complications remained difficult or impossible.

The first actual measurements of blood glucose became available in hospital or physicians' laboratories only about 70 years ago. However, during the 1970s and '80s new techniques have enabled patients to monitor their own blood glucose with electronic meters. Since then, patients have assumed greater responsibility in self-management skills in concert with other members of the team.[r28]

Insulins with prolonged action were developed to provide a baseline support and to avoid frequent injections. The first aim is an important one; the second too often results in unphysiologic control. Scott at Columbia University reported in 1936 that complexing with the basic fish protein, protamine, did prolong its action,[22] and Hagedorn[23] later produced the stable preparation NPH insulin.

In 1963, Hallas-Moller[24], in Denmark, developed sized zinc-insulin crystals with more prolonged action.

Indications for Treatment with Insulin in the Two Main Types of Diabetes Are:

(a) Demonstrable insulinopenia and/or underweight. If there is evidence of autoimmune beta cell destruction, early treatment with insulin, rather than with oral hypoglycemic agents, should be considered.

(b) Failure of optimal diet and exercise combined with oral hypoglycemic agents in patients with NIDDM.

(c) Diabetic ketoacidosis or hyperosmolar coma for any reason requires treatment with insulin at least temporarily, even in the obese.

(d) Diabetes in pregnancy, since close control is essential for protection of the fetus and hypoglycemic agents are contraindicated.

(e) Severe stress of infection, injury, or surgery.

Insulin Types, Dosage, and Administration

Insulin is not effective orally because it is inactivated by proteolytic enzymes in the GI tract. The usual route of administration is SQ, but, in special circumstances, clear or regular insulin may be administered IM or IV. It is essential that the response of each individual be closely monitored.

Forms of insulin of either intermediate or long durations of action, but shorter than intermediate, as listed in Table 41.3, have been developed by complexing the molecule with basic proteins or by altering the crystalline form to achieve the lengthened bioavailability. Unmodified regular insulin starts to act within 20 minutes and peaks at 2–3 hours, with duration of 6–8 hours. NPH insulin (Neutral Protamine Hagedorn or isophane suspension), which has onset at 1–2 hours, peaks at 6–8 hours, and duration of action of 16–22 hours. This unfortunately fostered the often inappropriate attempt to control diabetes with a single injection per day. Stable mixtures of 70 per cent NPH and 30 per cent regular insulin are available that have onset of action in less than an hour, peak activity at 4–6 hours and duration of action of 18–24 hours. The timing of the peak and the duration of action of the lente group of insulins varies with the size of the zinc-insulin crystals. Semilente, with small crystals, has a longer duration of action: 12–18 hours as opposed to 4–8 hours for regular insulin. The peak of action of ultralente insulin of animal origin is delayed to 4–6 hours, with duration of 24–36 hours, while the duration of action of human ultralente is much shorter, not beyond 26 hours. Lente insulin, more commonly used, contains 30 per cent of the former rapid-acting semilente, and 70 per cent of the ultralente. Thus various insulins can be combined with regular insulin or crystalline zinc insulin in many ways to meet the specific needs of individual work schedules and lifestyles. However, care must be taken to select combinations that are stable when mixed, to avoid modification of one by the other.

The Goals of Treatment of Diabetes with Insulin

The results of the recently completed Diabetes Control and Complications trial (DCCT)[25], a landmark project, demonstrate without doubt that near normalization of glucose concentration by three or more daily injections or by insulin pump delays the onset or slows the progression of diabetic retinopathy, nephropathy, and neuropathy in patients with insulin-dependent diabetes. In the primary prevention cohort of 726 patients there was a 76 percent reduction in the mean risk for development of retinopathy as compared with conventional therapy. In the secondary intervention cohort of 715 patients the reduction was 54 percent. Neuropathy was reduced 60 percent and microalbuminuria 39 percent. This striking demonstration of the value of intensive control is provoking discussion at all levels of health care as to whether and how this standard of

Table 41.3 Commonly Available Preparations of Insulin

Type[1]	Appearance	Action Profile (Hours)[2]		
		Onset	Peak	Duration
Rapid				
Regular crystaline	Clear	0.3–0.7	2–4	5–8
Semilente (zinc suspension)	Cloudy	0.5–1.0	2–8	12–16
Intermediate				
NPH (isophane)	Cloudy	1–2	6–12	12–16
Lente	Cloudy	1–2	6–12	12–16
Prolonged				
Ultralente	Cloudy	4–6	not well defined	20–36

[1]All are available as standard, recombinant, or semi-synthetic human insulin, and at pH buffered to 7.2–7.4. Only the NPH insulin contains protein. The peak action and the amplitude of the human insulins is earlier, but the total effect is comparable. See Figure 41.6 for peak action and duration in relation to site of administration.

care can be duplicated in the usual clinical setting and for what categories of patients it is safe and cost effective. The recommendations for therapy of IDDM in this chapter are presented in the light of these results.

The research Group of the DCCT trial have, however, warned that if the main conclusions of the trial with regard to the benefits of reduction of glycemia are extended to patients with NIDDM, careful regard for age, capabilities, and coexisting diseases will be necessary. They advise caution in the use of therapies other than diet that are aimed at achieving euglycemia. In the great majority of patients with NIDDM, insulin resistance is predominant and the hyperinsulinemia is known to be a factor in the complications. Therefore, intensive use of insulin or of agents that stimulate insulin secretion rather than increasing insulin sensitivity may be contraindicated.

The *overall goal* is, of course, to reproduce the normal pattern of insulin availability in order to optimize carbohydrate as well as lipid and protein metabolism. This requires availability of basal insulin and additional concentrations at the time of meals.

Specific goals are:

(a) Normalizing lifestyle with maintenance of body weight optimal for the individual and achieving good physical condition, along with a feeling of wellness.

(b) Minimizing chronic complications by reducing glycosylation of proteins and normalizing serum lipids.

(c) Achieving optimal ranges of plasma glucose while minimizing episodes of hypoglycemia. What is reasonable for the particular individual must be evaluated.

Complete normalization, however, is not always possible, for several reasons:

(1) We cannot reproduce the instantaneous monitoring of glucose and delivery of insulin by the beta cells of the normal pancreas.[r28]

(2) The needs for insulin vary from day to day and from hour to hour.

(3) Textbook diagrams to the contrary, the patterns of absorption of short- and long-acting insulins vary greatly between individuals and between injection sites (see p. 703).

(4) The extraportal route of delivery of insulin by injection bypassing the liver is unphysiologic, and portal delivery by a totally implantable pump would be ideal.[28] A recent clinical trial in France indicates that delivery via an external pump has both advantages and risks.[28]

Initiation and Modification of Insulin Treatment

Despite all of the above limitations, excellent results usually can be obtained if certain crucial elements are included in patient management. A team effort is optimal for guidance and education and ideally includes a physician, nurse or other health professional, and dietician working together with the patient and critical members of his or her family. A support group of fellow patients can be invaluable.[r28] Self blood glucose monitoring and periodic checks of plasma lipids and of increased glycosylation of proteins, as reflected in Hemoglobin-A1c or in the "fructosamine" assay of plasma proteins, provide essential feedback to members of the team.

The total daily requirement is variable, and initially requires an educated guess followed by clinical trial. A normal lean person produces 0.25 to 0.5 U of insulin/kg body weight per day, of which about one-half is basal secretion and the rest, the prandial component, is secreted in direct response to meals. Larger total amounts of exogenous insulin are usually required, and due to inactivity and increased counterregulatory hormones in the morning hours, the requirement for the breakfast period is usually about 1.5 times that for lunch and supper periods. A high requirement suggests that insulin resistance requires investigation.

Options for Providing Basal Insulin

A continuous supply of basal insulin can be provided in the various ways outlined in Table 41.4.

The most effective, but also the most demanding on the patient, is continuous SQ delivery of regular insulin by means of a programmable pump. Delivery first to the liver via the portal bed via a catheter seems more physiologic, but requires further clinical evaluation.[26] Associated risks are rapid development of ketoacidosis, if pump or catheter failure cuts off the supply of the short-acting insulin, or infection at the injection site.

A single dose of ultralente insulin of animal origin may be adequate, but human ultralente has too short an action. Regular and

Table 41.4

Schema	Basal Component	Prandial Component
1*	Constant infusion of regular insulin	Regular insulin—prior to meal ingestion
2**	Ultralente	Regular insulin before every meal
3	Intermediate acting insulin (NPH, lente) before bedtime	Regular insulin before every meal
4***	Intermediate acting insulin (NPH, lente) AM and PM	Regular insulin before breakfast and before supper

*A portable infusion pump delivers a constant rate of regular insulin (basal rate), which can be increased manually prior to every meal (prandial component).

**A single dose of ultralente insulin of animal origin usually is enough to provide sustained concentrations of insulin in blood to mimic the basal component; however, when using human ultralente insulin, 2 doses/d usually are necessary. Regular and ultralente should NOT be mixed in the same syringe.

***NPH and regular insulin CAN be mixed together or can be obtained premixed, thus providing a more acceptable regimen. The prandial component for lunch in this schema corresponds to the peak activity of the dose of AM NPH insulin. The peak of the PM NPH insulin dose may induce early morning hypoglycemia, which is correctable by administering the PM NPH insulin before bedtime.

ultralente insulin should not be mixed in the same syringe. Two doses of NPH or lente insulin allow greater flexibility. Evening intermediate-acting insulin alone may be of value as an aid in controlling hepatic glucose production overnight and obtaining a normal fasting values for serum glucose and lipids.[27]

If there is unusually prolonged action of short-acting or intermediate-acting insulin, long-acting insulin may not be necessary. Caution and close monitoring are required when substituting synthetic human for animal insulin preparations, since, as shown in Figure 41.6, A and B, its peak action may be earlier and greater than that of insulins of animal origin.

Provision of the Prandial Component of Insulin

This can be mimicked clinically by adding short-acting insulin (of which human insulin is the shortest) 15 to 30 minutes before meals (Fig. 41.6), or by mixing

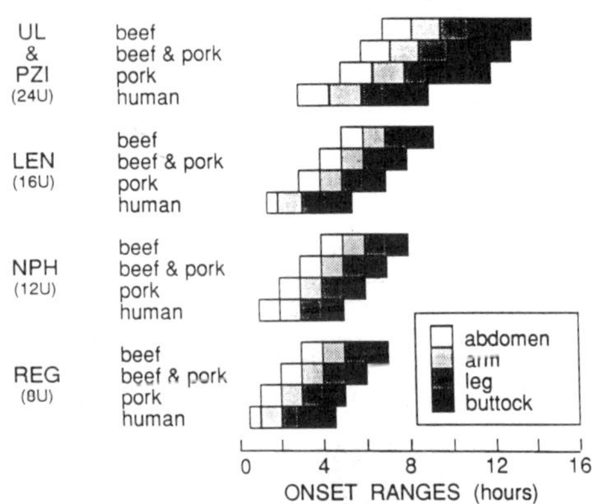

Figure 41.6A Typical ranges in *onset (time to peak action)* of the various insulins, according to formulation, species of origin, and site of injection at the nominal doses indicated. Time to peak action is inversely related to absorption rate. The ranges are relative and should serve only as a guide. (With permission from Albisser[17].)

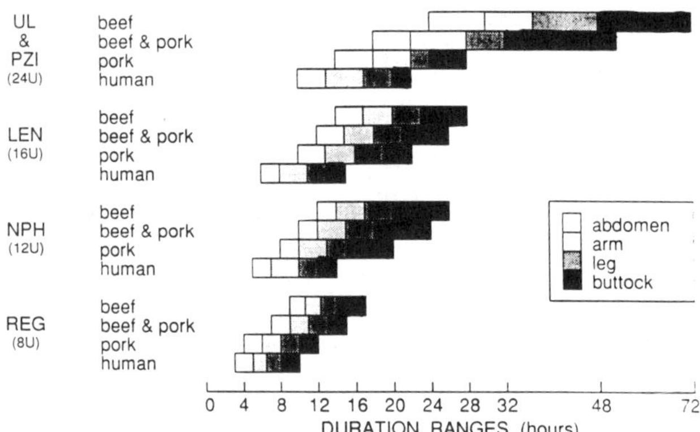

Figure 41.6B Typical ranges of the *duration of action*, under conditions similar to those in Figure 41.6A. Note the difference in time scale. Again, these should serve only as a guide. (With permission from Albisser[17].)

the basal and prandial components of insulin before injection (Table 41.4). Pump users can call for additional insulin as required. The selection of a regimen depends on the experience of the team and the circumstances and ability of the patient. Again, frequent self blood glucose monitoring and charting, with occasional checks in the small hours of the night, is essential.

The DCCT trial has shown that target ranges of glucose can be met in the large majority of patients. Each patient must learn by monitoring blood glucose his/her individual sensitivity to the type or types of insulin. When unexpected high or low glucose values appear, the patient must learn to recognize such variables as the effect of previous exercise, of stress, and particularly of previous hypoglycemia with reactive hypoglycemia and to adjust their insulin dose accordingly. When hyperglycemia is marked, urinary ketones must be checked. For a minority of patients it may be unwise to strive for the ideal target ranges in view of such variables as advanced age, extreme lability, unawareness of hypoglycemia, or associated renal, hepatic, or other disease.

Adjustment of Insulin Dosage and Self-Monitoring of Blood Glucose Steps in the Control of Diabetes with Insulin

Initial emphasis should be on gradually normalizing the fasting blood glucose, within a range of 70 to 120 mg/dl, as an index of the required basal component of insulin. Adjustments should be made in small steps, allowing 2–3 days to evaluate their effect and a daily record of insulin dosage, blood glucoses, symptoms, and activity should be encouraged. Once the basal component is adjusted, the prandial dosage can be similarly titrated, with a goal of 100–180 mg/dl within two hours after a meal. Patients should not be hurried, and should realize that their target ranges of glucose can eventually be reached.

Management of Hypoglycemic Reactions

Mild episodes of hypoglycemia are to be expected and accepted, but severe episodes, which may produce permanent brain damage, must be avoided. Many different mechanisms may account for so-called "brittle" diabetes.[32] These include diminished awareness secondary to neuropathy and diminished counterregulatory hormonal response, particularly when the autonomic and the glucagon responses are impaired. Delayed and unpredictable gastric emptying similarly increases the risk of hypoglycemia. More rapid correction of hypoglycemia is provided by ingestion of glucose, rather than complex carbohydrates. Glucose may be given IV as a 50 percent solution or absorbed from a retention enema in 5 percent solution. The use of glucagon is described in the following section.

Early morning hyperglycemia often is difficult to control as a result of either of two possible mechanisms.[r29]:

(1) The so-called "dawn phenomenon," attributed to waning of available insulin and the effect of nocturnal growth hormone secretion.[30] This requires careful adjustment of the dose of long-acting insulin during the evening on the basis of checks of the blood glucose during the early hours of the morning and avoiding escalation of the morning insulin dose. The possibility of using long-acting somatostatin to block early morning growth hormone secretion is described in Chapter 55.

(2) Following a period of hypoglycemia there may be a rise in blood glucose as a result of compensatory secretion of catecholamines, growth hormone, and adrenocorticoids, known as the Somogyi phenomenon. This is important to recognize, as it may lead to inappropriate escalation of the insulin dosage. Recent studies, however, indicate that asymptomatic nocturnal hypoglycemia does not lead to morning hyperglycemia.[31]

Diabetic Ketoacidosis[r30]

Diabetic ketoacidosia (DKA) is potentially fatal, particularly in the elderly. It is characterized by rampant gluconeogenesis, protein degradation, marked lipolysis with acidosis, and variable degrees of fluid and electrolyte depletion.

A critical need is to supply IV fluid and electrolyte, with or without insulin, as soon as possible, since dehydration is a major problem. Intravenous infusions of insulin of as little as 0.1 U/kg of body weight usually provide a serum insulin concentration of approximately 100 uU/ml (600 pM/L) and suffice for control of even severe DKA. An initial bolus of 0.1 U/kg (0.6 pM/kg) body weight of regular crystalline insulin should be given, but the mainstay is continuous infusion of insulin adjusted on the basis of the response of the ketosis and hyperglycemia.

The clinically available tests for ketosis, Acetest and Ketostix, measure only acetoacetate and acetone. Thus, the apparent concentration of ketones may not decrease even though the total amount of ketone declines, since the beta-hydroxybutyric acid is still being converted to acetoacetate. A flow sheet to record changes in metabolic parameters and fluid and electrolyte balance is essential. If there is no reduction in ketosis and hyperventilation and no rise in pH after 3–4 hours, larger doses of insulin must be administered promptly and their effect monitored. Glucose should not be given until the plasma concentration has fallen to about 250 mg/dl. Plasma concentrations should fall 50–100 mg/dl per hour, and reduction of hyperglycemia to 200–300 mg/dl usually can be achieved within 4–6 hours. In children, a slower rate of decline is desirable. Rarely, a patient with severe insulin resistance may require much larger amounts of insulin. Since the half-life of insulin in the serum is only 5–6 minutes, the shift to SQ injections should be made at least 30 minutes before IV insulin is discontinued.

It is essential to replace losses of body fluids and electrolytes.[r30] Replacement of sodium is critical. This should be in net hypotonic form, since both as a result of the osmotic diuresis and of the depletion of intracellular electrolyte the loss of water is in excess of that of sodium. The timing of replacement of potassium depends on the initial serum concentration, which may be monitored by both serum concentrations and EKG patterns. If low, replacement must start immediately; if elevated, infusion may be delayed for as long as four hours. Since potassium enters the cells along with glucose in response to the insulin infusion, and is also lost in the urine, potassium and glucose should be given together to replace losses, with monitoring of the EKG effect. Magnesium is another important electrolyte that may require replacement. When cations are given along with chloride as the only anion, a chloride acidosis is substituted for the ketoacidosis. With severe ketoacidosis with $pH < 7.0$, bicarbonate should be replaced. Rarely, phosphate may be required to correct hypophosphatemia.

Nonketotic Hyperglycemic Coma[r29,r30]

This life-threatening disorder typically develops insidiously in a patient with insulin reserve just adequate to prevent ketosis. In spite of typically higher glucose concentrations, smaller amounts of insulin are needed than for patients with ketoacidosis and, again, fluid and electrolyte replacement is critical, since dehydration can be even more severe than in DKA.

Patients with any type of diabetes who experience trauma or surgical procedures may require temporary treatment with insulin. Continuous infusion with close monitoring is often needed.[r32]

Undesirable Effects of Insulin

In patients with predominantly insulin-resistant diabetes, ill-advised use of insulin without control of caloric intake and physical activity leads to a vicious cycle in which increasing weight gain is associated with increased insulin resistance and, in turn, apparent increased need for insulin. The antilipolytic fat-storing action of insulin is unimpaired in those otherwise insulin-resistant,[r31] so that insulin injection or stimulation of the beta cells by a sulfonylurea drug may simply add to the obesity and insulin resistance and worsen the problem. Use of insulin in a manner that exaggerates hyperinsulinemia may be counterproductive.

Insulin resistance and the resulting hyperinsulinemia are now known to be closely related to four disorders prevalent in western society,[r33] namely obesity,[r34] NIDDM,[r35] dyslipidemia,[r35] and hypertension.[r36] The association is commonly referred to as "Syndrome X" or more appropriately the Syndrome of insulin resistance. Thus, it is not surprising that any regimen of treatment of patients with this syndrome with insulin or with an agent that exaggerates hyperinsulinemia may exacerbate obesity, lipid disorders, or hypertension.

Local and generalized allergic reactions to insulin, as well as lipoatrophy or hypertrophy at injection sites are much less frequent since highly purified insulins and human insulins came into wide use. Injection of purified insulin may correct local lipoatrophic areas. Antibodies to insulin ultimately develop in 70 per cent of patients taking insulin, and local or generalized eczematoid immune reactions may occur. The use of the less antigenic recombinant human insulin minimizes binding to anti-insulin antibodies, thus increasing effectiveness. However, the risk of severe allergic reactions is not entirely eliminated.

Insulin-induced edema may be encountered occasionally on

initiating treatment with insulin. It may be related to the antinatriuretic of insulin, and is usually self-limited.

Toxic Effects of Insulin

Frank overdose of insulin can produce irreversible brain damage secondary to hypoglycemia, and the person with repeated severe reactions may suffer permanent mental impairment. Concurrent use of propranolol and other beta-antagonists may blunt awareness of hypoglycemia by reducing tachycardia and other symptoms, leading to a damaging insulin reaction; and interactions with other drugs must be avoided.

Pharmacokinetics of Insulin Treatment

Differences in Individual Response to Insulin

Four major factors account for the variation between the responses of patients to insulin:[r38]

(1) Absorption of insulin injected SQ is a main variable. There is a wide range of variation between individuals in the uptake of injected insulin, in addition to the variation based on the site selected, which may be as much as 50 per cent. Differences in vascularity and fibrosis at the site of injection modify the rate of absorption. Also, the degree of glycosylation of capillary basement membranes may seriously impede the transfer of insulin from injection site to the blood stream as well as the distribution of insulin to target cells. All these factors may change in long-standing diabetes. Inadvertent injection into a muscle or, particularly, into a vein speeds absorption, increasing the peak effect, but shortening its action. Absorption is fastest from the abdominal wall, followed by the arm, thigh, and buttocks, so that consistency in the choice of sites of injection at corresponding times of day is in order (Fig. 41.6). Variations in ambient temperature will affect local circulation and absorption, and this change may be further modified by strenuous exercise involving the particular area of the body injected. Smoking also delays absorption as a result of the vasoconstriction it causes. The timing of peak action after SQ injection differs by 50 percent between individuals and by as much as 25 percent on different days in the same person.[r38] Thus, it is no wonder that the disorder is difficult to control and may be frustrating to patient and physician alike.

(2) Strenuous exercise has a sustained effect directly on increasing sensitivity of muscle to insulin, and indirectly by increasing blood flow. The direct effect may carry over to the following day and require a reduction of insulin dosage.

(3) In about 70 per cent of patients with long-standing diabetes, circulating antibodies to insulin may develop and unpredictably prolong its action and reduce its availability once it is absorbed. The clinical importance of this is controversial.

(4) Other factors that can unpredictably modify the response include degree of insulin resistance, variations in the antecedent diet, and counterregulatory hormonal response to stress.

Preparations of insulin available in the US are listed in Table 41.3.

Glucagon[r38]

Insulin-, glucagon-, and somatostatin-producing cells are closely related anatomically in the pancreatic islet and are capable of paracrine intercommunication. Their physiologic relationship is equally close, in that insulin is predominantly the hormone of carbohydrate, as well as protein and lipid metabolism and storage, whereas glucagon ensures that glucose and substrates for gluconeogenesis are mobilized in sufficient quantity in times of physiologic stress. The principal use of glucagon in the management of diabetes is to treat insulin-induced hypoglycemic coma. After 2–5 years of autoimmune insulin-dependent diabetes, the glucagon response to hypoglycemia usually becomes impaired. After 15 years or more, there may be diminished catecholamine response as well, with further severe hypoglycemic episodes. On the other hand, in NIDDM, hyperglucagonemia may contribute to hyperglycemia by promoting hepatic glucose production.

Glucagon is also used as a GI relaxing agent in radiology.

Chemistry, Occurrence, and Relative Potency

Glucagon, a single chain polypeptide of molecular weight 3483, is secreted by the alpha cells of the pancreas, with the amino acid sequence.

NH_2
His-Ser-Glu-Gly-Thr-Phe-Thr-Ser-

NH_2
Asp-Tyr-Ser-Lys-Tyr-Tyr-Leu-Asp-Ser-Agr-Arg-Glu-

NH_2 NH_2
Asp-Phe-Val-Glu Trp-Leu-Met-Asp-Thr

It is derived from a preprohormone, but unlike insulin, has no cross-linkages, since it contains no cysteine residues. Closely related peptides with similar but weaker actions are secreted by alpha-like cells of the intestine in response to common stimuli. Teleologically, during prolonged fasting, glucagon provides the CNS with fuels derived from fat by promoting ketosis, while sparing the breakdown of protein.

History of Glucagon

Glucagon was discovered by Murlin and Kimball in 1923, and its structure was clarified by Behrens several years after that of insulin. Since it lacked an immediate therapeutic application, it was not extensively studied or utilized until many years later. Only in recent years has it become apparent that the complete pattern of insulin deficiency with ketosis is dependent on a reciprocal relative increase in glucagon concentration.

The Regulation of Secretion of Glucagon

For insulin to carry out its various functions and to avoid development of hypoglycemia, a delicate balance of hormonal responses is necessary. Glucagon provides a hormonally mediated mechanism against hypoglycemia by promoting hepatic gluconeogenesis, lipolysis, and glycogenolysis. Its secretion is not only triggered by hypoglycemia, but is also stimulated by amino acids, particularly arginine; and this provides protection against hypoglycemia following a meal low in carbohydrate and rich in protein. Its secretion prior to release of insulin is brought about by a host of other signals, including several GI peptides released during meals and the hormones released during stress, epinephrine, cortisol, beta-endorphin, and growth hormone.[r39] In addition, when hypoglycemia triggers hypothalamic sensors, secretion of glucagon is stimulated by both adrenergic and cholinergic mechanisms. On the other hand, during carbohydrate feeding the rises in both plasma glucose and insulin suppress glucagon secretion. The microcirculation of the islet is such that the outward circulation of secreted insulin directly inhibits the alpha-cells lining its circumference. Glucagon is weakly suppressed by secretin and strongly suppressed by somatostatin and perhaps other signals.

Mechanisms of Action and Effects

Analogous to insulin, glucagon binds to the regulatory subunit of its receptor. This, in turn, activates adenylate cyclase, with generation of cyclic AMP. This further activates cAMP-dependent protein kinase, leading in turn to phosphorylation of key enzymes in glycogenolysis and gluconeogenesis. By a related series of actions, glucagon promotes ketogenesis, thus providing an alternative source of energy during stress. Its release is initiated by hypoglycemia and is accompanied by, but not totally dependent on, epinephrine secretion. A fall in insulin and a rise in glucose concentration limits further increase in glucagon secretion. The ratio of plasma glucagon to plasma insulin in the portal vein determines whether the liver stores or releases glucose. In both main types of diabetes, the relative lack of insulin leads to a relative increase in glucagon secretion that exaggerates the diabetic state by promoting release of glucose.

The bulk of the evidence to date indicates that glucagon is required for the overproduction of both glucose and ketone bodies during insulin deficiency. Even after pancreatectomy, glucagon immunoreactivity accounting for the entire molecule can be secreted by alpha-like cells in the gut or formed from closely related peptides.[33,34] Glucagon is produced in excess in relation to insulin in most patients with diabetes. In patients with NIDDM, glucagon is believed to mediate the increased basal hepatic glucose output, which falls when glucagon is suppressed. Deficiency of both glucagon and insulin produces only modest or absent hyperglycemia and hyperketonemia.[r39]

Clinically, a syndrome of glucagon excess is seen in the rare malignant glucagon-producing tumor of the pancreas (glucagonoma), which, not surprisingly, produces diabetes as well as eczematoid dermatitis, psychiatric disturbances, and diarrhea.

Therapeutic Uses, Pharmacokinetics, and Undesirable Effects

The main therapeutic use of glucagon is in treating severe hypoglycemia or coma in patients with diabetes when infusion of glucose is not feasible or when there is confusion or combativeness. Subcutaneous, IV, or IM injection of 0.5–1.0 Unit (mg.) usually restores normoglycemia to comatose patients with 5–20 minutes. It may also be given intranasally by insufflation.[33] The half-life of glucagon in the plasma is only 3–5 minutes, and the dose may be repeated 1–2 times. The injection should be followed promptly by oral or IV glucose. Prolonged, refractory coma must be treated, if possible, with IV glucose to avoid brain damage. Glucagon itself may provoke nausea and vomiting, with risk of aspiration; therefore, glucose administration IV or rectally is preferable. Where there is severe glycogen depletion or when brain damage has been extensive, coma may persist after treatment with glucagon.

Available Preparations

Glucagon is available in 1- or 10-mg amounts, either as a dry powder or in a form suitable for nasal aspiration. Since it is unstable in solution, it must be diluted before use. The lyophilized preparation for intranasal use is available commercially.[35]

The Sulfonylurea Oral Hypoglycemic Agents[r10,r11]

Two main classes of oral hypoglycemic agents used extensively are the sulfonylurea derivatives and the less frequently prescribed biguanides, of which metformin has gained the widest use (see p. 713). The sulfonylureas increase endogenous insulin secretion in the presence of glucose or certain amino acids, and may potentiate the action of insulin. The biguanides (see p. 714) do not stimulate insulin secretion, but increase glucose transport across the cell membrane of skeletal muscle, with secondary inhibition of hepatic gluconeogenesis, of lipogenesis, and to a lesser degree of intestinal absorption of carbohydrates. Each of these two main classes has disadvantages. Other oral agents with different mechanisms of action are being developed or are undergoing clinical trial, and may well eventually replace them (see p. 717).

Warning: When any oral hypoglycemic agent is prescribed, renal or hepatic insufficiency and possible interactions with other drugs must be excluded to avoid prolonged or fatal hypoglycemia (in the case of the sulfonylureas) or lactic acidosis (in the case of the biguanides).

The sulfonylurea oral hypoglycemic agents are widely used and effective in the management of predominantly insulin-resistant diabetes in the early stages, during which the secretory capacity for insulin is relatively well preserved. Initially, they act by further increasing insulin secretion, thus counteracting the insulin resistance.[r42] Correction of the hyperglycemia, in turn, further improves the responsiveness of the islet cell to glucose, and may account for much of the lessening of insulin resistance. Most evidence for a peripheral action involves in vitro studies and supraphysiologic concentrations of the drug.[36] The bulk of the often-contradictory evidence suggests that any extrapancreatic effect of these drugs involves potentiation of the action of insulin distal to the receptor on muscle and adipose tissue glucose transport and on the liver to decrease hepatic glucose production. Adequate caloric restriction and physical activity are prerequisites. The major adverse effects of these drugs are continued weight gain in obese patients, which further increases the insulin resistance, and, rarely, prolonged or fatal hypoglycemia.

Chemistry and Relative Potency of the Sulfonylureas

The sulfonylurea hypoglycemic agents are all arylsulfonylureas having the following basic structure:

R1—[Benzene Ring]-SO_2NHCONH—R2

The main effects and mechanism of action are essentially the same for all the variants containing this central structure. The so-called first-generation drugs had relatively simple substitutions at R1 and R2, as diagrammed in Table 41.4. As discussed below under Pharmacokinetics, the substitutions modify their hepatic metabolism, the potency of their metabolites, and the route of excretion.

The second-generation drugs have more complex substitutions at R1 and R2 that increase their potency per mole 100- to 150-fold relative to tolbutamide.

History

Quite by accident, Jambon in France in 1942 discovered during the treatment of typhoid fever the antidiabetic action of a sulfonamide antibiotic that produced severe hypoglycemia and seizures when given to soldiers. By 1946 Loubatières had demonstrated that the action of the sulfonamide derivative depended on intact pancreatic tissue. Not until 1956 was the hypoglycemic action of tolbutamide demonstrated in humans. First-generation agents were widely and enthusiastically used, until findings of the University Group Diabetes Project (UGDP) in the US caused a temporary reduction during the 1970s.[36] Tolbutamide was found to be associated with increased cardiac mortality, while dietary therapy alone proved of benefit. This multicenter, controlled prospective study raised serious doubts about the safety of tolbutamide that have not yet been completely resolved. Subjects treated with this drug had more adverse cardiac effects and mortality than untreated control subjects. In recent years, the use of the sulfonylureas has increased strikingly, but this increase has varied markedly from country to country. There is now an increasing interest in newer drugs that do not increase hyerinsulinemia and that tend to normalize plasma lipids.

Mechanisms of Action of Sulfonylurea Compounds

Loubatière and most others since have shown that the sulfonylureas are ineffective in the face of total pancreatectomy, suggesting that at least their initial effect is mainly on insulin secretion by increasing the sensitivity to glucose of the beta cells of the pancreas.[r42] After the drug binds to specific receptors on the beta cells, ATPase-sensitive potassium channels are closed and the cells are depolarized. Calcium channels are activated, and in turn the steps already described in relation to insulin secretion are initiated (Fig. 42.1). Since hyperglycemia itself impairs insulin secretion and blunts its peripheral action, its correction can explain many of the beneficial effects of the sulfonylureas.

Stimulation by the sulfonylurea drug glyburide of the synthesis and translocation of glucose transporters in cultured cells[38] has suggested a peripheral action of the sulfonylureas. However, in depancreatized animals[33] or patients with no residual insulin secretion,[39] no acute increase in insulin sensitivity can be demonstrated. On the other hand, an acute effect of glyburide in increasing insulin sensitivity during insulin infusion at physiologic and higher insulin concentrations has been shown in insulin-dependent patients.[40] This suggests that the sulfonylureas act to potentiate the action of insulin.[r36] A sulfonylurea-specific binding protein that mediates the increased glucose transport has been demonstrated in cultured rat adipocytes.[42] Preincubation with glyburide gave increased acetate incorporation into lipids.

Therapeutic Uses and Limitations

The sulfonylurea drugs are used throughout the world for the treatment of predominantly insulin-resistant diabetes mellitus. These agents are effective only if maximum benefits have been obtained from nonpharmacologic measures. Increasing physical activity and improving dietary control are essential, since both lessen insulin resistance. Physical training added to dietary restriction in patients with this type of diabetes can provide a more normal pattern of nonoxidative as opposed to oxidative glucose disposal and reduce excessive hepatic gluconeogenesis.[43] Together, these measures may restore normal tolerance to glucose, at least for a considerable period. Associated hypertension and hyperlipidemia usually lessen, since these disorders are closely linked to insulin resistance.[r37] In the obese person with diabetes, improved physical training and minimal weight loss may be all that is required. Obese patients poorly controlled while receiving very large doses of insulin may often be brought under control when their program is initiated by a period of total fasting or very low calorie diet and may be maintained without insulin.[43] This approach may show the patient that vigorous efforts to reduce insulin resistance can be effective.

In Figure 42.5B, the amount of insulin resistance and insulin secretory capacity at the various stages of predominantly insulin-resistant diabetes is related to options for treatment. The presence of such complications as hepatic or renal impairment that may affect the metabolism or excretion of sulfonylureas must be taken into consideration as well.[13]

Persons Likely to Benefit from the Sulfonylurea Drugs

Patients meeting the following criteria may be candidates for use of the sulfonylurea drugs, at least initially:

(a) Inability to respond to the non-pharmacologic measures.

(b) Insulin treatment not required to prevent ketosis.

(c) Fasting plasma glucose concentrations under 10 mM/L (180 mg/dl).

(d) Obese rather than lean.

(e) No evidence of predominant insulin deficiency, such as low insulin/glucose ratio.

(f) Metformin and the newer oral agents that more directly address insulin resistance and obesity not available.

Persons Not Likely to Benefit from the Sulfonylurea Drugs

Secondary failure in those responding initially occurs in approximately 5–10 per cent per year of uncharacterized patients, with ultimate failure in about 50 percent.[46,39] These include:

(a) Those who are not obese.

(b) Those with severe fasting hyperglycemia (>250 mg/dl-14 mM/L) and who fall in Stage IV of Figure 41.5B.

(c) Those with evidence of slowly developing autoimmune diabetes.[r23] Insulin dependence may be expected within a few years, and preventive measures or early introduction to insulin is preferable. Measurement of the antibody against the islet cell antigen glutamic acid decarboxylase, (antiGAD), now under refinement, provides a more practical and more predictive method of detecting immune destruction of islet cells.[18] Once identified, patients with this subtype of diabetes may be expected to progress to absolute insulin deficiency within a few years and must be monitored accordingly. When the methods of specifically blocking the involved autoimmune mechanisms become available, early identification of such patients before diabetes becomes overt will be essential.

Patients taking oral hypoglycemic agents frequently require other medication. Drugs that may significantly amplify or inhibit the action of the oral agent must be identified.[r46] Since the list of such drugs is extensive and there are many mechanisms for interraction, recourse to a computerized program of identifying such possible interactions in such patients is advisable.

Other causes of inadequate response to oral hypoglycemic agents include poor adherence to diet and primary endocrine disease with increased counterregulatory hormones. Since hyperglycemia per se increases insulin resistance and blunts insulin response, an intensive period of control may at least temporarily restore responsiveness. Simply shifting to a maximal dose of another sulfonylurea drug usually is not effective. Shifting to metformin (p. 715) may give satisfactory control in about 50 per cent of such patients.[39] When sulfonylurea or metformin treatment becomes marginal, however, it seems logical to adopt insulin treatment earlier rather than later. Results of a controlled clinical trial[45] suggests that, if the choice in such patients is between treatment with insulin or with a sulfonylurea drug, the former may be preferable because the pattern of postprandial carbohydrate metabolism more closely approximates that in nondiabetic subjects.

Possible Combined Treatment with Insulin and a Sulfonylurea Drug

Many studies have discussed whether, when a patient with so-called NIDDM fails to respond to insulin, a sulfonylurea drug should be added—or, conversely, whether insulin should be added to the regimen when response to a drug is unsatisfactory. Conclusions have varied, perhaps because the types and stages of the patients in the studies also varied. However, a number of carefully controlled studies[29,r43] indicate demonstrable benefit. Whether this warrants the increased cost and risk of adverse reactions remains to be established in more completely characterized patients. Hyperinsulinemia may contribute directly to atherosclerosis.[48] Adding a sulfonylurea drug to the regimen may reduce the insulin dose required, but the atherogenic risk presumably is not diminished if the hyperinsulinemia is unaltered.[46,47] It is preferable instead to intensify the nonpharmacologic measures, particularly in the obese and sedentary patient to consider the use of metformin (p. 713). A case can be made for providing bedtime long- or intermediate-acting insulin to a drug-treated patient with fasting hyperglycemia in order to suppress the increased hepatic glucose and fatty acid production.[27] Adding insulin during the daytime and/or replacing completely the oral agent by insulin resulted in equal improvement in control, but these maneuvers produce normalization in only a small percentage of patients.[48]

Available Sulfonylurea Drugs and their Advantages and Disadvantages[r44]

The characteristics of the first-generation tolbutamide and three of the second generation sulfonylurea drugs are listed in Table 41.5. They differ in peak and duration of action, in potency/mol of the parent drug and its various metabolites, in type and degree of binding to serum proteins, and in route of excretion. These features are critical to selection in relation to the various stages and complications of diabetes. Starting doses of all should be small and titrated upward at a rate appropriate to the individual patient or drug. Self-monitoring of blood glucose and measure of hemoglobin A1c and serum lipids is essential to confirm that the patient is obtaining adequate metabolic improvement, not just symptomatic relief.

Of the first-generation drugs, tolbutamide has a short half-life of about four hours and thus must be taken two to three times a day. Its metabolites are only weakly active and it causes minimal

Table 41.5 Structure of Sulfonylurea Oral Hypoglycemic Agents

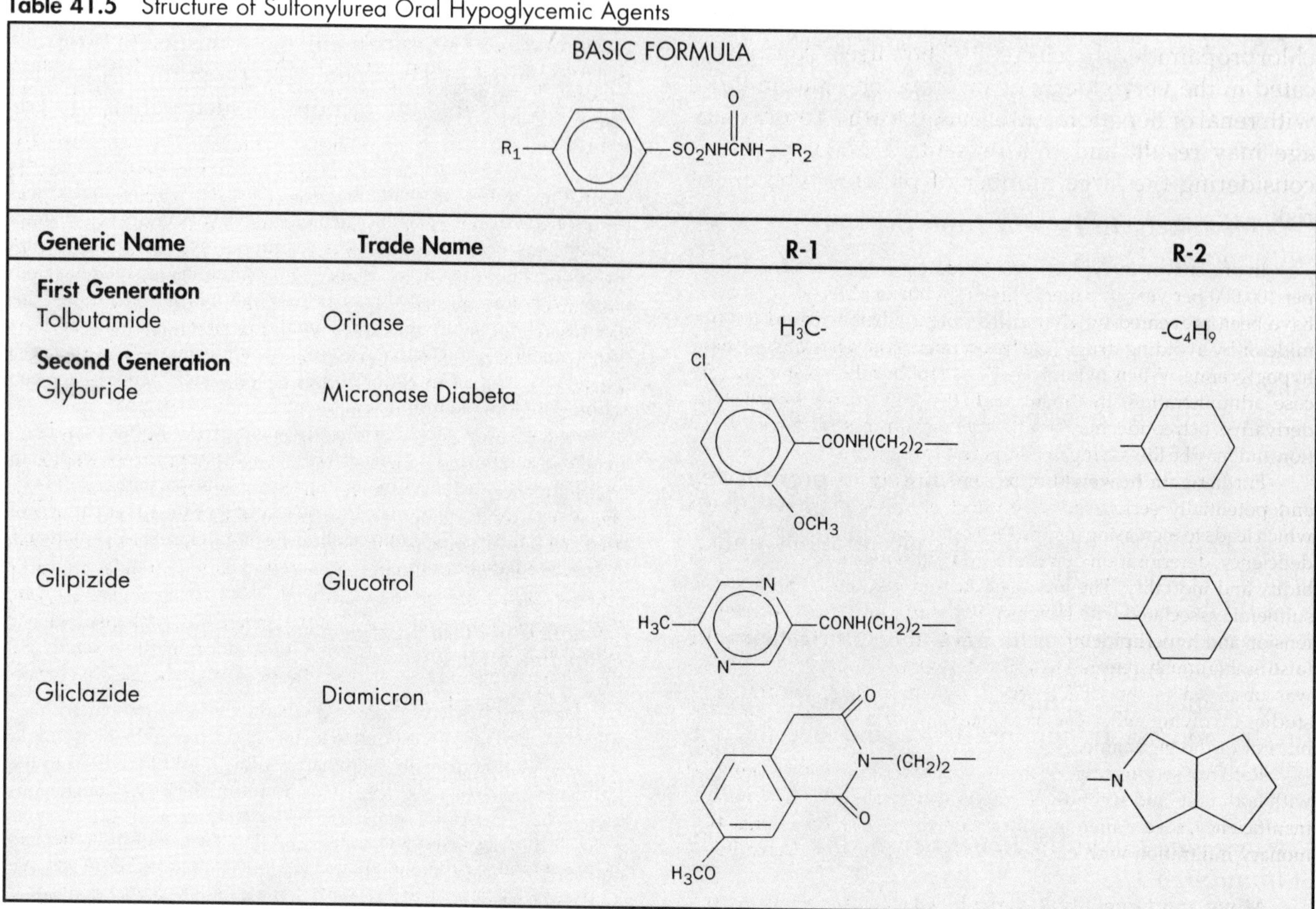

BASIC FORMULA

R_1–C₆H₄–$SO_2NHCONH$–R_2

Generic Name	Trade Name	R-1	R-2
First Generation			
Tolbutamide	Orinase	H_3C-	$-C_4H_9$
Second Generation			
Glyburide	Micronase Diabeta	Cl; $-CONH(CH_2)_2-$; OCH_3	
Glipizide	Glucotrol	N; H_3C-; $-CONH(CH_2)_2-$; N	
Gliclazide	Diamicron	O; $N-(CH_2)_2-$; O; H_3CO	$-N$

adverse reactions, although hyponatremia and hypoglycemia may occur. It is as effective in comparable dosage and currently cheaper, while the over-all risk of serious side-reactions and severe hypoglycemia is less.

Acetohexamide and tolazamide are rarely used today. Chlorpropamide, unfortunately still widely used, has a duration of action of up to 72 hours and a high proportion of adverse reactions. Its hepatic metabolites produce a disulfuram type of flushing reaction and hypotension when taken with alcohol. It has the highest incidence of side-effects of all the sulfonylureas, including hyponatremia, abnormal liver function tests, and severe prolonged hypoglycemia with associated high mortality. For these reasons it will not be considered further.

The second generation drugs have 100–150 times greater potency. There is a difference in their bioavailability, since their binding to serum proteins is nonionic rather than ionic. This also reduces the problem of displacement by other drugs. Superiority in efficacy to tolbutamide remains controversial, but they have a greater over-all incidence of serious side-effects, and minimal differences in mechanisms of hypoglycemic action have been demonstrated. The University Group Diabetes Project (UGDP) raised the possibility that tolbutamide increased mortality from cardiac malfunction. There is now some evidence that the second generation of oral agents actually improves cardiac function, at least in rats, and has antiarrhythmic properties.[49]

The peak concentration of glyburide (glibenclamide) in the plasma after ingestion is reached at approximately three hours.[49] Half is excreted in the feces and half in the bile, but this advantage is offset by the slow renal excretion of its active metabolite. Its effective action is 24 hours, so once-a-day dosage is possible, although larger doses should be divided. Its prolonged action accounts for a somewhat higher incidence of severe hypoglycemia, its main adverse effect.

Glipizide has a shorter plasma peak of one hour. It is converted in the liver to inactive metabolites. Fifteen percent is excreted in the feces, and only 3 per cent is excreted unchanged by the kidney. Gliquidone also has the advantage of predominantly biliary excretion. Thus both are preferred for patients with renal insufficiency.

Gliclazide is very widely used in Europe.[51] A specific anti-platelet-aggregation activity and an effect on the fibrinolytic system that might delay development of vascular complications has been claimed. A specific action on thromboxane synthesis and platelet aggregation independent of glycemic control has been reported.[52] A lack of weight gain attributed to the more natural contour of insulin secretion has been reported.[53]

Undesirable Effects of Sulfonylurea Drugs

Weight-gain with increasing insulin resistance, hypoglycemic coma, particularly by interaction with other drugs, and rare, but serious toxic or allergic reactions are the major adverse effects (See Table 41.5.)

Prolonged hypoglycemia is the major hazard of all of the agents, even when used appropriately, and occurs more frequently when the drugs with longer physiologic effect, such as glyburide and the older chlorpropamide, are selected.[r46] Their use is contraindicated in the very elderly or incompetent, and in those with renal or hepatic insufficiency. Death or brain damage may result, and this presents a major problem, considering the large number of patients who are at risk.

In one survey in 1979 in West Germany, there were 2.17 deaths per 100,000 per year in patients given glyburide. Most deaths could have been prevented by giving less potent agents such as tolbutamide or by avoiding drugs (see below) that synergistically promote hypoglycemia. When hypoglycemia is stubbornly resistant to glucose administration, treatment with the long-acting somatostatin derivative, octreotide, may be effective in suppressing insulin secretion and may be life-saving. It is superior to diazoxide in this regard.[54]

Further **gain in weight** of patients already obese is a common and potentially serious adverse effect of the sulfonylurea drugs, which leads to increasing insulin resistance, increased relative insulin deficiency, deterioration of morale, and ultimately to increased morbidity and mortality. The increased insulin resistance and hyperinsulinemia associated with increasing obesity contribute to the hypertension and hyperlipidemia of the **Syndrome of Insulin Resistance** (also ambiguously referred to as Syndrome X).[r36] Indeed, weight gain was observed in the UGDP study and in subsequent large-scale studies involving either use of the sulfonylureas and/or of insulin, but not of the biguanides.

Rare but serious toxic or immune reactions have been reported with both first- and second-generation drugs. These include hepatic insufficiency, severe anemias, thrombocytopenia or leukopenia, pulmonary infiltration with eosinophilia, and exfoliative dermatitis.[39]

Minor and Generally Reversible Adverse Reactions

Side-effects occur in approximately 6 percent of patients treated with chlorpropamide and 3.2 per cent of those treated with tolbutamide; the situation is essentially the same with second-generation agents. These include minor skin reactions and GI disturbances. Flushing following alcohol ingestion and varying degrees of fluid retention and hyponatremia from the syndrome of inappropriate ADH secretion are typical of chlorpropamide.

Pharmacokinetics

As indicated above in discussing individual agents, the various sulfonylureas differ in their duration of action, hepatic metabolism, bioactivity of metabolites, and route of excretion,[r45] as indicated in Table 41.5. In addition, there is variation between individuals in their pharmacokinetics. Thus, close self-monitoring of the profile of response of the blood glucose is essential.

There is much variation between individuals in the rate of absorption of sulfonylureas,[r45] and this may confound the results of clinical trials. Because of slower absorption, tolbutamide and glipizide are best given one half-hour before a meal. A diet high in fiber may further delay absorption to some degree.

Hypoglycemic Coma from Drug Interactions

All the first-generation sulfonylurea drugs are approximately 99 per cent bound ionically to serum proteins, mainly to albumin, and are readily displaced by other drugs. The second-generation drugs, given in hundred-fold smaller dosage, are less readily displaced, and, as noted previously, this has been attributed to nonionic binding. Many of these drugs potentiate the action of the sulfonylureas and may precipitate serious or fatal reactions by the wide range of mechanisms,[r46] as outlined in Table 41.5. The most important of these are ethanol, phenylbutazone, sulfinpyrazone, monoamine oxidase inhibitors, sulfonamides, the coumarin anticoagulants, allopurinol, chloramphenicol, salicylates, and cimetidine. The combination of a tricyclic antidepressant and a sulfonylurea drug can produce profound hypoglycemia.[55] Older patients with diabetes frequently are subject to polypharmacy and receive a variety of drugs. Since the list of possible interactions of drugs and their metabolites is extensive, the reader is referred to current indexes of such potential interactions, either in printed form or as one of the commercially available computerized versions.

The relative degree of **hepatic metabolism** and the formation of active metabolites are indicated in Table 41.5. Most are inactivated and eliminated by renal excretion, but some metabolites, such as those of acetohexamide, are more potent than the parent compound and increase the risk of hypoglycemia. As noted above, glyburide differs in that its metabolites are excreted equally in bile and urine, and glipizide is converted in the liver to inactive metabolites, making these drugs somewhat safer for patients with renal insufficiency. Gliquidone has the advantage that it is predominantly excreted via the biliary tract, and hence, like glyburide, might be cautiously used in the face of renal insufficiency.

Available Preparations and Usual Dosage

Of the four drugs surviving from the first generation, there are 116 proprietary preparations on the world market. There are over 14 second-generation drugs, with 83 proprietary preparations marketed. Eleven preparations combining a sulfonylurea with a biguanide drug are available worldwide, but not in the United States. The combined use is discussed on p. 715. Only two of the second generation, glyburide and glipizide, were approved for marketing in the US as of 1993. It is hoped that before the end of this century, all of these drugs will be replaced by members of the third generation of drugs, which more closely target the underlying mechanisms of this group of disorders.

The ranges of initial and maintenance dosage are given in Table 42.5.

The Biguanide Metformin in the Treatment of Predominantly Insulin-Resistant Diabetes

The dimethylbiguanide, metformin, is widely used throughout the world as a hypoglycemic agent, and has a number of advantages. It is not bound to plasma proteins and is not metabolized in the body. Insulin resistance and hyperinsulinemia are reduced by potentiating the receptor and postreceptor action of insulin in muscle with respect to nonoxidative glucose disposal and glucose transport. Hyperlipidemia is decreased, and the drug tends to raise HDL-cholesterol. Intestinal absorption of carbohydrates is reduced, and weight loss is promoted in the obese. There is no stimulation of insulin secretion. Metformin may be effective when sulfonylurea drugs are not. Adverse

Table 41.6 Characteristics of Selected Oral Hypoglycemic Agents[f]

	Tolbutamide	Glyburide	Glipizide
Relative Potency	1	150	100
Duration of Action (hrs)	6–10	18–24	16–24
Type of protein binding. (all 98%)	mainly ionic	part nonionic	part nonionic
Activity of metabolites	weak[c]	active[d]	inactive
% renal excretion (active forms)	85	50[d]	5
% fecal excretion	0	50	12
Adverse Effects:			
Weight gain	+	+	+
Gastrointestinal	0	2[e]	
% severe hypoglycemia	<1	4–6	2–4
Hyponatremia	+	0	0
% Over-all incidence adverse reactions	3%	6%	7%
Normalizing serum lipids	0[b]	0[b]	0[b]
Increase fibrinolytic activity	0	0	0
Dosage:			
Range mg.	500–3000	1.5–20	2.5–40
Initial/d mg	500	2.5	500
Doses/d	2–3	1–2	1–2

(a) clearance 500 ml/min by both filtration and secretion.
(b) Indirect effect only.
(d) 36% excreted as 4-hydroxyglyburide, which is 15% as active as parent drug.
(e) Rare cholestatic jaundice or hepatitis Modified from Gerich[38]

reactions may include GI distress and lactic acidosis in patients with underlying renal or hepatic insufficiency.

Chemistry and Relative Potency of Metformin

The molecular structure of metformin is diagrammed in Figure 41.7.

History of The Biguanides as Hypoglycemic Agents

Diguanides have been known as hypoglycemic agents in animals since 1929. In 1957 metformin, the N,N-bimethyldiguanide derivative, was first used in humans. When the prospective trial, the University Group Diabetes Project (UGDP), was initiated in the US in the 1960s, its related compound, phenformin (phenylethyldiquanide), was chosen as one of the agents to be tested for prevention of complications of NIDDM. Because of the incidence of lactic acidosis leading to cardiac failure and death, phenformin finally was withdrawn in 1977 from use in the US and most other countries. The related metformin was also withdrawn, although its incidence of lactic acidosis is 1/10th or 1/15th that of phenformin. Many other countries have continued to support the use of metformin, and some have also permitted phenformin, while urging that it not be given to patients with such definite contraindications as cardiac and renal disease. It is estimated that, in the 1980s, at least 600,000 patients worldwide were taking biguanides, and it is hoped that the drugs will be approved for use in the US in the near future. Meanwhile, clinical and basic studies are continuing.

Mechanism of Action of the Biguanide Metformin

The major actions of metformin are independent of weight loss and include: (a) stimulation of glucose uptake into skeletal muscle and adipocytes by increasing glucose transporters in the plasma membrane;[56,57] (b) increase in insulin-mediated glucose disposal;[58,59] (c) reduction of basal hepatic glucose production through inhibition of gluconeogenesis;[58] and (d) reduction of hyperlipidemia and increase in HDL-cholesterol.[58,60,61] Unlike the sulfonylurea drugs, metformin has no effect on the insulin secretory response. Midintestinal glucose absorption is inhibited in mice,[61] but is not considered a major action in humans.

As in the case of the sulfonylureas, it is often difficult to estimate whether a particular response to metformin in patients with diabetes is direct or is the result of lessening of hyperglycemia, hyperinsulinemia, and obesity. There is improvement in glucose transport in hyperglycemic, but not euglycemic subjects, suggesting that metformin increases glucose-mediated uptake. The increased insulin response in rats is in part related to an increase in receptor tyrosine kinase.[63] Metformin increases glucose transport and the translocation of the GLUT 1 and GLUT 4 isoforms of the glucose transporters from the intracellular pool in rat adipocytes[64] and in muscle.[65] There are conflicting conclusions from studies of the mechanism of action in humans, perhaps because of differences in subtypes of patients classed as NIDDM. In both obese and lean diabetic NIDDM patients in one study,[58] under hyperglycemic conditions there was augmented glucose uptake from metformin, but no increase in tissue sensitivity to insulin. In another recent study[66] in similar patients, suppression of hepatic glucose production and suppression of lipolysis was the predominant action.

Most important, metformin treatment improves plasma lipids, with a significant decrease in plasma triglyceride concentration and an increase in the beneficial HDL-cholesterol concentration.[67,61] The

Table 41.6 *Continued*

	Metformin	Gliclazide
Relative Potency	. . . .	125
Duration of Action (hrs)	12–24?	6–12[G]
Type of protein binding (all 98%)	not bound	part nonionic
Activity of metabolites	none formed	weak
% renal excretion (active forms)	85–100	60–70
% fecal excretion	0	10–20
Adverse Effects:		
Weight gain	(anorexic)	minimal
Gastrointestinal	20 (initial)[b]	<2%
% Severe hypoglycemia	0	2–4%
Hyponatremia % Incidence	0	0
% Over-all incidence	6–28[a]	<3%
Normalizing serum lipids	+	0[b]
Increase fibrinolytic activity	?	+[c]
Dosage:		
Range mg.	500–2500	80–240
Initial/d mg	500	80
Doses/d	1–2	1–2

(a) Mainly at onset of therapy and dose related. 20% incidence with <3 Gm starting dose, with 4% discontinuing treatment in published reports 1960–1980.
(b) Evidence inconsistent in published reports.
(c) For review, see Krall chapters number 6, 1988 and 1990 Diab Ann. [1]
(Modified from Gerich [38]

increased lactic acid production is mainly balanced by an increase in hepatic gluconeogenesis, which in turn provides a buffer against hypoglycemia.[r43]

In subjects treated with metformin without renal or hepatic insufficiency, there is only minimal increase in serum lactic acid.[56]

Recently, studies of relatively normal subjects without hyperglycemia have clarified some of the responses. In mildly hyperinsulinemic close relatives of persons with NIDDM the effect of chronic metformin on the increased insulin resistance was studied by means of the euglycemic hyperinsulinemic insulin clamp technique combined with indirect calorimetry.[68] Insulin-stimulated glucose disposal was significantly increased, primarily due to an increase in nonoxidative glucose disposal, while glucose oxidation was somewhat decreased. In a recent study, chronic treatment with metformin of a group of hypertensive patients reversibly lowered blood pressure without change in body weight.[69] Fasting serum insulin and C-peptide were reduced, while glucose disposal, measured by the euglycemic hyperinsulinemic clamp technique, was increased. Both total and LDL-cholesterol and triglycerides were lowered. HDL-cholesterol and fibrinolytic activity were both increased.

Therapeutic Uses

Many effects of metformin are similar to those of exercise, and a more active lifestyle with dietary restriction should be the first approach to prevention and treatment. In the real world, however, and in spite of sincere efforts by physician and patient, continued weight gain and increasing insulin resistance prove frustrating. The main advantages of metformin over those of the sulfonylureas or insulin in treatment of the obese patient with NIDDM, as diagrammed in Stage III of Figure 42.5B, are that weight gain does not occur and there is no risk of hypoglycemia.

In patients with other features of the syndrome of insulin resistance, namely hyperlipidemia and/or hypertension, an agent such as metformin has advantages in not increasing serum insulin and in the antihypertensive and lipid-lowering effects described above.

Metformin has been given as a single agent, in combination with a sulfonylurea, or with insulin when sulfonylurea drugs alone have not been effective.[r43] However, the gain in control is variable and, particularly in younger patients with primary failure, may not justify compounding the increased risk of adverse reactions and cost.[29]

As in the case of the sulfonylures, primary failure occurs when there is predominantly a deficiency of insulin secretion. The secondary failure rate appears to be comparable to that with the sulfonylurea drugs, and may vary according to whether there is autoimmune islet destruction or some other mechanism producing insulin deficiency.

Metformin may be of value in extreme insulin resistance. In a patient with Type B resistance secondary to anti-insulin-receptor antibodies, metformin increased insulin binding in vitro and in vivo.[70] The plasma glucose and insulin were decreased, and sensitivity to exogenous insulin was increased. Metformin was also effective in reducing the extreme insulin resistance of a patient with lipoatrophic diabetes,[71] but was ineffective in a patient with the insulin resistance of Mendenhall's syndrome.[72]

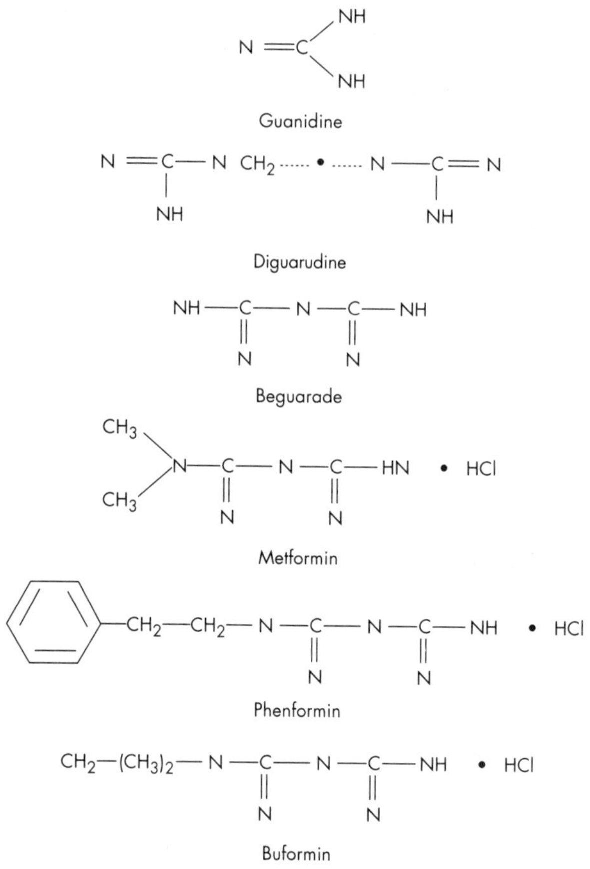

Guanidine

Diguarudine

Beguarade

Metformin

Phenformin

Buformin

Figure 41.7 The structure of guanidine, diguanidine, and biguanide with its derivatives: metformin, widely used except in the US, phenformin, and buformin, also widely used. Phenformin is contraindicated because of its tendency to produce lactic acidosis.

Undesirable or Toxic Effects

The incidence of severe lactic acidosis associated with metformin, which is not metabolized within the body, about equals the incidence of severe hypoglycemia produced by the longer-acting sulfonylurea derivatives, and the resulting mortality has been similar.[r47] In almost all the metformin cases there were contraindications to its use, such as renal or hepatic insufficiency. When used appropriately, there is minimal increase in basal serum lactate and only a modest increase in postprandial lactate production.[r48,58]

Gastrointestinal side-effects occur, including discomfort, occasional diarrhea, or vomiting. Nausea occurred in one large series in 75 percent of the cases during the first 3–4 days of treatment, but usually cleared within a week and only rarely disrupted the schedule of treatment. The incidence is in the range of 20–25 percent when initiation is gradual and the total dose is limited to 2.5 gm per day, in divided doses taken with or immediately after meals.

Metformin inhibits absorption of vitamin B-12 from the distal ilium. However, only one case of vitamin B-12 deficiency leading to megaloblastic anemia has been reported in a patient treated with metformin.[r48]

Finally, it may produce a metallic taste in the mouth.

Metformin does not produce hypoglycemia, major drug interactions, or cholestasis, and has a lower incidence of hypersensitivity reactions than do the sulfonylureas.

The list of contraindications is formidable: (a) Age over 65 or incompetence; (b) renal, hepatic, or cardiac disease; (c) alcohol ingestion in excess; (d) acute infection or other severe stress; (e) severe caloric restriction or exhausting exercise; (f) pulmonary insufficiency; and, of course, (g) pregnancy. Diagnostic angiography, which reduces renal clearance of the drug, is a temporary contraindication. However, only 28 fatalities directly attributable to the drug were recently reported out of 600,000 users worldwide, and in every incidence there was one of the above contraindications to its use.

Pharmacokinetics

Approximately 50 per cent of ingested metformin is bioavailable. It does not bind to serum proteins, and thus is not subject to displacement by competitive binding of other drugs. Unlike phenformin, it is not hydroxylated by the liver,[73] and 80 to 100 percent of an injected dose is excreted unchanged by both renal glomerular filtration and tubular secretion. There is no secretion into the intestinal tract. The half-life in serum is only 1.5 hour, as opposed to 12 hours for phenformin, and its duration of action is approximately 12 hours.

Available Preparations and Dosage

Metformin is supplied as 500-mg and 850-mg white tablets; it is marketed in all countries except the US under 28 different trade names. The daily maintenance dose is 0.5 to 3.0 g in-divided dosage, taken with meals.

New and Experimental Agents for the Prevention and Treatment of Diabetes Mellitus

The Immunosuppressive Approach to Prevention or Cure of Diabetes

Those at high risk for developing insulin deficient diabetes can now be more readily identified. However, for a number of reasons, attempts to arrest pancreatic islet cell destruction by broadly suppressing autoimmunity with cyclosporine and later with azathioprine have not been encouraging.[r49,r50] Remissions are generally not sustained; there is considerable toxicity and concern regarding risk of inducing malignancy. Of the many approaches to a more specific attack on the immune destruction, anti-T-lymphocyte therapy with diphtheria toxin linked to interleukin-2 has proven effective in mice.[74]

As this book goes to press another exciting possibility emerges.[r51] In the Non-Obese Diabetic (NOD) mouse model of IDDM and in humans, antibody against the enzyme glutamic acid decarboxylase (GAD) appears long before overt diabetes. The GAD enzyme forms gamma-aminobutyric acid, a probable paracrine signal molecule in the islets as well as an inhibitory neurotransmitter. Loss of tolerance to the main GAD enzyme apparently initiates T-cell responses, the first in a cascade of autoimmune reactions leading to destruction of beta cells of the pancreas. In the NOD mouse, IV or intrathymic injection of GAD 65 impairs the response of the T-cell subtypes most involved and prevents both ileitis and diabetes. Since patients at high risk for IDDM can be identified early by measurement of the serum anti-GAD65 antibody, it will be a major advance if diabetes can be prevented or ameliorated without adverse effects on the neuronal GAD in such humans by the technique that is effective in NOD mice.

Adjuncts to Dietary Restriction

Alpha-glucosidase inhibitors have been developed to block the absorption of sugars derived from starches and secondarily to reduce plasma lipids.[r51] Only one, acarbose, has achieved limited licensing to date, and it has been associated with a modest reduction in glycosylated hemoglobin.

Tetrahydrolipostatin, a drug that directly inhibits intestinal lipase and thus may counter the effects of a diet inappropriately high in fat, is undergoing clinical trials.[75]

The inevitable side-effects are flatulence and occasional diarrhea, which may prompt the patient to reduce food intake or which may require adjustment of the dosage.

Thermogenic Agents that Increase Lipolysis and Reduce Insulin Resistance

Beta-3 adrenoceptor agonists with minimal beta-1 and -2 stimulation have potential advantages for the person with obesity and insulin-resistant diabetes.[r43,r51]

In animal models of obesity with or without diabetes, weight loss is entirely due to lipolysis, without decrease in muscle mass. Thermogenesis is increased, in part due to stimulation of brown adipose tissue. The effect is greater in obese than in lean animals.[76] Chronic administration of a beta-3 agonist increases insulin sensitivity and decreases hyperinsulinemia.

In obese humans, short-term administration for 10 days increases glucose disposal solely by an increase in nonoxidative glucose disposal with a modest increase in thermogenesis.[76,r51] Dormant brown fat may be reactivated and stimulated. Weight loss of patients undergoing moderate caloric restriction is increased significantly. The main side-effect is tremor, apparently from some degree of beta-2 stimulation. Beta-1 cardiovascular effects have not been a problem with more recent analogues.[r51] Long-term studies are required to evaluate possible physiologic and psychologic effects.

The net metabolic effects of the agonists are similar to those of exercise.[42] Longer-term studies are in progress to estimate whether any of the agonists being developed have advantages over exercise in efficacy, cost effectiveness, and sense of well being

Agents that Minimize the Complications of Diabetes

Accumulation of sorbitol and depletion of myoinositol are established in animals as promotors of diabetic neuropathy, retinopathy, and capillary basement membrane thickening. A year-long multicenter trial of an aldose reductase inhibitor, tolrestat, involving 520 patients established that some improvement in symptomatic neuropathy was obtainable in those given the highest dosage level.[77] In a similar trial of 112 patients with chronic symptomatic sensorimotor neuropathy there was long-term benefit in approximately one-fourth of the subjects.[78] The benefits in those with more advanced neuropathy are minimal.[79] Whether longer term inhibition may prove a practical and safe method of preventing or treating neuropathy remains to be established. In a similar 41-month trial involving sorbinil, an aldose reductase inhibitor derived from spirohydantoin, there was noted a slight limitation of progression of retinal microaneurysms, but its clinical importance was considered uncertain.[80]

The glycosylation and cross-linking of proteins secondary to hyperglycemia and the subsequent development of irreversible advanced nonenzymatic glycosylation products that cannot be scavenged by monocytes is a major cause of microvascular and other complications of diabetes. In diabetic animals the linkages that produce the advanced glycosylation products can be blocked by administering aminoguanidine hydrochloride or its somewhat more effective diamino derivative,[81,82] with reduction of retinopathy, nephropathy, neuropathy, and cataract formation. Current clinical trials in normal subjects have given no evidence of toxicity, and further trials in patients are awaited with great interest.

Somatostatin was originally isolated from the hypothalmus as an inhibitor of release of growth hormone from the pituitary. It was later isolated from the delta cells of the pancreatic islets and other tissues, and was found to be a potent inhibitor of the release of both insulin and glucagon. As such, it has been a useful tool for research in diabetes. Analogues with a half-life in plasma of 8–12 hours have been produced that are valuable in management of several hormone-producing tumors. A potential use of these analogues in diabetes is in control of early morning hyperglycemia, the so-called "dawn phenomenon," which has been attributed to increased secretion of growth hormone during the late hours of the night.[30]

New Oral Hypoglycemic Agents

It seems likely that, soon after this book is published, the sulfonylureas will be replaced by agents with physiologic action more appropriate to the syndromes of insulin resistance and that metformin or its equivalent will be available for use in the US.

The thiazolidinedione derivatives, developed in 1983 in Japan, hold promise in that they improve insulin sensitivity and responsiveness peripherally, while circulating insulin concentrations decrease. The excessive hepatic glucose production of NIDDM is reduced, and, like the biguanides, these new drugs improve the serum lipid profile.[r43] Thus they hold promise of benefitting the syndrome of insulin resistance.

The structure of pioglitazone, a potent second-generation thiazolidinedione derivative, is

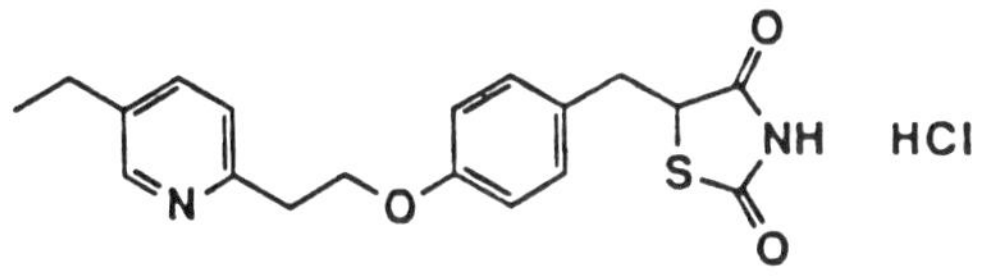

A host of studies in obese and insulin-resistant diabetic animals have shown that the drug (a) increases insulin sensitivity by increasing insulin-stimulated receptor kinase activity,[83] and is ineffective in the face of insulin deficiency; (b) reduces hepatic glucose output by increasing phosphoenolpyruvate carboxykinase and not by affecting GLUT2 in liver;[84] (c) increases glucose transport in muscle and adipocytes by increasing GLUT4 in the presence of insulin;[85] and (d) lowers plasma triglycerides and cholesterol.[86] Clinical trials are in progress, and the only adverse effect reported to date has been mild tremor.[86]

Another thiazolidinediol derivative, CS-045, has similar actions in patients. In a study employing the euglycemic, hyperinsulinemic clamp technique in a heterogeneous, uncharacterized group of patients with NIDDM, CS-045 produced a marked increase in glucose disposal rate and a decrease in hepatic glucose production.[87]

Drugs that Suppress Appetite and Also Have Direct Hypoglycemic and Lipid-lowering Activity

An available, safe, and effective appetite suppressant for the chronic treatment of obesity associated with diabetes would be valuable. Agents that suppress appetite by blocking reuptake of serotonin at the nerve terminal may be useful in this connection. Fenfluramine (see Chapter 64) given to insulin-resistant animals increases serotonin secretion and also increases insulin sensitivity independent of change in dietary intake and body weight.[r43,88] The action is distal to the insulin receptor. Dex-fenfluramine, the active isomer, has somewhat greater effectiveness, and those with central obesity and those who crave carbohydrates appear to benefit most. The antidepressant fluoxetine (Prozac) has similar effects.[89,r43,r51] The drugs are widely used outside the US for treatment of obesity.

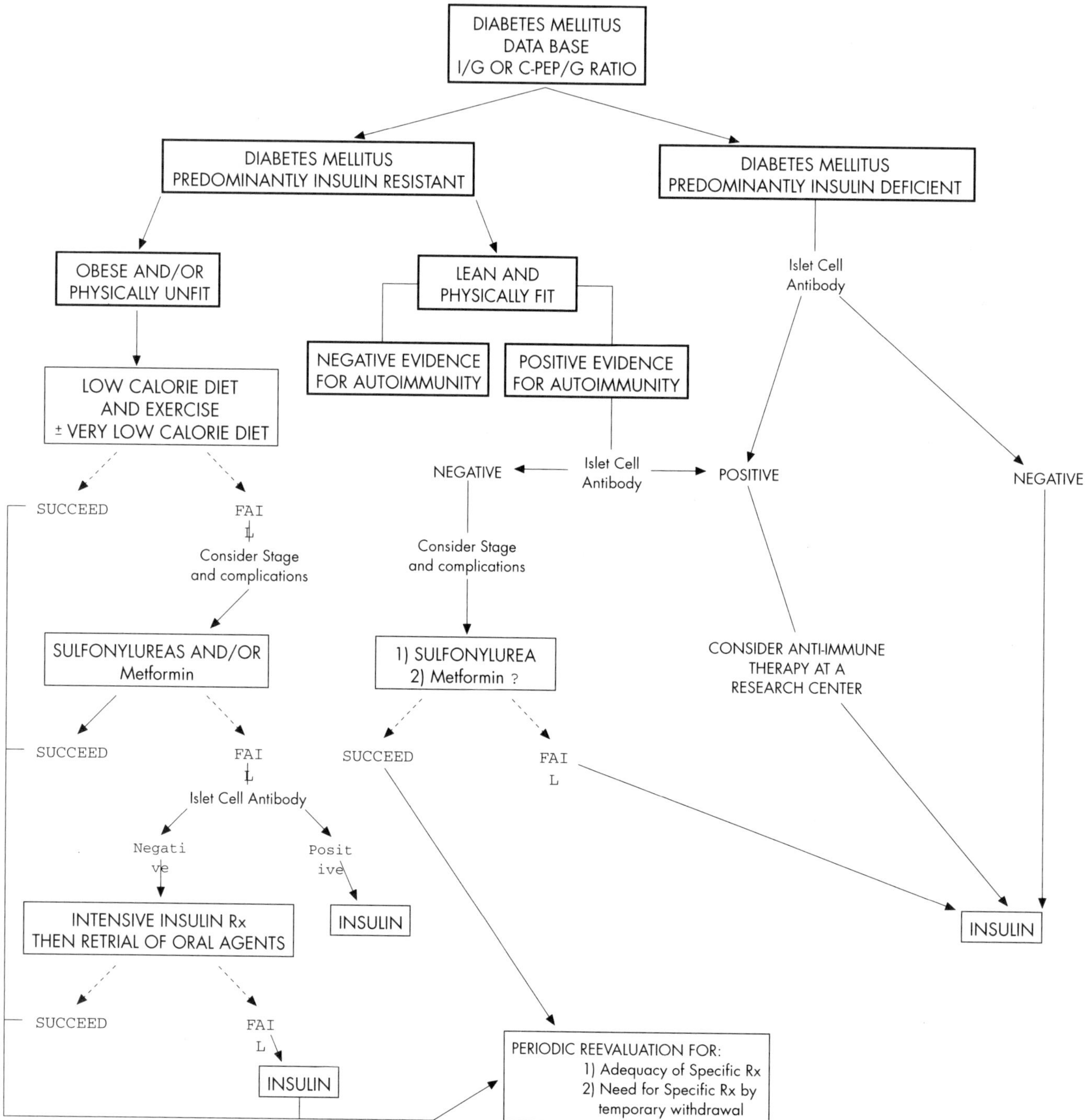

Figure 41.8 A Sumary of the options for management of the various subtypes and stages of diabetes. I/G and C-Pep/G are the ratios of fasting and stimulated insulin and C-peptide to glucose in plasma. See text for details.

A Hypolipidemic Agent that Reduces Hyperinsulinemia

A hypolipidemic agent, benflourex, which has been used since 1974, has properties that may make it uniquely suitable for treatment of the syndrome of insulin resistance.[43] It has the following structure:

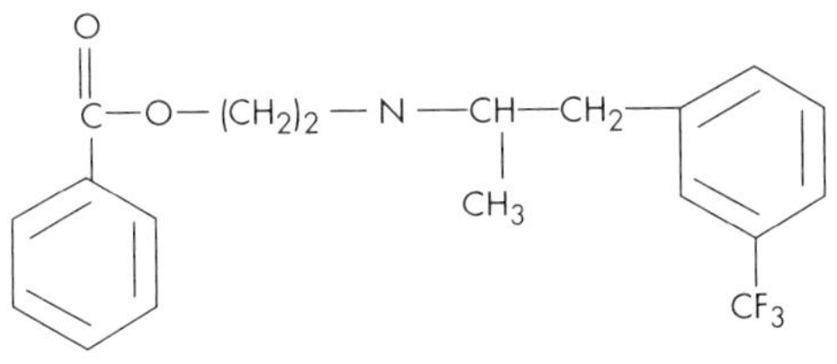

Studies in insulin-resistant animals have shown: (1) inhibition of hepatic fatty acid synthesis from acetate and an inhibition of triacylglycerol synthesis; (2) a decrease in plasma insulin concentrations; (3) a decrease in insulin resistance; (4) improvement in hypertension; and (5) improvement in hyperlipidemia—all in the absence of weight loss. No effect on carbohydrate metabolism has been noted in animals without insulin resistance. Clamp studies have shown normalization of basal glucose concentrations and almost complete suppression of hepatic glucose production, with less effect on peripheral insulin resistance. Gluconeogenesis from lactate plus pyruvate or from alanine is inhibited, and it has been suggested that the inhibition is located at the level of the mitochondrial pyruvate carrier. There is also an increase in the hepatic clearance rate of insulin. Chronic administration of the drug in humans significantly improves HgbA1c and fructosamine concentrations and the insulin/glucose ratio, without change in weight. In one study, the effect was greater than in a biguanide control.

Nonpharmacologic Treatment

Once again, it should be emphasized that if a sustained change in lifestyle can accomplish the same physiologic effects, it is preferable both with respect to prevention of complications and for cost effectiveness.

Summary: An Integrated Approach to the Management of Diabetes by Insulin and by Pharmacologic and Nonpharmacologic Means

The treatment at a given time of the heterogeneous group of disorders grouped as diabetes mellitus will depend on the subtype, the stage of the diabetes, and the previous response to available therapeutic measures. Figure 41.8 is an algorithm of the various options.

References

Research Reports

1. Vincent S. Nitric oxide and arginine-evoked insulin secretion. Science 1992;*258*:1376.
2. Calles-Escandon J, Robbins DC. Loss of early phase of insulin release in humans impairs glucose tolerance and blunts thermic effect of glucose. Diabetes 1987;*36*, 1167.
3. Bingley PJ. Loss of regular oscillatory insulin secretion in islet cell antibody positive non-diabetic subjects Diabetologia 1992;*35*:32–38.
4. Froguel P, Zouali H, Vionnet N, Velho G, Vaxillaire M, Sun F, Lesage S, Stoffel M, Takeda J, Passa P, Permutt A, Beckman JS, Bell GI, Cohen D. Familial hyperglycemia due to mutations in glucokinase Definition of a subtype of diabetes mellitus. N Engl J Med 1993;*328*:697–702.
5. Takasawa S, Nata K, Yonekura H, Okamato H. Cyclic ADP-Ribose in insulin secretion from pancreatic beta cells. Science 1993;*259*:370–373.
6. Ciaraldi TP, Gilmore A, Olefsky JM, Goldberg M, Heidenreich KA. In vitro studies on the action of CS-045, a new antidiabetic agent. Metabolism Clin & Exptl 1990;*39*:1056–1062.
7. Molina JM, Cooper GJS, Leighton B, Olefsky JM. Induction of insulin resistance in vivo by amylin and calcitonin gene-related peptide. Diabetes 1990;*39*:260–265.
8. Sowa R, Sanke R, Hirayama J, Tabata H, Furuta H, Nichimura S, Nanjo K. Islet amyloid polypeptide amide causes peripheral insulin resistance in vivo in dogs. Diabetologia 1990;*33*:118–120.
9. Bretherton-Watt D, Gilbey SG, Ghatei MA, Beacham J, Bloom SR. Failure to establish islet amyloid polypeptide (amylin) as a circulating beta cell inhibiting hormone in man. Diabetologia 1990;*33*:115–117.
10. Johansson B-L, Sjoberg S, Wahren J. The influence of human C-peptide on renal function and glucose utilization in Type I (insulin-dependent) diabetic patients. Diabetologia 1992;*35*:121–128.
11. Taira Masato, Taira Masanori, Hashimoto N, Shimada F, Suzuki Y, Kahasuka N, Nakamura F, Ebina Y, Tatibana M, Makino H. Human diabetes associated with a deletion of the tyrosine kinase domain of the insulin receptor. Science 1989;*245*:63–66.
12. Arner P, Pollare T, Lithell H, Livingston JN. Defective insulin receptor tyrosine kinase in human skeletal muscle in obesity and type 2 (non-insulin-dependent) diabetes mellitus. Diabetologia 1987;*30*:437–440.
13. Olefsky JM, Brillon DJ, Freidenberg GR, Henry RR. Mechanism of defective insulin-receptor kinase activity in NIDDM. Diabetes 1989;*38*:397–404.
14. Bogardus C, Ravussin E, Robbins DC, Wolfe RR, Horton ES, Sims EAH. Effects of physical training and diet therapy on carbohydrate metabolism and glucose tolerance in non-insulin-dependent diabetes. Diabetes 1984;*33*:311–318.
15. National Diabetes Data Group. Harris M, Cahill GF. Co-Chairpersons. Classification and diagnosis of diabetes mellitus and other categories of glucose intolerance. Diabetes 1979;*28*:1039–1057.
16. Zavala AV, Fabiano LE, Cardoso AI, Mota AI, Mota AH, Capucchio M, Poskus E, Fainboim L. Cellular and humoural autoimmunity markers in type 2 diabetic patients with secondary drug failure. Diabetologia 1992;*35*:1159–1164.
17. Christie MR, Tun RYM, Lo SSS, Cassidy D, Brown TJ, Hollands J, Shattock M, Bottazzo GF, Leslie DG Antibodies to GAD and tryptic fragments of islet 64K antigen as distinct markers for development of IDDM: studies with identical twins. Diabetes 1992;*41*:782–787.
18. Tuomi T, Groop LC, Zimmet PZ, Rowley MJ, Knowles W, Mackay Jr. Antibodies to glutamic acid decarboxylase reveal latent autoimmune diabetes mellitus in adults with a non-insulin-dependent onset of disease. Diabetes. 1993;*42*:359–362.

19. Thivolet C, Tappaz M, Durand A, Petersen J, Stefanutti A, Chatelain P, Vialettes B, Scherbaum W, Orgiazzi J. Glutamic acid decarboxylase (GAD) autoantibodies are additional predictive markers of type I diabetes mellitus in high risk individuals. Diabetologia 1992;*35*:570–576.

20. Hagopian WA, Karlsen AE, Gottsater A, Landin-Olsson M. Grubin CE, Sundkvist G, Petersen JS, Boel A, Durberg T, Lernmark A. Quantitative assay using recombinant human islet glutamic acid decarboxylase (GADS65) shows that 64K autoantibody positivity at onset predicts diabetes type. J Clin Invest 1993;*91*:368–374.

21. Eriksson KF, Lindgarde F. Prevention of Type 2 diabetes mellitus by diet and physical exercise. Diabetologia 1991;*34*:891–898.

22. Scott J, Poffenberger PL. Pharmacogenetics of tolbutamide metabolism in humans. Diabetes 1979;*28*:41–51.

23. Hagedorn HC. Modification of insulin. Phys Bull 1947;*12*:26–33.

24. Hallas-Moller K, Petersen K, Schlichtkrull J. Crystalline and amorphous insulin-zinc compounds with prolonged action. Science 1952;*116*:394–398.

25. The Diabetes Control and Complications Trial Research Group. The effect of intensive treatment of diabetes on the development and progression of long-term complications in insulin-dependent diabetes mellitus. N Engl J Med 1993;*329*:977–986.

26. Duckworth WC, Saudek CD, Henry RR. Why intraperitoneal delivery of insulin with implantable pumps in NIDDM? Diabetes 1992;*41*:657–661.

27. Taskinen M-R, Sane T, Helve E, Karonen S-L, Nikalla EA, Yki-Jarvinen H. Bedtime insulin for suppression of overnight free-fatty acid, blood glucose, and glucose production in NIDDM. Diabetes 1989;*38*:80–88.

28. Broussolle C, Jeandidier N, Hanaire-Broutin H, Raccah D, Renard E, Guerci B, Haardt MJ, Gilly F, Pinget M, Tauber JP, Lassman-Vague V, Bringer J, Drouin P, Selam JL, Vague Ph. Long term intraperitoneal insulin therapy with programmable implantable pumps: the French Multi Center Trial. The Endocrine Society. 75th Annual Meeting. Abstracts 1993; 230.

29. Schade DS, Mitchell WJ, Griego G. Addition of sulfonylurea to insulin treatment in poorly controlled type II diabetes: A double-blind, randomized clinical trial. JAMA 1987;*257*:2441–2445.

30. Perriello. G, De Feo P, Torlone E, Fanelli C, Santeusanio F, Brunetti P, Bolli GB. The dawn phenomenon in type 1 (insulin-dependent) diabetes mellitus: magnitude, frequency, variability and dependency on glucose counterregulation and insulin sensitivity. Diabetologia 1991;*34*:21–28.

31. Tordjman KM, Havlin CE, Levandoski LA, White NH, Santiago JV, Cryer PE. Failure of nocturnal hypoglycemia to cause fasting hyperglycemia in patients with insulin-dependent diabetes mellitus. N Engl J Med 1987;*317*:1552–1559.

32. Schade, DS, Eaton RP, Drumm DA, Duckworth WC. A clinical algorithm to determine the etiology of brittle diabetes care. 1985;*8*:5–11.

33. Boden G, Master RW, Rezvani I, Palmer JP, Lobe TE, Owen OE. Glucagon deficiency and hyperaminoacidemia after total pancreatectomy. J Clin Invest 1980;*65*:706–716.

34. Holst JJ, Pedersen JH, Baldiserra F, Stadil F. Circulating glucagon after total pancreatectomy in man. Diabetologia 1983;*25*:396–399.

35. Slama G, Reach G, Cahane M, Quetin C. Villanove-Robin F. Letter to the editor: Intranasal glucagon in the treatment of hypoglycemic attacks in children: experience at a summer camp. Diabetologia 1992;*35*:398.

36. Lebovitz HE, Pasmantier R. Combination insulin-sulfonylurea therapy. Diabetes Care, 1990;*13*:667–675.

37. University Group Diabetes Program. VIII. Evaluation of insulin therapy: final report. Diabetes 1982;*31*:(Suppl 5, pt 2)1–81.

38. Jacobs DB, Hayes GR, Lockwood DH. In vitro effects of sulfonylurea on glucose transport and translocation of glucose transporters in adipocytes from streptozocin-induced diabetic rats. Diabetes 1989;*38*:205–211.

39. Gerich JE. Oral Hypoglycemic Agents. N Engl J Med 1989;*321*:1231–1245.

40. Garrel DR, Pica R, Bajard L. Harfouche M, Tourniaire J. Acute effects of glyburide on insulin sensitivity in type I diabetic patients. J Clin Endocrinol Metab 1987;*65*:896–900.

41. Martz A. Jo I, Jung CY. Sulfonylurea binding to adipocyte membranes and potentiation of insulin stimulated hexose transport. J Biol Chem 1989;*264*:13672–13678.

42. Bogardus CE, Ravussin E, Robbins DR, Wolfe RR, Horton ES, Sims EAH. Effects of physical training and diet therapy on carbohydrate metabolism in patients with glucose intolerance and non-insulin-dependent diabetes mellitus. Diabetes 1984;*33*:311–318.

43. Davidson JK. The practical use of dietary techniques, including a 1-week total fast for weight reduction in patients with NIDDM. Diabetes Care 1986;*10*:639–644.

44. Singer DL, Hurwitz D. Long-term experience with sulfonylureas and placebo. N Engl J Med 1967;*9*:450–456.

45. Firth R, Bell P, Marsh M, Rizza RA. Effects of tolazamide and exogenous insulin on pattern of postprandial carbohydrate metabolism in patients with non-insulin-dependent diabetes mellitus. Results of randomized crossover trial. Diabetes 1987;*36*:1130–1138.

46. Stolar MW. Atherosclerosis in diabetes: the role of hyperinsulinemia. Metabolism 1988;*37*:1–9.

47. Peters AL, Davidson MB. Insulin plus a sulfonylurea agent for treating type 2 diabetes. Ann Intern Med 1991;*115*:45–53.

48. Groop LC, Widen E, Ekstrand A, Saloranta C, Franssila-Kallunki A, Shalin-Jantti C, Eriksson JG. Morning or bedtime NPH insulin combined with sulfonylurea in treatment of NIDDM. Diabetes Care. 1992;*15*:831–834.

49. Mozafarri MS, Allo S, Schaffer SW. The effect of sulfonylurea therapy on defective calcium movement associated with diabetic cardiomyopathy. Canad J Physiol Pharmacol 1989;*57*:1431–1435.

50. Simonson DC, Delprato S, Castellino P. 1987 Effect of glyburide on glycemic control, insulin requirement, and glucose metabolism in insulin-treated patients. Diabetes 1987;*36*:136–146.

51. Gram J, Jespersen J, Kold A. Effects of an oral antidiabetic drug (gliclazide) on the fibrinolytic system of blood in insulin-treated patients. Metabolism 1988;*37*:937–943.

52. Florkowski CM, Rowe BR, Nightengale S, Harvey TC, Barnett AH. Clinical and neurophysiological studies of aldose reductase inhibitor ponalrestat ion chronic symptomatic diabetic peripheral neuropathy. Diabetes 1991;*40*:129–33.

53. Hosker JP, Rudenski AS, Burnett MA, Matthews DR, Turner RC. Similar reduction of first- and second-phase B-cell responses at three different glucose levels in type II diabetes and the effect of gliclazide therapy. Metabolism 1989;*38*:767–772.

54. Boyle PJ, Justice K, Krentz AJ, Nagy RJ, Schade DS. Octreatide reverses hyperinsulinemia and prevents hyperglycemia induced by sulfonylurea overdoses. J Clin Endocrinol Metab 1993;.*76*:752–756.

55. True BL, Perry PJ, Burns EA. Profound hypoglycemia with the addition of a tricyclic antidepressant to maintenance sulfonylurea therapy. Am J Psychiatr 1987;*144*:1220–1221.

56. Serabia V, Lam L, Burdett E, Leiter LA, Klip A. Glucose transport in human skeletal muscle cells in culture. Stimulation by insulin and metformin. J Clin Invest 1992;*90*:1386–1395.

57. Hundal HS, Ramlal T, Reyes R, Leiter LA, Klip A. Cellular mechanism of metformin action involves glucose transporter translocation from an intracellular to the plasma membrane in L6 muscle cells. Endocrinology 1992;*131*:165–173.

58. DeFronzo RA, Barzilai N, Simonson DC. Mechanism of metformin action in obese and lean noninsulin-dependent diabetic subjects. J Clin Endocrinol Metab 1991;*73*:1294–1301.

59. H(ther-Neilsen O, Schmitz O, Anderson PH, Beck-Nielsen, Pedersen O. Metformin improves peripheral but not hepatic insulin action in obese patients with type II diabetes. Acta Endocrinologia (Copenh) 1989;*120*:257–265.

60. Schneider J, Erren T, Zofel P, Kaffarnik H. Metformin-induced changes in serum lipids, lipoproteins, and apoproteins in non-insulin-dependent diabetes mellitus. Atherosclerosis 1990;*82*:97–103.

61. Hollenbeck CB, Johnston P, Varasteh BB, Chen YD, Reaven GM. Effects on metformin on glucose, insulin and lipid metabolism in patients with mild hypertriglyceridaemia and non-insulin-dependent diabetes by glucose tolerance test criteria. Diabete et Metabolisme 1991;*17*:483–489.

62. Wilcox C, Bailey CJ Reconsideration of inhibitory effect of metformin on intestinal glucose absorption. J Pharm Pharmacol 1991;*43*:120–121.

63. Rossetti L, DeFronzo RA, Gherzi R. Effect of metformin treatment on insulin action in diabetic rats in vivo and in vitro correlations. Metabolism 1990;*39*:425–435.

64. Matthaei S, Hamann A, Klein HH, Benecke H, Kreyman G, Flier JS, Greten H. Association of metformin's effect to increase insulin-stimulated glucose transport with potentiation of insulin-induced translocation of glucose transporters from intracellular pool to plasma membrane in rat adipocytes. Diabetes 1991;*40*:850–857.

65. Klip A, Leiter L. Cellular mechanism of action of metformin. Diabetes Care 1990;*13*:696.

66. Perriello G, Misericordia P, Volpe E. Metformin reduces hyperglycemia in lean and obese NIDDM by suppressing hepatic glucose production and lipolysis without increasing glucose utilization. Diabetes 1991,*40*:(Suppl 1), 305A.

67. Wu M-S, Johnston P, Sheu W-H, Hollenbeck CB, Jeng C-Y, Goldfine LD, Chen Y-D, Reaven GM. Effect of metformin on carbohydrate and lipoprotein metabolism in patients with non-insulin-dependent diabetes. Diabetes Care 1990;*13*:1–8.

68. Widen EIM, Eriksson JG, Groop LC. Metformin normalizes non-oxidative glucose metabolism in insulin-resistant normoglycemic first-degree relatives of patients with NIDDM. Diabetes 1992;*41*:354–358.

69. Landin K, Tengborn L, Smith U. Treating insulin resistance in hypertension with metformin reduces both blood pressure and metabolic risk factors. J Intern Med 1991;*229*:181–187.

70. Di Paolo S. Metformin ameliorates extreme insulin resistance in a patient with anti-insulin receptor antibodies: description of insulin receptor and postreceptor effects in vivo and in vitro. Acta Endocrinologia 1992;*126*:117–123.

71. Labeille B, Lalau JD, Chouquais et al. 1988 Diabete lipoatrophique avec insulino-resistance controle par la metformine. Ann Dermatol Venereol 1988;*115*:1151–1152.

72. Quin JD, Fisher BM, Paterson KR, Inoue A, Beastall GH, MacCuish AC. Acute response to recombinant insulin-like growth factor I in a patient with Mendenhall's syndrome. (Letter). N Engl J Med 1990;1425–1426.

73. Bosisio E. Defective hydroxylation of phenformin as a determinant of drug toxicity. Diabetes 1983;*30*:644–649.

74. Pacheco-Silva A. Bastos MG, Muggia RA, Pankewycz O, Nichols J, Murphy JR, Strom TB, Rubin-Kelley VE. Interleuken 2 receptor targeted fusion toxin (DAB-486-IL2) treatment blocks diabetogenic autoimmunity in non-obese diabetic mice. Eur J Immunol 1992;*22*:697–702.

75. Hauptmann JB, Jeunet FS, Hartman D. Initial studies in humans with the novel gastrointestinal lipase inhibitor Ro 18-0647 (tetrahydrolipstatin). Am J Clin Nutr 1992;*55*:309S–313S.

76. Cawthorne MA, Sennit MV, Arch JRS, Smith SA. BRL 35135, a potent and selective atypical beta-adrenoceptor agonist. Am J Clin Nutr 1992;*55* (Suppl 1): 252S–257S.

77. Giugliano D, Marfalla R, Quatraro A, De Rosa N, Salvatore R, Cozzolino D, Ceriollo A, Torella R. Tolrestat for mild diabetic neuropathy. A 52-week randomized, placebo controlled clinical trial. Ann Int Med 1993;*118*:7–11.

78. Boulton, AJM, Levin S, Comstock J. A multicentre trial of the aldose-reductase inhibitor, tolrestat, in patients with symptomatic diabetic neuropathy. Diabetologia 1990;*33*:431–437.

79. Florkowski CM, Rowe BR, Nightingale S, Harvey TC, Barnett AH. Clinical and neurophysiological studies of aldose reductase inhibitor ponalrestat in chronic symptomatic diabetic peripheral neuroppathy. Diabetes 1991;*40*:129–133.

80. Sorbinol Retinopathy Trial Research Group. A randomized trial of sorbinil, an aldose reductase inhibitor, in diabetic retinopathy. Arch Ophthalmol 1990;*108*:1234–1244.

81. Kumkari K, Uma RS, Bansal V, Sahib MK. Inhibition of diabetes-associated complications by nucleophilic compounds. Diabetes 1001:*40*:1079–1084.

82. Oxlund H, Andreassen TT. Aminoguanidine treatment reduces the increase in collagen stability of rats with experimental diabetes mellitus. Diabetologia 1992;*35*:19–25.

83. Kobayashi M, Iwanishi M, Egawa K, Shigeta Y. Pioglitazone increases insulin sensitivity by activating insulin receptor kinase. Diabetes 1992;*41*:476–483.

84. Hofmann CA, Edwards CW 3d, Hillman RM, Colca JR. Treatment of insulin-resistant mice with the oral antidiabetic agent pioglitazone: evaluation of liver GLUT2 and phosphoenolpyruvate carboxykinase expression. Endocrinology 1992;*130*:735–740.

85. Hofmann CA, Lorenz K, Colca JR. Glucose transport deficiency in diabetic animals is corrected by treatment with the oral antihyperglycemic agent pioglitazone. Endocrinol. 1991;*129*:1915–1925.

86. Colca JR, Dailey CF, Palazuk BJ, et al. Pioglitazone hydrochloride inhibits cholesterol absorption and lowers plasma cholesterol concentrations in cholesterol-fed rats. Diabetes 1991;*40*:1669–1674.

87. Suter SL, Nolan JJ, Wallace P, Gumbiner B, Olefsky JM. Metabolic effects of new oral hypoglycemic agent CS-045 in NIDDM subjects. Diabetes Care 1992;*15*:193–203.

88. Pestell RC, Crock PA, Ward GM, Alford FP, Best AD. Fenfluramine increases insulin action in patients with NIDDM. Diabetes Care 1990;*12*:252–258.

89. Wise SD. Clinical studies with fluoxetine in obesity. Am J Clin Nutr 1992;*55*:181S–184S.

Reviews

r1. Daughaday WH and Rotwein P. Insulin-like growth factors I and II. Peptide messenger ribonucleic acid and gene structures, serum and tissue concentrations. Endocrin Rev 1989;*10*:68–91.

r2. Bliss M. The Discovery of Insulin. Chicago: University of Chicago Press. 1982.

r3. Luft R. Oskar Minkowski: Discovery of the pancreatic origin of diabetes 1889. Diabetologia 1989;*32*:399–401.

r4. Pfeiffer EF, Ed. Comparative endocrinology of the insulin family. A minisymposium. Horm Metab Res 1988;*20*:401–444.

r5. Zwalich WS, Rasmussen H. Control of insulin secretion: a model involving Ca^{2+}, cAMP and diacylglycerol. Mol Cell Endocrino 1990;*70*:119–137.

r6. Matschinsky FM. Glucokinase as glucose sensor and metabolic signal generator in pancreatic beta cells and hepatocytes. Diabetes 1990;*39*:647–652.

r7. Magnuson MA. Glucokinase gene structure. Functional implications of molecular genetic studies. Diabetes 1990: *39*:523–527.

r8. Schwartz MW, Figlewicz DP, Baskin DG, Woods SC, Porte D Jr. Insulin in the brain: A hormonal regulator of energy balance. Endocrin Rev 1992;*13*:387–414.

r9. Yamaguchi N. Sympathoadrenal system in neuroendocrine control of glucose: mechanisms involved in the liver, pancreas, and adrenal gland under hemorrhagic and hypoglycemic stress. Canad J Physiol Pharmacol 1992;*70*:167–206.

r10. Sims EAH. Energy balance in human beings: Problems of plenitude. In Auerbach GD, McCormick DB, Eds. Vitamins and Hormones. New York: Academic Press 1986;*43*:1–101.

r11. Hokfelt R, Bartfai T, Jacobowitz D, and Ottoson D. Eds. Galanin. A new multifunctional peptide in the neuro-endocrine system. London: Macmillan, Wenner-Gren International Symposium Series, vol. 58, 1992.

r12. Westermark P, Johnson KH, O'Brien TD, Betsholtz C. Islet amyloid polypeptide—a novel controversy in diabetes research. Diabetologia 1992;*35*:297–303.

r13. Steiner D, Yoshimasa Y, Seino S, Whittaker J, Karehi T. Is islet amyloid polypeptide a significant factor in pathogenesis or pathophysiology of diabetes? Diabetes 1991;*40*:305.

r14. Duckworth WC. Insulin degradation: mechanisms, products, and significance, Endocrin Rev 1988;*9*:319–356.

r15. Lev-Ran A, Hwang DL. C-Peptide in NIDDM. Diabetes Care 1993;*16*:76–81.

r16. Moller DE, Flier JS: Insulin resistance-mechanisms, syndromes, and implications. N Engl J Med 1991;*325*:938–948.

r17. DeFronzo R (Ed). Review articles on non-insulin-dependent diabetes. Diabetes Care 1992;*15*:317–455.

r18. DeFronzo RA, Ferrannini E. Insulin resistance: A multifaceted syndrome responsible for NIDDM, obesity, hypertension, dyslipidemia, and atherosclerotic cardiovascular disease. Diabetes Care 1991;*14*:173–194.

r19. Denton RM, Tavare JM. Insulin action: mechanisms involved in the rapid effects of insulin on lipid metabolism. Diabetes Annual 1988;*4*:546–564.

r20. McGarry JD. What if Minkowski had been ageusic? An alternative angle on diabetes. Science 1992;*258*:766–770.

r21. Granner DK, O'Brien RM. Molecular physiology and genetics of NIDDM. Importance of metabolic staging. Diabetes Care 1992;*15*:3; 369–395.

r22. Brownlee M, Cerami A, Vlassara H. Advanced glycosylation end products in tissue and the biochemical basis of diabetic complications. N Engl J Med 1988;*318*:1315–1321.

r23. Sims EAH, Calles-Escandon J. Classification of diabetes. A fresh look for the 1990s? Diabetes Care 1990;*13*:1123–1128.

r24. Björntorp P. Metabolic implications of body fat distribution. Diabetes Care 1991;*14*:1132–1143.

r25. Ruderman NB, Schneider SH, Berchtold P. The "metabolically-obese" normal weight individual. Am J Clin Nutr 1981;*34*:1617–1621.

r26. Yki-Jarvinen J. Glucose toxicity. Endocrin Rev 1992;*13*:415–431.

r27. Vranic M, Hollenburg, CH, Steiner G (Eds.). Comparison of type I and type II diabetes. New York: Plenum Press, 1985.

r28. Sims DF, Sims EAH (Eds). Motivation, adherence, and the therapeutic alliance. In: Diabetes Spectrum 1989;*2*:17–52.

r29. Cryer PE, Binder C, Bolli GB, Cherrington AD, Gale EAM, Gerich AE, Sherwin RS. Hypoglycemia in IDDM. Diabetes 1989;*38*:1193–1199.

r30. Foster DW, McGarry JD. The metabolic derangements and treatment of diabetic ketoacidosis. N Engl J Med 1983;*309*:159–170.

r31. Kitabshi AE, Murphy MB. Diabetic ketoacidosis and hyperosmolar hyperglycemic nonketotic coma. Med Clin N America 1988;*72*:1545–1563.

r32. Hirsch IB, McGill JB, Cryer PE, White PF. Perioperative management of surgical patients with diabetes mellitus Anaesthesiology 1991;*74*:346–359.

r33. Caro JF, Singha MK, Dohm BM. Insulin resistance in obesity. In Bray, GA, Ricquier D, Spiegelman BM. (Eds.). Obesity: Toward a molecular approach. New York, Wiley-Lisa 1990.

r34. Reaven, GM. Role of insulin resistance in human disease. Diabetes 1988;*37*:1595–1607.

r35. Björntorp P, Ottossom M, Rebuffe-Scrive M, Xuefan X. Regional obesity and steroid hormone interactions in human adipose tissue. In Bray GA, Ricquier DM, Spiegelman BM (Eds.) Obesity: Toward a molecular approach. (pp 147–157) New York: Alan R. Liss, Inc. 1990.

r36. Karam JH. Type II Diabetes and syndrome X, pathogenesis and glycemic management. Endocrinol Metabol Clin N America. Diabetes mellitus: Perspectives on therapy. Philadelphia: WB Saunders, 1992: 329–350.

r37. Sims EAH, Berchtold P. Obesity and hypertension: mechanisms and implicaitons for management. JAMA 1982;*247*:49–52.

r38. Binder C, Lauritzen T, Faber O, Pramming S. Insulin pharmacokinetics. Diabetes Care 1984;*7*:188–199.

r39. Unger RH, Orci L. The essential role of glucagon in the pathogenesis of diabetes mellitus. Lancet 1975;*1*:14–16.

r40. Yarborough M, Steil C. Oral hypoglycemic agents. Applications of current research. Diabetes Spectrum 1989;*2*:294–322.

r41. Lebovitz HE, Pasmantier R. Combination insulin-sulfonylurea therapy. Diabetes Care 1990;*13*:667–675.

r42. Boyd AE, Aquilar-Bryan L, Bryan J. Sulfonylurea signal transduction. Recent Prog Horm Res 1991;*47*:299–317.

r43. Bailey CJ, Flatt PR (Eds.). New antidiabetic drugs. Smith-Gordon Co. London, Nishamura Co. Ltd. Niigata-Shi, Japan 1990.

r44. Krall LP. The sulfonylureas. Diabetes Annual 1991;*6*:137–147.

r45. Scott J, Poffenbarger PL. Pharmacogenetics of tolbutamide metabolism in humans. Diabetes 1979;*28*:41–51.

r46. Hansen JM, Christensen LK. Drug interactions with oral sulfonylurea hypoglycemic agents. Drugs 1977;*13*:24–34.

r47. Luft D, Schmulling RM, Eggstein M. Lactic acidosis in biguanide treated diabetics. Diabetologia 1978;*14*:75–87.

r48. Bailey C. Biguanides and NIDDM. Diabetes Care 1992;*15*:755–770.

r49. Eisenbarth GS, Di Mario UD. Immunotherapy of insulin-dependent diabetes mellitus. Diabetes Spectrum 1992;*5*:269–305.

r50. Skyler JS, Marks JB. Immune intervention in type I diabetes mellitus. Diabetes Rev 1993;*1*:15–42.

r51. Bressler R, Johnson D. New pharmacological approaches to therapy of NIDDM. Diabetes Care 1992;*15*:792–805.

r52. Solimena M. and DeCamilli P. Spotlight on a neuronal enzyme. Nature 1993; 15–17.

r53. Bray GA, Inoue S. (Eds.). Pharmacological treatment of obesity. Satellite symposium to the 6th international congress of obesity. Am J Clin Nutr 1992; 55 (Suppl to vol 1):151S–319S.

r54. Guy-Grand B. Clinical Studies with d-Fenfluramine. Am J Clin Nutr 1992;*55* (Suppl 1):173S–176S.

Reviews Not Cited

Alberti KGMM, Krall LP (Eds). Annual The Diabetes Annual. New York, Amsterdam, London: Elsevier.
Contains useful annual updates of the field of diabetes.

Rifkin H, Porte D Jr. (Eds). Diabetes mellitus, Theory and practice, 4th Ed. New York, Amsterdam, London: Elsevier, 1990.
An up-to-date and authoritative textbook.

Davidson, JK (Ed.). Clinical diabetes—A problem oriented approach, 2d. Ed. Stuttgart, New York: Thieme-Stratton, 1991.
A book that provides a knowledge base and highlights the team approach as an essential component of delivery of optimal contemporary care.

Defronzo RA (Ed). Diabetes reviews.
A new publication of the American Diabetes Association.

CHAPTER 42

Parathyroid Hormone and Bisphosphonates

Paul L. Munson

Parathyroid Hormone

Parathyroid hormone (PTH),[r1–r3] so far the only known hormone of the parathyroid gland, is essential for good health. It is produced, secreted, and its secretion regulated by the chief cells of the parathyroid gland. The major function of PTH is to maintain within rather narrow limits a certain concentration of calcium (approximately 10 mg/dl) in the blood plasma that is ideal for efficient neuromuscular function and for the development and maintenance of a healthy skeleton.

Parathyroid hormone has not yet achieved any role as an established therapeutic agent. The treatment of choice for hypoparathyroidism is not PTH but, rather, vitamin D or a related compound because vitamin D is both more effective and more economical. Because of the anabolic actions of PTH on bone, its use in the treatment of osteoporosis is being considered, but this has not yet gone beyond the investigational stage.

Chemistry

Mammalian parathyroid hormones[r4] are single-chain polypeptides made up of 84 amino acid residues. They lack cysteine and substituted amino acid residues but contain two methionines. Neither terminus of the chain is blocked. The molecules do not contain carbohydrates or other nonamino acid cofactors. There is a preponderance of basic amino acid residues; over-all, the molecules are basic in character.

The amino acid sequences of PTHs from several mammalian species—ox,[1,2] pig,[3] human,[4] and rat[5]—have been determined.[r4,r5] The sequences are quite similar but not identical. The sequence of human PTH is shown in Figure 42.1. The sequence of chicken PTH also has been determined.[6,7] It is similar to the mammalian PTHs but differs in having a chain length of 88 residues instead of 84 and quite a few segments that differ from mammalian PTHs. The comparative sequences of all the known PTHs are shown in Figure 42.2.[r8]

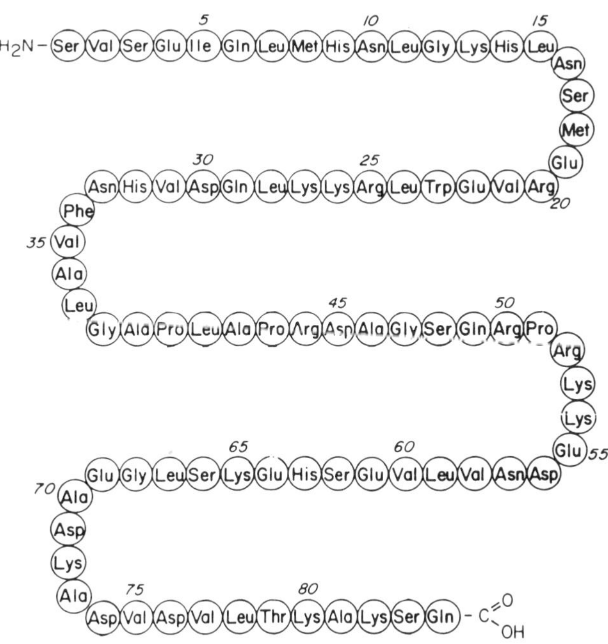

Figure 42.1 Amino Acid Sequence of Human Parathyroid Hormone (Courtesy of Dr. M. Rosenblatt)

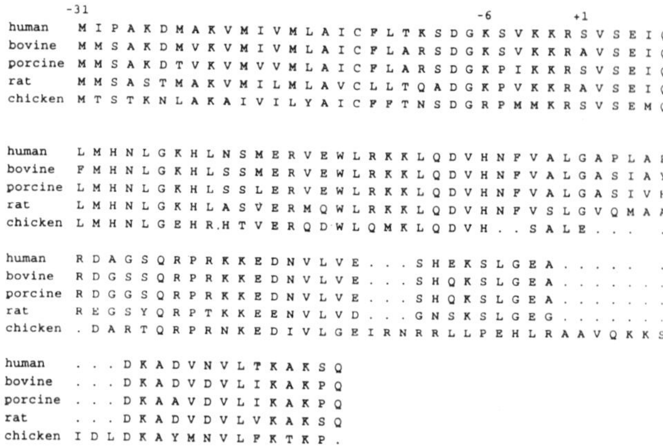

Figure 42.2 Amino acid sequences of preproPTH from mammalian and avian species. Residues from −31 to −7 constitute the "pre" sequences; residues −6 to −1 constitute the "pro" sequences. Dots in the mammalian sequences indicate residues in the chicken sequence not found in the mammalian sequences. Dots in the chicken sequence indicate residues in the mammalian sequences not found in the chicken sequence. Amino acid residues are indicated by the single letter code: ala A, arg R, asn N, asp D, cys C, gln Q, glu E, gly G, his H, ile I, leu L, lys K, met M, phe F, pro P, ser S, thr T, trp W, tyr Y, val V.

Biosynthesis[r7,r8]

The human gene for PTH is on the short arm of chromosome 11 at band 11p15.[8] After transcription of the DNA into mRNA in the nucleus of the chief cell, mature mRNA moves into the cytoplasm and mammalian PTH is biosynthesized as part of a larger 115 amino acid polypeptide known as "preproPTH." The synthesis of this larger molecule takes place on ribosomes bound to membranes of the rough endoplasmic reticulum of the chief cell.[9–11]

The next stage consists of two steps. In the first, 25 amino acids at the amino terminus (known as the signal or leader sequence) are removed by proteolytic enzymes in or near the rough endoplasmic reticulum.[r4] (The function of the signal sequence is to direct the protein across the membrane of the endoplasmic reticulum and into the secretory pathway.) The product, "proPTH", contains six more amino acids at the amino-terminus than PTH.[r4] (The function of the pro-sequence has not been established.) The proPTH then is moved to the Golgi apparatus, where it is converted, by another proteolytic enzyme, possibly furin,[12] to PTH.[r8] PTH(1-84) itself is the major form of the hormone contained in the mammalian gland; only 7 percent of the total is proPTH, and there is an even lower percentage of preproPTH. After biosynthesis, the PTH is transported to secretory granules, from which it is secreted, along with a variable amount of inactive carboxy-terminal PTH fragments.[r5]

Neither preproPTH nor proPTH is secreted, and neither has any significant biologic activity.[r5] Their biologic significance is confined to their role as biosynthetic precursors of PTH.

Structure-Activity Relationships for PTH[r6]

There is considerable cross-reactivity between the known mammalian PTHs, but their relative potencies differ considerably, depending on which assay method is used for the comparison. In an in vivo method (chick hypercalcemia), the ratio of bovine to porcine to human was 1: 2: 4. In an in vitro method (rat adenyl cyclase) the ratio was 9: 3: 1. Rat PTH (1-34) is considerably more active than all the rest according to the in vitro assay,[13] but the potency by an in vivo assay has not yet been reported. For human biology, the in vivo ratios would seem to be more meaningful.

If the methionine residues are subjected to mild oxidation to convert them to methionine sulfoxide, the ability to inhibit the renal reabsorption of phosphate in rats and to stimulate cAMP production in Japanese quail are lost, but the ability to produce hypercalcemia and hypocalciuria and to increase production of calcitriol are retained.[14]

Synthetic polypeptides that contain the amino acid sequence 1-34 of the human and bovine PTHs are about as active on a molar basis as the entire 1-84 sequence in most assay methods.[r6] In the adenyl cyclase assays, in vivo and in vitro, and the chick in vivo assay, the sequence 1-25 was the minimum for retaining any detectable biologic activity.[15] Removal of the two amino terminal acids resulted in complete loss of activity.[r7,r8] On the other hand, the amino terminus is less important for a cytochemical assay method. Even the synthetic 13-34 human peptide was active in this method.

The PTH receptor binding site is in the segment of ampiphilic alpha-helix (24-31).[16] The carboxy terminus of PTH is essential for hormone processing and secretion in the cell.[17]

The entire human PTH molecule (1-84) has been produced by solid-phase synthesis, and it was biologically active.[18]

Similar to PTH in its biologic effects but different in amino acid sequence is the so-called "PTH-related protein (PTHrP)".[r9] It is produced by certain malignant tumors, especially squamous, bladder, and ovarian (without bone metastases), and is associated with and responsible for hypercalcemia, "humoral hypercalcemia of malignancy (HHM)".[19] The amino acid sequence of PTHrP is homologous with but not identical to the first N-terminal sequence of PTH 1-13 and for sequence 14-34 there are a few identical residues. The rest of PTHrP is different from the PTH sequence, including size, three varieties of PTHrP being 139, 141, or 147 residues in length.[r9,r10] There are high concentrations of PTHrP in milk,[20] and PTHrP has been found in placenta, pregnant uterus, and some fetal tissues, as well as in mammary gland.[r9] Therefore, the possibility that PTHrP plays some role in normal physiology is being explored. The human gene for PTHrP is on the short arm of chromosome 12.[r12]

Research toward development of potent antagonists for PTH is in progress. A synthetic peptide patterned after a partial sequence (7-34) of PTHrP is six to eight times more potent than the comparable peptide from bovine PTH, but still not potent enough to be practical as a treatment for hyperparathyroidism.[21,r6]

Along with PTH, the parathyroid gland also secretes a larger polypeptide, the so-called "parathyroid secretory protein" (mol wt. 70,000).[22,23] It is secreted in response to calcium in a manner similar to that for PTH. Parathyroid secretory protein is a glycosylated protein similar or identical to chromogranin A found in secretory granules of the adrenal medulla.[24,r11] Current evidence suggests that it is a precursor of pancreastatin, which may affect the secretion of PTH. (Pancreastatin was discovered as a strong inhibitor of glucose-stimulated insulin release.[25])

History[r12]

The parathyroid gland was first identified by Owen in 1850 during the autopsy of a rhinoceros that had died in the London Zoo. The name parathyroid was first given to the gland in 1880 by the young Swedish histologist, Ivar Sandstrom, in 1880, who found the glands by dissection of human bodies—usually four glands in each body—as well as in oxen, dogs, cats, and rabbits. Sandstrom, however, did not suggest any physiologic significance of the glands. Later (1891), the French physiologist, Eugene Gley, who, like many others at the time, was studying the physiology of the thyroid, found that removal of the thyroid gland while preserving the external parathyroid glands intact was not fatal—contrary to the opposite view at the time that ignored the inadvertent removal of the small parathyroid glands during thyroidectomy. Gley, however, overlooked the hidden internal parathyroid glands and erroneously concluded that surgery in his rabbits was fatal only if both the thyroid and parathyroid glands were removed. It remained for Vassale and Generali (in 1894) to discriminate correctly between the effects of thyroidectomy and parathyroidectomy and to conclude correctly that tetany and death were the result of loss of the parathyroids, not of the thyroid. Vassale and Generali and others at the time thought that the importance of the parathyroid glands for survival was due to their detoxification of toxic metabolites.[r12]

The next major advance in the endocrinology of the parathyroid was provided by MacCollum and Voegtlin in 1909.[26] They found that the fatal tetany following parathyroidectomy was accompanied by severe hypocalcemia and that the tetany could be relieved by administration of a calcium salt. Nevertheless, it was not until the mid-1920s that the detoxification hypothesis was abandoned. In 1911, Greenwald discovered that parathyroidectomy led to a decrease in the urinary excretion of inorganic phosphate.[27] The next important advance in parathyroid endocrinology was the preparation, in 1924, by Hanson[28] and Collip,[29] independently, of extracts of parathyroid tissue that would reverse the effects of parathyroidectomy.[r12] These parathyroid extracts would relieve the tetany, raise serum calcium, increase urinary inorganic phosphate, and lower the hyperphosphatemia in parathyroidectomized animals. Many years later, in 1959, Aurbach isolated a substantially homogeneous bovine parathyroid polypeptide.[30] In 1970, Niall et al.[2] and, simultaneously, Brewer and Roner,[1] reported the amino acid sequence of the 84 amino acid bovine polypeptide. Determination of the amino acid sequences of the PTHs of other species followed.[r6]

Therapeutic Use and Physiologic Functions of PTH

Therapeutic Use

Although PTH would seem to be the logical treatment of hypoparathyroidism, it is not used for that purpose. As stated in the introduction, vitamin D or a related compound (dihydrotachysterol or calcitriol) is the drug of choice. These compounds all are active orally; they have a longer duration of action and are less expensive.[r13]

A less obvious therapeutic use for PTH now being investigated intensively in a number of centers, is in the prevention and treatment of osteoporosis.[r14,r15] This is based on the now well-recognized anabolic actions of PTH on bone under certain circumstances. The earlier emphasized catabolic actions of PTH on bone dominated thinking on the subject because of the hypercalcemia and bone loss of severe hyperparathyroidism and the effects of large doses of PTH in experimental animals. Differentiation between the catabolic and anabolic effects of PTH on bone is quite complex, but there is no longer any doubt that both actions are fundamental characteristics of PTH. Treatment of osteoporosis with PTH alone and in combination with other agents, estrogens, calcitonin, vitamin D, and bisphosphonates is being investigated.[r15]

Physiologic Functions[r17]

Calcium Homeostasis

A major function of PTH is to raise the concentration of calcium in the blood plasma to an optimum level of about 10 mg/dl and to keep it there. The rapid fall in plasma calcium after removal of the parathyroid glands is illustrated in Figure 42.3. In the absence of PTH, as shown in the figure, the plasma calcium may fall to as low as 5 md/dl, a concentration that reflects the apparent equilibrium between bone mineral and body fluids. To avoid an excess of PTH that would result in hypercalcemia, the rate of secretion is regulated by negative feedback, to be described later.[r16]

The calcium in blood is essentially all in plasma, where it is divided about equally between protein-bound and ionized calcium. (A small percentage, less than 10%), is complexed with organic acids, such as citrate.) Only the ionized calcium is physiologically active, but because the forms of plasma calcium are in rapid equilibrium in most situations, any change in total calcium is reflected in a corresponding change in the concentration of ionized calcium.[r15] Exceptions to this statement are: in humans with serum protein abnormalities, total serum calcium can change considerably without much change in ionized calcium; and in birds, during the normal egg-laying cycle, the total serum calcium may even double (by binding to phosvitin) without any change in ionized calcium.[r17]

Three organ systems affected by PTH contribute

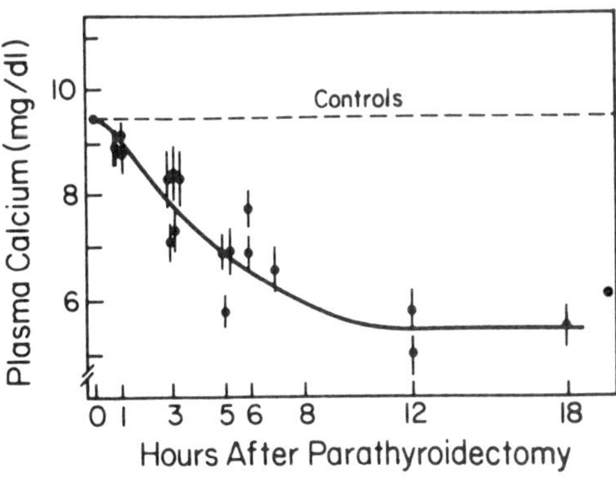

Figure 42.3 Rapid fall in plasma calcium after removal of the parathyroid glands in young male rats. Each point and vertical line represent the mean plus or minus the standard error of four to six rats. (Redrawn with permission from Tashjian AH Jr. Endocrinology 1966;*78*:1144–1153.)

to its ability to maintain the normal serum calcium concentration, bone, kidney, and intestine.

Bone.[r18,r19] The mineral phase of bone is predominantly hydroxyapatite, Ca10(PO4)6(OH)2. A part of the calcium in bone is adsorbed to the surface of bone in dynamic equilibrium with the calcium in plasma. PTH favors outflow of calcium from bone over inflow into bone and thereby prevents a fall in the plasma calcium when the over-all calcium balance is negative. In the absence of the hormone, inflow is favored, the result being a lowering of the plasma calcium. The action of PTH on a subpopulation of osteoblasts, including those that line bone surfaces, appears to be principally responsible for the minute-to-minute and hour-to-hour regulation of plasma calcium.

A second PTH-mediated process that affects plasma calcium is "bone remodeling," in which some areas of bone are being "resorbed" (matrix as well as mineral removed) and then replaced by new bone formation. The balance between the two activities of bone formation and bone resorption affects the plasma calcium concentration over the long term, but the changes are too slow to explain the rapid plasma calcium-raising activity of an injection of PTH under experimental situations.

Bone resorption is performed by the osteoclast, a large, multinucleated bone cell. Although PTH has a strong effect to increase the number of osteoclasts and their level of activity, it has been difficult to find PTH receptors on these cells. On the other hand, osteoblasts (the bone forming-cells) are rich in PTH receptors. It has been shown in in vitro experiments that PTH stimulates osteoclastic bone resorption most vigorously in the presence of osteoblasts. PTH acts on osteoclasts by stimulating osteoblasts to elaborate osteoclast-stimulating factors (interleukin 6 and probably others yet to be identified), and it is in this way that PTH effectively but indirectly stimulates bone resorption.[34] Some evidence for PTH receptors on osteoclasts has been obtained, however, and it seems likely that PTH affects osteoclasts by direct as well as indirect stimulation. A considerable amount of evidence has been accumulated to support the anabolic as well as catabolic effect of PTH on bone.[r13] This includes an effect of small or intermittent doses of PTH to increase net bone formation and the beneficial effects of endogenous PTH on bone at levels insufficient to raise serum calcium above the normal level. Attempts are being made to exploit this effect of PTH for the treatment of osteoporosis, as mentioned above.[r14]

Kidney. PTH also acts on the kidney to promote calcium homeostasis. It does so by: (1) reducing the renal excretion of calcium; and (2) stimulating the production of calcitriol, which increases intestinal absorption of calcium.

Most of the calcium in the glomerular filtrate is not excreted in the urine but is reabsorbed in the proximal tubule independent of PTH. Nevertheless, the added action of PTH to enhance reabsorption of calcium, which is on the thick ascending and granular portions of the distal tubule, is extremely important.[35,36] The additional calcium reabsorbed under the influence of PTH could account for as much as one-fifth to one-third of the total extracellular fluid calcium.

Intestine: Calcitriol. The third major organ system by which PTH affects calcium metabolism is the small intestine. Most, if not all of this effect is mediated through the hormonal metabolite of vitamin D, calcitriol (1-alpha, 25-dihydroxycholecalciferol), the production of which is increased by PTH.[37,r20,r21]

Calcitriol is produced in the kidney by the action of the enzyme, renal 25-hydroxyvitamin D 1-alpha-hydroxylase, on the precursor of calcitriol, calcifediol (25-hydroxycholecalciferol), produced by the liver from cholecalciferol. PTH affects the production of calcitriol by stimulating the renal 1-alpha-hydroxylase, which results in the supply of an adequate quantity of calcitriol or its analogue 1-alpha-25-dihydroxyergocalciferol, to promote a healthy rate of absorption of calcium by the small intestine (See the section on vitamin D in Chapter 58).

There also is evidence for some direct effect of PTH on the intestine for increasing absorption of calcium.[38]

Effect on Metabolism of Inorganic Phosphate[39,r22]

PTH also has an effect on the concentration of inorganic phosphate in the blood, which, like calcium, is located almost entirely in the plasma. Again, the effect is produced by actions of PTH on three organ systems—bone, kidney, and intestine—of which the kidney is predominant.

Kidney. About 75 percent of filtered phosphate is reabsorbed by the proximal tubule, the remainder by the distal tubule and cortical collecting loop. PTH depresses reabsorption of inorganic phosphate in both the proximal and distal tubules, thereby increasing the quantity of inorganic phosphate excreted in the urine and decreasing the concentration of inorganic phosphate in the plasma.

Bone. The effect of PTH to increase outflow of mineral from bone in the short term and during bone resorption in the long term tends to increase the concentration of inorganic phosphate as well as of calcium in the plasma, but the renal effect on phosphate predominates, so that, over-all, the result is a decrease in plasma inorganic phosphate, as is often seen in hyperparathyroidism.

Intestine. Inorganic phosphate, unlike calcium, is readily absorbed from the small intestine. Nevertheless, calcitriol increases its absorption; therefore, indirectly, by its effect on calcitriol production, PTH favors the absorption of phosphate as well as calcium from the intestine.

Importance. The effect of PTH on phosphate metabolism is secondary in importance to its effect on calcium metabolism. The supply of phosphate in food and its absorption from the intestine are ample, unlike the situation for calcium. Therefore, the loss of phosphate due to the action of PTH is not usually detrimental. On the other hand, excretion of phosphate protects the body from hyperphosphatemia, which tends to lower plasma calcium by several mechanisms.

The Adenylate Cyclase-Cyclic AMP System and Inositol 1,4,5 Triphosphate in the Mechanism of Action of PTH; G Proteins[r15,r23]

Much experimental evidence indicates that the increase in plasma calcium after an injection of PTH is mediated by an increase in cAMP. The same is true for the effect of PTH on the decrease in reabsorption of inorganic phosphate by the renal tubule. It is thought that after PTH binds to its receptor the receptor interacts with and activates a guanyl nucleotide-binding protein "G," which, in turn, activates adenyl cyclase and increases the hydrolysis of ATP to cAMP. G proteins are membrane-associated proteins that facilitate activation or inhibition of second-messenger effector systems in response to receptor activation. Although the concept that PTH acts through cAMP is well supported, there also is strong evidence for another second messenger, inositol, 1,4,5-triphosphate.

Regulation of Secretion of PTH[40,r15,r24]

The most important factor regulating the rate of secretion of PTH is the plasma concentration of ionized calcium. (This is unlike the situation in most endocrine cells, where an increase in calcium stimulates hormone secretion.) An increase in calcium inhibits the secretion of PTH and decreases ("stimulates") it by releasing the gland from inhibition. The interaction of ionized calcium and secretion of PTH constitutes a valuable feedback system that works to regulate the plasma calcium concentration within narrow limits between 8.0 and 10.4 mg/dl of total calcium. Figure 42.4 illustrates changes in the plasma concentration of PTH in response to changes in plasma calcium.[41]

The reaction of the feedback system is quite rapid. Observations in experimental animals indicate that the gland responds within one minute of an induced fall in serum ionized calcium to increase hormone secretion.

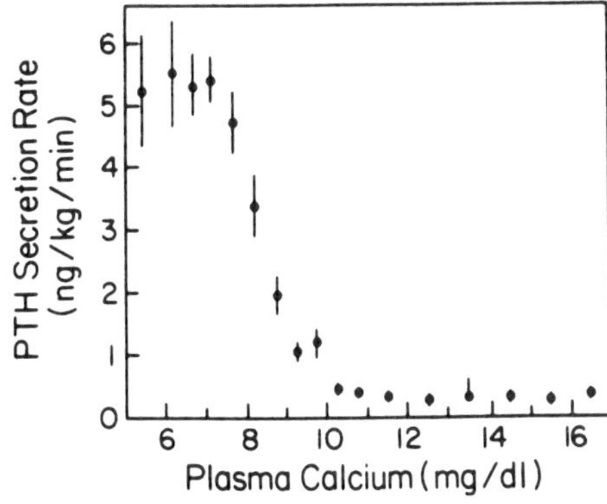

Figure 42.4 Changes in plasma concentration of parathyroid hormone in relation to induced changes in plasma calcium concentration in calves. Each point and vertical line represent the mean plus or minus the standard error of repeated measurements in two to twelve calves. (Redrawn with permission from data in Fig. 2 in Mayer GP, Horst JG. Endocrinology 1978; *102*:1036–1042.)

The first PTH released is that which has been stored in "mature" secretory granules. Later, if the calcium concentration stays low for a long time, with continuous release of PTH, a greater proportion of the secreted hormone is newly synthesized hormone. It has been calculated that there is enough PTH in the gland to last seven hours at normal serum calcium concentrations, but only two and one-half hours under protracted hypocalcemic conditions.

The fact that calcium and other agents that inhibit PTH secretion also inhibit accumulation of cAMP within parathyroid cells suggests that there is an intimate relationship between secretion of PTH and the adenyl cyclase-cAMP system.[43] On the other hand, cAMP affects secretion from a preformed hormone pool while calcium controls secretion of newly synthesized hormone, suggesting a certain independence of the two factors.[44]

Recently, Brown et al reported cloning of a protein from a cDNA library derived from bovine parathyroid cell mRNA with characteristics of a calcium sensor.[44a] The protein derived from this cDNA has a predicted topological structure that is similar to the seven membrane-spanning domains of the G-protein-coupled superfamily of receptors. The receptor responds to extracellular Ca and other polyvalent cations with increase in intracellular phosphaticylinositol turnover. Using the bovine calcium receptor cDNA, a similar nucleotide sequence was identified in human parathyroid adenoma cells. Thus, the transducing mechanism for hypocalcemic stimulation of PTH secretion is beginning to be elucidated.

Other factors have been shown to affect the secretion of PTH. An increase in the magnesium concentration inhibits the secretion of PTH in a manner similar to that of calcium, but the parathyroid is much less responsive to magnesium than to calcium. Paradoxically, severe and prolonged hypomagnesemia may occasionally lead to hypoparathyroidism. High concentrations of potassium, on the other hand, stimulate secretion of PTH.[45] Catecholamines also can increase the secretion of PTH, as can various other factors. Nevertheless, the feedback relationship between ionized calcium and PTH secretion is the dominating influence on hormone secretion and plasma calcium concentration.

There appears to be a modest circadian rhythm in the rate of secretion of PTH, with the rate during the night about twice that in the daytime.[46,47] In rats, the plasma PTH concentration is considerably elevated during lactation.[48–50,r25,r26] The phenomenon also has been seen in women secreting large amounts of milk, such as mothers nursing twins.[51] Both the circadian changes and the lactation-associated increase in PTH secretion in women appear to be related to factors other than plasma calcium.[47,51] In lactating rats the PTH increase may be related to hypocalcemia as well as other factors.[48,50]

Increasing the plasma concentration of calcitriol also decreases secretion of PTH, which suggests a feedback relationship between PTH and calcitriol, with PTH increasing the production of calcitriol and calcitriol decreasing the production of PTH. However, the physiologic significance of the interactions of the two feedback systems has not yet been worked out. In fact, in lactating rats the concentrations of both plasma calcitriol and plasma PTH are elevated,[52,53] and, in patients with secondary hyperparathyroidism of renal failure, administration of calcitriol can suppress PTH secretion.[51a]

Regulation of the Biosynthesis of PTH[54–56]

To supply enough PTH to reverse prolonged hypocalcemia, hormone production is increased. Evidence suggests that during hypocalcemia the PTH gene is nearly maximally active and that during hypercalcemia it is inhibited. Furthermore, during hypocalcemia most of the biosynthetic product is intact (1–84) nonfragmented PTH, whereas during hypercalcemia there is a high percentage of PTH fragments due to intraglandular cleavage. Finally, after prolonged hypocalcemia the number of chief cells is considerably increased. Taken together, this evidence supports the idea that a low concentration of plasma calcium increases net synthesis of PTH by stimulating both formation of new chief cells and hormone production within each cell. In contrast, a high concentration of calcium decreases the PTH supply.

Toxicity of PTH

Ordinary doses of PTH or secretory levels adequate to maintain the serum calcium in the neighborhood of 10 mg/dl have no toxic side-effects.

On the other hand, large continued doses of PTH or excessive secretion of PTH, as with parathyroid adenomas, parathyroid carcinoma, and parathyroid hyperplasia, are toxic and even may be fatal, as in some cases of acute primary hyperparathyroidism. The toxicity is due to severe hypercalcemia accompanied by initial polyuria (due to interference with the renal concentrating mechanism) followed by bone demineralization, osteitis fibrosis cystica, and leading to ectopic calcification usually of the kidney (nephrolithiasis or nephrocalcinosis), and sometimes of other tissues.[57,58]

Interactions with Other Hormones

Calcitriol

PTH and calcitriol work together in a poorly understood manner to promote the normal growth, development, and maintenance of the skeleton as well as to increase net outflow of calcium from bone to promote calcium homeostasis. In vitamin D-deficient animals, a larger amount of PTH is needed to produce the usual effect. Excessive treatment with calcitriol or related compounds can, like excessive PTH, result in extensive bone demineralization, with resulting bone fragility and soft tissue calcification.

Calcitonin

A second hormone that interacts with PTH is calcitonin. Adequate doses of calcitonin can antagonize the action of PTH by counteracting the effect of PTH on outflow of calcium from bone and by inhibiting resorption of bone by osteoclasts (see Chapter 43).

Estrogens

It was demonstrated recently that small doses of 17-beta estradiol increased PTH and calcitonin mRNAs fourfold in ovariectomized rats, suggesting that these effects may contribute to the beneficial effect of estrogens in osteoporosis.[59]

Glucocorticoids[60]

In a variety of experimental animals (dogs, cats, rats, and mice) it has been found that the hypocalcemia that occurs after parathyroidectomy is greatly reduced by adrenalectomy. According to recent experiments in rats, this effect of adrenalectomy is due to removal of the source of supply of glucocorticoid, which, in rats, is corticosterone. When corticosterone was given to parathyroidectomized adrenalectomized rats at physiological concentrations, the plasma calcium was reduced to the level after parathyroidectomy alone. Higher doses of corticosterone or of hydrocortisone can reduce the plasma calcium even further. In contrast glucocorticoids did not have an acute hypocalcemic effect in parathyroid-intact rats. Since substantial doses of the classic PTH in parathyroidectomized rats did not reverse the hypocalcemic effect of hydrocortisone, the possibility is being investigated that there is a second PTH that protects from glucocorticoid hypocalcemia.

Pharmacokinetics[r5]

Because of its polypeptide nature, PTH is not active by the oral route. Whether or not PTH is active by the nasal or rectal route has not been reported.

Varying amounts of N-terminal and C-terminal fragments are secreted by the parathyroid gland alone with intact PTH, but these fragments are, so far as known, biologically inactive.

Intact PTH, injected or secreted, is rapidly cleared from the circulation, with a disappearance half-time of about two minutes. Removal of PTH from the blood occurs mainly (60–70%) in the liver but also in the kidneys (20–30%). PTH also is bound to receptors on bone cells, but the amount bound, <1 percent, is quantitatively insignificant compared with the amount extracted by liver and kidney.[61,62] Clearance of PTH by the liver is mediated mainly by a high-capacity nonsaturable uptake by Kupffer cells[63] and is followed by rapid and extensive proteolysis. Renal clearance occurs almost entirely by glomerular filtration. The hormone is also reabsorbed by the renal tubules and then extensively degraded, so that little or no PTH appears in the final urine. This rapid metabolism in liver and kidney in normal individuals ensures that the concentration of hormone available to receptors in target tissues is dictated exclusively by the rate at which PTH is secreted by the parathyroid glands.

Preparations

The old-fashioned Extract Parathyroid is no longer available commercially.

Triparatide (brand name Parathar) is synthetic human PTH (1-34) for clinical use. It is available as a sterile lyophilized powder, 200 units per vial, to be reconstituted with diluent supplied.

Available for use in experimental animals, in amounts of 0.5 or 1 mg:

PTH (1-34), Human
PTH (1-34), Bovine
PTH (1-34), Rat
Biotinyl-PTH (1-34), Human
[Tyr^{3}]-PTH (1-34), Human
[Nle^{8,18}]-PTH (1-34), Human
[Nle^{8,18}, Tyr^{34}]-PTH (1-34), Human
[Nle^{8,18}, Tyr^{34}]-PTH (1-34), Amide, Bovine
[Tyr^{1}]-PTH (1-34), Rat
[Nle^{8,21}, Tyr^{84}]-PTH (1-34), Amide, Rat

Bisphosphonates

The bisphosphonates (also known as diphosphonates) are synthetic organic compounds analogous to pyrophosphate. In the bisphosphonates the two P atoms are joined through C (P-C-P) for greater stability, while in pyrophosphate they are joined through O (P-O-P). The bisphosphonates are used therapeutically in the treatment of Paget's disease of bone and hypercalcemia, especially the hypercalcemia of malignancy, and are being investigated for the treatment of other disorders of calcium metabolism, including osteoporosis[r28–r30] and renal stone-forming propensity associated with immobilization.[63a]

Chemistry and History

The classic bisphosphonate, etidronate, was first synthesized a century ago, but its use in medicine, following the recognition that it inhibited osteoclastic bone resorption in vitro, is quite recent, beginning in about 1974.

Many bisphosphonates have now been synthesized and are being studied for their pharmacologic properties and clinical potential, but only one, pamidronate, in addition to etidronate, has been approved for clinical use (for Paget's disease and hypercalcemia of malignancy) in the US.[r31,64]

The structures of etidronate, pamidronate, and some of the newer bisphosphonates are shown in Figure 42.5.[r32]

Study of the pharmacology of the bisphosphonates was inspired by the finding that pyrophosphate inhibited osteoclastic activity in vitro. However, pyrophosphate was inactive in vivo because it was hydrolyzed to phosphate too rapidly. The bisphosphonates, however, proved to be active in vivo as well as in vitro.[r33] Their plasma half-life is rather short, about two hours, but they are very avidly bound by hydroxyapatite. Fifty percent or more of the absorbed dose goes to the skeleton, and the half-life in bone may be as long as two years.

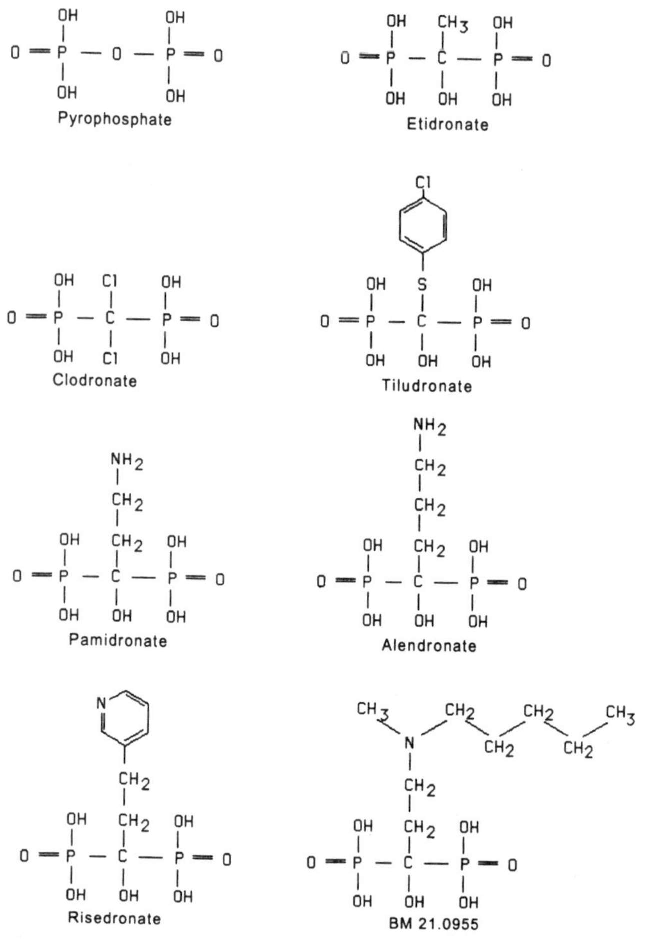

Figure 42.5 Structures of some of the bisphosphonate compounds. (Reprinted with permission from Ott SM J Bone Mineral Res 1993;*8* (Suppl 2):S597–S606.

Mechanism of Action

The mode of action, like that of calcitonin, is by inhibiting bone resorption. The bisphosphonates have the advantages over calcitonin of oral activity (although only about 1–5% absorbed) and lower cost. (Calcitonin also has advantages—lower toxicity, for one.)

The exact mechanism of action by which bisphosphonates inhibit bone resorption is not known, but there is new evidence that they act by stimulating osteoblasts to produce an osteoclast-inhibiting factor.[65]

Toxicity

Etidronate (disodium etidronate, EHDP) will reduce bone turnover in patients with Paget's disease of bone by about 50 percent within eight months when given in a dose of 5 mg/kg daily.[r34] Although larger doses are more effective in controlling very active disease, there is a risk of causing defective bone mineralization, which may result in the development of atraumatic bone fractures or diffuse bone pain. Combinations of EHDP with calcitonin at usual doses seem to result in an additive suppressant effect on bone turnover.[r35,66–68]

What is needed is a compound with as large a margin as possible between the desirable effect on resorption and the unwanted effect on mineralization by EHDP. Some of the newer bisphosphonates offer promise in this direction.[r35,69–71]

Preparations and Dosage

Etidronate disodium:
- Tablets: 200 mg, 400 mg
- Recommended dosage in Paget's disease of bone: 5–10 mg/kg/day, not to exceed six months or 11–20 mg/kg/day, not to exceed three months.

Pamidronate disodium for injection:
- 30-mg, 60-mg, and 90-mg vials
- Recommended dosage in hypercalcemia of malignancy: 60–90 mg by IV infusion over 24 hours

References

Research Reports

1. Brewer HG Jr, Ronan R. Bovine parathyroid hormone: Amino acid sequence. Proc Natl Acad Sci USA 1970;*67*:1862.
2. Niall HD, Keutmann HT, Sauer R. The amino acid sequence of bovine parathyroid hormone I. Hoppe Seylers Z Physiol Chem 1970;*351*:1586–1588.
3. Sauer RT, Niall HD, Hogan ML. The amino acid sequence of porcine parathyroid hormone. Biochemistry 1974;*13*:1994.
4. Keutmann HT, Sauer MM, Jacobs JW. The complete amino acid sequence of human parathyroid hormone. Biochemistry 1978;*17*:5723–5729.
5. Heinrich G, Kronenberg HM, Potts JT Jr, Habener JF. Gene encoding parathyroid hormone. Nucleotide sequence of the rat gene and deduced sequence of rat preproparathyroid hormone. J Biol Chem 1984;*259*:3320–3329.
6. Khosla S, Demay M, Pines M, Hurwitz S, Potts JT Jr, Kronenberg HM. Nucleotide sequence of cloned cDNAs encoding chicken preproparathyroid hormone. J Bone Mineral Res 1988;*3*:689–698.
7. Russell J, Sherwood LM. Nucleotide sequence of the DNA complementary to avian (chicken) preproparathyroid hormone mRNA and the deduced sequence of the hormone precursor. Mol Endocrinol 1989;*3*:325–331.
8. Zabel BU, Kronenberg HM, Bell GI, Shows TB. Chromosome mapping of genes on the short arm of human chromosome 11: Parathyroid hormone is at 11p15 with the genes for insulin, c-Harvey-ras 1, and b-hemoglobin. Cytogenet Cell Genet 1985;*39*:200–205.
9. Hamilton JW, MacGregor RR, Chu LLH, Cohn DV. The isolation and partial purification of a non-parathyroid hormone calcemic

fraction from bovine parathyroid glands. Endocrinology 1971;*89*:1440–1447.

10. Kemper B, Habener JF, Potts JT Jr, Rich A. Proparathyroid hormone: Identification of a biosynthetic precursor to parathyroid hormone. Proc Soc Natl Acad Sci USA 1972;*69*:643–647.

11. Kemper B, Habener JF, Mulligan RC, et al. Pre-proparathyroid hormone: A direct translation product of Parathyroid messenger RNA. Proc Soc Natl Acad Sci USA 1974;*71*:3731–3735.

12. Lindberg I. The new eukaryotic precursor processing proteinases. Mol Endocrinol 1991;*5*:1361–1365.

13. Keutmann HT, Griscom AW, Nussbaum JR, Reiner BT, Goud AN, Potts JT Jr, Rosenblatt M. The rat parathyroid hormone (1-34) fragment, renal adenylate cyclase activity, and receptor binding properties in vivo. Endocrinology 1985;*117*:1230–1234.

14. Miller SC, Kenny AD. Activation of avian medullary bone osteoclasts by oxidized synthetic parathyroid hormone (1-34). Proc Soc Exp Biol Med 1985;*179*:38–43.

15. Tregear GW, van Rietschoten J, Greene E, et al. Bovine parathyroid hormone: Minimum chain length of synthetic peptide required for biological activity. Endocrinology 1973;*93*:1349–1353.

16. Barden JA, Cuthbertson RN. Stabilized NMR structure of human parathyroid hormone (1-34). Eur J Biochem 1993;*215*:315–321.

17. Lim SK, Gardella, TJ, Baba H, Nussbaum SR, Kronenberg HM. The carboxy terminus of parathyroid hormone is essential for hormone processing and secretion. Endocrinology 1992;*131*:2325–2330.

18. Goud NA, McKee RL, Sardana NK, De Haven PA, Hueler E, Syed MM, Goud RA, Gibbons JW, Fisher JE, Levy JJ, et al. Solid-phase synthesis and biologic activity of human parathyroid hormone (1-84). J Bone Mineral Res 1991;*6*:781–789.

19. Broadus AE, Mangin M, Ikeda K, et al. Humoral hypercalcemia of cancer: Identification of a novel parathyroid hormone-like peptide. N Engl J Med 1988;*319*:556–563.

20. Budayr AA, Halloran BR, King JC, Diop D, Nissenson RA, Strewler GJ. High levels of a parathyroid hormone-related protein in milk. Proc Natl Acad Sci USA 1989;*86*:7183–7185.

21. Rosenblatt M. Peptide hormone antagonists that are effective in vivo. N Engl J Med 1988;*319*:556–563.

22. Kemper B, Habener JF, Rich A, Potts JP Jr. Parathyroid secretion: Discovery of a major calcium-dependent protein. Science 1974;*184*:167–169.

23. Cohn DV, Morrissey JJ, Hamilton JW, Shofstall RF, Smardo FC, Chen LLH. Isolation and partial characterization of secretory protein-1 from bovine parathyroid glands. Biochemistry 1981;*20*:4135–4140.

24. Kruggel W, O'Connor DT, Lewis RV. The amino terminal sequences of bovine and human chromogranin A and secretory protein. Biochem Biophys Res Commun 1985;*127*:380–383.

25. Tatemoto K, Efendic S, Mutt V, Makk G, Feistner GJ, Barcho JD. Pancreastatin, a novel pancreatic peptide that inhibits insulin secretion. Nature 1986;*324*:476–478.

26. MacCollum WG, Voegtlin C. On the relation of tetany to the parathyroid gland and to calcium metabolism. J Exp Med 1909;*11*:118–51.

27. Greenwald I. The effect of parathyroidectomy upon metabolism. Am J Physiol 1911;*28*:103–32.

28. Hanson AM. Parathyroid preparations. Mil Surgeon 1924;*54*:554–560.

29. Collip JB. Extraction of a parathyroid hormone which will prevent or control parathyroid tetany and which regulates the level of blood calcium. J. Biol Chem 1925;*63*:396–438.

30. Aurbach GD. Isolation of parathyroid hormone after extraction in phenol. J Biol Chem 1959;*234*:3179–81.

31. Tashjian AH Jr. Effects of parathyroidectomy and cautery of the thyroid gland on the plasma calcium level of rats with autotransplanted parathyroid glands. Endocrinology 1966;*78*:1144–1153.

32. Rodan GA, Martin TJ. Role of osteoblasts in hormonal control of bone resorption: a hypothesis. Calcif Tissue Intl 1981;*33*:349–351.

33. McSheehy PM, Chambers TJ. Osteoblast-like cells in the presence of parathyroid hormone release soluble factor that stimulates osteoclastic bone resorption. Endocrinology 1986;*119*:1654–1659.

34. Duong LT, Grasser W, DeHaven PA. Sato M. Parathyroid hormone receptors identified in avian and rat osteoclasts. J Bone Mineral Res 1991;*6*:85–93.

35. Nordin BEC, Peacock M. Role of the kidney in regulation of plasma calcium. Lancet 1969;*2*:1280–1283.

36. Bourdeau JE, Burg MB. Effect on PTH on calcium transport across the thick ascending limb of Henle's loop. Am J Physiol 1980;*239*:F121–F126.

37. Janulis M, Wong MS, Favus MJ. Structure-function requirements for stimulation of 1,25-dihydroxy D3 production by rat renal proximal tubules. Endocrinology 1993;*133*:713–719.

38. Nemere I, Norman AW. Parathyroid hormone stimulates calcium transport in perfused duodenum from normal chicks: Comparison with the rapid (transcaltachtic) effect of 1,25- dihydroxyvitamin D3. Endocrinology 1986;*119*:1406–1408.

39. Harrison HE, Harrison HC. Intestinal transport of phosphate: Action of vitamin D, calcium, and potassium. Am J Physiol 1961;*201*:1007–1012.

40. Sherwood LM, Potts JT Jr, Care AD, Mayer GP. Evaluation by radioimmunoassay of factors controlling the secretion of parathyroid hormone. Nature 1966, *209*:52–55.

41. Mayer GP, Horst JG. Sigmoidal relationship between parathyroid hormone secretion rate and plasma calcium concentration in calves. Endocrinology 1978;*102*:1036–1042.

42. Naveh-Many T, Silver J, Regulation of parathyroid hormone gene expression by hypocalcemia, hypercalcemia, and vitamin D in the rat. J Clin Invest 1990;*86*:1313–1319.

43. Brown EM, Gardner, DG, Windeck R, Aurbach GD. Relationship of intracellular 3′5′-adenosine monophosphate accumulation to parathyroid hormone release from dispersed parathyroid cells. Endocrinology 1978;*103*:2323–2333.

44. Brown EM, Fuleihan GEH, Chen CJ, Kifor O. A comparison of the effects of divalent and trivalent cations on parathyroid hormone release, 3′, 5′-cyclic adenosine monophosphate accumulation, and the levels of inositol phosphate in bovine parathyroid cells. Endocrinology 1990;*127*:1064–1070.

44a. Brown EM, Garuba G, Riccardi D, Lombardi M, Butters R, Kifer O, Sun A, Hediger MA, Lytton J, Hebert SC. Cloning and characterization of an extracellular Ca^{2+}-sensing receptor from bovine parathyroid. Nature 1993;*366*:575–580.

45. Brown EM, Adragna N, Gardner DG. Effect of potassium on PTH secretion from dispersed parathyroid cells. J Clin Endocrinol Metab 1981;*53*:1304–1306.

46. Jubiz W, Canterbury JM, Reiss E, Tyler FH. Circadian rhythm in serum parathyroid hormone concentration in human subjects: correlation with serum calcium, phosphate, albumin, and growth hormone levels. J Clin Invest 1972;*52*:2040–2046.

47. Perault-Staub AM, Tracqui P, Staub JF. Modeling of in vivo calcium metabolism I. Optimal cooperation between constant rhythmic behaviors. Acta Biotheor 1992;*40*:95–102.

48. Garner SC, Boass A, Toverud SU. Hypercalcemia fails to suppress elevated serum parathyroid hormone concentration during lactation in rats. J Bone Mineral Res 1989;*4*:577–583.

49. Garner SC, Boass A, Toverud SU. Parathyroid hormone is not required for normal milk composition or secretion or lactation-associated bone loss in normocalcemic rats. J Bone Mineral Res 1990;*5*:69–75.

50. Garner SC, Peng T-C, Hirsch PF, Boass A, Toverud SU. Increase in serum parathyroid hormone concentration in the lactating rat: Effects of dietary calcium and lactational intensity. J Bone Mineral Res 1987;*2*:347–352.

51. Greer FR, Lane J, Ho M. Elevated serum parathyroid hormone, calcitonin, and 1,25-dihydroxyvitamin D in lactating women nursing twins. Am J Clin Nutr 1984;*40*:562–568.

51a. Delmez JA, Tindiri C, Gromms P, Dusso A, Windus DW, Slatopolsky E. Parathyroid hormone suppression by intravenous $1,25(OH)_2D_3$. A role for increased sensitivity to calcium. Clin Invest 1989;*83*:1349–1355.

52. Pike JW, Parker JB, Haussler MR, Boass A, Toverud SU. Dynamic changes in the concentration of 1,25-dihydroxyvitamin D during reproduction in rats. Science 1979;*204*:1427–1429.

53. Schultz NL, Garner SC, Lavigne JR, Toverud SU. Determination of bioactive rat parathyroid hormone (PTH) concentration in vivo and in vitro by a II-site homologous radiometric assay. Bone Mineral, 1994, in press.

54. Henry HL, Midgett RJ, Norman AW. Regulation of 25-hydroxy vitamin D3-1-hydroxylase in vivo. J Biol Chem 1974;*249*:7584–7592.

55. Garabedian M, Holick MF, DeLuca HF, Boyle IT. Control of 25-hydroxycholecalciferol metabolism by parathyroid glands. Proc Natl Acad Sci USA 1972;*69*:1673–1676.

56. Hughes MR, Brumbaugh PF, Haussler MR, Wergedal JE, Baylink DJ. Regulation of serum 1alpha-25-dihydroxyvitamin D3 by calcium and phosphate in the rat. Science 1975;*190*:578–580.

57. Klugman VA, Favus MJ, Pak CYC. Nephrolithiasis in primary hyperparathyroidism. In Bilzekian et al (eds.) 1994, op cit: 505–517.

58. Davies M, Mawer EB. The pathogenesis of hypercalcemia in vitamin D poisoning. In Norman AW (ed): Vitamin D: A Chemical, Biochemical, and Clinical Update. Berlin: Walter de Gruyter, 1985, pp 57–58.

59. Naveh-Many T, Almogi G, Livni N, Silver S. Estrogen receptors and biologic response in rat parathyroid tissue and C cells. J Clin Invest 1992;*90*:2434–2438.

60. Nishino K, Hirsch PF, Mahgoub A, Munson PL. Hypocalcemic effect of physiological concentrations of corticosterone in adrenalectomized-parathyroidectomized rats. Endocrinology 1991;*128*:2259–2265.

61. Bringhurst FR, Stern AM, Yotts M, Mizrahi N, Segre GV, Potts JT Jr. Peripheral metabolism of PTH: Fate of biologically active amino terminus in vivo. Am J Physiol 1988;*225*:E886–893.

62. Martin KJ, Hruska KA, Freitag JJ, Klahr S, Slatopolsky E. The peripheral metabolism of parathyroid hormone. N Engl J Med 1979;*302*:1092–1098.

63. Bringhurst FR, Segre GV, Lampman GW, Potts JT Jr. Metabolism of parathyroid hormone by Kupffer calls: analysis by reverse-phase high-performance liquid chromatography. Biochemistry 1982;*21*:4252–4258.

63a. Ruml LA, Dubois SK, Robert ML, Pak CY. The effect of alendronate on immobilization-induced bone loss and stone-forming propensity. J Bone Mineral Res 1994;*9* (Suppl 1):S268.

64. Price RI, Gutteridge DH, Stuckey BG, Kent GN, Retallack RW, Prince RL, Bhagat CI, Johnston CA, Nicholson GC, Stewart GO. Rapid divergent changes in spinal and forearm bone density following short-term intravenous treatment of Paget's disease with pamidronate disodium. J Bone Mineral Res 1993;*8*:209–217.

65. Sahni M, Guenther HL, Fleisch H, Collin P, Martin TJ. Bisphosphonates act on rat bone resorption through the mediation of osteoblasts. J Clin Invest 1993;*91*:2004–2011.

66. Reasner CA, Stone MD, Hosking DJ, Ballah A, Mundy GR. Acute changes in calcium homeostasis during treatment of primary hyperparathyroidism with risedronate. J Clin Endocrinol Metab 1993;*77*:1067–1071.

67. Schweitzer DH, Zwinderman AH, Vermieij P, Bijvoet OL. Improved treatment of Paget's disease with dimethylaminohydroxypropylidene bisphosphonate (dimethyl-APD). J Bone Mineral Res 1993;*8*:175–182.

68. Ammann P, Rizzoli R, Caverzasio J, Shigematsu T, Slosman D, Bonjour JP. Effects of the bisphosphonate tiludronate on bone resorption, calcium balance, and bone mineral density. J Bone Mineral Res 1993;*8*:1491–1498.

69. Murakami H, Nakamura T, Tsurukami H, Abe M, Barbier A, Suzuki K. Effects of tiludronate on bone mass, structure, and turnover at the epiphyseal, primary, and secondary spongiosa in the proximal tibia of growing rats after sciatic neurectomy. J Bone Mineral Res 1994;*9*:1355–1364.

70. Adami S, Baroni MC, Broggini M, Carratelli L, Caruso I, Gnessi L, Laurenzi M, Lombardi A, Norbiato G, Ortolani S, et al. Treatment of postmenopausal osteoporosis with continuous daily oral alendronate in comparison with either placebo or intranasal salmon calcitonin. Osteoporosis Int 1993;*3* (Suppl 3):S21–27.

71. Reginster JY, Treves R, Renier JC, Sany J, Ethgen E, Picot C, Franchimont P. Efficacy and tolerability of a new formulation of oral tiludronate (tablet) in the treatment of Paget's disease of bone. J Bone Mineral Res 1994;*9*:615–619.

Reviews

r1. Aurbach GD, ed. Parathyroid gland. In: Greep RO, Astwood EB. Endocrinology. In: Handbook of Physiology. Washington: Am Physiol Soc (1976): Section 7, volume VII, 1–480.

r2. Munson PL. Parathyroid gland and hormone. In: Dulbecco R. Encyclopedia of Human Biology. San Diego: Academic Press (1991): Vol. 5, 657–666.

r3. Bilezikian JP, Marcus R, Levine MA. The Parathyroids. New York: Raven Press (1994):1–854.

r4. Rosenblatt M, Kronenberg HM, Potts JT Jr. Parathyroid hormone. In: DeGroot LJ op cit (1989) (r3):848–891.

r5. Kronenberg HM, Bringhurst FR, Segre GV, Potts JT Jr. Parathyroid hormone biosynthesis and metabolism. In: Bilezikian JP et al. op cit (1994) (r3):125–138.

r6. Chorev M, Rosenblatt HM. Structure-function analysis of parathyroid hormone and parathyroid hormone-related protein. In: Bilezikian JP et al. op cit (1994) (r3):139–156.

r7. Habener JF, Rosenblatt M, Potts JT Jr. Parathyroid hormone: Biochemical aspects of biosynthesis, secretion, action, and metabolism. Physiol Rev 1984;*64*:985–1053.

r8. Aurbach GD, Marx SJ, Spiegel AM. Parathyroid hormone, calcitonin, and the calciferols. In: Wilson JD, Foster GW. Williams Textbook of Endocrinology, 8th ed. Philadelphia: WB Saunders (1992):1397–1476.

r9. Broadus HE, Stewart AF. Parathyroid hormone-related protein. In: Bilezikian JP et al. op cit (1994) (r3):259–294.

r10. Grill V, Martin TJ. Parathyroid hormone-related protein as a cause of hypercalcemia of malignancy. In: Bilezikian JP et al. op cit (1994) (r3):295–310.

r11. Cohn CV, Fasciotto BH, Zheng J-X, Gorr SU. Chemistry and biology of chromogranin A (secretory protein I) of the parathyroid and other endocrine glands. In: Bilezikian JP et al. op cit (1994) (r3):107–120.

r12. Munson PL. Parathyroid hormone and calcitonin. In: McCann SM. Endocrinology: People and ideas. Bethesda: Am Physiol Soc (1988):239–284.

r12a. Li A, Collip JB. AM Hanson and the isolation of the parathyroid hormone, or endocrines and enterprise. J Hist Med 1992;*47*:405–438.

r13. Parfitt AM. Surgical, idiopathic, and other varieties of parathyroid hormone-deficient hypoparathyroidism. In: DeGroot LJ. op cit (1989) 2d ed. (r3):1049–1064.

r14. Dempster DW, Cosman F, Parisien M, Shen V. Anabolic actions of parathyroid hormone on bone. Endocrine Rev 1993;*14*:690–709.

r15. Marcus R. Parathyroid hormone and growth hormone in the treatment of osteoporosis. In: Bilezikian JP et al. op cit (1994) (r3):813–821.

r16. Brown EM. Homeostatic mechanisms regulating extracellular and intracellular calcium metabolism. In: Bilzekian JP et al. op cit (1994) (r3):15–54.

r17. McIndoe WA. Yolk synthesis. In: Bell DJ, Freeman DM (eds). Physiology and Biochemistry of the Domestic Fowl. New York: Academic Press, 1971.

r18. Talmage RV. Calcium homeostasis: calcium transport: parathyroid action. Clin Orthopaed 1969;*67*:210–224.

r19. Talmage RV, Meyer RA Jr. Physiological role of parathyroid hormone. In Aurbach GD (ed.) v.7. Parathyroid gland. In Greep RO, Astwood EB (eds). Endocrinology. Washington: American Physiological Society (1976), pp 343–351.

r20. DeLuca HF. The metabolism, physiology, and function of vitamin D. In Kumar R (ed): Vitamin D. Basic and clinical Aspects. The Hague: Niehoff (1984):1–68.

r21. Henry HL. Regulation of the synthesis of 1,25-dihydroxy-vitamin D3 and 24,25-dihydroxyvitamin D3 in kidney cell culture. In Kumar R (ed) (1984) op cit (r20):151–174.

r22. Agus ZS, Wassersteinn A, Goldfarb S. PTH, calcitonin, cyclic nucleotides, and the kidney. Ann Rev Physiol 1981;*43*:583.

r23. Chase LR. Parathyroid hormone and cyclic adenosine monophosphate. The early days. In Bilezekian (ed.) (1994) op cit (r3):121–124.

r24. Brown EM. Extracellular Ca2+ sensing, regulation of parathyroid function, and role of Ca2+ and other ions as extracellular (first) messengers. Physiol Rev 1991;*71*:371–411.

r25. Toverud SU, Boass A. Hormonal control of calcium metabolism in lactation. Vitamins Hormones 1979;*37*:303–347.

r26. Garel J-M. Hormonal control of calcium metabolism during the reproductive cycle in mammals. Physiol Rev 1987;*67*:1–66.

r27. Patel S, Lyons AR, Hosking DJ. Drugs used in the treatment of metabolic bone disease. Clinical pharmacology and therapeutic use. Drugs 1993;*46*:594–617.

r28. Lombardi A, Santora AC, Clinical trials with bisphosphonates. Bone Mineral 1993;*22* Suppl.:S59–S70.

r29. Bilezekian JP. Clinical review 5. Management of hypercalcemia. J Clin Endocrinol Metab 1993;*77*:1445–1449.

r30. Fleisch H. Bisphosphonates—history and experimental basis. Bone 1987;*8* (Suppl 1):523–528.

r31. Ott, SM. Clinical effects of bisphosphonates in involutional osteoporosis. J Bone Mineral Res 1993;*8* (Suppl 2):S597–S606.

r32. Fleisch H. Experimental basis for the use of bisphosphonates in Paget's disease of bone. Clin Orthop 1987;*217*:72–78.

r33. Patel S, Stone MD, Coupland C, Hosking DJ. Determinants of remission of Paget's disease. J Bone Mineral Res 1993;*8*:1467–1473.

r34. Hosking AJ. Paget's disease of bone. An update on management. Drugs 1985;*30*:156–173.

r35. Fleisch H. New bisphosphonates in osteoporosis. Osteoporosis Int 1993;*3* (Suppl 2):S15–S22.

CHAPTER 43

Calcitonin

Philip F. Hirsch

Calcitonin (CT), a hypocalcemic hormone discovered 30 years ago,[1,2,r1] is synthesized in and secreted by the thyroid gland of mammals and by the ultimobranchial body of lower vertebrates. Calcitonin is important in medicine for the treatment of certain bone diseases and for the diagnosis of medullary thyroid carcinoma (MTC). Sensitive assays of CT in blood are useful to detect MTC and to follow both its remission and its recurrence after tumor extirpation. The finding that the hormone lowers blood calcium in some bone diseases, inhibits bone loss, and relieves bone-associated pain has led to its increased use in therapy. Calcitonin is a useful drug in the treatment of hypercalcemia of various causes, especially those disorders that involve increased turnover of bone—for example, Paget's disease of bone, hypervitaminosis D, and osteoporosis. Salmon and other ultimobranchial calcitonins have been found to be more potent and to have a longer duration of action than mammalian calcitonians. Preparations of calcitonin that are effective when administered intranasally rather than by injection will increase their use in the treatment of osteoporosis and other disorders of calcium metabolism. A role for calcitonin in normal human physiology, originally proposed to be "fine tuning" of serum calcium or protection against hypercalcemia has not been well established.

Chemistry

Structure

Porcine calcitonin was the first to be purified,[3] sequenced,[4,5] and synthesized.[6] It was found to have 32 amino acids with a disulfide bond forming a 1-7 ring, connecting the amino-terminal cysteine to another cysteine. Soon after, human CT was purified, its sequence determined,[7,8] and it was synthesized.[9] Now, the sequences are known for calcitonins from a number of species (Fig. 43.1). All calcitonins from thyroid glands of mammals as well as those from ultimobranchial bodies of lower vertebrates have 32 amino acids with the 1-7 disulfide ring structure, and a prolinamide at position 32, the carboxy-terminal amino acid. Although there is considerable homology in the amino acid sequence within the ring structure, those sequences occurring in the 24 amino acids toward the carboxy-terminal end differ markedly between species. However, the sequence differences between some species are minor. For example, bovine and ovine calcitonin differ by just three amino acids and rat and human calcitonin differ by only two amino acids.

Assay and Units

The first biologic assay method to follow the purification of the hormone was developed by Hirsch et al.[10] It was based on the one-hour hypocalcemic response to a subcutaneous injection of porcine calcitonin into intact rats fed a low calcium diet. A unit was defined as an amount of test preparation that would decrease the serum calcium of a 165-g intact rat (fed a low calcium diet for 4 days) to the same extent as that produced by 10µg of nitrogen in a standard, partially purified porcine thyroid extract. Cooper et al. improved the hypocalcemic bioassay method by showing that using younger rats fed the low-calcium diet for only one day resulted in a dose-response curve with a steeper slope and a superior index of precision.[11] A number of other bioassay methods were developed and other units were defined, creating the need for a common standard. The British Medical Research Council undertook a collaborative study with seven laboratories to compare potencies of standard preparations distributed in sealed vials.[12] The result of this study led to the preparation and distribution of Research Standard B, a vial containing 1 MRC unit of porcine calcitonin. One MRC unit was approximately 100 Hirsch units. In 1972 the World Health Organization established the International Unit (IU) replacing the equivalent MRC unit. The most recent collaborative assays compared potencies of calcitonins of major clinical interest, salmon, and eel calcitonin

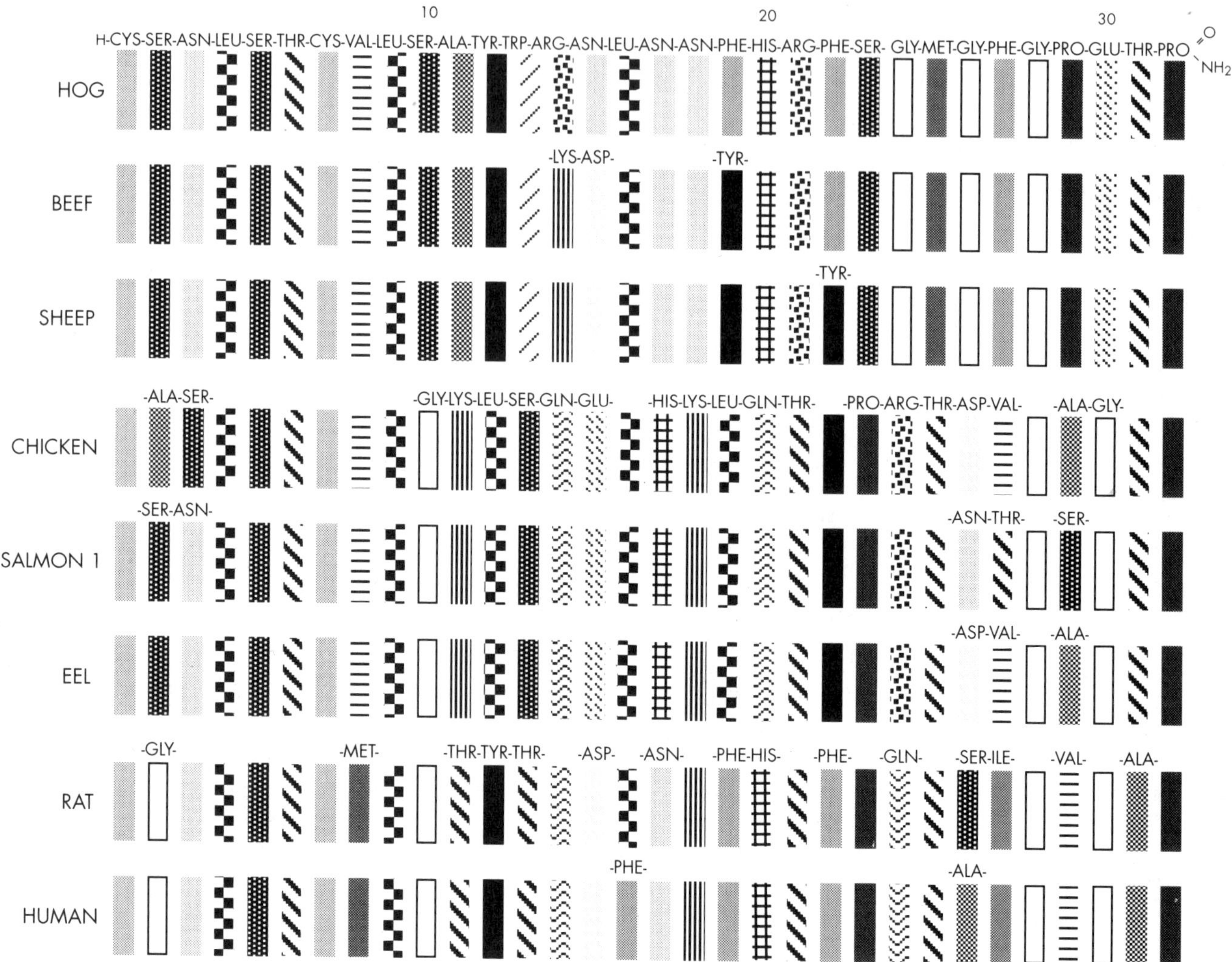

Figure 43.1 Amino Acid Sequences of Some Calcitonins

as well as the analogue [Asu^{1,7}]-eel calcitonin,[13] porcine, and human calcitonin.[14] Azria described many of the initial bioassays performed and compared units defined in different laboratories to the MRC unit and the IU.[r2]

Salmon calcitonin, the most widely used because of its high potency and longer duration of action, has a potency of about 5000 IU/mg. Human and porcine calcitonins contain 100 to 200 IU/mg. Eel calcitonin, isolated and characterized by Otani et al.,[15] is similar in structure and activity to salmon CT. It is of interest that the synthetic aminosuberic analogue of eel calcitonin, in which the two sulfurs forming the 1-7 disulfide bond are replaced with methyl groups, [Asu^{1,7}]-eel-calcitonin (elcatonin, Elcitonin), is equipotent to eel or salmon CT.[r2] Although the methyl groups are claimed to improve its stability,[16] purified forms of other CTs are also quite stable.

As purification of the hormone progressed, immunoassay procedures to measure rat[17] and human[18] CT were developed. Immunoassays and immunoradiometric (IRMA) assays are now sufficiently sensitive to measure concentrations of CT in blood. However, caution must be exercised in interpretation of these measurements as they do not always represent biologically active CT or equal only the monomeric calcitonin secreted by the thyroid gland.[r3] Three methods are currently employed to measure circulating levels of calcitonin.[r4] The first involves radioimmunoassays utilizing polyclonal antisera and has a sensitivity of 2–10 pg/ml. The second method involves an extraction of calcitonin by passing plasma through a silica cartridge; the calcitonin is then eluted, dried, and reconstituted in a small volume of buffer, and assayed by a sensitive radioimmunoassay method. Advantages include removing interfering substances in serum and lowering the detection limit to 0.5 pg/ml. A disadvantage is the extra steps involved. In a third method, a two-site IRMA utilizes affinity-purified polyclonal antibodies directed against two epitopes with the calcitonin monomer. This method is considered to be specific for the monomer and is adequately sensitive, 10 pg/ml. A similar technique uses monoclonal antibodies for a colorimetric ELISA to measure calcitonin. Also, a two-site IRMA specific for procalcitonin has been used to measure the monomer as well as the flanking region (ketacalcin, the carboxy-terminal adjacent peptide).[r4] These newer methods often give values for calcitonin in normal human serum less than 10 pg/ml.

Structure-Activity Relationships

Unlike parathyroid hormone (PTH), where most if not all of the biologic activity persists after a part of the secreted native hormone molecule has been removed, calcitonin loses most of its biologic activity with the loss of just one amino acid.[19] However, the S-S bond is not essential for biologic activity; as mentioned above, the S-S bond has been replaced with CH_2-CH_2 with no apparent loss of activity.[16] Changes in the amino acid sequence outside the ring structure, as occurs between structures from different species or by synthesis, do affect potency. Potts has described consequences of some alterations and substitutions of the structure of calcitonin and the complexities involved.[r5]

History

The discovery of calcitonin, unlike that of many other hormones, did not arise from the identification of a pathology caused by either over- or undersecretion. Rather, it was the result of serendipitous observations. While performing experiments on the regulation of secretion of PTH in dogs, Copp and coworkers[1] perfused the thyroid-parathyroid glands of the dog with blood high in calcium. When the perfusate reentered the systemic circulation, blood calcium fell more rapidly than it did after thyroparathyroidectomy. Thus, the fall in serum calcium could not be explained just by the loss of PTH, but had to involve the secretion of a hypocalcemic factor from the thyroid-parathyroid apparatus. On the basis of this and other experiments, Copp et al. concluded that a hypocalcemic hormone, which they named *calcitonin,* was secreted by the parathyroid gland.[1]

That calcitonin originated in the thyroid gland rather than in the parathyroid was first demonstrated by Hirsch et al.[2] They deduced that the greater hypocalcemic response to parathyroidectomy by hot-wire cautery than by surgical excision, reported earlier by Munson,[20] was due to the release of a hypocalcemic substance by the thyroid after cautery. Subcutaneous injection of a small volume of an extract of rat thyroid from which the parathyroid glands had been removed caused a marked hypocalcemic response in intact rats within one hour. The thyroid hypocalcemic substance was initially named *thyrocalcitonin* to distinguish it from the putative parathyroid *calcitonin.*[2] Soon thereafter, additional evidence was obtained showing that the thyroid, not the parathyroid, was the gland responsible for the fall in serum calcium after a high calcium infusion.[21-23] Identifying the thyroid as the source of calcitonin was important for rapid advancement of the field; it pointed to the appropriate gland to identify the cell of origin of the hormone and from which large quantities of active material could be obtained, purified, and its biologic activity determined.[r1]

The progress achieved during the subsequent six years was truly remarkable. The parafollicular cells of the thyroid, now more commonly called the C cells,[24] were identified as the source of CT. CT was found in the ultimobranchial glands of lower vertebrates, CT from porcine and human thyroid glands was purified, and the structures were determined. Copp et al.[25] and Tauber[26] independently and simultaneously were the first to show that calcitonin could be extracted from ultimobranchial glands of the chicken. In lower vertebrates the ultimobranchial gland remains as a separate gland, whereas in mammals it merges with the thyroid.[27] A hypersecretory syndrome, medullary carcinoma of the thyroid (MTC), was identified in humans.[28-30] That CT inhibited osteoclastic resorption in resorbing bone in tissue culture was convincingly shown by Friedman and Raisz[31] and Aliapoulios et al.[32]

Milhaud and Job[33] were the first to use calcitonin in therapy: it was used to treat idiopathic hypercalcemia. The lowering of calcium was ascribed, at least in part, to inhibition of osteoclastic activity. Later, Milhaud et al.[34] used calcitonin in the treatment of Paget's disease of bone. Milhaud[35] presented an interesting account of the brief period between the discovery of calcitonin and its first therapeutic use in their patients. A detailed review of the progress during the first six years after its discovery was published by Hirsch and Munson.[r6]

A little later, salmon calcitonin was isolated from ultimobranchial glands; its structure was determined,[36] and it was synthesized.[37] Salmon CT has become the most widely used therapeutic form because it is not only more potent but also has a longer duration of action than mammalian CTs. Evidence was soon obtained demonstrating that C cells originate in the neural crest. During embryogenesis, these cells migrate to the ultimobranchial body,[38,39] and, in mammals, they merge with the thyroid gland. Pearse introduced the term *APUD* to identify neural crest-derived cells, like the C cells, that have some characteristics common to neurones, namely *a*mine *p*recursor *u*ptake and *d*ecarboxylation, and that produce and secrete polypeptide hormones.[40] The PUD concept was criticized[42] because not all polypeptide-producing cells that fulfilled many of the neuroendocrine criteria established by Pearse synthesized, stored, or decarboxylated amines. Since some of these cells are not derived from the neural crest, but from common epithelial stem cells, the APUD concept has been modified.[r8] Use of the term *diffuse neuroendocrine system* (DNES) rather than APUD is often preferred to encompass the many diverse polypeptide or protein hormone-synthesizing cell types with neuroendocrine function.[r9]

Using an antibody with carboxyterminal recognition, Silva and Becker detected immunoreactive CT in many human tissues other than the thyroid, e.g., jejunum, thymus, urinary bladder, lung, rectum, and testis; some of these ectopic sites may secrete CT.[r10] Thus, it is not surprising that some of these sites have been found to be the source of the primary cells in ectopic CT-producing neoplasms.[r11]

Calcitonin Gene-Related Peptide (CGRP)

Using molecular biologic techniques, the calcitonin gene complementary to the 32-amino acid rat calcitonin mRNA was cloned by Amara et al.[41] Examination of the gene structure revealed the possibility of alternative splicing that would result in an mRNA different from calcitonin mRNA; the alternate mRNA would translate to a 128-amino acid precursor of a 37-amino acid peptide, named the calcitonin gene-related peptide (CGRP).[42,43] The presence of CGRP in rat tissues was confirmed in immunohistochemical studies with an antibody prepared from synthesized CGRP.[43] Two different CGRPs have now been identified, α and β, differing by only one amino acid but formed by two different genes.[44] CGRP has been localized in nerve endings, very often in the same sites as substance P—as, for example, in the gastric mucosa.[r12] In neural tissues, CGRP is formed, whereas in the thyroid gland, the processing leads predominantly to the mRNA for calcitonin synthesis. The mechanism responsible for the precise control of the alternate pathways is being actively pursued.[45,46] The physiologic functions of CGRP are not yet understood. However, evidence suggests that CGRP has a functional role at three primary sites: (1) at neuromuscular junctions in modulating cardiovascular homeostasis; (2) on GI motility and function; and (3) as a neurotransmitter or modulator of neural transmission in the central and peripheral nervous systems. The proceedings of a conference reviewing the first 10-year history of CGRP were published in 1992.[r13]

Effects and Actions of Calcitonin

Physiologic Functions of Calcitonin

Calcitonin is considered a calcium-regulating hormone. Its hypocalcemic effect is easily seen in experimental animals and in humans. The initial experiments that provided evidence for the existence of calcitonin led Copp and collaborators to propose that calcitonin acted in concert with parathyroid hormone to maintain a constant level of blood calcium.[1,r14] However, convincing evidence to support this hypothesis is lacking. Humans with functioning parathyroid glands but who are deficient in CT, such as after thyroidectomy, usually are normocalcemic.[r3]

The possibility that calcitonin protects against hypercalcemia was also proposed as an important physiologic function. Many animal experiments have demonstrated that the thyroid gland by secreting CT protects against the hypercalcemia caused by large doses of calcium,[21,47] vitamin D,[48,49] or parathyroid hormone.[50] But, such situations seldom occur in humans, so it does not seem reasonable to consider that the main physiologic function of calcitonin should be to intervene in such rare eventualities. Furthermore, the suppression of PTH secretion by hypercalcemia is already a powerful protective mechanism.

The conservation of calcium for the skeleton remains as a probable and important physiologic function for calcitonin. The first evidence pointing to this role was obtained by Gray and Munson.[51] They gave calcium chloride by gavage to two groups of rats with functional parathyroid transplants and found that serum calcium rose to higher levels and the hypercalcemia lasted longer in thyroidectomized rats than in rats with intact thyroid glands. A similar hypercalcemia was obtained 90 minutes after thyroparathyroidectomy, but not after a sham-operation, in rats voluntarily consuming a calcium-containing diet just after the operation.[51] These results led the authors to conclude that calcitonin, by restricting hypercalcemia after ingestion of calcium, minimize loss of calcium from blood into urine and feces, thereby conserving calcium for bone. Additional support for this function for calcitonin was provided by Talmage et al.[52] Using rats with functional parathyroid transplants, they found a sevenfold higher urinary excetion of calcium in thyroidectomized rats than in thyroid-intact rats when the diet was switched from a calcium-free to a calcium-containing diet. Administration of calcitonin prevented the increased urinary calcium excretion in thyroidectomized rats. These findings suggest strongly that there are environmental conditions where conservation of dietary calcium by calcitonin may help to maintain the structural integrity of the skeleton.

The cellular mechanisms to conserve ingested calcium have not yet been elucidated. Talmage et al. proposed that calcitonin increases intracellular phosphate, forming a complex with calcium postprandially to enhance calcium storage on bone surface.[53,54] Support for this hypothesis comes from the work of Ahmado et al.,[55] who found that physiologic doses of calcitonin, as well as of parathyroid hormone, increased the uptake of ^{32}Pi and the intracellular Pi concentration in osteoblast-like cells (UMR-106-06). Increased cytosolic calcium in cells treated with calcitonin[56,57] is due mostly to release of calcium from intracellular storage forms, and partly to increased calcium in flux from extracellular fluids,[58,59] an action that is rapid, beginning within two minutes compared with eight minutes for parathyroid hormone, and the influx may involve chloride channels.[59]

In contrast to the strong evidence obtained in rats for a role of CT in conservation of calcium, a similar role in humans has not yet been established.[r15] Evidence that bone density was lower in calcitonin-deficient humans who had undergone thyroid ablation has been reported.[60] However, more recent studies in long-term thyroidectomized patients relate bone loss to their use of doses of thyroxine that suppresses TSH secretion below normal.[61–64,r16]

Calcitonin Affects the Circadian Rhythms of Calcium

As methods for the determination of blood calcium improved, it became clear that in rats the concentration of blood calcium undergoes circadian rhythms and that these rhythms were influenced by calcitonin.[65] In rats kept on a 12-hour light/dark regimen and fed only at the beginning of the dark period, plasma calcium was higher during the light than the dark period. Interestingly, plasma calcium began to fall preprandially even before turning off the lights, leading Perault-Staub et al.[65] to suggest that it was an "anticipatory regulation." They also proposed that the fall in serum calcium was due to an increase in plasma CT since it did not occur if rats with functional parathyroid transplants were thyroidectomized just before the dark-fed period; in fact serum calcium rose. Results obtained when sensitive immunoassays for CT became available supported the "anticipatory regulation" concept proposed by Perault-Staub et al;[65] CT levels were low during the light-fasted period, increased before the beginning of the dark-fed period, and reached the highest concentrations during the dark period[66–68]. The pattern of the circadian rhythm of calcium in blood was essentially a mirror image of that for CT. Hirsch and Hagaman[67] reported that the light-dark circadian rhythms were similar whether the rats were on a fixed feeding schedule or fed ad libitum. Mühlbauer and Fleisch[69] measured 6-hour urinary excretion of [^{3}H]tetracycline in rats. They concluded that changes in bone resorption as indicated by changes in the diurnal rhythms in the excretion of [^{3}H]tetracycline were strongly diet-dependent but neither PTH- nor CT-dependent. These findings appear, at first, to conflict with those obtained by measuring circadian rhythms of serum calcium. However, circadian rhythms of blood calcium in rats reflect changes in fluxes of calcium from bone that are affected by CT and PTH.[54,70] Changes in circadian rhythms of blood calcium do not represent changes in bone resorption, so that the findings on bone resorption are not contradictory to those on blood calcium.

Circadian rhythms of blood levels of CT in humans have not been established. In one study variations were seen only in the daytime and appeared to be influenced by eating.[71] In another study evidence was found for circadian rhythms,[72] while in others rhythms have not been detected.[73,74]

Specific Receptor Sites for Calcitonin

Identification of cell membrane receptors for calcitonin is required to define target cells and tissues of interaction and mechanisms of action as well as to determine physiologic functions and therapeutic uses. Beginning with the studies of Marx et al.[75], calcitonin receptors have been found in many tissues, including bone and kidney. The presence of binding sites on osteoclasts was inferred by the finding that calcitonin in tissue culture inhibited osteoclastic bone resorption induced by parathyroid hormone.[31,32] Of interest to binding and receptors was the finding that the inhibition of parathyroid hormone-induced bone resorption by calcitonin in vitro disappeared in less than 36 hours to several days of treatment despite addition of fresh media. The loss of the inhibitory activity was termed "escape."[76,77] Binding of calcitonin to bone in vitro and its relation to the "escape" phenomenon was examined by Tashjian et al.[78] They described in vitro studies showing that high doses of sCT and hCT resulted in down regulation of calcitonin receptors in calvaria from 3–5 day old mice and concluded that down regulation accounted at least in part for the "escape phenomenon".[78] Whether or not the "escape phenomenon" plays any role in the often reported loss of responsiveness of calcitonin with continued use in the therapy of human osteoporosis[r17–r21] is still unanswered. Heersche,[r22] summarizing the experimental evidence for "escape," pointed out that the phenomenon is dose-dependent and varies markedly between species. He suggested that the loss of in vivo responsiveness of bone to CT in the treatment of osteoporosis has several components: the production of antibodies, the development of secondary hyperparathyroidism, and escape from the direct inhibitory action on osteoclasts.

Warshawksky et al.[79] used radioautography to demonstrate that labeled calcitonin administered IV to rats bound strongly to cells in bone and kidney. In bone the label was localized in resorptive sites, indicating strong binding to osteoclasts. In kidney the saturable, specific binding was localized over vesicles below the brush border of cells of the proximal convoluted tubules. Other investigators found that the formation of CT receptors was stimulated by 1α, 25-dihydroxyvitamin D_3 in osteoclast-like multinucleated cells derived from mouse bone marrow[80] and in osteoclasts derived from organ cultures of fetal mouse metatarsals.[81] Although these in vitro studies are interesting, they may not have physiologic relevance since the doses of 1α, 25-dihydroxyvitamin D_3, usually 10nM or 4ng/ml, were supraphysiologic. The effects of calcitonin on bone and kidney are known, whereas the action of calcitonin on other tissues with specific binding sites,[r3] as for example CNS, pituitary, lymph, and tumor cells, is not clear. With respect to the CNS sites, it is tempting to speculate that some of these identifiable receptors are involved in the analgesic action of calcitonin.

Lin et al. were the first to clone a calcitonin receptor (CTR) from porcine kidney cells.[82] Other studies have followed in which CTRs have been obtained from human ovarian cell lines,[83] a human CTR cloned and expressed in baby hamster kidney cells,[84] two rat CTR isoforms identified by cDNA cloning from a hypothalamic library,[85] and two CTRs cloned from rat brain.[86] Considerable structural homology exists between CT and PTH receptors[r5] as well as with receptors for parathyroid hormone-related peptide, secretin, vasoactive intestinal peptide, growth hormone releasing hormone, glucagon-like peptide, and glucagon.[83] The strong structural homology of this family of G protein-coupled receptors suggests evolution from an early ancestral form that has been modified to express specific affinity for individual hormones.[83,r5]

Calcitonin Action on Target Organs

Bone

Two easily measured actions of calcitonin, especially in rats, are its hypophosphatemic and hypocalcemic actions. The effects are attributed to the inhibition of release of calcium and phosphate from bone into extracellular fluid. Early after its isolation from the thyroid gland, CT was shown to inhibit bone resorption,[31,32] and the inhibition of osteoclastic activity by CT has been well documented. However, the hypocalcemic and hypophosphatemic effects of administered calcitonin in rats are too large and too rapid to be due entirely to inhibition of osteoclasts; other bone cells, osteoblast lining cells, osteoblasts, and osteocytes also participate. Wallach et al.[r23] reviewed studies on the effects of calcitonin on bone quality and osteoblastic function in experimental animals as well as in humans. They concluded that, in addition to its well known effect to inhibit bone resorption CT also enhances osteoblastic bone formation, and thereby improves bone quality. Calcitonin abolished cytoplasmic motility of osteoclasts isolated from rat long bones.[87] However, calcitonin also affected osteoblasts[r2,88–90] and osteocytes,[88] and calcitonin binds to osteocytes and periosteal osteoblasts.[91] CT receptors are numerous in osteoclasts, whereas receptors for parathyroid hormone are numerous on osteoblasts and, as yet, unidentified on osteoclasts. Considering that there are different receptors for parathyroid hormone and calcitonin, it is not surprising that calcitonin can act in the absence of parathyroid hormone.[r24]

Whereas exogenous CT induces a marked hypocalcemia in rats, a much smaller response has been seen in normal adult human subjects. The difference in the magnitude of the response between species was attributed by Milhaud et al.[34] to the ability of CT to reduce the rate of bone metabolism, much higher in rats than in humans. This concept has been borne out in studies on normal humans where IV administration of calcitonin to normal adult subjects has produced either no significant lowering[92] or only a small decrease in serum calcium with porcine CT—a decrease that was somewhat larger with human and salmon CT.[93] In patients with elevated blood calcium due to high rates of bone resorption, as occurs in Paget's or malignant bone diseases, CT is highly effective in reducing blood calcium. However, the calcium-lowering action of calcitonin in patients with other hypercalcemias has been shown to be related directly to the degree of hypercalcemia rather than elevated bone resorption. The mechanism of this action may be different from that occurring in bone diseases involving high rates of bone resorption. Regardless of the mechanism involved, calcitonin has proved to be an effective and useful hypocalcemic agent.

Kidney

High supraphysiologic doses of calcitonin increase the urinary excretion of ions and, hence, increase urinary volume. The marked natriuretic effect of CT in humans was shown first by Bijvoet et al.[94] The effects on sodium and other ions are thought to be due to inhibition of renal tubular reabsorption. Establishing with certainty that CT has a physiologic role in the renal handling of ions has been difficult because results in humans and in experimental animals have not been consistent and the effects occur only with large doses. In favor of a role for calcitonin is the presence in the kidney of large numbers of specific receptors for calcitonin that activate adenylate cyclase and that are distinctly different from those for PTH and vasopressin.[r2,r25]

There is now substantial evidence that high doses of calcitonin increase 1-α-hydroxylase activity, thereby increasing production of 1α,25-dihydroxyvitamin D_3.[95–97, 103–105] This action occurs at a site in the proximal tubule different from that affected by PTH and does not appear to involve stimulation of a cyclic AMP mechanism. Since calcitonin increases synthesis of 1α, 25-dihydroxyvitamin D_3, the hormone that enhances formation of calcitonin receptors,[80,81] a feedback mechanism is suggested.

Gastrointestinal Tract

Cooper et al.[98] and Care et al.[99] independently provided the first evidence that those GI hormones with the same penultimate carboxy-terminal tetrapeptide found in gastrin and cholecystokinin are potent calcitonin secretagogues. This finding led to a clinical study showing that pentagastrin evoked a larger, more rapid increase in CT secretion than did the administration of calcium in patients with surgically proven or a positive family history of medullary thyroid carcinoma (MTC).[100] Provocative tests to detect tumors in families with a history of MTC are now in wide use. Screening for MTC in children from families with multiple endocrine neoplasia Type 2 or to detect recurrence in patients who have undergone surgery for MTC is performed frequently with pentagastrin, either alone or in conjunction with calcium.[101,102] Progress in the search for gene defects in MTC and MEM 2 recently was summarized by Gagel et al.[r26] Important findings are that: (1) calcitonin reduces gastric acid secretion;[103] (2) gastrin and cholecystokinin stimulate calcitonin secretion; and (3) neural crest-derived cells that may secrete CT or CT-like peptides are present in the GI tract.[104] These findings suggest possible physiologic feedback mechanisms that may have importance in GI physiology.[r27]

In contrast to the effects of feeding on the circadian rhythms of CT, summarized above, feeding appears to play a more pronounced role in lactating rats. First, lactating rats have higher serum levels of calcitonin and lower serum calcium than do nonlactating females.[105] Fasting the lactating rats reduced serum calcitonin and refeeding caused a marked threefold increase in serum calcitonin. An increase in serum calcitonin was also observed in pups during suckling, possibly caused by increased serum calcium inducing secretion of calcitonin from the thyroid.[106] A detailed discussion of calcitonin in lactation has been provided in reviews by Talmage et al.[r28] and Garel.[r29] Whether there is a similar role of feeding in calcitonin secretion in humans has not yet been clarified.

Other effects of calcitonin on the GI tract include the finding by Gray et al.[107] that high therapeutic doses of calcitonin decrease net water and electrolyte absorption from the intestinal lumen. This action may explain the diarrhea that occurs in patients with medullary thyroid carcinoma.

Other Actions

A number of other actions have been ascribed to calcitonin, including an increase in parathyroid hormone secretion, increases in the secretion of vasoactive intestinal polypeptide, somatostatin, ACTH, and β-endorphin; inhibition of secretion of thyroid stimulating hormone; and an increase in the secretion of luteinizing hormone, growth hormone, ACTH, and prolactin.[r2] Many of these actions have not been adequately confirmed and some require very high (supraphysiologic) doses—in which case the effects may be indirect.[r3]

Therapeutic Uses of CT

Hypercalcemias

Calcitonin is used to treat hypercalcemias due to excessive osteoclastic activity, hyperparathyroidism, vitamin D toxicity, myelomas, Paget's disease of bone and bone malignancies.[r2,r3,r30] It is usually employed as an emergency first procedure, together with hydration and loop diuretics, to lower excessively high and dangerous levels of blood calcium.[r30] It is also used in combination with other calcium-lowering agents such as bisphosphonates or plicamycin.[108,r30] After the initial lowering with CT, other therapeutic procedures are employed to normalize blood calcium and restrict recurrence of high levels of blood calcium.[r30]

Paget's Diseases

Calcitonin, like the bisphosphonates, is of major importance in the treatment of Paget's disease of bone and bone metastases. It is the drug of choice to treat the pain of Paget's disease. Treatment should be initiated with low daily doses of 0.25 mg of human CT or 25 to 50 IU of salmon CT. If low doses are ineffective, they can be increased to 0.5 mg of human CT or 50 to 100 IU of salmon CT. Skin testing is advisable before using salmon CT; still, about 25 per cent of the patients on sCT develop antibody-mediated resistance over three years of treatment.[r31] CT is very effective in reducing the high turnover characteristic of the disease and in the relief of pain that can be extremely severe and debilitating. Some patients may develop resistance, especially to sCT.[r31] The resistance to CT may be due in part to the development of antibodies and in part to the "escape phenomenon."[76,77] When antibody resistance is suspected, replacement with another calcitonin, especially human CT, may suffice.

Osteoporosis

Calcitonin is widely used in the treatment of osteoporosis, especially in Europe and Japan. Its use in the US has increased since CT was approved for such treatment by the Food and Drug Administration in 1984. The evidence is now overwhelming that calcitonin is an effective drug in high turnover osteoporosis to slow or prevent bone loss and, in some cases, to increase bone mass.[r17,r21,r32] It is a relatively safe drug with few adverse reactions, usually not serious. For example, the most common side-effect, in about 10 to 15 percent of patients, is nausea with or without vomiting. Usually, the incidence of nausea decreases with continued therapy. The incidence of another adverse effect, flushing of the face and neck that affects 2 to 5 percent of patients, also decreases with repeated use. Local inflammation at the site of administration affects up to 10% of patients and may require administration at alternate sites. Current drawbacks to its continued long-term use are the need for frequent parenteral administration and the high cost.[r18–r20] Calcitonin, because of its analgestic property, is especially useful in osteoporotic patients with protracted pain. It is hoped that the FDA will approve the administration of calcitonin by the intranasal route, already shown to be effective and used therapeutically in Europe. In one double-blind study of early postmenopausal women with calcium supplementation 50 IU of calcitonin was given intranasally in the morning and in the evening. Calcitonin prevented bone loss in the lumbar spine after one and two years of treatment, whereas the placebo-treated controls lost bone from the spine. While the difference of spinal measurements at two years was highly significant, no difference was noted in peripheral bones.[109] Recent reviews are in general agreement that treatment with CT suppresses annual bone loss and may at certain doses increase vertebral and perhaps even long-bone mass. For example, Reginster[r21] has reviewed evidence that 100 IU/day of nasally administered salmon CT prevents trabecular bone loss during the first year of the menopause. Also emphasized is that half of the dose, 50 IU/day, may be sufficient to prevent bone loss, whereas twice the dose, 200 IU/day may increase bone mineral content. In an important study by Civitelli et al,[110] 53 postmenopausal women with radiologic evidence of osteoporosis were treated with salmon calcitonin, 50 IU SQ, every other day for one year. The bone turnover rate was assessed by measurement of whole body retention of ^{99m}Tc-methylene diphosphonate and subjects were divided into a high turnover (HTOP) and normal turnover (NTOP) groups. Examination by dual photon absorptiometry revealed a highly significant 22 percent increase in the HTOP group and no change in the NTOP group. These results suggest that calcitonin treatment is most effective in those postmenopausal patients with high-turnover osteoporosis.

Many studies both reported and in progress are examining combination as well as alternating therapies in the treatment of osteoporosis. Reports indicate loss of effectiveness of treatment after continued use for two years.

Therapeutic doses of corticosteroids, chronically, are known to cause loss of bone. Although the mechanism has not been adequately determined, it is likely a combination of decreased bone formation, an increase in osteoclastic activity, decreased intestinal absorption of calcium, and an increase in the urinary excretion of calcium. Calcitonin has been used as a safe and effective agent to prevent glucocorticoid-induced bone loss and to treat established bone loss in patients treated with glucocorticoids.[r33,r34] A large clinical study by Sambrook et al.[111] utilized calcitonin for one year in combination with calcitriol and calcium. Treatment with calcitriol and calcium alone or with calcitonin prevented corticosteroid-induced bone loss in the lumbar spine. However, measurements at the end of the second year indicated that only those subjects previously treated with calcitonin had no bone loss. Unfortunately, a group treated with calcitonin alone was not included. Because calcitriol can frequently cause hypercalcemia, Meunier[r34] questioned the risk-benefit ratio with this agent when other effective therapies,

Generic Name	Trade Name	Dosage Forms	Dose*
Calcitonin-salmon	Calcimar	200 IU/ml	100 IU/day** SQ or IM
Calcitonin-salmon	Miacalcin	200 IU/ml	100 IU/day** SQ or IM
Calcitonin human	Cibacalcin	0.5-mg/syringe 5 syringes	0.5mg/day# SQ
Salmon calcitonin	Salcatonin	Nasal spray+	
Salmon calcitonin	Miacalcin	Nasal spray+	50–100 IU 2–7 doses/week SQ IM or intranasal
Elcatonin	Elcitonin	10 or 20 IU/ml Vials	10 IU IM twice a week 20 IU IM once a week

* Initial dosages are often much lower and are increased when required to obtain the desired response.
** Skin tests are recommended before initiating treatment, especially when using salmon or porcine calcitonins.
\# Double-chambered syringe—each contains 0.5 mg of calcitonin for injection and 20 mg of mannitol.
\+ Not yet approved by the US FDA for use in treatment of osteoporosis.

such as estrogens, calcitonin, and biphosphonates, can be utilized. In another study intranasal calcitonin was considered beneficial in treating patients with established corticosteroid-induced osteoporosis.[r35]

Pain

Calcitonin has an antinociceptive action that deserves special consideration. There is little doubt that calcitonin relieves bone pain, in part by inhibiting elevated osteoclastic activity. CT has been useful as an analgesic agent in patients with bone pain due to Paget's disease and osteoporosis; the pain relief is often so complete as to rehabilitate the patient. CT is also useful in reducing the pain in patients with intractable bone cancer. Part of the analgesic effect involves interference with peripheral pain transmission as well as an action on the CNS, for which there is substantial evidence.[r36] The mechanisms involved are poorly understood and controversial.[r36,r37] CT is an effective analgesic agent, even with nonosteogenic pain such as phantom-limb pain.

Future Possible Uses

The possibility that calcitonin may be useful in the therapy of many conditions other than bone and mineral disorders has been suggested. The list includes diseases of the GI tract, and disorders of the endocrine, immune, and cardiovascular systems, as well as psychiatric disorders.[r2] One must approach these suggestions with skepticism and caution. Further and more definitive studies are needed before other uses can be justified.

Toxic Effects and Drug Interactions

The toxic effects of calcitonin are relatively minor at therapeutic dose levels. Less serious but still undesirable side-effects include flushing, nausea, and swelling and tenderness of the hands. Urticaria seldom occurs. Nasal CT can avoid most of these side-effects, but leads to nasal irritation, stuffiness, etc., due apparently to the agent added to enhance mucosal penetration of CT.[r32]

There are no serious interactions of CT with other drugs.

Absorption, Transport, and Excretion

The peptide nature of calcitonin has prevented its oral use. It is easily absorbed from subcutaneous or intramuscular sites and can be administered intranasally or by rectal suppositories. It is transported in blood as the monomeric active form. While blood proteases break down CT into inactive fragments, the proteases in tissues, especially kidney, are responsible for the major metabolism of CT. The half-life of sCT in the blood of dogs is about 20 minutes compared to about 2.2 minutes for pCT, findings that are offered as one explanation for the higher activity of sCT than pCT. CT has been identified in the urine of a patient with medullary thyroid carcinoma,[29] but is not usually found in normal urine.

Preparations

Listed above are some of the major preparations and the doses used either for the treatment of Paget's disease of bone or for osteoporosis.

References

1. Copp DH, Cameron EC, Cheney BA, Davidson AGF, Henze KG. Evidence for calcitonin—a new hormone from the parathyroid that lowers blood calcium. Endocrinology 1962;*70*:638–649.

2. Hirsch PF, Gauthier GF, Munson PL. Thyroid hypocalcemic principle and recurrent laryngeal nerve injury as factors affecting the response to parathyroidectomy in rats. Endocrinology 1963;*73*:244–252.

3. Potts JT Jr, Reisfeld RA, Hirsch PF, Wasthed AB, Voelkel EF, Munson PL. Purification of porcine thyrocalcitonin. Proc Natl Acad Sci USA 1967;*58*:328–335.

4. Potts JT Jr, Niall HD, Keutmann HT, Brewer HB, Jr, Deftos LJ. The amino acid sequence of porcine thyrocalcitonin. Proc Natl Acad Sci USA 1968;*59*:1321–1328.

5. Neher R, Riniker B, Zuber H, Rittel W, Kahnt FW. Thyrocalcitonin. II. Struktur von α-Thyrocalcitonin. Helv Chem Acta 1968;*51*:917–924.

6. Rittel W, Brugger M, Kamber B, Riniker B, Sieber P. Thyrocalcitonin III. Die Synthese des α-Thyrocalcitonins. Helv Chim Acta 1968;*51*:924–928.

7. Riniker B, Neher R, Maier R, Kahnt FW, Byfield PGH, Gudmundson TV, Galante L, MacIntyre I. Menschliches Calcitonin. I. Isolierung und Charakterisierung. Helv Chim Acta 1968;*51*:1738–1742.

8. Neher R, Riniker B, Rittel W, Zuber H. Menschliches Calcitonin. III. Struktur von Calcitonin M und D. Helv Chim Acta 1968;*51*:1900–1905.

9. Sieber P, Brugger M, Kamber B, Riniker B, Rittel W. Menschliches Calcitonin. IV. Die Synthese von Calcitonin M. Helv Chim Acta 1968;*51*:2057–2061.

10. Hirsch PF, Voelkel EF, Munson PL. Thyrocalcitonin: Hypocalcemic hypophosphatemic principle of the thyroid gland. Science 1964;*146*:412–413.

11. Cooper CW, Hirsch PF, Toverud SU, Munson PL. An improved method for the biological assay of thyrocalcitonin. Endocrinology 1967;*81*:610–616.

12. Parsons JA, Woodward PM. Report on collaborative bioassay of four preparations of porcine thyrocalcitonin in seven laboratories. In: Taylor S, ed. Calcitonon—Proceedings of the Symposium on Thyrocalcitonin and the C Cells. London: Heinemann, 1968:42–50.

13. Zanelli JM, Gaines-Das RE, Corran PH. International Standards for salmon calcitonin, eel calcitonin and the ASU[1-7] analogue of eel calcitonin: calibration by international collaborative study. Bone Miner 1990;*11*:1–17.

14. Zanelli JM, Gaines-Das RE, Corran P. Establishment of the second international standards for porcine and human calcitonins: report of the international collaborative study. Acta Endocrinol 1993;*128*:443–450.

15. Otani M, Yamauchi H, Meguro T, Kitazawa S, Watanabe S, Orimo H. Isolation and characterization of calcitonin from pericardium and esophagus of eel. J Biochem Japan 1976;*79*:345–352.

16. Morikawa T, Munekata E, Sakakibara S, Noda T, Otani M. Synthesis of eel-calcitonin and [Asu[1,7]]-eel-calcitonin: contribution of the disulfide bond to the hormonal activity. Experientia 1976;*32*:1104–1106.

17. Cooper CW, Obie JF, Hsu WH. Improvement and initial in vivo application of the radioimmunoassay of rat thyrocalcitonin. Proc Soc Exp Biol Med 1976;*151*:183–188.

18. Deftos LJ, Lee MR, Potts JT Jr. A radioimmunoassay for thyrocalcitonin. Proc Natl Acad Sci USA 1968;*60*:293–299.

19. Guttmann S. Chemistry and structure-activity relationship of natural and synthetic calcitonins. In: Pecile A, ed. Calcitonin 1980. Chemistry, Physiology, Pharmacology and Clinical Aspects. Amsterdam: Excerpta Medica, 1981:11–24.

20. Munson PL. Biological assay of parathyroid hormone In: Greep RO, Talmage RV, eds. The Parathyroids, Springfield, IL: Thomas, 1961:94–113.

21. Talmage RV, Neuenschwander J, Kraintz L. Evidence for the existence of thyrocalcitonin in the rat. Endocrinology 1965;*76*:103–107.

22. Foster GV, Baghdiantz A, Kumar MA, Slack E, Soliman HA, MacIntyre I. Thyroid origin of calcitonin. Nature 1964;*202*:1303–1305.

23. Care AD. Secretion of thyrocalcitonin. Nature 1965;*205*:1289–1291.

24. Pearse AGE. The cytochemistry of the thyroid C cells and their relationship to calcitonin. Proc Roy Soc Lond 1966;*164*:478–487.

25. Copp DH, Cockcroft DW, Keuh Y. Calcitonin from the ultimobranchial glands from dogfish and chickens. Science 1967;*158*:924–926.

26. Tauber SD. The ultimobranchial origin of thyrocalcitonin. Proc Natl Acad Sci. USA 1967;*58*:1684–1687.

27. Pearse AGE, Carvalheira AF. Cytochemical evidence for an ultimobranchial origin of rodent thyroid C cells. Nature 1967;*214*:929–930.

28. Milhaud G, Tubiana M, Parmentier C, Coutris G. Epithélioma de la thyröide sécrétant de la thyrocalcitonine. CR Acad Sci Paris 1968;*266*:608–610.

29. Melvin KEW, Tashjian AH Jr. The syndrome of excessive thyrocalcitonin produced by medullary carcinoma of the thyroid. Proc Natl Acad Sci USA 1968;*59*:1216–1222.

30. Meyer JS, Abdel-Bari W. Granules and thyrocalcitonin-like activity in medullary carcinoma of the thyroid gland. N Engl J Med 1968;*278*:523–529.

31. Friedman J, Raisz LG. Thyrocalcitonin: Inhibitor of bone resorption in tissue culture. Science 1965;*150*:1465–1467.

32. Aliapoulios MA, Goldhaber P, Munson PL. Thyrocalcitonin inhibition of bone resorption induced by parathyroid hormone in tissue culture. Science 1966;*151*:330–331.

33. Milhaud G, Job JC. Thyrocalcitonin: Effect in idiopathic hypercalcemia. Science 1966;*154*:794–795.

34. Milhaud G, Tsien-Ming L, Nesralla H, Moukhtar MS, Perault-Staub AM. Studies on the mode of action and the therapeutic use of thyrocalcitonin. In: Taylor SR, ed. Calcitonin. Proceedings of the Symposium on Thyrocalcitonin and the C Cells. London: Heinemann, 1968:347–370.

35. Milhaud G. First therapeutic use of calcitonin Bone Miner 1992;*16*:201–210.

36. Niall HD, Keutmann HT, Copp DH, Potts JT Jr. Amino acid sequence of salmon ultimobranchial calcitonin. Proc Natl Acad Sci USA 1969;*64*;771–778.

37. Guttmann St, Pless J, Huguenin RL, Sandrin Ed, Bossert H, Zehnder K. Synthese von Salm-Calcitonin, einem hochaktiven hypocalcämischen Hormon. Helv Chim Acta 1969;*52*:1789–1795.

38. Le Dourain N, Le Lièvre C. Démonstration de l'origine neurale des cellules à calcitonine du corp ultimobranchial chez l'embryon du poulet. C R Acad Sci Paris 1970;*270*:2857–2863.

39. Pearse AGE, Polak JM. Cytochemical evidence for the neural crest origin of mammalian ultimobranchial C cells. Histochemie 1971;*27*:96–102.

40. Pearse AGE. Common cytochemical and ultrastructural characteristics of cells producing polypeptide hormones (the APUD series) and their relevance to thyroid and ultimobranchial C cells and calcitonin. Proc Roy Soc London, Ser B 1968;*170*:71–80.

41. Amara SG, David DN, Rosenfeld MG, Roos BA, Evans RM. Characterization of rat calcitonin mRNA. Proc Natl Acad Sci USA 1980;*77*:4444–4448.

42. Amara SG, Jonas V, Rosenfeld MG, Ong, ES, Evans RM. Alternative RNA processing in calcitonin gene expression generates mRNAs encoding different polypeptide products. Nature 1982;*298*:240–244.

43. Rosenfeld MG, Mermod JJ, Amara SG, Swanson LW, Sawchenko PE, Rivier J, Vale WW, Evans RM. Production of a novel neuropeptide encoded by the calcitonin gene via tissue-specific RNA processing. Nature 1983;*304*:129–135.

44. Steenbergh PH, Höppener JWM, Zandberg J, Lips CJM, Jansz HS. A second human calcitonin/CGRP gene. FEBS Letter 1985;*183*:403–407.

45. Delsert CD, Rosenfeld MG. A tissue-specific small nuclear ribonucleoprotein and the regulated splicing of the calcitonin/calcitonin gene-related protein transcript. J Biol Chem 1992;*267*:14573–14579.

46. Horn DA, Suburo A, Terenghi G, Hudson LD, Ploak JM, Latchman DS. Expression of the tissue specific splicing protein SmN in neuronal cell lines and in regions of the brain with different splicing capacities. Brain Res Mol Brain Res 1992;*16*:13–19.

47. Harper C, Toverud SU. Ability of thyrocalcitonin to protect against hypercalcemia in adult rats. Endocrinology 1973;*93*:1354–1359.

48. Bugnon C, Maurat JP, Lenys D, Moreau N, Rousselet F. Etude de l'origine cyotologique de la thyrocalcitonine chez des rats en hypervitaminose D. Compt Rend Soc Biol 1967;*161*:2363–2366.

49. DeLuca HF, Morii H, Melancon MJ Jr. The interaction of vitamin D, parathyroid hormone and thyrocalcitonin. In: Talmage RV, Bélanger LF, eds. Parathyroid Hormone and Thyrocalcitonin (Calcitonin). Amsterdam: Excerpta Medica, 1968:448–454.

50. Hirsch PF, Munson PL. Importance of the thyroid gland in the prevention of hypercalcemia in the rat. Endocrinology 1966;*79*:655–658.

51. Gray TK, Munson PL. Thyrocalcitonin: Evidence for physiological function. Science 1969;*166*:512–513.

52. Talmage RV, Vanderwiel CJ, Decker SA, Grubb SA. Changes produced in postprandial urinary calcium excretion by thyroidectomy and calcitonin administration in rats on different calcium regimes. Endocrinology 1979;*105*:459–464.

53. Talmage RV. Comment on the physiological role of calcitonin. Bone Miner 1992;*16*:186.

54. Talmage RV, Grubb SA, Norimatsu H. VanderWiel CJ. Evidence for an important physiological role for calcitonin. Proc Natl Acad Sci USA 1980;*77*:609–613.

55. Ahmado A, Khouja HI, Kemp GJ, Guilland-Cumming DF, Russell RGG, Bevington A. Calciotropic hormones raise the chemically detectable [Pi] in UMR 106-06 osteoblast-like-cells. Cell Biochem Funct 1993;*11*:25–34.

56. Malgaroli A, Meldolesi J, Zallone AZ, Teti A. Control of cytosolic free calcium in rat and chicken osteoclasts. The role of extracellular calcium and calcitonin. J Biol Chem 1989;*264*:14342–14347.

57. Moonga BS, Alam ASMT, Bevis PJR, Avaldi F, Soncini R, Huang CL-H, Zaidi M. Regulation of cytosolic free calcium in isolated rat osteoclasts by calcitonin. J Endocrinol 1992;*132*:241–249.

58. Gesek FA, Friedman PA. Calcitonin stimulates calcium transport in distal convoluted tubule cells. Am J Physiol 1993;*264*:F744–751.

59. Paniccia R, Colucci S, Grano M, Serra M. Zallone AZ, Teti A. Immediate cell signal by bone-related peptides in human osteoclast-like cells. Am J Physiol 1993;*265*:C1289–1297.

60. Awbrey BJ, Rosenstein BD, Grubb SA, Talmage RV. The effect of chronic calcitonin deficiency after thyroidectomy on calcium regulating hormones and bone density in women. J Bone Joint Therap (Orthop Trans) 1985;*9*:229–230.

61. Hurley DL, Tiegs RD, Wahner HW, Heath H III. Axial and appendicular bone mineral density in patients with long-term deficiency or excess of calcitonin. New Engl J Med 1987;*317*:537–541.

62. Pioli G, Pedrazzoni M, Palummeri E, Sianesi M, Del Frate R, Vescovi PP, Prisco M, Ulietti V, Costi D, Passeri M. Longitudinal study of bone loss after thyroidectomy and suppressive thyroxine therapy in premenopausal women. Acta Endocrinol 1992;*126*:238–242.

63. Štěpán JJ, Límanová Z. Biochemical assessment of bone loss in patients on long-term thyroid hormone treatment. Bone Miner 1992;*17*:377–388.

64. Diamond T, Nery L, Hales I. A therapeutic dilemma: Suppressive doses of thyroxine significantly reduce bone mineral measurements in both premenopausal and postmenopausal women with thyroid carcinoma. J Clin Endocrinol Metab 1991;*72*:1184–1188.

65. Perault-Staub AM, Staub JF, Milhaud G. A new concept of plasma calcium homeostasis in the rat. Endocrinology 1974;*95*:480–484.

66. Roos BA, Cooper CW, Frelinger AL, Deftos LJ. Acute and chronic fluctuations of immunoreactive and biologically active plasma calcitonin in the rat. Endocrinology 1978;*103*:2180–2186.

67. Hirsch PF, Hagaman JR. Feeding regimen, dietary calcium, and the diurnal rhythms of serum calcium and calcitonin in the rat. Endocrinology 1982;*110*:961–968.

68. Lausson S, Segond N, Milhaud G, Staub JF. Circadian rhythms of calcitonin gene expression in the rat. J Endocrinol 1989;*122*:527–534.

69. Mühlbauer RC, Fleisch H. A method for continual monitoring of bone resorption in rats: evidence for a diurnal rhythm. Am J Physiol 1990;*259*:R679–689.

70. Talmage RV, Doppelt SH, Fondren FB. An interpretation of acute changes in plasma ^{45}Ca following parathyroid hormone administration to thyroparathyroidectomized rats. Calc Tiss Int 1976;*22*:117–128.

71. Eastell R, Calvo MS, Burritt MF, Offord KP, Russell RGG, Riggs BL. Abnormalities in circadian patterns of bone resorption and renal calcium conservation in Type I osteoporosis. J Clin Endocrinol Metab 1992;*74*:487–494.

72. Hillyard CJ, Cooke TJC, Coombes RC, Evans IMA, MacIntyre I. Normal plasma calcitonin circadian variation and response to stimuli. Clin Endocrinol 1977;*6*:291–298.

73. Manolagas SC, Deftos LJ. No diurnal variations in calcitonin and vitamin D_2. N Engl J Med 1985;*312*:122–123.

74. Tiegs RD, Heath H III. Effects of altered calcium intake on diurnal and calcium-stimulated plasma calcitonin in normal women. J Bone Miner Res 1989;*4*:407–412.

75. Marx SJ, Fedak SA, Aurbach GD. Preparation and characterization of a hormone-responsive renal plasma membrane fraction. J Biol Chem 1972;*247*:6913–6918.

76. Friedman J, Au WYW, Raisz LG. Responses of fetal rat bone to thyrocalcitonin in tissue culture. Endocrinology 1968;*82*:149–156.

77. Wener JA, Gorton SJ, Raisz LG. Escape from inhibition of resorption in cultures of fetal bone treated with calcitonin and parathyroid hormone. Endocrinology 1972;*90*:752–759.

78. Tashjian AH Jr, Wright DR, Ivey JL, Pont A. Calcitonin binding sites in bone: relationships to biological response and "escape." Rec Prog Hormone Res 1978;*34*:285–334.

79. Warshawsky H, Goltzman D, Rouleau MF, Bergeron JJM. Direct in vivo demonstration by radioautography of specific binding sites for calcitonin in skeletal and renal tissues of the rat. J Cell Biol 1980:*85*:682–694.

80. Takahashi N, Akatsu T, Sasaki T, Nicholson GC, Moseley JM, Martin TJ, Suda T. Induction of calcitonin receptors by 1α,25-dihydroxyvitamin D_3 in osteoclast-like multinucleated cells formed from mouse bone marrow cells. Endocrinology 1988;*123*:1504–1510.

81. Minkin C, Yu X. Calcitonin receptor expression and its regulation by 1α,25-dihydroxyvitamin D_3 during de nova osteoclast formation in organ cultures of fetal mouse metatarsals. Bone Miner 1991;*13*:191–200.

82. Lin HY, Harris TL, Flannery MS, Aruffo A, Kaji EH, Gorn A, Kolakowski LF Jr, Lodish HF, Goldring SR. Expression cloning of an adenylate cyclase-coupled calcitonin receptor. Science 1991;*254*:1022–1024.

83. Goldring SR, Gorn AH, Yamin M, Krane SM, Wang JT. Characterization of the structural and functional properties of cloned calcitonin receptor cDNAs. Horm Metab Res 1993;*25*:477–480.

84. Stroop SD, Thompson DL, Kuestner RE, Moore EE. A recombinant human calcitonin receptor functions as an extracellular calcium sensor. J Biol Chem 1993;*268*:19927–19930.

85. Sexton PM, Houssami S, Hilton JM, O'Keeffe LM, Center RJ, Gillespie MT, Darcy P, Findlay DM. Identification of brain isoforms of the rat calcitonin receptor. Mol Endocrinol 1993;*7*:815–821.

86. Albrandt K, Mull E, Brady EM, Herich J, Moore CX, Beaumont K. Molecular cloning of the two receptors from rat brain with high affinity for salmon calcitonin. FEBS Lett 1993;*325*:225–232.

87. Chambers TJ, Moore A. The sensitivity of isolated osteoclasts to morphological transformation by calcitonin. J Clin Endocrinol Metab 1983;*57*:819–824.

88. Matthews JL, Martin JH, Collins EJ, Kennedy JW III, Powell EL Jr. Immediate changes in the ultrastructure of bone cells following thyrocalcitonin administration. In: Talmage R. Munson PL, eds. Calcium, Parathyroid Hormone, and the Calcitonins. Amsterdam: Excerpta Medica, 1971:375–385.

89. Ferrier J, Ward-Kesthely A, Heersche JNM, Aubin JE. Membrane potential changes, cAMP stimulation and contraction in osteoblast-like UMR 106 cells in response to calcitonin and parathyroid hormone. Bone Miner 1988;*4*:133–145.

90. Jones SJ, Boyde A. Experimental study of changes in osteoblastic shape induced by calcitonin and parathyroid extract in an organ culture system. Cell Tiss Res 1976;*169*;449–465.

91. Rao LG, Heersche JNM, Marchuk LL, Sturtridge W. Immunohistochemical demonstration of calcitonin binding to specific cell types in fixed rat bone tissue. Endocrinology 1981;*108*:1972–1978.

92. Singer FR, Woodhouse NJY, Parkinson DK, Joplin GF. Some acute effects of administered porcine calcitonin in man. Clin Sci 1969;*37*:181–190.

93. Gennari C, Chierichetti SM, Vibelli C, Francini G, Maioli E, Gonnelli S. Acute effects of salmon, human and porcine calcitonin on plasma calcium and cyclic AMP levels in man. Curr Ther Res 1981;*30*:1024–1032.

94. Bijvoet OLM, Vander Sluys Veer J, deVries HR, van Koppen ATJ. Natriuretic effect of calcitonin in man. New Engl J Med 1971;*284*:681–688.

95. Horiuchi N, Takahashi H, Matsumoto T, Takahashi N, Shimazawa E. Suda T, Ogata E. Salmon calcitonin-induced stimulation of 1α,25-dihydroxycholecalciferol synthesis in rats involving a mechanism independent of adenosine 3′:5′-cyclic monophosphate. Biochem J 1979;*184*:269–275.

96. Kawashima H, Torikai S, Kurokawa K. Calcitonin selectively stimulates 25-hydroxyvitamin D_3-1α-hydroxylase in proximal straight tubule of rat kidney. Nature 1981;*291*:327–329.

97. Econs MJ, Lobaugh B, Drezner MK. Normal calcitonin stimulation of serum calcitriol in patients with X-linked hypophosphatemic rickets. J Clin Endocrinol Metab 1992;*75*:408–411.

98. Cooper CW, Schwesinger WH, Mahgoub AM, Ontjes DA. Thyrocalcitonin: stimulation of secretion by pentagastrin. Science 1971;*172*:1238–1240.

99. Care AD, Bruce JB, Boelkins J, Kenny AD, Conaway H, Anast CS. Role of pancreozymin-cholycystokinin and structurally related compounds as calcitonin secretogogues. Endocrinology 1971;*89*:262–271.

100. Hennessy JF, Wells SA, Jr, Ontjes DA, Cooper CW. A comparison of pentagastrin injection and calcium infusion as provocative agents for the detection of medullary carcinoma of the thyroid. J Clin Endocrinol Metab 1974;*39*:487–495.

101. Gagel RF, Jackson CE, Block MA, Feldman ZT, Reichlen S, Hamilton BP, Tashjian AH, Jr. Age-related probability of development of hereditary medullary thyroid carcinoma. J Pediatr 1982;*101*:941–946.

102. Barbot N, Calmettes C, Shuffenecker I, Saint-André JP, Franc B, Rohmer V, Jallet P, Bigorgne JC. Pentagastrin stimulation test and early diagnosis of medullary thyroid carcinoma using an immunoradiometric assay of calcitonin: comparison with genetic screening in hereditary medullary thyroid carcinoma. J Clin Endocrinol Metab 1994;*78*:114–120.

103. Doepfner WEH, Briner U. Calcitonin and gastric secretion. In: Pecile A, ed. Calcitonin 1980. Chemistry, Physiology, Pharmacology and Clinical Aspects. Amsterdam: Excerpta Medica, 1981:123–135.

104. Pearse AGE, Polak JM. Neural crest origin of the endocrine polypeptide (APUD) cells of the gastrointestinal tract and pancreas. Gut 1971;*12*:783–788.

105. Toverud SU, Cooper CW, Munson PL. Calcium metabolism during lactation: elevated blood levels of calcitonin. Endocrinology 1978;*103*:472–479.

106. Cooper CW, Obie JF, Toverud SU, Munson PL. Elevated serum calcitonin and serum calcium during suckling in the baby rat. Endocrinology 1977;*101*:1657–1664.

107. Gray TK, Bieberdorf FA, Fordtran JS. Thyrocalcitonin and the jejunal absorption of calcium, water and electrolytes in normal subjects. J Clin Invest 1973;*52*:3084–3088.

108. Fatemi S, Singer FR, Rude RK. Effect of salmon calcitonin and etidronate on hypercalcemia of malignancy. Calcif Tissue Int 1992;*50*:107–109.

109. Overgaard K, Riis BJ, Christiansen C, Hansen MA, Effect of salcatonin given intranasally on early postmenopausal bone loss. Brit Med J 1989;*299*:477–479.

110. Civitelli R, Gonnelli S, Zacchei F, Bigazzi S, Vattimo A, Avioli LV, Gennari C. Bone turnover in postmenopausal osteoporosis. Effect of calcitonin treatment. J Clin Invest 1988;*82*:1268–1274.

111. Sambrook P, Birmingham J, Kelly P, Kempler S, Nguyen T, Stat M, Pocock N, Eisman J. Prevention of corticosteroid osteoporisis. A comparison of calcium, calcitriol, and calcitonin. New Engl J Med 1993;*328*:1747–1752.

Reviews

r1. Munson PL. Parathyroid hormone and calcitonin. In: McCann SM. ed. Endocrinology: People and Ideas. Bethesda: American Physiological Society, 1988:239–284.

r2. Azria M, The Calcitonins, Physiology and Pharmacology. Basel: Karger, 1989:153.

r3. Austin LA, Heath H, III. Calcitonin: physiology and pathophysiology. New Engl J Med 1981;*304*:269–278.

r4. Mallette LE, Gagel RF. Parathyroid hormone and calcitonin. In: Favus MJ. ed. Primer on the metabolic bone diseases and disorders of mineral metabolism. Second Ed. New York: Raven Press, 1993:90–99.

r5. Potts JT, Jr. Chemistry of the calcitonins. Bone Miner 1982;*16*:169–173.

r6. Hirsch PF, Munson PL. Thyrocalcitonin. Physiol Rev 1969;*49*:548–622.

r7. Bennett HS. A review of "chromaffin, enterochromaffin and related cells," with some comments on the APUD and paraneuron concepts. Arch Histol Jap 1977;*40*:Suppl:317–325.

r8. Pearse AGE. Calcitonin and the C cells: Role models for the neuroendocrine system. Bone Miner 1992;*16*:166–168.

r9. Burkitt HG, Young B, Heath JW., 17. The endocrine glands. In: Burkitt HG, ed. Wheater's Functional Histology: a Text and Colour Atlas, 3d ed. Edinburgh: Churchill Livinstone, 1993:304–322.

r10. Silva OL, Becker KL. Immunoreactive calcitonin in extrathyroid tissues. In: Pecile A, ed. Calcitonin 1980. Chemistry, Physiology, Pharmacology and Clinical Aspects. Amsterdam: Excerpta Medica, 1981:144–153.

r11. Milhaud G. Ectopic secretion of calcitonin. In: Pecile A, ed. Calcitonin 1980. Chemistry, Physiology, Pharmacology and Clinical Aspects. Amsterdam: Excerpta Medica, 1981:154–169.

r12. Sundler F, Ekblad E, Håkanson R. Occurrence and distribution of substance P- and CGRP-containing nerve fibers in gastric mucosa: Species differences. Adv Exp Med Biol 1991;*298*:29–37.

r13. Taché Y, Holzer P, Rosenfeld MG, eds. Calcitonin gene-related peptide. The first decade of a novel pleiotropic neuropeptide. Ann NY Acad Sci 1992;*657*:1–561.

r14. Copp DH. Endocrine regulation of calcium metabolism. Ann Rev Physiol 1970;*32*:61–86.

r15. Deftos LJ. Calcitonin. In: Favus MJ, ed. Primer on the Metabolic Bone Diseases and Disorders of Mineral Metabolism. Second Ed. New York: Raven Press, 1993:70–76.

r16. Baran DT, Braverman LE. Editorial: Thyroid hormones and bone mass. J. Clin Endocrinol Metab 1991;*72*:1182–1183.

r17. Avioli LV, Gennari C. Calcitonin therapy in osteoporotic syndromes. In: Avioli LV, ed. The Osteoporotic Syndrome: Detection, Prevention, and Treatment, 3d ed. New York: Wiley-Liss, 1993;137–154.

r18. Peck WA, Riggs BL, Bell NH, Wallace RB, Johnston, CC Jr, Gordon SL, Shulman LE. Research directions in osteoporosis. Am J Med 1988;*84*:275–282.

r19. Raisz LG, Smith J-A. Pathogenesis, prevention, and treatment of osteoporosis. Ann Rev Med 1989;*40*:251–267.

r20. Recker RR. Current therapy for osteoporosis. J Clin Endocrinol Metab 1993;*76*:14–16.

r21. Reginster J-Y, Calcitonin for prevention and treatment of osteoporosis. Am J Med 1993;*95* Suppl 5A:44S–47S.

r22. Heersche, JNM. Calcitonin effects on osteoclastic resorption: The 'escape phenomenon' revisited. Bone Miner 1992;*16*:174–177.

r23. Wallach S, Farley JR, Baylink DJ, Brenner-Gati L. Effects of calcitonin on bone quality and osteoblastic function. Calc Tissue Int 1993;*53*:335–339.

r24. Munson PL, Hirsch PF. Thyrocalcitonin: newly recognized thyroid hormone concerned with metabolism of bone. Clin Orthop 1966;*49*:209–232.

r25. Agus ZS, Wasserstein A, Goldfarb S. PTH, calcitonin, cyclic nucleotides and the kidney. Ann Rev Physiol 1981;*43*:583–595.

r26. Gagel RF, Robinson MF, Donavan DT, Alford BR. Medullary thyroid carcinoma: Recent progress. J Clin Endocrinol Metab 1993;*76*:809–814.

r27. Cooper CW, Bolman RM, III, Linehan WM, Wells SA, Jr. Interrelationship between calcium, calcemic hormones and gastrointestinal hormones. Rec Prog Hormone Res 1978;*34*:259–283.

r28. Talmage RV, Cooper CW, Toverud SU. The physiological significance of calcitonin. In: Peck WA. ed. Bone and Mineral Research, Annual 1. Amsterdam: Excerpta Medica, 1983:74–143.

r29. Garel J-M. Hormonal control of calcium metabolism during the reproductive cycle in mammals. Physiol Rev 1987;*67*:1–66.

r30. Bilezikian JP. Management of acute hypercalcemia. N Engl J Med 1992;*326*:1196–1203.

r31. Bone HG, Kleerekoper M. Paget's disease of bone. J Clin Endocrinol Metab 1992:*75*:1179–1182.

r32. Carstens JH, Jr, Feinblatt JD. Future horizons for calcitonin: a U.S. perspective. Calc Tiss Int 1991;49(Suppl 2):S2–6.

r33. Sullivan SL. Editorial: Management of corticosteroid-induced osteoporosis: a clinician's perspective. Calcif Tissue Int 1992;*50*:101–103.

r34. Meunier PJ. Editorial: Is steroid-induced osteoporosis preventable? New Engl J Med 1993;*328*:1781–1782.

r35. Ringe JD. Intranasal salmon calcitonin in the treatment of steroid-induced osteoporisis. In: Christiansen C, Overgaard K, eds. Osteoporosis 1990. Copenhagen: Osteopress ApS, 1990:1868–1871.

r36. Pecile A.: Calcitonin and the relief of pain. Bone Miner 1992;*16*:187–189.

r37. Passeri M, Baroni MC, Pedrazzoni M, Vescovi PP. Protocols of treatment of chronic back pain in involutional osteoporosis. Bone Miner 1993;*22*Suppl:S23–52.

CHAPTER 44

Adrenal Corticosteroids, Corticotripin Releasing Hormone, Adrenoconticotropin, and Antiadrenal Drugs

David A. Ontjes

Introduction to Pharmacology of the Pituitary Gland and Related Endocrine Systems

The pituitary gland, together with the adjacent neural tissue of the hypothalamus, is the control center for the neuroendocrine system. Many hormones and neuroactive drugs affect this system through actions on the pituitary, the hypothalamus, or both. The anterior pituitary controls hormone production in several other endocrine glands through production of specific trophic hormones, including adrenocorticotropin (ACTH), thyroid-stimulating hormone (TSH), luteininzing hormone (LH), and follicle-stimulating hormone (FSH). Without the presence of these trophic hormones, the target organs, including the adrenal cortex, the thyroid, and the gonads fail to function and undergo atrophy. The anterior pituitary also produces hormones that act directly on nonendocrine target tissues to control their growth and function. Growth hormone, for example, acts on several peripheral tissues to stimulate the production of local growth factors causing mitosis and growth. Prolactin acts on breast tissue to stimulate the synthesis of milk proteins and to induce lactation. The posterior pituitary hormone, vasopressin, acts on the kidney to control the permeability of the tubular epithelium to water and to regulate water balance.

The anterior and posterior lobes of the pituitary are anatomically and functionally distinct although both ultimately are subject to control by the CNS. The relationships between the hypothalamus and the pituitary gland are shown in Figure 44.1. The posterior lobe or neurohypophysis represents an extension of the axons of neurons whose cell bodies lie in the floor of the third ventricle. The posterior pituitary hormones, vasopressin and oxytocin, are synthesized in these neurons and transported down the axons to the neurohypophysis where they are released adjacent to a capillary plexus. After being taken up by the circulation they are conveyed to distant target organs where they exert their characteristic effects.

The control of the hormone-producing cells of the anterior lobe (adenohypophysis) is quite different. The anterior pituitary hormones are produced by epithelial cells that are located in the anterior lobe. These cells have differentiated, probably from a common stem cell, so that each of the anterior pituitary hormones is produced by a specific cell type. The exception is in the cell producing gonadotropins. Both LH and FSH may be produced by the same differentiated cell. The growth and function of the anterior pituitary cells are controlled by the CNS through the mediation of hypothalamic releasing and inhibiting factors, as shown in Figure 44.1. These factors are neuropeptides produced in cell bodies located in the hypothalamus. In contrast to vasopressin and oxytocin, these neuropeptides are released into a localized portal system, originating in a capillary plexus in the median eminence of the hypothalamus and ending in another plexus in the adenohypophysis. From the capillaries of this plexus they diffuse to exert their effects locally on their target cells in the anterior pituitary.

The interactions between the CNS, the pituitary

gland, and the several endocrine glands under pituitary regulation are characterized by a hierarchy of feedback mechanisms. These mechanisms may involve both stimulatory and inhibitory effects by humoral messengers acting on specific receptors in target tissues. The messengers for these systems may be classic hormones, transported in the general circulation, hypothalamic hormones, transported in the localized portal circulation, or classic neurotransmitters released from nerve axons and diffusing across synaptic junctions. Some of the characteristics of the hypothalamic hormones and their effects on the secretion of pituitary hormones are outlined in Table 44.1.

The modern field of neuroendocrinology and much of the field of neuropharmacology depends on our understanding of how the CNS affects the pituitary and the endocrine glands dependent on pituitary hormones for their control. The hypothalamic neuropeptides are at the core of the relationships between the endocrine system and the CNS. Because of their central role in human physiology, they also have great potential as diagnostic and therapeutic agents in medicine. More detailed discussions of the pharmacology of these compounds are presented in the chapters that follow.

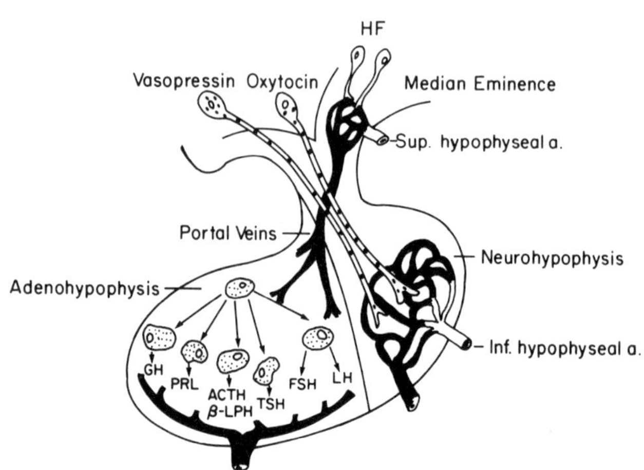

Figure 44.1 Functional Anatomy of the Hypothalamus and Pituitary. Hypophysiotrophic neurons in the hypothalamus secrete hypothalamic factors (HF) that either stimulate or inhibit the secretion of the individual anterior pituitary hormones. The hypothalamic factors reach the adenohypophysis via the hypophysial portal system as shown. Other neurons located primarily in the supraoptic and paraventricular nuclei of the hypothalamus secrete vasopressin and oxytocin from axons extending into the neurohypophysis. These hormones are released directly into the systemic circulation.

Adrenal Corticosteroids

The adrenal corticosteroids are a group of related compounds derived from cholesterol that are essential for life and widely used in medicine. Natural corticosteroids act directly on diverse cells and organs to serve many adaptive functions in the body. The physiologic effects of the adrenal corticosteroids fall into two major categories.

Glucocorticoid activities are those related to the regulation of energy metabolism and glucose homeostasis. *Mineralocorticoid activities* are related to sodium and potassium metabolism and the maintenance of salt and water balance. Both glucocorticoid and mineralocorticoid activities are important in maintaining an adequate blood pressure through effects on the vascular system and blood volume. In human physiology the principal glucocorticoid is *cortisol* and the principal mineralocorticoid is *aldosterone*. A large number of synthetic analogues of these naturally occurring steroids are used in clinical medicine, not only for replacement therapy in patients with adrenal insufficiency, but in supraphysiologic doses for the suppression of inflammation and the immune response.

The adrenal cortex itself is part of an integrated endocrine organ system that includes the pituitary gland and the hypothalamus. The physiologic role of the hypothalamic-pituitary-adrenal cortical system is to provide cortisol and aldosterone in sufficient quantities in the circulation to meet the changing needs of the body. Two peptide hormones, *corticotropin releasing hormone* (CRH) and *adrenocorticotropic hormone* (ACTH) are of critical importance in the control of the system, as shown in Figure 44.2. CRH is produced by neurons in the hypothalamus under the influence of afferent nerves from other sites in the CNS as well as negative feedback control from circulating cortisol. CRH is carried by portal vessels down the pituitary stalk to the anterior pituitary gland, where it stimulates the synthesis and release of ACTH and other peptides derived from a common biosynthetic precursor, pro-opiomelanocortin (POMC.) ACTH secretion is also regulated by the negative feedback of cortisol activity directly at the pituitary level. Once released into the systemic circulation, ACTH acts on the adrenal cortex to stimulate the synthesis of cortisol and related corticosteroids. The normal plasma concentrations of ACTH and cortisol vary widely depending on the time of day and the environment. The normal ranges for plasma cortisol, aldosterone, and ACTH are shown in Table 44.2.

Chemistry

All naturally occurring steroid hormones are derived from the biosynthetic transformation of cholesterol, as shown in Figure 44.3. In man the most active and important hormones produced by the adrenal cortex are the glucocorticoid, cortisol, and the mineralocorti-

Table 44.1

Hypothalamic Hormone	Effect on Secretion of Pituitary Hormone	Control Factors Mediated by CNS	Feedback by Peripheral Hormones
Thryrotropin Releasing Hormone (TRH)	Stimulates both Thyrotropin (TSH) and Prolactin	Cold exposure stimulates (newborn infants only)	Thyroid hormones inhibit by action on pituitary
Gonadotropin Releasing Hormone (GnRH) also known as Luteinizing Hormone Releasing Hormone (LHRH)	Stimulates both Luteinizing Hormone (LH) and Follicle Stimulating Hormone (FSH)	CNS inhibits GnRH secretion before puberty CNS inhibition decreases after puberty	Gonadal steriods (estrogens and androgens) inhibit by action on hypothalamus Estrogens enhance pituitary response to GnRH prior to ovulation
Corticotropin Releasing Hormone (CRH)	Stimulates Adrenocorticotropin (ACTH)	Stress and awakening stimulate	Adrenal glucocorticoids inhibit by action on both hypothalamus and pituitary
Growth Hormone Releasing Hormone (GHRH)	Stimulates Growth Hormone	Sleep, stress, and exercise stimulate. Increased blood glucose inhibits	Somatomedin (IGF-I) inhibits GHRH effects on pituitary
Somatostatin	Inhibits Growth Hormone	See above	Somatomedin increases somatostatin secretion by hypothalamus
Prolactin Inhibitory Factor (dopamine)	Inhibits Prolactin	Suckling stimulates by reducing hypothalamic dopamine release	Estrogens enhance prolactin secretion by causing hyperplasia of prolactin-secreting cells in pituitary

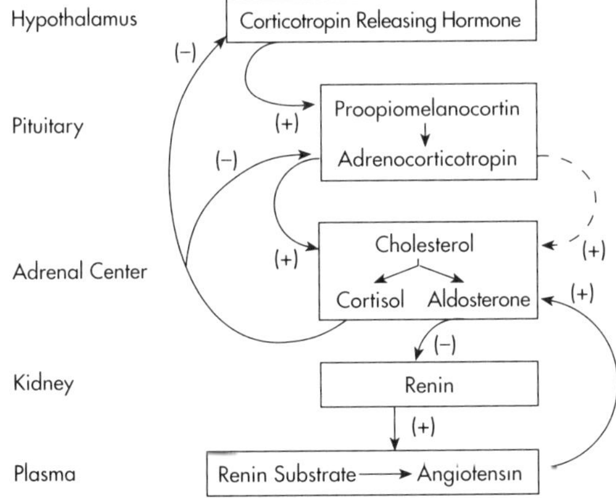

Figure 44.2 Relationship of the Hormones of the Hypothalamic-Pituitary-Adrenal System

coid, aldosterone. The weak androgens androstenedione and dehydroepiandrosterone are also produced in substantial quantities. The potent androgen, testosterone, and the potent estrogen, estradiol, are normally produced in physiologically insignificant amounts by the adrenal cortex, but in much larger amounts by the testis and ovary, respectively.

Biosynthetic Pathways

Steroid-producing tissues can synthesize cholesterol de novo or import cholesterol from the circulation by receptor-mediated endocytosis of low density lipoprotein (LDL). The pathways by which all steroids are produced from cholesterol are mediated by enzymatic conversions, as outlined in Figure 44.3. Most steroidogenic enzymes are members of a family of cytochrome P450 oxidases that contain heme and that catalyze electron transport from NADPH via flavoproteins serving as electron carriers.[12] The result is usually a hydroxylation of the substrate.

Each individual P450 enzyme is capable of handling more than one substrate, and several are multifunctional, being able to catalyze more than one reaction in a sequence. As shown in Figure 44.3, four distinct P450 enzymes are capable of catalyzing the transformations leading to over a dozen steroid products.

The Regulation of Biosynthesis

The adrenal cortex is traditionally divided into three concentric zones, an outer zona glomerulosa, a middle zona fasciculata, and an inner zona reticularis. These zones are defined morphologically by the varying arrangements of the cells within them. In addition to morphologic zonation, there also tends to be functional zonation according to the relative activities of the different steroidogenic enzymes and the predominant corticosteroids produced.[15] Hence, the synthesis of aldosterone is ordinarily confined to the glomerulosa layer, while in humans cortisol and androgens are produced in the fasciculata and reticularis layers. The distribution of some of the enzymes serving steroid biosynthesis varies according to the functional zone. In cells of the glomerulosa layer, the enzyme serving 17-hydroxylation is relatively inactive; but the multifunctional enzyme catalyzing the last three oxidative steps in the conversion of corticosterone to aldosterone is highly active. Cytochrome P450 c11 in the glomerulosa catalyzes not only 11-hydroxylation but also 18-hydroxylation and 18-methyloxidation. In some species there are

Table 44.2 Plasma Concentrations of Adrenal Corticosteroids and Hormones Regulating Their Secretion

Hormone	SI Units	Conventional Units
Cortisol		
8AM	220–660 nmol/L	8–24 μ/dL
4PM	50–410 nmol/L	2–15 μg/dL
Aldosterone		
supine, salt-loaded	<240 pmol/L	<8.5 ng/dL
upright, salt-depleted	415–1720 pmol/L	15–62 ng/dL
Dehydroepiandrosterone sulfate (DHEAS)	5.4–9.2 μmol/L	820–3380 ng/mL
17α-Hydroxyprogesterone		
Women	1–13 nmol/L	0.3–4.2 μg/L
Men	1.5–7.5 nmol/L	0.5–2.5 μg/L
Adrenocorticotropin		
8AM	4.5–18 pmol/L	20–80 pg/mL
4PM	<4.5 pmol/L	<20 pg/mL
Corticotropin-releasing hormone (in peripheral plasma only; may not correlate with levels in hypophyseal portal plasma[r32])	0.4–6.1 pmol/L	1.8–28 pg/mL

Values from Orth DN, Kovacs WJ, DeBold CR, The adrenal cortex. In Wilson JD, Foster DW, Textbook of Endocrinology, 8th edition. pp. 576–582, Philadelphia: WB Saunders, 1992.

two different cytochrome P450 c11 enzymes in different zones of the adrenal. Only the form in the glomerulosa layer can carry out the terminal step of 18-methyloxidation.[4] In cells of the fasciculata layer, where 17-hydroxylation occurs more readily, cortisol is the prevailing product. In the zona reticularis, where 3-β-hydroxysteroid dehydrogenase has a lower level of activity, the production of the weak androgen dehydroepiandrosterone (DHA) is favored. However, in rats and mice, experimental animals extensively used in adrenal research, cortisol is absent and corticosterone is solely responsible for glucocorticoid function.

The over-all rate of biosynthesis of adrenal steroids is determined by the rate of supply of cholesterol to the cytochrome P450 enzyme that cleaves it to yield pregnenolone. This step is stimulated rapidly by ACTH and is rate-limiting for steroidogenesis in general. Beyond pregnenolone formation, the relative size of the different zones of the adrenal cortex and the relative activities of the enzymes of the steroidogenic pathways determine the pattern of steroidogenesis. Thus, an important means of regulating the synthesis of a given steroid is the regulation of the mass of the tissue involved in its synthesis. The more chronic effects of ACTH involve regulation of synthesis of enzymes involved in the steroidogenic pathways.[r11] While ACTH is clearly the most important hormone governing overall adrenocortical mass, it probably functions as an indirect mitogen. ACTH can stimulate protein synthesis and hypertrophy, but not DNA synthesis and hyperplasia of adrenal cells in tissue culture. In vivo, where chronic ACTH administration does stimulate hyperplasia, the effects may be mediated by locally acting growth factors as well as by changes in vascular supply. Factors responsible for alterations in the mass of specific zones are probably important. For example, the increase in the number of cells in the glomerulosa layer under conditions of chronic salt deprivation may be mediated in part through increased activity of the renin-angiotensin system. The cells of the glomerulosa show a greater steroidogenic response to angiotensin II than do cells in the other zones because they are richer in angiotensin receptors.

Peripheral Conversions of Adrenal Steroids

The adrenal synthesizes relatively large quantities of weak androgens with 19-carbon atoms and much smaller quantities of estrogens with 18-carbon atoms. The adrenal androgens, dehydroepiandrosterone and androstenedione, can be converted by peripheral tissues, especially liver and adipose tissue, to more potent androgens and estrogens.[5] Peripheral metabolism of weak adrenal androgens is an important source of circulating testosterone in women, but not in men, where the testis is the major androgen source. When ovarian production of estrogens ceases at menopause, peripheral production of estrone and estradiol from adrenal androgen precursors becomes the chief source of residual estrogens. Such peripherally produced steroids become important in certain clinical situations, such as the evaluation of women with hirsutism due to excess androgens. A common characteristic of adrenal androgens and their peripherally produced derivatives is their ultimate dependence on ACTH for continued biosynthesis.

Natural and Synthetic Corticosteroids Used as Drugs

Today the number of corticosteroid compounds available for use as drugs is quite large. The structures of some of the most commonly used natural and synthetic corticosteroids are shown in Figure 44.4. Appropriate use of these compounds depends on an understanding of some of the effects of synthetic structural modifications on function.

In the early years of corticosteroid use no synthetic derivatives more active than cortisone itself were found. It soon became evident, however, that certain structural modifications could affect glucocorticoid and mineralocorticoid potency differentially, as shown in Table 44.3. For example, the introduction of an additional double bond at $C_{1,2}$ in hydrocortisone yields prednisolone, a compound with a fourfold increase in glucocorticoid activity but decreased sodium-retaining ac-

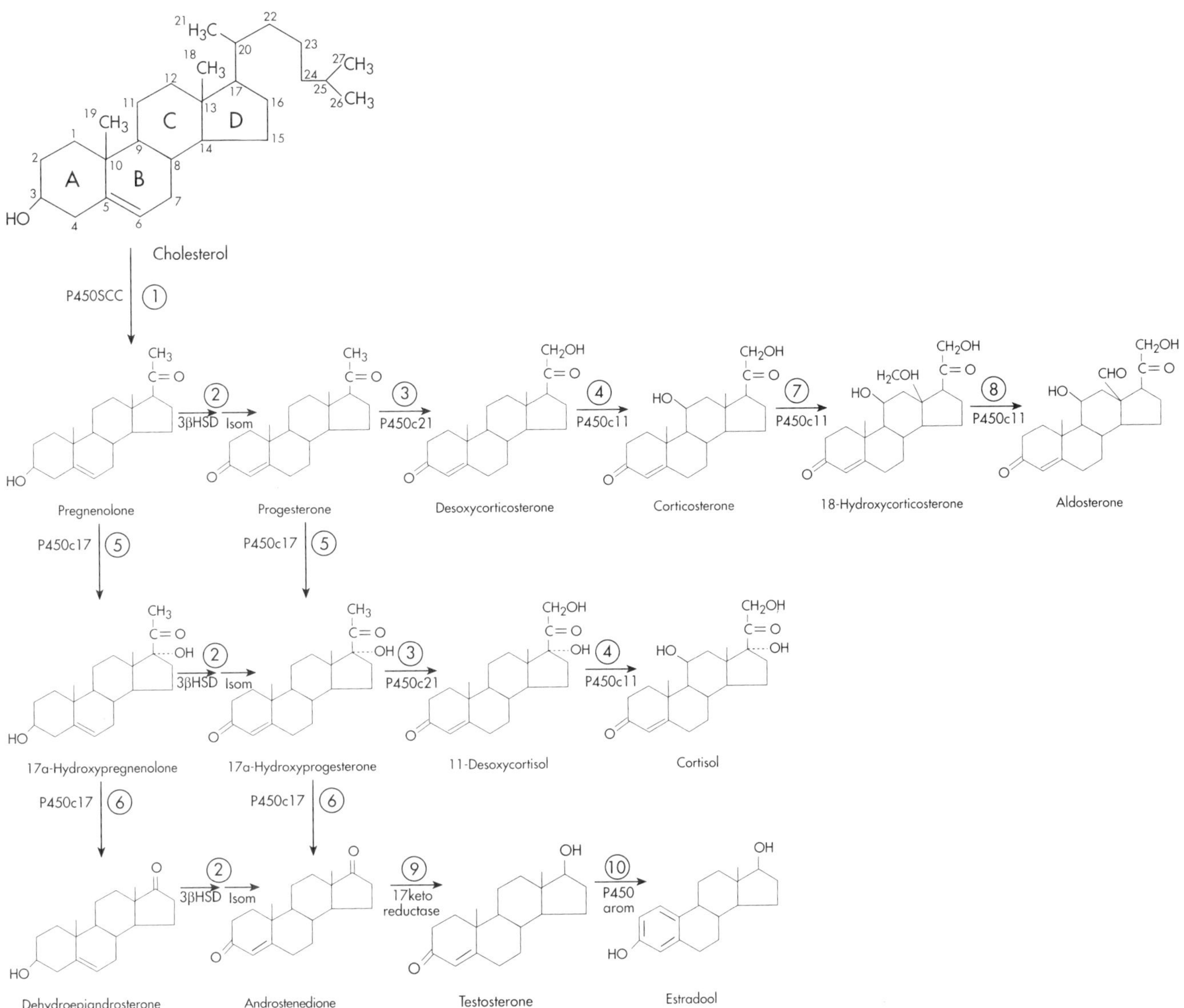

Figure 44.3 Principal pathways for human adrenal steroid synthesis. ***Reaction 1*** in the sequence occurs in mitotochondria where cholesterol is converted to pregnenolone. This step involves 20 α-hydroxylation, 22-hydroxylation and cleavage of the C20-22 carbon bond, all catalyzed by the side chain cleavage enzyme, cytochrone P450 scc. This reaction is rate limiting for the entire sequence and is stimulated by ACTH. ***Reaction 2*** is mediated by one or more non-P450 enzymes in the endoplasmic reticulum catalyzing dehydrogenation of the 3-β-hydroxy group and isomerization of the double bond from C5-6 to C4-5. ***Reaction 3***, mediated by cytochrome P450 c21 in the endoplasmic reticulum introduces the 21-hydroxyl group. ***Reactions 4, 7, and 8*** are all mediated by a single multifunctional enzyme in mitochondria, cytochrome P450 c11. This enzyme mediates 11 β-hydroxylation in the production of corticosterone and cortisol, and also mediates 18-hydroxylation and 18-methyl oxidase activity in the pathway to production of aldosterone. The latter two steps occur predominantly in cells of the glomerulosa layer of the adrenal cortex. ***Reactions 5 and 6*** are both mediated by cytochrome P450 c17 in the endoplasmic reticulum. This enzyme can catalyze both 17-α-hydroxylation, leading to 17-OH progesterone in the cortisol pathway, and cleavage of the C17-20 bond leading to the adrenal androgens dehydroepiandrosterone (DHEA) and androstenedione. ***Reactions 9 and 10*** occur mainly in the testis and ovary. ***Reaction 9*** mediated by 17 ketoreductase, a non P450 enzyme in the endoplasmic reticulum, produces testosterone. ***Reaction 10***, mediated by cytochrome P450 arom also in endoplasmic reticulum, produces estradiol through aromatization of ring A in the sterol nucleus.

tivity. Introduction of the 9-α-fluoro group into hydrocortisone yields fludrocortisone, a compound with a tenfold increase in glucocorticoid activity but an even greater increase in mineralocorticoid activity. The 16-α-methyl group, as introduced in methylprednisolone, further enhances glucocorticoid activity, but nullifies mineralocorticoid activity. The introduction of several modifications in a single compound can have additive and independent effects. Thus, dexamethasone, which possesses a $C_{1,2}$ double bond, a 9-α-fluoro group, and a 16-α-methyl group, has approximately 30 times the glucocorticoid activity of hydrocortisone but no sodium-retaining effects.

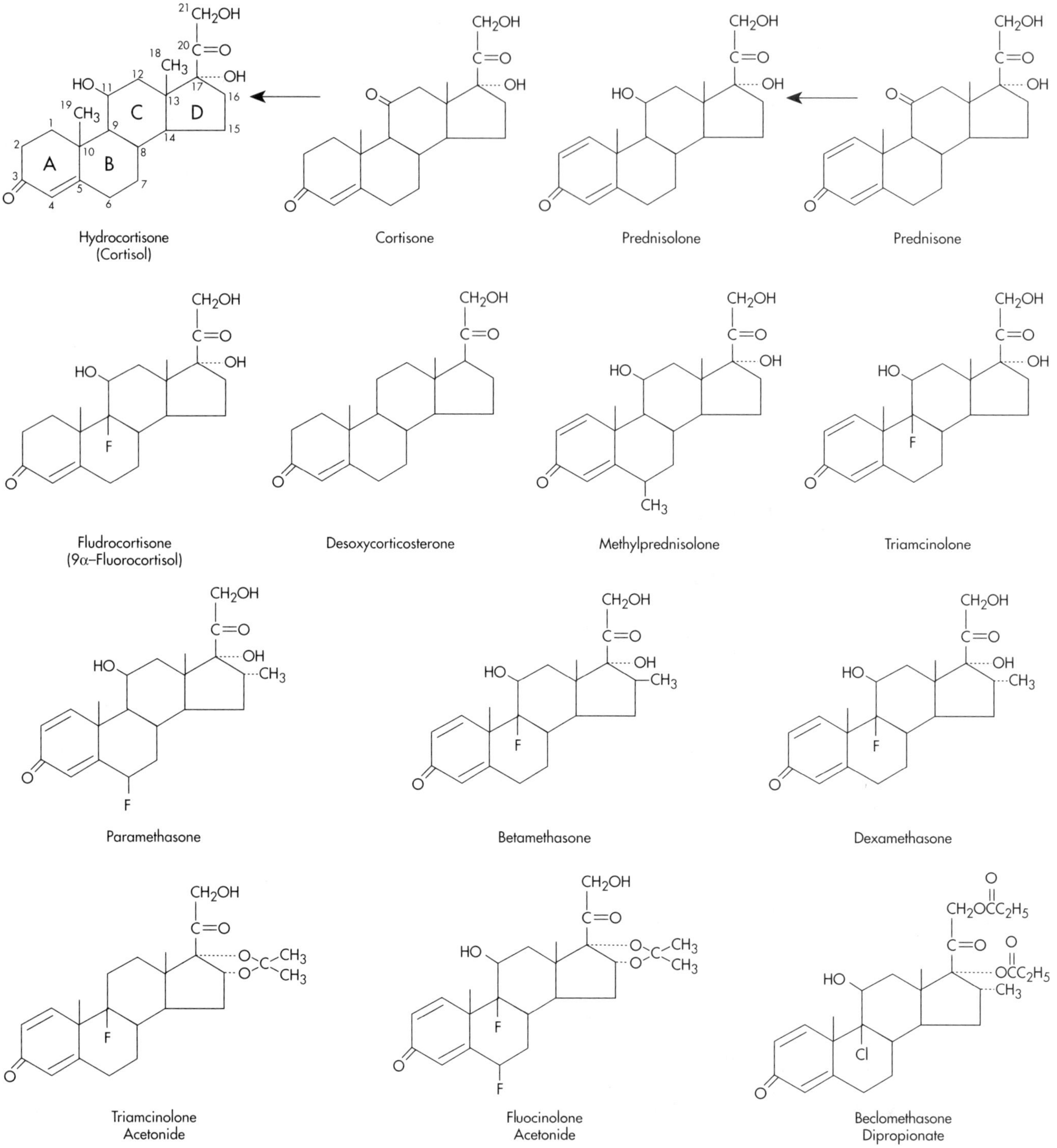

Hydrocortisone (Cortisol)

Cortisone

Prednisolone

Prednisone

Fludrocortisone (9α–Fluorocortisol)

Desoxycorticosterone

Methylprednisolone

Triamcinolone

Paramethasone

Betamethasone

Dexamethasone

Triamcinolone Acetonide

Fluocinolone Acetonide

Beclomethasone Dipropionate

Figure 44.4 Structures of Commonly Used Adrenocorticosteroids

History

The development of our knowledge about the hormones of the adrenal cortex is a story of the insights of physicians, physiologists, chemists, and, more recently, molecular biologists that extends over 100 years.[1,r1] Although the adrenal glands were described anatomically by Bartolomeo Eustacchio in 1563, their importance to health was not recognized until 1849, when Thomas Addison identified a clinical syndrome of weakness, wasting, hypotension, and hyperpigmentation resulting from their destruction. During the early 20th century physiologists recognized that the adrenal cortex, but not the medulla, was essential for life. Early attempts to identify the life-giving principle of the cortex were confounded by the presence of epinephrine in crude adrenal extracts. The catecholamines of the

Table 44.3 Relative Potency, Receptor Affinity, and Duration of Action of Commonly Used Corticosteroid Preparations

	Relative Potency		Relative Receptor Affinity		Plasma	Biologic
Steroid Compound	**Glucocorticoid**	**Mineralo-corticoid**	**Glucocorticoid**	**Mineralo-corticoid**	**Half-Life Minutes**	**Half-Life Hours**
Cortisol (Hydrocortisone)	1.0	1.0	1.0	1.0	80–120	8–12
Cortisone	0.8	0.8	0.1	1.0	80–120 as cortisol	8–12
Prednisolone	4.0	0.8	2.1	0.9	120–300 as prednisolone	12–36
Prednisone	3.5	0.7	0.1	0.1	120–300	12–36
Fludrocortisone	10	125	3.5	12	90	8–12
11-Desoxycorticosterone	0	100	0.3	—	30	8–12
Methylprednisolone	5	0.5	12	—	120–180	12–36
Triamcinolone acetonide	5	0	1.9	—	—	—
Dexamethasone	30	0	7.1	0.2	150–270	24–72
Betamethasone	25–30	0	5.4	0.8	130–330	24–72

adrenal medulla could temporarily raise the blood pressure of patients with Addison's disease, especially when given with large volumes of saline. By 1930, several investigators had developed methods for the extraction of "cortin," which was free of epinephrine and able to keep adrenalectomized animals and a few Addisonian patients alive. However, the cost and difficulty in preparing and standardizing large quantities of active material greatly limited clinical use. In 1932, Cushing described a syndrome of obesity, hirsutism, hypertension, adrenal hyperplasia, and pituitary adenoma. It later became clear that Cushing's syndrome was the direct result of excess adrenal corticosteroids.

The modern era of adrenal steroid pharmacology began in the period from 1930–1950, when Kendall in the United States and Reichstein in Switzerland purified and identified a series of pure adrenal corticoids, including corticosterone, 11-deoxycorticosterone, cortisone, and cortisol. By 1940 assays could clearly distinguish the relative potencies of these compounds, both in maintaining glucose homeostasis and sodium balance. Cortisone was more potent in elevating the blood glucose, while deoxycorticosterone was more potent in preventing urinary salt loss. With improving methods for synthesis using simple steroids such as deoxycholic acid or progesterone as starting materials, pharmaceutical chemists produced sufficient corticosteroids for clinical trials. In 1948, Hench, speculating that the course of rheumatoid arthritis might improve spontaneously in situations where endogenous corticoid levels were high, gave injections of cortisone to a patient and noted rapid and dramatic improvement. This period of rapid progress culminated in the award of the Nobel Prize in Medicine to Kendall, Reichstein, and Hench in 1950.[1]

The last physiologically important corticosteroid, aldosterone, was isolated in 1954 by Simpson and Tait, and was synthesized a year later.[6] This hormone, though present in extremely small amounts, was shown to account for much of the mineralocorticoid activity in the adrenal cortex. Physicians began to use cortisone and cortisol in high doses to ameliorate a growing number of inflammatory diseases. At the same time, the serious side-effects associated with corticosteroid therapy became clear. Pharmaceutical companies, realizing more efficient ways to synthesize cortisone, fortuitously discovered modifications in structure that could cause large increases in either the glucocorticoid or mineralocorticoid potency of synthetic steroids. A wave of research between 1950 and 1960 led to the synthesis of potent analogues clinically useful as either pure glucocorticoids or pure mineralocorticoids. While glucocorticoid and mineralocorticoid activities could be dissociated with appropriate structural modifications, glucocorticoid and anti-inflammatory activities could not. Thus, the metabolic complications of Cushing's syndrome were inextricably linked to the use of corticosteroids as anti-inflammatory drugs.

In the past 20 years attention to the pharmacokinetics of glucocorticoids has led to important improvements in therapy. Intermittent dosing regimens as well as the development of topical analogues have substantially reduced the severity of systemic side-effects. Finally, contemporary molecular biology has provided a detailed account of the mechanism of action of all steroid hormones through the structural analysis of steroid receptors and the genes coding for them. The identification of separate glucocorticoid and mineralocorticoid receptors in separate target cells, each capable of controlling the expression of certain genes within the cell, offers the possibility of new ways in which the therapeutic response to corticosteroids may be altered.

Therapeutic Uses and Limitations

Adrenal corticosteroids are among the most widely used drugs in the world. Their use varies from the treatment of mild self-limited conditions to life-threatening problems. A partial list illustrating some of the more common uses is shown in Table 44.4. These uses fall into two broad categories.

Corticosteroid Replacement

Adrenal corticosteroids are used for essential replacement therapy in patients with adrenal insufficiency. In patients with primary adrenal insufficiency due to loss of functioning adrenal cortical tissue, both glucocorticoids and mineralocorticoids are usually deficient and must be replaced in amounts sufficient to

Table 44.4 Some Therapeutic Uses of Adrenal Corticosteroids

Replacement Therapy	Hematologic and Neoplastic Diseases	Gastrointestinal Diseases

Primary adrenal insufficiency
Secondary Adrenal insufficiency
Congenital adrenal hyperplasia
Selective aldosterone deficiency
Musculoskeletal Diseases
Rheumatoid arthritis
Systemic lupus erythematosus
Mixed connective tissue syndromes
Polymyositis
Polymyalgia rheumatica
Pulmonary Diseases
Bronchoconstrictive diseases
  Acute asthma
  Chronic asthmatic bronchitis
Aspiration pneumonitis
Interstitial diseases
  Hypersensitivity pneumonitis
  Sarcoidosis
  Idiopathic pulmonary fibrosis
Pulmonary vasculitides
	Inflammatory bowel disease
	Aplastic anemias (some forms)
	Immune hemolytic anemia
	Immune thrombocytopenia
	Transfusion reactions
	Hematologic malignancies
	  Acute lymphoblastic leukemia
	  Lymphomas (some forms)
	  Multiple myeloma
	Complications of malignancy
	  Hypercalcemia
	Allergic and Immune Diseases
	Acute hypersensitivity reactions
	Anaphylaxis
	Angioedema and urticaria
	Insect venom allergy
	Allergic rhinitis
	Some drug allergies
	Serum sickness
	Transplantation rejection
	Cardiovascular Diseases
	Temporal arteritis
	Giant cell arteritis
	Myocarditis (some forms)
	Pericarditis (some forms)
		Crohn's disease
		Ulcerative colitis
		Nontropical sprue
		Chronic active hepatitis
		Neurologic Conditions
		Acute cerebral edema
		Multiple sclerosis
		Myasthenia gravis
		Eye Diseases
		Uveitis
		Exophthalmos
		Scleritis
		Allergic conjunctivitis
		Optic neuritis
		Skin Diseases
		Atopic dermatitis
		Contact dermatitis
		Seborrheic dermatitis
		Pemphigus
		Erythema multiforme
		Mycosis fungoides

restore normal physiologic regulation. Hydrocortisone or other glucocorticoids in appropriate amounts are essential for the maintenance of normal energy metabolism, including glucose homeostasis, and for maintenance of a normal blood pressure and circulation. Glucocorticoid deficiency leads to a profound systemic disorder manifested by weakness, nausea, hypoglycemia, and shock that may be fatal if untreated. Mineralocorticoids act primarily through the kidney to maintain a normal blood and ECF volume and to regulate body stores of sodium and potassium. Mineralocorticoid deficiency may cause hyponatremia, hyperkalemia, hypovolemia, and orthostatic hypotension.

In patients with secondary adrenal insufficiency there is a primary deficiency of ACTH, CRH, or both, due to disease of the pituitary or hypothalamus. Such individuals have glucocorticoid deficiency due to the absolute dependence of cortisol secretion on ACTH, but they may still produce adequate amounts of aldosterone through continued stimulation by the renin-angiotensin system. Thus, patients with secondary adrenal insufficiency commonly require replacement with glucocorticoids but not mineralocorticoids.

In patients with selective hypoaldosteronism, there is a deficiency of aldosterone but not of cortisol. This occurs most commonly with a primary deficiency of renin in patients with kidney disease, but may rarely result from isolated aldosterone biosynthetic defects. Patients with selective hypoaldosteronism suffer from hyperkalemia and metabolic acidosis due to failure to excrete potassium and hydrogen ions, but they do not usually have problems with salt-wasting or hypovolemia. Appropriate replacement therapy in this situation involves administration of synthetic mineralocorticoids, such as fludrocortisone. Patients with various forms of congenital adrenal hyperplasia have deficiencies in the activity of enzymes catalyzing one or more of the steps in the biotransformation of cholesterol to cortisol. Because the enzyme deficiency is often incomplete and may be overcome by an increased secretion of ACTH, many of these individuals have adequate production of cortisol and are not overtly glucocorticoid deficient. The undesirable effects of these syndromes are usually related to the overproduction of steroid products proximal to the defective biosynthetic step. These by-products are often weak androgens capable of causing virilization in women or sexual precocity in boys. Partial deficiency of 21-hydroxylation modulated by the enzyme P450 c21 occurs with varying severity in both infants and adults, and is the most common virilizing form of congenital adrenal hyperplasia. Androstenedione and dehydroepiandrosterone are the chief androgens that are overproduced. Partial blocks at other steps can cause overproduction of mineralocorticoids. For example, deficient 17-hydroxylation due to a deficiency of P450 c17 activity leads to an excess of deoxycorticosterone. The therapeutic goal in all forms of congenital adrenal hyperplasia is to provide adequate exogenous glucocorticoid replacement and to suppress endogenous ACTH secretion and steroid biosynthesis. The overproduction of unwanted androgens or mineralocorticoids can usually be suppressed by physiologic or only slightly supraphysiologic glucocorticoid replacement.

High-Dose Glucocorticoid Therapy

In addition to physiologic replacement, corticosteroids are often used at supraphysiologic doses to suppress various disease processes through their effects on inflammation or the immune response. The list of diseases that may be ameliorated in this way is extremely long and involves nearly every type of medical practice (Table 44.4). The limitations of high-dose glucocorticoid therapy are of two kinds. First, glucocorticoids are rarely curative for the underlying disorder. Usually, only the immediate consequences of the body's inflammatory response are reduced. Second, the action of excess glucocorticoids over time invariably creates a new disease. In some cases the consequences of iatrogenic hypercortisolism or Cushing's syndrome may be more disabling than the condition for which glucocorticoids were originally given. Unfortunately, the desired anti-inflammatory and immunosuppressant effects of high-dose corticosteroids are mediated by mechanisms similar to those mediating a myriad of other glucocorticoid effects throughout the body. While undesired mineralocorticoid effects can be eliminated by the choice of highly potent pure glucocorticoids, untoward glucocorticoid effects can be only partially reduced by judicious therapy.

Corticosteroid Effects and Their Mechanisms

Basic Mechanisms of Corticosteroid Action

Early functional assays classified the corticosteroids as having either glucocorticoid or mineralocorticoid effects according to their activity in promoting either liver glycogen deposition or sodium retention by the kidney.[r1] In spite of the diversity of potential effects in vivo there is now much evidence that all corticosteroids act by common mechanisms at the cellular level. In recent years two receptor systems have become increasingly well-defined in terms of molecular biology. A glucocorticoid receptor probably subserves the anti-inflammatory and immunosuppressive effects of the corticosteroids as well as their effects on glucose homeostasis.[r4,r12] A closely related but distinct mineralocorticoid receptor subserves the salt-regulating function of corticosteroids in the kidney. Both receptors are widely distributed in body tissues as shown in Table 44.5. Few of the physiologic functions governed by these receptors have yet been fully integrated with the growing knowledge of molecular events.

Both the human glucocorticoid receptor and the mineralocorticoid receptor are members of a supergene family of steroid hormone receptors[7,8,9] that also includes the thyroid hormone receptor. This family of proteins, each coded by a separate gene, shares certain homologies of structure and function that suggest evolutionary development from a common ancestral gene. The common structural features of several receptors in the family are shown in Figure 44.5.

The Glucocorticoid Receptor

The human glucocorticoid receptor is a phosphoprotein of 777 amino acids with a molecular weight of approximately 94,000. When isolated in free form it exists as an aggregate of approximately 330,000 molecular weight.[r12] It shares with receptors for other steroids certain functional domains in which there is a high degree of structural homology (Fig. 44.6.) Cortisol binds to the steroid-binding domain with an affinity of 20–40 nM, a value similar to the free cortisol concentration in plasma. Most synthetic glucocorticoids bind with similar or higher affinity, while aldosterone binds with slightly less affinity.

Most evidence now suggests that cortisol diffuses across the membrane of the target cell to reach its receptor in the cytoplasm. The sequence of events triggered by the binding of the steroid ligand is depicted in Figure 44.6. Binding of the steroid induces a conformational change in the receptor, causing the receptor to have a high binding affinity for DNA. In the course of activation of the receptor, the domain responsible for binding to DNA is unveiled and made available for binding to chromatin in the cell nucleus. The DNA-binding domain is responsible for the binding of the activated receptor to specific nucleotide sequences along the genome. These sequences are known as glucocorticoid response elements or GREs. The GREs located in various genes share common core sequences. These common sequences appear to be present, sometimes in multiple copies, near the promoter regions of genes known to be responsive to glucocorticoids.[r4,r12,9,10]

Once bound to the GRE of a specific gene, the activated receptor can regulate the rate of transcription of messenger RNA by altering the activity of the gene promoter. The promoter region, which is

Table 44.5 Actions of Adrenal Corticosteroids in Tissues Having Glucocorticoid or Mineralocorticoid Receptors

Tissue	Recepter Type	Predominant Biologic Effects
Liver	Glucocorticoid	Increased glycogen synthesis and storage Increased conversion of amino acids to glucose Increased glucose release
Striated Muscle	Glucocorticoid	Decreased synthesis of some Proteins Increased protein breakdown Increased amino acid release
Adipose Tissue	Glucocorticoid	Increased lipolytic response to catecholamines Increased fat stores (increased appetite)
Heart and Blood Vessels	Glucocorticoid	Increased pressor response to catecholamines Increased myocardial contractility Increased vascular tone
Bone and Connective Tissue	Glucocorticoid	Decreased synthesis of collagen Decreased synthesis of glycosaminoglycans non-collagen proteins Increased bone resorption Decrease bone deposition
Central Nervous System and Pituitary	Glucocorticoid	Decreased synthesis of CRH and ACTH Decreased synthesis of vasopression Increased secretion of growth hormone
	Mineralocorticoid	Decreased appetite for salt
Kidney	Glucocorticoid	Increased glomerular filtration and renal plasma flow Increased free water clearance Increased ammonia excretion (proximal tubule)
	Mineralocorticoid	Increased reabsorption of sodium (distal tubule) Increased potassium excretion (distal tubule) Increased excretion of calcium and magnesium Increased proton excretion (collecting duct)
Salivary and Sweat Glands	Mineralocorticoid	Decreased sodium content in sweat and saliva

the initial binding site for RNA polymerase, is usually located just upstream from the starting site for mRNA transcription. The GRE is considered to be one of a class of DNA regulatory elements called enhancers. Enhancers are capable of binding regulatory proteins, in this case glucocorticoid receptors, and controlling nearby promoters. The effects on transcription have been stimulatory in several carefully studied systems, but inhibitory effects are believed to prevail for other negatively regulated genes. The end-result of the interaction between the activated glucocorticoid receptor and the genome is increased (or decreased) accumulation of specific mRNAs within the target cell. Changes in these specific mRNAs lead to changes in the rate of synthesis of specific proteins that carry out the biologic actions of cortisol.

Many details of this currently accepted theory of steroid hormone action are yet to be understood. Some, but by no means all, of the functional proteins regulated by glucocorticoids are known. Some of these are known to be rate-limiting enzymes in important metabolic pathways. It is clear that gene regulation by cortisol involves more than binding to a glucocorticoid receptor and subsequent binding of the receptor to DNA. For example, levels of phosphoenol-pyruvatecarboxykinase, a critical enzyme in gluconeogenesis, are stimulated by cortisol in the kidney, but are inhibited in white adipose tissue, even though both cells have similar glucocorticoid receptors and DNA.[11] The role of the glucocorticoid receptor in the regulation of complex gene networks and in combination with other regulatory hormones or growth factors will continue to be actively explored.

The Mineralocorticoid Receptor

As with the glucocorticoid receptor, the gene for a human mineralocorticoid receptor has been cloned and sequenced.[12] This receptor of 984 amino acids has a steroid-binding domain that is 57 percent homologous and a DNA-binding domain 94 percent homologous with the corresponding domains of the human glucocorticoid receptor. In transfected cells, the mineralocorticoid receptor has an affinity for aldosterone of approximately 1 nM. In the kidney, autoradiographic studies with tritium-labeled aldosterone have demonstrated specific binding in the distal and collecting tubules.[13] Other corticosteroids with mineralocorticoid activity, such as corticosterone, deoxycorticosterone, and cortisol, are similar to aldosterone in affinity, but synthetic "pure" glucocorticoids such as dexamethasone show weaker binding.

As might be expected from the extensive homology of the DNA-binding domain, the human mineralocorticoid receptor is also capable of interacting with glucocorticoid response elements in the genome. It is not known whether there are distinct mineralocorticoid response elements that govern the transcription of mRNAs unique

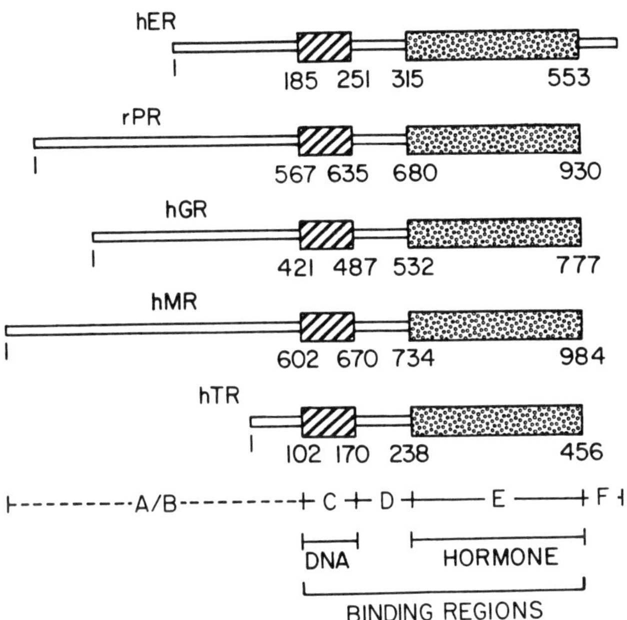

Figure 44.5 Structural Comparison of the Gene Family of Steroid Hormone Receptors. The amino acid sequences of the human estrogen receptor (hER), rodent progesterone receptor (rPR), human glucocorticoid receptor (hGR), human mineralocorticoid receptor (hMR), and human thyroid hormone receptor (hTR) have been deduced from their complimentary DNA sequences. The two highly conserved regions, representing the proposed DNA binding (region C) and hormone binding (region E) domains, are shown as shaded blocks. There is little or no homology when comparing other regions of the receptors (region A/B, region D, and region F.) The human glucocorticoid and mineralocorticoid receptors have 94% homology in region C and 57% homology in region E, but less than 15% homology in region A/B, which tends to be the immunogenic region of the receptor. Other members of the gene family include receptors for 1,25 dihydroxy vitamin D and retinoic acid (not shown.)

to the action of mineralocorticoids. Indeed, the connection between the actions of aldosterone at the cellular or tissue level and those at the level of the gene are still poorly understood.[r14,r15] Several proteins in kidney tubules, including citric acid cycle enzymes, Na^+-K^+ ATPase, and carbonic anhydrase have been reported to be influenced by aldosterone.

Another question about the physiologic significance of mineralocorticoid receptors relates to their distribution throughout the body, sometimes in tissues not recognized as being under mineralocorticoid control. For example, apparently identical receptors have been demonstrated not only in classic mineralocorticoid target tissues, such as kidney, but also in brain, pituitary, and heart. It has been proposed that the effective physiologic ligand for the mineralocorticoid receptor may depend on the tissue in which the receptor is located and the local concentration of free steroids available for binding. The relative concentrations of cortisol and aldosterone at various tissue sites may depend on the local activity of the enzyme 11β-hydroxysteroid dehydrogenase (11βHSD).[14] This enzyme inactivates cortisol by reversible dehydrogenation of the 11-hydroxyl group, forming cortisone, which lacks the ability to activate the mineralocorticoid receptor. Aldosterone is resistant to the action of 11βHSD. In tissues such as the kidney, where the enzyme is abundant, intracellular levels of biologically active cortisol are greatly reduced, thus preventing cortisol from competing effectively with aldosterone for the mineralocosticoid receptor. The colocalization of 11βHSD with corticosteroid receptors in the brain may be an important factor in determining whether the receptors are predominantely affected by cortisol or by aldosterone or other mineralocorticoids.

Homeostatic and Regulatory Functions of Adrenal Corticosteroids

It has been customary to designate the various in vivo effects of the corticosteroids as either "physiologic" or "pharmacologic", depending on the dose required to produce the effect. With increasing realization that essentially all corticoid activities are mediated by common receptors through similar mechanisms, this dichotomy may not be justified. Even activities such as anti-inflammatory effects that were thought to be limited to artificially high steroid concentrations can be demonstrated at physiologic concentrations if sensitive enough methods of detection are used. In physiologic terms, however, it is still useful to differentiate those effects that appear to be important for homeostasis under basal conditions from those that appear to be important under conditions of stress. In the latter situation endogenous glucocorticoid levels are normally much higher than in the basal state. This situation is similar to one in which high doses of glucocorticoids are administered to a patient to achieve anti-inflammatory effects. At low concentration, cortisol and aldosterone act in a number of different tissues to promote the maintenance of a constant internal environment. Among the processes dependent on adequate basal glucocorticoid levels are the maintenance of blood glucose, the regulation of energy metabolism during fasting and eating, the regulation of body water and sodium balance, and the feedback regulation of ACTH secretion. Most of these homeostatic processes depend on multiple hormones for their regulation. In some cases corticosteroids appear to play a "permissive" rather than a primary regulatory role. Some of the target tissues involved in the basal and regulatory activities of cortisol and aldosterone are listed in Table 44.5.

Effects on Energy Metabolism

Energy storage and utilization are broadly affected by the actions of glucocorticoids in concert with insulin, glucagon, and catecholamines.[r14] Insulin is the primary regulator of energy metabolism in most tissues, but cortisol is required to maintain adequate blood glucose levels during fasting. In the liver, glucocorticoids promote the formation of glucose from pyruvate or amino acids and promote the storage of energy

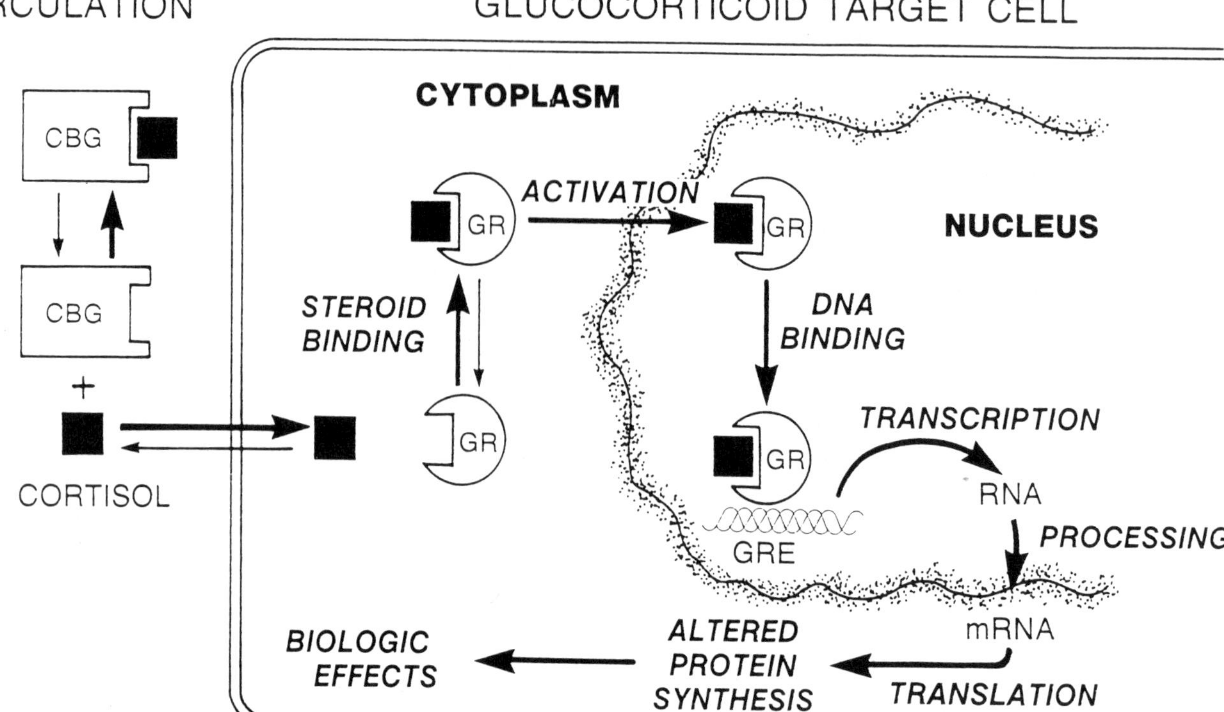

Figure 44.6 General mechanism of action of glucocorticoids through regulation of gene expression in the target cell. Cortisol circulates in plasma bound to the transport protein, corticosteroid binding globulin (CBG.) Unbound or free cortisol enters the target cell and binds to the glucocorticoid receptor (GR). The occupied receptor undergoes a conformational change that probably involves dimer formation with a second receptor (not shown) and exposure of a DNA binding domain capable of binding to specific genes having glucocorticoid response elements (GREs.) This process stimulates transcription of specific mRNAs that are translated to yield specific proteins. The binding of the active glucocorticoid receptor to a genre may also inhibit expression of the gene and result in reduced synthesis of specific proteins. Biologic effects are mediated by changes in the concentrations of the affected proteins.

as glycogen. In peripheral tissues, especially muscle, glucocorticoids act to decrease the utilization of glucose and to mobilize amino acids from the breakdown of protein. Amino acids are then carried to the liver, where they form the substrate for enhanced gluconeogenesis.

Some of these effects are probably due to the induction of new enzyme synthesis by glucocorticoids acting through the glucocorticoid receptor. For example, several liver enzymes mediating gluconeogenesis, such as phosphoenolpyruvate carboxykinase, and glucose-6-phosphatase, are increased within several hours after administration of cortisol to adrenalectomized animals. The abilities of glucagon and catecholamines to stimulate gluconeogenesis are enhanced by the presence of cortisol.

Other effects on energy metabolism are related to the inhibition of protein synthesis. In striated muscle as well as bone, adipose, and lymphoid tissues, glucocorticoids both decrease protein synthesis and enhance protein breakdown. There is an increase in plasma levels of alanine and branched chain amino acids available for gluconeogenesis.

In adipose tissue, glucocorticoids primarily enhance the lipolytic effects of catecholamines or cyclic AMP. Thus, mobilization of free fatty acids is increased. At the same time glucose utilization by both adipose tissue and muscle is inhibited. The resulting higher glucose levels lead to secondary hyperinsulinemia in the intact animal. Consequently, the net result of increased glucocorticoid levels is often an increase in total fat stores, because of the powerful effects of insulin in promoting triglyceride synthesis.

Effects on Salt and Water Metabolism

Electrolyte and fluid balance is regulated jointly by both glucocorticoids and mineralocorticoids. The most important effect mediated by mineralocorticoid receptors is in the collecting tubules of the renal cortex, where the reabsorption of sodium and the secretion of potassium and hydrogen ions are stimulated. These effects require mRNA and protein synthesis, although the precise identity of the proteins mediating the effect is not known. Under conditions of sodium depletion, aldosterone is normally stimulated through the renin-angiotensin system, leading to sodium retention by the kidney and a more positive body sodium balance. Hence, the ECF volume is expanded and maintained. The ability of aldosterone to stimulate potassium secretion is dependent on dietary sodium intake and the quantity of sodium delivered to the distal tubule, where the steroid acts. In the presence of adequate distal tubular sodium, aldosterone causes the reabsorption of large quantities of sodium, creating electronegativity within the tubular lumen and leading to the passive diffusion of potassium ion into the tubule to be excreted. In sodium-depleted states where little sodium is presented to the distal tubule for exchange, the kaliuretic effects of aldosterone are blunted. In contrast to potassium secretion, the hydrogen ion secretion induced by mineralocorticoids is independent of sodium reabsorption and occurs at a spatially distinct location in the outer portion of the medullary collecting duct.[r15] Mineralocorticoids decrease sodium excretion and increase potassium excretion by sweat and salivary glands, although these effects do not assume major homeostatic importance in humans.

Glucocorticoids are also required for maintenance of normal sodium and water balance, but their receptors mediate effects at other tissue sites distinct from those affected by aldosterone (Table 44.5). Glucocorticoids increase glomerular filtration and renal plasma flow. It is unclear whether these effects on renal hemodynamics are due to an increase in cardiac output or to a direct effect on the kidney. The result is an increase in the quantity of both sodium and water delivered to the distal renal tubule, and an increased capacity of the kidney to excrete both salt and water. Another important glucocorticoid effect on water balance is mediated through vasopressin, whose synthesis and secretion are inhibited by cortisol under basal conditions. In the absence of glucocorticoids, vasopressin levels rise, leading to excessive water retention by the distal collecting tubules. Even when aldosterone secretion is adequate, a deficiency of cortisol can lead to a dilutional hyponatremia due to the inability of the kidney to excrete a water load. Glucocorticoids also can increase the capacity of the kidney to excrete acid. This effect is not accomplished by decreasing the urinary pH, as is the case with mineralocorticoids, but by increasing the excretion of buffer as phosphate or ammonia. The effects of glucocorticoids on renal acid elimination are mediated by receptors in the proximal tubule, in contrast to those of mineralocorticoids, which are mediated in the distal collecting ducts.[15]

Circulatory and Hemodynamic Effects

Both glucocorticoids and mineralocorticoids are essential for the maintenance of a normal blood pressure and circulation. Mineralocorticoid actions are mediated indirectly through the regulation of sodium excretion by the kidney, as described above. When salt and water intake is sufficiently high, blood pressure and vascular volume may remain adequate even in the absence of aldosterone. Under conditions of dietary sodium restriction or of excessive salt and water loss by nonrenal routes (for example diarrhea or vomiting) increased levels of aldosterone are needed to promote renal sodium retention and adequate homeostasis.

Glucocorticoid effects on the cardiovascular system are more direct. In glucocorticoid-deficient states, there is typically hypotension with a reduced cardiac output and reduced vascular responsiveness to pressor stimuli.[r14] In this situation, the circulation may be adequate under resting or basal conditions, but stresses such as blood loss or infection can rapidly precipitate shock.

Direct glucocorticoid actions on the heart can increase the number and affinity of β-adrenergic receptors mediating the positive inotropic effects of catecholamines.[16] This is due to promoter sites on the β-adrenergic gene. Myocardial contractility is increased. Glucocorticoids are necessary for the maintenance of normal peripheral vascular tone, where a permissive effect on vasoconstriction mediated by catecholamines or angiotensin II is believed to be important. The mechanisms for this effect are not well understood. Part of the synergism between glucocorticoids and various physiologic vasoconstrictors may depend on the ability of glucocorticoids to inhibit the production of prostaglandins, particularly PGI_2. This prostaglandin is a potent vasodilator and the main product of arachidonic acid in peripheral vessels.[17]

Effects on Connective Tissue, Cartilage, and Growth

In addition to the general effects on energy metabolism described above, glucocorticoids have specific effects on the growth and function of skeletal and connective tissues. At higher levels, corticosteroids tend to have an inhibitory or catabolic effect on these tissues. At low basal levels, certain synthetic functions may be enhanced. Thus biphasic effects can be seen for a particular connective tissue cell type. Glucocorticoid receptors have been described in fibroblasts and osteoblasts, indicating that direct effects are likely. However, indirect effects, mediated through local cytokines and growth factors as well as traditional calciotropic hormones, are also important.

Glucocorticoids at high physiologic concentration have an inhibitory effect on both type I and type III collagen production by fibroblasts. They also inhibit glycosaminoglycan production. Thus, extracellular collagen and matrix formation is impaired by high-dose glucocorticoid therapy, and wound healing is slowed. Glucocorticoids inhibit the proliferative and chemotactic response of fibroblasts to various cytokines acting locally in the healing wound.[18]

The actions of cortisol on the synthesis of collagen have been studied in detail in isolated human fibroblasts.[19] Biosynthesis of type I collagen is a complex process involving transcription of two different procollagen genes, pro-A1 and pro-A2, processing of pre-mRNAs to the respective mRNAs, and translation of these into the corresponding prepro-A-collagen chains. The two types of procollagen chains are then modified in several post-translational steps to create a mature collagen molecule consisting of two A1 chains and one A2 chain coiled into a triple helix. Cortisol at physiologic concentration reduces cellular accumulations of mRNAs for both the pro-A1 and pro-a2 chains. This is not due to a decrease in gene transcription, but to an increase in the rate of degradation of the specific mRNAs. The effect may be mediated by a steroid-induced increase in ribonuclease activity.

In vivo administration of high-dose glucocorticoids to children causes a fall in serum levels of type I procollagen within 24 hours.[20] Chronic high-dose glucocorticoid therapy in children blocks linear growth, depending on the dose and interval of administration. The clinical impairment of cartilage, bone, and connective tissue growth correlates well with measurements of the inhibition of collagen synthesis, as seen by depressed serum levels of type I procollagen. A major mediator of linear growth in children is somatomedin C or insulin-like growth factor-I. Somatomedin C is a potent locally-acting mitogenic agent produced by liver, fibroblasts, and other peripheral tissues under the influence of growth hormone. Its action in causing normal growth of bone and cartilage is blocked by glucocorticoids. Clinical investigations of the mechanisms of the antagonistic effects of cortisol and growth hormone indicate that glucocorticoids do not significantly impair either growth hormone secretion or somatomedin production.[21] However, the cartilage growth-promoting activity of somatomedin assayed in the plasma of corticosteroid treated subjects is impaired. There is evidence that this may be due in part to a corticosteroid-induced suppression of the synthesis of somatomedin acting locally on skeletal cells.[22] It is likely that the antagonism between somatomedin and cortisol is also due to a direct effect on the chondrocyte that impairs its response to somatomedin and other mitogens.

Bone and Calcium Homeostasis

Therapeutic (supraphysiologic) doses of glucocorticoids continued for extended periods result in progressive bone loss. Yet, at physiologic levels, glucocorticoids may have beneficial effects on calcium metabolism and bone. Receptors for glucocorticoids have been identified in osteoblast-like bone cells, and may also be present in normal osteoblasts.[23] While high levels of glucocorticoids are associated with an overall increase in bone resorption and a decrease in bone formation, these effects are complex and dose-related. Short-term exposure of fetal rat bone to cortisol at low concentrations actually increases the production of collagen. Only later, or with higher doses, does there appear a dose-dependent suppression of the synthesis of type I and III collagen, as well as noncollagen protein.[r16] The enhancement of osteoblastic activity at low concentration may represent a physiologic effect of glucocorticoids in promoting bone cell differentiation and maturation.

In addition to collagen, mature osteoblasts characteristically synthesize osteocalcin and other noncollagen proteins. Osteocalcin synthesis is a useful marker of osteoblast activity because this protein is produced exclusively by osteoblasts and not by fibroblasts or precursors of differentiated bone cells.[r17] Serum osteocalcin concentrations show a diurnal variation, with a nadir corresponding to the usual peak of diurnal cortisol secretion. Single small doses of glucocorticoid given just before the peak in serum osteocalcin can reverse the rise.[24] Serum osteocalcin levels in subjects with chronic hypercortisolism are typically low. The osteocalcin gene is subject to control by both vitamin D and glucocorticoids. 1,25-dihydroxyvitamin D_3 binds to a receptor belonging to the same family as the glucocorticoid receptor. The activated vitamin D receptor binds to a DNA sequence in the promoter region of the gene, thus stimulating the transcription of osteocalcin mRNA. The cortisol receptor appears to interact with a separate DNA sequence to inhibit expression of the gene and block the promoting effects of vitamin D.[25]

Several of the effects of glucocorticoids on calcium homeostasis are indirect. With high doses there is a negative total body calcium balance. Serum calcium remains normal, while serum phosphorus tends to be reduced. The intestinal absorption of calcium, but not phosphorus, is decreased. Glucocorticoids have a direct suppressive effect on calcium transport in the gut, where they again oppose the actions of vitamin D. This effect is not due to alteration of the production of biologically active vitamin D metabolites, but may involve reduced synthesis of an intestinal calcium binding protein[26] and possibly inhibition of another gene controlled by vitamin D. Corticosteroids at high levels have more general depressive effects on intestinal function, including reduced sodium and iron transport and reduction in the height of intestinal villi.

Glucocorticoids promote increased urinary excretion of calcium and phosphorus. The phosphaturic effect is probably due largely to secondary hyperparathyroidism developing in response to the decrease in calcium influx from the gut. The characteristic hypercalciuria seen with glucocorticoid excess probably represents a direct glucocorticoid effect on the kidney. Conversely, glucocorticoid deficiency can cause impaired renal calcium clearance and predispose to hypercalcemia under conditions where the calcium flux from either gut or bone to blood is maintained. In contrast to parathyroid hormone, calcitonin secretion is usually suppressed under conditions where glucocorticoid levels are high.[r16] The mechanisms are unknown, but the combination of elevated parathyroid hormone and suppressed calcitonin levels probably accounts for the observed increase in bone resorption associated with high-dose corticosteroid therapy. Thus, the most important effects of high levels of glucocorticoids are the direct inhibition of bone formation and the indirect enhancement of bone resorption, both leading to progressive bone loss.

Suppression of Inflammation and the Immune Response

The high levels of endogenous glucocorticoids found during stress resemble the levels seen with high-dose glucocorticoid therapy of inflammatory or immune diseases. It now appears that many of the therapeutic effects of high-dose glucocorticoids used in treating various inflammatory diseases are also exerted by endogenous glucocorticoids at higher physiologic levels. Munck has proposed that endogenous glucocorticoids protect against stress by damping down normal defense reactions, preventing overshooting and damage due to the defense reactions themselves.[r5] Many of the therapeutic effects of glucocorticoids are exerted through modulation of the actions of humoral mediators of immunity and inflammation. Some of the more important effects are listed in Table 44.6. Consistent with a unified hypothesis of steroid action, these effects depend in most cases on the induction or inhibition of mRNA and protein synthesis by specific genes.

Distribution of Cells Mediating Immunity and Inflammation

The immune and inflammatory cells whose function is most affected by glucocorticoids are lymphocytes, macrophages, and neutrophils. Both the distribution and the function of these cells are altered. Glucocorticoids cause an increase in circulating neutrophilic leukocytes together with a decrease in circulating eosinophils, lymphocytes, and monocytes. In the first several hours after a large single dose of glucocorticoid to a normal human subject, both lymphocyte and monocyte counts fall in the blood as neutrophils rise. The numbers of circulating T-lymphocytes are reduced more than B-lymphocytes and helper T-cells more than suppressor T-cells. These acute effects are due to a redistribution of cells into extravascular compartments, rather than to cell death.[r18] The mechanisms of these effects on cell distribution in vivo are still unclear, but may involve steroid-induced changes in the properties of the cell surface. Within 24 hours after the discontinuation of high-dose glucocorticoid therapy, cell distribution tends to return to normal. The results of steroid-induced cell redistribution are probably most significant for neutrophil function. Glucocorticoids cause a decreased adherence of neutrophils to endothelial surfaces as well as an acute release of young neutrophils from the bone marrow. This results in an increase in the number of neutrophils in the

Table 44.6 Actions of Glucocorticoids on Immune and Inflammatory Responses

Cell or Tissue	Probable Primary Effects	Secondary Effects
T-lymphocytes	Decreased synthesis of γ-interferon	Decreased macrophage activity in killing tumor cells and removing opsonized cells. (MAF, FRAF)
		Decreased activity of natural killer cells
		Decreased production of macrophages and granulocytes from progenitor cells.
	Decreased synthesis of interleukin-2	Decreased proliferation of antigen-activated T cells (TCGF)
Macrophages Monocytes	Decreased synthesis of interleukin-1	Decreased T cell activation in response to antigens (LAF)
		Decreased pyrogenic response to inflammation (EP)
	Decreased response to migration inhibitory factor (MIF)	Decreased accumulation of macrophages at site of inflammation
B-Lymphocytes	Decreased interaction with T lymphocytes (T-helper)	Early activation in response to antigens inhibited
Neutrophils	Decreased adherance to endothelial cell surfaces	Increased circulating neutrophils and decrease tissue neutrophils
		Decreased release and activity of plasminogen activator and collagenase
		Decreased fibrinolysis, complement production and collagen destruction.
		Decreased tissue damage at inflammatory site
Diverse cell types	Decreased phospholipase A^2 activity and decreased arachidonic acid release	Decreased formation of prostaglandins and leukotrienes
	Decreased action of bradykinin and serotonin	Decreased vasodilatation and edema at inflammatory site
	Decreased release of histamine (basophils and mast cells)	Decreased immediate hypersensitivity response

circulation and a decrease in the tissue compartment. Thus, fewer neutrophils are available at sites of tissue injury to mediate the inflammatory process.[r18]

Glucocorticoids and the Immune Response

The immunosuppressive effects of the glucocorticoids may be detected at levels seen during physiologic stress as well as during high-dose corticosteroid therapy. Generally the effects on cellular immunity and delayed hypersensitivity are more marked than are those on humoral immunity. Some of the effects on cell-mediated immune responses are probably related to the changes in immune cell traffic and distribution, as noted above. More important, glucocorticoids can act directly on various kinds of immune cells to affect their function and their interactions with one another. At the cellular level many actions of the glucocorticoids appear to be mediated by a decrease in the synthesis of cytokines that act as critical intercellular signals in the normal immune response.

One of the pivotal direct effects of glucocorticoids on lymphocytes is an inhibition in the synthesis of *γ-interferon* or *immune interferon*.[r5] IFN-γ is a 146 amino acid protein normally produced by antigen-stimulated T-lymphocytes. As shown in Table 44.6, IFN-γ has several known functions and has been called by different names, depending on the system being studied. Macrophage activating factor (MF) and F γ-receptor activating factor activities pertain to the effects of immune interferon on macrophages. IFN-γ greatly stimulates the number of Fγ receptors for immunoglobulin on the surface of monocytes and macrophages. These receptors are involved in the recognition by macrophages of particulate antigens that have been opsonized by immunoglobulins, facilitating the clearance of immune complexes, bacteria, or antibody-tagged host cells. Fγ receptors may guide mononuclear phagocytes in the destruction of foreign cells, as well as their stimulation of immunoglobulin production and the release of inflammatory mediators.[27] In addition to the effects that depend on Fγ receptors, macrophages can be activated in the presence of immune interferon to lyse tumor cells in the absence of added antigens or antibodies. This experimental effect has been attributed to macrophage-activating factor, which is probably identical to IFN-γ. Other activities attributable to immune interferon in experimental systems include a mitogenic effect on the production of granulocytes and macrophages from immature progenitor cells or colony stimulating factor activity, and the stimulation of a T-cell subset having natural killer cell activity. Glucocorticoids thus may act to diminish the number of functional macrophages and natural killer cells.

A second T-cell derived protein whose synthesis is inhibited by glucocorticoids is interleukin-2 (IL-2). Human IL-2, also known as T-cell growth factor, is a protein of 153 amino acids that appears to provide a key signal for the proliferation of T-cells, once they have been exposed to an antigen.[46] IL-2 mediates the clonal expansion of T-lymphocytes that normally occurs after the antigen recognition phase of the normal immune response. The suppression of this process by glucocorticoids is important in explaining how glucocorticoids can suppress primary immune responses. The inhibition of T-cell proliferation in the clonal expansion phase may explain why corticosteroids are much more effective in suppressing an immune response when they are present early, rather than late, in the process.

Interleukin 1 production by macrophages can also be inhibited by glucocorticoids (Table 44.5). IL-1 is a macrophage protein of 12–15,000 molecular weight that has also been called lymphocyte activation factor or endogenous pyrogen.[6] An important role of IL-1 appears to be its stimulation of T-cells to produce IL-2. Glucocorticoid suppression of IL-1 production thus augments the direct effects of steroids on IL-2 production and the over-all suppression of immune responses mediated by T-cells. The suppression of endogenous pyrogen production is likely to explain the fever-suppressing effects of glucocorticoids in a variety of inflammatory disease states.

A second effect of glucocorticoids exerted on macrophages involves their tendency to congregate in increased numbers at a site of inflammation. Another cytokine, migration inhibition factor, is elaborated by lymphocytes at the inflammatory site and inhibits the movement of macrophages away from the site. Corticosteroids do not impair the generation of this factor but do inhibit its action on macrophages.[r18]

In contrast to effects on T-lymphocytes and macrophages, the direct effects of glucocorticoids on B-lymphocyte function are modest. High-dose corticosteroid therapy has little effect on over-all immunoglobulin levels or on the proliferation and function of B-cells once these cells are committed to production of antibody against a particular antigen. The earliest steps in B-cell activation, which depend on T-cell function, may be suppressed by corticosteroids. Thus, the antibody response to a new antigen may be suppressed if high levels of corticosteroids are present at the time of initial exposure to the antigen.[47]

Glucocorticoids and the Inflammatory Response

Glucocorticoids at high physiologic concentrations are capable of suppressing the inflammatory response, whether the initiating event is infection, physical or chemical injury, or an immune reaction. As in the case of the immune response, several types of cells and intercellular mediators are involved.

The glucocorticoid-induced redistribution of neutrophils mentioned above is undoubtedly important. Systemic administration of corticosteroids results in decreased numbers of leukocytes and monocytes appearing at sites of experimental tissue injury, as demonstrated by techniques such as the Rebuck skin window.[29] At the biochemical level, glucocorticoids inhibit either the production or actions of several humoral mediators of inflammation, as outlined in Table 44.6.

The prostaglandins, thromboxanes, and leukotrienes are all biologically active substances derived from fatty acids of the cell membrane in diverse tissues. The pharmacology of this group of compounds is described in detail in Chapter 9. The rate of formation of both prostaglandins and leukotrienes depends on the availability of free arachidonic acid, which acts as a common precursor to both groups of compounds. The glucocorticoids block the release of arachidonic acid from cellular phospholipids by inhibiting the activity of phospholipase A_2. The effects of glucocorticoids on this rate-limiting enzyme are not direct, but apparently are mediated by increased levels of a protein, lipocortin or macrocortin, that inhibits phospholipase A_2.[r20] A second effect of glucocorticoids in arachidonate metabolism is exerted through the activity of cyclo-oxygenase, leading to prostaglandin and thromboxane synthesis. The consequence is that glucocorticoids suppress the synthesis of cyclo-oxygenase by suppressing the formation of its specific mRNA. This probably occurs through regulation of the cyclo-oxygenase gene.[30] Thus, the generation of both prostaglandins and thromboxanes is further decreased. The thromboxanes generally cause thrombotic occlusion of small vessels in an area of inflammation. Prostaglandins of the E, F, and I series cause vasodilatation.

Perhaps the most important proinflammatory derivatives of arachidonic acid are the leukotrienes.[r21] Leukotriene B_4 promotes neutrophilic chemotaxis and adherence at the inflammatory site. Leukotrienes C_4 and D_4, also known as the slow-reacting substance of anaphylaxis, are produced by basophils and macrophages. These compounds cause bronchoconstriction, vasoconstriction, and increased vascular permeability, especially of venules. By inhibiting the formation of leukotrienes as well as prostaglandins, glucocorticoids can inhibit both the accumulation and activation of neutrophils and the formation of edema. Nonsteroidal anti-inflammatory drugs such as aspirin are less powerful than glucocorticoids because they reduce only the formation of prostaglandins, not leukotrienes.

Glucocorticoids inhibit either the generation or action of several other known mediators of inflammation (Table 44.6.) Some of these mediators are biogenic amines. The most important is histamine, which is released from mast cells in the early phase of inflammation. Serotonin, another biogenic amine, acts like histamine in causing local vasodilatation and increased capillary permeability. These vascular effects are reinforced by the action of bradykinin, a nonapeptide cleaved from circulating kininogen by kinin-forming enzymes (kallikreins) also activated during the early phase. Bradykinin, a vasodilator, also induces release of arachidonic acid, increasing the formation of prostaglandins and other arachidonic acid metabolites. It is likely that these mediators account for the cardinal signs of early inflammation—warmth, redness, pain, and edema.[r22]

Glucocorticoids decrease the release of histamine from mast cells and basophils under various experimental conditions and lower histamine levels in the blood if administered prior to an immediate hypersensitivity reaction. At high doses, corticosteroids administered to patients also suppress levels of bradykinin in inflamed tissues.[31] In experimental animals the prior administration of dexamethasone can block the development of foot-pad edema after local injection of both bradykinin and serotonin. This effect of dexamethasone is blocked by simultaneous administration of an inhibitor of mRNA synthesis (actinomycin D), suggesting that conventional glucocorticoid receptor mechanisms are involved.[32] The clinical observation that the early events of inflammation are most effectively blocked when corticoids are administered prior to the initial injury also coincides with a mechanism of gene modulation.

Table 44.7 Frequency of Undesirable Glucocorticoid Effects in Relation to Duration of Therapy

Early Effects (days/weeks)	
Common	*Sporadic*
Weight gain	Anaphylactoid reactions
Mood changes	Hypertriglyceridemia
Glucose intolerance	Peptic ulcers
Transient adrenal suppression	Acute pancreatitis
Later Effects (months/years)	
Common	*Sporadic*
Central obesity	Aseptic necrosis of bone
Cutaneous fragility	Cataracts
Myopathy	Glaucoma
Osteoporosis	Hypertension
Growth failure	Opportunistic infections
Prolonged adrenal suppression	

Later stages of the inflammatory response often involve the release of neutral proteases, such as plasminogen activator and collagenase, by a variety of participating cells. If the release of these enzymes is excessive or prolonged, extensive tissue destruction may result.[r23] Plasminogen activator, a serine protease produced by macrophages, converts plasminogen to plasmin and initiates fibrinolysis at the inflammatory site. Excessive plasminogen activator can lead to tissue damage and hemorrhage. Collagenase is one of several lysosomal enzymes, including elastase and cathepsins, released by macrophages, neutrophils, and other cells. These enzymes break down connective tissue, including collagen and cartilage. Glucocorticoids can markedly reduce the activity of plasminogen activator and collagenase released by these cell types, regardless of the initiating cause of inflammation.[r5,r23] The inhibition of plasminogen activator is through induction by glucocorticoids of a specific inhibitor of the enzyme. The production of the inhibitor is probably due to increased transcription of the gene for the inhibitor.[33]

Undesirable and Toxic Effects

Factors Determining Undesirable Effects

Most undesirable effects of corticosteroids are predictable from their known pharmacologic effects on various tissues. The likelihood of an undesirable effect is usually proportional to the dose of corticosteroid and the duration of time over which it is given. Untoward effects are rare when lower doses are used for physiologic replacement, but become increasingly common as the dose exceeds two or three times the daily replacement equivalent. Short-term therapy, even with very high doses of potent glucocorticoids, usually can be undertaken with little risk of serious consequences. However, the longer high doses are continued, the more inevitable are certain complications such as osteoporosis. Some untoward effects, including many of the physical changes of Cushing's syndrome, occur in virtually all patients given high doses of glucocorticoids over a prolonged period. Other less predictable effects, such as aseptic necrosis of bone or acute pancreatitis, seem to occur only in a small subset of treated patients either early or late during the course of therapy. The frequency and time relationships of a number of recognized effects are shown in Table 44.7.

Besides dose and duration of therapy, patient factors are also important in predicting therapeutic complications. Elderly patients tend to have an increased incidence of side-effects at lower doses because they are more likely to have pre-existing conditions such as glucose intolerance or muscle weakness that may be worsened by corticosteroids. Patients who are chronically ill or malnourished may tolerate glucocorticoids poorly because of decreased serum steroid-binding proteins and a proportionate increase in levels of active, unbound drug. Whenever corticosteroid therapy is chosen for an individual patient, the physician must carefully consider the balance of benefits and risks.

Complications and Their Management

Hypertension and Electrolyte Disorders

Salt and water retention, edema, hypertension, and hypokalemia are the expected untoward effects when high doses of mineralocorticoids are given. Hypertension, which occurs often with supraphysiologic doses of cortisone or hydrocortisone, is seldom a clinical problem with synthetic "pure" glucocorticoids. Prednisone and prednisolone seldom cause hypertension or fluid retention, although they may elevate the systolic blood pressure, especially in the elderly.[34] The relatively weak hypertensive side-effects of synthetic glucocorticoids may be mediated by mechanisms other than salt retention, including increased vasoconstrictor responsiveness.

Abnormalities in Glucose and Lipid Metabolism

Most patients treated with high-dose glucocorticoids will gain weight. Increased adipose tissue will be centrally deposited, producing a characteristic "moon face" and "buffalo hump." The basic alterations in energy metabolism have been discussed earlier. Increased gluconeogenesis and increased resistance to the glucose-lowering effects of insulin lead to a hyperinsulinemic state within hours of the initiation of glucocorticoid therapy in most subjects. Fasting hyperglycemia and overt diabetes mellitus occur only in subjects with pre-existing abnormalities in glucose tolerance and insulin reserve.[r24] Subjects who already have insulin-dependent diabetes ordinarily will require larger insulin doses to maintain glycemic control and to avoid ketoacidosis. Non–insulin-dependent diabetics may require insulin administration to maintain control while receiving glucocorticoids. Occasionally, patients with steroid-induced diabetes will also have marked hypertriglyceridemia.[r6,35] Impaired glucose regulation resulting from glucocorticoid therapy can usually be managed successfully with appropriate use of insulin or oral hypoglycemic drugs and is usually reversible, although recovery may require several months after steroids are withdrawn.[36]

Cutaneous and Connective Tissue Disorders

The inhibitory effects of glucocorticoids on the synthesis of collagen and other structural proteins can lead to thinning and fragility of the skin. Cutaneous problems occur in most patients treated with high-dose glucocorticoids over several months. Thinning of the dermal layer of skin and loss of supporting tissues surrounding small blood vessels leads to easy bruising and tearing of the skin. Poor healing of wounds can be a major problem in surgery, unless doses of corticosteroids can be reduced. Frequent bleeding from skin capillaries may occur with minimal trauma, causing purpura especially over the hands and forearms. The face may develop a plethoric appearance. These problems are more severe in elderly or debilitated patients, where the strength of connective tissues already is diminished.

Hair changes are also characteristic of long-term therapy. Unlike spontaneous Cushing's syndrome, iatrogenic Cushing's syndrome is not associated with excess adrenal androgens. Thus, true virilizing changes are not characteristic in treated women. Instead, high doses of glucocorticoids tend to produce an increase in downy hair on the sides of the face and an increase in dark hair between the lateral eyebrows and the temporal hairline. These changes, plus increased subcutaneous fat deposits in the face and neck, account for the undesirable changes in facial appearance that accompany prolonged glucocorticoid therapy.

Myopathy

Wasting and weakness of muscles, especially in the proximal muscles of the trunk and limbs, may occur in both spontaneous and iatrogenic Cushing's syndrome. Patients may complain of the insidious onset of weakness, may have progressive difficulty in climbing stairs, and finally may be unable to walk. Testing may reveal early difficulty in standing from a squatting position or in sitting up from a recumbent position. While the proximal muscles are most involved, a few patients show weakness of distal limb muscles as well. Muscles supplied by the cranial nerves are usually spared. Tendon reflexes, sensory modalities, and motor control of sphincters are normal.

Since steroid-induced myopathy may occur in patients having pre-existing connective tissue disorders, assessment of the principal cause of weakness may be difficult. Serum concentrations of enzymes derived from muscle, such as aldolase and creatinine kinase, are typically normal in steroid myopathy. Electromyographic findings are variable, but often show a myopathic pattern. Histopathologic studies of muscle biopsies have shown large aggregates of glycogen in subsarcolemmal sites, disarray and loss of myofibrils, and abnormalities in the distribution and structure of mitochondria.[37] Any glucocorticoid may be associated with myopathy, but alpha-fluorinated derivatives such as triamcinolone and dexamethasone have been particularly incriminated in a number of case reports.[37] The apparently greater tendency of these drugs to produce myopathy may be a result of the longer duration of their biologic effects in comparison with other glucocorticoids.

Steroid myopathy is reversible. Symptoms usually begin to improve within days or weeks after the glucocorticoid is withdrawn or its dose reduced. Concurrent administration of estrogens, androgens, or anabolic steroids is not helpful.

Steroid-induced Osteoporosis

Bone loss and pathologic fractures are among the most common and distressing side-effects of corticosteroid therapy. The incidence of atraumatic fractures in patients on long-term treatment has been estimated at 30 to 50 percent.[8] Trabecular bone is more affected than cortical bone. Therefore, the lumbar vertebrae, femoral neck, or distal radius, all having a preponderance of trabecular bone, are most weakened. Glucocorticoid doses exceeding 7.5 mg of prednisone per day are associated with diminished bone density, and the extent of bone loss increases with the cumulative dose of glucocorticoid. Short-term longitudinal studies have suggested that glucocorticoid-induced bone loss is most rapid in the first six months of therapy. If glucocorticoid administration is continued, the rate of bone loss tends to slow and to approach the rate seen in untreated subjects after one to two years.[r16] Bone loss leads to increased fractures only after a critically low mineral density is reached. Thus, patients who already have relatively low bone densities at the outset of steroid therapy will be more likely to suffer fractures. Older patients, especially postmenopausal women, are at highest risk.

The pathogenesis of steroid-induced osteoporosis reflects the basic effects of glucocorticoids on bone cells and calcium homeostasis discussed earlier. Decreased GI calcium absorption and increased urinary calcium excretion tend to promote a negative calcium balance. A compensatory secondary hyperparathyroidism is associated with increased bone mineral resorption. At the same time there is inhibition of the synthesis of collagen and other bone matrix proteins through direct effects of glucocorticoids on osteoblasts.[r7] The diminished bone density associated with a long course of glucocorticoid therapy usually persists after glucocorticoid administration is stopped. Thus, most strategies to ameliorate the problem are directed at slowing the rate of loss during ongoing steroid therapy. Lowering the dose of glucocorticoid to the minimum amount required and shortening the course of therapy as much as possible will help to minimize the problem. Assurance of an adequate dietary calcium intake of at least 1000 mg per day and a vitamin D intake of at least 400 units per day is prudent in all patients. Thiazide diuretics may be given to reduce urinary calcium excretion if hypercalciuria is present. Estrogen replacement should be given to postmenopausal women receiving glucocorticoids unless estrogens are contraindicated by other medical problems. Other agents that decrease bone resorption have been used to a limited extent in attempts to reduce steroid-induced bone loss. Short-term studies suggest that salmon calcitonin[38] and aminohydroxy-propylidene bisphosphonate[39] may help to preserve bone mass. More studies are needed to assess the usefulness of these agents.

Growth Failure

The predominant skeletal side-effect of prolonged high-dose glucocorticoid therapy in children is growth failure. The effects of glucocorticoids on growth hormone, insulin-like growth factors, and bone or cartilage cells have been discussed in an earlier section. Clinically, the degree of growth inhibition is roughly proportional to the dose used. The arrest of linear growth is accompanied by continuing weight gain, so that on a typical growth chart height will be retarded relative to both chronologic age and weight. Glucocorticoids delay epiphyseal closure as well as growth. Some amount of "catch-up growth" usually occurs if therapy is stopped or the dose reduced. Nevertheless, the extent of postglucocorticoid growth acceleration is often insufficient to restore the treated child to normal height. Intermittent high doses of glucocorticoids are less disruptive of growth than continuous therapy, and growth can be sustained in many cases if single larger doses can be given on alternate days.[40]

Change in Mental Status

Neuropsychiatric side-effects were recognized in the early years of corticosteroid therapy, with a reported incidence ranging from 4 to 36 percent.[65] These effects vary considerably in severity, ranging from slight mood changes, most often euphoria, to manic-depressive or schizophrenic psychoses, and suicidal tendencies. Some writers have suggested that a psychosis occurring during steroid treatment reflects an exaggeration of a pre-existing personality disorder. However, prospective surveillance of general hospital inpatients indicates that acute psychiatric reactions are relatively common in steroid-treated subjects without a prior history of neuropsychiatric disease. In a study by the Boston Collaborative Drug Surveillance Program, the probability of an acute reaction depended on the steroid dose, occurring in less than 2 percent of patients receiving 40 mg of prednisone per day or less, but in 18 percent of patients receiving more than 80 mg per day.[41] Remission of psychiatric symptoms generally followed reduction in the dose of prednisone.

Less is known about the longer-term psychiatric effects of chronic low-dose steroid administration, or whether permanent changes in mental status can occur. The biologic basis for glucocorticoid effects on mental status is also incompletely understood. There is evidence that high physiologic concentrations of glucocorticoids can impair the capacity of neurons to withstand coincident insults, such as ischemia or toxins. The hippocampus, which plays important roles in both cognitive and neuroendocrine function, is particularly sensitive to glucocorticoid-enhanced experimental injury.[42] Short-term administration of glucocorticoids to normal subjects can lead to subtle defects in memory and cognitive function by psychometric testing, even though most subjects do not complain of difficulty with memory or concentration.[43]

Infections

The multiple effects of high-dose glucocorticoids in suppressing host defenses lead to an increased incidence of infections in steroid-treated patients. As with other side-effects, increased susceptibility to infection tends to parallel glucocorticoid dose, duration of therapy, and the biologic half-life of the steroid being used.[r26] Because the steroid-induced defect in host defenses is broad, one cannot predict the kind of microorganism that will cause a complicating infection. However, steroid-treated patients are particularly likely to have problems with the infections shown in Table 44.8. Similar kinds of opportunistic infections, including *Pneumocystitis carinii* pneumonia, aspergillosis, nocardiosis, and cryptococcosis, are seen in patients with spontaneous Cushing's syndrome.[44] The incidence of infectious complications is decreased when alternate-day steroid therapy is used.

Most bacterial infections in steroid-treated patients will respond to appropriate antibiotics. Some opportunistic infections such as cryptococcal meningitis or *Pneumocystitis carinii* pneumonia tend to relapse as long as steroids are continued and will require long-term antibiotic maintenance. The possibility that inactive tuberculosis will reactivate during corticosteroid administration has been of particular concern. Patients receiving 15 mg or more of prednisone per day usually lose reactivity to intermediate strength tuberculin skin testing two to four weeks after therapy has begun. Therefore, it is best to assess tuberculin reactivity within the first week of therapy. Patients with initially positive tuberculin skin tests, but normal chest radiographs, do not appear to develop active tuberculosis on moderate doses of glucocorticoids.[45] However, patients with abnormal radiographs consistent with inactive pulmonary tuberculosis should be treated with antituberculous drugs for as long as corticosteroids are continued.

Other Sporadic Effects

A number of other serious complications may occur in a small minority of patients.

Table 44.8 Infections Occurring with Increased Frequency and Severity in Patients Treated with Glucocorticoids (ref)

Bacterial	Tuberculosis, staphylococcal, Listerial, Gram-negative organisms (especially proteus and pseudomonas)
Viral	Varicella-Herpes Zoster, Herpes Simplex, Vaccinia, Variola, Cytomegalovirus
Fungal	Candidal, Cryptococcal, Aspergillus, Nocardial
Parasitic	Toxoplasmosis, Pneumocystosis, Malaria, Amebic, Strongyloidiasis

Anaphylactoid reactions are rare but have been associated with IV administration of glucocorticoids.[46]

Peptic ulcer disease and GI hemorrhage are weakly associated with glucocorticoid therapy.[47] The combination of corticosteroids with NSAIDs causes a much higher risk than the use of corticosteroids alone.[74] The incidence of ulcers appears to vary directly with steroid dosage and may be an early or late complication. The added risk of corticosteroids alone, though significant, is small. Thus, prophylaxis with antacids or H2-receptor blockers is not indicated routinely in all patients who are receiving corticosteroids.

Acute pancreatitis is a rare but serious complication not clearly related to the duration or dose of corticosteroid used. Corticosteroid therapy may mask the symptoms of pancreatitis, making its clinical recognition more difficult. The mechanism by which glucocorticoids induce pancreatitis in man is unknown. In some cases an associated hypertriglyceridemia may contribute.[r6]

Aseptic necrosis of the femoral head is another uncommon but extremely debilitating complication, most often seen in patients who have received high doses of corticosteroids for more than three months.[49] Patients with concurrent hyperuricemia, alcoholism, hyperlipidemia, or polycythemia, who also receive corticosteroids, are at the highest risk. The most favored theory to explain this complication involves the occurrence of multiple fat microemboli that lodge in the subchondral end arterioles, ultimately causing the death of bone cells. This may explain why aseptic necrosis is bilateral in 40 percent of cases. Affected patients typically complain of hip pain and stiffness and later evolve characteristic radiographic changes. Once ischemic necrosis has occurred, a femoral head prosthesis offers the best possibility for restoring a normal gait.

Ocular effects, particularly *increased intraocular pressure,* are seen most commonly with topical corticosteroids applied to the eye, but also may occur with systemic therapy. The risk of glaucoma is highest in individuals with myopia or diabetes.[r27] The proposed mechanism involves increased production of aqueous humor and increased resistance to outflow through the trabecular meshwork in the drainage angle of the anterior chamber. Increased intraocular pressure usually subsides with cessation of steroid therapy. A small number of patients on long-term therapy will develop posterior subcapsular cataracts.[r27] For this reason regular ophthalmologic examinations should be recommended. A few patients, usually children or young women, will develop evidence of increased intracranial pressure, manifested by headache and papilledema, while their steroid dosage is being reduced. A temporary increase in dosage and more gradual reduction often will relieve this problem.[r27]

Pituitary-Adrenal Insufficiency with Glucocorticoid Withdrawal

High doses of glucocorticoids will predictably suppress endogenous secretion of both ACTH and cortisol in normal subjects. The degree and duration of suppression depends on the dose and duration of therapy.

For example, a three-week course of prednisolone at a dose of 20 mg twice a day will result in a reduction in basal serum levels of both ACTH and cortisol for up to three days after the drug is discontinued.[50] The responsiveness of the adrenals to a test done of exogenous ACTH is suppressed after the first 24 hours of the beginning of such short-term therapy, but usually recovers within a few days after its cessation. Abnormalities in other tests of the pituitary-adrenal axis, such as the response of ACTH and cortisol to hypoglycemic stress[51] or to CRH administration,[52] may show a similar or slightly longer period of post-treatment suppression. In contrast, patients receiving continuous high doses of corticosteroids for more than a year may require several months off corticosteroids before basal levels of cortisol and ACTH become normal.[53] Presumably, a defective adrenal response to stress may persist even longer. The concern in managing such patients is that stress may precipitate acute adrenal insufficiency if endogenous secretion of cortisol cannot be raised.

Pharmacokinetics

Role of Pharmacokinetic Behavior in Glucocorticoid Drug Effects

The biologic effect of a given dose of a corticosteroid depends not only on its affinity for the receptor (pharmacodynamics) but on its distribution in the body and its rate of metabolic breakdown (pharmacokinetics). Table 44.3 compares the receptor affinity and plasma half-life for a number of commonly used corticosteroids. The over-all biologic effect of the most active compounds is enhanced not only by a high receptor affinity but by a longer persistence of the compound in tissues. It is important to note that the biologic half-life for each corticosteroid in Table 44.3 greatly exceeds its plasma half-life. This property is inherent in the way corticosteroids act. Once the expression of a gene is modified by the presence of an activated steroid receptor, and once mRNA and protein synthesis have been altered, those changes will persist for hours or even days after the steroid has disappeared from the blood.

One consequence of this property of extended action is that seemingly small differences in pharmacokinetics can be magnified into large differences in the duration and extent of a given biologic effect. A good example of such magnification is seen in the comparison of the effects of a short-acting glucocorticoid, such as hydrocortisone, with a long-acting glucocorticoid, such as dexamethasone. According to the estimates of relative potency in Table 44.3, dexamethasone is about 30 times more potent than hydrocortisone. However, most published estimates of relative potency are based on observations in which both drugs are administered frequently so as to maintain a steady state. When doses are given less frequently, the differences in potency become much greater, favoring the drug with the longer biologic half-life. If an effect such as the suppression of endogenous adrenal cortical function is measured at varying intervals after a single oral dose of each glucocorticoid, the relative potencies are as shown in Table 44.9. While dexamethasone is approximately 17 times more potent than hydrocortisone when the responses are extrapolated to zero time, it is 154 times more potent at 14 hours.[54] Prednisone, having an intermediate biologic half-life, is nearly equivalent to hydrocortisone at zero time but five times more potent at 14 hours. Since most clinical dosing schedules involve

Table 44.9 Relative Potencies of Three Glucocorticoids in Suppressing Endogeneous Glucocorticoid Production When Given as a Single Oral Dose

	Potency Relative to Hydrocortisone Time After Dose		
	0 hr	8 hr	14 hr
Hydrocortisone	1	1	1
Prednisone	1.05	3	5.2
Dexamethasone	17	52	154

Estimates from Meikle and Tyler, Am J Med 1977, *63*:200–207.

intermittent administration in which a steady state of drug effect is not achieved, differences in the pharmacokinetic behavior of various synthetic glucocorticoids is of great clinical importance. These differences arise from variations in several pharmacokinetic parameters including bioavailability, distribution, and clearance. Some representative estimates of these parameters for commonly used glucocorticoids are summarized in Table 44.10.

Bioavailability

Oral preparations are most often used for systemic corticosteroid therapy because they are well absorbed from the GI tract by passive diffusion. After oral hydrocortisone administration, peak plasma levels occur at about one hour, and the extent of absorption ranges from 45 to 80 percent.[r8] Hydrocortisone administered as a retention enema is absorbed nearly as well as by the oral route. Prednisolone and dexamethasone are at least as well absorbed orally as hydrocortisone. Because of the requirement for conversion to active metabolites in the liver, the bioavailability of cortisone and prednisone is slightly less than for hydrocortisone and prednisolone. After an oral dose of cortisone acetate, peak plasma levels of the active metabolite, hydrocortisone, occur at one to two hours.[r8] Other glucocorticoids including methylprednisolone, betamethasone, and triamcinolone are systemically active by the oral route, although their pharmacokinetics are generally less well characterized. Parenteral formulations of the corticosteroids are designed either for IV use, where bioavailability approaches 100 percent, or for depot administration, where absorption into the systemic circulation is slow and often limited.

Distribution and Transport

The corticosteroids are lipophilic compounds that readily penetrate cell membranes and distribute freely in the intracellular as well as extracellular space. Cortisol and prednisolone both bind primarily in plasma to a high-affinity glycoprotein known as corticosteroid-binding globulin or CBG, but can secondarily also bind to albumin. At physiologic concentrations, approximately 75 percent of circulating cortisol will be bound to CBG, 15 percent to albumin, and 5–10 percent will be free. The free fraction is believed to be most capable of penetrating cells and combining with glucocorticoid receptors. At supraphysiologic concentrations of cortisol, the binding capacity

Table 44.10 Representative Pharmacokinetic Parameters for Glucocorticoids in Normal Adults

Drug	Plasma Clearance (ml/min)	Volume of Distribution (liters)	Plasma Half Life (hr)	Oral Bioavailability (fraction)	Bound Fraction in Plasma	Relative Oral Potency
Hydrocortisone	362	21	1.3	0.58	0.90	1.0
Prednisolone	111	24	2.7	0.90	0.90	4.0
Methylprednisolone	266	61	2.8	NA	0.50	5.0
Dexamethasone	247	63	3.5	0.78	0.23	30
Betamethasone	148	65	5.1	NA	0.38	30

Values are from Gustavson and Benet. Pharmacokinetics of natural and synthetic glucocorticoids. In *The Adrenal Cortex*. London: Butterworth, 1985, p. 248. Relative oral potencies are from Table 46.1.
NA = data not available.

of CBG is exceeded, so that the proportion of free, biologically active steroid increases.

In addition to simple diffusion, it is possible that the entry of cortisol into cells is mediated in part by the binding of CBG to target cell membranes. Specific high-affinity cell membrane binding sites have been described.[55] Prednisolone and cortisol compete for the same binding sites on CBG, and one may displace the other when added to plasma. Prednisone has a much lower binding affinity for CBG than prednisolone. There is only limited information available about the macromolecular binding of other synthetic glucocorticoids in plasma. In general, the more potent compounds appear to have a low affinity for CBG and to bind less extensively to plasma proteins, predominantly albumin.[r8] In comparison to cortisol and prednisolone, methylprednisolone and dexamethasone have higher circulating fractions of free drug and larger apparent volumes of distribution, as shown in Table 44.10.

Metabolism and Clearance

The rate at which corticosteroids are metabolized and thus inactivated is an important determinant of their over-all biologic potency. For the natural glucocorticoid cortisol, the most important inactivating step is normally A ring-reduction to form tetrahydrocortisol. Further reduction of the keto group at C-20 may occur, yielding cortol. Conjugation with glucuronic acid renders these inactive metabolites more water-soluble, so that they are excreted in the urine as 17-hydroxycorticosteroids. Synthetic modifications in the A ring, the B ring, or the AB ring angle decrease the ability of enzymes in the liver to reduce the A ring. For example, the metabolism of prednisolone, with its C1-2 double bond, and of dexamethasone and betamethasone with their additional 9-α-fluoro substitutions, is slowed relative to hydrocortisone. In these cases, degradative pathways other than A ring reduction become more important. The relative rates of metabolism of commonly used glucocorticoids are best appreciated by comparing the representative clearances shown in Table 44.10. Note that the plasma half-life is a function not only of metabolic clearance, but of the apparent volume of distribution. Those compounds with longer half-lives in plasma and more sustained biologic effects are those that distribute into a larger space as well as those that are metabolized and cleared more slowly.

Patient Factors and Diseases Affecting Pharmacokinetics

A large number of clinically encountered conditions may alter the biologic effects of corticosteroid drugs. With few exceptions, these recognized factors are exerted through alteration in one or more of the pharmacokinetic parameters discussed above. Variations in absorption, elimination, and compliance can lead to wide differences in drug effects among individuals. In some cases, evaluation of blood levels of administered corticosteroids may be worthwhile.[56] While glucocorticoid resistance due to genetically determined alteration in the glucocorticoid receptor is well characterized[r28,57] and of considerable interest, it is uncommon. Pharmacodynamic resistance based on acquired receptor defects or down-regulation is theoretically possible and may eventually be recognized when glucocorticoid receptor dynamics can be observed in clinical situations.

Age and Pregnancy

In general, clearance is similar in children and adults when normalized for body surface area.[r8] Clearance may decrease slightly in older women. Glucocorticoids diffuse freely across the placenta and, when measured, have shown significant concentrations in fetal compartments, together with suppression of fetal cortisol after maternal administration. Only minute quantities of glucocorticoids are found in breast milk when nursing women are given prednisone or prednisolone.[r8]

Liver Disease

Severe hepatocellular disease can lead to impaired conversion of prednisone to prednisolone in some patients. Therefore, many clinicians prefer to use hydrocortisone or prednisolone in preference to their 11-keto derivatives in patients with advanced liver failure. Plasma half-lives of cortisol may be prolonged in some patients, presumably because of reduced rates of metabolic inactivation. The hypoalbuminemia seen in many patients with chronic liver disease would be expected to lead to a higher unbound drug fraction, potentially increasing the biologic and toxic effects. There appears to be a positive correlation between hypoalbuminemia, hyperbilirubinemia, the unbound fraction of drug, and the likelihood of glucocorticoid side-effects in patients with chronic active hepatitis who are treated with prednisolone.[58]

Kidney Disease

The kidney is also a site of steroid metabolism, though less important than the liver. Most studies examining metabolic clearance rates of glucocorticoids in patients with renal disease have found insignificant effects.[r8] Patients undergoing active hemodialysis may show an increased clearance of drug via the dialysate and thus require an adjustment of steroid dose.

Other Diseases

Absorption of oral corticosteroids is not appreciably altered in patients with ulcerative colitis, Crohn's disease, or celiac disease.

Rectally administered corticosteroids, often used for treating ulcerative colitis, are as well absorbed from the diseased as from the normal colon. Patients with severely impaired GI motility or ileus do not absorb oral corticosteroids reliably and should be treated with parenteral preparations. Hypothyroidism and hyperthyroidism are associated with an increase and a decrease, respectively, in the plasma half-life of cortisol.[59] Treatment of a hypothyroid patient with thyroid hormone ordinarily causes an increased endogenous secretion of cortisol as normal serum cortisol levels are maintained. When adrenal reserve is limited, as it is in some patients with hypopituitarism or long-standing severe primary hypothyroidism, treatment of hypothyroidism may require glucocorticoid replacement as well.

Interactions with Other Drugs

Several drugs including phenytoin, carbamazepine, phenobarbital, and rifampin can increase the level of microsomal oxidation in the liver and promote the accelerated inactivation of corticosteroids by alternative oxidative pathways such as 6-beta-hydroxylation.[58] When such drugs are initiated, a previously established dosage schedule of corticosteroids may be rendered ineffective unless the dose of corticosteroid is increased. In patients with unrecognized Addison's disease or hypopituitarism, enzyme-inducing drugs can precipitate acute adrenal insufficiency. They may also confound the interpretation of standardized diagnostic tests for Cushing's syndrome by enhancing the metabolism of dexamethasone and hence reducing its suppressive effects on endogenous cortisol secretion. Estrogens and oral contraceptives affect the plasma binding of cortisol and prednisolone by increasing the hepatic synthesis of CBG. The clearance and volume of distribution of these corticosteroids is decreased and half-life is increased in women taking oral contraceptives. Measured plasma levels of cortisol are increased.[60] Patients receiving concurrent estrogen and corticosteroid therapy should be monitored carefully for possible side-effects. Reduced doses of hydrocortisone or prednisolone may be required.

Preparations and Doses of Corticosteroids for Therapeutic Use

Available Formulations

The clinician may choose from a large number of commercially available corticosteroid preparations, some of which are listed in Table 44.11. These preparations may be divided according to whether they are suitable for oral, parenteral, or topical use. The rate of absorption of parenteral formulations after IM injection varies widely depending on the solubility of the steroid derivative. Those listed as suitable for IV use are rapidly absorbed, while those denoted as suspensions are absorbed slowly from an IM or intralesional site. The IV preparations generally are soluble esters, such as hydrocortisone hemisuccinate or dexamethasone phosphate, in which systemic bioavailability is essentially 100 percent. These soluble preparations are also rapidly and efficiently absorbed when given IM.

Depot preparations such as cortisone acetate are slowly absorbed over two or three days after IM administration, with peak plasma levels much lower than those achieved by comparable oral doses. Formulations designed specifically for intrasynovial or intralesional injection, such as methylprednisolone acetate or triamcinolone acetonide, are poorly soluble and poorly absorbed. Hence their actions may be confined largely to an affected region of the body such as a joint space, with reduced or negligible systemic effects. Topical formulations are designed to concentrate the action of the corticosteroid at the site wherever it is applied, usually as a cream or lotion applied to the skin or mucous membranes. Some absorption of topical preparations always occurs, and there may be systemic effects such as suppression of adrenal function. Absorption from the skin is increased where the steroid preparation is applied to larger areas under occlusive dressings. Systemic absorption of corticosteroids applied as aerosols or solutions to the nasal mucosa, bronchial tree, or conjunctival sac may be high.

Choosing the Appropriate Dose and Formulation

In spite of the bewildering array of corticosteroid products on the market, a small number of preparations will meet most indications for which corticosteroids are given. The therapeutic purpose must first be clearly determined before a rational choice of formulation and dose can be made. The clinical treatment plan should include criteria for monitoring whether the corticosteroid is having its intended effects and, if large doses are being used, for monitoring adverse effects. The most unfortunate side-effects are those occurring in patients whose corticosteroid therapy is continued in spite of a lack of evidence for significant clinical benefit. The specific indications for corticosteroids and therapeutic goals involved in individual diseases are discussed in detail in textbooks dealing with those diseases. While other textbooks should be consulted for disease-related details, the pharmacologic principles underlying the major categories of therapy hold true whatever the disease. The body of clinical information dealing with the use of corticosteroids as anti-inflammatory or immunosuppressant agents is highly empirical.

Chronic Adrenal Insufficiency

In most patients with primary adrenal failure there is a deficiency of both cortisol and aldosterone. Thus, replacement with both glucocorticoids and mineralcorticoids is needed. For chronic maintenance, the natural corticosteroid hydrocortisone (cortisol) is usually given orally in a dose of 20 to 30 mg per day in adults or 15–20 mg/sq meter in children. In an attempt to recreate the natural diurnal rhythm, two-thirds of the

Table 44.11 Preparations of Adrenocorticosteroids

Generic Name (Trade Names)	Oral Forms	Injectable Forms	Other Forms
Beclomethasone dipropionate (Beclovent, Vanceril, others)	—	—	OI: 42 μg/dose TA
Betamethasone (Celestone)	0.6-mg tablets 0.6-mg/5ml syrup	—	—
Betamethasome sodium phosphate (Celestine)	—	IV, IM solution 4 mg/ml	—
Cortisone acetate (Cortone acetate)	5–25-mg tablets	IM suspension 25–50 mg/ml	Suspension also for IL, IA
Dexamethasone (Decadron, others)	0.25–6-mg tablets 0.5-mg/5 ml elixir	— —	— —
Dexamethasone acetate (Decadron LA)	—	IM suspension 8–16 mg/ml	Suspension also for IL, IA
Dexamethasone sodium phosphate (Decadron phosphate, others)	—	IV, IM solution 4–24 mg/ml	TA: 0.1% O: 0.05, 0.1% NA: 100 μg/dose
Fludrocortisone acetate (Florinef acetate)	0.1-mg tablets	—	—
Flunisoslide (Aerobid, Nasalide)	—	—	OI: 250 μg/dose N: 25 μg/dose
Hydrocortisone (Cortef, Hdyrocortone, others)	5–20-mg tablets	IM suspension 25, 50 mg/ml	TA: 0.25–2.5% Enema: 100 mg Otic soln: 1%
Hydrocortisone acetate (Hydrocortone acetate)	—	1A, 1L suspension 25, 50 mg/ml	TA: 0.5–1% Suppositories: 25 mg Rectal foam: 90 mg
Hydrocortisone cypionate	2-mg/ml susp.	—	—
Hydrocortisone sodium phosphate (Hydrocortone phosphate)	—	IV, IM 50 mg/ml	
Hydrocortisone sodium succinate (Solu-Cortef)	—	IV, IM powder for injection 100–1000 mg	—
Methylprednisolone (Medrol)	2–32-mg tablets	—	—
Methylprednisolone acetate (Depo-Medrol, Medrol acetate)	—	IA, IL, IM suspension 20–80 mg/ml	TA: 0.25–1% Enema: 40 mg
Methylprednislone sodium succinate (A-methapred, Solu-Medrol)	—	IV, IM, powder for injection 40–2000 mg	—
Paramethasone acetate (Haldrone)	2-mg tablets	—	—
Prednisolone (Delta-Cortef)	5-mg tablets 3-mgl/ml syrup	—	—
Prednisolone acetate (Key-Pred, Predcor, Others)	—	IA, IL, IM suspension 25–50 mg/ml	0.12–1%

continued

Table 44.11 *Continued*

Generic Name (Trade Names)	**Oral Forms**	**Injectable Forms**	**Other Forms**
Prednisolone sodium phosphate (Hydeltrasol, Pediapred, others)	5-mg/ml solution	IA, IL, IM solution 20 mg/ml	O: 0.125–1%
Prednisolone tebutate (Hydeltra T.B.A., others)	—	IA, IL suspension 20 mg/ml	—
Prednisone (Deltasone, others)	1–50-mg tablets 1, 5-mg/ml solution 1-mg/ml syrup	—	—
Triamcinolone (Aristocort, Kenacort)	1–16-mg tablets	—	—
Triamcinolone acetonide (Kenalog, others)	—	IA, IL, IM Suspension 3, 10, 40 mg/ml	TA: 0.025–0.5% OI: 100 μ/dose
Triamcinolone diacetate (Aristocort, Kenacort diacetate, others)	2, 4-mg/5 ml syrup	IA, IL, IM suspension 25, 40 mg/ml	—
Triamcinolone hexacetonide (Aristospan)	—	IA, IL suspension 5, 20 mg/ml	—

Preparations For Topical Use Only

Generic Name (Trade Names)	**Generic Name** (Trade Names)
Aclometasone dipropionate (Aclovate)	**Flumethasone pivalate (Locacorten)**
Amcinonide (Cyclocort)	**Fluocinolone acetonide (Fluonid, Synalar)**
Clobetasol propionate (Temovate)	**Fluocinonide (Lidex)**
Clocortolone pivalate (Cloderm)	**Flurandrenolide (Cordran)**
Desonide (Desowen, Tridesilon)	**Halcinonide (Halog)**
Desoximetasone (Topicort)	**Hydrocortisone butyrate (Locoid)**
Diflorasone diacetate (Florone, Maxiflor)	**Hydrocortisone valerate (Westcort)**
Diflucortolone valerate (Nerisone)	**Medrysone ophthalomic (HMS Liquifilm)**
	Mometasone furoate (Elocon)

Abbreviation:
IA = intrarticular; IL = intralesional; IM = intramuscular
IV = intravenous; NA = nasal aerosol; O = ophthalmic or otic;
OI = oral inhalation;
TA = topical application (sprays, creams lotions, ointments)

total dose may be administered in the morning and one-third in the evening. The equivalent dose of cortisone is 25 to 37.5 mg per day. Both hydrocortisone and cortisone acetate at these dosages have modest salt-retaining effects. However, most patients will require an additional mineralocorticoid to maintain normal sodium and potassium balance. The drug of choice for this purpose is fludrocortisone, given orally in a dose ranging from 0.05 to 0.2 mg per day. Synthetic glucocorticoids such as prednisone may also be used in replacement regimens, but concurrent administration of a mineralocorticoid becomes even more essential. Dexamethasone, because of its long duration of action, does not permit a restoration of the natural diurnal rhythm of ACTH as do the shorter-acting glucocorticoids.[61] This disadvantage may be of minor concern in adults. However, in children the greater tendency of long-acting glucocorticoids to suppress growth argues in favor of choosing the shorter-acting compounds. The maintenance dose of hydrocortisone or cortisone is usually adjusted based on careful observation of clinical signs and symptoms, not on laboratory tests. Maintenance of normal weight, energy, and sense of well-being indicate that an adequate dose is being given. The hyperpigmentation associated with Addison's disease will typically diminish, although plasma ACTH levels will often remain mildly elevated. Excessive replacement doses of glucocorticoids are accompanied by the subtle onset of signs of Cushing's syndrome, especially weight gain and bruising of the skin.

The maintenance requirement of fludrocortisone will vary inversely with dietary salt intake. Adjustments should be made by regular monitoring of supine and upright blood pressure as well as serum electrolytes. Undertreatment is associated with postural hypotension and hyperkalemia, while overtreatment is associated with the development of hypertension and edema. The patient with underlying essential hypertension is likely to require either lower doses of supplemental fludrocortisone or none.

Patients with secondary adrenal insufficiency should be treated with glucocorticoids in the same way as patients with primary adrenal disease, except that they usually do not require additional mineralocorticoids. This is more likely to be the case when hydrocortisone or cortisone is selected for glucocorticoid replacement. It is important to educate all patients with chronic insufficiency about their need to maintain adequate glucocorticoid replacement by parenteral administration whenever oral administration is not feasible. Patients should be advised to increase their usual oral dosage of glucocorticoid by two- or threefold during intercurrent minor illnesses and to contact their physicians immediately if they begin to vomit or if they note other symptoms of acute adrenal insufficiency. Family members should be made aware of the absolute need for maintaining adequate glucocorticoid therapy under all circumstances. Patients should also wear appropriate identification in the form of a necklace or bracelet identifying their need for glucocorticoids in the event of medical emergencies.

Acute Adrenal Insufficiency

Acute adrenal insufficiency usually occurs under conditions of stress when the patient's need for glucocorticoids greatly exceeds the supply. Most individuals developing acute insufficiency will have a known history of chronic adrenal disease or of iatrogenic adrenal suppression, but some will present with the features of adrenal crisis as the first manifestation of adrenal insufficiency. The clinical picture is one of volume depletion and vascular collapse accompanied by metabolic abnormalities, which may include hyperkalemia, acidosis, and hypoglycemia. Immediate high-dose glucocorticoid therapy should be given in any patient in whom the diagnosis of adrenal insufficiency is suspected or likely. Initially the IV administration of a soluble glucocorticoid such as hydrocortisone hemisuccinate, 100 mg every six hours, is combined with the infusion of normal saline and glucose to restore intravascular volume. Provided that adequate water and electrolytes are given, specific mineralocorticoid replacement is not required. Once the patient has responded and the factors precipitating the stress have been controlled, the dose of IV glucocorticoid may be tapered over several days before oral maintenance therapy is resumed. Treatment with an oral mineralocorticoid may also be initiated, if required.

The same principles of therapy are applicable when the precipitating stressful event is planned, as in elective surgery for a patient with chronic adrenal insufficiency. On the day before surgery the patient should be given two or three times his normal steroid replacement dose. On the day of surgery, hydrocortisone 50–100 mg is given IV every 4–6 hours while fluid and electrolyte status is monitored carefully. As the patient recovers from surgery, steroid doses may be tapered back to oral maintenance levels over several days.

Selective Aldosterone Deficiency

Patients may suffer from a relative deficiency of mineralcorticoids in several situations where glucocorticoid production is adequate. Hyporeninemic hypoaldosteronism or primary renin deficiency is relatively common, especially in elderly diabetic individuals, and may lead to hypoaldosteronism as a result of decreased activity of the renin-angiotensin system. Inherited disorders of aldosterone biosynthesis are rare causes of selective mineralocorticoid deficiency. More commonly encountered are drugs that can suppress the production of renin (β-blockers, NSAIDs) angiotension II (converting enzyme inhibitors), or aldosterone (heparin).

The most significant clinical problem in patients with aldosterone deficiency is hyperkalemia. At serum potassium levels exceeding 6 mEq per liter, the increased risk of serious cardiac arrhythmias requires vigorous measures such as the administration of IV saline and potassium-wasting diuretics or the oral or rectal administration of potassium-absorbing resins. Drugs blocking the activity of the renin-angiotension system should be stopped. Chronic therapy of selective aldosterone deficiency may be provided with oral fludrocortisone, 0.1 to 0.3 mg per day. A reasonable therapeutic goal is to control the serum potassium at a level not exceeding 5.5 to 6 mEq per liter while avoiding hypertension, edema, and pulmonary congestion due to excessive salt and water retention. This may be a delicate balancing act in the patients in which hyporeninemic hypoaldosteronism usually occurs, since they frequently have underlying cardiovascular and renal disease.

Congenital Adrenal Hyperplasia

The congenital adrenal hyperplasias are a family of inherited deficiencies in steroidogenesis involving deficiencies of specific enzymes necessary for cortisol production. The recognized forms are summarized in Table 44.12. The most common inherited deficiency is of 21-hydroxylase followed by 11-beta hydroxylase and 3-beta hydroxysteroid dehydrogenase. These disorders may cause a deficiency of cortisol, aldosterone, or both, and may thus present in infants and children with problems common to those of acute adrenal insufficiency. In addition there is a characteristic overproduction of the corticosteroid precursors prior to the deficient enzyme. In 21-hydroxylase deficiency and 3-beta hydroxysteroid dehydrogenase deficiency, these precursors are weak androgens. In 11-beta hydroxylase deficiency, they are mineralcorticoids. Depending on which precursors predominate, the clinical effects may involve virilization, precocious puberty, or hypertension, as shown in Table 44.11. The

Table 44.12 Features of the Congenital Adrenal Hyperplasias Relating to Cortiosteroid Replacement Therapy

Enzyme Deficiency	Corticosteroid Deficiency	Corticosteroids in Excess	Replacement Needs
21-hydroxylase (severe-salt losing)	Cortisol Aldosterone	17-OH progesterone Adrenal androgens	Hydrocortisone Fludrocortisone
21-hydroxylase (milder forms)	Cortisol or None	Same as in severe syndrome	Hydrocortisone or other glucocorticoids
11-β hydroxylase	Cortisol	Desoxycorticosterone Adrenal androgens	Hydrocortisone or other glucocorticoids
3-β hydroxysteroid dehydrogenase	Cortisol Androstenedione Testosterone	Dehydroepiandro sterone	Cortisol Testosterone (males only)

goal of corticosteroid replacement therapy in patients with congenital adrenal hyperplasia is twofold: to assure an adequate supply of glucocorticoids and mineralcorticoids; and to suppress the endogenous overproduction of deleterious corticosteroid precursors.

The choices of corticosteroids for treating the various forms of congenital adrenal hyperplasia are summarized briefly in Table 44.12. It is desirable to monitor the effectiveness of therapy by measuring one or more of the precursors that are characteristically overproduced. Undertreatment of these syndromes with replacement glucocorticoids will fail to suppress the biologic effects of the unwanted precursors. Overtreatment will produce the unwanted features of Cushing's syndrome, including growth suppression in children. For these reasons, most patients will be controlled best on short-acting glucocorticoids at doses approximating the normal daily production rate of cortisol. The therapeutic issues involved in managing both children and adults with congenital adrenal hyperplasia prenatal diagnosis and treatment are discussed in recent reviews.[r29,62]

Corticosteroids for the Suppression of Nonendocrine Diseases

The vast majority of corticosteroid therapy today is given in an empirical attempt to control one of the allergic, inflammatory, or neoplastic conditions listed in Table 44.4. In all cases the therapeutic benefit in these diseases is the result of a glucocorticoid effect, usually at doses exceeding those required for physiologic replacement. Textbooks and original articles dealing with each disease should be consulted for detailed information and opinion about specific glucocorticoid treatment regimens. Whatever the disease may be, certain principles should guide the clinician who wishes to provide the potential benefits of corticosteroid therapy while limiting the serious side-effects.

Defining the Therapeutic Goals

The decision to use corticosteroids should be made when a presumptive diagnosis has been made and when available information suggests a reasonable possibility of benefit. In each patient the potential benefits should be judged likely to outweigh the risks. The clinician should clearly identify the criteria that will be used to determine whether corticosteroids are having a beneficial effect. At least some of the selected criteria should be objective or quantifiable. Examples might include reduction in the serum calcium in the patient with suspected sarcoidosis, reduction in urinary protein excretion and improvement in creatinine clearance in the patient with nephritis due to systemic lupus, or improvements in spirometry or arterial blood gases in the patient with obstructive lung disease. Criteria based on subjective parameters such as the sense of well-being or even reduced pain can be misleading because of the tendency of corticosteroids to produce euphoria in many individuals. If objective evidence of a positive therapeutic response is lacking after an appropriate trial period, it is usually in the patient's best interest to discontinue therapy.

Minimizing Undesirable Effects

In many situations corticosteroids are best used as second-or third-line drugs rather than as initial therapy. This is the case when other modes of therapy with fewer side-effects are likely to be effective. An example is in the management of rheumatoid arthritis, where NSAIDs should be given a full trial before turning to corticosteroids or other more hazardous drugs. In other situations the need for long-term corticosteroid administration at high dosage may be reduced by using steroids in conjunction with a nonsteroidal drug having complementary effects. The use of intermittent corticosteroid therapy together with cyclosporine or other immunosuppressants to prevent transplant rejections is an example.

Short-term intensive therapy is often effective and safe. Initially, large doses may be required to control the disease, but after improvement has occurred it may be possible to taper and stop corticosteroid therapy quickly. After a desired therapeutic response the physician should test the need to continue steroids and should lower the dose to the minimum required to maintain essential benefits. An example is the use of short courses of high-dose corticosteroids to manage acute exacerbations of chronic asthma. In between the more severe attacks, patients may be maintained satisfactorily without steroids or on very low doses.

Short- or intermediate-acting forms of corticosteroids are preferable to long-acting forms for chronic maintenance. This is because side-effects are decreased when glucocorticoid effects are not continuously present. Many diseases can be controlled with intermittent dosing regimens once an initial response is obtained. In terms of side-effects, giving 40 mg of prednisone as a single large dose once a day is better than giving it in divided doses. Giving 80 mg on an every other day treatment regimen is even better if adequate control of the disease can still be maintained.[r30] Alternate-day steroids may be effective maintenance therapy in certain forms of nephrotic syndrome, ulcerative colitis, chronic dermatitis, rheumatoid arthritis, and other arthritic disorders. Before attempting to convert a patient to an alternate-day regimen, specific literature about the patient's condition should be reviewed. Some conditions, such as giant cell arteritis, may not be effectively controlled unless drug effects are maintained by more frequent dosage schedules.[63]

Topical or regional corticosteroid therapy is often preferable. In situations where topical or regional therapy is effective, the side-effects are usually fewer than for equivalent doses of systemic corticosteroids. For example, chronic symptomatic asthma may be effectively controlled with aerosolized beclomethasone at doses causing relatively fewer systemic side-effects than orally administered corticosteroids, which may then be reserved for use during more severe acute attacks.

Withdrawal of Glucocorticoids

The recognized effects of chronic glucocorticoid therapy have focused much interest on the various problems associated with glucocorticoid withdrawal.[2] Symptoms during the withdrawal period may be due to recrudescence of the underlying disease that was being controlled with corticosteroids, to clear-cut adrenal insufficiency, or both. Often patients may have subjective withdrawal symptoms, such as nausea, lethargy, weakness, and arthralgia, without objective or laboratory evidence of true adrenal insufficiency. Such symptoms may improve when the corticosteroid dosage is again raised to a supraphysiologic level. While these patients may have a form of drug dependence, the biologic mechanisms are unclear.[2]

In practice, the greatest difficulties in withdrawal are encountered when the underlying inflammatory or immune disease is still present. Disease activity may increase notably when corticosteroids are reduced to a dosage that is still well above that required for physiologic replacement. In that case, the lowering must be done very slowly over a number of weeks or months, and a dose equivalent to physiologic replacement may be difficult to reach. Some patients will remain controlled when the dose is gradually lowered only on alternate days, allowing a transition to an alternate-day treatment regimen. If it is possible to make such a transition, the side-effects will be less even if corticosteroids cannot be discontinued entirely.

In patients whose underlying inflammatory process has resolved or is in stable remission, the corticosteroid dose may be reduced more rapidly to a physiologic replacement equivalent. The rate of reduction beyond this point will then depend on whether there has been long-term pituitary-adrenal suppression. Pituitary-adrenal recovery can still occur while a patient is maintained on a once-daily replacement dose of a short-acting corticosteroid such as hydrocortisone. Measurement of the endogenous plasma cortisol level in the morning before the daily dose is administered can provide laboratory evidence of endogenous adrenal function if there is doubt. Plasma cortisol levels exceeding 10 μg/dL (275 nmol/L) usually indicate that cortisol production is adequate to meet basal needs, though not necessarily adequate to meet conditions of stress. In patients who have successfully discontinued corticosteroid therapy under basal conditions it is usually advisable to provide temporary "stress" coverage with additional glucocorticoids for problems such as major infections, trauma, or surgery. Although a normal endogenous cortisol response to ACTH or insulin-induced hypoglycemia may predict recovery of normal adrenal responsiveness to stress, these tests are not required in the majority of patients. They are most useful in distinguishing the patient with true pituitary-adrenal insufficiency from the "steroid-dependent" patient who has withdrawal symptoms and apparently normal endogenous adrenal function.[2]

Corticotropin Releasing Hormone

Chemistry and Biologic Effects

Corticotropin releasing factor was the first hypothalamic releasing factor to be demonstrated experimentally, but one of the last to be chemically characterized.[94] In 1981 a 41-amino acid peptide with the structure shown in Figure 44.6 was isolated from sheep hypothalamic tissue.[3] This peptide, termed CRF-41 or simply CRH, is the most potent substance known in releasing ACTH from the anterior pituitary. The structure of human CRH, as illustrated in Figure 44.6 is very similar to that of ovine CRH.

The CRH present in the hypothalamus is synthesized primarily in nerve cells in the paraventricular nucleus, a site where vasopressin is also synthesized. It now appears that CRH and vasopressin are produced by separate neurons, although they are released together by certain stressful stimuli. Once released from axons terminating in the median eminence, CRH enters the hypophyseal portal circulation and is carried to the cells of the anterior pituitary, where it acts on specific high-affinity receptors on corticotropin-producing cells. Ovine CRH increases cyclic AMP levels in cultured anterior pituitary cells as it brings about increased ACTH release, suggesting that cAMP serves as a second messenger in the action of CRH. Glucocorticoids can act directly on corticotropin-producing cells to block both the cAMP accumulation and ACTH release triggered by CRH.[64]

Vasopressin can act synergistically with CRH in stimulating ACTH release in vitro, and is present in hypophyseal portal blood in concentrations sufficient for producing an in vivo response in rats and monkeys.[r31] It is likely that vasopressin acts as an enhancer for CRH action in a number of physiologic situations involving stress. It is also possible that other hypothalamic peptides not yet characterized can contribute as CRFs in the over-all stress response. ACTH response to stress is effectively blocked by passive immunization of rats with anti-CRF-41 antibodies and partially blocked with anti-vasopressin antibodies.[65]

Peptides crossreacting to antisera against CRF-41 have been found in many areas of the brain other than the hypothalamus, although hypothalamic levels are highest. The role of CRF-like peptides in other parts of the nervous system is conjectural, but these CRFs appear to act as neurotransmitters, perhaps subserving responses to stress. CRF immunoreactive peptides are also found in the normal GI tract and in certain tumors, including gangliocytomas, pheochromocytomas, bronchial carcinoids, medullary carcinomas of the thyroid, and carcinomas of the prostate.[r32] In a few cases such tumors have been associated with Cushing's syndrome.

Therapeutic Uses and Limitations

Synthetic ovine CRH is currently available only for experimental use in human subjects. It shows promise as a diagnostic agent for the differential diagnosis of Cushing's syndrome and for the testing of pituitary ACTH reserve in cases of suspected pituitary disease. It is likely that it eventually will be approved for these uses by drug regulatory agencies. In theory, CRH might also be used to restore ACTH and cortisol secretion in situations where the pituitary gland is intact but hypothalamic function is deficient. The main limitations of CRH relate to its cost and the requirement for repeated parenteral administration to achieve sustained effects. These limitations should not preclude its use as a diagnostic agent.

Clinical Effects of CRH

Most clinical studies in humans have been carried out with synthetic ovine CRH rather than human CRH. The ovine hormone has a longer plasma half-life than human CRH in patients, probably because it is degraded more slowly by proteolytic enzymes. Hence it is more potent.[r32] In normal subjects a maximal rise in plasma ACTH occurs after short IV infusions of 1 to 10 μg/kg. Peak ACTH levels occur at 15 to 30 minutes, followed by peak cortisol levels at 60 minutes. Enhanced cortisol secretion may persist for several hours. Pretreatment with dexamethasone blocks both the ACTH and cortisol responses. Side-effects associated with CRH administration may include facial flushing and hypotension, particularly with doses exceeding 100 μg. Serious side-effects are unusual at doses not exceeding 1 μg/kg.[66]

The most promising diagnostic application of CRH at this time is in differentiating the several possible causes of spontaneous Cushing's syndrome. Compared with normal subjects, the majority of patients with ACTH-producing pituitary tumors (Cushing's disease) show an enhanced ACTH and cortisol response to a test dose of CRH. In contrast, patients having ACTH overproduction by nonpituitary tumors (ectopic ACTH syndrome) show a reduced or absent response. When ACTH and cortisol are measured serially in peripheral blood, the CRH test has a predictive value comparable to the dexamethasone suppression test in defining the cause of Cushing's syndrome.[r33] If blood from the petrosal sinuses, representing pituitary venous drainage, is sampled, the diagnostic accuracy of the test is increased.[67]

Adrenocorticotropin and Related Peptides

Chemistry

The pituitary gland was recognized as the source of adrenocorticotropin and melanotropic hormones in the early part of this century.[r34] Bioassays based on both corticotropic and melanotropic effects of pituitary extracts enabled Bell and coworkers to determine the primary structure of porcine ACTH in 1954. Subsequently the sequences of ACTH from humans and other mammalian and nonmammalian species were found to be remarkably similar, as reviewed in detail by Hofmann.[r13] The sequence of human ACTH is shown in Figure 44.7 The sequences of other species are identical in the first 24 amino acids and differ only in the identity of residues 25 to 39. $ACTH_{1-24}$ has the full biologic activity of native $ACTH_{1-39}$.

In the course of purifying ACTH from pituitary extracts, several other bioactive peptides with structural similarities to ACTH were isolated by several investigators. These peptides included α-MSH, which overlapped with residues 1–14 of ACTH, and β-lipotropin, a 91-amino acid peptide with melanocyte-stimulating activity. Finally, a peptide with potent opiate-like activity and corresponding to residues 61–91 of β-lipotropin was found and eventually designated β-endorphin, implying "endogenous morphine." This peptide contained within its sequence the structure of another potent opioid peptide, methionine enkephalin, that had been isolated from several areas of the brain.

The reason for these relationships became clearer when more was learned about the biosynthesis of ACTH. Pulse labeling experiments with cultured ACTH-secreting tumor cells showed that the earliest biosynthetic products with ACTH immunoreactivity had molecular weights of approximately 28–30 kiloDaltons, far larger than the molecular weight of $ACTH_{1-39}$.[r9] The labeled product proved

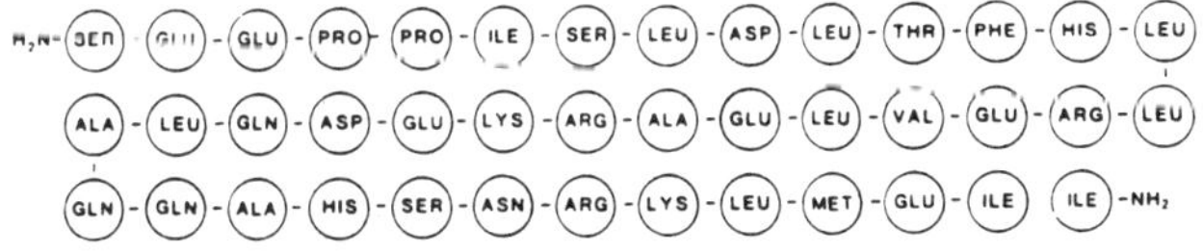

Human Corticotropin Releasing Hormone

H-SER-TYR-SER-[MET-GLU-HIS-PHE-ARG-TRP-GLY]-LYS-PRO-VAL-
1 2 3 4 5 6 7 8 9 10 11 12 13

GLY-LYS-LYS-ARG-ARG-PRO-VAL-LYS-VAL-TYR-PRO-ASN-GLY-
14 15 16 17 18 19 20 21 22 23 24 25 26

ALA-GLU-ASP-GLU-SER-ALA-GLU-ALA-PHE-PRO-LEU-GLU-PHE-OH
27 28 29 30 31 32 33 34 35 36 37 38 39

Human Adrenocorticotropin

Figure 44.7 Primary Structure of Corticotropin Releasing Hormone and Adrenocorticotropin

to be a high molecular weight precursor, not only for ACTH, but for β-LPH (lipotropic hormone), β-endorphin, and several peptides with melanocyte-stimulating activity. The pathways by which the precursor, termed pro-opiomelanocortin or POMC, is converted by proteolytic enzymes into smaller peptide products are shown in Figure 44.8. Cleavages generally occur between pairs of basic amino acids in the precursor peptides. Cleavage may vary, depending on whether the corticotropin-producing cells are located in the anterior or intermediate lobe of the pituitary. In the intermediate lobe, ACTH is processed further by cleavage into two smaller peptides, corticotropin-like intermediate peptide (CLIP) and α-MSH. The latter peptide is acetylated on its amino terminus and amidated at its carboxyl terminus. The enzymes necessary for these transformations are present only in intermediate lobe tissue. In human adults, where the intermediate lobe of the pituitary is only a vestigial structure, CLIP and α-MSH are not produced.

The major secretory products of the adult pituitary are predominantly ACTH and β-lipotropin. These peptides are normally secreted in equimolar amounts in response to CRH or a variety of physiologic stimuli. Smaller peptides derived from β-lipotropin, including β-endorphin, may also be measured in the circulation.[r34] The physiologic function of POMC peptides other than ACTH is still unclear.

Therapeutic Uses and Limitations

Adrenocorticotropin (ACTH, corticotropin) is the only peptide in the POMC family currently approved for clinical use. Corticotropin may be given to stimulate the adrenal cortex, and thereby increase endogenous levels of natural corticosteroids. The predominant therapeutic benefit is a result of increased cortisol production. In virtually all clinical situations, corticotropin administration is inferior to the direct administration of a selected glucocorticoid as a means of providing systemic glucocorticoid effects. Because the magnitude of the adrenal response varies among individuals and under differing clinical conditions, one cannot be confident that a desired concentration of cortisol will be achieved with a given dose of ACTH. If corticotropin treatment is continued, there will also be substantial increases in the production of adrenal androgens, such as androstenedione, and mineralocorticoids, such as deoxycorticosterone. Thus, virilization, salt retention, and hypertension are all more likely during therapy with ACTH than with pure glucocorticoids. Greater expense and the inconvenience of repeated injections are further drawbacks to ACTH therapy. For all of these reasons, corticotropin is seldom used today as a therapeutic agent.

The main use of corticotropin is in the diagnosis of adrenal disease. Given over the short term, it may be used to assess adrenal reserve in the production of cortisol and other corticosteroids. By making serial measurements of the plasma or urine concentrations of corticosteroids after a test dose of corticotropin, it is possible to make useful inferences about the clinical status of the adrenal-pituitary axis. Other POMC peptides may have future clinical utility through their effects on pain perception or behavior. β-endorphin, for example, is among the most potent analgesics known.

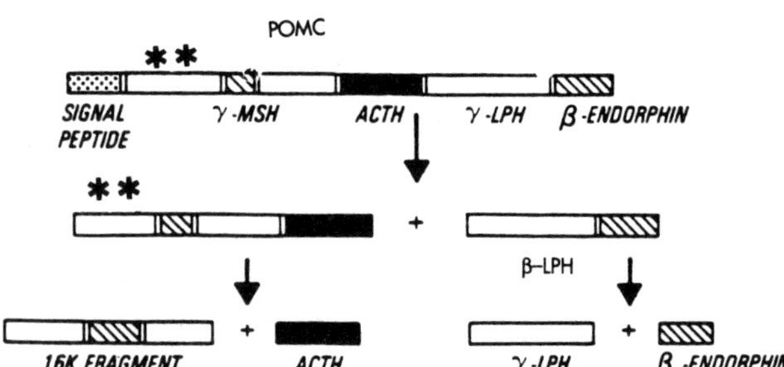

Figure 44.8 Biosynthesis of the ACTH-related peptides. The diagram indicates post translational processing in the anterior pituitary beginning with the prohormone pro-opiomelanocortin (POMC.) Asterisks indicate sites of attachment of carbohydrate side chains to the glycoprotein. In the intermediate lobe of the pituitary the 16K fragment is cleaved further to release α-MSH.

Corticotropin Effects

The primary action of ACTH is on the adrenal gland. It also shares melanocyte-stimulating and weak lipolytic activity with other active POMC peptides. Receptors for ACTH are present on cells in all three histologic layers of the adrenal cortex. The adrenal ACTH receptor is linked to adenylyl cyclase and employs cyclic AMP as a second messenger for many of its intracellular effects.

Like several other peptide hormone receptors, the ACTH receptor interacts first with the hormone ligand on the external cell surface. The activated hormone-receptor complex then interacts with a guanine nucleotide binding protein Gs, which consists of two subunits, (α) and (β).[r35] The binding of the hormone-receptor complex to Gs promotes the binding of GTP to α and the dissociation of β. The activated α subunit, α-GTP, then interacts with the inactive catalytic component of adenylyl cyclase to enhance its affinity for the substrate Mg ATP. As long as it remains in its activated state, this enzyme converts ATP to cAMP. In addition to the requirement for GTP, the coupling process requires Ca^{++}.[68] Shortened peptide analogues of natural ACTH, such as $ACTH_{6-39}$, are capable of high-affinity binding to the ACTH receptor without activating Gs and adenylate cyclase.[69] Such analogues can function as competitive inhibitors of ACTH under in vitro conditions.

The most critical effect of ACTH on steroidogenesis is a rapid increase in the rate of conversion of cholesterol to pregnenolone, as noted earlier in the discussion of steroid biosynthesis. Cyclic AMP and calcium ion can mimic the short-term effects of ACTH on steroidogenesis in adrenal cells. The steps by which increased concentrations of cAMP lead to increased steroidogenesis are incompletely understood. It is likely that cAMP activates one or more protein kinases that phosphorylate other regulatory proteins, but the identity of such proteins in the adrenal cortex is not known. There is evidence for ACTH-induced labile protein factors that may stimulate either the binding of cholesterol to the side-chain cleaving enzyme or the transfer of cholesterol to the inner mitochondrial membrane where cleavage occurs.[r3] ACTH also increases the activity of cholesterol esterase, possibly through a cAMP-dependent phosphorylation. This increases the critical concentration of free cholesterol available for conversion to pregnenolone by side-chain cleavage. It is also unclear how ACTH exerts its trophic effects on the adrenal. These effects are unlikely to involve the cAMP mechanism, and may require the action of growth factors other than ACTH itself. Other POMC peptides cosecreted with ACTH are candidates for a physiologic role in promoting adrenal growth. The amino terminal fragment of POMC, designated as a 16 K fragment in Figure 44.8, can stimulate adrenal cell DNA synthesis in vitro and mitosis in vivo.[r34]

The IV administration of corticotropin to a normal human subject causes a release of cortisol within two or three minutes. The peak cortisol response occurs within 30 to 60 minutes. As shown in Figure 44.9, peak plasma cortisol levels usually exceed 20 mg/dl. Subjects with primary adrenal insufficiency fail to respond to exogenous corticotropin, while those with secondary adrenal insufficiency show an incomplete response (Fig. 44.9). These differences in ability to respond rapidly to a test dose of ACTH are the basis of a rapid corticotropin stimulation test for the diagnosis of adrenal insufficiency.[70]

If corticotropin is administered repeatedly, there is also an increase in the secretion of adrenal androgens. Increases in adrenal protein, RNA, and DNA content begin to occur within 48 hours and progress through seven days of treatment. The over-all size of the gland can double. Patients with secondary adrenal insufficiency who show a subnormal cortisol response to the initial dose of corticotropin usually will show a normal response by the third day of continued administration. Patients with primary insufficiency, however, will fail to respond regardless of the duration of treatment.

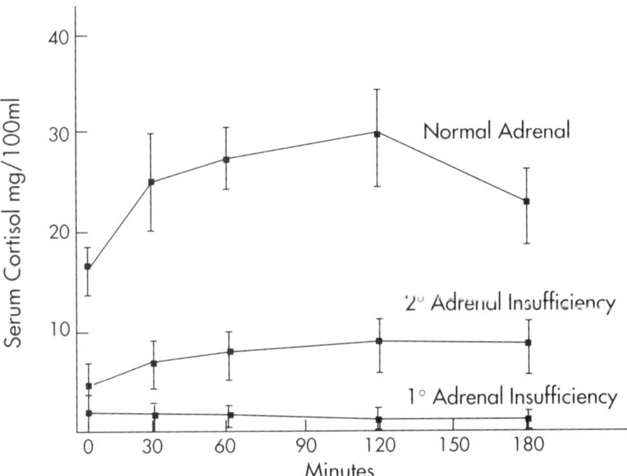

Figure 44.9 Serum cortisol response to an acute IV dose of corticotropin. Response curves show mean serum cortisol levels (± SE) after 0.25 mg of cosyntropin in normal subjects (n = 9), hypopituitarism (n = 8), and Addison's disease (n = 7) P <.01 between all means except zero times in primary and secondary adrenal insufficiency. From Speckart P, et al. Arch Int Med 1971; *128*:761–763, with permission.

Patients who have been exposed previously to moderately elevated levels of endogenous pituitary ACTH tend to show an exaggerated acute response to a test dose of exogenous corticotropin. Thus, patients with ACTH-producing pituitary tumors show further increases in already elevated cortisol levels. Most patients with Cushing's syndrome due to cortisol-producing adrenal tumors, where ambient levels of ACTH have been low, do not show an acute response to corticotropin. Patients with the various forms of congenital adrenal hyperplasia show an exaggerated response, not of cortisol, but of the steroid precursor proximal to the deficient biosynthetic enzyme. For example, patients with 21-hydroxylase deficiency will show an exaggerated rise in 17-OH progesterone. For this reason the rapid corticotropin stimulation test may be useful in diagnosing mild or incomplete forms of congenital adrenal hyperplasia.[r36]

Preparations and Doses

Cosyntropin (Cortrosyn) is a synthetic peptide corresponding to the first 24 amino acids of ACTH. This preparation is the drug of choice for diagnostic testing. It is given either IM or IV in a dose of 0.25 mg. One milligram of cosyntropin has approximately 150 USP units of biologic activity.

Corticotropin for injection (ACTHAR) is naturally-occurring ACTH purified from the pituitaries of swine and cattle obtained after slaughter. It is available as a lyophilized powder for SQ, IM, or IV use. Maximum adrenal secretion usually is stimulated by an 8-hour infusion of 25 units. Vials containing 25 and 40 units are available.

Repository corticotropin injection (ACTHAR GEL) is similarly purified beef or pork ACTH in a gelatin solution. It is absorbed slowly after SQ or IM injection. Vials containing 40 and 80 units are available. This material has been used for therapy in conditions responding to corticosteroids, but is not a drug of choice in situations where a defined corticosteroid dose is required.

Drugs Inhibiting the Synthesis or Actions of Adrenocorticoids

Chemistry and Therapeutic Uses

A diverse group of drugs acts as antiadrenal agents, either by impairing the ability of the adrenal cortex to synthesize corticosteroids or by blocking the effects of corticosteroids on their receptors in target tissues. The structures of several antiadrenal drugs are shown in Figure 44.10. Table 44.13 summarizes the therapeutic uses of these inhibitory drugs. Metyrapone, aminoglutethimide, and ketoconazole are reversible inhibitors of adrenal steroidogenesis. Ketoconazole also has prominent inhibitory effects on gonadal steroid production. All three drugs are used to block cortisol synthesis in treating patients with Cushing's syndrome. Aminoglutethimide and ketoconazole, but not metyrapone, also block adrenal androgen and mineralocorticoid production. Because of their broader effects on steroidogenesis, aminoglutethimide and ketoconazole have further use in reducing androgen and estrogen levels in patients with metastatic breast and prostate cancer, where tumor cells may depend on the presence of sex steroids for growth. Because of its more selective effect on cortisol synthesis by blocking the terminal 11-hydroxylation step, metyrapone is useful as a diagnostic drug. It is used primarily as an agent to test pituitary ACTH reserve. Mitotane differs from the other inhibitors of steroidogenesis by the irreversibility of its effects. Because it causes necrosis of both normal and neoplastic adrenocortical cells, its use is limited largely to the chemotherapy of inoperable or metastatic adrenal cortical carcinoma.

Two other drugs, spironolactone and mifepristone, act as reversible antagonists of mineralocorticoids and glucocorticoids, respectively, through competitive binding to steroid hormone receptors. Spironolactone is useful in treating patients with both primary and secondary hyperaldosteronism, where it can reverse excessive sodium retention, edema, and hypokalemia. Spironolactone also competes for binding to the androgen receptor and is used clinically as an antiandrogen in conditions such as hirsutism. Mifepristone (RU 486) is a competitive inhibitor of both the glucocorticoid receptor and the progesterone receptor. Though still an experimental drug in the US, it shows promise both in the treatment of Cushing's syndrome and as an antifertility agent.

Effects and Dosages of Drugs Inhibiting Corticosteroid Synthesis or Activity

Ketoconazole

Ketoconazole is an orally administered imidazole derivative used primarily as a broad-spectrum antifungal agent. Like other imidazole derivatives, it appears to interact with cytochrome P-450 at the iron site.[r37] The drug inhibits the 14-demethylation of lanosterol, preventing its conversion to ergosterol in fungi. At slightly higher concentrations it also inhibits the conversion of lanosterol to cholesterol in mammalian cells. The most sensitive site of action in humans is the cytochrome P-450-dependent C_{17-20} lyase step required for the production of androgens both in the adrenal and the testes.[r37] This explains why the secretion of testosterone and adrenal androgens is more readily affected than the secretion of cortisol in normal subjects. Ketoconazole is a reversible blocker of several other steps requiring cytochrome P450 enzymes in the adrenal. These include cholesterol side-chain cleavage, 11-beta-hydroxylation, and 18-hydroxylation. At low doses of 200–400 mg per day, the drug lowers testosterone and

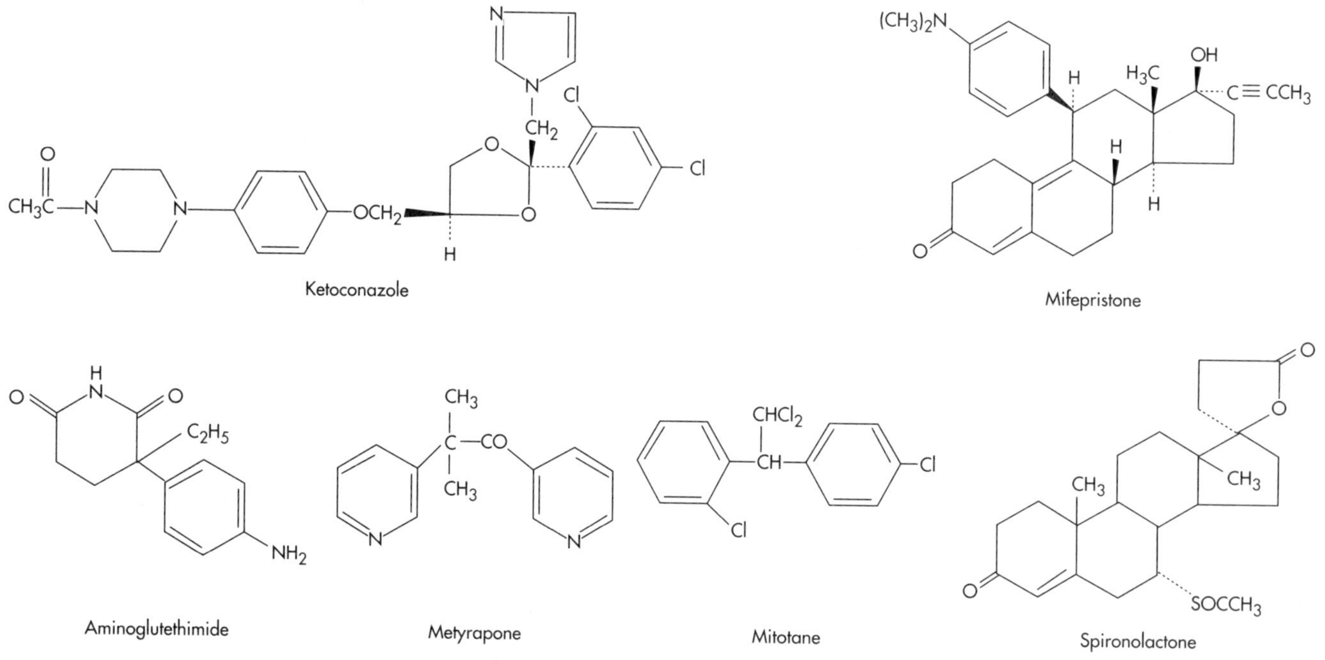

Ketoconazole Mifepristone Aminoglutethimide Metyrapone Mitotane Spironolactone

Figure 44.10 Structures of drugs inhibiting the synthesis or actions of corticosteroids.

Table 44.13 Drugs Inhibiting the Synthesis or Actions of Adrenocortical Steroids

Drug	Site of Inhibition	Clinical Effects	Applications
Metyrapone	Adrenalcortex 11-hydroxylation	Cortisol ↓ Adrenal androgens ↑ 11-desoxycorticosteroids (some mineralocorticoids) ↑	Diagnostic drug Therapy of Cushing's syndrome
Aminoglutethimide	Adrenal cortex Cholesterol side chain cleavage Peripheral aromatization of androgens	Cortisol ↓ Adrenal androgens ↓ Mineralocorticoids ↓	Therapy of Cushing's syndrome Reduction of adrenal androgens and peripheral estrogens
Ketoconazole	Adrenal cortex Gonads Cholesterol synthesis Cholesterol side chain cleavage; C17-20 lyase 11-hydroxylation	Cortisol ↓ Adrenal androgens ↓ and Mineralocorticoids ↓ Gonadal steroids ↓	Therapy of Cushing's syndrome Reduction of adrenal and gonadal androgens
Mitotane	Adrenal cortex Cholesterol side chain cleavage 11-hydroxylation Adrenocortical necrosis	Cortisol ↓ Adrenal androgens ↓ Mineralocorticoids ↓	Therapy of inoperable adrenal cortical carcinoma
Mifepristone	Peripheral tissues Glucocorticoid receptor Progesterone receptor	Reduced glucocorticoid and progesterone effects ACTH ↑ Cortisol ↑	Therapy of Cushing's syndrome Contraception and induction of abortion
Spironolactone	Kidney Peripheral tissues Mineralocorticoid receptor	Reduced mineralocorticoid and androgen effects	Therapy of mineralocorticoid dependent hypertension Therapy of hirsutism

androstenedione levels in normal men and tends to increase the ratio of estrogen to testosterone in the plasma. Higher doses cause a progressive blockade of cortisol synthesis. While basal cortisol levels are usually little affected in normal subjects, the plasma cortisol response to a test dose of corticotropin is blunted.

Ketoconazole is effective in reducing cortisol secretion in all forms of spontaneous Cushing's syndrome at doses ranging from 400–1200 mg per day. Patients with ectopic ACTH production[71] as well as patients with Cushing's disease due to pituitary tumors[72] have shown rapid declines in plasma cortisol with the onset of therapy and in some cases have been maintained for prolonged periods on the drug. Cessation of the drug results in a prompt increase in cortisol secretion and a return of symptoms. Because production of androgens and mineralocorticoids is also inhibited, ketoconazole is effective in reducing the hirsutism, sodium retention, and hypokalemia present in many patients with Cushing's syndrome.

Ketoconazole is readily absorbed after oral administration, with peak serum concentrations occurring two hours after a single dose.[r37] An acidic stomach pH is required for solubilization and absorption. Thus, concurrent administration of antacids or blockers of gastric acid secretion may impair bioavailability. The drug is bound extensively to albumin in the plasma, but distributes widely in body fluids. Serum clearance of the drug is biphasic, with a terminal half-life of eight hours. Metabolism to inactive compounds occurs mainly in the liver. The drug is usually well tolerated in doses up to 1200 mg per day. Its principal toxicity is hepatic, and hepatic insufficiency is a contraindication to its use. Up to 10 per cent of patients may have transient elevations in liver enzymes, but the incidence of true liver injury is probably not more than 1 per cent. Gastrointestinal symptoms and pruritus may also occur. Gynecomastia is a common side-effect in males. As with other inhibitors of steroid biosynthesis, ketoconazole can cause acute adrenal insufficiency, especially if given at high doses to patients who are unable to increase their rate of ACTH secretion. Although ketoconazole has been used successfully to treat Cushing's syndrome in the third trimester of pregnancy,[73] little is known about its passage across the placenta or whether it can influence sexual differentiation in the fetus.

Because of its relatively infrequent side-effects and its favorable profile of activity against synthesis of androgens and mineralocorticoids as well as glucocorticoids, ketoconazole is the drug of choice in many situations where the objective is reversible inhibition of excess corticosteroid production. The usual starting dose is 200 to 400 mg every 12 hours, with frequent monitoring of plasma and urinary cortisol levels. If necessary, the dose may be raised to 600 mg twice a day. If urinary cortisol is suppressed to less than 40 mg per day or plasma cortisol to less than 10 mg/dl the dose may be lowered or supplemental therapy with glucocorticoids begun. Patients should be monitored carefully for signs of adrenal insufficiency or liver dysfunction, particularly during the first two months of therapy.[r37] Ketoconazole has been given in a dose of 400 mg every eight hours to suppress adrenal androgen production in men with metastatic prostate cancer. It may be most effective for this purpose when used in castrated subjects or subjects with castrate testosterone levels due to concurrent administration of gonadotropin-releasing hormone analogues.[74,75] Ketoconazole (Nizoral) is available in 200-mg tablets for oral administration. The drug is approved in the US for use as a systemic antifungal agent.

Aminoglutethimide

This drug was introduced over 30 years ago as an anticonvulsant but was withdrawn because of a number of side-effects, including the induction of adrenal insufficiency. Later it was reintroduced as an adrenal blocking agent.[76] Its primary effect is competitive blockade of the conversion of cholesterol to pregnenolone, thus reducing the secretion of all classes of adrenal steroids. At doses from 0.5 to 1.5 g per day, the drug reduces cortisol secretion in normal subjects and in many patients with Cushing's syndrome for treatment periods up to a year.[77,78] ACTH levels in treated patients with pituitary-dependent Cushing's disease may rise further, leading to partial adrenal escape from the effects of the drug. Aminoglutethimide at doses of 1–2 g per day given together with dexamethasone causes essentially complete suppression of all adrenal steroid synthesis in subjects with a normal pituitary-adrenal axis. This combination has been proposed for "medical adrenalectomy" to block all remaining estrogen production in ovariectomized women with metastatic breast cancer.[79]

Aminoglutethimide causes relatively frequent side-effects, including rash, lethargy, headache, myalgia, and upper GI symptoms, especially at doses greater than 1.0 g per day.[77,79] Like other adrenal blocking drugs, it may cause acute adrenal insufficiency. It has the effect of inducing more rapid metabolism of certain synthetic glucocorticoids, such as dexamethasone,[79] so that larger replacement doses may be required to correct glucocorticoid deficiency.

Aminoglutethimide (Cytadren) is available as 250-mg tablets for oral administration. Therapy should be initiated with 250 mg every six hours and increased as needed by 250 mg per day up to a maximum dose of 2 g per day. Monitoring for drug effects and the possible need for corticosteroid replacement are similar to those for ketoconazole.

Metyrapone

This drug exerts its greatest inhibitory effect on the final step in glucocorticoid synthesis, the conversion of biologically inactive 11-deoxycortisol to cortisol.[80] Blockade of the 11-hydroxylation step leads to a compensatory increase in ACTH secretion in normal subjects and an increased synthesis of adrenal steroid precursors prior to the block. In addition to 11-deoxycortisol there is increased production of adrenal androgens and of 11-deoxycorticosterone, a potent mineralocorticoid. The drug may be used as adjunctive therapy in the management of Cushing's syndrome at doses of 0.5 to 2.5 g per day.[78,81] However, it fails to reverse and may actually increase the manifestations of hirsutism, amenorrhea, edema, and hypokalemia often associated with the syndrome. An additional disadvantage is that patients with pituitary-dependent Cushing's disease are capable of escaping metyrapone blockade through further increases in ACTH secretion.

Metyrapone is most useful as a diagnostic agent for testing pituitary-adrenal reserve. Given orally, either as a single dose of 1 gram, or in divided doses of 750 mg every six hours for four doses, it increases serum 11-deoxycortisol and urinary 17-hydroxycorticosteroids in normal individuals. Failure to elicit the expected response implies deficient reserve of the pituitary, the adrenal, or both. Further testing with corticotropin administration can distinguish these possibilities.[70]

When used as a short-term diagnostic drug, metyrapone can precipitate acute adrenal insufficiency in patients who actually do have limited ACTH reserve. Thus, all patients should be carefully observed when treatment is being initiated. In longer-term therapy, the side-effects in addition to those due to increased mineralocorticoids and adrenal androgens include GI symptoms and skin rashes.[78,80] Metyrapone (Metopirone) is available in 250-mg tablets for oral administration. In the US it is approved for use only as a diagnostic drug.

Mitotane

Originally marketed in the 1940s as an insecticide related to DDT, DDD (1,1-dichlorodiphenyldichlorethane) was withdrawn when it was found to cause adrenal necrosis and atrophy in dogs.[82] The o,p, isomer of DDD, or mitotane, was tested as an experimental drug for treating adrenal cortical cancer between 1959 and 1970, when it was approved for that use in the US. Its cytotoxic action on both normal and neoplastic adrenal cortical cells may depend in part on the availability of reduced triphosphopyridine nucleotide. In treated human subjects there is impairment in several steps in steroidogenesis, including the conversion of cholesterol to pregnenolone and the conversion of 11-deoxycortisol to cortisol. Secretion of aldosterone and adrenal androgens as well as cortisol is reduced.

Unlike ketoconazole and aminoglutethemide, which are rapidly acting and reversible, the action of mitotane is slow in onset with respect to steroidogenesis and often is irreversible. Consequently, replacement with both glucocorticoids and mineralocorticoids must be given. Mitotane is effective in reversing the symptoms of hyperadrenocorticism in patients with functioning malignant adrenal tumors, but causes regression of tumor size in only a minority of such patients.[82,r38] The drug does not have a consistent effect on survival. Thus, its use is limited largely to palliation in patients who have nonresectable or recurrent disease. Its use as an adjunct after apparently successful surgery for adrenocortical carcinoma is controversial.[r38]

Treatment with mitotane may be initiated at 3 to 4 g per day in four daily doses and increased over one or two weeks to a maximum dose of 8 to 10 g per day unless limited by toxicity. Adrenal replacement therapy is usually needed after the second or third week. Reduction in tumor size, if any, occurs after four to six weeks. Later, the disease may progress in spite of the continuation of therapy.

Most patients have side-effects from mitotane therapy, the most common being lassitude. Somnolence, depression, confusion, neurologic disturbances, and GI symptoms also are common. Abnormalities in liver function, hypercholesterolemia, toxic retinopathy, and skin rashes may occur.[82,r38] In a minority of patients, these side-effects necessitate withdrawal of the drug. Because of the greater severity of side-effects and its irreversible effects on normal adrenal tissues, mitotane is not the drug of choice for control of Cushing's syndrome due to benign adrenal tumors or adrenal hyperplasia.

Mitotane (Lysodren) is available as 0.5-g tablets for oral administration.

Mifepristone

Mifepristone (RU 486) is the most potent of a series of glucocorticoid antagonists modified in both the C-11 position and in the C-17 ketolic side-chain.[14] Mifepristone binds to the unactivated glucocorticoid receptor with an affinity similar to that of dexamethasone and other potent agonists. When the receptor is in the activated form, however, mifepristone dissociates more rapidly. Furthermore, the mifepristone-receptor complex has a much lower affinity for DNA than does the complex formed by potent glucocorticoid agonists. The result is that the glucocorticoid receptor interacting with mifepristone fails to translocate properly to the cell nucleus or to trigger a glucocorticoid response.[83] Mifepristone also has a strong affinity for the progesterone receptor, where it blocks the action of progesterone agonists in an analogous way.

Mifepristone can block a number of the physiologic effects of cortisol in man, including the negative feedback of cortisol on ACTH secretion. The normal pituitary-adrenal axis responds by increasing production of both ACTH and cortisol. When given as a single dose at 2 AM, for example, mifepristone will increase plasma cortisol levels measured between 7 AM and 4 PM.[84] These levels will return to normal by 8 AM the following day. The drug is absorbed efficiently after oral administration. Its half-life in the serum is approximately 20 hours.[85] Thus effective plasma levels can be obtained by administering the drug twice a day.

Mifepristone shows promise as an antiglucocorticoid in the treatment of spontaneous Cushing's syndrome. When treated with doses of 10–20 mg/kg day, patients have shown regression of the somatic features of Cushing's syndrome without a corresponding decline in cortisol production or ACTH levels.[86] There is also considerable interest in the use of mifepristone as an oral contraceptive and abortifacient.[r39] Because of continuing controversy surrounding the latter use, it is not available in the US. It is, however, licensed in the United Kingdom, France, Sweden, and China. The antiprogesterone effects of the drug appear to occur at a slightly lower dose level than the antiglucocorticoid effect.[87] Thus, use of the drug as an anti-infertility agent in women should not necessarily cause the side-effects due to cortisol blockade.

Spironolactone

Spironolactone is the most potent of a family of steroid derivatives, the spirolactones, all having a lactose ring at the C-17 position. Members of this family are competitive mineralocorticoid antagonists with little or no agonist activity. Their effects in vivo are exerted on tissues possessing mineralocorticoid receptors. In the kidney (see Chapter 38), spironolactone promotes a dose-dependent decrease in sodium reabsorption and an increase in net sodium excretion. There is also a net decrease in potassium and hydrogen ion excretion. These effects are not seen in adrenalectomized animals, implying that aldosterone or other mineralocorticoids must be present in order for an antagonist effect to be manifest. Spironolactone is an effective competitor for mineralocorticoid, but not glucocorticoid, receptors in the kidney. When ^{3}H-spironolactone is bound to mineralocorticoid receptor preparations, the complexes are ineffective in binding to chromatin. This suggests that spironolactone binds but fails to activate the receptor.[r40] The spirolactones also can inhibit aldosterone synthesis at high concentrations by interfering with both 18- and 11-hydroxylation. At doses commonly used in therapy, these effects are probably unimportant compared with the effects on the mineralocorticoid receptor. Indeed, after continued treatment with spironolactone, aldosterone secretion in normal subjects tends to rise owing to a compensatory increase in the activity of the renin-angiotensin system. In addition to its effects on mineralocorticoid action, spironolactone has predictable antiandrogenic effects at doses ordinarily used in human subjects. The drug interferes competitively with the binding of testosterone to its cytoplasmic receptor in various target tissues, including hair follicles.[r40] It also inhibits the biosynthesis of testosterone and other androgens by inhibiting the cytochrome P450 enzyme responsible for 17-hydroxylation and side-chain cleavage. The latter effect is demonstrable in boys but is minimal in adult men. In treated adults an increase in the ratio of circulating estradiol to testosterone is commonly seen.[88]

The main therapeutic uses of spironolactone are derived from its antimineralocorticoid effects. Its use as a diuretic and antihypertensive agent is discussed in detail in Chapter 38. Spironolactone is especially effective as an antihypertensive under conditions of aldosterone excess. In primary hyperaldosteronism due to an aldosterone-secreting tumor or to adrenal hyperplasia, spironolactone is the drug of choice. At doses of 100 to 400 mg per day, the elevated blood pressure and hypokalemia characteristic of primary hyperaldosteronism may be normalized. After initial control is achieved, the dose may often be lowered to a maintenance dose of 100 to 150 mg per day. Long-term spironolactone therapy is a reasonable alternative to surgery when surgical risk is high or where the presence of bilateral adrenal hyperplasia is suspected.

A secondary therapeutic application involves the antiandrogen effects of spironolactone. The drug is useful in treating hirsutism and other undesirable manifestations of hyperandrogenism in women, although it has no effect on the underlying cause of the problem. This is the case regardless of whether the androgens are primarily of adrenal or ovarian origin. At systemic doses of 100 to 200 mg per day, spironolactone is effective in reducing the quantity of facial and body hair growth in women with hirsutism.[89] Regression in hair diameter, density, and rate of growth may be seen after two to six months of therapy. Serum testosterone and androstenedione levels decrease transiently in the first two weeks of therapy, but soon return to baseline levels. This suggests that the main therapeutic effect is exerted at the level of the androgen receptor in the hair follicle. Topical spironolactone, applied directly to the skin, shows promise in treating localized acne that may be dependent on androgen-mediated sebaceous gland activity.[90]

Spironolactone is efficiently absorbed from the GI tract. The drug is metabolized in the liver to other spirolactone derivatives, including canrenone, which has weak activity as an aldosterone antagonist. The most serious toxic effect is hyperkalemia. This effect is predictable and occurs most often in the presence of a high potassium intake or when spironolactone is given with other potassium-sparing diuretics. Gynecomastia, and, occasionally, decreased libido and impotence may occur in men. Women may note menstrual irregularities and painful breast enlargement.[88,90] Spironolactone (Aldactone) is available in 25-, 50-, and 100-mg tablets. The initial daily dose is usually 100 mg given as a single or divided dose. Fixed-dose combinations of spironolactone with thiazides and other potassium wasting diuretics are also available.

References

Research Reports

1. Nobel Lectures for Medicine and Physiology, 1942–1962. Amsterdam: Elsevier, 1964. See lectures by Kendall EC. The development of cortisone as a therapeutic agent, pp 270–285; Reichstein T. Chemistry of the adrenal cortex hormones, pp 291–305; Hench, PS.: The reversibility of certain rheumatic and non-rheumatic conditions by the use of cortisone or the pituitary adrenocorticotrpic hormone, pp 310–355.
2. Dixon RB, Christy NP. On the various forms of cortiosteroid withdrawal syndrome. Am J Med 1980;*68*:224–230.
   Presents a rational analysis of a difficult problem in therapeutics.
3. Vale W, Spiess J, Rivier C, Rivier J. Characterization of a 41-residue ovine hypothalamic peptide that stimulates secretion of corticotropin and B-endorphin. Science 1981;*213*:1394–1397.
   Initial report on the structure of CRH
4. Ogishima T, Mitani F, Ishimura Y. Isolation of aldosterone synthase cytochrome P-450 from zona glomerulosa mitochondria of rat adrenal cortex. J Biol Chem 1989;*264*:10935–10938.
5. Baird DT, Horton R, Longcope C, Tait JF. Steroid dynamics under steady state conditions. Rec Progr Horm Res 1969;*25*:611–664.
6. Simpson SA, Tait JF, Wettstein A, Neher R, Euw JV, Schindler D, Reichstein T. Constitution des aldosterone, des neun mineralocorticoids. Experientia 1954;*X/3*:132–133.
7. Green S, Chambon P. A superfamily of potentially oncogenic hormone receptors. Nature 1986;*324*:615–617.
8. Evans RM. The steroid and thyroid hormone receptor superfamily. Science 1988;*240*:889–895.
9. Wahli W, Martinez E. Superfamily of steroid nuclear receptors: positive and negative regulators of gene expression. FASEB 1991;*5*:2243–2249.
10. Fuller PJ. The steroid receptor superfamily: mechanisms of diversity. FASEB 1991;*5*:3092–3099.
11. Feldman D. Glucocorticoid receptors and the regulation of phosphoenol-pyruvate-carboxykinase activity in rat kidney and adipose tissue. Am J Phyisol 1977;*233*:E147–E151.
12. Arriza JL, Weinberger C, Cerelli G, Glaser TM, Handelin BL, Housman DE, Evans RM. Cloning of human mineralocorticoid receptor complementary DNA: Structural and functional kinship with the glucocorticoid receptor. Science 1987;*23*:268–275.
13. Vandewalle A, Farman N, Bencsath P, Bonvalet JP. Aldosterone binding along the rabbit nephron: an autoradiographic study on isolated tubules. Am J Physiol 1981;*240*:F172–F179.
14. Mondy C. Corticosteroids, receptors and the organ-specific functions of 11 B-hydroxysteroid dehydrogenase. FASEB 1991;*5*:3047–3054.
15. Wilcox CS, Cemerikic DA, Giebisch G. Differential effects of acute mineralo- and glucocorticosteroid administration on renal acid elimination. Kidney Int 1982;*21*:546–556.
16. Davies DO, De Lean A, Lefkowitz RJ. Myocardial beta-adrenergic receptors from adrenalectomized rats: Impaired formation of high-affinity agonist-receptor complexes. Endocrinology 1981;*108*:720–722.
17. Axelrod L. Inhibition of prostacyclin production mediates premissive effects of glucocorticoids on vascular tone. Lancet 1983;*1*:904–906.
18. Hein R, Mauch C, Hatamochi A, Krieg T. Influence of corticosteroids on chemotactic response and collagen metabolism of human skin fibroblasts. Biochem Pharmacol 1985;*37*:2723–2729.

19. Hamalainen L, Dikarinen J, Kivirikko KI. Synthesis and degradation of type I procollagen mRNAs in clutured human skin fibroblasts and the effect of cortisol. Biol Chem 1985;*260*:720–725.

20. Hyams JS, Moore RE, Leichtner AM, Carey DE, Goldberg BD. Relationship of type I procollagen to corticosteroid therapy in children with inflammatory bowel disease. J Pediatr 1988;*112*:893–898.

21. Gourmelen M, Girard F, Binoux M. Serum somatomedin/insulin-like growth factor (IGF) and IGF carrier levels in patients with Cushing's syndrome or receiving glucocorticoid therapy. J Clin Endocrinol Metab 1982;*54*:885–892.

22. McCarthy TL, Centrella M, Canalis E. Cortisol inhibits the synthesis of insulin-like growth factor-I in skeletal cells. Endocrinology 1990;*126*:1569–75.

23. Chen TL, Aronow L, Feldman D. Glucocorticoid receptors and inhibition of bone cell growth in primary culture. Endocrinology 1977;*100*:619–628.

24. Nielsen HK, Charles P, Mosekilde L. The effect of single oral doses of prednisone on the circadian rhythm of serum osteocalcin in normal subjects. J Clin Endocrinol Metab 1988;*67*:1025–1030.

25. Morrison NA, Shine J, Fragonas J-C, Verkest V, McMenemy L, Eisman JA. 1,25-dihydroxy-vitamin D-responsive element and glucocorticoid repression in the osteocalcin gene. Science 1989;*246*:1158–1161.

26. Feher JV, Wasserman RH. Intestinal calcium-binding protein and calcium absorption in cortisol-treated chicks: effects of vitamin D_3. Endocrinology 1979;*104*:547–551.

27. Guyre PM, Bodwell JE, Munck A. Glucocorticoid actions on the immune system: inhibition of production of an Fc-receptor augmenting factor. J Steroid Biochem 1981;*15*:35–39.

28. Watson JD, Mochizuki DY, Gillis S. Molecular characteristics of interleukin 2. Fed Proc 1983;*42*:2747–2752.

29. Allison F, Smith MR, Wood WB. Studies on the pathogenesis of acute inflammation: the action of cortisone on the inflammatory response to thermal injury. J Exp Med 1955;*102*:669–676.

30. Bailey JM, Makheja AN, Pash J, Verma M. Corticosteroids suppress cycloxygenase messenger RNA levels and prostanoid synthesis in cultured vascular cells. Biochem Biophys Res Commun 1988;*157*:1159–1163.

31. Hargreaves KM, Costello A. Glucocorticoids suppress levels of immunoreactive bradykinin in inflamed tissue as evaluated by microdialysis probes. Clin Pharmacol Therap 1990;*48*:168–78.

32. Tsurufuji S, Sugio K, Takemasa F, Yoshizawa S. Blockade by antiglucocorticoids, actinomycin D and cycloheximide of anti-inflammatory action of dexamethasone against bradykinin. J Pharmacol Exp Ther 1980;*212*:225–231.

33. Coleman PL, Barouski PA, Gelehrter TD. The dexamethasone-induced inhibitor of fibrinolytic activity in hepatoma cells. A cellular product which specifically inhibits plasminogen activator. J Biol Chem 1982;*257*:4260–4264.

34. Jackson SHD, Beavers DG, Myers K. Does long-term low-dose corticosteroid therapy cause hypertension? Clin Sci 1981;*61*:381S–383S.

35. Bagdade JD, Porte D, Bierman EL. Steroid-induced lipemia. Arch Int Med *125*:129–134.

36. Miller SE, Neilson JM. Clinical features of the diabetic syndrome appearing after steroid-therapy. Postgrad Med 1964;*40*:660–664.

37. Afifi AK, Bergman RA, Harvey JC. Steroid myopathy: Clinical, histologic and cytologic observations. Johns Hopkins Med Bull 1968;*123*:158–174.

38. Ringe JD, Welzel D. Salmon calcitonin in the therapy of corticoid-induced osteoporosis. Eur J Clin Pharmacol 1987;*33*:35–9.

39. Reid IR, King AR, Alexander CJ, Ibberston HK. Prevention of steroid-induced osteoporosis with (3-amino-1-hydroxypropylidine)-1,1-bisphosphonate (APD). Lancet 1988;*1*:143–6.

40. Soyka LF. Treatment of the nephrotic syndrome in childhood: Use of an alternate-day prednisone regimen. Am J Dis Child 1967;*113*:693–701.

41. The Boston Collaborative Drug Surveillance Program. Acute adverse reactions to prednisone in relation to dosage. Clin Pharmacol Therap 1972;*13*:694–98.

42. Packan DR, Sapolsky RM. Glucocorticoid endangerment of the hippocampus: tissue, steroid and receptor specificity. Neuroendocrinology 1990;*51*:613–618.

43. Wolkowitz OM, Reus VI, Weingartner H, Thompson K, Brier A, Doran A, Rubinow D, Pickar D. Cognitive effects of corticosteroids. Am J Psychiatr 1990;*147*:1297–1303.

44. Graham BS, Tucker WS. Opportunistic infections in endogenous Cushing's syndrome. Ann Int Med 1984;*101*:334–338.

45. Schotz M, Patterson R, Klomer R, Falk J. The prevalence of tuberculosis and positive tuberculin skin tests in a steroid-treated asthmatic population. Ann Intern Med 1976;*84*:261–265.

46. Chan CS, Brown IG, Oliver WA, Zimmerman PV. Hydrocortisone-induced anaphylaxis. Med J Aust 1984;*141*:444–446.

47. Messer J, Reitman D, Sacks HS, Smith H, Chalmers TC. Association of adrenocorticosteroid therapy and peptic ulcer disease. Engl J Med 1983;*309*:21–24.

48. Piper JM, Ray WA, Daugherty JR, Griffin MR. Corticosteroid use and peptic ulcer disease: role of nonsteroidal anti-inflammatory drugs. Ann Int Med 1991;*114*:735–40.

49. Richards JM, Santiago SM, Klaustermeyer WB. Ascptic necrosis of the femoral head in corticosteroid-treated pulmonary disease. Arch Int Med 1980;*140*:1473–1475.

50. Webb J, Clark TJH. Recovery of plasma corticotropin and cortisol levels after a three-week course of prednisolone. Thorax 1981;*36*:22–24.

51. Livanou T, Ferriman D, James VHT. Recovery of hypothalamo-pituitary-adrenal function after corticosteroid therapy. Lancet 1967;*2*:856–859.

52. Schurmeyer IH, Tsokos GC, Avgerinos PC, Balow JE, D'Agata R, Loriaux DL, Chrousos GP. Pituitary-adrenal responsiveness to corticotropin-releasing hormone in patients receiving chronic alternate day therapy. J Clin Endocrinol Metab 1985;*61*:22–27.

53. Graber AL, Ney RL, Nicholson WE, Island DP, Liddle GW. Natural history of pituitary-adrenal recovery following long-term suppression with corticosteroids. J Clin Endocrinol 1965;*25*:11–16.

54. Meikle AW, Tyler FH. Potency and duration of action of glucocorticoids. Am J Med 1977;*63*:200–207.

55. Hryb DJ, Khan MS, Romas NA, Rosner W. Specific binding of human corticosteroid-binding globulin to cell membranes. Proc Natl Aca Sci 1986;*83*:3253–3256.

56. Hill MR, Szefler SJ, Ball BD, Bartoszek M. Brenner AM. Monitoring glucocorticoid therapy: a pharmacokinetic approach. Clin Pharmacol Ther 1990;*48*:390–8.

57. Karl M, Lamberts SWJ, Detera-Wadleigh SD, Encio IJ, Stratakis CA, Hurley DM, Accili D, Chrousos GP. Familial glucocorticoid resistance caused by a splice site deletion in the human glococorticoid receptor gene, J Clin Endocrinol Metab 1993;*76*:683–689.

58. Uribe M, Go VLW. Corticosteroid pharmacokinetics in liver disease. Clin Pharmacokinetics 1979;*4*:233–240.

59. Beisel WR, Diraimondo VC, Chao PY, et al. The influence of plasma protein binding on the extra-adrenal metabolism of cortisol in normal hyperthyroid and hypothyroid subjects. Metabolism 1964;*13*:942–951.

60. Boekenoogen SJ, Szefler SJ, Jusko WJ. Prednisolone disposition and protein binding in oral contraceptive users. J Clin Endocrinol Metab 1983;*56*:702–709.

61. Khalid BAK, Burke CW, Hurley DM, Funder JW, Stockigt JR. Steroid replacement in Addison's disease and in subjects adrenalectomized for Cushings disease: comparison of various glucocorticoids. J Clin Endocrinol Metab 1982;*55*:551–559.

62. Pang S, Pollack M, Marshall RN, Immken L. Prenatal treatment of congenital adrenal hyperplasia due to a 21-hydroxylase deficiency. N Engl J Med 1990;*322*:111–115.

63. Hunder GG, Sheps SG, Allen GL, Joyce, JW. Daily and alternate day corticosteroid regimens in treatment of giant cell arteritis. Ann Intern Med 1975;*82*:613–618.

64. Bilezekian LM, Vale W. Glucocorticoids inhibit corticotropin-releasing factor-induced production of adenosine 3′,5′-monophosphate in cultured anterior pituitary cells. Endocrinology 1983;*113*:657–662.

65. Linton EA, Tilderg FJH, Hodgkinson S, et al. Stress-induced secretion of ACTH in rats is inhibited by administration of antisera to ovine corticotropin-releasing factor and vasopressin. Endocrinology 1985;*116*:966–970.

66. Schulte HM, Chrousos GP, Chatterji DC, et al. Safety of corticotropin-releasing factor. Lancet 1983;*1*:1227.

67. Oldfield EH, Doppman JL, Nieman LK, et al. Petrosal sinus sampling with and without corticotropin-releasing hormone for the differential diagnosis of Cushing's syndrome. N Engl J Med 1991;*325*:897–905.

68. Mahaffee DD, Ontjes DA. Activation of adrenal adenylate cyclase by guanine nucleotides: promotion of nucleotide binding by calcium but not by ACTH. Mol Pharmacol 1983;*23*:369–377.

69. Ways DK, Mahaffee DD, Ontjes DA. An adrenocorticotropin analog (ACTH 6-39) which acts as a potent *in vitro* adrenocorticotropin antagonist at low calcium concentration and as a weak agonist at high calcium concentration. Endocrinology 1979;*104*:1028–1035.

70. Speckart JT, Nicoloff JT, Bethune. Screening for adrenocortical insufficiency with cosyntropin (synthetic ACTH). Arch Int Med 1971;*128*:761.

71. Shepherd F, Hoffert B, Evans WK, Emery G, Trachtenberg J. Ketoconazole: Use in the treatment of ectopic adrenocorticotropin hormone production and Cushing's syndrome in small-cell lung cancer. Arch Int Med 1985;*145*:863–864.

72. Sonino N, Boscaro M, Merola G, Mantero F. Prolonged treatment of Cushings disease by ketoconazole. J Clin Endocrinol Metab 1985;*61*:718–722.

73. Amado JA, Pesquera C, Gonzalez EM, Otero M, Freijanes J, Advarez A. Successful treatment with ketoconazole of Cushing's syndrome in pregnancy. Postgrad Med J 1990;*66*:221–223.

74. Williams G. Ketoconazole for prostate cancer. Lancet 1984;*2*:696.

75. Allen JM, Kerle DJ, Ware H, Doble A, Williams G, Bloom S. Combined treatment with ketoconazole and luteinizing hormone releasing hormone analog: a normal approach to resistant progressive prostatic cancer. Br Med J 1983;*287*:1766.

76. Fishman LM, Liddle GW, Island DP, Fleischer N, Kuchel O. Effects of aminoglutethimide on adrenal function in man. J Clin Endocrinol Metab 1967;*27*:481–490.

77. Misbin RI, Canary J, Willard D. Aminoglutethimide in the treatment of Cushing's syndrome. J Clin Pharmacol 1976;*16*:645–651.

78. Thoren M, Adamson V, Sjoberg HE. Aminoglutethimide and metyrapone in the management of Cushing's syndrome. Acta Endocrinol 1985;*109*:451–457.

79. Santen RJ, Lipton A, Kendall J. Successful medical adrenalectomy with amino-glutethimide. JAMA 1974;*230*:1661–1665.

80. Orth DN. Metyrapone is useful as adjunctive therapy in Cushing's disease. Ann Int Med 1978;*89*:128–130.

81. Jeffcoate WJ, Rees LH, Tomlin S, Jones AE, Edwards CRW, Besser GM. Metyrapone in long term management of Cushing's disease. Br Med J 1977;*2*:215–217.

82. Luton, J-P, Cerdas S, Billaud L, et al. Clinical features of adrenocortical carcinoma, prognostic factors, and the effect of mitotane therapy. N Engl J Med 1990;*322*:1195–1201.

83. Moguilewsky M, Philbert D. RU38486: Potent antiglucocorticoid activity correlated with strong binding to the cytosolic glucocorticoid receptor followed by impaired activation. J Steroid Biochem 1984;*20*:271–276.

84. Bertagna X, Bertagna C, Luton J-P, Husson J-P, Girard F. The new steroid analog RU486 inhibits glucocorticoid action in man. J Clin Endocrinol Metab 1984;*59*:25–28.

85. Kawai S, Nieman LK, Brandon DD, Peden GW, Loriaux DL, Chrousos GP. Pharmacokinetic properties of the glucocorticoid and progesterone antagonist RU486 in man. Clin Res 1986;*34*:401A.

86. Nieman LK, Chrousos GP, Kellner C, et al. Successful treatment of Cushing's syndrome with the glucocorticoid antagonist RU486. J Clin Endocrinol Metab 1985;*61*:536–540.

87. Gaillard RC, Riondel A, Muller AF, Heramann W, Baulieu EE. RU486: A steroid with antiglucocorticosteroid activity that only disinhibits the pituitary-adrenal system at a specific time of day. Proc Nat Acad Sci USA 1984;*81*:3879–3882.

88. Loriaux DL, Menard R, Taylor A, Pita JC, Santen R. Spironolactone and endocrine dysfunction. Ann Int Med 1976;*85*:630–636.

89. Cumming DC, Yang JC, Rebar RW, Yen SSC. Treatment of hirsutism with spironolactone. JAMA 1982;*247*:1295–1298.

90. Messina M, Manieri C, Musso MC, Pastorino R. Oral and topical spironolactone therapies in skin androgenization. Panminerva Med 1990;*32*:49–55.

Reviews

r1. Szpilfogel SA. Adrenocortical steroids and their synthetic analogs. In: Discoveries in pharmacology, Volume 2. Parnham MJ, Bruinvels J. Amsterdam: Elsevier, (1984); pp 253–284.
Good summary of the history of discovery and development of the corticosteroid drugs.

r2. Miller WL. Molecular biology of steroid hormone synthesis. Endocrine Rev 1988;*9*:295–318.

r3. Waterman MR, Simpson ER. Cellular mechanisms involved in the acute and chronic actions of ACTH. In Anderson DC, Winter JSD. The adrenal cortex. London: Butterworth (1985); pp 57–85.

r4. Gustafsson JA, Carlstedt-Duke J, Poellinger L, Okret S, Wikstrom AC, Bronnegard M, Gillner M, Dong Y, Fuxe K, Cintra A, Harfstrand A, Agnati L. Biochemistry, molecular biology and physiology of the glucocorticoid receptor. Endocrine Rev 1987;*8*:185–225.

r5. Munck A, Guyre PM, Holbrook NJ. Physiological functions of glucocorticoids in stress and their relation to pharmacological action. Endocrine Rev 1984;*5*:25–44.
Develops the hypothesis that corticosteroids function to limit over response to stress through effects on inflammation and the immune response.

r6. Dujovne CA, Azarnoff DL. Clinical complications of corticosteroid therapy; a selected review. In Azarnoff DL. Steroid therapy. Philadelphia: WB Saunders, (1975); pp 27–41.
This book contains chapters reviewig a variety of applications of corticosteroid therapy in medicine.

r7. Luckert BP, Raisz LG. Glucocorticoid-induced osteoporosis: Pathogenesis and management. Ann Int Med 1990;*112*:352–364.
Good review of a major complication of corticosteroid therapy.

r8. Gustavson LE, Benet LZ. Pharmacokinetics of natural and synthetic glucocorticoids. In Anderson DC, Winter JSD. The adrenal cortex. London: Butterworth, (1985); pp 235–281.

r9. Eipper BA, Mains RE. Structure and biosynthesis of proadrenocorticotropin/endorphin and related peptides. Endocrine Rev 1980;*1*:1–27.
Review of work delineating the biosynthesis of ACTH.

r10. Agarwal MK, Hainque B, Moustaid N, Lazer G. Glucocorticoid antagonists. FEBS Letters 1987;*217*:221–226.
Review of structure and function of glucocorticoid antagonists

r11. Hornsby P. The regulation of adrenocortical function by control of growth and structure. In Anderson DC, Winter JSD. The adrenal cortex. London: Butterworth (1985); pp 1–31.

r12. Feldman D. Mechanism of action of cortisol. In DeGroot LJ. Endocrinology, Vol. 2. Philadelphia: WB Saunders, 1989.

r13. Hofmann KH. Relations between chemical structure and function of adrenocorticotropin and melanocyte-stimulating hormones. In Greep RO, Astwood EB. Handbook of Physiology, Section 7: Endocrinology, Vol. IV, pp. 29–58. Washington Am Physiol Soc 1974.

r14. Orth DN, Kovacs WJ, Debold CR. The adrenal cortex. In Wilson JD, Foster DW. Textbook of endocrinology, 8th edition. Philadelphia: WB Saunders, (1992); pp 489–619.

r15. Crabbe J. Mechanism of action of aldosterone. In DeGroot LJ. Endocrinology, Vol. 2, pp. 1572–1581, Philadelphia: WB Saunders, 1989.

r16. Gennari C. Glucocorticoids and bone. In Peck, WA. Bone and mineral research, Vol. 3. Amsterdam: Elsevier (1985); pp 213–231.

r17. Hauschka PV, Lian JB, Cole DEC, Gundberg CM. Osteocalcin and matrix Gla protein: vitamin K-dependent proteins in bone. Physiol Rev 1989;*69*:990–1047.

r18. Fauci AS, Dale DC, Balow JE. Glucocorticoid therapy: mechanism of action and clinical considerations: NIH Conference: Ann Int Med 1976;*84*:304–315.

r19. Parrillo JE, Fauci AS. Mechanisms of glucocorticoid action on immune processes. Ann Rev Pharmacol Toxicol 1979;*19*:179–201.

r20. Flower RJ. Macrocortin and the antiphospholipase proteins. Adv Inflammation Res 1986;*8*:1–39.

r21. Samuelsson B. Leukoetrienes: mediators of immediate hypersensitivity reactions and inflammation. Science 1983;*220*:568–575.

r22. Larsen GL, Henson PM. Mediators of inflammation. Ann Rev Immunol 1983;*1*:335–359.

r23. Fahey JV, Guyre PM, Munck A. Mechanism of anti-inflammatory actions of glucocorticoids. Adv Inflammation Res 1981;*2*:21–51.

r24. Olefsky JM, Kimmerling G. Effects of glucocorticoids on carbohydrate metabolism. Am J Med Sc 1976;*271*:202–210.

r25. Ritchie EA. Toxic psychoses under cortisone and corticotrophin. J Ment Sci 1956;*102*:830–37.

r26. Dale DC, Petersdorf RG. Corticosteroids and infectious diseases. In Azarnoff DL. Steroid Therapy. Philadelphia: WB Saunders, (1975); pp 209–222.

r27. David DS, Berkowitz JS. Ocular effects of topical and systemic corticosteroids. Lancet 1969;*2*:149–151.

r28. Javier EC, Reardon GE, Malchoff CD. Glucocorticoid resistance and its clinical presentations. The Endocrinologist 1991;*1*:141–148.

r29. New MI, Karaviti L. Congental adrenal hyperplasia. in Barden CW. Current therapy in endocrinology and metabolism Philadelphia: BC Decker, (1991); pp 144–150.

r30. Fauci AS. Alternate-day corticosteroid therapy. Am J Med 1978;*64*:729–731.

r31. Gillies G, Linton E, Lowry P. The physiology of corticotropin-releasing factor. In De Groot LW. Endocrinology, New York: Grune & Stratton, (1989); pp 167–175.

r32. Orth DN. Corticotropin-releasing hormone in humans. Endocrine Rev 1992;*13*:164–191.

r33. Kaye TB, Crapo L. The Cushing syndrome: an update on diagnostic tests. Ann Int Med 1990;*112*:434–444.

r34. Hale AC, Rees LH. ACTH and related peptides. In De Groot LW. Endocrinology, New York: Grune & Stratton, (1989); pp 369–376.

r35. Gilman AG. G proteins and regulation of adenylyl cyclase. JAMA 1989;*262*:1819–1825.

r36. White PC, New MI, Dupont B. Congenital adrenal hyperpasia. N Engl J Med 1987;*316*:1519–1524, 1580–1586.

r37. Sonino N. The use of ketoconazole as an inhibitor of steroid production. N Engl J Med 1987;*317*:812–818.

r38. Schteingart DE. Treating ADRENAL cancer. Endocrinologist 1992;*2*:149–157.

r39. Spitz IM, Bardin CW. Clinical applications of the antiprogestin RU 486. Endocrinologist 1993;*3*:58–66.

r40. Corval P, Claire M, Oklin ME, Geering K, Rossier B. Mechanisms of the antimineralocorticoid effects of spirolactones. Kidney Int 1981;*20*:1–6.

CHAPTER 45

Thyroid Hormones, Thyroid Stimulating Hormone (TSH), Thyrotropin Releasing Hormone (TRH), and Antithyroid Drugs

Mark C. Lakshmanan
Jacob Robbins

The hypothalamic-pituitary-thyroid system (Fig. 45.1) is an integrated organ complex providing for the regulated production of the thyroid hormones.[r1,r2] The cascade begins in cells of the supraoptic nucleus with secretion of a tripeptide, the thyrotropin releasing hormone (TRH). This neuropeptide passes down the pituitary stalk to the anterior pituitary gland, causing release of a polypeptide, the thyroid stimulating hormone (TSH), into the general circulation. TSH has both trophic and tropic effects on the epithelial cells of the thyroid follicles, and ultimately induces release of thyroxine (T_4) and triiodothyronine (T_3). This is preceded by accumulation of iodine, a trace dietary element, and iodination of a unique protein, thyroglobulin, which is first secreted into the follicle lumen and then taken from storage in the colloid back into the thyroid cell. There, thyroglobulin is hydrolyzed to liberate the hormones from the polypeptide chain. The final step in thyroid hormone synthesis occurs in peripheral organs, where thyroxine, the major secretory product of the thyroid gland, is converted to T_3 by enzymatic monodeiodination. Some of this T_3 enters the circulation to reach and affect other organs.

There is a feedback control between thyroid and pituitary in which both T_4 and T_3 suppress TSH secretion.[1] T_4 is the more important inhibitor, although it accomplishes this by conversion to T_3 within the pituitary.[2] Dopamine and somatostatin also are inhibitory at the pituitary level.

Patients with failure of the hypothalamic-pituitary-thyroid system at any level are treated with a preparation of thyroid hormone(s). The only exception is in the relatively rare cases of peripheral resistance to thyroid hormones. TRH and TSH are not used for replacement therapy but only for testing the system or to stimulate iodine accumulation in thyroid cancer in preparation for therapeutic radioiodine. Similarly,

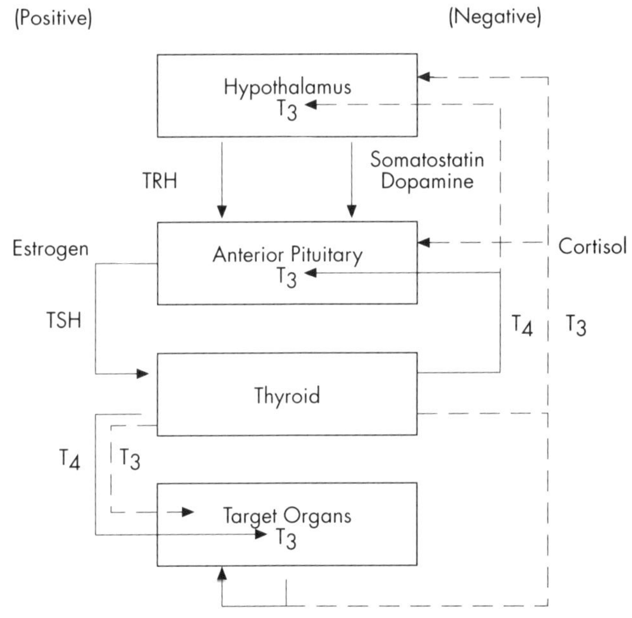

Figure 45.1 Hypothalamic-Pituitary-Thyroid System. Solid lines = major pathways; broken lines = minor pathways. Vertical lines = hypophyseal portal circulation; circuitous lines = peripheral circulation. Brain centers also impinge on the hypothalamus through various neurotransmitters.

overactivity is treated at the level of the thyroid gland with drugs that inhibit thyroid hormone production and/or secretion. For example, Graves' disease or diffuse toxic goiter, a common cause of thyroid overactivity, is an autoimmune disease often treated with agents that inhibit thyroid hormone production and/or destroy the gland's ability to synthesize and secrete thyroid hormone. Drugs that interfere with some thyroid hormone effects also are available.

Thyroxine and Triiodothyronine

Thyroid follicular cells produce the iodoamino acid hormones, T_4 and T_3, which occur naturally only as L-isomers. They are formed by the oxidative coupling of two iodinated tyrosine residues in thyroglobulin, a large protein molecule that constitutes the colloid of the thyroid follicles (Fig. 45.2). Thyroglobulin is reabsorbed and hydrolyzed, and T_4 and T_3 are released into the circulation in an approximate ratio of 10:1. While all T_4 is derived from the thyroid, 80 per cent of the body's T_3 is derived from peripheral conversion of T_4 to T_3.

Many structural analogues of the thyroid hormones have been synthesized, but efforts to separate effects such as cholesterol-lowering from tachycardia have not yet been successful. Thyroid hormones are critical for normal growth and development, are important in energy metabolism, and have a variety of effects on virtually every organ. Pharmacologically, therefore, they are used in hypothyroidism for thyroid hormone replacement. They are also used when clinically indicated to suppress pituitary TSH secretion.

Chemistry

T_4 and T_3 are iodinated derivatives of thyronine, a unique amino acid formed by post-translational modification of thyroglobulin (Fig. 45.2). After iodination and coupling of a limited number of tyrosyl groups, the polypeptide chain contains T_4, T_3, and inactive dehydroalanine residues derived from "donor" tyrosyls.[r3] Human thyroglobulin has 134 tyrosine residues of which only about 17 on the average are iodinated to form monoiodotyrosine or diiodotyrosine. The sites of iodothyronine formation from monoiodotyrosine and diiodotyrosine within the thyroglobulin molecule have been partially characterized. The donor and acceptor sites are not next to each other by primary sequence of the amino acids, but, owing to secondary and tertiary structure of the protein, they are in close proximity. Mature, iodinated thyroglobulin can be used medicinally, since the hormones are released by hydrolysis in the intestinal tract and probably elsewhere in the body as well. Because most of the soluble fraction of the thyroid gland consists of thyroglobulin, a simple or slightly purified thyroid extract is effective.

The pure hormones are obtained by chemical synthesis, usually as the sodium salt. Both are lipophilic, T_4 more than T_3, and minimally soluble in water at neutral pH. In alkaline aqueous solution they are more soluble and also more stable than in acid. The diphenyl ether bridge (see Fig. 45.3) has an angle of 110°, and the planes of the two phenyl rings are slightly twisted (minus 20° from perpendicular).[3]

The structure-activity relationships of substituted thyronines show that replacing the alanine side-chain by short-chain carbon acids, or changing the linkage between the phenolic rings from oxygen to methylene or sulfur, only slightly decreases pharmacologic potency.[r4] On the other hand, L-T_4 is ten times more potent then D-T_4, in which the side-chain is D-alanine. Phenolic ring substitutions cause significant changes in activity correlated with altered nuclear receptor affinity. In general, analogues lacking a 5′ group have greater affinity and potency. T_3, for example, is three to four times more potent than T_4. Active compounds have halogen or methyl groups at positions 3 and 5′, halogen, alkyl, or aromatic groups at positions 3′ or 5′; and a hydroxyl at the 4′ position.[4] The most active analogue is a 3′-isopropyl-3,5-diiodothyronine; the halogen-free analog, 3′-isopropyl-3,5-dimethylthyronine, is about one-fifth as active as T_3. The T_4 metabolite, 3,3′,5′-T_3 (reverse T_3, rT_3), on the other hand, is inactive. Biologic potency of thyroid hormone analogues correlates with their in vitro binding to nuclear receptors.[5]

History

The first recorded treatment of hypothyroidism was by a British surgeon, GR Murray, who in 1891 used injections of an extract of thyroid gland. Soon it became known that oral administration of thyroid preparations was also effective. Kendall in 1915 was the first to purify thyroxine from thyroid tissue, but not until 1926 was its structural formula elucidated by Harington. However, thyroxine did not account for all the metabolic activity in thyroid extracts, and triiodothyronine was discovered in 1952 by Gross and Pitt-Rivers. The higher potency of T_3 was quickly realized, and it was later shown that most circulating T_3 is derived from 5′ deiodination of T_4 in liver and other tissues. Brain and pituitary cells also have 5′ deiodinase activity, but this T_3 is used in the cells where it is generated. About one-third of the T_4 produced is converted to T_3, a similar amount is converted to the inactive reverse T_3 by 5-deiodinase.

Although the mechanisms whereby thyroid hormones affect their end-organs have not been fully elucidated, the discovery that nuclear receptors are the final common pathway for many of their actions has explained the delay of hours to days after administration before effects occur. The interaction with nuclear receptors was foreshadowed by the findings of Tata and Widnall in 1966 that RNA synthesis was increased by thyroid hormone. The next advance was the discovery by Oppenheimer et al., in 1972, of nuclear receptors that were highly specific and few in number. In 1986, Sap et al. and Weinberger et al. made the serendipitous and simultaneous discovery that the c-erb-A proto-oncogene gene product binds thyroid hormones specifically. Exactly how these interactions affect the transcription of DNA is currently under intensive study.[r5]

For more than 50 years, crude desiccated thyroid was the preferred treatment of hypothyroidism. Means, DeGroot, and Stanbury, in the 1963 edition of their textbook, stated for the first time that synthetic L-thyroxine "is the most generally satisfactory medication, and [we] now routinely prescribe it rather than desiccated thyroid." In part, this was because the USP standard for thyroid extract required only that it contain a fixed amount of iodine (between 0.17 to 0.23% by weight), and there were no specifications for metabolic potency. Even though extracts of beef or pork thyroid and purified hog thyroglobulin are commercially available and are now standardized for hormone content,[6] the preferred treatment of hypothyroidism today is with the synthetic hormones.

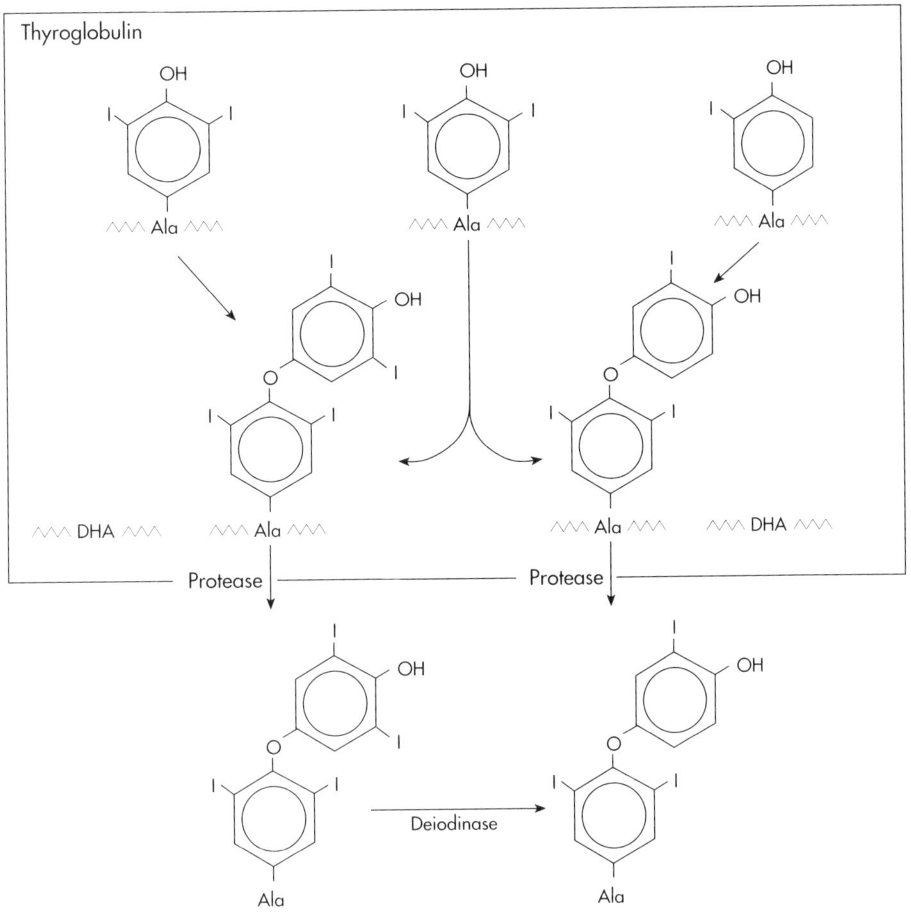

Figure 45.2 Formation of thyroxine (left) and 3,5,3′-triiodothyronine (right) by oxidative coupling of diiodotyrosine and monoidotyrosine residues in thyroglobulin, followed by proteolysis, release, and monodeiodination of thyroxine. Ala = alanine side chain, DHA = dehydroalanine.

Uses, Limitations, and Biologic Effects

Replacement therapy for hypothyroidism, one of the two major indications for giving thyroid hormone, is as obvious as it is effective. The second indication is suppression therapy for nodular thyroid disease and thyroid cancer and to prevent thyroid neoplasms following exposure to ionizing radiation. Based on the facts that thyroid cell division requires TSH and that excess thyroid hormone prevents TSH secretion, this use is theoretically sound; however, it is controversial. In recent prospective randomized studies of patients with solitary benign thyroid nodules, TSH suppression by levothyroxine for solitary, benign thyroid nodules did not alter nodule volume or diameter when compared to controls.[7,8,9] Although similarly controlled studies have not been carried out in thyroid cancer, the use of suppression therapy is generally still accepted for this indication. Both animal experiments and prospective studies on patients afford some support for this approach. The use of suppression therapy to prevent thyroid neoplasms following exposure to ionizing radiation remains controversial in part because of the effects of prolonged hyperthyroidism on skeletal mineralization (see below).[10,11] Finally, following the near-total thyroidectomy for nodular disease, the need for replacement thyroid hormone therapy is obvious; but even after partial thyroidectomy the prevention of enhanced TSH secretion is probably beneficial.

Thyroid hormones and some of their analogues lower serum cholesterol, but their use in hypercholesterolemia is limited by concomitant cardiac and metabolic effects. No thyromimetic agents have yet been found that can fully separate these effects. A controlled trial using D-T_4 was not completed because of unacceptable cardiac effects, including death. Nevertheless, the development of such an agent may be possible and is worth pursuing.

Even though thyroid hormones cross the placenta

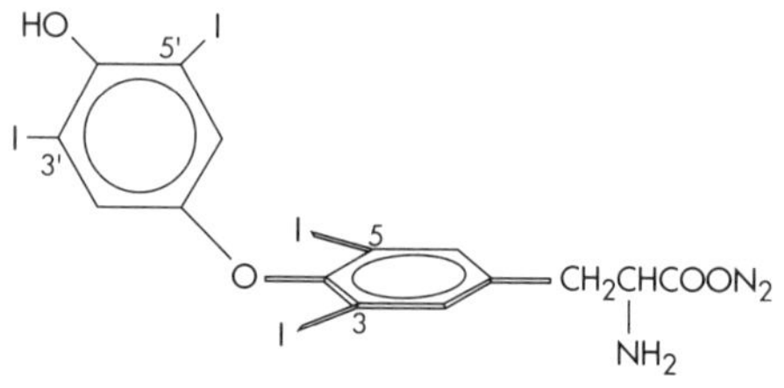

3, 5, 3', 5'–Tetraiodothyronine (Thyroxine, T_4)

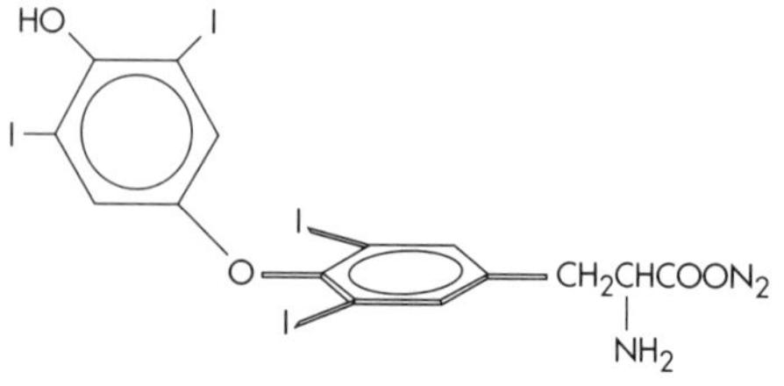

3, 5, 3'–Triodothyronine (Liothyronine, T_3)

Figure 45.3 Thyroid Hormones

only to a small extent,[12] maintaining their optimal replacement in the expectant mother is important for normal fetal development. Hyperthyroidism and hypothyroidism are associated with an increased frequency of spontaneous abortion; severe maternal hyper- or hypothyroidism may result in abnormal fetal development. Congenital hypothyroidism, whether endemic or sporadic, is a definite indication for early thyroid hormone replacement because irreversible defects in brain development will otherwise occur.[13,r6] For this reason, newborn screening for hypothyroidism is mandatory in many countries. Methods for detection and treatment of fetal hypothyroidism have not yet been perfected.

The use of thyroid hormones in euthyroid patients for weight reduction and to correct abnormalities of reproductive function such as menorrhagia or oligospermia is controversial and not recommended. Hyperthyroidism increases the appetite and is associated with cardiac arrhythmias and loss of lean body mass; elevated thyroid hormone has not been shown to reverse reproductive system abnormalities.

Thyroid hormones are essential for normal growth and development, particularly of the nervous system and skeleton. Lack of thyroid hormone in neonates leads to profound and irreversible changes known as cretinism.[13,r6] In the CNS, decreased neuronal interactions and a consequent decrease in neuropil, including decreased myelinization, may lead to mental retardation, spastic gait, strabismus, and occasionally to seizures. The bones and teeth are affected by a general delay in maturation involving ossification, epiphyseal unions, and dentition.

The stimulatory effect of thyroid hormones on the cardiovascular system is complex. Because of the increase in oxygen consumption in most tissues, there is an increase in cardiac output based on peripheral demand. Thyroid hormones also increase the number of beta-adrenergic receptors and, hence, increase the response of cardiac myocytes to catecholamines. Finally, thyroid hormones appear to increase cardiac myocyte contractility independent of catecholamines. The over-all effects of thyroid hormone absence are bradycardia, decreased cardiac output, and cardiomyopathy with dilatation. Hyperthyroidism has the opposite effects, may lead to high output cardiac failure, and causes tachycardia and arrhythmias.[14] The Qkd interval, the time between the initial wave of the QRS complex and the arrival of the systolic wave at the brachial artery, normally 200 milliseconds, is shortened in hyperthyroidism and increased in hypothyroidism. Because of the major effects of thyroid hormone on the heart when there is cardiac disease or when the hypothyroid state is of long duration or profound, therapy should be instituted gradually and monitored closely.

Before the availability of methods for measuring thyroid hormone in blood, the classic laboratory test of thyroidal status was the basal metabolic rate (BMR). This is estimated by measuring oxygen consumption under basal conditions, indexing this value to the body surface area, and reporting it as a percentage of normal for age and sex. While the BMR can be reliably performed and thyroid hormone excess or insufficiency has reproducible effects, the measurements are inconvenient and are affected by such other clinical states as febrile illness, pheochromocytoma, etc. The thyroid hormones increase oxidative metabolism in all but a few tissues (e.g., testes and ovaries). The calorigenic action is not fully understood but is dependent in part on increased synthesis of plasma membrane, Na^+–K^+ ATPase.[15,16] Enhanced ATPase activity seen in red blood cells, however, may not require new protein synthesis and may account for a substantial increase in the metabolic rate. Although high affinity binding sites had been found in mitochondria, and although pharmacologic doses of thyroid hormone cause uncoupling of oxidative phosphorylation, this mechanism's contribution to the calorigenic effect is uncertain.

Thyroid hormones do not alter oxygen metabolism in the adult brain, but hypothyroidism has profound but reversible effects on the mature nervous system. At its most profound it causes myxedema coma, a true medical emergency. Among the effects on higher cortical function is a decreased attention span that leads to impairment of short-term memory. Long-term memory is also impaired, with inability to recall and use vocabulary properly. Hyperthyroidism, however, does not improve memory. Hyperthyroid individuals are anxious, restless, and, even though tired, are unable to sleep, while hypothyroid individuals are usually complacent and somnolent. Muscle strength is decreased in hyperthyroidism; it is usually normal in hypothyroidism, but muscle cramps and stiffness (myalgias) are common and may worsen when replacement therapy is initiated. The characteristic slowing of the deep tendon reflex relaxation time in hypothyroidism can be used as a diagnostic tool although there is overlap with normal. Sensory changes are common in hypothyroidism: numbness; tingling; and painful paresthesias can result from nerve entrapment syndromes. These most commonly affect the median nerve at the carpal tunnel or the eighth cranial nerve.

Thyroid hormone replacement therapy increases calcium mobilization and bone remodeling in the mature skeleton, causing a net loss of calcium in urine; and hyperthyroidism is a risk factor for osteoporosis.[17] Because mild hyperthyroidism is associated with increased calcium loss,[18,r7] there is currently controversy concerning suppression therapy in nodular thyroid disease, which commonly involves women. It is important to maintain adequate calcium intake in such patients and to decrease other risk factors of osteoporosis.

Changes in facial appearance and in the integument are probably the most easily recognized diagnostic features of both hypothyroidism and hyperthyroidism. In the former, the face and in particular the eyelids are puffy and the tongue is swollen. These myxedematous changes, a nonpitting generalized edema, are the result of excessive production of hydrophilic ground substance in the subcutaneous tissues. Myxedema of the tongue, pharynx, and vocal cords leads to the husky, low-pitched voice. The eyelids appear to droop not only because of the myxedema but also from decreased sympathetic tone. This is the opposite of the lid retraction seen in hyperthyroidism, which is responsible for widening of the palpebral fissure, lid lag on upward or downward gaze, and a staring expression. These reversible changes occur in the absence of the infiltrative ophthalmopathy that may accompany Graves' disease.

The skin in hypothyroidism is thin, dry, cold, and pale. Occasionally, there is a pale yellow tinge, particularly in the palmar creases, due to alteration in the metabolism of beta-carotene. The hair becomes brittle, sparse, and coarse. In hyperthyroidism, in contrast, the skin is typically smooth, flushed, warm, and moist; the hair is fine, soft, and straight but tends to fall out easily. The nails grow slowly and are brittle in hypothyroidism, whereas in hyperthyroidism there is onycholysis. In its mildest form, the latter appears as "dirty nails" because the hyponychium is ragged.

Smooth muscle contractility is decreased in hypothyroidism, which may lead to decreased GI motility and urinary bladder atony. Anorexia, constipation, and distention are common symptoms. Conversely, increased appetite and hyperdefecation due to increased peristaltic activity are seen in hyperthyroidism.

Except for the developmental changes mentioned earlier, physiologic replacement levels of thyroid hormones reverse all of the effects of hypothyroidism. The only adverse effects occur when replacement therapy is too rapid, especially in severe hypothyroidism or in individuals with arterial sclerosis or myocardial disease. The increase in metabolic demands may exceed the cardiac capacity to respond. Overdosage of thyroid hormones, whether intentional as in suppression therapy or accidental, can lead to all the hyperthyroid symptoms and signs listed above. These include heat intolerance, nervousness, insomnia with fatigue, hyperdefecation, weight loss, increased perspiration, and the potentially dangerous cardiac effects. An acute overdose may warrant the use of gastric lavage and/or emetics followed by charcoal absorbents. Drugs that block thyroid hormone synthesis or release are not useful but beta-blockade and high dose glucocorticoids may be of benefit. If the offending agent contains thyroxine, a drug capable of inhibiting 5′-deiodinase activity, such as propylthiouracil or iopanoic acid, can be employed. Glucocorticoids and propranolol also have this effect.

Pharmacokinetics

Since thyroid hormones generally are administered by the oral route, the efficiency of their absorption from the intestinal tract is significant. T_3 is almost completely absorbed, but T_4 absorption does not exceed 80 per cent and may be considerably lower, depending on its formulation. Absorption can also be affected by food intake or drugs. Cholestyramine markedly decreases thyroid hormone absorption, and at least four to five hours should elapse between a dose of thyroid hormone and this drug. Recently, the effect of cholestyramine on thyroid hormone levels has been used to decrease the serum level of thyroxine in iatrogenic hyperthyroid patients awaiting urgent surgery.[r8] Iron sulfate has also been shown to decrease thyroxine absorption. Consistency in the brand of hormone that is used and the time of day it is taken may be required to overcome variations in therapeutic effect.

After entering the circulation and equilibrating with body pools, T_4 is distributed in a plasma equivalent volume of 10 L and normally disappears with a half-time of six to seven days. In contrast, T_3 is distributed in 40 L and has a half-life of one to two days. The hormone turnover is slowed in hypothyroidism and increased in hyperthyroidism. More than 99 per cent of circulating T_4 or T_3 is bound to plasma protein,[r9] the majority to thyroxine-binding globulin (TBG) and the remainder to prealbumin (transthyretin) and albumin. Only 0.03 per cent of T_4 and 0.3 per cent of T_3 are unbound in normal plasma, and biologic activity depends on the free T_4 and T_3 concentrations. These tend to remain constant in euthyroid individuals, whereas total plasma T_4 and T_3 vary with the concentration of binding protein (especially TBG) and the effect of drugs that compete for binding. The TBG concentration may be altered genetically[r10] or in response to physiologic (e.g., pregnancy)[r11] or pharmacologic (e.g., estrogen, phenytoin) determinants.[r12]

The thyroid hormones are conjugated, largely in the liver, to glucuronides and sulfates; but, because of enterohepatic recirculation, only approximately 20 per cent of thyroid hormone is excreted in feces as the conjugated compounds. The major metabolic fate is total deiodination. Intermediates resulting from the action of specific monodeiodinases, however, are of key importance. Approximately 35 per cent of T_4 entering the circulation is converted to T_3 in peripheral tissues by Type I and Type II deiodinases acting on the phenolic ring. This T_3 is in part available for delivery to other organs. The remainder is generated within cells as an intermediate in T_4 action, especially in the CNS and pituitary.[4] The large pool of T_4 in the body (approximately 800 μg) and its slow metabolism (approximately 10% of the T_4 pool per day) provides for the steady formation of T_3. In contrast, oral administration of T_3, superimposed on the low concentration in the circulation and its rapid clearance, results in major variations in blood levels and cellular entry, even when given in divided doses.

Preparations and Doses

Thyroid hormone preparations fall into four categories: synthetic T_4; synthetic T_3; mixtures of the two synthetic hormones; or natural products containing T_4 and T_3 (see Table 45.1). The latter are dried whole thyroid gland, or partially purified extracts containing thyroglobulin. For reasons discussed earlier, mainly the smoothness and reliability of the pharmacologic effect, the preferred therapy is synthetic T_4 (levothyroxine) as a single agent. Patients who have used thyroid tablets or thyroglobulin for many years and who are stable may be continued on this less expensive medication. Thyroid tablets are now required by the US Pharmacopeia to contain specified amounts of T_4 and T_3,[6] a more reliable index of potency than merely the previously required total iodine content.

Table 45.1 Thyroid Preparations

Generic Name	Substance*	Approximate Equivalent Doses	Some Brand Names
Levothyroxine	L-thyroxine sodium (T_4) - synthetic	100 μg	Synthroid Levothroid
Liothyronine	3,5,5′-triido-L-thyronine sodium (T_3) - synthetic	25 μg	Cytomel
Liotrix	$T_4 + T_3$ (4:1)	50 μg T_4 + 12.5 μg T_3 or 60 μg T_4 + 15 μg T_3	Thyrolar Euthroid
Thyroglobulin USP	Purified thyroid extract (porcine)	60 mg (contains 60 μg T_4 + 15 μg T_3)	Proloid
Thyroid USP	Dried thyroid (porcine)+	60 mg (contains 38 μg T_4 + 9 μg T_3)	Thyrar

*Almost all thyroid hormone preparations are supplied as tablets in a wide range of doses. Only Levothyroxine is available commercially for injection. Liothyronine for injection must be prepared by dissolving T_3 powder in dilute NaOH, and sterilizing by filtration (0.2 μm).
+ Some bovine thyroid preparations and some formulations other than the dried powder are available.

The quantitative assessment of thyroid hormone therapy is accomplished by measuring the concentrations of T_4, T_3, free T_4, and TSH in serum by immunoassay (see Table 45.2 for normal plasma values). Free T_4 assay is more subject to methodologic artifact than is total T_4, but it is not affected by variations in the binding proteins. Immunoassay of free T_4[r13] has largely replaced the standard but more complicated equilibrium dialysis method. Still in common use is the free T_4 index. In this test, ^{125}I-labeled T_3, test serum, and ion exchange resin are equilibrated, and the T_3 resin uptake is multiplied by the separately-determined total T_4. The normalized free T_4 index is proportional to the free T_4 concentration. The recently available supersensitive TSH immunometric assays[r14] can measure well below the lower limit of normal, and thus can differentiate between replacement and suppressive thyroid hormone therapy. Thus, it is no longer necessary to use the TRH stimulation test to assure complete TSH suppression.

Liothyronine (T_3) is occasionally preferred over levothyroxine when a quicker response or faster disappearance is desired, but the swings in T_3 blood levels are more likely to produce cardiovascular side-effects. Liotrix, a mixture of T_4 and T_3 comparable to that found in thyroglobulin USP, is equivalent in therapeutic effect to levothyroxine alone, because T_4 is converted to T_3 in peripheral tissues. Liotrix, therefore, offers no clinical advantage, even in athyrotic individuals.

The equivalent doses listed in Table 45.1 are only approximate because of variations in bioavailability. The proper use of all these agents requires that the effects be monitored by clinical response and laboratory testing. Levothyroxine from different sources and even within a given source can vary significantly in bioavailability.

Doses of levothyroxine used in replacement therapy are listed in Table 45.3. In young adults with mild to moderate hypothyroidism, who are otherwise in good health, therapy is initiated with nearly a full replacement dose. Until recently, 2.2 μg L-thyroxine per kg body weight was the recommended daily dose, but careful studies have shown this to be a slight overtreatment. Currently, 1.6 μg/kg is considered the average replacement dose.[19]

The first evidence of clinical benefit is diuresis with subsequent weight loss and decrease in puffiness, the time of onset depending on the initial level of thyroid hormone administered. Most of the other signs and symptoms regress over days to weeks, but hoarseness and the skin and hair changes may require months to resolve. The patient should be monitored for signs and symptoms related to thyrotoxicosis. Because loading with hormone is seldom used in uncomplicated hypothyroidism, steady state levels are not reached

Table 45.2 Plasma Concentrations in Normal Humans

Hormone	Reference Range
Total Thyroxine	5–10 μg/dl
Free Thyroxine	0.73–2.01 ng/dl
Total Triiodothyronine	40–181 ng/dl
Free Triiodothyronine	260–480 pg/dl
TSH	0.46–3.59 μIU/ml

Note: These values vary depending on the assay method; therefore, these ranges should be determined for the particular assay method used.

until four or more half-lives have elapsed. Therefore, laboratory assessments should be delayed until four weeks after initiation or change in dosage. An elevated TSH level indicates inadequate replacement, even when clinical assessments suggest euthyroidism and free T_4 is in the normal range. In patients with central hypothyroidism, of course, TSH levels cannot be used to monitor therapeutic effect.

Because bioavailability varies from brand to brand, the same preparation should be continued once a steady state has been achieved. Similarly, test results between laboratories may vary, even though standard assay kits are used. Finally, compliance with a chronic medication is imperfect even when as simple as one pill per day. Because the half-life of thyroxine is approximately one week, one can advise patients to count out the pills required for one week on a given day and to consume those remaining at the end of the week. Indeed, it is even possible to administer the full week's supply in a single weekly dose with good control and without adverse effects.

In elderly patients, or in those with severe hypothyroidism or associated heart disease, it is preferable to begin therapy at a lower level and to use smaller dose increments at longer intervals, as described in Table 45.3, because these patients are more sensitive to the hormone. Patients with possible adrenal insufficiency should have this assessed and corrected before beginning T_4 therapy.

The most extreme state of hypothyroidism is myxedema coma, recognized by mental obtundation and severe slowing of body func-

Tabld 45.3 Replacement Therapy with Levothyroxine

Initial Dose	**μg/d**	
myxedema coma	300–500 (IV)*	
young adult	100	
child > 10 yr	50	
child < 10 yr	25	
elderly	25	
severe hypothyroidism	25	
heart disease	12.5–25	
Dose Increment	**μg/d**	
usual	25 q 4–6 wks	
myxedema coma	75–100+	
child < 3 yr	12.5–25 q 2–4 wks	
elderly	12.5–25 q 6–8 wks	
severe hypothyroidism	12.5–25 q 6–8 wks	
heart disease	12.5–25 q 6–8 wks	
Maintenance Dose	**μg/kg/d**	**μg/d**
child < 6 mo	7–15	25–50
child 6–12 mo	6–10	50–75
child 1–5 yr	4–6	75–150
child > 5 yr	2–5	100–200
young adult	1.6++	100–150
elderly	< 1.6++	50–150
heart disease	< 1.6++	50–150

* Approximately 7 μg/kg body weight. May need to be repeated once.
\+ Maintenance dose beginning on 2nd or 3rd day.
++ Average maintenance dose.

tions. It is often precipitated by exposure to cold, infection, trauma (including surgical procedures), or CNS depressants. Because the mortality rate is high and delay in therapy worsens the prognosis, prompt and aggressive therapy, both specific and supportive, instituted before the results of laboratory tests are available, improve the patient's chances of survival.[20] Necessarily, this requires a high index of suspicion and clinical acumen in recognizing the triad of hypothermia, bradycardia, and hypotension. Initial thyroid hormone therapy should be administered IV because absorption in the GI tract or from IM or SQ sites is slow and unpredictable. Thyroxine should be given in one or more large doses, typically 500 μg, to replete circulating hormone levels and protein binding sites rapidly. Even though triiodothyronine has the advantage of quicker onset of action, the known deleterious effects on cardiac function and rhythm, and the fact that thyroxine therapy is effective, restricts its use in myxedema coma. Therapy should include "shock" doses of hydrocortisone administered IV every six hours (100 mg hydrocortisone), support of respiratory function, judicious administration of IV fluids until renal function normalizes, and passive preservation of body temperature. Search for and correction of the precipitating factor also should be performed.

When thyroid hormone therapy is used for suppression in the management of thyroid tumors, the objective is often complete suppression of serum TSH. This can be assessed by the ultrasensitive TSH immunoassay or by a blunted response to TRH, and usually is achieved with little or no symptoms of hyperthyroidism. The average dose of levothyroxine to produce this state of "chemical hyperthyroidism" is about 2.5 to 3 μg/kg/d.

Pediatric Therapy

Normal mental and physical development depends on the adequacy of treatment and the age of onset of the deficiency.[13] Most defects associated with cretinism can be prevented or minimized if therapy is begun shortly after birth. As in adult hypothyroidism, thyroxine is the medication of choice because of its long half-life and uniform potency. In neonates, therapy is usually initiated at 25 μg/d and increased by 25-μg increments until a total dosage of 7–15 μg/kg[21,22] is achieved in a period of weeks (see Table 45.3). Older children require less thyroxine per kilogram until about age 12 years, when normal adult dosages can be used. Therapy is monitored clinically by carefully observing that physical and developmental milestones are maintained and in the laboratory by measuring serum TSH and thyroxine levels. It should be noted that the TSH level may be mildly to moderately elevated when the child is euthyroid, apparently because the hypothalamic-pituitary system has not matured properly.[23] The free T_4 concentration is a better index of adequate replacement. If therapeutic efficacy is uncertain, radiologic examination for bone age may be of benefit.

Treatment in Pregnancy

During pregnancy, estrogen effects on the liver increase thyroxine-binding globulin serum levels until a plateau two to three times normal is reached in the second trimester.[r11,24] The thyroid, driven by TSH, increases its production of thyroid hormones to raise the serum T_4 concentration, while the free T_4 remains in the normal range. This causes, in many women, the benign goiter of pregnancy first recognized by the ancient Egyptians, who used it as a diagnostic test for pregnancy. Therefore, in hypothyroid patients who become pregnant, therapy may have to be altered in the first two trimesters.[25] Even though thyroid hormones do not freely cross the placenta,[12] the maintenance of optimal thyroid hormone replacement probably is important for normal fetal growth and development. Because signs and symptoms associated with pregnancy can simulate hyperthyroidism, clinical assessment is difficult. Frequent laboratory measurements may be required to keep the serum free T_4 and TSH levels in the normal range.

Indications and Contraindications For Using T_3

Because triiodothyronine has a rapid half-life, its onset and duration of action are short. Therefore, its plasma levels vary widely, and it is not as useful as thyroxine in chronic maintenance therapy. However, under certain circumstances its use is recommended. In the thyroid suppression test, 75–100 mg of triiodothyronine in divided doses is administered for one to two weeks, and TSH, T_4, and thyroid uptake of radioactive iodine are measured. In normal individuals, thyroid function should be suppressed, but not in hyperthyroid patients. This test can confirm the diagnosis of Graves' disease in individuals who are euthyroid. The syndrome of thyroid hormone resistance also can be evaluated in this way. T_3 is also used in patients with thyroid carcinoma who are maintained on suppressive doses of thyroxine and who are preparing for I-131 whole-body scanning. Thyroxine must be discontinued four to six weeks before I-131 is administered, but T_3, because of its short half-life, can be administered until two weeks before I-131 administration. Therefore, clinical hypothyroidism is prevented, except for the last two weeks before scanning. Its use requires care in individuals with cardiac disease.

When Liothyronine is used for suppression or replacement therapy, the only useful test is a serum TSH. The serum T_3 does not remain at a steady level because of the rapid turnover of T_3. T_4 and

T_3 levels achieved with the different thyroid hormone preparations at optimal dose levels also may vary, so that the TSH concentration is the best over-all criterion for monitoring therapy.

TRH and TSH

Thyroid stimulating hormone (TSH) and TSH-releasing hormone (TRH) have diagnostic but not therapeutic uses. TRH, a tripeptide released into the hypophyseal portal circulation by hypothalamic cells, stimulates the secretion of TSH from the pituitary. TSH, a glycoprotein consisting of two noncovalently linked polypeptides, stimulates the growth and function of the thyroid gland. While both can be used to test the integrity of the hypothalamic-pituitary-thyroid axis, TRH is more commonly used for this purpose. TSH occasionally is used to stimulate thyroid carcinoma metastases, particularly in hypopituitary patients prior to whole-body scanning with radioiodine.

Chemistry

The structure of TRH, L-pyroglutamyl-L-histidyl-2-proline amide (molecular weight 362) is identical in the human, porcine, and bovine species. Both terminal groups are blocked; the amino group of glutamic acid is cyclized with its gamma carboxyl, and the carboxyl group of proline is amidated.[26]

TSH is a glycoprotein heterodimer with a molecular weight of 28,000 to 30,000.[27] The alpha subunit, also present in pituitary LH and FSH and chorionic gonadotropin, has 89 amino acids, including 10 cysteine residues, all in disulfide linkage, and two carbohydrate chains attached to asparagine residues. Although the beta subunit is target-organ specific among this family of glycoprotein hormones, both subunits are needed for function. The TSH beta subunit has 112 amino acids and one asparagine-linked carbohydrate chain. The oligosaccharide units make up about 13 per cent of the TSH molecule, but their amount and their structures vary with the physiologic state. This heterogeneity is not fully understood, but the hormone's function and clearance rate depend on these N-linked sugars.

History

For their discovery of TRH, the first hypothalamic releasing factor to be identified, purified, and used clinically, Guillemin[28] and Schally[29] shared the Nobel Prize in physiology/medicine in 1977. Even though such factors, both positive and negative, had been predicted since the 1950s,[30] their discovery required the processing of enormous quantities of hypothalamic tissue and the application of sensitive, specific, and rapid assays. Synthesis of TRH in paraventricular and supraoptic chiasm nuclei of the hypothalamus from a precursor polypeptide and its storage in the median eminence have now been demonstrated, but TRH is also found in CNS sites other than the hypothalamus and in the endocrine pancreas. While its function outside the hypothalamic-pituitary axis is unknown at the present time, its clinical use is predicated on the well-documented stimulation of pituitary TSH and prolactin release[31] accompanied by few systemic effects.

TSH was discovered in the 1920s and 1930s along with the other pituitary hormones. Shortly after PE Smith demonstrated in the rat that hypophysectomy caused atrophy of the adrenals, thyroid, and gonads, Aron, Loeb, and Bassett in 1929 independently demonstrated that pituitary extracts reversed this effect in hypophysectomized guinea pigs. However, isolation of TSH and elucidation of its structure had to wait until more powerful methods of protein purification and more sensitive biologic assays became available. This achievement in 1969 by Pierce and colleagues was a culmination of 40 years of research by multiple investigators. Today, the complete amino acid and oligosaccharide structure is known.[r15]

Uses and Limitations

The use of TRH clinically is based on its stimulatory effect on both thyrotrophs and lactotrophs.[31] Even though TRH is very unstable in plasma, with a half-life of approximately five minutes, only a very small quantity is required to obtain a response. The TRH stimulation test[32] is performed by injecting 200 to 400 µg IV and sampling the serum TSH serially for up to one hour. The maximum response is elicited by 400 µg, usually occurs at 10 to 15 minutes, and averages 15 microinternational units/ml above baseline. In primary hypothyroidism, the TSH response is accentuated; in hyperthyroidism, the response is blunted because of the direct negative feedback of thyroid hormone on TSH secretion. Before ultrasensitive TSH assays were available, the TRH test was the only means to differentiate normal individuals with undetectable TSH levels from hyperthyroid patients. A blunted response also can result from pituitary failure. In hypothalamic insufficiency, however, the response to TRH may be quantitatively normal but the peak is usually delayed until 60 minutes. Although the test may not differentiate the precise cause of low TSH hypothyroidism, this is still the major use for the TRH test since it has been supplanted by the ultrasensitive TSH immunoassay in screening for thyrotoxicosis.

Because TRH has arousal, analeptic, and opiate antagonistic effects in the CNS, clinical research has been undertaken in patients with disorders in these areas. Results so far have been variable and inconclusive, perhaps in part because TRH crosses the blood-brain barrier slowly and has a short half-life in plasma. More stable analogues of TRH may, in the future, have therapeutic uses in depression, movement disorders, or as an opiate antagonist.

The TSH stimulation test of thyroid reserve was formerly a useful diagnostic test that utilized bovine TSH to distinguish primary hypothyroidism from secondary hypothyroidism. Today, the ease and dependability of serum TSH immunoassay has supplanted this time-consuming study, which required thyroid radioiodine uptake measurements before and after three days of daily hormone injection. Occasionally, the old test is useful in patients with toxic nodular goiter to verify the presence of normal paranodular tissue.

Although bovine TSH can be used in thyroid cancer to stimulate radioiodine uptake for detection and treatment of metastatic disease, the response to endogenous TSH is better. In addition, blocking antibodies are formed by repeated exposure to this foreign protein. In the rare thyroid cancer patient with coincident pituitary deficiency, however, bovine TSH is a useful agent. The same three-day regimen as in the TSH stimulation test is followed. Currently, recombinant human TSH is in clinical trials; when available it will supplant bovine TSH for these two indications.

Effects

The secretion of TSH is controlled primarily by the negative effects of thyroid hormones and the positive effects of TRH.[33] The action of TRH on thyrotrophs to release TSH from secretory granules and to synthesize new TSH is mediated by specific plasma membrane receptors. In response to TRH binding, intracellular calcium is mobilized to activate phospholipase C to give inositol 1,4,5-triphosphate. At the same time, production of diacyl glycerol activates protein kinase C.[r16] Cyclic AMP is also produced, but does not appear to be the second messenger for TRH action.[34] The number of receptors is decreased by thyroid hormones, which may also decrease the synthesis of TRH in the hypothalamus. TRH in nanomolar concentrations, the physiologic level in the hypophyseal portal system, is capable of inducing TSH release.

Mammotrophs also have specific, high-affinity receptors for TRH and respond to TRH by increasing the release and synthesis of prolactin.[31] Elevated thyroid hormone levels blunt this response while hypothyroidism enhances it, occasionally causing pathologic galactorrhea. The mechanism of action of TRH on mammotrophs is similar to that on thyrotrophs. These effects on TSH and prolactin release are the basis of the TRH stimulation test.

Because TRH is found in animals that lack pituitary gland in tissues as diverse as the cerebral cortex, the pineal, pancreatic islets, and the GI tract, it may have physiologic functions besides those on the pituitary. Pharmacologically, it has many effects on the CNS, including an increase in spontaneous motor activity, anorexia, hyperthermia, and protection from spinal shock.[r17] As mentioned above, none of these is clinically relevant, and their mechanisms of action are poorly understood. When used clinically in the usual test doses, the only systemic effects of TRH are transient and mild. They include a metallic taste, nausea, desire to micturate or defecate, chest tightness, dry mouth, and rarely a slight rise in blood pressure.

The action of TSH on thyroid follicular cells is mediated by binding to plasma membrane receptors followed by generation of cyclic AMP as the second messenger.[35] An increase in secretion of thyroid hormone occurs within minutes. Over time, all steps in the synthesis of thyroid hormone, including iodide uptake and organification, thyroglobulin synthesis, endocytosis, and proteolysis of colloid, are increased. There is also an increase in thyroid vascularity and in hypertrophy and hyperplasia of follicular cells, which eventually lead to the formation of a goiter. While many of the effects on follicular cells can be mimicked by cAMP, some actions may be mediated by the hydrolysis of phosphatidylinositol, which increases intracellular calcium through its product, inositol triphosphate.[36,37] TSH increases the hydrolysis of phosphatidylinositol independent of cAMP production. Adipocytes also have high-affinity receptors for TSH, but possible extrathyroidal physiologic effects of TSH are unclear. The major nonthyroidal effects of TSH are related to the fact that the only currently available form of TSH for medicinal use is bovine—and it is, therefore, a foreign protein. Although significant undesirable effects are rare, almost all patients develop discomfort at the injection site. Less common side-effects secondary to allergic reactions include nausea, vomiting, fever, urticaria, and even anaphylactoid reactions that may be fatal. Side-effects secondary to increased thyroid hormone secretion include angina or cardiac arrythmias. As with any foreign protein, antibody production may be induced by repeated exposure, increasing undesirable side-effects and decreasing the beneficial effects. It may be prudent to test with a small SQ dose before IM administration.

Pharmacokinetics

Even though TRH is effective in increasing TSH after oral or IM administration, the standard route is IV, and the standard dose is a single bolus of 400 μg/1.73m^2. Plasma and tissue TRH is rapidly metabolized to diamido-TRH, the cyclized metabolite, histidyl-proline-diketopiperazine, and then to the constituent amino acids. The plasma half-life is approximately five minutes, and is shortened in hyperthyroidism and lengthened in hypothyroidism. TSH may slow the degradation of TRH in hypothyroidism by inhibiting TRH amidase activity. TRH levels cannot be quantitated in peripheral plasma, in part because of high dilution in the systemic circulation and rapid degradation. In pharmacologic single doses from 6 μg to the maximum 400–500 μg, the amount of TSH secreted is correlated with the log of the TRH dose, as in most tropic hormone-target hormone interactions. Because TRH crosses the blood-brain barrier poorly, CNS uses may require intrathecal or intraventricular administration, but these uses are only experimental.

The half-life of native TSH, like other glycoproteins, is measured in hours and depends on the degree and type of glycosylation. Plasma levels normally follow a diurnal pattern, with the peak just prior to arising in the early morning and the nadir approximately 12 hours later. When bovine TSH is administered IM, the pharmacokinetics depend on absorption and immune phenomena. As with TRH, effects outlast measurable circulatory levels, and injections once daily will reliably stimulate the thyroid.

Preparations and Doses

Synthetic TRH (protireline) is available for IV use in 500-μg single dose vials. The proprietary names are Thypinone and Relefact-TRH. For the TRH stimulation test, 200 μg–500 μg is injected as an IV bolus. For children or small adults, the dose can be scaled to 7 μg/kg or 400 μg/1.73m² up to 500 μg total dosage.

Thyrotropin (thytropar) is available from bovine pituitary for IM or SQ administration in 10 international unit vials. For the thyroid stimulation test, baseline thyroid radioiodine uptake is measured. Then 10 international units are administered daily for one to three days, and the uptake measurement is repeated one day later. Three days of hormone administration should be used—especially for patients recently withdrawn or still taking thyroid hormones and for patients with suspected profound secondary or tertiary hypothyroidism. For the diagnosis and therapy of thyroid carcinoma, TSH is used only in those patients who lack a pituitary or an intact hypothalamic-pituitary axis because of the development of antibodies with repeated use. TSH is usually administered IM for three to seven days before ^{131}I is administered. Recombinant human TSH may eventually replace bovine TSH and make unnecessary the prolonged hypothyroid state presently needed to induce endogenous TSH production. Unlike growth hormone, TSH from human pituitary has not been used clinically; and is unlikely ever to be used because at least three individuals receiving growth hormone injections developed Creutzfeldt-Jakob disease.

Antithyroid Drugs

Strictly speaking, antithyroid drugs are agents that interfere with one of the steps in iodine metabolism, hormone formation, or hormone release by the thyroid gland (Fig. 45.4). Perchlorate and thiocyanate, drugs seldom used at present, inhibit the transport of iodide ion across the basal membrane of the thyroid follicular epithelium. Next are the more important inhibitors of iodide organification, the thiourylenes, and, finally, drugs that prevent secretion of the hormone: iodide and lithium ion. To these, we must add agents that destroy the integrity of the gland, i.e., radioactive isotopes of iodine, and monodeiodinase inhibitors that block the extrathyroidal production of T_3 from T_4. Still another group is represented by propranolol, agents that block thyroid hormone action at the target organ. These beta-adrenergic blockers are mentioned elsewhere and discussed more fully in Chapter 28.

The principal use of these drugs is in hyperthyroidism. Radioactive iodine also is used to destroy functioning thyroid nodules and thyroid cancer, to ablate residual thyroid tissue following surgical thyroidectomy, and for diagnostic studies. Perchlorate may be used in the diagnosis of defective organification, especially in congenital goiter. Other uses of iodide include protection of the thyroid gland against exposure to radioactive iodine and involution of the hyperemic thyrotoxic gland prior to surgery.

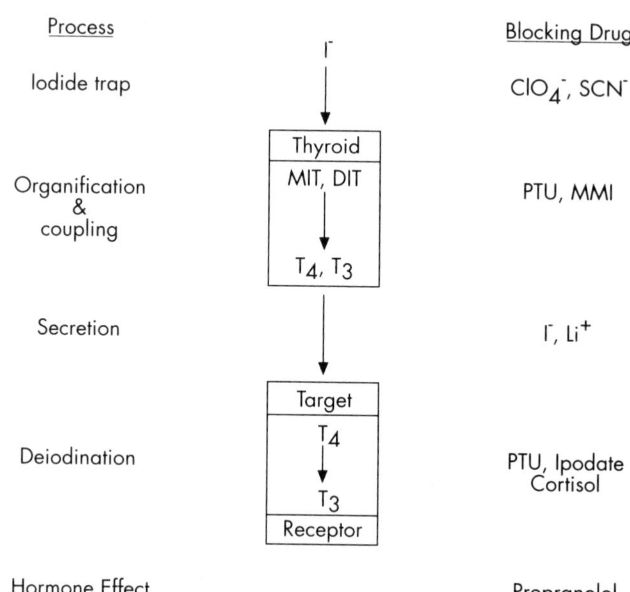

Figure 45.4 Sites of Action of Antithyroid Drugs

Iodine

The history and chemistry of stable iodine are covered in Chapter 61 on the nutritional pharmacology of microminerals. Very briefly, iodine was discovered by Courtois in 1812, its relationship to goiter was studied in Europe and the U.S. after 1819, and iodine deficiency was firmly established as a major cause of endemic goiter by 1920. Iodine in the thyroid gland was identified in 1895, and thyroxine was isolated in 1915 and its structure determined in 1926. Only nonradioactive, or stable, iodine (127I) is present in nature.

Uses, Limitations, and Mechanism of Action

Plummer is credited with the first report, in 1923, that iodide could reduce the thyrotoxicosis of Graves' disease in the perioperative period, thus introducing it as an antithyroid drug. At the present time, it is used only as an ancillary drug in the treatment of hyperthyroidism. Nevertheless, it has an important therapeutic role in several clinical situations: the preparation of patients with Graves' disease (diffuse toxic goiter) for thyroidectomy; the control of hyperthyroidism following low-dose ^{131}I therapy; the rapid control of thyrotoxicosis in thyroid storm (sudden onset of severe thyrotoxicosis as may occur after thyroid surgery); and in severe neonatal hyperthyroidism. It is also used to protect the thyroid gland against unwanted exposure to radioactive iodine, as in a nuclear reactor accident.

Before the advent of thiourylenes, iodide was the only drug available to reduce hormone secretion and thereby increase the safety of thyroid surgery. It does this by inhibiting hormone synthesis (the Wolff-Chaikoff effect),[38] and by inhibiting thyroid hormone release;[39] but the biochemical mechanism of neither of these actions is understood. Both effects occur rapidly and are incomplete (not more than 80 per cent). Both require high serum concentrations, although ingestion of as little as 1 mg of potassium iodide per day can block release. By comparison, approximately 100 μg of iodine is the minimum daily requirement to prevent goiter, approximately 500 μg per day is now the usual dietary intake in North America,[40] and 2–4 mg per day is consumed when iodine is used to purify water. Inhibition of synthesis may be transient (escape from the Wolff-Chaikoff effect) because a homeostatic mechanism within the gland decreases iodine trapping, thus lowering intracellular iodide below the required concentration.

The net result is to lower the serum T_4 and T_3 concentrations, beginning within 24 hours and reaching a minimum within a few days to a week or two. This rapid response depends mainly on inhibition of secretion, since even complete blockade of synthesis does not lower the serum level until the store of hormone within the gland is depleted.

It is the rapidity of the response that gives iodide an advantage in treatment of thyroid storm. Because the effect is transient and incomplete, however, a thiourylene drug is added to insure that synthesis is completely inhibited. This avoids the formation of a large quantity of hormone from the administered iodide. The sequence of administration is important: the thiourylene first, followed by iodide after an interval of one hour. An exception is when iodide is used to control hyperthyroidism after treatment with radioiodine, since the damaged gland is more sensitive to iodide and less likely to escape. In this setting, the usual dose of potassium iodide will often cause hypothyroidism, but this can be reversed by lowering the dose.

When used to protect the thyroid against unwanted radioiodine exposure, iodide is given at least 30 minutes and not more than 12 hours in advance (or at any time if exposure continues). The protective effect is derived mainly from saturation of the iodide trap and dilution of the radioisotope. The optimal dose, 130 mg potassium iodide or 100 mg iodine, reduces radioiodine uptake by at least 90 per cent and must be given daily.

When taken chronically, as little as 2 mg potassium iodide in children and 5 mg potassium iodide in adults will provide a comparable blockade after several weeks of administration. When iodide is used for a patient with diffuse toxic goiter for thyroidectomy, the inhibition of secretion results in retention of colloid within the follicles, and there is an involution of the cellular hyperplasia. This results in a less friable gland, making surgical manipulation much less difficult. In addition, there is a decrease in vascularity, so that bleeding is less of a problem. The biochemical mechanism(s) of these effects is also obscure.

Adverse Effects

Serious toxic effects of iodine occur very rarely. Susceptible individuals, such as those with hypocomplementemic vasculitis, may develop a serum sickness type syndrome with angioedema and hemorrhagic skin lesions. Less rare but less severe reactions include acneform skin lesions, sialoadenitis, coryza, conjunctivitis, and a metallic taste. Individuals with autonomous thyroid function, as in some cases of nodular goiter, may become hyperthyroid when given excess iodide. In areas of iodine deficiency, this is known as Jod-Basedow disease. A thyroid gland damaged by prior radiation or inflammation may be oversensitive to the blocking effects of iodine, leading to hypothyroidism.

Pharmacokinetics

Absorption of an oral dose of iodide is from the small intestine, and excretion is mainly renal, where the iodide is filtered but not secreted. Iodine intake can be evaluated by measuring the iodide: creatinine ratio in a random urine sample, although large day-to-day variations are common in areas of iodine sufficiency.[41] Several tissues other than the thyroid possess an iodide trapping mechanism closely related to that in the thyroid epithelium. These include the salivary glands, gastric mucosa, and the lactating mammary gland. They maintain an iodide concentration ratio of 20:1 to 60:1 in equilibrium with plasma iodide, which decays with a half-time of about eight hours. The ciliary body of the eye and the choroid plexus of the cerebrospinal space also transport iodide, but in the direction of the plasma.

Preparations and Doses

Two oral preparations are the most common dosage forms. Potassium iodide solution USP (saturated solution of KI, SSKI) contains one gram KI per milliliter and approximately 20 mg per drop. A calibrated dropper should be used; the viscous solution gives small diameter drops compared with water. Strong iodine solution USP (Lugol's solution) contains 5 per cent I_2, 10 per cent KI, and approximately 7 mg iodine per drop. For IV use, 10 per cent NaI is given by infusion. Although approximately 6 mg of KI probably is sufficient to control hyperthyroidism in most cases, the amount needed to bring about thyroid gland involution in the usual 10-day preoperative treatment period is not well defined. The customary dosage is much greater than 6 mg, and different amounts are used for different clinical indications. For treatment of hyperthyroidism, one drop of SSKI or three to five drops of Lugol's solution are given three times per day. When used after radioiodine treatment, the dose is titrated to obtain the desired effect. For thyroid storm, 0.5 to 1 gram NaI per day is given IV.

To protect the thyroid from radioiodine acutely, an optimal dose of 130 mg KI has been well characterized. It should be started not more than 12 hours before exposure and continued daily as long as required. Protection can also be achieved by giving 5 mg KI per day chronically, but requires several weeks to become effective. The ideal dosage form is in tablets that can be individually sealed and protected from light for convenient storage.

Radioactive Iodine and Technetium

Chemistry and Other Properties

Although several radioactive isotopes of iodine are available for diagnostic use, only two, ^{131}I and ^{125}I have been used for therapy. They are listed in Table 45.4. Others could be made available and might have desirable properties, such as improved tumor-to-body radiation exposure in thyroid cancer, or positron emission for tomographic scanning. Except for their differing emission properties, all iodine isotopes are chemically identical to ^{127}I.

Technetium-99m in the form of pertechnetate (TcO_4^-) is a popular diagnostic agent because of its low radiation dose coupled with emission properties that are excellent for imaging. TcO_4 is concentrated in the thyroid by the I^- trap but is not organified and leaves the gland in parallel with the fall in serum concentration. An iodine isotope must be used instead of $^{99m}TcO_4^-$ when organification is to be evaluated. ^{123}I is preferred over $^{131}I^-$ for use in imaging because of the lower radiation dose received by the thyroid. It also permits study at a later time than TcO_4^- (up to 24 hours).[42,43]

^{132}I is not commercially available at present in the US. ^{125}I and ^{131}I will be discussed below.

History

The first radioactive isotopes of iodine were produced by Fermi in 1934 by neutron bombardment. The first therapeutic medical use was in 1942, when ^{130}I produced in the cyclotron was employed by Hertz and Roberts and by Hamilton and Laurence for the diagnosis and treatment of hyperthyroidism. In 1946, when fission products from nuclear reactors became available in the US, ^{131}I was substituted for ^{130}I, and, because of its easy availability, longer half-life, and desirable emission properties, soon came into widespread usage. Beginning in 1969, another fission product, ^{125}I, generated much interest. The short path length of its low energy beta emissions originating in the colloid was expected to favor destruction of function in the apical region of the columnar epithelial cells of Graves' disease without damaging the basally located nuclei. This interesting hypothesis failed to materialize, and ^{131}I is now the only iodine isotope used in clinical practice.

Uses, Limitations, and Mechanism of Action

The goal of ^{131}I therapy is to deliver enough radiation to damage the thyroid cells. The intended extent of damage varies with the disease under treatment. In diffuse toxic goiter, the aim is to destroy enough function to restore euthyroidism but not enough to induce hypothyroidism. In toxic nodular goiter, the goal is to destroy the nodule(s) almost completely. In thyroid cancer, whether for ablation of thyroid remnant or treatment of recurrent or metastatic cancer, complete destruction is intended. Most of the radiation damage is produced by the beta particles, which have a range of 0.4 to 2 mm in tissue. This allows a more uniform effect than would otherwise be the case, since distribution of iodine among the thyroid follicles is irregular.

Radioiodine therapy of toxic goiter is widely available, easy to use, and relatively safe. Except for occasional exacerbation of hyperthyroidism, which is potentially serious in cardiac patients, there is no important acute toxicity. No induction of thyroid neoplasia has been documented, apparently because the cells undergo lethal rather than tumorigenic mutation. Deleterious effects of whole-body radiation, especially leukemia induction and germ cell mutation, are valid theoretically but have not been demonstrated. Potential damage to a fetus, however, is well recognized and obviously must be avoided. The danger to the fetus varies with the stage of pregnancy. The fetal thyroid gland is not subject to damage until the fourth month, when it begins to function. In the first trimester, a radiation dose to the fetus exceeding 5–10 rads increases the risk of nonthyroid developmental abnormalities. The usual treatment in toxic goiter, however, does not reach this level.

The major complication of ^{131}I therapy is the induction of hypothyroidism. The occurrence of early thyroid failure is dose-dependent, and may be acceptable

Table 45.4 Radioisotopes of Iodine (and Technetium) Used in Clinical Medicine

Isotope	Production	Chemical Form	Half-life	Major Emissions	Clinical Use
123_I	cyclotron	I^-	13 hr	γ	diagnosis
125_I	reactor	I^-	60 d	γ (low energy)	therapy
131_I	reactor	I^-	8.1 d	γ + β	diagnosis and therapy
132_I	reactor[a]	I^-	2.3 hr	γ + β	diagnosis
$99m_{Tc}$	reactor	TcO_{4-}	6 h	γ	diagnosis

[a]Derived from a Tellurium-132 generator ($t\frac{1}{2}$ = 77h)

when there is a need for early resolution of the toxic goiter. Late development of hypothyroidism is a characteristic of Graves' disease, regardless of the method of treatment, but radiation may increase the risk.[44] Whereas in treating toxic goiter, the limiting factor is the desired amount of thyroid destruction, in thyroid cancer ^{131}I dose is restricted by the toxic effects of whole-body radiation. Repeated high-dose radiation to the bone marrow can induce leukemia or irreparable bone marrow failure. In addition, treatment of miliary pulmonary carcinomatosis can result in respiratory failure if the radiation dose to the lung is excessive. Ablation of a thyroid remnant, especially when it retains the thyroid capsule, can cause painful radiation thyroiditis. Although there may be significant swelling, the airway is not usually compromised. Because almost all of the beta ray energy of ^{131}I is absorbed within the thyroid tissue, there is no significant damage to such surrounding tissues as the parathyroid glands. The exception is in miliary lung metastases, where the volume of the minute tumors is insufficient to absorb all the beta rays.

Pharmacokinetics

Even the largest dose of ^{131}I used for therapy is a trace quantity compared with dietary iodine. Consequently, the distribution and disposition of the isotope depends on the existing state of iodine metabolism. Since the therapeutic effect is proportional to the concentration of ^{131}I in the tissue, integrated over time, the rate of loss of the isotope is an important parameter. In the normal thyroid, the secretion rate is very slow ($t_{1/2}$ approximately 90 days), so that the disappearance of the isotope is governed by its eight-day half-life. In the toxic thyroid, the average biologic half-life is 20 days, and the combined or effective half-life is six days ($1/t_{eff} = 1/t_{biol} + 1/t_{I\text{-}131}$).

In some cases, however, the biologic half-time may be as rapid as two to three days, and thus becomes the determining factor in the residence time of the isotope. In thyroid cancer, the average biologic half-time is six days, and may be as rapid as two days. This is obviously an important factor in determining therapeutic effect.

Since the radiation dose is proportional to the integrated concentration of ^{131}I, it is obvious that, in addition to the rate of secretion, the volume of the gland or tumor and the maximum uptake are important factors. The maximum uptake is determined by the balance between the rate of uptake (which is always rapid), the ability of the tissue to organify iodine, and the rate of secretion. In the normal and toxic thyroid, iodide trapping is rate-limiting for the uptake of iodine, but in thyroid cancer the ability to organify may be the rate-limiting factor. The relation of the size of the iodide pool (i.e., iodine intake) to the amount of uptake is complex. Rapid fluctuations in iodide intake do not affect the uptake rate unless intake is high enough to dilute the isotope or saturate the iodide trap effectively. When the change in iodide intake persists for one to two weeks, homeostatic mechanisms within the normal thyroid gland tend to maintain a constant "absolute" rate of uptake (i.e., μg/d).

Preparations and Doses

The fission product, ^{131}I, is supplied as carrier-free Na^{131}I in solution or absorbed in gelatin capsules. The cyclotron product, ^{123}I, is supplied as NaI in solution for diagnostic use only. Their use in the US is restricted to physicians authorized by the Nuclear Regulatory Commission, and generally is carried out in nuclear medicine departments. Both agents have limited shelf life because of isotope decay. In addition, ^{123}I is not isotopically pure, and in a relatively short period will contain amounts of longer-lived isotopes that alter its chemical and safety properties.

As already stated, the therapeutic dose of ^{131}I varies according to the disease being treated, the goal of the treatment, and safety considerations. In addition, medical opinion is divided as to goals and procedures. In diffuse toxic goiter, the usual aim is to control the hyperthyroidism while preserving a normal amount of thyroid function. To minimize the incidence of hypothyroidism, a dose of 80 μCi in the gland per gram of tissue may be used.[45] The dose given orally is determined from the percent uptake at 24 hours and the estimated weight of the gland. For example, the oral dose is 5 to 6 mCi, if the gland is twice normal size and the 24-hour uptake is 50 per cent. Refinements of this technique include measurement of ^{131}I secretion rate to adjust for variations in this parameter and measurement of gland volume by three-dimensional imaging. If the combined biologic and physical half-time is average (i.e., 6 days), 80 μCi per gram will give approximately 7000 rads to the thyroid gland. Since control of hyperthyroidism is slow, adjuvant therapy with iodine, a thiourylene drug, or propranolol is required until the radiation takes effect. The ^{131}I dose is repeated if necessary after about six months. If the goal is to maximize early control of hyperthyroidism while still attempting to preserve thyroid function, a dose of 120 μCi per gram in the gland (approximately 12,000 rads) may be given. If the goal is to destroy thyroid function completely, a dose of 300 μCi per gram in the gland (approximately 27,000 rads) may be given. The latter may be more than required to destroy a diffuse toxic goiter, but it is the correct dose to destroy a toxic nodule and reduce the size as well as to control its function. Even in low-dose therapy[44] (80 μCi per gram) and in treatment of a solitary toxic nodule, it is important to test for hypothyroidism, which may develop in Graves' disease at the rate of approximately 2 per cent per year. Early onset of hypothyroidism occurs in about 10 per cent of patients with low-dose therapy and about 20 per cent of patients treated with a medium dose (120 μCi per gram). Late onset hypothyroidism may occur in any patient with Graves' disease, regardless of therapy, and requires continuous vigilance.

In thyroid cancer, ^{131}I therapy may be divided into three categories: ablation of normal thyroid remnant after initial thyroidectomy;[46] treatment of residual or recurrent thyroid cancer in regional lymph nodes or the thyroid bed; and treatment of metastases in lung, bone, or other organs.[47] In the US, where dietary iodine is relatively high and uptake is low, thyroid remnant ablation with a single dose of ^{131}I usually requires an oral dose of 100 mCi.[48] To minimize whole body radiation in young individuals with low risk papillary thyroid cancer, a dose of 30 mCi may be given. This can be done without hospitalization but requires repetition in about two-thirds of cases.

To treat residual cancers, cervical lymph node metastases, especially in low risk patients, 150 mCi may be given and repeated in six-month intervals if imaging shows persistent uptake. This dose is safe if there is no bone marrow depression from accumulated radiation.

To treat distant cancer metastases, larger doses are given, usually between 200 and 300 mCi. These doses may be empirical, with attention to possible lung damage from radiation of miliary pulmonary metastases; or they may be based on predicted whole body radiation calculated from a diagnostic study of ^{131}I retention. When such calculations are made, doses even greater than 300 mCi may be safely given.

Lithium

Chemistry and History

Lithium is the third element, an alkaline metal with atomic weight 6.9. Various lithium salts had been used medicinally since the late 19th century; but, in 1948, Cade, an Australian psychiatrist, accidentally discovered the antimanic effects of lithium ion. Its subsequent extensive employment in psychiatry was pioneered by Schou in Denmark, who also reported in 1968 that patients receiving lithium carbonate sometimes developed goiter and hypothyroidism. In 1968, Sedvall and colleagues suggested, on the basis of clinical studies, that the action of lithium was to impair the release of thyroid hormone from the thyroid gland.

Uses, Limitations, and Mechanisms of Action

At high drug levels, reached only in animal studies, lithium blocks thyroid iodine metabolism at multiple sites. In normal therapeutic usage, however, the dominant effect is to slow the release of hormone from the gland.[49] Lithium is the only agent other than iodide with this action. Unlike iodide, of course, lithium cannot serve as a substrate for hormone synthesis. This affords lithium a unique role as an adjuvant in radioiodine therapy in that it potentiates the effectiveness of the isotope without interfering with iodine uptake. This is a trivial advantage in treating hyperthyroidism since the same effect is achieved by increasing the dose of radioiodine. In thyroid cancer, however, where radiation to the bone marrow is limiting, there is a distinct potential advantage. This has been demonstrated in a number of cases, but its therapeutic utility is still under investigation.[r18] Lithium can enhance the radioiodine effect only if the half-time of release of thyroid iodine is short relative to the eight-day half-life of ^{131}I. This is the case in most thyroid cancers, but only in the minority of toxic goiters.

As an independent therapeutic agent in treating hyperthyroidism, lithium[50] has the same potential role as iodide, without the danger of supplying substrate for hormone synthesis. Its blockade of hormone release is also incomplete, but the actions of lithium and iodide are additive. This can be used to advantage in treating thyroid storm, but the potential toxic effects of lithium require caution. For the same reason, lithium is not a preferred therapeutic agent unless other drugs cannot be used.

Lithium has many effects on other tissues. A secondary action on the thyroid system is to slow the metabolic clearance of thyroxine from the circulation. This is seen in hyperthyroid but not in euthyroid subjects. Lithium interferes with the action of antidiuretic hormone on the kidney, causing increased water excretion; it also increases the production of granulocytes. Its potentially serious toxic actions are on the cardiovascular and nervous systems, causing arrhythmias and A-V block, confusion, and other neurologic symptoms, including seizures and coma. These occur at high serum levels and are avoided by monitoring the serum lithium level, particularly in the setting of renal failure.

The mechanism by which lithium blocks thyroid hormone release is unknown, except that it interferes with the response to TSH and cyclic AMP.[51] In normal subjects, the incomplete blockade coupled with continued hormone synthesis allows recovery from hypothyroidism to occur when the intrathyroid hormone pool increases sufficiently. This recovery does not usually occur in a toxic goiter or in a thyroid gland damaged by autoimmune thyroiditis or radiation.

Pharmacokinetics

Orally administered lithium ion reaches a peak blood level in two to four hours and disappears with an initial half-time of 12 to 24 hours and then more slowly. With a constant daily intake, equilibrium is reached in five to six days. Lithium is widely distributed in the body, substituting as a cation for sodium and potassium, and is reabsorbed by the kidney proximal tubule. It is selectively concentrated by the thyroid gland. Serum levels are measured by flame photometry.

Preparations and Doses

Lithium carbonate is given so as to maintain a serum concentration between 0.6 and 1.2 mEq/L, above which toxic side-effects are likely to occur. This level is similar to that used in psychiatric therapy. Administration usually begins with an oral loading dose of 600 mg, followed by 300 mg three or four times per day. The serum level is measured on a morning specimen obtained before the dose is given.

Thiourylenes

Chemistry

Although a large number of compounds are capable of inhibiting thyroid hormone synthesis, including thioamides, aniline derivatives, polyhydroxyphenols, and others, those used as therapeutic agents are cyclic derivatives of thiourea (Fig. 45.5). One, 6-n-propyl-2-thiouracil (propylthiouracil, PTU) is a less active and less toxic analogue of 2-thiouracil in humans, although it is ten times more active than 2-thiouracil in the rat. The second, 1-methyl-2-mercaptoimidazole (methimazole, MMI), is 50 times more active than PTU in man and only two times more active in the rat. The third, 1-methyl-2-thio-3-ethoxycarbonylimidazole (carbimazole, CMI), is rapidly converted to MMI in the body.[52] PTU is a pyrimidine derivative, freely soluble in dilute alkali while MMI and CMI are imidazoles, the former being freely soluble in water.

History

The identifications of substances having antithyroid activity dates from the chance observation of goiter developing during experiments with animals. In 1928 Chesney, et al., found goiters in rabbits on a diet of cabbage. In 1936 Hercus and Purves demonstrated goitrogen activity in seeds of the cabbage family. The causative agent was not identified, but in 1949 a goitrogen in the seeds of cruciferous plants was identified by Astwood, et al. This sulfur-containing compound, progoitrin, releases L-5-vinyl-2-thiooxazolidone, a cyclic thioamide. In 1941 McKenzie, et al., showed that goiter was caused by the antibiotic sulfaguanidine; and in 1942 Richter and Clisby in their studies on taste produced goiter with phenylthiourea. The following year, Astwood showed that inhibition of thyroid hormone synthesis was a common property of these goitrogens and that formation of the goiter resulted from the unopposed action of increased pituitary TSH. He went on to study a large number of unrelated compounds and to test their activity in humans, and ultimately in patients with thyrotoxicosis.

Uses, Limitations, and Mechanisms of Action

Thiourylenes are the major drugs currently used in the management of thyrotoxicosis, either alone or in combination with other treatment. They act by inhibiting the formation of thyroid hormones within the gland, and have no effect on iodide trapping or on hormone secretion. The mechanism is by inhibiting thyroid peroxidase,[53] a membrane-bound enzyme responsible for the iodination of tyrosines as well as the coupling of these iodotyrosines within the thyroglobulin molecule. The degree of inhibition is dose-related, allowing for a gradation of effect from complete blockade to restoration of a normal rate of hormone production. Also, the iodotyrosine coupling reaction[54] is more sensitive to the drugs than iodotyrosine formation, so a complete block of iodide organification is not required for significant inhibition of hormone synthesis.

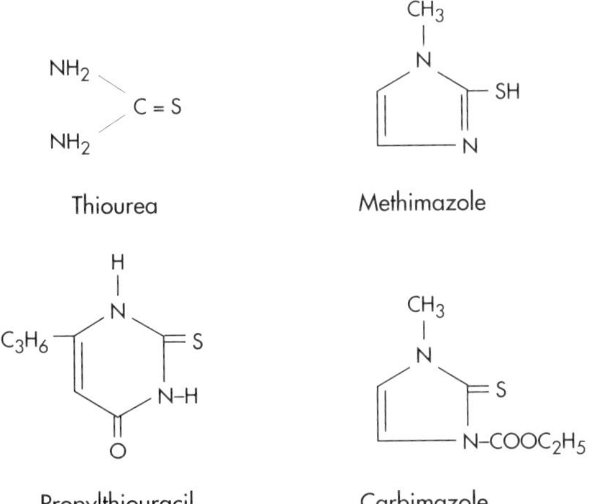

Figure 45.5 Antithyroid Drugs

For this reason, the use of perchlorate discharge to test for adequacy of blockade is only partially successful. Since secretion is not affected, control of hyperthyroidism is delayed until the preformed hormone pool in the gland is depleted. In a normal individual it could take months for the serum hormone level to fall, but in toxic goiter this begins within days and usually plateaus within a few weeks on a given dose. For more rapid control, it is necessary to add an agent that blocks secretion such as iodide or lithium. If iodide is used, it is important to initiate therapy with a dose of thiourylene that completely inhibits iodination in order to prevent potential synthesis of new hormone from the large load of substrate.

An additional pharmacologic action of some thiourylene derivatives can assist in controlling the thyrotoxic state. PTU,[55] but not MMI, inhibits the monodeiodination of thyroxine in peripheral tissues, leading to a decrease in formation of the active hormone, triiodothyronine. Although this effect is believed to be less important than the decrease in hormone synthesis by the thyroid gland, advantage is taken of this additional action in treating very severe thyrotoxicosis. Another drug that blocks the 5′-monodeiodinase, ipodate or iopanoic acid, can also be employed.

The thiourylenes are equally effective in diffuse or toxic nodular goiter, but of course are ineffective when hyperthyroidism is caused by thyroid destruction (e.g., in the thyrotoxic state of thyroiditis) rather than by increased hormone synthesis. In many patients, long-term control is achieved easily with low or moderate doses; and, after a year or so, about one-third to one-half of patients with Graves' disease will undergo spontaneous remission to euthyroidism.[56] There is some evidence that thiourylenes may hasten the remission by interfering with the production of thyroid stimulating immunoglobulin. If a remission does not occur, the decision can be taken to continue drug therapy or to use radioiodine or surgical ablation. Despite considerable effort, no fully reliable method to predict remission has been found. One possible technique is to demonstrate the return of suppressibility of radioiodine uptake when T_3 or T_4 is given, an indication that thyroid stimulating antibodies have disappeared. Another indication of remission is a decrease in the size of goiter. An enlarging gland, on the other hand, may only indicate an overdosage of thiourylene, resulting in pituitary TSH oversecretion. The goiter will then decrease when the dose is reduced or when thyroid hormone is administered.

An important use of the thiourylenes is to prepare the thyrotoxic patient for thyroidectomy. This is a reliable way to restore euthyroidism, and greatly reduces the hazard of perioperative thyroid storm. Iodide is added for ten days prior to surgery in order to involute the gland and thereby simplify the surgical procedure. In radioiodine therapy, pretreatment with thiourylene is used only when the hyperthyroidism is very severe; this may prevent an exacerbation following the radiation. The drug is discontinued 72 hours before ^{131}I is given to allow recovery of iodine organification. A more common use is in the period following low-dose radioiodine therapy in order to control the thyrotoxicosis until the radiation takes effect.

Pharmacokinetics

Both PTU and MMI are rapidly absorbed after oral administration, and inhibition of thyroid iodine organification begins within 20 to 30 minutes.[r19] The disappearance of PTU from plasma ($t_{1/2}$ is approximately 2 hours) is much faster than that of MMI ($t_{1/2}$ is 6 to 13 hours), both being recovered mainly in the urine. In pregnancy, the portion of PTU that crosses the placenta is one-tenth that of MMI. Both drugs are secreted in milk.

PTU and MMI are accumulated by the thyroid gland and are retained there longer than in the plasma. After administration of carbimazole, the thyroid contains only MMI (and other metabolites). The duration of action of PTU is considerably shorter than that of MMI. Following a single 10-mg of dose of MMI, almost complete blockade of organification of iodine persists for more than 12 hours in euthyroid subjects and for more than eight hours in most hyperthyroid subjects, whereas by eight hours after 100 mg PTU organification is only about 60 per cent inhibited.

Adverse Effects

Most toxic reactions to a thiourylene occur within two months of the beginning of therapy. The majority, affecting two to five per cent of patients are mild and include skin rash, urticaria, itching, loss of hair, and other rare events.[r19] They often are transient despite continued therapy. More severe reactions occur in two to three per 1000 patients. The most serious is agranulocytosis, with rapid onset and usually heralded by fever and a sore throat. Discontinuation of the drug almost always results in complete recovery. Arthralgias and the serum sickness syndrome also occur rarely. The incidence of reaction to PTU, MMI, and carbimazole is similar, and usually the patient will tolerate another of these drugs after developing a reaction to one of them.

Preparation and Doses

PTU and MMI (Tapazole) are the thiourylene drugs employed in the US, whereas carbimazole (neo-mercazole) is commonly used in Great Britain. It is usual to begin therapy with 100 mg of PTU, 10 mg of MMI, or 10 mg of carbimazole orally every eight hours. In case of lack of response or very severe hyperthyroidism, the PTU dose can be increased to as much as 300 mg every six hours and MMI to 30 mg every eight hours. When the hyperthyroidism comes under control, the maintenance dose is gradually reduced to the minimum required to keep the patient euthyroid. With PTU this may be 50–200 mg per day and with MMI 5–20 mg per day, in one or two doses per day. An alternative method is to keep the dose of thiourylene high and add thyroxine to maintain euthyroidism. Although this may be simpler, it has the disadvantage that toxic reactions may be dose-related and the onset of remission more difficult to detect.

For the rare situation requiring IV therapy, the more soluble MMI is dissolved in saline solution and sterilized.

Perchlorate

Perchlorate is one of a group of complex monovalent anions able to block the uptake of iodide by the thyroid. The earliest studies were with thiocyanate, a goitrogen derived from cabbage and other foods; but this compound has more complex effects, including interference with iodination. Its antithyroid action was discovered in 1936 by Barker during studies on the treatment of hypertension. The ability of nonmetabolized complex anions including perchlorate (ClO_4^-) to interfere with iodide transport was first shown by Wyngaarden, et al., in 1951. They include polyoxy anions, in some of which oxygen is replaced by fluorine and many containing elements of Periodic Group VII. Their blocking activity is related to ionic size, and several of them have a much greater affinity for the iodide trap than iodide itself. They are $TcO_4^- > ClO_4^- > ReO_4^- > BF_4^- > I^-$. The first of these, pertechnetate, in radioactive form ($^{99}mTcO_4^-$), is used in the nuclear medicine imaging of the thyroid gland. The second, perchlorate, is used to test the extent to which iodine accumulated by the thyroid gland is organified. When one gram of $NaClO_4$ is given orally, any iodide in the gland is almost immediately released.

In 1960 Morgans and Trotter reported that ClO_4^- could effectively control the rate of hormone synthesis in hyperthyroidism by limiting substrate availability. After a brief period during which this treatment was used successfully, the occurrence of serious toxicity (agranulocytosis and nephrosis) led to its discontinuation. It should be noted that no serious toxicity has been reported from single doses of perchlorate used in testing. It also should be noted that the blockade of thyroid hormone synthesis by perchlorate is counteracted by a high iodine intake. Thus, perchlorate could not be used in conjunction with iodide to prepare patients for thyroidectomy. In rare circumstances, short-term therapy with perchlorate may be clinically justifiable.[57]

Choices in the Treatment of Hyperthyroidism

There is no unanimity about the selection of therapy for hyperthyroidism.[58] The three principal methods are surgical thyroidectomy, radiation by isotopic iodine, and definitive antithyroid drug administration. In addition, antithyroid drugs are used in conjunction with either form of ablative therapy, and ancillary drugs are used with all three methods. In this section we present guiding principles that should underlie the choices that are made, recognizing that regional, cultural, and institutional differences in training, experience, and risk perceptions are significant considerations. In preceding sections we discussed how the use of each drug can be modified in relation to the clinical situation and the therapeutic goal; these variations must also enter into the treatment plan.

Etiology

Thyrotoxicosis can result from increased synthesis of hormone in the thyroid gland, increased release of hormone without increased synthesis, or an exogenous source of thyroid hormone. Increased synthesis due to thyroid-stimulating immunoglobulins (Graves' disease) is treated by thyroid ablation or an antithyroid drug. Increased synthesis due to excess TSH resulting from a pituitary neoplasm is treated primarily by excision of the neoplasm; but control at the level of the thyroid gland also may be required. Increased synthesis due to a defect in feedback control of the pituitary, in the absence of generalized thyroid hormone resistance, can be managed by thyroid ablation and replacement therapy or by antithyroid drugs; but additional control at the pituitary level is required. Treatment of this disorder is difficult and uncertain. Increased thyroid hormone release without increased synthesis (radiation thyroiditis, autoimmune thyroiditis, etc.) is usually self-limited. Antithyroid drugs are ineffective, and thyrotoxicosis is controlled by ancillary drugs: a beta-blocker such as propranolol or a monodeiodinase inhibitor such as ipodate. Thyrotoxicosis due to an exogenous hormone source (thyrotoxicosis facticia) is treated similarly, although obviously the source should be removed.

Severity

Extreme thyrotoxicosis (thyroid storm, thyrotoxic crisis) requires rapid, multimodality therapy. Hormone release is controlled by high-dose iodide (and/or lithium) preceded by a high dose of thiourylene drug. PTU is preferred because of its additional blocking effect on mondeiodination of T_4. A beta-blocker is used to provide additional antihormone effect. Supportive therapy and other measures discussed earlier also must be employed.

Severe thyrotoxicosis, short of thyroid storm, also warrants combined therapy and high drug doses at the onset. Therapy should not rely on radioiodine alone, or on a thiourylene drug alone, because of the time required for the therapeutic response. If surgical ablation is preferred as the definitive treatment, it should be delayed until the thyrotoxicosis is controlled by drug and supportive therapy. Most therapists also recommend full control by drugs and iodide for seven to ten days before surgery, regardless of the initial severity of the thyrotoxicosis.

Mild thyrotoxicosis, especially when accompanied by a small, diffuse goiter, often responds to low dose thiourylene therapy.[59] It is more likely to undergo remission after six to eighteen months of treatment.

A large goiter, whether diffuse or nodular, is less likely to remit, and surgery may be preferred for cosmetic reasons. Radioiodine therapy will also shrink the goiter but, of course, more slowly.

Age

Surgical ablation is particularly difficult in young children, and such treatment must depend on the availability of surgical expertise—which also should be a consideration at any age. Radiation-induced thyroid neoplasia in children, and ovarian effects of radiation in girls and young women, are factors to consider when using radioiodine; but strong evidence indicates that neither is sufficiently dangerous to preclude such therapy. In men and women, after the procreative period, radioiodine is clearly the definitive therapy with the lowest risk.

Pregnancy

Thiourylene drugs are safe, provided that the dose required for control is not very high (below 400 mg propylthiouracil, for example). Radioiodine should not be used, especially after the first trimester when the fetal thyroid gland begins to function. In early pregnancy, fetal radiation below 5 to 10 rads appears to be safe. Iodide should be avoided because of the risk of iodide goiter in the child.

Complicating Illness

Increased risk from protracted or recurrent hyperthyroidism, from exacerbation of hyperthyroidism after radioiodine or from surgery itself needs to be considered, especially in cardiovascular disease. An exacerbation after radioiodine or surgery can be minimized by prior control of the thyrotoxicosis by antithyroid drugs.

Patient Compliance

Although it is obvious that patient compliance is important for drug therapy, it must also be understood that Graves' disease will eventuate in hypothyroidism in many patients regardless of the method of treatment.[60] This is perhaps more likely after radioiodine, but depends on the treatment design (see p. 801). Hypothyroidism is more likely to occur early after high-dose radioiodine therapy.[61] The diagnosis and treatment of hypothyroidism after Graves' disease is important as patient compliance is variable. Communication between primary care physician and referral physician must include adequate safeguards for the patient's long-term follow-up.[62]

References

Research Reports

1. Silva JE, Larsen PR. Pituitary nuclear 3,5,3′-triiodothyronine and thyrotropin secretions: An explanation for the effect of thyroxine. Science 1977;*198*:617–620.

2. Silva JE, Larsen PR. Contributions of plasma triiodothyronine and local thyroxine monodeiodination to triiodothyronine to

nuclear triiodothyronine receptor saturation in pituitary, liver, and kidney of hypothyroid rats. J Clin Invest 1978;*611*:1247–1259.

3. Cody V, Duax WL. Distal conformation of the thyroid hormone 3,5,3′-triido-L-thyronine. Science 1973;*181*:757–758.
4. Money WL, Kumaoka S, Rawson RW, Kroc RL. Comparative effects of thyroxine analogues in experimental animals. Ann NY Acad Sci 1960;*86*:512–544.
5. Koerner D, Schwartz HL, Surks MI, Oppenheimer JH, Jorgensen EC. Binding of selected iodothyronine analogues to receptor sites of isolated rat hepatic nuclei. J Biol Chem 1975;*250*:6417–6423.
6. USPDI Drug Information for the Health Care Professional. Pharmacopeial Convention, Inc. 11th Ed 1991;*IB*:2509–2510.
7. Reverter JL, Lucas A, Salinus I, Audi L, Foz M, Sanmati A. Suppressive therapy with levothyroxine for solitary thyroid nodules. Clin Endocrinol 1992;*36*:25–28.
8. Cheung PSY, Lee JMH, Boey JH. Thyroxine suppressive therapy of benign solitary thyroid nodules: A prospective randomized study., WorLd J Surg 1989;*13*:818–822.
9. Gharib H, James EM, Charbonea W, Naessens JM, Offord KP, Gorman CA. Suppressive therapy with levothyroxine for solitary thyroid nodules. N Engl J Med 1987;*317*:70–75.
10. Robbins J. Thyroid suppression therapy for prevention of thyroid tumors after radiation exposure. In DeGroot LJ (Ed) Radiation-associated thyroid carcinoma. New York: Grune & Stratton. (1977); pp 419–431.
11. Fogelfeld L, Wiviott MBT, Shore-Freedman E, Blend M, Bekerman C, Pinsky S, Schneider AB. Recurrence of thyroid nodules after surgical removal in patients irradiated in childhood for benign conditions. N Engl J Med 1989;*320*:835–840.
12. Vulsma T, Gons MH, DeVijlder JJ. Maternal-fetal transfer of thyroxine in congenital hypothyroidism due to a total organification defect or thyroid agenesis. N Engl J Med 1989;*321*:13–16.
13. Klein AH, Meltzer S, Kenny FM. Improved prognosis in congenital hypothyroidism treated before age three months. J Pediatr 1972;*81*:912–915.
14. Woeber, KA. Thyrotoxicosis and the heart. N Engl J Med 1992;*327*:94–98.
15. Ismail-Beigi F, Edelman IS. The mechanism of the calorigenic action of thyroid hormone. J Gen Physiol 1971;*57*:710–722.
16. Lin MH, Akera T. Increased (Na^+, K^+) - ATPase concentrations in various tissues of rats caused by thyroid hormone treatment. J Biol Chem 1978;*253*:723–726.
17. Paul TL, Kerrigan J, Kelly AM, Braverman LE, Baran DT. Long term L-thyroxine therapy is associated with decreased hip bone density in premenopausal women. JAMA 1988;*259*:3137–3141.
18. Diamond T, Nery L, Hales I. A therapeutic dilemma: Suppressive doses of thyroxine significantly reduce bone mineral measurements in both premenopausal and postmenopausal women with thyroid carcinoma. J Clin Endocrinol Metab 1990;*72*:1104–1188.
19. Fish LH, Schwartz HL, Cavanaugh J, Steffes MW, Bantle JP, Oppenheimer JH. Replacement dose, metabolism, and bioavailability of levothyroxine in the treatment of hypothyroidism. N Engl J Med 1987;*316*:764–770.
20. Gavin LA. Thyroid crises. Med Clin North Amer 1991;*75*:179–193.
21. Rezuani I, Di George AM. Reassessment of the daily dose of oral thyroxine for replacement therapy of hypothyroid children. J Pediatr 1977;*90*:291–297.
22. Abassi R, Aldige C. Evaluation of sodium L-thyroxine requirement in replacement therapy of hypothyroidism. J Pediatr 1977;*90*:298–301.
23. Penny R, Spencer CA, Fraiser SD, Nicoloff JT. Thyroid stimulating hormone and thyroglobulin levels decrease with chronological age in children and adolescents. J Clin Endocrinol Metab 1983;*56*:177–180.
24. Glinoer D, DeNayer P, Bourdoux P, Lemone M, Robya C, Steirteghem AV, Kinthaert J, Lejuene B. Regulation of Maternal Thyroid During Pregnancy. J Clin Endocrinol Metab 1990;*71*:276–287.
25. Mandel SJ, Larsen PR, Seely EW, Brent GA. Increased need for thyroxine during pregnancy in women with primary hypothyroidism. N Engl J Med 1990;*323*:91–96.
26. Folkers K, Enzman F, Boler J, Bowers CY, Schally AV. Discovery of modification of the synthetic tripeptide sequence of the thyrotropin releasing hormone having activity. Biochem Biophys Res Commun 1969;*37*:123–126.
27. Pierce JG. The subunits of pituitary thyrotrophin. Endocrinol 1971;*89*:1331–1344.
28. Guillemin R. Peptides in the Brain: The new endocrinology of the neuron. Science 1978;*202*:390–402.
29. Schally AV. Aspects of hypothalmic regulation of the pituitary gland. Science 1978;*202*:18–28.
30. Greer MA. Evidence of the hypothalamic control of the pituitary release of thyrotrophin. Proc Soc Exp Biol Med 1951;*77*:603–608.
31. Noel GL, Dimond RC, Wartofsky L, Earll JM, Frantz AG. Studies of prolactin and TSH secretion by continuous infusion of small amounts of thyrotropin releasing hormone (TRH). J Clin Endocrinal Metab 1974;*39*:6–17.
32. Ormston BJ, Garry R, Cryer RJ, Besser CM, Hall R. Thyrotrophin-releasing hormone as a thyroid function test. Lancet 1971;*2*:10–14.
33. Jackson IMD. Thyrotropin-releasing hormone. N Engl J Med 1982;*306*:145–155.
34. Gershengorn MC, Rebecchi MJ, Geras E, Arevalo CO. Thyrotropin-releasing hormone (TRH) action in mouse thyrotropic tumor cells in culture. Endocrinal 1980;*107*:665–670.
35. Field JB. Thyroid-stimulating hormone and cyclic adenosine 3′5′-monophosphate in the regulation of thyroid gland function. Metabolism 1975;*24*:381–393.
36. Field JB, Ealey PA, Marhsall NJ, Cockcroft S. Thyroid-stimulating hormone stimulates increases in inositol phosphates as well as cyclic AMP in the FRTL-5 rat thyroid cell line. Biochem J 1987;*247*:519–524.
37. Laurent E, Mockel J, VanSande J, Graft I, Dumont JE. Dual activation by thyrotropin of phospholipase C and cyclic AMP cascades in human thyroid. Mol Cell Endocrinal 1987;*52*:273–278.
38. Wolff J, Chaikoff IL. Plasma inorganic iodine as a homeostatic regulator of thyroid function. J Biol Chem 1948;*174*:555–564.
39. Pisarev MA, DeGroot LJ, Hati R. KI and imidazole inhibition of TSH and c-AMP induced thyroidal iodine secretion. Endocrinal 1971;*88*:1217–1221.
40. Allegrini M, Pennington JAT, Tanner JT. Total Diet Study: Determination of iodine intake by neutron activation analysis. J Am Diet Assoc 1983;*83*:18–24.
41. Vought RL, London WT, Lutwak L, Dublin TD. Reliability of estimates of serum inorganic iodine and daily fecal and urinary iodine excretion from single casual specimens. J Clin Endocrinal Metab 1963;*23*:1218–1228.

42. Kusic Z, Becker DV, Saenger EL, Paras P, Gartside P, Wessler T, Spaventi S. Comparison of technetium-99m and iodine-123 imaging of thyroid nodules. J Nucl Med 1990;*31*:393–399.

43. Beierwaltes WH. Editorial: Comparison of technetium-99m and iodine-123 nodules: Correlation with pathologic findings. J Nucl Med 1990;*31*:400–402.

44. Glennon JA, Gordon ES, Sawin CT. Hypothyroidism after low-dose ^{131}I treatment of hyperthyroidism. Ann Int Med 1972;*76*:721–723.

45. Cevallos JL, Hagen GA, Maloof F, Chapman FM. Low-dosage ^{131}I therapy of thyrotoxicosis (diffuse goiters). N Engl J Med 1974;*290*:141–143.

46. Van De Velde CJH, Hamming JF, Gosling BM, Schelfhout LJDM, Clark OH, Smeds S, Bruining HA, Krenning EP, Cady B. Report of the consensus development conference on the management of differentiated thyroid cancer in the Netherlands. Eur J Cancer Clin Oncol 1988;*24*:287–292.

47. Robbins J, Merino MJ, Boice JD Jr, Ron E, Ain KB, Alexander HR, Norton JA, Reynolds J. Thyroid cancer: A lethal endocrine neoplasm. Ann Int Med 1991;*115*:133–147.

48. Beierwaltes WH, Rabbani R, Dmuchowski C, Lloyd RV, Eyre P, Mallette S. An analysis of "ablation of thyroid remnants" with I-131 in 511 patients from 1947–1984. J Nucl Med 1984;*25*:1287–1293.

49. Spaulding SW, Burrow GN, Bermudez F, Himmelhoch JM. The inhibitory effect of lithium on thyroid hormone release in both euthyroid and thyrotoxic patients. J Clin Endocrinal Metab 1972;*35*:905–911.

50. Temple R, Berman M, Robbins J, Wolff J. The use of lithium in the treatment of thyrotoxicosis. J Clin Invest 1972;*51*:2746–2756.

51. Forrest JJ. Lithium inhibition of cAMP-mediated hormones: A caution. N Engl J Med 1975;*292*:422–442.

52. Jansson R, Dahlberg PA, Lindstrom B. Comparative bioavailability of carbimazole and methimazole. J Clin Pharmacol Therap Toxical 1983;*21*:505–510.

53. Taurog A. The mechanism of action of thioureylene antithyroid drugs. Endocrinal 1976;*98*:1031–1046.

54. Taurog A, Lothrop ML, Estabrook RW. Improvements in the isolation procedure for thyorid peroxidase. Arch Biochem Biophys 1970;*139*:221–229.

55. Leonard JL, Rosenberg IW. Thyroxine 5′-deiodinase activity of rat kidney. Endocrinal 1978;*103*:2137–2144.

56. Schleusener H, Schwander J, Fisher C, Holle R, Holl G, Badenhoop K, Hensen J, Finke R, Bogner U, Mayr WR, Schernthaner G, Schatz H, Pichardt CR, Kotulla P. Prospective multicenter study on the prediction of relapse after antithyroid drug treatment in patients with Graves' disease. Acta Endocrinal 1989;*120*:689–701.

57. Martino E, Lombardi-Agnahi F, Mariotti S, Lenziardi M, Baschieri L, Braverman LE, Pinchera A. Treatment of amiodarone associated thyrotoxicosis by simultaneous administration of potassium perchlorate and methimazole. J Endocrinal Invest 1986;*9*:201–207.

58. Dunn JT. Choice of therapy in young adults with hyperthyroidism or Graves' disease. Ann Int Med 1984;*100*:891–893.

59. Laurberg P, Hansen PEB, Iversen E, Jansen SE, Weeke J. Goiter size and outcome of medical treatment of Graves' disease. Acta Endocrinol 1986;*111*:39–43.

60. Hirota Y, Tamai H, Hyashi Y, Matsubayashi S, Matsuzuka F, Kuma K, Kumasai LF, Nagataki S. Thyroid function and histology in forty-five patients with hyperthyroid Graves' disease in clinical remission more than ten years after thionamide drug treatment. J Clin Endocrinol Metab 1986;*62*:165–169.

61. Holm LE. Changing annual incidence of hypothyroidism after iodine-131 therapy for hyperthyroidism, 1951–1975. J Nucl Med 1982;*23*:108–112.

62. Safa AM, Skillern PG. Treatment of hyperthyroidism with a large initial dose of sodium iodide I131. Arch Intern Med 1975;*135*:673–675.

Reviews

r1. Morley JE. Neuroendocrine control of thyrotropin secretion. Endocrinol Rev 1981;*2*:396–436.

r2. Robbins J. The thyroid as a model endocrine system. Adv Exp Med Biol 1990;*261*:1–4.

r3. Taurog A. Hormone synthesis: Thyroid iodine metabolism. In: Braverman LE, Utiger RD (ed). Werner and Ingbar's The thyroid (6th ed) Philadelphia: Lippincott (1991) pp 51–97.

r4. Jorgensen EC. Structure activity relationships of thyroxine analogues. Pharmacol Ther B 1976;*2*:661–682. *An extensive summary of data on thyroid hormone analogues and thier biological effects.*

r5. Samuels HH, Forman BM, Horowitz ZD, Ye ZS. Regulation of gene expression by thyroid hormone. J Clin Invest 1988;*81*:957–967. *A current review of the working hypothesis of thyroid hormone action.*

r6. DeLong GR, Robbins J, Condliffe PG (eds.). Iodine and the brain. New York: Plenum Press, 1989.

r7. Harvey RD, McHardy KC, Reid IW, Patterson F, Bewsher PD, Duncan A, Robins SP. Measurement of bone collagen degradation in hyperthyroidism and during thyroxine replacement therapy using pyridinium cross-links as specific urinary markers. J Clin Endocrinol Metab 1991;*72*:1189–1194.

r8. Shakir KMM, Michaels RD, Hays JH, Potter BB. The use of bile acid sequestrants to lower serum thyroid hormones in iatrogenic hyperthyroidism. Ann Int Med 1993;*118*:112–113.

r9. Robbins J, Rall JE. Proteins associated with the thyroid hormones. Physiol Rev 1960;*40*:415–489.

r10. Refetoff S. Inherited thyroxine-binding globulin abnormalities in man. Endocrinol Rev 1989;*10*:275–293.

r11. Ain KB, Mori Y, Refetoff S. Reduced clearance rate of thyroxine-binding globulin (TBG) with increased sialylation. J Clin Endocrinol Metab 1987;*65*:689–696.

r12. Cavalieri RR, Pitt-Rivers R. The effects of drugs on the distribution and metabolism of thyroid hormones. Pharmacol Rev 1981;*33*:55–80.

r13. Ekins R. Measurement of free hormones in blood. Endocrinol Rev 1990;*11*:5–46.

r14. Nicoloff JT, Spencer CA. The use and misuse of the sensitive TSH assays. J Clin Endocrinol Metab 1990;*71*:553–558.

r15. Pierce JG, Parsons TF. Glycoprotein hormones. Ann Rev Biochem 1981;*50*:465–495.

r16. Gershengorn MC. Thyrotropin-releasing hormone action. Recent Prog Horm Res 1985;*41*:607–653.

r17. Horita A, Carino MA, Lai H. Pharmacology of thyrotropin-releasing hormone. Ann Rev Pharmacol Toxicol 1987;*26*:311–332.

r18. Movius EG, Robbins J, Pierce LR, Reynolds JC, Keenan AM, Phyillaier MA. The value of lithium in radioiodine therapy of thyroid carcinoma. In: Medeiros-Neto G, Gaitan E (ed). Frontiers in thryoidology, Vol 2. New York: Plenum (1986); pp 1269–1272.

r19. Marchant B, Lees JFH, Alexander WD. Antithyroid Drugs. Pharmacol Therap 1978;3:305–348. *This review contains detailed information on the pharmacokinetics of antithyroid drugs.*

r20. Kelley FC. Iodine in medicine and pharmacy since its discovery—1811–1961 Proc Roy Soc Med 1961;54:831–836. *The president's address to the library (Scientific Research) section contains an entertaining discussion of the early history of iodine and the thyroid, a calendar of events, and pictures of the protagonists.*

r21. Astwood EB. Thyroid and antithyroid drugs. In Goodman LS, Gilman A (ed). The pharmacological basis of therapeutics (4th ed). New York: Macmillan, 1965:1466–1500. *This classic pharmacology chapter was written by the physician-scientist who pioneered the development of antithyroid drug therapy.*

r22. Wolff J. Lithium interactions with the thyroid gland. In Cooper TB, Gershon S, Kline NS, and Schon M (eds). Lithium controversies and unresolved issues. Amsterdam: Excerpta Medica, 1979. *This article thoroughly reviews the literature on lithium and the thyroid.*

r23. Harbert JC. Nuclear medicine therapy. New York: *Thieme Medical Publishers,* 1987. *Includes a detailed account of the properties and uses of radioactive iodine.*

r24. DeGroot LS. Endocrinology (3d ed). New York: Grune & Stratton, 1989. *Comprehensive chapters on all aspects of basic and clinical thyroidology.*

r25. Bardin CW. Current therapy in endocrinolgy and metabolism (4th ed). Toronto: BC Decker, 1991. *Chapters by recognized experts on hypothyroidism in adults and children, myxedema coma, and hyperthyroidism.*

r26. Braverman LE and Utiger RD. Werner and Ingbar's The thyroid. A fundamental and clinical text (6th ed). Philadelphia: JB Lippincott, 1992. *The classic multi-authored textbook of thyroidology in all of its aspects.*

CHAPTER 46

Kenneth S. Korach
Silvia Migliaccio
Vicki L. Davis

Estrogens

Estrogens are a class of steroid hormones linked principally with the control of female sex organ responsiveness and of reproduction. However, males also produce measurable levels of estrogen. The hormones are produced biosynthetically in the female ovary or formed peripherally in both sexes by aromatization of circulating androgen steroid hormone precursors (eg., testosterone or androstenedione). The three principal native forms of known endogenous estrogens are 17 β-estradiol, estrone, and estriol (Fig. 46.1). The most potent biologic form is 17 β-estradiol, which elicits a variety of actions in a number of different tissues. An obvious therapeutic use of estrogens is for postmenopausal replacement therapy, where the hormones' beneficial role in slowing bone loss and stabilizing hot flashes has been well documented. In other cases, gonadal insufficiency requires the use of estrogen replacement or supplement. Another application has been the use of estrogen as a component of oral contraceptives for inhibiting gonadotropin secretion. Besides steroidal estrogen derivatives, a number of synthetic nonsteroidal estrogens have been formulated as pharmaceuticals. Currently, most estrogen formulations use steroidal compounds. Because research is presently underway to evaluate other possible sites of action of estrogen and its role in endocrine regulation, it is probable that other new therapeutic uses for estrogens will be discovered.

Chemistry (Fig. 46.1)

Estrogens are steroid hormones containing the cyclopentanoperhydrophenanthrene chemical ring structure. They differ from the other classes of steroid hormones because they are composed of an estrane steroid nucleus containing 18 carbons (C18). Most unusual is the phenolic A ring, rather than the nonaromatic cyclohexane ring seen with the steroids of the androstane (C19) or pregnane (C21) ring structures. The phenolic ring gives these steroids some unique chemical properties. In fact, the phenolic ring is an essential chemical requirement for hormonal activity mediated through binding to the estrogen receptor protein (discussed in a later section), and the oxygen at C17 is necessary for biologic activity. Biologic potency is influenced by the type of oxygen function present at C17. The biologic activity of estrogens classically is assayed by assessing the ability of the substance to stimulate or increase the weight of the rodent uterus. Other early assays evaluated their ability to induce vaginal cornification in rats or mice. For the endogenous estrogens, 17 β-estradiol has the greatest hormonal potency; this potency is reduced approximately tenfold when the 17-hydroxyl group is enzymatically or chemically oxidized to a keto group, as found in estrone. Estriol contains an additional 16α-hydroxyl group and has also a tenfold lower potency than estradiol. Most biologically active estrogens have similar effects in the major target tissues from different species. Recently, however, as more is known about estrogen effects, studies using synthetic compounds have suggested that there may be differential hormonal activities.[r1] A current research approach is to identify estrogenic componds that may elicit tissue-specific effects, such as bone-specific agonists with minimal side-effects in the uterus.

The chemical derivatization of estradiol at C17 has been a common synthetic and pharmacologic technique used to increase the biologic activity of a number of compounds. Derivatization occurs through the C17 oxygen function producing an ester linkage that provides a depot effect within the body. De-esterification of the compound occurs by a variety of esterases, thereby producing estradiol. A representative schematic of the common components of some

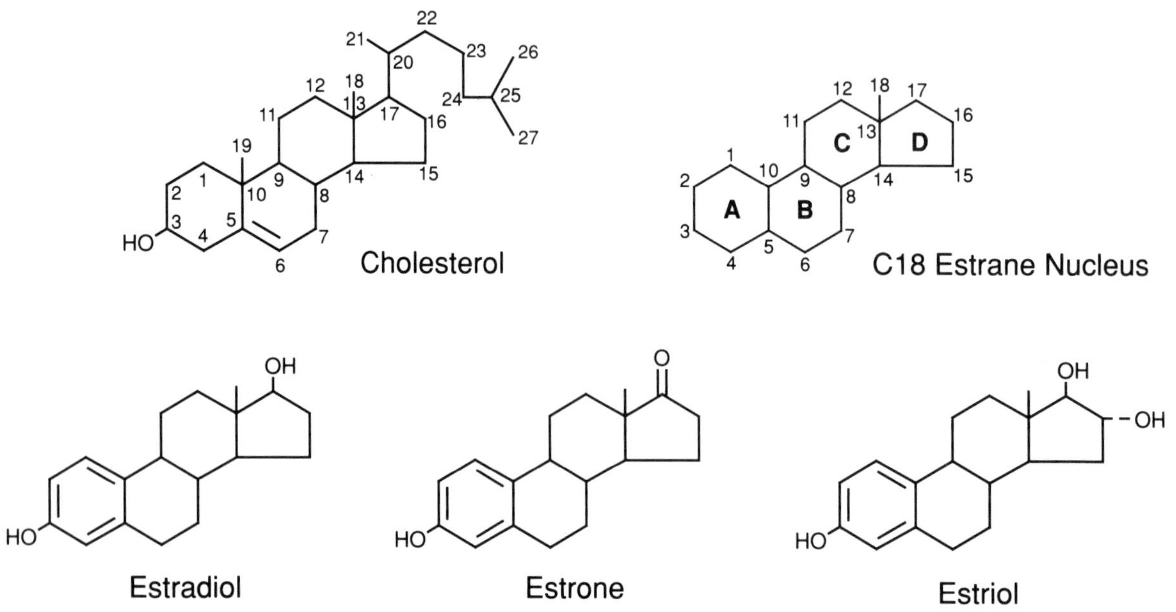

Figure 46.1 Chemical and Molecular Structures of Natural Steroidal Estrogens

estrogenic substances is shown in Figure 46.2, illustrating the variety of types of derivatives ranging from pentyl to benzoyl groups. Descriptions have been made of endogenous estrogens having fatty acid esters at C17 that are similar to the chemical derivatives. These fatty acid ester estrogens are regulated to be long-lived.[1] On the other hand, because of the phenolic ring structure, a number of synthetic compounds have been shown to mimic estrogens. These include stilbene estrogens such as diethylstilbestrol (E-DES), hexestrol, or E,E-dienestrol.[r1] Similarities to steroidal estrogens arise from a composite diphenolic ring structure, as shown in Figure 46.3. This stilbene ring structure is also the chemical basis of several triphenylethylene compounds that possess antiestrogenic activity.[r2]

History

The initial understanding of estrogenic hormones and their actions began in the early 1900s. In 1900, Knauer was the first to establish the endocrine functions of ovaries by transplanting the glands into animals and preventing symptoms after ovariectomy.[1a] Indeed, the biologic activity of estrogens was known far earlier than was their chemical structure. Seminal studies by Stockard and Papanicolaou in 1917 showed that accessory organs (i.e., vagina and uterus) of laboratory animals responded with cyclic changes similar to those in the ovary.[2] Estrogen was the first steroid hormone isolated and identified.[3] Allen and Doisy isolated lipoidal substances from large ovarian follicles from swine and reported in 1923 that components of this material could induce estrous changes in the vagina of rats.[2] A correlation had been drawn by reproductive physiologists that the ovaries were producing some agents that could affect other organs (i.e., vagina and uterus); however, the early efforts to identify the substance(s) chemically were unsuccessful. At this time, the first definition for an "estrogen" was given as a "substance that induced estrus." The whole face of hormone research changed in the late 1920s, when Ascheim and Zondek reported that urine from pregnant animals contained materials that could be termed hormones.[4] One component that was isolated mimicked the estrus-producing activity found in ovarian follicles. Separately, the laboratories of Doisy and Butenandt succeeded in crystallizing a low molecular weight lipophilic steroidal substance from urine of pregnant women.[5a] Doisy was awarded the 1943 Nobel Prize for this discovery, which he termed "Theelin," and which was later named estrone.[5] Isolation of estrogens directly from ovarian tissue did not occur until 1935 by Doisy. At the time, four tons of sow's ovaries were needed to isolate approximately 12 mg of 17 β-estradiol. Following the chemical isolation and characterization of estradiol and estrone, a search was initiated for an inexpensive synthetic estrogen that exhibited oral biopotency. In the mid-1930s, Dodds and associates produced some stilbestrol estrogens, diethylstilbestrol and hexestrol, that were quite effective and are still used in some therapeutic preparations.[6] Because estrogens induce phenomenal growth stimulation of reproductive tract tissues, studies attempting to understand the mechanism were initiated. A prevailing theory amongst biochemists and physiologists in the 1950s was that estrogens acted as cosubstrates to increase tissue metabolism, which resulted in proliferation. However, in 1960 the field of steroid hormone physiology changed when Jensen described "receptors" in estrogen target tissue.[r3] Those findings and subsequent investigations by other laboratories advanced our understanding of these proteins, which are present in vanishingly small amounts, and the mode of action of estrogen.[r4–r7] In fact, the presence of receptors for a particular steroid hormone partly defines the specificity of tissue response. The model that evolved over the past three decades for estrogen hormone action, depicted in Figures 46.6 and 46.7 (described in more detail later in the Molecular Mechanism section), indicates that the steroid binds to the receptor protein within the nucleus, producing a complex capable of binding to DNA, increasing gene transcription, and altering target tissue responses to the hormone. Research studies a half-century after the first realization of a physiologic estrogen response to the chemical characterization of a steroid agent, and subsequent cloning and identification of a receptor protein and specific regulated genes, have brought us closer to an understanding of the cell biology, physiology, and pharmacology of estrogens.

	R_1	R_2	R_3
17 β Estradiol	H	H	H
Estradiol 17 - Benzoate	H	$-C(=O)-C_6H_5$	H
Estradiol 3 - Benzoate	$-C(=O)-C_6H_5$	H	H
Estradiol 17 β- Cyclopentyl-propionate	H	$-C(=O)-CH_2CH_2-C_5H_9$	H
Estradiol Dipropionate	$-C(=O)-CH_2CH_3$	$-C(=O)-CH_2CH_3$	H
Estradiol 17-V alerate	H	$-C(=O)(CH_2)_3CH_3$	H
Ethinyl Estradiol	H	H	$-C\equiv CH$

Figure 46.2 Structures of the More Common Synthetic Steroidal Estrogenic Compounds

Synthesis of Estrogens

The naturally occurring estrogens are C18-steroids characterized by the presence of an aromatic A ring, a phenolic hydroxyl group at C-3, and either a hydroxyl (estradiol) or a ketone group (estrone) at position 17 of the D ring. Estradiol, the most important and potent endogenous estrogen, is produced mainly by the ovaries. Although estrone is also produced by the ovaries, the principal source of estrone is from extraglandular conversion of androstenedione in peripheral tissues. In certain tissues, estradiol dehydrogenase functions bidirectionally to interconvert estradiol to estrone. The less pharmacologically active estriol is the most abundant estrogen during pregnancy and was used as an index for fetal/placental functions. Most of the estriol during pregnancy is formed by placental aromatization of androgens (16 α dehydroepiandrosterone) produced by the fetal adrenal cortex and liver. The principal estrogenic compounds are shown in Figure 46.1.

Estrogens, as all the other steroid hormones, are synthesized starting from cholesterol, which is provided to the steroidogenic tissues by de novo synthesis from 2 C-units (acetyl coenzyme A) or by uptake of circulating cholesterol synthesized in the liver and transported in low-density lipoprotein (LDL) particles.[r8] The rate-limiting step in all steroid synthesis is the cleavage of the side-chain of cholesterol to generate pregnenolone (Fig. 46.3), by the enzyme P-450 side-chain cleavage ($P450_{scc}$). The major pathways of the estrogen biosynthesis in the ovary are outlined in Figure 46.4. In the ovaries, estrogen production depends on the cooperation of both granulosa and thecal cells.[r9] In fact, theca cells produce, by either the Δ4 or Δ5 pathways, both testosterone and androstenedione, which are then converted to estradiol and estrone in the granulosa cells by the P-450 aromatase ($P450_{arom}$), which catalyzes the unsaturation and aromatization in the A ring (Fig. 46.2). Additionally, the corpus luteum is able to generate dehydroepiandrosterone or 17-OH-progesterone by Δ4 and Δ5 pathways (Fig. 46.4). Estrogen biosynthesis and secretion are complicated by the constantly changing population of cells in the ovaries during the processes of follicular development, ovulation, and corpus luteum formation and regression. These processes are regulated by the gonadotropins FSH and LH through the menstrual cycle. In addition, some studies have also proposed a two-cell, two-gonadotropin hypothesis,[7,r10] postulating that LH stimulates thecal cells to produce androgen C19-steroids (androstenedione and testosterone) and FSH stimulates granulosa cells to aromatize these preformed C19-steroids. Moreover, during pregnancy estrogens are also produced by the fetal-placenta unit at very high levels. Other peripheral tissues, such as skin, adipose tissue, skeletal muscle, hair follicles, and bone tissue have been shown to aromatize circulating androstenedione to estrone. The production of estrogens by these "nonclassic" steroidogenic tissues is mainly responsible for the re-

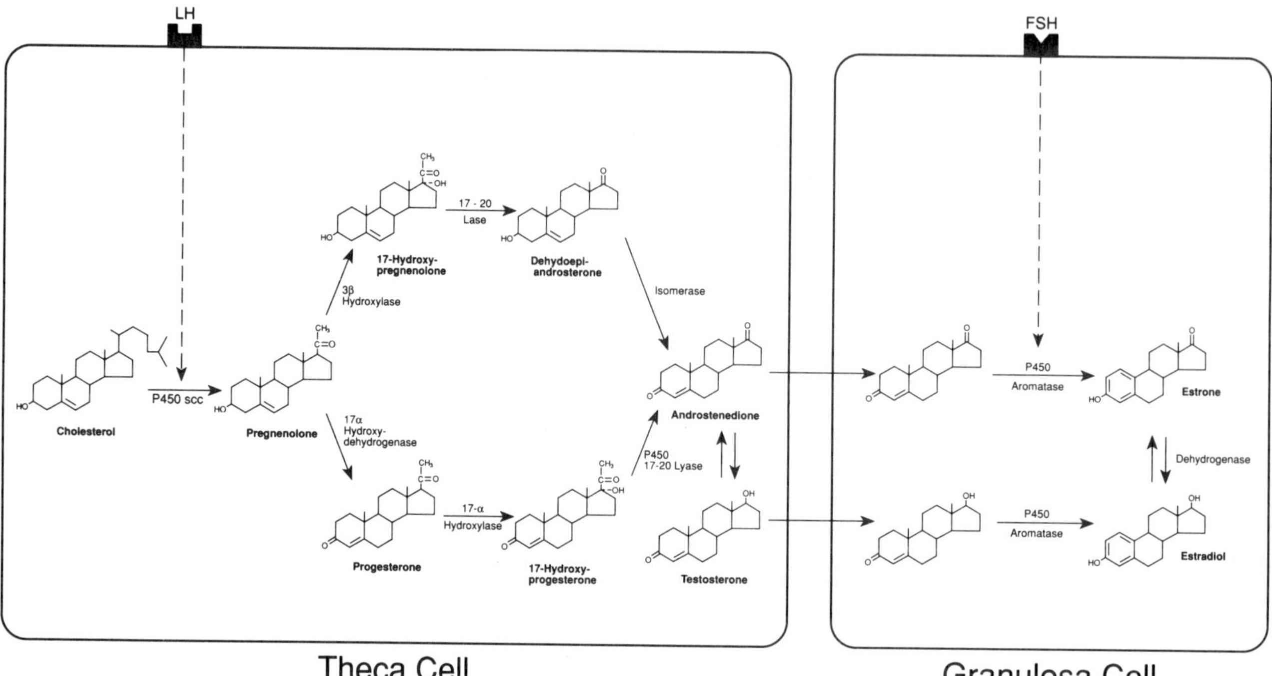

Figure 46.3 Biosynthetic pathways of ovarian steroidogenesis. Granulosa and theca cells cooperate to produce estrogens. Both Δ4 and Δ5 pathways are depicted. (Modified from Carr BR). In Wilson JD, Foster DW eds. Williams textbook of endocrinology. Philadelphia: Saunders, 1992; pp 1290–1350.

maining circulating estrogens in postmenopausal women when the ovaries have exhausted their follicular development.[8] This extraglandular aromatization is also responsible for the circulating estrogen levels in men (<20 pg/mL). The estrogen levels in women during different phases of life and during the menstrual cycle are listed in Table 46.1.

Transport and Metabolism of Estrogens

After secretion into the circulation, only 2–3 percent of the biosynthetic estrogen remains as unbound hormone. The bulk of estrogens (approx 60%) are weakly bound to albumin and (approx 38%) to the sex hormone binding globulin (SHBG), a glycoprotein made in the liver, also called testosterone-binding protein (TeBG). In fact, testosterone binds the same glycoprotein with higher affinity than estrogen, so that each steroid may influence the metabolism of the other. The free fraction of estrogen is responsible for the biologic responses in estrogen target tissues. These tissues, in particular the uterus, can interconvert free estradiol and estrone by estradiol dehydrogenase (Fig. 46.4); however, the oxidation of estradiol to estrone occurs more rapidly and is favored over the reverse reaction.[r11]

The circulating estrogens are quickly metabolized in the liver to water-soluble compounds, which are metabolically inactive. Both estrogens, but particularly estrone, are rapidly converted to estrone-3-sulfate, which is the most abundant circulating estrogen, but is not physiologically active because of its weak binding affinity for the estrogen receptor. The two most important hydroxylation pathways involve carbons in the A and D rings of the steroid nucleus. Hydroxylation in position 16 has been known for some time to be the major pathway and leads to estriol glucuronide as the prevalent urinary metabolite. However, hydroxylation at C-2 is also an important metabolic pathway, producing catechol estrogens. Catechol estrogens are substrates for catechol O-methyl transferase, producing methoxy forms that have a high metabolic clearance rate. Another catechol estrogen can be produced at C-4, but it is produced only in small amounts. Biologic studies have indicated that the catechol 4-hydroxyestradiol has activity in the uterus and neuroendocrine action involving LH suppression.[9] The findings suggest that some metabolism of estrogen may be directed toward producing certain hormonal responses only in specific target tissues. As a result of liver metabolism, 50 to 80 percent of estrone and estradiol are excreted in the urine, mainly as glucuronide conjugates, and up to 20 percent is recovered in the feces. It is important to remember these particular pathways for the conversion of estrogens, since disorders and diseases can significantly decrease the catabolism of these hormones and interfere with the normal physiology, creating conditions of hyperestrogenism. Furthermore, liver me-

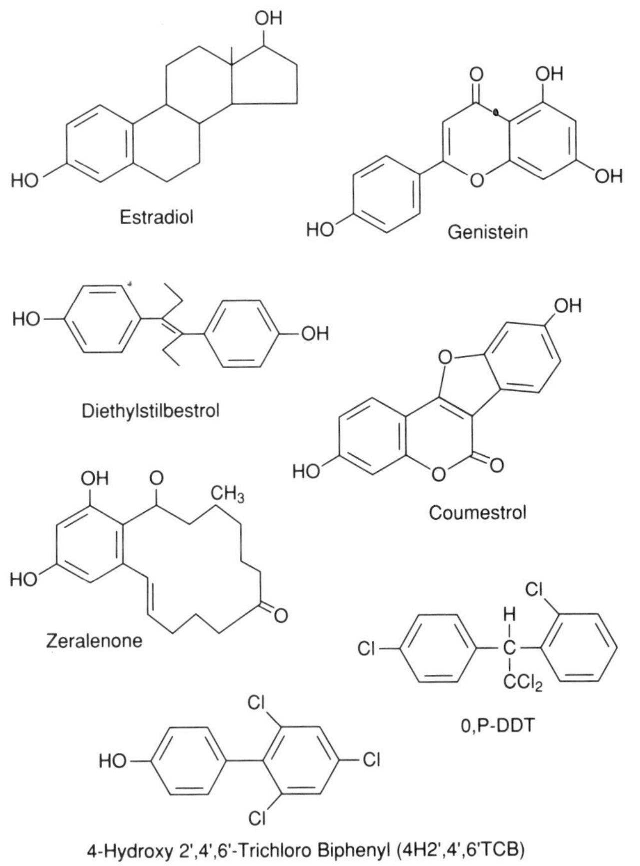

Figure 46.4 Chemical Structures of Different Environmental Compounds Reported to Exhibit Estrogenic Activity

tabolism becomes an important consideration when choosing the route of administration and dosages for estrogen replacement therapy (ERT), since it results in the conversion of estrogens to less pharmacologically active compounds (see below). It is interesting to know that modest steroid metabolism has also been described in the intestines, producing enterohepatic recirculation of estrogens by the intestinal flora.[10] This is a minimal factor with respect to estrogen metabolism, but may be considered more influential when antibiotic therapy is given, since alteration of the intestinal flora could then alter the normal estrogen metabolic cycle.

Phytoestrogens and Other Environmental Estrogenic Compounds

Estrone has also been identified in plants, leading to the further discovery that other estrogenic activity in plants is due to other nonsteroidal estrogenic compounds.[11–12,r12] Many of these molecules contain a hydroxyl group and a phenolic ring structure, which enable them to bind to the estrogen receptor in target tissues and exert estrogenic biologic activities. Environmental compounds having estrogenic activity are also called "xenoestrogens" to indicate their source and role in hormone action. These substances include estrogen analogues generated for clinical or veterinarian use, such as DES, and pesticides like DDT.[11] Moreover, industrial byproducts, like PCBs, or pesticides such as bisphenol A or nono-phenol, do manifest estrogenic activity.[11] All these compounds enter our environment as pollutants and can reach humans via food or water.

Estrogenic compounds derived from plants or fungal contaminants in stored grains are termed phytoestrogens. The major chemical groups of phytoestrogens are classified as flavonoids (flavones, flavonones, hydroxychalcones, and isoflavonoids) coumestrans, lignans, and mycoestrogens. Isoflavonoids, the most prevalent plant estrogens, are a common dietary source for estrogenic exposure (Fig. 46.3). Several phytoestrogens have been identified or detected in human urine.[r13–r14] These compounds, interacting with the estrogen receptor, exert estrogenic activity, such as uterotropic effects. However, the affinity of these molecules for the receptor can vary among the dissimilar compounds, so that a different EC_{50} is exhibited, defining these compounds as full or partial (weak) agonists. Although these compounds possess estrogenic activity, antiestrogenic effects also have been described. Sterility or disruption of normal reproductive processes occurs in farm animals grazing in pastures with plant sources high in phytoestrogens. In humans, cancer-protective properties have been associated with phytoestrogens, especially lignans and isoflavonoids, based on the fact that cultures consuming mainly vegetarian or soy-based diets have a lower risk of breast and prostate cancer.[r13–r15] It is postulated that in persons consuming small rather than large amounts of phytoestrogens, the properties of the compounds to change from estrogenic to antiestrogenic may possibly explain the antiproliferative or cancer-protective properties on hormonally responsive neoplasms.

Molecular and Cellular Mechanism of Estrogen Action

Estrogens exert their actions by inducing specific physiologic responses via the estrogen receptor (ER).[r5–r6] Although the ER has usually been described at the intracellular level,[r5–r7] estrogen-binding proteins located on plasma membranes have also been reported.[12a,r15a] The ER acts as an inducible transcription factor that can modulate expression of target genes after binding estrogen agonists.[r7] The ER resides in the nucleus, and the hydrophobic estrogenic compounds

Table 46.1 Estrogen Levels in Different Phases of Life and During the Menstrual Cycle

	Levels (pg/ml)	Production Rate* (μg/24 hr)	Secretion Rate (μg/24 hr)
Estradiol			
Woman: Basal	20–60	80	70
Late follicular	300–700	400–900	400–800
Midluteal	200	270	250
Postmenopause	<20	12	Insignificant
Estrone			
Woman: Basal	20–60	80	70
Late follicular	150–300	330–650	250–500
Midluteal	120	250	160
Postmenopause	20–30	40	Insignificant

*Production rate is the velocity at which the hormone enters into the blood both from glandular secretion and from extraglandular conversion.

readily diffuse through the cellular and nuclear membranes to bind and subsequently "activate" the ER (Fig. 46.5). The activated form of the ER can then stimulate the transcription of estrogen-responsive genes.

The ER is a member of the nuclear hormone receptor superfamily that includes the receptors for steroid hormones, thyroid hormones, vitamin D, and retinoic acid as well as orphan receptors with undiscovered ligands[r16] (Fig. 46.6). The human ER gene has been localized to chromosome 6q.[13] The ER protein is composed of six functional domains, designated A-F[14] (Fig. 46.7). The ligand binding domain (E) binds the estrogenic ligands. The DNA binding domain (C) has a zinc finger motif and recognizes DNA sequences termed "estrogen response elements" (ERE) housed within estrogen-regulated genes. Specificity for DNA sequence recognition resides in the alpha helical region of the first zinc finger. The consensus sequence for the ERE is an inverted repeat 5′ GGTCA-NNN-TGACC 3′.[15–16] This element is a perfect palindrome, composed of two half-sites separated by three nucleotides. Spacing between the half-sites is important for receptor/DNA interactions. The ERE half-sites can contain one or two base modifications, creating imperfect palindromic sequences that still retain ER binding. Other hormone receptors, such as thyroid (TR) and retinoic acid (RAR and RXR) receptors, also may recognize the half-site of an ERE, but cannot induce transcription; however, they may be able to act as inhibitors of ER transactivation.[17–18,r17] The ER can bind as a monomer to the half-site of a thyroid response element or an ERE, but it has a fastidious requirement for elements with the three nucleotide spacing between the two half-sites for transactivation functions.[19,r17–r23] ER binds to the response element as a dimer, with one ER molecule per half-site. At this time, the ER is only known to form homodimers, unlike other members of the nuclear receptor superfamily, which readily form heterodimers. The sequences that allow dimerization are within both the DNA and ligand binding domains; however, in vitro studies indicate that dimerization can occur prior to binding to DNA or ligand[20] and that ligand is not required for ER binding to an ERE.[21–22] It is not known at this time if these in vitro studies mimic the actual in vivo dynamics of ER dimerization and DNA binding. These data suggest that the ER may reside on the ERE of a target gene in the absence of ligand; however, the ER cannot activate transcription in the absence of hormone.

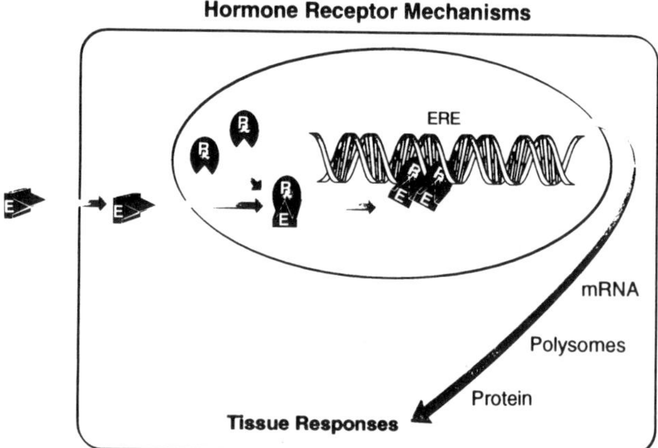

Figure 46.5 Graphic representation of an estrogen target cell depicting the estrogen interaction with the receptor and stimulation of the physiologic response.

Transcriptional activation is modulated by two regions of the ER protein, designated as activation functions AF 1 and AF 2. AF 1 and AF 2 are localized within the A/B and E domains of the receptor,[23–24] respectively, as shown in Figure 46.7. ER mutational studies

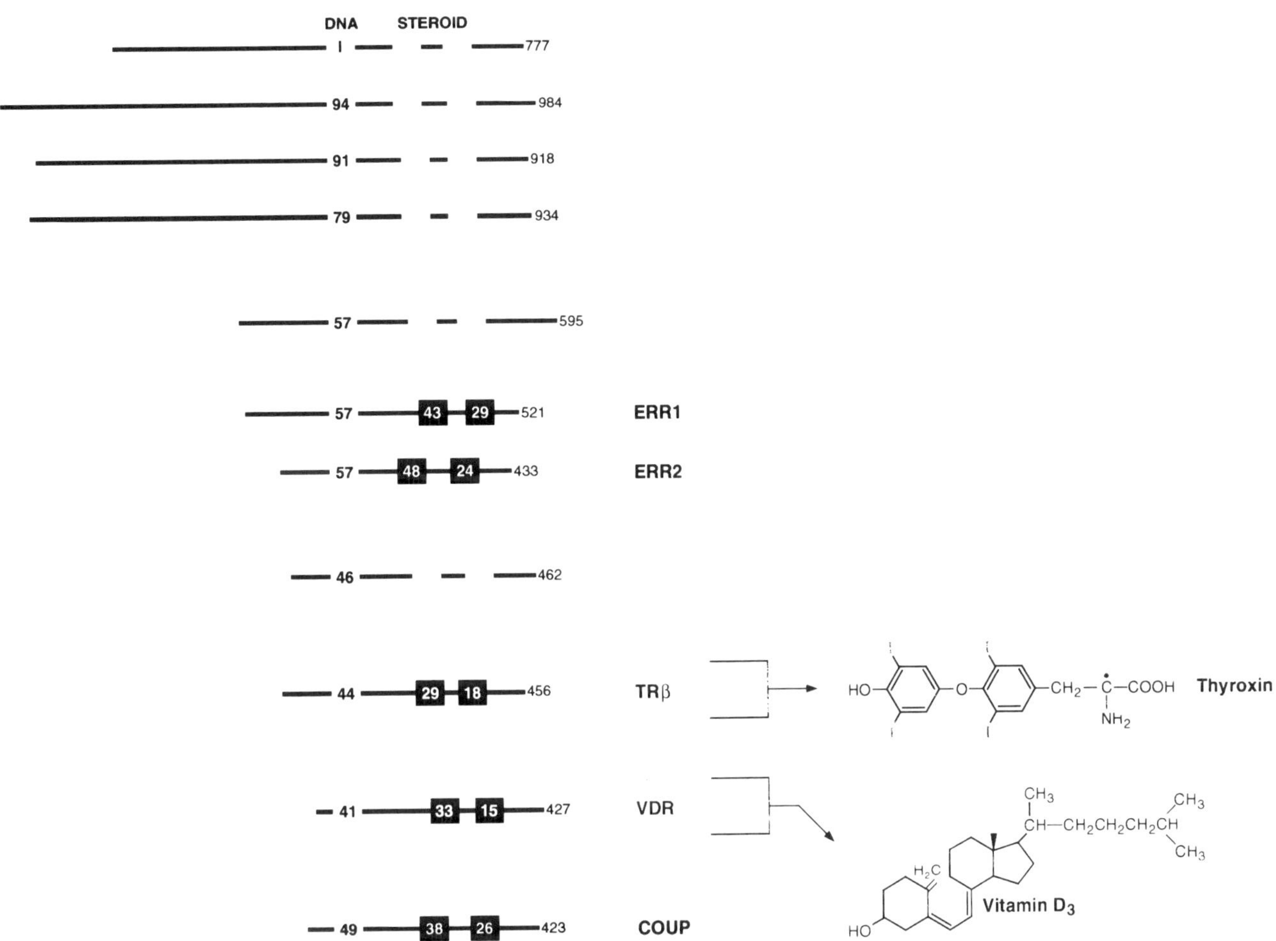

Figure 46.6 Diagram of the sequence homology for some of the various nuclear receptors. Domains for the DNA (yellow box) and steroid (blue box) binding are shown with the percentage homology of each receptor compared to the glucocorticoid receptor sequence. Lengths of the receptor proteins and the total amino acids are shown. Receptors are grouped by the types of steroids and vitamins which are bound. ERR1, ERR2, and COUP are orphan nuclear receptors and currently have no known ligand for activation. (Modified from Evans[r10] and Green and Chambon.[r44])

showed that the dominant transcriptional activation function of the ER arises from the AF 2 region and is estrogen-dependent. In receptors with AF 2 deletions, the AF 1 region can function independent of hormone, displays constitutive activity, and, therefore, may affect basal promoter activity of ERE-containing genes. The level of ER transcriptional activation depends on the promoter, cell-type, and ligand structure.

The mechanisms of transcriptional repression by estrogens are not clearly understood at this time. One physiologic example of negative regulation is the ability of estrogens to suppress gonadotropin secretion. Recent investigations with the neu proto-oncogene discovered a 140 bp region of the neu promoter responsible for transcriptional repression by estradiol.[25] In transfection assays in vitro, this promoter region, which does not contain an ERE-like sequence, required the presence of the ER as well as hormone to diminish expression of neu. Very likely, future studies will help delineate the mechanisms of negative transcriptional regulation to the equivalent understanding of positive activation by estrogens.

Specific growth factors can mimic estrogen biologic responses, just as EGF administration in ovariectomized mice can stimulate uterine growth, proliferation, and differentiation.[27] Moreover, several recent studies have indicated an interaction between the ER and other intracellular pathways, which can act in a synergistic or antagonistic manner.[26–29]

In transfection studies in vitro, IGF-1,[26] EGF,[27] and dopamine[28,r19] have been shown to require the presence of the ER, but not ER agonists, to induce transcription of ERE-reporter genes. Estrogen antagonists can block this induction. These data illustrate the presence of an interaction between the polypeptide growth factor signalling pathway and the ER nuclear receptor, and the prospect of novel mechanisms of "activation" of ER by nonclassic estrogenic ligands. Thus, it is possible that some compounds may have estrogenic activity by activating other signaling systems in the cell. However, the mechanisms are still under investigation and will require more extensive study to ascertain their relevance in human physiology.

All of this experimental evidence indicates that a normal ER

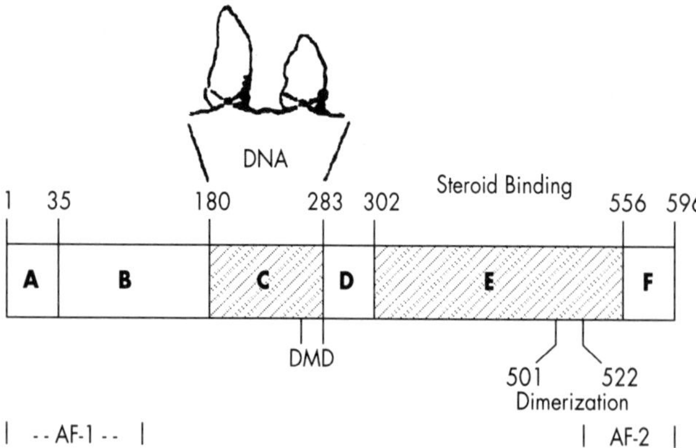

Figure 46.7 Diagram of the peptide structure of the estrogen receptor protein. Each functional domain is denoted by a letter (A-F) and the peptide size and position given above. Domain A and B contains region one of the transcription activation function (AF-1) in the N-terminus of the protein. Domain C is the DNA binding region of the receptor. Shown above the C domain is an illustration of the putative zinc finger motif indicating the zinc atoms coordinately bound with the cysteine residues in the domain. There is an alpha helical region in the C terminal end of each finger structure. DMD denotes a region in the second zinc finger which has been mapped as a secondary dimerization domain. Domain D is the hinge region with little prescribed function, as presently understood. Steroid binding occurs in the E domain and is most closely mapped to the C terminus. The major dimerization interaction occurs in the peptide region between residues 501–522. The F domain and the last portion of the E domain contains a region involved with ligand induced transcriptional activation (AF-2).

protein is required to trigger a typical physiologic cascade of biologic events upon activation. Interestingly, multiple mutant forms of the ER have been isolated from breast cancer tissue or cell lines. These forms include constitutively active receptors, which do not require estrogens for transactivation of promoters containing EREs; dominant negative mutants, which can prevent transactivation by wild-type ER; and nonfunctional ERs, which cannot induce transcription because at least one functional domain of the protein (i.e., DNA or ligand binding domains) has been inactivated.[r23–r25] The significance of these mutants in vivo is still unclear, but the existence of such forms of the ER in neoplastic breast tissues does suggest a plausible mechanism for the development of estrogen resistance seen in some breast cancers.

Furthermore, epidemiologic data have connected germline modifications of the ER with B region polymorphism associated with an increased incidence of spontaneous abortions.[30] In addition, recently, the first known patient exhibiting estrogen insensitivity and lacking functional ER has been discovered.[31] This adult male has osteoporosis, nonfusion of his epiphyseal plates, and no evidence of gynecomastia despite high circulating levels of estradiol and gonadotropin. Molecular analysis of the ER gene uncovered a homozygous point mutation in the second exon, resulting in a premature termination codon that would produce a truncated, nonfunctional ER protein that would not contain either the DNA or ligand binding domains. The phenotype in a female exhibiting null mutation for the estrogen receptor is not yet known.

The use of animal models has produced significant advances in our understanding of the physiologic roles and mechanisms of ER action. For instance, transgenic mice have provided a useful tool to evaluate and understand molecular mechanisms of different pathologies. A novel line of mice has been developed in which a germline mutation in the ER gene has been introduced into the second exon.[32] This mutation results in the disruption of the ER gene transcription; therefore, the homozygous mouse is lacking functional ER, much like the patient mentioned above. The uteri of the female homozygous mice are hypoplastic and unresponsive to estrogens, the ovaries are cystic and hemorrhagic, and the bones show decreased density, despite high circulating levels of estradiol. Fertility and bone density are also affected in the homozygous males. Sperm counts approximate only 10 percent of the wild-type male, and there is significant dysmorphogenesis of the seminiferous tubules. The seminal vesicle, prostate, and epididymis weights are similar to the wild-type male, indicating that the circulating androgen levels are adequate. This animal model should provide a significant contribution to the investigations into the biologic role of the ER in vivo. Another transgenic mouse model has been developed demonstrating overexpression of the wild-type ER.[33] The females display aberrant reproductive phenotypes, especially at parturition. As maternal age increases, so does the incidence and intensity of the delayed parturition, prolonged labor, stillborn litters, and severe dystocia. These mice may provide a novel animal model for investigating the role of the ER at parturition.

Biological Effects of Estrogens

Estrogen During Pregnancy and the Fetal Period

Fetal ovaries are not histologically distinguishable until about the tenth to eleventh week of gestational age. Although fetal ovaries cannot synthesize steroids de novo at this period, it is probable that small amounts of estrogens are produced by aromatization in the granulosa cells by the tenth week.[34] Their exact nature and local significance remain to be defined. Moreover, it appears that the female internal genital tract development does not depend on any hormonal or other influences from the ovary.[r26]

Nonetheless, the fetus, independently of its gender, is in a significantly high-estrogen environment, owing to the high levels of estrogens produced by the maternal placenta, along with progesterone, during this period. Especially during the last days of pregnancy, circulating placental levels of sex-steroid hormones reach adult amounts, but no visible estrogenic effects are observed in the neonate besides rare transient breast and clitoral enlargement. This is probably due to the high circulating levels of α-fetoprotein (αFP), which binds estrogen and protects the fetus from such high circulating levels of free hormone. AFP interacts only with endogenous steroidal estrogens and does not bind synthetic estrogens such as diethylstilbestrol (DES). Still, there are some differences between steroid secretion during pregnancy and the pattern present in nonpregnant women. In fact, the secretion of estrogen from the placenta is quite different than from the ovaries, since a large share of estrogen produced by the placenta is estriol, which, as mentioned above, is the weakest naturally-occurring estrogen. In fact, from the beginning to the end of pregnancy there is an approximately 1000-fold increase in estriol production, but only about a 100-fold increase in the production of estrone and estradiol. Furthermore, the placenta is not responsible for de novo synthesis of estrogens from basic substrates as described for the ovary. Instead, DHEA and 16OH-DHEA formed by the mother's adrenal glands and by the fetal adrenal glands are transported by the bloodstream to the placenta and then transformed to estradiol, estrone, and estriol. Thus, the fetus and the placenta work as the human fetoplacental unit in estrogen biosynthesis, as first characterized by Diczfalusy.[35] However, the complex physiologic role of this large amount of estrogen secretion during pregnancy both for the fetus and for the mother is not yet fully understood. Estrogen does stimulate uterine and mammary gland development during this period, and estriol also may have a role in the maintenance of the uteroplacental blood flow.

In addition, it is not definite, at present, what the optimal levels of maternal estrogens are for normal fetal development; but it is well known that alterations in the maternal estrogen levels during pregnancy can significantly affect both female and male fetuses, producing permanent changes in several estrogen target tissues. In fact, several decades ago pregnant women were given DES during pregnancy to avoid miscarriages and other potential side-effects induced by pregnancy. In the years following, a multitude of reports[36–37] described malformations and lesions of estrogen target organs in both female and male offspring. Several studies using animal models clearly provided evidence for a cause-and-effect relationship between abnormal levels of estrogenic compounds during gestation and the presence of alterations in several organ systems in the offspring in later stages of life.[38–39,r27]

Puberty

After the transient rise of estrogen levels in the first days of life, sex steroids remain at undetectable levels during childhood. In fact, if individuals are exposed to exogenous estrogens (e.g., contaminations in food) during these early years, abnormal endocrine conditions can develop with subsequent pathologic features, such as abnormal breast development, in both girls and boys.[40,41] Normally, when a girl reaches six to seven years of age, some ovarian follicles start to grow and develop (eg., 5- to 6-mm stage). At the same time, circulating levels of estradiol increase progressively, as well as the peripheral plasma levels of FSH and LH.[r9,r28,r29] The mechanism(s) underlying the control of the onset of follicular estrogen synthesis involves the stimulatory effects of gonadotropins, particularly the FSH induction of aromatase activity in the granulosa cells.

The increase, by the second decade of life, in the frequency of GnRH pulse stimulation seems to be the triggering signal for the onset of puberty.[r30] FSH and LH levels increase, and their secretion begins to be pulsatile as well. As a consequence, the ovaries show an increasing capacity for producing estradiol and for follicular growth, until the moment in which a dominant follicle is chosen, ovulation occurs, and a corpus luteum subsequently develops. Without fertilization, bleeding follows, and at this age menarche occurs. Pathologic aberrations in the timing of menarche occur, resulting in either precocious (before age 8 to 9) or delayed (after 16) puberty.[r31,r32] The menstrual cycles that follow through adult life are based on the sequence of these events. The augmented estrogen levels at puberty accelerate the linear growth spurt that affects the fusion of the epiphysis and diaphysis of the long bones. Development of female secondary characteristics involving growth of the breast, maturation of the responsiveness of the urogenital tract (i.e., cornification of vaginal epithelium), and female habitus are stimulated. Pigmentation of the skin of the nipples areolae, and genital area are also affected by this rise in estrogens.

Lack of this normal sequence of events often occurs in different genetic or endocrinologic disorders. These can result in precocious, delayed, or lack of the pubertal spurt, producing disorders later in life. Turner's syndrome, primary, secondary, and tertiary hypogonadism, as well as ovarian failure (also called hypergonadotropic amenorrhea) can be causes of abnormally low circulating levels of estrogens with accompanying menstrual irregularities. The former results in a condition that lacks the female sexual characteristics.[r31–r33]

Menopause

The depletion of the pool of primordial follicles in the ovaries is the basis for the permanent termination of menstruation. The last episode of menstrual bleeding is called menopause and must be considered a physiologic event of a woman's life, not a disease. The period of months during which these endocrine and biologic changes of the ovaries take place is called the climacteric period or perimenopause.[r34] As defined, this time span lasts until one year after the menses have ceased. The median age at menopause is about 52 years; during the climacteric a high percentage of women (95%) experience endocrine, somatic, and psychologic changes. As mentioned above, the principal endocrine change of menopause is the dramatic fall (90–95%) in estrogen secretion as a result of the loss of ovarian follicles.[42,r9] Owing to the lack of the physiologic steroidal negative-feedback, the gonadotropins levels increase strikingly after menopause. The increased LH levels produce an intense stimulation of the ovarian interstitial cells, which have retained their steroidogenic activity with subsequent increased synthesis of androstenedione and testosterone, but not of estradiol. Extraglandular aromatization of the circulating androgens occurs in places such as the adipose tissue and explains the persistent low circulating levels of estrone and estradiol still found in this period.[8] However, the ratio of the estrogenic hormones is totally different before and after menopause. In fact, the most important estrogen before menopause is estradiol, which can be readily metabolized to either estrone or estriol, both of which are less potent than estradiol, and the ratio between estradiol and estrone is ≥ 1. On the contrary, after menopause the major source of estrogen is estrone, produced from the extraglandular aromatization of androstenedione, produced by the theca in the ovary or by the adrenal. Some estrone can then be converted to estradiol; however, this results in a lower ratio of ≤ 0.3 estradiol to estrone.

Many of the undesiderable climacteric symptoms and postmenopausal problems derive from these hormonal fluctuations. In fact, the drop in plasma estrogens gives rise to vasomotor instability (hot flushes in 75% of women), with sensation of warmth and heat followed by profuse sweating. Further, it is believed that part of the vasomotor instability (flushes) is also associated with LH pulsatility.[43,44] It is now thought that the decrease in cathechol estrogens and change in neurotransmitter levels or activity may affect both the central thermoregulatory and GnRH centers. The reduced estrogen-stimulated maturation of the vaginal epithelium after menopause causes vaginal atrophy, with consequent dyspareunia, dryness, burning, and sometimes bleeding. The urethral mucosa atrophies at the same time as the vaginal epithelium (probably owing to their common embryologic derivation). Infections, prolapse, dysuria, and urinary urgency are some of the symptoms that can generate a urethral syndrome. Disruption of the rapid-eye movement (REM) phases of sleep and consequent fatigue are other possible symptoms women can experience during these months. Although there are no recent studies correlating estrogen levels and sleep disturbances, some investigators have suggested a highly positive correlation between these symptoms and hormonal levels.[45,46] In addition, osteoporosis and cardiovascular problems are long-term effects of the missing circulating estrogens that women can develop only a few years after menopause. It has been well known since the late 1940s that the decrease of estrogens plays a dramatic role in the onset of postmenopausal osteoporosis,[47] and several studies have shown that ovariectomy can dramatically influence bone turnover in both women and animal models.[48,49] Recent studies also have demonstrated the presence of the ER in bone cells[50,51] and have shown that estrogens can modulate bone cell homeostasis in vitro by a direct specific estrogen receptor mechanism.[50–52] All this evidence demonstrates a direct role arising from the lack of estrogens influencing the onset of postmenopausal osteoporosis. Moreover, since 1950 an increasing body of evidence has linked the fall of estrogen with increased cardiovascular problems, including heart attacks after menopause.[53,54] These effects are claimed to be linked to the different pattern of lipoprotein synthesis.[54,55] Women have higher levels of HDL (particularly HDL-2) than men, and this sex-difference pattern starts at puberty and ends at menopause. Conversely, low density lipoprotein (LDL) cholesterol increases (to levels even higher than in men) as HDL cholesterol decreases after menopause. There is increasing evidence that also suggests a direct beneficial effect of estrogens on blood vessel physiology independent of lipoprotein effects. In fact, ER has been recently demonstrated in endothelial cells of blood vessels; it has also recently been suggested that estrogens may play an inhibitory role in atheromatous plaque formation.[56,r35]

Therapeutic Uses of Estrogens

One of the main therapeutic uses of estrogens is in combination with progestins in order to inhibit ovulation. This contraceptive use of estrogen is discussed in further detail in Chapter 49.

In addition, estrogens are widely used in replacement therapy in patients with estrogen-deficiency status. The presence of an intact, unmutated functional ER protein is of fundamental importance for the success of such therapy.

Estrogen Replacement Therapy (ERT) After Menopause

Few medical interventions have had as extensive application as exogenous estrogen treatment in postmenopausal women. ERT has both short-term benefits in the treatment of postmenopausal symptoms and beneficial effects in the treatment of the long-term complications of menopause. However, few other therapies in the clinical field have led to so many controversies as this hormone replacement therapy.[57,58]

There are several types of indications for the use of ERT after menopause: (a) Early symptoms related to estrogen deficiency, such as vasomotor symptoms and atrophic changes in the vagina and urinary tract. These are usually the manifestations for which women first seek therapeutic intervention. (b) Osteoporosis prophylaxis and therapy. (c) Prevention of cardiovascular morbidity and mortality.

If ERT is provided to relieve vasomotor symptoms, three to five years of therapy usually are enough, since hot flashes usually decline with time. However, if therapy is pursued for symptoms related to vaginal and urinary tract atrophy, long-term or indefinite therapy may be needed, owing to the frequent recurrence of symptoms if ERT is discontinued. In addition, the sooner ERT is started after the onset of menopause, the more effective the protective action with respect to bone density. In fact, it has been observed in several clinical studies that ERT can conserve and even augment (not all clinical trials agree on this latter point) existing bone mass and significantly decrease the incidence of fractures of the hip and distal radius in postmenopausal women.[59–61] Nonetheless, if ERT plays a pivotal role in the protection of the bone mass in postmenopausal women, it must also be mentioned that other factors are important in undertaking postmenopausal osteoporosis therapeutic management. For instance, such endocrine factors as vitamin D, PTH, calcitonin (and probably also growth factors with a paracrine action) as well as nutritional, environmental, and genetic components must be considered along with estrogens. All can modulate bone homeostasis in a multifactorial fashion.[r36] Besides these dramatic positive effects of estrogens on bone mass after menopause, ERT also can effectively influence lipoprotein metabolism,[r36] decreasing circulating levels of LDL and augmenting HDL to premenopausal levels. In addition, an increasing amount of evidence has linked ERT to a protective effect on the cardiovascular system as well as an improved arterial blood flow and arterial pulsatility index,[62,63,r37] with an over-all decreased mortality from coronary artery disease, myocardial infarction, and stroke.[64–66,r38]

Oral administration is still the most common route for ERT. However, alternative routes are available. Different routes of estrogen administration exert similar effects, even though each route has different pharmacokinetics and different properties. A recently developed procedure, already extensively used, is estrogen administration by transdermal application.[r39,r40] However, clinical trials are still continuing in an attempt to verify whether the effects of the oral and transdermal routes can fully overlap.[r39,r40] An oral dose adequate to manage postmenopausal symptoms usually utilizes small doses of conjugated (i.e., valerate, sulfate) estrogens (0.625–1.25 mg). Equivalent doses of other estrogens and other routes of administration available are shown in Table 46.2. These are the currently reccommended dosages to control and manage postmenopausal symptoms and osteoporosis.[67,r40] ERT should be addressed differently, depending on whether a woman has had a hysterectomy. ERT in women with an intact uterus should always be administered in association with progesterone to protect the uterus from excessive hyperstimulation by the estrogen components. Currently, ERT is either administered in a cyclical manner, such as for the first 25 days of the month with the addition of a progestational agent (i.e., 5–10 mg of medroxyprogesterone acetate) for 10 to 14 days at the end of the month. This type of administration will maintain a monthly bleeding pattern. Alternatively, ERT can be given continuously (i.e., 0.625 mg conjugated estrogens) with the addition of progesterone (i.e., 2.5 mg Provera); the continuous pattern of administration will discontinue monthly bleeding. A clinical problem sometimes associated with this pattern is "breakthrough bleeding". Unopposed, continuous estrogens should be given only to women after hysterectomy who have no risk of developing endometrial hyperplasia, which increases the risk for uterine cancer. This issue is still debated with respect to potential increased risk of breast cancer.[68,69]

On the other hand, there is evidence that seems to suggest that the addition of progestogens diminishes some beneficial effects of estrogens on lipoprotein patterns and the cardiovascular system.[62,63] At the present time, there are no indications that suggest a decrease in the protective role of the estrogen on the skeleton. However, since these negative effects of progestational agents have been demonstrated to occur in a dose-dependent manner, the minimal effective dose (i.e., 5 mg for 12–14 days) should be added to the ERT. There are no findings, as yet, that can explain the mechanism of action of the effects of progesterone when added to ERT. However, some recent in vitro data suggest that progesterone can exert an inhibitory modulation of estrogen activity in cell cultures upon binding to the A form of the progesterone receptor instead or to the B form.[78] Activation of the A form of the progestrerone receptor antagonizes B form activity regarding the hormonal responsiveness of the cells. Further studies are needed, however, to evaluate the importance of these findings in vivo and to clarify the significance of these molecular mechanisms in estrogen target tissue homeostasis.

Table 46.2 Estrogens Used in the Replacement Therapy

Drug	Route	Dose (mg)	Interval
17b-estradiol (micronized)	Oral	1–2	5 days/week
17b-estradiol	SC	25	3–4 months
17b-estradiol	TD	0.5 (10 cm)	3–4 days
17b-estradiol	VC	0.625	daily
Estradiol benzoate	IM	0.5–1.5	2–3 days/week
Estradiol cypionate	IM	1–5	weekly
Estradiol valerate	IM	10–40	1–4 weeks
Estrone	IM	0.1–2	weekly
Estrone piperazine sulfate	Oral	0.3–1.5	daily
Conjugated estrogens	Oral	0.3–1.2	daily
Esterified estrogens	Oral	0.3–1.2	daily
Ethinyl estradiol	Oral	0.02–0.05	daily
Diethylstilbestrol	Oral	0.2–0.5	daily
Hexestrol	Oral	0.1–0.2	daily

SC: subcutaneous implant; TD: transdermal patches; IM: intramuscularly; VC: vaginal cream.

Estrogen Replacement Therapy in Hypogonadic Conditions

Estrogen replacement usually is necessary for the development of sexual secondary characteristics in ovarian deficiency conditions already present before puberty (i.e., Turner's or Kallman syndromes). Treatment in these hypogonadic conditions usually is started at the age of presumed puberty (13–14 years), with small doses of estrogens (i.e., ethinyl estradiol 0.01 mg) in cyclic patterns (e.g., 3 weeks every month), with a doubling of the dosages after approximately four months. After nine to 12 months, considering also the effectiveness of the treatment in developing sexual characteristics, progesterone is usually added during the last ten days of the estrogen treatment. This regimen will induce regular menstrual bleeding.

In ovarian insufficiency due to either secondary (pituitary) or tertiary (hypothalamic) causes, therapy can differ according to the desire of the woman to become pregnant. In fact, estrogen supplementation can be established as already described for postmenopausal management when pregnancy is not desired; otherwise, pulsatile therapy with GnRH-analogues or gonadotropin injections (Perganol) can be the treatments of choice. Continuous administration of GnRH-analogues is used to treat endometriosis, an estrogen-dependent pathology.

Hypoestrogenism is naturally associated with premature ovarian failure—for which the term "hypergonadotropic amenorrhea," is now preferred. This can include heterogeneous disorders, and it is not always associated with a permanent deterioration of ovarian function. In this case, ERT also is the therapy of choice.

Other Uses of Estrogens

Dysfunctional uterine bleeding may be caused by an estrogen and progesterone imbalance. When the condition is associated with a decrease in estrogen levels it is also correlated with an atrophic endometrial epithelium. Estrogen treatment usually is administered cyclically.

Vaginal atrophy is another indication for estrogen supplementation. Local treatment is usually chosen.

Estrogens also have been used to suppress postpartum lactation. However, the current treatment is bromocriptine, which is more effective in inhibiting secretion of prolactin and suppressing the postpartum lactation.

Another use is in the palliative treatment of hormone-dependent breast cancer. The effectiveness of this therapy is believed to involve a down-regulation of the estrogen receptor in the breast tissue by high doses of estrogen. The therapy of choice of this hormone-responsive breast cancer is anti-estrogen compounds (see Chapter 47).

Estrogens are also used in the hormonal treatment of androgen-dependent prostate cancer, along with other primary (GnRH-analogues, flutamide) or secondary treatments (ketokonazole, anti-androgens). High doses of estrogens (diethylstilbestrol, 1–3 mg daily) are directed to induce medical castration resulting in the suppression of testicular androgens.

Adverse Effects of Estrogens

All estrogen preparations, particularly during the first period of therapy, may exhibit some slight side-effects. Breast tenderness, vaginal spotting and/or bleeding, fluid retention, headaches, and nausea may all be present during ERT. However, the effects are dose-dependent and tend to decrease with time. Oral estrogens have been described to increase renin substrate levels or activity, with a subsequent increase in blood pressure;[r41] to induce a state of "hypercoagulability" by depressing antithrombin III and inducing hepatic synthesis of clotting factor;[71] to produce a rise in the biliary saturation index and to increase the risk of gallstone disease.[72] The use of transdermal estradiol appears, from all recent clinical trials, not to cause these side-effects. On the other hand, the transdermal route has been described to be, at least in the first months of therapy, not as effective as oral preparations in affecting the levels of HDL and LDL cholesterol lipoproteins.[r40,r41]

The major risk of unopposed estrogen replacement therapy is the induction of endometrial hyperplasia and carcinoma. Studies over the years have provided a large body of evidence of an increased relative risk, ranging from 1 to 12,[73] and have shown that unopposed therapy does induce endometrial proliferation with hyperplasia. Progestogen addition diminishes this risk.[r40,r41]

One point of debate is the association of estrogen replacement therapy with an increased risk of breast cancer. Some epidemiologic studies have demonstrated an increased risk in long-term users,[75,76] but others had shown little or no effect.[79] Currently, there is no unanimous consensus on this issue.[75,76]

Another point of controversy is the potential association of estrogen therapy with increased risk of liver cancer. In fact, animal studies seem to suggest the presence of the correlation[r42,43] between steroid exposure and benign and malignant neoplasia of the liver. Some clinical studies reported an association between oral estrogen intake and liver neoplasia.[77,78] However, some other clinical trials have not found a strong correlation between estrogen replacement and liver cancers.[79,80] More studies are needed to investigate such a link further.

Principal Preparations and Routes of Administration

As described earlier, several steroidal compounds that possess estrogenic activity have been produced through the years. All these preparations have comparable estrogenic activity, although potency will differ with the compounds and the routes of administration. Upon oral administration, conjugated equine estrogens or estradiol valerate pass through the intestinal mucosa into the portal circulation and the liver, where they undergo hepatic metabolism, resulting in a transient elevation in plasma estradiol. Hepatic metabolism requires the use of high doses of estrogens in order to obtain effective plasma levels of estradiol. Moreover, the passage through the liver may affect the production of lipoproteins, clotting factors, plasma proteins, and other liver products. When estrogens are given parenterally, this first pass through the liver will not occur. Thus, levels of circulating estrogens will closely reflect the administered estrogen. When administered intravaginally, however, circulating levels are only one-fourth those from the equivalent oral dosage. Finally, transdermal delivery of estrogen by "patches" has been approved for clinical use. The delivery occurs directly into the circulation, without first-pass hepatic metabolism, assuring that estradiol goes directly to the target organs before conversion to less active metabolites. As a consequence, transdermal ERT can produce an estradiol/estrone ratio that closely resembles the ratio during premenopausal years,[81] without further inducing hepatic enzymes.

Independently of the route of administration, the half-life of estrogens is approx one hour, with a plasma metabolic clearance of approx 650–900 L/day/m^2. Table 46.3 shows some of the compounds used in these preparations and their trade names.

Interference of ERT with Other Drugs and Diseases

Long-term administration of antibiotics can reduce or sometimes abolish estrogen effectiveness by inducing hepatic microsomal enzymes and accelerating the drug's metabolism. Antibiotics also can interfere with ERT, disrupting the microbial flora in the intestine;

Table 46.3 Estrogen Preparations: Major Trade Names Used in the US

Natural	
Estradiol	Estrace (tablets, cream)
Estradiol	Estraderm Transdermal
Estropipate	Ogen (tablets, cream)
Synthetic	
Diethylstilbestrol	Diethylstilbestrol
Ethynl estradiol	Estynil
Chlorotrianisene	Tace
Quinestrol	Estrovis
Equine	
Conjugated estrogens	Premarin

short-term antibiotic administration is not, presumably, an obstacle to estrogen therapy. Anticonvulsant and antacid drugs also can decrease the therapeutic effects of estrogens, decreasing the absorption by the stomach when the steroids are administered by the oral route. Conversely, estrogen therapy may alter the therapeutic effects of other drugs, such as antidiabetics, anticonvulsants, and such antihypertensives as guanethidine or alpha-methyldopa, when given simultaneously.

Summary

Estrogens are steroid hormones associated with the female phenotype and reproductive cycle. Steroidal estrogens have a unique aromatic ring structure different from other classes of steroid compounds. Their biologic activity can be mimicked by other chemicals having a phenolic ring structure from a variety of sources, including the diet and environment. Endogenous estrogens are synthesized in the ovaries of females and formed peripherally by aromatization from androgen in both sexes. During pregnancy the major site of estrogen synthesis is the placenta. Responsive estrogen tissues include the reproductive tract organs, liver, mammary glands, skeleton, pituitary, and hypothalamus. Specific estrogenic activity in each tissue varies, depending on the physiologic response. Because of the variety of actions and sites of response for estrogens, future therapeutic approaches will involve the development of tissue-specific estrogen agonists. Hormonal activity is mediated by interaction with a receptor protein found in responsive cells and tissues producing an increase in gene transcription. Untimely estrogen exposure, especially early in development, can cause alterations in fertility and reproductive tract lesions. Estrogen therapy principally involves replacement of estrogen, either due to conditions of hypogonadism or menopause resulting in low circulating levels of hormone. Use of chemically derivatized steroidal estrogens, combined in some cases with progesterone, are the most common formulations, although other synthetic estrogenic agents are also available. Side-effects of estrogens vary, but, if carefully controlled, do not outweigh the benefits produced from treatment of postmenopausal patients for retarding osteoporosis and possibly cardiovascular disease.

Acknowledgments

The authors wish to thank Russ Maxwell, Sue Edelstein and Steve Edgerton from Image Associates and the Photography and Graphics Department of NIEHS for their skilful help with the illustrations.

References

Research Reports

1. Larner JM, Pahuja SL, Shackleton CH, McMurray WJ, Giordano G. The isolation and characterization of estradiol-fatty acid esters in human ovarian follicular fluid. Identification of an endogenous long-lived and potent family of estrogens. J Biol Chem 1993;*268*(19):13893–13899.

1a. Knauer, E. Die Ovarientransplantation. Experimental Studie Arch f. Grynak Berl 1900;*LX*:322–376.

2. Stockard CR, Papanicolau GN. Diestrus cycle in guinea pig. Am J Anat 1917;*22*:225–230.

3. Allen E, Doisy EA. An ovarian hormone: A preliminary report on its localization, extraction, and partial purification, and action in test animals. JAMA 1923;*81*:819–821.

4. Ascheim S, Zondek B. Ovarialhormon. Wachstum der Genitalien, sexuelle fruhrelfe. Klin Wchnschr 1926;*5*:2199–2202.

5. Doisy EA, Veler CD, Thayer SA. The preparation of crystalline ovarian hormone from the urine of pregnant women. J Biol Chem 1930;*86*:499–509.

5a. Butenandt, A. When die Reindarstellung les follekelhormones aus schevangerenharn Ziachs f. Physiol Chem 1930;*191*:127–139.

6. Dodds EC. The significance of synthetic oestrogenic agents. Acta Med Scan (Suppl) 1938;*90*:141–145

7. McNathy KP, Makris A, De Grazia A. The production of progesterone, androgens and estrogens by granulosa and theca tissue and stroma from human ovaries in vitro. J Clin Endocrinol Metab 1979;*49*:687–699.

8. Grodin JM, Siiteri PK, MacDonald PC. Source of estrogen production in postmenopausal women. J Clin Endocrinol Metab 1973;*36*:207–214.

9. McChusky NJ, Naftolin F, Krey LC, Franks S. The cathecol estrogens. J Steroid Biochem 1981;*15*:111–124.

10. Adlercreutz HF, Martin P, Pulkkinen H. Intestinal metabolism of estrogens. J Clin Endocrinol Metab 1976;*43*:497–505.

11. McLachlan JA, Korach KS, Newbold RR, Degen GH. Diethylstilbestrol and other estrogen in the environment. Fundam Appl Toxicol 1984;*4*:686–692.

12. Armstrong BK, Brown JB, Clarke HT, Crooke DK, Hahnel R, Masarei JR, Ratajczak T. Diet and reproductive hormones: a study of vegetarian and non-vegetarian postmenopausal women. J Natl Cancer Inst 1981;*67*:761–767.

12a. Pietras RJ, Szego CM. Estrogen receptors in uterine plasma membranes. J Steroid Biochem 1979;*11*:1471–1483.

13. Gosden JR, Middleton PG, Rout D. Localization of the human oestrogen receptor gene to chromosome 6q24—q27 by in situ hybridization. Cytogenet Cell Genet 1986;*43*:218–220.

14. Green S, Walter P, Kumar V, Krust A, Bornert J-M, Argos P, Chambon P. Human oestrogen receptor cDNA; sequence, expression and homology to v-*erb* A. Nature 1986;*320*:134–139.

15. Klein-Hitpass L, Ryffel GU, Heitlinger E, Cato ACB. A 13 bp palindrome is a functional estrogen responsive element and interacts specifically with estrogen receptor. Nuc Acids Res 1988;*16*:647–663.

16. Klock G, Strahle U, Schutz G. Oestrogen and glucocorticoid responsive elements are closely related but distinct. Nature 1987;*329*:734–736.

17. Glass CK, Holloway JM, Devary OV, Rosenfeld MG. The thyroid hormone receptor binds with opposite transcriptional effects to a common sequence motif in thyroid hormone and estrogen response elements. Cell 1988;*54*:313–323.

18. Naar AM, Boutin J-M, Lipkin SM, Yu VC, Holloway JM, Glass CK, Rosenfeld MG. The orientation and spacing of core DNA-binding motifs dictate selective transcriptional responses to three nuclear receptors. Cell 1991;*65*:1267–1279.

19. Segars JH, Marks MS, Hirschfeld S, Driggers PH, Martinez E, Grippo JF, Wahli W, Ozato K. Inhibition of estrogen-responsive gene activation by the retinoid X receptor beta: Evidence for multiple inhibitory pathways. Mol Cell Biol 1993;*13*:2258–2268.

20. Sabbah M, Redeuilh G, Baulieu EE. Subunit composition of the estrogen receptor. J Biol Chem 1989;*264*:2397–2400.

21. Curtis SW, Korach KS. Uterine estrogen receptor interaction with estrogen-responsive DNA sequences in vitro: Effects of ligand binding on receptor-DNA complexes. Mol Endocrinol 1990;*4*:276–286.

22. Fawell SE, Lees JA, White R, Parker MG. Characterization and colocalization of steroid binding and dimerization activities in the mouse estrogen receptor. Cell 1990;*60*:953–962.

23. Bocquel MT, Kumar V, Stricker C, Chambon P, Gronemeyer H. The contribution of the N- and C-terminal regions of steroid receptor to activation of transcription is both receptor and cell-specific. Nuc Acids Res 1989;*17*:2581–2595.

24. Lees JA, Fawell SE, Parker MG. Identification of two transactivation domains in the mouse oestrogen receptor. Nuc Acids Res 1989;*17*:5477–5488.

25. Russell KS, Hung M-C. Transcriptional repression of the neu protooncogene by estrogen stimulated estrogen receptor. Cancer Res 1992;*52*:6624–6629.

25b. Ignar-Trowbridge DM, Nelson KG, Bidwell MC, Curtis SW, Washburn JF, McLachlan JA, Korach KS. Coupling of dual signaling pathways: Epidermal factor action involves the estrogen receptor. Proc Natl Acad Sci USA 1992;*89*:4658–4662.

26. Aronica SM, Katzenellenbogen BS. Stimulation of estrogen receptor-mediated transcription and alteration in the phosphorylation state of the rat uterine estrogen receptor by estrogen, cyclic adenosine monophosphate, and insulin-like growth factor I. Mol Endocrinol 1993;*7*:743–752.

27. Ignar-Trowbridge DM, Teng CT, Ross KA, Parker MG, Korach KS, McLachlan JA. Peptide growth factors elicit estrogen receptor-dependent transcriptional activation of an estrogen-responsive element. Mol Endocrinol 1993;*7*:992–998.

28. Smith CL, Conneely OM, O'Malley BW. Modulation of the ligand-independent activation of the human estrogen receptor by hormone and antihormone. Proc Natl Acad Sci USA 1993;*90*:6120–6124.

29. Migliaccio S, Wetsel WC, Fox WM, Washburn TF, Korach KS. Endogenous protein kinase C activation in osteoblast-like cells modulate the responsiveness to estrogen and estrogen receptor levels. Mol Endocrinol 1993;*7*:1133–1143.

30. Lehrer S, Sanchez M, Song HK, Dalton J, Levine E, Savoretti P, Thung SN, Schachter B. Oestrogen receptor B-region polymorphism and spontaneous abortion in women with breast cancer. Lancet 1990;*335*:622–624.

31. Smith EP, Boyd J, Frank GR, Takahashi H, Cohen RM, Specter B, Williams TC, Lubahn DB, Korach KS. Estrogen insensitivity syndrome in an adult man: caused by homozygous nonsense mutation of the estrogen receptor gene. New Engl J Med 1994 (submitted).

32. Lubahn DB, Moyer JS, Golding TS, Couse JF, Korach KS, Smithies O. Alteration of reproductive function but not prenatal sexual development after insertional disruption of the mouse estrogen receptor gene. Proc Natl Acad Sci USA 1993;*90*:11162–11166.

33. Davis VL, Couse JF, Goulding EH, Power SGA, Eddy EM, Korach KS. Aberrant reproductive phenotypes evident in transgenic mice expressing the wild-type estrogen receptor. Endocrinology 1994; (submitted).

34. George FW, Wilson JD. Conversion of androgen to estrogen by the human fetal ovary. J Clin Endocrinol Metab 1978;*47*:550–555.

35. Diczfalusy E. Endocrine functions of the human fetoplacental unit. Fed Proc 1964;*23*:791–798.

36. Herbst AL, Ulfeder H, Poskanzer DC. Adenocarcinoma of the vagina. Association of maternal stilbestrol therapy with tumor appearance in young women. N Engl J Med 1971;*284*:878–881.

37. Horwitz RI, Viscoli CM, Merino M, Brennan TB, Flannery JT, Robboy SJ. Clear cell adenocarcinoma of the vagina and cervix: Incidence, undetected diseased and diethylstilbestrol. J Clin Epidemiol 1988;*41*(6):593–597.

38. McLachlan JA, Newbold RR, Bullock BC. Long-term effects on the female mouse genital tract associated with the prenatal exposure to diethylstilbestrol. Cancer Res 1980;*40*:3988–3989.

39. Migliaccio S, Newbold RR, Bullock BC, McLachlan JA, Korach KS. Developmental exposure to estrogens induce persistent changes in skeletal tissue. Endocrinology 1992;*130*:1756–1758.

40. Fara GM, Del Corvo, Bernuzzi S, Biagetello A, DiPietro C, Scaglioni S, Schiumello G. Epidemic of breast enlargement in an Italian school. Lancet 1979;*2*:295–297.

41. Saenz de Rodriguez CA, Toro-Sola MA. Anabolic steroids in meat and premature thelarche. Lancet 1982;*1*:1300–1302.

42. Moore DC, Schlapfer LV, Paunier L, Sizonenko PC. Transient pubertal gynecomastia: Abnormal androgen-estrogen ratios. J Clin Endocrinol Metab 1984;*58*:492–499.

43. Casper R, Yen SC. Neuroendocrinology of menopausal flushes: an hypothesis of flush mechanisms. Clin Endocrinal 1985;*40*:553.

44. Tulandi T, Lal S. Menopausal hot flush. Obstet Gynecol Surv 1985;*40*:553.

45. Erlik Y, Tatryn IV, Meldrum DR, Lomax P, Bajorek JG, Judd HL. Association of waking episodes with menopausal hot flashes. JAMA 1981;*245*:1741–1744.

46. Thomson J, Oswald I. Effects of estrogen on the sleep, mood and anxiety of menopausal women. Br Med J 1977:1317–1319.

47. Albright F, Bloomberg F, Smith PH. Postmenopausal osteoporosis. Trans Assoc Am Physician 1940;*55*:298–305.

48. Heaney RP. Estrogens and postmenopausal osteoporosis. Clin Obstet Gynecol 1976;*19*:791–803.

49. Wronsky TJ, Cintron M, Doherty AL, Dann. Estrogen treatment prevents osteopenia and depresses bone turnover in ovariectomized rats. Endocrinology 1988;*123*:681–686.

50. Komm BS, Terpening CM, Benz DJ, Graeme KA, Gallegos A, Kore M, Greene GL, O'Malley BW, Haussler MR. Estrogen binding, receptor mRNA and biologic response in osteoblast-like cells. Science 1988;*241*:81–84.

51. Eriksen EF, Colvard DS, Berg NJ, Graham ML, Mann KG, Spelsberg TC, Riggs BL. Evidence of estrogen receptor in normal human osteoblast-like cells. Science 1988;*241*:84–86.

52. Migliaccio S, Davis VL, Gibson MK, Gray TK, Korach KS. Estrogens modulate the responsiveness of osteoblast-like cells (ROS 17/2.8) stably transfected with the estrogen receptor. Endocrinology 1992;*130*:2617–2624.

53. Robinson RW, Higano N, Cohen WD. Increased incidence of coronary heart disease in women castrated prior to the menopause. Arch Inter Med 1959;*104*:908–913.

54. Colditz GA, Willett WC, Stampfer MJ. Menopause and the risk of coronary heart disease in women. N Engl J Med 1987;*316*:1105–1110.

55. Sznajderman M, Oliver MF. Spontaneous premature menopause, ischemic heart-disease and serum lipids. Lancet 1963;*1*:962–965.

56. Adams MR, Clarkson TB, Koritnik DR, Nash HA. Contraceptive steroids and coronary artery atherosclerosis in cynomologous macaques. Fertil Steril 1987;*7*:1010–1018.

57. Notelovitz M. Estrogen replacement therapy: Indications, contraindications and age selection. Am J Obstet Gynecol 1989;*161*:1832–1941.

58. Weinstein MC. Estrogen use in postmenopausal women - costs, risks, benefits. N Engl J Med 1980;*303*:308–316.

59. Lindsay R, Aitkin JM, Anderson JB, Hart DM, MacConald EB, Clarke AC. Long-term prevention of postmenopausal osteoporosis by oestrogen. Lancet 1976;*1*:1038–1040.

60. Christiansen C, Christiansen MS, Transbol I. Bone mass in postmenopausal women after withdrawal of oestrogen/gestagen replacement therapy. Lancet 1981;*99*:459–461.

61. Notelovitz M. Estrogen replacement therapy: Indications, contraindications and age selection. Am J Obstet Gynecol 1989;*161*:1832–1841.

62. Wren BG, Routledge AD. The effect of type and dose of oestrogen on the blood pressure of post-menopausal women. Maturitas 1983;*5*:35–142.

63. Bourne T, Hilard TC, Whitehead MI. Oestrogen, arterial status and postmenopausal women. Lancet 1990;*335*:1470–1471.

64. Henderson BE, Paganini-Hill A, Ross RK. Estrogen replacement therapy and protection from acute myocardial infarction. Am J Obstet Gynecol 1988;*159*:312–317.

65. Burch JC, Byrd BF, Vaughn WK. The effects of long term estrogen on hysterectomized women. Am J Obstet Gynecol 1974;*118*:778–782.

66. Henderson BE, Paganini-Hill A, Ross RK. Decreased mortality in users of estrogen replacement therapy. Arch Intern Med 1988;*151*:75–78.

67. Lindsay R, Hart DM. The minimum effective dose of oestrogen for prevention of postmenopausal bone loss. Obstet Gynecol 1984;*63*:759–763.

68. Buring JE, Hennekens CH, Lipnick RJ, Willett W, Stamfer MJ, Rosner B, Peto R, Speizer FE. A prospective cohort study of postmenopausal hormone use and risk of breast cancer in US women. Am J Epidemiol 1987;*125*:939–947.

69. LaVecchia C, DeCarli A, Parazzini F, Gentile A, Liberati C, Franceschi S. Noncontraceptive estrogens and the risk of breast cancer: un update. Int J Cancer 1992;*50*:161–162.

70. McDonnell DP, Vegeto E, O'Malley BW. Identification of a negative regulatory function for steroid receptors. Proc Natl Acad Sci USA 1992;*89*:10563–10567.

71. Conrad J, Cazenave B, Samama M et al. AtIII content and antithrombin activity in oestrogen-progestogen and progestogen only treatment. Thrombosis Res 1980;*18*:675–686.

72. Petitti DB, Sidney S, Perlman JA. Increased risk of cholecystectomy in users of supplemental estrogen. Gastroenterology 1988;*94*:91–97.

73. Brinton LA, Hoover R, Fraumeni JF Jr. Menopausal oestrogens and breast cancer risk: an expanded case- control study. Br J Cancer 1986;*54*:825–832.

74. Hunt K, Vessey M. Long-term effects of postmenopausal hormone replacement therapy. Br J Hosp Medic 1987:450–460.

75. Dupont WF, Page DL. Menopausal estrogen replacement therapy and breast cancer. Arch Inter Medic 1991;*151*:67–72.

76. Steinberg K, Thacker SB, Smith SJ, Stroup DS, Zack M, Flanders WD, Berkelman RL. A meta-analysis of the effect of estrogen replacement therapy on the risk of breast cancer. JAMA 1991;*265*:1895–1990.

77. Mettlin C, Natarajan N. Studies on the role of oral contraceptive use in the etiology of benign and malignant liver tumors. J Surg Oncol 1981;*18*:74–82.

78. Palmer JR, Rosenberg L, Kaufman DW, Warshauer ME, Stolley P, Shapiro S. Oral contraceptive use and liver cancer. Am J Epidemiol 1989;*130*:878–882.

79. Adami HO, Persson I, Hoover R, Schairer C, Bergkvist L. Risk of cancer in women receiving hormone replacement therapy. Int J Cancer 1989;*44*:833–839.

80. Tavani A, Negri E, Parazzini F, Franceschi S, La Vecchia C. Female hormone utilisation and risk of hepatocellular carcinoma. Int J Cancer 1993;*48*:635–637.

81. Nichols KC, Schenkel L, Benson H. 17 β-estradiol for postmenopausal estrogen replacement therapy. Obstet Gynecol Survey 1984;*39*:230–236.

Reviews

r1. Korach KS. Stilbestrol estrogens: Molecular/structural probes for understanding estrogen action. In Bohl M, Duax WL. CRC Unicience report: Molecular structure and biological activities of steroids. Boca Raton: CRC Press, pp 1992; 210–227.

r2. Jordan VC. Biochemical pharmacology of antiestrogen action. Pharmacol Rev 1984;*36*:245–276.

r3. Jensen EV, Jacobson HI. Basic guides to the mechanism of estrogen action. Rec Prog Horm Res 1962;*18*:387–414.

r4. Jensen EV, De Sanbre ER. Mechanism of action of the female sex hormones. Ann Rev Biochem 1972;*41*:203–230.

r5. O'MAlley BW, Means AR. Female steroid hormones and target cell nuclei. Science 1974;*183*:610–620.

r6. Gorski J, Gannon F. Current models of steroid hormone action: A critique. Ann Rev Physiol 1976;*38*:425–450.

r7. Green S, Chambon P. The estrogen receptor: From perception to mechanism. In: MG Parker. Nuclear hormone receptors. London: Academic Press, 1991; pp 15–38

r8. Fotherby K Biosynthesis of oestrogens. In: Makin HLJ ed. Biochemistry of steroid hormones. Oxford: Blackwell, 1984; pp 207–229.

r9. Carr BR. Disorders of the ovary and female reproductive tracts. In: Wilson JD, Foster DW. eds. Williams' textbook of endocrinology. Philadelphia: Saunders, 1992; pp 1290–1350.

r10. Erikson GF. The ovary: basic principles and concepts. A. Physiology. In: Felig P, Baxter JD, Broadus AE, Frowman LA. Endocrinology and metabolism. New York: McGraw-Hill 1987; pp 905–950.

r11. Engel LL. The biosynthesis of estrogens. In: Greep RO, Astwood EB, Geiger SR. Handbook of physiology. Baltimore: Williams & Wilkins. 1973;*2*:463–483.

r12. Kaldas RS, Hughes CL Jr. Reproductive and general metabolic effects of phytoestrogen in mammals. Reprod Toxicol 1989;*3*:81–89.

r13. Adlercreutz H. Diet, breast cancer and sex hormone metabolism. Ann NY Acad Sci 1990;*595*:281–290.

r14. Setchell KDR, Adlercreutz H. In: Rowland IR. Role of the gut flora in toxicity and cancer. London: Academic Press 1988; pp 315–345.

r15. Rose DP. Diet, hormones and cancer. Annu Rev Publ Health 1993;*14*:1–17.

r15a. Szego C. Membrane recognition and effector sites in steroid hormone action. In Litwak G, ed. Biochemical actions of hormones. New York, Academic Press, vol. 8, 1981; pp 307–463.

r16. Evans RM. The steroid and thyroid hormone receptor superfamily. Science 1988;*240*:889–895.

r17. Gronemeyer H. Transcriptional activation by estrogen and progesterone receptors. Ann Rev Genet 1991;*25*:89–123.

r18. Green S. Modulation of oestrogen receptor activity by oestrogens and anti-oestrogens. J Steroid Biochem Molec Biol. 1990;*37*:747–751.

r19. Power RF, Conneely OM, O'Malley BW. New insights into activation of the steroid hormone receptor superfamily. Trends Pharmacol Sci 1992;*13*:318–323.

r20. King RJB. Effects of steroid hormones and related compounds on gene transcription. Clin Endocrinol (Oxf) 1992;*36*:1–14.

r21. Beniahmad A, Tsai MJ. Mechanisms of transcriptional activation by steroid hormone receptors. J Cell Biochem 1993;*51*:151–156.

r22. Truss M, Beato M. Steroid hormone receptors: Interaction with deoxyribonucleic acid and transcription factors. Endocrinol Rev 1993;*14*:459–479.

r23. Sluyser M. Role of estrogen receptor variants in the development of hormone resistance in breast cancer. Clin Biochem 1992;*25*:407–414.

r24. Fuqua SA, Chamness GC, McGuire WL. Estrogen receptor mutations in breast cancer. J Cell Biochem 1993;*51*:135–139.

r25. Wei LL. Trancriptional activation of the estrogen receptor. Clin Chem 1993;*39*:341–345.

r26. Sizonenko PC. Sexual differentiation. In: Bertrand J, Rappaport R, Sizonenko PC eds. Pediatric Endocrinology. Baltimore: Williams & Wilkins, 1993; pp 88–99.

r32. Bourguignon JP. Delayed puberty and hypogonadism. In: Bertrand J, Rappaport R, Sizonenko PC eds. Pediatric Endocrinology. Baltimore: Williams & Wilkins, 1993; pp 404–419.

r27. Bern HA, Talamantes FJ Neonatal mouse models and their relation to disease in the human female. In: Herbst AL, Mern HA. Developmental effects of diethylstilbestrol(DES) in pregnancy. New York: Thieme-Statton, 1981; pp 129–147.

r28. Ducharme JR. Normal puberty: Clinical manifestations and their endocrine control. In: Collu R, Ducharme JR, Guyda H. Pediatric endocrinology. New York: Raven Press, 1989; pp 307–330.

r29. Weitzman ED, Boyar RM, Kapen S, Hellman L. The relationship of sleep and sleep stages to neuroendocrine secretion and biological rhythms in man. Recent Prog Horm Res 1975;*31*:399–441.

r30. Bourguignon JR. Time-related neuroendocrine manifestations of puberty: a combined clinical and experimental approach extracted from the 4th Belgian Endocrine Society Lecture. Horm Res 1988;*30*:224–234.

r31. Sizonenko PC. Precocious Puberty. In: Bertrand J, Rappaport R, Sizonenko PC. Pediatric endocrinology. Baltimore: Williams & Wilkins, 1993;*28*:387–403.

r32. Bourguignon JP. Delayed puberty and hypogonadism. In: Bertrand J, Rappaport R, Sizonenko PC. Pediatric endocrinology. Baltimore: Williams & Wilkins, 1993;*29*:404–419.

r33. Rebar RW, Cedars MI. Hypergonatropic forms of amenorrhea in young women. Endocrinol Metab Clin North America, 1992;*21*(1):173–191

r34. Utian WA. The climacteric syndrome. In: van Keep PA, Greenblatt RB, Albeaux-Fernit M. Consensus on menopausal research. Lancaster: MTP Press, 1976: pp 1–12.

r35. Riggs BL. Pathogenesis of osteoporosis. Am J Obstet Gynecol 1987;*156*:1342–1346.

r36. Wren BG. The effects of estrogen on the female cardiovascular system. Med J Aust 1992;*157*:204–208.

r37. Hussman F. Long-term metabolic effect of estrogen therapy. In: Greenblatt RB, Heithecker R. A modern approach to the perimenopausal years: new developments in bioscience. New York: W de Gruyter. 1986; pp 163–175.

r38. Barrett-Connor E, Miller V. Estrogens, lipids and hearth disease. Clinics Geriat Med 1993;*9*(1):57–67.

r39. Corson SL. A decade of experience with transdermal estrogen replacement therapy: overview of key pharmacologic findings. Int J Fertil 1993;*38*(2):79–91.

r40. Balfour JA, McTavish D. Transdermal estradiol. A review of its pharmacological profile, and therapeutic potential in the prevention of postmenopausal osteoporosis. Drugs & Aging 1992;*2*(6):487–507.

r41. Anderson F. Kinetics and Pharmacology of estrogens in pre- and postmenopausal women. Int J Fertil 1993;*38*(1):53–64.

r42. Yager JD Jr, Yager R. Oral contraceptives steroids as promoters of hepatocarcinogenesis in female Sprague-Dawley rats. Cancer Res 1980;*40*:3680–3685.

r43. Lucier GW. Receptor-mediated carcinogenesis. In: Vainio H, Magee PN, McGregor DB, McMichael AJ. Mechanism of molecular carcinogenesis in risk identification. Lyon: International Agency for Research on Cancer 1992; pp 87–112.

r44. Green S, Chambon P. Nuclear receptors enhance our understanding of transcriptional regulation. Trends Genet 1988;*4*:309–314.

CHAPTER 47

V. Craig Jordan

Antiestrogens

Tamoxifen is a nonsteroidal antiestrogen with more than 5 million women-years' experience for the treatment of breast cancer. The drug is used primarily as long-term adjuvant therapy after surgery in selected patients with either node-positive or node-negative disease.[r1] Clinical trials are currently underway to evaluate the worth of tamoxifen in preventing breast cancer in high-risk women.[r2] At present, tamoxifen is the only antiestrogen available clinically in the US, but a range of new agents is being developed, with different pharmacologic properties to target specific estrogen-sensitive diseases.

Chemistry

The structure and major features of tamoxifen are illustrated in Figure 47.1. Tamoxifen is the *trans* isomer of a substituted triphenylethylene. The compound is a partial estrogen agonist in rat uterine weight and vaginal cornification assays, but it blocks the full action of estradiol in these target tissues.[1] Tamoxifen appears to exhibit some species-specific estrogenic effects because it is an estrogen in the mouse, an antagonist with partial agonist actions in the rat and human, but a pure antagonist in the chick.[r3] There is no adequate molecular explanation for these effects.

The key structural feature of the tamoxifen molecule that produces antiestrogenic and anticancer effects is the positioning of the alkylaminoethoxy side-chain. Loss of the side-chain or the movement of the side-chain to other phenyl rings in the molecule results in the loss of antiestrogenic activity. The *trans* structure appears to be essential for antiestrogenic activity because the *cis* geometric isomer has only estrogenic properties.

Tamoxifen is extensively metabolized. 4-Hydroxylation of the phenyl ring attached to carbon 1 of the butene chain results in an increased affinity for receptor binding in estrogen target tissues. 4-Hydroxytamoxifen has a relative binding affinity for the estrogen

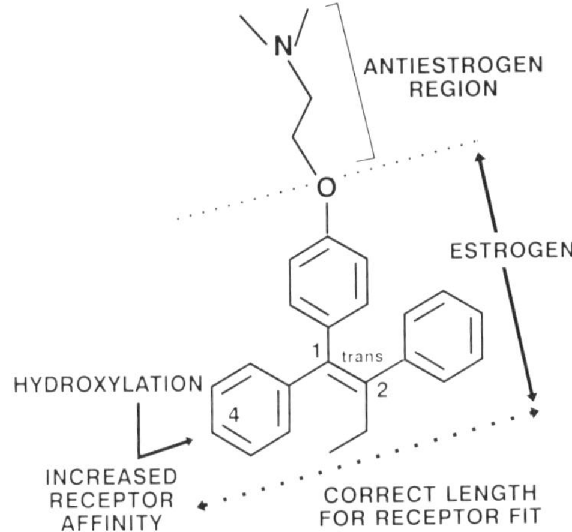

Figure 47.1 The principal structural features of the tamoxifen molecule to fit the estrogen receptor and cause estrogenic or antiestrogenic effects.

receptor equivalent to that of estradiol, whereas tamoxifen has a binding affinity only about 5 percent of that of estradiol.[2] Extensive laboratory studies have shown that tamoxifen is more potent as an antiestrogen if the molecule can be hydroxylated in vivo. However, hydroxylation is not a requirement for antiestrogenic efficacy, only an advantage for potency in vitro.

The successful development of tamoxifen for the treatment—and possibly the prevention—of breast cancer has proved a catalyst for the development of new antiestrogens. Each is a structural derivative of tamoxifen or its hydroxylated metabolites. All the new compounds have reached clinical testing.

Toremifene (Fig. 47.2) is a chlorinated derivative of tamoxifen marketed in Finland for the treatment of advanced breast cancer. The pharmacologic profile of toremifene is very similar to tamoxifen, but its potency in animal models is reduced to approximately one-

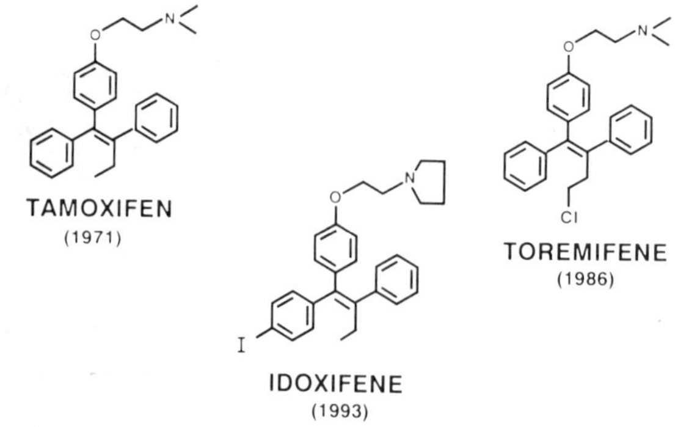

TAMOXIFEN (1971)

IDOXIFENE (1993)

TOREMIFENE (1986)

Figure 47.2 The tamoxifen derivatives that are in clinical trial. The date in parentheses indicates the year breast cancer studies were reported.

third.[3] Extensive clinical trials in Europe and the US have confirmed the reduced potency of toremifene (recommended dose 60–100 mg daily) and have also demonstrated cross-resistance with tamoxifen.[4]

The major route of metabolism for tamoxifen is N-demethylation and 4-hydroxylation, and it is reasoned that the metabolites of tamoxifen may be involved in promoting rat liver carcinogenesis (see Undesirable Effects). Idoxifene (Fig. 47.2) is designed to be metabolically stable. The iodine in the 4 position on the phenyl ring of Idoxifene is to prevent hydroxylation, and the pyrrolidino ring on the side-chain is to avoid demethylation and prevent metabolic degradation.[5] Idoxifene is being tested in the United Kingdom in the hope that the toxicity and resistance profile is significantly different from that of tamoxifen. Droloxifene (3-hydroxytamoxifen) (Fig. 47.3) has a high affinity for the estrogen receptor and is a weaker estrogen agonist than either 4-hydroxytamoxifen or the parent drug tamoxifen. The drug has been extensively tested in clinical trials, but its potency has been found to be less than half that of tamoxifen.[6] The derivative of 4-hydroxytamoxifen TAT-59 is being evaluated in Japan as a therapy for advanced breast cancer.[7] The 4-hydroxyl group is phosphorylated but must be dephosphorylated to produce the active antiestrogen.

A new series of pure estrogen antagonists is being developed as a second-line therapy after the failure of long-term tamoxifen treatment. It is reasoned that continuous tamoxifen treatment eventually could lead to tamoxifen-stimulated tumor growth. This principle has been demonstrated in the laboratory using human breast tumor cell lines grown in athymic mice, and pure estrogen antagonists have been shown to block tamoxifen-stimulated growth. The first compound in clinical trial, ICI 182,780 (Fig. 47.4), is an estradiol derivative that has been shown to reduce tumor proliferation in patients.[8] However, the principal drawback of the new compounds is that they are not administrated orally. The triphenylethylene antiestrogens have been noted to have target site-specific effects, i.e., tamoxifen has an antiestrogenic effect on breast tumors but has estrogenic actions on the maintenance of bone density. There are current research efforts in the pharmaceutical industry to exploit these unusual pharmacologic effects. Raloxifene (Fig. 47.4), a nonsteroidal compound with a high affinity for the estrogen receptor, was originally targeted as an anticancer agent (keoxifene).[9] However, laboratory studies demonstrate that the drug not only acts as an antiestrogen and weak antitumor agent, but will also preserve bone density. Preliminary clinical studies in postmenopausal women demonstrate the drug can reduce circulating cholesterol (an estrogenic effect) and could maintain bone density (an estrogenic effect). Clearly, an agent like raloxifene could potentially be used to treat osteoporosis but may also prevent the development of both breast and endometrial carcinoma as well as coronary heart disease in postmenopausal women.

4-HYDROXYTAMOXIFEN

metabolism

TAT-59

3,4-DIHYDROXYTAMOXIFEN

DROLOXIFENE

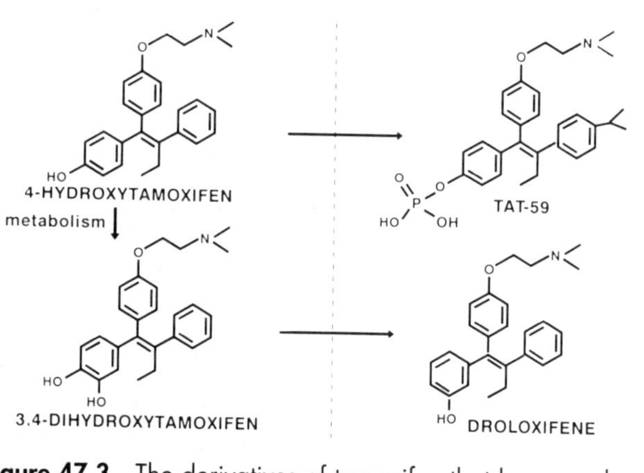

Figure 47.3 The derivatives of tamoxifen that have used metabolite mimicry to design an anti-breast-cancer agent.

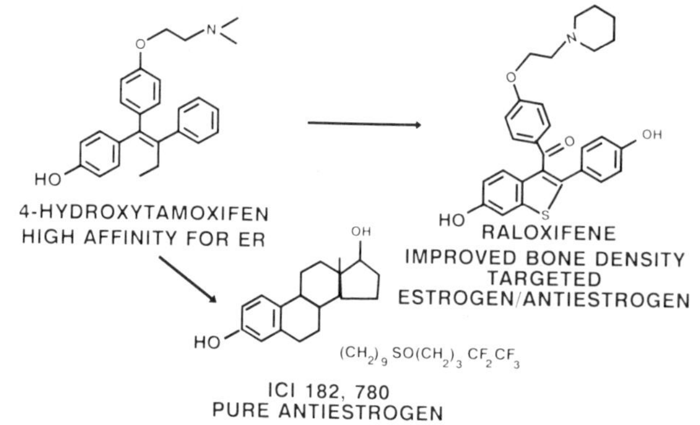

4-HYDROXYTAMOXIFEN
HIGH AFFINITY FOR ER

RALOXIFENE
IMPROVED BONE DENSITY
TARGETED
ESTROGEN/ANTIESTROGEN

$(CH_2)_9SO(CH_2)_3CF_2CF_3$

ICI 182, 780
PURE ANTIESTROGEN

Figure 47.4 New clinical concepts that are being developed that exploit the high-affinity binding of compounds for the estrogen receptor (shown in the shaded area) to produce a complete antagonist (pure antiestrogen) or to produce a compound that prevents bone loss.

History

In 1958 Lerner and coworkers[10] described the pharmacologic properties of the first nonsteroidal antiestrogen ethamoxytriphetol (MER25) (Fig. 47.5). The drug is an antiestrogen in all species tested and possesses no other hormonal or antihormonal activity. Unfortunately, MER25 has low potency, and clinical studies have demonstrated unacceptable CNS toxicity.[r4]

Clomiphene (Fig. 47.5) was discovered by the same research group at the William S. Merrell Company in Cincinnati, Ohio.[11] This triphenylethylene, a derivative of the clinically useful estrogen trianisylchlorethylene, is more potent as an antiestrogen than MER25, but also has more estrogen agonist properties. Initial interest in developing antiestrogens was aroused with the finding that drug administration on the morning after mating blocked subsequent implantation of the blastocyst in rats and mice. Clinical studies, however, demonstrated that clomiphene was unlikely to be a useful "morning-after" pill because it induced ovulation in women and guaranteed the very thing it was attempting to prevent![12] Clomiphene, a mixture of *cis* and *trans* geometric isomers, is marketed for the induction of ovulation in subfertile women with a functional hypothalmo-pituitary-ovarian axis. Tamoxifen (ICI 46,474) is the result of a systematic search by ICI Pharmaceuticals (UK) (now renamed Zeneca) to discover a clinically useful antiestrogen. Harper and Walpole, in the fertility control program at ICI Pharmaceuticals, were the first to describe the opposing pharmacologic properties of the *cis* and *trans* geometric isomers of triphenylethylenes.[13] The fertility control group then went on, in the late 1960s, to describe the anti-implantation properties of tamoxifen in the female rat. The clinical utility of tamoxifen was, however, poorly defined. Applications were demonstrated for the induction of ovulation and the treatment of gynecologic disorders, and preliminary studies demonstrated some activity for the treatment of advanced breast cancer in postmenopausal women.[r4]

The subsequent key to the success of tamoxifen for the treatment of advanced breast cancer was the low reported incidence of side-effects. This was despite the fact that the objective response rate (approximately 30%) for advanced breast cancer was similar to that observed with either diethylstilbestrol or high-dose androgen therapy, less expensive established treatments. Nevertheless, tamoxifen is only a palliative treatment. In the 1970s, a new concept of adjuvant therapy was proposed to destroy micrometastatic disease in a patient's body immediately after mastectomy, thereby improving chances of survival. At that time, tamoxifen was believed to act as a tumoristatic agent in rat mammary tumor models because tumors appeared when therapy was stopped. Continuous therapy was necessary to control tumor growth. Based on these findings, long-term adjuvant tamoxifen therapy was proposed as a potentially successful strategy for clinical trials.[r2] A recent overview analysis of randomized clinical trials conducted throughout the world over the past 15 years clearly demonstrates that long-term tamoxifen therapy (up to five years) provides a survival advantage for both node-positive and node-negative patient with breast cancer.[14] Longer therapy, i.e., more than two years, is more effective than shorter therapy, regardless of menopausal status.

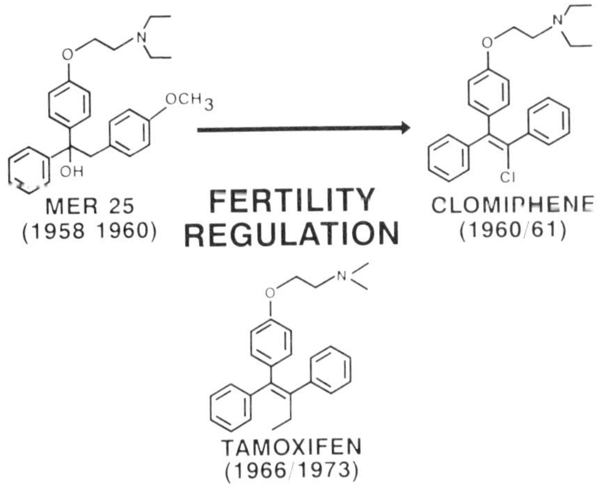

Regrettably, currently available therapies do not control disease in all women, so a new strategy of breast cancer *prevention* is being evaluated. This preemptive approach is based on two decades of laboratory testing and clinical experience with more than a million women. In the early 1970s, Jordan[15] demonstrated that tamoxifen will prevent the chemical induction of rat mammary tumors. Clinical experience subsequently demonstrated that tamoxifen is a safe and efficacious antibreast cancer drug, but most important, that tamoxifen prevents the appearance of 40 percent of contralateral breast cancer detected during adjuvant clinical trials. Large clinical studies are now being conducted in North America, the United Kingdom, and Italy to test the worth of tamoxifen as a breast cancer preventive in high-risk women. Each of the clinical trials is recruiting up to 20,000 high-risk women to be randomized to receive either tamoxifen (20 mg daily) or placebo for five years.

As the clinical development of tamoxifen has expanded, several analogues have been developed; but, in the main, the changes in structure of the compounds have been based on the emerging knowledge of structure-activity relationships and the pharmacologic properties of tamoxifen. New antiestrogens with high affinity for the estrogen receptor were designed based on the observation by Jordan and co-workers[2] that tamoxifen could be metabolically activated to the high-affinity antiestrogens 4-hydroxytamoxifen and 3,4-dihydroxytamoxifen. This discovery established the principle that affinity and efficacy of the antiestrogens could be manipulated as separate structural features

Figure 47.5 The first nonsteroidal antiestrogens that were initially shown to act as antifertility agents in laboratory animals but subsequently were shown to induce ovulation in humans (clomiphene and tamoxifen). The dates in parentheses indicate the first laboratory report followed by the first clinical report for fertility regulation.

of the molecule. The observation that tamoxifen and raloxifene (Fig. 47.4) could be beneficial in preserving bone density was first made in the laboratory in 1987[16] and later confirmed in the clinic.[17] It has become increasingly clear that the partial agonist actions of antiestrogens will mimic many of the physiologic functions of estrogen in postmenopausal woman and, potentially, these compounds will help prevent coronary heart disease (by lowering circulating cholesterol) and osteoporosis (by preserving bone density) in the elderly.

In contrast, the serendipitous discovery of the pure steroidal estrogen antagonists resulted from the knowledge that an antiestrogen could have high affinity for the estrogen receptor,[2] and that it was possible to substitute the 6 or 7 position of estradiol without affecting steroid-estrogen receptor interaction.[18] Wakeling and co-workers[19] made a systematic study of 7α substitutents in the early 1980s that resulted in ICI 182,780,[20] a compound with potential clinical use.[8] The idea is that a complete antiestrogen blocking drug will increase the initial response duration in advanced disease or that the drug will be valuable as a second-line agent if tamoxifen-stimulated growth occurs during long-term adjuvant therapy.

Therapeutic Uses and Limitations

In 1896, George Beatson demonstrated that removing the ovaries of women with advanced breast cancer could provide benefit in some cases. It was subsequently found that only about one-third of women will respond to oophorectomy. Similarly, in the 1950s about one-third of postmenopausal women were found to respond to adrenalectomy. However, it was unclear which patients would respond until Jensen and co-workers[21] suggested that the estrogen receptor, an extractable nuclear protein, could be used to identify hormone-responsive tumors. Jensen[22] had earlier found that estrogen target tissues, e.g., uterus and vagina, contain estrogen receptors, whereas non-target tissues, e.g., muscle, do not. He therefore proposed that those breast tumors with the estrogen receptor would be more likely to respond to estrogen deprivation than those tumors without the estrogen receptor. Extensive clinical testing has demonstrated that patients with estrogen receptor-rich tumors (>10 femtomoles/mg cytosol protein) have a 60 percent chance of responding to endocrine therapy, but those patients with estrogen receptor poor tumors (<10 femtomoles/mg cytosol protein) have only a 10 percent chance of responding to endocrine therapy.[r5]

Tamoxifen is the first-line endocrine therapy for postmenopausal patients with advanced breast cancer, and it is also approved by the Food and Drug Administratiion (FDA) for the treatment of premenopausal patients whose advanced disease is estrogen receptor-positive. As would be expected, the majority of responses to tamoxifen occur in patients with receptor-positive disease.

Adjuvant therapy following mastectomy or lumpectomy has revolutionized the treatment of breast cancer. In the 1970s it was normal practice to perform surgery and deliver local radiotherapy for patients with node-positive or node-negative breast cancer. Hormonal therapy and combination chemotherapy were administered only when there was a recurrence. The patient would then be classified as having advanced or metastatic breast cancer (Stage IV). However, it was found that patients whose tumors had metastasized to axillary nodes (determined after surgery) had a high probability of disease recurrence. Clinical experience during the past decade demonstrates[r2] that the administration of between two and five years of adjuvant tamoxifen therapy produces a highly significant increase in disease-free survival and improved over-all survival even out to 10 years after treatment.[14] Tamoxifen is recommended as the treatment of choice for postmenopausal women with node-positive estrogen receptor-positive breast cancer. It is usual to treat premenopausal node-positive patients with combination chemotherapy, but maintenance on tamoxifen can provide disease-free survival advantages over chemotherapy alone. Approximately 90,000 women are diagnosed each year in the US with node--negative breast cancer. Seventy per cent of these patients will be cured by surgery alone, but either pre- or postmenopausal women who have an estrogen receptor-positive primary tumor can benefit from up to five years of adjuvant tamoxifen therapy. What is particularly interesting about the therapeutic effects of tamoxifen is that a decrease in fatal myocardial infarction[23] and hospitalization for cardiac conditions[24] has been noted over and above the antitumor actions. These positive actions, coupled with a maintenance of bone density,[17] provide additional therapeutic security as a "hormone replacement therapy" for the postmenopausal woman with a diagnosis of breast cancer to reduce the risks of coronary heart disease and retard the development of osteoporosis. Women with a prior diagnosis of breast cancer are normally denied hormone replacement therapy, as it is reasoned that estrogen may reactivate tumor growth at micrometastatic sites.

It is, however, important to stress that tamoxifen treatment is FDA-approved only for women following a diagnosis of breast cancer. Tamoxifen *should not* be used outside the context of a clinical trial in women only at risk for breast cancer. The prevention trials are being extensively monitored for toxicity as well as effects on bones, lipids, and competing causes of death. Since it is not possible to predict with absolute certainty which women will develop breast cancer, and only two to six high-risk women per 1000 per year develop breast cancer, the benefits of tamoxifen as a preventive must be carefully balanced against any toxicologic risks. The results of these trials will not be available until the turn of the century.

Mechanism of Action

Estrogen is known to promote the development of breast cancer because women without functioning ovaries have an incidence similar to men. However, breast cancer incidence increases with age, and it must be pointed out that a postmenopausal woman produces sufficient estrogen from the peripheral aromatization of androstenedione from the adrenals to estrone to maintain the development and growth of a hormone-dependent breast tumor. The estrogen dependence of some breast tumors is therefore the key to the therapeutic intervention with antiestrogens. Estrogen action (Fig. 47.6) in estrogen target tissues—e.g., uterus, some breast cancers, vagina, and the hypothalmo-pituitary axis—is mediated by nuclear estrogen receptors that dimerize and activate estrogen-responsive genes through an estrogen response element in the promoter region of the estrogen-sensitive genes.[r6] The estrogen receptor should be viewed as a transcription factor that forms a transcription unit, with RNA polymerase and other as yet unknown transcription factors, that initiates RNA transcription.

Antiestrogens are competitive inhibitors of estrogen binding to the estrogen receptor, but different types of antiestrogen appear to have different molecular mechanisms.[r3,r6] The triphenylethylene type of antiestrogens bind to the estrogen receptor, but cause an imperfect conformational change that results in an inability of the complex to initiate *all* the necessary estrogenic responses. Growth is impaired, but some estrogen-regulated protein synthesis can be initiated, so triphenylethylenes are classified as partial estrogen agonists. In contrast, the pure steroidal antiestrogens bind to the estrogen receptor, but the shape of the molecular complex prevents binding to estrogen response elements, and the antiestrogen promotes a rapid degradation of the freed estrogen receptor protein. The loss of receptors in a target tissue denies all estrogen responsive genes any possibility of stimulation.

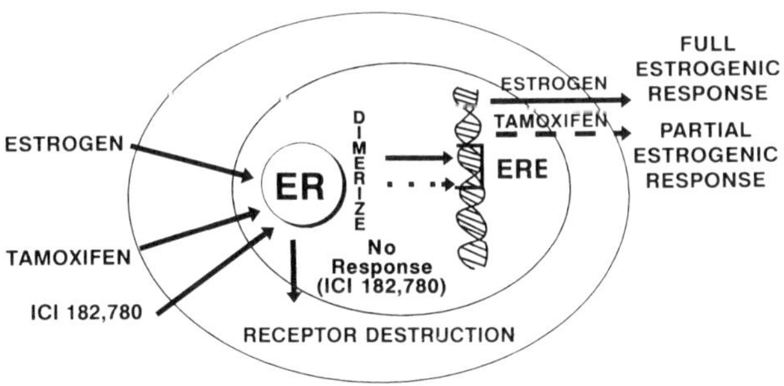

Figure 47.6 Subcellular actions of estrogens and antiestrogens at the nuclear estrogen receptor (ER). Estrogen causes the receptor to dimerize and interact with estrogen response elements (ERE) on the DNA that causes transcription of estrogen responsive genes. Tamoxifen and ICI 182,780 are competitive antagonists that either cause partial or no estrogenic responses respectively.

The theory for the mechanism of action of antiestrogens is based on experiments with human breast cancer cell lines in culture and immunocytochemistry to detect estrogen receptors in patients. However, a much more complex situation of intercellular growth control has now emerged to explain the responsiveness (or lack of responsiveness) of human breast tumors to hormonal therapies. The "estrogen receptor value" for a human tumor specimen is the average result of extracted proteins (cytosol) from a piece of tumor. Tumors are a heterogeneous mix of estrogen receptor-positive and estrogen receptor-negative cells, and the higher the proportion of tumor cells that contain estrogen receptor, the higher will be the "estrogen receptor value" for the tumor. A basic understanding of the cellular communication system is now considered to be essential to understand the mode of action of antihormonal agents.

Estrogen increases the levels of stimulatory growth factors (transforming growth factor (TGFα) but reduces the levels of inhibitory growth factors (TGFβ) within the tumor. Studies in patients have demonstrated that tamoxifen can reduce the level of TGFα in breast tumors[25] and causes a rise in TGFβ in tumor *stromal* cells.[26] It is known from laboratory studies that TGFβ can retard the growth of estrogen receptor-negative tumor cells; therefore, TGFβ from stromal cells could control the growth of receptor-negative tumors during tamoxifen therapy. This conversation between cells is referred to as paracrine growth control.

The mechanisms discussed to this point provide a model to describe growth control in a tumor, but do not explain the ability of adjuvant tamoxifen to increase patient survival. The over-all effects of tamoxifen on the homeostasis of tumors is illustrated in Figure 47.7. Metastases kill the cancer patient, and it may be that the ability of tamoxifen either to control metastatic spread or prevent the survival of micrometastases is the key to the success of tamoxifen as a therapeutic agent.[r1] Tamoxifen is known to reduce insulin-like growth factor-1 (a stimulatory growth factor) produced in normal tissues and also to prevent angiogenesis (the growth of new blood vessels) to a tumor. New micrometastases could be destroyed by denying growth factors and a blood supply to a tumor by appropriately timed adjuvant therapy.

Although the precise mechanisms of the antitumor action of tamoxifen are extremely complex in vivo, the actions of tamoxifen and related compounds to maintain bone density and reduce circulating cholesterol in animals and patients has focused intense interest on new drug development. The actions in bone and liver are expressions of estrogen-like activity. Hormone replacement therapy (estrogen plus an intermittent progestin) is often recommended to prevent osteoporosis and reduce the risk of coronary heart disease in postmenopausal women. Tamoxifen mimics the actions of estrogen in the relevant physiologic sites and has been found both to maintain bone density and to reduce circulating cholesterol. A reduction in fatal myocardial infarction has been noted in elderly women treated with five years of adjuvant tamoxifen.

Drug Interactions and Undesirable Effects

The wide use of tamoxifen within the oncology community has revealed only a few significant drug interactions. Most important, the administration of tamoxifen with combination chemotherapy can result in an increase in thromboembolic disorders.[27] Some episodes have resulted in death,[28] so great care needs to be exercised when considering this treatment strategy. This is especially true for the patient maintained on warfarin anticoagulants, because the extremely high

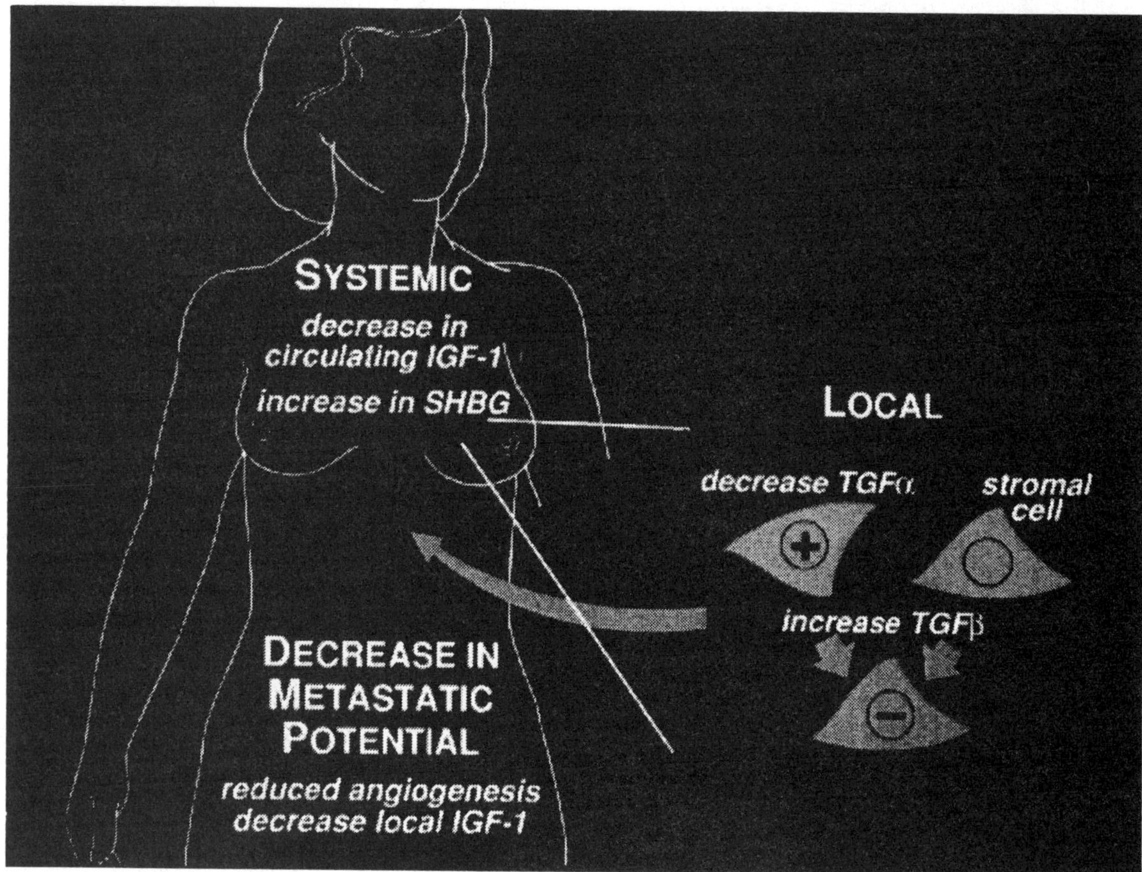

Figure 47.7 The range of pharmacologic actions of tamoxifen in the tumor tissue or within the woman's body. Tamoxifen decreases the tumor levels of the stimulatory peptide transforming growth factor (TGF)α in estrogen receptor positive (+) cells. The antiestrogen also increases the levels of the inhibitory growth factor TGFβ both in epithelial and in stromal cells. The TGFβ can control estrogen receptor negative (–) cell growth through a paracrine medium. The decrease of local and circulating levels of insulin-like growth factor –1 creates a hostile environment for the growth of either estrogen receptor positive or negative tumor cells. The ability of tamoxifen to prevent angiogenesis will deny small metastatic lesions the nutrients they need to grow.

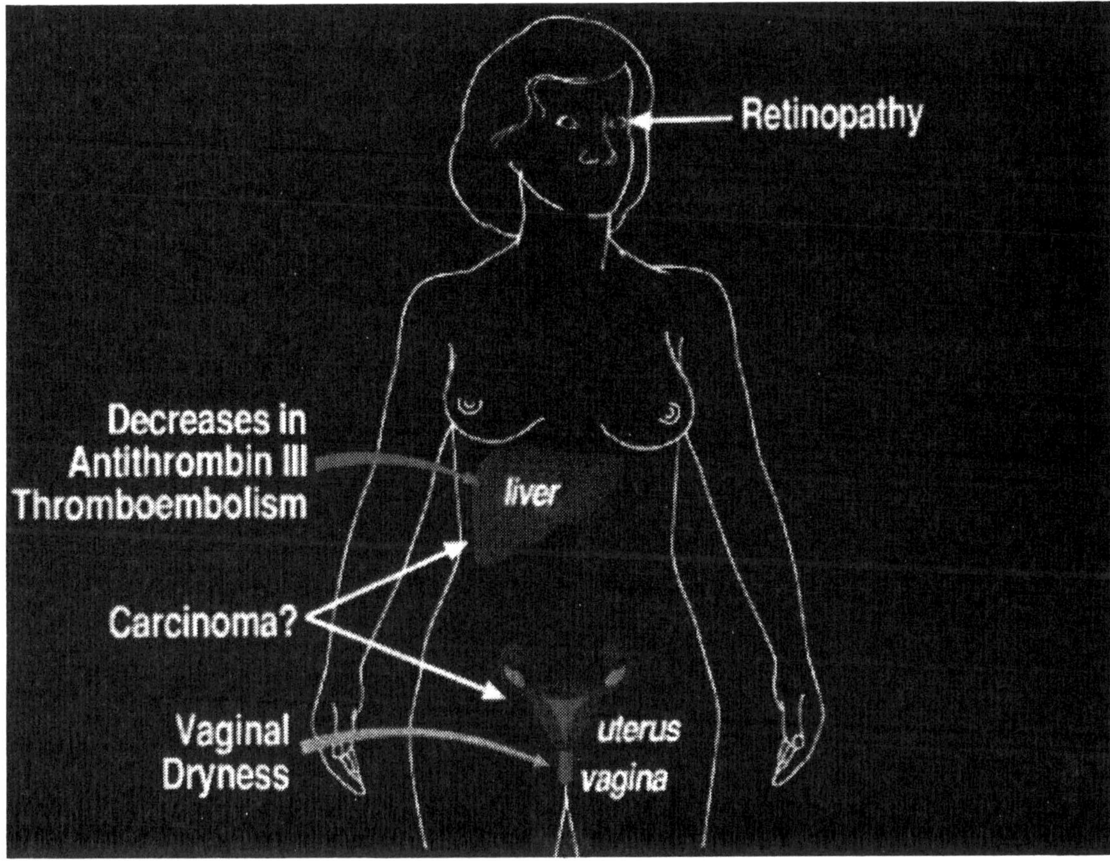

Figure 47.8 The principal toxicologic effects of tamoxifen that are of most concern during long-term (5 years) of therapy. See the text for a detailed description of the potential risks and incidence.

plasma protein binding of tamoxifen (>98%) leads to an alteration in the plasma transport of anticoagulants.[29] Patients must be monitored carefully.

Clinical trials to assess the combined value of tamoxifen and aminoglutethimide (an aromatase inhibitor that blocks estrogen biosynthesis) to treat advanced breast cancer show no improvement in responses. However, evaluation of the pharmacokinetics of the drugs demonstrates that aminoglutethimide promotes the rapid metabolism of tamoxifen,[30] probably by increasing liver P_{450} enzyme systems.

The short term undesirable effects of antiestrogens are manifestated as the menopausal symptoms of hot flashes and sweats. Most postmenopausal patients over the age of 60 are symptom-free, but up to 5 percent of younger women find some difficulty in continuing tamoxifen.[r2] As yet there are no therapies that can be recommended to avoid hot flashes.

The toxicologic side-effects of concern to all patients are illustrated in Figure 47.8. The incidence of each reported adverse effect of tamoxifen is very low compared with the benefits observed in survival for women with breast cancer.[r2] A number of case reports about ocular toxicity require increased vigilance by the physician. Tamoxifen has been reported to cause retinopathies and to exacerbate macular degeneration.[31] Although there are only about a dozen case reports, this toxicity must be monitored closely in women with pre-existing conditions.

Women who take two to five years' adjuvant tamoxifen therapy are at increasing risk (an estimated excess of 3 per 1000 women per year) of developing endometrial carcinoma. This is thought to be a consequence of the estrogenic actions of tamoxifen in the uterus. There are, however, only about 200 reported cases of endometrial carcinoma in women taking tamoxifen. Some of these cases are from women who may have had occult endometrial disease at the time of their treatment for breast cancer. Furthermore, the majority of women had been taking tamoxifen for less than two years or at higher doses than the recommended 10-mg twice daily when the endometrial carcinoma was diagnosed. While the true risk of tamoxifen-induced endometrial cancer is unknown, it is essential for physicians to order a gynecologic examination for any postmenopausal woman who is taking tamoxifen and reports spotting or bleeding. Early-stage endometrial carcinoma is curable with surgery.

There have been two reported cases of hepatocellular carcinoma in women who received 40 mg tamoxifen daily as an adjuvant therapy for breast cancer.[32] Laboratory research has demonstrated that tamoxifen can produce liver tumors in rats, but it is at present unclear whether these data are relevant to human treatment schedules. In the rat, tamoxifen produces DNA adducts in the liver, and also acts as a tumor promoter because of its estrogenic activity.[33]

With regard to overdose toxicities, there are no reports of life-threatening episodes. Up to a 100 mg daily dose of tamoxifen has been administered either as a therapy for advanced breast cancer or as an agent to reverse drug resistance to cytotoxic chemotherapy. High doses (>400 mg daily) can lead to CNS disturbances and alterations of gait.[r2] Tamoxifen causes an increase in ovarian steroidogenesis and, like its analogue clomiphene, it induces ovulation. The manufacturer recommends that tamoxifen should not be administered to the pregnant patient. There is little laboratory evidence that tamoxifen is teratogenic; but concerns mandate caution in premenopausal women, so the physician must recommend forms of barrier contraception. Finally, the stimulating effect of tamoxifen on the ovary may result in a subsequent increased risk for ovarian cancer. There is no evidence for this at present; however, since oral contraceptives prevent ovulation and reduce ovarian cancer, the converse could also be true.

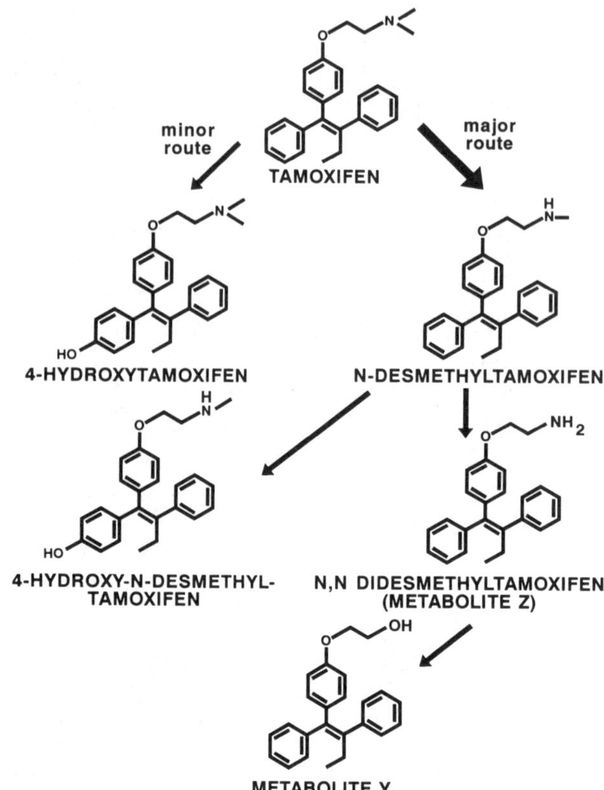

Figure 47.9 The antiestrogenic metabolites of tamoxifen identified in patient plasma.

Pharmacokinetics

A number of analytical methods are available to determine serum and plasma levels of tamoxifen and its metabolites. In the main, the current methodologies use high-performance liquid chromatography and a UV activation system that converts the triphenylethylenes to phenanthrenes for sensitive fluorescence detection.[r2,r3] Compounds that are not triphenylethylenes cannot use this detection system, and individualized methodologies have to be developed.

Tamoxifen is administered in tablet form and is almost completely absorbed, with peak levels occurring four hours after ingestion. Daily tamoxifen administration (20 or 40 mg) results in accumulation to steady-state levels within four weeks. The drug is almost completely protein-bound (>98%) and is metabolized by $P_{450's}$ via the pathways described in Fig. 47.9. The principal metabolite in humans is N-desmethyl tamoxifen, which accumulates to produce higher plasma levels than tamoxifen. At steady-state tamoxifen levels are 100 to 150 ng/ml, and those for N-desmethyltamoxifen are 200 to 250 ng/ml. N-Desmethyltamoxifen is demethylated and then deaminated to the minor metabolites—Metabolite Z and Metabolite Y respectively. 4-Hydroxytamoxifen and 4-hydroxy N-desmethyltamoxifen are minor metabolites of tamoxifen with high binding affinity for the estrogen receptor. The plasma levels are usually only 1 to 5 ng/ml for either metabolite. The hydroxylated metabolites are glucuronidated or sulfated, and the major route of excretion for tamoxifen and its metabolites is via the bile duct.

At steady state, tamoxifen has a long plasma half-life. The $t_{1/2}$ for the parent drug is seven days; for N-desmethyltamoxifen the $t_{1/2}$ is 14 days.[r2] Metabolic tolerance does not seem to occur, as patients have been monitored and found to produce stable tamoxifen plasma levels for up to a decade.[34] Most important, tamoxifen does not appear to be significantly converted to nonsteroidal estrogen that might promote tumor growth. As a general principle, any novel antiestrogen with phenolic hydroxyl groups will have low circulating levels, rapid clearance, and will require higher daily doses to maintain therapeutic effectiveness. The free phenolic hydroxyl group will be vulnerable to conjugation during phase II metabolism. For example, droloxifene is effective as an antitumor agent between 60–100 mg daily, and raloxifene is being tested as a drug to preserve bone at a daily dose of 200 and 600 mg.

Clinical testing of the pure antiestrogen is by IM injection because of concerns that the steroid will be converted to estrogens by first-pass metabolism and poor bioavailability by the oral route. A much higher daily dose is required to achieve adequate drug absorption. The daily injection of 18 mg ICI 182 780 (Fig. 47.4) produces serum levels of 25 ng/ml.[8] It is not known as yet whether this dosing schedule will produce optimal antitumor actions, but it clearly would be an advantage to develop a sustained release preparation that will last for up to a month.

Available Preparations

All clinical trials to establish the efficacy of tamoxifen have been conducted using Nolvadex (Zeneca Pharmaceuticals). The formulations are white tablets containing 10, 20, 30, or 40 mg tamoxifen citrate. Tablets should be stored in dark glass bottles to protect from sunlight. Tamoxifen is sold worldwide, and more than 50 generic versions are available with names ranging from alpha-tamoxifen (Genpharm) to Zitazonium (Hungary). Toremifene is marketed in Finland as Farestone (Farmos Pharmaceuticals). The tablets contain 20, 40, or 60 mg toremifene.

References

Research Reports

1. Harper MJK, Walpole AL. A new derivative of triphenylethylene: Effect on implantation and mode of action in rats. J Reprod Fertil 1967;*13*:101–119.
2. Jordan VC, Collins MM, Rowsby L, Prestwich G. A monohydroxylated metabolite of tamoxifen with potent antioestrogenic activity. J Endocrinol 1977;*75*:305–316.
3. Kangas L, Nieminen AL, Blaco G, Gronros M, Kallio S, Karjalainen A, Perila M, Sodervall M, Toivola R. A new triphenylethylene compound Fc1157a II. Antitumor effects. Cancer Chemother Pharmacol 1986;*17*:109–113.
4. Vogel CL, Shemano I, Schoenfelder J, Gams RA, Green MR. Multicenter Phase II efficacy trial of toremifene in tamoxifen-refractory patients with advanced breast cancer. J Clin Oncol 1993;*11*:345–350.
5. Chander SK, McCague R, Luqami Y, Newton C, Dowsett M, Jarman M, Coombes RC. Pyrrolidino-4-iodotamoxifen and 4-iodotamoxifen, new analogs of the antiestrogen tamoxifen for the treatment of breast cancer. Cancer Res 1991;*51*:5851–5858.
6. Bruning PF. Droloxifene, a new antiestrogen in postmenopausal advanced breast cancer. Preliminary results of a double-blind dose finding Phase II trial. Eur J Cancer 1992;*28A*:1404–1407.
7. Toko T, Sugimoto Y, Matsuo KI, Yamasaki R, Takeda S, Wiereba K, Asao T, Yamada Y. TAT-59, a new triphenylethylene derivative with antitumor activity against hormone dependent tumors. Eur J Cancer 1990;*26*:397–404.
8. DeFriend DJ, Howell A, Nicholson RL, Anderson E, Dowsett M, Mansel RE, Blamey RW, Bundred MJ, Robertson JF, Saunders C, Baum M, Walton P, Sutcliffe F, Wakeling AE. Investigation of a pure new antiestrogen (ICI 182,780) in women with primary breast cancer. Cancer Res 1994;*54*:408–414.
9. Black LJ, Sata M, Rowley ER, Magee DE, Bekele A, Williams PC, Cullinan GJ, Bendele R, Kauffman RF, Bensch WR, Frolik CA, Termine JD, Bryant HU. Raloxifene (LY139481 HCl) prevents bone loss and reduces serum cholesterol without causing uterine hypertrophy in ovariectomized rats. J Clin Invest 1994;*93*:63–69.
10. Lerner LJ, Holthaus FJ, Thompson CR. A nonsteroidal estrogen antagonist 1-(p-2 diethylaminoethoxyphenyl)-1-phenyl-2-p-methoxyphenyl ethanol. Endocrinology 1958;*63*:295–318.
11. Holtkamp DE, Greslin JG, Root CA, Lerner LJ. Gonadotrophin inhibition and anti-fecundity effects of chloramiphene. Proc Soc Exper Biol Med 1960;*105*:197–201.
12. Greenblatt RB, Barfield WE, Jungck EC, Ray AW. Induction of ovulation with MRL-41, preliminary report. JAMA 1961;*178*:101–104.
13. Harper, MJK, Walpole AL. Contrasting endocrine activities of *cis* and *trans* isomers in a series of substituted triphenylethylenes. Nature (London) 1966;*212*:87.
14. Early Breast Cancer Trialists' Collaborative Group. Systemic treatment of early breast cancer by hormonal, cytotoxic or immune therapy. 133 randomized trials involving 31,000 recurrences and 24,000 deaths among 75,000 women. Lancet 1992;*339*:1–15.
15. Jordan VC. Effect of tamoxifen (ICI 46,474) on initiation and growth of DMBA-induced rat mammary carcinomata. Eur J Cancer 1976;*12*:419–424.
16. Jordan VC, Phelps E, Lindgren JU. Effects of antiestrogens on bone in castrated and intact female rats. Breast Cancer Res Treat 1987;*10*:31–35.
17. Love RR, Mazess RB, Barden HS, Epstein S, Newcomb PA, Jordan VC, Carbone PP, DeMets DL. Effects of tamoxifen on bone mineral density in postmenopausal women with breast cancer. N Engl J Med 1992;*326*:852–856.
18. Bricourt R, Vignan M, Torelli V, Richard-Foy H, Geynet C, Jecco-Millete, Redeuclh G, Baulieu EE. New biospecific absorbents for the purification of estradiol receptors. J Biol Chem 1978;*253*:8221–8228.
19. Wakeling AE, Bowler J. Steroidal pure antiestrogens. J Endocrinol 1987;*112*:R7–R10.
20. Wakeling AE, Dukes M, Bowler J. A potent specific pure antiestrogen with clinical potential. Cancer Res 1991;*51*:3867–3873.
21. Jensen EV, Block GE, Smith S, Kyser K, DeSombre ER. Estrogen receptors and breast cancer response to adrenalectomy. Natl Cancer Inst Monograph 1971;*34*:55–70.
22. Jensen EV, Jacobson HI. Basic guides to the mechanism of estrogen action. Recent Prog Horm Res 1962;*18*:387–414.
23. McDonald CC, Stewart HJ. Fatal myocardial infarction in the Scottish adjuvant tamoxifen trial. BMJ 1991;*303*:435–437.
24. Rutqvist LE, Mattson A. Cardiac and thromboembolic morbidity among postmenopausal women with early-stage cancer in a randomized trial of adjuvant tamoxifen. J Natl Cancer Inst 1993;*85*:1398–1406.

25. Noguchi A, Motomora K, Inaji H, Imaoka S, Koyama H. Down regulation of transforming growth factor alpha by tamoxifen in human breast cancer. Cancer 1993;*72*:131–136.

26. Butta A, Maclennan K, Flanders KC, Sacks NPM, Smith I, Mc Kinna A, Dowsett M, Wakefield LM, Sporn MB, Baum M, Colletta AA. Induction of transforming growth factor β_1 in human breast cancer in vivo following tamoxifen treatment. Cancer Res 1992;*52*:4261–4264.

27. Saphner T, Tormey DC, Gray R. Venous and arterial thrombosis in patients who received adjuvant therapy for breast cancer. J Clin Oncol 1991;*9*:286–294.

28. Falkson HC, Gray R, Wolberg WH, Gillchrist KW, Harris JE, Tormey DC, Falkson G. Adjuvant trial of 12 cycles of CMFPT followed by observation of continuous tamoxifen versus four cycles of CMFPT in postmenopausal women with breast cancer: An Eastern Co-operative Oncology Group Phase III Study. J Clin Oncol 1990;*8*:599–607.

29. Lodwick R, McConkey B, Brown AM. Life-threatening interaction between tamoxifen and warfarin. Br Med J 1987;*295*:1141.

30. Lien EA, Anker G, Lonning PE, Solheim E, Veland PM. Decreased serum concentrations of tamoxifen and its metabolites induced by aminoglutethimide. Cancer Res 1990;*50*:5851–5857.

31. Pavlidis NA, Petris C, Briassoulis E, Klouvas G, Psilas C, Rempapis J, Petroutsos G. Clear evidence that long-term low dose tamoxifen treatment can induce ocular toxicity. Cancer 1992;*69*:2961–2964.

32. Fornander T, Rutqvist LE, Cedermark B, Glas U, Mattson A, Silverward C, Skoog L, Somell A, Theve T, Wilking N, Askergren J, Hjalman ML. Adjuvant tamoxifen in early breast cancer: occurrence of new primary cancers. Lancet 1989;*i*:117–120.

33. Greaves P, Goonetillebe R, Nunn G, Topham J, Orton T. Two year carcinogenicity study of tamoxifen in Alderley Park Wistar-derived rats. Cancer Res 1993;*53*:3919–3924.

34. Langan-Fahey SM, Tormey DC, Jordan VC. Tamoxifen metabolites in patients on long-term adjuvant therapy for breast cancer. Eur J Cancer 1990;*26*:883–888.

Reviews

r1. Jordan VC. A current view of tamoxifen for the treatment and prevention of breast cancer. Gaddum Memorial Lecture. Br J Pharmacol 1993;*110*:507–517.

r2. Jordan VC. Long-term tamoxifen treatment for breast cancer. Madison, University of Wisconsin Press, 1994.

r3. Jordan VC. Biochemical pharmacology of antiestrogen action. Pharmacol Rev 1984;*36*:245–276.

r4. Lerner LJ, Jordan VC. Development of antiestrogens and their use in breast cancer: Eighth Cain Memorial Award Lecture. Cancer Res 1990;*50*:4177–4189.

r5. McGuire WL, Carbone PP, Volmer EP. Estrogen receptor in human breast cancer. New York, Raven Press, 1975.

r6. Parker MG. Structure and function of the oestrogen receptor. Mortyn Jones Memorial Lecture. J Neuro Endocrinol 1993;*5*:223–228.

CHAPTER 48

H. Maurice Goodman

Progestins

Progesterone is a steroid hormone secreted by the corpus luteum during the postovulatory phase of the menstrual cycle and by the placenta. Progesterone and the synthetic progestins support pregnancy by preparing the endometrial lining of the uterus for implantation of the embryo and by promoting retention of the conceptus through suppression of myometrial contractions. They also block ovulation. The principal therapeutic uses of progestins are for contraception, for treatment of menstrual disorders (including dysfunctional uterine bleeding, dysmenorrhea, and endometriosis), and for palliative treatment of endometrial cancer.

Chemistry

Progesterone, the physiologically produced progestin, is a 21-carbon steroid that contains the keto group on carbon 3 and the 4,5 double bond that are characteristic of the progestins. It is produced by isomerization of pregnenolone, which is formed from cholesterol by oxidative cleavage of the bond linking carbons 20 and 22 of the side-chain (Fig. 48.1). Presumably because of its central position in the biosynthetic pathway of all steroid hormones, some progesterone is also formed by the adrenal glands and testes as well as by the corpus luteum and placenta. Hence, small amounts of progesterone are found in blood of men and postmenopausal women as well as women in their reproductive years. Concentrations of progesterone in normal human plasma are shown in Table 48.1. The closely related derivative, 17α-hydroxyprogesterone, is the only other naturally-occurring progestin, but it is biologically inactive unless the 17-hydroxyl group is esterified synthetically, typically with acetate. Addition of a methyl group to carbon 6 in the B ring of 17-acetoxyprogesterone increases progestational activity and yields the potent, orally-active compound medroxyprogesterone acetate (provera), or, after partial oxidation of the B ring, megestrol acetate (Fig. 48.1). The three-dimensional configuration of the A ring of the steroid nucleus is thought to be critical for binding to the progesterone receptor, but substituents on the D ring are also important determinants of progestational activity.[r1] Other naturally-occurring steroid hormones also have the requisite ketone group on carbon 3 and the 4,5 double bond, and derivatives of these, particularly the androgens, may also bind to the progesterone receptor and act as agonists or antagonists.[r2] Conversely, a number of synthetic progestins may bind to receptors for androgens and adrenal cortical hormones. Addition of an ethinyl group to carbon 17 of testosterone produced the first orally effective progestin, 17α-ethinyltestosterone (ethisterone).[1] Removal of the angular methyl group (C19) from carbon 10 of ethisterone decreased androgenic activity and led to the development of the nortestosterone series of progestins, including norethindrone and its exceedingly potent C-13 ethyl analogue, norgestrel.[2] All synthetic progestins used therapeutically are derivatives of progesterone or testosterone (Fig. 48.1).

History

In 1901 Fraenkel and Cohn demonstrated that the corpus luteum was needed for implantation of rabbit embryos.[3] Although it was recognized as early as 1906 that the secretion of the corpus luteum that sustained pregnancy was functionally different from the follicular secretion, it was not until 1929 that G.W. Corner and W.M. Allen produced extracts of the corpus luteum that could produce "progestational proliferation" of the estrogen-primed rabbit endometrium.[4] Their bioassay system and variations on it, particularly the Clauberg test,[5] guided subsequent efforts to isolate pure hormone. The isolation of the pure progestational hormone was announced independently and almost simultaneously by four groups in 1934.[6–9] Proof of the structural formula was obtained almost immediately, and the hormone was named progesterone in 1935. Two years later, Browne, Henry, and Venning[10] demonstrated that progesterone was also synthesized by the placenta. In 1936 Klein and Parkes[11] showed that methyl derivatives of a variety of andro-

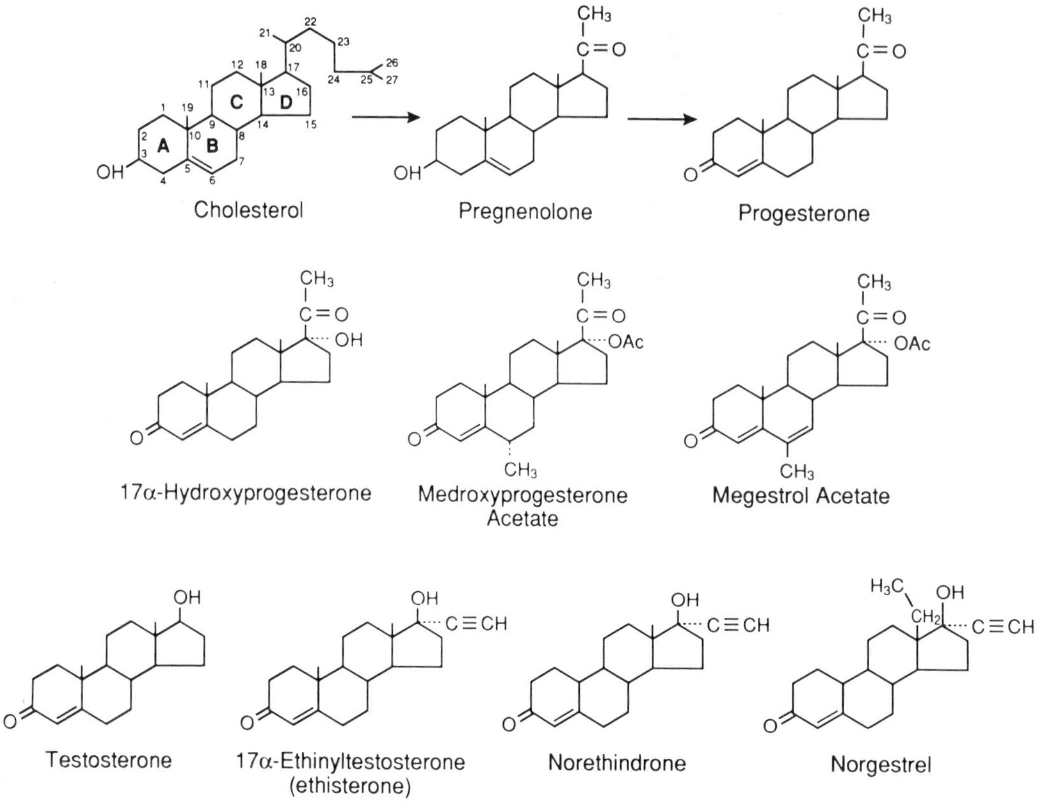

Figure 48.1 Structures of the progestins and related compounds. Top row: Biosynthesis of progesterone. Middle row: Synthetic progestins derived from progesterone. Bottom row: Testosterone and its progestational derivatives.

gens had progestational activity. The discovery in 1938 that addition of an ethinyl group to carbon 17 conferred oral potency to estradiol[12], followed several years later by the finding that removal of the C19 methyl group from testosterone increased progestational activity[13], led to the preparation of the ethinylated nortestosterone family of progestins that played a prominent role in development of the oral contraceptives (see Chapter 49). Nearly a half century later, a new class of nortestosterone derivatives with an aminophenyl substitution on C11 were developed as progesterone antagonists.[14]

Physiology of Progesterone

Understanding of the physiology of the natural progestin, progesterone, made possible the development of rational therapeutic applications of the progestins.

Table 48.1 Concentrations of Progesterone in Normal Human Plasma

Men	15–150 pmol/L
Women	
Follicular phase	25–134 pmol/L
Luteal Phase	6–64 nmol/L
Third trimester of pregnancy	300–450 nmol/L

Control of Progesterone Secretion

In the nonpregnant woman, secretion of progesterone depends on LH[15]. After binding to specific receptors on the luteal cell surface, LH triggers the production of cyclic adenosine monophosphate (cAMP), which activates enzymes that catalyze conversion of cholesterol to pregnenolone,[r3] the rate-determining reaction in progesterone synthesis. Sensitivity of the corpus luteum to LH is limited in duration, however. At about the ninth day after ovulation the corpus luteum begins to decline, and completely involutes by about the 13th day despite continued stimulation with LH. In pregnancy, secretion of human chorionic gonadotropin (hCG) by the conceptus is sufficient by the ninth day after ovulation to "rescue" the corpus luteum and support continued secretion of progesterone. Maintenance of pregnancy for about the first seven weeks depends on continued secretion of progesterone by the corpus luteum.[16] Thereafter, production of progesterone by the placenta is adequate to sustain pregnancy and continues to increase through the second trimester. At term, the placenta produces more than 200 mg of progesterone/day,[17] which is 10 to 15 times more progesterone than the corpus luteum produces at the time of implantation.[18] Control of progesterone synthesis by the placenta is poorly understood. Whereas synthesis of steroid hormones by other endocrine glands is limited by cAMP-dependent conversion of cholesterol to pregnenolone, the requisite enzyme(s) are constitutively active in the placenta.[19] The rate of progesterone production by the placenta may be limited by the rate of cholesterol uptake by endocytosis of low density lipoproteins (LDL) from the maternal circulation.[20] Indeed, progesterone production in late pregnancy is equivalent to about 25 percent of cholesterol turnover in nonpregnant women.

Effects of Progestins

Progesterone acts physiologically to support gestation. Its target tissues include the epithelial lining of the female reproductive tract, including the vagina, uterus, and oviducts, the lobular alveolar system of the mammary glands, certain cells in the hypothalamus and higher brain centers, and the pituitary gonadotropes. Progesterone modifies or reverses the effects of estrogen on all tissues in the female reproductive tract, but has little or no effect without prior stimulation with estrogen. Under the influence of progesterone, secretions of the estrogen-primed cervical glands change from watery to viscous. Spontaneous contractions of the myometrium and musculature of the oviducts are suppressed by progesterone. The epithelium of the oviducts, which thickens and becomes ciliated in response to estrogen, shrinks and loses its cilia under the influence of progesterone, even in the continued presence of estrogen.

During the preovulatory portion of the menstrual cycle, the endometrium proliferates and increases in thickness in response to estrogen secreted by the developing follicle. After ovulation and the resultant formation of the corpus luteum, blood levels of progesterone increase from virtually nil to about 10 ng/ml in midluteal phase of the cycle. Under the dominant influence of progesterone, the estrogen-primed endometrium thickens further and its epithelial glands differentiate and secrete a fluid rich in glycogen, lipid, and proteins. Vascularity increases as does the content of blood, and the stroma becomes edematous. Predeciduous cells appear in the perivascular stroma and condense to form the compact decidua. When the corpus luteum involutes, blood levels of estradiol and progesterone fall. Withdrawal of estrogen and progesterone results in sloughing of the endometrium and the menstrual flow.[r4]

In the hypothalamus, progesterone slows the frequency of pulsatile release of GnRH (gonadotropin releasing hormone)[21] and, in a manner not yet understood, blocks ovulatory surges of gonadotropin secretion. It is this action of progesterone that prevents surges of gonadotropin secretion during pregnancy and the luteal phase of the cycle and that accounts, at least in part, for the contraceptive efficacy of the progestins. Presumably, by acting on other cells in the hypothalamus, progesterone raises basal body temperature by about 1 degree F. in the postovulatory woman.

Progesterone, along with estrogens, prolactin, and other hormones, contributes to proliferation and differentiation of the lobuloalveolar tissues in the mammary gland. Although concentrations of prolactin are high during pregnancy, milk production does not begin until after parturition, when it is triggered by the decline in estrogen and progesterone concentrations in blood. Progesterone inhibits milk production in all species, possibly by interfering with production of prolactin receptors in the secretory acini.[22]

Other effects of progesterone include hyperventilation, possibly resulting from increased reactivity of the respiratory center to such stimulatory inputs as pCO_2 and hypoxia. Progesterone also antagonizes the sodium-retaining activity of mineralocorticoids and the effects of androgens on target tissues. This antihormonal activity is presumably due to the shared configuration of the A ring and has led to development of the potent antiandrogen, cyproterone acetate (see chapter 50) and the aldosterone antagonist, spironolactone (see chapter 44).

Mechanism of Action

The effects of progesterone and estrogen on the endometrium and other tissues are mediated by specific receptor molecules located primarily, and perhaps exclusively, in nuclei of target cells.[r5] Progesterone, which is lipid-soluble, readily penetrates the plasma membrane and binds to its receptor. The transformed hormone-receptor complex then binds to specific chromosomal loci and initiates transcription of certain portions of the genome, resulting in the synthesis of specific proteins. Receptors for estrogens are constitutively expressed in target cells, whereas expression of effective numbers of receptors for progesterone appears to require estrogen priming. The requirement of estrogen to induce progesterone receptors explains the failure of progesterone to act on uterine and other tissues that have not been exposed first to estrogen. The ability of progesterone to modify or antagonize actions of estrogen is due in part to a transient reduction of estrogen receptors,[23] in part to interference with some nuclear binding sites for the estrogen-receptor complex, and in part to accelerated estrogen degradation. Progesterone also causes a decline in abundance of its own receptors unless estrogen is also present.[24]

Therapeutic Uses

Fertility Control

The most frequent use of the progestins is for contraception, as discussed in chapter 49.

Dysfunctional Uterine Bleeding[r4]

Normal uterine bleeding occurs at regular intervals, usually lasts four to six days, and typically results in blood loss of about 30 ml. Dysfunctional uterine bleeding is characterized by episodes of irregular, prolonged, profuse, or scanty bleeding and commonly results from ovulatory failure or luteal inadequacy. This condition is frequently seen around the menarche before regular ovulatory cycles are established and preceding the menopause. In the absence of progesterone and the periodic desquamation that normally follows involution of the corpus luteum, the endometrium proliferates in response to estrogens secreted by anovulatory follicles and may reach abnormal thickness. Withdrawal of estrogens as follicles become atretic, or simply fragility of the tissue, leads to incomplete or asynchronous breakdown with the resulting loss of blood. In normal cycles, the action of progesterone provides some structural rigidity to the endometrium with the decidualization of the stroma so that, on progesterone withdrawal, desquamation is uniform and complete. The ischemic events that precede such desquamation are thought to culminate in prolonged vasoconstriction in the collapsing endometrium and stasis of flow, both of which promote sealing off of exposed bleeding sites.

Treatment of dysfunctional uterine bleeding with high doses of a progestin such as norethindrone (e.g., 10 mg every 4–6 hr) stops bleeding within 24 hours. Continuation of therapy (10–20 mg/d) for the next ten days to two weeks should prevent further bleeding and permit development of normal progestational changes in the endometrium. Flow may be copious on withdrawal. After ruling out other causes of abnormal bleeding (i.e., fibroids, neoplasia, endometriosis), repeated cyclical administration may be prescribed to achieve regular menses. Combined estrogen-progestin therapy as in birth control regimens (see chapter 49) may be desirable.

Dysmenorrhea

Primary dysmenorrhea is commonly encountered in otherwise normal cycles and is thought to be due to myometrial contractions in response to prostaglandins, especially $F_{2\alpha}$, released by the endometrium during the first day or two of menstruation. Inhibition of prostaglandin synthesis (see section on prostaglandins) is the treatment of choice, but beneficial effects are also obtained with progestins. Contraceptive formulations (see chapter 9) bring relief, probably by decreasing prostaglandin synthesis as a consequence of decreased endometrial tissue.

Endometriosis[r6]

Endometriosis, the growth of endometrial tissue in the abdominal cavity or other ectopic locations, may be encountered in as many as 10 percent of women in their reproductive years and may result in pain during menstruation, painful intercourse, and infertility. The ectopic endometrial tissue responds to estrogen and progesterone in the same manner as does endometrial tissue within the uterus: it undergoes proliferative changes during the follicular phase of the cycle, progestational changes during the luteal phase, and desquamation and bleeding when progesterone is withdrawn. Therapy is designed to reduce the mass of ectopic tissue and interrupt the cycle of proliferation and bleeding. Continuous administration of progestins, either alone or in combination with estrogens as in birth control pills (chapter 49) leads to regression of endometrial growths.[25] Oral (30–40 mg/d) and injectable depot medroxyprogesterone acetate (200 mg/month) or oral norethindrone (20–30 mg/d) given continuously suppress ovulation and produce the desired atrophy of the endometrium. Beneficial effects are encountered in the majority of women after six to nine months of treatment. Fertility returns after cessation of treatment in about 50 percent of cases.

Endometrial Carcinoma

Treatment with high doses of progestins may be of benefit in about one-third of patients with advanced endometrial carcinoma. A considerable fraction of such carcinomas retain receptors for estrogen and progesterone, and these are more likely to respond to therapy. Remission may be accompanied by relief of pain, increased appetite, and sense of well being. This response is usually of short duration, however. Doses of medroxyprogesterone acetate of 250–100 mg/week by injection or 40–160 mg/day of megestrol acetate by mouth have given good results.[r7]

Other Uses

Progesterone may also be used to increase fertility in women with inadequate luteal responses to gonadotropins.[26] However, there are potential risks to the fetus, including virilization and abnormal genital development. Progestins have also been used for suppression of lactation in women who choose not to nurse their babies. Both uses follow from the physiology of progesterone described above. Progestins have also been used for palliative therapy of disseminated breast cancer.[r8,r9] In addition, use of progestins as an adjunct to estrogen therapy is sometimes recommended, as discussed in other chapters.

Undesirable Side-Effects

Progestins may impair glucose tolerance and increase insulin resistance. The nortestosterone derivatives are more potent in this regard than the progesterone derivatives. The nortestosterone derivatives tend to decrease total triglyceride levels in blood plasma as well as the very low density (VLDL) and high density (HDL) lipoproteins. These effects appear to correlate with androgenic potency; the purely progestational progesterone derivatives appear to be relatively inert in this regard.[27] The resulting increase in ratio of LDL cholesterol to HDL cholesterol may increase risk of coronary heart disease, particularly in the presence of such other risk factors as smoking. The progestins may also affect blood clotting and increase risk of thromboembolic disease. These effects as well as the purely androgenic side-effects of some of the nortestosterones are considered further in Chapter 50.

Pharmacokinetics and Metabolism[r10]

Oral Administration

Progesterone and the synthetic progestins are readily absorbed from the digestive tract. However, orally administered progesterone is so rapidly degraded in passing through the liver as to make this route of administration impractical. Ethinylation or esterification of carbon 17 protects against first-pass inactivation. Orally active synthetic progestins derived from either progesterone or nortestosterone attain maximal blood concentrations within one to two hours after ingestion. Biologic activity decays with a half-time of about two to three hours during the first six hours, and with a half-time of about eight to nine hours thereafter. Metabolites may remain in the blood for several days after a single dose.

Intramuscular Injection

Progesterone may be given by injection dissolved in vegetable oil, and is rapidly absorbed and metabolized with a half-life of just a few minutes. The amount that can be injected at each site is limited because it is locally irritating. Injectable progestins in the form of microcrystals are used in long-acting preparations. The most widely used of these are medroxyprogesterone acetate (Depo-Provera) and norethindrone enanthate. Depending on dose, effective concentrations can be maintained for three to six months after a single administration. Maximum plasma concentrations are achieved after about 24 hours, and thereafter decline steadily, with a half-time on the order of about 10 weeks.

Metabolism

Progesterone circulates in the blood in association with the corticosteroid binding globulin and is destroyed principally in the liver, where the A ring and the ketone groups at carbons 3 and 20 are reduced to form the major metabolite, pregnane-3α,20α-diol. Pregnanediol is excreted in the urine as water-soluble sulfate or glucuronide esters. Synthetic progestins derived from progesterone have low affinity for either corticosterone-binding globulin or the sex hormone-binding globulin, but about 80 percent of the nortestosterone derivatives circulate bound to the sex hormone-binding globulin. The progesterone derivatives have a high affinity for the progesterone receptor and need not be metabolized to be activated. In contrast, many of the nortestosterone derivatives are converted to norethindrone before interacting with the progesterone receptor. The pattern of metabolic degradation for all of the progestins is similar and consists of reduction of the A ring and the ketone group at carbon 3 to a hydroxyl. The 3-hydroxyl group is then esterified with sulfate or glucuronide to produce the water-soluble urinary excretory products.

Preparations Available

Progesterone

Injection: (oily solution): 25, 50, 100 mg/ml
(aqueous suspension): 50 mg/ml
Suppositories: 25-mg/suppository

Hydroxyprogesterone Caproate Injection (Prodrox)

125 and 250 mg/ml

Medroxyprogesterone Acetate (Provera)

Oral: 2.5-, 5-, and 10-mg tablets
Injection: (aqueous suspension) 50, 100, and 400 mg/ml

Megestrol Acetate

Oral: 20- and 40-mg tablets

Norethindrone (Norethisterone)

Oral: 0.35- and 5-mg tablets

Norethindrone Acetate

Oral: 5-mg tablets

Norgestrel

Oral: 0.075-mg tablets

References

Research Reports

1. Djerassi C, Miramontes L, Rosencranz G, Sondheimer F. Steroids LIV. Synthesis of 19-Nor-17α-ethinyl testosterone and 17-Nor-17α-methyl testosterone. J Am Chem Soc 1954;*76*:4092–4097.
2. Douglas GH, Graves JMH, Hartley D. Hughes GA, McLoughlin BJ Siddall JB, Smight H. Totally synthetic hormones (I) Estrone and related estrapolyenes. J Chem Soc. 1963; (Nov.) 5072–5094.
3. Fraenkel L, Cohn F. Experimentalle Untersuchung über den Einfluss des Corpus luteum of die Insertion des Eies. Anat Anz 1901;*20*:294–300.
4. Corner GW, Allen WM. Physiology of the corpus luteum II. Production of a special uterine reaction (progestational prolifera-

tion) by extracts of the corpus luteum. Am J Physiol 1929;*88*:326–339.

5. Clauberg C. Zur Physiologie und Pathologie der Sexual Hormone, im Besonderen des Hormons des Corpus-luteum. I. Mitteilung. Der biologische Test für das Luteohormon (das spezifische Hormon des Corpus-luteum) am infantilen Kaninchen. Zentralblatt f Gynäk 1930;*54*:2757–2770.
6. Butenandt A, Westphal U, Hohlweg W. Über das Hormon des Corpus luteum. Z physiol Chem 1934;*227*:84–98.
7. Allen WM, Wintersteiner O. Crystalline progesterone. Science 1934;*80*:190–191.
8. Slotta KH, Ruschig H, Fels E. Reindarstellung der Hormon aus dem Corpus-luteum. Ber chem Ges 1934;*67*:1270–1273.
9. Hartmann M, Wettstein A. Ein krystallisiertes Hormon aus Corpus-luteum. Helv chim Acta 1934;*17*:878–882.
10. Browne JSL. Henry JS, Venning EM. The corpus luteum hormone in pregnancy. J Clin Invest 1937;*16*:678.
11. Klein M, Parkes AS. Progesterone-like activity of testosterone and certain related compounds. Proc Roy Soc Lond B 1938;*121*:574–579.
12. Inhoffen HH, Logemann W, Hohlweg W, Serini A, Untersuchung in der Sexualhormon-Reihe. Ber Dtsch Chem Ges 1938;*71*:1024–1032.
13. Inhoffen HH, Hohlweg W. Neue per os wirksame weiblische Keimdrüsenhormon-Derivate, Naturwissenschaften 1938;*26*:96.
14. Elger W, Bier S, Chwalisz K, Fänrich M, Hasan SH, Henderson D, Neef G, Rohde R. Studies on the mechanism of action of progesterone antagonists. J Steroid Biochem 1986;*25*:835–845.
15. Rice BF. Hammerstein J, Savard K. Steroid hormone formation in the human ovary. II. Action of gonadotropins *in vitro* in the corpus luteum. J Clin Endocrinol Metab, 1964;*24*:606–615.
16. Csapo Al, Pulkkinen MO, Ruttner B, Sauvage JP, Wiest WG. The significance of the human corpus luteum in pregnancy maintenance. I. Preliminary studies. Am J Obstet Gynecol 1972;*112*:1061–1067.
17. Lin TJ, Lin SC, Erlenmeyer F, Kline IT, Underwood R, Billiar RB, Little B. Progesterone production rates during the third trimester of pregnancy in normal women, diabetic women, and women with abnormal glucose tolerance. J Clin Endocrinol Metab 1972;*34*:287–297.
18. Lin TJ, Billiar RB, Little B. Metabolic clearance rate of progesterone during the menstrual cycle. J Clin Endocrinol Metab 1972;*35*:879–886.
19. Simpson ER, Miller DA. Cholesterol side-chain cleavage, cytochrome P-450, and iron-sulfur protein in human placental mitochondria. Arch Biochem Biophys 1978;*190*:800–808.
20. Winkel CA, Snyder JM, MacDonald PC, Simpson ER. Regulation of cholesterol and progesterone synthesis in human placental cells in culture by serum lipoproteins. Endocrinology 1980;*106*:1054–1060.
21. Van Vugt DA, Lan NY, Ferin M. Reduced frequency of pulsatile luteinizing hormone secretion in the luteal phase of the rhesus monkey. Involvement of endogenous opioids. Endocrinology 1984;*115*:1095–1101.
22. Goodman GT, Akers RM, Friderici KH, Tucker HA. Hormonal regulation of a-lactalbumin secretion from bovine mammary tissue cultured *in vitro*. Endocrinology 1983;*112*:1324–1330.
23. Hsueh AJW, Peck EJ, Clark JH. Control of uterine estrogen receptor levels by progesterone. Endocrinology 1976;*98*:438–444.
24. Walters MR, Hunziker W, Clark JH. Hydroxylapetite prevents nuclear receptor loss during the exchange assay of progesterone receptors. J Steroid Biochem 1980;*13*:1129–1132.
25. Hull ME, Moghissi KS, Magyar DF, Haves MF. Comparison of different treatment modalities of endometriosis in infertile women. Fertil Steril 1987;*47*:40–44.
26. Huang K-E. The primary treatment of luteal phase inadequacy: Progesterone versus clomiphene citrate. Am J Obstet Gynecol 1986;*155*:824–828.
27. Nikkilä EA, Tikkanen MJ, Kuusi T. Effects of progestins on plasma lipoproteins and heparin-releasable lipases. In: Bardin CW, Milgröm E, Mauvais-Jarvis P Progesterone and progestins. New York: Raven Press (1983); pp 411–420.

Reviews

r1. Duax WL, Griffin JF, Weeks CM, Wawrzak Z. The mechanism of action of steroid antagonists: Insights from crystallographic studies. J. Steroid Biochem 1988;*31*:481–492.

r2. Janne O, Hemminki S, Isomaa V, Kokko E, Torkkeli H, Torkkeli T, Vierikko P. Progestational activity of natural and synthetic androgens. Int J Andrology Suppl 1978;*2*:162–174.

r3. Niswender GD, Nett TM. The corpus luteum and its control. In: Knobil E, Neill JD eds. The physiology of reproduction. New York: Raven Press, (1988); pp 489–525.

r4. Speroff L, Glass RH, Kase NG. Dysfunctional Uterine Bleeding. In: Speroff L, Glass RH, Kase NG. eds. Clinical gynecologic endocrinology and infertility, 4th ed., Baltimore: Williams & Wilkins (1989); pp 265–282.

r5. Clark JH, Markaverich BM. Actions of ovarian steroid hormones. In: Knobil E, Neill JD The physiology of reproduction. New York: Raven Press, (1988); pp 675–724.

r6. Wilson EA. Endometriosis. New York: Alan R. Liss, Inc. 1987.

r7. Kistner RW. Therapeutic application of progestational compounds in gynecology. Adv Obstet Gynecol 1967;*1*:391.

r8. Santen RJ, Manni A, Harvey H, Redmond C. Endocrine treatment of breast cancer in women. Endocr Revs 1990;*11*:221–265.

r9. Horwitz KB, Wei LL, Sedlacek SM, D'Arville CN. Progestin action and progesterone receptor structure in human breast cancer: a review. Recent Progress Hormone Res, 1988;*41*:249–316.

r10. Goebelsmann U. Pharmacokinetics of contraceptive steroids in humans. In: Gregoire AT, Blye RT Contraceptive steroids pharmacology and safety. New York, London: Plenum Press, (1986); pp 67–111.

r11. Pramik MJ. Norethindrone, the first three decades, Palo Alto: Syntex Laboratories, 1978.

r12. Clarke, CL, Sutherland RL. Progestin regulation of cell proliferation. Endocrinal Rev 1990;*11*:266–301.

r13. Horwitz K. The molecular biology of RU486. Is there a role for antiprogestins in the treatmeny of breast cancer? Endocrinal Rev 1992;*13*:146–163.

CHAPTER 49

Ranjit Roy Chaudhury
Chandrima Shaha

Contraception

Contraception is prevention of conception. However, fertility control methods also involve postcoital contraception and termination of pregnancy. This chapter deals with methods of contraception that use distinct pharmacologic entities, most of which are hormones. Hormonal methods include oral contraceptives, long-acting injectables, hormonal implants, and vaginal hormonal devices. Currently available methods have some advantages or disadvantages relative to each other.

Some new methods now being developed are described under "New Methods Under Development."

Methods Currently in Use

Oral Contraceptives

Reports of the ability of progesterone to block ovulation led to the concept of the oral contraceptive pill.[r1] Synthesis of new progestational compounds like norethindrone and norethistrone in 1952 led to the biologic tests carried out by Pincus and coworkers. They were involved in the first clinical trials with these compounds at the high dose of 10 mg/day. Current formulations of this type of contraception provide a very popular method of birth control.[r2] They are a combination of the female sex hormones, estrogen and progesterone on their analogues. They are taken in constant amounts for 20, 21, or 22 days, followed by a pill-free interval of seven days during which "withdrawal bleeding" occurs.

The molecular structure of the synthetic steroidal contraceptives is related to that of natural estrogens and progesterones. Modifications are made in the basic steroid nucleus to render them effective at low dose and to make oral administration effective.

Estrogens

Synthetic steroidal estrogens used in oral contraceptives are either ethinyl estradiol (EE) or mestranol. Mestranol is the 3-methyl ester derivative of EE. It is promptly metabolized in the body to EE. The half-life of EE varies from 24 to 28 hours. Synthetic estrogens resemble natural estrogens in their actions on the reproductive tract and hypothalamus.

Progestagens

Synthetic progesterone-like substances are structurally related to four parent compounds: testosterone (T); 19-nortestosterone (NT); 17-hydroxyprogesterone; and progesterone (P) itself. NT derivatives are the most widely used progestagens in hormonal contraceptives. These include the norethistrone group: norethisterone; norethynodrel; ethynodiol diacetate; and lynestrenol. All these are converted to norethisterone in the body. Liver metabolism reduces bioavailability by 40 percent. A more potent 19-norsteroid, levonorgestrel (LN), is not affected by liver metabolism. Newer NTs include desogestrel, gestodene, and norgestimate. These compounds remain active for 24 to 36 hours. They suppress production of the luteinizing hormone, resemble progesterone in their effects on the endometrium, produce viscous cervical mucus, and inhibit ovulation. A naturally-occurring steroid in the female is 17-hydroxyprogesterone. Synthetic derivatives include chlormadinone acetate, megestrol acetate, and medroxyprogesterone acetate (MPA). These inhibit ovulation and have no androgenic, anabolic, or estrogenic effects. Chlormadinone acetate was withdrawn from the market because animal experiments demonstrated occurrence of breast nodules in beagle dogs.

Four types of oral contraceptive pills are currently in use: (1) combined low-dose pills; (2) phasic pills; (3) minipills; and (4) postcoital hormonal pills.

(1) Combined Low-Dose Pills

The amount of EE used in oral contraceptives has progressively decreased over the years. Combinations of two steroids are used in these pills. The most common combinations are: norethistrone acetate (NA, 1 mg) and EE (.05mg); norethistrone (NE, 1mg) and mestranol (.05mg); norgestrel 0.5mg and EE (.03mg); lynestrenol (1mg) and EE (.05mg); and ethynodiol diacetate and EE (.05mg). Somewhat higher dose combinations used are norgestrel (.05mg) and EE

(.05mg); NE (2.5mg) and EE (.05mg); NE (3 mg) and EE (.05mg). To minimize androgenic side-effects, the types of synthetic progestins have been changed. The newest, so-called third generation progestogens, block ovulation effectively.[1]

(2) Phasic Pills

Phasic pills have been designed to reduce the total intake of estrogen and progestagen in a whole cycle. For the first six days the phasic pills provide .05mg 1-norgestrel and .03mg EE per day, .075mg of 1- norgestrel and .04mg EE for the next five days, and 0.125 1-norgestrel and .03mg EE per day for the last ten days. This combination achieves a reduction of 35 percent in total dose of estrogen and progestin administered.

(3) Minipills

In those cases where estrogens are contraindicated, progestagen-only pills are taken daily without interruption to effect contraception. Progestagens used in these minipills are NE (0.3mg), norgestrel (.07mg), ethynodiol diacetate (0.5ng), and lynestrenol (0.5mg).

(4) Postcoital Hormonal Pills

Postcoital contraception is intended for emergencies. Estrogen–progestagen combinations have been found to be the most effective. The most popular regimen provides two tablets each of 50 ug of EE and 0.25 mg of LN taken as soon as possible after exposure to risk of pregnancy and another two tablets of the same composition taken 12 hours later. Treatment starts within 72 hours of exposure. The pregnancy rate in those treated varies between 1 and 4 percent, depending on the stage of cycle when coitus occurred.

Mechanism of Action

The combination pills and the minipills work by inhibition of ovulation.[r3] The inhibition results from suppression of the midcycle surge of gonadtropins. The steroids may act directly on the pituitary or on the hypothalamus. With sequential formulations, FSH is usually suppressed, but LH often shows multiple midcycle peaks. Thus, follicular and ovum maturation is likely to be inhibited. If not, ovulation may occur, especially when a pill is omitted. This could account for the somewhat impaired efficiency compared to the combination formulations.

Side-Effects

Oral contraceptives induce side-effects, but those effects do not constitute a significant medical risk. Besides spotting and breakthrough bleeding, nausea, cyclical weight gain from fluid retention, nonspecific vaginal discharge, premenstrual tension, irritability, and breast tenderness occur in women administered the estrogen-dominant pills. With progestagen-dominant preparations, depression, loss of libido, dryness of vagina, sustained weight gain, and acne occur.

Data from developed countries indicate that oral contraceptives may have an important deleterious effect, increasing the risk of some circulatory diseases in certain groups of women. The current formulations of oral contraceptives now employ the lowest effective doses of estrogen and progestin. The risk of disease was found to be higher in women who are smokers.[r4]

Some studies indicate a causal relationship between oral contraceptives and breast cancer; others do not. It has been suggested that certain groups of women may be at higher risk of developing breast cancer if they use pills for a long time. Some studies indicated that in a certain group of women the pill may actually provide protection from the risk of breast cancer.

Studies undertaken in the UK, the US, Sweden, and Denmark showed evidence of a relationship between the use of oral contraceptives and both venous and arterial thromboembolic complications. The risk of venous thromboembolism is limited to current users, and disappears soon after stopping the pill.

About 3 percent of women using the combined form of oral contraceptives suffer from diabetes, which is reversible on withdrawal of steroids. The insulin-antagonistic effect of the contraceptives may be a progestagen effect.

A list of currently available oral contraceptives with combinations of steroids is shown in Table 49.1.

Injectable Contraception

Immediately after widespread introduction of hormonal oral contraceptives in developed countries, it became evident that alternative steroid hormone delivery systems were required in some cultural settings, to eliminate the need for daily pill taking. This was the beginning of research needed to develop agents for long-acting contraception. Most of the research effort in this direction was focused on developing sustained-release formulations of steroids to be used either as injectable contraceptives (ICs) or as subdermal contraceptive implants.

Progestin-Only Injectable Contraceptives

The two most widely used hormonal preparations are depomedroxyprogesterone acetate (DMPA) and norethistrone–enanthate (NET-EN), which must be injected every two to three months. These are depot preparations given by deep IM injection; they provide contraception for eight to 12 weeks. The efficacy of these progestin-only preparations is higher than that of oral contraceptives.[r5]

DMPA

This microcrystalline suspension of 17-acetoxy-6-alpha-methyl-progesterone is closely related to the natural progesterone (Fig. 49.1A). Owing to the low solubility of this synthetic steroid in aqueous media, administration of DMPA by deep IM injection is followed by prolonged release from the depot site. Duration of its progestational effect is largely dependent on the crystal size of the molecule and its rate of absorption.[2]

Table 49.1 Types of Oral Contraceptives Available

Name of Pill	Dose of Progestin (mg)		Dose of Estrogen (μg)	
Micronor, Nor Q-D	NE	0.35	Nil	
Ovrette	NGR	0.075	Nil	
Loestrin	NEA	1.00	EE	20
Norinyl, Ortho	NE	1.0	ME	50
Triphasil, Trilevien	L-N	.0.05/.075/.125	EE	30/40/30
Nordette, Levien	L-N	.15	EE	30
Lo/Ovral	NGR	0.3	EE	30
Loestrin 1.5/30	NEA	1.5	EE	30
Ovcon 35	NE	0.4	EE	35
Brevicon, Modicon	NE	0.5	EE	35
Ortho 10/11	NE	0.5/1.0/0.5	EE	35
Trinorinyl	NE	0.5/.75/1.0	EE	35
Ortho 7/7/7	NE	0.5/0.75/1.0	EE	35
Norinyl, Ortho Genora, N.E.E.1/35	NE	1.0	EE	35
Demulen 1/35	ED	1.0	EE	35
Norinyl, Ortho 1/80	NE	1.0	ME	80
Ovcon 50	NE	1.0	EE	50
Noriestrin 1/50	NEA	1.0	EE	50
Norinyl 2, Ortho 2	NE	2.0	ME	100
Enovid - E	NE	2.5	ME	100
Noriestrin 2.5/50	NEA	2.5	EE	50
Ovral	NGR	0.5	EE	50
Demulen 1/50	ED	1.0	EE	50
Ovulen	ED	1.0	ME	100

Abbreviations: NGR = Norgestrel, NEA = Norethindrone Acetate, NE = Norethindrone, ME = Mestranol, L-N = Levonorgestrel, EE = ethinyl estradiol

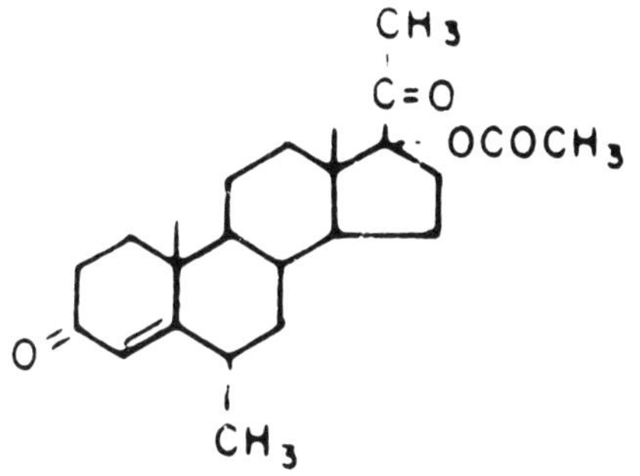

MEDROXYPROGESTERONE ACETATE

Figure 49.1A

Efficacy. DMPA administered at a dose of 150 mg every three months is a highly effective preparation.[76] Following IM injection of DMPA there is an initial rise of progestin delivery into the blood stream; the serum MPA concentrations then fall at a first-order release rate. MPA is the active molecule responsible for the contraceptive effect.

Mechanism of Action. The contraceptive effect of MPA is exerted mainly through ovulation inhibition mediated by the suppression of the cyclic release of pituitary gonadotropins. In addition, MPA exerts subsidiary contraceptive effects at the tubal, endometrial, and cervical levels. It has been shown that MPA has an antiproliferative effect on stromal cell proliferation in vitro. In the blood, MPA circulates tightly bound by albumin. At the target cell, MPA interacts with the progesterone receptor.

Side-Effects. DMPA received FDA approval under the trademarked name of Depo-Provera for use in the treatment of endometriosis, threatened abortion, precocious puberty, and acromegaly. Administration of DMPA for these noncontraceptive purposes in large doses was not accompanied by noticeable side-effects. Irregularity of menstruation was reported in some cases with administration of DMPA.

NET-EN

Net-En is a long-chain ester of norethistrone (Fig. 49.1B) formulated in castor oil benzyl benzoate solution (6:4). Net-En circulates both as an ester and as active free steroid.

Efficacy. This formulation is highly effective when administered at a dose of 200 mg every 60 ± 14 days to maximize contraceptive protection. Pharmacokinetic

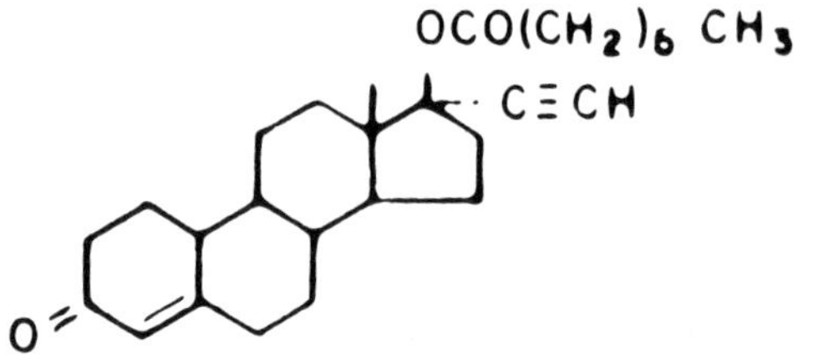

NORETHISTERONE ENANTHATE

Figure 49.1B

assessment shows that after the IM injection of Net-En at 200 mg, a peak of serum Net is noticed 1 week after administration, which is then followed by a gradual decline.[3] Pregnancy rates are less than 0.5 per 100 woman-years of use.

Mechanism of Action. The mechanisms of contraceptive action of Net-En are exerted at the central neuroendocrine and peripheral target organ levels; thus, it appears that in the first week after injection the main operating mechanism is ovulation inhibition through hypothalamic blockade of the estrogen-induced midcycle gonadotropin release.[4] Later effects are mediated by the production of a hostile type of cervical mucus.

Side-Effects. One of the major disadvantages associated with Net-En use is irregularities in menstruation in the form of vaginal bleeding or spotting or cessation of menstruation. Weight-gain, dizziness, and headache may occur also.

Combined Progestin-Estrogen Injectable Contraceptives

Combined injectable preparations are those in which estrogen esters are added to long acting progestins.[r7] This formulation shows no problem of endometrial bleeding in women.

Efficacy

The most widely used formulations include "Number 1" developed in the Peoples' Republic of China. This contains 250 mg 17-hydroxyprogesterone caproate (17-OHPC) and 5 mg estradiol valerate. The other combination contains 150 mg dihydroxyprogesterone acetophenide and 10 mg estradiol enanthate. The main feature of this long-acting contraceptive is that it produces a single defined and predictable bleeding episode every month and has high contraceptive efficacy.

Mechanism of Action

The mechanism of action is at the level of the hypothalamus, where the surge of pituitary gonadotropins is blocked by the steroid. It also renders the cervical mucus impenetrable to sperm.

Side-Effects

This preparation shares contraindications of oral contraceptives containing estrogens. Other preparations include one that is very popular in China and contains 250 mg 17 OHPC and 5 mg E_2. Deladroate (DHPA, 150 mg E_2 E 10 mg) has a great acceptance in Latin America. Two once-a-month injectable contraceptives underwent clinical trials by the World Health Organization. One is Mesigyna (HRP 102), containing 50 mg Net-En and 5 mg estradiol valerate. The other one is HRP 112, called Cyclofem, containing 5 mg estradiol cyprionate and 25 mg DMPA. These two preparations were extensively tested in women in various trials. They are almost ready for use.[r8]

Implants

In an effort to widen the choice and increase safety, research has focused on several new hormone delivery systems, such as subdermal implants and vaginal rings. Slow-release systems have definite advantages over daily administration. Daily administration involves regular fluctuation of blood levels, and pills may be forgotten. Slow-release systems have a steady state of release, allowing a single administration to last several months. Implants provide a metered system for delivery of steroids in the body so that a constant blood level can be maintained within a desired range.

Norplant

The most developed and most widely used implant today is "Norplant." This system consists of six flexible silastic capsules (2.4 mm diameter and 3.4 cm long), each containing crystalline levonorgestrel (LNG). Levonorgestrel (Fig. 49.1C) is regarded as pharmacologically safe at doses given in oral contraceptives. Immediately following implantation, the dose of LNG provided by Norplant is about 85 ug per day; it declines about 50 ug per day by nine months; it then falls to about 35 ug per day by 18 months and to about 30 ug per day over the remaining five years of use. Insertion of Norplant takes about five minutes, whereas removal takes about 15 minutes. Implants become surrounded by fibrous tissue and are easily palpable under the skin. After successful removal of the implants, plasma LNG disappears within 24 to 96 hours allowing a rapid return of fertility.[5]

Efficacy. Norplant provides protection within the first month and through five years.[r9] Protection against

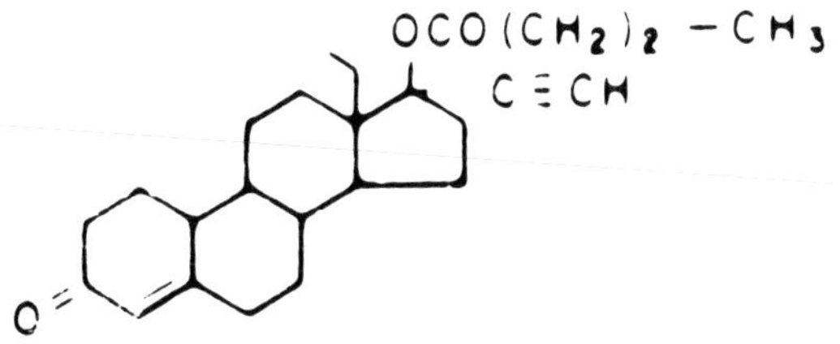

OCO(CH$_2$)$_2$ –CH$_3$
C≡CH

LEVONORGESTREL
BUTANOATE

Figure 49.1C

pregnancy with Norplant is quite high, the annual pregnancy rate being 0.5 to 1.0 pregnancy per 100 women-years of use.[r10]

Mechanism of Action. Norplant implants mediate their effects on fertility by a variety of mechanisms. These include suppression of ovulation and alteration of cervical mucus. Suppression of ovulation occurs through the inhibition of gonadotropins in the pituitary gonadal axis during the cycle. Basal estradiol levels and estradiol surges are not inhibited by Norplant. The cervical mucus becomes extremely thick in Norplant users, making it impenetrable to sperm.

Side-Effects. Except for menstrual problems, Norplant showed very few side-effects. However, women with a history of acne tend to develop more acne. This seems to be due to a direct effect on skin by LNG.

Vaginal Rings

Injectable contraceptives are not immediately reversible, and implants require a small operation to be made reversible. Vaginal rings, however, may be removed at will. Contraceptive vaginal rings (CVR) are silastic rings impregnated with hormones; they are highly effective, having many of the advantages of oral contraceptives. Steroids are released from the surface of the ring and are absorbed through the vaginal epithelium into the circulation at a constant rate.[r11]

CVRs are made of nontoxic dimethylpolysiloxane; they release steroids in proportion to their surface area and inversely in proportion to the thickness of the outer wall. The duration of action of the CVR is determined by the amount of steroid contained within the reservoir of the device.

There are four major designs of CVRs. One is a mixture of silastic and steroid. A second type of ring, called the core vaginal ring, has a central 3.5-mm core containing the steroid, which is surrounded by a 5-mm layer of nonmedicated silastic. In a third, the steroid is located in a band of collagen placed in a groove on the outer surface of the ring. The fourth and most successful design is the shell vaginal ring. In this type the steroid-containing portion is centered between a nonmedicated central core and an outer band.[6]

CVRs also vary in terms of the hormones they carry.

Progestin-Only CVRs for Continuous Use

(a) LNG-Only CVRs. The device releases 20 ug of LNG in 24 hours (a total of 600 ug in one month). The ring releases a constant amount of LNG over three months and is worn continuously through menstruation. The effect does not totally depend on ovulation inhibition; it also affects the cervical mucus.

(b) Progesterone-Only CVRs. A CVR releasing 5–10 mg of progesterone per day has been undergoing clinical trials and appears to be an acceptable method.

Estrogen Plus Progestin-CVRs for Discontinuous Use

(a) LNG Plus E_2 CVRs. The Population Council CVR, releasing 280–300 ug of LNG and 180 ug 17 beta E_2, is an excellent ring in terms of efficacy.[7] The ring is inserted and retained for three weeks and removed for one week to allow menstruation.

(b) NE Plus E_2 CVRs. A CVR releasing 800 ug NE plus 200 ug E_2 was associated with 10 percent nonsignificant decrease in LDL-cholesterol. The latest CVRs containing EE_2 and low androgenic progestins have overcome previous problems of lipoprotein changes and have excellent contraceptive efficacy.[8]

Safety and Efficacy. Absorption through the endometrium avoids many changes in hepatic proteins. However, these devices are contraindicated in people with genital infections. The LNG-releasing CVR is effective in blocking ovulation in 40 percent of cycles.

Side-Effects. The main side-effect is related to placement in the vagina, including increased discharge, expulsion, and sensations of a foreign object.

Intrauterine Devices

The intrauterine device (IUD) is a well-established method of contraception. First developed in 1909 by Richter, the IUD experienced brief popularity in the 1920s and 1930s. After a long period of disfavor, interest in them was rekindled in 1962; since that time many types of IUD were developed. IUDs may be medicated or nonmedicated. The most widely used contain copper; they may also contain progesterone or levonorgestrel. The nonmedicated IUD (Lippes loop) is associated with a high incidence of bleeding and spotting. The efficacy rate here was one to six pregnancies per 100 users.

A new device (LNG IUD) that releases levonorgestrel at the rate of 20 ug per day has shown high acceptability and high contraceptive efficacy in extensive trials.[7] The striking positive features of the LNG IUD compared with other IUDs are high effectiveness, reduction in both the amount and duration of menstrual bleeding, and reduction in menstrual pain. The return of fertility is immediate after discontinuation.

Today only two IUDs are available in the US, TCu-380A and the progesterone T device.

Efficacy

The progesterone-releasing device (Progestasert) has long been available, but has not reached widespread use owing to the short duration of protection it offers and the risk of ectopic pregnancy.

The plain plastic device, the same as that used in the copper-releasing IUD Nova T (Leiras Pharmaceuticals, Turku, Finland), has a steroid reservoir around the vertical stem. The reservoir consists of a cylinder made of a mixture of LNG and silastic. This mixture, containing 50 percent steroid by weight, forms an arm around the vertical stem of the IUD and is covered by a silastic membrane that regulates the daily release of LNG to 20 ug. The recommended duration of use of the device is five years, and the LNG-IUD should be removed during the sixth year of use. The intrauterine release of LNG results in absorption of the steroid into the systemic circulation. Absorption occurs through the endometrium to the capillary network in the basal layer of the mucosa. Fifteen minutes after insertion, the plasma level of LNG is detectable. The individual plasma LNG concentrations are relatively stable, but great variations exist between individuals.[9] In plasma, LNG binds to steroid hormone binding globulin (SHBG). In clinical trials, one study had two pregnancies out of 755 acceptors; in another, one woman became pregnant out of 1821 acceptors.[r6] The pearl index is .12 per 100 users.

Mechanism of Action

The action of inert IUDs may take place by preventing implantation through nonspecific foreign body reaction. The low dose of progesterone released by hormone-releasing devices may induce changes in endometrial receptivity, making the surface unsuitable for blastocyst implantation.

Side Effects

Adverse reactions like pain, bleeding, and expulsions reduce acceptability of these devices. The risk of ectopic pregnancy is also there. These complications have been reduced in IUDs that contain progesterone.

Spermicides

Spermicidal agents prevent normal function of spermatozoa in the reproductive tract. They are simple, medically safe, and reduce STD incidence rates. These preparations consist of two components: an inert base or carrier (foam, cream, jelly, suppository, or tablet) and a spermicidal agent. The most common spermicidal agents used today are monoxynol-9, octoxymol-9, and mentegol.[r12] Efficacy varies from 0.3 to eight pregnancies per 100 women years.

Methods Under Development

Transdermal Delivery Systems

The passive absorption of contraceptive drugs through skin is of interest now. Steroids can be delivered via the transdermal route.[r13,10]

ST 1435 (16-methylene-17-a-acetoxy-19-nor-4-pregnene- 3,20 dione) is a synthetic progestin derived from 19-norprogesterone. Silastic capsules containing this progestin implanted subdermally effectively suppressed follicular development and ovulation in women. Inhibition of ovulation was achieved by plasma concentrations of ST 1435 above 50 pg/ml. In one study, a single 4-cm subdermal 1435 with a lifetime of two years showed good contraceptive effect and suppressed ovulation. No significant side-effect was found.

Mifepristone (RU 486)

This compound, is a competitive antagonist of progesterone and may be used as an abortifacient (see Chapter 52). RU 486 (17β-hydroxy-11-[4-dimethylaminophenyl}-17a-1-{prop-1-ynyl;estra-4,9-dien-3-one) is a 19-norsteroid derivative lacking the C19-methyl group of natural progesterone and glucocorticosteroids. It binds to progesterone as well as glucocorticoid receptors and competes with natural steroids for their sites. The brief interruption of progesterone secretion achieved by this compound will induce dysfunction of the decidualized endometrium, leading to endometrial shedding and abortion. This compound also can be used for postcoital contraception in women. A single 600-mg dose appears to be highly effective as a postcoital contraceptive.[11]

GnRH Analogues

GnRH or gonadotropin releasing hormone (also known as LHRH, luteinizing hormone releasing hormone) is secreted by the hypothalamus and acts on the pituitary by controlling the release of FSH and LH. Both FSH and LH are released in a periodic fashion, with peaks at 1.5 to two hour. GnRH analogues suppress the pituitary-gonadal axis. These analogues may be antagonists or agonists. Buserelin, one of the agonists tested in normal menstruating women, inhibited ovulation and menses. Agonist analogues desensitize the gonadotroph cells, whereas antagonists compete with endogenous natural GnRH for its receptors on such cells. GnRH agonists require several days to switch off gonadotroph cells; antagonists have an immediate effect on the release of gonadotropins. The agonists have been found not to have sufficient contraceptive effect. GnRH antagonists also are not suitable for female contraception; however, they are remarkably effective in male contraception. Azoospermia is obtained by treatment with these antagonists.

Immunologic Methods

The concept of vaccination against pregnancy is a fairly new one. Antifertility vaccines are designed to work by generating immunity to one or more molecules involved in reproduction. The vaccine at the most advanced stage of development is human chorionic gonadotropin (hCG) vaccine. Titers above 20 mg/ml of hCG binding capacity are supposed to block hCG at the preimplantation stage. Phase 1 clinical trial has shown that it has no side-effects.

HCG is a glycoprotein secreted by the placenta as early as four days after conception that maintains corpora lutea that secrete the progesterone necessary for sustaining pregnancy. The vaccine produces anti-hCG antibodies that prevent action of the hormone.[12]

The hCG molecule consists of one alpha and one β subunit. The alpha subunit is common with other pituitary hormones, while the β subunit has a unique amino acid sequence. The improved vaccine consists of a β-subunit annealed to a heterospecies alpha subunit conjugated to tetanus toxoid or cholera toxin chain as carriers. Immunized women have so far not shown any side-effects. The vaccine is under Phase II clinical trial and has so far demonstrated efficacy in women when levels of antibodies remain high.

Hormonal Contraception in the Male

Two hundred milligrams of testosterone enanthate per week was used in 271 men in a multicentered clinical trial undertaken by the World Health Organization.[13] Azoospermia was achieved within six months in a substantial number of men. This study shows that suitable hormonal regimens could induce azoospermia with minimum side-effects.[24] DMPA was combined with one of two androgens, TE or the longer-acting 19-nortestosterone-hexyl-oxy-propionate. More than 97 percent of Indonesian men achieved azoospermia.

In summary, hormonal contraception remains the most reliable and effective form of contraception with minimal side-effects. Several new leads now being investigated also may lead to other forms of contraception that would be useful where hormonal contraception is contrandicated.

References

Research Reports

1. Rebar RW, Zeserson K. Characteristics of the new progestogens in combination oral contraceptives. Contraception. 1991;*44*:1–10.
2. Kirton KT, Cornette JC. Return of ovulatory cyclicity following an intramuscular injection of medroxyprogesterone acetate. Contraception 1974;*10*:39–45.
3. Fotherby K, Howard G, Shrimanker K. Effect of norethisterone enanthate on serum gonadotropin levels. Contraception 1977;*16*:591–604.
4. Ortiz A, Hiroi M, Stanczyk FZ, Goebelsmann U, Mishell DRJr. Serum MPA concentrations and ovarian function following intramuscular injection of Depo Provera. J Clin Endocrinal Metab 1977;*44*:32–38.
5. Olsson SE, Odlind V, Johansson EDB, Nordstrom ML. Plasma level of levonorgestrel and free levonorgestrel index in women using Norplant implants or two covered rods (Norplant - 2). Contraception 1987;*35*:215–228.
6. Jackanicz TM. Levonorgestrel and estradiol release from an improved contraceptive vaginal ring. Contraception 1981;*24*:323.
7. Sivin I, Mishell DRJr, Victor A. A multicenter study of levonorgestrel estradiol contraceptive vaginal rings. III Menstrual pattern. An international comparative trial. Contraception 1981;*24*:377.
8. Apter D, Caccaiatore B, Stenman UH, Alphlessa U, Assendorp R. Clinical performance and endocrine profiles on contraceptive vaginal rings releasing 3-keto-desogestrel and ethinylestradiol. Contraception 1990;*42*:563.
9. Luukkainen T, Allonen H, Haukkamaa M, Lahteenmaki P, Nilsson CG, Toivonen J. Five years' experience with levonorgestrel releasing IUD's. Contraception 1986;*33*:139–148.
10. Pang SC, Greendale GA, Cedars MI, Gambone JC, Lozano K, Eggenap LH. Long term effect of transdermal estrogen with and without MPA. Fertil Steril 1993;*59*:76–82.
11. Glasier A, Thong KJ, Dewar M, Mackie M, Baird DT. Mifepristone (RU 486) compared with high dose estrogens and progestogen for emergency postcoital contraception. N Engl J Med 1992;*327*:1041–1044.
12. Singh O, Rao LV, Gaur A, Sharma NC, Alam A, Talwar GP. Antibody response and characteristics of antibodies in women immunized with three contraceptive vaccines inducing antibodies against chorionic gonadotropin. Fertil Steril 1989;*52*(5),739–744.
13. World Health Organization: Task force on methods for regulation of male fertility: Contraceptive efficacy of testosterone-induced azoospermia in normal men. Lancet 1990;*336*:955.

Reviews

r1. Pincus G. The control of fertility. New York: Academic Press, 1965.

r2. Fathalla MF. Reproductive health in the world: two decades of progress and the challenge ahead. WHO Biennial Report. WHO Publications, 1992; pp 3–29.

r3. Harper MJ. (1983) Oral contraceptive steroids. In: Harper MJK ed. Birth control technologies. University of Texas Press. (1983); pp 18–30. 3.

r4. Kleinman RL. Hormonal Contraception. London: IPPF Medical Publishers, 1990.

r5. Flores-Garza J, Craviotto MD, Perez-Palacios G. Steroid injectable contraception: Current concepts and perspectives. In Sitruk-Ware R, Bardin CW. eds. Contraception, newer pharmacological agents, devices and delivery systems. Marcel Dekker (1992); pp 41–70.

r6. Hall PE. Long-acting injectable formulations. In: Diczfalusy E, Bygdeman M. eds. Fertility regulation today and tomorrow. New York: Serono Symposia publications, Raven Press (1987);*36*:119–141.

r7. Toppozada M. The clinical use of monthly injectable preparations. Obstet Gynaecol Surv 1977;*32*:335–347.

r8. d'Arcangues A. Long acting systemic agents for fertility regulation. WHO Annual Technical Report, 1991. Geneva (1992); pp 23–35.

r9 Bardin CW. Norplant contraceptive implants. Obstet Gynecol Rep 1990;2:96–102.

r10. Bardin CW. Long acting steroidal contraception—an update. Int J Fertil 1989;*34*:88–95.

r11. Shoupe D, Mishell DRJr. Contraceptive vaginal rings: Efficacy and acceptability. In: Sitruk-Ware R, Bardin CW. eds. Contraception: newer pharmacological agents, devices and delivery systems. New York: Marcel Dekker (1992); pp 71–89.

r12. Hatcher RA, Stewart F, Trussell J, Kowal D, Guest F, Stewart GK, Cates W. Vaginal Spermicides. In: Contraceptive Technology 1990–1992. New York: Irvington Publishers.

r13. Brown L, Langer R. Transdermal delivery of drugs. Ann Rev Med 1988;*39*:221–29.

r14. Fraser IS. Systemic hormonal contraception by nonoral routes. In: Filshie M, Guillebaud J. eds. Contraception: Science and practice. London: Butterworths. (1989); pp 109–25.

r15. Drife JO. Complications of combined oral contraception. In: Filshie M, Guillebaud J. eds. Contraception: Science and practice. London: Butterworths. (1989); pp 39–51.

r16. Koetsawang S. Present and future trends. Ann NY Acad Sci 1991;*626*:30–42.

r17. Luukkainen T. Levonorgestrel releasing intrauterine device. Ann NY Acad Sci 1991;*626*:43–49.

r18. Fathalla MF. New contraceptive methods and reproductive health. In Segal SJ, Tsui AO, Rogers SM. eds. Demographic and programmatic consequences of contraceptive innovations. New York: Plenum, (1989); pp 153–175.

r19. Baird DT, Glasier AF. Hormonal contraception. Drug Therapy N Engl J Med 1993;*328*:1543–1548.

CHAPTER 50

Androgenic and Anabolic Steroids and Antagonists

Richard A. Hiipakka
Shutsung Liao

Introduction

Androgens are the steroid hormones responsible, in part, for the expression of the male phenotype. The most important androgen circulating in the blood of males is testosterone, and it is the major androgen secreted by the testis. The clearest indication for the therapeutic use of these hormones is for treatment of men with low levels of circulating androgens due to dysfunction of the pituitary or testis. Androgens have been used in treating various disorders, but their virilizing effects can limit their usefulness in females and prepubertal males. Anabolic steroids are structurally modified androgens that show greater anabolic effects relative to virilizing effects; they were developed to overcome the clinical limitations of androgens like testosterone.

Chemistry

Naturally-occurring androgens and many synthetic ones are based on the 19-carbon parent steroid androstane (Fig. 50.1). Testosterone is a Δ^4-3-keto-17β-hydroxyandrostane. The oxygen groups at the C-3 and C-17 positions are essential for high androgenic activity.

Upon chemical or enzymatic reduction of the Δ^4-double bond, the C-5 becomes asymmetric, and two isomeric androstanes (5α and 5β) can be formed. Many active androgenic and anabolic steroids are derivatives of 5α-androstane (trans A/B ring junction), while all 5β-androstanes (cis A/B ring junction) are not androgenic. Many 5β-androstanes (also called etiocholanes) are, however, active as hematopoietic agents, stimulating the production of hemoglobins and formation of blood cells.[r1]

Androgenic activity is often evaluated by measuring the weight increase of the prostate and/or seminal vesicles of castrated rats given test compounds; anabolic activity is measured by following the growth of the levator ani (dorsal bulbocavernosus) muscle.[1] A chick comb growth test has also been employed as a bioassay for androgens. Potential androgen agonists and antagonists can be screened most readily by analyzing their ability to compete with radioactive androgens for binding to androgen receptors.

In many clinical situations measurements of blood levels of circulating androgens are required. Radioimmunoassays used with fractionation techniques allow quantitation of various androgens, their precursors, and their metabolites.

History

The effects of castration must have made it evident to humans early in history that the testis was related to virility. Convincing experimental evidence supporting the hypothesis that the testis secretes a virilizing factor came with the publication in 1849 of experiments by Berthold, who showed that transplantation of the testis into the abdomen of a castrated rooster prevented or reversed the effects of castration. The response of the capon's comb to exogenous androgenic factors provided a suitable bioassay, which was used by Walker in 1908 and by Pezard in 1911 to show that cell-free testicular extracts contained virilizing factors. McGee in 1928, in the laboratory of FC Koch, used the bioassay to develop methods to fractionate bovine testicular extracts and concentrate the virilizing factor with organic solvents. Then, in 1931, Butenandt purified and crystallized from human male urine an androgen that he named androsterone. Subsequently, David and coworkers in 1935 purified and crystallized from bovine testes an androgen that they named testosterone, an androgen more than ten times more potent than androsterone. An account of many of these early androgen studies was written by Koch.[r2]

An understanding of the mechanism by which androgens and other steroid hormones elicit their effects awaited the discovery, within cells that respond to steroid hormones, of proteins that act as specific, high-affinity receptors for a given class of steroid hormones. Androgen receptors were initially identified and characterized in

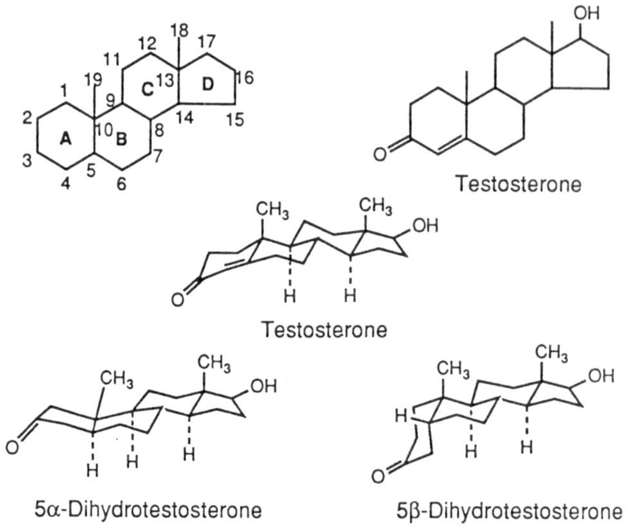

Figure 50.1 Structural representations and the carbon numbering system for androgens. Testosterone is a member of the androstane class of steroid hormones. A steroid structure can be displayed by simple two-dimensional drawings (top) or by more informative three-dimensional representations (bottom). 5α-Dihydrotestosterone is the active androgen in many target organs and is produced from testosterone by the enzyme 5α-reductase. 5β-Dihydrotestosterone is not an active androgen, but may have a role in controlling proliferation of certain blood stem cells.

extracts of prostatic tissue in 1969 by Fang, Anderson, and Liao,[2] by Mainwaring,[3] and by Unhjem and Tveter.[4] Prior to this discovery, Bruchovsky and Wilson[5] and Anderson and Liao[6] in 1968 showed that labeled testosterone was converted to 5α-dihydrotestosterone in prostatic tissue, and that this metabolite was selectively retained by prostatic nuclei. Androgen receptors also were found to have a higher affinity for 5α-dihydrotestosterone than testosterone. Therefore, it appeared that the active androgen in prostatic tissue was 5α-dihydrotestosterone, which produced its effects by binding to an intracellular receptor that interacted with components in the cell nucleus. However, in certain tissues (muscle, mouse kidney) that have low 5α-reductase activity, testosterone may be the active androgen, apparently interacting directly with the androgen receptor. Further research on various steroid receptor systems has led to a model of steroid hormone action that depicits steroid receptors as proteins that bind to their respective steroid hormones and then interact with specific DNA sequences controlling the expression of specific genes. Insight into the structure and function of androgen receptors was achieved in 1988 when the full-length cDNA for this receptor was cloned and sequenced in the laboratories of S. Liao[7] and of EM Wilson and FS French.[8]

Biosynthesis and Metabolism of Androgens

Various androgenic steroids are produced by the testes, adrenals, and ovaries from cholesterol by pathways[r3,r4] shown in Figure 50.2. There are two possible routes for the synthesis of testosterone: (1) one involving 5-ene-3β-hydroxysteroids, such as 17-hydroxypregnenolone and dehydroepiandrosterone (the Δ^5 pathway); and (2) another involving 4-ene-3-ketosteroids, such as progesterone and 4-androstenedione (the Δ^4 pathway). The Δ^5 pathway appears to predominate in the testis of man. Both pathways are functional in adrenals and ovaries. The secretion rates for androgenic steroids produced in these organs[r5] are summarized in Table 50.1. Plasma levels of various steroids[9] and blood production rates[r4] for these steroids are given in Table 50.2.

Testicular Androgens

Testosterone is the major androgen produced by Leydig cells and secreted by the testis. More than 95 percent of the testosterone in the plasma of men is derived from this source. Steroids, such as 4-androstenedione and dehydroepiandrosterone, also are secreted by the testis, but in much smaller amounts than testosterone. Testosterone also can be produced by metabolism of certain steroids—such as 4-androstenedione in organs besides the testis—but this route contributes to less than 5 percent of plasma testosterone in men. The production of testosterone by the Leydig cells of the testis is controlled by blood levels of luteinizing hormone (LH) released from the anterior pituitary.

The secretion of testosterone by the testis begins early in embryonic development. At approximately eight weeks of gestation, the human fetal testis can synthesize testosterone, and testicular levels of testosterone reach their peak at 10–15 weeks of development. Testosterone synthesis then begins to decrease by 13–15 weeks of gestation; at birth, circulating levels of testosterone are relatively high at 2 ng/ml. They then fall rapidly during the first week of life to about 0.3 ng/ml. The drop in testosterone levels shortly after birth may be due to the decrease in plasma hCG levels that occurs at this time. At the age of 1–3 months plasma testosterone levels increase again to about 2

Table 50.1 Secretion Rates of Various Steroids by the Testis, Adrenal, and Ovary

Steroid	Secretion Rate (mg/d)		
	Testis	Adrenal	Ovary
Testosterone	7	0.01	0.01
4-Androstenedione	0.2	2	1
Dehydroepiandrosterone	0.2	7	1
Dehydroepiandrosterone-SO_4	0	7	0

Table 50.2 Plasma Concentrations and Blood Production Rates of Various Steroids

Steroid	Plasma Concentration (ug/L)		Blood Production Rate* (mg/day)	
	Males	Females	Males	Females
Tesosterone	2–10	0.2–0.7	7	0.2
5α-Dihydrotestosterone	0.3–0.8	0.1–0.3	0.3	0.1
5α-Androstanediols	0.05–0.2	0.05–0.3	0.2	0.1
4-Androstenedione	1–2	0.2–2	1.5	3.4
Dehydroepiandrosterone	4–6	4–6	7	7
Dehydroepiandrosterone-SO_4	900–2000	400–2000	11	7

*Amount of steroid entering the peripheral blood de novo from all sources.

ng/ml, and then decline to prepubertal levels of about 0.05 ng/ml at 7–12 months of age. This burst of testosterone synthesis appears to be due to production of pituitary gonadotropin (LH) previously suppressed by the high estrogen levels present during the perinatal period. The production of testosterone by the neonatal testis then decreases with decreasing LH secretion and remains low until puberty, when increased secretion of LH leads to increased production of testosterone.

Adrenal Androgens

The normal human adrenal synthesizes and secretes large amounts of both dehydroepiandrosterone and dehydroepiandrosterone sulfate, and lesser amounts of 4-androstenedione, all of which have the potential to serve as precursors for the synthesis of more potent androgens, including testosterone. However, less than 1 percent of the testosterone in the blood of men is derived from dehydroepiandrosterone; under normal conditions, adrenal synthesis of androgens or their precursors is insufficient to maintain secondary sexual characteristics or accessory sex gland function in castrated men. The secretion rates for these androgenic steroids are similar in women, and again the rates of secretion are insufficient to produce virilization. However, conditions producing adrenal hyperplasia often lead to increased secretion of androgens and their precursors, causing virilization. Congenital adrenal hyperplasia (CAH), such as that associated with a deficiency in the enzyme 21-hydroxylase, leads to decreased cortisol synthesis and increased secretion of adrenocorticotrophic hormone (ACTH) by the pituitary, which is due to the loss of negative feedback control by cortisol. Elevated ACTH secretion causes increased production of adrenal steroids, such as 4-androstenedione and testosterone, and subsequent virilization. This condition can cause virlilization of the external genitalia of affected female fetuses, resulting in female pseudohermaphroditism. Development of CAH in adults also produces inappropriate virilizing effects in women. Excessive secretion of androgens by adrenal cortical tumors and the subsequent increase in circulating levels of androgens also causes virilization.

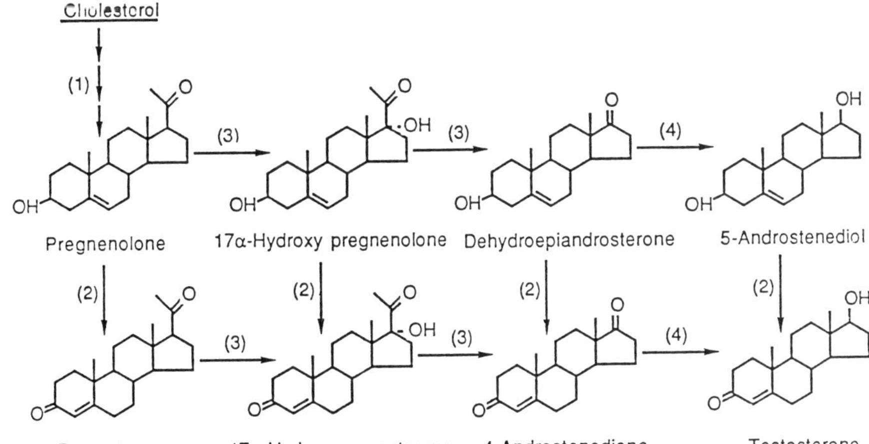

Figure 50.2 Pathway for the synthesis of testosterone in the testis, adrenal, or ovary. The enzymes involved are: (1) cytochrome P-450scc or 20,22 desmolase; (2) 3β-hydroxysteroid dehydrogenase; (3) cytochrome P-450c17 or 17α-hydroxylase; (4) 17β-hydroxysteroid dehydrogenase. In man, genetic defects in each of these enzymes have been described. Individuals with mutations in any of these enzymes that result in a loss of enzymatic activity exhibit incomplete male phenotypic development of varying severity.

Ovarian Androgens

The ovary also synthesizes and secretes dehydroepiandrosterone, 4-androstenedione, and testosterone. About 50 percent of plasma testosterone in normal women is derived from the peripheral conversion of 4-androstenedione to testosterone, and an equal amount comes from direct secretion by the ovary. Secretion of androgenic steroids by the ovary varies with the stage of the menstrual cycle and is regulated by LH and FSH (follicle-stimulating hormone), which control steroid synthesis by the various cell types (theca, granulosa, stroma) in the ovary. Normal secretion rates of androgenic steroids by the ovary are insufficient to induce virilization; however, the ovary can produce large amounts of androgenic steroids in certain pathologic conditions, causing virilization. One example is the polycystic ovary syndrome, in which increased secretion of ovarian 4-androstenedione and its peripheral conversion to testosterone and dihydrotestosterone causes hirsutism, sterility, and irregular menstrual cycles.

Metabolism of Androgens

Some androgenic steroids, such as 4-androstenedione and dehydroepiandrosterone, appear to produce androgenic responses only after their conversion to other potent androgenic steroids. In fact, testosterone itself is converted irreversibly by the enzyme 5α-reductase (Δ^4-3-ketosteroid-5α-oxidoreductase) to 5α-dihydrotestosterone in many androgen-responsive tissues.[10] 5α-Dihydrotestosterone is probably responsible for producing androgenic effects in these tissues, since this steroid has a high affinity for the androgen receptor. However, in tissues such as muscle that respond to androgens but have little or no 5α-reductase, testosterone may interact directly with the androgen receptor to produce a response.

Testosterone and androstenedione are also metabolized to the estrogens, estradiol and estrone, in peripheral tissues; and approximately 75–90 percent of the estrogens in the plasma of normal men are generated in this manner, the remainder coming from direct synthesis and secretion by the testis. Synthesis of estrogens from these androgens occurs predominantly in adipose tissue, with lesser amounts produced in muscle, kidney, liver, and hypothalamus. Estrogen formation from androgens in the hypothalamus may be important in the control of gonadotropin secretion. The synthesis of estrogens by adipose tissue of men may become medically relevant in obesity, where increased synthesis of estrogens from androgens can produce gynecomastia. The growth of the mammary gland in men depends on a balance between estrogenic stimulation and androgenic inhibition.[r6] Gynecomastia can be due to a testosterone deficiency, an increase in estrogen levels, or a combination of these two factors.

Biological Effects of Androgens

Embryonic Development

Testosterone and 5α-dihydrotestosterone play critical roles in male sexual differentiation during embryogenesis and in the development of secondary sexual characteristics that occurs at puberty.[r7,r8] Testosterone secreted by the fetal testis is responsible for differentiation of the Wolffian ducts into the epididymides, vas deferentia, and seminal vesicles. Testosterone appears to be directly responsible for Wolffian duct differentiation, since there is little or no 5α-reductase activity in the Wolffian ducts during the critical period of differentiation. Individuals with a 5α-reductase deficiency have normal virilization of the Wolffian ducts, but virilization of the external genitalia is impaired and prostatic development is lacking, indicating that these tissues require 5α-dihydrotestosterone for their differentiation. 5α-Reductase deficiency has been linked to mutations in the 5α-reductase type 2 gene.[11,12] In the absence of the testes or in some individuals with a disorder that impairs the function of the androgen receptor, there is no differentiation of the Wolffian duct or virilization of the external genitalia, which emphasizes the role of androgens and androgen receptors in this differentiation process.[r9] The descent of the testis into the scrotum, as well as continued growth of the external genitalia, depends on androgens, and these processes continue until shortly after birth, when declining production of testosterone by the testis leads to a cessation of androgen-dependent development until puberty.

Puberty

At puberty, synthesis and secretion of testosterone by the testis increases and blood levels of testosterone gradually rise over a 4–5 year period until adult levels are reached. During this time the dramatic changes characteristic of male development at puberty take place. The testis is one of the first organs to respond to the increase in testosterone synthesis at puberty. Testosterone in combination with FSH promotes the initiation of spermatogenesis and the maturation of the seminiferous tubules. 5α-Dihydrotestosterone is produced locally from testosterone in the testis by developing germ cells and Sertoli cells, and may be responsible for androgenic effects in the testis. 5α-Dihydrotestosterone also appears to be responsible for other changes at puberty, such as growth and pigmentation of external genitalia, growth and secretory activity of the accessory sex glands (prostate, seminal vesicle, epididymis), temporal hair line recession, development of characteristic facial and body hair patterns, and stimulation of sebaceous gland function. Puberty is also characterized by a rapid increase in height and weight, which appears to be due to androgens stimulating the growth of certain muscles as well as bones. Androgens also stimulate skeletal maturation by accelerating fusion of epiphyseal cartilages. It is not clear whether these androgenic effects on growth are mediated directly by testosterone or by 5α-dihydrotestosterone. The androgenic effect on bone growth may involve conversion of testosterone to estradiol, which alone or in conjunction with testosterone stimulates the synthesis and secretion of growth hormone and insulin-like growth factor I (somatomedin C). Androgens produce an enlargement of the larynx and thickening of the vocal cords, which lowers the pitch of the voice in males at puberty. Erythropoiesis is stimulated by androgens by increasing the production of erythropoietin, which results in the higher red blood cell mass seen in males. Studies in various animals showed that androgens have effects on the CNS.[r10] Testosterone, its aromatization product, estradiol, and 5α-dihydrotestosterone play important roles in producing sexual dimorphisms of neuronal architecture during the perinatal period and in the development and expression of male sexual behavior. The relevance of these laboratory results to human sexual behavior remains an open question.

Mechanism of Action

Cells containing androgen receptors have the potential to respond to androgens. Some cells lacking androgen receptors may respond indirectly to androgens by interacting with trophic factors that are synthesized and secreted by other cells that respond directly to androgens. Testosterone enters a cell by passive diffusion through the cell membrane and in many androgen-responsive cells is converted by 5α-reductase to 5α-dihydrotestosterone, which then binds to the androgen receptor. Both 5α-reductase and androgen receptor have been localized to nuclei of some androgen-responsive cells by immunocytochemical staining.[13,14] Colocalization of these two critical components of androgen action may be an important factor in some androgenic responses. Direct interaction of testosterone with the androgen receptor may occur in those cells that are deficient in 5α-reductase. A single gene for the androgen receptor is present on the X-chromosome,[15] and a single type of androgen receptor is thought to be present in the various cells that directly respond to androgens. The structure of the androgen receptor has been determined from cloning and sequencing of the mRNA for the receptor[7,8] (Fig. 50.3). Comparison of the sequence of the androgen receptor with other steroid receptors[r11] and structure-function analysis of the cloned androgen receptor[16,17] has revealed three functional domains. The amino acids in the amino-terminal half of the receptor form a domain that is important for modulation of gene transcription. A central DNA-binding domain is made up of a cysteine-rich region whose amino acids define secondary structures called zinc fingers. These structures form a complex with a zinc ion and participate in sequence-specific DNA binding. The steroid-binding domain is made up of amino acids comprising the carboxyl-terminal third of the receptor.

Men with partial or complete androgen resistance have been shown in many cases to have mutations in the androgen receptor

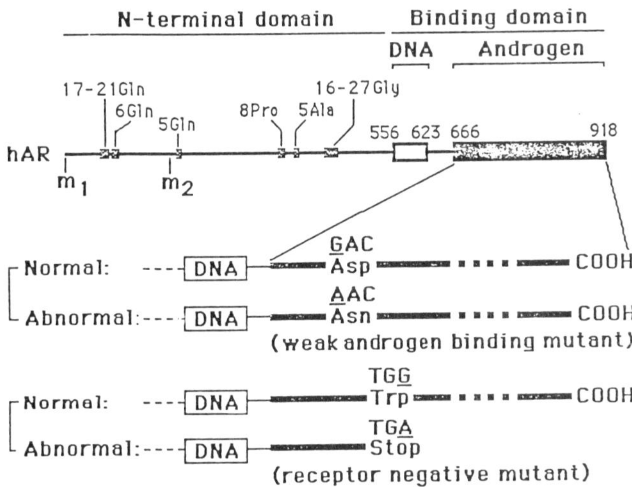

Figure 50.3 Schematic diagram of the structure of the normal and mutant human androgen receptors deduced from the nucleotide sequence coding for the androgen receptor. The normal androgen receptor shown at the top has 918 amino acids. The amino terminal domain (left) has several poly and oligo amino acid stretches consisting of glutamine, glycine, or other amino acids. Two amino-terminal region methionines (m_1 and m_2) represent potential terminal amino acids for two forms of the androgen receptor. The DNA and androgen-binding domains are in the center and carboxyl-terminal end of the receptor, respectively. An androgen-insensitive patient has a guanine (G) to adenine (A) mutation in the androgen-binding domain, causing a change in the coded amino acid from aspartic to asparagine.[29] The mutant receptor was not able to bind androgens tightly. Another androgen-insensitive patient has a G to A mutation that creates a stop codon.[30] The truncated receptor does not bind androgens.

gene.[r12] These individuals have a 46 X,Y genotype, testes, and adequate circulating levels of testosterone, but vary from phenotypic females to undervirilized or infertile men. Some cases of androgen insensitivity are due to total or partial gene deletions. In most cases, however, a single point mutation in the androgen receptor gene results in single amino acid replacements that affect receptor function (DNA or steroid-binding activity), or in the production of premature termination codons leading to truncated forms of the receptor that lack the DNA and/or steroid-binding domains. Kennedy disease (spinal and bulbar muscular atrophy) has been linked to a mutation in the length of a CAG repeat, coding for an amino-terminal polyglutamine stretch, of the human androgen receptor gene (Fig. 50.3).[18]

Receptor binding of steroid initiates a change in the receptor that enhances its affinity for components in the cell nucleus. The steroid-receptor complex interacts with specific DNA sequences, which usually are located in the 5′-noncoding region of a particular gene. This interaction modulates the transcription of the gene by a mechanism, presently unclear, that may involve interaction of the receptor with other regulatory factors and/or components of the transcriptional machinery. Steroids can stimulate as well as inhibit specific gene transcription. In addition, steroids affect gene expression through other processes that lead to changes in mRNA levels and protein synthesis, which produce some of the characteristic responses to a steroid hormone. The molecular mechanism of these effects are not as well-documented as the effects of steroids on gene transcription. The specific changes in gene transcription or other processes that lead to the characteristic response to androgens have not been described in many instances. A detailed discussion by the authors of various aspects of the mechanism of androgen action is available.[r13]

Therapeutic Uses of Androgens

Treatment of Androgen Deficiencies

Androgens are most appropriately used for the treatment of males who have circulating levels of testosterone insufficient for the androgen-dependent development and function of various tissues. Androgens are administered to these individuals to restore normal development of male secondary sexual characteristics, as well as to promote the effects of androgens on somatic growth. Androgen therapy also is used to normalize male sexual behavior and, in some cases, to restore fertility, although spermatogenesis may not return to normal levels. If the hypogonadal state develops prior to the normal time period for puberty, androgen replacement therapy can bring about, in a timely manner, the series of changes that usually take place at puberty. In these circumstances, it is important that androgen therapy be administered gradually over a period of several years, so that plasma testosterone levels increase slowly to adult levels, as normally occurs during puberty. Early exposure to adult levels of testosterone can lead to premature closure of the epiphysis and development of short stature. If androgenic therapy is started after the normal time period for puberty, the extent of virilization can vary, but often proceeds normally. When there is complete testicular failure, extended therapy with androgens usually is required. Since prolonged use of most orally active androgens is associated with hepatic toxicity, parenteral administration of testosterone esters, such as testosterone enanthate or cypionate should be used.

Androgen levels in men often decrease with old age. Treatment with androgens has been advocated to maintain strength and increase libido. However, the common occurrence of androgen-dependent disorders, such as benign prostatic hyperplasia and prostatic carcinoma in the elderly, are contraindications to the general therapeutic use of androgens in older men.

Other Clinical Uses of Androgens

Delayed Puberty/Short Stature

A controversial use of androgens is in the acceleration of growth of boys with delayed puberty. Therapy is initiated to minimize psychologic distress, even though puberty and associated growth usually will take place by the age of 20. Typically a six-month course of treatment will stimulate both growth and puberty modestly, and further therapy seldom is necessary. Treatments with low doses (50 mg/m^2/mo) of testosterone esters are effective and do not compromise the adult height potential.[19] Orally-active androgens have been recommended for treatment of this disorder. Since the duration of treatment is usually short, hepatic toxicity may not become evident during treatment.

Catabolic States

Androgens have been used to treat a variety of catabolic states, such as those involving acute and chronic illnesses, surgical trauma, osteoporosis unassociated with male hypogonadism, and undernourished, debilitated, or elderly individuals. The ability of androgens to promote a positive nitrogen balance, muscle and bone growth, and to increase body weight in androgen-deficient men appears to be the rationale for the use of androgen therapy in these situations. However, the degree and duration of effectiveness of androgen therapy in individuals with normal androgen levels is slight and has proved to be of little benefit in controlled studies.

Hematologic Disorders

Androgens enhance erythropoiesis by stimulating the production of erythropoietin. Because of this effect, androgens have been used in the treatment of some hematologic disorders, such as the anemia associated with bone marrow and renal failure, and with myelofibrosis.[r14] However, androgen therapy in these disorders is controversial; a number of uncontrolled studies have indicated a beneficial role for androgens, while other controlled studies have not. It remains uncertain to what degree spontaneous remissions account for improvements seen after androgen therapy. A positive response to androgen therapy may depend on the severity of the anemia. The presence of stem cells in bone marrow favorably influences the response and survivability of patients.

Both oral and parenteral androgens have been reported to be effective in treating these anemias. Long-term therapy would indicate a preference for parenteral androgens to avoid the hepatotoxicity of oral preparations. Recombinant human erythropoietin is effective in treating certain anemias, and should become the treatment of choice because of the lack of toxicity and virilizing side-effects associated with oral androgen therapy.

Etiocholanolone, a 5β-reduced metabolite of testosterone, stimulates heme synthesis and has few or no virilizing side-effects. It use in the treatment of anemia is currently under investigation. Because etiocholanolone is pyrogenic in man, it usually is administered in combination with a glucocorticoid to decrease local inflammation.

Hereditary Angioedema

Hereditary angioedema is an autosomal dominant disorder characterized by recurrent edema of the oropharynx and the extremities and by abdominal pain. Individuals afflicted with this disorder have decreased blood levels of C1-esterase inhibitor, the first component of complement. This leads to unimpeded activation of the complement cascade and generation of factors that increase the permeability of vessels, which produces attacks of angioedema. Various 17α-alkylated androgens are effective in the long-term management of this disorder. Testosterone and testosterone esters are not effective in its treatment. This fact and the ability of orally active androgens, but not the parenteral esters, to increase blood levels of the C1-esterase inhibitor and a variety of other proteins may indicate that the beneficial effects of certain androgens in this disorder are not due to the standard mechanism of action of androgens, but may be the result of their side-effects (e.g., hepatotoxicity).[r15]

Breast Carcinoma

Androgens have been used in the treatment of women with metastatic breast carcinoma, with regression of metastases in 10–30 percent of patients treated. The mechanism of this effect is unclear, but androgens may act as antiestrogens. Since metastatic breast carcinoma also can be treated with other forms of chemotherapy with remission rates higher than those achieved with androgen therapy, and since androgens have bothersome virilizing side-effects, androgens have a minor role in the management of this disease.

Enhancement of Athletic Performance

There has been extensive use of androgens over the last three decades by various individuals in attempts to improve their athletic performance.[r15–r17] Although steroid use has been banned at many levels of organized sport competition, the use of steroids by both amateur and professional athletes continues. Steroid use by athletes has taken place in the face of past statements by health professionals that androgens do not enhance athletic performance in men and that the amount of androgens taken by some athletes can lead to health problems. However, the athletic and financial success of some athletes using steroids has led only to more widespread use of steroids.

Many studies have been conducted to determine whether androgens enhance athletic performance; however, objective evidence for increased performance due to androgens remains inconclusive. Many factors are responsible for this continuing uncertainty. It is difficult to design, conduct, and evaluate studies to determine whether androgens have effects on athletic performance. Androgens produce side-effects, such as acne and testicular atrophy, that make it difficult to conduct a blinded study. A placebo effect has been documented in some tests on athletes. Different studies have used different preparations of androgens, dosage schedules, training programs, assessment criteria, diets, and training regimens, making it nearly impossible to evaluate the data as a whole. Many athletes take androgens in amounts much higher than those evaluated in published studies. Androgens are often self-administered by athletes in what is called a "stacked pyramid" regimen. Several androgens, both oral and parenteral preparations, are taken simultaneously, and the amounts increased over time. Use is often discontinued before competitive performances (to avoid detection) or as part of a routine and then reinitiated. The amount of androgens administered in these situations can be 10–100 times the amount evaluated in controlled studies. The use of similar stacking regimens in controlled studies is unethical because of potentially toxic side-effects.

Despite this continuing uncertainty, health and medical organizations have recently given statements recognizing that steroid use can have some benefits to athletic performance, including increases in lean muscle mass, but that steroid use carries the risk of potentially severe side-effects.[r17]

Undesirable Effects of Androgens

Administration of testosterone esters to normal men in amounts equivalent to the normal daily secretion rate of testosterone has no apparent side-effects. However, administration of similar doses to females or prepubertal boys, or administration of higher amounts to normal men, can produce a variety of unwanted effects.[r15,r16] All androgens, including those referred to as anabolic steroids, can cause virilization in women. Early symptoms of virlization include hirsutism, deepening of the voice, acne, and menstrual irregularities, which slowly disappear if androgen therapy is discontinued soon after symptoms appear. Continued use of androgens can result in irreversible effects, including more extensive hirsutism, further changes in the tone of voice, hypertrophy of the clitoris, and male pattern baldness. Androgens should not be given during pregnancy, since they may cause masculinization of female fetuses. Androgen treatment of prepubertal individuals also can produce virilization, as well as premature closure of the epiphyses. Androgens produce gynecomastia in both men and children. This effect is thought to be due to peripheral conversion of testosterone to estradiol. Gynecomastia is more likely to occur in individuals with liver disorders, where decreased clearance of androgens by the liver allows greater peripheral metabolism to estradiol. 5α-Reduced androgens are not metabolized to estrogens, and so preparations containing androgens such as 5α-dihydrotestosterone could be useful in some circumstances. The A-ring structure of many of the orally-active androgens prevents their conversion to estradiol and minimizes their feminizing side-effects. Large doses of androgens can produce salt and water retention, which can cause edema, especially in patients with congestive heart disease or renal failure.

Administration of androgens to men in amounts above that necessary to maintain normal virilization can decrease LH and FSH secretion, owing to the negative feedback control of androgens on the pituitary. Decreased secretion of gonadotropins leads to a decrease in spermatogenesis and testicular atrophy. The prolonged use of excessive amounts of androgens, as with some athletes, can lead to azoospermia.

All androgens with 17α-alkyl substitutions, in contrast to testosterone esters, cause disturbances in liver function. These hepatotoxic effects become more likely with increasing dosage or length of treatment. Symptoms of liver dysfunction include jaundice, increases in a variety of plasma proteins of liver origin, and retention of bromosulfophthalein. Orally-active androgens, at levels commonly used by athletes, also can decrease the level of high-density lipoproteins and increase the level of low-density lipoproteins, which may increase the user's risk of atherosclerosis. More severe but rare complications of administering 17α-alkylated androgens include peliosis hepatitis (blood-filled cysts in the liver) and hepatoma.

Antagonists of Androgens

Antiandrogens

The biologic actions of androgens can be counteracted by a variety of methods, including those that block the synthesis of androgens, stimulate conversion of active androgens to inactive metabolites, increase the level of high-affinity androgen-binding proteins in blood, or prevent the interaction of androgens with receptors in target cells or organs. The last category of compounds is called "antiandrogens."[r18] Antiandrogens compete for binding to the androgen receptor; however, once bound, they are unable to form a productive (transcriptionally active) complex.

Both steroidal and nonsteroidal antiandrogens are now known (Fig. 50.4). Many steroidal antiandrogens, such as cyproterone acetate, megestrol acetate, or chlormadinone acetate have progestational and/or glucocorticoid activity. Nonsteroidal antiandrogens, such as flutamide and anandron, are "pure antiandrogens" in the sense that they do not exhibit any agonist activity or interfere with other classes of steroid hormones at effective doses. Flutamide apparently acts in vivo after its conversion to hydroxyflutamide. Although these antiandrogens bind to androgen receptors with a low affinity (usually much less than 1/50th of natural androgens), they are clinically useful as chemotherapeutic agents because they do not show significant side-effects or toxicity at effective doses. A variety of compounds may act as antiandrogens because they can physically block androgen binding to receptors. For example, cimetidine, a histamine H_2 receptor antagonist,[20] and dihydrophenanthrene,[21] a simple polycyclic hydrocarbon devoid of oxygen groups, bind to androgen receptors and act as antiandrogens.

Antiandrogens have been employed for treatment of a variety of androgen-dependent disorders, such as hirsutism, acne, hyperseborrhea, hypersexuality, precocious puberty, and androgen-dependent tumors. Approximately 80 percent of prostatic tumors are responsive to androgen ablation therapies, which include surgical castration, administration of pharmacologic doses of estrogens, or inhibition of the synthesis and release of pituitary gonadotropins with the use of potent gonadotropin-releasing hormone analogues. To maximize the effects of androgen ablation and to counteract the possible effects of androgens of adrenal origin, antiandrogens are used in combination with gonadotropin-releasing hormone analogues.[22] Topically active antiandrogens without systemic activity are being developed for clinical use in treatment of androgen-dependent skin disorders in males and females.[23] Systemic administration of antiandrogens, such as cyproterone and spironolactone, can be effective in treatment of female androgenization, but there is the risk of feminization of a male fetus. Systemic administration of antiandrogens is not appropriate for treating pattern baldness, acne, or other skin diseases in males because antiandrogens can cause general inhibition of androgenic activity and induce various side-effects, including a decrease in libido, effects on spermatogenesis, and gynecomastia.

5α-Reductase Inhibitors

Inhibition of 5α-reductase would limit the availability of 5α-dihydrotestosterone but not testosterone. 5α-Reductase inhibitors, therefore, would be very useful in selective treatment of 5α-dihydrotestosterone-dependent abnormalities such as those associated with the prostate (benign prostatic hyperplasia), hair follicles (hirsutism and baldness), and sebaceous glands (acne). 5α-Reductase inhibitors that do not bind to androgen receptors would not seriously impede testosterone-dependent actions, such as growth of skeletal muscle, sexual differentiation, and male sex drive, some of which also may be dependent on aromatization of testosterone to estrogens, which cannot be formed from 5α-dihydrotestosterone. In contrast, hormonal therapies using gonadotropin-releasing hormone analogues, estrogens, receptor-binding antiandrogens, and orchiectomy, which impede all androgenic activities in the individual, can cause side-effects, such as impotence, gynecomastia, and alteration of sexual behavior in males.

Various inhibitors of 5α-reductase (Fig. 50.5) are under study, and of these the 4-azasteroidal compounds are the most extensively studied.[r19] These inhibitors are 3-oxo-4-aza-5α-steroids with a bulky functional group at the 17β-position. The prototype for this class of 5α-reductase inhibitors is 17β-N,N-diethyl-carbamoyl-4-methyl-4-aza-5α-androstan-3-one (4-MA), which decreases the prostatic con-

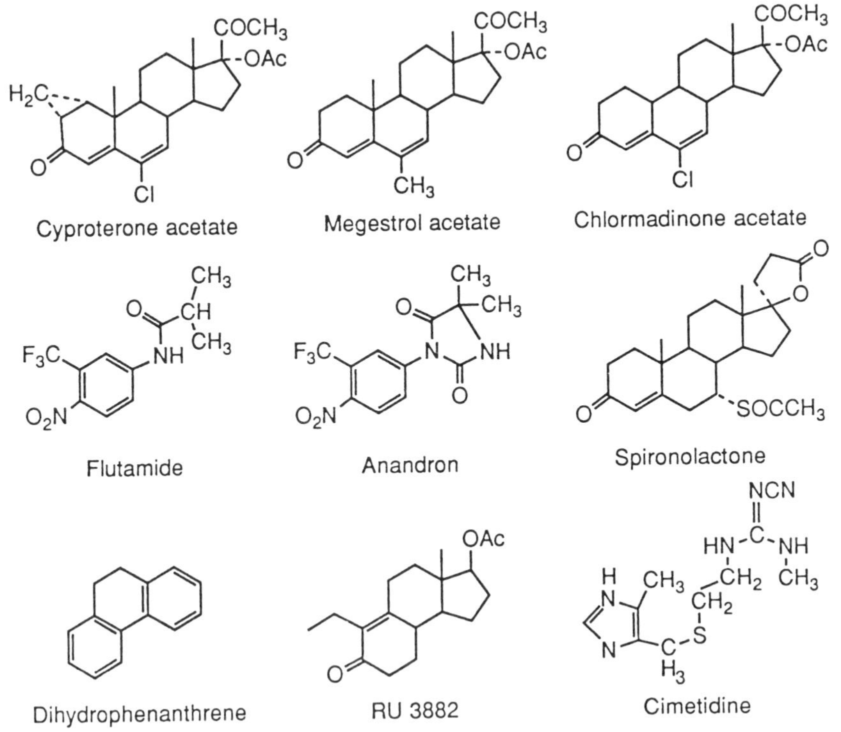

Cyproterone acetate, Megestrol acetate, Chlormadinone acetate, Flutamide, Anandron, Spironolactone, Dihydrophenanthrene, RU 3882, Cimetidine

Figure 50.4 Structure of various antiandrogens. Antiandrogens compete with androgens for binding to androgen receptors and in so doing block the ability of androgens to elicit a response. Some antiandrogens are used in the clinical treatment of androgen-dependent disorders.

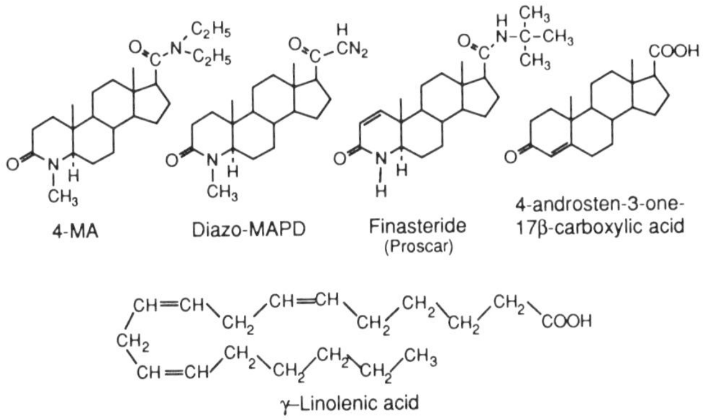

4-MA, Diazo-MAPD, Finasteride (Proscar), 4-androsten-3-one-17β-carboxylic acid, γ-Linolenic acid

Figure 50.5 Structure of inhibitors of 5α-reductase. Some androgenic effects depend on the conversion of testosterone to 5α-dihydrotestosterone by the enzyme 5α-reductase. Inhibitors of 5α-reductase may be of clinical use in the treatment of hirsutism, baldness, acne, and benign prostatic hyperplasia.

centration of 5α-dihydrotestosterone in male rats.[24] 4-MA attenuated the growth of the prostate of castrated rats induced by testosterone, but had much less of an effect in rats given 5α-dihydrotestosterone. When dogs are treated with 4-MA, the prostate size decreases.[25] Topical applications of 4-MA to the scalp of the stumptail macaque, a primate model of human male pattern baldness, also prevented the baldness that normally occurs at puberty in these monkeys.[26] These results also suggest that the prostate growth in rats and dogs and baldness in the stumptail macaque depend on 5α-dihydrotestosterone.

Finasteride (N-(2-methyl-2-propyl)-3-oxo-4-aza-5α-androst-1-ene-17β-carboxa mide, MK-906, or Proscar) is an orally-active inhibitor of 5α-reductase (K_i = 26 nM) in humans and is more potent than 4-MA in inhibiting the growth of the prostate. The inhibitor has no significant affinity for the rat prostate androgen receptor, and so can be used as a pure inhibitor that does not interfere with testosterone-dependent androgenic activities. A single oral dose of 0.5 mg of finasteride decreases the plasma level of DHT by 50 percent 24 hours after administration.[27] This compound is now under clinical testing for the treatment of benign prostate hyperplasia.[28] In one study, oral Proscar, 5 mg once a day for 24 weeks, reduced the prostate volume by 28 percent in 71 percent of men with BPH.

Absorption, Transport, and Excretion of Androgens

Blood steroid concentrations are of the order of 10–100 nM for androgens, glucocorticoids, and progestins, and of the order of 1 nM or lower for estrogens and mineralocorticoids. Most of the unconjugated testosterone and dihydrotestosterone in blood, even in amounts 100 times the physiologic concentration, is bound to a specific high-affinity testosterone-estradiol binding globulin (also known as sex hormone binding globulin),[r20] as well as to albumin, which binds steroids nonspecifically. Plasma steroid-binding proteins may be important for steroid distribution to target organs, protection of steroids from degradation, or slowing down metabolic clearance. The effective activity of androgens is probably exerted by the unbound form,[r21] which is only a small portion of the total blood androgen concentration.

Testosterone is rapidly absorbed into the portal

blood after oral administration and is metabolized in the liver to inactive products. Testosterone is also quickly absorbed from the site of parenteral injections and into the systemic circulation, where it is taken up by various tissues, metabolized, and inactivated. To attain therapeutically effective levels of active androgens in the systemic circulation, it has been necessary to modify testosterone and other active androgens chemically (Fig. 50.6). Three modifications most commonly used are: (1) esterification of the 17β-hydroxy group; (2) alkylation at the 17α position; and (3) various alterations of the steroid ring structure.

Esterification of the 17β-hydroxy group of an androgenic steroid decreases its polarity and increases its solubility in oil-based vehicles used for parenteral injection, and so decreases the rate of absorption into the systemic circulation. Most of these esters are not suitable for oral administration since they are still rapidly inactivated in the liver. The duration of effectiveness of a particular ester depends on the nature of the esterified acid. Esters with longer or less polar acids are effective for longer periods. Testosterone propionate is usually administered one to three times a week; whereas, testosterone cyprionate or enanthate are given in larger doses but at one- to three-week intervals. All esters are hydrolyzed in the body before the free steroid acts on a cell.

Methyl and ethyl substitutions at the 17α position on androgenic steroids decrease the rate of hepatic inactivation of these compounds and allow the oral administration of these drugs. Removal of the alkyl group at the 17α position does not appear to be necessary for these compounds to be effective androgens. Various other modifications of testosterone have been adopted empirically in the development of compounds that show androgenic and/or anabolic activity on oral administration. The effectiveness of these compounds may be due to a decrease in their rate of inactivation and/or enhancement of their potency.

Testosterone, secreted by various organs, produced from precursors in extraglandular tissues, or supplied by therapy, is metabolized in the liver to 4-androstenedione and then irreversibly converted to the 5α- and 5β-reduced metabolites, androstanedione and etiocholanolone (Fig. 50.7). Androstanedione is the precursor of urinary androsterone. These metabolites can be further metabolized by various liver cytochrome P450-dependent monooxygenases to a number of hydroxylated (C5α, C6α, C6β, C11β, C16α) products. These metabolites are conjugated to glucuronate and sulfate, and are excreted in urine. Only a small fraction of the 17-ketosteroids found in urine are derived from testosterone secreted by the testes. Most of these urinary 17-ketosteroids are derived from metabolism of adrenal steroids, such as dehydroepiandrosterone. 5α-Dihydrotestosterone, the active androgen in many tissues, can be locally metabolized to 3α- and 3β-androstanediols. 5α-Androstanediols bind very poorly to the androgen receptor, and any androgenic activity they display may reflect their conversion to 5α-dihydrotestosterone. These diols are substrates for conjugation or can be metabolized further and inactivated by cytochrome P450-dependent mono-oxygenases in various tissues.

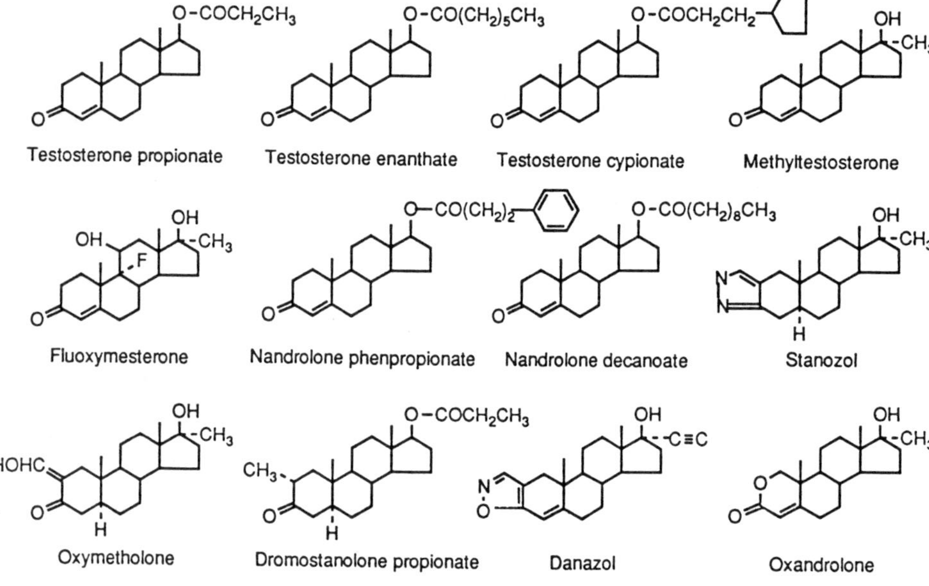

Figure 50.6 Androgenic and anabolic steroids in clinical use. Androgens such as testosterone must be structurally modified to delay metabolism (oral administration) or release from the injection site. This allows adequate blood levels of the androgenic compound to be attained for therapeutic purposes. The relative androgenic to anabolic activities for some of the steroids are shown.

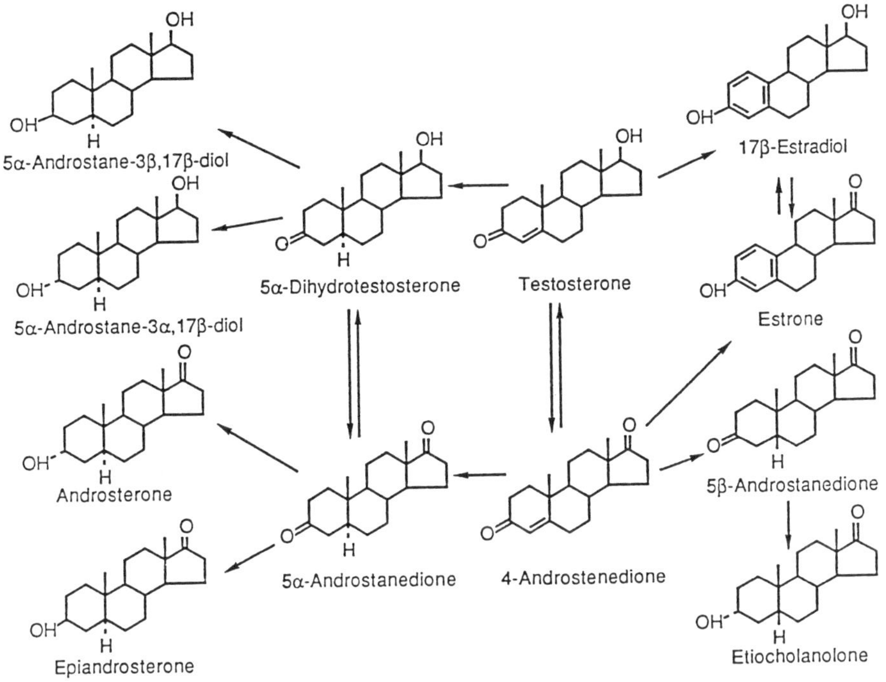

Figure 50.7 Metabolism of testosterone. Testosterone can be metabolized to more active androgens, such as 5α-dihydrotestosterone, or can serve as a precursor for estrogens such as estradiol. The 3-keto and 17β-hydroxy groups of testosterone and its metabolites undergo enzymatic oxidation/reduction in various tissues, producing less active steroids, which can be conjugated to sulfate and glucuronate and then excreted.

Preparations and Dosages

Some preparations of androgenic/anabolic steroids are listed in Table 50.3. The appropriate dosage may vary, depending on the individual, the condition being treated, and its severity. For development or maintenance of secondary sex characteristics, IM preparations (10 to 25 mg testosterone equivalent dose daily) are most effective. Since the use of orally active steroids may cause serious side-effects that usually are dose related, the lowest effective dose should be used for patients. The use of high doses of androgens in females may cause the undesirable side effects described earlier.

Other synthetic anabolic steroids (trade name) not listed in Table 50.3 include: androstanolone (Anaboleen); chlorotestosterone (Steranabol, Clostebol); chloromethyltestosterone (Turinabol tablet); chloro-1-dehydromethyltestosterone (oral Turinabol); chloro-19-nortestosterone (Steranabol); dimethyltestosterone (Myagen); dehydroepiandrosterone (Psicosterone); dehydroisoandrosterone (Diandrone); dehydrotestosterone (Boldenone); drostanolone (Drolban); mestanolone (Ermalon); mesterolone (Mestoran); methandienone (Abirol); methandrostenolone (Dianabol); methenolone (Nibol, Primbolan); methyl-19-nortestosterone (Methalutin); methyltestosterone (Oreton Methyl); 19-nortestosterone (Anabol); norbolethone (Genabol); norethandrolone (Nilevar); ethylnortestosterone (Norneutromone); exabolone (Steranabol-depot); oxymesterone (Oranabol); stanozolol (Adroyd, Stromba); thiomesterone (Emdobol); trenbolone (Quindenione).

Summary

Androgens are steroid hormones responsible, in part, for the expression of the male phenotype. Androgens virilize the urogenital tract during embryonic development and, at puberty, induce and maintain male secondary sexual characteristics and stimulate the growth and function of the accessory sex glands. Androgens also have systemic anabolic effects and increase nitrogen retention, muscle mass, and body weight in androgen-deficient subjects. Although androgens are noted for their role in male development, androgens also are present in females, serving as precursors for the biosynthesis of estrogens. Androgens are produced by the testes, adrenals, and ovaries. The major androgen secreted by the testis and the most important androgen circulating in the blood of males is testosterone. In many androgen-responsive tissues, testosterone is metabolized to 5α-dihydrotestosterone by the enzyme, 5α-reductase; and this metabolite produces the characteristic response to androgens. Androgens elicit their effects by interacting with intracellular receptors, which function as transcriptional regulators. The clearest indication for the therapeutic use of androgens is in men with low amounts of circulating androgens due to dysfunction of the pituitary or testis. Parenteral administration of testosterone esters is recommended for long-term therapy; whereas, orally active androgens are best suited for short-term treatment regimes. Androgens have been utilized in the treatment of various disorders, but the virilizing effects of androgens like testosterone often limit their usefulness in females and prepubertal males. Anabolic steroids are structurally modified androgens that show greater anabolic effects relative to virilizing effects and were developed to overcome the limitations to the use of

Table 50.3 Preparations of Androgenic Steroids

Generic name and TRADE NAME	Preparation and dosage for androgen deficiency	Relative activity *Androgenic* Anabolic
Testosterone TESTOJECT	Aqueous suspension for IM 10–50 mg 3 times/week	1/1
Testosterone propionate TESTEX	Oil solution for IM 10–25 mg 2–3 times/week	1/1
Testosterone enanthate DELATESTRYL	Oil solution for IM 50–400 mg/2–4 weeks	1/1
Testosterone cypionate DEPO-TESTOSTERONE	Oil solution for IM 50–400 mg/2–4 weeks	1/1
Methyltestosterone ANDROID METANDREN TESTRED	Oral: 10–40 mg or buccal: 5–20 mg daily 5-mg buccal tablets 10-, 25-mg oral tablets 5-, 10-mg buccal capsules 10-, 20-mg oral tablets 10-mg oral capsules	1/1
Fluoxymesterone HALOTESTIN	Daily dose: 2–20 mg 2, 5, and 10 mg oral tablets	1/1
Nandrolone phenpropionate DURABOLIN	Oil solution for IM 25–50 mg/week for breast carcinoma 25 mg/ml	1/2
Nandrolone decanoate DECA-DURABOLIN	Oil solution for IM, highly anabolic, 50 mg/ml in oil	1/3
Stanozolol WINSTROL	Highly anabolic 2-mg tablets, 6 mg daily	1/3
Oxymetholone ANADROL	Anabolic, 1–5 mg/kg daily for anemia 5-, 10, and 50 mg oral tablets	1/2
Dromostanolone propionate DROLBAN	Oil solution for IM 100 mg 3 times/week for breast carcinoma	1/3
Oxandrolone ANAVAR	Daily dose: 5–10 mg 2.5-mg tablets	
Danazol DANOCRINE	Anabolic, 200–800 mg daily for suppression of pituitary and treatment of angioneurotic edema	

androgens like testosterone. All anabolic steroids, however, have some virilizing side-effects.

Antiandrogens are compounds that compete with androgens for binding to androgen receptors and block the androgenic response. They are used in clinical treatment of certain androgen-dependent disorders. Inhibitors of 5α-reductase may be of clinical use in the treatment of androgen-dependent disorders induced by 5α-dihydrotestosterone.

References

Research Reports

1. Boris A, Stevenson RH, Trmal T. A comparison of the androgenic and myotrophic activities of some anabolic steroids in the castrated rat. J Steroid Biochem 1970;*1*:349–354.
2. Fang SF, Anderson KM, Liao S. Receptor proteins for androgens. On the role of specific proteins in selective retention of 17β-hydroxy-5α-androstan-3-one by rat ventral prostate in vivo and in vitro. J Biol Chem 1969;*244*:6584–6595.
3. Mainwaring WIP. A soluble androgen receptor in the cytoplasm of rat prostate. J Endocrinol 1969;*45*:531–541.
4. Unhjem O, Tveter KJ. Localization of an androgen binding substance from the rat ventral prostate. Acta Endocrinol 1969;*60*:571–578.
5. Bruchovsky N, Wilson JD. The conversion of testosterone to 5α-androstan-17β-ol-3-one by rat prostate in vivo and in vitro. J Biol Chem 1968;*243*:2012–2021.
6. Anderson KM, Liao S. Selective retention of dihydrotestosterone by prostatic nuclei. Nature 1968;*219*:277–279.
7. Chang C, Kokontis J, Liao S. Structural analysis of complementary DNA and amino acid sequences of human and rat androgen receptors. Proc Natl Acad Sci USA 1988;*85*:7211–7215.
8. Lubahn DB, Joseph DR, Sar M, Tan J, Higgs HN, Larson RE, French FS, Wilson EM. The human androgen receptor: Comple-

mentary deoxyribonucleic acid cloning, sequence analysis and gene expression in the prostate. Molec Endocrinol 1988;*2*:1265–1275.

9. Belanger A, Couture J, Caron S, Roy R. Determination of nonconjugated and conjugated steroid levels in plasma and prostate after separation on C-18 columns. Ann NY Acad Sci 1990;*595*:251–259.
10. Gloyna RE, Wilson JD. A comparative study of the conversion of testosterone to 17β-hydroxy-5α-androstan-3-one (dihydrotestosterone) by prostate and epididymis. J Clin Endocrinol Metab 1969;*29*:970–977.
11. Thigpen AE, Davis DL, Gautier T, Imperato-McGinley J, Russell DW. Brief report: The molecular basis of steroid 5α-reductase deficiency in a large Dominican kindred. N Engl J Med 1992;*327*:1216–1219.
12. Thigpen AE, Davis DL, Milatovich A, Mendonca BB, Imperato-McGinley J, Griffin JE, Francke U, Wilson JD, Russell DW. Molecular genetics of steroid 5α-reductase 2 deficiency. J Clin Invest 1992;*90*:799–809.
13. Hiipakka RA, Wang M, Bloss T, Ito K, Liao S. Expression of 5α-reductase in bacteria as a trpE fusion protein and its use in the production of antibodies for immunocytochemical localization of 5α-reductase. J Steroid Biochem Molec Biol 1993;*45*:539–548.
14. Liang T, Hoyer S, Yu R, Soltani K, Lorincz AL, Hiipakka RA, Liao S. Immunocytochemical localization of androgen receptors in human skin using monoclonal antibodies against the androgen receptor. J Invest Dermat 1993;*100*:663–666.
15. Brown CJ, Goss SJ, Lubahn DB, Joseph DR, Wilson EM, French FS, Willard HF. Androgen receptor locus on the human X chromosome: regional localization to Xq11–12 and description of a DNA polymorphism. Am J Hum Genet 1989;*44*:264–269.
16. Simental JA, Sar M, Lane MV, French FS, Wilson EM. Transcriptional activation and nuclear targeting signals of the human androgen receptor. J Biol Chem 1991;*266*:510–518.
17. Jenster G, van der Korput HAGM, van Vroonhoven C, van der Kwast TH, Trapman J, Brinkmann AO. Domains of the human androgen receptor involved in steroid binding, transcriptional activation, and subcellular localization. Molec Endocrinol 1991;*5*:1396–1404.
18. LaSpada AR, Wilson EM, Lubahn DB, Harding AE, Fischbeck KH. Androgen receptor gene mutations in X-linked spinal and bulbar muscular atrophy. Nature 1991;*352*:77–79.
19. Rosenfield RL. Low-dose testosterone effect on somatic growth. Pediatrics 1986;*77*;853–857.
20. Sivelle PC, Underwood AH, Jelly JA. The effects of histamine H_2 receptor antagonists on androgen action in vivo and dihydrotestosterone binding to the rat prostate androgen receptor in vitro. Biochem Pharmacol 1982;*31*:677–684.
21. Chang C, Liao S. Topographic recognition of cyclic hydrocarbons and related compounds by receptors for androgens, estrogens and glucocorticoids. J Steroid Biochem 1987;*27*:123–131.
22. Crawford ED, Eisenberger MA, McLeod DG, Spaulding JT, Benson R, Dorr FA, Blumenstein BA, Davis MA, Goodman PJ. A controlled trial of leuprolide with and without flutamide in prostatic carcinoma. N Engl J Med 1989;*321*:419–424.
23. Bouton MM, Lecaque D, Secchi J, Tournemine C. Effect of a new topically active antiandrogen (RU38882) on the rat sebaceous gland: comparison with cyproterone acetate. J Invest Derm 1986;*86*:163–167.
24. Brooks JR, Baptista CM, Berman C, Ham EA, Hichens M, Johnston DBR, Primka RL, Rasmusson GH, Reynolds GF, Schmitt SM, Arth GE. Response of rat ventral prostate to a new and novel 5α-reductase inhibitor. Endocrinol 1981;*109*:830–836.
25. Brooks JR, Berman C, Glitzer MS, Gordon LR, Primka RL, Reynolds GF, Rasmusson GH. Effects of a new 5α-reductase inhibitor on size, histologic characteristics, and androgen concentrations of the canine prostate. Prostate 1982;*3*:35–44.
26. Rittmaster RS, Uno H, Povar ML, Mellin TN, Loriaux DL. The effects of N,N-diethyl-4-methyl-3-oxo-aza-5α-androstane-17β-carboxamide, a 5α-reductase inhibitor and antiandrogen on the development of baldness in the stumptail macaque. J Clin Endocrinol Metab 1987;*65*:188–193.
27. Gormley GJ, Stoner E, Rittmaster RS, Gregg H, Thompson DL, Lasseter KC, Vlasses PH, Stein EA. Effects of finasteride (MK-906), a 5α-reductase inhibitor on circulating androgens in male volunteers. J Clin Endocrinol Metab 1990;*70*:1136–1141.
28. MK-906 (Finasteride) Study Group. One year experience in the treatment of benign prostatic hyperplasia. J Androl 1991;*12*:372–375.
29. Ris-Stalpers C, Trifiro MA, Kuiper GGJM, Jenster G, Romalo G, Sai T, van Rooij HCJ, Kaufman M, Rosenfield RL, Liao S, Schweikert HU, Trapman J, Pinsky L, Brinkmann AO. Substitution of aspartic acid-686 by histidine or asparagine leads to a functionally inactive protein with altered hormone-binding characteristics. Molec Endocrinol 1991;*5*:1562–1569.
30. Sai T, Seino S, Chang C, Trifiro M, Pinsky L, Mhatre A, Kaufman M, Lambert B, Trapman J, Brinkmann AO, Rosenfield RL, Liao S. An exonic point mutation of the androgen receptor gene in a family with complete androgen insensitivity. Am J Hum Genet 1990;*46*:1095–1100.

Reviews

r1. Gardner FH, Besa EC. Physiologic mechanisms and the hematopoietic effects of the androstanes and their derivatives. Curr Top Hematol 1983;*4*:123–195. The effects of 5α- and 5β-androstanes on hematopoiesis—experimental and clinical aspects.

r2. Koch FC. The male sex hormones. Physiol Rev 1937;*17*:153–238. A good account of early research into the discovery of androgens.

r3. Gower DB. Biosynthesis of androgens and other C19 steroids. In: Makin HLJ (ed.) Biochemistry of steroid hormones. Oxford: Blackwell (1984); Chap 5:170–206.

r4. Vermeulen A. The androgens. In: Gray CH, James VHT (eds.) Hormones in blood. New York: Academic Press (1979); Vol 3:355–361. A comprehensive review on androgen synthesis, metabolism, pharmacology, clinical disorders and analytical methods.

r5. Brooks RV. Androgens: physiology and pathology. In: Makin HLJ (ed). Biochemistry of steroid hormones. Oxford: Blackwell (1984); Chap 15:565–594.

r6. Wilson JD, Aiman J, MacDonald PC. The pathogenesis of gynecomastia. Adv Intern Med 1980;*25*:1–32.

r7. Rosenfield RL. Role of androgens in growth and development of the fetus, child and adolescent. Adv Pediatr 1972;*19*:171–213.

r8. George FW, Wilson JD. Hormonal control of sexual development. Vitam Horm 1986;*43*:145–196. Review of the role of androgens in sexual differentiation.

r9. Griffin JE, Wilson JD. The androgen resistance syndromes: 5α-reductase deficiency, testicular feminization and related disorders. In: Scriver CR, Beaudet AL, Sly WS, Valle D eds. The metabolic basis of inherited disease. New York: McGraw-Hill

(1989); Chap 75:1919–44. Basic science and clinical consequences of genetics defects in 5α-reductase and androgen receptors.

r10. Mooradian AD, Morley JE, Korenman SG. Biological actions of androgens. Endocrine Rev 1987;*8*:1–28. A survey of the effects of androgens on different organ systems.

r11. Evans RM. The steroid and thyroid hormone superfamily. Science 1988;*240*:889–895. A concise summary of the molecular biology of nuclear hormone receptors.

r12. McPhaul MJ, Marcelli M, Tilley WD, Griffin JE, Wilson JD. Androgen resistance caused by mutations in the androgen receptor gene. FASEB 1991;*5*:2910–2915.

r13. Hiipakka RA, Liao S. Androgen receptors and action. In: DeGroot LJ (ed). Endocrinology. Philadelphia, WB Saunders 1994 (In press) A review of the molecular mechanisms in androgen action.

r14. Ammus SS. The role of androgens in the treatment of hematologic disorders. Adv Intern Med 1989;*34*:191–208.

r15. Wilson JD, Griffin JE. The use and misuse of androgens. Metab 1980;*29*:1278–1295.

r16. Wilson JD. Androgen abuse by athletes. Endocrine Rev 1988;9:181–199.

r17. Strauss RH, Yesalis CE. Anabolic steroids in the athlete. Ann Rev Med 1991;*42*:449–457.

r18. Moguilewsky M, Bouton MM. How the study of the biological activities of antiandrogens can be oriented towards the clinic. J Steroid Biochem 1988;*31*:699–710. A review of the available antiandrogens and possible clinical applications.

r19. Liang T, Rasmusson GH, Brooks JR. Biochemical and biological studies with 4-azasteroid 5α-reductase inhibitors. J Steroid Biochem 1983;*19*:385–390.

r20. Petra PH. The plasma sex steroid binding protein (SBP or SHBG). A critical review of recent developments on the structure, molecular biology and function. J Steroid Biochem Molec Biol 1991;*40*:735–753.

r21. Mendel CM. The free hormone hypothesis: a physiologically based mathematical model. Endocrine Rev 1989;*10*:232–274.

CHAPTER 51

Irving M. Spitz

Gonadotropins

The pituitary gonadotropins, luteinizing hormone (LH) and follicle stimulating hormone (FSH), together with human chorionic gonadotropin (hCG), which is derived from the placenta, are glycoproteins that play a key role in reproduction. The hypothalamic releasing hormone, gonadotropin releasing hormone (GnRH), is secreted into the hypothalamic-portal system and acts on the pituitary gonadotrophs regulating LH and FSH synthesis and secretion. The gonadotropins stimulate the maturation and function of the testis and ovary, controlling gametogenesis and steroid hormone production. These steroids promote sexual development and act on the hypothalamic-pituitary system to control gonadotropin secretion in a closed feedback system. This is diagrammatically shown in Fig. 51.1. hCG is secreted from the placental trophoblast cells soon after implantation of the fertilized egg. It stimulates progesterone secretion from the corpus luteum and is crucial for the early maintenance of pregnancy. The principal therapeutic application of gonadotropins is in induction of ovulation and spermatogenesis in selected infertile subjects.

Chemistry[r1,r3,r5]

LH and FSH, together with hCG and thyrotropin, are glycoprotein hormones that have been purified and characterized. In the human, as well as in other species, these hormones contain two nonidentical and noncovalently linked peptide subunits designated α and β. Each subunit is internally cross-linked and stabilized by disulfide bonds. Individual subunits have little if any biologic activity. The α-subunits of each of these four glycoprotein hormones are nearly identical and differ only in carbohydrate structure. The β-subunits differ more extensively in both amino acid and carbohydrate composition, and are largely responsible for conferring different biologic activities on the hormones. The α-subunit of any of these glycoprotein hormones can be combined with the β-subunit of another to yield a hybrid molecule that has the biologic activity of the β-subunit donor. The molecular weight of LH and FSH is approximately 28,000–29,000; that of hCG is 37,000. The molecular weight of the common α-subunit is 14,000.

The first 121 amino-terminal amino acids of βhCG show about 80 percent sequence homology with βhLH; the carboxy-terminus of βhCG contains a 24-amino acid extension not present in βhLH. The sequence homologies between βhCG and the β-subunits of FSH and TSH are much lower than that between βhCG and βhLH. In view of the structural similarity between the β-subunits of LH and hCG, it is not surprising that the biologic actions of LH and hCG are similar.

The carbohydrate groups are found in specific locations in the structure of each subunit. The constituent monosaccharides are mannose, galactose, fucose, glucosamine, galactosamine, and neuraminic (sialic) acid. The carbohydrate groups influence the ability of the glycoprotein hormones to combine with and activate their receptor sites.

History[r1]

A relationship between the pituitary gland and the gonads was noted in 1921, when Evans and Long observed that pituitary extracts produced a marked increase in ovarian weight. Five years later, Smith in California and Zondek and Aschheim in Berlin independently showed that the pituitary was able to stimulate the gonads. Early on the question arose as to whether there was one or more than one distinct chemical entity in the pituitary gland. This was not easy to resolve, since early preparations were impure and there was synergism in different bioassay systems. Fevold and coworkers in 1931 were the first to separate pituitary extracts into two fractions,

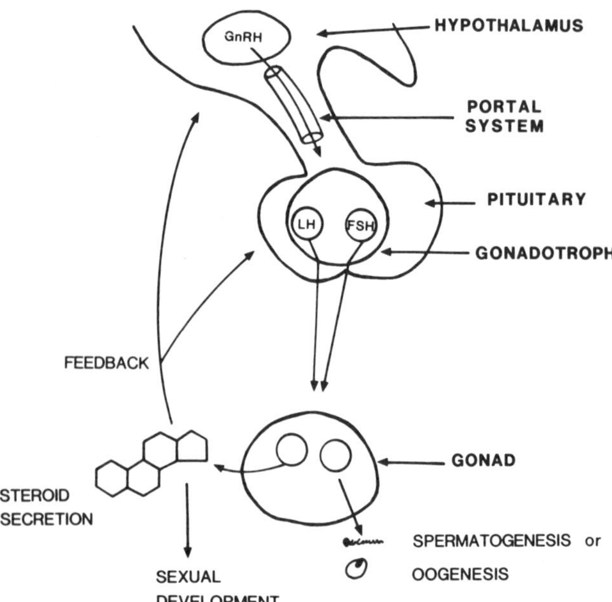

Figure 51.1 The hypothalamic-pituitary-gonadal axis. GnRH secreted from the hypothalamus into the hypothalamic-portal system stimulates the pituitary gonadotrophs to synthesize and release LH and FSH. The target organ for the gonadotropins is the gonad. There they promote gametogenesis (i.e., spermatogenesis or sperm formation in the male and oogenesis or formation and development of ova in the female). The gonadotropins also control steroidogenesis, which induces sexual development and also feed-back to the hypothalamus and pituitary.

one of which promoted growth of ovarian follicles (follicle stimulating hormone) and the other fraction, which induced luteinization of follicles (luteinizing hormone). When this latter hormone was first discovered in the male, it was called interstitial cell stimulating hormone (ICSH) because of its effect on testicular Leydig cells. Today it is recognized that LH and ICSH are identical, and the term LH is used in both sexes. Aschheim and Zondek detected gonadotropic activity in human pregnancy urine in 1927. Subsequently it was shown that this gonadotropin was not identical to the pituitary gonadotropins, and it was called human chorionic gonadotropin (hCG).

A significant impetus to the understanding of the physiology and pathology of gonadotropin secretion began with the advent of radioimmunoassay. This was applied initially to the measurement of serum insulin by Berson and Yalow. Later the same principle was adapted to measure serum gonadotropins and steroids. For the first time it was possible to determine the functional state of the gonads by taking a small sample of blood.

Progress in the isolation and purification of gonadotropins was slow and not achieved until the 1950s and 1960s, when ion exchange chromatography and gel filtration of proteins were developed. The amino acid sequences of TSH, LH, hCG, and FSH were determined in the 1970s. Currently, hCG is obtained from commercial concentrates of first-trimester pregnancy urine. Although LH and FSH may be obtained by purification of human pituitaries, for clinical use gonadotropins are isolated from the urine of postmenopausal women. This preparation is known as human menopausal gonadotropins (hMG) and contains both FSH and LH. With the availability of gonadotropins, it became possible to induce ovulation in women and spermatogenesis in men. Very recently, using DNA technology, human recombinant FSH has become available, and is now undergoing preliminary evaluation in humans.[1]

In 1971, Schally and coworkers published the primary structure of porcine GnRH. This step further advanced the understanding of gonadal physiology and pathology. Recently, therapy with pulsatile native GnRH has been used to stimulate sexual development in both men and women with decreased gonadotropin function.[r6] In a further therapeutic development, synthetic GnRH analogues with agonistic or antagonistic activity were synthesized that suppress gonadotropin and steroid secretion.[r7] These analogues have wide clinical application and are dealt with in Chapter 54.

Biosynthesis[r8,2,r9,3–6]

The genes for all four glycoproteins are thought to have evolved from a single precursor gene, although a separate gene codes for the synthesis of each subunit. The gene structures for the α- and β-subunits are known. A single gene located on chromosome 6 is responsible for coding all α-subunits. The β-LH subunit gene is located on chromosome 11. A total of seven genes on chromosome 19 code for βhCG. The human FSH beta gene is located on chromosome 11. Biosynthesis of gonadotropic hormones occurs by ribosomal synthesis of the peptide chains with post-translational cleavage of presequences from the amino terminus of the nascent α- and β-subunit polypeptides and the subsequent addition of carbohydrate residues. Precise details of formation and combination of the α- and β-subunits have not yet been clarified, but biosynthesis of the α-subunit occurs more actively than the β-subunit in both pituitary and placenta. Thus, it appears likely that formation of the β-subunits acts as the rate-limiting step in biosynthesis of the pituitary and placental glycoprotein hormones.

Regulation of Secretion

LH and FSH[r10,r11]

A pulse generator in the arcuate region of the medial basal hypothalamus governs the episodic secretory discharges of GnRH into the hypophyseal-portal system. An optimal frequency of GnRH pulsatility is essential to maintain appropriate circulatory levels of LH and FSH; gonadotropins decrease when GnRH pulse frequency is too low. Conversely, too-frequent or continuous native GnRH stimulation or use of an agonistic analogue results in a transient increase in LH and FSH secretion. This is followed by inhibition of gonadotropin release and a fall in sex steroid secretion.[r6]

In the human pituitary, LH and FSH coexist in the same population of gonadotrophs.[7] GnRH interacts with high-affinity cell surface receptor sites on the plasma membrane of the gonadotrophs, causing increased exocytosis and discharge of granules from the pituitary cells. The release of both LH and FSH occurs within minutes via a calcium-dependent mechanism independent of cAMP or cGMP.[r12,r13] GnRH also has a long-term effect on the regulation of gonadotropin synthesis. So far no separate hypothalamic hormone releasing FSH has been identified.

The amounts of LH and FSH secreted by the gonadotrophs are largely influenced by gonadal steroids in a classic negative feedback system. When sex steroids fall, as in menopause in women or after castration in men, a marked rise in FSH and LH secretion occurs. The inhibition of gonadotropins by sex steroids is probably exerted at both the pituitary and the hypothalamic level (Figs. 51.1 and 51.2). In the male, both testosterone and estradiol inhibit LH secretion. The negative feedback inhibition of testicular hormones on FSH secretion is less well understood. Serum FSH concentrations increase selectively in proportion to the loss of germinal elements in the testis. The main regulation of FSH secretion appears to be a nonsteroid peptide inhibitor known as inhibin, which is secreted by the Sertoli cell (Fig. 51.2). A similar material is present in ovarian follicular fluid. Inhibin has been purified and its structure elucidated. It serves to inhibit FSH preferentially, but not LH secretion. Other testicular proteins structurally related to inhibin, such as activin, serve to stimulate FSH secretion. Inhibin and activin are synthesized in the pituitary and other tissues as well as in the ovary and testes and are dealt with in Chapter 53. Another glycosylated single-chain polypeptide known as follistatin is also produced by the ovary. It is not a member of the inhibin family, but it selectively decreases FSH beta mRNA and inhibits FSH secretion in vitro.[8–10]

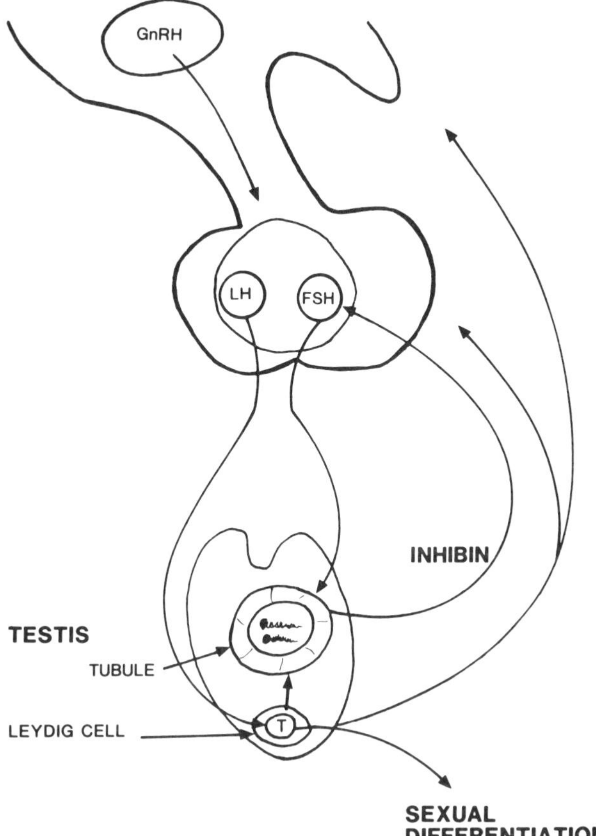

Figure 51.2 The hypothalamic-pituitary-testicular axis in the male. LH acts at the Leydig cells to produce testosterone (T). Testosterone feeds back at the hypothalamic-pituitary level. FSH and testosterone act on the tubule to promote spermatogenesis. Inhibin secreted by the Sertoli cells of the seminiferous tubule preferentially inhibits FSH secretion.

hCG[r2]

After implantation of the fertilized egg, hCG is secreted by the syncytiotrophoblast cells of the placenta. This serves to prolong the life of the corpus luteum and to maintain progesterone secretion in the early stages of pregnancy. The precise mechanism controlling hCG secretion is unknown. The placenta has been reported to synthesize GnRH, which may act locally to regulate hCG secretion. After the first trimester, the ovary and corpus luteum are no longer required for maintenance of pregnancy, since the placenta itself secretes adequate estrogen and progesterone. hCG is elaborated by all types of trophoblastic tissue, including that from hydatidiform mole and choriocarcinoma. It is also produced by the normal testis, ovary, and numerous other tissues.

Effects and Actions of Gonadotropins

LH and FSH[r4]

When LH and FSH are not secreted, the gonads are unstimulated. There is failure of steroid secretion as well as absence of ovulation in the female and spermatogenesis in the male. If this occurs before puberty because of the lack of sex steroid secretion, there is no development of secondary sex characteristics, and both males and females are tall with disproportionately long bones due to a delay in epiphyseal closure. Males have a high-pitched voice, sparse pubic and body hair with little beard, and small gonads. The universal feature in females is primary amenorrhea, but there is also infantilism of the female external and internal genitalia. If failure of gonadotropin secretion occurs after full sexual development has already occurred, the diagnosis may be more subtle. The presentation may be amenorrhea in females and infertility and decrease in libido in males.

In the ovary, the target cell for FSH is the primordial follicle. Under the influence of FSH, the follicle secretes estradiol. LH stimulates progesterone production by the corpus luteum and is required for ovulation (Fig. 51.3). In the testis, LH acts on the Leydig cell to produce testosterone (Fig. 51.2). Estradiol in females and testosterone in males are the steroid hormones that promote sexual development. In the male, the primary target cell for FSH is the Sertoli cell. Together with testosterone, FSH stimulates the synthesis of many testicular proteins, which leads to spermatogenesis. When hypophysectomy is performed, there is testicular regression; restoration of spermatogenesis requires both FSH and LH.

The Menstrual Cycle[r10,11]

The coordinated interactions of GnRH, LH, FSH, and steroids are required for ovulation in the female (Fig. 51.3). Unlike the male, sex steroids in the female exert both a positive and negative feedback on FSH and LH secretion. During the early or follicular phase of the menstrual cycle, successive groups of small follicles start to grow, the largest being known as the dominant follicle. This ovarian response represents the action of FSH, which stimulates estradiol secretion from the dominant follicle. During the later part of the follicular phase of the cycle, FSH levels show a progressive decline, a consequence of the rise of estradiol. LH levels during the follicular phase are generally stable or rise slightly. The progressive rise in plasma estradiol is followed by a brief preovulatory rise in progesterone. These latter hormonal changes trigger the surge of LH and FSH that precedes ovulation by 12–24 hours.[12]

At the time of ovulation, one area on the surface of the dominant follicle thins and then undergoes dissolution, leaving an aperture through which the ovum passes. The dominant follicle now becomes the corpus luteum, and the luteal phase begins (Fig. 51.3). Those follicles not destined to ovulate show regressive changes. The corpus luteum secretes progesterone under the influence of LH, which maintains the corpus luteum until estradiol and progesterone secretion decline. Menstrual bleeding commences with the slough-

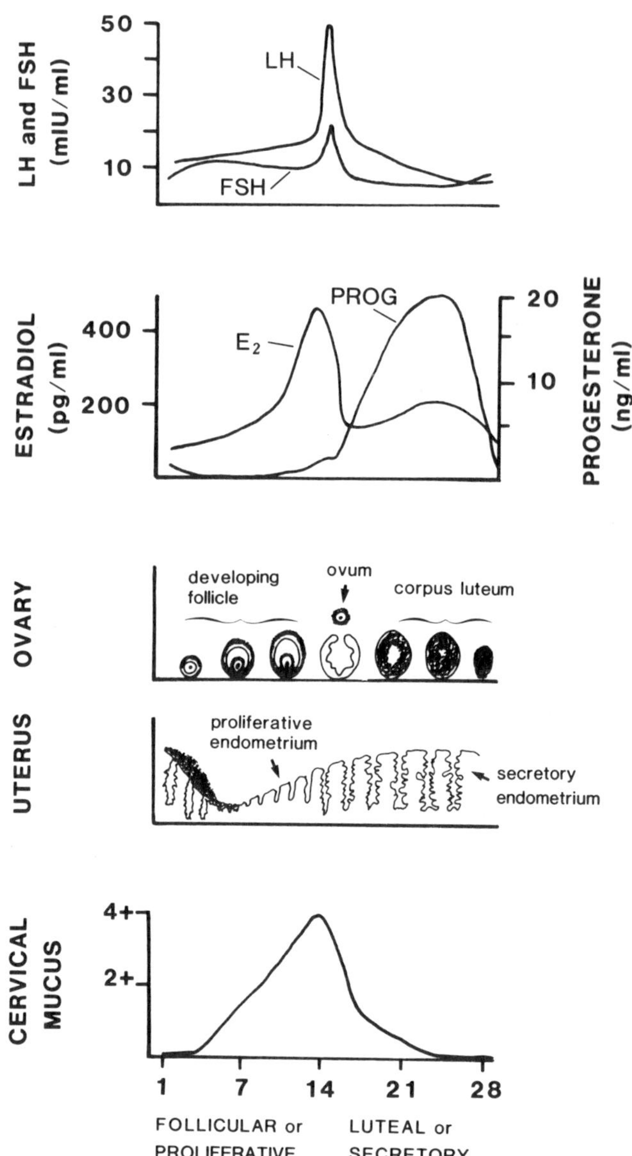

Figure 51.3 The menstrual cycle in the female. The upper panel shows serum LH and FSH; the second panel shows serum estradiol and progesterone. The third and fourth panels depict ovarian and uterine events, respectively. Following the onset of menses the follicular phase commences. Under the influence of FSH, there is progressive development of the follicle, which secretes estradiol. Shortly after the LH surge, ovulation occurs, and the luteal phase begins. The follicle is converted into the corpus luteum, which secretes progesterone. In the follicular phase, estradiol induces proliferation of the endometrium. This is also known as the proliferative phase of the cycle. Estradiol also produces an increase in the quantity and ferning of the cervical mucus, with increase in elasticity, i.e., spinnbarkeit (panel 5). After the LH surge, progesterone transforms the endometrium into a secretory organ. Hence the term "secretory phase." If pregnancy does not occur, the corpus luteum regresses. With the withdrawal of estradiol and progesterone support, the endometrium sloughs, bleeding occurs, and a new cycle begins.

ing of the endometrium owing to withdrawal of estrogen and progesterone support. Thereafter a new cycle begins.

hCG[r2]

hCG rescues the corpus luteum during the latter part of the luteal phase, resulting in the maintenance of luteal progesterone production well beyond the time when luteal regression occurs in nonfertile cycles. This action of hCG maintains pregnancy until placental progesterone production is well established. This takes about three months.

hCG also has other actions. It plays a role in the early masculinization and sexual differentiation of the male fetus by stimulating androgen secretion from the fetal testis. hCG is also required for steroidogenesis of the fetal adrenal gland, although it is not known for certain whether hCG is necessary for the control of placental steroidogenesis. hCG has also been shown to have very weak thyrotropic activity.

Mechanism of Action[r3,r4]

LH and hCG

The effects of LH and hCG are initiated by binding of the circulating hormone to specific high affinity receptors for LH and hCG in the cell membrane, resulting in activation of adenylate cyclase that mediates the action of the hormone on steroidogenesis. These receptors exhibit similar properties in testicular and ovarian target cells. At the target cell surface, LH reacts with a specific membrane receptor, which is coupled to adenylate cyclase by the guanyl nucleotide regulatory subunit (G). This is shown in Figure 51.4. Adenylate cyclase catalyzes the conversion of ATP to cAMP, which activates protein kinases. At the same time there is an increase in Ca^{++} permeability of the cell membrane and efflux of Ca^{++} from the mitochondria. This leads to a rise in cytosolic Ca^{++} concentration, which has various positive and negative feedback effects on the products of cAMP-dependent protein kinases. Some of the phosphorylated proteins are believed to facilitate the hydrolysis of cholesterol esters and the transport of free cholesterol into the mitochondrion, where it is metabolized to pregnenolone. In the ovary, pregnenolone is the precursor of progesterone synthesis in the corpus luteum and of estrogen synthesis in the thecal cells. Similar events occur in the Leydig cell. Following conversion of cholesterol to pregnenolone, there is enhanced synthesis of testosterone. The LH-receptor complexes undergo endocytosis and internalization, with subsequent degradation or recycling.

FSH

The biologic effects of FSH are exerted on the maturation and function of somatic cells associated with gametogenesis, i.e., granulosa cells of the ovary and Sertoli cells of the testis. Both of these cell types display many homologous features, including the possession of specific plasma membrane receptors for FSH and an associated adenylate cyclase system activated by the FSH-receptor interaction. In the testis, FSH augments the action of LH by causing an increase in the number of LH receptors. In the ovary, FSH stimulates the mitotic activity of granulosa cells in the follicle and converts the surrounding stroma into a layer of theca cells. Granulosa cells in small follicles contain only FSH receptors. As the follicle grows, FSH induces the appearance of LH receptors so that follicles bind both

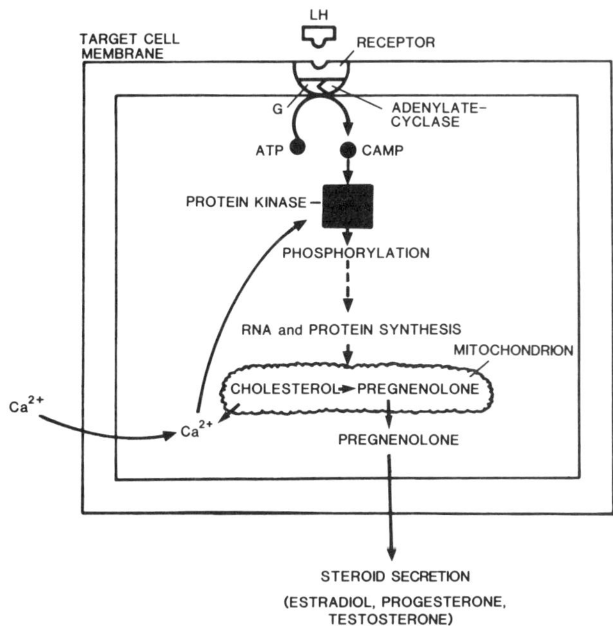

Figure 51.4 Schematic representation of a target cell for LH or hCG. LH binds to its receptor, which is coupled to adenylate cyclase by the guanyl nucleotide regulatory subunit (G). Adenylate cyclase catalyzes the conversion of ATP to AMP; activating protein kinases. These phosphorylated proteins synthesize RNA and protein, promote the conversion of cholesterol to pregnenolone, and stimulate steroidogenesis. There is also an increase in cytosolic Ca^{2+} due to efflux from the mitochondria and increase in calcium permeability of the cell membrane. The rise in cytosolic Ca^{2+} modulates the products of CAMP-dependent protein kinases.

gonadotropins. FSH also stimulates the aromatization of androgens to estrogen.

Therapeutic Use of Gonadotropins

The use of gonadotropins for treatment of infertility is costly, time-consuming, and requires careful monitoring to prevent complications. It should be undertaken only by an experienced physician who has full laboratory back-up.

Treatment of Females[13–19,r14]

Selection of Subjects

Any subject with decreased LH and FSH secretion of pituitary or hypothalamic origin who is desirous of fertility is a potential candidate for gonadotropin therapy. This includes patients with primary or isolated gonadotropin (LH and FSH) deficiency (hypogonadotrophic hypogonadism); but other causes of hypopituitarism also can be treated, as can women with secondary amenorrhea or anovulation (Fig. 51.5). Subjects with polycystic ovary syndrome and endogenous estradiol secretion unresponsive to clomiphene also are potential candidates. However, in this group, the incidence of the hyperstimulation syndrome is much higher.

Today, one of the most important uses of gonadotropin therapy is in programs utilizing in vitro fertilization (IVF) and embryo transfer. Originally, this treatment was restricted to subjects with fallopian tube obstruction. Today it is used in unexplained infertility, ovarian failure, and even in situations where infertility is due to oligospermia. The success of IVF is improved by transferring more than one embryo, and to achieve this hMG is frequently used.

Subjects with pituitary or hypothalamic tumors should not receive hMG until after treatment of their primary tumor. Gonadotropin therapy is of very limited value in subjects with high levels of FSH and LH consequent to primary ovarian failure and should not be used in subjects with abnormal uterine bleeding or those with marked ovarian enlargement due to polycystic ovary disease.

Treatment Schedule

The aim of therapy is to stimulate follicular growth for 10 to 15 days with hMG and then to administer hCG, which simulates

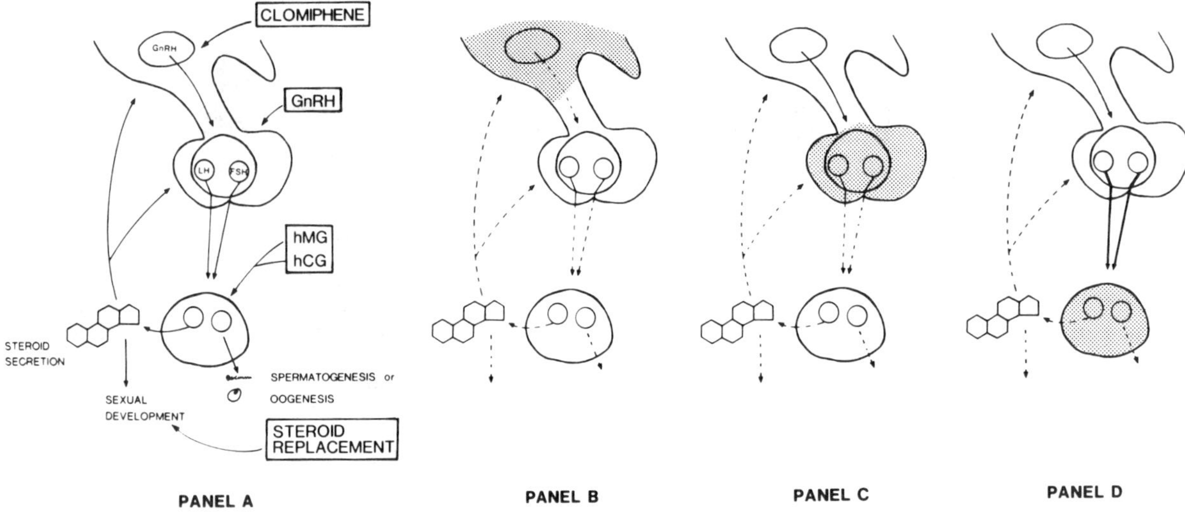

Figure 51.5 An approach to the diagnosis and treatment of hypogonadism. Panel A shows the normal hypothalamic-pituitary-gonadal axis and the various therapeutic agents that are available, together with their site of action. Clomiphene citrate acts at the level of the hypothalamus, pulsatile GnRH therapy at the pituitary, and exogenous gonadotropins (hMG and hCG) on the gonad. Steroid replacement will not induce gametogenesis, but will only maintain secondary sexual characteristics. Panel B shows the situation in hypothalamic amenorrhea, which is characterized by decreased secretion of gonadotropins and steroids. These subjects can respond to clomiphene, pulsatile GnRH, or exogenous gonadotropins. With a lesion in the pituitary (panel C), gonadotropins and steroids are again low. The subject will invariably respond to pulsatile GnRH therapy or a combination of hCG and hMG. The hypogonadism in panels B and C is secondary to hypothalamic-pituitary pathology. Primary hypogonadism occurs when the site of the lesion is at the level of the gonad (panel D). Because of the lack of steroid feedback, there is increased LH and FSH secretion. In primary hypogonadism, induction of gametogenesis is not possible, and the patient is treated with steroid replacement. However, with the advent of in vitro fertilization, ovum transfer can now be performed in female patients with primary hypogonadism.

an LH surge and induces ovulation. Because of differences in sensitivity to gonadotropins, the individual response varies considerably. This variability may even occur in the same individual during successive cycles of therapy. Subjects must be under close supervision and evaluated daily. Cervical mucus is a sensitive indicator of estrogen activity. When an increase in cervical mucus together with spinnbarkeit (i.e., spinnability or strongly elastic quality of the mucus) and ferning is apparent, daily serum estradiol or urinary estrogen determinations as well as daily ultrasound examinations are to be performed. Blood or urine samples should be taken in the morning and hormones measured before administration of the next dose of hMG, which is to be given in the evening. The usual commencing dose of hMG is 150 IU. If the estradiol level remains unchanged after three days, the dose of hMG should be increased by a factor of 0.5 and continued for a further three to four days. The dosage of hMG is increased in this stepwise fashion until serum estradiol or urinary estrogen levels increase. The dose is then maintained until the dominant follicle reaches 18 to 22 mm. This usually corresponds to an estradiol level of 700 to 1000 pg/ml and a urinary estrogen level of 60–100 μg/24 hours. At this stage, therapy with hMG is stopped. hCG is usually administered 24 hours after the last injection of hMG, provided the urinary estrogen or serum estradiol do not exceed these levels. The dose of hCG is usually 5000–10,000 IU, and further doses may be given at three-day intervals. Although this dose of hCG is adequate to maintain corpus luteum function, serum progesterone levels should be monitored during the luteal phase. Frequent sexual intercourse is advised at the time of the expected ovulation. A representative example of treatment with hMG and hCG is shown in Figure 51.6. If there is no response to hMG after 14 days of treatment, therapy should be stopped and recommenced after a rest period. It should be noted that patients with polycystic ovary disease who have high LH and low FSH levels often ovulate without the addition of hCG.

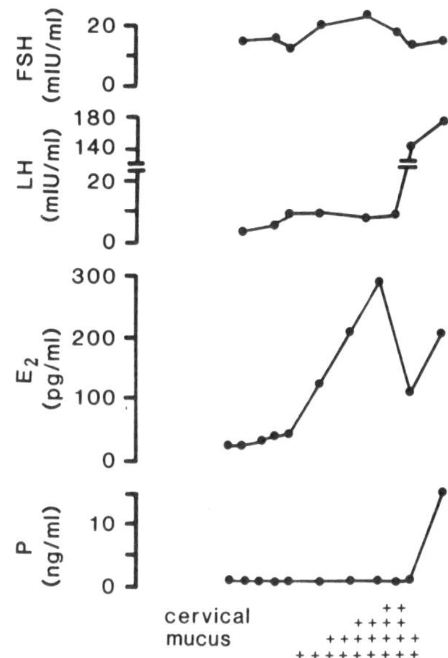

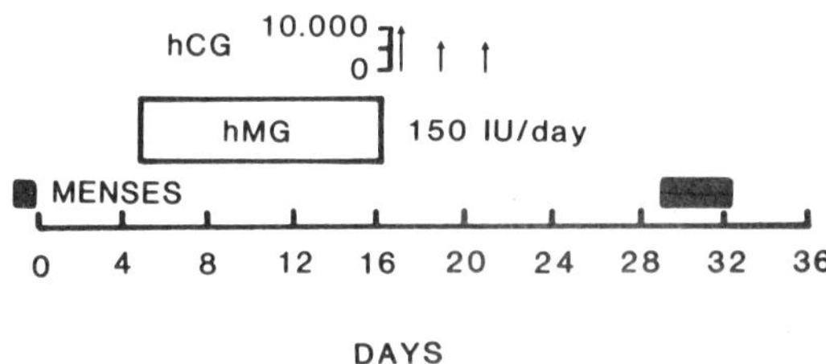

Figure 51.6 Ovulation induction with hMG and hCG in a patient with isolated gonadotropin deficiency. An increase in cervical mucus and estradiol occurs during hMG administration, and progesterone increases following hCG. The high levels of LH represent cross-reaction of exogenous hCG in the LH immunoassay.

Results

In carefully selected subjects, the ovulation rate should exceed 90 percent. Best results occur in those without endogenous estrogen activity, when pregnancy rates can reach over 90 percent. In those with endogenous estrogen activity, pregnancy rates at six months are usually about 40 percent.

Treatment of Males[r4,r6,20,21]

Selection of Subjects

Gonadotropin therapy is indicated in those who have hypogonadism consequent to decreased gonadotropin secretion. This can be primary isolated gonadotropin deficiency or part of generalized pituitary disease. These males can be rendered fertile by the administration of hMG and hCG. In those with only partial gonadotropin deficiency and some previous testicular development, it may be possible to induce spermatogenesis with the administration of hCG alone.

Subjects with hypogonadotrophic hypogonadism and bilateral cryptorchidism usually are unresponsive to hMG and hCG therapy. The use of gonadotropins in the treatment of azoospermia, oligospermia, or infertility other than gonadotropin deficiency has also been attempted; however, in general, the results have been poor. Gonadotropin therapy is contraindicated in men with prostatic carcinoma or with benign prostatic hypertrophy.

Treatment Schedule

LH is required to stimulate the Leydig cells to secrete testosterone and is given as hCG in a dose of 4000 to 5000 IU two to three times a week for up to six months. After adequate masculinization has been induced, hMG is added to the regimen in a dosage of 75–150 IU twice per week in combination with hCG (2000 IU). The FSH component present in hMG is required for spermatogenesis. Often 12–18 months of combined therapy are required before spermatozoa are present in the ejaculate. Despite the length of treatment required to induce spermatogenesis, patient compliance is usually good and the subjects can be taught to self-administer the injections.

In isolated gonadotropin deficiency, although sperm output only rarely rises above 10 million per ejaculate, this low level is usually adequate to impregnate an otherwise normal healthy ovulating spouse. Once maximal stimulation of the germinal tissue and sperm output has been achieved, FSH often can be stopped, and sperm production will continue as long as hCG is maintained. If fertility is not required, then testosterone therapy alone is adequate to induce or maintain secondary sex characteristics and libido. At a subsequent stage, if fertility is desired, hCG and hMG can be substituted for testosterone. Recently, pulsatile native GnRH has been used to promote gonadal and sexual development (Fig. 51.5). This therapy requires continuous use of a pump, and the results are similar to those obtained with combined hMG-hCG therapy.

hCG in the Treatment of Other Conditions

hCG therapy is also used in the treatment of cryptorchism, which is a failure of one or sometimes both testes to descend into the scrotum. If the condition is bilateral and the testes are below the inguinal ring, an attempt can be made to produce testicular descent by the administration of hCG, usually in doses of 500 to 4000 IU two or three times a week for several weeks. If the treatment is not successful, the undescended testis is placed into the scrotum surgically.

hCG also can be used to induce puberty in subjects with constitutional delay of puberty.

Finally, hCG may also be used as a diagnostic test to determine whether the testis produces testosterone. For example, in a prepubertal boy with undescended gonads, a rise in testosterone after a test dose of hCG indicates that the testes are present and functional.

Undesirable Effects of Gonadotropins

In Relation to Ovulation Induction[r14]

Hyperstimulation Syndrome

Moderate ovarian enlargement during hMG therapy is not uncommon and occurs in 7 to 10 percent of treated subjects. In the hyperstimulation syndrome, there is excessive ovarian stimulation by hCG. It usually presents 4 to 7 days after hCG administration. There is rapid ovarian enlargement associated with ascites, weight gain, and hydrothorax. The basic pathogenesis of the full-blown syndrome is a shift of fluid from the intravascular space into the abdominal cavity, leading to hypovolemia. As a consequence, there is oliguria, hemoconcentration, and often hypotension. There also may be fever, increased blood coagulability, and electrolyte imbalance. Arterial thromboembolism has been described.

With regard to management, if palpable ovarian enlargement does occur, hMG should be stopped. If ovarian enlargement is noted at the end of hMG treatment, no hCG should be given. In the full-blown syndrome, subjects must be hospitalized and treated by IV fluid replacement using colloidal volume expanders such as mannitol and dextran.

The incidence of this complication ranges from 0.5 to 2 percent. It is seen when estradiol levels exceed 1000 pg/ml and urinary estrogen rises above 150 μg/ml. hCG should be withheld under those conditions. Hyperstimulation syndrome is commonly observed in those subjects with endogenous estrogen activity, as in polycystic ovary syndrome, who have high serum LH and low FSH. It is believed that the use of urinary FSH as opposed to hMG is associated with a lower incidence of hyperstimulation syndrome in this group.

Multiple Pregnancies

This complication is due to stimulation of too many follicles. The incidence for twins ranges from 10 to 20 percent and for triplets from 5 to 10 percent.

Pregnancy Wastage

This occurs in up to 25 percent of subjects due to inadequate luteal stimulation or multiple gestation. The frequency of birth defects has not been increased in those subjects who carry to term.

Enlargement of an Existing Pituitary Tumor

In a normal pregnancy, there is physiologic enlargement of the pituitary gland due to the high levels of estrogens. When hMG is used to induce ovulation in women with a pre-existing untreated pituitary tumor, the rise in estradiol levels often produces enlargement of the pituitary tumor, and hMG is contraindicated.

Other Complications

Antibody Production[22,23]

Despite the fact that urinary preparations are injected, the incidence of antibody formation, which inhibits gonadotropin action, is very low. In the vast majority of subjects antibodies to hMG or hCG do not develop despite repeated courses of treatment. Anti-hCG antibodies occasionally have been documented in males and females with hypogonadotrophic hypogonadism following administration of hCG. There is also one documented female with isolated FSH deficiency who developed antibodies to FSH but not LH following hMG administration.

Gynecomastia

Gynecomastia may develop in male subjects given hCG therapy for the induction of spermatogenesis. This is due to hCG-induced estradiol secretion. If worrying to the patient this gynecomastia may be treated surgically.

Epiphyseal Closure

If excessive hCG is administered to young boys with cryptorchidism or for induction of puberty, the dramatic increase in serum testosterone can result in precocious sexual development and early epiphyseal fusion of the long bones. This may produce a sudden growth spurt, but the ultimate adult height is decreased.

Other Side-Effects

Other rare side-effects reported during hCG administration include fever, headache, depression, and edema. Very rarely, pain and swelling occur at the site of injection in some subjects.

Circulatory Levels

LH and FSH[r11,24,25]

Plasma levels of both LH and FSH rise shortly after birth to reach a peak at one to four months of age. Values of both hormones then decrease to low levels until puberty. The earliest sign of the onset of puberty is the nocturnal rise of LH. Episodic secretion of LH is present in postpubertal men and women, with peaks occurring every two to three hours. These peaks vary in magnitude (Fig. 51.7). Estradiol, progesterone, and testosterone alter both the frequency and amplitude of LH secretory pulses. Secretory bursts of FSH are less marked and more difficult to detect. This is presumably a consequence of the smaller amplitude of the FSH response to GnRH and its longer half-disappearance time. The free α-subunit has been identified in the circulation particularly in the post-menopausal state.

Because of the variable secretion of LH, single samples are of limited value in the evaluation of the gonadal secretory status. When gonadotropins are used in the diagnosis and management of patients with gonadal pathology, levels should be measured in multiple plasma samples obtained at 20–to 30–minute intervals for three to six hours; alternatively, timed urine samples may be used. Both these approaches give an estimate of mean or integrated LH secretion per unit of time.

In cases of gonadal failure or hypogonadism, levels of sex steroids are low. When the hypogonadism is due to gonadal disease (i.e., primary hypogonadism), plasma FSH and LH levels are elevated (Fig. 51.5, panel D). In secondary hypogonadism due to hypothalamic-pituitary pathology, plasma gonadotropins are inappropriately low in association with the low sex steroid levels (Fig. 51.5, panels B and C). This distinction between primary and secondary hypogonadism, which is based on measurement of circulating gonadotropins, is of great importance, because induction of spermatogenesis and ovulation is possible only in those subjects with secondary hypogonadism (Fig. 51.5, panels B and C). Today, however, subjects with ovarian failure (Fig. 51.5, panel D) on steroid replacement have been treated in IVF programs by oocyte donors and embryo transfer.

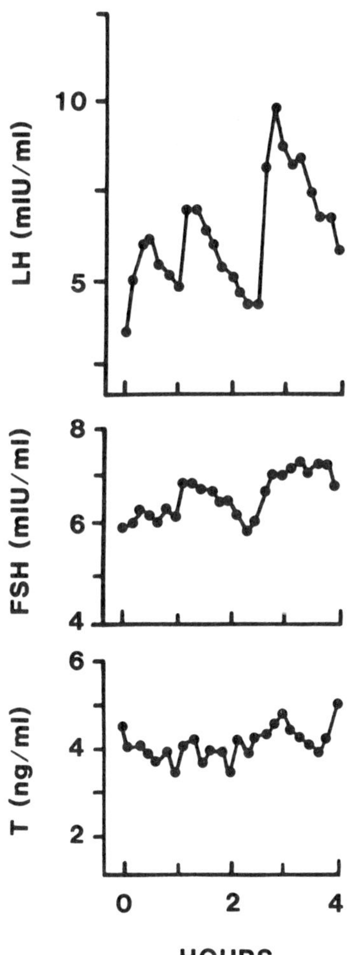

Figure 51.7 Pulsatile LH, FSH and Testosterone Secretion in a Normal Male Subject over a Four-Hour Time Period

hCG[r2]

hCG is detected in the maternal circulation as early as the ninth or tenth day after the midcycle LH surge. Its secretion begins with the period of implantation, and its concentration increases very rapidly to peak values by 60 to 90 days of gestation. Thereafter, there is a reduction in hCG levels to a plateau that is maintained during the remainder of pregnancy. Although large sporadic fluctuations are frequent, there is no circadian rhythm. Free βhCG is also released into the maternal circulation. hCG or its subunits are frequently secreted into the circulation by tumors of trophoblastic origin (hydatidiform mole and choriocarcinoma).

Metabolism and Excretion of Gonadotropins[r1,r5]

Gel filtration of plasma LH and FSH has shown that the molecular form in which the pituitary glycoprotein hormones circulate in plasma is similar to that of the hormones extracted from the pituitary. The survival time of glycoproteins in the circulation is strongly influenced by their sialic acid content, and is more prolonged for more highly sialated molecules. hCG, which contains approximately 10 percent sialic acid, has an initial half-life of about six hours, whereas the initial plasma half-life of FSH (5 percent sialic acid) is four hours, and that of LH (2% sialic acid) is approximately one hour. After desialation, most glycoproteins are rapidly removed from the circulation by hepatic extraction. The completely desialated hCG has a plasma half-life of only several minutes. Despite the relationship between metabolic clearance and sialic acid residues, there is little evidence concerning the role of desialation in the normal metabolism of gonadotropins. The liver and kidney play a major role in the clearance and excretion of circulating gonadotrophic hormones. The urinary excretion of LH and FSH is small; however, about 20 to 25 percent of hCG is excreted in the urine in an intact form.

Desialated preparations of LH, hCG, and FSH show reduced biologic activity in vivo but still bind to membrane receptors in vitro. However, their ability to stimulate adenylate cyclase is reduced. Such deglycosylated hormones can act in vitro as competitive antagonists of the actions of the intact hormone on steroid hormone biosynthesis.

Since gonadotropins are glycoproteins, they are subject to proteolysis. Consequently they are not absorbed from the GI tract and have to be given by parenteral injection.

Measurement of Gonadotropins[r3,r4]

Radioimmunoassays (RIAs)

Sensitive RIAs are available for measuring circulating levels of LH, FSH, and hCG. Assay specificity depends on the particular antigenic determinants recognized by the antisera. One of the major problems in the RIA of pituitary gonadotropins relates to the choice of standards. The most common reference preparation used for both LH and FSH originates from human urinary menopausal urine. This preparation, distributed by the Medical Research Council in England, is known as the Second International Reference Preparation (Second IRP-hMG). Many laboratories use the reference standard provided by the National Pituitary Agency known as LER 907, which is a partially purified pituitary extract calibrated against the second IRP-hMG. The use of different standards has resulted in a wide range of values for gonadotropins measured in individual laboratories. Absolute levels vary, making comparison between laboratories difficult; however, all assays show similar profiles of circulating hormones during the menstrual cycle and other physiologic states.

Because of the great similarity of the structures of LH and hCG, significant cross-reactivity is observed in these two assays. For this reason antisera to the hormone-specific β-subunit of hCG have been employed to improve the specificity of the hCG assay. This approach has been of value for the measurement of the low levels of hCG in both blood and urine in the early diagnosis of pregnancy, even in the presence of significant levels of LH.

In addition to its use in the diagnosis of early pregnancy, βHCG assays are used to diagnose and monitor treatment of tumors of trophoblastic origin that secrete hCG. Quantitation of hCG secretion by choriocarcinoma and hydatidiform moles provides an accurate index of tumor regression or recurrence.

The same RIAs are used to measure LH and FSH in urine. The quantity of LH and FSH in a three-hour urine sample has been shown to correlate well with the integrated value of plasma gonadotropins during the same period and can therefore provide a useful index of gonadotropin secretion.

In addition to radioimmunoassay, gonadotropins may also be measured by fluroimmunoassay (FIA) or enzyme-linked immunoabsorbent assay (ELISA).

Radioreceptor Assays

Radioligand receptor assays are readily able to measure LH or hCG concentrations. These assays are somewhat less sensitive than RIAs and more susceptible to nonspecific interference by plasma proteins. For these reasons, radioligand receptor assays have not been applied routinely to the measurement of plasma gonadotropin levels.

Bioassays

Early described bioassays were insensitive and time-consuming. They could be used only to measure urinary or pituitary gonadotropins. Recently more sensitive biologic assays for plasma LH and hCG have been employed using dispersed Leydig cells from the rodent testis. These cells are highly responsive to primate gonadotropins in vitro and show a sensitive dose-response curve for testosterone production. This Leydig cell assay has shown that immunoactive and bioactive LH profiles are closely correlated in many physiologic situations.

More recently a sensitive FSH bioassay system has been developed based on induction of aromatase activity in immature rat granulosa cells. This test utilizes the fact that FSH promotes aromatization of androgens to estrogens.[26]

Preparation and Doses

Because of their protein structure, the gonadotropins of either pituitary or placental origin are effective only if given by injection. The following preparations are available:

a. Human menopausal gonadotropins (hMG), also known as menotropins (Pergonal). This preparation is isolated from the urine of postmenopausal women and contains both FSH and LH. Each ampoule contains 75 IU of FSH and 75 IU of LH activity. The preparation is given by IM injection. The usual dose is one or two ampoules.

b. Human urinary follicle stimulating hormone or urofollitropin (Metrodin). This is also extracted from postmenopausal urine and contains 75 IU of FSH and less than 1.0 IU of LH. It is used in in vitro fertilization programs as well as in situations where endogenous gonadotropins and estradiol are present; e.g., polycystic ovary syndrome.

c. Human pituitary gonadotropin (hPG). This is prepared from human pituitary glands and contains both FSH and LH.

d. Human pituitary FSH. This preparation has a very low LH content. Previously both this pituitary preparation and human pituitary gonadotropin were available in limited supply for investigational use from the National Pituitary Agency. However, because of possible contamination with Jakob-Creutzfeldt virus, their distribution has been discontinued.[27]

e. hCG. This is obtained from the urine of pregnant women and is sold under various trade names (Pregnyl, A.P.L., etc.). The preparation is given IM in doses of 400 to 10,000 IU.

f. Gonadotropins from animal sources are immunologically incompatible and unsuitable for therapeutic uses. Previously a preparation known as Pregnant Mares' Serum was used to a limited extent; but there are no longer any indications for this preparation.

References

Research Reports

1. Schoot DC, Coelingh-Bennink HJT, Mannaerts BMJL, Lamberts SWJ, Bouchard P, Fauser BCJM Human recombinant follicle-stimulating hormone induces growth of preovulatory follicles without concomitant increase in androgen and estrogen biosynthesis in a woman with isolate gonadotropin deficiency. J Clin Endocrinol Met 1992;*74*:1471–1473.
2. Godine JE, Chin WW, Habener JF. Luteinizing and follicle-stimulating hormones. Cell-free translations of messenger RNAs coding for subunit precursors. J Biol Chem 1980;*225*:8780–8783.
3. Nilson JH, Thomason AR, Cserbak MT et al. Nucleotide sequence of a cDNA for the common alpha subunit of the bovine pituitary glycoprotein hormones. Conversion of nucleotides in the 3′-untranslated region of bovine and human pre-alpha subunit mRNAs. J Biol Chem 1983;*258*:4679–4682.
4. Fiddes JC, Goodman HM. Isolation, cloning and sequence analysis of the cDNA for the alpha-subunit of human chorionic gonadotropin. Nature 1979;*281*:351–356.
5. Fiddes JC, Goodman HM. The gene encoding the common alpha subunit of the four human glycoprotein hormones. J Mol Appl Genet 1981;*1*:3–18.
6. Talmadge K, Vamvakopoulos NC, Fiddes JC. Evolution of the genes for the beta subunits of human chorionic gonadotropin and luteinizing hormone. Nature 1984;*307*:37–40.
7. Phifer RF, Midgley AR, Spicer SS. Immunohistologic and histologic evidence that follicle-stimulating hormone and luteinizing hormone are present in the same cell type in the human pars distalis. J Clin Endocrinol Metab 1973;*36*:125–141.
8. Carroll RS, Corrigan AZ, Gharib SD et al. Inhibin, activin and follistatin: Regulation of follicle-stimulating hormone messenger ribonucleic acid levels. Mol Endocrinol 1989;*3*:1969–1976.
9. Ueno N, Ling N, Ying SY et al. Isolation and partial characterization of follistatin: a single-chain M, 35,000 monomeric protein that inhibits the release of follicle-stimulating hormone. Proc Natl Acad Sci USA 1987;*84*:8282–8286.
10. Ying SY, Becker A, Swanson G. Follistatin specifically inhibits pituitary follicle stimulating hormone release in vitro. Biochem Biophys Res Commun 1987;*149*:133–139.
11. Hodgen GD. Neuroendocrinology of the normal menstrual cycle. J Reprod Med 1989;*34*: Suppl 1, 68–75.
12. Hoff JD, Quigley MD, Yen SSC. Hormonal dynamics at midcycle: A re-evaluation. J Clin Endocrinol Metab 1983;*57*:792–796.
13. Lobo RA, Granger LR, Davajan V, Mishell DR. An extended regimen of clomiphene citrate in women unresponsive to standard therapy. Fertil Steril 1982;*37*:762–766.
14. O'Herlihy C, Pepperell RJ, Brown JB et al. Incremental clomiphene therapy: A new method for treating persistent anovulation. Obstet Gynecol 1981;*58*:535–542.
15. Thompson LR, Hansen LM. Pergonal (menotropins): A summary of clinical experience in the induction of ovulation and pregnancy. Fertil Steril 1970;*21*:844–853.
16. Garcea N, Campo S, Panetta V et al. Induction of ovulation with purified urinary follicle-stimulating hormone in patients with polycystic ovarian syndrome. Am J Obstet Gynecol 1985;*151*:635–640.
17. Schoemaker J, Wentz AC, Jones GS et al. Stimulation of follicular growth with "pure" FSH in patients with anovulation and relevant LH levels. Obstet Gynecol 1978;*51*:270–277.
18. Saffan D, Seibel MM. Ovulation induction with subcutaneous pulsatile gonadotropin releasing hormone in various ovulatory disorders. Fertil Steril 1986;*45*:475–482.
19. Miller DS, Reid RR, Cetel NS et al. Pulsatile administration of low dose gonadotropin releasing hormone ovulation and pregnancy in women with hypothalamic amenorrhea. JAMA 1983;*250*:2937–2941.
20. Hoffman AR, Crowley WF Jr. Induction of puberty in men by long-term pulsatile administration of low-dose gonadotropin-releasing hormone. N Engl J Med 1982;*307*:1237–1241.
21. Crowley WF, McArthur JW. Simulation of the normal menstrual cycle in Kallmann's syndrome by pulsatile administration of luteinizing hormone-releasing hormone (LHRH). J Clin Endocrinol Metab 1980;*51*:173–175.
22. Spitz IM, Bell J, Arad G, Benveniste R, Rabinowitz D. Development of anti-human FSH antibody in a patient with isolated FSH deficiency. J Clin Endocrinol Metab 1973;*36*:684–690.
23. Rabinowitz D, Spitz IM, Bercovici B, Bell J, Laufer A, Polishuk WZ. Isolated deficiency of follicle-stimulating hormone. Clinical and laboratory features. N Engl J Med 1972;*287*:1313–1317.
24. Santen RJ, Bardin CW. Episodic luteinizing hormone secretion in man. Pulse analysis, clinical interpretation, physiologic mechanisms. J Clin Invest 1973;*52*:2617–2628.
25. Veldhuis JD. Pathophysiological features of episodic gonadotropin secretion in man. Clin Res 1988;*36*:11–20.
26. Jia XC, Hsueh AJW. Sensitive *in vitro* bioassay for the measurement of serum follicle-stimulating hormone. Neuroendocrinol 1985;*41*:445–448.
27. Powell-Jackson J, Weller RO, Kennedy P et al. Creutzfeldt-Jakob disease after administration of human growth hormone. Lancet 1985;*2*:244–246.

Reviews

r1. Pierce JG. Gondatropins: Chemistry and biosynthesis. In: Knobil E, Neill J, (eds). The physiology of reproduction. New York: Raven Press (1988); pp 1335–1348.

r2. Talamantes F, Ogren L. The placenta as an endocrine organ: Polypeptides. In: Knobil E, Neill J, (eds). The physiology of reproduction. New York: Raven Press (1988); pp 2093–2144.

r3. Catt KJ, Pierce JG. Gonadotropic hormones of the adenohypophysis. In: Yen SSC, Jaffe RB, (eds). Reproductive endocrinology. Philadelphia: WB Saunders (1986); pp 75–114.

r4. Bardin CW. Pituitary-testicular axis. In: Yen SSC, Jaffe RB, (eds). Reproductive endocrinology. Philadelphia: WB Saunders (1986); pp 177–199.

r5. Parsons TF, Pierce JG. Glycoprotein hormones: structure and function. Ann Rev Biochem 1981;*50*:465–495.

r6. Crowley Jr WF, Filicori M, Spratt DI et al. The physiology of gonadotropin-releasing hormone (GnRH) secretion in men and women. Rec Prog Horm Res 1985;*41*:473–531.

r7. Karten MJ, Rivier JE. Gonadotropin-releasing hormone analog design: structure-function studies toward the development of agonists and antagonists. Rationale and perspective. Endocrinol Rev 1986;*7*:44–66.

r8. Gharib SD, Wierman ME, Shupnik MA et al. Molecular biology of the pituitary gonadotropins. Endocrine Rev 1990;*11*:177–179.

r9. Fiddes JC, Talmadge K. Structure, expression, and evolution of the genes for the human glycoprotein hormones. Rec Prog Horm Res 1984;*40*:43–78.

r10. Knobil E. The neuroendocrine control of the menstrual cycle. Rec Prog Horm Res 1980;*36*:53–88.

r11. Marshall JC, Kelch RP. Gonadotropin-releasing hormone: Role of pulsatile secretion in the regulation of reproduction. N Engl J Med 1986;*315*:1459–1468.

r12. Clayton RN, Catt KJ. Gonadotropin-releasing hormone receptors: characterization, physiological regulation, and relationship to reproductive function. Endocrine Rev 1981;*2*:186–209.

r13. Conn PM. The molecular basis of gonadotropin-releasing hormone action. Endocrine Rev 1986;*7*:3–10.

r14. Wentz AE. Amenorrhea: Evaluation and treatment. In: Jones HW, Wentz AC, Burnett LS, (eds). Novak's textbook of gynecology. Baltimore: Williams & Wilkins, 1988.

CHAPTER 52

Antiprogestins

Irving M. Spitz

RU 486, or mifepristone, is a synthetic steroid that is an antagonist of both progesterone and glucocorticoids. Since progesterone is essential for the initiation and maintenance of pregnancy, the principal use of RU 486 lies in its ability to induce abortion in early pregnancy; however, RU 486 has several other therapeutic indications.

Chemistry

RU 486 [11-[4-(dimethylamino) phenyl]-17-hydroxy-17-(1-propynyl)-(11β, 17β)-estra-4, 9-dien-3-one] differs structurally from progesterone and glucocorticoids in that it lacks the C19 methyl group and the 2-carbon side-chain at C17 of progesterone and glucocorticoids (Fig. 52.1). RU 486 possesses a 4-(dimethylamino) phenyl group at the 11β position and a 1-propynyl chain at the 17α position.[r1]

Although many other antiprogestins have been synthesized, RU 486 is the only one with which there has been extensive clinical experience. Recently, studies have commenced with ZK 98 299 (Onapristone) another antiprogestin.[1] The two-dimensional structure of ZK 98 299 is similar to RU 486, but has configurational inversions at the C13 and C17 positions (Fig. 54.1). Although this antiprogestin also has a high affinity for both progesterone and glucocorticoid receptors, ZK 98 299 is reported to have less antiglucocorticoid activity than RU 486.[1] These synthetic steroids also bind slightly to the androgen receptor but not to the estrogen or mineralocorticoid receptors.[r2]

History

In the late 1960s, following the demonstration of the progesterone receptor, it was realized that a significant advance in contraceptive technology would be the development of a progesterone receptor antagonist. The search for such an antiprogesterone extended over many years and culminated in 1982 with a report by scientists at Roussel-Uclaf in Paris of the synthesis of RU 486.[r3] Subsequently, it was shown by Herrmann et al.[2] that RU 486 could induce abortion when administered in early pregnancy.

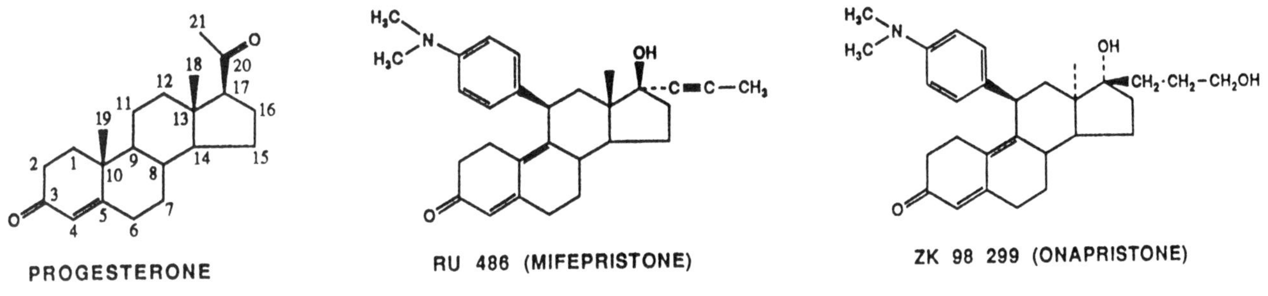

Figure 52.1 Structural Configuration of Progesterone, RU 486, and ZK 98299

Mechanism of Action

The action of progesterone in target tissues is mediated by a progesterone receptor, which has a domain for DNA binding, hormone binding, and transactivation. When progesterone combines with the receptor, it induces a dramatic change in the progesterone receptor, transforming it from a non-DNA binding form to one that will bind DNA. This is accompanied by a loss of associated heat-shock proteins and dimerization. In the presence of other nuclear factors, this activated receptor dimer then binds to progesterone-response elements in the promoter region of progesterone-responsive genes. This ultimately leads to biologic effects characteristic of progesterone. When RU 486 binds to the progesterone receptor, it also induces loss of heat-shock proteins and produces dimerization. However, unlike the situation with progesterone, the RU 486-receptor dimer fails to induce a biologic response in the presence of progesterone. Under these circumstances, RU 486 will act as a progesterone antagonist. In the absence of progesterone, however, RU 486 displays mild progesterone agonistic effects.[3,r4]

It is thus evident that RU 486 may function either as a progesterone antagonist or partial agonist. Its use as an antagonist is best illustrated in its action as an abortifacient. Under these conditions, the antiprogestin activity of RU 486 is targeted to the decidua, which contains a high concentration of progesterone receptors. The receptor blockade results in withdrawal of progesterone support and the onset of menstrual bleeding with disruption of placental function. The subsequent decline in βhCG is believed to be due to detachment of chorionic tissue of the blastocyst.

RU 486 may also act as a progesterone antagonist in the endometrium. When administered in doses of 50 mg or greater in the mid- or late luteal phase, it induces menstrual bleeding within three days. Doses of RU 486 as low as 5 mg will induce profound changes in endometrial morphology without inducing bleeding.[4]

Under certain conditions, RU 486 may also act on the endometrium as a partial progesterone agonist.[r4,5] This is evident when it is administered in situations where there is no progesterone activity, as in postmenopausal women or ovariectomized monkeys receiving only estrogen replacement. Under these conditions, low doses of RU 486 produced progesterone-like effects on the endometrium and induced secretory transformation of the endometrium. Higher doses of RU 486 inhibited both endometrial proliferation and secretory activity and thus demonstrated an antiestrogenic action. This also represents a progesterone agonistic effect, since high doses of progestins produce similar antimitogenic effects and endometrial atrophy. This effect of RU 486 is independent of the estrogen receptor since RU 486 does not bind to the estrogen receptor.[r2] It is possible that the partial progesterone agonistic effect of RU 486 might explain its benefit in the treatment of endometriosis and uterine leiomyomata, as well as its effect in breast carcinoma and meningioma.

In addition to its effect on the decidua and endometrium, RU 486 also acts to soften and dilate the cervix and it also increases myometrial contractility.[r4] Many studies have shown that it also inhibits gonadotropin secretion. It appears that the endometrium is the tissue most sensitive to RU 486. Doses can be administered that will induce dramatic changes in endometrial morphology without inducing bleeding or altering gonadotropin, estradiol, and progesterone levels. It is possible that this could have important contraceptive implications.[r4]

Therapeutic Uses

Abortion Induction

When administered to women with amenorrhea of up to seven weeks' duration, RU 486 has been shown to induce abortion in 64 to 85 percent. It failed to induce bleeding in 1 to 10 percent and resulted in incomplete expulsions in 10 to 30 percent.[2,3,6]

The reason why RU 486 is not successful in inducing abortion in 100 percent of women is not known with certainty, and may be related to several factors. It is possible that the drug might not have been administered early enough in pregnancy. Indeed, the ability of RU 486 to induce abortion decreases in more advanced pregnancies.[r4] However, there are well-documented instances of women at the earliest stage of gestation who fail to respond to RU 486. Nonresponsiveness does not appear to be related to dosage, and effectiveness appears similar with total doses ranging from 140 to 700 mg administered over one to seven days.[r4] It is conceivable that genetic mutations in the progesterone receptor could also explain some cases of nonresponsiveness. Indeed, it has been shown that glycine at position 722 in the hormone-binding domain of the human progesterone receptor (i.e., Gly 722) is critical for RU 486 binding. The chicken and hamster progesterone receptor, which possess cysteine at this comparable position in the hormone-binding domains of the progesterone receptor, does not bind RU 486; and substitution of glycine by cysteine at this critical position in the human progesterone receptor results in a receptor that does not bind RU 486.[7] It is also possible that nonresponsiveness to RU 486 could be related to variations in RU 486 metabolism in different women. This phenomenon has indeed been documented with the antiglucocorticoid response to RU 486 in dogs. However, to date, differences in the pharmacokinetics of RU 486 and its metabolites have not been detected in women who respond or those who fail to respond to RU 486.[r4]

Currently, it is believed that the most important factor explaining nonresponsiveness is an inadequate increase in the endogenous production of the prostaglandin PGF2α or in the uterine response to prostaglandins.[8] An increase of endogenous PGF2α production accompanies the onset of labor. It has also been shown that antiprogestins stimulate PGF2α synthesis and inhibit its metabolism. Many studies have shown that administration of prostaglandins by either the IM, vaginal, or oral route after RU 486 results in a markedly improved response. The initial prostaglandin used was sulprostone, a PGE analogue (16-phenoxy-tetranor-PGE_2 methylsufonyl amide) administered IM. Because cardiovascular complications were encountered in a few subjects, sulprostone is now no longer recommended as the prostaglandin of choice, and has been superseded by either gemeprost (16,16-dimethyl-trans-Δ2 PGE, methylester) administered as a vaginal pessary or misoprostol, (cytotec) methyl 11α,16-dihydroxy-16-methyl-9-oxoprost-13-E-en-1-oate], a prostaglandin E_1 analogue, which is administered orally.[9,10] The success rate with RU 486 and misoprostol is similar to that with parenteral or vaginal prostaglandin administration. Over 100,000 women have now received this RU 486 prostaglandin regimen, and the incidence of complete abortion in women with amenorrhea of up to 7 weeks' duration is 95 percent.[9] The usual recommended protocol is a single dose of 600 mg RU 486 followed in 48 hours by administration of a prostaglandin preparation.

Inhibition of Ovulation

Mid-or late-follicular phase RU 486 administration inhibits the LH surge and delays ovulation. Follicular growth is reinitiated after cessation of RU 486 administration; however, intermittent administration of RU 486 repeated at intervals of seven to ten days has been unsuccessful in consistently inhibiting ovulation.[r4] On the other hand, continuous administration of 2 mg to 10 mg daily for one month has resulted in ovulation inhibition with a delay in menstruation. Trials in unprotected women, however, have not been conducted.[r4] As already discussed, disruption of endometrium maturation is the most sensitive effect of RU 486. It is thus conceivable that RU 486 may be administered in a low dose that would permit ovulation and menstruation to continue yet render the endometrium hostile to implantation. Indeed, preliminary results have shown that a single dose of 200 mg RU 486 administered on the second day after the LH surge may well be an effective method of birth control. In a trial of 18 unprotected women treated for over 80 cycles, only one pregnancy resulted.[11] However, a drawback to this approach is that it is necessary to time the onset of the LH surge accurately. Currently this is not practical.

Menses Regulation

Several studies have been conducted in which different doses of RU 486 have been administered at the expected time of bleeding in repeated cycles, independent of whether the woman was pregnant. The aim has been to develop RU 486 as a monthly menses regulator. Results have shown that there is often a delay in onset of menstruation that causes disruption of the menstrual rhythm. In addition, there is often a failure of menstrual bleeding, especially in anovulatory cycles. For these reasons, compliance with this method was poor.[12] Moreover, in the three largest studies conducted in which βhCG levels were determined to document precisely the occurrence of pregnancy, 15 to 20 percent of proved pregnancies were not terminated by RU 486. Thus, at the current state of development, RU 486 cannot be recommended as an agent that will act as a monthly menses regulator.[r4]

Postcoital Contraception

RU 486 has been administered as a single dose of 600 mg within three days of unprotected intercourse. Under these circumstances, it has been shown to be as effective a postcoital method as standard high-dose estrogen-progestin administration. Moreover, RU 486 has significantly fewer of the side-effects (nausea, vomiting, and headache) seen when high-dose estrogen-progestin is used. On the other hand, disturbances in menstrual cycle occur more frequently with RU 486.[13]

Cervical Dilatation

In view of the marked ability of RU 486 to dilate the cervix and induce myometrial contractility, this agent has been found to be useful in the preoperative preparation of women for first or second trimester pregnancy interruption.[14] In France, RU 486 has been approved for therapeutic termination of first and second trimester pregnancies when used in conjunction with prostaglandins.

RU 486 is also very effective for the induction of labor following intrauterine fetal death.[15] Although it has also been used to induce labor at the end of the third trimester, it should be mentioned that RU 486 does cross the feto-placental barrier and that further studies are required to document its safety.[r4]

Other Gynecologic Indications

There has been a small preliminary trial of the use of RU 486 in the treatment of women with endometriosis.[16] There was an improvement in pelvic pain in all subjects, although no change in severity of the disease as determined by follow-up laparoscopy. RU 486 also has been shown to decrease the size of uterine leiomyomata.[17]

Treatment of Tumors

Animal studies have shown that combined treatment with RU 486 and antiestrogens or GNRH agonists may produce remission rates in breast carcinoma. Two preliminary studies have been conducted in women, but further studies are needed to determine whether antiprogesterones might be useful in human breast cancer.[r4]

Since many meningiomas have significant concentrations of progesterone receptors, RU 486 has also been used to treat patients with inoperable meningioma. In one preliminary study, five out of 14 subjects showed objective improvement.[18]

Antiglucocorticoid Applications

RU 486 is also a potent glucocorticoid antagonist, and has been used to treat patients with Cushing's syndrome due to ectopic ACTH secretion or adrenal carcinoma. High-dose RU 486 administration normalized the cushingoid appearance, improved clinical symptoms, and reversed the hypertension and eliminated carbohydrate intolerance in many of these subjects.[r5] In Cushing's disease, where the ACTH-cortisol axis is functional but reset at a higher level, RU 486 is not indicated, since ACTH secretion would be enhanced consequent to the glucocorticoid receptor blockade.

Side-Effects

In an evaluation of 16,173 subjects treated with RU 486 and a prostaglandin, only 11 subjects required a blood transfusion.[9] Excessive uterine bleeding requiring either vacuum aspiration or dilatation and curettage was seen in 0.8 percent of the subjects. The average duration of bleeding was eight days. Most women reported abdominal pain during the first four hours after prostaglandin administration.[9] Other side-effects reported during this time included nausea (33.8%), vomiting (15.3%), and diarrhea (7.5%). These symptoms generally do not necessitate any treatment, and it is often difficult to dissociate many of them from those occurring in normal pregnancy or spontaneous abortion. Thus, severe side-effects consequent to single dose RU 486 administration for abortion induction are rare.

Long-term RU 486 administration in doses of 100 to 200 mg per day are generally well tolerated. However, many subjects complain of fatigue, anorexia, nausea, and vomiting. Other side-effects reported during long-term administration include weight loss, cessation of menses in premenopausal women, hot flashes, transient thinning of the hair, development of Hashimoto's thyroiditis, decrease in libido, and gynecomastia.[18] Administration of high doses to normal males was also associated with the development of a generalized exanthem.[r4] Hypoadrenalism secondary to glucocorticoid antagonism during long-term RU 486 administration has been reported,[r5] but the diagnosis is often difficult to prove. Nevertheless, if the clinical picture does suggest hypoadrenalism, glucocorticoid replacement is indicated.[r4]

RU 486 has not been shown to be teratogenic in rats or monkeys. In rabbits, however, skull deformities were attributed to a mechanical effect of the uterine musculature due to decrease in progesterone activity. The situation is not known in humans, although misoprostol has been shown to be teratogenic.[r4] At this stage of development, if a woman takes RU 486 and prostaglandin and fails to abort, she should be warned about possible teratogenic effects and be offered surgical abortion.

Pharmacokinetics[r6]

RU 486 is administered by the oral route. The pharmacokinetics of RU 486 have been studied in humans, rats, and monkeys. The absorption rate after oral administration in humans is high, and the bioavailability is approximately 70 percent. In humans, serum RU 486 levels reach a maximum between one and four hours after administration of single doses ranging from 50 to 800 mg. Extravascular diffusion is greater in animal species than in humans. Thus the plasma clearance is higher in rats and monkeys than in humans. The half disappearance time in humans with a dose of 100 mg or less is approximately 24 hours. This long disappearance time is due to binding to an α_1 glycoprotein (or orosomucoid) in humans, but not in other species. In view of the protein binding, RU 486 need be administered only once daily.

The major route of excretion in all species is in feces; less than 10 percent of an administered dose is recovered from urine. RU 486 is metabolized by the liver to a mono-demethylated, di-demethylated, as well as an alcoholic derivative. These metabolites bind to both progesterone and glucocorticoid receptors and display antagonistic actions.

Available Preparations and Doses

RU 486 is given orally. Tablets of 50 mg and 200 mg are available. For pregnancy interruption the recommended dose is 600 mg, and a prostaglandin preparation should be given 36–48 hours after RU 486 administration. At the moment, RU 486 and a prostaglandin (gemeprost or misoprostol) is approved for pregnancy interruption in France, Britain, Sweden, and China.

References

Research Reports

1. Wiechert R, Neef G. Synthesis of antiprogestational steroids. J Steroid Biochem 1987;27:851–858.

2. Herrmann W, Wyss R, Riondel A, Philibert D, Teutsch G, Sakiz E, Baulieu EE. Effet d'un steroide antiprogesterone chez la femme: Interruption du cycle menstruel et de la grossesse au debut. CR Acad Sci Paris 1982;*294*:933–938.

3. Baulieu EE. Contragestion and other clinical applications of RU 486, an antiprogesterone at the receptor. Science 1989;*245*:1351–1357.

4. Li TC, Dockery P, Thomas P, Rogers AW, Lenton EA, Cooke ID. The effects of progesterone receptor blockade in the luteal phase of normal fertile women. Fertil Steril 1988;*50*:732–742.

5. Wolf JP, Ulmann A, Hsiu JG, Baulieu EE, Anderson TL, Hodgen GD. Noncompetitive antiestrogenic effect of RU 486 in blocking the estrogen-stimulated luteinizing hormone surge and the proliferative action of estradiol on endometrium in castrate monkeys. Fertil Steril 1989;*52*:1055–1060.

6. Couzinet B, Strat NL, Ulmann A, Baulieu EE, Schaison G. Termination of early pregnancy by the progesterone antagonist, RU 486 (mifepristone). N Engl J Med 1986;*315*:1565–1570.

7. Benhamou B, Garcia T, Lerouge T, Vergezac A, Gofflo D, Bigogne C, Chambon P, Gronemeyer H. A single amino acid that determines the sensitivity of progesterone receptors to RU 486. Science 1992;*255*:206–209.

8. Bygdeman M, Swahn ML. Progesterone receptor blockage. Effect on uterine contractility and early pregnancy. Contraception 1985;*32*:45–51.

9. Ulmann A, Lilvestre L, Chemma L, Rezvani Y, Renault M, Aguillaume CJ, Baulieau EE. Medical termination of early pregnancy with mifeprostone (RU 486) followed by a prostaglandin analogue. Acta Obstet Gynecol Scand 1992;*71*:278–283.

10. Aubeny E, Baulieu EE Contragestion with RU 486 and an orally active prostaglandin. CR Acad Sci Paris 1991;*312*, series III:539–545.

11. Swahn ML, Gemzell K, Bygdeman M. Contraception with mifepristone. Lancet 1991;*338*:942–943.

12. Couzinet B, Strat NL, Silvestre L, Schaison G. Late luteal administration of the antiprogesterone RU486 in normal women: Effects on the menstrual cycle events and fertility control in a long-term study. Fertil Steril 1990;*54*:1039–1044.

13. Glasier A, Thong KJ, Dewar M, Mackie M, Baird DT. Mifepristone (RU 486) compared with high-dose estrogen and progestogen for emergency postcoital contraception. N Engl J Med 1992;*327*:1041–1044.

14. Henshaw RC, Templeton AA. Pre-operative cervical preparation before first trimester vacuum aspiration: a randomized controlled comparison between gemeprost and mifepristone (RU 486). Brit J Obstet Gynaecol 1991;*98*:1025–1030.

15. Cabrol D, Dubois C, Cronje H, Gonnet JM, Guillot M, Maria B, Moodley J, Oury JF, Thoulon JM, Treisser A, Ulmann D, Correl S, Ulmann A. Induction of labor with mifepristone (RU 486) in intrauterine fetal death. Am J Obstet Gynecol 1990;*163*:540–542.

16. Kettel LM, Murphy AA, Mortola JF, Liu JH, Ulmann A, Yen SS. Endocrine responses to long-term administration of the antiprogesterone RU486 in patients with pelvic endometriosis. Fertil Steril 1991;*56*:402–406.

17. Murphy AA, Kettel LM, Morales AJ, Roberts VJ, Yen SSC. Regression of uterine leiomyomata in response to the antiprogesterone RU 486. J Clin Endocrinol Metab 1993;*76*:513–517.

18. Grunberg SM, Weiss MH, Spitz IM, Ahmadi J, Sadun A, Russell CA, Lucci L, Stevenson LL. Treatment of unresectable meningiomas with the antiprogesterone agent mifepristone. J Neurosurg 1991;*74*:861–866.

Reviews

r1. Teutsch G. Analogues of RU 486 for the mapping of the protestin receptor: synthetic and structural aspects. In: EE Baulieu, SJ Segal, eds. The antiprogestin steroid RU 486 and human fertility control. New York: Plenum Press, (1985); pp 27–47.

r2. Philibert D. RU 38486: An original multifaceted antihormone in vivo. In: MK Agarwal (Ed) Adrenal steroid antagonism. Berlin: Walter de Gruyter & Co., (1984); pp 77–101.

r3. Ulmann A, Teutsch G, Philibert D. RU 486. Sci Amer 1990;*262*:42–48.

r4. Spitz IM, Bardin CW. RU 486 A modulator of progestin and glucocorticoid action. N Engl J Med 1993;*329*:404–412.

r5. Chrousos GP, Laue L, Nieman LK, Udelsman R, Kawai S, Loriaux DL. Clinical applications of RU 486, a prototype glucocorticoid and progestin antagonist. In: Mantero F, Takeda R, Scoggins BA, Biglieri EG, Funder JW (eds). The adrenal and hypertension: From cloning to clinic. New York: Raven Press (1989); pp 273–284.

r6. Deraedt R, Bonnat C, Busigny M, Chatelet P, Cousty C, Mouren M, Philibert D, Pottier J, Salmon J. Pharmacokinetics of RU 486. In: Baulieu EE, Segal SJ, (eds). The antiprogestin steroid RU 486 and human fertility control. New York: Plenum Press (1985); pp 103–122.

CHAPTER 53

Wylie W. Vale
Catherine Rivier

Activins and Inhibins

Inhibins and activins were discovered by virtue of their effects on the gonadotropic cells of the anterior pituitary. The existence of inhibin had been proposed over 50 years ago by McCullagh[1] and others[r1] as a water-soluble proteinaceous substance extracted from gonads that could prevent changes that typically occur in rat pituitary after castration. However, the structurally and functionally related protein, activin, was unknown until recently. Although ligands that interact with the activin receptor show promise for the therapeutic regulation of the reproductive, hematopoietic, and central nervous systems, such applications have not yet been developed. The same can be said for inhibins.

Chemistry[r1,2]

Inhibin, which suppresses the production of pituitary follicle stimulating hormone, FSH, was isolated from ovarian fluids by four groups in 1985[r1] and characterized as a heterodimeric glycoprotein of approximately 32 kDaltons comprising an alpha subunit and one of two beta subunits, β_A or β_B. Activins, (molecular weight /26 kDaltons), which stimulate FSH production, were also purified from ovarian fluids, and are composed of two inhibin β subunits. The three subunits combine through disulfide bonds to form the five dimeric inhibins/activins: αβA, inhibin A; αβB, inhibin B; βAβA, activin A; βAβB, activin AB; βBβB, activin B. The α subunits apparently do not form homodimers. The three subunits are derived from the C-terminal region of three precursor proteins encoded by three separate genes. The mature human α subunit is a 132 amino acid protein with 2 potential N-linked glycosylation sites; the βA and βB subunits do not have consensus N-linked glycosylation sites and are 116 and 115 amino acids in length. The α and βB subunits are found on human chromosome 2, and βA has been localized on human chromosome 7. The inhibin subunits are structurally related to the TGF-beta superfamily of growth and differentiation factors.

Anatomic Distribution of Inhibin/Activin Subunits

Inhibin/activin subunits and their mRNAs have been detected in many tissues, including the ovary, testis, placenta, pituitary, CNS, adrenal, and bone marrow[3]. The amounts of subunits vary, as do the proportions of particular subunits. The ovary, for example, has high expression of α subunits and lower amounts of both βA and βB subunits and makes both inhibins and activins. The immature testis has all three subunits, but the adult testis contains mainly α and far lesser amounts of βB. The original concept was that inhibin was produced by the "nurse" cells of the gonads, namely ovarian granulosa cells and testicular Sertoli cells, but inhibin/activin subunits have been detected in a variety of additional gonadal cell types, including theca interna cells, luteal cells, unfertilized oocytes. Leydig cells, and spermatids. The bone marrow has predominantly βA subunits and presumably produces a predominance of activin A. The brain expresses α, βA, βB subunits; the pituitary has α and βB.

Inhibin-Like Activity in Plasma[r2]

Although the mature forms of inhibin and activin are those shown in Figure 53.1, variants of especially the α subunit have been found in gonadal fluids and in plasma. In fact, both the αβ dimers and free α subunits are secreted and have been detected in plasma of humans. Such variants complicate the measurement of inhibins and activins. Assays specific for the α subunit measure both free α (which is biologically inactive to modify FSH secretion) and assays directed toward the β subunit would detect both inhibins and activins. The measurement of biologically active inhibin would be best accomplished with two-site assays that require linked α and β subunits for detection; such assays are

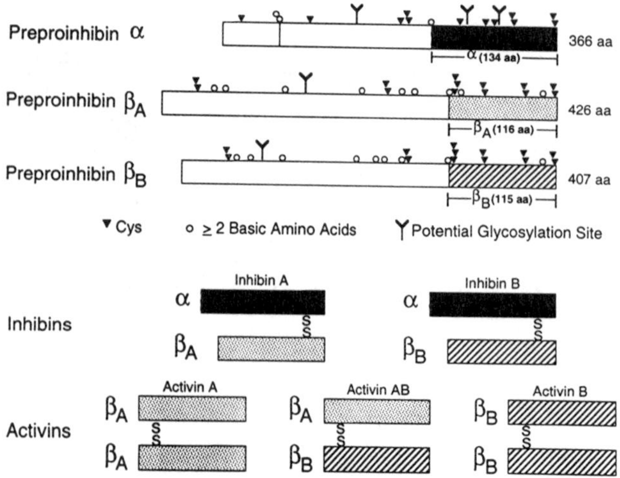

Figure 53.1 Schematic of the precursors of the human inhibin α-, βA-, and βB- subunits. Mature portions of each subunit as they appear in the putative M_r ~32000 inhibin A (αβA) and inhibin B (αβB) are shaded.

currently being validated. Most studies of circulating inhibin have been based on assays that measure the α subunit and are subject to the caveat mentioned above. The measurement of activin and inhibin is also complicated by the binding of activin and inhibin to α_2 macroglobulins and to follistatin, a specific activin binding protein. Nevertheless, it is clear from several lines of evidence, including in vitro studies where the inhibin dimers were monitored, that gonadal inhibin production is stimulated by FSH and modulated by many other hormones and growth factors. In female rats and humans, circulating inhibin α activity comes largely from the ovaries and varies as a function of the cycle, maturation, and pregnancy.

Regulation of Pituitary FSH by Inhibin and Activin

The pituitary gonadotropins, FSH and LH, are secreted by a single cell type, the gonadotrophs, that are controlled by the interaction of neural, local, and peripheral signals. The decapeptide, gonadotropin releasing hormone, GnRH, is secreted by the hypothalamus in a pulsatile manner and stimulates LH and FSH secretion with short latency. Sex steroids and other gonadal signals stimulated by gonadotropins feed back in turn at both the central and pituitary levels to modulate GnRH and/or gonadotropin production. Inhibin is a slow-acting but powerful inhibitor of pituitary FSH biosynthesis and secretion by the anterior pituitary. Under most circumstances, inhibin does not modify LH secretion. Studies with neutralizing antibodies indicate that in the female rat and immature male rat inhibin of gonadal origin exerts a tonic inhibitory effect on FSH production and may play the biologic role of limiting litter size. Activin B is produced locally by pituitary gonadotrophs themselves and provides an important autocrine stimulus for FSH biosynthesis and production (Fig. 53.2). It is possible that much, if not all, of the effects of inhibin depend on its ability to interfere with the actions of activin. Activin, under some experimental circumstances, can suppress the biosynthesis and secretion of corticotropin and growth hormone.

Activin and Inhibin Act Locally Within the Gonads and Placenta

In addition to a possible hormonal role for gonadal inhibin, both inhibin and activin have important local functions within the gonads to modulate steroidogenesis and gametogenesis. Likewise, locally produced inhibin and activin exert inhibitory or stimulatory effects, respectively, on the secretion of progesterone and human chorionic gonadotropin by the human placenta.

Effects of Activin on the Central Nervous System

Inhibin/activin subunits and their mRNAs are expressed in all major regions of the brain and have been identified in specific nuclei and fiber pathways. The best described system is a group of activin-positive cell bodies found in the nucleus tractus solitarius of the caudal brainstem and projecting to several hypothalamic areas including the oxytocin-positive cells in the magnocellular zone of the paraventricular and supraoptic regions. The injection of activin into the hypothalamus has been shown to stimulate oxytocin secretion; consistently, immunoneutralization of activin blocks sucking-induced oxytocin secretion. It is likely, therefore, that this activinergic pathway is a crucial component of the neuroendocrine reflex arc controlling milk letdown and perhaps parturition. Activin fibers are

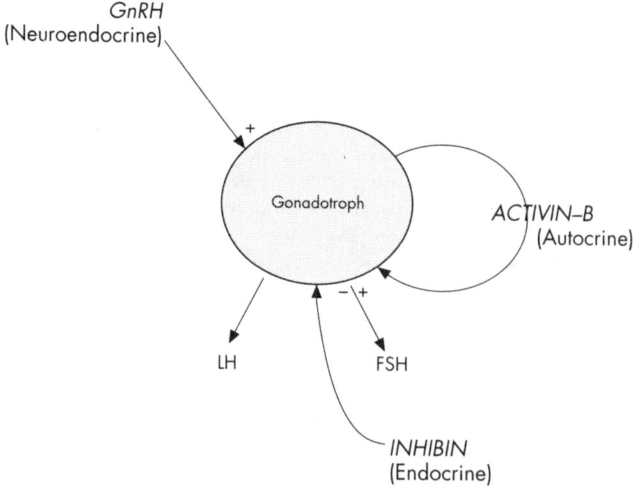

Figure 53.2 Neuroendocrine, Endocrine, and Autocrine Regulation of FSH Production by Anterior Pituitary Gonadotroph

also localized in the vicinity of GnRH positive cells in the preoptic region and of corticotropin releasing factor (CRF)-containing cells in the parvocellular hypothalamus. Initial studies have suggested that activin might stimulate the neurosecretion of both GnRH and CRF. In some neuronal cultures and cell lines, activin can replace other factors such as retinoic acid and promote survival and the development of the neuronal phenotype.

Activin Stimulates Erythropoiesis

The mRNA for activin A has been detected in the bone marrow and subsequently the protein was isolated from a leukemic cell line and from bone where it may contribute to the regulation of erythropoiesis and bone formation. Activin synergizes with erythropoietin to promote commitment of pleuripotent stem cells to the erythroid lineage and subsequently to stimulate proliferation of erythroid progenitors. In the latter stages, activin acts independently of erythropoietin to induce erythroid differentiation as measured by hemaglobin production and inhibits proliferation. All of these hematopoietic activities of activin are antagonized by inhibin.

Activin and Embryogenesis[4,5]

Activin subunits have been detected during all stages of amphibian and mammalian embryogenesis, including in sperm and unfertilized and fertilized oocytes. In latter stages, activin and inhibin subunits are associated with specific organs, including the brain, skin, and gonads. Most attention lately has been focused on the role of activin in the early development of the frog, where activin has been found to be a powerful inducer of mesodermal organs and may work in concert with at least one other candidate growth factor to initiate organogenesis.

Activin Receptor[6,7]

The initial step in the action of activin is its binding to plasma membrane receptors. Activin binds with high affinity to at least two classes of membrane proteins of molecular weights of ~50 kDa and ~70 kDa, referred to as the Type I and Type II receptors in keeping with the terminology developed for the TGF-β receptors. Recently, two distinct but closely related Type II activin receptors have been cloned, IIA and IIB, which were proposed to be transmembrane kinases with serine/threonine specificity. Subsequently, the Type II TGF-β receptor was also cloned and found to be a transmembrane serine/threonine kinase related to the known activin receptors. The Type II activin/TGF-β receptors are the first vertebrate transmembrane serine/threonine kinases; by contrast, many other growth factor receptors have been found to be tyrosine kinases. The activin receptor phosphorylates both itself and probably other proteins as part of its transduction mechanism, however, the heterologous targets are unknown at this time. Experiments have suggested that the intracellular signaling pathways mediating the effects of activin might involve $p21^{ras}$ and an interaction with the tissue-specific POU homeodomain transcription factors. The activin receptors are broadly distributed in adult and developing animals. Overexpression of the receptors increases cellular sensitivity to activin and can markedly alter activin-dependent processes such as development.

Receptor for Inhibin

Some but not all effects of activin can be reversed by inhibin. Inhibin can compete for the binding of activin with activin receptors but with much lower affinity, in contrast to the much higher potency of inhibin relative to activin in bioassays that respond to both substances. These indications that inhibin does not act, at least solely, through the activin receptor have led to investigation of the possibility that inhibin acts through a distinct receptor; as yet, however, no definitive conclusion has been reached.

References

Research Reports

1. McCullagh D. Dual endocrine activity of the testis, Science 1932;*76*:19–20.
2. Mason AS, Hayflick VS, Ling N, Esch F, Veno N, Ying SY, Guillemin B, Niall H, Seeburo PH. Complementary DNA sequences of ovarian follicular fluid inhibin show precursor structure and homology with transforming growth factor-beta. 1985; Nature 318:659–663.
3. DePaolo LV, Bicsak TA, Erickson GF, Shimasaki S, Ling N. Follistatin and activin: A potential intrinsic regulatory system within diverse tissues. Proc Soc Exper Biol Med 1991;*198*:500–512.
4. Jessell TM, Melton DA. Diffusible factors in vertebrate embryonic induction. Cell 1992;*68*:257–270.
5. Mathews LS, Vale WW, Kintner CR. Cloning of a second type of activin receptor and functional characterization in *Xenopus* embryos. Science 1992;*255*:1702–1705.
6. Mathews LS, Vale WW. Expression cloning of an activin receptor, a predicted transmembrane serine kinase. Cell 1991;*65*:973–982.
7. Robertson DM. Follistatin/activin-binding protein. Trends Endocrinol Metab 1992;*3*:65–68.

Reviews

r1. Vale W, Hsueh A, Rivier C, Yu J. The inhibin/activin family of growth factors. In Sporn MA, Roberts AB. Peptide growth factors and their receptors. Handbook of experimental pharmacology. Heidelberg: Springer-Verlag, (1990); 95/II, 211–248.

r2. Burger, HG. Clinical utility of inhibin measurements. J Clin Endocrinol Metab 1993;*76*:1391–1396.

CHAPTER 54

Gonadotropin-Releasing Hormone (GnRH), GnRH Superagonists, and GnRH Antagonists

Cyril Y. Bowers
Karl Folkers

The hypothalamic, hypophysiotropic hormone decapeptide, pGluHisTrpSerTyrGlyLeuArgProGlyNH$_2$, gonadotropin–releasing hormone (GnRH), releases both LH and FSH from the pituitary in varying ratios depending on conditions. It is also known as luteinizing hormone-releasing hormone (LHRH). McCann et al[1] have persuasively marshalled evidence for a separate FSH-releasing hormone produced by the hypothalamus, but chemical isolation of such a hormone has proved elusive and has not yet been accomplished.

GnRH is utilized diagnostically to assess pituitary gonadotropin function directly and gonadal function indirectly. Therapeutically, it is utilized primarily to regulate and/or enhance fertility.

Surprisingly, the primary therapeutic use of GnRH superagonists, which are 50 to 200 times more potent than GnRH, is to inhibit the function of the pituitary-gonadal axis and, thus, to produce a state of functional castration. GnRH antagonists also can induce a state of functional castration but, as will be discussed, GnRH superagonists and GnRH antagonists produce this effect by different molecular mechanisms. Another important difference between the superagonists and antagonists is that the inhibitory effect of the superagonists is delayed over a two- to three-week period, during which time release of LH, FSH, and the gonadal steroids is stimulated, while the inhibitory effect of the antagonists is relatively immediate, i.e., within hours. The increased testosterone and estradiol secretion induced during the first two to three weeks of GnRH superagonist therapy may produce an adverse clinical effect designated as "disease flare."

From the broadest viewpoint the GnRH agonists and antagonists should, in principle, allow detailed investigation, regulation, and/or treatment of any bodily function or pathologic process that is sex steroid hormone-dependent. This includes a variety of hormone-dependent processes such as precocious puberty, endometriosis, uterine fibroids, advanced metastatic breast and prostate cancer. They should potentially be useful as new types of contraceptive agents. Even though the effects of GnRH, the superagonists, and antagonists are relatively straightforward, simple, and direct, the disorders in which they will be utilized are complicated. Thus, an in-depth understanding as well as careful consideration of alternative therapies is required.

Chemistry

GnRH Analogue Superagonists

The GnRH superagonists of similar potency and long duration of action that have been utilized clinically are recorded in Table 54.1.

The amino acid residue(s) or the chemical functional group(s) of GnRH responsible for triggering the biologic response is still unknown. The fact that modification of Trp^3 of GnRH results in complete loss of activity while substitution of ornithine for Arg^8 of GnRH reduces agonist potency but nevertheless still has biologic activity indicates that the N-terminal amino acids are more critical than the C-terminal amino acids of GnRH for activation of the receptor. Additionally, avian and teleost GnRH molecules with conserved N-terminal amino acids of mammalian GnRH but different C-terminal amino acids have low but full biologic LH-releasing activity across species. Thus, the N-terminal part of the GnRH molecule again appears to be conserved for activation of the receptor while

Table 54.1 GnRH—Superagonists

	Sequence										Potency
	1	2	3	4	5	6	7	8	9	10	
GnRH	pGlu -	His -	Trp -	Ser -	Tyr -	Gly -	Leu -	Arg -	Pro -	$GlyNH_2$	1
Goserelin						D-Ser-(Bu)				Az-$GlyNH_2$	50–100
Leuprolide[b]						D-Leu				Ethylamide	50–100
Buserelin**						D-Ser				Ethylamide	50–100
Nafarelin[c]						D-3(2-Naphthyl)Ala					50–100
Trptorelin						D-Trp					50–100
Histrelin***[d]						D-His				Ethylamide	50–100

*Leuprolide = [desGlyNH_2^{10}, DLeu^6, Proethylamide^9]-GnRH
**Buserelin = [desGlyNH_2^{10}, Proethylamide^9]-GnRH
***Histrelin = [desGlyNH_2^{10}, TyrN'Benzyl^5, Proethylamide^9]-GnRH

the C-terminal part of the molecule is related to binding and appears to be responsible for species specificity.

It is amazing that such simple changes in the primary structure of GnRH at the achiral Gly^6 residue of GnRH convert this molecule into a long-acting, clinically valuable superagonist. Except for the C-terminal glyamide^{10}, none of the currently developed GnRH superagonists have modifications at sites other than position 6, indicating the rigid requirements for LH- and FSH-releasing activity in the remaining parts of the molecule. At position 10, the glyamide C-terminus has been replaced with the alkyl amine, ethylamide (NEt), i.e., desGly^{10}-GnRH Pro^9-NEt in some but not all current GnRH superagonists.

GnRH Analogue Antagonists

Some of the currently known potent and clinically directed GnRH antagonists are presented in Table 54.2.

Potent competitive receptor GnRH antagonists should bind to the GnRH pituitary receptor with high affinity without triggering a biological response and, thus, prevent endogenous GnRH from binding and activating the receptor. The amino acid residues most likely to be involved in receptor interactions as well as the type of interaction between the side chains of these amino acids and the receptor are His^2 (charge-transfer, ionic, aromatic stacking), Trp^3 (aromatic stacking, charge transfer, hydrogen bonding), and Arg^8 (ionic and hydrogen bonding). New GnRH antagonists have been designed based on consideration of the above types of interactions between the receptor and the antagonist, particularly at positions 1, 2, 3, 5, 6, 8, and 10. A recent summary by Janecka et al[r2] on the GnRH structure-activity relationships of these analogues describes 395 GnRH antagonist analogues we designed, synthesized, and studied over the past six years.

History

McCann et al, in 1960, were the first to publish evidence that injection of extracts of hypothalami released LH from the pituitary.[1] Subsequently, Nikitovich-Winer[2] induced ovulation in rats by direct intrapituitary infusion of median eminence extracts and G.W. Harris and coworkers reported similar results in rabbits.[3]

In 1971, the monumental accomplishment of isolation and structure determination of the decapeptide, GnRH (or LHRH) was achieved first by Schally's group[4] (from porcine hypothalami) and shortly thereafter by Guillemin's group[5] (from ovine hypothalami).

Within the next few years the first GnRH agonist and antagonist analogues were synthesized.[6,7] The chemical changes required for a desirably long duration of action were much simpler to establish for the agonists than for the antagonists.[8]

Current potent GnRH analogue antagonists[6,8] are greatly altered in structure, with as many as 7 of the 10 amino acid residues of GnRH being substituted with amino acids that have novel side chains and/or D-amino acid residues. A common favorable change for both potent agonist and antagonist activity has been D-amino acid substitutions at position 6.

The most precise and widely used method to monitor the activity of the agonist/antagonist analogues in vitro has been the dispersed pituitary cell culture method of Vale et al,[9] while an in vivo assay utilizes release of LH and FSH by the agonist or inhibition of the LH/FSH response to GnRH or a superagonist by the antagonist in 26 day-old immature female/male rats. Other methods utilized to determine potency are the pituitary incubate and GnRH radioreceptor in vitro assays as well as several different in vivo assays, i.e., prevention or interruption of pregnancy, disruption of the estrus cycle, inhibition of elevated serum levels of LH and FSH in the castrated rat, and inhibition of ovulation in the spontaneous cycling female rat.

Mechanisms of Action

GnRH is released in a pulsatile manner at different frequencies from the hypothalamus into the hypophyseal portal system in order to regulate the release and synthesis of LH and FSH for the purpose of initiating and maintaining the reproductive cycle in animals and humans.[r3] After GnRH binds to a seven transmembrane-spanning, guanine nucleotide-binding protein-coupled receptor on the peripheral membrane of the

Table 54.2 GnRH-Antagonists

AcDNal-DCpa-DPal-Ser-[ ]^5 - [ ]^6-Leu-[ ]^8-Pro-DAla-NH_2

Common Name	Position 5	6	8	Organization/Status
Nal-Arg[1]	Tyr	DArg	Arg	Salk/Withdrawn
Nal-Glu	Arg	DGlu(AA)	Arg	Salk/Phase II
SB-75	Tyr	DCit	Arg	Asta/Phase II
Ganirelix	Tyr	DhArg(Et_2)	hArg(Et_2)	Syntex/Phase II
A-75998	N-Me-Tyr	DLys(Nic)	Lys(Ipr)	Abbott/Phase I
Azaline B	Aph(Atz)	DAph(Atz)	Lys(Ipr)	Ortho/Phase I
Antide	Lys(Nic)	DLys(Nic)	Lys(Ipr)	Serono/Phase I
HOEO13[2]	Tyr	DSer(Rha)	Arg	Hoechst/Phase I

1 DFpa^2, DTrp^3,Gly^{10}
2 DTrp^3, AzaGly^{10}

DGlu(AA) = D-2-amino-5-oxo-5-(4-methoxyphenyl)pentanoic acid
DCit = citrulline
DhArg(Et_2) = N^g, $N^{g'}$-diethylhomoarginine
DLys(Nic) = N^ϵnicotinoyllysine
Aph(atz) = 4-(3′amino-1H-1,2′,4′-triazol-5′-yl)phenylalanine
Lys(Ipr) = N^ϵ = isopropyllysine
DSer(Rha) = L-rhamnose

pituitary gonadotrophs, several phospholipases (PL-C,D,A) are activated that produce water-soluble and insoluble factors that mediate the actions of GnRH.[10] PL-C generates inositol 1,4,5 triphosphate, which raises cytoplasmic free calcium levels and also generates diacylglycerol, which activates protein kinase C. Both the extracellular influx and intracellular mobilization of calcium play a role in the exocytotic release of LH and FSH.[r4,r5] PL-D appears to be sequentially activated by protein kinase-C, and it elevates phosphotidylethanol and phosphotidic acid intracellular levels. PL-A generates arachidonic acid, which in turn results in the formation of lipoxygenase metabolites such as the leukotrienes and 5-and 15-eicosatetraenoic acids. Thus, at least three different families of second messengers, Ca^{2+}, protein kinase-C, and arachidonate metabolites mediate the actions of GnRH. Gonadotropin gene expression has been increased by GnRH. This includes rapid increases in the gonadotropin subunit LHβ and FSHβ mRNA, possibly in part due to the effects of Ca^{2+} and protein kinase-C.

Several molecular mechanisms also are involved in the homologous desensitization or down-regulation of the GnRH effect on gonadotropin release.[11,12] These include a decrease of the GnRH receptor number, loss of the functional GnRH receptor-linked calcium ion channels and, more recently, revealed loss of ability to transfer gonadotropin from a non-releasable to a releasable pool. Also, probably applicable to the mechanisms involved in the GnRH receptor homologous desensitization, are the results of desensitization studies of the beta-adrenergic receptors because both of these receptors belong to the same superfamily of peripheral membrane receptors that consist of seven transmembrane-spanning helices. A combination of pharmacologic, biochemical, and genetic approaches has revealed molecular mechanisms involved in the latter desensitization. These have been found to involve receptor phosphorylation, sequestration, and down-regulation that last from seconds to minutes, minutes to hours, or hours, respectively.[12]

In contrast to the mechanism of action of the GnRH superagonists, down-regulation and desensitization of the receptor, that of the GnRH antagonists is much simpler. The latter act by binding specifically to the GnRH pituitary receptor with high affinity without triggering a biologic response, and thus the antagonists prevent endogenous GnRH binding to its own receptor.

It is by no means certain that GnRH, GnRH superagonists, and GnRH antagonists exert all their biologic effects only by way of stimulating or inhibiting gonadotropin secretion from the pituitary. Evidence is accumulating to support the presence of GnRH, the GnRH receptor, and extrapituitary biologic effects in both normal (ovary, testis, placenta, T-lymphocytes, CNS) and abnormal tissue (breast and prostate cancer) of humans. Some results indicate a possible paracrine, autocrine effect of GnRH and that GnRH analogues, both superagonist and antagonist, may produce some unexpected extrapituitary actions under both physiologic and pathologic conditions.

Pharmacokinetics

Pharmacokinetic human data recorded in Table 54.3 indicate that GnRH superagonists are more potent than GnRH in part because of a longer plasma half-life and a considerably smaller plasma clearance-rate.[r6,r7] In addition, the pharmacokinetic data for the GnRH antagonist, Detirelix, recorded in Table 54.3, very possibly reflect the pharmacokinetics of other antagonists because of a number of similar chemical properties with other antagonists, i.e., more "protected" peptide, increased hydrophobicity. Several GnRH antagonists have been demonstrated to be highly stable even when incubated in vitro with the nonspecific, broad-spectrum enzymes, pronase and subtilisin. The prolonged plasma half-life and low plasma clearance rate both help to explain the longer duration of action of the antagonists. In general, the results indicate how valuable these parameters can be for better understanding the actions of these peptides. These factors also might help to assess the differences between the various peptides and how they might be utilized most effectively.

Clinical Applications[13,14,r10]

Current and potential clinical uses of GnRH and of GnRH superagonists in various stages of clinical development are presented in Table 54.4 The biologic effectiveness of the GnRH peptides is independent of age and gender, and their effects may be induced either acutely or chronically. Key clinical advantages of the GnRH analogues, include high potency, long action, rapid onset, selectivity, and reversibility.

Clinical Uses of GnRH Itself

Low-dose pulsatile administration of the short-acting GnRH elicits a more physiologic pituitary and gonadal pattern of secretion, while with a two- to three-week period of frequent administration or high doses of GnRH (or similarly with a long-acting superagonist), gonadotropin and gonadal steroid secretion are markedly inhibited.

Table 54.4 Clinical Uses of GnRH and/or GnRH Superagonists

Clinical Uses of GnRH
- For diagnosis
- For treatment of idiopathic hypothalamic hypogonadism (IHH)
- For induction of ovulation
- For treatment of cryptorchidism

Clinical Uses of GnRH Superagonists
- For treatment of:
  - Cryptorchidism
  - IHH
  - Precocious puberty
  - Cancer of the prostate and of the breast
  - Benign prostatic hypertrophy
  - Endometriosis
  - Uterine fibroids

For Diagnosis

Determination of the LH and FSH responses to GnRH (usually 100 μg IV) is an established diagnostic procedure.[15,16] GnRH is utilized for grading the stages of centrally originating precocious puberty, for monitoring pituitary desensitization during chronic inhibitory therapy with an GnRH superagonist, and for determination of pituitary LH/FSH secretory reserve. The GnRH diagnostic test also has helped detect gonadotropin-secreting pituitary tumors.

For Idiopathic Hypothalamic Hypogonadism (IHH)[17]

A "physiologic" regimen for men with IHH would be administration of GnRH in very small amounts, i.e.,

Table 54.3 Plasma Pharmacokinetic Data Obtained in Normal Human Subjects

Peptide	Dose mg	Dose Route	$T_{1/2}$ (hr)	V_d (1)	Plasma Clearance (ml/min)
Leuprolide	1.0	IV	2.9±0.5	26.5±10.1	139±30
Leuprolide	1.0	SQ	3.6±1.2	37.1±16.8	151±43
Nafarelin	2.0	SQ	4.3±0.3	34.8±7.3	97±23
GnRH	*	IV	≈.33	≈12.0	≈1.4 (1)
Detirelix[1]	10.0	SQ	47.6±15.3		65.0±14.7

[1]= [N-acetylDpClPhe[1,2],DTrp[3],DLys[6], DAla[10]]GnRH (antagonist)
*Multiple Doses

24 ng/kg SQ every two hours over several months with a portable programmable pump in order to simulate the endogenous GnRH pulsatile secretory pattern from the hypothalamus. This approach, which has been studied in depth and established so elegantly by Crowley and coworkers,[17,r8] has resulted in near-normal episodic serum LH pulse patterns, normal serum FSH and testosterone levels and, in addition, has produced secondary sex characteristics, sexual behavior, spermatogenesis, and fertility. Usually, GnRH administered SQ at 10 ng/kg every two hours and/or 25 ng/kg administered hourly or at four-hour intervals is less effective than 25 ng/kg SQ every two hours. Patient variation is a factor because some patients required 50 to 200 ng/kg of GnRH every two hours. A problem for some patients is that GnRH administered SQ may be less effective because of local degradation at the injection site. Another consideration is the relative inability to deliver a short, sharp GnRH pulse by SQ administration that closely simulates the size and shape of the secretory pulses of endogenous GnRH released from the hypothalamus.[15]

The pattern of the GnRH secretory pulses is well established as the regulator of both the amplitude and frequency of LH secretion and as an important determinant of the LH/FSH ratio. Gonadal steroids not only govern the amplitude/frequency of the pulsatile secretion of GnRH from the hypothalamus but together with inhibin modulate the GnRH effect on the pituitary.

Induction of Ovulation

Induction of ovulation by pulsatile GnRH therapy in patients suspected of hypothalamic suppression has been well documented.[23-26] The principles for administration of GnRH for this purpose are the same as for IHH patients. It must be appreciated that the endogenous secretory pattern varies in frequency and amplitude at different stages of the menstrual cycle.[27,r10] For example, after ovulation has been induced, hormonal support during the luteal phase of the cycle should be provided and administration of the GnRH should be less frequent.

For Cryptorchidism[28]

GnRH or GnRH superagonists, especially administered intranasally (1–3% absorbed), have been as effective as HCG therapy for cryptorchidism, and androgenic effects with the GnRH peptides appear to have been less than with HCG. In order to stimulate LH release and prevent pituitary desensitization, the optimal regimen requires individualization. Successful regimens are more than 30 percent effective within four weeks.

Clinical Uses of GnRH Superagonists[29,30,r9]

For Cryptorchidism

See above under Clinical Uses of GnRH.

IHH

The superagonists were investigated for the treatment of IHH but the results were poor and currently they are not being used for this purpose. A tentative explanation by Crowley et al of the poor results was that the testis, like the pituitary, may respond better to episodic rather than to continuous trophic stimulation. Because of the long duration of action of the GnRH superagonists, LH and FSH secretion was also prolonged resulting in continuous stimulation of the gonads.

For Precocious Puberty

GnRH superagonists are drugs of choice for treatment of centrally stimulated precocious puberty.[r11] In fact, if puberty cannot be reversed by superagonist therapy it would be strong evidence of a pseudopuberty state mediated via a non-GnRH mechanism. The very favorable results with GnRH superagonists during and after prolonged chronic administration to children with precocious puberty validates the effectiveness of the treatment, its low toxicity, and the reversibility of the "medical castration" effect.

Administration of GnRH superagonists monthly with delayed release preparations has been particularly advantageous in children with precocious puberty who previously received the superagonist nasally (2–4 times/day) or SQ daily (1–2 times/day). Plasma estradiol, testosterone, and FSH decreased within three weeks. Breasts, uterus, ovaries, testes, growth velocity, and bone maturation all decreased within six months.[31] Evidence supported the reversibility of the endocrine effect even after two to four years of suppression. Still to be determined is the eventual gonadal germ cell and reproductive function once the therapy is stopped.

For Cancer of the Prostate and of the Breast[r12]

The GnRH superagonist leuprolide (Lupron) has been approved by the FDA for treatment of patients with prostate cancer.

GnRH superagonists are administered SQ or IM daily as well as nasally three to four times per day or as a slow-release IM depot preparation in order to inhibit the pituitary-gonadal axis. Formulations of the peptide dispersed in a biodegradable lactide-glycolide copolymer are administered monthly or even less frequently. GnRH superagonists rather than GnRH are utilized to inhibit function of the pituitary-gonadal axis. Superagonist therapy can lower serum testosterone[r13] and estradiol levels equivalent to surgical castration,[32] provided special consideration is given to frequency of administration, dosage, formulation, and route of administration. Measurements of immuno- and bioactive LH and FSH, estradiol, progesterone, and testosterone serum levels are used to assess changes in hormonal secretion. Measurement of the steroid responses shortly after rather than 24 hours after administration of a superagonist may be a more sensitive index for assessing small but significant rises and a more critical assessment of the degree of down-regulation.

A partial castration effect occurs more often after intranasal administration than after IM depot administration of the GnRH superagonist, but both are dose- and frequency-dependent.

Monthly injection of the superagonist, Zoldex (3.6 mg = 125 µg/day), in a slow-release depot formulation was equally as effective as orchidectomy in prostate cancer patients with bone and soft tissue metasteses. Serum testosterone was reduced below castrate levels (<2nmol/L) by 15 days and was maintained at this level for at least one year.

Combination therapy of a superagonist with a testosterone- or estradiol-blocking agent[34] has been advocated to prevent the effect of testosterone or estradiol that may arise from the adrenal or from adrenal steroid precursors. Noteworthy has been the combination of flutamide and, more recently, nilutamide with GnRH superagonists for prostate cancer.[35] Randomized double-blind trials supported the conclusion that flutamide plus leuprolide had a small but significant effect on over-all survival (35.6 vs 28.3 months increase in the median length of survival), and buserelin plus nilutamide prevented the clinical adverse effects ("disease flare") of the GnRH superagonist[33] that may occur because of the buserelin-induced transient rise in plasma testosterone levels in men with advanced prostate cancer.[36]

The completeness of ablation of estradiol and testosterone secretion and/or inhibition of the effects of these steroids at the receptor level arise as basic pathophysiologic and therapeutic issues in the utilization of the GnRH superagonists for patients with advanced prostate and breast cancer.

Benign Prostate Hypertrophy

Leuprolide (1 mg SQ daily) and nafarelin (0.4 mg SQ daily) have decreased prostate size in patients with benign prostate hypertrophy. Obstructive urinary symptoms may decrease within one month. Maximal decrease in prostate size (mainly epithelial) occurs within about six months of starting therapy and regrowth of the prostate to the initial size usually occurs about six months after stopping the superagonist. So far the main indication has been for poor surgical risk patients. Because of the major effect of the superagonist on the epithelium of a hyperplastic prostate and because of the cell morphologic heterogeneity of benign prostatic hypertrophy, i.e., stromal, muscular, fibromuscular, fibroadenoma, or fibromyoadenoma, the effects of the therapy will vary from patient to patient. In addition, three months' treatment with Zoldex may not completely abolish intraprostatic androgen concentration. Intraprostatic testosterone decreased to about 25 percent while dihydrotestosterone and 5 alpha-androstane 3 alpha, 17 beta diol decreased to about 10 percent of the values in untreated men. Prostate alpha reductase and androgen nuclear receptors also decreased.

Endometriosis

The favorable results of GnRH superagonist therapy for endometriosis (similar to effects of ovariectomy or the menopause) strongly supports the estrogen dependency of the disorder. Nearly one in 15 women of reproductive age have been benefited, emphasizing the important potential for a nonsurgical approach. Nafarelin (400–800 µg/day) administered for endometriosis for six months by nasal spray twice daily was just as effective in a multicentered double-blind comparative clinical trial as an established therapeutic agent, the 17-ethyl testosterone derivative, danazol.[37,38] Laparoscopy demonstrated 80 percent of the patients were improved. Symptoms of pelvic pain decreased rapidly and markedly (often within a month). The pregnancy rate after treatment was 39 percent. Bone loss from the spine was demonstrable in about 66 percent of the patients.[39] In other nafarelin studies in women, bone loss appeared reversible six months after stopping nafarelin. Consistently, amenorrhea and menopausal symptoms were induced but usually were well tolerated.

Uterine Fibroids

Rapid partial regression of uterine fibroids occurs within one month of starting superagonist therapy and will plateau after about three months of therapy. These benefits are rapidly reversed on stopping therapy, thus indicating that at present this approach usually is limited to patients in whom surgery is contraindicated or to perimenopausal patients. Superagonist therapy prior to surgery may decrease blood loss during surgery or facilitate removal of the fibroid because of the smaller size of the fibroid.[40,41] Superagonists in combination with other therapies will be a major future research objective.[33]

Clinical Use of GnRH Antagonists

Thus far, clinical use of GnRH antagonists has been quite limited. For one thing, GnRH and GnRH superagonists have been so successful for those conditions for which the antagonists might be considered that an antagonist has not been needed. In addition, the antagonists thus far developed have had undesirable side-effects. There has been difficulty in maintaining a good balance between high potency, long duration of action, and desirable physical chemical characteristics, including good solubility, lack of gel formation in normal saline, and low histamine-releasing activity along with ease and reasonable cost of synthesis. The histamine-releasing activities of Nal-Arg, Nal-Glu, and SB-75, for example, are high. Ganirelix and A-75998 also have relatively high histamine-releasing activity. Both Azaline B and Antide have low histamine-releasing activities, but a problem with Antide is that it forms a gel in normal saline solution; although to a lesser degree, so does Azaline B. A-75998 is more soluble in normal saline, but its potency is relatively low. It may be that an antagonist with a better combination of properties and higher potency will be developed in the future.

Antagonist as Male Contraceptive

Three weeks' administration of the NalGlu antagonist decreased spermatogenesis in normal younger men. In principle, this suggests that an GnRH antagonist might be useful as a male contraceptive agent.

Table 54.5 Available Preparations for Clinical Use in the U.S.

Preparation	Dose
Lutrepulse = gonadorelin acetate	1–20 µg every 90 min/ day via IV pump 50–200 µg IV
Lupron = leuprolide acetate	3.75 mg IM monthly 0.3 mg/kg IM monthly 7.5 mg IM monthly
Synarel = nafarelin acetate	200 µg bid intranasally
Supprelin = histrelin acetate	10 µg/kg/day SQ
Zoladex = goserelin acetate implant	= 3.6 mg goserelin

Adverse Effects

Most of the adverse effects of GnRH superagonists are related to steroid deficiency.

When 200 and 400 µg nafarelin was administered intranasally twice daily for six months to 25 premenopausal women with endometriosis (mean age ≈ 33 years) serum estrone and estradiol reached postmenopausal levels in three months at the 400-µg dosage and in six months at the 200-µg dosage. In two months all of these women had amenorrhea. Biochemical estimates of bone resorption (serum phosphorus, hydroxyproline/creatinine, or calcium/creatinine fasting urinary ratios) and bone formation (plasma Gla protein and serum alkaline phosphatase) were increased after three to six months of therapy in both treatment groups, indicating increased bone turnover. These parameters returned to normal three to six months after stopping nafarelin. Single/dual photon absorptiometry with a ^{153}Gd source demonstrated a 2 to six percent decrease in bone mineral content of the trabecular bone of the wrist and lumbar spine after six months of therapy with 400 µg nafarelin, which returned to pretreatment levels six months after stopping the agonist. Metacarpal cortical bone was not changed. No bone demineralization was demonstrated at the 200 µg dose.

Serum antibodies have very occasionally been reported for GnRH, but not for the GnRH superagonists. Ovarian hyperstimulation and multiple pregnancies have been reported, but usually may be avoided with low-dose GnRH therapy. This is more likely to occur in patients with polycystic ovarian syndrome than in patients with hypothalamic amenorrhea.

Women with endometriosis who were treated for six months intranasally with 400 µg nafarelin also experienced postmenopausal symptoms of hypoestrogenism. This included hot flashes (90%) emotional lability (30%), headaches (34%), vaginal dryness (25%), reduction of breast size (18%), and weight gain (20%). Rhinitis occurred in ≈ 12 percent of the patients. There was no change in the serum atherogenic index.

Seventy-six per cent of men treated with DTrp^6 GnRH for prostate cancer experienced vasomotor flushing and about 80 percent experienced decreased libido or erectile dysfunction. After six months of therapy there was less fatigue, anger, depression, and anxiety. Energy and cheerfulness were increased.

Two approaches have been proposed to prevent the possible adverse clinical effects that may occur from the increased secretion of LH-testosterone during the first two to three weeks after starting superagonist therapy that is designed for its eventual down-regulation effect. The superagonist has been administered with diethylstilbesterol to inhibit the stimulated release of gonadotropin or the superagonist has been administered with flutamide, nilutamide, or cyproterone acetate in order to inhibit the effect of testosterone on its peripheral receptors.

Preparations

Available preparations and dosages of GnRH (gonadorelin) and of GnRH superagonists (leuprolide, nafarelin, histrelin, and goserelin) are listed in Table 54.5.

References

Research Reports

1. McCann SM, Taleisnik S, Friedman U-M. LH-releasing activity in hypothalamic extracts. Proc Soc Exp Biol Med 1960;*104*:432–434.
2. Nikitovich-Winer MB. Induction of ovulation in rats by direct intrapituitary infusion of median eminence extracts. Endocrinology 1962;*70*:350–358.
3. Campbell HJ, Feuer G, Harris GW. The effects of intrapituitary infusion of median eminence and other brain extracts on anterior pituitary gonadotrophin secretion. J Physiol (London) 1964;*170*:474–486.
4. Matsuo H, Balea Y, Nair RM, Arimura A, Schally AV. Structure of the porcine LH- and FSH-releasing hormone. I. The proposed amino acid sequence. Biochem. Biophys. Res. Commun 1971;*43*:1334–1339.
5. Burgus R, Butcher M, Amoss M, Ling N, Monahan MW, Rivier J, Fellos R, Blackwell R, Vale W, Guillemin R. Primary structure of the ovine hypothalamic luteinizing hormone releasing factor (LRF). Proc. Ntal. Acad. Sci. 1972;*69*:278–282.
6. Vale W, Grant G, Rivier J, Monahan M, Amoss M, Blackwell R, Burgus R, Guillemin R. Synthetic polypeptide antagonists of the hypothalamic luteinizing hormone releasing hormone factor. Science 1972;*176*:933–934.
7. Monahan MW, Amoss MS, Anderson HA, et al. Synthetic analogs of the hypothalamic luteinizing hormone releasing hormone releasing hormone with increased agonist or antagonist properties. Biochemistry 1973;*12*:4614.
8. Rivier J, Porter J, Hoeger C, Theobald P, Craig AG, Dykert J, Corrigan A, Perrin M, Hook WA, Siraganian RP, Vale W, Rivier C. Gonadotropin-releasing hormone antagonists with N-triazolylornithine, -lysine, or p-aminophenylalanine residues at positions 5 and 6. J. Med. Chem 1992;*35*:4270–4278.
9. Vale, W., Grant, G. In vitro pituitary hormone secretion assay for hypophysiotropic substances. Methods in Enzymology, Eds: BW. O'Malley and JG. Hardman, 1975, Volume XXXVII:82–93.
10. Naor A, Shraga A, Limor R, Marantz Y, Ben-Menahem D. Signal transduction cascade of the GnRH receptor. Third International Pituitary Congress 1993 (in press).
11. Janovick JA, Conn PM. A cholera toxin-sensitive guanyl nucleotide binding protein mediates the movement of pituitary luteinizing hormone into a releasable pool: Loss of this event is associated with the onset of homologous desensitization to gonadotropin-releasing hormone. Endocrinology 1993;*132*:2131–2135.
12. Hawes BE, Barnes S, Conn PM. Cholera toxin and pertussis toxin provoke differential effects on luteinizing hormone release, inositol phosphate production, and gonadotropin-releasing hormone (GnRH) receptor binding in the gonadotrope: evidence for multiple guanyl nucleotide binding proteins in GnRH action. Endocrinology 1993;*132*:2124–2130.
13. Pippig S, Andexinger S, Daniel K, Puzicha M, Caron MG, Lefkowitz RJ, Lohse MJ. Overexpression of β-arrestin and β-adrenergic receptor kinase augment desentization of β_2-adrenergic receptors. J. of Biol. Chem 1993;*268*:3201–3208.
14. Pavlou SN, Wakefield G, Schlechter NL, Lindner J, Souza KH, Kamilaris TC, Konidaris S, Rivier JE, Vale WW, Toglia M. Mode of suppression of pituitary and gonadal function after acute or prolonged administration of a luteinizing hormone-releasing hormone antagonist in normal men. J Clin Endocrinol Metab 1989;*68*:446–454.
15. Pavlou SN, Brewer K, Farley MG, Lindner J, Bastias MC, Rogers BJ, Swift LL, Rivier JE, Vale WW, Conn PM, Herbert CM. Combined administration of a gonadotropin-releasing hormone antagonist and testosterone in men induces reversible asoosperimia without loss of libido. J Clin Endocrinol Metab 1991;*73*:1360–1369.
16. Monroe S, Blumenfeld Z, Andreyko JL, Schriock E, Henzl M, Jaffe RB. Dose-dependent inhibition of pituitary-ovarian function during administration of gonadotropin releasing hormone agonistic analog (nafarelin). J Clin Endocrinol Metab 1986;*63*:1334–1341.
17. Mais V, Kazer RR, Cetel NS, Rivier J, Vale W, Yen SSC. The dependency of folliculogenesis and corpus luteum function on pulsatile gonadotropin secretion in cycling women using a gonadotropin-releasing hormone antagonist as a probe. J Clin Endocrinol Metab 1986;*62*:1250–1255.
18. de Ziegler D, Cedars MI, Randle D, Lu JD, Judd HL, Meldrum DR. Suppression of the ovary using a gonadotropin releasing-hormone agonist prior to stimulation for oocyte retrieval. Fertil Steril 1987;*48*:807–810.
19. Cuttler L, Rosenfield RL, Ehrmann DA, Kreiter M, Burstein S, Cara JF, Levitsky LL. Maturation of gonadotropin and sex steroid responses to gonadotropin-releasing hormone agonist in males. J Clin Endocrinol Metab 1993;*76*:362–366.
20. Smals AG, Hermus AR, Boers GH, Pieters GF, Benraad TJ, Kloppenborg PW. Predictive value of luteinizing hormone releasing hormone (LHRH) bolus testing before and after 36-hour pulsatile LHRH administration in the differential diagnosis of constitutional delay of puberty and male hypogonadotropic hypogonadism. J Clin Endocrinol Metab 1994;*78(3)*:602–608.
21. Spratt DI, Crowley WF Jr, Butler JP, Hoffman AR, Conn PM, Badger TM. Pituitary luteinizing hormone responses to intravenous and subcutaneous administration of gonadotropin-releasing hormone in men. J Clin Endocrinol Metab 1985;*61*:890–895.
22. Hoffman AR, Crowley WF Jr. Induction of puberty in men by long-term pulsatile administration of low-dose gonadotropin-releasing hormone. N Engl J Med 1982;*307*:1237–1241.
23. Crowley WF Jr, McArthur JW. Simulation of the normal menstrual cycle in Kallmann's syndrome by pulsatile administration of luteinizing hormone-releasing hormone (LHRH). J Clin Endocrinol Metab 1980;*51*:173–175.
24. Reid RL, Leopold GR, Yen SS. Induction of ovulation and pregnancy with pulsatile luteinizing hormone releasing factor: dosage and mode of delivery. Fertil Steril 1981;*36*:553–559.
25. Martin KA, Hall JE, Adams JM, Crowley WF Jr. Comparison of exogenous gonadtropins and pulsatile gonadotropin-releasing hormone for induction of ovulation in hypogonadotropic amenorrhea. J Clin Encrinol Metab 1993;*77(1)*:125–129.

26. Filicori M, Flamigni C, Meriggiola MC, Ferrari P, Michelacci L, Campaniello E, Valdiserri A, Cognigni G. Endocrine response determines the clinical outcome of pulsatile gonadotropin-releasing hormone ovulation induction in different ovulatory disorder. J Clin Endocrinol Metab 1991;*72(5)*:965–972.

27. Apter D, Butzow TI, Laughlin GA, Yen SSC. Gonadotropin-releasing hormone pulse generator activity during pubertal transition in girls: pulsatile and diurnal patterns of circulating gonadotropins. J Clin Endocrinol Metab 1993;*76*:940–949.

28. Christiansen P, Muller J, Buhl S, Hansen OR, Hobolth N, Jacobsen BB, Jorgensen PH, Kastrup KW, Nielsen K, Nielsen LB, et al. Hormonal treatment of cyrptorchidism—hCG or GnRH—a multicentre study. Acta Paediatrica 1992;*81(8)*:605–608.

29. Muse K, Cetel NS, Futterman LA, Yen SSC. The premenstrual syndrome: Effects of "medical ovariectomy", N Engl J Med 1984;*311*:134–139.

30. Hussain SY, Massil JH, Matta WH, Shaw RW, O'Brien PM. Buserelin in premenstrual syndrome. Gynecological Endo 1992;*6(1)*:57–64.

31. Partsch CJ, Hummelink R, Peter M, Sippell WG, Oostdijk W, Odink RJ, Drop SL. Comparison of complete and incomplete suppression of pituitary-gonadal activity in girls with central precocious puberty: influence on growth and predicted final height. Hormone Research 1993;*39(3–4)*:111–117.

32. Kaisary AV, Tyrrell CJ, Peeling WB, Griffiths K. Comparison of LHRH analogue (Zoladex) with orchiectomy in patients with metastatic prostatic carcinoma. Br J Urol 1991;*67(5)*:502–508.

33. Wada I, Matson PL, Troup SA, Lieberman BA. Assisted conception using buserelin and human menopausal gonadotrophins in women with polycystic ovary syndrome. British Journal of Obstetrics and Gynaecology 1993;*100(4)*:365–369.

34. Mechain C, Cedrin I, Pandian C, Lemay A. Serum FSH bioactivity and response to acute gonadotropin releasing hormone (GnRH) agonist stimulation in patients with polycystic ovary syndrome (PCOS) as compared to control groups. Clinical Endocrinology 1993;*38(3)*:311–320.

35. Kunh JM, Billebaud T, Navratil H, Moulonguet A, Fiet J, Grise P, Louis JF, Costa P, Husson JM, Dahan R, Bartagna C, Edelstein R. Prevention of the transient adverse effects of a gonadotropin-releasing hormone analogue (buserelin) in metastatic prostatic carcinoma by administration of an antiandrogen (nilutamide). N Engl J Med 1989;*321*:413–418.

36. Labrie F, Dupont A, Belanger A, Lachance R. Flutamide eliminates the risk of disease flare in prostatic cancer patients treated with a luteinizing hormoen-releasing hormone agonist. J Urol 1987;*138*:804–806.

37. Surrey ES, Judd HL. Reduction of vasomotor symptoms and bone mineral density loss with combined norethindrone and long-acting gonadotropin-releasing hormone agonist therapy of symptomatic endometriosis: a prospective randomized trial. J Clin Endocrinol Metab 1992;*75*:558–563.

38. Hoshiai H, Ishikawa M, Sawatari Y, Noda K, Fukaya T. Laparoscopic evaluation of the onset and progression of endometriosis. American J of Obstetrics and Gynecology 1993;*169(3)*:714–719.

39. Johansen JS, Rus BJ, Hassager C, Moen M, Jacobson J, Christansen C. The effect of a gonadotropin-releasing hormone analog (nafarelin) on bone metabolism. J Clin Endocrinol Metab 1988;*67*:701–706.

40. Friedman AJ, Daly M, Juneua-Norcross M, Rein MS, Fine C, Gleason R, Leboff M. A prospectice randomized trial of gonadotropin-releasing hormone agonist plus estrogenprogestin or progestin "ad-back" regimens for women with leiomyomata uteri. J Clin Endocrinol Metab 1993;*76*:1439–1445.

41. Vollenhoven BJ, McCloud P, Shekleton P, McDonald J, Healy DL. An open study of luteinizing hormone releasing hormone agonists in infertile women with uterine fibroids. Gynecological Endocrinology 1993;*7(1)*:57–61.

Reviews

r1. McCann SM, Mizanuma H, Samson WK. Differential hypothalamic control of FSH secretion: a review. Psychoneuroendocrinology 1983;*8*:299–308.

r2. Janecka A, Janecki T, Bowers C, Folkers K. The structural features of effective antagonists of the luteinizing hormone releasing hormone. International Journal of Peptide and Protein Research (submitted).

r3. Evans WS, Sollenberger MJ, Booth RA, Rogol AD, Urban RJ, Carlsen EC, Johnson ML, Veldhuis JD. Contemporary aspects of discrete peak-detection algorithms. II. The paradigm of the luteinizing hormone pulse signal in women. Endocrine Reviews 1992;*13*:81–104.

r4. Naor Z. Signal transduction mechanisms of Ca^{2+} mobilizing hormones: The case of gonadotropin-releasing hormone. Endocrine Reviews 1990;*11*:326–353.

r5. Stojilkovic SS, Catt KJ. Calcium oscillations in anterior pituitary cells. Endocrine Reviews 1992;*13*:256–280.

r6. Handelsman DJ, Swerdloff RS. Pharmacokinetics of gonadotropin-releasing hormone and its analogues. Endocrine Reviews 1986;*7*:95–105.

r7. Chan RL, Nerenberg CA. Pharmacokinetics and metabolism of LHRH analogs. In: LHRH and its analogs, part 2; MTP Press Limited 1987:577–593.

r8. Santoro N, Filicori M, Crowley WF. Hypogonadotropic disorders in men and women: diagnosis and therapy with pulsatile gonadotropin-releasing hormone. Endocrine Reviews 1986;*7*:11–23.

r9. Conn PM, Crowley WF Jr. Gonadotropin-releasing hormone and its analogues. N Engl J Med 1991;*324*:93–103.

r10. Yen SS. Female hypogonadotropic hypogonadism. Hypothalamic amenorrhea syndrome. Endocrinol Metab Clin of N Am 1993,*22(1)*:29–58.

r11. Boepple PA, Mansfield MJ, Wierman ME, Rudlin CR, Bode HH, Crigler JF Jr, Crawford JD, Crowley JF Jr. Use of a potent long-acting agonist of gonadotropin-releasing hormone in the treatment of precocious puberty. Endocr Rev 1986;*7*:24–33.

r12. Santen RJ, Manni A, Harvey H. Gonadotropin releasing hormone (GnRH) analogs for the treatment of breast and prostatic carcinoma. Breast Cancer Res Treat 1986:129–145.

r13. Labrie F, DuPont A, Belanger A, St-Arnaud R, Giguere M, Lacourciene Y, Emond J, Monfette G. Treatment of prostate cancer with gonadotropin-releasing hormone agonists. Endocr Rev 1986;*7*:67–74.

CHAPTER 55

Growth Hormone and Insulin-Like Growth Factors (IGFs)

Louis E. Underwood

Growth Hormone

Growth hormone (GH) is a peptide secreted from the anterior pituitary gland under the stimulus of the hypothalamic peptide, growth hormone releasing factor (GRF).[r1] GH secretion is inhibited by another hypothalamic peptide, somatostatin. GH is one of the principal stimulators of somatic growth, exerting many (or all) of its effects on growth through the insulin-like growth factors. In addition, GH is important in regulating protein, carbohydrate, and fat metabolism. In clinical medicine, the principal use of GH is in the promotion of growth in short children.

Chemistry

The predominant human GH species is a 191-amino acid single-chain peptide with two intrachain disulfide bonds (Fig. 55.1). Multiple forms of GH have been described, and the chemical structure and biologic specificity of these forms vary somewhat from one species to another. For example, 90 percent of the GH secreted by the human pituitary is a 22,000-dalton molecule. The remaining 10 percent is secreted as a 20,000-dalton (175-amino acid) peptide, produced by differential splicing of the GH mRNA. Various forms of GH in the circulation result from N-acylation, deamidation, noncovalent association or binding to a GH carrier protein, and fragmentation of the mature GH molecule. Growth hormones from other mammalian species have only modest differences in structure from human GH, but are generally ineffective in promoting growth and in producing anabolic effects in humans.

History

Following experiments in the 1920s, first by Evans and Long,[1] in which bovine pituitary extracts were observed to have anabolic effects in rats, human GH was purified from pituitary glands in the late 1950s. Between 1960 and 1985, most GH therapy was directed at the treatment of statural growth failure in GH-deficient children.

Biosynthesis, Metabolism, and Regulation of GH

GH is encoded in the human by one member of the hGH/human placental lactogen gene family. This cluster of genes, on the long arm of chromosome 17, is composed of the GH 1(GHN) gene, which encodes pituitary GH; the GH 2 (GHV) gene, which encodes a placental GH-like peptide that differs by 13 amino acids from pituitary GH; the CSH1 and CSH2 genes, which encode placental lactogen; and the CSH P1 gene, which encodes a peptide that differs by 13 amino acids from placental lactogen. Each of these five gene loci has five exons with short introns at identical positions. The genes are over 90 percent identical to each other. The human GH (GH I) gene encodes a prehormone of 217 amino acids. The 26 amino acids at the N-terminus compose the leader sequence, which is essential for transporting the molecule to the rough endoplasmic reticulum where it is cleaved, a process that precedes its secretion. A 191-amino acid GH peptide is secreted.[r2,r3,2]

Human GH has a half-time in the circulation of approximately 20 minutes, and only minimal amounts are excreted in urine or other body fluids. The kidney is believed to be its major site of degradation.

The regulation of GH secretion is a complex process, with a host of factors exerting effects on the hypo-

Table 55.1 Factors that Stimulate GH Secretion in Humans

Physiologic	Pharmacologic
deep sleep strenuous exercise emotional stress physical stress protein meal decline of blood glucose post-prandially fasting	hypoglycemia (insulin) amino acid infusion (arginine, ornithine, leucine, etc.) peptides (GRF, glucagon) Nonpeptide hormones (estrogens) Monoaminergic substances (1-dopa, bromocriptine clonidine, propranalol)

thalamus to stimulate the secretion of either growth hormone releasing hormone (GRH) or somatostatin, the inhibitor of GH secretion. Under physiologic conditions, GH secretion occurs after strenuous exercise, during deep sleep, after physical or emotional stress, and after ingestion of protein (Table 55.1). During any 24-hour period, humans normally experience six to eight surges of GH secretion. During these surges serum concentrations rise from low values (a few ng/ml) to concentrations of 10–40 ng/ml. The ventromedial and arcuate nuclei in the hypothalamus are involved in the stimulation of GH secretion, and the ventromedial nucleus, in particular, is believed to be important in the integration of signals provided by the glucoregulatory hormones. Specific neurotransmitters appear to act as specific stimuli to GH secretion. For example, GH release is often blunted by alpha adrenergic blockers and stimulated by beta$_2$-adrenergic agonists; dopamine is believed to stimulate GRF directly and, after being converted to norepinephrine, to stimulate GH through alpha-adrenergic receptors. Serotonin and acetylcholine also stimulate GH release.

Growth hormone inhibits its own secretion through a short loop feedback mechanism and IGF-I inhibits GH secretion by stimulating somatostatin secretion by the hypothalamus and by directly inhibiting GH secretion by the pituitary.[3]

Physiologic Function of GH

The principal physiologic actions of GH fall into two categories: (1) those that are direct and (2) those that are indirect, mediated by the insulin-like growth factors (IGFs) (Fig. 55.2).[4,r4] Those actions believed to be mediated by the IGFs are mainly anabolic and include the stimulation of amino acid transport; stimulation of DNA, RNA, and protein synthesis; and the induction of cell proliferation and growth.[r5] These actions, which are the most important expressions of GH,

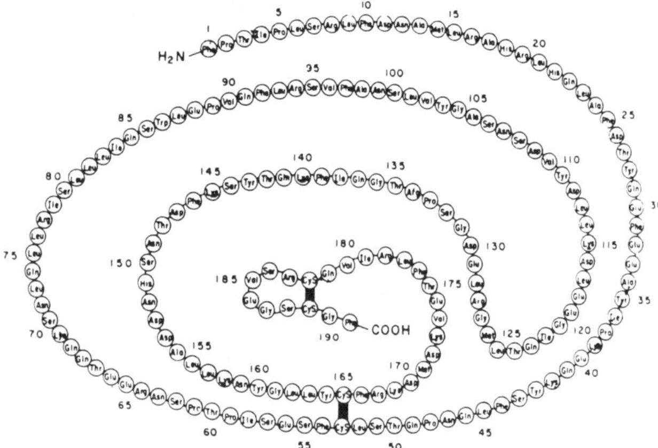

Figure 55.1 Amino acid sequence of the predominant human growth hormone.

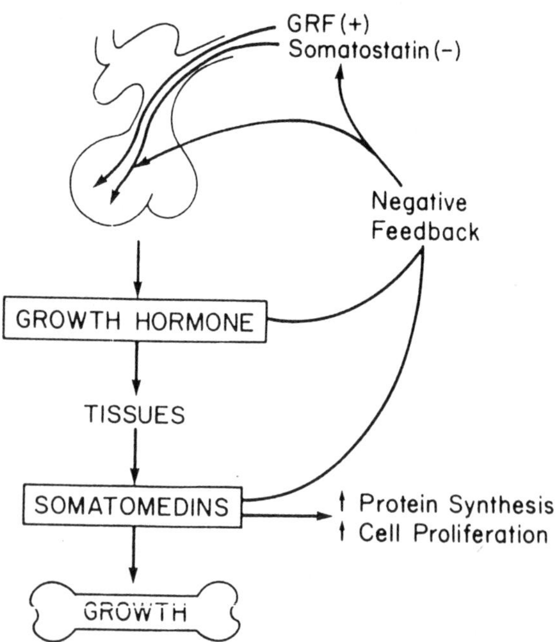

Figure 55.2 The growth hormone-somatomedin (IGF) cascade. Most of the growth-promoting anabolic actions of GH are exerted through the Insulin-like Growth Factors (IGFs). The IGFs, in turn, modulate the secretion of GH.

will be discussed in more detail in the section on IGFs. The actions of GH that are presumed to be direct include antagonism of the peripheral action of insulin and the subsequent stimulation of insulin secretion (diabetogenic effects); stimulation of various hepatic enzymes; stimulation of lipolysis, with net loss of body fat; induction of a positive calcium balance and increased urine calcium; and retention of sodium and potassium.

Hypopituitarism—GH Deficiency[r6]

GH deficiency may occur at any age, but its effects are most dramatic in children, in whom absent or inadequate GH secretion results in failure of linear growth.[r7,r8] The causes of GH deficiency range from disorders that impair the ability of the hypothalamus to secrete GRF to processes that cause destruction of the pituitary gland itself (Table 55.2). The single most common form of GH deficiency is referred to as "idiopathic hypopituitarism." This form of the disease has an early onset and is characterized by slowing of statural growth in the first few months of life. A large proportion of affected children have histories of perinatal trauma, including hypoxic injury to the CNS during the birth process. Breech delivery among these patients is much more common than in the population as a whole. The most common tumor associated with GH deficiency is craniopharyngioma, which arises from embryonic rests of cells derived from Rathke's pouch in the roof of the embryonic pharynx. Craniopharyngiomas are nonmalignant tumors that usually grow slowly and damage the hypothalamus and pituitary by direct pressure. In recent years the occurrence of GH deficiency following cranial irradiation for leukemia and various solid tumors has increased.

The principal consequence of GH deficiency in children, which occurs with a frequency of about 1:5000, is growth failure.[5] Affected children grow slowly and, depending on the duration and severity of disease, may fall several years behind their peers in growth. Depending on etiology and severity, affected individuals may have deficiencies of pituitary hormones other than GH. Deficiency of TSH can result in low serum concentrations of thyroid hormone, and occasionally can cause clinically significant hypothyroidism. Deficiency of ACTH results in impaired secretion of adrenal corticosteroids. This becomes problematic when the patient is physically or emotionally stressed and is unable to raise the serum cortisol concentration appropriately. Deficiency of gonadotropic hormones usually is not apparent during childhood, but causes impairment of sexual maturation and fertility later in life.

When GH deficiency is severe or accompanied by other pituitary hormone deficiencies, the diagnosis is relatively easy. Diagnosis is more difficult, however, when the deficiency of GH is only partial.[r9] Because GH is normally secreted episodically, it usually is not possible to diagnose (or exclude) GH deficiency by measurement of the levels of GH in serum samples drawn randomly. Rather, it is necessary to administer a provocative stimulus for GH secretion to the patient and observe the GH response in the serum in the 1 to 1.5 hours that follow. A variety of stimuli that act via the hypothalamus can be used for this purpose (Table 55.3). An alternative to provocative testing is the measurement of GH on blood samples drawn frequently (every 10–20 min) over prolonged periods (i.e., 12–24 hr). Using these technique it is possible to determine whether GH secretory bursts occur. In normal individuals, there are six to eight secretory bursts of GH over a 24-hour period.

Table 55.2 Causes of Pituitary Deficiency

Primary Pituitary Disease
Familial—aplasia, hypoplasia, deleted or mutant GH gene.
Destruction of Anterior Pituitary
Craniopharyngioma or other intrasellar tumor
Trauma
Histiocytosis-x
Midline Cranial Anomalies
Pituitary Deficiency Secondary to Hypothalamic Dysfunction
Suprasellar, hypothalamic tumors (Craniopharyngioma, dysgerminoma, etc.)
Congenital malformations of the forebrain
Septo-optic dysplasia
Holoprosencephaly
Irradiation damage to hypothalamus
Idiopathic hypopituitarism
Psychosocial dwarfism

Acromegaly, Gigantism—GH Excess[r7]

GH excess in children who have not fused their bony epiphyses causes statural overgrowth, but GH excess after epiphyseal fusion produces acromegaly. In most patients, GH excess is caused by a GH-producing adenoma of the pituitary.

The course of acromegaly is insidious, and many years may elapse between the onset of the disease and its diagnosis. Characteristic findings include coarsening of facial features, soft tissue thickening of the hands and feet, thickening of skin, development of skin tags, and excessive sweating. The bones of the hands and feet undergo cortical thickening and distal tufting. The mandible increases in size, causing protrusion of the jaw and a marked underbite. Long-standing disease is accompanied by arthritis, hypertension, glucose intolerance and diabetes mellitus, entrapment and damage to nerves by overgrowth of tendon sheaths, and visceromegaly.

The diagnosis of GH excess is made by showing that serum GH concentrations are high and fail to sup-

Table 55.3 Clinical Tests of Growth Hormone Secretion*

	Test Conditions	Time of Growth Hormone Response
Screening Tests		
Exercise	Patient should be fasting; 15 min moderate exercise, then 5 min vigorous exercise	40 min after exercise is begun
Sleep	GH rise occurs with deep sleep (EEG stages 3,4); with EEG monitoring and frequent sampling, may be used as a more definitive test	Initial peak within 1 hr after onset of deep sleep; awaken patient for sample
Formal Tests		
Insulin	Regular crystalline insulin 0.05–0.1 U/kg (IV). 50% fall in blood sugar is necessary for adequate test. Nadir blood sugar occurs 20–30 min after insulin is given	45–75 min
Arginine	L-Arginine mononhydrochloride, 5–10% solution, 0.5 g/kg (30 g for adults) infused over 30 min	60–120 min
L-Dopa	0.5 g/1.73 m^2 orally; GH responses are often improved by administering priming doses (0.25 g/1.73 m^2 of L-dopa for 1 or more days prior to test dose)	45–120 min
Glucagon	0.03 mg/kg IM or SC (maximum of 1 mg)	120–180 min
Clonidine	4 μg/kg orally	60–120 min
Propranol (used to augment responses to primary stimulus)	30–40 mg (children 0.75 mg/kg) orally 30–60 min before glucagon, insulin, arginine, or exercise tests	As with primary stimuli

*In general, measurement of GH in serum during any two of these tests is considered sufficient. Most experts agree that no one of these tests provides significant diagnostic advantage over another.

press to below 2–3 ng/ml after the patient is given a glucose load orally. Diagnosis is aided by showing that the serum concentration of IGF-I is elevated.[6,7] Therapy is directed at removing the pituitary tumor causing the GH excess. Complete relief of the GH excess by surgical means, however, is not always possible. Suppression of GH secretion by treatment with bromocriptine or a somatostatin analogue often is helpful in reducing the complications of the disease.

Therapeutic Use of GH

Daily or every other day injections of recombinant human GH are used for treatment of the growth failure that results from GH deficiency.[r10] Two recombinant GH preparations are available: methionyl-GH (methionyl group attached at the N terminus of molecule) and natural GH. These generally are given at a dose of 0.05 mg/kg/day subcutaneously. Such treatment in children in whom the bony epiphyses are open often accelerates the rate of growth two- to threefold (pretreatment growth rate of 4 cm/yr, to growth rates of 8–12 cm/yr during treatment). Early diagnosis and aggressive treatment may result in normalization of the stature of affected children (Fig. 55.3). If other pituitary hormones are deficient, the respective target gland products (thyroid hormone, cortisol, estrogen, or testosterone) should be replaced as well. While GH secretion continues after statural growth is complete, there is little information on the possible benefit of GH therapy in GH-deficient adults.

Because some short children have no readily definable cause for their short stature, and because the diagnosis of GH deficiency may be difficult to make with certainty, many short children who may not be GH-deficient are being treated with GH. A significant proportion of such children will experience accelerated growth with GH treatment. However, it is not possible to predict whether a particular child will respond nor is it possible to predict the effect of treatment on adult stature.[8–10,r11]

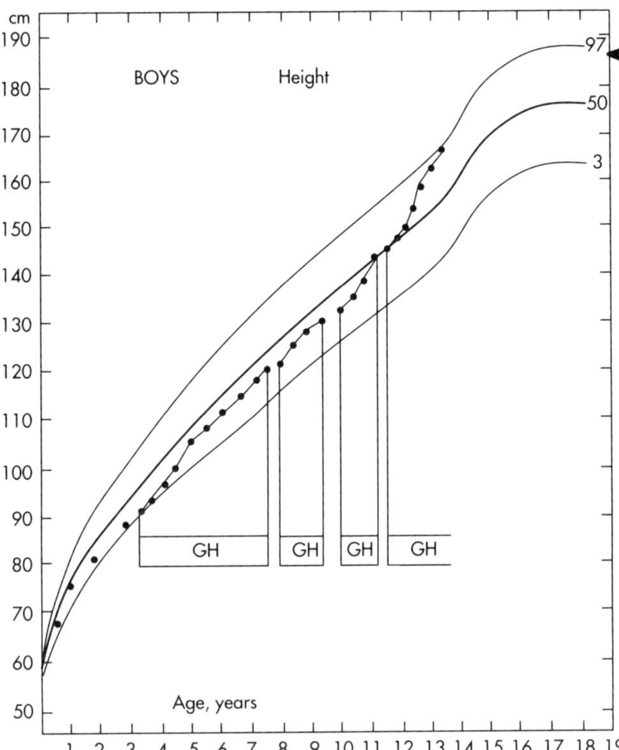

Figure 55.3 Height-attained curve of a boy with GH deficiency who began treatment with GH before he fell below his peers in growth. The smoothed growth curve lines are the 97th, 50th, and 3rd centiles. The curve of the patient shows rapid growth early in GH therapy and at puberty. The arrowhead at the right margin depicts the patient's adult target height.

Insulin-Like Growth Factors (IGFs)

Most or all of the growth-promoting effects of GH are probably mediated through the IGFs (somatomedins).[r12,r13] Two structurally-related IGFs, IGF-I and IGF-II, have been characterized in humans and in other species where they have been studied: IGF-I (somatomedin-C)[14] is highly GH-dependent and more potent in assays for promotion of growth, and IGF-II is less GH-dependent and more potent in assays for insulin-like activity. The IGFs were isolated on the basis of three properties: their GH-like activities in cartilage (sulfation or thymidine factor activity); their insulin-like activity in adipose tissue and muscle (nonsuppressible insulin-like activity); and their mitogenic effect in cell cultures (multiplication stimulating activity).

Chemistry

IGF-I is a 70-amino acid straight-chain basic (pI. 8.1–8.5) peptide that is homologous with proinsulin (Fig. 55.4). IGF-II is a 67-amino acid neutral peptide homologous to IGF-I. The structures of the IGFs are highly conserved across species, with the respective peptides of many species exhibiting differences in only a few amino acids.

History

The biologic phenomenon produced by the IGFs were first described in 1957 by William Salmon and William Daughaday.[r13] Purification of IGF-I and IGF-II was achieved by Rinderknecht and Humbel[11] in Zurich and that of IGF-I by Van Wyk in Chapel Hill.[r6] Much of the early work on the IGFs was done by Froesch, Zaopf and colleagues[r4,12] in Zurich, Van Wyk and colleagues in Chapel Hill,[r7] and Hall et al. in Stockholm.

Biosynthesis, Metabolism, and Regulation

Both IGFs are encoded by single copy genes, with the gene for prepro-IGF-I located on the long arm of chromosome 12 and the gene for prepro-IGF-II on the short arm of chromosome 11. A variant form of IGF-II in which the tetrapeptide Arg-Leu-Pro-Gly is substituted for the serine at residue 29 probably represents another allelic form. The prepro-IGF-II gene is in close physical proximity to the gene for prepro-insulin. Analysis of cDNAs coding for the IGFs reveal that both IGF-I and IGF-II are synthesized like other secreted proteins, with leader sequences of 25 and 24 amino acids, respectively, at the amino termini. In addition, IGF-I has an extension of 35 amino acids and IGF-II an extension of 89 residues at their respective carboxy termini. Variant forms of the cDNAs for IGFs arising from alternate splicing provide a variety of mecha-

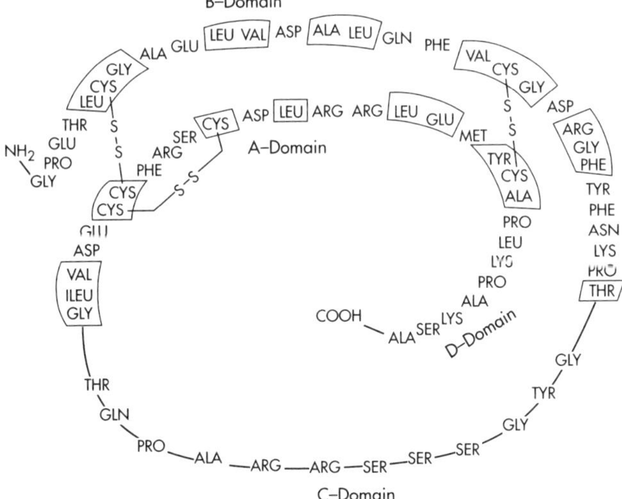

Figure 55.4 The primary structure of human Insulin-like Growth Factor I. (IGF-I; Somatomedin-C). The amino acid residues enclosed in boxes are identical with amino acid residues at the same position in human proinsulin.

nisms by which gene expression can be modified in different tissues under different circumstances.

The mean concentration of IGF-I in serum of adults is approximately 200 ng/ml. Because of the presence of specific IGF binding proteins in serum, these relatively high values remain constant throughout the day.[r13] The concentration of IGF-I is low in newborns and rises progressively after the first year of life, reaching concentrations that are 2.5 times adult values during mid- to late puberty. There is an age-dependent decline in serum IGF-I; by the seventh decade, values are only half those of young adults.

The principal hormonal regulator of IGF-I is GH. In individuals with severe GH deficiency, IGF-I values are 10 to 15 percent of normal; in states of GH excess, they may be several times normal. IGF-I is also often reduced in thyroid hormone deficiency, owing in part to diminished GH secretion.

The other major regulator of IGF-I is nutritional status.[13,14] Fasting reduces IGF-I to values 10 percent of normal after 10 days of fasting. Chronic undernutrition is also accompanied by low IGF-I, and refeeding restores values to normal. Both dietary protein and energy are important determinants of IGF-I concentrations in serum. Studies in animals suggest that the decrease in serum IGF-I that occurs in malnourished patients or in individuals subjected to short-term nutrient deprivation is mediated at several levels. In severe diet restriction, GH receptors on cell membranes are decreased, and there is evidence of GH resistance. In less severe restriction, GH receptors may be normal, but post-receptor resistance to GH persists; IGF-I mRNA is decreased when nutrients are restricted; and one of the IGF binding proteins (IGFBP-3) also is reduced. This causes a secondary reduction in serum IGF-I concentration.

Most of the IGF-I in the serum probably is produced by the liver. However, IGF mRNAs and IGF peptides are found in almost all tissues. IGF-I production in tissues is differentially regulated. Although growth hormone controls production of IGF-I by liver and certain other tissues, estrogen controls IGF-I production in the endometrium, a tissue in which growth hormone has no effect. Similarly, IGF-I synthesis in the adrenal is stimulated by ACTH, angiotensin II, and fibroblast growth factor and is stimulated by gonadotrophic hormones in the gonads. The varied sites of origin and the multiplicity of cells on which the IGFs act have led to the proposal that these peptides act by autocrine and/or paracrine mechanisms (Fig. 55.5). In the proposed paracrine model, IGFs act on cells that are in close proximity to the cells of secretion. In the autocrine model, IGFs act on the cells from which they are secreted.

Serum concentrations and actions of the IGFs are also regulated by the IGF binding proteins (IGFBPs). These IGFBPs are high-affinity carrier proteins found in blood and extracellular fluids that control IGF transport, efflux from the vascular compartment, and association with cell surface receptors. Multiple IGFBPs exist, and three have been isolated and characterized in humans. Each is structurally distinct and has different mechanisms of regulation. IGFBP-1 is a 25 kDa protein whose serum concentrations fluctuate widely through the day. One of its principal regulators is insulin, which causes IGFBP-1 concentrations to decline. During even brief periods of fasting, when insulin values are low, IGFBP-1 concentrations rise dramatically. IGFBP-2 is a 31-kDa protein whose serum concentrations fluctuate less than IGFBP-1. It is present in higher concentrations in fetal than in postnatal life. IGFBP-2 concentrations are lowered by GH and raised by IGF-I. Both IGFBP-1 and 2 are believed to facilitate the movement of IGFs across the vascular endothelium and to regulate binding of IGFs to the cell surface. IGFBP-3 is a 53-kDa glycoprotein that associates with an acid-labile non-binding subunit and IGF-I or IGF-II in serum to form a 150-kDa complex. This complex appears to prevent the removal of IGF from the vascular compartment and stabilizes the concentrations of IGFs in blood. It is generally accepted that the primary function of IGF-BP-3 is to serve as a reservoir for IGF in blood. IGFBP-3 is increased by GH and by IGF-I and is decreased with nutrient restriction.

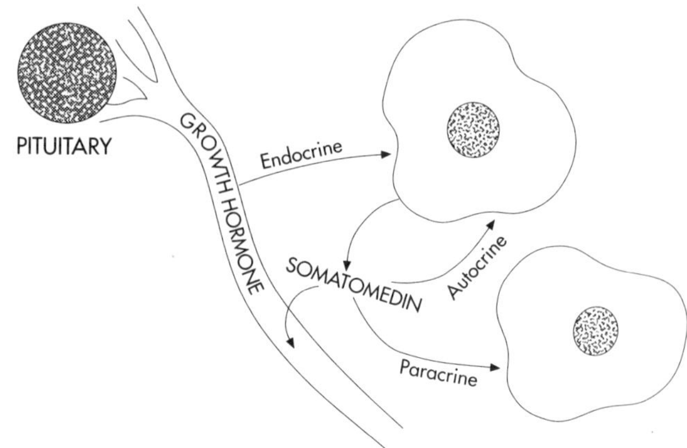

Figure 55.5 Proposed models for the action of Insulin-like Growth Factors. GH binds to its receptor and stimulates IGF production in liver and many other tissues. These IGFs then may act on the cell that produced them (autocrine action) or on nearby cells (paracrine action). Neither of these modes of action excludes the classic endocrine model, in which IGF enters the bloodstream and eventually acts on cells at distant sites.

Physiologic Functions of the IGFs

The IGFs stimulate DNA synthesis and cell proliferation in a variety of cell types from phyla as low as the invertebrates. The stimulation of cellular proliferation by IGFs requires the participation of other growth factors, such as platelet derived growth factor (PDGF). Because IGF receptors are ubiquitous, it appears that they are important in the growth, development, and function of most tissues. They also may regulate the body's response to injury. IGF-I acts in concert with erythropoietin to stimulate erythropoiesis. In the ovary, IGF-I enhances FSH-stimulated production of progesterone and accumulation of cyclic AMP (Fig. 55.6). In the adrenal gland, IGF-I acts in concert with ACTH and angiotensin II to promote steroidogenesis. IGF-I potentiates the action of LH on steroidogenesis in theca-interstitial cells of the ovary and Leydig cells of the testis. In cultured thyroid cells, IGF-I and TSH enhance one another's mitogenic effects, and in muscle IGF-I stimulates proliferation of myoblasts and their differentiation into myotubes.

When given in vivo by IV infusion or SQ injection, IGF-I produces a variety of GH-like effects, including reduction in blood and urinary urea nitrogen, urinary phosphate, and urinary sodium. It increases creatinine clearance, promotes hypercalciuria and, by virtue of its insulin-like action,[15] causes a reduction in blood glucose. Because of its anabolic effect, IGF-I may prove useful in the treatment of catabolic disorders but much research on possible clinical uses remains to be done.[r15]

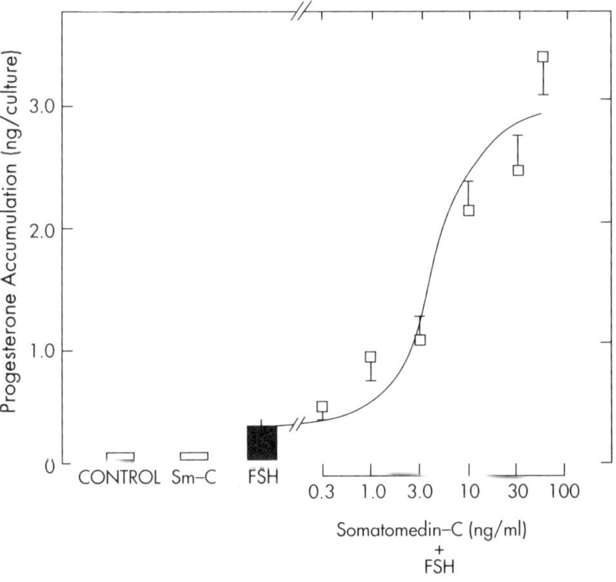

Figure 55.6 Effect of treatment with Sm-C/IGF-I on basal and FSH-stimulated progesterone accumulation by cultured rat granulosa cells. Cells were obtained from immature, hypophysectomized, diethylstilbestrol-treated female rats. Granulosa cells (1×10^5/dish) were cultured for 72 hours under serum free conditions in the absence or presence of FSH (20 ng/ml) with or without increasing concentrations (0.1–50 ng/ml) of IGF-I (Sm-C). The concentration of progesterone in the medium was measured by RIA. (From Adashi EY, Resnick GE, Svoboda ME, Van Wyk JJ. Endocrinology, 1984; *115*:1227–1229, with permission.)

Growth Hormone Releasing Hormone (GRH) and Somatostatin

GRF (or GH releasing hormone; GHRH), a 44-amino acid peptide that is synthesized and released from the hypothalamus, is the principal stimulator of GH release from the pituitary.[r16] Active GRF has been purified and sequenced as 44-, 37-, and 29-amino acid peptides, each of the latter representing a C-terminal shortened form of GRF-44. The principal site of production of GRF is the arcuate nucleus, and only scattered GRF-producting neurons are found elsewhere. GRF stimulates GH synthesis and release through cyclic AMP/calcium–calmodulin interactions. The amplitude and frequency of GH secretion by the pituitary are determined by the positive influence of GRF in synchrony with the inhibitory effect of somatostatin. The pulsatile release of GH appears to be caused by pulsatile secretion of GRF associated with a temporary decline in somatostatin release.

In normal humans, GRF (1 ug/kg) given IV stimulates GH secretion. The response is blunted by increased blood glucose, increased free fatty acids, prolonged corticosteroid excess, cholinergic-muscarenic antagonists, infusions of somatostatin, and injections of GH itself.[r17,r18]

GRF has been used in the assessment of short children and individuals suspected to be GH deficient. Because other provocative tests of GH secretion act via the hypothalamus and GRF acts directly on the pituitary, GRF has the theoretical advantage of discriminating between a hypothalamic defect versus a lesion involving the pituitary directly. While appealing in theory, the practical application of GRF testing has been somewhat disappointing. In some patients with pituitary lesions a response to GRF is observed, probably because the pituitary has residual capacity to secrete GH. On the other hand, patients with hypothalamic lesions may not respond to GRF until after a prolonged period of priming.

GRF has been used to promote GH secretion and linear growth in GH-deficient children. In general, the growth rates achieved are less impressive than those produced by GH. Presumably this is because GRF has a half-life of only a few minutes and would need to be administered several times daily to exert its full effect on GH secretion. It seems likely that until long-acting analogues of GRF (or alternate forms of delivery) are developed, this agent will not be widely accepted for long-term therapy.

Somatostatin

Somatostatin is a cyclic peptide of 14 amino acids that inhibits GH and TSH secretion by the pituitary. Somatostatin was characterized, chemically isolated and sequenced in 1973 in Roger Guillemin's laboratory.[16] Somatostatin is distributed in neurons throughout the body and is present in such extraneuronal tissues as gut and pancreas, where it exerts a variety of effects distinct from those affecting GH secretion (Table 55.4). A larger 28-amino acid somatostatin peptide has been isolated from various animal tissues, and this is 10 times as potent in inhibiting growth hormone and insulin secetion. This 28-amino acid peptide may be the parent, physiologically active, compound.

A therapeutically useful derivative of somatostatin is a cyclic octapeptide (D Phe-Cys-Phe-DTrp-Lys-Thr-Cys-Thr-ol; octreotide acetate [Sandostatin]). Unlike somatostatin, which has a serum half-life of 1–3 minutes, octreotide is resistant to degradation by serum proteolytic enzymes, has a half-life of about 1.5 hours and can be given SQ. This agent has proved useful in the treatment of patients with secretory diarrhea secondary to tumors that produce vasoactive intestinal peptide (VIPoma). Octreotide also has been used to decrease GH secretion in patients with acromegaly, to decrease the insulin requirement in diabetes mellitus, and to alleviate the hypoglycemia that accompanies insulin-secreting tumors.

Somatostatin may be useful in diabetics because it inhibits the secretion of hormones (glucagon and GH) that oppose the action of insulin. Long-acting analogues of somatostatin reduce the requirement for exogenous insulin by as much as 30 to 50 percent and, in some instances, reduced brittleness of the diabetes.

Table 55.4 Some Biological Effects of Somatostatin

Organ	Inhibitory Effect
Pituitary	GH, TSH (occasionally prolactin and ACTH) secretion
GI Tract	Gastrin, secretin, gastrointestinal polypeptide, enteroglucagon secretion
Pancreas	Insulin secretion Glucagon, bicarbonate, and enzymes secretion
GU Tract	Renin secretion
Stomach	Gastric acid and gastric fluid secretion gastric emptying

References

Research Reports

1. Evans HM, Long JA. The effect of the anterior lobe administered intraperitoneally upon growth, maturation, and oestrous cycles of the rat. Anat Rec 1921;*21*:62–63.
2. Clemmons DR, Underwood LE, Ridgway EC, Kliman B, Van Wyk JJ. Hyperprolactinemia is associated with increased immunoreactive somatomedin-C in hypopituitarism. J Clin Endocrinol Metab 1981;*52*:731–735.
3. Berelowitz M, Szabo M, Frohman LA, Firestone S, Chu L, Hintz RL. Somatomedin-C mediates growth hormone negative feedback by effects on both the hypothalamus and the pituitary. Science 1981;*212*:1279–1281.
4. Salmon WD Jr, Daughaday WH. A hormonally controlled serum factor which stimulates sulfate incorporation by cartilage in vitro. J Lab Clin Med 1957;*49*:825–836.
5. Vimpani GV, Vimpani AF, Lidgard GP, Cameron EH, Farquhar JW. Prevalence of severe growth hormone deficiency. Br Med J 1977;*2*:427–430.
6. Clemmons DR, Van Wyk JJ, Ridgway EC, Kliman B, Kjellberg RN, Underwood LE. Evaluation of acromegaly by radioimmunoassay of somatomedin-C. N Engl J Med 1979;*301*:1138–1142.
7. Barken A, Beitins IZ, Kelch RP. Plasma insulin-like growth factor I/somatomedin C in acromegaly: Correlation with the degree of growth hormone hypersecretion. J Clin Endocrinol Metab 1988;*67*:69–73.
8. Hagenas L. Clinical tests as predictors of growth response in GH treatment of short normal children. Acta Paediatr Scand 1989;*362*:36.
9. Ivarsson SA. Can growth hormone increase final height in constitutional short stature? Acta Paediat Scand 1989;*362*(suppl):56–60.
10. Underwood LE, Rieser PA. Is it ethical to treat healthy short children with growth hormone? Acta Paediatr Scand 1989; Suppl *362*:18–23.
11. Rinderknecht E, Humbel RE. Primary structure of human insulin-like growth factor II. FEBS Lett 1978;*89*:283–286.
12. Schoenle E, Zapf J, Humbel RE, Froesch ER. Insulin-like growth factor I stimulates growth in hypophysectomized rats. Nature 1982;*296*:252–253.
13. Clemmons DR, Underwood LE, Dickerson RN, Brown RO, Hak LJ, MacPhee RD, Heizer WD. Use of plasma somatomedin-C/insulin-like growth factor I measurements to monitor the response to nutritional repletion in malnourished patients. Am J Clin Nutr 1985;*41*:191–198.
14. Unterman TG, Vazquez RM, Slas AJ, Martyn PA, Phillips LS. Nutrition and somatomedin. XIII Usefulness of somatomedin-C in nutritional assessment. Am J Med 1985;*78*:228–234.
15. Guler H-P, Schmid C, Zapf J, Froesch ER. Effects of recombinant insulin-like growth factor I on insulin secretion and renal function in normal human subjects. Proc Natl Acad Sci USA 1989;*86*:2868.
16. Brazeau P, Vale WW, Burgus R, Ling N, Butcher M, Rivier J, Guillemin R. Hypothalamic polypeptide that inhibits the secretion of immunoreactive pituitary growth hormone. Science 1973;*179*:77–79.

Reviews

r1. Bercu BB. (ed), Basic and clinical aspects of growth hormones. New York: Plenum Press, 1988.

r2. Chawla RK, Parks JS, Rudman D. Structural variants of human growth hormone: biochemical, genetic and clinical aspects. Annu Rev Med 1983;*34*:519–547.

r3. Baumann G. Heterogenity of growth hormone. In: Bercu B Basic and clinical aspects of growth hormone. New York: Plenum Press, 1988; pp 13–31.

r4. Zapf J, Froesch ER, Humbel RE. The insulin-like growth factors (IGF) of human serum: chemical and biological characterization and aspects of their possible physiological role. Curr Top Cell Regul 1991;*19*:257–309.

r5. Isakkson OG, Lindahl A, Nilsson A, Isgaard J. Mechanism of the stimulatory effect of growth hormone on longitudinal bone growth. Endocr Rev 1987;*8*(4):426–438.

r6. Underwood LE, Van Wyk JJ. Normal and Aberrant Growth. In Foster DW and Wilson JD (eds). Williams Textbook of Endocrinology, 8th Ed. Philadelphia. WB Saunders 1992; pp 1079–1138.

r7. Brook CGD, Hindmarsh PC, Smith PJ, Stanhope R. Clinical Features and Investigation of Growth Hormone Deficiency. Clin Endocrinol Metab 1986;*15*:479–493.

r8. D'Ercole AJ, Underwood LE. Anterior pituitary gland and hypothalamus: Disorders affecting anterior pituitary function. In: Rudolph Am (ed) Pediatrics, 19th ed. New York: Appleton-Century-Crofts 1991; pp 1566–1577.

r9. Preece MA. Diagnosis and treatment of children with growth hormone deficiency. Clin Endocrinol Metab 1982;*11*:1–24.

r10. Ranke MB, Bierich JR. Treatment of Growth Hormone Deficiency. Clin Endocrinol Metab 1986;*15*:495–510.

r11. Underwood LE, Sherman BM. Controversies in the treatment of short stature. In: Underwood LE (ed), Human Growth Hormone: Progress and Challenge. New York: Marcel Dekker, 1988; pp 145–191.

r12. Van Wyk JJ. The somatomedins: Biological actions and physiologic control mechanisms. In: Li CH ed. Hormonal Proteins and Peptides, Vol 12. New York: Academic Press, 1984; pp 81–125.

r13. Doughaday WH. Growth hormone: Normal synthesis, secretion, control and mechanisms of action. In De Groot LJ. Endocrinology 22nd ed Vol 1 Philadelphia: WB Saunders 1989; pp 318–329.

r14. Underwood LE, Smith EP, Van Wyk JJ, Clemmons DR, D'Ercole AJ, Pandian MR, Preece MA, Moore WV. Somatomedin-C/insulin-like growth factor I: regulation and clinical applications. In: Raiti S, Tolman RA, eds. Human Growth Hormone. Baltimore: Raven Press, 1986; pp 609–619.

r15. Froesch ER, Guler H-P, Schmid C, Binz K, Zapf J. Therapeutic potential of insulin-like growth factor I. Trends Endocrinol Metab 1990;*1*:254–260.

r16. LeRoith D, Raizada MK. Molecular and cellular biology of insulin-like growth factors and their receptors. New York: Plenum Press, 1989.

r17. Thorner MO, Vance ML. Regulation of growth hormone secretion in men and the therapeutic implications of GHRH. In Frisch H, Thorner MO, (eds). Hormonal regulation of growth. New York: Raven Press, 1989; pp 19–29.

r18. Frohman LA, Jansson J-O. Growth-hormone releasing hormone. Endocr Rev 1986;*7*:223–253.

CHAPTER 56

Prolactin and Treatment of Hyperprolactinemic States with Bromocriptine

Marsha L. Davenport

Prolactin

Prolactin is a polypeptide hormone secreted by the acidophilic cells (lactotropes) of the anterior pituitary, although extrapituitary sites of prolactin synthesis such as the decidua basalis of the placenta have recently been discovered. Prolactin's primary function in humans is to stimulate mammary gland development and lactation. Its biologic effects, however, are extraordinarily diverse and vary from species to species. Included among its actions are promotion of gonadal function, salt and water balance, parental solicitude, and immune responses.[r1]

Chemistry

Prolactin is a 198 amino acid polypeptide that shares significant homology to growth hormone (GH) and placental lactogen (PL) (Fig. 56.1). Based on analyses of their amino acid composition and gene organization, prolactin, GH, and PL are proposed to have arisen from a common ancestral gene.[1] Human prolactin is found in the serum in different molecular sizes, the predominant form of immunoreactive prolactin being "little" prolactin, with a MW of 23,000 daltons. Forms with other MWs probably result from phosphorylation, glycosylation, dimerization, and aggregation. The biologic significance of these different forms is not clear.[2] Currently, there is no established therapeutic use for prolactin.

History

Prolactin was discovered in 1928 by Stricker and Greuter, who demonstrated that an extract from the anterior pituitary caused lactation in pseudopregnant rabbits.[2,r2] Riddle et al. demonstrated that similar extracts stimulate the growth and differentiation of the pigeon crop sac, leading to the formation of "crop milk," a secretion used by brooding pigeons to feed their young. Injection of prolactin-containing solutions into pigeons and examination of the crop sac for mucosal proliferation served as a standard bioassay for prolactin for many years.[3] In 1932, prolactin was isolated from sheep pituitaries, but it was not until 1971 that Lewis et al. isolated human prolactin[4] and showed that it has lactogenic properties and is distinct from growth hormone, which is roughly 100-fold more abundant in pituitary tissue. Hwang, Guyda, and Friesen developed a specific radioimmunoassay for human prolactin shortly thereafter.[5] In the early 1980s, Cooke et al. sequenced the gene for prolactin and identified it as a member of the superfamily containing GH and PL.[6]

Biosynthesis, Metabolism, and Regulation of Prolactin

Biosynthesis and Metabolism

Prolactin is synthesized in the pituitary as a prehormone on the ribosomes of the rough endoplasmic reticulum, and its 28-amino acid signal peptide is cleaved prior to transport to the Golgi apparatus. There, the prolactin molecule is variably glycosylated and packaged into large, dense secretory granules. Like all the anterior pituitary hormones, prolactin is secreted episodically, being carried in the bloodstream to target organs. Its half-life is about 15 minutes.[r1] During pregnancy, prolactin is also produced by the decidua and secreted into the amniotic fluid. At midgestation, concentrations of prolactin in amniotic fluid are 100-fold higher than those of maternal or fetal serum and may serve to help regulate amniotic fluid volume and osmolarity.[r3] Although the kidney is the main site of

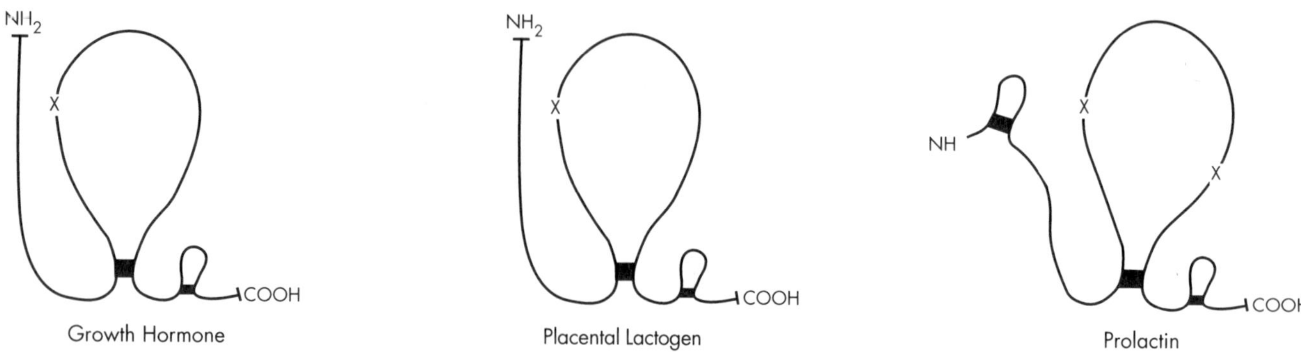

Figure 56.1 Structural relationships of human placental lactogen and prolactin to growth hormone. X indicates the position of constant tryptophan residues and the bars represent disulphide bridges. Overall sequence homologies are 84% for hPL and hGH and only 16% for hPRL and hGH.

prolactin elimination, the exact mechanism for clearance is not known.

Regulation

Prolactin can first be identified in the pituitary and serum of human fetuses at 11 weeks' gestation. By late gestation, prolactin values in cord blood are extremely high (about 250 ng/ml); with the withdrawal of the hormones of pregnancy they decline over the first six postnatal weeks to the normal prepubertal values of 3–7 ng/ml. During puberty, prolactin concentrations rise in both sexes, but to a greater degree in females. Maternal serum prolactin levels begin to rise from 7–10 ng/ml during the first trimester of pregnancy and increase to an average of 200 ng/ml by term (Fig. 56.2). Postpartum, serum prolactin declines, reaching prepregnancy values by about four weeks.[7]

Regulation by Estrogens

Estrogens regulate prolactin secretion at several points, acting at the level of gene transcription, lactotrope differentiation, and neuroendocrine modulation. Estrogen affects prolactin gene transcription directly by binding to its 5′ regulatory region.[8] Primary pituitary cell cultures incubated with physiologic amounts of 17β-estradiol increase prolactin mRNA levels two- to threefold after two days in culture. Estrogen also increases the number of prolactin-secreting cells in the pituitary, an effect evident during pregnancy, when the pituitary increases in size and weight as the lactotropes increase in number. Finally, estrogen acts at the level of the hypothalamus to suppress dopamine secretion, allowing sustained prolactin secretion.

Regulation by Neuroendocrine Factors

A variety of neuroendocrine factors and reflexes cause wide swings in prolactin secretion over brief time periods (Fig. 56.3). When serum prolactin is measured at frequent intervals over a 24-hour period, 4 to 11 peaks are seen, with slightly more frequent and higher peaks occurring during sleep. Bursts of prolactin secretion occur following surgery, exercise, hypoglycemia, needle puncture, and other types of stress.[r4] Suckling causes an increase in maternal prolactin levels within ten minutes, with peak values approximately eight times greater than baseline occurring at about 30 minutes (Fig. 56.2).[9] This response to suckling is most intense shortly after delivery, and declines over the ensuing months despite continuation of suckling.

Prolactin-Inhibiting Factors (PIFs)

Although prolactin secretion from the anterior pituitary is controlled by both stimulatory and inhibitory hypothalamic substances, secretory control is predominantly one of tonic inhibition. Separation of the pituitary gland from the hypothalamus, e.g., by stalk section, releases the lactotrophs from the tonic inhibition exacted by the hypothalamus, and allows increased prolactin production while causing a dramatic decrease in the secretion of other anterior pituitary hormones.

The principal hypothalamic factor responsible for inhibition of prolactin synthesis and release appears to be dopamine, a catecholamine secreted by hypothalamic neurons and transported by the hypophyseal portal blood to the anterior pituitary, where it binds to dopamine receptors on the surface of the lactotropes and inhibits prolactin secretion.[r5] Nondopaminergic prolactin-inhibiting factors include GABA, a GnRH-associated peptide, and possibly α-MSH.

Because prolactin does not stimulate the secretion of a target organ hormone, it is not regulated by a traditional long-loop feedback system. Instead, prolactin serves as its own inhibiting factor by binding to

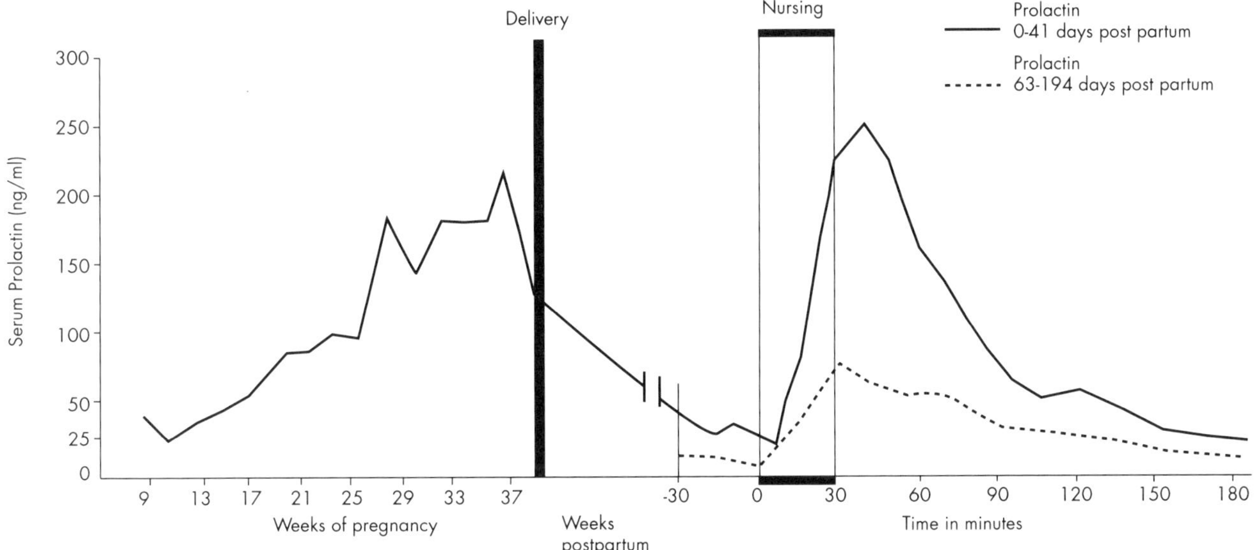

Figure 56.2 Human prolactin in maternal serum (mean ± SEM) throughout pregnancy and in response to nursing in the postpartum period. Redrawn from Metzky OA et al. Am J Obstet Gynecol 151:878–884, 1985 and Noel GL et al. J Cl Endo Metab 38:413–423, 1974.

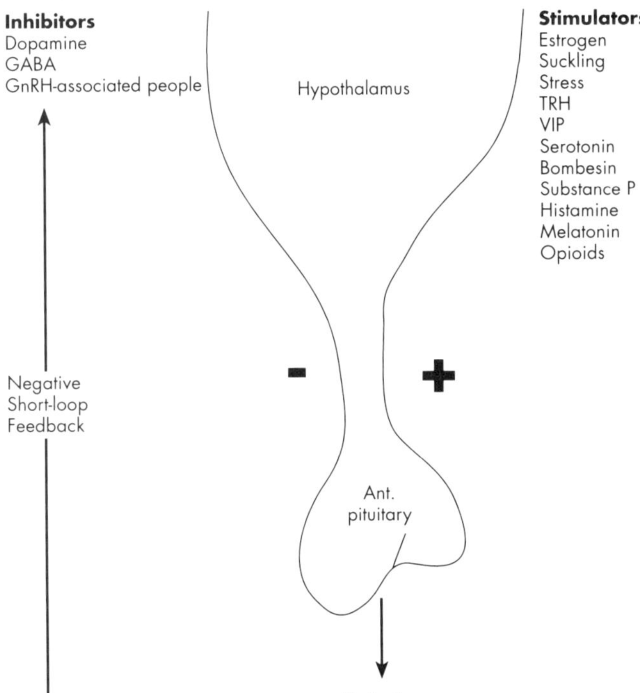

Figure 56.3 Principal Regulators of Prolactin Production in Mammals

receptors in the median eminence and causing increased dopamine synthesis.

Prolactin-Releasing Factors (PRFs)

The two best understood prolactin-releasing factors are thyrotropin-releasing hormone (TRH) and vasoactive intestinal peptide (VIP). Each is secreted by the hypothalamus into the hypophyseal portal blood to stimulate the lactotropes in the pituitary directly. TRH administered IV causes a brisk increase in serum prolactin that peaks within 30 minutes at levels roughly eight times baseline in women and half that level in men.

Although VIP originally was isolated from intestinal extracts, it is also present in both the central and peripheral nervous systems. Intravenous injection of VIP elevates prolactin concentrations and can totally block the stress-induced prolactin response in rats.

Other factors considered as neurotransmitters for the neuronal release of PRFs such as serotonin, histamine, bombesin, substance P, cholecystokinin, neurotensin, galanin, gonadotropin releasing hormone, growth hormone releasing hormone, and melatonin have been reported to stimulate prolactin secretion. The opiates and their synthetic agonists may mediate the increase in prolactin release during stress by decreasing dopamine synthesis by the hypothalamus. This effect is abolished by pretreatment with antagonists such as naloxone.

Physiologic Functions

Breast

In mammals, the primary function of prolactin is to promote lactation.[r6] During pregnancy, prolactin stimulates mammary tissue growth in conjunction with estrogen, progesterone, placental lactogen, cortisol, and insulin. True glandular acini begin forming in the third month of pregnancy, and alveolar secretion begins in the second trimester. Despite high levels of prolactin during pregnancy, lactation does not begin until postpartum, when the inhibitory effects of estrogen on lactation are removed and there is also a 20-fold induction of prolactin receptors. Prolactin stimulates the synthesis of the milk proteins, such as casein, as well as the enzymes, such as α-lactalbumin, necessary for milk production. Each surge in prolactin that occurs with suckling stimulates milk formation, which prepares the breast for the next feeding and maintains an active state of lactogenesis.

Gonadal Function

Suckling and persistent elevations of prolactin suppress ovulation by decreasing the frequency and amplitude of LH pulses. In addition, high levels of prolactin disrupt ovarian function and lead to hypoestrogenism by directly suppressing ovarian androgen synthesis and aromatase activity.[r7] In rats, but apparently not in humans, prolactin is also important in maintaining the corpus luteum.

In human males, prolactin increases the number of LH receptors in the testis, helping to sustain testosterone levels, and, in rodents, prolactin potentiates the effects of androgens on the growth and secretory activity of the male accessory glands. High levels of prolactin, however, decrease libido and potency.

Osmoregulation

Prolactin is involved in osmoregulation in many species. It allows fish that migrate from salt to fresh water to conserve salt; in rats, it has salt-conserving effects on the kidneys and small intestine. It has been proposed that prolactin in amniotic fluid decreases the diffusion of fluid from the fetus to the mother.

Other Effects

The immune functions of prolactin include promoting the migration of IgA-secreting plasma cells into the breast during pregnancy and serving as a mitogen for the Nb2T-cell-derived lymphoma line. In some species, but not in humans, prolactin is important in stimulating nurturing parental behavior.

Bromocriptine in the Treatment of Hyperprolactinemia

A state of "physiologic" hyperprolactinemia occurs in all mammals during pregnancy and in the postpartum period. However, elevations of prolactin (greater than 25 ng/ml in most laboratories) in the nonpregnant or nonlactating state are pathologic, require investigation, and often require treatment. Bromocriptine, a dopamine agonist, is the prototype of drugs used to lower prolactin in "physiologic" hyperprolactinemia as well as in pathologic states. It has become the mainstay of treatment for prolactinomas, although it is also used in conjunction with surgical or radiation therapy.[r8,r9]

Chemistry

Bromocriptine (2-bromo-alpha-ergocryptine mesylate) is a derivative of lysergic acid and one of several ergot alkaloids that are direct dopamine receptor agonists with preference for D2 receptors (dopamine receptors found primarily in the pituitary whose effects are not mediated through cAMP). Other ergot derivatives, such as lisuride, pergolide, and mesulergine, have undergone trials as antiprolactin drugs. The structural relationships of these derivatives to dopamine are illustrated in Figure 56.4.[r10]

History

In the 1950s, Shelesnyak observed that ergot alkaloids prevented the decidualization of rat endometrium by decreasing prolactin concentrations. Subsequently, large numbers of ergot alkaloids were screened for clinical use before bromocriptine was identified in 1967. It was introduced into clinical medicine in 1971 and has become the principal therapeutic agent for the treatment of physiologic as well as pathologic hyperprolactinemic states.[r11] It has supplanted the use of estrogens to suppress postpartum lactation, not only because it is more effective, but also because it does not increase the risk of thromboembolism.

Therapeutic Uses

Postpartum "Physiologic" Hyperprolactinemia

Bromocriptine is prescribed in the immediate postpartum period to stop lactation in mothers who do not wish to breastfeed. When the drug is taken under these circumstances, prolactin concentrations decline within hours to nonpregnant values, and lactation ceases.

Pathologic Hyperprolactinemia

Hyperprolactinemia is the most frequently encountered hypothalamic-pituitary disorder in clinical endocrinology.[r4] The most common pathologic processes that produce hyperprolactinemia are prolactin-secreting tumors (prolactinomas) or processes that interfere with the synthesis, transport, or binding of dopamine to its receptor on the lactotrope (Table 56.1). Bromocriptine is also the mainstay of therapy for pathologic hyperprolactinemia.

The most common presenting symptoms of chronic hyperprolactinemia are amenorrhea, oligomenorrhea, and infertility. In both males and females, it may also be associated with decreased libido. Galactorrhea occurs in 30 to 80 percent of females with hyperprolactinemia.

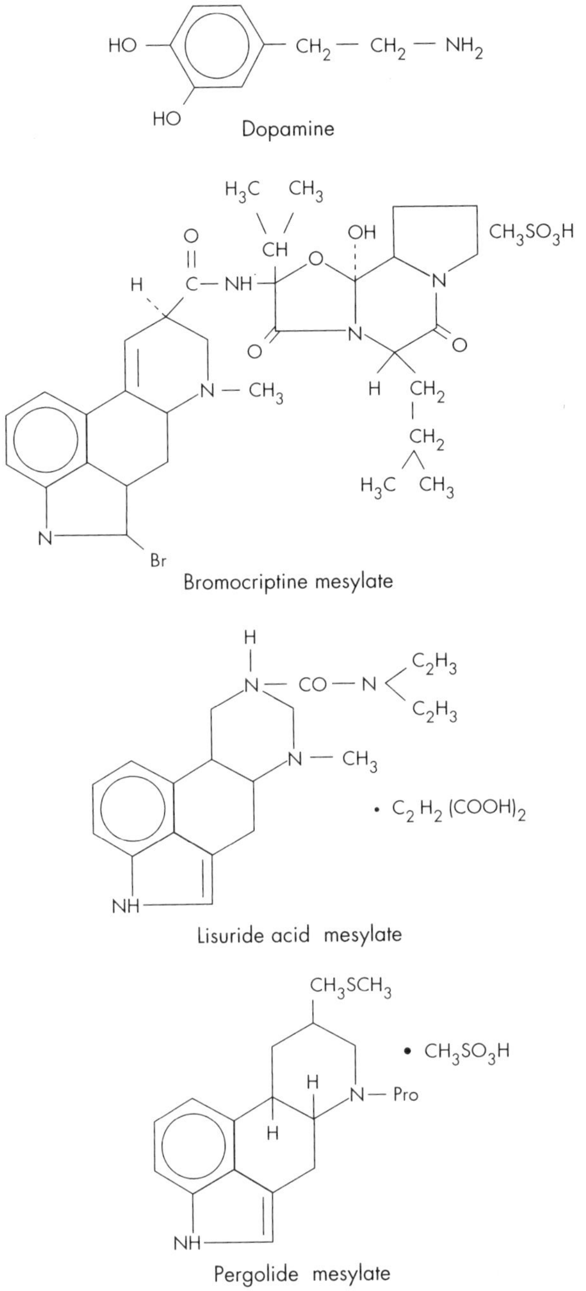

Dopamine

Bromocriptine mesylate

Lisuride acid mesylate

Pergolide mesylate

Figure 56.4 Structural Formulas of Dopamine and 3 Commonly Used Dopamine Receptor Agonists

Medications

Numerous antipsychotic drugs, including phenothiazines (e.g., chlorpromazine), butyrophenone (e.g., haloperidol), benzodiazapines (e.g., clozapine), and the substituted benzamides (e.g., metochlopramide) can produce hyperprolactinemia by blocking the binding of dopamine to its receptor. Tricyclic antidepressants interfere with dopamine action by blocking its reuptake by the presynaptic neuron and enhancing its degradation; alpha-methyldopa inhibits synthesis of DOPA; reserpine depletes hypothalamic dopamine stores.[r10,r12]

Tumor

Prolactinomas are the most common cause of hyperprolactinemia other than drugs. Evidence of a pituitary tumor by CT scan or MR imaging is present in at least 30 percent of women with hyperprolactinemia. Pituitary tumors other than prolactinomas that prevent dopamine transport by disrupting the hypophyseal blood supply and hypothalamic tumors that interfere with dopamine synthesis may also cause elevated prolactin levels. If the hyperprolactinemia is due to a macroadenoma, such symptoms as headache, visual field disturbances, and ophthalmoplegia may be exhibited due to the mass effect; and other pituitary hormonal deficits may be present.

Other Causes

In longstanding hypothyroidism, excessive TRH induces prolactin secretion, which resolves with appropriate thyroid replacement. Hyperprolactinemia also occurs in 20 to 75 percent of men and women with chronic renal failure, and is not improved with hemodialysis. Twenty to 25 percent of women with polycystic ovary syndrome have mildly elevated prolactin levels, perhaps due to elevated estrone concentrations. Chronic nipple or chest wall stimulation also can lead to stimulated prolactin levels.

Other Uses

Bromocriptine is useful as an adjunct to the surgical and radiation treatments of GH-secreting tumors, as well as in the treatment of Parkinson's disease.

Table 56.1 Etiologies of Pathologic Hyperprolactinemia

1. Medications
   Dopamine-receptor blocking agents (phenothiazines, butyrophenones, benzamines)
   Dopamine-depleting agents (tricyclic anti depressants, α-methyl dopa, reserpine)
2. Hypothalamic-Pituitary Disease
   Hypothalamic disease (tumor, inflammation, irradiation)
   Pituitary disease (prolactinoma, other pituitary tumors, stalk section, empty sella)
3. Primary Hypothyroidism
4. Renal failure
5. Neurogenic (chest wall lesions, nipple stimulation)
6. Stress
7. Polycystic Ovarian Disease

Effects of the Drug

Bromocriptine acts directly at the dopamine receptor on the lactotrope to inhibit prolactin release, and in most patients causes prolactin levels to return to normal, galactorrhea to resolve, and menses to return. In patients with prolactinomas, bromocriptine appears to bind preferentially to tumor tissue to inhibit both prolactin synthesis and secretion. Bromocriptine reduces serum prolactin concentrations within hours and tumor size within days to weeks. The latter is due to diminished prolactin synthesis rather than direct tumoral activity. If bromocriptine is discontinued, hyperprolactinemia and attendant symptoms usually recur.

Undesirable Effects

Almost 70 percent of bromocriptine-treated patients experience side-effects. These usually are mild-to-moderate, dose-dependent, and often subside with continued use. Nausea is the most common side-effect, followed by headache, dizziness, fatigue, lightheadedness, and vomiting. Orthostatic hypotension is seen in some patients. High doses of bromocriptine have been associated with hallucinations, confusion, seizures, and stroke. Side-effects seem to be worst in patients given bromocriptine for indications other than hyperprolactinemia. The side-effects can be minimized by taking the drug with meals, starting at a subtherapeutic dose, and gradually increasing. When given during pregnancy, bromocriptine does not appear to increase the rate of birth defects, abortion, or multiple births.

Use of bromocriptine in conjunction with dopamine antagonists may decrease the efficacy of both drugs.

Pharmacokinetics

Forty to 90 percent of an oral dose of bromocriptine is rapidly absorbed from the GI tract. First-pass metabolism is extensive, so that only a small fraction of the dose is available to the tissues. Peak plasma concentrations and biologic action occur two to three hours after a single oral dose, but effects on serum prolactin persist for eight to 12 hours. Bromocriptine is highly protein bound in plasma and is metabolized in the liver. The metabolites do not appear to be active, and most are excreted in the bile.[r11]

Preparations and Doses

Bromocriptine

Bromocritine mesylate (Parlodel) is available for oral use in tablets of 2.5 mg or capsules of 5 mg.

For treatment of hyperprolactinemia, the usual adult dose is 2.5 mg every eight hours with meals. To minimize side-effects, therapy can be initiated with 1.25 mg at bedtime and increased by 1.25 mg every two to three days. Doses as high as 30 mg per day have been employed to suppress prolactin levels in poorly-responsive tumors.

For suppression of postpartum lactation, bromocriptine 2.5 mg twice daily initiated immediately postpartum for two weeks followed by 2.5 mg daily for the third week is now the treatment of choice.

An injectable form of bromocriptine (Parlodel) is now available. A single 50-mg IM dose decreases prolactin concentrations within 24 hours, exhibits peak effect at three weeks, and wears off by six weeks. Unlike oral bromocriptine, it does not appear to cause significant GI side-effects.

Other Dopamine Receptor Agonists

These agents are currently under study but not yet approved for treatment of hyperprolactinemia in the US. Pergolide mesylate (Permax) has a duration of action approximately three times longer than that of bromocriptine, appears to be comparable to bromocriptine in efficacy, and has similar or fewer side-effects. Hyperprolactinemia unresponsive to bromocriptine may respond to pengolide, and vice versa. Pergolide has been approved by the FDA for the treatment of Parkinson's disease only. Other drugs under study include quinagolide, mesulergin, lisuride, terguride, and carbergoline, which also have longer durations of action than bromocriptine.

References

Research Reports

1. Niall HD, Hogan ML, Sauer R, Rosenblum IY, Greenwood FC. Sequences of pituitary and placental lactogenic and growth hormones: Evolution from a primordial peptide by gene reduplication. Proc Natl Acad Sci USA 1971;*68*:866–869.
2. Stricker S, Grueter F. Action du lobe antérieur de l'hypophyse sur la montée laiteuse. Compt Rend Soc Biol 1928;*99*:1978–1980.
3. Riddle O, Bates RW, Dykshorn SW. The preparation, identification and assay of prolactin—a hormone of the anterior pituitary. Am J Physiol 1933;*105*:191–216.
4. Lewis UJ, Singh RNP, Seavey BK. Human prolactin: Isolation and some properties. Biochem Biophys Res Commun 1971;*44*:1169–1176.
5. Hwang P, Guyda H, Friesen HG. A radioimmunoassay for human prolactin. Proc Natl Acad Sci USA 1971;*68*:1902–1906.
6. Cooke NE, Coit D, Weiner RI, Baxter JD, Martial JA. Structure of cloned DNA complementary to rat prolactin messenger RNA. J Biol Chem 1980;*255*:6502–6510.
7. Tyson JE, Hwang P, Guyda H, Friesen HG. Studies of prolactin secretion in human pregnancy. Am J Obstet Gynecol 1972;*113*:14–20.
8. Shull JD, Gorski J. Estrogen regulates the transcription of the rat prolactin gene in vivo through at least two independent mechanisms. Endocrinology 1985;*116*:2456–2462.
9. Noel GL, Suh HK, Frantz AG. Prolactin release during nursing and breast stimulation in postpartum and nonpostpartum subjects. J Clin Endocrinol Metab 1974;*38*:413–423.

Reviews

r1. Cooke NE. Prolactin: Normal synthesis, regulation, and actions. In: DeGroot LE (ed). Endocrinology, 2d ed. Philadelphia: WB Saunders (1989); pp 384–407.

r2. Meites J. Prolactin. In: McCann SM (ed). Endocrinology: People and ideas. Bethesda: American Physiological Society (1988); pp 117–148.

r3. Handwerger S, Richards R, Markoff E. The physiology of decidual prolactin and other decidual protein hormones. TEM 1992;*3*:91–95.

r4. Molitch ME. Pathologic hyperprolactinemia. Endocrinol Metab Clin North Am 1992;*21*:877–901.

r5. Ben-Jonathan N. Dopamine: A prolactin-inhibiting hormone. Endocr Rev 1985;*6*:564–589.

r6. Friesen HG, Cowden EA. Lactation and galactorrhea. In: DeGroot LE (ed). Endocrinology, 2d ed. Philadelphia: WB Saunders (1989); pp 2074–2086.

r7. Blackwell RE. Hyperprolactinemia. Evaluation and management. Endocrinol Metab Clin North Am 1992;*21*:105–124.

r8. Bevan JS, Webster J, Burke CW, Scanlon MF. Dopamine agonists and pituitary tumor shrinkage. Endocr Rev 1992;*13*:220–240.

r9. Archer DF. Current concepts and treatment of hyperprolactinemia. Obstet Gynecol Clinc North Am 1993;*14*:979–998.

r10. Muller EE, Locatelli V, Cella S, Penalva A, Novelli A, Cocci D. Prolactin-lowering and -releasing drugs. Drugs 1983;*25*:399–432.

r11. Ho KY, Thorner MO. Therapeutic applications of bromocriptine in endocrine and neurological diseases. Drugs 1988;*36*:67–82.

r12. Hell K, Wernze H. Drug-induced changes in prolactin secretion. Med Toxicol Adverse Drug Exp 1988;*3*:463–469.

SECTION VII

Pharmacology of Nutrients and Nutritional Diseases

Editor:
Robert E. Olson

CHAPTER 57

Pharmacology of Nutrients and Nutritional Diseases

Robert E. Olson

Introduction to Pharmacology of Nutrients

Nutrition is the science of food and its relationship to health. Nutrition science deals with the nature and distribution of nutrients in foods and their metabolic effects. Nutrients may be defined as chemical compounds in food that are absorbed and utilized to promote health.

Only some nutrients are essential. Furthermore, essentiality varies from species to species. Essential nutrients are those required by each organism that it cannot synthesize. Hence, these nutrients must be derived from food. If they are not supplied in adequate amounts, deficiency diseases result. Conversely, an excess of some essential nutrients may cause toxicity and even death. Essential nutrients vary in nature and amount in the diet, from vitamins like thiamine and riboflavin, amino acids like leucine and threonine, fatty acids like linoleic and linolenic acid, and ions like sodium and potassium. Nonessential nutrients are those that the body can synthesize from other compounds but that also can come from the diet. Total nutrients in the average diet for humans exceed 300, whereas only 45 are essential.

Nutrients are generally divided into two classes. The macronutrients constitute the bulk of the food consumed and supply the energy needed for growth, maintenance, and activity. Macronutrients are required in gram quantities and include proteins, fats, carbohydrates, and some mineral salts. Micronutrients are required in milligram (mg) or microgram (ug) quantities per day. These are the vitamins and trace minerals that catalyze the utilization of the macronutrients.

Many other useful components of the food supply are not digested or metabolized to any appreciable extent. These include some fibers, e.g., cellulose, hemicelluloses, pectins, and gums. In addition, trace components, such as spices, flavors, odors, additives, and many natural products, improve the taste and stability of the diet. As many as 100,000 individual substances can be found in the daily human food supply.

Pathophysiology of Nutritional Disease

If the food supply fails to supply the energy and nutrients needed for health, or if the individual cannot utilize them, deficiency diseases result. Nutritional deficiency diseases can occur by virtue of: (1) a dietary inadequacy (primary malnutrition); (2) GI malabsorption; (3) abnormal systemic loss of nutrients through hemorrhage, diarrhea, or excessive sweating; (4) failure to reabsorb and retain nutrients by the kidney. Items 2–4 are considered causes of secondary malnutrition. In some cases, both primary and secondary events contribute to the malnourished state.

What is the sequence of events leading to a deficiency disease? When nutrients are either not received or not retained by the body, plasma and tissue levels decline. This is the first, usually asymptomatic phase, which must be called the preclinical stage of malnutrition. It is followed in time by loss of cellular stores of the nutrient, which in turn is followed by reduction in all functions that depend on a given nutrient, e.g., synthesis of hemoglobin from iron, plasma proteins from amino acids, coenzyme synthesis from B-complex vitamins, or changes in the expression of genes controlled by the active forms of vitamins A and D (Fig. 57.1).

If the deficiency persists, these biochemical changes are followed by impairment of physiologic functions in given cells and their organs. This can result in failure of hematopoiesis, muscular contraction, skin protection, nerve conduction, night vision, and replacement of tissues required in normal cellular turnover. At this point clinical signs and symptoms occur, and the patient usually seeks medical advice.

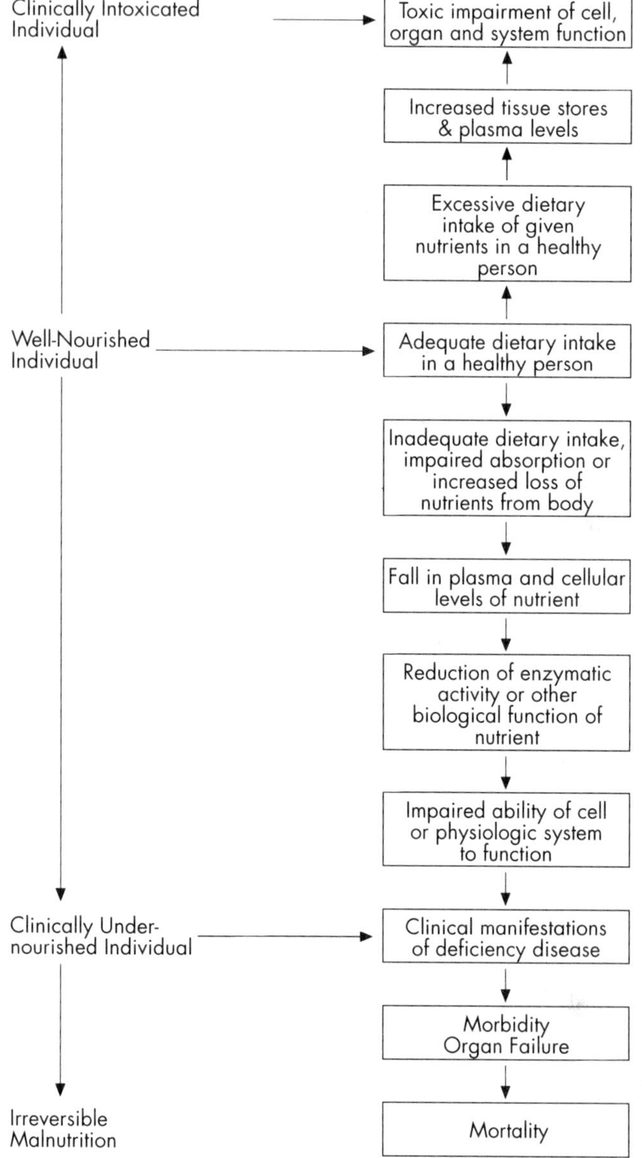

Figure 57.1 Stages of Malnutrition Caused by Excessive or Inadequate Intake of Nutrients

A careful history and analysis of systems usually will help the physician identify the deficiency. For example: anemia may be due to iron, copper, pyridoxine, folic acid, or vitamin B_{12} deficiency; cardiac failure and peripheral neuropathy to thiamine or vitamin B_6 deficiency; failure to thrive in infants may be due to energy and protein deficiency; diarrhea, dementia, and dermatitis to pellagra (niacin deficiency); failure of night vision and xerophthalmia to vitamin A deficiency; failure to develop proper bony structure to lack of vitamin D, calcium, and/or phosphorus; hypotension to sodium deficiency; hemorrhage to vitamin C and/or vitamin K deficiency. The final result of these various nutritional diseases is weakness, lassitude, weight loss, increased morbidity and, if neglected, death. Malnutrition also can reduce immune function, so that infection and its deleterious effects can contribute to both morbidity and mortality.

Nutritional Requirements

One of the essential questions in nutrition science is "Which nutrients are required for normal growth and development and in what amounts at different times during the life cycle?"[r2] The human organism requires about 45 distinct chemical substances that represent the ultimate monomers (unit chemicals) of various components of the diet. For example, nutritionists talk about fat, carbohydrate, and protein as nutrients. In fact, they are sources of nutrients, since they are not used in their polymerized form. These substances are broken down to their component parts in digestion and then absorbed as their monomers. For example, dietary carbohydrates, like starch, mannans, and pentosans, are digested to the simple sugars, glucose, mannose, and pentose. These simple sugars are absorbed and utilized. Dietary proteins are broken down to their 20 individual amino acids before being utilized and resynthesized into proteins required by humans. Likewise, lipids are changed by digestion to a myriad of fatty acids, glycerol, phosphate, and bases such as choline. These are absorbed and resynthesized in the gut to lipoproteins, which are vehicles for transporting lipids to the organs where they are taken up and utilized.

Primitive organisms like blue-green algae have nutritional requirements for only mineral elements, water, carbon dioxide, and ammonia, from which they build up all the constituents of their protoplasm. In the course of evolution, the ability to use elemental substances from the environment has been partly lost, and nutritional requirements for organic compounds developed. The human can synthesize most of the amino acids, all purines and pyrimidines, sugars, and most fats. Essential nutrients for humans include oxygen, water, energy, 8–9 amino acids (children need 9), an additional source of nitrogen (e.g. NH_3), two essential fatty acids, 15 minerals, and 13 vitamins. The actual requirements for a sedentary adult male are shown in Table 57.1. Women and children require less.

Recommended Dietary Allowances

The recommended dietary allowances (RDA) are defined as the levels of nutrients required to meet the requirements of practically all healthy persons in a population.[2] Since the dietary requirements vary among individuals, these recommendations, termed "allowances," take this variability into account by setting the allowance at the level corresponding to the highest requirement for any nutrient. In this way, the RDAs cover the needs for almost all healthy persons and are used in planning diets for groups of people. In most populations the range of requirements may vary as much as two- to threefold.

It should be pointed out that the requirements of persons with illnesses involving changes in metabolism, absorption, and utilization of nutrients are not encompassed by the RDA. The intakes of sick persons should be set individually by a health practitioner.

The RDAs are set by expert committees in 41 countries. In the US RDAs are set by the Food and Nutrition Board of the National Research Council/National Academy of Sciences. The first edition was published in 1943; the 10th edition appeared in 1989. As time has passed, more information has become available about the essential nature of nutrients, so that the number of recommendations has increased since 1943. In the first edition of the RDA, recommendations were made for only four vitamins, protein (as a source of amino acids), energy as calories, and two minerals. In the 10th edition (1989), there were recommendations for 11 vitamins, eight minerals, two essential fatty acids, protein, and energy. The RDAs are given by age, sex, pregnancy, and lactation in Table 57.2, which presents data for 1989.

Table 57.1 Adult Human Daily Requirements for Nutrients (Reference 70-kg man)

A. Macronutrients
1. Water; 1,600 ml/m²/d; 2,400 ml/d
2. Energy; 1,600 kc/m²/d; 2,400 kc/d
3. Protein (supplying the essential amino acids) 60 g/d
4. Fat (the essential fatty acids) 3 g/d
5. Carbohydrates (supplying energy and a minimum of 1 g/kg of glucose equivalents) ~ 100 g/d
6. Minerals (Na, K, Cl, Ca, P, Mg) (Range is (0.5–2.0 g/d)

B. Micronutrients
1. Trace minerals (Fe, Zn, Cu, Mn, Se, F, Mo, I) Range is .05 (for Se) to 10 mg/d (for Fe and Zn)
2. Vitamins
   a. Water-soluble: vitamin C, thiamin, riboflavin, niacin, folate, biotin, pantothenate, pyridoxine, vitamin B_{12} (Range is 2 μg, (for B_{12}) to 60 mg (for ascorbic acid)
   b. Fat-soluble (vitamins A, D, E, K) Range is 5 μg (D) to 8 mg (E)

The usual intake of vitamins is at the preventive level in the range of 0.5 to 1.5 times the RDA. When vitamins are administered as pure compounds for the treatment of severe deficiency diseases, in malabsorption, to counteract genetic conditions, for vitamin deficiency states, or when given at megadoses to achieve other effects, they become "drugs," and their use constitutes therapeutics.[2] Examples of nutrients used to treat specific diseases are: vitamin A for acne; nicotinic acid for hyperlipidemia; and vitamin D for hypoparathyroidism or osteoporosis.

Appraisal of Nutritional Status

The appraisal of nutritional status should be a part of every general health evaluation. It involves all the techniques of the clinical method—taking a history, doing a physical examination, and ordering selected laboratory tests. Appraisals of nutritional status may relate to rate of growth and development of infants and children, to the body composition of both children and adults, and to evidence of specific essential nutrient deficiencies or excesses.

History

History taking generally begins with inquiry of the patient's "chief complaint." Examples of a chief complaint are: (1) headache; (2) weakness; (3) chronic cough; (4) shortness of breath; (5) joint pain; (6) a lump, rash, or sore on the skin that doesn't heal; (7) recent changes in body weight or failure to grow.

The nutritional history is inevitably intertwined with the medical history, and clues of the nature of the nutritional disease are often obtained from the medical history. For instance, a history of GI bleeding can account for iron-deficiency anemia, treatment of acne with vitamin A can lead to vitamin A intoxication man-

Table 57.2 Food and Nutritional Board, National Academy of Sciences—National Research Council Recommended Dietary Allowances,[a] Revised 1989

Designed for the maintenance of good nutrition of practically all healthy people in the United States

		Weight[b]		Height[b]			Fat-Soluble Vitamins				Water-Soluble Vitamins							Minerals						
Category	Age (years) or Condition	(kg)	(lb)	(cm)	(in)	Protein (g)	Vitamin A (μg RE)[c]	Vitamin D (μg)[d]	Vitamin E (mg α-TE)[e]	Vitamin K (μg)	Vitamin C (mg)	Thiamin (mg)	Riboflavin (mg)	Niacin (mg NE)[f]	Vitamin B_6 (mg)	Folate (μg)	Vitamin B_{12} (μg)	Calcium (mg)	Phosphorus (mg)	Magnesium (mg)	Iron (mg)	Zinc (mg)	Iodine (μg)	Selenium (μg)
Infants	0.0–0.5	6	13	60	24	13	375	7.5	3	5	30	0.3	0.4	5	0.3	25	0.3	400	300	40	6	5	40	10
	0.5–1.0	9	20	71	28	14	375	10	4	10	35	0.4	0.5	6	0.6	35	0.5	600	500	60	10	5	50	15
Children	1–3	13	29	90	35	16	400	10	6	15	40	0.7	0.8	9	1.0	50	0.7	800	800	80	10	10	70	20
	4–6	20	44	112	44	24	500	10	7	20	45	0.9	1.1	12	1.1	75	1.0	800	800	120	10	10	90	20
	7–10	28	62	132	52	28	700	10	7	30	45	1.0	1.2	13	1.4	100	1.4	800	800	170	10	10	120	30
Males	11–14	45	99	157	62	45	1,000	10	10	45	50	1.3	1.5	17	1.7	150	2.0	1,200	1,200	270	12	15	150	40
	15–18	66	145	176	69	59	1,000	10	10	65	60	1.5	1.8	20	2.0	200	2.0	1,200	1,200	400	12	15	150	50
	19–24	72	160	177	70	58	1,000	10	10	70	60	1.5	1.7	19	2.0	200	2.0	1,200	1,200	350	10	15	150	70
	25–50	79	174	176	70	63	1,000	5	10	80	60	1.5	1.7	19	2.0	200	2.0	800	800	350	10	15	150	70
	51+	77	170	173	63	63	1,000	5	10	80	60	1.2	1.4	15	2.0	200	2.0	800	800	350	10	15	150	70
Females	11–14	46	101	157	62	46	800	10	8	45	50	1.1	1.3	15	1.4	150	2.0	1,200	1,200	280	15	12	150	45
	15–18	55	120	163	64	44	800	10	8	55	60	1.1	1.3	15	1.5	180	2.0	1,200	1,200	300	15	12	150	50
	19–24	58	128	164	65	46	800	10	8	60	60	1.1	1.3	15	1.6	180	2.0	1,200	1,200	280	15	12	150	55
	25–50	63	138	163	64	50	800	5	8	65	60	1.1	1.3	15	1.6	180	2.0	800	800	280	15	12	150	55
	51+	65	143	160	63	50	800	5	8	65	60	1.0	1.2	13	1.6	180	2.0	800	800	280	10	12	150	55
Pregnant						60	800	10	10	65	70	1.5	1.6	17	2.2	400	2.2	1,200	1,200	320	30	15	175	65
Lactating	1st 6 months					65	1,300	10	12	65	95	1.6	1.8	20	2.1	280	2.6	1,200	1,200	355	15	19	200	75
	2nd 6 months					62	1,200	10	11	65	90	1.6	1.7	20	2.1	260	2.6	1,200	1,200	340	15	16	200	75

[a] The allowances, expressed as average daily intakes over time, are intended to provide for individual variations among most normal persons as they live in the United States under usual environmental stresses. Diets should be based on a variety of common foods in order to provide other nutrients for which human requirements have been less well defined. See text for detailed discussion of allowances and of nutrients not tabulated.

[b] Weights and heights of Reference Adults are actual medians for the U.S. population of the designated age, as reported by NHANES II. The median weights and heights of those under 19 years of age were taken from Hamill et al. (1979) (see pages 16–170). The use of these figures does not imply that the height-to-weight ratios are ideal.

[c] Retinol equivalents. 1 retinol equivalent = 1 μg retinol or 6 μg β-carotene. See text for calculation of vitamin A activity of diets as retinol equivalents.

[d] As cholecalciferol. 10 μg cholecalciferol = 400 iu of vitamin D.

[e] α-Tocopherol equivalents. 1 mg d-α tocopherol = 1 α-TE. See text for variation in allowances and calculation of vitamin E activity of the diet as α-tocopherol equivalents.

[f] 1 NE (niacin equivalent) is equal to 1 mg of niacin or 60 mg of dietary tryptophan.

ifested by headache, nausea, and diplopia, and an enlargement of the thyroid gland may be due to iodine deficiency.

What are some of the high risk states that may identify patients with nutritional disorders? Table 57.3 presents a number of conditions that predispose to nutritional disease, such as gross underweight, gross overweight, recent weight loss, alcoholism, malabsorption, hyperthyroidism, protracted fever, and/or sepsis. A diet history should be part of the medical history, and physicians should be acquainted with its use. The methods employed for diet history-taking include: (1) a 24-hour recall of foods eaten; (2) a food frequency questionnaire that asks about foods or food groups frequently taken; (3) a food diary in which the patient reports in writing what is eaten over a three-day period; (4) a weighed ad libitum diet that is selected by the patient and weighed each day. This last method, which can extend from three days to a week, is the most accurate but also the most labor-intensive.

Table 57.3 Nutritionally High-Risk Patients

- Gross underweight: weight-for-height (or BMI) below 80% of standard
- Gross overweight: weight-for-height (or BMI) above 120% of standard
- Recent loss of 10% or more of usual body weight
- Persons with a high alcohol intake
- No oral intake (npo) for over 10 days
- Protracted nutrient losses due to
  - Malabsorption syndromes
  - Short-gut syndromes/fistulae
  - Renal dialysis
  - Draining abscesses, wounds
- Increased metabolic needs
  - Extensive burns, infection, trauma
  - Protracted fever
  - Hyperthyroidism
- Intake of drugs with antinutrient or catabolic properties: appetite depressants, steroids, immunosuppressants, antitumor agents

Physical Examination

The physical examination should be an objective evaluation of the patient's appearance, manner, and organ functions as appraised by inspection, palpation, auscultation, and sensory stimulation. Every body system can be involved in nutritional disease. For example, the CNS is involved in pellagra, beri beri, pyridoxine deficiency (and excess), and vitamin B_{12} deficiency. Taste and smell are affected by zinc deficiency and in diseases related to obesity, hypertension, and coronary artery disease. The GI system can be altered through malnutrition and alcoholism. The oral cavity (lips, tongue, teeth, gums, and buccal mucosa) is affected by vitamin B-complex deficiency and scurvy. The thyroid gland is enlarged in iodine deficiency, and the skin may reveal a variety of changes due to malnutrition, including rashes, petechial hemorrhages, ecchymoses, pigmentation, edema, and dryness. Bones and joints are diseased in rickets, osteomalacia, osteoporosis, and scurvy and are studied by radiographs.

Anthropometric Measurements: Height and Weight

Measurements of height and weight generally are considered part of the physical examination. Other anthropometric measurements include measurements of skin fold thickness and mid-arm muscle circumference. Height and weight are critical to estimations of desirable weight and optimal body proportions. Desirable weights, which are approximately equal to average weights at age 25, are shown in Table 57.4. Desirable weights for height also can be determined by computing the body mass index, or BMI, which is the weight in kilograms divided by the height in meters squared and is a guide to desirable body composition. The general accepted normal range of BMI for males and females is 20 to 25, a variation of 10 percent around the mean of 22.5. The relationship of the BMI to various degrees of undernutrition and overnutrition is shown in Table 57.5. These standards for the growth and weight gain of infants up to the age of 18 are available in pediatric textbooks and other manuals.[r2]

Table 57.4 Weight-Height Reference Chart (Adults)*

Height (no shoes)		Reference weight			
		Women		Men	
Feet/ inches	Centimeters	Pounds	Kilograms	Pounds	Kilograms
4 10	147	101	46	—	—
4 11	150	104	47	—	—
5 0	152	107	49	—	—
5 1	155	110	50	—	—
5 2	157	113	51	124	56
5 3	160	116	53	127	58
5 4	162	120	54	130	59
5 5	165	123	56	133	60
5 6	167	128	58	137	62
5 7	170	132	60	141	64
5 8	172	136	62	145	66
5 9	175	140	63	149	68
5 10	178	144	65	153	69
5 11	180	148	67	158	71
6 0	183	152	69	162	74
6 1	185	—	—	167	76
6 2	188	—	—	171	78
6 3	190	—	—	176	80
6 4	193	—	—	181	82

*Data adapted from Metropolitan Life Insurance Company: Build and Blood Pressure Study, 1959.

Table 57.5 Standards for Desirable Weight and Abnormal Weight Using Body Mass Index (BMI)

Nutritional Status	BMI (Wt in Kg/(Ht m)^2)	Percent Change From Desired Weight
Undernutrition		
Grade 2	16	−30
Grade 1	16–17.9	(−21) to (−30)
Thin	18–19.9	(−11) to (−20)
Normal	20–25	±10
Fat	25.1–26.9	+11 to +20
Obesity		
Grade 1	27–29.9	+21 to +32
Grade 2	30–40	+33 to +77
Grade 3	40	+77

Creatinine: Height Index

The creatinine-height index is a measure of lean body mass. Creatinine is the spontaneous decomposition product of creatine phosphate, a high-energy component of muscle. The amount of creatinine coefficient, i.e., milligrams of creatinine excreted per kilogram body weight is 10 to 25 in women and 18 to 32 in men, reflecting their variations in muscle mass. Average values for urinary creatinine as a function of height are presented in Table 57.6. The creatinine-height index diminishes as the lean body decreases. When the lean body mass is decreased 60 to 80 percent of normal, the patient is considered malnourished; when it reaches 60 percent of normal, the patient is regarded as severely malnourished.[r2]

Triceps Skin Fold

The triceps skin fold (TSF) provides an estimate of fat stores. About 50 percent of the average person's adipose tissue is beneath the skin. The skinfold consists of a double layer of skin and subcutaneous fat, which is measured with a special large skin fold caliper at several sites. Subscapular, lower thoracic, ileac, and abdominal sites can be used, although the deltoid triceps is used most often because of its easy accessibility and the usual absence of edema at this site. The triceps skin fold (TSF) averages about 12 millimeters in males

Table 57.6 Ideal Urinary Creatinine Values (mg), Adults*

Male*		Female**	
Height (cm)	Ideal Creatinine (mg)	Height (cm)	Ideal Creatinine (mg)
157.5	1288	147.3	830
160.0	1325	149.9	851
162.6	1359	152.4	875
165.1	1386	154.9	900
167.6	1426	157.5	925
170.2	1467	160.0	949
172.7	1513	162.6	977
175.3	1555	165.1	1006
177.8	1596	167.6	1044
180.3	1642	170.2	1076
182.9	1691	172.7	1109
185.4	1739	175.3	1141
188.0	1785	177.8	1174
190.5	1831	180.3	1206
193.0	1891	182.9	1240

*Creatinine coefficient (males)—23 mg/kg of ideal body weight
**Creatinine coefficient (females)—18 mg/kg of ideal body weight.

and about 23 in females (Table 57.7). A wide range on either side of the standard is considered an acceptable TSF measure, since large variances are found for fatfold thicknesses in the normal population. A patient whose TSF thickness is less than 50 per cent of the HANES standard is considered to have depleted body fat stores; those with TSF 50 percent above the standard are considered obese.[r3]

Midarm Muscle Area

This derived value is used to estimate lean body or skeleton muscle mass. To calculate this value, the midarm circumference must first be measured at the same site as the triceps fatfold with the patient's right arm in a relaxed posture. The average midarm circumference for males is about 26 cm and for females about 23 cm. The formula to calculate bone-free, upper-arm midarm muscle area in mm^2 is:

$$\frac{[\text{midarm circumference (cm)} - (3.14 \times \text{TSF cm})]^2}{4\pi}$$
$$- 10 \text{ (males)}$$
$$- 6.5 \text{ (females)}$$

This formula corrects the area of the upper arm for fat and bone. Median values are shown in Table 57.7. A value 30 to 35 per cent below this standard (depending on age) is indicative of a depletion of lean body mass.[r4]

Laboratory Studies

Both biophysical and biochemical laboratory studies are useful in appraising nutritional status. In addition to the usual radiographs, imaging techniques such as computer assisted tomography (CAT scans) and magnetic resonance imaging (MRI) are useful in viewing soft tissues. Radiographs of both the thorax and the skeleton are important to determine cardiopulmonary function and bone density. Gastrointestinal disturbances secondary to malnutrition can be studied radiographically with contrast media. Laboratory tests are designed to measure given physiologic systems, such as the hematopoietic and endocrine systems. The plasma proteins, lipids, electrolytes, trace minerals and vitamins can provide evidence about body stores of these nutrients. Modern analytical instrumentation with high-pressure liquid chromatography or enzyme radio immunoassays or flame photometry has greatly improved the sensitivity and specificity of biochemical tests for nutritional status. The body stores of some vitamins, particularly the B-complex, can be estimated by measurement of urinary excretion before and after load tests. There are nutrient-dependent enzymatic tests that can be applied to both red and white blood cells. The immune status can be appraised by studying lymphocyte counts, immunoglobulin levels, and the response of lymphocytes to mitogens. Delayed hypersensitivity reactions can be studied by applying selected antigens to the skin. A summary of the cellular and biochemical examinations applicable to determination of nutritional status is shown in Table 57.9.

In conclusion, evaluation of nutritional status em-

Table 57.7 Some Anthropometric Criteria for Normal and Abnormal Nutritional Status

Measurement	Standard		At Risk for Malnutrition
	Men	Women	%
Tricep Skinfold (mm)	12	23	50
Midarm Muscle area (cm^2)	54	33	70

*Values for men and women 18–74 years old from NHANESI (1971–74) and NHANESII (1976–1980) ref Fransancho 1990. The values for those at risk correspond to less than the 15 percentile of those measured.

Table 57.8 Quantitative Values Commonly Used to Stratify Nutritional Status

Method of Assessment	Normal	Moderately malnourished	Severely malnourished
Ideal weight,%*	90–110	60–80	60
Creatinine-height index: (24-h urine creatinine) Actual/Ideal × 100 %	90–110	60–80	60
Serum albumin, (g/dL)	3.5–5.5	2.1–3.0	< 2.1
Serum transferrin, (mg/dL)	200–400	100–150	< 100
Total lymphocyte count, (per mm^3)	1500–3000	800–1200	< 800
Delayed hypersensitivity index***	2	1	0

*See Table 57.4 for data
**See Table 57.6 for data
***Delayed hypersensitivity index quantitates the amount of induration elicited by skin testing with a common antigen such as Candida, Trichophyton, or mumps. Induration grade 0 = 0.5 cm 1 = 0.5 cm 2 = 1.0 cm.

Table 57.9 Cellular and Biochemical Examinations

1. Complete blood count including hematocrit, hemoglobin, RBC, red cell indices; WBC, lymphocytes and differential.
2. Plasma proteins including albumin, globulin, prealbumin, transferrin and retinal binding protein.
3. Plasma nitrogen, BUN, creatinine, uric acid.
4. Plasma lipids including total cholesterol, triglycerides, LDL-cholesterol and HDL-cholesterol.
5. Plasma electrolytes: Na^+, K^+, Cl^-, HCO_3^-, Mg^{2+}, Ca^{2+}, HPO_4^{2-}.
6. Vitamins: plasma vitamin A, vitamin E, 25-OH-D, vitamin K, vitamin C, folate and vitamin B_{12}, urinary thiamin, riboflavin, N-methylnicotinamide; RBC transketolase and glutathione reductase.
7. Minerals: a) plasma: iron, zinc, copper, manganese.
   b) urine: sodium, zinc, copper, manganese, phosphorus.
8. Urinary nitrogen, urea, creatinine, uric acid, hydroxyproline, 3-methylhistidine.
9. Skin tests for antigens (to assess cell-mediated immunity).

ploys the age-old methodology of the physician, upgraded by scientific advances, in arriving at a diagnosis. Data from the medical and dietary history, the physical examination, and laboratory tests must be integrated into a scenario that will produce a differential diagnosis that can be refined by treatment and follow-up.

Dietary Pharmacology

According to G.A. Spiller,[4] dietary pharmacology is the study of the pharmacologic consequences of ingestion of particular dietary components (usually not essential) that may exceed amounts usually found in diets. P.B. Dews,[5] in his definition of dietary pharmacology, adds behavioral consequences to the pharmacologic result of a dietary component, but points out that it may be in concentrations within the range of reasonable dietary practices. For example, fiber is present in low amounts in some diets and high amounts in others, but supplements of fiber often exceed usual dietary practices. Large variations in the relative amounts of protein, carbohydrate, and fats are within the range of reasonable dietary practices, but the use of complex carbohydrates to change bowel habits or amino acid supplements to change behavior constitutes dietary pharmacology.

According to Dews,[5] the province of dietary pharmacology stretches from the study of alcohol, caffeine, and herbal hallucinogens (where it overlaps with ordinary pharmacology) to the effects of modest changes in the content of amino acids and fatty acids to achieve a therapeutic effect.

One good example of dietary pharmacology is the effect of elevating linoleic acid from its essential level as a source of polyunsaturated fatty acids (about 3% of calories) to 15 percent of calories, at which level it exerts a hypolipidemic effect on plasma cholesterol and lipoprotein levels. A recommendation to reduce saturated fats and cholesterol has become part of the prudent diet for controlling certain types of hyperlipidemia. In other words, linoleic acid has a new activity in controlling lipid synthesis that gives it the properties of a drug, although it is within the dietary range of the composition of foods. Likewise, the use of supplementary tryptophan (2–3 g/d) to change its ratio to other amino acids in the hope that it will alter behavior by increasing the synthesis of serotonin, a neurotransmitter, is another example of dietary pharmacology. The most obvious effect of this dietary change is sleepiness, in fact, tryptophan has been recommended as a sleeping potion.

Parenteral nutrition (TPN) is a form of nutritional therapeutics. The IV infusions contain amino acids in doses that exceed the normal requirements but can be considered to be in the dietary range. Vitamins and minerals are also given in high doses because of the portal of entry, namely the venous circulation, which bypasses the normal regulatory mechanisms of the gut and the enterohepatic circulation. Sometimes it is the only satisfactory way to deliver nutrients to an individual whose gut is inactive, blocked, or absent.

Parenteral nutrition should be considered part of pharmacology and therefore part of nutritional pharmacology for several reasons: (1) nutrients are administered by vein; (2) the doses of nutrients employed are usually considerably higher than those present in the diet; (3) the handling of nutrients given in the general circulation is often different from those administered via the GI route.

Other examples of dietary pharmacology include the administration of lecithin and choline to affect cholinergic neural transmission, the administration of branched-chain amino acids to cause changes in anabolism in patients with liver failure, portocaval shunts, burns, or serious injuries.

The use of plant and marine sterols to reduce cholesterol absorption is a form of dietary pharmacology. These sterols are not well absorbed by the animal GI tract, but nonetheless compete with cholesterol for its absorption. This is an example of the pharmacologic use of a substance normally present in the diet at higher than normal concentrations. The same is true of dietary fiber, particularly guar gum, used to slow glucose absorption and reduce the glycemic index. This fiber, normally found in foodstuffs, can be used at higher levels as a pharmacologic agent for selected patients.

Lactulose, a synthetic disaccharide of galactose and fructose, has been used in the treatment of portocaval encephalopathy, which takes advantage of the fact that lactulose is not digestible in the small bowel and is fermented in the large bowel. It is thought that lactulose reduces ammonia production in the GI tract, ammonia being a cerebral toxin, particularly for patients with severe liver disease.

Vitamins in therapeutic amounts (normally 5–10 times the RDA) are indicated only for the treatment of deficiency states or pathologic conditions in which absorption and utilization of vitamins is reduced or requirements increased. In addition, vitamins are used for the treatment of non-nutritive disease, in which large doses have unique effects independent of their nutritional activity. The decision to employ vitamin preparations in therapeutic amounts clearly rests with the physician, and the importance of medical supervision under these conditions cannot be overestimated.

When nicotinic acid is administered at the RDA level of 15–20 mg/day, it is a nutritional supplement. On the other hand, nicotinic acid at 1500 to 3000 mg/d (150 times the RDA) to control hyperlipidemia is functioning as a drug. Nicotinic acid at gram levels has an entirely different physiologic activity than when administered at the RDA level. Under these conditions, nicotinic acid suppresses free fatty acid release from adipose tissue acid and tends to reduce lipoprotein secretion by the liver.

Vitamin D and its derivatives are used for the pharmacologic treatment of certain bone diseases, such as osteoporosis and renal osteodystrophy. In the case of vitamin A, the small physiologic dose of retinol of 10 ug/kg/d, prevents xerophthalmia. As a drug, 2 mg/kg/d of retinol (200 times the physiologic dose), however, may exert an antiproliferative effect in the skin. At or beyond this therapeutic dose, frank toxicity may occur, including embryotoxicity and birth defects.[r1] Nonetheless, the retinoids have also been used to combat certain types of cancer.

Since the margin of safety for vitamins A and D (between physiologic activity and toxicity) can be as low as five times the RDA in some persons, severe disease of the skin, liver, kidneys, and bones can occur and represent a risk to be considered in using these vitamins as drugs.

Alcohol ingestion is a form of dietary pharmacology. Ethyl alcohol in humans is a metabolite of glucose in traces, a food in moderation, and a drug at high doses. Endogenous alcohol is produced in minute amounts through shunts in the pyruvate dehydrogenase system[6]; at that level (<1 mg/dl), it has no pharmacologic effect.

If one consumes alcohol in moderation, i.e., two glasses of wine per day, which provides about 20 g of ethanol and equals about 140 calories (around 6% of total calories), such use usually does not intoxicate. Under these conditions, alcohol can be considered a food. Moderate drinking is defined as two to four whisky ounce equivalents per day (17–34 g of alcohol per day), which enters the zone of use as a drug. Higher intake, i.e., 40 g of alcohol per day in men and 20 g in women, over long periods is the minimum effective dose for cirrhosis of the liver. Some alcoholics take as much as 750 ml of 80 proof (40%) (around 200 g of alcohol per day), which causes serious intoxication, reduces dietary intake of protective foods, and causes injury to many tissues, particularly of the CNS, liver, and GI tract.

The major chapters to follow include those on vitamins, minerals, starvation, and undernutrition and obesity. Each nutrient considered will be discussed under: (1) history; (2) chemistry; (3) physiology; (4) requirements; (5) deficiency disease; (6) therapeutic uses; (7) toxicology; and (8) preparations.

Nutrients used in doses exceeding 5 times the RDA will be considered drugs; in some instances such doses create novel effects in the organism not related to the primary function of the nutrient.

References

Research Reports

1. Olson RE. Clinical nutrition: An interface between human ecology and internal medicine. Nutr Rev 1978;*36*:161–177.
2. Food and Nutrition Board, National Research Council. Recommended dietary allowance, 10th Ed. Washington: National Academy Press, 1989.
3. Council on Scientific Affairs American Medical Association. Vitamin preparations as dietary supplements and as therapeutic agents. JAMA 1987;*257*:1929–1936.
4. Spiller, GA. Defining nutritional pharmacology. In Nutritional pharmacology. New York: Liss, 1981; pp 1–30.
5. Dews PB. Dietary pharmacology. Nutr Rev 1986;*44*:(Supplement) 246–251.
6. McManus IR, Contag AO, Olson RE. Studies on the identification and origin of ethanol in mammalian tissues. J Biol Chem 1966;*241*:349–356.
7. Blackburn GL et al. A nutritional and metabolic assessment of the hospitalized patient. J Parent Enter Nutr 1977;*1*:11–15.
8. Frisancho AR. New norms of upper limb fat and muscle areas for assessment of nutritional status. Am J Clin Nutr 1981;*34*:2540.

Reviews

r1. DiPalma JR, Ritchie DM. Vitamin toxicity. Ann Rev Pharmacol Toxicol 1977;*17*:133–148.

r2. Weinsier RL, Butterworth CE. Handbook of Clinical Nutrition. St. Louis: CV Mosby, 1981.

r3. Gibson RS. Nutritional assessment: A laboratory manual. New York: Oxford University Press, 1993.

r4. Russell RM. Nutritional assessment in: Wyngaarden JB, Smith LH: Cecil Textbook of Medicine 18th Ed., Philadelphia: WB Saunders, 1988, pp 1208–1211.

CHAPTER 58

Robert E. Olson
Paul L. Munson

Fat-Soluble Vitamins

A vitamin is defined as an organic dietary substance required in trace amounts (μg to mg per day) by animals and humans for health. The history of research on the vitamins extends back to Hippocrates, the first Greek physician, who recognized the power of food to cure certain illnesses. The classic vitamin deficiency diseases have been recognized as diseases of unknown etiology by physicians since the time of Christ. In the early years of this century the five classic vitamin deficiency diseases were related to their specific causes: xerophthalmia (vitamin A); beriberi (thiamine); rickets (vitamin D); pellagra (niacin); and scurvy (vitamin C). In addition, modern nutritional investigations have recently revealed additional deficiency diseases related to other vitamins. All of these developments will be discussed in detail.

Thirteen vitamins are required by humans. These include four fat-soluble vitamins: A (retinol); D (cholecalciferol); E (α-tocopherol); and K (phylloquinone). There are nine water-soluble vitamins: thiamine; riboflavin; niacin; pantothenic acid; folic acid; pyridoxine; biotin; vitamin B_{12}; and ascorbic acid.

Fat-Soluble Vitamins

The fat-soluble vitamins, vitamins A, D, E, and K, were discovered between 1917 and 1929, subsequently isolated, chemically characterized, and then synthesized. Their chemical names, precursors, and biologic active forms are shown in Table 58.1. The fat-soluble vitamins differ from the water-soluble vitamins in more than solubility.

Fat-soluble vitamins, as a class, deal with the regulation of protein synthesis, although some have collateral actions. This is in contrast to the B-complex vitamins, which form coenzymes and catalyze the oxidation of small molecules in the production of energy.

The active forms of vitamins A and D are now identified as ligands for two transcription factors that belong to the superfamily of steroid and thyroid hormone receptors. These receptors interact with DNA and control gene expression. Vitamin E is an antioxidant but, in addition, controls the synthesis of a number of biologically significant proteins. Vitamin K controls at the posttranslational level the synthesis of a number of proteins involved in coagulation and in the metabolism of bone.

Fat-soluble vitamins also have some interesting chemical properties. In common with the steroid hormones, they all possess an isoprenoid structure. These vitamins also require carrier proteins for transport, as is true of all lipids in the body. Vitamins A and D are carried by specific plasma proteins, whereas vitamins E and K are carried by plasma lipoproteins.

All fat-soluble vitamins are converted to active forms. The active forms of vitamin A are oxidation products of retinol, namely retinal, which functions as a photosensitive pigment in the eye, and two isomers of retinoic acid, which interact with genomic receptors. α-Tocopherol must be ionized before its electrons become available for antioxidation, and vitamin K must

Table 58.1 Characteristics of the Fat-Soluble Vitamins

Vitamin	Date of Discovery	Chemical Name	Precursor	Active Form
Vitamin A	1917	Retinol	β-Carotene	Retinal, retinoic acid
Vitamin D_2	1919	Ergocalciferol	Ergosterol	1,25-Dihydroxyergocalciterol
Vitamin D_3	1919	Cholecalciferol	7-Dehydrocholesterol	1,25-Dihydroxycholecalciferol
Vitamin E	1925	α-Tocopherol	None	α-Tocopherol anion
Vitamin K	1929	Phylloquinone	Menadione	Dihydrophylloquinone

be reduced to the hydroquinone in order to catalyze the formation of protein-bound (gamma)-carboxy-glutamic acid.

Although these vitamins are not required by lower forms, e.g., bacteria and other unicellular organisms, they are needed by higher organisms to regulate the synthesis of proteins concerned with differentiation, bone and mineral metabolism, reproduction, and the proliferation of various cell types.

The fat-soluble vitamins will be discussed here as follows: (1) history; (2) chemistry; (3) physiology; (4) nutritional requirements; (5) deficiency diseases; (6) therapeutic uses; (7) toxicology; and (8) preparations.

Vitamin A

History

Night blindness, a manifestation of vitamin A deficiency, was first described in Egypt around 1500 BC. Although it was not then linked to a dietary deficiency, liver extracts were originally applied to the eyes and later ingested in order to cure the disease. Xerophthalmia was first described in the mid-nineteenth century in Brazil and Africa. Vitamin A was discovered in 1913 by McCollum and Davis[1] in experiments that showed that butterfat and egg yolk but not lard or olive oil promoted growth in rats and prevented eye signs. In 1917, McCollum[r1] suggested that human xerophthalmia was a manifestation of vitamin A deficiency. Carotene was identified as a precursor of vitamin A by Moore in 1930,[2] and the isolation, structure, and synthesis of vitamin A were accomplished by Karrer and Morf[3] in 1931. In 1934 Wald discovered that the photosensitive pigment of the eye was retinal.[4]

Chemistry

Vitamin A refers generically to all compounds structurally related to retinol that have its biologic activity. In addition, there is a large number of synthetic compounds related to retinol, which are called retinoids. Some retinoids are devoid of vitamin A activity, but have anticancer and anticell differentiation activities. In addition to the all-transretinol, five other isomers (7-cis, 9-cis, 11-cis, 13-cis, and 9,13-cis) have vitamin A activity. The 11-cis isomer of retinol is of particular importance in vision. Of some 400 known cartenoids, all-trans β-carotene is the most widely distributed and the most effective precursor of vitamin A. (Fig. 58.1)

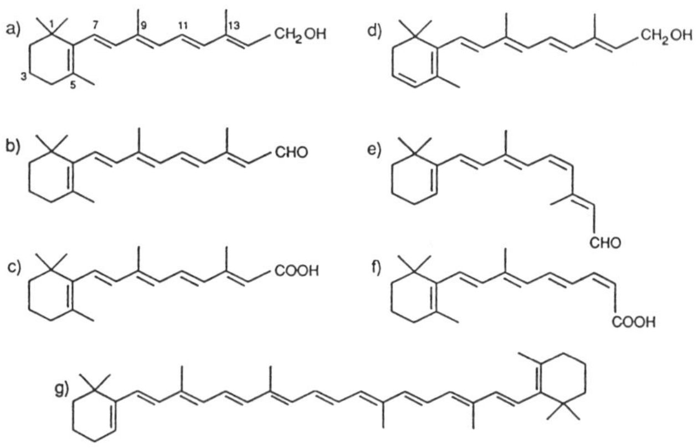

Figure 58.1 Structures of selected retinoids and β-carotene: a) all-trans retinol; b) all-trans retinal; c) all trans retinoic acid; d) all-trans dehydroretinol (vitamin A_2); e) 11-cis retinol; f) 13-cis retinoic acid (isotretinoin); and g) all-trans β-carotene.

Physiology

Vitamin A is present in food mainly as the palmitate ester. It is hydrolyzed in the small intestine by a pancreatic esterase and an intestinal brush border hydrolase. Bile salts are required for activation of these enzymes and the formation of the mycelle conducive to vitamin A absorption. Retinol is absorbed as the free alcohol by an active transport system containing a cellular retinol binding protein (CRBPII).[r2] The yellow beta carotene also requires bile salts for absorption and is converted to vitamin A mainly in the small bowel.

Beta carotene is converted enzymatically to retinal in the enterocyte and then reduced to retinol by an alcohol dehydrogenase. The product is then esterified with palmitic acid and enters the chylomicron as retinyl palmitate. (Fig. 58.2) Chylomicrons are reduced in size by lipoprotein lipase, and the chylomicron remnant is taken up principally by the liver. After uptake, the retinyl ester is hydrolyzed to free retinol, incorporated into retinol-binding protein (RBP molecular weight 21,000), and secreted as a complex into the plasma, where it combines with transthyretin (molecular weight 55,000) to form a ternary complex (of molecular weight 76,000) resistant to glomerular filtration in the kidney (Fig. 58.3). The retinol in plasma is distributed to peripheral cells by the RBP-TT carrier system, where it is taken up via cell surface RBP receptors.[5]

The body pool of vitamin A in well-nourished humans is about 10 mg/kg of body weight, with 90% in the liver. It is distributed between hepatocytes and stellate cells, the latter being a storage depot for vitamin A. In the steady state the daily intake of 1 mg of retinol equivalents equilibrates with various retinol tissue pools that ultimately are oxidized to retinoic acid and other chain-shortened acids. These acid metabolites are excreted in the urine as free acids or via the bile as glycuronides.

There are three main physiologic functions of vitamin A: (1) maintenance of vision, particularly night vision; (2) maintenance of epithelial tissues; and (3) differentiation of many other tissues, particularly during reproduction, gestation, and growth. In vision, all trans-retinol is taken up by an RBP receptor in the eye, the retinol is endocytosed, oxidized to retinal, and isomerized to the 11 cis-derivative. 11 cis-retinal then condenses with opsin to form rhodopsin (MW 40,000). When light strikes rhodopsin, it causes an isomerization of the 11 cis-retinal and a conformational change in rhodopsin to produce metarhodopsin II. This photoexcited rhodopsin triggers an enzymatic cascade that results in the hydrolysis of cyclic GMP. This event closes sodium channels in the plasma membrane, results in hyperpolarizaton of the membrane, and sends an impulse to the brain that is registered as light.[r3]

The other functions of vitamin A are somatic and are accomplished by retinoic acid interacting with the genome. In vitamin A-responsive tissues, plasma RBP-retinol is internalized and the retinol is bound to retinol-binding protein CRBPI (MW 15,000). The retinol is oxidized to retinoic acid, which is quickly bound to a retinoic acid cellular binding protein (CRABP), which is part of the shuttle system for delivering retinol to its final DNA-binding receptor, RAR or RXR. These act as transcription factors and result in the expression of a variety of genes. The vitamin A receptors (RAR and RXR) are part of a family of steroid, thyroid, and fat-soluble vitamin receptors that have related structures and that result in the expression of genes specific for each ligand.[6] (Fig. 58.4)

All the retinoic acid receptors contain 462 amino acids distributed in conventional domains, i.e.: (a) short-enhancer region; (b) a DNA-binding region; and (c) a retinoic acid-binding region. The RAR- and RXR-

Figure 58.2 Metabolism of β-carotene in the intestinal mucosa. Carotene is oxidized to retinaldehyde, which is reduced to retinol and esterified with palmitate via its coenzyme A (CoA) thioester.

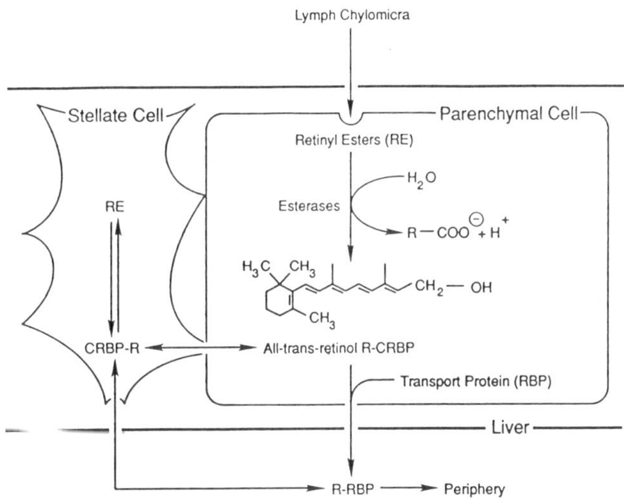

Figure 58.3 Metabolism of retinol esters in the liver. Retinol palmitate is delivered to the hepatocyte via the chylomicron remnant. The ester is hydrolyzed and the free retinol is taken up by a cellular retinol-binding protein (CRBP). If retinol is in excess of hepatocyte needs for secretion to the plasma, the retinol is transferred to the stellate cell for storage, which can return retinol to the hepatocyte as needed. The hepatocyte, and possibly the stellate cell, secrete plasma retinol-binding protein (RBP) complexed with retinol for delivery to peripheral tissues. RBP-specific receptors exist on the membranes of most cells.[r5]

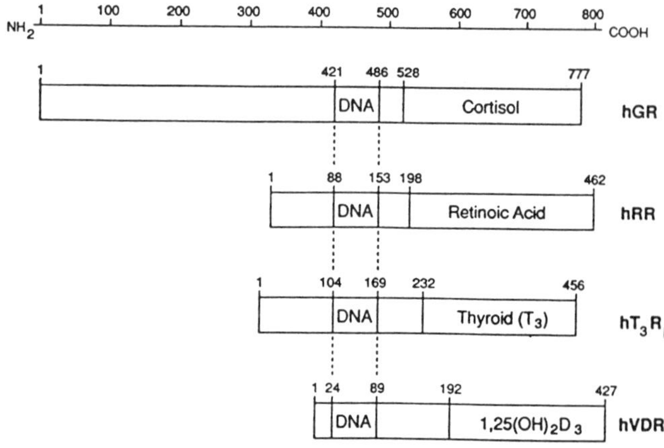

Figure 58.4 Structures of human genomic receptors for glucocorticoids (hGR), retinoic acid (hRR), thyroid hormones (hT_3R_β) and 1,25$(OH)_2$-vitamin D_3 (hVDR). The amino acid content of each receptor is shown by numbers at the right of each bar. The receptors are aligned to show the constancy of the highly conserved DNA-binding domain. The enhancer domain, which provides immuno-logic specific and maximum activity, is at the N-terminal portion of the receptor and is highly variable. The hormone- or vitamin-binding domain averages about 250 amino acids in length and is at the C-terminal end of the receptor. When the hormone or vitamin combines with the receptor it alters its confirmation, promotes DNA binding, and affects gene expression.[r6]

activated genes produce enzymes for glycoprotein synthesis, proteins required for epithelial cell integrity, and a variety of proteins essential for normal reproduction and differentiation of the fetus.[r4]

Nutritional Requirements

Requirements for vitamin A intake by humans are based on studies of dark adaptation, electroretinograms, and the ability of dietary vitamin A to maintain plasma concentrations in excess of 20 µg/dL in the plasma. The vitamin A requirement for humans ranges from 10 to 50 µg of retinol equivalents/kg body weight per day, with infants having the highest requirement. RDAs[7] are shown in Table 58.2. As regards precursors of vitamin A, 6 µg of β-carotene is considered equal to 1 µg of retinol because of the poor absorption of β-carotene and its inefficient conversion to retinol.

Deficiency Diseases

Xerophthalmia and night blindness have been known to physicians for many centuries. The term "xerophthalmia" means dry eyes. The syndrome of vitamin A deficiency consists of night blindness, Bitot spots, xerophthalmia, keratomalacia, corneal opacities, hyperkeratosis, growth failure, and death. Other findings include infertility, metaplastic bone disease, and general keratinization of epithelial tissue, particularly of the skin, genitourinary tract, and lung. Urinary calculi are common, and fetal abnormalities have been seen in pregnant mothers who are vitamin A deficient.[r5]

Diets consisting of polished rice with little or no vegetables or fruits increased the risk of xerophthalmia and, hence, its high prevalence in Asia. Thirty per cent of children admitted to a pediatric clinic in Thailand with protein energy malnutrition had xerophthalmia. Laboratory tests relevant to the diagnosis of vitamin A deficiency are a reduced level of serum retinol (15 ug/dL or less; normal is 20–80 ug/dL).

Therapeutic Uses

It is generally accepted that the dose of a vitamin required to prevent a deficiency disease and maintain health in an otherwise normal individual is 0.5–1.5 × the RDA. For the treatment of vitamin A deficiency, 10 mg/day (10 × the RDA) usually is required. At this dose, vitamin A is being used as a drug for the treatment of a disease. In India, vitamin A has been given at high spaced doses to prevent vitamin A deficiency. Because dietary supplementation is practically impossible, 60 mg of retinol as retinol palmitate (50 × the RDA) is administered orally to children between one and five years of age every six months. There were a few instances of nausea and vomiting at this high dose, but these symptoms were transient.

Another therapeutic use of vitamin A or vitamin A metabolites such as retinoic acid or 13 cis-retinoic acid is in globular acne. The dose is massive, i.e., 1–2 mg/kg/day, which is, again, equivalent to 50–100 × the RDA and, although effective in the treatment of globular acne, it also may induce hypervitaminosis A.

Vitamin A and related retinoids can also influence carcinogenesis in experimental animals.[r6] Retinoic acid is effective in inhibiting tumor development in skin, lymphopoietic cells, and bladder in appropriate experimental animals and is now being tested in humans. Other retinoids, which are not convertible to retinoic acid (deoxyretinol and the retinamines), exert chemopreventive activity against breast cancer, presumably by a pathway different from that employed by retinoic acid via the RAR receptor.

Toxicology

Hypervitaminosis A has been observed in children and adults ingesting more than 50,000 IU/day (12 × the RDA) for several months. This means that all persons receiving therapeutic doses of vitamin A for such indications as acne and cancer are at risk for hypervitaminosis A. The presenting symptoms are fatigue, malaise,

Table 58.2 Recommended Daily Dietary Allowances for Vitamins A, D, E, and K

Group	Age (yr)	Vitamin A (μg RE)[a]	Vitamin D (μg)[b]	Vitamin E (mg α-TE)[c]	Vitamin K (μg)
Infants	0–0.5	375	7.5	3	5
	0.5–1.0	375	10.0	4	10
Children	1–3	400	10.0	6	15
	4–6	500	10.0	7	20
	7–10	700	10.0	7	30
Males	11–24	1,000	10.0	10	65
	25–51+	1,000	5.0	10	80
Females	11–24	800	10.0	8	55
	25–51+	800	5.0	8	65
Pregnant		800	10.0	10	65
Lactating		1,300	10.0	12	65

From ref.[7]
[a]Retinol equivalents. 1 retinol equivalent = 1 μg retinol or 6 μg β-carotene of vitamin A activity of diets as retinol equivalents.
[b]As cholecalciferol. 10 μg cholecalciferol = 400 IU of vitamin D.
[c]α-Tocopherol equivalents. 1 mg d-α-tocopherol = 1 α-TE.

anorexia, vomiting, headache, and diplopia, related to elevated CSF pressure. Other findings are bone pain, dermatitis, hepatomegaly with liver abnormalities, hypercalcemia, hypoprothrombinemia, and fetal abnormalities. Women considering pregnancy should avoid megadoses of vitamin A because retinoic acid is an established teratogen.[r7,r8]

Preparations

Retinol

There are many multivitamin preparations that contain retinol in doses of 1.2 to 3.0 mg per day (4000–10,000 I.U.) Capsules supplying megadoses of 7.5 to 15 mg retinol (25,000–50,000 I.U.) are also available.

Tretinoin

(All trans-retinoic acid - Retin-A) is available for topical use as a solution (0.05%) or a cream (0.05 to 0.10%) for the treatment of acne and other skin ailments.

Isotretinoin

(13-cis-retinoic acid, Accutane) is available for oral use as 10, 20, and 40 mg. capsules for the treatment of globular acne.

Vitamin D and the Vitamin D-Related Hormones

History

Rickets is a disease of antiquity first described clinically by Glisson in London in 1650 and characterized by inadequate mineralization of the bones.[r9] Despite the fact that Darby in Manchester recommended cod liver oil for the prevention and treatment of rickets as an empirical remedy in 1789, the prevalence of rickets in children in cloudy Britain in the late 19th century was more than 50%. In 1890 Palm recommended sunlight as a preventative for rickets because of its comparative rarity in the tropics.

In 1919 Edward Mellanby produced experimental rickets in puppies by feeding them diets free of animal fat and found that he could prevent or cure the rickets by adding cod liver oil to the diet.[8] McCollum repeated his study at Johns Hopkins University and concluded that the active constituent could not be fat-soluble vitamin A, which he had discovered earlier, because the antirachitic substance was less sensitive to oxidation than vitamin A.[9] Therefore, McCollum named the antirachitic factor vitamin D. (The letters B and C had already been used for water-soluble vitamins discovered since the naming of vitamin A.)

Coincidentally with the discovery of the antirachitic vitamin in 1919, Huldschinsky in Vienna cured spontaneous rickets in children by exposing their skin to ultraviolet light.[10] In 1924, Steenbock and Black[11] at the University of Wisconsin and Hess and Weinstock[12] at Columbia University discovered that UV irradiation of various foods had the same antirachitic effect when fed to experimental animals as direct irradiation of the animals. It was therefore concluded that the antirachitic constituent of fish liver oils and the product of irradiation of foods and the skin are the same or similar substances.

The irradiation of ergosterol, the principal sterol of yeast and ergot, led to antirachitic products from which a crystalline material was obtained in 1931 by Windaus et al[13] and named vitamin D_1. Subsequently this group discovered that the crystalline substance, though antirachitic, was impure and contained lumisterol, an intermediate in the irradiation process. A year later, the pure vitamin, now named D_2 (ergocalciferol), was isolated from irradiated ergosterol by Windaus et al[14] in Gottingen and by Askew et al[15] in London.

The structure of ergosterol, the sterol precursor of vitamin D_2, was determined by Bernal[16] by x-ray diffraction in 1932. It showed a much more extended molecule than that postulated by Wieland and Windaus in their Nobel lectures in 1928. The extended structure postulated by Bernal in which rings A, B, C, & D are in tandem was consistent with all the previous chemical data and a revised formula for deoxycholic acid, and by inference, cholesterol and ergosterol, was published in 1932 by Wieland and Dane[17] in Munich and Rosenheim and King[18] in London.

The structure of vitamin D_2 was ultimately established by Windaus and Thiele[19] in Göttingen and Heilbron et al[20] in London. (Fig 58.5) The structure of vitamin D_2 features a rupture in ring B induced by irradiation which makes it even more extended than its precursor ergosterol as shown in Fig 58.6. The structure of crystalline vitamin D_3 (cholecalciferol), derived from 7-dehydrocholesterol, was ultimately determined by Schenck[21] in Windaus' laboratory in 1937.

The biological inactivity of the D vitamins in vitro and the long lag period between administration of vitamin D and its first detectable effect in vivo suggested that vitamin D must act through endogenous biotransformation products.[22] DeLuca and associates at the University of Wisconsin prepared tritium-labeled vitamin D_3 with a specific radioactivity high enough so that picomolar amounts of metabolites could be detected in tissues.[23] In 1968, Blunt, DeLuca, and Schnoes discovered that vitamin D_3 is hydroxylated in the liver to a more polar metabolite, 25-hydroxyvitamin D_3, which acted more rapidly in vivo and was also active in vitro.[24,25] In 1970, Fraser and Kodicek in Cambridge, England discovered that a more potent vitamin D metabolite is produced by the kidney.[26] In 1971 this powerful metabolite was independently identified as 1-alpha,25-dihydroxyvitamin D_3 by DeLuca and coworkers in Madison[27], by Lawson, Kodicek, and associates in Cambridge,[28] and by Norman et al,[29] University of California, Riverside. These findings led to the view that the most active form of vitamin D_3 is the 1,25 dihydroxy-derivative, which was named calcitriol. It was recognized as a renal hormone essential for normal calcium metabolism.

Calcitriol can be formed by step-wise hydroxylation of either vitamin D ingested in the diet or by hydroxylation of the irradiation product of 7-dehydrocholesterol, an intermediate in cholesterol biosynthesis in the skin. Thus vitamin D is a facultative vitamin that is required in the diet when insufficient sunlight is available to convert 7-dehydrocholesterol in the skin to vitamin D_3. The multiple actions of the hydroxylated forms of vitamin D that prevent rickets in children and osteomalacia in adults will be discussed.

Chemistry

Vitamin D is a generic term for a family of secosteroids with antirachitic activity. In the secosteroids, rings A, C, and D are intact whereas the ring B is opened and the molecule converted into a conjugated system of double bonds (Fig. 58.5). All molecules with vitamin D activity have the same interrupted ring system but vary in their side chains.

The chemical structures of the two forms of vitamin D used in medicine, vitamin D_2 (ergocalciferol) and vitamin D_3 (cholecalciferol), are shown in Fig. 58.5 Their precursor molecules are ergosterol (7-dehydro-22-dehydro-24-methyl-cholesterol) and 7-dehydrocholesterol, both having conjugated double bonds in ring B. Ergosterol was first isolated from the fungus ergot, and is widely distributed in plants, fungi, moulds, lichens, and lower inverterbrates such as snails and worms. Ergosterol does not occur in higher vertebrates. 7-dehydrocholesterol is an intermediate in the biosynthesis of cholesterol in animals that accumulates in the skin to the extent of about 10 ug/gm. Cholecalciferol (vitamin D_3) is widely distributed in animals, but is usually absent from plants. The one exception is the plant Solanum malocoxylon in Argentina, in which calcitriol occurs as a glycoside and is responsible for the poisoning of animals that ingest this plant. It can produce hypercalcemia, hypophosphatemia, and soft tissue calcification in domestic animals.[30]

The concentration of vitamin D_3 in human plasma ranges from 2 to 10 nanograms/ml depending on the exposure to sunlight. The most prevalent vitamin D metabolite in human plasma, however, is 25-hydroxyvitamin D, whose concentration ranges from 4–50 ng/ml. The body pool of vitamin D secosteroids is small, about 5 ug/kg, of which 25-hydroxyvitamin D_3 makes up 90% of the total. These plasma values are presented in Table 58.3.

Vitamin D_3 is most concentrated in the livers of fish. Cod liver oil contains about 5 ug/g of oil whereas halibut liver oil contains

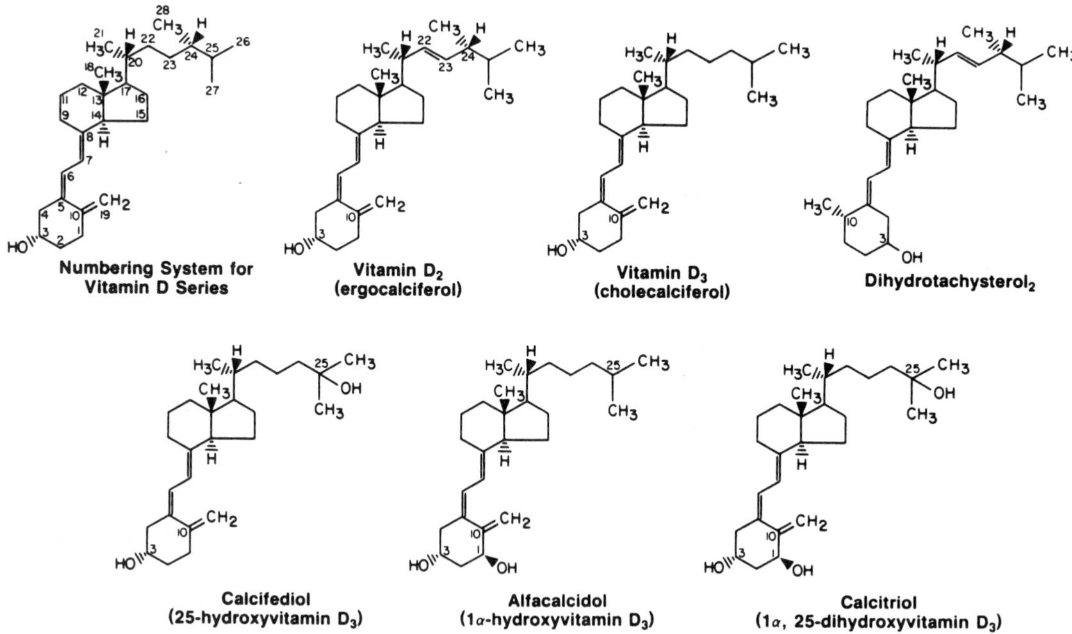

Figure 58.5 Structures of vitamin D and related secosteroids used in medicine. The very similar *vitamins D_2 and D_3* each have a single hydroxyl group, at the 3-position. The only chemical differences are: the C_{22-23} double bond in D_2 is saturated in D_3 and the methyl group (C-28) at C-24 in D_2 is absent in D_3. The single hydroxyl group in *dihydrotachysterol* at position 3 is in approximately the same geometrical position as the 1α-hydroxyl of calcitriol, which contributes to its potential activity. *Calicifediol, alfacalcidol,* and *calcitriol* are active, hydroxylated derivatives of vitamin D_3.

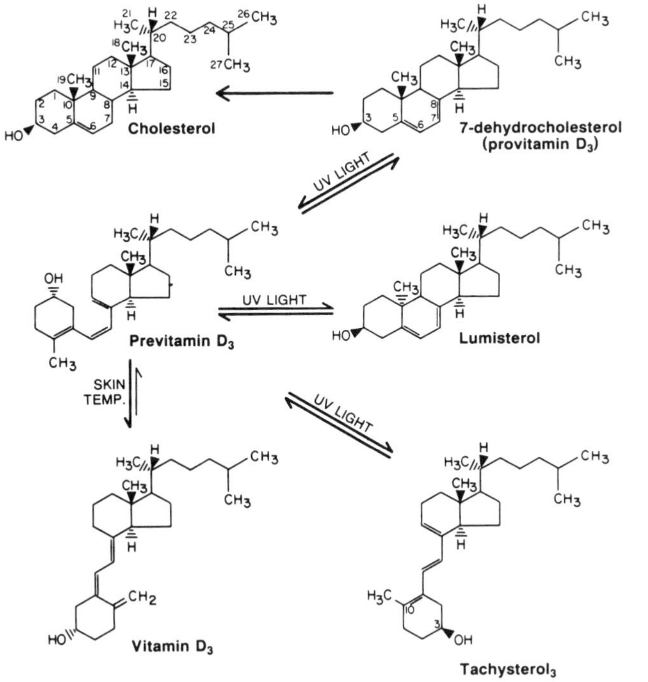

Figure 58.6 Biosynthesis of vitamin D_3 in the skin. In all layers of the *epidermis*, *7-dehydrocholesterol*, an intermediate in the biosynthesis of cholesterol, is photolyzed by UV light to *previtamin D_3*, which spontaneously isomerizes to vitamin D_3. Additional UV irradiation converts previtamin D_3 to *lumisterol* and *tachysterol*, thereby protecting people who have been overexposed to the sun from toxic effects.

about 50 ug/g and the vitamin D_3 content of tuna liver oil ranges from 500 to 1000 ug/g of oil.

The photochemical formation of vitamin D is a multistage process. It requires ultraviolet light in the range of 290 to 315 nm, which unfortunately is screened out by window glass and atmospheric smog. The 5-7 diene of the provitamin absorbs energy in this band of light and causes cleavage of 9-10 bond in Ring B of the sterol, with the formation of a conjugated triene called previtamin D. This intermediate undergoes a thermal-dependent rearrangement to form vitamin D.[r10,r11] Side reactions of previtamin D catalyzed by UV light may yield such products as lumisterol and tachysterol shown in Fig. 58.6.[r11] Tachysterol can be reduced chemically to dihydrotachysterol (shown in Fig. 58.5), which appears to be 25-hydroxylated in the liver and has proved useful in the treatment of hypoparathyroidism.

The melanin in the epidermis absorbs UV light and thereby decreases the efficiency of vitamin D synthesis in dark-skinned persons. Nevertheless, prolonged exposure to the sun produces essentially the same amount of previtamin D3 in dark skin as in light skin; regardless of skin color, previtamin D3 reaches a maximum and plateaus at about 15% of the original 7-dehydrocholesterol concentration.[31]

Several metabolites of vitamin D_3 that have already been discussed include 25-hydroxyvitamin D_3 (calcifediol) synthesized in the liver, and 1,25-dihydroxyvitamin D_3 (calcitriol) synthesized in the kidney from 25-hydroxyvitamin D_3. 1 α-hydroxyvitamin D_3 (alfacalcidol) is a synthetic secosterol that can be converted to calcitriol by 25-hydroxylation in the body. Both the active hormone calcitriol and its hepatic precursor 25-hydroxyvitamin D_3 are hydroxylated further in the 24R position to produce inactivation, and thus control the concentration of the active forms (Fig 58.7).

Vitamins D_2 and D_3 are about equally effective in the prevention and treatment of rickets in most mammalian species, including humans. In chicks and New-World monkeys, however, vitamin D_2 is only one tenth as potent than vitamin D_3.[32,33] In vitro, calcifediol is only about 1/1000 as potent as calcitriol, but in vivo the relative potency of calcifediol is about 1/10 that of calcitriol. The higher potency of calcifediol in vivo is due to its partial metabolic conversion to calcitriol. In antirachitic assays, calcifediol is about 1.4 times as active as vitamin D_3,[r12] whereas 1 α-hydroxyvitamin D_3 is about one half the activity of calcitriol.[34]

The synthetic 22-oxacalcitriol is of interest for the treatment of secondary hyperparathyroidism because it is equal in potency to calcitriol in reducing PTH mRNA but very much less potent in producing hypercalcemia. 22-oxacalcitriol is also much more potent than calcitriol in inducing the primary immune response.[35,36]

Physiology

The Absorption and Metabolism of Vitamin D

Vitamin D is absorbed in the small intestine, mainly in the duodenum, by an active transport system that delivers vitamin D to the enterocyte. Even in the presence of bile salts and dietary fat, the overall efficiency of absorption is about 50%.[37,38] In the enterocyte, it is incorporated into chylomicrons for delivery to the liver and other tissues. In the liver, vitamin D is hydroxylated to 25-hydroxyvitamin D and secreted in association with an alpha globulin of molecular weight 60,000. This carrier protein transports all forms of vitamin D, of which 25-hydroxyvitamin D_3 is in the highest concentration in plasma (20–40 ng/ml), whereas vitamin D itself is present in a concentration of only 2–4 ng/ml. The vitamin D hormone 1,25-dihydroxyvitamin D_3 is present at 1/1000 of the concentration of 25-hydroxyvitamin D, namely 20–40 picograms/ml of plasma.[39,40] (Table 58.3)

The liver contains a vitamin D-25 hydroxylase that converts most of the vitamin D delivered to it by chylomicrons to 25-hydroxyvitamin D, which is then quantitatively secreted into the plasma. The enzyme appears to be located in the endoplasmic reticulum of the liver and consists of NADPH, a flavoprotein, and cytochrome P450, which inserts an oxygen atom into vitamin D at the 25 position. This enzyme is inhibited by its substrate, vitamin D_3 which at high levels tends to down regulate the output of 25-hydroxyvitamin D_3 by the liver.

In the mitochondria of the tubular cells of the kidney, a 1 α-hydroxylase converts 25-hydroxyvitamin D into 1,25-dihydroxy vitamin D_3, the active hormone, which is secreted into the plasma. Like the 25-hydroxylase in liver, the enzyme in kidney is a mixed function oxygenase requiring NADPH, a flavoprotein, and cytochrome P450. This enzyme is more tightly regulated

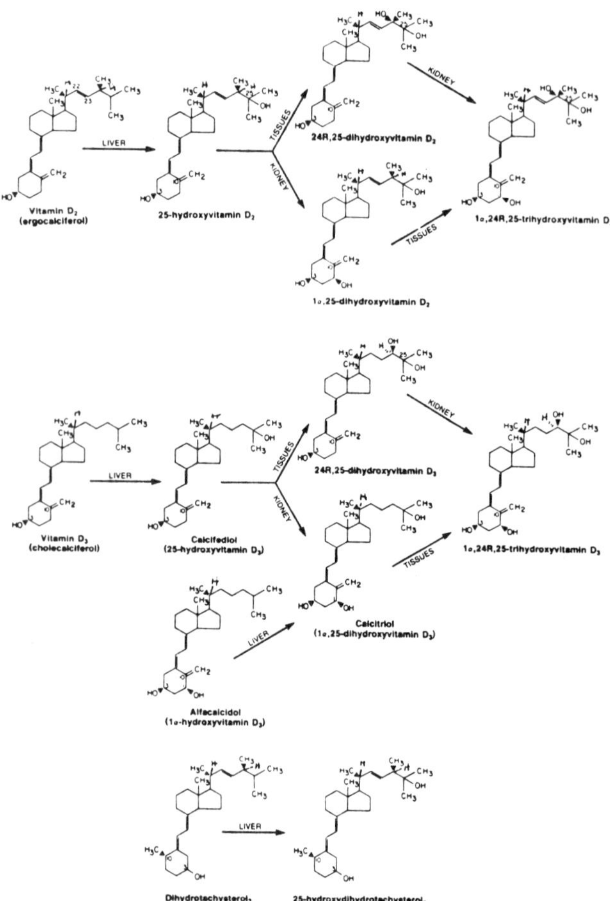

Figure 58.7 Metabolic products of vitamin D-related compounds used in medicine. Vitamin D_2 and Vitamin D_3 are converted in the liver to the weakly active 25-hydroxy metabolites. They, in turn, are converted in the kidney either to the highly potent 1α,25-dihydroxy metabolites or to the very weak 24R,25-dihydroxy metabolites. (The 24R,25-dihydroxy compounds may also be produced in extrarenal tissues.) The activity of the 24R,25-dihydroxy metabolites, such as it is, is probably due to conversion to the 1α,24R,25-trihydroxy vitamin D's. The liver 25-hydroxylates the synthetic *alfacalcidol* to the highly active *calcitriol*. The activity of *dihydrotachysterol* is due to its conversion in the liver to 25-hydroxydihydrotachysterol.

than the 25-hydroxylase in liver. The kidney enzyme is stimulated by parathyroid hormone (PTH), and low levels of plasma inorganic phosphate. It is inhibited by its product, calcitriol. There also is evidence that the plasma concentration of calcium inhibits the production of calcitriol by a direct effect on the kidney in addition to its indirect effect by inhibition of PTH secretion.[41]

There are also enzymes that inactivate active forms of vitamin D. For example, 25-hydroxyvitamin D_3 is hydroxylated to 24R,25-dihydroxyvitamin D_3 by another cytochrome P-450 mixed function oxygenase. A related (or the same) enzyme hydroxylates 1,25-dihydroxyvitamin D_3 to inactivate the hormone and control its duration of action, which computes to an average half-life of about 80 minutes.[r10] 24R25-dihydroxyvitamin D_3 is the second most abundant metabolite of vitamin D_3 in human plasma, being present in amounts of 1–4 ng/ml. PTH decreases the production of 24R, 25(OH)$_2$ vitamin D_3. The 24-hydroxylase is more widely distributed than the 1 α-hydroxylase; it has been found in intestine and bone as well as in the kidney. Other minor metabolites of 1,25-dihydroxyvitamin D include 1,25,26(OH)$_3$D$_3$, and side chain shortened products like 1-hydroxy,25,26,27 trinor 24-(COOH) vitamin D. These products are excreted principally in the bile as glucuronides.[r13]

Vitamin D and Calcium Homeostasis

The actions of vitamin D in various systems are the actions of its 1,25-dihydroxy derivative calcitriol, the vitamin D hormone. The classic actions of vitamin D relate to the maintenance of calcium homeostasis and normal bone metabolism. It is now clear that these effects are the results of changes in gene expression that are under the control of calcitriol and mediated by a vitamin D receptor protein that is a transcription factor.[r14,r15] The gene for the vitamin D receptor has been cloned and its product characterized in respect to amino acid sequence and 3 domains: an enhancer region, a DNA binding domain, and 1,25-dihydroxy vitamin D_3 binding domain. It contains 427 amino acids and has a molecular weight of 47,000.[r16]

Years before the discovery of calcitriol, Nicolaysen (1943) observed that after experimental animals and humans had been fed a low-calcium diet long enough to result in considerable demineralization of the skeleton, intestinal calcium absorption became more efficient, whereas an excess of dietary calcium decreased the percent calcium absorbed. As an explanation of these results, Nicolaysen postulated that an under-mineralized skeleton produced a vitamin D-dependent "endogenous factor" that increased calcium absorption.[42] This "endogenous factor" may be the PTH-calcitriol system, as suggested by DeLuca,[r16] in combination with yet unknown factors.

The organs affected by calcitriol are principally the intestine, kidney, and bones. In the intestine, the hormone induces a calcium transport system involving transport proteins and an intracellular calcium binding protein named calbinden (CBP), which aids in the transport of calcium from the gut across the enterocyte to the circulation. In the kidney, calcitriol enhances calcium reabsorption in the proximal tubule by a mechanism similar to that in the gut. In bone, calcitriol stimulates bone-forming cells (osteoblasts) to produce

Table 58.3 Vitamin D and Metabolites in Plasma.
Approximate Values for Healthy Children and Adults with Average Exposure to Sun and Average Oral Intake of vitamin D[39,40]

	Plasma Concentration		
	Total	**Free**	**Half-life**
Vitamins $D_2 + D_3$	1–5 ng/ml		2 or more months
Calcifediol + ercalcifediol	20–40 ng/ml	6–12 pg/ml	14–24 days
Calcitriol + ercalcitriol	25–50 pg/ml	0.1–0.4 pg/ml	ca. 24 hours
24R,25-dihydroxy-vitamins D_2 & D_3	1–4 ng/ml	0.3–1.2 pg/ml	

The prefix "er" indicates metabolite of vitamin D_2.
All the plasma concentrations of vitamin D_3 and its metabolites, except for calcitriol, are increased by exposure to the sun and, for this reason, tend to be higher in the summer than in the winter. Calcitriol is relatively unaffected because of regulation by feedback inhibition. The plasma concentration of the free (unbound) metabolite is the fraction that is directly available to target tissues.
An assay method that measures the sum of calcifediol and ercalcifediol in plasma is a generally useful index of the total vitamin D supply.

more alkaline phosphatase and less collagen, all of which favor bone formation. At higher doses, calcitriol stimulates mononuclear cells (including HL-60 leukemia cells) to differentiate into macrophages. Macrophages are then transformed into osteoclasts, which stimulate bone turnover and calcium mobilization. If hypercalcemia occurs, the C-cells of the thyroid gland secrete calcitonin, a peptide hormone, that acts opposite to the action of calcitriol. Calcitriol also stimulates the synthesis of vitamin K-dependent bone matrix proteins (osteocalcin and matrix-GLA-protein) that further control bone remodeling. These events are pictured in Figure 58.8.

Calcitriol localizes in the nucleus of the intestinal epithelial cell, where it, like other steroid hormones, interacts with its receptor, which is a transcription factor to induce synthesis of proteins that mediate its actions. The best authenticated of these is the vitamin D-induced intestinal calcium-binding protein (CaBP) discovered by Wasserman and Taylor in 1966[43], now known as calbindin. The mammalian intestinal form of calbindin has a molecular weight of 9500 and is termed calbindin-9K. The avian intestinal form has a molecular weight of 28,000 and is known as calbindin-28K. Calbindin-9K binds two atoms of calcium. Calbindin, undetectable during severe vitamin D deficiency, begins to appear in both the crypt and the villus cell within two to three hours after administration of calcitriol. The role of calbindin is to bind and translocate calcium from the mucosal region of the enterocyte across the cell to the site of the calcium pump on the basolateral membrane. There is also evidence that calbindin may be an activator of the ATP-dependent basolateral calcium pump to facilitate the exchange of Ca^{2+} for Na^{+} which is responsible for transferring Ca^{2+} from the intracellular to the extracellular space. (Fig. 58.9)

There also appears to be a paracellular diffusion process that occurs at higher concentrations of calcium (>2.5 mM), a nonsaturable process in which the energetics favor diffusion directly from lumen to blood.)[r17]

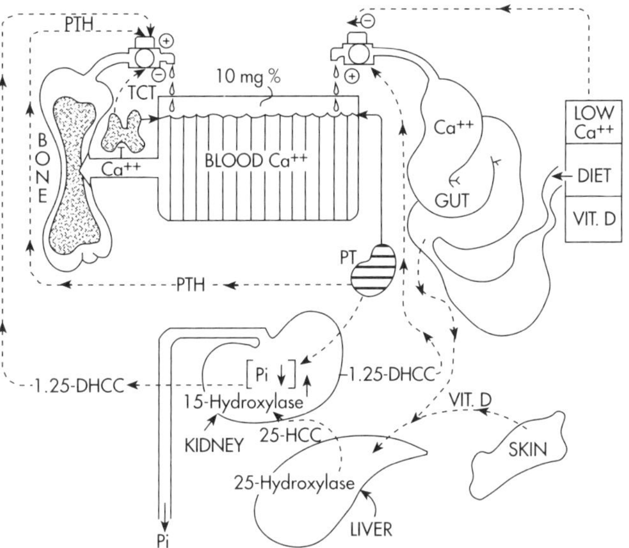

Figure 58.8 Endocrine regulation of calcium metabolism. The organs involved are the gut, the skin, the liver, the kidney, the bones, and the parathyroid and thyroid glands. PT= parathyroid gland; T= thyroid gland; PTH= parathyroid hormone; TCT= thyroid calcitonin; Both the parathyroid and thyroid glands sense the plama calcium level. The chief sources of calcium for the plasma are 1) the gut from dietary calcium and 2) the bones from matrix calcium. 25-HCC = 25-hydroxycholecalciferol; 1,25-HCC = 1,25-dihydroxycholecalciferol. The faucets shown at the top of the diagram can be turned on or off by humoral events. Modifed from Deluca, H. F. Nutr. Rev 37, 161–193, 1979.[r13]

A nongenomic effect of calcitriol has been reported by Nemere and Norman,[r18,44,r19] which occurs in vitamin D-replete animals within a few minutes, as in contrast

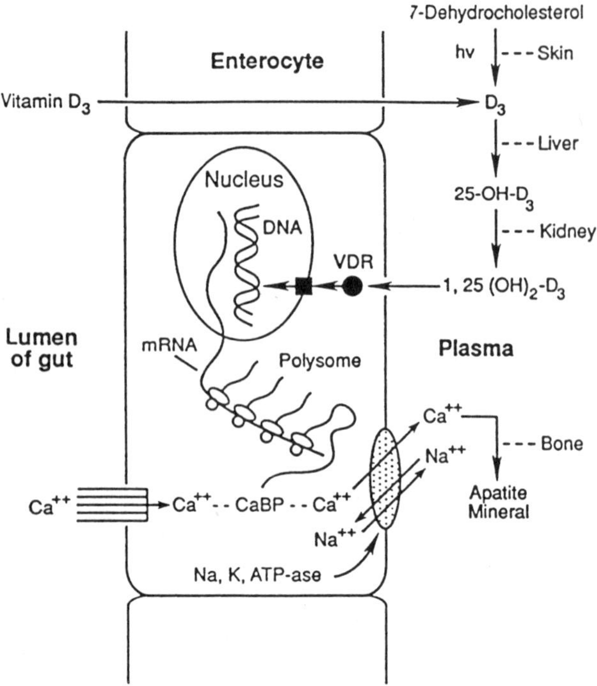

Figure 58.9 The production of 1,25(OH)$_2$-vitamin D$_3$ and its action in stimulating calbindin (CaBP) synthesis in the intestinal mucosa. VDR is a vitamin D receptor protein (●) whose conformation is changed by the uptake of 1,25(OH)$_2$-vitamin D$_3$ (■). The holoprotein migrates to the nucleus and combines with the hormone receptor element of the genome, which initiates transcription of the calbindin gene. The resulting mRNA is translated into a protein by interaction with ribosomes.

to a lag period of several hours for the genomic process. This rapid effect has been termed "transcaltachia". It involves endocytotic-exocytotic vesicular flow in which Ca2+ is moved from the brush border membrane (endocytosis) to the basolateral membrane (exocytosis) without Ca2+ entering the cell.

Calcitriol also increases active absorption of phosphate by a sodium-dependent process in the enterocyte[45]. In the kidney, calcitriol enhances calcium reabsorption in the proximal tubule by a mechanism similar to that in the gut. In bone, calcitriol and related compounds stimulate the outflow of calcium from bone into the circulation, in synergy with parathyroid hormone (PTH). These actions are summarized in Fig. 58.9.

It also is to be noted that the vitamin D endocrine system has other effects on the body than the control of calcium homeostasis. Calcitriol receptors have been found in skin, muscle, most endocrine tissues, thymus, lymphocytes and monocytes, as well as intestine, bone, and kidney. Clear effects of vitamin D deficiency upon endocrine secretion, immunity, and oncogene expression have been demonstrated in animals.[r17]

Requirements

Since vitamin D$_3$ is produced endogenously in the skin through the action of sunlight on 7-dehydrocholesterol, the human does not have a nutritional requirement for vitamin D when sufficient sunlight is available. However, when shielded from sunlight, both infants and adults will develop vitamin D deficiency, which presents as rickets in infants and osteomalacia in adults.

In 1970, an expert committee of the FAO/WHO concluded that full-term infants required 400 I.U.s (10 micrograms/day) for optimum absorption of calcium and satisfactory growth rates. It was concluded that after age 6, the requirement dropped to 5 micrograms daily. The RDAs shown in Table 58.2 give an allowance of 10 ug/day for children, adolescents, adult men and women, and pregnant and lactating women.

In 1989, an expert committee of the Food and Nutrition Board of the U.S. National Research Council (FNB/NRC) published daily dietary allowances for vitamin D: for fullterm infants (birth to 0.5 year) 7.5 ug; (300 IU); for infants, children, and adolescents (0.5–24 years) 10 ug (400IU), and for adults 5 ug (200 IU), except during pregnancy and lactation, when 10 ug (400 IU) was recommended.

Human milk is deficient in vitamin D and contains only 22 I.U.s per liter (0.55 micograms), mostly from 25-hydroxyvitamin D$_3$. If breastfed, the infant must receive an additional source of vitamin D; cows' milk and milk formulae are enriched to the level of 400 I.U.s, i.e., 10 ug/l, but there has been a problem with the reliability of vitamin additions.[46]

Deficiency Diseases

Rickets in infants and osteomalacia in adults are vitamin D deficiency diseases. Clinical manifestations of rickets include skeletal deformities with bone pain, muscle weakness, failure to grow, hypocalcemia, and hypophosphatemia. The failure to mineralize osteoid tissue at the epiphyseal-diaphyseal junction of bone causes a variety of deformities, e.g., craniotabes, enlargement of the joints, "rachitic rosary" at the costochondral junctions, bow legs, and knock knees. X-ray examination of long bones in rickets shows rarified shafts and uneven blurred ends. Fractures occur not infrequently.

When vitamin D intake is inadequate, vitamin D hormone levels fall, and calcium absorption is reduced. This causes plasma calcium concentrations to fall, which in turn increases PTH output. The increased PTH causes a fall in plasma phosphate by stimulating increased phosphate excretion, which directly or indirectly causes an increase in 1-(alpha)-hydroxylase activity in the kidney. These events collectively increase the synthesis and output of 1,25-dihydroxy vitamin D_3, which increase calcium absorption and calcium deposition in growing bones.

Calcitriol stimulates bone-forming cells (osteoblasts) to produce more alkaline phosphatase and osteocalcin and less collagen, all of which favor bone formation. In the absence of a continual supply of vitamin D these homeostatic mechanisms fail to protect the bones and rickets or osteomalacia results.

Laboratory studies of rachitic children show that they usually have hypocalcemia, hypophosphatemia, and elevated alkaline phosphatase. 25-Hydroxyvitamin D_3 levels in plasma are reduced to below normal. Adequate mineralization of bone requires normal values of serum Ca++ and inorganic phosphate to form bone hydroxyapatite, $(Ca_{10}(PO4)_6(OH)_2$. A guideline to normal plasma values for bone mineralization is a Ca $\times$ P product of 40 when both are expressed as mg/dl. The treatment of rickets requires high levels of vitamin D by mouth (100 ug/day for 10 days).

Osteomalacia, the counterpart of rickets in adults, causes less severe clinical signs and symptoms. In adults, a deficit in skeletal mineralization takes several years to develop and is usually part of a malabsorption syndrome. The most characteristic symptom is pain when weight or pressure is applied to the decalcified bones. There also may be muscle weakness. Vitamin D also cures this deficiency disease when administered at high doses (100–400 ug per day).

There are several types of vitamin D-resistant rickets, all of which are genetic disorders, which will be described in the next section on the therapeutic uses of vitamin D and its derivatives.

Therapeutic Uses

The major therapeutic uses of vitamin D and its homologues as drugs may be divided into 3 categories: 1) treatment of nutritional rickets and osteomalacia, 2) treatment of genetically conditioned metabolic bone disease, and 3) treatment of hypoparathyroidism.

As already indicated, the curative dose for rickets is about 10 times the RDA or about 4,000 I.U.s (100 ug/day) and will produce normal plasma calcium and phosphorus levels in 2 to 3 weeks. In malabsorption, megadoses of vitamin D may be necessary to obtain a therapeutic result. This can occur in steatorrhea, biliary obstruction, short bowel syndrome, and other abnormalities of gastrointestinal function. Doses needed for these cases are shown in Table 58.4.

Calcitriol is also used in the treatment of renal osteodystrophy associated with renal failure, which is due to the inability of the diseased kidney to convert 25-hydroxyvitamin to the vitamin D hormone, 1,25-hydroxyvitamin D_3. The compound 1α-hydroxy D_3 (alfacalcidol), a synthetic derivative of vitamin D_3, is also hydroxylated in the body in the 25 position by the hepatic microsomal system to form 1,25-dihydroxyvitamin D_3. This compound has been found to be very useful in the treatment of renal osteodystrophy.

There are several types of vitamin D-resistant rickets, all of which are genetic disorders requiring special therapies. Vitamin D-resistant rickets may involve 1) the loss of the system for the renal reabsorption of phosphate; 2) absence of the 1(α)hydroxylase in kidney; 3) mutations in the vitamin D receptor gene.[r20]

Familial X-linked hypophosphatemia rickets is the most common inherited abnormality of renal tubular transport. The most common features are short stature and femoral and tibial bowing presenting at 1–2 years of age. Laboratory findings include low serum phosphate, increased alkaline phosphatase, increased PTH, normal calcifediol, and low normal calcitriol. The most effective therapy for X-linked familial hypophosphatemic rickets consists of phosphate supplements 1.0 to 1.5 grams phosphate in divided doses and calcitriol initially in doses of 0.5 to 0.75 ug, increasing to the dose necessary to suppress PTH.[r21]

Vitamin D-dependent rickets Type I (vitamin D pseudo-deficiency) is a rare autosomal recessive disorder, usually appearing at 4 to 12 months of age. The defect in this disorder is the absence of the 1-alpha hydroxylase in the kidney. Infants diagnosed with this disorder do not respond to preventive doses of vitamin D but require high doses of calcitriol, 0.5–1.5 ug per day.

Vitamin D-resistant rickets Type II is due to a variety of defects in the calcitriol receptor protein. This disease presents in childhood with hypocalcemia, rickets, alopecia, and very high levels of calcitriol, which may exceed 1000 pg/ml.

Studies of the molecular biology of this disease have identified defects in different patients of all three domains of the genomic calcitriol receptor including the enhancer region, the DNA-binding region, and the calcitriol binding region. The treatment includes high levels of calcitriol (5–60 ug/d) and doses of oral calcium salts of 1000 mg calcium per day. Some patients respond to this regimen (if their receptor protein is partially active) and some are totally refractory to treatment.

Hypoparathyroidism is characterized by a low serum calcium and an elevated serum inorganic phosphate. Both are corrected by high doses of vitamin D

Table 58.4 Average Recommended Daily Doses of Vitamin D and Related Compounds and Approximate Relative Potencies

	Vitamin D_2 or D_3		*Dihydrotachysterol (DHT)*		*Calcifediol*		*Alfacalcidol*		*Calcitriol*	
	Dose	**Rel. Pot**	**Dose**	**Rel. Pot**	**Dose**	**Rel. Pot**	**Dose**	**Rel. Pot**	**Dose**	**Rel. Pot**
Prophylaxis	2.5–10μg (100–400 IU)	1	[20–100μg]	0.1	[1μg]	10			[0.1μg]	100
D-deficiency rickets	100μg (4000 IU)	1			5μg	20	2μg	50	1μg	100
Refractory rickets										
a) 1α-hydroxylase deficiency	1.25–3.75μg (50,000–150,000 IU)	1	0.4–1mg	3	50–200μg	20	1–2.5μg	1250	0.5–1.5μg	2500
b) target organ insensitivity	0.625–2.5 mg (25,000–100,000 IU)	1	0.125–1mg	3	50–300μg	10	10–30μg	60	5–20μg	125
Hypoparathyroidism	1.25–3.75mg (50,000–150,000 IU)	1	0.4–1mg	3	50–150μg	20	1–3μg	1250	0.5–1.5μg	2500
Renal osteodystrophy	1.25–2.5mg (50,000–100,000 IU)	1	0.2–1mg	3	50–100μg	20	1–2μg	1250	0.5–1μg	2500

Blank spaces and bracketed numbers indicate where medication is not used or recommended. The potency of each derivative is compared to vitamin D in each case.

Calcitriol and alfacalcidol are much more potent than vitamin D, DHT, and calcifediol. They are still more potent, relatively, in conditions involving 1α-hydroxylase deficiency (including hypoparathyroidism and renal osteodystrophy). The comparatively low cost of vitamin D is its principal advantage.

Relative to vitamin D, DHT is less potent in preventing rickets (increase in intestinal calcium absorption) and more potent in treatment of refractory rickets,hypoparathyroidism, and renal osteodystrophy (mobilization of calcium from bone).

or related compounds. Vitamin D in high doses, 1.25 to 3.75 mg/day, with a calcium supplement, is widely used for this purpose. The effective dose varies considerably from patient to patient. A limitation is the tendency of the patients to develop hypercalcemia during treatment. The patient must be carefully monitored for hypercalcemia and the calcium dose adjusted to normalize the serum calcium. Dihydrotachysterol (DHT) (0.4–1.0 mg/d) has been used as a substitute for vitamin D in the treatment of hypoparathyroidism because it has a more rapid onset of action, a shorter duration of action, and a relatively large effect on the mobilization of bone calcium. If it becomes necessary to discontinue treatment because of hypercalcemia, the serum calcium will return to normal more quickly with DHT than with vitamin D because of the shorter half life of DHT.

Therapy of pseudohypoparathyroidism is similar to that of hypoparathyroidism per se although in some cases calcitriol may be more effective.

Secondary hyperparathyroidism observed in renal failure is treated with Vitamin D or calcitriol. A new synthetic analogue of vitamin D, 22-oxa-1 alpha, 25-dihydroxy vitamin D3, is being studied as a possible therapeutic agent for secondary hyperparathyroidism. This compound is equipotent with calcitriol in inhibiting the production of parathyroid hormone but very weak as an agent for increasing serum calcium.[35]

Studies of treatment of osteoporosis with calcitriol have yielded conflicting results.[47,48] Both topical and systemic treatment of psoriasis with calcitriol have been reported to be of benefit,[r22,r23] which is not surprising, because of the well established use of UV light for treating psoriasis and the recent demonstration of therapeutic effects of calcitriol on skin cells in vitro.[52]

Parturient paresis (milk fever) is an acute hypocalcemic disorder associated with the onset of lactation in some dairy cows. The usual treatment is iv administration of calcium salts, which may require repetition in some of the cows. In these relapsing cows, plasma calcitriol does not increase normally in response to the hypocalcemia.[49] Recently it has been found that treatment with a vitamin D analogue is more effective than calcium alone.[50,51]

Toxicology

The daily preventive intake of vitamin D (400 I.U., 10 ug) recommended for growth and maintenance of normal bone has no undesirable side effects. A typical dose to cure D-deficiency rickets, 100 ug/day, although ten-fold higher than needed for prevention, is not toxic when used to treat established rickets. On the other hand, the ratio between the preventive dose and the toxic dose of vitamin D-related compounds is a low 5 to 10 fold. It is prudent to avoid giving children more than 1000 I.U. (25 ug) of vitamin D prophylactically including that supplied as additive to milk or other foods. Some children may already receive an adequate supply of vitamin D3 from the skin. In Britain inadvertant overdosage with vitamin D as a food additive 2000–3000 I.U. (50–75 ug) caused failure to thrive, hypercalcemia, anorexia, hypertension, and renal insufficiency in a large percent of the children studied.[53]

The major toxic effect of overdosage of vitamin D is hypercalcemia, which, even at the moderate hypercalcemic level of 11.5 mg/dl of plasma, may lead to ectopic calcification of and serious damage to the kidneys, blood vessels, and other vital tissues.[54] The extra calcium may come both from the intestine, because of increased absorption of calcium, and from the skeleton. Hyperphosphatemia is not recognized as a separate problem in vitamin D toxicity but, in the hypercalcemic state, an elevated plasma phosphate concentration can contribute to the production of ectopic calcification.

The beneficial effect of glucocorticoids in combating hypercalcemia also points to one of the relatively few interactions of the vitamin D group of compounds with other medications. Continued high doses of an adrenal glucocorticoid, as in the treatment of inflammatory disease, reduce intestinal absorption of calcium. Another suspected drug interaction is that with the anticonvulsant drugs, phenytoin and phenobarbitol. The incidence of osteomalacia is high in epileptic patients on long-term therapy with these drugs and the plasma level of 25-hydroxyvitamin D is low. It is still uncertain, however, whether these effects are caused by an effect of the drugs on vitamin D metabolism or mainly represent vitamin D deficiency in the patients. The classic often cited drug interaction of vitamin D with the digitalis glycosides applies only in case overdosage with vitamin D results in hypercalcemia, in which the sensitivity of the heart to the glycosides is increased.

The main route of excretion for vitamin D and related compounds is through the bile. Some of the unmetabolized compounds and metabolites are conjugated to form glucuronides and sulfates and excreted as such in the feces. There is some enterohepatic circulation but it is not regarded as pharmacologically significant.

Calcitroic acid, cholecalcioic acid, products of side-chain cleavage of the vitamin D molecule, and the 25-hydroxyvitamin D-26,23-lactone are among the inactive products that are formed and appear in the excreta.

Preparations

Vitamin D_2 and vitamin D_3 may be used interchangeably in humans. Vitamin D is labeled in units of weight and in international units (IU). One IU = 0.025 ug; 1 ug = 40 IU.

Vitamin D_2 is available for oral use in tablets of 1.25 mg, capsules of .625 and 1.25 mg, and in a solution containing 200 ug/ml. It is also supplied as one of the components of multivitamin preparations (examples: infant drops, chewable tablets) at the level of 10 ug per dosage unit.

Both vitamin D2 and vitamin D3 are used as food supplements but, in the U.S.A., only vitamin D2 is readily available as a medication.

Dihydrotachysterol (DHT)

Available in tablets and capsules of 125, 200, or 400 ug.

Calcifediol

Available in capsules of 20 or 50 ug.

Alfacalcidol

Available in capsules of .25 or 1 ug in Canada, Europe, Japan, and the U.K. but not at all in Australia and the U.S.A.

Calcitriol

Available in capsules of 0.25 or 0.5 ug.

Vitamin E

History

Vitamin E was discovered in 1922 by Evans and Bishop[55] as essential for reproduction in the rat. Although the deficient animals, reared on a diet containing only lard as a fat, ovulated and conceived normally, their pups died during gestation and were resorbed. Addition of wheat germ oil prevented these fetal deaths. Later these investigators named the vitamin tocopherol, from the Greek *tokos* (childbirth) and *pherein* (to bring forth). Vitamin E was isolated by Evans et al.[56] in 1936 and synthesized by Karrer et al.[57] in 1938.

The diseases caused by tocopherol deficiency vary widely according to the affected species. Disorders of reproduction, abnormalities of muscle, liver, bone marrow, and brain function, defective embryogenisis, and exudative diathesis, a disorder of capillary permeability, have been observed. Skeletal muscle dystrophy has been noted as well and, in certain species, is accompanied by cardiomyopathy. In ruminants, the cardiac disease is severe, but is mild in rabbits and nonexistent in primates. Hematopoiesis is affected only in monkeys and pigs; hepatic necrosis occurs only in rats and pigs. This bewildering and unpredictable array of manifestations has impeded an in-depth understanding of the vitamin's function at the cellular and molecular level. A number of enzymes are controlled by α-tocopherol in animals. These include xanthine oxidase, creatine kinase, cytochrome oxidase, lipoxygenase, glutathione reductase, aldolase, and arylsulfatase.[58]

In humans, the main manifestations of vitamin E deficiency are: (a) mild hemolytic anemia associated with increased erythrocyte hemolysis; and (b) spinocerebellar disease, mostly observed in children who have fat malabsorption due to abetalipoproteinemia, chronic biliary disease with cholestasis, or a genetic abnormality in vitamin E metabolism.

Chemistry

Vitamin E is a generic term for compounds that have a 6-chromanol ring, an isoprenoid side chain, and the biologic activity of α-tocopherol. The tocols have a phytyl side-chain, whereas the trienols have a classic isoprenoid side-chain with double bonds at the 3′, 7′, and 11′ positions (Fig. 58.10). Both tocols and trienols occur as a variety of isomers that differ by the number and location of methyl groups on the chromanol ring. α-Tocopherol is the most active form of vitamin E.

The only naturally-occurring stereoisomer of α-tocopherol, formerly known as d-α-tocopherol, should be designated RRR-α-tocopherol. The totally synthetic α-tocopherol, formerly known as dl-α-tocopherol, should be designated *all-rac*-α-tocopherol (for all racemic-α-tocopherol). Esters of tocopherols should be designated as esters of the parent vitamin (e.g., α-tocopherol acetate).

α-Tocopherol is practically insoluble in water and is completely soluble in oils, fats, and fat solvents. Tocopherols are stable to heat and alkali in the absence of oxygen and are unaffected by acids up to 100°C. They are, however, slowly oxidized by atmospheric oxygen. Oxidation is accelerated by exposure to light, heat, and alkali and by the presence of iron and copper salts. Oxidation products include tocopheroxide, tocopherol quinone, and tocopherol hydroquinone, as well as dimers and trimers. Since the esters of the free phenolic hydroxyl group are much more stable in the presence of oxygen, tocopherol usually is provided commercially as the acetate ester. The esters, however, cannot function as antioxidants.

Physiology

The tocopherols are poorly absorbed to the extent of only 20 to 40 percent of the administered vitamin E. Tocopherol esters are almost completely hydrolyzed by a duodenal mucosal esterase prior to absorption. The absorption of vitamin E is maximal in the median portion of the small intestine. Unlike cholesterol and vitamin A, α-tocopherol is not reesterified prior to its incorporation into the chylomicron and its delivery to the liver with the chylomicron remnant. From the liver it is secreted with VLDL and delivered to LDL and HDL via exchange and most likely delivered to peripheral tissues via the LDL receptor. Plasma tocopherol levels vary with the total lipid concentration in the plasma as they are carried in the lipoproteins, including VLDL.[r24]

Free tocopherol is concentrated in the membranes of cells, including the plasma membrane and those of mitochondria and the plasma reticulum. RRR-alpha

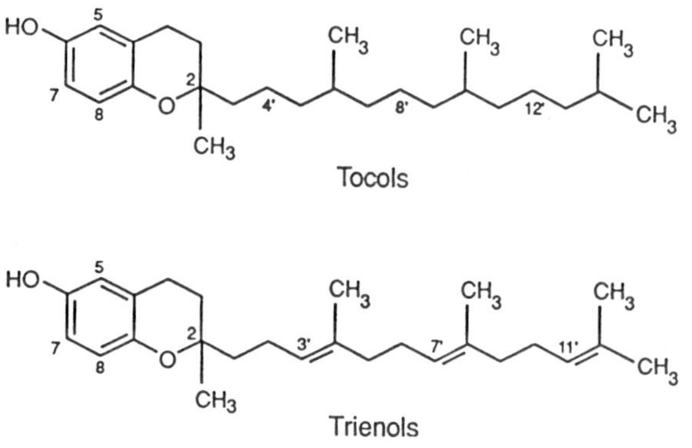

HO 5 7 8 2 O 4' 8' 12' CH_3 CH_3 CH_3 CH_3 CH_3

Tocols

HO 5 7 8 2 O 3' 7' 11' CH_3 CH_3 CH_3 CH_3 CH_3

Trienols

Figure 58.10 Basic structures of molecules with vitamin E activity. The tocols have a phytol side-chain, whereas the tocotrienoids have a classic isoprenoid side-chain.

tocopherol, the natural form, is well retained in tissue membranes, whereas its stereoisomers are not so well retained and are more rapidly metabolized. Adipose tissue, adrenal, testis, and the pituitary contain the highest concentrations of alpha tocopherol in the animal body. The human body stores about 40 mg/kg of vitamin E, the greatest amount of any fat-soluble vitamin, of which 77 percent is in adipose tissue.

Vitamin E is oxidized to a variety of chain-shortened products in the body. Less than 1 percent of orally ingested vitamin E is excreted in the urine as metabolites. Most of it is found in the feces, where excretion ocurrs via the hepatobiliary system.

The principal function of vitamin E is to serve as a physiologic membrane antioxidant. Since free radicals catalyze lipid peroxidation, this continual biologic process damages cellular and intracellular structures. Vitamin E appears to promote health by inhibiting this process and terminating radical chain reactions.[r24]

The antioxidant function of vitamin E is supported by seven lines of evidence: (a) α-tocopherol in vitro is a lipid antioxidant; (b) a high intake of polyunsaturated fat increases the vitamin E requirement; (c) tissues of vitamin E-deficient animals are usually more peroxidized than those of normal animals; (d) ceroid pigments, which are polymerization products of peroxidized fats, accumulate in vitamin E deficiency; (e) several labile polyunsaturated lipids like vitamin A and carotene are protected from destruction by vitamin E; (f) synthetic antioxidants can protect against certain signs of vitamin E deficiency in certain species; and (g) the metabolic products of tocopherol are consistent with its antioxidant function.

There are certain features of vitamin E deficiency, however, that are not consistent with the antioxidant hypothesis and that have led to the view that, like vitamins A and D, vitamin E may affect the expression of some genes.[55,59] Evidence in favor of a genetic regulatory function for vitamin E includes the following: (a) defective embryogenesis observed in vitamin E deficiency; (b) alteration of sexuality and morphology has been induced by vitamin E in the rotifer, *Asplanchna,* a carnivorous metazoan; (c) the rate of synthesis of the creatine kinase and xanthine oxidase are increased four to eight times in vitamin E-deficient animals; (d) a cytoplasmic binding protein for α-tocopherol has been identified; and (e) DNA and RNA turnover are altered in dystrophic muscle from vitamin E-deficient rabbits.

Nutrition Requirements

The vitamin E requirement of the normal infant was estimated from the amount needed to prevent peroxidative hemolysis and is approximately 0.4 mg/kg body weight/day or about 2 mg of RRR-α-tocopherol per day. For premature infants the requirement is higher (10–15 mg/d) because placental transport of vitamin E is slow, and hence the tissues of the premature infant are nearly devoid of vitamin E. The requirement in adult humans is about 6–8 mg of RRR α-tocopherol/day and the RDAs are appropriately higher. (Table 58.2)

Deficiency Disease

As already noted, vitamin E deficiency is expressed in various ways in different species. In the human, the expression of vitamin E deficiency is confined to the bone marrow,[60] muscle, and the CNS.[61] Infants are born in a state of relative tocopherol deficiency with plasma α-tocopherol levels below 5 ug/ml. The smaller and more premature the infant, the greater the degree of deficiency. Term infants who are breastfed quickly attain adult blood tocopherol values. The vitamin E-deficient state of premature infants persists during the first few weeks of life and can be attributed to limited placental transfer of vitamin E, low tissue levels at birth, relative dietary deficiency in infancy, intestinal malabsorption, and rapid growth. As the digestive system matures, tocopherol absorption improves, and blood vitamin E levels rise. Infants weighing less than 1500 g at birth may, however, have tocopherol malabsorption until two to three months of age.

Hemolytic anemia in premature infants is a manifestation of vitamin E deficiency.[61,62] The anemia presents with hemoglobin levels in the range of 7 to 9 g/dl, and is accompanied by low plasma vitamin E levels, reticulocytosis, and hyperbilirubinemia. In these children, administration of iron may exacerbate red blood cell destruction unless vitamin E is administered also.

In children and adults, fat malabsorption generally underlies vitamin E deficiency; in its most severe manifestation, spinal cerebellar ataxia. Abetalipoproteinemia, caused by the genetic absence of apolipoprotein B, causes serious fat malabsorption and steatorrhea, with progressive neuropathy and retinopathy in the first two decades of life. Plasma vitamin E levels are sometimes undetectable. High-dose vitamin E has improved symptoms in young patients and arrested the neurologic disorder in older patients.

In 1981, children with chronic cholestatic hepatobiliary disease and cystic fibrosis were also found to manifest the neurologic syndrome of vitamin E deficiency.[61,r25] It consists of spinal cerebellar ataxia with loss of deep tendon reflexes, truncal and limb ataxia, loss of vibration and position sense, ophthalmoplegia, muscle weakness, ptosis, and dysarthria. (Table 58.5) In adults with malabsorption, spinal cerebellar ataxia due to vitamin E deficiency is extremely rare, no doubt because of heightened vitamin E stores in adipose tissue in adults.

Another rare genetic form of vitamin E deficiency without fat malabsorption has been described.[63] In these patients the liver appears to lack a tocopherol transfer protein that normally transfers RRR alpha tocopherol from the hepatocyte to VLDL. These patients are thus unable to maintain normal α-tocopherol concentrations in plasma. Megadoses of α-tocopherol of the order of 100 to 200 IU/d are effective in ameliorating the deficiency and preventing the development of the neurologic sequelae.

Therapeutic Uses

In cases of malabsorption, megadoses of vitamin E in the range of 100 to 200 mg/kg are administered to retard the spinal cerebellar syndrome and correct excessive red cell hemolysis. Also, such doses have been found to be useful in patients with genetic deficiency diseases involving glutathione peroxidase and superoxide dismutase.

Intermittent claudication has been reported to respond to daily doses of 400 mg/day after 18 months of therapy, but the effects have been variable. Improvement in blood flow to the extremities has been noted in some patients. It has also been claimed that retrolentalfibroplasia and bronchial pulmonary dysplasia may improve with vitamin E therapy. The administration of megadoses of vitamin E to middle aged persons in an attempt to prevent the occurence of such chronic diseases as cancer and coronary heart disease has given mixed results[64,r26]

Toxicology

Relatively large amounts of vitamin E in the range of 400 to 800 mg/day have been taken by humans for months to years without causing any apparent harm. Occasionally muscle weakness, fatigue, nausea, and diarrhea have been reported by persons taking vitamin E in excess of 1000 to 3200 IU/day. The most significant toxic effect of vitamin E at doses exceeding 1000 IU/day is antagonism to vitamin K action and enhancement of the effect of oral coumarin anticoagulant drugs with overt hemorrhage.[65]

Preparations

One international unit of vitamin E is equivalent to the activity of dl-α-tocopherol acetate (now described as all-rac-α tocopherol acetate) synthesized from triethyl hydroquinone and isophytol. The natural product, d-a-tocopherol has about 150% of the biological activity of the synthetic isomer, and is the preferred product. Multivitamin preparations contain about 10 I.U/capsule. Both the dl and the d isomers are available in amounts ranging from 50–1000 mg in capsules. Intravenous preparations are also available.

Table 58.5 Clinical Features of Vitamin E Deficiency Disorders[r21]

	Abetalipoproteinemia	Chronic Childhood Cholestasis	Other Fat Malabsorption Disorders	Isolated Vitamin E Deficiency
Hypo/areflexia	++	++	++	±
Cerebellar ataxia	++	++	++	++
Loss of position sense	++	++	+	±
Loss of vibratory sense	++	++	++	++
Loss of touch, pain	+	±	+	–
Ophthalmoplegia	+	+	+	–
Ptosis	+	+	±	–
Muscle weakness	+	+	+	+
Pigmented retinopathy	++	±	+	–
Dysarthria	+	±	+	±

++, always present; +, commonly present; ±, inconsistently present; –, absent.

Vitamin K

History

In 1929 Dam observed subcutaneous and intraperitoneal hemorrhages in chicks fed a fat-free diet. He then demonstrated that these hemorrhages were the result of a dietary deficiency of a previously unrecognized fat-soluble substance.[66] Further investigation showed that this new factor was widely distributed in the plant kingdom, particularly in green leafy vegetables. Dam named the new substance "vitamin K" for its "koagulation" activity.[67]

In 1939 Doisy and his colleagues in St. Louis[68] and Dam and his colleagues in Copenhagen[69] announced the isolation of vitamin K from alfalfa. In addition, Doisy's group reported the isolation of a related, but not identical, vitamin K from putrified fishmeal. They named the compound from alfalfa vitamin K_1 and the one from fishmeal vitamin K_2.[70]

It was soon discovered by Dam and coworkers that the hemorrhagic disease in chicks was due to absence of prothrombin activity in the plasma, and that was also found to be the case in vitamin K-deficient humans. Additional vitamin K-dependent coagulation factors were discovered during the next 20 years. These included proconvertin (Factor VII), Stuart-Prower factor (Factor X), and Christmas factor (Factor IX). In the past 15 years, three more coagulation factors dependent on vitamin K have been discovered. They are protein C, protein S, and protein Z, all of which are anticoagulants. In addition, two bone matrix proteins necessary for normal bone metabolism have been found to be vitamin K-dependent.

Chemistry

Vitamin K is a generic term for derivatives of 2-methyl-1,4-naphthoquinone with coagulation activity. The natural forms are substituted in position 3 with an alkyl side-chain. Vitamin K_1, now called phylloquinone, has a phytyl side-chain in position 3 and is the only homologue of vitamin K found in plants. Vitamin K_2 is a family of homologues with 2-methyl-1,4-naphthoquinone substituted in position 3 with isoprenyl side-chains containing from 4 to 13 isoprenyl units. These are called menaquinones-n, the suffix noting the number of isoprene units in the side-chain. For example, menaquinone-7 was the first member of the vitamin K_2-family isolated from fermented fishmeal by Doisy et al.[70] The menaquinones are synthesized by bacteria in the intestinal tract and can contribute to the vitamin K requirement of animals. Vitamin K is essential because the 1,4-naphthoquinone nucleus cannot be synthesized in animal cells. Menaquinone-4 is synthesized in animals and birds from the provitamin menadione (2-methyl-1,4-naphthoquinone), formerly known as vitamin K_3 (Fig. 58.11) by enzymatic alkylation with digeranyl pyrophosphate.[71] The enzyme has been partially purified and characterized in chicken and rat liver microsomes. The other menaquinones are products of bacterial biosynthesis, and range from menaquinone 6 to menaquinone 13.

Physiology

The absorption of the various vitamin K homologues requires bile and pancreatic juice for maximal effectiveness. Dietary vitamin K is absorbed in the small bowel, incorporated into chylomicrons, and delivered to the circulation via the lymph. The efficiency of absorption has been measured from 40 to 80% de-

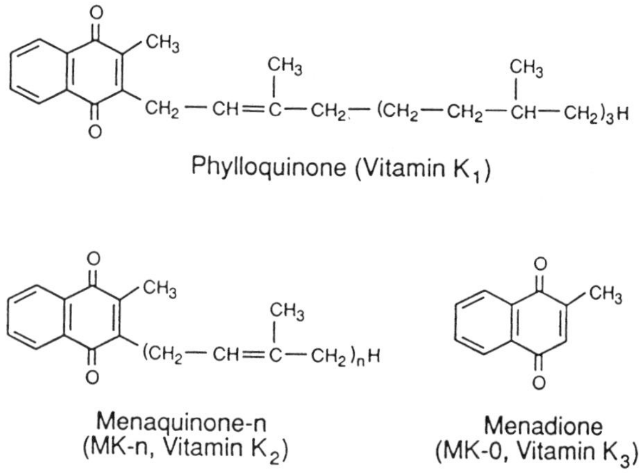

Phylloquinone (Vitamin K_1)

Menaquinone-n (MK-n, Vitamin K_2)

Menadione (MK-0, Vitamin K_3)

Figure 58.11 Structures of vitamin K homologues, which are derivatives of 1,4-naphthoquinone, Phylloquinone (vitamin K_1), menaquinone (vitamin K_2), and menadione (vitamin K_3) are shown.

pending on the vehicle with which vitamin K is administered and the extent of the enterohepatic circulation.

During the action of lipoprotein lipase, vitamin K remains in the chylomicron remnant, is taken up by the liver and resecreted into the plasma with VLDL, which ultimately is converted to LDL. It is likely that vitamin K is delivered to cells via the LDL receptor. No specific carrier proteins for vitamin K have been identified in plasma. The postabsorptive plasma concentration of phylloquinone is 0.3–1.2 ng/ml, with an average of 0.5 ng/ml. Menaquinones are present in normal human plasma in much lower concentrations.

After oral administration of vitamin K, the liver may contain as much as 20 percent of the administered dose at 2 hour, which then declines to low values after 24 hours. The principal sites of uptake, after liver, are skin and muscle. The total body pool of vitamin K in animals and humans is surprisingly small, approximately 1 to 3 ug/kg, of which 80 percent is in the liver. In omnivorous animals like humans, both phylloquinone and the higher molecular weight menaquinones (MK-7 to MK-13) of bacterial origin are found in the liver.[72] Haroon and Hauschka[73] have found phylloquinone levels in rat liver to vary between 8 and 44 ng/g fresh weight (20 to 100 pmol/g) and Shearer[74] has found somewhat lower levels in human liver, i.e., 1 to 21 ng/g. Taggart and Matschiner[75] estimated that 10 pmol/g (4.5 ng/g) of vitamin K is the minimum hepatic concentration required to sustain normal prothrombin synthesis in the rat, and it is probably lower in the human.

The terminal oxidation of vitamin K and its epoxides involves chain shortening and excretion of the products in urine and stool, mainly as glucuronides of vitamin K lactones.

Vitamin K-dependent Carboxylase

The physiologic function of vitamin K is to carboxylate selected glutamic acid residues in the vitamin K-dependent proteins to produce gamma carboxyglutamate (Gla) residues.[76] The number of Glas/mole of protein ranges from 10 to 12. Factors II, VI, IX, and X are procoagulant proenzymes, whereas proteins C, S, and M are anticoagulant proenzymes.

The function of Gla in these proteins is to facilitate the chelation of calcium ions to Gla residues and platelet phospholipids, which are essential for the operation of the coagulation cascade.

The vitamin K-dependent carboxylase system is a membrane-bound component of the endoplasmic reticulum.[r27,r28] The carboxylase has been solubilized from microsomes and isolated in pure form. This system requires preprothrombin as a substrate oxygen, carbon dioxide, and vitamin K hydroquinone. ATP is not required. As noted, the active form of the vitamin is the reduced form of vitamin K, which acts as an electron donor for a mixed-function carboxylase-epoxidase, which results in the reduction of oxygen to one mole of vitamin K epoxide and one mole of water. During this reaction, CO_2 is fixed in peptide-bound glutamic acid. The carboxylase is an integral membrane glycoprotein (MW 95,000), whose cDNA has been cloned and the enzyme expressed in the kidney 293 cells.[77]

The mechanism of the vitamin K-dependent carboxylation is discussed below.

$$KH_2 + O_2 + Glu_p + CO_2 \xrightarrow[\text{carboxylase}]{Mn^{++}} Gla_p + KO + H_2O$$

It is visualized that this carboxylation reaction is ordered in which O_2 combines with vitamin K hydroquinone to produce an alkoxide anion,[78] which is sufficiently basic to remove the proton from the gamma carbon of glutamate. The resulting carbanion then attacks CO_2 and produces Gla, as shown in Figure 58.12.[79]

Vitamin K Cycle

In 1970, Matchiner et al.[80] reported the isolation and characterization of phylloquinone 2,3-epoxide as a metabolite of phylloquinone in the rat. Normally found in small amounts, the epoxide was demonstrated to accumulate in the presence of warfarin. Approximately 30 years earlier, Fieser et al.[81] had synthesized the 2,3-epoxide of phylloquinone and showed that it was rapidly converted to vitamin K in animals and humans.

The vitamin K cycle shown in Figure 58.13 is a salvage pathway for vitamin K, a vitamin present in only nanomolar quantities in liver and other tissues. The cycle postulates that the vitamin K-dependent carboxylase converts vitamin K hydroquinone to its 2,3-epoxide, usually in excess of the carboxylation rate. The epoxide is then reduced to vitamin K by a dithiothreitol-dependent epoxide reductase, and the vitamin K quinone is then reduced to the vitamin K hydroquinone by several enzymes, at least two of which are driven by a dithiol and others by NADPH. The dithiol-

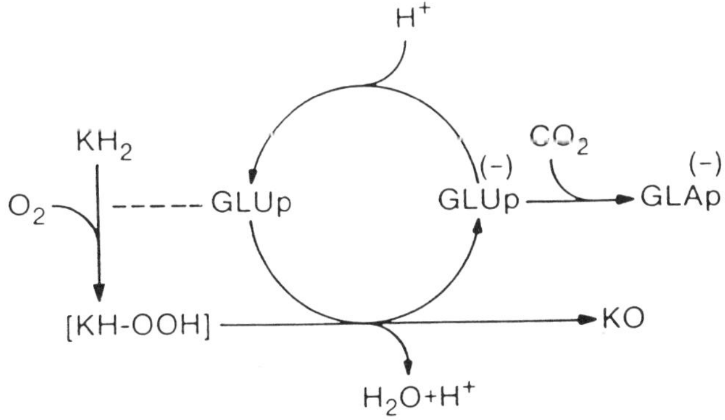

Figure 58.12 Hypothetical mechanism for the coupling of carboxylation and epoxidation in vitamin K-dependent Gla synthesis. Vitamin K hydroquinone is KH_2; vitamin K hydroperoxide is KH-OOH; vitamin K-2,3-epoxide is KO; peptide-bound nate is GLUp; peptide-bound γ-carboxyglutamate is GLAp.

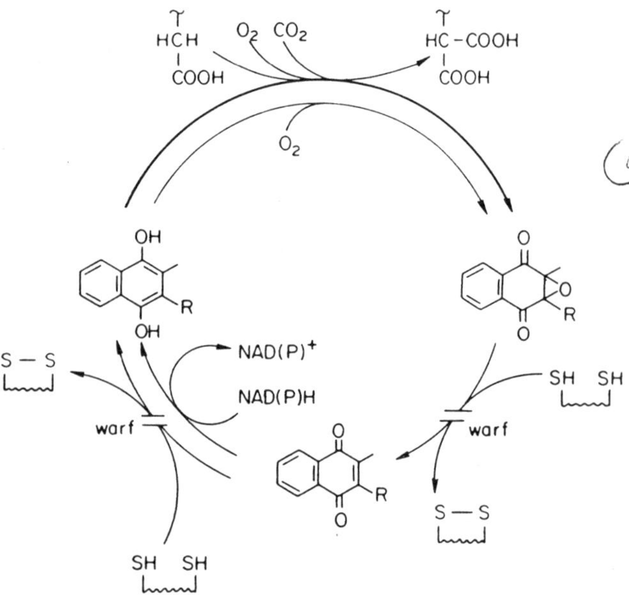

Figure 58.13 The vitamin K cycle occurs in the hepatic endoplasmic reticulum. The carboxylation and expoxidation activities are catalyzed by the same enzyme. The dithiol-dependent reductions of the vitamin K epoxide and of vitamin K are extremely sensitive to the action of coumarin anticoagulants such as warfarin (warf). NADPH-dependent dehydrogenases, however, are not inhibited by warfarin (68).

dependent epoxide reductase and the quinone reductase are strongly inhibited by warfarin and other coumarin anticoagulants, whereas the NADPH-dependent dehydrogenases are relatively insensitive to warfarin. Relatively large amounts of vitamin K are required to regenerate the hydroquinone in the presence of coumarin drugs.

The vitamin K cycle thus regenerates vitamin K from the product of the carboxylation reaction, the 2,3-epoxide, which in turn is reduced by a quinone reductase. Inasmuch as this vitamin K-dependent multienzyme system regenerates the hydroquinone from its reaction product, vitamin K may be considered to be a coenzyme for the system.

Nutritional Requirements

The vitamin K requirement of mammals is met by a combination of dietary intake and microbiologic biosynthesis in the gut. Phylloquinone seems to be the most active source of vitamin K in meeting the requirements of humans. Genetic factors play a role, as shown by the higher requirement of vitamin K by males compared with females. Microbiologic flora play an undetermined role in meeting human requirements. In germ-free rats the vitamin requirement in the diet is twice that of conventional rats.

Vitamin K-dependent coagulation factors are depressed to 30 percent of normal adult levels at birth in full-term infants and even lower in premature newborns.[82] The vitamin K requirement for the normalization of prothrombin and other factor levels in newborn infants is 3–5 ug phylloquinone per day. Since breast milk contains only 2 ug of phylloquinone/liter, breast-fed infants are at risk for hemorrhagic disease and must be fortified with vitamin K in order to prevent this complication. In adults, studies in volunteers have shown that prothrombin levels can be maintained on intakes of 10–30 ug of phylloquinone/day for as long as eight weeks.

From these data it may be concluded that the requirement for adults is in the range of 10–30 ug/day or 0.2–0.5 ug/kg/day. The usual diets in the US contain between 100 and 300 μg phylloquinone per day. Green leafy vegetables are rich in phylloquinone, as already mentioned; animal foods are intermediate, and cereals are low in this vitamin.

The RDAs, for vitamin K are shown in Table 58.2. The allowance for infants increases from 5 ug/day at birth to 10 ug/day at two years. For adults the recommended amounts are 65 ug/day for females and 80 ug/day for males.

Deficiency Diseases

The vitamin K nutrition of newborn infants warrants special attention because: (1) the placenta is a relatively poor organ for the maternal-fetal transmission of lipids; (2) the neonatal liver is immature with respect to prothrombin synthesis; and (3) the gut is sterile during the first few days. In normal newborns, the plasma prothrombin concentration and that of the other vitamin K-dependent factor and may be as low as 30 percent of adult levels, gradually climbing, if dietary vitamin K levels are adequate, to normal adult values over a period of weeks.[82]

If vitamin K-dependent factors fall to less than 10 percent of adult values, hemorrhagic disease of the newborn may appear. In this disease, bleeding is spontaneous and may occur in the skin and subcutaneous tissues, the GI tract, umbilical cord, or, most seriously, in the brain or meninges. Birth injuries aggravate bleeding in these infants. Plasma vitamin K levels in these deficient newborns have been as low as 40–50 pg/ml, and liver concentrations of phylloquinone are also very low, on the order of 1 ng/g tissue with menaquinones absent. Since most breast-fed infants are at higher risk of hemorrhage than formula-fed babies, it is recommended that breast-fed infants receive 1 mg of phylloquinone IM at birth.

Infants of mothers on hydantoin anticonvulsants should have prophylactic vitamin K because diphenylhydantoin is an antagonist to vitamin K. Neonatal complications, such as diarrhea, malabsorption, cystic fibrosis, idiopathic cholestosis, atresia of the bile duct, and prolonged parenteral nutrition are all indications for IM vitamin K administration to infants. Adults are relatively resistant to vitamin K deficiency unless they have some acquired illness such as biliary obstruction, malabsorption, liver disease, or total parenteral nutrition, or receive coumarin anticoagulant drugs.[r28]

Therapeutic Uses

Vitamin K is used in milligram quantities to treat hemorrhagic disorders due to K deficiency or coumarin drug excess. Phylloquinone is also of some value in treating the hemorrhage associated with severe liver disease. If, however, 10 mg of parenteral phylloquinone does not change the coagulation factor profile within 48 hours, it means that the liver is nonresponsive to vitamin K because of the loss of endoplasmic reticulum and its associated vitamin K-dependent carboxylase. Menaquinone has been administered in large doses to cancer patients as an aid to chemotherapy and radiation.

Toxicology

Menadione, a provitamin K, unsubstituted in the 3 position, causes toxicity in children that is expressed by jaundice, hemolysis, and kernicterus. This provitamin combines with sulfhydryl groups in membranes. Less than 1% is converted to MK-4. Phylloquinone is essentially nontoxic and is the drug of choice when therapy with vitamin K is necessary.

Preparations

Phylloquinone is marketed in 5mg. tablets for oral use and in ampules containing 2 or 5 mg/ml of phylloquinone together with an emulsifier such as polyoxyethylated fatty acids or polysorbate and propylene glycol. The solubilized form can be given intramuscularly or intravenously, some times as part of total parenteral nutrition. Anaphylactic reactions to intravenous administration have been observed, but they are rare. Phylloquinone is the preferred form of vitamin K therapy.

Menadione in 5 mg. tablets is available but is not recommended 1) because the yield of active menaquinone-4 is very small and 2) menadione, unlike phylloquinone, can be toxic by virtue of its reaction with sulfhydryl groups in membranes, as mentioned above. Menadiol sodium diphosphate is a water-soluble derivative for parenteral use, but its use is not recommended.

References

Research Reports

1. McCollum EV, Davis M. The necessity of certain lipids in the diet during growth. J Biol Chem 1913;*15*:167–175.
2. Moore T. The conversation of carotene to vitamin A in vivo. Biochem J 1930;*24*:682–702.
3. Karrer P, Morf R. The constitution of β-carotene. Helv Chim Acta 1931;*14*:1033–1040.
4. Wald G. Carotenoids and vitamin A cycle in vision. Nature 1934;*134*:65.
5. Blomhoff R, Green H, Berg T, Norum KR. Transport and storage of vitamin A. Science 1990;*250*:399–403.
6. Evans RM. The steroid and thyroid hormone receptor superfamily. Science 1988;*240*:889–894.
7. Food and Nutrition Board. Recommended dietary allowances, 10th ed. Washington, DC: National Research Council/National Academy Press, 1989.
8. Mellanby E. An experimental investigation on rickets. Lancet 1919;i:407–412.
9. McCollum EV, Simmonds N, Becker JE, Shipley PG.: Studies on experimental rickets. XXI. An experimental demonstration of the existance of a vitamin which promotes calcium deposition. J Biol Chem 1922;*53*:293–312.
10. Huldschinsky K. Heilung von rachitis durch kunstliche hohensonne. Dtsch Med Wochenschr 1919;*45*:712–713.
11. Steenbock H, Black A. Fat-soluble vitamins. XVIII. The induction of growth-promoting and calcifying properties in a ration by exposure to ultra-violet light. J Biol Chem 1924;*61*:405–422.
12. Hess AF. Weinstock, Antirachitic properties imparted to lettuce and to growing wheat by ultraviolet irradiation. Proc Soc Exp Biol Med 1924;*22*:5–6.
13. Windaus A, Luttringhaus A, and Deppe M, Crystalline Vitamin D_1 Ann 1931;*489*:252–269.
14. Windaus A, Linsert O, Luttringhaus A, Weidlich G. Crystalline vitamin D_2. Ann 1932;*492*:226–241.
15. Askew FA, Bourdillon RB, Bruce HM, Callow RK, Philpot JS, Webster TA. Crystalline vitamin D. Proc Roy Soc Lond 1932;*B109*:448–506.
16. Bernal JD. Crystal structures of vitamin D and related compounds. Nature 1932;*129*:277–278.
17. Wieland H, Dane E. Untersuchen über die Konstitution der Gallensauren XXXIX. Zur kenntnis der 12-oxy-cholansaure. Z. Physiol Chemie 1932;*210*:268–281.
18. Rosenheim O, King H. The ring system of sterols and bile acids Nature, 1932;*130*:315.
19. Windaus A, Thiele W. The structure of vitamin D_2 Ann 1936;*521*:160–165.
20. Heilbron IM, Jones RN, Samant KM, Spring FS. Constitution of calciferol. J Chem Soc 1936:905–907.
21. Schenck F,: Uber das kristallisierte Vitamin D_3. Naturwissenschaften 1937;*25*:159–164.
22. Kodicek E. Vitamin D in Vitamin Metabolism, W. Umbert and M. Molitan, Ed., Vol. XI, Pergamon Press, London, 1960.
23. Neville PF, DeLuca HF. The synthesis of [1,23-H]^{3}H-vitamin D_3 and the tissue localization of a 0.25 ug (10 IU) dose per rat. Biochemistry 1966;*5*:2201.

24. Blunt JW, DeLuca HF, Schnoes HK. 25-hydroxycholecalciferol. A biologically active metabolite of vitamin D_3. Biochemistry 1968;*7*:3317–3322.

25. Olson EB, DeLuca HF. 25-Hydroxycholecalciferol: direct effect on calcium transport. Science 1969;*165*:405–407.

26. Fraser DR, Kodicek E. Unique biosynthesis by kidney of a biologically active vitamin D metabolite. Nature (Lond.) 1970;*22*:764–766.

27. Holick MF, Schnoes HK, DeLuca HF. Identification of 1,25-dihydroxycholecalciferol, a form of vitamin D_3 metabolically active in the intestine. Proc Nat Acad Sci 1971;*68*:803–804.

28. Lawson DEM, Fraser DR, Kodicek E, Morris HR, Williams DH. Identification of 1,25-dihydroxycholecalciferol, a new kidney hormone controlling calcium metabolism. Nature (Lond.) 1971;*230*:228–230.

29. Norman AW, Myrtle JF, Midgett RJ, Nowicki HF, Williams V, Popjak G. Identification of 1,25-dihydroxy cholecalciferol as the active form of vitamin D_3. Science 1971;*173*:51–54.

30. Mautalen CA.: Mechanism of action of Solanum malacoxylon upon calcium and phosphate metabolism in the rabbit. Endocrinology 1972;*90*:563–567.

31. Holick MF, MacLaughlin JA, Doppelt SH. Regulation of cutaneous previtamin D_3 photosynthesis in man: skin pigment is not an essential regulator. Science 1981;*211*:590–593.

32. Steenbock H, Kletzein SWF, Halpin JG.: The reaction of the chicken to irradiated ergosterol and irradiated yeast as contrasted with the natural vitamin D of fish liver oils. J Biol Chem 1932;*97*:249–264.

33. Hunt RD, Garcia FG, Hegsted DM.: A comparison of vitamin D_2 and D_3 in new world primates. I. Production and progression of osteodystrophia fibrosa. Lab Anim Care 1967;*17*:222–234.

34. Holick MF, Kasten-Schraufrogel K, Tavela T, DeLuca HF.: Biological activity of 1 α-hydroxyvitamin D_3 in the rat. Arch Biochem Biophys 1975;*166*:63–66.

35. Finch JL, Brown AJ, Mori T, Nishii Y, Slatopolsky E. Suppression of PTH and decreased action on bone are partially responsible for the low calcemic activity of 22-oxacalcitriol relative to 1,25-(OH)2D3. J Bone Miner Res 1992;*7*:835–839.

36. Abe J, Takita Y, Nakano T, Miyaura C, Suda T, Nishii Y. A synthetic analogue of vitamin D_3, 22-oxa-l alpha, 25-dihydroxyvitamin D_3, is a potent modulator of in vivo immunoregulating activity without inducing hypercalcemia in mice. Endocrinology 1989;*124*:2645–2647.

37. Norman A, DeLuca HF. The absorption of vitamin D_3. Biochemistry 1963;*2*:1160–1165.

38. Schachter D, Finkelstein JD, Kowarski S. Metabolism of vitamin D. J Clin Invest 1964;*43*:787–791.

39. Rosen JF, Chesney RW.: Circulating calcitriol concentrations in health and disease. J Pediatr 1983;*103*:1–17.

40. Porteous CE, Coldwell RD, Trafford DJH, Makin HLJ.: Recent developments in measurement of vitamin D and its metabolites in human body fluids. J Steroid Biochem 1987;*28*:785–801.

41. Fox J. Hypocalcemia, but not PTH or hypophosphatemia induces a rapid incrase in $1,25(OH)_2$ D_3 levels in rats. Am J. Physiol 1992;*262*:E211–215.

42. Nicolaysen R. The absorption of calcium as a function of body saturation with calcium. Acta Physiol Scand 1947;*5*:200–211.

43. Wasserman RH, Taylor AN.: Vitamin D_3-induced calcium-binding protein in chick intestinal mucosa. Science 1966;*152*:791–793.

44. de Boland AR, Nemere I. Rapid actions of vitamin D compounds. J Cell Biochem 1992;*41*:231–240.

45. Lee DB, Walling MW, Corry DB. Phosphate transport across the rat jejunum: influence of sodium, pH and 1,25-dihydroxyvitamin D_3. Am J Physiol 1986;*251*:G90–95.

46. Holick MF, Shao Q, Liu WW, Chen TC. The vitamin D content of fortified milk and infant formula. N Engl J Med 1992;*326*:1178–1181.

47. Ott SM, Chesnut CH 3d. Calcitriol treatment is not effective in postmenopausal osteoporosis. Am Intern Med 1989;*110*:262–274.

48. Chapuy MC, Arlot ME, Duboeuf F, Brun J, Crouzet B, Arnaud S, Delmas PD, Meunier PJ. Vitamin D_3 and calcium to prevent hip fractures in the elderly women. N Engl J Med 1992;*327*:1637–1642.

49. Goff JP, Reinhardt TA, Horst RL. Recurring hypocalcemia of bovine parturient paresis is associated with failure to produce 1,25-dihydroxyvitamin D. Endocrinology 1989;*125*:49–53.

50. Barlet JP, Davicco MJ. 1 alpha-hydroxycholecalciferol for the treatment of the downer cow syndrome. J Dairy Sci 1992;*75*:1253–1256.

51. Hodnett DW, Jorgensen NA, DeLuca HF. 1 alpha-hydroxyvitamin D3 plus 25-hydroxyvitamin D3 reduces parturient paresis in dairy cows fed high dietary calcium. J Dairy Sci 1992;*75*:485–491.

52. Abe J, Kondo S, Nishii Y, Kuroki T. Resistance to 1,25-dihydroxyvitamin D_3 of cultured psoriatic epidermal keratinocytes isolated from involved and uninvolved skin. J Clin Endocrinol Metab 1989;*68*:851–854.

53. Forfar JO, Balf CL, Maxwell GM, et al. Idiopathic hypercalcemia of infancy: clinical and methodological studies with special reference to the etiological role of vitamin D. Lancet 1956;*1*:982–985.

54. Howard JE, Meyer RJ. Intoxication by vitamin D. J Clin Endocrinol Metab 1948;*8*:895–910.

55. Evans HM, Bishop K. On the relation between fertility and nutrition. Am J Physiol 1922;*63*:396–402.

56. Evans HM, Emerson OH, Emerson, GA. Isolation from wheat germ oil of alcohol, α-tocopherol, having properties of vitamin E. J Biol Chem 1936;*113*:319–332.

57. Karrer P, Fritzsche H, Ringier BH, Salomon H. α-Tocopherol. Helv Chim Acta 1938;*21*:520–525.

58. Olson RE. Vitamin E and its relation to heart disease. Circulation 1973;*48*:179–184.

59. Olson RE. Creatine kinase and myofibrillar proteins in hereditary muscular dystrophy and in vitamin E deficiency. Am J Clin Nutr 1974;*27*:1117–1129.

60. Kayden HJ, Silben R, Kossman CE. The role of vitamin E deficiency in the abnormal autohemolysis and acanthocytosis. Trans Assoc Am Physicians 1965;*78*:334–342.

61. Rosenblum JL, Keating JP, Prensky AL, Nielson JS. Progressive neurological syndrome in children with chronic liver disease. N Eng J Med 1981;*304*:503–508.

62. Oski FA, Barness LA. Hemolytic anemia in vitamin E deficiency. Amer J Clin Nutr 1968;*21*:45–50.

63. Harding AE, Muller DPR, Thomas PK, Willison JH. Spinocerebellar degeneration associated with a selective defect in vitamin E absorption. N Engl J Med 1985;*313*:32–35.

64. The Alpha-tocopherol, Beta carotene Cancer Prevention Group The effect of vitamin E and beta carotene on the incidence of lung cancer and other cancers in male smokers New England J Med 1994;*330*:1029–1035.

65. Corrigan JJ, Marcus FI. Coagulopathy associated with vitamin E ingestion. JAMA 1974;*230*:1300–1301.

66. Dam H. Colesterinstoffwechsel in Huhnereiern und Hugnchen. Biochem Zeitschr 1929;*215*:475–492.

67. Dam H. The antihemorrhagic vitamin of the chick. Biochem J 1935;*29*:1273–1285.

68. Binkley SB, MacCorquodale D, Thayer SA, Doisy EA. The isolation of vitamin K_1. J Biol Chem 1939;*130*:219–234.

69. Dam H, Geiger A, Glavind J, Karrer P, Karrer W, Rothschild E, Salomon H. Isolierung des vitamins K in hochgereinigter form. Helv Chim Acta 1939;*22*:310–313.

70. McKee RW, Binkley SB, Thayer SA, MacCorquodale DW, Doisy EA. The isolation of vitamin K_2. J Biol Chem 1939;*131*:327–344.

71. Dialameh GH, Yekundi KG, Olson RE. Enzymatic alkylation of menaquinone-O to menaquinones by microsomes from chick liver. Biochim Biophys Acta 1970;*223*:332–338.

72. Duello TJ, Matschiner JT. Characterization of Vitamin K from human liver. J Nutr 1972;*102*:331–335.

73. Haroon Y, Hawschka PV. Application of high pressure liquid chromatography to the assay of phylloquinone in rat liver. J Lipid Res 1983;*24*:481–484.

74. Shearer MJ. Vitamin K and vitamin K-dependent proteins. Br J Haematol 1990;*75*:156–162.

75. Taggart WV, Matschiner JT. Metabolism of menadione-6,7-^{3}H in the rat. Biochem J 1969;*8*:1141–1146.

76. Stenflo J, Fernlund P, Egan W, Roepstorff P. Vitamin K-dependent modification of glutamic acid residues in prothrombin. Proc Natl Acad Sci USA 1974;*71*:2730–2733.

77. Wu S-M, Cheung W-F, Frazier D, Stafford DW. Cloning and expression of the cDNA for human γ-glutamyl carboxylase. Science, *254*:1634.

78. Dowd P, Ham SW, Geib SJ. Mechanism of Action of vitamin K J. Amer Chem Soc 1991;*113*:7734–7743.

79. Olson RE, Hall AL, Lee FC, Kappel WK. Properties of vitamin K-dependent α-glutamyl carboxylase for rat liver. Chemica Scripta 1987;27A:187–192.

80. Matschiner JT, Bell RG, Amelotti JM, Knauer TE. Isolation and characterization of a new metabolite of phylloquinone in the rat. Biochim Biophys Acta 1970;*201*:309–315.

81. Fieser LF, Tishler M, Sampson WL. Vitamin K activity and structure. J Biol Chem 1941;*137*:659–692.

82. Bleyer WA, Hakami N, Shepard TH. The development of hemostasis in the human fetus and newborn infant. J Pediatrics 1971;*79*:838–853.

Reviews

r1. McCollum EV. The supplementary dietary relationship among our natural foodstuffs. Harvey Lect 1917;*12*:151–180.

r2. Ong DE. Vitamin A-binding proteins. Nutr Rev 1985;*43*:225–232.

r3. Stryer L. Cyclic GMP cascade of vision. Ann Rev Neurosci 1986;*9*:87–119.

r4. Blomhoff R, Green MH, Norum KR. Vitamin A: Physiological and biochemical processing, Ann Rev Nutr 1992;*12*:37–57.

r5. Anonymous, Vitamin A deficiency—a global disease. Nutr Rev 1985;*43*:240–243.

r6. Hill DL, Grubbs CJ. Retinoids and cancer prevention. Ann Rev Nutr 1992;*12*:161–182.

r7. DiPalma JR, Ritchie DM. Vitamin Toxicity. Ann Rev Phamacol and Toxicol, 1977;*17*:133–148.

r8. Kamm JJ. Toxicology, carcinogenicity and teratogenicity of some orally administered retinoids. J Amer Acad Dermatology 1982;*6*:652–659.

r9. Hess AF, Rickets Osteomalacia and Tetany, Lea and Febiger, Philadelphia, 1929; pp 28–61.

r10. Lawson E. Vitamin D in Fat-soluble vitamins Ed. A.T. Diplock, Technomic Publishing Co., Lancaster, PA 1985; pp 76–142.

r11. Holick MF. Vitamin D in Modern Nutrition Health and Disease Eds. Shils M, Olson J, Shike M. Vol. 1 Eighth Edition pp 308–325 Lea & Febiger, Philadelphia, 1994.

r12. Stern PH. The D vitamins and bone. Pharmacol Rev 1980;*32*:47–80.

r13. Deluca HF. The Vitamin D system in the regulation of calcium and phosphorus metabolism. Nutr Rev 1979;*37*:161–193.

r14. DeLuca HF. The transformation of a vitamin into a hormone: the vitamin D story. Harvey Lecture Series 75; pp 333–379, 1979–80.

r15. Haussler MR. Vitamin D receptors: nature and function. Annu Rev Nutr 1986;*6*:527–562.

r16. Pike JW. Vitamin D_3 receptors: structure and function in transcription. Ann Rev Nutr 1991;*11*:189–216.

r17. Wasserman RH, Fullmer CS. Calcium transport proteins, calcium absorption and vitamin D. Ann Rev Physiol 1983;*43*:375–390.

r18. Nemere I, Norman AW. Transcaltachia, vesicular calcium transport, and microtubule-associated calbindin 28-k; emerging views of 1,25-dihydroxyvitamin D_3-mediated intestinal calcium absorption. Miner Electrolyte Metab 1990;*16*:109–124.

r19. Norman AW, Nemere I, Zhou LX, Bishop JE, Lowek E, Malyar AC, Collins ED, Taoka T, Sergeev I, Farach-Carson MC. 1,25(OH), a steroid hormone that produces biologic effects via both genomic and nongenomic pathways. J Steroid Biochem Mol Biol 1992;*41*:231–240.

r20. Miller BE, Norman AW. Vitamin D In Handbook of Vitamins Ed. LJ Machlin pp 45–97, Marcel Dekker, New York, 1984.

r21. Rasmussen H, Tenenhouse HS. Hypophosphatemias In the Metabolic Basis of Inherited Disease. 2581–2604, Vol. II Ed. RC Scriva, AL Beaudit, WS Sly, Valle, D. McGraw Hill, New York, 1989.

r22. Holick MF. Will 11,25-dihydroxyvitamin D_3, MC903, and their analogues herald a new pharmacologic era for the treatment of psoriasis? Arch Derm 1989;*125*:692–697.

r23. Kragballe K. Vitamin D analogues in the treatment of psoriasis. J Cell Biochem 1992;*49*:46–52.

r24. Burton GW, Traber MG. Vitamin E: antioxidant activity, biokinetics and bioavailability. Ann Rev Nutr 1990;*10*:357–382.

r25. Sokol RJ. Vitamin E deficiency and neurologic function. Ann Rev Nutr 1988;*8*:351–373.

r26. Byers T. Vitamin E supplements and coronary heart disease. Nutr Rev 1993;*51*:333–336.

r27. Olson RE. The function and metabolism of vitamin K. Ann Rev Nutr 1984;*4*:28k–337.

r28. Olson RE. Vitamin K in Modern Nutrition in Health and Disease, Eds. Shils M, Olson J, Shike, M. Eighth Edition, Lea and Febiger, Philadelphia, 1994; pp 342–357.

CHAPTER 59

Water-Soluble Vitamins

Robert E. Olson

Three of the traditional deficiency diseases known since antiquity, beriberi, pellagra, and scurvy, are due to the absence from the diet of three water-soluble vitamins, namely thiamine, niacin, and ascorbic acid (vitamin C). Another ancient disease, pernicious anemia, finally was shown to be caused by the absence of vitamin B_{12}.

These diseases were intensively studied at the turn of the 20th century and linked to experimental findings by Casimir Funk in London and F.G. Hopkins in Cambridge, England. The idea that disease would be caused by the lack of an essential nutrient was revolutionary in 1912 when Hopkins published his classic paper on "accessory food factors," describing a new set of trace nutrients for which Funk coined the name "vitamine." From 1912 to 1935 one of the main concerns of biochemists was to identify the vitamins required for growth and health.

There are nine water-soluble vitamins: thiamine, riboflavin, niacin, pyridoxine, pantothenic acid, biotin, folic acid, vitamin B_{12}, and ascorbic acid (Fig. 59.1). In the early period of discovery of the vitamins, thiamine was identified as vitamin B_1 and shown to be heat-labile. There were, however, other chemicals in cereals also necessary for growth of animals; these were heat-stable and were denoted vitamin(s) B_2. Subsequently it was shown that the remaining seven substances identified by further research as vitamins were heat-stable, and these were classified as part of the B_2-complex. All of them function as coenzymes in biochemical reactions, as shown in Figure 59.2.

Vitamin C (ascorbic acid) is also water-soluble and was shown to be a component of citrus fruits in the 18th century. It was isolated in 1930 independently by Szent-Gyorgy in Hungary and King in the US. Vitamin C is an antioxidant, but also plays a specific role in the hydroxylation of selected compounds.

Thiamine

History

Beriberi is an ancient disease; it was described in Oriental medical writings about the time of Christ and has been associated with rice diets since antiquity. Beriberi has both neurologic and cardiologic manifestations associated with the "dry" and "wet" forms of the disease. The disease was particularly prominent among sailors in the Japanese and other Far Eastern navies at the turn of the century. In 1884, Takaki,[1] a surgeon in the Japanese navy, fortified the rice diet aboard his ship with milk and meat and observed a dramatic decrease in the prevalence of beriberi. This was the first evidence that beriberi was a nutritional disease.

In 1897, a Dutch medical officer, Christian Eijkman, stationed in Java, Dutch East Indies, discovered that a form of neuritis resembling dry beriberi could be produced in chickens fed polished rice.[2] Furthermore, he showed that the disease could be prevented or cured by feeding the chickens rice bran. His associate, Grijns, noted that addition of green peas, green beans, and meat could also prevent beriberi in fowl; and he correctly deduced that such natural foodstuffs contained a factor needed for the prevention of beriberi. In 1911, Casimir Funk, a chemist at the Lister Institute in London, isolated a crystalline nitrogen-containing substance from rice bran and was convinced he had isolated the antiberiberi factor. He named it *vitamine* (for life-giving amine), but alas it had little antineuritic activity and turned out to be nicotinic acid!

It was not until 1926 that Jansen and Donath, working in Java, succeeded in obtaining the crystalline antiberiberi vitamin.[3] Jansen suggested the name aneurine, which has since been replaced by *thiamine.*

Figure 59.1 Thiamine and Related Compounds. *A*, Thiamine; *B*, Thiamine pyrophosphate; *C*, Thiamine (cyclic form); *D*, Thiochrome; *E*, Oxythiamine; *F*, Pyrithiamine

It was noted by Neuberg and Karczag[4] in 1911 that yeast extracts would decarboxylate pyruvate to acetaldehyde. In 1932, Auhagen showed that a heat-stable cofactor was involved in the decarboxylation of pyruvate by yeast. He named the cofactor cocarboxylase.[5] Thiamine itself was not isolated until 1934 by R.R. Williams et al.,[6] who determined its structure in 1936.[7] In 1936, R.A. Peters[8] and his coworkers at Oxford showed that thiamine would correct a defect in pyruvate metabolism in brain tissue from thiamine-deficient pigeons. In the same year, Lohmann and Schuster[9] isolated cocarboxylase from yeast and determined its structure to be the pyrophosphate of thiamine.

Chemistry

Thiamine is a pyrimidyl-substituted thiazole that has the structure of 3(2′-methyl-4′amino-5′-pyrimidylmethyl)-5-(2-hydroxyethyl)-4-methylthiazolium chloride, as shown in Figure 59.1. Thiamine is a white crystalline substance soluble in water, partially soluble in alcohol, and insoluble in fat solvents. Thiamine is stable to boiling, freezing, and ultraviolet light. Below pH 5.0 it is stable to heat, but in alkaline solution it is labile to heat and sulfite ions. At pH 6.0, thiamine is cleaved into its pyrimidine and thiazole components by bisulfite. The free vitamin is a base; it is isolated or synthesized as a solid thiazolium salt, e.g., thiamine chloride hydrochloride. The principal coenzymic form of thiamine is the pyrophosphate ester (TPP), in which pyrophosphate is esterified with the hydroxyl of the β-hydroxyethyl side-chain, as shown in Figure 59.1. The enzyme thiamine pyrophosphokinase catalyzes the formation of TPP from thiamine and ATP.

The 4-amino group on the pyrimidyl position of thiamine can attack the 2-position of the thiazole ring to form a tricyclic isomer of thiamine, which can be oxidized to thiochrome by ferricyanide. Thiochrome gives a blue fluorescence and has been used to measure thiamine in biologic materials. Numerous analogues of thiamine have been made, including those used as experimental antithiamines, e.g., oxythiamine first produced by Bergel and Todd[10] and pyrithiamine synthesized by Tracy and Elderfield.[11]

Physiology

The small intestine absorbs thiamine by two mechanisms.[r2] At high concentrations, thiamine is absorbed by passive diffusion; at low concentrations, it is absorbed by an active process involving a Na^+-dependent, ATP-dependent mechanism. Thomson and Leevy[12] reported that the intestinal absorption of thiamine in humans can be described by Michaelis-Menten kinetics. Thiamine is phosphorylated to its esters soon after entering the intestinal cells and then is hydrolyzed before secretion into the blood stream. Thiamine is carried via the portal blood to the liver, where the "first pass" delivers a large portion of the vitamin to hepatocytes that serve as a buffer for thiamine stores in the body. The body pool in humans varies from 30 to 70 mg. Most of the thiamine in the body is associated with mitochondria, where it participates in cellular oxidation.

Thiamine has a relatively high turnover in the body, with a half-time of about nine to 18 days. The concentration of thiamine is highest in heart muscle, high in liver and kidney, low in brain, and lowest in muscle. The over-all range, as shown in Table 59.1, is from 1 to 10 μg/g fresh tissue. Although muscles contain only 1 to 2 μg/g of thiamine, they make up a large

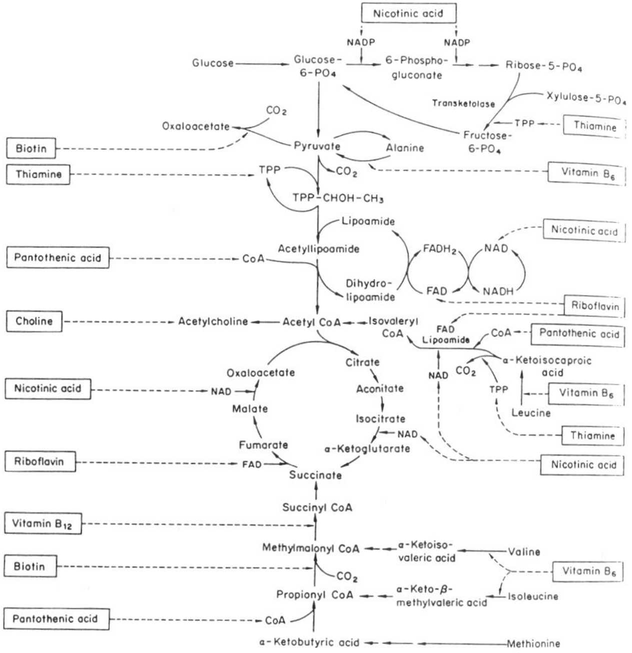

Figure 59.2 Some major metabolic pathways involving coenzymes formed from water-soluble vitamins. (Abbreviations are defined in the text.) (From r1)

percentage of body weight and account for 40 percent of the total body thiamine. The main storage organ for thiamine is the liver, where thiamine is stored as coenzymes and mobilized as needed. In tissues, thiamine is distributed as 80 percent TPP, 11 percent TMP, 5 percent TTP, and 4 percent free thiamine. Thiamine triphosphate plays a role in the polarization of membranes in the CNS.

As regards the catabolism of thiamine, thiamine phosphate esters are hydrolyzed by their respective phosphatases in cells, partially metabolized, and thiamine released into the plasma. Thiamine and its metabolic products are all excreted in the urine. There are 20 metabolites of thiamine observed in the urine of animals and humans; most have both rings still intact. Such compounds as 2-methyl-4-amino-5-pyrimidine carboxylic acid, 4-methyl thiazole-5-acetic acid, and 2-methyl-4-amino-5-hydroxymethyl-pyrimidone, have been identified in the urine.

The biochemical function of thiamine pyrophosphate is the transfer of an acyl carbanion ($R\text{-}CO^-$), also denoted as an "active aldehyde," from one compound to another. Indeed, thiamine and its pyrophosphate were found to catalyze nonenzymatically not only the decarboxylation of pyruvate but also acyloin-type condensations.[13] The discovery by Breslow[14] that the hydrogen at the C-2 position of the thiazole ring readily exchanged with ^2H_2O led to the proposal that this C-2 position of the thiazole ring was the reaction center of the coenzyme and reacted with "active aldehydes." The intermediate in pyruvate decarboxylation, 2-α-hydroxyethylthiamine, postulated by Breslow, was synthesized and found to form acetaldehyde with yeast pyruvate carboxylase.[15] 2-α-Hydroxyethylthiamine pyrophosphate subsequently was isolated from yeast by Holzer and Beauchamp.[16]

There are two general types of reactions in which TPP functions as the Mg^{2+}-coordinated coenzyme for active aldehyde transfers. There are the oxidative decarboxylation of α-keto acids catalyzed by dehydrogenase complexes and the formation of α-ketols (ketoses) catalyzed by transketolase.[18]

The multienzymic dehydrogenase complexes that affect oxidative decarboxylation of α-keto acids to *acyl-CoA* derivatives, (e.g., pyruvate dehydrogenase and α-ketoglutarate dehydrogenase), are localized in the mitochondria. Three types of subunit proteins comprise these dehydrogenase complexes: (1) a TPP-dependent decarboxylase, which converts the α-keto acid to α-hydroxyalkyl-TPP derivative (e.g. 2-α-hydroxyethyl-TPP from pyruvate); (2) dihydrolipoyl transacetylase, which contains lipoyl residues that are acylated by the α-hydroxyalkyl-TPP; and (3) a FAD-dependent dihydrolipoyl dehydrogenase, which reoxidizes the reduced lipoyl residues produced after transfer of their acyl functions to CoA.

Table 59.1 Thiamine Content of Animal Tissues*

Tissue	Range of Thiamine Concentration in μg/gram fresh weight
Heart	6–10
Liver	5–8
Kidney	4–6
Brain	2–5
Muscle	1–2

*These data are taken from various animal studies. The thiamine concentration in human tissues is about 50% of the values cited above. Thiamine pyrophosphate makes up about 80% of the total for each tissue.

Transketolase is a TPP-dependent enzyme found in the cytosol of many tissues, especially liver and blood cells. This enzyme catalyzes the reversible transfer of a glycolaldehyde moiety (2-α-dihydroxyethyl-TPP) from the first two carbons of a donor ketose phosphate of the pentose phosphate pathway, which additionally supplies NADPH needed for biosynthetic reactions.[17] The role of thiamine in metabolic reactions is shown in Figure 59.2.

Although TPP contributes to nervous system function by catalyzing energy production and biosyntheses of lipids and acetylcholine, it appears that there is another incompletely understood role, particularly for the triphosphate. Thiamine and its phosphate esters are located in axonal membranes of nerves; electrical stimulation leads to hydrolysis and release of both the di- and triphosphate.[18] The enzymes involved in formation and cleavage of thiamine triphosphate are in nervous tissue. Moreover, a subacute necrotizing encephalomyelopathy in patients with Leigh's syndrome results from the presence of an inhibitor of TPP-ATP phosphoryl transferase.[r3]

Various biochemical tests have been devised to measure the thiamine status of humans. These include measurement of blood thiamine, blood pyruvate, blood alpha-ketoglutarate, blood lactate, blood glyoxalate, urinary thiamine (usually as thiochrome), urinary thiamine metabolites before and after a thiamine loading test, and transketolase in red cells. Red cell transketolase seems to be the most sensitive test for thiamine nutritional status. In thiamine deficiency, erythrocyte transketolase activity is low, and enhancement of enzyme activity, with TPP added in vitro, is observed. A TPP effect of greater than 20 percent usually indicates a deficiency state. In severe deficiency states, all tests of thiamine status show reduced activities.

Nutritional Requirements

The main dietary sources of thiamine are cereal grains, yeast, organ meats, pork, legumes, and nuts. In the Western countries, many processed cereals are fortified with thiamine. In the US the average intake of thiamine is 1.75 mg/day in men and 1.08 mg/day in women. In men the intake is about 0.67 mg/1000 kcal, whereas in adult women and children the value is about 0.75 mg/1000 kcal. Many studies in human subjects have shown that the minimum thiamine requirement is about 0.25 mg/1000 kcal. There is a range around this number, which is probably about 0.25 ± 0.10—i.e., from approximately 0.15 to 0.25 μg/1000 kcal. Thiamine requirements vary with caloric expenditure because of its key role in energy production. The RDA is set at approximately 0.5 mg/1000 kcal (1.5 mg/day for men and 1.1 mg/day for women.) Infants should receive 0.5 mg/day and children about 1.0 mg/day. The stratified values for infants, children, adults, and pregnant and lactating women are given in Table 57.2.[r4]

Deficiency Diseases

Thiamine lack in animals and humans affects the cardiovascular, muscular, nervous, and gastrointestinal systems. The pathophysiology of thiamine deficiency involves the consequences of reduction in energy production and causes creatine phosphate (CP) and ATP concentrations in tissues to decrease. As a result, cellular work cannot be performed at a normal rate. Thiamine deficiency also affects the hexose-shunt pathway that produces the NADPH required in many synthetic reactions. Finally, there are poorly understood events in the nervous system that impair both peripheral and central nerves.

Table 59.2 Flavoprotein Enzymes

Name	Source	Flavin	Other Cofactor
Glucose-6-phosphate dehydrogenase	Yeast	FMN	NADH
Aldehyde oxidase	Liver	FAD	Mo
Xanthine oxidase	Milk	FAD	Mo
Sarcosine dehydrogenase*	Liver	FAD	
L-amino acid oxidase	Liver	FMN	
D-amino acid oxidase	Kidney	FAD	
Lactic dehydrogenase	Yeast	FMN	
Acyl CoA dehydrogenase	Liver	FAD	
Succinate dehydrogenase*	Heart	FAD	Fe

*Covalently bound to their apoenzymes through histidyl (N3)-8α-FAD

The major manifestations of thiamine deficiency in humans are peripheral neuropathy, beriberi heart disease, and Wernicke's encephalopathy, an often fatal acute cerebral disorder.[r3] Peripheral neuropathy (dry beriberi) is a symmetrical impairment or loss of sensory, motor, and reflex function affecting the distal segments of limbs more severely than the proximal ones. In developing countries, peripheral neuropathy can occur because of dietary thiamine deficiency. It can also occur as a result of the presence of thiaminase, an enzyme in raw fish that splits thiamine in the gut. In developed countries, peripheral neuropathy is commonly associated with alcoholism, where it is most likely to be of nutritional rather than toxic etiology. It is also the most chronic and difficult to treat.

Beriberi heart disease (wet beriberi) is characterized by enlargement of the heart, tachycardia, systemic venous hypotension, sodium retention, bounding arterial pulsations (wide pulse pressure), and the classic phenomena of high-output cardiac failure with both generalized and pulmonary edema. It responds dramatically to the administration of thiamine.

Wernicke's encephalopathy is characterized by altered mental state, including hallucinosis and disorientation, nystagmus, ophthalmoplegia, and ataxia. Wernicke's encephalopathy is the severest form of thiamine deficiency and constitutes a medical emergency. It occurs most frequently in alcoholics who have been drinking continuously for a very long period without food. In the absence of alcoholism, isolated reports of Wernicke's encephalopathy have been reported in association with parenteral nutrition, use of IV glucose solutions for long periods, GI problems involving restriction of food, starvation, chronic infection, and chronic hemodialysis. Following treatment with sedatives, thiamine, and food, this neurologic disease may be followed by Korsakoff's syndrome, which is an amnesic confabulatory disorder. Wernicke-Korsakoff's disease may result in bilateral damage to diencephalic structures, including the dorsal medial nucleus of the thalamus and the hyperthalamic mammillary bodies. The consistent presence of these lesions in Korsakoff's amnesia established that the diancephalon is a crucial component of the memory-related network.

Therapeutic Uses

When used to treat severe deficiency, thiamine is used at a supraphysiologic level ten times the RDA or more. In Wernicke's disease it is important to give as much as 100 times the RDA (100 mg) of thiamine IV, followed by oral treatment at about ten times the RDA/day until the patient has recovered. In vitamin deficiency diseases, it's generally useful to give the other

B-complex vitamins as well because of the likelihood that a secondary deficiency may be revealed by treating the first. Also, several other conditions may be thiamine-dependent states: (1) subacute necrotizing encephalitis; (2) a rare form of megaloblastic anemia. In branched-chain ketoaciduria, a genetic disorder, large amounts of thiamine are needed (10–20 mg/d). In malabsorption, high doses of thiamine may also be needed.

Toxicology

There is no evidence that oral thiamine is toxic, even at doses 500 times the RDA.

Preparations

Thiamine is available in doses with multivitamins of 1 to 5 mg/day, plus other forms.

Riboflavin

History

In 1794, Shoepf reported the occurrence of a fluorescent yellow pigment in milk; in 1879, Blyth obtained this pigment from whey in the form of an impure orange pigment and named it "lactochrome." Later it was renamed lactoflavin.[r1] In 1926, Smith and Hendrick[19] showed that the vitamin B-complex consisted of a heat-labile portion, the antineuritic factor (thiamine), and a heat-stable portion, a group of B vitamins that included riboflavin. In 1932, Warburg and Christian[20] isolated a yellow pigment from yeast, a cofactor for glucose-6-phosphate dehydrogenase, which turned out to be flavin mononucleotide (FMN). In 1933, the yellow pigment from whey was identified by Kuhn[21] as riboflavin and was shown to be identical to lactoflavin from milk.

Chemistry

The structure of riboflavin, solved by Kuhn and coworkers,[21] was found to be 6,7-dimethyl-9-(1 -D-ribityl) isoalloxazine. It is shown in Figure 59.3. The vitamin was named riboflavin because of the presence of ribose in the structure. The synthesis of riboflavin was accomplished by Kuhn et al.[22] and Karrer et al.[23] in 1935. Riboflavin is only slightly soluble in neutral aqueous solutions. The biologically active forms of riboflavin are its coenzyme forms. First, flavin mononucleotide (FMN), is the phosphorylated form of riboflavin. Flavin adenine dinucleotide (FAD) involves the addition of adenine monophosphate (AMP) to FMN to form a flavin adenine dinucleotide. Both reactions involve blood kinases and ATP as shown:

1. Riboflavin + ATP → FMN + ADP
2. FMN + ATP → FAD + PP

FAD is a coenzyme for many dehydrogenases, as shown in Table 59.2. Although some flavoproteins are formed by noncovalent attachment of FAD and FMN to the protein, some involve a covalent linkage from histadine through a methylene bridge to the 8 position of riboflavin.[r6,r7]

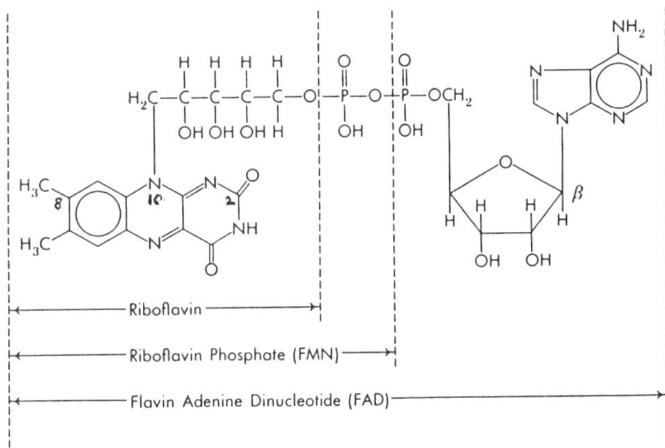

Figure 59.3 Structure of Riboflavin and the Flavin Coenzymes

Physiology

Both FMN and FAD are present in foods and must be degraded to riboflavin by proteases and phosphatases before being absorbed. Riboflavin is absorbed in the upper GI tract by a specific, saturable active transport process. Enterocytes in the upper small bowel absorb riboflavin by a sodium-dependent mechanism that is hindered by ouabain, reflecting the involvement of the Na^+, K^+, ATP pump. Riboflavin is converted to FMN and FAD in enterocytes, but the coenzymes are split before the release of the vitamin to the circulation. Small amounts of FMN may accompany riboflavin to the liver via the portal circulation.

The transport of riboflavin by blood plasma is known to involve both loose association with albumin and tighter association with some globulins. The immunoglobins have been identified as major binding proteins. The rate of uptake of flavins from the blood by cells varies considerably. Hepatocytes exhibit an initial rapid uptake followed by a slower phase of diffusion of the vitamin, which becomes metabolically trapped by flavokinase plus secondary phosphorylations. The uptake process in liver reflects facilitated transport, is relatively insensitive to sodium and ouabain, and thus is different from the uptake by enterocytes.

In the renal tubule flavin uptake exhibits sodium dependence and operates in both directions, i.e., riboflavin can be reabsorbed from the tubular filtrate or can be excreted in urine. In fact, the major metabolite of the flavin coenzymes is riboflavin itself, although other metabolites are detectable. The rate of excretion of riboflavin in the urine is about 10 percent of intakes of 1.0 mg/day or less. If the dietary intake is increased above 1.5 mg/day, the urinary output rises to 20 percent. This relatively low excretion fraction suggests that the remainder appears in the feces after extensive enterohepatic circulation. For normal adults eating varied diets, riboflavin comprises 60 to 70 percent of urinary flavins, 7-hydroxymethyl riboflavin—10 to 15%; 8(alpha)-sulfonyl riboflavin—5 to 10 percent; 8-hydroxymethyl riboflavin—4 to 7 percent; riboflavinyl peptide ester—5 percent; and 10-hydroxyethyl flavin—1 to 3 percent.

All cells require the activity of flavoproteins in both mitochondria and cytosol and are under control by the thyroid, particularly triiodothyronine. In hypothyroidism, flavokinase is not expressed and FMN phosphatase has its usual activity. This greatly inhibits FMN synthesis. On the other hand, in hyp*er*thyroidism, flavokinase, FAD synthetase, and the catabolic enzymes are all increased. The hydrolytic enzymes for FMN and FAD are located in lysosomes in the cell.

Erythrocyte glutathione reductase is an FAD-requiring enzyme that is sensitive to nutritional status; it is one enzyme used to detect riboflavin deficiency.[r1]

Nutritional Requirements

Good sources of riboflavin are milk and dairy products, which supply about half the daily intake. Meat, fish, poultry, and eggs provide another 30 percent. The remainder comes largely from fruits, vegetables, and grains. In 1985, adult men in the US consumed about 2 mg/day, women ate 1.34 mg/day, and children 1 to 5 years 1.57 mg/day.

Clinical signs of deficiency in adults can be prevented with intakes of riboflavin above 0.4 mg/1000 kcal, but over 0.5 mg/1000 kcal may be required to maintain tissue reserves in adults and children as reflected in urinary excretion, red cell riboflavin, and erythrocyte glutathione reductase. From these considerations, the riboflavin allowances are now computed as 0.6 mg/1000 kcal for people of all ages. This leads to RDAs ranging from 0.4 mg/day in early infants to 1.7 mg/day for young adult males. However, for elderly people and others whose daily calorie intake may be less than 2000 kcal, a minimum of 1.2 mg/day is recommended. Since pregnancy imposes extra demands, reflected by decreased excretion and an elevated FAD stimulation of erythrocyte glutathione activity, an additional 0.3 mg/day is recommended. The lactating woman secretes approximately 40 μg/100 ml of milk for an output of about 0.34 mg/day. Since the utilization of the additional riboflavin for milk production is assumed to be 70 percent, an additional intake of 0.5 mg is recommended.

The RDA for riboflavin in adult males is 1.4 to 1.8 mg/day and for adult females 1.2 to 1.3 mg/day, depending on age. Allowances are increased during pregnancy and lactation to 1.6 to 1.7 mg/day.[r4]

Deficiency Disease

Riboflavin deficiency in humans is uncommon, and when seen is generally associated with other nutritional deficiencies, including protein, energy, and other vitamins. Reported signs of deficiency include oral buccal cavity lesions, cheilosis, angular stomatitis, photophobia, generalized seborrheic dermatitis, scrotal and vulvar skin changes, and normocytic anemia. Because riboflavin is essential to the function of vitamins B_6 and niacin, some signs attributed to riboflavin deficiency may be due to the failure of the proper utilization of these other nutrients. Riboflavin intake of 0.5 mg or less per day (0.2 mg/1000 kcal) results in clinically recognizable signs of riboflavin deficiency.

Important in diagnosing riboflavin deficiency is the correlation of dietary history with clinical laboratory findings. Urinary excretion of riboflavin of less than 50 μg/day and changes in EGR activity and response to in vitro FAD suggest riboflavin deficiency. Bates[24] has recently reported that riboflavin-deficient rats have a block with oxidation of adipic acid that is relieved by enhanced oxidation after dosing with riboflavin. Application of this test to humans would be of interest.

Therapeutic Use

Riboflavin deficiency is treated with 10 to 15 mg/day of riboflavin, usually supported with other vitamins in patients with multiple vitamin deficiencies. It is noted that this dose of riboflavin will result in healing of skin lesions within days to weeks. Riboflavin in large doses has been utilized to treat several rare inborn errors in metabolism, including congenital methemoglobinemia, pyruvate kinase deficiency, and glutaryl Co-A dehydrogenase deficiency.

Toxicology

No adverse effects of riboflavin ingestion at 100 to 1000 times the RDA have been reported.

Preparations

Riboflavin is packaged in multivitamin capsules at doses of 1.7 to 10 mg/capsule.

Niacin (Nicotinic Acid)

History

Pellagra is one of the classic deficiency diseases known since antiquity and associated with maize-eating populations. The disease was first described by Gasper Casal, physician to King Philip V of

Spain in 1735 and by Antonio Pugati in Italy in 1755. The term pellagra comes from the Italian, *pelle agra* or rough skin. During the 19th century the disease was observed in many countries besides Italy and Spain, including France, Egypt, Romania, and the southern US.[r7] In 1912, coincident with the classic animal work of F.G. Hopkins referred to earlier, Casmir Funk postulated that pellagra, along with beriberi and scurvy, were diseases due to a deficient diet.

In the early 1900s pellagra became epidemic in the southern US, particularly in mental hospitals. The epidemiologic studies of pellagra by Joseph Goldberger, a physician in the US Public Health Service in the 1920s, showed that pellagra was not an infectious disease but was due to an unknown dietary deficiency. Subsequently Goldberger carried out two experiments. First, he fed diets on which humans developed pellagra to dogs; this produced black tongue, the analogue of pellagra in dogs, which had been described by Chittenden in 1907. Next, Goldberger fed diets rich in animal protein to patients in one of the mental institutions of the south who normally exhibited pellagra in the spring. This prevented the appearance of pellagra. Goldberger concluded correctly that their maize diet, known to be deficient in tryptophan, was responsible for the disease.

In 1937, however, Elvejhem et al. at the University of Wisconsin, demonstrated that nicotinic acid, which had been known as an oxidation product of nicotine since 1867, would cure canine black tongue. Nicotinic acid also had been isolated from yeast by Casimir Funk in 1911, who thought it was the anti-beriberi factor, when in fact it was the pellagra-preventive factor. Within a year, Spies et al.[26] demonstrated that nicotinic acid would also cure pellagra in humans. For the moment the discovery distracted attention from tryptophan as a pellagra preventative.

In 1945, Krehl et al.[27] at the University of Wisconsin, discovered that tryptophan could replace niacin in sustaining the growth and preventing dermatitis in rats on a corn diet. By 1948, Heidelberger[28] et al. at the University of California showed that animals fed $3^{14}C$-DL-tryptophan excreted radioactive nicotinic acid in their urine. When tryptophan was labeled with N-15 in the indole nucleus, ring-labeled nicotinic acid was also excreted. In 1940, Vilter[31] showed that tryptophan would cure pellagra. Thus, the linkage between niacin (the term adopted for nicotinic acid) and tryptophan was finally solved by biochemists. Looking back at the epidemiologic studies of Goldberger, who thought that an amino acid deficiency was the most likely cause of pellagra, it became clear why maize was causative. Maize is low in tryptophan, pyridoxine, and riboflavin. Both pyridoxine and riboflavin are required for the biosynthesis of nicotinic acid from tryptophan. Thus, the poor diets of the southern blacks, many confined in mental institutions because of the dementia of pellagra, were ideal for perpetuating pellagra.

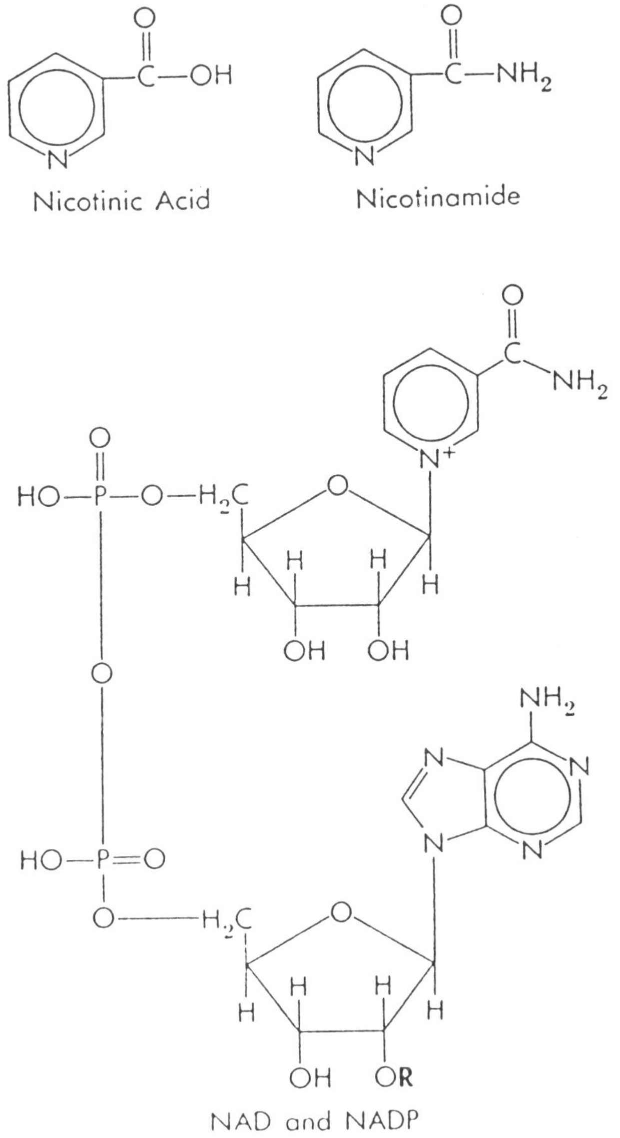

Figure 59.4 Niacin and NAD(P)

Chemistry

Nicotinic acid, which is pyridoxine-3-carboxylic acid (MW = 123), initially was produced by the oxidation of nicotine. Nicotinamide is the amide of nicotinic acid, which is the functional group in the pyridine nucleotide coenzymes. Niacin is a generic term that encompasses both nicotinic acid and its amide. The conversion of tryptophan to nicotinic acid involves the degradation of tryptophan to kynurenine, then to quinolinic acid, and finally to nicotinic acid (Fig. 59.6). Nicotinic acid crystallizes as white needles from alcohol. It is freely soluble in water and stable to boiling. Nicotinamide adenine dinucleotide (NAD^+) and nicotinamide adenine dinucleotide phosphate (NADP) with the phosphate on the 2′ position of ribose are the coenzyme forms of niacin are shown in Fig. 59.4.

The synthesis of the nicotinamide adenine dinucleotides is accomplished by the reaction of nicotinic acid with phosphoribose pyrophosphate (PRPP) to form nicotinic acid ribonucleotide plus inorganic pyrophosphate (PP). Nicotinic acid ribonucleotide then reacts with ATP to form desamino NAD plus PP; desamino NAD then reacts with glutamine plus ATP to produce nicotinamide adenine dinucleotide plus glutamate plus ADP plus phosphate. For the synthesis of NADP, an NAD kinase plus ATP attach the third phosphate to the 2′ position of ribose. It was Warburg and associates[29] who in 1935 first obtained nicotinic amide from NADP isolated from red blood cells of the horse. This finding further stimulated studies on the nutritional value of nicotinic acid.

Physiology

NAD and NADP are the major dietary forms of niacin. They are hydrolyzed by enzymes in the intestinal mucosa to yield nicotinamide as the major end-product.[r9] Both vitamers are absorbed by facilitated diffusion at low concentrations and by passive diffusion at higher concentrations, and both appear in blood plasma. Even large doses (3 g or more) of niacin are efficiently absorbed from the intestine. Niacin is rapidly removed from blood plasma by the tissues, particularly the liver and red cells. Although most tissue cells absorb niacin by passive diffusion, facilitated diffusion also takes place in the kidney and the erythrocyte. Plasma levels range from 5 to 50 μg/ml.

In the liver, any excess of free niacin that accumulates is methylated to (NMN) N-methyl nicotinamide by N-methyl transferase. NMN is the major niacin metabolite excreted in the urine. Other metabolites found in urine include the oxidized derivatives of NMN, 2- and 4-methyl pyridone, and nicotinuric acid, the conjugate of nicotinic acid and glycine. The oxide and hydroxyl forms of niacin are also excreted in small amounts.[21]

Niacin is biosynthesized from quinolinate in all organisms studied. In mammals, quinolinic acid arising from dietary Trp through the kynurenine pathways is converted to nicotinic acid ribonucleotide. This conversion apparently is regulated by the enzyme quinolinate phosphoribosyltransferase. In humans the biosynthesis of niacin from Trp is an important route for meeting the body's niacin requirement. The efficiency of conversion of dietary Trp to niacin is affected by nutritional factors (protein, energy, pyridoxine, riboflavin, and niacin) and hormonal factors. To estimate nutritional intake or niacin equivalents (NE) from Trp, and average conversion ratio of 60 mg Trp to 1 mg niacin was recommended by the Food and Nutrition Board of the National Research Council,[r3] although it is known that the rate of conversion of Trp to niacin is increased three times in pregnant women.

As regards its biochemical function, over 200 enzymes require nicotinamide as part of either NAD or NADP. Most of these oxidoreductases function as dehydrogenases and catalyze such diverse reactions as the conversion of alcohols (often sugars and polyols) to aldehydes or ketones, hemiacetals to lactones, aldehydes to acids, and certain amino acids to keto acids. The common mechanism of operation, as generalized in Figure 59.5, involves the stereospecific abstraction of a hydride ion from substrate, with para addition to one or the other side of carbon 4 in the pyridine ring of the nucleotide coenzyme. The second hydrogen of the substrate group oxidized is concomitantly removed as a proton and ultimately exchanges as hydronium ion.

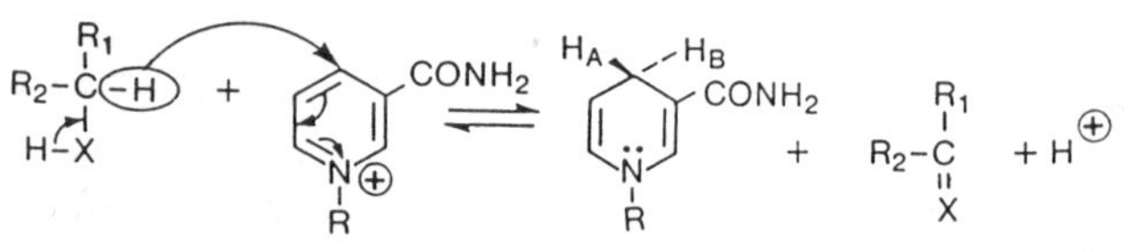

Figure 59.5 The Common Mechanism of Operation for Niacin

Most dehydrogenases utilizing NAD or NADP function reversibly. Glutamate dehydrogenase, for example, favors oxidation, whereas others, like glutathione reductase, prefer reduction. A further generality is that most NAD-dependent enzymes are involved in catabolic reactions, whereas NADP systems are more concerned with biosynthetic reactions. The discovery that some NAD glycohydrolases have the ability to transglycosidate, i.e., transfer the ADPR moiety of NAD to macromolecules, has led to recognition of nonredox functions of the coenzyme. ADP-ribosyl transferases catalyze the transfer of ADPR to such macromolecules as elongation factor 2, diphtheria toxin, and cholera toxin. Some ADP-ribosylated protein appear to function in DNA repair, DNA replication, and cell differentiation.

Nutritional Requirements

The calculated average daily intake of niacin in the US is 27 mg of niacin equivalents (NE) for women and 41 mg for men. The corresponding values for preformed niacin are 16 mg/day for women and 24 mg/day for men. Niacin deficiency has been observed in people receiving 8.8 mg NE per day.[32] The RDA for adults,[r4] based on the conversion factor of 60 mg Trp to 1 mg of niacin, ranges from 15 to 20 mg NE for males and 13 to 15 mg NE for females. In terms of energy, recommendations are for 6.6 mg NE/1000 kcal, but the total niacin intake should not be less than 13 mg per day for adults of all ages. Most of the evidence for these allowances was derived from studies of adult men and women conducted during the 1950s.[33] There are no data on niacin requirements of children through adolescence. Because milk from well-nourished mothers appears to be adequate to meet niacin needs of infants, however, the RDA for infants up to six months of age is set at 8 mg NE/1000 kcal, which is the average content of niacin in human milk. Because the energy requirement is increased by 300 kcal per day in pregnancy, the RDA was increased to 17 mg/day for pregnant women. The RDA for lactating women is 20 mg/day, which includes an additional allowance of 5 mg NE per day, based on the calculated content of 750 ml breast milk, 1.0 to 1.3 mg, plus the energy increment required to support lactation.

Deficiency Disease

Pellagra generally is a disease of poor people subsisting on marginal diets based on corn products. The

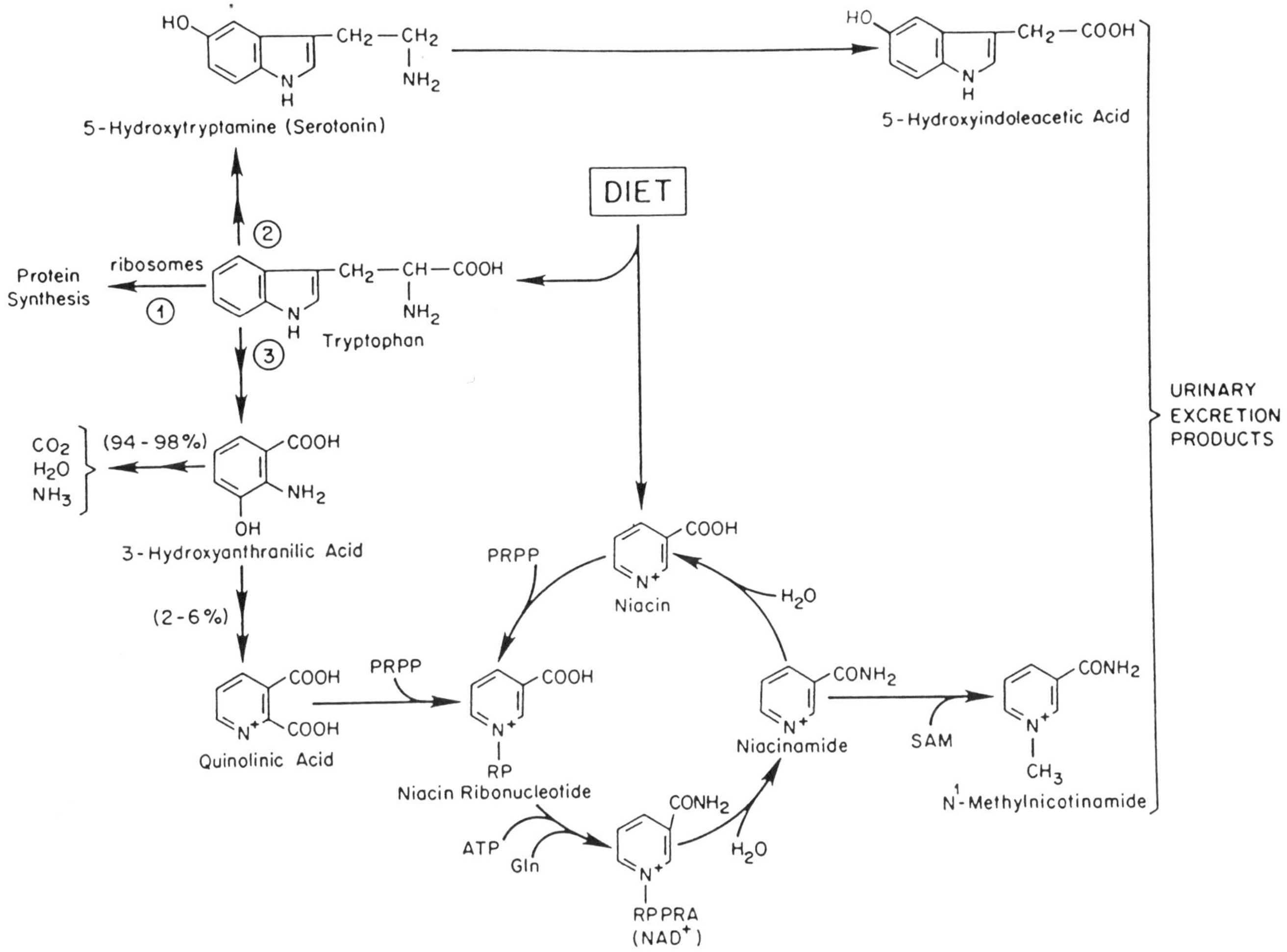

Figure 59.6 The metabolism of tryptophan and niacin in humans. Dietary tryptophan is absorbed and distributed to various tissues. It may be ① incorporated into protein via ribosomes, ② metabolized to serotonin and 5-hydroxyindoleacetic acid via the serotonin pathway, or ③ converted to NAD^+ or CO_2, H_2O, and NH_3 via the kynurenin pathway. Dietary niacin is converted to NAD^+ via a different phosphoribosyl transferase than the one acting on quinolinate. All N^1-methylnicotinamide appearing in the urine is derived from the catabolism of NAD^+. PRPP: phosphoribosylpyrophosphate; SAM: *S*-adenosylmethionine; RPPRA: ribose pyrophosphoryladenosine; Gln: glutamine.

disease is seasonal and appears in the spring and lasts through the summer. It is recurrent in populations on poor diets. The first symptom is a symmetrical, photosensitive erythema that resembles a sunburn but does not disappear, making the erythematous area brown (pigmented), scaly, and ugly. Casals necklace is the dermatitis appearing on sun-exposed skin around the neck.

The erythema is usually followed by GI disturbances, such as nausea, anorexia, and diarrhea, consisting of fetid fatty stools, sometimes with blood. The whole GI tract is affected, and may result in achlorhydria, glossitis, stomatitis, and vaginitis. Pigmentation around the vulva is not uncommon.

Finally, mental changes occur, which include fatigue, insomnia, and apathy—a prodrome for encephalopathy characterized by confusion, disorientation, hallucinations, amnesia, and even manic-depressive psychosis. These neurologic symptoms were the reason that pellagrins found their way into mental hospitals in the southern US in the early 1900s.

In summary, pellagra can be summarized as the syndrome of the 3 Ds: dermatitis, diarrhea, and dementia. In the Western world chronic alcoholics are at high risk for pellagra. In addition, Hartnup's disease is a rare genetic disorder in which impairment of neutral amino acid transport occurs in intestine and kidney. Because tryptophan is neither absorbed by the gut nor retained by the kidney, these patients develop pellagra and require large doses of niacin to prevent symptoms.

Biochemical tests of humans with suspected niacin deficiency include reduced levels of niacin and niacin metabolites in blood and urine. Reduced levels of N-methyl nicotinamide (NMN) and its pyridone in urine are useful markers for niacin deficiency. A guideline for making the diagnosis of niacin deficiency is NMN levels less than 0.8 mg/day. Tryptophan metabolites such as xanthurenic and kynurenic acid are also reduced in the urine in pellagra.[r8]

Therapeutic Uses

Pellagra should be treated with 100 mg of niacin per day for several weeks. In Hartnup's disease, 50 to 300 mg of nicotinamide are required to control the pellagra. Nicotinic acid, but not the amide, at megadoses of 3 to 6 grams/day has a hypocholesteremic effect in humans. The most significant adverse effect of this dose is serious flushing, although some patients develop liver disease.

Toxicology

The large doses of nicotinic acid required for the control of hypercholesterolemia (3–6 g/day) may cause liver disease.

Preparations

Nicotinamide is available as part of multivitamin capsules in amounts of 20 to 80 mg/capsule. Nicotinic acid is available in doses of 100 to 300 mg/capsule.

Pyridoxine (Vitamin B_6)

History

After the identification of thiamine as vitamin B_1 and riboflavin as vitamin B_2, evidence mounted that a cluster of unknown water-soluble vitamins in bran and yeast remained to be discovered.[r4] In 1926, Paul Gyorgy showed that rats on a vitamin B_2-complex-deficient diet developed a dermatitis not unlike human pellagra, which he postulated was due to the absence of a new "acrodynia factor." In 1935, Gyorgy[33] showed that the "acrodynia factor" was distinct from riboflavin, and he christened it vitamin B_6. Shortly afterwards, in 1938, this vitamin was isolated from extracts of rice bran and yeast by several independent groups of investigators, which included Gyorgy,[34] Lefkosky,[35] and Kerestezy and Stevens.[36] In 1939, the synthesis of this new vitamin, now called pyridoxine, was accomplished by Harris and Folkers.[37] Soon it became evident that the vitamin B_6 family was composed of more than one chemical form. By 1944, Snell[38] identified pyridoxal and pyridoxamine derivative forms of the vitamin, and also identified pyridoxyl-5-phosphate as the active coenzyme form of vitamin B_6.[39]

Chemistry

Pyridoxine is 2-methyl-3-hydroxy-4,5-dihydroxymethylpyridine. Its structure and two other vitamers and their coenzyme forms are shown in Figure 59.7. They differ only in the nature of the functional group attached to position 4 of the pyridine ring. They are, furthermore, interconvertable in metabolism in the body. In fact, the aldehyde, which is the major active form, is converted to the amine in transamination and then returned to the aldehyde during the enzyme action. In the process, an amino group from one amino acid is transferred to another.

The conversion of the vitamin to its coenzyme form is accomplished by a kinase that phosphorylates the alcoholic group in the 5 position. The mechanism of action of pyridoxyl phosphate involves the formation of a Schiff base with an amino group of an amino acid. With the aid of a metal and the phenolic group on the pyridine ring, a planar structure is formed that permits the electron sink of the pyridine ring to pull electrons into the ring and shift the double bonds in the amino acid-pyridoxyl adduct. This labilizes the alpha carbon and permits transfer of the amino group to the coenzyme to form pyridoxamine.

The major degradation product of B_6 homologues is pyridoxic acid which as a carboxyl in position 4. Vitamin B_6 compounds absorbs light in the UV and are fluorescent. Microbiologic assays, HPLC measurements, and enzyme bioassays are used to determine the amount of the pyridoxal and related homologues in biologic materials.

Antimetabolites of pyridoxine have been synthesized that are capable of blocking the action of the vitamin and producing symptoms of vitamin B_6 deficiency. The most active is 4-deoxypyridoxine, shown in Figure 59.7, in which the substituent on carbon atom 4 is a methyl group. It has therefore no functionality as a reactant, and, as 4-deoxypyridoxine phosphate, is a competitive inhibitor of several pyridoxyl phosphate-dependent enzymes.

Physiology

Pyridoxine (PN), pyridoxal (PL), and pyridoxamine (PM) are readily absorbed from the GI tract. Their coenzyme forms, which make up the bulk of the vitamin B_6 in foods, are split by an intestinal alkaline phosphatase. The enterocytes take up the B_6-vitamins by a nonsaturable mechanism with intracellular ATP-

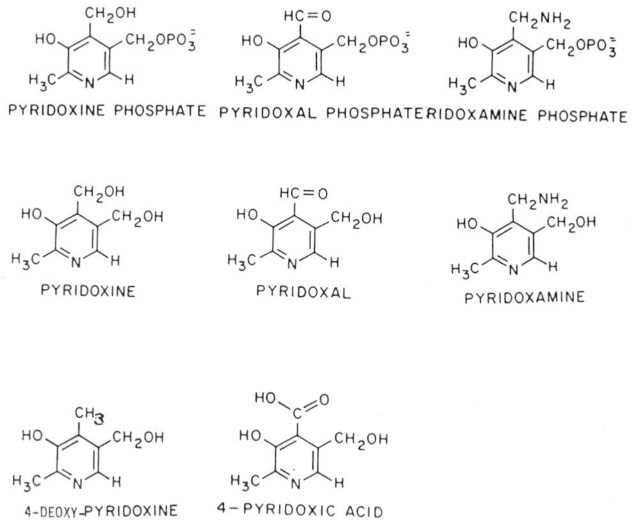

Figure 59.7 Structures of the Vitamin B_6 Vitamins and Their Coenzymes

dependent phosphorylation of all three vitamers in the cytosol, a phenomenon known as metabolic trapping. The cofactors are dephosphorylated before secretion into the portal blood, where they travel to the liver and are taken up by facilitated transport and again converted to coenzyme forms. The kidney, it appears, has a saturable sodium-dependent mechanism for reabsorbing the B_6 vitamins.

Plasma levels of vitamin B_6 compounds in healthy persons range from 5 to 15 μg/L. PLP accounts for 60 percent of plasma vitamin B_6, PN and PL 15 percent each. Erythrocytes take up both PL and PN. The remainder is pyridoxic acid, a degradation product that is rapidly excreted in the urine and serves as a marker for B_6 adequacy. PLP in plasma is tightly complexed to protein, mostly albumin.

Intracellularly, pyridoxine is oxidized to pyridoxal by a FMN-dependent oxidase and then converted to pyridoxal phosphate by a kinase. The coenzyme can enter directly into subcellular organelles such as mitochondria. The erythrocyte traps PLP as the conjugate Schiff's base with lysine in hemoglobin. Glycogen phosphorylase contains most of the PLT in Schiff's combination with a lysine, where it appears to exercise an allosteric effect on the enzyme. Glycogen phosphorylase accounts for about half the body pool of B_6, which is of the order of 25 mg in an adult human.

Pyridoxal 5′-phosphate is utilized by over 60 enzymes. They typically bind the coenzyme tightly in a Schiff's base linkage with the γ-amino group of an active-site lysine. Listed below are the categories of enzymes that are B_6-dependent.[r10]

Aminotransferases

The interconversions of amino acids and their respective α-ketoacids by aminotransferases (e.g., alanine aminotransferase, aspartate aminotransferase, etc.) are central to the biosynthesis and catabolism of essential and nonessential amino acids. In many instances they provide a simple link between the amino acid and intermediates of glycolysis (e.g., alanine and pyruvate) and the tricarboxylic acid cycle (e.g., aspartate and oxaloacetate, glutamate and α-ketoglutarate). Not all aminotransferases act on the α-amino group, however, as illustrated in the conversion of ornithine to pyrroline-5-carboxylate by ornithine-γ-aminotransferase.

Decarboxylases

The synthesis of polyamines, serotonin, tyramine, histamine, and γ-amino butyric acid (GABA), for example, involves the decarboxylation of precursor amino acids. The de novo formation of phosphatidylethanolamine (which is also an intermediate in the synthesis of choline and phosphatidylcholine) by decarboxylation of phosphatidylserine is thought to utilize a PLP-dependent enzyme. Sometimes decarboxylation occurs with carbon-carbon bond formation. The initial and regulatory enzymes of heme (δ-amino levulinate synthetase) synthesis, and sphingolipid (serine palmitoyltransferase) synthesis condense glycine with succinyl-CoA and serine and palmitoyl-CoA, respectively.

Side-chain Cleavage Enzymes

The key step in initiation of one-carbon metabolism is the transfer of a hydroxymethyl group from serine to tetrahydrofolate (catalyzed by serine hydroxymethyltransferase) to form glycine and N^5, N^{10}-methylenetetrahydrofolate. Another example of a side-chain cleavage reaction is the splitting of cystathionine (by cystathionase) in cysteine biosynthesis from methionine. Tryptophan catabolism and its utilization in nicotinamide biosynthesis also proceed via an intermediate that is cleaved by a PLP-dependent enzyme; the accumulation of various intermediates and side-produts of this pathway in response to a tryptophan load has been used as a test of vitamin B_6 status.

Dehydratases

Another type of side-chain modification reaction (β-elimination) is exemplified in the deamination and dehydration of serine to pyruvate, ammonia, and water by L-serine dehydratase.

Racemases

There are also PLP-dependent enzymes that catalyze the interconversion of D- and L-amino acids.

Nutritional Requirements

Essentially all bacterial and animal forms require vitamin B_6 for survival. In humans the requirement ranges from 1 to 2 mg/day and is dependent on protein intake. It is estimated that 0.01 to 0.015 mg of vitamin B_6/g of protein is necessary to prevent vitamin B_6 deficiency. Biochemical tests include direct measurement of vitamin forms of B_6 in the blood and urine. For example, the concentration of PLP in plasma or urine and the excretion of 4-pyridoxic acid are useful indicators. The administration of 2 to 5 gram of L-tryptophan followed by measurement of xanthurenic and kynurenic acids is also a useful test. There are also indirect functional tests that measure the activity of several B_6-dependent enzymes; for example, erythrocyte alanine aminotransferase.

In healthy infants, B_6 intake of 0.3 mg/day protects against abnormal excretion of tryptophan metabolites following the load test. The 1989 RDAs for pyridoxine are 0.3 to 0.6 mg/day for infants, 1 to 1.4 mg/day for children, 2.0 mg/day for adult males, and 1.6 mg/day for adult females. In pregnancy the allowance is increased to 2.2 mg/day and for lactating women to 2.1 mg/day.

Good sources of vitamin B_6 in the diet are chicken, fish, kidney, liver, pork, and eggs—each of which provides more than 0.4 mg per 100-g serving. Other good sources are unmilled rice, soybean, oats, whole wheat products, peanuts, and walnuts. Dairy products and red meats are relatively poor sources.

Deficiency Disease

Signs referrable to pyridoxine deficiency have been produced in all mammalian species studied, including humans. These include skin disease, mostly hyperkeratosis, acanthosis, seborrhea-like skin lesions, particularly in humans, which can be produced either by a severe deficiency or by using the antagonist 4-deoxypyridoxine. Another manifestation of vitamin B_6-deficiency observed in lambs, pigs, dogs, and humans are convulsive seizures.

In 1954, when some infant formulas were not properly constituted with adequate B_6, convulsions were observed in a number of infants. It has been determined that this effect was probably due to the lack of formation of γ-amino butyric acid (GABA), a neurotransmitter formed as a result of decarboxylation of glutamic acid. In some case the vitamin B_6-dependency syndrome characterized by severe convulsions and retarded mental and psychomotor development responded to early and continuous treatment with large doses of 10 to 20 mg/day of pyridoxine. In addition to the CNS symptoms, B_6 deficiency can cause deterioration of the dorsal roots and cause peripheral neuropathies.

Pyridoxine deficiency also has been shown to cause microcytic anemia in the dog, pig, and monkey. This apparently is due to the failure to synthesize heme in adequate amounts. While dietary deficiency of pyridoxine may rarely cause anemia in humans, there are genetically-conditioned pyridoxine dependencies for sideroblastic anemias.

Therapeutic Uses

The treatment of vitamin B_6 deficiency requires about 10 times the RDA (25 mg) daily until signs remit. Vitamin B_6 dependency states may require 50 to 200 mg of pyridoxine/day. One of these is hereditary sideroblastic anemia. Sideroblasts are nucleated red cell precursors containing excess iron. The genetic lesion is not certain, but may relate to defective heme synthesis,

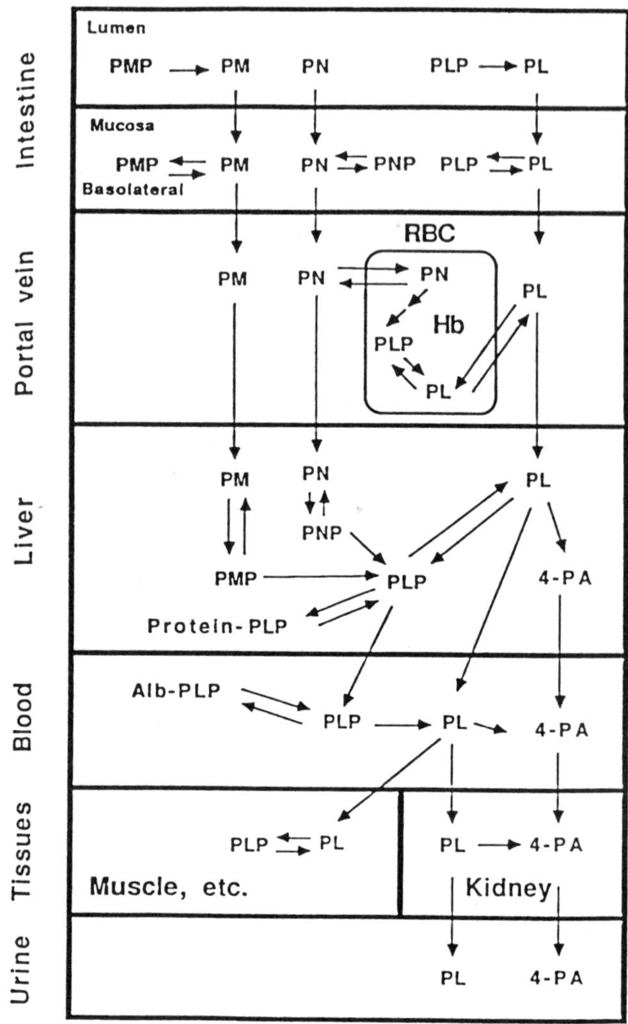

Figure 59.8 Overview of vitamin B_6 transport and metabolism. PN = pyridoxine; PL = pyridoxal; PM = pyridoxamine; PLP = pyridoxal-5-phosphate; PA = pyridoxic acid; Hb = hemoglobin; Ald = albumin; RBC = red blood cells.[r10]

which occurs in bona fide vitamin B_6 deficiency, particularly in swine. Most but not all patients with this disorder respond to megadoses of pyridoxine.

Isonicotinic acid hydrozide (isoniazid) is an antibiotic prescribed for tuberculosis and other acid-fast bacterial diseases. This drug also can combine with pyridoxyl to form a hydrazone that is a potent inhibitor of pyridoxyl kinase. Thus, isoniazid can produce a B_6-deficiency. Patients given the drug should also receive supplementary vitamin B_6 in doses of 10 to 20 mg/day.

Toxicology

Although acute toxicity of vitamin B_6 is low, when high doses of pyridoxine in the range of 2 to 6 g/kg were given to rats and mice, convulsions and death occurred. When vitamin B_6 is taken in gram quantities for months or years (1–2 grams daily), as it might be when self-administered or when prescribed by physicians to treat premenstrual syndrome, Schaumberg et al.[40] observed that vitamin B_6 can cause ataxia and a severe sensory neuropathy due to necrosis of the dorsal roots of the spinal cord (a site where vitamin B_6 deficiency also attacks). This was not immediately reversed by cessation of the megadoses. In another study by Dalton and Dalton,[41] pyridoxine toxicity was the apparent cause of neurologic symptoms in 103 women at a private clinic. These women took an average dose of 117 ± 92 mg vitamin B_6 for more than six months to more than five years. They recovered completely from their symptoms within six months of discontinuing the supplements.

Preparations

Multivitamin capsules contain 2 to 5 mg/capsule of B_6. Higher amounts in the range of 10 to 50 mg also are available.

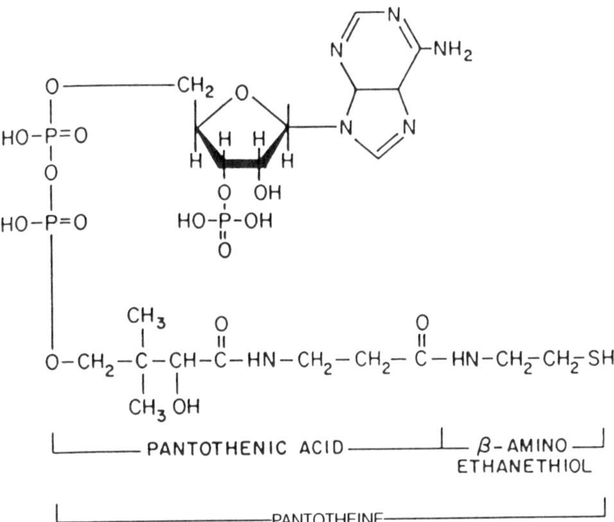

Figure 59.9 Structure of Coenzyme A

Pantothenic Acid

History

Pantothenic acid was recognized as a growth factor for yeast in 1933 by R.J. Williams and his co-workers,[42] isolated in 1939,[43] and its structure determined and synthesized in 1940.[44,45] In 1939, Jukes[46] and Wooley[47] independently showed that the "antidermatitis factor" in chickens and the "filtrate factor" in rat liver were identical with pantothenic acid. Afterwards, D(+)-pantothenate was shown to be an essential nutrient for a wide range of animals and birds. In 1947, Lipmann et al.[48] showed that pantothenic acid was an essential component of coenzyme A, the coenzyme for acetylation. Pantothenic acid deficiency in a variety of animals causes growth failure, dermatitis, achromotrichia (graying), spectacle eyes, spastic gait, adrenal necrosis and hemorrhage, anemia, leukopenia, impaired antibody production, infertility, and duodenal ulcer.

In World War II a new deficiency disease was described in prisoners in the Philipines, Japan, and Burma described as the "burning foot syndrome." Therapy with thiamine and niacin relieved some of the symptoms, but pantothenic acid was required to relieve the burning foot syndrome, later called nutritional erythromelalgia.[r11]

Chemistry

Pantothenic acid (MW 219) consists of pantoic acid (2,4-dihydroxy-3,3-dimethyl butyric acid) joined to beta alanine in an amide linkage. The biologically active form of pantothenic acid (coenzyme A) was discovered by Lipmann and co-workers in 1947[48] as a cofactor for acetylation. The structure of coenzyme A is shown in Figure 59.9. In coenzyme A the vitamin is derivatized at its carboxyl end by β-mercaptoethylamime, and at its alcoholic end by phosphate. This moiety, known as 4-phosphopantotheine, is the active form of pantothenic acid in all of its coenzymes.

Physiology

Dietary pantothenate occurs primarily in the form of CoA and pantotheine derivatives. Tomatoes contain a glycoside of pantothenate, 4′0 (α-D-glucopyranosyl)-D-pantothenic acid. Coenzyme A is hydrolyzed to pantetheine and then to pantothenate by enzymes in the intestinal lumen.

Pantothenate is then absorbed in the jejunum by a specific transport system that is saturable and sodium ion dependent.[49] After absorption, the free vitamin is transported to various tissues in plasma, from which it is taken up by most cells via another active transport process involving cotransport of pantothenate and sodium in a 1:1 ratio.[50] Plasma concentrations of pantothenic acid range from 32 to 160 μg/L in various species. Because of the coA present in blood cells, total pantothenate concentrations in blood range from 199 to 600 μ/L.

The synthesis of CoA begins with the ATP phosphorylation of pantothenic acid by a kinase, a reaction that appears to be rate-limiting for coenzyme A synthesis. The 4′-phosphopantothenate is then converted to 4′-phosphopanthenyl cysteine by an ATP-requiring synthetase. Decarboxylation of the cysteine derivative produces 4-phosphopantetheine, which is coupled with ATP to generate dephospho Co-A. The dephospho CoA is then phosphorylated in the 3′ position by a ribose by ATP to form CoA.

In normal tissues, CoA undergoes constant turnover. The degradation of CoA is accomplished by phosphatases, amidase, and oxygenase to yield pantothenic acid and hypotaurine. The pantothenic acid is then recycled to CoA. The hypotaurine is further metabolized to sulfate and excreted.

CoA, an acyl carrier protein, and other pantetheine-containing enzymes all employ the free sulfhydryl group of pantetheine as the site for acyl transfer reactions. These acyl derivatives participate in a number of metabolic reactions involving condensation and addition reactions, acyl group exchange, acyl group transfers, and nucleophilic reactions. In this manner CoA is enzymatically involved in acylation of alcohols, amines, and amino acids (including choline, sulfonamides, p-aminobenzoate, and proteins); oxidation of pyruvate and α-ketoglutarate; and fatty acid β-oxidation. Pantetheine derivatives also are involved in the synthesis of fatty acids, cholesterol, sphingosine, citrate, acetoacetate, 3-hydroxy-3-methylglutarate (HMG), and porphyrins. A selected group of coA-dependent enzymes is presented in Table 59.3.

4′-Phosphopantetheine is incorporated into an acyl carrier protein (molecular weight 10,000), which acts as an acyl carrier in fatty acid synthesis. 4′-Phosphopantetheine also is the prosthetic group of an enzyme system that synthesizes peptide antibiotics, such as gramicidin in bacteria. In the transport of fatty acyl groups across the mitochondrial membrane, fatty acyl coenzyme esters in the cytoplasm react with carnitine to form fatty acyl carnitine esters that reacylate coA in the mitochondrial matrix where β-oxidation occurs.

Antimetabolites of Pantothenic Acid

Omega-methyl pantothenate has been used to induce pantothenic acid deficiency in both animals and humans. In this compound the terminal hydroxymethyl group is replaced by a methyl group, which prevents phosphorylation of the analogue and inhibits the action of pantothenic acid kinase. Desthio-CoA, in which the terminal sulfhydryl group is replaced by a hydroxyl, is also inactive as a coenzyme. Another homologue of pantothenic acid is hopantenate, in which the β-alanine moiety containing three carbons is replaced by the four-carbon γ-aminobutyric acid (GABA) to produce pantoyl-GABA. This compound was synthesized first in 1964 by Fuerst and Li[51] and shortly thereafter was discovered to be a pantothenic acid antagonist.[52] GABA is a central inhibitory neurotransmitter. Mitsuma and Nogimori[53] found that hopantenate inhibited the secretion of the thyrotropin-releasing hormone from rat hypothalamus in vivo.

Schaefer et al.[54] reported that pantothenic acid deficiency in dogs is characterized by sudden prostration, vomiting, convulsions, hypoglycemia, and fatty liver. These symptoms are typical of Reye's syndrome. Reye's syndrome also was noted in three elderly patients who were treated with hopantenate for four months as an aid to memory.[55] Whether Reye's syndrome is a manifestation of pantothenic acid deficiency in humans is open to further study.

Nutritional Requirements

Pantothenic acid is one of the few water-soluble vitamins for which there is no recommended dietary allowance. This omission occurred because of the widespread distribution of pantothenate in foods and

Table 59.3 Selected Biochemical Reactions Catalyzed by Coenzyme A

Enzyme	Pantothenate derivative	Reactant	Product	Site
Pyruvic dehydrogenase	CoA	Pyruvate	Acetyl CoA	Mitochondria
α-Ketoglutarate dehydrogenase	CoA	α-Ketoglutarate	Succinyl CoA	Mitochondria
Fatty acid oxidase	CoA	Palmitate	Acetyl CoA	Mitochondria
HMG CoA synthetase	CoA	Acetyl CoA Acetoacetyl CoA	HMG CoA	Microsomes
Acyl CoA transferase	CoA	Protein + acyl CoA	Acylproteins + CoA	Cytoplasm
Propionyl CoA carboxylase	CoA	Propionyl CoA Carbon dioxide	Methylmalonyl CoA	Microsomes
(ATP) Acyl CoA synthetase	CoA	ATP + acetate + CoA	Acetyl CoA + ADP + P_i	Cytoplasm
(GTP) Acyl CoA synthetase	CoA	Succinate GTP + CoA	Succinyl CoA GDP + P_i*	Mitochondria
Fatty acid synthetase	Acyl carrier protein	Acetyl CoA Malonyl CoA	Palmitate	Microsomes

*Reaction moves in the opposite direction in tricarboxylic acid cycle.

the lack of evidence of significant deficiencies in world populations. In fact, as mentioned earlier, the only evidence for pantothenic acid deficiency in humans is the erythromyalgia observed under extreme conditions of food deprivation in prison camps during World War II.

Eissenstat et al.[56] studied the nutritional status of 63 healthy adolescents. Dietary intakes of pantothenic acid, which ranged from 1.7 to 12.7 mg/d, were calculated from four-day diet records. Pantothenic acid concentrations in urine, whole blood, and erythrocytes were determined by radioimmunoassay. Although 49 percent of females and 15 percent of males consumed 4 mg/day of pantothenate, average blood concentrations for both groups were in the normal range of 20 to 60 μg/dl. Urinary excretion varied from 1.99 to 7.99 mg/day and was highly correlated with dietary intake. The 1989 report of the Food and Nutrition Board of the National Research Council[r3] set 4 to 7 mg/day for adults and 2 to 5 mg/day for infants and children as safe and adequate daily intakes.

Deficiency Disease

The syndrome of pantothenate deficiency in animals and birds has been described. In humans, pantothenic acid deficiency is rare, principally because of the widespread distribution of pantothenic acid in foods. As noted above, a new deficiency disease was observed in malnourished World War II prisoners, particularly in the Philippines, Japan, and Burma, described as the burning-foot syndrome. The symptoms consisted of numbness and tingling toes, and burning and shooting pains in the feet. These cardinal symptoms were associated with other neurologic and mental symptoms. Therapy with thiamine and niacin relieved some of the symptoms, but pantothenate was required to relieve the burning-foot syndrome, which was later called nutritional erythromelalgia.[57] Furthermore, subjects with this disorder had reduced ability to acetylate p-aminobenzoic acid and a low urinary concentration of pantothenic acid, both of which are suggestive of pantothenic acid deficiency.

Human volunteers fed 1 g/day of the antimetabolite ϖ-methyl pantothenic acid for 12 weeks developed vomiting, malaise, abdominal distress, burning cramps, fatigue, insomnia, and parethesias of hands and feet. The eosinopenic response to ACTH was reduced in these subjects, but adrenocortical function remained within normal limits.[58,59] Three elderly patients receiving 37 mg/kg/d of hopantenate developed Reye's syndrome, which includes hepatomegaly, fatty liver, and encephalopathy with coma.[55]

Therapeutic Use

There are no indications for administering pantothenic acid to humans except in cases of deficiency, which are very rare. The dose should be ten times the recommended intake, of the order of 50 mg/day.

Toxicology

There is no evidence that pantothenic acid is toxic even at 1000 times the recommended levels.

Preparations

There are multiple-vitamin capsules containing 2 to 10 mg of pantothenate per capsule.

Biotin

History

Experiments performed by Leibig in the 19th century showed that an unknown factor from an extract of natural materials was necessary for the growth of yeast. This was christened "bios" by Wilders in 1901. Further work showed that "bios" was composed of three fractions. Bios I was identified as meso-inositol; bios II turned out to be a mixture of pantothenic acid and Bios IIA; the third component, Bios IIB, was eventually identified as biotin.[r5]

In the 1930s, the Bios IIB was found to be related to a respiration-promoting factor, *Rhizobium trifolii* (coenzyme R) and a factor essential in rat nutrition to neutralize the toxic effects of uncooked egg white, the so "anti-egg white injury factor,"[60] also called vitamin H by P. Gyorgy.[r15] In 1936, biotin was isolated in crystalline form from egg yolk using the yeast bioassay by Kogl and Tonnis.[61] It was then shown that coenzyme R and vitamin H were identical to biotin.[62] The structure of biotin was solved by Hoffman et al[62,69] in 1942, and it was synthesized by Folkers and his colleagues in 1944.[65]

Subsequently, the role of biotin in CO_2-fixation reactions[r14] and the function of avidin (MW 70,000) as the biotin-binding protein in egg white were established. The dermatitis of egg white injury in rats can be duplicated in humans fed large amounts of raw eggs, but primary biotin deficiency is extremely rare in humans. It occasionally occurs in persons receiving biotin-free parenteral nutrition. Genetic disorders in infants that block biotin metabolism present with dermatitis, failure of neurologic development, and organic acidosis.

Chemistry

Biotin is an optically active dextrorotatory organic acid with a pKa of 4.51. It has a bicyclic structure consisting of a ureido ring fused with a tetrahydrothiophene ring bearing a valeric acid side-chain, as shown in Figure 59.10. Most of the biotin found in natural materials is bound to peptides. Biocitin (epsilon biotinyl-L-lysine) is an amide derived from biotinyl proteins, which illustrates the linkage of biotin to enzymes (Fig. 59.10). Only the (+) stereoisomer of biotin has significant biologic activity. Biotin is soluble in water (0.82 mmol/L at 25° C). It is more soluble in hot water and in dilute alkali and four times more so in 95 percent ethanol than in cold water. It is not soluble in other organic solvents. Various biotin derivatives, analogues, and antagonists are known. Dethiobiotin,

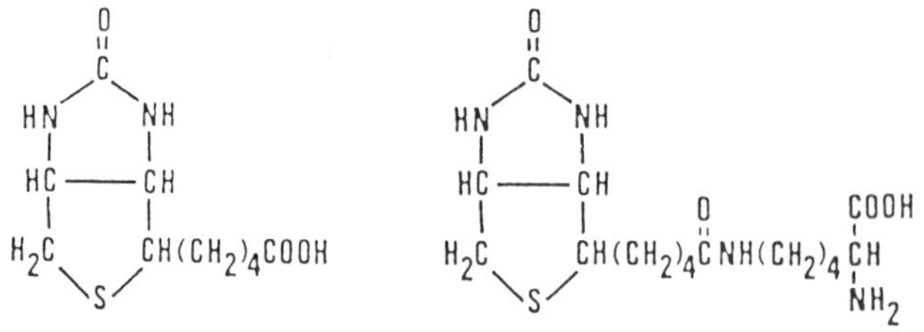

Biotin   Biocytin

Figure 59.10 Structures of Biotin and Biocytin

a sulfur-free analogue of biotin is the direct precursor of biotin in microorganisms.

Physiology

Most of the biotin in natural products is protein-bound. The digestion of dietary proteins containing biotin by proteolytic enzymes in the gut produces biocytin, which is converted to biotin by biotinidase. Biotin is absorbed at low concentrations by a specific saturable transport system and at higher concentrations by diffusion. Biotin is then taken up from the blood by an active transport system in liver and other tissues, which is more rapid in deficient animals than in normal ones. Intracellular biotin is then converted to its active form first by reaction with ATP to form a biotineal 5-adenylate followed by condensation of the biotineal moiety with epsilon amino groups of specific lysine residues in the biotin-dependent apoenzymes. The enzymes responsible for catalyzing the formation of the biocytinyl moiety of proteins are holoenzyme synthetases.

Biotinyl proteins in the cell function as catalysts for carboxylation, transcarboxylation, and decarboxylation.[r12] Nine biotin-dependent enzymes are listed in Table 59.4. Biotin catalyzed carboxylation depends on ATP as a source of energy, as shown in Figure 59.11. It appears that ATP-dependent carboxylases operate via the phosphorylation of biocarbonate to form carbonyl phosphate, a mixed acid anhydride that is suitably electrophilic to attack the sterically less-hindered nitrogen of the nucleophilic isourea-like tautomer of the biotinyl moiety. The resulting N^1-carboxybiotinyl enzyme can then exchange the carboxylate function with a reactive carbon or nitrogen center in a substrate. The overview of this process is shown in Figure 59.11. It now seems likely that the hydrogen on the isoamide oxygen of biotin exchanges from an amino acid residue in the enzyme during consecutive reactions rather than by a concerted mechanism in which a substrate hydrogen would concomitantly participate.[r12]

From the list of enzymes in Table 59.4 it is clear that biotin is crucial for implementing major pathways in fat, carbohydrate, and amino acid metabolism. The carboxylation of acetyl CoA is essential for fatty acid synthesis; the carboxylation of pyruvate is essential for gluconeogenesis and the continued activity of the TCA cycle; and the carboxylation of propionate is necessary for the catabolism of the branched-chain amino acids and threonine.

The final carboxylase of interest, namely β-methyl crotonyl CoA carboxylase, is needed for the catabolism of leucine. The product of this carboxylation is β-methyl glutaconyl CoA, which is the immediate precursor of HMG-CoA of importance in sterol synthesis. Biotin is catabolized to oxidized end-products containing sulfoxides and sulfones and these products are excreted mainly in the urine.

Table 59.4 Biotin-Dependent Enzymes (r12)

- I. Carboxylases
  - A. Acyl-CoA carboxylases
    1. Acetyl-CoA ⇌ malonyl-CoA
    2. Propionyl-CoA ⇌ D-methylmalonyl-CoA
    3. β-Methylcrotonyl-CoA ⇌ β methylglutaconyl-CoA
    4. Geranyl-CoA ⇌ carboxygeranyl-CoA
  - B. α-Ketocarboxylase
    Pyruvate ⇌ oxalacetate
  - C. Amidocarboxylase
    Urea ⇌ allophanate
- II. Transcarboxylase
  - A. D-Methylmalonyl-CoA + pyruvate ⇌ propionyl-CoA + oxalacetate
- III. Decarboxylases
  - A. D-Methylmalonyl-CoA → propionyl-CoA
  - B. Oxalacetate → pyruvate

Nutritional Requirements

Good sources of biotin include yeast, liver, kidney, pancreas, eggs, milk, fish, and nuts. No definitive studies on human biotin requirements have been conducted. Hence, there is no specific recommended dietary allowance.[10] In adults receiving total parenteral nutrition, daily administration of 60 μg prevented signs of deficiency.

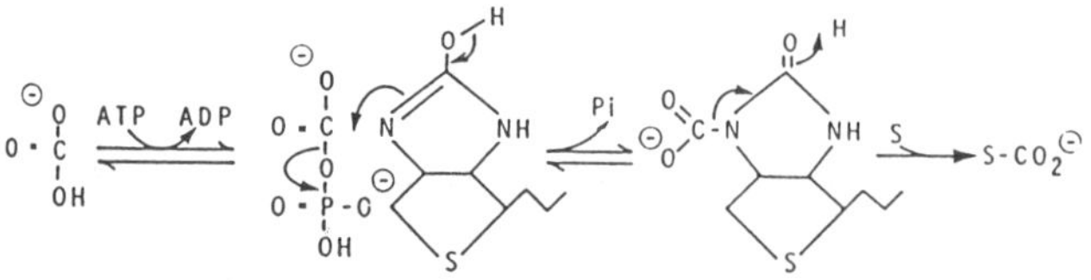

ATP ADP Pi

Figure 59.11 Mechanism of Biotin Carboxylation

An RDA for biotin has not been developed because of wide distribution of the vitamin and lack of evidence of a significant primary deficiency disease. Safe and adequate daily dietary intakes noted by the RDA Committee for the 10th Edition (1989) are 10 to 15 μg/day for infants, 20 to 30 μg/day for children, and 30 to 100 μ/day for adults.

Although blood biotin levels fall progressively throughout gestation, such low biotin values are not associated with low-birth weight infants. Hence, no increment for pregnancy and lactation has been recommended. Based on the biotin content of human milk, which is all in the free, available form, and assuming a daily milk consumption of 750 ml by the infant, the daily biotin intake of breast-fed infants would be in the range of 2 to 15 μg per day. For formula-fed infants, an intake of 10 to 15 μg biotin per day has been recommended during the first year.

Deficiency Disease

A biotin deficiency has been observed in several animal species, ranging from small animals such as mice, rats, and cats to large animals such as swine and humans. Clear evidence of the biotin deficiency syndrome in humans has been found in studies of total parenteral nutrition. Egg white injury was first described in 1927 by Boas,[60] who observed that feeding raw egg white to rats produced an eczematous dermatitis accompanied by loss of hair. In 1942, Sydenstricker et al.[66] fed seven adult volunteers 200 g of dehydrated egg white per day with an otherwise balanced diet. Lassitude, somnolence, hallucinations, and anxiety with muscle pain and hyperesthesia occurred during the study. After eight weeks, anorexia and a striking grayish pallor with a "brauny" dermatitis and desquamation occurred. The experiment was terminated because of the marked fall in food intake. Within five days of treatment with 75 to 300 μg per day of parenteral biotin, symptoms and signs disappeared.

The biotin-dependent enzymes of importance in mammalian metabolism are pyruvate carboxylase (PC), which converts pyruvate to oxalacetic acid; propionyl-CoA carboxylase (PCC), which converts propional-CoA to methylmalonyl-CoA; β-methylcrotonyl-CoA carboxylase (MCC), which converts β-methylcrotonyl-CoA to β-methylglutaconyl-CoA; and acetyl-CoA carboxylase (ACC), which forms malonyl-CoA.

Some of the early cases of genetic PCC and MCC deficiencies associated with neurologic manifestations were not responsive to biotin, presumably because the apoenzyme was so altered by the gene mutation that no association of biotin with the carboxylase apoenzyme could occur.[67] Subsequent cases of MCC deficiency in infants were intriguing in that the patients did not show neurologic disease but had an extensive skin rash, irritability, and withdrawn behavior with persistent vomiting. Furthermore, these patients did respond to large doses of biotin,[68,69] suggesting a defect in the linking enzyme, holocarboxylase synthetase, which could be overcome by large doses of the vitamin.[70]

A more recent case of genetic disease was an infant presenting with an erythematous rash over her face and eyelids followed by delayed neuromotor development, nystagmus, hypotonia, and reduced antibody response to pneumococcal polysaccharide. Intradermal skin tests to Candida and streptokinase/streptodornase showed a failure of the delayed hypersensitivity response. She showed an accumulation of abnormal acids, including 3-hydroxyisovalerate, 3-methylcrotinylglycine, and 3-hydroxypropionate—all associated with interruption in the catabolism of leucine, isoleucine, and valine. This patient responded to oral administration of 10 mg or more of biotin per day with normalization of the clinical and biochemical abnormalities.[71]

Although primary biotin deficiency has been associated heretofore only with egg white injury,[60,66] the advent of total parenteral nutrition has ushered in a new challenge to the physician. A number of new deficiency diseases in humans, including biotin deficiency, have been discovered because of the mistaken belief that what is adequate for human nutrition by mouth is also adequate by vein.

Therapeutic Uses

In the rare case of dietary biotin deficiency due to ingestion of raw eggs, 10 times the recommended dose of 50 to 300 μg should be given. There is no indication for the use of biotin as a drug except in genetic diseases, where 10 to 20 mg/day are administered.

Toxicology

Biotin has no known toxicity.

Preparations

Biotin is available as a dose of 50 μg/capsule in multivitamin products and there are preparations available for both oral and parenteral administration.

Folic Acid

History

In 1937, Wills et al.,[72] described a macrocytic anemia in Hindu women in Bombay, usually associated with pregnancy, which responded to therapy with a commercial preparation of autolyzed yeast called Marmite. Although megaoblastic anemia is also found in vitamin B_{12} deficiency, it was recognized by Osler[73] that the megaloblastic anemia of pregnancy was caused by an agent different from that which causes Addisonian pernicious anemia. By feeding the same type of Indian diet that was ingested by her pregnant patients, Wills et al.[77] produced in monkeys a similar macrocytic anemia that responded to crude, but not purified, liver extracts. This came to be known as the Wills factor.

In 1940, Snell and Peterson[75] reported that a factor in crude liver extract that could be absorbed on and then eluted from charcoal (Norite LU8 factor) was essential for the growth of *Lactobaccillus caseii*. It came to be known as the *L. caseii* factor. About the same time, Day[76] and his associates reported that a factor from dried brewer's yeast, which they called vitamin M, could correct the anemia, leukopenia, and diarrhea of monkeys fed a purified diet devoid of the factors in brewer's yeast.

It became clear that all of these factors were related following the purification of pteroylglutamic acid in 1943 by Stokstad[77] and its crystallization from liver in the same year by Pfillner and associates.[78] The term folic acid was coined by Mitchell and coworkers[79] because this factor was found in green leafy vegetables. It was also recognized by Hogan and Parrot[80] that an anemia in chicks caused by feeding a B_2-complex-deficient diet could be due to a lack of folic acid (Norite eluate factor).

Although it was not known at the time of discovery of folic acid that it was different from the factor that prevented the megaloblastic anemia of Addison, time has proved that folate and cobalamin are not identical but closely related in metabolism.

Chemistry

The structure of pteroylglutamic acid is shown in Fig. 59.12. Major portions of the molecule include a pteridine ring linked by a methylene bridge to p-aminobenzoic acid, which in turn is joined by an amide linkage to glutamic acid, whereas the pteroylglutamic acid is a basic building block for coenzymes in the body and is the monomeric form of folic acid. It crystallizes in yellow-orange plates, is slightly soluble in water, and is acidic, with a pH in water of 4.0. The molecular weight is 441. It is a precursor of the active coenzymes needed for intracellular metabolism.

Folacin is a generic term used to describe folic acid and related compounds that exhibit the biologic activity of folic acid. Three features of the structure should be emphasized. First is the oxidation state of the pteridine portion of the molecule. Folic acid (Pte) is the completely oxidized form of the molecule and is probably never found as such in nature. The molecule must be reduced to the dihydro- and tetrahydro forms to be biologically active. Reduced folates accomplish their metabolic function as carriers of one-carbon units.

The second structural feature concerns the type of one-carbon unit that is carried and the site of attachment to the folate molecule. It can be seen in Figure 59.13 that the one-carbon units are attached to positions 5 or 10 or may bridge between positions 5 and 10. The one-carbon units are either derivatives of formate [5-formyl-, 10-formyl, 5,10-methylidene- (previously called 5,10-methylenyl) or 5-formimino-], derivatives of formaldehyde (5,10-methylene-), or derivatives of methanol (5-methyl-). Thus the one-carbon units themselves may be at different levels of oxidation from formate to methanol when attached to the folate molecule.

The third important feature of the structure is that folic acid as the monoglutamate has no biologic activity. Additional glutamic acid residues must be added in metabolism to give it potential coenzyme activity. Most natural folates are polyglutamates.[r15]

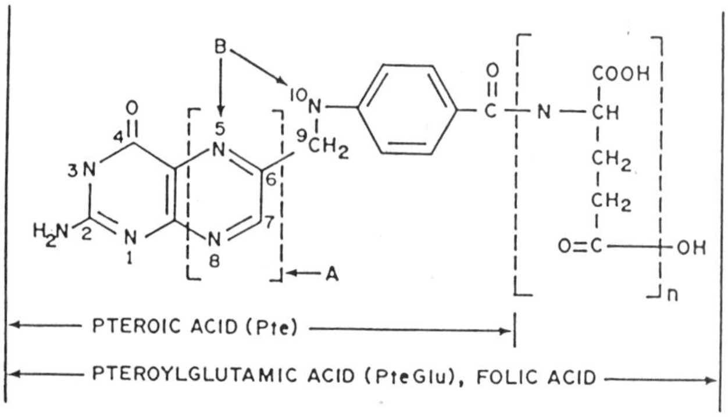

Figure 59.12 Structure of Folic Acid (pteroylglutamic acid, PteGlu)

A. *State of Reduction*
   7,8-dihydro—e.g., dihydrofolic acid, H_2PteGlu
   5,6,7,8-tetrahydro—e.g., tetrahydrofolic acid, H_4PteGlu
B. *One-Carbon Substituent*
   5-formyl—e.g., 5-formyltetrahydrofolic acid, 5-HCO-H_4PteGlu
   10-formyl—e.g., 10-formyltetrahydrofolic acid, 10-HCO-H_4PteGlu
   5,10-methylidene—e.g., 5,10-methylidenetetrahydrofolic acid, 5,10-CH=H_4PteGlu
   5,10-methylene—e.g., 5,10-methylenetetrahydrofolic acid, 5,10-CH_2-H_4PteGlu
   5-methyl—e.g., 5-methyltetrahydrofolic acid, 5-CH_3-H_4 PteGlu
n; *Number of Glutamates*
   n = 1—e.g., 5-formyltetrahydrofolic acid, 5-formyltetrahydropteroylglutamic acid, 5-HCO-H_4PteGlu
   n = 5—e.g., 5-methyltetrahydropteroylpentaglutamic acid, 5-CH_3-H_4PteGlu$_5$

Physiology

Because the natural folacin present in foods is primarily in the polyglutamate form and the absorbed folate in the portal circulation is exclusively the monoglutamate, it is clear that hydrolysis of the polyglutamates occurs as part of the absorption process. The enzyme activity responsible for hydrolysis of the polyglutamates is referred to as conjugase, which is actually a family of enzymes that hydrolyzes the γ-glutamyl bond. They should properly be called γ-glutamylcarboxypeptidases, but the designation as conjugase is widespread and generally accepted. Several conjugase enzymes in the gut are responsible for the hydrolysis of the long-chain folate polyglutamates to the monoglutatamates, which are then taken up by the mucosal cell. It appears that there is a single transport system at the brush border surface for the uptake of different forms of folate. Since most of the folate that appears in the portal circulation is 5-methyl-H_4PteGlu, the intestinal cells are very active in conversion of both oxidized and reduced folates to 5-methyl-H_4PteGlu. When PteGlu or 5-formyl-H_4PteGlu is fed, 5-methyl-H_4PteGlu is found in the serum in significant amounts. The usual folate concentration in the serum of humans is 6 to 15 ng/ml. Red blood cells concentrate folate and contain 160 to 300 ng/ml. The average intake of folate by humans is about 200 μg/day, of which 40 μg is excreted in the urine and 160 μg in the stool. There is a vigorous enterohepatic circulation of folate that attempts to conserve the vitamin. The body pool of folate in humans is estimated to be 7.5 ± 2.5 mg, most of which is in the liver.

The function of folates in animal tissues is to transfer one-carbon units in metabolism. These one-carbon units are generated primarily during amino acid metabolism and are used in the metabolic interconversions of amino acids and in the biosynthesis of the purine and pyrimidine components of nucleic acids needed for cell division. The folates are a family of coenzymes and function in association with their respective enzymes. It has become clear that the polyglutamate forms of the folates are the natural coenzymes.

Figure 59.13 summarizes the transfer and oxidation-reduction reactions of one-carbon fragments that require folate coenzymes.[r16] Names of the enzymes catalyzing each reaction are listed in the legend. Two crucial groups of reactions compete in the cell for available folates, i.e., the reactions of nucleotide biosynthesis and a large number of S-adenosylmethionine-requiring methylation reactions that are dependent on a steady supply of methionine.

Conversion of the internalized monoglutamates to polyglutamates (Reaction 3) locks the folates inside the cell at concentrations of one or two orders of magnitude greater than the extracellular concentrations. Polyglutamylation requires prior reduction of folic acid to tetrahydrofolic acid (Reaction 2) or demethylation of the circulating for 5-methyl-tetrahydrofolic acid by the vitamin B_{12}-requiring Reaction 7. Reaction 4, going in the direction of glycine synthesis, is the main de novo generator of one-carbon fragments. Note that serine, the one-carbon donor molecule, is a nonessential amino acid biosynthesized from glucose in unlimited amounts by most cells. The products of Reaction 5, the 5-CH_3-THFAGlu$_n$, are trapped in that form and can only re-enter the pool of metabolically active unsubstituted tetrahydrofolates via the vitamin B_{12}-requiring Reaction 7. They may provide: (1) a stable storage form for reduced folates that can be mobilized as needed by activation of Reaction 7; (2) a mechanism for suppressing the synthesis of purines and thymidylate by sequestering reduced folates; or (3) a route for the production of methionine when the latter is unavailable from external sources.

These three possible roles are not mutually exclusive; in fact all three probably occur simultaneously. This conclusion is suggested by the multiple and complex regulatory influences to which methylene tetrahydrofolate reductase (the enzyme catalyzing Reaction 5) is subjected. It is inhibited by S-adenosyl methionine (SAM) and by polyglutamyl derivatives of dihydrofolic acid. If the former decreases, more folates are committed to the remethylation of homocysteine (Reaction 7) as required by Role 3; if thymidylate synthesis (Reaction 14) increases, formation of the other products of that reaction, the DHFAGlu$_n$, also increases, leading to inhibition of Reaction 5 and the commitment of additional folate to the nucleotide biosynthesis pathways as required by Role 2. The putative storage role presumably served also by the 5-CH_3-THFAGlu$_n$ is supported by observations suggesting that the ratio of total folates made up by these forms decreases during folate deficiency. In contrast, the 5-CH_3-THFAGlu pool increases in vitamin B_{12} deficiency, because the methyltransferase is blocked causing the so-called "methyl trap".[r14]

Reaction 14 is the sole de novo pathway for thymidylate synthesis and the only folate-requiring reaction in which the cofactor serves a dual purpose of one-carbon donor and reducing agent. Inhibition of Reaction 2 by methotrexate or other dehydroreductase inhibitors effectively blocks thymidylate and hence DNA synthesis and stops cell replication. The same can occur with folate or vitamin B_{12} deficiency, because of their metabolic interactions. All of these events lead to inhibition of the bone marrow and the resultant leukopenia and megaloblastic anemia. Other reactions in the scheme presented in Figure 59.13 lead to purine biosynthesis and various methylations.

Nutritional Requirements

Folates are widely distributed in foods; liver, yeast, green leafy vegetables, and legumes are rich sources. The average intake of folate in the US in the past 20 years has been 280 to 300 μg/capita/day. In Canada in 1977 the mean intake of folate for men was 205 μg/day and for women 149 μg/day. It has been demonstrated that 100 μg of folate per day will prevent a deficiency and maintain liver stores at 3 μg/g. Less than 1 μg/gram in the liver and 3 ng/ml plasma results in production of macrocytic anemia. Thus the minimum intake of folacin to prevent deficiency is about 1 μg/kg body weight.

The Food and Nutrition Board of the NRC/NAS

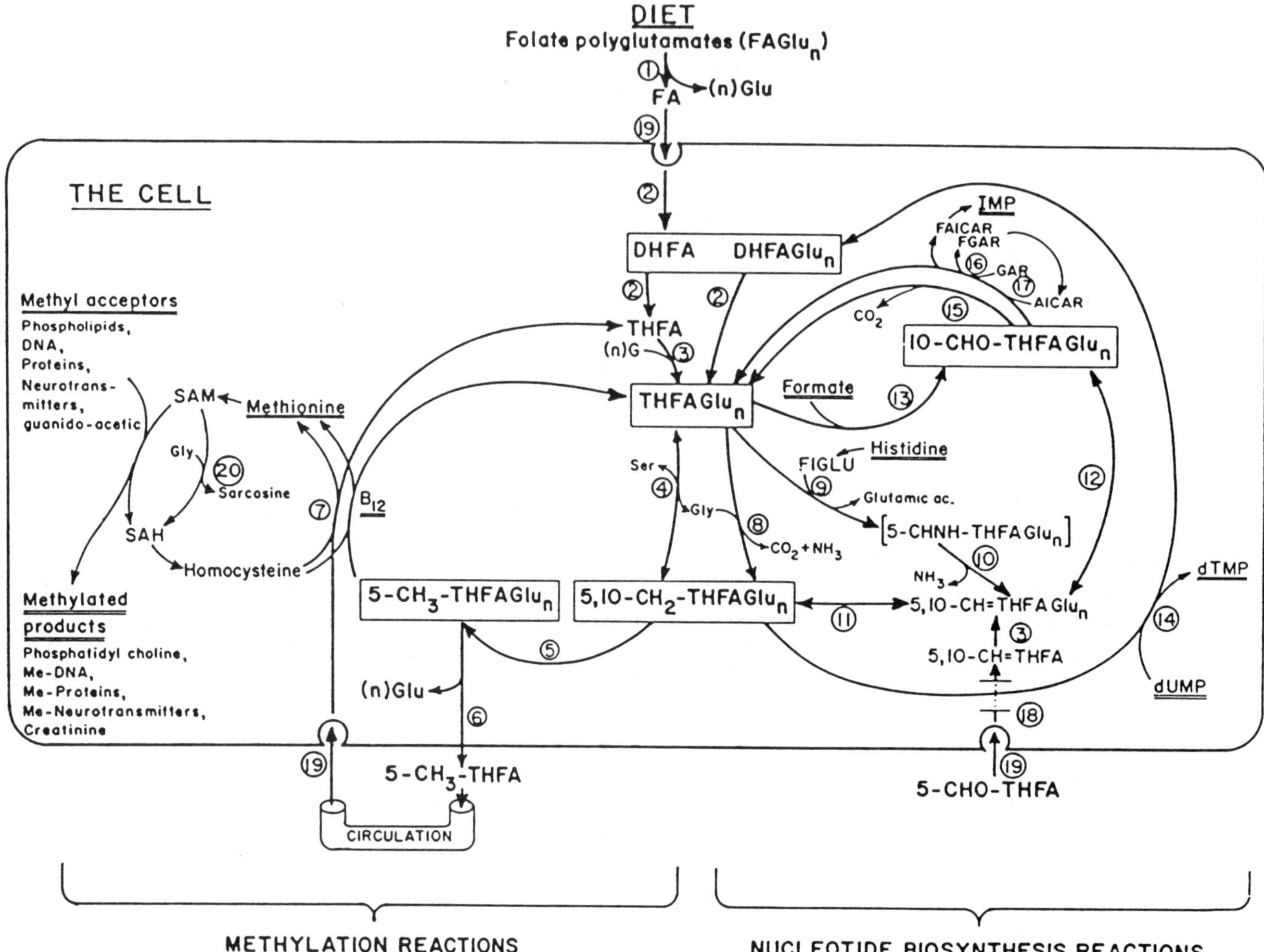

Figure 59.13 Enzymes and reactions of folate metabolism: (1) γ-glutamyl hydrolase (brush border ?) (EC 3.4.22.12), (2) dihydrofolate reductase (EC 1.5.1.3), (3) folyl poly-γ-glutamate synthase (EC 6.3.2.17), (4) serine hydroxymethyl transferase (EC 2.1.2.1), (5) methylene tetrahydrofolate reductase (EC 1.7.99.5), (6) γ-glutamyl hydrolase (lysosomal ?) (EC 3.4.22.12), (7) cobalamin-dependent methionine synthase (EC 2.1.1.13), (8) glycine cleavage enzyme system (EC 1.4.4.2; 2.1.2.10), (9) glutamate formiminotransferase (EC 2.1.2.5), (10) formiminotetrahydrofolate cyclodeaminase (EC 4.3.1.4), (11) methylene tetrahydrofolate dehydrogenase (EC 1.5.1.5), (12) methenyl tetrahydrofolate cyclohydrolase (EC 3.5.4.9), (13) formyl tetrahydrofolate synthetase (EC 6.3.4.3), (14) thymidylate synthase (EC 2.1.1.45), (15) formyl tetrahydrofolate dehydrogenase (EC 1.5.1.6), (16) phosphoribosyl glycinamide (GAR) formyl transferase (EC 2.1.2.2), (17) phosphoribosyl aminoimidazole carboxamide (AICAR) formyl transferase (EC 2.1.2.3), (18) 5-formyl tetrahydrofolate cycloligase (EC 6.3.3.2), (19) folate/MTX transport mechanism, and (20) glycine methyl transferase (EC 2.1.1.20). (ref r[16])

in 1989 set the recommended dietary allowance at 200 μg/day for men and 180 μg/day for women. In pregnancy, 400 μg/day were recommended and during lactation 280 μg/day were recommended. For infants from birth to 1 year, 3.6 μg/kg were specified and for older children about 2.5 μg/kg were recommended.

Deficiency Disease

Folic acid deficiency occurs in malnourished children, pregnant women, alcoholics, and patients with malabsorption. Diarrhea usually is present, accompanied by cheilosis, glossitis, GI distress, and macrocytic anemia. The megaloblastic bone marrow is similar to that seen in pernicious anemia, but the neurologic consequences of vitamin B_{12}-deficiency are absent. In fact, if patients with B_{12}-deficiency are mistakenly given folate to treat their anemia, the neurologic disease gets worse. It is estimated that 40 to 87 per cent of alcoholics in this country have low serum folate and 40 to 61 percent have megaloblastic anemia. Herbert[81] put himself on a folate-deficient diet for 20 weeks, during which he observed reductions in serum folate, hypersegmentation of granulocytes, increased urinary formimino-glutamic acid macrocytosis, and a megaloblastic bone marrow just before discontinuing the regimen.

Because of the demand of the marrow for folate, patients with chronic hemolytic anemia who have a hyperactive bone marrow may become folate-deficient and require oral supplementation. Drugs such as direct inhibitors of DNA synthesis (e.g., 5-fluorouracil and 6-thioquanine), folate antagonists (e.g., methotrexate pentamidine, triamterene), and anticonvulsants (e.g., phenytoin and phenobarbital) can produce a megaloblastic anemia that requires rescue by folate derivatives.

Finally, three genetic diseases of folate metabolism should be mentioned. These are: (1) methylenetetrahydrofolate reductase deficiency (Reaction 5); (2) glutamate formiminotransferase deficiency (Reaction 4); and (3) hereditary folate malabsorption (Reaction 19). The first two, which have homocystinuria as the cardinal sign, are resistant to treatment with folate. The third causes florid megaloblastic anemia, which requires megadoses of oral folic acid (ca 100 mg/day) or parenteral folates.

Therapeutic Uses

The dose for treatment of folic acid deficiency is 0.5 to 1 mg/day. In hereditary folate dependency states, the dose of folate required may range from 50 to 100 mg/day. Folate as an agent for preventing neural tube defects in susceptible women has required folate fortification during pregnancy in the range of 0.4 to 4.0 mg/day.[82]

Toxicology

Folate is toxic at 50 to 100 times the RDA in very special circumstances. In epileptics treated with phenytoin, it may increase seizure frequency.[13] In patients with pernicious anemia it will mask the hematologic signs and enhance the neurologic signs. In one study, no untoward effects were reported in women given 10 mg/day of folic acid continuously for four months. However, without evidence of benefit and with some potential for toxicity, excessive intakes of supplemental folate are not recommended.

Preparations

Folate is available in multivitamin capsules at a dose of 0.3 to 0.4 mg/capsule.

Vitamin B_{12}

History

The first clinical description of pernicious anemia is attributed to Thomas Addison in 1855, but earlier case reports of macrocytic anemia were made in 1823 by Combe and Andral and in 1837 by Hall. In 1860, Flint described the severe gastric atrophy associated with the anemia and called attention to the possible relationship of this GI disorder to the anemia. By 1870, pernicious anemia was known to include megaloblastic anemia, GI dysfunction, and neurologic disease.[83]

In the 1920s Whipple[86,87] in Rochester, New York, in studying the efficacy of various foods for the treatment of iron-deficiency in animals, demonstrated the value of liver, which led Minot and Murphy in Boston to use liver as a therapeutic agent for pernicious anemia. The dramatic results obtained by Minot and Murphy ushered in a new era in hematology and led to a Nobel Prize for Minot, Murphy, and Whipple.[84] Castle, a pupil of Minot, then demonstrated that both an extrinsic factor in liver, subsequently identified as vitamin B_{12}, and an intrinsic factor derived from the stomach were essential for the prevention of this megaloblastic anemia.[85] Twenty years later in 1948, Rickes and co-workers[99] and Smith and Parker[89] isolated and crystallized vitamin B_{12}. In 1956, Dorothy Hodgkin and her co-workers[90] at Oxford determined the crystal structure of vitamin B_{12} by X-ray diffraction and subsequently received the second Nobel awarded for the study of this disease. The structure of vitamin B_{12} is shown in Fig. 59.14.

Chemistry

Vitamin B_{12}, known as cobalamin, forms dark red crystals from water (MW = 1355). It has three chemical components; (1) a planar corrin nucleus, embracing a cobalt atom in the center; (2) a 5-6 dimethylbenzimidazole nucleotide linked at right angles to the corrin nucleus and bonded through a coordinate covalency to the cobalt atom; (3) a d-amino-2-propanol moiety which links the phosphate of the benzimidazole nucleotide to the propionic acid side-chain of Ring D. The corrin ring system resembles a porphyrin ring structure, with four reduced pyrrole rings extensively substituted with methyl, acetamide, and propionamide residues linked to a central cobalt atom. The corrin ring differs from the porphyrin ring in having an absent branching methylene group between rings A and D, as shown in Fig. 59.14. The central cobalt has six coordinate covalencies, which bind the four pyrrole rings, the benzymidazole nucleotide, and the functional group of the coenzyme, which can be CN^-, $O\bar{H}$,H_2O, CH_3, or 5-deoxyadenosyl.

The main commercial product is cyanocabalamin (CNCbl), with cyanide as the R group. (CNCbl) is an analogue and must be metabolized to hydroxyl Cbl before the two coenzyme forms of vitamin B_{12}, namely 5-deoxyadenosylcobalamin and methylcobalamin, can be formed.

Physiology

The absorption of vitamin B_{12} from the gut is a receptor-mediated event. It has several phases. In the gastric phase, Cbl is liberated from proteins in food by the action of pepsin. This initial peptic digestion is important since patients with achlorydria or partial gastrectomy fail to absorb cobalamins at normal rates. In the second phase after release from food proteins in the stomach, cobalamin is bound to non-intrinsic

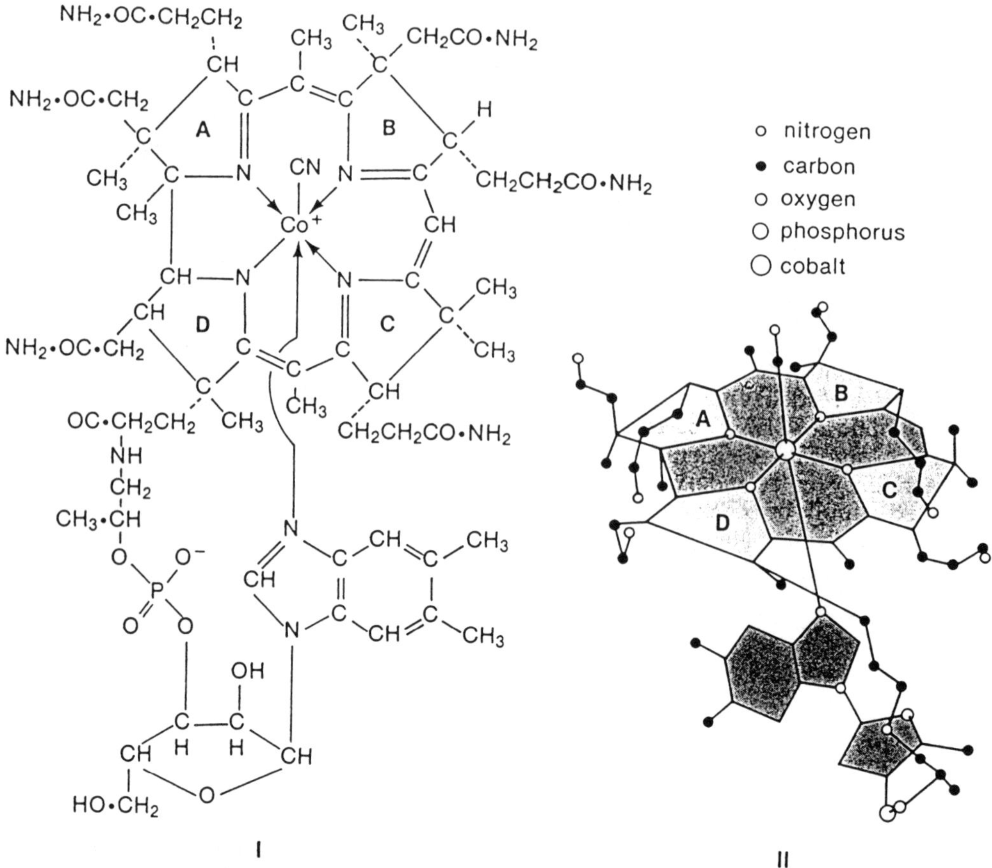

Figure 59.14 Structures of Vitamin B_{12}. I = Planar View; II = Three-Dimensional View

factor proteins called R-proteins, which have a high affinity for cobalamin. Intrinsic factor (IF), a glycoprotein (MW = 44,000) with a high affinity for cobalamin, is secreted with HCl by the parietal cells of the stomach. Cobalamin bound to R-proteins in the stomach, however, is transferred to IF only after R-protein degradation by pancreatic proteases. Failure to degrade the R protein-CBL complex due to the lack of pancreatic proteases may explain the cobalamin malabsorption observed in patients with pancreatic insufficiency.

The third phase of cobalamin absorption is the mucosal uptake of cobalamin in the ileum. The IF-CBL complex attaches to receptors located in the ileum in humans and most other species. The ileal receptor, which recognizes the IF-CBL complex has been identified in humans and several other mammalian species (see Figure 59.15).[91]

The IF CBL complex is internalized by cells in the ileum where it enters lysosomes. The IF is degraded but cobalamin is released to the intracellular milieu and exported in association with transcobalamin II. TCII is the primary transport protein for vitamin B_{12} in plasma and accounts for about 20 percent of total plasma B_{12}. TCII turns over rapidly and is the principal vehicle for transporting cobalamin to various tissues. Transcobalamin I and III, which account for a greater percentage of cobalamin present in plasma, but are not so specific for vitamin B_{12}, have slower turnover times and bind cobalamin analogues as well as cobalamin itself.

In the TC-II-cobalamin complex the cobalt is in the 3+ valence state. Receptors in target cells recognize the TC-II cobalamin complex and internalize the complex, which enters lysosomes that in turn digest IF and free cobalamin. This cobalamin^{3+} is reduced by an NADH-dependent system to CBL^{2+}. Subsequently CBL^{2+} is reduced to CBL^{1+} by either NADH or glutathione (GSH) to form adenosylcobalamin^{1+} from ATP or methyl cobalamin from $MeFH_4$. It is clear that cobalamin^{1+} is the reactive form of cobalamin in biochemical reactions. In fact, nitrous oxide inhibits cobalamin metabolism by oxidizing cobalamin^{1+} to cobalamin^{3+}.

Thus, in cells there are two cobalamin-dependent reactions. One is a mutase for converting methyl malonyl CoA to succinyl coA and requires deoxyadenosyl cobalamin^{1+} as a coenzyme. The other is methionine synthetase, which mediates the methyl transfer from methyl tetrahydrofolic acid ($MeFH_4$) to homocysteine

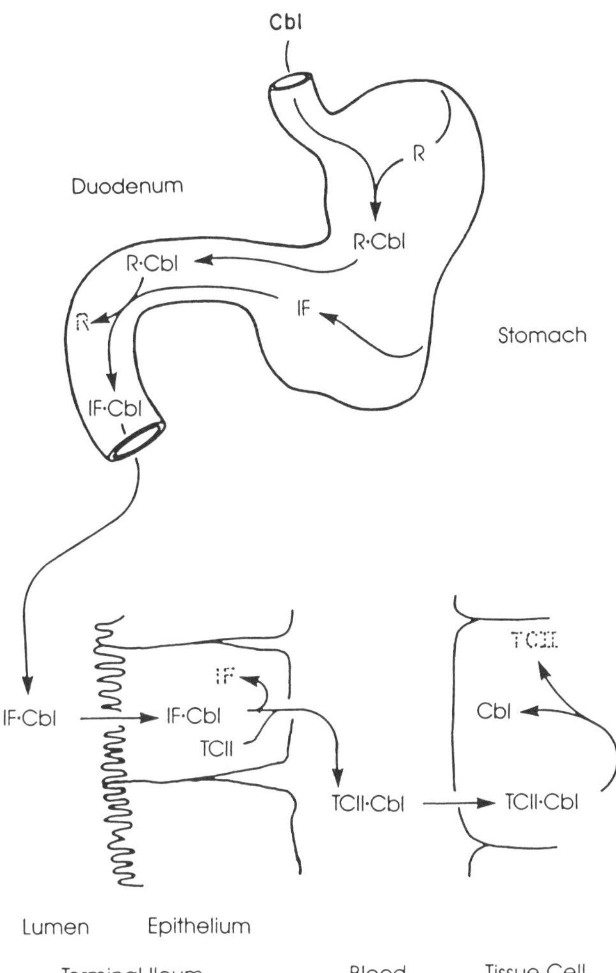

Figure 59.15 The assimilation of cobalamin. On entering the stomach dietary cobalamin (Cbl) forms a complex with R binding protein. As this protein is digested, cobalamin is transferred to intrinsic factor (IF). This complex passes through the intestine until it reaches specific receptors on the mucosa of the distal ileum. The internalized Cbl is then transferred to transcobalamin II (TCII) which circulates in the plasma until it is binds to receptors on cells throughout the body and is internalized. (r18)

to form methionine. Impairment of DNA synthesis in the bone marrow in vitamin B_{12} deficiency is the result of the blockade of methionine synthesis which sequesters folic acid as N-methyl-FH_4, and prevents its conversion to $N^{5,10}$ methylene FH_4 required for the synthesis of thymidylic acid (see Fig. 59.12).

In summary, there are several diseases that block the various steps in the absorption, transport, or metabolism of cobalamin. A decrease in the activity or synthesis of intrinsic factor by parietal cells in the stomach will impair the absorption of cobalamin and result in pernicious anemia. This occurs in most PA patients because of neutralization of IF by autoantibodies. In pancreatic insufficiency there is impaired transfer of CBL from R-proteins to IF. Intestinal disease can contribute to decreased ileal binding. Competition for the ileal receptor can also occur from bacterial overgrowth or fish tapeworm infestation and can impair attachment of IF cobalamin to the ileal receptor.

Genetic disease can also block access of CBL to cobalamin-dependent enzymatic reactions. Hereditary transcobalamin II deficiency will inhibit transport of CBL. At the metabolic level, six mutations have been identified that affect the biochemical fate of vitamin B_{12}. The cobalamin A mutation is due to lack of a reductase of Cbl in the methylmalonyte coA mutase pathway and results in methylmalonic aciduria. Cobalamin B deficiency is the result of the absence of the Cbl-adenosyl transferase, the enzyme that synthesizes deoxyadenosyl cobalamin. Cobalamin C and D diseases result from the absence of reductases that convert Cbl^{3+} and Cbl^{2+}, thus blocking both the activity of the mutase and the methionine synthetase, resulting in both methylmalonic aciduria and homocystinuria. Cobalamin E disease is due to an abnormality in $MeFH_4$-homocysteine transferase. The mutase is normal. The signs of this disease are anemia, homocystinuria, and mental retardation. Cobalamin F disease seems to be the result of the failure to convert cobalamin to hydroxy cobalamin, probably due to a lysosome defect. Although cyanocobalamin is

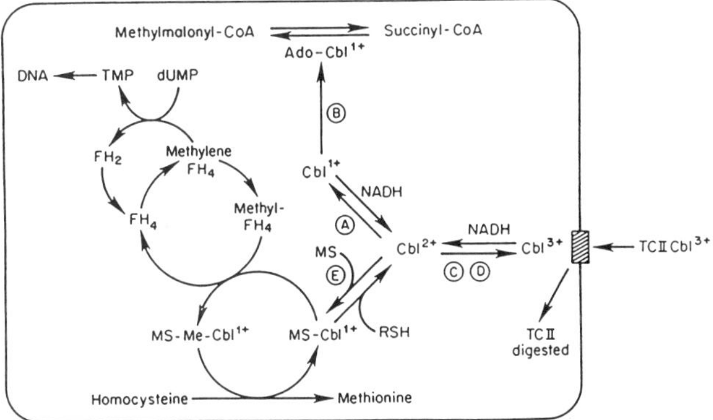

Figure 59.16 Conversion of vitamin B_{12} (cbl) to its active coenzyme forms. Cbl^{3+} is introduced into cells by receptor-mediated transfer form TCII to intracellular lysosomes from which, after digestion of TCII, cbl^{3+} is transferred to the cytoplasm. Cytoplasmic NADH, or another reductant in equilibrium with NADH, then converts cbl^{3+} to cbl^{2+} and then to cbl^{1+}, at which valence it can react with adenosine triphosphate to form adenosyl cbl^{1+} (Ado-cbl) and triphosphate. Genetic blocks have been noted at all stages in this pathway (cbl A,B,C,D diseases) and produce methylmalonic aciduria. The reaction that reduces cbl^{2+} to cbl^{1+} in association with methionine synthetase apparently requires a thiol (RSH) which permits the transfer of a methyl group from $MeFH_4$ to MS-cbl^{1+} to form Me-cbl^{1+}, which is the cofactor of the synthesis of methionine from homocysteine. If this reaction is blocked, homocysteine and $MeFH_4$ accumulate, and FH_4 declines. As a result, the thymidylate synthetase reaction is inhibited, DNA is not synthesized, and megaloblastic anemia occurs. In cobalamin E disease, methionine synthetase is uniquely inhibited to produce megaloblastic anemia and homocystinuria, but not methylmalonic aciduria. (ref r20)

the most available chemical derivative of cobalamin, CNCBL is an analogue and must be converted to the hydroxy form.[21]

Nutritional Requirements

Since cobalamin is synthesized only by bacteria, plants are devoid of this vitamin and vegetarians are at risk of vitamin B_{12} deficiency. The vitamin B_{12} in animal foods is due to their ingestion of bacteria in soil, sewage, rumen, or flora indigenous to their intestines. Foods high in vitamin B_{12} are meat, liver, fish, eggs, and milk. The average daily Western diet contains from 5 to 30 μg, of which only 1 to 5 μg is absorbed. The total body content of an adult, however, is 2 to 3 mg of which 1 mg is in the liver. If body stores are in the normal range and vitamin B_{12} is excluded from the diet, it will take about seven years to develop symptoms of pernicious anemia. The minimum IV dose required to support normal hematopoiesis is 0.1 μg/day—equivalent to about 0.5 μg by mouth. The recommended dietary allowance for adults is 2 μg/day, with lesser amounts for infants and children. The RDA for infants up to one year is 0.5 μg/day, for young children 0.7 to 1.0 μg/day, and for adolescents 1.4 μg/day.

Deficiency Disease

Pernicious anemia (PA) is the most frequent effect of vitamin B_{12} deficiency in humans. Because of advances made in understanding the pathophysiology of vitamin B_{12} deficiency, the once-fatal disease and its variants now can be treated successfully. The incidence of PA is age-related, most cases occurring after age 40. It typically affects northern Europeans of fair complexion, but paradoxically, young black women also are vulnerable. In many patients it relates to autoimmunity and is higher in persons with achlorhydria. Normal plasma contains 200 to 800 picograms/ml of vitamin B_{12}. In pernicious anemia, clinical signs appear when the plasma B_{12} value falls below 100 pg/ml. These signs include megaloblastosis, slowly progressing macrocytic anemia, glossitis, weakness, achlorhydria, methylmalonic aciduria, and neurologic abnormalities, the latter being due to demyelination of the dorsolateral columns of the spinal cord but also spotty areas of myelinated nerves in the cerebral white matter. The neurologic symptoms include symmetrical paraesthesias and reduced vibration sense and position sense in the feet and hands, progressing to ataxia with subacute combined system disease of the spinal cord.

The diagnosis of vitamin B_{12} deficiency is aided by immunoassays for plasma vitamin B_{12} and the Schilling test, which quantitates the ileal absorption of vitamin B_{12}. In this test, isotopically-labeled vitamin B_{12} is administered orally and the radioactivity in the urine is quantitated after a parenteral flushing dose of nonisotopically-labeled vitamin B_{12}.

The neurologic manifestations of vitamin B_{12} deficiency appear to be due to a failure to form methionine and S-adenosylmethionine from $MeFH_4$ in the brain and spinal cord.

Therapeutic Uses

For vegans, a daily oral dose of 1–5 μg is preventive. For pernicious anemia and other B_{12}-deficiency states 100 μg of of cobalamin parenterally per month is sufficient. For genetically conditioned disorders as much as 1 mg/d of B_{12} parenterally has been given.

Toxicology

Vitamin B_{12} is not known to cause adverse effects at 100 times the RDA. It must be realized, however, that CNCBL is an analogue and must be converted to hydroxy CBL to be used. There is a rare metabolic disorder where this reaction does not occur, and adverse affects of CNCBL should be investigated.

Preparations

Oral preparations of vitamin B_{12} are available in doses of 4 to 80 μg/capsule. Parenteral preparations of vitamin B_{12} contain from 4 to 1000 μg/ml.

Ascorbic Acid

History

Scurvy is an ancient disease. It was first recognized by the Egyptians before 1515 BC. Later, the Greeks and the Romans described it as the scourge of their armies and navies. Military rations at that time seldom contained adequate amounts of vitamin C, because they were composed of dessicated meat and flour. Armies from the crusaders to the forces of the US Civil War were menaced by scurvy. The clinical syndrome of scurvy is dominated by hemorrhagic manifestations—petechiae, perifollicular hemorrhage, subperiosteal hemorrhage, ecchymoses, bleeding and rotten gums, and swollen joints, associated with psychologic depression, vasomotor instability, fatigue, and lassitude. In infants, discrete changes in bone development are observed, owing to failure to form collagen at the epiphyseal:diaphyseal junction.

The early American explorers noted beneficial effects of bark, berries, and citrus fruits in the treatment of scurvy. The investigation of James Lind, a military surgeon aboard the Salisbury in May 1747, documented unequivocally the role of citrus fruits in treating scurvy.[92] He separated sailors with severe scurvy into several groups and treated them differently. The basic diet was water-gruel, sweetened with sugar; fresh mutton broth for dinner; puddings and biscuits with sugar; and barley and raisins, rice and currants, sago, and wine for supper. The controls received either a quart of cider a day, 25 gutts of elixir vitriol three times a day, or two spoonfuls of vinegar

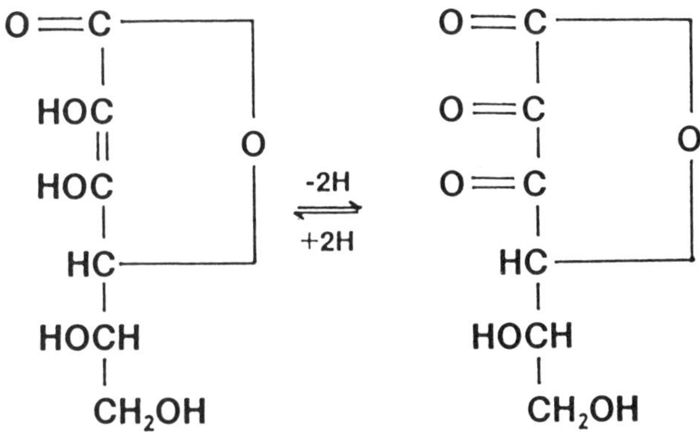

Figure 59.17 The Structures of Reduced and Oxidized Ascorbic Acid.

three times a day. The experimental group received two oranges and one lemon each day. The effect of citrus fruits was dramatic—one seaman was ready for duty at the end of six days after being so sick that he was unable to rise from his bed. This was the first controlled therapeutic trial in clinical medicine, and it established citrus fruits as curative of scurvy. Not until 1907 was an experimental model of scurvy produced in the guinea pig by Holst and Frohlich[93]; finally, in 1920, the antiscorbutic factor was recognized as a dietary essential and was given the name of vitamin C.[96]

In 1932 the active principle of citrus fruits, L-ascorbic acid, was isolated independently by two research groups, Szent-Gyorgy and Svirbely[94] in Szeged, and King and Waugh[95] in Pittsburgh. The structure of ascorbic acid was determined by the Haworth group[97,98] in London and its synthesis was accomplished by Reichstein et al.[99] in Zurich. The biochemical function of ascorbic acid is to act as a mandatory or facultative reductant for a series of hydroxylation reactions, the most vital of which is the hydroxylation of proline and lysine. These hydroxylations are important for the synthesis of collagen, the reduction of which accounts for much of the pathophysiology of scurvy.

Persons at risk for scurvy include infants fed from the bottle, military personnel eating dried rations, alcoholics during binges, and elderly people, usually living alone and subsisting on soup, tea, and bread.

Chemistry

Ascorbic acid is the enolic form of L-3-ketothreohexurenic acid lactone (MW = 176) with a formula of $C_6H_8O_8$. It is a white crystalline powder with a melting point of 192°C. It is a powerful reducing agent and a monobasic acid with a pKa of 4.17. It is freely soluble in water, slightly soluble in ethanol, and quite insoluble in most nonpolar lipid solvents. L-Ascorbic acid is reversibly converted to dehydroascorbic acid, and together these compounds have redox characteristics that influence the biologic activity of vitamin C. L-Ascorbic acid and dehydroascorbic acid together constitute the active form of vitamin C because they are equally antiscorbutic and biologically inseparable (Fig. 59.17).

Several analytical procedures for estimating the amount of vitamin C in biologic materials are available. They include colorimetric, fluorometric, chromatographic, and electrochemical techniques. The commonest method is to determine levels of ascorbic acid by measuring its ability to reduce chromogens such as 2,6-dichlorophenol-indophenol. To measure total ascorbic acid and dehydroascorbic (DHAA) requires oxidation of ascorbic acid to DHAA followed by derivatization with phenylhydrazine.

Physiology

Vitamin C is readily absorbed from the digestive tract of humans when ingested in physiologic amounts. Apparently, absorption of L-ascorbic acid, like that of glucose, is an energy-dependent process, although undoubtedly some diffusion also occurs. When progressively larger doses of L-ascorbic acid are ingested, the increment of increased absorption falls. Thus, a dose of less than 100 mg will be almost completely absorbed, but a dose of 180 mg will be only about 70 percent absorbed. When the dose is increased to 1500 mg, only about half of the total is absorbed. At a level of 12,000 mg, only 16 percent of the total is absorbed. The unabsorbed ascorbic acid remaining in the lumen of the bowel exerts an osomtic effect and causes loose watery diarrhea.

Once L-ascorbic acid is absorbed, it is distributed throughout the water space of the body. The metabolically active pool in adult humans has been found to be approximately 1500 mg, which is approximately at half-saturation. The rate of utilization in depletion-repletion studies has been found to be approximately 3 percent of the existing metabolic body pool/day. Thus, an individual whose body pool is 1500 mg will catabolize 3 percent, or 45 mg/day (Fig. 59.18). The concentration of this vitamin was found to be highest in the pituitary, adrenal gland, brain, liver, spleen, kidneys, and lesser amounts in lung, skeletal muscle, testes, thyroid, and saliva as shown in Table 59.5. The rate of loss of ascorbate at the scorbutic level of 300 mg is still 3 percent per day, or 9 mg/day.

The dose-dependent absorption of vitamin C (AA) is one mechanism to maintain homeostasis. A second mechanism is renal action to conserve or excrete ascorbate (AA). The amounts of AA cleared by glomerular filtration depends on the plasma AA level and the glomerular filtration rate. As this amount increases, the ability of the renal tubules to reabsorb AA reaches a maximum, and the unresorbed excess AA is excreted in the urine. This point, called the renal threshold, occurs in humans at plasma AA levels of about 1.2 mg/dl. Hence renal regulation of AA operates to conserve body AA stores during low AA intakes through renal tubular reabsorption, and to eliminate unneeded AA by urinary excretion at high intakes of 100 mg/day or more.

At the usual intakes of 50 to 100 mg/day, AA is not subject to significant oxidation, and homeostasis depends entirely on controlling the rates of absorption from the gut and excretion by the kidney. Only with

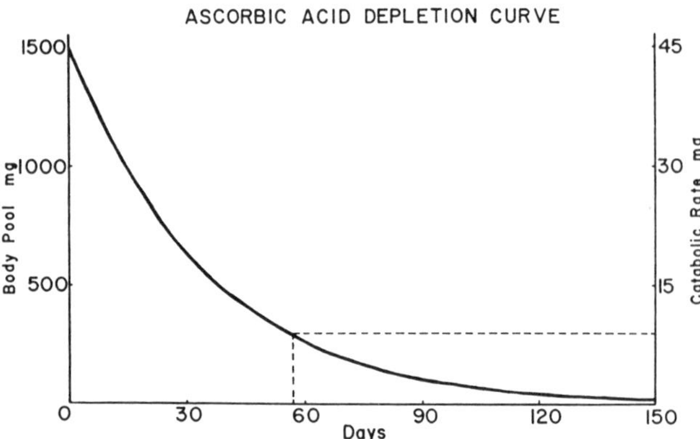

Figure 59.18 Curve of ascorbate pool derived from data of 9 men whose body pool of ascorbate was labeled with ^{14}C L-ascorbic acid. They were then fed a diet devoid of vitamin C. Initially the body pool averaged 1500 mg. The average daily rate of catabolism was 3 per cent of the existing body pool. Thus, the maximal rate of catabolism approximated 45 mg per day. When the body pool fell below 300 mg total and the catabolic rate below 9 mg per day, signs of scurvy began to appear (about 55 days). From this curve the approximate body pool size can be estimated from the dose. Thus, with a daily intake of 30 mg, the pool size should be about 1,000 mg. (r22)

Table 59.5 Vitamin C Content of Human Tissues and Fluids

Specimen	Vitamin C (μmol/100 g wet*)
Pituitary gland	227–284
Adrenal glands	170–227
Eye lens	142–176
Brain	75–85
Liver	57–91
Spleen and pancreas	57–85
Kidneys	28–85
Heart muscle	28–85
Semen (whole)	20–60
Lungs	40
Skeletal muscle	17
Testes	17
Thyroid	11
Plasma	1.7–8.5
Saliva	0.01–0.5

*μmol/100 g wet × 0.176 = mg/100 g wet.

megadoses does the body treat AA like a xenobiotic, degrading it to oxalate and other products excreted in the urine.

Most mammals synthesize AA from glucose by way of D-glucuronic acid, L-gulonic acid, L-gulonolactone, and L-gulonolactone oxidase, which is absent from the tissues of humans, monkeys, guinea pigs, and the ruby throated hummingbird. In fact the vulnerability of the human race to scurvy is due to a mutation in DNA that eliminated functional L-gulonolactone oxidase from human cells. This genetic defect has not yet been mapped to a specific chromosome in any of the animals incapable of synthesizing AA.

The biochemical functions of ascorbate are based on its properties as a reversible biologic reductant. Eleven enzyme systems dependent to a greater or lesser extent on ascorbate as a reductant are shown in Table 59.6. All ascorbate-dependent enzymes are metalloenzymes utilizing either Cu or Fe as a cofactor, which suggests that ascorbate is required to maintain the metal in a reduced state. Enzymes 1 and 2 are monooxygenases in which one atom of O_2 is transferred to the product and the other to water. Enzyme 3 is a deoxygenase requiring Fe in which both oxygens enter into the single product, homogentisic acid. Enzymes 4-11 are deoxygenases that require Fe and for which the following typed reaction occurs:

$$O_2 + \text{substrate} + \alpha\text{-ketoglutarate} \xrightarrow[\text{AA}]{Fe^{2+}}$$
$$\text{hydroxylated substrate} + \text{succinate} + CO_2$$

In this type of dioxygenase, one oxygen atom of O_2 enters the substrate and the other is incorporated into succinate. The activities of all these enzymes are reduced to a greater or lesser degree in vitamin C deficiency. The consequences are that the hydroxylation of proline and lysine, essential for collagen synthesis, is reduced; the oxidation of tyrosine is impaired; pyrimidine metabolism is altered; and carnitine synthesis is inhibited. In addition, there may be other biochemical reactions blocked in vitamin C deficiency that are required to explain the full pathophysiology of scurvy.

Nutritional Requirements

Fruits and vegetables are the principal source of vitamin C in the diet. Green and red peppers, collard greens, broccoli, spinach, tomatoes, potatos, strawberries, oranges, lemons, and other citrus fruits contain high concentrations of ascorbic acid. Meat, fish, poultry, and eggs contain smaller amounts, and grains contain none. The average intake of vitamin C by adult men and women in the US in 1985 was 109 mg and 77 mg, respectively.

Studies of volunteers by the British Medical Research Council scientists during World War II[102] demonstrated that 10 mg of L-ascorbate/day was sufficient to protect their subjects for 427 days, and to cure scurvy once it appeared in those receiving no vitamin. A similar study in Canada revealed that 7.9 mg of L-ascorbate per day would prevent scurvy for 240 days.[103] A group at the US Army Medical Research and Nutrition Labo-

Table 59.6 Enzymes Requiring Ascorbate for Maximal Activity

Class	Enzyme	Product
Monoxygenases	1) Dopamine-β-hydroxylase (Cu)	Norepinephrine
	2) Peptidyl-α-amidating enzyme (Cu)	C-terminal peptide amide
Deoxygenases	3) 4-hydroxy phenyl pyruvate hydroxylase (Fe)	Homogentisate
	4) Prolyl-4-hydroxylase (Fe)	Peptidyl-4-trans-hydroxy 2-proline
	5) Prolyl-3-hydroxylase (Fe)	Peptidyl-3-trans-hydroxy proline
	6) Lysyl-hydroxylase (Fe)	Peptidyl-S-erythro-hydroxy-L-lysine
	7) Thymine-7-hydroxylase (Fe)	5-hydroxy-methyl ???
	8) Pyrimidine deoxyribonucleoside 2'hydroxygenase (Fe)	Uridine
	9) Deoxy uridine hydroxylase (Fe)	Uracil
	10) 6-N-trimethyl-L-lysine Hydroxylase (Fe)	Erythro-5-Hydroxy-6-N-Trimethyl-L-lysine
	11) α-Butyrobetaine Hydroxylase (Fe)	R-carnitine

ratory[105] carried out a number of studies to determine the vitamin C requirement in several young male volunteers by feeding them a formula diet containing vitamin-free casein, corn oil, and starch but no ascorbic acid. This diet was fed for 90 days, during which the subjects plasma ascorbate fell from 1.2 mg/dl to an average of 0.1 mg/dl. Petechial hemorrhages and follicular hyperkeratosis appeared after 40 days, followed by swollen and bleeding gums, joint effusions, edema, neuropathy, and xerophthalmia (Sjögren's syndrome). During depletion, the body pool of ascorbate had decreased from 1500 mg to about 100 mg. After the depletion period, some of these volunteers were given 6.5 mg of L-ascorbate, which relieved all their signs and symptoms over the next 90 days, during which time their body pools increased to about 350 mg. Others receive higher doses up to 66 mg per day, and their symptoms disappeared more rapidly. All volunteers were restored to prestudy values at the end of the seven-month study.[104] Table 59.7 shows the relationship between the ascorbic acid content of plasma, whole blood, leukocytes, and the metabolic body pool in human adults (16 μg/10^8 WBC = 24 mg/dl of WBC).

The allowance for vitamin C has been the subject of extensive and continuing debate among expert committees. The RDAs in various countries have an unusual range of 20 to 200 mg/day for adults. The debate has been concerned with the issue of whether, as with other deficiency disease, the RDA is set at 2 to 3 times the minimum preventable dose or at some higher and arbitrary level to approach tissue saturation.

The Canadians and the British have recommended 30 mg/day for years (three times the minimum required dose to protect against scurvy). The FAO/WHO in 1974 also recommended 30 mg/day for adults. The US Food and Nutrition Board has varied from 75 mg/day for men and 70 mg/day for women in 1943 to a minimum of 45 mg/day for men and women in 1974. The current (1989) RDA for ascorbic acid in the US is 60 mg/day for both men and women which will maintain a body pool size of 1500 mg and will protect against scurvy with no further intake for six weeks. The amount of 30 to 40 mg/day was recommended for infants, 45 for older children, and 70 to 95 mg/day for pregnant and lactating women.

Table 59.7 Evaluation of Vitamin C Status

	Plasma (mg/dl)	Whole blood (mg/dl)	Leukocytes (μg/10^8 cells)	Metabolic body pool (mg)
High	0.60–1.40	>1.0	>16	1500
Normal	0.40–0.59	0.60–0.99	11–15	600–1499
Low	0.20–0.39	0.30–0.59	2–10	300–599
Deficient	<0.20	<0.30	<2	<300

Deficiency Disease

The symptoms and signs of scurvy have already been described in this chapter. They include systemic, hemorrhagic, secretory, psychologic, neurologic, hematologic, and arthritic manifestations which, are summarized in Table 59.8.[100,101] The biochemical activities of ascorbate are lost, and inhibition of over-all protein synthesis appears to occur. Moreover, this syndrome is not only observed in areas of the world where ascorbate is lacking (including US alcoholics) but also in healthy volunteers observed under metabolic ward conditions.

Vitamin C is a nutrient that is poorly retained (losing 3–4%/day) and probably only loosely bound to intracellular proteins, and can be almost completely lost from the body (pool size of less than 50 mg from a normal pool of 1500 mg) before the death of the subject. In fact, an intake of 10 mg per day will maintain

Table 59.8 Manifestations of Ascorbic Acid Deficiency in Man

1. Systemic
   - Fatigability
   - Lassitude
2. Hemorrhagic
   - Petechiae
   - Perifollicular hemorrhages
   - Ecchymoses
   - Bleeding gums
3. Psychologic
   - Depression
   - Hypochondriasis
   - Hysteria
4. Secretory
   - Dry skin, Xerophthalmia, Xerostomia } Sjögren's syndrome
   - Follicular hyperkeratosis
5. Vasomotor instability
   - Altered metabolism of neurotrophic amines
6. Hematologic
   - Impaired iron absorption
   - Impaired folate metabolism
7. Connective tissues
   - Scorbutic arthritis
   - Impaired wound healing

a pool of about 400 mg, well above the scorbutic level of 300 mg. The RDA for the US of 60 mg/day will maintain a pool size of 1500 mg/day.

Therapeutic Use

Probably no other required nutrient for humans has had so much promotion as a cure-all for medical illness if taken in megadoses—e.g., 500 to 10,000 mg/day—as vitamin C. Various claims have been made for the effectiveness of large doses of vitamin C in preventing (1) the common cold; (2) schizophrenia; (3) various types of cancer; (4) hypercholesterolemia and atherosclerosis. At present, most of these claims have not been convincingly validated, although there is continuing study of vitamin C as an "antioxidant."

The giving of megadoses of vitamin C changes the metabolism of vitamin C from nutrient to drug. Not only is absorption reduced, but oxidation of vitamin C, which is essentially nil on protective doses, becomes greatly increased. As a result, oxalate and other metabolites of vitamin C appear in the urine in large amounts. Large oral doses of vitamin C also cause diarrhea from osmotic effects and will acidify the urine, which may precipitate calcium salts and water. Thus, high levels of ascorbate in excretion will give a false-positive result for urinary tests for glucose and a false-negative for tests of occult blood in the stool.

Toxicology

Many adverse effects have been reported for persons taking over 1 gram of ascorbate daily. Besides diarrhea, stone-formers experience more renal calculi. There have been reports of altered menstrual periods and interruption of pregnancy in some women taking megadoses of vitamin C. It has been reported that vitamin C may be a pro-oxidant in the presence of high iron intake. Finally causes of "rebound scurvy" have been described in persons who abruptly stop taking megadoses of vitamin C.

Preparations

Preparations are available as multivitamins containing 50–100 mgs vitamin C/capsule and as single constituents containing 250 to 1000 mg/capsule.

References

Research Reports

1. Takaki K. Special report of the Kakke patients in the Imperial Navy from 1878 to 1886. Trans Sei-1-Kwai. Lancet 1887;*6*:73–95.
2. Eijkman C. Eine beriberi-ahnliche Kraukheit der Huhner. Virch Arch 1897;*148*:523–535.
3. Jansen BCP, Donath WF. Isolation of the chemically pure, antineuritic substance. Proc Konink Acad Wetenschap, Amsterdam. 1926;*29*:1390–1400.
4. Neuberg C, Karczag L. Carboxylase, ein neues Enzym der Hefe. Biochem Zeit 1911;*36*:68–76.
5. Auhagen EZ. Cocarboxylase, a new coenzyme of alcoholic fermentation. Physiol Chemie. 1932;*204*:149–167.
6. Williams RR, Waterman RE, Keresztesy JC. Larger yields of crystalline antineuritic vitamin J Am Chem Soc 1934;*56*:1187–1191.
7. Williams RR, Cline JK, Finkelstein J. Synthesis of vitamin B_1. J Am Chem Soc 1936;*58*:1504–1505.
8. Peters RA. Biochemical lesions in vitamin B_1 deficiency. Application of biochemical analysis in its diagnosis. Lancet 1936;*1*:1161–1164.
9. Lohmann K, Schuster P. Cocarboxylase. Naturwischft 1937;*25*:26–27.
10. Bergel F, Todd AR. A synthesis of aneurin. J Chem Soc 1937;*30*:1557–1559.
11. Tracy AH, Elderfield RC. Synthesis of 2-methyl-3-(2-hydroxyethyl pyridine and the pyridine analog of thiamine (vitamin B_1) J Org Chem 1941;*6*:54–62.
12. Thompson AD, Leevy CM. Observation of the mechanism of thiamin hydrochloride absorption in man. Clin Sci 1972;*43*:153–163.
13. Ukai T, Tanaka S, Dokawa S. A new catalyst for acyloin condensation. J Pharm Soc Japan 1943;*63*:269–272.

14. Breslow R. On the mechanism of thiamine action. J Am Chem Soc 1958;*80*:3719.

15. Krampitz LO, Greull G, Miller CS, Bicking JB, Skeggs HR, Sprague JM. An active acetaldehyde-thiamine intermediate. J Am Chem Soc 1958;*80*:5893–5894.

16. Holzer H, Beauchamp K. Detection of intermediates of the decarboxylation and oxidation of pyruvate. Angew Chemie 1959;*71*:776.

17. Horecker BL, Smyrniotis PZ, Klenow H. The formation of sedo-keptulose phosphate from pentose phosphate. J. Biol. Chem. 1953;*205*:661–682.

18. Itokawa Y, Cooper JR. Ion movements and thiamine The release of the vitamin from membrane fragments. Bioch Biophys Acta 1970;*196*:274–284.

19. Smith MI, Hendrick EG. Some nutrition experiments with brewers yeast with special reference to its value in supplementing certain deficiencies in experimental rations. Pub Health Rep 1926;*41*:201–210.

20. Warburg O, Christian W. The yellow oxidation enzyme. Biochem Zeit 1933;*263*:128–341.

21. Kuhn R, Gyorgy P, Wagner-Jauregg T. A new class of natural pigments. Ber 1933;*66*:317–320.

22. Kuhn R, Reinemund K, Kaltschmitt H. Synthesis of 6,7-dimethyl-9-d-riboflavin. Naturwischf 1935;*23*:260–265.

23. Karrer P, Schopp K, Benz F: Synthesis of flavins Helv Chim Acta 1935;*18*:426–429.

24. Bates CJ. Liberation of $^{14}CO_2$ from [^{14}C]-adipic acid [^{14}C]octanic acid by adult rats during riboflavin deficiency and reversal. Br J Nutr 1990;*63*:553–562.

25. Elvehjem CA, Madden RJ, Strong FM et al. Isolation and identification of anti-black tongue factor. J Biol Chem 1938;*123*:137–149.

26. Spies TD, Cooper C, Blankenhorn MA. Use of nicotinic acid in treatment of pellagra. JAMA 1938;*110*:622–627.

27. Krehl WA, Tepley LJ, Sarma PS, Elvehjem CA. Growth retarding effects of corn in nicotinic acid-low rations and its counteraction by tryptophane. Science 1945;*101*:489–492.

28. Heidelberger C, Gilbert Morgan F, Lefkovsky. Tryptophan metabolism. J Biol Chem 1948;*179*:151–155.

29. Warburg O, Christian W, Griese. Hydrogen-transferring coenzyme, its composition and mode of action. Biochem Zeit 1935;*282*:157–165.

30. Goldberger J, Tanner WF. Amino acid deficiency probably the primary etiological factor in pellagra. Pub Health Rep 1922;*37*:462–486.

31. Vilter RW, Mueller JF, Bean WB. The therapeutic effect of tryptophane in human pellagra. J Lab Clin Med 1949;*34*:409–413.

32. Goldsmith GA, Gibbens J, Unglaub WG, Miller ON. Rat pellagra. Bioch J 1935;*29*:741.

33. Goldsmith GA, Gibbens J, Unglaub WG, Miller ON. Studies on niacin requirement in man. Am J Clin Nutr 1956;*4*:151–160.

34. Gyorgy P. Crystalline vitamin B_6. J Am Chem Soc 1938;*60*:983–984.

35. Lepkowsky S. Isolation of factor one in crystalline form. J Biol Chem 1938;*124*:125–128.

36. Keresztesy JC, Stevens JR. Vitamin B_6. J Am Chem Soc 1938;*60*:1267–1268.

37. Harris SA, Folkers K. Synthesis of vitamin B_6. J Am Chem Soc 1939;*61*:1245–1247.

38. Snell EE. The vitamin B_6 group: I. Formation of additional members from pyridoxine and evidence concerning their structures. J Am Chem Soc 1944;*66*:2082–2088.

39. Snell EE, Guirade BM, Williams RJ. Occurrence in natural products of a physiologically active metabolite of pyridoxine. J Biol Chem 1942;*143*:519–530.

40. Schaumberg H, Kaplan J, Windebank A, Vick N, Rasmus S, Pleasure D, Brown MJ. Sensory neuropathy from pyridoxine abuse. N Engl J Med 1983;*309*:445–448.

41. Dalton K, Dalton MJT. Characteristics of pyridoxine overdose neuropathy syndrome. Acta Neurol Scand 1987;*76*:8–11.

42. Williams RJ, Lyman CM, Goodyear GH, Truesdail JH, Holliday D. Pantothenic acid: A growth determinant of universal biological occurrence. J Am Soc 1933;*55*:2912–2927.

43. Williams RJ. Pantothenic acid—A vitamin. Science 1939;*89*:486.

44. Williams RJ, Weinstock HH Jr, Rohrmann E, Truesdail JH, Mitchell HK, Meyer CE. Pantothenic acid. III: Analysis and determination of constituent groups. J Am Chem Soc 1939;*61*:454–458.

45. Williams RJ, Major RT. The structure of pantothenic acid. Science 1940;*91*:246.

46. Jukes TH. Pantothenic acid requirement of chick. J Am Chem Soc 1939;*61*:975–978.

47. Wooley DW, Waisman HA, Elvejhem CA. Nature and partial synthesis of the chick antidermatitis factor. J Am Chem Soc 1939;*61*:977–978.

48. Lipmann F, Kaplan NO, Novelli, GD, Tuttle LC, Guirard BM. Coenzyme for acetylation, a pantothenic acid derivative. J Biol Chem 1947;*167*:869–870.

49. Fenstermacher DK, Rose RC. Absorption of pantothenic acid in rat and chick intestine. Am J Physiol 1986;*250*:G155–G160.

50. Smith CM, Milner RE. The mechanism of pantothenate transport by rat liver parenchymal cells in primary culture. J Biol Chem 1985;*260*:4823–4831.

51. Fuerst R, Li L. A study of the synthesis of γ-pantothenate by Neurospora. Biochim Biophys Acta 1964;*86*:26–32.

52. Matsuzaki F. Antagonistic action of homopantothenate against panthothenic acid. Vitamin (Japan) 1965;*32*:245–259.

53. Mitsuma T, Nogimori T. Effects of calcium hopantenate on the hypothalamic-pituitary-thyroid axis in rats. Horm Res 1983;*18*:210–214.

54. Schaefer JM, McKibbin JM, Elvehjem CA. Pantothenic acid deficiency studies in dogs. J Biol Chem 1942;*143*:321–330.

55. Noda S, Umezaki H, Yamamoto K, Araki T, Murakami T, Ishii N. Reye-like syndrome following treatment with the pantothenic acid antagonist calcium hopantenate. J Neurol Neurosurg Psychiatry 1988;*51*:582–585.

56. Eissenstat BR, Wyse BW, Hansen RG. Pantothenic acid status of adolescents. Am J Clin Nutr 1986;*44*:931–937.

57. Glusman M. The syndrome of "burning feet" (nutritional malalgia) as manifestation of nutritional deficiency. Am J Med 1947;*3*:211–223.

58. Hodges RE, Ohlson MA, Bean WA. Pantothenic acid deficiency in man. J Clin Invest 1958;*37*:1642–1657.

59. Hodges RE, Bean WB, Ohlson MA, Bleiler R. Human pantothenic acid deficiency produced by omega-methyl pantothenic acid. J Clin Invest 1959;*38*:1421–1425.

60. Boas MA. Effect of desiccation upon the nutritional properties of egg white. Biochem J 1927;*21*:712–724.

61. Kogl F, Tonnis B. Isolation of crystalline biotin from egg yolk. Zeit Physiol Chemie 1936;*242*:73–74.

62. Gyorgy P. Possible identity of vitamin H with biotin and coenzyme R. Science 1940;*91*:243–245.

63. du Vignaud V, Hofmann K, Melville DB, Rachele JR. The preparation of free crystalline biotin. J Biol Chem 1941;*140*:765–

64. Hofmann K, Melville DB, du Vigneaud VJ. Characterization of the functional groups of biotin. Biol Chem 1941;*141*:209–

65. Harris SA, Folkers K, Heyl D. Synthesis of biotin. J Am Chem Soc 1944;*66*:2088–2092.

66. Sydenstryker VP, Segal SA, Briggs AP, DeVaughn NM, Isbell H. Observation of "egg white injury" in man and its cure with a biotin concentrate. JAMA 1942;*118*:1199–1200.

67. Tanaka K. New light on biotin deficiency. N Engl J Med 1981;*304*:839–840.

68. Gompertz D, Draffan GH, Watts JL, Hull D. Biotin-responsive β-methyl-crotonylglycinuria. Lancet 1971;*2*:22–24.

69. Sweetman L, Bates SP, Hull D, Nyhan WL. Propionyl-CoA carboxylase deficiency in a patient with biotin-responsive 3-methylcrotonylglycinuria. Pediatr Res 1977;*11*:1144–1147.

70. Bartlett K, Gompertz D. Combined carboxylase defect: Biotin-responsiveness in cultured fibroblasts. Lancet 1976;*2*:804.

71. Cowan JM, Wara DW, Packman S, Ammann AJ, Yoshino M, Sweetman L, Nyhan W. Multiple biotin-dependent carboxylase deficiencies associated with defects in T cell and B cell immunity. Lancet 1979;*2*:115–118.

72. Wills L, Contab MA, Lond BS. Folate deficiency. Brit Med J 1931;*1*:1059–1064.

73. Osler W. The severe anemias of pregnancy. Brit Med J 1919;*i*:1–3.

74. Wills L, Bilimoria HS. Studies in pernicious anemia of pregnancy: Production of macrocytic anemia in monkey by deficient feeding. Indian J Med Res 1932;*20*:391–402.

75. Snell EE, Peterson WH. Growth factors for bacteria X. Additional factors required by certain lactobacilli. J Bact 1949;*39*:273–285.

76. Day PL, Langston WC, Darby WJ. Failure of nicotinic acid to prevent nutritional cytopenia in the monkey. Proc Soc Exp Biol Med 1938;*60*:860–863.

77. Stokstad ELR. Some properties of growth factor for Lactobacillus casei. J Biol Chem 1943;*149*:573–574.

78. Pfiffner JJ, Binkley SB, Bloom ES, Brown RA, Bird OD, Emmett AD, Hogan AG, O'Dell BL. Isolation of antianemia factor in crystalline form from liver. Science 1943;*97*:404–405.

79. Mitchell HK, Snell EE, Williams RJ. Concentration of folic acid. J Am Chem Soc 1941;*63*:2284–2285.

80. Hogan AG, Parrott EM. Anemia in chicks caused by vitamin deficiency. J Biol Chem 1940;*132*:507–517.

81. Herbert V. Experimental nutritional folate deficiency in man. Trans Assoc Am Phys 1962;*75*:307–320.

82. Czeizel A, Dudas I. Prevention of the first occurrence of neural-tube defects by periconceptual vitamin supplementation. N Engl J Med 1992;*327*:1832–1835.

83. Castle WB. The conquest of pernicious anemia. In MM Blood, pure and eloquent. A story of discovery of people and of ideas. New York: McGraw-Hill, 1983, pp 316–331.

84. Minot GR, Murphy WP. Treatment of pernicious anemia by special diet. JAMA 1926;*87*:470–476.

85. Castle WB, Townsend WC. Observations on the etiologic relationship of achylia gastrica to pernicious anemia. II. The effect of the administration to patients with pernicious anemia of beef muscle after incubation with normal human gastric juice. Am J Med Sci *178*:764–777.

86. Whipple GH, Robscheit-Robbins FS. Blood regeneration in severe anemia: Favorable influence of liver, heart and skeletal muscle in diet. Am J Physiol 1925;*72*:408–418.

87. Whipple GH, Robscheit-Robbins FS. Iron and its utilization in experimental anemia. Am J Med Sci 1936;*191*:1124–1143.

88. Rickes EL, Brink NG, Koniuszy FR et al. Crystalline vitamin B-12, Science 1948;*107*:396–397.

89. Smith EL, Parker LFJ. Purification of anti-pernicious anemia factor. Biochem J 1948;*43*:vii–ix.

90. Hodgkin DC, Kayser J, Mackay M, Pickworth J, Trueblood N, White JG. Structure of vitamin B_{12}. Nature 1956;*178*:64–66.

91. Seetharam B, Alpers DH, Allen PH. Isolation and characterization of the ileal receptor for intrinsic factor-cobalamin. J Biol Chem 1981; 256:3785–3790.

92. Lind J. A treatment of the scurvy. Sands, Murray and Cochran, Edinburgh 1753; reproduced in part in Nutr Rev 1983;*41*:155–157.

93. Holst A, Frolich T. Experimental studies relating to ship-beriberi and scurvy. J Hyg (London) 1907;*7*:634–671.

94. Svirbely and Szent-Gyrogy A. The chemical nature of vitamin C. Biochem J 1932;*26*:865–870.

95. King CG, Waugh WA. Chemical nature of vitamin C. Science 1932;*75*:357–358.

96. Drummond JC. The nomenclature of the so-called accessory food factors (vitamins). Biochem J 1920;*14*:660–669.

97. Percival EGV, Smith F. Constitution of ascorbic acid. Nature 1933;*131*:617.

98. Haworth WN, Hirst EL. The constitution of ascorbic acid. J Soc Chem Ind (London)*52*:482–484.

99. Reichstein T, Grussner A, Oppenauer R. Synthesis of d-ascorbic acid (d-form of vitamin C). Helv Chim Acta 1933;*16*:561–565.

100. Hodges RE, Hood J, Canham JE, Sauberlich HE, Baker EM. Clinical manifestations of ascorbic acid deficiency in man. Am J Clin Nutr 1971;*24*:432–433.

101. Hood J, Burns CA, Hodges RE. Sjögren syndrome in scurvy. N Engl J Med 1970;*282*:1120–1124.

102. Bartley W, Krebs HA, O'Brien JRP. Vitamin C requirements of human adults. Medical research council special report. Series No. 280 HM Stationery Office, London, 1953.

103. Johnstone WM, Drake TGH, Tisdale FF, Harvie FF. A study of the ascorbic acid metabolism of healthy young Canadians. Can Med Assoc J 1946;*55*:581–585.

104. Schaffer CF. The diuretic effect of ascorbic acid. JAMA 1944;*124*:700–701.

105. Hodges RE, Baker EM, Hood J, Sauberlich HE, March SC. Experimental scurvy in man. Am J Clin Nutr 1969;*22*:535–548.

Reviews

r1. Marcus R, Coulston AM. Water-soluble vitamins; the vitamin B complex and ascorbic acid. In Gilman AG, Goodman LS, Rall TW, Murad F., eds. The Pharmacological Basis of Therapeutics, 7th ed. New York: Macmillan, 1985.

r2. Rindi G, Ventura U. Intestinal transport of thiamine. Physiol Rev 1972;*52*:821–827.

r3. Tanphaichiter V, Wood B. Thiamin in present knowledge. In Olson RE. ed. Nutrition, 5th ed. Washington: Nutrition Foundation, 1984.

r4. Recommended Dietary Allowances NRC/NAS Food and Nutrition Board, 10th Edition. Washington: National Academy Press, 1989.

r5. McCollum EV, Orent-Keiles E, Day HG. The Newer Knowledge of Nutrition, 5th ed. New York: MacMillan, 1939.

r6. Decker KF. Biosynthesis and function of enzymes with covalently bound flavin. Ann Rev Nutr 1993;*13*:17–41.

r7. McCormick DB. Riboflavin. In Shils ME, Young VR, eds. Modern Nutrition in Health and Disease, 7th ed. Philadelphia: Lea & Febinger, 1988.

r8. Swenseid ME, Jacob RA. Niacin. In Shils ME, Olson JA, Shike M. eds. Modern Nutrition and Health and Disease, 8th ed. Philadelphia: Lea & Febiger, 1994.

r9. Henderson LM. Niacin. Ann Rev Nutr 1983;*3*:289–307.

r10. Merrill AH, Burnham FS. Vitamin B-6. In Brown M. ed. Present Knowledge in Nutrition, 6th ed. ILSI-NF, Washington, 1990.

r11. Olson RE. Pantothenic acid. In Brown M. ed. Present Knowledge of Nutrition, 6th ed. ILSI-NF Washington, D.C. 1990.

r12. McCormick DB, Olson RE. Biotin. In Olson RE. ed. Present Knowledge of Nutrition, 5th ed. Washington: Nutrition Foundation, 1984.

r13. Gyorgy P. Vitamin H. Handbook of Pediatrics. 1935;*10*:45, Pfandler-Schossman, Berlin.

r14. Lardy HA, Peanasky R. Biotin enzymes. Physiol. Rev 1953;*33*:560–580.

r15. Wagner C. Folic acid. In Olson RE. ed. Present Knowledge of Nutrition, 5th ed. Washington: Nutrition Foundation, 1984.

r16. Krumdieck CC. Folic Acid. In Brown M. ed. Present Knowledge of Nutrition 6th ed. ILSI-NF, Washington, D.C. 1990.

r17. Herbert V, Colman N. Folic acid and vitamin B-12. In: Shils ME, Young VR. Modern nutrition in health and disease. Philadelphia: Lea & Febiger, 1988, pp 388–416.

r18. Seetharam B, Alpers DH. Absorption and transport of cobalamin (vitamin B_{12}. Ann Rev Nutr 19082;*2*:343–369.

r19. Herbert V, Daj K. Folic acid and vitamin B_{12}. In Shils ME, Olson JA, Shike IM. eds. Modern Nutrition in health and disease, 8th ed. Philadelphia: Lea & Febiger, 1994.

r20. Olson RE. Cobalamin E disease in an infant. Nutr Rev 1986;*44*:239–241.

r21. Fenton WA, Rosenberg LE. Inherited disorders of cobalamin transport and metabolism. In The Metabolic Basis of Inherited Diseases, New York: McGraw-Hill, 1989.

r22. Sauberlich HE. Ascorbic acid. In Olson, RE.Present Knowledge in Nutrition, 5th ed. Nutr. Foundation, Washington DC, 1984.

CHAPTER 60

Robert E. Olson

Macrominerals

The macrominerals required by the human body are distinguished from micro minerals only by the magnitude of their requirement and to a lesser extent by their position in the periodic table. The daily requirements for these minerals range from about 0.3 gm for sodium and magnesium to 2.0 grams for potassium. Sodium and potassium and alkali metals, calcium and magnesium are alkali earths, and chloride and phosphate are accompanying anions. Water is not a mineral, but it is the oxide of hydrogen, which is in Group I in the periodic table and is considered in this chapter on minerals. Water makes up about 60 percent of body weight and should be grouped with other substances that contribute to the matrix portion of the body. It has the highest requirement of any essential nutrient namely 1 ml/kcal of energy expended, which for most persons exceeds 2 kilograms per day.

These minerals will be discussed under the topics of: 1. history; 2. chemistry; 3. physiology; 4. nutritional requirements; 5. deficiency disease; 6. therapeutic uses; 7. toxicity; and 8. preparations.

Water

History

All life on this planet, and all the evolutionary forms that preceded the present array of plants and animals in the world, required water as an essential nutrient. Empedocles of Agrigentum, a Greek philosopher and physician (504–432 B.C.) formulated the first theory of matter, namely that there were four elements: fire; air; earth; and water. Empedocles appreciated what is now so obvious—that water was the basic element of living things and its motion through the body from drink to urine via the blood (and he postulated the heart at the center of man) was the basis of physiology. Sanctorius, an Italian physician (1561–1636), did the first balance studies on humans (including himself) and discovered that "insensible perspiration" was mostly expired water vapor. Lavoisier, a French chemist (1743–1794), discovered the true nature of animal combustion and found that CO_2 and water were the ultimate products.[r1]

Water is required by all animals in the amount of 1 liter per square meter per day (equivalent to 1 ml/kcal expended per day). Its principal role is that of a solvent for inorganic and organic substances in both intracellular and extracellular spaces. Cells are enclosed by and partitioned into spaces by membranes made of lipids and proteins, insoluble in water, that create compartments in which metabolism and other life processes occur. Water is not a static substance since it turns over each day and is a reactant and product in many biochemical reactions.

Chemistry

Water is composed of two atoms of hydrogen and one of oxygen to form H_2O (MW=18). It is the most important of all oxides. Water is both a weak acid and weak base with a pKa = 7.0. It has a high specific heat of 1 cal/ml.

The water molecule is nonlinear with the H ⁄O∖ H angle equal to 104.5°. Each bond is covalent, but is polarized so that a residual positive charge is on each H and a negative one is on each O. This polarity results in hydrogen bonding between different water molecules to produce a large network of loosely attached water molecules. When water freezes, these bonds form a tetrahedral crystalline structure with four H atoms around each O.

When ice melts, this structure becomes less orderly but is not destroyed. In fact, at 4°C, water has its maximum density; for this reason, ice (at 0°C) floats on water. As the temperature is raised above 4°C, the density again decreases, because more hydrogen bonds are broken and H_2O molecules move farther apart. The heat of fusion for water at 0°C is 80 calories/gram and the heat of vaporization at 100°C is 539 calories/gram. These heats are entropic and are needed to change the hydrogen bonding of water at its freezing and boiling points. Because of these properties of water, life forms are not active at temperatures below 4°C or above 100°C.

Water is the universal solvent for living organisms, but not all biochemicals are soluble in water. Since water is a polar solvent, charged substances like electrolytes (NaCl, KCl, $NaHCO_3$) and nonelectrolytes with comparable polar groups (sucrose, glucose, ethanol, amino acids, hydrophilic proteins like albumin) are water-soluble. Uncharged lipid-soluble substances like N_2, CH_4, triglycerides, and hydrophobic proteins like collagen are insoluble in water.

The movement of water between different body fluid compartments is related to the concentration of osmotically active particles regardless of their size or valence. Solute concentration can be expressed in terms of osmoles/L or in terms of the reciprocal (ml/osmole). NaCl, being totally dissociated into Na^+ and Cl^- in aqueous solutions has two osmoles per mole. Glucose (MW=180) and albumin (MW=69,000) each have one osmole/mole. Most cell membranes are semipermeable, i.e., permeable to water but not to some solutes, so that water will move toward the compartment with the higher osmolarity.

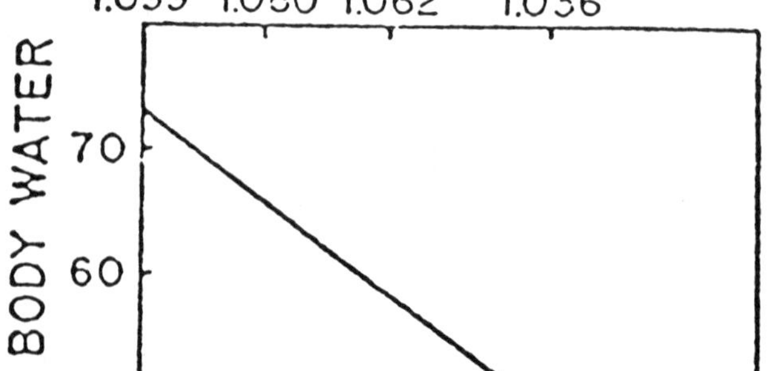

Figure 60.1 Relationships between body fat, specific gravity, and percentage of water. (Adapted from Behnke, A.R., Jr.: Harvey Lect *37*:198, 1941–42.)[1]

Physiology

Water is the most abundant constituent of the human body, accounting for 50 to 70 percent of body weight, depending mainly on the body fat content of the individual. The ratio is higher in adult males and lower in females because of females' higher fat content. The percentage of water also tends to fall with age (Fig. 60.1).

Approximately two-thirds of the total body water is found in the intracellular compartment, whereas the remaining one-third is found in the extracellular space. The extracellular space is composed of plasma, interstitial fluid, and a small transcellular fluid volume (Fig. 60.2).

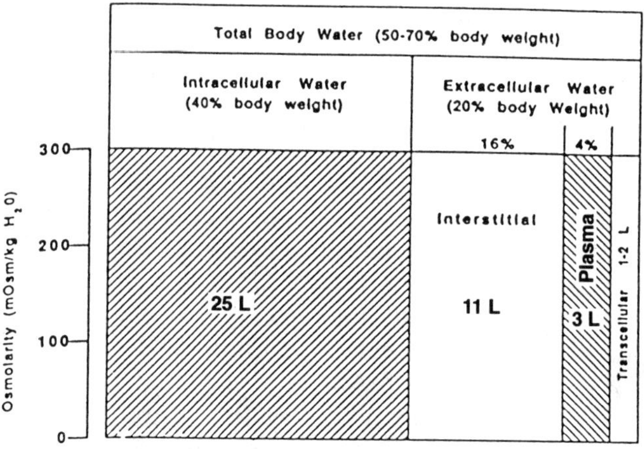

Figure 60.2 Distribution of water in a normal human. Approximately 60% of body weight results from total body water. Intracellular water volume is equal to ~40% of body weight, whereas extracellular water is ~20% of body weight.[r2]

Water is absorbed from the GI tract by simple diffusion, governed by osmotic gradients. Dietary water for an average adult will vary from 1800 to 3000 ml/day. In addition the GI tract secretes and resorbs about 8000 ml of saliva, gastric fluid, bile, pancreatic fluid, and intestinal secretions per day. The stool normally contains only 100 to 200 ml/day. The balance of input and output of water for a healthy adult is shown in Table 60.1. Water from oxidation of food ranges from 300 to 400 ml/day; outputs from insensible loss range from 800 to 1000 ml and urinary output is 1000 to 2000 ml/day.

Because the body is unable to prevent obligatory losses of water, such as insensible water loss, sweat, fecal loss, and a minimum urine volume of 500 to 600 ml required to excrete osmotically active catabolites like creatinine, urea, and minerals, the output side ordinarily must drive the input side in achieving water balance.

The water homeostatic system depending on a neurohypophyseal axis is designed to keep the ratio

Table 60.1 Major Inputs and Outputs of Water[a]

Inputs	Average Volume per Day, ml/day	Outputs	Average Volume per Day, ml/day
Water content of food	800–1000	Insensible loss	800–1000
Water generated during oxidation of food	300–400	Sweat	200
Water consumed as a liquid	1000–2000	Feces	100–200
		Urine	1000–2000
Total	2100–3400	Total	2100–3400

*Adapted from Weitzman and Kleeman (1980).[r3a] Inputs and outputs represent average basal values for an adult in a cool environment.

of water to solutes in body fluids within range of 3.5 to 3.7 ml for each milliosmole (equivalent to 280 mOsm/L). This is an important physiologic variable because elevation of the water-solute ratio by as little as 10 percent to 3.9 or 4.0 ml per mOsm is apt to result in water intoxication. Contrariwise, reduction of the ratio by 5 to 10 per cent to 3.3 ml per moSm, or less, tends to produce symptoms and signs of dehydration.

The system functions like a feedback circuit. A tendency to abnormal lowering of the ratio of water solutes in body fluids is recognized by osmoreceptors in the hypothalamus. As the ratio falls, the body responds by creating a sensation of thirst and by causing the neurohypophysis to secrete antidiuretic hormone. The renal tubules react to this hormone by reducing the quantity of water accompanying each milliosmole of solute excreted in the urine. Passage of urine, which is so concentrated that it contains less water for each milliosmole of solute than the plasma from which it was derived, tends to raise the water-solute ratio of the body fluids, but usually additional water input is necessary. When the water-solute ratio approaches a physiologically satisfactory level, the sensation of thirst abates and the secretion of antidiuretic hormone ceases. On the other hand, the reverse of these homeostatic reactions follows an abnormal rise in the water-solute ratio of the body fluids after water loading. Then the ratio in the body fluids falls as the ratio in the urine rises. These mechanisms are summarized in Figure 60.3.

The water homeostatic system, while closely concerned with the stability of the water-solute ratio of body fluids, also is involved in the preservation of a satisfactory vascular volume. Available evidence suggests that there are stretch- or pressure-sensitive elements, possibly in the left atrium, that can promote thirst and antidiuretic hormone production irrespective of the water-solute ratio of body fluids should the vascular volume become abnormally reduced. In patients suffering from blood loss, hypoalbuminemia,

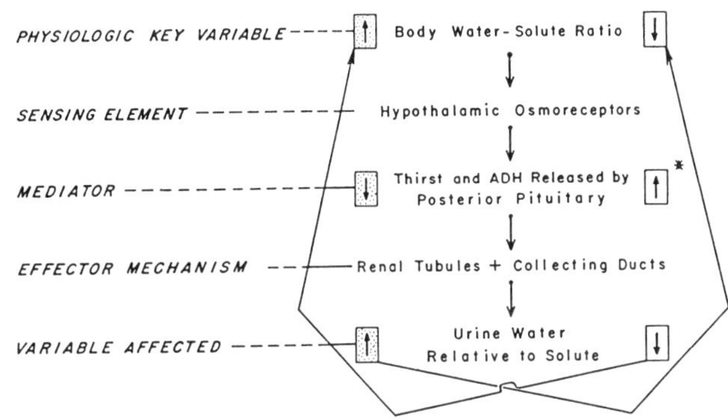

Figure 60.3 Water Homeostatic System[r4]

or extracellular electrolyte deficiency, this response can result in the retention of enough water to increase the water-solute ratio of body fluids above the normal level and to cause water intoxication with convulsions.[r3]

Nutritional Requirements

The guideline for water intake by adult humans is 1 ml/kcal of energy expended or 2000 ml on average. For older persons, infants, and those exposed to a hot environment the recommendation is for 1.5 ml/kcal of energy. In pregnancy the need for water intake increases because of needs of the mother, fetus, and placenta, so 1.5 ml/kcal is a satisfactory guideline. In lactating mothers, additional water is needed for milk formation, and the recommendation increases to 2 ml/kcal.

Deficiency Disease

Dehydration or hypohydration is the deficiency disease associated with water lack. In water deprivation, the water-solute ratio in the plasma can drop to below 3 ml/milliosmole. This dehydration results in thirst, concentrated urine, (up to the maximum level of 1400 mOsm/L), fever, irritability, lethargy, muscle twitching, EEG changes, acidosis, and even respiratory and circulatory failure. In this situation, serum sodium may rise as high as 170 mEq/L and chloride to 130 mEq/L. Total water deprivation will cause death in a few days. It is, no doubt, man's most essential nutrient. The treatment is restoration of water, by mouth, in relatively small increments to repair the deficit of 8 to 10 liters in body water.

Therapeutic Uses

Water is used to repair dehydration and as a vehicle for countless substances administered as drugs.

Preparations

Tap water is the cheapest form of water preparation, but there are others that are bottled, including sterile water for IV administration.

Sodium, Potassium, and Chloride

History

Sodium and potassium are widely distributed in the oceans and land masses of this planet. Many scientists believe that life began in a salty marine environment. Although the sodium and chloride contents of human blood plasma are much lower than the concentrations of these ions in today's oceans, it is believed that primeval oceans were less briny. It is possible that the present concentrations of sodium, chloride, and potassium in our plasma resemble those that existed in the oceans in ancient geologic times.

Potassium and sodium were discovered in 1807 by electrolysis of their fused chlorides by Sir Humphrey Davy (1778–1829), an English chemist. Claude Bernard (1813–1878), the great French physiologist, was the first to appreciate the importance of the internal environment, the *milieu intérieur*, by which he meant the blood plasma and extracellular fluid, for the health of cells and their intracellular activities. He recognized that the extracellular fluid approximated 0.9 percent sodium chloride and that the predominant cation within cells was potassium. In 1873, Forster discovered that salt was a nutritional requirement for dogs. More recently Homer Smith, the American physiologist, observed that the kidney was the guardian of our internal environment by regulating the extent to which sodium, potassium, and chloride were reabsorbed by the kidney tubule.[r6]

Chemistry

Sodium and potassium are alkali metals in group I of the periodic table. Sodium is in the third period and potassium is in the fourth. Chlorine is a halogen in Group VII of the fourth period. Sodium has an atomic weight of 23 and an atomic number of 11; chlorine has an atomic weight of 35.5 and an atomic number of 17. Sodium has no natural isotopes but 13 radioisotopes, including $_{11}Na^{22}$, a beta and gamma-emitter with a half-life of 2.6 years, and $_{11}Na^{24}$ with a half-life of 15 hours. Potassium has two naturally-occurring isotopes, $_{19}K^{40}$ and $_{14}K^{41}$, of which $_{19}K^{40}$ (half-life = 10^9 years) is the most useful in biology. Potassium has 12 radioactive isotopes, all short-lived. Chloride has one naturally-occurring isotope $_{17}Cl^{37}$ and eight radioactive isotopes $_{17}Cl^{36}$ a beta-emitter, which is the most useful (half-life = 3×10^5 years).

Sodium and potassium are strong reducing agents and give up electrons with great ease, e.g.,

$$2Na + 2H_2O \rightarrow 2Na^+ + OH^- + H_2$$

Sodium hydroxide formed in the above reaction makes an alkaline, caustic (pH = 14), soapy solution. Potassium hydroxide has similar properties. Sodium chloride (NaCl), the most important compound of sodium, and comprises common table salt. It is the major ionic component of plasma, occurs in sea water to the extent of 3 percent, and is found in salt deposits. Potassium chloride, an important compound of potassium, also occurs in earth deposits.

Chloride, on the other hand, an electronegative element, is a good oxidizing agent; and in typical reactions is reduced to chloride ion (^-Cl). For example, when hydrogen and chlorine react, hydrochloric acid, a strong acid, is formed

$$H_2 + Cl_2 \rightarrow 2H^+Cl^-$$

and is completely dissociated to give protons (H^+) and chloride ions (Cl^-). Sodium hydroxide reacts with HCl to form NaCl, a neutral salt, but one that is completely ionized—as in fact it is in the body. Such soluble ions as Na^+, K^+, and Cl^- are commonly called *electrolytes*.

Physiology

In most foods, Na, K, and Cl are present as ions and enter the GI tract as electrolytes, where they are readily absorbed by the small intestine. Sodium is actively transported, linked to an exchange with H^+ in the jejunum and ileum and with Cl^- and HCO_3^- in the ileum. Na^+ transport is enhanced by glucose absorption in the jejunum (via the glucose-Na^+ carrier on the microvillus membrane) and by water. Some Na^+ also moves down a gradient across the mucosa, i.e., by passive diffusion. Changes in the concentration of sodium in the lumen depend on relative rates of exchange of both sodium and water with blood and lumen. Potassium passively diffuses from the lumen of the proximal small intestine and into the lumen in the distal small intestine.

Simultaneous absorption of Na^+ is required for absorption of glucose, amino acids, and certain vitamins. The Na^+ that enters the cell as a co-transporter is ejected on the serosal side of the cell in exchange for potassium by the Na^+, K^+ ATPase. In general the Na^+, K^+ ATPase enzyme maintains the gradients between Na^+ and K^+ in the intracellular and extracellular compartments. As already noted, Na^+ is high in plasma and low inside cells, whereas K^+ is high inside cells and low in plasma, as shown in Figure 60.4.[r5] The pH of the blood is maintained at 7.4 by virtue of the HCO_3^- ion present in plasma. The pH of the intracellular compartment is about pH 6.9, and that is buffered by the protein and organic phosphates (metabolic intermediates) present in cells.

The homeostasis of sodium, potassium, and chloride is accomplished by the renin-angiotensin-aldosterone system shown in Figures 60.5 and 60.6. Renin is an enzyme (MW=40,000) secreted by the juxtaglomerular cells of the kidney in response to decreases in blood pressure, plasma volume, or plasma sodium. Angiotensin II is an octapeptide that is a potent vasoconstrictor and trophic hormone for the glomerulosa of the adrenal cortex, which secretes aldosterone, a potent mineralocorticoid that promotes the reabsorption of sodium and excretion of potassium by the kidney. The structures of aldosterone (in two forms) together with the synthetic steroid deoxycorticosterone, which has less potent sodium-retaining properties than aldosterone, are shown in Figure 60.6. Angiotensinogen is a prohormone globulin synthesized by the liver. The interaction of these various factors in promoting sodium and potassium homeostasis is shown in Figure 60.7.

Low-sodium diets lead to constriction of the extracellular space. In fact, 7.2 ml of extracellular water are excreted for each milliosmole of sodium lost. This, in turn, turns on the renin-angiotensin-aldosterone system to enhance sodium retention, not only in the kidney but also in the sweat glands. The lower the sodium intake, the higher the plasma aldosterone level. On the other hand, the higher the potassium intake, the lower the aldosterone level.

The primary role of sodium chloride is its contribution to osmolarity of extracellular fluid. It also contributes to acid-base balance, membrane potential of cells, and to the active transport of many metabolites across cell membranes. Potassium is the principal intracellular cation required by some enzymes for optimal activity; it contributes to nerve impulse transmission and to muscle contractility.

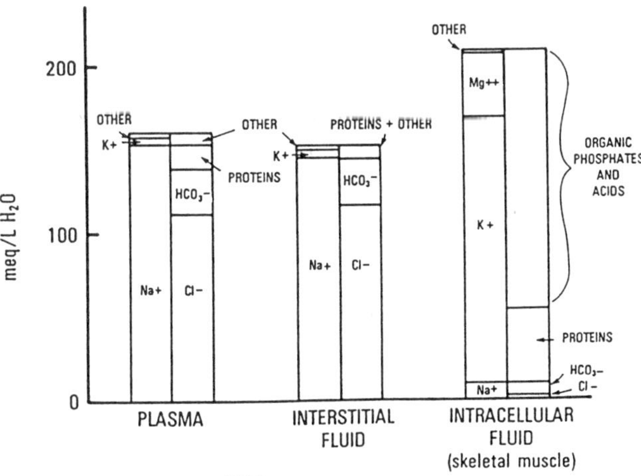

Figure 60.4 Electrolyte Composition of the Major Body Fluids

Nutritional Requirements

The average intake of sodium chloride in the US is about 11 grams per day (190 mEq/d) (range 4–24 gm). For every gram of sodium chloride, 39 percent is sodium. Of this total, about 7 grams of salt is nondiscretionary, added to food to improve taste and enhance preservation of processed foods. The remaining 4 grams from the salt shaker is discretionary.

Potassium is widely distributed in all foods, particularly foods from plants. The average intake in the US ranges from 4 to 8 grams/day, which averages about 6 grams (234 mEq)/day. Healthy persons can maintain sodium balance on 230 mg (10 mEq) per day and potassium balance on 1560 mg (40 mEq) per day. The 1989 US RDA recommended 500 mg (22 mEq) of sodium and 2000 mg (51 mEq) of potassium as "minimum" allowances for adults.[r9]

It is clear that average intakes of sodium in the Western world greatly exceed minimum requirements. In view of the relationship between sodium intake and hypertension in *susceptible* persons, it might be wise for populations to approximate more closely their minimum need for salt.

Deficiency Diseases

Sodium

Most of the symptoms and signs of sodium deficiency are the result of depletion of extracellular sodium stores with contraction of the plasma volume and circulatory collapse. This has been well documented in patients with aldosterone deficiency plus sodium lack, but also occurs in unadapted persons exposed to high temperatures who develop heat stroke and sodium deficiency from loss of salt in sweat. Also at risk are patients with pyloric obstruction, diarrhea, and salt-losing nephritis. The syndrome of sodium deficiency includes dehydration, soft eyeballs, tachycardia, hypotension (to the level of shock), hemoconcentration, azotemia, and circulatory failure.

Potassium

Potassium deficiency in the presence of a usual sodium intake results in a reduction of potassium content of cells, which is replaced by sodium and hydrogen ions. The change in K/Na ratio and intracellular pH causes muscle weakness, ileus and/or diarrhea,

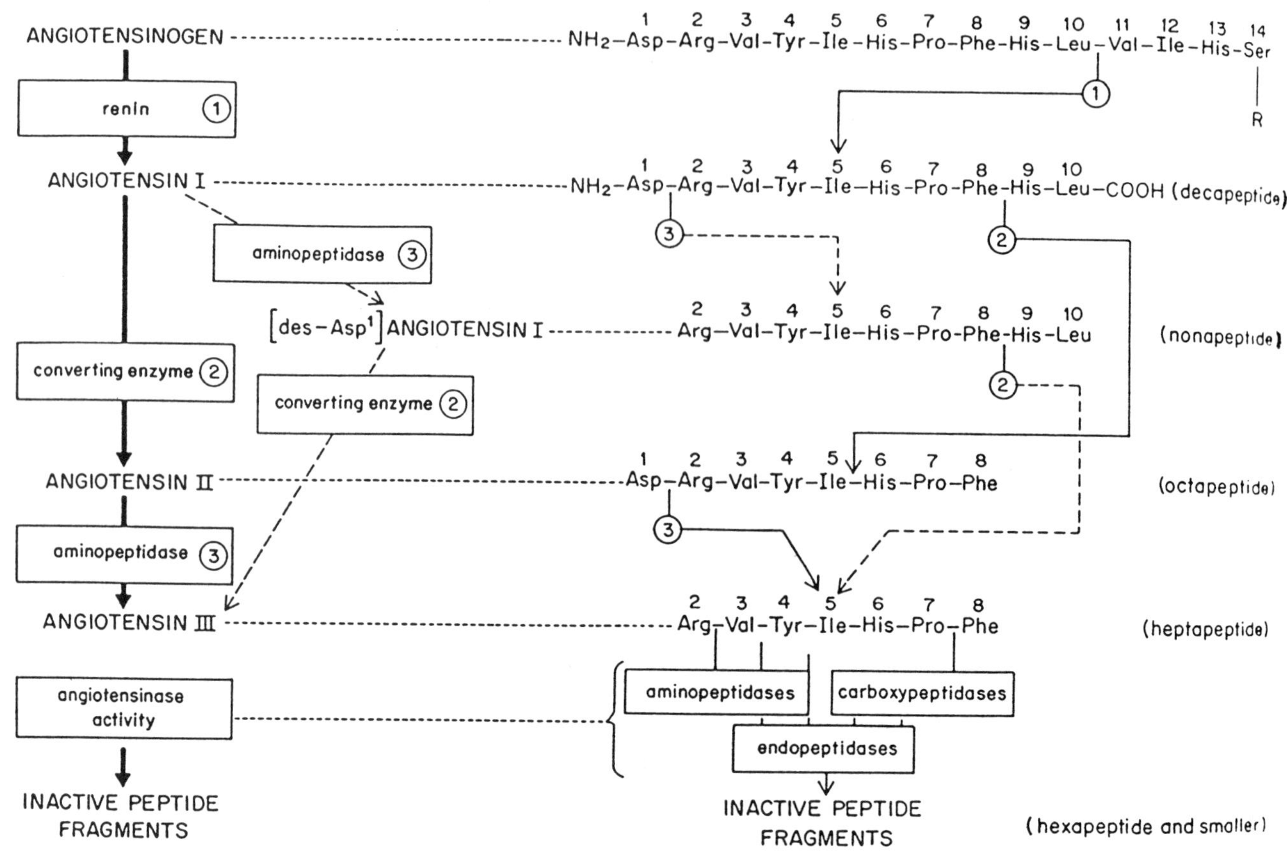

Figure 60.5 Formation and Destruction of Angiotensins[17]

Deoxycorticosterone

Aldosterone

Aldosterone (hemiacetal structure)

Figure 60.6 Salt-Retaining Steroids

loss of ability to concentrate urine, abnormal electrocardiogram, and hypokalemic alkalosis.

Chloride

Another cause of hypochloremic, hypokalemic alkalosis is chloride deficiency. In 1979, Roy and Arant[2] reported that three infants five to six months of age, who had been given the soy-protein based formula, Neo-Mull-Soy, had failed to thrive and had been found on admission to the hospital to have severe hyponatremic, hypochloremic, hypokalemic metabolic alkalosis with increased plasma renin activity. Bartter first observed this syndrome in three patients with growth failure and hypokalemia due to a defect in chloride reabsorption in the ascending limb of Henle's loop in the kidney.[3] Earlier, in 1965, Kassirer et al.[4] demonstrated in humans on low-chloride intakes given acidifying agents like sodium nitrate, that a hypokalemic hypochloremic alkalosis developed (as a defense

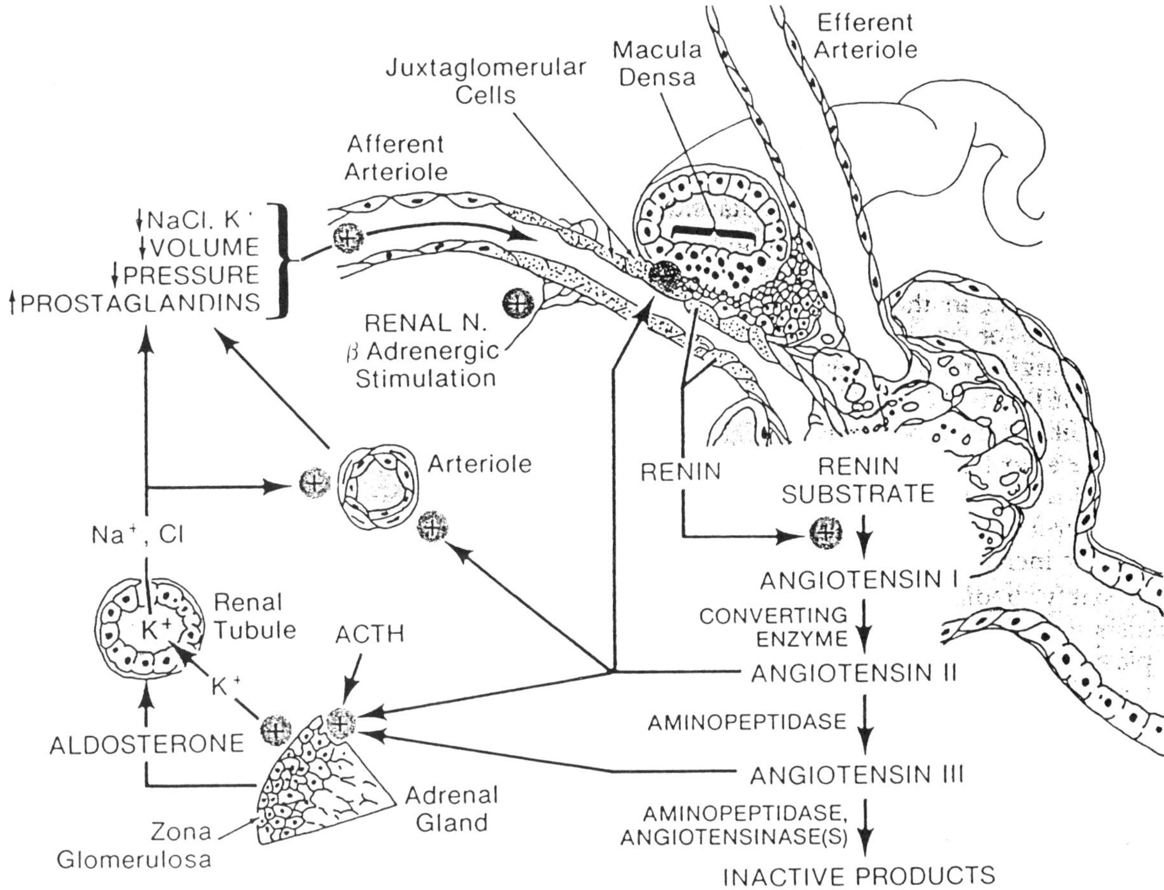

Figure 60.7 The Integrated Activities of the Renin-Angiotensin-Aldosterone System[r8]

against the treatment) that could not be corrected by the administration of potassium but only by restoring chloride. Further, they showed that the elevation of the renal threshold for biocarbonate is due to the unavailability of chloride and the heightened sodium-hydrogen ion exchange. Chloride ion, therefore, apart from sodium is an essential nutrient for humans.

Therapeutic Uses

Sodium, potassium, and chloride are given at high doses to correct their respective deficiency diseases whether for dietary lack or renal insufficiency. In situations of hemorrhagic shock, sodium chloride is infused to restore the blood volume.

Toxicology

Rapid IV infusion of sodium chloride may lead to over-expansion of the vascular volume and the onset of congestive heart failure. Hypertension and edema also may follow overdosage with sodium.

High levels of plasma potassium from rapid infusions or oral loads or concurrent kidney disease will cause paresthesias, muscle weakness, and EKG changes with possible cardiac arrest.

Preparations

Oral preparations of Na^+ and K^+ in mineral supplements are available. Table salt is the most available source of NaCl. Intravenous preparations of sodium and potassium salts are available.

Magnesium

History

Magnesium is the eighth most common element in the earth's crust, making up about 2 percent of its mass. Magnesium was discovered by Sir Humphry Davy in 1807 by electrolysis of fused magnesium chloride. This element is widely distributed, principally in silicate minerals such as asbestos ($CaMgSi_4O_{12}$), but also as magnesite ($MgCO_3$) and dolomite ($Mg\ CO_3 \times Ca\ CO_3$). The volcanic ash from Mount Vesuvius was rich in periclase (MgO) and was actually eaten by the Italians as a "health food." Geophagy is still practiced by some Third World populations to compensate for mineral deficiencies in their diet—but also, paradoxically, it may cause them (see section on zinc).

The requirement for magnesium in animals was first studied by McCollum and co-workers in rats and dogs in the 1930s.[5] They observed that neuromuscular and vasomotor signs including flushing of the skin, cardiac arrhythmias, and tonic-clonic seizures were associated with low serum magnesium. In 1954, Flink et al.[6] reported that alcoholics were at risk for magnesium deficiency, and the extent of depression of serum magnesium correlated with the presence of delirium tremens. More recently Shils[10] has documented a syndrome of magnesium deficiency in humans consisting of hypomagnesemia, hypokalemia, and hypocalcemia associated with neurologic abnormalities, personality changes, anorexia, tetany, and convulsions. Magnesium plays a role in energy production as MgATP, as a cofactor for many enzymes, as a bone salt, and as a modulator of endocrine function, particularly of the parathyroid gland. In plants it is the metal coordinated within the porphyrin moiety in chlorophyll that is essential for photosynthesis.

Chemistry

Magnesium is an alkaline earth metal with an atomic weight of 24 and an atomic number of 12. It occupies a position in Group II of the third period in the periodic table. Magnesium has two naturally-occurring isotopes $_{12}Mg^{25}$ (10%) and $_{12}Mg^{26}$ (11%) and seven radioactive isotopes, of which $_{12}Mg^{28}$ with a half-life of 21 hours is the most useful for biologic studies. Mg is a good conductor of heat and electricity and is used extensively as an alloy with aluminum, zinc, and manganese in the aircraft industry. Finely divided Mg burns in air to produce a flash and MgO. Mg reacts with boiling water to produce $Mg(OH)_2$, an alkali. Magnesium sulfate, as the heptahydrate $MgSO_4 \times 7H_2O$ or epsom salt, is a well-known purgative. $MgCO_3$ is a source of hardness in drinking water. Mg forms salts with phosphates, pyrophosphates, and adenosinetriphosphate in biologic systems. It is part of the hydroxyapatite crystal in bone ($Ca_8Mg_2\ (PO_4)_6(OH)_2$).

Physiology

The adult human body contains 20 to 28 grams of magnesium, of which about 64 percent is in bone (where it makes up 0.5% of bone ash), 27 percent in muscle, 7 percent in other cells, and less than 1 percent in extracellular water. In plasma the normal range for Mg is 1.6 to 2.1 mg/dl (0.65–0.88 mmol/L), and in red blood cells the values are 4 to 6.5 mg/dl. In plasma, 55 percent of the Mg is free, 13 percent is complexed with citrate and phosphate, and 32 percent is bound to proteins, mainly albumin.

Magnesium is absorbed both by active transport and by simple diffusion. The gut can also secrete Mg, and net absorption is the algebraic sum of the two processes. In the duodenum, secretion is greater than in the jejunum, ileum, and colon (which has a small capacity for absorbing Mg). Humans given magnesium in the form of a standard meal absorbed 65 to 70 percent of intakes of 40 mg, which decreased to 11 to 14 percent with intakes of 960 mg. At usual intakes of about 300 mg per day, the efficiency of absorption is about 33 percent. This figure is also influenced by such substances as phytate and fatty acids, which can make dietary Mg more insoluble and less well absorbed.

Magnesium homeostasis does not appear to be regulated by hormonal mechanisms but by mechanisms intrinsic to kidney tubules. Plasma magnesium levels are therefore believed to be regulated primarily by the kidney. Approximately 70 percent of plasma magnesium is not bound to protein and is therefore filterable. About 30 percent of filtered magnesium is reabsorbed in the proximal tubule; another 65 percent is reabsorbed in the loop of Henle, the site at which major adjustments in response to plasma concentrations appear to take place. A portion of bone magnesium is in passive equilibrium with that in the plasma and acts as a buffer against fluctuations in extracellular magnesium concentrations. When magnesium in the diet is lowered to 10 mg/day, the kidney adjusts to the lower intake by reducing output to about 0.5 mm (12 mg)/day with only a small initial change in serum Mg.

Magnesium secreted into the gut is efficiently reabsorbed. Only 25 to 50 mg of endogenous magnesium are normally excreted in the feces; on a 300-mg intake, the fecal output will be about 200 mg and the daily urinary output will be equivalent to the absorbed amount, namely 100 mg.

Magnesium is principally an intracellular cation, accounting for 38 mM/L of total magnesium, most of which is complexed with phosphates and organic phosphate metabolites. Only 1 mM is free Mg^{++}. Magnesium plays a critical role in energy storage and utilization. Magnesium ATP is the substrate for phosphatase (ATPases) essential for the regulation of the flow of potential energy from mitochondria and cytoplasm. MgATP plays a role in glycolysis, in the citric acid cycle, in pentose synthesis, in RNA and DNA synthesis, and in the phosphorylation and nucleotide derivatization of vitamins. Magnesium ATPases include Mg(NaK) ATPase, ($Mg + HCO_3^-$) ATPase, and MgCa ATPase, which are associated with the control of sodium, proton, and calcium pumps. Magnesium also is involved in protein synthesis through its action on nucleic acid polymerization, its role in ribosomal binding to ribonucleic acid (RNA), and in the synthesis and degradation of deoxyribonucleic acid (DNA). In addition to its role in phosphorylation of glucose, magnesium may also control mitochondrial oxidative metabolism. Protein kinases that phosphorylate proteins in signalling cellular events require MgATP. Adenylate cyclase, critical in the generation of intracellular secondary messenger cyclic AMP, has also been shown to be dependent on magnesium. More recently, intracellular magnesium has been shown to have an important regulatory function on both K^+ and Ca^{2+} membrane channels. Magnesium is essential for activation of the K^+ channel by ACh and GTP.

Bone magnesium but not soft tissue magnesium varies with magnesium intake from 116 to 390 mmoles/kilogram (2.8 to 9.4 gm/kg) of bone ash, the average being about 5 grams/kg bone ash. Mg also is required for the physiologic response of the parathyroid gland to hypocalcemia and the release of Ca^{++} from the bones in response to the vitamin D hormone (calcitriol).

Nutritional Requirements

Magnesium is widely distributed in natural foods, and levels are particularly high in nuts, legumes, and unmilled grains. Green leafy vegetables are another good source because of Mg complexed with chlorophyll. Dairy products, grains, vegetables, and animal foods each supply about 15 percent of the daily intake of Americans, for a total of 60 percent, the remainder being distributed among other components of the diet. Estimates of average national intakes for 1949 to 1982 have ranged from 368 to 326 mg/day. In 1985, mean Mg intakes for males was 329 mg; for adult women and children 1 to 5 years of age, 207 mg and 193 mg, respectively.

Magnesium balance can be obtained in healthy males on intakes of 210 to 320 mg/day. The RDA for adults set by the Food and Nutrition Board (NRC/NAS) in 1989 was 4.5 mg/kg or 350 mg/day for men and 280 mg/day for women. The RDA for pregnant women was set at 320 mg/day; for lactating women, 340 to 355 mg/day. The recommendation for infants up to one year is 40 to 60 mg/day; for children 1 to 5, 80 to 120 mg/day.

Deficiency Disease

Mg deficiency can occur in individuals with malabsorption, intestinal fistulae, alcoholism, renal dysfunction with failure to reabsorb cations, or iatrogenic overzealous nasogastric or intestinal suctioning. All the signs and symptoms of Mg deficiency were observed in a classic clinical investigation by Shils,[r10] in which he maintained volunteers on very low intakes of Mg (10 mg per day) for 40 days. Urine and fecal Mg fell to trace levels within seven days. As shown in Figure 60.8, plasma Mg fell from control levels of 2.5 mEq to values of 0.3 mEq after 40 days. Surprisingly, both plasma Ca and K levels also fell to significantly lower values. Hypomagnesemia, hypocalcemia, and hypokalemia were found in all subjects, despite adequate amounts of potassium and calcium in the diet. Plasma sodium levels remained within physiologic limits, accompanied by a positive sodium balance, whereas the subjects were in negative potassium balance.

Trousseau's and Chvostek's signs suggesting impending tetany were present in the 25th day of the study. On day 41, anorexia, nausea, paresthesias, and general muscle spasticity developed. The parenteral administration of PTH was given on day 35 without effect. On day 41, 17 mEq of Mg was given IV, followed by 40 mEq daily for the next month. Following the first IV treatment, the response was dramatic; with restoration of plasma Mg and Ca levels, parathyroid hormone levels were low at the end of 40 days and responded to Mg supplementation. It appears that Mg deficiency inhibits both the release and peripheral activity of PTH. The peripheral resistance to PTH may actually be resistance to calcitriol, which under normal conditions mobilizes bone Ca^{++} for secretion into plasma. 1,25-$(OH)_2D_3$ levels also were depressed during the period of Mg restriction, so these conclusions seem reasonable.

Therapeutic Uses

The therapeutic use of Mg is principally to treat Mg^{++} deficiency in the various clinical situations al-

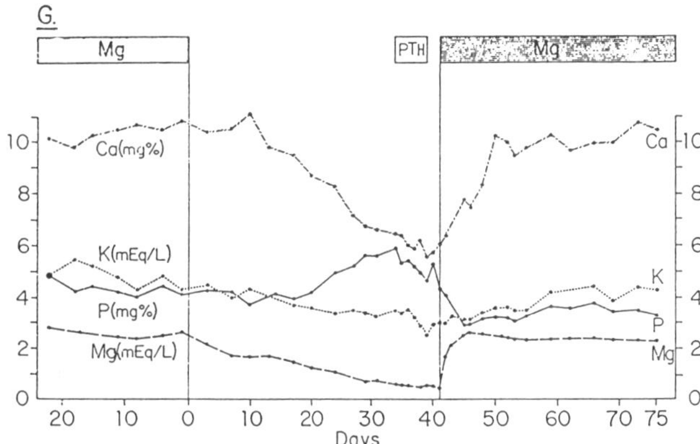

Figure 60.8 Blood chemistries in subject on experimental magnesium (Mg) depletion. Mg was omitted after the patient was one month on the control diet. The rise in serum inorganic phosphate (P) with Mg depletion in this patient was unique among the depleted subjects. On depletion day 25, Trousseau's and Chvostek's signs first occurred, and the former became progressively stronger as plasma calcium (Ca), Mg, and potassium (K) continued to decline. On depletion day 35, parathyroid hormone (PTH) was given IM at 50 units t.i.d. for 5 days; this had no effect on plasma Ca but appeared to decrease P. On day 41, anorexia, nausea, paresthesias, and generalized muscle spasticity developed; 17 mEq of Mg IV was then given with rapid improvement. This was followed by similar amounts of Mg IM 12 and 15 hours later. Dietary Mg (40 mEq daily) was resumed on the third repletion day.[r10]

ready discussed. In addition, Mg salts are used in leavening breads and are used as antacids and purgatives. Healthy persons can tolerate 4 to 6 grams of Mg per day, with the total amount being excreted by the kidney.

Toxicology

Because the kidney controls Mg homeostasis, persons with kidney failure are at risk for hypermagnesemia. Mg concentrations in the plasma of patients with renal disease frequently rise above the normal range of 1.6 to 2.4 mEq/L. Even women with toxemias of pregnancy with transient renal failure may develop hypermagnesemia if treated with Maalox ($Mg(OH)_2$) or Mg salts. Uncommon causes of high plasma Mg are hypothyroidism, hyperparathyroidism, milk-alkali syndrome, and acute diabetic ketoacidosis.

The toxic effects of hypermagnesemia shown in Figure 60.9 are a function of increasing plasma concentrations. The earliest observations are hypotension, nausea, and vomiting at concentrations of 3 to 9 mEq/liter. Because these early symptoms of hypermagnesemia are not dissimilar from those of uremia, the diagnosis may easily be overlooked. Urinary retention due to failure of micturition reflexes is also observed at these levels. Bradycardia also may be observed at this concentration, as may cutaneous vasodilation. Electrocardiographic changes, hypoflexia, and secondary CNS depression are the next major manifestations at 5 to 10 mEq/liter. Respiratory depression and coma are observed above 9 to 10 mEq/liter; asystolic arrest may occur above 14 to 15 mEq/liter. These effects are not dissimilar to the effects of hyperkalemia. Transient reversal of these toxic events can be effected with IV calcium, but dialysis is the treatment of choice.

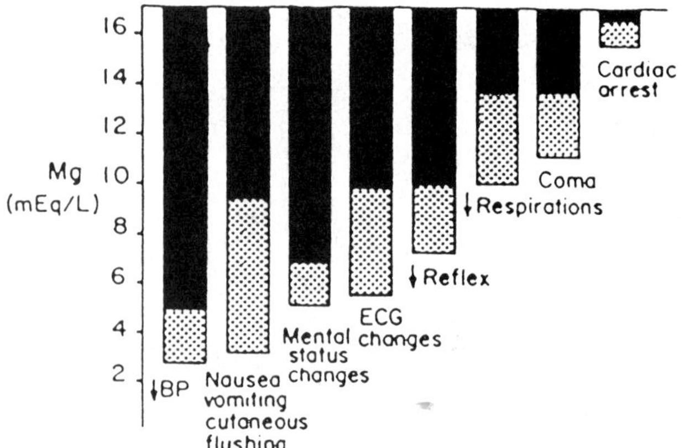

Figure 60.9 Relationship of signs and symptoms of magnesium intoxication to serum magnesium levels. The bottom line of each bar is the minimum concentration of Mg at which a specified symptom will occur. The stippled areas represent levels of inconstant symptomatology, and the solid portion of each bar represents the range of Mg levels at which the specified symptom is usually present.[r10]

Preparations

One-a-day type vitamin/mineral supplements contain about 100 mg of Mg, but Mg-based antacids contain much more. Maalox tablets contain 200 mg of Mg(OH) per tablet, with accompanying instructions to users to take two to four tablets four times a day. The Maalox liquid contains 450 mg (Mg(OH)) per 5 ml. Other antacids are comparable; for example, Philip Milk of Magnesia contains 405 mg $Mg(OH)_2$ per 5 ml. Intravenous solutions of Mg are also available.

Calcium and Phosphate

History

Calcium and phosphate are considered together in this chapter because of their chemical relationship to each other, to the bony skeleton, and to a common endocrine system that regulates the concentration of their ions in the body. They are also unusual macronutrients in the sense that not only is $Ca_3(PO_4)_2$ the principal structure element of bone, but both elements play functional roles as micronutrients in all living forms.

The adult human body contains about 1200 gm of calcium (1.7%) and about 750 gm of phosphate (1.0%). Ninety-nine per cent of the calcium and 80 percent of the phosphorus are in the skeleton. Powerful hormonal mechanisms exist to achieve calcium and phosphate homeostasis in the body and to maintain constant extracellular concentrations of these ions.

The essentiality of calcium for life was recognized in the 17th century, when rickets was first described. Ringer discovered that Ca^{++} was essential for the heartbeat in 1883. The importance of the parathyroid glands in controlling serum Ca^{++} levels was recognized in the late 19th century. Vitamin D was discovered by Mellanby in 1920, and the value of ultraviolet irradiation in forming vitamin D was discovered by Steenbock four years later. Calcitonin was discovered by Copp in 1961, and the mode of action of calcitriol was established only within the last decade.[r13]

Much progress has been made in the past few decades in both understanding the mechanisms of calcium and phosphorus homeostasis and the pathophysiology of metabolic bone disease. Adenosine triphosphate (ATP) has an established role in energy transduction and the cyclic nucleotides (cAMP and cGMP) have been shown to serve as second messengers in a variety of endocrine responses. Finally, variations in intracellular Ca serve as second messengers for muscular contraction and, via inositol phosphates, the induction of a variety of growth factors.

Chemistry

Calcium is an alkaline earth element in Group II in the fourth period of the periodic table. It has an atomic number of 20 and an atomic weight of 40. Calcium has five natural isotopes amounting to a total of only 3 percent of abundance, the most important one being ${}_{20}Ca^{44}$ (2.09%), and 10 radioactive isotopes, of which the most important is the beta-emitter ${}_{20}Ca^{45}$ (half-life = 164 days).

Calcium is the fourth most prevalent element in the earth's crust, making up 3.6 percent of its mass. The most important compound of calcium is calcium carbonate ($CaCO_3$). This substance occurs in the beautiful birefringent crystals of calcite. Marble is a microcrystalline form of $CaCO_3$. This salt also occurs in pearls, coral, seashells, and vertebrate bones. Other calcium salts of importance are the silicates, fluorides, sulfates, and phosphate. $CaSO_4$ occurs in nature as the mineral gypsum, $CaSO_4 \cdot 2H_2O$, the main component of wall-board. Calcium phosphate $Ca_3(PO_4)_2$, the main salt in bone, also occurs in large deposits of phosphate rock. Phosphate-like calcium is also a major element on the earth's crust.

Calcium is a silvery white metal that is fairly hard. It reacts with water to liberate H_2 and to yield alkaline $Ca(OH)_2$. Ca burns in air to form CaO (quicklime), which reacts with water to form slaked lime ($Ca(OH)_2$) Ca reacts with hydrogen to form calcium hydride (CaH_2), which will react with water to form H_2, and as such is a portable source of H_2. $CaCl_2$ is a dehydrating agent because of its great affinity for water.

Phosphorus is a member of Group V in the 4th period of the periodic table. Its atomic number is 15 and its atomic weight is 31. Phosphorus has no naturally-occurring isotopes, but has nine radioactive ones, of which ${}_{15}P^{32}$ is the most useful in biology. It is a ? emitter with a half-life of 14.3 days. Its principal valences are +3 and +5.

The principal chemical form of P is $Ca_3(PO_4)_2$, which is found in earth deposits. At high temperatures, $Ca_3(PO_4)_2$ can be reduced with sand and coke to produce gaseous P_2, which is condensed in water to yield P_4 (red phosphorus). When P_4 is burned in air, phosphorus pentoxide (P_2O_5) is formed, which is the anhydride of phosphoric acid. Phosphoric acid (H_3PO_4) has three protons, which dissociate with Ka_1 of 7.5×10^{-3}, $Ka_2 = 6.2 \times 10^{-8}$ and $Ka_3 = 1 \times 10^{-12}$. Na_3PO_4 is very basic. The only forms of P that are important in cell biology are phosphates and their derivatives.

Pyrophosphate ($H_4P_2O_7$), which is the anhydride of two molecules of orthophosphate, is an important metabolite in the cell. Phosphate esters are important metabolic intermediates in glycolysis, the hexomonophosphate shunt, and in phosphorylated proteins of biologic importance. Adenosine triphosphate (ATP) is composed of one ester phosphate (with ribose) and an anhydride bond to form a terminal pyrophosphate linkage. On hydrolysis of the anhydride bond, about 12 kcal/mole are released, which is the energy that drives most chemical reactions in the cell. The monomers in the synthesis of ribonucleic acid (RNA) and deoxyribonucleic acid (DNA) are all nucleoside triphosphates that condense to form their respective polymers.

Physiology

There are two routes of calcium absorption in the intestine. One is an active saturable, transcellular process that occurs mainly in the duodenum and jejunum and to a lesser extent in the ileum. It is regulated by vitamin D-hormone, which stimulates the synthesis of a calcium-binding protein, calbindin, and also promotes changes in the brush border of the enterocyte to promote calcium absorption. Calbindin aids Ca absorption by ferrying Ca across the enterocyte to the basolateral membrane, where a Ca-activated ATPase pumps Ca out of the cell into the circulation. Intracellular free Ca concentrations are very low, of the order of 0.1 μM, which is 10,000 times lower than the free Ca concentration of plasma (Table 60.2). The second is a minor pathway operating by simple diffusion. The overall efficiency of Ca absorption is low, of the order of 15 to 20 percent. This low efficiency is not only due to competing ions and inhibitors of Ca absorption in the diet, but also because of endocrine control of Ca absorption, which is responsive to the state of body stores of Ca.

Phosphate is absorbed mainly by an active, saturable Na-dependent mechanism and is much more efficient than Ca absorption. In addition, a minor nonsaturable diffusion pathway exists. Calcitriol increases phosphate absorption as well as calcium absorption. It has been suggested that a ratio of Ca to P in the diet of 1.2 makes for optimal calcium absorption.

Ca and P are present in blood plasma in various forms. The total concentration of calcium in plasma is 2.5 mmole/L (10 mg/dl). One-half of this is free; the other half is bound to protein and other complexing anions. Most of the phosphate in plasma is phospholipid P (8 mg/dl), which is bound in covalent linkage to the lipid; another 0.5 mg/dl is bound to protein. The remaining 3.5 mg/dl (1.1 mmole/L) is inorganic P, of which about half is complexed with Ca^{++} and Mg^{++} and half ionized in the form of $H_2PO_4^-$ and HPO_4^{2-} in the ratio required to give pH 7.4. Most laboratories report total Ca in plasma but only the acid soluble phosphate as P. The constancy of Ca and P levels in plasma is essential for normal neuromuscular excitability and metabolic exchange with both soft tissues and bones.

The control of Ca and P levels in plasma and indirectly those in the tissues is due to the activity of three hormones. These are: 1. parathyroid hormone (PTH) secreted by the chief cells of the parathyroid gland; 2.

Table 60.2 Distribution of Calcium and Phosphorus in the Body and a Summary of their Intake and Absorption

Calcium	Grams	Concentration
Body pool (70 kg)	1,210	
Bones (6 kg)	1,200	5.0 M.
Extracellular	1	2.5 mM.
Intracellular	9	0.1 uM. (free)
Daily intake	1.0	
Absorption	0.15	
Urinary excretion	0.15	
Phosphorus	**Grams**	**Concentration**
Body pool	750	
Bones (6 kg)	600	2.7 M
Extracellular	1	1.1 mM.
Intracellular	150	200.0 mM.
Daily intake	1.0	
Absorption	0.7	
Urinary excretion	0.7	

calcitriol (1,25-$(OH)_2D_3$) secreted by the kidney; and 3. calcitonin secreted by the C-cells of the thyroid gland. They and their functions are described in Table 60.3 (see also Chaps. 42 and 59).

The over-all flux of calcium and phosphate per day in a healthy young adult in mineral balance is shown in Figures 60.10 (for calcium) and 60.11 (for phosphorus). The intake of both Ca and P is set at 1.0 gram, which is within the usual limits.[r13]

In the case of Ca, absorption is 36 percent, but enterohepatic circulation returns 19 percent to the lumen of the GI tract and 0.83 grams appears in the stool. The net absorption of calcium of 17 percent is matched by the urinary excretion of 17 percent of the dietary intake, which again is within normal limits. About 10 grams of Ca pass through the glomeruli of the kidneys each day; all but 170 mg is reabsorbed. It is estimated that about one-half gram of Ca exchanges with the skeleton each day and that a minimum of 2 grams of Ca/day exchange with the lean body mass mediated by Ca transporters. PTH inhibits Ca excretion and promotes Ca mobilization from bones. PTH also stimulates the synthesis of calcitriol in the kidney, which stimulates Ca absorption by the gut and is cooperative with PTH in mobilizing Ca from bones.

As regards P, the enterocyte absorption is Na-dependent, and is more complete, reaching 90 percent in the upper GI tract. Twenty per cent of the intake, however, is resecreted into the gut through the bile and pancreatic secretions, leaving a net absorption of 70 percent. Calcitriol increases both Ca and phosphate absorption. This net absorption is matched by urinary excretion. The kidney is the crucial organ for P homeostasis. Its reabsorption of P is regulated by PTH, which promotes renal excretion of P, and calcitriol, which promotes retention of P. The intracellular P is about 150 grams, which includes phospholipids, organic

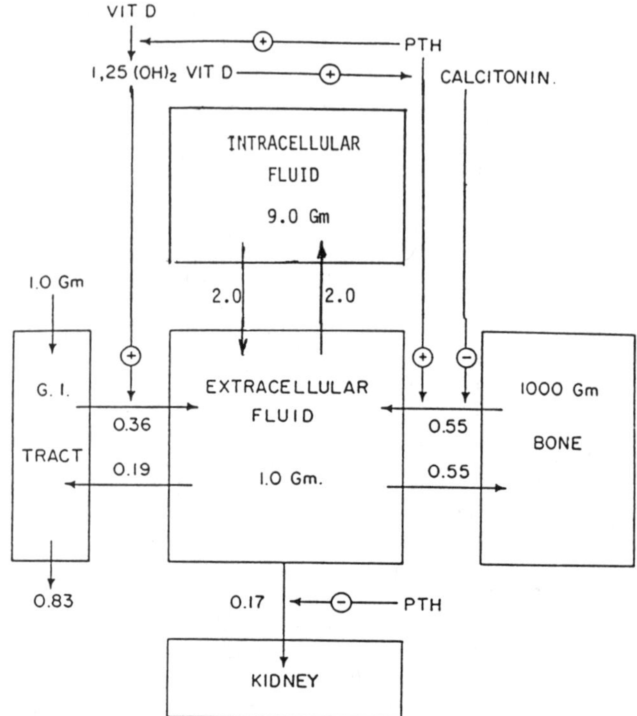

Figure 60.10 Hormonal control of calcium homeostatis. Not shown are complex effects of PTH on bone formation, which is discussed in text. (Numbers [grams] modified from Auerbach GD, Marx SJ, Spiegel AM, in Wilson JD, Foster DW [eds]: *Williams Textbook of Endocrinology*, ed. 7. Philadelphia, WB Saunders Co, 1985.).[r19]

phosphate esters, and inorganic P. The exchange between extracellular phosphate and intracellular phosphate has not been accurately quantitated, but there are a variety of P-transporters that affect entry and exit of P from the extracellular fluid.

The intracellular flux of Ca is illustrated in Figure

Table 60.3 Substances that Affect Calcium Metabolism

Substance	Source	Chemical Nature	Site of Action	Effect
Vitamin D	Diet	Steroid	Intestinal Mucosa, kidney, bones (increases absorption Ca and mobilization from bone)	Increases Ca^{2+} binding protein facilitating absorption of Ca^{2+} & retention of Ca^{++} in kidney.
Calcitonin	Thyroid	Polypeptide MW = 3700 (33 amino acids)	Bone (increases deposition of calcium salts)	Decreases serum Ca^{2+}, Mg^{2+}, urinary hydroxyproline, and PO_4^{3-}
Parathyroid hormone	Parathyroid	Polypeptide (84 amino acids) MW=9500	Bone (activates osteoclastic cells, causing resorption of bone) Kidney (increases reabsorption of Ca^{2+})	Increases serum Ca^{2+} and urinary PO_4^{3-}

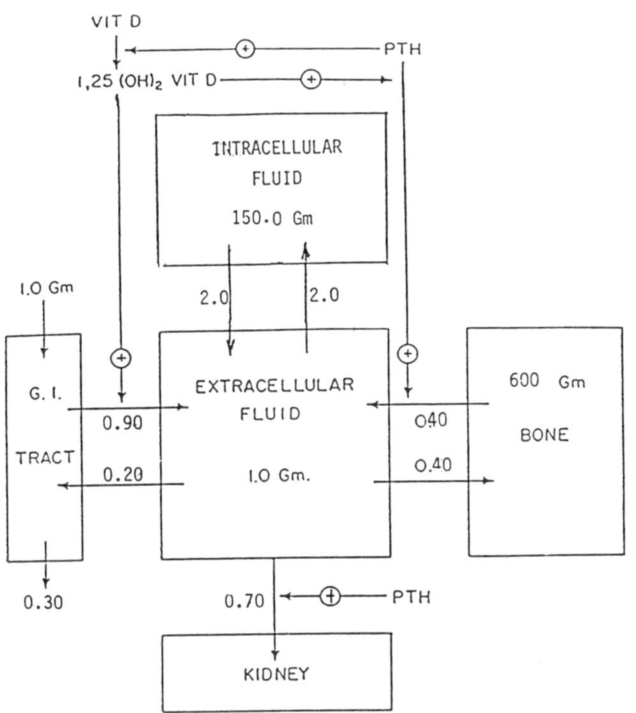

Figure 60.11 Hormonal control of phosphorus homeostasis. Not shown are complex effects of PTH on bone formation, which is discussed in text. (Numbers [grams] are from Auerbach GD, Marx SJ, Spiegel AM, in Wilson JD, Foster DW [eds]: *Williams Textbook of Endocrinology*, ed. 7. Philadelphia, WB Saunders Co., 1985.)[r19]

60.12. Although intracellular free Ca is of the order of 0.1 μM, total cellular Ca is 1 to 4 mM. This difference is represented by Ca storage in intracellular Ca-binding proteins like calmodulin and troponin and organelles like mitochondria and endoplasmic reticulum. Entry of calcium from the extracellular space to cells is achieved by the Ca^{2+} channel. Two additional systems, shown in Figure 60.12 export Ca^{++} from the intracellular to the extracellular space. These are the Na^+/Ca^{2+} exchange and the Ca^{2+}/ATPase. Both pump Ca^{++} out the cell against a concentration gradient of 10.[4,r14] Borle[r15] concluded from the kinetic study of a variety of animal tissues with Ca^{45} that the Ca^{++} flux in and out of cells averaged about 100 pmol/mg protein/minute; if extrapolated to a 70-kg man, this would suggest a flux in excess of 10 grams Ca/day. In other words the isotopically exchangeable Ca^{++} in humans (which is about 10 gm) represents the daily exchange of most of the intracellular pool with the extracellular pool, and a small fraction (2 gm) of the skeletal pool.

The mobilization of Ca from intracellular stores like the endoplasmic reticulum (ER) is important in muscular contraction and for the induction of growth factors. In the case of muscle, the action potential activates Ca release from the ER, which combines with troponin (MW = 45,000) to relieve its inhibition of the actomyosin ATP-ase and produce a contraction.

In noncontractile tissues like lymphocytes, fibroblasts, kidney, pancreas, and liver cells, phosphatidylinositol phosphate in the membrane, when acted on by phospholipase C, liberates inositol triphosphate (Ins P_3) and diacylglycerol. $InsP_3$ then becomes a second messenger for the liberation of calcium from the ER. The diacylglycerol + Ca^{++} then act on protein kinase C, which phosphorylates other proteins, leading to growth factor induction and, in some cases, cell proliferation. Phosphorylation-dephosphorylation as a device for activating and deactivating proteins and enzymes, together with the Ca as an initiator of the process, is another example of the overlapping functions of Ca and P in biology.

A final example of the importance of phosphorylation is the mode of action of insulin in achieving its

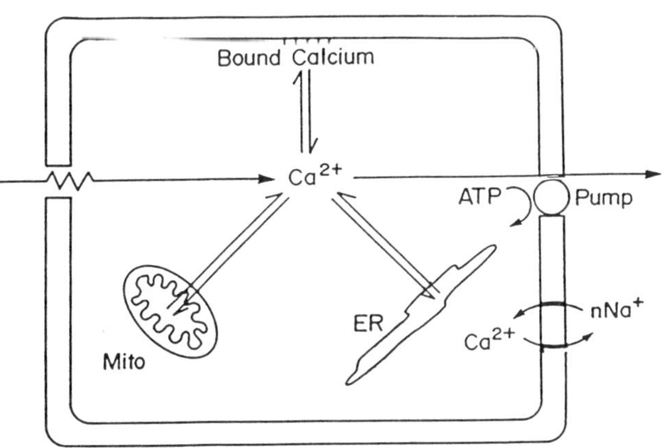

Figure 60.12 The Distribution of Intracellular Calcium[r14]

Table 60.4 Regulations of Ca^{++}Flux

Hormone	ACTION			
	Gut Ca++, P In	Kidney Ca++, P Out	Bone Ca++, P Out	Blood Ca++, P Conc.
PTH	↑* ↑*	↓ ↑	↑* ↑*	↑ ↓
Calcitonin	⇀ ⇀	⇀ ⇀	↓ ↓	↓ ↓
Vitamin D	↑ ↑	↓* ↓*	↑ ↑	↑ ↑

*Vit. D-dependent
**PTH-dependent

biologic effects. Insulin, a small two-chain peptide (MW = 5700) can bind to a membrane receptor that is a much larger heterotetramer consisting of two extracellular α-chains (MW = 135,000) linked by disulfide bonds to two intracellular β chains (MW = 95,000). When insulin reacts with the receptor it converts the receptor to an active enzyme capable of phosphorylating tyrosine residues, not only in its β chains, but also in tyrosines in intracellular proteins, which become the second messengers for insulin action. These actions include the transportation of glucose receptors from an intracellular site to the membrane and the induction of a variety of enzymes, which include glucokinase, malic enzyme, pyruvate kinase, and fatty acid synthetase.

The incorporation of Ca into bones and its release from bones is a cellular event under the control of osteoblasts and osteoclasts[9] (see Fig. 60.13) These bone cells, which make up only 2 percent of the weight of bone, appear to be interconvertible under the influence of the peptide hormones that regulate calcium metabolism. Osteoblasts are relatively small cells with an active reticulum that synthesizes collagen, alkaline phosphatase, and apparently excretes glucose-6-phosphate. Glucose-6-phosphate is a substrate for alkaline phosphatase, which produces locally high phosphate concentrations at initiation foci in bone matrix, providing for the local deposition of calcium phosphate and calcium carbonate. The bone salts are apatites, which can vary in composition from $3Ca_3(PO_4)_2$. $Ca(OH)_2$. (Often written $Ca_{10}PO_4)_6(OH)_2)$, $3Ca_3(PO_4)_2 \cdot CaCO_3$ and $3Ca_3(PO_4)_2{\cdot}CaF_2$. Osteoclasts are multinucleated giant cells containing many mitochondria and lysosomes with degradative enzymes, which labilize both protein and mineral matrix from bone. Under the stimulus of parathyroid hormone, osteoblasts may be transformed into osteoclasts.

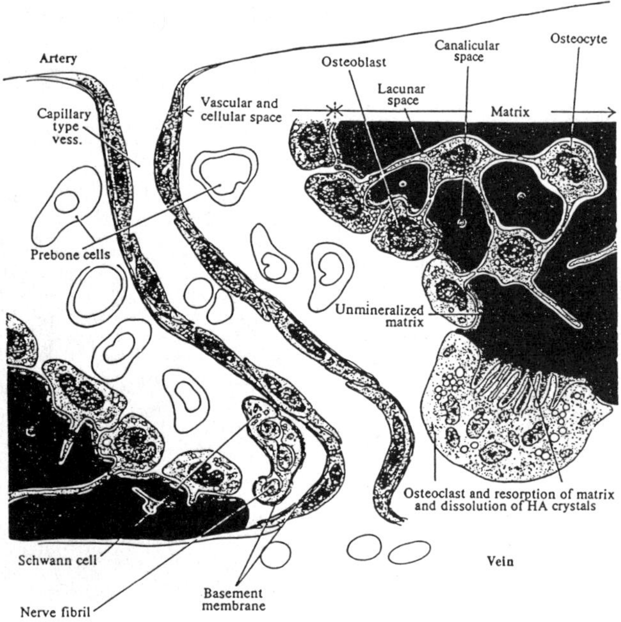

Figure 60.13 Schematic representation of a physioslogical unit of bone tissue showing the osteocytes, osteoblasts, and osteoclasts. (From Doty and Schofield, 1976.)

Calcitriol stimulates osteoblasts to produce more alkaline phosphate and less collagen, which favors bone formation. The inorganic P formed locally in the presence of free calcium in plasma results in the precipitation of $Ca_3(PO_4)_2$ and the other salts in the bone matrix. It is commonly said that the plasma is "saturated" with Ca and P and that the "solubility product" of Ca × P expressed in mg/dl to give a value of 40 is optimal for bone formation. If the product exceeds 40, calcification of soft tissues may occur; if it falls below 20, as in rickets, bone salt formation is difficult. Thus, the process of bone deposition and resorption in the normal individual represents a balance between the activity of osteoblasts, which deposit bone matrix, and osteoclasts, which resorb bone matrix. As indicated in Figure 60.10, this flux of calcium may be as much as 550 mg/day, which is three times the net absorption of Ca from the GI tract in one day. If the Ca intake is inadequate to maintain calcium balance, bone Ca will be mobilized to meet the needs of the soft tissues.

Nutritional Requirements

The nationwide food consumption survey of the USDA in 1977–1978 reported an average intake of Ca for all people of 743 mg/day. Women 35 to 50 years of age ingested only 530 mg/d, whereas adolescent boys took an average of 1179 mg/day. Dairy products accounted for 55 percent of the intake noted; lesser amounts were due to green leafy vegetables and soft fish bones. Bone mass reaches a maximum in the mid-20s, and then declines at variable rates into old age. The rate of loss accelerates in postmenopausal women. High calcium intake increases bone density in adolescents and reduces the rate of loss in middle age. The postmenopausal rate of decline in bone mineral is strongly dependent on estrogen status. High-protein, low-phosphorus intakes promote Ca loss via the kidney, which is prevented by increasing dietary phosphorus. Many Third World populations, furthermore, appear to maintain calcium balance and preserve bone matrix on intakes of 400 to 500 mg/day of dietary calcium.

The US Food and Nutrition Board in 1989 recommended that the RDA for adolescent and young adult men and women be 1200 mg of Ca per day until age

24, to maximize bone density during the growth period, and 800 mg/day Ca for men and women from 25 to 75 years. No increase in allowance was given to postmenopausal women. The recommendation for infants from birth to one year was 400 to 600 mg/day; for children, it was 800 mg/day. Pregnant and lactating women were allowed 1200 mg/day.[r9]

Phosphorus is widely distributed in all foods. The intake of P by US males in 1986 was 1500 mg/day; for females, 1000 mg/day. The main sources of P in the American diet are milk, meat, poultry, and fish. Some soft drinks contain appreciable phosphorus. The 1989 RDA of the Food and Nutrition Board (NRC/NAS) recommended essentially the same intake of P as Ca throughout all age/sex groups.

Deficiency Diseases

Calcium

Osteoporosis is the principal manifestation of calcium deficiency in humans.[r17] This disease has a long latent period and is affected by other contributing factors. The sequence of events arises because of the dual role of calcium in bone and soft tissue metabolism particular that of the neuromuscular system. The regulation of Ca levels in plasma takes priority over retention of calcium in bone. If the intake of calcium is inadequate to compensate for obligatory losses in the urine, stool, milk, or feces, PTH and calcitriol cooperate to mobilize Ca from bones. Since the calcium salts stored in the bone matrix represent 99 percent of body calcium, a long-standing dietary deficiency is necessary to deplete the bones of mineral matrix until the syndrome of osteoporosis occurs with its syndrome of back pain; spinal kyphosis; vertebral fractures; and radiographic evidence of reduction in bone density. The loss of estrogen at menopause contributes to the osteopenia, but is not of itself sufficient to cause the disease. The levels of Ca, P, and alkaline phosphatase in plasma do not change in osteoporosis because it is a normal adaptation to diminished dietary Ca intake.

Osteoporosis differs from rickets and the osteomalacia caused by vitamin D deficiency. In vitamin D deficiency, the hypercalcemic action of vitamin D in promoting intestinal absorption and bone salt deposition and mobilization is absent. In this situation, Ca and P levels fall, and alkaline phosphatase levels increase. Tenany is the result of acute reduction in serum Ca, and may be considered a symptom of a plasma deficit in Ca.

Phosphorus

Dietary phosphate deficiency is extremely rare in children and adults. The exception is a premature infant fed human milk low in phosphorus (150 mg P/L vs 1000 mg P/L in cows' milk). The premature infant is retarded in skeletal development and needs more P/Kcal than does a full-term infant. As a result, overall growth and skeletal growth are impaired, and low-phosphate rickets occurs.

In adults, a low-phosphate diet plus the use of aluminum oxide antacids that bind dietary phosphate are necessary to deplete plasma phosphorus to below 0.3 mol/L (1.0 mg/dl). At this level of hypophosphatemia, symptoms of P deficiency ensue, namely anorexia, weakness, debility, and bone pain. Urinary P is greatly reduced and the excretion of urinary Ca, Mg, and K is increased.[8]

Phosphate deficiency occurs in medical disorders of genetic (X-linked hypophosphatemic rickets, Fanconi syndrome), endocrine (diabetic acidosis), nutritional (long-term total parenteral nutrition), and GI (malabsorption) origin. The syndrome of extreme phosphate deficiency seen in these medical diseases includes tissue abnormalities due to the lack of ATP, anoxia due to depletion of red cell diphosphoglycate, seizures and coma, hemolysis, insulin resistance, ileus, rickets/osteomalacia, glycosuria, and renal tubular acidosis.[r18] Many of these signs and symptoms are the result of an energy deficit in several organs. The rickets/osteomalacia and bone pain occur because the low serum P will not support the usual deposition of Ca by osteoblasts in bones. The treatment in these cases requires replacement of the phosphate deficit.

Therapeutic Uses

Calcium is used in the treatment of deficiency states and as a dietary supplement when intake may be inadequate. Calcium salts are specific in the immediate treatment of low-calcium tetany regardless of etiology.

In severe manifest tetany, the symptoms are best brought under control by IV medication. Five to 20 ml of 10 percent calcium gluconate is injected slowly. For the control of milder symptoms or latent tetany, oral medication suffices. Average doses are calcium gluconate, 15 gm daily in divided doses; calcium lactate, 4 gm, calcium carbonate or calcium phosphate, 1 to 2 gm with meals.

Toxicology

No adverse effects have been observed in healthy persons taking 2500 mg of Ca/day; high intakes in special cases, however, may increase the risk of urinary stores. A high calcium intake also may inhibit the absorption of iron and zinc. Intakes of phosphate greater than two times the Ca intake may lower serum calcium and increase the risk of secondary hyperparathyroidism.

Preparations

In the treatment of hypocalcemia, several preparations are available. Calcium gluconate contains 9 percent calcium. It is available as calcium gluconate tablets, containing 500, 650, or 1000 mg of the salt (equivalent to 2.3, 3.0, or 4.5 mEq Ca^{2+}, respectively). It is nonirritating to the GI tract. For IV injection, calcium gluconate injection is administered as a 10 percent solution (0.45 mEq Ca^{2+}/ml). The IV administration of this salt is the treatment of choice for severe hypocalcemic tetany. The IM route should not be employed in children, as abscess formation at the site of injection may occur.

Calcium lactate contains 13 percent calcium. Its physical properties are similar to those of the gluconate. Tablets (325-mg or 650-mg) are available for oral administration. In the treatment of tetany, absorption apparently is enhanced by simultaneous administration of lactose.

Calcium carbonate is an insoluble, fine, white microcrystalline powder containing 40 percent calcium; it is available in tablets containing 350 mg to 1.5 g. $CaCO_3$ is also used as an antacid.

Phosphate is available in oral capsule in doses of 100 to 250 mg/capsule. Intravenous solutions can be prepared in any pharmacy.

References

Research Reports

1. Behnke AR Jr. Body fat and percent of water. Harvey Lect 1941;*37*:198–204.
2. Roy S, Arant BS. Alkalosis from chloride-deficient Neo-Mull-Soy. N Engl J Med 1979;*301*:615–620.
3. Bartter FC, Pronove P, Gill JR Jr, MacCardle RC. Hyperplasia of the juxtaglomerular complex with hyperaldosteronism and hypokalemic alkalosis. Am J Med 1962;*33*:811–828.
4. Kassirer JP, Berkman PM, Lawrenz DR, Schwartz WB. The critical role of chloride in the correction of hypokalemic alkalosis in man. Am J Med 1965;*38*:172–189.
5. Kruse HD, Orent ER, McCollum EV. Studies on magnesium deficiency in animals' symptomatology resulting from magnesium deprivation. J Biol Chem 1932;*96*:519–536.
6. Flink EB, Stutzman, Anderson, Konig, Fraser. Magnesium deficiency after prolonged parenteral fluid administration and after chronic alcoholism complicated by delirium tremens. J Lab Chem Med 1954;*43*:169–175.
7. Randall RE, Cohen D, Spray CC, Rossmeisel EC. Hypermagnesmia in renal failure. Ann Int Med 1964;*61*:73–88.
8. Lofz M, Zisman E, Bartter FC. Phosphorus deficiency in man. N Engl J Med 1968;*278*:409–415.
9. Doty SD, Schofield BH. Enzyme histochemistry of bone and cartilage cells. Progr Histochem Cytochem 1976;*8*:1–38.

Reviews

r1. McCollum EV, Orent-Keiles Day. The Newer Knowledge of Nutrition, 5th ed., New York: MacMillan, 1939.

r2. Janssen HF. Water. In: Brown M. Present Knowledge of Nutrition, 6th ed. Washington: ILSI-NF, 1990.

r3. Weitzman R, Kleeman CR. Water metabolism and neurohypophyseal hormones. In Maxwell MH, Kleeman CR: Clinical Disorders of Fluid and Electrolyte Metabolism. New York: McGraw-Hill, 1980.

r4. Talbot NB, Richie RH, Crawford JD. Metabolic Homeostasis. Cambridge: Harvard University Press, 1959.

r5. Laiken N, Fanestil DD. Physiology of body fluids; Regulation of volume and osmolarity of the body fluids. In West JB, Best and Taylor Physiological Basis of Medical Practice; 11th ed. Baltimore: Williams and Wilkins, 1985.

r6. Smith H. From Fish to Philosophy: The Study of Our Internal Environment. Summit NJ. CIBA Pharmaceutical Products, 1959.

r7. Douglas WW. Polypeptides-angiotensin, plasma kinins and others. In Gilman AG et al. Goodman and Gilman's The Pharmacologic Basis of Therapeutics, 7th ed. New York: MacMillan, 1985.

r8. Baxter JD, Perloff D, Hseuh W, Biglieri EG. The endocrinology of hypertension. In Felig D et al.: Endocrinology and Metabolism, 2d ed New York: McGraw-Hill, 1987.

r9. Recommended Dietary Allowances, Food and Nutrition Board (NRC/NAS), 10th ed. Washington: National Academy Press, 1989.

r10. Shils ME. Magnesium. In: Shils ME, Olson JA, Shike M. Modern Nutrition in Health and Disease, 8th ed. Philadelphia: Lea & Febiger, 1994.

r11. Alfrey AC. Disorders of magnesium metabolism. In: Seldin DW, Giebisch G. The Kidney, Physiology and Pathophysiology, 2d ed. New York: Raven Press, 1992.

r12. Mordes JP, Wacker EC. Excess magnesium. Pharmacol Rev 1978;*29*: 274–300.

r13. Tepperman J, Tepperman HM. Hormone regulation of calcium homeostasis. In: Metabolic and Endocrine Physiology, 5th ed. Chicago: Year Book, 1987.

r14. Carafoli E. Intracellular calcium homeostasis. Ann Rev Biochem 1987;*56*:395–433.

r15. Borle AB. Control, modulation and regulation of cell calcium. Rev Physiol Biochem Pharmacol 1981;*90*:14–153.

r16. Arnaud CD. Mineral and bone homeostasis. In: Wyngaarden JB, Smith LH. Cecil Textbook of Medicine, 18th ed. Philadelphia: WB Saunders, 1988.

r17. Nordin BEC, Morris HA. The calcium deficiency model for osteoporosis. Nutr Rev 1989;*47*:65–72.

r18. Berner YN, Shike M. Consequences of phosphate imbalance. Ann Rev Nutr 1988;*8*:121–148.

r19. Auerback GD, Marx SJ, Spiegel AM. Parathyroid hormone, calcitonin, and the calciferols. In: Wilson JD, Foster DW (eds). Williams Textbook of Endocrinology 7th ed., Philadelphia, WB Saunders, 1985) pp 1137–1217.

CHAPTER 61

Robert E. Olson
Carolyn D. Berdanier

Microminerals

In addition to the macrominerals already described as nutrients needed by humans in gram quantities per day, there is a second group of minerals needed by humans in far smaller amounts. Included in this trace metal group are iron, zinc, copper, selenium, manganese, molybdenum, iodide, and fluoride. These minerals are required in small quantities, (micrograms to milligrams per day) and are listed in Table 61.1. Although recommended daily allowances have been made for only four, the others are listed as required and daily amounts specified as adequate and safe.

Other microminerals have been studied for their requirements and activities in animals, but the need by humans has not been established. These minerals are arsenic, chromium, cobalt, nickel, silicon, and vanadium. All microminerals are toxic at high levels, and some (arsenic, nickel, and chromium) have been implicated in human carcinogenesis. Each of the trace minerals required by humans will be discussed under the headings of: (1) history; (2) chemistry; (3) physiology; (4) nutritional requirements; (5) deficiency disease; (6) therapeutic uses; (7) toxicology; and (8) preparations.

Iron

History

Iron is the fourth most prevalent element on earth, making up about 5 percent of the earth's crust. Neolithic man learned to forge tools from iron, and the Romans used iron potions as tonics. In the 17th century Sydenham was the first to propose that chlorosis (the green pale sickness of adolescent women) is due to iron deficiency anemia, and he showed that iron salts were a specific remedy. In 1713, Lemery and Geoffrey showed that iron is present in blood by chemical analysis of the ash; in 1852, Funke crystallized hemoglobin from blood and showed that it contained iron.[1] Thereafter, microscopic methods were developed for measuring the number of red cells in blood. In 1892, Bunge recognized the vulnerability of infants to iron deficiency because of the low concentration of iron in milk.[r1]

During this past century the structure of the major iron-containing proteins has been elucidated, and iron absorption and utilization have been quantitated. In 1943, Hahn et al.[2] introduced the use of radioactive isotopes of iron, which greatly aided the study of iron metabolism.

Chemistry

Iron is a transition element in the fourth period of the periodic table. Its atomic number is 26; its atomic weight is 55.85. Fe^{56} has 15 isotopes, three natural-occurring and 12 radioactive. The natural ones are ${}_{26}Fe^{54}$ (5.8%), ${}_{26}Fe^{57}$ (2.2%), and ${}_{26}Fe^{58}$ (0.3%). The main radioactive ones are ${}_{26}Fe^{55}$ ($t_{1/2}$ = 2.7 yr), ${}_{26}Fe^{59}$ ($t_{1/2}$ = 44.5 d), and Fe^{60} ($t_{1/2} = 10^5$ yr). ${}_{26}Fe^{55}$ and ${}_{26}Fe^{55}$ and ${}_{26}Fe^{59}$ are the isotopes used most often in iron absorption studies. Iron occurs in two common oxidation stats, Fe^{2+} (ferrous) and Fe^{3+} (ferric). Ferrous salts are stable in acid solution but are oxidized to the ferric state in alkaline solutions exposed to air. The yellow-brown color characteristic of ferric salts is due to the formation of $FeOH^{2+}$ by hydrolysis. In both the Fe^{2+} and Fe^{3+} states, iron tends to form complex ions. Ferric ion combines with thiocyanate ion to form $FeCNS^{2+}$, which has a dark wine color. Both ferric and ferrous ions form complexes with CN^- ions to form an octahedral configuration with six cyanide groups coordinated with the iron in ferrocyanide $Fe(CN)_6^{-4}$ and ferricyanide $Fe(CN)_6^{-3}$. The same type of structure occurs in heme, in which the four pyrrole rings of the porphyrin moiety are coordinated with Fe^{2+} to form heme. Heme occurs in hemoglobin, a tetramer of four peptide subunits ($\alpha_2\beta_2$) (MW = 64,500), in myoglobin (MW = 16,000), and the cytochrome enzymes (MW = ca. 12,000). Each polypeptide unit contains one atom of iron. In addition to heme iron, ferrous and ferric salts occur in the diet, but only heme-iron and the ferrous salts are absorbed by the GI tract.

Table 61.1 Microminerals with Established Nutritional Requirements of Humans, Their Functions and Toxicities

Microminerals	Function	Daily Allowance	Remarks
Copper[2]	Essential cofactor for a variety of enzymes involved in iron use, collagen synthesis, and antioxidants	1.5–3.0 mg	Wilson's disease results from failure to excrete copper; anemia, leukopenia and osteoporosis are the principal signs of copper deficiency; Menkes disease is due to lack of copper transportation
Fluoride[2]	Increases the hardness of bones and teeth, activates adenylate cyclase	1.5–4.0 mg	Fluorosis (mottling of teeth) results from excess intake
Iodine[1]	Essential for thyroid hormone synthesis	120–150 μg	Goiter and cretinism result from inadequate intake
Iron[1]	Essential for hemoglobin synthesis, cytochrome activity, activity lipogenesis and cholesterogenesis	10–15 mg	Anemia is the major sign of inadequate intake; hemochromatosis results from excess intake
Manganese[2]	Cofactor in a wide variety of enzymes; essential for reactions using ATP or UTP	2–5 mg	Widely distributed in foods; deficiency is unlikely
Molybdenum[2]	Activates adenylate cyclase; cofactor for sulfite oxidase and xanthine oxidase	75–250 μg	Widely distributed in foods. Deficiency is unlikely except with total parenteral nutrition
Selenium[1]	Needed for activity of glutathione peroxidase and thyroid hormone deiodinases	50–70 μg	Toxicity is common in regions of the world where the soil is rich in this element
Zinc[1]	Essential to the function of over 70 enzymes; important to activity of DNA and RNA polymerase	10–15 mg	Deficiency may occur with use of diuretics and trauma. Megadose may cause copper deficiency

[1]A Recommended Daily Allowance has been set for this mineral by the Food and Nutrition Board (NAS/NRC).
[2]Estimated safe and adequate daily dietary intake has been set by the Food and Nutrition Board (NAS/NRC).

Physiology

The total iron content of the adult body averages 4.0 g in men and 2.6 g in women.[r1] As shown in Table 61.2, these iron-containing compounds can be considered as essential and storage forms. The first category of essential iron compounds contains hemoglobin, myoglobin, cytochromes, iron-sulfur proteins, and other enzymes. Hemoglobin is the most abundant and most easily sampled of the heme proteins, and accounts for more than 65 percent of body iron. The red cell and the hemoglobin it contains have a lifetime of about 120 days.[3]

Ferritin is the iron storage protein, with a molecular weight of 450,000.[4] It is composed of 24 subunits that form an outer shell within which there is a storage cavity for polynuclear hydrous ferric oxide phosphate. Over 30 percent of the weight of ferritin is iron. It is present in the liver, gut, reticuloendothelial cells, and bone marrow. Hemosiderin is a denatured form of ferritin that constitutes about one-third of the body's iron stores.

Cytochromes, enzymes involved in electron transport, are located principally in the mitochondria. Cytochrome P-450, a specialized cytochrome used to hydroxylate organic compounds, is located in the endoplasmic reticulum. Other enzymes in which iron is not bound to heme include iron sulfur proteins, metalloflavoproteins, and certain glycolytic enzymes.

Transferrin is an α-glycoprotein (MW = 76,000) that binds two atoms of ferric iron per mole and has a half-life of eight days in humans. Iron is transferred from the intestinal mucosa to transferrin, which carries it through the blood to peripheral tissues containing transferrin receptors. Transferrin is synthesized in liver, brain, testes, and other tissues.[5,6] The expression of the transferrin gene is related inversely to the iron supply. Tissue iron compounds, which include the cytochrome enzymes and a variety of other non-heme enzymes, are heterogeneous with respect to life span

Table 61.2 The Content of Iron in Men and Women

Types of Iron	Male 70-kg	Female 60-kg
Essential Iron	3.100 g	2.100 g
Hemoglobin	2.700	1.800
Myoglobin, cytochromes and other enzymes	0.400	0.300
Storage and transport iron	0.900	0.500
Ferritin, Hemosiderin	0.897	0.497
Transferrin	0.003	0.003
Total Iron	4.000	2.600

and dependent, in part, on the subcellular organelle with which they are associated. For example, in rats, mitochondrial cytochrome C has a half-life of about six days, whereas hemoglobin has a life of about 100 days. The metabolism of iron is summarized in Figure 61.1.

Absorption

The regulation of iron absorption takes place at the mucosal cell of the small intestine,[r3] but the mechanism by which iron absorption is regulated remains controversial.[7] If iron stores are low, as is true for most women and children, the intestinal mucosa takes up iron readily. Conversely, the high-iron stores typical of men and postmenopausal women reduce the percentage of iron absorbed, thereby offering some protection against iron overload. In infancy the abundance of lactoferrin, an iron-binding protein in human milk, and the presence of lactoferrin receptors on the surface of the intestinal mucosa may explain why iron is so well absorbed from human milk.[8] The bioavailability of iron—that is, the amount absorbed from food—can vary from 1 to 50 percent.[9,10] The percentage absorbed depends both on the nature of the diet and on regulatory mechanisms in the intestinal mucosa that reflect the body's physiologic need for iron.

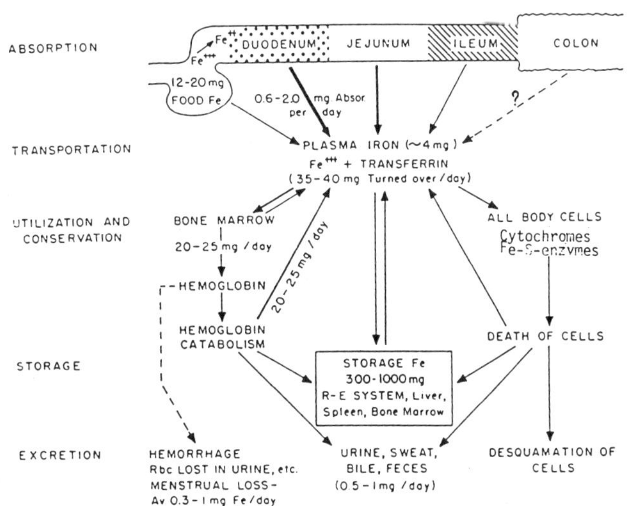

Figure 61.1 Schematic Outline of Iron Metabolism in Adults (Hillman & Finch[r4])

Two types of iron are present in the food—namely, heme iron, which is found principally in animal products, and non-heme iron, which is inorganic iron bound to various proteins in the plant. Most of the iron in the average diet, usually more than 85 percent, is present in the non-heme form. The absorption of the non-heme iron is strongly influenced by its solubility in the upper part of the intestine, depends on the composition if the meal, and is affected by enhancers of absorption such as animal protein and vitamin C. On the other hand, heme iron is absorbed much better (to the extent of 15–30%), is not subject to these enhancers, and normally accounts for a smaller proportion of iron in the diet but plays a quantitatively more important role in delivering iron to the body.

Since the lifetime of a red cell is about 120 days in humans, the flow of iron through the plasma space amounts to about 25 to 30 mg/day in the adult (about 0.5 mg/kg body weight). This amount of iron corresponds to the degradation of about 1 percent of the circulating hemoglobin per day. Iron is conserved in the body in males to a great degree. Only 10 percent is lost *per year* in normal men, or about 1 mg/day. This loss of 1 mg/day is made up by absorption of 1 mg of iron from the diet, which in men without blood loss is only about 10 percent efficient, requiring about 10 mg of dietary iron/day. In menstruating females the loss is increased to 2 mg/day, and the absorption of iron is increased proportionately to prevent the development of iron deficiency. The pathway of iron absorption is shown in Figure 61.2.

In order to be absorbed, iron must be in the ferrous state. Upon entry into the enterocyte, part is incorporated into ferritin in the ferric state, but most is transported via cytoplasmic proteins from the mucosal to the serosal side of the enterocyte in the ferrous state. After the iron is pumped out of the enterocyte it must be oxidized to the ferric state in order to bind to transferrin. This is accomplished by ceruloplasmin (MW = 160,000) a plasma protein that contains eight copper ions in the divalent state. Ceruloplasmin copper is reduced by the iron, resulting in the formation of cuprous ions in ceruloplasmin and ferric iron in transferrin. As mentioned earlier, transferrin is recognized in the periphery by cells with transferrin receptors. The num-

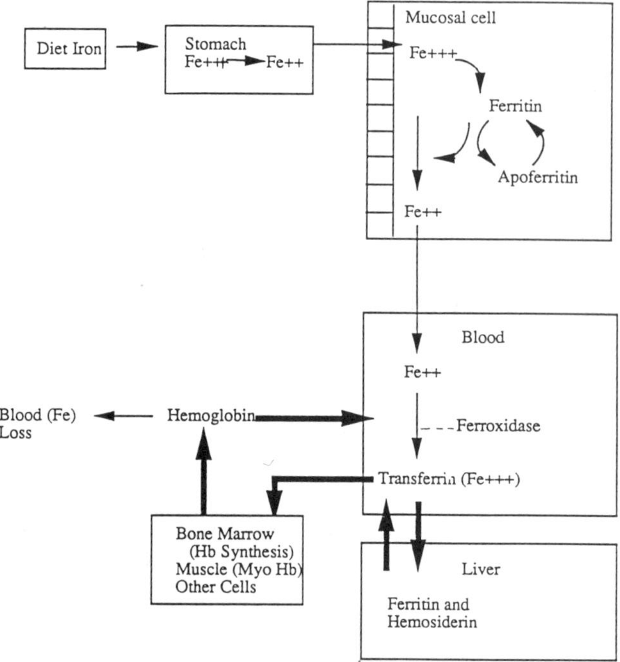

Figure 61.2 Overview of iron uptake and use showing the apparent closed system that indicates the recycling and conservation of iron once absorbed from the gut.

ber of transferrin receptors varies, depending on the tissue and the condition. Tissues such as erythroid precursors, placenta, and liver, which have a large number of transferrin receptors, have a proportionally high uptake (and turnover) of iron. When these cells are in an iron-rich environment, the number of receptors decreases; conversely, when they are in an iron-poor environment, the number of receptors increases.

The regulation of transferrin receptors is accomplished at the genetic level. The measurement of messenger RNA for the transferrin receptor, indicates that there can be as much as a 20-fold change in mRNA and, presumably, as much as a 20-fold difference in transcription of the transferrin receptor gene, depending on iron availability. There is an *iron responsive element* present in the promotor region of the ferritin gene and in the 3-untranslated region of transferrin receptors mRNA, which inhibits the synthesis of transferrin mRNA when iron is in excess. There is an increase in the synthesis of ferritins and a decrease in the synthesis of transferrin receptors.[11,12]

When the iron is delivered to an erythroid precursor cell in the bone marrow, the ferric iron is reduced to the ferrous state in order to be incorporated into the heme prosthetic group. The reduction is accomplished by an NADH-dependent reductase and the insertion of iron in the heme ring is accomplished by the enzyme chelatase. After the ferrous iron is inserted into heme associated with the α and β subunits, the four subunits polymerize to form hemoglobin.

The presence of oxygen in oxyhemoglobin tends to oxidize a small percentage of the iron each day to ferric iron, which converts hemoglobin to methemoglobin, which has no capacity to take up and release oxygen. In order to minimize this effect, methemoglobin reductase, an NADH-dependent enzyme, reduces the ferric iron in methemoglobin back to the ferrous state, which regenerates ordinary hemoglobin.

Nutritional Requirements

The average daily intake of iron by persons in North America and Europe is between 10 and 30 mg, or about 5 to 7 mg/1000 calories.[13] Iron utensils can contribute some iron to the diet, but fluids (water, wine, and other beverages) contribute little. As already noted, there are two types of iron in the food supply—namely, heme and non-heme iron. Heme iron does not contribute more than 2 to 4 mg of iron to the food supply per day, but it is absorbed to the extent of 20 to 30 percent. Vegetarians, of course, receive no heme iron, and non-heme iron is absorbed much more poorly (5–10%). Healthy persons absorb about 10 percent of dietary iron, but iron-deficient patients, for reasons already cited, absorb about 20 percent.

A normal red cell lasts about 120 days in the circulation of a human. It is then taken up by the reticuloendothelial system and degraded into bile pigments and ferric iron, which enters the transferrin pool and is recirculated to the extent of about 25 mg/day. Thus, the turnover of iron within the body is 10 to 20 times the amount absorbed. A similar small amount 1 mg/day is lost by the sloughing of GI cells and skin cells. Fecal losses of iron are about 0.6 mg/day. Urinary losses are essentially nil. In women who bleed periodically, or in individuals with hemorrhage, iron losses can be considerable and anemia can occur as a result of bleeding. This is the basis for chlorosis in adolescent girls, who were first identified as iron-deficient in the 17th century, and for the pallor of adults after severe hemorrhage.

During the child-bearing years, females must replace the iron lost in pregnancy and during ordinary menstruation. Loss in the menses amounts to about 1.4 mg/day. The needs of the pregnant woman are great because in pregnancy a total of about 1.0 gm of iron is needed to cover both fetal and maternal needs during the course of pregnancy and delivery. There is no way that one can obtain this amount of iron from dietary intake. It is estimated that about 30 mg/day of elemental iron is needed in the diet to provide 4 mg/day for absorption. During infancy and childhood, about 40 mg of iron are required for the production of essential iron compounds associated with weight gain of 1 kg of new tissue.

The RDA for iron varies between 10 and 15 mg/day for different groups, except in pregnancy, when it is 30 mg/day. This 30 mg/day cannot be supplied from foods and must be given as a medication. If it is not given during pregnancy, iron stores are diminished and must be replenished after the pregnancy.[r5]

Deficiency Disease

Iron deficiency is the most common nutritional deficiency in the world. Iron is poorly absorbed, particularly from the diet consumed in the Third World, which consists primarily of whole-grain cereals and legumes that contain only non-heme iron but also contain phytates and other inhibitors of iron absorption. Furthermore, women and children are at constant risk for iron deficiency.

The appearance of clinical iron deficiency anemia occurs in three stages. The first involves depletion of iron stores as measured by decrease in serum ferritin, which reflects the ferritin supply in the body. At this point there is minimal loss of essential iron compounds and no evidence of anemia. The second stage is characterized by biochemical changes that reflect the lack of iron sufficient for the normal production of hemoglobin and other iron compounds. This is indicated by an increase in transferrin levels, a decrease in transferrin saturation levels, and an increase in erythrocyte protophyrin. This second stage is called iron deficiency without anemia. In the final stage, iron deficiency anemia occurs with depressed hemoglobin production, a reduction in hematocrit, and a change in the mean corpuscular volume of the RBC to produce a microcytic hypochromic anemia. Iron deficiency anemia is expressed clinically as pallor, spoon nails, and weakness. Muscular performance is also impaired in severe iron deficiency, presumably because of a decrease in the heme enzymes in mitochondria. This evolution of iron deficiency is depicted in Figure 61.3.

It is also believed that in some individuals iron deficiency causes a change in cognitive behavior (impaired psychomotor development and intellectual performance) because of depletion of iron in the CNS.[r4] This abnormality is corrected when the iron deficiency is corrected. Also, in some persons, an impaired capacity to maintain body temperature in a cold environment appears to be related to decreased secretion of thyroid stimulating hormone (TSH) in iron deficiency.

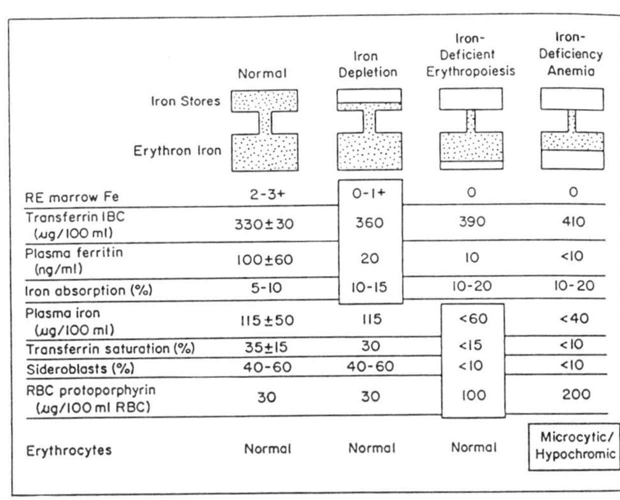

	Normal	Iron Depletion	Iron-Deficient Erythropoiesis	Iron-Deficiency Anemia
Iron Stores				
Erythron Iron				
RE marrow Fe	2-3+	0-1+	0	0
Transferrin IBC (μg/100 ml)	330±30	360	390	410
Plasma ferritin (ng/ml)	100±60	20	10	<10
Iron absorption (%)	5-10	10-15	10-20	10-20
Plasma iron (μg/100 ml)	115±50	115	<60	<40
Transferrin saturation (%)	35±15	30	<15	<10
Sideroblasts (%)	40-60	40-60	<10	<10
RBC protoporphyrin (μg/100 ml RBC)	30	30	100	200
Erythrocytes	Normal	Normal	Normal	Microcytic/Hypochromic

Figure 61.3 Sequential changes (from left to right) in the development of iron deficiency in the adult. (From Hillman & Finch 1974[4])

Therapeutic Uses

The treatment of iron deficiency anemia requires large doses of iron, usually 60 mg of elemental iron equivalent to 300 mg of ferrous sulfate, once or twice a day. The iron usually is given between meals to minimize GI side-effects. Fortunately, the smaller the dose and the more severe the anemia, the greater will be the percentage of iron absorbed, so it is not necessary to give more than 120 mg of elemental Fe per day. This treatment should be continued for two to three months to normalize hemoglobin levels and iron stores.

Toxicology

Excess iron is toxic. Sometimes children will ingest iron pills accidentally, resulting in severe iron poisoning, characterized by damage to the intestine with bloody diarrhea, vomiting, acidosis, and sometimes liver failure. Effective treatment includes inducing emesis, food and electrolyte treatment to prevent shock, and the use of iron-chelating agents to bind the excess iron. This treatment has substantially decreased mortality from about 50 percent in 1950 to only a small percentage in recent years.

Chronic overload of iron results primarily from a variety of factors, including excessive medication with iron compounds, chronic alcoholism with chronic liver disease terminating in cirrhosis, frequent and chronic transfusions for treatment of anemia, and hereditary hemachromatosis (HH).[r5] Hemochromatosis is a genetic disease caused by a recessive gene on chromosome 6 that nullifies the regulation of iron absorption and increases iron uptake.[14] The frequency of the disease is 3/1000, with about 10 percent of North Americans carrying one copy of the recessive gene. In this disease, iron-binding proteins are increased in liver and gut. The homozygotes for HH have skin pigmentation, cirrhosis, diabetes, cardiomyopathy, and degeneration, and CNS manifestations. The homozygous state is manifested after puberty in males and after the menopause in females. Both serum iron and percentage saturation of transferrin are increased. Other major clinical features of HH are fatigue, cardiac arrythmias, cardiac arthropathy, hepatoma, hypothyroidism, and gonadal failure—all from iron deposition on the affected tissues. Patients with HH are susceptible to infection, sepsis and coronary heart disease. The treatment of HH is by repeated phlebotomy. Heterozygotes for HH show increased iron absorption and higher than normal saturation of transferrin. Even the heterozygotes appear to be more vulnerable to myocardial infarction than do normal persons.[15,16]

Preparations

A typical set of iron preparations available for the treatment of iron deficiency anemia is shown in Table 61.3.[r5]

Zinc

History

Zinc was recognized as an element in 1509 and as an essential nutrient for plants in 1869.[17] It was not until 1934, however, that zinc was established as an essential factor for the growth and health of rats by Todd et al.[18] Underwood[r5] has reviewed the subsequent progress in identifying zinc as an essential nutrient for animals and birds. The first enzyme shown to be a zinc metalloenzyme was carbonic anhydrase.[19] Since this discovery in 1940, there have been more than 100 zinc metalloenzymes identified, which include dehydrogenases, phosphatases, phosphorylases, DNA and RNA polymers, peptidases, superoxide dismutase, and a variety of transcription factors that bind to DNA.

The first evidence that zinc is essential in humans was obtained by Prasad and his coworkers in the study of dwarfism, hypogonadism, splenomegaly, and anemia in children in Iran in 1961.[20–22] Genetic disorders of zinc absorption are known in humans (acrodermatitis enteropathica)[23] in Friesian cattle (Adema disease), and in mice (lethal milk mutation.)[r7]

Chemistry

Zinc is the last transition element in the series of the fourth period of the periodic table. It has an atomic number of 30 and a molecular weight of 65.4. For a metal, it has a relatively low melting point of 419°C. Fifteen isotopes of zinc have been described, ranging from ${}_{30}Zn^{57}$ to ${}_{30}Zn^{72}$. Five of these isotopes are naturally occurring; the principal one is ${}_{30}Zn^{64}$, with 48.6 percent prevalence. The second most abundant is ${}_{36}Zn^{66}$, 27.9 percent prevalence and with two to three minor isotopes, ${}_{30}Zn^{67}$, ${}_{30}Zn^{68}$, and ${}_{30}Zn^{70}$. The rest are radioactive isotopes, of which ${}_{30}Zn^{65}$, with a 244-day half-life has been the most useful for biologic experiments.

Metallic zinc is a good reducing agent, particularly in acid solution. It is amphoteric and will dissolve in both mineral acids and strong bases. Ionic zinc exists in only one oxidized state, namely Zn^{2+}, and forms stable complex ions such as $Zn(NH_3)_4{}^{2+}$. Zinc forms a large range of soluble salts including the chloride, bromide, iodide, acetate, sulfate, nitrate, and others. Insoluble salts include carbonate, sulfate, hydroxide, ammonium phosphate, oxalate, and phytate. The most common mineral is zinc sulfide, known as sphalerite and sometimes called zinc blende. The metal is prepared from zinc sulfide by roasting in air to convert it to the oxide and then reducing the oxide with finely divided carbon. Because $zinc^{2+}$ cannot be oxidized or reduced under physiologic conditions, zinc in biologic materials (enzymes and various proteins forms complexes) does not provide for the donation or uptake of electrons.

Physiology

Absorption occurs primarily in the small intestine, although the relative contributions of the duodenum and ileum are not clear. Of the 6 to 15 mg of zinc in the average diet, only 10 to 40 percent is absorbed. Dietary factors inhibiting zinc absorption include clay, fiber, phytate, and chelating agents. Unbound zinc is absorbed rapidly, and the transport process is energy-dependent. Absorption involves two kinetic processes—a carrier-mediated component saturable at higher luminal zinc concentrations and a nonsaturable diffusion component. The site of absorption is the brush border membrane of the enterocyte.[r8] The absorption of zinc is like that of copper and iron in the sense that as zinc content of the food increases the absorption decreases.

The absorption of zinc is regulated by metallothionein (MT) a 6500 KD cysteine-rich protein, induced by zinc, other heavy metals, and by certain hormones. The high thiol content of MT binds metals with variable affinity, copper being more tightly bound than zinc. High zinc intakes increase the level of intestinal MT and nutrient zinc absorption. High intakes of zinc also tend to displace copper from MT (by mass action) and may induce copper deficiency. After absorption, the zinc is transferred to the liver via the portal system, where some is stored and the remainder distributed to extrahepatic tissues. Since there is no specific plasma transport protein for zinc, most of the metal (~80%) is attached to albumin and the rest to α–2 macroglobulin and to a lesser extent to transferrin and amino acids. About 5 percent is ultrafiltrable and appears in the urine to the extent of 0.5 to 0.8 mg/day. The remainder of the oral intake (~12 mg) is excreted via the feces, of which at least 50 percent has undergone enterovisceral circulation via the pancreas, liver, and gut.

Table 61.3 Comparison of Iron Content and Costs of Some Oral Iron Medications*

Name	Manufacturer	Iron Content (Mg per tablet)	Cost ($) Per 100 Tablets or Capsules	Cost ($) Per Gram of Iron
Plain iron tablets or capsules				
Ferrous sulfate				
Feosol	Manly & James	66	8.50	1.28
Generic	Golding†	66	2.29	0.35
Ferrous fumarate				
Ircon	Kenwood	66	7.26	1.10
Generic	Nature-Made	20	3.97	1.98
Ferrous gluconate				
Fergon	Winthrop-Breon†	37	7.92	2.14
Simron	Marion Merrell Dow	10	44.69	44.69
Generic	Nature-Made	37	3.97	1.07
Enteric-coated tablets				
Generic	Goldine	66	3.00	0.45
"Delayed-release" capsules				
Fero-Gradumet‡	Abbott	105	30.39	2.90
Ferro-sequels	Lederle	50	29.25	5.85
Feosol Spansules	Manly & James	50	22.86	4.57
Combination tablets or capsules				
Geritol	Beecham	50	14.52	2.91
Trinsicon	Russ	90	56.70	6.29
Unicap Plus Iron	Upjohn	18	9.75	5.38
Vitron-C	Fisons	66	10.98	1.66

*Figures are based on average retail price in the United States in June 1991. Prices vary slightly among pharmacies. Numerous other iron preparations are available and many other manufacturers produce generic iron preparations. Those shown are selected only as examples, and their listing does not imply endorsement.

†Sugar-coated. Potentially dangerous in households with young children.

‡Although the manufacturer represents Fero-Gradumet as a "slow release" form of iron, independent studies indicate that it actually releases iron rapidly, a desirable property. In this regard, it resembles many of the medications listed as "plain iron tablets." (From Fairbanks, V.F.[r5])

The total body zinc in an adult varies from about 1.4 to 2.4 grams (about half that of iron). Plasma concentrations of zinc range 80 to 130 μg/dl. The red cells contain 42 ± 6 μg per gm hemoglobin or about 630 μg/dl of red cells, about 6 times the concentration in plasma. The portion of zinc in erythrocytes is associated primarily with isoenzymes of carbonic anhydrase and to a lesser extent with superoxide dismutase and MT. Other tissue levels are even higher, ranging from 2 to 10 mg/100 gm fresh tissue. The highest amounts are in liver, kidney, muscle, prostate, and testes. The turnover of zinc in the body is shown in Figure 61.4.

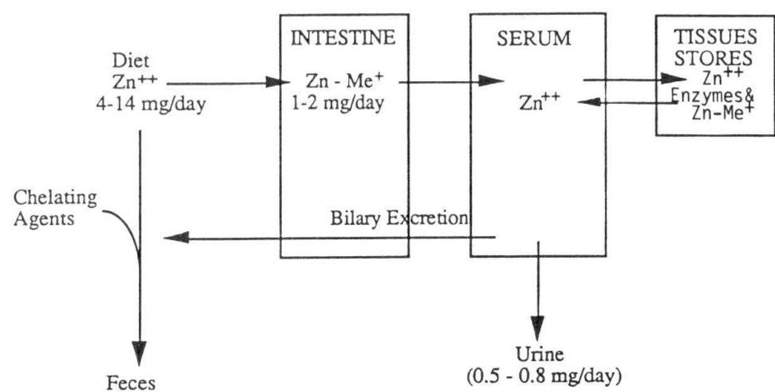

Figure 61.4 Zinc Balance in a Normal Adult Human

The biologic activity of zinc is the result of its combination with a wide range of biochemically active proteins, which include enzymes (as already mentioned), plus a variety of transcription factors that regulate gene function and gene expression. Of particular importance is the fact that zinc is a component of many enzymes that catalyze nucleotide phosphate ester formation. This metal is well-suited for this role in nucleic acid metabolism because Zn^{2+} does not exhibit any direct redox activity, thus precluding the generation of DNA-damaging free radicals. Present evidence suggests that zinc is vital for certain DNA polymerases,

RNA polymerases I, II, and III, and a variety of nuclear transcription factors through the formation of *zinc fingers* (via chelation with cysteine and histidine), which forms a structure essential for binding to DNA. Zinc also assists in the binding of proteins to membranes, e.g., protein kinase C to plasma membranes.[r8] Finally, zinc plays a role in antioxidation via its structural contribution to cystolic superoxide dismutase, a copper:zinc protein of MW 31,200, and the free-radical suppression observed by MT induced by zinc.

Of interest is the demonstration that MT exists as two distinct yet related compounds, MT-1 and MT-2. As already noted, these proteins are hydrophylic, low molecular weight proteins (6–7 k Da) containing a high percentage of cysteine residues (23–22 mol %). The synthesis of MTs is regulated by zinc, other heavy metals, glucocorticoids, and bacterial endotoxin through its action on the expression of the genes for these proteins.[r11,r12] The MT cDNA and genes were identified by Hager and Palmiter et al.[24–26] and by Shay and Cousins.[27] By combining the results of DNA sequence information with the results of deletion mapping studies, unique short sequences of DNA were found that mediated the role of zinc in this process. The metal response units were sites for transacting transcription factors that bind and enhance the basal rate of transcription of the genes for MT.[r11] In the absence of dietary zinc, gene transcription is impaired and MT levels are low. In addition, zinc-deficient animals demonstrate numerous breaks in single-stranded DNA.[28] This can be reversed when dietary zinc is restored. The cytokine, interleukin 1, has been shown to direct and regulate zinc metabolism in the traumatized or septic individual by increasing the expression of the MT gene. As a result, zinc uptake is increased by the gut and its transport to and uptake by the various tissues in the body is expedited.[27]

Nutrition Requirements

The intake of zinc by healthy humans ranges from 6 to 15 mg/day.[30] The bioavailability of zinc in different foods varies widely. Meat, liver, eggs, and seafood (especially oysters) are good sources of available zinc, whereas whole-grain products contain the element in a less available form. Of the various factors believed to affect zinc availability adversely, high concentrations of dietary phytate, polyphosphate, calcium, and fiber have practical importance worldwide. The ingestion of clay by children in Iran (geophagia) contributed to their zinc deficiency.

Because the bioavailability of zinc varies so much in various diets, estimates of endogenous losses in healthy males from urine, dermal losses, and semen ranged from 2.2 to 2.8 mg/day, with an average of 2.5 mg. Assuming an average absorption of 20 percent, the oral requirement in adult males was calculated to be 12.5 mg/day. An additional safety factor of 20 percent was added for unknown changes in bioavailability. The final RDA was thus set at 15 mg for males and 12 mg for females, based on average body weight.[31] These estimates agree with balance studies of Sandstead, who determined the requirement of zinc in adult males to be 12.7 mg/day.[32]

Deficiency Disease

Zinc deficiency has been documented in both animals and humans. The signs and symptoms that have been observed in humans include anorexia, growth retardation, delayed sexual maturation, hypogonadism and hypospermia, alopecia, immune disorders, dermatitis, night blindness, impaired taste (hypogeusia), and impaired wound healing. The first signs of zinc deficiency in marginally nourished children are suboptimal growth, anorexia, impaired taste and low zinc content of hair. The administration of 0.4 to 0.8 mg/kg of zinc in this population resulted in marked improvement of these problems.[33] The most serious manifestations of zinc deficiency were reported in Iranian dwarfs by Prasad et al.[22,r8] These adolescent boys, who consumed large amounts of clay, were retarded in growth and sexual development and had anemia, hypogonadism, hepatosplendomegaly, rough skin, and mental lethargy. Following treatment with a well-balanced diet containing adequate amounts of zinc for one year, public hair appeared; there was an increase in the size of sexual organs, linear growth was resumed, and the skin became normal. The anemia responded to iron supplements. Subsequent studies in Egypt and Turkey revealed similar persons with zinc deficiency.[r9]

The biochemical signs associated with zinc deficiency included reduced plasma zinc, decreased alkaline phosphatase, decreased alcohol dehydrogenase in the retina (which accounts for night blindness), decreased plasma testosterone levels, impaired T-lymphocyte function, decreased collagen synthesis (poor wound healing), and decreased RNA polymerase activity in several tissues.

The clinical assessment of mild zinc deficiency is difficult because of the nonspecific nature of many of the signs and symptoms. Nonetheless a malnourished person with a borderline low plasma zinc level, reduced taste sensitivity, impaired response of lymphocytes to mitogens, and altered gonadic hormone function should be suspected of zinc deficiency and given a clinical trial with zinc supplements. Persons at high risk for zinc deficiency include those with acrodermatitis enteropathica, an autosomal recessive genetic disease in which zinc absorption is greatly reduced. Large doses of oral zinc (30–45 mg/d) bypass the mucosal lesion and provide a remission. Others at high risk are chronic alcoholics, children with protein-calorie malnutrition, pregnant and lactating women on marginal diets, patients on long-term total parenteral nutrition who are inadequately fortified with zinc, patients with uremia, and patients with malabsorption syndromes. Persons at somewhat lesser risk of zinc deficiency are those with sickle-cell anemia, vegetarians on high cereal intakes, patients with chronic infections, and the aged. Zinc deficiency has also been induced by penicillamine therapy in Wilson's disease.[34,35]

Therapeutic Uses

Persons being treated for zinc deficiency with doses of 0.5 to 5.0 mg Zn/kg body weight are receiving the high doses necessary to replete zinc stores and restore normal physiologic functions. Zinc has also been given to patients with sickle-cell anemia, not only to repair the zinc deficiency accompanying that disease, but also to increase the affinity of sickle cell hemoglobin for oxygen.[r9] The doses used in these studies were 660 mg $ZnSO_4$ per day by mouth (~5 mg Zn/kg/d). Zinc in doses of 150 mg/day also has been used to remove copper from patients with Wilson's disease.[35]

Toxicity

Zinc is acutely toxic when given in high doses. Doses in excess of 200 mg per day are emetic; doses of 1 gram per day may be fatal. Metal fume fever with sweating, hyperpnea, and weakness has been reported in workers exposed to ZnO fumes.[37] Impairment of copper status of human volunteers taking 18.5 to 25 mg of Zn/day has been reported. Patients given 150 to 300 mg Zn/day developed hypocupremia, microcytosis, and neutropenia.[38] Other healthy adults receiving zinc in this dose range for six weeks developed abnormalities in immunity and a decline in high-density lipoprotein (HDL) concentration. Excess zinc also can interfere with ferritin synthesis and the sequestration of iron in that substance.[36]

Preparations

Zn SO_4 is available in various high-potency vitamin mineral supplements in doses of 80 mg per capsule.

Copper

History

Since the Bronze Age, copper alloyed with tin has been used by humans to fabricate a vast array of useful items. However, only in the last half-century has copper been recognized as an essential nutrient for man and other animals. In 1928, Hart[39] recognized that iron-deficient rats were responsive to iron only when copper was also available. Wilson, in 1912, described a hereditary disease characterized by hepatocellular degeneration which later was found to be a copper storage disease and focused attention on copper as a nutrient.[40] Menke's disease due to an abnormality in copper absorption and distribution was first described in 1962.[41] Evidence of copper deficiency in humans was not forthcoming until the studies of Graham and coworkers in malnourished children in Lima, Peru, were published in 1964.[42] In 1968, Cartwright[43] and his associates showed the synergistic relationship between copper and iron in the biosynthesis of heme. Other enzymatic roles for copper and mechanisms of its transport have since been elucidated.

Chemistry

Copper is a transition metal in the fourth period of the periodic table. Its atomic number is 29 and its atomic weight 63.4. Copper has two naturally occurring isotopes $_{29}Cu^{63}$ and $_{29}Ca^{65}$ and two radioactive isotopes $_{29}Cu^{64}$ ($t_{1/2}$ = 12.7 h) and $_{29}Cu^{67}$ ($t_{1/2}$ = 62 h) that have been used as biologic tracers. Copper exists in two oxidation states, Cu^{+1} (cuprous) and Cu^{2+} (cupric). The blue hydrated cupric ion is an oxidizing agent used, for example, in the detection of glucose in biologic fluids in which Cu^{2+} is reduced to Cu^{1+} which precipitates as the red Cu_2O. The redox properties of copper are utilized in many copper enzymes.

Physiology

Copper absorption takes place in the stomach and small intestine.[r12] The amount absorbed depends on dietary intake. If the dietary intake is low (ca 0.8 mg), absorption is high (56%); contrariwise, at high intakes of Cu (8 mg/d) absorption is reduced to about 12 percent. High levels of dietary zinc inhibit copper absorption.[44] Copper is subject to extensive enterohepatic circulation. It is estimated that the biliary excretion is about 2 mg/day, which finds its way with unabsorbed copper into the feces. The urinary excretion is very small, amounting to only 10 to 50 µg/day.

When copper is absorbed by the intestinal cell, it is bound by serum albumin and to a lesser extent transcuprein (MW = 270,000) and is delivered to the liver, which incorporates it into the protein ceruloplasmin, α-2-glycoprotein (MW = 150,000). Ceruloplasmin contains six copper atoms, is the main carrier of copper in the plasma, and has ferroxidase activity. The concentration of copper in plasma is about 1 µg/ml and that of ceruloplasmin is 15 to 60 mg/dl. As a ferroxidase, ceruloplasmin is an active participant in the conversion of Fe^{2+} to Fe^{3+} and promotes its incorporation into transferrin, the iron transport protein. Metallothionein

(MW = 6500), a cysteine-rich metal-binding protein, serves as a buffer for Cu in cells, is induced by copper, and thus plays a role in the homeostasis of Cu.

Copper transport into cells from the plasma appears to involve ceruloplasmin and membrane transporter proteins. Studies of the kinetics of copper transport show the Km values to be in the low micromolar range, whereas the Vmax is highly variable, depending on cell type, incubation conditions, and the media used.[44] Both copper and zinc stimulate the expression of the gene for MT, which is a major ligand for copper in cells, and provides a normal reservoir for cellular copper.

Enzymes containing copper are generally oxidoreductases in which copper is situated at the active site. Monoamine oxidase (MW = 290,000) inactivates biologically active amines such as serotonin, tyramine, and polyamines by converting them to aldehydes. Lysyloxidase deaminates lysine in nascent collagen and elastin and promotes the cross-linking of chains essential for the maturation of connective tissue. Copper deficiency, like scurvy, causes a failure in the synthesis of collagen and, among other things, impedes wound healing. Cytochrome oxidase, the terminal and limiting enzyme in the electron transport chain of mitochondria, contains seven subunits, one of which, cytochrome a (MW = 26,000) contains two copper atoms per molecule and reduces O_2 to water. It is a key enzyme in the synthesis of ATP. Dopamine β-hydroxylase (MW = 290,000) catalyzes the conversion of dopamine to norepinephrine. It contains eight atoms of copper per molecule and requires ascorbic acid as a reducing agent. Superoxide dismutase (MW = 31,200) is a cystolic enzyme containing one atom of copper and one atom of zinc per molecule. It is required for the efficient conversion of superoxide ions to oxygen and hydrogen peroxide, the latter being converted to oxygen and water by catalase, an iron-containing enzyme. Tyrosinase, a copper-containing monophenol oxygenase (MW = 120,000) converts tyrosine to dopamine and dopaquinone, which are intermediates in the synthesis of melanin. Copper-containing enzymes in humans are shown in Table 61.4. The copper content of the adult human body ranges from 100 to 150 mg.

Two well-recognized genetic diseases affecting copper metabolism are Menkes' disease[46] and Wilson's disease.[r14] Menke's disease is a fatal, X-linked disorder characterized by abnormal (kinky) hair, maldistribution of copper in cells, and mental retardation. Serum copper and ceruloplasmin levels are low, as are the levels of copper in liver and brain. In contrast, copper levels accumulate in the intestinal mucosa, muscle, spleen, and kidney. The synthesis of most copper enzymes, however, is impaired, which causes defects in connective tissue, brain neurons, and energy exchange (with hypothermia). The gene responsible for Menke's disease has recently been cloned[47] and its product identified as a membrane-bound ATP-dependent copper transport protein. Its absence prevents the normal intracellular distribution of Cu and its incorporation into Cu-containing enzymes. No treatment has been found for this disease.

Wilson's disease, first described by Kinear-Wilson in 1912,[40] is an uncommon autosomal recessive disease of copper storage. Copper accumulates in the liver, the brain, and the cornea of the eye (Kayser-Fleisher rings). Urinary copper excretion is abnormally high, despite the fact that ceruloplasmin values are usually low. The principal defects in this disease are the failure of the liver to incorporate copper into ceruloplasmin for export to plasma and an inability to excrete copper into the bile, which is the major normal excretory pathway for copper. If the disease goes untreated, non-ceruloplasmin plasma copper accumulates in the liver and brain, resulting in neurologic damage and severe disease, including cirrhosis. Hepatitis, hemolytic crisis, and hepatic failure may ensue. The most effective treatment is chelation therapy, usually with D-penicillamine, which was introduced by Walshe in 1956[47] and facilitates the excretion of copper in the urine. The exact molecular defect has not yet been discovered, although the gene for Wilson's disease is on chromosome 13.

Nutritional Requirements

The copper requirement for adults ranges from 0.5 to 1.3 mg/day. In 1989 the Food and Nutrition Board[31] stated that the estimated safe and adequate daily dietary intakes of copper for adults are 1.5 to 3.0 mg/day. For infants less than 1 year old they recommended 0.6 to 0.7 mg/day.

Copper is present in nearly all foods in varying amounts. Although dairy products are poor sources of copper, liver, legumes, and nuts are rich in this mineral. Raisins, whole grains, shellfish, and shrimp are excellent sources as well. Surveys of foods consumed by a variety of population groups in the US indicate a range of intake of copper from 0.7 to 7.5 mg/day. As noted, at low intakes, absorption efficiency is markedly higher than when intake is high. Zinc, tin, ascorbic acid, and iron adversely affect copper absorption.[r10]

Copper Deficiency

Copper deficiency is rare in healthy persons but occurs most commonly in infants who are either premature or recovering from protein-calorie malnutri-

Table 61.4 Copper Enzymes in Humans

Common Name	Functional Role	Known or Expected Consequence of Deficiency
Cytochrome oxidase	Electron transport chain	Muscle weakness; neurologic effects; hypothermia
Superoxide dismutase	Free radical detoxification	Uncertain
Tyrosinase	Melanin production	Failure of pigmentation
Dopamine β-hydroxylase	Catecholamine production	Neurologic effects; possible hypothermia
Lysyl oxidase	Cross-linking of collagen and elastin	Arterial abnormalities; bladder diverticulae; loose skin and joints
Ceruloplasmin	Ferroxidase; copper transport	Anemia; secondary copper deficiency
Enzyme not known	Cross-linking of keratin (disulfide bonds)	Pili torti

tion. Patients receiving long-term parenteral nutrition also are at risk for copper deficiency. Frank copper deficiency is associated with lassitude, hypocupremia (0.3 Cu μg/ml) and low serum ceruloplasmin values (3.5 mg/dl). Anemia, leukopenia, neutropenia, and osteoporosis are regularly observed. Small petechial hemorrhages and arterial aneurysms also are signs of copper deficiency.[r15]

The failure to observe normal wound healing in copper deficiency emphasizes the vital role copper plays in the synthesis of connective tissue. Central nervous system degeneration can be related to a decline in respiratory chain activity, although, in the hierarchy of enzymes requiring copper for function, cytochrome oxidase is the last to be affected. Other signs of the Cu-deficient state include moderately elevated levels of plasma cholesterol,[49] and reduced levels of catecholamines. The most severe copper deficiency is seen in Menke's disease, which displays most of the above signs plus "kinky hair" and severe cerebral and cerebellar disease.

Therapeutic Uses

Ceruloplasmin is generally regarded as the most reliable index of copper status in otherwise healthy persons. Plasma ceruloplasmin, however, is an acute phase reactant, and will rise under conditions of trauma and sepsis regardless of the status of copper stores. In view of this, some consider erythrocyte superoxide dismutase a more reliable indicator. The treatment of copper deficiency is accomplished with a dose of 0.1 mg/kg for several weeks. Occasionally copper salts are used as emetics in doses of 1 mg per kg body weight, but this borders on a toxic dose.

Toxicity

As little as 10 mg of oral copper in an adult can cause nausea, although chronic intakes of 10 to 35 mg/day have been observed in some humans without adverse effects.[r10] The lethal dose of Cu in humans ranges from 3.5 to 35 grams.[r16]

Preparations

One-a-day type vitamin and mineral supplements may contain 2 mg of copper per capsule.

Selenium

History

The element selenium was discovered by Berzelius in 1817.[r17] Metallic selenium occurs in a variety of allotropic forms, which appear silver gray, black, or dark red. Selenium on earth is about as rare as gold—although it was named for the moon. It occurs admixed with sulfur as selenides of heavy metals. Selenium first attracted the attention of biologists in the 1930s because plants high in selenium were found to cause chronic poisoning of livestock.[r17] The research on selenium by biologists between 1930 and 1950 was devoted to attempts to understand the mechanism of selenium toxicity and to prevent it in areas where soils were rich in selenium.

The preoccupation with selenium as a toxic material changed with the discovery in 1957 by Schwartz and Foltz[50] that traces of selenium as selenite or selenate would prevent the hepatic necrosis that occurred in vitamin E-deficient rats fed a torula yeast diet. Soon thereafter deficiencies of selenium and vitamin E were shown to be involved in several economically important nutritional diseases in cattle, sheep, swine, and poultry. The interaction with vitamin E was interesting because it suggested that both nutrients had antioxidant potential, although the degree of protection afforded by vitamin E and selenium varied from species to species. Some of these differences and similarities are shown in Table 61.5.[51] Vitamin E deficiency disease in animals affects the reproductive, muscular, vascular, hepatobiliary, and central nervous systems. Selenium deficiency, on the other hand, affects the reproductive, muscular, vascular, and hepatobiliary systems. The exchangeability of dietary selenium and vitamin E as protective nutrients is most conspicuous in hepatic necrosis in rat and pig and exudative diathesis in chicks. In 1973, Rotruck et al.[52] demonstrated that selenium was an intrinsic component of the enzyme glutathione peroxidase (GSHPx), which clarified the overlapping activities of α-tocopherol and selenium in some combined deficiency diseases.[53]

Selenium deficiency is rare in humans, although it has been associated with Keshan disease, an endemic cardiomyopathy that primarily affects children and women of child-bearing age in some areas of China. Selenium deficiency with muscle disease has also been observed in a patient on long-term total parenteral nutrition.

Chemistry

Selenium is a allotropic metal in group six of the fourth period of the periodic table. Its atomic number is 34, and its molecular weight is 78.96. Selenium has 26 isotopic forms, of which four occur naturally. These are $_{34}Se^{76}$ 9 percent, $_{34}Se^{77}$ 7.6 percent, $_{34}Se^{78}$ 23.5 percent, $_{34}Se^{80}$ 49.6 percent, and $_{34}Se^{82}$ 9.4 percent. The principal naturally occurring form of the element is $_{34}Se^{80}$, even though the average molecular weight is 78.96. Of the 22 radioactive isotopes, $_{34}Se^{75}$ is a weak gamma emitter widely used in biology with a half-life of 118 days. The other isotopes are short-lived except for $_{34}Se^{79}$, which is a weak beta emitter with a half-life of 6×10^4 years. Of the allotropic forms of selenium metal, the gray form has measurable photoconductivity and has been used in photocells.

The chemistry of Se is similar to sulfur. It reacts with metals to form selenides. H_2Se is toxic and burns to give SeO_2, which dissolves in water to form selenious acid H_2SeO_3. H_2SeO_3 can be oxidized to H_2SeO_4, but is a weaker acid than H_2SO_4. It is, however, a stronger oxidizing agent than H_2SO_4. H_2Se is also a better reducing agent than H_2S. The valences of selenium are +2, +4, and +6. The forms of selenium in biologic materials, both plant and animal, include selenides, selenate, selenomethionine, selenocystine, methyl selenocysteine, and such volatile forms as dimethyl selenide. Soils high or low in inorganic selenium compounds determine the selenium content of plants, which in turn can produce nutritional states that range from the deficient to the toxic in animals, including humans.

Physiology

Free selenium compounds are well-absorbed from the diet by animals. Unlike some of the transitional metals like iron, copper, and zinc, there seems to be no gate for absorption. Nonetheless the bioavailability of selenium from foods is related to the digestibility of the over-all foodstuff. In one study the bioavailability of selenium from mushrooms, tuna, and wheat was 5, 57, and 83 percent compared to sodium selenite.[r18] The uptake of selenium by the gut is thus not regulated by the size of the body pool of Se, which can vary four to fivefold in healthy adult humans. After absorption, inorganic selenium and selenoamino acids are distributed to all tissues in the plasma. There is no established transport protein for selenium; it therefore is likely that the low molecular weight forms of selenium are either free or loosely attached to plasma proteins. The kidney is the main organ for excretion of selenium, with lesser amounts appearing in sweat, desquamating epithelial cells, and the feces. There is no significant enterohepatic circulation of selenium.

Blood values of selenium vary with intake, as shown in Figure 61.5 and can vary from 16 to 25 μg/dl in the US and Canada to values of 5 to 8 μg/dl in Finland and New Zealand. Erythrocytes have two to three times as much Se as plasma owing to the presence of large amounts of GSHPx in the erthyrocyte. Seleno-

Table 61.5 Interaction of Vitamin E with Other Nutrients in Treatment of Various Deficiency Diseases[51]

I. Chemical antioxidant-responsive diseases
   A. Encephalomalacia (chicks, turkeys)
   B. Abortion-resorption (rats)
   C. Erythrocyte hemolysis (rats, man)
   D. Ceroid pigmentation (rats, mink, pigs)
II. Principally vitamin E-responsive diseases
   A. Muscular dystrophy (rabbits, guinea pigs, monkeys, chicks)
   B. Testicular degeneration (rat)
III. Principally selenium-responsive diseases
   A. Embryogenesis defect (cow)
   B. Muscle dystrophy (lamb, calf, kid, turkey)
IV. Vitamin E and selenium-responsive diseases
   A. Hepatic necrosis (rat, pig)
   B. Exudative diathesis (chicken)

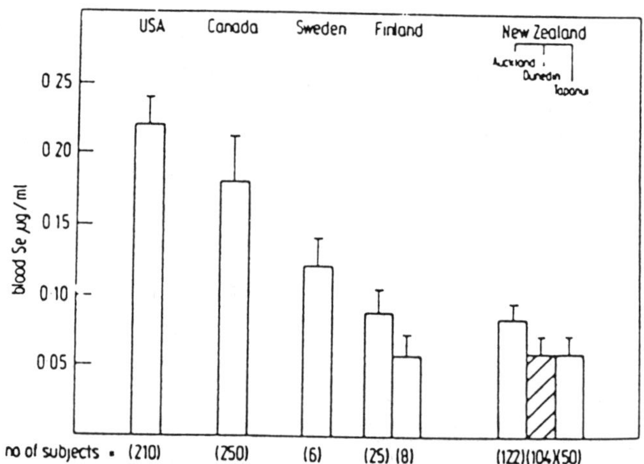

Figure 61.5 Blood selenium levels reported in healthy adults in various countries. (0.1 μg Se/ml = 1.27 μmol Se/L). (From ref [55]).

protein P may account for up to 50 percent of plasma selenium.[r20] The body pool of selenium can vary from 20 mg in persons residing in the US to less than 6 mg in women living in New Zealand.[55]

Approximately 10 selenoproteins have been identified in animals and man. Four have been shown to have enzymatic activity, and three are isoforms of glutathione peroxidase (GSHPx). The classic cellular GSHPx was discovered in 1957 and was shown to contain Se in 1973.[52] It occurs in all cells. Approximately 25 percent of body selenium is in liver cGSH-Px. It is a tetramer containing four identical subunits (MW = 23,000). Each contains one residue of selenocysteine. The reaction is shown below:

$$2GSH + H_2O_2 \xrightarrow{GSHPx} GSSG + 2H_2O$$

The enzyme prevents the accumulation of peroxide or other hydroperoxides and their precursors in cells and thus preserves labile protein and lipid groups from oxidation.

Extracellular glutathione peroxidase (eGSHPx), an isoform of cGSHPx with similar properties, is found in plasma. Its activity is a convenient index of selenium status. Phospholipid hydroperoxide glutathione peroxidase is the third GSHPx that has been characterized. Unlike the two enzymes discussed above, it is a monomer of MW 20,000; it also contains selenocysteine at its active site, and is present in testes and other endocrine organs. It reduces fatty acid hydroperoxides esterified to phospholipids.

Type I Iodothyronine 5′-deiodinase (5′DI) converts thyroxine to triiodothyronine, the most active thyroid hormone. The enzyme is a selenium homodimer with each subunit (MW = 27,000) containing one selenocysteine moiety.[56] Selenoprotein (SeP) is a glycosylated plasma selenoprotein (MW = 41,000) that has ten selenocysteine residues in its primary structure. Its function is unknown, but it appears to protect the body against prooxidant xenobiotics. Some believe it is a transporter of Se.

Finally, selenomethionine proteins are a large group of proteins formed in the body when selenomethionine is in the diet. Dietary selenomethionine simply follows the metabolic pathways of methionine, including its incorporation into tissue protein via SeMet-$tRNA^{met}$ at positions specified by the Met codon. These Se proteins have no enzymic activity peculiar to Se, but may have other activities peculiar to the peptide such as thiolase or β-galactosidase. Selenomethionine cannot be synthesized from selenite in the animal body. The metabolism of selenium, including its incorporation into the above proteins, is shown in Figure 61.6.

[Se]Met degradation is shown to follow the usual methionine transamination pathway. An enzyme like the L-methionine-β-lyase might release methane selenol in animals. [Se]Cys metabolism does not follow cysteine metabolism (with oxidative release of selenite); instead, the [Se]Cys-specific enzyme selenocysteine lyase directly releases elemental Se, which is reduced to selenide. Selenite is also reduced to selenide and the methylation of selenide leads to the formation of various species that are excreted in urine and breath.

The biosynthesis of Se-specific proteins involves a unique pathway by which a special tRNA for serine is modified to provide a t-RNA for selenocysteine. The special t-RNA for serine, furthermore, is complementary to a UGA codon in the mRNA for GSHPx. Thus, UGA, which is ordinarily a termination codon, becomes the codon for selenocysteine. The reaction by which serine is converted to selenocysteine involves phosphorylation of the tRNA-bound serine followed by reaction with H_2Se to displace the phosphate and form the [Se]Cys-$tRNA_{UGA}$. All of the Se-specific selenoproteins described use this mechanism for incorporation of Se into their peptide backbone.[r21]

Nutritional Requirements

Dietary intake of selenium by adults worldwide varies from 10 to 15 µg per day in parts of China to 28 to 56 µg in New Zealand and Finland to 100 to 250 µg/day in the US and Canada. Seafoods, kidney, liver, and selected grains are good sources of Se. Adequate diets generally contain not less than 0.1 µg/gram of dry foods or 50/µg/day. In the Keshan study in China, workers given selenite supplements increased their intake to about 40 µg per day, which prevented the cardiomyopathy. This "requirement" turns out to be about 0.8 µg/kg body weight. In the 1989 RDA, the Food and Nutrition Board of the USA recommended 55 µg/d for women and 70 µg/day for men. Recommendations for infants were 2 µg/kg; for children, about 1 µg/kg. The allowance for pregnant women was 65 µg and for lactation 75 µg/day.[31,r19]

Deficiency Disease

As already noted, a deficiency of selenium produces well-recognized syndromes in animals, including growth failure and hepatic necrosis in rats and pigs, white muscle disease in sheep, gizzard myopathy in turkeys, and exudative diathesis in chicks. Since glutathione peroxidase is an antioxidant enzyme, it is not surprising that the pathophysiology of selenium deficiency includes enhanced lipid peroxidation, disorganized membranes and organelles in cells, and specific necrotic changes in muscle and liver.

The only clinical deficiency disease responsive to

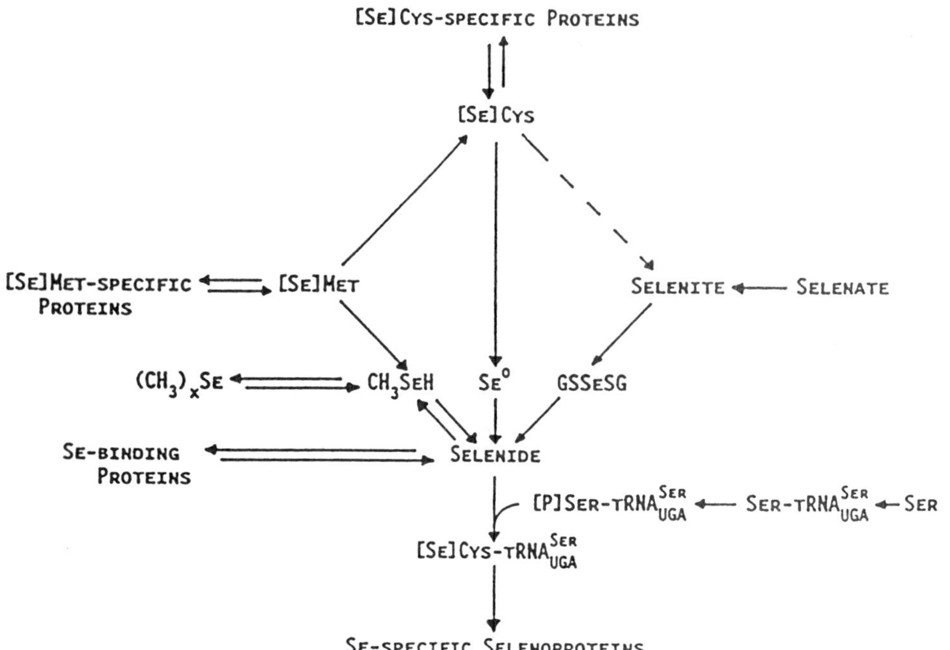

Figure 61.6 Selenium metabolism and the four classes of selenoproteins. The diagram shows the various pathways of selenium metabolism and the Se precursors that lead to the synthesis of each class of selenoproteins.[r21]

selenium in human beings is Keshan disease, a cardiomyopathy observed in China, afflicting only about 1 per cent of the exposed population and preventable by selenite supplements.[57,58] Epidemiologic studies have linked the potential for selenium deficiency in animals and human beings to low selenium content in soil and local cereal grains. The effect of Se intake on plasma level is shown in Table 61.6. Low plasma selenium levels also have been noted in colonic, gastric, and pancreatic carcinoma and cirrhosis, in burns, and in two groups of children with kashiorkor.[r22]

Premature infants[60] and adults sustained by parenteral or enteral solutions[61] devoid of this mineral are at risk of deficiency. Symptoms characteristic of deficiency include cardiomyopathy, growth retardation, cataract formation, abnormal placenta retention, deficient spermatogenesis, and necrotic and dystrophic changes in skeletal muscle.

Total parenteral nutrition (TPN) is known to be a risk factor for a variety of deficiency diseases involving micronutrients not included in the fluids infused. In 1979, Van Rij et al.[59] reported the case of a 37-year-old New Zealand woman who was admitted to hospital with a performated small bowel, and underwent subsequent surgery requiring TPN for 60 days. On admission she was hypoalbuminemic and anemic, with elevated liver enzymes and a plasma Se of 2.5 μg/dl (normal 5–25 μg/dl). Her urinary Se was 10.4 μg/day. She developed fever due to sepsis, and TPN was started 10 days after admission to the hospital. The solution given contained 25 per cent glucose, 500 ml crystalline amino acids, 500 ml Intralipid per day, electrolytes and vitamins—but no additional trace minerals. During the next 20 days she showed general improvement, with a 6-kg weight gain. Thirty days after commencement of TPN, however, the patient complained of increased bilateral discomfort in her quadriceps and hamstring muscles. Muscle pain was present at rest, and there was tenderness on palpation. Her pain was aggravated by walking, which became increasingly difficult. A generalized muscle wasting of all limbs was observed, despite the TPN. No muscle fasciculation or neurologic deficits were observed. Her plasma selenium had fallen to 0.9 μg/dl, and urinary Se excretion was down to 6 μg/day. A tentative diagnosis of selenium deficiency was made and selenium supplementation of 100 μg selenium as selenomethionine was infused daily with the TPN solution. During the next week, muscle pain at rest, tenderness to palpation, and pain on active and passive movement disappeared. A return to full mobility followed. After seven days of supplementation, her plasma Se rose to 2.2 μg/dl, and urinary losses increased to 9.4 μg Se per day, representing a markedly positive balance. After another 17 days she was discharged, and has remained well at home on an ordinary diet.

This is the first published case of selenium depletion associated with myopathy in which symptomatic response to selenium supplementation was noted. Cumulative selenium loss by one of the New Zealand patients in this study during one month of TPN amounted to 312 μg Se, or about 5 per cent of the total body content of healthy New Zealand residents. It is clear that long-term withdrawal of selenium from the

Table 61.6 Selenium Levels in Selected Populations

Country	Dietary Intake μg per day	Plasma Level μg/dl
United States	60–216	15–20
New Zealand	28–56	5–10
Finland	25–50	3–12
China	<30	<1

regimen of a patient who is conditioned by low body stores of Se and the stress of a surgical procedure with sepsis produces a clinical syndrome of selenium deficiency consistent with the biologic function of Se.

Therapeutic Uses

The only acceptable therapeutic use of selenium at a supraphysiologic level is treatment of selenium deficiency. Claims of selenium as a chemoprotectant against cancer have not been validated. Selenium compounds may both promote and inhibit experimental cancers in animals.[62,63]

Toxicology

The selenium poisoning of livestock was noted in 1856 in Nebraska by a veterinarian who described a fatal disease characterized by loss of hair, nausea, tender feet and unsteady gait called "blind staggers." Selenium poisoning in humans from intakes of 5 to 50 mg Se per day results in nausea and vomiting, loss of hair and nails, skin lesions, tooth decay, and abnormalities of the peripheral CNS. The biochemical effects of these toxic doses appear to relate to disturbances of sulhydryl function and inhibition of protein synthesis. Even 750 to 900 μg/day have been shown in China to result in chronic toxic changes in hair, nails, and Se distribution in the body.

Preparations

Oral preparations of selenium containing 200 μg/tablet are available, as are solutions for IV use containing 33 μg/ml.

Manganese

History

The essentiality of manganese for animals was first reported in 1931[64,65] by investigators who demonstrated that diets devoid of manganese would not support normal growth and reproduction in mice and rats. Subsequently, manganese was reported to be essential for a variety of domestic animals and birds. Abnormalities found in manganese-deficient animals relate to the skeleton and include growth failure, perosis (slipped tendon disease), chondrodystrophy, metabolic bone disease, decreased glucosaminoglycan synthesis in skeletal cartilage, reduced uptake of radioactive sulfate into fetal cartilage, and impaired mucopolysaccharide synthesis.[r23] Furthermore, the *pallid* mouse mutant, which has defective otolith formation, also demonstrates a failure to transport manganese normally.

Despite these clear-cut findings in animals, there is little evidence of a deficiency syndrome in humans. Attempts have been made to deplete manganese stores in human volunteers, but the reduction in the body manganese pool has not led to a unique deficiency syndrome. This result is unexpected, since manganese is implicated in a number of important enzyme systems. These Mn-containing metalloenzymes include pyruvate carboxylase, arginase, one of the superoxide dismutases, glutamine synthetase in brain, and some glycosyl transferases. In addition Mn^{2+} can activate a variety of enzymes that are not manganoproteins.[68]

Chemistry

Manganese is a transition element in period 4 of the periodic table. It has a molecular weight of 54.9 and an atomic number of 25. Manganese has nine radioactive isotopes, ranging from ${}_{25}Mn^{49}$ to ${}_{25}Mn^{62}$. The most useful isotope for biologic studies is ${}_{25}Mn^{54}$ ($t_{1/2}$ = 312 days). The concentration of manganese in the earth's crust is about 0.08 percent, but it is as abundant as carbon and more abundant than sulfur. The most important compounds of manganese are its oxides: MnO_2 (pyrolusite); Mn_2O_3 (braunite), and Mn_3O_4 (hausmannite). Manganese forms alloys with iron to the extent of as much as 80 percent manganese. Manganese exhibits oxidation states of +2, +3, +4, +6, and +7. Most of these compounds are colored and paramagnetic. In enzymes the valence of Mn is either +2 (manganous) or +3 (manganic). Unlike its neighbor chromium, manganese^{2+} is a very poor reducing agent; also unlike Cr^{3+}, Mn^{3+} is a very powerful oxidizing agent. The permanganate ion $(MnO_4)^-$ is a good oxidizing agent especially in acid solution, where it can be reduced to the manganous ion.

Physiology

The absorption of manganese, which is relatively low, is believed to occur throughout the small intestine and is not thought to be under regulatory control. With the aid of ${}_{25}Mn^{54}$, manganese absorption in adults has been reported to range from 2 to 15 percent.[66,67] Manganese homeostasis is accomplished by control of its excretion via the bile and to a much lesser extent by the kidney. For example, 50 percent of a manganese salt injected IV can be recovered in the feces within 24 hours. Manganese entering into the portal blood from the GI tract becomes associated with alpha2- macroglobulin before transversing the liver, where it is almost completely removed. A small fraction enters the systemic circulation after oxidation to Mn^{3+} and is bound to transferrin. Manganese uptake by the liver is a saturable process mediated by a carrier. After uptake by the liver, manganese enters at least five metabolic pools: (1) lysosomes; (2) the bile canaliculi; (3) the mitochondria; (4) the nucleus; (5) the cytoplasm. Various body turnover rates of Mn vary from 1 to

56,100 minutes. Several phases in Mn metabolism have been recognized by using Mn^{54} and are presented in Table 61.7. In addition the concentration of Mn is estimated for several of the components.

The average human body contains between 200 and 400 micromoles of manganese, equivalent to 11 to 22 mg. Manganese tends to be high in tissues rich in mitochondria (related to the content of Mn containing superoxide dismutase). Bone, liver, pancreas, and kidney tend to have higher concentrations of manganese (10 to 50 nmol/g) than other tissues. Concentration of manganese in brain, heart, lung, and muscle are typically less than 20 nanomoles per gram. Blood and serum concentrations are 200 and 20 nanomoles per liter (10 and 1 μg/L), respectively. Typical milk concentrations are of the order of 1 micromole per liter. Bone can account for up to 65 percent of the total body manganese because of its mass.

Manganese can replace magnesium (and vice versa) for a variety of enzymes that are activated by magnesium ion, including hydrolases, kinases, decarboxylases, and transferases. Two cases where manganic ion is specific for activation are (1) manganese-specific glycosyl transferases and (2) phosphoenolpyruvate carboxykinase. Low activities of both of these enzymes have been reported in manganese-deficient animals. Thus, three kinds of manganese-dependent enzymes can be identified: (1) metalloenzymes in which Mn is intrinsic to the enzyme (arginase, pyruvate carboxylase, manganese superoxide dismutase, and glutamine synthetase in brain); (2) enzymes in which Mn is specifically required for activation; (3) enzymes for which Mn^{2+} and Mg^{2+} are interchangeable for activation.

Evidence has been reported[r24] that manganese deficiency in experimental animals causes the down-regulation of the mitochondrial superoxide dismutase at the genetic level. Superoxide dismutases are a class of metalloproteins that catalyze the dismutation of the superoxide radical (O_2) to oxygen (O_2) and hydrogen peroxide (H_2O_2). These enzymes play a critical role in protecting cells against oxidative stress, particularly that produced by drugs. Most mammalian cells contain two forms of this enzyme—one requiring iron and the other requiring manganese. It is generally thought that the latter, present in mitochondria, protects that organelle from potential damage by the superoxide radical produced by the respiratory chain.

Other genetic interrelationships with Mn have been discovered. Congenital ataxia caused by missing or absent otoliths occurs as the result of a mutant gene called *pallid* in mice. This gene also affects pigmentation giving the animals a pale color.[7] The effect of the pallid gene on development of otoliths can be prevented during pregnancy by giving manganese in the diet at approximately 50 times the normal level. In pallid mice, the basic defect responsible for abnormal development of otoliths also appears to be defective mucopolysaccharide synthesis, since incorporation of radioactive sulfate was reduced in the otolithic membrane. Sulfate metabolism in cartilage, however, is not as greatly affected in pallid mice as in manganese-deficient animals.

Mutant pallid mice demonstrate slower transport of manganese, L-dopa (deoxyphenylalanine), and L-tryptophan into bone and brain than do control mice. The possible relationships among manganese, L-dopa, tryptophan, and melanin are of special interest because of the role of manganese in the metabolism of biogenic amines and brain function. The occurrence of the mutant gene *screwneck*, analogous to *pallid*, has recently been reported in mink.

Nutrition Requirements

Manganese is widely distributed in foods, being particularly high in nuts, whole cereals, dried fruits, and leafy vegetables. Several studies of manganese requirements in children and adults have been carried out. Both Everson and Daniels and Engel et al. found that about 1 mg of manganese per day would sustain manganese balance in children five to ten years old. Freeland-Graves and co-workers have recently ob-

Table 61.7 Components Involved in Turnover of ^{54}Mn in Humans

Component of Decay Curve	Half-Time (min)	Probable Store or Action	Pool Size* mg/Kg
1.	0.88	Transcapillary	0.01 (blood)
2.	2.85	Liver mitochondria	2.00 (liver)
3.	36.5	Liver nuclei	
4.	5760.	Soft tissue	0.50 (viscera)
5.	56,160.	Bone	3.50 (bone)

*Amounts estimated from analytical data

served that an intake of about 2 milligrams will maintain manganese balance in healthy college students.[70] The 1980 recommended dietary allowances of the Food and Nutrition Board NAS/NRC[R] state that safe and adequate intakes of manganese for infants range from 0.5 to 1 mg per day and for adults from 2.5 to 5.0 mg per day.

Deficiency Disease

No well-documented case of manganese deficiency in a human subject has ever been reported, although there have been studies of manganese depletion in humans that have not resulted in a specific deficiency syndrome.

The effect of chronic manganese deficiency in young men was investigated by Friedman et al.[70] As part of a manganese balance study, seven male subjects were fed manganese-deficient diets (0.11 mg Mn/d) for 39 days. During the depletion period all the subjects were in negative manganese balance and five developed a fleeting dermatitis (milaria crystallina, i.e., prickly heat) at the end of the study. Diet, feces, urine, and blood were analyzed for manganese. The following data are typical of the group. As shown in Figure 61.7, which depicts the results in a 19-year-old male student of 39 days of depletion, urinary manganese decreased from 8 μg per day to about 1. Associated with this fall, the manganese balance, which was negative to the extent of 1.8 mg per day for the first week came to zero.

On the low-Mn diet, fecal losses accounted for 99 per cent of all measured losses. Urinary and integumental losses were trivial by comparison and were measured in μg/L. The negative balance of Mn persisted for only two weeks on an intake of 0.11 mg/day and accounted for loss of 13.5 mg of an estimated body pool of 20 mg, or a 66 per cent reduction. Urinary Mn values decreased from about 2.1 to 0.21 μg/L, and total blood Mn values declined from 9.3 to 6.6 μg/L. Despite the low intake, there was no further loss of Mn during the remaining four weeks of the depletion period. Body weight was not changed during depletion. At the end of the depletion period, the subject developed an itchy erythematous rash on the upper torso, groin, and thighs. It was diagnosed as miliaria crystallina, sometimes called "prickly heat." Serum calcium and phosphorus increased slightly but significantly during the depletion period, as did alkaline phosphatase, suggesting that Mn depletion caused mobilization of bone salts. Changes in red blood cell count, hemoglobin, and hematocrit were negligible. Serum cholesterol and HDL cholesterol decreased 27 and 8 mg/dl, respectively. There is some evidence that Mn deficiency in rats affects HDL synthesis.[10] The subject was then given a Mn-repletion diet, which brought about the disappearance of his rash, but no significant change in biochemical indices.

On negligible intake, fecal Mn decreased from 1.77 mg/day the first week to 0.2 mg/day the second week, and to less than 0.1 mg/day for the remaining four weeks, indicating that the feces are the main route of excretion. Upon repletion, fecal Mn output increased to 0.60 mg/day the first week and to 1.5 the second week on intakes of 1.5 and 2.5 mg Mn, respectively. Mean Mn intake, output, balance, and mean urinary values for all seven volunteers in this study are presented in Figure 61.7. The plasma values of Mn in the control period were 1.02 ± 0.57 μg/L (SD) in the seven healthy college students, which did not change significantly with depletion or repletion.

It would appear that Mn (the name is derived from mangania, the Greek word for magic or voodoo) is appropriately designated. As a biochemical it is unpredictable, its apoenzymes are promiscuous, and its mul-

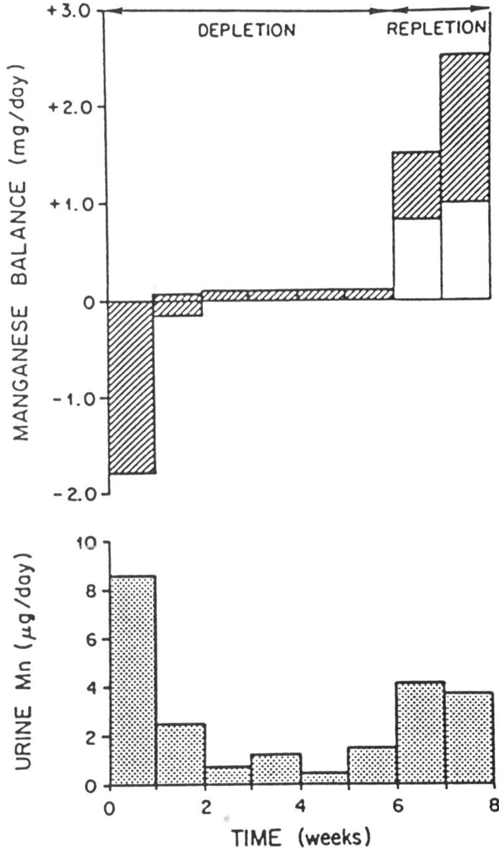

Figure 61.7 Manganese (Mn) intake, output, and balance and urinary excretion in a subject undergoing Mn depletion over 6 weeks and repletion over 10 days. Mn intake is plotted upward from zero, and Mn output is plotted downward from the intake value. The resulting line indicates the balance. Urinary Mn is shown in μg/day.[70]

tiple activities in vitro create illusions that do not exist in vivo. The precise pathophysiology of Mn deficiency in humans remains a challenge to scientists and pediatricians, who will someday identify a real case of Mn deficiency.[69]

Therapeutic Uses

The main use of Mn as a therapeutic agent is the treatment of Mn-deficiency acquired from the use of drugs. Of special interest is hydralazine, an antihypertensive drug with chelating properties, which dilates arteriolar smooth muscle and binds Mn. It was introduced into clinical practice over 30 years ago and has a range of serious side-effects, including the appearance of a lupus erythematosus-like syndrome with neuralgia, arthralgia, fever, antinuclear antibodies, and occasionally rash, lymphadenopathy, chest pain, and hepatosplenomegaly in 10 percent of treated patients. Comens[72] first suggested that this "hydralazine disease" in humans was a conditioned Mn deficiency and showed that Mn supplements would reduce the symptoms in these patients. To substantiate this hypothesis, Comens fed hydralazine to ten-day-old cockerels at a dose of 10 mg/day and induced perosis (slipped tendon disease), a classic sign of Mn deficiency in chicks. When Mn citrate was given with the hydralazine at 5 mg/day, the perosis did not occur and tendon development was normal. The recommended therapeutic dose of Mn for adult humans in 10 mg/day, given as a manganic salt.

Toxicology

Industrial toxicity from inhalation exposure, generally to manganese dioxide in mining or manufacturing, is of two types: The first is manganese pneumonitis, which results from acute exposure. Men working in plants with high concentrations of manganese dust show an incidence of respiratory disease 30 times greater than normal. Pathologic changes include epithelial necrosis followed by mononuclear proliferation. The second and more serious type of disease resulting from chronic inhalation exposure to manganese dioxide over a long period involves the CNS. Those who develop chronic manganese poisoning (manganism) exhibit a psychiatric disorder characterized by irritability, difficulty in walking, speech disturbances, and compulsive behavior that may include running, fighting, and singing. If the condition persists, a masklike facies, propulsion, and a parkinson-like syndrome develop.[73] The outstanding feature of manganese encephalopathy has been classified as severe selective damage to the subthalamic nucleus and palladium. These symptoms and the pathologic lesions, degenerative changes in the basal ganglia, make the analogy to Parkinson's disease plausible. In addition to the CNS changes, liver cirrhosis is frequently observed. Victims of chronic manganese poisoning tend to recover slowly, even when removed from the excessive exposure. Metal-sequestering agents have not produced remarkable recovery; L-dopa, used in the treatment of Parkinsons disease, is of some value.[73]

Preparations

Manganese salts are available for IV use (0.1 mg/ml) and for oral intake in chelated form in doses of 5, 10, 15, and 50 mg/tablet.

Molybdenum

History

The essentiality of molybdenum for N-fixation in bacterial systems was recognized in 1930. Shortly afterward, molybdenum was found to be widely distributed in plants and necessary for their growth. Unequivocal evidence for the importance of the element in human health, however, has been more difficult to obtain. Nutritional studies of Richert and Westerfeld in 1953[74] provided the first evidence that molybdenum was required by animals and was essential for the development and maintenance of tissue xanthine oxidase. Additional research has revealed that the biologic functions of molybdenum in animals can be traced to its role as a prosthetic group in three enzymes, xanthine oxidase/dehydrogenase, aldehyde oxidase, and sulfite oxidase. All these enzymes catalyze oxidation reduction reactions and contain in addition to molybdenum other cofactors such as flavin adenine dinucleotide (FAD), heme, and iron sulfur complexes.[r25]

Genetically-conditioned sulfite oxidase deficiency was first described in 1967 by Mudd, Irreverre, and Laster[75] in a child who had mental retardation, seizures, opisthotonus, and lens dislocation. Subsequently it was found that other children with this syndrome had a combined deficiency of xanthine oxidase and sulfite oxidase owing to the absence of a molybdenum cofactor, a pterin derivation complexed with molybdenum.[76] In ruminants, molybdenum, sulfur, and copper interact to form cupric thiomolybdate complexes.[r28] If molybdenum and sulfate exceed copper intake on a molar basis, copper deficiency can occur. In humans copper deficiency due to molybdenum excess is rare, since ordinary diets contain more copper than molybdenum.

Chemistry

Molybdenum is a transition metal in the fifth period of the periodic table. It has an atomic weight of 95.94 and an atomic number of 42. Molybdenum has naturally occurring isotopes ranging from ${}_{42}Mo^{92}$ to ${}_{42}Mo^{100}$, but the most significant normal ${}_{42}Mo^{96}$ has a prevalence of only 16.7 percent. Molybdenum also has eight radioactive isotopes, ranging from ${}_{42}Mo^{88}$ to ${}_{42}Mo^{93}$. Molybdenum is found in nature as MoS_2 (molybdemite), a blue-gray material of metallic luster. Molybdenum metal is exceedingly hard, melts at 2620°C, and forms complex ions including oxyanions. When heated in air, molydenum sulfide is oxidized to the trioxide MoO_3, which is then reduced to the metal by heating with hydrogen. Mo has four oxidation states: +3; +4; +5; and +6, the most common being the +6 state. The trioxide, MoO_3, dissolves in basic solutions to form a complicated series of oxyanions called molybdates, the simplest of which is $^{-}MoO_4$. In the enzymatic molybdate cofactor, the valence of Mo oscillates from +6 to +4 with oxidation-reduction.

Physiology

Molybdenum is readily and rapidly absorbed from the GI tract. Unlike copper, iron, and zinc, which have highly regulated absorption rates, molybdenum, particularly in the form of hexavalent molybdate, is unregulated and can be absorbed up to 90%. Also unlike many trace minerals, the blood level of Mo in both animals and humans is proportional to dietary intake. Blood molybdenum in the US ranges from 0.5 to 15 μg/dl. Molybdenum levels in tissues vary from 0.1 to 1.0 μg/g. Liver, kidney, adrenal, and bone contain the highest tissue Mo levels and are also responsive to dietary intake.[r23]

Molybdenum must be incorporated into its coenzyme before becoming active in metabolism. The molybdenum coenzyme is a 6-substituted pterin, similar to the pterin moiety in folic acid, which, together with some metabolites, is shown in Figure 61.8. Molybdopterin, which is tetrahydropterin with a 4-carbon side-chain at position 6, which contains an ene-thiol that binds Mo and has a terminal phosphate ester. All tissue molybdenum appears to be complexed with molybdopterin. The molybdenum center of the oxidases is directly involved in oxidative hydroxylation of the substrates. The transfer of electrons from the substrate leads to the reduction of Mo^{+6} to Mo^{+4} and the electrons are then transported to FAD before eventual transfer to the final electron acceptor (NAD, oxygen, or ferredoxin).

The metabolic end-product of molybdenum cofactor is urothione (formula C in Fig. 61.8) in which the cofactor is oxidized to form a thiophene adduct to molybdopterin with loss of molybdenum, hydrolysis of the phosphate, and methylation of the second thiol.

The physiology of molybdenum is related to the three enzymes for which it is a cofactor.[25,26] Sulfite oxidase, an enzyme (MW = 110.00) located in the mitochondrial intermembrane space, catalyzes the terminal step in the metabolism of methionine and cystine. It consists of two identical subunits, one containing the molybdenum cofactor and one a cytochrome b-5 type heme. Cytochrome C is the final electron acceptor in the oxidation of sulfite. The genetic deficiency of sulfite oxidase[75] first described in an infant, was characterized by seizures, mental retardation, dislocation ocular lenses, and, ultimately, death. It is believed that these signs are the result of the toxicity of sulfite and possibly the absence of sulfate for macromolecular syntheses. Sulfate is incorporated into sulfate esters in sulfolipids, sulfated polysaccharides, and glycoproteins via 3'phophoadenosine-5'-phosphosulfate.

Xanthine dehydrogenase is a dimer of 300,000 MW and contains one FAD, two Fe_2S_2 clusters and one molybdenum center per subunit. Xanthine dehydrogenase catalyzes the hydroxylation of hypoxanthine and xanthine to produce uric acid as the final product. The reaction mechanism involves the abstraction of a hydride ion from the substrate and replacement with

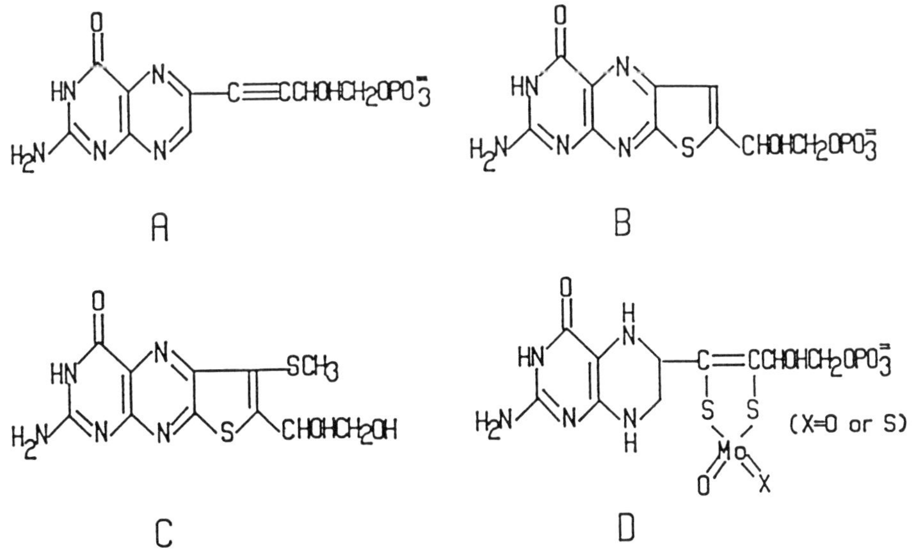

A: HN, H2N, N, C≡CCHOHCH2OPO3=
B: HN, H2N, N, S, CHOHCH2OPO3=
C: HN, H2N, N, S, SCH3, CHOHCH2OH
D: HN, H2N, N, H, C=CCHOHCH2OPO3=, S S, Mo, O, X, (X=O or S)

Figure 61.8 Various derivates of the Mo cofactor. Structures A and B are fluorescent derivatives of a 6-substituted pterin isolated from oxidized samples of sulfite oxidase and xanthine oxidase. C is urothione, which contains a thienopterin ring system and was identified from human urine. D has been proposed for the active Mo cofactor.[r25]

a hydroxyl ion ultimately derived from water substrate binding and oxidative hydroxylation involves the molybdenum center with concomitant reduction of Mo^{6+} to Mo^{4+}, and the electrons are then transferred to FAO. Mo^{6+}. Molybdenum is reoxidized as electrons are transferred to FAD and then to NAD or O_2. Because hypoxanthine and guanine can be reclaimed to a large extent by the action of hypoxanthine guanine phosphoribosyl transferase and because hypoxanthine and xanthine are not highly toxic compounds, deficiencies of xanthine dehydrogenase in humans are largely benign. Xanthinuria is the major sign of the deficiency, which can cause renal stones in some patients.

The molybdoprotein aldehyde oxidase (MW = 270,000) is an enzyme distinct from the group of other aldehyde-metabolizing enzymes, the aldehyde dehydrogenases. The enzyme seems to be restricted to animal cells. The highest activity is present in the liver, but information on the tissue distribution of the enzyme is not available. Aldehyde oxidase is very similar to xanthine oxidase/dehydrogenase in size, cofactor composition, and substrate specificity but does not use NAD or NADP as electron acceptors, and presumably functions as a true oxidase, using only oxygen as its physiologic electron acceptor. Aldehyde oxidase will hydroxylate hypoxanthine to xanthine but converts the latter to uric acid. It metabolizes xenobiotics and appears to be part of the body's general detoxification system. It has been reported that molybdenum will activate adenyl cyclase in some tissues.[78]

The pathway of biosynthesis of molybdenum cofactor appears to involve the pathway already identified for other pterin cofactors, such as tetrohydrobiopterin, the cofactor for phenylalanine hydroxylase.[r27] The precursor of the pterin molecule is guanosine triphosphate, which is converted by a GTP cyclohydroxylase to dihydroneopterin triphosphate. In plants and microorganisms this intermediate is converted to folic acid, in animals to tetrohydrobiopterin. It is likely that the four-carbon side-chain, which is one carbon longer than that of tetrahydrobiopterin, is derived from some component in GTP, possibly the formate carbon lost in dihydrobiopterin synthesis. Finally, the hydroxyl groups in the side-chain can exchange with sulfydryl groups to yield molybdopterin.

Nutritional Requirements

The molybdate requirement of most animals is very low. Even on diets containing 0.02 μg/g of Mo, rats grow normally, reproduce, synthesize xanthine oxidase, and oxidize xanthine normally. When a metabolic competitor of Mo, is added to low-Mo diets, growth depression is seen in chicks, goats, and minipigs. Molybdenum deficiency has not been observed in humans unless they: (1) have a genetic disease that blocks the synthesis of molybdopterin essential for molybdenum retention and action in tissues; or (2) they are on long-term total parenteral nutrition without molybdenum supplements.

The range of intake of molybdenum by Americans is 76 to 240 μg/day, with an average of about 180 μg/day.[77] Cows' milk contains about 40 μg/liter, but human milk is lower, i.e., 2 μg/liter. The molybdenum content of vegetables is influenced by the content of molybdenum in the soil. The foods that contribute most to dietary levels of molybdenum are milk, beans, breads, and cereals. The Food and Nutrition Board of the NRC/NAS in the US has set the adequate and safe levels for adults at 75 to 250 μg/day. For infants, the recommendation is 15 to 40 μg/day; for children, 25 to 75 μg/day.[31]

Deficiency Disease

Clinical molybdenum deficiency has not been achieved in experimental animals. Conditional molybdenum deficiency following the addition of sulfate or copper to diets low in Mo has reduced growth of chickens and goats and reduced fertility and fetal survival. Molybdenum deficiency in a 24-year-old male with Crohn's disease was reported by Abumrad et al.[79] This patient, who had had previous malabsorption for 12 years, had been on TPN 18 months following multiple small bowel resections for his Crohn's disease. After 12 months on TPN, the patient developed symptoms of intolerance to the TPN solution fortified only with zinc, copper, manganese, and iodide as sources of micronutrients. This was expressed as tachycardia, tachypnea, headache, nausea, and vomiting, leading to disorientation and coma. A metabolic study of urinary metabolites showed high levels of sulfite and thiosulfite and low sulfate, symptomatic of sulfite oxidase deficiency, and high levels of hypoxanthine and xanthine and low uric acid, symptomatic of xanthine oxidase deficiency. His plasma, furthermore, had high levels of methionine, marginal levels of taurine, and low levels of urate. A diagnosis of molybdenum deficiency was made and supplementation of the TPN solution with 300 μg/day of Mo led to a dramatic decrease in the urinary content of the abnormal metabolites and the capacity to tolerate the TPN treatment. These important findings provide a convincing argument for supplementation of TPN regimes with Mo, particularly when there is a long history of previous malabsorption and malnutrition.

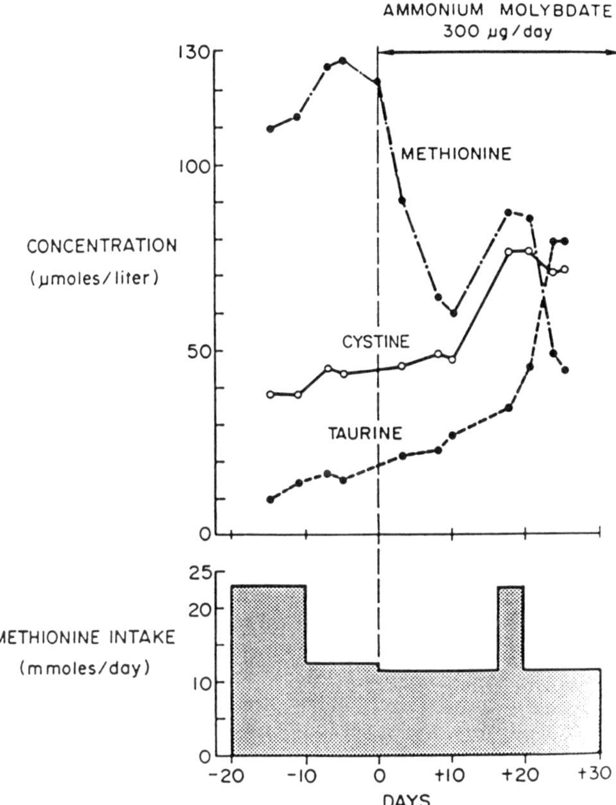

Figure 61.9 Plasma levels of methionine, cystine, and taurine in response to TPN solution containing different loads of methionine, before and after treatment with 300 µg/day of ammonium molybdate. Each *point* represents a mean of two determinations.[79]

Low molybdenum intakes in Chinese farmers in Hunan province showed an inverse relationship of Mo intake and plasma Mo levels to mortality from esophageal cancer. In a preliminary report these same authors stated that Mo supplementation inhibited the esophageal cancer induced in male rats given N-nitrosarcosine ethyl ester.[80] Molybdenum supplementation of the genetically induced molybdopterin deficiency has no effect on the metabolic disorders observed because Mo *per se* cannot function as a coenzyme in these diseases.

Therapeutic Uses

Mo given to deficient animals or humans corrects the deficiency and restores normal metabolism.[6,r23] It has no other known function. It must be emphasized, however, that molybdenum deficiency is rare in animals and unknown in humans with normal intestinal absorption receiving a mixed diet. Its possible function in the chemoprevention of cancer is a hypothesis requiring much additional study.

Toxicology

The effect of molybdate intake on tissues depends on the age and species of the animal. Relative amounts of molybdenum in the diet induce copper deficiency by the formation of thiomolybdates in the gut, which inhibits the absorption of copper. This effect is most prominent in ruminants, but also is seen in nonruminants to a lesser extent. Molybdenum toxicity in humans has been reported rarely. Persons on diets high in molybdenum (10–15 mg/day) in the 1950s were reported to develop arthralgias, deformities, and edema associated with high urate (81 ± 4 mg/dl) and high Mo (31 ± 2 µg/dl). Miners exposed to dusts of the order of 10 mg/day developed only nonspecific complaints.[r25]

Preparations

The only preparations of Mo available are solutions of about 25 µg/ml for administration to patients on TPN.

Iodine

History

Iodine was discovered by the French chemist, Courtois, in 1812 while he was engaged in the manufacture of gunpowder for the Napoleonic wars. Some seaweed ash was being used in the process, which volatilized a violet vapor that Cortois collected and studied. In 1819, Fyfe discovered iodine in the sea sponge; in the same year, Coindet, a Swiss physician, claimed that goiter, very common in the Alps, could be cured by iodine. Its use by physicians in the therapy of goiter, however was abandoned because of alleged deleterious side-effects.[r29] Between 1820 and 1876, Chatin, a French chemist, analyzed food and water for iodine and postulated a negative correlation between iodine intake and goiter, but his conclusions were neglected until 1910–1920, when David Marine made the same observations in the Great Lakes region of the United States.[81] Baumann identified iodine in the thyroid gland in 1895,[82] and thyroxine was isolated by the American chemist Kendall in 1915,[83] followed by the elucidation of its structure in 1926 by Harington and Barger[84] in London. Plummer first reported in 1923 that iodide could reduce the thyrotoxicosis of Graves' disease in the perioperative period, thus introducing it as an antithyroid drug.

Chemistry

Iodine is a halogen (Group VII) in the fifth period of the periodic table. It has an atomic number of 53 and an atomic weight of 127. It has no naturally-occurring isotopes but has 33 radioactive isotopes, ranging from ${}_{53}I^{110}$ to ${}_{53}I^{140}$, of which the most useful in biology are ${}_{53}I^{125}$, a β-emitter with a half-life 60 days, and ${}_{53}I^{131}$, a γ-emitter with a half-life of eight days. Iodine occurs in soil and sea as iodide, which is oxidized by sunlight to iodine and vaporizes into the air.

The concentration of iodide in sea water is 50 to 60 μg/L; in the air it is 0.7 μg/m^3. Some of this iodide is returned to the soil by rain, but much is lost in the stratosphere. This photolysis of iodine accounts for the continuing depletion of iodide in soil, its lack of capture by plants, and continuing iodine deficiency in humans, particularly at higher altitudes in the Third World. Iodine-deficient areas have iodide levels less than 2 μg/L in drinking water (Andes, Alps, Himalayas), whereas in iodide-replete areas the drinking water contains 4 to 10 μg/L.

Fortunately, iodine also is present as sodium iodide in salt wells and as sodium iodate in Chile saltpeter ($NaNO_3$). Iodine crystallizes as black leaflets with a metallic luster. It is only slightly soluble in water, but readily soluble in solutions of iodide to form a brown solution. Iodine vapor is violet, but iodide solutions are colorless. I_2 forms a deep blue color with starch. It is the only halogen that can occur in a positive oxidation state, +5 in iodate and +7 in periodate. Iodine solutions are antiseptic. Traces of sodium iodide (70 μg/gm) are added to table salt as a preventative for iodine deficiency and goiter.

Physiology

The primary function of iodine in the body is to provide substrate for the synthesis of the thyroid hormones, thyroxine (3,5,3′,5′-tetraiodothyronine also known as T_4) and triiodothyronine (3,5,3′-triiodothyronine [T_3]). The hormones are crucial for normal growth and development of mammals. The thyroid gland weighs 15 to 20 grams and contains 80 percent of the body iodine pool of about 15 mg.[r30]

Iodine is rapidly absorbed from the GI tract and distributed in extracellular water. The fasting plasma concentration is about 1 μg/L. Of about 100 μg absorbed, 80 μg is trapped by the thyroid gland through

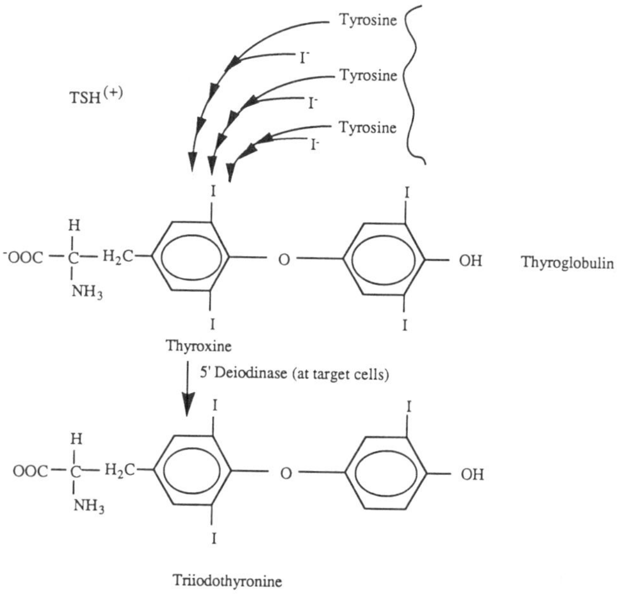

Figure 61.10 Schematic Representation of Thyroid Hormone Synthesis

an ATP-dependent iodide pump that concentrates the I^- 100 or more times in the cytoplasm of the thyroid follicular cell. Thyroglobulin, a glycoprotein (MM = 650,000) rich in tyrosine residues, is synthesized by the thyroid cell, undergoes iodination of selected tyrosine residues by I_2 produced by a thyroperoxidase located at the apical membrane of the cell, and is stored in the lumen of the follicle. The thyroperoxidase also couples individual iodinated tyrosines into iodothyronines.

In the secretory process, follicular cells internalize thyroglobulin and introduce it into lysosomes, which digest the peptide-bound thyronines and release them as T_3 and T_4 into the circulation. About 60 μg of iodine is released daily from the gland in the form of T_4 (60%) and T_3 (40%). Plasma levels of T_4 are normally 50 to 120 μg/L; of T_3, 0.7 to 1.9 μg/L. The hormones are deiodinated in the target cells after exerting their hormonal effects. This event returns iodide to the circulation. About 90 percent of the absorbed dose of iodide is excreted in the urine and 10 percent in the feces.

The power of the thyroid gland to concentrate I^- is enhanced in iodine deficiency about fourfold, and the gland hypertrophies under the influence of thyroid stimulating hormone (TSH) of the pituitary. The circulating level of iodothyronines, which decrease in iodine deficiency, stimulates the hypothalamus to secrete thyrotropin-releasing hormone, which acts on the pituitary to secrete TSH.

Thyroid hormones are transported in the plasma bound to several proteins. These are thyroxine binding protein (TBG), thyroxine binding prealbumin (transthyretin), and albumin. Thyroxine should be regarded as a prohormone, since the most active form in cells is T_3. T_4 is transferred to target cells from its carrier protein, diffuses through the cell membrane, is converted to T_3, and reacts with a carrier protein that ferries it to the nuclear receptor for action. The thyroid hormone receptors (THRα and THRβ) are part of a family of steroid, thyroid, and fat-soluble vitamin receptors that have related structures and that result in the expression of genes specific for each ligand.[86] All thyroid hormone receptors contain 410 amino acids distributed in conventional domains, i.e., (a) short enhancer region, (b) a DNA-binding region, and (c) a thyroid hormone binding region. T_3 is bound much more tightly than T_4. These receptors are transcription factors, which find response elements in the promoter of each gene expressed.[r30]

Thyroid hormones are required for normal growth and development of humans, including cerebral development. One of the tragedies of iodine deficiency in pregnancy is the failure of the fetus to develop a normal brain, which results in cretinism. The calorigenic effects of thyroid hormone appear to be due to expression of the gene for the Na^+, K^+, ATPase and its electron cou-

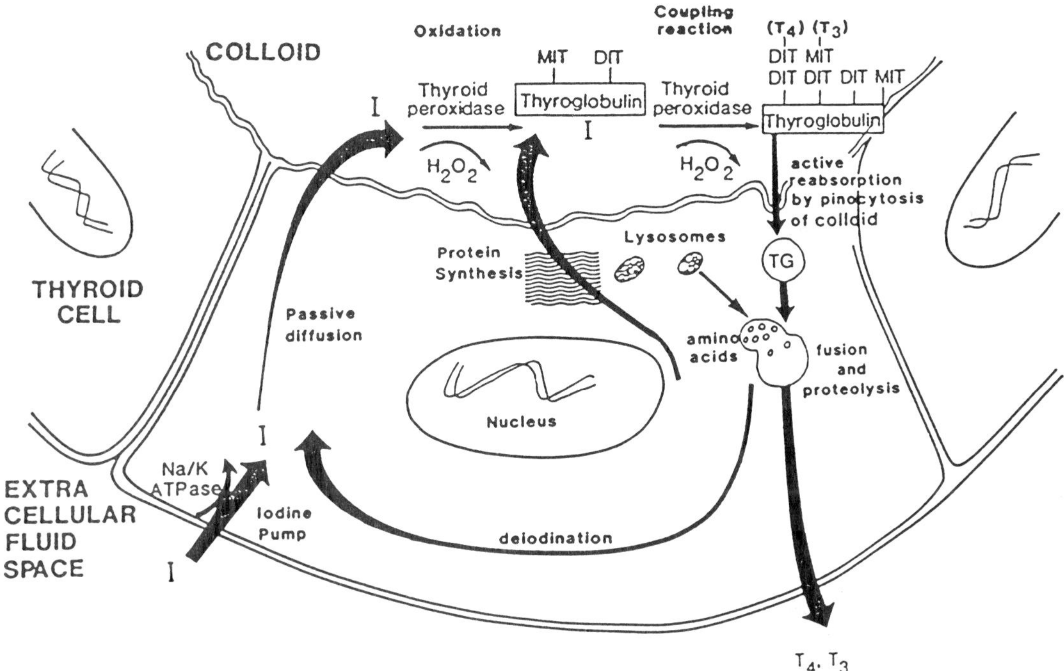

Figure 61.11 Diagram Showing Pathways of Synthesis of Thyroid Hormones From Iodine Within the Thyroid Gland.[32]

pling enzyme, α-glycerophosphate dehydrogenase. Other enzymes known to be affected by T_3 include malic dehydrogenase and many involved in protein synthesis.

Nutrition Requirements

It is estimated that 10 percent of the world population live on diets providing only 25 μg of iodine per day and thus are heir to all the consequences of iodine deficiency. Adding iodized salt to provide another 70 μg/gram of salt per day prevents the onset of goiter. In 1985–86 the iodine intake in the US was 250 μg/d for males and 170 μg/d for females. The Pan American Health Organization (PAO) considered 50 μg of urinary iodine/gram of creatinine as adequate, 25 to 50 μg/gram of creatinine borderline, and less than 25 μg/g as indicative of serious risk for iodine deficiency. Hetzel[r31] recommends 1 to 2 μg/kg for adults. The Food and Nutrition Board of the NAS/NRC recommends 150 μg/day for both men and women, 6 μg/kg/day for infants, 5 μg/kg for young children, and 4 μg/kg for older children. Pregnant and lactating females should take 175 to 200 μg/day.[31]

Deficiency Disease

Iodine deficiency reduces production of thyroid hormones, especially T_4, and reduces the rate of energy metabolism. Iodine deficiency (and the resulting reduction in iodothyronines) mobilize TSH and increase iodine retention by the body. TSH also stimulates synthesis of thyroglobulin and plasma TBG. This directly or indirectly causes hypertrophy and/or hyperplasia of thyroid follicles and increases the extent to which the thyroid can capture iodine. If this adaptation fails, hypothyroidism occurs, causing cretinism in newborns and myxedema in adults. The resulting enlarged thyroid, or goiter, usually can be treated by dietary iodine.

While iodine deficiency is always present to some extent in goiter, it is not the only factor precipitating this disease. Genetic tendencies, including defects in enzymes involving iodine and thyroid metabolism, as well as intake of "goitrogens," play a role. Goitrogens are present to a variable degree in many foodstuffs, notably rutabagas, turnips, and cabbages, and some of these (e.g., goitrin) have been isolated. The drug proplthiouracil is also a goitrogen. Goitrogens cause goiter by inhibiting the synthesis of thyroid hormones.

As already pointed out, iodine deficiency of the fetus is the result of iodine deficiency in the mother.

The condition is associated with a greater incidence of stillbirths, abortions, and congenital abnormalities. Iodine deficiency in children is characteristically associated with goiter. The goiter rate increases with age so that it reaches a maximum with adolescence. Girls are more affected than boys. Goiter rates in 8- to 14-year-old school children are a convenient indicator of iodine deficiency in a community. School children living in iodine-deficient areas from a number of countries show impaired school performance and lower IQs compared with matched groups from areas not iodine-deficient. The iodine deficiency disorders are shown in Table 61.8.

Therapeutic Uses

The treatment of iodine deficiency requires about 10 times the RDA or 1.5 mg/day for several weeks to restore the iodine content of the depleted gland. The output of T_4 returns to normal and remains at that level. In hyperthyroidism, 1 to 2 mg/day will inhibit hormone release and ameliorate the symptoms. This use of megadoses of I^- is well established in the preparation of hyperthyroid patients for surgery.

Table 61.8 The Spectrum of Iodine Deficiency Disorders (IDD)

Fetus	Abortions Stillbirths Congenital anomalies Increased perinatal mortality Increased infant mortality Neurologic cretinism (Mental deficiency, deaf mutism, spastic diplegia, squint) Myxedematous cretinism (dwarfism, mental deficiency) Psychomotor defects
Neonate	Neonatal goiter Neonatal hypothyroidism
Child and Adolescent	Goiter Juvenile hypothyroidism Impaired mental function Retarded physical development
Adult	Goiter with its complications Hypothyroidism Impaired mental function Iodine induced hyperthyroidism

Data from Hetzel BS, Potter BJ, Dulberg EM: World Rev. Nutr. Diet., 62:59–119, 1990; and Hetzel BS, Dunn JT, Stanbury JB (eds.): The Prevention and Control of Iodine Deficiency Disorders. Amsterdam, Elsevier, 1987).

The use of even larger doses of iodide in normal persons (100–200 mg/day) can shut off T_4 synthesis for a time and cause hypothyroidism. Most persons adapt to these megadoses, but some do not. In vulnerable patients two extremes may occur: (1) they may develop myxedema; or 2) they may develop hyperthyroidism (Jod-Basedow's disease). The reason for these idiosyncrases is not fully understood.

Toxicology

In some coastal areas in Japan, inhabitants may get as much as 50 to 80 mg I/day with high plasma levels (200–400 mg/LO and massive excretion of 20–30 mg/day. Some of these persons develop goiters, but many remain euthyroid. As noted, after medical treatment with megadoses of iodide, a few develop myxedema and some develop hyperthyroidism.

Preparations

Multivitamin mineral capsules may contain 150 μg iodide. Certain cough syrups may contain 150 μg per 5 ml.

References

Research Reports

1. Christian HA. A sketch of the history of the treatment of chlorosis. Med Lab Hist J, 1903:*1*:176–180.
2. Hahn PF, Bale WF, Ross JF, Balfour WM, Whipple GH. Radioactive iron absorption by the gastrointestinal tract: Influence of anemia, anoxia, and antecedent feeding; distribution in growing dogs. J Exp Med 1943;*78*:169–188.
3. Dalman PR, Yip R, Johnson C. Prevalence and causes of anemia in the United States. Am J Clin Nutr 1984;*39*:437–445.
4. Munro HN, Kikinis Z, Eisenstein RS. Iron dependent regulation of ferritin synthesis. In Berdanier CD, Hargrove JH, Nutrition and Gene Expression. Boca Raton, FL, CRC Press, 1993.
4. Hubers HA, Finch CA. The physiology of transferrin and transferrin receptors. Physiol Rev 1987;*67*:520–581.
5. Zakim MM. Regulation of transferrin gene expression. FASEB J 1992;*6*:3253–3258.
6. Peters JJ, Raja KB, Simpson RJ, Snape S. Mechanisms and regulation of iron absorption. Ann NY Acad Sci 1988;*526*:141–147.
7. Davidson LA, Lonnerdal B. Specific binding of lactoferrin to brush-border membrane: Ontogeny and effect of glycon chain. Am J Physiol 1988;*254*:G580–G585.
9. McCance RA, Widdowson EM. Absorption and excretion of iron. Lancet 1937;*233*:680–684.
10. Hallberg L. Bioavailability of iron in man. Ann Rev Nutr 1981;*1*:123–147.
11. Casey JL, Mentze MW, Koeller DM. Iron-responsive elements: Regulatory RNA sequences that control mRNA levels and translation. Science 1988;*240*:924–928.

12. Theil EC. Regulation of ferritin and transferrin receptor mRNAs. J Biol Chem 1990;*265*:4771–4774.

13. Johnson MA. Iron: Nutrition monitoring and nutrition status assessment. J Nutr 1990;*120*:1486–1491.

14. Bothwell TH, Charlton RW. A general approach to the problems of iron deficiency and iron overload in the population at large. Sem in Hematol 1982;*19*:54–67.

15. Salonen JT, Nyysson K, Korpela H, Tuomilehto J, Seppanen R, Salonen R. High stored iron levels are associated with excess risk of myocardial infarction in Eastern Finnish men. Circulation 1992;*86*:803–811.

16. Crosby WH. The safety of iron-fortified food. JAMA 1978;*239*:2026–2027.

17. Raulen MJ. Chemical studies on vegetation. Ann Sci Nat Bot Biol Veg (Ser. 5) 1969;*11*:93–299.

18. Todd WR, Elvejhem CA, Hart EB. Zinc in the nutrition of the rat. Am J Physiol *107*:146–156.

19. Keilin D, Mann T. Carbonic anhydrase. Nature (London) 1939;*144*:442–444.

20. Prasad AJ, Halsted JA, Nadami M. Syndrome of iron deficiency anemia, splenomegaly, hypogonadism, and geophagia. Am J Med 1961;*31*:532–546.

21. Prasad AS, Meali A Jr, Faid Z, Shulert A, Sandstead HH. Zinc metabolism in patients with a syndrome of iron deficiency anemia, hepatomegaly, hypogonadism and dwarfism. J Lab Clin Med 1963;*61*:537–549.

22. Prasad AS, Meali A Jr, Farid Z, Sandstead HH, Schulert AR, Darby WJ. Biochemical studies in dwarfism, hypogonadism and anemia. Arch Int Med 1963;*111*:407–428.

23. Nelder KH, Hambridge KM. Zinc therapy of acrodermititis enteropathica. N Engl J Med 1975;*292*:879–882.

24. Durnam DM, Palmiter R. Transcriptional regulation of the mouse metallothionine-I gene by heavy metals. J Biol Chem 1981;*256*:6712–6716.

25. Durnam DM, Hoffman JS, Quaife CJ, Palmiter RD. Induction of mouse metallothionine in RNA by bacterial endotoxin Proc Nat Acad Sci 1984;*81*:1053–56.

26. Hager LJ, Palmiter RD. Transcriptional regulation of mouse liver metallothionein I by glucocorticoids. Nature 1981;*291*:340–342.

27. Shay NF, Cousins RJ. Dietary regulation of metallothionein expression. In: Berdanier CD, Hargrove JL, eds. Nutrition and Gene Expression. Boca Raton, FL: CRC Press, 1993.

28. Castro CE, Kaspin LC, Chen SS, Nolker SG. Zinc deficiency increases the frequency of single strand DNA breaks in rat liver. Nutr Res 1992;*12*:721–736.

29. Cousins RJ, Leinhart AS. Tissue specific regulation of zinc metabolism and metallothionine genes by interleukin 1. FASEB J 1988;*2*:2884–2890.

30. Halstead JA, Smith JC Jr, Irwin MI. A conspectus of research on zinc requirements of man. J Nutr 1974;*104*:345–378.

31. Recommended Dietary Allowances, NAS, NRC. Washington: National Academy Press, 1989.

32. Sandstead HH. Are trace element requirements meeting the needs of the user? In Trace Elements in Man and Animals. Mills CF, Bremner J, Chester JK. FEMA 5 Agricultural Bureau, Royal Commission, UK 1985.

33. Hambidge KM, Hambidge C, Jacobs M, Baum JD. Low levels of zinc in hair, anorexia, poor growth and hypogeusia in children. Pediatr Res 1972;*6*:868–874.

34. Mahajan SK, Prasad AS, Rabbani P, Briggs WA, McDonald FD. Zinc deficiency: A reversible complication of uremia. Am J Clin Nutr 1982;*36*:1177–1183.

35. Hill GM, Brewer GJ, Prasad AS, Hydrick CR, and Hutmann DE. Treatment of Wilson's disease with zinc. I. Oral zinc therapy regimens. Hepatology 1987;*7*:822–826.

36. Price D, Joshi JG. Ferritin: A zinc detoxicant and a zinc ion donor. Proc Natl Acad Sci USA 1982;*79*:3116–3119.

37. Beethof RL. Zinc toxicity. In Handbook on Toxicity of Inorganic Compounds. Ed. H.G. Seiler & H. Sidel, Marcel Dekker, 1988, NY, NY.

38. Prasad AS, Brewer GJ, Schoomaker EB, Rabbania P. Hypocupremia induced by zinc therapy in adults. JAMA 1978;*240*:2166–2168.

39. Hart EB, Steenbock J, Waddel J, Cartwright G. Iron in nutrition VII. Copper as a supplement to iron for hemoglobin building in the rat. J Biol Chem 1928;*77*:797–812.

40. Gibbs K, Walshe JN. Biliary excretion of copper in Wilson's disease. Lancet 1980:2:538–541.

41. Menkes JH, Alter M, Steigleder GK, Weakley DR, Sung JH. A sex-linked recessive disorder with retardation of growth, peculiar hair and focal cerebral and cerebellar degeneration. Pediatrics 1962;*29*:764.

42. Cordano A, Baertl JM, Graham GG. Copper deficiency in infancy. Pediatrics 1964;*34*:324–336.

43. Lee GR, Cartwright GE, Wintrobe MM. Heme biosynthesis in copper deficient swine. Proc Soc Exp Biol Med 1968;*127*:977–981.

44. Fischer PWF, Giroux A, L'Abbe MR. Effect of dietary zinc on intestinal copper absorption. Am J Clin Nutr 1981;*34*:1670–1675.

45. Harris EO. Copper transport. Proc Soc Exp Biol Med 1991;*196*:130–146.

46. Menkes JH, Alter M, Steigleder GK, Weakley DR, Sung JH. A sex-linked recessive disorder with retardation of growth, peculiar hair and focal cerebral and cerebellar degeneration. Pediatrics 1962:*29*:764–770.

47. Davies K. Cloning the Menkes disease gene. Nature 1993;*361*:98.

48. Walshe JM. Copper chelation in patients with Wilson's disease. Q J Med 1973;*29*:764–779.

49. Klevay LM, Inman L, Johnson LK, Lawler M, Mahalko JR, Milne DB, Lukaski HC, Bolochuk W, Sandstead HH. Increased cholesterol in plasma in a young man during experimental copper deficiency. Metab 1984;*33*:1112–1118.

50. Schwartz K, Foltz CM. Selenium as an integral part of factor 3 against dietary chronic liver degeneration. J Am Chem Soc 1957;*79*:3292–3293.

51. Olson RE. Vitamin E and its relationship to heart disease. Circulation 1973;*48*:179–184.

52. Rotruck JT, Pope AL, Ganther HE, Swanson AB, Hafeman DG, Hoekstra WG. Selenium: Biochemical role as a component of glutathione peroxidase. Science 1973;*179*:588–591.

53. Burk RF, Lane JM. Modification of chemcial toxicity by selenium deficiency. Fund. Applied. Toxicol. 1983;*3*:218–221.

54. Yang JG, Geo K, Chen J, Chen X. Selenium-related endemic diseases and the daily selenium requirement of humans. World Rev Nutr Diet 1988;*55*:98–152.

55. Thomson CD, Robinson MF. Selenium in human health and disease with emphasis on these aspects peculiar to New Zealand. Am J Clin Nutr 1980;*33*:303–323.

56. Berry MJ, Banu L, Larson PR. Type I iodothyronine deiodinase is a selenocysteine containing enzymes. Nature 1991;*349*:438–40.

57. Keshan Disease Research Group of the Chinese Academy of Medical Sciences, Beijing: Epidemiologic studies on the etiologic relationship of selenium and Keshan disease. Chinese Med J 1979;*92*:477–482.

58. Keshan Disease Research Group of the Chinese Academy of Medical Sciences, Beijing. Observations on effect of sodium selenite in prevention of Keshan disease. Chinese Med J 1979;*92*:471–476.

59. van Rij AM, Thomson CD, McKenzie JM, Robinson MF. Selenium deficiency in total parenteral nutrition. Am J Clin Nutr 1979;*32*:2076–2085.

60. Amin S, Cheasy RA, Collipp PJ, Castro-Masana M, Maddariah, VT, Klein SW. Selenium in premature infants. Nutr Metab 1980;*24*:331–340.

61. Cohen HJ, Brown MR, Hamilton D, Lyons-Patterson J, Avissar N, Liegy P. Glutathione peroxidase and selenium deficiency in patients receiving home parenteral nutrition: Time course for development of deficiency and repletion of enzyme activity in plasma and blood cells. Am J Clin Nutr 1989;*49*:132–139.

62. Clark LC. The epidemiology of selenium and cancer. Fed Proc 1985;*44*:2584–2589.

63. Schranzer GN. Selenium and cancer. Bioorganic Chem 1976;*5*:275–285.

64. Kemmerer AR, Elvenhjem CA, Hart EB. Studies on the relationship of manganese to the nutrition of a mouse. J Biol Chem 1931;*92*:623–630.

65. Orent EE and McCollum EV. Effects of deprivation of manganese in the rat. J Biol Chem 1931;*92*:651–678.

66. Mena I, Marin O, Fuenzalida S, Cotzias GC. Chronic manganese poisoning: Clinical picture and manganese turnover. Neurology 1967;*17*:128–136.

67. Davidson G, Cedarblad A, Hagel E, Lonnerdal B. Intrinsic and extrinsic labeling for studies of manganese absorption in humans. J Nutr 1988;*118*:1517–1521.

68. Utter ME. Manganese dependent enzymes. Med. Clinics North America 1976;*60*:713–727.

69. Manganese Deficiency in Humans: Fact or Fiction? Nutr Rev 1988;*46*:348–352.

70. Friedman BJ, Freeland-Graves JH, Bales CW, Behmardi F, Shorey Kutche RL, Willis RA, Crosby JB, Trickett PC, Houston SD, Manganese balance and clinical observations in young men fed a manganese-deficient diet. J Nutr 1988;*118*:764–773.

71. Kawano J, Neg DM, Keen CL, Schneeman BO. Altered high density lipoprotein composition in manganese-deficient Sprague-Daivley and Wistan rats. J Nutr 1987;*117*:902–906.

72. Comens P. Manganese depletion as an etiological factor in hydralazine disease. Am J Med 1956;*20*:944–945.

73. Mena I, Kazuko H, Burke K, Cotzias GC. Chronic manganese poisoning. Neurology 1969;*19*:1000–1006.

74. Richert D, Westerfeld WW. Isolation and identification of the xanthine oxidase factor as molybdenum. J Biol Chem 1953;*203*:915–923.

75. Mudd SH, Irreverre F, Laster L. Sulfite oxidase deficiency in man. Demonstration of the enzymatic defect. Science 1967;*156*:1599–1602.

76. Johnson JL, Rajagopalan DV. Human sulfite oxidase deficiency characterization of the molecular defect in a multicomponent system. Proc Natl Acad Sci 1982;*79*:6856–6860.

77. Tsongas TA, Meglen RR, Uabravens PA, Chappell WR. Molybdenum in the diet: An estimate of average daily intake in the U.S. Am J Chem Nutr 1980;*33*:1103–1107.

78. Richards JM, Sunslocki NI. Activation of adenylate cyclase by molybdate. J Biol Chem 1979;*254*:6857–6860.

79. Abumrad NM, Schnieder AJ, Steel D, Rogers LS. Amino acid intolerance during prolonged total parenteral nutrition reversed by molybdate therapy. Am J Clin Nutr 1981;*34*:2551–2559.

80. Luo XM, Wei HJ, Yang SP. Inhibitory effects of molybdenum on esophageal and forestomach carcinogenesis in rats. J Nat Cancer Inst 1983;*17*:75–80.

81. Kimball OP, Marine D. Iodine-lack as a cause of goiter. Arch Intern Med 1918;*22*:41–48.

82. Baumann H. Iodine in the thyroid gland. Physiol Chemie 1896;*21*:329–334.

83. Kendall EC. Isolation of thyroxine. JAMA 1915;*64*:2042–2044.

84. Harington OR, Barger G. Thyroxine III Constitution of thyroxine. Biochem J 1927;*21*:169–183.

85. Evans RM. The steroid and thyroid receptor family. Science 1988;*244*:889–894.

Reviews

r1. Fairbanks VF, Fahey JL, Beutler E. History of iron in medicine. In Clinical Disorders of Iron Metabolism, 2d ed. New York: Grune and Stratton, 1971.

r2. Dallman PR. Iron. Ed. M. Brown. In present knowledge in nutrition. 6th ed. pp 241–250 ILSI Nutr. Foundation Washington DC, 1990.

r3. Charlton RW, Bothwell TH. Iron absorption. Ann Rev Med 1983;*34*:55–68.

r4. Hillman RS, Finch CA. Drugs effective in iron deficiency and other hypochronic anemias. In Goodman & Gilman Pharmacologic Basis of Therapeutics, pp. 1308–1322, MacMillan, NY, NY.

r5. Fairbanks VF, Iron in medicine and nutrition. In Olson JA, Shils ME. Modern Nutrition in Health and Disease, 8th ed. Philadelphia: Lea & Febiger, 1994.

r6. Underwood EJ. Zinc. In Trace Elements in Humans and Animal Nutrition 2d ed. New York: Academic Press, 1962.

r7. Hansen MA, Fernandez G, Good RA. Nutrition and immunity and the role of zinc in the immune response. Ann Rev Nutr 1982;*2*:151–178.

r8. Cousins RJ, Hempe JM. Zinc. In Present Knowledge in Nutrition. Washington: ILSI Nutr. Foundation, 1990.

r9. Prasad AS. Deficiency of zinc in man and its toxicity. In Prasad A, Oberles D. eds. Trace Elements in Human Health and Disease, Vol. I. New York: Academic Press, 1976.

r10. Solomons NW. Zinc and Copper. In Shils ME, Young V. eds. Modern Nutrition in Health and Disease, 6th ed. Philadelphia: Lea & Febiger.

r11. Bremner, I, Beattie JH. Metallothionein and the trace minerals. Ann Rev Nutr 1990;*10*:63–83.

r12. Hamer DH. Metallothionein. Ann Rev Bioch 1986;*55*:913–951.

r13. Danks, D.M. Disorders of copper transport. In Metabolic Basis of Inherited Disease 6th Ed; Ed. Scriver CR, Beaudet AL, Sly WS, Valle D. eds. pp 1411–1431, McGraw Hill, NYC, 1989.

r14. Scheinberg IH, Sternlieb I. Wilson's Disease. Philadelphia, WB Saunders, 1984.

r15. Turnland JR, Copper, Shils ME, Olson JA, Shike M. eds. Modern Nutrition in Health and Disease, 8th ed. Philadelphia: Lea & Febiger, 1994.

r16. Gosselin RE, Hodges HC, Smith RP. Clinical Toxicology of Commercial Products, 4th ed., Baltimore: Williams & Wilkins, MD, 1977.

r17. Wilbur CG. Toxicology of selenium: A review. Clin Toxicol, *17*:171–230.

r18. Levander OA, Burk RF. Selenium. In Brown M. eds. Present Knowledge of Nutrition 6th ed. Washington: ILSI-NUTR. Rev. 1990.

r19. Levander OA, Burk RF. Selenium. In Shils ME, Olson JA, Shike M. Modern Nutrition in Health and Disease, 8th ed. Philadelphia: Lea & Febiger, 1994.

r20. Burk RF, Hill KE. Regulation of selenoproteins. Ann Rev Nutr 1993;*13*:65–81.

r21. Sunde RA. Molecular biology of selenoproteins. Ann Rev Nutr 1990;*10*:451–474.

r22. Anonymous. Selenium deficiency in a woman given total parenteral nutrition. Nutr Rev 1985;*43*:339–341.

r23. Underwood EJ. Molybdenum. In Trace Elements in Human and Animal Nutrition, 2d ed. New York: Academic Press, 1962.

r24. Keen CL, Zidenberg-Cher S. Manganese. In Brown M. Present knowledge in nutrition, 6th ed. New York. ILSI Nutr Foundation, 1990.

r25. Rajagopalan KW. Molybdenum, an essential trace element in humans. Ann Rev Nutr 1988;*8*:401–427.

r26. Johnson JL, Wadman SK. Molybdenum Cofactor, 6th ed. Ed. Scriver CR, Beaudet AL, Sly WS, and Valle D, New York: McGraw-Hill, 1989.

r27. Nicol CA, Smith GK, Duch DS. Biosynthesis and metabolism of tetrahydrobopterin and molybdopterin. Ann Rev Biochem 1985;*54*:729–764.

r28. Suttle NF. The interaction between copper, molybdenum and sulfur in ruminant nutrition. Ann Rev Nutr 1991;*11*:121–140.

r29. Hirsch J. Handbook of Geographical and Historical Pathology, Vol. II. London: The New Sydenham Society, 1885.

r30. Clugston GA, Hetzel BS. Iodine. In Shils ME, Olson JA, Shike M. eds. Modern Nutrition in Health and Disease, 8th ed. Philadelphia: Lea & Febiger, 1994.

r31. Hetzel BS, Dunn JT, Stanburg JB Editors. The Prevention and Control of Iodine Deficiency Disorders, Amsterdam, Elsevier, 1987.

r32. Hetzel BS, Maberly GF. Iodine. In Trace Elements in Human and Animal Nutrition. 5th ed. Ed. W. Mertz. Vol 2. New York, NY. Academic Press, 1986, pp 139–208.

CHAPTER 62

Svein U. Toverud
James W. Bawden

Fluorides

Introduction

Fluoride is the ionic form of fluorine, which is the halogen in the second period of the periodic table, and is widely distributed in nature. Fluorides have been used extensively since the 1930s to prevent dental caries. Both systemic administration and topical application to the dentition have been shown to be effective in numerous epidemiologic and clinical trials.[r1,r2] The effectiveness of relatively large doses of fluorides to halt or reverse the progress of postmenopausal osteoporosis is not as well documented, and this therapy remains experimental and controversial. Finally, fluorides at high doses may give rise to both acute and chronic toxicities.

Sources

Natural sources of F include F^-, HF_2^-, or HF in low concentrations [less than 1 mg/L=1 ppm (parts per million)] in surface waters. Underground or subsoil waters often have higher F content. Natural foods obtained from seawater (0.8–1.4 ppm F), such as fish, have a relatively high F content, particularly if the bones are eaten, as in sardines and canned salmon. Other foods containing significant amounts of F include vegetables (spinach, asparagus, and onions, in particular), grains, and meats. The bioavailability of F in the diet is in the range of 50–80 percent. Most adults in the US and Europe have an average daily intake of approximately 1 mg F from foods and up to 1.5 mg from water and beverages, depending on the F content of the drinking water and bottled beverages. The F intake of young children is closer to 0.5 mg per day.

Other sources may be fluoride ions released from F-containing drugs and fluorides in dentifrices (1000–2000 ppm F) and mouthwashes (200 ppm F). Inadvertent ingestion of fluoride from the latter products by young children on a regular basis may increase the likelihood of dental fluorosis. Finally, occupational exposure to high concentrations of F may occur as a result of industrial accidents, where the source may be hydrofluoric acid (HF), which is highly corrosive, or through chronic exposure to F-containing vapors and dust-borne particles (e.g., bauxite factories).

Pharmacokinetics

Fluoride appears to cross the gastric mucosa primarily as HF rather than F^-.[1] The acid environment of the stomach favors rapid and extensive absorption of fluoride. Following a fluoride dose on an empty stomach, plasma levels peak in about 30 minutes and return to baseline over a period of three to six hours. Foods containing relatively large amounts of Ca^{2+} and Mg^{2+} slow the rate and limit the extent of absorption.

Clearance of fluoride from the ECF compartment occurs almost entirely by two mechanisms.[2] In adults, uptake by the skeleton (incorporation into the mineral) accounts for approximately half of the clearance. In children, skeletal uptake may amount to 80 percent of the clearance of fluoride. Nearly all remaining fluoride clearance from the ECF occurs through the renal system. Fluoride is freely filtered through the glomerular capillaries, but various levels of tubular reabsorption occur. Reabsorption apparently is influenced by urine pH and flow rate. Minor amounts of F are excreted in the sweat and into the colon.

In subjects who consume fluoridated water (1 ppm F) from early childhood, plasma levels are relatively constant, because of the ingestion of frequent, small increments. The skeletal and renal clearance mechanisms effectively dampen fluctuations in the extracellular concentration. Baseline plasma fluoride levels in subjects drinking water containing <0.1 ppm are approximately 0.01 ppm. In subjects drinking fluoridated water (1 ppm) plasma levels are about 0.02 ppm. Fluoride levels in milk (human and cow) are typically <0.02 ppm, even when maternal fluoride intake is high. Parotid duct saliva fluoride levels are 70–80 percent of those found in plasma, and the levels fluctuate directly with the plasma concentration.

Effects on Bone

High doses of sodium fluoride (40–75 mg NaF = 18–34 mg F daily) combined with calcium supplements have been used experimentally to treat primary idiopathic osteoporosis in postmenopausal women.[r3] Results of several uncontrolled open studies of moderate duration (3 years or less) have indicated that the fluoride-calcium combination can lead to increased bone formation, increased bone mineral mass, and a decrease in vertebral crush fracture rate. However, FDA approval in the US of high-dose fluoride in osteoporosis has been delayed not only because of uncertainty of the clinical efficacy, especially in the long term, but also because of several adverse effects: increased risk of wrist fractures; osteoarticular pain; and GI irritation. The latter has been alleviated by the use of enteric-coated NaF tablets or a slow-release preparation of NaF.[3] However, the authors of a four-year double-blind, prospective study did not find an acceptable risk-benefit ratio of high doses of fluoride: even though the treatment increased trabecular bone mass, there was no significant decrease in vertebral fracture rate.[4] On the other hand, results from a long-term, retrospective study with lower doses of fluoride (30 mg/day) indicate that as the bone density increases the vertebral fracture rate decreases.[5] Administration of daily doses of 60 mg NaF to osteoporotic patients for 1–2 years resulted in abnormal bone mineralization, revealed by ultrastructural analyses of bone biopsies.[6] Such abnormal mineralization may render the bone more brittle in spite of the higher mineral density.[6]

The mechanisms underlying the beneficial effect of fluoride treatment on trabecular bone mass in osteoporosis appear to involve an effect on osteoblasts to increase their rate of proliferation and synthetic (bone matrix-forming) activity, possibly by increasing the sensitivity of the cells to transforming growth factor β.[7] In addition, the higher percentage of fluoride incorporated into the bone mineral renders the mineral more stable and less soluble.

Use in Dental Caries Prevention

Systemic

Fluorides ingested regularly during tooth formation render the teeth more resistant to dental caries. Enamel formation begins in some primary teeth prenatally and in the permanent first molars and incisors at or shortly after birth. Postnatal systemic administration of fluorides is most effectively and inexpensively accomplished through fluoridation of public water supplies (usually at 1 ppm F). The first definitive evidence of an association between fluoride content of water supplies and increased resistance to dental caries was provided in 1938 by H. Trendley Dean, who also noted the occurrence of dental fluorosis (see Chronic Toxicity below) with high water fluoride concentrations. Subsequently, over 100 studies have demonstrated significant caries reductions. In early studies, 40 to 60 percent reductions in caries were achieved by water fluoridation. More recent studies report reductions from 18 to 30 percent.[8] The change is due to the extensive use of topical fluorides and the distribution of beverages and foods processed in fluoridated communities to non-fluoridated populations. Where such changes have not occurred, caries reductions resulting from water fluoridation are still over 50 percent.[9] In spite of claims to the contrary by antifluoridationists, all studies published in recognized, refereed scientific journals indicate that no harmful side-effects occur from drinking water fluoridated at the recommended level. The cost per capita is minimal, and patient cooperation is not required to deliver the optimal dose on a daily basis.

Many children drink water containing low levels of fluoride from wells or other sources that cannot be fluoridated. In some circumstances these children can be provided with systemic fluoride by use of a school-water fluoridator. The recommended fluoride concentration is then controlled at 4.5 ppm. This level, which is higher than that used in municipal water supplies, compensates for late starting exposure (typically age 5), limited exposure each day, and lack of exposure on week-ends and vacations. Controlled studies report caries reductions of approximately 40 percent.

Children at moderate or high risk for caries who do not drink municipally fluoridated water, naturally fluoridated water at optimum or above levels, or water from a school fluoridator should receive a daily supplement in the form of drops for infants and tablets for children who have erupted teeth. The fluoride concentration of the home water supply should be established by assay before prescribing supplements. Other significant sources to which the child may be exposed should be considered as well (time at school, day care center, etc). The dose schedule published by the American Dental Association should be followed.

Currently, infants from birth to two years of age should receive 0.25 mg F daily, children two to three years of age 0.5 mg, and three years of age and older 1 mg. Significant levels of fluoride naturally occurring in the home water (>0.2 ppm) require reduction of the dose. This dose schedule is currently under review and may be modified. The review was prompted by documented changes in patterns of fluoride ingestion.[r4,10]

Topical

Several means of topical applications of fluorides to teeth have been shown to be effective in caries prevention. Concentrated agents (1.23% F) are applied to the teeth, usually in trays, for four minutes at six-month intervals. Such applications must be made by professional personnel, and care should be taken to avoid ingestion of excessive amounts of fluoride, which can cause gastric distress and vomiting. Sodium fluoride (0.2%) rinses used in schools for one minute weekly have shown positive results, as has the daily use of over-the-counter 0.05 percent sodium fluoride rinses. Over 90 percent of the dentifrice used in the US contains approximately 0.1% fluoride as sodium fluoride or disodium-monofluorophosphate. The caries-preventive effect of daily use has been documented in clinical trials.

The mechanisms by which systemic and topical fluorides prevent dental caries are not clearly defined. Three hypotheses are supported by significant data: (1) fluorides reduce enamel solubility in acid; (2) fluorides enhance remineralization of early caries lesions; and (3) fluorides reduce acid production by cariogenic plaque bacteria. It is likely that these mechanisms work in combination.

Acute Toxicity

Acute toxicity may occur after accidental swallowing of F-containing products or NaF tablets, or as a result of an industrial accident. Initial symptoms after excess F ingestion are due to irritation of the GI tract and include salivation, nausea, vomiting, and pain. Evidence of systemic involvement includes hypocalcemia, hyperkalemia, hyperreactive reflexes, parasthesias, hypotension, convulsion, and polyuria.[11] The estimated lethal dose in humans is 50–100 mg/kg. Death may result from respiratory paralysis or cardiac failure. The use of the general anesthetic methoxyflurane, which is extensively metabolized, has resulted in blood F concentrations of 3–4 ppm, leading to polyuria refractory to antidiuretic hormone. Accidental exposure of the skin to high concentrations of hydrofluoric acid (widely used in the manufacture of ceramics, in electropolishing of metals, and in etching of glass) causes severe burns and marked hypocalcemia from the percutaneous entry of F, which may give rise to potentially lethal blood levels of 6–7 ppm.[11] The primary goal of treatment is to prevent the potentially fatal hypocalcemic tetany by administering calcium IV. Fluoride overdoses occur most frequently in young children who use fluoride supplements at home. However, acute ingestion of up to 8 mg F appears to lead only to mild GI symptoms.[r5]

Chronic Toxicity

Dental Fluorosis

The process of tooth enamel formation is most sensitive to toxic effects of F, and very mild mottled enamel of permanent teeth is therefore the earliest sign of F toxicity. This degree of mottled enamel consists of small, white (chalk-like) spots on the enamel visible only to the trained clinician; it has no functional or esthetic significance. It will occur in 10 to 28 percent of all children who have consumed drinking water with 1.0–1.2 ppm F since birth.[r6] Children under seven years of age who use fluoridated toothpastes have an increased risk of developing mild mottled enamel, because they tend to swallow some of the paste and therefore inadvertently increase their daily fluoride intake.[r7]

In moderately mottled enamel the spots are larger, more numerous, and may be discolored. In the severe form there are pitted, discolored areas in the enamel. The moderate and severe forms occur when the drinking water has contained F in the range of 2–10 ppm.[r6]

Skeletal Fluorosis

Osteosclerosis is usually an asymptomatic, moderate form of chronic toxicity consisting of radiologically detectable bone changes with increased mineral density. It may occur after chronic ingestion of water with more than 2–3 ppm F for decades. Crippling fluorosis is a severe, disabling form of chronic toxicity occurring after ingestion for many years of water with more than 10 ppm F. It is characterized by marked thickening of cortical bone, numerous exostoses, and calcification of ligaments and tendons.

Chronic skeletal fluorosis also may result from inhalation of fluoridated gases or dust by industrial workers or from long-term treatment with F-containing drugs that are slowly metabolized, such as niflumic acid. This anti-inflammatory drug has been used in patients with rheumatoid arthritis in Europe, Asia, Africa, and South America, but not in the US.

References

Research Reports

1. Whitford GM, Pashley DH. Fluoride absorption: The influence of gastric acidity. Calcif Tissue Int 1984;*36*:302–307.
2. Whitford GM. The physiological and toxicological characteristics of fluoride. J Dent Res 1990;*69*:539–549.
3. Pak CYC, Sakhaee K, Zerwekh JE, Parcel C, Peterson R, Johnson K. Safe and effective treatment of osteoporosis with intermittent slow release sodium fluoride: augmentation of vertebral bone mass and inhibition of fractures. J Clin Endocrinol Metab 1989;*68*:150–159.
4. Riggs BL, Hodgson SF, O'Fallon WM, Chao EYS, Wahner HW, Muhs JM, Cedel SL, Melton JL III. Effect of fluoride treatment on the fracture rate in postmenopausal women with osteoporosis. N Engl J Med 1990;*322*:802–809.
5. Farley SM, Wergedal JE, Farley JR, Javie GN, Schulz EE, Talbot JR, Libanti CR, Lindegren L, Bock M, Goette MM, Mohan SS, Kimball-Johnson P, Perkel VS, Cruise RJ, Baylink DJ. Spinal fractures during fluoride therapy for osteoporosis: relationship to spinal bone density. Osteoporosis Int 1992;*2*:213–218.
6. Fratzl P, Roschger P, Eschberger J, Abendroth B, Klaushofer K. Abnormal bone mineralization after fluoride treatment in osteoporosis: a small-angle X-ray-scattering study. J Bone Miner Res 1994;*9*:1541–1549.
7. Reed BY, Zerwekh JE, Antich PP, Pak CYC. Fluoride-stimulated [^{3}H]thymidine uptake in a human osteoblastic osteosarcoma cell line is dependent on transforming growth factor β. J Bone Mineral Res 1993;*8*:19–25.
8. Brunelle JA, Carlos JP. Recent trends in dental caries in U.S. children and the effect of water fluoridation. J Dent Res 1990;*69*:723–727.
9. O'Mullane DM. The future of water fluoridation. J Dent Res 1990;*69*:756–759.
10. Pang DTY, Phillips CL, Bawden JW. Fluoride intake from beverage consumption in a sample of North Carolina children. J Dent Res 1992;*71*:1382–1388.
11. Greco RJ, Hartford CE, Haith LR, Patton ML Hydrofluoric acid-induced hypocalcemia. Trauma 1988;*28*:1593–1596.

Reviews

r1. Murray JJ, Rugg-Gunn AJ. Water fluoridation update. In: Stewart RW, Barber TK, Troutman KC, Wei SHY (Eds.). Paediatric dentistry. St. Louis: Mosby, 1982.

r2. Stooky GK. Critical evaluation of the composition and use of topical fluorides. J Dent Res 1990;*69*:805–812.

r3. Kleerekoper M, Mendlovic DB. Sodium fluoride therapy of postmenopausal osteoporosis. Endocrine Rev 1993;*14*:312–323.

r4. Bawden JW (ed). Proceedings of workshop on changing patterns of fluoride intake. J Dent Res 1992;*71*:1212–1265.

r5. Augenstein WL, Spoerke DG, Kulig KW, Hall AH, Hall PK, Riggs BS, El Saadi M, Rumack BH. Fluoride ingestion in children: A review of 87 cases. Pediatrics 1991;*88*:907–912.

r6. Moller IJ. Fluorides and dental fluorosis. Int Dent J 1982;*32*:135–147.

r7. Pang DTY, Vann WF Jr. The use of fluoride-containing toothpastes in young children: The scientific evidence for recommending a small quantity. Pediatr Dentistry 1992;*14*:384–387.

CHAPTER 63

Starvation, Undernutrition, and Trauma

Carolyn D. Berdanier
Robert E. Olson

The basic metabolic response of an otherwise healthy individual to starvation is conservation.[r1,r2] As the patient's gut receives less food, it slowly empties. First the stomach, then the duodenum, the jejunum, the ileum, and the large intestine lose their contents and shrink in size. Simple mono- and disaccharides are the first to disappear, followed by the products of the progressively more complex nutrients: polysaccharides; proteins; and lipids. As the sugars disappear, there is less stimulus for insulin release, and basal insulin levels are approached. As glucose becomes less available from the gut, the body begins to mobilize its glycogen stores; when they are nearly depleted, the body will begin to mobilize its stores of triacylglycerol from adipose tissue and, to a lesser extent, its muscle protein. It can use certain of the amino acids and glycerol from the triacylglycerols to synthesize glucose via gluconeogenesis and to utilize the carbon skeletons of other deaminated amino acids plus the fatty acids liberated from the triacylglycerols for fuel. As fasting continues, insulin levels fall even lower, and glucagon and corticosteroid levels increase with concomitant fatty acid release from depot fat and gluconeogenesis from amino acids derived principally from muscle.

In 1915 Benedict[1] reported a study of a man (Levanzin) who fasted under medical surveillance for 31 days. Over that period he lost 13 kg of body weight (from 60–47 kg), and his oxygen consumption and urinary nitrogen excretion decreased about 30 percent. Benedict concluded that over 75 percent of the calories utilized after the first few days came from adipose tissue and that the decrease in urinary nitrogen represented an attempt to conserve body protein.

Cahill[2] later estimated that a 70-kg man had approximately 75 grams of glycogen stored in the liver, which could provide approximately 300 Kcalories during the first 24 hours of starvation. The glycogen plus the glucose synthesized via gluconeogenesis, which provides an additional 400 Kcal, contribute only 30 percent of the 2000 to 2500 calories needed per day for maintenance. After the first day, the contribution of stored carbohydrate to energy expenditure is negligible. The fuel stores of the human body are shown in Table 63.1. Benedict estimated that mobilizable body protein could provide about 15 percent of the body's fuel needs and that the fat in adipose tissue provided the rest. Although Benedict did not have today's sophisticated technology at his disposal, his estimates were remarkably close to those of Cahill. Cahill estimated that a "normal" 70-kg man required about 2000

Table 63.1 Fuel Composition of 70-Kg Man[r1]

Fuel	Kg	Calories
Tissues:		
Fat (adipose triglyceride)	15	141,000
Protein (mainly muscle)	6	24,000
Glycogen (muscle)	0.150	600
Glycogen (liver)	0.075	300
Total		165,900

calories per day to maintain his body composition and that he had sufficient stores of fuel to sustain life for about 80 days. Toward the end of a 30-day fast about 90 percent of the energy expenditure is derived from fat.

These lipids, primarily triacylglycerols, are hydrolyzed to fatty acids and glycerol through the action of a hormone-sensitive lipase. This enzyme, on the interior aspect of the fat cell membrane, is activated by the catabolic hormones glucagon, epinephrine, and the glucocorticoids. Its lipolytic activity is increased when glucagon is high and insulin is low. The glycerol is converted to glucose via gluconeogenesis in the liver and kidney. The fatty acids are oxidized to ketones and to carbon dioxide and water. During fasting, both the liver and muscle depend increasingly on fatty acids for energy. In fact, the mobilization of fatty acids from adipose tissue exceeds the capacity of the liver to oxidize them completely to CO_2 and water, and ketosis results. A reduction in the activity of the tricarboxylic cycle in the liver is due to the diversion of oxaloacetic acid to gluconeogenesis through induction of PEP-carboxykinase. As a result, ketone bodies (acetoacetate and β-hydroxybutyrate) are secreted into the circulation to provide fuel for many tissues, including the brain. After about 40 days of starvation, the brain obtains nearly 65 percent of its energy from the ketones that it extracts from plasma in proportion to their concentration.[3] These fuel fluxes are diagrammed in Figure 63.1.

Under normal (i.e., fed) conditions, the CNS uses 115 g of glucose/day, while erythrocytes, bone marrow, renal medulla, and peripheral nerves use about 36 g of glucose/day. In the first few days of fasting, most of this glucose is synthesized via gluconeogenesis from glycerol, lactate, and selected amino acids. However, as starvation continues, the body attempts to protect its protein component by reducing gluconeogenesis and the corresponding mobilization of amino acids from muscle. Proteolysis in muscle, initially increased to provide amino acids to protein synthesis in viscera and gluconeogenesis, is suppressed by rising levels of growth hormone after 48 hours of fasting. Once these mechanisms are implemented, body protein is conserved.

Thus, during starvation the human undergoes a series of enzymatic and hormonal adaptations to derive energy from adipose tissue (which visibly shrinks in mass) and to conserve body protein. Death from starvation does not occur from loss of body fat, but from loss of tissue protein. Body protein stores are not just a reserve supply of nitrogen, but constitute the enzymatic machinery of the body. When body protein is reduced to a critical level of 70 percent, muscular contraction, protein synthesis, hormonal secretion, antibody protection, and tissue respiration are all imperiled.

In summary, the metabolic adaptations to preserve life in starvation are: (1) the elimination of glucose as a source of fuel for many tissues; (2) the augmentation of the Cori-cycle, which returns lactate, the product of glycolysis in muscle, red cells, white cells, and bone marrow, back to the liver for resynthesis into glucose; and (3) the induction of enzymes in brain that enable it to subsist on ketone bodies instead of glucose. The fall in insulin levels and the rise in glucocorticoids, glucagon, and growth hormone are responsible for this adaptation.

Protein-Energy Malnutrition

As already noted, starvation is the extreme state of malnutrition that occurs when no food is provided to nourish the body. Between starvation and adequate nourishment, there are various levels of inadequate nutrient intake. Although infants and children of Third-World nations dramatically exemplify such malnutrition, people of all ages in all countries are vulnerable. Where the intake of macronutrients is inadequate, the syndrome is called protein-calorie malnutrition (PCM) or protein energy malnutrition (PEM). Chronic PCM is characterized not only by an energy deficit but also by a deficit in the required intake of protein and micronutrients. The requirements for energy and these nutrients are determined by the age and health of each individual. Rapid growth, infection, injury, and chronic debilitating disease can increase the need for food and the nutrients it contains, particularly in infants and young children.[r2]

PCM presents clinically as three types.[r3] At the extremes it is recognized either as "wet", i.e., edematous, or "dry" i.e., thin and desiccated. The "wet" form is referred to as kwashiokor, an African word meaning "first child–second child." It refers to the observation that the first child suffers from PCM when the second child is born and replaces the first child at the breast. The weaned child is fed a thin gruel of poor nutritional quality (compared to mother's milk) and fails to thrive. The energy, protein, and micronutrient content of the weaning food is poor and does not meet the nutrient needs of the child. Children with kwashiorkor tend to be older and to develop their disease in the postweaning period.

The "dry" form of PCM, marasmus, results from almost total starvation. The marasmic child is not edematous and is very thin from loss of both muscle and body fat. While the child with kwashiorkor may be consuming subobtimal amounts of food poor in

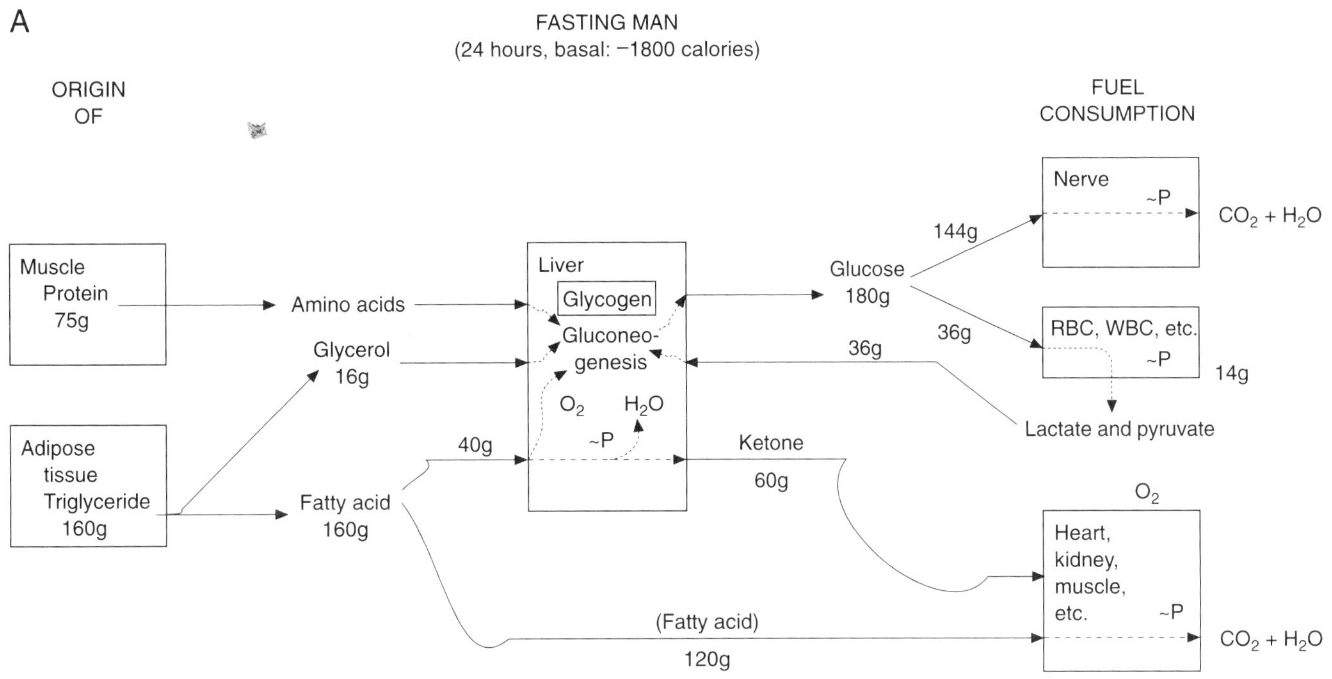

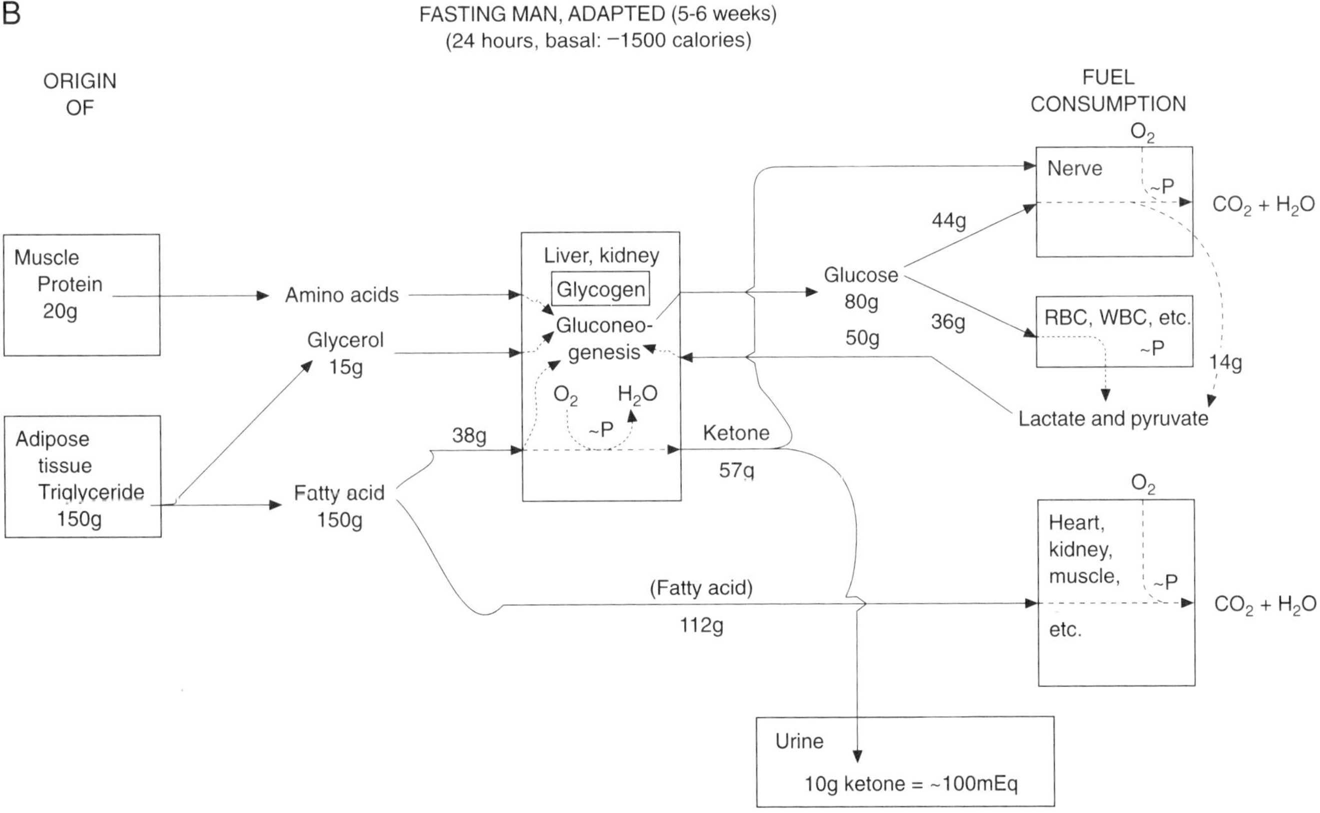

Figure 63.1 General scheme of fuel metabolism in a normal man, fasted for 24 hours (A) and 5–6 weeks (B). The two primary sources of fuel, muscle and adipose tissue, are shown together with three types of users: nerve, red and white blood cells, and the rest of the body (heart, kidney, skeletal muscle). The liver modulates the type of fuel that reaches the periphery. ~ P is high-energy phosphate. (Reproduced from [r1]).

protein, the child with marasmus consumes little or no food. Almost invariably there is infection; sometimes there is trauma and sepsis, which worsens the prognosis and jeopardizes the life of the child. The intermediate state between marasmus and kwashiorkor is represented by children who have some edema and more body fat. This state is called marasmic kwashiorkor. PCM is the leading cause of death in Third-World countries.

Olson and colleagues studied about 200 children with PCM in northern Thailand.[r4] Approximately 30 percent had marasmus, 30 percent had kwashiorkor, and the remaining 40 percent had marasmic kwashiorkor. As expected, the marasmic children were younger, shorter, and lighter (54 percent of expected weight for age) than the children with kwashiorkor, who were six months older, taller, and heavier (76 percent of weight for age) than the marasmic ones. The biochemical findings in these patients are presented in Table 63.2.[4] The anemia was mild, with hemoglobin values averaging about 10 g/dl on admission. Only 67 out of 195 showed values less than 10 g/dl on admission, although after one week of treatment with rehydration, about 50 percent had hemoglobin values below 10 g/dl. The transferrin content was measured by total iron-binding capacity and was below normal in all children, but markedly reduced in kwashiorkor. Plasma iron was in the low-normal range in all three groups, which gave a higher percentage saturation of transferrin in the kwashiorkor group. Serum folate was low-normal in all groups, but megaoblastic anemia was rare. Serum cholesterol generally was low, being lowest in the kwashiorkor group. Plasma vitamin E was low, again most markedly reduced in the kwashiorkor group. Serum vitamin A levels were depressed in all groups, with about 30 percent of children showing frank vitamin A deficiency. Retinol-binding protein was decreased from a normal value of 40 µg/ml to about 20 µg/ml in the children with PCM.

In marasmus, the symmetrical decrease in all dietary nutrients, including calories, causes the child to consume his own tissues as a source of nutriment. Body tissue is a nutritious fare that prevents development of specific deficiency signs, although total energy expenditure falls as the total body mass shrinks.[5] All of the endocrine adjustments to fasting occur. Under the influence of somatotropin, corticoids, and glucagon, fatty acids are mobilized from adipose tissue and amino

Table 63.2 Biochemical and Hematologic Data in Protein-Calorie Malnutrition[4]

	Units	Marasmus (n = 62)	Marasmus-kwashiorkor (n = 72)	Kwashiorkor (n = 61)	Control (n = 50)
Hemoglobin	g/dl	10.0 ± 0.3	9.0 ± 0.3	9.7 ± 0.31	1.7 ± 0.3
Hematocrit	g/dl	34.0 ± 0.7	33.0 ± 0.8	31.5 ± 0.8	36.2 ± 0.6
Total Serum Protein	g/dl	7.0 ± 0.8	4.9 ± 0.1[a]	3.9 ± 0.1[a]	7.2 ± 0.1
Albumin	g/dl	2.8 ± 0.1	1.9 ± 0.1[b]	1.5 ±0.1[c]	3.7 ± 0.1
Globulin	g/dl	3.4 ± 0.1	3.1 ± 0.1[b]	2.5 ± 0.8[a]	3.5 ± 0.1
α -1-Globulin	g/dl	0.3 ± 0.1[a]	0.3 ± 0.1[b]	0.3 ± 0.1[b]	0.2 ± 0.1
α -2-Globulin	g/dl	0.9 ± 0.1	0.7 ± 0.1[a]	0.6 ± 0.1[a]	0.9 ± 0.1
β -Globulin	g/dl	0.7 ± 0.1[a]	0.5 ± 0.1[a]	0.5 ± 0.1[a]	0.9 ± 0.1
γ -Globulin	g/dl	1.6 ± 0.1	1.6 ± 0.1	1.2 ± 0.1	1.5 ± 0.1
Iron	ug/dl	70.7 ± 9.5	54.1 ± 3.9[b]	70.9 ± 5.7	69.0 ± 4.0
Total iron binding Capacity	ug/dl	239.2 ± 14.7[a]	138.4 ± 7.3[a]	110.7 ± 7.9[a]	357.0 ± 7.0
Cholesterol	mg/dl	109.3 ± 5.9[c]	92.9 ± 6.0[a]	81.5 ± 5.0[a]	129.0 ± 5.0
Cholesterol ester	mg/dl	60.2 ± 6.5	35.8 ± 4.0[a]	35.4 ± 3.4[a]	73.1 ± 5.0
Triglyceride	mg/dl	67.5 ± 7.9	70.8 ± 8.4	103.6 ± 13.3	98.3 ± 15.8
Vitamin A	ug/dl	38.2 ± 4.5[b]	21.2 ± 2.0[a]	23.6 ± 4.0[a]	54.0 ± 5.0
β -carotene	ug/dl	18.1 ± 1.8[a]	15.3 ± 1.1[a]	18.0 ± 3.1[a]	57.0 ± 3.0
Retinol-binding protein	ug/ml	23.1 ± 2.6	21.5 ± 3.0[c]	19.7 ± 5.7[a]	28.0 ± 1.6
Prealbumin	ug/ml	62.0 ± 5.7[a]	49.1 ± 2.3[a]	43.0 ± 0.1	125.0 ± 12.5
Vitamin E	mg/dl	0.3 ± 0.1[a]	0.3 ± 0.1[a]	0.2 ± 0.1[a]	0.4 ± 0.1
Serum Folate	ng/ml	9.4 ± 1.2[a]	7.5 ± 0.9[a]	5.1 ± 0.6[a]	25.0 ± 1.0
Vitamin B_{12}	pg/ml	711.6 ± 82.0	1,306 ± 295	906 ± 203	443.0 ± 60.0

Mean ± SEM
a = $p < 0.001$ compared with controls.
b = $p < 0.01$ compared with controls.
c = $p < 0.05$ compared with controls.

acids from muscle tissue. Hepatic gluconeogenesis is enhanced, and plasma proteins are maintained near normal concentrations. No edema occurs as long as the cardiac index is sufficient to provide adequate renal perfusion. When relative cardiac output falls to the point where renal perfusion is no longer adequate, sodium retention occurs, and the extracellular space expands.[6] When this expansion of extracellular fluid becomes clinically evident as edema, the diagnosis of marasmic kwashiorkor is made.

When children consume diets in which calories are less limiting than protein, kwashiorkor occurs. Because of different endocrine adjustments to this type of diet, mobilization of fatty acids from depot fat and amino acids from muscle does not occur to the same extent as in marasmus, and the hepatic synthesis of plasma proteins falls. With the fall of oncotic pressure, extracellular water accumulates, tissue pressure rises, and cardiac output falls. These events reduce perfusion pressure in the kidney, with a resulting fall in glomerular filtration and increased sodium retention. The ischemic juxtaglomerular apparatus produces more renin, and the resulting aldosterone further enhances sodium retention[7] and further dilutes the plasma proteins. As in all edematous states, the increased salt and water retention assists in maintaining the plasma volume and blood pressure within normal limits.

In the face of the limited amino acid supply, rates of synthesis and catabolism of most plasma proteins are reduced. James and Hay[8] showed that in both well-nourished and malnourished children the rate of albumin synthesis is very sensitive to the amino acid supply. With reduction of dietary protein, the turnover rate of serum albumin decreased from 200 mg/kg per day to less than 100 mg/kg per day. The reduction in the synthetic rate was followed in a few days by the reduction in the catabolic rate. Hoffenberg and his coworkers[9,10] also showed that dietary protein deficiency in both rats and human subjects, which produces a fall in concentration of serum albumin by 25 percent, reduces both the rate of synthesis and catabolism of albumin by 70 percent. In children with severe PCM, serum glucocorticoids are high (marasmus > kwashiorkor), somatotropin levels are high (kwashiorkor > marasmus),[11,12] and insulin levels are low.[13,r3] These endocrine changes promote mobilization of fatty acids from adipose tissue and amino acids from muscle, which accounts for the extreme wasting of both fat depots and muscle in PCM. In the liver, the enzymes regulating gluconeogenesis are induced, and triglyceride tends to accumulate because the rate of β-lipoprotein apopeptide synthesis does not keep pace with the flux of fatty acids. On low-protein diets the urea cycle enzymes fall, but the hepatic tRNA aminoacyl ligases increase, which improves the hepatic recycling of amino acids to as high as 95 percent.[14] This high reutilization of amino acids by liver exceeds the release of amino acids by muscle; as a result, plasma amino acid concentrations fall. The essential amino acids decrease in concentration more than the nonessential ones, particularly in kwashiorkor.[15]

An interesting feature of the endocrine response to PCM is the elevated somatotropin (growth hormone) level, which is refractory to glucose and albumin infusions, but is immediately responsive to protein feeding or the IV infusion of amino acids. Normally, hyperglycemia causes somatotropin levels to fall, and hyperaminoacidemia causes somatotropin levels to rise. Both Pimstone et al.[16] and Suskind et al.[12] have proposed that this paradoxical response of growth hormone in PCM may be explained by the assumption that a depression of essential amino acids in the plasma may be the most powerful positive stimulus to the secretion of somatotropin by the hypothalamus that exists. In protein deficiency, such a powerful signal may be necessary to the attempt to conserve nitrogen and modulate the catabolic effects of corticosteroids in muscle and bone, where somatotropin exerts its maximum anabolic effects.

In contrast to most plasma proteins, all classes of immunoglobulins are increased in severe PCM.[17,18] Studies in Thailand showed, furthermore, that despite high IgG, IgM, IgA, and IgD levels children had a depressed response to typhoid antigen,[19] an observation also made by Reddy and Skrikantia.[20] Studies by Cohen and Hansen[21] showed that γ-globulin turnover was in the normal range in PCM, and preliminary studies in Thailand with ^{125}I-labeled IgG showed, if anything, an increased turnover in PCM. These data indicate that the plasma cell is extraordinarily competitive with other cell types for the limited amino acid supply. The reduction in specific humoral immunity suggests, furthermore, that the immunoglobulins synthesized may, in part, be "nonsense immunoglobulins" and hence wasteful of the limited amino acids available. It has been suggested that this paradox is associated with a defect in cell-mediated immunity that may be due to associated zinc deficiency.[r5]

In the PCM reported from northern Thailand, the plasma levels of cholesterol, retinol, and α-tocopherol were depressed. The fall in the concentrations of these lipids has two possible causes: (1) a fall in their respective carrier proteins; (2) an actual deficiency of the lipid. One can distinguish between these two possibilities by observing the response to the feeding of either dietary protein or lipid. The feeding of protein alone increased the concentrations of these lipids and their carrier proteins to normal values.[22] Cholesterol and α-tocopherol are carried mainly by β-lipoproteins, the apoproteins of which are limiting for the hepatic secretion of all the lipids associated with them. Vitamin A is carried by retinol-binding protein (RBP) and, like cholesterol, is not secreted by the liver unless its carrier protein is present. Vitamin A-deficient rats with adequate protein intake have been shown to accumulate RBP in their livers. When vitamin A is given, the accumulated RBP is released within an hour.[23] Vitamin A-deficient patients with PCM, however, show no increase in RBP 24 hours after a parenteral dose of the vitamin.[24] This result provides further evidence for the depressed synthesis of RBP in patients with PCM.

As pointed out in the introduction to the discussion of PCM, infants are particularly vulnerable to this type of malnutrition, but people of all ages, particularly those in low socioeconomic groups and the chronically ill, are also at risk. Bistrian et al in 1974[25,26] studied a series of hospitalized patients in a Boston hospital and concluded that 44 percent of general medical patients and 50 percent of surgical patients had protein-calorie malnutrition. Similar observations were made by Smith and Corli[27] in a London hospital in 1977. Weinsier et al in 1977[28] studied 134 medical service patients at the University Hospital in Birmingham, Alabama. They reported that protein-calorie malnutrition developed in 37 patients hospitalized for more than two weeks. They suggested that one of the "skeletons in the hospital closet" is malnutrition and that clinicians in general should be more alert to the problems of malnutrition in their patients.

Effect of Biologic Stress on Nutrient Requirements

Biologic stress can be defined as the sum of all nonspecific biologic reactions elicited by adverse external influences. Such adverse external influences include: (1) trauma; (2) infection; (3) sepsis; (4) burns; (5) cold; (6) heat; (7) severe exercise; and (8) malnutrition.

The effects of starvation and other forms of malnutrition have been discussed earlier in this chapter. Many of the metabolic effects elicited by starvation are magnified in humans subjected to serious injuries and/or infection. When they occur to already malnourished persons, these metabolic effects are further exaggerated.

In the 1930s Cuthbertson[29–33] studied patients with long bone fractures and observed that, following these fractures, patients lost large quantities of nitrogen, potassium, and phosphate into the urine. This effect could not be reversed by oral feeding. In addition, Cuthbertson observed that immediately following injury the patients seemed to be in shock, with reduced blood pressure, cardiac output, body temperature, and oxygen consumption. After 12 to 24 hours, however, this "ebb" condition was replaced by one of "flow," in which cardiac output, oxygen consumption, nitrogen loss, glucose intolerance, body temperature, and blood pressure increased. This was probably a result of ACTH and corticoid secretion coupled with low insulin and high glucagon levels. In addition, many patients demonstrated sodium and water retention during this period, with heightened secretion of aldosterone and pituitary antidiuretic hormone. Hypermetabolism is characteristic of serious injury and infection, with the usual patient showing an increase of 25 to 50 percent in oxygen consumption. In severe burns, the metabolic rate may be double the usual basal rate. The effect of endocrine changes in the trauma on physiologic events is shown in Figure 63.2.

Parenteral and enteral feeding of patients during serious injury have minimized, but not entirely abolished, the catabolic response to trauma or infection. In fact, Francis Moore,[r6] Chief of Surgery at the Peter Bent Brigham Hospital in Boston, used to advise his colleagues not to attempt to feed patients increased amounts of food until the hormonally stimulated hypermetabolism, hyperglycemia, and nitrogen losses began to recede and anabolic hormones—principally insulin and growth hormone—replaced the counterregulatory hormones mentioned above. Moore argued that the hormonal responses to injury serve as initiators or inducers of metabolic events that must occur if recovery is to proceed. As relief from the trauma occurs, these hormonal responses recede and other metabolic control mechanisms assume command.

Energy Metabolism

Kinney[r7] has shown that basal energy requirements increase by as much as 100 percent to twice the normal

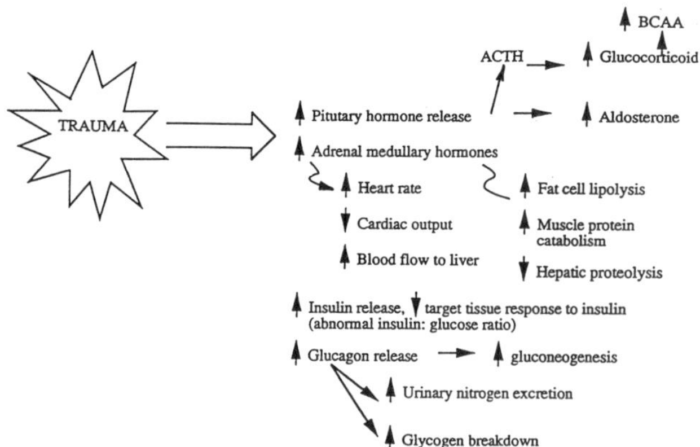

Figure 63.2 Effects of trauma on hormone release and the subsequent effects on heart rate, cardiac output, blood flow to the liver and urinary nitrogen. ACTH = adrenocorticotropic hormone; BCAA = branched-chain amino acids.

in traumatized patients. Elective operations increase resting energy expenditure by 10 percent, multiple fractures and gunshot wounds by 30 percent, severe sepsis by up to 60 percent, and third-degree burns by up to 100 percent. Part of this increase can be attributed to the thermogenic effects of the catecholamines and cytokines released in response to injury. The increased energy expenditure is accompanied by an increase in the body core temperature due to a resetting of the hypothalamic thermostat. The precise mechanism by which this is accomplished is not settled, but it appears to be the combined result of prostaglandin E_2 and two cytokines, interleukin-1 and cachectin (also known as the tumor necrosis factor). A general increase in body temperature, mediated by the CNS, must involve activation of a variety of "futile biochemical cycles" that convert the energy of adenosine triphosphate (ATP) into heat. A good example from normal physiology is the shivering response to cold. This mechanically ineffective form of muscular contraction converts most of the energy of ATP into heat. Since most of the ATP formed in the human body is linked to concomitant oxygen uptake (P/O ratio = 3), useful as well as futile ATP expenditure accounts for the increase in oxygen consumption noted in injured and/or septic patients. A maximum of 30 percent of the energy of ATP is conserved in useful work and a minimum of 70 percent appears as heat.[r8]

Carbohydrate Metabolism

Reduced glucose tolerance is usually observed in the post-tramatic period (Fig. 63.3). Studies of burned and septic humans[34–36] have revealed a difference in the time-frame for this insulin resistance, but both conditions have similar effects on insulin-stimulated glucose uptake. The insulin dose required by the traumatized patient for the maintenance of normoglycemia is five times that required by the nontraumatized individual. This increased insulin resistance in the periphery is due to the presence of catabolic hormones and the greatly increased hepatic glucose production via glycogenolysis and gluconeogenesis.[37] In the normal nontraumatized state the gluconeogenic pathway is regulated by insulin. In traumatized patients, however, this regulation is minimized because of the inadequate insulin response and the elevated glucagon and corticoids that support continued gluconeogenesis from amino acids. If the patient is diabetic, the effect of trauma or sepsis on glucose tolerance and enhanced gluconeogenesis is additive.

The traumatized diabetic patient will require more rigorous nutritional support and closer monitoring of blood glucose levels than will the nondiabetic. Aging

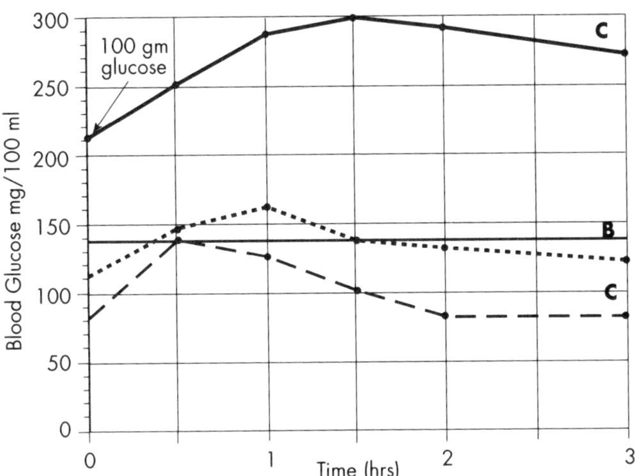

Figure 63.3 Glucose tolerance curves. *A* depicts a normal glycemic response to an oral dose of 100 g glucose. *B* shows the glucose tolerance curve commonly found after severe trauma. *C* is the glucose tolerance curve of an uncontrolled diabetic patient. Glycosuria is commonly observed in persons whose glucose level exceeds 140 mg/dl.

patients and children also will have an exaggerated metabolic response to trauma compared with otherwise healthy adults. Although the sequence of hormonal and metabolic responses will be similar, the time frame and intensity of response will differ. Sometimes these differences can be life-threatening if close monitoring is not accomplished. The elderly may already have peripheral tissue insulin resistance that is made worse by the trauma. The child is likely to exhaust fuel stores more quickly because of smaller reserves. In each instance, the difference between death and survival may depend on the provision of adequate nutritional support, including adequate amounts of energy, glucose, and amino acids plus appropriate amounts of insulin to facilitate the return to normal fuel homeostasis.

Fat Metabolism

With trauma, free fatty acid levels in the plasma rise. These increases correlate well with the increases in serum catecholamines and indicate an increased mobilization of adipose tissue lipids. While this mobilization initially occurs in response to increases in epinephrine, the increased lipolysis continues long after serum epinephrine levels have fallen and is probably due to continuing secretion of glucagon and glucocorticoids. With the increase in plasma free fatty acids, there is a concomitant increase in hepatic triglycerides. Since more fatty acids are released from the adipose tissue than can be utilized directly as fuel, deposition of triglycerides in the liver and ketogenesis occur. Cortisol has been shown to enhance hepatic (but not adipocyte) lipogenesis in the recovering stressed animal. Trauma also reduces the rate at which triglycerides are released from the liver in the form of very low density lipoproteins (VLDL). Thus, increased deposition of triacylglycerols formed from glycerol and the fatty acids released by the peripheral tissues, increased de novo lipogenesis, and decreased triacyglycerol release all contribute to the development of the fatty liver frequently observed in the traumatized patient during the early phases of recovery. In thermal injury these changes are maximized, mostly because the endocrine response to injury is enhanced and prolonged.

Most of the substrate oxidized under stressful conditions is fatty acid, which is liberated from adipose tissue by the counter-regulatory hormones, epinephrine, glucagon, and the corticosteroids. The glut of fatty acids produced tends to inhibit glucose utilization further via the glucose-fatty acid cycle.[39] Ketone bodies synthesized in the liver compete successfully with glycolysis in most tissues for the TCA cycle and inhibit glycolysis. Another factor aggravating the insulin insensitivity in these septic patients is their anorexia. This further lowers effective insulin levels, increases the levels of glucagon and corticoids, and promotes gluconeogenesis in the liver.

Protein Metabolism

Injury, infection, and sepsis cause a net catabolism of body protein, the amount being dependent on the severity of the insult and, to a lesser extent, on dietary intake.[r10] Urinary nitrogen excretion for normal subjects and patients with various diseases receiving only 5 percent glucose infusion is shown in Figure 63.4. The nitrogen excretion of healthy persons on zero protein intake is about 50 mg/kg (3.5 g/day). In burned patients it can rise to 400 mg/kg or 27 g per day—an eight-fold increase. With intermediate degrees of injury, lesser amounts of nitrogen are lost.[r10]

Nitrogen balance is improved in stress patients in response to both N and energy intake. At any given level of N and energy intake, however, N balance in stressed patients is more negative than in normal patients, and the size of the difference depends on the degree of stress. Malnourished patients not otherwise stressed are in more positive N balance than are injured patients. Even after moderate abdominal surgery (vagotomy, pyloroplasty, or cholecystectomy), an apparently obligatory N loss of 5 g per day occurs despite what would normally be considered adequate intake. By the fourth day on either enteral or parenteral feeding, N balance returns to zero.[r10]

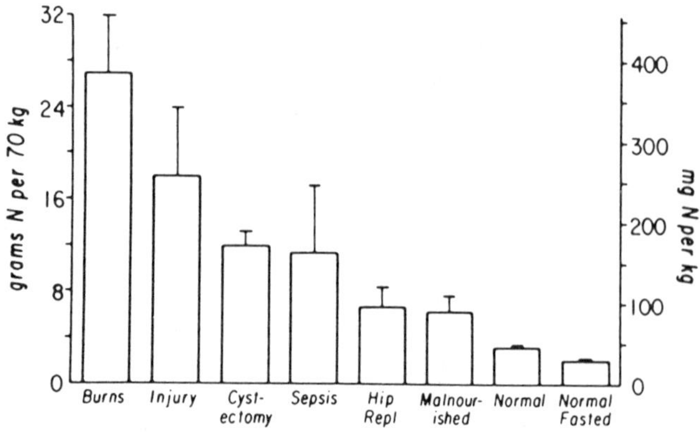

Figure 63.4 Total nitrogen excretion in fasting injured, septic, burned, or malnourished patients and normal subjects receiving only 5% glucose by vein during the 24-hr period of observation. Data are presented for patients with 47% whole-body burns, severe accidental injury, post-radical cystectomy, sepsis, post-total hip replacement, normal subjects, normal subjects after a 10–14 day fast. (Reproduced from [r10].)

In addition to the elevated total protein requirement, there is also an increase in the need for certain amino acids. Investigators have shown that the branched chain amino acids (leucine, isoleucine, and valine) are lost more readily than are the other essential amino acids,[39,40] and must be replaced proportionately by feeding. Arginine also appears to be needed in larger amounts after trauma. If the energy intake of the traumatized patient is inadequate, dietary protein will be catabolized to meet this energy need rather than being used for tissue repair—to the detriment of the patient. Protein synthesis is highly dependent on energy intake. New proteins are needed for tissue repair and for the inflammatory and immunologic responses of the body to infection or injury or both. The amino acids not used for protein synthesis are deaminated, and the resulting ammonia converted to urea. Urea production likewise is energetically expensive. Thus, large increases in both protein synthesis and ureogenesis represent an increase in the basal energy requirement and an increase in the protein requirement.

In injured or traumatized patients, protein catabolism is accelerated without a concomitant increase in over-all protein synthesis in the immediate postinjury period. During the "ebb phase" of the individual's response to trauma, where shock is the primary response, it has been estimated that the oxidation of the carbon chain of the amino acids released from muscle protein and of muscle glycogen produces almost all of the respired CO_2. In normal subjects, protein and muscle glycogen account for approximately one-third of the respired CO_2 and fatty acids the remainder.

The increase in protein catabolism is characterized by a rise in urinary urea, sulfate, and phosphate and by a depletion of tissue levels of potassium, copper, and manganese. Zinc stores are sequestered in the liver. All organs contribute to the protein loss except the brain and nervous tissue. Because muscle comprises about 70 percent of lean body mass, the bulk of proteolysis after injury occurs in muscle. The total peripheral output of amino acids rises from 7 g N/day to 23 g N/day, and all amino acids participate in the exodus from muscle. Notable are glutamine and alanine, which account for 9 grams N/day or 40 percent of the total. Also conspicuous in the drain are the branched-chain amino acids (leucine, isoleucine, and valine) and methionine. Much of the output of amino acids from the periphery is taken up by the visceral organs, so plasma amino acid levels actually may fall.[r11] Pearl et al[40] observed that a vigorous transfer of amino acids from muscle to liver and other splanchnic organs is a good prognostic sign for recovery from trauma. The negative nitrogen balance that accompanies this muscle proteolysis usually lasts for several days.

In a study of the effects of tularemia on food intake and protein catabolism, Beisel[41] found that only a fraction of the nitrogen loss by the patient studied (compared to the food-restricted control) could be accounted for by illness-induced reduction in food intake. Figure 63.5 presents Beisel's findings diagrammatically. Besides reduced food intake and secretion of counter-regulatory catabolic hormones, the inflammatory response to necrosis and sepsis involves prostaglandins and a range of cytokines, including cachetin, interleukin-1, and interleukin 6. These factors enhance both proteolysis and the hepatic uptake of amino acids, zinc, and iron, and stimulate RNA and the synthesis of acute-phase proteins. These include C-reactive protein, α-1 acid glycoprotein, hepatoglobin, α-1-antitrypsin, α-2-macroglobulin, ceruloplasmin, and fibrinogen. These changes reflect the activation of the body's defense mechanisms needed to repel invading pathogens and combat tissue injury, and contribute to the over-all negative nitrogen balance.[r10]

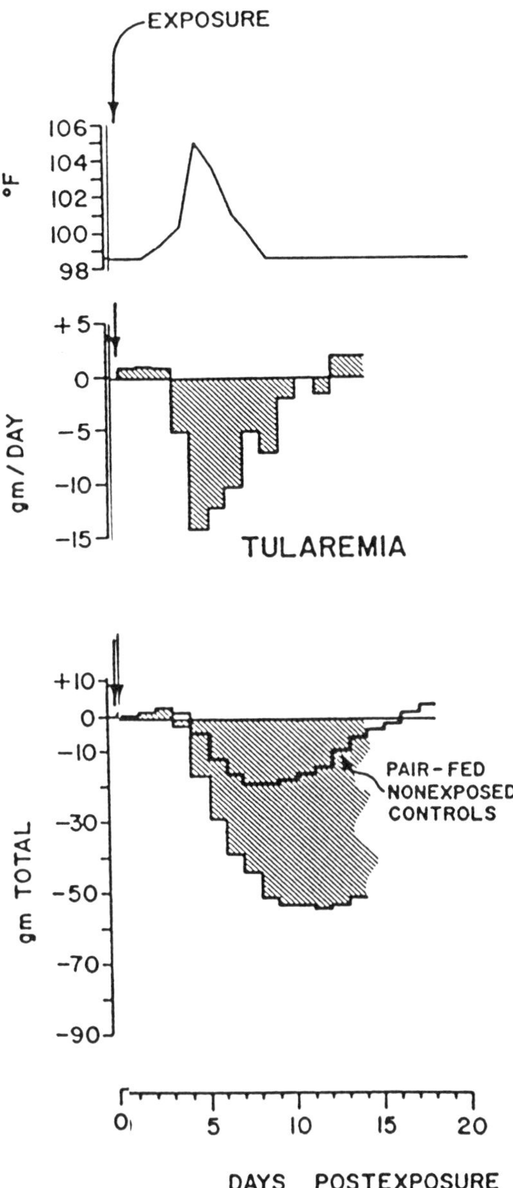

Figure 63.5 Comparison of nitrogen balance data in a patient developing a febrile illness due to tularemia with healthy persons pair-fed the same intake as the ill patient. (Reproduced from [41])

Most micronutrient requirements are based on the need for cofactors in protein and energy metabolism. Thus, as the energy and protein requirements are increased, the requirements for these nutrients are increased as well. These relationships are summarized in Table 63.3.

Severe tissue damage frequently is followed by losses in sodium, potassium, nitrogen (amino acids), calcium, phosphorus, and zinc due to destruction of the muscle and other cells and the loss of cell components.[42,43] These constituents must be provided when the malnourished tissues are repleted and destroyed cells are replaced. Thus, as recovery proceeds and protein anabolism overtakes catabolism, the needs for such nutrients as amino acids, essential fatty acids, sodium, potassium, calcium, phosphorus, iron, zinc and other trace minerals will exceed the basal requirements and even the RDA. In addition, both the prior increased catabolism and the current anabolism will increase the needs for vitamins that serve as coenzymes in metabolic processes. For example, riboflavin, which serves as a cofactor in several steps in biologic oxidation, is needed in greater amounts when there is an increase in protein turnover or when the energy requirement

Table 63.3 Effect of Trauma on the Basal Requirements for Selected Nutrients

Nutrient	Basal Requirement[a]	Stress effect
Calories	833 cal/m^2 body surface	Up to 200% increase
Protein[b]	2 mg N/basal calorie	60–500% increase
Calcium	~1% basal protein requirement	Increase[c]
Phosphorus	~2% basal protein requirement	Increase[c]
Zinc	5–22 mg/day[d]	Increase[c]
Vitamin A (retinol equivalents)	0.5–1.2 mg/day	Increase[c]
Vitamin C	10 mg/day	Increase[c]
Thiamin	0.2–0.5 mg/1000 calories	Increase[c]
Riboflavin	0.55–1.1 mg/day	Increase[c]
Niacin equivalents[e]	4.4 mg/1000 calories	Increase[c]

[a]Requirement is defined as that intake below which deficiency symptoms can occur. The figure makes no allowance for increments due to age, activity or bioavailability.
[b]Assumes a good quality protein.
[c]Percent increase unknown; research is needed to establish the needs for these and other nutrients in traumatized persons.
[d]Broad range given due to insufficient data (Halsted et al., 1974).
[e]Includes tryptophan, which is available for conversion to niacin.

is increased. Studies of riboflavin excretion following severe trauma, which is characterized by both an increase in protein turnover and an increase in energy requirement, show that excretion of riboflavin metabolites is increased.[44,45]

Factors such as disturbed renal function in the immediate post-trauma period and increased heat production also will affect energy, water, and electrolyte requirements. Wound healing, in addition, imposes special requirements for nutrients involved in the synthesis of collagen and the maintenance of the integrity of the skin. Thus, in the post-trauma and convalescent period requirements for all essential nutrients increase. Unfortunately, the degree to which requirements for these nutrients are increased during convalescence is unknown. As a guideline, they should be given at two to three times the RDA.

A further consideration in the determination of the nutrient needs of the injured or infected patient is the effect on nutrient utilization of the various drugs used to combat pain and infection. Drug-nutrient interactions as well as drug-hormone and drug-metabolite interactions may decrease the availability of some nutrients while potentiating the biologic effects of others. Table 63.4 lists some of these interactions.

As described above, patients who have experienced significant trauma, be it thermal, microbiologic, or mechanical, have greatly increased nutrient needs. Yet, these patients have no desire to eat, or may be unable to eat. In fact, many of the hormonal and metabolic changes in traumatized people are similar to those signals proposed as suppressors of appetite. Because of trauma, the signals for hunger are muted, even though nutrient needs may be increased. The patient may have nausea, vomiting, and extensive injury or disease affecting the gastrointestinal tract, or may even be unconscious. Under these circumstances, patients must be nutritionally supported through the use of solutions administered by nasogastric tube into

Table 63.4 Some Drugs That Affect Nutrient Intakes and Use

Drug	Effect
Phenethylamine and related compounds	Anorexia
Amphetamine	Anorexia
Ethanol	Inhibits intestinal absorption of folate and B_{12}; increases need for niacin, riboflavin, thiamin, and pyridoxine
Diphenylhydantoin (Dilantin)	Impairs use of folate
Oral Contraceptives	Increased folate turnover
Azulfidine	Decreases folate absorption, B_{12} and fat soluble vitamins
Neomycin	Decreases lipid absorption
P-aminosalicylic acid	Promotes diarrhea and results in decreased absorption of almost all nutrients
Colchicine	Promotes diarrhea and results in decreased absorption of almost all nutrients
Biguanides (phenformin, metformin)	Decreased absorption of B_{12}
Bile salt sequestrants	Decreased fat and fat-soluble vitamin absorption

the GI tract or, if that is not feasible, by IV infusion. The details of enteral and parenteral nutrition support are presented in Chapter 66.

References

Research Reports

1. Benedict FC. A study of prolonged fasting. Washington: Carnegie Institute, Publication #203, 1915.
2. Cahill GF Jr, Herrera MG, Morgan AP, Soeldner JS, Levy PL, Reichard GA, Kipnis DM. Hormone fuel relationships during fasting. J Clin Invest 1966;*45*:1751–1769.
3. Saudek CD, Felig P. The metabolic events of starvation. Am J Med 1976;*60*:116–126.
4. Suskind RM, Thanangkul O, Darwongsak D, Leitzmann C, Suskind L, Olson RE. The malnourished child: Clinical, biochemical and hematological changes. In: Suskind RM. Malnutrition and the Immune Response. New York: Raven Press, 1977, pp 4–8.
5. Olson RE. The role of hormones in protein metabolism. JAMA. 1957;*164*:1758–1765.
6. Alleyne GAO. Mineral metabolism in Protein-Calorie Malnutrition, edited by R.E. Olson, pp 201–212, Academic, N.Y., N.Y. 1975.
7. Kritzinger EE, Kanengoni E, Jones JJ. Effective renin activity in plasma of children with kwashiorkor. Lancet 1972;*1*:412–413.
8. James WPT, Hay AM. Albumin metabolism: Effect of the nutritional state and the dietary protein intake. J Clin Invest 1968;*47*:1958–1972.
9. Hoffenberg R, Black E, Borck JA. Albumin and gamma-globulin tracer studies in protein depletion states. J Clin Invest 1966;*45*:143–152.
10. Kirsch R, Frith L, Black E, Hoffenberg, R. Regulation of albumin synthesis and catabolism by alteration of dietary protein. Nature 1968;*217*:578–579.
11. Hansen JDL. Endocrines and malnutrition. In: Olson RE. Protein-Calorie Malnutrition. New York: Academic Press, 1975, p 229.
12. Suskind R, Amatayakul K, Lietzmann C, Olson RE. Interrelationships between growth hormone and amino acid metabolism in protein-calorie malnutrition. In: Gardner LJ, Amacher P. Endocrine Aspects of Malnutrition. Santa Ynez, CA: KROC Foundation, 1973, pp 99–113.
13. Pimstone BL, Becker D, Weinkove C, Mann M. Insulin secretion in protein-calorie malnutrition In: Gardner LI, Amacher P. Endocrine Aspects of Malnutrition. Santa Ynez, CA: KROC Foundation, 1973, pp 289–305.
14. Stephen JML, Waterlow JC. The effect of malnutrition on activity of two enzymes concerned with amino acid metabolism in human liver. Lancet 1968;*1*:118–121.
15. Holt, LE Jr,Snyderman SE, Norton PM, Roitman E, Finch J. The plasma aminogram in kwashiorkor. Lancet 1963;2:1343–1348.
16. Pimstone BL, Wittmann W, Hansen JDL, Murray P. Growth hormone and kwashiorkor: Role of growth hormone in protein homeostasis. Lancet 1966;*2*:779–780.
17. Alvarado J, Luthringer DG. Serum immunoglobulins in edematous protein-calorie malnourished Guatemalan children at INCAP. Clin Pediatr 1971;*10*:174–179.
18. Najjar, S.S., Stephan, M, Astour, R.Y. Serum levels of immunoglobulins in marasmic infants. Arch Dis Child 1969;*44*:120–124.
19. Suskind RM, Sirisinha S, Vithayasai V, Edelman R, Damrongsak D, Charuptana C, Olson RE. Immunoglobulins and antibody response in children with protein-calorie malnutrition. Am J Clin Nutr 1976;*29*:836–841.
20. Reddy V, Srikantia SG. Antibody response in kwashiorkor. Indian J Med Res 1964;*52*:1154.
21. Cohen S, Hansen JDL. Metabolism of albumin and γ-globulin in kwashiorkor. Clin Sci 1962;*23*:351.
22. Scrimshaw N, Behan M, Arroyave G, Tyada G, Viteri F. Kwashiorkor in children and its response to protein therapy. JAMA 1957;*164*:555–561.
23. Muto Y, Smith JE, Milch PO, Goodman DS. Regulation of retinol-binding protein metabolism by vitamin A status in the rat. J Biol Chem 1972;*247*:2542–2545.
24. Smith FR, Suskind RM, Thanangkul O, Leitzmann C, Goodman DS, Olson RE. Plasma vitamin A, retinol binding protein, and prealbumin concentrations in protein calorie malnutrition. III. Response to varying dietary treatments. Am J Clin Nutr 1975;*28*:732–738.
25. Bistrian B, Blackburn G, Hallowell E, Hedle R. Protein status of general surgical patients. JAMA 1974;*230*:856–886.
26. Bistrian BR, Blackburn GL, Vitale J, et al. Prevalence of malnutrition in general medical patients. JAMA 1976;*235*:1567–1570.
27. Smith T, Corli A. Hospital malnutrition. 1977; Lancet *1*:689–693.
28. Weinsier RL, Hunker EM, Krumdieck CL, Butterworth CE Jr. Hospital malnutrition: A prospective evaluation of general medical patients during the course of hospitalization. Am J Clin Nutr 1979;*32*:418–426.
29. Cuthbertson DP. The disturbance of metabolism produced by bony and non-bony injury, with notes on certain abnormal conditions of bone. Biochem 1930;*24*:1244–1249.
30. Cuthbertson DP. Observations on the disturbance of metabolism produced by injury to the limbs. Quart J Med 1932;*25*:233–245.
31. Cuthbertson DP. Post-shock metabolic response. Lancet 1942;*i*:433–434.
32. Cuthbertson DP, Tilstone WJ. Nutrition of the injured. Am J Clin Nutr 1957;*21*:911–920.
33. Cuthbertson DP. Post traumatic metabolism: A multidisciplinary challenge. Surg Clin North Am 1978;*58*:1045–1054.
34. Shangraw RE, Jahoor F, Miyoshi H, Neff WA, Stuart CA, Herndon DN, Wolfe RR. Differentiation between septic and post burn insulin resistance. Metabolism 1989;*38*:983–989.
35. Lang CH, Dobrescu C. Sepsis induced changes in in vivo insulin action in diabetic rats. Am J Physiol 1989;*257*:E301–E308.
36. Clemens MG, Chandry IH, McDermott PH, Bave AE. Regulation of glucose production from lactate in experimental sepsis. Am J Physiol 1983;*244*:R794–R800.
37. Lang CH. Sepsis-induced insulin resistance in rats is mediated by a β adrenergic mechanism. Am J Physiol 1992;*263*:E703–E711.
38. Berdanier CD. Role of glucocorticoids in the regulation of lipogenesis. FASEB J. 1989;*3*:2179–2183.
39. Randle PJ, Hales CN, Garland PB, Neisholme EA. The glucose-fatty acid cycle: Its role in insulin sensitivity and the metabolic disturbances of diabetes mellitus. 1963; Lancet *1*:785–789.

40. Pearl RH, Clover GHA, Hirsch EF, Loda M, Grindlinger GA, et al. Prognosis and survival as determined by visceral amino acid clearance in severe trauma. J Trauma 1985;*25*:777–83.

41. Beisel WR. Effect of infection on human protein metabolism. Fed Proc 1966;*25*:1682–1686.

42. Moser PB, Borel J, Majerus P, Anderson RA. Serum zinc and urinary zinc excretion in trauma patients. Nutr Res 1985;*5*:253–261.

43. Shippee RL, Mason AD, Burleson DG. The effect of burn injury and zinc nutriture on fecal endogenous zinc, tissue zinc distribution, and T-lymphocyte subset distribution using a murine model. Proc Soc Exp Biol Med 1988;*189*:31–38.

44. Andreae WA, Schenker V, Browne JSL. Riboflavin metabolism after trauma and during convalescence in man. Fed Proc 1946;*5*:3A.

45. Goldsmith G. Riboflavin. In: Progress in Food and Nutritional Science (1975); *1*:559–609.

Reviews

r1. Cahill GF. Starvation in man. N Engl J Med 1970;*282*:668–678.

r2. Hoffer LJ. Starvation. In: Shils M, Olson J, Shike M. eds. Modern Nutrition in Health and Disease. Philadelphia: Lea & Febiger, 1994, pp 927–949.

r3. Torun B, Viteri FE. Protein-energy malnutrition. In: Shils M, Young V. eds. Modern Nutrition in Health and Disease, 7th ed. Philadelphia, Lea & Febiger, 1988, pp 746–773.

r4. Olson RE. Protein Calorie Malnutrition. New York: Academic Press, 1975.

r5. Hansen MA, Fernandez G, Good RA. Nutrition and immunity: The influence of diet on autoimmunity and the role of zinc in the immune response. Ann Rev Nutr 1982;*2*:151–177.

r6. Moore FD. Metabolic Care of the Surgical Patient. Philadelphia: WB Saunders, 1959.

r7. Kinney JM. Energy requirements for the surgical patient. In: Ballinger WF, Collings JA, Drucker WR, Dudrick SJ, Zeppa R. eds. Manual of Surgical Nutrition. Philadelphia, WB Saunders, 1975, pp 223–235.

r8. Frayn KN. Substrate turnover after injury. Br Med Bull 1985;*41*:232–239.

r9. Kinney JM, Elwyn DH. Protein metabolism and injury. Ann Rev Nutr 1983;*3*:433–466.

r10. Goldstein SA, Elwyn DH. The effects of injury and sepsis on fuel utilization. Ann Rev Nutr 1989;*9*:445–473.

r11. Wolfe RR, Jahoor F, Hartl WH. Protein and amino acid metabolism after injury. Diabetes Metab Rev 1989;*5*:149–164.

CHAPTER 64

Hyperphagia, Anorexia, and Regulation of Food Intake

Carolyn D. Berdanier
Robert E. Olson

The signals for hunger and satiety are diverse and, as yet, not well understood. Animals that have been overfed will undereat (or abstain from eating) until they attain the body weight of their untreated cohorts. Contrariwise, animals that have been underfed will subsequently overeat to obtain a proper body composition. Humans, likewise, will often self-regulate their food intake so as to attain a desired body weight. There are numerous reports in the literature that support the existence of both short-term (minutes to hours) and long-term (days to months) controls of food intake that, in turn, affect the regulation of body weight.[r1,r2] The regulation of food intake is a very active area of research at present, and includes the study of the role of the CNS in determining satiety and hunger as well as the study of the effects of food and food components on these behaviors and on food use.

A number of hormones, diet ingredients, metabolites, and drugs have been shown to influence food intake and feeding behavior. Some of the more important ones are shown in Table 64.1. Hormones that can enhance food intake at one level can suppress it at another level. Insulin is a prime example; thyroxine is another. Normal individuals given a low dose of insulin will experience hunger. However, large doses of insulin can provoke a serious hypoglycemia that will have the opposite effect. Campfield and Smith[1] have studied the signals for feeding that occur in a free-feeding rat. They have shown that feeding is initiated when the brain perceives a fall in blood glucose. Transient declines of blood glucose levels within the normal range were found to precede meal initiation. This feeding response could be attenuated if blood glucose levels were elevated via an IV infusion of glucose. Preceding the transient fall in blood glucose was a transient insulin spike that probably was responsible for the transient fall in glucose. Soon after a high glucose meal individuals will feel satiated; their blood and brain glucose levels have risen, as has blood insulin, and their appetite is suppressed. Other hormones are involved as well. At low levels of thyroxine, hunger signals are poorly perceived. The patient, although not anorexic, does not have a strong drive to eat. In contrast, hyperthyroidism is characterized by strong, almost unremitting hunger.

Within this framework are a number of afferent and efferent systems that influence food intake by providing information to the brain and relaying instructions via neuronal signals from the brain to the rest of the body. Bray[2] has recently reviewed the actions of peptides that affect the intake of specific nutrients and the sympathetic nervous system. Food intake can be increased or decreased with reciprocal effects on the CNS when these peptides are administered. Galanin, neuropeptide Y, opioid peptides, growth hormone releasing hormone, and desacetyl-melanocyte stimulating hormone increase food intake, whereas insulin excess, glucagon, cholecystokinin, anorectin, corticotropin-releasing hormone, neurotensin, bombesin, cyclo-his-pro, and thyrotropin-releasing hormone reduce food intake. Several of these hormones or peptides have specific actions with respect to the intake of given food components. For example, increases in neuropeptide Y result in increased carbohydrate intake, while increases in the levels of galanin and opioid peptides increase fat intake. Fat intake is suppressed when the blood level of enterostatin rises. Rising blood levels of glucagon suppress protein intake. All of the above are short-term signals that appear to regulate food selection as well as the amount of food consumed.

Table 64.1 Factors That Affect Food Intake

Enhancers	Suppressors	
Insulin	Cachectin (tumor necrosis factor)	Anorectin
Testosterone	Estrogen	Corcicotropin-releasing hormone
Glucocorticoids	Phenylethylamines[1]	
Thyroxine	Mazindol	Neurotensin
Low serotonin levels	Substance P	Bombesin
Dynorphin	Glucagon	Cyclo-his-pro
Bendorphin	"Satietin" (a blood-borne factor)	High-protein diets
Neuropeptide Y	High-fat diet	High blood glucose
Galanin	Serotonin	
Opioid peptides	Fluoxetine	
Growth hormone-releasing hormone	Pain	
Desacetyl-melanocyte stimulating hormone	Histidine (precursor of histamine)	
Antidepressant[2]	Amino acid imbalance in diet	
	Tryptophane (precursor of serotonin)	
	Cholecystokinin	
	Somatostatin	
	Thyrotropin-releasing hormone	

[1]All these drugs except phenylpropanolamine are controlled substances. Many have serious side-effects. They are structurally related to the catecholamines. Most of them are active as short-term appetite suppressants and act through their effects on the CNS particularly through the β adrenergic and/or dopaminergic receptors. This group includes amphetamine, methamphetamine, phenmetrazine, phentermine, diethylpropion, fenfluramine, and phenylpropanolamine. Phenylpropanolamine-induced anorexia is not reversed by the dopamine antagonist haloperidol.
[2]All these drugs are controlled substances and their use must be carefully monitored. This group includes amitriptyline, buspirone, chlordiazepoxide, chlorpromazine, cisplatin, clozapine, ergotamine, fluphenazine, impramine, iprindole, and others that block 5-HT receptors.

Although most of these studies have been done in carefully prepared experimental animals (usually rats), there is sufficient indirect evidence to suggest that short-term food intake is similarly regulated in humans. In humans serotoninergic agents are being developed for use as treatment for obesity and eating disorders. These agents are successful because they either block the binding of serotonin (5-hydroxytryptamine, 5-HT) to its receptor, or upregulate the receptors' binding affinity. 5-HT receptors are widespread throughout the cerebral cortex, the limbic system, the striatum, the brain stem, the choroid plexus, and almost every other region of the CNS. Because serotonin suppresses feeding, blocking the receptor enhances feeding. Thus, drugs that block these receptors are useful in treating anorexia (decreased desire to eat), especially the anorexia that accompanies anxiety, depression, obsessive-compulsive disorders, panic disorders, migraine, and emesis due to chemotherapy. In contrast, drugs that potentiate the binding of 5HT to its receptor will result in a suppression of appetite and may be useful in treating the hyperphagia of Prader Willi syndrome[6] and that associated with genetic obesity.

Drugs, particularly those used in cancer chemotherapy, frequently have appetite suppression as a side-effect. In part, this reduction in food intake may be due to disease and/or drug-induced changes in taste and aroma perception and in part due to the effects of the disease and/or drugs on the CNS, particularly the adrenergic and serotonergic receptors. Several of the drugs listed in Table 64.1 are appetite suppressants and are chemically related to the catecholamines. As indicated, some of these drugs can be addictive and are therefore controlled substances. It appears that none of the drugs listed in Table 64.1 are free of side-effects.

Some steroids affect food intake. Adrenalectomized animals or humans with Addison's disease, both glucocorticoid-deficient states, do not perceive normal hunger signals. If without food for extended periods, they are difficult to realiment. However, once eating commences, a normal feeding pattern will be maintained. In excess, glucocorticoid stimulates feeding, and patients with Cushing's disease (excess glucocorticoid production) or those on long-term glucocorticoid treatment report increased hunger and food intake. Patients with Cushing's disease often have increased fat depots across the shoulders and in the abdomen. In addition, obese patients are frequently characterized by excess blood levels of both glucocorticoids and insulin. As noted above, these hormones stimulate appetite, and feeding commences.

Within the normal range, doses of the steroids testosterone and estrogen, have opposite effects on food intake. In experimental animals day-to-day variations in food intake by females will follow the same pattern as their day-to-day variations in estrogen level. When estrogen is high, food intake is suppressed, and vice versa. Women who are anestrus owing to ovariectomy or who are postmenopausal frequently lose their day-to-day estrogen-mediated food intake pattern. With this loss is a more even (and somewhat increased) food intake and subsequent body fat gain. This has been found as well in castrated female rats[6] and is explained by the loss in food intake control exerted by the estrogens rather than by an estrogen-inhibiting effect on lipogenesis.[8] Testosterone tends to increase food intake, but because it also stimulates protein synthesis and spontaneous physical activity, changes in food intake are marginal. As testosterone levels decline in males with age, protein synthesis declines and fat synthesis increases. This results in a change in body composition, with an increase in body fat stores. The age-related decline in testosterone production is not accompanied by a decline in food intake.

Although food intake can vary from day to day in response to minor day-to-day variations in food supply, activity, and hormonal status, body weight is relatively constant. The mechanisms that control body weight are complex, and the fine details of this regulation are far from clear. However, major deviations in either food intake or physiologic state can affect body weight or energy balance. If food intake (energy intake) is curtailed for days to months, body weight will fall; similarly, if food intake is dramatically increased, body weight will increase. This relationship assumes no change in body energy demand. As described in the chapter on undernutrition, energy requirements can be increased up to tenfold by major illness even when the patient is recumbent and perhaps sedated. Similarly, an individual who has markedly changed his or her activity level will affect his or her energy balance. If strenuous exercise is added without an increase in food intake, weight loss will occur. In most individuals, therefore, changes in energy balance, whether through changes in intake or expenditure, will result in a body weight change.

Anorexia Nervosa

That food intake can be consciously controlled is evident in the condition known as anorexia nervosa. This condition is frequently observed in adolescent females and is related to their inaccurate perception of their body fatness. They become obsessed with the desire to be thin, and either refuse to eat and adequately nourish their bodies or do eat but, after eating, force themselves to regurgitate food. Self-induced vomiting is called bulimia. Additional behaviors related to an obsession with body image include the regular use of laxatives and diuretics and extensive participation in exercise designed to increase energy expenditure. Although the patients may be eating some food, they do not consume enough to meet their macro- and micronutrient requirements.[8] Because of this they are in negative energy and protein balance. These patients are characterized by greatly reduced body fat,[9] amenorrhea, hypothermia, and hypotension, if untreated, they will starve to death. In many respects, these patients' physiologic/biochemical features are similar to those patients described in the chapter on starvation. Their catabolic hormone levels are high, and their body energy stores are being raided as a result.[10,11] Insulin resistance due to the catabolic hormones is observed.[12] Liver and muscle glycogen levels are low. Fat stores are minimal. As the weight loss proceeds further, these individuals develop a reduced bone mass,[9] a decreased metabolic rate, decreased heart rate, hypoglycemia, hypothyroidism, electrolyte imbalance, reduced levels of gonadotropic and gonadal hormones, elevated free fatty acid and cholesterol levels, peripheral edema, and, lastly, cardiac and renal failure. When their fat stores fall below 2 percent of total body weight they will die, although many die earlier from protein depletion. This 2 percent represents the lipids essential to the structure and function of membranes as well as those complex lipids that comprise the CNS.

When a physician encounters such a patient, he faces the challenge of reversing the condition. Just as it is difficult to reverse starvation-induced changes in metabolism of unintentionally starving humans (see chapter on starvation, protein-calorie malnutrition, trauma, and on enteral and parenteral feeding), reversing the weight loss of anorexic patients presents some special challenges. The caloric requirements for weight regain in anorexic patients are highly variable[13] and depend largely on the physiologic status of the patient at the time of treatment and on the preanorexia body weight. Patients who had been obese prior to their self-induced anorexia regain their lost weight faster than those patients whose body weight had been normal.[13–14] Dietary treatment should be initiated with a liquid diet of 1200–1400 kc/day containing all essential nutrients. After a week it should be increased to 3000 kc/day and eventually replaced by solid foods.

Pharmaceutical agents to stimulate appetite and reverse depression (if present) can be used. Frequently, if the person is clinically depressed, treatment of the depression will often have a positive effect on food intake. Treatment of the anorectic person with appetite-stimulating drugs, nutritional support, and counseling can usually reverse the condition of weight loss and, secondarily, positively affect the depression. The outcome of the treatment depends on when it is initiated. If anorexia nervosa is recognized early in the disease, chances of success are much greater than if treatment is initiated after irreversible tissue changes have occurred. While there is controversy about the success of treatment as well as the accuracy of diagnosis, it is generally agreed that aggressive treatment can achieve reversal in 50 percent of cases. Mortality is estimated at 6 percent. This leaves approximately 42 percent who recover spontaneously without medical intervention. Treatment success also depends on the degree of self-prescribed food intake restriction. Total food abstinence is far more threatening than mild abstinence. Included in the mortality figure of 6 percent are those who commit suicide. This implies a relationship between the development of depression and anorexia—two self-destructive behavioral abnormalities.

Restoring the weight loss of the anorectic patient follows a slightly different pattern from the regain of fat by traumatized or formerly obese individuals. In the latter two groups the regain of fat precedes the regain of protein. In fact, when the reduced genetically obese individual is refed, restoration of fat stores takes precedence over restoration of protein levels.[r1] In the recovering anorectic patient resynthesis of protein keeps pace with resynthesis of fat. As both synthetic processes utilize micronutrients, these must be provided at levels similar to those prescribed for growing children. Recovering anorectic patients are "growing" new tissue to replace that which was "raided" during the energy deficit period. They must consume balanced diets to support this regrowth.

Bulimic and nonbulimic anorectics differ in their weight recovery.[14] Those who were bulimic recover lost weight more rapidly than do those who were anorectic only. This is probably due to the difference in rate of weight loss. Those anorectics who were also bulimic were more severely starved and lost weight faster than did nonbulimic anorectic subjects. Thus, they are more likely to be diagnosed and treated sooner than nonbulimic anorectics patients. In anorexia, as with prolonged starvation, gut absorptive capacity is compromised owing to a loss of cells lining the GI tract. In the early phase of treatment, malabsorption is likely to occur. Because of the development of malabsorption, the recovering anorectic person requires more food than the recovering bulimic-anorectic patient. The recovering anorectic person has lost more absorptive cells than has the bulimic anorectic person. Of interest is the report that even after weight regain, the recovered person with anorexia has a higher than normal energy requirement; and, if this requirement is not met, will begin to lose weight again. This suggests that not all of the anorexia nervosa is self-inflicted. It may begin with a conscious effort to consume less food, but then may continue because of a change in the signals for food intake initiation and cessation and a change in the efficiency with which the body uses the food consumed.

References

Research Reports

1. Campfield LA, Smith FJ. Transient declines in blood glucose signal meal initiation. Int J Obesity 1990;*14*:15–33.
2. Bray GA. Peptides affect the intake of specific nutrients and the sympathetic nervous system. Am J Clin Nutr 1992;*55*:265S–271S.
3. Blundell JE. Serotonin and the biology of feeding. Am J Clin Nutr 1992;*55*:155S–159S.
4. Yen TT, Fuller RW. Preclinical pharmacology of fluoxetine, a serotonergic drug for weight loss. Am J Clin Nutr 1992;*55*:177S–180S.
5. Zipf WB, Berntson GG. Characteristics of abnormal food intake patterns in children with Prader-Willi Syndrome and study of effects of naloxone. Am J Clin Nutr 1987;*46*:277–281.
6. Shutte M, Parente J, Berdanier CD. Ovariectomy results in increased fat gain in weight cycled female BHE/cdb rats. Nutrition 1993; (in press).
7. Berdanier CD. Effects of estrogen on the responses of male and female rats to starvation-refeeding. N Nutr 1981;*111*:1425–1429.
8. Huse DM, Lucas AR. Dietary patterns in anorexia nervosa. Am J Clin Nutr 1984;*40*:251–254.
9. Mazeso RB, Barden HS, Ohlrich ES. Skeletal and body composition effects of anorexia nervosa. Am J Clin Nutr 1990;*52*:438–441.
10. Johnston JL, Leiter LA, Burrow GN, Garfinkel PE, Anderson GH. Excretion of urinary catecholamine metabolites in anorexia nervosa: Effect of body composition and energy intake. Am J Clin Nutr 1984;*40*:1001–1006.
11. Casper RC, Chatterton RT, Davies JM. Alterations in serum cortisol and its binding characteristics in anorexia nervosa. J Clin Endocrinol Metab 1979;*49*:406–411.
12. Wachslight-Rodbard H, Gross HA, Rodbard D, Ebert MH, Roth J. Increased insulin binding to erythrocytes in anorexia nervosa. N Engl J Med 1979;*300*:882–887.
13. Walker J, Roberts SL, Halmi KA, Goldberg SC. Caloric requirements for weight gain in anorexia nervosa. Am J Clin Nutr 1979;*32*:1396–1400.
14. Kaye WH, Gwirtsman HE, Obarzanek E, George TR, Jimerson DC, Ebert MH. Caloric intake necessary for weight maintenance in anorexia nervosa: nonbulimics require greater caloric intake than bulimics. Am J Clin Nutr 1986;*44*:435–443.

Reviews

r1. Anderson GH. Regulation of food intake, in Modern Nutrition in Health and Disease 8th Edition, Shils M, Olson J, Shike M eds. Lea and Febiger, Philadelphia, 1994:524–536.

r2. Martin RJ, White BD, Hulsey MG. The regulation of body weight. Am Scientist 1991;*79*:528–541.

r3. Harrington MA, Zhong P, Garow SJ, Ciaranello RD. Molecular biology of serotonin receptors. J Clin Psychiatr 1992;*53*:8–27 (Supplement 10).

r4. Wellman PJ. Overview of adrenergic anorectic agents. Am J Clin Nutr 1992;*55*:193S–198S.

CHAPTER 65

Carolyn D. Berdanier

Obesity

Obesity, excess body fatness, is one of the leading nutritional disorders in the developed world. It is one of the prime contributors to the development of cardiovascular disease, hypertension, and diabetes.[1,r1,2,3,r2] Obesity is more prevalent in lower socioeconomic groups[r3] than in higher socioeconomic groups and is associated with a shortened lifespan.[1,r1,2,3,r2] Men in their third and fourth decades of life are more vulnerable to the adverse effects of obesity than are women of the same age or than men and women over 70. Mortality due to cardiovascular disease or to other obesity-related disease is greater in this population segment (30–50-year-old males) than in other segments. One survey reported a 12-fold increase in mortality among obese men aged 25–34 compared with normal-weight men. The prevalence of adult-onset diabetes is about three times higher in overweight individuals than in normal weight individuals. Hypercholesterolemia and hypertension are two and six times higher, respectively, for overweight Americans between the ages of 20 and 45, compared to nonoverweight Americans of the same age group. The 1988 Surgeon General's Report on Nutrition and Health identified "Energy and Weight Control" as one of the five major diet-related health issues for Americans. This report and many others recommended that people should achieve and maintain a desirable body weight.

It is the excess body fat store and its distribution that concerns health professionals, not the excess body weight.[r4] Body builders and other athletes can have greater than average body weight, but a larger than average percentage of their body weight is bone and muscle, not stored fat. As people age, their body composition changes, but their body weight may not. They may decrease their physical activity, losing muscle mass while gaining fat mass.

Body Fat Estimates

Fat mass cannot be measured directly in humans. However, a number of indirect methods are available and have been used to estimate the extent of the body fat store. Sophisticated techniques using ultrasound, computer-assisted tomography, magnetic resonance imaging, or bioelectrical impedance are available, but none of these is really practical in the clinical setting. Underwater weighing is used by researchers and is based on the difference in density of the different body components. The subject is weighed both before immersion and while immersed in water. The body water, which comprises approximately 60 percent of total body weight, has a density of 1; body fat has a density of less than 1. Thus, the ratio of the weight in air to that of the immersed weight will be a reflection of extent of body fat store. The larger the ratio, the smaller the fat store, and vice versa. Estimating fat stores in this way is cumbersome and/or not feasible in most clinical settings. Researchers using this method have made some correlations between this estimate and estimates of body fatness using the measurement of skinfold thicknesses at key locations. These are sites where subcutaneous fat can be assessed using calipers to estimate the skinfold thickness. The fold below the upper arm (triceps fold) and the fold at the iliac crest are frequently used. Equations have been derived to calculate body fatness from these measurements.

Even simpler estimates of body fatness can be derived using the patient's body weight and height and comparing these values to those considered desirable for men and women. The first such tables were developed by the Metropolitan Life Insurance Company. This company made the assumption that young (age 20–30) people applying for life insurance (and found insurable) were healthy. They then took the body weights of these people and their heights and arranged the weights according to height for both males and females. They called these weights "desirable" weights because they were associated with the lowest mortality. Because the weight range for each height was so large, they later subdivided each weight for height range into thirds and presented these thirds as being representative of small, medium, and large frame sizes. This table has been found useful by many in estimating desirable body weight, but the user must remember that it was not based on actual measurements of body composition, nor was the frame size categorization based on actual measurements of skeletal size. The table is based only on heights and weights of individuals in the third decade of life who wanted (and could afford) life insurance. In this respect there is a bias. The heights and weights were from those affluent enough to buy life insurance. Minority groups were largely underrepresented in the data base.

A broader data base using subjects of all ages, economic status, both sexes, and from minority and majority cultural/ethnic groups was obtained by the National Health and Nutrition Examination Survey (NHANES) that has been conducted at ten-year intervals by the Center for Disease Control of the US Public Health Service. These surveys have collected data not only from young adult men and women, but also from children and older adults. These weights and heights have been used to create tables giving desirable weight ranges for males and females. In addition, NHANES made more detailed measurements of skinfold thickness, skeletal size, and density and a variety of biochemical and physiologic features using a representative subset of the population assessed. The NHANES tables, therefore, have a broader data base. Despite the difference in data bases used to construct the tables, both are useful in evaluating the patient in terms of desirable body weight.

Perhaps more popular now is the use of body mass index (BMI). This useful index is obtained by dividing the body weight (kg) by the height in meters (m) squared (wt/ht^2). BMI correlates with body fatness and with the risk of obesity-related disease or diseases. The BMI varies with age in that a desirable BMI for people aged 19–29 is between 19 and 24; that for people aged 55–64 is between 23 and 28.[r4] Overweight is defined as a BMI between 25 and 30; obesity is a BMI over 30.

While total body fatness is an important risk factor for several degenerative diseases, the distribution of the stored fat may impact on these diseases as well. Males and females differ in the pattern of body fat stores. Males tend to deposit fat in the abdominal area, while females tend to deposit fat in the gluteal area and thighs. Measuring the waist and hip circumference allows one to compute the waist to hip ratio (WHR); as this ratio increases, so too does the risk for cardiovascular disease, diabetes mellitus, and hypertension.[2,4,5] In men, if the WHR is greater than 0.90 and in women if the WHR is greater than 0.80, the risk for cardiovascular disease increases significantly.

Although excess body fat stores, or obesity, is considered a risk factor in a number of diseases, no permanent cure for the disorder has yet been discovered. The key words in the above sentence are "permanent cure." The lack of an appropriate lasting treatment for this disorder is due to our lack of understanding of why people become overfat. Diet restriction is recommended but seldom followed in the long term. Listed in Table 65.1 are some of the reasons why excess body fatness develops.

Research on the genetic basis for excess body fatness has been stimulated by the reports of Stunkard et al.[6,7], Bouchard et al.[8–11] and Borjeson[12], who have shown that a familial trait for body fatness has a much stronger influence on body composition than do food intake patterns. Studies of monozygotic and dizygotic twins reared by their biologic parents or by adoptive parents have been conducted. In one study, adopted children and their biologic and adoptive parents were compared with respect to body weight and body fatness; in other studies twins reared together or apart were compared. In all these studies it is clear that the genetic influence far outweighs environmental influences, all other factors being equal. Further, a number of genetically obese rats, mice, dogs, and desert animals have been described.[r5,r6,13] In the rodent species, the mode of inheritance and, in some instances, the chromosomal location of the relevant gene has been identified. Obesity can be inherited via an autosomal recessive or dominant or sex-linked trait. The X chromosome and chromosomes 2, 4, and 6 have been identified as loci for aberrant genes that are related to obesity.[13] All these reports show that there is more than one genetic error that can result in obesity. Thus, the obesity syndrome may develop for a variety of reasons. In each of these mutations, an error in metabolism that affects energy balance has been suggested. Errors in the regulation of food intake[14,15] can explain excess food intake (hyperphagia) that characterizes several of these mutants. Both inappropriate hunger signals and satiety signals have been implicated. Higher than normal food intake also may characterize the genetically obese human. Yet, there are many overweight people who are not hyperphagic. There are some who can not dissipate their surplus energy as heat, i.e., stimulate thermogenesis. These individuals also do not tolerate cold well. The common thread to these two conditions is the apparent inability of the brown fat mitochondria to uncouple their electron transport, so as to release heat rather than synthesize ATP, which is required for the synthesis of fat. Failure to produce heat in the brown fat cell in response to cold or overeating is a feature of genetically obese rats and mice.[r7] This failure is attributed to a genetically determined failure to make thermogenin, the uncoupling agent responsible for brown fat thermogenesis.[r7,r8] It has also been attributed to a failure of the brown fat cell to respond to the stimulatory effects of epinephrine and is associated with an anomalous central regulation of the sympathetic input to this tissue. The function of brown fat in normal, overweight, and obese people has been studied,[r9] but it is not clear whether humans have defects in this tissue similar to those found in animals.

As mentioned in the section on anorexia in chapter 64, hormonal balance is important to the regulation of energy balance and normal body weight. Hypercortisolism[16] and hyperinsulinism[4] are associated with obesity. Cortisol and its related compounds corticosterone and cortisone play an important role in the regulation of lipogenesis.[17] These hormones are usually catabolic, but there are circumstances when they stimulate anabolic processes. This is found, for example, in the early phase of recovery from stress or trauma.

Last, there are social and cultural influences that can ensure or potentiate genetic tendencies to develop obesity. Anthropologists[r10]

Table 65.1 Suggested Reasons Why Obesity May Develop

Genetic Errors
(a) Satiety signal not sent or perceived
(b) Inability to utilize stored energy
(c) Inability to increase brown fat thermogenesis to get rid of excess intake energy
Hormonal Imbalance
(a) Excess glucocorticoids
(b) Hypothyroidism
(c) Hyperinsulinism
(d) Inappropriate neuropeptide levels
Other Causes
(a) Injury to hypothalamus
(b) Sociocultural feeding behaviors

and medical historians[r11] have identified countless examples of cultural groups that consider excess body fat as a mark of beauty as well as an indication of economic status within their society. Examples of this can be seen in statuary of different ages all the way from the upper Paleolithic period through the Renaissance to the 18th and 19th century. Women have been represented with large bellies and breasts; they are to the eye of today's observer, overfat. Men too, are of ample proportions. In fact there is an old German expression that indicates the desire of men to have as wives overweight women: "A fat wife and a full barn never did a man harm." Even today there are cultures, notably in Africa, that have customs that include preparing girls for marriage by fattening them. Malcom,[18] for example, described this practice for elite Efik girls in traditional Nigeria as well as the custom in Kenya of demanding high prices for fat brides. In these cultures, female fatness may not only be a testament to the families' wealth; it may also be a symbol of maternity and nurture. This is important to the woman if she gains status only through motherhood.

With respect to societally perceived fatness and the value of fatness, it can be assumed that the fatter a person is in a society that values fatness, the more likely that person will be married and produce children carrying genetic tendencies to fatness who will be similarly taught to eat enough to be fat. Lean people will be less likely to contribute to the gene pool because they will be considered as less desirable mates. While people in the US as well as other developed nations may not have these values, there is no doubt that eating behaviors can be taught. If young children are constantly reminded and coached to overeat, there may be a continuing stimulus to overconsume food. Added to this may be cultural and social dictates with respect to physical activity. A decrease in energy expenditure ensures a positive energy balance, which in turn may well result in excess body fatness.

Frequently, those who are overfat are told that they could become lean by reducing food intake. However, simply restricting intake does not cure the problem; it merely treats the result of the positive energy balance: excess body fat. Once this fat is lost, the formerly obese person frequently abandons the restricted diet and returns to the eating habits that result in a return to the prior weight. In some, there may be an increase in body fatness, not just a return to the prior body weight.

Set Point Theory in Body Weight Regulation

The idea that each body has its own unique size and weight has been discussed, denied, and supported by a wide variety of researchers. The hypothesis that adult body weight is closely regulated at its own unique level developed from observations of both humans and animals.[19,r12] The mechanism(s) that serve to regulate this steady state body weight are not fully known.

Healthy adult humans vary little over the years in their body weight. They may be overweight and/or overfat but, for most, that weight is maintained for years until some event occurs that results in change. In women, pregnancy, a perfectly normal physiologic event, may perturb the system sufficiently to establish a new steady-state body weight (or new set point) that, again, will be defended tenaciously. A change in the endocrine system, an insult to the body, or a conscious decision to eat more (or less) over a prolonged period (months to years) are other examples of events that might perturb the system sufficiently to result in a new set point—a new body weight that tends to be maintained from that time on.

Similarly, animals appear to regulate their body weight within fairly tight limits. Much of the research on the set-point hypothesis has been based on studies of rats and mice.[19,r12] Studies using rats that were either overfed or underfed revealed that these rats had a body weight related to their food intake. That is, if they were forced to consume more calories than they would voluntarily, they would become overfat. If they were underfed they would be leaner than normal. After these feeding treatments were discontinued, the rats that were overfed significantly reduced their food intake and used their fat stores to provide their energy needs, while those that were underfed dramatically increased their intake until they gained the weight they would have gained had they not been food-restricted. When both groups attained the weight of their untreated controls they resumed normal feeding behavior.

Although the body weight returned to normal in these overfed or underfed rats after the treatment was terminated, the composition of the body was not the same as their untreated counterparts. The percentage of body fat was affected. Underfed rats recovered by significantly increasing the synthesis and deposition of body fat. This recovery was faster than the recovery of body protein. In overfed rats, the carcass protein normalized within days of cessation of overfeeding, yet carcass fat content remained elevated weeks after overfeeding ended. Other studies have used parabiotic rats or mice to study the consequences of overfeeding or underfeeding on body weight and composition. Parabiosis is a technique where two weanling animals are joined together surgically at the skin so that they have a common circulation. Hervey, Harris, and others[19,r12] have used this technique to answer the question of whether there are blood borne factors that are involved in the regulation of feeding and body weight. Genetically obese animals have been joined to genetically lean ones, as have normal weight partners in which one partner was either overfed or underfed or was lesioned in either the feeding center of the hypothalamus or the satiety center. In each of these instances the feeding behavior of both as well as their body weight and composition were monitored. In each instance, where one partner overate and became obese, the other underate or starved and subsequently lost its body fat as well as its lean body tissue. These results were interpreted as indications that there are blood-borne factors generated by the overfed animal that signaled his feeding behavior. Further, the results of studies using genetically obese animals suggested that these obese animals did not either receive these signals or were not able to respond to them by decreasing their food intake. Likely the nonresponsivity (that is, a lack of receptor recognition of the signal) is the explanation since parabiotic pairs using genetically lean and obese animals behaved like the force-fed and voluntary feeding pairs. When the genetically obese partner was hyperphagic and obese, the lean partner ceased eating and eventually starved to death.

It is apparent that although there may be controls that influence feeding these controls may not fully regulate body fatness. Both food intake and physical activity influence lean body weight and fatness. This may explain why aging humans may gain body fat while decreasing food intake to maintain their body weight. As humans age, they decrease their physical activity, and their body composition changes; they lose muscle mass and gain body fat. Their body shape changes as well. They may observe an increase in fat mass in the abdomen and on the thighs and buttocks. Again, as already discussed, epidemiologists have noted the differences in health risks associated with the location of the excess fat stores. In humans, studies of cells isolated from the femoral, gluteal, and omental (thigh, buttocks, abdomen) depots revealed significant differences in free fatty acid release. On the basis of the rate of free fatty acid release and the size of the depot, the half-life of the fat depot in the femoral area was calculated to be 305 days. For the gluteal depot it was 326 days, and for the omental depot it was 134 days. Estimates of the half-life of the fat in the other depot sites have not been made. As the human uses stored lipid, more lipid is synthesized to replace it. Hence, the term "fatty acid turnover" means that fatty acids are both used and replaced. If they are used at a greater rate than they are replaced, net fat loss will occur. As can be seen, however, different depots will shrink at different rates, depending on their location. In addition to the aforementioned differences in depot fat use, there are also genetic and sex differences in the extent and location of the fat depots. Women, for example, have larger subcutaneous fat stores than men. Men tend to have larger omental fat depots than women of the same age and weight.

Treatment of Obesity

In almost no other area of medicine have there been so many failures as in the treatment of obesity. Fully 90 percent of all those who lose weight regain it. Data from the Chicago Gas and Electric Study[20] suggest that one cycle of loss and regain is a risk factor for death from coronary heart disease independent of body fatness. The gain-loss group when compared with subjects who neither gained nor lost weight had 1.8 times the risk of death from heart disease. This suggests that weight cycling is not a healthy behavior. If weight is to be lost it must stay lost if health benefits are to be gained. Weight cycling consists of intermittent periods of food restriction followed by periods of "normal" eating patterns. These patterns may include periods of gorging or binge eating. One of the major effects of calorie restriction on metabolism is a reduction in resting metabolic rate (RMR).[21] This lowers the overall energy requirement and increases energy efficiency, thus allowing a greater percentage of dietary calories to be partitioned into fat synthesis upon refeeding.[22,23]

The effects of weight cycling on energy efficiency may be due to the composition of the weight loss during calorie restriction. One of the consequences of rapid weight loss, especially when induced by very low-calorie, low-carbohydrate diets, is the loss of body protein or lean body mass.[24] This is especially true when the individuals are physically inactive. Maintenance of LBM is an energy-expensive process. Lean body mass is the most metabolically active tissue in the body with respect to energy demands, accounting for the majority of calories used to support the basal energy requirement (i.e., 60–70% of daily energy requirements for adults). Therefore, the less body protein, the lower the energy requirement. If weight loss includes significant amounts of body protein, the formerly overfat person will have a lower basal energy requirement and increased energy efficiency in terms of the weight regain as fat.

One of the responses of cycled humans is the tendency to overeat during the initial few days of the refeeding period. This suggests that the regulation of food intake is affected by the weight loss. Signals sent to the brain by the starved body must set the stage for hyperphagia (food intake above normal) once food becomes available for consumption. These signals must be fairly enduring because this hyperphagia is of about the same duration as the restriction period. The origin of these signals is not known, but no doubt they exist because food intake is an event regulated by the CNS. Further studies of realimented rats that have been starved or food-restricted showed that they had a preference for dietary fat if given a choice of several energy sources. As a result of this selection, cycled rats regain more body fat than if the food offered were less energy-dense. Again, this suggests the involvement of signals from the brain directing the individual toward calorically rich food. This signal, coupled with increased efficiency in retaining ingested energy, helps explain why regain of fat occurs in those who have restricted their energy intake to lose weight. Food restriction puts into place a metabolic machinery geared to save as much energy as possible and to stimulate the brain to signal the body to consume energy-rich foods. Thus, even though the patient tries to control eating and food intake, the body seeks to return to its prior overfat state Constant vigilance is required to override biological signals that direct the body to be fat. However, even when the patient carefully monitors food energy intake and consciously decides to regulate it, weight regain may occur owing to the body's increased energetic efficiency and its tendency to synthesize and store fat in preference to protein. In this situation a good exercise program is generally useful. Exercise, on a regular basis, stimulates muscle protein development and increases energy expenditure. Exercise can be a useful adjunct to energy intake restriction because it redirects energy loss from the lean body mass. In the sedentary individual, weight loss occurs at the expense of both fat and protein components of the body. In the exercising food-restricted individual, the weight loss is primarily fat loss. Further, mild to moderate exercise seems to suppress food intake. Thus the benefits of food restriction with exercise are additive.

Morbidity of Severely Obese People

Health care professionals have observed countless instances of the codevelopment of overweightness or obesity with diabetes mellitus, hypertension, and cardiovascular disease. Epidemiologists have reported that obesity and overweight are risk factors in the development of these diseases. However, there are some inconsistencies with respect to the relationship of obesity to cardiovascular disease and total mortality. Studies by Sjostrom[25] suggest that weight loss by the obese person does not affect lifespan. On the other hand, long-term studies of mortality of formerly obese people conducted by Williamson et al. of the CDC[r13] suggest that the mortality in people who have consciously reduced their body weight and remained lean is increased. These reports have raised serious questions about the efficacy of weight loss with respect to lifespan extension.

Drug Treatments

Because the problem of overweight and obesity is so pervasive in developed nations, research on possible drug therapies is quite active.[26–28,r14] Drugs that safely control food intake by correcting aberrant hunger and satiety signals, drugs that decrease energy efficiency or increase energy expenditure, and drugs that affect emotional states that have an effect on energy balance are being developed. Few have made it past the preclinical testing phase. All seem to have unpleasant and/or undesirable side-effects. Anorectic drugs work on the feeding center of the CNS, while drugs that decrease energetic efficiency do so by increasing peripheral fat cell lipolysis and increasing energy lost as heat. In this latter category are the β-adrenergic and the serotonergic drugs. Several reviews and books are available that list and describe these drugs.[23–25,r13,26] Those that affect food intake are discussed in the previous chapter 64, on Hyperphagia, Anorexia, and Regulation of Food Intake.

References

Research Reports

1. Everhart JE, Pettitt EJ, Bennett PH, Knowler WC. Duration of obesity increases the incidence of NIDDM. Diabetes 1992;*41*:235–240.
2. Fontbonne A, Thibult N, Eschwege E, Ducimetiere P. Body fat distribution and coronary heart disease mortality in subjects with impaired glucose tolerance or diabetes mellitus: The Paris prospective study, 15-year follow-up. Diabetologia 1992;*35*:464–468.
3. Sjostrom LV. Morbidity of severely obese subjects. Am J Clin Nutr 1992;*55*:5085–5155.
4. Haffner SM, Fong D, Hazuda HP, Pugh JA, Pallerson JK. Hyperinsulinemia, upper body adiposity and cardiovascular risk factors in non-diabetics. Metabolism 1988;*37*:333–345.
5. Despres JP, Moorjani S, Lupien PJ, Tremblay A, Nadeau A, Bouchard C. Regional distribution of body fat, plasma lipoproteins and cardiovascular disease. Arteriosclerosis 1990;*10*:497–511.
6. Stunkard AJ, Harris JR, Pedersen NL, McClearn GE. The body mass index of twins who have been reared apart. N Engl J Med 1990;*322*:1483–1487.
7. Stunkard AJ, Sorensen TIA, Harris C, Teasdale TW, Chakraborty R, Schull WJ, Schulsinger F. An adoption study of human obesity. N Engl J Med 1986;*314*:193–198.
8. Bouchard C. Genetic factors in obesity. Med. Clin. North America 1989;*73*:67–81.
9. Bouchard C, Savard R, Despres JP. Body composition in adopted and biological siblings. Human Biol 1985;*57*:61–75.
10. Bouchard C, Perusse L, Leblanc C. Using MZ twins in experimental research to test for the presence of a genotype-environment interaction effect. Acta Genet Gemellol 1990;*39*:85–89.
11. Despres J-P, Moorjani S, Lupin PJ, Tremblay A, Nadeau A, Bouchard C. Genetic aspects of susceptibility to obesity and related dyslipidemias. Mol Cell Biochem 1992;*113*:151–169.
12. Borjeson M. The aetiology of obesity in children. Acta Pediatr Scand 1976;*65*:279–287.
13. Coleman DL. Diabetes and obesity: thrify mutants? Nutr Rev 1978;*36*:129–132.
14. Jeanrenaud B. An hypothesis on the aetiology of obesity: Dysfunction of the central nervous system as a primary cause. Diabetologia 1985;*28*:502–513.
15. Morley JE. The neuroendocrine control of appetite: The role of the endogenous opiates, cholecystokinen TRH, gamma amino butyric acid and the diazepam receptor. Life Sci 1980;*27*:355–368.
16. Hollifield G. Glucocorticoid-induced obesity—a model and a challenge. Am J Clin Nutr 1968;*21*:1471–1474.
17. Berdanier CD. Role of glucocorticoids in the regulation of lipogenesis. FASEB 1989;*3*:2179–2183.
18. Malcolm LWG. Note on the seclusion of girls among the Efik at Old Calabar. Man 1925;*25*:113–120.
19. Harris RBS. Role of set point theory in regulation of body weight. FASEBJ 1990;*4*:3310–3318.

20. Hamm P, Shakelle RB, Stamler J. Large fluctuations in body weight during young adulthood and twenty-five year risk of coronary death in men. Am J Epidemiol 1989;*129*:312–318.

21. Welle SL, Amatruda JM, Forbes GB, Lockwood DH. Resting metabolic rates of obese women after rapid weight loss. J Clin Endocrinol Metab 1984;*59*:41–44.

22. Dulloo AG, Girardier L. Influence of dietary composition on energy expenditure during recovery of body weight in the rat: Implications for catch-up growth and obesity relapse. Metab 1992;*41*:1336–1342.

23. Dulloo AG, Girardier L. 24 Hour energy expenditure several months after weight loss in the underfed rat: Evidence for a chronic increase in whole body metabolic efficiency. Int J Obesity 1993;*17*:115–123.

24. Kreitzman SN. Factors influencing body composition during very low calorie diets. Am J Clin Nutr 1992;*56*:217S–223S.

25. Bray GA. Drug treatment of obesity. Am J Clin Nutr 1992;*55*:538S–544S.

26. Wellman PJ. Overview of adrenergic anorectic agents. Am J Clin Nutr 1992;*55*:193S–198S.

27. Yen TT, Fuller RW. Preclinical pharmacology of fluoxetine, a serotonergic drug for weight loss. Am J Clin Nutr 1992;*55*:177S–180S.

Reviews

r1. Bray GA. Complications of obesity. Ann Intern Med 1985;*103*:1052–1062.

r2. Björntorp P, Brodoff BN. Obesity. Philadelphia: JB Lippincott (1992); pp 805.

r3. Epstein FH, Higgins M. Epidemiology of obesity. In: Bjorntorp P, Brodoff BN eds. Obesity. Philadelphia: JB Lippincott 1992;330–342.

r4. Bray GA. An approach to the classification an evaluation of obesity. In: Bjorntorp P, Brodoff BN eds. Obesity. Philadelphia: JB Lippincott 1992;294–308.

r5. Bray GA, York DA. Hypothalamic and genetic obesity in experimental animals: An autonomic and endocrine hypothesis. Physiol Rev 1979;*59*:719–809.

r6. York DA. Genetic models of animal obesity. In: Bjorntorp P, Brodoff BN eds. Obesity. Philadelphia: JB Lippincott 1992;223–240.

r7. Himms-Hagen J. Brown adipose tissue metabolism. In: Bjorntorp P, Brodoff BN eds. Obesity. Philadelphia: JB Lippincott 1992;15–34.

r8. Lean MEJ. Evidence for brown adipose tissue in humans. In: Björntorp P, Brodoff BN eds. Obesity. Philadelphia: JB Lippincott 1992;117–129.

r9. Jequier, E. Regulation of thermogenesis and nutrient metabolism in the human: Relevance for obesity. In: Bjorntorp P, Brodoff BN eds. Obesity. Philadelphia: JB Lippincott 1992.

r10. Brown PJ. The biocultural evolution of obesity: An anthropological view. In: Bjorntorp P, Brodoff BN eds. Obesity. Philadelphia: JB Lippincott 1992;320–329.

r11. Bray GA. Obesity: Historical development of scientific and cultural ideas. In: Bjorntorp P, Brodoff BN eds. Obesity. Philadelphia: JB Lippincott 1992;281–293.

r12. Martin RJ, White DB, Hulsey MG. The regulation of body weight. Am Scientist 1991;*79*:528–541.

r13. Williamson D. NIH technology assessment conference report. 1992; Office of Medical Applications of Research, NIH, Federal Building, Rm. 618, Bethesda, MD 20892.

r14. Brodoff BN, Nathan C. Pharmacologic treatment of obesity. In: Bjorntorp P, Brodoff BN eds. Obesity. Philadelphia: JB Lippincott 1992;745–750.

r15. Surgeon General's Report on Nutrition and Health (1988) US Dept Health & Human Services Publication NR 88-50210 Washington, D.C.

CHAPTER 66

Enteral and Parenteral Feeding

Robert E. Olson
Carolyn D. Berdanier

Enteral and parenteral nutrition are part of nutritional pharmacology. Special feeding of patients through tubes either inserted into the upper portion of the GI tract or by tubes inserted into the venous circulation is necessary to support life in patients who are either unwilling or unable to eat or are unable to digest and absorb nutrients taken by mouth.

Enteral feeding is indicated in patients who cannot ingest adequate amounts of food. Reasons may include persistent anorexia, moderately severe burns, partial obstruction of the stomach or small bowel, malabsorption secondary to inflammatory disease of the bowel, hepatic failure, and increased metabolic needs that cannot be supplied by oral feeding (e.g., severe burns) and fistulas of the alimentary tract. Persons with at risk for inhalation plus trauma are prime candidates for enteral nutrition before parenteral nutrition is considered, since the gut is the preferred organ for the absorption of nutrients. Enteral feeding is contraindiated in severe nausea and vomiting and in intestinal obstruction.

The primary objective of parenteral nutrition, on the other hand, is improved nutritional status in patients who for a critical period cannot be adequately nourished by oral or enteral tube feeding. These indications include severe malabsorption not amenable to enteral tube feeding (e.g., anomalies of the GI tract, obstruction with delayed surgery, radiation enteritis, intractible diarrhea or high volume fistulas, paralytic ileus, persistent vomiting due to CNS disease or cancer chemotherapy), heavy sedation with danger of aspiration, pancreatitis, and very severe burns.

Enteral Feeding

Enteral feeding requires the administration of nutrient solutions through a tube into the upper GI tract and may be divided into two categories: those entering the GI tract through the nose (nasal-gastric); and those entering the abdominal wall through an incision (gastrostomies, duodenostomies, or jejunostomies). The tubes are generally made of silicon or polyurethane and vary in length depending on the site at which the nutrient solution is to be introduced. Long-term enteral feeding gastrostomy or jejunostomy tubes are advantageous for several reasons: (1) they have a large diameter and hence do not clog; (2) they permit quicker and easier administration of feeding solutions and medications; (3) the risk of aspiration is decreased; and (4) they are more convenient and esthetically acceptable to most patients.[r1]

The United States Food and Drug Administration defines enteral nutrition products, as distinguished from other foods for special dietary purposes, by the requirement that they be used under medical supervision and be specified for oral tube feeding. These products, furthermore, are labeled for the dietary management of a medical disorder, disease, or condition. Foods used in enteral feeding include: (1) blenderized natural foods; (2) polymeric solutions containing macronutrients in the form of intact protein, triglycerides, and starch or dextrin; (3) monomeric solutions containing protein as peptides and/or amino acids, fat as long-chain triglycerides or a mixture of long-chain triglycerides and medium-chain triglycerides (MCT), and carbohydrates as partially hydrolyzed maltodextrins, polysaccharides, or free sugars. Aqueous solutions providing minerals and vitamins also are available. Recommended intakes for these oral preparations are those of the Food and Nutrition Board NAS/NRC embodied in the RDA and the "Estimated Safe and Adequate Intakes of Selected Vitamins and Minerals".[r2]

Enteral feedings can be administered by either a bolus or continuous drip. The bolus sometimes is preferred because it takes less time, gives the patient more freedom, is easier to use, and does not require pump control. The bolus method is reserved for feedings into the stomach. Continuous drip with a closed sterile system, preferably pump-controlled, is used to avoid intestinal distension and the dumping syndrome. The advantages of the continuous feeding include: ability to administer larger volumes; greater reliability; less chance of abdominal distension; and less chance for bacterial overgrowth.

These enteral solutions contain all the nutrients required by humans, including proteins, usually administered intact or partially hydrolyzed to avoid overly high osmotic pressure, and carbohydrates, which are in general partially hydrolyzed starches and dextrins—again to avoid the osmotic impact of high concentrations of glucose. The lipids range from 2 to 45 percent of total calories from fat, which is usually corn oil or soy oil with or without lecithin. Some have medium-chain triglycerides containing fatty acids from six to 12 carbon atoms in various proportions. The gut has a high capacity for lipolysis. Even patients with exocrine pancreatic insufficiency may absorb more than 50 percent of dietary fat administered through the enteral tube. Likewise, patients with short bowel syndrome that is not extreme also can absorb roughly 50 percent of dietary fat administered enterally.

Enteral solutions are designed to provide the RDA of vitamins and trace elements with an intake of 1500 to 2000 calories (which include vitamins for which there are not as yet stated RDAs, such as pantothenic acid and biotin). As regards the trace elements, most enteral solutions contain iron, zinc, copper, and iodine. Other established required elements, like manganese, molybdenum, and selenium, probably should be added in amounts regarded as safe and adequate. Most enteral solutions do not contain fiber, but recently some manufacturers have been adding such fibers as soy polysaccharides, oat fiber, or guar gum.

Enteral feeding can be a safe and effective nutritional support method. Its safety depends on: (1) the choice of an appropriate formula; (2) the delivery of the formula into the appropriate part of the GI tract; and (3) metabolic evaluation of the patient prior to and during enteral feedings. The most severe potential complication of enteral feeding is aspiration. This can be avoided by appropriate positioning of the feeding tube, elevating the upper body to 30 to 45 degrees, and avoiding enteral feeding in the presence of impaired gastric emptying or the absence of the gag reflex.

Nausea and vomiting have been reported in as many as 20 percent of patients. There are, in addition, nonspecific symptoms of cramps, distensions, and bloating. Diarrhea occurs in 5 to 30 percent of patients, and can be controlled either by slowing the rate of enteral feeding or changing the medication regimen. Patients intolerant of enteral feeding who do not take adequate food by mouth should be recommended for parenteral feeding. Constipation can occur in as many as 10 to 15 percent of patients receiving long-term enteral feeding, in which case the addition of fiber may be indicated.

Preparations

There are over one hundred commercial formulas promoted for enteral feeding. A selected few are presented in Table 66.1.[r3]

Parenteral Nutrition

Glucose solutions have been infused into humans IV and IM for centuries, but the use of hypertonic glucose in peripheral venous infusions is limited to a concentration of 10 percent by volume because of possible osmotic damage to tissues, including the veins. The maximum infused into a human via a peripheral vein in one day is 3L of a 10 percent solution of glucose. This provides only 1200 kc, which is insufficient to support the metabolic needs of even a healthy adult. In order to provide more energy, infusions of emulsified lipids were found necessary. Early attempts to develop such lipid emulsions for IV use were unsuccessful. After World War II efforts were redoubled to develop a safe and effective intravenous fat preparation. Intravenous Lipomul was developed by a group at Harvard University[1] and marketed in the 1950s but was withdrawn in the early 1960s because of many adverse reactions.[r4] In 1961, however, Schuberth and Wretlind[2] developed a safe and effective lipid emulsion for IV use in humans. Named Intralipid, it contained 100 g of soybean oil, 12 g of egg yolk phosphatides, 25 grams of glycerol, and pyrogen-free distilled water to a volume of 1000 ml. In 1966, Wretlind and coworkers reported the results of 2781 infusions of Intralipid in humans without significant side-effects,[3] and in 1977 it was approved for general use in the US. At

Table 66.1 Composition of Complete Diet Formulas[r3]

Product	Description and use	kcal/ml	N:kcal	Osmolality (mOsm/kg H_2O)	Lactose	Composition/L Protein gm	Protein % cal	Fat gm	Fat % cal	CHO gm	CHO %cal	Na mg	Na mEq	K mg	K mEq	Ca (mg)	P (mg)	Comment
Citrotein (Doyle)	Orange flavor; oral feeding; can use in clear liquid diets	0.7	1:100	500	–	43	24	2	2	130	74	740	32	740	19	1,110	1,110	Low fat, calorie, and residue; high protein
Compleat B (in bottle) (Doyle)	Standard diet; blenderized for tube feeding	1.1	1:160	405	+	43	16	43	36	128	48	1,680	72	1,400	36	680	1,480	High sodium, phosphorus; fiber content of average U.S. diet
Compleat B (in can) (Doyle)	Standard diet; blenderized for tube feeding	1.0	1:160	490	+	40	16	40	36	120	48	1,560	68	1,310	37	625	1,690	High sodium, phosphorus; fiber content of average U.S. diet
Ensure (Ross)	Liquid, flavored; oral or tube feeding	1.1	1:180	450	–	37	14	37	32	145	55	740	32	1,270	33	420	420	
Ensure Plus (Ross)	Liquid, flavored; oral or tube feeding	1.5	1:170	600	–	55	15	53	32	200	53	1,060	46	1,900	49	630	630	High calorie, potassium
Flexical (Mead Johnson)	Powder, flavored; oral or tube feeding	1.0	1:280	723	–	22	9	34	30	155	61	350	15	1,500	39	500	450	Relatively unpalatable; partially elemental; low sodium
Isocal (Mead Johnson)	Liquid; tube feeding	1.0	1:200	350	–	33	12	44	38	130	50	520	23	1,300	23	620	520	Low osmolality, sodium
Lonalac (Mead Johnson)	Milk-type beverage; Oral or tube feeding	0.6	1:120	NA*	+	34	21	35	49	48	30	25	1	1,200	31	1,100	1,100	Very low calorie; low sodium
Meritene Liquid (Doyle)	Flavored; oral or tube feeding	1.0	1:100	539	+	60	24	33	30	115	46	920	40	1,670	43	1,250	1,250	High protein, calcium, phosphorus
Meritene Powder (whole milk) (Doyle)	Mixed with milk; oral or tube feeding	1.1	1:100	NA	+	75	26	38	30	130	45	1,040	45	3,200	82	2,500	2,090	High protein, potassium, calcium, phosphorus
Nutri-1000 (Cutter)	Liquid, flavored; oral or tube feeding	1.1	1:190	400	+†	34	14	55	47	106	40	500	72	1,500	38	1,300	950	Low osmolality, sodium; high calcium
Osmolite (Ross)	Liquid, milk flavor; oral or tube feeding	1.1	1:180	300	–	37	14	38	32	143	54	540	24	875	22	540	540	Isotonic; low sodium
Portagen (Mead Johnson)	Powder, unflavored; oral or tube feeding	1.0	1:100	354	+	35	14	44	40	115	46	600	26	1,500	38	1,000	800	Low osmolality; fat largely as MCT oil
Precision High Nitrogen (Doyle)	Powder, flavored; oral or tube feeding	1.0	1:150	557	–	42	18	<1	<1	207	83	933	41	867	22	333	333	Low fat
Precision Low Residue (Doyle)	Powder, flavored; oral or tube feeding	1.1	1:280	525	–	24	10	<1	<1	224	90	670	27	833	21	555	555	Low fat
Precision isotonic (Doyle)	Powder, flavored; oral or tube feeding	1.0	1:210	300	–	29	12	30	28	144	60	800	35	1,000	26	680	680	Low residue, isotonic
Sustacal Liquid (Mead Johnson)	Flavored; oral or tube feeding	1.0	1:100	625	+	60	24	23	21	138	55	1,100	48	1,700	44	1,500	1,300	High osmolality, protein, calcium, phosphorus
Sustacal Powder (+ whole milk) (Mead Johnson)	Mixed with milk; oral or tube feeding	1.3	1:100	NA	+	80	24	33	22	179	54	1,200	53	3,370	86	2,800	2,520	High protein, potassium, calcium, phosphorus

continued

Table 66.1 *Continued*

Product	Description and use	kcal/ml	N:kcal	Osmolality (mOsm/kg H_2O)	Lactose	Protein gm	Protein % cal	Fat gm	Fat % cal	CHO gm	CHO %cal	Na mg	Na mEq	K mg	K mEq	Ca (mg)	P (mg)	Comment
Sustagen Powder (+ water) (Mead Johnson)	Flavored; oral or tube feeding	1.8	1:100	1200	+	105	24	15	8	300	68	1,200	52	3,600	92	3,200	2,300	High calorie, protein, osmolality, potassium, calcium, phosphorus; low fat
Sustacal Pudding (Mead Johnson)	In flavors; oral feeding	1.6	1:220	NA	+	45	11	63	36	213	53	800	35	1,930	49	1,470	1,470	Alternative to liquid feeding
Vital (Ross)	Powder, flavored; oral or tube feeding	1.0	1:150	450	+‡	42	17	10	9	185	74	380	17	1,290	30	667	667	Pleasant taste; partially elemental; low fat, sodium
Vipep (Cutter)	Powder, flavored; oral or tube feeding	1.0	1:250	520	–	25	10	25	22	175	68	750	33	850	22	600	500	Palatable; low residue; partially elemental
Vivonex High Nitrogen (Eaton)	Powder, unflavored; crystalline amino acids; oral or tube feeding	1.0	1:150	810	–	41	16	<1	<1	210	84	770	34	700	34	333	333	Gelatin form palatable; fully elemental; low fat
Vivonex Standard (Eaton)	Powder, unflavored; tube feeding	1.0	1:310	550	–	20	8	1.5	1	226	90	859	37	1,170	30	555	555	Relatively unpalatable; fully elemental; low fat
W.T. Low Residue (Warren Teed)	Powder, flavored; crystalline amino acids; oral or tube feeding	1.0	1:290	500	–	22	9	<1	<1	227	91	1,600	70	1,170	30	560	560	Relatively unpalatable; fully elemental; low fat, high sodium

*NA, No information available.
†Lactose free available (Nutri-1000 LF).
1% of carbohydrates.

present, Intralipid is used in both central and peripheral parenteral nutrition.

In addition to the problem of supplying enough energy to humans, the other unknowns in total parenteral nutrition were the nutritional requirements for humans nourished by vein, and the overall safety of the method with respect to bacterial infections, allergic reactions, and other adverse effects. One of the important questions was the absolute requirements for the essential nutrients for humans when given by vein. When they are taken orally, the absorption of many nutrients is controlled by transporters in the intestinal wall that serve as gates whose opening is determined by the body pool of the nutrient. Part of this system is the recycling of nutrients between liver and gut—so-called "enterohepatic" circulation. In addition, intestinal bacteria either use or export nutrients, which modifies the oral requirement. None of these controls exist when nutrients are introduced in high doses directly into the systemic circulation.

Many of these questions were answered by the pioneering work of Dudrick and his collaborators at the University of Pennsylvania.[4–8] These investigators introduced use of a central venous catheter through which highly concentrated glucose solutions could be

Table 66.2 ISPN Recommendations for Parenteral Intake of Energy and Protein

Subject	Energy (Kcal/kg/d)	Protein (g/kg/d)
Growing children	100–150	1.6–2.0
Normal adults	25–30	0.8–1.6
Adults in catabolic states	35–55	1.9–2.0

introduced to supply more calories. They found that 25 to 35 percent glucose solutions could be introduced into the vena cavae where the blood flow was very high. Dilution was almost instantaneous, causing no injury to that vein. This procedure allowed 5400 mOsmol of nutritionally complete, fat-free formula containing 3600 kcal to be administered daily to patients. Dudrick et al. showed that beagle puppies nourished solely by the central venous route for up to eight months grew normally to healthy adulthood.[4] Likewise, human infants, with congenital disorders of the GI tract grew normally during six months of total parenteral nutrition (TPN).[5] In 1969, Dudrick et al.[6] reported that TPN for up to seven months achieved nutritional repletion and maintenance of 100 undernourished adults with GI fistulas. In 1973, Wilmore et al. from Dudrick's group reported that the addition of Intralipid to the fat-free glucose-amino acid formula was particularly useful in the treatment of patients with extensive burns.[8,r5]

Early TPN preparations were composed of 5 percent protein hydrolysates (fibrin, casein, lactalbumin) plus an equal volume of 50 percent glucose to which was added KCl, NaCl, $MgSO_4$, KH_2PO_4 (optional) and calcium gluconate plus selected vitamins and trace minerals.[r6] These preparations resulted in the occurrence of a number of deficiency diseases in persons give TPN for months or years.[r7,9,10] Deficiencies of

Table 66.3 Recommendations for Daily Enteral (EN) and Parenteral (PN) Intakes of Essential Fatty Acids, Minerals and Vitamins (Modified from Ref [31,r10])

Nutrient	Daily Intake By 70-kg Adult EN*	PN
Essential fatty acids % Kcal (Ratio n–6/n–3 = 5.0)	1–2	2–4
Calcium g	0.8–1.2	0.4–0.6
Phosphorus g	0.8–1.2	0.4–0.8
Potassium g	2.0–5.0	4.0–5.0
Sodium g	2.0–3.0	1.0–2.0
Chloride g	2.0–5.0	1.5–3.0
Magnesium g	0.3–0.4	0.3–0.4
Iron mg	10.0–15.0	1.0–2.0
Zinc mg	12.0–15.0	3.0–5.0
Copper mg	2.0–3.0	0.5–1.5
Iodine mg	0.15–0.20	0.05–0.10
Manganese mg	2.0–5.0	0.15–0.80
Molybdenum mg	0.15–0.30	0.01–0.05
Selenium mg	0.05–0.20	0.05–0.10
Chromium mg	0.05–0.20	0.01–0.02
Ascorbic acid mg	50–60	100–
Thiamine mg	1.1–1.5	3.0***
Riboflavin mg	1.3–1.8	3.6
Pyridoxine mg	1.6–2.0	4.0
Niacin mg	15–20	40.0
Panthothenic acid mg	4–7	15.0
Biotin ug	30–100	60.0
Folic acid ug	150–200	400
Cobalamin ug	2.0–3.0	5.0
Retinol ug	800–1000	1300.0
Cholecalciferol ug	5–10	5.0
-Tocopherol mg	8–10	10.0
Phylloquinone ug+	45–80	200

*The enteral recommendations are the range of RDA for men and women.
**Parenteral iron is usually given as the dextran complex IM.
***These vitamin recommendations come from an Expert Committee of the FDA (Fed Reg *44*: 40933–40936, 1979).
+Vitamin K, as phylloquinone, is usually given in a dose of 2 mg/week IM.

Table 66.4 Composition of Single-Formula TPN Solution* (Modified from Shils[r9])

Item	Volume (ml)	Kcal	Na (mEq)	K (mEq)	Cl (mEq)	Mg (mEq)	Ca (mg)	P (mg)	Zn (mg)
Crystalline amino acids/water (7.0%)	1000	280	10					225	
Dextrose/water (50%)	1000	1700							
Dextrose/saline (10%)	250	85	39						
KCl (4 mEq/ml)	20			80	40				
NaCl (2.5 mEq/ml)	10		25		25				
Na acetate (2 mEq/ml)	10		20						
$MgSO_4 \times 7H_2O$ (50%)	4					17			
Ca gluconate (10%)	40						372		
K phosphate	3			13				279	
Trace minerals	1								4
Totals	2338	2065	94	93	65	17	372	504	4
IV supplements during week: Intralipid 10%—500 ml once weekly; Vitamins—see below; Trace elements**—1 ml twice weekly									

*An example of an inpatient or home TPN formula for a stable 62-kg man with moderate gastrointestinal losses following bowel resection. It is prepared in a plastic bag of 2.8-L volume or in two 1-L bags connected by Y tubing.
Vitamins: MVI (conc) 5 ml twice/wk; Berocca C 2 ml/twice/wk; vitamin K_1 5 mg/wk; folic acid 1.5 mg twice/wk; vitamin B_{12} 50 ug once/wk.
**Trace element solution (MH #3) containing $ZnCl_2$, $CuSO_4 \times 5\ H_2O$, $MnSO_4\ H_2O$ and NaI in sterile saline. One ml provides 4.0 mg Zn^{++}, 1.0 mg Cu^{++}, 0.1 Mn^{++} and 0.056 mg 1. For patients on TPN for more than 6 months, 1 ml of $CrCl_3\ 6H_2O$ in sterile saline (= 38 ug of Cr^{+++}) and 1 ml of $NaNoO_4$ containing 50 ug Mo may be added once or twice weekly.

phosphate with hypophosphatemia,[11] essential fatty acids,[12-14] copper,[15-17] zinc,[18,19] folic acid,[20] selenium,[21] vitamin A,[22] biotin,[23] molybdenum,[24] and glucose intolerance alleged to be due to chromium deficiency.[25,r8]

Of the problems encountered when a glucose-amino acid solution was infused, perhaps the more serious was an essential fatty acid deficiency. Essential fatty acids are integral components of the membranes within and around cells; they affect the intra- and intercellular transport of metabolites and nutrients. If the essential fatty acids are not provided in the diet, the membranes will gradually lose their ability to exchange nutrients and metabolites within the cell compartments and between the cell and its surrounding fluid. Fortunately, the adult body has a large reservoir of essential fatty acids stored in adipose tissue, but the growing infant is more vulnerable. Two studies of infants on TPN in the 1970s[12,13] reported that after five months on TPN these patients developed dermatitis, alopecia, thrombocytopenia, and poor wound healing associated with an increase in the level of 5,8,11-eicosatrienoic acid and a decrease in the levels of linoleic and arachidonic acids in the serum. The symptoms disappeared after the addition of linoleic acid to the daily infusions. Not only is linoleic acid (n-6) required by humans, but also linolenic acid (n-3), as indicated by the report of Holman et al.,[14] who observed a six-year old girl who received only linoleic acid in her TPN and developed neurologic signs and symptoms after five months on TPN that were promptly relieved by linolenic acid. Burn patients, because of their particularly high catabolic rate, appear to develop essential fatty acid deficiency far sooner than do surgical or septic patients, who still develop the deficient state more quickly than normal subjects.

A great deal has been learned about human requirements for essential nutrients given IV since the early experiments by Dudrick et al.[r6] and Wretlind et al.[r5] in the 1960s. During the last three decades the composition and techniques for administering TPN have improved greatly. Currently, most TPN solutions are made up from crystalline amino acids, 50 percent glucose, mineral salts, essential fatty acids, and all of the vitamins, including pantothenate and biotin. The recommendations of the International Society for Parenteral Nutrition for energy and protein are shown in Table 66.2, and the recommended values for essential fatty acids, minerals, and vitamins are shown in Table

Table 66.5 Monitoring the Patient on Total Parenteral Nutrition[r10]

Clinical data checked daily	
Patient's sense of well being: (symptoms suggesting fluid overload, high or low blood glucose, electrolyte imbalance)	
Patient's strength as judged by graded activity, getting out of bed, walking, stair climbing.	
Vital signs: temperature, blood pressure, pulse rate, and respiratory rate,	
Fluid balance: weight, fluid input (intravenous ± enteral) venous fluid output (urine, stool, gastric suction, etc.).	
Delivery equipment for parenteral nutrition: composition of nutrient solution, tubing, pump, filter, catheter, dressing (skin checked for local infection at time of dressing change).	
Laboratory data	
Urine quantitative glucose	Four times daily
Blood glucose Na^+, K^+, Cl^-, HCO_3^- Blood urea nitrogen	Daily until glucose infusion rate and patient stable, then twice weekly
Serum albumin, transferrin Liver function studies Serum creatinine Ca^{2+}, PO_4^{2-}, Mg^{2+} Hb/Ht, WBC	Baseline, then twice weekly
Prothrombin time	Baseline, then weekly
Micronutrient tests as indicated	

66.3. The composition of a single formula TPN solution with supplements for a 62-kg patient is shown in Table 66.4. The use of IV fat for persons with hyperlipidemia must be carefully monitored.[26]

It should be noted from Table 66.3 that although the electrolytes, sodium, potassium, chloride, and magnesium are recommended at the same doses for oral and parenteral nutrition, calcium, phosphorus, iron, zinc, copper, iodine, manganese, and molybdenum are recommended for lower intakes when given parenterally. This is because the absorption of the latter set of minerals is tightly regulated. The water-soluble vitamins are recommended at higher doses for parenteral administration, mostly because exact requirements are unknown and toxicity is minimal at the doses recommended. The fat-soluble vitamins are recommended at approximately the same dose by both routes.

It must be recognized that central parenteral nutrition carries a significant risk to the patient. It should be used only when the benefit outweighs the risk. Some possible adverse effects are related to: (1) placing the central catheter (sepsis, thrombophlebitis, artery and vein lacerations, pneumothorax) (<5%); (2) metabolic complications (hyperglycemia, postinfusion hypoglycemia, hyperammonemia, prerenal azotemia, electrolyte imbalance such as hypophosphatemia, hypercalciuria, hypomagnesemia, and liver dysfunction); (3) vitamin and mineral deficiencies (already discussed) of vitamin A, biotin, folate, copper, zinc, molybdenum if these substances are not added to the parenteral solutions; (4) reactions to IV fat, which are uncommon (<3%), but which may occur and present as fever, chills, nausea, thrombocytopenia, hyperlipemia, dyspnea, and increased coagulability of the blood.

In order to prevent these side-effects and to maximize the benefits to the patient on TPN, careful monitoring is essential. Guidelines for clinical and biochemical studies are presented in Table 66.5.

Special modifications are made to the TPN formula in cases of renal failure, hepatic failure, pancreatitis, pulmonary insufficiency, metabolic bone disease, and diabetes mellitus.[r1] Also, administration of the conditionally essential nutrients, tyrosine, taurine, choline, cysteine, and carnitine may be needed in some cases.[r7]

Stress, trauma, sepsis, and diabetes can result in an impairment of glucose utilization. The insulin responses of individual patients during the initial period of adaptation to parenteral infusions must be studied. In most patients the initial rise in serum insulin is followed by a fall in both blood glucose and insulin. A new steady state of insulin secretion to control the glucose load, however, may not be attained in some patients; and metabolic acidosis, glycosuria, and hyperglycemia may occur in traumatized or diabetic patients. The prevention of this complication requires careful monitoring.[27–29] In fact, diabetic or prediabetic patients may require exogenous insulin beyond the initial adaptation period. In addition, hyperosomolar nonketotic hyperglycemia may result if the hypertonic glucose solution is administered too rapidly. The syndrome can be avoided by careful adjustment of the rate of the glucose infusion according to the patient's ability to respond with a rise in insulin secretion.[29,30]

In summary, the availability of TPN represents a new era in clinical nutrition. At present, thousands of nutritionally handicapped patients receive a mixture of essential nutrients by vein for months or even years. It represents a triumph in the application of the principles of nutritional pharmacology to special problems of malnutrition.

Much of the early difficulties resulting from the use

Table 66.6 Compositions of Crystalline Amino Acid Infusions (per 100 ml) (From Ref [r3])

	Aminosyn 7% (Abbott)	Aminosyn 10% (Abbott)	FreAmine II 8.5% (McGraw)	Nephramine 5.1% (McGaw)	Travasol 5.5% (Travenol)	Travasol 8.5% (Travenol)	Veinamine 8% (Cutter)
Protein (gm)	7	10	8	5	5.5	8.5	8
Nitrogen (gm)	1.1	1.6	1.2	0.6	0.9	1.4	1.3
Potassium (mEq)	0.5	0.5	—	—	—	—	3.0
Sodium (mEq)	—*	—	1.0	0.6	—	—	4.0
Phosphate (mmole)	—	—	2.0	—	—	—	—
Magnesium (mEq)	—	—	—	—	—	—	0.6
Chloride (mEq)	—	—	—	—	2.2	3.4	5.0
Acetate (mEq)	—	—	—	—	3.5	5.2	5.0
Osmolarity (mOsm/L)	700	1,100	850	420	—	—	950
pH	5.3	5.3	6.6	6.0	6.0	6.0	6.2–6.6
Amino acids (mg)							
Essential							
Isoleucine	510	720	590	560	263	406	493
Leucine	660	940	770	880	340	526	347
Lysine	510	720	870	640	318	492	667
Methionine	280	400	450	880	318	492	427
Phenylalanine	310	440	480	886	340	526	400
Threonine	370	520	340	400	230	356	160
Tryptophan	120	160	130	200	99	152	80
Valine	560	800	560	650	252	390	253
Nonessential							
Tyrosine	44	44	—	—	22	34	—
Alanine	900	1280	600	—	1,140	1,760	
Arginine†	690	980	310	—	570	880	749
Histidine†	210	300	240	—	241	372	237
Proline	610	860	950	—	230	356	107
Serine	300	420	500	—	—	—	—
Glycine	900	1,280	1,700	—	1,140	1,760	3,387
Cysteine†	—	—	20	—	—	—	—
Aspartic acid	—	—	—	—	—	—	460
Glutamic acid	—	—	—	—	—	—	426
Trace elements (μg)							
Zinc	12–14	3–6	82–404	NA	NA	14	13–15
Copper	—	—	0.9–8.5	NA	NA	—	1.3–1.5
Chromium	NA	—	0.2	NA	NA	NA	0.8–2.4
Manganese	NA	NA	0.3	NA	NA	NA	NA

*—, Not detectable or negligible; NA, No information available.
†Considered nonessential for adults but essential for infants.

of incomplete TPN formulas with resulting deficiency diseases have been avoided by routine supplementation of all essential trace nutrients. Nonetheless, centrally administered TPN is still risky and must be monitored carefully to prevent all adverse effects. The physiologic impact of presenting a patient his "food" by vein instead of by mouth is still not fully understood, and further research is necessary to explain the different metabolic results obtained in animals from oral vs. IV nutrition.[r7]

Preparations

There are many commercially available amino acid solutions for preparing solutions for total parenteral nutrition. Seven of them are presented in Table 66.6. The two main fat emulsions are Intralipid (Cutter) and Lipsyn (Abbott).

References

Research Reports

1. McKibbon JM, Pope A, Thayer S, Ferry RJ Jr, Stare FJ. Parenteral nutrition: Studies on fat emulsion for intravenous alimentation. J Lab Clin Med 1945;*30*:488–497.
2. Schubert O, Wretlind A. A fat emulsion for parenteral use. Acta Chirung Scandinavica. 1961;*278*:Suppl, 1–21.
3. Hallberg D, Schubert O, Wretlind A. Experimental and clinical studies with fat emulsion for intravenous nutrition. Nutrio et Dieta 1966;*8*:245–281.
4. Dudrick SJ, Wilmore DW, Vars HM, Rhoads JE. Long-term parenteral nutrition with growth, development and positive nitrogen balance. Surgery 1968;*64*:134–145.
5. Wilmore DW, Dudrick SJ. Growth and development of an infant receiving all nutrients exclusively by vein. JAMA 1968;*203*:860.
6. Dudrick SJ, Wilmore DW, Vars HM, Rhoads JE. Can intravenous feeding as a sole means of nutrition, support growth in a child an restore weight loss in an adult? An affirmative answer. Ann Surg 1969;*169*:974–984.
7. Dudrick SJ, Macfadyen VB, Van Buren CT, Rubert RT, Maynard AT. Parenteral hyperalimentation, metabolic problems and solutions. Ann Surg 1972;*176*:259.
8. Wilmore DW, Moylan JA, Helmkamp GM, Pruitt BA. Clinical evaluation of a 10% intravenous fat emulsion for parenteral nutrition in thermally injured persons. Ann Surg 1973;*178*:503–513.
9. Rudman D, Millikan WJ, Richardson TJ, Bixler TJ III, Stackhouse WJ, McGarrity WC. Elemental balances during intravenous hyperalimentation. J Clin Invest 1955;*55*:94–97.
10. Solomons NW, Layden TJ, Rosenberg IW, Vo-Khactu K, Sandstead H. Plasma trace minerals during total parenteral alimentation. Gastroenterol 1976;*70*:1022–1027.
11. Lichtman MA, Miller DR, Cohen J, Waterhouse, C. Phosphate deficiency in a patient given total parenteral nutrition. Ann Int Med 1971;*74*:562–568.
12. Caldwell MD, Jonsson HT, Othersen HB. Essential fatty acid deficiency in an infant receiving prolonged parenteral alimentation. J Pediatr 1972;*81*:894–898.
13. Paulsrud JR, Pensler L, Whilten CF, Stewart S, Holman RT. Essential fatty acid deficiency in infants induced by fat-free intravenous feeding. Am J Clin Nutr 1972;*25*:897–904.
14. Holman RT, Johnson, Hatch TF. A Case of human linolenic acid deficiency involving neurological abnormalities. Am J Clin Nutr 1982;*35*:617–623.
15. Karpel JT, Peden VH. Copper deficiency in long term parenteral nutrition. J Pediatr 1972;*80*:32–36.
16. Dunlap WM, James JC, Hume DM. Anemia and neutropenia caused by copper deficiency. Ann Int Med 1979;*80*:470–472.
17. Vilter RW, Bozian RC, Hess EV. Manifestations of copper deficiency in a patient with systemic sclerosis on intravenous hyperalimentation. J Clin Invest 1974;*55*:94–98.
18. Fleming CR. Trace element metabolism in adult patients requiring total parenteral nutrition. Am J Clin Nutr 1989;*49*:573–579.
19. Kay RG, Tasman-Jones C, Pybus J, Whiting R, Black H. A syndrome of acute zinc deficiency during total parenteral alimentation in man. Ann Surg 1976;*183*:331–340.
20. Steinberg D. Folic acid deficiency: Early onset of megaloblastosis. JAMA 1972;*222*:490–493.
21. Vanrij AM, Thomson CD, McKenzie JM, Robinson MF. Selenium deficiency in total parenteral nutrition. Am J Clin Nutr 1979;*32*:2076–2085.
22. Howard L, Chu R, Feman S, Mintoz H, Oversen L, Wolf B. Vitamin A deficiency from long-term parenteral nutrition. Ann Int Med 1980;*93*:576–577.
23. Mock DM, deLorimer AA, Liebman WM, Sweetman L, Baker H. Biotin deficiency: An unusual complication of parenteral alimentation. N Engl J Med 1981;*304*:820–823.
24. Abumrad NN, Schneider AJ, Steel D, Rogers LS. Amino acid intolerance during prolonged total parenteral nutrition reversed by molybdate therapy. Am J Clin Nutr 1981;*34*:2551–2559.
25. Jeejeebhoy KN, Chu RC, Marliss EB, Greenberg GR, Bruce-Robertson A. Chromium deficiency, glucose intolerance and neuropathy reversed by chromium supplementation in a patient receiving long term parenteral nutrition. Am J Clin Nutr 1977;*30*:531–538.
26. Toisvik H, Feldman HA, Fischer JE, Lees RS. Effects of intravenous hyperalimentation on plasma-lipoproteins in severe familial hypercholesterolemia. Lancet 1975;*2*:601.
27. Sanderson I, Deital M. Insulin response in patients receiving concentrated infusions of glucose and casein hydrolysate for complete parenteral nutrition. Ann Surg 1974;*179*:387–394.
28. Genuth S. Insulin response to intravenous alimentation N Engl J Med 1973;*289*:107.
29. Knopf RJ, Conn JW, Floyd JC Jr, Frajans SS, Rull JA, Guntsche EM, Thiffault CA. The normal endocrine response to ingestion of protein and infusions of amino acids. Sequential secretion of insulin and growth hormone. Trans Assoc Am Phys 1966;*79*:312–321.
30. Hinton P, Allison SP, Littlejohn S, Lloyd J. Insulin and glucose to reduce catabolic response to injury in burned patients. Lancet 1971;*1*:767.
31. AMA Department of Foods and Nutrition: Guidelines for essential trace element preparations for parenteral use. JAMA 1979;*241*:2051–2054.

Reviews

r1. Shils ME. Enteral (tube) and parenteral nutrition support. In Shills ME, Young V. eds. Modern Nutrition in Health and Disease, 7th ed. Philadelphia: Lea & Febiger, 1988, 1023–1065.

r2. National Research Council: Recommended Dietary Allowances Food and Nutrition Board, 10th ed. Washington, National Academy Press, 1989.

r3. Weinsiger RL, Butterworth CE Jr. Handbook of Clinical Nutrition. St. Louis, C.V. Mosby, 1981.

r4. Geyer RP. Parenteral Nutrition. Physiol Rev 1960;*40*:150–186.

r5. Wretlind A. Parenteral nutrition. Surg Clin North Am 1978;*58*:1055–1070.

r6. Dudrick SJ, Ruberg RL. Principles and practice of parenteral nutrition. Gastroenterol 1971;*61*:901–930.

r7. Rudman D, Williams PJ. Nutrient deficiencies during total parenteral nutrition. Nutr Rev 1985;*43*:1–13.

r8. Anonymous. Is chromium essential for humans? Nutr Rev 1988;*46*:17–20.

r9. Shils, ME. Parenteral nutrition. In Goodhart R, Shils ME. eds. Modern Nutrition in Health and Disease, 6th ed. Philadelphia, Lea & Febiger, 1980.

r10. Howard LJ. Parenteral and enteral nutrition therapy. In Wilson, J., Braunwald E, Isselbacher KJ, Petersdorf RJ, Martin JB, Fauci AS. Harrison's Principles of Internal Medicine, 12th Ed. New York, McGraw-Hill, 1991, pp 427–434.

SECTION VIII

Drugs Affecting Gastrointestinal Function

Editor:
Thomas F. Burks

CHAPTER 67

Therapy of Acid Peptic Diseases

Thomas F. Burks

Peptic ulcer and related acid peptic diseases affect up to 10 percent of the population with sufficient severity to prompt victims to seek medical attention. The vast majority of people, on the other hand, suffer occasional, transient episodes of acute upper GI discomfort involving acid pepsin aggression. The most significant disorders requiring medical attention are peptic ulcer and gastroesophageal reflux disease (reflux esophagitis). Fortunately, modern drugs provide relief for most persons suffering from these disorders.

Peptic ulcer results from lesions in the gastric or duodenal mucosa caused or exacerbated by gastric acid and pepsin. Although the role of pepsin in the etiology of peptic ulcer is uncertain, successful therapeutic strategies are directed toward reduction of acid secretion, neutralization of acid, or protection of the mucosa from acid.[1] Because pepsinogens are activated by acid and the proteolytic activity of pepsin is reduced at high pH, successful strategies of treatment address pepsin activity as well as acid. Peptic ulcer may be viewed as the result of a confrontation between acid aggression and mucosal defense. The healthy mucosa withstands acid attack and prevents back-diffusion of H^+ into the mucosa. The specific biologic mechanisms involved in mucosal defense are not known, but probably include a mucous coat provided by surface epithelial cells that secrete mucus and bicarbonate, maintenance of adequate blood flow in the mucosa, and production of prostaglandins by the mucosa. Prostaglandins themselves stimulate mucus and bicarbonate production and increase blood flow. Excessive secretion of acid may overwhelm the mucosal defense and result in mucosal lesions and ulcers that penetrate the mucosa. About one-third of patients with duodenal ulcer display above-normal rates of basal and stimulated gastric acid secretion. Patients with gastrin-secreting tumors, usually pancreatic gastrinomas, secrete large amounts of acid and invariably develop duodenal ulcers. By contrast, patients with gastric ulcers often display normal or below-normal rates of basal or stimulated acid secretion. It is presumed that ulcers in these cases reflect deficient mucosal defense mechanisms rather than excessive acid secretion. In any event, peptic ulcer disease recurs naturally, and patients may require intermittent or continuous therapy for many years.

The role of *Helicobacter pylori* infections in the etiology of peptic ulcer disease has recently received much attention.[2] There is a close association between chronic *H. pylori* infection of the mucosa and development of gastritis and peptic ulcer. The inflammation produced by *H. pylori* may disrupt normal mucosal defense mechanisms, thereby predisposing the mucosa to ulceration. The evidence favoring an etiologic role of *H. pylori* is sufficiently strong to warrant antibacterial therapy in patients resistant to antiulcer drugs.

Nonulcer dyspepsia is characterized by burning epigastric pain, especially after meals and at night. Endoscopy in patients with nonulcer dyspepsia fails to reveal the mucosal lesions characteristic of peptic ulcers. Nevertheless, the symptomatology closely resembles that of peptic ulcer, even though acid/pepsin aggression is difficult to demonstrate.

Gastroesophageal reflux disease results from inflammation of the esophageal mucosa caused by reflux of gastric contents into the esophagus. Limited gastroesophageal reflux occurs episodically in normal subjects. In patients with gastroesophageal reflux disease, the reflux of acid and other gastric contents occurs frequently and leads to prolonged, painful inflammation of the esophageal mucosa. Strategies for treatment of gastroesophageal reflux disease include measures that decrease secretion of gastric acid, neutralize acid, improve esophageal clearance, protect the esophageal mucosa, or increase the competence of the lower esophageal sphincter to prevent reflux.

Normal Regulation of Acid Secretion

Secretion of gastric acid is accomplished by activity of an ion-motive ATPase that exchanges cytosolic H^+ for luminal K^+, resulting in acidification of the extracellular surface of the parietal cell.[r1] Parietal cell H^+,K^+-ATPase, often designated the gastric "proton pump," derives its energy for transport of H^+ and K^+ from the hydrolysis of ATP. In the secreting parietal cell, the enzyme has access to the canalicular membrane that provides a pathway for inward K^+ transport in exchange for outward H^+ transport. The transport activity of H^+,K^+-ATPase is regulated by levels of intracellular second messengers, either cAMP or calcium ion (Fig. 67.1). Levels of second messengers are regulated by three receptor pathways: histamine; acetylcholine; and gastrin.

Histamine is now regarded as the primary regulator of acid secretion by the parietal cell.[3] Histamine is released from nearby paracrine cells, either mast cells or histamine-containing enterochromaffin-like cells. There are marked quantitative differences in the content of the glandular mucosa of mast cells and enterochromaffin-like cells among species, but both types of cells occur in the human mucosa. Histamine that is released from the paracrine cells acts at histamine H_2 receptors on the plasma membrane of the parietal cell. The H_2 receptor is coupled by means of a G_s protein to adenylyl cyclase that catalyzes conversion of ATP to cAMP. The cAMP, either directly or through a protein kinase, activates the H^+,K^+-ATPase and initiates secretion of H^+ into the canaliculus. The central role of histamine as the critical regulator of gastric acid secretion is demonstrated by the efficacy of H_2 receptor antagonists in inhibiting acid secretion induced by stimulation of the vagus nerve, presence of food in the stomach, or by gastrin.

Acetylcholine is the mediator of neural secretory influences on the parietal cell. Acetylcholine acts both directly on the parietal cell and indirectly through release of histamine from histamine-containing paracrine cells. The direct effect of acetylcholine on the parietal cell occurs from acetylcholine actions on M_3 muscarinic receptors on the plasma membrane of the parietal cell. The indirect component of acetylcholine action occurs by effects at M_1 receptors of paracrine cells that result in release of histamine. The histamine released from the paracrine cells acts at H_2 receptors of the parietal cell. Neural stimuli arising from the sight, smell, and taste of food, the cephalic phase of gastric secretion, depends on activity of cholinergic motor fibers in the vagus pathway. Parietal cell M_3 muscarinic receptors are coupled by means of G_p protein to phospholipase C, which produces hydrolysis of phosphatidylinositol to form inositoltrisphosphate that in turn causes release of intracellular calcium from stores in the endoplasmic reticulum. The increased level of free intracellular calcium activates the H^+,K^+-ATPase. Possibly because they act through distinct intracellular second messengers, the effects of acetylcholine and histamine on the parietal cell are mutually enhancing.

Gastrin is the major hormonal regulator of gastric acid secretion. Gastrin is a peptide hormone released from gastrin cells in the gastric antral mucosa. Gastrin is active in multiple molecular forms that circulate through the bloodstream to the glandular mucosa of the stomach. Parietal cells are thought to possess gastrin receptors coupled with phospholipase C pathways that increase intracellular levels of calcium to activate the H^+,K^+-ATPase. In addition, gastrin may act indirectly by releasing histamine from mucosal paracrine cells. Stimuli for release of gastrin include the presence of food and elevated pH in the gastric antrum.

The three regulatory mechanisms that stimulate gastric secretion, paracrine (histamine), neural (acetylcholine), and endocrine (gastrin), interact to produce activation of parietal cell H^+,K^+-ATPase. Inhibitory influences on gastric secretion include prostaglandins and somatostatin. Prostaglandins, formed by the cyclooxygenase pathway of arachidonic acid metabolism, interact with parietal cell prostaglandin receptors that are negatively coupled by means of a G_i protein to adenylyl cyclase. Prostaglandins inhibit formation of cAMP and reduce activity of the H^+,K^+-ATPase. Somatostatin, which inhibits gastric secretion, can be released by gastrin; but somatostatin release is inhibited by acetylcholine. The cholinergic neural pathway can prevent somatostatin inhibition of gastric secretion.

Histamine H_2 Antagonists

The histamine H_2 receptor antagonists are among the most effective antisecretory drugs available for management of acid peptic diseases. This class of drugs was developed with the aim of producing agents for the treatment of peptic ulcer.[3] They have been among the most successful therapeutic agents in the history of medicine.

Histamine H_2 antagonists are competitive antagonists at the parietal cell H_2 receptor.[r2] They reduce basal secretion of acid and also secretion stimulated by food, neural, and hormonal influences. They increase the incidence and rate of healing of peptic ulcers and, taken prophylactically, decrease recurrence of ulcers. The positive therapeutic benefits of H_2 antagonists are accomplished with minimal side-effects. H_2 antagonists are among the safest drugs presently available, although they are not totally free of adverse effects.

Cimetidine (Fig. 67.2) is generally considered the prototype of the histamine H_2 antagonists, although a newer product, ranitidine, currently enjoys more widespread use.[r3] The pharmacodynamic and pharmacoki-

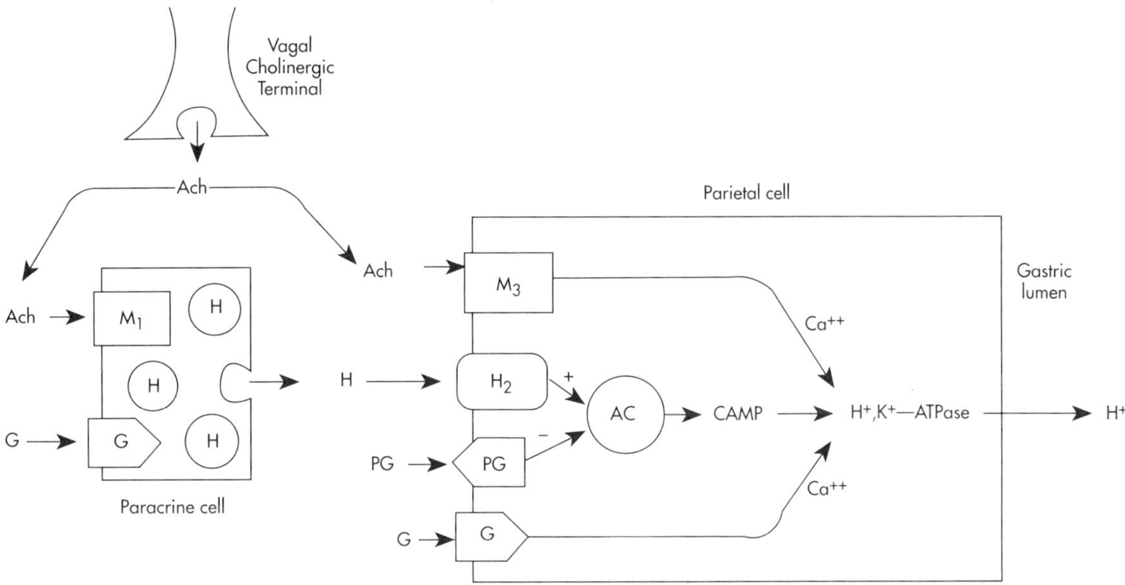

Figure 67.1 Chemical regulation of the gastric parietal (oxyntic) cell. Neurally secreted acetylcholine (ACh) acts at M_1 muscarinic receptors of histamine-containing paracrine cells to release histamine (H), which acts a parietal cell H_2 receptors that are positively coupled with intracellular adenylyl cyclase (AC). cAMP serves as a second messenger to activate the proton pump, H^+, K^+-ATPase. Acetylcholine also acts at parietal cell M_3 muscarinic receptors to increase intracellular concentrations of Ca^{++}, presumably through a phosphatidylinositol pathway. Food and gastric distension promote release of histamine, which acts at parietal cell H_2 receptors. Gastrin (G), a peptide hormone released from the antral mucosa, releases histamine from paracrine cells and also acts directly on parietal cell gastrin (G) receptors. Prostaglandins (PG), formed locally, act at PG receptors of the parietal cell that are negatively coupled with adenylyl cyclase, thus decreasing intracellular levels of cAMP.

netic properties of the marketed H_2 receptor antagonist drugs are similar (Table 67.1).

The rapidity and efficacy of ulcer healing with H_2 receptor antagonists can be predicted by the degree and duration of the inhibition of acid secretion achieved. Nevertheless, peptic ulcers may recur rapidly after cessation of antiulcer therapy with H_2 receptor antagonists. Recurrences are effectively suppressed by continued maintenance therapy with the H_2 blockers. Typically, it is possible to prevent recurrence with reduced doses of antagonists in maintenance therapy. Long-term studies with ranitidine indicate that little tolerance to antisecretory effects occurs during five months of maintenance therapy.

The H_2 antagonists do not directly suppress secretion of pepsinogen, but the total amount of pepsinogen

Histamine

Cimetidine

Ranitidine

Famotidine

Nizatidine

Figure 67.2 Structures of histamine and four histamine H_2 receptor antagonists. Histamine and cimetidine contain imidazole nuclei. Ranitidine contains a furan nucleus. Famotidine and nizatidine contain thiazole nuclei. All four H_2 antagonists posses side-chains that differ from the ethylamine side-chain of histamine.

secreted is reduced in proportion to the over-all decrease in volume of gastric secretions. Moreover, the increase in intragastric pH associated with suppression of acid secretion reduces formation and activity of pepsin, which has a pH optimum of 2. Pepsin is essentially inactive at pH higher than 5. H_2 receptor antagonists may reduce secretion of intrinsic factor, but absorption of vitamin B_{12} is generally not impaired. Plasma levels of gastrin may increase, especially after meals, in patients treated with H_2 antagonists, but no specific adverse effects have been associated with a modest increase in plasma gastrin. In fact, gastrin may promote healing of ulcers by virtue of its trophic effects on gastrointestinal mucosa.

Pharmacokinetics

The H_2 antagonists are rapidly absorbed after oral administration, with peak serum concentrations occurring generally within one to three hours.[r4] All of the agents are subject to significant presystemic clearance, and bioavailability ranges from 43 percent for famotidine to 72 percent for nizatidine. The drugs distribute throughout the body, except into fat. Binding to plasma proteins is generally less than 30 percent. The drugs can appear in breast milk.

All H_2 antagonists are eliminated by renal clearance of intact drug and metabolites. Some 25 to 60 percent of the drug may be metabolized in the liver, primarily to N- and S-oxides. Unchanged drug appears to undergo tubular secretion in the kidneys. The serum half-life is approximately two hours for cimetidine and ranitidine, less for nizatidine, and longer for famotidine (Table 67.1). Dosage reduction is generally recommended in patients with severe renal disease.

Adverse Effects

The incidence of adverse effects with H_2 antagonist drugs is low, affecting fewer than 5 percent of patients, and the effects are usually transient and mild. The most common include diarrhea, headache, fatigue, drowsiness, and constipation. Mental confusion is a rare complication. The low incidence of side-effects reflects the fact that H_2 antagonist drugs interfere with few physiologic functions other than secretion of gastric acid.

Cimetidine, like some other drugs that possess an imidazole nucleus, may bind to liver cytochrome P-450 mixed-function oxidases to inhibit metabolism of several other drugs. Clinically significant drug interactions may occur owing to interference with metabolism of warfarin, theophylline, or phenytoin; and significant inhibition of metabolism of over 40 drugs by cimetidine has been documented.[r4] Ranitidine, which contains a furan nucleus, and famotidine and nizatidine, which contain thiazole nuclei, do not significantly inhibit the activity of cytochrome P-450.

When given in high doses, cimetidine and ranitidine increase blood levels of prolactin. Cimetidine also exerts antiandrogenic effects in high doses by inhibiting binding of dihydrotestosterone to androgen receptors. Moreover, cimetidine can inhibit the metabolism of estradiol and increase plasma levels of estradiol in normal men. Cimetidine in high doses, especially when administered over long periods, can induce gynecomastia in men, and can induce impotence and loss of libido. These effects probably are related to hyperprolactinemia, antiandrogenic effects, and increases in plasma levels of estradiol. After substitution of another H_2 antagonist for cimetidine, the feminizing effects gradually resolve.

The elevation of intragastric pH produced by the H_2 antagonist can alter absorption of other drugs, such as ketoconazole. Cimetidine may increase absorption of ethanol from the stomach because it can inhibit gastric alcohol dehydrogenase.

Therapeutic Uses

Cimetidine and the other H_2 receptor antagonists decrease acid secretion and promote healing of both duodenal and gastric ulcers. Some four to eight weeks of treatment is required. Without further treatment, ulcers may recur; therefore, maintenance therapy usually is prescribed. Patients with Zollinger-Ellison syndrome, a condition caused by pancreatic gastrin-secreting tumors, may require very high doses of H_2 antagonists to achieve adequate suppression of acid secretion. These patients receiving high doses of H_2 receptor antagonists are more likely to show side-effects than are patients with idiopathic peptic ulcers receiving lower doses of drug.

H_2 antagonists are also employed to prevent development of peptic ulcers induced by aspirin and NSAIDs, including indomethacin. The reduction of acid and pepsin output by H_2 antagonists reduces mucosal damage induced by NSAIDs. There is evidence that H_2 receptor antagonists reduce the incidence and severity of stress ulcers and GI bleeding that can occur in severely ill hospitalized patients, such as patients with extensive burns.

H_2 receptor antagonists are also useful in the management of reflux esophagitis. The decrease in acid production and elevation in pH of the gastric contents reduces the irritating properties of material refluxed into the esophagus and allows healing of the mucosa.

H_2 antagonists generally are of no benefit in management of nonulcer dyspepsia.

Table 67.1 H_2 Receptors Antagonists

Variable	Cimetidine	Ranitidine	Famotidine	Nizatidine
EC-50 (μg/L)[a]	250–500	60–165	10–13	150–180
Daily dose (mg/d)				
Heal ulcers	800–1200	300	40	300
Prevent recurrence	400	150	20	150
Bioavailability (%)	60	50	43	72
Peak serum concentration (hr)[b]	1–2	1–3	1–3.5	1–3
Volume of distribution (L/kg)	0.8–1.2	1.2–1.9	1.1–1.4	1.2–1.6
Half-life in serum (hr)	1.5–2.3	1.6–2.4	2.5–4	1.1–1.6

[a]Serum concentration necessary to inhibit secretion of acid stimulated by pentagastrin by 50%.
[b]Time required to attain peak concentration in serum after oral administration.

Preparations and Doses

The H_2 receptor antagonists available at present are cimetidine (Tagamet), famotidine (Pepcid), nizatidine (Axid), and ranitidine (Zantec). All are available in tablets for oral use; cimetidine, ranitidine, and famotidine are available in liquid formulation for oral use; and cimetidine and ranitidine are available in sterile solutions for parenteral use. Average doses are listed in Table 67.1.

Because of the low level of toxicity or other adverse effects produced by the H_2 receptor antagonists, they can be given in relatively large doses that provide extended antisecretory activity, despite their relatively short half-lives in plasma. They are generally administered orally two to four times per day for the acute phase of peptic ulcer healing and once at bedtime as maintenance therapy to prevent recurrence. Famotidine, which has a longer plasma half-life than the other three drugs, may be given once daily for acute ulcer therapy.

H^+,K^+-ATPase Inhibitors

Inhibitors of H^+,K^+-ATPase are presently the most efficacious antisecretory drugs available. Because the H^+,K^+-ATPase of the parietal cell is the ultimate mechanism by which acid is secreted, its inhibition can lead to total cessation of H^+ transport. Only one inhibitor of H^+,K^+-ATPase, omeprazole (Fig. 67.3), is presently marketed. It is capable of producing almost complete suppression of acid secretion.

The mechanism of action of omeprazole is such that it binds very specifically to a single subunit of the H^+,K^+-ATPase at the secretory surface of the parietal cell.[r5] Omeprazole is, in essence, a prodrug that is converted in the parietal cell secretory canaliculus to its active form, which both binds with and inhibits the enzyme responsible for H^+ secretion. Omeprazole is a weak base with a pK_a of 4.0 that can accumulate in acidic spaces. Only the secretory canaliculus of the parietal cell has a pH low enough to accumulate omeprazole. The pK_a of omeprazole therefore targets the drug to the functioning parietal cell. In low pH, such as that of the secretory canaliculus, the omeprazole molecule undergoes rearrangement to form a sulfenamic acid, which can then interact with a critical site on the enzyme to form a covalent bond and inactivation of the enzyme (Fig. 67.3). It is thought that the covalent bonding of the omeprazole sulfenamine adduct forces the enzyme into an inactive conformation. As a covalently bound, noncompetitive inhibitor of H^+,K^+-ATPase, omeprazole produces long-lasting inhibition of the enzyme. Recovery from omeprazole inhibition requires 72 hours or more after cessation of drug treatment. Once-daily dosing with omeprazole suppresses acid secretion both day and night. Because omeprazole effectively inhibits the proton pump of the parietal cell, it reduces acid secretion regardless of the source of secretory stimulation. It reduces basal acid secretion and that stimulated by food, muscarinic agonists, gastrin, histamine, and other pharmacologic agents. By increasing intragastric pH through inhibition of acid secretion, omeprazole inhibits activation of pepsin.

Pharmacokinetics

Omeprazole is rapidly absorbed after oral administration in a formulation that dissolves mainly in the small intestine and its bioavailability is 50 to 70 percent. It is over 95 percent bound to plasma proteins and is delivered to gastric parietal cells from the blood stream. Onset of antisecretory activity occurs within one hour. Because of its mechanism of action, the duration of suppression of acid secretion attained with omeprazole is far longer than the plasma half-life of less than one hour.[4] Omeprazole is metabolized extensively in the liver, and the metabolites are excreted primarily in the urine.[r6]

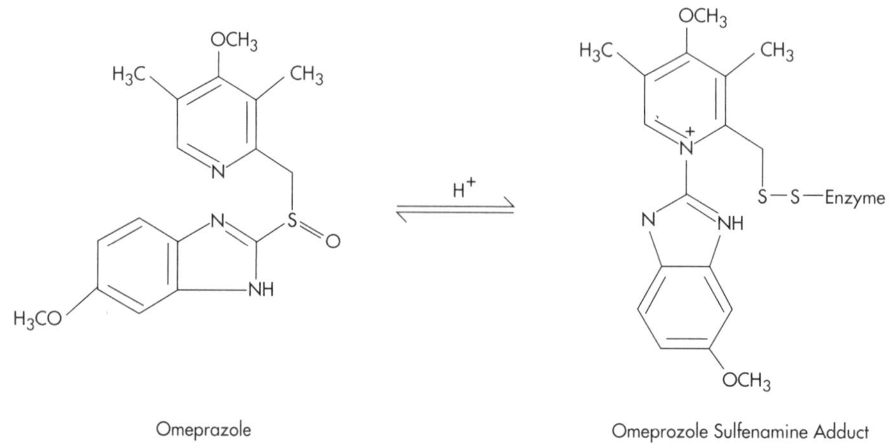

Omeprazole

Omeprozole Sulfenamine Adduct

Figure 67.3 Structure of omeprazole and its active sulfenamine product that interacts irreversibly with the enzyme, H^+,K^+-ATPase. The sulfenamine product results from rearrangement of omeprazole in the highly acidic environment of the secretory canaliculus of the parietal cell.

Therapeutic Uses

Therapy with omeprazole increases both the incidence and rate of healing of duodenal and gastric ulcers. The time required for healing is somewhat shorter than that necessary with H_2 receptor antagonists. Because of its high degree of efficacy in suppressing secretion of gastric acid, it is considered the drug of choice for management of Zollinger-Ellison syndrome associated with pancreatic gastrinoma. Omeprazole is also effective in the management of reflux esophagitis because of suppression of acid secretion.

In clinical practice, optimal suppression of acid secretion is achieved after three daily doses. Because it requires an acidic environment for activation, omeprazole affects only parietal cells that are actively secreting acid. Because of its short plasma half-life, only those proton pumps actually secreting acid within a few hours of drug administration will be inhibited, and several days of therapy are required to inhibit most of the enzyme. Preliminary clinical studies indicate that omeprazole is effective in long-term therapy in the prevention of peptic ulcer recurrence.

Adverse Effects

Because omeprazole is active only in acid-secreting canaliculi, coadministration of an H_2 antagonist or muscarinic antagonist will prevent conversion of omeprazole to its active form and will prevent its antisecretory actions. Therefore, other agents that suppress acid production should not be given with omeprazole. Omeprazole can prolong the elimination of certain drugs metabolized by oxidation in the liver, including diazepam, warfarin, and phenytoin. The clinical importance of these drug interactions remains to be established.

Omeprazole causes profound inhibition of acid secretion and consequent alkalinization of the gastric antrum. Plasma levels of gastrin therefore are often elevated during treatment with omeprazole. Gastrin exerts trophic effects on the gastric mucosa and there has been concern that the hypergastrinemia associated with omeprazole might result in mucosal hyperplasia. To date, however, mucosal hyperplasia in humans has not been found to occur consistently.

Omeprazole is well tolerated in most patients. A few (less than 3 percent) patients may experience headache, nausea, or diarrhea.[5] Even lower incidences of skin rash, dizziness, and constipation have been reported.

Preparations and Doses

Omeprazole (PriLosec) may be administered orally for peptic ulcers or reflux esophagitis in doses of 20 or 40 mg once daily, usually in the morning. Therapy is recommended for up to eight weeks, although ulcer healing often occurs within four weeks. Higher doses may be required for ulcer healing in patients with hypersecretory states such as Zollinger-Ellison syndrome.

Sucralfate

Sucralfate is composed of sucrose octasulfate complexed with aluminum hydroxide (Fig. 67.4). At low pH (below pH 4), there is extensive polymerization of sucralfate to form a viscous gel. The gel adheres strongly to the proteinaceous slough of the mucosal ulcer crater to provide a barrier between the acid gastric contents and the ulcer base.[r7] The gel adheres more strongly to the ulcer crater than to the surface of mucosal epithelial cells. Sucralfate has no significant acid neutralizing properties.

The antiulcer properties of sucralfate appear to occur from coating of the ulcer crater. The gel remains adherent to the ulcer crater for several hours. In addition, sucralfate inhibits pepsin activity in gastric juice and adsorbs bile acids. The primary antiulcer mechanism probably results from coating the ulcer crater and preventing access by H^+ and possibly by decreasing aggression by pepsin and bile acids.[6]

Pharmacokinetics

Sucralfate is poorly absorbed from the intestine and is excreted primarily in the feces. The small amounts of sucralfate absorbed systemically from the GI tract are excreted primarily in the urine. The duration of action is six to 12 hours.

Therapeutic Uses

Sucralfate displays healing efficacy in duodenal ulcer comparable to that of the H_2 receptor antagonists after four to eight weeks of therapy. Relief of ulcer pain achieved with sucralfate is similar to that provided by H_2 antagonists, although the onset of pain relief is less rapid. Long-term efficacy and safety for maintenance therapy to prevent ulcer recurrence have not been clearly established, but limited data indicate that sucralfate given in twice-daily doses may be comparable with H_2 receptor antagonists for prevention of recurrence.

Healing rates of gastric ulcers treated with sucralfate are similar to those obtained with cimetidine, but no convincing data have been presented to support use of sucralfate in preventing recurrence of gastric ulcer.[r8]

Sucralfate has shown promise in management of reflux esophagitis. Its mechanism of action in gastroduodenal reflux disease is presumably similar to that in duodenal ulcer: coating of the mucosal lesions and craters to prevent access by H^+.

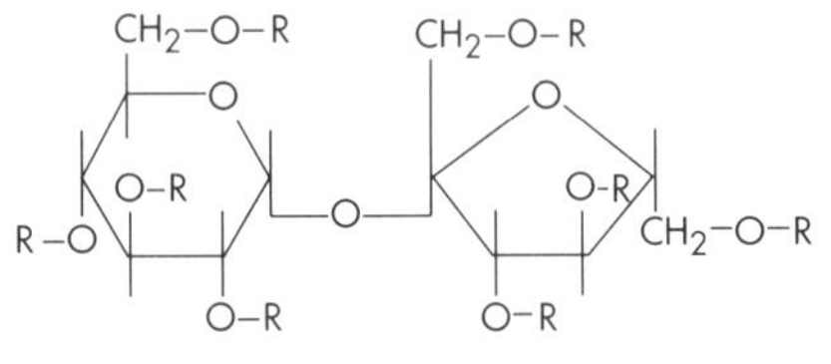

$R = SO_3[Al_2(OH)_5 \cdot (HOH)_2]$

Figure 67.4 Structure of sucralfate, an aluminum hydroxide complex with sucrose octasulfate.

Adverse Effects

Constipation is the most frequent side-effect of sucralfate therapy and occurs in approximately 2 percent of patients. Other side-effects are infrequent and mild. Sucralfate may bind theophylline, tetracycline, phenytoin, and certain other drugs and reduce their bioavailability after oral administration.[r8]

Preparations and Dose

Sucralfate (Carafate) is administered orally in a dose of 1 g two to four times daily.

Muscarinic Antagonists

Muscarinic cholinergic antagonists inhibit gastric acid secretion by competitive antagonism of acetylcholine at paracrine cell M_1 receptors and parietal cell M_3 receptors.[7] They can significantly reduce acid secretion and promote healing of peptic ulcers. Unfortunately, the muscarinic antagonists presently available produce intolerable side-effects at antisecretory doses, and thus fail to achieve the patient acceptance necessary for effective therapy of peptic ulcer disease. The unacceptable side-effects occur because these agents are antagonists at all three types of muscarinic receptors, M_1, M_2, and M_3, and therefore produce side-effects characteristic of nonspecific muscarinic antagonists.

At the doses necessary to bring about significant inhibition of gastric acid secretion, muscarinic antagonists typically reduce salivary secretion and induce dry mouth, tachycardia, and visual disturbances, and may interfere with urination. Moreover, muscarinic antagonists may interfere with normal contractions of GI smooth muscle by blockade of neurotransmission in the enteric nervous system, resulting in hypomotility and constipation. Patients find these effects objectionable and, even prior to the introduction of histamine H_2 receptor antagonists for treatment of peptic ulcer, the antimuscarinic drugs did not find favor in patients with peptic ulcer disease. After introduction of the H_2 receptor antagonists, the use of muscarinic antagonists in peptic ulcer disease declined even more. The conventional muscarinic antagonists serve as examples of drugs that are effective for the treatment of a disorder, but that have side-effects that greatly limit their practical utility. This observation suggests that antimuscarinic drugs that could act selectively on mechanisms that control gastric acid secretion might be practical therapeutic agents.

Pirenzepine (Fig. 67.5) is the prototype of newly developed selective M_1 receptor antagonists. Laboratory experiments and clinical experience with this drug suggest that it can inhibit gastric acid secretion without producing the spectrum of uncomfortable side-effects associated with muscarinic antagonists that block all three subtypes of the muscarinic receptor. Pirenzepine is thought to act by antagonism of the muscarinic receptors at histamine-containing paracrine cells in the gastric mucosa that release histamine when activated by neurally-secreted acetylcholine. According to this concept, pirenzepine inhibits vagally-induced gastric acid secretion by acting in the pathway responsible for release of histamine, which in

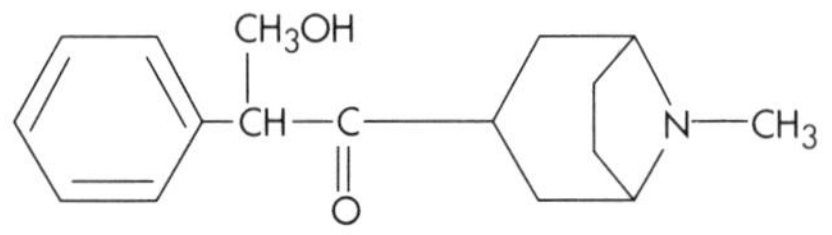

Figure 67.5 Structures of prototype muscarinic receptor antagonists. Atropine, dicyclomine, and pirenzapine are tertiary amines. Propantheline and glycopyrrolate are quarternary amines.

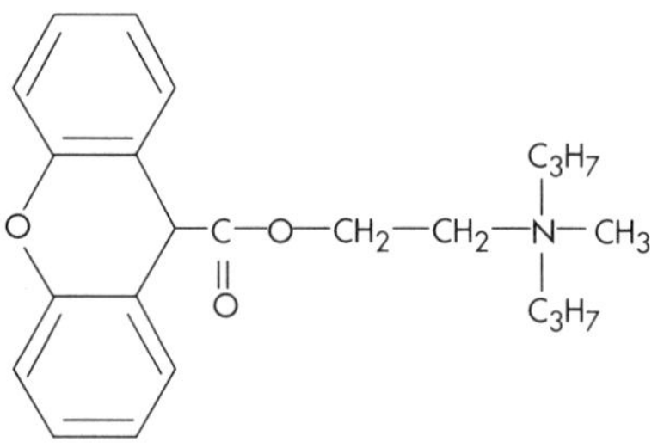

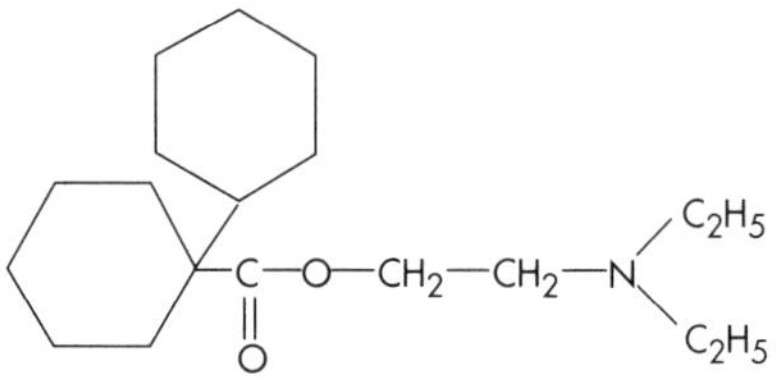

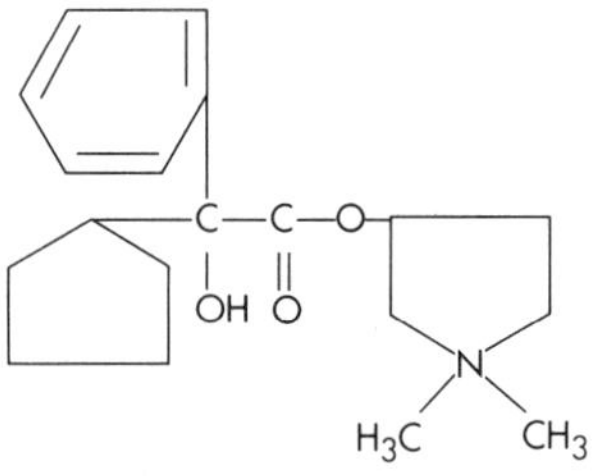

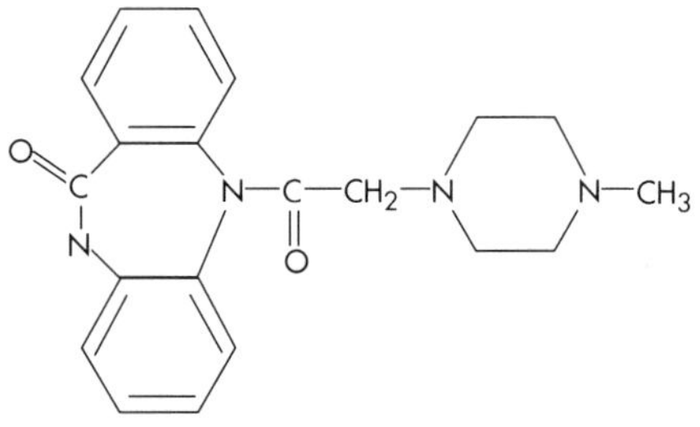

turn acts at the parietal cell H_2 receptor to stimulate acid production. Consistent with this concept, pirenzepine is more effective in blocking vagally-stimulated acid secretion than in blocking histamine-induced secretion. Pirenzepine has enjoyed significant use in the European countries where it is marketed. However, pirenzepine appears somewhat less effective than H_2 receptor antagonists or omeprazole in management of peptic ulcer disease. It is possible that a selective M_3 muscarinic antagonist would provide even more selective blockade of gastric acid secretion than pirenzepine. Efforts are underway to develop drugs with suitable selectivity for muscarinic M_3 receptors.

The muscarinic antagonist drugs are used occasionally as primary or adjunctive agents in the management of peptic ulcer disease. While they are effective in reducing gastric secretion and increasing the rate of healing of peptic ulcers, side-effects resulting from blockade of muscarinic receptors limit their use. Antimuscarinic drugs are not used in the treatment of gastroesophageal reflux disease because they decrease esophageal clearance, delay gastric emptying, and relax the lower esophageal sphincter. These effects can contribute to reflux of gastric contents into the esophagus and exacerbate reflux esophagitis.

Pharmacokinetics

The tertiary amine muscarinic antagonists (see Fig. 67.5), including atropine, dicyclomine, and pirenzepine, are rapidly absorbed from the GI tract after oral administration. Atropine has a plasma half-life of three to five hours. It is eliminated by renal excretion of intact drug and hepatic metabolites. The tertiary amine compounds, especially atropine, readily cross the blood-brain barrier and in high doses can produce CNS effects.

The quaternary amine muscarinic antagonists (see Fig. 67.5), such as propantheline and glycopyrrolate, are poorly absorbed from the GI tract. The plasma half-life of propantheline is one to two hours, and the drug is excreted primarily in the urine, mainly as metabolites.

Adverse Reactions

The most common side-effects associated with the nonspecific muscarinic antagonists include decreased salivary secretions, decreased sweating, and ocular side-effects including blurred vision, mydriasis, cycloplegia, and increased intraocular pressure. These drugs are generally contraindicated in patients with glaucoma. The drugs may produce urinary hesitancy and retention. They should be avoided in patients with urinary obstruction and used cautiously in the elderly. Another side-effect associated with muscarinic antagonists is constipation. These drugs should not be used in patients with intestinal hypomotility.

Preparations and Doses

Propantheline (Pro-Banthine) has been one of the most widely used of the muscarinic antagonist drugs. It is a quaternary amine and does not effectively cross the blood-brain barrier. The usual dose (15 mg) has a four- to six-hour duration of effect; it usually is administered four times daily. Dicyclomine (Bentyl) is given in doses of 10 to 20 mg four times daily. Glycopyrrolate (Robinul), a quaternary amine, is given four times daily in doses of 10 or 20 mg. Pirenzepine is not marketed in the US.

Prostaglandins

Prostaglandins, products of the cyclooxygenase pathway of arachidonic acid metabolism, occur naturally in the gastric and intestinal mucosa. Experience with NSAIDs that block the cyclooxygenase pathway suggests that prostaglandin production may be necessary for maintenance of healthy GI mucosa. Nonsteroidal anti-inflammatory and salicylate drugs, such as aspirin, indomethacin, and others, can damage the gastric and duodenal mucosa. Such damage, often resulting in ulcers, is a major side-effect associated with therapeutic use of NSAIDs. Moreover, mucosal damage induced by NSAIDs can be prevented by prior exposure of the GI mucosa to prostaglandins. This observation led to the concept that peptic ulcers associated with NSAID therapy represent a prostaglandin deficiency disease and that replacement of prostaglandins would prevent the mucosal damage. Subsequent laboratory and clinical experiments supported this concept. Several prostaglandins were found to increase epithelial cell secretion of mucus and bicarbonate and to improve mucosal blood flow, which may remove H^+ that diffuses through the mucosal barrier. Moreover, many prostaglandins decrease gastric acid secretion. Prostaglandin receptors on the parietal cell plasma membrane are negatively coupled by means of a G_i protein to adenylyl cyclase of the parietal cell. Activation of the prostaglandin receptor results in a decreased activity of adenylyl cyclase and decreased generation of intracellular cAMP. Thus, the prostaglandin receptor functions in the parietal cell in a manner opposite to functions of the histamine H_2 receptor. These discoveries promoted great interest in prostaglandins as potential antiulcer drugs.

Natural prostaglandins, including prostaglandins E_1 and E_2, protect against mucosal damage and decrease secretion of gastric acid. Unfortunately, the natural prostaglandins are extremely unstable in the GI tract and other biologic tissues because they are substrates for the enzyme, prostaglandin 15-hydroxydehydrogenase, that oxidizes the 15-hydroxyl group in prostaglandins to the corresponding ketone. Other enzymatic transformations can occur subsequently. In addition to biologic instability, prostaglandins of the E-type produce other serious side-effects. They act on intestinal and colonic epithelial cells to induce secretion of salt and water into the intestinal lumen, thus inducing diarrhea. The diarrhea is frequently associated with severe abdominal cramps. Moreover, E-type prostaglandins cause contractions of the uterus and abortion.

A number of synthetic analogues of prostaglandin E_1 and E_2 have been evaluated for potential use as antiulcer drugs. Misoprostol was recently introduced for therapeutic use.[r9] Misoprostol is 16-hydroxyl, 16-methyl prostaglandin E_1 methyl ester (Fig. 67.6). Because the 16-hydroxy group is protected by the 16-methyl substitution, misoprostol is resistant to prostaglandin 15-hydroxydehydrogenase. As a result, misoprostol is orally active, resistant to metabolism, and shows an increased duration of action compared with natural prostaglandin E_1. Misoprostol is also somewhat less likely than the natural prostaglandin E_1 to induce such side-effects as diarrhea. However, diarrhea is nevertheless one of the most frequent side-effects associated with administration of misoprostol.

Pharmacokinetics

Orally administered misoprostol is rapidly de-esterified to form 16-hydroxy, 16-methyl prostaglandin E_1, the active form of the drug. It penetrates the gastric mucosa to act at prostaglandin receptors of the oxyntic cell. It is also absorbed from the stomach and small intestine into the bloodstream. It is excreted in the urine primarily as hepatic metabolites. The duration of action of misoprostol is approximately six hours.

Therapeutic Uses

Misoprostol is used primarily to prevent peptic ulcers in patients with rheumatoid arthritis who are being treated with NSAIDs. The hazard of peptic ulcers in patients undergoing treatment with high doses of such drugs is greatest in the elderly, especially if prior episodes of GI bleeding have occurred. Misoprostol treatment has been shown in clinical trials to decrease the incidence of gastric ulcers associated with NSAID therapy.

Misoprostol also shows efficacy in idiopathic peptic ulcer disease.[r11] The antiulcer activity of this drug, however, is somewhat less than can be obtained with histamine H_2 antagonists, sucralfate, and omeprazole. In addition, misoprostol therapy is associated with a significantly greater incidence of side-effects. For this

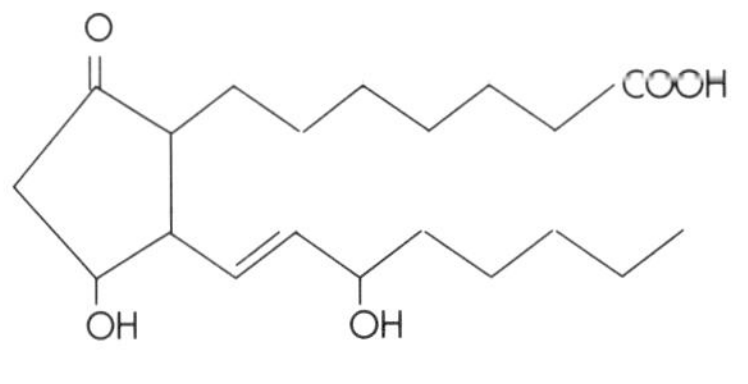

O COOH OH OH

Prostaglandin E_1

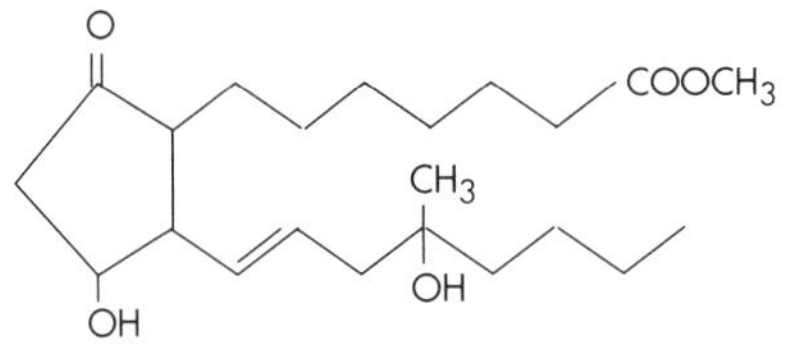

O $COOCH_3$ CH_3 OH OH

Misoprostol

Figure 67.6 Structures of Natural Prostaglandin E_1 and Synthetic Misoprostol

reason, its use is limited largely to prevention of ulcers during treatment with NSAIDs.

Adverse Effects

The most common side-effect associated with misoprostol is diarrhea. The diarrhea results from net secretion of fluid and electrolyte from intestinal crypt cells into the intestinal lumen. The increased secretory activity of the epithelial cells leads to accumulation of fluid in the bowel lumen, thus exceeding the absorptive capacity of the small intestine and colon. Watery diarrhea can follow. The over-all incidence of diarrhea complicating misoprostol therapy is as high as 10 per cent of patients. Dosage reduction can decrease the incidence and severity of the diarrhea. Diarrhea also tends to diminish after several days of therapy with misoprostol.

Because of its uterotonic activity, misoprostol is not administered to women who may become pregnant. Misoprostol can induce uterine contractions that result in complete or incomplete abortion. Misoprostol therapy is generally reserved for males and postmenopausal females. Many therapists prefer to use histamine H_2 antagonists as first-line treatment of gastric or duodenal ulcers associated with NSAID therapy because of their more favorable safety profile.

Preparations and Doses

Misoprostol (Cytotec) is available as a 200-mg tablet for oral administration for prevention of peptic ulcers induced by NSAIDs. The recommended frequency of dosing is four times daily. This may be reduced in patients exhibiting significant side-effects, including nausea, abdominal cramps, or diarrhea.

Antacids

Prior to the introduction of histamine H_2 receptor antagonists, antacids were the primary therapeutic agents used in treatment of acid peptic diseases, including peptic ulcer, gastroesophageal reflux disease, and dyspepsia. In view of the safety and efficacy of the modern drugs now available, antacids are prescribed less frequently for these disorders. However, lay use remains popular for self-medication of upper GI disturbances and as adjunctive therapy in patients undergoing treatment for peptic ulcer, reflux esophagitis, or occasional dyspepsia. In general, the risk-to-benefit ratio of antacids is less favorable than that with other pharmacologic agents for therapy of ulcers.

Antacids are simply basic compounds that neutralize acid in the gastric lumen (Fig. 67.7), thereby raising the pH of stomach contents, decreasing the acid load delivered to the duodenum, and reducing the activity of pepsin. Antacids are generally divided into two classes, systemic and nonsystemic. The systemic antacids are those that are absorbed from the GI lumen and that can raise the pH of blood and urine. Nonsystemic acids are poorly absorbed from the GI tract and do not elevate blood or urine pH. Nevertheless, small amounts of nonsystemic antacids can be absorbed and produce deleterious effects in susceptible individuals. Sodium bicarbonate is an example of a systemic antacid. Orally administered sodium bicarbonate is absorbed into the bloodstream and excreted in the urine. Salts of aluminum and magnesium are the most frequently used nonsystemic antacids. Aluminum- or magnesium-containing antacids are excreted mainly in the feces.

Antacids are bases that interact with gastric acid to form salt plus water. Antacid preparations differ in both rapidity of neutralization and neutralizing capacity (Table 67.2). Most recommended antacid preparations contain aluminum or magnesium hydroxide. Magnesium hydroxide is the most rapidly acting of the nonsystemic antacids. Magnesium trisilicate reacts very slowly with acid and is a poor antacid for therapeutic purposes. Aluminum hydroxide reacts more slowly with acid than does magnesium hydroxide, but is sufficiently rapid to be an effective gastric antacid. The effect of aluminum hydroxide is more sustained than that of magnesium hydroxide. Moreover, magnesium hydroxide is laxative, and aluminum hydroxide is constipating. Many commercial antacid preparations contain mixtures of aluminum hydroxide and magnesium hydroxide to achieve rapid and sustained neutralization of gastric acid and to balance laxative and constipating effects on bowel function.

Calcium compounds, such as calcium carbonate and calcium hydroxide, are rarely used at present in the management of acid peptic disorders. Calcium compounds provide adequate initial neutralization of gastric acid, but they are more likely than magnesium or aluminum compounds to stimulate excess secretion of acid that may persist after the antacid leaves the stomach and can no longer neutralize the gastric contents. The excess secretion that occurs after antacids leave the stomach, known as "acid rebound," can provoke symptoms of dyspepsia. Antacids that contain calcium are most likely to cause acid rebound because

$$Mg(OH)_2 + 2HCl \longrightarrow MgCl_2 + 2H_2O$$

$$Al(OH)_3 + 3HCl \longrightarrow AlCl_3 + 3H_2O$$

Figure 67.7 Neutralization of Gastric HCl by Two Nonsystemic Antacids, Magnesium Hydroxide and Aluminum Hydroxide

Table 67.2 Composition and Acid-Neutralizing Capacity of Representative Liquid Antacids

	Content (mg/5mL)				
Product	**$Al(OH)_3$**	**$Mg(OH)_2$**	**Simethicone**	**Na**	**Acid-Neutralizing Capacity (mEq/ml)**
Alternagel	600	0	0	<2.5	16
Aludrox	3	103	0	<3.0	12
Amphojel	320	0	0	<0.1	10
Gaviscon	95	412[a]	0	13	4
Gelusil	300	200	25	<2.0	15
Kolantyl Gel	150	150	0	<5.0	10
Maalox	225	200	0	1.4	13
Milk of magnesia	0	390	0	<1.0	14
Mylanta	200	200	20	<1.0	12

[a]Magnesium carbonate

the calcium ion can increase acid secretion by direct and indirect mechanisms. Calcium can directly increase acid secretion by parietal cells, presumably by activation of H^+, K^+-ATPase, and can indirectly stimulate secretion by increasing release of gastric secretagogues, such as gastrin and histamine. Some over-the-counter antacids intended for occasional lay use contain calcium carbonate.

Pharmacokinetics

The gastric antacids are administered orally as tablets or liquid suspensions. The liquid preparations are generally thought to provide more effective neutralization of acid. Antacids containing magnesium hydroxide quickly neutralize gastric acid, whereas antacids containing aluminum hydroxide neutralize acid more slowly. Once they leave the stomach, magnesium and aluminum chloride salts may interact with intestinal luminal contents to form hydroxide salts, carbonate salts, or soaps with fatty acids. These insoluble salts and soaps are excreted in the feces. Aluminum chloride may interact with luminal phosphates and be excreted as phosphate salts.

Adverse Effects

The major adverse effect of magnesium hydroxide is laxation and diarrhea. Aluminum hydroxide may produce constipation. Other adverse effects include systemic toxicity in patients with impaired renal function who cannot adequately excrete aluminum or magnesium. Despite the small amounts of these cations absorbed from the intestine, accumulation in plasma can occur in patients with renal failure. Because they form salts with luminal phosphate, chronic use of aluminum-containing antacids can lead to phosphate depletion and bone resorption. Excessive accumulation of magnesium can result in muscular weakness and CNS effects.

By raising gastric pH, antacids may alter dissolution and bioavailability of other drugs. Moreover, the basic compounds may adsorb other drugs, including tetracyclines, benzodiazepines, and ranitidine.

Antacids containing calcium are rarely prescribed, although they may be present in some lay remedies. Calcium-containing antacids have been found to produce "acid rebound" as discussed above. However, calcium-containing antacids have been used as inexpensive calcium supplements in women to prevent osteoporosis.

Therapeutic Uses

The major medical use of antacids at present is for self-medication during the acute phase of treatment of peptic ulcers, for occasional dyspepsia, and in management of reflux esophagitis. When taken in conjunction with histamine H_2 antagonists, antacids can provide additional relief from peptic ulcer pain. Their main value is for symptomatic relief of symptoms of dyspepsia.[8]

Preparations and Dosage

Preparations of representative antacids are listed in Table 67.2. The usual recommended doses are 10 to 20 ml four times daily. Many preparations are flavored to mask a chalk-like taste. Some preparations contain simethicone, an antifoaming agent intended to reduce gas bubbles.

Antimicrobial Therapy

Persistent infection with *H. pylori* may represent an etiologic factor in peptic ulcer disease. In some cases of recalcitrant ulcers resistant to conventional therapy, antimicrobial therapy has been attempted with varying success. Colloidal bismuth preparations, alone or in combination with antibiotics, have been employed to eradicate *H. pylori* infections.[9] Colloidal bismuth subcitrate is the subject of current investigation because of its bactericidal effects on *H. pylori*. It also provides a barrier between the gastric contents and the ulcer base, and mucosal protective properties have been ascribed to this preparation. Significant amounts of bismuth may be absorbed from some colloids, raising concerns about systemic toxicity. Triple therapy with bismuth, metronidazole, and amoxicillin or tetracycline has been suggested in some cases for the initial healing of duodenal ulcers associated with mucosal colonies of *H. pylori*. However, this approach to treatment should be viewed as highly experimental and is not recommended in most cases of peptic ulcer.

References

Research Reports

1. Soll AH. Pathogenesis of peptic ulcer and implications for therapy. N Engl J Med 1990;*322*:909–916.
2. Peterson WL. Helicobacter pylori and peptic ulcer disease. N Engl J Med 1991;*324*:1043–1048.
3. Black JW, Duncan WAM, Durant CJ, Ganellin CR, Parsons EM. Definition and antagonism of histamine H_2 receptors. Nature 1972;*236*:335–391.
4. Walon A. The clinical utility and safety of omeprazole. Scan J Gastroenterol 1989;*24*:140–144.
5. Simon TJ, Bradstreet DC. Comparative tolerability profile of omeprazole in clinical trial. Dig Dis Sci 1991;*36*:1384–1389.
6. Shea-Donohue T, Steel L, Montcalm E, Dubois A. Gastric protection by sucralfate. Gastroenterology 1986;*91*:660–666.
7. Goyal RK. Identification, localization and classification of muscarinic receptor subtypes in the gut. Life Sci 1988;*43*:2209–2220.
8. Kumar N, Vy JC, Karol A, Anand BS. Controlled therapeutic trial to determine the optimum dose of antacids in duodenal ulcer. Gut 1984;*25*:1199–1202.
9. Rauws EAJ, Tytgot GNJ. Cure of duodenal ulcer associated with eradication of *Helicobacter pylori*. Lancet 1990;*335*:1233–1235.

Reviews

r1. Schubert ML, Shamburek RD. Control of acid secretion. Gastroenterol Clin North Amer 1990;*19*:1–25.

r2. Richardson CT. Effect of H_2 receptor antagonists on gastric acid secretion and serum gastrin concentration: A review. Gastroenterology 1978;*74*:366–370.

r3. Brogden RN, Carmine AA, Heel RC, Speight TM, Avery GS. Ranitidine: A review of its pharmacology and therapeutic use in peptic ulcer disease and other allied diseases. Drugs 1982;*24*:267–303.

r4. Feldman M, Burton ME. Histamine$_2$—receptor antagonists. N Engl J Med 1990;*323*:1672–1680.

r5. Wallmark B, Lorentzon P, Larsson H. The mechanism of action of omeprazole: a survey of its inhibitory actions in vitro. Scand J Gastroenterol 1985;*20*(Suppl. 108):37–51.

r6. Maton PN. Omeprazole. N Engl J Med 1991;*324*:965–975.

r7. Nagashima R. Mechanisms of action of sucralfate. J Clin Gastroenterol 1981;*3*(Suppl. 2):117–127.

r8. McCarthy DM. Sucralfate. N Engl J Med 1991;*325*:1017–1025.

r9. Monk JP, Clissold SP. Moprostol: A preliminary review of its pharmacodynamic and pharmacokinetic properties, and therapeutic efficacy in the treatment of peptic ulcer disease. Drugs 1987;*33*:1–30.

r10. Aly A. Prostaglandins in clinical treatment of gastroduodenal mucosal lesions: A review. Scand J Gastroenterol 1987;*22*:(Suppl. 137):43–49.

CHAPTER 68

Timothy S. Gaginella

Laxative Drugs

Laxatives are intended for use in the therapy of constipation. Arriving at a clear definition of constipation is difficult because physicians and patients often have differing opinions about it. While physicians understand that normal bowel habits vary widely among individuals (from five to 15 bowel movements per week), patients often complain that they are "constipated" if they do not have a bowel movement every day, if the bowel movement is incomplete, or if it is painful. A working definition of constipation among clinicians is fewer than three spontaneous bowel movements per week.

There is no question that constipation is a real phenomenon. It may idiopathic, due to neurologic disorders, to hyperparathyroidism, hypothyroidism, or hypercalcemia, or due to drugs such as the opiates, anticholinergics, aluminum-containing antacids, and iron (Table 68.1). Unfortunately, the easy availability of over-the-counter laxative preparations, and the belief by so many in the general population that anything less than one bowel movement a day is unhealthy, have led often to the inappropriate use of laxatives.[2] There are approximately 200 laxative products on the market; and about $368 million is spent annually on over-the-counter laxatives in the US. Although mechanisms of action vary among different laxatives, as a group they result in an increase in frequency of bowel movements. It is important to establish the cause of the constipation before choosing a particular laxative for therapy.[3]

The term "laxative" will be used throughout this chapter, although readers may see the terms *cathartics* or *purgatives* (sometimes even *aperients* or *drastics*) elsewhere. Laxatives are often thought to produce a milder effect than cathartics, but generally it is simply a matter of dose; many laxatives can have a more pronounced (cathartic) effect if given in a higher dose. Exceptions are inert substances, such as mineral oil.

Table 68.1 Causes of Constipation

Diseases	Drugs
Paraplegia	Aluminum-containing antacids
Multiple Sclerosis	Barium and bismuth salts
Hypothyroidism	Anticholinergics, tricyclic antidepressants
Intestinal Carcinoma	Ganglionic blockers
Strictures	Ferrous sulfate
Hyperparathyroidism	Morphine, codeine, other opieates
Hemorrhoids	Antiparkinson drugs

Laxatives are often classified as irritant (or stimulant), lubricant, saline, and bulk-forming agents. Although such classification has been employed in various textbooks, it is often misleading. In this chapter we will deal with each drug or group of drugs rather than attempt to characterize them strictly according to presumed pharmacologic action. For example, castor oil is often stated to produce its laxative action by "irritating" the intestine by contact with the mucosa, thereby "stimulating" motility and a peristaltic reflex. These assumptions are inaccurate, as the active ingredient in castor oil alters mucosal electrolyte transport[4–7] and either inhibits intestinal circular muscle activity or causes a nonpropulsive coordination of muscular contraction of the gut wall.[8–9]

Sources and Chemistry of Laxatives

At least two of the most commonly used laxatives are from botanical sources. Castor oil (the active ingredient of which is ricinoleic acid) is expressed from the seeds of *Ricinus communis;* anthraquinones come from aloe leaves and cascara sagrada bark. Synthetic laxatives with actions similar to these natural products are danthron (1,8-dihydroxyanthraquinone), the diphenylmethanes (diphenols) phenolphthalein and bisacodyl, and the surfactant compound dioctyl sodium (or potassium) sulfosuccinate (Fig. 68.1). Poorly absorbable polyvalent salts such as magnesium sulfate ($MgSO_4$) and phosphates also are components of commonly used laxative preparations. Lactulose is a synthetic disaccharide composed of galactose and fructose. Its mechanism of action is unique among laxatives, in that it depends mostly on intestinal bacteria for its action. Mineral oil is inert and acts as a physical barrier to water, thus serving as a lubricant for the movement of luminal contents. Thus, laxatives represent a diverse group of chemicals, the actions of which result in an increase in intestinal luminal fluid accumulation and/or changes in motility.

The laxative with perhaps the richest history is castor oil. Castor oil has been recognized and used therapeutically as a laxative for centuries.[10] The oil, obtained from the seeds of *Ricinus communis,* was known to ancient cultures. The Ebers Papyrus (16th century BC) records the use of the *Ricinus* plant by the Egyptians. The Aztecs also utilized a variety of the plant for medicinal purposes. Other terms applied to the Ricinus seeds signify its laxative properties; in the 1600s it was variously referred to as "seeds of spurge" and "purgative beans". Reference to the oil was made in the 1788 edition of the London Pharmacopeia and the Edinburgh New Dispensatory in 1797. In the 1800s castor oil was even thought to be effective in dysentery, being said to act by providing an oily protective effect over the mucosa.

The active component of castor oil was identified as ricinoleic acid in 1890. Ricinoleic acid is an 18-carbon C_{9-10} monounsaturated fatty acid that is hydroxylated at the C_{12} position (Fig. 68.1). This aliphatic fatty acid is present as the triglyceride in the oil, to the extent of about 90 percent.[11]

Laxatives of the anthraquinone class include sennosides, emodin, and barbaloin. The anthraquinones may occur in the free form or as glycosides in plants. Aloe, a member of the lily family, is the source of emodin, aloin (barbaloin), and other anthraquinones that are not fully characterized but may contribute to the laxative properties of the crude plant material. Aloe was known by ancient civilizations to have beneficial dermatologic and GI effects.

The sennosides are derived from the dried leaflets and pods of *Cassia acutifolia,* introduced into medicine by the Arabs in about 800 BC. Sennoside A and sennoside B are the major components of the plant material. Cascara sagrada contains anthraquinone glycosides and aglycones (ring structure without sugar attached) present in the dried bark of *Rhamnus purshiana.* This plant grows along the coast of Oregon and Washington. The laxative activity of cascara is attributed to hydroxymethylanthraquinones, many of which are also found in aloe, senna, and the rhubarb plant. Emodin (1,6,8-trihydroxy-3-methyl-anthraquinone), isoemodin, and chrysophanol (1,8-dihydroxy-3-methylanthraquinone) are the primary active principles (see Fig. 68.1 for example). The anthraquinone laxatives vary considerably in enteral potency.[12]

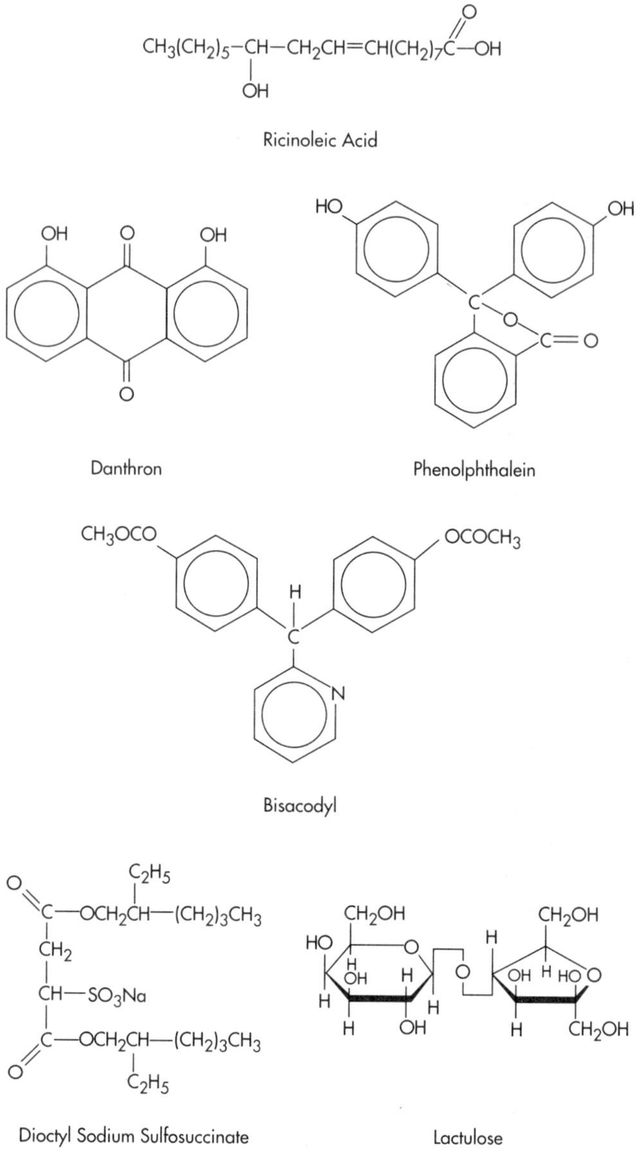

$CH_3(CH_2)_5-CH(OH)-CH_2CH=CH(CH_2)_7C(=O)-OH$

Ricinoleic Acid

Danthron

Phenolphthalein

Bisacodyl

Dioctyl Sodium Sulfosuccinate

Lactulose

Figure 68.1 Chemical Structures of Common Laxatives

Mineral oil (liquid paraffin), poorly absorbable inorganic salts, and water-retaining plant fibers such as bran and psyllium are also natural products with laxative effects.

The synthetic compound phenolphthalein [3,3-bis(p-hydroxyphenylphthalide)] was first used in 1902 as a laxative. Its effects on the intestinal tract were noted during an investigation of its pharmacology. Phenolphthalein is in many over-the-counter laxative preparations because of its relatively pleasant taste, its efficacy, and its lack of significant side-effects or toxicity. The popularity of phenolphthalein led to the rational synthesis of this bisacodyl [4,4-(pyridylmethylene)diphenol diacetate] (Fig. 68.1), which has been used successfully in suppository and oral tablet form.

Lactulose is a disaccharide (4-O-β-galactopyranosyl-D-fructofuranose) synthesized from galactose and fructose. This substance was originally used in portal-systemic encephalopathy in patients with chronic liver disease. It is not available in the US as an over-the-counter preparation, but can be obtained with a prescription.

Therapeutic Uses and Actions

Castor Oil

Historically, castor oil has been the stalwart among the laxatives. Ancient practitioners recommended crude, and later, more refined forms of the oil for its effects on the intestinal tract. Today, castor oil is still used by some as a general laxative. Its principal application in medicine is to evacuate the bowel prior to GI radiographs. Attempts have been made to mask the unpleasant odor and taste of castor oil by mixing it with peppermint flavoring, emulsifying it into a white creamy mixture that is flavored, or simply stirring it into orange juice prior to administration.

Upon oral ingestion the oil mixes with bile and pancreatic enzymes to liberate ricinoleic acid from the triglyceride. A small amount of ricinoleic acid is absorbed from the GI tract and metabolized like other fatty acids, but most remains in the intestine where it produces an action on the mucosa. The ricinoleic acid readily forms ricinoleate salts with sodium and potassium in the lumen of the intestine, which act as soaps (surfactants) within the gut and at the mucosal surface. Contrary to what previously was taught as dogma, castor oil is not an "irritant" to the intestinal lining, and it does not "stimulate" the coordinated movement of GI propulsion to bring about its laxative effect. Thus, it is inappropriate to classify castor oil in this manner. However, its categorization as a "contact laxative" is not totally incorrect, since castor oil and ricinoleic acid act luminally through direct or reflex mechanisms involving the mucosa.

Modern experimental techniques have allowed detailed investigation of the mechanism of action of ricinoleate on the mucosa and smooth muscle of the gut. Contractility in vitro of longitudinal muscle from the small intestine of rodents is not stimulated but depressed by ricinoleate.[8,13] This effect also occurs with the anthraquinones and dioctyl sodium sulfosuccinate.[14]

The rhythmic pattern of electrical activity that drives the coordinated movement of intraluminal contents through the bowel is altered by castor oil and other laxatives.[9] This effect, which may be prominent in the fasted state, facilitates the movement of fluid from the small intestine into the colon; this is not due to an enhancement of peristalsis. Since the colon has the capacity to absorb water at about six liters per 24 hours,[15] fluid accumulation in excess of this amount will result in loose or watery stools and laxation.

The best documented effects of ricinoleic acid are on the intestinal mucosa. Exposure of the mucosa to a concentration of ricinoleic acid of 5 mM or more, which can be achieved in the lower bowel after a normal therapeutic dose (30 ml)[6] of castor oil, causes inhibition of water and electrolyte movement into the jejunal[16] and ileal lumina, as also commonly observed in diarrheal diseases. The electrolytes, through osmotic forces, carry water with them, causing increased fluidity of the luminal contents. This effect, coupled with the effects of the ricinoleate on intestinal smooth muscle, causes an increase in the rate of flow through the small intestine, further reducing the opportunity for absorption. Ricinoleate affects the colonic mucosa in the same manner as it does the small intestinal mucosa.[17,18]

The mechanism responsible for the effects on the mucosa is still somewhat a mystery. Depending on the study consulted (experimental animal or human, etc.), at concentrations from 2 to 10 mM, ricinoleate has several actions that could account for its antiabsorptive/secretory effect on the mucosa. It inhibits the enzyme sodium-potassium ATPase,[19] and increases permeability[7,20] of the intestinal epithelium, produces a cytotoxic effect on isolated enterocytes,[21] and inhibits epithelial cell mitochondrial metabolism.[22] It also may stimulate epithelial cell adenylyl cyclase,[23] release prostaglandins[24] (or other metabolites of arachidonic acid), and platelet activating factor.[25] Most recently, nitric oxide has been claimed to contribute to the laxative action of castor oil.[26] Another hypothesis is that ricinoleate acts as a calcium ionophore, increasing the influx of extracellular calcium,[27] which activates calmodulin-dependent secretory mechanisms. Such diverse effects might be expected from the mucosal injury and enhanced cell membrane permeability produced by ricinoleate, and may account for stimulation of adenylyl cyclase, since prostaglandins released by injury may activate this and other enzymes in the intestinal mucosa. All of these effects are probably the result of the surfactant properties of ricinoleic acid, above its critical micellar concentration (approximately 2–5 mM).

The normal laxative dose of castor oil is 30 ml orally. It is usually administered on an empty stomach and acts within two to six hours. It is available as castor oil, USP, the flavored emulsion Neoloid, and various other flavored formulations. The side-effects from castor oil are intestinal pain and griping. Long-term use (abuse) can alter normal motility of the bowel and may result in systemic electrolyte depletion.

Anthraquinones

Anthraquinones, including sennosides, cascara, and aloe, are widely used by the public as all-purpose laxatives and also as recommended by physicians for bowel evacuation prior to diagnostic radiographs. The anthraquinones as a class have no well defined activity on intestinal smooth muscle. Some studies indicate that they depress contractility of the gut muscle,[28] although other studies indicate that propulsive waves of contraction in the rectum and colon can be evoked in man by their topical application.[29] A well-documented effect of anthraquinones is inhibition of intestinal electrolyte absorption.[12,30] This effect, as in the case of ricinoleic acid, leads to fluid accumulation in the intestinal lumen and a more rapid movement of material to and through the colon. Part of the action of these laxatives (and others) may be a reflex stimulation of colonic motility due to the mass of fluid accumulation. In this sense, the observed mass movements of the material through the colon upon administration of anthraquinones may be due more to an indirect rather than a direct effect on the colonic muscle.

It is generally believed that the anthraquinones act in part through an activating effect on the myenteric neurons that innervate the gut. This contention is supported by studies indicating that anthraquinones taken on a chronic basis can cause degeneration of myenteric neurons[31] and colonic muscle flaccidity, resulting in what is termed "cathartic colon." This condition can arise particularly in the elderly from abuse of the anthraquinone laxatives.[32] Overuse leads to constipation and dependency, making continued use necessary to produce normal bowel movements.

The anthraquinones are usually present in laxative preparations as the glycosides. Being large polar molecules, the glycosides are poorly absorbed in the small intestine. As they reach the colon, bacteria hydrolyze the glycoside linkage, liberating the active molecule, which must be reduced from the quinone to the alcohol (anthrol).[33] Thus, the primary action of the anthraquinones is believed to be on the colon.

Danthron is a synthetic nonglycoside anthraquinone and therefore does not require hydrolysis by intestinal bacterial. Danthron probably has more of an action on the small intestine than do the glycosidic anthraquinones.

The mechanism by which the anthraquinones alter fluid transport across the intestinal mucosa is believed to be through inhibition of sodium absorption,[12] through a nonspecific metabolic effect on the epithelial cells,[34] or inhibition of sodium-potassium ATPase. They do not appear to stimulate adenylate cyclase or produce mucosal injury, but an aloe preparation has been reported to stimulate prostaglandin synthesis.[35] An effect on the release of neurotransmitters from the myenteric plexus, which in turn may alter fluid absorption by the gut, cannot be ruled out.

The natural glycosidic anthraquinones usually produce their effect after five to six hours, while danthron may produce laxation in about half that time. The most common side-effects from anthraquinones are intestinal cramping and potential excessive electrolyte loss if the drugs are used at a high dosage or for prolonged periods. Patients who have been exposed to the anthraquinones on a chronic basis develop pigmentation of the colonic mucosa termed "melanosis coli." This is usually reversible after the medication has been discontinued. Its presence does not seem to be associated with pathology, but can help the gastroenterologist confirm suspected laxative abuse by colonoscopy.

Another interesting property of the anthraquinones is that they can be secreted into human milk during lactation. Whether the secreted drug has any effect on the nursing infant is not clear. The urine may also be discolored by excreted anthraquinones.

Danthron is available as 37.5- and 75-mg tablets and in water solution form. Various other preparations of aloe, senna, and cascara sagrada are available as tablets or fluid extracts and syrups for oral use. Sennosides A and B (USP) are available as 12-mg tablets. One or two tablets is the usual dose. Cascara is administered orally at a dose of 30 mg in tablet form or as extract or syrup.

Diphenylmethane Laxatives

The best-known and most widely used diphenylmethane laxative is phenolphthalein. Used since the turn of the 20th century, when its laxative properties were first recognized, this drug is now in many over-the-counter preparations (e.g., Ex-Lax). Phenolphthalein, like castor oil and the anthraquinones, is often classified as a stimulant or contact laxative, but there is no evidence of a direct stimulating effect on intestinal motility in humans. However, phenolphthalein does exert an antiabsorptive/secretory effect on electrolytes and water in the small intestine.[36] Just as for the previously-discussed laxatives, this leads to fluid accumulation in the lumen, a less viscous stool, and laxation. It is not entirely clear how, on a cellular basis, phenolphthalein induces this effect, but it is believed to be partly through inhibition of active transport of sodium across the basal-lateral aspect of the epithelial cells.[37] Phenolphthalein is also associated with mucosal prostaglandin E release[38] and exfoliation of small intestinal villus tips,[39] implying possible epithelial injury. Such an effect, however, might also be due to hydraulic flow as a result of the movement of fluid from the interstitium to the lumen.

Phenolphthalein acts mainly on the small intestine; up to 15 percent of the therapeutic dose is absorbed, and the remainder is excreted in the feces. Once in the systemic circulation, it is metabolized by the liver and cleared in the conjugated (glucuronide) form by the kidney.

Some of the conjugated phenolphthalein is secreted back into the small intestine in the bile (Fig. 68.2). This enterohepatic "recycling" of the drug probably contributes to its pharmacologic effect. The glucuronide is poorly absorbed throughout the smaller intestine, thus delivering the conjugated drug to the lower ileum and colon, where bacteria hydrolyze the glyco-

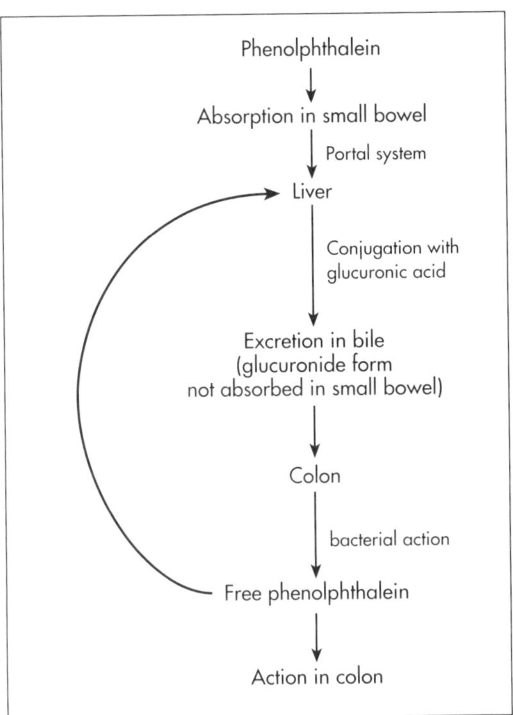

Figure 68.2 The Enterohepatic Circulation of Phenolphthalein

sidic linkage and liberate the phenolphthalein. In this form it may act on the colonic mucosa and possibly alter colonic neuromuscular function.

Phenolphthalein is relatively nontoxic, but large doses may result in watery diarrhea and excessive loss of electrolytes. Allergic reactions have been reported, and these usually take the form of skin lesions. Deaths have been attributed to allergic reactions to phenolphthalein. It is a favorite of laxative abusers, but surreptitious abuse of this drug can be unveiled by simply alkalinizing the urine or feces; a red color indicates the presence of phenolphthalein.

Phenolphthalein is available in numerous over-the-counter preparations, including Ex-Lax, Correctol, Phenolax, Feen-A-Mint. The usual dose is 30 to 270 mg. The action of the drug is usually noted within six to eight hours.

Bisacodyl is another diphenolic laxative, and has been used since 1953. It was synthesized in an effort to produce a rational approach to new drugs related to phenolphthalein. Originally introduced as a formulation for rectal administration, bisacodyl is now also available as oral tablets.

Only a small amount (approximately 5%) of an orally-administered dose of bisacodyl is reported to be absorbed in humans. Some of the absorbed drug appears in the urine as the glucuronide. Its action can occur within minutes after rectal administration, suggesting that in some manner it may evoke a neural reflex upon contact with rectal mucosa[40] that induces a response and defecation. The mechanism of action on the epithelium after oral administration is complex,[41,42] being partly due to inhibitory effects on Na^+/K^+-ATPase, release of prostaglandin E_2, stimulation of phosphodiesterase and adenylyl cyclase, and mucosal injury.

The usual oral dosage is 10 to 15 mg for children. Tablets should be swallowed without chewing or crushing to avoid gastric irritation and should be taken at least one hour prior to antacid in order to protect the enteric coating. If this is destroyed, GI upset and vomiting may result. The laxative effect occurs six to eight hours after oral administration.

Sulfosuccinate Salts

Dioctyl sodium sulfosuccinate (DSS) is commonly referred to as a fecal softener, wetting agent, or emollient. Originally thought merely to soften the stool by helping incorporate water, it is now known that DSS can produce mucosal injury and epithelial cell toxicity.[21,43] It inhibits fluid absorption by the intestine; thus, its effects are not merely the result of physical penetration into the stool and reduction of the surface tension of the fecal material. It does not act as a mucosal lubricant.

DSS is generally used alone to promote laxation whenever straining needs to be avoided. This includes use in pregnant or postpartum women and in patients with heart disease or cardiovascular weakness and after rectal or anal surgery. Many combination products (e.g., with anthraquinones) also contain DSS.

Hepatotoxicity has been reported with combination products containing DSS, possibly because it may enhance the absorption of the other ingredients. If given with a lubricant agent such as mineral oil, absorption of the oil may produce systemic toxicity.

Colace and doxinate are over-the-counter formulations of DSS. The usual dosage is 50 to 400 mg daily, as a single or divided dose. Oral solutions are also supplied containing 10 or 50 mg/ml. The calcium form of the drug is available as Surfak, with the same action as DSS.

Mineral Oil

Heavy mineral oil has been employed as a mucosal coating or lubricating agent to ease bowel movements in patients who have had abdominal or rectal surgery. The principal problem with mineral oil is leakage from the rectum leading to discomfort and retarded healing after rectal and anal surgery. The oil also may act as a solvent for lipid-soluble vitamins such as A, D, E, and K, and drugs. Some mineral oil can be absorbed by the intestine and can deposit in liver cells. There is also the danger of aspiration of the oil, resulting in lipoid pneumonia. This is especially a problem when the oil is taken at bedtime, in infants, and in the elderly.

The usual dosage of mineral oil is 15 to 45 ml. Emulsions of the oil also are available to overcome objections to its taste or consistency.

Natural Fibers

Fiber in the form of bran or psyllium has been widely used to promote normal bowel activity. Bran imbibes water like a sponge and swells in the intestinal lumen, thereby forming a semisolid material that keeps the contents moist and tends to enhance reflex contractile activity of the small bowel and colon. Fecal water and bulk increase after bran administration.[44]

Psyllium is a hydrophilic colloid that forms a muciláginous mass when mixed with water in the intestinal tract, increasing the rate of transit.[45] Bulk-forming agents, also, particularly those containing psyllium, may bind bile acids (which have a laxative effect). It is believed that sufficient quantities of these bile acids may reach the colon, induce fluid secretion, and thus contribute to the laxative effect.[46]

Although there is no known toxicity or side-effect associated with bran or psyllium, each dose should be taken with several glasses of water to prevent the material from becoming impacted. The absorption of some drugs may be impaired by these bulk-forming agents. Common psyllium-containing products include Metamucil, Petro-Syllium, and Serutan.

Lactulose

The disaccharide of galactose and fructose, lactulose, is a unique laxative. The small intestine lacks a specific disaccharidase to hydrolyze lactulose into its constituent monosaccharides. Thus, it remains nearly unaltered and nonabsorbed until it reaches the colon, where bacteria metabolize it to lactic and acidic acids and carbon dioxide. It is believed that laxation is produced by virtue of the effects of these acids on the colon, either direct or through alteration of colonic pH.[47] No doubt the osmotic activity of the unabsorbed lactulose in the small intestine also contributes.

Lactulose causes abdominal discomfort and flatulence in about 20 percent of patients. Nausea and vomiting are also common, especially with higher dosage.

Cephulac and Duphalac are syrup preparations of lactulose. Because of their higher sugar content, they must be administered with care to diabetics. Laxation usually occurs with a dose of 10 to 15 ml (7–10 g lactulose, comprised of 2.2 g of galactose, 1.2 g of lactose, and 1.2 g of other sugars). Several days may be required for the full effect of this laxative to be produced.

Inorganic Salts

Magnesium sulfate (also known as Epsom Salts) is a potent saline laxative. Magnesium hydroxide (milk of magnesia) has antacid and laxative properties. Magnesium ion and poorly absorbed anions such as sulfate and phosphate, through osmotic actions, hold or draw fluid into the intestinal lumen. This is the result of an osmotic gradient. Tartrates and citrates (e.g., Citrate of Magnesia USP) also are believed to act in this manner, although it is not possible to rule out completely an intrinsic effect of some of these ions on the gut.

When taken as a laxative, the usual dose of magnesium hydroxide is 15 to 30 ml. A usual dose of 15 g of magnesium sulfate yields a greater number of moles of osmotically active cations so that $MgSO_4$ is a more potent laxative than is magnesium hydroxide.

Magnesium ions are absorbed poorly (only to about 20% of the dose). This is usually of no consequence to individuals with normal kidneys, but may be a threat to those with impaired renal function. Excess plasma levels of magnesium can produce CNS depression, cardiovascular irregularities, and muscle weakness.

Table 68.2 Doses and Approximate Times to Onset of Commonly Used Laxatives

Class	Example(s)	Trade name(s)	Adult Dose	Approximal Time to Onset (hr)
Anthraquinone	Senna	Cascara Sagrada extract	5 ml	6–8
Bulk forming	Psyllium	Metamucil, Serutan	4–30 g	12–72
Diphenylmethane	Bisacodyl	Dulcolax	5–15 mg	6–10
	Phenolphthalein	Ex-Lax, Feen-A-Mint	30–270 mg	6–8
Fatty Acid	Ricinoleic acid	Caster oil USP	15–60 ml	2–6
	Neoloid			
Lubricant	Mineral Oil, USP	Various		
Saline	$Mg(OH)_2$; $Mg(SO_4)$	Milk of Mag; Epsom Salt	2–4 g; 10–30 g	0.5–3
	Sodium phosphate	Fleet's Phospho-Soda	4–8 g	
Surfactant	Sulfosuccinate salts	Surfak; Colase	50–400 mg	12–72
Miscellaneous	Lactulose	Duphalac; Cephalac	10–15 ml	8–72

Tartrate salts are rarely used today, but phosphates are found in oral products and in renal enemas. Oral phosphate solutions also contain large amounts of sodium and should be used with caution in patients with hypertension. Fleet's Phospho-Soda and Fleet's enema are perhaps the most popular of the phosphate-containing products.

Summary

Constipation is a real phenomenon. Although often more imagined than real, constipation is widely treated by self-medication with over-the-counter laxative products. Laxatives represent one of the oldest classes of therapeutic agents. Table 68.2 summarizes the most common laxatives in terms of their usual dosage and time to response. Their mechanisms of action involve principally the accumulation of fluid in the intestinal lumen, making the contents more liquid and providing a more frequent passage of the stool. Motility undoubtedly also plays a role in the action of most laxatives. This may be due to a direct effect of some laxatives on the nerves or muscle of the gut, or through an indirect reflex mechanism in response to the accumulation of fluid and distention of the gut wall. Nevertheless, the universal notion that laxatives act by stimulating intestinal motility is not rational and should be viewed with caution.

As a class, laxatives are relatively nontoxic. However, patients with impaired renal function, infants, or the elderly are especially susceptible to untoward effects. In general, the side-effects associated with laxatives are intestinal cramping and excessive electrolyte loss, if the drugs are administered for prolonged periods or at an excessively high dosage. Individuals can become "dependent" on laxatives, especially the anthraquinones. The lack of muscular responsiveness requires continued use of the drugs in order to maintain normal bowel movements.

References

Research Reports

1. Thompson WG. The irritable gut. In: Functional disorders of the alimentary canal. Baltimore: University Park Press, 1979.
2. Cummings JH. Laxative abuse. Gut 1974;*15*:758–766.
3. Thompson WG. Laxatives: Clinical pharmacology and rational use. Drugs 1980;*19*:49–58.
4. Racusen LC, Binder HJ. Ricinoleic acid stimulation of active anion secretion in colonic mucosa of the rat. J Clin Invest 1979;*63*:743–749.
5. Gaginella TS, Stewart JJ, Olsen WA, Bass P. Actions of ricinoleic acid and structurally related fatty acids on the gastrointestinal tract. II. Effects on water and electrolyte absorption in vitro. J Pharmacol Exper Therap 1975;*195*:355–361.
6. Ammon HV, Thomas PJ, Phillips SF. Effects of oleic and ricinoleic acids on net jejunal water and electrolyte movement: Perfusion studies in man. J Clin Invest 1974;*53*:374–379.
7. Gaginella TS, Chadwick VS, Debongnie JC, Lewis JC, Phillips SF. Perfusion of rabbit colon with ricinoleic acid: Dose related mucosal injury, fluid secretion and increased permeability. Gastroenterology 1977;*73*:95–101.
8. Stewart JJ, Gaginella TS, Bass P. Actions of ricinoleic acid and structurally related fatty acids on the gastrointestinal tract. I. Effects on smooth muscle contractility in vitro. J Pharmacol Exper Therap 1975;*195*:347–354.
9. Stewart JJ, Bass P. Effects of ricinoleic and oleic acids on the digestive contractile activity of the canine small and large bowel. Gastroenterology 1976;*70*:371–376.
10. Gaginella TS, Phillips SF. Ricinoleic acid: Current view of an ancient oil. J Dig Dis 1975;*20*:1171–1177.
11. Binder RG, Applewhite TH, Kohler GO, Goldblatt LA. Chromatographic analysis of seed oils. Fatty acid composition of castor oil. J Am Oil Chem Soc 1962;*39*:513–517.
12. Van Os FHL. Some aspects of the pharmacology of anthraquinone drugs. Pharmacology 1976;*14* (Suppl.1): 18–29.
13. Stewart JJ, Gaginella TS, Olsen WA, Bass P. Inhibitory actions of laxatives on motility and water and electrolyte transport in the gastrointestinal tract. J Pharmacol Exper Therap 1975;*192*:458–467.
14. Gaginella TS, Stewart JJ, Gullikson GW, Olsen WA, Bass P. Inhibition of small intestinal mucosal and smooth muscle cell function by ricinoleic acid and other surfactants. Life Sci 1975;*167*:1595–1606.
15. Debongnie JC, Phillips SF. Capacity of the human colon to absorb fluid. Gastroenterology 1978;*74*:698–703.
16. Ammon HV, Phillips SF. Inhibition of ileal water absorption by intraluminal fatty acids. J Clin Invest 1974;*53*:205–210.
17. Ammon HV, Phillips SF. Inhibition of colonic water and electrolyte absorption by fatty acids in man. Gastroenterology 1973;*65*:744–749.
18. Bright-Asare P, Binder JH. Stimulation of colonic secretion of water and electrolytes by hydroxy fatty acids. Gastroenterology 1973;*64*:81–88.
19. Phillips RA, Love AHG, Mitchell TG, Neptune EM. Cathartics and the sodium pump. Nature 1965;*206*:1367–1368.
20. Cline WS, Lorenzsonn V, Benz L, Bass P, Olsen WA. The effects of sodium ricinoleate on small intestinal function and structure. J Clin Invest 1976;*58*:380–390.
21. Gaginella TS, Haddad AC, Go VLW, Phillips SF. Cytotoxicity of ricinoleic acid (castor oil) and other intestinal secretagogues on isolated intestinal epithelial cells. J Pharmacol Exper Therap 1977;*201*:259–266.
22. Gaginella TS, Bass P, Olsen W, Shug A. Fatty acid inhibition of water absorption and energy production in the hamster jejunum. FEBS Lett 1975;*53*:347–350.
23. Racusen LC, Binder JH. Ricinoleic acid stimulation of active anion secretion in colonic mucosa of the rat. J Clin Invest 1979;*63*:743–749.
24. Beubler E, Juan H. Effect of ricinoleic acid and other laxatives on net water flux and prostaglandin E release by the rat colon. J Pharm Pharmacol 1979;*31*:681–685.
25. Pinto A, Calignano A, Mascolo N, Autore G, Capasso F. Castor oil increases intestinal formation of platelet-activating factor and

acid phosphatase release in the rat. Br J Pharmacol 1989;*96*:872–874.

26. Mascolo N, Izzo AA, Capasso F. Castor oil-induced diarrhea: Involvement of nitric oxide. In: Capasso F, Mascolo N. Natural drugs and the digestive tract. Rome: EMSI, (1992), pp 123–128.

27. Maenz DD, Forsyth GW. Ricinoleate and deoxycholate are calcium ionophores in jejunal brush borders. J Memb Biol 1982;*70*:125–133.

28. Garcia-Villar R, Leng-Peschlow E, Rukebusch Y. Effects of anthraquinone derivatives on canine and rat intestinal motility. J Pharm Pharmacol 1980;*32*:323–329.

29. Hardcastle JD, Wilkins JL. The action of sennosides and related compounds on human colon and rectum. Gut 1970;*11*:1038–1042.

30. Lemmens L, Borja E. The influence of dihydroxyanthracene derivatives on water and electrolyte movement in rat colon. J Pharm Pharmacol 1976;*28*:498–501.

31. Smith B. Effect of irritant purgatives on the myenteric plexus in man and the mouse. Gut 1968;*9*:139–143.

32. Riemann JF, Schmidt H, Zimmerman W. The fine structure of colonic submucosal nerves in patients with chronic laxative abuse. Scan J Gastroent 1980;*15*:761–768.

33. Lemli J, Lemmens L. Metabolism of sennosides and rhein in the rat. Pharmacology 1980;*20* (Suppl.1):50–57.

34. Verhaeren E. Mitochondrial uncoupling activity as a possible base for a laxative and antipsoriatic effect. Pharmacology 1980;*20* (Suppl.1):43–49.

35. Collier HO-J, MacDonald-Gibson WJ, Saeed SA. Stimulation of prostaglandin biosynthesis by drugs: Effects in vitro of some drugs affecting gut function. Br J Pharmacol 1976;*58*:193–199.

36. Powell DW, Lawrence BA, Morris SM, Etheridge DR. Effect of phenolphthalein on in vitro rabbit ileal electrolyte transport. Gastroenterology 1980;*78*:454–463.

37. Chignell CF. The effect of phenolphthalein and other purgative drugs on rat intestinal ($Na^+ + K^+$) adenosine triphosphatase. Biochem Pharmacol 1968;*17*:1207–1212.

38. Beubler E, Juan H. PGE-mediated laxative effect of diphenolic laxatives. Naunyn Schmiedeberg's Arch Pharmacol 1978;*305*:241–246.

39. Saunders DR, Sillery J, Surawica C, Tytgat GN. Effect of phenolphthalein on the function and structure of rodent and human intestine. Dig Dis 1978;*23*:909–913.

40. Preston DM, Lennard-Jones JE. Pelvic motility and response to intraluminal bisacodyl in slow-transit constipation. Dig Dis Sci 1985;*30*:289–294.

41. Saunders DR, Sillery J, Rachmilewitz D, Rubin CE, Tytgat GN. Effect of bisacodyl on the structure and function of rodent and human intestine. Gastroenterology 1977;*72*:849–856.

42. Rachmilewitz D, Karmeli F, Okon E. Effects of bisacodyl on cAMP and prostaglandin E_2 contents, ($Na^+ + K^+$) ATPase, adenyl cyclase, and phospodiesterase activities of rat intestine. Dig Dis Sci 1980;*25*:602–608.

43. Saunders DR, Sillery J, Rachmilewitz D. Effect of dioctyl sodium sulfosuccinate on structure and function of rodent and human intestine. Gastroenterology 1975;*69*:380–386.

44. Eastwood MA, Kay RM. A hypothesis for the action of dietary fiber along the gastrointestinal tract. Am J Clin Nutr 1979;*32*:364–367.

45. Spiller GA, Shiplley EA, Chernoff MC, Cooper WC. Bulk laxative efficacy of a psyllium seed hydrocolloid and of a mixture of cellulose and pectin. J Clin Pharmacol 1979;*19*:313–320.

46. Stanley MM, Paul D, Gacke D, Murphy J. Effect of cholestyramine, metamucil and cellulose on fecal bile salt excretion in man. Gastroenterology 1973;*65*:889–894.

47. Bass P, Dennis S. The laxative effects of lactulose in normal and constipated subjects. J Clin Gastroenterol 1981;*3* (Suppl.1):23–29.

Reviews

r1. Gaginella TS, Bass P. Laxatives: An update on mechanism of action. Life Sci 1978;*23*:1001–1010.
An overview of the comparative mechanisms of action of commonly used laxatives. Brief, with emphasis on intestinal secretion as the primary action of laxation.

r2. Binder HJ. Pharmacology of laxatives. Ann Rev Pharmacol Toxicol 1977;*17*:355–367.
A discussion of the effects of substances that stimulate intestinal secretion. Major treatment of bile acids and fatty acids as laxatives. A different perspective than R1, with more emphasis on intracellular mediators.

r3. Gullikson GW, Bass P. Mechanisms of action of laxative drugs (Chapter 28) In: Csaky TZ. Handbook of experimental pharmacology, pharmacology of intestinal permeation 2d ed. Berlin: Springer-Verlag, (1984); pp 419–459.
Very complete review. Thorough discussion of motility and secretory effects of all classes of laxatives. Good section on bulk forming agents and on lactulose.

CHAPTER 69

Antidiarrheal Drugs: Pharmacologic Control of Intestinal Hypersecretion

David R. Brown

The major role of the intestines is to absorb ingested electrolytes, nutrients, and water: approximately 9 liters of fluid, isosmotic with plasma, are absorbed daily from the intestinal tract. Ions and water are also secreted continuously into the intestinal lumen, although in normal individuals absorption slightly exceeds secretion. The secretory process aids in lubricating the digestive tract for the efficient movement and solubilization of food material. Because the intestine is often exposed to ingested microorganisms, allergens, and noxious chemicals, it serves a protective function in defending the body from infection and poisoning. In addition to mobilizing a number of immunologic defense processes, the intestine may actively secrete large amounts of electrolytes and fluid that act in concert with increased contractions in gut smooth muscle to dilute and purge foreign substances from the lumen effectively. In many cases, this occurs at the level of the small intestine, and fluid and electrolyte losses can be partially recovered through colonic absorption. Diarrhea, if self-limiting, is a protective mechanism designed to prevent systemic infection or toxicity. If uncontrolled, however, diarrhea can be debilitating because it may lead to rapid dehydration and disturbances in electrolyte and acid-base homeostasis (i.e., metabolic acidosis).

Mechanisms of Intestinal Ion and Water Transport

Transport Processes in the Intestinal Epithelium Maintain Fluid and Electrolyte Balance

There is considerable evidence supporting the hypothesis that absorption and secretion occur in spatially separated epithelial cell types, notably the superficial villous cells and cells lining the intestinal crypts, respectively. A simple (but not all-inclusive) model depicting these different processes is illustrated in Figure 69.1. The passive diffusion of water between cells of the intestinal mucosa occurs in response to local osmotic gradients produced by net electrolyte movements.

Ion transport pathways in the luminal and contraluminal membranes of villous and crypt cells are organized in an asymmetric fashion. In the absorptive cells of the small intestine, Na^+ ions are transported from the lumen to the blood either alone or coupled with Cl^- ions or nutrients, such as glucose, amino acids, or small peptides. Sodium entering the cell is actively transported across the contraluminal membrane (and into the small intracellular space lying below the cell) by the action of Na^+, K^+-ATPase, a membrane-bound enzyme whose activity is inhibited by digitalis and other cardiotonic glycosides (Fig. 69.1, top).

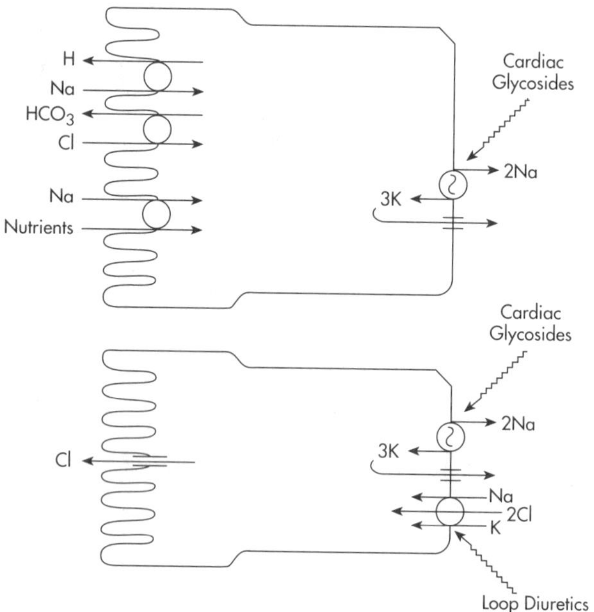

Figure 69.1 Schematic model depicting ion transport in an absorptive cell (top) and a secretory cell (bottom) of the small intestinal epithelium. Active transport in both cell types is mediated by Na^+, K^+-ATPase, a membrane-bound enzyme inhibited by cardiotonic glycosides. (Top) Sodium absorption occurs through secondary active transport coupled to nutrients (electrogenic process) or protons (electroneutral process). A portion of Cl^- absorption may be mediated by a Cl^-/HCO_3^- antiport pathway, but most Cl^- absorptive flux may be through paracellular routes. (Bottom) Chloride ions enter the secreting cell by secondary active transport of Na^+, Cl^-, and possibly K^+ ions; this process can be inhibited by loop diuretics. The exit of Cl^- down its electrochemical gradient and into the intestinal lumen is mediated through the opening of Cl^- channels in the luminal membrane. In some cases, HCO_3^- ions may pass through these channels as well. Potassium efflux through membrane K^+ channels hyperpolarizes the resting membrane potential of the cell, which is necessary to sustain active anion secretion.

In secreting cells, Cl^- ions enter the cytoplasm by means of a cotransport protein located in the contraluminal cell membrane; this secondary active transport process is electrically neutral and involves the inward movement of Cl^-, Na^+, and K^+. It is inhibited by loop diuretics, such as bumetanide and furosemide. This influx of Cl^- ions is energized by Na^+, K^+-ATPase, which functions, in this case, to recycle Na^+ across the contraluminal membrane. Chloride ions accumulate in the electronegative cell interior (≈ -40 mV relative to lumen); in response to an appropriate intracellular stimulus (see below), anion channels in the luminal membrane open, Cl^- leaves and enters the intestinal lumen. Potassium channels situated in the contraluminal membrane open simultaneously with Cl^- channels; K^+ exit through these channels maintains intracellular electronegativity, which provides an electrical driving force for continued Cl^- efflux (Fig. 69.1, bottom). In addition to Cl^- secretion, the cytoplasmic pH in enterocytes is maintained through transport processes involving H^+ and HCO_3^- ions; the colon actively secretes K^+ ions.[r1,r2]

Receptors Coupled to Intracellular Second Messengers Modulate Ion Transport in the Intestinal Mucosa

The activity of membrane-associated proteins mediating epithelial ion transport and smooth muscle contractility is regulated by intercellular second messengers, including cyclic nucleotides (AMP and cyclic GMP), elements of the phosphoinositide-diacylglycerol pathway, and free intracellular [Ca^{2+}]. A wide variety of neurotransmitters, gut hormones, and inflammatory mediators can alter second messenger levels by acting on G protein-coupled receptors in the contraluminal membrane of gut myocytes and enterocytes. Some of these receptors may be coupled directly to ion channels. Toxins produced by enteric bacteria also can act through receptors and other recognition molecules associated with the luminal membrane of these cells to affect intracellular levels of second messengers.[r2]

Pathophysiology of Diarrhea

Diarrhea occurs as a sign of an underlying disease condition and usually reflects a disruption in the bidirectional transport of Na^+ and Cl^- ions through intestinal epithelial cells. A decrease in net ion absorption or an increase in net secretion without a proportional change in the opposing flux can result in diarrhea if luminal ions cannot be absorbed in sufficient amounts by the intestinal mucosa distal to the site of transport impairment. Most secretory diarrheas result in a stool volume exceeding 1 liter/day in nonfasting patients.[r1] Alterations in gut motility or blood flow also may play some role in the pathogenesis of diarrhea, but their involvement is not well defined.

Diarrhea Can be Evoked by Intestinal Infections

The delicate balance between net transcellular absorption and secretion can be disturbed by microorganisms. Pathogenic bacteria entering the gut lumen can: (1) release enterotoxins that provoke anion secretion, such as *Escherichia coli* and *Vibrio cholerae;* (2) release cytotoxins that destroy enterocytes, such as *Clostridium difficile* or enterohemorrhagic *E. coli;* (3) penetrate the gut epithelium and stimulate inflammation, which leads to net secretion, such as *Shigella dysenteriae, E. coli, Campylobacter jejuni*, or *Salmonella;* or (4) adhere to the intestinal brush border, decreasing net absorption, such as *E. coli*. Overgrowth of resident microflora in the gut or fungal infestations in immunocompromised patients also impair absorption and produce diarrhea.[r3] Viruses may diminish net ion absorption by processes that selectively destroy the villus epithelium, but leave secretory cells intact.[r2]

Noninfectious Causes of Diarrhea

Diarrhea may also occur as a manifestation of noninfectious disease. First, the malabsorption of nutrients, as occurs in celiac disease, may lead to the accumulation of osmotically active particles or prosecretory substances (e.g., bile acids) in the intestinal lumen; water may diffuse into the lumen as a result of the standing osmotic gradient. Second, the immune system of the gut may be activated, as in cases of food allergy or chronic inflammation, resulting in the release of histamine, eicosanoids, and other prosecretory substances from mucosal mast cells and immunocytes. Third, diarrhea can occur secondary to disturbances in the endocrine system. Tumors involving endocrine-type cells may produce excessive amounts of circulating hormones that can subsequently act on the intestinal mucosa to promote secretion. Malignant carcinoid tumors, for example, may release serotonin, substance P or related peptides, and other gut secretagogues. Tumors involving the GI tract and pancreas, adrenal glands, lungs, or thyroid gland may secrete such diverse substances as vasoactive intestinal peptide (VIP), gastrin, prostanoids, and other substances known to stimulate intestinal secretion. Patients with diabetes mellitus may report bouts of watery diarrhea and nocturnal fecal incontinence, symptoms that have been attributed to a degeneration of adrenergic nerves regulating intestinal ion transport.[r2]

Therapeutic Considerations in the Management of Diarrhea

In managing the patient with diarrhea, one must define and treat the underlying cause of this disease sign. Thus, the judicious use of antibiotics or vaccines may relieve bacterial infections of the gut, surgical resections of tumors may arrest diarrheas due to carcinoids, VIPomas, and other hormone-producing tumors, and dietary alterations will prevent diarrheas associated with celiac disease and other malabsorptive states. Oral rehydration therapy (ORT) may have beneficial effects in rapidly replacing ongoing losses of electrolytes and water that occur in diarrheal states. Sodium absorption by the small intestinal mucosa is accelerated by the addition of glucose, complex carbohydrates, amino acids, or small peptides to oral electrolyte solutions; these mixtures bypass anion secretory processes by facilitating sodium absorption that is coupled to nutrient transport.[r4] Of course, the efficacy of ORT is dependent on the presence of a functional villous brush border, which may be destroyed or severely compromised in the course of some enteric infections. In severe cases of dehydration (≥ 10% of body weight), the IV administration of fluids and electrolytes is indicated in order to afford rapid replacement of excreted water and ions.

In the absence of contraindications, acute and chronic diarrheas may respond to intestinal antisecretory drugs. These drugs are generally used in treating specific types of diarrheas and, as a class, produce a wide variety of effects on intestinal function. Although a number of substances have been purported to alleviate diarrhea,[r1] we will consider those that have a defined mechanism of action and have been proven effective in diarrheal states.

Antidiarrheal Drugs

Potential Sites of Antidiarrheal Drug Action

An antidiarrheal drug effective in noninfectious diarrheas would inhibit secretion or promote absorption, and produce some decrease in intestinal motility to permit a longer contact time of luminal fluids with epithelial cells. On the other hand, it is desirable that a drug capable of inhibiting intestinal secretion produced by enteric microorganisms have little or no effect on gut motor function.[r5] Drugs that inhibit intestinal motility may compromise the luminal removal of diarrheagenic microorganisms. Furthermore, intestinal stasis may promote the pooling of fluids within the intestinal lumen, resulting in the underestimation of body fluid losses and possibly in bowel strangulation. In addition to this major consideration, it would be desirable that the "ideal" antidiarrheal agent act rapidly to attenuate fluid losses, be compatible with ORT, have no effects on CNS activity and limited actions on normal digestive system function, and possess a high therapeutic index.[r5,r6] Drugs designed to tip the balance of intestinal ion transport selectively in favor of net absorption could potentially act at a variety of intestinal and extraintestinal sites to inhibit diarrhea. These sites include: (1) nervous pathways underlying the intestinal mucosa that serve to regulate epithelial function; (2) the immune cells synthesizing and releasing inflammatory and allergic mediators; (3) the epithelial cell receptors for neurohumoral substances, immune mediators, and luminal enterotoxins; (4) elements of the intracellular signal transduction pathways linked to these receptors; and (5) the ion-transporting processes (i.e., cotransport proteins, ion channels) themselves. Although some drugs act at one or two of these sites, no antisecretory drug yet identified fulfills the criteria of an "ideal", broad-spectrum antidiarrheal agent. Indeed, some drugs produce serious side-effects that limit their therapeutic usefulness to particular diarrheal disease states.

Drugs Affecting the Synthesis of Inflammatory Mediators

Anti-inflammatory Agents Alleviate Diarrhea in Chronic Inflammatory States

Severe, chronic inflammation of the small and large bowel, as manifested in Crohn's disease or ulcerative colitis, often is associated with bloody diarrhea. Although the pathophysiologic mechanisms underlying inflammatory bowel disease have yet to be defined, the lipoxygenase products of arachidonic acid metabolism, especially leukotrienes, may be involved. Kinins, cytokines, and some enteric neuropeptides also may play a role in this multifaceted disorder. It is now becoming apparent that these and other classes of inflammatory mediators may affect the function of neurons, myocytes, epithelial cells, and immunocytes in the intestine.[r7] Pharmacotherapy of inflammatory bowel disease is palliative and generally directed toward limiting the production of inflammatory mediators. To this end, anti-inflammatory and immunosuppressive agents have formed the mainstay of drug treatment for many years.

Sulfasalazine, a sulfonamide that is poorly absorbed from the GI tract, has been used for several decades in the treatment of ulcerative colitis and other enteritides. The drug is cleaved to the 5-aminosalicylic acid (5-ASA or mesulamine), its biologically active form, by an azoreductase enzyme produced by intestinal microflora.

At high luminal concentrations, 5-ASA acts locally in the intestine to block the synthesis of prostanoids and leukotrienes from arachidonic acid by inhibiting the enzymes cyclooxygenase and 5-lipoxygenase, respectively. The ability of 5-ASA to inhibit lipoxygenase seems to account for its effectiveness in treating bowel inflammation and the associated diarrhea.[1] Both cyclooxygenase and lipoxygenase products have been shown to produce active anion secretion and are present at high concentrations in the inflamed bowel. Common NSAIDs such as aspirin or indomethacin, which inhibit the production of prostanoids via the cyclooxygenase pathway, have been used in treating diarrheas produced by enteropathogenic bacteria. However, they are ineffective in inflammatory bowel disease and may actually exacerbate the disorder.[r8] Selective blockers of leukotriene receptors or synthesis may constitute new approaches in the future therapy of inflammatory bowel disease.

In patients whose disease is severe or otherwise remains refractory to 5-ASA treatment, the administration of glucocorticoids may be indicated. By inducing the protein lipocortin, anti-inflammatory steroids act to inhibit phospholipase A_2. Phospholipase A_2 catalyzes the release of arachidonic acid from the phospholipid pool in cell membranes and thus constitutes the rate-limiting step of prostanoid and leukotriene biosynthesis; lipocortin inhibits the activity of this enzyme. In addition to this and other inflammatory and immunosuppressive actions, glucocorticoids may directly enhance Na^+ absorption across the epithelia of the small and large intestines.[2–4]

In inflammatory states involving the distal large bowel, poorly-absorbed steroids, sulfasalazine, or 5-ASA can be administered in the form of a topical enema to achieve effective luminal concentrations and reduce the possibility of systemic toxicity. After peroral administration, 5-ASA is rapidly absorbed in the upper small intestine. To prevent systemic drug absorption and increase 5-ASA concentrations in the lumen of the small intestine (for therapy of Crohn's disease) or proximal colon, two general approaches have been taken in formulating the drug. These include the application of enteric coatings that slowly release the drug into the intestinal lumen, or a chemical modification of the 5-ASA structure, which allows the free drug to be liberated after diazo bond reduction by colonic microflora.[r8] Depending on the preparation employed, these orally-administered 5-ASA derivatives can be useful in patients manifesting inflammation involving either the small intestine or colon.

Sulfasalazine (Azulfidine) is available in 500-mg tablets and an oral suspension containing 250 mg/5 ml. The usual dose is 3–4 g daily in divided doses.

Olsalazine (Dipentum) is available in 250-mg capsules. The usual dose is 1 g per day in divided doses.

Hydrocortisone (Cortenema and other brands) is most often employed as a cream or retention enema for distal forms of ulcerative colitis. It is available in single-dose bottles containing 100 mg hydrocortisone/60 mL or as a cream containing 2.5 percent hydrocortisone.

Bismuth Subsalicylate and Acute Diarrheas

Bismuth subsalicylate (BSS; the active ingredient in Pepto-Bismol) has been used since 1900 to treat diarrheas resulting from infections and acute inflammation of the bowel. The drug is administered orally and is hydrolyzed in the stomach to salicylate ions and bismuth oxychloride.[r9] BSS not only inhibits preexisting diarrheas, but prevents traveler's diarrhea caused by enterotoxigenic strains of *E. coli* during short periods of risk. The antidiarrheal action of BSS has been attributed to the bactericidal activity of bismuth oxychloride and perhaps other bismuth salts. In addition, salicylate ions have antisecretory and antiinflammatory actions that may arise from their ability to inhibit the biosynthesis of prostanoids, potent mediators of intestinal secretion.[r10] BSS is used for the short-term prevention and management of acute and relatively mild diarrheal states.

Bismuth subsalicylate (Pepto-Bismol) is available as tablets containing 262 mg of bismuth subsalicylate or liquid containing 262 mg of bismuth subsalicylate/5 ml. The usual dosage is 520 mg every hour for up to eight doses/24 hr. The maximum dosage provides the equivalent of 1632 mg of salicylate/24 hr.

Drugs Affecting the Neuroregulation of Intestinal Ion Transport

The Enteric Nervous System: A Prominent Site of Action for Intestinal Antisecretory Agents

Cells in the intestinal tract are contraluminally innervated by nearly 100 million nerves whose perikarya lie either within (intrinsic neurons) or outside (extrinsic neurons) the intestinal wall. A simple schematic diagram of intestinal neural circuitry appears in Figure 69.2. Extrinsic neurons constitute a minority of intestinal nerve cells and are believed to subserve a modulating influence on the activity of intrinsic nerves; indeed, the intestine is able to function independently of its extrinsic neural input. The extrinsic innervation of the intestine includes sympathetic nerves that originate in prevertebral ganglia lying in the thoracolumbar region of the spinal cord and co-contain norepinephrine and at least one neuropeptide (either somatostatin or neuropeptide Y). Moreover, vagal nerves projecting to and from the gut wall contain acetylcholine together with several neuropeptides. Sensory neurons whose cell bodies lie in the dorsal root ganglion of the spinal cord convey afferent information to and from the intestine and contain substance P and other peptides.

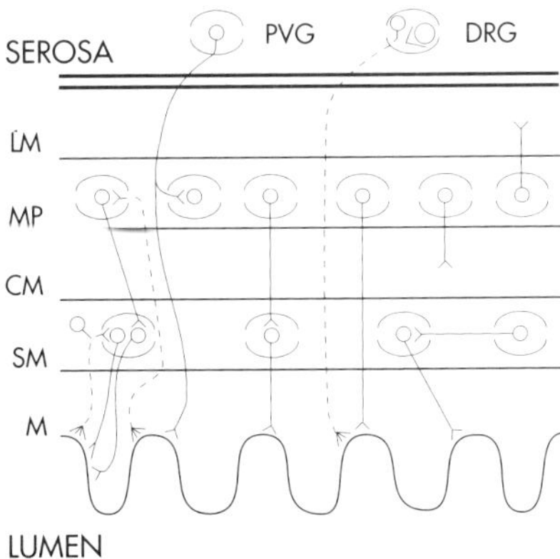

Figure 69.2 Some neuronal circuits modulating the transport function of the intestinal mucosa. Efferent or motor neurons are shown by solid lines; afferent or sensory neurons are depicted by stippled lines and are bipolar. Note reflex arcs formed between mucosa and the two major ganglionated plexuses at far left, as well as interactions of submucous and myenteric neurons with each other and with the mucosa. Abbreviations: PVG, prevertebral ganglion; DRG, dorsal root ganglion; LM, longitudinal muscle; MP, myenteric plexus; CM, circular muscle; SM, submucous plexus; M, mucosa.

The intrinsic nervous system of the gut is organized into two discrete but interconnected ganglionated plexuses that lie beneath the longitudinal and circular muscles, respectively, namely the myenteric (or Auerbach) and the submucous (or Meissner) plexuses. In humans and other large animals, a third ganglionated plexus (the external submucous or Schabadasch plexus) may be present between the Meissner plexus and circular muscle layer.[r11] Smooth muscle and epithelial cells form synapses with myenteric and submucous neurons primarily, but may also be innervated by extrinsic neurons. As with extrinsic neurons, the chemical characteristics of the intrinsic gut neurons are complex; often a classic neurotransmitter (e.g., acetylcholine or serotonin) is co-contained with one or more peptide transmitters. The conditions of neural activity under which these different substances are released and how they contribute to the overall absorptive and motor tone of the intestine remain largely unknown.

The role of gut neurons in the control of intestinal epithelial transport has been studied in isolated sheets of intestinal mucosa with attached submucosa obtained from a variety of animal species, including humans. The results of these experiments, conducted with tissues mounted in Ussing flux chambers, suggest that ongoing activity in submucosal neurons of the small intestine and colon tends to suppress electrolyte absorption. Furthermore, depolarization of neurons in the gut submucosa evoked by electrical field stimulation is frequently associated with anion secretion.[r12] Thus, it appears that the intrinsic nervous system of the gut functions to reduce maximal absorption. Several classes of drugs indicated below may exert their antidiarrheal effects in part through their ability to inhibit basal and stimulated activity in subpopulations of submucous neurons; in so doing, they enhance absorption and attenuate secretion of electrolytes and water.

Alpha$_2$-Adrenergic Agonists

Clonidine and lidamidine manifest antidiarrheal activity as a result of selective agonist interactions with G protein-coupled α_2-adrenoceptors within the gut wall. Presynaptic α_2-adrenergic receptors have been detected in association with vagal nerves terminating in the gut wall and appear to decrease neuronal acetylcholine release. Moreover, several lines of evidence suggest that α_2-adrenergic receptors are associated with myenteric and submucous neurons that mediate a decrease in intestinal transit and an increase in mucosal absorption produced by α_2-adrenergic agonists. Electrophysiologic experiments using single intracellular electrodes or whole-cell patch clamp have been performed to characterize these neuronal α_2-adrenergic receptors. Receptor activation is associated with an increased K^+ conductance and hyperpolarization of the resting membrane potential.[5,r13] In addition, a decrease in a voltage-activated Ca^{2+} conductance has been detected in submucous neurons.[6] These drug effects on ionic conductances lead to an inhibition of neuronal activity. Measurements of messenger RNAs encoding α_2-adrenergic receptors and receptor binding assays using selective α_2-adrenergic radioligands confirm that these receptors are associated with neuronal membranes.[7,8] At least in the porcine small intestine, these neuronal receptors appear to be of the α_{2A} subtype[8] and are associated with an increase in transepithelial Cl^- absorption in Cl^--secreting mucosal sheets.[9]

In some animal species, such as the rabbit, postsynaptic α_2-adrenoceptors may be present on ion-transporting epithelial cells where they decrease secretion and enhance absorption.[10]

In humans, lidamidine seems to possess a modest antisecretory action that is dependent on the nature of the initiating secretory stimulus. For example, the drug reduces secretion induced by prostaglandin E_2, but not by VIP or cholera toxin.[11–13] Although the antimotility actions of α_2-adrenergic agonists preclude their use in the treatment of secretory diarrheas induced by infectious agents, these drugs may be useful in arresting idiopathic diarrheas occurring in diabetes mellitus and other noninfectious disease states.[r14] At therapeutic doses, clonidine produces sedation and hypotension through its interaction with α_2-adrenoceptors in the CNS; these and other side-effects limit its general utility as an antidiarrheal agent. Lidamidine may cause less sedation and hypotension at oral doses effective in treating diarrhea.[r15]

Clonidine (Catapres) is used primarily as an antihypertensive drug, but has beneficial effects in some cases of diarrhea. It is available in tablets containing 0.1, 0.2, or 0.3 mg of clonidine hydrochloride for oral use. The usual dose is 0.1 mg twice daily. Side-effects include hypotension, sedation, dry mouth, and dizziness.

Lidamidine is not marketed in the U.S.

Somatostatin and a Synthetic Derivative

Octreotide (Sandostatin) is a synthetic analogue of the endogenous gut hormone and neurotransmitter somatostatin. This cyclic octapeptide has a greater biologic potency and longer half-life when compared to its natural counterpart. Moreover, it can be administered SQ, rather than by continuous IV infusion as is necessary for native somatostatin. Following its injection, octreotide reaches peak levels in plasma within 30 to 60 minutes and undergoes extensive metabolism in the liver.

Like the α_2-adrenergic agonists (and opiates, see below), somatostatin and octreotide decrease intestinal motility and promote ion and water absorption by the gut mucosa, probably by activating specific G protein-coupled receptors present on enteric neurons.[r16] In both myenteric and submucous neurons, somatostatin increases a K^+ conductance and hyperpolarizes the resting membrane potential.[5,r13] Furthermore, it decreases a voltage-activated Ca^{2+} conductance in submucous neurons.[6] Somatostatin may augment the release of the myorelaxant transmitter VIP from myenteric neurons, an effect mediated by interneurons containing endogenous opioids or γ-aminobutyric acid.[r17] It has no direct contractile or relaxant effect on isolated smooth muscle cells from human intestine.[r17]

Neural conduction blockade inhibits the antisecretory or proabsorptive actions of somatostatin and octreotide in isolated mucosal sheets from some animals, such as the pig,[14] peptide activity remains unaffected in intestinal preparations from other species, such as the rabbit.[15] Thus, the precise site (i.e., neuron or enterocyte) mediating the antisecretory actions of octreotide seems to vary according to the species examined; conclusive information bearing on this issue is not yet available for human intestine.

At present, octreotide is indicated for the treatment of diarrheas caused by the excessive release of gut hormones from endocrine tumors. These diarrheas, although rare, are generally resistant to conventional antidiarrheal drugs. Octreotide is effective, for example, in inhibiting the release of prosecretory hormones from serotonin-, kinin-, and substance P-producing carcinoid tumors and VIPomas.[r18] It has been recommended for the treatment of diarrheas associated with the acquired immunodeficiency syndrome, particularly if a treatable enteropathogen cannot be identified.[r2] Moreover, it may be useful for treatment of diarrheas associated with ileostomy, diabetes, irritable bowel disease, and the dumping syndrome.[r19]

Octreotide (Sandostatin) is administered by SQ injection and is available in sterile solution for injection.

Opioids

Extracts from the opium poppy have been used for centuries to treat dysentery. Endogenous opioid peptides, which are present in gut neurons, and their exogenous counterparts, such as the alkaloids morphine and codeine, have complex effects on intestinal motor and secretory function. Opiates capable of penetrating the blood-brain barrier may exert antidiarrheal effects at sites within the intestine and the CNS.[16] Like intestinal α_2-adrenoceptors and somatostatin receptors, μ-opiate receptors present on the postsynaptic membranes of myenteric and submucous neurons are coupled to a G protein that appears to be linked to an increase in a neuronal K^+ conductance; this results in membrane hyperpolarization.[5,r13] The K^+ channels involved in these effects appear to be the same as those mediating the neuronal inhibitory actions of somatostatin and α_2-adrenergic agonists. Radioligand binding and electrophysiologic studies indicate that there are δ-opiate receptors in the submucous plexus and that they mediate an increase in neuronal K^+ conductance.[7,17] In addition, the opioids appear to act at κ-opiate receptors to decrease a voltage-activated Ca^{2+} conductance in both myenteric and submucous neurons.[6,18]

Opiate agonists act at μ-opiate receptors on myenteric plexus to decrease acetylcholine release and accordingly reduce propulsive movements of the longitudinal smooth muscle; these opioid receptors have been shown to coexist with α_2-adrenoceptors on myenteric neurons, but not submucous neurons.[19] Moreover, opiates reduce the release of VIP from myenteric neurons innervating the circular smooth muscle; these actions appear to be mediated by δ-opiate receptors.

Finally, μ-, δ-, and κ-opiate receptors residing on myocytes mediate circular muscle contraction.[r17] The latter two effects underlie the ability of the opiates to increase intestinal segmentation. Enhanced segmentation with a decrease in peristalsis results in a slowing of intestinal transit. It has been proposed that the ability of opiates to reduce stool volume may stem principally from this effect on transit, which lengthens the contact time of luminal fluid with absorptive epithelial cells.[20–22]

In addition to their effects on motor function, δ- (and possibly μ-) opiate receptors on submucosal neurons mediate an increase in salt and water absorption by the mucosa.[23–25] Opiates have been shown to inhibit ongoing secretion induced by a variety of intestinal secretagogues.[r20] The synthetic, peripherally-acting opiates diphenoxylate (Lomotil) and loperamide (Imodium) may possess an additional action to inhibit Ca^{2+}-dependent signal transduction systems in enterocytes that promote secretion.[26,r21] The use of diphenoxylate in children is limited by the drug's ability to penetrate the immature blood-brain barrier, resulting in CNS depression and other adverse reactions. Diphenoxylate is biotransformed to an active metabolite, difenoxin (an ingredient in Motofen), which extends its duration of action.

Because they inhibit intestinal propulsion, opiates are contraindicated in the therapy of profuse diarrheas of infectious etiology. In addition, they should not be used for treatment of diarrheas caused by bowel inflammation, because they may aggravate colonic ulceration. Loperamide and diphenoxylate are administered orally for the treatment of diarrhea in the absence of fever or bloody stools.[r22] Moreover, loperamide is used in the management of intractable diarrheas associated with the irritable bowel syndrome.[r23]

Diphenoxylate is available in Lomotil liquid and tablets in combination with a subtherapeutic amount of atropine. Each tablet and each 5 ml of liquid contains 2.5 mg of diphenoxylate and 0.025 mg of atropine. The usual dose of diphenoxylate is 5 mg administered four times daily.

Loperamide (Imodium) is available in 2-mg capsules to be taken orally in divided doses not to exceed 16 mg/day.

Conclusions

Diarrhea is a sign common to a diverse number of disease entities and represents a normal protective mechanism. Mild to moderate forms of diarrhea (one to five unformed stools/day), in the absence of other important symptoms, are most common and can at the very least be bothersome and disconcerting to patients. In these cases, the patient may require oral fluid and electrolyte therapy, and antidiarrheal drugs may be administered if it can be established that enteroinvasive microorganisms are not involved. Although acute diarrheas of this magnitude may resolve spontaneously, chronic diarrheas resulting from systemic disease may demand additional therapeutic interventions. In cases of severe diarrhea (≥ 6 unformed stools/day), that are accompanied by symptoms or test results indicative of enteric infection, rehydration and antimicrobial therapy are preferred. Because they correct imbalances in electrolyte secretion and absorption that underlie many forms of diarrhea, antisecretory drugs modulating the inflammatory process or neuronal activity in the intestine continue to occupy an important place in palliative antidiarrheal therapy.

References

Research Reports

1. Peskar BM, Dreyling KW, Peskar BA, May B, Goebell H. Enhanced formation of sulfidopeptide leukotrienes in ulcerative colitis and Crohn's disease: Inhibition by sulfasalazine and 5-aminosalicylic acid. Agents Actions 1986;*18*:381–383.
2. Sellin JH, Field M. Physiologic and pharmacologic effects of glucocorticoids on ion transport across rabbit ileal mucosa in vitro. J Clin Invest 1981;*67*:770–778.
3. Foster ES, Zimmerman TW, Hayslett JP, Binder HJ. Corticosteroid alteration of active electrolyte transport in rat distal colon. Am J Physiol 1983;*245*:G668–G675.
4. Sellin JH, DeSoignie RC. Steroids alter ion transport and absorptive capacity in proximal and distal colon. Am J Physiol, 1985;*249*:G113–G119.
5. Tatsumi H, Costa M, Schimerlik M, North RA. Potassium conductance increased by noradrenaline, opioids, somatostatin, and G-proteins: whole-cell recording from guinea pig submucous neurons. J Neurosci 1990;*10*:1675–1682.

6. Surprenant A, Shen K-Z, North RA, Tatsumi H. Inhibition of calcium currents by noradrenaline, somatostatin and opioids in guinea-pig submucous neurones. J Physiol (London) 1990;*431*:585–608.

7. Ahmad S, Allescher HD, Manaka H, Manaka Y, Daniel EE. Biochemical studies on opioid and α_2-adrenergic receptors in canine submucosal neurons. Am J Physiol 1989;*256*:G957–G965.

8. Hildebrand KR, Lin G, Murtaugh MP, Brown DR. Molecular characteristics of α_2-adrenergic receptors regulating intestinal electrolyte transport. Mol Pharmacol 1993;*43*:23–29.

9. Hildebrand KR, Brown DR. Norepinephrine and alpha$_2$-adrenoceptors modulate active ion transport in porcine small intestine. J Pharmacol Exp Therap 1992;*263*:510–519.

10. Chang EB, Field M, Miller RJ. Enterocyte α_2-adrenergic receptors: yohimbine and *p*-aminoclonidine binding relative to ion transport. Am J Physiol 1983;*244*:G76–G82.

11. Edwards CA, Read NW. Effect of lidamidine, a proposed alpha$_2$-adrenoceptor agonist, on salt and water transport in human jejunum. Dig Dis Sci 1986;*31*:817–821.

12. Edwards CA, Cann PA, Read NW, Holdsworth CD. Effect of two new antisecretory drugs on fluid and electrolyte transport in a patient with secretory diarrhoea. Gut 1986;*27*:581–586.

13. Rabbani GH, Butler T, Patte D, Abud RL. Clinical trial of clonidine hydrochloride as an antisecretory agent in cholera. Gastroenterology 1989;*97*:321–325.

14. Brown DR, Overend MF, Treder BG. Neurohormonal regulation of ion transport in the porcine distal jejunum. Actions of somatostatin-14 and its natural and synthetic homologs. J Pharmacol Exp Therap 1990;*252*:126–134.

15. Dharmsathaphorn K, Binder HJ, Dobbins JW. Somatostatin stimulates sodium and chloride absorption in the rabbit ileum. Gastroenterology 1980;*78*:1559–1565.

16. Shook JE, Lemcke PK, Gehrig CA, Hruby VJ, Burks TF. Antidiarrheal properties of supraspinal mu and delta and peripheral mu, delta, and kappa opioid receptors: inhibition of diarrhea without constipation. J Pharmacol Exp Therap 1989;*249*:83–90.

17. Mihara S, North RA. Opioids increase potassium conductance in submucous neurones of guinea-pig caecum by activating δ-receptors. Br J Pharmacol 1986;*88*:315–322.

18. Cherubini E, North RA. Mu and kappa opioids inhibit transmitter release by different mechanisms. Proc Natl Acad Sci (USA), 1985;*82*:1860–1863.

19. Surprenant A, North RA: μ Opioid receptors and α_2 adrenoceptors coexist on myenteric but not submucous neurones. Neuroscience 1985;*16*:425–430.

20. Schiller LR, Davis GR, Santa Ana CA, Morawski SG, Fordtran JS. Studies of the mechanism of the antidiarrheal effect of codeine. J Clin Invest 1982;*70*:999–1008.

21. Schiller LR, Santa Ana CA, Morawski SG, Fordtran JS. Mechanism of the antidiarrheal effect of loperamide. Gastroenterology 1984;*86*:1475–1480.

22. Kachel G, Ruppin H, Hagel J, Barina W, Meinhardt M, Domschke W. Human intestinal motor activity and transport: Effects of a synthetic opiate. Gastroenterology 1986;*90*:85–93.

23. Kachur JF, Miller RJ, Field M. Control of guinea pig electrolyte secretion by a δ-opiate receptor. Proc Natl Acad Sci (USA), 1980;*77*:2753–2756.

24. Binder HJ, Laurenson JP, Dobbins JW. Role of opiate receptors in regulation of enkephalin stimulation of active sodium and chloride absorption. Am J Physiol 1984;*247*:G432–G436.

25. Quito FL, Brown DR. Neurohormonal regulation of ion transport in the porcine distal jejunum. Enhancement of sodium and chloride absorption by submucosal opiate receptors. J Pharmacol Exp Therap 1991;*256*:833–840.

26. Stoll R, Ruppin H, Domschke W. Calmodulin-mediated effects of loperamide on chloride transport by brush border membrane vesicles from human ileum. Gastroenterology 1988;*95*:69–76.

Reviews

r1. Krejs G. Secretory diarrhea. Triangle, 1988;*27*:143–148.

r2. Field M, Rao MC, Chang EB. Intestinal electrolyte transport and diarrheal disease. Parts I and II. N Engl J Med 1989;*321*:800–806, 879–883.

r3. Simon D, Weiss LM, Brandt LJ. Treatment options for AIDS-related esophageal and diarrheal disorders. Am J Gastroenterol 1992;*87*:274–281.

r4. Sack DA. Use of oral rehydration therapy in acute watery diarrhoea. A practical guide. Drugs 1991;*41*:566–573.

r5. Edelman R. Prevention and treatment of infectious diarrhea. Speculations on the next 10 years. Am J Med 1985;78 (Suppl. 6B):99–106.

r6. Ludan AC. Current management of acute diarrhoeas. Use and abuse of drug therapy. Drugs 1988;36 (Suppl. 4):18–25.

r7. Powell DW. Immunophysiology of intestinal electrolyte transport. In: Handbook of Physiology. Section 6: The Gastrointestinal System. Vol. 4: Intestinal Absorption and Secretion, chapter 25, Bethesda: American Physiological Soc. (1991); pp 591–641.

r8. Ruderman WB: Newer pharmacologic agents for the therapy of inflammatory bowel disease. Med Clin North Amer 1990;*74*:133–153.

r9. Bierer DW. Bismuth subsalicylate: history, chemistry, and safety. Rev Infect Dis 1990;12 (Suppl. 1):S3–S8.

r10. DuPont HL. Bismuth subsalicylate in the treatment and prevention of diarrheal disease. Drug Intell Clin Pharm 1987;*21*:687.

r11. Timmermans J-P, Scheuermann DW, Stach W, Adriaensen D, de Groot-Lasseel MHA. Functional morphology of the enteric nervous system with special reference to large mammals. Eur J Morphol 1992;*30*:113–122.

r12. Brown DR, Miller RJ. Neurohormonal control of fluid and electrolyte transport in intestinal mucosa. In: Handbook of Physiology. Section 6: The Gastrointestinal System. Vol. 4: Intestinal Absorption and Secretion, Bethesda: American Physiological Soc. (1991); pp 527–589.

r13. North RA. Drug receptors and the inhibition of nerve cells. Br J Pharmacol 1989;*98*:13–28.

r14. Fedorak RN, Field M. Antidiarrheal therapy. Prospects for new agents. Dig Dis Sci 1987;*32*:195–205.

r15. DiJoseph JF, Mir GN. Lidamidine's effects on the lower gastrointestinal tract: A review. Drug Develop Res 1986;*7*:101–109.

r16. Gyr K, Meier R. Pharmacodynamic effects of Sandostatin in the gastrointestinal tract. Metabolism 1992;41 (Suppl. 2):17–21.

r17. Grider JR. Peptidergic regulation of smooth muscle contractility. In: Brown DR. Gastrointestinal Regulatory Peptides [Handbook of Experimental Pharmacology, vol. 106], Heidelberg: Springer-Verlag, 1993.

r18. Battershill PE, Clissold SP. Octreotide. A review of its pharmacodynamic and pharmacokinetic properties, and therapeutic potential in conditions associated with excessive peptide secretion. Drugs 1989;*38*:658–702.

r19. Burroughs AK, McCormick PA. Somatostatin and octreotide in gastroenterology. Aliment Pharmacol Therap 1991;*5*:331–341.

r20. Awouters F, Neimegeers CJE, Janssen PAJ. Pharmacology of antidiarrheal drugs. Ann Rev Pharmacol Toxicol 1983;*23*:279–301.

r21. Ruppin H. Loperamide: A potent antidiarrhoeal drug with actions along the alimentary tract. Aliment Pharmacol Ther 1987;*1*:179–190.

r22. Okhuysen PC, Ericsson CD. Travelers' diarrhea. Prevention and treatment. Med Clin North Amer 1992;*76*:1357–1373.

r23. Pattee PL, Thompson WG. Drug treatment of the irritable bowel syndrome. Drugs 1992;*44*:200–206.

CHAPTER 70

Drugs Affecting Gastrointestinal Motility and Antiemetic Agents

Thomas F. Burks

Gastrointestinal motility is regulated by mechanisms intrinsic and extrinsic to the GI tract. The most critical regulation of contractile activity is provided by the enteric nervous system, but over-all patterns of activity are coordinated by the CNS, which is linked to the enteric nervous system by efferent and afferent pathways over the sympathetic and parasympathetic divisions of the autonomic nervous system. In addition, the endocrine system, especially the endocrine cells of the GI tract itself, provides important regulatory influences. Each regulatory component is subject to modification by drugs. It is becoming increasingly possible to bring about very specific changes in contractile activity by means of pharmacologic agents. Many of these drugs offer significant promise of benefit in the management of disorders of GI motility.

Normal Factors in Gastrointestinal Motility

Intrinsic Regulation of Motility

The enteric nervous system provides a rich innervation of GI smooth muscle and mucosa. Intrinsic nerves are grouped into two major nerve plexuses, the myenteric (Auerbach's) plexus, and the submucosal (Meissner's) plexus, plus other, more diffuse plexuses. The myenteric and submucosal plexuses receive extrinsic innervation over sympathetic and parasympathetic autonomic pathways from the CNS. Afferent fibers that terminate in all regions of the wall of the gut travel over autonomic pathways to the CNS. Both the myenteric plexus and the submucosal plexus provide innervation to smooth muscle and regulate contractile activity. In addition, the submucosal plexus provides innervation to the mucosa to regulate transport of fluid and electrolytes across the intestinal epithelium. The enteric nervous system represents the third major division of the autonomic nervous system; in total, it comprises a number of neurons equalling that of the spinal cord. Each plexus consists of nerve cell bodies with processes that make synaptic connections with other neurons or that innervate smooth muscle, mucosa, or sensory receptors. Some sensory neurons are totally intrinsic to the enteric nervous system and serve as the afferent limbs of intrinsic reflexes. Enteric neurons may project in the oral or aboral directions to provide ascending and descending excitation and inhibition or may travel in the transverse plane of the gut wall. All the neurotransmitter substances identified in the CNS appear to function as neurotransmitters in the enteric nervous system, giving rise to a complex neural network that is semiautonomous in its regulation of GI functions.

Extrinsic Innervation

The major extrinsic innervation of the GI tract is provided by the sympathetic and parasympathetic divisions of the autonomic nervous system. The parasympathetic innervation occurs over the VII, IX, and X cranial nerves and over the pelvic nerve from the sacral spinal cord. The esophagus, stomach, small intestine, and proximal colon are innervated by the vagus (X) nerve. The distal colon and rectum are innervated by the pelvic nerve. The sympathetic innervation occurs from postganglionic sympathetic fibers that originate in the paravertebral and prevertebral sympathetic ganglia. It is important to note that extrinsic nerves rarely provide direct innervation of GI smooth muscle or mucosa. Instead, extrinsic autonomic fibers terminate at neurons of the enteric nervous system to modulate neural activity within intrinsic circuits. It is the processes of the enteric nerves that provide direct motor control over smooth muscle and mucosa.

The CNS plays a critical role in regulation of GI motility. Central processing of sensory information results in selection of coordinated patterns of GI motility. Drugs may act in the CNS to alter motility patterns, and many GI effects result from actions in the CNS. Sites in the brain and in the spinal cord, involving both ascending and descending pathways, may be involved.

The mucosa of the GI tract represents the largest endocrine organ in the body. A number of hormones, notably cholecystokinin, gastrin, secretin, motilin, and gastric inhibitory peptide, play important roles in regulation of specific motility functions. For example, cholecystokinin is the major regulator of gall bladder emptying after ingestion of fat. Gastric inhibitory peptide plays a role in regulation of the rate of gastric emptying. Motilin is thought to play a role in initiation of the fasting pattern of GI motility.

Patterns of Motility

Specific patterns of contractile activity of GI smooth muscle are precisely coordinated by the enteric and CNS. For example, the propulsion of a bolus of swallowed food through the smooth muscle part of the esophagus is controlled by carefully programmed activity of vagal and enteric neurons. As the bolus approaches the distal esophagus, neurally-mediated relaxation of the tonically contracted lower esophageal sphincter occurs in carefully timed sequence with the arrival of the bolus to allow the bolus to pass into the stomach. Immediately after passage of the bolus through the lower esophageal sphincter, the sphincter contracts to prevent reflux of gastric contents into the esophagus. Failure of the lower esophageal sphincter to relax in the act of swallowing leads to pathologic abnormalities of swallowing. Failure of the lower esophageal sphincter to contract properly after swallowing can lead to gastroesophageal reflux. In the stomach and small intestine, patterns of motility depend on feeding status, as distinct patterns occur during fasting and after feeding.

The fasting pattern of motility in the upper GI tract consists of bands of contractions that may begin in the stomach or proximal small intestine and slowly migrate down the small intestine to the ileocecal junction, where they terminate. These bands of intense contractile activity are known as the migrating motor complex (MMC) that occurs with a periodicity of approximately 150 minutes.[r1] That is, a new MMC wave is initiated in the stomach or duodenum, moves slowly down the small intestine, and reaches the terminal ileum two to three hours later. As the MMC activity reaches the terminal ileum, another MMC band of contractions begins in the upper GI tract and starts its progression down the small intestine. The cycles repeat constantly until feeding occurs. The presumed purpose of the MMC is to sweep debris out of the stomach and small intestine in preparation for a future meal. The intense contractions of the stomach in association with MMC activity, often noticed as hunger pangs, can cause emptying of large particles that are not emptied during the fed pattern of motility. The hormone motilin is thought to play a role in initiation of the fasting motility pattern and development of MMC activity.[1]

Immediately upon ingestion of a meal, the pattern of GI motility changes from the fasting pattern to the fed pattern. The fed pattern in the intestine is characterized by frequent, random segmenting or mixing contractions of circular muscle. These contractions occur at a maximum frequency dictated by the frequency of electrical slow waves (basic electrical rhythm) of the smooth muscle. Myoelectric slow waves occur with higher frequency in the upper small intestine than in the lower small intestine, thus providing an aboral gradient of contractile frequency. Coincident with or after the appearance of mixing contractions in the small intestine, coordinated propulsive contractions begin in the stomach after food ingestion. These contractions mix the gastric contents with acid and pepsin to initiate digestion. As large amplitude pressure waves pass over the stomach antrum toward the pylorus, there is coordinated relaxation of the duodenum to facilitate passage of gastric contents into the duodenal bulb. Effective gastric emptying depends on development of high amplitude pressure waves in the stomach and coordinated relaxation of the duodenum. Once gastric contents begin to enter the duodenum, segmenting contractions of the circular muscle coat mix the contents with digestive enzymes contained in pancreatic secretions and intestinal fluids. The intestinal contents are brought into contact with the intestinal mucosa for absorption. Intestinal contents move slowly through the small bowel, propelled primarily by the frequency gradient of mixing contractions.

The presence of content in the terminal ileum causes distention of the ileum and relaxation of the ileocecal junction, permitting ileal content to flow into the proximal colon. In the colon, mixing contractions, observed as haustrations, mix the colonic content as water is extracted. Contents are moved through the colon primarily by mass movements consisting of coordinated propulsive contractions of the colon.[r2] The presence of material in the rectum increases rectal pressure and signals the urge to defecate. Defecation requires simultaneous relaxation of the smooth muscle internal anal sphincter and the skeletal muscle external anal sphincter.

If the ingested meal contains fat, the hormone cholecystokinin is released from the intestinal mucosa into the circulation. It circulates to the gall bladder to produce contractions, thus emptying the gall bladder's content of bile into the duodenum. Intraluminal bile acids facilitate the absorption of fats.

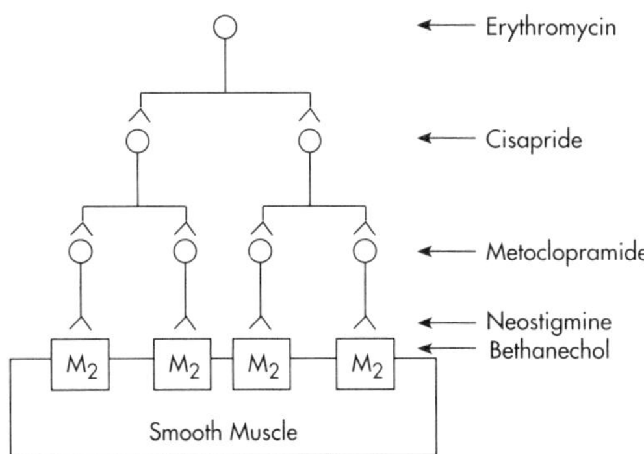

Figure 70.1 Postulated sites of action of prokinetic drugs in the neuronal hierarchy of enteric motor neurons. Erythromycin, cisapride, and metoclopramide appear to act at secondary or tertiary level motor neurons to produce coordinated patterns of propulsive activity. Neostigmine increases transmission only at the nerve-muscle junction. Bethanechol acts directly on smooth muscle muscarinic receptors.

Prokinetic Drugs

Prokinetic drugs are those that increase propulsive activity in the GI tract, including the esophagus, stomach, small intestine, and colon. A variety of agents is presently available to increase propulsion and overcome pathologic hypomotility of the GI tract. These agents are of value in management of gastroesophageal reflux disease, diabetic gastroparesis and gastric stasis, intestinal atony, pseudo-obstruction, and adynamic colon.[r3] Several of the agents also show promise in management of irritable bowel syndrome.

All the agents presently available share an ultimate mechanism of action: they act through the smooth muscle M_2 muscarinic cholinergic receptors, either directly or indirectly (Fig. 70.1).

Cholinergic Agents

Direct muscarinic cholinergic receptor agonists were among the first useful prokinetic drugs. Muscarinic agonists, such as bethanechol, act directly at the smooth muscle M_2 receptor to induce contractions. Muscarinic agonists can increase the incidence and amplitudes of contractions in the stomach, small intestine, and colon. They thus increase muscle tone, strength of propulsive contractions, and can enhance the rate of gastric emptying.[2] Unfortunately, muscarinic agonists do not improve antroduodenal coordination and are not as effective as some other drugs in promoting gastric emptying. Moreover, muscarinic agonists produce a variety of undesired side-effects, such as increasing the volume of salivary and gastric secretion, inducing diarrhea, and causing sensations of abdominal cramping. The indirectly-acting prokinetic drugs offer advantages over the directly-acting agonists.

Reversible inhibitors of acetylcholinesterase, such as neostigmine, were used to increase contractile activity and propulsion in the GI tract. These drugs were especially popular for management of postoperative intestinal and colonic atony. By reducing hydrolysis of neurally-secreted acetylcholine, neostigmine and related drugs enhance the excitatory effects of cholinergic motor neurons on GI smooth muscle. However, like the directly acting muscarinic agonists, inhibitors of acetylcholinesterase can induce a number of undesired effects, such as increased secretory activity in the GI tract.

Metoclopramide

Several peripherally- and centrally-acting dopamine receptor antagonists produce GI prokinetic effects. The prototype of this group of drugs is metoclopramide (Fig. 70.2). Metoclopramide is a benzamide drug with significant dopamine receptor antagonist actions. It is also a weak antagonist at $5\text{-}HT_3$ receptors and has modest ganglionic stimulating properties (Table 70.1). Metoclopramide blocks presynaptic dopamine receptors that inhibit release of acetylcholine from cholinergic motor neurons of the enteric nervous system. Metoclopramide thereby promotes release of neural acetylcholine that interacts with smooth muscle cell M_2 muscarinic receptors to induce contractions (Fig. 70.1). Because it merely facilitates normal cholinergic neurotransmission in cholinergic neurons firing in a programmed sequence, metoclopramide enhances

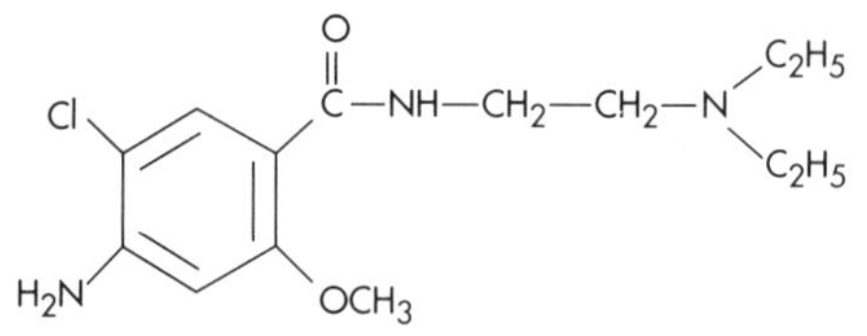

Metoclopramide

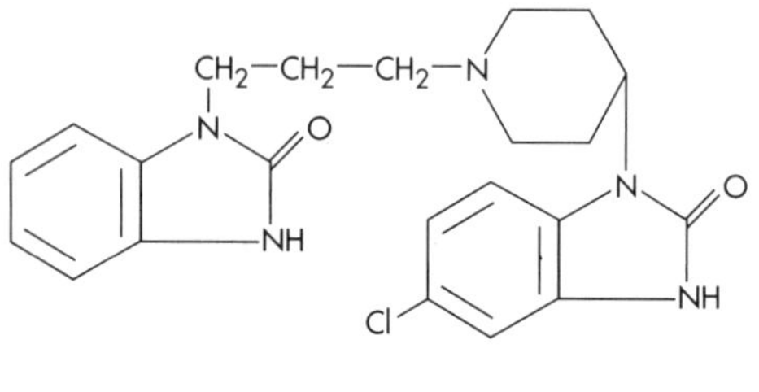

Domperidone

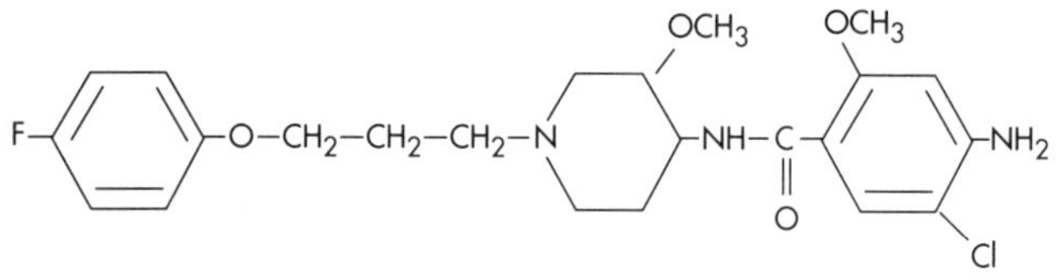

Cisapride

Figure 70.2 Structures of Prokinetic Drugs

normal propulsive activity in a coordinated manner. It thus increases muscle tone, strength of propulsive contractions, and gastric emptying. It also enhances antroduodenal coordination, the relaxation of the proximal duodenum in close time sequence to arrival of antral contractions at the pylorus. Metoclopramide stimulates motility of the upper GI tract without stimulating gastric, biliary, or pancreatic secretions. It increases the resting tone of the lower esophageal sphincter. It has little effect on the motility of the colon or gall bladder.

Metoclopramide crosses the blood-brain barrier and exhibits CNS effects characteristic of dopamine receptor blockade.[3] Because it acts by increasing release of acetylcholine from enteric cholinergic motor neurons, the prokinetic effects of metoclopramide are blocked by atropine and other muscarinic antagonists.

A drug related chemically (Fig. 70.2) and pharmacologically to metoclopramide, domperidone, is a dopamine receptor antagonist that does not cross the blood-brain barrier.[4] Domperidone has modest prokinetic properties, but does not produce adverse CNS effects.[5] Domperidone can increase tone of the lower esophageal sphincter, increase the incidence and amplitude of gastric contractions, increase gastric emptying, and increase transit in the small intestine. Like metoclopramide, domperidone does not produce significant changes in colonic or gall bladder motility, nor does it alter secretions of the upper GI tract. Domperidone is not marketed in the US.

Pharmacokinetics

Orally administered metoclopramide is rapidly absorbed with peak plasma concentrations occurring one to two hours after the oral dose. The average plasma half-life is five to six hours. Metoclopramide is excreted in the urine, partly as free drug and partly as conjugates or other products of hepatic metabolism. The drug is not extensively bound to plasma proteins.

Therapeutic Uses

Clinical studies have shown the utility of metoclopramide in diabetic gastroparesis. Metoclopramide decreases vomiting, persistent feelings of fullness, anorexia, and dyspepsia associated with gastroparesis. Laboratory studies indicate that metoclopramide increases the rate of emptying of both solids and liquids from the stomach.[r4]

Metoclopramide is also useful in management of gastroesophageal reflux disease. The beneficial effects probably include improved clearance of refluxed gastric contents from the esophagus, improved tone of the lower esophageal sphincter, and more rapid emptying of gastric contents after meals. Healing of esophageal erosions has been demonstrated endoscopically after several weeks of treatment with metoclopramide.

The use of metoclopramide as an antiemetic drug is discussed below.

Adverse Effects

Many of the adverse responses to metoclopramide result from blockade of dopamine receptors in the CNS.[3] Approximately 10 per cent of patients receiving metoclopramide display CNS effects, including restlessness, drowsiness, and fatigue. Extrapyramidal reactions, including acute dystonic reactions, occur in fewer than 1 per cent of patients. Dystonic reactions can include involuntary movements, Parkinsonism-like symptoms, tardive dyskinesia, and motor restlessness. Metoclopramide also increases release of prolactin from the pituitary. Adverse events relating to hyperprolactinemia include galactorrhea, amenorrhea, and gynecomastia.

Prokinetic drugs should be avoided in patients with GI hemorrhage, perforation, or mechanical obstruction.

Preparations and Dosage

Metoclopramide (Reglan) is available in tablets and syrup form for oral administration and as a sterile solution for injection. The usual doses are 10–15 mg three to four times daily orally for gastroesophageal reflux disease, or 10 mg orally, 30 minutes before each meal and at bedtime, for diabetic gastroparesis.

Table 70.1 Profiles of Prototype Prokinetic Drugs

Activity	Metoclopramide	Cisapride	Erythromycin
Cellular mechanism			
Dopamine antagonist	+++	0	0
5-HT_3 antagonist	++	+	0
5-HT_4 agonist	0	+++	0
Motilin agonist	0	0	+++
Inhibited by muscarinic antagonists	+++	+++	+
Prokinetic effect			
Proximal bowel	+++	+++	+++
Distal bowel	±	++	+++

+++ = pronounced activity, ++ = activity, + = weak activity, ± = possible activity, 0 = no activity.

Cisapride

Cisapride is the prototype of several substituted benzamide drugs (Fig. 70.2) that produce GI prokinetic effects without blockade of dopamine receptors.[r5] Cisapride is a weak antagonist at 5-HT_3 receptors and is unique among the benzamide compounds that have been adequately studied in that it is a full agonist at the recently recognized 5-HT_4 receptors.[6,7] Its activity as a prokinetic drug appears to result primarily from agonist actions at 5-HT_4 receptors in the enteric nervous system.[8] Agonist actions at 5-HT_4 receptors may be of primary importance in prokinetic effects, whereas antagonist actions at 5-HT_3 receptors may be of primary importance for antiemetic effects.[9] Cisapride increases esophageal clearance, increases tone of the lower esophageal sphincter, increases gastric emptying, and increases propulsion in the small intestine and colon. Like metoclopramide, cisapride enhances antroduodenal coordination to enhance gastric emptying.[10] It is more effective than metoclopramide in enhancing propulsion in the distal small intestine and colon.

Cisapride (Propulsid), recently marketed in the US, was introduced for management of gastroesophageal reflux disease, diabetic gastroparesis, intestinal atony, and adynamic colon. Because it can stimulate propulsive activity in the colon, cisapride may find use for chronic idiopathic constipation and other diseases related to functional adynamic colon. As it does not block dopamine receptors, cisapride produces fewer side-effects than metoclopramide. The major side-effect of cisapride is diarrhea. It is not as effective as metoclopramide as an antiemetic agent.

The prokinetic effects of cisapride appear to result from activation of 5-HT_4 receptors in the enteric nervous system to increase release of acetylcholine from cholinergic motor neurons that innervate GI smooth muscle.[8] As the final effects of cisapride occur by means of acetylcholine activation of smooth muscle M_2 receptors, the prokinetic effects of cisapride can be blocked by muscarinic receptor antagonists (Fig. 70.1). Several other substituted benzamide derivatives, including zacopride and renzapride, appear to possess pharmacologic properties similar to those of cisapride and may be shown beneficial in management of disorders of GI motility.[r6] However, cisapride may be unique among the existing benzamide agents in that it seems to be a full agonist at 5-HT_4 receptors, whereas other drugs may be partial agonists.

Cisapride is rapidly absorbed after oral administration, reaching peak plasma levels one to two hours later. The bioavailability is 40 to 50 per cent, with significant first-pass metabolism occurring in the liver.[r5] Cisapride is extensively metabolized by oxidative N-dealkylation and aromatic hydroxylation. Cisapride metabolites are excreted in the urine and feces. The plasma half-life is approximately eight hours. Cisapride is available in 10 mg tablets and recommended dosing is 10 or 20 mg four times daily.

Erythromycin

Erythromycin, an antibiotic long known to induce GI side-effects, was recently discovered to produce GI prokinetic effects. It has been shown that erythromycin can stimulate GI motility, and it has been employed with some success in the treatment of diabetic gastroparesis. The prokinetic actions of erythromycin are known to be unrelated to its antimicrobial activity because structural analogues that are not antibiotic nevertheless possess prokinetic actions. The mechanism by which erythromycin stimulates GI motility has not been conclusively established. There is evidence, however, to suggest that erythromycin is a motilin receptor agonist and acts in part through activation of GI motilin receptors.[11] Motilin is a GI hormone believed to be involved in the initiation of the MMC activity characteristic of the fasting pattern of motility. Erythromycin and structurally-related analogues mimic the actions of exogenously administered motilin by initiating MMC activity in the proximal bowel in dogs and humans.[12] Erythromycin also displaces iodinated motilin from high-affinity binding sites in preparations of GI tissues. However, in dog intestine in vivo, erythromycin displays a number of excitatory and inhibitory effects on GI motility that are only partially mimicked by motilin.[13] In isolated preparations of GI smooth muscle, erythromycin produced inhibitory effects not mimicked by motilin.[14]

Whether or not the prokinetic effects of erythromycin can be attributed solely to actions at GI motilin receptors in nerve and muscle, erythromycin is presently of great interest for treatment of GI hypomotility syndromes, especially those involving the stomach, distal small intestine, and the colon. Initial clinical studies indicate that erythromycin is more effective than metoclopramide or cisapride as a prokinetic agent in the distal small intestine and colon. Like other prokinetic drugs, erythromycin improves esophageal clearance, increases the rate of gastric emptying, and increases propulsion in the small intestine.

Pharmacokinetics

Orally administered erythromycin is incompletely absorbed from the GI tract. Different esters of erythromycin (stearate, estolate, and ethylsuccinate) have been employed in attempts to improve oral bioavailability. However, various formulations of erythromycin have been evaluated primarily with the aim of improving antimicrobial activity, not prokinetic activity. It is not certain which drug formulation is optimal for prokinetic actions. The plasma half-life of erythromycin is one to two hours. Erythromycin is extracted by the liver and excreted in active form in the bile. Only a small fraction of orally administered erythromycin is excreted in the urine.

Therapeutic Uses

Erythromycin has become increasingly popular as a prokinetic drug, especially to improve gastric emptying and to increase propulsion in the distal small intestine and colon. Although adequate well-controlled clinical trials have not yet been conducted, it is noted that erythromycin produces powerful contractions of the gastric antrum and rapid gastric emptying in humans. It should be useful in the management of gastroparesis and intestinal pseudoobstruction in acute settings and for distal intestinal hypomotility conditions in acute and chronic settings.

Adverse Effects

Orally administered erythromycin, especially in large doses (greater than 500 mg) can produce acute epigastric pain, probably associated with powerful contractions of gastric smooth muscle. Similar symptoms may occur after IV administration. Nausea, vomiting, diarrhea, and abdominal cramps may be noted. These adverse effects are thought to be dose-related.

In its use as an antibiotic, cholestatic hepatitis has been induced by erythromycin estolate, and is characterized by nausea, vomiting, and abdominal cramps beginning one to three weeks after treatment. The symptoms may be followed by jaundice, fever, and eosinophilia. Cholestatic hepatitis may result from a hypersensitivity response to erythromycin estolate. Fortunately, it is a rare complication of erythromycin treatment.

Preparations and Doses

Erythromycin is available in a variety of preparations for oral or parenteral administration. Both liquid and solid dosage forms for oral administration are available. Tablets typically contain 250 mg, 400 mg, or 500 mg. Erythromycin lactobionate is available for IV administration.

Gonadotropin-Releasing Hormone Agonists

Leuprolide acetate, a synthetic analogue of gonadotropin-releasing hormone, has been found in preliminary studies to improve symptoms of gastroparesis, abdominal pain, and nausea in patients suffering from severe chronic GI motor dysfunction. Leuprolide is a GnRH agonist that transiently increases pituitary secretions of gonadotropins in males and females, then causes prolonged suppression of gonadotropin release through desensitization of GnRH receptors on pituitary gonadotrophs. Leuprolide has been used primarily for palliative treatment of prostatic cancer in males or suppression of fertility in females.[r7] Its mechanism of action in improvement of symptoms of gastroparesis is not known. A large percentage of patients with nondiabetic gastroparesis, however, are premenopausal females with symptoms often correlating with stages of the menstrual cycle. Leuprolide may improve symptoms by suppression of the ovulatory and menstrual cycles. Appropriate controlled clinical trials will be necessary to establish the efficacy and safety of leuprolide in management of GI motility disorders.

Antiemetic Drugs

Emesis is a complex pathophysiologic event requiring coordinated actions of the enteric nervous system, autonomic nervous system, somatic nervous system, and CNS. Emetic stimuli may arise from the GI tract, from the chemoreceptor trigger zone (CTZ) of the medulla, from the cerebral cortex, or from the vestibular system (Fig. 70.3). Emesis is associated with a complex series of GI motor changes.

In the GI tract, vomiting involves initial inhibition of gastric contractions, relaxation of the lower esophageal sphincter, and orally migrating contractions of the small intestine (reverse peristalsis) that move into the stomach to produce gastric contractions.[15] Feelings of intense nausea are usually associated with the aborally progressing intestinal contractions. Muscles of the diaphragmatic dome contract along with muscles of the abdominal wall to expel gastric contents. Respiration is reflexly inhibited during emesis. Coordination of vomiting occurs in the CNS. The emetic response can be induced by stimulating afferent nerves from the viscera to the CNS and by stimulation of sites within various regions of the brain. Vagal afferent fibers from the GI tract travel to the nucleus and tractus solitarius (NTS), the primary visceral sensory receiving center in the brain. The NTS projects fibers to the CTZ, to the vomiting center, and to the dorsal motor nucleus of the vagus. Emetic stimuli can arise in the GI tract and may be induced by chemicals or by bacterial toxins. Emetic stimuli also arise from the cerebral cortex and from the vestibular system, both of which are thought to project to the medullary vomiting center. The vomiting center also receives input from the CTZ. The blood-brain barrier in the region of the CTZ is relatively permeable to emetic substances in the circulation, including opiate drugs, nicotine, cardiac glycosides, many cancer chemotherapeutic agents, and others. Emetic substances activate the CTZ, which, in turn, stimulates the vomiting center. The vomiting center coordinates activity of the dorsal motor nucleus (DMN) of the vagus to produce characteristic patterns of GI motility during vomiting and also coordinates activity of the phrenic nerves and the spinal innervation of the abdominal musculature.

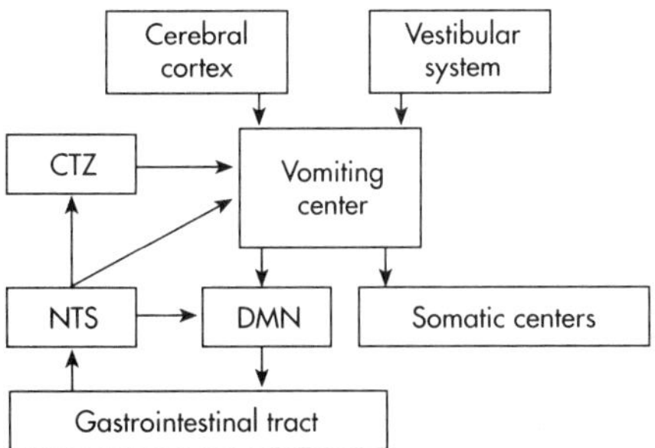

Figure 70.3 Primary neural circuits responsible for regulation of vomiting. Antiemetic drugs act at one or more sites to suppress the vomiting reflex.

Several types of drugs possess antiemetic activity (Table 70.2). They differ in their sites of action, mechanisms of action, relative efficacy against different emetic stimuli, and in the profile of side-effects associated with their use.

Antimuscarinic and Antihistaminic Drugs

Scopolamine, a natural alkaloid with pronounced antagonist activity at muscarinic cholinergic receptors, has significant efficacy in the prevention of motion sickness. Scopolamine is a tertiary amine that readily crosses the blood-brain barrier and is distributed throughout the brain. Administered prophylactically, it reduces the incidence and severity of motion sickness, but can be associated with unpleasant side-effects. When given by the oral route, scopolamine plasma levels increase rapidly to produce the full panoply of side-effects associated with antagonism at muscarinic receptors: dry mouth; blurred vision; decreased sweating; urinary hesitancy; and constipation. When administered by transdermal patch, more sustained, lower plasma levels of scopolamine are achieved that are adequate to suppress motion sickness but generally are not sufficient to produce significant side-effects. Nevertheless, scopolamine patches may be associated with dry mouth, blurred vision, sedation, or other antimuscarinic side-effects.

The beneficial effects of scopolamine in preventing the nausea and vomiting of motion sickness are thought to result from blockade of muscarinic receptors in the vestibular apparatus and cells innervated by cholinergic fibers projecting from the vestibular system to the vomiting center. Scopolamine is generally regarded as the most effective of all drugs for the prophylaxis and treatment of motion sickness. However, other drugs with muscarinic antagonist properties and histamine H_1 receptor antagonists properties also show activity in suppression of motion sickness. Several H_1 antagonists, such as diphenhydramine or its chlorotheophylline salt, dimenhydrinate, also posses significant antagonist activity at muscarinic receptors. Indeed, promethazine, a phenothiazine H_1 antagonist, has the most significant muscarinic antagonist activity among the H_1 antagonists and is the most effective H_1 antagonist in the management and prevention of motion sickness. It is likely that the pharmacologic properties of

Table 70.2 Summary of Sites and Mechanisms of Action of Selected Antiemetic Drugs

Antiemetic	Sites of Action	Mechanisms
Scopolamine	Vestibular, VC	Block muscarinic receptors
Diphenhydramine	Vestibular, VC	Block muscarinic, H_1 receptors
Prochlorperazine	CTZ, VC	Block D_2 receptors
Metoclopramide	CTZ, VC	Block D_2, 5-HT_3 receptors
Nabilone	CTZ, VC, cortex	Activate THC receptors
Ondansetron	Vagal afferents, CTZ	Block 5-HT_3 receptors
Cisapride	Gastric efferents	Activate 5-HT_4 receptors

VC = vomiting center, CTZ = chemoreceptor trigger zone

antagonism at both muscarinic receptors and H_1 receptors contribute to the therapeutic effect of the H_1 antagonists useful for motion sickness. These drugs block muscarinic and H_1 receptors in the vestibular apparatus and block the effects of cholinergic and histaminergic fibers projecting from the vestibular system to the vomiting center. Diphenhydramine (Benadryl), dimenhydrinate (Dramamine), and promethazine (Phenergan) are useful for prevention of motion sickness, postoperative nausea and vomiting, and often are of value in treatment of vestibular disturbances, such as Meniere's disease. These drugs are less useful against the nausea and vomiting associated with chemotherapy or radiation treatment.

Phenothiazine Drugs

The antiemetic properties of promethazine, an H_1 and muscarinic antagonist, were described above. Several other phenothiazine derivatives, such as prochlorperazine (Compazine), possess useful antiemetic properties of benefit in various disorders associated with vomiting. Prochlorperazine can prevent or reduce vomiting induced by gastroenteritis, drug-induced emesis, and radiation sickness. Although prochlorperazine should not be given to pregnant women for this purpose, it can reduce the nausea and vomiting of pregnancy. Like other phenothiazines (except for promethazine), prochlorperazine is not useful in preventing motion sickness.

Prochlorperazine and several other phenothiazines (chlorpromazine, triethylperazine, and triflupromazine) as well as the butyrophenone, droperidol, tend to produce significant sedation in antiemetic doses and occasionally precipitate dystonias.

These drugs are thought to produce their antiemetic actions in the chemoreceptor trigger zone and the vomiting center by virtue of their antagonist effects at dopamine D_2 receptors. It is known that dopamine agonists, such as apomorphine, produce emesis by actions at dopamine receptors in the CTZ. The emetic effects of apomorphine and related dopamine agonists are readily blocked by the phenothiazine antiemetic drugs.

Metoclopramide

Metoclopramide (Reglan) is a substituted benzamide with significant prokinetic properties. It is an effective antiemetic drug especially useful for the management of nausea and vomiting associated with administration of cancer chemotherapeutic drugs.[16] It is used widely to control emesis during cancer chemotherapy, especially when highly emetogenic drugs are used, such as cisplatin or cyclophosphamide.[17] Controlled clinical trials have provided evidence that metoclopramide is more effective than diphenhydramine, prochlorperazine, or promethazine in prevention of chemotherapy-associated nausea and vomiting.[18] Metoclopramide has become a standard agent for use in management of an extremely unpleasant side-effect associated with certain anticancer drugs.

Metoclopramide possesses pronounced antagonist activity at dopamine D_2 receptors, and its antiemetic effects probably result primarily from blockade of D_2 receptors in the CTZ and the vomiting center. Unlike the phenothiazines, metoclopramide also possesses weak antagonist activity at 5-HT_3 receptors. 5-HT_3 receptors probably are located on vagal afferent fibers and contribute to the nausea and vomiting associated with gastroenteritis and other GI emetic stimuli.

Cannabinoids

Tetrahydrocannabinol (THC), the active ingredient of marijuana, is known to exert significant antiemetic effects. Marijuana itself has been used occasionally under medical supervision as an antiemetic drug. Synthetic analogues of THC with similar activity at the brain THC receptor have been introduced into medicine as antiemetic agents. Nabilone (Cesamet) is a synthetic cannabinoid administered orally for management of nausea and vomiting. It is indicated for the treatment of nausea and vomiting associated with cancer chemotherapy in patients who have failed to respond adequately to conventional antiemetic treatments.[18] Nabilone produces the full spectrum of mental effects associated with marijuana or THC. Patients receiving nabilone may experience changes in mood, decrements in cognitive performance, loss of memory, decreased ability to control impulses, and alterations in the experience of reality. Occasional patients may suffer psychosis. Use of nabilone is restricted for these reasons and because a substantial proportion of patients treated with nabilone experience disturbing psychic reactions not associated with other antiemetic drugs. Nabilone should be used only in circumstances that permit close supervision of the patient; it is highly abusable and is controlled under Schedule II of the Controlled Substances Act.

5-*Hydroxytryptamine*$_3$ *Antagonists*

Ondansetron (Zofran) is the prototype of antiemetic drugs that act by blocking 5-HT_3 receptors (Fig. 70.4). Ondansetron is a potent, highly selective 5-HT_3 receptor antagonist.[19] It is not a dopamine receptor antagonist. Receptors of the 5-HT_3 type are present both peripherally on vagal nerve terminals and centrally in the CTZ.[20] The peripheral vagal receptors appear to be associated with afferent fibers that serve sensory receptors in the gastric wall and project to the tractus and nucleus solitarius (NTS) of the brain stem. Chemotherapy with cytotoxic drugs appears to be associated with release of 5-HT from the enterochromaffin cells of the small intestine. Urinary levels of 5-HT metabolites increase, for example, after administration of cisplatin in parallel with the onset of emesis. The 5-HT released by chemotherapy may stimulate the vagal afferents through 5-HT_3 receptors and initiate the vomiting reflex. 5-HT_3 receptors also occur in the CTZ of the area postrema and appear to be involved in initiation of emesis provoked by cisplatin.[21] Controlled clinical studies indicate that ondansetron was more effective than placebo or metoclopramide in preventing emesis associated with administration of highly emetogenic chemotherapeutic drugs, including cisplatin.

Side-effects of ondansetron appear to be mild and transient. The major adverse effect observed in clinical trials was headache, which occurred in some 10 per cent of patients.

Ondansetron is intended for IV administration. Volume of distribution is 1.9–2.6 L/kg, indicating that much of the drug is taken up by body tissues. Ondansetron is moderately (70%) bound to plasma protein and crosses membranes readily. It is excreted in the urine (approximately 65%) and feces (35%) after extensive hepatic metabolism involving hydroxylation and conjuration reactions. The plasma half-life of ondansetron is 3.5 hours. Studies in animals indicate that ondansetron does not affect the efficacy of anticancer drugs.

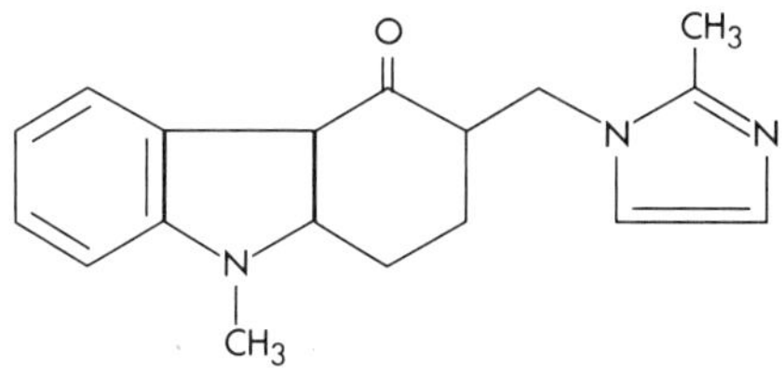

Preparation and Doses

Ondansetron is given by IV administration. The recommended IV dosage of ondansetron is three 0.15 mg/kg doses infused over 15 minutes, beginning one-half hour before the start of chemotherapy, with subsequent doses four and eight hours after the first dose. It may be administered according to the same schedule daily for up to five days in patients receiving chemotherapy for multiple days. Ondansetron is supplied in 20-ml multidose vials.

Ondansetron

Figure 70.4 Structure of Ondansetron

Cisapride

The general pharmacologic and therapeutic effects of cisapride are discussed above. Cisapride and other prokinetic drugs may display modest efficacy in the management of emesis of certain etiologies. For example, the prokinetic drugs, presumably by increasing the rate of gastric emptying, decrease nausea and vomiting associated with gastroparesis. They may offer modest effects as general antiemetic drugs if a component of delayed gastric emptying or gastric stasis contributes to the underlying pathophysiology. Cisapride and related drugs are generally not effective in management of emesis associate with cancer chemotherapeutic drugs.

Drugs that Inhibit Gastrointestinal Propulsion

The propulsive activity of the GI tract can be inhibited in two ways: by inhibition of contractions necessary for movement of luminal contents and by increasing the occurrence of segmenting contractions that retard flow of luminal content. Drugs that inhibit GI contractions in humans include alpha and beta adrenergic receptor agonists and muscarinic antagonists.

Drugs that inhibit propulsion by increasing segmenting contractions include the mu opioid agonists.

Opiate Drugs

Opiate drugs act as agonists at opioid receptors. Opiates can act at opioid receptors in the enteric nervous system and in the brain and spinal cord to affect GI contractile activity and propulsion.[r9,r10] The effects of opiates on GI motility differ by species. In the human and most higher mammals, opiates that are agonists at mu opioid receptors increase the incidence and amplitude of segmenting contractions of the small intestine.[r11] By contrast, mu opiates inhibit contractions in the rodent small intestine. Opiates appear to exert two opposing neural effects with differing consequences in terms of GI motility: they act at presynaptic mu opioid receptors on excitatory cholinergic motor neurons to inhibit release of acetylcholine, thereby inhibiting contractions; and they act presynaptically at inhibitory neurons, probably those releasing nitric oxide (NO) or vasoactive intestinal peptide (VIP), to inhibit release of the inhibitory neurotransmitter, thereby promoting contractions through the process of disinhibition.[22] Inhibition of release of acetylcholine may result in decreased propulsive contractions, especially those involving longitudinal muscle, whereas inhibition of release of inhibitory neurotransmitter may promote segmenting contractions of the circular muscle. The major effect of opiate agonists in humans is to increase segmenting, nonpropulsive contractions of the circular muscle and to inhibit propulsive contractions. The increase in segmenting contractions increases luminal resistance to flow and retards propulsion of intestinal contents. Gastric emptying is reduced; small intestinal and colonic propulsion are inhibited.

The antipropulsive effect of opioids appears to contribute to their antidiarrheal effects and certainly explains their constipating effects.[23] Opiates increase tone of GI sphincters, especially the ileocecal sphincter and the sphincter of Oddi. Contraction of the ileocecal sphincter may contribute to the antipropulsive effects of opiates. Contraction of the sphincter of Oddi decreases flow of bile into the duodenum.

As indicated above, the effects of opiates on GI motility appear to be mediated largely by actions on neural structures, both in the CNS and in the enteric nervous system. In the small intestine, opioid receptors are located primarily or exclusively on nerves and are primarily of the mu and delta types.[24] Activation of mu and delta, but not kappa, opioid receptors produces contractions of the small intestine.[25,26] Tolerance to the intestinal stimulating effect of opiates can occur, but develops slowly.[27] As described in Chapter 20, the primary use of opiates in GI disorders is in the management of diarrhea. The antidiarrheal effects of opioids probably result primarily from their ability to inhibit secretion of fluid into the lumen of the intestine. However, decreases in propulsion may contribute to the antidiarrheal effects of opiates.

Morphine and codeine are natural opiate alkaloids used in the management of diarrhea. These drugs induce segmenting contractions of the small intestine. Morphine has been shown to induce MMC activity as well.[28] Diphenoxylate and loperamide (Fig. 70.5) are synthetic opiates related to meperidine that are used exclusively for management of diarrhea. Like morphine and codeine, diphenoxylate and loperamide stimulate contractions of intestinal circular muscle and delay gastric emptying and intestinal propulsion.[29] The antipropulsive effects of these drugs appear to be mediated by GI opioid receptors as their effects are blocked by naloxone, an opioid antagonist.[30]

Loperamide (Imodium) is absorbed after oral administration, with peak plasma levels occurring 2.5. to 5 hours after dosing. The elimination half-life is 11 hours. The drug is excreted primarily in the feces. It is supplied in 2-mg capsules. The recommended initial dose is 4 mg, followed by 2 mg after each unformed stool, with daily dosage not to exceed 16 mg. Diphenoxylate with atropine is available as Lomotil liquid and tablets. Each tablet and each 5 ml of liquid contains 2.5 mg of diphenoxylate and 0.025 mg of atropine. The atropine is present in a subtherapeutic dose to prevent abuse. The elimination half-life of diphenoxylate is approximately 12 hours. It is extensively metabolized to difenoxin, which is biologically active. Diphenoxylate metabolites are excreted largely in the feces. The recommended dosage of diphenoxylate is 5 mg administered orally four times daily until symptoms subside.

In contrast to morphine and codeine, diphenoxylate and, especially, loperamide cross the blood-brain barrier poorly and exhibit low abuse liability. Their

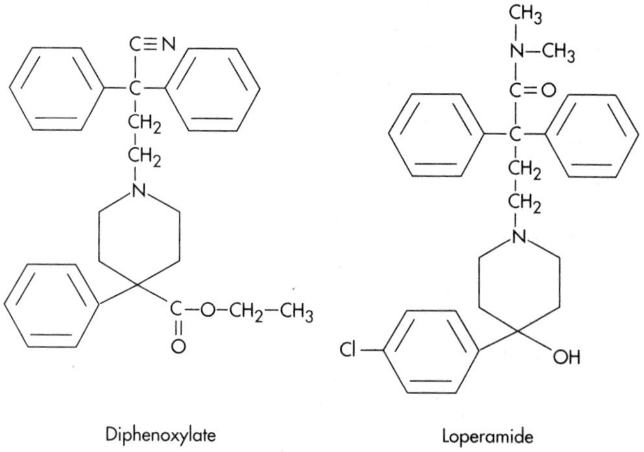

Diphenoxylate   Loperamide

Figure 70.5 Structures of Peripherally-Acting Antidiarrheal Opiates

actions on GI motility result exclusively from peripheral effects.

References

Research Reports

1. Lee KY; Kim MS, Chey WY. Effects of a meal and gut hormones on plasma motilin and duodenal motility in the dog. Am J Physiol 1980;*238*:G280–G283.
2. Euler AR. Use of bethanechol for the treatment of gastroesophageal reflux. J Pediatr 1980;*96*:321–324.
3. Bateman DN, Rawlins MD, Simpson JM. Extrapyramidal reactions with metoclopramide. Br Med J 1985;*291*:930–932.
4. Schuurkes JAJ, Helsen LFM, Ghoos ECR, Eelen JGM, Van Nueten JM. Stimulation of gastroduodenal motor activity: dopaminergic and cholinergic modulation. Drug Dev Res 1986;*8*:233–241.
5. Sowers JR, Sharp B, McCallum RW. Effect of domperidone, an extracerebral inhibitor of dopamine receptors, on thyrotropin, prolactin, renin. aldosterone, and 18-hydroxycorticosterone secretion in man. J Clin Endocrinol Metab 1982;*54*:869–871.
6. Craig DA, Clarke DE. Pharmacological characterization of a neuronal receptor for 5-hydroxytryptamine in guinea pig ileum with properties similar to the 5-hydroxytryptamine$_4$ receptor. J Pharmacol Exp Therap 1990;*252*:1378–1386.
7. Dumuis A, Seben M, Backstreet J. The gastrointestinal benzamide derivatives are agonists at the non-classical 5-HT receptor (5-HT$_4$) positively coupled to adenylate cyclase neurons. Naunyn-Schmiedeberg's Arch Pharmacol 1989;*340*:403–410.
8. Taniyama K, Nakayama S, Takeda K, Matsumaya S, Shirakawa J, Sano I, Ranaka C. Cisapride stimulates motility of the intestine via the 5-hydroxytryptamine receptors. J Pharmacol Exp Therap 1991;*258*:1098–1104.
9. Nemeth PR, Gullikson GW. Gastrointestinal motility stimulating drugs and 5-HT receptors on myenteric neurons. Eur J Pharmacol 1989;*166*:387–391.
10. Schuurkes J, Van Nueten JM, Van Daele P, Reyntjens AJ, and Janssen P. Motor-stimulating properties of cisapride on isolated gastrointestinal preparations of the guinea pig. J Pharmacol Exp Therap 1985;*234*:775–783.
11. Peeters TG, Matthys G, Depoortere I, Cachet T, Hoogmartins J, Vantrappen G. Erythromycin is a motilin receptor agonist. Am J Phsiol 1989;*257*:G470–G474.
12. Itoh Z, Nakaya M, Suzuki T, Arai H, Wakabayashi K. Erythromycin mimics exogenous motilin in gastrointestinal contractile activity in the dog. Am J Physiol 1984;*247*:G688–G694.
13. Otterson MF, and Sarna SK. Gastrointestinal motor effects of erythromycin. Am J Physiol 1990;*259*:G335–G363.
14. Minscha A, Galligan JJ. Erythromycin inhibits contractions of nerve-muscle preparations of the guinea pig small intestine. J Pharmacol Exp Therap 1991;*257*:1248–1252.
15. Stewart JJ, Burks TF, Weisbrodt NW. Intestinal myoelectric activity after activation of the central emetic mechanism. Am J Physiol 1977;*233*:E131–E137.
16. Allen JC, Gralla R, Reilly L, Kellick M, Young C. Metoclopramide dose-related toxicity and preliminary antiemetic studies in children receiving cancer chemotherapy. J Clin Oncol 1985;*3*:1136–1141.
17. Cunningham D, Soukap M, Gilchrist NL, Forrest GJ, Hepplestone A, Calder IT. Randomized trial of intravenous high dose metoclopramide and intramuscular chlorpromazine in controlling nausea and vomiting induced by cytotoxic drugs. Br Med J 1985;*290*:604–605.
18. Einhorn LH, Nagy C, Furnas B, Williams SD. Nabilone: An effective antiemetic in patients receiving cancer chemotherapy. J Clin Pharmacol 1981;*21*:64S–69S.
19. Butler A, Hill JM, Ireland SJ, Jordan CC, Tyers MB. Pharmacological properties of GR38032F, a novel antagonist at 5-HT$_3$ receptors. Br J Pharmacol 1988;*94*:397–412.
20. Kilpatrick GJ, Jones BJ, Tyers MB. The distribution of specific GR76630 binding in the brains of several species. Characterization of binding to rat area postrema and vagus nerve. Eur J Pharmacol 1989;*159*:157–164.
21. Higgins GA, Kilpatrick JG, Bunce KT, Jones BJ, Tyers MB. 5-HT receptor antagonists injected into the area postrema inhibit cisplatin-induced emesis in the ferret. Br J Pharmacol 1989;*97*:247–255.
22. Bauer AJ, Sarr MG, Szurszewski JH. Opioids inhibit neuromuscular transmission in circular muscle of human and baboon intestine. Gastroenterology 1991;*101*:970–976.
23. Schiller LR, Davis RR, Santa Ana CA, Morawski SG, Fordtran JS. Studies of the mechanism of the antidiarrheal effect of codeine. J Clin Invest 1982;*70*:999–1008.
24. Allescher HD, Ahmad S, Kostka P, Kwan CY, Daniel EE. Distribution of opioid receptors in canine small intestine: implications for function. Am J Physiol 1989;*256*:G966–G974.
25. Hirning LD, Porreca F, Burks TF. μ, But not κ, opioid agonists induce contractions of the canine small intestine ex vivo. Eur J Pharmacol 1985;*109*:49–54.
26. Vaught JL, Cowan A, Jacoby HI. μ And δ, but not κ, opioid agonists induce contractions of the canine small intestine in vivo. Eur J Pharmacol 1985;*109*:43–48.
27. Weisbrodt NW, Thor PJ, Copeland EM, Burks TF. Tolerance to the effects of morphine on intestinal motility of unanesthetized dogs. J Pharmacol Exp Therap 1980;*215*:515–521.
28. Sarna S, Northcott P, Belbeck L. Mechanism of cycling of migrating myoelectric complexes: effect of morphine. Am J Physiol 1982;*242*:G588–G595.
29. Dajani EZ, Roge EAW, Bertermann RE. Effect of E prostaglandins, diphenoxylate and morphine on intestinal motility in vivo. Eur J Pharmacol 1975;*31*:105–113.
30. Basilisco G, Camboni G, Bozzani A, Paravicini M, Bianchi PA. Oral naloxone antogonizes loperamide-induced delay of orocecal transit. Dig Dis Sci 1987;*32*:829–832.

Reviews

r1. Sarna SK, Otterson MF. Small intestinal physiology and pathophysiology. Gastroenterol Clin No Amer 1989;*18*:375–404.

r2. Sarna SK. Physiology and pathophysiology of colonic motor activity. Dig Dis Sci 1991;*36*:827–862.

r3. Reynolds JC. Prokinetic agents: a key in the future of gastroenterology. Gastroenterol Clin No Amer 1989;*18*:437–457.

r4. Schulze-Delrieu K. Metoclopramide. Gastroenterology 1979;*77*:768–779.

r5. McCallum RW, Prakash C, Campoli-Richards DM, Goa KL. Cisapride: A preliminary review of its pharmacodynamic and pharmacokinetic properties, and therapeutic use as a prokinetic agent in gastrointestinal motility disorders. Drugs 1988;*36*:652–681.

r6. Demol P, Ruoff HJ, Weihrauch TR. Rational pharmacotherapy of gastrointestinal motility disorders. Eur J Pediatr 1989;*148*:489–495.

r7. Conn PM, Crowley WF. Gonadotropin-releasing hormone and its analogues. N Engl J Med 1991;*324*:93–103.

r8. Gralla RJ. Metoclopramide: A review of antiemetic trials. Drugs 1983;*25*(Suppl.1):63–73.

r9. Burks TF. Central sites of action of gastrointestinal drugs. Gastroenterology 1978;*74*:322–324.

r10. Manara L, Bianchetti A. The central and peripheral influence of opioids on gastrointestinal propulsion. Ann Rev Pharmacol Toxicol 1985;*25*:249–273.

r11. Kromer W. Endogenous and exogenous opioids in the control of gastrointestinal motility and secretion. Pharmacol Rev 1988;*40*:121–162.

SECTION IX

Drugs Affecting Blood, the Immune System, and Inflammation

Editor:
James W. Fisher

CHAPTER 71

Drugs that Act on Blood and Blood-Forming Organs

James W. Fisher

Introduction

The most important pharmacologic agents that affect blood and blood-forming organs are iron, cyanocobalamin (Vitamin B12), folic acid, erythropoietin and a few other hematopoietic growth factors, and several hormones that affect blood formation. When the patient presents with shortness of breath, lack of usual energy, and easy fatigability, the physician must consider that these may be signs and symptoms of anemia. Anemia is a signal that some organ is in distress; it is diagnosed by finding a low hemoglobin or hematocrit or red cell count. The physician should search for the underlying cause of the anemia and make a correct etiologic diagnosis. For example, an iron deficiency anemia may signal GI bleeding that have such disparate causes as chronic use of an irritant drug such as aspirin or a bleeding carcinoma of the colon. The use of "shot-gun" hematinics—for example, preparations that contain a large number of minerals, vitamins, and other hematinic agents—is to be condemned. These mixtures, some of which contain 20 to 30 agents, may obscure the diagnosis, are expensive, and are unneeded. The appropriate single agent should be used for each particular deficiency. Anemia is defined as a decrease in the hemoglobin, red cell count, and total circulating red cell mass. In some instances when plasma volume expansion occurs, such as during pregnancy, this cannot be true anemia, since total red cell mass is unchanged, but it is a physiologic hemodilution. There are two major causes of anemia[r1]: (1) diminished production of red blood cells—caused by a deficiency of erythropoietin, iron, vitamin B12, folic acid, hematopoietic growth factors, or some essential hormone; (2) excessive loss of red cells—from hemolysis, a decrease in red cell life span, or chronic blood loss. Agents included in this chapter that are effective in the various types of anemia include several other hematopoietic growth factors, such as interleukin 3, granulocyte-macrophage colony stimulating factor (GM-CSF), granulocyte colony stimulating factor (G-CSF), colony stimulating factor (CSF-1 or M-CSF), and thrombopoietin (TSF), as well as iron, vitamin B12, folic acid, and erythropoietin.

Hematopoietic Growth Factors

Growth and differentiation of blood cells are regulated by a large number of known hematopoietic growth factors.[r2] Clinical trials of six growth factors have been carried out recently, and the indications and guidelines for their use in the treatment of cytopenias have been defined.[r3,1] They are erythropoietin (Epo, Ep), granulocyte/macrophage colony stimulating factor (GM-CSF), multipotent colony stimulating factor (IL-3 or multi-CSF), colony stimulating factor (CSF-1 or M-CSF), granulocyte stimulating factor (G-CSF), and thrombopoiesis stimulating factor (TSF, thrombopoietin) (Table 71.1). Figure 71.1 illustrates the sites of action of the hematopoietic growth factors on the proliferation, differentiation, and maturation of several marrow cell lines.

Table 71.1 Biologic Actions of Hematopoietic Growth Factors

Erythropoietin (Epo, Ep)
— Stimulates the proliferation and maturation of the committed erythroid progenitor cell (CFU-E).
— Acts synergisticaly with IL-3 and GM-CSF to stimulate the formation of BFU-E.
— Increases heme synthesis in nucleated erythroid cells.
— Stimulates the early release of reticulocytes from the bone marrow compartment.

Granulocyte/Macrophage colony Stimulating Factor (GM-CSF)
— Acts synergistically with IL-3 to stimulate the formation and proliferation of colony forming cells CFU-GEMM, BFU-E, CFU-Meg, CFU-GM, CFU-M and CFU-Eo
— Increases cytotoxic and phagocytic activity of mature granulocytes.
— Reduces motility and clearance of granulocytes from the peripheral circulation.
— Enhances cytotoxicity and leukotriene synthesis in mature eosinophils.

Interlukin-3 (ILK-3 or Multi-CSF)
— Acts synergistically with GM-CSF to stimulate the formation of granulocytes, macrophages, eosinophils and megakaryocytes.
— Acts synergistically with erythropoietin to stimulate formation of BFU-E colonies.
— Induces pluripotent stem cells (CFU-S) and leukemic blast cells into cell cycle.

Colony Stimulating Factor-1 (CSF-1 or M-CSF)
— Acts synergistically with GM-CSF and, IL-3 to stimulate monocyte/macrophage colony formation and function.
— Increases anti-tumor activity of macrophages and their secretion of O_2 reduction products and plasminogen activation.

Granulocyte Colony Stimulating Factor (G-CSF)
— Acts synergistically with IL-3, GM-CSF and CSF-1 to stimulate formation of megakaryocytes, granulocyte-macrophage and high proliferative potentital (HPP) colonies.
— Induces release of granulocytes from marrow.
— Enhances phagocytic and cytotoxic action of mature granulocytes.

Thrombopoietin (TSF)
— Increases the size and number of megakaryocytes.
— Increases the concentration of early megakaryocytic cells (SACHE+ cells) in bone marrow.
— Produces an increase in megakaryocyte endomitosis.
— Increases platelet size and number in plasma.

Erythropoietin

Erythropoietin (Epo, Ep) is a glycoprotein hormone produced by the kidney in adult mammals.[r3,1,r4] Epo is produced in the liver in the fetus and switches over about six weeks after birth to the kidney.

The liver maintains its ability to produce small amounts of erythropoietin in anephric adults suffering from renal disease whose anemia is severe. A more severe hypoxic stimulus is required for extrarenal liver erythropoietin production than for kidney production of erythropoietin. Erythropoietin has a molecular weight of 30,400 D, is heavily glycosylated, and is made up of 165 amino acids in human plasma and urine.[2] The hormone contains a 27-amino acid leader sequence that is cleaved off in the endoplasmic reticulum before erythropoietin is secreted. Removal of the sialic acid constituent of erythropoietin results in its rapid clearance from plasma. Two forms of erythropoietin are available for clinical use: the alpha form, which contains 34 percent carbohydrate, and the beta form, which contains 26 percent carbohydrate. No difference in the pharmacokinetics of the alpha and beta forms has been demonstrated. Both are capable of potent stimulation of early erythroid cells in the marrow.

The target cell for erythropoietin in the bone marrow is the erythroid colony forming unit erythroid (CFU-E) (Table 71.1). Erythropoietin acts synergistically with IL-1, IL-3, IL-4, and GM-CSF to cause a differentiation of the burst forming unit erythroid (BFU-E), which is a progenitor cell for the CFU-E. EPO and IL-9 are required for the differentiation of CFU-E into the recognizable nucleated erythroid series. High levels of erythropoietin may produce direct effects on the nucleated erythroid series and an early release of reticulocytes.

Regulation of Erythropoietin Production

Erythropoietin production is regulated by hypoxia. Reduced oxygen delivery (hypobaric hypoxia, anemia, ischemia, or cobalt) creates an oxygen deficit in the kidney to trigger production of erythropoietin. Goldberg et al[3] proposed that a heme protein senses an oxygen deficit, assuming a deoxy conformation in hypoxia, to stimulate Epo mRNA and an oxy confor-

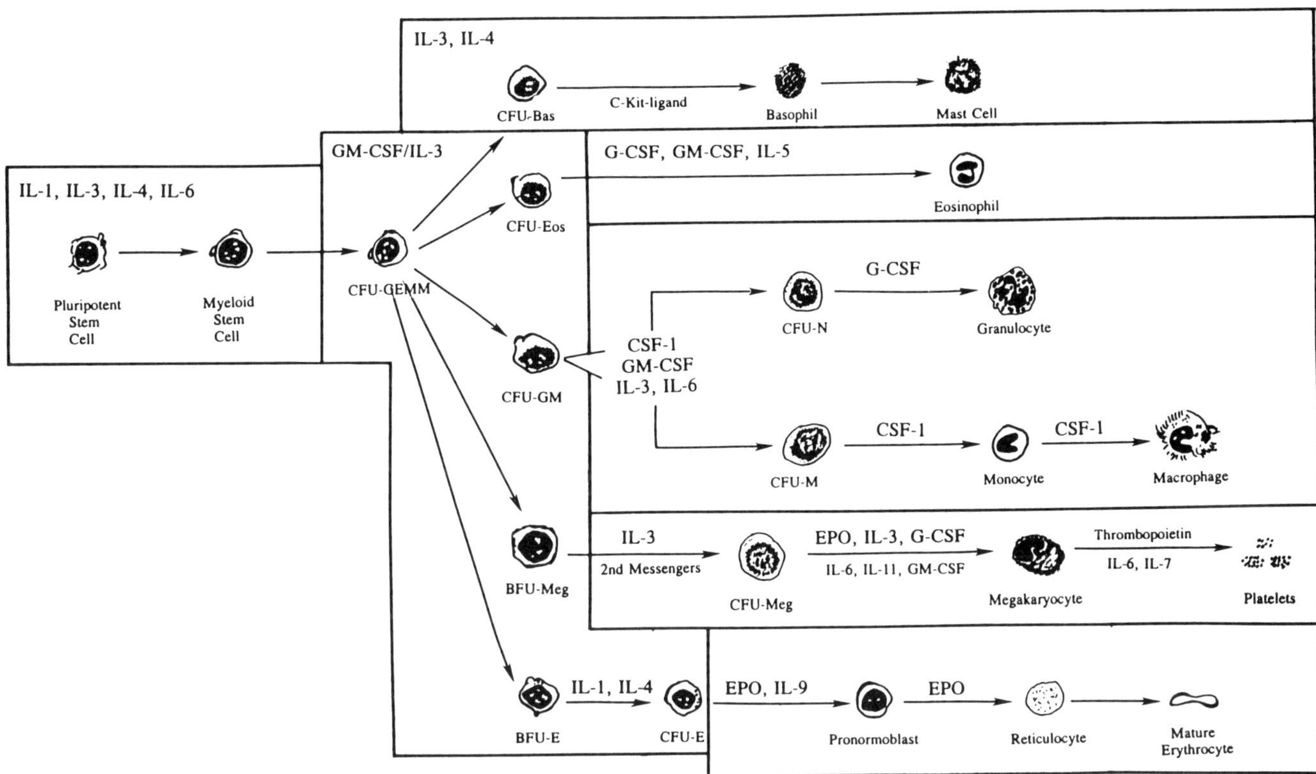

Figure 71.1 Hematopoietic growth factor sites of action on differentiation and maturation of cells of the erythropoietic, myelocytic, megakaryocytic, and thrombopoietic lineages. Interleukins-1, 3, 4, and 6 provide the stimulus for the differentiation of the pluripotent stem cells into a myeloid stem cell. Granulocytic-macrophage-colony stimulating factor (GM-CSF) and interleukin-3 (IL-3) trigger the myeloid stem cell to differentiate the colony forming unit precursor cell, the CFU-GEMM, which gives rise to specific colony forming units for the erythrocyte burst forming unit erythroid (BFU-E) and colony forming unit erythroid (CFU-E); megakaryocytes (BFU-Meg); CFU-GM, which gives rise to both precursors for granulocytes (CFU-N) and monocytes and macrophages (CFU-M), which also requires CSF-1, GM-CSF, IL-3, and IL-6. In addition, granulocytes require G-CSF. CFU-Eos requires G-CSF, GM-CSF, and IL-5 for its differentiation into eosinophils. IL-3, IL-4, and c-kit ligand are required for CFU-Bas differention into basophils; IL-1 and IL-4 act on the BFU-E to form the CFU-E; and EPO and IL-9 act on the CFU-E to form the nucleated erythroid series; IL-3 and second messengers are required for the differentiation of BFU-Meg into CFU-Meg and Epo, IL-3, G-CSF, IL-6, IL-11, and GM-CSF are required for the CFU-Meg to differentiate into megakaryocytes; thrombopoietin, IL-6 and IL-7 act on megakaryocytes to produce thrombocytes (platelets).

mation under normal oxygen tension to express Epo mRNA. We propose that there is an oxygen sensing cell in the kidney that is probably closely adjacent to the erythropoietin-producing cell. This cell that senses an oxygen deficit responds to produce a humoral agent that activates a cascade of events leading to increased synthesis of erythropoietin following an elevation in erythropoietin messenger RNA. Adenosine is postulated to amplify the effects of hypoxia on erythropoietin production through an adenylyl cyclase-dependent mechanism. Nitric oxide may also be released during hypoxia by the oxygen sensing cell to diffuse into the Epo producing cell and enhance Epo mRNA production. Nitric oxide synthase is the rate-limiting enzyme for the production of nitric oxide and causes the conversion of L-arginine to L-citruline and nitric oxide.[r7] Nitric oxide is rapidly metabolized to NO_2 and NO_3 in the presence of oxygen, which are less effective in triggering guanylyl cyclase than is NO. NO diffuses out of the oxygen-sensing cell and passes into the erythropoietin-producing cell to bind to guanylyl cyclase. NO may change the conformation of guanylyl cyclase, causing its activation and the production of cyclic GMP from GTP. Cyclic GMP activates a cGMP-dependent protein kinase that produces phosphoproteins that are important in the transcription of erythropoietin messenger RNA. Epo gene expression could be regulated by several kinases: kinase A, C, and G. Once erythropoietin mRNA is produced, it diffuses out of the nucleus and lays down a translation code on the ribosome in the cytoplasm to produce a specific erythropoietin protein.

Therapeutic Uses of Erythropoietin

The primary use of erythropoietin is in the anemia of end-stage renal disease.[4] The primary mechanism of anemia of end-stage renal disease (ESRD) is a deficiency of erythropoietin. Apparently insufficient amounts of erythropoietin are produced in response to the anemic stimulus to meet the demands for new red blood cell production in ESRD. In the severely uremic patient who is not well dialyzed, uremic toxins such as polyamines produce a suppression of the bone marrow, perhaps by suppressing the effects of erythropoietin on the CFU-E compartment.[r7] Shortened red cell life span also may be present in these patients. In addition to its use in the anemia of ESRD, erythropoietin has recently been approved by the FDA for use in the anemia of the immune deficiency syndrome (AIDS) in patients receiving AZT treatment, who usually are more anemic. It is possible to use AZT for antiviral therapy and still alleviate the anemia with Epo in these patients. The FDA has also approved Epo for the anemia associated with cancer chemotherapy.

Thus, approved indications for Epo by the FDA are the anemia of ESRD, anemia related to AZT therapy in HIV infection, and the anemia related to cancer and/or chemotherapy.[1] The guidelines for erythropoietin therapy are outlined in Table 71.2.

The nonapproved investigational use of erythropoietin are: bone marrow transplantation; anemia related to chronic inflammatory disease; myelodysplastic syndromes; anemia of prematurity; idiopathic aplastic anemia and Fanconi's anemia; sickle cell anemia; anemia in surgical patients.

Table 71.2 Guidelines for EPO Therapy

Guidelines
I. Currently approved indications
A. Anemia* of chronic renal failure (creatinine ≥ 1.8 mg/dl)
B. Anemia with HIV infection, in patients undergoing treatment with AZT
C. Anemia in cancer patients undergoing chemotherapy
II. Indications under investigation
A. Anemia of chronic disease, including rheumatoid arthritis and cancer
B. Donation of blood for autologous use
C. Surgical blood loss
D. Bone marrow transplantation
E. Anemia of prematurity
F. Myelodysplastic syndromes
G. Sickle cell anemia
III. Current contraindications
A. Patients in whom therapy will result in polycythemia
B. Patients with uncontrolled hypertension

*Anemia is defined as reduced RBC volume for which a blood transfusion is anticipated or needed.
(With permission of Transfusion, 1993;*33*:944.)

Preparations Available. Human recombinant erythropoietin is marketed as epoietin alpha (Epogen, Amgen) (Procrit, ortho Biotech). Single-use solution (sterile) vials containing 2000, 3000, 4000, and 10,000 IU of erythropoietin in 1.0 ml/vial for either IV or SQ use are available in buffered saline (pH 6.9) containing human albumin (2.5 mg/ml). These vials should not be frozen or shaken. The plasma half-life of epoietin alpha after IV injection in the patient with anemia of ESRD is approximately 10 hours. However, peak plasma levels of erythropoietin are reached between 5 and 24 hours after a SQ injection. The recommended dose-range initially in the patient with anemia of ESRD is between 50 and 100 units/kg, 3 times per week, usually given IV at the time of dialysis. When the hematocrit and hemoglobin levels rise too rapidly, it may be necessary to provide a supplement with oral iron as ferrous sulfate. After the hematocrit has reached approximately 30 percent, a reduction in the erythropoietin dose is advised until the hematocrit reaches a target level of 35 percent. The dose of erythropoietin to sustain a normal hematocrit can be reduced once the target hematocrit is reached.

Side-Effects of Recombinant Erythropoietin

There have been no reported allergic manifestations from either SQ or IV administration of epoietin alpha. No antibodies or other growth factors have been reported to be elevated. The only complications appear to be: (1) an approximately 10-mm rise in diastolic pressure when the hematocrit and red cell mass are elevated too rapidly in the hemodialysis patient; (2) iron deficiency because of the rapid increase in hemoglobin synthesis. This increase in diastolic blood pressure is associated with an increase in peripheral vascular resistance, in part secondary to increased blood viscosity. This elevation in blood pressure is usually found only when erythropoietin is administered to anemic patients with ESRD. The increase in diastolic pressure has been reported to be due to the vasoconstriction induced by the release of endothelin from endothelial cells along the wall of the blood vessel.[8] This increase in diastolic pressure can be avoided by attempting a more gradual increase in red cell mass, which would allow sufficient time for sympathetic nervous system adjustment in the peripheral vasculature, thus preventing the rise in peripheral resistance with an increasing red cell mass. It may be necessary in some patients who are on medication for hypertension to have the dosage regimen of antihypertensive agent changed and oral ferrous sulfate administered when iron deficiency occurs. Its recent abuse by world-class cyclists has led to several deaths from thrombosis related to excess red cells clogging blood flow.

Granulocyte/Macrophage Colony Stimulating Factor (GM-CSF)

GM-CSF acts synergistically with IL-3 (multi-colony stimulating factor) to stimulate colony formation and proliferation of granulocytes, monocyte/macrophages, megakaryocytes, and erythroid precursors (Table 71.1). In conjunction with erythropoietin, GM-CSF will promote BFU-E formation. GM-CSF has a broad range of target cells. It appears to be the most promising growth factor clinically.

GM-CSF increases the phagocytic and cytotoxic potential of mature granulocytes and reduces their motility and clearance in the circulation. It stimulates proliferation of small cell carcinomas in culture and the cytotoxicity of eosinophils. GM-CSF increases leukotriene synthesis. In general, GM-CSF produces an immediate transient fall in circulating neutrophils, eosinophils, and monocytes, followed by a marked leukocytosis with an increase in neutrophils, eosinophils, monocytes, and, in some instances, lymphocytes. A significant effect on platelets and red cells has been reported in some clinical trials of GM-CSF, but these findings have not been consistent. Idiopathic thrombocytopenia purpura has been reported in one patient taking GM-CSF. GM-CSF has been reported to be effective in relative or absolute neutropenia secondary to neoplasia, congenital cyclic neutropenia, aplastic anemia, myelodysplasia, and AIDS.[9–11] It also has an application in preventing the neutropenia associated with chemotherapy and autologous bone marrow transplantation.[12]

The side-effects of GM-CSF include local induration after SQ administration and thrombophlebitis at sites of infusion. Some patients have developed fever, myalgia, fatigue, skin rashes, GI distress, pericarditis, pleural effusion, and emboli that represent dose-limited toxicities. Similar to G-CSF, GM-CSF has been shown to be effective in ameliorating the myelosuppressive effects of chemotherapy. When used in bone marrow transplantation patients, GM-CSF was found to be useful in enhancing neutrophil recovery. GM-CSF has produced a modest increase in granulocytes, monocytes, and reticulocytes (at high doses) in patients with aplastic anemia.[11] The responses to GM-CSF in aplastic anemia are only transient. Groopman and colleagues[10] showed in 16 AIDS patients that GM-CSF produced a dose-dependent increase in circulating leukocytes, neutrophils, eosinophils, and monocytes. The combination of GM-CSF and erythropoietin is currently being studied in AIDS patients with azidovudine (AZT)-induced marrow suppression to ameliorate the dose-limited marrow toxicity of AZT and allow for continued antiviral therapy.

Multi-CSF (IL-3)

Multi-CSF stimulates colony formation in most of the hematopoietic cell lines. It acts synergistically with GM-CSF to increase the numbers of neutrophils, monocytes, and eosinophils in peripheral blood. It acts with erythropoietin to expand the BFU-E compartment and also acts jointly with erythropoietin to stimulate CFU-E proliferation. IL-3 stimulates pulmonary macrophages to proliferate and, with CSF-1, stimulates peritoneal macrophages. Multi-CSF produces significant shortening of postchemotherapy reduction in neutrophils and also appears to accelerate platelet recovery. Absolute eosinophil and basophil counts increased in

Table 71.3 Guidelines for Myeloid Recombinant Growth Factor Therapy

Currently approved indications
GM-CSF to accelerate myeloid recovery in patients with non-Hodgkin's lymphoma, acute lymphoblastic leukemia, and Hodgkin's disease who are undergoing autologous BMT
G-CSF to decrease the incidence of infection, as manifested by febrile neutropenia, in patients with nonmyeloid malignancies receiving myelosuppressive anticancer drugs associated with a significant incidence of severe neutropenia with fever
Indications under investigation
To accelerate myeloid recovery in patients with myelodysplastic syndrome. AIDS, marrow graft failure, PBSC transplantation, congenital agranulocytosis, or malignancies not mentioned above
Current contraindications
GM-CSF in patients with excessive leukemia myeloid blasts in the bone marrow or peripheral blood (>10%) with known hypersensitivity to GM-CSF, yeast-derived products, or any component of the product G-CSF in patients with known hypersensitivity to E. coli-derived proteins

(With permission of Transfusion 1993;*33*:944.)

postchemotherapy patients after treatment with multi-CSF. Human clinical trials have been carried out that are promising in patients with progressing neoplasms. Dose-related increases in white blood cells, platelets, neutrophils, and eosinophils were observed in all patients. Toxic reactions in some patients included fever, flushing, headache, and local erythema at the injection site.

Colony-Stimulating Factor (CSF-1 or M-CSF)

CSF-1 stimulates monocytes/macrophage colony formation alone and will act synergistically with GM-CSF and IL-3. It induces synthesis of G-CSF and IL-1 and enhances the production of interferon and tumor necrosis factor (TNF). There is a good relationship between the receptors for M-CSF and the VFMS oncogene product and cotransfection of cells with the genes for M-CSF receptor, and M-CSF itself will cause the transformation of fibroblasts.

CSF-1 was one of the first colony stimulating factors to be discovered that predominantly affects the myeloid lineage. CSF-1 has been purified from human urine preparations and has undergone clinical trials. Komiyama[13] has reported that nine children responded to a one-week course of therapy with human CSF-1 (M-CSF) with a small increase in white blood cells and total neutrophil counts. There was no significant effect on any other hematologic parameters. The gene for human CSF-1 has been cloned and expressed and has provided large amounts of purified recombinant CSF-1 for clinical trials. Unfortunately, thrombocytopenia is a common side-effect of CSF-1 infusion, despite the increase in megakaryocytes in the bone marrow. In all likelihood, the primary clinical use of CSF-1 may lie in combination with other growth factors, such as GM-CSF. The enhancement of macrophage function may provide a clinical role for CSF-1 in enhancing the immune system and could be an adjunct for immunostimulation therapy in malignancy.

Granulocyte Colony Stimulating Factor (G-CSF)

The most extensively studied clinical application of G-CSF has been to ameliorate the side-effects of myelosuppression produced by cancer chemotherapeutic agents.

It has recently been shown that G-CSF treatment may shorten the duration of neutrophil suppression after melphalan chemotherapy.[14] Another report of the effects of G-CSF in patients with transitional cell carcinoma of the bladder being treated with chemotherapy has indicated a 91 percent reduction in the number of neutropenic days when compared to subsequent cell cycles where G-CSF was similar to GM-CSF. G-CSF has been reported to be beneficial, and significantly reduced the duration of neutropenia after autologous bone marrow transplantation. Several other applications of G-CSF currently being explored are the amelioration of the myelosuppressive effects of azidovudine in AIDS patients where G-CSF treatment is being combined with erythropoietin therapy. G-CSF shows promising increases in neutrophil counts and a decrease in the incidence of infection in chronic neutropenias. G-CSF has also been demonstrated to produce a rapid increase in leukocyte counts in five patients with myelodysplasia and pancytopenia. Other areas where G-CSF has shown to be potentially beneficial include hairy cell leukemia and neutropenia.[15] Generally, G-CSF has been well tolerated by most patients, but in some instances has been associated with bone pain. However, this can be alleviated by administering the drug SQ, which does not seem to affect its efficacy adversely.

Human granulocyte colony stimulating factor (G-CSF) is marketed as filgastrim (Neupogen) produced by recombinant DNA technology as recombinant methionyl human granulocyte colony stimulating factor (τ-metHuG-CSF) and is a glycoprotein with 175 amino acids. It is recommended primarily to decrease the incidence of infection, as manifested by febrile neutropenia, in patients with non-myeloid malignancies receiving myelosuppressive anti-cancer drugs associated with a significant incidence of severe neutropenia with fever.

Thrombopoietin (TSF)

Thrombopoiesis stimulating factor (TSF) or thrombopoietin is well documented to be a factor that controls megakaryocytopoiesis and, thus, thrombocytopoiesis. Increased thrombopoietin production apparently is not the result of a panic mechanism but is required for the day-to-day maintenance of platelet counts. The site of production of thrombopoietin has not been completely elucidated, but kidney cells have been reported to produce TSF. Thrombopoietin is just now beginning to be studied clinically.

Evidence indicates that it may play a critical role in many patients with platelet production disorders. Thrombopoietin apparently acts in conjunction with megakaryocyte colony stimulating factor (Meg-CSF) to regulate megakaryocytopoiesis and enhanced production of platelets. It now seems well established that megakaryocytopoiesis is regulated by two factors that appear to affect the proliferation of progenitor cells in the development of megakaryocytes. Meg-CSF acts on megakaryocytes colony-forming units (CFU-Meg) and controls the proliferation of these progenitor cells; whereas thrombopoietin and possibly other potentiators control megakaryocyte development and platelet production. Clinical trials of thrombopoietin have been undertaken, but it is not yet clear in which diseases thrombopoietin might prove useful.

Iron

Iron deficiency anemia affects hundreds of millions of people throughout the world and is one of the most common health problems worldwide.[r8] In this book, the causes of iron deficiency anemia are covered in the section on nutritional agents. Iron has been known to be of value in the treatment of iron deficiency anemia since the time of the Roman physicians, who administered water from blacksmith shops where hot iron utensils were cooled. This iron-containing water was known to be of value in the so-called "green pallor" or chlorosis in young women beginning menstruation. Some common causes of iron deficiency anemia include blood loss due to hookworms, nutritional deficiencies, pregnancy, and various chronic blood losses. The average human female loses approximately 50 ml of blood each month during the menstrual cycle, causing a negative iron balance usually corrected by enhanced absorption. As indicated in Figure 71.2, there is approximately 15 mg of iron/day in the average US diet and 1 mg of ferrous iron is absorbed each day from iron-containing foods.

Iron is split off in the gastric juice from chelates and the gastric acid keeps the iron in a soluble form. Ascorbic acid and SH groups from amino acids are reducing agents that convert iron from the poorly absorbed ferric to the well-absorbed ferrous form. As shown in Figure 71.2, the ferrous (Fe^{2+}) form of iron is absorbed from the duodenum and jejunum. In contrast, the ferric (Fe^{3+}) form of iron is preferred for absorption across the intestinal mucosal cells in the dog.

The mechanism of iron absorption across the intestinal mucosal cell is controversial and still not well understood. Only a small fraction of heme iron is absorbed by the intestinal mucosal cell. Inorganic iron absorption by the mucosal cell apparently involves an active process. This mechanism involves endocytosis. When iron enters the mucosal cell, it is combined with apotransferrin and is carried as transferrin to the submucosal surface; it passes through the mucosal cell membrane and is delivered into the circulation. It is again taken up by plasma transferrin and is transported to the hemoglobin synthesizing erythroid cells. Transferrin, a 678-amino acid glycoprotein with an M_r of 79,570 daltons, migrates electrophoretically with beta-1-globulins. Ceruloplasmin, a ferroxidase present in plasma, is involved in the conversion of Fe^{2+} to Fe^{3+} when the iron is bound to plasma transferrin. There is a physiologic mechanism in the intestinal mucosal cell for trapping iron when body iron stores are high. In iron deficiency and when iron stores are low, very little trapping of iron occurs, and it passes, combined with apotransferrin as transferrin, rapidly from the intestinal lumen through the mucosal cell into the circulation. Macrophages often become loaded with iron and are involved in the passage of some iron into the intestinal lumen. The intestinal mucosal cell contains ferritin, which is incorporated into the so-called "F" bodies in the cytoplasm.[16]

Intestinal mucosal cell regulation of iron absorption operates normally as an active process when small amounts of iron pass directly through the mucosal cell into the circulation while certain amounts may be retained by the intestinal mucosal cell. In iron overload, however, very little iron will be taken up by the intestinal mucosal epithelial cell. In states of iron deficiency, increased amounts of iron will traverse the intestinal mucosal cell and pass into the circulation; while very little iron is trapped in the intestinal mucosal cell in iron deficiency states. Normal physiologic day-to-day iron absorption probably is regulated by transferrin or a transferrin-like protein when intestinal mucosal cell iron concentration is low. However, when the intestinal lumen contains high concentrations of iron, as when iron salts are administered therapeutically or in iron intoxication, when large amounts of iron are ingested accidentally by children, there is no mechanism to regulate iron absorption at such high concentrations. Thus, in iron overload increased amounts of iron rapidly traverse the mucosal cell to reach the plasma, perhaps by a passive process of mass action.

Iron plays a unique role in regulating the proteins ferritin and transferrin through messenger RNA for ferritin and transferrin receptors. There is a mRNA regulatory sequence called the iron responsive element (IRE)[17] present in the 5′-untranslated region of ferritin mRNAs and in the 3′-untranslated region of transferrin receptor mRNA. When iron is in excess, there is an increase in the synthesis of ferritin and an increase in iron storage. Concurrently, transferrin receptor synthesis is decreased and is correlated with a decrease in iron uptake. The translation of ferritin mRNA is enhanced by excess iron when the IRE is in the 5′-untranslated region. On the other hand, the presence of IRE in the 3′-untranslated region of the transferrin receptor mRNA apparently leads to an iron-dependent decrease in transferrin receptor mRNA. The mechanism by which iron acts in the ferritin and transferrin receptor mRNA is not known.[17]

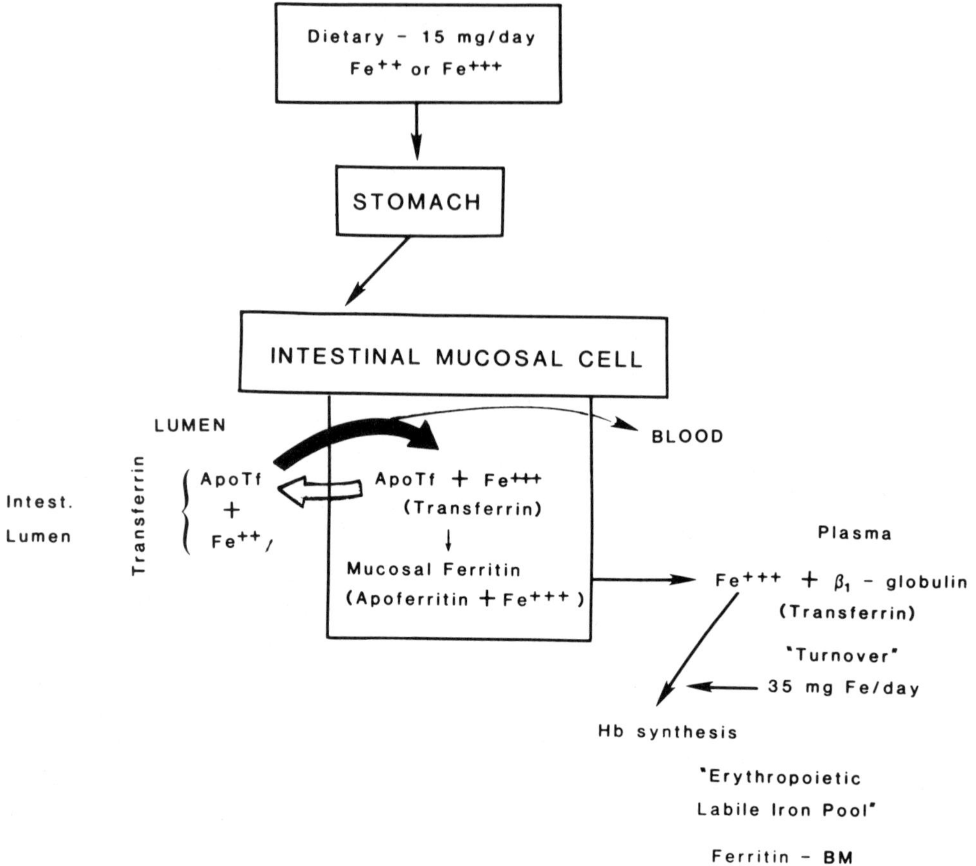

Figure 71.2 Absorption, Transport, Storage and Metabolism of Iron in the Normal Human Subject

One hypothesis for the mechanism of iron absorption is that the protein apotransferrin is involved[1F] (Fig. 71.2). This protein is present in the mucosal cell membrane and reacts with the ferrous form of iron to form transferrin in the mucosal cell. This increased amount of apotransferrin in the mucosal cell in iron deficiency signals a need for an increased amount of iron and enhanced iron absorption. Iron is partly stored in the form of ferritin, which is a high molecular weight protein complexed with the ferric form of iron in the mucosal cell. When ferritin levels are high in the mucosal cells, less iron is absorbed. When ferritin levels are low and apotransferrin levels are high in mucosal cells, this is a signal for increased iron absorption. Once iron reaches the blood stream in the ferric form, it combines with a beta-1-globulin in plasma to form a complex known as plasma transferrin, a transport form of iron in the blood stream. Iron is also stored in the liver and bone marrow as ferritin. Approximately 35 mg of iron is turned over through new hemoglobin synthesis each day in the average adult human. Day-to-day absorption of iron probably is regulated by apotransferrin, which is an active transport system operative at low doses of iron. However, when GI levels of iron are high, as when medicinal iron preparations are taken orally, glycine and serine may be involved in a second mechanism for iron absorption, which is a mass action effect involving passive diffusion. Even though the shuttle hypothesis for transferrin-mediated intestinal luminal cell uptake is very attractive, this mechanism has not been supported by some investigators.[19] Transferrin mRNA has not been demonstrated in mucosal epithelial cells from the small intestine of either normal or iron deficient rats.[20] Transferrin receptors have not been demonstrated on the brush border of mucosal epithelial cells.[21]

Transferrin is also important in the delivery of iron to hemoglobin-synthesizing normoblasts in the bone marrow along the following lines: (1) iron that is absorbed by the intestinal mucosal cell is deposited in the liver when transferrin reaches saturation; and (2) in certain congenital anomalies where transferrin is absent, iron absorption by the intestinal mucosal cell is increased and accumulates in such organs as the spleen, pancreas, and liver, and very little will ever have a chance to reach the bone marrow—which eventually leads to microcytic hypochromic anemia.

Iron Preparations

Ferrous sulfate (Feosol), which contains 20% Fe^{++} iron, is the least expensive and most often used of the oral iron preparations. Some common adverse effects of oral iron are nausea, upper abdominal pain, constipation, and diarrhea. Iron dextran (Imferon), is an IV form of iron. Intravenous iron may be necessary in severe iron deficiency anemia, iron malabsorption syndromes, dialysis patients, prolonged oral use of salicylates, lack of compliance with oral iron preparations, or when a GI disease such as ulcerative colitis is present. The dosage of IV iron must be calculated very carefully according to several formulae that are available.

Iron Toxicity

Approximately 5000 cases of iron overdose occur in the US every year.[22] Most iron toxicity occurs following accidental ingestion of iron-containing pills by children. The acute symptoms of iron intoxication are nausea, vomiting, and diarrhea. Those who survive an iron overdose will suffer from scarring of the pyloric sphincter and erosion of the stomach. The treatment of choice for iron overdose is gastric lavage with a phosphate solution to remove the unabsorbed iron. A specific antidote, such as deferoxamine (Desferal), is indicated in iron poisoning. Deferoxamine is administered in the gastric lavage to chelate any unabsorbed iron. The deferoxamine-iron complex is not absorbed from the GI tract.

Intravenous or IM deferoxamine may be used if systemic iron levels are high causing cardiovascular collapse due to the free form of iron present in plasma. The deferoxamine-complexed iron is less toxic to the vascular system and more readily excreted in the urine. Deferoxamine is also useful in the treatment of hemosiderosis or other iron storage diseases to remove the tissue storage form of iron. Deferoxamine will remove iron stored in organs such as the liver, spleen, and pancreas. British antilewisite (BAL) should never be used for iron poisoning because it forms a highly toxic complex with iron.

Sources of Iron

Foods that are high in iron (5< mg/gm) are liver, heart, wheat germ, egg yolk, oysters, and dried beans. The World Health Organization has reported hundreds of millions of people in the world with iron deficiency anemia: 10 to 20 percent of premenstrual females are iron-deficient, and 5 percent of males and postmenopausal females are iron-deficient. The minimum daily requirement of iron absorbed is 1 mg per day.

Therapeutic Uses of Iron

The sole therapeutic use of iron is significant iron depletion or deficiency, which can be caused by pregnancy, prematurity, blood loss, hookworm infestation, malabsorption syndrome, or GI bleeding due to such medications as aspirin. Recently it has been reported that excessive consumption of coffee (4 to 6 cups per day) can chelate sufficient iron to cause iron deficiency in people with low iron stores, as excessive tea consumption has long been known to do.

Vitamin B_{12} (Cyanocobalamin) and Folic Acid in Megaloblastic Anemias

The Nobel prize winning discovery of Vitamin B12 by Minot and Murphy[23] is one of the most interesting stories in the history of medicine. Whipple made the observation in 1925 that the liver was the source of some hematopoietic substance useful in iron-deficient dogs. Minot and Murphy[23] carried out their Nobel prize-winning experiments by feeding liver to patients with pernicious anemia. After several years, Castle labeled this liver factor as the "extrinsic factor," later discovered to be vitamin B12 (cyanocobalamin), and he identified a protein that he called "intrinsic factor" which was secreted by the parietal cells of the gastric mucosa and which made possible absorption of the "extrinsic (food) factor." Castle demonstrated that intrinsic factor deficiency was the cause of pernicious anemia.

Metabolic Interrelationships between Cyanocobalamin and Folic Acid

Vitamin B12 is present intracellularly as two active coenzymes: methylcobalamin (Fig. 71.3,*A*) and deoxyadenosylcobalamin (Fig. 71.3,*B*). Deoxyadenosylcobalamin is a cofactor that catalyzes the isomerization of L-methylmalonyl CoA, a critical event for the mutase reaction to form succinyl CoA, which is very important in both carbohydrate and lipid metabolism. There is a metabolic interrelationship between folic acid and vitamin B12 in this reaction. However, the methylcobalamin form of vitamin B12 is critical for the support of the methionine synthetase reaction, which is essential for the normal metabolism of folic acid. 5-methyltetrahydrofolic acid (CH3H4PTEGLU1) provides methyl donors in intermediary metabolism. The methyl groups contributed by 5-methyltetrahydrofolic acid are used to form methyl cobalamin and this methyl group from methylcobalamin methylates homocysteine to form methionine. Methionine is very important for normal DNA synthesis, which is outlined in Figure 71.3,*A*. Tetrahydrofolic acid is the acceptor of 1-carbon groups in the conversion of serine to glycine, with the resulting formation of 5–10 methylene tetrahydrofolate (5,10-CH2H4PTEGLU). This methylated form of tetrahydrofolic acid donates the methylene group to deoxyuridylate for the synthesis of thymidylate, an important reaction in DNA synthesis (Fig. 71.3,*A*). It is important to note here that the folic acid antagonist methotrexate, which is an inhibitor of dihydrofolate reductase used in cancer chemotherapy, will block this reaction and produce a folic acid deficiency and a megaloblastic anemia.

The mechanism of the peripheral neuropathy created by vitamin B12 deficiency has, over the years, been

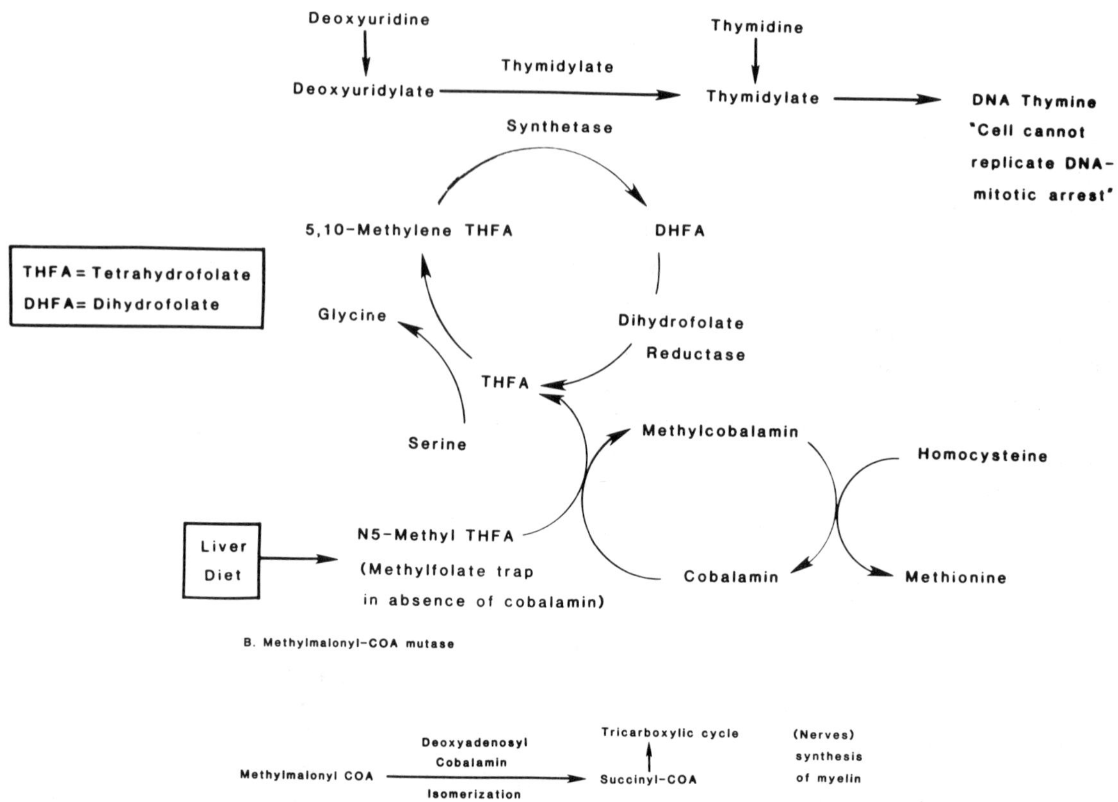

Figure 71.3 The Two Cobalamin-Dependent Reactions in Humans

unclear. However, it is clear that damage to myelin is the primary lesion in this neuropathy. A concept that has been held for several years involved the conversion of L-methylmalonyl CoA to succinyl CoA (Fig. 71.3,*B*). Deoxyadenosylcobalamin plus mutase is required for this conversion. However, a recent proposal that a deficiency in methionine synthetase (a homocysteine methyl transferase), which results in a blockade of the conversion of methionine to adenosylmethionine in the absence of deoxyadenosylcobalamin, is an important reaction that may also be involved in the decreased myelinization of nerves and peripheral neuropathy in B-12 deficiency.[24]

Both vitamin B12 and folic acid are essential in the human diet. A deficiency of either will lead to a defect in DNA synthesis. Thus, the necessary DNA synthesis for cells to divide and to replicate requires both cyanocobalamin and folic acid. Cells that are turned over rapidly, such as bone marrow and GI cells, are especially sensitive to the deficiency of these two agents. The damaged DNA synthesis in either vitamin B12 or folic acid deficiency results in a megaloblastic anemia. Large macro-ovalocytic red blood cells appear in peripheral blood in the severely anemic patient with B12 or folic acid deficiency. It is very important to understand in the management of pernicious anemia patients that folic acid will correct only the hematologic lesion, not the neurologic damage. Vitamin B12, when sufficient amounts of folic acid are present, will correct both the hematologic and the neurologic lesions in pernicious anemia.

Sources of Vitamin B12

Vitamin B12 is synthesized by organisms in the intestinal tract of humans. Humans do not produce vitamin B12 systemically.[r9] Foods that are high (>10 μg per 100 μg) in vitamin B12 are liver, clams, kidneys, and oysters. All animal foods contain B12; no plant foods do. Man requires 3 to 5 μg vitamin B12 per day from animal byproducts in the diet.

Gastrointestinal Absorption of Vitamin B12

Vitamin B12 is absorbed primarily in the lower ileum after oral intake. Gastrointestinal absorption depends on two mechanisms: (1) Intrinsic factor, a glycoprotein secreted by the parietal cells, is required for physiologic day-to-day (low-dose) absorption of vitamin B12. Intrinsic factor increases absorption of Vitamin B12 from the ileum, a process that requires calcium. (2) Approximately 1 percent of any oral dose of vitamin B12 is absorbed by a mass action mechanism (diffusion). This second mechanism is, of course, the mechanism by which the early observations that the ingestion of large amounts of liver by patients with pernicious anemia cured their megaloblastic anemia.

Vitamin B12 is required for normal growth of all cells, particularly cells that turn over rapidly, such as erythroid and myelocytic cells in the bone marrow and epithelial cells in the GI tract, cervix, and vagina. Vitamin B12 also is required for the maintenance of normal myelin in nerve sheaths. Transport of vitamin B12 in plasma is complexed to a plasma beta-1-globulin (transcobalamin II) for transport to tissues. Approximately 90 percent of vitamin B12 storage is in the liver. Pernicious anemia has the following symptoms: (1) megaloblastic macro-ovalocytic anemia; (2) soft raw smooth tongue due to the decrease in epithelial cell growth; (3) atrophy of gastric mucosa with no production of intrinsic factor by the parietal cells; (4) myelin degeneration and peripheral neuropathy, leading to numbness and tingling in the hands.

Therapeutic Indications for Vitamin B12

Vitamin B12 deficiency occurs in such impaired GI absorption states as malabsorption syndromes, pernicious anemia, following gastrectomy, after corrosive injury to the GI mucosa, and infestation with fish tapeworm. Fish tapeworm siphons vitamin B12 from the GI tract. Many claims for vitamin B12 are supported by no reliable data—such as its use in multiple sclerosis and trigeminal neuralgia. The widespread use of vitamin B12 solution as a tonic or placebo is to be deplored.

Vitamin B12 Preparations. Cyanocobalamin injection (Redisol; Rubramin PC). These are clear aqueous solutions with a reddish color. Most aqueous solutions available are in concentrations of 30, 100, and 1000 μg/ml. No adverse reactions have been reported after IM or SQ use of cyanocobalamin injection. It should never be given IV. There have been some rare anaphylactoid reactions after injection. Cyanocobalamin is administered in dosages of 1 to 1000 μg per day. A number of multivitamin preparations are marketed as nutritional supplements. They are "shot-gun" preparations, some containing vitamin B-12 and as many as 20 to 30 other nutritional supplements. These compounds are not indicated in vitamin B12 deficiency because they obscure the diagnosis, are expensive, and are unneeded medication.

Folic Acid

Wills described in 1939 a macrocytic anemia in pregnant females in India that responded to yeast ("marmitz"). Folic acid deficiency is usually the result of: (1) a decrease in folic acid in the diet (often by simply cooking it out); (2) impaired folic acid absorption from the GI tract; or (3) increased folic acid requirements. Folic acid deficiency due to decreased intake usually is due to poor nutrition—examples are the elderly in poverty, alcoholism, hemodialysis, premature infants, children on synthetic diets, and goat's milk anemia. Eating one fresh uncooked piece of fruit twice daily would eliminate the deficiency. Impaired folic acid absorption can occur in nontropical or tropical sprue, or in almost any other disease of the small intestine.

There may be an increased requirement for folic acid in pregnancy and such increased cell turnover states as chronic hemolytic anemia and exfoliative dermatitis. Megaloblastic anemia occurs in chronic liver disease and usually is at least partly a folic acid deficiency resulting from poor diet and decreased liver storage of folic acid. Ethyl alcohol itself may acutely depress serum folate levels, even in a subject with normal folate stores; it greatly accelerates the appearance of megaloblastic anemia in individuals with folate deficiency. Ethyl alcohol in large quantities has an effect on hematopoiesis, causing an acute marrow suppression and reduced numbers of circulating reticulocytes, platelets, granulocytes, reversible vacuolization of marrow red cells and white cell precursors, and functional impairment of granulocytes. These changes can occur even when pharmacologic doses of folate are administered with alcohol.

Sources of Folic Acid in Food

Sources of folic acid in food include yeast, egg yolk, liver, leafy vegetables, and many fruits.[r10] Protracted cooking can destroy up to 90 percent of the folate content of food. In general, a standard US diet provides 50 to 500 μg of absorbed folate per day. In the normal adult, the minimal daily requirement has been estimated at 50 μg; however, pregnant or lactating females and any patient with an increased cell turnover, as in hemolytic anemia, may require as much as 100 to 200 μg or more per day.

Absorption and Pharmacokinetics of Folic Acid

Folic acid is absorbed mainly from the proximal half of the small intestine. Folates in food are largely conjugated with reduced polyglutamates. Absorption requires transport and the action of carboxypeptidases associated with mucosal cell membranes. These carboxypeptidases split folic acid from its conjugated form in food. The mucosa of the duodenum and the upper part of the jejunum have high levels of dihydro-

Table 71.4 Clinical Parameters For Anti-Anemia Drugs

Generic Name	Proprietary Names	Preparations	Approx Dose and Routes
Filgrastrim (G-CSF)	Neupogen	Sterile, clear injectable solution 300mcg Filgastrim in water for injection with 0.59 mg mannitol, .004% Tween 80 and .035 mg sodium per ml, bufferol at pH 4.0 (single dose vial)	IV or SQ starting dose 5 mcg/kg/day as a per ml single injection. Admin no earlier than 24 hr. after cytotoxic chemotherapy
Sargramostim (GM-CSF)	Leukine	Provided as a freeze dried powder 250 and 500 mcg with 40 mg manitol, 10 mg sucrose and 1.2 mg tromethanine per vial. Add 1 ml water (sterile) to single dose vial for injection	The freeze dried powder should be dissolved in sterile water at a conc. of 500 mcg/ml no more than 6 hr. before use. Can be further diluted for IV infusion with 0.9% saline. When conc. is <10 μ/ml. Human albumin (0.1%) should be added to prevent adsorption of the cytokine to the wall of the vial.
Erythropoietin (Epoietin alpha)	Epogen, Procrit	Supplied in 1.0 ml containers with water for injection buffered at pH 6.9 and human albumin (2.5 mg/ml single use vials solution (sterile 2000, 3000, 4000 or 10,000 Units for IV or SQ use	50–100 Units/kg in patients with human albumin. Single use vials 2000, ESRD $T_{1/2}$ *Hours* for IV or 10 hr. in ESRD, SQ 5–24 hr.
Ferrous Sulfate (iron sulfate)	Feosol, others	Hydrated salt, FES04.7$H_2$0 with 20% iron per tablet, 200 mg dried ferrous sulfate (65 mg elemental iron); capsule, 159mg dried ferrous sulfate (50 mg elemental iron); Elixir, 5 ml (1 tsp.) contains 220 mg ferrous sulfate (44 mg elemental iron) in 5% alcohol	Adults—1 tablet 3 or 4 times daily, after meals; children 6–12 years old 1 tablet 3 times daily after meals 1–2 capsules per day; Elixir adult 1–2 tsp. 3 times daily, children 1–2 tsp. 3 times daily
Iron Dextran	Imferon	Viscous sterile–liquid complex of ferric oxyhydroxide and low m.v. dextran derivative in 0.9% W/V sodium chloride for uses; contains equiv. iron (as an dextran complex) per ml.	IV test dose ferric of 0.5 ml for possible anaphylactic reaction; IV or IM calculate dosage contains of 50 mg IV by formula: Total Gms Iron = If no allergic reaction to test dose, a total of 100 mg (2 ml) of undiluted drug may be given daily at a rate not exceeding 50 mg (1 ml)/min.

continued

folic acid reductase, which methylates most of the absorbed reduced folic acid. Some folic acid is absorbed from the proximal portion of the small intestine; when the jejunum is diseased, folic acid deficiency may occur.

Folic acid is rapidly transported and is absorbed as CH_3H_4PteGlu1. It is carried in plasma bound to proteins. In certain disease states such as uremia, cancer, and alcoholism, increased binding capacity of the plasma proteins occur that might affect folic acid metabolism. The enterohepatic cycle provides for a constant supply of CH3H4PETGLU1, which is maintained in food. After uptake in the cells by a process of receptor-mediated endocytosis CH3H4PTEGLU1 donates a methyl group for the formation of methylcobalamin that has as its source H4PTEGLUE. Folate is stored within cells as polyglutamates.

Table 71.4 *Continued*

Generic Name	Proprietary Names	Preparations	Approx Dose and Routes
Deferoxamine Mesylate	Desferal	Each vial contains–500 mg sterile, lyophilized deferoxamine mesylate; desferal is dissolved by adding 2 ml sterile water into injection vial to give 250 mg/ml	IM preferred route-1.0 gm initially then followed by 500 mg (1 - vial) every 4 hr. for 2 doses subsequent doses of 500 mg every 4–12 hr. depending on response; IV—only use in patients with cv collapse–rate of infusion not to exceed 15 mg/kg/hr; SQ daily 1.0–2.0 gm (20–40 mg/kg day) every 8–24 hr.
Cyanocobalamin	Redisol Rubramin PC	Solution-30 mcg/ml in 30 ml containers 100 μg/ml in 10 and 30 ml containers; 120 μg/ml in 30 ml ml containers; 1,000 μg/ml in 10 ml and 30 ml containers; oral-tablets 500 and 1,000 μg (nonprescription)	IM or SQ (deep) Adults–100 mcg daily for 5–10 days followed by 100–200 μg monthly until remission is complete; thereafter, 100 μg monthly will maintain remission; children–total of 1,000 to 5,000 μg given in divided doses of 30 to 50 μg/day for 2 or more weeks—thereafter, 100 μg every 4 weeks will maintain remission; oral–adults and children–6 μg daily (in vegans) for oral dietary supplements.
Hydroxocobalamin	Codroxomin	Solution—1,000 μg/ml in 10 and 30 ml containers (IM only)	oral–Adults and children 30 ml for maintenance of remissions in pernicious anemia–1,000 mcg twice weekly; 100 μg IM more sustained effect than cyanocobalamin- single dose maintains plasma levels for 3 months.
Folic Acid	Folvite solution	Solution–(injection equivalent to folic acid 5 mg/ml in 10 ml containers; tablets-Generic - 0.1, 0.4, 0.8 and 1 mg Folvite - Tablets 1 mg	IV, IM, SQ–adults 0.5–1.0 mg daily for most deficiencies—maintenance dose of 0.1–0.25 mg daily given orally; oral—adults and children—0.25–1.0 mg daily
Leucovorin Calcium (Folinate calcium) (citrovorum factor)	Wellcovorin	Generic - Powder - for injection –50 mg; solution (injection) 3 mg/ml in 1.0 ml containers; Wellcovorin solution (injection) 5 mg/ml in 1 and 5 ml containers tablets 5 and 25 mg.	Adults and children, for megaloblastic anemia, no more than 1 mg daily.

Drug Interactions and Folic Acid

A number of drugs may interfere with folic acid utilization. Dihydrofolate reductase inhibitors, such as methotrexate and pyrimethamine, produce folic acid deficiency because folic acid is not reduced and methylated and thus cannot donate a methyl group for intermediary metabolism. Ingestion of such drugs as phenytoin and the progestin/estrogen oral contraceptives may inhibit intestinal folic acid conjugases and decrease intestinal absorption of folic acid. Decreased absorption of folic acid also occurs in sprue, celiac disease, and after partial gastrectomy. In rheumatoid arthritis there is an increased demand for or utilization of folic acid.

Metabolic Function of Folic Acid

Major portions of the molecule of folic acid includes a methylene bridge to para-aminobenzoic acid with a linkage to glutamic acid (Fig. 71.4: chemical structure of folic acid). After absorption, pteroylglutamic acid is rapidly reduced at the 5, 6, 7 and 8 positions to form tetrahydrofolic acid (H4PTEGLU1), which then acts as an acceptor of a number of 1-carbon fragments. The intracellular metabolism and metabolic functions of folic acid are as follows: (1) Conversion of homocysteine to methionine. This reaction requires CH_3H_4PTEGLU for the donation of a methyl group in order for vitamin B12 to be utilized as a cofactor. (2) In the synthesis of thymidylate, CH_3H_4PETGLUE donates a methyl group to deoxuridylic acid, according to the scheme in Figure 71.3,*A* for the synthesis of thymidylate, which is rate-limiting in DNA synthesis. This cycle provides for a constant supply of CH_3H_4PteGlu1 that is maintained by food. After uptake by the mucosal cells by a process of receptor-mediated endocytosis, CH_3H_4PteGlu1 donates a methyl group for the formation of methylcobalamin. (3) Conversion of serine to glycine. This reaction also requires tetrahydrofolic acid as an acceptor of a methylene group from the serine and utilizes pyridoxal phosphate as a cofactor. (4) Histidine metabolism. Tetrahydrofolic acid acts as an acceptor of formimino groups. (5) Folic acid is also involved in the synthesis of purines and for the utilization or generation of formate.

Clinical Features of Folic Acid Deficiency

The clinical picture of folic acid deficiency includes megaloblastic anemia, glossitis, cytologic abnormalities of various epithelial cells, and elevated serum lactic dehydrogenase (LDH). Attempts to find the underlying cause usually will disclose a history of such circumstances as nutritional anemia and the absence of neurologic changes of the type seen in vitamin B12 deficiency. A full response after a physiologic dose of folate (200 μg daily) usually distinguishes folate deficiency from cobalamin deficiency, in which a response to folate occurs only at pharmacologic dosages (e.g., 500 mg or more daily). An early laboratory feature of folate deficiency is a low serum folate level. Low serum folate levels, below about 3 ng per ml, may indicate only negative folate balance, due to a drop in folic acid intake over the preceding few days, as might occur in the alcoholic. A good indicator of tissue folic acid reserves is the red cell folate concentration.

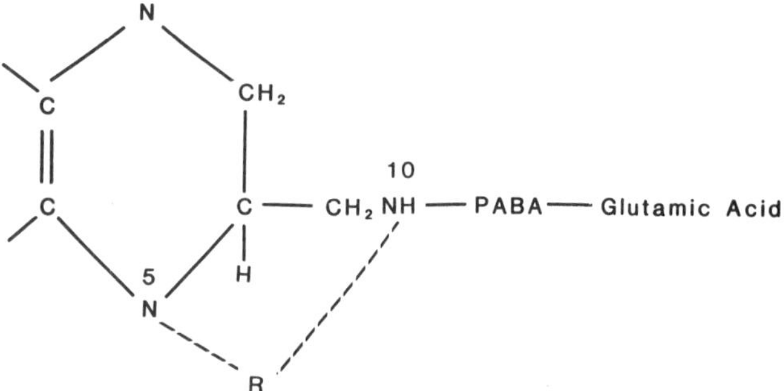

Figure 71.4 Chemical Structure of Pteroylglutamic Acid (Folic Acid)

Therapy of Folic Acid Deficiency

Folic acid usually is given orally in dosages of 1 to 5 mg daily. However, 1 mg is nearly always sufficient, and a hematologic response is seen even if malabsorption of folic acid is present. An injectable preparation of 5 mg per ml of the vitamin is also available. Oral folic acid of 1 mg two to three times per day usually will correct folic acid deficiency anemia. Folinic acid (N5-formyl-FH4) can be used specifically in treating toxicity due to the folic acid antagonist drugs used for cancer chemotherapy, which may block dihydrofolic acid reductase. Folic acid itself is not effective in the folic acid deficiency anemia produced by folate antagonist drugs because the block in reductase prevents the conversion of folic acid to the tetrahydro form. Folinic acid is already in the tetrahydro form and therefore is effective in spite of the dihydrofolate reductase blockade. The usual dose of folinic acid (citrovorum factor) is 3 to 6 mg per day IM. Larger doses may be required in chemotherapeutic regimens in which folinic acid is used to rescue patients deliberately treated with high dosages of methotrexate. This is called "citrovorum rescue." It should be understood that therapeutic doses of folate will partly correct the hematologic abnormality in cobalamin deficiency, but the neurologic manifestations of this disease will be improved only by B12 and not by folate. Folic acid alone is contraindicated in pernicious anemia because it will correct the hematologic but not the neurologic lesion, and large doses may actually accelerate the neurologic damage.

Preparations of Folic Acid Available

Folic acid (Folvite) is an oral preparation. Tablets of folic acid contain 0.8 or 1 mg of pteroylglutamic acid. Folic acid injection is available in an aqueous solution as the sodium salt of pteroylglutamic acid. Leucovorin (folinic acid, citrovorum factor) is available as an oral preparation or in a parenteral injection form as the calcium salt (Wellcovorin). The tablets contain 5, 10, 15, or 25 mg of leucovorin. The primary indication for citrovorum factor is to bypass the metabolic block produced by inhibitors of dihydrofolic reductase, such as methotrexate. Folic acid itself is not effective, since the inhibitors block it. Leucovorin should not be used in the treatment of pernicious anemia or other megaloblastic anemias caused by vitamin

B12 deficiency, because, like folic acid, it will produce a hematologic response but will not correct the neurologic damage.

References

Research Reports

1. Goodnough LT, Anderson KC, Kurtz S, Lane TA, Pisciotto PT, Sayers, Silverstein LE. Indications and guidelines for the use of hematopoietic growth factors. Committee Report. Transfusion 1993;*33*:(11), 944–959.
2. Recny MA, Scoble HA, Kim Y. Structural characterization of natural human urinary and recombinant DNA-derived erythropoietin. J Biol Chem 1987;*262* (No. 35):17156–17163.
3. Goldberg MA, Dunning, SP, Bunn HF. Regulation of the erythropoietin gene: Evidence that the oxygen sensor is a heme protein. Science 1988;*242*:1412–1415.
4. Eschbach JW, Kelly MR, Haley NR, Abels RI, Adamson JW. Treatment of the anemia of progressive renal failure with recombinant human erythropoietin. N Engl J Med 1989;*321*:158–163.
5. Kushner D, Beckman B, Nguyen L, Chen S, Della Santina C, Husserl F, Rice J, Fisher J. Polyamines in the anemia of end stage renal disease (ESRD). Kid Intl 1991;*39*:725–732.
6. Adamson JW, Eschbach JW. The use of recombinant human erythropoietin (RHUEPO) in humans. Cancer Surveys 1990;*9*:157–167.
7. Goodnough LT, Rudnick S, Price TH, Ballas SK et al. Increased preoperative collection of autologous blood with recombinant human erythropoietin therapy. N Engl J Med 1989;*321*:1163–1168.
8. Takahaski K, Totsune K, Imai Y, Sone M, Nozaki M, Murakami O, Sekino H, Mouri T. Plasma concentrations of immunoreactive endothelin in patients with chronic renal failure treated with recombinant human erythropoietin. Clin Sci 1993;*84*:47–50.
9. Vadhan-Raj S, Buescher S, LeMaistre A, Keating M, Walters R, Ventura C, Hittleman W, Broxmeyer HE, Gutterman JU. Stimulation of hematopoiesis in patients with bone marrow failure and in patients with malignancy by recombinant human granulocyte-macrophage colony-stimulating factor. Blood 1988;*72*:134–141.
10. Groopman JE, Mitsuyasu RT, DeLeo MJ, Oette DH, Golde DW. Effect of recombinant human granulocyte-macrophage colony-stimulating factor on myelopoiesis in the acquired immunodeficiency syndrome. N Engl J Med 1987;*317*:593–598.
11. Antin JH, Smith BR, Holmes W, Rosenthal DS. Phase I/II study of recombinant human granulocyte-macrophage colony-stimulating factor in aplastic anemia and myelodysplastic syndrome. Blood 1988;*72*:705–713.
12. Brandt SJ, Peters WP, Atwater SK, Kurtzberg J, Borowitz MJ, Jones RB, Shpall EJ, Bast RC Jr, Gilbert CJ, Oette DH. Effect of recombinant human granulocyte-macrophage colony-stimulating factor on hematopoietic reconstitution after high dose chemotherapy and autologous bone marrow transplantation. N Engl J Med 1988;*318*:869–876.
13. Komiyama A, Ishiguro A, Kubo T, Matsuoha T, Yasukokihi T. Increases in neutrophil counts by purified human urinary colony-stimulating factor in chronic neutropenia of childhood. Blood 1988;*71*:41–45.
14. Morstyn G, Campbell L, Souza LM, Alton NK, Keech J, Green M, Sheridan W, Metcalf D, Fox R. Effect of granulocyte colony stimulating factor on neutropenia induced by cytotoxic chemotherapy. Lancet 1988;*1*:667–672.
15. Glaspy JA, Baldwin GC, Robertson PA, Souza L, Vincent M, Ambersley J, Golde DW. Therapy for neutropenia in hairy cell leukemia with recombinant human granulocyte colony stimulating factor. Ann Int Med 1988;*109*:789–795.
16. Hartman RS, Conrad ME Jr, Hartman RE. Ferritin containing bodies in human small intestinal epithelium. Blood 1963;*22*:397.
17. Theil EC. Regulation of ferritin and transferrin receptor in RNAs. J Biol Chem 1990;*265*(9):4771–4774.
18. Huebers HA, Heubers E, Csiba E, Rummel W, Finch C. The significance of transferrin for intestinal iron absorption. Blood 1983;*61*:283–290.
19. Cook JD. Adaptation in iron metabolism. Am J Clin Nutr 1990;*51*:301–308.
20. Idzerda RL, Huebers H, Finch CA, McKnight GS. Rat transferrin gene expression: Tissue-specific regulation of iron deficiency. Proc Nat Acad Sci USA 1986;*83*:3723–3727.
21. Banerjce D, Flanagan PR, Cluett J, Valberg LS. Transferrin receptors in the human gastrointestinal tract. Relationship to body iron stores. Gastroenterology 1986;*91*:861–869.
22. Litovitz T, Normann JA, Veltri JC. 1985 annual report of the American Association of Poison Control Centers National Data Collection System. Am J Emerg Med 1986;*4*:427–458.
23. Minot GA, Murphy WP. Treatment of pernicious anemia by a special diet. JAMA 1926;*87* (Part 1):470–476.
24. Scott JM, Dinn JJ, Wilson P, Weir DG. Pathogenesis of subacute combined degeneration: A result of methyl group deficiency. Lancet 1981;*2*:334–337.

Reviews

r1. Finch CA, Huebers H. Perspectives in iron metabolism. N Engl J Med 1982;*306*:1520–1528.

r2. Robinson BE, Quensenbery PJ. Hematopoietic growth factors: Overview and clinical applications, Part III. Am J Med Sci 1990;*300*(5):311–321.

r3. Grosh WW, Quesenberry PJ. Recombinant human hematopoietic growth factors in the treatment of cytopenias. Clin Immunol Immunopath 1992;*62*:525–538.

r4. Fisher JW. Pharmacologic modulation of erythropoietin production. Ann Rev Pharmacol Toxicol 1988;*28*:101–122.

r5. Krantz JB. Erythropoietin. Blood 1991;*77*:419–434.

r6. Pagel H, Weiss C, Jelkman W. Pathophysiology and pharmacology of erythropoietin. Heidelberg: Springer-Verlag, 1992; pp 1–1328.

r7. Moncada S, Palmer MJ, Higgs EA. Nitric oxide physiology, pathophysiology and pharmacology. Pharmacol Rev 1991;*43*:109–142.

r8. Scrimshaw NJ. Iron deficiency. Sci Am 1991; October, 46–52.

r9. Herbert V. Vitamin B12, Chap. 20 In: Brown ML. Present knowledge in nutrition, 6th Ed. 170–178, Harper, Int. Life Sci. Inst. Nutri. Found., Washington, D.C., 1990.

r10. Herbert V. Development of Human Folate Deficiency, Chapter 11, pp 195–210, In: Picciano MF, Stokstard ELR, Gregory JF. Folic acid metabolism in health and disease. New York: Wiley-Liss, 1990.

r11. Mertelsmann R, Herrmann F. Hematopoietic growth factors in clinical applications. New York: Marcel Dekker, 1990.

r12. Metz J. Cobalamin deficiency and the pathogenesis of nervous system disease. Ann Rev Nutr 1992;*12*:59–79.

r13. Jelkamnn W. Erythropoietin: Structure, control of production and function. Physiol Rev 1992;*72*:449–489.

r14. Fisher JW. Regulation of erythropoietin production. Handbook of physiology, Section 8, Renal physiology, Vol. II, Chapter 51, pp 2407–2438. Oxford: Oxford University Press, 1992.

r15. Lee RG. Nutritional factors in the production and function of erythrocytes. In Chap. 7, Vol. 1, 9th Ed. pp 158–194, Lee GR, Bithell TC, Foerster J, Athens JW, John N. Lukens JN. Wintrobes Clinical Hematology Lea & Febiger, Philadelphia: London, 1993.

r16. Finch CA, Huebers HA. Iron metabolism. Clin Physiol Biochem 1986;*4*:5–10.

r17. Fisher, James W. Recent Advances in Erythropoietin Research. In Progress in Drug Research, Vol. 41, pp 293–311, Ed. Ernst Jucker, Birkhauser Verlag Basel (Switzerland), 1993.

CHAPTER 72

Roy L. Silverstein

Drugs Affecting Hemostasis

Hemostasis refers to a complex homeostatic mechanism within blood and on blood vessels that serves to maintain the patency of vessels after injury, while preserving the fluidity of blood. The hemostatic process is initiated immediately after vascular injury, and involves, in addition to contraction of the injured vessel, three sets of complicated, interrelated events:

(1) Adhesion and accumulation of blood platelets at the site of injury. This process forms a platelet plug and is called primary hemostasis.

(2) Activation of the coagulation enzyme cascade to generate a protein clot, of which the primary component is cross-linked fibrin. This process is called secondary hemostasis.

(3) Activation of an enzymatic system to solubilize the fibrin clot and eventually restore blood flow. This process is called fibrinolysis.

Each of these three systems is tightly regulated at multiple levels by interconnecting control mechanisms consisting mainly of enzymes (proteases) and protease inhibitors. Decades of clinical and basic research, much of which is still ongoing, have led to an understanding of these hemostatic mechanisms in fine molecular detail. Drugs affecting the hemostatic system can be categorized, as seen in Table 72.1, according to which of these three systems they influence and whether they inhibit or promote its activity.

Abnormal Hemostasis

Disorders of these systems or their regulatory mechanisms may result in increased bleeding (hemorrhage), either spontaneously or in response to trauma; or inappropriate clot formation (thrombosis). Thrombosis rarely occurs spontaneously; rather it is more likely on a background of diseased blood vessels (e.g., atherosclerosis or vasculitis) or diminished blood flow (e.g., stasis or atherosclerosis). Thrombi in the arterial side of the circulation tend to be platelet-rich (so-called white thrombi), while thrombi in the venous system tend to be platelet-poor (red thrombi). Embolism is the term used to describe vascular occlusion caused by fragmentation or dislodgement of thrombi from their site of origin, with subsequent migration to a more distal part of the circulation. Emboli from the venous circulation tend to become trapped in the pulmonary vasculature, causing the clinical syndrome termed pulmonary embolism; whereas arterial emboli tend to become lodged in the cerebral or extremity circulation, causing the clinical syndromes of stroke and gangrene.

Drugs Affecting Platelet Function (Primary Hemostasis)

Normal Platelet Physiology

After vascular injury, platelets quickly adhere to exposed subendothelial connective tissue matrix.[r1] This adhesion, as shown in Figure 72.1, is mediated by the binding of von Willebrand factor, a protein in plasma and subendothelial matrix, to a platelet membrane receptor termed the glycoprotein lb complex. Patients lacking this glycoprotein (Bernard-Soulier disease) or von Willebrand factor (von Willebrand disease) suffer

Table 72.1 Drugs Affecting Hemostasis

I. Drugs affecting platelet function
  A. Antiplatelet agents
    1. cyclo-oxygenase inhibitors
       aspirin
       sulfinpyrazone
       other nonsteroidal anti-inflammatory agents
    2. phophodiesterase inhibitors (dipyridamole)
    3. ticlopidine
    4. phospholipase inhibitors
    5. thromboxane synthetase inhibitors
    6. thromboxane receptor blockers
    7. prostacyclin
  B. Platelet promoting agents
    1. desmopressin
    2. conjugated estrogens
II. Drugs affecting coagulation
  A. Anticoagulant agents
    1. heparin
    2. vitamin K antagonists
       coumarins (warfarin and dicoumarol)
       indanediones
    3. ancrod
  B. Pro-coagulant agents
    1. vitamin K
    2. desmopressin
    3. danazol
III. Drugs affecting fibrinolysis
  A. Antifibrinolytic agents
    1. lysine analogues (EACA and tranexamic acid)
  B. Profibrinolytic agents
    1. urinary plasminogen activator (uPA; urokinase)
    2. streptokinase
    3. tissue plasminogen activator
    4. single-chain urinary plasminogen activator (scuPA)
    5. anistreplase

from a life-long bleeding tendency of variable severity. Interactions of other subendothelial glycoproteins, in particular collagen and fibronectin with their platelet surface receptors, also contribute to platelet adhesion. Coincident with adhesion, agonists such as collagen, ADP, or thrombin at the site of injury interact with specific platelet surface receptors to initiate a series of events termed "activation." These result in a change in the shape of the platelets from round and discoid to irregular and pseudopodal, secretion of granular contents (including calcium, ADP, fibrinogen, and serotonin), and surface expression of a functional receptor for the circulating protein, fibrinogen.[r2] As shown in Figure 72.1, each fibrinogen molecule can bind two platelets, thereby linking one platelet to another to cause the phenomenon termed "aggregation." Patients deficient in fibrinogen or the platelet fibrinogen receptor (the integrin molecule known as glycoprotein IIb/IIIa) may bleed excessively. ADP secreted by activated platelets activates other nearby platelets, resulting in the recruitment of more platelets into the site of injury. The net result of this activation, recruitment, and aggregation is the formation of a platelet plug adherent to the site of injury.

Among the earliest events after an agonist interacts with its platelet receptor is activation of phospholipase A_2, which cleaves membrane phospholipid to liberate arachidonic acid.[r3] Arachidonic acid is then converted by the action of cyclooxygenase to the cyclic endoperoxides, prostaglandins H_2 and G_2. Thromboxane synthetase then converts these cyclic endoperoxides to the primary prostanoid metabolite of platelets, thromboxane A_2 (TXA_2). TXA_2 is a potent vasoconstrictor and platelet agonist and is necessary for the platelet release reaction. Phospholipase C is also activated on platelet stimulation. This enzyme liberates inositol phosphate (IP_3) and diacylglyceride (as well as some arachidonic acid) from platelet membrane phospholipid. IP_3 is an important intracellular messenger and is involved in raising the intracellular calcium level, essential for platelet secretion and expression of the functional fibrinogen receptor. This intracellular activation cascade is summarized schematically in Figure 72.2. It is counterbalanced within the platelet by inhibitory systems mediated by cAMP and cGMP. Adenylyl cyclase, an enzyme within the platelet membrane, can be activated by certain platelet inhibitory substances, such as prostacyclin (PGI_2), to convert ATP to cAMP, which inhibits TXA_2 generation and platelet release. Similarly guanylyl cyclase, which converts GTP to cGMP, can be activated by endothelial relaxing factor (nitric oxide). Within the platelet, cyclic nucleotides are inactivated by the enzyme, phosphodiesterase.

Antiplatelet Therapy

The pharmacologic approach to inhibit platelet function can be understood in the context of the paradigms of platelet function described above. Two general approaches have been taken: (1) interrupting the complicated sequence of events by which a stimulus effects platelet "activation", for example by inhibiting the enzymes phospholipase A_2 or C, cyclooxygenase, thromboxane synthetase, or phosphodiesterase; or by activating adenylate cyclase; or (2) inhibiting function at the level of the cell membrane, for example by blocking fibrinogen binding to its receptor $GPII_b/III_a$ or vWF binding to its receptor GPI_b. Unfortunately, laboratory evaluation of antiplatelet therapy is unreliable and in-

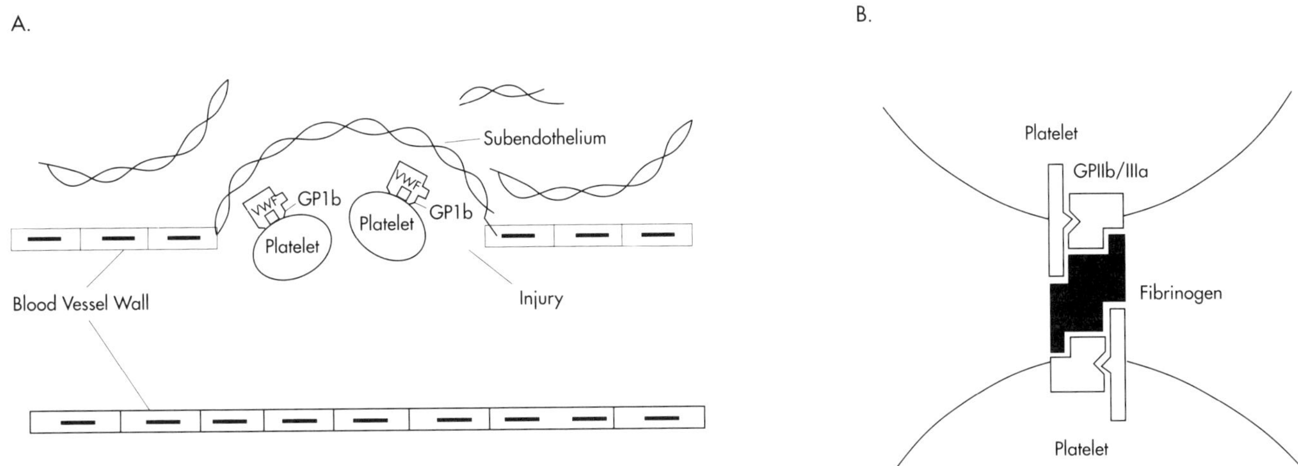

Figure 72.1 Molecular models of platelet adhesion and aggregation. (A) At sites of vessel injury, platelets adhere to exposed subendothelium in a reaction mediated by platelet surface glycoprotein Ib (GPIb) and von Willebrand factor (vWF), a glycoprotein present in the plasma and the subendothelium. (B) Upon activation, platelets express a surface receptor (GPIIb/IIIa) for fibrinogen. Each fibrinogen molecule has two independent binding sites for platelets so that adjoining platelets are bridged by the fibrinogen molecule.

exact. The best test of platelet function is the bleeding-time test, which measures the time taken for a standardized skin wound to stop bleeding. This test may be useful as a screen for platelet dysfunction, but is not, in general, useful to follow when planning therapy.

Inhibitors of Thromboxane Generation or Activity

Cyclooxygenase Inhibitors

These drugs, which are the most important antiplatelet agents,[r4] prevent generation of both the cyclic endoperoxides and TXA_2 and thus inhibit platelet release and the secondary phase of platelet aggregation. Aspirin (acetylsalicylic acid) is the most widely used and best understood of these drugs. Because aspirin irreversibly inactivates the enzyme by covalent acetylation, and because platelets cannot synthesize new proteins, the effect of aspirin persists for the life of the platelet (7–10 days). A single oral dose of 5 to 7 mg/kg, or one 325-mg tablet produces near total inhibition of TXA_2 synthesis lasting approximately two days, with slow recovery over seven to ten days.

Other NSAIDs, such as ibuprofen and indomethacin (but not the nonacetylated salicylates) also inhibit cyclooxygenase, although not irreversibly. Sulfinpyrazone (Anturane) is a pyrazole uricosuric compound structurally related to the NSAID phenylbutazone. At recommended doses of 200 mg four times per day it is a weak inhibitor of cyclooxygenase and platelet function.

It is important to realize that prostaglandin metabolism is not restricted to platelets. Many cells and tissues, including the vascular endothelium, also have phospholipase A_2 and cyclooxygenase; therefore, in response to stimuli, they generate cyclic endoperoxides. Endothelial cells, however, do not have thromboxane synthetase, and therefore do not produce TXA_2. Rather, they have an enzyme that converts the cyclic endoperoxides to PGI_2 (prostacyclin), a potent vasodilator and activator of platelet adenylyl cyclase. Thus, the effect of PGI_2 is opposite to that of TXA_2: it inhibits platelet function and relaxes vascular tone. A potential problem with the cyclooxygenase inhibitors is that production of both platelet TXA_2 and endothelial PGI_2 are inhibited. Thus the beneficial (antiplatelet and vasodilating) effects of PGI_2 are lost along with the anti-TXA_2 effect. This problem can be addressed by taking advantage of differences in sensitivity between platelets and endothelium to aspirin.[1,r5] Low doses of aspirin (1–2 mg/kg/d; 20–100 mg/d) seem to inhibit platelet TXA_2 generation selectively, while preserving endothelial PGI_2 production. This may be because nucleated endothelial cells have full protein synthetic capability and thus can synthesize new enzyme after the aspirin-induced acetylation reaction.

Phospholipase Inhibitors

Agents with antiphospholipase activity prevent the intracellular generation of arachidonic acid and thus inhibit platelet thromboxane synthesis. Local anesthetics and β-adrenergic blockers are weak inhibitors, while corticosteroids are more potent inhibitors. These drugs have been shown to decrease thromboxane generation and inhibit platelet release in vitro; however, in vivo no increase in platelet survival or in bleeding time ensues, and they are not considered good antiplatelet agents.

Thromboxane Synthetase Inhibitors and Receptor Blockers

To eliminate the problem of PGI_2 inhibition by cyclooxygenase inhibitors, selective TXA_2 inhibitors have been developed. Thromboxane synthetase inhibitors (imidazole and dazoxiben) have been disappointing in early clinical trials, probably because accumulation of the intermediary cyclic endoperoxides PGG_2 and PGH_2 stimulate platelet activation. Also being studied are agents that competitively inhibit the TXA_2 receptor, which has recently been identified and cloned.

Agents that Raise Intracellular Nucleotide Levels

Prostacyclin and Prostacyclin Agonists

Any agent that activates platelet adenylyl cyclase will raise intracellular cAMP levels and thereby inhibit platelet activation. PGI_2 and PGE_1 are natural prostanoids with potent antiplatelet effects. Although PGI_2 infusions have been used to decrease platelet activation on artificial surfaces (such as during extracorporeal hemodialysis), the instability of these natural prostanoids and their very short circulating $t_{1/2}$ limits their potential use as antiplatelet drugs. Stable analogues are currently under development and show great promise of being useful vasodilators and platelet antagonists.

Nitric Oxide

Nitric oxide (NO) or pharmacologic agents that generate NO in vivo also may have utility as antiplatelet agents by raising intracellular cGMP concentrations. The antiplatelet effect of inhaled NO gas may contribute to its beneficial action in the treatment of adult respiratory distress syndrome (ARDS).[2]

Phosphodiesterase Inhibitors

Phosphodiesterase inhibitors inhibit platelet function by preventing the breakdown of intracellular cAMP and cGMP (Fig. 72.2). Dipyridamole (Persantin), a pyrimido-pyrimidine derivative, is the best-studied of these drugs and is widely used as an adjunct to cyclooxygenase inhibitors.[r6] Alone, it is a weak inhibitor of platelet function, although it also has vasodilating activity by raising circulating adenosine levels. Some evidence suggests that dipyridamole inhibits platelet activation by artificial surfaces more effectively than by biologic agonists. It is usually given in oral doses of 75 mg three times daily, although absorption is highly variable. Metabolism is primarily biliary, with a component of enterohepatic recirculation. Although this drug is widely prescribed for its antiplatelet activity, clinical studies comparing aspirin alone to aspirin plus dipyrimidole have not clearly shown increased efficacy by the addition of the second drug.

Ticlopidine

Ticlopidine is a potent but poorly understood inhibitor of platelet function. It is a thienopyridine derivative with little in vitro activity, suggesting that its in vivo effect may be due to one of numerous hepatic metabolites. At recommended doses of 250 mg twice daily, platelet aggregation is inhibited by 50 to 70 percent and bleeding time prolonged by two to five times

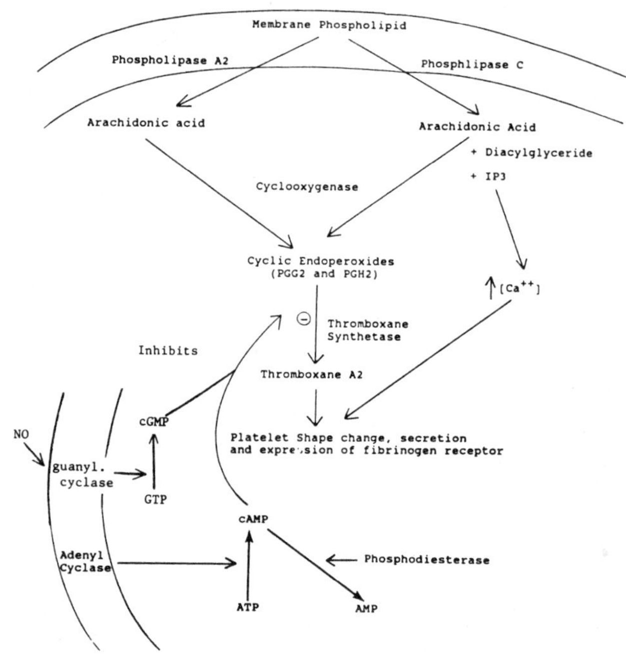

Figure 72.2 Intracellular signal cascades involved in platelet activation. Upon interaction of a stimulus with its receptor on the platelet surface, phopholipases in the cell membrane are activated. Phospholipase A2 liberates arachidonic acid which then undergoes sequential enzymatic modifications by cyclooxygenase and thromboxane synthetase to generate thromboxane. Phospholipase C liberates some arachidonic acid, as well as diacylglyceride (DAG) and inositol triphosphate (IP3). IP3 production leads to an increase in intracellular calcium concentration, which, along with TXA2 and protein kinases activated by calcium and DAG (not shown), bring about platelet shape change, secretion, and expression of the fibrinogen receptor. Counterbalancing this activation scheme is an inhibitory system mediated by cAMP. An inhibitory stimulus acting on the cell surface activates adenylyl cyclase within the membrane, converting ATP to cAMP, which inhibits thromboxane generation and platelet activation. Similarly, nitric oxide can activate guanylyl cyclase, producing cGMP, which also inhibits platelet activation. Phosphodiesterase within the cytoplasm metabolically inactivates cyclic nucleotides.

baseline. Platelets from patients taking this drug do not bind fibrinogen in response to most agonists, suggesting that they are incapable of generating a functional fibrinogen receptor. Although the plasma half-life of ticlopidine is eight to 12 hours, like aspirin, its antiplatelet effect persists for the lifetime of the platelet. While some studies have reported that this drug might be slightly more effective in preventing stroke than aspirin,[3] serious blood cytopenias have been reported, so that it is generally recommended only for patients who cannot tolerate aspirin or who do not respond to aspirin. Large studies have reported ~ 2 to 3 percent incidence of neutropenia occurring three to 12 weeks after initiation of therapy, with 0.8 percent of the episodes severe. In addition, thrombocytopenias and elevations of liver enzymes have also been reported.

Other Inhibitors of Platelet Function

Many drugs in common clinical practice, including β-adrenergic blockers, nitrates, calcium channel blockers, and local anesthetics can inhibit platelet function in vitro.[r4] In practice, most of these agents have no utility as antiplatelet therapy.

Indications and Benefits

Platelets are important mediators of pathologic thrombus formation, in particular thrombi that form on the arterial side of the circulation. Arterial thrombus formation is important in the pathophysiology of cerebral vascular disease, including stroke and transient ischemic attack (TIA); coronary disease, including angina pectoris and acute myocardial infarction (AMI); and peripheral vascular insufficiency.[r6] Platelets also play an important role in the development of the atherosclerotic vessel lesions that ultimately lead to heart attacks and strokes. These lesions develop slowly over many years (decades) and result from a complicated set of factors including heredity, hypercholesterolemia, hypertension, and tobacco smoke. Platelet activation at the vessel wall may be an early pathogenic event in atherosclerosis. Clinical studies examining whether long-term pharmacologic inhibition of platelet function could interrupt or lessen the atherosclerotic process are currently ongoing.

Platelet activation and consumption also have been reported in association with septic shock, ARDS (adult respiratory distress syndrome), membranoproliferative glomerulonephritis, and cancer metastasis. Antiplatelet therapy has been shown to benefit some patients with membranoproliferative glomerulonephritis,[4] while studies with animal models have suggested that some clinical aspects of shock and ARDS can be ameliorated by antiplatelet therapy, and certain types of tumor metastasis slowed. Adequate studies in humans have not been carried out. Antiplatelet therapy has been studied, however, in a variety of vascular diseases, and probable benefit demonstrated in at least six clinical situations:

(1) Secondary prevention of coronary or cerebral vascular events (i.e., stroke, TIA, MI, sudden cardiac death) in patients who have already had such an event. Trials involving well over 10,000 patients worldwide using mainly aspirin ± dipyridamole, or sulfinpyrazone[5] have demonstrated significant reduction in nonfatal MI (as much as 50%) and nonfatal stroke, as well as significant though smaller reductions in total vascular mortality (fatal stroke and MI). One aspirin/day (325 mg), with or without dipyridamole, is now recommended for most patients with angina[6] or who have had recent MI, stroke, or TIA. Unfortunately most of these studies showed significantly less benefit to women than men. For patients who can not tolerate aspirin, or who have a stroke while on aspirin, ticlopidine may be indicated.

(2) Primary prevention of coronary or cerebral vascular disease; i.e., for patients who have no clinical evidence of underlying atherosclerotic disease. Two prospective clinical trials have recently been reported: one in Britain and one in the US. Although the American study showed that, compared to placebo, aspirin-treated men (one 325-mg tablet every other day) had 47 percent fewer fatal and nonfatal MIs,[7] the British study showed no such reduction. In both studies a trend toward an increase in hemorrhagic stroke was observed.[8] At this point it is premature to recommend aspirin for all healthy middle-aged men.

(3) Improvement in postoperative graft patency in coronary artery bypass surgery.[9] Dipyrimidole begun preoperatively and aspirin begun immediately postoperatively improved graft patency after saphenous vein coronary artery bypass grafting. Benefit was significant both for short-term (30-day) patency and long-term (12-month) patency. The role of antiplatelet therapy in the prevention of reocclusion of nongrafted vessels after angioplasty or fibrinolytic therapy remains to be defined.

(4) Antiplatelet therapy has been used successfully as an adjuvant to thrombolytic therapy in the treatment of acute MI[10] to increase vessel patency and improve survival.

(5) Improvement in platelet survival and blood flow during extracorporeal circulation. Platelet activation on artificial surfaces during extracorporeal circulation (e.g., during hemodialysis, hemoperfusion, and heart bypass) contributes to both hemorrhagic and thrombotic complications of these therapies. Generally, blood is anticoagulated with heparin for these procedures, but prostacyclin has been used as a successful alternative for some patients during hemodialysis. The short biologic half-life of this drug minimizes the sys-

temic anticoagulant effect, particularly in patients with ongoing hemorrhage, as from peptic ulcer.

(6) Prevention of thrombotic complications in patients with valvular heart disease. The addition of antiplatelet therapy to systemic anticoagulation may decrease the risk of thromboembolic events in patients with prosthetic heart valves or stenosed native valves who have had emboli while on warfarin alone. Because the combination of aspirin plus warfarin is associated with a very high incidence of bleeding complications, dipyridamole is the most common choice of antiplatelet therapy in this setting.[11]

Complications of Antiplatelet Therapy

In large scale clinical trials of aspirin in the prevention and treatment of thrombotic disease, the major side-effects were dose-related GI symptoms, in particular epigastric pain, heartburn, and nausea. Gastrointestinal blood loss was common, and although mostly occult, frank hemorrhage was not rare. Aspirin-related gastritis and ulcer disease might result from inhibition of "cytoprotective" prostaglandin synthesis by gastric mucosal cells, while the propensity for these lesions to bleed is undoubtedly the result of inhibition of platelet function. Aspirin and the other nonsteroidal cyclooxygenase inhibitors, therefore, should not be used in patients with active or strong histories of peptic ulcer disease and/or GI bleeding. Gastrointestinal bleeding risk with these agents is substantially greater in elderly patients and those with disorders of coagulation; they should be used with caution in these groups. Unfortunately, commercially available buffered preparations of aspirin (Bufferin, Alka-Seltzer) do not have enough buffering capacity to be effective. Coated tablets ("enteric-coated") are absorbed more slowly and therefore expose the gastric mucosa to less aspirin than do standard preparations. Whether they reduce the risk of gastric symptoms or bleeding has not been well studied.

Other side-effects of aspirin are described in detail in other chapters. These include rash, nasal polyps, gout, and, with severe overdosage, tinnitus and acid-base disturbances. Sulfinpyrazone and the NSAIDs are associated with fewer GI side-effects than aspirin. The major side-effects of dipyrimidol are nausea and epigastric pain, which may occur in up to 10 percent of patients. Because it is a weak vasodilator, headaches are not uncommon. Side-effects of ticlopidine are described above.

Future Directions

Approaches to antiplatelet therapy are currently at an exciting frontier stage, both in terms of the design of new agents and in their broadening use. The development of new agents based on better understanding of the molecular mechanisms of platelet function should yield compounds of greater specificity and therefore fewer side-effects. This should be followed by broadening of the use of antiplatelet therapy to limit the morbidity and mortality of vascular disease as well as adjuncts to the treatment of other diseases in which platelets play a contributing role. Certain monoclonal antibodies to the platelet fibrinogen receptor, $GPII_b/III_a$, developed as a research tool, inhibit fibrinogen binding and are therefore potent inhibitors of platelet function.[12] Current trials in both animal models and humans are underway to test their utility in preventing platelet thrombi after occluded vessels are opened by angioplasty or fibrinolytic therapy. Fibrinogen binds to its platelet receptor via at least two domains in the fibrinogen molecule, one of which contains the "universal" integrin recognition sequence RGD (arg-gly-asp). Synthetic peptides containing this amino acid sequence also inhibit fibrinogen binding and platelet aggregation and are being studied. Similarly, a large class of anticoagulant peptides isolated from snake venoms also contain this sequence and are being studied.[13] A similar approach to inhibit platelet adhesion with monoclonal antibodies to GPI_b and synthetic peptides mimicking the vWF binding domain for GPI_b may also be of value as antiplatelet therapy.

Therapy Promoting Platelet Function

Desmopressin

Disorders of platelet function are very common. Most are acquired, usually due to drugs (especially aspirin and the NSAIDs), uremia, or cardiopulmonary bypass. Platelets from these patients share, in part, a defect in ability to secrete granular contents in response to agonists. This type of "storage pool" defect can also be inherited, resulting in a mild to moderate bleeding disorder associated with moderate prolongation of the bleeding time test. Recently it was found that the synthetic vasopressin analogue, desmopressin (1-desamino-8-D-arginine vasopressin or dDAVP), shortens the bleeding time in a large percentage of these patients.[14,15] The drug is administered IV over 30 minutes at a dose of 0.3 to 0.4 μg/kg body weight and has a rapid effect, shortening the bleeding time within one hour. The duration of effect is highly variable, but almost always lasts at least four to six hours, making it an ideal agent for preoperative prophylaxis. Because it is not possible to predict which patients will not respond to this drug, the bleeding time is usually checked one hour after administration to verify efficacy. The mechanism of its effect is unknown but probably relates to stimulation (via specific receptors on vascular endothelial cells) of von Willebrand factor (vWF) release.[r8] The released vWF is in a high molecular weight form that binds preferentially to the platelet surface and thereby facilitates adhesion and activation. This agent also causes release and elevation of coagulation Factor VIII levels, which will be discussed in greater detail below (see Procoagulant Drugs). Even though this drug has potent antidiuretic activity, side-effects are remarkably infrequent. Rarely, patients report mild, transient headache or facial flushing. Investigators have recently demonstrated that the use of desmopressin preoperatively or intraoperatively in patients with no known platelet dysfunction may decrease operative blood losses and transfusion requirements. This approach was used in complicated cardiothoracic surgery and in Harrington Rod spinal fusions with success,[16] but because of the preliminary nature of the studies it cannot yet be recommended for general use. Unfortunately, enhanced risk of thrombophlebitis has also been reported, probably as a result of the procoagulant effect.

Conjugated Estrogens

Infusions of conjugated estrogens at a dose of 0.6 mg/kg for five days (total dose 3 mg/kg) significantly shortened the bleeding time in patients with platelet dysfunction associated with uremia.[17] The mechanism of action of estrogens is not known. The effect was detectable six hours after the first infusion but reached maximum between days 5 and 7. The effect lasted ~ 14 days. This treatment was associated with no side-effects and thus may be a useful alternate to desmopressin.

Drugs Affecting Coagulation (Secondary Hemostasis)

Normal Coagulation

Circulating in blood plasma is an enzyme system, termed the "coagulation cascade," poised on activation by vascular injury to generate an active enzyme called thrombin. Thrombin, in addition to activating platelets and endothelial cells, converts the large soluble glycoprotein, fibrinogen, into insoluble polymeric fibrin (called a "soft" clot) by cleavage of two peptide bonds. Thrombin also converts another enzyme, Factor XIII, to its active form, a transglutaminase that crosslinks fibrin into a sturdier clot. The coagulation system is an excellent example of the type of physiologic regulatory mechanism known as a "sequential proteolytic cascade." In this type of system an inactive precursor (proenzyme) is activated by a stimulus to an active enzyme that then proteolytically converts a second proenzyme into an active enzyme. This second enzyme then acts on a third proenzyme, which acts on a fourth, etc. The advantage of this kind of system is amplification: a minimal localized stimulus can quickly generate a maximal response. By convention, the proenzymes of the coagulation cascade are designated by Roman numerals (e.g., Factors I through XIII) and the active enzymes by the subscript "a".

Thrombin is generated from its precursor, prothrombin (Factor II), by one of two different cascade mechanisms, termed the "intrinsic" system and the "extrinsic" system.[r9] The intrinsic system was so-named because all its components are contained within blood plasma; the extrinsic system can operate in tissues outside the circulation. Both cascades terminate in the formation of the active prothrombinase complex, which consists of an active enzyme (Factor X_a) and two cofactors (Ca^{++} and a protein, Factor V) assembled on a cellular surface (Fig. 72.3).

The intrinsic system can be activated in vitro by glass or highly charged surfaces, resulting in the sequential activation of Factors XII, XI, and IX. Factor IX_a, like the prothrombinase complex, forms an active enzymatic complex on cellular surfaces consisting of the enzyme plus two cofactors (Ca^{++} and a protein, Factor VIII). This Factor IX_a complex then activates Factor X so that it in turn can form the prothrombinase complex. It is not yet known exactly how the intrinsic system is activated in vivo, but recent studies suggest that Factor XI may in fact be activated by thrombin,[18] providing an additional amplification loop in the system. It is also possible that contact of blood with exposed charges on the injured vessel wall may be involved in activating the intrinsic pathway. The in vitro activation of this system by kaolin forms the basis of the clinically useful partial thromboplastin time (PTT) assay.

The extrinsic system is probably the more important in vivo activator of coagulation. After injury, blood is exposed to nonvascular surfaces, allowing a circulating protein, Factor VII, to interact with an integral membrane protein found on many cells, termed Tissue Factor.[r10] As shown in Figure 72.4A, a cell surface associated complex of Tissue Factor, Factor VII, and Ca^{++} then activates Factor X, allowing the formation of the prothrombinase complex. The Tissue Factor/Factor VII complex is also able to activate Factor IX, thus involving the "intrinsic" system in "extrinsic" activation. The in vitro activation of the extrinsic system by exogenous tissue factor forms the basis of the clinical Prothrombin Time (PT) assay.

The coagulation system is tightly regulated on multiple levels (Fig. 72.4B). Three of the critical blood clotting enzymes (Factors X_a, IX_a, and VII_a) are effective on a physiologic time scale only when assembled in complexes on membrane surfaces with protein cofactors (Factors V, VIII, and Tissue Factor respectively), thus speeding their activity where needed and limiting it where not needed. Calcium ions have a critical role in that many of the component reactions are either calcium-dependent or require calcium for the interaction of proteins with membrane surfaces.

Just as the amplifying cascades and proper presentation of enzymes on cellular surfaces have evolved to lead to rapid and efficient thrombin generation in response to injury, a protective mechanism has evolved to terminate thrombin activity and generation rapidly.[r11] This is very important since there is more than enough circulating prothrombin to clot the entire circu-

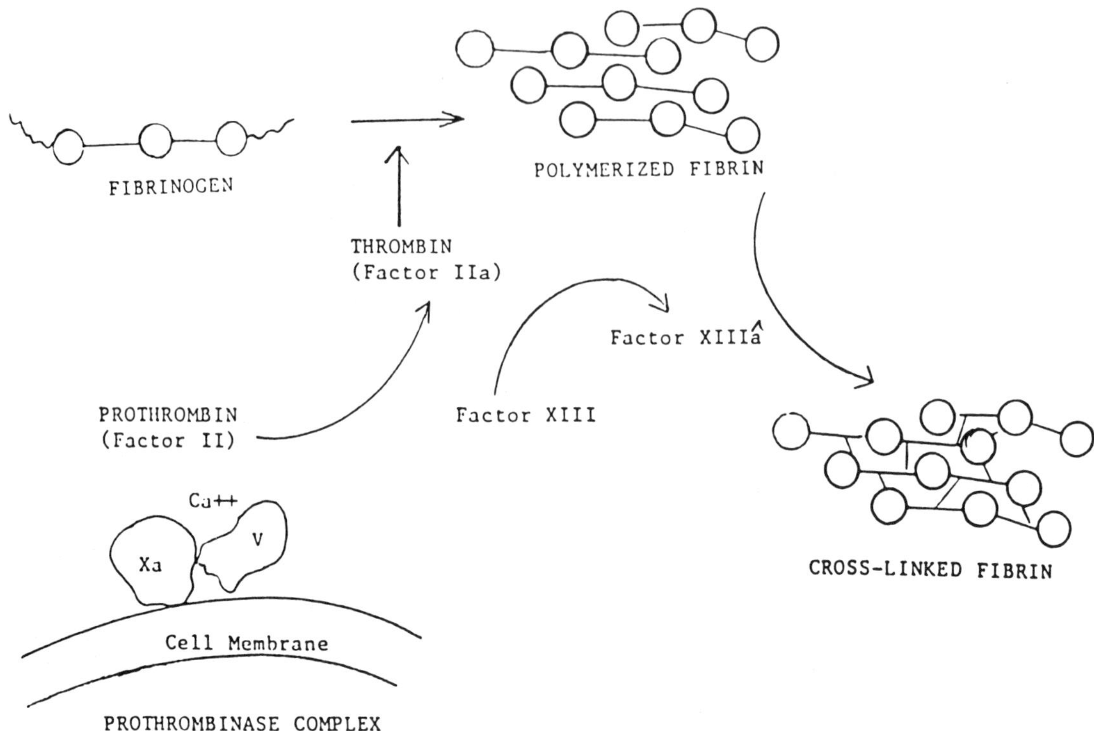

Figure 72.3 Terminal events of clot formation. The prothrombinase complex, made up of Factor Xa, Factor V, and Ca^{++}, associated with a cell membrane converts prothrombin to the active enzyme thrombin (Factor IIa). Thrombin then cleaves two peptide bonds in the soluble glycoprotein fibrinogen, resulting in its self-assembly into an insoluble fibrin polymer. Thrombin also activates the transglutaminase, Factor XIII, which cross links the polymerized fibrin into a hard clot.

lation. The primary mechanism to terminate clot formation is protease inhibition. Active proteases can be quickly inhibited by other proteins, termed protease inhibitors, via the formation of tight inhibitor-enzyme complexes. The major protease inhibitors of the coagulation cascade are anti-thrombin III (ATIII)[r12] and the Tissue Factor Pathway Inhibitor (TFPI). ATIII is one of a family of so-called "serpins" (*ser*ine *p*rotease *in*hibitors) that circulate in high concentrations in plasma. In the presence of heparan sulfate proteoglycans on vessel surfaces, ATIII effectively inhibits thrombin and Factors IX_a, X_a and XI_a. Other circulating heparin-binding proteins, including histidine-rich glycoprotein and heparin cofactor II, have the capacity to inhibit thrombin in vitro, although their role as in vivo anticoagulants has not been defined.

TFPI[r13] is a member of the so-called Kunitz family of inhibitors. It circulates in an inactive form in association with plasma lipoproteins. When Factor X_a is formed it enters a complex with TFPI, which then becomes a potent inhibitor of the Tissue factor/Factor VII_a complex.

In addition to these protease inhibitors, the Protein C (PC) enzyme system[r11] in blood, when activated, down-regulates coagulation by proteolytically inactivating the two essential protein cofactors of the cascade, Factors V and VIII. Activation of PC to PC_a occurs by the proteolytic action of thrombin. Thus, thrombin is not only responsible for forming fibrin and activating platelets, but also for turning off its own production. Circulating thrombin, however, does not activate PC; rather, thrombin binds to thrombomodulin, a protein on the surface of vascular endothelial cells, changing its specificity so that it no longer cleaves fibrinogen but instead activates PC. PC_a, in conjunction with a cofactor on cell surfaces, Protein S, then inactivates Factors V and VIII (Fig. 72.5).

Most proteins of the coagulation system are synthesized in the liver. The zymogens of six of them, Factors II, VII, IX, and X, and Proteins C and S, contain an unusual modified amino acid, gamma-carboxylated glutamic acid or "gla".[r14] Approximately 40 of these amino acids are clustered near the amino terminal ends of the molecules, where they serve to bind calcium ions and facilitate the interaction of the enzymes with phospholipid on cell surfaces. In the absence of the "gla" residues, these factors are inactive. As shown in Figure 72.6, the post-translational modification of glu to gla is accomplished by a vitamin K-dependent carboxylase.

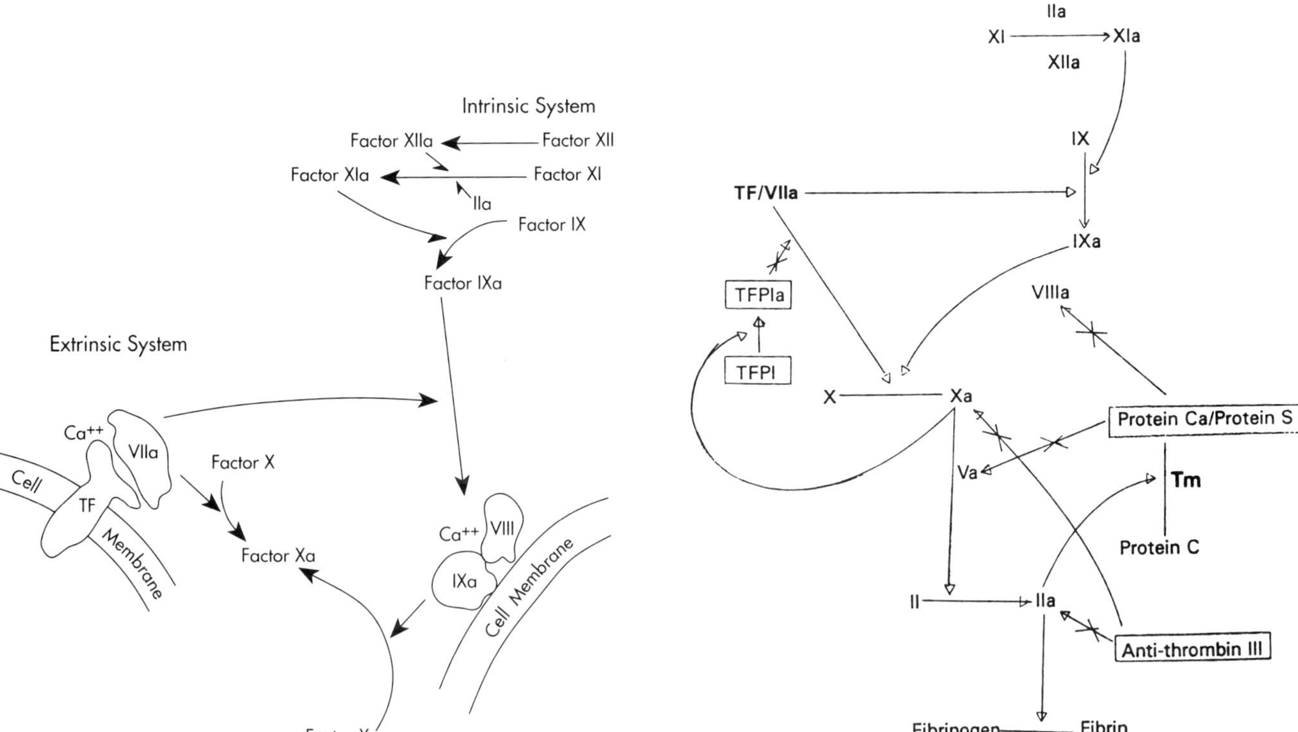

Figure 72.4 Coagulation cascades. (A) The extrinsic system consists of an enzyme complex made up of Factor VII (a plasma protein) in association with Ca^{++} and the transmembrane protein Tissue Factor (TF). This complex activates Factor X to form Factor X_a. Factor X is also activated by an intrinsic system via a membrane associated complex of IX_a and VIII. The major pathway of activation of IX is through the tissue factor/VII_a complex, although IX also can be activated through the intrinsic cascade by XI_a. Factor XI can be activated by thrombin (II_a) or by activated Factor XII. (B) The Factor X_a formed via these pathways then assembles on a cell membrane with Ca^{++} and Factor V and in turn generates thrombin (II_a) from the inactive zymogen prothrombin. Three major inhibitory systems (boxes) regulate the coagulation cascade. The Tissue Factor Pathway Inhibitor (TFPI) inhibits TF/VII_a and X_a; Antithrombin III (ATIII) in conjunction with heparin sulfate proteoglycans inhibits primarily II_a and X_a; and the Protein C system inhibits V_a and VIII_a.

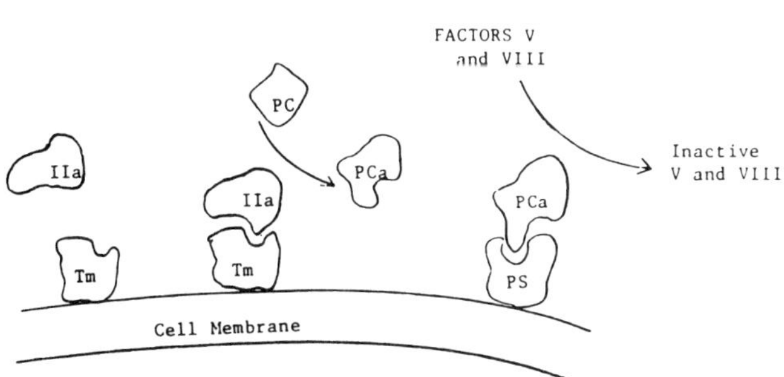

Figure 72.5 The protein C system. Thrombin (II_a) at the site of thrombus formation interacts with thrombomodulin (Tm), a protein on the surface of endothelial cells. When complexed to Tm, thrombin loses its ability to activate platelets and clot fibrinogen, but gains the ability to activate protein C (PC). Activated PC (PC_a) then forms a complex with protein S (PS) on a cellular surface and proteolytically inactivates coagulation factors V and VIII, thus down-regulating clot formation.

Abnormalities of the coagulation system can lead to excessive bleeding or thrombosis. Deficiencies of coagulation factors, either inherited (such as hemophilia A) or acquired (such as severe liver disease) cause excessive bleeding. Deficiencies of protease inhibitors, such as ATIII, or within the Protein C system cause inappropriate thrombosis.

Anticoagulant Drugs

Heparin

Heparin[r15] is a naturally-occurring acidic carbohydrate produced commercially from extracts of animal tissues, most commonly bovine lung or porcine intestine. It was discovered by J. McLean in 1916, a medical student at Johns Hopkins, first characterized structurally several years later by researchers in Toronto, and administered clinically for the first time in 1936. Heparin, as shown in Figure 72.7, is a polymer of O- and N-linked sulfated glucosamines and hexuronic acids (iduronic and glucuronic) joined by glycoside linkages. It is the most acidic organic acid in the body. The anticoagulant activity of heparin is the result of its high affinity interaction with antithrombin III.[r12] This induces a conformational change in

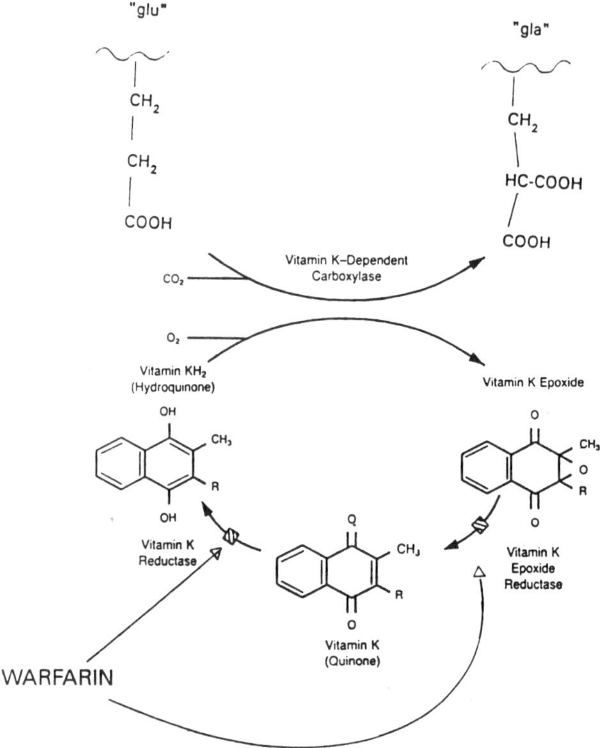

Figure 72.6 The vitamin K cycle. Glutamic acid ("glu") residues on coagulation factors II, VII, IX, X, PC, and PS are gamma-carboxylated to the "gla" form by the vitamin K-dependent enzyme gamma-carboxylase. In this reaction vitamin K is oxidized to a 2,3-epoxide form, which is inactive. The active reduced vitamin is then regenerated enzymatically by two enzymatic reductions. The coumarin anticoagulant drugs block this regeneration reaction.

ATIII and confers activity on the complex as a potent inhibitor of coagulation Factors II_a (thrombin) and X_a. In addition, Factors IXa, XIa, and XIIa are inhibited by the ATIII-heparin complex. Heparin is highly heterogeneous in size; commercial preparations contain heparins ranging from 2000 to 40,000 MW, with means ranging from 15,000 to 18,000 MW. Fractionation experiments have shown that most of the anticoagulant activity of commercial heparin is in the lower molecular weight forms. At least 16 to 20 monosaccharide units per molecule are required for full expression of anti-thrombin activity. This activity requires formation of trimolecular complexes of heparin, ATIII and II_a. In contrast, a bimolecular complex can form between ATIII and heparin that contains less than 16 monosaccharide units. This complex is an effective X_a inhibitor, and synthetic pentasaccharides have been produced that have anti-Factor X_a activity but no anti-Factor II_a activity.[r16] This is the molecular basis for the development of low-molecular heparin preparations as a therapeutic modality (see below).

Heparin: Indications and Benefits

Administration of heparin leads to the immediate prolongation of plasma clotting time, both in vivo and in vitro, lasting from three to four hours. Because of this immediacy of action, heparin is the anticoagulant of choice for acute thromboembolic disease. Its benefits are well-documented in four types of clinical situation:

(1) Venous thromboembolic disease. Deep vein thrombosis (DVT) of the lower extremities with pulmonary embolism results in ~ 50,000 deaths/year in the US. Anticoagulant therapy prevents clot propagation, decreases recurrent embolization, speeds recovery of pulmonary function, and decreases mortality of this disease.[19] Generally, patients are treated with heparin for three to five days for DVT and seven to ten days for pulmonary embolism. Oral anticoagulant therapy is usually initiated at the same time.

(2) Arterial thromboembolic disease. Heparin is used in the treatment of unstable angina and the clinical syndrome of stroke-in-evolution to prevent MI or stroke.[20] As discussed below in the section on fibrinolytic therapy, heparin is also used after thrombolytic therapy in acute MI[10] to prevent reocclusion of recently opened vessels. In addition acute anticoagulation with heparin is used in treating arterial embolism to the extremities and kidneys. Use of heparin in treating completed strokes and MI is controversial.

(3) Extracorporeal circulations. Heparin is used to maintain blood fluidity through extracorporeal tubing, as during hemodialysis, plasmapheresis, and heart-lung bypass. In these situations, the heparin is administered regionally; i.e., as blood leaves the patient and enters the tubing. Certain indwelling diagnostic and therapeutic catheters are maintained free of clots with regional heparin infusions.

(4) Prophylaxis of DVT. Low doses of heparin are administered to patients at forced bed rest to prevent formation of stasis-related DVT of the lower extremities. In particular, clinical studies have shown benefit for patients with acute MI[21] and for patients undergoing elective abdominal surgery and orthopaedic surgery involving the lower extremities.[22]

Heparin: Dosage and Monitoring

Heparin is available as both a calcium and sodium salt of bovine lung or porcine intestine preparations. It is prescribed based on units of activity, rather than mass, with 1 unit being defined as the amount of heparin required to prevent 1 ml of citrated sheep plasma from clotting for 1 hr after the addition of calcium. In clinical preparations, 1 mg is ~ 100 units of activity. Heparin is not absorbed through the GI tract, but can be given either IV or SQ. IM injections are not recommended because of the propensity to form hematomas at injection sites. When given IV, the onset of action is immediate; when given SQ, it is within 20 to 60 minute. The circulating $t_{1/2}$ is variable and depends on the dose administered. At doses of 100 U/kg, 200 U/kg, and 400 U/kg the $t_{1/2}$ are 1 hour, 1.5 hour, and 2.5 hour respectively. Metabolism is primarily hepatic and reticuloendothelial. No ideal laboratory test is completely satisfactory for monitoring doses, both in terms of efficacy of anticoagulation and risk of unwanted bleeding. Most physicians use a global test of coagulation, the activated partial thromboplastin time (aPTT), and adjust dosages to maintain the aPTT at a defined level, usually 1.5 to 2 times normal. In treating acute DVT or pulmonary embolism, a loading dose of

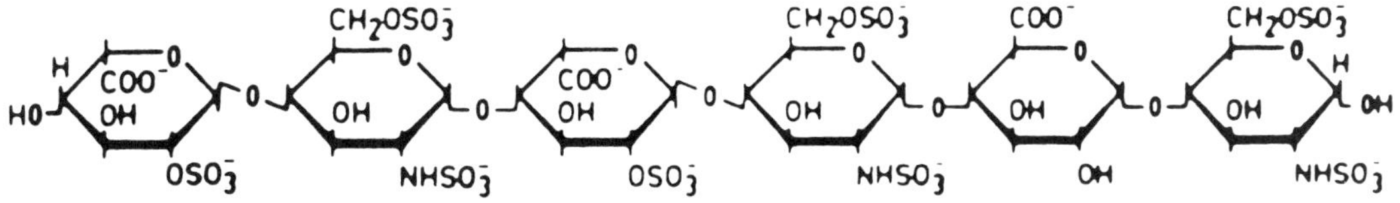

Figure 72.7 Biochemical structure of a representative subunit of heparin. Shown is a hexasaccharide made up of several different N- and O-linked sulfated sugars, polymerized via glycoside bonds.

50 to 100 U/kg (generally 5000–10,000 U) is given IV, followed by 20,000 to 50,000 U per day, either by continuous IV infusion[19] or as bolus injection every four to six hours.[23] The constant infusion method may be associated with fewer complications. Pediatric dosages are 50 U/kg IV bolus followed by 100 U/kg per four hour period, or 20,000 U/M^2/d. Heparin can also be used for long-term chronic prophylaxis of pulmonary embolism and DVT in patients who cannot take oral anticoagulants (see below). Doses of 10,000 to 15,000 U/day SQ in two or three divided doses, adjusted to maintain the mid-dosage aPTT in "therapeutic range" are as effective as warfarin.

The use of "mini-heparin"—that is, doses of 5000 units every 12 hours—is effective in preventing lower extremity DVT in certain hospitalized patients, as described above. This dose results in plasma concentrations < 1/5 those required to increase the aPTT by 1 1/2- to twofold, but is an effective inhibitor of thrombin generation.

Low molecular weight heparin preparations (4000 to 6000MW) isolated from commercial heparins by hydrolysis and chromatographic methods are now readily available.[r16] These preparations have greater anti-X_a activity per unit of anti-II_a activity than do standard heparins; in animal studies they have produced less bleeding for equivalent antithrombotic activity. Studies in humans have shown efficacy in the treatment of DVT and in the prophylaxis of DVT in patients undergoing general and orthopedic surgery.[22] Plasma half-lives of low-molecular heparins average approximately twice that of standard heparin.

Heparin: Complications and Contraindications

The most common and worrisome complication of heparin therapy is unwanted bleeding. Unfortunately, careful monitoring of dose to keep the aPTT in "therapeutic range" does not guarantee safety. Older patients, patients with coexisting renal disease, alcoholics, and patients with platelet dysfunction (e.g., thrombocytopenia or aspirin treatment) have a higher risk of bleeding complications.[24,25] Although bleeding is unusual during the initial 24 to 48 hours of therapy, as many as 8 to 10 percent of patients will bleed some time during their course of treatment. Heparin should not be given to patients with active GI bleeding, recent CNS trauma or surgery, or malignant hypertension; and should be used with caution in the high-risk patients described above. Recent clinical studies suggest that low molecular weight heparin preparations may be associated with fewer bleeding complications than standard heparin, with no loss of anticoagulant function. These studies are being continued on a larger scale in preparation for eventual marketing.

Should hemorrhage occur while a patient is being treated with heparin, stopping the drug is usually sufficient, since its $t_{1/2}$ is brief. For severe bleeding or overdosage, protamine sulfate can be given as a specific antidote. This is an arginine-rich mixture of basic peptides that binds to and inactivates heparin. It is available as a 10-mg/ml sterile injection and is given as a slow IV injection (no more than 5 mg/min). Each milligram of protamine will neutralize ~ 100 units of heparin. The $t_{1/2}$ of protamine is less than heparin, so repeated doses are sometimes required for massive overdoses of heparin. At doses above 100 mg in excess of heparin binding requirements, protamine has anticoagulant effects. Anaphylactoid reactions have been reported, as has thrombocytopenia.[26] Protamine is significantly less effective in blocking low molecular weight heparin preparations than standard heparin.

A frequent and sometimes serious complication of heparin therapy is thrombocytopenia.[r17] Up to 5 percent of patients experience a mild drop in platelet count within the first few days of treatment. This rapidly reverses when the drug is stopped. Bovine heparin is more frequently associated with this complication, so switching from bovine to porcine preparations is often sufficient to reverse the thrombocytopenia. A smaller number of patients experience a profound and rapid drop in platelet count in association with paradoxical acute arterial or venous thrombosis. This usually occurs after eight to ten days of heparin administration and can be life-threatening. Current evidence suggests that antiheparin antibodies are responsible for this syndrome, and that the antigen-antibody complexes may bind to and activate platelets, causing inappropriate aggregation and thrombus formation.[27,28] The thrombocytopenia is due to platelet consumption within these thrombi.

In addition to antithrombin III, heparin also binds numerous other biologically active molecules, including growth factors, matrix proteins, and enzymes. In practice, however, little effect other than that seen on blood coagulation is apparent. Heparin interaction with endothelial cell surfaces causes the release of TFPI and lipoprotein lipase, an enzyme that "clears" lipemic plasma. The physiologic significance of these effects is unknown. With prolonged heparin administration (> 6 months of at least 15,000 U/d) reversible osteoporosis leading to pathologic bone fractures can occur. Rare complications of heparin therapy include neuropathy and skin necrosis.

Oral Anticoagulants

In 1922 Schofield described a mysterious bleeding disorder in cattle fed rotting sweet clover. Seventeen years later Karl Paul Link and colleagues isolated and characterized a hemorrhagic agent from this material as bishydroxycoumarin (dicoumarol). This compound was then shown to exert its anticoagulant function by inhibiting Vitamin K, which had been described and characterized earlier by Heinrik Dam. Subsequently it was shown that Vitamin K is an essential cofactor in the biosynthesis of the gamma-carboxylated clotting factors II, VII, IX and X.[r14,r18] A large number of 4-hydroxycoumarins were synthesized in Link's lab at the University of Wisconsin, including warfarin (named for *W*isconsin *A*lumni *R*esearch *F*oundation), which has become the most widely used oral anticoagulant. Kabat, in 1944, synthesized another group of anticoagulant vitamin K antagonists, the indanediones. These agents have more untoward effects than warfarin and are not in widespread use.

Figure 72.6 shows the mechanism by which these agents inhibit vitamin K action.[r14] Dietary vitamin K is active only in the reduced hydroxylated or hydroquinone form, which participates, in the presence of O_2, CO_2 and a carboxylase enzyme, in the carboxylation of glutamic acid residues on the clotting factors to the gamma-carboxylated "gla" form. The carboxylase enzyme responsible for these post-translational modifications is an integral membrane protein. During this reaction the Vitamin K is oxidized to a 2,3-epoxide. The epoxide then undergoes two successive enzymatic reductions to regenerate the active vitamin. Both reduction steps are inhibited by the coumarins, resulting in "trapping" of vitamin K in an inactive oxidized form. Rarely patients are resistant to oral anticoagulant drugs because of a congenital deficiency of the vitamin K reductase.

Dosage

The development of the one-stage Prothrombin Time (PT) assay by Quick increased the therapeutic index of these drugs by allowing individualization of therapy via regular monitoring of the level of anticoagulation. This test measures the time for citrated plasma to clot after the addition of calcium and a source of tissue factor ("thromboplastin"), usually rabbit brain or lung extracts. It is a sensitive assay for coagulation factors II, VII, and X, and thus is very sensitive to the presence of vitamin K antagonists. Results will vary, however, depending on the source of the tissue factor. The WHO has introduced a standardized system of reporting prothrombin time values based on the determination of an International Normalized Ratio (INR) of thromboplastins against an international reference standard of human brain thromboplastin. It is now recommended to individualize oral anticoagulant therapy to keep the PT in a range so that the INR is two to three times control. In the US, with current preparations of rabbit brain thromboplastin, this represents PT values of 1.3 to 1.5 times control. With British thromboplastin, PT ratios are kept at 2.0 to 2.5 times control. For certain clinical situations, including patients with mechanical mitral valve prostheses, or patients who have had arterial emboli while on standard doses, INRs of 3 to 4.5 are recommended.[29] Table 72.2 summarizes current recommended INR levels for individual therapeutic indications.

Warfarin (coumadin) is rapidly and totally absorbed from the GI tract, whereas dicoumarol is erratically absorbed and hence not as reliably administered. Because of their mechanism of action, the anticoagulant effect is not immediate. Generally, two to three days will be required to achieve therapeutic anticoagulation. Usually 10 to 15 mg/day of warfarin or 200 mg/day of dicoumarol is administered until the PT reaches the desired level. The dose is then varied until daily determinations of PTs are stable at the desired level. Because of this delay in establishing effective anticoagulation, most patients are begun on oral therapy while still being treated with heparin. The heparin is stopped when a stable oral dose is achieved, providing continuous anticoagulation for the transition period. There is no increased bleeding risk with the concomitant use of heparin and oral agents. Most patients require 2 to 10 mg/day of warfarin or 25 to 150 mg/day of dicoumarol as maintenance. Phenindione, the only indandione in frequent clinical use, is given as 100 to 200 mg/d

Table 72.2 Drugs Affecting Response to Coumarin Anticoagulants

I. Drugs that depress response
   A. Stimulation of hepatic microsomal enzymes
      1. barbiturates
      2. diphenylhydantoin
      3. rifampin
      4. griseofulvin
      5. glutethemide
      6. other sedatives (chloral hydrate, ethchlorvynyl, meprobamate)
   B. Stimulation of clotting factor synthesis
      1. vitamin K
      2. estrogens
II. Drugs that increase response
   A. Inhibition of hepatic microsomal enzymes
      1. disulfiram (antabuse)
      2. methylphenidate
      3. phenyramidol
      4. chloramphenicol
      5. alcohol (chronic use)
      6. allopurinol
      7. phenothiazines
      8. tricyclic antidepressants
      9. cimetidine
      10. quinidine
   B. Displacement from plasma proteins
      1. phenylbutazone
      2. clofibrate
      3. thyroid hormone
      4. salicylates
   C. Increase in "receptor site" affinity
      1. d-thyroxine
   D. Reduction in availability of vitamin K
      1. broad-spectrum antibiotics
      2. mineral oil and other laxatives

loading dose and 25 to 100 mg/d maintenance. It is used infrequently in the US.

These agents have a long circulating $t_{1/2}$ (40 hours for warfarin) secondary to binding by plasma proteins (principally albumin). They are inactivated by hepatic microsomal enzymes. Because of their microsomal metabolism and protein binding, circulating levels are prone to change dramatically by coadministration of other drugs or superimposed medical illnesses that alter the availability of protein binding sites. For these reasons patients must be monitored periodically, even after a stable dose is defined, and other drugs must be prescribed with care. Table 72.3 outlines some of the more important drug interactions with the oral anticoagulants. Drugs that decrease response to oral anticoagulants include those that induce hepatic microsomal enzymes (barbiturates and dilantin). Those that increase the response to anticoagulants include those that inhibit microsomal enzymes (antabuse, chloramphenicol) and those that displace them from albumin (clofibrate, phenylbutazone). Broad-spectrum antibiotics or decreased food intake can increase response by reducing availability of Vitamin K, while exogenous Vitamin K can have the opposite effect.

Indications and Benefits

Because of their effective GI absorption and long $t_{1/2}$, warfarin and dicoumarol are the anticoagulants of choice for long-term (weeks to years) treatment and prevention of thromboembolic disease. Oral anticoagulant therapy is highly effective in preventing recurrent DVT and pulmonary embolism. Recurrent thrombosis is 70 to 80 percent less common in patients treated initially with heparin and then for several months with oral agents. Generally, treatment is continued for three to six months. Should thrombosis recur, treatment usually is extended to at least one year. These agents are also effective in preventing arterial emboli associated with cardioversion of atrial arrhythmias, and in preventing recurrent arterial emboli in patients with supraventricular tachyarrhythmias, in particular these associated with valvular heart disease.[30] In addition, oral anticoagulation therapy is used in women who have had TIAs and in patients with vertebrobasilar TIAs, conditions where aspirin may not be effective. Life-long anticoagulation with oral agents is necessary for patients with prosthetic heart valves to prevent thrombotic valve failure and systemic emboli. Controversial indications for oral anticoagulation include acute MI and dilated cardiomyopathy.[31]

Patients undergoing elective hip replacement surgery are at exceedingly high risk of developing thrombosis of the deep venous system of that extremity. Warfarin begun immediately preoperatively is effective in preventing these intra- and postoperative thromboses.[32] Recent interest has focused on long-term treatment with "mini" doses of warfarin in prophylactic settings. Studies are ongoing on the effects of 1 mg/day doses, which are well below those required to prolong the prothrombin time, in prevention of MI.

Complications and Contraindications

The major complication of oral anticoagulant therapy, as with heparin, is unwanted bleeding. This occurs in up to 25 percent of patients treated for long periods, with up to 7 percent of the episodes being severe. Risk is increased in patients with pre-existing hemostatic defects, so that these agents should be used with extreme caution in patients with thrombocytopenia or platelet dysfunction, and concomitant aspirin use should be avoided. Contraindications include recent neuro- or ophthalmic surgery, active peptic ulcer disease, active GI bleeding, and bacterial endocarditis.

Table 72.3 Recommended Anticoagulation Levels[28]

Indication	Minimal INR	Upper Limit INR
Acute DVT/PE	2.0	3.0
Long-Term DVT/PE Prophylaxis	1.5	3.0
Prevent systemic embolism		
Atrial Fibrillation	1.5	3.0
Mechanical heart valves	2.0	4.0
Tissue heart valves	2.0	3.0
Cardiomyopathy	1.5	3.0
Post-Myocardial Infarction	1.5	3.0

Use in patients with a propensity to fall, for example alcoholics or the debilitated elderly, is also not recommended.

Accidental or intended overdosage with these agents is not uncommon and can lead to severe spontaneous hemorrhage, including disastrous intracranial bleeding. Treatment of overdosage depends on the degree of overdose (as estimated by the prothrombin time), the presence of bleeding or neurologic symptoms, and the severity of the condition for which the anticoagulant drug was given. For mild overdosage (no symptoms, prothrombin time modestly increased) the anticoagulant drug can be withheld while the patient is closely observed until the PT is back to normal or back to therapeutic range. For more severe overdosage with no or mild symptoms, vitamin K can be given as a specific antidote (see below). For overdosage with more severe bleeding, fresh frozen plasma can be given along with Vitamin K to replete coagulation factors II, VII, IX, and X. For life-threatening hemorrhage or intracranial bleeding, lyophilized "Prothrombin Complex" concentrates (PCC) can be given while the frozen plasma is being thawed. These products contain Factors II, VII, and X, in addition to Factor IX. The use of blood-derived products, however, should be avoided if at all possible because of the risk of allergic reactions and of transmitting infections.

An unusual complication of the oral anticoagulants is skin necrosis, due to thrombotic occlusion of small dermal vessels, usually in the extremities, buttocks, abdominal wall, or breasts. This usually occurs early in the course of administration and may be due to the transient generation of a "hypercoaguable" state induced by rapid falls in protein C levels prior to the decrease in factors II, VII, IX, and X.[33] Patients with hereditary deficiency of protein C are at higher risk of developing this complication. To minimize the risk of skin necrosis, it is now recommended that therapy be started slowly; the older approach of administering a single "loading dose" (e.g., 30 mg of warfarin) is no longer used. Rather, a lower dose of 5 to 10 mg/d is given to establish therapeutic levels slowly. Other nonhemorrhagic complications of the coumarins, including allergic, are uncommon. The indandiones, however, are associated with significant side-effects, including rash, diarrhea, neutropenia, and thrombocytopenia. The coumarins cross the placenta and are teratogenic in the 6th through 12th weeks of gestation. They are therefore contraindicated during the first half of pregnancy. They do not appear in milk.

Ancrod

Ancrod is a defibrinogenating enzyme isolated from the venom of the Malaysian pit viper. It has been shown to be effective for the treatment of acute DVT, and, most recently, has been recommended for treatment of patients with the syndrome of heparin-induced thrombocytopenia with thrombosis who require immediate anticoagulation.[34] It is given at doses of 1 to 2 units/kg per 24 hours by IV infusion, with daily dose adjustment to keep plasma fibrinogen levels at 0.5 to 1.0 gm/L. Ancrod currently is not approved for use in the US.

Future Directions

As with antiplatelet treatment, advances in molecular and cellular biology have led to rapid development of new agents of potential benefit as anticoagulants and/or antithrombotics. These include recombinant proteins designed to mimic hirudin, a potent antithrombin found in the saliva of the leech. Purified or recombinant active Protein C is also being studied, as is a Factor X_a inhibitor discovered in tick secretions (Tick Anticoagulant Protein). Dermatan sulfate, like heparin a glycosoaminoglycan, has been shown to bind and activate heparin cofactor II, a thrombin-inactivating plasma protein. Dermatan sulfate has been successfully used in one clinical trial as a prophylactic antithrombotic during orthopedic surgery.[35]

Pro-Coagulant Drugs

Vitamin K

Vitamin K deficiency is associated with abnormal coagulation tests (prothrombin time) and increased risk of bleeding.[r14] Since this vitamin is primarily a product of enteric microorganisms, deficiency is commonly seen in hospitalized patients, particularly elderly, poorly nourished patients receiving broad-spectrum antibiotics. In addition, neonates and chronic alcohol abusers are frequently Vitamin K deficient, as, of course, are patients treated with oral anticoagulant drugs. Replacement therapy of Vitamin K deficiency is simple; Vitamin K_1, a synthetic, lipid-soluble form of Vitamin K is available in oral and parenteral preparations (Aquamephyton, phylloquinone (phytonadione)). Although oral absorption is slow and erratic, if the coagulation defect is mild, oral doses of 10 to 20 mg/day will correct the deficiency and normalize coagulation tests in two to three days. If more rapid correction is required, as in the preoperative state or in the presence of bleeding or severe prolongation of the PT, doses of 5 to 10 mg can be given SQ every six hours. This regimen will normalize levels in 6 to 12 hours. Intramuscular injections are not recommended because of the tendency to form hematomas at the injection site. Intravenous administration in the past was associated with hypotension and shock, but if given slowly by IV push, Vitamin K_1 can be given safely. Menadiol sodium diphosphate (Vitamin K_3) is a water-soluble derivative that can be administered either orally or parenterally. It is converted in the body by isoprenylation to the active form (Vitamin K_4). Since the alkylation step is inefficient, this form is not recommended for reversal of coumarin toxicity. For severe bleeding associated with Vitamin K deficiency or coumarin administration, fresh frozen plasma is given along with Vitamin K to replace missing coagulation factors. In treating overdosage of oral anticoagulants, Vitamin K therapy should be given every six hours for several days because the $t_{1/2}$ of Vitamin K is shorter than that of warfarin.

Drugs that Raise Coagulation Factor Levels

Desmopressin

This drug is discussed in detail above[r8] (see section on drugs promoting platelet function). In addition to its effects on platelet function, desmopressin (dDAVP or 1-desamino-8-D-arginine vasopressin), in IV doses of 0.3–0.04 μg/kg increases circulating levels of coagulation factor VIII and von Willebrand Factor by causing their release from endothelial cell stores. Intranasal administration of 150 μg in each nostril may be equivalent to IV infusions.[36] The increase is maximal at 90 to 120 minutes and persists for > 4 to 6 hours. Repeated doses at 12 to 24 hours are also effective, although a diminished response can be seen after 24 to 48 hours. This is presumably because of exhaustion of endothelial cell stores of these proteins. The degree of increase of von Willebrand Factor is usually two to threefold, while Factor VIII increases by four to sixfold. Response rates are high (64 of 68 patients in one study), but confirmation of efficacy by measuring postinfusion factor levels is suggested. This drug has been of substantial benefit in treating Type I von Willebrand disease and mild to moderate hemophilia, dramatically lowering or eliminating the need for plasma products for some patients.[37,38] Since purified clotting factors are generally prepared from pooled human blood plasmas, their use is associated with high risks of infectious complications, in particular hepatitis B and AIDS. Desmopressin has gained widespread use in the surgical management of patients with von Willebrand's disease.

Danazol

Danazol is an attenuated androgen derivative used for its anabolic and erythropoietic effects. Danazol affects the plasma levels of many proteins, including coagulation factors VIII and IX, protein C and antithrombin III. Current studies are underway to test this drug in patients with hypercoagulable states associated with Protein C, or antithrombin III deficiencies. Recent studies have shown that short-term administration of 600 mg/day for 14 days increased clotting factor levels in patients with mild to moderate hemophilia.[39] The increase induced by danazol, on average, was up to 15% of normal, a level adequate for hemostasis under many conditions, including mild trauma and dental work. The chronic use of danazol in these diseases is limited because of toxicity associated with long-term use, primarily hepatic and renal. Desmopressin is preferred for short-term or acute use.

Drugs Affecting the Fibrinolytic System

Normal Fibrinolysis

The fibrinolytic system[r19,r20] generates, in response to clot formation, the broadly active protease, plasmin, from its inactive precursor, plasminogen. Plasmin cleaves and solubilizes fibrin, thus restoring flow to the area of injury. In addition, plasmin may help disaggregate platelets and digest connective tissue during wound healing. Plasminogen circulates in high concentrations and can be activated by one of two enzymes, tissue plasminogen activator (tPA) or urinary plasminogen activator (uPA or urokinase). tPA, which is secreted by endothelial cells, is the more important intravascular activator, while uPA may be important in nonvascular plasmin production, such as by leukocytes during an inflammatory response. Activation of plasminogen by tPA is controlled at the kinetic level by the presence of its substrate, fibrin. In the fluid phase (i.e., blood plasma), tPA activates plasminogen very slowly because the K_M of the reaction is well above plasma plasminogen concentrations. In the presence of fibrin, as shown in Figure 72.8, a trimolecular complex forms between plasminogen, tPA and fibrin, increasing the reaction rate by several orders of magnitude. This complex formation is mediated by structures on plasminogen, called lysine binding sites (LBS) because of their affinity for lysine residues exposed on the fibrin molecule. uPA is less affected by the presence of fibrin and works better in blood plasma. uPA, however, is

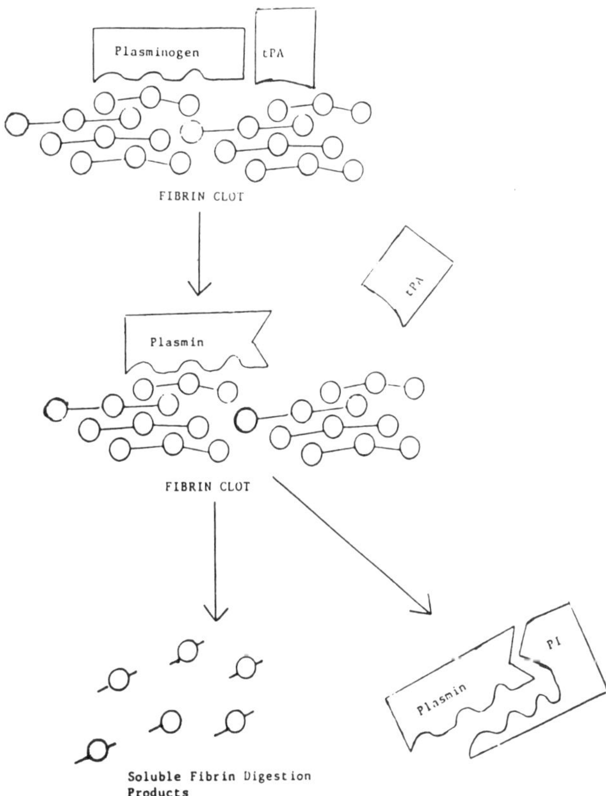

Figure 72.8 The fibrinolytic system. Plasminogen, the zymogen of the fibrinolytic system, binds to a fibrin clot via structures called lysine binding sites. TPA also binds to the clot (and to plasminogen) forming a trimolecular complex that then brings about rapid and efficient activation of plasminogen to plasmin. Plasmin remains bound to the clot, where it degrades the fibrin into soluble fibrin digestion products. On the clot the plasmin is protected from its physiologic inhibitor α2-plasmin inhibitor (PI), but once the clot is digested the plasmin is liberated and is quickly inactivated by α2-PI.

secreted from some cells in a single-chain form (scuPA or pro-urokinase), which is cleaved by plasmin into a more active two-chain molecule. This activation is facilitated by fibrin. The fibrinolytic system is also regulated by two specific classes of protease inhibitors. α2-plasmin inhibitor binds to and inhibits circulating plasmin, whereas plasminogen activator inhibitors 1 and 2 rapidly inhibit circulating tPA and uPA. Plasmin bound to a fibrin clot via its LBS cannot be inhibited by α2-plasmin inhibitor. This effectively limits the activity of the enzyme to the locale of the clot.

Profibrinolytic (Thrombolytic) Therapy

The major morbidity and mortality of thrombotic disease is due to vascular occlusion, with resultant tissue ischemia and infarction. While anticoagulant or antiplatelet agents can prevent clot extension and propagation, re-establishment of blood flow depends on the relatively slow processes of fibrinolysis and repair. The idea that rapid reperfusion and thus tissue salvage could be attained by infusion of plasmin or plasminogen activators, either systemically or directly into the occluded vessel, was proposed when the biochemistry of the fibrinolytic system was initially described. With the development of methods to purify and isolate pharmacologic quantities of plasminogen activators, large-scale clinical trials were undertaken throughout the world to test this hypothesis.[r21] Initial studies treated patients with venous thromboembolic disease (proximal DVT of the lower extremity and pulmonary embolism) with streptokinase or urokinase. More recently, multiple studies have tested fibrinolytic therapy with streptokinase, anistreplase (a derivative of streptokinase), urokinase, or tPA in arterial thrombotic disease, in particular, acute MI. These drugs are now an established and rapidly growing part of clinical therapeutics.

Indications and Benefits

Venous Thromboembolic Disease

If used within seven days of symptoms, approximately 65 percent of clots in the proximal deep venous system of the lower extremities can by lysed. Compared to heparin therapy, this is associated with more rapid symptomatic relief and fewer late complications (e.g., recurrent edema).[40] Large pulmonary emboli can also be lysed effectively with this therapy.[r22] Studies have shown greater reperfusion and faster improvement in pulmonary function, compared to heparin, if these drugs are given within one to two days of symptoms. Other venous thromboses have also been treated successfully with fibrinolytic therapy, including hepatic vein and renal vein thrombosis.

Arterial Thromboembolic Disease

A major advance in the treatment of acute MI was the introduction of fibrinolytic therapy. If administered within the first two to four hours of symptoms, either systemically or locally into the occluded coronary vessel, reperfusion can be established in as many as 80 percent of thrombosed vessels.[41,42] This is associated with improvement in left ventricular function and in over-all patient survival at both one month and one year after the infarction. Improvement in survival measured in several large studies ranged from 18 percent to > 50 percent in some subgroups of patients.[r20] Thrombolytic therapy has also been used successfully in treating patients with acute occlusion of renal, mesenteric, and extremity arteries.

Shunts and Catheters

Occluded indwelling venous and arterial catheters as well as arteriovenous shunts created for chronic hemodialysis can be successfully reopened by local infusion of fibrinolytic therapy.

Principles and Complications of Treatment

Because of the inherent danger of precipitating unwanted bleeding by the use of these potent agents, attention to three important principles of management is required for their best use:[r20] proper timing of drug administration; achievement of the "lytic state;" and minimization of bleeding risk. Because of cross-linking and other events, thrombi become more resistant to enzymatic lysis as they age. For this reason fibrinolytic therapy generally is not effective unless instituted soon after the occurrence of symptoms. As described above, clinical studies have shown that this is within two days of pulmonary embolism or five to seven days of DVT. In addition, irreversible tissue injury occurs within several hours of arterial occlusion, narrowing even further the "window of opportunity" for these clots. Fibrinolytic therapy is most effective when administered within four hours (preferably two hours) of symptoms of MI. To be assured that sufficient fibrinolytic therapy has been administered, it is necessary to demonstrate that the blood plasma has been converted to a "lytic state." This is verified by assuring that laboratory tests of coagulation are prolonged. Since "premature" destruction of intravascular clots is the mechanism by which these agents work, bleeding at sites of recent vascular trauma is their major side-effect. Unfortunately, neither efficacy nor bleeding risk correlate well with degree of abnormality of laboratory coagulation tests, although circulating fibrinogen levels < 80 percent of normal are clearly associated with some increased risk of bleeding. Minimization of invasive procedures and careful patient observation are thus essential to the proper use of this therapy.

Bleeding complications of fibrinolytic therapy are caused by more than the premature lysis of clots overlying damaged vessels. Infusion of plasminogen activators results in the generation of circulating active plasmin, which cleaves many proteins important in hemostasis. Fibrinogen is rendered unclottable and Factors V and VIII are inactivated, resulting in a hemophilia-like coagulopathy. In addition, platelet adhesion and aggregation may be inhibited by plasmin cleavage of platelet surface glycoproteins. The actual bleeding risk associated with fibrinolytic therapy therefore depends on many factors in addition to recent vascular injury. Dose and duration of treatment are perhaps the major variables. High doses given over short periods (for example in treating MI) cause more bleeding than low doses, even if given over longer periods (such as in treating pulmonary embolism). Underlying medical diseases and associated use of anticoagulants and antiplatelet therapy also raises the risk of bleeding. Most recent studies have reported minor bleeding complications in 3 to 5 percent of patients and major bleeding in 0.5 to 1 percent.

Because of the risk of intracranial hemorrhage,[43] contraindications to the use of fibrinolytic therapy include recent cerebrovascular accident, intracranial neoplasm, or recent cranial trauma or surgery (within 10 days). It should be noted, however, that clinical studies are now in progress to test the use of these agents during acute cerebrovascular occlusion. The risk of major localized bleeding contraindicates these agents during ongoing severe GI hemorrhage or recent major surgery. The presence of severe thrombocytopenia or coagulopathy also prevents their use. Should serious bleeding occur during fibrinolytic therapy there is no specific antidote. Since all currently available agents have short plasma half-times (see below), cessation of treatment is usually adequate. For life-threatening emergencies, fresh frozen plasma can reverse the coagulopathy and the lytic state by repleting coagulation factors and $\alpha 2$-plasmin inhibitor.

Nonhemorrhagic complications of fibrinolytic therapy are quite unusual. Since all these agents are proteins, allergic reactions are possible. In practice, only streptokinase and anistreplase are associated with allergic reactions, which are of three types. Serum-sickness-like symptoms (fever, rash, and nausea) are common, but true anaphylaxis is rare (< 0.1% of patients). Some patients have neutralizing antistreptokinase antibodies in their plasma, making them refractory to this agent.

Fibrinolytic Agents

Streptokinase

Streptokinase, the first fibrinolytic drug to be used clinically, is a 46 kD protein extracted from Group C β-hemolytic streptococci. It is not a direct activator of plasminogen. A stable 1:1 stoichiometric complex, however, forms between streptokinase and plasminogen, which then acts enzymatically to cleave free plasminogen to its active form. As described above, a unique feature of this drug is its antigenicity. Streptokinase is administered either IV or directly into an occluded vessel and has a $t_{1/2}$ in the circulation of ~ 23 min. Typical dosages for venous or pulmonary thrombosis are a loading dose of 250,000 units followed by an infusion of 100,000 units/hr for 12 to 24 hours. For MI, 1.5 million units are given IV over 1 hour or 10 to 30,000 units directly into the occluded coronary artery, followed by 2 to 4000 units/hr.[41,42]

Urokinase

Urokinase (uPA) is a 34 kD protein prepared either by recombinant technology or from human fetal kidney cells in tissue culture. It is also administered either IV or directly into an occluded vessel and has a $t_{1/2}$ in the circulation of ~ 16 min. Urokinase is more potent than streptokinase and is not antigenic. Typical dosages for venous and pulmonary disease are 4 to 5000 units/kg as an IV bolus (over 20 minutes), followed by a continuous infusion of 4 to 5000 units/kg/hr for 12 to 24 hours.[40] For MI, doses of 2 to 3 million units IV have been used.[44]

Tissue Plasminogen Activator (Alteplase)

The pharmacologic preparation of human tPA is a 65 kD single-chain enzyme produced by recombinant technology.[r23] An earlier version was a two-chain version of the same enzyme. Since efficient tPA activation of plasminogen occurs only in the presence of fibrin (see above), tremendous enthusiasm was generated for this drug by the medical and financial communities. This fibrin dependence led to predictions that tPA would be a "clot specific" drug; i.e., it would lead to efficient local clot lysis but would not generate circulating plasmin, with its attendant coagulopathy and bleeding risks. Unfortunately, clinical studies have shown little difference in bleeding complications when tPA is used, compared to streptokinase or urokinase. This may relate to the doses of tPA used as well as to emerging evidence that other biologic surfaces (such as leukocyte, platelet, and endothelial cell membranes) in addition to fibrin can facilitate plasminogen activation by tPA.[45] TPA has a short $t_{1/2}$ in the circulation of 3.6 to 4.6 min, and therefore should be given as a continuous infusion, either IV or directly into the occluded vessel. The current recommended dosage for MI[41–44] is 100 mg (if body weight is > 65Kg) or 1.25 mg/kg (if body weight is < 65kg) given IV over a three-hour period. Higher doses led to only slightly greater reperfusion rates, with a significantly higher risk of bleeding complications, including a 1.6 percent incidence of intracranial hemorrhage in one study (compared with ~ 0.5% for the lower dose). Dosages for treatment of pulmonary embolism or DVT have not yet been established.

Anistreplase

A derivatized streptokinase-lys-plasminogen complex (anisoylated lysplasminogen-streptokinase complex; APSAC) is now available and is approved by the FDA for the treatment of acute MI.[46] It is inactive, and resistant to inhibitors, but binds fibrin where it is deacylated and becomes active. Since the deacylation proceeds at a slow, controlled rate, the drug has a prolonged effective $t_{1/2}$ of 105 to 120 minutes. Therefore, unlike other fibrinolytic drugs, it can be given as a single bolus, usually 30 units over 2 to 5 min. It may have somewhat greater fibrin selectivity than streptokinase.

scuPA

Recombinant forms of single-chain urokinase (scuPA) have been produced and used in limited clinical trials for treatment of acute MI.[47] Since the conversion of the poorly active scuPA to highly active uPA is facilitated by fibrin, this drug may be more fibrin-specific than urokinase.

Agents Under Development

Much research effort is being put into the development of new fibrinolytic agents, in particular ones that might be safer (less bleeding) and more effective (e.g., lyse older clots). One goal is to make a truly fibrin-specific agent with recombinant technology by combining the enzymatic domain of a plasminogen activator with highly specific fibrin binding moieties, such as monoclonal antifibrin antibodies. Attempts to create activators that can be administered by routes other than intravenous or with longer circulating $t_{1/2}$ are also underway.

Clinical Agents of Choice

Results of multiple large clinical trials of fibrinolytic agents in the treatment of both venous and arterial thromboembolic disease do not clearly favor the use of one agent over another. In acute MI, reperfusion rates, preservation of left ventricular function and improvements in over-all survival have been similar with streptokinase, anistreplase, urokinase, and tPA, although clots may lyse more rapidly with tPA.[r24] In spite of predictions based on in vitro observations, bleeding complications have not differed among the available agents. Table 72.4 summarizes the key differences among these agents; cost, antigenicity, circulating $t_{1/2}$, and theoretical fibrin specificity.

Antifibrinolytic Therapy

Complex formation between plasminogen and fibrin, mediated by the plasminogen lysine binding sites, is a critical feature in normal fibrinolysis. Lysine is a competitive inhibitor of this interaction and thereby inhibits fibrinolysis.[48] Two amino acid analogues of lysine, ε-amino caproic acid (EACA, aminocaproic acid) and tranexamic acid, have been developed for clinical use as antifibrinolytic agents.[49] Both are rapidly absorbed through the GI system, although tranexamic acid is ten times more potent than EACA. At high concentrations ($> 5 \times 10^{-2}$M) EACA, unlike tranexamic acid, also directly inhibits the active enzyme plasmin. This concentration, however, is 100 to 500 times that necessary to effect inhibition of plasminogen activation.

Indications and Benefits

The antifibrinolytic amino acids are used mostly to help control bleeding either due to excessive fibrinolysis or deficient coagulation. In the latter case their efficacy reflects the importance of an ongoing balance between clot formation and dissolution in normal hemostasis. In particular, these drugs are useful adjuncts to factor replacement therapy for patients with hemophilia or von Willebrand's Disease who are undergoing dental surgery. Their use is associated with less blood loss and less required factor replacement. Similar efficacy has been shown for patients with artificial heart valves chronically anticoagulated with warfarin.[49] Excessive bleeding after prostatic or uterine surgery often responds to these drugs. Since these tissues are rich in plasminogen activator, bleeding may be the result of pathologic activation of the fibrinolytic system. Bleeding disorders precipitated by extracorporeal heart-lung bypass, burns, and heat stroke may also be associated

Table 72.4 Comparison of Available Fibrinolytic Agents

Agent	$t_{1/2}$	Fibrin Specificity	Antigenicity	Cost AMI*/ PE**
uPA	16 min	+	–	$2300/$290
SK	23 min	–	++	$340/$95
tPA	<5 min	++++	–	$2230
scuPA	7 min	++	–	NA
anistreplase	90 min	+	++	$1675

*Approximate cost to hospital pharmacy of treating acute myocardial infarction using recommended doses of 1.5 million units SK, 100mg tPA or 2 million units urokinase.

**Approximate cost to hospital pharmacy of treating pulmonary embolism with recommended doses of 750, 000 units of SK or 250,000 units of urokinase. Costs are per event.

with primary fibrinolysis and may respond to these agents. Although EACA has been used to prevent rebleeding in patients with subarachnoid hemorrhage due to ruptured aneurysms, controlled clinical trials have shown no benefit.

Dosage

Both EACA and tranexamic acid can be given orally, IV, or topically (as a mouthwash). EACA is administered by giving a 4 to 6-gm loading dose followed by 2 to 4 gm every four hours or 1 gm/hr as a constant infusion. Pediatric dosages are 100 mg/kg or 3 gm/M^2 as a loading dose then 33 mg/kg/hr or 1 gm/M^2/hr, not to exceed 18 gm/24h. Tranexamic acid is given as 30 to 50-mg/kg loading dose followed by 10 mg/kg three times per day. Treatment for dental surgery is usually given orally and continued for seven to ten days, although mouthwashes four times per day have also been used successfully.

Complications

These drugs have relatively few side-effects, although they have rarely caused GI upset, muscle necrosis, or impotence. Their greatest risk is precipitating unwanted thrombosis by tipping the coagulation-lysis balance in favor of clot formation. This has been noted, in particular, within the renal collecting system if these agents are given during active hematuria. Patients with compensated ("masked") disseminated intravascular coagulation are at risk of systemic thrombosis if given these drugs. At high doses (> 24 gm/d) EACA inhibits platelet function and can cause bleeding.

References

Research Reports

1. Weksler BB, Pett SB, Alonso D, Richter RC, Stelzer P, Subramanian V, Tack-Goldman K, Gay WA. Differential inhibition by aspirin of vascular and platelet prostaglandin synthesis in atherosclerotic patients. N Engl J Med 1983;*308*:800–805.
2. Rosasaint R, Falke KJ, Lopez F, Slama K, Pison U, Zapol WM. Inhaled nitric oxide for the adult respiratory distress syndrome. N Engl J Med 1993;*328*:399–405.
3. Hass WK, Easton JD, Adams HP, Pryse-Phillips W, Molony BA, Anderson S, Kamm B. A randomized trial comparing ticlopidine hydrochloride with aspirin for the prevention of stroke in high-risk patients. N Engl J Med 1989;*321*:501–507.
4. Donadio JV, Anderson CF, Mitchell III JC. Membranoproliferative glomerulonephritis. A prospective clinical trial of platelet-inhibitor therapy. N Engl J Med 1984;*310*:1421–1426.
5. The Anturane Reinfarction Trial Research Group. Sulfinpyrazone in the prevention of sudden death after myocardial infarction. N Engl J Med 1980;*302*:250–256.
6. Ridker PM, Manson JE, Gaziano JM, Buring JE, Hennekens CH. Low-dose aspirin therapy for chronic stable angina. Ann Intern Med 1991;*114*:835–839.
7. Steering Committee of the Physicians' Health Study Research Group. Final report on the aspirin component of the ongoing physicians' health study. N Engl J Med 1989;*321*:129–135.
8. Peto R, Gray R, Collins R, Wheatley K, Hennekens C, Hafner B, Jamrozik K, Warlow C, Thompson E, Norton S. Randomised trial of prophylactic daily aspirin in British male doctors. Brit Med J 1988;*296*:313–316.
9. Chesebro JH, Fuster V, Elveback LR, Clement IP, Smith HC, Holmes DR Jr, Bardsley WT, Pluth JR, Wallace RB, Puga FJ, Oraszulak TA, Piehler JM, Danielson GK, Shaff HV, Frye RL. Effect of dipyridamole and aspirin on late vein-graft patency after coronary bypass operations. N Engl J Med 1984;*310*:209–214.
10. Hsia J, Hamilton WP, Kleiman N, Roberts R, Chaitman BR, Ross AM. A comparison between heparin and low-dose aspirin as adjunctive therapy with tissue plasminogen activator for acute myocardial infarction. N Engl J Med 1990;*323*:1433–1437.
11. Petersen R, Boysen G, Godtfredsen J, Andersen B. Placebo-controlled, randomised trial of warfarin and aspirin for prevention of thromboembolic complications in chronic atrial fibrillation: the Copenhagen AFASAK study. Lancet 1989;*1*:175–179.
12. Coller BS, Scudder LE. Inhibition of dog platelet function by in vivo infusion of $F(ab')_2$ fragments of a monoclonal antibody to the platelet glycoprotein IIb/IIIa receptor. Blood 1985;*66*:1456–1459.
13. Huang TF, Holt JC, Kirby EP, Niewiarowski S. Tigramin: Primary structure and its inhibition on von Willebrand factor binding to glycoprotein IIb/IIIa complex on human platelets. Biochemistry 1989;*28*:661–666.
14. Mannucci PM, Remuzzi G, Pusineri F, Lombardi R, Valsecchi C, Mecca G, Zimmerman TS. Desamino-8-d-arginine vasopressin shortens the bleeding time in uremia. N Engl J Med 1983;*308*:8–12.
15. Nieuwenhuis HK, Sixma JJ. 1-Desamino-8-d-arginine vasopressin (desmopressin) shortens the bleeding time in storage pool deficiency. Ann Intern Med 1988;*108*:65–67.
16. Kobrinsky NL, Letts RM, Patel LR et al. 1-desamino-8-d-arginine vasopressin (desmopressin) decreases operative blood loss in patients having harrington rod spinal fusion surgery. Ann Intern Med 1987;*107*:446–450.
17. Livio M, Mannucci PM, Vigano G, Mingardi G, Lombardi R, Mecca G, Remuzzi G. Conjugated estrogens for the management of bleeding associated with renal failure. N Engl J Med 1986;*315*:731–735.
18. Naito K, Fujikawa K. Activation of human blood coagulation factor XI independent of factor XII. J Biol Chem 1990;*266*:7353–7358.
19. Hull RD, Raskob GE, Rosenbloom D, Lemaire J, Pineo GF, Baylis B, Ginsberg JS, Panju AA, Brill-Edwards P, Brant R. Optimal therapeutic level of heparin therapy in patients with venous thrombosis. Arch Intern Med 1992;*152*:1589–1595.
20. Neri Serneri GG, Rovelli F, Gensini GF, Pirelli S, Carnovali M, Fortini A. Effectiveness of low-dose heparin in prevention of myocardial reinfarction. Lancet 1987;*1*:937–942.
21. Collins R, Scrimgeour A, Yusuf S, Peto S. Reduction in fatal pulmonary embolism and venous thrombosis by preoperative administration of subcutaneous heparin. N Engl J Med 1988;*318*:1162–1172.
22. Levine MN, Hirsh J, Gent M, Turpie AG, Leclerc J, Powers PJ, Jay RM, Neemen J. Prevention of deep vein thrombosis after elective hip surgery; a randomized trial comparing low molecu-

lar weight heparin with standard unfractionated heparin. Ann Intern Med 1991;*114*:545–551.

23. Hommes DW, Bura A, Mazzolai L, Buller HR, ten Cate JW. Subcutaneous heparin compared with continuous intravenous heparin administration in the initial treatment of deep vein thrombosis. Ann Intern Med 1992;*116*:279–284.

24. Mant MJ, Thong KL, Birtwhistle AV, O'Brien BD, Hammond GW, Grace MG. Haemorrhagic complications of heparin therapy. Lancet 1977:1133–1135.

25. Nieuwenhuis HK, Albada J, Banga JD, Sixma JJ. Identification of risk factors for bleeding during treatment of acute venous thromboembolism with heparin or low molecular weight heparin. Blood 1991;*78*:2337–2343.

26. Wakefield TW, Bouffard JA, Spauding SA, Petry NA, Gross MD, Lindblad B, Stanley JC. Sequestration of platelets in the pulmonary circulation as a consequence of protamine reversal of the anticoagulant effects of heparin. J Vasc Surg 1987;*5*:187–193.

27. Chong BH, Pitney WR, Castaldi PA. Heparin-induced thrombocytopenia; association of thrombotic complications with heparin-dependent IgG antibody that induces thromboxane synthesis and platelet aggregation. Lancet 1982:1246–1248.

28. Kelton JG, Sheridan D, Santos A, Smith J, Steeves K, Smith C, Brown C, Murphy WG. Heparin-induced thrombocytopenia: laboratory studies. Blood 1988;*72*:1988;925–930.

29. Hirsh J. Substandard monitoring of warfarin in North America. Arch Intern Med 1992;*152*:257–258.

30. Ezekowitz MD, Bridgers SL, James KE. Warfarin in the prevention of stroke associated with nonrheumatic atrial fibrillation. N Engl J Med 1992;*327*:1406–1412.

31. Smith P, Arnesen H, Holme I. The effect of warfarin on mortality and reinfarction after myocardial infarction. N Engl J Med 1990;*323*:147–152.

32. Stulberg BN, Insall JN, Williams GW, Ghelman B. Deep vein thrombosis after total knee arthroplasty. J Bone Joint Surg 1984;*66*:194–201.

33. Broekmans AW, Bertina RM, Loeliger EA, Hoffman V, Klingmann HG. Protein C and development of skin necrosis during anticoagulant therapy. Thromb Haemost 1983;*49*:251.

34. Demers C, Ginsberg JS, Edwards PB, Panju A, Warkentin TE, Anderson DR, Turner C, Kelton JG. Rapid anticoagulation using ancrod for heparin-induced thrombocytopenia. Blood 1991;*78*:2194–2197.

35. Agnelli G, Cosmi B, Di Filippo P, Ranucci V, Veschi F, Longetti M, Renga C, Barzi F, Gianese F, Lupattelli L. A randomised, double-blind, placebo-controlled trial of dermatan sulphate for prevention of deep vein thrombosis in hip fracture. Thromb Haemost 1992;*67*:203–208.

36. de la Fuente B, Kasper CK, Rickles FR, Hoyer LW. Response of patients with mild and moderate hemophilia A and von Willebrand's disease to treatment with desmopressin. Ann Intern Med 1985;*103*:6–14.

37. Rodeghiero F, Castaman G, DiBona E, Ruggeri M. Consistency of responses to repeated DDAVP infusions in patients with von Willebrand's disease and hemophilia A. Blood 1989;*74*:1997–2000.

38. Rose EH, Aledort LM. Nasal spray desmopressin (DDAVP) for mild hemophilia A and von Willebrand Disease. Ann Intern Med 1991;*114*:563–568.

39. Gralnick HR, Rick ME. Danazol increases factor VIII and factor IX in classic hemophilia and Christmas disease. N Engl J Med 1983;*308*:1393–1395.

40. Urokinase-streptokinase embolism trial. Phase 2 results. A cooperative study. JAMA 1974;*229*:1606–1613.

41. White HD, Rivers JT, Maslowski AH, Ormiston JA, Takayama M, Hart HH, Sharpe DN, Whitlock RM, Norris RM. Effect of intravenous streptokinase as compared with that of tissue plasminogen activator on left ventricular function after first myocardial infarction. N Engl J Med 1989;*320*:817–821.

42. The International Study Group. In-hospital mortality and clinical course of 20,891 patients patients with suspected acute myocardial infarction randomised between alteplase and streptokinase with or without heparin. Lancet 1990;*336*:71–75.

43. Maggioni AP, Franzosi MG, Santoro E, White H, Van de Werf F, Tongnoni G. The risk of stroke in patients with acute myocardial infarction after thrombolytic and antithrombotic treatment. N Engl J Med 1992;*327*:1–6.

44. Neuhaus KL, Tebbe U, Gottwik M et al. Intravenous recombinant tissue plasminogen activator (rt-PA) and urokinase in acute myocardial infarction: results of the German Activator Urokinase Study (GAUS). J Am Coll Cardiol 1988;*12*:581–587.

45. Miles LA, Plow EF. Binding and activation of plasminogen on the platelet surface. J Biol Chem 1985;*260*:4303–4311.

46. Anderson JL, Rothbard RL, Hackworthy RA, Sorensen SG, Fitzpatrick PG, Dahl CF, Hagan AD, Browne KF, Symkoviak GP, Menlove RL. Multicenter reperfusion trial of intravenous anisoylated plasminogen activator complex (APSAC) in acute myocardial infarction: controlled comparison with intracoronary streptokinase. J Am Coll Cardiol 1988;*11*:1153–1163.

47. Diefenbach C, Erbel, R, Pop T, Mathey D, Schofer J, Hamm C, Ostermann H, Schmitz-Hubner U, Bleifeld W, Meyer J. Recombinant single-chain urokinase-type plasminogen activator during acute myocardial infarction. Am J Cardiol 1988;*61*:966–970.

48. Green D, Ts'ao C-H, Cerullo L, Cohen I, Ruo TI, Atkinson AJ. Clinical and laboratory investigation of the effects of ε-aminocaproic acid on hemostasis. J Lab Clin Med 1985;*105*:321–327.

49. Sindet-Pedersen S, Ramström G, Bernvil S, Blombäck M. Hemostatic effect of tranexamic acid mouthwash in anticoagulant-treated patients undergoing oral surgery. N Engl J Med 1989;*320*:840–843.

Reviews

r1. Shattil SJ, Bennett JS. Platelets and their membranes in hemostasis: physiology and pathophysiology. Ann Intern Med 1980;*94*:108–118.

r2. Leung L, Nachman R. Molecular Mechanisms of Platelet Aggregation. Ann Rev Med 1986;*37*:179–86.

r3. Kroll MH, Schafer A. Biochemical Mechanisms of Platelet Activation. Blood 1989;*74*:1181–1194.

r4. Weiss HJ. Antiplatlet therapy. N Engl J Med 1978;*298*:1344–1347 (Part I) and 1403–1406 (Part II).

r5. Oates JA, FitzGerald GA, Branch RA, Jackson EK, Knapp HK, Roberts LJ. Clinical implications of prostaglandin and thromboxane A2 formation. New Engl J Med 1988;*319*:689–698.

r6. FitzGerald GA. Dipyridamole. N Engl J Med 1987;*316*:1247–1256.

r7. Willar JE, Lange RA, Hillis LD. The use of aspirin in ischemic heart disease. N Engl J Med 1992;*327*:175–181.

r8. Richardson DW, Robinson AG. Desmopressin. Ann Intern Med 1985;*103*:228–239.

r9. Furie B, Furie BC. The molecular basis of blood coagulation. Cell 1988;*82*:505–518.

r10. Nemerson Y. Tissue factor and hemostasis. Blood 1988;*71*:1–8.

r11. Esmon CT. The regulation of natural anticoagulant pathways. Science 1987;*235*:1348–1352.

r12. Rosenberg RD. Biochemistry of heparin antithrombin interactions, and the physiological role of this natural anticoagulant mechanism. Am J Med 1989;*87*(suppl 3B):2S–9S.

r13. Rapaport S. Inhibition of factor VIIa/tissue factor-induced blood coagulation: With particular emphasis upon a factor Xa-dependent inhibitory mechanism. Blood 1989;*73*:359–365.

r14. Furie B, Furie BC. Molecular basis of vitamin K-dependent gamma-carboxylation. Blood 1990;*75*:1753–1762.

r15. Hirsh, J. Heparin. N Engl J Med 1991;*324*:1565–1574.

r16. Hirsh J, Levine MN. Low molecular weight heparin. Blood 1992;*79*:1–17.

r17. King DJ, Kelton JG. Heparin-associated thrombocytopenia. Ann Intern Med 1984;*100*:535–540.

r18. Hirsh J. Oral Anticoagulant Drugs. N Engl J Med 1991;*324*:1865–1875.

r19. Lijnen HR, Collen D. Interaction of plasminogen activators and inhibitors with plasminogen and fibrin. Sem Throm Hemost 1982;*8*:2–10.

r20. Collen D, Lijnen HR. Basic and clinical aspects of fibrinolysis and thrombolysis. Blood 1991;*78*:3114–3124.

r21. Marder VJ, Sherry S. Thrombolytic therapy: Current status. N Engl J Med 1988;*318*:1512–1520 (Part I) and 1585–1595 (Part II).

r22. Marder VJ. Guidelines for thrombolytic therapy of deep-vein thrombosis. Progress Cardiovascular Dis 1979;*XXI*:327–332.

r23. Loscalzo J, Braunwald E. Tissue plasminogen activator. N Engl J Med 1988;*319*:925–931.

r24. Sherry S, Marder V. Streptokinase and recombinant tissue plasminogen activator (rt-PA) are equally effective in treating acute myocardial infarction. Ann Intern Med 1991;*114*:417–423.

CHAPTER 73

Drugs that Act on the Immune System: Immunopharmacology and Immunotherapy

John W. Hadden
Elba M. Hadden

Immunopharmacology is the study of the regulation of the immune system and of therapeutic methods that can selectively modify immune function in human diseases.[r1] The origin of immunotherapy lies in the development of the vaccines that today are the mainstay of specific immunizations for poliomyelitis, smallpox, tetanus, diphtheria, measles, mumps, pertussis, and influenza. With the discovery of the immunoglobulins, the administration of gammaglobulins in agammaglobulinemia and for hepatitis prophylaxis followed in the 1950s. The discovery of the severe combined immunodeficiency disease brought bone marrow transplantation, now also an accepted treatment for bone marrow aplasia and certain leukemias. The elucidation of the cellular immune system and the mechanisms of allograft rejection in the early 1960s brought the use of immunosuppression for renal transplantation and for selected autoimmune diseases. In the last 15 years, the demonstration of the prevalence of cellular immune deficiencies in cancer, aging, autoimmunity, and infectious disease such as acquired immunodeficiency syndrome (AIDS) has generated interest in the clinical use of immunotherapeutic agents. Finally, the recent development of monoclonal antibodies and genetically engineered cytokines has brought us a wealth of new agents for immunotherapy. At the present time this field is largely experimental, yet the work to date suggests that in the future a variety of biologicals and drugs will be used in the treatment of several human diseases.

Immunosuppressive Agents (Figs. 73.1, 73.2; Table 73.1)

Immunosuppressive therapy is used to inhibit graft rejection in transplantation[2] and to reduce autoimmunity.[2] Transplantation of the kidney is accepted therapy for most forms of renal failure, and heart and liver transplants are under experimental development. In these settings, the use of immunosuppressive agents is well accepted. Their use in autoimmune disorders is restricted to patients with severe and progressive disorders unresponsive to other treatments. Their use in both transplantation and autoimmunity is associated with an increased incidence of secondary infections with viruses and a higher but tolerated rate of cancer, especially lymphoma and leukemias. The immunosuppressive agents in use are glucocorticosteroids, azathioprine, cyclophosphamide, methotrexate, cyclosporin A, and antilymphocyte globulin.

Glucocorticosteroids

Steroid hormones have been widely employed in aberrant immune responses like allergy and autoimmunity, as well as organ allograft rejection, graft-vs-host disease, and certain leukemias. Many different steroid preparations are available, and they vary in their potency and side-effects (see Chapter 43). All can induce Cushingoid side-effects (fluid accumulation,

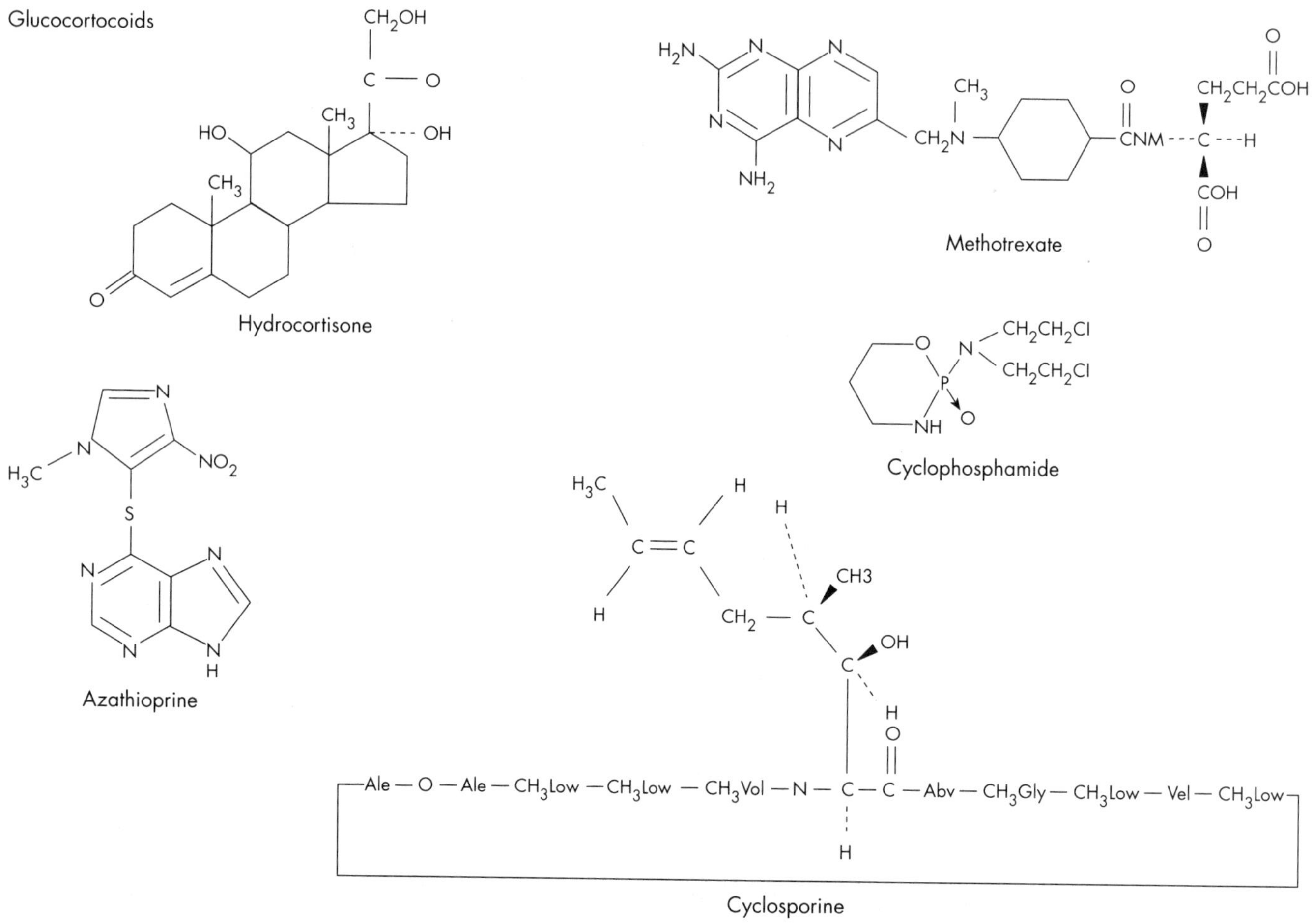

Glucocortocoids

Hydrocortisone

Methotrexate

Cyclophosphamide

Azathioprine

Cyclosporine

Figure 73.1 Immunosuppressive Drugs

euphoria, hirsutism, "buffalo hump," "moon" facies, striae, etc.) and peptic ulcers. In addition, they suppress the pituitary-adrenal axis, resulting in hypoadrenalism on withdrawal. The latter effect may be diminished, where clinically permissible, by alternate-day therapy.

The mechanisms of action of glucocorticoids on the immune system are not entirely clear.[3] Steroids influence the circulation of white blood cells, and administration results in monocytopenia, eosinopenia, lymphopenia, and neutrophilia. These effects result from altered release from the bone marrow and exodus from the circulation. Macrophage and granulocyte mediator release is impaired, which probably accounts for the anti-inflammatory and antiallergic actions of steroids at lower doses. Glucocorticoids do not inhibit antibody production to any great extent. They do inhibit proliferation, lymphokine production, cytotoxicity, and helper and suppressor activity of T cells. The major mechanism of immunosuppression at higher doses is thought to be on T-lymphocyte and macrophage collaboration through inhibition of proliferation and cytokine release and action. Immunosuppressive side-effects generally involve infection with viruses (*Herpes zoster* and *simplex*), fungi (*Candida albicans*), and intracellular bacterial pathogens (*Mycobacteria tuberculosis*). Long-term steroid treatment is sufficiently hazardous in terms of these and other side-effects to be employed only when the original disease is debilitating or life-threatening.

Glucocorticoids are used in transplantation in combination with azathioprine and/or cyclosporin A. They are used alone in autoimmune conditions like lupus erythematosus, polymyositis, dermatomyositis, polyarteritis nodosa, polymyalgia rheumatica, mixed connective tissue diseases, and hematologic autoimmune disorders like hemolytic or aplastic anemia, and autoimmune thrombocytopenia or neutropenia. When the disease is particularly severe and life-threatenting, as is lupus vasculitis or nephritis, steroids are employed in combination with azathioprine or cyclophosphamide. In rheumatoid arthritis, oral or intra-articular steroids may be used in conjunction with NSAIDs and other immunomodulating agents.

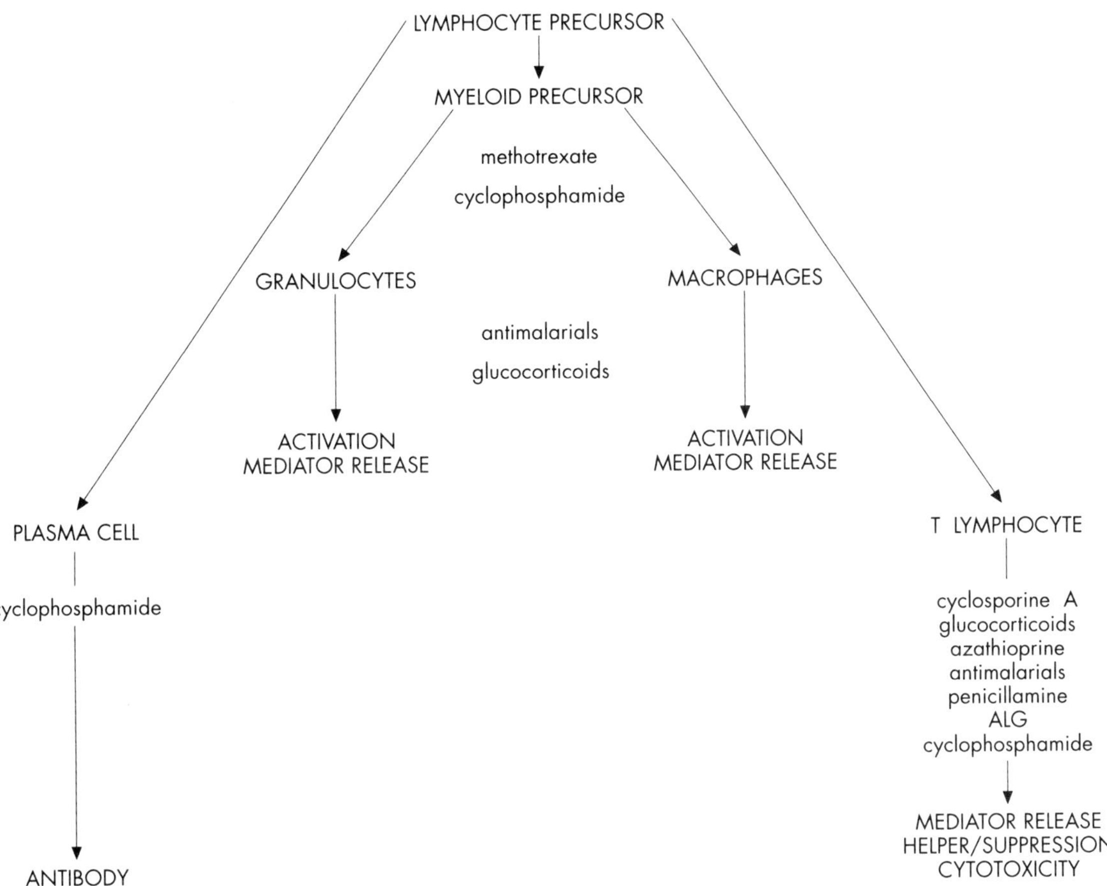

Figure 73.2 Cellular Sites of Actions of Immunomodulators and Immunosuppressive Agents Used in Transplantation and Autoimmunity

Azathioprine

Azathioprine is a nitroimidazole derivative of 6-mercaptopurine that acts as an antagonist of cellular replication through inhibition of de novo purine synthesis. This drug is only moderately suppressive for the hematopoietic system, and at clinical doses of 1 to 5 mg/kg/day its major side-effects are neutropenia and monocytopenia. Lymphopenia is minimal, and suppression of lymphocyte function in vitro and in vivo is reversed by discontinuance of therapy. Azathioprine is relatively selective for T-cell responses. At clinically employed doses, antibody responses remain intact. Its inhibitory effects on T-cell function induce allograft acceptance and anergy but also increase susceptibility to infection and lead to an increased incidence of cancer. Azathioprine is generally employed clinically in combination with glucocorticosteroids in transplantation or severe autoimmune disorders. Its use in rheumatoid arthritis is reserved for patients unresponsive to NSAIDs and second line disease modifying antirheumatic drugs (DMARDs).

Cyclophosphamide

Cyclophosphamide is an alkylating cyclic mustard with potent effects to kill both B and T lymphocytes at high doses. Treatment with high doses is associated with bone marrow suppression, pancytopenia, and hemorrhagic cystitis. At lesser doses, B lymphocytes appear to be more inhibited than T lymphocytes, providing a basis for preferential use of the agent in such autoimmune diseases as severe rheumatoid arthritis and systemic lupus erythematosus with nephritis and vasculitis. Low doses of cyclophosphamide act preferentially on T suppressor precursor cells. This action is the rationale for its experimental clinical application in cancer therapy, particularly in conjunction with interleukin 2, to prevent T suppressor cell development.

Methotrexate

Methotrexate is a cell cycle-specific antifolate compound developed for cancer. It is active in suppressing

Table 73.1 Immunosuppressive Agents

Cytotoxic Agent	Disease Indication	Toxic Effects
Glucocorticoids	Rheumatoid Arthritis SLE Autoimmunity Transplantation	Cushing's Syndrome Ulcers
Cyclophosphamide	Rheumatoid Arthritis SLE ITP	Myelosuppression Alopecia GI Symptoms Cystitis Infertility
Azathioprine	Rheumatoid Arthritis SLE Polymyositis Collagen Diseases Transplantation	Myelosuppression GI Symptoms Hepatotoxicity
Methotrexate	Psoriasis Arthritis, RA Dermatomyositis	Myelosuppression Ulcerative Pulmonary Fibrosis
Cyclosporine A	Experimental in RA SLE Type I diabetes Psoriasis Uveitis Transplantation	Hepatotoxic Renotoxic Neurotoxic Hypertension

both B and T lymphocyte proliferation and at high doses induces lymphopenia and bone marrow suppression. Methotrexate occasionally is used in organ transplantation, graft-versus-host diseases, severe rheumatoid arthritis, polymyositis, dermatomyositis, and psoriasis. Low-dose methotrexate is now used in rheumatoid and psoriatic arthritis.[2] Clinical studies indicate that low dose methotrexate may have anti-inflammatory effects independent of its immunosuppressive actions. The fact that intra-articular injection is ineffective suggests that these anti-inflammatory actions are indirect; however, their mechanisms remain obscure at present. At low doses the side-effects of methotrexate are minimal.

Cyclosporin A

Cyclosporin A is a fungus-derived hexadecapeptide that selectively inhibits proliferation, cytotoxicity, and lymphokine production of T cells by blocking critical early activation events.[r2] It impairs renal allograft rejection alone and in combination with glucocorticoids. It inhibits graft-vs-host disease after bone marrow transplantation. Clinical side-effects include hepatic and renal toxic reactions. It has a steroid-sparing activity that allows the use of less toxic doses of steroids. A significant incidence of secondary malignancies is seen with cyclosporin A, comparable with that after the use of azathioprine and steroids. Recently, there have been encouraging results in autoimmune diseases like lupus erythematosus and type I diabetes.

Antilymphocyte Globulin (ALG)

ALG is currently an adjunctive therapeutic agent in allograft recipients intolerant to steroids or to other agents, and is sometimes used experimentally in autoimmune disorders. It impairs reactivity of both T and B cells and produces lymphocytopenia that is reversible on discontinuance of therapy. The major side-effects are infections and allergic reactions to heterologous proteins in the ALG.

New Agents

Irradiation, thoracic duct drainage, anti-T-cell monoclonal antibodies, and high-dose interferon have all been used experimentally to induce immunosuppression, yet none is generally accepted clinically. Two fungus-derived cyclosporin A-like compounds, FK506 and rapamycin, are currently in development for transplantation and other uses.[6,7] Growth factor toxin conjugates like interleukin 2-dipheria toxin are under study for more selective approaches to T cell suspension.[8]

Immunotoxic Drugs

Anticancer Drugs

Cancer chemotherapeutic drugs, like the immunosuppressive agents in general, inhibit proliferation of lymphoid and marrow cells. Consequently, secondary infections with common pathogens as well as opportunistic organisms are frequent in cancer patients treated with these drugs. These infections are often the cause of death. Tumor-produced immunosuppressive factors and malnutrition are clearly contributory. Recent studies indicate that anticancer agents differ in their immunosuppressive effects.[r3] Intensive radiotherapy and such drugs as glucocorticosteroids, chlorambucil, busulfan, thioguanine, cyclophosphamide, hydroxyurea, daunorubicin hydrochloride, cytarabine, methotrexate, doxorubicin, bleomycin, and asparaginase, when used in combined protocols, are potently immunosuppressive and place patients at great risk for infection. Use of these agents singly is generally less immunosuppressive.

Studies indicate that these chemotherapeutic agents affect differentially the various components of the immune system and in some cases stimulate certain cells and functions. Some agents, e.g., low-dose cyclophosphamide and doxorubicin, may restore the immune response by reducing tumor-related immunosuppression.[4,9] The status of the immune system after cytoreductive therapy is important to the ultimate prognosis. As the immunopharmacologies of the individual anticancer agents become better understood, strategies may be devised to reduce immunosuppression while not compromising their anticancer activity.

Abused Drugs

Ethanol, cannabis, and opiates have been implicated directly and indirectly through abnormal lifestyles and malnutrition to contribute to impaired immune response and resistance.[r4]

Prescribed Drugs

Independent of allergenic potential, an increasing number of drugs have been demonstrated to modulate immune response. Examples include NSAIDs, cimetidine, antiepileptic drugs, diethyl stilbesterol, anesthetics, antimicrobial agents, and tranquilizers. More studies of most of the currently employed medications are needed.

Immunomodulating Compounds (Fig. 73.2, Table 73.2)

A number of compounds used as disease-modifying antirheumatic drugs (DMARDs) in rheumatoid arthritis are not anti-inflammatory by inhibiting prostaglandin production. They modify autoimmune inflammation by indirect ways, involving the immune mechanisms central to the pathogenesis of autoimmunity.[10]

Gold Salts

Two parenteral gold salt preparations (aurothioglucose and gold sodium thiomalate) and an oral form (auranofin) are active in severe forms of rheumatoid arthritis. The mechanism of this latter action is not well understood. While not generally immunosuppressive, gold salts modulate a spectrum of immune and inflammatory responses. The primary cellular targets appear to be phagocytic cell populations.

Table 73.2 Immunomodulators

Agent	Disease Indication	Toxic Effects
Gold Salts	Rheumatoid Arthritis	Dermatitis GI Symptoms Protenuria
Penicillamine	Rheumatoid Arthritis	Dermatitis GI Symptoms Protenuria
Antimalarials	Rheumatoid Arthritis SLE	Retinopathy
Interferons	Hairy Cell Leukemia Kaposi's Sarcoma Venereal & Laryngeal Warts	Fever Flu-like Syndrome

After administration, gold is taken up in "aurosomes" of these cells in the synovium and elsewhere in the reticuloendothelial system (liver, spleen, bone marrow, and lymph nodes). A decrease in leukotactic and phagocytic activity results; while the cells are capable of degranulating, the activities of various lysosomal enzymes are reduced. Reduced lymphoproliferative responses likely result in great part from impaired accessory macrophage function and perhaps cytokine release. In addition, complement activation is directly impaired by gold salts. It has been inferred that the molecular basis of these many actions involves binding of sulfur by gold and an interference in sulfhydryl (SH-SS) exchange. Gold salts are employed in patients with relatively severe rheumatoid arthritis who cannot be controlled by NSAIDs alone. The majority of these patients will improve, and approximately 15 percent will remit for varying periods. In responding patients, gold salts are thought to slow the joint destructive process. The turnover of gold is slow, allowing infrequent administration but favoring cumulative toxicity. The most common problems involve dermatitis and mucous membrane lesions (stomatitis, enteritis). Gastrointestinal disturbances progressing to diarhhea are also common. Nephrosis with proteinuria, hematologic and allergic reactions, and hepatitis also limit therapy.

D-Penicillamine

D-penicillamine is a dimethyl analogue of d-cysteine that chelates such trace metals as copper, lead, and mercury—thus its clinical use in Wilson's disease and heavy metal poisoning. D-penicillamine is used in severe rheumatoid arthritis generally after patients have failed on NSAIDS and gold salts (see Chapter 74). D-penicillamine is also considered a disease-modifying agent in RA. The basis for its activity in rheumatoid arthritis from an immunopharmacologic standpoint is not clear. It is not overtly anti-inflammatory nor immunosuppressive. Two types of actions have been focused upon. The first relates to a direct action to dissociate rheumatoid factor and antigen-antibody complexes in vitro. This action is associated with decreased immune complexes in serum and synovia; yet, in many patients, increased glomerular deposition with associated nephropathy has been observed. The second action relates to modulation of T lymphocyte proliferative and helper and/or suppressor cell function. These actions are favored in explaining decreased autoimmune phenomena. A parallelism of the immunopharmacology of d-penicillamine and related agents like bucillamine with those of the thymic hormones and the thymomimetic drugs, levamisole and diethyldithiocarbamate, discussed in the next section, make if likely that T cell immunomodulation is central to the action of all these agents. A variety of studies indicate complex immunodulatory effects of d-penicillamine. The major toxicity of d-penicillamine is nephropathy with proteinuria, skin rash, GI symptoms, and hematologic findings. D-penicillamine is not used in other autoimmune diseases.

Antimalarial Drugs

Chloroquine and hydroxychloroquine, are orally active anti-inflammatory agents. The mechanisms of their actions from an immunopharmacologic standpoint are unclear. Accumulated evidence indicates that the drugs act both in vitro and in vivo to suppress leukocyte responses, including leukotaxis, interleukin 1 (IL1) production by macrophages, lymphoproliferative responses of T lymphocytes, and cytotoxic responses of T lymphocytes and natural killer (NK) cells. While these agents inhibit RNA and DNA synthesis at high doses, the therapeutic effects appear to result from an attenuation of activation events of leukocytes, perhaps through the inhibition of sulfhydryl systems or membrane phospholipases. At therapeutic levels these agents are not clinically immunosuppressive and are relatively nontoxic (mild GI and CNS effects). Their use is complicated by slow turnover and excretion. Their capacity to accumulate in pigmented tissues such as the retina occasionally can lead to a sometimes irreversible retinopathy. They are used as second-line therapy in rheumatoid arthritis and in related inflammatory connective tissue diseases like systemic lupus erythematosus.

Interferons

Alpha-interferons are produced by leukocytes of various types, and as many as 20 distinct genetic types

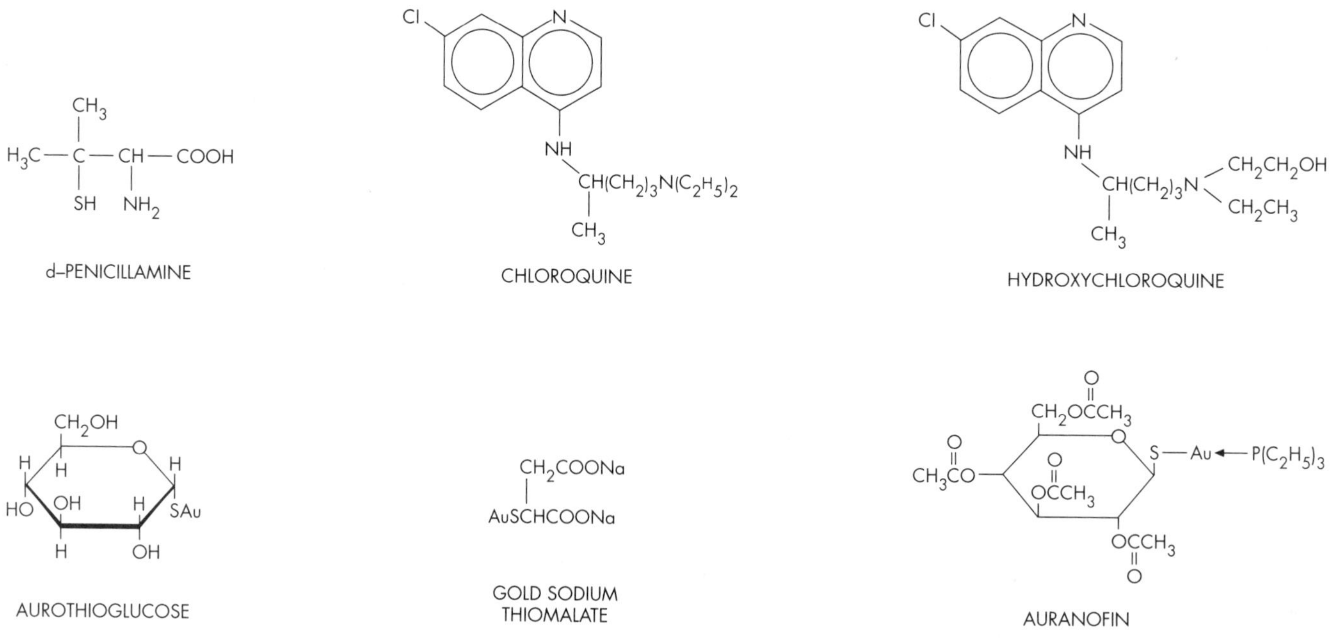

d–PENICILLAMINE: $H_3C—C(CH_3)(SH)—CH(NH_2)—COOH$

CHLOROQUINE: 7-Cl-quinolin-4-yl–NH–$CH(CH_3)(CH_2)_3N(C_2H_5)_2$

HYDROXYCHLOROQUINE: 7-Cl-quinolin-4-yl–NH–$CH(CH_3)(CH_2)_3N(CH_2CH_2OH)(CH_2CH_3)$

AUROTHIOGLUCOSE: CH_2OH, H, H, HO, OH, H, SAu, H, OH

GOLD SODIUM THIOMALATE: CH_2COONa / $AuSCHCOONa$

AURANOFIN: CH_2OCCH_3 (=O), CH_3CO (=O), $OCCH_3$ (=O), $OCCH_3$ (=O), $S—Au \leftarrow P(C_2H_5)_3$

Figure 73.3 Immunomodulating Drugs

have been identified with some heterogeneity of action.[11] Beta-interferon is produced by nonlymphocytes. Gamma or immune interferon is produced by activated T lymphocytes (see immunopotentiators). All interferons share the capacity to inhibit replication of DNA and RNA viruses; alpha and beta interferons inhibit the replication of both normal and malignant cells. They both modulate the immune system and are, therefore, classified as immunomodulators. High doses of interferons inhibit both B- and T-cell proliferation and can decrease humoral and cellular immune responses. At lower doses interferons stimulate the immune system by increasing the cytocidal activity of natural killer cells, macrophages, and T lymphocytes.

Interferons also appear to enhance microbicidal function. The administration of interferons produces a "flu-like" syndrome with fever, malaise, and myalgias. Interferons given nasally or parenterally can prevent certain virus infections; however, they are less active therapeutically for established infections. They have shown clinical activity in virus infections such as chronic active hepatitis (Hb +) and Herpes zoster and in virus-related disorders such as laryngeal and venereal papillomas. Gamma interferon is licensed for clinical use in chronic granulomatous disease.[12] Interferons have not been effective in the treatment of the immunodeficiency of AIDS and related conditions; however, they are active in Kaposi's sarcoma seen in AIDS[13] (see below). Purified and recombinant interferons have been employed in high doses as a monotherapy with positive results in a number of cancers.[14] Significant palliation (approximately 30% response rates) has been observed in hairy cell leukemia, non-Hodgkin's lymphoma, and multiple myeloma; in nasopharyngeal, renal cell, and bladder carcinomas; in osteogenic and Kaposi's sarcoma; and in malignant melanoma. Complete regression has been observed occasionally in hairy cell leukemia, renal cell carcinoma, and Kaposi's sarcoma. Little or no effect has been observed in carcinomas of the lung, pancreas, or breast.

Because the antitumor effect of the interferons results, in part, from immune modulation, their efficacy will probably improve when they are combined with cytoreductive therapy or other forms of immune therapy.

Immunostimulation (Figs. 73.4, 73.5)

The initial development, 20 years ago, of immunostimulating agents occurred for use in a limited number of primary and secondary immunodeficiency diseases.[r5] Dialyzed leukocyte extract or transfer factor therapy has been employed experimentally with limited success in Wiskott-Aldrich syndrome and mucocutaneous candidiasis. The thymic hormone preparations were employed in DiGeorge's syndrome and severe combined immunodeficiency with B cells with some effect on T cell number and function. However, since most genetically defined primary immunodeficiencies involve the lack of cellular populations or immunologically active molecules and small nonspecific immunostimulants offer an augmentation of intact systems, limited clinical benefit of these therapies should be expected.

With the progressive development in our understanding of cellular immune deficiencies, it has become apparent that many diseases, cancers in particular, are associated with this type of deficiency and that the immune status of the patient is of prognostic importance. Initial efforts to stimulate the immune system nonspecifically to improve prognosis in cancer began with bacterial products like Bacille Calmette-Guerin (BCG) and *Corynebacterium parvum*. Early encouraging results in often antigenic animal tumors led to widespread clinical trials.

The last 15 years have seen intensive clinical application of immunotherapy in human cancers. Although responses with BCG were noted in cutaneous malignant melanoma, bladder carcinoma, and osteogenic sarcoma, the side-effects of such bacterial preparations, their antigenicity, and their limited efficacy have shifted emphasis to chemically defined agents.

A number of other bacterial preparations including Klebsiella, Brucella, and mixed bacterial vaccines are under evaluation and probably face the same fate. Endotoxins, lipopolysaccharide endotoxin, and lipid A are immunologically active components of gram-negative organisms. Recent reports of their detoxification through chemical modification without loss of immunologic activity may warrant a resurgence of interest in this area. In any case, the rarity of clinical responses and the clinical toxicity, using crude bacterial products, has led to a general moratorium on these efforts and emphasis has shifted to the biologicals derived from the immune system and chemically defined drugs.

Biologicals (Table 73.3)

Thymic Hormones

The thymus is thought to produce several hormones that regulate the maturation of immature T-cells and modulate the functions of mature T-cells. Of these putative hormones, only zinc thymulin has been demonstrated to circulate in the blood at levels that decline with thymectomy or involution and whose secretion has been shown to be regulated from thymic epithelial cells.[15] Recent data also indicate that interleukins play important roles complementary to thymic hormones in promoting T lymphocyte development.[16]

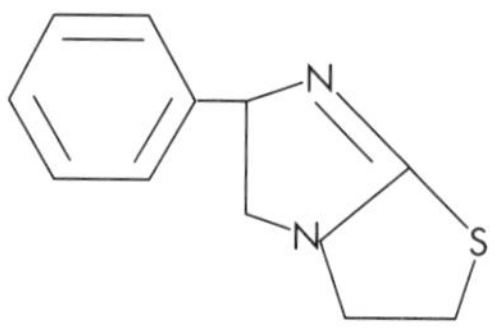

LEVAMISOLE

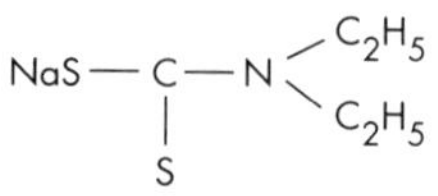

DTC

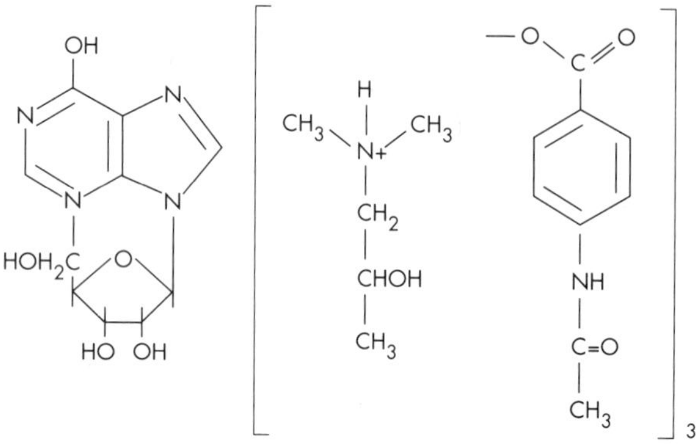

ISOPRINOSINE

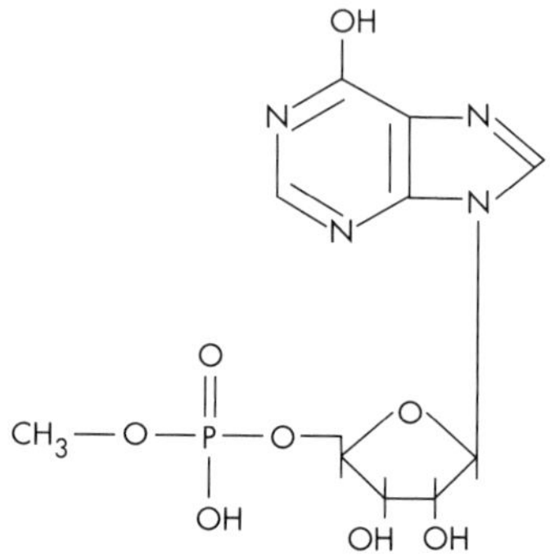

METHYL INOSINE MONOPHOSPHATE (MIMP)

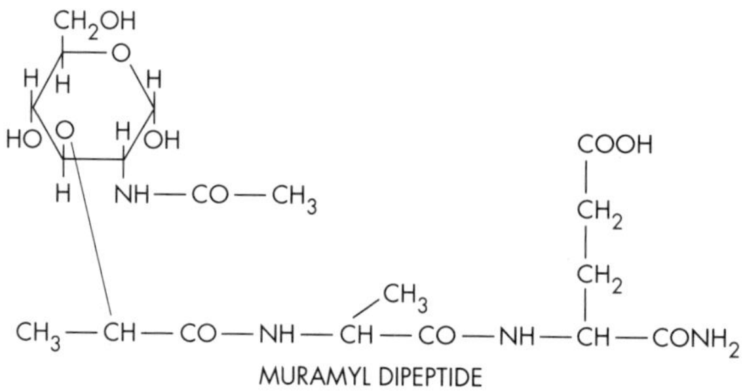

MURAMYL DIPEPTIDE

Figure 73.4 Immunostimulating Drugs

Thymosin fraction V and thymostimulin are two thymic extracts in widespread clinical use in Europe. Three purified peptides, thymosin α_1, thymopoietin, and thymic humoral factor are also in experimental clinical use. These have been synthesized chemically or produced by genetic engineering. Each of these purified peptides is chemically distinct, yet they all modulate the function of T-cells in vitro and cell-mediated immunity in vivo.

The extracts derived form bovine sources produce allergic reactions. The purified preparations are not immunogenic and are apparently free of side-effects. Animal studies indicate that these hormone preparations will partially restore immune defects in aging, cancer, autoimmunity, and after immunosuppressive therapy and will increase survival with various pathogen and tumor challenges. Clinical administration of these preparations has been shown to increase T-cell number, function, or receptor display and certain aspects of cell-mediated immunity.

The clinical administration of thymosin fraction V, thymostimulin TP-1, thymopentin, and thymic humoral factor in patients with the AIDS-related complex (ARC) have improved T lymphocyte function but have so far failed to demonstrate beneficial clinical effects. Thymosin fraction V and α_1 are currently in cancer trials. Initial studies indicate benefit in lung, head and neck, and renal cell cancer. Recent studies[16] point to potent synergy of thymic peptides and interleukins and future application of thymic hormones in combination with interleukins in cancer and age-related immunodeficiency seems logical.

Leukocyte Extracts

A number of products extracted from lymphocytes have been employed experimentally in immunotherapy. Such operational terms as "dialyzed leukocyte extract" and "transfer factor" have been applied to them. Both nonspecific immunoenhancement and specific transfer of delayed-type hypersensitivity have been claimed. Their chemical definition and mechanisms of action are unclear. Better chemical definitions and more reliable in vitro assays to assess cell targets and mechanisms of action are needed to provide the basis for improved clinical results and more general acceptance.

Lymphokines-Monokines

These cytokines (also called interleukins) are products of activated lymphocytes and macrophages and

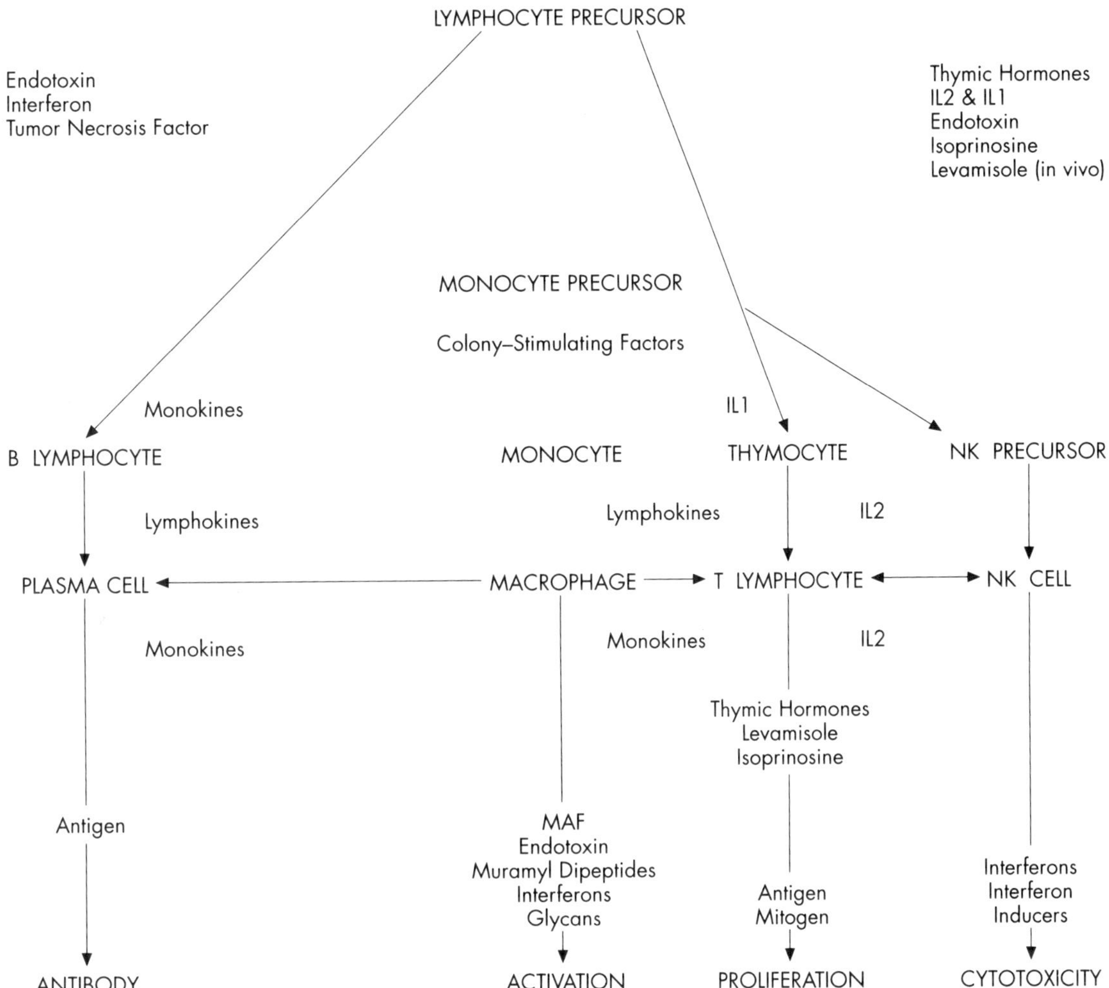

Figure 73.5 Cellular Sites of Action of Immunostimulating Drugs and Biologicals

are thought to play central regulatory roles in the cellular immune response. Examples are T-cell growth factor (interleukin 2), lymphocyte activating factor (interleukin 1), colony-stimulating factors (CSFs), tumor necrosis factor (TNF), and gamma interferon. Many cytokines have been cloned in bacteria and their therapeutic potentials are currently being actively explored. Interleukin 2 (IL2) acts to promote T lymphocyte development and, in concert with IL1, to expand antigen triggered T lymphocytes. Interleukin 1 also activates natural killer (NK) and lymphokine-activated killer (LAK) cells. The side-effects of high doses of IL2 in humans include "flu-like" symptoms and a capillary leak syndrome leading to fluid accumulation and respiratory distress. Initial trials of IL2 in patients with AIDS produced positive effects to increase lymphocyte counts; however, high doses by continuous infusion were required. Lower doses of IL2 with antiviral therapy are under study.

Interleukin 2 has also been introduced in cancer trials. It showed mild-to-moderate effect when given IV alone and in conjunction with LAK cells with considerable toxicity, particularly in renal cell cancer and malignant melanoma and was recently licensed for clinical use.[14] When applied in moderate doses regionally by the peri- or intralymphatic route or with low-

Table 73.3 Biologicals Acting on the Immune System

Gammaglobulin
Antilymphocyte globulin
Transfer factor
Thymic hormones (thymosin α_1, thymulin, thymopentin)
Interferons (alpha, beta & gamma)
Interleukins
Tumor necrosis factor
Colony stimulating factor
Monoclonal antibodies
Immunotox

dose cyclophosphamide, more significant palliative responses have been observed with interleukin 2 preparations in human malignant melanoma and head and neck cancer.[18,19] IL2 has also been combined with tumor infiltrating lymphocytes (TILs) and early results are encouraging.[20,21] IL2 has great potential for increasing the number and function of T lymphocytes and should yield beneficial clinical results especially when combined with antigen.

Interleukin 1 (α & β) and the colony-stimulating factors for granulocytes (CSF-G), monocytes (CSF-M), and both granulocytes and macrophages (CSF-GM) are potent growth promoters for the lymphoid and myeloid systems. Several CSFs have been cloned and are now licensed for use to restore bone marrow function following marrow destruction, such as that during bone marrow transplantation or after intensive cancer chemotherapy.[22] The side-effects so far include fever and "flu-like" symptoms.

Tumor necrosis factor (TNF) is a product of macrophages that has been cloned by genetic engineering techniques. It has been effective against a number of mouse tumors, with an efficacy comparable with that of chemotherapy. Its initial testing in humans with cancer has yielded acceptable toxicity but only negligible clinical effect. Its future use in combination with other lymphokines like gamma interferon or with chemotherapy is expected to improve its efficacy to reduce tumors in humans. TNF has also been implicated in the pathogenesis of septic shock, via production of the vasodilator, nitric oxide.

The development of recombinant cytokines will continue to be an area of rapid progress, and one can expect their use in a large variety of diseases besides cancer. It is important to recognize that these molecules normally act in vivo in complicated molecular scenarios that involve synergistic interactions with both positive and negative feedbacks; therefore, learning to harness these molecules as single entities and more importantly as mixtures poses a great immunopharmacologic challenge.

Monoclonal Antibodies

These antibodies are prepared by fusing lymphocytes immunized against antigens like human cancers with immortalized antibody-producing cells established in culture. The result is a clone of cells that all make the same antibody. These clones have been scaled up to produce large vats of pure antibody. When these antibodies fix complement, they can effectively kill human and murine tumors in vivo.[23,24] These monoclonal antibodies have been armed with isotopes like I^{131}, toxins like ricin, and anticancer drugs to make immunotoxins, and their efficacy to kill cancer cells has been improved in the experimental setting. The attachment of isotopes to these antibodies has also allowed imaging techniques capable of localizing small amounts of cancer in animals.[25] Mouse monoclonal antibodies have demonstrated diagnostic and therapeutic efficacy in a number of human tumors. The side-effects are generally related to allergic responses to the heterologous mouse proteins. A number of humanized monoclonals are under development and appear to be free of this side-effect. This area of experimentation is in a very early phase; the potential of these monoclonals for the diagnosis and treatment of human cancers appears to be great.

Immunostimulating Drugs (Fig. 73.3)

Levamisole

This compound is a phenylimidothiazole antihelminthic drug that was found to reverse anergy in human cancer patients, a response that correlates with poor prognosis. This finding led to intensive study of its immunopharmacology and to extensive evaluation in cancer and other diseases.[r6] The compound potentiates the stimulation of lymphocytes, granulocytes, and macrophages by such stimuli as antigen, mitogen, lymphokine, and chemotactic factors. Proliferation, secretion, and motility are thus modified. Enhancement of cell-mediated immunity is more manifest than enhancement of humoral immunity. The effects of levamisole on the T-cell system appear to be the central feature of its action and this effect has been postulated to result from the induction of a thymic hormone-like factor from liver. For this reason levamisole has been classified as an indirect-acting thymomimetic drug (i.e., mimicking the thymus). Its side-effects include nausea and vomiting, rash, a "flu-like" syndrome, and a reversible agranulocytosis.

Levamisole has been used experimentally with some success in brucellosis, tuberculosis, leprosy, candidiasis, aspergillosis, and recurrent Herpes I, II, and zoster. Levamisole has been reported to be active in recurrent aphthous stomatitis, a presumed infectious disease. It has proved as effective as d-penicillamine in reducing the signs and symptoms of rheumatoid arthritis, yet the incidence of agranulocytosis is high in RA patients. In humans, levamisole has shown a significant effect to increase survival in DUKES C colon cancer after cytoreductive therapy with 5-fluorouracil[18] and is now licenced for this use.

The low efficacy and side-effects of levamisole have prompted a search for alternative, more active agents. Based on the demonstration that the sulfur moiety in the levamisole is immunologically active to induce the liver factor, a number of other similar compounds have been under study, including diethyldithiocarbamate (DTC), NPT 16416, bucillamine, ADA202-718, and thiazolobenzimidazoles. More consistent activity with lower toxicity makes these compounds of interest. Of the above compounds, DTC has shown clinical activity in initial studies in rheumatoid arthritis and AIDS-related complex patients.[28]

Isoprinosine

This inosine complex is licensed in 80 countries (but not in the US and Japan) as an antiviral and immunostimulating agent.[r7] The compound shows mild antiviral activity at high concentrations. The immunopharmacology of isoprinosine includes actions to induce T-lymphocyte differentiation in a way comparable with that of thymic hormones and actions to augment lymphocyte, macrophage, and natural killer cell functions in a potentiator mode of action. The action of isoprinosine on T-cells appears central to its efficacy; therefore, it has been classified as a direct-acting thymomimetic drug.[29] In general, the activity of isoprinosine, both in vitro and in vivo, has been more consistent than that of levamisole. It is virtually nontoxic, with only mild hyperuricemia as a side-effect. Data indicate that it augments virus-specific immune responses, including mitogen and lymphokine responses, active T lymphocyte rosettes, and delayed skin test responses in humans. In controlled or double-blinded studies, significant mild to moderate efficacy of isoprinosine to reduce symptoms and/or shorten the disease period or recurrences has been reported in subacute sclerosing panencephalitis and in Herpes simplex types I and II, influenza, rhinovirus infections, and in human immunodeficiency virus (HIV) infection.[30] While antiviral activity might explain these clinical results, it seems likely that known effects of this compound on the immune system are the explanation. Other purines, like PCF 39 and MIMP[22] are currently under development to improve on the action of this class of thymomimetic drug.

Muramyl Dipeptide (MDP)

Muramyl dipeptide is the smallest component of the mycobacterial cell wall that has adjuvant activity and induces protection against pathogen challenge.[r8] Muramyl dipeptide is active when administered by mouth. Many analogues have been prepared by various pharmaceutical firms, and it appears that the immunopharmacology of the MDP analogues depends on their particular structure. Muramyl dipeptides induce fever, which can be prevented by inhibition of prostaglandin synthesis or obviated by the use of analogues.

Muramyl dipeptide promotes secretion of enzymes and monokines by macrophages. The effect of MDP is a direct one not requiring lymphokine or other influence. With oil and antigen, MDP augments both humoral and cellular immunity. The MDPs have both adjuvant potential when mixed or particularly when coupled with antigen and their experimental use in synthetic vaccines is very encouraging. They are protective against a variety of viral and bacterial challenge yet are poorly or not effective in treatment. Their use in conjunction with antimicrobial therapy seems logical. By nature of the induction of marrow stimulating cytokines (IL1, CSFs) MDPs are useful to promote marrow recovery.

While the major focus of MDP has been as an adjuvant with vaccines, its immunopharmacology strongly suggests useful application in cancer to prevent tumor recurrence and in infections where the macrophage plays a central role in resistance. Several derivatives (murabutide and MTP-PE) have recently been introduced into humans for toxicologic evaluation and clinical trials. One preparation (MDP 18 Lys-muroctasin) is in use in Japan as a marrow and immunorestorative agent after cancer chemotherapy.[r9]

Fungal Products

A number of fungi have yielded 1-3-β-linked glycans, often termed glucans. In general, these high-molecular-weight glucans expand the reticuloendothelial system and activate macrophages. Two preparations, krestin and lentinan, are licensed in Japan and have been used extensively in gastric cancer following surgery.

The foregoing represent only a partial list of biologicals and chemically-defined agents under development potentially useful in immunotherapy of a number of diseases.

Immunotherapy: Prospects for the Future

Infectious Diseases

In general, immunotherapy is applicable where antimicrobial therapy is not available, as in viral infections, or ineffective due to an immunocompromised host.[r10] In the future, serotherapy with antimicrobial monoclonal antibodies will offer adoptive immunotherapy particularly relevant in immunoprophylaxis and treatment of high-grade pyrogenic pathogen infections. The interferons, interferon inducers, fungal glycans, and the MDPs have all shown activity in preventing infection in pretreated hosts and should provide a degree of immunoprophylaxis in immunosuppressed patients as in those treated with cancer chemotherapy. The thymic hormone preparation and the thymomimetic drugs levamisole and isoprinosine have been useful in treatment of a number of different infections. The clinical experience to date suggests that use of immunotherapy for human infections will increase.

The major clinical experience with immunotherapeutic agents in infections has been in the secondary immunodeficiency diseases like AIDS and the AIDS-related complex (ARC).[r11] In general, except for minor effects on T-cell number and function in ARC patients, interleukin 2, the thymic hormone preparations, and the various thymomimetic drugs have failed to reduce symptoms, to decrease the conversion from ARC to AIDS, or to decrease mortality in AIDS. Thus the immunotherapy for AIDS and ARC is clearly a limited effort. Its use in asymptomatic or lymphodenopathic HIV+ individuals remains to be determined. Combinations of immunotherapeutic agents (e.g., isoprinosine and interferon, thymic hormones and interleukin 2, or MDP and lymphokines) may prove to be more effective and need to be studied. Immunotherapeutic approaches have to focus on both the immune defects and the nature of host-virus interactions. Antiviral therapy (e.g., zidovudine or dideoxycytidine) in the absence of effective immunity is associated with inhibition of viral replication during therapy. It is reasonable to postulate that only immune reconstitution *plus* antiviral therapy can be effective in patients with AIDS or ARC.

Autoimmune Diseases

Immunomodulator therapy has been one approach to autoimmune disorders resistant to NSAIDs.[r12] One experimental approach has been immunorestorative therapy with thymic hormone preparations and drugs having thymomimetic action (levamisole, diethyldithiocarbamate, bucillamine, lobenzarit, and isoprinosine). Thymopentin and thymulin given parenterally have shown both clinical and laboratory benefit in experimental use in rheumatoid arthritis (RA). Levamisole has received extensive use in RA with effects on clinical and laboratory values approximately similar to those of penicillamine but with more severe side-effects. Other sulfur-containing drugs, like diethyldithiocarbamate and bucillamine, would appear to offer similar clinical benefit with fewer side-effects and, therefore, would represent more likely candidates. The successful use of immunomodulators alone and in conjunction with NSAIDs offers the prospect of less toxic therapy and can be, on occasion, remission-inducing, indicating that these drugs are capable of addressing a yet-to-be-defined primary immunologic defect in RA, not merely reducing inflammation.

Another interesting class of immunomodulators not previously discussed in this chapter are the sex steroids.[r12] Animal experiments indicate that the female sex hormones promote and male hormones inhibit experimental autoimmune disease. The use in human autoimmune disease seems feasible, particularly in conjunction with other modalities of treatment.

Finally, immunosuppressive treatment of autoimmunity, like transplantation, is benefitting from the introduction of more selective and less toxic agents (e.g., cyclosporin A) and their use in combination with lower doses of other immunosuppressive agents. It is hoped that the future will bring a clearer view of the causes of autoimmunity, for example, hidden pathogens like retroviruses will perhaps allow curative strategies with antimicrobial or synthetic vaccine treatments. In any case, more selective therapies may well derive from cytocidal monoclonal antibodies for specific subsets of T or B lymphocytes critical to the autoimmune or rejection processes. Antibodies for the IL2 receptor may be useful in turning off an ongoing response.

Cancer

In human cancer, extensive trials of immunorestorative therapy with levamisole, lentinan, krestin, and thymosin have been performed and have shown activity.[r13] In each of these cases the immunotherapy has been effective only after cytoreductive procedures such as chemotherapy, surgery, or irradiation. Thus, nonspecific immunostimulants may produce a small increase in survival of patients who can be potentially cured by a primary cytoreductive therapy. This effect is one of "remission stabilization," and such therapy has little or no role as a single therapy in active, progressive cancer. The effect of immunotherapy on the incidence of infection in treated cancer patients has not been adequately assessed.

Interferons have been used in human cancers because of their ability to modulate immune functions, on the one hand, and to inhibit malignant cell growth on the other. Purified and recombinant interferons have been used as a monotherapy in a variety of late stage cancers with positive results. Unfortunately, the clinical responses observed have not been analyzed to demonstrate whether the antitumor or immunomodulatory effects or both account for the responses. Such information is crucial in determining whether future strategies should see interferons employed with chemotherapy or other forms of immunotherapy or both.

The demonstrated efficacy of interleukin 2 with LAK cell, TILs, or low dose cyclophosphamide in active progressive human cancer more clearly demonstrates that the immune system can be mobilized in late stage cancer therapy. The demonstration of therapeutic activity of monoclonal antibodies and immunotoxins is another important first.

In addition, cancer vaccines have been recently employed to prevent recurrence in lung cancer and with adjuvants like detoxified endotoxin to induce regression in malignant melanoma, thus opening up another avenue of immunotherapy.

In cancer, no single immunotherapeutic agent used as a monotherapy offers meaningful potential capable of cure. These agents can be used in combination with chemotherapy, surgery, or radiation to reduce the frequency of recurrence and of infection resulting from immunosuppression.[r14,33] Their successful use in active, progressive cancer will depend on the development of new strategies. Combinations of immunotherapeutic agents offer synergistic interactions that need to be more fully explored. In addition, prospective cancer therapies will include tumor vaccines and in vitro expansion of tumor-responsive clones. With more potent immunorestoration and activation, and with strategies to overcome tumor-related immunosuppression, more successful cancer immunotherapies will develop and provide an encouraging therapy frontier.

Dosage Summary Table

	Dosage			Pharmacokinetics			
Drugs	**Route**	**Size**	**Dose Protocol**	**Pk**	**$t_{1/2}$**	**V_D**	**CL or Duration of Response**
Immunosuppresant Cyclosporin Sandimmune	Oral Capsule Solution Parenteral	25, 100mg 100 mg/ml 50 mg/ml	15 mg/kg q.d.	3–5 hrs immed.	19–27 hrs	13 1/kg	
Immunostimulants Interleukin-2 Aldesleukin Proleukin	Parenteral	22 × 10⁶ units	0.6 × 10⁶ units/kg				
Interferon Alfa-2a Roferon-A	Parenteral	3–36 × 10⁶ units	q8hr for 14 doses 3 × 10⁶ units	1–8 hrs post IM		0.2–0.6 1/kg	2–4 ml/kg/min
Interferon Alfa-2b Intron	Parenteral	3–50 × 10⁶ units	2 × 10⁶ units qd		4–9 hrs.		
Interferon Alfa-N3 Alferon	Parenteral	5 × 10⁶ units					

References

Research Reports

1. Stratta RJ, D'Alessandro AM, Hoffman RM, Sollinger HW. Kalayoglu M, Lorentzen DF, Pirsch JD, Belzer FO. Cadaveric renal transplantation in the cyclosporine and OKT3 eras.
2. Bach J-F. The new era of immunosuppressive therapy in autoimmune diseases. Transplant Proc 1991;*23*(6):3319–3321.
3. Claman HN. Glucocorticosteroids, I: anti-inflammatory mechanisms. Hosp Prac 1983;*18*:123–134.
4. Turk JL, Parker D. Effect of cyclophosphamide on immunological control mechanisms. Immunol Rev 1982;*65*:99–113.
5. Feutren G. The optimal use of cyclosporin A in autoimmune disease. J Autoimmunity 1992;*5*(SA):183–195.
6. Nossal GJ. Summary of first international FK506 congress: Perspectives and prospects. Transplant Proc 1991;*23*(6):3371–3375.
7. Eng CP, Gullo-Brown J, Chang JY, Sehgal SN. Inhibition of skin graft rejection in mice by rapamycin: A novel immunosuppressive macrolide. Transplant Proc 1991;*23*:868–869.
8. Strom TB, Kelley VR, Murphy JR, Nichols J, Woodworth TG. Interleukin-2 receptor-directed therapies: antibody-or cytokine-based targeting molecules. Ann Rev Med 1993;*44*:343–353.
9. Maccubbin DL, Wing KR, Mace KF, Ho RLX, Ehrke MJ, Mihich E. Adriamycin-induced modulation of host defenses in tumor-bearing mice. Cancer Res 1992;*52*:3572–3576.
10. Wilke WS, Clough JD. Therapy for rheumatoid arthritis: combinations of disease-modifying drugs and new paradigms of treatment. Semin Arth Rheumatol 1991;*21*(1):21–34.
11. Steinmann GG, Rosenkaimer F, Leitz G. Clinical experiences with interferon-alpha and interferon gamma. Int Rev Exp Path 1993;*34*:183–207.
12. Todd PA, Goa KL. Interferon gamma-1b. A review of its pharmacology and therapeutic potential in chronic granulomatous disease. Drugs 1992;*43*(1):111–122.
13. deWit R. AIDS-associated Kaposi's sarcoma and the mechanisms of interferon alpha's activity: A riddle with a puzzle. J Int Med 1992;*231*(4):321–325.
14. Goldstein D, Laszlo J. The role of interferon in cancer therapy: A current perspective. CA 1988;*38*(5):258–277.
15. Coto JA, Hadden EM, Sauro MD, Zorn N, Hadden JW. Interleukin-1 regulates secretion of zinc-thymulin by thymic epithelial cells and its action on T lymphocyte proliferation and nuclear protein kinase C. Proc Natl Acad Sci 1992;*89*:7752–7756.
16. Hadden EM, Malec PH, Sosa M, Hadden JW. Mixed interleukins and thymosin fraction V synergistically induce T lymphocyte development in hydrocortisone-treated aged mice. Cell Immunol 1992;*144*:228–236.
17. Kolitz JE, Mertelsmann R. The immunotherapy of human cancer with interleukin 2: Present status and future directions. Cancer Invest 1991;*9*(5):529–542.
18. Mitchell MS, Kempf RA, Harel W, Shau H, Boswell WD, Lind S, Dean G, Moore J, Bradley EC. Efficacy of low-dose cyclophosphamide and interleukin-2 in melanoma. **In**: Advances in Immunopharmacology 4, Hadden JW, Spreafico F, Yamamura Y, Austen KF, Dukor P, Masek K, eds. Oxford: Pergamon Press, pp 105–118, 1989.
19. Hadden JW, Endicott J, Baekey P, Skipper P, Hadden EM. Interleukins and contrasuppression induce immune regression of head and neck cancer. Int Arch Otolaryngol, 1994;*120*:395–403.
20. von Rohr A, Thatcher N. Clinical applications of interleukin-2. Prog Growth Factor Res 1992;*4*(3):229–246.
21. Kurnick JT, Kradin RL. Adoptive immunotherapy with recombinant interleukin 2, LAK and TIL. Allergologia Immunopathologia 1991;*19*(5):209–214.
22. Donahue RE, Clark SC. Granulocyte colony-stimulating factors as therapeutic agents. Immunol Series 1992;*57*:637–49.
23. Schwartz MA, Scheinberg DA, Houghton AN. Monoclonal antibody therapy. Cancer Chemother Biolog Res Mod 1992;*13*:156–174.
24. Frankel AE. Immunotoxin therapy of cancer. Oncology 1993;*7* (5):69–78.
25. Reilly RM. Immunoscintigraphy of tumors using 99Tcm-labelled monoclonal antibodies: a review. Nucl Med Communications 1993;*14*(5):347–359.
26. Moertel CG, Fleming TR, McDonald JS, Haller DG, Laurie JA, Goodman PJ, Ungerleider JS, Emerson WA, Tormey DC, Glick JH, Veeder MH. Levamisole and fluorouracil for adjuvant therapy of resected colon carcinoma. N Engl J Med 1990;*322*:352–358.
27. Rougier P, Nordlinger B. Large scale trial for adjuvant treatment in high risk resected colorectal cancers. Rationale to test the combination of loco-regional and systemic chemotherapy and to compare 1-leucovorin + 5-FU to levamisole + 5-FU. Ann Oncol 1993;*4*(2):21–28.
28. Hersh EM, Brewton G, Abrams D, Bartlett J, Galpin J, Gill P, Gorter R, Gottlieb M, Jonikas JJ, Landesman S, Levine A, Marcel A, Petersen EA, Whiteside M, Zahradnik J, Negron C, Boutitie F, Caraux J, Dupuy J-M, Salmi LR. Ditiocarb sodium (diethyldithiocarbamate) therapy in patients with symptomatic HIV infection and AIDS. A randomized double-blind placebo-controlled multicenter study. JAMA 1991;*265*:1538–1544.
29. Hadden JW. Thymomimetic drugs. **In**: Serono Symposium on Immunopharmacology, Miescher PA, Bolis L, Ghione M, eds. Vol 23, New York: Raven Press, pp 183–192, 1985.
30. Pedersen C, Sandstrom E, Petersen CS, Norkrans G, Gerstoft J, Karlsson A, Christiansen KC, Hahansson C, Pehrson PO, Nielsen JO, Jurgensen HJ, and the Scandinavian Isoprinosine Study Group. The efficacy of inosine pranobex in preventing the acquired immunodeficiency syndrome in patients with human immunodeficiency virus infection. N Engl J Med 1990;*322*:1757–1763.
31. Hadden JW, Giner-Sorolla A, Hadden EM. Methyl inosine monophosphate (MIMP), a new purine immunomodulator for HIV infection. Int J Immunopharmacol 1991;*13*(S1):49–54.
32. DeJesus A, Talal N, Practical use of immunosuppressive drugs in autoimmune rheumatic diseases. Crit Care Med 1990;*18* (S2):132–137.
33. Hadden JW, Spreafico F. New strategies of immunotherapy. **In**: Springer Seminars in Immunopathology, Hadden JW, Spreafico F, eds. Vol. 8, Heidelberg: Springer Verlag, pp 321–326, 1985.

Reviews

r1. Hadden JW, Smith DL. Immunomodulation and immunotherapy. JAMA 1992;*268*:2964–2969.

r2. Fox DA, McCune WJ. Immunological and clinical effects of cytotoxic drugs used in the treatment of rheumatoid arthritis and systemic lupus erythematosis. **In**: Cruse JM, Lewis RE. Therapy of autoimmune disease. Basel: Karger, Switzerland. 1989; pp 20–78.

r3. Mihich E, Ehrke MJ. Immunomodulation by anti-cancer compounds. **In**: Chedid L, Hadden JW, Spreafico F, Dukor P, Willoughby D. Advances in immunomodulation III. Elmsford, NY: Pergamon Press, 1986; pp 257–265.

r4. Friedman H, Specter S, Klein T. Drugs of abuse, immunity and immunopharmacology. New York: Plenum Press, 1991.

r5. Hadden JW. Immunostimulants. Immunology today 1993;*14*(6):275–280.

r6. Renoux G. The general iummunopharmacology of levamisole. Drugs 1980;*19*:89–99.

r7. Tsang KY, Fudenberg HH, Hoehler FK, Hadden JW. Immunostimulating compounds: Isoprinosine and NPT15396. **In**: Fenichel RL, Chirigos MA. Immunomodulation agents and their mechanisms. New York: Marcel Dekker, 1984; pp 79–95.

r8. Lederer E. Natural and synthetic immunomodulators derived from the mycobacterial cell wall. **In**: Bizzini B. Bonmassar E. Advances in immunomodulation. Rome: Pythagora Press, 1988; pp 9–36.

r9. Azuma I. Review: Inducer of cytokines in vivo: Overview of field and romurtide experience. Int J Immunopharmacol 1992;*14* (3):487–496.

r10. Madje JA. Immunopharmacology of infectious diseases-vaccine adjuvants and modulators of non-specific resistance. New York: Alan R. Liss, 1987.

r11. Hadden JW. Immunotherapy of human immunodeficiency virus. Trends Pharmacol Sci 1991;*12*:107–111.

r12. Talal N, Hadden JW. New approaches to the drug treatment of inflammation with particular reference to murine autoimmune models and rheumatoid arthritis. **In**: Bonta IL, Bray MA, Parnham MJ. Handbook of inflammation. Amsterdam: Elsevier North Holland, 1895; pp 5–12.

r13. Taylor CW, Hersh EM. Immunotherapy and biological therapy of cancer: Current clinical status and future prospects. **In**: Immunopharmacological reviews I. New York: Plenum Press, 1990; pp 89–136.

r14. Hadden JW, Spreafico F. New strategies of immunotherapy. **In**: Springer Seminars in Immunopathology. Heidelberg: Springer-Verlag, 1985;*8*:321–443 and 1986;*9*:1–116.

r15. Fenichel RL, Chirigos MA. Immune modulation agents and their mechanisms. New York: Marcel Dekker, Vol 25, 1984.

r16. Bizzini B, Bonmassar E. Advances in immunomodulation. Rome: Pythagora Press, 1988.

r17. Hadden JW, Spreafico F, Yamamura Y, Austen KF. Dukor P, Masek K. Advances in immunopharmacology. Oxford: Pergamon Press, Vol 4, 1989.

r18. Masihi KN, Lange W. Immunotherapeutic prospects of infectious diseases. Berlin: Springer-Verlag, 1990.

r19. Hadden JW, Szentivanyi A. Immunopharmacology reviews. New York: Plenum Press, Vol. 1. 1990.

CHAPTER 74

Dennis B. McNamara
Philip R. Mayeux

Nonopiate Analgesics and Anti-Inflammatory Drugs

Nonopiate analgesics differ from the opiate analgesics in both their mechanism of action and the type of pain they alleviate. Morphine and other opiate analgesics stimulate opiate receptors in the CNS and inhibit the perception of pain. Nonopiate analgesics act by inhibiting the synthesis of endogenous compounds that sensitize and stimulate pain fibers. It is for this reason that the nonopiate analgesics are effective in alleviating the dull throbbing pain associated with such pathologic processes as inflammation, and not the sharp pain associated with direct mechanical stimulation of pain fibers. Nonopiate analgesics for the most part are anti-inflammatory and are, therefore, divided into two broad groups of drugs: the anti-inflammatory steroids and the nonsteroidal anti-inflammatory drugs (NSAIDs).

Inflammation

Inflammation is an extremely complex process. It may be initiated by tissue damage, immunologic reactions, microorganisms, or other phenomena leading to the infiltration of inflammatory cells, such as leukocytes. Local release of histamine, 5-hydroxytryptamine (serotonin), leukotrienes (the "slow-reacting substance of anaphylaxis"), various chemotactic factors, chemical mediators derived from plasma (bradykinin, complement, lysosomal enzymes, and prostaglandins [PGs]) may all contribute to the inflammatory process. The cell membrane damage associated with inflammation results in leukocyte release of lysosomal enzymes that can be injurious to nearby cells and cause the release of arachidonic acid and other precursor compounds, leading to the formation and release of prostaglandins, thromboxane, leukotrienes, kinins, and histamine.[r1,1,r2] Stimulation of neutrophils can lead to the production of oxygen-derived free radicals that can produce further cellular damage.[2] Clinical signs of the inflammatory process include erythema, heat, edema, hyperalgesia, pain, and altered function of the affected tissue or organ. It is important to remember that whereas all the NSAIDs share the ability to suppress the signs and symptoms of inflammation, they do not alter the underlying causes.[3] It should also be remembered that suppression of the signs and symptoms of inflammation by NSAIDs may mask an ongoing inflammatory process.

Anti-Inflammatory Actions of the NSAIDs (Table 74.1)

The inflammatory process is often associated with erythema and edema formation at the site of inflammation. The reddening and swelling are results of microvascular dilation and increased water permeability, respectively. The prostaglandins, PGE_2 and PGI_2, are potent precapillary vasodilators, but have relatively weak ability to increase vascular permeability. Histamine and bradykinin are the primary mediators of edema formation during the inflammatory process. The presence of vasodilator prostaglandins at the site of inflammation can potentiate the effects of histamine and bradykinin to produce edema by increasing flow to the region. It is for this reason that NSAIDs are effective in reducing erythema and edema. Increased heat at the site of inflammation is also mediated by increased flow to the region.

Pyresis or fever is a result of a resetting of the temperature regulator center in the hypothalamic region of the brain.[r3] Bacteria and other microorganisms can release pyrogens, which effect an elevation in the temperature set point. Endotoxins, lipopolysaccha-

Table 74.1 Classification and Therapeutic Uses for Nonsteroidal Antiinflammatory Drugs

	Plasma Half-life (hr)	Indication and Usage	Most Frequently Reported Adverse Reaction
Salicylates			
Aspirin*	3–5	F,P,RA,JA,AS	GI, Reye's syndrome, tinnitus, hypersensitivity, inhibit uric acid excretion
Diflunisal	8–12	P,RA,JA,AS,OA not an effective antipyretic	GI, rash, headache, somnolence, dizziness
Phenylproprionic Acid			
Ibuprofen*	2	F,P,RA,OA,D	GI, dizziness, rash
Fenoprofen	2	F,P,RA,OA,D	GI, dizziness, somnolence, nervousness, palpitations
Flurbiprofen	3	RA,OA	GI, headache, edema
Ketoprofen*	Variable	F,P,RA,OA,D	GI, headache, renal toxicity
Suprofen	2–4	D	GI, flank pain, renal toxicity
Naproxen*	13	F,P,RA,JA,AS,OA, D,AG,EAI	GI, headache, dizziness, drowsiness, dermatologic, tinnitus, edema
Oxaprozin	>20	OA,RA	GI, rash
Phenylacetic Acid Derivative			
Diclofenac*	1–2	RA,OA,AS	GI, dizziness, rash, tinnitus, edema, cramps
Pyrrole Acetic Acid			
Indomethacin	4	AG,AS,RA,OA,EAI	GI, severe frontal headache, dizziness, tinnitus, somnolence
Sulindac*	18	RA,OA,AS,EAI,AG	GI, dizziness, headache, nervousness, tinnitus, rash, edema
Tolmetin	1 acid	RA,JA,OA	
Ketorolac	2–9	P (only up to 5 days of therapy)	GI, edema, hypertension, rash, purpura, dizziness, drowsiness, headache
Etodolac	1–2	P,OA	GI, chills, fever, asthenia/malaise, nervousness, depression, rash, blurred vision, tinnitus, urinary frequency, dysuria

continued

rides released from gram-negative bacteria, can produce fever in humans in the absence of any microorganisms. Fever may result from infection, but tissue damage occurring as a result of inflammation also can produce fever. Stimulated neutrophils can release an endogenous pyrogen (interleukin-1) that acts at the hypothalamus to trigger an elevation in the temperature set point. Three lines of evidence suggest that prostaglandins are responsible, at least in part, for the elevation in the temperature set point: (1) NSAIDs, in particular aspirin, are very effective antipyretics; (2) some prostaglandins, namely, PGE_1, PGE_2, and $PGF_{1\alpha}$, are themselves pyrogenic; and (3) levels of PGs in the hypothalamus increase after the injection of bacterial endotoxin.

Physiologic concentrations of the prostaglandins do not produce pain. Their release at the site of inflammation results in an increased sensitivity of the pain nerve nociceptors to algesic stimuli.[r4] Substances released during the inflammatory process, such as organic acids, potassium, kinins, histamine, and acetylcholine, are direct stimulators of nociceptors. Prostaglandins, particularly PGE_2, sensitize pain receptors to these mediators, resulting in hyperalgesia or a reduction in the pain threshold.[r5] The analgesic action of the NSAIDs is through the inhibition of prostaglandin

Table 74.1 *Continued*

	Plasma Half-life (hr)	Indication and Usage	Most Frequently Reported Adverse Reaction
Napthylacetic Acid Derivative			
Nabumetone	20–30	RA,OA	GI, dizziness, headache, rash, tinnitus, edema
Pyrazolone			
Apasone	20–24	P,F,G	GI, agranulocytosis,
Phenylbutazone	50–100	not generally recommended (see text)	GI, blood dyscrasia, edema
Anthranilic Acid			
Meclofenamate	2	RA,OA,P,D	GI, edema, rash, headache, dizziness, tinnitus
Mefenamic acid	2–4	P (less than 1 week of treatment), D	GI, dizziness, agranulocytosis
Oxicam			
Piroxicam*	30–90	RA,OA	GI, renal toxicity, decreased hemoglobin, leucopenia, eosinophilic, rash, dizziness, somnolence, vertigo, BUN and creatinine elevations, headache, malaise, tinnitus, edema
Paraaminophenol			
Acetaminophen	1–3	P,F	Hepatic damage

RA, rheumatoid arthritis; JA, juvenile arthritis; OA, osteoarthritis; AS, ankylosing spondylitis; AG, acute gout; EAI, extra-articular inflammation; D, dysmenorrhea

*Indicates that drug is listed in the National Prescription Audit as one of the 200 most commonly prescribed drugs in the US in 1989.

synthesis not through receptor antagonism, since NSAIDs do not prevent hyperalgesia when PGE_2 is administered directly. Therefore, NSAIDs act by returning abnormally hypersensitive nociceptors to their normal sensitivity. Such an effect can be quite dramatic. There is evidence that, in postoperative dental pain, the use of NSAIDs is even preferable to the use of centrally acting analgesics. Postpartum pain associated with prostaglandin-induced uterine cramping is effectively treated with NSAIDs. This type of pain associated with prostaglandin-induced smooth muscle contraction may be more effectively treated with NSAIDs than with centrally acting narcotics, since NSAIDs alleviate the cause of the pain.

The enzyme prostaglandin endoperoxide H (PGH) synthase exhibits both cyclooxygenase and peroxidase activities.[4] Cyclooxygenase converts arachidonic acid to the cyclic endoperoxide PGG_2; peroxidase converts PGG_2 to the pivotal substrate for the prostaglandins and thromboxane, PGH_2[5] (Fig. 74.1). An interesting property of cyclooxygenase is its requirement of low levels of peroxide for activation. PGG_2 generated in the first step may keep cyclooxygenase activated and serve as a positive feedback control mechanism. However, high concentrations of lipid peroxides will inhibit cyclooxygenase. It is likely that cellular peroxidases can maintain the levels of peroxides low enough to preserve cyclooxygenase activity.[4] It has been proposed that infiltrating cells, such as neutrophils and monocytes, at the site of inflammation may, when stimulated, produce hydrogen peroxide, and lipid peroxides that could stimulate cyclooxygenase activity.[1,r2]

NSAIDs exert their anti-inflammatory activity by the inhibition of cyclooxygenase and thus the inhibition of the formation of the prostaglandins.[6,7] However, at concentrations higher than those required to inhibit cyclooxygenase activity, some NSAIDs have been reported to inhibit differentially the activity of enzymes that metabolize PGH_2.[8] As prostaglandins and thromboxane are synthesized de novo and released in response to stimuli rather than stored after synthesis,

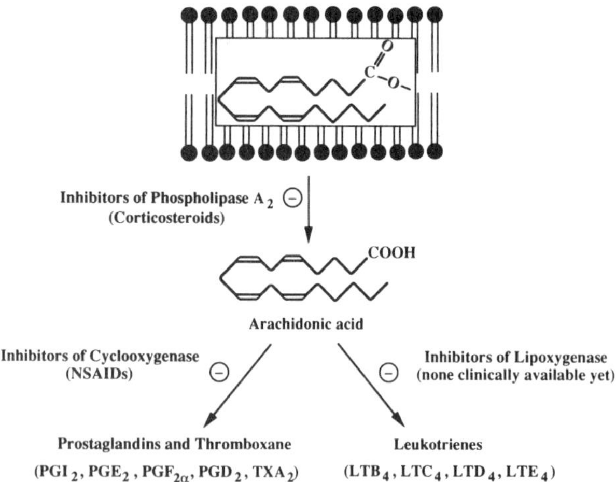

Figure 74.1 Arachidonic acid as precursor for prostaglandins, thromboxane, and leukotrienes. Arachidonic acid, part of the membrane phospholipid pool, is released by the action of phospholipase A_2 (PLA_2). Once released from the membrane fatty acid pool, arachidonic acid can proceed along two proinflammatory pathways. The cyclooxygenase pathway leads to the formation of the prostaglandins and thromboxane; the lipoxygenase pathway leads to the formation of the leukotrienes. Certain anti-inflammatory drugs act at the level of arachidonic acid release by inhibiting PLA_2 activity; the corticosteroids act at this step. Other drugs act by inhibiting cyclooxygenase and thus the formation of the prostaglandins and thromboxane; the NSAIDs act at this step. Another potential site of action might be at the level of lipoxygenase thus inhibiting the formation of the leukotrienes. The development of selective inhibitors of lipoxygenase is an area of intense research.

inhibition of cyclooxygenase activity removes the influence of cyclooxygenase products on cellular events. A unique property of aspirin is its ability to form a covalent bond with a serine residue on the enzyme. This acetylation irreversibly inactivates cyclooxygenase and results in loss of cyclooxygenase activity until a new enzyme is synthesized.[9] The platelet, being anucleate, is unable to synthesize new cyclooxygenase; therefore, aspirin treatment inhibits the formation of the principal cyclooxygenase metabolite formed by the platelet, thromboxane A_2 (TXA_2). TXA_2 is a potent stimulator of platelet aggregation and vascular smooth muscle contraction. The other NSAIDs inhibit cyclooxygenase through reversible competitive inhibition. These drugs bind to the active site of the enzyme and compete with the natural substrate, arachidonic acid. Their effectiveness is reduced as their concentration decreases. These NSAIDs are a heterogeneous class of compounds, and the structure-activity relationship for inhibition of cyclooxygenase is not fully understood.[7,9]

It has been shown recently that there are at least two isoforms of cyclooxygenase (PGHS-1 and PGHS-2). PGHS-1 is a constitutive enzyme, whereas the expression of PGHS-2 appears to be triggered by mediators of inflammation and the inflammatory process.[10–13] Interestingly, selective inhibition of PGHS-2 may become clinically useful and represent selective inhibition of prostaglandin biosynthesis during the inflammatory state.[12,14]

Shared Toxic Side-Effects of NSAIDs

The toxic side-effects shared by the NSAIDs discussed here are a result of their activity to inhibit prostaglandin synthesis. Toxicities specific to individual drugs will be discussed later under each drug heading.[r6]

Inhibition of Platelet Aggregation

Since the NSAIDs have therapeutic usefulness as inhibitors of platelet aggregation, their use as anti-inflammatory drugs can lead to prolonged bleeding times.[15–17] Inhibition of platelet-derived TXA_2 production removes an important stimulus for platelet aggregation and local vasoconstriction—events necessary for rapid, effective cessation of blood flow.[18] It must be pointed out that TXA_2 is not the only mediator of platelet aggregation. Other endogenous compounds, such as thrombin, generated in the plasma, and platelet-activating factor, released by neutrophils and other cells, are potent activators of platelets through mechanisms independent of TXA_2 generation. Inhibition of cyclooxygenase not only inhibits TXA_2 generation by the platelet but also inhibits prostaglandin generation by the vascular endothelium and smooth muscle cell. However, as the endothelial cell contains much more cyclooxygenase than the vascular smooth muscle cell, the endothelial cell is a more important source for vascular prostacyclin (PGI_2).[19] PGI_2 synthesized and released by vascular endothelial and smooth muscle cells is a potent inhibitor of platelet aggregation and vasoconstriction.[20] Therefore, inhibition of PGI_2 generation would tend to lessen the effects of reduced TXA_2 generation by the platelet. Nevertheless, long-term treatment with NSAIDs generally leads to a prolonged bleeding time, particularly in patients with a pre-existing bleeding disorder. Great care must be taken when administering NSAIDs to patients taking anticoagulants, as inhibition of hemostatis at multiple sites may result in serious bleeding.

The inability of the platelet to synthesize new cyclooxygenase is exploited in low-dose aspirin anticoagulant therapy.[6,16,17] While the platelet loses its ability to generate TXA_2, the vascular endothelial cells can synthesize new cyclooxygenase and regain PGI_2 synthetic activity.[21] The interactions between platelets and the vascular wall with respect to arachidonic acid metabolism during aspirin therapy are not fully understood;[19,22] however, low-dose aspirin (as little as 50 mg/day) may selectively inhibit platelet TXA_2 generation and thus be therapeutically beneficial in some forms of coronary artery disease.[16,17]

Acute Renal Failure (ARF)

Treatment with NSAIDs for conditions such as rheumatoid arthritis has resulted in documented cases of nephrotoxicity. Although the incidence of nephrotoxicity is relatively rare, patients with compromised renal function or hemodynamic instability are particularly susceptible to NSAID-induced nephrotoxicity. In humans or animals with normal hemodynamic control, NSAIDs have little if any effect on renal function. Patients with CHF, underlying renal disease, hypertension, shock, septicemia, volume depletion, or those undergoing diuretic therapy are at greatest risk of NSAID-induced ARF.[23] Under conditions of elevated renin, angiotensin, and sympathetic outflow to the kidney, the prostaglandins exert a moderating effect to lessen the vasoconstriction and sodium and water retention.[r7] Inhibition of PGI_2 and PGE_2 formation by NSAIDs appears to be the primary cause of ARF under these conditions. Renal synthesis of PGI_2 and PGE_2 oppose the actions of angiotensin and norepinephrine by dilating the renal vasculature, increasing renal blood flow, increasing glomerular filtration rate, and decreasing renal vascular resistance. PGI_2 and PGE_2 can promote natriuresis by promoting blood flow to the inner cortical and medullary regions of the kidney, thereby reducing the hypertonicity of the medullary interstitium and decreasing passive water reabsorption in the descending loop of Henle. Moreover, this effect could lead to a reduction in the osmotic forces driving passive sodium reabsorption in the ascending limb and result in a decrease in sodium and water excretion. In addition, these prostaglandins are thought to have a direct effect in inhibiting sodium transport and can antagonize vasopressin-induced water reabsorption.

Inhibition of prostaglandin synthesis can, therefore, exacerbate renal hypertension through increased sodium reabsorption in predisposed patients and lead to ARF. Patients with predisposing factors undergoing NSAID therapy should have frequent monitoring of serum creatinine levels. NSAID-induced renal failure is usually reversible on discontinued use. Much research has been devoted to the development of NSAIDs that do not inhibit renal cyclooxygenase ("renal sparing" NSAIDs). The approach is to develop a drug that is specifically metabolized by the kidney to an inactive form. One such NSAID in use is sulindac. It is expected that the active form of the drug (the sulfide derivative formed in the liver and kidney) will be converted to an inactive form by the mixed function oxidases in the kidney and spare renal cyclooxygenase activity. The protective effect of sulindac is still in question and it should be used with the same caution used for all NSAIDs. A number of NSAIDs have been reported to interfere with the diuretic effects of furosamide and thiazides. Patients on concurrent use of these agents should be closely observed to determine whether the desired therapeutic effect is obtained.

Gastrointestinal Ulceration

As a class, the NSAIDs are weak organic acids, meaning that at physiologic pH they are predominantly in the ionized form. In the acidic pH of the stomach, the unionized form predominates and absorption is facilitated; however, high concentrations can develop in the gastric mucosa as the drugs become ion-trapped at the higher pH of the intracellular space. This can lead to damage of the gastric mucosa and ulcerations.[24] Damage to the mucosa can lead to diffusion of acid into the cells of the mucosal lining and cause necrosis and bleeding. The cyclooxygenase inhibitory activity of the NSAIDs increases their potential for GI ulceration by inhibiting the synthesis of prostaglandins.

PGE_2 is very effective in reducing gastric acid secretion and may serve to protect and heal the mucosa as well. PGE_2 and PGI_2, at concentrations lower than those that inhibit gastric acid secretion, and $PGF_{2\alpha}$, which is not acid-antisecretory, can prevent mucosal necrosis if administered just prior to necrotizing agents. This property is referred to as cytoprotection or, more accurately, as mucosal protection, as the cells and blood vessels situated in the mucosa rather than the surface cells are protected.[25] The mechanism(s) underlying this phenomenon are uncertain. Both PGE_2 and PGI_2 help to maintain blood flow to the mucosa and affect removal of the drug, as well as acid that might escape the stomach. Therefore, inhibition of prostaglandin synthesis that leads to increased acid secretion coupled with decreased blood flow and perhaps even local ischemia results in further damage of the mucosa. During the ulcerative process blood vessels can become damaged and the ulcer may begin to bleed. Inhibition of TXA_2 synthesis, as discussed earlier, can prolong bleeding time. While all NSAIDs have the potential to produce GI ulceration, aspirin, the irreversible inhibitor of cyclooxygenase activity, is the most notable. Chronic treatment with anti-inflammatory doses of aspirin (4 gm per day) will almost certainly produce some degree of gastric ulceration. Even systemic administration of NSAIDs can result in damage to the gastric mucosa. The use of these drugs in patients with preexisting GI damage must be with caution and under supervision. The concurrent use of NSAIDs with inhibition of gastric acid secretion, such as a stable analogue of PGE_1 or PGI_2, an inhibitor of the histamine$_2$ receptor or an inhibitor of the proton pump, is a therapeutic approach that may be useful in patients with GI damage or sensitivity to NSAIDs.[26]

Delayed Labor

At parturition PGE_2 and $PGF_{2\alpha}$ contribute to the rhythmic uterine contraction necessary for birth.[27] Because of their effect on uterine smooth muscle, PGE_2 and $PGF_{2\alpha}$ can be used as abortifacients. NSAIDs administered during the last trimester have been used therapeutically to prolong gestation and delay the onset of labor. Information regarding the potential for fetal malformations resulting from NSAID therapy during pregnancy is still incomplete; however, chronic ingestion of NSAIDs may result in reduced birth weight. The major complications of NSAID therapy (in particular aspirin) are prolonged gestation, delayed labor, complications during delivery, and postpartum bleeding and hemorrhage likely resulting from inhibition of TXA_2 synthesis.

Ophthalamic Symptoms

As a class, NSAIDs have been reported to produce adverse eye findings in animal studies. It is generally recommended that ophthalamic studies be conducted if any change or disturbance in vision occurs.

Drug Interactions

Because many NSAIDs avidly bind to plasma proteins, they will compete at this site with other drugs that also bind to the plasma proteins. This may result in the displacement of a previously bound drug from the plasma protein to the serum, raising the concentration and increasing the biologic effects or produce the toxic effects of that drug. Examples of drugs that interact with NSAIDs in this manner are coumarin-type anticoagulants, hydantoin, sulfonamides, or sulfonylureas. Many NSAIDs are metabolized by the hepatic microsomal enzyme system, and drug interactions may occur with concomitant use of other drugs with NSAIDs owing to competition for metabolism at this site. Moreover, concomitant use of NSAIDs with drugs that induce the de novo synthesis of this enzyme system may be associated with a decrease in the plasma half-life of NSAIDs. In all cases where the potential for drug interaction exists, close monitoring of patients is required.

Therapeutic Uses of NSAIDs

Rheumatoid Arthritis

Rheumatoid arthritis is a systemic, inflammatory disease that can develop at any age. The highest incidence, however, occurs between 40 and 60 years of age. Synovial tissues are primarly involved, and progression can lead to destruction of cartilage and bone. Other tissues and organs also can become involved. Examples of extra-articular involvement are anemia, peripheral neuropathy, pericarditis, and vasculitis.

A therapeutic pyramid has been widely used in the treatment of rheumatoid arthritis. At the base of the pyramid are the NSAIDs, with aspirin usually the first-line drug, as salicylates are rapidly effective and low in cost. Members of this class of drugs have a relatively rapid onset of action (days to weeks) and produce similar analgesic and anti-inflammatory effects. There is no evidence that any one differs significantly from the others clinically. While NSAIDs can provide symptomatic therapy, they do not treat the underlying causes (see "Disease-Modifying Antirheumatic Drugs", below). Drug choice is based on the avoidance of particular side-effects and desired pharmacokinetics and half-life of action. Often several NSAIDs are systematically tried before one is found to produce the desirable therapeutic benefit with the least toxicity. Because of the frequency of serious GI toxicity, long-term use of NSAIDs in the treatment of rheumatoid arthritis must be re-evaluated frequently.

Anemia is frequently observed in rheumatoid arthritis, and this condition can be aggravated by NSAIDs that may produce minor GI blood loss owing to inhibition of platelet aggregation and local GI irritation. Therefore, patients with initial hemoglobin values of 10 g/dL or less receiving or about to receive long-term therapy with NSAIDs should have hemoglobin values determined periodically.

Rarely does treatment with NSAIDs alone provide enough therapy. The second-line drug and the second step in the therapeutic pyramid includes gold compounds, chloroquine, and penicillamine. Unlike the NSAIDs these drugs may actually alter the course of disease and even induce remission. These drugs are referred to as "disease modifying antirheumatic drugs" (DMARDs). Their onset of action is much delayed (weeks to months) and their therapeutic effect may last long after discontinuing treatment. DMARDs are not analgesics; therefore, their use at least initially is in combination with NSAIDs. As their effectiveness is realized, the NSAIDs may slowly be withdrawn as symptoms allow. In aggressive disease, third-line drugs may be required. These DMARDs include the cytotoxic and immunosuppressive drugs, azathioprine, methotrexate, and cyclophosphamide.[28] NSAIDs have been reported to displace bound methotrexate from serum proteins, thus increasing its therapeutic effects, but this may also increase its plasma concentration to toxic levels. When such concomitant therapy is employed, careful monitoring is required.

The pyramid approach has recently come under re-evaluation.[29,30] Early aggressive therapy may best serve to arrest the progression and prevent permanent joint damage. One strategy is early combination drug therapy. A definitive diagnosis of rheumatoid arthritis is crucial. The failure of NSAID therapy may well imply the presence of aggressive disease and warrant the addition of one or more DMARDs. These drugs are most effective if implemented before erosive joint disease and/or deformities develop. Early inclusion into the therapeutic regime, if warranted, may begin with lower doses thereby reducing toxicity. Another factor considered in the therapeutic regime is the therapeutic/toxicity ratio. In general, NSAIDs are less toxic than DMARDs. However, in the treatment of rheumatoid arthritis, long-term high-dose therapy with NSAIDs can produce severe and life-threatening side-effects. When one considers that NSAIDs provide only symptomatic relief, the therapeutic/toxicity ratio of DMARDs is far more desirable. It may be possible to manipulate this ratio by altering the time of drug administration.[31] For example, NSAID GI toxicity may be less when the drugs are administered at night.

Glucocorticoids have been demonstrated to exhibit an attenuating influence on the inflammatory response associated with rheumatoid arthritis. However, they are not drugs of first choice nor should they be considered for monotherapy in rheumatoid arthritis (Table 74.2). Steroids inhibit leukocyte infiltration and accumulation at the site of inflammation. This action most likely is a reflection of their inhibition of the formation of lipid chemokinetic and chemotactic factors (e.g., leukotriene B_4, hydroxyeicosatetraenoic acids [HETEs] or lipoxins). These lipid mediators of the inflammatory response are products of arachidonic acid metabolism. Arachidonic acid, a constituent of the phospholipids of cell membranes, is released from the storage depot by phospholipase A_2. Glucocorticosteroids stimulate the de novo synthesis of a protein, lipocortin, that inhibits the activity of phospholipase A_2, thus attenuating the release and subsequent metabolism of arachidonic acid.[32] In addition, steroids attenuate polymorphonucleocyte and macrophage phagocytoic activity. Moreover, they inhibit fibroblast proliferation and deposition of both collagen and the ground substance of connective tissue. However, owing to the wide range of biologic effects, corticosteroids are not used for initial therapy of rheumatoid arthritis. In particular, their immunosuppressive activity limits their use, especially in an infected joint or in instances in which there is a possibility of infection. In the treatment of bursitis or tendonitis, a smaller dose of a repository steroid is indicated where other approaches have proved ineffective.

Juvenile Arthritis

Juvenile arthritis, occurring by age 16, may manifest itself as multisystemic (even without symptomatic joint involvement), monarticular (usually the knee), which develops to pauciarticular (fewer than five joints), or polyarticular (five or more joints involved) similar to the arthritis seen in the adult. Aspirin again is the drug of choice. Because of potential serious side-effects of indomethacin and phenylbutazone, these drugs should not be administered to children under 14 years of age. The therapeutic approach to treating juvenile arthritis has become more aggressive and often includes the use of level 3 disease-modifying drugs.[18]

Ankylosing Spondylitis

Ankylosing spondylitis most often occurs in individuals between 20 and 40 years of age. It is characterized by involvement of the sacroiliac joints, the spinal apophyseal joints, and the paravertebral soft tissues. Aspirin has limited efficacy in relieving pain associated with severe flare-ups. Indomethacin has been considered the drug of choice for the symptomatic treatment of ankylosing spondylitis. Due to the potential for serious side-effects with indomethacin, piroxicam may be used instead. Piroxicam can provide good relief of pain with less severe side-effects and usually with once-daily dosing.

Osteoarthritis

This disorder is characterized by degeneration of articular cartilage and proliferative changes within the joint. The onset is most common in middle- or more advanced age. This disorder was thought to be noninflammatory; however, an inflammatory component is now recognized. NSAIDs are employed in treatment. As the patient population is older and frequently more sensitive to side-effects, it may be necessary to try several drugs to determine which is best tolerated. Indomethacin has proved particularly efficacious in the treatment of degenerative disease (osteoarthritis) of the hip. Since the therapeutic aim is to reduce pain, acetaminophen or codeine has been used; however, these drugs exert no anti-inflammatory action. Physical therapy in combination with appropriate drug therapy is an important adjunct in the management of osteoarthritis.[33]

Closure of the Ductus Arteriosus

Alterations in the profile and quantity of prostaglandin metabolites have been reported to affect the patency of the ductus arteriosus and perinatal breathing movements. PGE_2 has been reported to produce decreased fetal breathing movements in late term and apnea in newborn animals, and PGE_1 maintains ductal patency.[34,35] Indomethacin and other NSAIDs have been used to reverse these effects.[36]

Table 74.2 Comparisons of Selected Corticosteroids

	Relative Potency (anti-inflammatory)	Relative Potency (mineralo-corticoid)	Equivalent Dose (mg)	Available Dosage Form
Short duration				
Cortisone	0.8	0.8	25	oral, injectable, topical
Hydrocortisone	1	1	20	
Intermediate duration				
Methylprednisolone	5	0.5	5	oral, injectable, topical
Prednisolone	4	0.8	5	oral, injectable, topical
Prednisone	4	0.8	5	oral
Triamcinolone	5	0	4	oral, injectable, topical inhalation
Long duration				
Betamethasone	25	0	0.75	oral, injectable, topical
Dexamethasone	25	0	0.75	oral, injectable, topical inhalation
Paramethasone	10	0	2	oral

Nonsteroidal Anti-Inflammatory Drugs

Salicylates (Table 74.3)

Members of this class of NSAIDs include aspirin (acetylsalicylic acid), sodium salicylate, salicylic acid, methylsalicylate, and diflunisal.

Aspirin (Fig. 74.2)

Aspirin is widely used to reduce inflammation, fever, and mild-to-moderate pain. Aspirin is listed in the National Prescription Audit as one of the 200 most commonly prescribed drugs in the US in 1989. Aspirin is the drug of first choice for rheumatoid arthritis, a disorder marked by inflammatory changes in the synovial membranes and articular structures.[r9] This disorder can be controlled with aspirin alone in most patients. It should be emphasized that the cause of this disorder is unknown (viral infection and antiimmune mechanisms have been suggested), and NSAIDs only slow the progression and alleviate the symptoms. The most common reason for failure to obtain a therapeutic response to aspirin in the treatment of RA is the administration of an inadequate dose. This is generally due to the side-effects of NSAIDs, as discussed above. Aspirin is also used to treat ankylosing spondylitis and acute rheumatic fever. However, aspirin does not affect the endocarditis or permanent cardiac valvular damage associated with acute rheumatic fever. Aspirin is contraindicated in gout because it inhibits the elimination of uric acid by the kidney.

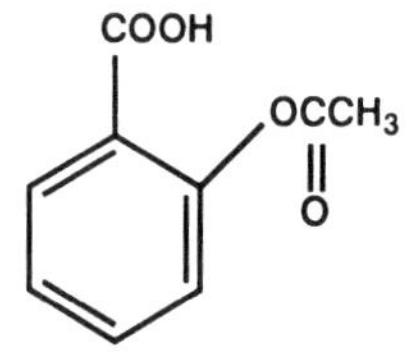

COOH

$OCCH_3$

O

Figure 74.2 Aspirin

Sodium Salicylate

Sodium salicylate is a less potent anti-inflammatory agent than aspirin, as it cannot irreversibly inhibit prostaglandin formation by acetylating the cyclooxygenase enzyme. While it may produce fewer GI side-effects than an equal amount of aspirin, the amount needed to produce a similar anti-inflammatory response is greater. Acetylsalicylate (aspirin) is rapidly metabolized to salicylate after ingestion.

Salicylic Acid

Salicylic acid is keratolytic and its primary use is to remove corns and warts. It is an organic acid that is corrosive to the mucosal lining of the GI tract and should not be taken internally.

Methylsalicylate (Fig. 74.3)

Methylsalicylate is a lipid soluble oil that is very irritating to tissues it contacts. Methylsalicylate is absorbed through the skin and produces effects similar to oral sodium salicylate. It is for external use only and is used primarily as a rubefacient to produce cutaneous vasodilation. It is also known as oil of wintergreen and is found in over-the-counter preparations employed topically to alleviate local

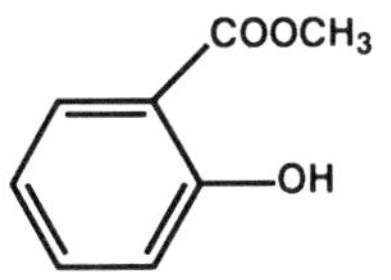

COOCH3 / OH

Figure 74.3 Methyl Salicylate

muscle soreness and to produce local vasodilation (heat). Because it is absorbed through the skin, methylsalicylate contributes salicylate toward total plasma salicylate, and thus can be a factor in salicylate toxicity.

Diflunisal (Fig. 74.4)

Diflunisal is a difluorophenyl derivative of salicylic acid. Absorption of diflunisal after oral administration is complete with peak plasma concentration reached in two to three hours. The plasma half-life is eight to 12 hours, with greater than 99 percent bound to plasma proteins. Because of its long half-life and nonlinear pharmacokinetics, several days of dosing are required before plasma levels reach steady-state and the therapeutic usefulness can be evaluated. An initial loading dose can shorten the time to reach steady-state. Diflunisal is eliminated primarily by the kidneys as two soluble glucuronidase conjugates. It is not metabolized to salicylic acid.

Diflunisal is indicated for acute or long-term therapy for mild to moderate pain, osteoarthritis, and RA.[r10] Diflunisal is not recommended for use as an antipyretic owing to its low efficacy. In the symptomatic treatment of osteoarthritis, diflunisal is as effective as aspirin at one-fourth the dose. Similarly, in the acute and chronic treatment of RA diflunisal is as effective as aspirin with fewer intolerable side-effects. There is a lower incidence of dyspepsia, GI pain, and tinnitus. In addition, at therapeutic doses diflunisal exhibits a much lower platelet-inhibitory activity than aspirin; unlike aspirin, the activity is reversible. Cross-sensitivity may occur in patients with aspirin hypersensitivity. Diflunisal, when administered at 500 or 700 mg daily in divided doses, has a uricosuric effect. It increases the renal clearance of uric acid and decreases serum uric acid. A severe and potentially life-threatening hypersensitivity syndrome has been associated with diflunisal. This syndrome is a multisystem with symptoms that may include fever, chills, cutaneous and hepatic changes, jaundice, leukopenia, thrombocytopenia, and renal failure. Upon evidence of hypersensitivity, diflunisal therapy should be discontinued.

Reye's Syndrome

Reye's syndrome is characterized by acute encephalopathy in association with fatty degeneration of the liver and mitochondrial dysfunction. The disease occurs primarily in children between the ages of 4 and 16 and is usually associated with viral infection, such as influenza and/or chickenpox.[r11] For as yet unknown reasons, aspirin administration is closely associated with the development of Reye's syndrome.[37] Juveniles are at higher risk with even relatively low doses of aspirin. The use of salicylates should be avoided in all children with viral infection, particularly varicella and/or influenza.

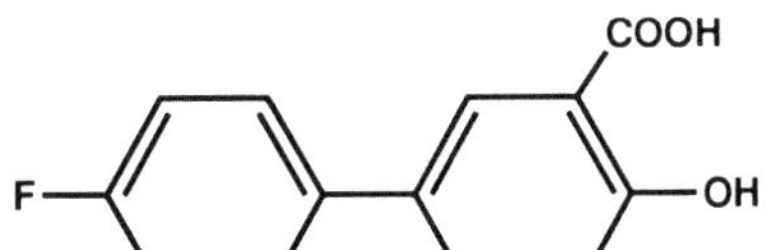

COOH / F / OH / F

Figure 74.4 Diflunisal

Salicylate Toxicity

Aspirin has a wide safety margin at therapeutically active doses. However, at the higher end of the therapeutic dose spectrum and with prolonged medication, toxicity can and most probably will develop, but side-effects are generally mild. One tablet of aspirin contains 325 mg of acetylsalicylic acid. The usual dose to alleviate inflammation or the pain associated with headache is two to three tablets (0.650–0.975 g). The dose used to treat RA is 15 to 25 tablets/day (4.9–8.1 g); generally, GI upset and tinnitus are associated with this regimen. More severe side-effects as described below are associated with a toxic overdose resulting from acute ingestion of 20 to 30 tablets (6.5–9.8 g). Such an overdose usually produces a serum salicylate level of 30 mg/dl or greater. The acute ingestion of 60 to 100 tablets (19.5–32.5 g) can produce death subsequent to respiratory depression. It should be noted that both sodium and methyl (absorbed through the skin) salicylate can contribute to the serum salicylate levels. Accidental salicylate overdose can result from concomitant use of aspirin and one or more of many over-the-counter preparations that contain aspirin or soldium salicylate.

In general, salicylate toxicity presents a complex and confusing clinical picture due to the effects of salicylates on multiple body functions.[38]

Gastrointestinal symptoms (nausea, vomiting, and gastric pain) can result from local direct irritation and back diffusion of gastric acid into the mucosa, as well as from decreased prostaglandin formation. The GI symptoms associated with the reduction in formation of PGE_2 and PGI_2 require several hours for onset. These symptoms are a result of increased secretion of gastric HCl and decreased cytoprotection subsequent to decreased prostaglandin formation.

The effects of salicylism on the CNS are profound and life-threatening. The initial symptoms of dizziness, headache, dimness of vision, auditory problems (tinnitus), irritability, confusion, hyperventilation (due to direct stimulation of the medullary respiratory center), thirst, fever, and dehydration are a result, at least in part, of stimulation of the CNS. In the adult, tinnitus is one of the earliest and most reliable signs of salicylate intoxication; however, this is not always the case with children. These symptoms are reversible within two to three days after cessation of aspirin or salicylate intake. If, however, the quantity of acutely ingested salicylate is high enough, depression of the respiratory center follows the initial symptoms resulting from stimulation of the CNS. This central depression of respiration can result in death.

Aspirin toxicity can also affect blood coagulation. One to two aspirin tablets can roughly double bleeding time for several days. The mechanism underlying this prolongation is at least twofold. One, a decrease in the formation of thromboxane A_2, the platelet proaggregatory metabolite formed by the platelet, subsequent to inhibition of cyclooxygenase activity; and, two, decreased prothrombin synthesis in the liver resulting in a hypoprothrombinemia subsequent to altered metabolism of vitamin K.

Salicylate toxicity is associated with stimulation of the metabolic rate, which results in an increase in body temperature. The increase in temperature is secondary to the uncoupling of mitochondrial oxidative phosphorylation. While mitochondrial respiration proceeds, the formation of adenosine triphosphate (ATP) does not occur, and the free energy of respiration is dissipated as heat rather than stored in the high-energy phosphate linkage of ATP. In addition, there is an increase in plasma and urine glucose concentration secondary to stimulation of glycogenolysis. Moreover, there is a decrease in plasma-free fatty acid concentration secondary to the inhibition of the incorporation of acetate into fatty acid.

Salicylate toxicity is also characterized by an acid/base imbalance. Initially, respiratory alkalosis is produced. This state results from the direct stimulation of the respiratory center by salicylate-producing hyperventilation. The increase in depth and rate of breathing results in a loss of CO_2, which results in an increase in plasma pH. A pattern of decreased pCO_2, increased pH, and normal plasma potassium concentration (K^+) and bicarbonate HCO_3^- concentration is a reliable and persistent sign of moderate salicylate toxicity-induced respiratory alkalosis in adults. The fall in pCO_2 alters the $[HCO_3^-]/[H_2CO_3]$ balance. The balance is restored toward normal by renal excretion of HCO_3^-. This is renal compensation of respiratory alkalosis and is generally characterized by a plasma pattern of decreased pCO_2, slightly increased pH, decreased plasma HCO_3^- concentration, and decreased plasma K^+ concentration (as K^+ usually follows HCO_3^-). This pattern is mirrored by an increase in urinary pH and increased HCO_3^- and K^+ concentrations. In adults on intensive salicylate therapy, these patterns produced by renal compensation of respiratory alkalosis are common, are well maintained, and seldom proceed further. However, in children, infants, and a small number of adults, depression of the medullary respiration center occurs after the above-outlined stimulation of that center. This phase of salicylism is characterized by hypoventilation, which produces a respiratory acidosis. This phase is characterized by a pattern of increased plasma pCO_2, decreased plasma pH, as well as decreased plasma HCO_3^- and K^+ concentrations. This respiratory acidosis remains uncompensated as plasma HCO_3^- concentration cannot be increased by reducing renal HCO_3^- excretion, because a large amount of HCO_3^- was excreted during renal compensation of respiratory alkalosis. In addition to respiratory acidosis developing, metabolic acidosis also develops. The development of metabolic acidosis is mediated by the presence of salicylic acid, a salicylate-induced increase in hepatic ketone production, and an accumulation of organic acids (sulfuric and phosphoric) subsequent to depressed hepatic and renal function associated with uncoupling of oxidative phosphorylation. The plasma profile presented in these individuals is decreased pH, HCO_3^- and K^+ concentrations, and nearly normal pCO_2.

In addition to the disturbances in water/electrolyte balance associated with renal compensation, other disturbances in water and electrolyte balance are also observed in salicylate toxicity. Hyperventilation, sweating associated with fever, and vomiting and diarrhea associated with GI upset all contribute to loss of water. The sweating, vomiting, and diarrhea are also associated with loss of electrolytes. Dehydration, as evidenced by decreased skin turgor, dry mucous membranes, increased urine specific gravity, decreased urine output, loss of body weight, and thirst, is observed. Dehydration in children is rapid in onset.

Treatment of Salicylate Toxicity

The immediate goal is to eliminate salicylate from the body.[38] Depending on the clinical presentation, the steps to be taken include: induction of vomiting, gastric lavage with water or 3 to 5 percent solution of $NaHCO_3$, and IV $NaHCO_3^-$. The latter intervention is an attempt to increase the ionized species of salicylate (as compared to the unionized acid) to promote renal excretion and to "trap" the ionized salicylate in alkaline urine. However, if the urine is already alkaline, the use of IV HCO_3^- is contraindicated. In addition, supportive actions to maintain renal function should be undertaken. These actions may include rehydration and the use of an osmotic diuretic (e.g., mannitol; however, this is not indicated in the presence of hypokalemia).

Phenylpropionic Acid Derivatives (Table 74.3)

Members of this class of NSAIDs—ibuprofen, fenoprofen, flurbiprofen, ketoprofen, naproxen, and suprofen—are all derivatives of phenylpropionic acid; however, their individual chemical structures are quite diverse. All members of this class of NSAIDs are effective both as anti-inflammatory drugs and as analgesics. They are used in inflammatory disorders, such as osteoarthritis and ankylosing spondylitis. As analgesics, they are used to relieve postpartum pain and postsurgical pain, as well as pain associated with dysmenorrhea.[39]

Ibuprofen (Fig. 74.5)

Ibuprofen in lower doses is available as an over-the-counter medication in Advil, Nuprin, and Motrin. Ibuprofen is listed in the National Prescription Audit as one of the 200 most commonly prescribed drugs in the US in 1989. At these lower doses, ibuprofen is more effective as an analgesic rather than as an anti-inflammatory drug. At prescribed doses of 2 g per day, ibuprofen is as effective in anti-inflammatory activity as 4 g of aspirin. Its absorption is complete after oral administration and is usually well tolerated, even by patients who cannot tolerate the gastric irritation caused by aspirin. Food does not generally affect the bioavailability of ibuprofen. The concomitant use of ibuprofen with aspirin has not been investigated in clinical trials. Thus, it is not recommended.

Peak plasma levels occur one to two hours after oral administration. Serum half-life is only two hours; therefore, multiple daily dosing is necessary. At higher doses, gastric irritation and bleeding can occur. Rash, peripheral edema, decreased appetite, tinnitus, dizziness, and some CNS effects, such as anxiety, headache, nervousness, or blurred vision, have been reported.[40] More serious side-effects include agranulocytosis, aplastic anemia, acute renal failure, interstitial nephritis, and nephrotic syndrome. Do not exceed 3200 mg total daily dose. Ibuprofen has been reported to elevate plasma lithium levels, reduce renal excretion of methotrexate, and inhibit the natriuretic effects of furosemide.

Fenoprofen (Fig. 74.6)

Fenoprofen is only slightly more potent in anti-inflammatory acitvity than ibuprofen and comparable to aspirin in rheumatoid arthritis or osteoarthritis. However, the occurrence of GI reactions and tinnitus is more frequent with aspirin. Absorption after oral administration may be incomplete if taken with food. Its serum half-life is three to four hours; therefore, it must be given in repeated doses. It is excreted in the urine as glucuronide metabolites formed in the liver. Side-effects of fenoprofen are similar to those of ibuprofen. Concurrent use of fenoprofen and aspirin is not indicated, as this results in decreases in the biologic half-life of fenoprofen owing to

Table 74.3 Suggested Dosages for Specific Indications

Class and Generic Name	Proprietary Name	Indication	Route and Approximate Dose (mg)
Salicylates			
Aspirin	Various	Antipyresis Analgesia RA,OA	650–950 qid 4900–8100 daily in divided doses
Diflunisal	Dolobid	Analgesia	oral; 1000 initially followed by 500 every 12 hours
		RA,OA	oral; 500–1000 daily in divided doses
Phenylproprionic Acid Derivatives			
Ibuprofen	Advil Medipren Motrin Nuprin Rufen Trendar	Analgesia,D	oral; 400 every 4–6 hours oral; 400 every 4 hours
		RA	oral; 1,200–3,200 daily (300 qid, 400, 600, or 800 tid or qid)
Fenoprofen	Nalfon	Analgesia RA,OA	oral; 200 every 4–6 hours; 300–600 tid or qid; RA therapy generally requires higher doses than OA but do not exceed 3,200 daily
Flurbiprofen	Ansaid	RA,OA	oral; 200–300 total daily, administered in divided doses bid, tid or qid; 100 is largest recommended single dose
Ketoprofen	Orudis	RA, OA	oral; 75 (tid) or 50 (qid)
Suprofen	Suprol	Analgesia	oral; 200 every 4–6 hours
Naproxen	Anaprox Naproxyn	Analgesia	oral; 550 initially followed by 275 every 6–8 hours; do not exceed 1,375
		RA,OA,AS	oral; 275 or 550 tid; do not exceed 3,200 daily
		AG	oral; 825 initially followed by 275 every 8 hours
		JA	oral; 10 given in 2 divided doses; do not exceed 15 mg/kg/day in children over 2 years of age
Oxaproxin	Daypro	RA, OA	oral; 1,200 in 2 divided doses
Phenylacetic Acid Derivative			
Diclofenac	Voltaren	OA	oral; 100–150 in divided doses 59 (bid or tid) or 75 (bid)
		RA	oral; 150–200 in divided doses 50 (tid or qid) or 75 (bid)
		AS	oral; 100–125 as 25 qid

continued

Table 74.3 *Continued*

Class and Generic Name	Proprietary Name	Indication	Route and Approximate Dose (mg)
Pyrrole Acetic Acid Derivatives			
Indomethacin	Indocin	RA,OA,AS	oral; 25 bid or tid; this may be increased until a total daily dose of 150–200 is achieved
Sulindac	Clinoril	RA,OA,AS	oral; 150 bid; do not exceed 400 daily
		AG,EAI	oral; 200 bid
Tolmetin	Tolectin	RA,OA	oral; 400 tid initially followed by 600–1800 daily in divided doses (tid) after control is achieved
		JA	oral; 20 mg/kg/day initially in divided doses (tid or qid) followed by 15–30 kg/day in divided doses (tid or qid) after control is achieved
Ketorolac	Toradol	Analgesia	IM; 30–70 as a loading dose followed by half of the loading dose every 6 hours; maximal daily dose is 150 for first day and 120 subsequently; not recommended for use beyond 5 days
Etodolac	Lodine	Analgesia	oral; 200–400 every 6–8 hours; do not exceed 1200/day
		OA	oral; 800–1200/day initially followed by 600–1200/day in divided doses
Napthyl Acetic Acid Derivative			
Nabumetone	Relafen	OA,RA	oral; starting dose is 100 daily; can increase to 1500–2000 daily in either single or twice daily doses
Pyrazolone Derivatives			
Apazone		RA,OA	oral; 1200 per day in divided doses
		AG	oral; 2400 on first day in divided doses; tid followed by 1800 daily until attack subsides followed by 1200 per day until symptoms disappear
Phenylbutazone	Azolid Butazolidine	AS	oral; 300 mg daily in 3–4 equally divided doses; not generally recommended, see text
Anthranilac Acid Derivatives			
Meclofenamate	Meclomen	Analgesia	oral; 50–100 every 4–6 hours; do not exceed 400 daily
		RA, OA	oral; 200–400 in divided doses tid or qid
Mefenamic Acid	Ponstel	Analgesia, D	oral; 500 initially followed by 250 every 6 hours

continued

Table 74.3 *Continued*

Class and Generic Name	Proprietary Name	Indication	Route and Approximate Dose (mg)
Oxicam Derivative			
Piroxicam	Feldene	RA, OA	20/day
Disease Modifying Antirheumatic Drugs			
Aurothioglucose	Solganal	RA	IM; adult: 1st dose, 10; 2nd & 3rd doses, 25; 4th + dose, 50. Dosing interval, 1 week; if no improvement after 1.0 g given, discontinue IM; children (6–12 years old): 1/4 of adult dose (varying with body weight); do not exceed 25/dose
Gold Sodium Thiomalate	Myochrysine	RA	IM; adult: 1st dose, 10; 2nd dose, 25; 3rd + doses, 25–50; dosing interval, 1 week; continue until 1 g given
		JA	IM; children: proportional to adult on a weight basis; after initial test dose of 10, follow with 1/kg; do not exceed 50/single injection
Auranofin	Ridaura	RA	oral; adult: 6 daily, given as 3 (bid) or 6 once; if response inadequate after 6 months, increase to 9 (3 tid); if still inadequate after 3 months, discontinue
Dimercaprol		Gold antidote see "Other" below	
Azathioprine	Imuran	RA	oral or IV; initial dose, 1/kg as single dose or divided bid dose may be increased slowly after 6–8 weeks to a maximum of 2.5/kg/day
Choloroquine	Aralen	RA	oral; initial dose, 1000 (the equivalent of 600 mg base) followed by 500 daily
Hydroxychloroquine	Plaquenil	RA	oral; 400–600 (310–465 mg base) daily; within 5–10 days increase dose to optimal response level; maintenance dose, 200–400 (155–310 mg base) daily
Penicillamine	Cuprimine Depen	RA	oral; initially daily single dose of 125 or 250; increase at 1–3 month intervals by 125 or 250/day up to 500–750/day; after 2–3 months, can increase by 250/day up to 1000 to 1500/day; maintenance therapy must be individualized

continued

Table 74.3 *Continued*

Class and Generic Name	Proprietary Name	Indication	Route and Approximate Dose (mg)
Disease Modifying Antirheumatic Drugs *continued*			
Methotrexate	Methotrexate Rheumatrex	RA	oral; 7.5/week
Nonsteroid Analgesic and Antipyretic			
Acetaminophen	Anexsia, Atarin, Aspirin-free Excedrin, Feverall, Fioricet, Hycomine Compound, Hydrocet, Isocom, Midrin, Phrenilin, Tylenol, Tylox, Vicodin, Zydone	Fever, analgesia	oral; adults and children over 12 years of age 500 tid (maximum of 4000/day)
Drugs for Treatment of Gout			
Allopurinol	Zyloprim	Gout	oral; 200–300/day for mild gout; 400–600/day for moderately severe tophaceous gout
		Inhibit acute gouty flare-up	oral; initially 100/day with weekly increases of 100
Sulfinpyrazone	Anturane	Gout	oral; 200–400 daily in 2 divided doses, increasing to maintenance dose (400) within 1 week
Probenecid	Benemid	Gout	oral; 0.25 g bid for 1 week followed by 0.5 g bid thereafter
Colchicine	—	Acute gouty arthritis	IV; initially 2 followed by 0.5 every 6 hours until satisfactory response
	Colbenemid tablet (0.5 g probenecid + 0.5 g colchicine)	"	oral; one tablet daily for a week followed by one table bid thereafter
Other			
N-acetylcysteine	Acetylcysteine Mucomyst Mucosil Acetylcysteine	Acetaminophen antidote	oral; loading dose 140/kg; additional doses of 70/kg at 4 hour intervals IV; loading dose 150/kg over 15 minutes, followed by 50/kg in 500 ml 5% dextrose solution over 4 hours and 100/kg in 1000 ml 5% dextrose solution over the next 16 hours; total dose 300/kg in 20 hours
Dimercaprol	Bal in Oil Ampules	Gold antidote	IM; mild poisoning, 2.5/kg qid for 2 days, bid on third day and one daily for next 7 days; severe poisoning, 3/kg qid for 2 days, 4 times on third day and bid for next 7 days

RA, rheumatoid arthritis; OA, osteoarthritis; DF, dysmenorrhea; AG, acute gouty arthritis; JA, juvenile arthritis; EAI, extraarticular inflammation; AS, ankylosing spondylitis

Figure 74.5 Ibuprofen

Figure 74.6 Fenoprofen Calcium

an increase in metabolic clearance. Do not exceed total daily usage of 3200 mg. Pediatric dose not established.

Flurbiprofen (Fig. 74.7)

Flurbiprofen is more potent than ibuprofen in anti-inflammatory activity. It is completely absorbed after oral administration, reaches peak blood levels in approximately 1.5 hours, has a serum half-life of four hours, and achieves high concentration in synovial fluid. If taken with food, the rate of absorption is slowed, but bioavailability is not affected. More than 99 percent is bound to serum proteins. It is metabolized in the liver and excreted primarily in the urine. Its side-effects include nausea, diarrhea, and general stomach upset. Concurrent use with aspirin is not recommended, as this produces a 50 percent lower serum flurbiprofen concentration. Flurbiprofen pretreatment has been reported to reduce the hypotensive effect of propranolol. Flurbiprofen may be used in combination with gold salts or corticosteroids in the treatment of RA. Safety and efficacy in children have not been studied.

Ketoprofen (Fig. 74.8)

Ketoprofen is listed in the National Prescription Audit as one of the 200 most commonly prescribed drugs in the US in 1989. Ketoprofen is similar in potency to flurbiprofen; it is absorbed rapidly and completely after oral administration, but has a more variable serum half-life (2–4 hours). The rate of absorption but not bioavailability is decreased by food. In vitro, ketoprofen inhibits both cyclooxygenase and lipoxygenase enzyme activities. It is excreted primarily in the urine as the glucuronide metabolite. As with other drugs in this class, concurrent use with aspirin is not recommended. Probenecid increases both free and bound ketoprofen; therefore, concurrent therapy with probenecid is not recommended. It is also not recommended for use with methotrexate. The major side-effects

Figure 74.7 Flurbiprofen

Figure 74.8 Ketoprofen

of ketoprofen are on the GI tract and the CNS. Safety and efficacy in children have not been established.

Suprofen (Fig. 74.9)

Suprofen exhibits analgesic and antipyretic properties. It is rapidly and completely absorbed after oral administration. Plasma half-life is two to four hours; more than 99 percent is bound to plasma proteins. Although suprofen is more potent than ibuprofen, its potential for serious side-effects (flank pain and renal dysfunction) limits its use to the treatment of pain associated with dysmenorrhea, but not as initial therapy.

Naproxen (Fig. 74.10)

Naproxen, which is listed in the National Prescription Audit as one of the 200 most commonly prescribed drugs in the US in 1989, is a naphthylpropionic acid with intermediate potency. It is well absorbed after oral administration; however, antacids can reduce its rate of absorption. Naproxen has a long serum half-life of 13 hours, which may provide an advantage in situations in which patient compliance is a problem.[41] Do not exceed 3200 mg per day in adults. However, based on clinical studies, this drug is useful in the treatment of juvenile arthritis. Its safety and efficacy in other pediatric conditions or below the age of 2 has not been studied.

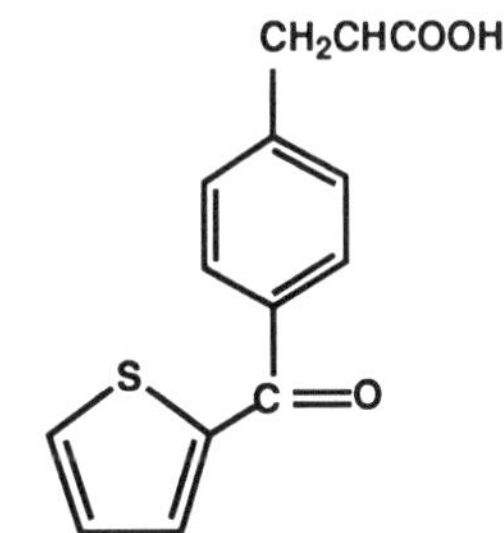

Figure 74.9 Suprofen

Figure 74.10 Naproxen

Oxaprozin (Fig. 74.11)

Oxaprozin exhibits analgesic and antipyretic properties. It is rapidly and essentially completely absorbed after oral administration. Plasma half-life is greater than 20 hours, and analgesic but not anti-inflammatory effects are produced acutely after a single dose; this is related to the long half-life. The long half-life may provide an advantage where compliance is a problem. Food may reduce the rate but not the extent of absorption. Oxaprozin exhibits a high degree of protein binding and primarily metabolic route of elimination (hepatic cytochrome P450 and glucuronic acid conjugation). Reported adverse reactions include constipation, diarrhea, dyspepsia, nausea, and rash. Somewhat less frequent reactions include CNS inhibition, disturbance of sleep, and tinnitus.

Phenylacetic Acid Derivative (Table 74.3)

Diclofenac (Fig. 74.12)

Diclofenac, which is listed in the National Prescription Audit as one of the 200 most commonly prescribed drugs in the US in 1989, is a very potent inhibitor of cyclooxygenase. It is rapidly and completely absorbed after oral administration, reaching peak plasma concentration within two to three hours. Diclofenac is extensively bound to plasma proteins (99%) and has a plasma half-life of one to two hours.

Diclofenac is approved for the chronic symptomatic treatment of rheumatoid arthritis, osteoarthritis, and ankylosing spondylitis. Its apparent accumulation in synovial fluid provided a longer duration of action than would be expected from its plasma half-life.

Because of its potent cyclooxygenase-inhibitor activity, the most common side-effects are GI bleeding and ulceration. Diclofenac undergoes substantial first-pass effect; moderate elevation of serum hepatic transaminase activities has been reported, but rarely is associated with any clinical evidence of hepatic injury. It is not recommended for use in patients with hepatic porphyria. Until more clinical studies are performed, diclofenac is not recommended for use in children, pregnant women, or nursing mothers. Concomitant use with aspirin is not recommended.

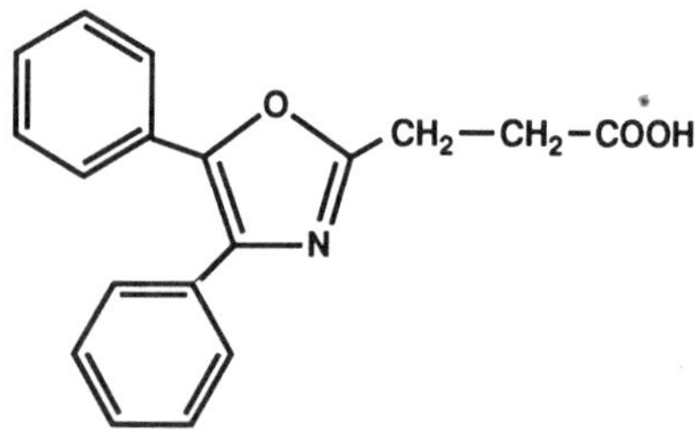

Diclofenac may have a dual mechanism of action with regard to its analgesic efficacy. In addition to inhibiting cyclooxygenase activity, it may also downregulate ongoing hyperalgesia.[42]

O, N, $CH_2—CH_2—COOH$

Figure 74.11 Oxaprozin

$HOOCCH_2$, Cl, NH, Cl

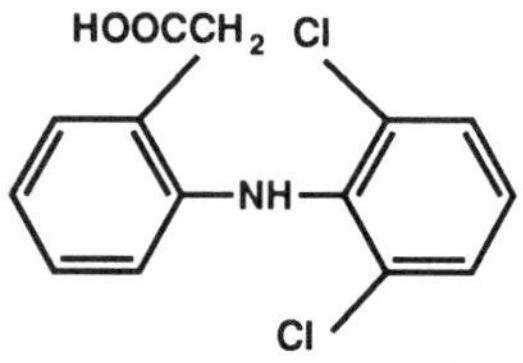

Figure 74.12 Diclofenac

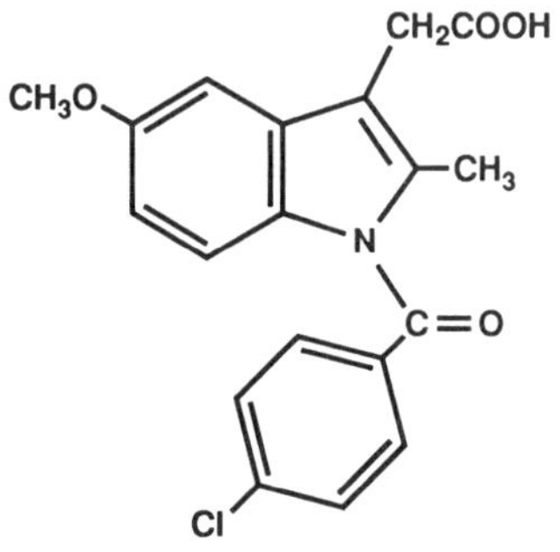

CH_2COOH, CH_3O, CH_3, N, C=O, Cl

Figure 74.13 Indomethacin

Pyrrole Acetic Acid Derivatives (Table 74.3)

This group of compounds contains diverse structures with a common link of pyrrole, indol, or indene ring systems containing acetic acid molecules.

Indomethacin (Fig. 74.13)

Indomethacin is a very potent NSAID absorbed well after oral administration. It is metabolized in the liver and has a relatively short serum half-life of four hours.

Although effective, indomethacin is not recommended for general use as an analgesic. Its use is primarily as an anti-inflammatory drug for the treatment of ankylosing spondylitis, osteoarthritis of the hip and hands, and extra-articular inflammatory conditions, such as pericarditis and pleurisy. A component of the anti-inflammatory activity of indomethacin is its ability to inhibit polymorphonuclear leukocyte chemotaxis. These properties make indomethacin very effective in the treatment of acute gouty arthritis and it is often the first line treatment of acute gout. While indomethacin should not normally be used in infants and children, it has been used in the treatment of patent ductus arteriosus, a condition thought to be dependent on the synthesis of endogenous vasodilator prostaglandins. Indomethacin is very effective in relieving the pain of dysmenorrhea and has been used to prevent spontaneous labor.

Indomethacin therapy is associated with a high incidence of intolerable side-effects, which can be irreversible and possibly fatal. Thus, careful observation and instruction of the patient are essential. The most frequent of these are GI complaints consisting of abdominal pain, nausea, diarrhea, and ulceration of the upper GI tract. Concomitant use with aspirin is not recommended, owing to a significant increase in GI adverse reactions. CNS effects include severe frontal headache, vertigo, dizziness, depression, and psychosis. The severity of these side-effects limits indomethacin to short-term therapy. The acute use of indomethacin has been reported to increase plasma growth hormone levels. As such, it may complicate the diagnosis of acromegaly and be contraindicated in diabetes mellitus. Whether chronic use produces a sustained increase in plasma growth hormone is uncertain.

Sulindac (Fig. 74.14)

Sulindac is structually related to indomethacin and is also listed in the National Prescription Audit as one of the 200 most commonly prescribed drugs in the US in 1989. It is a prodrug, having little if any anti-inflammatory activity prior to its biotransformation to the active sulfide metabolite in the liver. This active metabolite is only about half as potent as indomethacin. Sulindac is well absorbed after oral administration, although absorption will be delayed if taken with food; however, it is recommended that it be adminstered with food. The serum half-life of sulindac itself is about seven hours; however, the active sulfide metabolite has a half-life as long as 18 hours. Although the active sulfide is metabolized to an inactive compound by the kidney, a true "renal sparing" effect of sulindac is still in question.

Sulindac has been used as treatment for rheumatoid arthritis, osteoarthritis, and ankylosing spondylitis. A fairly rapid therapeutic response can be expected (about 1 week) in 50 percent of the patients. Sulindac is also indicated for treatment of bursitis, supraspinatus tendinitis, and acute gouty arthritis. Therapy for seven to 14 days is usually adequate for bursitis and tendinitis, whereas one week is adequate for acute gouty arthritis.

Sulindac shares many of the side-effects observed with indomethacin, although these are generally less severe. Since sulindac itself has little anti-inflammatory activity, oral administration results in infrequent GI distress. Safety and efficacy in children have not been determined.

Tolmetin (Fig. 74.15)

Tolmetin is a pyrrole-acetic acid derivative and is effective in juvenile and adult RA and osteoarthritis. It is about equally effective as aspirin, but exhibits fewer side-effects. A therapeutic effect can be expected within a few days to a week. It has been reported to increase the efficacy of corticosteroids or gold therapy. However, it must be taken frequently (e.g., 400 mg 3–4 times a day) as it has a half-life of about 60 minutes. Gastrointestinal side-effects comprise the most frequent complaints. The incidence of tinnitus is less than with aspirin. The concurrent use of tolmetin with anticoagulants or hypoglycemic agents is warranted if monitored. Tolmetin produces pseudoproteinuria in tests involving acid precipitation. The drug is eliminated by the kidney; therefore, it must be used with caution in patients with impaired renal function. Caution is also advised in patients with peptic ulcers. Safety and efficacy in children under two years of age have not been established.

Ketoralac (Fig. 74.16)

Ketoralac exhibits analgesic and antipyretic properties. It is completely absorbed after oral administration. Intramuscular preparations are also available. Plasma half-life following oral administration is two to nine hours; more than 99 percent is bound to plasma proteins. A high-fat meal may decrease the rate but not the extent of absorption. More than 90 percent of ketoralac and its metabolites is excreted in the urine. Ketoralac does not penetrate the blood-brain barrier very well. Clinical studies indicate that ketoralac produces analgesia following general or oral surgery. Based on the percentage of patients who did not remedicate, ketoralac (30 or 90 mg IM)

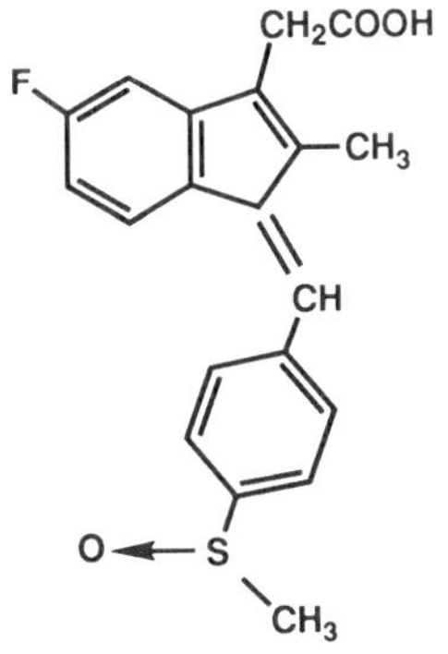

Figure 74.14 Sulindac

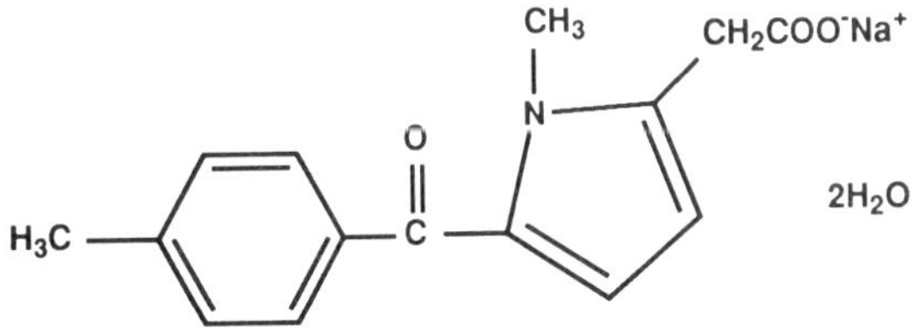

Figure 74.15 Tolmetin Sodium

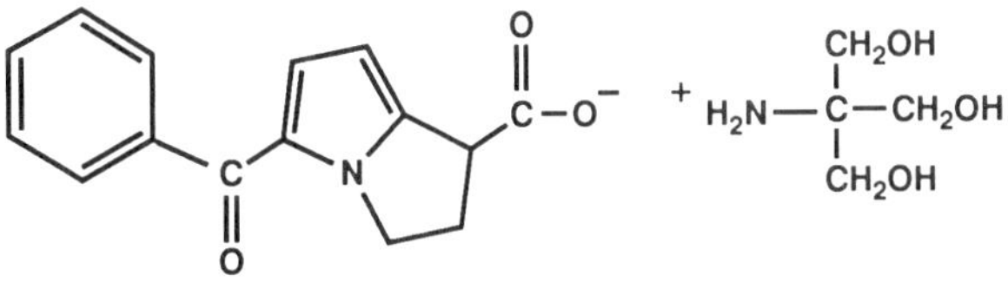

Figure 74.16 Ketorolac Tromethamine

compared favorably with meperidine (100 mg) or morphine (12 mg). Ketoralac is recommended only for therapy not exceeding five days; adverse reactions may increase with longer use at recommended doses. It is not recommended for use with other NSAIDs because of potential for additive side-effects. Adverse reactions include ulcerations, bleeding proliferation, interstitial nephritis, ARF, hemorrhage, and hypersensitivity reactions.

Etodolac (Fig. 74.17)

Etodolac exhibits anti-inflammatory, analgesic, and antipyretic activities. It is well absorbed (80%), bound more than 99 percent to plasma proteins, and is metabolized in the liver with the urinary route as the primary excretion of etodolac and its metabolites. Food does not affect the extent of absorption; however, it reduces the peak concentration by about one-half, as well as the time to peak concentration.

Etodolac is indicated for the treatment of pain and osteoarthritis. It is not recommended for RA; the results of clinical trials indicate it is generally not as effective as other NSAIDs. The dose for analgesics is 200–400 mg every six to eight hours, not to exceed 1200 mg/day. The dose for osteoarthritis is 800–1200 mg/day initially, followed by 600–1200 mg/day in divided doses. Concomitant administration with aspirin is not recommended. Concomitant administration with warfarin does not require dose adjustment for either drug. Gastrointestinal side-effects are the most frequent complaints (dyspepsia, abdominal pain). Asthenia/malaise, dizziness, tinnitus, blurred vision, and rash have also been reported. The safety and efficacy in children have not been established.

Napthylacetic Acid Derivative (Table 74.3)

Nabumetone (Fig. 74.18)

Nabumetone exhibits anti-inflammatory, analgesic, and antipyretic activities. It is a prodrug that is rapidly biotransformed by the liver to the active compound, 6-methoxy-2-naphthylacetic acid. It is well absorbed by the GI tract. About 80 percent is excreted in the urine following oral administration. More than 99 percent of the active compound is bound to plasma proteins. Concomitant administration with food increases the rate of absorption, as reflected by an increase in peak plasma concentration of about a third. Food does not affect the extent of conversion (about 35%) of nabumetone to the active compound. The effect of hepatic impairment on the conversion to active compound is uncertain, but conversion may be reduced. Nabumetone therapy has been reported to be associated with less GI blood loss than with aspirin. Moreover, 1000 mg daily of nabumetone has been reported not to affect platelet aggregation nor to prolong bleeding time.

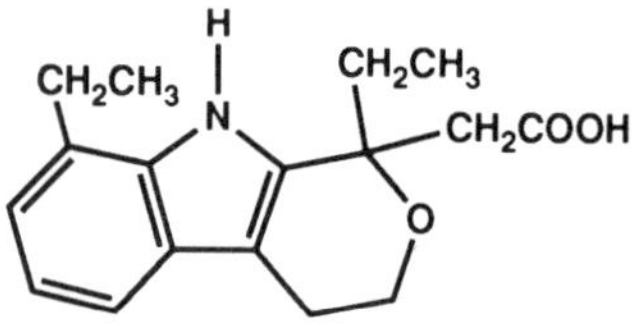

CH_2CH_3 H N CH_2CH_3 CH_2COOH O

Figure 74.17 Etodolac

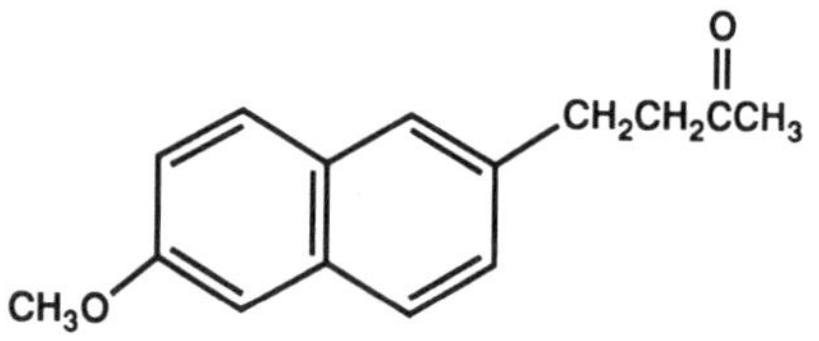

O $CH_2CH_2CCH_3$ CH_3O

Figure 74.18 Nabumetone

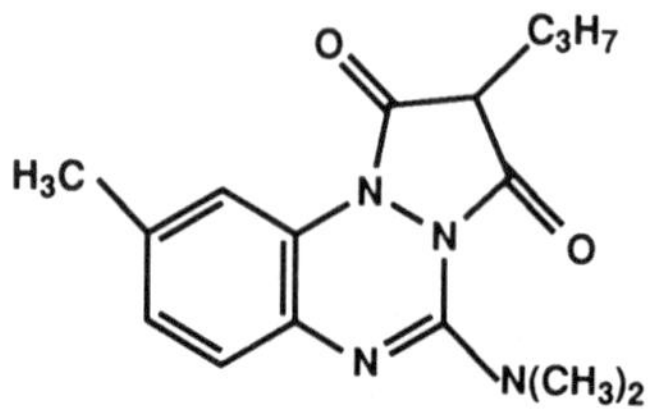

C_3H_7 O H_3C N N O N $N(CH_3)_2$

Figure 74.19 Apazone

Nabumetone therapy is indicated in the treatment of osteoarthritis and RA. For both conditions, the recommended starting dose is 1000 mg as a single dose with or without food. This may be increased to 1500 to 2000 mg per day in either single or twice daily doses.

Adverse reactions include diarrhea, dyspepsia, abdominal pain, constipation, flatulence, nausea, dizziness, headache, pruritus, rash, tinnitus, and edema.

Pyrazolone Derivatives (Table 74.3)

This group of drugs include apasone, oxyphenbutazone, phenylbutazone, and sulfinpyrazone. As a class, these drugs are effective anti-inflammatory agents; however, their antipyretic and analgesic activities are inferior to those of aspirin. Their use is primarily in the treatment of inflammatory disorders; owing to their toxicity, therapy is usually for the short term.

Apasone (Fig. 74.19)

Apasone is anti-inflammatory, analgesic, and antipyretic. It is also a potent uricosuric agent (inhibiting tubular reabsorption of uric acid), and may be of use in the treatment of gout. Apasone is rapidly and completely absorbed after oral administration. Because apasone is extensively bound to plasma proteins, its half-life is 20 to 24 hours. Another consequence of its extensive protein binding is the displacement of other protein-bound drugs. Apasone increases the levels of free phenytoin and warfarin by competing for their protein binding sites. The toxicity of apasone is similar to that of the other members of this class; however, it appears much less likely to produce agranulocytosis.

Phenylbutazone (Fig. 74.20)

Phenylbutazone is rapidly and completely absorbed after oral administration. It is extensively protein bound and has a very long half-life of 50 to 100 hours. Phenylbutazone is slowly metabolized into hydroxyphenylbutazone and oxyphenbutazone, both of which have activities similar to phenylbutazone. These metabolites contribute to the prolonged pharmacologic effects of phenylbutazone administration.

Phenylbutazone is an effective anti-inflammatory drug; however, its toxicity limits its use to short-term therapy, and only after other drugs have failed. The most effective and safe use of this drug is in acute flare-ups of RA and related disorders, and it should never be used as an analgesic or antipyretic. Phenylbutazone also inhibits tubular reabsorption of uric acid. This uricosuric activity, along with its anti-inflammatory activity, make phenylbutazone an effective treatment in acute gout; but owing to its toxicity, it should never be used prophylactically. The most serious adverse reaction is blood

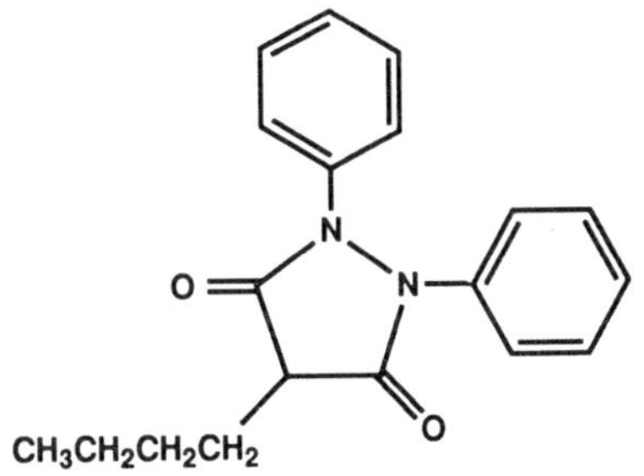

Figure 74.20 Phenylbutazone

dyscrasia. Other side-effects include rashes, water retention, edema, and hepatic and renal necrosis. Phenylbutazone should not be used in patients with borderline or overt CHF and is contraindicated in children under 14 years of age and in senile patients. Both phenylbutazone and oxyphenbutazone have been either withdrawn or their use faces restrictions in a number of countries.

Anthranilic Acid Derivatives (Table 74.3)

Members of this class include meclofenamate and mefenamic acid. Although both drugs exhibit analgesic, antipyretic, and anti-inflammatory activities, meclofenamate is used as an anti-inflammatory drug while mefenamic acid is used as an analgesic.

Meclofenamate (Fig. 74.21)

Absorption of meclofenamate is complete after oral administration, reaching peak plasma concentration in one-half to one hour. Plasma half-life is two hours. Meclofenamate is highly bound to plasma proteins and displaces warfarin. This effect combined with its inhibition of platelet TXA_2 generation requires that prothrombin time be monitored during simultaneous use with warfarin.

Meclofenamate is indicated for the symptomatic treatment of acute and chronic rheumatoid arthritis and osteoarthritis. It is not, however, recommended for initial therapy due to its potential for severe side effects.

Gastrointestinal toxicity is the most frequent complication of meclofenamate therapy. Diarrhea, nausea, and vomiting occur usually during early therapy and are reversed when the dose is reduced or discontinued. Meclofenamate can exacerbate preexisting gastric or duodenal ulcers and should be used with caution in these patients. CNS toxicity include headache and dizziness. Overdose may produce CNS stimulation and seizures. Safety and efficacy in children have not been established.

Mefenamic Acid (Fig. 74.22)

After oral administration, preferably with food, mefenamic acid reaches peak plasma concentration in two to four hours and has a

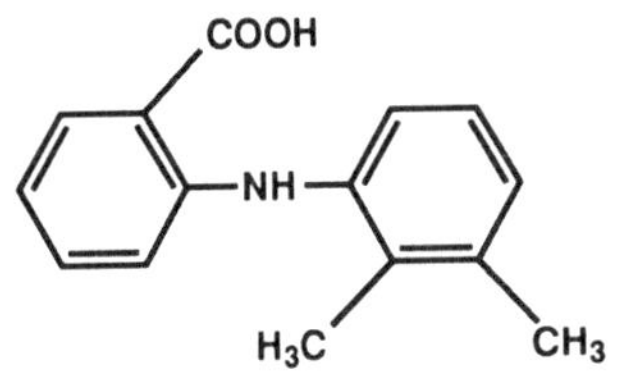

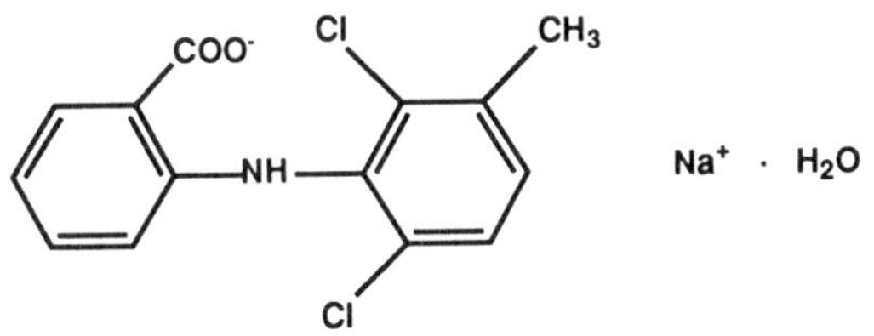

Figure 74.21 Meclofenamate Sodium Monohydrate

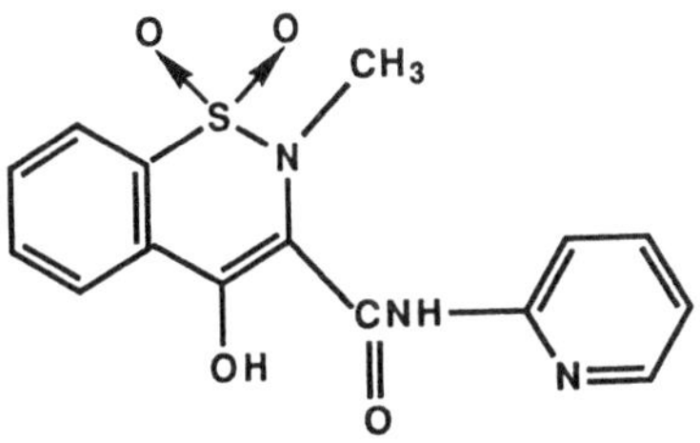

Figure 74.22 Mefenamic Acid

plasma half-life of two to four hours. Like meclofenamate, it is extensively bound to plasma proteins.

Mefenamic acid has anti-inflammatory and antipyretic activities; however, its use is limited to the treatment of mild to moderate pain. It is indicated in the treatment of primary dysmenorrhea, but its use should not exceed one week. Comparative studies have shown that mefenamic acid is no more effective than aspirin or other NSAIDs in relieving mild pain. Safety and efficacy in children under 14 years of age have not been established.

Gastrointestinal distress is the most common complaint. Diarrhea, nausea, vomiting, and abdominal pain are frequent symptoms. Megaloblastic anemia, hemolytic anemia, agranulocytosis, and thrombocytopenic purpura have also been reported. Mefenamic acid is contraindicated in patients with GI ulceration and impaired renal function.

Oxicam Derivative (Table 74.3)

Piroxicam (Fig. 74.23)

Oxicams are structurally different from other NSAIDs in that they are not carboxylic acids. Like other NSAIDs, piroxicam possesses anti-inflammatory, antipyretic, and analgesic activities by virtue of its ability to inhibit cyclooxygenase. Piroxicam also inhibits chemotaxis, release of lysosomal enzymes, and neutrophil aggregation. These properties increase its efficacy as an antiarthritic. It is listed in the National Prescription Audit as one of the 200 most commonly prescribed drugs in the US in 1989. Piroxicam is well absorbed after oral administration, with peak plasma concentration achieved within three to five hours. It is highly bound to plasma proteins and has a very long half-life of 30 to 86 hours. Dosing is once per day, and steady-state levels of the drug are reached in seven to 12 days. Doses in children have not been established.

Piroxicam is used in the acute and chronic symp-

Figure 74.23 Piroxicam

tomatic treatment of RA and osteoarthritis. At a dose of 20 mg/day, piroxicam is as effective as aspirin in the treatment of these conditions with lower incidence of minor GI effects and tinnitus. However, combination therapy with piroxicam and aspirin should not be undertaken, since the concomitant administration of aspirin reduces the plasma level of piroxicam by as much as 80 percent.

As with all NSAIDs, piroxicam can produce GI toxicity. Diarrhea, nausea, vomiting, abdominal pain, and ulceration are all potential side-effects, particularly with chronic use. Piroxicam can produce serious renal toxicity. Its elimination is primarily via the kidney, with up to 5 percent excreted unchanged. There have been reports of acute interstitial nephritis with hematuria, proteinuria, and nephrotic syndrome. At particular risk are patients with reduced renal blood flow (hypertension) or blood volume (CHF), where inhibition of prostaglandin synthesis may further reduce kidney perfusion. Owing to extensive plasma protein binding, piroxicam can displace other protein-bound drugs. It should be used with careful monitoring in patients receiving anticoagulant therapy.

Disease-Modifying Antirheumatic Drugs (Table 74.3)

Gold Compounds

Disease-modifying antirheumatic drugs have the potential for severe toxicity. They should not be used as first-line drugs in the treatment of RA.[43–45] Several months of use may be required before therapeutic efficacy can be evaluated.

The mechanism of action of the gold compounds (aurothioglucose, gold sodium thiomalate, and auranofin) is unknown. They are both anti-inflammatory and immunosuppressive. Unlike the other antiarthritic drugs, these gold compounds may actually alter the course of disease by retarding the progression to other uninfected joints, even inducing remission. Their use is indicated in active adult and juvenile RA responding poorly to or progressing despite NSAID therapy. The use of NSAIDs should be continued unless remission occurs. While most patients respond favorably to gold therapy, remission is usually temporary. The recurrence of disease is often less severe and should respond well to repeated therapy.

The usefulness of gold therapy is limited by the potential for severe toxicity experienced by as many as 25 percent of the patients. Toxicity can occur any time during therapy or even after therapy has been discontinued. Incidence of toxicity appears unrelated to plasma levels of these drugs. Total body accumulation of gold is the likely determinant of most toxicities. Gold salts should not be used concomitantly with penicillamine.

Aurothioglucose (Fig. 74.24)

As a suspension in sesame oil, aurothioglucose is administered as an IM injection once per week. Dosage is gradually increased until, by week four, 50 mg is administered. This dose may be continued in the absence of toxicity, or reduced. If no improvement is noted after the total administration of 1 g, therapy should be discontinued and re-evaluated. Aurothioglucose is indicated as adjunctive therapy for early active adult and juvenile RA. Concomitant NSAID therapy may be gradually withdrawn as the condition improves.

Aurothioglucose is contraindicated in patients with known hypersensitivity or severe toxicity to gold or other heavy metals, as well as those with uncontrolled diabetes mellitus, renal disease, hepatic dysfunction, CHF, hypertension, or blood dyscrasias. Because of its immunosuppressive activity, aurothioglucose should not be administered to patients who have recently received radiation therapy or those receiving other immunosuppressive drugs. Gold crosses the placenta and does appear in breast milk; therefore, aurothioglucose therapy is contraindicated during pregnancy and nursing of infants.

Dermatitis is the most common side-effect of therapy and may be aggravated by exposure to sunlight. Also common is stomatitis and the development of ulcers on the buccal membranes, tongue, and palate, often preceded by a metallic taste. The development of nephrotic syndrome or glomerulitis with proteinuria or hematuria can occur. Baseline values for protein excretion should be established before beginning therapy and monitored after each injection. If proteinuria or hematuria develop, therapy must be discontinued immediately and a gold chelating agent, such as dimercaprol, may be needed. These toxicities usually subside once therapy is discontinued.

Gold Sodium Thiomalate (Fig. 74.25)

Gold sodium thiomalate is administered as an IM injection once per week. The initial dose is 10 mg followed by an increase in dose until, by the third dose

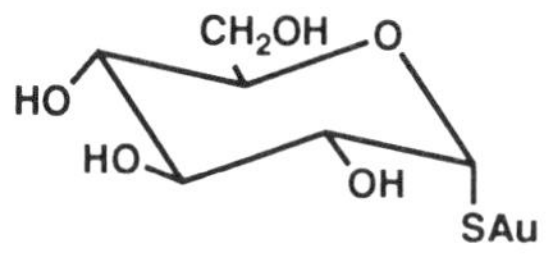

Figure 74.24 Aurothioglucose

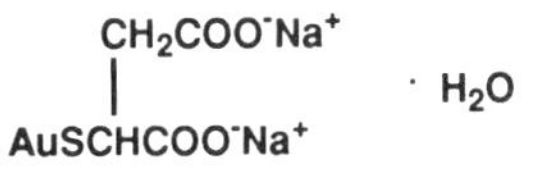

$$\begin{array}{l} CH_2COO^-Na^+ \\ | \\ AuSCHCOO^-Na^+ \end{array} \cdot H_2O$$

Figure 74.25 Gold Sodium Thiomalate

(third week), 50 mg is administered. This dose is continued unless toxicity develops. If no clinical improvement is observed after a total administration of 1 g, the patient should be considered refractory. Gold sodium thiomalate is indicated in the treatment of selected cases of both adult and juvenile active rheumatoid arthritis. Full benefit can be realized only in the early active stages, before structural damage has occurred. Because gold salts cannot repair damage, if therapy is started in the later stages after the involvement of cartilage and bone, they may succeed only in halting the progression of disease and preventing further damage. Salicylates or other NSAIDs, as well as corticosteriods, may be continued and then slowly withdrawn when there is no longer need for analgesic and anti-inflammatory therapy. Penicillamine should not be given with gold salts.

Gold sodium thiomalate is contraindicated in patients with known hypersensitivity to gold or other heavy metals. Clinical signs of gold toxicity include a rapid reduction of hemoglobin, leukopenia, decreased platelet count, or increased eosinophil count. Therapy should be discontinued with the development of albuminuria, hematuria, pruritus, skin eruption, stomatitis, or persistent diarrhea. It is critical that before therapy is started baseline hemoglobin, erythrocyte, white blood cell, and platelet counts be determined and used as reference. A baseline urinalysis for protein excretion also should be performed. It is recommended that a urinalysis be performed before each injection and a complete blood count performed at every second injection. In patients with a history of blood dyscrasias, kidney, or liver disease, gold sodium thiomalate must be used cautiously. The most common toxic reaction is dermatitis, which can be aggravated by exposure to sunlight. Severe reactions can lead to alopecia or nail loss. Stomatitis is also a common reaction that can develop into glossitis or gingivitis. A metallic taste should be considered a sign of impending development of this condition. In general, discontinuing treatment is enough to reverse these reactions; however, in cases of severe reactions, the use of corticosteroids may be required. The use of gold sodium thiomalate during pregnancy is generally contraindicated, as is its use during the nursing of infants. Gold salts do cross the placenta and are found in breast milk.

Auranofin (Fig. 74.26)

Auranofin is a gold-containing compound active when administered orally. It is indicated in the treatment of adult active rheumatoid arthritis insufficiently treated with full doses of NSAIDs. As with other forms of gold therapy, the greatest benefit of auranofin is realized only if therapy is initiated early in the course of disease. Approximately 65 percent of the gold in the administered dose is absorbed.

While blood concentrations of gold are proportional to the dose, they are not indices of therapeutic benefit or toxicity. The onset of patient response may be as long as three to six months after initiating therapy. The usual adult dose is 6 mg, given as a single dose or 3-mg dose twice daily. If after six months response is inadequate, the dose may be increased to 9 mg per day. If, after an additional three-month period at 9 mg per day, response is still inadequate, auranofin should be discontinued.

Auranofin is contraindicated in patients with known sensitivity to gold or heavy metals or with hematologic disorders. As with other forms of gold therapy, baseline hemoglobin, erythrocyte, white blood cell, and platelet counts should be determined and used as reference, as well as a baseline urinalysis for protein excretion. These tests should be repeated at regular intervals during therapy. Because auranofin is administered orally, GI toxicity is the most common side-effect. It may become severe enough to require that therapy be discontinued. Mild diarrhea, nausea, vomiting, anorexia, or abdominal cramps are usually controlled by reducing the dose. Patients with GI complaints should be monitored for GI bleeding. Dermatitis is also common and is usually aggravated by exposure to sunlight. Stomatitis, also common, is usually preceded by a metallic taste in the mouth. Nephrotic syndrome or glomerulitis with proteinuria and hematuria also has been associated with gold therapy. If recognized early, discontinuing treatment is usually enough to reverse these conditions. Most adverse reactions occur within, but are not limited to, the first six months of therapy. Generally, these patients were concomitantly taking NSAIDs or low-dose corticosteroids.

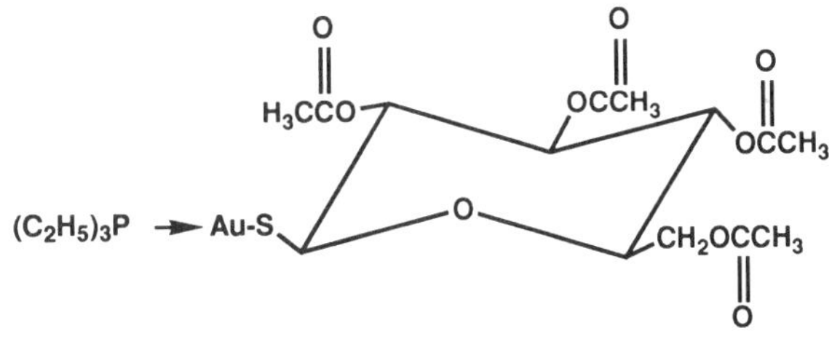

$(C_2H_5)_3P \rightarrow Au\text{-}S$ — pyranose ring with $H_3CC(=O)O$, $OC(=O)CH_3$, $OC(=O)CH_3$, $CH_2OC(=O)CH_3$ substituents

Figure 74.26 Auranofin

Because gold salts cross the placenta and appear in breast milk, auranofin is contraindicated during pregnancy and in nursing mothers. Auranofin is not recommended for pediatric use.

Azathioprine (Fig. 74.27)

Azathioprine is an immunosuppressive purine antimetabolite. It is well absorbed after oral administration and moderately bound to plasma proteins (30%). Azathioprine is metabolized to the parent compound, mercaptopurine, both of which have similar activities. Clearance of the blood and plasma is rapid. Tissue levels, not plasma levels, are an indicator of therapeutic level and duration of action. The effects of azathioprine may persist long after administration has been discontinued.

Azathioprine is indicated only in adult patients with clearly defined RA. Its use is restricted to patients with severe, active, and erosive disease not responsive to conventional management, including rest, NSAID therapy, or gold therapy. The mechanism of action of azathioprine in the treatment of RA is unclear. Azathioprine is usually given on a daily basis as a single or twice-daily dose. Several weeks of treatment usually are required before a therapeutic response is seen. Patients unresponsive after 12 weeks should be considered refractory. Azathioprine may be used for long-term therapy in responding patients with careful monitoring. During long-term therapy, an attempt should be made to reduce the dose and thus the risk of toxicity. Salicylate therapy should be continued concomitantly. The dose of corticosteroids may possibly be reduced. No information is available on the combined use with penicillamine, gold, or antimalarials.

Hematologic and GI toxicity is the most frequent and potentially serious side-effect of azathioprine therapy. Incidence during RA therapy, however, is lower than, for example, in the treatment of renal homograft recipients. Nausea and vomiting can occur early in azathioprine therapy and usually is managed by administering lower divided doses. The drug is contraindicated during pregnancy. Azathioprine is mutagenic and teratogenic. Because of its immunosuppressive activity, chronic use may increase the risk of neoplasia. This risk is increased in immunosuppressed patients or those on chronic immunosuppressive therapy. The principal metabolic pathway toward the degradation of azathioprine is by the enzyme xanthine oxidase. This enzyme is inhibited by the drug, allopurinol, an agent also used in the treatment of gout. In patients receiving both drugs, the dose of azathioprine should be reduced by one-third to one-fourth. Concomitant therapy with angiotensin-converting enzyme inhibitors has been reported to produce severe leukopenia. The safety and efficacy of azathioprine in the pediatric population has not been studied.

Chloroquine and Hydroxychloroquine (Figs. 74.28, 74.29)

Chloroquine and hydroxychloroquine are antimalarial drugs shown to be useful in the treatment of acute and chronic rheumatoid arthritis in adults. Their mechanism of action is unknown. Several months of therapy usually are required to produce beneficial effects. If after six months no improvement is observed (reduced joint swelling and increased mobility), therapy should be discontinued. Generally, an initial oral dose (equivalent to 300 mg base) once per day is taken after a meal or with milk to reduce stomach upset. Once symptoms have improved (4 to 12 weeks), the

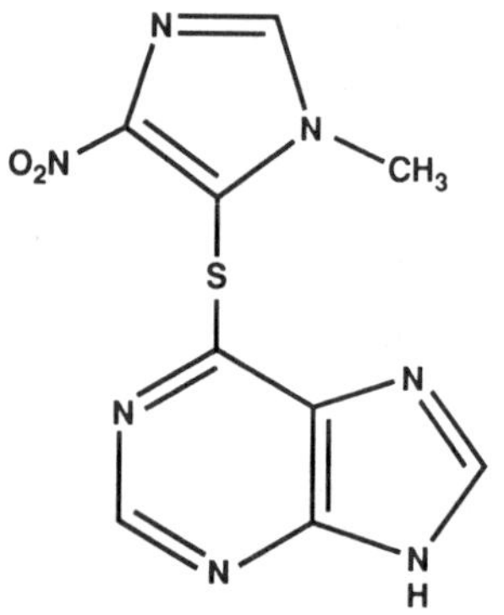

Figure 74.27 Azathioprine

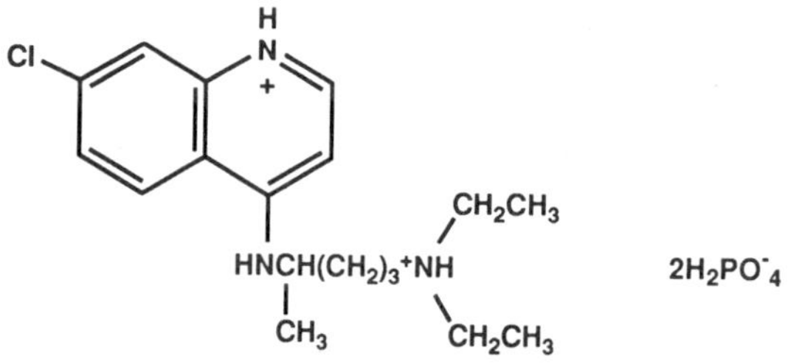

Figure 74.28 Chloroquine Phosphate

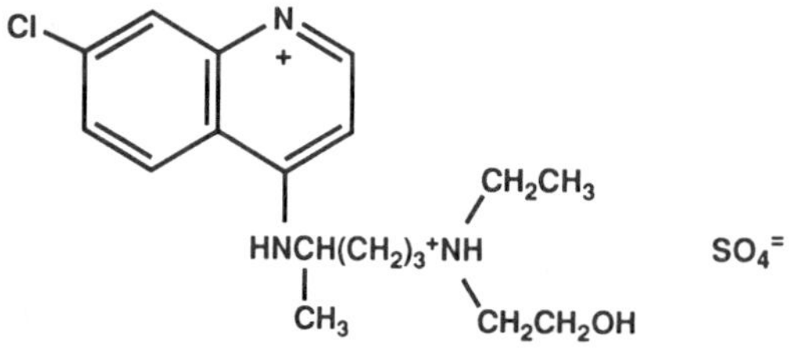

Figure 74.29 Hydroxychloroquine Sulfate

dose is reduced by half. Corticosteroids and salicylates may be used concomitantly during initial therapy and gradually withdrawn as symptoms permit.

All 4-aminoquinoline compounds are potentially toxic to the retina. If long-term therapy is planned, a baseline ophthalmologic examination must be performed. Retinopathy is dose-related and may result in irreversible retinal damage.

A complete ophthalmologic examination, including visual acuity, funduscopic, and visual fields tests should be performed every three months during therapy. Toxicity to the retina may be manifested by edema, atrophy, abnormal pigmentation, or a loss of foveal reflex. Patients may complain of blurred vision, difficulty in reading, photophobia, or light flashes. Retinopathy may progress even after discontinuing the drug. Toxicity to the ciliary body may result in disturbance of accommodation, with symptoms of blurred vision. Corneal changes (edema, decreased sensitivity, and corneal deposits) also may occur. Ciliary body and corneal toxicity is usually reversible upon discontinuing the drug. Other toxic reactions to these compounds include dermatologic reactions (skin eruptions, pruritus, alopecia), hematologic reactions (blood dyscrasias and hemolysis in individuals with glucose-6-phosphate dehydrogenase deficiency), GI reaction (anorexia, nausea, vomiting, diarrhea, abdominal cramps), and neuromuscular reactions (skeletal muscle weakness, absent or hypoactive deep tendon reflexes). The use of these drugs is contraindicated in patients with psoriasis, hepatic disease, or alcoholism, a deficiency in glucose-6-phosphate dehydrogenase, or during pregnancy.

Penicillamine (Fig. 74.30)

Penicillamine is a metal chelating agent used for the removal of excess copper in patients with Wilson's disease. Penicillamine also has been shown to be useful in the treatment of RA. It is indicated in the treatment of severe, active RA not responding to conventional therapy. Penicillamine appears ineffective as a treatment for ankylosing spondylitis. The mechanism through which it suppresses this disease is unknown. As with many of the other antiarthritic drugs, penicillamine has a delayed onset of action. Beneficial effects may not be seen for several months.

Initial therapeutic dosing is 125 or 225 mg once per day given on an empty stomach for the first month. The dose is then increased 125 or 225 mg at one- to three-month intervals. If required, this stepwise increase in dose is continued until a maximum tolerated or 1000 to 1500 mg per day dose is reached. If after three to four months on a 1000- to 1500-mg dose there is no sign of remission, the patient should be considered unresponsive and treatment discontinued. Continued use of salicylates or corticosteroids is recommended.

Penicillamine has a very high potential for serious side-effects and should be used in the treatment of RA only when conventional therapy has failed. It should not be used in patients with a history of renal insufficiency, and its use is contraindicated during pregnancy. The potential for serious hematologic (bone marrow depression) and renal (nephrotic syndrome) adverse reactions requires that routine urinalysis, white blood cell differential count, hemoglobin determination, and direct platelet count be performed every two weeks for at least the first six months of therapy and every few months thereafter. Gastrointestinal reactions (nausea, vomiting, anorexia, epigastric pain) are frequent, but usually can be controlled by lowering the dose or reversed by discontinuing therapy.

Methotrexate (Fig. 74.31)

Methotrexate is a folic acid antagonist; therefore, it affects DNA synthesis and cell replication. It is used an as antimetabolite in the treatment of some neoplastic diseases, and severe psoriasis.[45] It is also used as second-line therapy in selected adults with severe RA. It does not appear to modify the disease process in RA; however, it reduces swelling and tenderness in the joints, as well as attenuating the symptoms of inflammation. NSAIDs or corticosteroids may be continued concomitantly with methotrexate treatment.

Methotrexate can cause fetal death or teratogenic defects and is, therefore, contraindicated in pregnancy. Pregnancy should be avoided if either partner is on methotrexate therapy. It can cause hepatotoxicity, fibrosis, and cirrhosis. These effects are generally associated with long-term use. Alcoholism, chronic liver disease, or immunodeficiency preclude the use of this drug. The most frequent adverse reactions include nausea, leukopenia, ulcerative stomatitis, and abdominal distress.

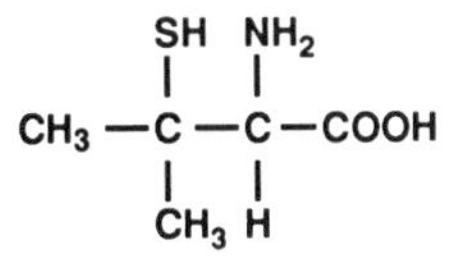

Figure 74.30 Penicillamine

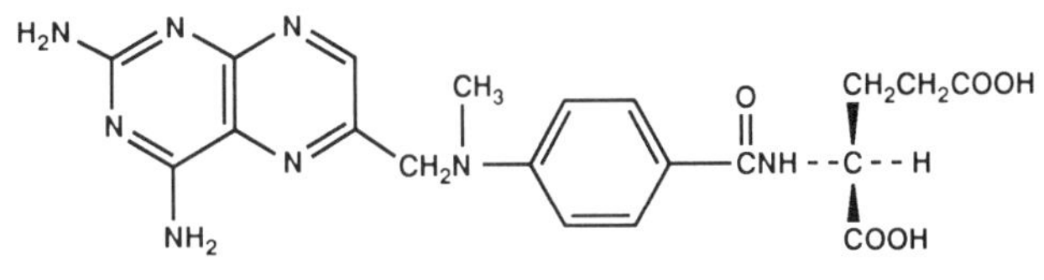

Figure 74.31 Methotrexate

Therapy for RA is weekly. All schedules should be individualized for these patients. The recommended starting dose is a single oral dose of 7.5 mg once a week. The dose can be lowered as much as possible after the response is achieved.

CD4 Monoclonal Antibody Therapy

It is clear that the accumulation of T lymphocytes, in particular the CD4+ subset, in the synovium plays a very important role in the pathogenesis of rheumatoid arthritis in both experimental animals and humans.[46,47] Monoclonal antibodies raised against the T4 antigen, CD4, are now undergoing clinical trials for the treatment of rheumatoid arthritis. Initial short-term trials have indicated a favorable clinical picture with significant reduction in disease activity.[48,49] The mechanisms responsible for the clinical effects are not yet understood. Response is poorly correlated with the degree of CD4+ T-cell depletion and is not associated with general systemic immune suppression. Clearly, additional studies must be performed. Nevertheless, immunotherapy is likely to gain an important role in the management of rheumatoid arthritis in the future.

Acetaminophen (Fig. 74.32) (Table 74.3)

Acetaminophen is the active metabolite of phenacetin and acetanilid. In Europe, acetaminophen is known as paracetamol. Acetaminophen exhibits far less toxic side-effects than the parent drugs. Although acetaminophen is not an NSAID, it is an effective analgesic and antipyretic. It is listed in the National Prescription Audit as one of the 200 most commonly prescribed drugs in the US in 1989. Its mechanism of action has been extensively studied, but still remains unclear. The low potency for inhibitory activity toward peripheral prostaglandin synthesis makes acetaminophen an ineffective anti-inflammatory drug.

Acetaminophen is rapidly absorbed after oral administration and reaches peak plasma concentration in 0.5 to one hour. Serum half-life is from one to 2.5 hours. Unlike the NSAIDs, acetaminophen displays little protein binding. It is metabolized in the liver primarily to glucuronide and sulfate conjugates; however, hydroxylate and deacetylate metabolites are also formed in minor amounts.

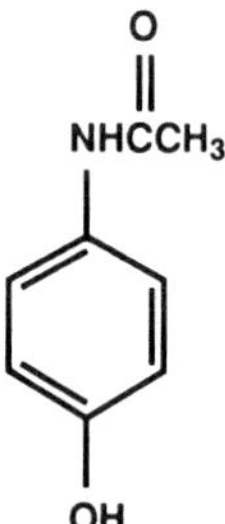

Figure 74.32 Acetaminophen

Acetaminophen is as effective as aspirin as an antipyretic and analgesic in the treatment of headache, postpartum, postoperative, and musculoskeletal pain. Acetaminophen is clearly the drug of choice in patients with bleeding disorders or those undergoing anticoagulant therapy, since acetaminophen does not inhibit platelet TXA_2 synthesis or affect prothrombin time, nor does it produce GI ulceration or bleeding. Because acetaminophen does not antagonize the effects of uricosuric drugs, it may be used in patients undergoing therapy for gouty arthritis. It is preferred over aspirin for children in treating the fever and pain associated with the common cold or flu. There appears to be no direct relationship between acetaminophen therapy and the incidence of Reye's syndrome.

Used as directed, acetaminophen rarely causes severe toxicity or side-effects. Incidences of skin eruption, thrombocytopenia, neutropenia, leukopenia, and hemolytic anemia have been reported. Chronic treatment with high doses can lead to hypoglycemia, jaundice, and hepatic necrosis. Acetaminophen is primarily metabolized in the liver by sulfation and conjugation and to a lesser degree by by the cytochrome P-450 mixed-function oxidases. The reactive hydroxylate metabolite of acetaminophen, which has arylating properties, is usually detoxified by oxidation of hepatic glutathione. The hepatoxicity observed with a large overdose is associated with a decrease in hepatic glutathione levels followed by the covalent binding of the reactive metabolite(s) to macromolecules, resulting in necrosis. Children appear to be less susceptible to toxicity than adults. Tubular necrosis and myocardial damage may also occur. Acute poisoning from overdose is divided into four clinical stages:

Stage 1: (12–24 hours)—nausea, vomiting, abdominal pain, excessive perspiration, anorexia
Stage 2: (24–48 hours)—clinical improvement; SGOT (serum glutamic-oxaloacetic transminase), SGPT (serum glutamic-pyruvic transaminase), bilirubin, and prothrombin levels rise
Stage 3: (72–96 hours)—peak hepatotoxicity
Stage 4: (7–8 days)—recovery

Administration of N-acetylcysteine is an effective antidote for acetaminophen overdose but must be administered within 16 hours of overdose. It serves to replace and preserve liver glutathione and is effective in preventing further liver damage.[50,r12] Because of the potential for liver damage, acetaminophen should not be used in patients with known liver damage or in chronic alcoholics.

Drugs for the Treatment of Gout (Table 74.3)

Gout is a metabolic disorder characterized by hyperuricemia and resultant deposition of monosodium urate in the tissues, particularly the joints and kidneys (Fig. 74.33). Proper diagnosis is critical because clinical signs often resemble those of other forms of arthritis. The presence of monosodium urate in synovial fluid leukocytes is diagnostic of gout. The therapeutic approach is to reduce serum levels of uric acid in order to prevent its precipitation.[51,52] Overproduction of uric acid and/or the reduced ability to excrete it can result in gout. This disorder can, therefore, be treated either by reducing the production of uric acid or by increasing its elimination in the urine. Inflammation and pain associated with acute gouty arthritis are treated with anti-inflammatory drugs.[53]

Allopurinol

Allopurinol is a xanthine oxidase inhibitor that can be administered orally. By inhibiting xanthine oxidase, allopurinol inhibits the conversion of hypoxanthine to xanthine and of xanthine to uric acid. Allopurinol

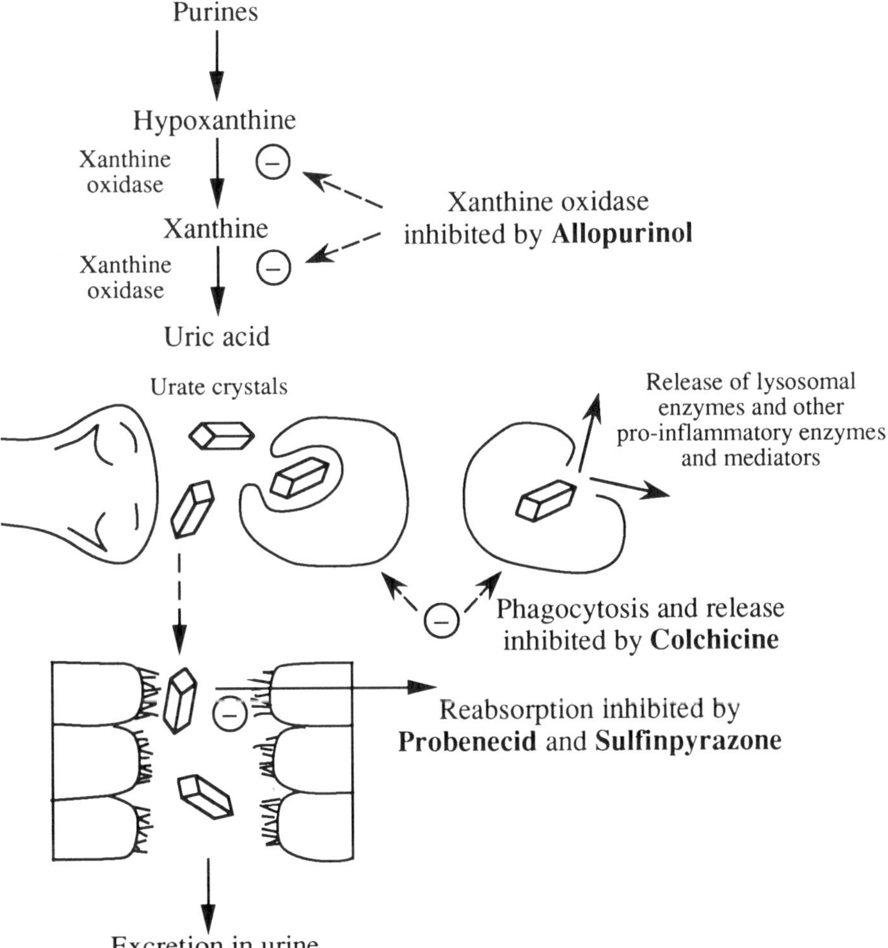

Figure 74.33 The development of gout and the sites of pharmacologic therapy. Uric acid, derived from purine metabolism, may deposit in joints as urate crystals. This can initiate an inflammatory reaction mediated by inflammatory cells as they phagocytize the urate crystals and release proinflammatory enzymes and mediators. The drug, allopurinol, can reduce the production of uric acid by inhibiting purine metabolism (xanthine oxidase). The drug, colchicine, can inhibit the progression of the inflammatory process by inhibiting inflammatory cell activity. The drugs, probenecid and sulfinpyrazone, allow for more uric acid excretion by inhibiting kidney tubule reabsorption.

thereby reduces the production of uric acid by inhibiting the enzymatic steps preceding its formation. Allopurinol is rapidly metabolized to oxipurinol, which also is an inhibitor of xanthine oxidase. After oral administration 90 percent of the allopurinol is absorbed. Plasma half-life for allopurinol is one to two hours; however, plasma half-life for its metabolite, oxipurinol, is 15 hours. Because oxipurinol is also active, xanthine oxidase inhibition is maintained over a 24-hour period, allowing for single daily dosing. Allopurinol is indicated in the treatment of primary or secondary gout. Initial therapeutic benefit is usually observed two to three days after initiating therapy, with full benefit occurring within one week. Its actions differ from those of uricosuric agents in that both serum and urinary uric acid levels are reduced owing to the inhibition of uric acid formation. Uricosuric agents increase the excretion of uric acid and have the potential of producing renal tubular damage due to the increase in urinary uric acid. Because the uric acid lowering effects of allopurinol do not depend on uric acid excretion, it can be used in patients with compromised renal function. In addition, allopurinol can be used in patients undergoing salicylate antirheumatoid therapy. While salicylates will reduce the effectiveness of uricosuric agents, they have no effect on the action of allopurinol. Allopurinol inhibits the metabolism of mercaptopurine, a metabolite of azathioprine. Dose adjustments must be made in concomitant therapy. Allopurinol also increases the toxicity of cyclophosphamide and vidarabine. Concomitant use with probenecid reduces the inhibitory effect of allopurinol on xanthine oxidase.

The most frequent adverse reaction to allopurinol is skin rash, which can be severe. Gastrointestinal distress, including diarrhea and nausea, may occur. Acute attacks of gout have been reported during the early stages of therapy.

Sulfinpyrazone

Sulfinpyrazone is an orally active uricosuric agent. Its use is indicated for the treatment of chronic gouty arthritis and intermittent gouty arthritis. Sulfinpyrazone is rapidly and completely absorbed after oral administration and has a plasma half-life of one to three hours. Initial dosing is 100 to 200 mg twice daily taken with meals or milk. The dose can be increased gradually until a full therapeutic dose is obtained. Sulfinpyrazone lowers serum uric acid by increasing the urinary excretion of uric acid. A lower initial dose reduces the incidence of acute gouty arthritis, as urate crystals begin to dissolve and redistribute. These acute attacks can be managed with concomitant administration of colchicine or indomethacin. Although sulfinpyrazone is related structurally to phenylbutazone, it does not exhibit anti-inflammatory or analgesic activity. Because salicylates antagonize the action of uricosuric agents, sulfinpyrazone will be ineffective in patients undergoing salicylate therapy for RA.

Sulfinpyrazone is contraindicated in patients with active peptic ulcers or GI ulceration, since it is irritating to the gastric lining and has been shown to inhibit platelet function. The most frequent complaints are upper GI upset accompanied by nausea and vomiting. Because sulfinpyrazone is related structurally to phenylbutazone, its use is contraindicated in patients with known hypersensitivity to phenylbutazone or those with blood dyscrasias. In patients with reduced renal function, sulfinpyrazone must be used with caution. As a uricosuric drug, sulfinpyrazone may cause urolithiasis and renal colic. Fluid intake should be increased and the urine alkalinized to reduce the potential for urate precipitation in the kidney, particularly during initial therapy. Sulfinpyrazone may potentiate the actions of certain sulfonamides as well as insulin and hypoglycemic sulfonylureas.

Probenecid

Probenecid is a uricosuric agent indicated for the treatment of gout and gouty arthritis. It is absorbed well after oral administration and has a plasma half-life of four hours. The recommended dosage is 0.5 g taken four times daily. Therapy should not be started until the acute gouty attack is over. However, if acute attack occurs during probenecid therapy, it may be continued with colchicine to control the attack. Probenecid increases urinary excretion of uric acid by inhibiting tubule reabsorption, thereby lowering serum uric acid levels. Because the site of action is the renal tubule lumen, the effectiveness of probenecid depends on renal function. In patients with reduced glomerular filtration rate (less than 30 ml/min), the dose should be increased. Salicylates antagonize the action of probenecid. If analgesics are required during therapy, indomethacin could be used if tolerated.

Probenecid is contraindicated in patients with blood dyscrasias or uric acid kidney stones. Uricosuric drugs can increase the urinary concentration of uric acid to levels that may result in precipitation of urate crystals in the kidney. Urolithiasis and renal colic may result. Fluid intake should be increased and the urine alkalinized to reduce the potential for urate precipitation in the kidney particularly during initial therapy. Acute gouty arthritis may occur during initial therapy as urate crystals begin to dissolve and redistribute. Colchicine or indomethacin can be used to manage these acute attacks. Probenecid inhibits the renal excretion of penicillin, indomethacin, and sulfonylureas. Doses of these drugs, when administered with probenecid, should be adjusted accordingly.

Colchicine

Colchicine is indicated for the treatment of acute gout. Although not generally considered an anti-inflammatory drug, colchicine reduces the inflammation and pain associated with acute gout. It is considered a first-line drug in acute gout. Its use may be continued in smaller doses in combination with uricosuric drugs to reduce the incidence of acute gouty arthritis. It is administered either orally or IV. The oral form is available as a combination of colchicine (0.5 g) and probenecid (0.5 g) in one tablet (Colbeneimid). As with probenecid alone, this combination should not be initiated until after the acute attack. It can be continued if an acute attack occurs during therapy. Onset of action is 24 to 48 hours after oral administration and 6 to 12 hours after IV administration.

Colchicine should be used with caution in patients with hepatic, renal, and cardiovascular diseases. Gastrointestinal reactions are the most common side-effect when administered orally. Nausea, vomiting, abdominal pain, and diarrhea occur in 80 percent of patients, and often require discontinuation of oral colchicine. Toxic doses by the oral route produce severe diarrhea. While IV administration does not produce GI toxicity, extravasation can result in inflammation and necrosis of the skin and soft tissue. This route of administration is contraindicated in patients with leukopenia or severe hepatic or renal disease. Toxic doses by the IV route produce generalized vascular damage. Colchicine toxicity also includes bone marrow depression, aplastic anemia, agranulocytosis, peripheral neuritis, muscular weakness, and dermatitis. Since colchicine can arrest cell division, its use is contraindicated during pregnancy.

References

Research Reports

1. Henson PM. Pathologic mechanisms in neutrophil-mediated injury. Am J Pathol 1972;*68*:593–612.
2. Holliwell B, Hoult JR, Blake DR. Oxidants, inflammation, and anti-inflammatory drugs. FASEB J 1988;*2*:2867–2873.
3. Vane J, Botting R. Inflammation and the mechanism of action of anti-inflammatory drugs. FASEB J 1987;*1*:89–96.
4. Ohki S, Ogino N, Yamamoto S, Hayaishi O. Prostaglandin hydroperoxidase, an integral part of prostaglandin endoperoxide synthetase from bovine vesicular gland microsomes. J Biol Chem 1979;*254*:829–836.
5. Hamberg M, Svensson J, Wakabayashi T, Samuelsson B. Isolation and structure of two prostaglandin endoperoxides that cause platelet aggregation. Proc Natl Acad Sci USA 1974;*71*:345–349.
6. Smith WL. The eicosanoids and their biochemical mechanisms of action. Biochem J 1989;*259*:315–324.
7. Flower JR, Vane JR. Inhibition of prostaglandin biosynthesis. Biochem Pharmacol 1974;*23*:1439–1450.
8. Mayeux PR, Kadowitz PJ, McNamara DB. Differential effects of ibuprofen, indomethacin and meclofenamate on prostaglandin endoperoxide H_2 metabolism. Molec Cell Biochem 1989;*87*:41–46.
9. Roth GR, Siok CJ. Acetylation of NH_2-terminal serine of prostaglandin synthetase by aspirin. J Biol Chem 1978;*253*:3782–3784.
10. Maier JAM, Hla T, Maciag T. Cyclooxygenase is an immediate-early gene induced by interleukin-1 in human endothelial cells. J Biol Chem 1990;*265*:10805–10808.
11. Fu J-Y, Masferrer JL, Seibert K, Raz A, Needleman P. The induction and suppression of prostaglandin H_2 synthase (cyclooxygenase) in human monocytes. J Biol Chem 1990;*265*:16737–16740.
12. Masferrer JL, Seibert K, Zweifel B, Needleman P. Endogenous glucocorticoids regulate an inducible cyclooxygenase enzyme. Proc Natl Acad Sci USA 1992;*89*:3917–3921.
13. Mansferrer JL, Zweifel BS, Seibert K, Needleman P. Selective regulation of cellular cyclooxygenase by dexamethasone and endotoxin in mice. J Clin Invest 1990;*86*:1375–1379.
14. Meade EA, Smith WL, DeWitt DL. Differential inhibition of prostaglandin endoperoxide synthase (cyclooxygenase) isozymes by aspirin and other non-steroidal anti-inflammatory drugs. J Biol Chem 1993;*268*:6610–6614.
15. Oates JA, FitzGerald GQ, Branch RA, Jackson EK, Knapp HR, Roberts LJ. Clinical implications of prostaglandin and thromboxane A_2 formation. N Engl J Med 1988;*319*:689–698.
16. Willard JE, Lange RA, Hillis LD. The use of aspirin in ischemic heart disease. N Engl J Med 1992;*327*:175–181.
17. Chesebro JH, Fuster V. Thrombosis in unstable angina. N Engl J Med 1992;*327*:192–194.
18. Hamberg M, Svensson J, Samuelsson B. Thromboxanes: A new group of biologically active compounds derived from prostaglandin endoperoxides. Proc Natl Acad Sci USA 1975;*72*:2994–2998.
19. Mayeux PR, Kadowitz PJ, McNamara, DB. Evidence for a bidirectional prostaglandin endoperoxide shunt between platelets and the bovine coronary artery. Biochim Biophys Acta 1989;*1011*:18–24.
20. Bunting S, Gryglewski R, Moncada S, Vane JR. Arterial walls generate from prostaglandin endoperoxides a substance (prostaglandin X) which relaxes strips of mesenteric and coeliac arteries and inhibits platelet aggregation. Prostaglandins 1976;*12*:897–913.
21. Jaffe EA, Weksler BB. Recovery of endothelial cell prostacyclin production after low dose aspirin. J Clin Invest 1979;*63*:532–535.
22. Marcus AJ, Weksler BB, Jaffe EA, Broekman MJ. Synthesis of prostacyclin from platelet-derived endoperoxides by cultured human endothelial cells. J Clin Invest 1980;*66*:979–986.
23. Clive DM, Stoff JS. Renal syndromes associated with nonsteroidal antiinflammatory drugs. N Engl J Med 1984;*310*:563–572.
24. Konturek SJ, Piastucki L, Przozowski T, Radecki T, Dembinska-Kiec K, Zmuda A, Gryglewski R. Role of prostaglandins in the formation of aspirin-induced gastric ulcers. Gastroenterology 1981;*80*:4–9.

25. Robert A. Cytoprotection by prostaglandins. Gastroenterology 1979;*77*:761–767.

26. Johansson C, Killberg B, Nordemar R, Samuelsson K, Bergstrom S. Protective treatment of prostaglandin E_2 in the gastrointestinal tract during indomethacin treatment of rheumatic patients. Gastroenterology 1980;*78*:479–483.

27. Wikland M, Lindblom B, Wilhelmsson L, Wiqvist N. Oxytocin, prostaglandins and contractility of the human uterus at term pregnancy. Acta Obstet Gynecol Scand 1982;*61*:467–472.

28. Ward JR. Role of disease-modifying antirheumatic drugs versus cytotoxic agents in the therapy of rheumatoid arthritis. Am J Med 1988;*85*:39–44.

29. Schenkier S, Golbus J. Treatment of rheumatoid arthritis. New thoughts on the classic pyramid approach. Postgrad Med 1992;*91*:285–289.

30. Wilske KR, Healey LA. Remodeling the pyramid—a concept whose time has come (editorial). J Rheumatol 1989;*16*:565–567.

31. Vener KJ, Reddy A. Timed treatment of the arthritic disease: A review and hypothesis. Semin Arthritis Rheum 1992;*22*:83–97.

32. Sebaldt RJ, Sheller JR, Oates JA, Roberts LJ. Inhibition of eicosanoid biosynthesis by glucocorticoids in humans. Proc Natl Acad Sci USA 1990;*87*:6974–6978.

33. Pinals RS. Pharmacologic treatment of osteoarthritis. Clin Ther 1992;*14*:336–346.

34. Guerra FA, Savich PD, Wallen LD, Lee CH, Clyman RI, Mauray FE, Kitterman JA. Prostaglandin E_2 causes hypoventilation and apnea in newborn lambs. J Appl Physiol 1988;*64*:2160–2166.

35. Sideris EB, Yokochi K, Coceani F, Olley PM. Prostaglandins and fetal cardiac output distribution in the lamb. Am J Physiol 1985;*248*:HB853–HB858.

36. Douidar SM, Richardson J, Snodgrass WR. Role of indomethacin in ductus closure: An update evaluation. Develop Pharmacol Ther 1988;*11*:196–212.

37. Pinsky PR, Hurwitz ES, Schonberger LB, Gunn WJ. Reye's syndrome and aspirin. Evidence for a dose-response effect. JAMA 1988;*260*:657–661.

38. Brenner BE, Simon RR. Management of salicylate intoxication. Drugs 1982;*24*:335–340.

39. Hart FD, Huskisson EC. Non-steroidal antiinflammatory drugs: current status and rational therapeutic use. Drugs 1988;*27*:232.

40. Avila HM, Walker AM, Romiere I, Spiegelman DL, Perera DR, Jick H. Choice of non-steroidal anti-inflammatory drug in persons treated for dyspepsia. Lancet 1988 (Sept 3):556–559.

41. Todd PA, Clissold SP. Naproxen: A reappraisal of its pharmacology and therapeutic use in rheumatic diseases and pain states. Drugs 1990;*409*:91–137.

42. Tonussi CR, Ferreira SH. Mechanism of diclofenac analgesia: Direct blockade of inflammatory sensitization. Eur J Pharmacol 1994;*251*:173–179.

43. Fries JF, Williams CA, Ramey D, Bloch DA. The relative toxicity of disease-modifying antirheumatic drugs. Arthritis Rheum 1993;*36*:2657–306.

44. Ward JR. Role of disease-modifying antirheumatic drugs versus cytotoxic agents in the therapy of rheumatoid arthritis. Am J Med 1988;*85*:12–17.

45. Weinblath ME, Coblyn JS, Fox DA, Fraser PA. Holdsworth DE, Glass DN, Trentham CB, Trentham DE. Efficacy of low-dose methotrexate in rheumatoid arthritis. N Engl J Med 1985;*13*:818–822.

46. Watts RA, Isaacs JD. Immunotherapy of rheumatoid arthritis. Ann Rheum Dis 1992;*51*:577–579.

47. Williams RO, Mason LJ, Feldmann M, Maini RN. Synergy between anti-CD4 and anti-tumor necrosis factor in the amelioration of established collagen-induced arthritis. Proc Natl Acad Sci USA 1994;*91*:2762–2766.

48. van der Lubbe PA, Reiter C, Breedveld FC, Krüger K, Schattenkirchner M, Sanders ME, Riethmüller G. Chimeric CD4 monoclonal antibody cM-T412 as a therapeutic approach to rheumatoid arthritis. Arthritis Rheum 1993;*36*:1375–1379.

49. van der Lubbe PA, Reiter C, Miltenburg AM, Krüger K, de Ruyter AN, Rieber EP, Bijl JA, Riethmüller G, Breedveld FC. Treatment of rheumatoid arthritis with a chimeric CD4 monoclonal antibody (cM-T412): immunopharmacological aspects and mechanisms of action. Scand J Immunol 1994;*39*:286–294.

50. Smilkstein MJ, Knapp GL, Kulig KW, Rumack BH. Efficacy of oral N-acetyl-cysteine in the treatment of acetaminophen overdose. N Engl J Med 1988;*319*:1557–1562.

51. Wallace SL. Colchicine: clinical pharmacology in acute gouty arthritis. Am J Med 1986;*314*:1001–1005.

52. Boss GR, Seegmiller JE. Hyperuricemia and gout: Classification, complications, and management. N Engl J Med 1979;*300*:1459–1468.

53. Vawter RL, Antonelli MAS. Rational treatment of gout. Postgrad Med 1992;*91*:115–127.

Reviews

r1. Janoff A. Neutrophil proteases in inflammation. Ann Rev Med 1972;*23*:177–190.

r2. Larsen GL, Henson PM. Mediators of inflammation. Am Rev Immunol 1983;*1*:335–359.

r3. Dascombe MJ. The pharmacology of fever. Prog Neurobiol 1985;*25*:327–373.

r4. Perl ET. Synthetization of nociceptors and its relation to sensation. In: Bonica JJ, Albe-Fersard D Advances in Pain Research and Therapy, Vol 1. New York: Raven Press (1976); pp 17–34.

r5. Davies P, Bailey PJ, Goldenberg MM. The role of arachidonic acid oxygenation products in pain and inflammation. Ann Rev Immunol 1984;*2*:335–357.

r6. Brooks PM, Day RO. Nonsteroidal antiinflammatory drugs: differences and similarities. N Engl J Med 1991;*324*:1716–1725.

r7. Henrich WL. Nephrotoxicity of nonsteroidal antiinflammatory agents. In: Disease of the Kidney. 4th ed, Vol 2. Boston: Little, Brown, 1988.

r8. Rose CD, Doughty RA. Pharmacological management of juvenile rheumatoid arthritis. Drugs 1992;*43*:849–863.

r9. Lasagna L, McMahon FG (editors). New perspectives on aspirin therapy. Am J Med, Suppl 6A, *74*, 1983.

r10. Brogden RN, Heel RC, Pakes GE, Speight TM, Avery GS. Diflunisal: A review of its pharmacological properties and therapeutic use in pain and musculoskeletal strains and sprains and pain in osteoarthritis. Drugs 1980;*19*:84–106.

r11. Hurwitz ES. Reye's syndrome. Epidemiol Res 1989;*11*:249–253.

r12. Prescott LF, Critchley JAJH. The treatment of acetaminophen poisoning. Ann Rev Pharmacol Toxicol 1983;*23*:87–101.

r13. Halushka PV, Mais DE, Mayeux PR, Morinelli TA. Thromboxane prostaglandin and leukotriene receptors. Ann Rev Pharmacol Toxicol 1989;*29*:213–239.

A compilation of location, characterization, and second messenger systems for the thromboxane, prostaglandin, and leukotriene receptors.

r14. Willard JE, Lange RA, Hikllis LD. The use of aspirin in ischemic heart diseases. N Engl J Med 1992;*327*:175–181.
A review of clinical studies addressing the therapeutic benefit of low-dose aspirin therapy in ischemic heart disease.

r15. Vane J, Botting R. Inflammation and the mechanism of action of anti-inflammatory dugs. FASEB J 1987;*1*:89–96.
Discusses mediators of inflammation and compares the mechanism of action of several classes of anti-inflammatory drugs. Also presents a historical perspective of the development of aspirin as an anti-inflammatory drug.

r16. Bloomfeld SS. Analgesic management of mild to moderate pain. Ration Drug Ther 1985;*19*:1–14.
An overview of pain management.

r17. Clive DM, Stoff JS. Renal syndromes associated with nonsteroidal antiinflammatory drugs. N Engl J Med 1984;*310*:563–572.
Reviews the potential renal toxicity of the NSAIDs.

r18. Rose CD, Doughty RA. Pharmacological management of juvenile rheumatoid arthritis. Drugs 1992;*43*:849–863.
Current concepts in the specific treatment of juvenile rheumatoid arthritis.

r19. Schenkier S, Golbus J. Treatment of rheumatoid arthritis: New thoughts on the classic pyramid approach. Postgrad Med 1992;*91*:285–292.
A review of the therapeutic benefit of the pyramid approach to rheumatoid arthritis therapy.

r20. Fries JF, Williams CA, Ramey D, Bloch DA. The relative toxicity of disease-modifying antirheumatic drugs. Arthritis Rheum 1993;*36*:297–306.
A survey of the clinical toxicities of the disease-modifying antirheumatic drugs. An excellent source for comparing clinical toxicities.

r21. Hess EV, Tangnijkui Y. A rational approach to NSAID therapy. Ration Drug Ther 1986;*20*:77–73.
An overview of choices to be made in NSAID therapy.

r22. Henrich WL. Nephrotoxicity of nonsteroidal anti-inflammatory agents. In: Schrier RW, Gottschalt CW Diseases of the Kidney, 4th Ed, Vol 2. (eds), Boston: Little, Brown, 1988.
Review of renal toxicity associated with NSAID therapy.

r23. Feldman M. Prostaglandins and gastric ulcers: From seminal vesicle to misoprostol. Am J Med Sci 1990;*300*:116–132.
A review of the relationships between prostaglandins, inhibition of prostaglandin synthesis by NSAIDs and gastric ulcers.

r24. Fries JF, Ramey DR, Singh G, Morfeld D, Bloch DA, Raynauld J-P. A reevaluation of aspirin therapy in rheumatoid arthritis. Arch Intern Med 1993;*153*:2465–2471.
A retrospective study of the safety of aspirin therapy in rheumatoid arthritis.

r25. Singh G, Fries JF, Williams CA, Zatarain E, Spitz P, Bloch DA. Toxicity profiles of disease modifying antirheumatic drugs in rheumatoid arthritis. J Rheumatol 1991;*18*:188–194.
A retrospective study of the toxicities of seven disease modifying antirheumatic drugs.

r26. Paulus HE. Current medicinal approaches to the treatment of rheumatoid arthrits. Clin Orthop Rel Res 1991;*265*:96–102.
Stresses the importance of individualized therapy and the role of pharmacokinetics in therapy design.

r27. Weinblatt ME, Maier AL. Disease-modifying agents and experimental treatments of rheumatoid arthritis. Clin Orthop Rel Res 1991;*265*:103–115.
A review of mechanisms of action and toxicities.

r28. Skeith KJ, Brocks DR. Pharmacokinetic optimisation of the treatment of osteoarthritis. Clin Pharmacokinet 1994;*26*:233–242.
Stresses the importance of the pharmacokinetic/pharmacodynamic response in designing a dosing regimen.

CHAPTER 75

Plasma Lipid Modifying Agents

Rodolfo Paoletti
Cesare R. Sirtori

Plasma lipid modifying agents are pharmacologic compounds that affect the levels of major circulating lipids, i.e., cholesterol and triglycerides. This effect is generally exerted through changes in absorption, synthesis, or catabolism of the lipid vectors in plasma, the lipoproteins. The rationale of plasma lipid modifying treatments is that abnormal levels of lipids/lipoproteins in plasma are associated with an increased prevalence of cardiovascular disease. Atherosclerosis-related disorders are, in fact, a major cause of death in western countries and clear evidence has been collected to indicate that drug treatments that correct abnormal plasma lipid levels can reduce the risk of arterial disease associated with dyslipidemia.

Treatment with lipid lowering drugs is, therefore, of growing significance in cardiovascular preventive medicine. Prescription of such agents is necessary both for patients poorly responsive to dietary management, and for those whose plasma lipid/lipoprotein abnormalities coexist with an increased genetic risk of atherosclerosis. Alterations of the lipoprotein spectrum, particularly a reduction of the apparently protective high-density lipoproteins, and/or increased levels of specific apolipoproteins (B,E), also carry a significant risk. The possibility of managing these last, more complex biochemical disorders is presently the object of investigation.

Lipids, Lipoproteins and Cardiovascular Disease

The major circulating lipids—cholesterol, triglycerides, and phospholipids—derive, to a variable extent, from the diet and from endogenous synthesis. The dietary intake of triglycerides, in particular, is rather conspicuous. Western humans have a mean daily intake between 80 and 100 g of triglycerides in the diet, versus an intake of around 4–6 g of phospholipids and 0.5 g of cholesterol. After reaching the intestine, dietary lipids undergo a variety of handling processes, both enzyme and nonenzyme regulated, finally being transported into the lymph and later into plasma, as globular particles, the lipoproteins.

Intestinal lipid transport requires the passage of lipids across the intestinal wall, a non-energy-regulated process, in the presence of intestinal pancreatic lipase, breaking up the complex micelles of dietary fat. Transfer through the intestine requires the additional presence of at least one major protein component, apolipoprotein B-48 (apo B-48). This is incorporated, together with dietary triglycerides (and to a lesser extent other dietary lipids) into large lipoprotein particles, the chylomicrons. These particles, with diameters up to 500 nm, enter the lymph and, through the thoracic duct, reach the general circulation.

Chylomicrons, upon reaching the periphery, in particular muscle and adipose tissue, are digested by the enzyme lipoprotein lipase, bound to the surface of endothelial cells in capillaries. Lipoprotein lipase (LPL), which can be released into plasma by mucopolysaccharides (in particular heparin), breaks the ester bonds in triglycerides, thus allowing fatty acids to reach tissues, either providing energy or being re-esterified into storage triglycerides (Fig. 75.1).

The remainder of chylomicron particles, so-called chylomicron remnants, are then taken up by the liver through specific receptors for the apolipoproteins E and B-48 and digested in the lysosomes. This process allows the liver to obtain free cholesterol from the chylomicron cholesteryl esters. Exogenous cholesterol is then eliminated through the bile or, most frequently, used for either membrane synthesis or lipoprotein production.

The liver is responsible for endogenous lipoprotein synthesis, partly regulated and partly independent from the exogenous pathway. The liver synthesizes triglycerides, particularly under the stimulus of dietary fat and carbohydrates and produces very low density lipoproteins (VLDL) (diameter 200 nm), similar in composition to chylomicrons, except for the presence of apo B-100 instead of apo

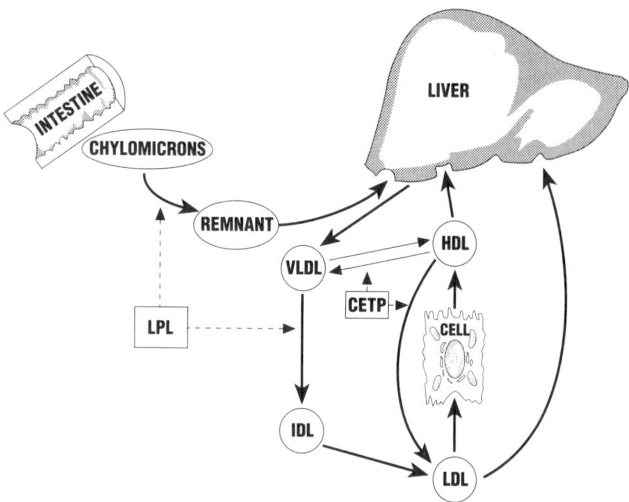

Figure 75.1 Major pathways of lipoprotein metabolism. Both the intestine and the liver produce large lipoproteins, rich in triglycerides, respectively chylomicrons and very low density lipoproteins (VLDL). Both are hydrolyzed in plasma by lipoprotein lipase (LPL) to remnants and to intermediate density lipoproteins (IDL). Chylomicron remnants are taken up by the liver by way of specific receptors. IDL are further lipolysed, in normolipidemic individuals, to low density lipoproteins (LDL). LDL are also taken up by the liver, as well as by peripheral cells, by way of high affinity receptors (absent in homozygous type II hypercholesterolemia). Finally, high density lipoproteins (HDL) remove free cholesterol from cells and also from lipolysed VLDL, converting it into cholesterol esters. Cholesterol esters in HDL have a dual fate: they are either transferred to the liver, by way of a binding protein, or back to VLDL and LDL by way of a cholesteryl ester transfer protein (CETP).

B-48. VLDL undergo a fate similar to chylomicrons, being acted on by LPL and producing a VLDL-remnant, also known as intermediate density lipoprotein (IDL). After having provided peripheral tissues with triglycerides as a source of energy, IDL can again re-enter the liver or be transformed into low density lipoproteins. These now contain minimal amounts of triglycerides, but a large load of cholesteryl esters and B-100 as the sole apolipoprotein.

Low density lipoproteins (LDL), with a far smaller diameter (around 20–50 nm) than chylomicrons or VLDL, have a relatively long circulation in the periphery (half-life of about 1.5 days) and constitute the major source of cholesterol for body tissues. A major fate of LDL, besides that of reaching extrahepatic tissues, is a return to the liver as the cholesterol source for the production of steroid hormones, bile acids, and cell membranes. In both the liver and extrahepatic tissues, LDL uptake is regulated by high affinity receptors, whose presence is genetically determined and whose number may increase or decrease, according to the metabolic demands of the different tissues or of the liver itself. In normal subjects, receptor biosynthesis is increased in all conditions where the tissue needs cholesterol for its metabolic tasks.

Accumulation of cholesterol in peripheral cells is prevented by continuous removal via high density lipoproteins (HDL). These very small particles (diameter around 10 nm) have apolipoprotein A-I and A-II as the major protein components. HDL are capable of efficiently absorbing free cholesterol from peripheral cells, with consequent esterification by the enzyme lecithin:cholesterol-acyltransferase (LCAT). HDL have a constant mobility from tissues to liver, where possibly part of the lipoprotein-free cholesterol may be used as the precursor of bile acids. In addition, HDL interact with VLDL and LDL in plasma, transferring back their cholesteryl esters to the lower density lipoproteins by way of a cholesteryl ester transfer protein (CETP) (Fig. 75.1). Excess cholesteryl esters in LDL are then disposed of by the high affinity receptor pathway. HDL may in this way act as an important defensive mechanism against excessive deposition of cholesterol in body tissues, particularly in the arterial wall.

Under conditions where the influx of both VLDL and LDL is steadily raised, there is the possibility that these lipoproteins, and particularly their metabolic derivatives in the circulation (oxidized products, acetyl or malondialdehyde conjugates) are not cleared by the receptor pathway but are taken up by macrophages or other cells in the reticuloendothelial system. This secondary or "scavenger" pathway of lipoprotein metabolism allows lipid deposition in different sites, particularly the arterial wall (thus inducing atheromas), tendons, and skin (with resulting xanthomas).

Hyperlipoproteinemias and Dyslipoproteinemias

Abnormalities in the physiologic mechanisms regulating plasma lipid/lipoprotein levels may result in a significant elevation of cholesterol, triglycerides or both. These are generally associated with a corresponding rise in the mass of the associated lipoprotein/s. A commonly used term for these disorders is "hyperlipoproteinemias". However, more recently, different syndromes have been described where the abnormality is a lower level of a protective lipoprotein such as HDL or of a qualitative nature, reflecting an altered distribution of either the lipids or of the protein (apolipoprotein) components. Thus the terms of "dyslipidemias" or "dyslipoproteinemias" are being applied more recently. Dyslipidemias may be either secondary or primary.

Secondary Hyperlipoproteinemias

(Table 75.1A) are relatively less frequent and may be associated with any endocrine or parenchymal disease affecting lipid/lipoprotein metabolism. A typical cause of secondary hyperlipoproteinemia is diabetes mellitus, generally with increased triglyceride and VLDL levels as a consequence of diabetic hyperglycemia or of the increased insulinemia resulting from insulin or drug treatments. Insulin is a powerful stimulator of triglyceride biosynthesis, while also increasing LPL activity. Hypothyroidism is, instead, associated with hypercholesterolemia (increased LDL) because of a reduced receptor regulated catabolism. Another endocrine disorder associated with hypercholesterolemia/hypertriglyceridemia is Cushing's disease, because corticosteroid hormones can reduce lipoprotein lipase activity.

Treatment with oral contraceptives may provoke

Table 75.1 **a—Secondary Forms of Hyperlipoproteinemia**

	Plasma Lipid/Lipoproteins Changes	Mechanism/s	Notes
Prevalent Hypertriglyceridemia			
Diabetes Mellitus	Raised VLDL, occasionally LDL	Increased VLDL secretion, reduced catabolism	Also correctable with sulfonylureas and biguanides
Alcoholic Hyperlipidemia	Raised VLDL	Increased VLDL secretion	Particularly in predisposed individuals (10–15% of the adult populations)
Uremia	Raised VLDL	Impaired VLDL catabolism (inhibited lipoprotein lipase)	Sensitive to treatment with fibric acids
Oral contraceptives	Raised VLDL, occasionally reduced HDL	Impaired VLDL catabolism (inhibited liver lipase by estrogens)	Expression may depend both on the estrogen and progestogen components
Beta-blockers	Raised VLDL, reduced HDL	Impaired activation of lipoprotein lipase	Less marked for cardioselective agents and for drugs with ISA
Hypercholesterolemia + hypertriglyceridemia			
Nephrotic syndrome	Raised VLDL + LDL	Compensatory for urinary albumin loss; partial inhibition of lipoprotein lipase	Responds to treatment with HMG CoA reductase inhibitors
Corticosteroids (Cushing syndrome)	Raised VLDL + LDL	Inhibited lipoprotein lipase	
Prevalent hypercholesterolemia			
Hypothyroidism	Raised LDL, occasionally also VLDL	Reduced LDL receptors	
Primary biliary cirrhosis	Increased lipoprotein X (abnormal LDL)	Interaction of bile acids with LDL in the circulation	
b—Primary Forms of Hyperlipoproteinemia (Fredrickson - WHO Classification)			
Type I	Raised chylomicrons, reduced HDL	Absence of lipoprotein lipase; deficiency of apo CII	
Type II-A	Raised LDL	Decreased catabolism of LDL (receptor deficiency or polygenic)	
Type II-B	Raised VLDL + LDL, often reduced HDL	Increased production of VLDL + impaired LDL catabolism	
Type III	Raised IDL (elevated cholesterol + triglycerides dysbetalipoproteinemia)	Abnormal apolipoprotein E, impairing catabolism of IDL	
Type IV	Raised VLDL, often reduced HDL	Impaired VLDL catabolism plus, frequently, dietary indiscretions	
Type V	Raised chylomicrons + VLDL, reduced HDL	Reduced lipoprotein lipase + VLDL hypersecretion	

an iatrogenic endocrine disorder, occasionally resulting in increased triglyceridemia, stimulated by the estrogen content of the pill. Similarly, beta-blockers may be associated with hypertriglyceridemia and at times also with reduced HDL-cholesterol.

Other causes of secondary hyperlipoproteinemias are: alcoholism, because of the potent stimulatory activity of ethanol on VLDL secretion; uremia, also resulting in increased VLDL levels because of a reduced catabolism of these lipoproteins; nephrotic syndrome with increased secretion of both VLDL and LDL, and finally biliary cirrhosis, where the increased formation of an abnormal lipoprotein, lipoprotein X, results from the interaction of bile acids with LDL in the circulation.

Primary Hyperlipoproteinemias

The more common hyperlipoproteinemias are primary, i.e., dependent on an altered intra-extravascular metabolism of lipoproteins. Generally, most patients with primary hyperlipoproteinemias do not show any clear-cut alteration in the endocrine system or at the gene level, their only abnormality being excess cholesterol or triglycerides in plasma, arbitrarily above the 90 to 95th percentile of that population on a free-choice diet.

Determination of the fasting total levels of cholesterol and triglycerides already provides a cue for the diagnosis of hyperlipoproteinemia. The classification proposed in 1967 by Fredrickson et al.,[1] identifying lipoprotein disorders according to five phenotypes, is still very helpful. Of these phenotypes the even-numbered are very common (more than 95% of those clinically observed), whereas of the odd-numbered I, III, and V are rare—not more than 1 to 2 percent in large samples of hyperlipoproteinemic patients. Primary hyperlipoproteinemias characterized, respectively, by excess levels of either cholesterol or triglycerides, are classified as Fredrickson's type II and IV. A more recent modification of the Fredrickson typing system, carried out by the WHO (1970),[2] recognized two subtypes, II-A and II-B, according to the presence, together with excess cholesterol, of either a normal triglyceridemia (II-A), or a hypertriglyceridemia (II-B) (Table 75.1B).

In Type II hyperlipoproteinemias high LDL levels are always present. In a small number of these individuals, the abnormality is related to an absence (total or partial) of high-affinity receptors for LDL. The total absence of receptors (homozygous Type II) occurs in about one individual per million, whereas partial absence (heterozygous Type II) can be found in approximately one out of 500 subjects. These typical familial hypercholesterolemias are associated with markedly elevated cholesterol (above 600 mg/dl in homozygotes and above 350 mg/dl in heterozygotes) and increased risk of early coronary disease. The majority of hypercholesterolemias, both II-A and II-B do not, however, recognize a distinct pathogenetic defect and may be linked to a variety of abnormalities in cholesterol absorption and handling and in LDL production and catabolism.

Hypertriglyceridemias are defined by the common Fredrickson's Type IV and the rare Types I and V. These latter are characterized by the presence, in fasting conditions, of a large load of chylomicrons, in Type I constituting the majority of circulating lipoproteins. Both in Type I and V the pathogenic mechanism is related to a deficient regulation of lipoprotein lipase. The very common Type IV is instead mostly found in adult individuals, frequently associated with "diabetic" traits, i.e., hyperinsulinemia, abnormalities in glucose handling, and elevated uricemia. In the case of Type IV, the distinction between a primary and secondary form may at times be difficult, particularly for the peculiar sensitivity of these individuals to ethanol. Hypertriglyceridemias (except Type I) carry a significant risk of early coronary and peripheral arterial disease, also for the concomitant presence of abnormalities in HDL formation and function, with a consequent deficient removal capacity for atherogenic lipoproteins.

Finally, combined elevations of cholesterol and triglycerides, besides the case of the common II-B hyperlipoproteinemia, can also be found in Fredrickson's type III disease. In this clinical condition an abnormal VLDL particle, poorly catabolized by lipoprotein lipase, is present, carrying both cholesterol and triglycerides. Type III disease is occasionally associated with the presence of palmar xanthomas, and definitive diagnosis requires the use of preparative ultracentrifugation and possibly of the electrophoretic separation of apoprotein E isoforms.

Dyslipoproteinemias

More recently-described lipid associated mechanisms for the development of arterial disease are abnormalities in the distribution/composition of lipoproteins. Dyslipoproteinemias are clinical conditions not strictly associated with quantitative abnormalities of lipid levels, but rather with increases/decreases of specific lipoproteins or even of apolipoproteins.[3] The most common is hypo-α-lipoproteinemia, characterized by low HDL-cholesterol levels. This abnormality may be present in as many as 10 percent of atherosclerotic patients, and is rated as an independent risk factor for arterial disease. Low HDL-cholesterol may be the consequence of different biochemical abnormalities and of some acquired disorders (physical inactivity, intake of some β-blockers). Hyper-apo B-lipoproteinemia has been described in numerous cohorts of coronary patients. It is characterized by an enrichment of apolipoprotein B in LDL, otherwise of relatively normal composition, except for a slight excess of triglycerides; mild hypertriglyceridemia occurs also in plasma.

The accumulation in plasma of a newly described form of lipoprotein, lipoprotein (a), Lp(a) (previously, "sinking pre-β lipoprotein," slow migrating pre-β lipoprotein, and others) has recently stimulated considerable interest. Lp(a) is separated in the density range of LDL and is composed of apolipoprotein B and of an apoprotein (apo a) of variable molecular weight (from 400 KD to 700 KD). It is considerably homologous with plasminogen.[4] About 30 percent of adults have elevated levels of Lp(a) (>35 mg/dl) and an enhanced risk of cardiovascular diseases, possibly owing to an interaction of the particles with arterial plasminogen binding sites, followed by local deposition of cholesteryl ester.[5] Treatment of such elevated Lp(a) levels has thus far had discouraging results.

Hyperlipoproteinemias may also be linked to mutations in the major apolipoproteins (apo Al, apo B, apo E). These mutants show amino acid changes in the sequence of the apoprotein, which may lead to an increase in some lipoprotein fractions. The list of mutants is now large and still growing: it includes apo B abnormalities linked to arterial disease, as well as mutations in apo A-I, one of which (apo A-I Milano) apparently is associated with protection from atherosclerotic disease.

Lipid Lowering in Preventive and Therapeutic Medicine

The "lipid hypothesis", the theory that links worsening or improvement of arterial disease risk to changes in plasma lipids, particularly cholesterol, has been supported by animal and human data since the beginning of this century. Anitschkow[6] first showed that feeding cholesterol to rabbits induced severe arterial disease; at a similar time, also in Russia, Ignatowsky[7] provided epidemiologic evidence that wealthy citizens who consumed fat and animal protein were more frequent victims of complications of arterial disease than were poor ones.

In the 1950s the first "intervention trials," based on a reduction in the dietary intake of (particularly) saturated fat, showed both a reduction of cholesterolemia and a lower incidence of coronary heart disease (CHD) in the treated groups. Classic studies in this field were carried out in New York (Anti-Coronary Club), Los Angeles, and Helsinki (Psychiatric Hospital Study). More definitive proof of the lipid hypothesis in man, has however, been obtained from two drug studies, both carried out very recently, the Lipid Research Clinics (LRC) Study in the US and the Helsinki Heart Study in Finland.

The LRC Study was carried out in 3806 middle-aged men with primary hypercholesterolemia (mean cholesterol 290 mg/dl) and no symptoms of arterial disease. These subjects received 24 grams per day of cholestyramine, a bile acid binding resin, or a corresponding placebo for an average of 7.4 years. Although compliance with the demanding drug regimen was erratic, the treated group experienced a mean reduction of LDL cholesterol concentrations around 20 percent (13% greater than the placebo group). Cholestyramine-treated subjects had a 24 percent reduction in death due to myocardial infarction (MI) and a 19 percent reduction in nonfatal MI (both $p < 0.05$). Also other endpoints of arterial disease (angina pectoris and coronary bypass surgery) were reduced by respectively 20 and 21 percent in the cholestyramine group, compared with the placebo-treated group.[8]

Analysis of the results of the LRC study provides some interesting additional conclusions. As noted, compliance to drug treatment was not good; only 25 percent took the full prescribed dose of cholestyramine. Extrapolation of data from fully compliant patients indicates that LDL-cholesterol levels in these were reduced up to 35 percent, with a nearly 50 percent decrease of coronary disease incidence.

Whereas the LRC study was carried out in primarily hypercholesterolemic individuals, the Helsinki Heart Study (HHS) evaluated employees of Finnish public services with a non-HDL cholesterol (VLDL + LDL) level of over 200 mg/dl.[9] Therefore, Finnish subjects had a lower cholesterolemia (mean 250 mg/dl) vs the LRC participants, and hypertriglyceridemia was rather common (mean plasma triglycerides: 175 mg/dl), 36 percent showing either type II-B or IV hyperlipoproteinemia. 2051 of the subjects received gemfibrozil (600 mg bid) and 2030 a corresponding placebo for a period of five years. In this study, significant reductions were noted in both cholesterol (–11% total and –10% LDL) and particularly triglycerides (–43%); treated subjects also experienced a rise of HDL-cholesterol (+14%). The HHS confirmed a striking reduction in the incidence of coronary heart disease (–34% in the gemfibrozil group), evident from the second year of the study onward; nonfatal MI was reduced by 37 percent.

Both the LRC and the Helsinki studies indicate that a reduction of plasma lipids, both cholesterol and triglycerides, as well as possibly a rise of HDL-cholesterol levels, are major goals in the prevention of cardiovascular disease. The benefit from these therapeutic measures appears to be more significant than that resulting from lowering elevated blood pressure.

In the past decade, emphasis has also been placed on the possible role of lipid lowering in the therapy of established cardiovascular conditions. Such studies, both in animals and in human disease, have described the potential for "regression" of atherosclerotic lesions. Studies in animals, both monkeys and pigs, clearly indicate that high-fat diets can induce the formation of severe atherosclerotic lesions and that, by replacing such diets with low fat regimens, lesions can "regress".[10] Regression may be further accelerated by the addition of different lipid-lowering drugs. Data in humans have recently been generated.[11] In general, angiographically-documented lesions are less likely to progress when patients are placed on low-fat regimens with drugs; the possibility of regression has recently been firmly established, although energetic combined drug regimens, including inhibitors of HMG CoA reductase or high-dose nicotinic acid combined with anion binding resins,[12] or the application of an apheretic treatment for LDL,[13] are necessary to induce regression of some lesions. In patients presenting with arterial lesions and elevated lipid levels, treatment with diet and drugs is a reasonable option.

Therapeutic Strategies

Recommendations in the US and in Europe

Following the LRC and Helsinki trials, major specialists in the US and in Europe convened to prepare documents outlining the most appropriate strategies for reducing the risk of cardiovascular disease. The first US document summarized present-day evidence supporting the lipid hypothesis. In particular, levels of cholesterolemia requiring different treatments were outlined (Table 75.2). This first US document also gave general ideas on the more proper approach to diet and/or drug therapy. Three successive European documents, published in 1987–1992,[14–16] provided more details, indicating at least five subgroups of patients with cholesterol and/or triglyceride elevations (Table 75.3). More recently, within the US National Cholesterol Education program, a report has been prepared for practicing physicians mainly related to the correction of elevated cholesterol levels, but also listing low HDL levels as a risk factor. This, as well as a further, more recent report, also deals with evaluation criteria for elevated triglyceride levels.[18]

The general therapeutic strategy of intervention in the US and European documents involves:

(1) *Assessment of the risk status of patients* (lipid and nonlipid variables, e.g., smoking, hypertension, sedentary life, etc.) and of the dietary status (excess consumption of saturated fat, total calories, animal proteins, etc.).

(2) *Dietary guidelines,* eventually correcting errors.

(3) *Addition of drugs,* when the dietary approach (e.g., correcting body weight) has not achieved the desired change in the abnormal lipid pattern. Bile-acid sequestrants, nicotinic acid, probucol, fibric acids, and the HMG CoA reductase inhibitors can be indicated.

The above-mentioned Policy Statements of the European Atherosclerosis Society call for a more detailed evaluation of plasma lipid/lipoprotein patterns in individuals. Moreover, the documents comment on other risk factors, e.g., smoking, hypertension, lack of physical activity, alcohol, etc. In terms of the guidelines for managing hyperlipidemia, they summarize five conditions, with graded levels of cholesterol/triglycerides, classified from A to E (Table 75.3) with differing risk, indicating where specific strategies of treatment should be advised.

Both the US and European Policy Statements encourage "population strategies," i.e., based on the assumption that the majority of individuals are exposed to moderately elevated levels of risk factors. They do not discourage, however, an individual or "high-risk" strategy that aims to identify the minority within the population whose risk of disease is particularly high.

Both the US and European documents, in their different versions, had a considerable impact, particularly on physicians, but also on the general population. It is expected that they should result in a considerable improvement in the detection and treatment of hyperlipidemia and, hopefully, in a consequent reduction of arterial disease.

Table 75.2 US Recommendations for the Management of Hypercholesterolemia (adults, 20 years and over)[17]

A. Classification	
<200 mg/dl	Desirable Blood Cholesterol
200–239 mg/dl	Borderline-High Blood Cholesterol
≥240 mg/dl	High Blood Cholesterol
B. Recommended Followup	
Total Cholesterol <200 mg/dl	Repeat within 5 yrs
Total Cholesterol 200–239 mg/dl	
Without definite CHD or two other CHD risk factors (one of which can be male sex)	Dietary information and recheck annually
With definite CHD or two other CHD risk factors (one of which can be male sex)	Lipoprotein analysis: further action based on LDL-cholesterol level
Total Cholesterol ≥ 240 mg/dl	Lipoprotein analysis: further action based on LDL-cholesterol level

Clinical Treatment of Hyperlipoproteinemias

The therapeutic approach to patients with elevated lipids is generally a combination of different strategies, i.e., dietary changes and the elimination of other risk factors that may worsen the prognosis of the metabolic disorder. Among these are cessation or reduction of smoking, proper management of hypertension, physical exercise, etc.

The major dietary changes aim at the reduction of excess body weight and at the controlled intake of nutrients generally linked to rises in plasma lipids. Reduction of body weight may lead to an improved control of several forms of hypertriglyceridemia; the same goal can be achieved by a reduction of ethanol intake. In the case of hypercholesterolemia, the total amount of dietary fat is correlated with raised cholesterol: saturated fats (of animal origin) are among the most potent causative factors in hypercholesterolemia.[19] In addition to these, animal protein intake may be a significant factor in many hypercholesterolemic patients; the change from animal to vegetable proteins as the major dietary protein may frequently lead to the correction of hypercholesterolemia.[20]

Drugs are to be administered when all of the above therapeutic approches have been exhaustively carried

Table 75.3 Guidelines for the Management of Lipid/Lipoprotein Disorders—European Atherosclerosis Society Policy Statements[14–16]

Treatment Group	Diagnosis Levels	Investigation	Management
A	Cholesterol 200–250 mg/dl Triglycerides < 200 mg/dl	Assess overall CHD risk (family history, habits, BP, body weight, etc.)	Restrict food energy if overweight, correct other risk factors if present. Consider additional therapy in individuals at high risk
B	Cholesterol 250–300 mg/dl Triglycerides < 200 mg/dl	Assess overall risk of CHD as under A	Same as for A, but if dietary control is inadequate consider lipid lowering drug therapy
C	Cholesterol < 200 mg/dl Triglycerides 200–250 mg/dl	Seek possible secondary causes (diabetes, ethanol etc.)	Reduce dietary energy if necessary; monitor strict lipid lowering diet, correct other risk factors, if present
D	Cholesterol 200–300 mg/dl Triglycerides 200–250 mg/dl	Assess overall risk of CHD as in A. Seek underlying causes of hypertriglyceridemia as in C	Same as in B and C; if serum lipid response is inadequate and CHD risk high, consider lipid lowering drug therapy
E	Cholesterol > 300 mg/dl and/or Triglycerides > 500 mg/dl	Make full diagnosis with laboratory and clinical data	Dietary and generally drug treatment. Consider referral to specialized center for complete diagnosis.

out. Drugs for hyperlipoproteinemia are not numerous, and some belong to other therapeutic classes. From a pharmacologic point of view, lipid-lowering agents can be classified into nonsystemic and sytemic agents. The former generally act at the intestinal level, by affecting the absorption/excretion of neutral and acidic steroids; the latter act by a variety of mechanisms, from activation of lipoprotein catabolism (e.g., fibric acid derivatives) to antagonism of cholesterol biosynthesis (hydroxymethylglutaryl CoA reductase inhibitors). The different drug groups may share, to a large extent, their major indications, but specific targets of activity are manifest for each drug. Moreover, the pattern of side-effects and/or contraindications may favor the selection of one or the other agent in specific clinical syndromes.

Lipid Lowering Drugs

Nonsystemic Lipid Lowering Drugs

The major nonabsorbable agents are the anion exchange resins, which bind bile acids in the intestine, and the antibiotic neomycin, stimulating the intestinal loss of both bile acid and neutral sterols. The prime bile acid binding resin, cholestyramine, was initially developed for the control of itching in cholestatic patients. More recently, it has been the first pharmacologic agent clearly shown to reduce the incidence of coronary disease in asymptomatic hypercholesterolemic patients.[8]

Anion-Exchange Resins

Two products are approved for use in most countries; others are less widely available. Cholestyramine and colestipol, with different chemical structures, exert a similar activity on intestinal bile acid reabsorption.

Cholestyramine is the 3-methylbenzylammonium derivative of styrene, a chemically stable, widely used polymer. The average molecular weight of the resin is in excess of 1 million (Fig. 75.2).

Colestipol is a copolymer of diethylpentamine and epichlorohydrin; its structural formula is depicted in Figure 75.3. The average molecular weight of colestipol is less than that of cholestyramine; neither product is water-soluble, and both are poorly absorbed by the intestine (less than 5% of the dose of radioactively-labeled drug may appear in urines). In some European countries, DEAE-Sephadex is used with similar indications; the product is equiactive to cholestyramine.

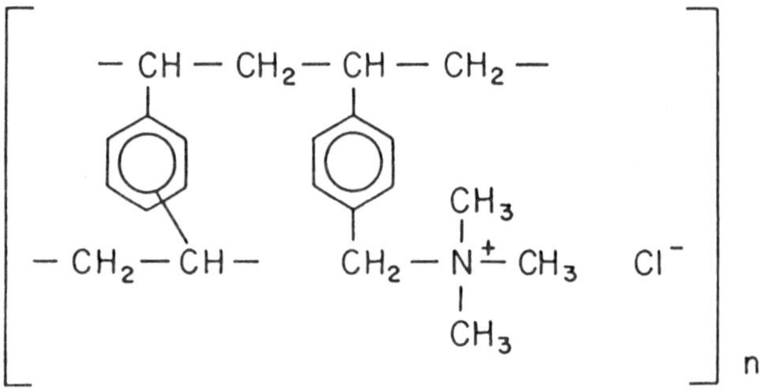

Figure 75.2 Chemical structure of the monomeric unit of cholestyramine. Bile acids are bound after interaction with the positive charge of the ammonium ion.

Because resins are practically not absorbed, they can bind bile acids in the intestine, favoring their loss in feces. Normally, daily intestinal loss of bile acids is seldom above 1 gram; following treatment with cholestyramine, the loss goes up to 2 to 3 grams per day. Besides impairing dietary sterol absorption, the marked loss of bile acids leads to a reduction of the cholesterol body pools. This may bring about a regression of tendon xanthomas and possibly of atherosclerotic lesions.[21] Another consequence of the bile acid loss is a compensatory increase in cell-surface LDL receptors in the liver, together with an increased activity of hydroxymethylglutaryl Coenzyme A (HMG CoA) reductase, the key enzyme in cholesterol biosynthesis. Increased receptor activity leads to an enhanced uptake of LDL from plasma, with a reduction of LDL-cholesterol levels.[22] This effect is somewhat counteracted by the increased HMG CoA reductase activity. However, in general, with the exception of homozygous Type II patients, who have no LDL-receptors, the LDL-cholesterol reduction is consistent and therapeutically effective.

Anion exchange resins significantly reduce the concentration of total and LDL-cholesterol, particularly in hypercholesterolemic patients. These effects are rapid in onset (within one week of treatment) and usually in the range of 20 to 30 percent vs starting levels. In some patients, a transient increase of VLDL-triglycerides may be seen early in the treatment. During the LRC study, significant rises of HDL-cholesterol levels were also noted.[23] This last finding may be linked to the increased cholesterol mobilization from tissues during therapy. Resins are contraindicated in patients with significant hypertriglyceridemia, where a further rise of plasma triglycerides and VLDL is not desirable. Clinical evidence also has been provided showing that cholestyramine treatment may consistently slow the progression (in some cases eliciting a moderate regression) of pre-existing coronary lesions. The combination of cholestyramine and nicotinic acid (CLAS study) also has shown that the long-term prognosis of coronary bypass grafts can be markedly improved.[11] Colestipol gave excellent results when combined with either nicotinic acid or lovastatin in the FATS study that evaluated coronary progression in mildly hypercholesterolemic patients with angina or previous MI.[12]

Adverse Effects and Interactions of Anion Exchange Resins

The use of anion exchange resins has always been hampered by the unpleasant taste and sandy feeling of these pharmaceutical preparations. In addition, cholestyramine, colestipol, and analogues are frequently associated with constipation, abdominal distress, and occasional nausea. Such unpleasant feelings are difficult to control. Good advice may be that of administering cholestyramine after mixing with fruit juices and crushed ice in a shaker, thus minimizing the sandy feeling. Constipation may be difficult to control in individual patients. Biochemical changes, occurring particularly after cholestyramine, are transient transaminase or alkaline phosphatase rises; rarely, the absorption of the chloride ion of the molecule may lead to hyperchloremic acidosis.

Interaction with different drugs and vitamins may be common after cholestyramine; in the case of vitamins it is generally slight. Drugs commonly bound by resins are: ferrous sulfate, acidic anti-inflammatory drugs, phenobarbital, thyroxine and the different digitalis molecules. In this last case, cholestyramine may provide a useful antidote in overdoses. Aside from the chemical interactions, anion exchange resins may also delay the absorption of some medications, just because of their bulk forming properties. For this reason, it is advisable to administer cholestyramine or other resins at least four hours before or two hours after intake of other drugs. There are no specific contraindications to resins during pregnancy.

Preparations and Doses

Cholestyramine is available in most countries in packets containing 4 g of resin (Questran, usually in a total of 9 g of powder). In some European countries different pharmaceutical preparations of cholestyramine are available, in packet, suspension, or also tablet form (Colestrol: Italy; Spain). A new candy-bar preparation has recently become available in the US (Cholybar). Colestipol (Colestid and others) is instead available in packets containing 5 g of resin. Daily doses for both resins range from 8 to 24 g (cholestyramine) or from 10 to 30 g (colestipol), divided into two or three portions. Some patients find it beneficial to take the resins in one single administration in the morning. DEAE-Sephadex is available in some countries in tablet form (0.5 or 1 g). Newer preparations of resins are presently being tested; among these are chitosan derivatives, formulated in water-soluble preparations.

Neomycin

Neomycin is an aminoglycoside antibiotic, generally used for the prevention of hepatic coma. A significant cholesterol reduction was noted as a side action in treated patients. Such activity can be of therapeutic interest in hypercholesterolemic patients with normal liver function. It appears that the cholesterol reduction is independent of the antimicrobial activity. Neomycin seems to perturb the formation of micelles of bile acids and neutral sterols, thus leading to a significant loss, particularly of neutral sterols, from the feces.[24]

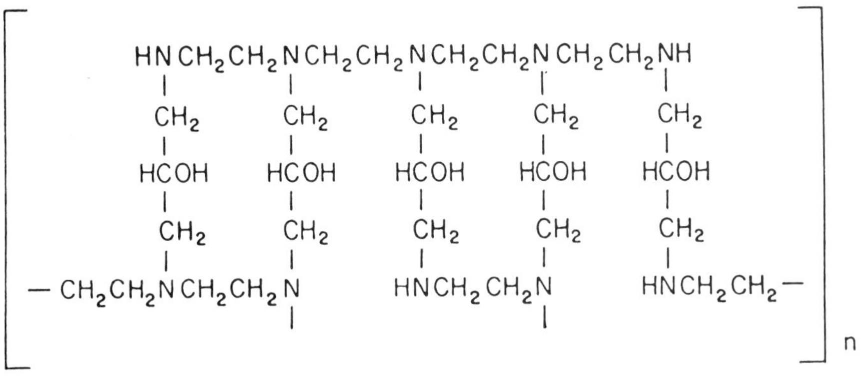

Figure 75.3 Chemical structure of the monomeric unit of colestipol. Positive charges (interacting with the bile acids) are distributed on the different nitrogens.

Administration of neomycin is not always well tolerated. Absorption of the compound, although small, may lead to a possible damage of kidney function; subjective side-effects also are often reported (itching and abnormalities in intestinal function).

Neomycin (numerous commercial names) is usually given in divided doses, ranging from 0.5 to 2 g/day. Cholesterol and LDL reductions may be observed—up to 20 percent or more in responsive patients. Neomycin may be the best available agent for the reduction of Lp(a), particularly when used in association with nicotinic acid.[21]

Systemic Lipid Lowering Drugs

Systemic lipid lowering agents include a variety of chemical structures with widely different mechanisms of action. Some of the agents, e.g., fibric acids, have been in use for many years and are still the mainstay of therapy in most countries; others, e.g., the HMG CoA reductase inhibitors, are relatively new, and their long-term activity and safety may still need evaluation. Finally, others, e.g., nicotinic acid, are slowly losing their share of therapeutic use.

Fibric Acid Derivatives

Fibric acid derivatives or "fibrates" constitute a rather large series of compounds characterized by the presence of an aryloxy acidic moiety. The prototype fibrate, clofibrate, was initially tested more than 25 years ago and found to be effective in numerous animal models of hyperlipidemia. Following clofibrate, several other fibrates have been made available, most notably bezafibrate, fenofibrate, gemfibrozil, and ciprofibrate.

Clofibrate is the ethyl ester of p-chlorophenoxyisobutyric acid (CPIB). The other major fibrates show a similar basic structure (gemfibrozil does not have the chlorine atom in the para position) (Fig. 75.4).

BEZAFIBRATE

CIPROFIBRATE

FENOFIBRATE

GEMFIBROZIL

CLOFIBRATE

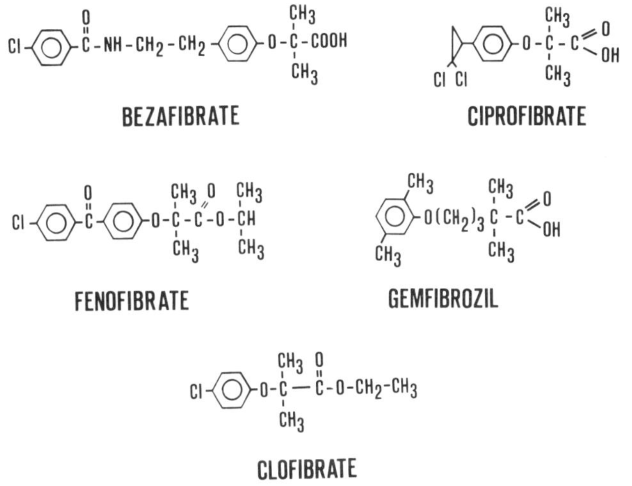

Figure 75.4 Chemical Structures of the Major Fibric Acid Derivatives So-called "Fibrates"

Mechanism of Action of Fibrates. Fibrates belong to a series of molecules that activate a catabolic system for fatty acids in liver cells by interacting with a nuclear receptor (PPAR) responsible for a coordinate stimulation of cytochrome P-450 IVA and mitochondrial/peroxisomal β-oxidation.[26] These abnormal or "fraudulent" fatty acids are a relatively large series of compounds, including fibric acids, ω-3 fatty acids from fish oil, and a variety of other chemicals, some of which are undergoing pharmacologic or clinical development.[27] Probably as a consequence of the stimulated fatty acid catabolism, there is an increased degradation in the periphery of triglyceride-rich lipoproteins (VLDL). This is exerted by way of an increased activity of the enzyme lipoprotein lipase, responsible for triglyceride hydrolysis in VLDL.[28] Besides the increased catabolism, the rate of direct removal of VLDL, HDL, and LDL also may be increased. Although depressive effects on the hepatic synthesis and release of cholesterol and lipoproteins have been shown in experimental animals, similar conclusions have not been consistently reached in humans.

By activating lipoprotein catabolism, fibrates can effectively reduce VLDL triglycerides in patients with elevated levels. This effect occurs in over 80 percent of treated patients and may bring triglyceridemia to normal values in the large majority. Consequences of increased VLDL catabolism are a rise of HDL-cholesterol (Fig. 75.1), occurring in most patients, and, in some hypertriglyceridemic patients, also a paradoxical rise of LDL-cholesterol.[29] Whereas this latter effect is not of major significance, the HDL-cholesterol rise is likely to be associated with lowered cardiovascular risk in treated patients.[9]

The activities of fibrates on total serum cholesterol levels are less clear-cut. These compounds significantly reduce cholesterolemia, particularly in patients with relatively marked elevations (familial Type II-A) and normal triglyceridemia. Pharmacokinetic studies have shown that, in these patients, plasma levels of CPIB, may be significantly higher than in normolipidemics or hypertriglyceridemics.[30] Another hypothesis links the activity on LDL-cholesterol levels to the improved delipidization of LDL because of the increased lipase, thus leading to a better interaction with the LDL receptors.[31]

Whatever the mechanism, there is no doubt that, in treated patients, fibrates can reduce the body cholesterol pool, thus leading to a significant reduction of cholesterol deposits in tissues, occasionally with regression of xanthomas. These clinical observations are particularly dramatic in patients with familial dysbetalipoproteinemia (Fredrickson's Type III). In these, the reduction of cholesterol and triglycerides is accompanied by clear-cut improvements in vascular disease and tissue lipid deposition.

New aspects of the activity of fibrates are related to nonlipid parameters. In particular, it has become clear that some fibrates display a potent plasma fibrinogen reducing activity.[32] This finding has particular significance in view of the clear-cut correlation between fibrinogenemia and cardiovascular risk. In addition, scattered reports indicate a potential activity on platelet aggregation, reducing sensitivity to different aggregants in treated patients. Finally, fibric acids may correct the reduced fibrinolytic activity in diabetes and Type IV hyperlipoproteinemia.[33] Whether this last observation may contribute to the preventive activity of fibrates against arterial disease is presently the object of investigation.

Clinical Activity of Fibrates. The major indication for fibrates is the treatment of hyperlipoproteinemias. The best activity is achieved in Type IV hyperlipoproteinemia, with a reduction of triglycerides in the range of 40 to 60 percent and concomitant increases of HDL-cholesterol levels. As indicated, in these patients an elevation of LDL-cholesterol may occur after treatment.

Hypercholesterolemias (Type II-A, II-B) show a less clear-cut response. In general, plasma cholesterol response is more marked in severe hypercholesterolemia (familial Type II), possibly because of a more prolonged elimination half-life and higher blood levels in these patients. Probably for the same reason, fibrates with a longer elimination half-life (fenofibrate, ciprofibrate) may be more effective in severe Type II hyperlipidemics. The most sensitive hyperlipoproteinemia is, however, Type III, because of the potent stimulation to lipoprotein clearance induced by fibrates.

Although it is difficult to point out specific sensitivities or activity patterns of different fibrates, several differences have become apparent. Long-acting fibrates are generally more effective in hypercholesterolemia, whereas compounds with a shorter half-life are more effective in Type IV. Gemfibrozil seems to be the most effective in raising HDL and apo AI, fenofibrate in reducing apo B concentrations. Clinical experience suggests, however, that resistance to treatment with one fibrate does not exclude sensitivity to another.

The clinical evidence for the efficacy of fibrates in the prevention of ischemic heart disease has not been obtained in a straightforward way. Initial controlled and open studies with clofibrate had indicated that this drug might reduce the incidence of ischemic heart disease and/or angina in patients with normal lipids, but not reduce mortality in post-infarction patients (Coronary Drug Project).[34] In 1978, a World Health Organization (WHO)-supported study compared clofibrate with placebo in 15,000 males with plasma cholesterol levels in the upper third of the population distribution. This study, showed that, after five years, clofibrate could lower cholesterol about 9 percent vs placebo.[35] To this reduction of cholesterolemia corresponded a 25 percent fall in the incidence of nonfatal MI. Unfortunately, a higher noncardiac mortality occurred in the clofibrate group, with a statistically significant (although not marked, from the numerical point of view) increase in malignant tumors and complications of cholecystectomy.

The recent study, carried out with gemfibrozil in Finland (Helsinki Heart Study) has been summarized previously.[9] Of interest, and different from the WHO study, the Helsinki Study failed to show any significant increase in the incidence of either neoplasms or gallstone operations. The administration of gemfibrozil to subjects with moderately increased cardiovascular risk led to the expected biochemical changes: significant drop of triglyceridemia; rise of HDL-cholesterol; small

(–10%) but significant reduction of LDL-cholesterol; and a dramatic fall in cardiovascular morbidity (–34%).

Absorption, Fate, and Excretion of Fibrates. The pharmacodynamic activity of fibrates is only partially linked to their kinetics, since the activation of lipoprotein lipase may be independent of a continued presence of the drug in plasma. On the other hand, fibrates with a long elimination half-life have the advantage of single daily administration (in some cases, patients may skip one or both week-end treatments without changes in the effects on plasma lipids). The major kinetic characteristics of the more widely available fibrates are summarized in Table 75.4. All fibrates, with the exception of gemfibrozil, are prodrugs, being deesterified to the active acid. The deesterification of clofibrate to clofibric acid (CPIB) is shown in Fig. 75.5.

The major metabolite patterns of fibric acids are also indicated in Table 75.4. Metabolite formation differs with the different agents, major metabolites including hydroxylated products, phenol metabolites, etc. In general, most of the transformation products are then excreted into the urine in the form of glucuronide conjugates. Fibric acids are extensively bound to plasma proteins, particularly albumin. A portion is also bound to lipoproteins, and it has been suggested that this latter binding may partly influence the pharmacodynamic properties.

Adverse Effects and Interactions of Fibrates. The administration of fibrates is generally well tolerated by most patients. Subjective side-effects, e.g., GI, skin, etc., are quite uncommon (2% or less in large series). Impotence and/or loss of libido have been reported occasionally but never clearly substantiated. Some of the newer agents, particularly those with the longest

Table 75.4 Fibric Acid Derivatives—Major Metabolic and Kinetic Parameters

Compound	Absorption	Protein Binding	Daily Dose	Metabolism	Elimination: $t_{1/2}$	Site	Notes
Clofibrate	99%	97%	1 g bid	de-ethylation, minor metabolite formation, conjugated with glucuronide	15–22h	renal	
Bezafibrate	95%	94–96%	400–600 mg qd	50% unchanged; 22% glucuronide conjugates; 22% other polar metabolites (hydroxy and others)	3–9h	renal	
Fenofibrate	90%	99%	250–300 mg qd	de-ethylation; 50% conjugated; 50% polar metabolites (phenol, benzhydrol)	20–26h	renal	Not removable by hemodialysis
Gemfibrozil	90%		900–1200 mg qd	40% unchanged; 60% numerous metabolites (conjugated, benzoic acid, phenol, etc.)	2–3h for the unchanged drug	renal	
Ciprofibrate	90%	90%	100 mg qd	de-ethylation; 73% glucurunide conjugates	42 h	renal	

half-life, e.g., fenofibrate, have been associated with increased transaminase levels in plasma. Clinical myositis was described in early patient series with clofibrate, associated with a flu-like syndrome and marked increases of plasma CPK; such findings are rarely encountered with the newer agents.

Fibrates may increase the elimination of cholesterol by way of bile and lead to an increased risk of lithogenicity. Such risk was clearly noted only in the WHO study with clofibrate[35]: reports on other agents are contradictory and do not seem to support a similar risk. In spite of the observation of an increased incidence of liver tumors in rodents due to a species-specific response (peroxisomal proliferation) and index of enhanced β-oxidation of fatty acids, there is no convincing evidence of an increased risk of tumors of any kind in humans receiving currently available fibrates.

It may be generally concluded that the profile of risk attributed to fibric acid derivatives after the Coronary Drug Project and the WHO studies with clofibrate (gallstone disease, increased incidence of tumors, liver toxicity, etc.), does not appear to be shared to a significant extent by any of the newer derivatives. This difference from clofibrate may be linked to the particular reactivity of the CPIB molecule, i.e., secondary to the vicinity between the Cl atom and the aliphatic side-chain.[36] In view of the differences between clofibrate and the other agents, a similar risk profile should not be automatically attributed to any new fibrate.

Major interactions between fibric acids and other drugs have been observed. The most significant clinically is the potentiation of coumarin anticoagulants. This interaction usually requires a halving of the dose of concomitantly given coumarins. The mechanism of this interaction, after an initial hypothesis of protein binding displacement, is as yet undefined. Fibric acids with tighter binding may also displace thyroxine from its binding globulin, leading in some cases to increased free thyroxine. These same agents may also reduce uric acid by competing for reabsorption.

Preparations and Therapeutic Use of Fibrates. Fibric acid derivatives are available in a wide range of doses, with different therapeutic schedules. Clofibrate is usually available in 500-mg capsules, given as 1000 mg bid (major name Atromid). Bezafibrate is usually given in two daily doses of 300 mg; a slow-release form is also available in some countries (major names, Bezalip, Cedur). Fenofibrate can be given in three divided doses of 100 mg or, because of the long half-life, as a single daily administration of 250 to 300 mg (major commercial name Lipanthyl); gemfibrozil is generally given as 600 mg bid, in some countries as 900 mg qd (major name Lopid) in tablet or sachet form. Less widely available are ciprofibrate (Lipanor), clinofibrate (Lipoclin), and others.

$$\text{Cl-C}_6\text{H}_4\text{-O-C(CH}_3)_2\text{-COOCH}_2\text{CH}_3 \longrightarrow \text{Cl-C}_6\text{H}_4\text{-O-C(CH}_3)_2\text{-COOH}$$

Clofibrate → Clofibric acid (CPIB)

Figure 75.5 Cleavage of the Ethyl Group of Clofibrate, Leading to the Active Compound Clofibric Acid

Although comparative data on the different fibrates may be difficult to analyze, clinical experience suggests the following:

(1) The use of clofibrate is now probably to be restricted only to the very sensitive Type III hyperlipoproteinemic patients.

(2) The hypotriglyceridemic effect of all the fibrates is rather similar, possibly somewhat better for bezafibrate and gemfibrozil.

(3) The HDL and apo A-I raising properties are most marked with gemfibrozil and fenofibrate.

(4) The most effective cholesterol reduction is usually achieved with the long-acting fibrates, ciprofibrate, and particularly fenofibrate, although the other agents are not much less effective. Interestingly, severe Type II hypercholesterolemic patients are generally more sensitive to fibrates vs patients with only marginally elevated cholesterolemia.

(5) The selective activity of some fibrates on plasma fibrinogen levels suggests possible use in patients with elevated fibrinogenemia; a potential use in the induction of fibrinolysis has also been suggested.

(6) The risk profile of the newer agents in particular is generally reassuring; more data are needed on the relative antithrombotic effectiveness of these drugs.

Nicotinic Acid

Nicotinic acid (niacin) is one of the B vitamins. Its activity on plasma lipids at very high doses (in excess of 0.2 g/d) was shown more than 30 years ago. Nicotinic acid since then has been found effective in numerous forms of hyperlipoproteinemia.[37]

The mechanism of action of nicotinic acid occurs through:

(1) Inhibition of lipolysis in adipose tissue, preventing utilization of free fatty acids for the synthesis of triglyceride-rich lipoproteins.

(2) A consequent decrease in the hepatic release of VLDL.

(3) Activation of hepatic lipase, preventing the transformation of the more efficient HDL_2 subfraction to the less efficient HDL_3.

Other mechanisms, e.g., reduced LDL synthesis, are less clearly demonstrated. The primary indications for nicotinic acid (NA) are, therefore, combined hyperlipidemias and isolated hypercholesterolemia. Typical changes after standard doses of nicotinic acid (2–8 g/d) are reductions of plasma triglycerides and cholesterol, of 30 to 40 percent and of 15 to 20 percent, respectively. LDL-cholesterol levels may be reduced by 20 percent or more. Increased levels of HDL-cholesterol may be the highest response among lipid-lowering agents; some patients may in fact, achieve elevations of 30 percent or greater. Unlike most other lipid-lowering agents, high-dose NA can reduce plasma levels of Lp(a).[38] For this reason, NA has, potentially, the widest range of therapeutic activity.

Unfortunately, these beneficial effects are counteracted by serious side-effects, ranging from impaired glucose tolerance, to hyperuricemia and GI intolerance, gastritis, abnormal liver function tests, and the occasional development of severe toxic hepatitis. Subjectively, the administration of NA is accompanied by severe skin flushing and, occasionally, by nausea. Both possibly are related to an enhanced vascular release of prostacyclin. These side-effects have curtailed the use of nicotinic acid in warmer countries. In these, some NA derivatives, such as nicotinyl alcohol, niceritrol, or acipimox, have been marketed with some success. Apparently, however, the newer agents do not share the remarkable activity of the parent compound in all forms of hyperlipidemia.

The interest in NA has been maintained because of the positive results obtained in the Coronary Drug Project,[34] a trial that examined hypolipidemic drugs in the secondary prevention of CHD. In this study, NA was the only drug that reduced the recurrence of nonfatal myocardial infarction. Interestingly, nine years after discontinuing treatment, men who had taken nicotinic acid still experienced a significant reduction in coronary mortality compared with the placebo group.[39] In the FATS Study,[12] the best results in terms of coronary regression/inhibited progression were achieved with a NA-colestipol combination.

Nicotinic acid, when available, is usually prepared in tablets of 100 to 500 mg. Treatment should be started with low doses (100 mg once or twice daily), gradually reaching the effective dose. If NA is given concomitantly with a bile acid binding resin, daily doses of 3 g generally are adequate. Niceritrol (Liposolvin in some countries), acipimox (Olbetam), nicotinyl alcohol (Ronicol) and others are given in different doses (tablets of 250–500 mg) and do not usually require gradual dose adjustments.

Probucol

Probucol was first developed as a potent antioxidant compound about 30 years ago. Lipid lowering properties in animals have been described more recently.[40] Probucol has rather unusual properties, not shared by other lipid lowering agents; it is, in fact, carried mainly by lipoproteins (LDL) and, because of its lipophilicity, may persist for a long time in adipose tissue. Moreover, it can cause a marked reduction of HDL-cholesterol. This mechanism may prove crucial for the understanding of the drug's therapeutic activity. Probucol is chemically related to the potent antioxidant β-hydroxy-toluene (BHT) and has the structural formula in Figure 75.6.

Mechanism of Action of Probucol. Initial studies on probucol showed that this compound may affect cholesterol absorption and, by unknown mechanisms, increase the catabolism of LDL and decrease the synthesis of HDL apolipoproteins.[41] Other studies show that probucol, being incorporated into LDL, may affect their metabolic properties, i.e., improving receptor and nonreceptor clearance. For this reason, probucol may also be effective in patients with no available LDL receptors, such as homozygous Type II.

More recent studies have been focused in two directions. Because of the similarity with BHT, it has been suggested that a potent antioxidant activity in plasma may reduce LDL peroxidation, a major factor increasing atherogenicity.[42] This hypothesis has been confirmed by in vitro findings as well as by a study in a mutant rabbit strain lacking LDL receptors, where probucol reduced atherosclerosis without markedly affecting plasma lipids.[43]

Another hypothesis relates to the remarkable reduction in HDL-cholesterol after probucol. This reduction, paradoxically, occurs in the face of very evident decreases in the size of tendon xanthomas and xanthelasmas in treated patients.[44] Recent clinical data indicate that probucol may improve the function of the cholesteryl ester (CETP) system (Fig. 75.1), delivering cholesteryl esters from HDL to lower density lipoproteins.[45] The reduction of HDL is, in fact, accompanied by a similar increase of the transfer reaction, suggesting that this may be a major mode of action.[46] Recently, clinical findings have confirmed that probucol may improve vascular lesions at various sites.

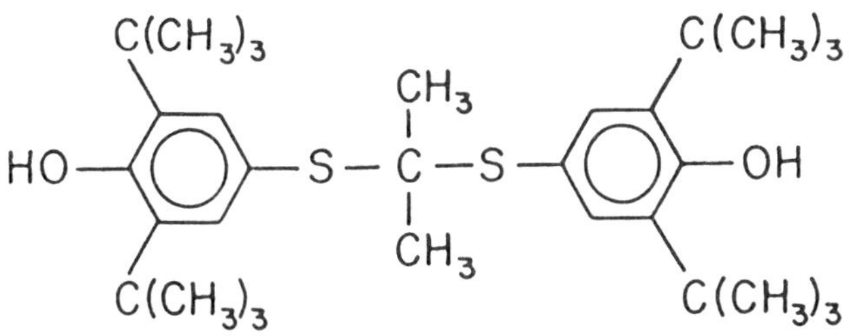

Figure 75.6 Chemical Structure of Probucol

Clinical Activity of Probucol. Probucol lowers LDL-cholesterol levels by 10 to 15 percent and HDL-cholesterol by 25 percent or more. The maximal effect on plasma cholesterol (LDL plus HDL) occurs after one to three months of treatment. Other effects (on triglycerides or VLDL) are minimal.

Adverse Effects and Interactions of Probucol. Subjectively, probucol is generally well tolerated. Abdominal side effects (diarrhea, flatulence, nausea) are transient and do not occur in more than 10 percent of patients. The safety of probucol has not been established for children or during pregnancy. Since probucol tends to remain in the body for prolonged periods, it is prudent to discontinue the drug at least six months before attempting pregnancy.

The only major described side-effect of probucol occurs in the cardiac conduction system. Probucol may cause arrhythmias in experimental animals, particularly when they are fed a cholesterol-rich diet. In patients, prolongation of Q-T electrocardiographic interval occasionally can occur, but reports of other arrhythmias or of syncope have been rare. Care should be taken in patients with EKG findings suggestive of ventricular irritability.

Absorption, Fate, and Excretion of Probucol. Probucol is absorbed to a limited extent into the general circulation (10% or less). This may have to do with the demonstrated activity on intestinal apolipoprotein biosynthesis. When, however, the drug is taken with food, peak plasma concentrations are definitely higher. Probucol may accumulate in adipose tissue, where it may persist for several months (up to six) after the last dose. A major pathway for elimination is via bile and feces. The persistence of the drug in body tissues does not lead to permanence of the hypocholesterolemic activity, which generally fades away within one month or so.

Preparations and Therapeutic Use of Probucol. Probucol (Lorelco, Lurselle, and other commercial names) is available in 250-mg or 500-mg tablets. The recommended dose is 500 mg twice daily, taken with meals. The general indications for the drug, besides the treatment of hypercholesterolemia (including the homozygous form), have now been expanded to patients with mild hypercholesterolemia associated with xanthomas or xanthelasmas. The drug is generally ineffective in hypertriglyceridemias.

HMG CoA Reductase Inhibitors

Inhibitors of hydroxymethylglutaryl coenzyme A reductase (HMG CoA reductase) constitute a novel class of lipid-lowering agents, with a very selective activity on cholesterol biosynthesis. These agents were initially extracted from the Penicillum species[47] and, later on, from Aspergillus and Monascus. The initial fungal derivative, compactin, markedly lowered cholesterol in normolipidemic and hyperlipidemic individuals. The original product did not undergo complete clinical development because of serious toxic effects in rodents.

Three new derivatives of compactin: lovastatin (previously mevinolin), simvastatin (previously synvinolin) and pravastatin (eptastatin) have undergone extensive clinical development in recent years; all are now available on the US market; lovastatin is not available in a number of European countries nor in Japan.

All semisynthetic HMG CoA reductase inhibitors have a chemical structure with a moiety resembling hydroxymethylglutaric acid (Fig. 75.7). Recently, a totally synthetic HMG CoA reduction inhibitor, flavastatin, has become available in the US and other markets. The HMG resembling moiety may be present in a closed (lactone) or in an open (hydroxyacid) form. The lactone ring is present in lovastatin and simvastatin, the open acid in pravastatin. Lactones are prodrugs, the open-ring hydroxyacids being the active compounds. Ring opening occurs at alkaline pH or in the liver.

Mechanism of Action of HMG CoA Reductase Inhibitors. Probably because of the structural similarity between these molecules and HMG, they have a unique profile of competitive, specific, and reversible inhibition of the HMG CoA reductase enzyme. Interestingly, their affinity for the enzyme (Ki = 10nM) is more than 1000-fold higher than the affinity of the natural substrate, HMG CoA (Km = 10μM). For this reason, even the apparently inactive metabolites of the three drugs (activities 10- 100-fold lower) may significantly contribute to the pharmacodynamic effect.

In vitro and in vivo, HMG CoA reductase inhibitors reduce sterol synthesis from ^{14}C-acetate at nM concentrations. In the cell, inhibition of reductase leads to two consequences:

(1) Marked increase of HMG CoA reductase with, however, no significant production of cholesterol.

(2) Increase of LDL receptors on the cell surface, draining LDL from the circulation, and providing the cell with the necessary cholesterol.

The major biochemical effect on the body economy is thus a dramatic reduction of circulating LDL-cholesterol. This occurs at drug concentrations requiring minimal daily dosages (generally from a minimum of 5 to a maximum of 80 mg/d).

The hypothesis that LDL receptor activity may be induced following treatment with reductase inhibitors has been shown clearly from both animal and human data, indicative of an increased rate of removal of labeled LDL after therapy.[48] The ineffectiveness of the raised production of HMG CoA reductase is supported by the observation of an unchanged total body synthe-

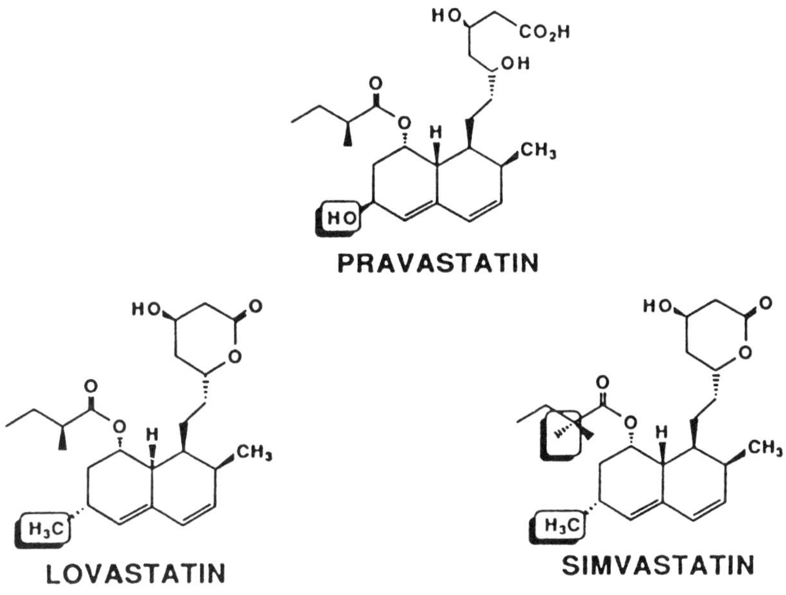

PRAVASTATIN

LOVASTATIN

SIMVASTATIN

Figure 75.7 Chemical structure of the major hydroxymethylglutaryl coenzyme A (HMG CoA) reductase inhibitors. The upper ring in all three molecules (chemically an analog of HMG) is in the open form in pravastatin (active *per se*) and in the closed lactone form in the other two compounds (which need ring opening for activation).

sis of cholesterol in treated patients. More recent studies suggest that, in addition to reducing cholesterol biosynthesis, HMG CoA reductase inhibitors may also somewhat reduce cholesterol absorption.

The selectivity in the mode of action is also confirmed by lipoprotein data in humans, indicating that, aside from a small increase of HDL-cholesterol, lipoprotein structure and composition is only moderately affected.[49] These findings allow one to conclude that the mode of action of HMG CoA reductase inhibitors in lowering plasma cholesterol is by reducing biosynthesis and, as a consequence, decreasing the number of circulating LDL particles.

Clinical Activity of HMG CoA Reductase Inhibitors. HMG CoA reductase inhibitors provide the most potent drug treatment for hypercholesterolemia up to now. In large clinical series of patients with Type II hyperlipoproteinemia (both II-A and II-B), total and LDL-cholesterol reductions were generally in the order of 25 to 30 and 30 to 40 percent, respectively. These results, at low daily doses, are generally very encouraging for the patients and are followed by excellent compliance. Other lipoprotein changes, as above indicated, are minimal. Triglyceride reduction seldom exceeds 20 percent and is mostly related to a decrease of triglycerides in the LDL fraction. Changes in HDL-cholesterol, although statistically significant in large series, are often unpredictable and not dose-related. Although it can be excluded that the mild microsomal enzyme inducing properties of these compounds are in play, the mechanism and clinical significance of HDL rises are difficult to evaluate. Possibly the rise of HDL may be only the consequence of improved removal of cholesterol from tissues.

Clinical and animal experience has suggested that the association of reductase inhibitors with other drugs may prove extremely effective in patients with severe hypercholesterolemia (e.g., familial heterozygous cases). The association with anion binding resins is among the most widely tested and achieves maximal effectiveness.[50] Plasma cholesterol and LDL reductions with this association may go up to 40 to 50 percent or more. This association was used in the previously described FATS Study.[12] A good activity has also been shown by associating probucol and also fibrates, in the case of Type II-B hyperlipoproteinemia. This last association, however, may carry considerable risk in terms of an increased incidence of myalgia.

Absorption, Fate, and Excretion of HMG CoA Reductase Inhibitors. Information on the kinetic behavior of the three reductase inhibitors is still incomplete, mostly because of the difficulty of direct measurements in plasma of the unchanged drugs or of major metabolites (e.g., lovastatin and simvastatin).[51] This is not the case with pravastatin, which remains more than 90 percent unchanged in plasma.

All reductase inhibitors are cleared quite rapidly, because of an efficient first pass metabolism at the liver or intestinal wall levels (the latter particularly for pravastatin).[52] While lovastatin and simvastatin need liver metabolism for activation (opening of the lactone ring), pravastatin is active per se. This last compound undergoes presystemic metabolism in the gut. Both lovastatin and simvastatin have four to six active metabolites, whereas only one such metabolite is known for pravastatin.

There is still question on the "selectivity" of action of the three agents in different tissues. Apparently, pravastatin's chemical and physical characteristics do result in a higher affinity for liver cells,[53,r9] and this may be associated with a reduced incidence of side-effects.

All three drugs have plasma elimination half-lives in the order of 1.4 to 1.9 hours, with complete disappearance of all the drug or of the active metabolites within 24 hours. All three are highly bound to plasma proteins, and the major elimination route is generally fecal.

Adverse Effects and Interactions of HMG CoA Reductase Inhibitors. Experience with lovastatin involving several thousands of patients treated for six years or longer does not show increased incidence of severe side-effects. Simvastatin and pravastatin studies are similar, but have a shorter follow-up. Theoretically, all reductase inhibitors should influence the refractory system of the eye to some extent because the lens, not having contact with the general circulation, is heavily dependent on local cholesterol biosynthesis. The development of cataracts in dogs with very high doses of both lovastatin and simvastatin has been described. Similar side-effects, in spite of intensive monitoring, have not been seen in patients.

In treated patients, a small incidence of liver (ALT, AST rises) and muscular (CPK rises) toxicities has been described with all inhibitors. Clinical myalgia occurs with higher frequency (5 percent or more) in patients concomitantly treated with lovastatin and a fibrate derivative.[54] Such side-effect definitely occurs more rarely with pravastatin.[55]

Both lovastatin and simvastatin seem to some extent to potentiate coumarin anticoagulants by an unknown mechanism. Simvastatin also increases steady-state digoxin levels in volunteer studies. Whereas caution needs to be applied in concomitant administration of lovastatin or simvastatin with warfarin, data on the digoxin interaction need further clarification.

At present, it is probably unwise to administer reductase inhibitors to patients over 65 years of age, with early lens opacities. Because of the critical role of HMG CoA reductase in embryogenesis, these compounds should not be given to pregnant women and should be withheld for several months before a planned pregnancy.

Preparations and Therapeutic Use of HMG Co A Reductase Inhibitors. Lovastatin (Mevacor) is commercially available in the US, Canada, and some European countries (20- and 40-mg tablets); the daily dose should not exceed 80 mg. Simvastatin and pravastatin are available in most countries (numerous commercial names). Simvastatin (Zocor, etc.) is available in tablets of 10 and 20 mg (maximal daily dose 40 mg), whereas pravastatin (Pravachol, Selectin, and others) is available in 10-, 20-, and 40-mg tablets (maximal dose, 80 mg).

The only clinical indication for these drugs is hypercholesterolemia, especially familial cases. Suggested drug combinations are with bile acid binding resins and possibly with probucol. None of the three agents is useful for the treatment of hypertriglyceridemia.

Other Drugs

Numerous other agents are available, in different countries, for the management of hyperlipoproteinemias. Most of these are absorbable and a few are of natural origin. Among the most widely used, the following may be listed:

β-sitosterol is a plant sterol, available in some countries (as Cytelline and others) for the treatment of hypercholesterolemia. It exerts a selective lowering of LDL-cholesterol at daily doses of 6 g or higher. It may occasionally induce nausea with mild laxative effects. β-sitosterol has generally been superseded by the newer anion exchange resins.

Metformin, a biguanide antidiabetic exerts a significant hypotriglyceridemic activity in nondiabetic patients.[56] The mechanism is linked to a reduced liver intestinal biosynthesis of VLDL and to stimulated activity of the glucose transporter mechanisms in peripheral cells.[57] Metformin (Glucophage and others) generally is used in daily doses of 1000 to 2550 mg. Although, in nondiabetic patients, the risk of lactic acidosis with this compound is negligible, care should be taken in the management of elderly people.

Tiadenol is a substituted decane affecting both cholesterol and triglyceride levels in different forms of hyperlipoproteinemia.[58] The mechanism is probably linked to an increased lipoprotein catabolism, as in the case of fibrates, but, in addition, the drug apparently reduces liver lipoprotein secretion. Although short-term trials have clearly indicated a potent activity of tiadenol in numerous patient series, long-term results are less satisfactory. Recent animal data indicate that chronic administration may lead to the activation of the liver microsomal enzyme system, thus lowering activity.[59] Tiadenol is otherwise generally well tolerated and cautionary notes are similar to those of fibric acids. Tiadenol is available in 800-mg tablets (Fonlipol and others) to be taken tid.

Pantethine is the disulfide dimer of pantetheine, the amide conjugate of pantothenic acid with cysteamine. Pantethine, in numerous clinical trials, has been shown to reduce significantly, although not markedly, serum total (10–12%) and LDL-cholesterol (12–15%) levels; some activity is also exerted in hypertriglyceridemias.[60] The mechanism of pantethine is rather unique, being linked to a reduced activation of HMG CoA reductase in the presence of high concentrations of cholesterol precursors.[61] Pantethine is well tolerated, and reported side-effects are minimal. It is available in 250- or 500-mg tablets for total daily doses of 750 to 1000 mg.

References

Research Reports

1. Fredrickson DS, Levy RI, Lees RS. Fat transport in lipoproteins: an integrated approach to mechanisms and disorders. N Engl J Med 1967;*276*:37–44, 94–103, 148–156, 215–226, 273–281.

2. WHO-Classification of hyperlipidaemias and hyperlipoproteinaemias. Bull Wld Hlth Org 1970;*43*:891–915.

3. Eisenberg S. Dyslipoproteinaemia and atherosclerosis. In: Olsson A (ed) Atherosclerosis—Biology and clinical science. Edinburgh; Churchill Livingstone, (1987); pp 275–280.

4. McLean JW, Tomlinson JE, Kuang W-J, Eaton DL, Chen EU, Fless GM, Scana AM, Lawn RM. cDNA sequence of human apolipoprotein(a) is homologous to plasminogen. Nature 1987;*330*:132–137.

5. Scanu AM, Lawn RM, Berg K. Lipoprotein(a) and atherosclerosis. Ann Int Med 1991;*115*:209–218.

6. Anitschkow NN, Chalatow S. Über experimentelle Cholesterinsteatose und ihre Bedeutung für die Entstehung einiger pathologischen Prozesse. Zentbl Allg Pathol Pathol Anat 1913;*24*:1–19.

7. Ignatowski A. Über die Wirkung des tierischen Eiweisses auf die Aorta und die parenchymatösen Organen der Kaninchen. Wirchows Arch Pathol Anat Physiol Klin Med 1909;*198*:248–270.

8. Lipid Research Clinics Coronary Primary Prevention Trial Results. I and II. JAMA 1984;*252*:351–374.

9. Frick MH, Elo O, Haapa K, Heinonen OP, Heinsalmi P, Helo P, Huttunen JK, Kaitaniemi P, Koskinen P, Manninen V, Mäenpää H, Mälkönen M, Mänttäri M, Norola S, Pasternack A, P.K. Pikkarainen J, Romo M, Sjöblom UF, Nikkilä E.A. Helsinki Heart Study: Primary-prevention trial with gemfibrozil in middle-aged patients with dyslipidemia. N Engl J Med 1987;*317*:1237–1245.

10. Blankenhorn DH, Kramsch DM. Reversal of atherosis and sclerosis. Circulation 1989;*79*:1–7.

11. Blankenhorn DH, Nessin SA, Johnson RL, Sanmarco ME, Azen SP, Cashin-Hemphill L. Beneficial effects of combined colestipol/niacin therapy on coronary atherosclerosis and coronary venous bypass grafts. JAMA 1987;*257*:3233–3240.

12. Brown G, Albers JJ, Fisher LD, Shaefer SM, Lin J-T, Kaplan C, Zhao K-Q, Bisson BD, Fitzpatrick UF, Dodge HT. Regression of coronary artery disease as a result of intensive lipid-lowering therapy in men with high levels of apolipoprotein B. N Engl J Med 1990;*323*:1289–1298.

13. Tatami R, Inoue N, Itoh H, Kishino B, Koga N, Nakashima H, Nishide T, Okamura K, Saito U, Teramoto T. Regression of coronary atherosclerosis by combined LDL-apheresis and lipid-lowering drug therapy in patients with familial hypercholesterolemia: a multicenter study. Atherosclerosis 1992;*95*:1–13.

14. Study Group, European Atherosclerosis Society. Strategies for the prevention of coronary heart disease: A policy statement of the European Atherosclerosis Society. Eur Heart J 1987;*8*:77–88.

15. Study Group, European Atherosclerosis Society. The recognition and management of hyperlipidaemia in adults: A policy statement of the European Atherosclerosis Society. Eur Heart J 1988;*9*:571–600.

16. EAS: Prevention of coronary heart disease: Scientific background and new clinical guidelines. NMCD 1992;*2*:113–156.

17. Report of the Expert Panel on: Detection, Evaluation and Treatment of High Blood Cholesterol in Adults, NIH Publ No 88-2925, 1988.

18. NIH Consensus Conference: Triglyceride, high-density lipoprotein, and coronary heart disease. JAMA 1993;*269*:505–510.

19. Anderson JT, Grande F, Keys A. Independence of the effects of cholesterol and degree of saturation of the fat in the diet on serum cholesterol in man. Am J Clin Nutr 1985;*29*:1184–1189.

20. Sirtori CR, Agradi E, Conti F, Gatti E, Mantero O. Soybean protein diet in the treatment of type II hyperlipoproteinaemia. Lancet 1977;*i*:275–277.

21. Kuo PT, Hayase K, Kostis JB, Moreyra AE. Use of combined diet and colestipol in long term (7–7½ years) treatment of patients with type II hyperlipoproteinemia. Circulation 1979;*59*:199–211.

22. Shepherd J, Packard CJ, Bicker S, Lawrie TDV, Morgan HG. Cholestyramine promotes receptor mediated LDL catabolism. N Engl J Med 1980;*302*:1219–1222.

23. Levy RI, Brensike JF, Epstein SE, Kelsey SF, Passamani ER, Richardson JM, Loh IK, Stone NJ, Aldrich RF, Battaglini JW, Moriarity DJ, Fisher ML, Friedman L, Friedwald W, Detre KM. The influence of changes in lipid values induced by cholestyramine and diet on progression of coronary artery disease: Results of the NHLBI Type II Coronary Intervention Study. Circulation 1984;*69*:325–327.

24. Sedaghat A, Samuel P, Crouse JR, Ahrens EH Jr. Effects of neomycin on absorption, synthesis and/or flux of cholesterol in man. J Clin Invest 1985;*55*:12–21.

25. Gurakar A, Hoeg JM, Kostner G, Papadoupulos NM, Brewer HB Jr. Levels of lipoprotein(a) decline with neomycin and niacin treatment. Atherosclerosis 1985;*57*:293–301.

26. Issemann I, Green S. Activation of a member of the steroid hormone receptor superfamily by peroxisome proliferators. Nature 1990;*347*:645–650.

27. Intrasuksri U, Feller DR. Comparison of the effects of selected monocarboxylic dicarboxylic and perfluorinated fatty acids on peroxisome proliferation in primary cultured rat hepatocytes. Biochem Pharmacol 1991;*42*:184–188.

28. Boberg J, Boberg M, Gross R, Grundy S, Augustin J, Brown VW. The effect of treatment with clofibrate on hepatic triglyceride and lipoprotein lipase activities of post-heparin plasma in male patients with hyperlipoproteinemia. Atherosclerosis 1977;*27*:499–503.

29. Wilson DE, Lees RS. Metabolic relationships among the plasma lipoproteins—Reciprocal changes in the concentrations of very low and low density lipoproteins in man. J Clin Invest 1972;*51*:1051–1057.

30. Pichardo R, Boulet L, Davignon J. Pharmacokinetics of clofibrate in familial hypercholesterolemia. Atherosclerosis 1977;*26*:573–582.

31. Kleinman Y, Oschry Y, Eisenberg S. Abnormal regulation of LDL receptor activity and abnormal cellular metabolism of hypertriglyceridaemic low density lipoprotein: normalization with bezafibrate therapy. J Clin Invest 1987;*17*:538–543.

32. Niort G, Bulgarelli A, Cassader M, Pagano G. Effect of short term treatment with bezafibrate on plasma fibrinogen, fibrinopeptide A, platelet activation and blood filterability in atherosclerotic hyperfibrinogenemic patients. Atherosclerosis 1988;*71*:113–119.

33. Andersen P, Smith P, Seljeflot I, Brataker S, Arnesen H. Effects of gemfibrozil on lipids and haemostasis after myocardial infarction. Thromb Haemost 1990;*63*:174–177.

34. Stamler J, et al. Clofibrate and niacin in coronary heart disease. The Coronary Drug Project Research Group. JAMA 1975;*231*:360–381.

35. Committee of the Principal Investigators. A cooperative trial in the primary preventive of ischaemic heart disease using clofibrate. Brit Heart J 1978;*40*:1069–1108.

36. Sirtori CR. Mechanism of action of absorbable hypolipidemic agents. In: Kritchevsky D, Holmes WL, Paoletti R: Drugs affecting lipid metabolism. New York Plenum Press, 1983; pp 241–252.

37. Carlson LA, Örö L. Effect of treatment with nicotinic acid for one month on serum lipids in patients with different types of hyperlipoproteinemia. Atherosclerosis 1973;*18*:1–9.

38. Carlson LA, Hamsten A, Asplund A. Pronounced lowering of serum levels of lipoprotein Lp(a) in hyperlipidaemic subjects treated with nicotinic acid. J Int Med 1989;*226*:271–276.

39. Canner PL, Berge KG, Wenger NK, Stamler J, Friedman L, Prinecs RJ, Friedewald W. Fifteen year mortality in Coronary Drug Project patients: Long-term benefit with niacin. JACC 1986;*8*:1245–1255.

40. Drake JW, Bradford RH, McDearmon M, Furman RH. The effect of [4,4(isopropylidenedithio) bis (2,6-di-t-butylphenol)] (DH-581) on serum lipids and lipoproteins in human subjects. Metabolism 1969;*18*:916–925.

41. Atmeh RF, Stewart JM, Boag DE, Packard CJ, Lorimer AR, Shepherd J. The hypolipidemic action of probucol: a study of its effects on high and low density lipoproteins. J Lipid Res 1983;*24*:588–595.

42. Partasarathy S, Young SG, Witztum JL, Pittman RC, Steinberg D. Probucol inhibits oxidative modification of low density lipoprotein. J Clin Invest 1986;*77*:641–644.

43. Kita T, Nakano Y, Yokoda M, Ishi K, Kume N, Ooshima A, Yoshida H, Kawai C. Probucol prevents the progression of atherosclerosis in Watanabe heritable hyperlipidemic rabbit, an animal model for familial hypercholesterolemia. Proc Natl Acad Sci USA 1987;*85*:5928–5931.

44. Yamamoto A, Matsuzawa Y, Yokoyama S, Funahashi T, Yamamura T, Kishino B. Effects of probucol on xanthomata regression in familial hypercholesterolemia. Am J Cardiol 1986;*57*:29S–35S.

45. Franceschini G, Sirtori M, Vaccarino V, Gianfranceschi G, Rezzonico L, Chiesa G, Sirtori CR. Mechanism of HDL reduction after probucol—Changes in HDL subfractions and increased reverse cholesteryl ester transfer. Arteriosclerosis 1989;*9*:462–469.

46. Chiesa G, Michelagnoli S, Cassinotti M, Gianfranceschi G, Werba JP, Pazzucconi F, Sirtori CR, Franceschini G. Mechanisms of HDL reduction after probucol. Changes in plasma cholesterol esterification/transfer and lipase activities. Metabolism 1993;*42*:229–235.

47. Endo A, Kuroda M, Tanzawa K. Competitive inhibition of 3-hydroxy-3-methylglutaryl coenzyme A reductase by ML-236A and ML-236B, fungal metabolites having hypocholesterolemic activity. FEBS Lett 1976;*72*:323–326.

48. Bilheimer DW, Grundy SM, Brown MD, Goldstein JL. Mevinolin and colestipol stimulate receptor-mediated clearance of low density lipoprotein. Proc Natl Acad Sci USA 1983;*80*:4124–4128.

49. Franceschini G, Sirtori M, Vaccarino V, Gianfranceschi G, Chiesa G, Sirtori CR. Plasma lipoprotein changes following treatment with pravastatin and gemfibrozil in patients with familial hypercholesterolemia. J Lab Clin Med 1989;*114*:250–259.

50. Vega GS, Grundy SM. Treatment of primary moderate hypercholesterolemia with lovastatin (mevinolin) and colestipol. JAMA 1987;*257*:33–38.

51. Pentikainen PJ, Saraheim M, Schwartz JI, Amin RD, Schwartz MS, Brunner-Ferber F, Rogers JD. Comparative pharmacokinetics of lovastatin, simvastatin and pravastatin in humans. J Clin Pharmacol 1992;*32*:136–140.

52. Pan HY, De Vault AR, Swites BJ, Whigan D, Ivashlav E, Willard DA, Brescia D. Pharmacokinetics and pharmacodynamics of pravastatin alone and with cholestyramine in hypercholesterolemia. Clin Pharmacol Ther 1990;*48*:201–207.

53. Koga T, Shimada Y, Kuroda M, Tsujita Y, Hasegawa K, Yamazaki M. Tissue-selective inhibition of sterol synthesis in vivo by pravastatin sodium, a 3-hydroxy-3-methylglutaryl coenzyme A reductase inhibitor. Biochim Biophys Acta 1990;*1045*:115–120.

54. Pierce LR, Wysowski DK, Gross TP. Myopathy and rhabdomyolysis associated with lovastatin-gemfibrozil combination theraphy. JAMA 1990;*265*:71–78.

55. Schalke BB, Schmidt B, Toyka K, Hartung H-P. Pravastatin associated inflammatory myopathy. N Engl J Med 1992;*327*:649–650.

56. Sirtori CR, Tremoli E, Conti F, Paoletti R. Treatment of hypertriglyceridemia with metformin: effectiveness and analysis of results. Atherosclerosis 1977;*26*:583–591.

57. Hundhal HS, Ramlal T, Reyes R, Leiter LA, Klip A. Cellular mechanism of metformin action involves glucose transporter translocation from an intracellular to the plasma membrane in L6 muscle cells. Endocrinology 1992;*131*:1165–1173.

58. Sirtori M, Montanari G, Gianfranceschi G. Clofibrate and tiadenol treatment in hyperlipoproteinemias. A comparative trial of drugs affecting lipoprotein catabolism and biosynthesis. Atherosclerosis 1983;*49*:149–161.

59. Maffei Facino R, Carini M, Tofanetti O. Metabolism of the hypolipidemic agent tiadenol in man and in the rat. Arzneimittelforsch/Drug Res 1986;*36*:722–728.

60. Gaddi A, Descovich GC, Noseda G Fragiacomo C, Colombo L, Craveri A, Montanari G, Sirtori CR. Controlled evaluation of pantethine, a natural hypolipidemic compound, in patients with different forms of hyperlipoproteinemia. Atherosclerosis 1984;*50*:73–83.

61. Cighetti G, Del Puppo M, Paroni R, Galli Kienle M. Modulation of HMG CoA reductase activity by pantetheine/pantethine. Biochim Biophys Acta 1988;*963*:389–393.

Reviews

r1. Assman G. Lipid metabolism and atherosclerosis. Stuttgart: Schattauer, 1982.
Overview on the relationship between lipid/lipoprotein changes in arterial disease, with special emphasis on epidemiology and lipoprotein structure.

r2. Classification of hyperlipidemias and hyperlipoproteinemias. Bull Wld Hlth Org 1970;*43*:891–915.
Updated classification (dividing Type II hyperproteinemias into Type II-a and II-b), of current use in the management of clinical lipoprotein disorders.

r3. Durrington PN. Hyperlipidaemia: Diagnosis and management. London: Butterworth, 1989.
Recent textbook, with excellent overview of the clinical aspects of lipoprotein disorders and novel approaches to treament.

r4. Eisenberg S. High density lipoprotein metabolism. J Lipid Res 1984;*25*:1017–1059.
Careful description of the metabolism of high density lipoproteins, with an evaluation of their role in protection vs arterial disease.

r5. Fredrickson DS, Levy RI, Lees RS. Fat transport in lipoproteins—An integrated approach to mechanisms and disorders. N Engl J Med 1967;*276*:32–44, 94–103, 148–156, 215–226, 273–281.
"Classical" overview of lipid disorders, with introduction of the concept of "hyperlipoproteinemia".

r6. Goldstein JL, Brown MS. The low density lipoprotein pathway and its relation to atherosclerosis. Annu Rev Biochem 1977;*46*:897–930.
A detailed summary of the original findings pointing to a specific receptor disorder in type II hyperlipoproteinemia.

r7. Miller NE, Miller GJ. Clinical and metabolic aspects of high density lipoproteins. Amsterdam: Elsevier, 1984.
Multi-authored textbook examining HDL structure, composition, including an in-depth analysis of the possible dietary and pharmacological influences on the HDL system.

r8. Scriver CR, Beaudet AL, Sly WS, Valle D. The metabolic basis of inherited disease, 6th Ed. New York: McGraw-Hill 1989.
Classic textbook on metabolic disorders. Numerous chapters deal with lipid/lipoprotein metabolism, particularly Part 7, providing an update on the metabolic bases on hyper- and dys-lipoproteinemias.

r9. Sirtori C. Tissue selectivity of hydroxymethylglutaryl coenzyme A (HMG CoA) reductase inhibitors. Pharmacol Ther 1993;60:431–459.
A detailed review article pointing out the potential advantages of tissue selectivity of HMG CoA reductase inhibitors.

SECTION X

Pharmacology of Skin

Section Editors:
Ronald Marks
Richard J. Motley

Associate Editor:
Andrew Y. Finlay

CHAPTER 76

Structure and Function of the Skin; Percutaneous Penetration

Ronald Marks

Skin is a complex layered composite of several tissues that function cooperatively to support and protect the deeper body structures. It is important to bear in mind the particular qualities and characteristics of skin when considering the action of drugs on the skin. This is especially the case with topical preparations because the drug has to be released from the vehicle in which it is formulated and then must penetrate into the part of the skin where its action is required.

The Stratum Corneum and Percutaneous Penetration

The stratum corneum is the outer horny structure composed of flattened horn cells tightly bonded together by interdigitations and an intercellular cement material that derive from the epidermis beneath. Its primary function is that of a protective barrier. It impedes the evaporation of water from the tissues beneath it and acts as a barrier to water and foreign substances with which the skin comes in contact. In most trunk and limb sites the stratum corneum is approximately 15 to 20 cell layers thick (15–20 μ), but is much thicker over the palms and soles (approximately 500 μ).

The stratum corneum is also the prime barrier to the penetration of substances into the skin from topical applications. Many factors govern the rate at which drugs penetrate the skin from topical applications. These include:

(a) The size of the molecule. Substances over molecular weight 500 penetrate the skin very slowly and with difficulty.

(b) The lipophilicity of the molecule. In general, the more lipophilic the molecule, the easier it is for it to cross the stratum corneum barrier.

(c) The physical format of the formulation containing the molecule. Substances in a solution of some sort penetrate more easily than from solid formulations.

(d) The presence of certain substances, when added to the preparation containing the molecule that is intended to cross the skin, will accelerate the penetration process. These molecules, known as "penetration enhancers," include such organic solvents as dimethyl sulfoxide and sundry other compounds, including urea, salicylic acid, and Azone.

(e) The state and site of the stratum corneum under consideration. Disordered stratum corneum such as occurs in psoriasis, the eczematous disorders, or congenital disorders of keratinization (e.g., the ichthyoses) is an inefficient barrier. There is a much increased rate of transepidermal water loss, and the rate of penetration of topically applied drugs through this abnormal horny layer is similarly much increased.

The rate of percutaneous penetration varies according to the anatomic site under consideration. Penetration from sites where the stratum corneum is especially thin and from moist flexural areas is greater than from skin with thick stratum corneum and extensor sites. Percutaneous penetration is notoriously rapid from the genitalia, the eyelids, and the retroauricular zone. Moist stratum corneum is a much less efficient barrier to penetration. Occlusion of the skin surface with plastic film—or for that matter a greasy ointment—by increasing the water content of the horny layer will enhance the rate of penetration manyfold.

Desquamation, Keratinization, Scaling, and Hyperkeratosis

Normally, single horn cells (corneocytes) lose contact with the corneocytes below and around about and drop off from the surface of the skin in a controlled manner. This process of desquamation is disturbed in many skin diseases, resulting in a failure of the corneocytes to separate properly, so that they fall off in clumps or aggregates. This results in visible scaling. If the process is even more disturbed, the corneocytes just stay stuck together and pile up in horny, hyperkeratotic masses.

Desquamation is the ultimate step in the process of epidermal differentiation or keratinization. During keratinization epidermal cells change in shape from ovoid or cuboidal through a number of steps to thin, flat, five-sided, shield-like structures as the basal cells ascend and ultimately reach the surface of the stratum corneum. The change in shape is accompanied by other structural alterations, including the loss of the nucleus and cytoplasmic organelles and thickening of the cell wall by the laying down of a protein band just inside the plasma membrane.

There is a complex intercellular substance, containing ceramides and glycoproteins, between the tough flattened corneocytes. It appears to be important both in the permeability function of the stratum corneum and in the process of desquamation. This intercellular material derives from minute organelles (lamellar bodies) in the granular cell layer of the epidermis.

The granular cell layer is so-called because these cells contain irregular basophilic granules that carry the precursor of a histidine-rich protein (filaggrin) responsible for the aggregation of keratin polypeptide tonofilaments into oriented bundles within the keratinocytes. The granular layer differs from the rest of the epidermis in that there are associated strong hydrolytic enzyme activity and transglutaminase activities. The first enzymes are needed to remove the epidermal cellular organelles; the transglutaminase cross-links the protein band that forms just within the plasma membrane, so that it contains tough cross-linked protein species (involucrin, loricrin, and keratolinin).

From the above it can be seen that epidermal differentiation is a complex and orderly affair and that there are many opportunities for abnormalities to wreck the process and result in scaling and/or hyperkeratosis. This can occur in both the genetically determined disorders of keratinization, such as the ichthyoses, and in the acquired inflammatory dermatoses. Treatments for the primary disorders of keratinization are unsatisfactory, probably because much of the detailed biochemistry has only recently been elucidated. Pharmacologic ways of manipulating the process, such as the retinoids and vitamin D analogues, are only just becoming available.

Epidermal Cell Production

Epidermal cells are produced in the basal layer of the epidermis and then ascend upward through the malpighian layer (also known as the prickle cell layer) and into the granular cell layer, where maturation into corneocytes starts to take place. The corneocytes formed ascend to the surface of the stratum corneum where they desquamate (see above). The normal thickness of the epidermis of the trunk and limbs is approximately 35 μ, so that with the 15-μ thickness of the stratum corneum the basal epidermal cell has to travel in total some 50 μ before it sees the light of day. This journey takes some 28 days, 14 days each in the epidermis and stratum corneum.

In psoriasis and in inflammatory diseases in which the epidermis becomes involved, there is accelerated epidermal cell production and usually epidermal hypertrophy as well. Thus, the usual epidermal thickness of three to five cells is increased to perhaps 20 to 25 cells. Despite this thickening there is a greatly accelerated rate of travel, so that in psoriasis it may take only four or five days before an epidermal cell produced at the basal layer is shed in scale from the surface. The decreased time that the epidermal cells spend within the epidermis means that there is less time for keratinization, so that the epidermal nuclei are retained in the abnormal scale that forms (parakeratosis). Many of the drugs used in psoriasis and in chronic eczema damp down the increased rate of epidermal cell division and slow down this process.

The Dermoepidermal Junction

The dermoepidermal junction is a quite complex structure that has only recently been characterized structurally and biochemically. Histologically a homogeneous pink-purple band is seen subepidermally when stained with periodic acid Schiff reagent, but this does not seem to identify a particular structure electron microscopically or represent any one substance or particular functional unit. Ultrastructurally, the epidermal cells can be seen to be attached by thin anchoring filaments (containing collagen VII) to an electron dense membrane—the lamina densa part of the basal lamina, consisting of Type IV collagen. Between the lamina densa and the keratinocytes there is an electron lucent zone known as the lamina lucida, containing among other things, the proteins laminin and nidogen.

The dermoepidermal junction is of great importance functionally, helping ensure that the skin behaves as an integrated, mechanically intact unit. Separation between the epidermis and dermis occurs in a number of blistering disorders, so that this site has particular pathophysiologic importance for the dermatologist.

The Dermis

The dermis consists of fibrous elements with amorphous ground substance between the fibers in addition to the fibroblasts that produce all these proteinaceous components. Blood vessels,

Table 76.1 Composition of Structurally Distinct Collagens

Collagen Type	Chain Composition	Tissue Distribution
I	α1 I, α1 I, α2	Skin, bone, tendon, ligament, fascia, arteries, uterus
II	α1 II, α1 II, α1 II	Hyaline cartilage
III	α1 III, α1 III, α1 III	Skin, arteries, uterus
IV	α1 IV, α1 IV, α1 IV	Basement membranes

lymphatics, and nerves course through the dermal structure; and the epidermally-derived appendageal structures that are really invaginations of the surface epidermis also sit amidst the acellular dermal components. The collagen fibers are composed of three peptide chains wrapped around each other as a triple helix. The peptide chains are of three types, and each of the different types of collagen has a specific composition of these chains (see Table 76.1).

Elastic fibers are arranged in a curious net immediately subepidermally as well as being irregularly wound around the collagen fibers. These structures consist of microfibrils set in an amorphous component.

The dermis functions as a protective and enveloping structure that, because of its mechanical qualities, permits body parts to move effectively. The bulk of the mechanical properties of the skin are in fact due to the dermal collagen. The bundles of collagen have a particular spatial orientation that determines the in vivo tissue tensions and the way the skin responds to a mechanical stimulus.

References

Reviews

r1. Scott RC, Guy RH, Hadgraft J. Prediction of percutaneous penetration, methods, measurements, modelling. London, IBC Technical Services Ltd., 1990.

r2. Shaw JE, Prevo M, Gale R, Yum S. Percutaneous absorption. In: Goldsmith LA, ed. Physiology, biochemistry and molecular biology of the skin, 2d ed. Oxford, Oxford University Press, 1991; pp 1447–1479.

r3. Odland GF. Structure of the skin. In: Goldsmith LA, ed. Physiology, biochemistry and molecular biology of the skin, 2d ed. Oxford, Oxford University Press, 1991; pp 3–62.

CHAPTER 77

Special Features Concerning Treatment for Skin Diseases

Andrew Y. Finlay

Introduction

The skin is said to be the largest organ in the body; its unique configuration and positioning at the interface between the outside world and the internal organs provides both special opportunities and challenges in the effective delivering of drugs. Opportunities arise from the skin's unique accessibility, which offers the chance to treat specifically, in high concentrations, the affected areas of this "spread out" organ. Difficulties arise from the skin's main barrier function: in protecting the body from penetration by outside chemicals, beneficial drugs also may be kept from reaching their target.

Although most patients with skin disease are treated with topical agents applied directly to the affected area, many other approaches to therapy are used in dermatology. Systemic drugs are used for systemic disorders in which the skin is also affected, and for their convenience of delivering the drug to all areas of the skin. Surgery is widely used to manage skin tumors, and various destructive techniques such as cryotherapy, radiotherapy, and laser therapy have specific purposes. More sophisticated combinations of therapy have been developed; PUVA is a good example (see Chapter 83), where the effect of a combined systemic (psoralens) and external (ultraviolet "A" radiation) therapy is localized to the skin by its being the only site where the two halves of the therapy are combined.

Topical Therapy

Introduction

To understand the complexities of topical therapy one must consider the variations in properties of the skin with age, site, hydration, and blood supply. Specialized structures such as hair or nails have their own additional problems of drug delivery. The disease process on the skin and its appendages will itself alter the way topical preparations can be delivered and will affect the absorption of the drug once it is applied to the surface.

Topical drugs can be formulated in a wide variety of ways, including creams, ointments, lotions, or gels. Once applied, the use of dressings or occlusion will further influence the effectiveness of therapy.

Guidance must be given to both prescriber and patient concerning how much topical application should be used, and some simple rules are given later in this chapter.

The Modulating Influence of Age

An important consideration in young children is that the ratio of body volume to skin surface area is lower than in adults, and so the potential for side-effects from systemic absorption are likely to be greater. This should be remembered when treating large areas of skin with salicylic acid preparations, as may be indicated, for example, in congenital disorders of keratinization. The same is true for topical steroids, which, if used over wide areas of skin in atopic eczema for an extended period, can more easily result in systemic effects in infants than in adults. The use of lindane in scabies, which is potentially neurotoxic, is also more hazardous in infancy.

In the elderly, the stratum corneum may be, surprisingly, a slightly more effective barrier, although the differences, compared to a younger adult, are only marginal and of no great clinical significance. What is of practical importance is the major difficulty that very elderly people may have in correctly applying topical agents. It is not easy for the elderly and infirm to apply therapy to the back or the scalp. This age group may also have difficulties in hearing, understanding, or remembering detailed instructions. The economic constraints and social constrictions of the retired older members of the community also make following dietary advice or special washing and bathing instructions very difficult to follow.[r1]

Site Considerations

There are wide skin variations in the anatomy of different body sites that should influence topical therapy decisions; the effectiveness of the same drug applied to the groin or to the palm may be very different.

In flexural areas, two skin surfaces frequently are either closely opposed or actually in contact with each other. Normally there is a slow movement of water across the stratum corneum, but when the overlying air becomes fully saturated with water, as in a flexure, the water content of the stratum corneum increases and it becomes swollen and less efficient as a barrier. Its barrier function for other chemicals then also becomes compromised. Topically applied drugs in this area must be creams, not ointments; ointments do not stick so easily to a moist area, and aggravate the tendency for the stratum corneum to become overhydrated. Any drug applied will be much more easily absorbed from these hydrated flexural sites. This, on the one hand, may increase efficacy, but on the other also increases the risk of an irritant reaction. A practical example of this is the irritant effect of anthralin, which is much greater in a flexural area than on an open area of body or limb. The enhanced penetration that occurs when hydration reduces the stratum corneum's barrier function is used therapeutically in the techniques of occlusion or frequent wet dressings.[r2]

Where the stratum corneum is very thick—as it is on the palms and soles—topical drugs have a much harder job crossing into the underlying epidermis. This is a situation where a very inflamed area from which the normal stratum corneum has largely been lost is markedly easier to treat topically. Where topical preparations are available in a range of concentrations or potencies, a high concentration should be used for the palms and soles.

Some considerations are specific to the face. Facial skin has tremendous importance to its owner with regard to communication and self-esteem. Its obvious visibility dictates that topical applications that stain or that are cosmetically unacceptable simply will not be used. A second consideration is the skin around the eyes: potentially irritating preparations easily may be smeared or rubbed into the eyes, causing chemical conjunctivitis. Some caution also should be exercised when applying topical treatments to the lips; ingestion of the treatment can result in unwanted systemic effects.

Most areas of the skin are readily accessible whatever application is chosen; the scalp and other hair-bearing areas are more difficult because, short of shaving the patient, the hair interferes with easy application and removal of drugs. Ointment-based preparations are therefore very difficult to use.

Effectively treating hair and nails requires a different approach. If there is an infection of hair shaft or nail plate, the drug must penetrate the site of infection, but many abnormalities are caused by a disease process that alters initial production of the hair or nail. The hair bulb and nail matrix are relatively protected, and systemic therapy often is more effective in reaching these sites.

Stratum Corneum Integrity and Cutaneous Blood Supply

Although the stratum corneum acts as a very effective barrier, this barrier function usually is severely compromised in inflammatory conditions of the epidermis. Although this is one of the most important adverse physiologic effects of skin disease, conversely it can provide an important therapeutic aid. Where the integrity of the stratum corneum is disturbed, topically applied drugs penetrate much more easily, and so there is a natural enhancement of the effect of the "natural" topical drug that often is applied to a wider area than necessary. As the epidermis heals and the stratum corneum returns to normal, this window of enhanced penetration for the topical drug closes. There would be some logic, therefore, in using a mild or low concentration of a topical drug in the acute inflammatory phase, and increasing the drug concentration as healing progresses. In practice many dermatologists use different drug concentrations in the reverse order.

The effects of stratum corneum hydration by occlusion on drug penetration of skin already has been mentioned.

Some areas of the skin, such as the face and scalp, have a particularly good blood supply. It might be expected therefore that topical drugs applied to these areas, once they had penetrated the epidermis, would be rapidly taken up by the systemic circulation. This consideration usually is of little practical importance, but becomes potentially a matter of life and death in the occasional patient with total body skin inflammation. In erythrodermic psoriasis or eczema, for example, the combination of "porous" stratum corneum and an increase in blood supply to the skin equalling up to 30 percent of the cardiac output results in a capability of massive systemic absorption of any drug applied widely and frequently to the skin. If, for example, salicylic acid is applied frequently under these circumstances, enough can be absorbed to result in severe toxic effects or even death.

Reservoir Effect and Frequency of Application

As a drug moves through a barrier, such as the stratum corneum, a concentration gradient of drug builds, with a high concentration on the outer surface and a lower concentration deeper down. The dermis and epidermis beneath act as a "sink"—with the dermal blood supply acting as the open "plughole." When there is no further topical preparation on the surface either because excess has been rubbed off or because it has been entirely absorbed, significant amounts of the drug remain in high concentration in the outer layers of stratum corneum. This persisting bulk of drug acts as a "reservoir" (perversely within the wall of the dam!), from which the drug continues to be slowly released. Occlusion at this stage may enhance this release process. The duration of effect of topical drugs therefore is not simply switched on and off by applying or wiping off a drug, but is "smoothed out" by the reservoir effect.

When considering how frequently topical therapy is needed, and how long the agent needs to be on the skin surface before the excess is removed, both the reservoir effect and the differential barrier function of normal and abnormal stratum corneum must be considered. The concept of short-contact therapy has been popularized for the use of anthralin in psoriasis, but also is applicable to other drugs and other skin disease. The concept of short-contact therapy is based on the supposition that a sufficiently large amount will be absorbed in a short time (half an hour) through the affected skin where barrier function is poor. The surrounding normal skin is relatively protected from the irritant effect of the anthralin by the normal adjacent stratum corneum barrier function.

The traditional timing of topical applications often is based on habit and convenience rather than on sound pharmacokinetic principles; this area is, however, being examined more critically in the clinical research of several new topical applications. For example, it has been demonstrated that once-daily application of some topical corticosteroids (e.g., methyl prednisolone aceponate) is as effective as twice-daily application. The same is true for the antifungal agent econazole—once-daily usage is enough.[1,2]

Different Types of Topical Application to the Skin

Most active drugs are applied to the skin in apparently low concentrations, such as 0.1 to 1 percent. There are exceptions of course—e.g., azelaic acid for acne is used in a concentration of 20 percent. The remaining 99 percent, the vehicle, takes a variety of different forms, ointment, cream, paste, lotion, or gel. The choice of the most appropriate vehicle depends primarily on the site and nature of the skin disease, but usually is limited by the chemical nature of the drug and its solubilities. An essential requirement for a vehicle is that the drug remain stable and active within it and capable of moving from the vehicle into the epidermis.

Most topical applications are either liquid or semi-solid preparations. The liquids include solutions, suspensions, and emulsions; the semi-solid preparations include water-free single phase ointments or water containing preparations. Pastes are stiff, very concentrated suspensions, usually of powder in ointment.

Creams remain the most popular form of topical application and are suspensions of oil in water for the most part but some water-in-oil creams are also used. The water evaporates, leaving an oily film behind—the basis of the "vanishing cream" concept. Ointments are single-phase oily materials that tend to be used for chronic dermatoses.

The oils and fats used in topical preparations can be derived from animal, vegetable, mineral, or synthetic sources. White soft paraffin, arachis oil, dimethicone, and lanolin are examples of oily materials used.

It should be remembered that, besides the vehicle, other excipients must be included in the preparation, including antimicrobial preservatives, emulsifying agents, colorants, and fragrances. The formulation of modern topical pharmaceuticals is a complex operation requiring experienced and expert pharmacists. This must be borne in mind if the question of extemporaneous formulation crops up. For example, formulated applications must not be diluted without due reference to the dilution of the excipient materials that occurs at the same time—and that may render the application ineffective or even dangerous.

In practice, aqueous creams are used on oozing, inflamed areas, whereas oily creams or ointments are used on dry areas. Lotions, gels, or creams are used in the scalp in present-day practice, but pastes are still sometimes used to apply a substance to a localized area.

How Much to Apply and How Much to Prescribe

It is very difficult both to explain to a patient how much ointment or cream should be applied, and to judge how much ointment will be needed. There are some simple guidelines that can be of practical value in a clinic.[3]

The patient can be instructed to use a simple approximate measure of ointment or cream: this is the amount of ointment that, when squeezed out of a tube onto the palmar aspect of the index finger, covers the distal third of the finger from the distal skin crease to the end of the finger. If a tube with a standard 5-mm nozzle is used, this amount, a "fingertip unit," is approximately 0.47g in men or 0.42g in women—for ease of remembering, approximately half a gram.

When this fingertip unit is spread on the skin it covers an area of 282 square cm. This is approximately the area covered by two hands, if the hands are placed (fingers together) on the skin surface. The area covered by a hand (approximately 140 cm^2, approximately 0.8% of the body surface) can be used as a rapid rough guide to estimating the area needing treatment. As two fingertip units are equivalent to one gram, which is equivalent to four "hand" areas, both the requirements for prescribing can easily be calculated and clear and simple instructions to the patients given.

A guide to the weights of ointment required, and the equivalent fingertip units to be applied, is given in Table 77.1.

Table 77.1 A Guide to the Weight of Ointment Required and the Equivalent Fingertip Units (FTU) to be Applied to Different Body Areas in Adults

Face and neck	1.3 g = 2.5 FTU
Front of trunk	3.5 g = 7 FTU
Back of trunk	3.5 g = 7 FTU
One arm	1.5 g = 3 FTU
One hand (front and back)	0.5 g = 1 FTU
One leg	3.0 g = 6 FTU
One foot	1.0 g = 2 FTU

References

Research Reports

1. Marks R, Dykes PJ, Williams DL, Thorne EG, Lufrano L. In vivo stratum corneum pharmacokinetics of econazole following once daily and twice daily application to human skin. J Dermatol Treatment 1990;*1*:195–197.
2. Zaumseil R-P, Kecskés A, Täuber U, Töpert M. Methylprednisolone aceponate (MPA)—a new therapeutic for eczema: A pharmacological overview. J Dermatol Treatment 1992;*3*(Suppl 2):3–7.
3. Long CC, Finlay AY. The fingertip unit: A new practical measure. Clin Exp Dermatol, 1991;*16*:444–446.

Reviews

r1. Marks R. Skin disease in old age. London: Martin Dunitz, 1987.
r2. Scott RC, Guy RH, Hadgraft J. Prediction of Percutaneous Penetration. London: IBC Technical Services, 1990.
r3. Polano MK. Topical Skin Therapeutics. New York: Churchill Livingstone, 1984.

CHAPTER 78

Adjuvant Treatments and Other Medicaments in the "Gray" Area between Medicine and Toiletries

Ronald Marks

There are a number of substances that appear to have little in the way of formal pharmacologic effect but are nonetheless very useful in the treatment of skin disease. They are mostly (but not exclusively) traditionally used materials that have been found empirically to improve the symptoms and signs of skin disorders. Such treatments sometimes are prescribed alongside more active agents, or may in themselves provide sufficient relief for the condition in question. In this category we include emollients, barrier creams, keratolytics, shampoos, sunscreens, and antiperspirants.

Emollients

Mode of Action

Emollients, also known as "moisturizers," soften and smooth the surface of the skin (the term emollient derives from the Latin *molle,* meaning soft). They do this by occluding the skin surface with an oily film, making it impervious to water. This prevents the normal water loss from the skin surface, causing a "build-up" of moisture in the stratum corneum. This increased water content smoothes the skin surface and softens the horny layer. This softening effect is accompanied by important changes in the physical properties of the stratum corneum. Scaling and hyperkeratotic stratum corneum is less flexible and elastic than normal, leading to superficial cracks and fissures during normal movements. Increased moisture content increases the elasticity and diminishes the tendency to fissure.

All forms of scaling are the result of increased internal binding forces within the stratum corneum, which prevent individual corneocytes from separating from each other, with the "stuck together" horn cells producing the appearance of scaling. Increased hydration reduces the increased binding forces and improves the tendency to scaling.

Apart from these beneficial actions on the abnormal stratum corneum, emollients have other therapeutic effects that may be summarized as "anti-inflammatory". How these effects are mediated is not entirely certain, although it appears that some emollients do have a prostaglandin synthetase inhibitory activity as well as an antimitotic effect for hyperplastic epidermis. In addition they have a weak vasoconstrictor activity, which is evident when they are used as "inactive controls" in tests of the vasoconstrictor activities of topical corticosteroids to assess anti-inflammatory potency.

Emollients also have an antipruritic and a "soothing" effect that may be related in part to their anti-inflammatory action and in part to the cooling effect of the evaporation of the water in the emollient.

Constituents

Emollients are either two-phase preparations, in which there are both oily and aqueous phases, or more commonly a single-phase preparation containing only an oily material. The two-phase preparations usually are oil-in-water emulsions, although uncommonly may be water-in-oil emulsions. The emulsions can be presented as lotions or creams of various consistencies.

The oil content of emollients may be animal, vegetable, mineral, or synthetic. Oily substances commonly used include lanolin, paraffin oils, whale oil, peanut oil, and polyethylene glycol. Emulsions containing these substances must contain stabilizers to prevent them from separating (often some detergent substance) and antimicrobial substances to prevent any bacterial contamination from establishing itself in the preparation. They also contain colorants and fragrances—so that it will be evident that modern emollients can be quite complex formulations. In addition, some emollients contain "humectants"—substances claimed actually to attract water into the stratum corneum. These include salts of pyrrolidine, carboxylic acid, and glycerine.

As pointed out above, single-phase oily substances are not often used because their greasiness is not often appreciated by patients who have to use them. Nonetheless, white soft paraffin is probably the most efficient emollient, both in the extent of the moisture build-up within the stratum corneum caused by its occlusive action and in the length of time over which this action persists. Peanut oil and olive oil also are used occasionally as single-phase emollients.

An emollient action is also obtained by use of emollient-containing cleansing preparations and bath oils.

Use

Emollients are used in both inflammatory and non-inflammatory dermatoses. Thus, they are used in eczema and psoriasis to relieve symptoms, to reduce scaling and fissuring, and to assist in damping down the inflammatory disease process. They reduce the amount of topical corticosteroid that need be prescribed for these disorders. They are of particular use in patients with atopic dermatitis, as there appears to be a background of roughness and "dryness" of the entire skin surface in many affected by this disorder that predisposes to the development of eczematous lesions.

Some patients with mild atopic dermatitis or very localized psoriasis may be managed by the use of emollients alone.

Patients with one of the disorders of keratinization such as the ichthyoses need to use emollient materials frequently to make their skin supple, to prevent fissures, and to reduce the appearance of scaling.

Side-Effects

Side-effects may be observed from the constituents of emollients. These include allergic contact dermatitis due to lanolin or to a paraminobenzoic acid ester employed as a preservative or to many other of the preservatives, emulsifiers, stabilizers, or fragrances employed. Infant dermatitis due to inclusion of high concentrations of propylene glycol, cetyl stearate, or sodium lauryl sulfate is less common but may be seen occasionally. Some of the oily constituents, such as cocoa butter and white soft paraffin, may provoke the formation of comedones or a folliculitis by irritating the follicular orifices.

Barrier Creams

Definition and Mode of Action

Barrier creams are substances designed to remain on the skin surface after application in order to prevent the skin from damage by contact with injurious substances. The injurious substances concerned are generally organic solvents, alkalis, minute particulate materials that can mechanically abrade the skin, or just plain water, which can macerate the skin and injure the skin's barrier after frequent contact.

Constituents

Substances that are impervious to water, resistant to organic solvents, are chemically inert, that are retained on the skin surface or better still substantive to it, and that are acceptable as topical applications are required. The formulations employed often contain silicone oils and waxes and inert oils (white soft paraffin) and tend to be thick, viscid substances. They may also contain preservatives and other adjuvant substances.

Uses

Barrier creams are used industrially to minimize injury to the skin from a variety of potentially toxic substances. They are not very popular because gloves give much better protection. They are not pleasant to wear on the skin, and their effectiveness is sometimes in doubt. The same factors apply to their domestic use. A further use claimed for them concerns protection of the skin against maceration and damage from urine, feces, and secretions. They are used in infants and in incontinent patients in the "napkin area".

Keratolytics

Keratolytics are agents that facilitate desquamation and, because of this, reduce scaling and hyperkeratosis. The modes of action of these agents are not clear, but they seem to alter the intercorneocyte binding forces either by changing the chemistry of the intercellular cement or by modulating the process of epidermal differentiation.

Agents Used

The most frequently used keratolytic agent is salicylic acid. This is employed in concentrations of 1 to 20 percent in creams, lotions, collodions, and ointments. Preparations containing concentrations above 6 percent are mostly used for the treatment of viral warts or callosities. For removal of scale in psoriasis, seborrhoeic dermatitis of the scalp, and hyperkeratotic eczema of the palms and soles, concentrations of 2 to 6 percent are used. The only local adverse side-effect is irritation of the skin, which is observed mainly at concentrations above 6 percent. A serious side-effect is the percutaneous penetration of sufficient salicylic acid to cause systemic toxicity (salicylism). This is unlikely at concentrations of 2 percent or below, but higher concentrations used on large areas of skin can cause this potentially serious and avoidable problem.

Other organic hydroxy acids also appear to have some keratolytic effect, but not as great as that of salicylic acid. Lactic, glycolic, and tartaric acids are among the hydroxy acids that appear to have some keratolytic effects. Lactic acid is used either with salicylic acid or alone in the same kind of concentrations as salicylic acid. Glycolic acid is also used in high concentrations as a "peeling agent."

Topical tretinoin (all-trans-retinoic acid) (see also Chapter 81) is sometimes used in concentrations of 0.01 to 0.1 percent as an agent to enhance desquamation.

Uses

Keratolytics are employed to reduce scaling in psoriasis, chronic eczema, and the ichthyotic disorders. They are also used in high concentrations in localized warty disorders such as viral warts, solar keratoses, and seborrhoeic warts.

Sunscreens

Sunscreens are preparations that filter out or reflect off the harmful radiations in the solar spectrum. Older, conventional sunscreens filter out only the "burning" rays in the ultraviolet part of the spectrum. The entire ultraviolet spectrum (UVR) runs from 200 to 400 nm and is conventionally divided into long wave or UVA (320–400 nm), the medium wave or UVB segment (290–320 nm), and the short wave UVR portion or UVC (200–290 nm), which mostly doesn't reach the earth's surface. The UVB portion is believed to be the most damaging with regard to photocarcinogenesis and causing sunburn, but the UVA segment certainly contributes to the production of skin cancers and may also be particularly responsible for chronic solar damage to the skin, giving rise to the appearance of aging.

The effectiveness of a sunscreen is measured in terms of its ability to prolong the time it takes to sustain a sunburn and is known as the sun protection factor (SPF). The SPF is the ratio:

$$\frac{\text{time to sustaining a burn with the sunscreen}}{\text{time to sustaining a burn without the sunscreen}}$$

The ratio usually is determined using special artificial sunlamps known as solar simulators. Protection against UVA cannot be determined in this way, and is either determined in vitro using a monochromator and a thermopile, or in vivo using the physiologic phenomenon of "immediate pigment darkening."

Sunscreens are of great importance in preventing sunburn and other acute reactions in sensitive individ-

Table 78.1 Examples of Substances Used in Sunscreens

Group	Specific Example	Type	Protects Against
Esters of para-aminobenzoic acid	Padimate	Filter	UVB
Esters of cinnamic acid	Ethylhexyl-*p*-methoxycinamate	Filter	UVB + some UVA
Benzophenones	Oxybenzone	Filter	UVB + some UVA
Titanium dioxide	Micronized titanium	Reflectant	UVB and UVA
Salicylates	Homomenthyl salicylates	Filter	UVB
Anthranilates	Menthyl anthranilate	Filter	UVA
Physical blocker	Red petrolatum	Reflectant	UVB and UVA

From: Marks R, *Sun Damaged Skin,* Martin Dunitz, London, 1992.

uals. They are also important in reducing the likelihood of developing some form of skin cancer.

Sunscreens differ greatly in their protective capacity and Table 78.1 contains the major constituents of sunscreens and their abilities to prevent skin damage.

Shampoos

Shampoos are often prescribed for patients with psoriasis affecting the scalp, patients with seborrhoeic dermatitis, and others with scaling dermatoses that affect the scalp. They contain a mild detergent to help loosen the scale and other detritus as well as "actives," such as coal tar extracts and antimicrobial agents. They are rarely sufficient as the only treatment for scalp disorders but are useful adjuncts.

Antiperspirants

These agents inhibit sweat secretion and are at present virtually restricted to preparations containing aluminum chlorhydrate. Deodorants are specifically designed to reduce body odor and are usually antimicrobials that reduce the bacterial flora responsible for breaking down sweat products causing this problem.

References

Reviews

r1. Lim HW, Soter NA. Clinical Photomedicine. New York: Marcel Dekker, (1993).

r2. Lowe NJ, Shaath NA. Sunscreens: Development, Evaluation and Regulatory Aspects. New York: Marcel Dekker, (1990).

r3. Marks R. Methods to evaluate effects of skin surface texture modifiers. In Frost P, Horwitz SN, eds. Principles of Cosmetics for the Dermatologist. Horwitz CV Mosby (1982), pp 50–58.

r4. Marks R. Effects of emollients on inflammatory dermatoses. In: Frost P, Horwitz SN, eds. Principles of Cosmetics for the Dermatologist, St. Louis: CV Mosby (1982), pp 334–336.

r5. Marks R. Sun-damaged skin. London: Martin Dunitz (1992).

CHAPTER 79

Topical Corticosteroids: Treatment of Eczematous Disorders

Ronald Marks

Corticosteriods are the most frequently prescribed and arguably the most important class of topical pharmaceutical agent for such common inflammatory skin disorders as eczema and psoriasis. The topical corticosteroid era began more than 40 years ago with the introduction of topical hydrocortisone; since then, new analogues with increased potency, improved delivery to the diseased tissue, and decreased potential for toxicity have been introduced in a steady stream. Despite the large numbers of such analogues it is possible to describe their actions, uses and side-effects together. Apart from differences in potency and some small differences in side-effects profile in more recently introduced compounds, they are very similar both pharmacologically and therapeutically.

Essentially they act as anti-inflammatory agents, as do systemic corticosteroids, but are able to achieve high tissue concentrations of the corticosteroid agent locally without the inevitable toxic side-effects seen when the systemic route is used.

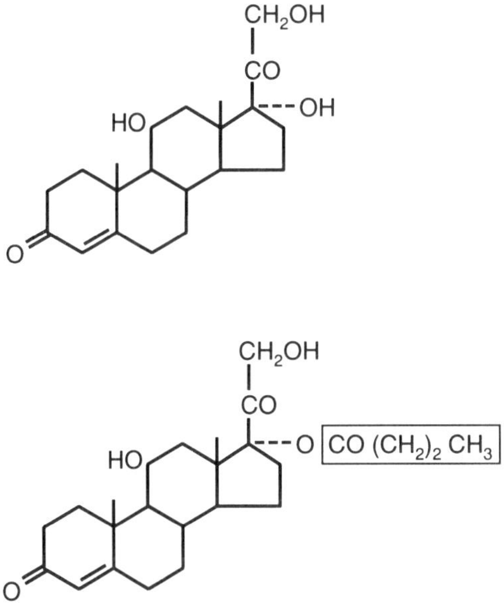

CH_2OH / CO / HO / OH / O

CH_2OH / CO / HO / O / $CO\ (CH_2)_2\ CH_3$ / O

Figure 79.1 Steroid penetration may be enhanced by esterification. In this example, hydrocortisone (top) is esterified to hydrocortisone 17-butyrate (bottom).

Corticosteroid Analogues for Topical Use

Several routes have been adopted to try to improve the therapeutic potential of hydrocortisone. Esterification of the corticosteroid molecule was an early device adopted to enhance skin penetration. Hydrocortisone-17-butyrate is an example of this approach, in which the ester has greatly enhanced potency compared to the parent compound (Fig. 79.1).[r1] "Double esterification" is a more recent technique employed to try to enhance penetration and at the same time decrease the potential for local side-effects (as with methylprednisolone aceponate).[1]

Increased potency has also been attained by the introduction of double bonds into the steroid nucleus (see Fig. 79.2)—as in corticosteroids used systemically, e.g., prednisolone. Another extremely effective technique for enhancing potency has been fluorination of the corticosteroid molecule—the most successful example being betamethasone-17-valerate.[r2] Introduction of the chlorine atom also has been effective in enhancing corticosteroid potency, as with one of the most potent topical corticosteroid agents yet developed—clobetasol-17-propionate (see Fig. 79.3).[r3]

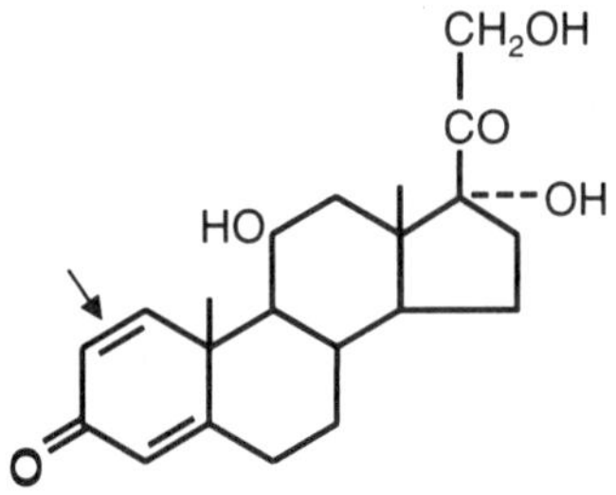

Figure 79.2 Steroid potency is enhanced by the introduction of a double bond (arrow) into the hydrocortisone molecule to produce prednisolone.

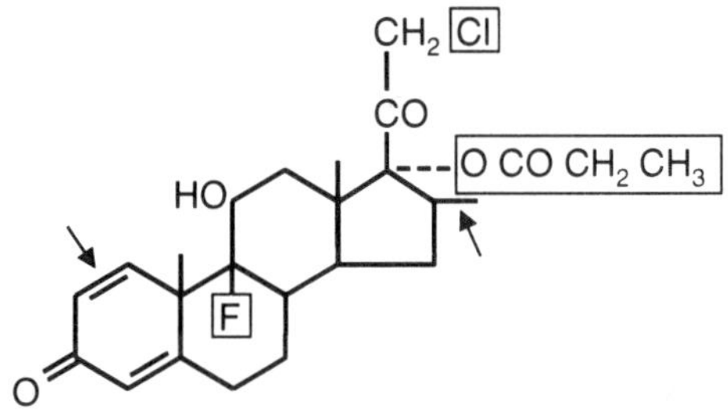

Figure 79.3 Clobetasol-17-propionate combines an additional double bond and fluoridation of the steroid nucleus, which increases potency, with esterification to enhance penetration, producing a very potent topical steroid.

Preparations Available

Apart from the inclusion of one or the other of the large number of different corticosteroid analogue molecules, there are several other ways of modulating the clinical efficacy of a topical preparation of a corticosteroid. One quite obvious way is by choosing the most appropriate vehicle. Corticosteroid preparations currently are available in single-phase greasy ointments, oil in water emulsions (mostly creams and lotions), alcoholic lotions (for scalp application), impregnated tapes, and sprays. Different corticosteroids are soluble to different extents in different vehicles, and these factors will influence both the concentration that can be obtained and the ease with which the molecule can cross the skin barrier.

Apart from variations in the vehicle, topical corticosteroids also may be formulated together with other pharmacologically active compounds. These include such antimicrobial agents as neomycin, aureomycin, clotrimazole and miconazole, and tars and salicylic acid. Purists disapprove of these "polypharmacy" combinations, but many clinicians (and their patients) are grateful for them. Combinations with antimicrobials are of particular value in the treatment of patients whose eczema has become secondarily infected. These combinations also are of undoubted value in the treatment of seborrhoeic dermatitis—particular combinations in which the antimicrobial agent is one of the "broad spectrum" compounds that can deal with pityrosporon ovale—such as imidazoles. Penetration enhancers are another class of agent sometimes included in corticosteroid preparations. These range from 2 percent acid (used with betamethasone propionate) and urea, to azone.

Mode of Action

As far as is known, the bulk of the pharmacologic actions of the corticosteroids are mediated via a nuclear receptor for hydrocortisone to which the other steroids also bind. In general, the stronger the affinity of the compound for the receptor, the more potent the compound.

The anti-inflammatory action of the corticosteroids depends on the induction of peptides known as lipocortins. These are antagonists of phospholipase A_2—an enzyme released from lysosomes that causes the breakdown of membrane phospholipids to release arachidonic acid, initiating the prostanoid cascade.

Other effects that contribute to the anti-inflammatory activity of the corticosteroids include lysosomal and cellular membrane stabilization, reduction in numbers of Langerhans cells, the modulation of the movement of inflammatory cells, a vasoconstrictor effect, and an antimitotic effect for many cell types, including epidermal cells.

Indications for Use

The major indication for topical corticosteroids is the group of skin disorders embraced by the term "eczema." In some eczematous dermatoses the causative agency can be removed and a topical corticosteroid is then necessary only for symptomatic relief during the defervescence of the condition. Unfortunately, in most instances it is not possible to remove the basic underlying cause of the eczematous disorder; to obtain continuing relief, patients with atopic dermatitis, for example, need to use these agents continuously or at least persistently. This long-term use clearly has important implications from the point of view of unwanted side-effects (see later).

The other major use for topical corticosteroids is psoriasis. There are two major considerations with regard to this clinical use. First, psoriasis does not respond adequately to weak corticosteroids—although, having said this, hydrocortisone is of some use for flexural, facial, and scalp psoriasis. The other point is that psoriasis is a chronic inflammatory skin disorder and that, as with atopic dermatitis, there is a serious risk of unpleasant side-effects. The additional risk of precipitating pustular psoriasis must also be remembered (see below).

Potent topical corticosteroids certainly produce a rapid response; the difficulty is that there is also a rapid relapse after treatment has stopped—in general, relapse (or "rebound") seems to be more rapid than with other treatments. Furthermore the relapse often appears to be more inflamed than the original lesions. For these reasons the use of topical corticosteroids in psoriasis is quite controversial—dermatologists in the UK and in some other parts of Europe in general are not in favor of their use for this indication.

Topical corticosteroids are also used with some success for other inflammatory skin conditions, including sunburn and thermal burns. They have also been employed for the inflammatory component of less common skin disorders, such as lichen planus, mycosis fungoides, and pityriasis lichenoides.

They should ***not*** be used for pruritus in the absence of an inflammatory skin problem as they are not in themselves antipruritic. Their use in acne is hardly ever warranted and is potentially hazardous. In rosacea, topical corticosteroids aggravate the disorder in the long term and should not be used. They also should not be used for skin infections, such as ringworm (see below).

Some Practical Hints Concerning Usage

After an initial response to topical corticosteroids, it is not unusual for the dermatosis to relapse and become refractory to further treatment with the same agent. Treatment with other similar corticosteroid preparations may, however, be successful. This situation is known as tachyphylaxis. Although common and important, it is inadequately researched.

The question of to which potency of topical corticosteroid to use is a further contentious issue. Some have advocated that potent agents should be employed initially and that less potent agents should be substituted as the condition improves. For the most part, the best advice is to use the least potent agent that obtains the therapeutic effect needed.

The most potent preparations (e.g., clobetasol-17-propionate 0.05%; Halcinonide) should be reserved for the most recalcitrant conditions, including keloid and hypertropic scars, discoid lupus erythematosus, hypertrophic lichen planus, lichen sclerosus et atrophicus, and lichen simplex chronicus.

The potency of a preparation can be enhanced by occlusion of the area to be treated with polythene film. However, the enhanced potency is matched by an increased risk of side-effects as well as the inconvenience.

Adverse Effects

Adverse effects from the use of topical corticosteroids are either local or systemic due to the absorption of the corticosteroid molecule. They are predominantly the result of using potent corticosteroids topically and are rarely evident after the use of hydrocortisone or clobetasone butyrate. Adverse side-effects are also mainly due to prolonged and/or unsupervised usage.

Systemic Side-Effects (see Table 79.1)

Pituitary-adrenal axis suppression may occur if more than 30 g of clobetasol-17-propionate (0.05%) or 50 g of betamethasone-17-valerate (0.1%) preparations are used per week. If this occurs and then the agent is withdrawn, adrenal failure may result. Fatalities have been recorded because of this. Iatrogenic Cushing's syndrome, with all the usual stigmata of this disease, from the use of potent topical corticosteroids is uncommon but unfortunately does still occur with unsupervised use. Arrested growth as a side-effect may result from continuous use in children but it is possible that the growth failure of atopic individuals is a result of the disease itself rather than its treatment. Atopy is an inherited condition in which individuals are predisposed to eczema, asthma, hay fever, and perennial rhinitis.

Local Side-Effects (see Table 79.2)

Potent topical corticosteroids regularly cause skin thinning and at sites of tissue tension will cause striae distensae—especially in young adults. Skin thinning also "exposes" the dermal vasculature and often results

Table 79.1 Systemic Side-Effects from the Use of Potent Topical Corticosteroids

- Pituitary adrenal axis suppression
- Iatrogenic Cushing's syndrome
- Arrested growth

Table 79.2 Local Adverse Side-Effects from Use of Topical Corticosteroids

- Masked infection—altered ringworm in particular (tinea incognito)
- Striae distensae
- Skin thinning
- Bruising and telangiectasia
- Aggravation of rosacea
- Acne
- Hirsutes

(Striae distensae, skin thinning, bruising and telangiectasia, aggravation of rosacea: from dermal thinning and skin atrophy)

in aggravation of rosacea (potent topical corticosteroids should ***not*** be used on the face!) as well as bruising and telangiectasia. Tinea incognito describes the odd clinical appearance of ringworm treated inappropriately with these agents—the rash spreads but becomes less inflamed.

Treatment of Eczema

Eczema is not a disease but a reaction pattern due to a large number of noxious agents and immunologic influences. There is skin inflammation and epidermal edema and abnormal keratinization as a result. The disorder is invariably itchy, and mostly pink and scaling. In the acute phase there is often vesiculation, and the broken skin surface may become infected. A primary principle is to remove the underlying cause if this is possible—often it is not.

Atopic dermatitis is marked by severe itching with obvious results on the skin, including lichenification and excoriation. It is also true that such patients often have widespread dryness and scaliness of the skin surface. For this reason, emollients are an important part of the treatment plan—both topical applications and oily bath preparations.

Topical corticosteroids are the most important form of treatment, but care must be taken to avoid the adverse side-effects by using the weakest dose consistent with relief. Lichenified areas may benefit from zinc or weak tar preparations, and bandaging is advocated by some. For severely affected patients whose lives are made miserable by the persistent scratching and sleeplessness, systemic therapy with PUVA or cyclosporin may be required. Systemic steroids should be given only as a last resort.

Seborrhoeic dermatitis may benefit from combinations of topical corticosteroids (e.g., hydrocortisone) and antimicrobial compounds such as miconazole, clotrimazole, or econazole. An 8 percent lithium succinate ointment also has been shown to be effective.

References

Research Reports

1. Zaumseil R-P, Kecskés A, Täuber U, Töpert M. Methylprednisolone aceponate (MPA)—a new therapeutic for eczema: A pharmacological overview. J Dermatol Treatment 1992;*3*(Suppl 2):3–7.
2. Long CC, Finlay AY. The fingertip unit: A new practical measure. Clin & Exp Dermatol, 1991;*16*:444–446.
3. Marks R, Dykes PJ, Williams DL, Thorne EG, Lufrano L. In vivo stratum corneum pharmacokinetics of econazole following once daily and twice daily application to human skin. J Dermatol Treatment 1990;*1*:195–197.

Reviews

r1. Christophers E, Schöpf E, Kligman AM, Stoughton RB. Topical corticosteroid Therapy: A novel approach to safer drugs. New York, Raven Press, 1988.

r2. Yohn JJ, Weston WL. Topical glucocorticoids. Curr Probl Dermatol 1990;*II*(2):34–63.

r3. Maibach HI, Surber Ch. Topical corticosteroids. Basel, Karger, 1992.

r4. Marks R. Skin Disease in Old Age. London: Martin Dunitz, 1987.

r5. Scott RC, Guy RH, Hadgraft J. Prediction of Percutaneous Penetration. London: IBC Technical Services Ltd., 1990.

r6. Polano MK. Corticosteroids for topical use. In: Topical skin therapeutics. New York: Churchill Livingstone, 1984; pp 101–139.

CHAPTER 80

Tars, Dithranol (Anthralin), Vitamin D Analogues, and Zinc Preparations—The Treatment of Psoriasis

Richard J. Motley

Introduction

Psoriasis is a common inherited inflammatory skin disorder of unknown cause in which hyperproliferation of the epidermis leads to well-defined, thick, scaly, erythematous plaques typically over the extensor aspects of the limbs and in the scalp. Tars and dithranol are traditional, effective, empirical topical remedies that inhibit the proliferative process by unknown mechanisms. In severe psoriasis, systemic therapy with retinoids, methotrexate, cyclosporin, or PUVA may be required.

Tar

Prior to the development of topical corticosteroids, tars were among the most valuable treatments the dermatologist had to offer. Tars are a complicated mixture of both aliphatic and aromatic hydrocarbons; they derive from the destructive distillation of one of three different but similar materials: shale; wood; and coal. Wood tars are of little value and will not be considered further. Ichthamol is a shale tar prepared by distillation of shale minerals. It is a black viscous liquid that may be mixed with glycerin to form a preparation with anti-inflammatory and vasoconstrictive properties; it is used for eczema and local inflammatory conditions of the skin. Its efficacy has not been established, although it has been a traditional treatment for boils and cellulitis.

Coal tar preparations are distilled from coal, and there are differences between the composition of coal tar obtained from different sources. It is effective in both chronic eczema and psoriasis, but is messy and has a strong, distinctive smell. Coal tar may be formulated in various vehicles to produce creams, ointments, gels, and pastes of varying strengths. Typical preparations include coal tar 10 percent, zinc oxide 30 percent, and yellow soft paraffin 60 percent; or coal tar 2 percent, salicylic acid 2 percent in polysorbate 80, emulsifying wax, white soft paraffin, coconut oil, and liquid paraffin. Liquor picis carbonis is a coal tar solution that may be added to a variety of formulations. It is difficult to assess adequately the therapeutic differences between the myriad different tar preparations, but it is clear that some vehicles produce a cosmetically more acceptable preparation than others, notwithstanding the fact that tars are messy to use. Certainly, some proprietary cream preparations are well accepted by patients.

Tar preparations may be applied to normal skin, usually without ill-effect, although occasional irritation or true allergy develops. This makes tar preparations the treatment of choice for the small-plaque variety of psoriasis in which hundreds of small plaques are scattered over the whole body area.

Side-effects from the use of tar preparations are few and far between. Irritation of the follicles, causing a folliculitis, is probably the commonest. "Tar smarts" are uncommon with newer preparations—the term refers to the stinging sensation at the site of application after sun exposure, and is the result of phototoxicity.

Dithranol (Anthralin)

Dithranol (anthralin) is a synthetic analogue of chrysarobin, a substance derived from the tropical tree *Vouacopoua araroba*. Chemically, it is 1,8-dihydroxy anthracenone. Although it has antimycotic actions and is also effective in chronic eczema, the main use of dithranol is in psoriasis. Some 80 percent of psoriatics respond to dithranol in a six-week period. Dithranol is irritant to normal skin, and when used in the treatment of psoriasis must be carefully localized to the affected areas. Its use is limited by its irritating effects, and it is customary to begin treatment with concentrations of 0.1 percent and to increase the concentration according to tolerance and therapeutic results. The drug stains the skin (and clothes) a brownish mauve. One of the most popular formulations of dithranol was in Lassar's paste—2 percent salicylic acid, 25 percent starch, 25 percent zinc oxide made up to 100 percent with soft paraffin. Dithranol in concentrations from 0.1 to 10 percent or more may be added to this. Dithranol is inactivated by oxidation to danthron when added to zinc oxide pastes, but the presence of salicylic acid in Lassar's paste prevents this. Lassar's paste is stiff and has little tendency to run. This facilitates localization of the treatments to affected areas of skin.

Stable proprietary dithranol preparations have been produced up to 2 percent, but higher strengths are unstable and a ready-mixed commercially available dithranol cream of more than 2 percent is not yet available.

Dithranol in paraffin ointment has a longer shelf life than dithranol in Lassar's paste. It is easily applied to affected skin, but also tends to spread onto normal skin and may lead to considerable irritation. One way to avoid this is to "fix" the ointment after application by using starch or talcuum powder.

Lassar's paste has given way in popularity to proprietary dithranol cream preparations. Short contact treatment in which the preparation is used for 30 to 60 minutes before being washed off was introduced in the 1970s and has proved a useful way of applying this agent. Patients can be treated at home and can live a normal life after washing off the material.[1,2,3]

Zinc Preparations

Zinc oxide and zinc carbonate in ointments, creams, and lotions are long-established, mildly anti-inflammatory preparations that are now mainly employed to help irritation (calamine lotions—aqueous and oily). It is also claimed that they accelerate wound healing, but evidence for this is slim.

Calcipotriol

Calcipotriol is a synthetic derivative of vitamin D. It induces cellular differentiation and suppresses keratinocyte proliferation. It is prepared as a colorless ointment that contains 50 μg of calcipotriol per gram and is applied to affected skin twice daily. It is non-staining and irritates skin less than dithranol; for these reasons, it has become extremely popular in the treatment of mild to moderate psoriasis. Hypercalcemia is rare but may occur in patients who apply more than the recommended weekly dose of 100g of the ointment to the skin; dermatitis occasionally may occur following application to the face. A recent study reported that topical calcipotriol was as effective as dithranol.[4] Other vitamin D analogues are being developed and will be available soon.

Systemic Therapies for Psoriasis

Severe psoriasis may require systemic treatment with methotrexate, etretinate, PUVA, or cyclosporin.

Methotrexate

Methotrexate is a folic acid analogue that interferes with normal cellular metabolism. It is given once weekly as an oral dose of between 7.5 and 30mg (and may also be given IM or IV). The dosage is titrated according to response. It is employed mainly for elderly patients who find difficulty in applying topical preparations to multiple patches of psoriasis, but may be used in milddle-aged and young adults who have failed to respond to other therapies. Its long-term use in these patients is limited by cumulative hepatotoxicity.

Methotrexate is an antimetabolite, and overdosage leads to bone marrow suppression. In the low doses used to treat psoriasis the main concern, however, is liver damage. A dose-related hepatotoxicity may develop and the liver must be monitored by regular examination of liver biopsies—typically every two years. Mild GI discomfort is a common side-effect. Hepatotoxicity is more likely to occur in those with previous liver disease and in those who drink alcohol—which therefore should be prohibited.[5]

A number of drugs interfere with methotrexate by displacing it from protein binding sites, by diminishing its excretion, or by also interfering with folate metabolism. Concurrent administration of these agents should be avoided or used only with extreme caution. These drugs include trimethoprim-sulfonamide antibiotics, NSAIDs, phenytoin, and certain antibiotics.

Etretinate

The retinoid etretinate is discussed in detail elsewhere (see Chapter 81). Etretinate is an effective treatment for psoriasis and is particularly useful for psoriasis of palms and soles. It causes a generalized drying of the skin that some patients find unpleasant, and may produce an elevation in serum triglycerides. Its main disadvantage is its potent teratogenicity and long half-life. This effectively excludes it as a treatment for women in the childbearing years because a two-year washout period is required following therapy before conception can be attempted.

Typical doses of 0.5–1.0 mg/kg per day are used.

PUVA

PUVA is a combination treatment of a naturally-occurring psoralen and UVA light. The psoralen may be taken orally or applied directly to the skin. Typically, 8-methoxypsoralen is taken orally two hours before UV light treatment. Exposure to UVA light then activates the drug which has an antiproliferative action. Care must be taken to shield the eyes from light and to avoid further sun exposure for a 24-hour period after taking the drug. Treatment is given two or three times weekly. Long-term PUVA therapy is associated with an increased risk of skin cancer, particularly squamous cell carcinoma.

Cyclosporin

Cyclosporin was isolated from a soil fungus *Tolypocladium inflatum* but is now produced synthetically. It is a cyclic polypeptide that appears to act principally by inhibiting the production of cytokines by T-helper cells. It is given orally in doses of 2 to 5 mg/kg per day for psoriasis. Its main side-effects are dose-related hypertension and renal impairment. It does not interfere with bone marrow production.[r3,r4,7]

References

Research Reports

1. Whitefield M. Pharmaceutical formulations of anthralin. Br J Dermatol 1981;*105*(S.20):28–32.
2. Bohlen P, Grove J, Beya MF et al. Skin polyamine levels in psoriasis: the effect of dithranol therapy. Eur J Clin Invest 1978;*8*:215–218.
3. Gay MW, Moore WJ, Morgan JM, Montes LF. Anthralin toxicity. Arch Dermatol 1972;*105*:213–215.
4. Hutchinson PE, Berth-Jones J, Chalmers RJC, Chu AC, Griffiths WAD, Klaber MR. A comparison of calcipotriol ointment and short contact dithranol in the treatment of chronic plaque psoriasis. Br J Dermatol 1992;*127*:(Suppl 40) 17.
5. Fairris GM, Dewhurst AG, White JE, Campbell MJ. Methotrexate dosage in patients aged over 50 with psoriasis. Br Med J 1989;*298*:801–802.
6. Tanew A, Guggenbichler A, Hönigsmann H, Geiger JM, Fritsch P. Photochemotherapy for severe psoriasis without or in combination with acitretin: A randomized, double-blind comparison study. J Am Acad Dermatol 1991;*25*:682–684.
7. Bos JD, van Joost TH, Powles AV, Minhardi MMHM, Heule F, Fry L. Use of cyclosporin in psoriasis. Lancet 1989;*2*:1500–1502.

Reviews

r1. Fry L. Psoriasis. Br J Dermatol 1988;*119*:445–461.

r2. Zelickson BD, Muller SA. Generalised pustular psoriasis—a review of 63 cases. Arch Dermatol 1991;*127*:1339–1345.

r3. Wolff K. Cyclosporin A and the Skin. London/New York: Royal Society of Medicine Services, 1992.

r4. Fry L. The Therapeutic Potential of Cyclosporin in Severe Psoriasis. London/New York: Royal Society of Medicine Services, 1990.

r5. British Photodermatology Group Guidelines for PUVA. Br J Dermatol 1994;*130*:246–255.

r6. Studniberg HM, Weller P. PUVA, UVB, psoriasis and non melanoma skin cancer. J Am Acad Dermatol 1993;*29*:1013–1022.

CHAPTER 81

Retinoids

Alex Anstey

Introduction

Vitamin A (retinol) is an essential nutrient for animal cells. It has diverse actions on cellular growth and differentiation that go far beyond its classically defined role in vision. In common with vitamin D, these actions are mediated through hormone-like nuclear receptors. The recognition of the prominent effects of vitamin A on epithelia has led to the development of a number of synthetic analogues of vitamin A that have important therapeutic applications.

Vitamin A is a polyisoprenoid alcohol that exists in several forms. Retinol (vitamin A_1) is a primary alcohol present in esterified form in the tissues of animals and sea-water fishes; 3-dehydro-retinol (vitamin A_2) is present in fresh-water fishes and usually occurs mixed with retinol; retinoic acid and retinol ethers and esters share some but not all of the actions of retinol. The term retinoid refers to compounds that resemble retinoic acid in structure but may or may not react with the vitamin A nuclear receptor.

Oxidation of the alcohol group on retinol produces retinoic acid (vitamin A acid), a compound potent in the promotion of growth and the control of differentiation in epithelial tissue. Isomerization of retinoic acid yields 13-cis-retinoic acid (isotretinoin), which has similar potency in its effects on epithelial tissue but is much less potent in producing the toxic symptoms of hypervitaminosis A. Retinoids also include a number of structurally related synthetic analogues. These include the prodrug etretinate, the ethyl ester of the active compound acitretin, and the arotinoids, highly potent "third-generation" retinoids that feature two aromatic rings.[r1]

Chemistry

Vitamin A (all-trans-retinol) (Fig. 81.1) acts as the precursor for the synthesis of its metabolites. Its metabolism is central to retinoid physiology and is summarized in Figure 81.2. Vitamin A in the body is derived from dietary sources of the compound or its pro-form beta-carotene, which is oxidized to retinol.

Retinoic acid (Fig. 81.3) is produced by oxidation of trans-retinal, which is itself the product of oxidation of the polar head of retinol. Isomerization of trans-retinoic acid at the 13–14 double bond of the side-chain produces 13-cis-retinoic acid (isotretinoin) (Fig. 81.4). All-trans-retinoic acid has several routes of metabolism, including oxidation to 4-oxo-retinoic acid, dehydrogenation to 3,4-didehydroretinoic acid, and glucuronidation to retinoyl glucuronide. Etretinate is the ethyl ester of acitretin (Fig. 81.5).

Alterations in the structure of vitamin A metabolites are responsible for dramatic differences in binding affinity to retinoid receptors and in turn influence the biologic consequences of such binding. Comparative studies on potency and binding affinity of retinoids reveal wide variation. The low retinoid-receptor binding affinity of acitretin yet high potency is probably explained by the transformation of acitretin to metabolites with binding activity.[r2]

History

Early studies on the nutritional importance of vitamins established the concept of a regulatory role for the fat-soluble vitamins (termed vitamin A), with the reversal of growth arrest and immaturity in animals deprived of an adequate dietary intake of fat.[1] The

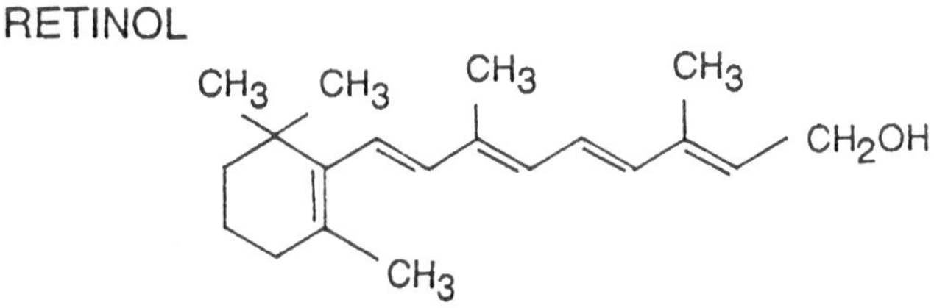

RETINOL

CH_3 CH_3 CH_3 CH_3 CH_2OH CH_3

Figure 81.1 Vitamin A (all-trans-retinol)

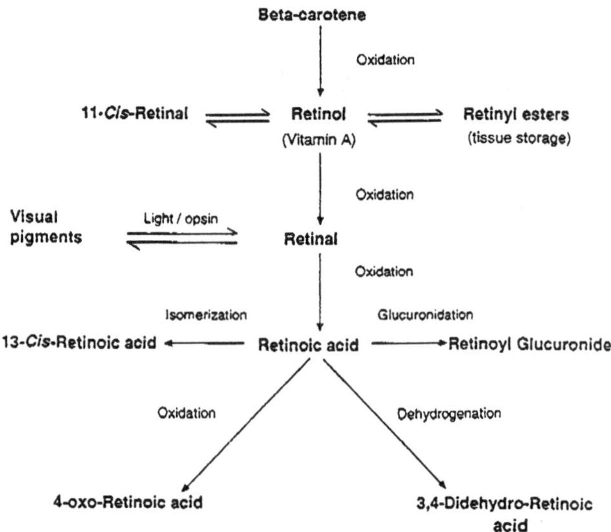

Figure 81.2 Metabolism of Vitamin A

RETINOIC ACID

Figure 81.3 Retinoic Acid (trans-retinoic acid)

ISOTRETINOIN

Figure 81.4 Isotretinoin (13-cis-retinoic acid)

ETRETINATE

Figure 81.5 Etritinate

observation by Steenbock[2] that the vitamin A content of vegetables varied according to degree of pigmentation led to its isolation in 1931 by Karrer et al,[3] who demonstrated it to be a cyclic polyisoprenoid alcohol, now known as all-trans-retinol. In the mid-1930s Wald[r3] showed that a vitamin A derivative was involved in phototransduction, but it was not until the 1940s when the aldehyde form of vitamin A, retinaldehyde, was identified by Morton.[4] Retinaldehyde (11-cis-retinal) is a prosthetic group that is covalently bound to the visual pigment known as rhodopsin. The photo-induced isomerization of this compound is the first step in the visual transduction pathway. Retinaldehyde was the first of the vitamin A metabolites to be recognized as important in its own right, and was soon joined by retinoic acid.

Van Dorp et al[5] synthesized retinoic acid in the 1940s and demonstrated it to be biologically more potent in its effects on epithelial cell maturation and reversal of growth arrest than retinol. It could not, however, support visual function because retinoic acid cannot be metabolized to retinaldehyde; neither could it support normal male reproductive function. The biologic potency of retinoic acid in the reversal of the extensive cutaneous manifestations of severe vitamin A deficiency led to the recognition of a potential therapeutic role for this compound. The beneficial effects of oral vitamin A in acne were first reported in 1943, but it subsequently became clear that very large doses were required to achieve a response. Topical retinoic acid was used in the early 1960s for the local treatment of a number of skin disorders[6] and was subsequently reported to be beneficial in acne in 1969. Retinoic acid is now accepted as a standard therapy for comedonal and papulopustular acne. Kligman in the 1980s observed reversal of photodamage in older women with acne whom he had treated for long periods with topical retinoic acid. This observation led to double-blind, placebo-controlled trials that confirmed that topical retinoic acid could improve the signs of photodamage.

The development of the aromatic retinoid etretinate in the early 1970s was the decisive breakthrough that followed the introduction of the first generation retinoids. Etretinate was first used successfully in the treatment of psoriasis and the congenital disorders of keratinization in the mid-1970s, and is now established as an important treatment for some of the more severe and chronic forms of psoriasis. The efficacy of isotretinoin in the treatment of cystic and conglobate acne was first demonstrated by Peck et al[7] in 1979 and is now established as the treatment of choice for the most severe variants of acne.

Therapeutic Uses

Vitamin A has a number of important physiologic functions. These include photoreception by the chromophore 11-cis-retinal, the promotion of bone and muscle growth, the promotion of growth and differentiation of epithelial tissue, and the maintenance of male reproductive function and embryonic development. Retinol deficiency leads to retardation of growth and development, impaired keratinization of the skin, night blindness, infertility, and abortion. The main dietary sources of vitamin A are eggs, milk, vitamin enriched margarine, fish oil, and vegetables containing the pigment beta-carotene, a proform of vitamin A.

Topical Retinoids

The diversity of effects of topical retinoids has resulted in their use in a wide range of dermatologic conditions. In addition to treating acne, beneficial effects have been reported in the reversal of solar elastotic degeneration—resulting in notoriety as an "anti-aging" cream.

Retinoic Acid

Retinoic acid has now been used for the treatment of acne for more than 20 years. The effectiveness of this compound is explained by its ability to stimulate epidermal activity and expel comedones through its desquamation-promoting effect. This also partly explains the beneficial effects of retinoic acid in the treatment of photoinduced epidermal dysplasia and solar keratoses, which have been confirmed by several double-blind placebo-controlled studies. Epidermal and dermal thickening with long-term application of retinoic acid both contribute to decreased wrinkling and have earned it the reputation as an "anti-aging" cream. Other uses include the treatment of senile lentigines, conditions characterized by hyperpigmentation, actinic keratoses, hyperkeratotic disorders, the promotion of re-epithelialization, and the treatment of keloid scars.

Isotretinoin

Isotretinoin has only recently become available for topical use. In Europe it is licensed for the treatment of acne, and it is anticipated that it will be licensed for the treatment of photodamage in the near future. The effects of topical isotretinoin are similar to those of retinoic acid, which is partly explained by the substantial photoisomerization that occurs between these two compounds on exposure to sunlight.[8]

Other Topical Retinoids

Several other retinoid drugs are being developed for topical use. These include CD271, which has been shown to be therapeutically active in acne, and AGN190168, an acetylenic retinoid shown to be clinically useful in psoriasis.

Systemic Retinoids

Isotretinoin

Isotretinoin is now prescribed for clinical conditions that go beyond the only approved use of this drug, the treatment of severe recalcitrant acne.[9] Increasing experience has led to its use in: (a) severe acne unresponsive to conventional therapy; (b) moderately severe acne showing only partial response to 18 months of conventional therapy; (c) moderately severe acne that rapidly relapses following several successful courses of conventional therapy; (d) intractable gram-negative folliculitis; (e) severe rosacea unresponsive to conventional therapy with long-term antibiotics; (f) dysmorphophobic acne; and (g) acne fulminans. Residual acne continues to improve after treatment is stopped, and most patients show a remission that lasts for two years or more; in fact many patients need no further treatment.

Isotretinoin is contraindicated in pregnancy and must not be taken by female patients of child-bearing potential who are not taking effective contraceptive measures. The full range of side-effects is discussed later.

Etretinate/Acitretin

Following oral administration, etretinate is metabolized to acitretin, the therapeutically active form of the drug. Acitretin has now been developed as a drug for therapeutic use in its own right, and for most purposes will replace etretinate. Both drugs can produce striking changes in the skin and mucous membranes through their effects on cell differentiation. Etretinate has proved to be effective in the treatment of erythrodermic and generalized pustular psoriasis,[10] but is somewhat less effective in chronic plaque psoriasis when used as monotherapy. It may be used alone in these conditions or in combination with psoralen and ultraviolet A radiation (PUVA). Several clinical trials have confirmed that the efficacy and side-effect profile of acitretin are similar to those of etretinate.[11]

A wide range of congenital disorders of keratinization respond to treatment with etretinate. These include many ichthyotic conditions, pityriasis rubra pilaris, nonbullous ichthyosiform erythroderma, and Darier's disease. Both drugs may also be helpful in the treatment and prophylaxis of widespread epidermal dysplasia and malignancy seen in chronic solar damage and in the chronically immunosuppressed. The inflammatory disorders discoid lupus erythematosus and lichen planus also may respond to etretinate and acitretin. For most of these conditions, long-term treatment is required, as prolonged remissions following treatment withdrawal are uncommon.

As with isotretinoin, both drugs are contraindicated in pregnancy and in female patients of child-bearing potential who are not taking effective contraceptive measures. The side-effects are considered later.

Retinoid Effects and Mode of Action

The fundamental role of retinoids in influencing cell growth and differentiation and the wide variety of these effects in different biologic systems is explained by the presence of a number of nuclear retinoic acid receptors that mediate these actions. Gene cloning has revealed homology for these receptors with nuclear receptors for steroid and thyroid hormones and vitamin D_3, confirming their inclusion in the nuclear receptor superfamily.[12] Differences in the expression of retinoic acid receptors in different tissues and in binding of retinoids to them has revealed a complex cell regulatory system whose control and over-all integration have yet to be fully established. It has been suggested that cytoplasmic retinoic acid-binding proteins (CRABPs) may bind free retinoic acid within cells and thereby provide fine regulation of the amount of biologically potent free retinoic acid.

Topical Retinoids

Topical retinoic acid has comedolytic actions mediated by loosening the adhesion of corneocytes and by induction of proliferation of the follicular epithelium. Topical retinoic acid is a skin irritant, and there is overlap for therapeutically effective concentrations with irritant concentrations. During the first few days of treatment, stinging, burning, pinkness, and scaling are common. Sometimes pustules develop, caused by the rupture of follicular epithelia and the expulsion of microcomedones. Provided treatment is continued throughout this period, an improvement usually occurs with clearance of comedones. Such improvement can then be maintained with less frequent application of retinoic acid.

Systemic Retinoids

Differentiation

It is well known that vitamin A deficiency results in epithelial squamous metaplasia that can be fully reversed by retinol supplements. These properties are shared by most retinoids that cause hyperplasia and reduced epithelial differentiation. Retinoid effects on cell differentiation also have been demonstrated in other cell types, including human myeloid leukemia cells, metaplastic bronchial epithelium, and connective tissue.

Malignancy

There is great variation in the effectiveness of given retinoids for treatment of given tumors.[r4] Epidermal neoplastic disorders such as solar keratoses, Bowen's disease, and basal cell carcinomas respond to systemic retinoids, which are particularly useful when there are large numbers of such lesions. Despite the inhibitory effects of retinoids on a number of human tumor-cell lines in vitro, retinoids have not yet proved to be important in nonepidermal cancer treatment.[r5] However, in combination with PUVA, etretinate has proved helpful in the management of mycosis fungoides, and in immunosuppressed transplant recipients etretinate is helpful in preventing malignant transformation of the multiple premalignant lesions commonly seen in such patients. Retinoids inhibit ornithine decarboxylase—an enzyme known to be associated with polyamine synthesis and carcinogenesis. The importance of this inhibition is uncertain.

Immune Effects

Retinoids exhibit immune-modulating effects at both the humoral and cellular level. They may act as an adjuvant and stimulate antibody formation to antigens not previously immunogenic. Effects on cellular immunity include inhibition of T-cell function by isotretinoin in a dose-dependent manner, suppressive effects on macrophages, and stimulation of Type IV hypersensitivity.

Anti-inflammatory Activity

Retinoids vary in their capacity to influence inflammatory processes. There is a reduction in blood sedimentation rate and acute phase reactants in treatment of severe inflammatory acne with isotretinoin. Both isotretinoin and etretinate have inhibitory effects on neutrophil and monocyte function, but these effects are less prominent for retinoic acid.

Sebosuppression

Isotretinoin is clinically the most potent sebosuppressive retinoid, and this effect is probably the most important of its various therapeutic actions on nodulocystic acne.[r6] In contrast, topical application of isotretinoin causes skin irritation at concentrations that are insufficient to produce any sebosuppressive effects. Etretinate has virtually no sebosuppressive properties and is of no therapeutic use in acne.

Connective Tissue Effects

Retinoids enhance the synthesis of some proteins derived from fibroblasts, such as fibronectin, and reduce the synthesis of others, such as collagenase. Retinoic acid is considerably more potent than retinol in mediating these effects.

Undesirable Effects of Retinoids. Retinoid Drug–Drug Interactions

Topical Retinoids

Topical retinoids have few adverse effects other than being mildly irritant to some patients during the first few days of treatment. Less than 5 percent of patients are unable to tolerate topical retinoids; in such patients prolonged application may induce an irritant eczema. More commonly, reduction in concentration, decrease in frequency of application, and the use of emollients can overcome the mild irritant effects experienced with topical retinoids. A degree of erythema and a drying effect are often experienced as normal therapeutic effects of topical retinoids, which are well tolerated when mild, but if more severe may be less acceptable. Topical retinoids have a low potential for inducing contact allergy. Patients using topical retinoids sometimes complain of increased sensitivity to the sun. This appears to be due to reduction in thickness of the stratum corneum rather than a true chemical photo-irritancy.

There is no evidence that topical retinoids are responsible for human fetal abnormalities.

Systemic Retinoids

Systemic retinoids are potent teratogens, and their most significant adverse effects are dysmorphogenesis and embryotoxicity. They are not, however, mutagenic, as demonstrated by negative results in various test systems of mutagenicity, including the Ames test. Mild abnormalities in sperm numbers and morphology have been reported in animals treated with high doses of retinoids, but no impairment of male reproductive capacity or alterations in sperm have been identified in humans, despite detailed investigation. Systemic retinoids cause transient minor abnormalities in liver function in approximately 10 percent of patients, and 25 to 30 percent of patients develop increases in cholesterol and triglyceride values. Rarer side-effects are myalgias and arthralgias, which occur in about 10 percent of patients, and skeletal dangers, which occur in less than 5 percent of patients. Mucocutaneous side-effects occur in nearly all patients treated with systemic retinoids (95%) and seldom require modification or discontinuation of therapy.

Teratogenicity

Doses of vitamin A in excess of 25,000 IU daily are reported to be associated with an increased rate of fetal abnormality, which has led to the recommendation in some countries for pregnant women to avoid foods that are particularly rich in vitamin A. Inadvertent exposure to retinoids during human pregnancy constitutes a more serious risk, and has resulted in a spectrum of malformations in the progeny, in addition to an increased rate of spontaneous abortion.[17] Abnormalities include craniofacial defects, cardiovascular malformations, CNS defects, and thymic anomalies. The relative risk of malformation in fetuses that survive to 20 weeks' gestation is 25 percent following maternal exposure to 13-cis retinoic acid at therapeutic doses. Etretinate is potentially as much as seven times more teratogenic than 13-cis-retinoic acid, and its extremely long half-life makes its use in women of child-bearing potential contraindicated. Neither all-trans-retinoic acid nor 13-cis-retinoic acid is absorbed to a significant degree in humans following topical application, and their teratogenic potential is therefore very low.

Experimental evidence suggests that retinoid-induced embryopathy is largely attributable to a major effect on neural crest cells that occurs during the fourth week of gestation. The consistent pattern of malformations following human exposure to isotretinoin suggests a narrow "window" of vulnerability. In contrast, retinoids that are more teratogenic, such as etretin, cause a broader spectrum of malformations. The basis for retinoid sensitivity of some embryonic cells remains uncertain, but, as with the therapeutic effects of retinoids, a direct action on the genome resulting in altered regulation of differentiation seems likely.

Lipids

Isotretinoin, etretinate, and acitretin may all cause increases in serum triglycerides and cholesterol. The mechanisms underlying this retinoid-induced alteration in serum lipids probably are the same for all three drugs—that is, by interference with the complex lipoprotein metabolic system. Intestinal absorption of lipids is not increased by synthetic retinoids.

However, retinoids interfere with lipoprotein metabolism by increasing the synthesis of triglycerides or very low density lipoprotein, or by inhibiting their elimination from the circulation. Isotretinoin-induced hyperlipidemia is caused by decreased uptake and degradation of very low density lipoproteins by parenchymal liver cells.[13] Fat elimination and degradation are impaired to a lesser degree by etretinate and acitretin. Alterations in lipid metabolism induced by retinoids are reversible on withdrawal of treatment. However, the raised serum lipid levels with acitretin, etretinate, and isotretinoin imply an augmented risk for the development of atherosclerosis in patients on long-term therapy. It is recommended that fasting lipids be measured before commencing treatment with systemic retinoids in order to detect occult cases of hyperlipidemia. Triglyceride and cholesterol levels should then be repeated after one month's therapy; if no increase is observed, a check-up every two to four months should suffice. If serum lipids are raised, the dose of retinoid may need to be reduced or, rarely, even stopped altogether. Another approach is to use a low-fat diet. In the more severe cases in which stopping the retinoid is inadvisable, use of fish oil supplements or lipid-lowering drugs has been advised.

Liver Function Abnormalities

About 10 percent of patients treated with oral retinoids develop transient abnormalities in liver function, as indicated by small rises in liver enzymes and bilirubin. Isotretinoin, etretinate, and acitretin may all cause such temporary changes, which are reversible on reduction or withdrawal of therapy. Studies on oral retinoids that have included liver biopsy have confirmed the lack of drug-induced hepatotoxicity. However, there have been isolated reports of toxic liver damage in patients treated with retinoids, most commonly in patients with pre-existing liver disease, although occasionally such a history was absent.

Bone Changes

Skeletal effects of overdosage with vitamin A have been well known since the 1940s. Following the introduction of synthetic retinoids for the treatment of dermatologic conditions, skeletal abnormalities have been reported, including premature closure of epithyses, periosteal-cortical hyperostosis, bony spurring at sites of ligamentous and tendon insertions, and osteoporosis. Premature epiphyseal fusion and serious bony changes with alteration of function have proved rare, but there has been considerable debate as to the prevalence and relevance of disseminated interstitial skeletal hyperostosis (DISH syndrome) in patients on retinoids. Present evidence on bony changes associated with retinoids does not warrant their restriction, although where long-term therapy is anticipated base line radiographs of a particular area such as the ankles may prove helpful subsequently.

Mucocutaneous Side-Effects

Retinoid-induced mucocutaneous side-effects occur in nearly all patients treated with oral retinoids and are generally well-tolerated. Cheilitis and dry nose are present in most patients and may be used to assess dosage and patient compliance. Ocular involvement is rare with etretinate and acitretin, but is commoner with isotretinoin, which affects the function of the meibomian glands, leading to alteration in the composition of the tear film. Increased rate of hair loss is of particular concern to women. It is reversible and usually transient and mild, but has led a few patients to stop treatment.

Cutaneous side-effects of retinoids include transient worsening of acne with isotretinoin, desquamation, xerosis, retinoid-dermatitis, and retinoid-induced facial erythema. Etretinate may rarely induce a rosacea-like eruption, and etretinate and isotretinoin occasionally increase photosensitivity, which probably has a phototoxic mechanism, due to thinning of the stratum corneum. Painful paronychial granulation tissue is an occasional problem. A much rarer side effect is the appearance of granulation tissue at sites of healing hemorrhagic nodulocystic acne in patients taking isotretinoin.

The mechanisms underlying the mucocutaneous side-effects of retinoids are the same as the mechanisms for the desirable effects on the skin, and are covered in the section on Retinoid Effects and Mode of Action.

Drug Interactions

Oral retinoids have few interactions with other drugs. Combination treatment with vitamin A increases the risk of symptoms of overdosage of vitamin

Table 81.1 Available Preparations and Usual Doses

	Tablet Dosages/Formulation and Concentration of Topicals	Recommended Initial Dosage	Method of Administration	Dose Range
Oral agents				
Isotretinoin	5mg; 20mg	0.5mg/kg/day	Divided dose with food	0.1mg/kg/day-1mg/kg/day
Etretinate	10mg; 25mg	0.75mg/kg/day	Divided dose with food	0.25mg/kg/day-1mg/kg/day
Acitretin	10mg; 25mg	25–30mg daily	Divided dose with food	25–75mg/day
Topical agents				
Retinoic acid	Cream: 0.025%; 0.05%; 0.1% Gel: 0.01%; 0.025% Lotion: 0.025%	Applied once or twice daily	Thin topical administration	0.01%–0.05%
Isotretinoin	Gel: 0.05%	Applied once or twice daily	Thin topical administration	Not relevant

A and should therefore be avoided. Both isotretinoin and etretinate rarely may cause benign intracranial hypertension, and concomitant use of other drugs that also induce this unusual side-effect, such as tetracyclines, may produce an additive effect and should therefore be avoided. Phenytoin and barbiturates may both interact with retinoids to produce altered serum concentrations of either drug, and caution should be exercised in cases where concomitant treatment is considered.

A number of drugs adversely affect the pathologic processes underlying psoriasis and may therefore work against the beneficial effects of oral retinoids in this context. Examples of such drugs are aspirin (particularly in high doses), lithium, β-blockers, antimalarials, and tetracyclines. Nonsteroidal anti-inflammatory drugs are often used in psoriatic arthropathy, which affects about 10 percent of patients, and may impair the efficacy of retinoids used for the skin disease.

Toxic Effects of Overdoses of Retinoids

Overdosage of retinoids greatly in excess of therapeutic requirements results in a syndrome known as hypervitaminosis A. Some of these features are manifest during the therapeutic use of synthetic retinoids in the treatment of dermatologic conditions. The toxicity of retinol depends on the age of the patient, the daily dose, and the duration of administration. During infancy, as little as 7.5 to 15 mg of retinol daily for 30 days can induce toxicity, whereas in adults toxicity is uncommon with consumption of less than 30 mg of retinol per day. Mild symptoms of hypervitaminosis A may, however, occur in adults who consume 10 to 20 mg of retinol daily for six months or more. Acute toxicity also may occur with large doses of retinol: more than 500 mg of retinol in an adult, 100 mg in a young child, and 30 mg in an infant frequently results in acute toxic effects. It is recommended that daily ingestion of retinol should not exceed 7.5 mg; however, as many as 5 percent of those who take vitamin A supplements in the USA exceed this dose.

Signs of acute poisoning with retinol are partly explained by raised intracranial pressure. These include drowsiness, irritability, headache, dizziness, vomiting, and papilledema, and constitute a medical emergency. Later effects are acute enlargement of the liver with abdominal pain and, after 24 hours, generalized peeling of the skin. Mucocutaneous changes are often the first features on chronic retinoid toxicity, and include facial dermatitis, desquamation of the skin, dry fissured lips and nostrils, altered hair texture, and sometimes generalized hair loss. Less common effects are aching in the muscles, bones and joints, and headaches, anorexia, fatigue, and irritability secondary to raised intracranial pressure manifest early with a bulging fontanelle, irritability, and vomiting.

Pharmacokinetics

Vitamin A

Dietary vitamin A is mainly in the form of esters, usually retinyl palmitate. Most of these retinyl esters are hydrolyzed in the intestinal lumen by pancreatic enzymes before absorption. Uptake of retinol by tissues is facilitated by a carrier-protein that specifically binds retinol with high affinity (cellular retinol-binding protein II or CRBO II). Most of the retinol is then re-esterified and incorporated into chylomicrons. The concentration of esterified retinol reaches a peak about four hours after ingestion of retinol. Most of the retinyl esters are taken up by the liver and stored, where the half-life of stores in the presence of a vitamin A-free diet is approximately 50 to 100 days. Before entering the circulation from the liver, hepatic retinyl esters are hydrolyzed; then most are bound to an alpha$_1$-globulin (retinol binding protein or RBP). This retinol complex then circulates until it binds to specific sites on the target cell surface. Retinol is then transferred from the RBP to a membrane-bound protein and converted into a retinyl ester. This in turn is cleaved by a membrane-associated hydrolase and free retinol is then taken up by free cytosolic CRBP. Retinol is in part conjugated in the liver to form a beta-glucuronide, which undergoes enterohepatic circulation and is in turn oxidized to retinal and retinoid acid. A number of other water-soluble metabolites are excreted in the urine and feces. The pharmacokinetics of vitamin A are reviewed in detail by Goodman.[r8]

Isotretinoin

The bioavailability of isotretinoin in fasting subjects is approximately 25 percent following oral administration.[r9] It is rapidly absorbed to give peak concentrations in the blood after one to four hours. The presence of food substantially increases the extent of systemic absorption. About six hours after administration the main metabolite of isotretinoin, 4-oxo-isotretinoin, is present in a higher concentration than the parent compound. Isotretinoin is almost completely (> 99.5%) bound to albumin in plasma. It is not stored in the tissues and its concentration is generally lower outside the circulation than within. Experimental evidence suggests that isotretinoin is transferred across the placenta and is secreted into breast milk, although this has not been corroborated with human studies. The half-life of isotretinoin is between 10 and 20 hours, whereas that of the main metabolite is 29 hours. After repeated administration, stable concentrations are established within 5–7 days. Isotretinoin is cleared almost entirely by metabolism with negligible urinary elimination of the intact drug. There are several metabolites that are cleared from the circulation rather slowly and in view of the general concern about teratogenicity with retinoids it is recommended that effective contraception is maintained for at least two months after isotretinoin is stopped. A pharmacodynamic study has confirmed that isotretinoin does not impair the activity of oral contraceptive drugs. Excretion is via the bile and urine. Assessment of isotretinoin levels in biologic fluids may be performed by HPLC with ultraviolet detection, but is not useful in the routine monitoring of patients.

Acitretin

Acitretin is variably and incompletely absorbed after oral dosage and is then about 98 percent bound to albumin.[r10] Absorption is increased when given with food, which produces an absolute bioavailability of approximately 60 percent. As with isotretinoin, peak plasma concentrations are reached within four hours and then rapidly decline over the next eight hours to below assay sensitivity. Considerable variability has been observed in the peak plasma concentrations, which may show up to twofold differences within a subject and 15-fold differences between subjects. Such variability is reduced by administering acitretin with food. Plasma concentrations reach a steady state within two to three weeks of repeated oral administration, which is consistent with a half-life for acitretin of approximately 50 hours. Following absorption into the blood, acitretin is rapidly isomerized and/or metabolized to up to 12 possible metabolites. The isomer of acitretin, cis-acitretin, has a longer half-life than the parent drug with which it is in equilibrium. The kinetics of acitretin on withdrawal of therapy are therefore formation rate-limited from the metabolite cis-acitretin, and both compounds are eliminated at similar rates. In common with etretinate, acitretin is very lipophilic, but owing to a relatively polar carboxyl group, acitretin is some 50 times less lipophilic than etretinate and therefore less likely to accumulate in adipose tissue. However, the formation of trace levels of etretinate from acitretin has meant that advice concerning avoidance of conception in females for two years after treatment withdrawal is the same as etretinate. Excretion is via the bile and urine. Acitretin can be measured in plasma by HPLC but this is not used in clinical practice, where appropriate dosage is determined by titration against therapeutic response.

Etretinate

The bioavailability of etretinate following oral dosage is approximately 40 percent, although there is considerable interindividual variation (30–70%). Etretinate reaches peak plasma concentrations after two to four hours, where it is largely (98%) bound to lipoproteins. The high lipophilicity of etretinate results in its substantial storage in the "deep tissue compartment" and accounts for a long elimination half-life after maintenance administration of 80–100 days. Etretinate may continue to be detectable in the blood 12 months after withdrawal of therapy. In women in the reproductive age group, contraception should be practiced for two years after stopping treatment. Animal studies have confirmed that etretinate crosses the placenta and also is excreted in breast milk. Etretinate is rapidly metabolized to its main metabolite, the free aromatic acid (acitretin). Excretion is via the bile and urine. Etretinate is detected in plasma by HPLC, but is not measured in routine clinical practice, where dosage is determined by titration against therapeutic response.

References

Research Reports

1. McCollum EV, Davis M. The necessity of certain lipids in the diet during growth. J Biol Chem 1913;*15*:167–175.
2. Steenbock H. White corn vs yellow corn, and a probable relation between the fat-soluble vitamin and yellow plant pigments. Science 1919;*50*:352–353.
3. Karrer P, Morf R, Schopp K. Zur kenntnis des Vitamin A aus fischtranen. Helv Chim Acta 1931;*14*:1036–1040.
4. Morton RA. Chemical aspects of the visual process. Nature (London) 1944;*153*:69–71.
5. van Dorp DA, Arens JF. The synthesis of vitamin A acid, a biologically active substance. Rec Trav Chim 1946;*65*:338–345.
6. Stuttgen D. Zur lokalbehandlung von keratosen mit Vitamin A - saure. Dermatologica 1962;*124*:65–80.
7. Peck GL, Olsen TG, Butkus D et al. Isotretinoin versus placebo in the treatment of cystic acne. J Am Acad Dermatol 1982;*6*:735–745.
8. Elbaum DJ. Comparison of the stability of topical isotretinoin and topical tretinoin and their efficacy in acne. J Am Acad Dermatol 1988;*19*:486–491.
9. Farrell LN, Strauss JS, Stanieri AM. The treatment of severe cystic acne with 13-cis-retinoic acid. Evaluation of sebum production and clinical response in a multiple dose trial. J Am Acad Dermatol 1980;*3*:602–611.

10. Orfanos CE, Runne U. Systemic use of a new retinoid with and without local dithranol treatment in generalized psoriasis. Br J Dermatol 1976;*95*:101–103.

11. Goldfarb MT, Ellis CN, Gupta AK, Tincoff T, Hamilton TA, Voorhees JJ. Acitretin improves psoriasis in a dose-dependent fashion. J Am Acad Dermatol 1988;*18*:655–662.

12. Petkovich M, Brand NJ, Krust A, Chambon P. A human retinoic acid receptor which belongs to the family of nuclear receptors. Nature 1987;*330*:444–450.

13. Kingston T, Marks R, Cunliffe WJ et al. Isotretinoin and serum lipids. Lancet 1983;*II*:471–472.

Reviews

r1. Apfel C, Crettaz M, Siegenthaler G, Hunziker W. Synthetic retinoids: Differential binding to retinoic acid receptors. In: Saurat J-H, ed. Retinoids: 10 years on. Basel, Karger, 1991, pp 110–120.

r2. Orfanos CE, Ehlert R, Gollnick H. The retinoids: A review of their clinical pharmacology and therapeutic use. Drugs 1987;*34*:459–503.

r3. Wald G. Carotenoids and the visual cycle. J Gen Physiol 1935;*19*:351–371.

r4. Hill DL, Grubbs CJ. Retinoids and cancer prevention. Ann Rev Nutr 1992;*12*:161–181.

r5. Editorial. Retinoids and control of cutaneous malignancy. Lancet 1988;*II*:545–546.

r6. Hughes BR, Cunliffe WJ. The effects of isotretinoin on the pilosebaceous duct in patients with acne. In: Marks R, Plewig G, eds. Acne and related disorders. London: Martin Dunitz, 1989, pp 223–226.

r7. Benke EP. The isotretinoin teratogen syndrome. JAMA 1984;*251*:3267–3269.

r8. Goodman DS. Vitamin A and retinoids in health and disease. N Eng J Med 1984;*310*:1023–1031.

r9. Brazzell RK, Colburn WA. Pharmacokinetics of the retinoids isotretinoin and etretinate. J Am Acad Dermatol 1982;*6*:643–651.

r10. Wiegand U-W, Jensen BK. Pharmacokinetics of acitretin in humans. In: Saurat J-H, ed. Retinoids: 10 years on. Basel, Karger, 1991, pp 192–203.

CHAPTER 82

Antimicrobial Compounds: The Treatment of Chronic Ulcers

Andrew Y. Finlay

Antimicrobial Compounds

Introduction

The antimicrobial compounds covered by this section include antibacterial (antibiotics and antiseptics) and antifungal agents. The commonest indication for the use of antibiotics in dermatology in the developed world is in the therapy of acne, and this is dealt with in a separate chapter. The use of antibiotics for their prime indication of treating infection is of course of great importance in the therapy of impetigo, erysipelas, and cellulitis.

Some skin diseases such as atopic eczema may have secondary infection as a contributing factor to their persistence and/or severity, and here antibiotics combined with anti-inflammatory agents may be of value. Antibiotics are given topically where the infection is superficial, affecting mainly the stratum corneum or epidermis, but systemically if the infection is dermal or subcutaneous. There are a number of antibiotics (e.g., mupirocin) and antifungal agents for which there is no simple method of systemic administration. These agents are therefore by definition reserved for the therapy of cutaneous problems.

A variety of specific systemic antimicrobial compounds are used in such infective skin diseases as leishmaniasis or cutaneous tuberculosis. These disorders are common in the developing world, but may of course occasionally present at a dermatology clinic in the affluent West. Other occasional uses for antibiotics in the practice of dermatology include prophylaxis in skin surgery when a patient has a heart valve problem, although in recent years doubt has been expressed as to the necessity of this in most cases.

The treatment of fungal infections of the skin was transformed by the advent of griseofulvin in the 1960s; over the last 15 years the introduction of various members of the "imidazole" group and more recently the "allylamine" group of antifungal agents for topical and systemic use has resulted in further clinical benefit.

Microbiology of Skin

To understand the impact of antimicrobial compounds on the skin it is necessary to review briefly the microbiology of normal skin. There are large numbers of "resident" bacteria, such as *Propionibacterium acnes* and *Staphylococcus epidermidis;* these organisms grow and multiply on the skin surface and are always present, but their populations are greater in specific areas. Some fungi, such as the yeastlike microorganism *Pityrosporum ovale,* also are resident. Other organisms are transient; they are contaminant and nonreproducing, and may be either harmless or pathogenic. Pathogenic organisms include *Staphylococcus aureus,* which may be carried in the nose or at the perineum.[r1,1]

Antiseptics

Disinfectants are used to kill microorganisms in the general environment. When applied to the skin surface—for example, in a cleansing agent or soap—

they are termed "antiseptics." Antiseptics ideally have a wide range of bactericidal activity that persists for some time after application.

Povidone Iodine

This antiseptic is an iodine complex from which iodine is slowly released. Iodine even in low concentrations rapidly kills bacteria and also may be virucidal. Povidone iodine is used widely to reduce postoperative sepsis. It also may be of value in the therapy of leg ulcers. It is useful in treating the crusted areas of herpes zoster.

It should not be used frequently over large areas in pregnant patients or during breast feeding; rarely, it can cause allergic sensitization.

Povidone-iodine is available in a range of different forms: as an antiseptic spray (5%); paint (10% alcohol solution); aqueous solution (10%); dry powder spray (2.5%); and as a scalp and skin cleanser (7.5%). It is most often used as a skin cleanser solution (4%) and as a surgical scrub (7.5%).[2]

Potassium Permanganate

Potassium permanganate is a time-hallowed dermatologic preparation, prepared as an aqueous solution of 1 in 8000 or 1 in 10,000. It is mildly antiseptic, and is used either in wet dressings applied to infected eczematous areas or to cleanse wounds. The main practical problems are that it stains clothing and other materials and is also irritant to the eyes and other mucous membranes. It is available as a 0.1 percent solution, which has to be further diluted, or as a 400-mg "solution tablet" to be dissolved in 4 liters of water.

Chlorhexidine

This antiseptic is very popular now that hexachlorophane is "out of favor" because of its rare neurotoxic potential with inappropriate use in neonates. Chlorhexidine is used for skin disinfection preoperatively and in obstetrics. It is effective in preventing neonatal skin colonization by staphylococci.

Sensitivity to chlorhexidine occasionally may occur, but this is unusual. It is available in a wide range of preparations as a hydrochloride, gluconate, or acetate salt, and in a range of concentrations. For direct cleansing of wounds a 0.015 or 0.05 percent solution is used; much more concentrated preparations are available for dilution for a range of disinfectant and antiseptic purposes. Eyes and mucous membranes must be avoided.

Topical Antibiotics

The topical antibiotics used in acne, clindamycin, erythromycin, and tetracycline, are described in Chapter 83. Other topical antibiotics used for the treatment of skin infection include mupirocin, neomycin, fusidic acid, and silver sulfadiazine. In addition, topical metronidazole is now available for use in rosacea. There are multiple additional preparations available with wider combinations of antibiotics, antifungal agents, and topical steroids.[r2]

Mupirocin

Mupirocin is pseudomonic acid, an antibiotic that works by interfering with bacterial protein synthesis. There is no cross-resistance with other antibiotics. It can be given only as a topical preparation, and is indicated for staphylococcal and streptococcal impetigo as well as in infected atopic eczema and to stop nasal carriage of staphylococci. It may cause some stinging but is otherwise well tolerated. It is given as a 2 percent ointment applied up to three times daily.[3]

Neomycin

Neomycin is an aminoglycoside too toxic for parenteral use—its application is therefore confined to the skin or to the bowel to reduce the bacterial population of the colon before bowel surgery. It has found its way into a wide variety of creams, ointments, powders, and sprays for skin antisepsis, often as one ingredient of a mixture. As it is an effective antibiotic against many gram-negative and some gram-positive organisms, it is valuable both in treating local skin infections and in preventing infection occuring postoperatively. It is unfortunately a well recognized cause of allergic hypersensitivity, and it is often in this context that patients using this drug are seen by dermatologists. As an ointment or cream, neomycin sulfate 0.5 percent is used once or twice daily.

Silver Sulfadiazine

This preparation is a sulfonamide that acts on the bacterial cell membrane and cell wall. Up to 10 percent may be absorbed. It is widely used in the management of infected burns, being particularly active against *Pseudomonas aeruginosa;* it is also of potential value in the treatment of infected ulcers and pressure sores. The 1 percent cream preparation is well tolerated, and is usually applied daily or on alternate days.

Fusidic Acid

This antibiotic inhibits bacterial protein synthesis. It is available both for topical and systemic use, and is specifically indicated for staphylococcal skin infections and abscesses. When used topically there may be hypersensitivity reactions, but these are rare. To prevent the emergence of resistant organisms it is recommended that when used orally, fusidic acid be used along with other antibiotics such as penicillin. As an oral preparation it is given in a dose of 500 mg every eight hours.

Metronidazole

Metronidazole is a derivative of 5-nitroimidazole that works by a metabolite of the metronidazole interfering with DNA. It is active against anaerobic protozoa and anaerobic bacteria. In recent years it has been of interest in dermatology because of its value as a second-line systemic agent for rosacea and because of its recently advocated use as a topical agent (in a 0.75% gel) for this disease. It has also been advocated topically as a "deodorizing agent" for infected, sloughy, intractable ulcers. The main problem with its oral use is that when alcohol is taken at the same time a disulfuram-like reaction may be induced, but the likelihood of this occurring with topical applications is remote.

Topical Antifungal Agents

Candida, dermatophytes, and pityrosporum ovale are all causative agents in human fungal disease of the skin. Systemic antifungal agents used to treat skin fungal infections include griseofulvin, the imidazoles such as ketoconazole, itraconazole, and fluconazole, and the allylamine terbinafine. Topical antifungal agents include a range of imadazoles such as miconazole, econazole, clotrimazole, and ketoconazole, and the polyene antibiotic nystatin. In addition, topical selenium sulfide is effective in pityriasis versicolor.[r3,r4]

Nystatin

Nystatin is a polyene antibiotic produced by the growth of *Streptomyces noursei.* Its fungistatic and fungicidal actions result from interference with fungal cell membrane permeability by its binding to ergosterol. It is effective against a range of yeasts and fungi, including Aspergillus species and *Cryptococcus neoformans,* but its main indication is for the treatment of *Candida albicans* infection of the skin and mucous membranes. It is not effective against dermatophyte infections. There are very few problems with its topical use, although allergic contact dermatitis rarely may occur. It is prescribed as a cream, ointment, or powder; these preparations are usually at a strength of 100,000 units per mg. The application is repeated two to four times daily until clinical cure.[5]

Miconazole

Miconazole is an imidazole antifungal that works, as do all imidazoles, by interfering with ergosterol synthesis, thereby affecting fungal cell wall permeability. It is effective against most common dermatophytes, and also against pityrosporum ovale and *Candida albicans.* Its broad spectrum of activity makes it a very useful topical agent in the treatment of fungal infections of the skin. It is well tolerated. Available usually as a 2 percent cream, powder, or ointment, it is applied twice daily to affected areas, usually for four weeks to allow time for complete renewal of the stratum corneum.

Ketoconazole

Ketoconazole is an imidazole antifungal agent; its main use has been as a systemic therapy in the treatment of a wide range of different systemic and cutaneous fungal infections. The rare occurrence of hepatotoxicity has now severely restricted the indications for its systemic use, but in dermatology there has been a revival of interest in this drug as a topical agent. Although active topically also against dermatophytes, its main use has been as a therapy for seborrhoeic dermatitis, which is thought to be at least exacerbated, or possibly caused, by *Pityrosporum ovale.* It is well tolerated topically, but should not be used on areas previously treated with topical steroids (especially the face) until there has been a "rest period" of about two weeks, or a transient irritant reaction may occur. It is available as a 2 percent cream or 5 percent shampoo and should be applied once or twice daily until a few days after clinical signs of infection have settled.[6]

Other Topical Antifungal Agents

Clotrimazole is a widely used imidazole antifungal agent. It is very effective against candida as well as against dermatophytes and is available as a 1 percent cream, solution, or powder; it is applied twice daily. Econazole has a spectrum of activity similar to ketoconazole and miconazole. Other topical imidazoles include isoconazole and sulconazole. Belonging to a different class of drugs, naftifine is a topical allylamine, which, in addition to its fungicidal actions, has an anti-inflammatory effect.

Treatment of Chronic Ulcers

The management of a chronic ulcer depends on a wide range of factors; this review will concentrate on the topical applications and dressings used. Diagnosis of the cause of the ulcer is, of course, the most crucial initial step. Leg ulcers are most commonly venous ulcers caused by long-term increased venous pressure and fibrinogen deposition around dermal blood vessels, but may be arterial in origin. Other causes of ulceration include infections, vasculitis, malignancy, and neurologic disease; initial therapy should, of course, be aimed at removal of the cause. Treatment of venous ulceration must include attention to the general medical state of the patient and edema and anemia must be corrected. Elevation of the leg is said to be of importance in promoting healing, but this in practice is very difficult to achieve for any significant length of time daily. The single most important aspect of management is regular and effective compression of the leg from the toes to above the knee using a graduated pressure stocking or compression bandage. Application of a bandage must be carried out evenly and by a trained person to ensure graduated pressure and to avoid any uneven constriction. Crepe bandages or simple support stockings are of no value because the pressures exerted are usually not great enough. While emphasizing the importance of compression in the management of venous ulceration, it must be stressed that compression is contraindicated in ulcers of arterial origin; differentiation between the two may be aided by the use of Doppler ultrasound, but some ulcers may be multifactorial.

Topical Applications for Ulcers

The functions of topical applications in the management of ulcers include treatment of infection, clearance of debris, crust, exudate, or scar, and the provision of a comfortable and protective dressing.

Treatment of Infection

All areas of skin ulceration are rapidly colonized by a host of different organisms, some potentially pathogenic. A swab from any ulcer will therefore grow many different bacteria. The presence of bacteria by itself however is not an indication for antimicrobial therapy—any attempt to eradicate all bacteria is doomed to failure and will carry the risk of encouraging the development of resistant organisms and the possible hazard of inducing allergic hypersenitization.

It is more logical to restrict the use of antibiotics to their systemic applications, and only when there is clinical evidence of the bacteria causing disease by inducing local cellulitis. On first presentation, however, when faced with an oozing, purulent, superficially inflamed ulcerated area, it does make sense to use antiseptic agents to control rapidly any superficial overgrowth of organisms. The antiseptics described above such as povidone iodine or potassium permanganate are appropriate.

Clearance of Debris: Desloughing Agents

Where there has been an accumulation of thick crust this may often be loosened and removed by simply soaking the ulcer in saline or potassium permangenate dressings for a few days. Where a thick, tough eschar has built up, local surgical debridement may be the most effective way of removal, but usually this is not necessary and the eschar can be loosened and eventually removed by using topical agents. Preparations that may be helpful in this situation include:

1. Hydrogen peroxide (1.5%) cream.
2. Steptokinase, streptodornase powder (100,000 units of each enzyme per gm powder).
3. Dextranomer beads.

Dressings

A vast range of topical dressings and applications are available for the treatment of ulcers. Most have not been adequately evaluated in long-term controlled double-blind trials. Probably the most important function of ulcer dressings is to provide some comfort and protection for the wound, and to provide an optimal local environment to allow natural re-epithelialisation. Claims that ulcer dressings actually actively promote healing beyond this role should be examined critically. The widespread use of hydrocolloid dressings has occurred largely because there is some evidence that the local environment created by these dressings at the wound site promotes growth of granulation tissue. In addition they are generally comfortable and can be left in place for two or three days. The main objection to their use is the odor and unpleasant appearance of the fluid that collects beneath the dressing and often seeps out—but this is obvious only at the time of redressing and in the initial stages of therapy.

Other hydrogel dressing preparations introduced over the last decade include microbeads of starch gel containing iodine, multilayered charcoal cloth dressings to absorb odor, and calcium alginate dressings derived from seaweed.

References

Research Reports

1. Marples RR. In: Maibach HI, Aly R: Skin microbiology—Relevance to infection. New York: Springer-Verlag, 1981, pp 45–61.
2. McClusky B. A prospective study of providone iodine solution in the prevention of wound sepsis. *Aust NZ J Surg* 1976;*44*:254–256.
3. Mertz PM, Marshall DA, Eaglstein WH, Piovanetti Y, Montalvo J. Topical mupirocin treatment of impetigo is equal to oral erythromycin therapy. Arch Dermatol 1989;*125*:1069–1073.

4. Rosenblatt JE, Edson RS. Metronidazole. Mayo Clin Proc 1983;*53*:154–162.

5. Clayton YM:, Connor BL. Comparison of clotrimazole cream, Whitfield's ointment and nystatin ointment for topical treatment of ringworm infections, pityriasis versicolor, erythrasma and candidiasis. Br J Dermatol 1973;*89*:297–303.

6. Carr M, Price D, Ive FA. Treatment of seborrhoeic dermatitis with ketoconazole: response of seborrhoeic dermatitis of the scalp with topical ketoconazole. Br J Dermatol 1986;*116*:213–216.

Reviews

r1. Noble WC. Microbiology of human skin. London:Lloyd-Luke Medical Books, 1981.

r2. Hirschmann JV. Topical antibiotics in dermatology. Arch Dermatol 1988;*124*:1691–1700.

r3. Davies RR. Griseofulvin. In:Speller DCE. Antifungal chemotherapy, Chichester:John Wiley, 1980, pp 149–182.

r4. Hay RJ. New oral treatments for dermatophytosis. Ann NY Acad Sci 1988;*544*:580–585.

r5. Philpot CM. Geographic distribution of the dermatophytes: A review. J Hyg 1978;*80*:301–313.

CHAPTER 83

Topical Treatments for Acne

Andrew Y. Finlay

Introduction

Acne is an extremely common disorder—in its mildest form it is virtually universal in late teenage. Very effective therapy with long term oral antibiotics and oral isotretinoin is available for moderate to severe acne, but common mild to moderate acne can be treated adequately in most young people with the correct use of topical agents.

Simple skin cleansers may have some marginal value, but the effective topical acne preparations contain active agents, usually benzoyl peroxide, antibiotics, or retinoic acid. Azelaic acid is an interesting new compound that also may prove beneficial for this group of patients. The biggest single cause of failure of acne therapy is lack of compliance, and patients need encouragement to continue on regular therapy over extended periods.

Benzoyl Peroxide

Benzoyl peroxide ($C_{14}H_{10}O_4$) is a strong oxidizing agent and is used as a bleaching agent in the food industry—curiously, in its pure powder form it may decompose violently! It has been used in acne for about 20 years, being one of the first effective topical agents for this condition. Since then, in higher concentrations of 20 percent or more, it has been used as a cleansing agent in gravitational leg ulcers and pressure sores.

The mode of action of benzoyl peroxide in acne is through its effect on comedones and its action as an antimicrobial agent against *Propionibacterium acnes*. When measured, its effect on comedogenesis is very slight, but clinically it appears to reduce the number of visible comedones.[1] Benzoyl peroxide reduces duct colonization and drastically reduces the population of *Propionibacterium acnes* and *Staphylococcus epidermidis* on the skin surface. It also may have a direct anti-inflammatory effect.[2]

The addition of sulfur to benzoyl peroxide reflects a hallowed tradition of the use of sulfur in topical remedies that stretches back many centuries. Good evidence of its value is lacking, and there is controversy over whether topical sulfur may even promote the production of comedones.

Benzoyl peroxide should be used for patients with the common form of mild inflammatory acne, and it is clinically helpful for most patients with mild acne; as with most acne therapies, however, it needs to be continued on a regular basis and its unsupervised intermittent use as a preparation available "over the counter" may not result in optimal benefit.

Benzoyl peroxide can have an irritant effect, resulting in a scaling "drying" effect; for this reason it needs to be used with care initially. Its bleaching effect can be a nuisance on hair and skin as well as on clothing.

Benzoyl peroxide is usually applied twice daily; initially 2.5 percent preparations are used to reduce the chances of the patient's developing an irritant reaction. The strength is then increased to 5 or 10 percent. Various bases are used; water as a base is better tolerated than alcohol. It should be applied to the whole of the affected area, not just to "the spots"—this is to prevent the appearance of new lesions.

Topical Antibiotics

A variety of topical antibiotics are claimed to be of value in the therapy of acne; there is good evidence that erythromycin,[3] clindamycin, and tetracycline are all of benefit.

Topical antibiotics in acne presumably work by their effect on reducing the population of *Propionibacterium acnes* and *Staphylococcus epidermidis* on the skin surface and within the pilo-sebaceous apparatus; the best evidence for this is with clindamycin. Although a separate anti-inflammatory effect has been proposed as one of the modes of action of antibiotics given systemically for acne, there is less evidence for this in their topical use.

The indications for topical antibiotics in acne are the same as those for benzoyl peroxide—mild to moderate pustular or inflammatory acne. Topical erythromycin 2 percent has been shown to reduce acne severity by 40 percent over a 12-week study and to be significantly superior to placebo.[4] Similar results have been obtained for topical clindamycin.

One advantage of giving antibiotics topically is the resulting reduction in systemic side-effects. Clindamycin, for example, would not be appropriate given orally because of the poor risk-benefit ratio concerning the possibility of pseudomembranous colitis; topical preparations are of course absorbed, but only in extremely small amounts, and so the likelihood of this side-effect is extremely low with topical application.[1] Topical tetracyclines have the disadvantage of staining yellow and fluorescing under UV radiation—a potential hazard at discotheques! Although not usually a disadvantage for the individual patient, there is a concern that the widespread use of topical antibiotics for acne will result in resistant organisms being selected in the community. The use of topical erythromycin for six months encourages the development of multiply-resistant staphylococci and resistant propionibacteria.[r1]

Topical antibiotics usually are applied twice daily to the affected areas for three to four months. Clindamycin 1 percent, erythromycin 2 percent, or tetracycline 2.2mg/ml are given most often in an alcoholic base. In some preparations, the constituent powder and alcoholic bases have to be freshly mixed at the time of dispensing.

Retinoic Acid (see also Chapter 81)

Retinoic acid has a variety of alternative names including Vitamin A acid, all-trans-retinoic acid, tretinoin, and Retin-A. This retinoid has been used topically for the treatment of mild to moderate acne for more than 20 years but should not be confused with isotretinoin (13 cis-retinoic acid), which is extremely effective orally in the therapy of severe acne. Topical isotretinoin gel (0.05%) is now also available in some countries and appears as effective as tretinoin in treating acne. Recently there has been great interest in the effects of topical retinoic acid in reversing some aspects of photodamage, and although this is not a licensed indication for its use in the US or UK, much retinoic acid is actually being used for this purpose. It is also used in the treatment of some hyperkeratotic conditions.

Retinoic acid works in acne by its effects on epidermal proliferation and differentiation, restoring abnormal keratinization processes in the follicular duct to normal. This results in softening and removal of comedones initially present, and stops new comedones forming. As well as its direct effect on comedone production, there may be a reduction in the ductal *P. acnes* population by an alteration in the local environment of the duct.

As would be expected from its prime effect on the process of keratinization, retinoic acid is of particular value in the treatment of acne where comedones obviously predominate; it is, however, of benefit in all presentations of mild to moderate acne. Its effectiveness is equivalent to that of benzoyl peroxide.

The side-effects of retinoic acid are noticeable by most people who use it—an initial inflammatory response of redness and soreness that settles with continued use. This effect is seen whatever the underlying problem, and therefore is not simply an exacerbation of the acne. During therapy there may be increased sensitivity to UV radiation as the protective effect of the stratum corneum may be lessened.

Topical tretinoin is available as a 0.05 percent cream, and 0.025 percent gel or lotion. It is applied twice daily for several weeks. Topical isotretinoin is available as an 0.05 percent gel.

Azeleic Acid

Azeleic acid is a dicarboxylic acid produced when the fungus pityrosporum is cultured. It was first noted to be of interest therapeutically when it was shown to inhibit tyrosinase competitively in vitro. Clinical testing followed in patients with melanoma—and a coincidental improvement in acne was noted.[6] As so often in medicine, clinical advances are made by astute clinical observation and intelligent follow-up of events that others might dismiss. Further clinical studies have confirmed its effectiveness[7] in acne.

The mode of action of azeleic acid may be twofold;

it may alter keratinization within the follicle, possibly by an effect on reducing filaggrin formation, and it has an antibacterial action, decreasing the population of *P. acnes*. It has no effect on sebum excretion.

The main indications for the use of azeleic acid are in comedonal acne and for low to moderate grades of acne. It also may be used in more severe forms of acne, but should then be combined with systemic antibiotic therapy.[7]

It is claimed that the clinical effectiveness of azeleic acid is comparable to that of topical tretinoin, benzoyl peroxide, or oral tetracycline. Clinical improvement may not be obvious for the first four weeks.

Azeleic acid appears to be well tolerated, with a low incidence of recorded side-effects. There may be initial local irritation, and after application slight but quickly fading redness, prickling, and some burning in 5 to 10 percent of patients.[7]

Azeleic acid is currently available for prescription in the UK and some other countries of Europe. It will be introduced into the US shortly. It is formulated as a 20 percent cream, and initially applied once daily for two weeks, and then twice daily for up to six months.[8]

References

Research Reports

1. Burke B, Eady EA, Cunliffe WJ. Benzoyl peroxide versus topical erythromycin in the treatment of acne vulgaris. Br J Dermatol 1983;*108*:199–204.
2. Schutte H, Cunliffe WJ, Forster RA. The short-term effects of benzoyl peroxide lotion on the resolution of inflamed acne lesions. Br J Dermatol 1982;*106*:91–94.
3. Dobson RL, Belknap BS. Topical erythromycin solution in acne. J Am Acad Dermatol 1980;*3*:478–482.
4. Lesher JL, Chalker DK, Smith JG. An evaluation of a 2% erythromycin ointment in the topical therapy of acne vulgaris. J Am Acad Dermatol 1985;*12*:526–531.
5. Parry MF, Rha CK. Pseudomembranous colitis caused by topical clindamycin phosphate. Arch Dermatol 1986;*122*:583–584.
6. Nazzaro-Porro M, Passi S, Picardo M, Breathnach A, Clayton R, Zina G. Beneficial effect of 15% azelaic acid cream on acne vulgaris. Br J Dermatol 1983;*109*:45–48.
7. Gollnick H, Graupe K. Azeleic acid for the treatment of acne: Comparative trials. J Dermatol Treat 1989;*1*(Suppl.1):27–30.
8. Zina S, Colonna S. The long term treatment of acne with azelaic acid cream. J Dermatol Treat 1989;*1*(Suppl.1):21–26.

Review

r1. Eady EA, Ross JI, Cove JH, et al. The effects of oral erythromycin therapy for acne on the development of resistance in cutaneous staphylococci and propionibacteria. In Marks R, Plewig G. Acne and related disorders. London: Martin Dunitz, 1989; pp 265–270.

CHAPTER 84

Treatment of Disorders of Keratinization

Caroline M. Mills

As part of its terminal differentiation, the epidermal cell, or keratinocyte, undergoes a complex process of "cornification" or "keratinization." This leads to changes in cell proteins, membranes, and lipids. The process is essential to the normal structure and function of skin, but may be disrupted under a variety of circumstances, giving rise to abnormalities of the most superficial layer, the stratum corneum.

Primary disorders of keratinization may be due to abnormal retention of the stratum corneum or to disordered production of the epidermal cells. The defect may be congenital or acquired. In addition it may be associated with various disease states. Clinical presentation may vary from mild scaling of the skin to a gross thickening of the epidermis that may be functionally disabling. Treatment depends not only on the severity of the disease but also on the disability suffered by the patient.

Topical treatment may be required for mild disease, whereas more severe skin disease may require systemic therapy.

Topical Therapy

Emollients (see also Chapter 78)

Emollients are hydrating agents. They work by altering the physical properties of the stratum corneum and by influencing formation of the epidermis.[1] The emollients add water to the dry, scaly epidermis that fills the intercellular spaces, making the skin softer, more pliable, and elastic. These factors tend to increase the efficiency of the epidermis. Oily preparations provide an occlusive film at the skin surface, which decreases water loss by transepidermal evaporation. Emollients are available in the form of an oil, emulsion of oil and water, cream, or lotion, and are most effective when applied to damp skin after bathing.

Bath additives are a useful adjunct to the treatment of dry scaly skin. These are usually oily preparations that form an emulsion when added to bathwater, covering the whole body surface with an oily film. Patients should be advised that bathing in water at lower temperatures has less detrimental effect on the skin. Soaps with added detergents should be avoided, and a soap substitute used.

Urea may be added to emollients to reduce scaliness further and to increase the hydration of the stratum corneum. Urea is a simple organic compound that has weak bacteriostatic action, is nonpathogenic, and at high concentrations has the ability to break hydrogen bonds and denature keratin. Urea-containing creams can increase water binding by up to 100 percent[2] and have been shown to reduce the mitotic rate of epidermal cells.[3]

Keratolytics

Many organic α-hydroxy and keto acids appear to promote normal keratinization and assist desquamation in ichthyotic disorders.[4] These include salicylic, lactic, pyruvic, and malic acids at a concentration of 2 to 5 percent in a suitable hydrophilic base. The precise mechanism by which these acids work is not fully understood. They promote desquamation of the stratum corneum. They appear to have no effect on epidermal cell production, but do appear to reduce cohesion between keratinocytes. Salicylic acid is the most frequently used of these compounds, usually at a concentration of 2 percent in a vehicle such as white soft paraffin. Part of the drug's action is due to the dissolving of the intercellular cement.[5] Extensive use of salicylic acid is limited by absorption, which may produce symptoms of salicylism.

Topical Retinoids (see also Chapter 81)

Topical retinoids enhance DNA synthesis in the germinal epithelium and increase mitotic activity, promoting normal differentiation of the epidermis. Both all-trans retinoic acid (tretinoin) and 13-cis retinoic acid (isotretinoin) used in creams, lotions, and gels at concentrations of 0.01 to 0.1 percent are effective. Retinoic acid has also been reported to increase the water holding capacity of the stratum corneum but does not reduce the transepidermal water loss.[6] Adverse effects of treatment include redness, irritation, and an eczematous reaction. Relapse will invariably occur after discontinuation of treatment.

Systemic Retinoid Treatment (see also Chapter 81)

These drugs usually are reserved for congenital disease that is physically and socially disabling. Retinoids modulate epidermal differentiation and cell production and normalize keratinization.[7] These attributes make these agents invaluable in the management of a number of skin diseases, including disorders of keratinization.[8] The following oral preparations of retinoids are currently available: isotretinoin; etretinate; and acitretin.

Clinical improvement tends to occur after several weeks. The major side-effect of all systemic retinoid drugs is teratogenicity, and therefore caution must be exercised in women of child-bearing age. Adequate contraception must be continued for at least two months after treatment with isotretinoin, but this must be extended to two years following discontinuation of treatment with etretinate on account of slow elimination from the body and storage of the drug in body fat. Acitretin is the major metabolite of etretinate, but, owing to reverse metabolism back to the parent compound when this drug is given, similar precautions are required.

Other major side-effects include hyperlipidemia, hepatotoxicity, and extraosseous ossification. Efforts must be made to monitor for these problems. Luckily serious problems with these drugs are uncommon, but minor side-effects are very common. Dry lips occur in most patients. Drying of other mucosal surfaces is less common but annoying. An additional side-effect that may occur is transient hair loss.

Specific Disorders

The Ichthyoses

Autosomal Dominant and X-linked Ichthyosis[9,10]

Mild disease requires no more than emollients and sometimes such keratolytics as urea, lactic acid, and salicylic acid preparations. Severe disease is uncommon, but rarely symptoms may warrant treatment with systemic retinoid drugs. Acitretin 10 to 35 mg/kg/day has proved beneficial in X-linked ichthyosis.

Lamellar Ichthyosis, Epidermolytic Hyperkeratosis, Non Bullous Ichthyosiform Erythroderma, Collodion, and Harlequin Baby[11–13]

These severe disorders of keratinization are more commonly treated with systemic retinoids, although topical emollients and keratolytics may produce short-lived clinical improvement.

Etretinate 0.5 to 1 mg/kg/day is the most widely used drug, although isotretinoin 2 mg/kg/day and acitretin 0.5 mg/kg/day also are effective.

Darier's Disease[14–16]

Mild disease may require no more than simple emollient therapy, or topical retinoic acid preparations. Moderate to severe disease requires systemic treatment with isotretinoin 0.5 to 2 mg/kg, etretinate 2 mg/kg, or acitretin 0.5 mg/kg. These are all effective, although response is often less marked with flexural disease. Lasting remissions are not seen following discontinuation of therapy. Comparison studies of etretinate and acitretin showed equal effectiveness in the disorder.

Sunscreens, antibacterial cleansers, and oral antibiotics may be helpful.

Pityriasis Rubra Pilaris[17,18,r1]

Spontaneous resolution occurs in about 80 percent of patients with this disorder. In the erythrodermic phase of the disease, rest and emollient therapy are required. The most consistently useful systemic therapy during the acute phase of the disease is with the retinoids. Isotretinoin 0.5 to 2 mg/kg, etretinate 0.75 to 1 mg/kg and acitretin 10 to 35 mg/day have proved to be effective in this disorder.

Methotrexate, PUVA, systemic and topical steroids, and cyclosporin are associated with as many failures as successful reports of treatment.

Keratosis Pilaris[6]

Emollients are not effective unless used in combination with 2 percent salicylic acid or 20 percent urea. Topical retinoic acid also may be useful.

The Keratodermas[19,20]

Emollients are used, as are such keratolytics as salicylic acid under occlusion to increase efficacy. Topical retinoids are not effective, but the systemic retinoids isotretinoin 2 mg/kg, etretinate 1.5 mg/kg, and acitretin 0.5 mg/kg are very effective.

References

Research Reports

1. Tree S, Marks R. An explanation for the "placebo" effect of bland ointment bases. Br J Dermatol 1975;*92*:195–198.
2. Swanbeck G. A new treatment of ichthyosis and other hyperkeratotic conditions. Acta Dermatol 1968;*48*:123–127.
3. Wohlerab W, Schiemann S. Unterschugen zum machanisms der harnstoffwirkung auf die haut. Arch Dermatol Res 1976;*255*:23–27.
4. Van Scott EJ, Yu RKJ. Control of keratinization with α-hydroxy acids and related compounds: topical treatment of ichthyotic disorders. Arch Dermatol 1974;*100*:586–590.
5. Davies MG, Marks R. Studies on the effect of salicylic acid on the normal skin. Br J Dermatol 1976;*95*:187–192.
6. Grice K, Sattar H, Bacien H. Urea and retinoic acid in ichthyosis and their effect on transepidermal water loss and water holding capacity of stratum corneum. Acta Dermatol 1973;*53*:114–118.
7. Pearce AD, Gaskell SA, Marks R. The effects of an aromatic retinoid (etretinate) on epidermal cell production and metabolism in normal and ichthyotic patients. Br J Dermatol 1986;*114*:285–294.
8. Marks R, Finlay AY, Holt PJA. Severe disorders of keratinization: Effects of treatment with Tigason (etretinate). Br J Dermatol 1981;*104*:667–673.
9. Blair C. The action of a urea-lactic acid ointment in ichthyosis: With particular reference to the thickness of the horny layer. Br J Dermatol 1976;*94*:145–153.
10. Bruckner-Tuderman N, Gigg C, Geiger JM, Gilandi S. Acitretin in the symptomatic therapy for severe recessive X linked ichthyosis. Arch Dermatol 1988;*124*:529–532.
11. Baden HP, Buxman MM, Weinstein GD, Yoder FW. Treatment of ichthyosis with isotretinoin. J Am Acad Dermatol 1988;*6*:716–720.
12. Blanchet-Bardon C, Nazzaro V, Rognin C, Geiger JM, Puissant A. Acitrein in the treatment of severe disorders of keratinisation. Results of an open study. J Am Acad Dermatol 1991;*24*(6pt1):982–986.
13. Nayar M, Chin GY. Harlequin fetus treated with etretinate (letter). Paed Dermatol 1992;*3*:311–314.
14. Steijlen PM, Happle R, Van Muijen GN, Van de Kerkhof PC. Topical treatment with 13-cis-retinoic acid improves Dariers disease and induces the expression of a unique keratin pattern. Dermatologica 1991;*182*:178–183.
15. Dicken CH, Baker EA, Hazen PG, Kruger GG, Maib JG, McGuire JS, Schachner LA. Isotreinoin treatment of Dariers disease. J Am Acad Dermatol 1982;*6*:721–726.
16. Christophensen J, Geiger JM, Danneskiold-Samsoe P, Kragballe K, Larsen FG, Laurberg G, Serup J, Thomsen K. A double-blind comparison of acitrein and etretinate in the treatment of Dariers disease. Acta Derm Venereol 1992;*72*(2):150–152.
17. Goldsmith LA, Weinrich AE, Shupach J. Pityriasis rubra pilaris response to 13-cis-retinoic acid (isotreinoin). J Am Acad Dermatol 1986;*6*:710–715.
18. Kanerva L, Lauharanta J, Niemi RM, Lassus A. Ultrastructure of pityriasis rubra pilaris with observations during retinoid (etretinate) treatment. Br J Dermatol 1983;*108*:653–663.
19. Bergfeld WF, Deubes VJ, Elias PM, Frost P, Greer KC, Shipach JL. The treatment of keratosis palmaris and plantaris with isotreinoin. J Am Acad Dermatol 1982;*6*:727–731.
20. Fritsch P, Honigsmann H, Jaschke E. Epidermolytic hereditary palmoplanter keratoderma: report of a family and treatment with an oral aromatic retinoid. Br J Dermatol 1978;*99*:561–568.

Review

r1. Griffiths WAD, Leigh I, Marks R. Disorders of keratinization. In: Champion RH, Burton JL, Ebling FJG. *Rook/Wilkinson/Ebling, Textbook of Dermatology, 5th edition*, Oxford: Blackwell, 1991, ch.30, pp 1361–1362.

CHAPTER 85

Viral Skin Disease and its Treatment

Richard J. Motley

Introduction

Viruses are obligate intracellular parasites that utilize enzyme systems of the host cell to replicate their own genetic material. The close integration between host cell and virus systems has presented a formidable challenge to the development of antiviral therapy.

Herpes Simplex

Herpes simplex produces one of the commonest viral infections of humans. Two antigenically distinct forms of the virus are recognized; Type 1 is usually associated with orofacial infections, Type 2 with genital infections. Both types, however, may give rise to infection in any area of the skin. Herpes infection starts with multiple small vesicles that rapidly develop into erosions and ulcers. Primary Type 1 herpes simplex infection usually occurs in childhood, but may pass unrecognized. Following primary infection the virus becomes dormant within the sensory nerve ganglia, a site at which it is shielded from the host's immune system. Reactivation of the latent virus leads to recurrent infections within the skin supplied by the sensory nerve. Both local and systemic factors appear to be capable of triggering a recurrence, and infections may be associated with a diverse range of conditions from sunburn to pneumonia. Patients with atopic dermatitis and those with deficient cell-mediated immunity may develop a severe, widespread, and potentially fatal form of herpes simplex infection—eczema herpeticum.

Genital Herpes

Genital herpes usually is associated with herpes virus hominis Type 2 and is acquired through sexual activity. Primary infections may be severe, especially in women, and may lead to dysuria and urinary retention. Recurrent infections may be a problem and, when frequent, are an indication for prophylactic oral acyclovir. Sexual partners should abstain from unprotected intercourse during clinically evident disease, but the virus may also be shed asymptomatically and thus transmitted to sexual partners. Previous Type 1 herpes simplex infection does not confer immunity to Type 2 genital herpes simplex.

Keratoconjunctivitis

Primary herpes infection of the eye may lead to corneal ulceration.

Recurrent Herpes Simplex

Recurrent herpes simplex may be precipitated by high fever in many patients. A small proportion develop recurrences following minor infections, in response to sunlight exposure, emotional stress or menstruation. The eruption usually is preceded by an itching or burning sensation. Recurrences are most frequently seen around the mouth. The diagnosis of herpes simplex is confirmed by culturing the virus from the lesions.

Treatment

Acyclovir

Systemic acyclovir is the treatment of choice for extensive, severe, or frequently recurrent infection. Although the drug is very effective in acute infection it does not eradicate latent virus in the sensory ganglia.

Acyclovir is phosphorylated after entry into herpes-infected cells to the active compound acyclovir triphosphate. This process is dependent on the presence of the herpes simplex virus-coded thymidine kinase. Acyclovir triphosphate acts as an inhibitor of, and substrate for, the herpes-specific DNA polymerase preventing further viral synthesis. The drug is effective against both herpes simplex and herpes zoster virus and has a low toxicity against mammalian cells.

Intravenous administration is recommended in severe disease. The recommended oral dose is 200 mg five times per day. Acyclovir cream may attenuate minor herpes simplex infections. Topical acyclovir ointment is effective for herpetic keratitis. In all instances therapy should be commenced as soon as possible.[r1]

Idoxuridine

This is an antimetabolite antiviral compound usually employed as a 0.5 percent ointment for ocular use and a 5 percent solution in DMSO for use in cutaneous herpes simplex.

Varicella—Zoster

Varicella (chickenpox) and Herpes zoster (shingles) are caused by the same virus—*Herpesvirus varicellae*. Varicella is transmitted by droplet infection from the nasopharynx and occurs in epidemics at irregular intervals, with the highest incidence in children aged 2 to 10 years. Following primary infection the virus remains latent in sensory neural ganglia, from where it may present as a recurrent infection—herpes zoster—typically distributed in the area of the sensory nerve.

Varicella

Varicella has an incubation period of 14 to 17 days. After this time mild fever and malaise develop in the child and are followed by papules that rapidly progress to become tense vesicles. These appear in several crops over a four-day period, particularly on the trunk. Characteristically, crops of lesions at different stages of evolution are present. The lesions dry up and resolve over several days. The duration of the condition depends on the severity of the eruption. Primary varicella in adults is uncommon and may be severe.

Herpes Zoster

Recurrent infection may occur spontaneously or may be precipitated by systemic disease or immune deficiency. The first manifestation usually is pain in the sensory nerve root. This may be accompanied by fever and malaise. After three to four days papules develop in the area of nerve distribution, and these rapidly become vesicular. New vesicles appear over several days. Involvement of the ophthalmic division of the trigeminal nerve may lead to herpetic keratitis. Secondary bacterial infection and extensive skin necrosis may develop. The most distressing complication, however, is a persisting neuralgia that may occur in up to 30 percent of patients over 40, and may be severe.

Diagnosis is established by culturing viral particles in fluid from the blister. The best bedside diagnostic test is the Tzank smear—material from the blister is stained with Giemsa and examined for the presence of typical multinucleate cells containing eosinophilic inclusions within their nuclei.

Treatment

Acyclovir (see above) is the treatment of choice for herpes zoster infections, particularly in the elderly or immunocompromised. There is currently debate as to its value in treating primary varicella infection. The varicella virus is less sensitive than herpes simplex to the drug, and higher doses therefore are needed. Intravenous administration is recommended in the immunosuppressed, but when oral therapy is considered adequate a dose of 800 mg five times per day should be given.[1,2]

Viral Warts

Skin infection with one of the many antigenic strains of papilloma virus leads to warts. These are usually treated with local destructive methods such as salicylic and lactic acid mixtures. Other topical treatments that are sometimes effective are podophyllin preparations. Podophyllin is a crude plant extract that contains cytotoxic alkaloids. Paints and resins containing 5 to 20 percent of the extract often are effective for genital warts. Care must be taken; the preparations are very irritant, and application must be to the warts alone. Care also must be taken to treat only small areas to prevent percutaneous absorption and serious sytemic toxicity. In recent years a purified alkaloid has been obtained from the crude extract (podophyllotoxin) and is now available for topical treatment (0.5% in alcohol solution). Podophyllin preparations are of undoubted activity. Numerous other materials have been employed, including formalin, glutaraldehyde solution, and copper sulfate. It is doubtful that these materials have much more than a placebo effect.[3–6]

Interferon

Interferons are naturally-occurring glycoproteins with antiproliferative, immunomodulatory, and antiviral properties. Alpha 2b interferon is synthesized using recombinant DNA technology and is useful for treating severe genital warts. One million units are injected intralesionally three times per week for three weeks. Up to 15 million units of interferon may be given weekly.

AIDS

A number of skin problems develop in patients with HIV infection, including seborrheic dermatitis, impetigo, severe herpes simplex, herpes zoster, Kaposi's sarcoma, and extensive cytomegalovirus (CMV) infection. Treatment with zidovudine 3.5 mg/kg four-hourly may improve all the cutaneous conditions associated with AIDS. Zidovudine is active against HIV. It is phosphorylated in infected cells, and as the triphosphate acts as an inhibitor of, and substrate for, the viral reverse transcriptase. The formation of further proviral DNA is blocked by incorporation of zidovudine triphosphate into the chain and subsequent termination.[r2,r3]

References

Research Reports

1. Dunkle LM, Arvin AM, Whitley RJ, Rotbart HA, Feder Jr HM, Feldman S, Gershon AA, Levy ML, Hayden GF, McGuirt PV, Harris J, Balfour HH. A controlled trial of acyclovir for chickenpox in normal children. N Engl J Med 1991;*325*:1539–1544.
2. Rothe MJ, Feder HM Jr, Grant-Kels JM. Oral acyclovir therapy for varicella and zoster infections in pediatric and pregnant patients: A brief review. Ped Dermatol 1991;*8*:236–242.
3. Bunney MH, Nolan MW, Williams DA. An assessment of methods of treating viral warts by comparative treatment trials based on a standard design. Br J Dermatol 1976;*94*:667–679.
4. Bentner Kr, Frieyman-Kien AE, Artmann NN et al. Patient-applied pudofilox for treatment of genital warts. Lancet 1989;*1*:831–833.
5. Gelmetti C, Cerri D, Schuima AA, Menni S. Treatment of extensive warts with etretinate: a clinical trial in 20 children. Paediatr Dermatol 1987;*4*:254–258.
6. Williams H, Potties A, Stracham D. Are viral warts seen more commonly in children with eczema? Arch Dermatol 1993;*129*:717–720.

Reviews

r1. King DH. History, Pharmacokinetics and pharmacology of acyclovir. J Am Acad Dermatol 1988;*18*:176–178.

r2. Dover JS, Johnson RA. Cutaneous manifestations of human immunodeficiency virus infection. Part I. Arch Dermatol 1991;*127*:1549–1558.

r3. Dover JS, Johnson RA. Cutaneous manifestations of human immunodeficiency virus infection, Part II. Arch Dermatol 1991;*129*:717–720.

CHAPTER 86

Ectoparasites and Their Treatment

Richard J. Motley

Introduction

It is human nature to suspect infestation whenever a previously unrecognized rash appears on the skin. This instinct may become extreme in "parasitosis," a monodelusional state in which the individual believes himself to be infested with parasites. Despite (or because of) our instinctive suspicions, human ectoparasites developed to be inconspicuous to their host, and it is not unusual for those suffering with ectoparasite infestation to fail to recognize its cause.

Two major types of infestation are seen: pediculosis or louse infestation and human scabies. In addition, a large number of other animal ectoparasites may bite human contacts, although their breeding cycle remains restricted to the animal host.

Pediculosis

Two species of blood-sucking louse are parasitic to man, *Phthirus pubis* and *Pediculus humanus*. The latter occurs in two distinct forms: *P. humanus capitis* (the head louse) and *P. humanus corporis* (the body louse). The body louse appears to have evolved from the head louse, adapting itself as humans began to wear clothing.

Pubic Lice

Pubic lice are predominantly transmitted through sexual contact, although they may be transferred on items of clothing, towels, or bedding. Predominantly infesting pubic hair, the lice may occasionally colonize the hairs of the abdomen, axillae, eyebrows, and eyelashes. Infestation leads to intense pruritus and irritation. Secondary eczema and infection may supervene and obscure the true diagnosis, but close inspection usually reveals the lice, which are easily visible with a hand lens.

Head Lice

In developed countries head louse infestation is mainly seen in schoolchildren and mentally and physically-handicapped individuals in institutions. However, in primitive societies where no treatment is available, a high proportion of the population may be infested.

The head louse is usually confined to the scalp, where there may be only six to 12 adult insects. Egg capsules, or "nits," are cemented to the hair shafts and provide visible evidence of infestation. Detection of the "nits" is facilitated with the use of Wood's light illumination and a hand lens. Infestation leads to severe pruritus, and bacterial infection may supervene.

Body Lice

In developed countries pediculosis corporis is seen mainly in itinerants with limited opportunity for personal hygiene. The eggs of the body louse are laid in the clothing, tending to be distributed along the seams.

The adult louse feeds off the human host who, after a period of sensitization, develops itchy papules. Scratching may lead to secondary bacterial infection.

The diagnosis is made by the demonstration of lice and their eggs in the seams of the clothes. It is the clothing and bedding, not the patient, that require treatment. Malathion dusting powder and permethrin are effective means of killing the lice and eggs. High-temperature washing, dry-cleaning, and tumble-drying are also suitable.

Treatment of Louse Infestation

Malathion and Carbaryl

The anticholinesterases malathion and carbaryl are effective treatments for louse infestation. Malathion is applied as a 0.5 percent lotion to the affected area and allowed to dry. Drying with hairdryers should be avoided as the drug is inactivated by heat. Lice are killed after two hours, but a more prolonged duration of action is obtained if the preparation remains on the skin for about 12 hours. This allows the drug to be absorbed onto keratin, producing a residual protection. Ovicidal activity is incomplete and repeat application after seven to ten days is recommended.

In an attempt to prevent the emergence of resistant strains of lice the use of malathion may be alternated with carbaryl by local agreement with public health departments.

Permethrin

Permethrin, a recently developed synthetic pyrethroid, is an effective treatment for lice and scabies. It was one of the first thermostable and photostable insecticides to be developed following elucidation of the structure of natural pyrethrins in 1947.[1] It has extremely low toxicity to mammals and even higher insecticidal activity than natural pyrethrins. It occurs as a racemic mixture of cis and trans isomers. The cis isomer has a higher potential for mammalian toxicity than the trans isomer, which is more rapidly metabolized and excreted. For human use, cis:trans ratios of 25:75 are preferred.

Permethrin applied to the skin is poorly absorbed, and the fraction that is absorbed is rapidly metabolized and excreted. It is available as a 1 percent lotion for treating head lice and a 5 percent cream for treating scabies.

Strains of lice resistant to DDT and gamma benzene hexachloride are commonly found, and these are therefore less suitable treatments.

Scabies

Scabies is caused by infestation with the mite *Sarcoptes scabiei.* The female mite measures about 0.4×0.3 mm and has a hemispherical body marked by transverse corrugations, spines, hairs, and eight short legs. The female burrows through layers of the epidermis, laying eggs along her track and finally dying in the burrow. Larvae emerge after three or four days and migrate across the skin surface to find a resting place, where they undergo three moults before reaching maturity about 14 days later. The male mite dies soon after copulation, and the female mite prepares a burrow in the skin, thus completing the life-cycle.

The mite prefers certain areas of the body—mainly peripheral sites such as the finger webs, wrists, and ankles, and the scrotum and penis. The total number of mites is usually small—on average 12 mites in adults and 20 in children. An exception occurs in the florid type of infestation "Norwegian scabies" seen in patients who are immunosupressed (see below).

An allergic sensitivity to the mite and its products develops in the human host about three weeks after primary infestation. This leads to an eczema-like eruption and large numbers of papules on the thighs, buttocks, and abdomen. Indurated papules may be seen in the axillae and groin. Pruritus is severe, and scratching may lead to secondary bacterial infection, which is a cause of considerable morbidity in primitive communities lacking medical services. The diagnosis is confirmed by finding typical burrows on the anterior surface of the wrists, between the fingers, and on the medial aspect of the feet and ankles. The adult mite may be just visible as a small dot at the end of its burrow. It can be extracted using a needle and the diagnosis confirmed by examining the material under a low-power microscope. It is also possible to visualize the mite in situ using high power surface microscopy.

Scabies is transmitted between human hosts by intimate contact. The mite cannot survive for more than a few days outside the skin. Norwegian scabies (so-called because it was first described in Norway) is characterized by infestation with enormous numbers of mites and is mostly seen in immunosupressed patients—those with leukemias or HIV infection, presumably reflecting the inability of the host to mount an immunologic defense against the mite. Patients typically develop crusted warty lesions on the hands and feet containing hundreds of mites. Pruritus may be minimal. Because of the large number of mites present this type of scabies is highly contagious.

Any patient who presents with sudden onset of pruritus with no previous history of skin disease, particularly if other members of the family have developed an itchy rash, should be considered likely to have contracted scabies until proved otherwise.[2,3]

Treatment of Scabies

Several effective preparations are available. The single most important aspect of treatment is that all intimate contacts of the patient should be treated simultaneously. Following treatment, itching will persist for several days but usually resolves within two weeks.

Gamma Benzene Hexachloride

Gamma benzene hexachloride (lindane) 1% as a single application washed off after 24 hours is effective. The lotion should be applied to all areas of the body below the neck. There have been reports neurologic toxicity from excessive or inappropriate use of lindane in children, and the duration of application should therefore be restricted to two hours in infants. Although uncommon, lindane-resistant strains of scabies have been reported.[4,5]

Benzyl Benzoate

Benzyl benzoate 25% emulsion is effective treatment after two to three applications over a 24-hour period. It is, however, irritant to the skin and patients should be warned against over-use. Special care should be taken in young children because of this.

Malathion

Malathion 0.5% is effective against scabies, but penetrates poorly and must be left on the skin for 24 hours and reapplied after a few days.

Monosulfiram

Monosulfiram 25% in alcohol, diluted with water to form an emulsion and applied daily for two to three days is effective. Monosulfiram-impregated soap has been used as a prophylactic measure. Percutaneous absorption of this material can produce an Antabuse-like effect after ingestion of alcohol.

Permethrin

Permethrin 5% cream is an effective scabicide when applied to the skin for eight to 12 hours. It does not have the potential neurologic toxicity associated with lindane and is safe for use on infants.[6,7]

Sulfur

Sulfur preparations have been used for centuries and are still the main form of treatment for scabies in many parts of the world. An ointment prepared using 2.5 to 10.0 percent sulfur in an oily vehicle—such as animal fat or soft paraffin—is applied twice daily to all areas of the skin for three days. Sulfur preparations such as this are very inexpensive (at least 200 times less expensive than lindane or benzyl benzoate) and may be the only affordable treatment in the primitive communities where scabies extracts its greatest toll. Sulfur preparations are unpleasant to use and tend to irritate the skin.

References

Research Reports

1. Taplin D, Meinning TL, Porcelain SL, Castillero PM, Chen JA. Permethrin 5% dermal cream: a new treatment for scabies. J Am Acad Dermatol 1986;*15*:995–1001.
2. Carslan RW. Scabies in a spinal injuries ward. Br Med J 1975;*2*:617.
3. Bernstein B, Mihan R. Hospital epidemic of scabies. J Paediatr 1973;*83*:1086–1087.
4. Rasmussen JE. Lindane. A prudent approach. Arch Dermatol 1987;*123*:1008–1010.
5. Ginsburg CM, Lowry W, Reisch JS. Absorption of lindane (gamma benzene hexachloride) in infants and children. J Paediatr 1977;*91*:998–1000.
6. Schultz MW, Gomez M, Hansen RC, Mills J, Menter A, Rodgers H, Judson FN, Mertz G, Handsfield H. Comparative study of 5% permethrin cream and 1% lindane lotion for the treatment of scabies. Arch Dermatol 1990;*126*:167–170.
7. Taplin D, Porcelain SL, Meinning TL, Athey RL, Chen JA, Castillero PM, Sanchez R. Community control of scabies: a model based on use of permethrin cream. Lancet 1991;*337*:1016–1018.

Review

Burns DA. The treatment of human ectoparasite infection. *Br J Dermatol* 1991;*125*:89–93.

CHAPTER 87

Treatment of Localized Neoplastic Disorders of Skin

Ronald Marks

For the most part, treatment of localized neoplastic lesions of skin is by surgical excision or ablation by electrodesiccation and cautery or cryotherapy. Nonetheless, the frequency of these disorders and the availability of pharmacologic methods of treatment necessitates a short commentary on this subject. Many agents used for localized skin cancer have also been tried for recalcitrant viral warts.

Topical 5-Fluorouracil (5-FU)

This compound is an antimetabolite that inhibits DNA synthesis and is tumoricidal. It is employed in a 5 percent concentration in an ointment. A treatment cycle usually involves once-daily application over a 10-day period, but some clinicians prefer a twice-daily schedule lasting 14 days. Because the treatment often causes soreness and even erosion of the lesion, it has become customary also to supply a corticosteroid-antimicrobial preparation (e.g., hydrocortisone-miconazole or triamcinolone acetonide–Aureomycin) to use for a 10 to 14-day period subsequent to the application of the 5-FU preparation. For small, superficial skin tumors—in particular solar keratoses or lesions of Bowen's disease (intraepidermal epithelioma)—it has a success rate of approximately 50 percent after one treatment cycle and perhaps 65 to 70 percent after two treatment cycles. It is also often successful for superficial basal cell carcinoma, but not for nodular and other deeper types, where it seems unlikely that the 5-FU will penetrate to the tumor cells in sufficient concentration.[1]

Adverse Side Effects

Soreness and erosion have already been mentioned, and are not usually a problem. If treated areas are exposed to the sun, a photosensitivity develops in some patients, and this possibility should be communicated to the patients. Caution should be exercised if multiple lesions are to be treated at the same time, because sufficient 5-fluorouracil may be absorbed percutaneously to cause systemic toxicity.

Interferons

Interferons are peptide cytokines that have an important role to play in recovery from infections. Three classes are recognized: alpha, produced by neutrophils; beta, produced by fibroblasts; and gamma, produced by lymphocytes. They have a variety of biologic properties, but the only one that concerns us here is their tumoricidal activity for neoplastic disease of skin. Molecular biology techniques have made recombinant forms of human interferon available.

Intralesional interferons have been employed to treat large solar keratoses and areas of Bowen's disease, and with considerable success. Unfortunately, multiple injections are required—1 million units of interferon alpha-2β twice weekly over a four-week period is a typical regimen. Treatment of basal cell carcinoma by interferons has also been reported on several occasions; although successful, it appears less so than for keratoses and Bowen's disease lesions.[2,3] Other interferons have also been used in this way. Intralesional interferons have also been used in the treatment of recalcitrant warts and other persistent infections.

Systemic infusions of interferons have also been used, usually in combination with other drugs or radiation schedules, to treat patients with mycosis fungoides and metastatic melanoma.

Podophyllum

Podophyllum resin is the name given to a crude plant extract containing several cytotoxic alkaloids. Traditionally, preparations of this have been used for the treatment of anogenital and other types of wart. They have also been used on occasion to treat skin tumors. More recently one of the alkaloids—podophyllotoxin—has been isolated and employed systemically to treat visceral neoplastic disease as well as viral warts by topical application.[r1]

Other Cytostatic Agents Used Occasionally

Bleomycin

This cytostatic agent, usually employed for large solid tumors, also has been employed intralesionally (1–2 mg) for recalcitrant plantar warts and cutaneous metastatic deposits.[4]

Nitrogen Mustard

Solutions of nitrogen mustard have been pricked onto the surface of recalcitrant warts and localized lesions of nonmelanoma skin cancer. They have also been painted on to the flat lesions of mycosis fungoides. They sensitize the skin very easily; whoever applies this solution must be very careful not to get it on their own skin.[5]

Photochemotherapy

Some success has been reported with the experimental use of long-wave UVR after exposure of the tumor to sensitizing porphyrins. One such porphyrin precursor is delta-aminolevulinic acid, which is apparently concentrated and metabolized to porphyrins in neoplastic tissue.[6,7]

Topical Retinoids (see also Chapter 81)

Both topical tretinoin (0.05%) and isotretinoin (0.1%) have been used to treat multiple solar keratoses. The treatment needs to be continued for long periods before reduction in size and number of lesions is seen. Use in conjunction with topical 5-fluorouracil has been recommended.

References

Research Reports

1. Ashton H, Beveridge GW, Stevenson CJ. Topical treatment of skin tumours with 5-fluorouracil. Br J Dermatol 1970;*82*:207–209.
2. Grob JJ, Collet AM, Munoz MH, Bonerandi JJ. Treatment of large basal cell carcinomas with intralesional interferon α-2β. Lancet 1988;*1*:878–879.
3. Shuttleworth D, Marks R. A comparison of the effects of intralesional interferon α-2β and topical 5% 5-fluorouracil cream in the treatment of solar keratoses and Bowen's disease. J Derm Treatment 1989;*1*:65–68.
4. Ames M, Diab N, Ramadan A, Galal A, Salam A. Therapeutic evaluation for intralesional injection of bleomycin sulfate in 143 resistant warts. J Am Acad Dermatol 1988;*18*:1313–1316.
5. Hoppe RT, Abel EA, Deneau DG, Price NM. Mycosis fungoides. Management with topical nitrogen mustard. J Clin Oncol 1987;*5*:1796–1803.
6. Lui H, Anderson RR. Photodynamic therapy in dermatology. Arch Dermatol 1992;*128*:1631–1636.
7. Wilson BD, Mang TS, Stoll H, Jones C, Cooper M, Dougherty TJ. Photodynamic therapy for the treatment of basal cell carcinoma. Arch Dermatol 1992;*128*:1597–1601.

Review

r1. Beutner KR. Podophyllotoxin in the treatment of genital human papilloma virus infection: a review. Semin Dermatol 1987;*6*:10–18.

CHAPTER 88

Antihistamines and Management of Urticaria

Richard J. Motley

The effect of histamine on skin, as seen in urticaria, is mediated for the most part via type 1 histamine receptors. Although there are other histamine receptors in the body, only the H_1 receptor antagonists will be discussed here.

More than 50 H_1 receptor competitive antagonists have been synthesized. All have the basic structure of histamine modified by substitution on the imidazole ring. In contrast to the newer antihistamines, earlier agents were lipid soluble and crossed the blood-brain barrier, where many caused a pronounced sedative effect, limiting their clinical usefulness. Other effects of these drugs included blockade of cholinergic (muscarinic), adrenergic, and 5-hydroxytryptaminergic receptors, and a local anaesthetic action. Some of these effects were of benefit in the treatment of motion sickness and, occasionally, Parkinson's disease.

The more recently developed antihistamines are nonsedating, have far fewer nonspecific effects, and are very potent inhibitors of the H_1 receptor; but, because their action is competitive and reversible, they are more effective if given before histamine release occurs. The new agents differ mainly in their half-lives, which vary greatly from 1.8 hours for acrivastine to more than nine days for astemizole. However, serum half-lives and half-lives for the biologic effect are not necessarily the same. Many antihistamines undergo extensive first-pass hepatic metabolism, and some form active metabolites. An example of this is the metabolism of the older agent hydroxyzine to cetirizine. Identification of the active metabolite led to its synthesis and independent use.

The absence of sedative side-effects with the newer antihistamines is partly due to these agents' not readily crossing the blood-brain barrier and partly to their more specific activity. Occasionally, however, individuals report sedation with these newer agents. It is important to be aware that the sedative effects of the older antihistamines are greatly potentiated by alcohol or other CNS depressant drugs.[r1,r2]

Terfenadine

This is the most established of the modern antihistamines. It is taken orally, a typical adult dose being 60 mg BD or 120 mg OD, and undergoes first-pass hepatic metabolism in which 99 percent of the drug is transformed into two major metabolites, only one of which has antihistaminic activity. Peak blood levels are achieved two hours after oral ingestion. The metabolites are excreted in the feces. In extensive tests of psychomotor function, subjects receiving terfenadine did not perform significantly differently from those taking placebo. Terfenadine is potentiated by concurrent administration of drugs such as ketoconazole and erythromycin, which inhibit hepatic oxidation; such combinations should therefore be avoided. Although adverse effects are extremely rare, prolongation of the Q-T interval, cardiac arrhythmias (torsades de pointes), and cardiac arrests have been reported in association with massive overdosage of both terfenadine and astemizole. For this reason the recommended daily doses should not be exceeded, and the dose should be reduced in circumstances that may alter hepatic metabolism.

Cetirizine

Cetirizine reaches peak plasma levels 30 minutes after oral ingestion, and is excreted unchanged in the urine. It is nonsedating at recommended therapeutic doses, but causes some signs of sedation when these doses are exceeded. Its main benefit is a relatively rapid onset of action; the usual adult dose is 10 mg at bedtime.

Astemizole

Astemizole is the longest acting nonsedative antihistamine and for this reason may be preferred when long-term therapy is required; the adult daily dose (which should not be exceeded) is 10 mg.

Sedative Antihistamines

Older types of antihistamine are still used in patients with atopic eczema in which the main antipruritic effect seems related to their sedative action. The newer antihistamines appear not to have an antipruritic effect. Chlorpheniramine and hydroxyzine continue to be popular choices, but drugs such as promethazine and trimeprazine have much greater sedative activity and may give additional benefit at night. (In larger doses, these latter drugs may be used for preoperative sedation).

Topical antihistamines do not have general antipruritic properties but may give symptomatic relief in insect bites. They may cause allergic contact dermatitis.

Antihistamines in the Treatment of Urticaria

The management of patients with urticaria requires experience and skill. Initially efforts should be made to determine whether there is an identifiable cause but the diligence with which this should be sought is a matter of debate. As it is uncommon to unearth an unequivocal cause in the majority of patients (some would say 90%) it is pointless to try to exclude every last cause of the disorder. Antihistamines provide important symptomatic relief in this disease.

The actions of histamine are typified by the triple response of Lewis: a firm scratch to the skin leads to an erythematous flare, itch, and edema due to local increased capillary permeability. This, and the response to intradermal histamine injection are greatly reduced by pretreatment with antihistamines. Although histamine is undoubtedly a cause of urticarial skin reactions, it is not the only mediator involved and the reaction may occur despite the use of potent antihistamines.[r3,r4] Nevertheless, antihistamines are often beneficial in urticaria, and it is usual to recommend a therapeutic trial of antihistamines for symptomatic relief of this condition. It is worth trying more than one agent because individual responses vary; however, caution is advised against the formerly popular practice of prescribing very high doses of these drugs, because this has been associated with cardiac arrhythmias.[r5]

Acute Urticaria

Acute urticaria and angioedema may at times be a true dermatologic emergency. Where there is massive facial swelling with swelling of the faucial mucosa and difficulty in breathing, intracutaneous adrenalin and IV hydrocortisone may be needed. Fresh plasma concentrates should be given for congenital C1 esterase deficiency.

The identification of histamine as a mediator of the inflammatory response, the characterization of its receptors, and the development of specific antagonists of its action has been one of the major pharmacologic achievements of the 20th century. Unfortunately, with the ability to inhibit the action of histamine in the skin completely has come the realization that histamine is but one of many mediators involved in cutaneous allergic reactions and that antihistamines are the answer to relatively few dermatologic problems.

Reviews

r1. Rimmer SJ, Church MK. The pharmacology and mechanisms of action of histamine H1-antagonists. Clin and Exp Allergy 1990;*20*:(suppl 2) 3–17.

r2. Estelle F, Simons R, Simons KJ. Pharmacokinetic optimisation of Histamine H1 receptor antagonist therapy. Clin Pharmacokinetics 1991;*21*:327–393.

r3. Kobza Black A, Grattan CEH. The mediators involved in acute and chronic urticaria and their therapeutic implications. In: Champion RH, Pye RJ, eds. Recent advances in dermatology 9. London: Churchill-Livingstone, 1992;119–133.

r4. Kennard CD, Ellis CN. Pharmacologic therapy for urticaria. J Am Acad Dermatol 1991;*21*:176–189.

r5. Kemp JP. Antihistamines—Is there anything safe to prescribe. Annals of Allergy 1992;*69*:276–280.

r6. Champion RH, Greaves MW, Kobza Black A, Pye RJ. The Urticarias. London: Churchill-Livingstone, 1985.

r7. Garnetski BM. Urticaria. Berlin: Springer-Verlag, 1986.

CHAPTER 89

The Treatment of Blistering Disorders of the Skin

Richard J. Motley

Fluid-filled vesicles or blisters may have a variety of causes, and careful diagnosis is essential to provide appropriate and sometimes specific treatment. The diagnosis may be evident from clinical examination, but frequently it is necessary to biopsy a recently formed blister for histologic examination. General measures for the care of blistered skin are regular cleansing and topical antiseptics such as povidone iodine 10% paint to prevent bacterial superinfection. Large blisters may be punctured with a sterile needle to release their contents, but the skin of the roof of the blister should not be removed. It provides natural protection for the regenerating wound surface.

Blisters are formed by disruption of the intercellular bridges within the epidermis or components of the dermoepidermal junction. The dermoepidermal junction is a complex zone composed of several layers and structural proteins. Blisters formed within the epidermis tend to be fragile; they rupture easily compared with subepidermal blisters that arise from abnormalities of the dermoepidermal junction.

The causes of blistering may be broadly divided into congenital, antibody-mediated, and others. The various types of epidermolysis bullosa are examples of the first; pemphigus, pemphigoid, and dermatitis herpetiformis are typical of antibody-mediated diseases. Miscellaneous causes of blistering include bullous impetigo, herpes infections, porphyria, drug reactions, heat, and friction. The following investigations may be necessary to determine the cause of blistering: culture of blister fluid for bacteria and viruses; biopsy of a recently formed blister for routine histology to establish whether the blister is intra- or subepidermal (blisters of more than 2–3 days duration may show re-epithelialization, confusing the histologic appearance); antibody studies to detect the presence of various antibodies; and electron microscopy to examine the precise level of any damage to the dermoepidermal junction.[r1]

Pemphigus, Pemphigoid, and Dermatitis Herpetiformis

Pemphigus, pemphigoid, and dermatitis herpetiformis are chronic blistering conditions in which an immunologically-meditated destruction of the skin occurs. Immunologic studies using fluorescent labeled antihuman immunoglobulin antibodies make possible detection of the type and site of antibody deposition and a precise diagnosis.

Pemphigus

Pemphigus typically occurs in middle-age. It is characterized by fragile blisters and erosions developed in the skin and mucosa. Histologically blisters are seen within the epidermis, and immunofluorescent studies reveal the deposition of IgG and C_3 around the epidermal cells. Before the advent of corticosteroids pemphigus frequently was fatal; systemic corticosteroids are now the mainstay of treatment and may be required in high dosage (up to 120 mg prednisolone per day). Azathioprine (2.5 mg/kg/day) or cyclophosphamide (1–3 mg/kg/day) may be added as a "steroid-sparing" agent. Methotrexate and systemic gold (sodium auriothiomalate by IM injection) also have been used. Once control of the condition is established—as evidenced by an absence of new blister formation—the dose of steroids is gradually reduced.[1–3,r2]

Pemphigoid

Pemphigoid is usually a condition of the elderly. The blisters are more robust than those of pemphigus, and they commonly appear on the trunk and limbs. Mucosal involvement is unusual. Histologically the condition is characterized by a blister developing at the dermoepidermal junction, and immunofluorescent studies demonstrate the deposition of IgG and C_3 at this site.

Pemphigoid responds to systemic corticosteroids at doses lower than those necessary for pemphigus, typically 40 to 60 mg prednisolone per day. However, as patients are often elderly, the side-effects from corticosteroids can be more troublesome. Azathioprine may be required as an additional immunosuppressive agent for its steroid-sparing effect. Steroid dosage is reduced when new blister formation ceases.[r3]

When corticosteroids are contraindicated, dapsone may be an effective alternative. It also may be used as a steroid-sparing agent, enabling more rapid withdrawal of the corticosteroids. Both pemphigus and pemphigoid may have circulating antibodies, and these may be useful in monitoring treatment and progression of the disease.

Dermatitis Herpetiformis

Dermatitis herpetiformis is characterized by small, intensely pruritic vesicles over the extensor aspects of the limbs and trunk. The vesicles develop at the dermoepidermal junction and immunofluorescent studies demonstrate a granular pattern of IgA deposition at this site. Most patients with dermatitis herpetiformis have histologic evidence of gluten-sensitive enteropathy, although very few have symptoms of malabsorption. Dapsone 50 to 150 mg per day is the treatment of choice and is effective within one to two days. (Its effectiveness in this condition was a serendipitous observation made while treating otitis media in a patient with dermatitis herpetiformis.) Dapsone has been shown to have many activities other than its antibiotic action, and it seems likely that its effect in this condition is due to an inhibition of antigen-antibody-induced complement activation. A gluten-free diet is recommended because this often enables the condition to be controlled with lower doses of dapsone. Dapsone is a sulfonamide antibiotic and should not be given to patients with sulfonamide sensitivity. It also causes hemolysis, which occurs to some degree in all individuals but may be severe in patients with glucose 6-phosphate dehydrogenase deficiency, in whom low doses should be employed. Dapsone also causes methemoglobinemia, which accounts for the "gray" appearance of patients taking the drug long-term.[4,5]

Bullous Impetigo

Bullous impetigo is a common cause of blistering in children and is due to infection with a toxin-producing strain of *Staphylococcus aureus*. The diagnosis is suggested by evidence of cutaneous infection and the presence of blistering in a restricted area of the skin surface. Treatment is with systemic antibiotics, such as penicillin V or flucloxacillin (floxacillin).

Epidermolysis Bullosa

There are more than 20 types of this inherited disorder. All are characterized by a tendency to develop blisters after minimal trauma. The most common form, epidermolysis bullosa simplex, is inherited as a autosomal dominant trait and presents with blistering on hands and feet and at points of friction. Treatment consists of ensuring appropriate foot wear and minimizing trauma to the skin.

Other forms of epidermolysis bullosa all demonstrate considerable skin fragility and lead to large areas of skin loss that may be fatal. Systemic steroids are ineffective; the minor degree of success reported with phenytoin and dantrolene—drugs with membrane-stabilizing activity—has not been substantiated in controlled trials.[6]

Porphyria Cutanea Tarda

This condition is seen in men with a history of excessive alcohol consumption, and may reflect an inherited predisposition. Patients develop blisters on exposed parts of the face and the backs of the hands in response to sunlight or minimal trauma. Treatment consists of alcohol avoidance and regular venesection—which appears to improve the condition by depleting hepatic iron stores.[7]

Eczema

Blisters are commonly seen in contact allergic eczema, e.g., following contact with poison ivy. They are also a prominent feature of eczema when it occurs on the palms and soles, so-called pompholyx (Greek for blister) eczema. Treatment consists of allergen avoidance and topical corticosteroids.

References

Research Reports

1. Levene GM. Treatment of the immunological bullous diseases. In: Wojnarowska F, Briggaman RA, eds. Management of Blistering Diseases. London: Chapman & Hall Medical, 1990; pp 35–42.
2. Younger IR, Harris DWS, Colver GB. Azathioprine in dermatology. J Am Acad Dermatol 1991;*25*:281–286.
3. Westerhof W. Treatment of bullous pemphigoid with topical clobetasol propionate. J Am Acad Dermatol 1989;*20*:458–461.
4. Stern RS. Systemic Dapsone. Arch Dermatol 1993;*129*:301–303.
5. Hall RP. The pathogenesis of dermatitis herpetiformis: Recent advances. J Am Acad Dermatol 1987;*16*:1129–1244.
6. Fine JD, Bauer EA, Briggaman RA, Carter DM, Eady RAJ, Esterly NB, Holbrook KA, Hurwitz S, Johnson L, Lin A, Pearson R, Sybert VP. Revised clinical and laboratory criteria for subtypes of inherited epidermolysis bullosa. J Am Acad Dermatol 1991;*24*:119–135.
7. Lim HW. Pathophysiology of cutaneous lesions in porphyrias. Semin Hematol 1989;*26*(2)(April):114–119.

Reviews

r1. Wojnarowska F, Briggaman RA. Management of Blistering Diseases. London: Chapman & Hall Medical, 1990.

r2. Korman N. Pemphigus. J Am Acad Dermatol 1988;*18*:1219–1238.

r3. Ahmed AR, Kurgis BS, Rogers RS. Cicatricial pemphigoid. J Am Acad Dermatol 1991;*24*:987–1001.

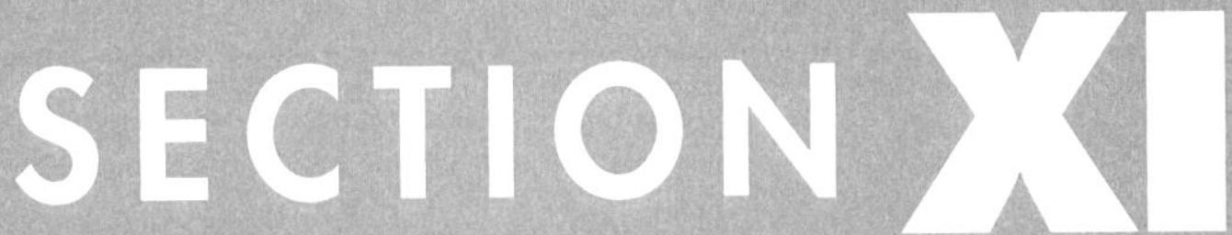

SECTION XI

Chemotherapeutic Drugs

Editors:
Yung-Chi Cheng
George H. Hitchings

Associate Editors:
Nitya Anand
Emil J. Freireich
L. A. Salako

CHAPTER 90

The Principles of Antimicrobial Chemotherapy

Adrien Albert (deceased)
Nitya Anand

Introduction

Ehrlich, around the turn of the 20th century, coined the term "chemotherapy" for agents that would selectively attack a parasite in preference to its host; he proposed some of the basic concepts of such drug use. The modern era of chemotherapy, however, began with the discovery in the 1930s of the antibacterial activity of sulfonamides, followed soon after by the isolation of penicillin from *Penicillium notatum* culture. This compound demonstrated an unprecedented high therapeutic index. These two discoveries, coming from different streams, had dramatic effects. New agents, both synthetic and of microbial origin, were introduced in quick succession—a process that has continued ever since. With chemotherapeutic agents now available it is possible to treat and control most of infectious disease. Knowledge of the mode of action of these drugs has greatly advanced our understanding of microbial physiology and biochemistry and of host-parasite relationships. These developments in chemotherapy have revolutionized the practice of medicine. However, widespread and often indiscriminate use of these drugs has also led to some problems, e.g., drug resistance and drug toxicity. Some broad principles and guidelines have emerged for the practice of chemotherapy to help physicians obtain optimal benefits from available drugs. It is the purpose of this chapter to highlight some of these issues and to present the principles that have emerged for chemotherapeutic practice.

Historical Development

Although the drug treatment of infectious diseases goes back to antiquity, the concept of a direct and selective action of a drug on the infective agent was first clearly enunciated by Paul Ehrlich (Fig. 90.1) around the turn of the 20th century.[r1,r2] While still a medical student, Ehrlich was struck by a report on lead poisoning by Heubel claiming that organs in which lead accumulated could also fix the

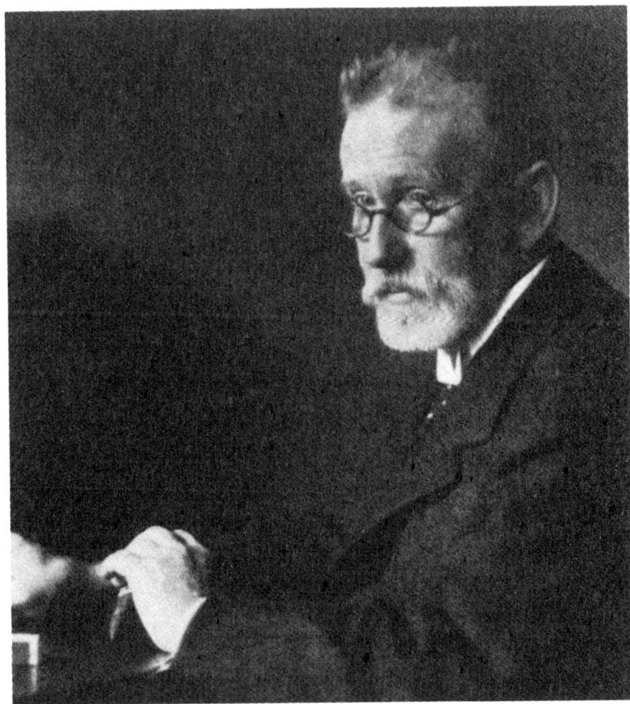

Figure 90.1 Portrait of Paul Ehrlich aged 56 by E. Spiro.

metal from lead salt solution after death. The study of selective uptake and distribution of chemicals by living systems became a major research concern for Ehrlich. He began his studies by using dyes that could be detected visually. Quite early, he examined the distribution of dyestuffs, first in blood and then in living animals.[1] His technique and his division of stained leukocytes into acidophil, basophil, neutrophil, and nongranular is used by clinical pathologists to this day. Following this, Ehrlich carried out his well-known experiments on vital staining, using methylene blue and neutral red, and ranking different body tissues by their comparative oxygen requirements. On killing an animal some time after injection of methylene blue, he found that the only tissues dyed were those of the nervous system and that nerves were sharply defined along their whole length. Using different dyes he found that he could demonstrate differential staining of different organs and cell types.

Ehrlich then turned his attention toward staining bacteria and protozoa. In 1891, he found that bacteria and the malaria parasite were stained by methylene blue, and that methylene blue also had activity—though weak—against tertiary malaria. These studies marked the beginnings of his chemotherapeutic research. Simultaneously, Ehrlich had made some outstanding discoveries in immunochemistry. He showed in vitro neutralization of toxin by antitoxin and of antigen by antibody. He went on to state his side-chain theory, a chemical interpretation of the immune process, as follows: an antigen has two active areas, namely the haptophore (anchorer) and the toxophile. Mammalian cells, he proposed, have side-chains that contain chemoreceptors complimentary to the haptophores and hence "anchor" them, bringing the toxophile close enough to the cell to poison it. He believed that the normal function of these receptors was the uptake of nutrients.[r19]

In 1904, drawing on these experiments, Ehrlich undertook his studies on the chemotherapy of trypanosomiasis,[2] and began to seek synthetic chemicals that would exhibit greater affinity for parasites than for host cells (*nihil agit nisi fixatur*). For this selective action he coined the word "chemotherapy," and defined it as "the use of drugs to injure an invading organisms without affecting the hosts".[3,4] He emphasized in chemotherapy the direct action on invading organisms by substances of low molecular weight, differentiating the process from immunotherapy derived from antibodies, which are much larger protein molecules produced by the host in response to the antigens of some infecting organisms. When Ehrlich moved from Berlin to Frankfurt in 1899, he switched his research totally from immunotherapy to chemotherapy and continued these studies until his death in 1915. In 1910, Ehrlich and his young Japanese collaborator, Hata, discovered the first drug that radically cured syphilis.[5] This agent, arsphenamine (Praparat 606) was promptly introduced into clinical practice (under the trade name Salvarsan) and achieved worldwide use. The discovery of arsphenamine is regarded as the opening event in a chemotherapeutic revolution that was to transform the management of infectious diseases. Ehrlich also introduced many of the basic concepts on which chemotherapy rests.[r3] Apart from introducing the concepts of selective toxicity and of chemoreceptors, Ehrlich also discovered the phenomenon of drug resistance, and introduced the concept of a therapeutic index. In seeking highly selective drugs, i.e., those that would have a great affinity for the invading organism but little for the host, Ehrlich saw the need to quantify the selectivity by observing the ratio of the lowest curative dose to the greatest tolerated dose.

Today, Ehrlich's therapeutic index concept is much used in the following form:

$$\frac{\text{Maximal tolerated dose}}{\text{Minimal effective dose}}$$

Another term for the maximal tolerated dose, usually written LD_{50}, was introduced by Trevan,[6] a mathematician, who showed that members of a set of cells (or animals) responded to a fixed dose of a drug according to a log normal distribution curve as shown in Figure 90.2; when such responses were summed for a series of logarithmically-increased doses, a sigmoid curve usually was obtained (Fig. 90.3). This represents a cumulative log normal distribution.

Although Ehrlich had introduced some very basic concepts of chemotherapy that are still valid, arsphenamine remained the only systemically-acting antibacterial that he could introduce; it also acted on only one microbe species, the spirochete of syphilis. Only one other significant development occurred during this period in chemotherapy, the discovery by Browning and Gilmour[7] of the selective antibacterial action of aminoacridines, such as proflavine, which

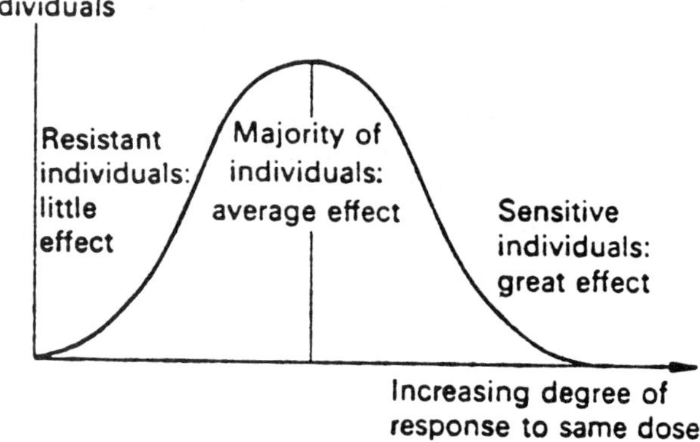

Figure 90.2 A Log Normal Distribution Curve

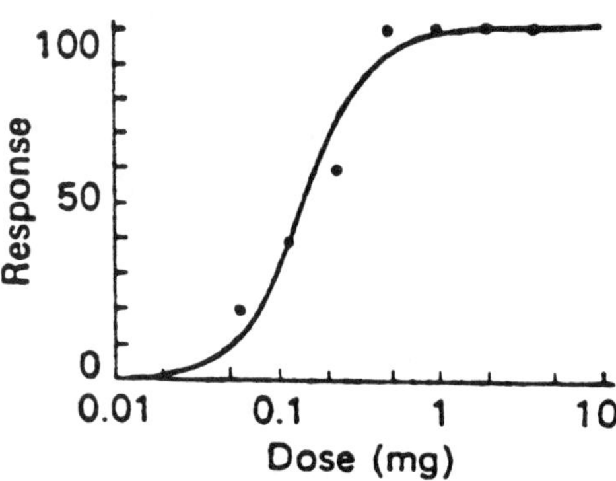

Figure 90.3 A cumulative normal distribution curve. The response has been plotted against the logarithm of the dose.

selectively eliminated bacteria from deep wounds—a discovery that saved the lives of many severely injured soldiers in the two world wars. Physicians had to wait another two decades for major antimicrobial drugs that could act safely and effectively in the circulatory system and deep tissues. In the early 1930s Domagk, a pathologist, reported the systemic antibacterial action in mice of sulfachrysoidine (Prontosil), a dye containing a sulfamide group.[8,r20] The first large and controlled clinical trial with this drug was reported in 1936 by Colebrook and Kenny[9] for puerperal sepsis caused by streptococci; this firmly established the agent's clinical usefulness. Soon both this drug and its more potent modifications came into wide use, mainly orally, for a wide range of bacterial infections. This discovery not only established firmly that direct attack on the microbe was possible by chemotherapeutic agents, but also led to the establishment in quick succession of many other important basic concepts of chemotherapy.[r4]

The demonstration that prontosil was metabolized in the body to sulfanilamide, the active species,[10] was the first clear establishment of the concept of prodrugs, which has been an important development in drug design. The improvement achieved in potency of sulfanilamide by introducing electron-withdrawing groups/heterocycles at the N^1-position, which produced such highly potent drugs as **sulfadiazine** established the power of molecular modification in drug discovery.[r5] The relationship uncovered between the pK_a of sulfonamides and, their potency and transport by Bell and Roblin[11] and others,[12,13] established the value of physicochemical properties in structure-activity relationship studies. The standardization of a simple method for the assay of sulfonamides in body fluids and tissues permitting precise determination of absorption, distribution, and excretion of the drugs,[14] provided a rational basis for calculating proper dosage regimens;[15] pharmacokinetic studies have now become an integral part of drug development programs.

Wood's (1940) observation of the competitive reversal of the action of sulfanilamide by p-aminobenzoic acid (pABA) was the first definitive demonstration of metabolite antagonism as a mechanism of drug action.[16] The elucidation of this relationship provided the long sought-after mechanistic basis for a rational approach to chemotherapy, and led Fildes (1940) to propose his classic theory of antimetabolite action.[17] This hypothesis formed the basis of numerous and intensive studies in chemotherapy and pharmacology and established the fundamental concepts of metabolite antagonism as an approach to drug design. Between the original contributions of Ehrlich and those resulting from early studies on sulfonamides, most of the basic concepts of chemotherapy, valid to this day, were established.

The success of sulfonamides also renewed interest in antibiotics—antimicrobial agents of microbial origin—reported occasionally in the literature since the first report of Pasteur in 1877 of the antagonistic effect of some bacteria against the anthrax bacilli.[r6] Following Fleming's report in 1929 that a contaminating colony of the mold Penicillium notatum lysed adjacent colonies of staphylococci,[18] Chain, Flory and their associates[19] in the early 1940s isolated the active material from this culture, and named it penicillin. It proved to have a therapeutic index favorable beyond any known before. Penicillin began to be widely used in clinical practice in the early 1940s, and was responsible for saving millions of lives in World War II.

These two discoveries—sulfonamides and penicillin—ushered in the modern era of chemotherapy. New agents, both synthetic and of microbial origin, were introduced in quick succession; and this process has continued ever since.

The success of penicillin sparked a worldwide search for other antibiotics. The more important antibiotics with some special features discovered in the early years were: (a) **streptomycin,**[20] with a high order of activity against Mycobacterium tuberculosis; (b) **chloramphenicol**[21] (Chloromycetin), with a high activity against Salmonella sp., and (c) **chlortetracycline,**[22] the first of the tetracyclines, which have a broad spectrum of antibacterial activity.

The spectacular achievements of antibiotics pushed the antibacterial sulfonamides into the background for several years. However, the problems encountered with widespread use of antibiotics, especially of drug resistance and of superinfection, caused sulfonamides to re-emerge strongly around 1970. Two other factors responsible for this resurgence were: (a) the discovery of second-generation sulfonamides with a long half-life (> 24 hrs); and (b) the discovery of synergisms between sulfonamides and dihydrofolate reductase inhibitors, e.g., between **sulfamethoxazole** and **trimethoprim.**[r21] The demonstration of the biochemical rationale for this synergism, which involved sequential blocking on the same metabolic pathway, added a new dimension to antimicrobial chemotherapy,[r7] and sharply focused attention on the usefulness of combination therapy to overcome/delay microbial resistance and to enlarge the antimicrobial spectrum. The successes achieved with multi-drug therapy (MDT) for leprosy and tuberculosis, both to avoid development of resistance and to cut down on time of treatment, are outstanding examples of the usefulness of this approach.

With a view toward improving the activity of penicillins, side-chain modification was introduced by incorporating the precursor acids into the culture medium; but this approach offered only limited possibilities. Major advances in this direction came when convenient enzymatic and chemical deacylation of natural penicillins to 6-aminopenicillanic acid (6-APA) could be achieved, and side-chains could be added by synthesis. Soon, semisynthetic penicillins with greatly improved pharmacokinetic characteristics, acid and β-lactamase stability, and a broadened antibacterial spectrum became available; this greatly enhanced the therapeutic usefulness of penicillins.[r8] A similar sequence happened with cephalosporins; and now first-, second-, and third-generation cephalosporins with special features are available in clinical practice.[r8] Improving the activity profile of antibiotics by synthetic modification has since become an established practice. **Rifampicin,** obtained by synthetic manipulation on rifamycin B obtained by fermentation is an important illustration of the success of this approach.[r9]

One of the major problems encountered during the clinical use of penicillins was the production of β-lactamases by many organisms, which could destroy these drugs. This problem has been overcome in two ways: (a) by using a β-lactamase inhibitor, of synthetic (**sulbactam**)[r21] or microbial (**clavulanic acid**)[23] origin in combination with penicillins; and (b) by using β-lactamase-resistant β-lactam antibacterials rich as in some of the more recent penicillins and cephalosporins.[r8] These drugs are preferred in clinical practice where β-lactamase-producing strains are expected as pathogens. A more significant development has been the discovery of carbapenem antibiotics, such as **thienamycin,** which are β-lactamase resistant, and of their synthetic analogues, such as **imipenem,** with a greatly improved antibacterial spectrum.[r22] Imipenem is active against both aerobic and anaerobic organisms, including β-lactamase-producing strains and those that are resistant to penicillins and aminoglycosides. Imipenem is a major addition to β-lactam antibacterials. The drug is hydrolyzed by a dehydropeptidase on the brush border of the proximal renal tubular cells, producing high concentrations of active drug to fight urinary tract infections. These developments have not only enlarged the scope of the clinical usefulness of β-lactam antibacterials, but have added new dimensions to combination therapy by using inhibitors of microbial or host enzymes that deactivate a drug by destroying its chemotherapeutic activity. To overcome the problem of destruction of imipenem, a dehydropeptidase inhibitor, **cilastatin,** is administered at the same time.[r23]

Concurrently, several other synthetic antibacterials were discovered that filled some troublesome gaps in antibacterial chemotherapy. Outstanding among these was **isoniazid** (INH),[24] which played the leading part in reducing tuberculosis from a dreaded scourge to a treatable condition. Other additions were the nitrofurans, such as **nitrofurantoin,**[r24] which proved specially useful for eliminating staphylococcal urinary tract infections frequently acquired in hospitals and resistant to treatment with antibiotics and sulfonamides. **Nalidixic acid** and its analogues were found useful to combat resistant Gram-negative organisms in the urinary tract.[25]

Following extensive research carried out in Japan on nalidixic acid analogues, the fluoroquinolone-carboxylic acid,[r10] such as **norfloxacin,**[r25] emerged in the 1980s as a major new group with an unprecedentedly wide antimicrobial spectrum that includes both gram-positive and gram-negative bacteria and mycobacteria. These agents inhibit virtually all the enterobacteriaceae at concentrations below 1 μg/ml, and have varying activity against Pseudomonas, Haemophilus, Branhamella, and methicillin resistant staphylococci. Carboxyquinolones have a novel mode of action and inhibit DNA gyrase (Topoisomerase II), which is involved in DNA replication. Thus they do not have cross-resistance with existing antimicrobial agents. These drugs are widely distributed in the body tissues and fluids, including the CSF, bone, respiratory tract, and urine. The discovery of carboxyquinolones has highlighted the continuing possibility of finding antimicrobial drugs with both novel modes of action and a broad spectrum of antimicrobial coverage.

Antiviral Chemotherapy

Progress in chemotherapy of viral diseases has been rather poor compared with that achieved in bacterial diseases.[r11] Viruses are intracellular and depend largely on the host's cellular machinery for multiplication. These attributes pose problems for transport of drugs and achieving selectivity of action. Synthetic antiviral agents discovered so far also tend to be specific for a limited range of viruses. Antiviral action of any significance has rarely been found among antibiotics. Most of the synthetic compounds have been designed as antimetabolites that interfere at some point of nucleic acid biology. The two more commonly used prophylactic agents are **amantadine** for the prevention of influenza, and **methisazone** for preventing smallpox infection. Following the elimination of smallpox from the world, methisazone is little used. Amantadine has only a rather limited usefulness, being active only against A strains of influenza virus. The more successful therapeutic agents are **idoxuridine** and **trifluridine** for herpes infection of the eye, **ribavirin** (Virazole) for the treatment of viral pneumonia, **vidarabin** (Ara-A) for herpes simplex encephalitis, and **acyclovir** (Zovirax) found effective against all types of herpes infections. The more active agents now used against HIV infection are **azidothymidine** (Zidovudine) and didedeoxy nucleosides, such as **dideoxycytidine** (DDC), although their efficacy is rather limited.[26]

Antifungal Chemotherapy

There have been significant developments in chemotherapy of fungal infections.[r12] Most nonsystemic fungal infections, such as ringworm, athelete's foot, and vulvogenital candidiasis, yield to **miconazole** or **clotrimazole,** which are about equally active. These interfere with the incorporation of ergosterol into the cytoplasmic membrane of fungi. Polyene macrolide antibiotics, such as **nystatin,** are not active against ringworm, but are effective against candidiasis of the skin and mucous membranes, e.g., oral thrush or vulvogenital candidiasis. Among the older but less effective topical antifungals are **tolnaftate** and **undecylenate,** which are active against ringworm but not candidiasis. Keratolytic agents, such as salicylic acid, are helpful as accessory drugs for some hyperkeratotic skin lesions.

Systemic antifungal chemotherapy started with the discovery of the antibiotic griseofulvin, which is useful in treating some kinds of ringworm infections but ineffective against candidiasis. It is particularly useful for infections of the nails, where it is still probably the best drug available. Systemic fungal diseases such as histoplasmosis and blastomycosis are uncommon, but if untreated, are often fatal. **Amphotericin B,** administered IV, was till recently the only treatment available. A useful recent addition is **ketoconazole,**[26] which is orally active and can be used for these infections.

Flucytosine[27] (5-fluorocytosine) is a synthetic oral drug useful in cryptococcosis, candidiasis, and chromomycosis. But drug resistance develops rather rapidly when flucytosine is used alone. The drug is therefore generally used in combination with amphotericin B, permitting a lower dose of the latter.

Antiprotozoal Chemotherapy

The treatment of protozoal diseases remains rather unsatisfactory.[r13] The number of drugs available remains small, and for some infections, such as cryptosporidiosis, satisfactory drugs have yet to be discovered; for others, such as leishmaniasis and trypanosomiasis (for both Chagas' disease and sleeping sickness), the available drugs are very inadequate. For exoerythrocytic stage parasites of vivax malaria, **primaquine** (by no means a safe drug to use) is the only drug available; there is urgent need for alternative non-8-aminoquinoline drugs. Drug resistance is further depleting the already rather inadequate stock of antiprotozoal drugs. This is particularly serious among the antimalarials.[r14] Chloroquine-resistant *Falciparum malaria,* present earlier in Southeast Asia and South America, has now spread to the African continent as well, and some of the chloroquine-resistant strains are now resistant to **pyrimethamine** and **sulfadoxine**—and some even to **mefloquine.** Much of this spread of resistance has been due to rather ill-designed and poorly executed field chemotherapy programs. It is important that available drugs be carefully used, both for the individuals and in the community, so that their usefulness is preserved and optimally exploited.

Antihelminth Chemotherapy

Worms that parasitize humans belong to widely separated zoologic families, and differ widely in their anatomy, physiology, biochemistry, and susceptibility to drugs. In spite of these limitations, impressive gains in the discovery and availability of antihelminth drugs have made it possible to manage and treat effectively the major human helminthic diseases.[r14,r15]

The modern era of antihelminth chemotherapy started around 1950 with the discoveries of the microfilaricidal activity of **diethylcarbamazine** (DEC; Hetrazan) and the anti-roundworm activity of piperazine. DEC was found effective against both lymphatic filariasis and onchocerciasis, but it is active only against microfilareae. There was no other significant addition to the drugs for treating filariasis until the late 1980s, when **ivermectin,** a 22,23-dihydro derivative of avermectin B, a fermentation product, was introduced.[28]

DEC does not act directly on the microfilareae; therefore, no resistance to **DEC** has been encountered, and even after 45 years of use its effectiveness has not been affected. **DEC** does appear to be a suitable drug for chemoprophylaxis, and the data available on this aspect are quite impressive. Ivermectin is active at extremely low concentrations against both lymphatic filariasis and onchocerciasis;

it offers a single-dose oral treatment compared with the multiple doses over many days required with DEC. The activity of ivermectin, however, is also confined only to microfilareae. Lack of a suitable macrofilaricide continues to be a big gap in the chemotherapy of filariasis. As DEC and ivermectin act by different mechanisms, combinations of the two may offer a cost-effective chemotherapy regimen for treating filariasis.

Both hookworms (*Necator* and *Ancylostoma* sp.) and roundworms (*Ascaris lumbricoides*) are rapidly eliminated by **mebendazole** (or its analogues) and pyrantel. The pinworm (*oxyuris*), common among young children world over, and whipworm (*Trichuris*) are also eliminated by **mebendazole** or **pyrantel.** Another broad-spectrum anthelmintic is **thiabendazole,** which is active against these worms but is also the treatment of choice for threadworms (*Strongyloides* and *Trichinella spiralis*).

For schistosomiasis, **niridazole** followed by **matrifonate** provided the early effective oral treatment, but these drugs were limited to *S. haematobium* infections. Next came **oxamniquine,** which was introduced as a single oral dose to cure *S. mansoni* infections and is well-tolerated. A major advance took place with the introduction of **praziquentel,** which can eliminate all three species of schistosomes, including the more recalcitrant *S. japonica* by a single oral dose. It is also highly effective against cestodes, and it has more or less replaced all the earlier drugs for these infections. Praziquentel is rapidly absorbed from the GI tract, and diffuses well into most tissues, including the CNS. The drug is practically free from side-effects, and is presently the treatment of choice for schistosomiasis, neurocysticercosis, Hymenolepsis infections, and most infections caused by hermaphroditic flukes.

Interface with Immunity

Accumulating experience with chemotherapy over recent decades resulted in a growing realization that the host immune system plays an important role in the outcome. Some of the facts that have enhanced this realization are: (a) the increasing incidence of opportunistic infections and increased severity of normal infections in immunocompromised and immunodeficient patients; (b) greater efficacy of chemothrapeutic agents in immune populations. Immunomodulation in conjunction with chemotherapy therefore has emerged as a useful means of treating infectious diseases. In leprosy it has been shown that a heterologous vaccine can greatly augment the response and hasten bacillary clearance.[29] In experimental filarial infection it has been shown that muramyl peptides, known immunomodulators, can both prevent infections when given prophylactically and modify their course when given along with DEC.[30,31] It is interesting that, although originally the term "chemotherapy" was coined by Ehrlich to distinguish it from immune prophylaxis, after almost 100 years the two are being considered in tandem. This will have special relevance in infections that usually cause immunosupression, such as many parasitic infections; it is also important in the use of drugs that depress the immune response, such as primaquine.

Factors Affecting Chemotherapy

The outcome of antimicrobial chemotherapy is determined by a set of interactions between the drug, the host, and the offending microbe (Fig. 90.4).

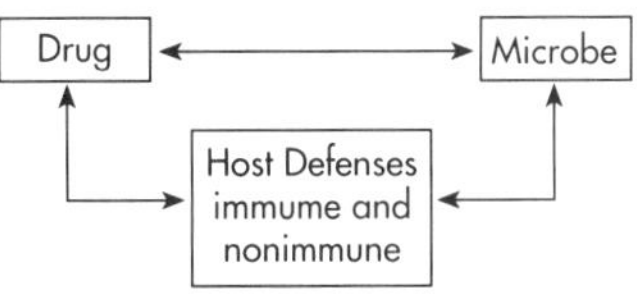

Figure 90.4

The Drug

The chemotherapeutic agent has a direct action on the microbe. In bacterial infections the drug either reversibly inhibits growth of bacteria, allowing no increase in viable organisms (**bacteriostatic**), or is irreversibly lethal to them (**bactericidal**). Though this distinction is more functional than absolute and is often concentration-dependent, it helps the clinician choose an agent and determine the dosage to be used. A close correspondence between **minimal inhibitory concentration** (MIC) and **minimal lethal concentration** (MLC) indicates a potential for lethal effects; as cure invariably requires the use of bactericidal agents, such agents are preferred. There is a dictum in chemotherapy: "Use an agent (or combination of agents) with potential for lethal activity in preference to a drug that is primarily only inhibitory" (-static).

Some chemotherapeutic agents, such as antifolates (sulfonamides and dihydrofolate reductase inhibitors), tetracyclines, and chloramphenicol are **broad spectrum:** they are therapeutically useful against more than one of the major groups of infectious agents. Besides bacteria, these agents are also active against chlamydiae, mycoplasma, and rickettsias. Others, such as penicillins and cephalosporins, are active only against some bacteria. The choice of a specific agent is determined by the bacterial sensitivity.

Chemotherapeutic agents, apart from their direct antimicrobial action, also may affect host defenses, acting as biologic response modifiers. Such agents can be classed into four categories:[32,r26] (a) those that have no effect on host defenses, e.g., most β-lactams; (b) those that depress immune functions, e.g., tetracylcines; (c) those that display synergy with the immune system, e.g., some macrolides and quinolones; (d) those that enhance the immune function, e.g., certain cephalosporins.[r27] Since the immune system has an important role to play in the final elimination of the infectious agent, drugs that enhance the immune function are preferred over those that depress this function; the development and availability of drugs that combine antibacterial activity with an ability to restore or enhance the immune system have opened up new avenues and put additional demands on the development of antimicrobial agents.

Microbes can also affect chemotherapeutic agents, as exemplified by the inactivation of penicillins by microbial β-lactamases (penicillinases), a matter of great concern in chemotherapy with β-lactam antimicrobials. The fate of the drug in the host and side-effects on the host of the parent drug or its metabolites are important in deciding the dosage regimen and are a part of clinical pharmacology studies.

The Microbe

A wide variety of viruses, bacteria, protozoa, fungi, and helminths have been demonstrated to infect humans. They vary enormously in their pathogenicity—i.e., their ability to cause disease. Most are nonpathogenic and commonly stay in ecologic balance in and with the host. In contrast, at the other end of the spectrum, are some organisms that are highly virulent and that usually or always produce disease when they infect. The ability of a specific pathogen to cause disease depends on the interaction between its intrinsic pathogenic potential, or virulence, and the defensive measures used by the host to contain or neutralize the infectious thread. A distinction is therefore often made between **infection** and **disease;** infection implies invasion of the host by a pathogen, whereas instances of impaired resistance of the host may shift the balance to the establishment of the disease state. In severe impairment of host resistance, organisms normally of low virulence can cause severe disease, and are called **opportunistic pathogens.** The virulence of a pathogen is thus a relative term. Infections with opportunistic pathogens have become more common and have assumed a serious dimension as a result of increasing use of cytotoxic drugs and radiation in cancer therapy, of immunosuppressives in transplantation surgery, of corticosteroids in inflammatory conditions, and because of the high prevalence of immunodeficiency disorders. Their treatment, therefore, has assumed special importance.

Superinfections

One of the more serious and common complications of antimicrobial therapy is superinfection with organisms insensitive/resistant to the drug being used and often resistant to many other drugs as well. This may arise from the outgrowth of indigenous commensal organisms (bacteria or fungi) that normally are held in check and in ecologic balance by other organisms. For example, bacterial enteritis, candidal stomatitis, and delayed gram-negative septicemia after severe burns are common complications of antibacterial chemotherapy and need special attention.

Extracellular and Intracellular Parasitism

It is useful to consider these two groups separately on account of their relevance to the outcome of chemotherapy. Most bacteria are extracellular, are harmful to the host as long as they remain outside the phagocytic cells, and cause mainly acute, short-lived diseases. Some others, e.g., *M. tuberculosis, M. leprae,* and *Salmonella typhi,* are intracellular, survive in phagocytic cells for long periods, are slow to respond to chemotherapy, and cause such chronic diseases as tuberculosis, leprosy, and typhoid. Their treatment therefore, poses special problems.

Drug Resistance

The term "drug resistance" refers not to the lack of sensitivity of a microbe species to a particular agent, but to acquired genotypic resistance, with or without exposure to the drug, which persists during cultivation even in the absence of the drug.

Ehrlich was the first to report the emergence of drug-resistant microbes. In 1905, he observed that mice suffering from trypanosomiasis when treated with a subcurative dose of a drug could not subsequently be cured with a curative dose of the same drug. This resistance in the trypanosomes proved to be hereditary and irreversible; thus, it was concluded that a genetic effect was operant. Later, similar phenomena have been reported in bacteria, viruses, cancer cells, and even insects.

It is now recognized that resistance may arise by a mutation, or insertion of a foreign DNA by recombination. Resistance genes are commonly carried on short lengths of extrachrosomal DNA, known as plasmids or resistance factors (R Factors) that can be transferred from other bacteria, even from those of another species, by conjugation, transduction, and transformation. Resistance to several antibiotics may exist on a single plasmid, e.g., in the form of information for producing acylating enzymes. These genes may even be packaged in units of DNA called transposons that allow them to jump from one DNA site to another, thus further facilitating the spread of resistance. Resistance may develop through stepwise increments by successive mutations or by one-step mutation to high-level resistance.

Resistance to drugs depends on different mechanisms,[33] and more than one mechanism may operate for the same drug. Five principal mechanisms are recognized by which organisms bring about resistance. In Type 1, the mutant develops a decreased permeability to the drug by a chemical change in the cytoplasmic membrane. Ehrlich found that the arsenic-containing growth medium, which surrounded his resistant trypanosomes without their suffering any harm, was rapidly lethal to the original, susceptible strain of trypanosomes. Similarly, *Staphylococcus aureus* can alter T membrane from the configuration that normally facilitates uptake of this drug. In that way, the bacteria are protected from the drug's action, even though the drug's target (the ribosomes) remains as susceptible as ever.[34]

In Type 2 resistance, the amount of a drug-destroying enzyme is increased. An example is provided by the treatment of acute leukemia with cytosine arabinoside. In this instance sensitivity to the drug falls in proportion to the appearance of malignant cells with a high concentration of cytosine deaminase. Again, response of this disease to 6-mercaptopurine lapses if the cells manufacture enough alkaline phosphatase to degrade all of the tumor-inhibiting nucleotide to which the cell normally converts this prodrug.

In Type 3, the amount of a target enzyme is increased many fold by gene amplification. This type comes to the fore when an enzyme is the receptor for a drug that has been designed to inhibit it. The now widespread resistance of malarial parasites to drugs acting on dihydrofolate reductase has this origin. For example, the Ugandan strain of pyrimethamine-resistant *Plasmodium falciparum* was found to contain 30 to 80 times as much of this enzyme as the susceptible strain.[35] In human leukemia, the malignant white blood cells can develop resistance to methotrexate by manufacturing a great excess of dihydrofolate reductase, the enzyme that this drug is employed to block.[36]

In Type 4 resistance, the target enzyme is replaced by one with less affinity for the drug. For example, the dihydrofolate reductase extracted from a normal strain of *P. berghei* had a 600-fold higher affinity for pyrimethamine than did a highly resistant strain. Moreover, the in-vitro concentration of this drug necessary to produce a 50 percent reduction in enzyme activity was increased 40-fold.[37]

Type 5 resistance is characterized by synthesis of excess of the metabolite to which the drug is a planned antagonist. Thus, staphylococci, gonococci, and pneumococci can become resistant to the usual effective concentrations of sulfonamide antibacterials by secreting an extra amount of p-aminobenzoic acid.

Another mechanism of drug resistance recently identified is the active extrusion of drugs from the target cell. This was first reported in relation to cancer chemotherapy, and involves for extrusion the mediation of a cell membrane glycoprotein, P-glycoprotein. The phenomenon was termed **multidrug resistance** (mdr).[r16] Similar extrusion as a mechanism of drug resistance also was observed subsequently in microbial cells and may be of common occurrence.[38]

The emergence of resistant bacterial strains is the most serious limitation of chemotherapy. Resistance development has many consequences, the most important being that the patient is compelled to use a more toxic (often also more expensive) alternative drug, posing greater danger to life. Since spontaneous mutation is an inherent characteristic of bacterial multiplication, the origin of mutants, including drug-resistant mutants, cannot be stopped. Sooner or later, microbes will develop resistance to virtually any antimicrobial agent. However, the survival and selection of resistant mutants can be prevented or delayed, and this is the main concern of research in chemotherapy. Although there is no general procedure for preventing or overcoming drug resistance, various useful strategems are available.

Anaerobic Infections

Anaerobic bacteria require reduced oxygen tension for growth, and are responsible for deep-seated infections in the body. Anaerobes can be grouped broadly into two classes, sporulating and nonsporulating. Sporulating organisms of clinical importance are the clostridia, which include *Clostridium perfringens, C. botulinum,* and *C. tetanus:* these organisms produce the most potent bacterial toxins known. The most important nonsporulating organisms belong to bacteroides, fusibacteria, and gram-positive cocci; the most common organism of this class in the body is *B. fragilis.* In general, anaerobes associated with human infection are aero-tolerant and can survive up to 72 hours in the presence of oxygen, although they will not multiply in this environment. This property gives them a survival advantage. The nonsporulating anaerobic bacteria are present as normal organisms on the mucosal surfaces, such as in mouth, GI tract, skin, and the female genital tract; clostridia are present in humans mainly in the normal intestinal microflora and are widely distributed in the soil. Most anaerobic bacteria thus exist in the human system as commensals, and anaerobic infections occur when the harmonious relationship between the host and the bacteria is disrupted. Any site in the body is susceptible to infection with these indigenous organisms when mucosal or skin barriers are compromised by surgery, trauma, tumor, or situations that reduce local tissue redoxpotentials, such as ischemia or necrosis. Because the sites that are colonized by anaerobic bacteria contain many other species of bacteria, disruption of anatomic barriers causes penetration by many other organisms as well, resulting frequently in mixed infections involving multiple species of these anaerobes with micro-aerophilic organisms. Such infections include sinusitis, chronic otitis media, Ludwig's angina, periodontal abscesses, brain abscesses, subdural empyema, aspiration pneumonia, necrotizing pneumonia abscesses, peritonitis, liver abscesses, and some female genital tract infections such as salpingitis, pelvic peritonitis, tubo-ovarian abscess, vulvogenital abscess, and septic abortion. These infections thus arise at sites of trauma, tissue destruction, compromised vascular supply, or as complications of preexisting infections that produce necrosis. Thus, abscesses of organs or tissues should first call to mind possible anaerobic infections.

The Host

A number of different host factors have an important influence on the efficacy and toxicity of antimicrobial agents. The age, renal and hepatic status, and nutritional and genetic factors of the host have a singificant effect on the metabolism, pharmacokinetics, and propensity to side-effects of drugs. Host defenses, both nonimmune and immune, complement chemotherapy and have an important role in the elimination of infecting organism. Persistant microbes, that arise from phenotypic resistance of microbes subjected to bacteriostatic action are finally eliminated by immune and phagocytic responses. The ultimate outcome of an infection is thus a result of the joint assault by the host and the chemotherapeutic agent. If the immune system is suppressed, deranged, or compromised, special care has to be taken in chemotherapy, as regards both dosage and duration of treatment.

Local Tissue Factors

When bacteria reach a high enough extracellular population density in a localized tissue site, the surrounding host cells die and suppuration results, forming an abscess; antibacterial chemotherapy in such areas becomes ineffective owing to several factors, such as impairment of circulation in the dead tissue, with reduced flow of antibodies, leukocytes, oxygen, and normal parenchymal cell nutrients, as well as slower removal of waste products, and a resultant build-up of acids and bacterial toxins. Since acidity, lack of oxygen and nutrients impair bacterial multiplication, drugs that require bacterial multiplication for their action (such as penicillins or aminoglycosides) cannot act. Tissue autolysis releases certain metabolites that antagonize the action of some chemotherapeutic agents, such as sulfonamides. The action of some agents is affected directly by tissue destruction. Such abscesses are cured only after surgical drainage, which permits the bacteriostatic pus to be replaced by fresh serous exudate, providing nutrients as well as a wave of new leukocytes and chemotherapeutic drugs.

Chemotherapy is also relatively ineffective when there is a foreign body in the lesion, e.g., sutures, splinters of wood, spicules of dead bone, or an artificial prosthesis. These provide foci protected from leukocytes but a site where bacteria may accumulate in a dormant state or accumulate bacterial products. Similarly, bacterial infections associated with obstructions of the urinary, biliary, or respiratory tract with impaired circulation also result in accumulation of quiescent bacteria and toxic products within the cavity. Both types of lesions are rarely cured by chemotherapy unless the foreign body or obstruction is removed.

Many disease states that depress natural resistance also impair the response to chemotherapy. Some reduce the number of effective phagocytic cells available at the infected site, (corticosteroid therapy, cytotoxic antitumor drugs, leukemia, radiation injury, or ethanol). Others may cause immunosuppression and impair antibody formation (e.g., multiple myeloma, chronic lymphocytic leukemia). Still others may depress resistance to the host by mechanisms not fully understood (e.g., uncontrolled diabetes or uremia). All these conditions require special consideration for the treatment of infection.

As a result of the foregoing considerations some general principles have emerged for the practice of chemotherapy, and these are discussed below.[r17,r18]

Basic Principles of Antimicrobial Chemotherapy

Initiation of Treatment

The earlier the treatment is begun in an infection episode, the more likely it is to be effective. Some of the special reasons for this are: (a) actively metabolizing and multiplying bacteria are more susceptible to the antibacterial action of most drugs, and some bacteria in a stationary phase become refractory to bactericidal drugs; (b) once suppurative lesions are formed, they require surgical drainage and may cause irreversible tissue damage; (c) the number of resistant mutants formed would be proportional to the total number of bacteria, so the earlier the cycle is interrupted the fewer resistant mutants are encountered; (d) lesions discovered late are more likely to become superinfected with resistant organisms.

Choice of Drug

Several factors bear directly on the selection of antimicrobial agents; these include the affected organ/site of infection, the microbe(s) causing the disease, the status of the host physiology, and other drugs being administered to the patient.

Infecting Organism

The basic aim of diagnosis in any infection episode is to determine which organ system is affected, identify the offending microbe, and determine the susceptibility of the strain causing the disease. Direct methods of identification typically include staining and culture of body fluids, secretions, and tissues or assay for microbial antigens using IFA, ELISA, or RIA techniques. DNA probes are also now becoming available for identification of organisms, and should be useful for organisms difficult to culture, such as protozoa or mycobacteria. These methods, however, are unlikely to replace culture tests for most conventional bacteria because culture tests are more direct and dependable.

In view of the high incidence of drug resistance in bacterial infections it is useful to know the drug susceptibility of the strain causing the disease. This can be determined semiquantitatively by the disk diffusion method, and quantitively by serial dilution techniques. The latter provides the lowest concentration (MIC) of antimicrobial agents that prevents visible growth after 18 to 24 hour of incubation, and has relevance with the pharmacokinetic data; an organism is considered susceptible when the MIC is no more than one-fourth of the readily obtainable peak serum level of the antimicrobial agent.

Susceptibility testing has special relevance for malaria because *Plasmodium falciparum*, which causes about 85 per cent of all cases of malaria and much of the mortality, has become resistant in many parts of the world not only to **chloroquine,** but also to some of the alternative drugs, such as **pyrimethamine** and **sulfonamides** and even to the recently introduced **mefloquine.** It is important to know the sensitivity of the isolates in these regions in order to institute an appropriate therapeutic regimen. Some field kits designed by the World Health Organisation are now available for determining sensitivity to commonly used drugs.

Knowledge of the infecting microbe, however, may not be available when therapy is initiated—or not at all because of the nonavailability of testing facilities in many regions. Antimicrobial therapy in such situations would be started empirically. Empiric selection of the antimicrobial agent should be based on a knowledge of the likely pathogens and their expected antimicrobial susceptibility. For example, the most common cause of urinary tract infections is *Escherichia coli;* therefore, normal urinary tract infection therapy should be directed to *E. coli.* Similarly, it is known that group *A. streptococci* and most strains of streptococcus pneumonia have remained susceptible to β-lactam antimicrobials and can be so treated empirically. However, in such cases a close watch should be kept on the clinical progress of the patient, and the treatment adjusted if the condition deteriorates.

Route and Dose of Administration

The site of infection is one of the most important factors in determining both dose and route of administration. Adequate concentrations of the drug must be delivered to the site of the infection, and concentrations above MIC achieved in all tissues. The pharmacokinetics of the antimicrobial agent and the clinical condition of the patient have to be considered in selecting therapeutic regimens that are both effective and safe. Data on the pharmacokinetics of most of the important antimicrobial agents are available in standard textbooks, providing a useful reference guide to the best route and best dose. Normally the oral route is preferred because of the ease of administration. In certain situations, however, alternative routes may be indicated. Rectal administration, though often leading to iregular/incomplete absorption, is useful if the patient is vomiting or unconscious or in cases of GI sensitivity to a drug; this route does lessen the first-pass effect since absorbed drug does not all pass through the hepatic portal circulation. Parenteral administration is necessary when the patient is unconscious, has difficulty in swallowing, for agents not absorbed from the GI tract, and for serious infections in which a high concentration of the antimicrobial agent is needed immediately, such as suspected bacteremia/meningitis and gram-negative pneumonia. Similarly in cases of cerebral malaria IV chloroquine or quinine must be given, and can be followed by oral administration when the patient has improved; IV infusion of a single dose can spread the release over several hours, whereas an IV bolus gives the most rapid elevation of blood levels possible.

The blood-brain barrier is an important factor in

the choice of agents for CNS infections; agents known to cross this barrier are preferred, e.g., sulfadiazine among sulfonamides.

Host Factors

As stated earlier, a number of host factors have a significant effect on the efficacy and toxicity of antimicrobial agents and must be considered while choosing the drug and its dosage regimen. A history of hypersensitivity and adverse reactions to certain groups of drugs should be considered. Similarly, genetic traits determine side-effects and rate of metabolism of drugs and should be considered before the administration of some agents. A number of antimicrobial agents will produce hemolysis in patients with glucose-6-phosphate dehydrogenase deficiency and adequate precautions have to be taken in the use of these drugs in such patients; these include primaquine, sulfonamides and sulfones, nitrofurantoin, and chloramphenicol. Similarly, 50 to 60 per cent of US and north European citizens are slow acetylators/inactivators of isoniazid, and polyneuritis is a common complication of isoniazid therapy in such individuals.

The age, nutritional, and physiologic status of the host has a marked effect on drug disposition and thus on its dosage and side-effects. Sulfonamides should not be administered to pregnant women or to newborns because they bind to serum albumin, displacing bilirubin, which may result in kernicterus. Tetracyclines should not be administered to pregnant females and to newborn infants or to children less than eight years of age because these drugs bind to developing bone and tooth structure and cause a permanent brown discoloration of the teeth.

Many antimicrobial agents are removed from the body by renal excretion. Where urinary excretion is an important route of elimination, renal failure causes slower removal of the drug; thus, administration of usual doses would lead to greater accumulation of drug and increased likelihood of toxicity. In infants, glomerular and some tubular functions do not develop to adult levels until up to two months of age. Similarly, with advancing age renal function decreases, and 1 per cent of glomerular clearance is lost per year after the age of 30. In these cases it becomes necessary to modify the dosage schedule to obtain the concentration-time profile of a patient with normal renal clearance. This becomes particularly important with drugs with a narrow therapeutic index, such as gentamycin.

Some antimicrobial drugs, including macrolides, isoniazid, rifamycins, and quinolones, are metabolized primarily by hepatic mechanisms. In patients with severe hepatic disease drug concentrations may reach toxic levels, and dose adjustment would be necessary. Some drugs, such as cimetidine, cause inhibition of drug metabolizing enzymes; others, such as barbiturates and rifampicin, induce mixed-function oxidases in the liver, thus affecting the bioavailability and clearance of the other drugs from the body. The rate of drug metabolism is also age-related; with advancing age there is an increase in the half-life of many drugs, and suitable dose adjustment becomes necessary.

The rate at which isoniazid (and some other drugs) is inactivated by acetylation in the liver is genetically determined, and the population can be categorized into "rapid" and "slow" acetylators. Polyneuritis is seen more frequently as a complication of isoniazid therapy in individuals who are slow acetylators, and dose adjustment is necessary in such cases.

Food intake can affect the absorption of some antimicrobials and it is best to administer them on an empty stomach except where contraindicated, such as NSAIDs, which can cause gastric irritation. Aluminum ions present in antacids form insoluble chelates with tetracyclines and carboxyfluoroquinolones, preventing their absorption. Similarly, tetracyclines, which form chelates with calcium ions, should not be administered with milk.

Drug-Drug Interaction

In treatment planning one must consider the possibility of drug interactions that may affect pharmacokinetics and metabolism—and thus the toxicity of drugs. A dangerous situation can arise when a potent drug adsorbed on albumin is displaced by another drug of higher affinity. A common example is a patient medicated with an anticoagulant drug such as warfarin and then given aspirin; the displaced anticoagulant will raise free warfarin in blood (and thus in liver), and subsequently will lower the level of circulating prothrombin, leading to a crisis of bleeding. Similarly, in young patients being treated for leukemia with methotrexate, self-administration of aspirin has often released a toxic concentration of this anticancer agent into the circulation. Rifampicin greatly stimulates the P-450-dependent mixed oxidases in the liver, thus increasing the rate of elimination of many drugs being administered simultaneously, including oral contraceptives, thus necessitating dose adjustment.

Combating Drug Resistance

Development of drug resistance is the most serious problem faced in antimicrobial chemotherapy. Though there is no one general procedure available to overcome drug resistance, various useful strategems have evolved that help to overcome/delay the development of resistant mutants and treat resistant organisms.

Some of these measures are: (a) initiating therapy early and with bactericidal drugs; (b) using combination therapy, where indicated, right from the beginning of the treatment; (c) proper compliance with chemotherapeutic regimens with proper dosage for an adequate period.

Antimicrobial Combination Therapy

Although the goal of chemotherapy is to use the most selectively acting drug that produces the least side-effects, and most infections can be treated with a single antimicrobial agent, there are definite situations when therapy with a combination of antimicrobial agents is indicated. Combination therapy can be of two types: **additive,** when the activity in combination equals the sum of their individual activities; and **synergistic,** when combined activity is presumed to be greater than the sum of their drugs' individual activities. The emergence of a rationale for combination therapy has been an important development in antimicrobial chemotherapy. Situations in which combination therapy is indicated are described below:

Preventing/Delaying the Emergence of Resistant Organisms

This is the most important indication for combination therapy. It is particularly indicated in conditions where a population of organisms of varying susceptibility is expected, as in the case of tuberculosis.

The most effective combinations are those for which there is a biochemical basis. For example, sulfonamides and dihydrofolate reductase inhibitors block consecutive steps on the metabolic pathway to folate coenzymes, and their combination thus causes **sequential blocking** that is very effective.[r28] If the first of the two enzymes is blocked to the extent of 90 per cent, 10 per cent of the product can reach the next enzyme; if the second drug blocks this enzyme, also by 90 per cent, only 1 per cent of the final product can emerge—usually too little to sustain the life of the microbe.

One of the earliest applications of sequential blocking was reported in 1953, when it was shown that the protozoan Toxoplasma was killed by a mixture of pyrimethamine and sulfadiazine, but not by either drug separately.[39] This combination has become the preferred treatment for human toxoplasmosis.

Sequential blocking also has produced excellent results in bacterial infections since the early 1970s, when a mixture of trimethoprim and sulfamethoxazole was introduced under the generic name co-trimoxazole. This combination is frequently, and very successfully, used in the treatment of bacterial dysentery, acute bronchitis, and long-standing infections of the urinary tract, whether due to gram-positive or gram-negative organisms.[40] Mixtures of trimethoprim with dapsone or sulfadoxine have given good results in drug-resistant malaria.[41]

Various forms of cancer commonly are treated with mixtures of cytostatic drugs. This strategy delays emergence of resistant cells. It also lessens side-effects (which vary from drug to drug, whereas cytostatic effects are additive), and it allows for sequential blocking.[r29]

A new concept in combination antimicrobial therapy has emerged with the development of β-lactamase inhibitors (clavulanic acid[23] and sulbactam[r21]), which themselves have little or no antimicrobial activity but are useful in combination with β-lactam antibiotics that are susceptible to β-lactamases (ampicillin, amoxicillin). For example, infections caused by β-lactamase-producting *H. influenzae* may be treated with a combination of ampicillin and clavulanic acid. **Imipenem,**[r22] a new carbepenem β-lactam antimicrobial is hydrolyzed in the kidney by a dehydropeptidase, and this problem has been overcome by administering a dehydropeptidase inhibitor, cilastatin,[r23] along with imipenem. Similarly, allopurinol has been shown to reduce the effective dose of 6-mercaptopurine several-fold in refractory leukemia patients by inhibiting xanthine oxidase, which destroys this purine.[42] This concept of using in combination an inhibitor of the drug deactivating enzyme along with the active drug is likely to find even broader application.

For Treatment of Polymicrobial Infections

Some infections, including intra-abdominal, intraperitoneal and pelvic infections and brain abscesses, usually are due to a mixture of anaerobic and aerobic flora. Combination therapy is strongly indicated for these. Brain abscesses are frequently caused by *Bacteroides* and anaerobic or microaerophilic streptococci. **Metronidazole** penetrates the abscess extremely well and has excellent activity against the *Bacteroides* species; however, it has poor activity against streptococcal species. Penicillin will penetrate the abscess well to kill the streptococci, but is destroyed by β-lactamases produced by Bacteroides strains. This is the rationale for combined use of metronidazole and penicillin.

To Lower Concentration of Individual Component Drugs

A theoretical reason for the use of drug combinations is to lower dosage/concentrations of drugs with toxic potential. Although this looks quite acceptable, especially in cases where synergism is expected, there are so far very few clinical reports to support this. Hurly[41] reported that in human falciparum malaria less then one-tenth of a median effective dose (ED_{50}) of pyrimethamine plus one-quarter of an ED_{50} of sulfadiazine was as effective as one ED_{50} of either drug alone. In subsequent studies it has been shown that sulfadiazine can be replaced by dapsone or sulfadoxine, which have a better matched half-life with pyrimethamine, and that this combination is effective for both suppression and treatment of falciparum malaria.

For Neutropenic Patients

An important indication for combined antimicrobial therapy is to provide a broad spectrum of coverage for the patient who is neutropenic and has compromised host defenses. This is done by combining a broad-spectrum anti-pseudomonas β-lactam with an aminoglycoside as initial therapy for the febrile neutropenic patient.

For Life-Threatening Emergencies

Combination therapy is often used to provide optimal effective therapy in life-threatening emergencies before an etiologic diagnosis can be established with certainty.

Drugs used in combination therapy should preferably be: (i) non-cross-resistant and act by different mechanisms; (ii) have well matched half-lives to decrease the need for frequent dosing.

There are certain risks also in the use of combinations of antimicrobial agents. The most important is toxicity. Certain drugs can be antagonistic, and their combinations should be avoided. Bacteriostatic drugs, such as tetracyclines and sulfonamides, may block the bactericidal action of drugs that attack only the growing organism (penicillins, cephalosporin, and vancomycin); chloramphenicol blocks the lethal action of aminoglycosides on *E. coli*.[42]

Chemoprophylaxis

The purpose of chemoprophylaxis is to avoid the need for chemotherapy by preventing an individual from acquiring a likely infection, or to prevent a dormant or localized infection from becoming more general. Chemoprophylaxis is, however, too often used indiscriminately and haphazardly, and may have deleterious effects on both the individual and the community.

Although antibacterials are quite commonly used for prophylaxis, this is recommended only in some special situations. Chemoprophylaxis should be used mainly to prevent infection by a specific microorganism or to eradicate an infection soon after it has become established. It has been used effectively in: (i) preventing recurrent streptococcal infections in patients with rheumatic fever; (ii) prevention of gonorrhea or syphilis after contact with an infected person; (iii) preventing subacute bacterial endocarditis in patients with valvular heart disease undergoing surgical procedures; (iv) preventing recurrent urinary tract infections caused by *E. coli;* (v) in terminating epidemics of meningococcal infections and of shigellosis in closed populations; (vi) to prevent bacterial diseases in neutropenic patients.

Chemopropylaxis has been used quite effectively to prevent malaria for visitors from nonmalarious regions to malaria endemic regions by using chloroquine or sulfonamide-pyrimethamine, keeping mefloquine in reserve for multiply-resistant strains of the parasite.

In areas where amebic dysentery is highly endemic, a monthly mass treatment with metronidazole has brought about a marked decrease in incidence. Chemoprophylaxis has also been quite effectively used to prevent helminth infections.

Use of Long-Acting Drugs

Long-acting drugs should be used carefully because, toward the end of a treatment protocol when the drug level is falling, the blood level may decrease below MIC. During this period resistant mutants may be selected before eradication of infection has been achieved. Long-acting drugs should, therefore, preferably be used in combination to ensure early achievement of bacterial death for chemoprophylaxis.

Use of Broad-Spectrum Drugs

Drugs with a broad antimicrobial spectrum need to be used carefully; otherwise, resistant strains of the organism for which the drug was not intended may become the predominant organism. For example, trimethoprim, active against both bacteria and protozoa, when used against protozoa may result in development of bacterial resistance, possibly losing its effectiveness for future antibacterial use in the bargain. The converse is also true for pyrimethamine, which should be reserved only for antiprotozoal use.

Rationale for Use of New Drugs

Newly discovered agents should be reserved for cases when there is a lack of sensitivity or resistance to known and commonly used drugs. Otherwise the new drugs also will become ineffective very quickly. Wherever possible a sensitivity test of the infecting organism should be carried out, and then only those agents should be used for treatment that are effective against that organism. For example, fluoroquinolones should not be the first line of treatment for common urinary tract infections or for gonococcal infections, and should be reserved for situations where other drugs have failed or there is established drug resistance.

Treatment of Anaerobic Infections

Because of the time and difficulty involved in the isolation of anaerobic bacteria, diagnosis and treatment of these infections has frequently to be made on an empirical basis. Certain clinical settings such as avascular necrotic tissues with lowered redox potential indicate anaerobic infection. Similarly, infections contiguous or in proximity to the mucosal surface are more likely to be anaerobic, as in the GI tract, the female genital tract, and the oropharynx. A foul odor or presence of gas in tissues is also highly suggestive of anaerobes. Successful management of anaerobic infections requires chemotherapy along with judicious surgical resection and drainage; either alone is inadequate. As most of these infections are caused by mixed flora, it is advisable to use combinations of antimicrobials, active both against aerobes and anaerobes, though not necessarily directed against all the organisms. The principle is that chemotherapy, combined with drainage, disrupts any interdependant relationship among the infecting organisms, and that species that may be resistant to the antimicrobial do not survive without the coinfective organisms; only some species such as *B. fragilis* require specific therapy. Penicillins, cephalosporins, erythromycin, clindamycin, tetracycline, and chloramphenicol are the drugs of choice for most anaerobes of clinical importance, but as its spectrum is confined only to anaerobes, the drug selected must be used in conjunction with an antibacterial active against facultative organisms. Prophylaxis and treatment by active and passive immunization with chemotherapy is advocated in clostridial infections.

Antihelminth Chemotherapy

The principles governing the treatment of helminth infections differ significantly from those employed for the management of bacterial and protozoal infections. Most worms do not multiply within the human host; they produce prodigous numbers of offspring, however, that mature to their infectious state outside the body and then infect the host to produce adult worms. There is a direct correlation between the total number of worms harbored by the human host and the disability incurred; clinical disease is manifest only with heavy worm burden resulting from repeated acquisition of the infectious stage of parasites. With this background, the main goal should be to lower the burden of the infection in the community in endemic areas, and treatment should be focused mainly on the clinically ill. This will cut costs dramatically. The drugs available do offer short-course treatment for practically all worm infections, which will decrease the worm burden, and decrease the transmission of the disease by targeting the major reservoir of the helminths. For example, for major intestinal helminths mebendazole (or related drugs) and pyrantel pamoate offer single-dose safe treatment, including for mixed infections. Repeated at intervals of four weeks they have been found to reduce greatly the burden of infection in the community.[r15]

The Individual and the Community

It cannot be sufficiently emphasized that the recommended dose range for a drug worked out during clinical trial is a median figure that refers to the average patient. However, every community contains a fraction of its population who under-react to a drug, and a fraction who over-react. This fact is represented graphically in Figure 90.2. This situation calls for a cautious approach when exposing a patient to any new drug that the body has not previously encountered. Equally important, enough supervision is needed to ensure that the patient is not seriously underdosed. One reason why individuals or even whole races, show different responses to identical doses of commonly prescribed drugs resides in genetics. As discussed earlier, many drugs are metabolized and deactivated by acetylation controlled by two different acetyl transferases, specified by different genes. These genes occur in different ratios in different individuals/races. Therefore, different people may require different doses of acetylatable drugs to achieve the same blood level of the free drug. The tendency to hemolysis in individuals with an inherited deficiency of glucose-6-phosphate dehydrogenase when exposed to certain drugs such as primaquine has also been discussed earlier.

Another cause for different chemotherapeutic responses of different individuals to the same drugs resides in differences in immune status. It is known, for example, that the therapeutic dose of chloroquine for treatment of malaria is lower in an immune population in an endemic area than in nonimmune people.

Nongenetic aberrant responses to standard doses of drugs are often seen in the newborn, the undernourished, and the elderly—all of whom metabolize drugs more slowly, as is also the case when renal or hepatic dysfunction is present. More rarely, drugs may combine with endogenous macromolecules to form allergens, as seems occasionally to occur when diethylcarbamazine is used in filariasis. A few drugs seem to form toxic material from the parasite they are killing. Thus, the use of melarsoprol in trypanosomiasis of the CNS produces what is called a Jarisch-Herxheimer encephalopathy in about 6 percent of cases, and about 3 percent of patients actually die from this reaction.

Finally, the problem of drug resistance has highlighted the need to follow appropriate dosage schedules. Inappropriate dosing is most often the cause of the emergence of drug-resistant mutants, affecting not only individual patients, but also the spread of resistant organisms in the community. This puts considerable civic responsibility on the physician and patient to follow the correct drug administration regimen.

References

Research Reports

1. Ehrlich P. Das Sauerstoff-Bedurfniss des Organismus: eine farben-analytische Studie. Berlin: A. Hirschwald 1885.
2. Ehrlich P. Chemotherapeutische Trypanosomen Studien. Berl Klin Wschr 1907;*44*:233–236.
3. Ehrlich P. Uber den jetzigen Stand der Chemotherapie. Ber dtsch Chem Ges 1909;*42*:7–47.
4. Ehrlich P. Chemotherapy. Lancet 1913;*2*:445.
5. Ehrlich P, Hata S. The experimental chemotherapy of spirilloses. London: Ribman 1911.
6. Trevan JW. The error of determination of toxicity. Proc Roy Soc 1927;*B101*:485–514.
7. Browning CH, Gilmour W. Bactericidal action and chemical constitution with special reference to basic benzene derivatives. J Path Bact 1913;*18*:144–146.
8. Domagk G. Ein Beitrag zur Chemotherapie der Bakteriellen Infektionen. Dtsch Med Wschr 1935;*61*:250–253.
9. Colebrook L, Kenny M. Treatment of human puerperal infections and of infections in mice, with prontosil. Lancet 1936;*1*:1279–1286.
10. Trefouel J, Trefouel MJ, Nitti F, Bovet D. Activité du p-aminophenylsulfamide sur les infections streptococciques expérimentales de la souris et du lapin. CR Soc Biol Paris 1935;*120*:756–758.
11. Bell PH, Roblin RO Jr. Studies in Chemotherapy VIII. A theory of the relation of structure and activity of sulfanilamide type compounds. J Am Chem Soc 1942;*64*:2905–2917.
12. Brueckner AH. The effect of pH on sulphonamide activity. Yale J Biol Med 1943;*15*:813–821.
13. Cowles PB. Ionization and the bacteriostatic action of sulfonamides. Yale J Biol Med 1942;*14*:599–604.
14. Marshall EK Jr. Determination of sulfanilamide in blood and urine. J Biol Chem 1937;*122*:263–273.
15. Kruger-Thaimer E, Wempe E, Topfor M. Die antibakterielle Wirkung des nicht eiweibgebundenen. Anteils der Sulfanilamide in menschlichen Plasmawassar. Arzneim Frosch 1965;*15*:1309–1317.
16. Woods DD. Relation of p-aminobenzoic acid to mechanism of action of sulphanilamide. Br J Exp Pathol 1940;*21*:74–90.
17. Fildes P. A rational approach to research in chemotherapy. Lancet 1940;*I*:955–957.
18. Fleming A. On the antibacterial action of cultures of a Penicillium, with special reference to their use in the isolation of B. influenzae. Br J Exp Path 1929;*10*:226–236.
19. Chain E, Florey HW, Gardner AD, Heatley NG, Jennings MA, Orr-Ewing J, Sanders AG. Penicillin as a chemotherapeutic agent. Lancet 1940;*2*:226.
20. Schatz A, Begie E, Waksman SA. Streptomycin, a substance exhibiting antibiotic activity against gram-positive and gram-negative bacteria. Proc Soc Exp Biol Med 1944;*55*:66–69.
21. Bartz QR. Isolation and characterisation of chloromycetin. J Biol Chem 1948;*172*:445–450.
22. Duggar BM. Aureomycin: A product of the continuing search for new antibiotics. Ann NY Acad Sci 1948;*51*:177–181.
23. Brown AG, Butterworth D, Cole M, Hauscomb G, Houd JD, Reading C. Naturally-occurring β-lactamase inhibitors with antibacterial activity. J Antibiotics 1976;*29*:668–669.
24. Offe HA, Siefken W, Domagk G. The tuberculostatic activity of hydrazine derivatives from pyridine carboxylic acids and carbonyl compounds. Z Naturforsch 1952;*7b*:462–468.
25. Lesher GY, Froelich EJ, Gruett MD, Bailey JH, Brundage RP. 1,8-Naphthyridine derivatives. A new class of chemotherapeutic agents J Med Pharm Chem 1962;*5*:1063–1065.
26. Clercq ED. Chemotherapeutic approaches to the treatment of the acquired immune deficiency syndrome (AIDS). J Med Chem 1986;*29*:1561–1569.
27. Chabala JC, Mrozik H, Tolman RL, Eskola P, Lusi A, Peterson LH, Woods MF, Fisher MH. Ivermectin, a new broad-spectrum antiparasitic agent. J Med Chem 1980;*23*:1134–1136.
28. Thomas B, Nutman MD, Miller KD, Mulligan M, Reinhardt GN, Currie BJ, Steel C, Ottesen EA. Diethylcarbamazine prophylaxis for human loaisis. Results of a double blind study. N Engl J Med 1988;*319*:752–756.
29. Deo MG, Chaturvedi RM, Kartikeyan S. A candidate anti-leprosy vaccine from ICRC bacilli. Trop Med Parasitol 1990;*41*:367–368.
30. Chatterjee RK, Fatma N, Jain RK, Gupta CM, Anand N. Litomosoides carinii in Rodents: Immunomodulation in potentiating action of diethylcarbamazine. Japan J Exp Med 1988;*58*:243–248.
31. Misra S, Singh DP, Gupta CM, Chatterjee RK, Anand N. Acanthocheilonema vitae in Mastomys natalensis: Effect of immunomodulation on establishment and course of infection. Med Sci Res 1991;*19*:53–55.
32. Ritts RE. Antibiotics as biological response modifiers. J Antimicrob Chemother 1990;*26*(Suppl C):31–36.
33. Jacoby GA, Archer GL. New Mechanisms of Bacterial Resistance to Antimicrobial agents. T N Engl J Med 1991;*324*(9):601–612.
34. Franklin TJ. The inhibition of the incorporation of leucine into protein of the cell-free systems from rat liver and Escherichia coli by chlortetracycline. Biochem J 1963;*87*:449–453.
35. Kan S, Siddiqui WA. Comparative studies of dihydrofolate reductases from Plasmodium falciparum and Aotus trivirgatus. J Protozool 1979;*26*:660–664.
36. Bertino JR, Cashmore A, Fink M, Calabresi P, Lefkowitz ER. The induction of leucocyte and erythrocyte dihydrofolate reductase by methotrexate. Clin Pharmacol Ther 1965;*6*:763–770.
37. Ferone R. Burchall JJ, Hitchings GH. Plasmodium berghei dihydrofolate reductase. Mol Pharmacol 1969;*5*:49–59.
38. Lomovaskaya O, Leis K emr. An Escherichia coli locus for multidrug resistance. Proc Natl Acad Sci 1992;*89*:8938–8942.

39. Eyles D, Colman N. Synergistic effect of sulfadiazine and Daraprim against experimental toxoplasmosis in the mouse. Antibiot Chemother 1953;*3*:483–490.

40. Cattell WR, Chamberlain DA, Fry IK, McSherry MA, Broughton C, O'Grady F. Long-term control of bacteriuria with trimethroprim-sulfonamide. Br Med J 1971;*1*:377–379.

41. Hurly MGD. Potentiation of pyrimethamine by sulfadiazine in human malaria. Tr Roy Soc Trop Med Hyg 1959;*53*:412–413.

42. Wyngaarden JB, Hitchings GH, Elion GB, Silberman HR. Effects of a xanthine oxidase inhibitor on thiopurine metabolism, hyperuricemia and gout. Trans Assoc Amer Physicians 1963;*76*:126–133.

Reviews

r1. Ehrlich P. The collected papers: Compiled and edited by Himmelweit F. Vol III. Chemotherapy. New York: Pergamon Press. 1960.

r2. Minor RW. Paul Ehrlich Centennial Issue. Ann NY Acad Sci 1954;*59*:141–276.

r3. Albert A. Selective toxicity: The physico-chemical basis of therapy, 7th edn. New York: Chapman & Hall 1985.

r4. Anand N. Sulfonamides and Sulfones.

r5. Molecular modification in drug design. Advances in Chemistry Series 45. Washington: Am Chem Society 1964.

r6. Waksman SA. Bacteria as antagonists in microbial antagonism and antibiotic substances. The Commonwealth Fund (1947).

r7. Hitching GH. Inhibition of folate metabolism in chemotherapy: The origins and uses of co-trimoxazole. Berlin: Springer-Verlag (1983).

r8. Mandell GL, Sande MA. Penicillins, cephalosporins and other beta-lactam antibiotics. In: Goodman et al. Goodman and Gilman's the pharmacological basis of therapeutics. (1991); Chapter 46: pp 1065–1097.

r9. Sensi P. Rifampicin. In Bindra JS, Lednicer D. Chronicles of drug discovery, Vol 1. New York: John Wiley (1982).

r10. Andriole VT. The quinolones. London: Academic Press (1988).

r11. WHO Scientific Group on progress in the development and use of antiviral drugs and interferons: Tech Report Series (1987); 754.

r12. Bennett JE. Antifungal therapy. Wilson JD et al. Harrison's Principles of Internal Medicine, 12th ed New York: McGraw Hill (1991); Chapter 87, pp 497–498.

r13. Plorde JJ. Therapy of parasitic infections. Wilson JD et al. Harrison's Principles of Internal Medicine, 12th ed New York: McGraw Hill (1991); Chapter 88, pp 498–502.

r14. WHO Scientific Group: Practical Chemotherapy of malaria. Technical Report Series 805 (1990). Geneva: World Health Organization.

r15. Webster LT Jr. Drugs used in the chemotherapy of helminthiasis. In Gilman et al. Goodman and Gilman's The pharmacological basis of therapeutics. New York: Pergamon Press. (1991); pp 959–978.

r16. Kartner N, Ling V. Multidrug resistance in cancer. Scientific American 1989; March: 26–33.

r17. Davis BD. The basis of chemotherapy. In Davis et al Microbiology, 3d ed. Harper International Edition (1980).

r18. Neu HC. Therapy and prophylaxis of bacterial infections. In: Wilson JD et al. Harrison's principles of internal medicine, 12th ed. New York: McGraw Hill (1991); Chap. 85, pp 478–493.

r19. Ehrlich P. On partial functions of the cell. Nobel Lecture (English Translation). In Himmelweit F. The collected papers of Paul Ehrlich, Vol 3. Chemotherapy. New York: Pergamon Press (1960); pp 183–194.

r20. Domagk G. Twenty five years of sulfonamide therapy. Ann NY Acad Sci 1957;*69*:380–384.

r21. Campoli-Richards DM, Brogden RN. Sulbactam/Ampicillin. A review of its antibacterial activity, pharmacokinetic properties and therapeutic use. Drugs 1987;*33*:577–609.

r22. Birnbaum J, Kahan FM, Kropp H, Macdonald JS. Carbapenems: A new class of antibiotics. Am J Med 1985;*78*:3–21.

r23. Neu HC. Summary of imipenem/cilastatin symposium. Am J Med 1985;*78*:165–167.

r24. Cadwallader DE, Jun WH. Nitrofurantoin. In Florey K. Analytical profiles of drug substances. New York: Academic Press 1976; Vol 5: pp 345–373.

r25. Holmes B. Norfloxacin: A review of its antibacterial activity. Drugs 1985;*30*:482–513.

r26. Labro MT. Cefodizine as a biological response modifier: A review of its in-vivo, ex-vivo and in-vitro immunomodulatory properties. J Antimicrob Chemother 1990;*26*(Suppl c):37–47.

r27. Antibiotics as biological response modifiers. Editorial, Lancet 1991;*337*:400–401.

r28. Wormser GP, Keusch GT. Trimethoprim/sulfamethoxazole: An overview. In Hitchings GH. Inhibition of Folate Metabolism in Chemotherapy. Berlin: Springer-Verlag, 1983.

r29. Schabel FM. Synergism and antagonism among antitumor agents. In Cumley RW. Pharmacological basis of cancer chemo therapy, Baltimore: Williams & Wilkins, (1975); pp 595–623.

CHAPTER 91

Nitya Anand

Sulfonamides and Sulfones

Introduction

The discovery in the early 1930s of the antibacterial activity of prontosil, the first effective chemotherapeutic agent employed for the systemic treatment of bacterial infections, was the beginning of the modern era of chemotherapy.[1,2] The expectations then aroused for the therapy of microbial infections have been amply fulfilled. Some of the other developments resulting from this important discovery had far-reaching effects on future progress, not only in the field of sulfonamides but on chemotherapy and drug research in general. The recognition of the inhibition of the action of sulfonamides by yeast extracts,[3,4] shown to be due to p-aminobenzoic acid (PABA),[3] was the first demonstration of metabolite antagonism as a mechanism of drug action; it led Fildes[5] (1940) to propose his classic theory of antimetabolites as a basis for chemotherapy. The development of dihydrofolate reductase inhibitors as antimicrobial agents was a direct result of this interest in antimetabolites. That the antibacterial action of prontosil that was of consequence was sulfanilamide formed in vivo focused attention on the importance of drug metabolism and blood levels of the active species for drug action, which provided a rational basis for calculating dosage regimens. Pharmacokinetic studies thus became an integral part of drug development programs. Studies on sulfonamides also led to their use as carbonic anhydrase inhibitors, diuretics, hypoglycemics, and antithyroid agents;[r4,r7] however, this chapter is limited to antimicrobial sulfonamides (and sulfones), all of which act by competitively antagonizing the uptake of p-aminobenzoic acid (PABA antagonists) by the organism, resulting in inhibition of the biosynthesis of the folate coenzyme systems.

Historical Development

Sulfonamides

The history of the development of sulfonamides as a major class of chemotherapeutic agents is one of the most fascinating chapters in drug research, highlighting the roles of skillful planning and serendipity. The synthesis of prontosil was a carry-over of the interest generated in dyes in general as possible antimicrobials following Ehrlich's studies[r8] on the relationship between selective staining by dyes and their antimicrobial activity, and in the sulfonamide group as contributory to fastness for acid wool dyes as a result of the work of IG Farbenindustrie (see Mietzch)[6] which led Mietzsch and Klarer[7] to synthesize a group of azo dyes containing a sulfonamide group, including prontosil. The lack of correlation between in vitro and in vivo antibacterial tests prompted Domagk[2] to resort to in vivo testing, a very fortunate decision, since otherwise the fate of sulfonamides might have been different. In fact, similar dyes had been synthesized almost a decade earlier, such as p-sulfonamidobenzeneazodihydrocupreine by Heidelberger and Jacobs,[8] but tested in vitro, thus understandably showing rather poor activity. Domagk[1] observed that prontosil protected mice against streptococcal infections and rabbits against staphylococcal infections, but had no effect on pneumococcal infections and was without action in vitro on bacteria. Foerster[9] soon after reported the first clinical success with prontosil in a case of staphylococcal septicemia. Trefouel et al,[10] working at the Pasteur Institute in Paris, prepared a series of azo dyes by coupling diazotized sulfanilamide with phenols, with and without amino or alkyl groups. They observed that variations in the structure of the phenolic moiety had very little effect on in vitro antibacterial activity, whereas even small changes in the sulfanilamide component reduced or abolished the activity. These and other[11] observations pointed to the sulfanilamide component as the active structural unit; sulfanilamide was tested and found as effective as the parent dye-stuff in protecting mice against meningococcal and streptococcal infections. Fuller's demonstration[12] of the presence of sulfanilamide in the blood and its isolation from urine of patients (and mice) under treatment with prontosil firmly established that prontosil is reduced in the body to form sulfanilamide, a compound synthesized as early as 1908 by Gelmo.[13] The era of modern chemotherapy had begun. These epoch-making results published between 1933 and 1937 aroused world-wide interest, and further development took place at a very rapid rate. The demonstration that the antimicrobial activity of prontosil was due to its metabolic reduction product, sulfanilamide, was a most important event. Sulfanilamide, being easy to prepare, cheap, and not covered by patents, became available for widespread use and brought a new hope for the treatment of microbial infections. Recognizing the potential of sulfonamides in chemotherapy, almost all major research organizations the world over initiated programs for the synthesis and study of analogues and derivatives of sulfanilamide with a view to: (i) enlarging its antmicrobial spectrum; (ii) increasing its transport and distribution in the body fluids and tissues; (iii) increasing its half-life to reduce the frequency of administration; (iv) increasing the water solubility, both of the parent compound and its metabolites in order to reduce a tendency toward crystalluria, a serious side-effect observed with early sulfonamides; (v) delaying the emergence of resistant bacterial forms and improving the activity against resistant organisms. New sulfonamides with improved spectra of activity were thus introduced in quick succession until about 1945; the more important ones were sulfapyridine (M&B 693), sulfathiazole, sulfacetamide, sulfadiazine, sulfamerazine, sulfamethazine, and sulfisoxazole, some of which are still used in clinical practice. The work of this period has been reviewed in a very exhaustive monograph by Northey.[rl]

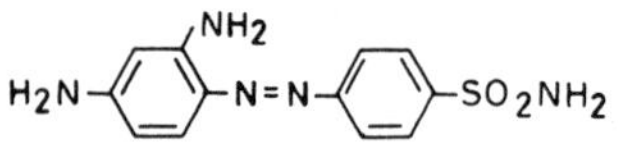

PRONTOSIL

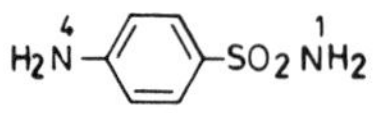

SULFANILAMIDE

With the introduction of penicillin in the early 1940s, emphasis in the development of antibacterials gradually shifted to antibiotics. However, after the initial flush of enthusiasm with antibiotics was over, owing to problems encountered with their use such as easy emergence of resistant strains, superinfection, and allergic reactions, a revival of interest in sulfonamides occurred around 1955. Knowledge gained during the intervening period about the selectivity of action of sulfonamides on the parasite, the relationship between their solubility and toxicity, pharmacokinetics and dose regimens (that some sulfonamides were rapidly absorbed and slowly excreted, resulting in maintenance of adequate blood level for a long period and thus requiring less frequent administration), and about their mode of action and therapeutic synergism with dihydrofolate reductase inhibitors, gave a new direction to further developments in this field. Soon sulfonamides with modified properties began to appear; the more important ones of the post-1955 period widely used in clinical practice are sulfamethoxypyridazine,[14,r9] sulfadimethoxine,[15,17] sulfamethoxypyrazine,[18] and sulformethoxine.[19,20] Although no major new sulfonanamide has been added in recent years, these and some of the earlier sulfonamides have continued to be used extensively. Their present status in therapeutics is discussed later. Following the initial observation of their powerful antibacterial activity, sulfonamides were tested against other organisms, and it was found that some large viruses, protozoa, and fungi also are inhibited by sulfonamides and sulfones. Some commonly used sulfonamides and their special features are described in Table 91.1.

Sulfones

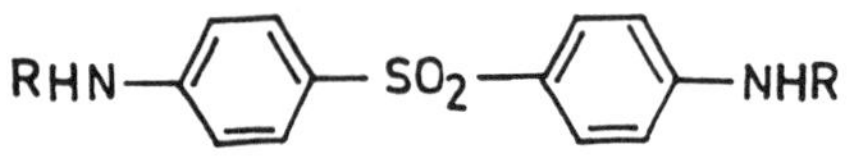

Dapsone, R = H

Acedapsone, R = $COCH_3$

Diphenylsulfones first attracted attention because of their structural similarity to sulfonamides. It was reported in the early 1940s that experimentally-induced tuberculosis could be controlled by 4,4'-diaminodiphenylsulfone (dapsone, Rist et al,[21] and by its N,N' didextrose sulfonate (promin, Feldman et al[22]). This was a major advance in the chemotherapy of mycobacterial infections. Although dapsone and promin proved disappointing in human tuberculosis, the latter showed a favorable response in rat leprosy.[23] This was soon followed by successful treatment of leprosy patients, first with promin and later with dapsone itself.[24] Despite the study of a large variety of sulfones, dapsone has remained the drug of choice for leprosy, and none of its analogues has so far surpassed it in activity. All the sulfones of clinical value are derivatives of dapsone. An important advance in the use of dapsone took place with the demonstration that certain N,N'-diacyl derivatives and Schiff's bases of dapsone have a repository effect[25,26] and release dapsone slowly. N,N'-Diacetamidodiphenylsulfone (acedapsone) is particularly useful as a repository form; after a single IM injection of 225 mg of acedapsone, a therapeutic blood level of dapsone is maintained for as long as 68 to 80 days.[27]

Antimicrobial Action

Antimicrobial Spectrum

The biologic activity of sulfonamides and sulfones extends to a number of microbial species possessing a folic acid pathway; these include many gram-negative and gram-positive cocci and bacilli, mycobacteria, some large viruses, protozoa, and fungi. In all cases action is related to PABA antagonism. In general, sulfonamides exert only a bacteriostatic effect, and cellular and humoral defense mechanisms of the host are essential for the final eradication of the infection. Minimal inhibitory concentrations range from 0.1 µg/ml for *C. trachomatis* to 4–64 µg/ml for *E. coli*; peak plasma drug concentrations achievable in vivo are approximately 100–200 µg/ml. Owing to extensive clinical use, many isolates of common organisms are now resistant. For example, many *E. coli* strains isolated from patients with urinary tract infections (community acquired) are often resistant to sulfonamides; these drugs are no longer the therapy of choice for such infections. Table 91.2 illustrates broadly the antimicrobial spectrum of

Table 91.1 Commonly Used Sulfonamides and Sulfones

$H_2N-C_6H_4-SO_2NHR$

Generic Name	R	pKa	Plasma $T_{1/2}$ hr (man)	In vitro activity against E. coli (umol/1)	Special Features
Sulfaguanidine	-NH-C(=NH)-NH2	Basic	—	—	Poorly absorbed, locally acting, used earlier in GI infections
Sulfamethizole	5-methyl-1,3,4-thiadiazol-2-yl-NH–	5.5	2.5	—	Rapidly absorbed, rapidly excreted mainly unmetabolised, used mainly for urinary tract infections
Sulfisoxazole	3,4-dimethylisoxazol-5-yl-NH–	5.0	6.0	2.15	Rapidly absorbed, rapidly excreted, excellant antibacterial activity, high solubility, 76.5% plasma protein bound, only infrequently produces hematuria or crystalluria, excreted mainly unmetabolised, employed for urinary tract infections
Sulfamethazine	4,6-dimethylpyrimidin-2-yl-NH–	7.4	7	1.7	Well absorbed, rapidly excreted mainly as N^4-metabolite
Sulfacetamide	–NHCON	5.4	7	2.3	Well absorbed, sodium salt makes high concentration non-irritant solution, used extensively in the management of eye infections, low plasma protein binding
Sulfisomidine	2,6-dimethylpyrimidin-4-yl-NH–	7.4	7.5		Well absorbed, rapidly excreted mainly unmetabolized, used for urinary tract infections
Sulfanilamide	H	10.5	9	128	Parent compound, low antibacterial activity
Sulfamethoxazole	5-methylisoxazol-3-yl-NH–	6.0	11	0.8	Well absorbed, half-life matched with trimethoprim, combined with latter (named cotrimaxazole) widely used in therapy for systemic infections
Sulfadiazine	pyrimidin-2-yl-NH–	6.52	17	0.9	Rapidly absorbed, moderate rate of excretion, well distributed in all body tissues including CNS, occupies a pre-eminent position among sulfonamides, 55% plasma protein bound, silver sulfadiazine inhibits in vitro nearly all pathogenic bacteria and fungi, used topically to reduce microbial colonization, one of the most effective sulfonamides

continued

sulfonamides and sulfones. The synergism observed between sulfonamides and dihydrofolate reductase inhibitors has further enlarged the antimicrobial range of sulfonamides.[48,r6]

Structure Activity Relationship

Antimicrobial sulfonamides and sulfones are characterized by their ability to interfere with the biosyn-

Table 91.1 *Continued*

Generic Name	R	pKa	Plasma $T_{1/2}$ hr (man)	In vitro activity against E. coli (umol/1)	Special Features
Sulfamerazine	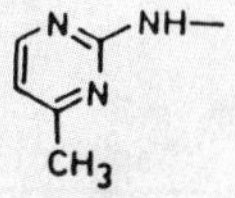 [structure: 4-methylpyrimidin-2-yl–NH–]	6.98	24	0.95	Rapidly absorbed, high solubility, and high antibacterial activity, component of "triple sulfa" combination employed earlier
Sulfamethoxypyridazine	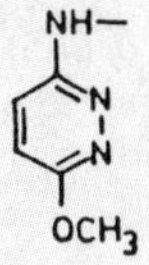 [structure: 6-methoxypyridazin-3-yl–NH–]	7.2	37	1.0	First long-acting sulfonamide discovered requiring once a day administration, 77% plasma protein bound
Sulfamethoxypyrazine	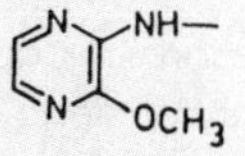 [structure: 3-methoxypyrazin-2-yl–NH–]	6.1	65	1.85	Well absorbed, sparingly soluble, 65% plasma protein bound, used for chronic infections and for chemoprophylaxis
Sulformethoxine Sulfamethoxine	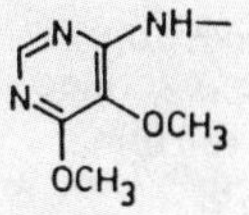 [structure: 5,6-dimethoxypyrimidin-4-yl–NH–]	6.1	150	0.8	Well absorbed, highly protein bound (95%), long half-life, matched with pyrimethamine and this combination (named fansidar) commonly used for prophylaxis & treatment of parasitic protozoal infections, particularly for malaria due to chloroquine resistant P. falciparum and Pneumocystis carinii pneumonia in AIDS patients, side-effects can be severe and should be carefully monitored
Dapsone	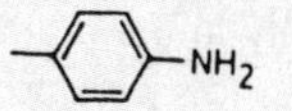 [structure: –C₆H₄–NH₂ (p-aminophenyl)]	13	20	44	Well absorbed, well distributed in all body tissues, moderate rate of excretion, retained in the circulation for a long time because of intestinal reabsorption from bile, M. *leprae*, very sensitive to it and is drug of choice for leprosy

thesis of folate coenzymes by competing with PABA at the enzyme site. The following generalizations regarding their structure-activity relationships to antimicrobial potency were arrived at quite early in their development and guided subsequent work. These generalizations, which still hold, are:[r4,r5]

1. Replacement of the benzene ring by other ring systems markedly reduces or abolishes the activity.
2. Introduction of additional substituents in the benzene ring decreases or abolishes the activity.
3. The amino and sulfonyl radicals on the benzene ring should be in 1,4-disposition for activity.
4. The 4′-amino group should be unsubstituted or have a substituent that is removed readily in vivo.
5. Replacement of the SO_2NH_2 by $SO_2C_6H_4$-p-NH_2 retains the activity, while that of SO_2 by CO markedly reduces it.
6. N^1-monosubstitution results in more active compounds with greatly modifed pharmacokinetic properties while N^1-disubstitution in general leads to inactive compounds.
7. These generalizations also apply broadly to sulfones, so that only N-monosubstituted derivatives of dapsone (or those which hydrolyze to it in vivo) retain the full activity.

The presence of the p-aminophenylsulfonyl radical thus seems essential for full activity, and practically all important drugs are N^1-substituted. These substituents seem to affect mainly the physicochemical characteristics and as a consequence the pharmacokinetic properties of the drugs.

Physicochemical Properties and Antimicrobial Activity

Quite early in the development of sulfonamides, possible correlation(s) between physicochemical prop-

Table 91.2 Antimicrobial Spectrum of Sulfonamides and Sulfones

Gram-Positive, Acid Fast	Gram-Negative	Other
	Highly Sensitive	
Bacillus anthracis (some strains)	Calymmatobacterium granulomatis	Chlamydia trachomatis,
Corynebacterium diphtheriae (some strains)	Hemophilus ducreyi	Lymphogranuloma venereum
Mycobacterium leprae (to Sulfones)	H. influenzae	Trachoma viruses
Staphylococcus aureus	Neisseria gonorrheae	Plasmodium falciparum*
Streptococcus pneumoniae	N. meningitidis	P. malariae*
S. pyogenes (group A)	Pasteurella pestis	Toxoplasma
	Proteus mirabilis	Coccidia
	Shigella flexneri S. sonnei	Actinomyces bovis
	Vibrio cholerae	Nocardia asteroides
	Weakly Susceptible	
Clostridium welchii	Aerobacter aerogenes	Plasmodium vivax*
Mycobacterium tuberculosis	Proteus vulgaris	
Streptococcus viridans	Pseudomonas aeruginosa	
	Salmonella	
	Brucella abortus	
	Escherichia coli	
	Klebsiella pneumoniae	

*Only blood schizontocide

erties and bacteriostatic activity attracted attention, and the parameters that have been most studied are the degree of ionization, protein binding, and lipid/water solubility.

As it was realized quite early in the development of sulfonamides that substitution in the benzene ring of sulfanilamide led to a lowering or loss of activity, studies to find a correlation between structure, physicochemical properties, and antimicrobial activity focused attention primarily on the amino and sulfonamido groups. The primary amino group in sulfonamides (and sulfones) is apparently vital for affinity to the enzyme and bacteriostasis,[28] since its substitution causes a loss of activity; all active compounds have a basic dissociation constant of about 2, which is close to that of PABA. It has been found by the molecular orbitals method that N^1-substituents did not vary the electronic charge on the 4-amino group.[29] Thus, attention has been focused mainly on the acidic dissociation constant, which varies widely from about 3 to 11.

Several groups of investigators in the early 1940s, almost simultaneously, noted the relationship between bacteriostatic activity and degree of ionization of sulfonamides. Bell & Roblin[31] in a comprehensive study of the action of a wide range of sulfonamides against *E. coli* in vitro found that there was a parabolic relationship between pKa and log 1/MIC, and that the highest point of this curve lay between pKa 6 and 7.4; the maximal activity was thus observed in compounds whose pKa approximated the physiologic pH. Increasing the pH of the growth medium increased the relative activity of a particular sulfonamide up to the point at which its degree of ionization reached 50 percent (Cowles,[31] Brueckner[32]). This effect was explained on the basis that the compounds penetrated the cell in the unionized form; once inside the cell, the bacteriostatic action is due to the ionized species. Therefore, for optimal activity, the compound should have a pKa that gives a proper balance between activity and penetration; a half-dissociation state appears to present such a balance. This would also explain the fact that in cell-free systems the most active agents are those that are ionized.

Yamazaki et al,[33] in a study of the relationship between antibacterial activity and pKa of 14 N^1-heterocyclic sulfanilamides, found that whereas the relationship between pKa and activity is parabolic when total concentration is considered, it is linear for ionized and unionized states, giving two lines with opposite slopes and intersecting each other, the point of intersection corresponding to the pH of the culture medium. They found the pKa for optimal activity to be between 6.61 and 7.4.

Another parameter of the sulfanamide group that has attracted some attention is the negative charge density on the SO_2 group. It has been shown by Coates et al[34] that an increase in the negative charge at the SO_2 group is produced by electron-releasing groups for sulfones, whereas for sulfonamides, ionization increases with electron attracting N^1-substituents, which provides a unifying picture for the activity of sulfonamides and sulfones.

Lipid solubility of different sulfonamides varies over a wide range. Several studies[35,36] on hydrophobic effects have shown these to be relatively unimportant for intrinsic activity at the enzyme, but of importance with respect to optimizing transmembrane transport into the cells. It has been shown that, in general, as the lipid solubility increases, so does the half-life; long-acting sulfonamides with high renal tubular reabsorption are generally characterized by high lipid solubility.[35] Serum protein binding of sulfonamides also varies over a wide range, from about 9.5 percent for sulfanilamide to about 95 percent for sulfadoxine; the structural features that favor protein-binding are the same that increase lipophilicity and favour transport across membranes. In general, the more lipophilic the sulfonamides, the stronger the protein binding and the longer the half-life (Table 91.1).

Mechanism of Antimicrobial Action

The sulfonamides are bacteriostatic and inhibit growing bacterial organisms. The discovery that sulfonamides act by inhibiting folic acid synthesis in microorganisms was the result of many lines of investigation proceeding simultaneously, which included identification of PABA as the factor in yeast extract and other biologic fluids responsible for antagonizing the action of sulfonamides, and elucidation of the structure, function, and biosynthesis of folic acid.[37]

In the biosynthesis of folic acid (Fig. 91.1), hydroxymethyldihydropterin either couples with PABA, via an ATP-activated process, leading to dihydropteroic acid, which in turn conjugates with glutamic acid to give dihydrofolic acid, or the latter is accomplished from the dihydropterin and PABA-glutamic acid conjugate via an ATP-activated process. The same enzyme system seems to be involved in the incorporation of either PABA or its glutamic acid conjugate,[37-39] and sulfonamides (and sulfones) compete with PABA for this enzyme. Using cell-free systems it has been shown that the relationship between sulfonamides and PABA is strictly competitive when incubation is carried out with all substrates present together and with normal concentrations of pteridines. Under these conditions the inhibitory effect of the sulfonamide can be reversed by addition of more PABA. It has also been shown that sulfonamides (and sulfones) can compete with PABA, not only for binding to the particular enzyme but they also get incorporated to form false folic acid analogues.[40,41] The latter have been shown to be inactive as C-1 carriers. It has, however, been shown that this incorporation is not relevant to the antimicrobial action of sulfonamides: binding strongly to dihydropteroate synthetase and thus inhibiting its coupling to PABA is their primary mode of action. The consequent reduction in the rate of dihydropteroate synthesis decreases the concentration of tetrahydrofolate cofactors in the cell, thus gradually turning off the normal supply of the one carbon metabolic pool involved in the biosynthesis of amino acids and purine and pyrimidine bases. This action explains why sulfonamides act only against growing microorganisms and why the onset of bacteriostasis is preceded by a lag phase, during which stores of PABA and folic acid are consumed. The length of the lag phase depends on the level of these stores; the inhibitory effect of sulfonamides can be reversed by addition of more PABA.

The mechanism of action of dapsone and other diarylsulfones is similar to that of sulfonamides, and their action is antagonized by PABA in mycobacteria,[42,43] as in other bacteria[44] and malarial parasites.[45,46] It has been suggested by Moriguchi and Wada[47] that there are two binding sites on the enzyme, dihydropteroate synthetase. One is specific for 4′-amino group and the other is nonspecific, where the acidic group of PABA or a highly polarized sulfonyl group can bind.

De novo folic acid synthesis takes place in a wide range of microorganisms, including bacteria, protozoa, yeasts, fungi, and large viruses; the action of sulfonamides on them is competetively antagonized by PABA. It appears that microorganisms are usually not able to assimilate the folic acid or its precursors present in humans, and the level of PABA in the host is too low to reverse the inhibition by sulfonamides.

Sulfonamides can thus in principle inhibit all organisms dependent on de novo folic acid synthesis for their survival. Higher organisms, such as humans, do not synthesize their own folic acid but obtain it from their diets; folic acid is produced by plants. This explains the selective antimicrobial action of sulfonamides and sulfones.

Synergism with Dihydrofolate Reductase Inhibitors

In the folic acid pathway, dihydrofolic acid undergoes reversible reduction by a dihydrofolate reductase (DHFR) to tetrahydrofolic acid, which is the active form of the coenzyme, and is involved in the enzyme catalyzed transfer of the one-carbon units (formyl, methyl, or hydroxymethyl) to various substrates. This dihydrofolate reduction step is inhibited by agents such as methotrexate, trimethroprim, and pyrimethamine. Thus, blocking of folic acid biosynthesis by both sulfonamides and dihydrofolate reductase inhibitors—but at different sequential sites—provided a suitable rational combination for synergistic action[48] (See Chapter 92). This synergistic interaction between sulfonamides and DHFRI is predictable, and was in fact demonstrated in the early 1950s.[49-51] It is now recognized as of general occurrence. Therapy with a combination of DHFRIs and sulfonamides has added a new dimension to treatment with these agents. The usefulness of such combinations may be due to one or more of the following factors; (i) several-fold increases in chemotherapeutic index; (ii) better tolerance of individual drugs; (iii) delayed development of resistance to individual drugs; and (iv) ability to cure microbial infections where the curative effects of the individual drugs are borderline owing to low sensitivity or resistance. For example, methicillin-resistant strains of *Staph. aureus* usually are susceptible to the combination.

Combinations of pyrimethamine and sulfonamides are now widely used for the treatment of plasmodial, toxoplasmal, and coccidial infections; and a combination of trimethoprim and sulfonamide is used for a number of bacterial infections. The choice of the component drugs is based both on their antimicrobial spectrum and on their matched half-life characteristics; the ratio of the two components depends on their pharmacokinetic characteristics. There is an optimal ratio of concentration of the two agents for synergism, and this is equal to the ratio of the minimal inhibitory concentrations of the drugs acting independently. The most effective ratio for the largest number of microorganisms is 20 parts of sulfamethoxazole to one part of trimethoprim. The quantities of the individual drugs formulated in the combination are such as would achieve sulfamethoxazole concentration in vivo 20 times greater than that of trimethoprim (5:1 ratio of sulfamethoxazole to trimethoprim achieves this). The more widely used combination for antibacterial che-

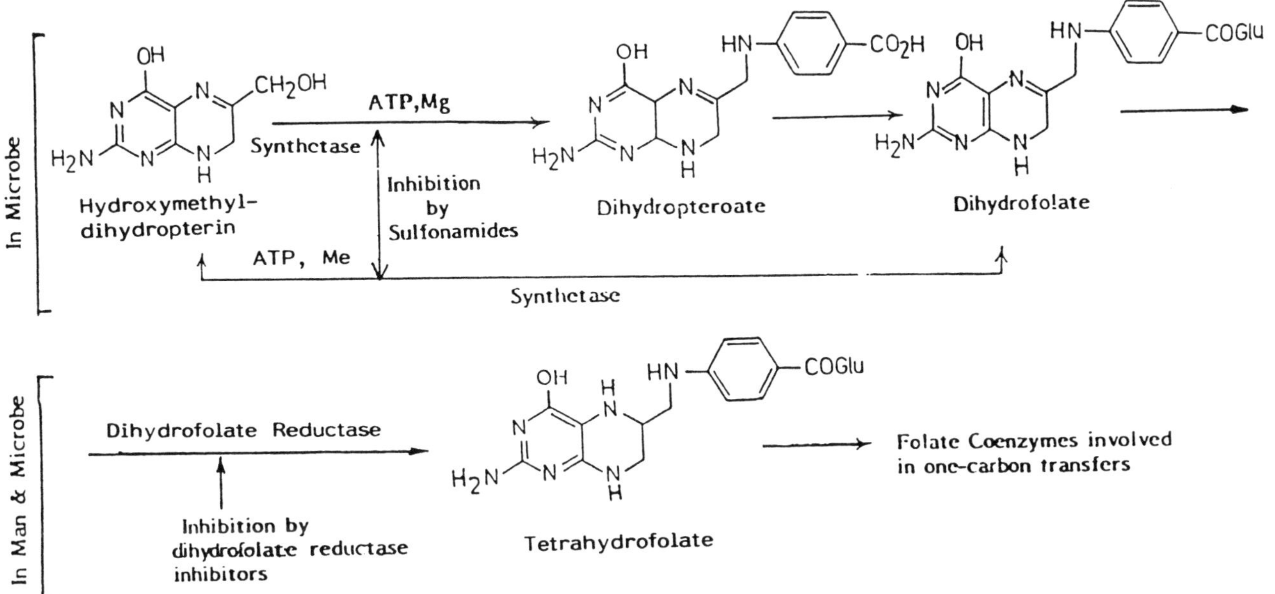

Figure 91.1 Folate metabolism and sites of action of sulfonamides, sulfones, and dihydrofolate reductase inhibitors.

motherapy is of trimethoprim and sulfamethoxazole (commonly named co-trimoxazole) and for antiprotozoal chemotherapy of pyrimethamine and sulformethoxine (commonly named Fansidar; 1:20 ratio) and occasionally of pyrimethamine and dapsone (named maloprim, 1:8 ratio).

Drug Resistance

Emergence of drug-resistant strains is a problem with sulfonamides as with many other antimicrobials. Such resistance can arise by one or more of the following mechanims: (i) altered permeability of the cell wall so that less sulfonamide is transported inside;[52,53] (ii) increased production of PABA by the pathogen;[54,55] (iii) changes in the target enzyme, making it more selective to the natural substrate;[53,56,57] (iv) gene amplification of the enzyme so that more copies of it are produced, thus rendering its saturation by antagonist difficult; (v) bypass mechanisms by which the microorganism develops an ability to utilize more effectively the folic acid present in the host.[58] These types of resistance can arise by random mutation[53] and selection or transfer of resistance by plasmids from other resistant organisms. Such resistance,[59] once it is maximally developed, usually is persistent and irreversible. Since the mode of action of sulfonamides involves the same basic mechanism, different sulfonamides usually show cross-resistance, but not to chemotherapeutic agents of other classes. To minimize the problem of development of resistance, well-accepted principles of antimicrobial therapy have to be followed, such as initial treatment with an adequate dose for an adequate period and treatment with a combination of drugs.

Pharmacokinetics and Metabolism

The sulfonamides in clinical use vary widely in their pharmacokinetic characteristics, which adds greatly to their spectrum of clinical usefulness. Except for those having additional ionizable groups, sulfonamides as a class, after oral intake, are rapidly absorbed from the GI tract—some from the stomach, but mainly from the small intestine—and excreted mainly in the urine. Those which are highly ionized are poorly absorbed build up high local concentrations in the gut and are thus considered useful for GI infections. In general those that are well absorbed are distributed throughout all tissues of the body. Those that are highly water-soluble, such as sulfisomidine, are largely confined to the extracellular space and do not attain a high tissue concentration, show no tendency to crystallize in the kidneys, are more readily excreted, and are useful in treating urinary tract infections. The relatively less soluble ones, such as sulfadiazine, build up high levels throughout the total body water and are useful for treating systemic infections. This wide range of solubilities and pharmacokinetic characteristics of sulfonamides permit their access to almost any site in the body.

Half-lives of different sulfonamides in clinical use

vary widely from 2.5 hour to 150 hour (Table 91.1); they also show marked differences in different animal species. Long-acting sulfonamides are in general more lipid-soluble than are short-acting compounds; factors such as tubular secretion and resorption also seem to affect the half-life. The half-life of sulfonamides is of great importance because the dosage regimen must be related to it. The Doseage schedule is a function of the inhibitory index and pharmacokinetic parameters. Kruger-Thiemer[59,60] has developed mathematical models for describing the relationship between these parameters and evolved a computer program for calculating them.

The sulfonamides may be classified on the basis of their pharmacokinetic characteristics as follows; these determine the clinical situation in which the drugs would be employed:

1. Absorbed rapidly and excreted rapidly, mainly unmetabolized (e.g., sulfisoxazole and sulfamethoazine), and are useful in urinary tract infections.
2. Absorbed rapidly, but have a medium rate of excretion and high tissue distribution (e.g., sulfadiazine); useful for systemic infections.
3. Absorbed very poorly when administered orally, and hence active in the bowel (e.g., sulfaguanidine and sulfasalazine).
4. Absorbed rapidly but excreted very slowly (long-acting) (e.g., sulfamethoxypyrazine and sulformethoxine); apart from other situations can be useful for chemoprophylaxis.
5. Sulfonamides mainly for topical use, such as sodium sulfacetamide and silver sulfadiazine.

Metabolism of sulfonamides takes place primarily in the liver and involves mainly N^4-acetylation, to a lesser extent N′-glucuronidation, and to a very small extent C-hydroxylation. All these metabolites are inactive.[61,r11] There is considerable genetic polymorphism in the ability to N-acetylate, and this has important implications for therapeutic regimens. In a leprosy population, almost 50 percent of patients have been reported to be slow acetylators.[62] Renal clearance rates of the metabolites are generally higher than those of the parent drugs. N^1-substituents markedly influence the metabolic fate of the sulfonamides. Some of the sulfonamides, such as sulfisomidine and sulfamethizole, are excreted almost unchanged and are especially useful for urinary tract infections; in most of them N^4-acetylation takes place to a substantial degree, along with varying degrees of N^1-glucuronidation

Dapsone is well absorbed after oral administration and is evenly distributed in almost all body tissues. It is excreted mainly through the kidney. Less then 5 percent is excreted unchanged, and most of it is present as the mono-N-glucuronide and as mono-N-acelyl derivatives. It has a half-life of about 20 hour.[63–65]

Present Status in Therapeutics

Sulfonamides, discovered almost six decades ago, still constitute an important group of antimicrobials. The number of conditions for which sulfonamides are drugs of first choice has declined on account of a gradual increase in resistance to them and the addition of more effective antimicrobials, but they still have a distinct place in therapeutics. They are useful because of the choice they provide of agents with greatly differing half-lives and pharmacokinetic characteristics, meeting the requirements of varied clinical situations, their wide spectrum of antimicrobial action, their synergistic action in combination with dihydrofolate reductase inhibitors, their highly selective action on the microbe and relative freedom from problems of superinfection, ease of administration and relatively low cost. About 15 sulfonamides and one sulfone are still widely used.

Nocardiosis

Sulfonamides, alone or combined with trimethoprim, are the drugs of choice in the treatment of infections due to Nocardia species,[66,67,r12] including cerebral nocardiosis.[68] Sulfisoxazole, sulfamethoxazole, and sulfadiazine are the commonly used drugs. Treatment may need to be continued for some months for complete cure, and in advanced cases may need to be combined with another antibiotic.

Toxoplasmosis

Combined with pyrimethamine, sulformethoxine or sulfadiazine remain the drugs of choice for toxoplasmosis,[r13] including materno-fetal toxoplasmosis.[69]

Lymphogranuloma Venereum and Chancroid

Sulfonamides remain the drug of choice for these conditions.[r14]

Eye Infections, Trachoma, and Inclusion Conjunctivitis

Sulfacetamide sodium eyedrops are employed extensively for the management of ophthalmic infections; a combination of topical and systemic application is of value in some conditions.

Leprosy

Dapsone remains the choice drug for all forms of leprosy and is an essential component of all multidrug therapy regimens used.[70]

Malaria

Combined with pyrimethamine, sulformethoxine, sulfamethoxypyridazine, and, more recently, dapsone have been used both for the treatment and chemoprophylaxis of chloroquine-resistant falciparum malaria.[r15,71]

Rheumatic Fever

Sulfonamides are commonly used in preventing streptococcal infections and recurrence of rheumatic fever among susceptible subjects, especially in patients who are hypersensitive to penicillin. Sulfisoxazole or sulfadiazine are the commonly used agents.

Urinary Tract, Gastrointestinal, Meningococcal, and Pulmonary Infections

Sulfonamides combined with trimethoprim are of value in the treatment of urinary tract infections,[72–75] bacillary dysentery (particularly that caused by Shigella),[76] salmonellosis,[77,78] and chronic bronchitis.[79,80] In meningococcal infections, sulfonamides are of value only if the strains of *N. meningitidis* or *H. influenzae* are sensitive to them.

Other Conditions

Silver sulfadiazine is very useful for the treatment of burn wounds. Sulfonamides have been found useful for the treatment of arterial infections due to *Listeria monocytogenes*[81] and for prophylaxis of otitis media in children.[82] Dapsone has also been reported to cure some cases of Crohn's disease, which may have a mycobacterial species origin.[83] A combination of sulfamethoxazole and trimethoprim has been found useful both for the prophylaxis[84,85] and treatment[86] of pneumocystis carinii pneumonia, a common sequelae in patients with AIDS.

Shortly after the introduction of sulfa drugs, sulfapyridine was found to have unique beneficial effects on some inflammatory conditions, especially dermatologic, unrelated to their antibacterial activity;[82] later dapsone was found to share the same properties, but at a much lower dose and thus with an improved therapeutic index.[87,88] The disorders that respond are dermatitis herpetiformis, pyoderma gangrenosum, subcorneal pustular dermatosis, acrodermatitis continua, impetigo herpetiformis, ulcerative colitis, and cutaneous lesions of patients with lupus erythematosus.[87–91] Salazosulfapyridine is the treatment of choice for ulcerative colitis.[92,93] These disorders are characterized by edema followed by granulocytic inflammation or by vesicle or bullae formation. The mechanism of action is not fully understood, but it has been proposed that these drugs enter or influence the protein moiety of glycosaminoglycans and decrease tissue viscosity, resulting in prevention of edema, dilution of tissue fluid, and decrease in inflammation and vesicle and bullae formation.[87]

Adverse Reactions

Though adverse drug reactions are numerous and varied, most are not serious. The over-all incidence of reactions is about 5 percent.[r2] Crystalluria, one of the earliest serious toxic reactions reported with sulfonamides, has been more or less overcome since the discovery of agents more soluble at the pH of urine, that require low dosage, or are excreted mainly as water-soluble metabolites.

Blood dyscrasias are quite uncommon; when they do occur, drug administration may need to be discontinued. Hemolytic anemia is relatively more common with sulfone therapy in leprosy patients, but discontinuation of treatment is not necessary; it may be related to the undernourished status of these patients.

Administration of sulfonamides, particularly long-acting, can lead to hypersensitivity reactions, such as urticaria, exfoliative dermatitis, photosensitization erythema nodosum, and, in its most severe form, erythema multiforme exudativum (Steven-Johnson type); the latter condition is a particularly serious hazard of long-acting sulfonamides; when it occurs, drug administration must be discontinued immediately.

References

Research Reports

1. Domagk G. Ein Beitrag zur Chemotherapie der bakteriellen Infektionen. Dtsch Med Wochenschr 1935;*61*:250–253.
2. Domagk G. Twentyfive years of sulfonamide therapy. Ann NY Acad Sci 1957;*69*:380–384.
3. Woods DD. Relation of p-aminobenzoic acid to mechanism of action of sulphanilamide. Br J Exp Pathol 1940;*21*:74–90.
4. Ratner S, Blanchard M, Coburn AF et al. Isolation of a peptide of p-aminobenzoic acid from yeast. J Biol Chem 1944;*155*:689–690.
5. Fildes PA. rational approach to research in chemotherapy. Lancet 1940;*I*:955–957.
6. Mietzsch F. The chemotherapy of bacterial infections. Chem Ber 1938;*71A*:15–28.
7. Mietzsch F, Klarer J. Verfahren zur Herstellung von Azoverbindungen. Deutsches Reichspatent 1935; 537–607.

8. Heidelberger M, Jacobs WA. Synthesis in the Cinchona series. III. Azodyes derived from hydrocupreine and hydrocupreidine. J Am Chem Soc 1919;*41*:2131–2147.
9. Foerster R. Sepsis im AnschluB an ausgehende Peritoritis Heilung durch Streptozon. Zentral Haut Geschlechtsker 1933;*45*:549–550.
10. Trefouel J, Trefouel MMe J, Nitti F et al. Activité du p-aminophenylsulfamide sur les infections streptococciques expérimentales de la souris et du lapin. CR Soc Biol 1935;*120*:756–758.
11. Fuller AT. Is p-aminobenzensulfonamide an active agent in prontosil therapy? Lancet 1937;*II*:194–198.
12. Geimo P. Uber Sulfamide der p-Amidobenzolsulphonsaure. J Prakt Chem 1908;*77*:369–382.
13. Buttle GAH, Grey WH, Stephenson D. Protection of mice against streptococcal and other infections by p-aminobenzene sulfonamide and related substances. Lancet 1936;*I*:1286–1290.
14. Nichols RL, Jones WF Jr, Finland M. Sulfamethoxypyridazine: preliminary observations on absorption and excretion of a new long-acting antibacterial sulfonamide. Proc Soc Exp Biol Med 1956;*92*:637–640.
15. Bretschneider H, Klotzer W, Spiteller G. Zweitsynthese des 6-sulfanilamido-2,4-dimethoxypyrimidins und Synthese des 6-sulfanilamide-2-methoxy-4,5-dimethylpyrimidins. Monatsh Chemie 1961;*92*:128–134.
16. Fust B, Bohni E. Tolerance and antibacterial properties of 2,4-dimethoxy-6-sulfanilamido-1,3-diazine (Madribon) and some other sulfonamides. Antibiot Med 1959;*6*(I):3–10.
17. Bohni E, Fust B, Reider J. Comparative toxocological, chemotherapeutic, and pharmacokinetic studies with sulformethoxine and other sulfonamides in animals and man. Chemotherapy 1969;*14*:195–226.
18. Camerino B, Palamidessi G. Derivati della parazina II. Sulfonamdopir. Gazz Chim Ital 1960;*90*:1802–1815.
19. Hitzenberger G, Spitzky KH. Experimental studies of a new sulfonamide with depot character: sulfamethoxydiazine. Med Klin 1962;*57*:310–313.
20. Reber H, Rutishauser G, Tholen H. Untersuchungen am Menschen mit Sulfamethoxazol und Sulforthodimothoxin. In: Kuemmerle HP, Preziosi 3d Int Congr Chemother Stuttgart 1963, Vol I. Stuttgart: Thieme 1964; p 648.
21. Rist N, Bloch F, Hamon V. Inhibiting action of sulfonamide and of a sulfone on the multiplication in vitro and in vivo of tubercle bacillus. Ann Inst Pasteur 1940;*64*:203–237.
22. Feldman WH, Hinshaw HC, Moses HE. Promin in experimental tuberculosis. Am Rev Tuberc Pulm Dis 1942;*45*:303–308.
23. Cowdry EV, Ruangsiri C. Influence of promin, starch, and heptaldehyde in experimental leprosy in rats. Arch Pathol 1941;*32*:632–640.
24. Lowe J, Smith M. The chemotherapy of leprosy in Nigeria. Int J Lepr 1949;*17*:181–195.
25. Elslager Ef. New perspectives on the chemotherapy of malaria, filariasis and leprosy. Prog Drug Res 1974;*18*:99–172.
26. Elslager EF, Worth DF. Repository antimalarial drugs: N, N′-diacetyl-4,4′-diaminodiphenylsulfone and related 4-acylaminodiphenylsulfones. Nature 1965;*206*:630–631.
27. Shepard CC, Tolentino JG, McRae DN. The therapeutic effect of 4,4′-diacetyldiaminodiphenylsulfone (DADDS) in leprosy. Am J Trop Med Hyg 1968;*17*:192–201.
28. Seydel JK. Molecular basis for the action of chemotherapeutic drugs: Structure-activity studies on sulfonamides. In: Ariens EJ Physico-chemical aspects of drug action. New York: Pergamon 1968; p 169.
29. Foernzler EC, Martin AN. Molecular orbital calculations on sulfonamide molecules. J Pharm Sci 1967;*56*:608–615.
30. Bell PH, Roblin RO Jr. Studies in chemotherapy. VII. A theory of the relation of structure to activity of sulfanilamide type compounds. J Am Chem Soc 1942;*64*:2905–2917.
31. Cowles PB. Ionization and the bacteriostatic action of sulfonamides. Yale J Biol Med 1942;*14*:599–604.
32. Brueckner AH. The effect of pH on sulphonamide activity. Yale J Biol Med 1943;*15*:813–821.
33. Yamazaki M, Kakeya N, Morishita T et al. Biological activity of drugs. X. Relation of structure to the bacteriostatic activity of sulfonamides (1). Chem Pharm Bull (Tokyo) 1970;*18*:702–707.
34. Coates EA, Cordes HP, Kulkarni VM et al. Multiple regression and principal component analysis of antibacterial activities of sulphones and sulphonamides in whole cell and cell-free system of various DDS sensitive and resistant bacterial strains. Quant Struct Act Relat 1985;*4*:99–109.
35. Rieder J. Physikalisch-chemische und biologische Untersuchungen an Sulfonamiden. Arzneim Forsch 1963;*13*:81–103.
36. Biagi GL, Barbaro AM, Guerra MC, Forti GC, Francasso ME. Relationship between π and Rm values of sulfonamides. J Med Chem 1974;*17*:28–33.
37. Brown GM. The biosynthesis of folic acid. Inhibition by sulfonamides. J Biol Chem 1962;*237*:536–540.
38. Weisman RA, Brown GM. The biosynthesis of folic acid. V. Characteristics of the enzyme system that catalyses the synthesis of dihydropteroic acid. J Biol Chem 1964;*239*:326–331.
39. Shiota T, Baugh CM, Jackson R. The enzymatic synthesis of hydroxymethyl-dihydrofolate. Biochemistry 1969;*8*:5022–5028.
40. Bock L, Miller GH, Schaper KJ et al. Sulfonamide structure activity relationships in a cell-free system. 2. Proof for the formation of a sulfonamide-containing folate analog. J Med Chem 1974;*17*:23–28.
41. Roland S, Ferone R, Harvey RJ, Styles VL, Morrison RW. The characteristics and significance of sulfonamides as substrates for E coli dihydropteroate synthase. J Biol Chem 1979;*254*:10337–10345.
42. Brownlee G, Green AF, Woodbine M. Sulphetrone. A chemotherapeutic agent for tuberculosis. Pharmacology and chemotherapy. Br J Pharmacol 1948;*3*:15–28.
43. Donovick R, Bayan A, Hamre D. The reversal of the activity of antituberculous compounds in vitro. Am Rev Tuberc Pulm Dis 1952;*66*:219–227.
44. Levaditi C. Woods phenomenon and N-containing sulfonamides, sulfoxides, and sulfones. CR Soc Biol 1941;*135*:1109–1111.
45. Maier J, Riley E. Inhibition of antimalarial action of sulfonamides by p-aminobenzoic acid. Proc Soc Exp Biol Med 1942;*50*:152–154.
46. Seeler AO, Graessle O, Dusenbery ED. The effect of PABA on the chemotherapeutic activity of sulfonamides in lymphogranuloma venereum and in duck malaria. J Bacteriol 1943;*45*:205–209.
47. Moriguchi I, Wada S. Protein binding IV. Relations of an index for electronic structure of binding constant with serum albumin and bacteriostatic activities of sulfonamides. Chem Pharm Bull (Tokyo) 1968;*16*:734–748.

48. Hitchings GH, Burchall JJ. Inhibition of folate biosynthesis and function as a basis for chemotherapy. Adv Enzymol 1965;*27*:417–468.

49. Greenberg J. The antimalarial activity of 2,4-diamino-6,7-diphenylpterin: Its potentiation by sulphadiazine and inhibition by pteroylglutamic acid. J Pharmacol Exp Ther 1949;*97*:484–487.

50. Greenberg J, Richeson EM. Potentiation of the antimalarial activity of sulfadiazine by 2,4-diamino-5-aryloxypyrimidines. J Pharmacol Exp Ther 1950;*99*:44–449.

51. Greenberg J, Richeson EM. Effect of 2,4-diamino-5-(p-chlorophenoxy) -6-methylpyrimidine and 2,4-diamino-6,7-diphenylpteridine on chlorguanide resistant strain of Plasmodium gallinaceum. Proc Soc Exp Biol Med 1951;*77*:174–176.

52. Akiba T, Yokota T. Studies on the mechanism of transfer of drug resistance in bacteria 18. Incorporation of ^{35}S-sulfathiazole into cells of the multiple resistant strain and artificial sulfonamide resistant strain of E coli. Med Biol 1962;*63*:155–159.

53. Pato ML, Brown GM. Mechanisms of resistance of E coli to sulfonamides. Arch Biochem Biophys 1963;*103*:443–448.

54. Landy M, Larkum NW, Oswald EJ et al. Increased synthesis of p-aminobenzoic acid associated with the development of resistance in Staph aureus. Science 1943;*97*:265–267.

55. White PJ, Woods DD. The synthesis of p-aminobenzoic acid and folic acid by staphylococci sensitive and resistant to sulphonamides. J Gen Microbiol 1965;*40*:243–253.

56. Wolf B, Hotchkiss RD. Genetically modified folic acid synthesising enzymes of pneumococcus. Biochemistry 1963;*2*:145–150.

57. Ho RI, Corman L, Morse SA, Artenstein MS. Alterations in dihydropteroate synthetase in cell free extracts of sulfanilamide resistant Neisseria meningitidis and Neisseria gonorrhoeae. Antimicrob Agents Chemother 1974;*5*:388–392.

58. Bishop A. Drug resistance in protozoa. Biol Rev 1959;*34*:445–500.

59. Kruger-Thiemer E. Die Losung pharmakologischer Probleme durch Rechenautomaten. Arzneim Forsch 1966;*16*:1431–1442.

60. Kruger-Thiemer E, Wempe E, Topfor M. Die antibakterielle Wirkung des nicht eiweiscbgebundenen Anteils der sulfanilamide im menschlichen Plasmanwasser. Arzneim Forsch 1965;*15*:1309–1317.

61. Yamazaki M, Aoki M, Kamada A. Biological activities of drugs. III. Physicochemical factors affecting the excretion of sulfonamides in rabbits. Chem Pharm Bull (Tokyo) 1968;*16*:707–714.

62. Eze LC, Okpogba AN, Ogan AU. Acetylation polymorphism and leprosy. Biochem Genet 1990;*28*(1–2):1–7.

63. Bushby SRM, Woiwood AJ. Excretion products of 4:4′-dimino-diphenylsulfone. Am Rev Tuber Pulm Dis 1955;*72*:123–125.

64. Bushby SRM, Woiwood AJ. The identification of the major diazotizable metabolite of 4:4′-diaminodiphenylsulphone in rabbit urine. Biochem J 1956;*63*:406–408.

65. Ellard GA. Absorption, metabolism and excretion of di-(p-aminophenyl) sulphone (dapsone) and di (p-aminophenyl)-sulphoxide in man. Br J Pharmacol 1969;*26*:212–217.

66. Smego RA, Moeller MB, Gallis HA. Trimethoprim-sulfamethoxazole therapy for Nocardia infection. Arch Intern Med 1983;*143*:711–718.

67. Hassan A, Erian MM, Farid Z et al. Trimethoprim-sulphamethoxazole in acute brucellosis. Br Med J 1971;*3*:159–160.

68. Herkes GK, Fryer J, Rushworth R et al. Cerebral nocardiosis: Clinical and pathological findings in three patients. Aust NZ J Med 1989;*19*(5):475–478.

69. Fortier B, Ajana F, Pinto de Sousa MI et al. Prevention and treatment of materno-fetal toxoplasmosis. Press Med 1991;*20*(29):1374–1383.

70. Ellard GA. Chemotherapy of leprosy. Br Med Bull 1988;*44*:775–790.

71. Phillips-Howard PA. Efficacy of drug prophylaxis. J Roy Soc Med 1989;*82*(17):23–29.

72. Fihn SD, Johnson C, Roberts PL et al. Trimethoprim-sulfamethoxazole for acute dysuria in women with a single dose or 10-day course. Ann Intern Med 1988;*108*:350–357.

73. Gleckman, RA. Trimethoprim-sulfamethoxazole vs. ampicillin in chronic urinary traci infections. JAMA 1975;*233*:427–431.

74. Stamm WE, Counts GW, Wagner KF et al. Antimicrobial prophylaxis for recurrent urinary tract infections. Ann Intern Med 1980;*92*:770–775.

75. Stein GE, Mummaw N, Goldstein EJC et al. A multicenter comparative trial of three-day norfloxacin vs ten-day sulfamethoxazole and trimethoprim for the treatment of uncomplicated urinary tract infections. Arch Intern Med 1987;*146*:1760–1762.

76. Chang MJ, Dunkle LM, Van Reken D, Anderson D, Wong ML, Feigin RD. Trimethoprim-sulfamethoxazole compared to ampicillin in the treatment of shigellosis Pediatrics 1977;*59*:726–729.

77. Scragg JN, Rubidge CJ. Trimethoprim and sulphamethoxazole in typhoid fever in children. Br Med J 1971;*3*:738–741.

78. Ramachandran S, Godfrey JJ, Lionel NDW. A comparative trial of co-trimoxazole and chloramphenicol in typhoid and paratyphoid fever. J Trop Med Hyg 1978;*81*:36–39.

79. Tandon MK. A comparative trial of co-trimoxazole and amoxycillin in the treatment of acute exacerbations of chronic bronchitis. Med J Aust 1977;*2*:281–284.

80. Carroll PG, Krejci SP, Mitchell J, Puranik J, Thomas R, Wilson B. A comparative study of co-trimoxazole and amoxycillin in the treatment of acute bronchitis in general practice. Med J Aust 1977;*2*:286–287.

81. Gauto AR, Cone LA, Woodard DR, Mahler R, Lynch RD, Stoltzman DH. Arterial infections due to Listeria monocytogenes: Report of four cases and review of world literature. Clin Infect Dis 1992;*14*(1):23–28.

82. Paradise JL. Antimicrobial prophylaxis for recurrent acute otitis media. Ann Otol Rhinol Laryngol Suppl 1992;*155*:33–36.

83. Prantera C, Bothamley G, Levenstein S, Mangiarotti R., Argentier R. Crohn's disease and mycobacteria: two cases of Crohn's disease with high antimycobacterial antibody levels cured by dapsone therapy. Biomed Pharmacother 1989;*43*(4):295–309.

84. Fischl MA, Dickinson GM, La Voie L. Safety and efficacy of sulfamethoxazole and trimethoprim chemoprophylaxis for pneumocystis carinii pneumonia in AIDS. JAMA 1988;*259*:1185–1189.

85. Montgomery AB. Prophylaxis of pneumocystis carinii pneumonia in patients infected with the human immunodeficiency virus type 1. Semin Respir Infect 1989;*4*(4):311–317.

86. Ileana M, John M, Grifford L et al. Oral Therapy for pneumocystis carinii pneumonia in the acquired immunodeficiency syndrome. N Engl J Med 1990;*323*:776–782.

87. Stone OJ. Sulfapyridine and sulfones decrease glycosaminoglycans viscosity in dermatitis herpetiformis, ulcerative colitis, and pyoderma gangrenosum. Med Hypotheses 1990;*31*(2):99–103.

88. Bernstein JE, Lorincz A. Sulfonamides and sulfones in dermatologic therapy. Int J Dermatol 1981;*20*:81–88.

89. Venning VA, Millard PR, Wojnarowska F. Dapsone as first line therapy for bullous pemphigoid. Br J Dermatol 1989;*120*(1):83–92.

90. Callen JP. Treatment of cutaneous lesions in patients with lupus erythematosus. Dermatol Clin 1990;*8*(2):355–365.

91. Oranje AP, Van Joost T. Pemphigoid in children. Pediatr Dermatol 1989;*6*(4):267–274.

92. Riis P, Anthonisen P, Wulff R et al. The prophylactic effect of salicylazosulphapyridine in ulcerative colitis during long-term treatment. Scand J Gastroenterol 1973;*8*:71–74.

93. Peliskova Z, Trnavsky K. Salazosulfapyridine (sulfasalazine) in inflammatory rheumatic diseases. Cas-Lek-Cesk 1989;*128*(30):949–951.

Reviews

r1. Northey EH. The sulfonamides and allied compounds. ACS Monograph Series. New York: Reinhold, 1948.

r2. Weintein L, Madoff MA, Samet CA. The sulfonamides. N Engl J Med 1960;*263*:793–800, 842–849, 900–907, 952–957.

r3. Struller T. Progress in sulfonamide research. Prog Drug Res 1968;*12*:389–457.

r4. Anand N. Sulfonamides and sulfones. In: Wolff ME Burger's Medicinal Chemistry, 4th Ed, Vol. II. New York: Wiley-Interscience, 1979; 1–40.

r5. Anand N. Sulfonamides: Structure activity relationship and mechanism of action. Handbook Exp Pharmacol 1983;*64*:25–54.

r6. Wormser GP, Keusch GT. Trimethoprim/sulfamethoxazole: An overview. Handbook Exp Pharmacol 1983;*64*:1–8.

r7. Sammes PG. Sulfonamides and sulfones. In: Hansch C Comprehensive medicinal chemistry, 1st Ed, Vol. II. Oxford: Pergamon Press 1990; pp 255–270.

r8. Ehrlich. The collected Papers, Vol III. Chemotherapy. Ed. by F. Himmelweit. Early studies with dyes and arsenical compounds. Pergamon Press, 1960; pp 9–234.

r9. Weinstein L, Madoff MA, Samet CM. The sulfonamides. N Engl J Med 1960;*263*:793–800, 842–849, 900–907.

r10. Watanabe T. Infective heredity of multiple drug resistance in bacteria. Bacteriol Rev 1963;*27*:87–115.

r11. Fujita T. Substituent effect analysis of the rates of metabolism and excretion of sulfonamide drugs. In: Gould RF Biological correlations the Hansch approach. Washington: American Chemical Society 1972b; p 80.

r12. Boiron P. Nocardiosis. Rev Prat 1989;*39*(9):1983–1987.

r13. McCabe RE, Oster S. Current recommendations and future prospects in the treatment of toxoplasmosis. Drugs 1989;*38*(6):937–987.

r14. Centers for Disease Control. Antibiotic-resistant strains of Neisseria gonorrhoeae: policy guidelines for detection management and control. MMWR 1987;*36*:Suppl 1S–18S.

r15. Keystone JS. Prevention of malaria. Drugs 1990;*39*(3):337–354.

CHAPTER 92

Trimethoprim-Sulfamethoxazole

David P. Baccanari

Introduction

Trimethoprim is a broad-spectrum antibacterial agent that shows significant clinical activity without frequent toxicity or serious side-effects. The biochemical target of trimethoprim, the enzyme dihydrofolate reductase, plays a central role in intermediary metabolism, and its inhibition ultimately affects the biosynthesis of DNA, RNA, and protein, resulting in stasis or cell death. Although dihydrofolate reductase is found in almost all organisms, the enzymes from bacterial and mammalian sources differ in their amino acid sequences, tertiary structures, and their ability to bind inhibitors. Thus, trimethoprim is a selective folate antagonist, even though its target is common to both infecting organism and host.

Trimethoprim was discovered by George Hitchings and his colleagues and has been heralded as the first rationally designed drug in the field of antibacterial chemotherapy. In contrast to a hit-or-miss method of randomly screening compounds for biologic activity, trimethoprim was developed through a systematic study of a series of compounds known to interfere with nucleotide synthesis.

The mechanism of action of another class of compounds, the sulfonamides, differs from that of trimethoprim. Sulfonamides inhibit the folate biosynthetic enzyme dihydropteroate synthase and derive their selectivity from the fact that *de novo* folate synthesis occurs in bacteria but not in humans. The combination of trimethoprim and a sulfonamide shows greater antibacterial activity than that expected from either agent acting alone. This phenomenon, called synergy, is one of the reasons that the first antibacterial preparations of trimethoprim contained sulfamethoxazole.

The trimethoprim-sulfamethoxazole combination was first marketed in the United Kingdom in 1968 and was introduced into the US five years later. It is currently used for the treatment of genitourinary, respiratory, and GI infections and for *Pneumocystis carinii* pneumonia.

As with other antibacterial drugs, extensive use of trimethoprim-sulfamethoxazole has led to the development of resistant organisms. In most cases the resistance is plasmid-mediated, and the bacteria synthesize a trimethoprim-insensitive dihydrofolate reductase and/or a sulfamethoxazole-insensitive dihydropteroate synthase in addition to the normal chromosomal enzymes. The incidence of trimethoprim-sulfamethoxazole resistance can be high (especially in developing countries), but it is not a major problem in the US.

Mechanism of Action

Agents that affect folate metabolism are called antifols or folic acid antagonists; their inhibitory activity is dependent on the central role of reduced folates in cellular metabolism. Tetrahydrofolate cofactors are required for the synthesis of purine ribotides, thymidylate, methionine, glycine, histidine, N-formylmethionyl tRNA, and pantothenate. The specific cofactors involved in each pathway are listed in Table 92.1. In general, the tetrahydrofolate reactions are catalyzed by transferases that shuttle a one-carbon unit between cofactor and a precursor to form the product. The carbon unit transferred by tetrahydrofolate can be substituted on position 10 (as a formyl group) or position 5 (as a methyl group), or it can bridge positions 5 and 10 (as a methylene or methenyl group). For example, 10-formyltetrahydrofolate transfers its carbon unit to glycinamide ribonucleotide and aminoimidazolecarboxamide ribonucleotide during *de novo* purine biosynthesis. Since the cofactor forms are interconvertible (via reactions not shown), agents that decrease the cellular level of tetrahydrofolate affect the cofactor pools and inhibit the formation of all the critical DNA, RNA, and protein components listed in Table 92.1.

Most bacteria synthesize tetrahydrofolate cofactors *de novo,* whereas humans obtain preformed tetrahydrofolates (as a vitamin) from food. Bacterial tetrahydrofolate biosynthesis starts with guanosine triphosphate (GTP, Fig. 92.1). The first few steps involve rearrangement, cyclization, fragmentation, and pyrophosphorylation to yield 2-amino-4-hydroxy-6-hydroxymethyldihydro pteridine pyrophosphate, which condenses with p-aminobenzoic acid (PABA) to form dihydropteroic acid. The latter reaction is catalyzed by the enzyme dihydropteroate synthase and is the site of action of the antibacterial sulfamethoxazole (Fig. 92.2). The discovery of the sulfonamide class of inhibitors in the mid-1930s and their use as selective antibacterial agents marked the beginning of the modern era in chemotherapy. Numerous sulfonamides with different

Table 92.1 Tetrahydrofolate Cofactors in Intermediary Metabolism

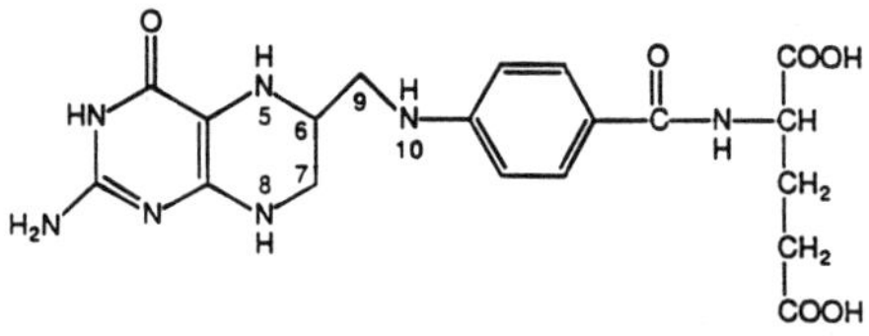

Product	Cofactor Required for Synthesis
purine ribotides	10-formyltetrahydrofolate
thymidylate	5, 10-methylenetetrahydrofolate
methionine	5-methyltetrahydrofolate
glycine	tetrahydrofolate
histidine	10-formyltetrahydrofolate[a]
formylmethionyl tRNA	10-formyltetrahydrofolate
pantothenate	5,10-methylenetetrahydrofolate

[a] 10-formyltetrahydrofolate is an indirect precursor (via ATP) of the imidazole ring of histidine

physical and pharmacokinetic properties have been prepared (see Chapter 91). Sulfonamides are structural analogues of PABA that compete with PABA for the substrate binding-site on dihydropteroate synthase. They are specific and exhibit low clinical toxicity because mammals lack the sulfonamide target enzyme, dihydropteroate synthase.

The last reaction in the tetrahydrofolate biosynthetic pathway, the NADPH-dependent reduction of dihydrofolic acid, is catalyzed by the enzyme dihydrofolate reductase. This and the subsequent tetrahydrofolate interconversion reactions are common to humans and bacteria. Dihydrofolate reductase is the site of action of the antibacterial trimethoprim, 2,4-diamino-5-(3′,4′,5′-trimethoxybenzyl)pyrimidine (Fig. 92.2). Trimethoprim is not a close structural analogue of dihydrofolate, yet it is a high-affinity inhibitor that competes with dihydrofolate for the substrate binding site.[1]

The development of trimethoprim as an antibacterial agent had its roots in a research program initiated by Dr. George Hitchings of the Burroughs Wellcome Co. He believed that basic biochemical and physiologic studies of nucleic acid biosynthesis would lead to the discovery of selective chemotherapeutic agents. When this work was started in 1942, it was a radical departure from the then well-entrenched empirical approach, where chemicals were randomly screened for biologic activity. Dr. Hitchings worked closely with Gertrude Elion, and their first chemotherapeutic successes with inhibitors of nucleic acid biosynthesis were the antileukemic purine analogues thioguanine and 6-mercaptopurine. Later, the 2,4-diaminopyrimidines were discovered and shown to be antifolates rather than thymine analogues. Trimethoprim and the antimalarial pyrimethamine (2,4-diamino-5-p-chlorophenyl-6-ethylpyrimidine) arose from this work.[2] Additional studies on nucleic acid metabolism led to the discovery of allopurinol and the immunosuppressant azathioprine. Drs. Hitchings and Elion shared (with Sir James Black) the 1988 Nobel Prize in Medicine for their discoveries of important principles in drug treatment.

Recent advances in molecular genetics and x-ray crystallography are allowing an unprecedented view of the inhibitor binding site and are heralding yet another era in the rational design of drugs. Gene cloning and expression can produce large amounts of protein for three-dimensional structure determinations, and inhibitors can be designed to fit the binding site. The process of inhibitor modeling, enzyme testing, and structure determination are then repeated until a high-affinity inhibitor is found.

The ability to custom-design new inhibitors is just the first step in drug development. Usually, only a subset of the good enzyme inhibitors cross the cell membrane and show the desired *in vitro* antibacterial activity. And of these, only a smaller number are found to be specific inhibitors of bacteria. Other factors such as pharmacokinetics, bioavailability, distribution, and metabolism must all be optimized to develop a safe and efficacious drug. In a worst case situation, the very inhibitor substituents that promote high enzyme affinity could also be responsible for poor cell permeability, rapid metabolism, etc. Therefore, the current state-of-the-art of drug development involves a mixture of molecular design techniques, empirical testing, and luck.

Dihydrofolate reductase is one of the first chemotherapeutic receptors to be studied on the molecular level. The three-dimensional structures of bacterial and mammalian dihydrofolate reductase and

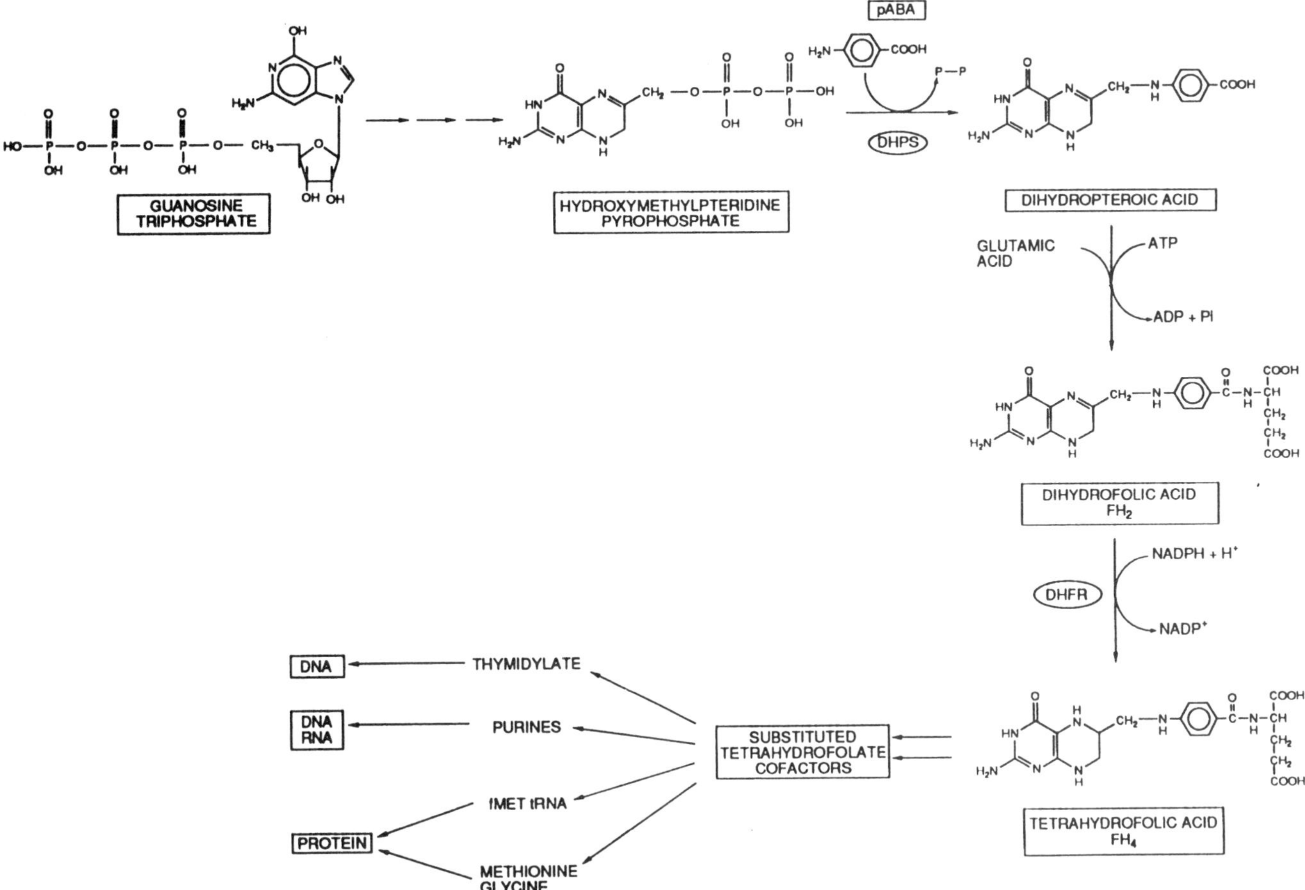

Figure 92.1 Simplified scheme of the bacterial tetrahydrofolate biosynthetic pathway showing positions of dihydropteroate synthase (DHPS) and dihydrofolate reductase (DHFR).

the conformation of trimethoprim in the enzyme active-site are known from x-ray crystallographic analyses.[r1] High trimethoprim binding-affinity to *Escherichia coli* dihydrofolate reductase is due to multiple enzyme-ligand interactions. A ribbon structure illustration of the conformation and positioning of trimethoprim in the *E. coli* enzyme active site is shown in Figure 92.3. The trimethoxyphenyl group of trimethoprim binds in a hydrophobic pocket formed by the side-chains of amino acid residues Met, Leu, Phe, and Ile. The drug forms five hydrogen bonds with the enzyme, including an ionic interaction between the pyrimidine ring of trimethoprim (which is protonated at N-1 when bound to dihydrofolate reductase) and the acidic side-chain of Asp-27. This ionic enzyme-ligand interaction does not occur with the substrate dihydrofolate (which is unprotonated at N-1) and is, in part, responsible for the enhanced binding of trimethoprim to the enzyme.[3,4]

Since dihydrofolate reductase is found in both infecting organism and host, it would seem to be a poor target for chemotherapy. However, trimethoprim has the unique ability to bind selectively to the bacterial enzyme. When binding affinity is measured by inhibitor K_i values, the *E. coli* enzyme (K_i = 1.3 nM) is about 3000-fold more sensitive to trimethoprim inhibition than is the human dihydrofolate reductase (K_i = 3.7 μM).[5] The relative ability of trimethoprim to inhibit bacterial and mammalian cell growth parallels enzyme inhibition. The minimum inhibitory concentration (MIC) of trimethoprim for *E. coli* is about 0.3 μM, whereas 100 μM trimethoprim does not inhibit the growth of cultured mammalian cells. X-ray crystallographic studies of bacterial (*E. coli* and *Lactobacillus casei*) and vertebrate (mouse, chicken, and human) dihydrofolate reductases are beginning to provide a rationale for these differences. The over-all three-dimensional structures of the two enzyme types are not fundamentally different, even though the enzymes only share about 35 percent amino acid sequence homology. One rationalization for the enhanced binding of trimethoprim to bacterial dihydrofolate reductase involves a "two-site" hypothesis,[r2] and this is illustrated in Figure 92.4. The similarities in protein structure and NADPH binding position in the *E. coli* and chicken enzymes are obvious, and the large difference in trimethoprim binding affinity may arise, in part, from the slightly different conformation of inhibitor in

SULFAMETHOXAZOLE

TRIMETHOPRIM

Figure 92.2 Structures of Trimethoprim and Sulfamethoxazole

the two enzymes.[r3] However, the binding interactions of trimethoprim with mouse liver dihydrofolate reductase are more closely similar to the *E. coli* model, and the physical basis of selectivity is still a controversial issue.[6] Nevertheless, the insights gained from these types of structural studies already have been used to design trimethoprim analogues with increased binding affinity for the *E. coli* enzyme.[7,r4]

Sulfamethoxazole and trimethoprim affect bacterial growth kinetics differently,[8] and their onsets of inhibition (Fig. 92.5) are dependent on the relative positions of dihydropteroate synthase and dihydrofolate reductase in the tetrahydrofolate pathway. The pathway has two major segments; a *de novo* sequence that includes dihydropteroate synthase and a cofactor interconversion portion that includes dihydrofolate reductase (Fig. 92.6). Sulfamethoxazole-mediated growth inhibition develops slowly because normal cellular metabolism does not consume tetrahydrofolates. *De novo* cofactor biosynthesis is needed only to replenish the tetrahydrofolate pools diluted by growth and cell division. As a consequence, the effects of dihydropteroate synthase inhibition are not evident until intermediary metabolism is limited by the diluted tetrahydrofolate cofactor pools. This process requires four or five cell doublings. In contrast, the rapid inhibition of bacterial growth by trimethoprim stems from the position of dihydrofolate reductase in the cyclic portion of the tetrahydrofolate pathway. This sequence contains the thymidylate synthase reaction, in which 5,10-methylenetetrahydrofolate serves as both a carbon donor and a reducing agent in the conversion of deoxyuridine monophosphate (dUMP) to deoxythymidine monophosphate (dTMP). As result, one molecule of tetrahydrofolate is oxidized to dihydrofolate for each turnover of thymidylate synthase. The molecule of dihydrofo-

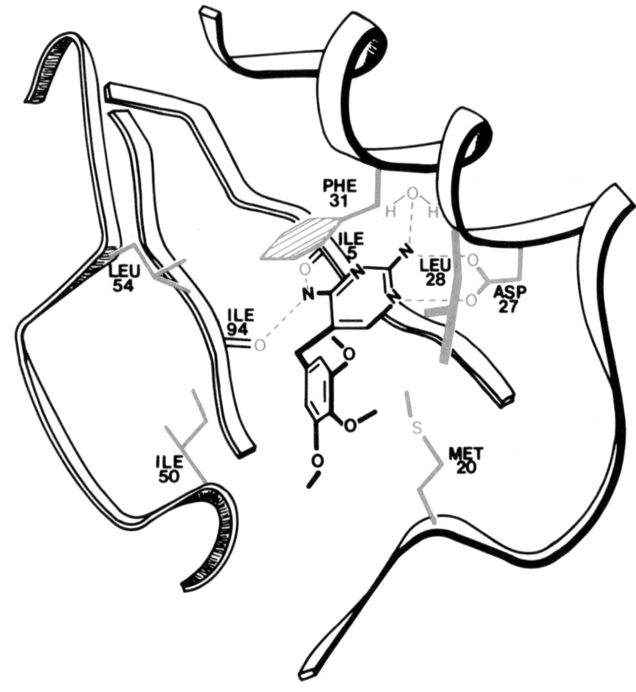

Figure 92.3. The active-site of *E. coli* dihydrofolate reductase with bound trimethoprim. The ribbon represents the amino acid backbone of the enzyme and shows regions of alpha helix, beta structure, and random coil. Two backbone carbonyl oxygens (ILE 5 and ILE 94), a water molecule, and the specific amino acid side-chains that interact with trimethoprim are shown in red. Five hydrogen bonds contribute to the tight binding of trimethoprim, and these are shown as dashed lines. NADPH has been omitted for clarity. (Structure provided by L. Kuyper)

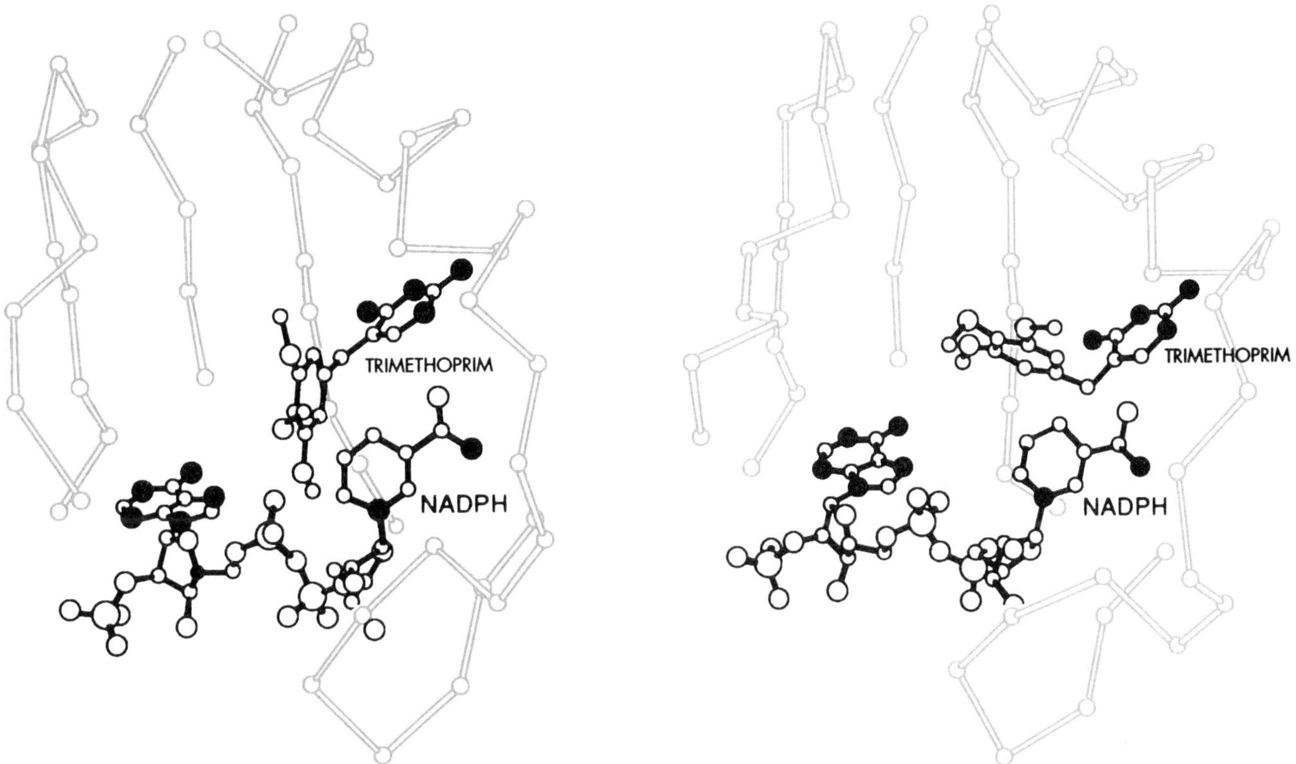

Figure 92.4 Comparison of trimethoprim binding to the active site of dihydrofolate reductase from *E. coli* (left) and chicken (right). The alpha-carbon backbones of the protein active sites are in red, and the structures of NADPH and trimethoprim are shown with filled bonds. Carbon atoms are represented by small open circles, oxygen atoms are large open circles, and nitrogen atoms are filled circles. In the *E. coli* enzyme, the trimethoxyphenyl group of trimethoprim binds in a hydrophobic region in the lower part of the cleft, and its diaminopyrimidine forms five hydrogen bonds deep within the protein (shown in Fig. 92.3). The chicken enzyme has a somewhat wider binding site, and the upper potion of the cleft interacts most favorably with the trimethoxyphenyl group. However, this conformation alters the position of trimethoprim's pyrimidine ring and results in the formation of one less hydrogen-bond than in *E. coli* dihydrofolate reductase. In addition, solvent (water) must be stripped from trimethoprim in order for its methoxy groups to bind the deeper (more hydrophobic) chicken enzyme site. Since the removal of water (desolvation) is an energy-requiring step, desolvation energy contributes to the decreased inhibitor binding affinity of the chicken enzyme. (Structures provided by L. Kuyper)

late must then be reduced by dihydrofolate reductase in order to re-enter the cofactor pool. Serine hydroxymethyltransferase completes the cycle by catalyzing the transfer of a carbon unit from serine to tetrahydrofolate to regenerate 5,10-methylenetetrahydrofolate. Since cellular demand for thymidylate forces a high flux through this pathway, inhibition of dihydrofolate reductase rapidly leads to the build-up of dihydrofolate, the depletion of tetrahydrofolate cofactors, and inhibition of cell growth.[9] Methotrexate is a tight-binding inhibitor of mammalian dihydrofolate reductase that is used extensively in cancer chemotherapy. Recent studies with methotrexate-inhibited mammalian cells indicate that the increased cellular levels of dihydrofolate also may have a direct inhibitory effect on thymidylate synthase activity and on *de novo* purine biosynthesis.[10] However, this effect may be cell-specific in mammalian cells.[11] It is not known if similar phenomena occur in bacteria inhibited by trimethoprim.

Thymineless Death

The cellular effects of folate antagonists depend on the extracellular environment. In minimal medium, high concentrations of trimethoprim inhibit DNA, RNA, and protein biosynthesis and stop bacterial growth. However, cell viability is not affected, and the inhibition is bacteriostatic.[12,13] Since this stasis results from decreased synthesis of purines, thymidylate, and (some) amino acids, the addition of these compounds or their precursors to the medium bypasses the trimethoprim blockade, and cell growth resumes even though dihydrofolate reductase remains inhibited. Similarly, a dihydrofolate reductase-deficient *E. coli* requires amino acids (methionine and glycine), a purine, and thymidine for growth.[14]

Nutritional reversal of trimethoprim inhibition obviously depends on the ability of the cell to transport and utilize exogenous precursors. There are a number

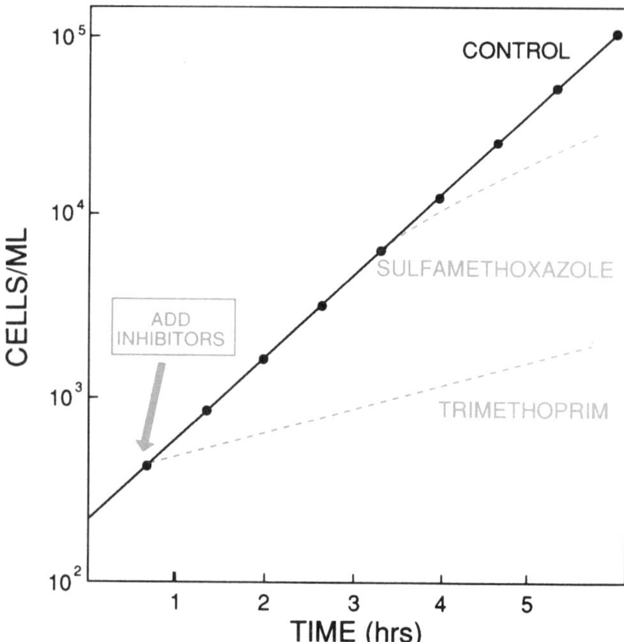

Figure 92.5 Relative onsets of inhibition by trimethoprim and sulfamethoxazole. Bacterial growth is monitored as a function of time after the addition of inhibitors.

of generalities and exceptions. (1) Most pathogenic bacteria that synthesize folates are unable to take up exogenous folates.[15] If this were not true, the pools of folate cofactors normally present in human tissues would reverse the activities of both sulfamethoxazole and trimethoprim. *Streptococcus faecium* is an exception and has the ability to bypass the metabolic blocks by utilizing exogenous folates.[16] (2) Bacteria generally take up and utilize the nucleoside thymidine (but not the nucleobase thymine), and the inhibitory activity of trimethoprim can be compromised by media thymidine levels as low as 0.25 μg/ml.[17] Fortunately, the concentration of thymidine in humans is too low to reverse inhibition by antifols. (3) *S. faecium* and *Streptococcus faecalis* are unusual because they can utilize thymine as well as thymidine, and this property is of concern in susceptibility testing. Since media often contain fairly high concentrations of thymine, trimethoprim-sensitive enterococci can appear to be resistant in vitro.[16] (4) Some bacteria (like *Neisseria meningitidis*) lack the enzymes required to take up and incorporate either thymidine or thymine,[18] and for them the antibacterial effect of trimethoprim is irreversible. (5) The initiation of bacterial protein biosynthesis by N-formylmethionyl tRNA poses an interesting physiologic problem for bacteria growing in the presence of trimethoprim. N-formylmethionyl tRNA is a large, complex molecule that cannot be supplied exogenously, yet trimethoprim-inhibited *E. coli* grow in medium supplemented with purines, thymidylate, and amino acids. It was discovered that under these conditions *E. coli* initiates protein synthesis with unformylated formylmethionyl-tRNA.[19] (6) Finally, the growth requirement for pantothenate is not readily apparent in trimethoprim-inhibited bacteria because normal cellular stores of the vitamin are adequate for several cell doublings.

The bacteriostatic activity of trimethoprim is not affected in minimal medium supplemented with either thymidine or purines or amino acids (methionine plus glycine).[12,13] However, a unique situation occurs when trimethoprim is added to cells growing in medium containing both a purine source and amino acids, but no thymidine (Fig. 92.7). Under these "thymineless" conditions, measurements of cell mass indicate that there is a significant time delay before the inhibitory effect develops, whereas cell viability determinations show a rapid onset of growth inhibition followed by cell kill. These conflicting observations can be reconciled by examining cell morphology (Fig. 92.8). In the presence of methionine, adenine, and glycine (but not thymidine), trimethoprim causes the transformation of *E. coli* from short cylindrical rods into swollen, elongated cells. Therefore, the increase in the mass of trimethoprim-inhibited cells does not represent normal cellular growth and division, and the viability determinations show that the aberrant cells rapidly lose their ability to form colonies when plated on trimethoprim-free medium. Under similar conditions, mammalian cells treated with a potent dihydrofolate reductase inhibitor such as methotrexate also swell and fail to divide.[20]

The process by which trimethoprim kills bacteria, called thymineless death, involves a series of biochemical alterations that ultimately result in irreparable damage to DNA. Thymineless death also can be induced by other dihydrofolate reductase inhibitors, by sulfonamides and thymidylate synthase inhibitors, and by transferring thymine-requiring bacteria into media lacking thymine. This latter observation was made in 1954 by Cohen and Barner who popularized the term "unbalanced growth" to describe the physiologic state in which the biosynthesis of DNA (but not RNA and protein) is inhibited.[21]

The mechanism of thymineless death is not completely understood, but the common features in prokaryotes and eukaryotes include an increase in cell mass, loss of viability within one generation, the need for protein synthesis and a functioning DNA apparatus, and the generation of fragmented DNA. The metabolic perturbations that will be described occur in mutant strains of *Bacillus subtilis*[22] and in some (but not all) mammalian cells.[23, 24] However, the same principles are assumed to apply to the bactericidal activity of trimethoprim. Inhibition of thymidylate synthase causes dramatic changes in the pyrimidine deoxynucleoside triphosphate pools; deoxyuridine triphosphate (dUTP) concentration increases several hundred-fold, and deoxythymidine triphosphate (dTTP) decreases. The pathway

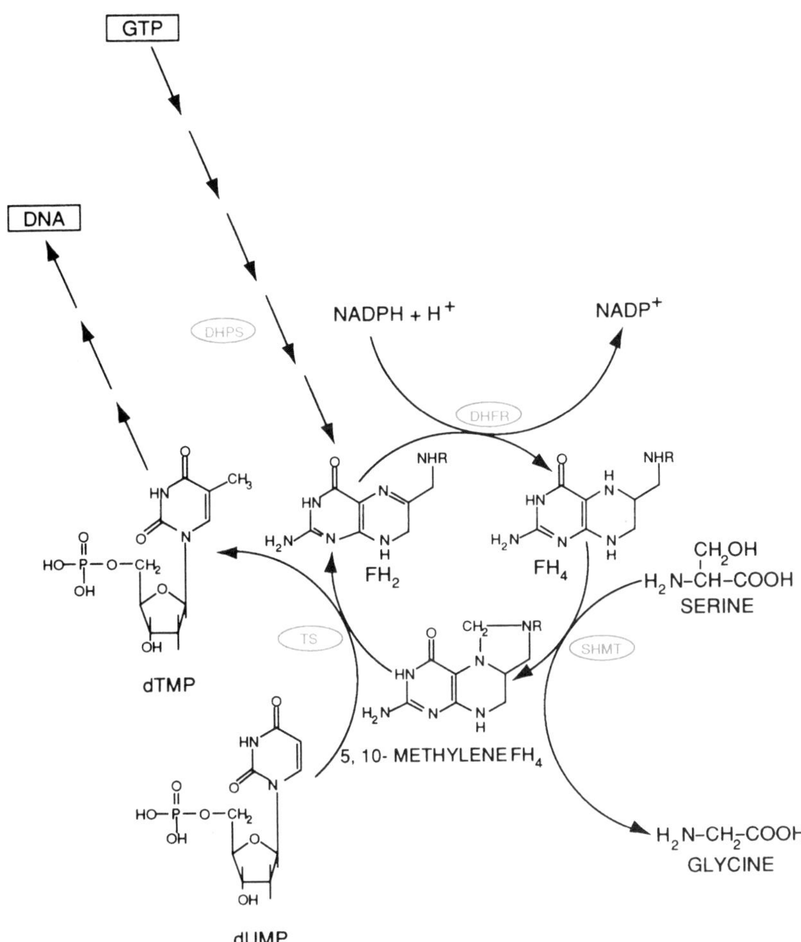

Figure 92.6 Role of dihydrofolate reductase (DHFR) and serine hydroxymethyl transferase (SHMT) in the biosynthesis of thymidylate. Dihydrofolate originates from two sources, de novo synthesis, and as a product of the thymidylate synthase (TS) reaction.

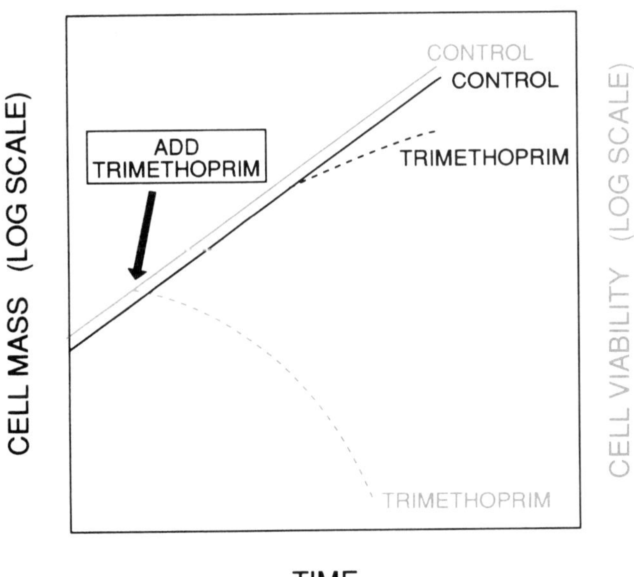

Figure 92.7 Trimethoprim inhibition under thymineless conditions. Cells are in medium containing methionine, adenine, and glycine. Growth was monitored by determinations of viability (shown in red) and mass (i.e., turbidity, shown in black).

responsible for these changes is illustrated in Figure 92.9. Inhibition of thymidylate synthase activity can be either direct (by an agent such as 5-fluorodeoxyuridine monophosphate) or indirect (by inhibition of dihydrofolate reductase or dihydropteroate synthase). Since the thymidylate synthase reaction is the only synthetic route for dTMP, substrate flow through the phosphorylation reactions to dTTP is blocked. The opposite effects are seen on the deoxyuridine nucleotide side. Thymidylate synthase inhibition causes dUMP levels to increase (up to several orders of magnitude), and flow through the deoxyuridine phosphorylation reactions is increased. Although an active deoxyuridine triphosphatase (dUTPase) breaks down dUTP to dUMP, the enzyme becomes saturated at extremely high dUTP levels, and degradation cannot keep pace with synthesis. DNA polymerase does not differentiate between dUTP and dTTP, but under normal conditions the ratio of dUTP/dTTP is so small that misincorporation is minimal. However, when thymidylate synthase is inhibited, this ratio is increased, and a significant amount of the dUTP is incorporated into DNA. Since misincorporated uracil bases destroy the integrity of the DNA template, cells have developed a process to repair such defects. Several steps mediated by specific enzymes are involved (Fig. 92.10). First uracil-DNA glycosylase cleaves the glycosidic bond and excises the uracil base, leaving what is termed an apyrimidinic (AP) site. The deoxysugar with a missing base is then recognized by the enzyme AP endonuclease, which cleaves the DNA phosphodiester backbone, and a small region on both sides of the AP site is excised by an exonuclease. DNA polymerase synthesizes a new strand, which is finally joined by a DNA ligase. However, under thymineless conditions, more U replaces T during repair, resulting in a futile cycle that enhances the damage. Eventually

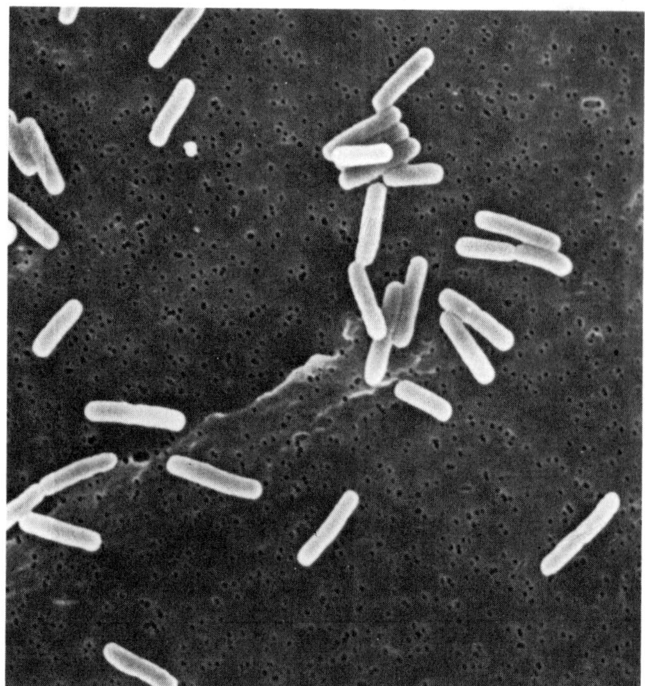

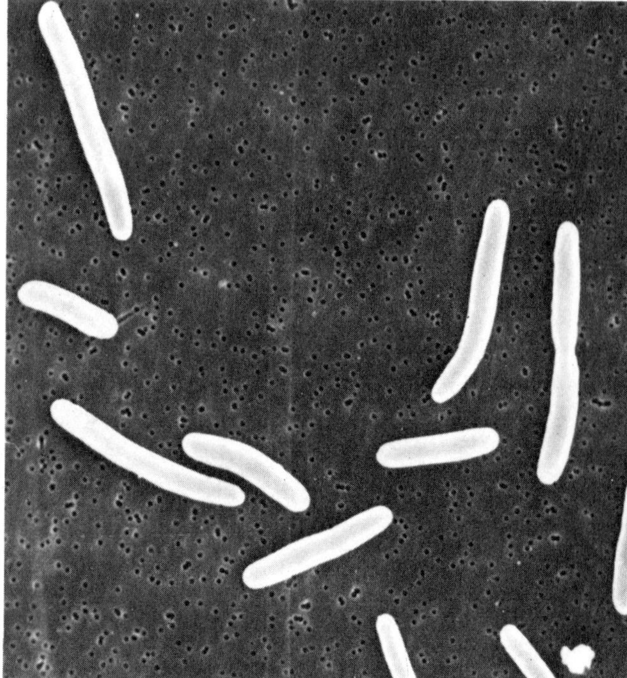

Figure 92.8 Scanning electron micrograph of *E. coli* grown under thymineless conditions in the absence (a) and presence (b) of trimethoprim. Note, the small irregular circles are pores in the polycarbonate filters used to collect the cells. (Photomicrograph provided by M. Dykstra- 6240-fold magnification)

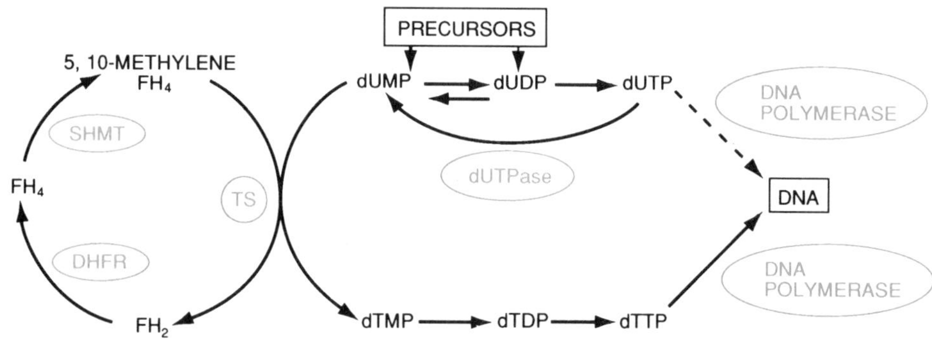

Figure 92.9 Pathway responsible for the incorporation of uracil into DNA when the synthesis of thymidylate is blocked. DNA polymerase can utilize dUTP instead of dTTP for DNA biosynthesis. See text for details.

thymidylate deprivation leads to irreparable fragmentation of newly synthesized DNA and cell death.

Synergy

Combinations of two antibiotics are used clinically for a number of reasons. The most common practices are to provide broad initial coverage in patients with sepsis of unknown etiology and to treat mixed bacterial infections. Antibiotics may also be combined to minimize the development of resistance to the individual agents. Trimethoprim is most often used in conjunction with sulfamethoxazole because that combination shows more activity than would be expected from either agent acting alone.[15] This enhanced activity, called synergy, can be qualitatively demonstrated by increased zones of inhibition in a disc diffusion assay (Fig. 92.11, top). Synergy is best described in terms of a deviation from the independent activity of two drugs.[25] Therefore, a quantitative analysis of synergy requires us to calculate the effect expected from a mixture of two agents acting independently. For example, if drug A (at a concentration that inhibits bacterial growth by 40%) is combined with drug B (which inhibits growth by 60%), what percent inhibition by the mixture would constitute independence? The fractional product concept is a widely used theory that addresses this question.

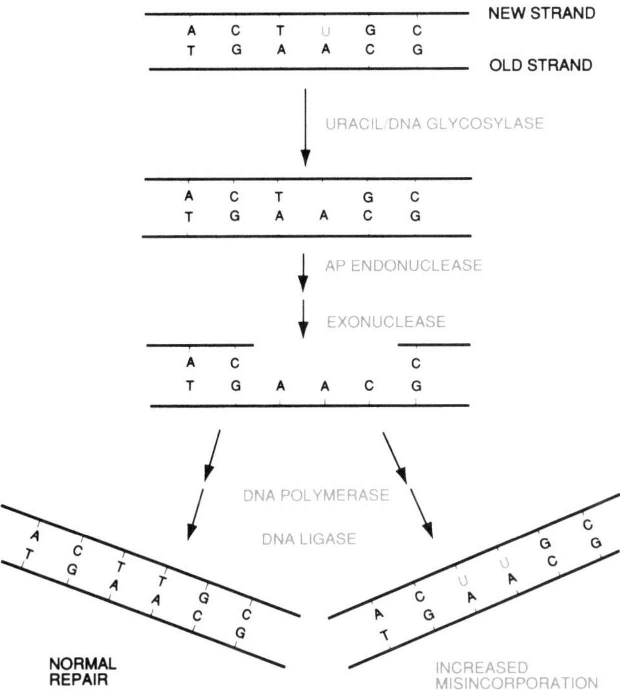

Figure 92.10 DNA repair. A multistep pathway is used to remove misincorporated bases (in this case a single U) from newly synthesized double-stranded DNA. The final step shows how this process can actually increase the extent of misincorporation under conditions where DNA polymerase continues to utilize dUTP as an alternative substrate for dTTP.

If we consider the extent of bacterial growth inhibition by a fixed concentration of a single drug:

$$\text{fractional inhibition} = 1 - \frac{\text{growth in presence of drug}}{\text{growth of control}}$$

where growth is a measurable parameter such as change in culture turbidity, cell number, etc. For two drugs acting independently,

$$\text{fractional inhibition} = 1 - \frac{\text{growth in the presence of drug A}}{\text{growth of control}} \times \frac{\text{growth in the presence of drug B}}{\text{growth of control}}$$

Therefore, for a concentration of drug A that produces 60 percent of control growth and a concentration of drug B that produces 40 percent of control growth, the expected fractional inhibition for the combination acting independently is 76% ({1−[0.6×0.4]}×100). Greater inhibition indicates synergism. If the combination is antagonistic, inhibition would be less than 76 percent. These circumstances are illustrated with growth rate determinations in Figure 92.11 (bottom).

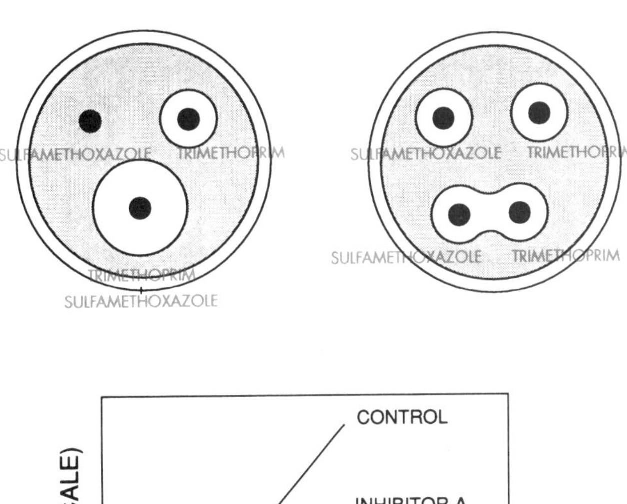

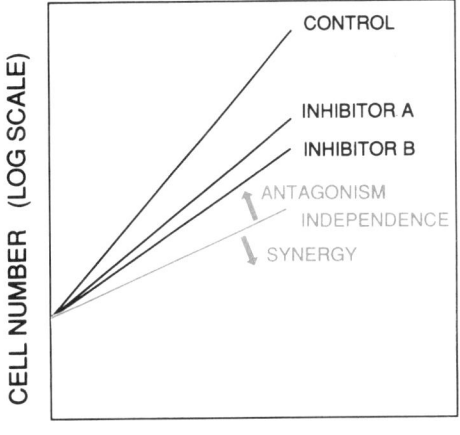

Figure 92.11 Demonstration of antibacterial synergy. Top: Diffusion of inhibitor from discs (shown as black circles) creates concentration gradients in the agar, and bacterial growth is inhibited (as shown by a cleared zone) wherever the drug concentration is greater than its MIC. In the left plate, a subinhibitory amount of sulfamethoxazole significantly enlarges the zone of inhibition produced by trimethoprim. In the right plate, discs containing the individual drugs develop fused zones of inhibition as they are placed close together. The distortion of the zones is caused by the antibacterial effect extending into areas that do not contain an inhibitory concentration of either drug alone. Bottom: The fractional inhibitions of antibacterials A and B acting alone are used to calculate the expected growth curve for independence of an A/B combination. Antagonism or synergy occurs when the measured growth rate of the combination is greater than or less than that calculated for independence.

The isobologram is a classic method of analyzing two-drug interactions.[26] In this technique, it is assumed that the inhibitors produce linear concentration-response curves and that they have different mechanisms of action. To generate an isobologram, MIC values are determined for each compound alone and for mixtures of the two drugs combined in fixed ratios (Table 92.2). At the MIC of each ratio mixture, fractional inhibitory concentrations (FIC) are calculated by dividing the concentration of the drug in the combination by its MIC when acting alone. In the example, trimethoprim and sulfamethoxazole have MICs of 0.32 μg/ml and 5 μg/ml, respectively. The MIC of the 1:1 mixture was 0.32 μg/ml, and the calculated FIC values are 0.5 (0.16/0.32) for trimethoprim and 0.03 (0.16/5) for

Table 92.2 Synergy with Combinations of Trimethoprim and Sulfamethoxazole[a]

Mixture *Trimethoprim* Sulfamethoxazole Ratio	Mixture MIC (μg/ml)	Individual Components in the Mixture			
		Trimethoprim		Sulfamethoxazole	
		MIC (μg/ml)	FIC	MIC (μg/ml)	FIC
—	—	0.32	1.00	—	0.00
1:1	0.32	0.16	0.5	0.16	0.03
1:4	0.4	0.08	0.25	0.32	0.06
1:15	0.67	0.04	0.12	0.63	0.13
1:125	1.26	0.01	0.06	1.25	0.25
—	—	—	0.00	5.00	1.00

[a]adapted from reference 15.

sulfamethoxazole. Thus, the MIC of trimethoprim was reduced twofold when sulfamethoxazole was present at a level of one-thirtieth of its MIC. At each of the other ratios, the total drug required for inhibition was less with the combination than with either drug alone. When the total data set is plotted as FIC of trimethoprim versus FIC of sulfamethoxazole, the resulting curve is concave upward (Fig. 92.12). This shape is diagnostic of synergy, and its symmetry signifies that the maximal reduction in the MIC values of both drugs occurs in a mixture with proportions corresponding to their respective MIC when acting alone. Isobolograms exhibiting a straight line are indicative of independence, whereas antagonism produces a concave downward curve.

Although maximal synergy is observed when trimethoprim and sulfamethoxazole are present in the ratio of their individual MIC's, significant synergy is seen over a wide range of ratios.[15] This is important because tissue trimethoprim-sulfamethoxazole ratios

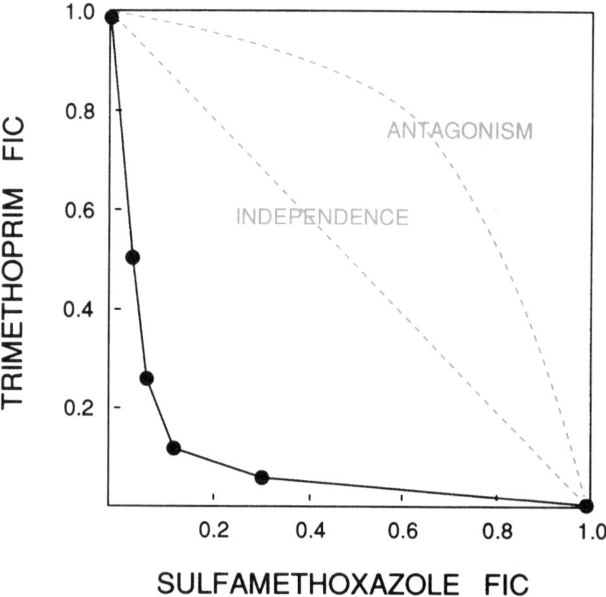

Figure 92.12 Isobologram showing synergy between trimethoprim and sulfamethoxazole. Data are from Table 92.2. Results expected from independence or antagonism are shown as dashed lines.

are often less than the ideal. Synergy is also observed in strains with elevated trimethoprim and/or sulfamethoxazole MIC values.

Enhanced activity of trimethoprim-sulfonamide combinations is also observed *in vivo*. Doses of trimethoprim or a sulfonamide that gave little or no protection to mice infected with *Proteus vulgaris* or *Stahpylococcus aureus* become completely protective when the drugs are administered simultaneously.[15] Similarly, trimethoprim or sulfonamides are inactive (or marginally active) as single agents in male patients with uncomplicated urethral gonorrhea, but the drugs are highly active when administered in combination.[27]

Kinetic analyses of multienzyme pathways indicate that the biochemical mechanism of trimethoprim-sulfamethoxazole synergy is based, in part, on the cyclic configuration of the tetrahydrofolate route (shown in Fig. 92.6). Sulfamethoxazole inhibition of tetrahydrofolate biosynthesis reduces the concentration of all of the cycle cofactors. Under these conditions, the increased concentration of dihydrofolate caused by inhibition of dihydrofolate reductase is balanced by a further decrease in the level of other substrates in the cycle, and the reaction rates of thymidylate synthase and serine hydroxymethyl transferase become more sensitive to the decrease in substrate concentration produced by sulfamethoxazole. As a result, trimethoprim and sulfamethoxazole act synergistically to inhibit the synthesis of thymidylate and all other products of the cycle. This theory leads to two predictions that have been experimentally verified.[r5] In thymine-requiring, thymidylate synthase-negative mutants, the cyclic portion of the pathway is broken, and the tetrahydrofolate biosynthesis pathway becomes a linear sequence. Since multiple inhibitions of a simple linear chain are (in general) incapable of producing an effect greater than that of a single inhibitor, trimethoprim and sulfamethoxazole should no longer be synergistic. In fact, the two agents were found to be antagonistic in a thymidylate synthase-negative mutant. Another prediction of the kinetic theory is that inhibition of any two enzymes within the cycle will result in antagonism. Dihydrofolate reductase and thymidylate synthase inhibitors have been shown to be antagonistic when simultaneously added to mammalian cells in culture.[28] However, there are examples where the combination acts synergistically, and this point is still controversial.[r6]

Activity Spectrum

In Vitro

Rich media cannot be used for susceptibility determinations with trimethoprim or sulfamethoxazole[29] because the antibacterial activities of these drugs are reversed by purines, thymidine, and amino acids (methionine and glycine). However, removal of any one of the "folate end-product groups" will result in a suitable test medium. In the early days of sulfonamides, it was discovered that *in vitro* inhibition can be improved dramatically if lysed horse blood is added to media.[30] It is not unusual to see the MIC of a trimethoprim-sensitive organism decrease from >50 μg/ml to 0.1 μg/ml in treated medium. The blood factor responsible for this effect was later shown to be the enzyme thymidine phosphorylase, and its mechanism of action is to catalyze the breakdown of thymidine to a much less active product (thymine).[31] Today, purified thymidine phosphorylase, rather than horse blood, is used to prepare media for inhibitor testing.

The *in vitro* activity spectrum of trimethoprim and sulfamethoxazole includes most common bacterial pathogens,[15] and MIC values for bacteria that are of particular importance for the clinical utility of the combination are shown in Table 92.3. Of the two agents, trimethoprim is the more potent. When large numbers of isolates are assayed, average trimethoprim MIC values are often in the range of 0.1 to 1 μg/ml, whereas sulfamethoxazole MIC values are usually 20-fold higher or more. With the trimethoprim-sulfamethoxazole combination in a 1/20 ratio, the MIC for the trimethoprim component of the mixture is often <0.1 μg/ml, and the MIC of the sulfamethoxazole component decreases to 1–5 μg/ml.

Several pathogens are either relatively insensitive or resistant to trimethoprim. *N. gonorrhoeae* and *N. meningitidis* exhibit increased trimethoprim MICs (about 2 to 70 μg/ml) because their dihydrofolate reductases have a 30-fold weaker trimethoprim binding affinity than the *E. coli* enzyme.[33] Consequently, high doses of trimethoprim-sulfamethoxazole are needed to see good clinical activity against gonorrhea.[27] Decreased enzyme affinity also renders *Bacteriodes sp.* relatively insensitive to trimethoprim (MIC> 4 μg/ml),[34] and patients treated with trimethoprim-sulfamethoxazole show little reduction in gut *Bacteroides*.[35] This may account for the low incidence of GI upsets during therapy. In contrast, the resistance of *Pseudomonas aeruginosa* to trimethoprim (MICs > 100 μg/ml) is probably due to poor membrane transport of trimethoprim rather than weak binding affinity to dihydrofolate reductase.[r7] Additional organisms relatively insensitive to trimethoprim-sulfamethoxazole include *Mycobacterium tuberculosis, Nocardia* species, and *Brucella* species.[r8]

Table 92.3 *In Vitro* Activity of Trimethoprim and Sulfamethoxazole Against Multiple Clinical Isolates of Various Species[a]

	Range of MIC Values (μg/ml)	
	Trimethoprim	Sulfamethoxazole
Escherichia coli	0.05–1.5	1–245
Proteus sp. (indole pos.)	0.5–5.0	7–300
Morganella morganii	0.5–5.0	7–300
Proteus mirabilis	0.5–1.5	7–30
Klebsiella sp.	0.15–5.0	2–245
Enterobacter sp.	0.15–5.0	2–245
Hemopilus influenzae	0.15–1.5	3–95
Streptococcus pneumoniae	0.15–1.5	7–25
Shigella flexneri	<0.01–0.04	<0.16–>320
Shigella sonnei	0.02–0.08	0.6–>320

[a]adapted from reference 32

Clinical Uses

Trimethoprim-sulfamethoxazole has been tested against a wide variety of infections, including prostatitis, gonorrhea, typhoid fever, and cholera, among others.[r9] In the US, the combination has been approved by the Food and Drug Administration for the treatment of: chronic urinary tract infections; acute otitis media in children; acute exacerbations of chronic bronchitis in adults; travelers' diarrhea in adults; enteritis (shigellosis) caused by *Shigella flexerni* and *Shigella sonnei;* and *Pneumocystis carinii* pneumonitis. Trimethoprim-sulfamethoxazole also was recently approved in the US for the prophylaxis of *P. carinii* pneumonia in immunocompromised patients. Trimethoprim (as a single agent) is approved for initial episodes of uncomplicated urinary tract infections.

Uncomplicated urinary tract infections caused by sensitive strains of *E. coli, Klebsiella* species, and *Enterobacter* species (among others) are effectively treated by either trimethoprim alone, sulfamethoxazole alone, or trimethoprim-sulfamethoxazole.[r10] Recurrent urinary tract infections in females are usually reinfections that arise from fecal bacteria colonizing the vaginal vestibule. Therapy with trimethoprim-sulfamethoxazole prevents reinfection by reducing both vaginal and fecal *E. coli*.[35]

Otitis media is the most commonly diagnosed disease in infants and children in the US. Approximately 25 percent of the estimated 120 million prescriptions written for oral antimicrobial agents each year in the US are for the treatment of otitis media.[r11] *Streptococcus pneumoniae* and *Hemophilus influenzae* are the predominant causative organisms, and most strains (including ampicillin-resistant, penicillinase-producing *H. in-*

fluenzae) are susceptible to trimethoprim-sulfamethoxazole. In addition, the pharmacodynamics of the combination are such that both agents are well-distributed in middle ear fluid.[36] Chronic bronchitis is characterized by the excessive production of sputum, which often becomes infected during exacerbations. Trimethoprim is also concentrated in sputum (relative to plasma) and trimethoprim-sulfamethoxazole is effective in treating acute exacerbations of chronic bronchitis.[37] However, the combination should not be used for the treatment of streptococcal pharyngitis.

Patients with shigellosis derive benefit from antimicrobial therapy; both the severity and duration of diarrhea can be reduced.[38] Trimethoprim-sulfamethoxazole is active against *Shigella in vitro,* including those strains resistant to ampicillin, and shigellosis is effectively treated by the drug.[39] However, the emergence of some *S. flexneri* and *S. sonnei* strains resistant to trimethoprim-sulfamethoxazole has recently been noted.[r12] In addition, travel to developing countries often results in diarrheal illness caused by the ingestion of enterotoxigenic *E. coli,* and treatment with trimethoprim-sulfamethoxazole significantly reduces the duration of traveler's diarrhea.[40]

P. carinii is an organism that commonly causes asymptomatic infections in humans. However, *P. carinii* pneumonia (PCP) is a major cause of illness and death in patients with human immunodeficiency virus (HIV) infection and in other immunocompromised individuals.[41] Trimethoprim-sulfamethoxazole is indicated for the treatment of PCP. In addition, prophylaxis is warranted in subgroups of HIV-infected patients known to be at high risk for developing PCP. The goal of prophylaxis is to reduce the frequency both of initial episodes of PCP (primary prophylaxis) and of relapses (secondary prophylaxis). Oral trimethoprim-sulfamethoxazole is recommended for both primary and secondary prophylaxis.[42]

The IV formulation of trimethoprim-sulfamethoxazole is used to treat PCP in adults and children, enteritis caused by *S. flexneri* and *S. sonnei,* and severe or complicated urinary tract infections.

The synergy of the trimethoprim-sulfamethoxazole combination is of therapeutic importance when the concentration of either component is near its (single agent) MIC at the site of the infection. However, this is probably not the case in simple, uncomplicated infections of the bladder because trimethoprim (a single 100 mg oral dose) attains urine concentrations of 50 to 100 μg/ml[r13] (i.e., 1000-fold greater than the MIC of *Enterobacteriaceae*). For this reason, trimethoprim alone is effective in treating acute urinary tract infections. It is a useful alternative to sulfisoxazole, sulfamethoxazole, nitrofurantoin, and amoxicillin.

The trimethoprim-sulfamethoxazole combination is well-tolerated in the vast majority of instances. Its principal common adverse reactions are mild GI distress (such as nausea and vomiting) and skin reactions (such as rash and urticaria).[32,43,r14] Severe reactions are rare, but, even so, serious reactions and fatalities have been associated with administration of the drug. These include Stevens-Johnson syndrome (a severe inflammatory eruption characterized by bullae on the oral mucosa, pharynx, anogenital region, and conjunctiva) and toxic epidermal necrolysis (a life-threatening skin disease characterized by peeling of the epidermis). Therefore, trimethoprim-sulfamethoxazole should be discontinued at the first appearance of skin rash. With prolonged or high-dose use, patients may develop folate-related blood dyscrasias, such as increased neutrophil lobe counts, pancytopenia, and megaloblastic marrow, caused by inhibition of human dihydrofolate reductase. The drug should be given with caution to patients with impaired renal or hepatic function or to those, such as the elderly and chronic alcoholics, with a potential for folate-mediated megaloblastic anemia and is contraindicated for pregnancy at term and during the nursing period. It should not be used concurrently with other antifolates like pyrimethamine or methotrexate. An increased incidence of side-effects such as rash and neutropenia on treatment with trimethoprim-sulfamethoxazole has been reported in AIDS patients.[44]

Adverse reactions with trimethoprim alone, in general, are similar to those of trimethoprim-sulfamethoxazole.[32,r10] Rash, pruritus, and phototoxic skin eruptions are seen, but there are only rare reports of hypersensitivity and GI, hematologic, or neurologic toxicities.

Clinical Pharmacology

Trimethoprim-sulfamethoxazole (in a 1/5 ratio) is available in the US either under the brand names Bactrim or Septra or in generic form. Among the many sulfonamides available, sulfamethoxazole was selected, in part, on the basis of its pharmacokinetic behavior, which is similar to that of trimethoprim. The combination can be administered in tablet, suspension, and IV infusion form, and, in some countries, an IM injectable formulation is also available. Its dose and schedule of administration vary with the patient and the infection. With oral formulations, adults receive 160 mg trimethoprim and 800 mg sulfamethoxazole, and children receive 4 mg/kg trimethoprim and 20 mg/kg sulfamethoxazole every 12 hours for 10 to 14 days for the treatment of urinary tract infections, shigellosis, and acute otitis media. Higher doses are given to patients with *P. carinii* pneumonia; five days of therapy are used in the treatment of traveler's diarrhea.[32] Trimethoprim-sulfamethoxazole is not recommended for children <2 months of age.

Trimethoprim, as a single agent, is available under the brand names Proloprim and Trimpex and in generic form. The usual oral adult dose in 100 mg every 12 hours or 200 mg every 24 hours, each for 10 days. The effectiveness of trimethoprim has not been established in children under 12 yrs of age.

Trimethoprim and sulfamethoxazole are well-absorbed following oral administration, and plasma concentrations are maintained at levels greater than the MIC of most pathogens for at least six to eight hrs.[45] Steady-state levels in adults are reached after dosing for two to three days. About 45 percent of trimethoprim and 65 percent of sulfamethoxazole are bound to plasma proteins. Peak blood levels after a single oral dose of 160 mg trimethoprim and 800 mg sulfamethoxazole are about 1.5 μg/ml and 50 μg/ml, respectively.[r11] At these concentrations the trimethoprim-sulfamethoxazole ratio (1/33) is near the optimal ratio seen for synergy *in vitro,* even though the drugs are administered at a 1/5 part mixture. Since both compounds are well-absorbed and have similar half-lives (10 to 12 hr), the final blood ratio reflects differences in distribution volume. As a consequence of its lipophilic properties, trimethoprim concentrates in most tissues, including kidney, liver, and lung. It also distributes into sputum, vaginal and urethral secretions, and prostatic fluid. These distributions may be an important factor in the efficacy of trimethoprim in bronchitis, urethritis, and prostatitis. Tissue concentrations of sulfamethoxazole are lower than serum concentrations and, as a result, tissue trimethoprim-sulfamethoxazole ratios vary from about 1 to 8.

Both drugs are excreted mainly by the kidney. Within 96 hours after a single dose, 80 percent of the trimethoprim and >95 percent of the sulfamethoxazole are recovered in the urine as free drug, metabolites, and/or conjugates.[r13] The majority of excreted trimethoprim is unchanged drug; its clearance is dependent on kidney function. The plasma half-life of trimethoprim increases as kidney impairment becomes severe, and the dose of trimethoprim (whether administered alone or in combination with sulfamethoxazole) should be adjusted accordingly. Sulfamethoxazole is more extensively metabolized than trimethoprim. Only 20 percent of the total urine sulfamethoxazole is in the form of parent compound. Urine concentrations of unmetabolized (active) trimethoprim and sulfamethoxazole 12 hours after a single dose are nearly equal and in the range 80 to 100 μg/ml,[45] considerably higher than the MIC of common urinary tract pathogens. These high urine concentrations result in the effective treatment of uncomplicated urinary tract infections by either agent alone.

Resistance

The widespread use of antibacterial agents commonly leads to the emergence of resistant strains. One potential advantage of a two-drug combination is that there might be a slower development of clinical resistance than with either agent alone. Nevertheless, several years after the introduction of the trimethoprim-sulfamethoxazole combination, strains with trimethoprim resistance were identified among clinical isolates, and a number of resistance mechanisms have been identified. Overproduction of the normal chromosomal enzyme imparts insensitivity because more drug is needed to inhibit the additional enzyme. Other mutational events, such as an altered chromosomal enzyme with reduced trimethoprim affinity, a decrease in membrane permeability, and loss of thymidylate synthase activity (thymine auxotrophy), also can result in trimethoprim resistance. However, all of these mechanisms account for a relatively low proportion of trimethoprim resistance in clinical isolates.[r15]

The most extensive and interesting form of trimethoprim resistance is mediated by plasmids and/or transposons. Plasmids are independently replicating DNA molecules that exist apart from the chromosome. They usually do not encode essential proteins, but their gene products often carry out accessory functions, including antibiotic resistance. Some plasmids occur in multiple copies per cell and produce large amounts of the enzymes responsible for resistance. Transposons (transposable elements) are segments of DNA that can transfer from plasmids to nonhomologous sites on the chromosome or on other plasmids; they can carry multiple genes and have developed into efficient repositories for antibiotic resistance. One of the first discovered antibiotic-resistance plasmids contains a transposon encoding for streptomycin, sulfonamide, and ampicillin resistance.[46] In addition, resistance genes are often joined to the genes required for plasmid replication and conjugal transfer. This is an important property that allows for the rapid spread of antibiotic resistance traits from bacterium to bacterium. An organism incorporating an antibiotic-resistance plasmid can become, in one step, resistant to multiple antibacterial agents without ever having been exposed to a single drug.

Plasmid-encoded trimethoprim resistance is mediated by the production of dihydrofolate reductase enzymes that are less sensitive to inhibition than is the chromosomal enzyme. The resistant dihydrofolate reductase allows the cell to maintain normal tetrahydrofolate cofactor pools when exposed to concentrations of trimethoprim that completely inhibit the chromosomal enzyme. High-level trimethoprim resistance (MIC values > 1 mg/ml) is common with this mechanism. Unlike the situation with penicillins and beta lactamases, there are no examples of plasmid-mediated trimethoprim resistance caused by drug metabolism.

Most plasmid-encoded trimethoprim resistance has been associated with *Enterobacteriaceae,* but multi-resistant strains of other gram-negative and gram-positive organisms have been isolated. At least 14 types of resistant enzymes have been identified.[47] Several that have been well-characterized are listed in Table 92.4; the enzymes markedly differ in molecular weight, trimethoprim K_i and specific activity (turnover). Trimethoprim resistance in *Enterobacteriaceae* has been dominated by the spread of Type I and Type II dihydrofolate reductase. The Type I enzyme is the most common. It is a dimer of identical 17500 molecular weight subunits. This subunit and the chromosomal *E. coli* enzyme are similar in size and share 40 percent amino acid sequence homology. However, the Type I enzyme is 10,000-fold resistant to trimethoprim, and bacteria expressing this enzyme have trimethoprim MICs of about 1 mg/ml.[48] The gene for the Type I enzyme is located along with streptomycin and spectinomycin resistance genes on transposon Tn7.

The Type II plasmid-encoded enzyme is the only known tetrameric dihydrofolate reductase. It is composed of four identical 8500 molecular weight subunits and does not share significant sequence homology with any other known dihydrofolate reductase. The Type II enzyme has a trimethoprim K_i value 15 million times greater than that of the chromosomal enzyme.[49] Bacteria expressing this enzyme have MIC values >2 mg/ml. Unlike the Type I gene, transposition has not yet been shown to be an important factor in the dissemination of Type II resistance.

The origins of the plasmid-encoded dihydrofolate reductase enzymes are not known, but there has been speculation about several obvious possibilities. For example, the monomeric structure and moderate trimethoprim resistance of Type III dihydrofolate reductase suggest that its gene may have arisen from the chromosome of an obscure bacterial species intrinsically insensitive to trimethoprim.[50] The unique tetrameric structure and low specific activity of Type II dihydrofolate reductase suggests that this enzyme may have been derived from an (as yet unidentified) oxidoreductase completely unrelated to dihydrofolate reductase. The plasmid-mediated transfer of DNA between the putative donors and *E. coli* could have taken place in the gut or some other environment where the two organisms coexist. Since trimethoprim (in combination with sulfadiazine) is used in veterinary medicine, the fecal flora of animals can act as a reservoir of resistant organisms.

Sulfonamide resistance is also an important consideration in chemotherapy. As was seen with trimethoprim, the major mechanism of sulfonamide resistance involves the expression of plasmid-encoded dihydropteroate synthase. Two resistant enzymes have been identified, and both exhibit about 10000-fold less sensitivity to sulfonamide inhibition than the chromosomal *E. coli* enzyme.[51] These resistance genes can reside on transposons and are frequently linked to ampicillin, chloramphenicol, tetracycline, streptomycin, and/or kanamycin resistance. In addition, the use of the trimethoprim-sulfamethoxazole combination has resulted in increased linkage of trimethoprim and sulfamethoxazole resistance determinants, with rates of cotransfer varying from 20 percent to nearly 100 percent, depending on the institution and its geographical location.[r16]

Plasmid- and/or transposon-mediated resistance is a significant problem in many developing countries where the consumption of trimethoprim is extensive and largely uncontrolled. For example, the incidence of trimethoprim-sulfamethoxazole resistance among *E. coli* isolates in Brazil, Chile, Costa Rica, Honduras, and Thailand was reported to be 40 to 50 percent during 1983–84.[52] Trimethoprim resistance in industrialized countries is, in general, less of a problem, even in persons receiving drug for long-term prophylaxis. However, the incidence of resistance varies among geographic regions and even among hospitals within a region. For example, several studies from Sweden, the UK, and the US showed trimethoprim-sulfamethoxazole resistance to be 3–8 percent, whereas other studies showed incidences up to 15 percent and higher.[r15,r16] Resistance has been managed by avoiding cross-infection and by temporarily restricting use of the drug during outbreaks.

In summary, trimethoprim and the trimethoprim-

Table 92.4 Properties of Chromosomal and Plasmid *E. Coli* Dihydrofolate Reductase

Enzyme	Molecular Weight	Trimethoprim $K_i(\mu M)$	Specific Activity[a] units/mg
Chromosomal	18000	0.0004	110
Type I	35000 (17500)[b]	6.4	250
Type II	34000 (8500)	6100	1
Type III	16900	0.019	10

[a]specific activity values are for the homogeneous enzymes
[b]values in parentheses are the subunit molecular weights

Summary Table

Trade Name	Dose Size/Form	Typical Dose*
Trimethoprim Proloprim, Trimpex	100 mg tablet; 200 mg tablet	100 mg every 12 hr; 200 mg every 24 hr
Trimethoprim/ Sulfamethoxazole Septra, Bactrim	80 mg trimethoprim; 400 mg sulfamethoxazole tablet	1 double strength tablet; two regular strength tablets; or 20 ml suspension every 12 hr
	160 mg trimethoprim; 800 mg sulfamethoxazole double strength tablet	For treatment of *P. carinii* pneumonia: 20 mg/kg trimethoprim and 100 mg/kg sulfamethoxazole per 24 hr in four equally divided doses
	40 mg trimethoprim; 200 mg sulfamethoxazole in 5 ml oral suspension	
	16 mg/ml trimethoprim; 80 mg/ml sulfamethoxazole i.v. infusion	For i.v. infusion: 8–15 mg/kg total daily dosage based on trimethoprim component in two to four equally divided doses

*For adults with normal renal function

Summary Table

	Dosage			Pharmacokinetics			
Drug	Route	Size	Dose	Peak	V_D	$t_{1/2}$	Clearance or Duration of Response
Trimethoprim Proloprim Trimpex	Oral	100, 200 mg	100 mg b.i.d. 200 mg q.d.	1–4 hours	1.5 l/kg	8–11 hrs	
Co-trimoxazole Bactrim, Septra	Oral	40 mg trimethoprim with 200 mg sulfamethoxazole/5 ml as suspension	160 mg trimethoprim every 12 hours (for adult indications other than the treatment of *P. carinii* pneumonia)				
	Oral	80 mg trimethoprim 400 mg sulfamethoxazole as tablet					
	Parenteral	16 mg/ml trimethoprim 80 mg/ml sulfamethoxazole					
	Oral	160 mg trimethoprim 800 mg sulfamethoxazole as tablet					

sulfamethoxazole combination have a unique mechanism of action compared to other antibacterials. They have a broad spectrum of activity and show minimal toxicity and side-effects. Even though resistance can be a problem, its occurrence has not prevented trimethoprim-sulfamethoxazole from being the drug of choice throughout the world for the treatment of urinary tract and lower respiratory tract infections.

References

Research Reports

1. Burchall JJ, Hitchings GH. Inhibitor binding analysis of dihydrofolate reductases from various species. Mol Pharmacol 1965;*1*:126–136.
2. Hitchings GH. Nobel lecture in physiology or medicine-1988: Selective inhibitors of dihydrofolate reductase. *In Vitro* Cell Develop Biol 1989;*25*:303–310.
3. Matthews DA, Bolin JT, Burridge JM, Filman DJ, Volz KW, Kaufman BT, Beddell CR, Champness JN, Stammers DK, Kraut J. Refined crystal structures of *Escherichia coli* and chicken liver dihydrofolate reductase containing bound trimethoprim. J Biol Chem 1985;*260*:381–391.
4. Baker DJ, Beddell CR, Champness JN, Goodford PJ, Norrington FEA, Smith DR, Stammers DK. The binding of trimethoprim to bacterial dihydrofolate reductase. FEBS Lett 1981;*126*:49–52.
5. Baccanari DP, Daluge S, King RW. Inhibition of dihydrofolate reductase: effect of reduced nicotinamide adenine dinucleotide phosphate on the selectivity and affinity of diaminopyrimidines. Biochemistry 1982;*21*:5068–5075.
6. Groom CR, Thillet J, North ACT, Pictet R, Geddes AJ. Trimethoprim binds in a bacterial mode in the wild-type and E30D mutant of mouse dihydrofolate reductase. J Biol Chem 1991;*266*:19890–19893.
7. Kuyper LF, Roth B, Baccanari DP, Ferone R, Beddell CR, Champness JN, Stammers DK, Dann JG, Norrington FEA, Baker DJ, Goodford PJ. Receptor-based design of dihydrofolate reductase inhibitors: comparison of crystallographically determined enzyme binding with enzyme affinity in a series of carboxy-substituted trimethoprim analogues. J Med Chem 1982;*25*:1120–1122.
8. Seydel JK, Wempe E, Miller GH, Miller L. Kinetics and mechanisms of action of trimethoprim and sulfonamides, alone and in combination, upon *E. coli*. Chemother 1972;*17*:217–258.
9. Nixon PF, Slutsky G, Nahas A, Bertino JR. The turnover of folate coenzymes in murine lymphoma cells. J Biol Chem 1973;*248*:5932–5936.
10. Chu E, Drake JC, Boarman D, Baram J, Allegra CJ. Mechanism of thymidylate synthase inhibition by methotrexate in human neoplastic cell lines and normal human myeloid progenitor cells. J Biol Chem 1990;*265*:8470–8478.
11. Rhee MS, Coward JK, Galivan J. Depletion of 5,10-methylenetetrahydrofolate and 10-formyltetrahydrofolate by methotrexate in cultured hepatoma cells. Mol Pharmacol 1992;*42*:909–916.
12. Aymes SGB, Smith JT. Trimethoprim action and its analogy with thymine starvation. Antimicrob Agents Chemother 1974;*5*:169–178.
13. Angehrn P, Then R. Nature of trimethoprim-induced death in *Escherichia coli*. Arnzeimittel-Forsch 1973;*23*:447–455.
14. Singer S, Ferone R, Walton L, Elwell L. Isolation of a dihydrofolate reductase-deficient mutant of *Escherichia coli*. J Bacteriol 1985;*164*:470–472.
15. Bushby SRM, Hitchings GH. Trimethoprim, a sulphonamide potentiator. Br J Pharmacol Chemother 1968;*33*:72–90.
16. Hamilton-Miller JMT, Purves D. Enterococci and antifolate antibiotics. Eur J Clin Microbiol 1986;*5*:391–394.
17. Koch AE, Burchall JJ. Reversal of the antimicrobial activity of trimethoprim by thymidine in commercially prepared media. Appl Microbiol 1971;*22*:812–817.
18. Jyssum S. Utilization of thymine, thymidine and TMP by *Neisseria meningitidis*. Acta Pathol Microbiol Scand Sect B 1971;*79*:778–788.
19. Harvey RJ. Growth and initiation of protein synthesis in *Escherichia coli* in the presence of trimethoprim. J Bacteriol 1973;*114*:309–322.
20. Rueckert RR, Miller GC. Studies on unbalanced growth in tissue culture: induction and consequences of thymidine deficiency. Cancer Res 1960;*20*:1584–1591.
21. Cohen SS, Barner HD. Studies on unbalanced growth in *Escherichia coli*. Proc Natl Acad Sci US 1954;*40*:885–893.
22. Makino F, Munakata N. Deoxyuridine residues in DNA of thymine-requiring *Bacillus subtilis* strains with defective N-glycosidase activity for uracil-containing DNA. J Bacteriol 1978;*134*:24–29.
23. Goulian M, Bleile BM, Dickey LM, Grafstrom RH, Ingraham HA, Scott A, Neynaber SA, Peterson MS, Tesng BY. Mechanism of thymineless death. Adv Exp Med Biol 1986;*195*:89–95.
24. Canman CE, Tang H-Y, Normolle DP, Lawrence TS, Maybaum J. Variations in patterns of DNA damage induced in human colorectal tumor cells by 5-fluorodeoxyuridine: implications for mechanisms of resistance and cytotoxicity. Proc Natl Acad Sci USA 1992;*89*:10474–10478.
25. Harvey RJ. Interaction of two inhibitors which act on different enzymes of a metabolic pathway. J Theor Biol 1978;*74*:411–437.
26. Elion GB, Singer S, Hitchings GH. Antagonists of nucleic acid derivatives VIII: Synergism in combinations of biochemically related antimetabolites. J Biol Chem 1954;*208*:477–488.
27. Csonka GW, Knight GJ. Therapeutic trial of trimethoprim as a potentiater of sulphonamides in gonorrhoeae. Brit J Ven Dis 1967;*43*:161–165.
28. Jackson RC, Harrap KR. Studies with a mathematical model of folate metabolism. Arch Biochem Biophys 1973;*158*:827–841.
29. Bushby SRM. Trimethoprim-sulfamethoxazole: *in vitro* microbiological aspects. J Infect Dis 1973;*128* (Suppl):S442–S462.
30. Harper GJ, Cawston WC. *In vitro* determination of sulphonamide sensitivity of bacteria. J Pathol Bacteriol 1945;*57*:59–66.
31. Ferone R, Bushby SRM, Burchall JJ, Moore WD, Smith D. Identification of Harper-Cawston factor as thymidine phosphorylase and removal from media of substances interfering with susceptibility testing to sulfonamides and diaminopyrimidines. Antimicrob Agents Chemother 1975;*7*:91–98.
32. Physicians' Desk Reference, 48 edition, Montvale, NJ: Medical Economics Data, 1994.
33. Averett DA, Roth B, Burchall JJ, Baccanari DP. Dihydrofolate reductase from *Neisseria* sp. Antimicrob Agents Chemother 1979;*15*:428–435.
34. Then RL, Angehrn P. Low trimethoprim susceptibility of anaerobic bacteria due to insensitive dihydrofolate reductases. Antimicrob Agents Chemother 1979;*15*:1–6.
35. Stamey TA, Condy M, Mihara G. Prophylatic efficacy of nitrofurantoin macrocrystals and trimethoprim-sulfamethoxazole in urinary infections. N Engl J Med 1977;*296*:780–783.
36. Klimek JJ, Bates JR, Nightingale C, Lehmann WB, Ziemniak JA, Quintiliani R. Penetration characteristics of trimethoprim-sulfamethoxazole in middle ear fluid of patients with chronic serous otitis media. J Pediatr 1980;*96*:1087–1089.
37. Hughes DTD. Co-trimoxazole in chest infections including its long-term use in chest infections. pp 397–410 *In* (Hitchings GH.

Inhibition of folate metabolism in chemotherapy; the origins and uses of co-trimoxazole ed.) New York: Springer-Verlag, 1983.

38. Bennish ML, Salam MA. Rethinking options for the treatment of shigellosis. J Antimicrob Chemother 1992;*30*:243–247.

39. Nelson JD, Kusmiesz H, Shelton S. Oral and intravenous trimethoprim-sulfamethoxazole therapy for shigellosis. Rev Infect Dis 1982;*4*:546–550.

40. Ericsson CD, Nicholls-Vasquez I, DuPont HL, Mathewson JJ. Optimal dosing of trimethoprim-sulfamethoxazole when used with loperamide to treat traveler's diarrhea. Antimicrob Agent Chemother 1992;*36*:2821–2824.

41. Masur H. Prevention and treatment of pneumocystis pneumonia. N Engl J Med 1992;*327*:1853–1860.

42. Recommendations for prophylaxis against *Pneumocystis carinii* pneumonia for adults and adolescents infected with human immunodeficiency virus. MMWR Morb Mortal Wkly Rep 1992;*41*(RR-4):1–11.

43. Frisch JM. Clinical experience with adverse reactions to trimethoprim-sulfamethoxazole. J Infect Dis 1973;*128*(Suppl):S607–S611.

44. Wofsy CB. Use of trimethoprim-sulfamethoxazole in the treatment of *Pneumocystis carinii* pneumonitis in patients with acquired immunodeficiency syndrome. Rev Inf Dis 1987;*9*(Suppl 2):S184–S191.

45. Bach MC, Gold O, Finland M. Absorption and urinary excretion of trimethoprim, sulfamethoxazole, and trimethoprim-sulfamethoxazole: results with single doses in normal young adults and preliminary observations during therapy with trimethoprim-sulfamethoxazole. J Infect Dis 1973;*128*(Suppl):SS584–SS598.

46. Kopecko DJ, Brevet J, Cohen SN. Involvement of multiple translocating DNA segments and recombinational hotspots in the structural evolution of bacterial plasmids. J Mol Biol 1976;*108*:333–360.

47. Amyes SGB, Towner KJ, Young H-K. Classification of plasmid-encoded dihydrofolate reductases conferring trimethoprim resistance. J Med Microbiol 1992;*36*:1–3.

48. Smith SL, Stone D, Novak P, Baccanari DP, Burchall JJ. R plasmid dihydrofolate reductase with subunit structure. J Biol Chem 1979;*254*:6222–6225.

49. Novak P, Stone D, Burchall JJ. R plasmid dihydrofolate reductase with a dimeric subunit structure. J Biol Chem 1983;*258*:10956–10959.

50. Joyner SS, Fling ME, Stone D, Baccanari DP. Characterization of an R-plasmid dihydrofolate reductase with a monomeric structure. J Biol Chem 1984;*259*:5851–5856.

51. Swedberg G. Organization of two sulfonamide resistance genes on plasmids of gram-negative bacteria. Antimicrob Agents Chemother 1987;*31*:306–311.

52. Murray BE, Alvarado T, Kim K-H, Vorachit M, Jayanetra P, Levine MM, Prenzel I, Fling M, Elwell L, McCracken GH, Madrigal G, Odio C, Trabulsi LR. Increasing resistance to trimethoprim-sulfamethoxazole among isolates of *Escherichia coli* in developing countries. J Infect Dis 1985;*152*:1107–1113.

Reviews

r1. Kraut J, Matthews DA. Dihydrofolate reductase. pp 1–71. *In* Jurnak F. McPherson A. Biological macromolecules and assemblies, Vol III. New York: Wiley 1987.

r2. Freisheim JH, Matthews DA. The comparative biochemistry of dihydrofolate reductase. pp 69–131. *In* Sirotnak FM, Burchall JJ, Ensminger WB, Montgomery JA, Folate antagonists as therapeutic agents, Vol. 1. New York: Academic Press, 1984.

r3. Kuyper LF. The potential role of solvation in the dihydrofolate reductase species selectivity of trimethoprim. *In* Bugg CE, Ealich SF, Crystallographic and modeling methods in molecular design. New York: Springer-Verlag, 1990.

r4. Kuyper LF. Inhibitors of dihydrofolate reductase. pp 327–369. *In* Perun TJ, Propst CL, Computer-aided drug design: methods and applications. New York: Marcel Dekker, 1989.

r5. Harvey RJ. Synergism in the folate pathway. Rev infect Dis 1982;*4*:255–260.

r6. Galivan J. Biochemical mechanisms of the synergistic interaction of antifolates acting on different enzymes of folate metabolic pathways. pp 339–362 *In* Chou T-C, Rideout DC, Synergism and antagonism in chemotherapy. New York: Academic Press, 1961.

r7. Burchall JJ. Enzyme inhibitors as antimicrobial agents. pp 285–293. *In* Drews J, Hahn FE, Topics in infectious diseases Vol 1. New York: Springer-Verlag, 1975.

r8. Bushby SRM. Antibacterial activity. pp 75–105. *In* Hitchings GH, Inhibition of folate metabolism in chemotherapy; the origins and uses of co-trimoxazole. New York: Springer-Verlag, 1983.

r9. Wormser GP, Keusch GT. Trimethoprim-sulfamethoxazole in the United States. Ann Intern Med 1979;*91*:420–429.

r10. Barry DW, Pattishall KH. Trimethoprim alone: clinical uses. pp 261–291, *In* Hitchings GH. Inhibition of folate metabolism in chemotherapy; the origins and uses of co-trimoxazole. New York: Springer-Verlag, 1983.

r11. Bluestone CD. Current therapy for otitis media and criteria for evaluation of new antimicrobial agents. Clin Infect Dis 1992;*14*(Suppl 2):197–203.

r12. Salam MA, Bennish ML. Antimicrobial therapy for shigellosis. Rev Infect Dis 1991;*13*(Suppl 4):S332–S341.

r13. Patel RB, Welling PG. Clinical pharmacokinetics of co-trimoxazole (trimethoprim-sulfamethoxazole) Clin Pharmacokinet 1980;*5*:405–423.

r14. Gutman LT. The use of trimethoprim-sulfamethoxazole in children: a review of adverse reactions and indications. Pediat Infect Dis 1984;*3*:349–357.

r15. Elwell LP, Fling ME. Resistance to trimethoprim. pp 249–290. *In* Bryan LE, Handbook of Experimental Pharamcology, Vol. 91. Berlin Heidelberg: Springer-Verlag, 1989.

r16. Huovinen P. Trimethoprim resistance. Antimicrob Agent Chemother 1987;*31*:1451–1456.

CHAPTER 93

Aminoglycosides, Tetracyclines, Chloramphenicol, Erythromycin and Related Macrolides, and Other Protein Synthesis Inhibitors

John L. Egle, Jr.

All the agents discussed in this chapter act through the general mechanism of inhibition of bacterial protein systhesis, although at different specific sites. The tetracyclines and chloramphenicol are characterized by a very broad spectrum of antimicrobial activity. The macrolides, while having a narrower over-all spectrum, are useful against many types of organisms; the aminoglycosides are employed only against certain infections caused by gram-negative bacteria. All these antibiotics are given orally except the aminoglycosides, which must be administered parenterally for systemic effect. With regard to potential for adverse effects, the macrolides, except for the estolate form of erythromycin, are among the safest antimicrobials in use today. The tetracyclines frequently cause minor adverse effects, but serious reactions are rare. Chloramphenicol is generally well tolerated, but causes dose-related bone marrow depression and, in rare instances, a fatal aplastic anemia unrelated to dose. The aminoglycosides have high potential for adverse reactions, particularly ototoxicity and nephrotoxicity. Although overused in the past, the tetracyclines remain the treatment of choice for several types of infections. Erythromycin is also the preferred therapy against several organisms. The role in therapy of two newer macrolides, clarithromycin and azithromycin, still is being defined, but they appear to be useful against *Mycobacterium avium* complex in AIDS patients. The therapeutic role of the aminoglycosides has diminished considerably owing both to their disadvantages and to the emergence of many newer alternatives. Chloramphenicol, also used indiscriminately in the past, now is recommended only as an alternative drug for selected infections because of its potential for serious toxicity. Other antibiotics acting by inhibition of bacterial protein synthesis include clindamycin and spectinomycin. Clindamycin is an orally administered agent especially useful for treating infections caused by anaerobic bacteria, but it frequently causes gastrointestinal distress. Spectinomycin is given by IM injection only for the treatment of gonorrhea.

Aminoglycosides

The aminoglycoside antibiotics are protein synthesis inhibitors with a wide spectrum of antibacterial activity. Because of their relatively low therapeutic index and the need for parenteral administration, their use largely has been restricted to infections caused by gram-negative organisms. The recent emergence of many alternatives exhibiting higher selective toxicity for gram-negative infections and more desirable pharmacokinetics—particularly from the cephalosporin and fluoroquinolone classes—has further diminished the usefulness of the aminoglycosides. Major adverse effects with aminoglycosides include impairment of eighth cranial nerve functions and nephrotoxicity.

This group includes gentamicin, amikacin, tobramycin, netilmicin, kanamycin, neomycin, streptomycin, and paromomycin.

Chemistry

All drugs of this class have a central hexose (aminocyclitol) nucleus with two or more amino sugars attached by glycosidic bonds. They are water soluble and stable in solution. The fact that they are polycationic, highly polar molecules, provides the basis for their undesirable pharmacokinetic properties. The aminoglycosides may be grouped structurally as the gentamicin family (gentamicin and netilmicin), the kanamycin family (kanamycin, amikacin, and tobramycin), and the neomycin family (neomycin and paromomycin). Amikacin is a semisynthetic derivative of kanamycin. Streptomycin differs from the other aminoglycosides in that it contains streptidine rather than 2-deoxystreptidine, and its aminocyclitol is not in a central position. Aminoglycosides can form complexes with beta lactam antibiotics, with resultant loss of activity. Their structures are shown in Figure 93.1.

History

Streptomycin, the first member of this series to be introduced, was also the second antibiotic to be discovered, preceded only by penicillin. The observation by Waksman in 1943 that *Streptomyces griseus* produced a powerful antibacterial substance led to the first use of streptomycin a year later. Its activity against the organism causing tuberculosis was of particular significance. Over the next three decades, several other aminoglycosides were isolated from species of Streptomyces and Micromonaspora and approved for clinical use. Netilmicin, the most recent addition to the series, was introduced in 1983.[r1] In view of their disadvantages and the introduction of many antibacterials with superior properties, it appears unlikely that additional aminoglycosides will be developed.

Antimicrobial Spectrum

The spectrum of activity of all aminoglycosides is similar, but there are some major differences noted below. They are most active against aerobic gram-negative bacteria, although activity against certain gram-positives such as Enterococcus and Staphylococcus is good. Activity against Streptococci and most anaerobes is poor. Some members of the group (gentamicin, tobramycin, amikacin, and netilmicin) possess a high degree of activity against *Pseudomonas aeruginosa*. Streptomycin, amikacin, and kanamycin are noted for activity against species of Mycobacterium.

Mechanism of Action and Resistance

Aminoglycosides bind irreversibly to the 30S bacterial ribosome inhibiting protein synthesis. Each aminoglycoside has a different binding site. Intracellular penetration of the bacteria by passive and active transport is essential before binding to the ribosome can occur. The passive process is facilitated by antibiotics acting on the cell wall, e.g., the beta-lactams. This active transport is energy- and oxygen-dependent and cannot occur under anaerobic conditions, accounting for the lack of efficacy of aminoglycosides against anaerobes.[1] As a result of irreversible inhibition of protein synthesis, aminoglycosides, unlike other inhibitors of protein synthesis, are bactericidal. Aminoglycosides appear to have several effects on ribosomal protein synthesis, including interference with the initiation complex of peptide formation, induction of misreading of the code on the mRNA template, and a break-up of polysomes into nonfunctional monosomes. Physical damage to the cell membrane, with efflux of vital cell constituents, e.g., potassium and sodium, may contribute to the bactericidal effect of the aminoglycosides. (Fig. 93.2)

Resistance to the aminoglycosides involves several mechanisms.[2] The most clinically important (except for amikacin) is acquisition by bacteria of the ability to elaborate enzymes that inactivate the drugs by phosphorylation, acetylation, or adenylation.[r2] There is increasing incidence of resistance mediated by plasmids transferred during conjugation that code for aminoglycoside-inactivating enzymes. Other mechanisms include alterations in the ribosomal binding site, with loss of affinity for the drug and loss of the ability to transport the drug into the bacterial cell. The latter mechanism is probably the most important for amikacin, which is resistant to degradation reactions.

Pharmacokinetics

Administration and Absorption

Owing to their highly polar cationic structure, aminoglycosides are not sufficiently absorbed from the normal GI tract to make oral administration for systemic use effective. However, the fact that the drugs remain in the intestine is a positive factor when these agents are used for prophylaxis in the GI tract or for treatment of infection at this site. It must be kept in mind that significantly greater intestinal absorption may occur in the presence of inflammatory disease. Aminoglycosides are well absorbed following IM injection. They are also administered IV. Neomycin, in particular, is applied topically, where its lack of ability to penetrate the skin becomes an advantage.

Distribution

Because of inability to cross membranes readily, distribution of aminoglycosides is relatively poor. The volume of distribution approximates the extracellular space. Only low levels are reached in the CSF and the eye. CSF levels are less than 10 percent of those in plasma in the absence of meningitis, but may reach 20 percent of plasma levels if the meninges are inflamed. Intrathecal or intraventricular injection may be employed to attain higher CSF levels. The drugs accumulate in the renal cortex, where concentrations may reach 10 to 50 times those in serum. Plasma protein binding with aminoglycosides is low, about 10 percent.

Disposition

Over 90 percent of a dose of all aminoglycosides undergoes rapid renal excretion by means of filtration—again characteristic of drugs with high polarity and low lipid solubility. Half-lives of all aminoglycosides are two to three hours. Urine concentrations may reach 100 times serum levels in persons with normal kidney function. The half-lives increase markedly in

Amikacin

Gentamicin

Kanamycin

Neomycin

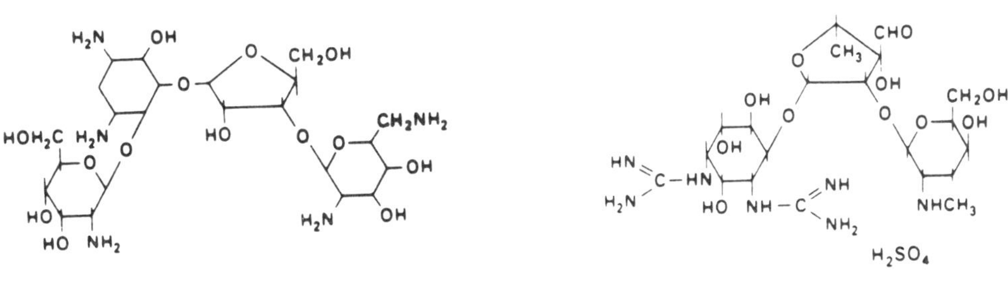

Paromomycin

Streptomycin

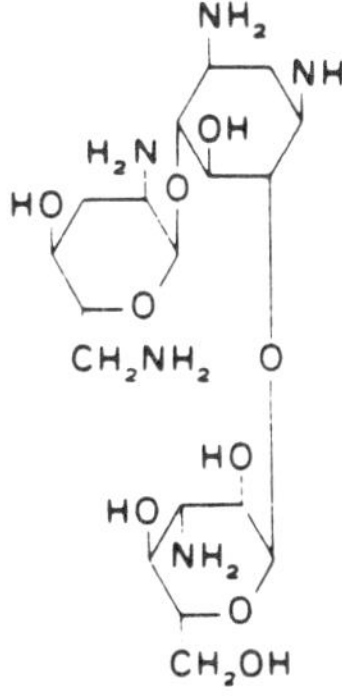

Tobramycin

Figure 93.1 Structures of the Aminoglycosides

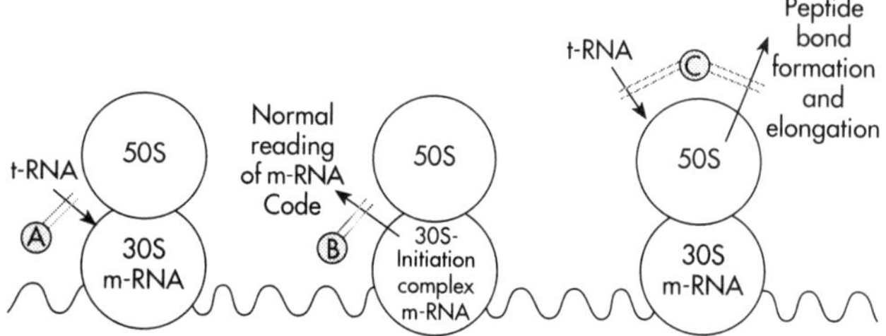

Figure 93.2 Sites of action of drugs inhibiting bacterial protein synthesis. (A) Tetracyclines attach to the 30S ribosomal subunit and prevent binding of t-RNA and formation of the initiation complex. (B) Aminoglycosides bind to a receptor on the 30S subunit blocking the normal activity of the initiation complex and causing misreading of m-RNA. (C) Chloramphenicol and the macrolides bind to the 50S ribosomal subunit. Chloramphenicol prevents the binding of t-RNA to the ribosome and interferes with peptide bond formation and the binding of new amino acids to the peptide chain. The macrolides interfere with translocation reactions and peptide elongation.

patients with renal failure and exceed 24 hours in cases of end-stage renal disease. Thus, it is quite important to adjust the treatment regimen in renal failure by either decreasing the amount administered or increasing the dosage interval, particularly since there is little margin between therapeutic and toxic levels. Nomograms and formulas are available for making adjustments based on serum creatinine concentrations.[3] Also, prolonged half-lives can be substantially shortened by hemodialysis, by which approximately 50 percent of a dose can be removed in 24 hours.[4,r3] Peritoneal dialysis is much less effective.[5] Monitoring of blood levels is advisable, especially when high doses are being administered.

Adverse Effects

In comparison to other classes of antibacterials, e.g., penicillins, fluoroquinolones, and erythromycins, the aminoglycosides possess considerable intrinsic toxicity and a low therapeutic index. Major adverse effects include auditory, vestibular, and renal toxicity and neuromuscular blockade.

Impairment of Eighth Cranial Nerve Function

Ototoxicity results from the destruction of outer hair cells in the organ of Corti with the degeneration of the auditory nerve fibers.[6] The aminoglycosides concentrate and persist for long periods within the endolymph and perilymph of the inner ear.[7] The ototoxicity manifests itself as hearing loss due to cochlear damage or as vestibular disturbances characterized by vertigo, ataxia, and loss of balance. A high-pitched tinnitus often is the initial symptom of developing ototoxicity. High-frequency hearing loss is common, but is often undetected until it progresses to a more severe stage. The auditory damage is often irreversible. The extent of permanent injury is related to the number of affected sensory hair cells and to sustained exposure to the aminoglycosides. Substantial recovery from the vestibular effects usually occur, but one to two years may be required, and most patients have permanent residual damage. Adverse effects involving eighth cranial nerve function are related to advanced age, prior aminoglycoside administration, and high dosage and levels. Other ototoxic agents, such as the loop diuretics ethacrynic acid and possibly furosemide, can potentiate the effects of the aminoglycosides. Vestibular toxicity is more frequently associated with gentamicin and streptomycin, whereas auditory impairment is more typical of kanamycin and amikacin. Tobramycin affects both to an equal degree.

Nephrotoxicity

Aminoglycosides are the most frequent cause of drug-induced renal failure and are responsible for about 10 percent of all cases of renal failure. Toxicity, primarily involving the proximal tubular cells, is thought to result from binding of aminoglycosides to phospholipids such as polyphosphoinositides in the brush border.[8] Elevation of cytosolic free calcium and inhibition of phospholipases probably play a role in mediating the toxicity. Aminoglycoside nephrotoxicity correlates with the total amount of drug administered. Streptomycin has lower potential for renal damage than do other members of the series. Studies of relative nephrotoxic potential of the other aminoglycosides have yielded conflicting results and no clear differences. Concurrent administration of other nephrotoxic drugs such as amphotericin B, cyclosporin, cisplatin, and vancomycin may increase the risk of aminoglycoside nephrotoxicity. The nephrotoxic effects produced by the aminoglycosides are generally reversible because the proximal tubular cells possess considerable regenerative capacity.

Neuromuscular Blockade

Aminoglycosides produce a nondepolarizing or curare-like blockade in skeletal muscle by both inhibiting the presynaptic release of acetylcholine and blocking postjunctional receptor sites.[9] Inhibition of calcium influx into neurons may be an underlying mechanism, since the blockade can be antagonized by calcium administration. These actions can result in skeletal muscle weakness and respiratory depression. This reaction is unlikely to manifest itself as a problem in the absence of predisposing factors such as presence of myasthenia gravis, the concurrent use of drugs intended to act as muscle relaxants, or very high doses.

Other Adverse Effects

Aminoglycosides, especially streptomycin, may produce dysfunction of the optic nerve and effects involving the peripheral nervous system, e.g., parathesias. Pain at the injection site is common. Hypersensitivity reactions are relatively rare with the aminoglycosides, but may occur. This has been particularly true with long-term exposure to streptomycin, both in patients receiving the drug and personnel who prepare or handle solutions (gloves should be worn to avoid this problem).

Therapeutic Uses

For many years after their introduction, the aminoglycosides were major agents for gram-negative bacterial infections, particularly for use against such organisms as *Psueudomonas aeruginosa,* for which there were few choices. Within the past decade, many newer drugs (e.g., extended spectrum penicillins, third-generation cephalosporins, and fluoroquinolines) with far superior selective toxicity and in some cases a much more favorable pharmacokinetic profile (oral administration and better distribution) and greater efficacy have greatly reduced the importance of the aminoglycosides as antibacterial agents. Despite these limitations, they are still useful alternatives for several gram-negative infections, especially in severe infections such as sepsis and pneumonia. Some agents in the group, particularly streptomycin, neomycin, and paromomycin have unique uses. On the other hand, kanamycin is rarely used today

Gentamicin, tobramycin, amikacin, or netilmicin, coadministered with an extended spectrum penicillin (ticarcillin, mezlocillin, or piperacillin) are considered first-choice therapy for *Pseudomonas aeruginosa* infections at sites other than the urinary tract,[10] although resistance is an increasing problem. These aminoglycosides and penicillins should not be mixed in the same solution because of the possibility of interaction and loss of activity. Cross resistance to these aminoglycosides by Pseudomonas is not complete, so infections failing to respond to one agent may be sensitive to another, e.g., amikacin often is effective in treating infections resistant to gentamicin or tobramycin. The same is true of netilmicin, which amikacin resembles in that it is not susceptible to inactivation by bacterial enzymes.

Gentamicin, amikacin, and tobramycin are alternative agents for the following infections:[10]

Enterobacter (alternate to imipenim)
E. coli (alternate to cephalosporins)
Klebsiella (alternate to cephalosporins)
Proteus [other than mirabilis] (alternate to cephalosporins)
Serratia (alternate to cephalosporins)

Streptomycin is considered the drug of choice for infections caused by *Yersinia pestus* (plague), tularemia, and *Pseudomonas mallei* (in combination with a tetracycline).[10] Patients with tularemia may respond dramatically to streptomycin.[11] As noted previously, streptomycin was the first effective agent against tuberculosis. It was part of the standard combination regimen for tuberculosis for several decades, despite requiring IM administration. Owing to resistance and the development of other effective agents with lower toxicity and the ease of oral administration, streptomycin has not been considered a first-choice agent for this infection for many years. However, the recent resurgence in the incidence of tuberculosis, because of its occurrence as a secondary infection in AIDS patients, and other factors may increase the importance of this use of streptomycin once again.

Neomycin is not used systemically because of its high potential for toxicity. However, owing to its lack of absorption from the GI tract, it can be administered orally for a prophylactic or therapeutic action against intestinal bacteria. Intestinal malabsorption and superinfection are a complication of oral administration. Neomycin is used in combination with erythromycin for reduction of bowel flora before surgery.[12] It is also employed for irrigation of the urinary bladder to prevent infections associated with indwelling catheters.

Because of its activity against many gram-negative pathogens and poor dermal absorption, neomycin is included in a wide variety of products for topical application. It is frequently combined with bacitracin, an antibiotic with excellent activity against gram-positive organisms, and polymyxin, another antibiotic highly active against gram-negatives. Such a combination of three agents with different mechanisms of action provides a broad spectrum of antibacterial activity that may be advantageous in some instances, but that also carries risk of destruction of normal flora and superinfection. Hypersensitivity reactions also may occur. It must be kept in mind that while absorption of neomycin is minimal from the normal intestine or skin, inflammation or injury (burns and abrasions in the case of the skin) may result in significant absorption and the systemic toxicity characteristic of the aminoglycoside class.

Paromomycin is an alternate to metronidazole and iodoquinol for treatment of intestinal infections caused by the protozoan *Entamoeba histolytica.* It exhibits characteristics typical of the aminoglycoside class, including poor absorption from the GI tract. Thus, it is not effective in extraintestinal, e.g., hepatic, forms of amebiasis. Nausea and abdominal pain are the primary adverse effects.

Preparations

Amikacin (Amikan)
Vials for injection containing 100, 500, and 1000 mg

Gentamicin (Garamycin)
Injectable forms containing 20, 60, 80, and 800 mg, including intrathecal, IV piggyback, and pediatric formulations, 0.1% cream, 0.1% ointment, ophthalmic ointment and solution.

Kanamycin (Kantrex)
500-mg oral capsules; 1-gram vials for injection; and 75-mg vial for injection (pediatric).

Neomycin
500-mg oral tablets; numerous products for topical application (creams, ointments, ophthalmic solutions and ointments).

Netilmicin (Netromycin)
Vials for injection containing 100 mg/ml.

Paromomycin (Humatin)
250-mg oral capsules.

Streptomycin
Ampules containing 1 gm.

Tobramycin (Nebcin)
Vials containing 20 (pediatric), 40, 60, and 80 mg for injection.

Tetracyclines

The tetracyclines, a group of very broad spectrum antibiotics, are closely related in terms of chemical structure. The spectrum of activity of all these agents is nearly identical. Differences in adverse effects are minor, but there is very marked variation in pharmacokinetics between members of the tetracycline group.

Chemistry

Tetracyclines are derivatives of the polycyclic substance naphthacenecarboxamide. Since solubility of the free form is limited, the more soluble hydrochloride form is used. Tetracycline solutions are acidic, and most (except chlortetracycline) exhibit good stability. Structures of the tetracyclines are shown in Figure 93.3.

History

The tetracyclines were derived from Streptomyces species, beginning with the isolation of chlortetracycline from *Streptomyces aureofaciens* in 1948. Several other members of the series followed within a few years, and the tetracyclines were a major component of the "wonder drug" era of the late 1940s and early 1950s. Doxycycline and minocycline are more recent additions to the group, but no new tetracyclines have been developed in the past few decades.

Antimicrobial Spectrum

The tetracyclines exhibit activity against a wide variety of gram-positive and gram-negative bacteria, with gram-positives generally being inhibited by lower concentrations than gram-negatives. Also included in their spectrum are some anaerobic bacteria and other organisms such as Rickettsiae, Chlamydia, Mycoplasma, spirochetes (Treponema and Borrelia), and certain protozoa, e.g., *Balantidium coli.* However, tetracyclines lack activity against viruses and fungi, the latter often thriving as superinfections secondary to destruction of the normal bacterial flora by these drugs.

Mechanism of Action and Resistance

Tetracyclines enter the bacterial cell by a combination of passive diffusion through hydrophilic pores in the outer cell membrane and an energy-dependent active transport mechanism that pumps the drug through the inner cytoplasmic membrane.[r4] This active transport system allows tetracyclines to be concentrated in bacteria because the system is not present in human cells. The tetracyclines inhibit bacterial protein synthesis by binding to the 30S ribosome and preventing access of aminoacyl tRNA to the acceptor site on the mRNA-ribosome complex Figure 93.2. This action prevents the addition of new amino acids to the growing peptide chain. Mammalian cell protein synthesis is inhibited by high concentrations of the tetracyclines, but they exhibit considerable selective toxicity. The tetracyclines are considered to have a bacteriostatic effect.

Resistance results primarily from plasmids, transmitted by conjugation or transduction, coding for proteins that allow organisms to develop the ability to interfere with the active transport of tetracyclines through the cytoplasmic membrane.[13] Loss of ability to penetrate by passive diffusion also may play a role in the development of resistance. Organisms are usually cross-resistant to all teteracyclines.

Pharmacokinetics

There are major differences in the pharmacokinetic properties of the various tetracyclines. Pharmacokinetic characteristics of individual tetracyclines are summarized in Table 93.1.

Administration and Absorption

All tetracyclines are sufficiently absorbed from the GI tract to be administered orally. However, the rate and extent of absorption varies with the individual agent (Table 93.1), ranging from 30 percent for chlortetracycline to nearly 100 percent for minocycline. The portion not absorbed has high potential for disrupting the normal flora of the colon, giving rise to superinfections. Absorption tends to be reduced by the presence of food and is markedly diminished by divalent or trivalent metal cations. These ions form a complex with tetracycline that causes the drug to be excreted in the feces rather than absorbed. Cation-containing products that must not be administered concurrently with tetra-

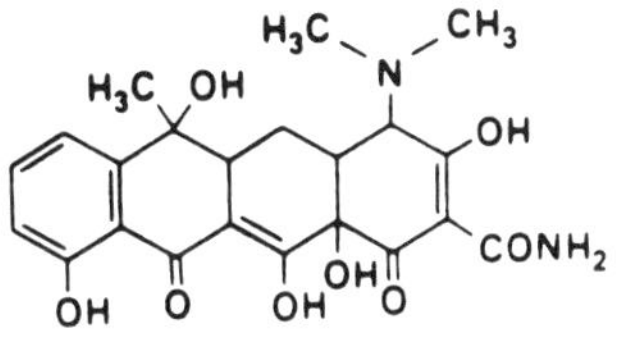

Tetracycline

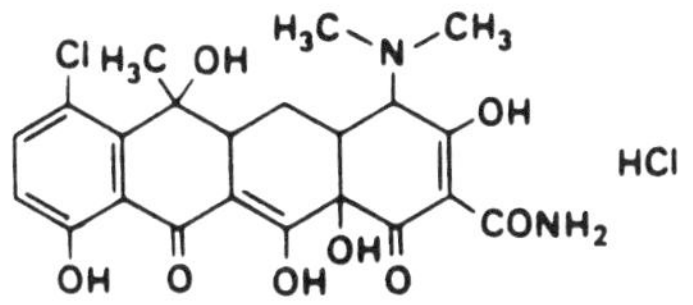

Chlortetracycline

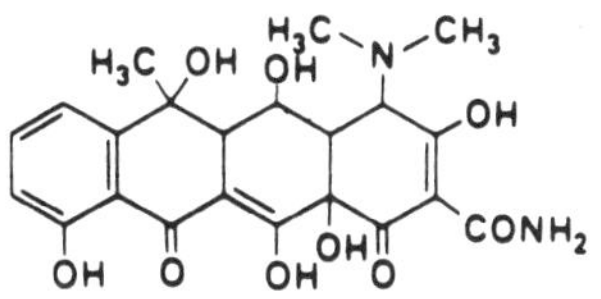

Oxytetracycline

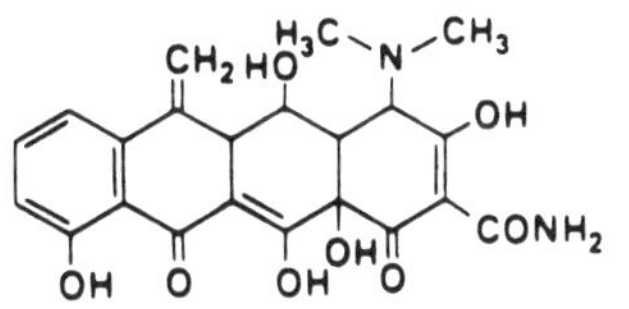

Methacycline

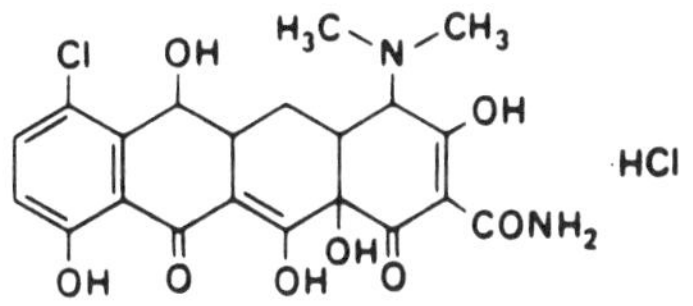

Demeclocycline

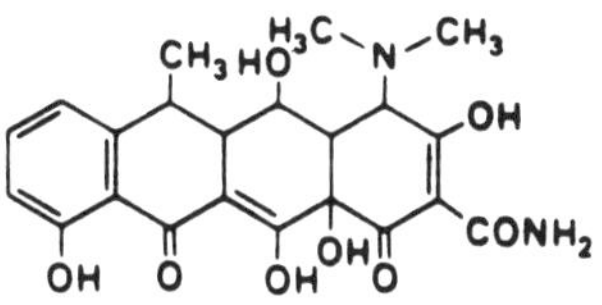

Doxycycline

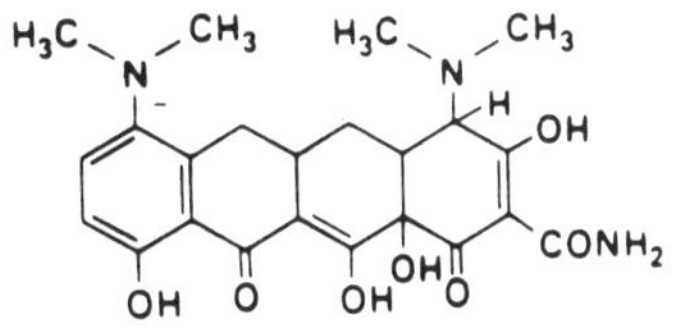

Minocycline

Figure 93.3 Structures of the Tetracyclines

Table 93.1 Pharmacokinetic Properties of the Tetracyclines

Drug	GI Absorption %	Plasma Protein Binding %	$T_{1/2}$ Hours	% Excreted in Urine	Major Nonrenal Elimination Route
Tetracycline	80	25–60	10	60	—
Chlortetracycline	30	40–70	7	20	Bile
Oxytetracycline	60	20–35	9	70	—
Demeclocycline	70	40–90	15	40	Metabolism
Methacycline	65	75–90	15	50	—
Doxycycline	93	25–90	15	35	Intestine
Minocycline	100	70–75	17	10	Metabolism

cyclines include dairy products (calcium), calcium supplements, antacids (aluminum and magnesium), and iron supplements. Preparations are available for topical use (including ophthalmic preparations) and for IV and IM administration.

Distribution

Tetracyclines are well distributed to body fluids and tissues. Oral administration results in low levels in the CSF, but about 25 percent of serum levels can be reached over a period of six hours if tetracyclines are given IV. Inflammation of the meninges does not increase CSF penetration to the extent seen with many other antibacterials. Penetration of tissues and fluids tends to be better with the more lipid-soluble tetracyclines, doxycycline and minocycline. Plasma protein binding varies considerably between agents (Table 93.1). Tetracyclines cross the placenta, with relatively high concentrations being found in human milk. Minocycline is unique in reaching high concentrations in tears and saliva. Plasma protein binding ranges from 40 to 80 percent.

Disposition

As indicated in Table 93.1, there are marked differences among the tetracyclines in both the route and rate of disposition. All undergo renal excretion by filtration to some degree, and all concentrate in the liver and appear in the bile, sometimes in concentrations higher than in the plasma. The bile is a particularly important route of elimination for chlortetracycline. At least 50 percent of a dose of tetracycline, oxytetracycline, and methacycline undergoes renal excretion. Doxycycline is handled by apparently unique, incompletely understood nonrenal mechanisms that appear to include metabolism and excretion of conjugates and chelates in the feces. It has low potential for accumulation in renal failure. Minocycline is mainly metabolized, with only about 10 percent of the free drug appearing in the urine. Thus, the pharmacokinetics of minocycline are not greatly altered in renal failure. The half-life of extensively metabolized tetracyclines may be decreased by the administration of a drug that induces hepatic microsomal enzymes, e.g., barbiturates. Half-life values for tetracyclines range from approximately seven to 17 hours, with chlortetracycline having the shortest half-life and minocycline the longest.

Adverse Effects

Tetracyclines are associated with numerous adverse effects, ranging from relatively frequent but minor to rare, serious complications of therapy. In addition to the following direct toxic effects, hypersensitivity reactions also occur.

Gastrointestinal Effects

Diarrhea, nausea, and vomiting are the most frequent complaints of patients receiving tetracyclines orally, and most often cause termination of therapy. Initial effects may result from irritation of the GI tract. Symptoms may be alleviated by taking tetracyclines with food (not dairy products) or antacids that do not contain aluminum, magnesium, or calcium. After a few days to a week of use, diarrhea, anal pruritus, and other symptoms may appear as a result of modification of the normal bacterial flora of the gut by tetracyclines, with resultant superinfection by opportunistic organisms not affected by the drug. The fungal organism, *Candida albicans,* is the most frequent cause of this problem. Less frequently, more serious superinfections may be caused by nonsusceptible or resistant bacteria, e.g., coliforms, Staphylcocci, Proteus, or Pseudomonas. Pseudomembraneous colitis secondary to *Clostridium difficile* has been associated with tetracyclines as a rare but serious effect.

Hepatotoxicity

Liver damage with tetracyclines involving jaundice and fatty infiltration is unlikely, but poses a particular hazard during pregnancy, when fatal reactions progressing to acidosis and irreversible shock have occurred. Pre-existing hepatic disease and administration of large doses (4 g/day), particularly IV, raise the potential for hepatotoxicity. In the absence of these predisposing factors, there is relatively little risk of hepatic damage with tetracycline use. Oxytetracycline and tetracycline appear to be the least likely to cause hepatotoxicity.

Developing Teeth

Tetracyclines have high affinity for calcium in newly formed teeth in children. This results in such effects as brown mottling, enamel defects, and inhibition of growth of the underlying bone structure. The period of greatest danger is from midpregnancy to about one year of age for the deciduous teeth and six months to five years for the permanent teeth. Thus, if alternatives are available, tetracyclines should not be given to children under eight years of age. This is also another reason for avoiding their use in pregnancy.

Renal Toxicity

The use of outdated tetracyclines containing degradation products has been associated with the Fanconi syndrome, which includes renal tubular acidosis and other manifestations of nephrotoxicity. Increased awareness of this potential problem and refinements in tetracycline formulations have decreased the likelihood of this problem. In addition, tetracyclines may aggravate uremia by inhibition of protein synthesis and a catabolic effect, leading to azotemia. Severe renal failure associated with calcium oxalate crystal formation has been reported in patients who received tetracycline after general anesthesia with methoxyflurane.[14]

Doxycycline appears to be least likely to cause kidney damage.

Phototoxicity

Tetracyclines can induce sensitivity to sunlight or ultraviolet light. The lighter the individual's skin, the greater the likelihood of this reaction. This effect is particularly associated with demeclocycline (in comparison with other tetracyclines) although the incidence is probably less than 5 percent.

Superinfections

In addition to the GI superinfections noted above, tetracyclines can cause other superinfections. Oral, pharyngeal, and genital candidiasis are particularly likely to occur.

Vestibular Disturbances

Initial administration of minocycline results in vestibular toxicity characterized by dizziness, ataxia, nausea, and vomiting in 70 percent or more of patients. These effects disappear rapidly if the drug is discontinued, and often sufficient tolerance develops so that drug administration can continue.

Effects Related to Administration Sites

In addition to irritation of the GI tract, tetracyclines cause thrombophlebitis when given IV and severe pain when injected IM without a local anesthetic.

Contraindications

In view of the adverse effects described, there are three major instances in which tetracyclines should be avoided unless a serious infection with no suitable alternative is present. These contraindications are: pregnancy; hepatic disease; and patients less than eight years of age.

Therapeutic Uses

The broad spectrum of the tetracyclines has led to widespread indiscriminate use. Among other problems, this has resulted in the extensive development of resistant strains. Also, while tetracyclines have a reasonably good safety profile, they have often been employed when agents with less potential for toxicity could be used. However, the tetracyclines are considered the drugs of choice for the following organisms and infections:[10]

Gram-Negative Bacilli

Brucella
Calymmatobacterium granulomatis (granuloma inguinale)
Helicobacter pylori
Pseudomonas mallei (in combination with streptomycin)
Vibrio cholerae (cholera)
Vibrio vulnificus

Acid Fast Bacilli

Mycobacterium fortuitum (doxycycline)
Mycobacterium marinum (minocycline)

Chlamydiae

Chlamydia trachomatis (urethritis, cervicitis, lymphogranuloma venereum)
Chlamydia psittaci (psittacosis, ornithosis)
Chlamydia pneumoniae

Mycoplasma

Mycoplasma pneumoniae

Rickettsia

(Rocky Mountain spotted fever, Q fever, typhus)

Spirochetes

Borrelia burgdorferi (Lyme disease)
Borrelia recurrentis (relapsing fever)

Protozoa

Balantidium coli

Tetracyclines are important alternatives to the treatment of choice for the following organisms or infections: *Moraxella catarrhalis; Clostridium perfringens; Clostridium tetani; Campylobacter jejuni; Acinetobacter* (doxycycline or minocycline); *Eikenella corrodens; Leptotrichia buccalis; Pasturella multocida; Spirillum minus* (rat bite fever); *Streptobacillus moniliformis* (Haverhill fever); *Yersinia pestis* (plague); *Actinomycetes israelii;* the Mycoplasma organism *Ureaplasma urealyticum;* the spirochetes Leptospira, *Treponema pallidum* (syphilis), *Treponema pertenue* (yaws), and *Rochalimaea henselae* (Bacillary angiomatosis).[10]

Since all members of the tetracycline class have a virtually identical antimicrobial spectrum, the selection of an agent from the group is based largely upon pharmacokinetic factors and individual patient characteristics. For example, doxycycline and especially minocycline would be rational choices in the presence of renal insufficiency since dependence upon the kidneys for disposition is relatively low. On the other hand, these agents would be relatively ineffective in urinary tract infections. Minocycline is useful for the eradication of meningococci from the nasopharynx, thus eliminating the carrier state.

Tetracyclines are used both systemically and topically in the treatment of acne owing to their activity against *Proprionbacterium acnes*, an anaerobic organism involved in the pathogenesis of the disease. With respect to the use of tetracyclines against *Helicobacter pylori*, it should be noted that there is considerable interest in this organism as a causative agent for peptic ulcer and hence in antibacterial therapy as a supplement or replacement for traditional modes of ulcer prevention and treatment.

On a quantitative basis, perhaps the major use of tetracyclines is as a supplement to livestock feed to increase growth rate in the animals. This practice is very controversial as it is a factor in the spread of organisms resistant to tetracyclines. This concern has resulted in the ban of such use of tetracyclines in Britain, but the practice continues in the US.

Preparations

Chlortetracycline (Aureomycin):
Topical: Ophthalmic ointment 1%, ointment 3%

Demeclocyline (Declomycin):
Oral: 150- and 300-mg tablets; 150-mg capsules

Doxycycline (Vibramycin)
Oral: 50- and 100-mg tablets and capsules; powder to reconstitute for 5 and 10 mg/ml suspension;
Parenteral: powder to reconstitute for injection (100 and 200 mg/vials)

Methacycline (Rondomycin):
Oral: 150- and 300-mg capsules

Minocycline (Minocin):
Oral: 50- and 100-mg capsules; 10 mg/ml oral suspension
Parenteral: powder to reconstitute for injection (100 mg/vial)

Oxytetracycline (Terramycin):
Oral: 250-mg capsules
Parenteral: 50, 125 mg/ml for ampules IM injection;
Topical: ophthalmic suspension (5 mg/ml) and ophthalmic ointment (5 mg/g)

Tetracycline (Achromycin V):
Oral: 250- and 500-mg capsules; 25 mg/ml suspension
Topical: ophthalmic ointment (1%), ophthalmic solution (1%), Topicycline topical solution (2.2 mg/ml)

Chloramphenicol

Chloramphenicol, a nitrobenzene-containing derivative of dichloroacetic acid, is a broad-spectrum protein synthesis inhibitor. While effective against a wide variety of gram-positive and gram-negative bacteria and other organisms such as rickettsiae, it is not the agent of first choice for any infection, owing to its potential for producing a serious adverse effect, aplastic anemia.

Chemistry

Chloramphenicol is a stable, colorless crystalline substance with low water solubility. The levorotatory form exhibits biologic activity. It has a bitter taste and is quite stable. The comparatively simple chemical structure (Fig 93.4) contains a nitrobenzene moiety and is a derivative of dichloroacetic acid.

History

This antibiotic is produced by *Streptomycin venezuelae* and was first isolated in 1947 from a soil sample collected in Venezuela.[15] Chloramphenicol was synthesized two years later, becoming the first major antibiotic to be produced in this manner. Its availability, ease of administration, broad spectrum, and initial apparent lack of toxicity resulted in widespread usage. An estimated 8 million persons received the drug between 1948 and 1951. However, association of chloramphenicol with often fatal adverse effects, such as aplastic anemia and the gray syndrome in infants, made it a very controversial drug. Demands were made that it be removed from the market. It remains a valuable alternative agent, but it is now understood that it must not be used indiscriminately.

Antimicrobial Spectrum

The very broad spectrum of chloramphenicol is quite similar to that of the tetracyclines. It is effective against a wide variety of both gram-positive and gram-negative bacteria as well as rickettsiae, Chlamydia and Mycoplasma. It is active against most anaerobic bacteria including *Bacteroides fragilis*; however, it lacks activity against *Pseudomonas aeruginosa*. Major differences in spectrum from the tetracyclines include lack of activity against Chlamydia and protozoan organisms.

Mechanism of Action and Resistance

Following penetration into cells by both passive and facilitated diffusion, chloramphenicol inhibits bacterial protein synthesis by binding reversibly to a receptor site on the 50S ribosomal subunit. This is very close to the site of action of the macrolides antibiotics. Thus, it prevents the binding of the amino acid-containing end of aminoacyl tRNA to its binding site on the ribosome and the subsequent association of peptidyltransferase with the amino acid substrate. Ultimately, peptide bond formation and the incorporation of amino acids into newly formed peptides is inhibited.[r5] Chloramphen-

$$O_2N-C_6H_4-\underset{\displaystyle OH}{\overset{|}{CH}}-\underset{\displaystyle CH_2OH}{\overset{|}{CH}}-NH-\overset{\displaystyle O}{\overset{\|}{C}}-CHCl_2$$

Figure 93.4 Structure of Chloramphenicol

icol also inhibits mitochondrial protein synthesis in mammalian cells, especially those involved with erythropoiesis. It is generally considered to be a bacteriostatic agent, although it may be bactericidal for certain organisms, e.g., *Haemophilus influenzae*.[16]

Bacterial resistance to chloramphenicol is due primarily to production of an enzyme that inactivates the drug. A plasmid, acquired during conjugation, produces a specific acetyltransferase resulting in the formation of acetylated derivatives which are not able to bind to bacterial ribosomes.[17,18] Resistance due to decreased permeability to the drug and loss of ribosomal sensitivity also has been reported.[19,20]

Pharmacokinetics

Chloramphenicol is a lipid-soluble molecule, and thus its pharmacokinetics reflect its ability to cross body membranes readily.

Administration and Absorption

Orally-administered chloramphenicol is rapidly and completely absorbed from the GI tract. Unlike some antibiotics, neither food nor metal ions reduce absorption of chloramphenicol. Chloramphenicol palmitate, used in an oral suspension, is hydrolyzed to the active form by pancreatic lipases in the small intestine.[21] Parenteral administration of chloramphenicol is seldom required, usually being reserved for such situations as treatment of meningitis or when vomiting precludes oral administration. The succinate form, used for IM or IV injection, undergoes hydrolysis to the free drug.

Distribution

Reflecting high lipid solubility, chloramphenicol is widely distributed, readily reaching essentially all tissues and body fluids, including the aqueous humor. Penetration into the CSF is better than with any other antibiotic, with levels often exceeding 50 percent of serum values, even in the absence of meningitis.[22] Chloramphenicol crosses the placenta and is secreted into milk. Binding to plasma protein is approximately 30 percent.

Disposition

Typical of a lipophylic drug, only a small proportion of chloramphenicol (5–10% of a dose) is excreted unchanged by the kidney. The major route of disposition is hepatic conjugation to an inactive glucuronide. Metabolites are excreted in the urine by a combination of filtration and secretion. Unlike many antibiotics, the disposition of chloramphenicol is not markedly altered by renal failure, so dosage adjustments are not necessary. However, hepatic disease, e.g., cirrhosis, may decrease metabolic clearance. The half-life is four hours.

Adverse Effects

Much of the toxicity produced by chloramphenicol can be attributed to inhibition of the synthesis of proteins of the inner mitochondrial membrane, probably by blocking the action of ribosomal peptidyl transferase.[r6] A common and important adverse effect of chloramphenicol is bone marrow suppression. This is a dose-related reaction particularly associated with daily doses above 4 grams and serum levels above 25 μg/ml. Duration of administration also appears to be a factor. Effects usually occur within five to seven days of initial administration and are characterized by reticulocytopenia, anemia, leukopenia, neutropenia, thrombocytopenia, and an increase in serum iron concentration. Recovery from dose-related bone marrow suppression usually occurs within three weeks after discontinuation of chloramphenicol. Complete blood cell and platelet counts should be obtained at least three times a week in patients who are receiving chloramphenicol therapy.

Aplastic anemia is a rare (approximately one case per 25,000 to 40,000 courses of therapy) adverse effect with chloramphenicol. It is unrelated to dose and is thought to be an idiosyncratic reaction. It can occur while the drug is being taken or days to months after administration ceases. The aplastic response involves all cellular elements of the marrow and is usually fatal. The longer the interval between the last dose of chloramphenicol and the onset of anemia, the greater the mortality rate. When bone marrow aplasia is complete, a high frequency of development of acute leukemia occurs in those patients who recover.[23] Exposure to the drug on more than one occasion also appears to be a risk factor.

Chloramphenicol is also associated with a fatal reaction in neonates, especially premature infants, known as the gray syndrome. This condition usually begins within the first week of therapy and is characterized by an ashen gray skin, vomiting, irregular and rapid respiration, abdominal distension, flaccidity, hypothermia, and vasomotor collapse. The mortality rate in affected infants is approximately 40 percent. The underlying mechanism is an inability of infants to conjugate chloramphenicol with glucuronic acid, owing to limited glucuronyl transferase activity during the first several weeks of life. Reduced renal excretion of unconjugated drug in the newborn also plays a role.

Common, but less serious adverse effects include GI disturbances and candidiasis of mucous membranes secondary to disruption of the normal flora, particularly in the mouth and vagina. Superinfection in the colon is less likely than with other broad spectrum antibacterials because of the excellent absorption of chloramphenicol from the small intestine. Hypersensitivity reactions, digital paresthesias, and optic neuritis (3–5% of children with mucoviscidosis) may occur.

Drug Interactions

Chloramphenicol irreversibly inhibits hepatic microsomal enzymes and thus raises blood levels and prolongs the half-life of many drugs metabolized by this system, including warfarin, phenytoin, tolbutamide, and chlorpropamide. Chronic administration of enzyme-inducing agents such as phenobarbital may result in lower than expected levels of chloramphenicol.

Therapeutic Uses

Because of the risk of serious toxicity and the availability of other usually effective agents, chloramphenicol is not the agent of first choice for infections caused by any organism.[10] Indiscriminate use must be avoided, and whenever the drug is used it should be determined that the potential benefit outweighs the risk involved. However, chloramphenicol is a valuable alternative in certain selected instances. Its excellect penetration of the CSF makes it an important drug for therapy of meningitis caused by *Haemophilus influenzae, Neisseria meningitides, Streptococcus pneumoniae,* and other organisms. It is also valuable for therapy of infections at other sites in the CNS, e.g., brain abscesses caused by various bacteria including anaerobes. It is a former drug of choice and is now a major alternative to the cephalosporins for infections caused by *Salmonella typhi* (typhoid fever), and can be used for treating other *Salmonella infections.* It is sometimes used as an alternative against anaerobic organisms such as *Bacteroides fragilis.* It is clearly the second best choice to tetracyclines for rickettsial infections such as Rocky Mountain spotted fever, and should be utilized in treating these infections when tetracyclines are contraindicated by pregnancy or other factors.

Preparations

Chloramphenicol (Chloromycetin) is available in capsules for oral administration containing 250 mg (Kapseals/Chloromycetin), an oral suspension (Chloromycetin Palmitate), 100-mg vials for injection (Chloromycetin Sodium Succinate), a 1% ointment containing fibrinolysin and desoxyribonuclease (Elase-Chloromycetin) a 1% cream for topical application (Chloromycetin Cream), a suspension with hydrocortisone for ophthalmic use (Chloromycetin Hydrocortisone Ophthalmic), an ophthalmic solution (Chloromycetin Ophthalmic Solution), an ophthalmic ointment (Chloromycetin Ophthalmic Ointment, 1%) and a solution for use in the ear (Chloromycetin OTIC).

Erythromycin and Related Macrolides

For many years erythromycin has been the only significant antibiotic in the macrolide class in terms of clinical usefulness. Seldom used macrolides include spiromycin and oleandomycin. Recently two new macrolides, azithromycin and clarithromycin, have been introduced. The macrolides are characterized by good activity against many gram-positive bacteria, a low degree of serious toxicity, and a high potential for interaction by alteration of the metabolism of such agents as theophylline and terfenadine.

Chemistry

Macrolides contain a many-membered (usually 14–16) lactone ring to which are attached one or more deoxy sugars. Erythromycin consists of a 14-member ring and the sugars desosamine and cladinose. Clarithromycin is 6-methoxy-erythromycin and demonstrates higher stability to acidic conditions than erythromycin. Azithromycin, an azalide, has a 15-member macrolide ring and is also more acid-stable. Erythromycin is unstable in an acid medium, undergoing an intramolecular cycling reaction that destroys the activity of the antibiotic. Considerable effort has been spent to produce compounds with greater acid stability and oral bioavailability. These efforts have included the development of water-insoluble acid-stable salts (stearate) and esters (ethyl succinate and propionate) of erythromycin, or derivatives and related compounds (clarithromycin and azithromycin). The structures of the macrolides are shown in Figure 93.5.

History

In 1952 erythromycin was isolated from *Streptomyces erythreus* derived from a soil sample collected in the Philippines. Azithromycin and clarithromycin were introduced in 1991.

Antimicrobial Spectrum

The spectrum of erythromycin resembles that of penicillins G and V in that the drug exhibits high activity against many gram-positive organisms (which accumulate much higher concentrations), but relatively few gram-negative bacteria. However, erythromycin is very active against certain gram-negative pathogens. In addition to activity against such gram-positives as Staphylococci, Streptococci, and Corynebacterium, of particular importance is the antibiotic's effectiveness against such gram-negatives as Legionella and Campylobacteria and other organisms, e.g., Chlamydia, Mycoplasma, and the spirochete Borrelia. Erythromycin is generally inactive against anaerobes and lacks action against fungi and viruses. The spectrum of clarithromycin generally resembles that of erythromycin. Clarithromycin is two- to fourfold more active than erythromycin against most Streptococci and Staphylococci.[24] It also has better activity than erythromycin against

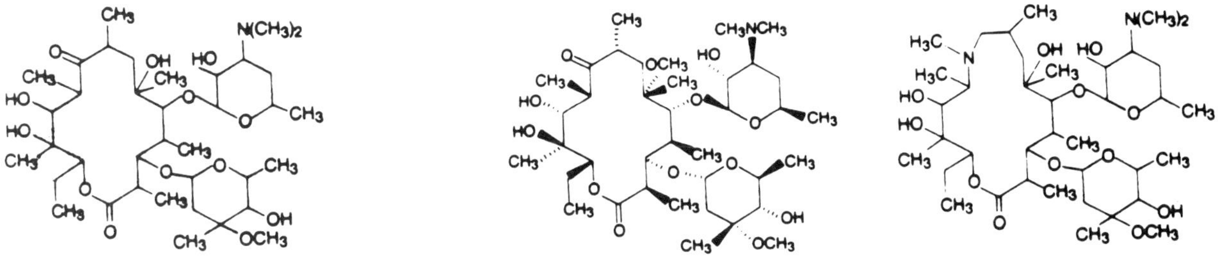

Erythromycin

Clarithromycin

Azithromycin

Figure 93.5 Structures of the Macrolides

Helicobacter pylori and Chlamydia.[r7] Azithromycin's spectrum is also similar to erythromycin, but it is somewhat less active than erythromycin against gram-positive cocci.[24] However, it is more active than erythromycin against gram-negative bacteria, possibly due to an additional positive charge created by the presence of a methyl-substituted nitrogen in the macrolide ring.[r8] The two newer agents have good activity against some species of Mycobacterium.[25]

Mechanism of Action and Resistance

Erythromycin and other macrolide antibiotics inhibit bacterial protein synthesis by reversible binding to the 50S ribosomal subunit.[26,r8] The 14-hydroxy active metabolite of clarithromycin acts in the same manner.[27] The specific receptor for the macrolides appears to be a 23S rRNA on the 50 S subunit. This location is similar to the site of action of chloramphenicol, and each drug can inhibit the binding of the other. Binding to the ribosome takes place at a site near peptidyltransferase, leading to inhibition of translocation, peptide bond formation, and dissociation of oligopeptidyl tRNA from the ribosome. Activity is enhanced by an alkaline pH. The macrolides may be bactericidal or bacteriostatic, depending on the concentration of the drug and the organism involved (greater bactericidal activity against rapidly-dividing bacteria). The influence of pH is probably based on the fact that increased pH results in more of the unionized form of the drug, which penetrates bacterial cells more readily.[28,29]

Resistance to the macrolides results primarily from modification of the receptor site on the ribosome, probably through a methylation reaction. The newer macrolides exhibit cross resistance with erythromycin.[r7] Other mechanisms of resistance to erythromycin shown experimentally with selected organisms, but of unclear clinical sigificance, include reduced drug movement through the cell envelope and bacterial production of an esterase capable of hydrolyzing the drug.

Pharmacokinetics

There are important differences in the pharmacokinetics of the macrolides, particularly with respect to mode of disposition and half-life. Pharmacokinetic properties are summarized in Table 93.2.

Administration and Absorption

The three macrolides are sufficiently absorbed from the GI tract to permit oral administration. Erythromycin base is susceptible to inactivation by gastric acid and therefore must be given in an enteric-coated form resistant to destruction by acidity in the stomach. Dissolution and absorption then take place in the duodenum. The presence of food inhibits absorption of erythromycin. Several esters of erythromycin that are more acid-stable have been used. The estolate ester is particularly acid resistant and is well absorbed. However, it must be hydrolyzed by bacterial enzymes after penetrating into the cell before binding to bacterial ribosomes can occur. Erythromycin is also administered parenterally, rectally, and topically. Clarithromycin is well absorbed from the GI tract, with or without food. Azithromycin is also well absorbed, but food decreases its bioavailability. Aluminum- and magnesium-containing antacids reduce the peak serum levels, but not the extent of azithromycin absorption.

Distribution

The macrolides generally penetrate well into body tissues and fluids, except the brain and CSF. Erythromycin is one of the few antibiotics that penetrates readily into prostatic fluid, where levels can reach 40 percent of those in serum. Erythromycin crosses the placental barrier and is present in maternal milk. Approximately 40 percent is bound to plasma protein. Clarithromycin and azithromycin also distribute well. Clarithromycin and azithromycin are 50 to 70 percent and 40 to 50 percent bound, respectively. The newer agents reach high concentrations in macrophages and polymorphonuclear leukocytes.[30]

Disposition

Erythromycin is excreted primarily in the liver and bile. The drug is concentrated in the bile to an extent

Table 93.2 Pharmacokinetic Properties of the Macrolide Antibiotics

Drug	GI Absorption %	Plasma Protein Binding %	$T_{1/2}$ Hours	% Excreted in Urine	Major Nonrenal Elimination Route
Erythromycin	35[a]	70–80	1.5	5–15	Bile
Clarithromycin	55	50–70	3–7[b]	30	Metabolism
Azithromycin	40	40–50	10–50[c]	5–15	Bile & Metabolism

[a] Value for enteric-coated erythromycin base
[b] Half-life is somewhat dose-dependent: 3–4 hours for 250-mg bid dose and 5–7 hours for 500-mg bid dose.
[c] Half-life is polyphasic: 10 hours within 24 hours of administration increasing to 50 hours or more 72 hours after administration.

that biliary levels may reach 50 times blood levels. Only 5 percent or less of an oral dose appears unchanged in the urine. With parenteral administration, urine excretion is somewhat higher, but still not greater than 15 percent. Hepatic demethylation is a minor route of disposition. Erythromycin is not readily removed by either hemodialysis or peritoneal dialysis. The half-life of erythromycin is approximately 1.5 hours.

The disposition of azithromycin resembles that of erythromycin. Only 6 percent of an oral dose can be recovered from the urine. Elimination in the bile, metabolism in the liver, and perhaps transintestinal elimination account for most of the clearance. Azithromycin has a relatively long, polyphasic half-life (see Table 93.2).

Clarithromycin undergoes a higher degree of renal excretion and hepatic metabolism than do the other two macrolides. Metabolism includes conversion to an antibacterially-active form, 14-hydroxyclarithromycin. Since 30 to 40 percent of a dose is excreted unchanged in the urine, patients with a creatinine clearance < 30 ml/min may require an adjustment in dosage regimen. The half-life of clarithromycin is three to seven hours and may vary with the dose administered.

Adverse Effects

Erythromycin has a relatively low potential for producing untoward effects. This is true of both direct toxicity and hypersensitivity reactions. It is one of the safest antibiotics ever developed. Mild GI distress characterized by diarrhea and nausea is the most common complaint. Similar symptoms may occur even with IV administration, presumably due to biliary secretion of the drug into the intestine. Less frequently, epigastric distress may be more severe, especially in children and young adults.[31] The estolate ester is associated with liver damage in the form of cholestatic hepatitis, resulting in fever, jaundice, abdominal pain, dark urine, and impaired hepatic function, as indicated by elevated serum bilirubin and transaminase levels. This reaction tends to develop 10 to 20 days after initiation of therapy and is possibly a hypersensitivity reaction.[32] It appears more likely to occur in adults than children, and fortunately is reversible, usually within a few days after drug administration ceases. Other relatively rare effects include allergic reactions, thrombophlebitis with IV administration, and transient hearing loss with very large doses of the gluceptate, lactobionate, and estolate forms.[33] Adverse effects with clarithromycin and azithromycin are mild to moderate in severity and reversible upon discontinuation of therapy. Gastrointestinal reactions are the most common problem, but neither causes the severe nausea that occurs with erythromycin. Reversible dose-related hearing loss has been reported with the high doses of both drugs used to treat *Mycobacterium avium* infections.

Erythromycin can inhibit cytochrome P450 and thus retard the metabolism of other drugs inactivated by this mechanism.[34,35] Of particular concern has been the potential for increased blood levels and cardiac arrhythmias when the antihistamine terfenadine has been administered concurrently with erythromycin. Theophylline, a drug with a narrow therapeutic range, may reach toxic levels due to an interaction with erythromycin. Concentrations of many other drugs including warfarin, digoxin, and cyclosporin can be elevated by erythromycin. Clarithromycin also raises terfenadine levels and may interact with other drugs. Azithromycin does not appear to inhibit the P450 system. However, aluminum and magnesium-containing antacids reduce the peak serum levels, but not the extent of azithromycin absorption.

Therapeutic Uses

The combination of excellent activity against many bacterial pathogens, low incidence of adverse effects (including allergy) and ease of administration make erythromycin a very valuable agent. In contrast to other antibiotics, e.g., the tetracyclines and chloramphenicol, which have been overused, erythromycin has actually been underutilized. It is widely used in pediatrics for treating otitis media and sinus infections, such as those caused by *H. influenzae* and *Streptococcus pneumoniae.* It is used topically and systemically for the treatment of acne. Erythromycin may be thought of as a general alternative to penicillin G and the first generation cephalosporins in instances where resistance and allergy preclude the use of these antibiotics, e.g., Staphylococcal infections.

Erythromycin is considered the drug of choice for infections caused by the following organisms:[10]

- Corynebacterium diptheriae (diphtheria)
- Campylobacter jejuni [co-choice with a fluoroquinolone]
- Bordetella pertussis (whooping cough)
- Legionella species (Legionnaires' disease)
- Mycoplasma pneumoniae [co-choice with a tetracycline]
- Ureaplasma urealyticum
- Chlamydia trachomatis (inclusion conjuctivitis, pneumonia, urethritis or cervicitis [co-choice with a tetracycline], and lymphogranuloma venereum [co-choice with a tetracycline]

Erythromycin is a major alternative agent for infections caused by:[10]

- *Streptococcus pyogenes,* Group B, and *pneumoniae*
- *Bacillus anthracis* (anthrax)
- *Eikenella corrodens*
- *Leptotrichia buccalis*
- *Mycobacterium fortuitum*
- *Borrelia burgdorferi* (Lyme disease)

Since clarithromycin and azithromycin are relatively new agents, their role in therapy is still being defined. Their most established use is in the treatment of *Mycobacterium avium* complex as a secondary infection to HIV.[36,r7,r8] Clarithromycin has shown promising activity against *Mycobacterium leprae* and *Helicobacter pylori* in clinical trials.[r7] Azithromycin has been used effectively in the treatment of urethritis and cervicitis caused by Chlamydia and Neisseria. It has been recommended as first-line therapy for these infections.[r8] Clarithromycin appears to be an effective alternative for treating infections caused by *Chlamydia pneumoniae* and *Mycoplasma pneumoniae.* Both agents are useful against *Streptoccus pyogenes* and *Borrelia burgdorferi.* The longer half-lives of the newer macrolides permit less frequent dosing than with erythromycin.

Preparations

Erythromycin is available as the base and the esters and salts indicated below. These in turn are supplied in a wide variety of products intended for oral (250 and 500 mg tablets, chewable tablets, 250 mg capsules, suspensions), topical (including ophthalmic), rectal, and parenteral administration. Chemical forms of erythromycin and brand names representing numerous dosage forms and products include:

- Erythromycin (Ilotycin, E-Mycin, Ery-Tab, others)
  - Erythromycin ethylsuccinate (E.E.S. 400 Filmtab, E.E.S. 400 Liquid, Pediazole, EryPed)
  - Ethromycin estolate (Ilosone)
  - Erythromycin gluceptate (Ilotycin Gluceptate)
  - Erythromycin lactobionate (Erythrocin Lactobionate-IV)
  - Erythromycin stearate (Erythrocin Stearate Filmtab, Wyamycin S)
  - Clarithromycin (Biaxin) is available as 250- and 500-mg tablets.
  - Azithromycin (Zithromax) is supplied as 250-mg capsules.

Clindamycin and Lincomycin

Lincomycin is an antibiotic derived from *Streptomyces lincolnensis.* Because of its association with severe diarrhea and potentially fatal colitis, its use is no longer recommended and its pharmacology will not be described here. Clindamycin, a 7-chloro derivative of lincomycin, often causes GI distress also, but is clearly better tolerated than lincomycin and is particularly useful for the treatment of infections caused by anaerobic bacteria such as Bacteroides and Clostridium. It acts by inhibiting bacterial protein synthesis at the 50S ribosomal subunit and can be administered orally for systemic effects. The chemical structure of clindamycin is shown in Figure 93.6.

Antimicrobial Spectrum

Clindamycin has a spectrum quite similar to that of erythromycin. However, it is more active than erythromycin against anaerobic bacteria, particularly *Bacteroides fragilis* and Clostridium. Clindamycin's good activity against gram positive organisms such as Staphylococcus and Streptococcus provides the basis for its use as an alternative against these organisms. Clindamycin is inactive against aerobic gram-negative bacteria, but has activity against the protozoal organ-

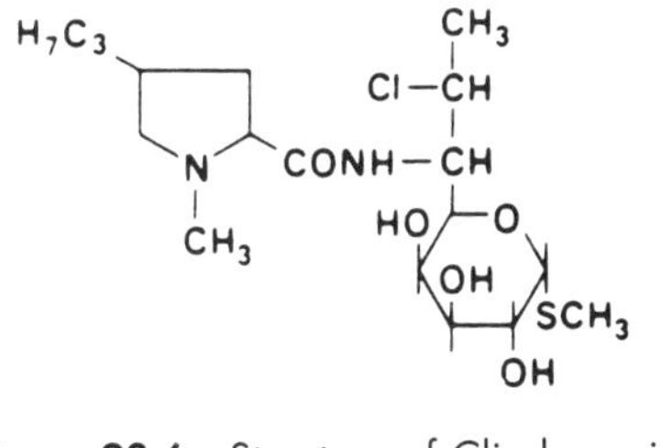

Figure 93.6 Structure of Clindamycin

isms *Toxoplasma gondii* and *Plasmodium falciparum* and *vivax*.

Mechanism of Action and Resistance

Clindamycin binds exclusively to a receptor on the 50S subunit of bacterial ribosomes (23S rRNA) and inhibits protein synthesis, blocking peptide bond formation by interference at either the A or P site on the ribosome. Erythromycin and chloramphenicol act at the same site, and the binding of one of the antibiotics to the ribosome may inhibit the binding of the others. Plasmid-mediated resistance to clindamycin may be due to methylation of bacterial RNA found in the 50S ribosomal subunit.[r9]

Pharmacokinetics

Administration and Absorption

Clindamycin is well absorbed from the GI tract and the presence of food does not appreciably impair absorption. Clindamycin palmitate, an oral preparation for pediatric use, is an inactive prodrug ester that undergoes rapid hydrolysis to the active form. Clindamycin is also applied topically and administered parenterally as a phosphate ester which is hydrolyzed to the parent drug.

Distribution

Clindamycin is generally well distributed, but significant concentrations are not achieved in the brain and CSF, even if the meninges are inflamed. Bone and joint infections caused by susceptible organisms respond well to clindamycin therapy. Clindamycin concentrates in phagocytic cells and readily crosses the placental barrier. Plasma protein binding is high, approximately 90 percent.

Disposition

Clindamycin undergoes hepatic metabolism to N-demethylclindamycin and clindamycin sulfoxide. In patients with impaired renal function, excretion in the feces is increased. Blood levels may be higher than anticipated in cases of severe hepatic failure. The half-life is three hours.

Adverse Effects

The incidence of diarrhea associated with administration of clindamycin ranges from 2 to 20 percent. In as many as 10 percent of patients receiving clindamycin,

Table 93.3 Aminoglycosides Summary Table

	Dosage			Pharmacokinetics			
Drug	**Route**	**Size**	**Dose**	**Peak**	**V_D**	**$t_{1/2}$**	**Clearance**
Amikacin							
Amikin	IM/IV	50–250 mg/ml	15 mg/kg/day divided in 3 doses	45 minutes–2 hours after IM	0.3	2–3 hrs	90 ml/min
Gentomicin							
Garamycin	IM/IV	2, 10, 40 mg/ml	3 mg/kg/d in 3 divided doses	1/2–1 1/2 hrs after IM	0.3	2–3 hrs	>90% renal
Kanamycin							
Kantrex	Oral IM/IV	500 mg capsule 37,250,333 mg/ml	1 g every 6 hrs. 15 mg/kg/day divided into 3 doses	1 hr. after IM	0.3	2–4 hrs	—
Netilmycin							
Netromycin	IM/IV	100 mg/ml	4–6.5 mg/kg/d in 3 divided doses	1/2–1 hrs	0.2	2–3 hrs	90 ml/min
Paromomycin							
Humatin	Oral	250 mg capsule	4 g daily in 2–4 divided doses	very poorly absorbed	—	—	—
Streptomycin	IM	1 g	15 mg/kg/d in 2 divided doses	1–2 hrs	0.25	2–3 hrs	85 ml/min
Tobramycin							
Nebcin	IM/IV	10, 40 mg/ml	3 mg/kg/d in 3 divided doses	1/2–1 hrs	0.3	2–3 hrs	77 ml/min

Table 93.4 Tetracycline Summary Table

	Dosage			Pharmacokinetics			
Drug	Route	Size	Dose	Peak	V_D	$t_{1/2}$	Clearance
Tetracycline							
Achromycin	Oral	125 mg/5ml suspension 250, 500 mg capsules	1–2 g/d in 2–4 divided doses	2–4 hrs	1.5	6–12 hrs	120 ml/min
Oxytetracycline							
Terramycin	IM	50, 125 mg/ml	250 mg/day	2–4 hrs		6–10 hrs	
	Oral	250 mg capsule	1 g/d in 4 divided doses				
Demeclomycin							
Declomycin	Oral	150, 300 mg tablets	600 mg/d in 4 divided doses	3–4 hrs		10–17 hrs	
Doxycycline							
Vibramycin	IV	100, 200 mg	100 mg q 12 hrs		0.8	14–17 hrs	37 ml/min
	Oral	50, 100 mg capsules		1.5–4 hrs			
Minocycline							
Minocin	IV	100 mg	200 mg initially; then 100 mg q 12 hrs	1–4 hrs	1.3	17 hrs	70 ml/min
	Oral	50, 100 mg capsule					

pseudomembraneous colitis characterized by diarrhea, abdominal pain, fever, and mucus and blood in the stools has developed. This potentially fatal reaction has been attributed to the production of an exotoxin elaborated by clindamycin-resistant strains of *Clostridium difficile.* Agents that inhibit gut motility, such as opioids, may prolong and worsen the condition. Clindamycin should be discontinued promptly if diarrhea occurs. Hypersensitivity reactions occur with some frequency. Impaired liver function and neutropenia have been rarely associated with clindamycin use.

Therapeutic Uses

The major indication for clindamycin use is as an alternative to penicillin for severe infections caused by Bacteroides and other anaerobes, such as Clostridium. It is also used as an alternative to penicillin G for treatment of infections caused by *Staphylococcus aureus*, *Streptococcus pyogenes*, Peptostreptococcus, Fusobacterium and Leptotrichia buccalis.[10] Owing to its activity against the anaerobic organism *Proprionbacterium acnes*, clindamycin is used topically in the treatment of acne. Some reports have indicated that clindamycin may be useful in the treatment of infections caused by the protozoan, *Toxoplasma gondii.*[37]

Preparations

Clindamycin hydrochloride (Cleocin): 75-, 105-, and 300-mg tablets for oral administration

Clindamycin palmitate hydrochloride (Cleocin Pediatric): flavored granules for solution to a concentration of 75 mg/5ml.

Clindamycin phosphate (Cleocin): 150 mg/ml vials for IM or IV use clindamycin phosphate (Cleocin T): topical solution, gel and lotion

Clindamycin phosphate (Cleocin) vaginal cream

Spectinomycin

Spectinomycin is an aminocyclitol antibiotic derived from *Streptomyces spectabilis.* Since the aminocyclitol is linked to a neutral sugar rather than an amino sugar, it is not an aminoglycoside. The structure of spectinomycin is shown is Figure 93.7. It is active against several gram-negative bacteria, but is used clinically only against *Neisseria gonorrhoeae.*

Table 93.5 Macrolides and Other Antibiotics Summary Table

Drug	Dosage			Pharmacokinetics			
	Route	Size	Dose	Peak	V_D	$t_{1/2}$	Clearance
MACROLIDES							
Erythromycin	Oral	250–500 mg tablets	250 mg q 6 hrs	3 hrs	0.8	1.5–2 hrs	640 ml/min
	IV	1g	15–20 mg/kg/d				
Azithromycin Zithromax	Oral	250 mg capsule	250–500 mg/d	2.5 hrs	31.1	10–50 hrs	
Clarithromycin Biaxin	Oral	250 + 500 mg tablets	250–500 mg b.i.d.	3 hrs	3.5	3–7 hrs	880 ml/min
OTHERS							
Chloramphenicol Chloromycetin	Oral	250 mg tablets 150 mg/5 ml suspension		1–3 hrs	0.9	4 hrs	
	IV	1 g	50 mg/kg/d divided in 4 doses				170 ml/min
Clindamycin Cleocin	Oral	75, 150, 300 mg capsules	150–450 mg q 6 hrs	3/4–1 hrs	1.1		330 ml/min
	IV	150 mg/ml	0.6–2.7 g/d divided into 4 doses				
Spectinomycin Trobicin	IM	2 or 4 g	Single 2 g IM	1 hr		1.2–2.8 hrs	

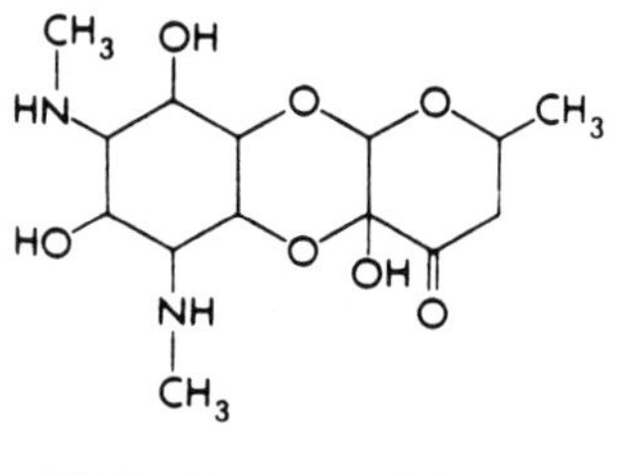

Figure 93.7 Structure of Spectinomycin

Spectinomycin binds to the 30S ribosomal subunit to inhibit translocation and protein synthesis in gram-negative bacteria. It binds to a specific site, designated P4, inhibiting translocation. Its site of action is similar to that of the aminoglycosides, but it is bacteriostatic rather than bactericidal. Resistance to spectinomycin by Neisseria has not been a major problem. Spectinomycin is not absorbed from the GI tract and is administered only by IM injection with rapid absorption occurring from this site. The drug does not penetrate into the CSF or the aqueous humor. It does not bind appreciably to plasma proteins. Disposition is almost entirely by glomerular filtration and renal excretion.

The major adverse effect with spectinomycin is pain at the IM injection site. Dizziness, nervousness, insomnia, nausea, urticaria, chills, and fever have been infrequently associated with use of the drug.

Spectinomycin is used as an alternative to ceftriaxone and other beta-lactam antibiotics for the treatment of gonorrhea, particularly in patients allergic to the cephalosporins or those with infections resistant to the beta-lactam agents. It is administered as a single 2- to 4-gram dose and achieves a cure rate of 95 percent in genital and rectal gonorrhea. It is useful, but less effective in treating pharyngeal gonococcal infections. It is not effective for the treatment of other sexually transmitted infections. Spectinomycin hydrochloride (Trobicin) is available as a sterile powder (2-gram vial) to be reconstituted for IM injection.

References

Research Reports

1. Moellering RC Jr, Weinberg AN. Studies on antibiotic synergism against enterococci. II. Effect of various antibiotics on the uptake of ^{14}C-labeled streptomycin by enterococci. J Clin Invest 1971;*50*:2580–2584.
2. Bryan LE, Kwan S. Roles of ribosomal binding membrane potential and electron transport in bacterial uptake of streptomycin and gentamicin. Antimicrob Agents 1983;*23*:835–845.
3. Hull JH, Sarubbi FA Jr. Gentamicin serum concentrations: pharmacokinetic predictions. Ann Intern Med 1976;*85*:183–189.
4. McHenry MC, Wagner JG, Hall PM, Vidt DG, Gavan TL. Pharmacokinetics of amikacin in patients with impaired renal function. J Infect Dis 1976;*134* (Suppl.):S343–S348.
5. Regeur L, Colding H, Jensen H, Kampmann JP. Pharmacokinetics of amikacin during hemodialysis and peritoneal dialysis. Antimicrob Agents Chemother. 1977;*11*:214–218.
6. Theopold HM. Comparative surface studies of ototoxic effects of various aminoglycoside antibiotics on the organ of Corti in the guinea pig. A scanning electron microscopic study. Acta Otolaryngol (Stockholm). 1977;*84*:57–64.
7. Huy PTB, Meulmans A, Wassef M, Manuel C, Sterkers O, Amiel C. Gentamicin persistence in rat endolymph and perilymph after a two-day constant infusion. Antimicrob Agents Chemother. 1983;*23*:344–346.
8. Tulkens PM. Experimental studies on nephrotoxicity of aminoglycosides at low doses: mechanisms and perspectives. Am J Med 1986;*80*(Suppl B):105–114.
9. Sokol MD, Gergis SD. Antibiotics and neuromuscular function. Anesthesiology 1981;*55*:148–159.
10. The choice of antibacterial drugs. Medical Letter 1992;*34*:49–56.
11. Evans ME, Gregory DW, Schaffner W, McGee ZA. Tularemia: A 30-year experience with 88 cases. Medicine 1985;*64*:251–269.
12. Clarke JS, Condon RE, Bartlett JG, Gorbach SL, Nichols R, Ochi S. Preoperative oral antibiotics reduce septic complications of colon operations: Results of prospective, randomized, double-blind clinical study. Ann Surg 1977;*186*:251–259.
13. Park BH, Hendricks M, Malamy MH, Tally FP, Levy SB. Cryptic tetracycline resistance determinant (class F) from Bacteroides fragilis-mediated resistance in Escherichia coli by actively reducing tetracycline accumulation. Antimicrob Agents Chemother 1987;*31*:1739–1743.
14. Kuzucu EY. Methoxyflurane, tetracycline and renal failure. JAMA 1970;*211*:1162–1164.
15. Bartz QR. Isolation and characterization of chloromycetin. J Biol Chem 1948;*172*:445–450.
16. Rahal JJ Jr, Simberkoff MS. Bactericidal and bacteriostatic action of chloramphenicol against meningeal pathogens. Antimicrob Agents Chemother 1979;*16*:13–18.
17. Gaffney DF, Foster TJ. Chloramphenicol acetyltransferase determined by R plasmids from gram negative bacteria. J Gen Microbiol 1978;*109*:351–358.
18. Piffaretti JC, Froment Y. Binding of chloramphenicol and its acetylated derivatives to Escherichia coli ribosomal subunits. Chemotherapy 1978;*24*:24–28.
19. Baughman GA, Fahnestock SF. Chloramphenicol resistance mutation in Escherichia coli which maps in the major ribosomal protein gene cluster. J Bacteriol 1979;*137*:1315–1323.
20. Sompolinsky D, Samra Z. Mechanisms of high-level resistance to chloramphenicol in different Escherichia coli variants. J Gen Microbiol 1968;*50*:55–66.
21. Kauffman RE, Thirumoorthi MC, Buckley JA, Aravind MK, Dajani AS. Relative bioavailability of intravenous chloramphenicol succinate and oral chloramphenicol palmitate in infants and children. J Pediatr 1981;*99*:963–967.
22. Friedman CA, Lovejoy FC, Smith AL. Chloramphenicol disposition in infants and children. J Pediatr 1979;*95*:1071–1077.
23. Shu XO, Linet MS, Gao RN, Gao YT, Brinton LA, Jin F, Fraumeni JF Jr. Chloramphenicol use and childhood leukemia in Shanghai. Lancet 1987;*2*:934–937.
24. Clarithromycin and azithromycin. Medical Letter 1992;*34*:45–47.
25. Dautzenberg B, Truffol C, Legris S. Activity of clarithromycin against Mycobacterium avium complex infection in patients with acquired immune deficiency syndrome: a controlled clinical trial. Am Rev Resp Dis 1991;*144*:564–569.
26. Brisson-Noel A, Trieu-cuot P, Courvalis P. Mechanism of action of spiromycin and other macrolides. J Antimicrob Chemother 1988;*22* (Suppl B):13–23.
27. Kakegawa T, Hirose S. Mode of inhibition of protein synthesis by metabolites of clarithromycin. Chemotherapy 1990;*38*:317–323.
28. Sabath LD, Gerstein DA, Loder PB, Finland M. Excretion of erythromycin and its enhanced activity in urine against gram-negative bacilli with alkalinization. J Lab Clin Med 1968;*72*:916–923.
29. Vogel Z, Vogel T, Elson D. The effect of erythromycin on peptide bond formation and the termination reaction. FEBS Lett 1971;*15*:249–253.
30. Schentag JJ, Ballow CH. Tissue directed pharmacokinetics. Am J Med 1991;*91*(Suppl 3A):5–11.
31. Seifert CF, Swaney RJ, Bellanger-McCleery RA. Intravenous erythromycin lactobionate-induced severe nausea and vomiting. Drug Intell Clin Pharm 1989;*23*:40–44.
32. Tolman KG, Sannella JJ, Freston JW. Chemical structure of erythromycin and hepatotoxicity. Ann Intern Med 1974;*81*:58–60.
33. Karmody CS, Weinstein L. Reversible sensorineural hearing loss with intravenous erythromycin lactobionate. Ann Otol Rhinol Laryngol 1977;*86*:9–11.
34. Ludden TM. Pharmacokinetic interactions of the macrolide antibiotics. Clin Pharmacokinet 1985;*10*:63–79.
35. Martell R, Heinrichs D, Stiller CR, Jenner M, Keown PA, Dupre J. The effects of erythromycin in patients treated with cyclosporin. Ann Intern Med 1986;*104*:660–661.
36. Horsbaugh CR. Mycobacterium avium complex infection in the acquired immune deficiency complex. N Engl J Med 1991;*324*:1332–1338.
37. Luft BJ, Remington JS. Toxoplasmic encephalitis. J Infect Dis 1988;*157*:1–6.

Reviews

r1. Price KE. Mini-review: aminoglycoside research 1975–1985: prospects for development of improved agents. Antimicrob Agents Chemother 1986;*29*:543–548.

r2. Kucers A, Bennett NM. Gentamicin. In Kucers A, Bennett NM The use of antibiotics, 4th ed. Philadelphia: Lippincott (1987); pp 619–674.

r3. Alexander DP, Gambertoglio JG. Drug overdose and pharmacologic considerations in dialysis. In Cogan MG Garovnoy MR Introduction to dialysis. New York: Churchill Livingstone, (1985); pp 261–292.

r4. Chopra I, Howe TGB. Bacterial resistance to the tetracyclines. Microbiol Rev 1978;*42*:707–724.

r5. Pratt WB, Fekety R. The antimicrobial drugs. New York: Oxford University Press, (1986); pp 205–208.

r6. Smith AL, Weber A. Pharmacology of chloramphenicol. Pediatr Clin North Am 1983;*30*:209–236.

r7. Peters DH, Clissold SP. Clarithromycin: A review of its antimicrobial activity, pharmacokinetic properties and therapeutic potential. Drugs 1992;*44*:117–164.

r8. Peters DH, Fridel HA, McTavish D. Azithromycin: A review of its antimicrobial activity, pharmacokinetic properties and clinical efficacy. Drugs 1992;*44*:750–799.

r9. Steigbigel NH. Erythromycin, lincomycin and clindamycin. Mandel GL, Douglas RG Jr, Bennett JE In Principles and practice of infectious diseases, 3d ed. New York: Wiley (1990); pp 308–317.

r10. Sturgill MG, Rapp RP. Clarithromycin: Review of a new macrolide antibiotic with improved microbiologic spectrum and favorable pharmacokinetic and adverse effect profiles. Ann Pharmacother 1992;*26*:1099–1108.

r11. Omura S. Macrolide antibiotics. New York: Academic Press, 1987.

r12. Edson RS, Terrell CL. The aminoglycosides. Mayo Clin Proc 1991;*66*:1158–1164.

r13. Smilack JD, Wilson WR, Cockerill FR III. Tetracyclines, chloramphenicol, erythromycin, clindamycin, and metronidazole. Mayo Clin Proc 1991;*66*:1270–1280.

CHAPTER 94

Fluoroquinolones, Quinolones, Nitrofurans, and Methenamine

John L. Egle, Jr.

Fluoroquinolones

The fluoroquinolones are a relatively new class of orally administered synthetic antibacterial agents. They were derived from the quinolones, a group of older nonfluorinated agents such as nalidixic acid, used since the early 1960s exclusively for the treatment of urinary tract infections. The fluoroquinolones differ significantly from the earlier agents in having a broader spectrum of antibacterial activity, increased potency, decreased potential for emergence of resistance, and a more favorable adverse effects profile. These properties, combined with efficacy by oral administration and relatively long half-lives, allow the fluoroquinolones to be used successfully for outpatient treatment of some infections that previously required hospitalization for parenteral therapy. The introduction of the fluoroquinolones is generally regarded as the most significant development in the field of antibacterial chemotherapy in several decades. In addition to norfloxacin, introduced in 1986, ciprofloxacin, ofloxacin, lomefloxacin, and enoxacin are available in the US. An additional agent, temafloxacin, was marketed for a short time before being withdrawn because of reports of serious adverse reactions, including hemolytic anemia, renal and hepatic dysfunction, and allergic reactions. The usefulness of norfloxacin, lomefloxacin, and enoxacin is limited to fewer types of infections than ciprofloxacin and ofloxacin, which have many indications in bacterial infections, including chronic osteomyelitis, chronic prostatitis, complicated urinary tract infections, and bacterial GI infections. Fluoroquinolones also are useful when patients are allergic or when bacteria are resistant to the usual agent or choice. Other fluoroquinolones currently in development include perfloxacin, fleroxacin, and sparfloxacin.[1]

Chemistry and Structure-Activity Relationship

The fluoroquinolones differ in structure from the quinolones in having a fluorine atom at position 6 and a piperazinyl or pyrrolidinyl substitution at position 7 of the quinolone nucleus. The fluoroquinolones differ among themselves primarily in the nature of substituents attached to the nitrogen at the one position and presence of a carbon or nitrogen at position 8 of the quinolone nucleus. Structures of the fluoroquinolones and nalidixic acid as a reference compound are shown in Figure 94.1.

The carboxyl group at position 3 and the keto group at position 4 are thought to be necessary for the inhibition of bacterial DNA gyrase.[1] The 3-carboxyl and 4-keto groups also may promote passage through bacterial outer membranes through chelation with magnesium ions.[2,3] The key structural difference between the quinolones and the fluoroquinolones is the fluorine atom at position 6. The piperazine group at the 7 position is thought to be responsible for the anti-Pseudomonal activity of the fluoroquinolones. Ofloxacin contains a 4-methylpiperazine group at C 7, which is thought to improve oral bioavailability and increase activity against Enterobacteriaceae, and a fused oxazine heterocycle to improve gram-positive and antianaerobic activity as well as reduce metabolic lability. Enoxacin contains a naphthyridine ring system instead of the quinoline ring structure.

Antimicrobial Spectrum

The fluoroquinolones have a broad spectrum of antibacterial activity. Fluoroquinolones exhibit good activity against most gram-negative aerobic bacilli,

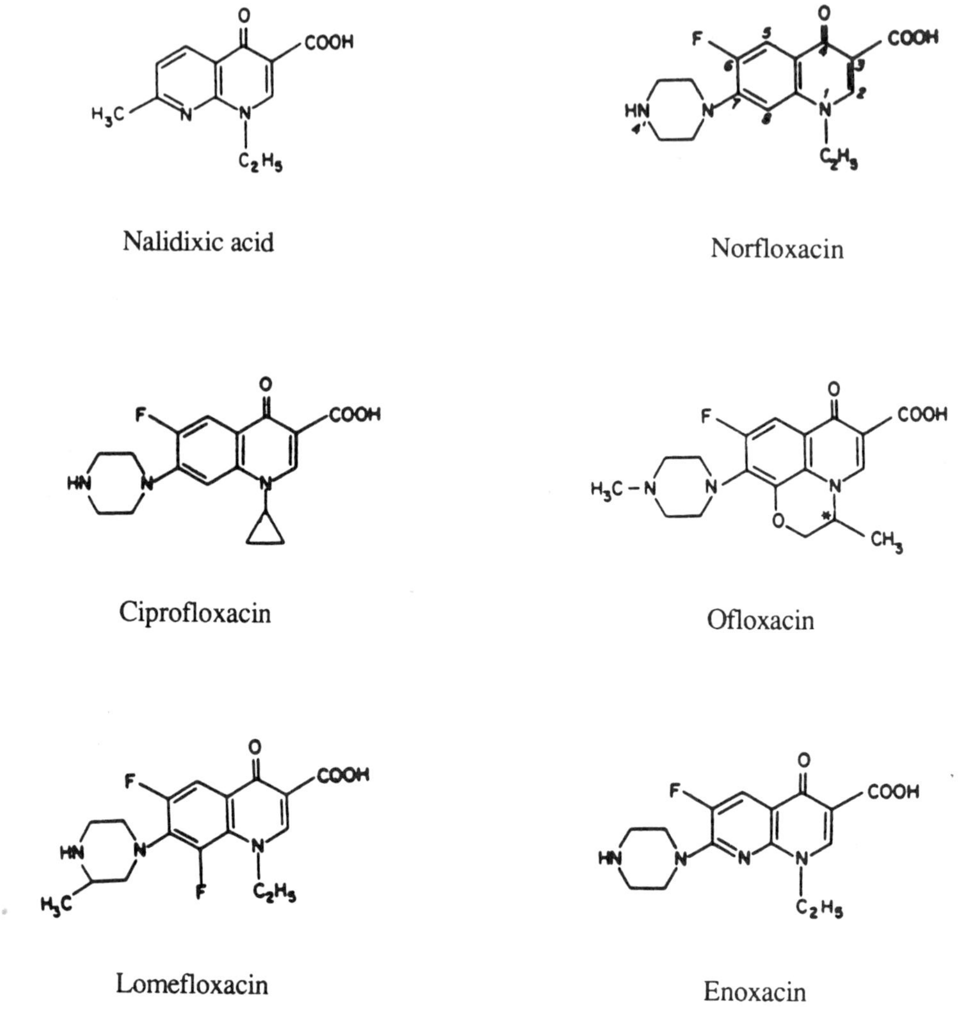

Nalidixic acid

Norfloxacin

Ciprofloxacin

Ofloxacin

Lomefloxacin

Enoxacin

Figure 94.1 Structures of the Fluoroquinolones and Nalidixic Acid

particularly against members of the family Enterobacteriaceace. They possess good activity against *Pseudomonas aeruginosa,* but are less active against other species of Pseudomonas. Other susceptible gram-negative organisms include *Haemophilus influenzae, Neisseria gonorrhoeae* and *meningitidis,* Brucella, Legionella, Branhamella, Campylobacter, Vibrio, and Aeromonas. Among gram-positive bacteria, Staphylococci exhibit moderate sensitivity to fluoroquinolones. Initially, methicillin-resistant *S. aureus* was generally susceptible to the fluoroquinolones, but widespread resistance to ciprofloxacin among these strains has been reported.[r1] Streptococci and Enterococci are less susceptible than Staphylococci. Fluororquinolones are active against *Mycobacterium tuberculosis, fortuitum kansasii,* and *xenopi,* but less active against *Mycobacterium avium* complex. *Chlamydia trachomatis, Mycoplasma hominis, Gardnerella vaginalis,* and Rickettsia are susceptible to these agents. Ofloxacin is more active against Chlamydia than the other agents in the class. The fluoroquinolones have little activity against anaerobic organisms and Nocardia.

Mechanism of Action and Resistance

The major target of the fluoroquinolones is DNA topoisomerase II or DNA gyrase, an essential bacterial enzyme. DNA gyrase is a tetramer, composed of two A-subunits and two B-subunits, which catalyzes supercoiling of cellular DNA by a nicking, pass-through, and resealing process.[r2] DNA gyrase is responsible for the generation of negative superhelical twists and is necessary for initiation and propagation of the DNA replication fork. Fluoroquinolones bind to the A subunits of DNA gyrase, rapidly arresting replicative DNA synthesis; they interrupt fork propagation, transcription, chromosome segregation, and other cell processes. By binding to and inhibiting DNA gyrase, the fluoroquinolones induce cleavage of the DNA backbone, thus exerting an antibacterial effect.[2] Eukaryotic cells do not contain DNA gyrase, but possess a conceptually and mechanistically similar type-II DNA topoisomerase that removes positive supercoils from eukaryotic DNA to prevent its tangling during replication. Eukaryotic topoisomerase is inhibited by fluoroquinolones only at much higher concentrations than those affecting the bacterial enzyme. The fluoroquinolones are considered to be bactericidal since they kill bacteria at concentrations only severalfold higher than inhibitory concentrations.

Resistance to the fluoroquinolones has been particularly noted in Staphylococci.[r1] This resistance has been associated with point mutations of the genes for either of two subunits of DNA gyrase (A proteins and B proteins).[r3,4] This results in the elaboration of DNA gyrase with lower affinity for the fluoroquinolones or changes in the outer membrane that reduce drug accumulation. Such resistance develops infrequently for most bacteria, but occurs often in *Pseudomonas aeruginosa*[7] and Mycobacteria.[6] Exposure to gradually increasing levels of fluoroquinolones can result in resistance that is probably attributable to changes in the outer membrane proteins of bacteria that lead to reduced permeability to the drugs.[r3] Resistance has also been attributed to efflux of fluoroquinolones from the cell.[7] Plasmid-mediated resistance to the fluoroquinolones has not yet been found.

Pharmacokinetics

There are some important differences in the pharmacokinetic properties of the individual fluoroquinolones. Pharmacokinetic properties are summarized in Table 94.1.

Administration and Absorption

All fluoroquinolones are administered orally. Absorption from the GI tract is nearly complete for ofloxacin, lomefloxacin, and enoxacin, approximately 70 percent for ciprofloxacin, but less for norfloxacin, for which 35 to 70 percent of an oral dose is absorbed. Owing to its more limited absorption, norfloxacin does not achieve sufficiently high serum concentrations relative to its minimal inhibitory concentration for most bacteria to be used for infections outside the genitourinary or intestinal tracts.[r4] Peak serum concentrations of all fluoroquinolones occur one to two hours after administration. The presence of food in the GI tract does not markedly reduce the bioavailability of the fluoroquinolones, but the time required to attain peak levels may be increased, except for ofloxacin. Ciprofloxacin and ofloxacin are also available in forms for IV administration, and there is a preparation of ciprofloxacin for ophthalmic use.

Distribution

Binding of fluoroquinolones to plasma proteins is generally low, ranging from 10 to 40 percent, being highest with ciprofloxacin and enoxacin. Volumes of distribution are relatively high, a favorable characteristic with regard to achieving high drug levels at infection sites. The drugs penetrate well into body tissues and fluids, including bone and prostate tissue.[8] Ofloxacin displays the best penetration into the CNS, with CSF levels 40 to 90 percent of those in serum having been reported.[9] For CSF obtained from patients with meningitis, concentrations 10 to 40 percent of those in serum have been reported for ciprofloxacin.[10] The fluoroquinolones accumulate in leukocytes to levels ten times the serum concentration. This may enhance the killing of such intracellular pathogens as Legionella, Brucella, Salmonella, and Mycobacterium.[11] Penetration of the eye is relatively poor.

Disposition

Inactivation of the fluoroquinolones occurs by both renal and nonrenal (GI and hepatic) routes, with considerable variability among the individual agents. Recovery of unchanged drug from the urine is highest for ofloxacin (70–90%) and relatively high for lomefloxacin (80%) and enoxacin (60–70%). Renal excretion values for the other available fluoroquinolones are 30 to 40 percent for norfloxacin and 40 to 60 percent for ciprofloxacin. Renal clearance of all fluoroquinolones exceeds the glomerular filtration rate, suggesting that tubular secretion plays a role in the renal excretion of these drugs. This is supported by the finding that probenecid reduces the renal clearance of ciprofloxacin[12] and norfloxacin.[13] High levels of fluoroquinolones, ranging from 25 to many hundredfold serum concentrations, are achieved in the urine.[r5] Because of extensive enterohepatic circulation, norfloxacin, ciprofloxacin, and enoxacin achieve high fecal concentrations. Metabolism accounts for less than 20 percent of the disposition of the fluoroquinolones.[14] Thus, alterations in metabolism are unlikely to markedly affect their clinical efficacy or toxic potential. However, fluoroquinolones can significantly alter the metabolism of other drugs, as described below. Half-lives of most fluoroquinolones range from three to five hours. However, lomefloxacin has a somewhat longer half-life of eight hours, which allows once- or twice-daily dosing, depending on the pathogen or site of infection.[15]

Table 94.1 Pharmacokinetic Properties of the Fluoroquinolones

	Norfloxacin	Ciprofloxacin	Ofloxacin	Lomefloxacin	Enoxacin
Gastrointestinal absorption (%)	35–70	70–80	85–95	95–98	80–90
Time to peak (hr)	1.5	1.1	1.4	1.3	1.6
Plasma protein binding (%)	15	20–40	15–25	10	35
Half-life (hr)	4	4	6	8	4
Renal clearance (L/hr)	14.0	21.4	10.4	11.5	12.0
Disposition (% of dose):					
Renal	30–40	40–60	70–90	80	60–70
Fecal/biliary	30	15	4	<5	18
Metabolized	20	10–15	6	5	7–15

Factors Influencing Pharmacokinetics

Renal failure (creatinine clearance of less than 20 ml/min per 1.73 m^2) decreases the disposition and increases the half-life of all fluoroquinolones. Since clearance of oxfloxacin is almost entirely by the renal route, it is affected to the greatest extent (4–5-fold increase in the half-life). For others, such as ciprofloxin and norfloxacin, the half-life would roughly double. Neither hemodialysis nor peritoneal dialysis eliminates the fluoroquinolones.[16] Liver disease appears to have relatively little effect on kinetics, even in the case of norfloxacin.[17] In elderly patients, 1.3- to threefold or greater increases in peak serum concentrations of fluoroquinolones may occur because of increased GI absorption, decreased renal elimination, or both.[r5]

Adverse Effects

One of the major reasons for regarding the fluoroquinolones as a significant advance in antibacterial chemotherapy is their relatively low incidence of adverse effects and their low potential for serious toxicity. Fluoroquinolones are well tolerated when used for a prolonged period, allowing oral administration for four to eight weeks or even long-term suppressive treatment.[r4]

The most frequent adverse effects with the fluoroquinolones are GI distress, but this occurs in only 1 to 5 percent of patients. The most common symptom is nausea followed in frequency by abdominal discomfort, vomiting, and diarrhea. *Clostridium difficile* cytotoxin enterocolitis rarely has been associated with use of the fluoroquinolones.

Symptoms involving the CNS (headache, dizziness, confusion, restlessness, sleep disturbance, tremors, hallucinations and seizures) have been reported in 1 to 4 percent of patients. Reports of more severe effects such as seizures have been rare, and in most cases were associated with such predisposing factors as a history of epilepsy or cerebrovascular accidents. Quinolones competitively inhibit binding of gamma-aminobutyric acid to specific receptors on rodent synaptic plasma membranes, and it has been suggested that this may be responsible for the apparent epileptogenic potential of this class of drugs.[18]

The fluoroquinolones occasionally cause allergic reactions (0.5–2% of patients). These reactions are most often characterized by rashes and pruritus. Fever, urticaria, angioedema, photosensitivity, and anaphylaxis have been uncommon. Serious hypersensitivity reactions involving the fluoroquinolones are very unlikely. One study has indicated that IV ciprofloxacin can cause transient erythema or sensations of burning and itching at the site of infusion.[19]

Infrequently (0.2–3%), abnormal laboratory values have been reported in patients receiving fluoroquinolones.[r6] These have included elevations in serum transaminases, leukopenia, and eosinophilia. These changes are transient and usually do not require termination of treatment.

Preclinical toxicity testing indicated that the fluoroquinolones produce irreversible damage to developing cartilage in the weight-bearing joints of young animals. As a result of this finding, these drugs are not recommended for use in children under 18 years of age or in nursing women. In children receiving older quinolones, such as nalidixic acid, for extended periods, joint toxicity has not been reported. One of 30 children receiving high doses of ciprofloxacin developed a reversible arthritis.[r7] In adults receiving fluoroquinolones, cartilage erosions have not been detected, and tendonitis and other joint problems have been rare.

Drug Interactions

Many drug classes interact with the fluoroquinolones, potentially requiring alteration of either agent in the regimen or a change in dosage.[20]

Gastrointestinal absorption of the fluoroquinolones can be reduced by the concurrent administration of products containing metal cations, e.g., aluminum or magnesium-containing antacids, calcium and iron supplements, and zinc in multivitamin preparations. This effect apparently is due to the formation of insoluble salts of the drugs and to reduced absorption. A six- to tenfold decrease in maximum levels of ciprofloxacin has been reported when the drug is administered concomitantly with magnesium and aluminum-containing antacids. Histamine-2 receptor blockers such as ranitidine delay but do not affect the extent of fluoroquinolone absorption. Cimetidine, but not ranitidine, has been reported to decrease the clearance of enoxacin. Sucralfate also interferes with absorption of the fluoroquinolones.

Coadministration of some fluoroquinolones (particularly enoxacin and to a somewhat lesser extent ciprofloxacin) with theophylline result in decreased hepatic clearance of theophylline.[21] This leads to increased half-life and serum levels of theophylline, a drug with a relatively narrow therapeutic range. It has been recommended that theophylline doses be reduced by 40 percent if these drugs must be used concurrently. The mechanism of the interaction appears to be interference by an oxoquinolone metabolite of the fluoroquinolones with the demethylation of theophylline by hepatic P450 enzymes. Ofloxacin and lomefloxacin are not metabolized to oxoquinolones and therefore do not increase theophylline levels. Clinically significant changes in theophylline do not appear to be caused by norfloxacin. Serum levels of caffeine, a methylxanthine structurally related to theophylline, can be elevated two- to fourfold by enoxacin and slightly raised by ciprofloxacin.

Coadministration of the nonsteroidal antiinflammatory agent fenbufen with enoxacin has been associated with the development of seizures.[22] Probenecid blocks the renal secretion of fluoroquinolones, but this action does not appreciably alter the pharmacokinetics of the antibacterials. Enoxacin has been shown to decrease the hepatic clearance of the R-enentiomer of warfarin, but not the S-enantiomer. Since R-warfarin has only one-fifth of the anticoagulant potency of S-warfarin, there is little alteration of the pharmacologic effect of warfarin by the fluoroquinolones. Increased levels of cyclosporine have been attributed to ciprofloxacin.

Therapeutic Uses

Ciprofloxacin and ofloxacin have many indications, including nearly all uses described below. The use of the other three available fluoroquinolones is more limited, owing to pharmacokinetic factors and lower activity against certain organisms. Norfloxacin is marketed only for urinary tract infections. Lomefloxacin is recommended for urinary tract infections and bronchitis caused by *Haemophilus influenzae* or *Moraxella catarrhalis.* Enoxacin is approved for treatment of urinary tract infections and uncomplicated urethral or cervical gonorrhea. Therapeutic uses of the fluoroquinolones are described in more detail below based on classes of organisms and sites of infections in the body. Again, it is emphasized that many of these indications apply only to ciprofloxacin and ofloxacin.

A fluoroquinolone is considered to be the drug of choice for infections caused by *Campylobacter jejuni,* Shigella, *Pseudomonas aeruginosa* (urinary tract infection) and *Afipia felis* (cat scratch bacillus).[23]

Fluoroquinolones are recommended as alternative therapy for infections due to the following organisms:[23]

Gram-positive cocci:
- Enterococcus (urinary tract infection)
- *Staphylococcus aureus* or *epidermidis*

Gram-negative cocci:
- *Neisseria gonorrhoeae*
- *Moraxella catarrhalis*

Enteric gram-negative bacilli:
- Enterobacter
- *Escherichia coli*
- *Klebsiella pneumoniae*
- *Proteus mirabilis*
- Proteus (indole-positive)
- *Providencia stuartii*
- *Salmonella typhi* and other Salmonella
- Serratia
- *Yersinia enterocolitica*

Other gram-negative bacilli:
- *Haemophilis ducreyi*
- *Pseudomonas aeruginosa* (other than urinary tract infections)
- *Vibrio cholerae*
- *Xanthomonas maltophilia*

Acid fast bacilli:
- *Mycobacterium tuberculosis*

Mycobacterium leprae

Chlamydiae:

Rickettsia (Rocky Mountain spotted fever, endemic typhus (murine), epidemic typhus (louse-borne), scrub typhus, trench fever, Q fever, human ehrlichiosis)

Indications for the fluoroquinolones are discussed below based on the site of the infection in the body. With the exception of infections of the urinary tract, only ciprofloxacin or ofloxacin are recommended in most situations.

Genitourinary Tract Infections

Their properties of high activity against gram-negative bacteria and high concentrations in the urine make fluoroquinolones effective for treating uncomplicated infections of the urinary tract, including cystitis and pyelonephritis. However, since the fluoroquinolones are more expensive and not clearly superior to trimethoprim-sulfamethoxazole, and to delay the development of resistance, it is recommended that they be reserved for infections in which organisms resistant to the usually administered antibiotics are present. Fluoroquinolones are recommended for the treatment of complicated urinary tract infections (due to structural or functional abnormalities of the tract) often caused by *Pseudomonas aeruginosa*.[r5] In therapy of other genitourinary infections, e.g., prostatitis, vesiculitis, and epididymitis, the fluoroquinolones compare favorably with other antibacterials such as trimethoprim-sulfamethoxazole.[24] The fact that fluoroquinolones penetrate into prostatic tissue in concentrations approaching or exceeding by severalfold those in serum helps account for their efficacy in the treatment of bacterial-induced acute and chronic prostatitis, particularly chronic prostatitis refractory to other orally administered agents.

With regard to sexually transmitted diseases, the fluoroquinolones are effective as single-dose therapy against urethral, cervical, rectal, and pharyngeal gonorrhea, including those caused by penicillin-resistant strains.[25] A single oral dose of ofloxacin is as effective as an injection of ceftriaxone for treatment of uncomplicated gonorrhea. Infections caused by *Chlamydia trachomatis* respond best to ofloxacin administered for seven to ten days. Fluoroquinolones are extremely effective against *Haemophilus ducreyi*, the causative agent of chancroid. However, the fluoroquinolones are not active against *Treponema pallidum*, the spirochete causing syphilis.

Gastrointestinal Tract Infections

The combination of excellent activity against enteric gram-negative pathogens, high concentrations in the colon (owing to incomplete absorption and biliary secretion), and preservation of the normal anaerobic intestinal flora (owing to lack of antibacterial activity) make the fluoroquinolones highly effective agents for treating infections caused by Salmonella, *E. coli*, Shigella, Campylobacter, and other organisms. Fluoroquinolones are recommended for empiric therapy of suspected bacterial GI infections.[r1] These agents are effective against typhoid fever and can eradicate Salmonella from chronic carriers. Fluoroquinolones have been found to be as effective as trimethoprim-sulfamethoxazole in preventing or treating traveler's diarrhea.[26] Despite their ability to achieve high concentrations in the bile, fluoroquinolones have not been particularly effective in biliary tract infections, perhaps because of the frequent presence of anaerobic organisms, against which the fluoroquinolones have little activity.

Respiratory Tract Infections

While fluoroquinolones are useful in treating selected infections of the respiratory tract, their relatively weak action against Streptococci precludes their use for the empiric treatment of community-acquired pneumonia because *Streptococcus pneumoniae* is the most frequent causative organism. Infections caused by such other common respiratory pathogens as *Haemophilus influenzae* and *Klebsiella pneumoniae* usually respond well to the fluoroquinolones. They are useful in the management of lower respiratory tract infections associated with cystic fibrosis and the acute bacterial exacerbations of chronic bronchitis. Ciprofloxacin has been used concurrently with other drugs for treatment of *Mycobacterium avium* infections and multiple drug-resistant tuberculosis. The value of the fluoroquinolones in treating infections caused by Legionella is not well established.

Osteomyelitis

The fluoroquinolones are recommended for the treatment of chronic osteomylitis due to gram-negative organisms because of their excellent activity against commonly involved pathogens, their ability to achieve adequate levels in bone, their ease of administration, and their relative lack of toxicity, even with long-term administration. Studies of ciprofloxacin in patients with gram-negative osteomyelitis have demonstrated clinical cure rates of 75 percent, a rate at least comparable with parenteral regimens.[r1] Ofloxacin also appears effective for the therapy of gram-negative chronic osteomyelitis. The efficacy of fluoroquinolones in the therapy of osteomyelitis due to gram-positive organisms such as *Staphylococcus aureus* or *epidermidis* has not been established.[27]

Other Uses

Fluoroquinolones are considered primary treatment for necrotizing external otitis, a rare and potentially fatal infection usually caused by *Psuedomonas aeruginosa* and often seen in elderly patients with diabetes. A 90 percent cure rate of this infection has been reported with oral ciprofloxacin.[28] Ciprofloxacin has been used successfully to eradicate the nasopharyngeal carriage of *Neisseria meningitidis*. Fluoroquinolone treatment of skin and soft-tissue infections has been limited largely to ciprofloxacin, which appears to have efficacy comparable to cefotaxime in infections caused by aerobic gram-negative bacteria.[r5] However, because of failures in infections caused by *Pseudomonas aeruginosa* and inconsistent results in Staphylococcal infections, the fluoroquinolones are not recommended for empiric use in the treatment of community-acquired skin and soft-tissue infections.[29] Fluoroquinolones have been found to be superior to other antibacterials in preventing bacteremia in patients with neutropenia.[30]

Preparations

Ciprofloxacin

Cipro: 250-, 500- and 750-mg tablets
Cipro: IV: vials containing 200 mg in 20 ml and 400 mg in 40 ml; flexible containers with 200 mg in 100 ml and 400 mg in 200 ml
Ciloxan: 2.5 and 5 ml sterile ophthalmic solution in plastic dispensers

Ofloxacin

Floxin: 200-, 300- and 400-mg tablets
Floxin IV: vials containing 400 mg in 10 ml and 400 mg in 20 ml; Premixed bottles with 400 mg in 100 ml; Flexible containers with 200 mg in 50 ml and 400 mg in 100 ml

Enoxacin

Penetrex: 200- and 400-mg tablets

Lomefloxacin

Maxaquin: 400-mg tablets

Norfloxacin

Noroxin: 400-mg tablets

Quinolones

The quinolones are an older group of synthetic antibacterials from which the fluororquinolones have been derived. The quinolones do not achieve systemic antimicrobial levels and therefore have been useful only in the treatment of urinary tract infections. Rapid development of resistance and prominent adverse effects—particularly involving the nervous system—severely limit the utility of the quinolones. Agents in this group include nalidixic acid, cinoxacin, and oxolinic acid.

Chemistry, Mechanism of Action, and Antimicrobial Spectrum

These compounds are 4-quinolones containing a carboxylic acid moiety in the 3 position of the basic ring structure. The structures of the quinolones are shown in Figure 94.2. The mechanism of action of the quinolones is the same as that of the fluoroquinolones—inhibition of bacterial DNA gyrase. The quinolones are active against gram-negative organisms likely to cause urinary tract infections such as *E. coli*, Klebsiella and Proteus. The quinolones generally lack activity against gram positive bacteria.

Pharmacokinetics

The quinolones are administered orally and are well absorbed. The presence of food in the GI tract may delay absorption, especially of oxolinic acid. Nalidixic acid is about 95 percent bound to plasma protein. Disposition of nalidixic acid and oxolinic acid is primarily by hepatic metabolism. Naladixic acid is largely converted initially to an active metabolite, hydroxynalidixic acid, and then to an inactive glucuronide. Oxolinic acid primarily undergoes glucuronide conjugation. Approximately 60 percent of a dose of cinoxacin is excreted unchanged in the urine. The quinolones have a short half-life, about 1.5 hours.

Adverse Effects

Adverse effects with the quinolones most frequently involve GI distress: nausea, vomiting, diarrhea, and abdominal pain. Allergic reactions also occur. However, a wide variety of symptoms involving the CNS are a major factor limiting the usefulness of the quinolones. These effects include headache, drowsiness, weakness, dizziness, visual disturbances, hallucinations, seizures, and toxic psychosis. The quinolones are contraindicated in patients with epilepsy.

Therapeutic Uses

The quinolones are useful in the treatment of urinary tract infections caused by most gram-negative bacteria, *Pseudomonas aeruginosa* being a notable exception. However, considering the numerous agents available with superior selective toxicity profiles and the tendency for organisms resistant to the quinolones to emerge, particularly against oxolinic acid, there is very limited rationale for the use of the quinolones.

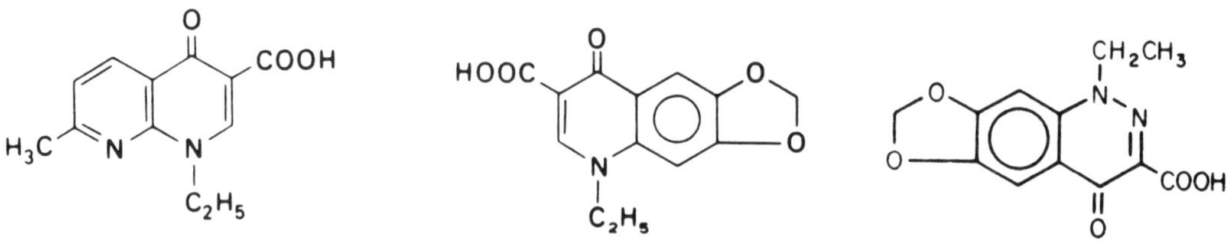

Naladixic acid

Oxolinic acid

Cinoxacin

Figure 94.2 Structures of the Quinolones

Preparations

Nalidixic acid (NegGram) is available as 250- and 500-mg and 1-gram tablets and as a suspension containing 250 mg/ml. Cinoxacin (Cinobac) is supplied as 250- and 500-mg capsules.

Nitrofurans

Chemistry and Mechanism of Action

Several 5-nitro-2-furaldehyde derivatives possess antibacterial activity and are referred to as the nitrofurans. The structures of the three compounds in clinical use are shown in Figure 94.3. The mechanism of their action is unclear, but appears to require reduction of the 5-nitro group to the nitro anion, which in turn undergoes recycling and production of superoxide and other toxic oxygen compounds, whose effects include damage to DNA. While similar reactions occur in human cells, the nitrofurans exhibit selective toxicity—apparently because concentrations remain relatively low in human cells, partly owing to hepatic inactivation. The antibacterial activity of the nitrofurans is enhanced at a pH of 5.5 or below. Clinical resistance to the nitrofurans is rare and develops slowly.

Antimicrobial Spectrum

The nitrofurans are active against a wide range of gram-positive and gram-negative bacteria. Nitrofurantoin has been used effectively against the protozoan *Giardia lamblia*.

Pharmacokinetics

Orally administered nitrofurans are well absorbed from the GI tract. Nitrofurazone is not appreciably absorbed through the skin following topical application. Disposition of nitrofurans is about 40 percent by renal filtration and secretion with significant metabolism also occurring. The half-life of nitrofurantoin is 20 minutes to one hour. The rapid disposition precludes achieving systemic levels sufficiently high for antibacterial action. The macrocrystalline form of nitrofurantoin is absorbed and excreted more slowly.

Adverse Effects and Drug Interactions

The most frequent adverse effect associated with systemic use of the nitrofurans is GI distress. Nausea, vomiting, and diarrhea with nitrofurantoin may be reduced by use of the macrocrystalline formulation. Both nitrofurantoin and furazolidone can cause hemolytic anemia in individuals with a deficient form of glucose-6-phosphodehydrogenase. Allergic reactions to both drugs occur. Nitrofurantoin has been associated with sensorimotor peripheral neuropathy, sometimes involving demyelination and degeneration.[31] Both acute pneumonitis, soon after initial administration, and interstitial pulmonary fibrosis, following chronic use, have been reported with nitrofurantoin. Elderly patients are particularly at risk for the pulmonary effects.[32] Chronic active hepatitis is a rare but serious adverse effect associated with nitrofurantoin.[33] Nitrofurantoin should be avoided in severe renal failure because of increased risk of toxic blood levels and reduced efficacy with lower urinary levels. Nitrofurantoin produces a harmless brown discoloration of the urine. Rarely, persons receiving furazolidone have exhibited a disulfiram-like reaction to ethanol.

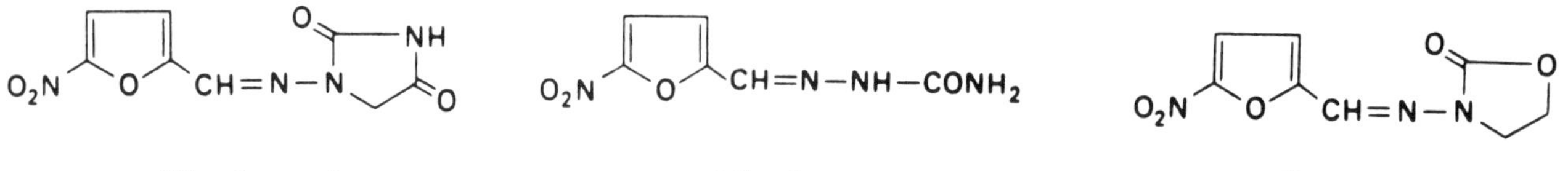

Nitrofurantoin

Nitrofurazone

Furazolidone

Figure 94.3 Structures of the Nitrofurans

Therapeutic Uses

Nitrofurantoin is used exclusively as an alternative agent for the treatment of urinary tract infections. Nitrofurazone is applied topically in the treatment of burns or in conjunction with skin grafts to prevent the development of bacterial infection. Furazolidone is used in the treatment of diarrhea and enteritis caused by susceptible bacteria and the protozoan *Giardia lamblia*.

Preparations

Nitrofurantoin (Furadantin) is available in tablets and capsules containing 50 or 100 mg and in an oral suspension containing 25 mg/5ml. Nitrofurantoin macrocrystals (Macrodantin) are available as 25-, 50-, and 100-mg capsules.

Nitrofurazone (Furacin) is used as a cream, topical solution, and soluble dressing (all containing 0.2%).

Furazolidone (Furoxone) is supplied as 100-mg tablets.

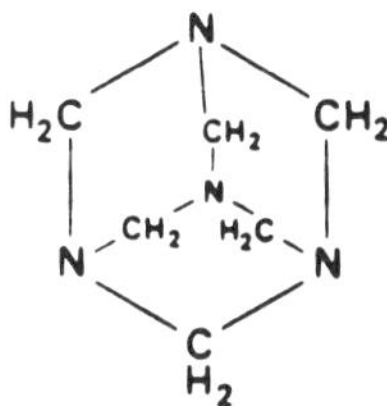

Figure 94.4 Structure of Methenamine

Methenamine

Chemistry and Mechanism of Action

Methenamine is often referred to as a urinary tract antiseptic, reflecting its exclusive use. Methenamine is a hexamethylenetetramine (shown in Fig. 94.4) that undergoes hydrolysis to liberate formaldehyde as a decomposition product. The formaldehyde formed denatures protein and is bactericidal. The rate of formaldehyde formation is related to the acidity of the medium, increasing from minimal at a pH of 7 or above to significant amounts at a pH of 5.5 or below. Therefore, acidification of the urine enhances formaldehyde formation and antibacterial action. This is accomplished by using the mandelate or hippurate salts, administering acidifying agents, such as ammonium chloride, and by increased dietary intake of acid-containing substances, e.g., cranberry juice. The lowered urinary pH itself results in an additional bacteriostatic action.

Antimicrobial Spectrum

A wide range of bacteria are susceptible to formaldehyde. Some organisms such as Proteus tend to produce ammonia from urea and raise urinary pH, thus reducing formaldehyde formation. Otherwise, bacteria do not develop resistance to methenamine.

Pharmacokinetics

Methenamine is well absorbed from the GI tract, but is subject to degradation by stomach acidity unless protected by enteric coating. Nearly all the absorbed

Table 94.2 Summary Table

	Dosage			Pharmacokinetics			
Drug	Route	Size (mg)	Dose (mg)	Time to Peak (h)	V_D (L)	$t_{1/2}$ (h)	Renal Clearance L/h
Norfloxacin	Oral	400 mg	400 mg q 12 h	1.5	—	4	14.0
Ciprofloxacin	Oral/IV	Oral: 250, 500, 750 IV: 200 & 400	Oral: 250–500 q 12 h IV: 400 q 12 h	1.1	348	4	21.4
Ofloxacin	Oral/IV	Oral: 200, 300, 400 IV: 200 & 400	Oral: 200–400 q 12 h IV: 200–400 q 12 h	1.4	102	6	10.4
Lomefloxacin	Oral	400	400/day	1.3	168	8	11.5
Enoxacin	Oral	200 & 400	400–800/day	1.6	175	4	12.0
Nalidixic acid	Oral	250, 500, 1000	100 qid	1.5	25	1.5	—
Cinoxacin	Oral	250 & 500	500 bid	1.5	23	2	10.5
Nitrofurantoin	Oral	25, 50, 100	50–100 qid	—	—	0.3	—
Furazolidone	Oral	100 mg	100 qid	—	—	—	—
Nitrofurazone	Topical	0.2%	Apply daily	—	—	—	—
Methenamine	Oral	1000 mg	1000 bid or qid	—	—	—	—

drug appears in the urine, where the conversion to formaldehyde occurs.

Adverse Effects and Drug Interactions

The most frequent adverse effect associated with methenamine is GI distress, particularly with doses exceeding 2 grams per day. Bladder irritation resulting in painful and frequent urination, albuminuria, and hematuria may result if high doses are administered for long periods. Rashes have been associated with methenamine use. Methenamine mandelate is contra-indicated in renal failure as the mandelate moiety can produce crystalluria. Sulfonamides cannot be given at the same time as methenamine because they may form an insoluble complex with the formaldehyde that is released.

Therapeutic Uses

Methanamine is used only as an alternative agent in urinary tract infections. The formaldehyde produced is particularly active against *E. coli* and is also effective against other bacteria likely to cause infections of the urinary tract. While there are many other drugs that would generally be considered to be superior choices, resistance or other factors resulting in chronic recurrence of an infection sometimes lead to methenamine being employed.

Preparations

Methenamine mandelate (Mandelamine) and methenamine hippurate (Urex) are available in oral dosage forms.

References

Research Reports

1. Chu DTW, Fernandes PB. Structure-activity relationships of the fluoroquinolones. Antimicrob Agents Chemother 1989;*33*:131–135.
2. Diver M. Quinolone uptake by bacteria and bacterial killing. Rev Infect Dis 1989;*11*(Suppl 5):S941–S946.
3. Neu HC. Chemical evolution of the fluoroquinolone antimicrobial agents. Am J Med 1989;*87*(Suppl 6C):2S–9S.
4. Piddock LJV, Hall MC, Wise R. Mechanism of action of lomefloxacin. Antimicrob Agents Chemother 1990;*34*:1088–1093.
5. Suzuki K, Nagata Y, Naide Y, Horiba M. Clinical study of strains of Pseudomonas aeruginosa and Serratia marcesans resistant to new quinolones in complicated urinary tract infections. Rev Infect Dis 1989;*11*(Suppl 5):S969–S970.
6. Wallace RJ, Bedsole G, Sumter G, Sanders CV, Steele LC, Brown BA, Smith J, Graham DR. Activities of ciprofloxacin and ofloxacin against rapidly growing mycobacteria with demonstration of acquired resistance following single drug therapy. Antimicrob Agents Chemother 1990;*34*:65–70.
7. Kaatz GW, Seo SM, Ruble CA. Efflux-mediated fluoroquinolone resistance in Staphlylococcus aureus. Antimicrob Agents Chemother 1993;*37*:1086–1094.
8. Gerding DN, Hitt JA. Tissue penetration of the new quinolones in humans. Rev Infect Dis 1989;*11*(Suppl 5):S1046–S1057.
9. Drancourt M, Gallais H, Raoult D, Estrangin E, Mallet MN, Micco PDe. Ofloxacin penetration into cerebrospinal fluid. J Antimicrob Chemother 1988;*22*:263–265.
10. Wolff M, Boutron L, Singlas E, Clair B, Decazes JM, Regnier B. Penetration of ciprofloxacin into cerebrospinal fluid in patients with bacterial meningitis. Antimicrob Agents Chemother 1987;*31*:899–902.
11. Pocidalo J-J. Use of fluoroquinolones for intracellular pathogens. Rev Infect Dis 1989;*11*(Suppl 5):S979–S984.
12. Bergan T, Dalhof A, Rohwedder R. Pharmacokinetics of ciprofloxacin. Infection 1988;*16*(Suppl 1):3–13.
13. Shimada J, Yamaji T, Veda Y, Uchida H, Kusajima H, Irikura T. Mechanism of renal excretion of AM-715, a new quinolonecarboxylic acid derivative, in rabbits, dogs and humans. Antimicrob Agents Chemother 1983;*23*:1–7.
14. Sorgel F. Metabolism of gyrase inhibitors. Rev Infect Dis 1989;*11*(Suppl 5):S1119–S1125.
15. Freeman CD, Nicolau DP, Belliveau PP, Nightingale CH. Lomefloxacin clinical pharmacokinetics. Clin Pharmacokinet 1993;*25*:6–19.
16. Wolfson JS, Hooper DC. Pharmacokinetics of quinolones: Newer aspects. Eur J Microbiol Infect Dis 1991;(special issue):47–54.
17. Eandi M, Viano I, Di Nola F, Leone L, Genazzani E. Pharmacokinetics of norfloxacin in healthy volunteers and patients with renal and hepatic damage. Eur J Clin Microbiol 1983;*3*:253–259.
18. Tsuji A, Sato H, Kume Y, Tamai I, Okezaki E, Nagata O, Kato H. Inhibitory effects of quinolone anticbacterial agents on gamma-aminobutyric acid binding to receptor sites in rat brain membranes. Antimicrob Agents Chemother 1988;*32*:190–194.
19. Thorsteinsson SB, Bergan T, Johannesson H, Thorsteinsson HS, Rodwedder R. Tolerance of ciprofloxacin at injection site, systemic safety and effect on electroencephalogram. Chemotherapy (Basel) 1987;*33*:448–451.
20. Stein G. Drug interactions with fluoroquinolones. Am J Med 1991;*91*(Suppl 6A):81S–85S.
21. Koup JR, Toothaker RD, Posvar E, Sedman AJ, Colburn WA. Theophylline dosage adjustment during enoxacin coadministration. Antimicrob Agents Chemother 1990;*34*:803–807.
22. Christ W, Lehnert T, Ulbrich B. Specific toxicologic aspects of the quinolones. Rev Infect Dis 1988;*10*(Suppl 1):141–146.
23. The choice of antibacterial drugs. The Medical Letter 1992;*34*:49–56.
24. Naber KG. Use of quinolones in urinary tract infections and prostatitis. Rev Infect Dis 1989;*11*(Suppl 5):S1321–S1337.
25. Covino JM, Cummings M, Smith B, Benes S, Draft K, McCormack W. Comparison of ofloxacin and ceftriaxone in the treatment of uncomplicated gonorrhea caused by penicillinase-producing and non-penicillinase-producing strains. Antimicrob Agents Chemother 1990;*34*:148–149.
26. Ericsson CD, Johnson PC, Dupont HL, Morgan DR, Bitsura JAM, de la Cabada FJ. Ciprofloxacin or trimethoprim-sulfamethoxazole as initial therapy for travelers' diarrhea: a placebo-controlled randomized trial. Ann Intern Med 1987;*106*:216–220.

27. Gentry LO, Rodriguez-Gomez GG. Oral ciprofloxacin versus parenteral therapy for chronic osteomyelitis. Antimicrob Agents Chemother 1991;*35*:538–541.

28. Lang R, Goshen S, Kitzes-Cohen R, Sade J. Successful treatment of malignant external otitis with oral ciprofloxacin: Report of experience with 23 patients. J Infect Dis 1990;*161*:537–540.

29. Gentry LO. Review of quinolones in the treatment of infections of the skin and skin structure. J Antimicrob Chemother 1991;*28*(Suppl C):97–110.

30. Bow EJ, Rayner E, Louie TJ. Comparison of norfloxacin with cotrimoxazole for infection prophylaxis in acute leukemia. The trade-off for reduced gram-negative sepsis. Am J Med 1988;*84*:847–854.

31. Toole JF, Parrish ML. Nitrofurantoin polyneuropathy. Neurology 1973;*23*:554–559.

32. Holmberg L, Boman G, Bottoger LE, Eriksson BA, Spross R, Wessling A. Adverse reactions to nitrofurantoin. Am J Med 1980;*69*:733–738.

33. Black M, Rabin L, Schatz N. Nitrofuran-induced chronic active hepatitis. Ann Intern Med 1980;*92*:62–64.

Reviews

r1. Sable CA, Scheld WM. Fluoroquinolones: How to use (but not overuse) these antibiotics. Geriatrics. 1993;*48*(6):41–51.

r2. Hooper DC, Wolfson JS. Mode of action of the quinolone antimicrobial agents: Review of recent information. Rev Infect Dis 1989;*11*(Suppl 5):S902–S911.

r3. Wolfson JS, Hooper DC. Bacterial resistance to quinolones: mechanisms and clinical importance. Rev Infect Dis 1989;*11*(Suppl 5):S960–S968.

r4. Walker RC, Wright AJ. The fluoroquinolones. Mayo Clin Proc 1991;*66*:1249–1259.

r5. Wolfson JS, Hooper DC. Fluoroquinolone antimicrobial agents. Clin Microbiol Rev 1989;*2*:378–424.

r6. Patterson DR. Quinolone toxicity: Methods of assessment. Am J Med 1991;*91*(Suppl 6A):355S–375S.

r7. Raeburn JA, Govan JRW, McCrae WM, Greening AP, Collier PS, Hodson, ME, Goodchild MC. Ciprofloxacin therapy in cystic fibrosis. J Antimicrob Chemother 1987;*20*:295–296.

r8. Andriole VT (ed). The Quinolones. New York: Academic Press, 1988.

r9. Bryson HM. Fourth international symposium on new quinolones. Drugs 1993;*45*(Suppl 3):1–475.

r10. Greenfield RA. Symposium on antimicrobial therapy. VII. The fluoroquinolones. J Okla State Med Assoc 1993;*86*:166–174.

r11. Just PM. Overview of the fluoroquinolone antibiotics. Pharmacotherapy 1993;*13*(2 Pt 2):4S–17S.

r11a. Paton JH, Reeves DS. Fluoroquinolone antibiotics: microbiology, pharmacokinetics and clinical use. Drugs. 1988;*36*:193–228.

r12. Tartaglione TA. The role of fluoroquinolones in sexually transmitted diseases. Pharmacotherapy 1993;*13*:189–201.

r13. Todd PA, Faulds D. Ofloxacin: A reappraisal of its antimicrobial activity, pharmacology and therapeutic use. Drugs 1991;*42*:825–876.

r14. Wadworth AN, Goa KL. Lomefloxacin: A review of its antibacterial activity, pharmacokinetic properties and therapeutic use. Drugs 1991;*42*:1018–1060.

CHAPTER 95

Robert A. Nicholas
Holli Hamilton
Myron S. Cohen

β-Lactam Antibiotics

Penicillins and cephalosporins are the main constituents of a class of drugs known as β-lactam antibiotics. These drugs display many similar properties, including mechanism of action, pharmacokinetics, and adverse side-effects. They share a common structure, the β-lactam ring, and can have a multitude of chemical substitutions at several key positions in the parent molecule. These substitutions determine both the pharmacologic properties of the antibiotic and its spectrum of action, i.e., whether its antimicrobial activity is restricted to a small number of organisms (narrow spectrum), or whether it is active against a wide variety of organisms (broad spectrum). The antibacterial activity of β-lactam antibiotics is due to the inhibition of bacterial cell wall synthesis, and this inhibition ultimately leads to cell death. Because of the high selective pressure placed on bacteria by these antibiotics, microorganisms have devised several mechanisms that lead to increased resistance to β-lactam antibiotics, and resistance has become a very important clinical problem. This chapter will outline the mechanism of action of β-lactam antibiotics and the various modes of resistance that are encountered in the treatment of bacterial infections.

Chemistry

The chemical structures of the penicillins, cephalosporins, monobactams, and carbapenems are shown in Figure 95.1. The basic nucleus of the penicillins (6-aminopenicillanic acid) consists of two fused ring structures: the thiazolidine ring (A) and the β-lactam ring (B), as per figure format. The attachment of different chemical moieties (R) through the amino group of 6-aminopenicillanic acid gives rise to a myriad of derivatives that possess useful clinical properties. The basic nucleus of the cephalosporins consists of the β-lactam ring fused with a six-membered ring structure that contains an additional substitution site (R_2). Monobactams contain only a substituted β-lactam ring and an ionizing acid moiety, indicating that this is the minimal structure required for antibiotic activity. The structures of the carbapenems resemble those of the penicillins, but with two important differences: (1) the stereochemistry at the α-carbon in the β-lactam ring is reversed; and (2) there is no heteroatom (e.g., S) in the equivalent position of the A ring. The β-lactam ring is absolutely required for antibiotic efficacy; hydrolysis of the β-lactam ring, whether by chemical or enzymatic means, destroys the antibiotic activity of the compound.

The immune response to β-lactam antibiotics is thought to be mediated through the derivatization of protein molecules that serve as carriers for the small molecules.[1] The major route of derivatization of penicillin G appears to be an isomerization of the thiazolidone ring structure (A in Fig. 95.1) to produce D-benzylpenicillenic acid. This highly reactive compound can react with lysine amino groups on the surface of proteins, which results in covalent linkage and the formation of an immunohapten molecule. The intact penicillin G molecule can also react with free amino groups on proteins, but this pathway is thought to be a minor route of antigen formation. Hypersensitivity to cephalosporins is less pronounced than with the penicillins, although cross-reactivity of antibodies to both penicillins and cephalosporins has been demonstrated. This cross-reactivity of cephalosporins in patients hypersensitive to penicillin may be more pronounced in cephalosporins with side-chains similar to benzyl penicillin than with those that contain very different side-chain structures. Interestingly, hypersensitivity and cross-reactivity to aztreonam, a monobactam, appears to be very rare, and thus this β-lactam antibiotic may be used sometimes in patients hypersensitive to penicillin G.[2]

The penicillins can be conveniently grouped by their spectrum of action. Table 95.1 shows the structures of some of the members of each group, their spectrum of action, and some of the defining characteristics of the individual antibiotics. The clinical uses of the

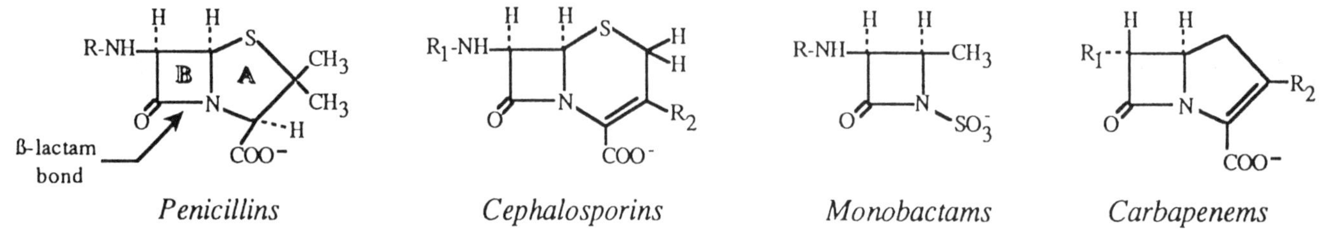

Figure 95.1 General Structures of β-Lactam Antibiotics. The basic structures of the four classes of β-lactam antibiotics are shown. The thiazolidine ring in the penicillins is designated by A; the β-lactam ring is designated by B. Note the stereochemistry at the α carbon in the β-lactam ring in the carbapenems as compared to the other classes of antibiotics. Substitutions at various positions (R, R_1, or R_2) leads to large number of potent antibiotics that differ in their antibacterial spectrum and their pharmacologic properties. An intact β-lactam bond is absolutely required for antibiotic activity.

penicillins and their pharmacokinetic properties are discussed more thoroughly in later sections of this chapter. Most cephalosporin antibiotics traditionally have been grouped into three generations, which were defined based on the time of their introduction into clinical usage. However, these generations can also be considered in terms of their spectrum of action: (a) the first-generation cephalosporins have the greatest activity against gram-positive organisms and much less activity against gram-negative bacteria; (b) the second-generation cephalosporins have expanded activity against gram-negative bacteria; (c) the third-generation drugs are even more active than the second-generation antibiotics against gram-negative organisms, but less active against gram-positive organisms. Clinically useful antibiotics from each of the three generations are listed in Table 95.2, along with their spectrum of action and defining characteristics.

History

One of the most fortuitous discoveries in the history of science was the observation by Alexander Fleming in 1928 that bacterial growth on an agar plate was inhibited in the vicinity of contaminating penicillium mold. Fleming attempted to purify the compound responsible for this antibiotic activity, but gave up after a year of failed attempts. In 1940, as the need for antibiotics became intensified during World War II, Sir Howard Florey, Ernst Chain, and their collaborators at the fermentation laboratories in Peoria, IL, began the laborious task of isolating the labile antibiotic from huge cultures of mold. They finally succeeded in isolating a small amount that was at best 10 percent pure and used this preparation to treat a sick London policeman who had a mixed staphylococcal and streptococcal bacteremia. Immediate improvement in the patient was noted, but they quickly ran out of penicillin and had to reisolate the antibiotic from the patient's urine in order to continue treatment. Although the patient died from the lack of more antibiotic, it was clear that penicillin was a powerful antibacterial agent with tremendous potential.

When the purification of penicillin G was finally achieved on a large scale, the full power of this potent antibiotic was realized. The use of penicillin G during those early years, however, was compromised by two different problems: (1) penicillin G was very susceptible to hydrolysis by β-lactamases; and (2) it was relatively inactive against gram-negative bacteria. In 1959, 6-aminopenicillanic acid was isolated from cultures of penicillium mold. This compound allowed the development of hundreds of new compounds by synthetic substitutions at the amino functionality, which greatly increased the spectrum of action for penicillins.

Cephalosporins were discovered in 1948 by G. Brotzu, who isolated the mold *Cephalosporium acremonium* from a sewer pipe draining into the sea on the coast of Sardinia. Crude filtrates of the mold, which contained three different cephalosporins, displayed antibiotic activity against *Staphylococcus aureus* both in vitro and in vivo. As with the penicillins, the manipulation of different side-chains onto the cephalosporin nucleus (Fig. 95.1) has produced a wide range of potent antibiotics. The constant search for new and useful antibiotics also led to the discovery of both monobactams and carbapenems, which are only now beginning to have a defined clinical role in antibacterial therapy.

During this time, interest in the mechanisms of action of these antibiotics intensified. It was known from very early morphologic studies that penicillin interfered with cell wall synthesis, killed only growing cells, and killed cells by inducing cell lysis. Research interests soon turned to the elucidation of the biosynthesis and structure of the bacterial cell wall, which culminated with the determination of the mechanism of action of penicillin.

Mechanism of Action of β-Lactam Antibiotics

The Bacterial Cell Wall

Almost all bacteria are surrounded by a cell wall that confers rigidity and stability on the cell. Since bacteria have no mechanism to regulate osmolarity, they must utilize a supporting structure around the cell to withstand the inherent high osmotic pressure. A notable exception to this is the bacterium *mycoplasma*, which has no cell wall and thus is susceptible to changes in osmotic pressure. Bacteria are classified as either gram-negative or gram-positive, based on absorption of crystal violet dye. The two groups of bacteria have a common structure known as peptidoglycan, which is composed of parallel polysaccharide chains cross-linked by peptide chains. The peptidoglycan completely surrounds the cell, and functions to contain a swelling bacterium and to prevent its lysis. The organization of the cell walls in gram-negative and gram-positive bacteria is quite different (Fig. 95.2), even though the basic mechanisms of cell wall synthesis are very similar. Gram-negative bacteria have both an inner membrane and an outer membrane, with a thin

Table 95.1 Structures and Properties of the Penicillins

Structure (R group)	Antibiotic	Distinguishing Features	Main Clinical Uses
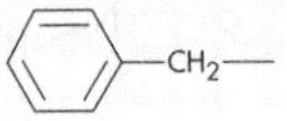 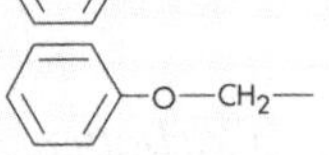 $-CH_2-$ $-O-CH_2-$	Penicillin G Penicillin V	β-lactamase sensitive β-lactamase sensitive Oral administration	Non β lactamase-producing strains of: *Streptococci* *Neisseria gonorrhoeae* *Neisseria meningitdis*
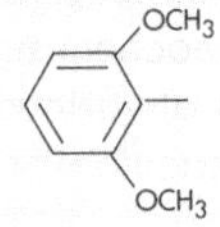 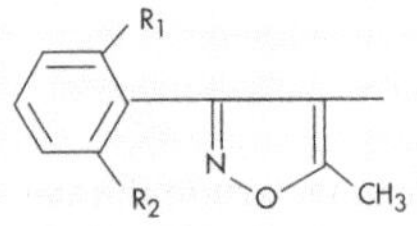 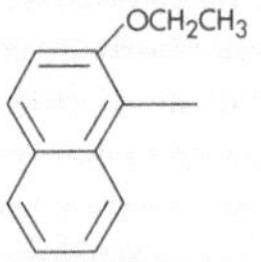 OCH_3, OCH_3 R_1, R_2, N, O, CH_3 OCH_2CH_3	Methicillin Oxacillin ($R_1 = R_2 =$ H) Cloxacillin (R_1 = Cl; R_2 = H) Dicloxacillin ($R_1 = R_2$ = Cl) Floxacillin (R_1 = Cl; R_2 = F) Nafcillin	(Not given orally) Resistant to β-lactamase Oral administration Resistant to β-lactamase Oral administration Resistant to β-lactamase	β-lactamase-producing strains of *Staphylococcus aureus* (but not MRSA)
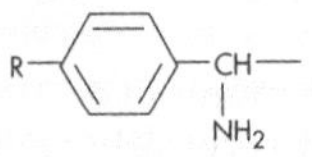 R– –CH–, NH_2	Ampicillin (R = H) Amoxicillin (R = OH)	Oral administration Sensitive to β-lactamase Often combined with clavulanic acid or sulbactam (Augmentin or Unasyn)	Same as penicillin G plus *Haemophilus influenzae* *Escherichia coli* *Proteus mirabilis* *Shigella* *Salmonella typhi*
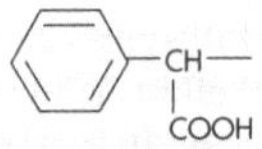 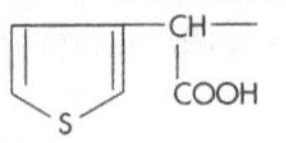 –CH–, COOH –CH–, COOH, S	Carbenicillin Ticarcillin	Hydrolyzed by β-lactamase Often combined with clavulanic acid = Timentin	*Pseudomonas aeruginosa* *Escherichia coli* *Proteus mirabilis*
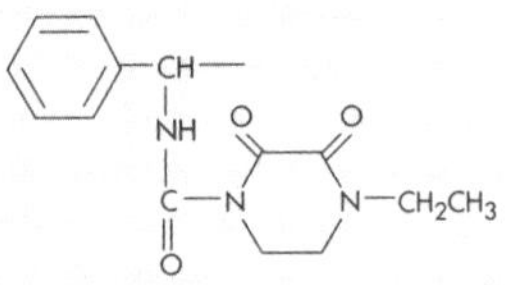 –CH–, NH, C=O, N, O, O, $N-CH_2CH_3$	Piperacillin	Rarely used alone to treat serious gram negative infections → usually combined with an aminoglycoside	*Pseudomonas aeruginosa* *Escherichia coli* *Proteus mirabilis* *Serratia marcescens*
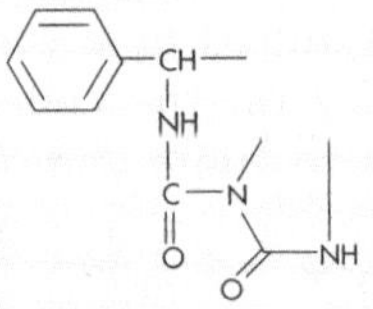 –CH–, NH, C–N, O, NH, O	Azlocillin	Rarely given as a single agent	Most active against *Pseudomonas* species
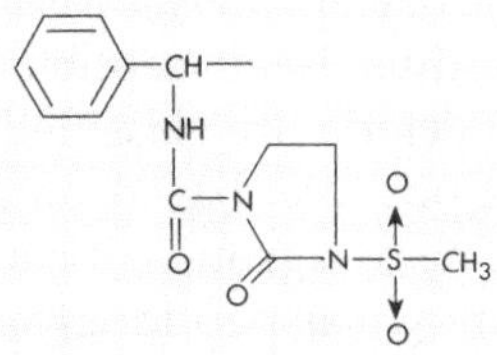 –CH–, NH, C–N, O, O, $N-S-CH_3$, O, O	Mezlocillin	Rarely given as a single agent	Most active against following species: *Proteus* *Enterobacter* *Klebsiella*

layer of peptidoglycan sandwiched between the two membranes. Gram-positive bacteria have only one membrane that is surrounded by a thick wall composed of peptidoglycan and teichoic acid, a polyol phosphate polymer. The unraveling of the synthesis of the peptidoglycan was deciphered mainly by the work of Jack Strominger and his colleagues.

Structure of Peptidoglycan

The structure of the peptidoglycan matrix is shown in Figure 95.3. It consists of glycan chains, which run in one plane, and peptide chains, which extend outward from the saccharide polymer. The glycan chains consist of the repeating amino sugars N-acetylglucosamine

Table 95.2 Structures and Properties of the Cephhalosporins

Structure R₁	Structure R₂	Antibiotic	Distinguishing Features	Spectrum of Action & Clinical Uses
		First-Generation Cephalosporins		
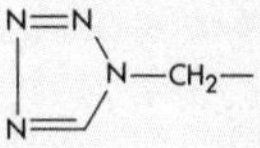 N=N, N—CH_2—, N (tetrazole ring)	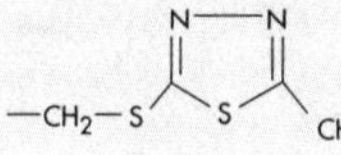 —CH_2—S—(N—N, S ring)—CH_3	Cefazolin	Parenteral use only	
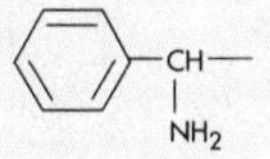 (benzene ring)—CH—, NH_2	—CH_3	Cephalexin	Oral administration	Very Active against gram-postiive cocci with the exception of enterococci and MRSA; limited activity against gram-negative organisms
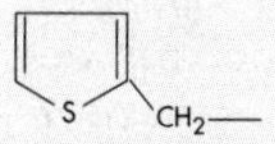 (thiophene ring, S)—CH_2—	—CH_2—O—C(=O)—CH_3	Cephalothin	Parenteral use only	Used for preoperative surgical prophylaxis to prevent wound infections
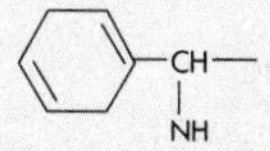 (cyclohexadiene ring)—CH—, NH	—CH_3	Cephadrine	Oral or parenteral administration	
		Second-Generation Cephalosporins		
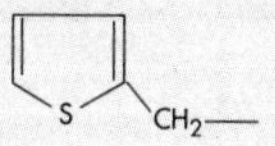 (thiophene ring, S)—CH_2—	—CH_2—O—C(=O)—NH_2	Cefoxitin	Highly Active against anaerobes such as *Bacteroides fragilis*	
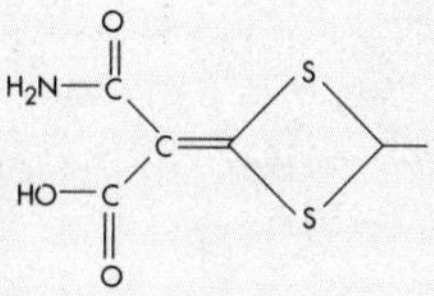 H_2N—C(=O)—C(—C(=O)—HO)=C(S, S ring)—	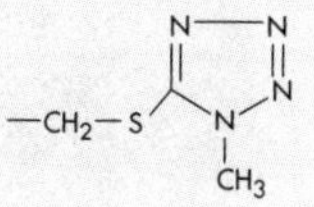 —CH_2—S—(N—N, N, N ring)—N—CH_3	Cefotetan	Highly Active against anaerobes such as *Bacteroides fragilis*	Increased activity against gram-negative infections caused by *H. influenzae* *N. meningitidis* *N. gonorrheae* *S. pneumoniae*
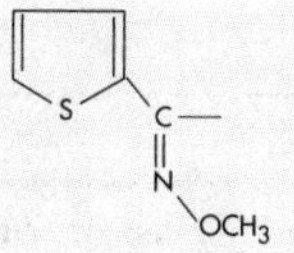 (thiophene ring, S)—C(=N—OCH_3)—	—CH_2—O—C(=O)—NH_2	Cefuroxime	Can be given orally Crosses blood-brain barrier Useful for treatment of childhood and adult meningitis	
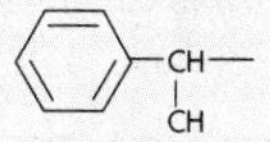 (benzene ring)—CH—, CH	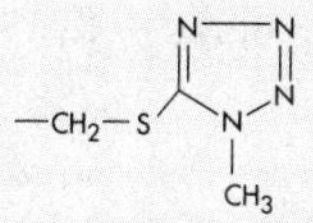 —CH_2—S—(N—N, N, N ring)—N—CH_3	Cafamandole		
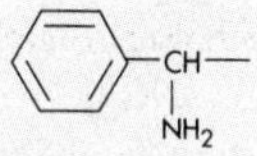 (benzene ring)—CH—, NH_2	—Cl	Cefaclor	Oral administration	
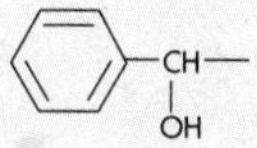 (benzene ring)—CH—, OH	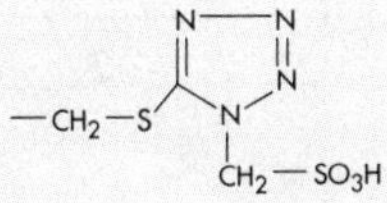 —CH_2—S—(N—N, N, N ring)—N—CH_2—SO_3H	Cefonicid		

continued

(GlcNAc) and N-acetylmuramic acid (MurNAc; the 3-O-D-lactic acid ether of GlcNAc) in a β-1,4-linkage. The peptide chains of the peptidoglycan are linked to the glycan chains via the carboxyl group of the lactic acid moieties of MurNAc. In *Staphylococcus aureus,* the peptide chain has the sequence L-alanyl-D-γ-isoglutamyl-L-lysyl-D-alanyl-D-alanine. The peptide chains are cross-linked to other peptide chains, which makes the macromolecule rigid and insoluble. In *Staphylococcus aureus,* the peptide chains are cross-linked by a pentaglycine "bridge," which extends from the amino group of a lysine residue of one peptide chain to the

Table 95.2 *Continued*

Structure: R_1	Structure: R_2	Antibiotic	Distinguishing Features	Spectrum of Action & Clinical Uses
		Third-Generation Cephalosporins		
H_2N–(thiazolyl)–C(=N–OCH_3)–	–CH_2–S–(triazinedione, H_3C–N, NH, =O, =O)	Ceftriaxone	Treatment of choice for *N. gonorrhoeae* infections and meningitis caused by *H. influenzae, N. meningitidis,* and *S. pneumoniae*	
H_2N–(thiazolyl)–C(=N–OCH_3)–	–CH_2–O–C(=O)–OCH_3	Cefotaxime	Also crosses blood-brain barrier; used to treat adult meningitis	Highly active against wide variety of gram-negative organisms, e.g., enteric gram-negative bacilli
H_2N–(thiazolyl)–C(=N–OCH_3)–	–H	Ceftizoxime		*H. influenzae* *N. gonorrhoeae*
H_2N–(thiazolyl)–C(=N–C(CH_3)(CH_3)–COOH)–	–CH_2–$N^{\oplus}$(pyridinium)	Ceftazidime	Crosses blood-brain barrier Active against *P. aeruginosa*	Some limited activity against gram-positive organisms, notably *S. aureus* Are generally β-lactamase-resistant, although some resistant strains have been noted
(phenyl)–N(piperazinedione, O, O)N–C(=O)–NH–CH–(phenyl–CH)	–CH_2–S–(tetrazolyl, N–CH_3)	Cefoperazone		
		Other β-Lactam Antibiotics		
H_2N–(thiazolyl)–C(=N–O–C(CH_3)(CH_3)–COOH)–		Aztreonam	Cross-reactivity in patients with penicillin hypersensitivy is extremely rare	Highly active against aerobic gram-negative rods No activity against gram-positive organisms
HO–CH(H_3C)–	–S–CH_2–CH_2–NH–CH=NH	Imipenem	β-lactamase-resistant, although some resistant strains beginning to appear Marketed with cilastin, a renal dipeptidase inhibitor	Very broad spectrum—has significant activity against a variety of gram-positive and gram-negative organisms. Not useful for MRSA

carboxyl group of a D-alanine residue from another peptide chain (Fig. 95.3). Although the amino acid at the third position of the peptide chain (Lys in Fig. 95.3) and the cross-linking bridge ($(Gly)_5$ in Fig. 95.3) varies among species, these differences are unimportant in the context of antibiotic efficacy. The unvarying portions of the peptidoglycan matrix, the repeating disaccharide and the D-alanyl-D-alanine carboxyl terminus of the peptide chains, are regions where almost all antibiotic action occurs.

Cell Wall Biosynthesis

The synthesis of the peptidoglycan matrix can be conveniently thought of as occurring in three stages in different regions of the cell: the cytoplasmic, membrane, and extracytoplasmic regions, respectively. In Stage I, the synthesis of UDP-MurNAc-pentapeptide occurs. In Stage II, GlcNAc is condensed with the MurNAc-pentapeptide, which is then attached to a grow-

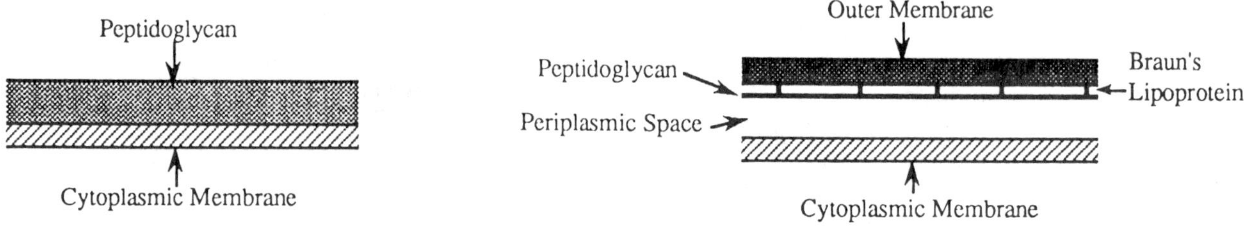

Figure 95.2 Bacterial Physiology. The organization of the cell walls in both gram-positive and gram-negative bacteria is shown. In gram-positive bacteria, a thick layer of peptidoglycan and teichoic acid surrounds the cell. Gram-negative organisms have two membranes, a cytoplasmic membrane and an outer membrane, with a thin section of peptidoglycan attached to the outer membrane by Braun's lipoprotein.[46]

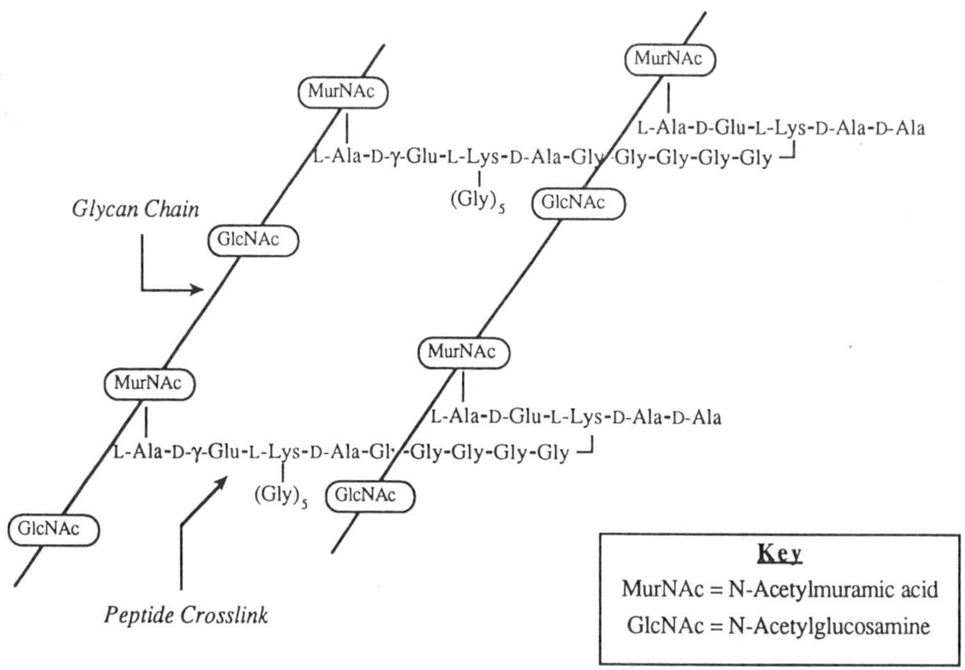

Figure 95.3 Cell wall structure of *Staphylococcus aureus*. A schematic representation of the cell wall peptidoglycan in *S. aureus*. The glycan chains run parallel to the cytoplasmic membrane and are composed of the repeating GlcNAc-MurNAc disaccharide. Peptide chains are present on the MurNAc residues, some of which are crosslinked to peptide chains from other glycan stands. (Adapted from Ghuysen et al., Fig. 1[47]).

ing chain of nascent peptidoglycan. In Stage III, the peptide chains are cross-linked. Each of these stages will be discussed separately, and the antibiotics that interfere with the reactions at each stage will also be presented.

Stage I of Cell Wall Synthesis

The reactions of cell wall synthesis in *Staphylococcus aureus* are shown in Figure 95.4. In Stage I, the cell synthesizes UDP-MurNAc-pentapeptide, which is the major compound that accumulates in penicillin-treated cells. Stage I synthesis starts with the phosphate ester of N-acetylglucosamine (GlcNAc-1-P), which is condensed with UTP to yield UDP-GlcNAc. Phosphoenolpyruvate is condensed onto the 3-hydroxyl of UDP-GlcNAc, and the enol group is subsequently reduced to yield UDP-MurNAc, a substituted lactic acid. The next series of reactions build the pentapeptide chain that is present in the final substrate. First, the amino group of L-alanine is condensed with the carboxyl group of the lactic acid moiety of UDP-MurNAc; this reaction is followed by the condensation of D-glutamic acid onto the new carboxyl terminus of the alanine residue. The next amino acid, L-lysine (m-diaminopimelic acid in *E. coli*), is condensed onto the γ-carboxyl group of D-glutamic acid to form an isopeptide bond. In the last step of Stage I synthesis, the dipeptide D-alanyl-D-alanine is added by the enzyme D-alanyl-D-alanine–adding enzyme to yield UDP-N-acetylmuramylpentapeptide.

The synthesis of D-alanyl-D-alanine is a site of antibiotic action. In the first reaction, L-alanine is isomerized to D-alanine by the enzyme alanine racemase. In the second step, D-alanine:D-alanine ligase condenses two D-alanine residues to give D-alanyl-D-alanine. Both of these enzymes are inhibited by the antibiotic D-cycloserine, which is produced by *Streptomyces orchidaceus*. This antibiotic appears to have at least two modes of action. There was initially some controversy over the mechanism of action of D-cycloserine, but it now appears that D-cycloserine is a suicide substrate that irreversibly inactivates alanine racemase by forming a stable product with the enzyme-bound pyridoxal phosphate moiety.[3] D-Cycloserine also may function as a competitive inhibitor of D-alanine:D-alanine ligase. D-Cycloserine is occasionally used in the retreatment of tuberculosis due to drug-resistant infections, in the treatment of various urinary tract infections, and in cases where traditional β-lactam antibiotic therapy is refractory.

Stage II of Cell Wall Synthesis

Once the synthesis of UDP-MurNAc-pentapeptide is completed, the next series of reactions shift from the

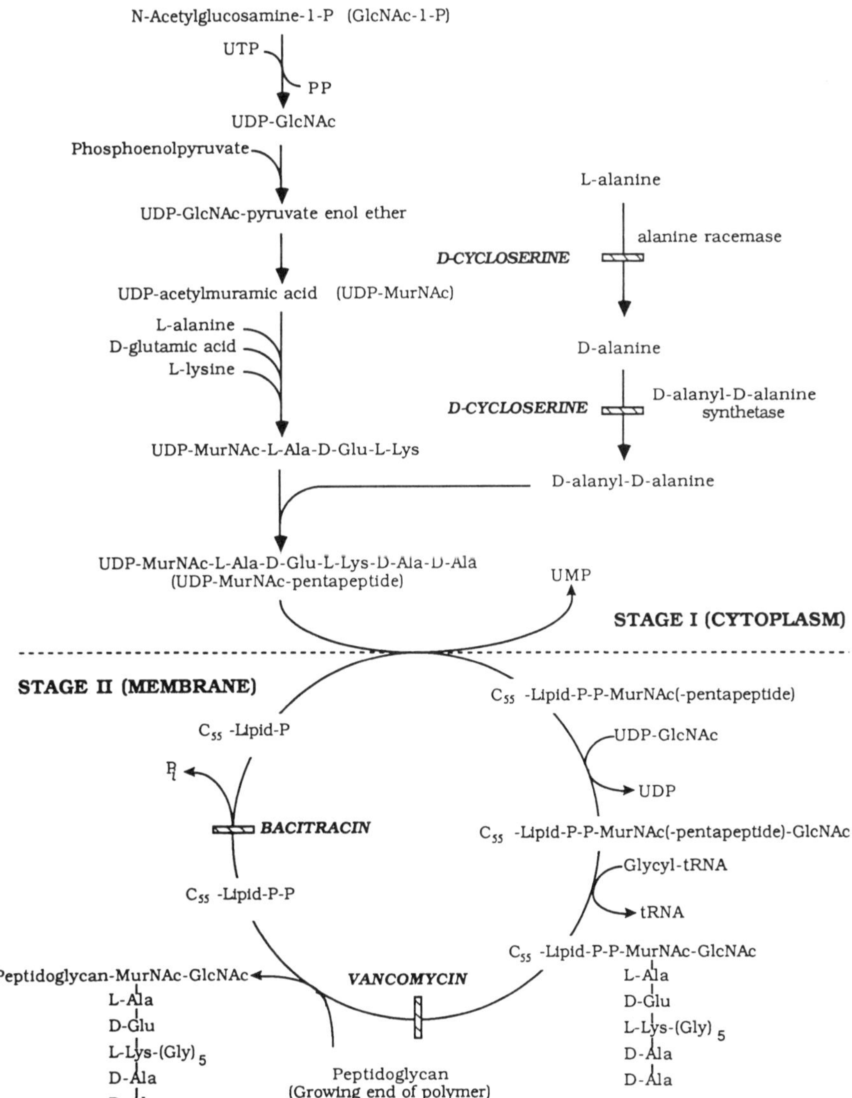

Figure 95.4 Cell wall synthesis in *Staphylococcus aureus.* The biosynthetic reactions of Stage I and Stage II cell wall synthesis are shown here. Stage I occurs in the cytoplasm of the bacterium, whereas the reactions of Stage II occur on the membrane surface. The locations of the inhibition by different non β-lactam antibiotics are shown by ____. (Modified from Strominger et al.[48]).

cytoplasm to the membrane. The first reaction of Stage II biosynthesis condenses the UDP-MurNAc-pentapeptide with the phosphate ester of the highly conjugated lipid, undecaprenol, which is also known as C_{55}-isoprenol phosphate. This compound is similar to dolichol phosphate, which is found in mammalian cells and is involved in the maturation of glycoproteins during their transport to the cell surface. Once the MurNAc-pentapeptide is covalently bound to C_{55}-isoprenol phosphate, it is further modified by the addition of GlcNAc. The next modification is different in various species: whereas in *E. coli* no modification occurs, in *Staphylococcus aureus* a pentaglycine bridge is linked to the free amino group of L-lysine in the pentapeptide by the repeated addition of glycine from glycyl-tRNA. The peptidoglycan substrate, C_{55}-isoprenol diphosphate-disaccharide pentapeptide $(Gly)_5$, is now ready to condense with an actively growing end of a glycan chain. Enzymes located in the cytoplasmic membrane catalyze the transglycosylation of the disaccharide pentapeptide $(Gly)_5$ onto nascent peptidoglycan. This transglycosylation step is inhibited by vancomycin, an antibiotic isolated from *Streptomyces orientalis.* It is an amphoteric glycopeptide that forms a high affinity noncovalent complex with the D-alanyl-D-alanine portion of the pentapeptide, and thus prevents the utilization of the substrate in peptidoglycan synthesis.[4] Vancomycin is now the drug of choice for methicillin-resistant *Staphylococcus aureus* (MRSA) and is also commonly used to treat pseudomembraneous colitis caused by the outgrowth of *Clostridium difficile.* Although resistance to vancomycin in the past was considered a rare event, recently clinical isolates of *Enterococcus faecium* and *Enterococcus faecalis* resistant to vancomycin have emerged.[5,6] This resistance is induced by vancomycin, and appears to involve at least two enzymes. One of these enzymes synthesizes a D-α-hydroxycarboxylic acid (probably D-lactate); the other protein is a D-alanine:D-alanine ligase with altered specificity that synthesizes D-alanyl-D-lactate.[7,8] This depsipeptide is then added onto the UDP-MurNAc-tripeptide to form a novel peptidoglycan substrate. The substitution of the ultimate D-alanine residue with D-lactate results in the loss of high-affinity binding by vancomycin (which requires D-alanyl-D-alanine for production of a high-affinity complex) and leads to high-level resistance to this antibiotic.[9]

Following the polymerization of the disaccharide pentapeptide $(Gly)_5$ into existing peptidoglycan, the C_{55}-isoprenol diphosphate must be dephosphorylated to its monophosphate form in order to react with a new molecule of UDP-N-acetylmuramylpentapeptide. This dephosphorylation reaction is inhibited by bacitracin, a cyclic peptide antibiotic produced by both *Bacillus subtilis* and *Bacillus licheniformis.* Bacitracin appears to bind to the diphosphate form of C_{55}-isoprenol in the presence of Mg^{2+} and prevents the regeneration of the monophosphate lipid carrier.[10] Its relatively severe toxicity limits its use to topical ointments.

Stage III of Cell Wall Synthesis

Stage III of cell wall synthesis occurs outside the cell. Once the disaccharide pentapeptide$(Gly)_5$ is attached to the growing end of a glycan chain, enzymes located in the cytoplasmic membrane catalyze the cross-linking of the peptide chains. Cross-linking of the cell wall peptidoglycan renders it insoluble and rigid, and β-lactam antibiotics inhibit the cross-linking reaction (Fig. 95.5). In 1965, Tipper and Strominger proposed that penicillin was a substrate analogue of the D-alanyl-D-alanine carboxyl terminus of the pentapeptide, and that penicillin bound to the transpeptidase enzymes that cross-link the peptidoglycan, thereby blocking their activity.[11] The hallmark of this proposal was that during the cross-linking reaction the transpeptidase enzymes react with the D-alanyl-D-alanine moiety of the pentapeptide chain to form an acyl-enzyme covalent complex, resulting in the release of the carboxyl terminal D-alanine. An amino group from the glycine bridge of another peptide chain then displaces the enzyme and a transpeptide bond is formed between two peptide chains (Fig. 95.5). Penicillin and other β-lactam antibiotics exert their antimicrobial activity by virtue of their similarity to D-alanyl-D-alanine (Fig. 95.6). β-lactam antibiotics, which are mistaken for substrate by cell wall synthesizing enzymes, also react to form an acyl-enzyme intermediate. Because of the long life of the acyl-enzyme intermediate, the antibiotics effectively block the cross-linking of the cell wall by occupying the active sites of the transpeptidase enzymes (Fig. 95.7).

There are two penicillin-sensitive reactions, transpeptidation and carboxypeptidation, that are known to occur in Stage III of cell wall synthesis (Figs. 95.5, 95.7). As mentioned above, transpeptidation results in the exchange of the carboxyl terminal D-alanyl-D-alanine bond for an transpeptide bond between the penultimate D-alanine residue and the glycine bridge from another strand of peptidoglycan. The other reaction, carboxypeptidation, results in the formation of a tetrapeptide. The enzymes that catalyze these reactions are known as penicillin-binding proteins or PBPs. The blockade of cell wall synthesis by β-lactam antibiotics is thought to activate enzymes known as autolysins that degrade the peptidoglycan. These autolysins hydrolyze the peptidoglycan and result in the eventual lysis of the bacterium.

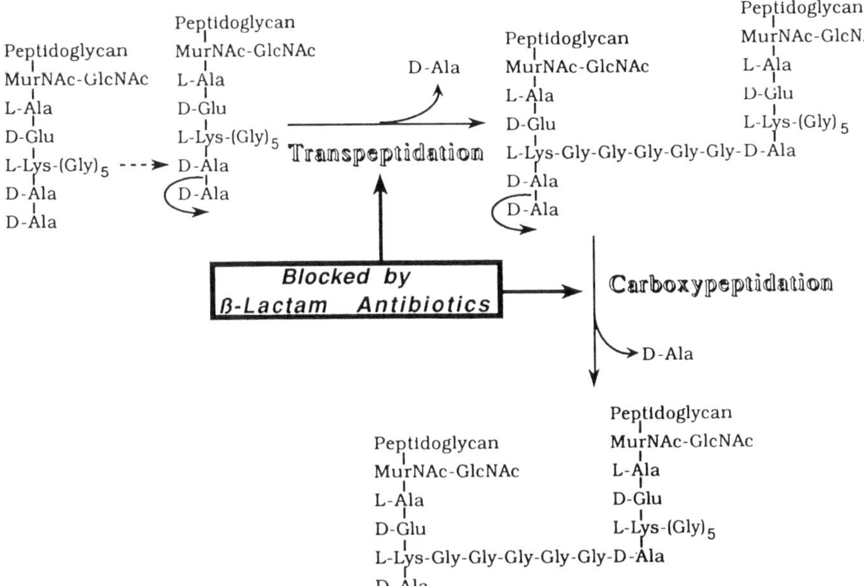

Figure 95.5 Inhibition of Stage III of cell wall synthesis by β-lactam antibiotics. The two reactions of Stage III synthesis are inhibited by β-lactam antibiotics. Transpeptidation is the cross-linking of two peptide chains from adjacent glycan strands. In the process, the ultimate D-alanine residue is replaced with glycine to form a cross-link. In carboxypeptidation, the ultimate D-alanine residue is hydrolyzed from the pentapeptide chain. (Modified from Strominger et al. [48]).

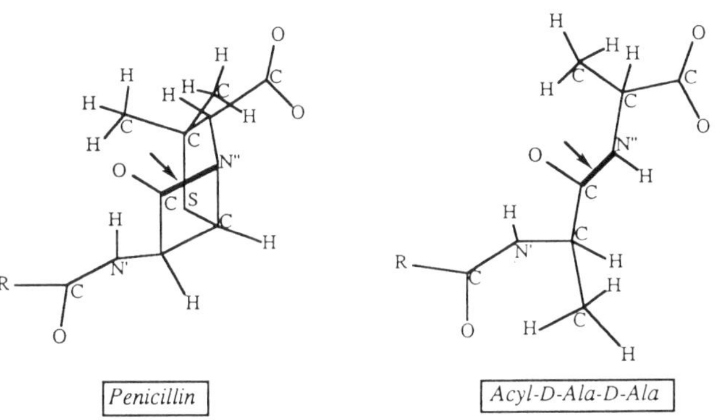

Figure 95.6 Similarity of penicillin and acyl-D-ala-D-ala. Dreiding stereomodels of penicillin (left) and the carboxyl terminal acyl-D-ala-D-ala of the pentapeptide chain (right). The arrows designate the β-lactam bond in penicillin and the D-alanyl-D-alanine peptide bond, respectively. (From Strominger et al.[48])

The Targets of β-Lactam Antibiotics

The study of penicillin-binding proteins has greatly increased our understanding of the mechanism of action of β-lactam antibiotics. PBPs are found in the cytoplasmic membrane of every bacterial species examined to date, although the total number of PBPs and their sizes may vary. The PBPs of *Escherichia coli* are the best studied, and most of what we know about the functions of PBPs has been determined in this organism. Because penicillin binds covalently, individual PBPs can be detected by incubation of cell membranes with radioactive penicillin G, followed by separation of the protein constituents on polyacrylamide gels and subsequent fluorography.[12] In *E. coli,* there are at least seven PBPs detected in this manner (Fig. 95.8). Using a combination of genetic analysis, in which temperature-sensitive mutations in specific PBPs produce morphologic changes of the bacteria at the restrictive temperature, and biochemical analysis, in which morphologic changes elicited by particular β-lactam antibiotics were correlated with their binding to specific PBPs, the role of these proteins in cell growth has been ascertained. This type of analysis also has determined that the high molecular weight PBPs, PBPs 1A/1B, 2, and 3, are essential for cell viability, whereas the low molecular weight PBPs, PBPs 4, 5, and 6, are not essential by themselves. The roles of each specific PBP in the maintenance of normal cell morphology and viability, which include cell elongation, cell shape, and cell division, are shown in Figure 95.8.

Inhibition of both PBPs 1A and 1B leads to rapid cell lysis; thus, these PBPs are believed to be involved in cell elongation and probably catalyze the majority of cell wall synthesis in this organism.[13,14] Inhibition of PBP 2 leads to the formation of large, spherical cells (instead of the normal rod shape),[15] and inhibition of PBP 3 results in filamentation, in which cells cannot separate from one another during cell division.[16] Interestingly, at least some of the high molecular weight PBPs, especially PBP 1B, are known to catalyze the penicillin-insensitive reaction of transglycosylation[17–19] (this is the same step that is inhibited by vancomycin; see Fig. 95.4). Thus, these high molecular weight enzymes are bifunctional and carry out both reactions of

Figure 95.7 Mechanism of penicillin inhibition of cell wall synthesis. Penicillin-binding proteins (PBP-OH) react with acyl-D-ala-D-ala to form a reactive acyl-enzyme intermediate (top), which can then react with the amino group from another peptide chain to yield a cross-link (transpeptidation) or with water to yield a tetrapeptide (carboxypeptidation). The reaction of penicillin with a PBP (bottom) leads to the accumulation of a stable acyl-enzyme complex that inactivates the PBP, whereas β-lactamases (BLA-OH) efficiently hydrolyze the acyl-enzyme complex. This last reaction opens the β-lactam ring of the antibiotic and destroys its antimicrobial activity. (Adapted from Waxman and Strominger[49])

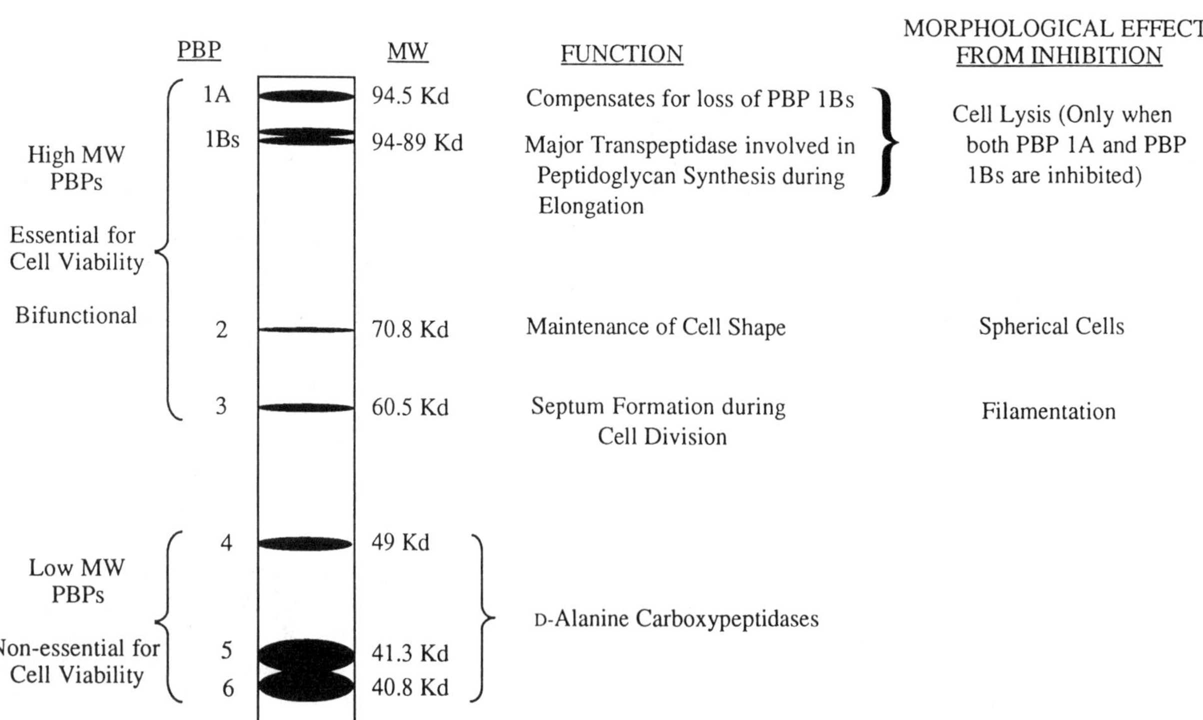

Figure 95.8 The penicillin-binding proteins of *E. coli*. This schematic illustrates the relative amounts of the seven PBPs in *E. coli* membranes and their functions in cell morphology and viability. (Compiled in part from the data of Spratt[12])

cell wall synthesis. PBP 4 is thought to catalyze either D-alanine carboxypeptidase activity or a secondary transpeptidation reaction (further cross-linking during maturation of the cell wall) in vivo,[20,21] whereas PBPs 5 and 6 are known to catalyze D-alanine carboxypeptidase activity both in vivo and in vitro.[22,23] It was initially believed that this activity serves to limit the amount of cross-linking of the growing cell, since the resulting tetrapeptide is no longer able to react with PBPs. However, recent evidence in *E. coli* suggests that D-alanine carboxypeptidase activity is necessary for the subsequent production of tripeptide chains (pentapeptide chains lacking D-ala-D-ala) that appear to be preferentially utilized as peptide acceptors during cell division.[24]

The efficacy of a particular β-lactam antibiotic in inhibiting the growth of an organism in vitro depends on several properties. In gram-positive bacteria, the antibacterial effect depends on the affinity of that antibiotic for the essential PBPs of that organism, since the cell wall peptidoglycan offers no resistance to the diffusion of small molecules. In gram-negative bacteria, the antibiotic efficacy also depends on the ability of the antibiotic to diffuse through pores in the outer membrane and reach its targets (PBPs) in the periplasmic space. The contribution of outer membrane diffusion in determining antibiotic efficacy is underscored by the example of penicillin G and ampicillin in the inhibition of growth of *E. coli.* Although penicillin G is known to have a high affinity for all the essential PBPs of *E. coli,* it is clinically ineffective in the treatment of *E. coli* infections (MIC = 16 μg/ml). The addition of an amino group in the side-chain of penicillin to form ampicillin (see Table 95.1) has virtually no effect on its affinity for the essential PBPs of *E. coli,* but it lowers the MIC more than fourfold (MIC = 3.2 μg/ml), making ampicillin an effective antibiotic for the treatment of *E. coli* urinary tract infections. The increased antibacterial effectiveness of ampicillin is due to the increased diffusion of ampicillin through the pores in the outer membrane to reach the PBP targets. The increased diffusion is correlated with the increase in the hydrophilic character of the antibiotic due to the addition of a positively charged amino group.

Mechanisms of Resistance

The antibacterial action of β-lactam antibiotics in all bacteria depends on the presence or absence of resistance. Bacteria have evolved several mechanisms to become resistant to the action of β-lactam antibiotics, and these ultimately can lead to clinical failure in the treatment of certain infections. Resistance to β-lactam antibiotics (and all other antibiotics) is a major problem in clinical settings worldwide, and is especially prevalent in hospitals. Every year, more and more organisms are isolated that have become resistant to β-lactam antibiotics. The major cause of this resistance is due to the production of β-lactamase (discussed below) that inactivates the drug, but recently new mechanisms of resistance have emerged that signals the need to observe prudent medical guidelines in the use of these antibiotics and for physicians to be aware of the problems of resistance. A striking example of the ability of bacteria to become resistant to β-lactam antibiotics is shown in Table 95.3, which indicates the onset of resistance to penicillin G and other β-lactam antibiotics by strains of *Staphylococcus aureus.*

It is clear from this table that bacterial resistance to antibiotics is a growing trend that is occurring with increasing frequency. Even more alarming is the realization that methicillin-resistant *S. aureus* are not only resistant to all β-lactam antibiotics currently in clinical use, but that there is significant resistance to other classes of antibiotics as well.[25] It is likely that resistance to β-lactam antibiotics will continue to be a major clinical problem in the future; therefore, it is important to understand the various ways in which bacteria have become resistant to these drugs. Five different mechanisms have been described for resistance to β-lactam antibiotics; these mechanisms are discussed in detail below. A schematic depicting the different mechanisms of resistance in both gram-negative and gram-positive bacteria is shown in Figure 95.9.

Table 95.3 The Onset of Resistance in β-Lactam Antibiotics by *Staphylococcus Aurues*

Resistance to Penicillin and Methicillin by Strains of *Staphylococcus Aureus*	
Year	**Resistance in *Staphylococcus Aureus***
1940	~100% of *S. aureus* susceptible to penicillin
1944	First description of β-lactamase in *S. aureus*
1951	73% of nosocomial *S. aureus* isolates resistant to penicillin
1967	82–84% of total *S. aureus* isolates (both community and nosocomial) resistant to penicillin. First report of nosocomial methicillin-resistant *S. aureus* (MRSA) in US
1981–93	MRSA widely disseminated

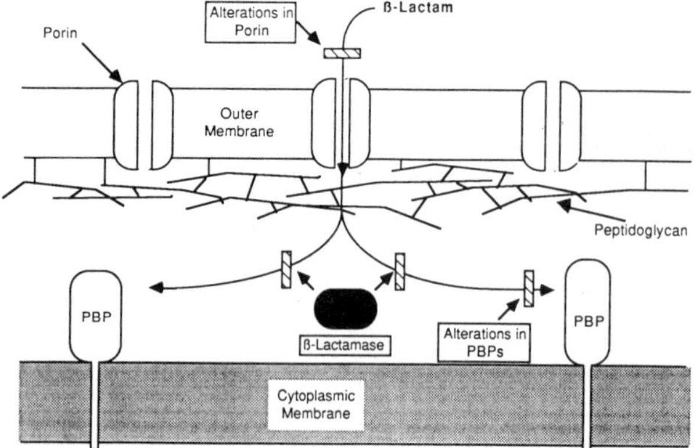

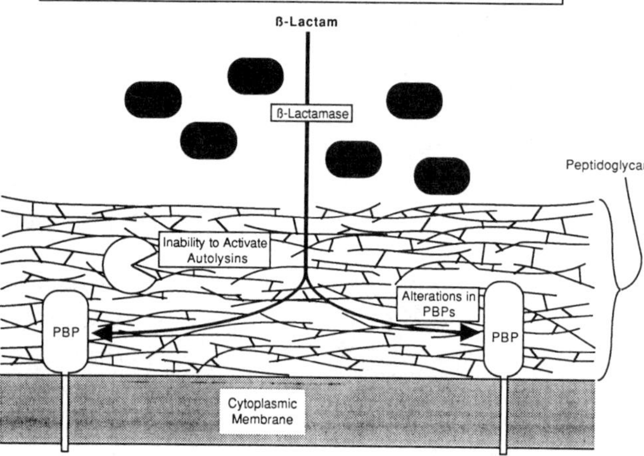

Figure 95.9 The modes of resistance in gram-negative and gram-positive bacteria. The various mechanisms by which bacteria become resistant to β-lactam antibiotics in each class of bacteria are illustrated. Note that in gram-negative bacteria, the β-lactam antibiotic must cross the outer membrane through proteins called porins, which can present a formidable barrier to the diffusion of the drug to reach the PBPs. The effectiveness of an antibiotic for gram-negative bacteria depends upon: (1) its ability to diffuse across the outer membrane; (2) the presence of a β-lactamase that can hydrolyze the β-lactam bond; (3) its affinity for the essential PBPs of the organism. There is no diffusional barrier in gram-positive bacteria, and thus in these organisms the efficacy of an antibiotic depends on: (1) the presence of a β-lactamase that can hydrolyze the drug; (2) the affinity of that antibiotic for the essential PBPs of the organism; (3) whether the autolysins of the organism are activated.

(1) Production of a β-Lactamase

By far the most common form of resistance is the production of an enzyme called a β-lactamase, which hydrolyzes the β-lactam bond of β-lactam antibiotics and renders the drug inactive. Much like the penicillin-binding proteins, β-lactamases react with β-lactam antibiotics to form an acyl-enzyme complex; however, this complex is rapidly hydrolyzed by the addition of water to yield free enzyme and hydrolyzed antibiotic (see Fig. 95.7). β-lactamases are thought to have evolved from the low molecular weight penicillin-binding proteins, since their three-dimensional structures are very similar.[26,27] There are a multitude of characterized β-lactamases, each with different activities on various β-lactam antibiotics.[28,29] For example, the well-known TEM-1 β-lactamase from *E. coli* hydrolyzes the β-lactamase-sensitive penicillins without displaying much activity toward cephalosporins. In contrast, the β-lactamase produced by *Enterobacter cloacae* has high activity toward cephalosporins. An alarming trend in resistance to cephalosporins is the appearance of a novel β-lactamase that hydrolyzes previously β-lactamase-resistant cephalosporins,[30] as well as the mutation of existing β-lactamases that extend their activity to include previously β-lactamase-resistant antibiotics. For example, two-point mutations in a β-lactamase that normally hydrolyzes only penicillins greatly increases the hydrolysis of several third-generation cephalosporins.[31]

β-lactamase-producing strains are often found in *Staphylococcus aureus, Haemophilus influenzae, Neisseria gonorrhoeae,* and most gram-negative enteric rods. Resistance to β-lactam antibiotics due to the production of a β-lactamase can be either chromosomally-mediated or plasmid-mediated; plasmid-mediated resistance can be transferred to other organisms by R-factors.[32] In gram-positive bacteria, the β-lactamase is transported out of the cytoplasm into the extracellular medium. Because this results in a significant dilution, β-lactamases from these organisms have a relatively high affinity for their target antibiotics and generally are produced in large amounts. In gram-negative bacteria, the outer membrane presents a barrier to large molecules, and the β-lactamase is confined to the periplasmic space (the space between the inner and outer membranes). This localization of the β-lactamase results in a high local concentration in the region where β-lactam antibiotics exert their action. The production of β-lactamases can either be constitutive or inducible; the production of these latter β-lactamases can be induced by the presence of many (but not all) β-lactam antibiotics. This induction is thought to require a cell surface receptor that is very similar to a PBP; this receptor covalently binds antibiotic and triggers an intracellular response that results in the rapid production of β-lactamase.[33]

(2) Mutations that Affect Outer Membrane Permeability

In gram-negative bacteria, proteins called porins form hydrophilic channels or pores in the outer membrane through which small substances can diffuse (including β-lactam antibiotics). Mutations in porins can reduce the permeability of a normally efficacious antibiotic, which leads to a higher level of resistance, since β-lactam antibiotics must diffuse into the periplasmic space to exert their action by binding to the PBPs.[34] These mutations often can be observed in conjunction with a β-lactamase, in which case reasonable levels of resistance can be achieved, even when the β-lactamase has a reduced affinity for the antibiotic. This is due to the interplay of the diffusion of the antibiotic across the outer membrane and the efficiency of the β-lactamase.

(3) The Inability to Activate Autolytic Enzymes

As mentioned previously, the inhibition of peptidoglycan synthesis is thought to activate autolysins that degrade the existing peptidoglycan.[35] Isolates from some species, such as *Staphylococcus, Streptococcus,* and *Listeria,* have lost the ability to activate these enzymes, and thus are tolerant to β-lactam therapy. These strains are inhibited but not killed, and can grow back following the cessation of β-lactam treatment.

(4) Mutations in PBPs that Lower Their Affinity for β-Lactam Antibiotics

Another widespread mechanism in the resistance to β-lactam antibiotics is the production of altered forms of PBPs. These new PBPs can be either entirely new gene products not present in susceptible bacteria, or they can arise through mutation or transformation/recombination, which subtly remodel the β-lactam binding sites of essential PBPs to result in lower affinities for β-lactam antibiotics. Methicillin-resistant *Staphylococcus aureus* (MRSA) strains, for example, have acquired a new PBP, PBP 2′, that displays very low affinity for virtually all β-lactam antibiotics, and is responsible for at least part of the resistance of this strain.[36] However, several other gene products also contribute to the resistance in this organism in an undetermined manner. In contrast, chromosomally-mediated resistant *Neisseria gonorrhoeae* or CMRNG have alterations in both essential PBPs and changes in their outer membrane permeability that results in a 1000-fold decrease in their sensitivity to penicillin.[37] The alterations in essential PBPs in *Neisseria meningitidis* and *N. gonorrhoeae* is a result of the horizontal transfer of genes from related Neisseria species that are incorporated by transformation and recombination.[38,39] In *Streptococcus pneumoniae,* resistant strains have been isolated that display a large increase in penicillin resistance due to multiple mutations in the sequences of essential PBPs,[40] which again appear to be the result of horizontal transfer.[41] These changes can cause a 200-fold decrease in the affinity of the antibiotic for an altered PBP. It should be noted that these changes must still preserve the substrate-binding site of the PBP, which must function in cell wall synthesis for the cell to survive.

(5) The Lack of Cell Walls or Metabolically Inactive Cells

Under certain conditions, cells can exist as spheroplasts (or L forms) that lack cells walls.[42] This is caused not by the acquisition or alteration of genetic information, but occurs when cells are challenged with β-lactam antibiotics in a region of high osmolarity (which prevents cell lysis by osmotic pressure). These forms can persist for some time, and the bacteria can grow back (with resynthesis of the cell wall) following the removal of antibiotic. Once the cells begin to grow again, they become susceptible to the antibiotic. Other bacteria, such as *Mycoplasma,* can exist in a metabolically inactive state for extended periods, and during that time are refractory to β-lactam antibiotic therapy.

β-*Lactamase Inhibitors*

As discussed above, the presence of a β-lactamase that hydrolyzes susceptible antibiotics is the major clinical form of resistance. The isolation of a naturally occurring β-lactamase inhibitor, clavulanic acid, from *Streptomyces clavuligerus* was a major step in the formulation of new antibiotic combinations that extend the spectrum of action of the parent antibiotic. Clavulanic acid has a β-lactam ring structure (Fig. 95.10) very similar to penicillins, but has poor antibacterial activity; it is, however, a very potent inhibitor of certain types of β-lactamases. Another β-lactamase inhibitor currently in use is sulbactam (Fig. 95.10). Important structural properties of clavulanic acid appear to be an oxygen atom at the usual position of the sulfur atom in penicillin and the ability to form a reactive conjugated intermediate during the enzymatic reaction. The mechanism of β-lactamase inhibition by clavulanic acid is shown in Figure 95.11, and has been worked out by Jeremy Knowles and his colleagues.[43]

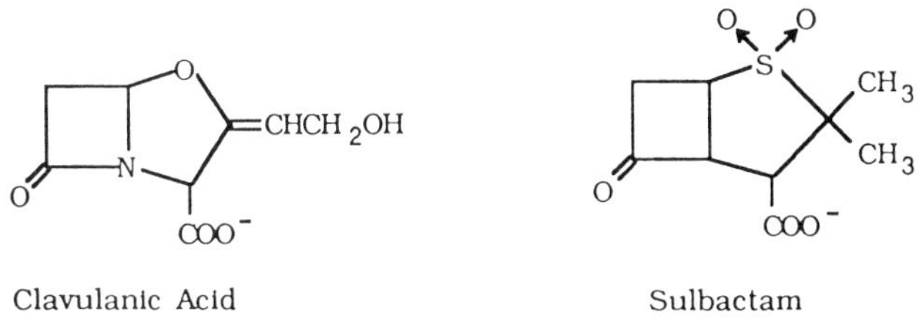

Clavulanic Acid — Sulbactam

Figure 95.10 Inhibitors of β-lactamases. The structure of clavulanic acid and sulbactam are shown. Both of these compounds are β-lactam antibiotics with very poor antibacterial activity, but are potent inhibitors of certain types of β-lactamases.

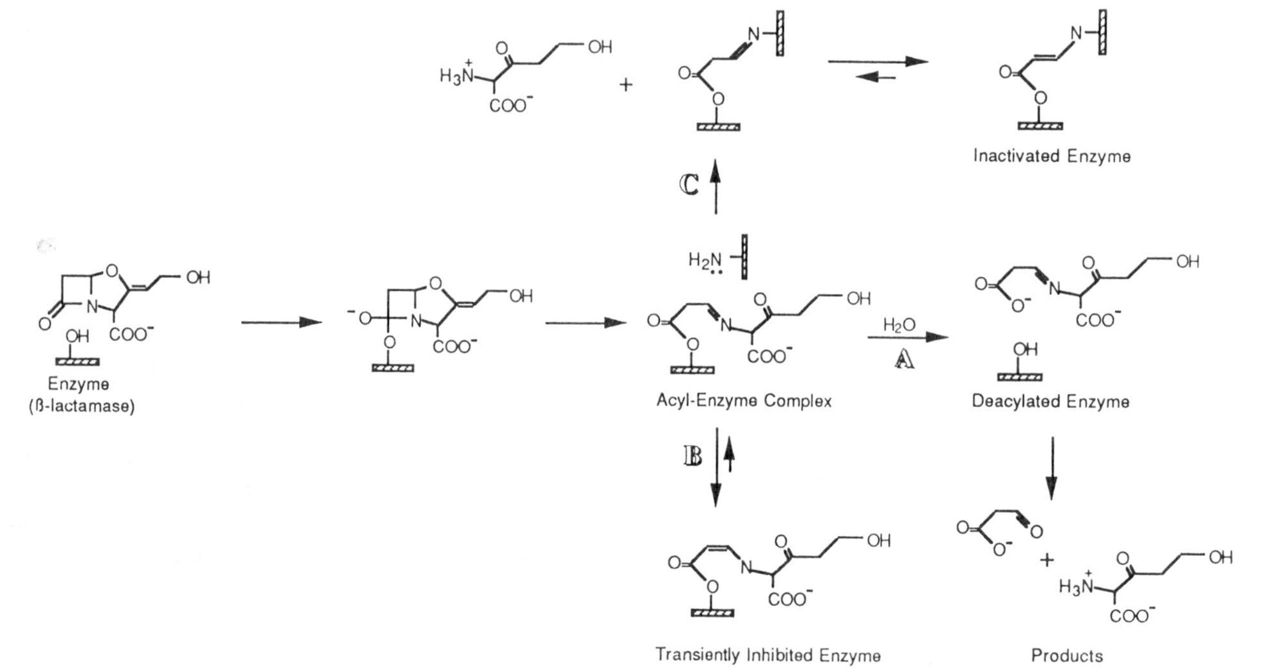

Figure 95.11 The mechanism of inhibition of β-lactamase by clavulanic acid. Upon reaction with β-lactamase, the acyl enzyme complex can go in one of three directions. In pathway A, the complex can undergo deacylation, which regenerates free enzyme and hydrolysis products. The complex can also undergo rearrangement (pathway B) to a transiently inhibited enzyme, or it can undergo a second modification (pathway C) to result in an irreversibly inactivated enzyme. Any free enzyme generated by pathway A will react further with the inhibitor until all molecules are inactivated. (Adapted from Charnas and Knowles[43])

Clavulanic acid interacts with the β-lactamase to form an acyl-enzyme complex; although some of this complex is hydrolyzed to free the enzyme (Pathway A), the rest of the complex can follow one of two reaction pathways, both of which result in inhibition. In the first pathway, the rearrangement of the acyl-enzyme results in a transiently inhibited enzyme (Pathway B), whereas in the second pathway (Pathway C) the attack of an active site amino group on the complex results in further covalent modification and an irreversibly inactivated enzyme. The free enzyme formed by hydrolysis of the complex reacts with another molecule of the inhibitor and undergoes the same cycle; eventually, all the β-lactamase molecules are inactivated. Both of these inhibitors have been combined with β-lactamase-susceptible antibiotics to extend their spectrum of action. Some examples of these combinations are Augmentin (amoxicillin + clavulanic acid), Timentin (ticarcillin + clavulanic acid), and Unasyn (ampicillin + sulbactam).

Carbapenems

Carbapenems are β-lactam antibiotics with some unique chemical and structural features. Imipenem is the major clinical antibiotic in this class, and this drug displays the broadest spectrum of antibacterial action of all currently available β-lactam antibiotics. It is considered β-lactamase-resistant, although the occurrence of β-lactamases that hydrolyze the antibiotic have been noted.[44] An interesting mechanism of resistance occurs in the treatment of certain strains of *Pseudomonas aeruginosa*. These strains become resistant during therapy by the alteration of an outer membrane channel that blocks the diffusion of the antibiotic into the periplasm.[45] The ability of other β-lactam antibiotics to inhibit these strains is unaffected, however, which suggests that imipenem diffuses through a different channel than other β-lactam antibiotics. During the initial trials of imipenem, it was noted that the antibiotic was hydrolyzed by an enzyme called dihydropeptidase II present in renal brush border cells. To prevent this hydrolysis, an inhibitor of dihydropeptidase II, cilastin, was synthesized; this compound is structurally similar to β-lactam antibiotics but possesses no antibacterial activity. Imipenem is now marketed as a mixture of cilastin and imipenem (Primaxin).

Therapeutic Uses and Limitations

The penicillins and cephalosporins are the most commonly prescribed antibiotic agents worldwide.

Since the original development of penicillin, several trends have emerged that delineate the utilization and limitations of these agents. The key issues regarding therapeutic use are as follows:

Spectrum of Action

What bacteria are killed by these antibiotics? Often the physician uses clinical information, laboratory data, and intuition to anticipate pathogens responsible for infection. The antibacterial agent or combination of agents must kill offending pathogens in vitro and have demonstrated efficacy in vivo. The latter point is important since there are many examples (e.g., treatment of infection with *Salmonella typhi*) in which antibiotics that might be predicted to be effective based on their activity in vitro have limited success in vivo.

Clinical Pharmacology

Absorption and peak levels in tissue often determine the usefulness of some antibacterial agents. For example, the ability of some of the newer cephalosporins to penetrate the CNS blood brain barrier has had a dramatic effect on the treatment of meningitis and other CNS infection.[48] Conversely, an important issue to emerge over the last few years focuses on the limitations of antibiotic pharmacokinetics in predicting clinical efficacy. There is very little information available that predicts the minimal frequency with which antibiotics can be administered and still be effective. A complex interaction involving the antibiotic and host defenses and the susceptible pathogen determines this outcome.

Historically, agents were used on a dosing schedule entirely determined by their half-life, and thus more frequent doses were used for antibiotics with very short half-lives. Because the cost of therapy has become an important issue, infrequency of dosing (a reductionist approach) has been emphasized. Initially, antibiotic agents with relatively long half-lives were explored for their usage once or twice each day. Since these drugs proved effective in such dosing schedules, antibiotics with shorter half-lives were also tried on similar dosing schedules, and some of these antibiotics were demonstrated to be effective at a low dosing schedule. Several possible explanations for the success of short half-life drugs in reduced frequency dosing schedules have been offered: (1) the partial damage to the bacterial cell wall renders them more susceptible to subsequent doses of antibiotics (the postantibiotic effect); (2) host defenses contribute sufficiently to the erradication of the infection; or (3) metabolic derivatives of the β-lactam compounds (e.g., the desacetyl derivative of cefotaxime) are active against bacteria. Any combination of these hypotheses is also plausible.

Similar issues surround the actual concentration of the drug to be used. A correlation can be made between in vitro susceptibility of the bacteria and the peak serum concentration achieved by a certain antibiotic dosage. Historically, antibiotics were used in concentrations that often greatly exceeded the minimal concentration predicted to be therapeutic. In recent years not only has the dosage frequency been reduced, but the concentrations of drugs used have decreased as well.

Penicillins and cephalosporins compare favorably with respect to efficacy and low side-effect profiles. Consequently, some favor double lactam therapy over a combination of a penicillin or cephalosporin with an aminoglycoside in the treatment of certain infections. This is surprising when one considers that the class of antibiotics works by the same mechanism and synergy would not be expected.

Undesirable Effects of β-Lactam Antibiotics

Although penicillin and cephalosporin antibiotics are among the safest therapeutic agents available, a wide array of side-effects (some severe) have been demonstrated.[49] Such effects often will determine the physician's choice of agents and must be carefully considered. A summary of the major side-effects observed with penicillin and cephalosporin agents is shown in Table 95.4. In general, the most serious reaction encountered is anaphylaxis. This reaction is more com-

Table 95.4 Potential Side Effects of Cephalosporins and Penicillins

Allergic
Anaphylaxis
Rash, including dermolysis
Fever
Hematologic
Anemia (Coombs positive or hemolytic)
Thrombocytopenia
Thrombocytosis
Coagulopathy
Renal
Interstitial nephritis
Gastrointestinal
Nausea and vomiting
Diarrhea, including pseudomembranous colitis
Elevations in liver enzymes
Local
Phlebitis

mon with penicillins than cephalosporins; the incidence is estimated to be two per 100,000 and the subsequent fatality rate to be one in 2000 among those so affected. Unfortunately, the patient's history of allergy is not highly predictive, and most fatalities from anaphylaxis occur in patients with no prior history of penicillin allergy.[50] Penicillins, perhaps more that cephalosporins, also frequently cause skin reactions that range from a mild self-limited rash to a generalized and sometimes fatal dermolysis.[51] Peculiarly, when patients with Epstein-Barr infection are administered ampicillin, almost all develop a papillary skin rash.

Other side-effects include liver enzyme abnormalities, thrombocytosis, thrombocytopenia, hemolytic anemia, and clinically significant coagulopathy. Cephalosporin-induced coagulopathy is a specific entity that has received a great deal of attention. Bacterial production of vitamin K is adversely affected by antibiotics, and it is impossible to produce vitamin K deficiency in voluntary subjects without concomitant treatment with antibiotics. In addition, some cephalosporins, such as cefotetan and cefoperazone, possess a methylthiotetrazole side-chain that interferes with prothrombin formation and can lead to clinical bleeding.[52] Supplemental vitamin K therapy can prevent this undesirable side-effect. Coagulopathy occurs more frequently and is more severe in patients with renal failure and elevated creatinine. Disulfiram-like reactions to alcohol have been reported with cephalosporins containing a methylthiotetrazole side-chain. The route of antibiotic elimination also has an impact on side-effects. Penicillins excreted renally can produce interstitial nephritis; methicillin has been most associated with this side-effect, and consequently is now rarely used.

Another common side-effect of antibiotic therapy with all penicillins and cephalosporins is diarrhea. A specific type of diarrhea produced by toxic from *C. difficile*, pseudomembraneous colitis, can also be a result of therapy with these agents. Drugs such as ceftriaxone and cefoperazone are excreted via the gallbladder and thus are more commonly associated with diarrhea than are the other cephalosporins. A syndrome mimicking cholecystitis has also been described with ceftriaxone. However, these symptoms abate when the antibiotic is discontinued. Sludging of bile has been observed in some children receiving ceftriaxone therapy.[53]

All β-lactam antibiotics, with the exceptions of nafcillin, ceftriaxone, and cefaperazone, are excreted in the urine. Consequently, care must be taken to adjust the dosing schedule properly in patients with renal failure. Elevated levels of penicillin G and ampicillin, which can be secondary to impaired elimination, are associated with seizures, but this is uncommon. Even very large doses of most cephalosporins and penicillins are well tolerated, and serious consequences from overdose are rarely encountered, even in renal failure. Although any β-lactam antibiotic can be linked to seizures, imipenem has been implicated more frequently. Seizures most often occur in patients with renal insufficiency or when the antibiotic is used at a high dose.

Pharmacokinetics

Oral absorption of β-lactam antibiotics varies widely with the particular agent and preparation. For example, Penicillin G is poorly absorbed orally, but a similar preparation (Penicillin V) is appropriate for oral administration because it is acid-resistant. Penicillin G can be administered IM to provide therapeutic blood levels for three to four weeks. Thus, one injection can be used to treat infections such as streptococcal pharyngitis or syphilis.

Once administered, penicillins and cephalosporins have a wide volume of distribution and penetrate most body cavities. However, certain compartments, such as the CSF, the eye, and the prostate, are penetrated by penicillins only in the presence of inflammation. In the intravascular space, penicillins reversibly bind to albumin, and only the unbound form is active. The half-lives of some penicillins may be as short as one-half hour owing to rapid elimination through the kidneys. To prolong the half-life of a penicillin or cephalosporin, probenecid may be administered concomitantly. Probenecid acts by blocking excretion in renal tubular cells and also by displacing a portion of the antibiotic from its albumin binding sites. The half-lives of cephalosporins tend to be longer than those of the penicillins. The $t_{1/2}$ varies from 0.6 hours for cephalothin to eight hours for ceftriaxone. As mentioned earlier, nafcillin, ceftriaxone, and cefoperazone are the only β-lactam antibiotics excreted via hepatic elimination. Penicillin and cephalosporin antibiotic levels are not routinely measured clinically because the therapeutic dose greatly exceeds the minimal dose required to cure infection.[54,55,56]

Clinical Usage of β-Lactam Antibiotics

Penicillins

Even though penicillin G has a limited spectrum of activity and resistance has developed in many pathogens, it is still the drug of choice for many infections. It is widely recommended to treat infections due to streptococci, susceptible staphylococci, *Pasteurella multocida, Neisseria meningiditis, Bacillus anthracis, Clostridium tetani,* and *perfringens, Spirillum minus, Streptobacillus moniliformis, Erysipelotrix rhysiopatheae,* and some treponemas, such as those causing syphilis, leptospirosis, and yaws.[57] As mentioned earlier, *Staphylococcus aureus* has developed resistance at a rapid rate (see Table 95.3). Similar experience has occurred with coagulase-negative staphylococci and *Neisseria gonorrhoeae.* Although penicillin has long been the gold standard for the treatment of infections with *Streptococcus pneumoniae,* within the past several years decreased sensitivity has been reported. Intermediate susceptibility and outright resistance has developed.[58] Penicillin G has very poor activity against aerobic gram-negative rods, including *Pseudomonas aeruginosa.*

The development of penicillins resistant to the β-lactamases of *Staphylococcus aureus* was the next event in the penicillin family. These antibiotics include methicillin, dicloxacillan, and nafcillin. Among these agents methicillin is the prototype drug; it was first introduced in the early 1960s to combat staphylococci, but is rarely used now because of its association with interstitial nephritis. These agents are effective against most staphylococci and are useful alone or in combination with other antimicrobials to treat infections commonly caused by *Staphylococcus aureus*, but not against MRSA. Nafcillin and methicillin are administered IV; only oxacillin is available as an oral preparation.

The next class of penicillins to emerge were the aminopenicillins, which are broader spectrum agents with activity against many aerobic gram-negative rods, such as *Escherichia coli, Haemophilus influenza, Proteus mirabilis, Salmonella* and *Shigella* species. These agents are also clinically useful against enterococcus and streptococcus. Uncomplicated urinary tract infections often are treated with aminopenicillins. Amoxicillin and ampicillin are the prototype drugs and most widely used. Unlike the β-lactamase-resistant penicillins, these agents preserve the efficacy of penicillin G against anaerobes. Unfortunately, many aerobic gram-negative rods originally sensitive to these agents now are inhibited marginally or not at all. It is necessary to evaluate each susceptibility profile individually to ensure adequate bacteria coverage. For instance, only about one quarter of the *Haemophilus* species currently isolated from childhood infections in the US are sensitive to these agents; this is usually the result of the production of a β-lactamase. Ampicillin and amoxicillin have both IV and oral forms; however, the superb oral absorption of amoxicillin makes it preferable to oral ampicillin in just about all infections but intestinal shigellosis, where the antibacterial effect of the unabsorbed ampicillin in the intestinal lumen is beneficial. Penetration of ampicillin into the CSF is excellent, and ampicillin is the drug of choice in the treatment of meningitis due to *Listeria monocytogenes*.

The most recent penicillin agents, the so-called "third generation penicillins," include ticarcillin, mezlocillin, piperacillin, carbenicillin, and azlocillin. These antibiotics are even broader in spectrum than any of the previously discussed penicillins, and possess activity against anaerobic bacteria including *Bacteroides fragilis* and many aerobic gram-negative rods including *Pseudomonas aeruginosa, Enterobacter*, indole-positive *Proteus*, and *Morganella*. These penicillins are not effective against β-lactamase-producing *Staphylococcus aureus* or MRSA. Individual agents within the group have superior action against certain pathogens. Piperacillin and azlocillin are most active against *Pseudomonas*, and mezlocillin and piperacillin are most active against enteric species such as *Proteus, Enterobacter*, and *Klebsiella*. Unfortunately, aerobic gram-negative rods can acquire resistance to these penicillin agents during therapy in vivo, which limits their usefulness as single agents.[59]

Penicillins and β-Lactamase Inhibitors

The production of different β-lactamases by anaerobic organisms, staphylococci and gram-negative rods has limited the efficacy of the penicillins. A recent approach to overcoming this problem has been development of preparations that include a β-lactam antibiotic in combination with a β-lactamase inhibitor such as clavulanic acid, sulbactam, or tazobactam (Fig. 95.10). Combination drugs that include β-lactamase inhibitors have excellent activity against methicillin-sensitive staphylococci, *Haemophilus influenza, Klebsiella, Escherichia*, and all anaerobic organisms including *Bacteroides* species. These drugs are useful in the treatment of upper and lower respiratory tract infections, skin and soft tissue infections, urinary tract infections, and certain mixed infections. However, efficacy in many serious infections such as *Staphylococcus aureus* endocarditis or osteomyelitis has not been established. The use of β-lactamase inhibitors lowers the minimal concentration of the β-lactam antibiotic required to kill the organism. Currently available agents use fixed dosages of these inhibitors.[60,61]

Cephalosporins

The development of cephalosporins has resembled the development of penicillins with respect to some key features: the newer agents are more specialized or broader in spectrum and require less frequent administration. For example, ceftriaxone can be administered once daily and still provide adequate therapy for most infections. Cephalosporins are very effective against aerobic gram-negative rods, but they are not active against *Enterococcus* or MRSA. Cephalosporins are an alternative to aminoglycosides when single agent therapy is required for infections with aerobic gram-negative bacilli.

First-Generation Cephalosporins

Cefazolin, the prototype of the first-generation cephalosporins, was among the first truly broad-spectrum antibiotic agents available; it is effective against methicillin-susceptible staphylococci, oral anaerobic organisms, and many aerobic gram-negative rods, including indole-negative *Proteus, Klebsiella*, and *Escherichia*. Cefazolin is effective as a single agent for a wide variety of infections, and it is unusual for gram-negative bacteria to acquire resistance during therapy. First-generation cephalosporins are widely used for preoperative surgical prophylaxis to prevent wound infections, where activity against *Staphylococcus aureus* is of great importance. Other first-generation cephalosporins include cephradrine and cephapirin. Oral preparations include cephradrine; all others mentioned above are IV preparations.[62] First-generation cephalosporins are older agents; many newer cephalosporins have a much broader spectrum of activity than the first-generation agents. However, it should be emphasized that broader spectrum is not necessarily better. First-generation cephalosporins are still useful in skin and soft tissue infections and in urinary tract infections. When compared with other antibiotics, they are often a cost effective alternative.

Second-Generation Cephalosporins

Second-generation cephalosporins have significantly greater activity against aerobic gram-negative rods than first-generation cephalosporins. Two members of the class, cefoxitin and cefotetan, display excellent activity against anaerobes including *Bacteroides fragilis* subspecies. Thus, these two cephalosporins are useful in abdominal infections, pelvic inflammatory disease, aspiration pneumonia, and some soft tissue infections such as diabetic foot infections. Because of their activity against anaerobes, cefoxitin and cefotetan are also used for prophylaxis in pelvic and abdominal procedures, where anaerobic infections are possible sequelae.

Cefamandole is a second-generation cephalosporin also active against certain aerobic Gram-negative rods such as ampicillin-sensitive *Haemophilus influenza*, indole-positive *Proteus, Escherichia coli, Enterobacter*, and *Klebsiella*, while maintaining efficacy against gram-positive cocci comparable to first-generation cephalosporins. It exhibits inconsistent activity against ampicillin-resistant *Haemophilus influenza*. It was introduced in the early 1980s with an aggressive advertising campaign, but it is used less often now. Other agents are either less expensive or more effective in treating these infections.

Although other second-generation cephalosporins do not exhibit significant anaerobic activity, many have expanded activity against aerobic gram-negative rods when compared with first generation agents. For example, cefuroxime has excellent activity against β-lactamase-producing *Haemophilus influenza* that is resistant to ampicillin. Cefuroxime also has increased penetration of the blood-brain barrier, which makes it very useful in the treatment of meningitis caused by the major agents of childhood and adult meningitis, *Haemophilus influenza, Neisseria meningiditis*, and *Streptococcus pneumoniae*. However, it has been supplanted in the therapy of meningitis because of the superior activity of the third-generation cephalosporins (see below). Cefuroxime is still widely used in treatment of pneumonia, sinusitis, otitis, and bronchitis, and an oral preparation appropriate for outpatient therapy is available.[62] Cefaclor and loracarbef have a similar spectrum of activity, but are available only in oral preparations.

Third-Generation Cephalosporins

Third-generation cephalosporins in general have excellent gram-negative activity and much less activity against gram-positive organisms. However, some of these agents have good activity against gram-positive cocci such as streptococci and *S. aureus*. Thus, ceftazidime and cefoperazone have activity against *Pseudomonas aeruginosa*, whereas cefoperazone, cefotaxime, and ceftizoxime have moderate activity against *Staphylococcus aureus*. Ceftriaxone and cefotaxime have excellent activity against *Haemophilus influenza* and most *Streptococcus pneumoniae*. As a result, these agents are often used to treat meningitis and respiratory tract infections due to these pathogens.[63,64]

Unlike the penicillins, third-generation cephalosporins demonstrate stable activity against aerobic gram-negative rods, and resistance only occasionally develops during the course of therapy. Cefotaxime, ceftizoxime, ceftazidime, and cefoperazone are generally reserved for treatment of infections with aerobic gram-negative rods resistant to the usual therapy, which often occurs in institutional and nosocomial settings. Third-generation cephalosporins are not active against *Bacteroides* species. Cefotaxime, ceftriaxone and ceftazidime have good penetration into the CSF and are useful in the treatment of meningitis. They are drugs of choice in the treatment of meningitis—ceftazidime is used to treat meningitis due to susceptible aerobic gram-negative rods, Cefotaxime and ceftriaxone are also useful is the treatment of infections due to *Streptococcus pneumoniae, Haemophilis influenza, Haemophilus ducreyi*, and *Neisseria meningiditis*. Ceftriaxone has an eight-hour half-life that makes it suitable for once-a-day dosing. Ceftriaxone is also the drug of choice in infections caused by *Neisseria gonorrhoeae* because of widespread penicillin resistance due to β-lactamases or chromosomally-mediated alterations in PBPs and outer membrane permeability. Third-generation cephalosporins are costly drugs; because side-effects are low and efficacy may be comparable in certain situations (i.e., ceftriaxone or cefotaxime in the treatment of meningitis due to susceptible *Streptococcus pneumoniae*), the specific choice of an antibiotic will often depend on cost. Cefotaxime is usually cited as the most cost-effective third-generation cephalosporin.[63,64]

Cefixime and cefpodoxime are oral third-generation cephalosporins useful against infections caused by certain pathogens such as pneumococci, group A streptococci, *Moraxella catarrhalis, Haemophilus influenza, Neisseria gonorrhoeae* and many other aerobic gram-negative rods. These agents may be used to treat pharyngitis, otitis, and urinary tract infections. In addition, cefpodoxime has approval for treatment of skin and soft tissue infections; however, cost precludes widespread use of these drugs for usual outpatient therapy, since equally effective, less expensive alternatives are available. Cefixime and cefpodoxime may find a niche in single-dose oral treatment of uncomplicated cervicitis and urethritis due to β-lactamase-producing strains of *Neisseria gonorrhoeae*.

Cephalosporins and β-Lactamase Inhibitors

Although the cephalosporins are considerably more stable to β-lactamases than the penicillins, cephalosporinases are produced and the β-lactamase inhibitors may be clinically useful. It is also possible that sulbactam or a similar agent will be marketed independently, so that a physician might choose to use this agent in combination with any other antibiotic. However, it should be noted that not all β-lactamases are inhibited by these agents, and thus the use of these combinations will not always be successful in the advent of infections caused by β-lactamase-producing organisms.[60,61]

Monobactams

Aztreonam is the only monobactam presently commercially available. Like the penicillins and cephalosporins, aztreonam is bactericidal and is active only against aerobic gram-negative rods. Consequently, it has a spectrum similar to ceftazidime, but no activity against streptococci or staphylococci. The clearest indication for its use is in patients who require specific therapy for infections due to aerobic gram-negative rods and who have life-threatening anaphylactic reactions to penicillin.[65,66]

Carbapenems

Imipenem is the only currently approved carbapenem available in the US. It has the broadest spectrum of any antibiotic now available. Because it is approved for many indications, it can also be broadly misused. Such a potent drug is best reserved for those situations where it is really necessary to preclude development of resistance. The most practical uses of imipenem include treatment of serious nosocomial infections with organisms resistant to other drugs and as an alternative to combination therapy in mixed or multiple infections. In addition, it is valuable in therapy against *Acinetobacter* infections and in combination therapy for infections with *Pseudomonas aeruginosa*. Others have advocated its use as monotherapy for patients with febrile neutropenia. It is not active against MRSA.[65,66]

Summary

β-Lactam antibiotics remain very effective drugs in the treatment of bacterial infections. Their low toxicity and high efficacy have made them among the most heavily prescribed drugs in world. Their spectrum of action can vary from very narrow to the most powerful and broadest spectrum antibiotic agents available. The development of these agents has focused on their use as a single agent with minimal doses and as infrequently as possible. The strong selective pressure put on bacteria by the constant presence of antibiotics, especially in nosocomial settings, has brought about the emergence of different forms of resistance to these drugs. This resistance can be mediated by the production of a β-lactamase, by changes in the permeability of the outer membrane (for gram-negative organisms), and alterations in the targets of β-lactam antibiotics, PBPs. Although the production of β-lactamase is the most important clinical form of resistance, all these mechanisms can result in clinical failure of the antibiotic treatment. Thus, resistance to these agents is a serious public health threat, and will continue to be an extremely important issue for years to come.

References

Research Reports

1. Levine BB, Ovary Z. Studies on the mechanism of the formation of the penicillin antigen. J Exp Med 1961;*114*:875–880.
2. Saxon A, Swabb EA, Adkinson NF Jr. Investigation into the immunologic cross-reactivity of aztreonam with other beta-lactam antibiotics. Am J Med 1985;*78*:19–26.
3. Wang E, Walsh CT. Suicide substrates for the alanine racemase of *Escherichia coli* B. Biochemistry 1978;*17*:1313–1320.
4. Sheldrick GM, Jones PG, Kennard O, Williams DH, Smith G. Structure of vancomycin and its complex with acetyl-D-alanyl-D-alanine. Nature 1978;*27*:223–224.
5. Shlaes DM, Bouvet A, Devine C, Shlaes JH, al Obeid S, Williamson R. Inducible, transferable resistance to vancomycin in *Enterococcus faecalis* A256. Antimicrob Agents Chemother 1989;*33*:198–203.
6. Williamson R, al Obeid S, Shlaes JH, Goldstein FW, Shlaes DM. Inducible resistance to vancomycin in *Enterococcus faecium* D366. J Infect Dis 1989;*159*:1095–1104.

7. Bugg TDH, Dutka-Malen S, Arthur M, Courvalin P, Walsh CT. Identification of vancomycin resistance protein VanA as a D-alanine:D-alanine ligase of altered substrate specificity. Biochemistry 1991;*30*:2017–2021.

8. Bugg TDH, Wright GD, Dutka-Malen S, Arthur M, Courvalin P, Walsh CT. Molecular basis for vancomycin resistance in *Enterococcus faecium* BM4147: Biosynthesis of a depsipeptide peptidoglycan precursor by vancomycin resistance proteins VanH and VanA. Biochemistry 1991;*30*:10408–10415.

9. Walsh CT. Vancomycin resistance: Decoding the molecular logic. Science 1993;*261*:308–309.

10. Storm DR, Strominger JL. Complex formation between bacitracin peptides and isoprenyl pyrophosphates: the specificity of lipid-peptide interactions. J Biol Chem 1973;*248*:3940–3948.

11. Tipper DJ, Strominger JL. Mechanism of action of penicillins: a proposal based on their structural similarity to acyl-D-alanyl-D-alanine. Proc Natl Acad Sci USA 1965;*54*:1133–1141.

12. Spratt BG. Distinct penicillin-binding proteins involved in the division, elongation, and shape of *Escherichia coli*. Proc Natl Acad Sci USA 1975;*72*:2999–3003.

13. Spratt BG. Properties of the penicillin-binding proteins of *Escherichia coli* K12. Eur J Biochem 1977;*72*:341–352.

14. Tamaki S, Nakajima S, Matsuhashi M. Thermosensitive mutation in *Escherichia coli* simultaneously causing defects in penicillin-binding protein-1Bs and in enzyme activity for peptidoglycan synthesis in vitro. Proc Natl Acad Sci USA 1977;*74*:5472–5476.

15. Spratt BG, Pardee AB. Penicillin-binding proteins and cell shape in *E. coli*. Nature 1975;*254*:516–517.

16. Spratt BG. Temperature-sensitive cell division mutants of *Escherichia coli* with thermolabile penicillin-binding proteins. J Bacteriol 1977;*131*:293–305.

17. Ishino F, Mitsui K, Tamaki S, Matsuhashi M. Dual enzyme activities of cell wall peptidoglycan synthesis, peptidoglycan transglycosylase and penicillin-sensitive transpeptidase, in purified preparations of *Escherichia coli* penicillin-binding protein 1A. Biochem Biophys Res Commun 1980;*97*:287–293.

18. Nakagawa J, Tamaki S, Tomioka S, Matsuhashi M. Functional biosynthesis of cell wall peptidoglycan by polymorphic bifunctional polypeptides. J Biol Chem 1984;*259*:13937–13946.

19. Ishino F, Matsuhashi M. Peptidoglycan synthetic enzyme activities of highly purified penicillin-binding protein 3 in *Escherichia coli*: A septum-forming sequence. Biochem Biophys Res Commun 1981;*101*:905–911.

20. Tamura T, Imae Y, Strominger JL. Purification to homogeneity and properties of two D-alanine carboxypeptidases I from *Escherichia coli*. J Biol Chem 1976;*251*:414–423.

21. dePedro MA, Schwarz U. Heterogeneity of newly inserted and preexisting murien in the sacculus of *Escherichia coli*. Proc Natl Acad Sci USA 1981;*78*:5856–5860.

22. Matsuhashi M, Tamaki S, Curtis SJ, Strominger JL. Mutational evidence for identity of penicillin-binding protein 5 in *Escherichia coli* with the major D-alanine carboxypeptidase 1A activity. J Bacteriol 1979;*137*:644–647.

23. Amanuma H, Strominger JL. Purification and properties of penicillin-binding proteins 5 and 6 from *Escherichia coli* membranes. J Biol Chem 1980;*255*:11173–11180.

24. Begg KJ, Takasuga A, Edwards DH, Dewar SJ, Spratt BG, Adachi H, Otta T, Matsuzawa H, Donachie WD. The balance between different peptidoglycan precursors determines whether *Escherichia coli* cells will elongate or divide. J Bacteriol 1990;*172*:6697–6703.

25. Brumfitt W, Hamilton-Miller J. Methicillin-resistant *Staphylococcus aureus*. N Engl J Med 1989;*320*:1188–1196.

26. Samraoui B, Sutton BJ, Todd RJ, Artymiuk PJ, Waley SG, Phillips DC. Tertiary structural similarity between a class A β-lactamase and a penicillin-sensitive D-alanyl carboxypeptidase-transpeptidase. Nature 1986;*320*:378–380.

27. Kelly JA, Dideberg O, Charlier P, Wery JP, Libert M, Moews PC, Knox JR, Duez C, Fraipont CI, Jorris B, Dusart J, Frere JM, Ghuyson JM. On the origin of bacterial resistance to penicillin: Comparison of a β-lactamase and a penicillin target. Science 1986;*231*:1429–1431.

28. Philippon A, Labia R, Jacoby G. Extended-spectrum β-lactamases. Antimicrob Agents Chemother 1989;*33*:1131–1136.

29. Jacoby GA, Medeiros AA. More extended-spectrum β-lactamases. Antimicrob Agents Chemother 1991;*35*:1697–1704.

30. Sirot J, Chanal C, Petit A, Sirot D, Labia R, Gerbaud G. *Klebsiella pneumoniae* and other Enterobacteriaceae producing novel plasmid-mediated b-lactamases markedly active against third-generation cephalosporins: epidemiologic studies. Rev Infect Dis 1988;*10*:850–859.

31. Sougakoff W, Goussard S, Gerbaud G. Courvalin P. Plasmid-mediated resistance to third-generation cephalosporins caused by point mutations in TEM-type penicillinase genes. Rev Infect Dis 1988;*10*:879–884.

32. Mitsuhashi S. Drug resistance plasmids. Mol Cell Biochem 1979;*26*:135.

33. Zhu Y, Englebert S, Joris B, Ghuysen JM, Kobayashi T, Lampen JO. Structure, function, and fate of the BlaR signal transducer involved in induction of beta-lactamase in *Bacillus licheniformis*. J Bacteriol 1992;*174*:6171–6178.

34. Nikaido H. Bacterial resistance to antibiotics as a function of outer membrane permeability. J Antimicrob Chemother 1988;*22*, Suppl. A:17–22.

35. Tomasz A, Albino A, Zanati E. Multiple antibiotic resistance in a bacterium with a suppressed autolytic system. Nature 1970;*227*:138.

35a. Georgopapadakou. Penicillin-binding proteins and bacterial resistance to β-lactams. Antimicrob Agents Chemother 1993;*37*:2045–2053.

36. Chambers HF, Hartman BJ, Tomasz A. Increased amounts of a novel penicillin-binding protein in a strain of methicillin-resistant *Staphylococcus aureus* exposed to nafcillin. J Clin Invest 1985;*76*:325–331.

37. Dougherty TJ, Koller AE, Tomasz A. Penicillin-binding proteins of penicillin-susceptible and intrinsically resistant *Neisseria gonorrhoeae*. Antimicrob Ag Chemother 1980;*18*(5):730–737.

38. Spratt BG, Zhang QY, Jones DM, Hutchison A, Brannigan JA, Dowson CG. Recruitment of a penicillin-binding protein gene from Neisseria flavescens during the emergence of penicillin resistance in *Neisseria meningitidis*. Proc Natl Acad Sci USA 1989;*86*:8988–8992.

39. Spratt BG, Bowler LD, Zhang QY, Zhou J, Smith JM. Role of interspecies transfer of chromosomal genes in the evolution of penicillin resistance in pathogenic and commensal Neisseria species. J Mol Evol 1992;*34*:115–125.

40. Dowson CG, Hutchison A, Spratt BG. Extensive re-modelling of the transpeptidase domain of penicillin-binding protein 2B

of a penicillin-resistant South African isolate of *Streptococcus pneumoniae*. Mol Microbiol 1989;*3*:95–102.

41. Dowson CG, Hutchison A, Brannigan JA, George RC, Hansman DH, Linares J, Tomasz A, Smith JM, Spratt BG. Horizontal transfer of penicillin-binding protein genes in penicillin-resistant clinical isolates of *Streptococcus pneumoniae*. Proc Natl Acad Sci USA 1990;*86*:8842–8846.

42. Feingold DS. Biology and pathogenicity of microbial spheroplasts and L-forms. N Engl J Med 1969;*281*:1159.

43. Charnas RL, Knowles JR. Inactivation of RTEM β-lactamase from *Escherichia coli* by clavulanic acid and 9-deoxyclavulanic acid. Biochemistry 1981;*20*:3214–3219.

44. Cuchural GJJr, Malamy MH, Tally FP. β-Lactamase-mediated imipenem resistance in *Bacteroides fragilis*. Antimicrob Agents Chemother 1986;*30*:645–648.

45. Büscher K-H, Cullmann W, Dick W, Opferkuch W. Imipenem resistance in *Pseudomonas aeruginosa* resulting from diminished expression of an outer membrane protein. Antimicrob Ag Chemother 1987;*31*:703–708.

46. Braun V, Wolff H. The murein-lipoprotein linkage in the cell wall of *Escherichia coli*. Eur J Biochem 1970;*14*:387–391.

47. Strominger JL, Izaki K, Matsuhashi M, Tipper DJ. Peptidoglycan transpeptidase and D-alanine carboxypeptidase: Penicillin-sensitive enzymatic reactions. Fed Proc 1967;*26*:9.

48. Spector R. Advances in Understanding the Pharmacology of Agents Used to Treat Bacterial Meningitis. Pharmacology 1990;*41*:113–118.

49. Fekety FR. Safety of parenteral third-generation cephalosporins. Am J Med 1990;*88*(suppl 4A):38S–43S.

50. Saxon A, Beall GN, Rohr AS, Adelman DC. Immediate hypersensitivity reactions to β-lactam antibiotics. Ann Int Med 1987;*107*:204–215.

51. Lin RY. A perspective on penicillin allergy. Arch Intern Med 1992;*152*:930–937.

52. Grasela TH Jr, Walawander CA, Welage LS, Wing P, Scarafoni DJ, Caldwell JW, Noguchi JK, Schentag JJ. Prospective surveillance of antibiotic-associated coagulopathy in 970 patients. Pharmacotherapy 1989;*9*(3):158–164.

53. Lee SP, Lipsky BA, Teefy SA. Gallbladder sludge and antibiotics. Pediatr Infect Dis J 1990;*9*(6):422–423.

54. Christ W. Pharmacological properties of cephalosporins. Infection 1991;*19*(supp 5):S244–S252.

55. Wright AJ, Wilkowske CJ. The Pencillins. Mayo Clin Proc 1991;*66*:1047–1063.

56. Neu HC. The in vitro activity, human pharmacology, and clinical effectiveness of new β-lactam antibiotics. Ann Rev Pharmacol Toxicol 1982;*22*:599–642.

57. MacGowan AP. When is penicillin monotherapy the antibiotic treatment of choice? J Antimicrob Chemoth 1992;*29*:239–243.

58. John CC. Treatment Failure with use of a Third Generation Cephalosporin for Penicillin-Resistant Pneumococcal Meningitis: Case Report and Review. Clin Infect Dis 1994;*18*:188–193.

59. White GW, Malow JB, Zimelis VM, Pahlavanzadeh H, Panwalker AP, Jackson GG. Comparative in vitro activity of azlocillin, ampicillin, mezlocillin, piperacillin, and ticarcillin alone and in combination with an aminoglycoside. Antimicrob Agents Chemoth 1979;*15*:540–543.

60. Gould IM, Wise R. Beta-lactamase inhibitors. In Peterson PK, Verhoef J. The antimicrobial agents annual, 3. Amsterdam: Elsevier (1988); pp 63–76.

61. Bush K. Beta-lactamase inhibitors from laboratory to clinic. Clin Micro Reviews 1988;*1*:109–123.

62. Wise R. Oral Cephalosporins. J Antimicrob Chemoth 1992;*29*:91–96.

63. Third Generation Cephalosporins: A decade in the progress in the treatment of severe infections. Am J Med 1990;*88*(4A):1–45S.

64. Donowitz GR. Third generation cephalsporins. Infect Dis Clin North Am 1989;*3*:595–612.

65. Sobel JD. Imipenem and Aztreonam. Infect Dis Clin North Am 1989;*3*:613–624.

66. Neu HC. New antibiotics: areas of appropriate use. J Infect Diseases 1987:403–410.

Reviews

r1. Bush LM, Calmon J, Johnson CC. Newer penicillins and β-lactamase inibitors. Infect Dis Clin North Am 1989;*3*.

r2. Gustaferro CA, Steckelberg JM. Cephalosporin Antimicrobial Agents and Related Compounds. Mayo Clin Proc 1991;*66*:1064–1073.

r3. Donowitz GR, Mandell GL. Beta-lactam antibiotics 1. N Engl J Med 1988;*318*(7):419–426.

r4. Donowitz GR, Mandell GL. Beta-lactam antibiotics 2. N Engl J Med 1988;*318*(8):490–500.

r5. Rev Infect Dis 1986; 8Suppl3:S235–358. Supplement dedicated to the β-lactam antibiotics.

r6. Ghuysen JM, Frere JM, Leyh Bouille M, Nguyen-Disteche M, Coyette J, Dusart J, Joris B, Duez C, Dideberg O, Carlier P, Dive G, Lamotte-Brasseur J. Bacterial wall peptidoglycan, DD-peptidases and beta lactam antibiotics. Scand J Infect Dis 1984; Suppl. *42*:17–37.

r7. Waxman D, Strominger JL. Penicillin-binding proteins and the mechanism of action of β-lactam antibiotics. Ann Rev Biochem 1983;*52*:825–869.

CHAPTER 96

Bacterial Infections: Antibiotics Acting on Membrane Permeability

Jacques Bolard

The bacterial cytoplasm is separated from the external medium by membranes that control nutrients influx and intracellular ions equilibrium. Antibacterial antibiotics therefore may act through selective disruption of these barriers, by producing specific changes in transmembrane permeability or inhibition of membrane-bound enzymes. Their direct action may lead then to a lethal alteration of the fluxes of essential components or an indirect action that will facilitate the incorporation of the drug itself (or other compounds) into the bacteria.

All bacteria possess a cell wall, and the cell wall component common to all of them is murein, the peptidoglycan that contributes to mechanical rigidity. All gram-negative bacteria contain an additional layer in the cell wall structure, i.e., the outer membrane. This outer membrane has a very important role in the physiology of gram-negative bacteria in making them resistant to host defense factors that are very toxic to gram-positive bacteria. At the same time, the outer membrane of enteric and some other gram-negative bacteria acts as a strong permeability barrier to many antibiotics that are effective against other bacteria (macrolides, novobiocin, rifamycins, etc.). This is obviously related to the high prevalence of gram-negative infections.

Bacterial outer membranes show unusual functional properties: very low permeability toward lipophilic solutes and high permeability toward hydrophilic solutes. These particular functional attributes can certainly be linked to the presence of unusual structural components such as lipolysaccharides (LPS) and porins, and to the precise molecular organization of these components.

Membrane Disrupting Agents

Polymyxins

These closely related antibiotics are active principally against gram-negative bacteria, including *Pseudomonas aeruginosa, Enterobacter, Escherichia coli, Klebsiellia, Salmonella, Pasteurella, Bordetella, and Shigella.*

They are produced by various strains of *Bacillus polymyxa*. They are cyclic compounds with a short polypeptide tail terminated by a fatty acid. Polymyxin B (a mixture of polymyxin B_1 and B_2) and colistin or polymyxin E (a mixture of colistin A and B) are the only polymyxins clinically used (Fig. 96.1).

Although polymyxin B was discovered over 40 years ago, its mode of action against gram-negative bacteria is still not precisely known; however, the antibacterial action is certainly related to membrane-damaging activity.[r3] It seems probable that the polymixins promote their own access to the inner membrane by first binding to and then disrupting the outer membrane,[r4] because they are too large to go through the narrow porin channels. Indeed polymyxin causes extensive, electron microscopically visible alterations and favors the intracellular transfer of other agents.

The proximal portion of the saccharide chain of LPS found in the outer membrane has a number of

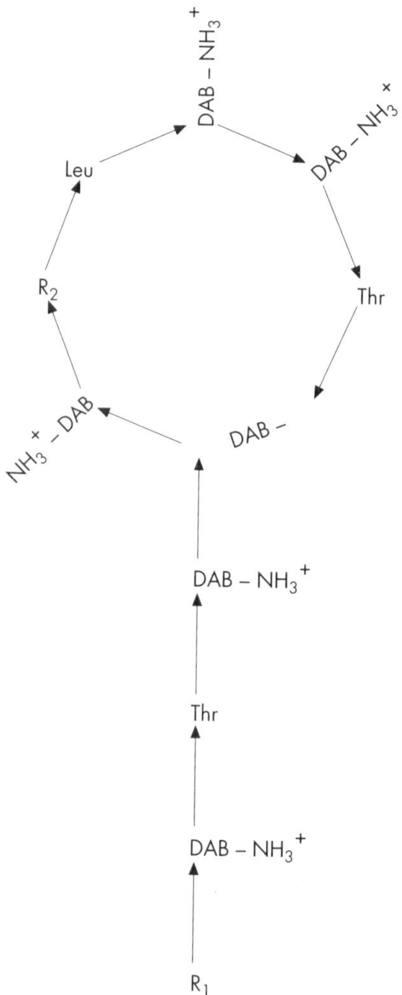

Figure 96.1 Structure of Polymyxins;

		R_1	R_2
Polymyxin B	B_1	MOA	Phe
	B_2	MHA	Phe
Polymyxin E	Colistin A	MOA	Leu
	Colistin B	MHA	Leu

DAB-NH_3^+, Thr, Leu, Phe are symbols for the amino acids side-chains of respectively: L-α,γ - diaminobutyric acid, L-threonine, L-leucine, L-phenylalanine, MOA and MHA are symbols for the acyl chains of respectively 6 - methyloctanoic acid and 6 - methylheptanoic acid. The arrows represent the peptide bond

$$-\underset{\underset{O}{\parallel}}{C}-\underset{\underset{H}{|}}{N}-$$

negatively charged groups. The counter ions (or cations) in particular Ca^{2+} and Mg^{2+}, play a crucial role in the organization of the LPS monolayer. The outer membrane can be disorganized by removing divalent cations with chelators. The presence in polymyxins of five positively charged groups without any negatively charged group at all has therefore been thought to be important. It has been proposed that polymyxin B interacts with a divalent cation-binding site and thus cross-bridges adjacent LPS molecules. Since the polycationic cyclopeptide is much larger than Mg^{2+} or Ca^{2+}, normal packing between lipid polar head-groups would necessarily be perturbed, probably leading to an expansion of the outer monolayer and its disruption by a mechanism related to that of detergents.[1]

Interactions between outer membranes and polymyxins have been extensively studied. Unfortunately, interactions between the antibiotics and cytoplasmic membranes have not been characterized to the same extent. The involvement of electrostatic interaction with the negatively charged phospholipids has, however, been supported by a number of different studies.[2] There are arguments that favor the view that the lethality of polymyxin B for gram-negative bacteria arises as a consequence of cytoplasmic membrane disruption. However, the consecutive leakage of amino acids, uracil, and K^+ is not itself lethal. This is evident from comparison of the effects of polymyxin B and of the deacylated derivative polymyxin B nonapeptide (PMBN). PMBN has very low intrinsic antibacterial activity, but still interacts with LPS, and so significantly expands the surface area of the outer leaflet of the outer membrane; it is also able to induce a loss of amino acids, uracil, and K^+ from *E. coli* to an extent similar to that of the parent compound. In contrast, however, polymyxin B rapidly renders the *E. coli* cytoplasmic membrane permeable to periplasmic and cytoplamic proteins, in particular murein hydrolases, a feature not shared by PMBN. Under normal conditions, the murein hydrolases are prevented from causing gross digestion of the murein—which would lead to cell lysis by the cytoplasmic membrane that separates them from the cell wall. Disruption of this barrier could account for the bactericidal properties of the antibiotic.

The basis for the selective toxicity of polymyxins has not been well defined. It has been supposed that these drugs have a lower affinity for the phosphatidylcholine molecules of the host cells than for the phosphatidyl ethanolamine of the bacteria. The presence of cholesterol in the host cell membranes would also decrease their sensitivity. It also is not clear why gram-negative bacteria are more sensitive than gram-positive ones.

The polymyxin resistance of some gram-negative strains is apparently attributable to their outer membranes and their impermeability to the drug. For example, *Proteus mirabilis* is normally quite resistant to polymyxin B. Conversion of a polymyxin-resistant strain to L-forms increased sensitivity to polymyxin 400-fold. In *Pseudomonas cepacia* it has been proposed that the resistance comes from the arrangement of the outer membrane which would be such that the divalent cation binding sites are hidden or protected.

Therapeutic Uses

With the development of more effective and less toxic antibiotics, indications for the polymyxins have become limited. Actually they are used mostly for infections caused by *Pseudomonas aeruginosa,* which is resistant to the antipseudomonal penicillins, to the third generation cephalosporins, and to the aminoglycosides. They are also used against other gram-negative bacterial infections resistant to the preferred antibiotics.

Topical preparations of polymyxin or colistin are indicated for external otitis since *P. aeruginosa* and *Escherichia* commonly infect the ear. However they are not active against Proteus or gram-positive bacteria often found in these infections. Local application of polymyxin B is often curative of corneal ulcers commonly caused by *P. aeruginosa.*

Combinations of bacitracin, neomycin, and polymyxin B are widely used in ocular therapy because of their broad spectrum of activity.

Infections of the skin are sensitive to polymyxin B, but, as multiple organisms are often associated with these infections, mixtures of topical antibiotics also are used.

Colistin sulfate is given to treat diarrhea caused by enteropathogenic or pathogenic *E. coli* in children with acute or refractory enteritis.

Preparations

Polymyxin sulfate can be administered by all parenteral routes and by topical application. It can be used for meningitis but must be given intrathecally, which may be hazardous.

Colistin sulfate, the water-soluble salt of colistin, is only slightly absorbed from the GI tract and is used orally to treat diarrheas in children.

Colistimethate sodium is the sodium salt of the sulfomethyl derivative of colistin. This parenteral preparation is seldom used.

Pharmacokinetics

Polymyxins are poorly absorbed when given orally. They do not pass readily into CSF or other body compartments. Once absorbed, their half-life is around five hours. They are excreted principally by glomerular filtration. Animal studies have shown that tissue binding is the major determinant of the distribution and persistence of these antibiotics in the body.

Adverse Reactions

Topical application causes no systemic reactions because of the poor absorption of the drug. Nausea, vomiting, and diarrhea are caused by large doses taken orally. Adverse effects that follow the parenteral administration are neurologic and renal. Transient neurologic disturbances have been observed: these reactions disappear as the drugs are excreted; however, they may be potentially dangerous for patients with neuromuscular diseases or patients receiving a neuromuscular blocking drug, since the paralytic effects of the neuromuscular blockers may be prolonged. Nephrotoxicity is observed in patients with impaired renal function.

The Aminoglycosides

These antimicrobial agents are known to inhibit protein synthesis at the ribosome. However, in order to explain the rapidity of their lethal action, a multistep model has been proposed in which the uptake of aminoglycosides leads first to outer membrane damage and only subsequently to ribosomal blockade.[r5] The sequence of the first events would be as follows:

(1) A small amount of antibiotic penetrates, by an unknown mechanism, into the cell, where its contact with chain-elongating ribosomes causes misreading of messenger RNA;

(2) Some of the misread and thus abnormal proteins are incorporated into the membrane, creating channels that permit influx of more antibiotic and thus initiating an autocatalytic process of increasing influx, misreading, and defective channel formation;

(3) The intracellular antibiotic eventually reaches a concentration that blocks all initiating ribosomes.

Others

Several treatments have been proposed to break off the outer membrane barrier, in particular the addition of EDTA in the presence of Tris buffer. Recently low doses of local anesthetics have also been shown to decrease the MIC of several antibiotics which penetrate very poorly into intact *E. coli.*[5]

It must be noted that polymyxin B is also considered as neutralizing endotoxin through its detergent-like activity: upon incubation with polymyxin, organized complexes of purified endotoxin become disaggregated.

Ionophores

Several antibiotics called "*ionophores*" have been shown to cause specific changes in the cation permeability of membranes. Most of these agents are too toxic to be clinically useful. We shall, however, briefly describe them because they are widely used in biologic studies as a tool in membrane research. The ionophores are generally extremely hydrophobic and have molecular sizes greater than 500 daltons. Therefore the outer membrane of gram-negative bacteria serves as a protective barrier and these bacteria are generally ionophore resistant. In contrast, gram-positive bacteria, which lack this protective outer membrane, are sensitive to these molecules.

It is possible to distinguish two classes of ion transport systems: channels and carriers. The main representative of ion channels is gramicidin A, an open-chain polypeptide of chemical structure HCo - Val - Gly - Ala - D Leu - Ala - D Val - Val - D Val - Trp - D leu - Trp - D Leu - Trp - D Leu - Trp - NHC_2H_4OH. Gramicidin A, in combination with tyrocidine A (a cyclic decapeptide), has been used topically as thyrotricin. There is a general agreement that the active structure of gramicidin A, through which leak cellular monovalent cations, is a dimer with head to head helices, although a double helical form has also been suggested. This structure spans the entire membrane and contains in its interior a tunnel-like pathway for ion translocation.[4]

In recent years, antimicrobial peptides have been isolated from species ranging from insects to mammals. Among them are defensins, a family of cysteine-rich peptides, 29 to 34 residues in length, cecropins, a family of amphipatic non hemolytic peptides, 37 amino acids long, and magainins, peptides 21 to 26 amino acids in length and basic (lysine-rich).[5] An interesting feature of magainins is that they are not generally toxic to eukaryotic cells, i.e., erythrocytes are not lysed and peripheral blood lymphocytes remain viable at concentrations toxic to sensitive cells. The probable mechanism of action of magainins is interference with membrane-linked free-energy transduction by making the membrane permeable to certain ions. Presumably, this involves a multimer of magainins forming ion-channel pores that span the membrane without specific interaction with chiral receptors or enzymes. Whether specificity is accomplished by differences in membranes composition or proteolytic defense of the target cells remains to be elucidated.

Among the class of ion carriers neutral ionophores and carboxylic ionophores may be described.[r6] These molecules bind the ion and transport it in its bound form through the membrane. Valinomycin, nonactin and synthetic cryptates are the best known neutral ionophores. Carboxyl polyether antibiotics act primarily by causing preferential leakage of K^+ (nigericin, lasalocid), or Na^+ (monensin). A 23 187 and ionomycin transport divalent cations and have been proved extremely useful in studying the physiologic and pharmacologic regulation of Ca^{2+} fluxes in mammalian cells as well.

It should be noted that other channel-forming drugs, the polyene macrolide antibiotics (in particular amphotericin B and Fungizone), are not active against bacteria, but have important antifungal toxicity. Actually, their activity depends on the presence of sterols in the cytoplasmic membrane (ergosterol in fungi); therefore, their effects are weak against bacteria (see Chapter 98).

Antibiotics Inhibiting Transport Processes of the Plasma Membrane

Membrane active drugs often act by impairment of the active transport processes or alteration of membrane coupling mechanisms. No antibacterial antibiotic has been developed in this direction. However several synthetic antibacterial agents used as antiseptics and disinfectants are known to inhibit the transport of low-molecular weight hydrophilic substances into bacteria. Such is the case of hexachlorophene. The synthetic cyclohexane triones, a novel group of antibacterial agents, seem to act similarly.[r7]

Vancomycin

The development of resistance by bacteria to antibiotics with minimal side effects is unfortunately very common. For this reason another less widely used antibiotic is often required to find a drug to which the bacteria are still sensitive. Vancomycin is infrequently used in common infections, but is often sought out for use in managing patients with persistent infections since resistance is quite rare to this drug.

Vancomycin is a tricyclic glycopeptide antibiotic initially isolated from Nocardia orientalis. The drug is water soluble, producing an acid solution (pH 3–4 at 5% concentrations). It has a bitter taste and is given by the intravenous route or as an oral capsule, since it is quite stable chemically. The drug is thought to block endogenous bacterial glycopeptide polymerization. Vancomycin appears to form a hydrogen bonded complex with the peptideglycan precursor UDP-N-acetylmuramyl pentapeptide[6], increasing cellular content of this metabolite, probably due to underutilization. This effect, at a locus not involved with the antibacterial action of penicillin, secondarily yields defects in the organism's cell wall which persumably make it more easily destroyed by host defense mechanisms. Many gram positive bacteria are susceptible at concentrations below 5 μg/ml (Staphylococci, Clostridia, Corynebacterium, Enterococci and Streptococci) but gram negative bacteria, yeasts, viruses and fungi are not inhibited. The drug may be given alone or in combination with an aminoglycoside (e.g. gentamycin).

Vancomycin is poorly absorbed from the gut, but is used in management of some enteric infections. After intravenous administration, the drug is poorly bound to plasma proteins, and it diffuses readily into many body fluids except the cerebral spinal fluid. However, during CNS surgery or infection effective concentrations may be found in the brain as well. While the serum $t_{1/2}$ for elimination may be as short as 4–6 hours after initial dosing in patients with normal renal function, the drug's nephrotoxic potential and dependence upon glomerular filtration for elimination, may produce a $t_{1/2}$ as long as several weeks in patients with impaired renal function. For these reasons, plasma level measurements are sometimes essential in order to maintain therapeutic plasma concentrations yet avoid the toxic effects of high levels. For the great majority of patients however, measurement of plasma levels is probably not necessary.[7] Conversely, in patients with increased glomerular filtration such as burn patients, the increased apparent volume of distribution and more rapid renal elimination require higher vancomyin doses than normal to reach equivalent plasma concentrations.[8]

The two most serious systemic side effects of vancomycin are its ability to produce ototoxicity or nephrotoxicity. In general, both of these difficulties are common (10%) and frequently occur in patients receiving other oto-nephrotoxic drugs or whose disease process may involve renal function impairment. Prolonged, high dose (high blood level) therapy appreciably increases the likelihood of those side effects. Intravenous administration must be done with care due to the severe local irritation or even necrosis that may follow extravasation. Rapid administration may produce a hypotensive response, often visable as a cutaneous flush or rash on the upper torso and extremeties. Patients who evidence this response despite a reduced infusion rate may respond to corticosteroids and antihistamines as well as I.V. fluids. Such a reaction does not, however, necessarily indicate an allergic response, and the drug may be begun again, often without incident if it is administered slowly. Bone marrow depression is a rare side effect with neutropenia most prominent.

The drug should not be used in patients with hearing loss or decreased renal function. Concurrent use with aminoglycosides, bacitracin, cisplatin, colistin etc., that have similar side effect profiles, should be done with caution.

Teichoplanin is a new glycopeptide antibiotic structurally related to vancomycin. It appears to have a lower incidence of side effects/toxicity, can be given by the I.M. route, and requires less frequent dosing.[9] Unfortunately there is some concern that resistance may develop to this drug, and that its clinical therepeutic/toxic dose ratio is not consistently higher than that of vancomycin.

Table 96.1 Summary Table

Drug	Dosage			Pharmacokinetics			
	Route	Size	Dose	Peak	V_D	$t_{1/2}$	Clearence or Duration of Response
POLYMIXIN B SULFATE Aerosporin	Parenteral	5×10^5 units	0.15×10^5 units/kg/day				
COLISTIMETHATE Coly-Mycin	Parenteral	150 mg	2.5–5 mg/kg/day in 4 divided doses				
COLISTIN SULFATE Coly-Mycin	Oral	25 mg/5 ml suspension	5–15 mg/kg/day in 5 divided doses				
VANCOMYCIN Vancocin	Oral Parenteral	125 and 250 mg 0.5, 5, 10 g pkg	0.5–2 g qd 50 mg/ml in 100 ml total volume 0.5–1 g q6hr over 1 hr minimum				$t_{1/2}$4–32 hrs
BACITRACIN Baci IM Ak-Tacin Baciquent	Parenteral IM Topical Ophthalmic Ointment Topical Skin Ointment	25,000 units per dose 500 units/g 500 units/g	10–25,000 units q6 hrs tid	1–2 hr	wide		1 day

Whereas vancomycin and teichoplanin block polymerization of cell wall precursors, another newer drug, ramoplanin inhibits transfer of the UDP-muramyl N acetyl pentapeptide to a lipid carrier in the cell wall required for polymerization, achieving the same result of inhibiting cell wall synthesis but by a different mechanism.[10]

Bacitracin

This mixture of 3 polypeptide antibiotics was first identified from Bacillus subtilis isolated from a child named Tracy, hence its name. The drug is very water soluble with a slightly acidic pH (5–7), probably accounting for its poor absorbtion and membrane penetration.

Depending upon the concentration the drug may be bacteriocidal (high) or bacteriostatic (low). The peptides inhibit mucopeptide insertion into the growing cell wall probably by inhibiting the insertion of amino acids and nucleotides via quenching of the final dephosphorylation sequence in the phospholipid carrier cycle. The drug inhibits or kills many gram positive organisms (e.g. Clostridia, Streptococci, Corynebacteria, and Staphyllococci), but only a few gram negative ones (e.g. Meningococci, Fusobacteria, Gonococci), and some Treponemes. (T. pallidum and T. vincenti). Though no crossresistance with other antibiotics develops, some penicillin resistent staphylococci are also bacitracin resistent. The drug is now used parenterally only in management of systemic infections with penicillin reisitant staphylococci. Occasionally, oral bacitacin is used in Clostridium difficile diarrhea or as an oral intestinal antiseptic, since it is not appreciably absorbed. By far the greatest use of the drug is as a topical antibiotic, since it is poorly absorbed through the skin.

The most serious side/toxic effect of the drug is renal tubular and glomerular necrosis. The onset of this complication is directly related to the dose and duration of administration, but uncharacteristically is rare in children given the drug. Maintaining the urine pH above 6%, administration of large volumes of intravenous fluids, and avoidence of coadministration with other nephotoxic drugs may be useful to decrease the incidence of renal toxicity. Local pain and swelling may follow IM administration, and neuromuscle paralysis may develop in patients with subclinical myasthenia. The drug prolongs the neuromuscle blocking action of general anesthetics and non-depolarizing muscle relaxants.

References

Research Reports

1. Schröder G, Brandenburg K, Seydel U. Polymyxin B induces transient permeability fluctuations in asymmetric planar lipopolysaccharide/phospholipid bilayers. Biochem 1992;*31*:631–638.

2. Dixon RA, Chopra I. Polymyxin B and polymyxin B nonapeptide alter cytoplasmic membrane permeability in Escherichia coli. J Antimicrob Chemother 1986;*18*:557–563.

3. Labedan B. Increase in permeability of Escherichia Coli outer membrane by local anesthetics and penetration of antibiotics. Antimicrob Ag Chemother 1988;*32*:153–155.

4. Jordan P. Microscopic approaches of ion transport through transmembrane channels. The model system gramicidin. J Phys Chem 1987;*91*:6582–6591.

5. Moore KS, Bevins CL, Brasseur MM, et al. Antimicrobial peptides in the stomach of Xenopus laevis. J Biol Chem 1991;*266*:19851–19857.

6. Freeman CD, Quintiliani R, Nightingale CH. Vancomycin therapeutic drug monitoring: is it necessary? Ann Pharmacother 1993;*27*:594–598.

7. Boucher BA, Kuhl DA, Hickerson WL. Pharmacokinetics of systemically administered antibiotics in patients with thermal injury. Clin Infect Dis 1992;*14*:458–463.

8. Casetta A, Bingen E, Lambert-Zechovsky N. Vancomycin in 1991: current status and perspectives. Pathol Biol Paris 1991;*39*:700–708.

9. Janknegt R. Teicoplanin in perspective. A critical comparison with vancomycin. Pharm Weekbl 1991;*13*:153–160.

10. Reynolds PE, Somner EA. Comparison of the target sites and mechanisms of action of glycopeptide and lipoglycodepsipeptide antibiotics. Drugs Exp Clin Res 1990;*16*:385–389.

Reviews

r1. Nikaido H, Vaara M. Molecular basis of bacterial outer membrane permeability Microbiol Rev 1985;*49*:1–32.
An extensive description of all the molecular components of bacterial outer membrane responsible for its permeability and its alteration by polymyxins.

r2. Hancock REW. Alterations in outer membrane permeability Ann Rev Microbiol 1984;*38*:237–264.

r3. Storm DR, Rosenthal KS and Swanson PE. Polymyxin and related peptide antibiotics. Ann Rev Biochem 1977;*46*:723–763.

r4. Vaara M, Vaara T. Polycations as outer membrane-desorganizing agent. Antimicrob Ag. Chemother 1983;*24*:114–122.

r5. Davis BD. Mechanism of bactericidal action of aminoglycosides Microbiol Rev 1987;*51*:341–350.

r6. Pressman BC. Biological Applications of ionophores Ann Rev Biochem 1976;*45*:501–530.

r7. Lloyd WJ, Broadhurst AV, Hall MJ et al. Cyclohexanone triones, novel membrane-active antibacterial agents. Antimicrob Ag Chemother 1988;*32*:814–818.

CHAPTER 97

Therapy of Mycobacterial Infections

Nitya Anand

Introduction

The developments during the last fifty years in the chemotherapy of tuberculosis and leprosy, the two most important chronic human diseases caused by mycobacteria, form a most instructive chapter in the history of the chemotherapy of infectious diseases. The modern era of their chemotherapy started around 1940, with the discovery of the antimycobacterial activity of 4,4′-diaminodiphenylsulfone (dapsone, DDS), a synthetic drug, and of the antituberculosis activity of streptomycin, an antibiotic. Following these discoveries, some very effective drugs were added for the chemotherapy of tuberculosis and leprosy, which brought about a dramatic decrease in the morbidity and mortality from these diseases. Even more important, these drugs totally changed the outlook for treatment; further, treatment changed from hospital-based to ambulatory. However, problems of the emergence of drug-resistant organisms and the high cost of the drugs, particularly for target groups in developing countries, posed serious limitations to the effective use of the new agents.

Much attention and research was then devoted to find out the best ways to use the available drugs to suit the medical needs and the socioeconomic situations prevalent in different countries. Some of the international agencies involved in health research, such as the Special Programme for Research and Training in Tropical Diseases (TDR) of WHO and the International Union Against Tuberculosis and Lung Diseases (IUATLD), have played a major role in these efforts. Based on the recognition that, in active infection, there are different populations of bacilli[1] with different sensitivity to different drugs, combination therapy regimens have been developed that make optimal use of the antibacterial potential of the available drugs.

With the short-course chemotherapy (SCC) regimen of six to nine months for tuberculosis, and six to twenty-four months' multidrug therapy (MDT) for leprosy now prescribed, it has become possible to treat practically all forms of tuberculosis and leprosy. These regimens are probably the most cost-effective interventions available in infectious diseases.[2,3] These modalities, even with the limited number of available drugs, have the potential of containing and reducing the burden of tuberculosis,[4] and, in the case of leprosy even of eradicating the disease.[15]

There are still fresh challenges for the chemotherapy of mycobacterial diseases. The most serious is posed by the emergence of HIV infection,[4,6–8] which has led to worsening of the tuberculosis situation in the developing countries[6,19] and re-emergence of the tuberculosis threat in developed countries[9–11] and all its associated problems. Multidrug-resistant tuberculosis spread in this manner is a particularly serious problem, because there is poor response to treatment, substantial mortality, and danger of spread of multidrug resistance in the community.[12,13] This underscores the need for new antituberculosis drugs with novel modes of action and without cross-resistance to existing drugs. Atypical mycobacteriosis,[14–16] particularly that caused by *M. avium* complex, the most common cause of disseminated bacterial infections in patients with AIDS, is another serious problem. Most of the atypical mycobacteria are not susceptible to most of the commonly used antimycobacterial agents, and new agents and suitable regimens for their use are needed for the management and treatment of opportunistic infections caused by atypical mycobacteria. In view of these developments, new concepts of the epidemeology, diagnosis, and treatment of mycobacterial infections are evolving,[4,17] with new demands on chemotherapy.

The association of lowered immunity and mycobacterial infections and the poor response of such patients to standard chemotherapy has also highlighted the important role that immunity plays in the outcome of chemotherapy. Thus, the possible use of immunoregulators along with chemotherapy needs to be studied in these infections. Leprosy vaccines prepared from atypical mycobacteria have been shown to potentiate the chemotherapy action in leprosy,[18] and this immunotherapeutic application of vaccines would add a new dimension to their use. There are also big gaps in our knowledge concerning the mode of action and mechanism of resistance of antimycobacterial drugs; these must be filled to design better drugs and find new strategies for overcoming the problems of drug resistance.

Mycobacterial Diseases

Mycobacteria are believed to be transition forms between bacteria and fungi. They are characterized by nonmotile, nonsporulating rods that, after staining with dyes, resist decolorization with acidified organic solvents; hence, they are also called "acid-fast" bacteria (AFB). Among the mycobacteria pathogenic to humans, the most important are: *Mycobacterium tuberculosis* hominis and *M. tuberculosis* bovis, the causative organisms for tuberculosis; and *M. leprae,* the causative organism for leprosy. Some *atypical mycobacteria* may also infect and cause disease in humans such as *M. avium* and *M. intracellulare,* especially when associated with HIV infection. These are discussed later under "Other mycobacterial diseases."

Tuberculosis

Tuberculosis is the leading cause of death among infectious diseases.[19] Each year there are an estimated 8 million new cases of TB and 2.9 million deaths from the disease. Around one-third of the world's population harbors *Mycobacterium tuberculosis* and is at risk of developing the disease. TB accounts for 6.7 per cent of all deaths in the developing world.[19] The steadily declining incidence of TB in the developed countries, such as in the UK and US has been reversed since 1985,[9,10] with a large proportion of the patients affected by drug-resistant mutants.[12,13,20] This high incidence of the disease despite significant advances made in its chemotherapy is a paradox.

M. tuberculosis is a slow-growing aerobic organism with a growth-doubling time of about 12 hours. In unfavorable conditions it will grow only intermittently or remain dormant for a prolonged period. There is a high rate of mutation with resistance to antituberculosis drugs; a wild strain will have one of every 10^5 to 10^8 bacilli resistant to any single antituberculosis drug.

Tuberculosis is primarily a chronic, occasionally acute, communicable disease that normally affects the respiratory tract but also may involve other organs, particularly the lymphatic, nervous, urogenital or GI systems and the bones.[21] The tubercle bacillus is an intracellular parasite, living and multiplying inside macrophages. It is generally ingested through inhalation. In the majority of individuals, inhaled bacilli ingested by macrophages are either directly killed, or grow intracellularly to a limited extent in localized lesions called tubercles. Within two to six weeks after infection, cell-mediated immunity develops with infiltration into the lesion of immune lymphocytes and activated macrophages, resulting in the killing of most bacilli, and the sealing-off of this primer of infection, providing the picture of a healed, calcified lesion. However, dormant but viable bacilli persist in the lesions, and can become activated by processes not fully understood. Alternatively, in about 10 per cent of cases the infection can result in active disease. The virulent bacilli in the tubercles and in the macrophages constitute a reservoir for invasion into other parts of the affected organs or into other organs. The bacilli spread from the initial site of infection in the lung through the lymphatics or blood to the apex of the lung, the lymph nodes, and other parts of the body. Although many bacilli are killed along with the infiltrating phagocytes and lung parenchymal cells, characteristic solid caseous necrosis develop in which bacilli may survive in a dormant state. If a protective immune response dominates, the lesion may be arrested, but with some damage to the lung or other tissue. If the necrotic reaction expands, breaking into a bronchus, a cavity is produced in the lung, allowing a large number of bacilli to spread with coughing to the outside. Occasionally the necrosed lesion may liquefy, creating a rich medium for the proliferation of the bacilli, which may reach as high a number as 10^9/ml. As a result of the spread of the bacilli, in about 15 per cent of TB patients extrapulmonary TB may develop in the pleura, lymphatics, genitourinary system, meninges, peritoneum, skin, or bone. The accompanying pathologic and inflammatory processes produce the characteristic weakness, fever, chest pain, and cough, and, when a blood vessel is eroded, bloody sputum.

Tuberculosis and HIV Infection

The association between tuberculosis and HIV infection is now well recognized and accepted.[4,6–8,22] In fact tuberculosis is a sentinel disease for AIDS because, in contrast to other opportunistic infections, it is very frequently the first indication of HIV infection. Patients infected with HIV show a much greater incidence of tuberculosis. According to WHO estimates in 1992, around 4 million people worldwide have been infected with both HIV and tuberculosis, with about 95 per cent in the developing world.[6] TB in HIV cases is quite often due to reactivation of earlier infections.

The course of TB in individuals infected with HIV is dramatically different, and so is the course of HIV infection in tuberculosis patients;[4,7] both affect cell-mediated immunity (CMI); *M. tuberculosis* affects the activation of T-helper lymphocytes.[23] It is the tropism of HIV for the CD4$^+$ T-helper/inducer lymphocytes that underlines the mechanism of reactivation or increased susceptibility to mycobacterial infections.[24] Therefore, in patients with advanced immunodeficiency, a disseminated extrapulmonary form of the disease, miliary TB, lymphadenitis, and meningitis, coexisting with pulmonary form of the disease is a more common form of TB.

This increase in morbidity among persons with HIV as a result of tuberculosis increases the risk of nosocomial transmission of tuberculosis. As HIV-induced immunosupression may amplify the spread of TB in hospitals, multi-drug-resistant TB is readily transmitted among hospitalized patients with AIDS.[12] Thus, multi-drug-resistant turberculosis and host immune deficiency may act in tandem to potentiate the transmission of tuberculosis among patients with HIV infection in hospitals. This poses a very serious threat both to the patient and for spread of multi-drug-resistant tuberculosis in the community. A number of foci of multi-drug-resistant tuberculosis among HIV patients have been reported from many countries.[13]

Leprosy

Leprosy is still one of the major infectious diseases in Asia and Africa, though the estimated 5.5 million leprosy cases in 1991,[25] represents a significant decline from the 10 to 12 million cases of earlier estimates. This is in large measure due to the effective drugs available and the ability of the multi-drug therapy (MDT) to cure almost all forms of leprosy.[5,26]

M. leprae is an obligate intracellular parasite, with low pathogenicity and infectivity; less than 1 per cent of the exposed subjects get the disease. *M. leprae,* perhaps the first major bacterial pathogen to be recognized as the cause of human disease (by Hansen in 1879—hence the name Hansen's disease), and yet it is one of the very few bacteria that still has not been cultured in vitro. *M. leprae* is extremely slow growing, much slower than *M. tuberculosis,* with a generation time of around 20 days.

Leprosy[27,28] is essentially a chronic disease. Principally, it affects the skin, mucous membrane, and peripheral nerves; occasionally, the eyes, bone, muscle, endocrine, reticuloendothelial, and hematopoietic systems may be involved. The sequalae of leprosy may be extensive and damaging. Lepra bacilli are considered to be transmitted principally via mucosal discharges from the nose and mouth; and nasal mucosa or skin seems to be the primary site of attack by *M. leprae.* The disease has a long incubation period, generally put at two to five years.

Leprosy—clinically, bacteriologically, and immunologically—presents a very varied picture.[29] At one end of the spectrum is **tuberculoid leprosy** (TT), characterized by skin macules with clear centers and well-defined margins, which are invariably anesthetic. *M. leprae* are rarely found in the smears. The patients' cell-mediated immune responses are normal, and the lepromin test is invariably positive. Patients may develop "reversal reaction," a manifestation of delayed hypersensitivity to bacterial antigens with periodic reactivation. At the other and of the spectrum is the widely disseminated **lepromatous leprosy** (LL), with markedly impaired cell-mediated immunity. These patients are frequently anergic; the lepromin test is negative. The disease is characterized by diffuse or ill-defined localized infiltration of the peripheral skin organs, which become thickened, glossy, and corrugated with areas of decreased sensation. Granulomas with bacteria-laden histiocytes (Virchow cells) are present, and smears are swarming with *M. leprae.* Occasionally there is a severe reaction, **erythema nodosum leprosum,** which is Arthus-type and characterized by the appearance of raised, tender, intracutaneous nodules, severe constitutional symptoms, and high fever. It is considered to be related to the release of microbial antigens. With the progression of the disease, the nerve trunks become involved, and anesthesia, atrophy of skin and muscle, resorption of small bones, ulceration, and spontaneous amputation may occur. The intermediate forms include the borderline tuberculoid (BT) and borderline (BB) to borderline lepromatous (BL).

The defect in cell-mediated immunity in lepromatous leprosy is extremely specific. The patients do not suffer increased risk for other infections for which cellular immunity is important. Tuberculin reactivity may be suppressed in untreated patients, but usually returns with treatment—unlike the lepromin response. Patients with lepromatous leprosy have been shown to have an increased number of circulating CD8+ ("suppressor") lymphocytes, which can be specifically activated by *M. leprae* antigens; the lymphocytes in their cutaneous granulomas are exclusively CD8+. In contrast, CD4+ 4B4+ ("helpers") predominate among the T-cells in the cutaneous lesions of tuberculoid patients. Intense bacillemia is very common in lepromatous leprosy; yet, high fever or signs of systemic toxicity are absent.

Other Mycobacterial Infections

Mycobacteria other than the tubercle and lepra bacilli, commonly termed "atypical mycobacteria," are of low virulence and have been shown to be agents of human disease only occasionally.[14] It is only since the advent of HIV infection in the 1980s, resulting in impaired immunity, that the more common occurrence of infections with atypical mycobacteria has brought these infections under sharp attention.

These bacteria are widely distributed in nature as saprophytes, primarily in soil and water. Animals can be infected and are considered reservoirs for infection of humans. Person-to-person transmission has not been documented. The atypical mycobacteria found in association with AIDS,[30] grouped according to their colonial morphology and growth characteristics are: photochromogens: *M. asiaticum, M. simiae,* and *M. kansasii;* nonchromogens: *M. avium, M. intracellulare;* the scotochromogens: *M. flavescens, M. xenopi, M. scrofulaceum, M. gordonae;* and rapid growing: *M. fortuitum, M. abscassus,* and *M. smegmatis.* Most of them share antigens with *M. tuberculosis* and respond to the tuberculin test.

The more important atypical mycobacteria and the diseases caused by them are briefly described below.[14]

M. Avium-Intracellulare

These two organisms, though distinguishable by ELISA, are difficult to differentiate by other means. Often they are treated as a complex (MAIC). These ubiquitous organisms are the most commonly isolated mycobacteria other than *M. tuberculosis.* Colonization and inapparent infection are common. The lungs are most often involved, and the clinical picture is similar to pulmonary tuberculosis. MAIC is a major cause of lymphadenitis in children. Profound diarrhea with intestinal pathology due to macrophages packed with MAIC is present. In other organs these macrophages resemble lepra cells.

M. Avium Complex

M. avium complex is one of the most common opportunistic infections in AIDS patients; of the 5.5 per cent incidence of disseminated nontuberculous mycobacteriosis, over 95 per cent is attributable to MAC.[15,16,31] The latter consists of 28 well-characterized serovars, of which the most common, both in AIDS and in nonAIDS cases, are serovars 4, 8, and 1, and a mixture of serovar 4 with *M. xenopi.* The occurrence of different serovars also may explain the variability of sensitivity to chemotherapy of different isolates. The marked association between organisms of MAC and AIDS have made this infection a matter of much public health concern.

M. Fortuitum and M. Chelonei

These are the fastest growing mycobacteria. The initial growth may take one to five weeks, but subsequent subcultures grow within five days. *M. fortuitum* is more frequently associated with posttraumatic and postsurgical skin and soft tissue infections; *M. chelonei* is a more common cause of pulmonary and disseminated infections. These are important nosocomial pathogens, and infections have followed major surgeries and dialysis.

M. Kansasii

This is a photochromogen, and is more common in the central US, England, and Wales among the white population. Its normal manifestation resembles pulmonary tuberculosis, although signs and symptoms are milder. However, in AIDS and in bone marrow and renal transplantation cases, the disease may be more disseminated; soft tissue and skin involvement also may be seen.

M. Scrofulaceum

This bacillus forms pigment even in the dark, and is a major cause of lymphadenitis in children. Cervical nodes are usually involved, and associated systemic symptoms are rare.

M. Marinum

This organism is usually associated with some aquatic activity and enters abraded skin; it forms a nodule, which can either spread along lymphatics, or ulcerate.

M. Ulcerans

It is present mainly in Australia and Africa in tropical regions. It grows only at 30 to 33°C and is a slow grower. It forms granulamatous ulcers, usually affecting the extensor surfaces of extremities. *M. ulcerans* is the etiologic agent of Buruli or Bairnsdale ulcers.

Antimycobacterial Agents

Since the discovery around 1940 of the antimycobacterial activity of dapsone, a synthetic compound, and of streptomycin, an antibiotic, large numbers of synthetic compounds and natural products/antibiotics have been screened for their antimycobacterial activity. However, rather small numbers of compounds have emerged that have therapeutic indices favoring their introduction into clinical practice. The drugs commonly used clinically are described below (Table 97.1), giving the salient features that bear on their clinical application. As the requirements of drugs for tuberculosis and leprosy are quite similar, and because some drugs find use in both diseases, the agents are described together in the order in which they were introduced into therapy. The laboratory models/methods commonly used for screening and evaluating antimycobacterial agents are first briefly described.

Table 97.1 Antimycobacterial Drugs in Therapeutic Use: Some Important Parameters[d]

	Year of Discovery	Dose (mg)	C_{max} ug/ml	t_{max} hr.	$t_{1/2}$ hr.	CSF_b %	Antimicrobial	Action
TUBERCULOSIS (administered orally)							EARLY BACTERIAL ACTIVITY	STERILIZING ACTIVITY
First line drugs								
Isoniazid	1952	300	3–5	1.5	1–3	90–100	+++	+
Rifampicin	1965	600	7	2–4	3	0,4[c]	++	+++
Pyrazinamide	1952	500	9–12	2	9	100	+	+++
Ethambutol	1961	1200	2–5	2–4	3	10[c]	++	±
Streptomycin[a]	1944	1000	40	2	2.3	poor	+	±
Thiacetazone	1946	150	1–2	4–5	12	—	+	±
Second line drugs								
Kanamicin[a]	1957	750	22	1	2–4	—	+	±
Cycloserine	1955	250	10	1–4	10	30–100	+	±
Capreomycin[a]	1960	1000	20–45	1–2	4–6	—	+	±
LEPROSY						Bactericidal		
First-line drugs								
Dapsone	1939	100	10–15	2–3	18	—	+++ (bacteriostatic)	
Rifampicin	1965	600	7	2–4	3	0,4[c]	+++	
Clofazimine	1957	100	—	—	70 d	—	++	
Ofloxacin	1984	400	3	2–3	5–8		+++	
Second-line drugs								
Ethionamide	1957	1000	20	3	3	100	++	
Atypical mycobacteriosis								
Rifampicin/Rifabutine								
Rifapentine								
Isoniazid								
Amikacin					In investigational stage			
Ethambutol								
Minocycline/doxycycline								
Fluoroquinolones:								
Ciprofloxacin, ofloxacin								
pefloxacin, Sparfloxacin								
Clarithromycin, azithromycin								

[a] not absorbed orally and administered parenterally; [b] percent of plasma concentration; [c] inflamed meninges; [d] data compiled from different sources
— definite data not available

Screening of Antimycobacterial Agents

Tuberculosis

Screening of drugs for tuberculosis is quite straightforward. The commonly used primary screen is demonstration of in vitro activity against virulent strains of *M. tuberculosis* $H_{37}Rv$. This test may give some false-negative or false-positive results, but over-all this is quite a dependable primary screen, and is widely used.

This study is followed by in vivo quantitative evaluation of the short-listed compounds in animal models against virulent strains of *M. tuberculosis*. There are a variety of procedures for performing these tests; they differ with respect to animal species, mycobacterial strain, size of inoculum, route of drug administration, etc. The mouse model is most commonly used, employing human virulent strain and evaluating the results in terms of ED_{50}, survival time, pathology of the lung, and bacterial count.[r2] The products active in mice are then evaluated in more sophisticated animal model, preferably primates.

Leprosy

In the case of leprosy where an in vitro culture is still not available and where no really satisfactory animal model is available, the in vitro antituberculosis screening or testing against *M. lepraemurium* in rodents are often used as the first screens. This rodent model, however, does not show much correlation with human activity, and is not very dependable; DDS shows no activity in this test, and isoniazid is highly active—opposite what is true in human leprosy.

The first unequivocally successful and reproducible transmission of a limited infection in animals, though limited in its scope, was achieved by Shepard in the mouse footpad[32] in 1960. As the generation time of lepra becilli is much too long (over 15 days), this model is not very convenient for general screening. Still, with various procedural modifications,[33,34] it is the best model available and has been used widely for screening and evaluation of drugs. The most important contribution of the foodpad model has been to the study of dapsone resistance, not only in establishing for the first time (1964) the isolation of dapsone-resistant strains of *M. leprae* from treated/relapsed patients,[35] but eventually for use in investigating the serious and ever-increasing worldwide prevalence of dapsone resistance.[36]

Thymectomy and body irradiation of mice inoculated with *M. leprae* provokes dissemination of bacilli, and this also may be used as a model for generalized infection.[37] As an alternative to use the thymectomized mouse, the congenitally athymic nude mouse to a lesser extent has been used as an immune-deficient model to study leprosy.[38]

However, nude mice, generally are very fragile and require specific pathogen-free housing, which is not easy for many laboratories to provide.

Another significant development took place with the demonstration that a progressive and generalized *M. leprae* infection resulted in the nine-banded armadillo inoculated IV with *M. leprae;* aramadillo was the first and remains one of the few animal species shown to have a natural susceptibility to *M. leprae.*[39] Armadillos cannot be bred in captivity, and therefore are not convenient for general screening; however, they have been used for supplying large quantities of *M. leprae.*

Atypical Mycobacteria

These mycobacteria are easy to grow in vitro, and products against them can be tested in vitro, followed by in vivo screening. The great increase in infections caused by atypical mycobacteria following HIV infection has focused attention on their chemotherapy, which until recently was a relatively neglected field. A number of atypical mycobacteria are now included in antimycobacterial screening programs, and new classes of compounds are showing up for activity against these infections (Table 102.1). As infections due to atypical mycobacteria take serious dimensions, and because many of them are not sensitive to known drugs, there is certainly a need to increase screening efforts against them and to focus on the study of their biochemistry, physiology, and pathogenic behavior in laboratory animals to achieve better drug design.

Antimycobacterial Drugs in Common Use[r1,r2,r3]

Dapsone

Following the demonstration of the promising activity of dapsone (DDS) in human leprosy in the 1940s,[40] a number of N-substituted and ring-substituted derivatives and analogues of dapsone were synthesized, but none surpassed the activity of dapsone.[r2,r4] Dapsone has occupied a pre-eminent position in the treatment of human leprosy ever since; all multidrug (MDT) regimens include dapsone. The only derivative used is N,N′-diacetamidodiphenylsulfone (acedapsone, DADDS), which acts as a repository form of DDS; after a single IM injection of 225 mg acedapsone, a therapeutic level of dapsone is maintained in the blood for a long as 68 to 80 days.[41]

Dapsone is a bacteriostatic agent, and *M. leprae* are highly sensitive to it; in vitro MIC is 0.01–0.02 μg/ml; in mice, levels in feed of 0.0003 to 0.00001 per cent are bacteriostatic, and the MIC in mouse plasma is less than 5 ng/ml, indicating that *M. leprae* are 100 times more sensitive to dapsone than are other mycobacteria so far tested. *M. leprae* became resistant to dapsone; in some areas of dapsone monotherapy, 15 to 20% of isolates show primary dapsone resistance; dapsone resistance has become a major problem in mass chemotherapy programs. In the case of sulfones, however, a small increase in dose can help to overcome resistance, unlike the sulfonamides.

Dapsone acts primarily as a p-aminobenzoic acid (PABA) antagonist, and blocks the synthesis of dihydrofolic acid in much the same way as do the sulfonamides.[42] That its action in mycobacteria, as in other bacteria, is antagonized by PABA was shown quite early. More definitive information on the mode of action was provided by Seydel et al., using whole cell and cell-free systems *E. coli, M. lufu* and *M. leprae.*[43] It was shown that dapsone competes with PABA for pteroate synthetase. It is incorporated into "false" dihydrofolate precursors by *E. coli,* though mycobacteria do not utilize DDS this way. In any case, this is not a rate-limiting step in folate biosynthesis; therefore, it is not of much consequence for mode of action of DDS. Synergistic effects of dapsone with certain dihydrofolate reductase inhibitors, bromdimaprin, have been demonstrated both in cell-free systems of *M. lufu* and in clinical testing.[44]

In addition, DDS modulates the immune response,[r4] acting as a scavenger of the active oxygen species known to have an important role in inflammation.[45,46] This property may explain its beneficial effects in some immune skin disorders;[47] some of the beneficial effects in leprosy also may result from this action. Overall, the action of dapsone may be twofold; a direct bactericidal action, and modulation of the host-response.

Dapsone is usually administered orally at a daily dose of 100 mg, even when used as a part of multiple-drug therapy (MDT). It is almost completely absorbed from the GI tract, reaching a peak blood level one to three hours after administration. After multiple dosing a steady state blood level of 10–30 ng/ml is reached. Dapsone is well distributed in all body tissues and is excreted primarily in the urine, mainly as the glucuronide or sulfonate. The drug remains in the circulatory system for a long period because it is reabsorbed from the bile; it is detectable even eight to 12 days after single-dose administration. It has a half-life of about 20 hour.

The drug seldom causes serious side-effects; hemolysis is the most common and is dose-dependent. In malnourished patients the "sulfone" syndrome may develop, which is characterized by fever, malaise, exfoliative dermatitis, jaundice, lymphadenopathy, methaemoglobinemia, and anemia. Such patients are helped when given iron and folic acid along with dapsone treatment.

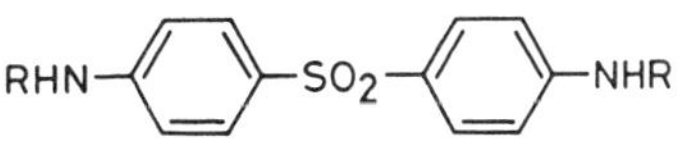

RHN–C_6H_4–SO_2–C_6H_4–NHR

Dapsone: R=H
Acedapsone: R=$COCH_3$

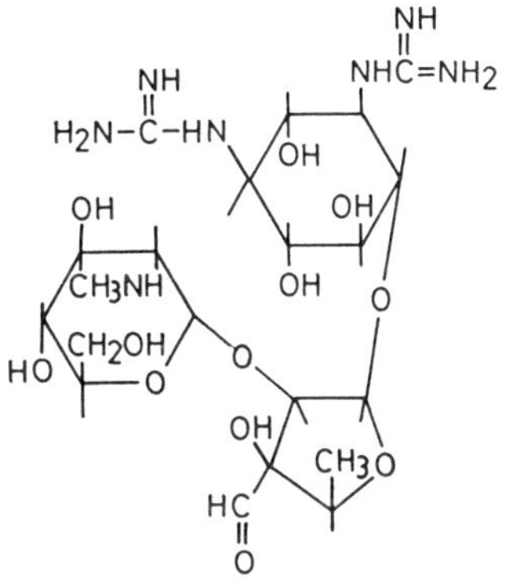

Streptomycin

Streptomycin

Streptomycin (SM), an antibiotic discovered in 1944, was found to inhibit the growth of *M. tuberculosis*, among other organisms, both in vitro and in vivo. Within a short time it became the first clinically available drug for the treatment of tuberculosis. It maintained a preeminent position until very recently, but is now gradually losing ground to more effective drugs. Structural modifications have not been successful in improving its activity. The changes carried out have included reduction of the aldehyde group to the primary alcohol to give dihydrostreptomycin. This compound is about as active as SM and is less toxic to the vestibular apparatus, but is more toxic to the auditory branch.

SM shows both bacteriostatic and bactericidal activities in vitro, depending on its concentration. Resistance to this drug emerges rapidly, and can develop spontaneously by mutation or by transfer of R factors through plasmids. The mechanism of resistance involves changes in the sensitivity of the P10 protein and in the ability of streptomycin to reach the ribosomes, or induction of metabolic enzymes that inactivate the drug.

SM, and the other aminoglycoside antibiotics, irreversibly block protein synthesis, which was at one time considered to be the cause of its lethal action.[48] However, much evidence has accumulated over the last three decades to show that the mode of action of SM is more intricate; blockade of protein synthesis is a sequela of these actions, not the primary mode of action. It was shown by Anand and Davis[49] that *E. coli* growing in the presence of SM become permeable in both directions to a variety of small molecules, resulting in increased uptake of SM itself, indicating the involvement of the cell membrane. This effect is prevented when protein synthesis is reversibly inhibited by chloramphenicol.[50] Subsequently, Plotz and Davis[51] showed that pretreatment of growing *E. coli* with penicillin, which distorted cell-wall synthesis, increased sensitivity to subsequent killing by SM, presumably by inducing some membrane damage. Meanwhile, Gorini[52] discovered that SM at sublethal levels causes misreading of the code, rather than blockage of protein synthesis, which was also confirmed in in vitro experiments as due to misreading of one base as another. A major step toward enhancing the understanding was provided by the study of Davis, Tai, and Wallace,[53] separating the step of initiating free ribosomes from chain-elongation polysomes, which lack initiating factors and can only complete the already growing chains on which SM causes misreading. Therefore, it appeared that the misreading effect of SM probably is involved in its mode of action. Based on all this evidence it has been proposed[54] that on first encounter with a bacterial cell a few SM molecules stray into the essentially impermeable cell, where they encounter the chain-elongating ribosomes that predominate in growing cells. This results in misreading, leading to formation of "abnormal" proteins. Abnormal membrane proteins may be the cause of membrane damage and its leakiness. This results in increased uptake of the antibiotic, which then saturates the ribosome populaton; the ribosomes are thus fixed in initiation complexes, blocking protein synthesis. Killing by SM thus appears to depend not on one key step but on a cycle of multiple steps, each equally important, and misreading of the code is at the center of all these events.

When SM is administered orally, almost none is absorbed; it is stable in the GI environment and is excreted unchanged in the feces. Therefore, it must be administered parenterally. After SQ or IM injection, peak blood level is reached in one to two hours; a peak of 15–27 μg/ml is attained after administration of 1 g. Its half-life is two to three hours. It diffuses slowly into the pleura, and more quickly into the peritoneal, pericardial, and synovial fluids. It does not penetrate the spinal fluid unless the meninges are involved.

The most important side-effects of SM involve the peripheral nerves and CNS; the most common is a vestibular disturbance resulting in vertigo. Damage to the auditory function of the eighth cranial nerve results in decreased hearing. This damage is dose-related; 2 to 3 g per day for two to four months produces this damage in about 75 percent of patients, but the incidence is much less when the dose is 1 g a day. Other side-effects are a hypersensitivity reaction and, rarely, renal damage.

Other aminoglycoside antibiotics have since then been discovered, the most important being neomycin, kanamycin, gentamycin, amikacin, and tobramycin. Of these kanamycin has been used to some extent to treat tuberculosis (although it does not offer any major advantage over streptomycin), and amikacin is used in some atypical mycobacterial infections.

Thiacetazone (Thioacetazone, Amithiozone)

Benzaldehyde thiosemicarbazone, prepared for the synthesis of sulfathiadiazoles, showed weak antituberculosis activity; this led to the development of its p-acetamido derivative, thioacetazone (THI), the most active member of the series, as an antituberculosis agent.[55]

The mechanism of action of thioacetazone is not known, but mycolic acid and lipid synthesis probably is involved. Its activity is not antagonized by PABA. Thiacetazone has no significant bactericidal action, and resistance to the drug develops rapidly. There is no cross resistance with isoniazid or streptomycin, with which it has been used in combination therapy. A dose of 300 mg isoniazid plus 150 mg of thioacetazone is a cheap and acceptable combination for long-term treatment after the initial treatment with three drugs. The drug is also reported to be effective in leprosy, but is of limited use in view of ready emergence of resistant strains of *M. leprae*.

The drug at the initially used daily dose of 300 mg showed a high incidence of side-effects, such as GI disorders, liver damage, and anemia, but it has acceptable toxicity at the lower daily dose of 150 mg now used. Hemolytic anemia, leukopenia, and agranulocytosis may occur in some patients.

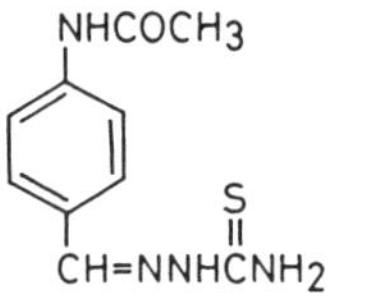

$NHCOCH_3$

$CH{=}NNHC(=S)NH_2$

Thioacetazone

$CONH_2$

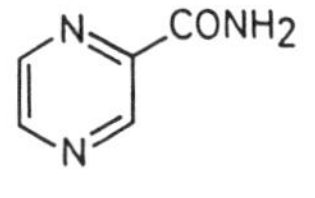

Pyrazinamide

Pyrazinamide

Investigation of heterocyclic analogues of nicotinamide led to the development of pyrazinamide (PZA) as an antituberculosis agent.[56] None of the structural modifications of PZA has provided an analogue with an improved therapeutic index.

In vivo studies show that PZA is bactericidal and has a specific sterilizing action against *M. tuberculosis* in the intracellular acid environment of lysosomes and phagosomes of phagocytes and the macrophages, where the dormant bacilli reside and where they must be killed to prevent relapses.[57] PZA, therefore, occupies a special position in chemotherapeutic regimens.[58] Resistance to PZA, however, develops readily, but there is no cross-resistance to isoniazid and streptomycin. PZA should, therefore, always be used in combination with other antituberculosis drugs.

Atypical mycobacteria are by and large resistant to PZA, except for *M. avium*-intracellular complex, against which infection it has sometimes been used.

The mode of action of PZA on tubercle bacilli is not known. It is more active in an acid environment, and some have suggested that its metabolites, though less active in vitro, may be involved in the in vivo activity of PZA.

The oral daily dose of PZA is 30–35 mg/kg. It is absorbed well from the GI tract and widely distributed throughout the body. PZA appears to penetrate the CSF, at least in patients with tuberculous meningitis; oral administration of 1 g in an adult produces plasma concentration of 45 μg/ml at two hour and 10 μg/ml at 15 hour. The drug is excreted rapidly, mainly in the urine, partly as the unchanged drug and partly as the inactive metabolites, pyrazinoic acid and 5-hydroxypyrazinoic acid. PZA is also suitable for intermittent therapy of tuberculosis; recommended doses are 45 mg/kg three time a week or 70 mg/kg twice a week.

The most common side-effect is hepatotoxicity. It also affects the excretion of urates, and thus might precipitate gout. Other common side-effects include anorexia, nausea, and vomiting.

Initially, pyrazinamide was used at rather high doses that gave rise to side-effects; as more effective drugs were discovered, it was relegated to a "reserve drug." Gradually, as its sterilizing action in acidic intracellular environment even at lower doses was recognized, its position has changed; it now has an important role, particularly in the short-course treatment of tuberculosis.

Isoniazid

Following reports of the tuberculostatic activity of nicotinamide and some thiosemicarbazones, thiosemicarbazones of isonicotinaldehyde and some related compounds, which included isonicotinyl hydrazid (isoniazid), an intermediate in the preparation of the aldehyde, were synthesized and tested for their antituberculosis activity in the early 1950s. Among these, isoniazid exhibited an unprecedented high order of antituberculosis activity in vitro and in experimental infections—more potent than that of any other known agent.[r3,59] This activity was soon confirmed in clinical trials. This was the beginning of a new chapter in the chemotherapy of tuberculosis. None of the congeners of this molecule has surpassed its activity, and isoniazid has remained the main anchor for the treatment of tuberculosis.

Isoniazid is bacteriostatic for resting bacilli, but is bactericidal for rapidly dividing microorganisms; its MIC is 0.025 to 0.05 μg/ml. The bacteria undergo one or two divisions before multiplication is arrested. The drug is just as effective against intracellular bacilli as it is against those growing in culture media. Isoniazid is equally effective for the treatment of experimentally-induced tuberculosis in animals. It is remarkably selective for tubercle bacilli, and concentrations in excess of 500 μg/ml are required to inhibit the growth of other microorganisms. Among the atypical mycobacteria, only *M. kansasii* is usually susceptible to isoniazid. It shows only marginal activity against *M. leprae* in the mouse footpad model and is essentially inactive in human leprosy.

Isoniazid, though active against *M. tuberculosis* strains resistant to other antimycobacterial agents, when administered alone results in quick emergence of resistant strains. Approximately one in 10^6 bacilli are genetically resistant to isoniazid; since tuberculous cavities may contain as many as 10^7 to 10^8 microorganisms, it is not surprising that monotherapy with isoniazid alone leads to ready emergence of resistant bacteria. Therefore, the drug always should be used in combination with other antituberculosis agents. Current evidence suggests that the development of resistance is related to the failure of the drug to penetrate or be taken up by the bacterial cell.

Though mycolic acid biosynthesis, NAD^+, pyridoxal phosphates, and catalase-peroxidase have all been proposed as possible targets for isoniazid action, no one mechanism is yet firmly established. Isoniazid inhibits the biosynthesis of mycolic acids,[60,61] which are unique to mycobacteria, and this action would explain the high degree of selectivity of the antimicrobial activity of isoniazid. This inhibition leads to a decrease in the quantity of methanol-extractable lipids of the bacilli, resulting in loss of acid fastness and deformation of the cell membrane. Only in isoniazid-sensitive cells do these changes take place.

Many isoniazid-resistant isolates of *M. tuberculosis* have decreased catalase activity, with the most highly resistant isolates being completely catalase-negative. Zhang et al[62] have shown that a single *M. tuberculosis* gene, *kat G*, encoding both catalase and peroxidase, restored sensitivity to isoniazid in a resistant mutant of *M. smegmatis* and conferred isoniazid susceptibility in some strains of *Escherichia coli*. It has also been shown that deletion of *kat G* gene from the chromosome was associated with isoniazid resistance in two patient isolates of *M. tuberculosis*. Based on these results, Zhang et al proposed that the catalase-peroxidase enzyme may be important in converting isoniazid to a metabolically active form in the cell, or in the isoniazid-dependent generation of reactive oxygen radicals. Gene deletion represents an unusual mechanism for development of drug resistance.[62]

Isoniazid is rapidly absorbed following oral or parenteral administration, passing readily into all body fluids and cells; peak blood level is reached in one to two hours. The drug is detectable in significant quantities in pleural and ascitic fluids; concentrations in the CSF are similar to those in plasma. Isoniazid penetrates well into the caseous material. The drug is excreted primarily in the urine, either unchanged, as the acetyl derivative, or as isonicotinic acid. The rate of excretion depends on the rate of metabolism, which varies greatly in different individuals. This difference appears to be race-related and seems to be under genetic control. Individuals can be slow or rapid acetylators of the drug; the half-life of isoniazid in rapid acetylators ranges from 45 to 110 minutes, and in slow acetylators from two to 4.5 hours. The commonly used total daily dose of the drug is 5 mg/kg, with a maximum of 300 mg; oral and IM doses are identical. The drug usually is given orally in a single daily dose, but may be given in two divided doses.

Isoniazid is one of the most effective antituberculosis drugs with minimal side-effects. Peripheral neuritis, occasional optical neuritis, and stimulation of the nervous system are the most common side-effects. Neuritis is very likely due to competition of the drug with the coenzyme pyridoxal phosphate, and the concurrent administration of the latter has been reported to prevent neural toxicity. Allergic reactions, though rare, may result in fever, skin eruptions, and hepatitis.

INH is still the most important drug for the treatment of all types of tuberculosis, with minimal side-effects, particularly when pyridoxine is used prophylactically. Isoniazid should always be used in combination therapy, except when used for chemoprophylaxis.

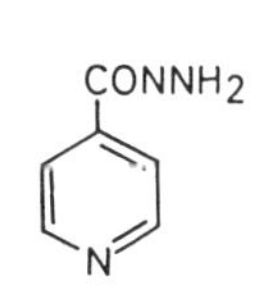

$CONNH_2$

Isoniazid

$C(=S)NH_2$

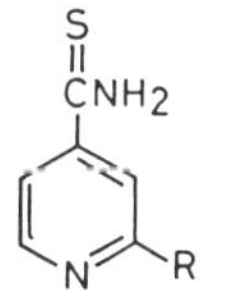

Ethionamide: $R=C_2H_5$
Prothionamide: $R=C_3H_7$

Ethionamide/Prothionamide

Following the reports of antituberculosis activity in nicotinamide and thionicotinamide, thioisonicotinamides were screened, and 2-alkyl derivatives showed increased in vivo activity. 2-Ethylthioisonicotinamide (ethionamide) and the 2-n-propyl analogue (prothionamide) were selected for clinical trials, and the former has been more extensively studied.[63]

In vitro MIC of ethionamide against *M. tuberculosis* including strains resistant to isoniazid and streptomycin is 0.6–2.5 μg/ml. It shows activity against atypical mycobacteria, especially those belonging to the photochromogenic group, and also against *M. leprae.* Bacterial resistance develops quickly when ethionamide is used alone in tuberculosis; therefore, it is used in combination with other antimycobacterial drugs. *M. tuberculosis* strains resistant to isoniazid and streptomycin remain ethionamide-sensitive, but ethionamide may show cross-resistance with thiacetazone.

Ethionamide is rapidly absorbed after oral administration and widely distributed in the body, with peak blood level being reached in about three hours (plasma level of about 20 μg/mg after 1 g of drug). The drug has a relatively short half-life and is rapidly excreted in the urine, with a small percentage in unaltered form and the rest as metabolites, the active sulfoxide, and the inactive 2-ethylisonicotinic acid and its amide. The drug is administered orally, mainly 250 mg twice daily to begin and reaching a maximum of 1 g/day.

Ethionamide, like isoniazid, inhibits mycolic acid and other long-chain fatty acid synthesis. It also inhibits peptide synthesis in mycobacteria by blocking incorporation of the sulfur-containing amino acids (cysteine and methionine) into growing peptide chains.

The drug is not tolerated well when administered orally; it causes severe GI reactions, and, in about 5 percent of cases, some hepatic toxicity has been reported. Other side-effects include olfactory disturbance, acne, dizziness, numbness of feet, and some symptoms indicative of ganglionic blockage. The symptoms disappear on withdrawal of the drug.

Ethionamide, both for tuberculosis and leprosy, is a secondary drug, and is used only when first-line drugs are ineffective owing to resistance or contraindicated because of toxicity.

Clofazimine

In a continuing interest in dyes as antimicrobial agents, Barry et al synthesized a series of substituted iminophenazines (often referred to as riminophenazines as a contraction of R-imino), and found that some of these had a high order of antimycobacterial activity.[64] Clofazimine (B 663) was selected as the best compound of the series for further development. Its high in vitro activity was confirmed in experimental infections in mice, hamsters, and rats, though a much higher dose was needed for a comparable effect in guinea pigs and monkeys. Limited clinical trial in human pulmonary tuberculosis at doses up to 10 mg/kg proved disappointing. Subsequently, however, clofazimine was found to be many times more active against *M. lepraemurium* and *M. leprae,* even in dapsone-resistant organisms. Clofazimine was found to have a pronounced bacteriostatic action at concentrations of 0.0001 to 0.001 per cent in mouse chow. These studies led to its introduction for the treatment of leprosy in 1962.[65–67] Clofazimine is now established as a front-line drug for the treatment of all lepromatous leprosy cases as a part of MDT and for treatment of dapsone-resistant leprosy. Clofazimine is more active against atypical mycobacteria than is isoniazid, particularly against *M. kansasii, M. ulcerans, M. chelonei,* and *M. avium* complex.[68]

Clofazimine has an anti-inflammatory action,[69] because of which, when used in treatment of lepromatous leprosy, without or in combination with dapsone, the characteristic "erythema nodosum leprosum" (ENL) seldom develops, thus avoiding need for corticosteroid or other anti-ENL drugs such as thalidomide.

Clofazimine is a very highly hydrophobic compound, with a measured log P in isoctane/buffer pH 5.15 of 5.01. It has pKa values of 8.35; it is 90 percent ionized under physiologic conditions and totally ionized at pH 5.15. The drug is slowly and poorly absorbed from the GI tract, unless presented in micronized form; the GI absorption ranges from 40 to 70 percent of the oral dose. It accumulates in the body in macrophages of the GI tract, skin, and eye. Clofazimine appears to accumulate in crystalline form in many organs, particularly in fatty tissues. The drug does not appear to enter the brain and CSF. It is extremely slowly excreted, mainly in an unaltered form, primarily by the fecal route. A two-compartment pharmacokinetic model giving $t_{1/2}$ of seven and 70 days has been proposed. In patients taking clofazimine 100–300 mg/daily, the steady-state serum concentration of 0.7 to 1.0 μg/ml is obtained only after about 30 days.

Although the mechanism of action of clofazimine is not established, it has some characteristic structural features indicative of its possible mode(s) of action. The molecule has a planar area with suitably positioned imino and amino groups for DNA bases interaction. It has been shown to bind in vitro to guanine of cytosine-guanine (CG) DNA base pairs, and DNA of *M. leprae* is rich in C-G content.[70] Another important structural feature is its quinonoid character, making it suitable for electron transfer reactions. It has been shown that redox properties of clofazimine can divert up to 20 percent of cellular oxygen and disrupt normal mitochondrial oxidation processes; as a consequence, cytotoxic oxygen species, hydrogen peroxide, and superoxide are generated, which would enhance the killing of the bacilli in macrophages.[71] Clofazimine is a lysosomotropic agent, and is actively transported into the lysosomes of macrophages. This may explain its anti-inflammatory activity.

Clofazimine is used in doses ranging from 50 mg/day or 100 mg on alternate days for chemotherapy and at 400 mg for ENL control. Despite the fact that clofazimine has been used for many years as a monotherapy in leprosy, there are only two reports of possible clofazimine-resistant leprosy cases.[72,73] However, persistent organisms remain unaffected even after prolonged treatment.

Clofazimine is well tolerated and shows few side-effects. Hyperpigmentation of the skin, which occurs in all patients, appears to be the main side-effect, which may be distressing in light-skinned people. Eosinophilic enteritis has also been described as an adverse drug reaction in some cases.

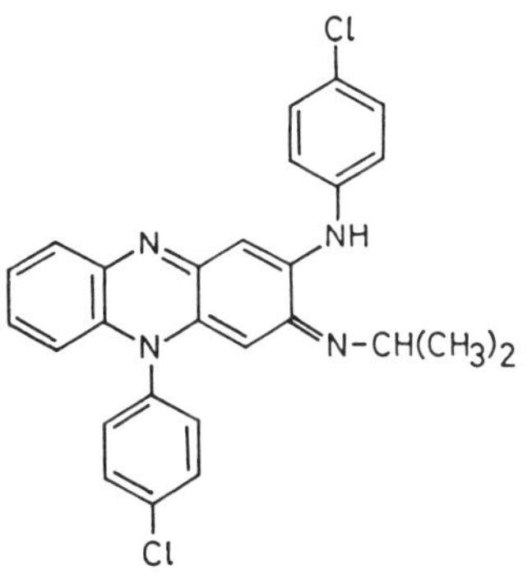

Clofazimine

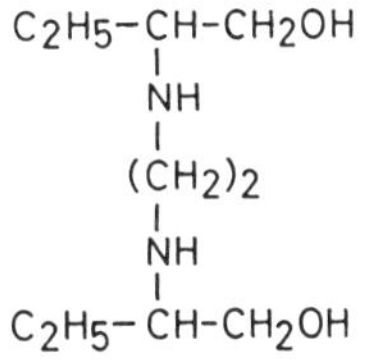

$C_2H_5-CH-CH_2OH$ | NH | $(CH_2)_2$ | NH | $C_2H_5-CH-CH_2OH$

Ethambutol

Ethambutol

Following the lead that alkylene diamines possess antimycobacterial activity, (+)-2,2′-(ethylenediamino)-*d*-1-butanol (ethambutol) was synthesized and found to exhibit a high order of antituberculosis activity; the meso isomer was less active and the levo isomer almost inactive.[74] The efficacy of ethambutol against *M. tuberculosi* in vivo was tested in experimental animal models and confirmed in clinical trials in human tuberculosis.

Ethambutol is active against most human strains of *M. tuberculosis* with an MIC of 0.5–2.0 μg/ml; there is no cross resistance to other drugs, and strains resistant to other antimycobacterial agents are just as sensitive to ethambutol. Ethambutol is not active in experimental *M. leprae* infection in mouse. As for atypical mycobacteria, *M. kansasii* and a number of strains of *M. avium* complex are sensitive to it; others show variable response. Ethambutol has no effect on other bacteria.

Though resistance to ethambutol develops slowly compared to other antimycobacterial agents, combination use with other antimycobacterial agents is preferred to prevent emergence of resistant strains.

The drug is well absorbed after oral administration, and its activity is the same whether given orally or parenterally. It does not seem to enter the CSF of patients with normal meninges. It concentrates in the red blood cells, from which it is slowly released. It penetrates both extracellular and intracellular environments of tuberculosis lesions. It is excreted in the urine mainly in the unaltered form along with minor quantities of two inactive metabolites, the dialdehyde and the dicarboxylic acid.

The mechanism of action of ethambutol is not yet clearly understood. Ethambutol inhibits protein and DNA synthesis in mycobacteria, and it has been proposed that it interferes with the role of polyamines and divalent cations in RNA metabolism.[75] Studies with *M. smegmatis* show that ethambutol inhibits the transfer of mycolic acids into the cell wall, possibly by competitive inhibition of an enzyme.[76] Other authors have observed an inhibitory effect on phosphorylation of some intermediary metabolites.

Ethambutol produces very few side-effects and reactions at the daily doses of 15 mg/kg normally used. The most important side-effect is optic neuritis, resulting in a decrease of visual acuity and loss of ability to differentiate red from green. The incidence of this side-effect is related to dosage and duration of therapeutic use.[77] Recovery occurs when ethambutol is withdrawn. Ethambutol is not recommended for children under five years of age because of the difficulty of testing their visual acuity reliably.

Ethambutol has been used with notable success in different forms of tuberculosis when used in combination therapy. Although originally considered as a "first-line" drug, its position has now been reassessed. Because it does not add any special effects on bacterial growth, its main use now is as a reserve drug for treatment of patients with special problems, including those with diabetes, pregnancy, severe liver disease, or with disease due to suspected or proved resistance to other antituberculosis drugs.

Rifampicin (Rifampin)

Rifamycines, produced by *Nocardia mediterranei* the first group of antibiotics with an ansa structure (an aromatic moiety spanned by an aliphatic bridge), were found to exhibit a broad antimicrobial spectrum, including antimycobacterial activity.[r2,r3,78] Their semisynthetic analogues showed an improved antimicrobial spectrum. This led to extensive investigation of derivatives of rifamycin B, one of the first naturally occurring rifamycines to be isolated, for obtaining analogues that would have the desired characteristics, such as oral absorption, long half-life, and high antimycobacterial activity. Rifampicin (rifampin) was the product of these studies, and was introduced for clinical use in 1968.[79]

Rifampicin has a broad antibacterial spectrum. It inhibits the growth of most gram-positive bacteria, as well as many gram-negative microorganisms, such as *E. coli,* Pseudomonas, Proteus, and Klebsiela. It is highly active against *Neisseria meningitidis* and *Haemophilus influenzae.* Rifampicin is active in vitro against *M. tuberculosis* at concentrations of 0.005 to 0.2 μg/ml in semisynthetic media; its bacteriostatic and bactericidal concentrations are quite close to each other. It is also active against isoniazid-resistant strains. There is no cross resistance to other antimycobacterial drugs. The antituberculosis activity is also seen in different experimental animal models. Rifampicin shows a high bactericidal effect and a therapeutic efficacy comparable to that of isoniazid and superior to that of all other known antituberculosis agents. A combination of rifampicin and isoniazid produces a more rapid bacterial negativity than any other combination.

Rifampicin is highly active against *M. leprae* in the mouse footpad model; suppression of multiplication and loss of viability of the organisms showed its rapid bactericidal action.[80,81] A single dose of 20 mg/kg has been shown to kill about 99.9 per cent of the viable bacilli in the mouse foot pad.[81,82] In previously untreated leprosy patients, a 600-mg single dose rendered bacilli taken four days later noninfectious for mice,[83] suggesting that such a dose had killed at least 99 per cent of the viable *M. leprae.* Rifampicin is by far the most potent antileprosy drug at present.[83–85]

Rifampicin is also active against a number of atypical mycobacteria; *M. kansasii* and *M. marinum* are the most sensitive and are inhibited by 0.25 to 1 μg/ml; the majority of strains of *M. avium intracellulare* and *M. scrofulaceum* are suppressed by concentrations of 4 μg/ml. However, *M. fortuitum* is highly resistant to the drug.

Rifampicin blocks transcription and thus inhibits RNA synthesis. It inhibits specifically the DNA-dependent RNA-polymerase (DDRP)[86] of sensitive bacteria at rather low concentrations. As a consequence of the block of RNA synthesis, the protein synthesis in the bacterial cell ceases, leading eventually to the death of the cell. It has no effect on the mammalian RNA-polymerase, which gives it the required selectivity of action against the pathogens. It has been shown that rifampicin forms a rather stable 1:1 noncovalent complex with DDRP by binding with the β-subunit of the enzyme; it appears to abort the initiation of RNA synthesis by interfering with the binding of the newly formed RNA chains. Bacterial mutants resistant to rifampicin possess an altered RNA polymerase not inhibited by rifampicin. Change in permeability to rifampicin has also been reported in some mycobacteria, which may also contribute to development of resistance.

Rifampicin is well absorbed following oral administration. It is distributed throughout the body tissues and fluids; it crosses the blood-brain barrier, and reaches good antibacterial levels in many organs and body fluids, including the CSF, cavern exudate, and pleural fluid. Its half-life is about three hours, and is higher in patients with biliary obstruction or liver disease. About 30 percent of the oral dose is excreted in the urine, but the major route of excretion is in bile. Part of that is reabsorbed from the GI tract. The drug may impart an orange color to body fluids. Rifampicin has a stimulating effect on microsomal drug metabolizing enzymes,[87] which is of consequence while administering rifampicin with other drugs, such as oral contraceptives,[88] where blood levels are critical for efficacy. The dose of oral contraceptive may need to be increased.

Rifampicin is generally well tolerated when given in doses of 10 mg/kg (with a daily maximum of 600 mg). The most notable problem is the development of jaundice, which occurs only in patients with chronic liver disease, alcoholism, or in the elderly. Administration of rifampicin on an intermittent schedule is associated with more incidence of side-effects.

Rifampicin at present occupies a special status in the treatment of mycobacterial infections. It is one of the two essential drugs for short-course chemotherapy regimens for tuberculosis,[r5,r6] and is also the essential drug on whose strong bactericidal action the success of the MDT for leprosy stands.[r7,85]

Newer Rifamycin Analogues

The important position that rifampicin has come to occupy in the chemotherapy of tuberculosis and leprosy focused attention on the possibility of further improving its therapeutic profile, particularly against some atypical mycobacteria. A number of new derivatives have been explored in recent years,[89–92] of which rifabutin (ansamycin) and rifapentine (MDL-473) were more active than rifampicin (MIC of 0.04 and 0.08 as compared to 0.3 mg/L of rifampicin), and seem the most promising. Rifabutine showed only partial cross resistance to rifampicin; it is active against 30 percent of the rifampicin-resistant *M. tuberculosis* strains.[89] Rifapentine is even more active in vitro than rifabutine, and much longer acting, with $t_{1/2}$ of 20 hours.[91] Rifapentine however, has complete cross resistance with rifampicin. Because of its long half-life and high activity, rifapentine may be useful for intermittent therapy.[90] Rifabutine is more active than rifampicin against *M. avium* complex infection, with a lower MIC and a lower natural resistance rate. In a study of the action of rifapentine and rifabutine in combination with other antimycobacterial agents against *M. avium* in the beige mouse model it has been found that combination with clofazimine appears most promising.[92]

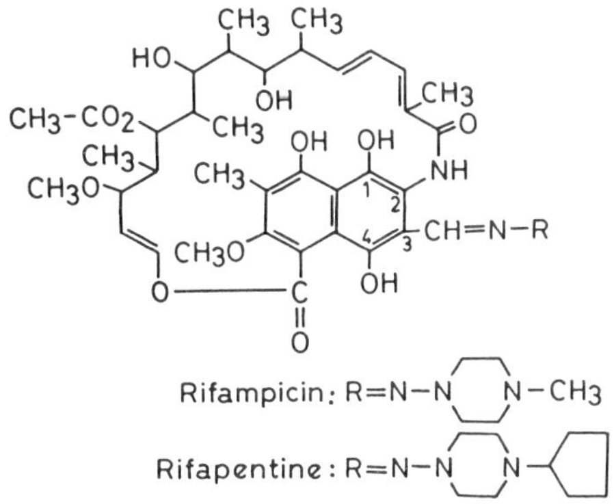

Rifampicin: R=N−N N−CH3

Rifapentine: R=N−N N−

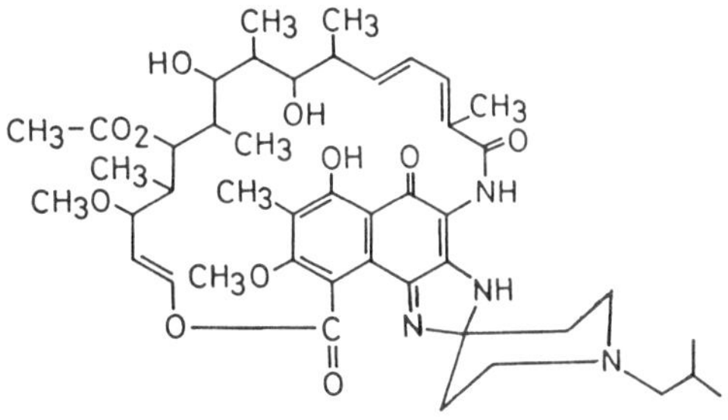

Rifabutine

Fluoroquinolones

Fluoroquinolones are a relatively new class of antimicrobial agents characterized by an unusually broad spectrum of antibacterial, activity including against mycobacteria. Fluoroquinolones have special pharmacokinetic and pharmacodynamic features that led to their detailed exploration as antimycobacterial agents. Fluoroquinolones in general are well absorbed after oral administration, with relatively long half-lives in serum, exellent penetration into many tissues and human cells, including macrophages, resulting in antimicrobial activity against intracellular pathogens. Fluoroquinolones inhibit the bacterial DNA gyrase, a target that had never before been exploited in chemotherapy. These special features made fluoroquinolones attractive molecules for exploration as antimycobacterial agents. Tests in the mouse footpad model showed that of the commonly available fluoroquinolones ciprofloxacin and norfloxacin had poor activity. Pefloxacin, however, had good activity: 50 mg/kg daily pefloxacin showed bacteriostatic activity, while 150 mg/kg displayed bactericidal activity by kinetic methods. Ofloxacin was found to be even more active than pefloxacin, displaying bactericidal activity at 50 mg/kg and profound killing at 150 mg/kg.[93] Ofloxacin was shown to have in vitro antituberculosis activity as well. These findings provided a very welcome new lead for antimycobacterial investigations.

Subsequently, a clinical trial in previously untreated lepromatous leprosy patients comparing 400 mg daily ofloxacin against 800 mg daily pefloxacin administered from Days 1 to 56 alone and from Days 57 to 180 with standard WHO MDT regimen was reported.[94–96] The bactericidal activities of the treatments were monitored by serial mouse footpad inoculation and by inoculation in congenitally athymic (nude) mice. The two treatments have been found equally effective; definite clinical improvement with drastic decrease of morphologic index to the baseline were observed in all patients two months from beginning of treatment; about 99.99 percent of organisms viable on Day 0 were killed by 22 doses of either of the drugs. The two drugs thus seem to have very powerful bactericidal activity, even against rifampicin-resistant mutants. The side-effects observed were mild and the drugs seemed to be well tolrated. It is possible that combination of ofloxacin and rifampicin may shorten the time required for MDT. Thus, fluoroquinolones in combination with other antimycobacterial agents seem to hold considerable promise for the treatment of these infections. With studies now going on, their proper position will be established. In a study of ofloxacin vs. ethambutol, used in combination with rifampicin and isoniazid in pulmonary tuberculosis for nine months, equally good results were obtained in both groups; ofloxacin thus appears to be as useful as ethambutol in the treatment of pulmonary tuberculosis.[97]

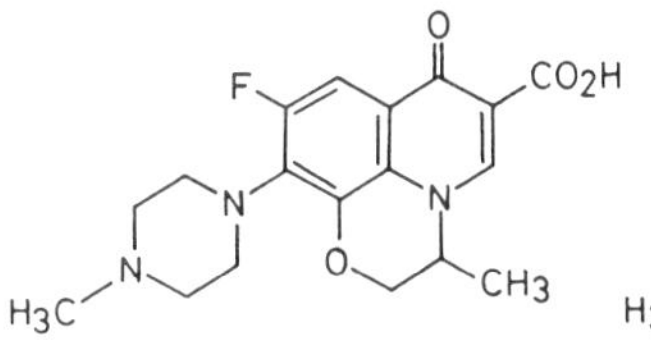

Ofloxacin

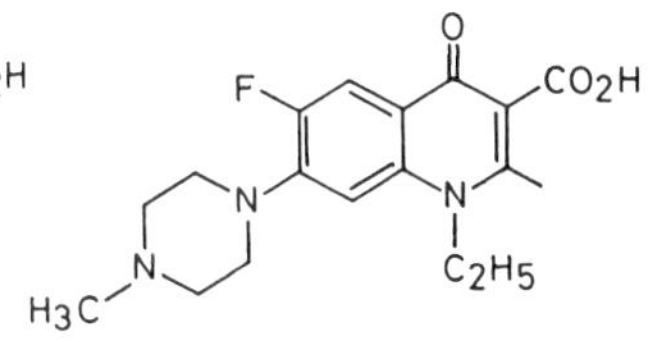

Pefloxacin

Other Drugs

Second-Line Drugs

There are a number of drugs, which though not very safe, have occasionally been used in chemotherapy. But, as more careful assessment was made of each drug's usefulness in combination therapy, these were assigned second-line status. They are not normally used, but may be helpful in some special situation, such as suspected or observed multiple-drug resistance to front-line drugs. For tuberculosis these agents include:

(i) Cycloserine:[r1,r3] It is a broad-spectrum antibiotic produced by *Streptomyces orchidaceus;* it was first isolated from fermentation broths, but later obtained by synthesis. It is inhibitory for *M. tuberculosis* in concentrations of 5 to 20 μg/ml in vitro. There is no cross resistance between cycloserine and other antimycobacterial agents. Its action in vitro is antagonized by D-alanine, and its mode of action seems to be to inhibit steps in bacterial cell wall synthesis involving D-alanine. When given orally, cycloserine is rapidly absorbed, distributed throughout the body tissues and fluids, including the CSF, and reaches a peak concentration in plasma three to four hours after a single administration. Its usual dose for adults is 5–20 mg/kg per day up to a maximum of 500 mg twice a day. Its side-effects involve mainly the CNS, and include somnolence, headache, tremor, vertigo, confusion, psychotic states, and suicidal tendencies. These tend to appear within two weeks of therapy and disappear when the drug is withdrawn. Cycloserine is now used to a very limited extent when microorganisms are resistant to other drugs, and then is used in combination with other drugs.

(ii) Capreomycin.[r1,r3] This agent, an antimycobacterial cyclic peptide, contains four closely related components, 1A, IB, IIA, IIB. The drug is given IM 15–30 mg/day, up to 1 g for 60 to 120 days. It is used primarily in cases of resistance or treatment failure. Undesired reactions associated with capreomycin are hearing loss, tinnitus, proteinurea, and nitrogen retention.

In leprosy, apart from thiacetazone and ethionamide described earlier, thiambutosine, belonging to the thiourea group, is another second-line drug. It has, however, a poor pharmacokinetic profile, low bactericidal action, and exhibits a variety of toxic side-effects. It should be used only in cases of resistance to both rifampicin and DDS. Thalidomide has an established place for the treatment of erythema nodosum leprosum at doses of 100–300 mg/day. Marked teratogenicity of thalidomide limits its use. The ability of clofazimine to control ENL, apart from its chemotherapeutic response, has further limited the need for thalidomide.

New Drugs[96,98,r6]

In view of the possibility of present drugs losing their prime position because of drug resistance or adverse reactions, there is a need to add new drugs constantly. Some new drugs identified in recent years, but still in an exploratory stage, are briefly described below.

Macrolides

A number of macrolides have shown promising antimycobacterial activity, particularly against atypical mycobacteria. A new erythromycin analogue, roxithromycin (RU-28965) seems promising in the treatment of tuberculosis. It has a more prolonged half-life and better tissue penetration than erythromycin, and is a candidate for further studies. Clarithromycin[99] and azithromycin[100] have shown promise in clinical trials in AIDS patients for treatment of infections caused by *M. avium* complex; clinical results with clarithromycin alone were better than even with a combination of rifampicin, isoniazid, and ethambutol.

β-Lactam Antibiotics

Since *M. tuberculosis, M. bovis,* and *M. kansasii* produce β-lactamase, β-lactam antibiotics were not considered suitable for mycobacterial infections. The recent development of β-lactamase-resistant β-lactam antibiotics has renewed interest in them as antimycobacterial agents. Some cephalosporins, such as ceforamide, have sufficient intrinsic antituberculosis activity to be explored as antituberculosis agents. Cephaloridine has shown activity against experimental leprosy.[80,101] β-Lactam antibiotics with β-lactamase inhibitors[102,103] such as augmentin (amoxicillin plus clavulanic acid) have been shown to inhibit and kill most strains of *M. tuberculosis* and some atypical mycobacteria.[102,103] The stage is thus set to explore the potential of β-lactam antibiotics as antimycobacterial agents.

Dihydrofolate Reductase Inhibitors (DHFRI)

From earlier studies it appeared that mycobacteria are not sensitive to DHFRIs. However, using cell-free extracts of *M. lufu* and *M. leprae,* Seydel et al showed that dihydrofolates of mycobacteria are inhibited by DHFRIs, and that this action was synergized by DDS.[43] Bromdimaprim was especially designed for its activity against *M. leprae;*[44] it has shown promising results in leprosy patients when used in combination with DDS. K-130 is another DHFRI developed more recently by Seydel et al and also in clinical development;[104] K-130 has structural features of both a DHFRI and a pterin-synthetase inhibitor, and it is likely that it may act at both these sites.

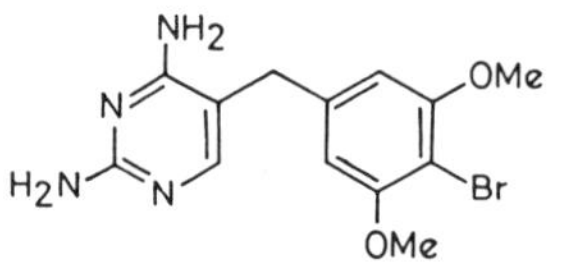

Brodimoprim

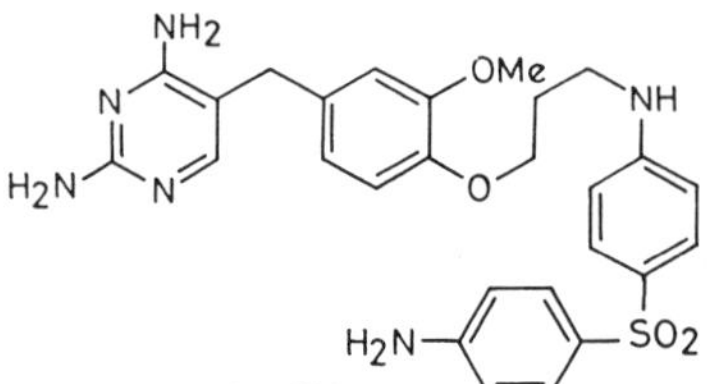

K−130

Present Status of Chemotherapy

Tuberculosis[r5,r6]

Short-Course Combination Therapy

Starting with the discovery in the 1940s that streptomycin could greatly reduce mortality in patients with pulmonary tuberculosis, there have been great advances in the chemotherapy of tuberculosis. The intensive short-course chemotherapy (SCC) regimens now prescribed have brought down the period of treatment to six to nine months from the 18 to 24 months of earlier regimens. This SCC can effectively control and treat practically all forms of tuberculosis, including that associated with HIV infection. Multi-drug-resistant tuberculosis now remains the most worrisome problem in the chemotherapy of tuberculosis. This shortening of the course of chemotherapy has had three major effects: the compliance rate is raised; drug toxicity is reduced; and cost of treatment is reduced and brought within the reach of larger numbers in the developing countries. The SCC antituberculosis regimens are considered to be the most cost-effective interventions available in infectious disease.[2–4] An even more significant contribution of SCC is the enhanced understanding it has provided of the dynamics of tuberculous infection versus the antibacterial potential of different drugs, which has led to more rational use of drug combinations.

Bacteriologic Basis for Current Chemotherapy Regimens

Grosset[1,105] and Mitchison[106,107] have suggested a theoretical basis for correlation of tuberculous infection with the antibacterial effect of the different drugs used in combination therapy, and have classified the drugs on this basis. They argued that since, in active human tuberculosis, the bacilli exist in several subpopulations, each with a distinct metabolic status, they would have varying susceptibility to different antituberculosis drugs. The largest population consists of rapidly growing metabolically active extracellular organisms—especially in the walls of cavitary lesions, where growth conditions are favorable because of high oxygen content and a neutral pH. This subpopulation was rapidly killed by the early bactericidal drugs such as isoniazid, and to a lesser degree by rifampicin, streptomycin, and ethambutol. A second subpopulation, which is slow growing or dormant, exists in the acidic intracellular environment in phagosomes and lysosomes and in sites of inflammation. This group is particularly susceptible to the sterilizing action of pyrazinamide. The third subpopulation is found mainly in the caseous material, where the pH is neutral but the oxygenation is poor, and these organisms grow very slowly with ocasional spurts of active metabolism. They are killed most effectivly by rapidly acting bactericidal drugs, such as rifampicin. Finally, there may be a small population of metabollically inactive, completely dormant organisms, often termed "persisters," which are not affected by any agent, but are eliminated over time by the host's immune system and need coverage by drugs to prevent reactivation and relapses. The active tuberculous infection viewed this way underscores the logistic need for the simultaneous use of different drugs acting on different subpopulations of bacteria to achieve effective control and cure. Another reason for the use of combinations of drugs is to overcome resistant strains, for which there is a statistical logic. If the mutation rate for resistance to a single drug is of the order of 10^{-6}, then the theoretical probability of developing resistance simultaneously to three drugs, assuming that they act independently and have similar pharmacokinetics, would be 10^{-18}—a very remote probability. Isoniazid and rifampicin are considered the most effective in resistance-preventing activity, followed by ethambutol and streptomycin. Pyrazinamide and thiacetazone are least effective in this regard.[106]

Based on these considerations the general guidelines that have emerged for successful therapy require the administration of at least two active drugs (to which organisms are not resistant), at least one of which should be bactericidal and the second sterilizing. The two together should be able to prevent the emergence of resistant organisms. The second principle of therapy requires the treatment to be continued well after the amelioration of the clinical disease to eliminate the "persistent" bacilli; inadequate treatment leads to the increased possibility of relapse months or years later.

Standard Therapy Regimens[108–112,r5,r6]

The goals of antituberculosis chemotherapy are to convert sputum cultures to negative in the shortest time possible, with low rates of adverse reactions, without allowing the emergence of resistant organisms, and with low rates of relapse following therapy. The various standard therapeutic regimens prescribed at present are described in Table 97.2; the six-month regimen is now most commonly prescribed. With the SCC regimens thus prescribed, most patients will be sputum culture regative within two months, virtually all by three months, and less than 5 per cent completing therapy will relapse.

Nine-Month Regimens

This regimen relies on the combination of isoniazid and rifampicin administered throughout, with or without streptomycin or ethambutol, given daily throughout or daily for the first one month, followed by twice-weekly administration. It was found that while a nine-month course was highly effective, shortening of this regimen to six months could result in an unacceptably high relapse rate. Treatment failure can be expected if primary resistance is present to one or both of these drugs. As isoniazid resistance is becoming quite common, it has been suggested to include ethambutol for all patients on this regimen until susceptibility results are available.

Six-Month Regimens

The addition of pyrazinamide, a sterilizing drug, in the first two months of combination therapy followed by isoniazid and rifampicin for the next four months provided a major advance in short-course therapy and helped to cut down the total treatment period to six months.[108] In some of these studies, drugs were given daily throughout therapy; in others, the drugs were given twice or thrice weekly after an initial two months of daily therapy. It is recommended that for patients with a chance of primary drug resistance, a fourth drug (ethambutol or streptomycin) should be added initially until drug susceptibility studies are available.

Table 97.2 Regimens Commonly Prescribed for Chemotherapy of Tuberculosis

Drug	Phase 1	Phase 2
6 Months Regimen (Short Course Chemotherapy)	**2 Months**	**4 Months**
Isoniazid	5 mg/kg/d	5 mg/kg/d or 15 mg/kg 3 times weekly
Rifampicin	10 mg/kg/d	10 mg/kg/d or 3 times weekly
Pyrazinamide	35 mg/kg/d	—
Supplemented in cases of suspected or observed primary resistance to INH or RIF by:		
Streptomycin or	15–20 mg/kg/d	
Ethambutol	25 mg/kg/d	
9 Months Regimen	**2 months**	**7 months**
Isoniazid	5 mg/kg/d	5 mg/kg/d
Rifampicin	10 mg/kg/d	10 mg/kg/d
Thiacetazone	4 mg/kg/d	4 mg/kg/d
with either:		
Streptomycin or	15–20 mg/kg/d	
Ethambutol	25 mg/kg/d	
12 Months Regimen	**2 months**	**10 months**
Isoniazid	5 mg/kg/d	5 mg/kg/d
Rifampicin	10 mg/kg/d	—
with either:		
Streptomycin or	15–20 mg/kg/d	4 mg/kg/d
Ethambutol	25 mg/kg/d	15 mg/kg/d

Alternative Regimens

If isoniazid or rifampin cannot be used because of drug intolerance/toxicity, or may not be effective because of drug resistance, ethambutol may replace either drug. As this is a less effective combination, treatment must be continued over a longer period, for 12–24 months. The addition of pyrazinamide for the first two months to a rifampicin-ethambutol regimen permits shortening of the treatment period to nine months; it also may help to cut down the treatment period in an isoniazid-ethambutol combination.

Side-Effects

The most common side-effect and most serious toxicity seen in TB therapy is drug-induced hepatitis. This is more frequent among older patients, those having pre-existing liver disease, and among those who abuse alcohol. Of the commonly used drugs, isoniazid is the most common cause of hepatotoxicity, and rifampin potentiates it. In such cases the drug intake must be stopped and substitute therapy started; rifampicin-ethambutol is suitable.

Special Clinical Situations

Human Immunodeficiency Virus (HIV) Infection

Most HIV-infected TB patients respond well to standard therapy, except for greater prevalence of drug reactions. The Center for Disease Control (US) has recommended an isoniazid-rifampicin and initial pyrazinamide regimen for a minimum of nine months, including six months beyond the timing of bacteriologic culture conversion.[113]

Smear-Negative but Culture-Positive and Smear-Negative Culture-Negative Cases

It is likely that in such cases the bacillary load will be lower than in smear-positive cases. Several studies have suggested[114] that in these patients the treatment period may be reduced to four months, with a cure rate of 98 per cent and a bacteriologic relapse rate of 1 per cent.

Drug Resistant Tuberculosis

Patients with isoniazid- or rifampicin-resistant disease should be treated with ethambutol added to the standard SCC regimen or substituted for the resistant drug. Results with both are quite satisfactory.[115]

When initial resistance to both isoniazid and rifampicin occurs, treatment is more difficult and failures more common. In such cases, substitute treatment with a minimum of two new bactericidal drugs should be started and the treatment guided by drug susceptibility studies. A single drug should never be added to a failing regimen. A three-drug regimen containing pyrazinamide, ethambutol, and ethionamide (if these have not previously been used) and an injectable drug, usually streptomycin or capreomycin, should be used. A combination of rifabutin and ofloxacin has also been used successfully for retreatment of patients resistant to isoniazid, rifampicin, and streptomycin.[116]

In cases where there is increased chance of primary resistance, the best protection against treatment failure is to add ethambutol in a short course regimen right from the beginning.

Pregnancy

Of the first-line drugs, isoniazid, rifampicin, and ethambutol can be given safely. Isoniazid-rifampicin, with or without ethambutol, is the treatment of choice. Streptomycin may cause ototoxicity to the fetus, and pyrazinamide is considered toxic. Both these drugs should be avoided.[117]

Chemoprophylaxis

Primary chemoprophylaxis has occasionally been used in infants who are being breastfed by a mother with pulmonary tuberculosis; isoniazid 10 mg/kg body weight is given to the infant for as long as the mother remains infectious.[118]

Secondary chemoprophylaxis has been used in infected tuberculin-positive individuals who have no clinical evidence of disease with the objective of preventing the development of tuberculosis. Both isoniazid and rifampicin have been used for this purpose. Generally, secondary prophylaxis has been used for the following groups: (a) recent tuberculin converters, in close contact with infectious tuberculosis; (b) tuberculin-positive children under five years of age with high risk of developing a serious form of tuberculosis, such as miliary or meningitis; (c) immunosupressed patients who are on long-term immunosupressant drugs and who were strongly tuberculin-positive or have evidence of old turberculous lesions.

Leprosy[r7,96,119–122]

Dapsone, first reported for the treatment of leprosy in 1947, was a cheap, safe, and easy-to-use drug. It was introduced for mass treatment in many areas of the world from the early 1950s. The success achieved brought about a dramatic change in the outlook for controlling leprosy. During the early period not many reports of dapsone-resistant cases appeared, which could be partly due to the nonavailability of convenient laboratory methods for detecting resistance of lepra bacilli to drugs. The first case of dapsone-resistant leprosy was reported in 1964[35] after Shepard had reported the footpad mouse model for testing. By the mid-1970s the phenomenon of relapses with DDS-resistant *M. leprae* and of infection with primary resistant bacilli was well established. In some countries the prevalence of DDS-resistant infection had reached a level as high as 10–20 percent. By end of 1970s it was quite clear that monotherapy with dapsone could not be continued.[36]

When sulfone resistance was encountered on such a large scale, the WHO special Program for Research and Training in Tropical Diseases, through its Leprosy Research Program, launched a series of surveys of both primary and secondary dapsone resistance in countries all over the world. Also convened was a Study Group on the Chemotherapy of Leprosy for Control Programs, which recommended combination therapy—what is often called the multi-drug treatment (MDT)[119] program. The MDT program drew heavily on the experience of the combination therapy regimens already used successfully in the chemotherapy of tuberculosis. The choice of drugs in leprosy, apart from DDS, was limited to rifampicin, clofazimine, and to some extent ethionamide/prothionamide. But still within this limited choice each drug had a different spectrum of antibacterial response and seemed to supplement each other's action. It was recognized[120,121] that as in the case of tuberculosis there would be different subpopulations of bacilli with varying susceptibilities to different drugs, ranging from those bacilli fully sensitive to all drugs to a small proportion, 1×10^5 to 10^6 that would be inherently resistant to one or the other drug and would respond only to the sensitive drug. There also would be a very small proportion of drug-sensitive, but dormant nonmultiplying bacilli that would not respond to any drug normally, but that might get eliminated over time by the host's immune responses acting in tandem with chemotherapy. The multi-drug therapy requires the use of at least two drugs to which *M. leprae* are sensitive, and the regimen used was determined by the antibacterial action of the drug. If the drug is bacteriostatic, like DDS, it will be essential to maintain continuous concentrations in excess of its MIC for *M. leprae;* for drugs that are highly bactericidal (or bacteriopausal), such as rifampicin, it may not be essential to maintain continuous inhibitory levels. Such drugs could be given intermittently under supervision. Clofazimine is the third most important antileprosy drug; it has an additional valuable property of aiding the control of 'erythema nodosum leprosum'. Based on these considerations the WHO recommended the multi-drug therapy (MDT) regimens given in Table 97.3. The main objectives of MDT are:[119,120] (i) to render all infectious cases noninfectious in as short a period as possible so as to interrupt transmission and prevent spread of leprosy; (ii) to give adequate and regular treatment to all existing and new cases and to cure them in as short a time as possible; (iii) to prevent emergence of drug-resistant strains of *M. leprae;* (iv) to ensure early detection and initiation of treatment to prevent development of abnormalities. In the initial studies in some cases where skin pigmentation caused by clofazimine appeared to be a problem, prothionamide (or ethionamide) was used as an alternative. Compliance in such cases was poor, however, owing to GI and hepatotoxic side-effects.

Table 97.3 WHO Recommended Multi-drug Therapy Regimens for Leprosy

1. Multibacillary leprosy (LL, BL, BB, BI = 2 or more at any site)		
Rifampicin	600 mg once monthly	Supervised
Clofazimine	300 mg once monthly	Supervised
Dapsone	100 mg daily	Self-administered
Clofazimine	50 mg daily	Self-administered
For a minimum of two years and wherever possible until skin smear are negative		
2. Paucibacillary leprosy (I, TT, BT, BI = less than 2 at all sites)		
Rifampicin	600 mg once monthly	Supervised
Dapsone	100 mg daily	Self-administered
For six months, if treatment is interrupted, the regimen should be recommenced where it was left off to complete the full course.		

The MDT regimens proved highly effective in all cases of leprosy, irrespective of whether resistance to one drug was present before the treatment was started.

Recent reports of the antileprosy activity of ofloxacin (and other fluoroquinolones) and of its ability to shorten further the period required to achieve bacterial negativity is an important addition to antileprosy drugs. Addition of ofloxacin is likely to add to the usefulness of combination therapy in the control and treatment of leprosy.

Chemoprophylaxis

The place of chemoprophylaxis in leprosy is not yet clearly delineated. In view of the uncertainty of the duration of the prophylactic treatment required and the small but definite drug toxicity risk, the use of dapsone as a prophylactic drug in large-scale control programs is not recommended.[119] Prophylactic dapsone is recommended for those at real risk because of prolonged and intimate contact with a person who had been shedding viable lepra bacilli. The usual weekly divided doses were: up to four year, 25 mg; four to seven year, 50 mg; seven to 12 year, 75 mg; 12 to 15 year, 100 mg; and over 15 year, 200 mg.

Multi-drug therapy has brought about a major change in the outlook for leprosy treatment and control and has raised hopes of considerably reducing leprosy in the next decade and finally eradicating it.

A new short-term therapy regimen using a combination of rifampicin, isoniazid, and co-trimoxazole has been reported recently on seven patients with lepromatous leprosy, with a relapse-free cure within two to four months.[123]

Atypical Mycobacteriosis

Nontuberculous mycobacterial infections are a heterogeneous group with different drug susceptibilities.[14,124–126] Each infection, therefore, has to be considered separately for response to chemotherapy by in vitro and in vivo testing. As in tuberculosis, the treatment depends on the use of a combination of drugs chosen from among: rifampicin (and its new analogues), isoniazid, ethambutol, clofazimine, ofloxacin (pefloxacin and sparfloxacin), kanamycin, amikacin, clarithromycin, and azithromycin. Over-all new macrolide and a fluroquinolone antibacterials have significant activity against atypical mycobacteria,[127] and they are being used increasingly in the treatment of such infections. Chemotherapy is more effective when accompanied with surgical cleaning-up, debridement, and drainage to reduce the load of the pathogen, when required. The treatment modalties for these infections are still in an exploratory stage. The over-all sensitivity of common atypical mycobacteria is indicated in Table 97.4.

M. kansasii, M. xenopi, and *M. marinum* respond well to treat-

Table 97.4 Sensitivity of Atypical Mycobacteria to Commonly Used Antibacterial Drugs

	Response to Drugs	RIF	CLO	INH	EMB	FQ	CLA AZI	AMIK	PZA	COT	MIN	CEF	SM
M. avium intracellulare	poor	✓	✓		✓	✓	✓	✓					
M. chelonei	poor					✓	✓	✓		✓	✓	✓	
M. fortuitum	poor	✓				✓	✓	✓	✓		✓		✓
M. kansasii	good	✓		✓	✓	✓						✓	✓
M. scrofuloceum	poor												
M. marinum	good	✓			✓					✓	✓		
M. ulcerans	variable												
M. xenopei	v. good	✓	✓	✓	✓	✓			✓				

RIF = rifamycins rifampicin, rifabutin, rifapentin; CLO = Clofazimine; INH = isoniazid; EMB = Ethambutol; FQ = Olfloxacin, sparfloxacin; CLA = Clarithromycin; AZI = azithromycin; AMIK = amikamycin; PZA = pyrazinamide; COT = co-trimoxazole (trimethoprin + sulfamethoxazole); MIN = minocycline; CEF = Cefazolin; SM = streptomycin

ment. Rifampicin appears to be the most effective drug, and should be an essential component of all regimens; rifampicin combined with isoniazid and ethambutol appears to be the combination of choice.[14] In *M. marinum* infections, minocycline and co-trimaxazole also have been reported to give good results.

Treatment of *M. avium intracellulare* infection was not satisfactory because the organisms are not very sensitive to known antimycobacterial drugs. However, with the introduction of new macrolides and fluoroquinolones to which the organisms are more susceptible, and with the use of drug combinations, the chemotherapy of these infections has greatly improved. It has been reported recently that clarithromycin and azithromycin, alone and in combination with ciprofloxacin and amikacin[99,100,128] and a combination of amikacin, ethambutol, and rifabutin[129] cleared bacteremia in patients within two to eight weeks of treatment. Clofazimine also seems a promising drug for these infections.

M. fortuitum and *M. chelonei* are generally resistant to most of the antimycobacterial drugs. Other drugs of value include amikacin, gentamycin, cefoxitin, doxycycline, sulfonamides (against *M. fortuitum*) and erythromycin (against *M. chelonei*); a combination of drugs is recommended.[14]

References

Research Reports

1. Grosset J. Bacteriological basis for the treatment of tuberculosis. Rev Prat 1990;*40*:715–718.
2. Murray CJL. World tuberculosis burden. Lancet 1990;*335*:1043–1044.
3. Joesoef MR, Remington PL, Jiptoherijanto PT. Epidemiological model and cost-effectiveness analysis of tuberculosis treatment programmes in Indonesia. Int J Epidem 1989;*18*:174–179.
4. Bloom BR, Murray CJL. Tuberculosis: Commentary on a reemergent killer. Science 1992;*257*:1055–1062.
5. Noordeen SK. A look at world leprosy. Leprosy Rev 1991;*62*:72–86.
6. Raviglione MC, Narain JP, Kochi A. HIV associated tuberculosis in developing countries: Clinical features, diagnosis and treatment. Bull WHO 1992;*70*:515–526.
7. Barnes PF, Bloch AB, Davidson PT, Snider DE Jr. Tuberculosis in patients with human immunodeficiency virus infection. N Engl J Med 1991;*324*:1644–1650.
8. Chaisson RE, Schechter GF, Theuer CP, Rutherfors GW, Eschenburg DF, Hopewell PC. Tuberculosis in patients with AIDS: Clinical features, response to therapy and survival. Am Rev Respir Dis 1987;*136*:570–574.
9. Watson JM. Tuberculosis in Britain today. Br Med J (Indian Ed) 1993;*9*:101–102.
10. Rieder HL, Cauthen GM, Comstock GW, Snider DE Jr. Epidemiology of tuberculosis in the United States. Epidemiol Rev 1989;*11*:79–98.
11. Morbidity Mortality Wkly Rep 1991;*39*:944.
12. Edlin BR, Tokars JI, Grieco MH et al. An outbreak of multidrug-resistant tuberculosis among hospitalised patients with the acquired immuno-deficiency syndrome. N Engl J Med 1992;*326*:1514–1521.
13. Fischl MA, Daikos GL, Uttam Chandani RB, Poblete RB, Moreno JN, Reyes RR, Boota AM, Thompson LM, Cleary TJ, Oldham SA. Clinical presentation and outcome of patients with HIV infection and tuberculosis caused by multiple drug-resistant bacilli. Ann Int Med 1992;*117*:184–190.
14. Freedman SD. Other mycobacterial infections, In Wilson JD et al: Harrison's principles of internal medicine, 12th Ed New York: McGraw Hill, (1990); pp 649–650.
15. Ellner JJ, Goldberger MJ, Parent DM. Mycobacterium avium infection with AIDS: A therapeutic dilemma in rapid evolution. J Infect Dis 1991;*63*:1326–1335.
16. Young LS. Mycobacterium avium complex infection. J Infect Dis 1988;*157*:863–867.
17. Schweinle JE. Evolving concepts of epidemiology, diagnosis and therapy of M. tuberculosis infection. Yale J Biol Med 1990;*63*:565–579.
18. Deo MG, Chaturvedi RM, Kartikeyan S. A candidate antileprosy vaccine from ICRC bacilli. Trop Med Parasitol 1990;*41*:367–368.
19. Sudre P, ten Dam G, Kochi A. Tuberculosis a global overview of the situation today. Bull WHO 1992;*70*:149–159.
20. Frieden TR et al. Abstract 41st Annual Epidemic Intelligence Service Conference, CDC Atlanta, April 6 1992.
21. Canetti G. Present aspects of the bacterial resistance in tuberculosis. Am Rev Respir Dis 1955;*92*:687–703.
22. Pitchenik AE, Cole C, Russell BW, Fischi MA, Spira TJ, Snider DE. Tuberculosis atypical mycobacteriosis and the acquired immunodeficiency syndrome among Haitian and non-Haitian patients in south Florida. Ann Intern Med 1984;*101*:641–645.
23. Edwards D, Kirkpatrick C. The immunology of mycobacterial diseases. Am Rev Respir Dis 1986;*134*:1062–1071.
24. Klatzmann D, Gluckman JC. HIV Infection: Facts and hypothesis. Immunology Today 1986;*7*:291–296.
25. Leprosy in the World Today. Lep News WHO 1992;*1*:2.
26. Leprosy situation in the world and multidrug therapy coverage. Weekly Epidemiological Record 1992;*21*:153–160.
27. Bullock WE. Mycobacterium leprae. In: Mandel GL, et al. Principles and practice of infectious diseases, 2d ed. New York: Wiley (1985); pp 1406–1413.
28. Hastings RC (ed) Leprosy. New York: Churchill Livingstone (1985).
29. Ridley DS, Joping WH. Classification of leprosy according to immunity: A five group system. Int J Lep 1966;*16*:437–465.
30. Nunn PP, McAdum KP. Mycobacterial infections with AIDS. Br Med Bull 1988;*44*:801–813.
31. Tsang AY, Denner JC, Brennan PJ, McClatchy JK. Clinical and epidemiological importance of typing of Mycobacterium avium complex isolates. J Clin Microbiol 1992;*30*:479–484.
32. Shepard CC. The experimental disease that follows the infection of human leprosy bacilli into footpads of mice. J Exp Med 1960;*112*:445–454.
33. Shepard CC. A kinetic method for the study of the activity of drugs against Mycobacterium leprae in mice. Int J Lepr 1967;*35*:429–435.
34. Shepard CC. Statistical analysis of results obtained by two methods for testing drug activity against Mycobacterium leprae. Int J Lep 1982;*50*:96–101.
35. Pettit JHS, Rees RJW. Sulphone resistance in leprosy: An experimental and clinical study. Lancet 1964;*ii*:673–674.
36. Ji B. Drug resistance in leprosy: A review. Lepr Rev 1985;*56*:265–278.

37. Lowe C, Rees RJW. Production of thymectomized-irradiated mice. In: WHO publication: Laboratory Techniques for leprosy. WHO/CDS/LEP/86.4. Geneva: WHO (1987); pp 54–57.

38. Kohsaka K, Mori T, Ito T. Lepromatoid lesion developed in nude mouse inoculated with Mycobacterium leprae. Leprosy 1976;*262*:399–401.

39. Kircheimer WF, Storrs EE. Attempts to establish the armadillo (Dasypus novemcinctus Linn.) as a model for the study of leprosy. 1. Report of lepromatoid leprosy in an experimentally infected armadillo. Int J Lepr 1971;*39*:693–702.

40. Lowe J, Smith M. The chemotherapy of leprosy in Nigeria. Int J Lep 1949;*17*:181–195.

41. Russell DA, Worth RM, Jano B, Fasal P, Shepard CC. Acedapsone in the prevention of leprosy: Field trial in three high prevalence villages of Micronesia. Am J Trop Med Hyg 1979;*28*:559–563.

42. Donovick R, Bayan A, Hamre D. The reversal of the activity of antituberculosis compounds in vitro. Am Rev Tubercul Pulm Dis 1952;*66*:219–227.

43. Seydel JK, Wempe EG. Bacterial growth kinetics of M. lufu in the presence and absence of various drugs alone and in combination. A model for the development of combined chemotherapy against M. leprae. Int J Lep 1982;*50*:20–30.

44. Seydel JK, Wempe EG, Rosenfeld M, Jaganathan R, Mahadevan RP, Dhople AM. In vitro and in vivo experiments with the new inhibitor of Mycobacterium leprae, Bromdimoprim alone and in combination with dapsone. Arzneim Forsch 1990;*40*:69–75.

45. Tsutsumi S, Gidoh M. On a role of antileprotic agents as the scavengers of active oxygen radicals. Int J Lep 1985;*53*:714–715.

46. Rosi F, Dri P, Bellavite P, Zabbuchi G, Berton G. Oxidative metabolism of inflammatory cells. In Weissimann G, Samuelson B, Paoletti R. Advances in inflammation research, (1979); Vol 1: p 139.

47. Martindale Extra Pharmacopoeia, 28th Edn. Reynolds JF (ed). Pharmaceutical Society Press (1982); p 1492.

48. Spotts CR, Stanier RY. Mechanism of streptomycin action on bacteria: A unitary hypothesis. Nature (London) 1961;*192*:633–637.

49. Anand N, Davis BD. Damage by streptomycin to the cell membrane of Escherichia coli. Nature (London) 1960;*185*:22–23.

50. Anand N, Davis BD, Armitage AK. Uptake of streptomycin by Escherichia coli. Nature (London) 1960;*185*:23–24.

51. Plotz PH, Davis BD. Synergism between streptomycin and penicillin: A proposed mechanism. Science 1962;*135*:1067–1068.

52. Gorini L, Kataja E. Phenotypic repair by streptomycin of defective genotypes in E. coli. Proc Natl Acad Sci (USA) 1964;*51*:487–493.

53. Davis BD, Tai PC, Wallace BJ. Complex interactions of antibiotics with the ribosome. In: M. Nomura A. Tissieres and P. Lengyel (ed.) Ribosomes. Cold Spring Harbor NY: Cold Spring Harbor Laboratory, 1974; pp 771–789.

54. Davis BD. Mechanism of bactericidal action of aminoglycosides. Microbiol Rev 1987;*51*:341–350.

55. Leading Article: Thiacetazone in tuberculosis. Lancet 1963;*2*:817–818.

56. Kushner S, Dalalian H, Sanjurjo JL, Bach FL, Safir, SR, Smith VK, Williams JH. Experimental chemotherapy of tuberculosis II: The synthesis of pyrazinamides and related compounds. J Am Chem Soc 1952;*74*:3617–3621.

57. Fergan-Smith R, Ellard GA, Newton D, Mitchison DA. Pyrazinamide and other drugs in tuberculous meningitis. Lancet 1973;*2*:374.

58. Crowle AJ, Sbarbaro J, May MH. Inhibition by pyrazinamide of tubercle bacilli within cultured human macrophages. Am Rev Respir Dis 1986;*134*:1054–1055.

59. Winder FG, In: Ratledg C, Stanford J. The Biology of the mycobacteria. New York: Academic Press (1982); Vol 1: pp 353–438.

60. Winder FG, Collins PB. Inhibition by Isoniazid of synthesis of mycolic acids in Mycobacterium smegmatis. J Gen Microbiol 1970;*63*:41–48.

61. Quemard A, Lacave C, Laneele G. Isoniazid inhibition of mycolic acid synthesis by cell extracts of sensitive and resistant strains of *Mycobacterium aurum*. Antimicrob Ag Chemoth 1991;*35*:1035–1039.

62. Zhang Y, Heym B, Allen B, Young D, Cole S. The catalase-peroxidase gene and isoniazid resistance of Mycobacterium tuberculosis. Nature 1992;*358*:591–593.

63. Riddell RW, Stewart SM, Somner AR. Ethionamide. Br Med J 1960;*2*:1207.

64. Barry VC, Conalty M. Antituberculosis activity in the phenazine series. Am Rev Tubercul 1958;*78*:62–73.

65. Browne SG, Hogerzeil LM. 'B663' in the treatment of leprosy: Preliminary report of a pilot trial. Lep Rev 1962;*33*:6–10.

66. Levy L. Pharmacologic studies of clofazimine. Am J Trop Med Hyg 1974;*23*:1097–1104.

67. Collaborative effort of the US leprosy panel (US Japan Cooperative Medical Science Program) and the Leonard Wood Memorial. Spaced Clofazimine therapy of lepromatous leprosy. Am J Trop Med Hyg 1976;*25*:437–444.

68. Fattorini L, Hu CQ, Jin SH, Santoro C, Tsang AY, Mascellino MT, Mandler F, Orefici G. Activity of antimicrobial agents against M. avium-intracellulare complex (MAIC) strains isolated in Italy. Int J Microbiol Virol Parasitol Infect Dis 1992;*276*:512–20.

69. Brown SG. B 663. Possible antiinflammatory action in lepromatous leprosy. Lep Rev 1965;*36*:9–11.

70. Zeis BM, Anderson R, O'sullivan JF. Peroxidative activities of 10′-phenazine derivatives related to that of clofazimine. Antimicrob Ag Chemoth 1987;*31*:789–793.

71. Niwa Y, Ozaki M. Oxygen-metabolism in phagocytes of nephrotic patients: Enhanced superoxide dismutase activity and hydroxyl radical generation by clofazimine. J Clin Microbial 1984;*20*:837–842.

72. Warndorff-Van Diepen T. Clofazimine-resistant leprosy: A case report. Int J Lep 1982;*50*:139–142.

73. Kar HK, Bhatia VN, Harikarishnan S. Combined clofazimine and daposone-resistant leprosy: Case report. Int J Lep 1986;*54*:389–391.

74. Karlson AG. The in vitro activity of ethambutol [dextro-2,2′-(ethylenediamino)-di-1-butanol] against tubercle bacilli and other microorganisms. Am Rev Respir Dis 1961;*84*:905–906.

75. Poso H, Paulin L, Brander E. Specific inhibition of spermidine synthase from mycobacteria by ethambutol. Lancet 1983;*2*:1418.

76. Takayama K, Armstrong EL, Kunugi KA, Kilburn JO. Inhibition by ethambutol of mycolic acid transfer into the cell wall of Mycobacterium smegmatis. Antimicrob Ag Chemother 1979;*16*:240–242.

77. Adel A. Ophthalmological side-effects of ethambutol. Scand J Respir Dis (Suppl) 1969;*69*:55.

78. Sensi P. Rifampicin. In: Bindra JS, Lednicer D. Chronicles of drug discovery. New York: Wiley Interscience (1982); Vol 1: pp 201–221.

79. Davidson PT, Goble M, Laster W. The antituberculosis efficacy of rifampin in 136 patients. Chest 1972;*61*:574–578.

80. Shepard CC, Walker LL, Van Landingham RM, Redus M. Kinetic testing of drugs against Mycobacterium leprae in mice. Activity of cephaloridine, rifampin, streptovaricin, and viomycin. Am J Trop Med Hyg 1971;*20*:616–620.

81. Pattyn SR. A comparison of the bactericidal activity of a series of rifampicins against Mycobacterium leprae. Arzneimittelforsch/Drug Res 1982;*32*:15–17.

82. Shepard CC, Levy L, Fasal P. Further experience with the rapid bactericidal effect of rifampin on Mycobacterium leprae. Am J Trop Med Hyg 1974;*23*:1120–1124.

83. Levy L, Shepard CC, Fasal P. The bactericidal effect of rifampicin on M. leprae in man: (a) Single doses of 600, 900 and 1200 mg; (b) Daily doses of 300 mg. Int J Lepr 1976;*44*:183–187.

84. Rees RJW, Pearson JMH, Waters MFR. Experimental and clinical studies on rifampicin in the treatment of leprosy. Br Med J 1970;*1*:89–92

85. Waters MFR, Rees RJW, Pearson JMH, Laing ABG, Helmy HS Gelber RH. Rifampicin for lepromatous leprosy: Nine years experience. Br Med J 1978;*1*:133–136.

86. Wehrli W. Rifampin: Mechanism of action and resistance. Rev Infect Dis 1983;*5*(Suppl 3):S407–S411.

87. Ohnhaus EE, Kirchoff B, Peheim E. Effect of enzyme induction on plasma lipids using antipyrine, phenobarbital and rifampicin. Clin Pharmacol Therap 1979;*25*:591–597.

88. Skolnik JL, Stoler BS, Katz DB, Anderson WH. Rifampin, oral contraceptives and pregnancy. JAMA 1976;*236*:1382.

89. Dickinson JM, Mitchison DA. In vitro activity of new rifamycins against rifampicin-resistant M. tuberculosis and MAI complex mycobacteria. Tubercle 1987;*68*:177–182.

90. Dickinson JM, Mitchison DA. In vitro observations on the suitability of new rifamycins for the intermittent chemotherapy of tuberculosis. Tubercle 1987;*68*:183–193.

91. Dickinson JM, Mitchison DA. In vitro properties of rifapentine (MDL473) relevant to its use in intermittent chemotherapy of tuberculosis. Tubercle 1987;*68*:113–118.

92. Klemens SP, Cynaman MH. In vivo activities of newer rifamycin analogis against Mycobacterium avium infection. Antimicrob Ag Chemther 1991;*35*:2026–2030.

93. Young LS, Berlin OGW, Inderlied CB. Activity of ciprofloxacin and other fluorinated quinolones against mycobacteria. Am J Med 1987;*82*(Suppl 4A):23–26.

94. Grosset JH, Ji B, Guelpa-Lauras CC, Perani EG, N'Deli L. Clinical trial of pefloxacin and ofloxacin in the treatment of lepromatous leprosy. Int J Lep 1990;*58*:281–295.

95. Chanteau S, Cartel JL, Perani E, N'Deli L, RouxJ, Grosset JH. Relationship between PGL-1 antigen in serum, tissue and viability of mycobacterium leprae as determined by mouse footpad assay in multibacillary patients during short term clinical trial. Lep Rev 1990;*61*:330–340.

96. Ji B, Grosset JH. (Editorial) Recent Advances in the chemotherapy of Leprosy. Lep Rev 1990;*61*:313–329.

97. Kohno S, Koga H, Kaku M, Maesaki S, Hara K. Prospective comparative study of ofloxacin or ethambutol for the treatment of pulmonary tuberculosis. Chest 1992;*102*:1815–1818.

98. Mitchison DA, Ellard GA, Grosset J. New antibacterial drugs for the treatment of mycobacterial disease in man. Br Med Bull 1988;*44*:757–774.

99. Dautzenberg B, Truffot C, Legris S, Meyohas MC, Berlie HC et al. Activity of clarithromycin against Mycobacterium avium infection in patients with the acquired immune deficiency syndrome. Am Rev Respir Dis 1991;*144*:564–569.

100. Young LS, Wiviott L, Klonoski P, Bolan R, Wu M, Inderlied CB. Azithromycin for treatment of Mycobacterium avium-intracellulare complex infection in patients with AIDS. Lancet 1991;*338*:1107–1109.

101. Shepard CC, Van Landingham RM, Walker L, Good RC. Activity of selected beta-lactam antibiotics against Mycobacterium leprae. Int J Lept 1987;*55*:322–327.

102. Casal M, Rodrigues F, Benavente M, Luna M. In vitro susceptibility of Mycobacterium tuberculosis, Mycobacterium fortuitum and Mycobacterium chelonei to augmentin. Eur J Clin Microbiol 1986;*5*:453–454.

103. Sorg TB, Cynamon MH. Comparison of four beta-lactamase inhibitors in combination with ampicillin against Mycobacterium tuberculosis. J Antimicrob Chemother 1987;*19*:56–64.

104. Czaplinsky Kh, Kansy M, Seydel JK. Design of a new substituted 2,4-diamino-5-benzylpyrimidine as inhibitor of bacterial dihydrofolate reductase inhibitor assisted by molecular graphics. Quant Struct Act Relat 1987;*6*:70–72.

105. Grosset J. Bacteriologic basis for short course chemotherapy for tuberculosis. Clin in Chest Med 1980;*1*:231–241.

106. Mitchison DA. Mechanism of drug action in short course Chemotherapy. Bull Int Union Against Tuberc 1985;*60*:34–37.

107. Mitchison DA. The action of antituberculosis drugs in short-course chemotherapy. Tubercle 1985;*66*:219–225.

108. Antituberculosis Regimens of Chemotherapy. Recommendations from the Committee on Treatment of the International Union against Tuberculosis & Lung Disease. Int J Tuberc 1980;*33*:150.

109. World Health Organization: Tuberculosis Control Report of a Joint International Union Against Tuberculosis/WHO Study Group. WHO Tech Rep Ser Geneva, 1982; No. 671.

110. Grosset JH. Present Status of chemotherapy for tuberculosis. Rev Infect Dis 1989;*11*(Suppl 2):S347–S352.

111. Perer-Stable EJ, Hopewell PC. Current tuberculosis treatment regimens. Choosing the right one for your patient. Clin Chest Med 1989;*10*:323–339.

112. Combs DL, O'Brien RJ, Geiter LJ. USPHS Tuberculosis short-course chemotherapy trial 21: Effectiveness, toxicity and acceptability, the report of final results. Ann Int Med 1990;*112*:397–406.

113. Tuberculosis and human immunodeficiency virus infection: Recommendations of the Advisory Committee for the Elimination of Tuberculosis (ACET). MMWR 1989;*38*:236–250.

114. Dutt AK, Moers D, Stead DD. Smear and culture negative pulmonary tuberculosis; Four month short-course chemotherapy. Am Rev Respir Dis 1989;*139*:867–870.

115. Davidson PT. Drug resistance and the selection of therapy for tuberculosis. Am Rev Respir Dis 1987;*136*:255–257.

116. Hong Kong Chest Service/British Medical Res Council. A controlled study of rifabutin and an uncontrolled study of ofloxacin in the retreatment of patients with pulmonary tuberculosis resistant to INH, streptomycin and rifampicin. Tub-Lung-Dis 1992;*73*:59–67.

117. Snider DE Jr, Layde PM, Johnson MW, Lyle MA. Treatment of tuberculosis during pregnancy. Am Rev Respir Dis 1980;*122*:65–79.

118. Citron MK. Control and prevention of tuberculosis by chemoprophylaxis in Britain. Br Med Bull 1988;*44*:711–712.

119. WHO Study Group. Chemotherapy of leprosy for control programmes. WHO Tech Rep Ser. (1982); 675.

120. Ellard GA. Rationale of the multidrug regimens recommended by a WHO Study Group on Chemotherapy of Leprosy for Control Programmes. Int J Lep 1984;*52*:395–501.

121. Ellard GA. Chemotherapy of Leprosy. Br Med Bull 1988;*44*:775–790.

122. Wheate HW. Management of leprosy. Br Med Bull 1988;*44*:791–800.

123. Freerksen E, Alvarenga AE, Lagnizamon O, De-Morra MV, Von Ballestrem W, Reyes LA. A new short-term chemotherapy of leprosy using vifampicin, isoinazid and co-trimaxazole. Med Klin 1991;*86*:441–448.

124. Sanders WE Jr, Horowitz EF. Other mycobacterium species. In: Mandell G, Donglas RG Jr, Bennett JE. Principles and practise of infections diseases, 3d ed. New York: Churchill Livingstone (1990); pp 1914–1926.

125. Dautzenberg B. Treatment of atypical mycobacterium infections: Current state and therapeutic perspectives (editorial). Rev Pneumol Clin 1992;*48*:139–141.

126. Brodt HR. Current therapy of atypical mycobacterial infections. Immune Infect 1992;*20*:39–45.

127. Ogawa K, MIWA T, Sasamoto M et al. In vitro susceptibilities of M. avium and M. intracellulare to new macrolides, new quinolones and antituberculous drugs on Dubos agar medium. Kakkaku 1992;*67*:735–738.

128. deLalla F, Maserati R, Scarpellini P, Marone P, Nicolin R, Caccamo F, Rigoli R. Clarithromycin ciprofloxacin-amikacin for therapy of M. avium intracellular bacteremia in patients with AIDS. Antimicrob Ag Chemother 1992;*35*:1567–1569.

129. Jorup-Ronstrom C, Julander I, Petrini B. Efficacy of triple drug regimen of amikacin, ethambutol and rifabutin in AIDs patients with symptomatic mycobacterium avium complex infection. J Infect 1993;*26*:67–70.

Reviews

r1. Antimycobacterial Agents. In Wade A. Martindale: The Extra Pharmacopoeia, 29th ed. London: Pharmaceutical Press, (1989); pp 546–577.
This review presents an account of the main characteristics of the mycobacteria and infections caused by them, including opportunistic infections caused by atypical mycobacteria, problems connected with their treatment and up-to-date accounts of the antimycobacterial agents in therapeutic use.

r2. Sensi P. Gialdroni-Grassi G. Antimycobacterial Agents. In Wolff ME. Berger's medicinal chemistry, 4th Ed. New York: Wiley Interscience (1979); Part II, 289–332.
This is a comprehensive review of the status of antimycobacterial agents in 1979 as viewed from the medicinal chemistry view-point.

r3. Kucers A, Bennet NM. Drugs mainly for tuberculosis. In: The use of antibiotics, 4th Ed. London: Heinemann Medical (1988); pp 1350.
This is an exhaustive account with extensive documentation of the history, antibacterial spectrum, clinical use, metabolism, mode of action, adverse drug reactions, and dosage-forms available of the drugs commonly used in the chemotherapy of tuberculosis.

r4. Hooper, M. The medicinal chemistry of antileprosy drugs. Chem Soc Rev 1987;*16*:437–465.
This review presents a brief account of leprosy as a disease, its epidemiology, characteristics, and the important features of Mycobacterium leprae. The historical development of the antileprosy drugs, their structure-activity relationship studies (including QSAR) and mode of action are then described.

r5. O'Brien RJ. Present chemotherapy of tuberculosis. Sem Res Inf 1989;*4*:216–224.
This review provides a brief account of the principles of short-course chemotherapy for tuberculosis and the regimens presently prescribed, including special clinical situations.

r6. Davidson PT, Le HQ. Drug treatment of tuberculosis: 1992. Drugs 1992;*43*:651–673.
Starting with a presentation of the bacteriologic basis of currently used chemotherapeutic regimens, this review provides a concise account of important pharmacokinetic and pharmacodynamic characteristics of drugs currently used in chemotherapy of tuberculosis, including some new drugs in the clinical development stage.

r7. Hastings RC, Franzblau SG. Chemotherapy of leprosy. Ann Rev Pharmacol Toxicol 1988;*28*:231–245.
This review describes the characteristics of Mycobacterium leprae experimental methods used to find antileprosy agents, important features of the drugs used in therapy, and the chemotherapeutic regimens used in leprosy.

r8. Sanders WE Jr, Horowitz EA. Other mycobacterial species. In: Mandell GL, Donglas RG (Jr), Bennott JE. Principles and Practice of Infections Diseases. 3d ed. New York: Churchill Livingstone (1990); pp 1914–1926.
This review presents an informative account of the atypical mycobacteria that cause disease in humans, their associated clinical problems, and their treatment.

CHAPTER 98

Ralph H. Raasch
Roy L. Hopfer

Antifungal Agents

Introduction

Background

Fungi are a highly diverse group of eukaryotic organisms that comprise their own kingdom. Fungi grow in two distinct morphologic types: single-celled budding yeasts and multiple-celled filamentous (hyphal) mold forms. There are more than 100,000 different species of fungi, many of which are beneficial to the food and fermentation industries; however, hundreds are pathogens to plants, causing tremendous economic damage every year. A few hundred also have been shown to cause infections in humans. Fewer than 20 species of fungi cause greater than 90 percent of all human infections. Fungal infections in humans can range in severity from easily treated superficial infections of the skin and hair to asymptomatic pulmonary infections requiring no treatment to difficult to treat life-threatening disseminated infections that involve multiple organ systems. Patients in the latter group typically are highly immunosuppressed cancer patients or immunologically debilitated patients, such as AIDS patients and transplant recipients.

Although fungi have existed for millions of years, their role in causing infections in humans was not recognized until the 1830–40s with the elegant work of Remak, who investigated favus of the scalp (ringworm). Early treatment modalities of human infection were based on the plant mycologists' experience and included use of such toxic agents as copper, mercury, and iodide. Other toxic reagents, such as Whitfield's ointment (a combination of benzoic and salicylic acids), were designed to dissolve the skin (keratin), rendering less substrate available to the fungus. Interestingly, Whitfield's is still used occasionally, and potassium iodide solution is still used to treat sporotrichosis. Systemic antifungals such as amphotericin B were not introduced until the 1950s. There has been considerable activity in the pharmaceutical industry during the last two decades following the introduction of the imidazole class of antifungals in 1969. These agents are much less toxic than the polyenes, but they are also less effective. Although much progress has been made toward developing an effective, yet nontoxic agent, the goal of finding an ideal antifungal agent is far from being realized. In fact, amphotericin B, a highly toxic agent, remains the "gold standard" for treating disseminated life-threatening fungal infections; however, the imidazoles are currently being evaluated for these patients with increasing success and optimism for the future.[1]

Fortunately, the fungi that cause most serious infections are susceptible to clinically achievable concentrations of polyenes and imidazoles. Clinical response to antifungal treatment is, however, directly related to recovery of the patient's cell-mediated immunity in the seriously infected immunosuppressed patient. Unfortunately, the value of antifungal susceptibility testing of fungal isolates is questionable for a number of reasons: (1) in vitro susceptibility test methods are not standardized (variables affecting results include inoculum preparation, test medium used, time and temperature of incubation); (2) results are often in disagreement if performed in different laboratories; (3) most importantly, there is poor correlation between in vitro test results and clinical response or outcome. This latter problem is most likely the result of earlier mentioned difficulties inherent in testing these organisms, the inability to effectively deliver the drug to the site of infection, and the host's immune status. Therefore, at the present time if susceptibility testing is warranted, isolates should be sent to a reputable reference laboratory familiar with fungal susceptibility test methods. With the introduction of effective less toxic antifungals, there may soon be an increasing justification for routine antifungal susceptibility testing.[2]

Polyenes

The polyenes are a group of chemically related antibiotics produced by soil bacteria, the Streptomycetaceae. There are around 100 of these compounds described, but only four or five are used with any frequency to treat human fungal infections. All polyenes contain unconjugated double bonds in a macrolide ring structure. The number of such bonds generally ranges from three to seven, i.e., trienes to heptaenes—hence the name polyenes. Polyenes used clinically include amphotericin B, nystatin, candicidin, pimaricin, and mepatricin. Since they have similar chemicophysical properties and mechanisms of action, the polyenes will be considered here as a group rather than singly. In spite of its toxicity, amphotericin B is still the "drug of choice" for treating most life-threatening fungal infections. Evaluations of the efficacy of newer antifungals are performed using amphotericin B as the "gold standard."

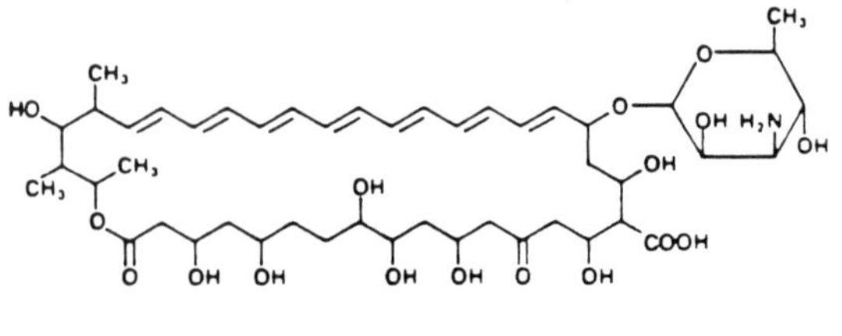

amphotericin B

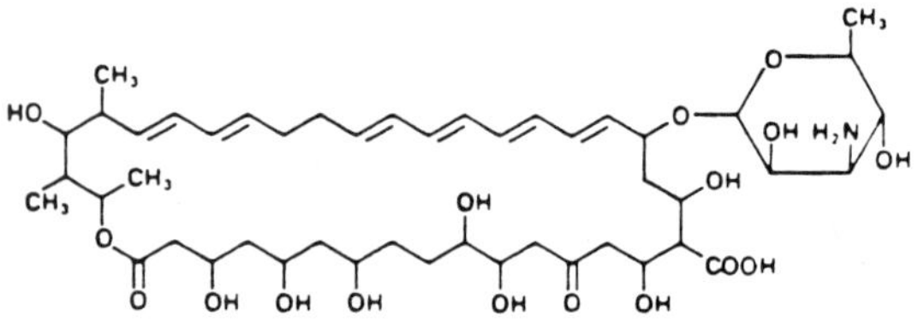

nystatin

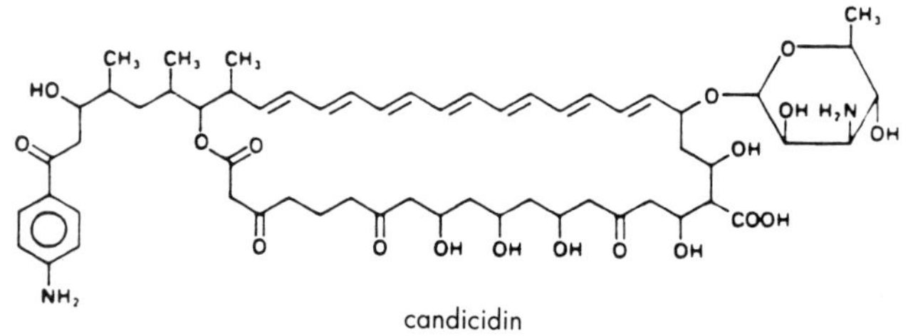

candicidin

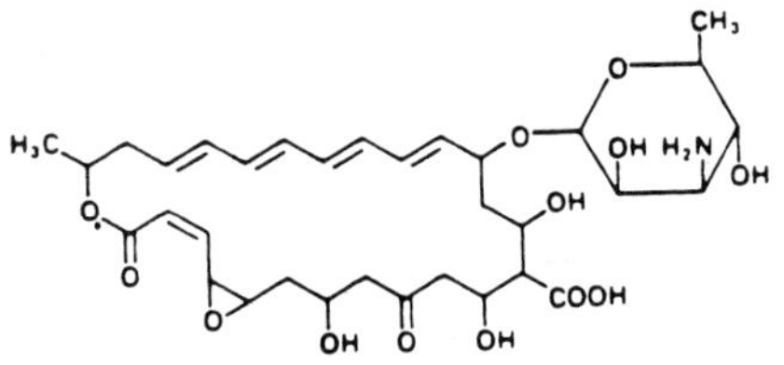

natamycin

Figure 98.1

Chemistry

The structural relatedness of the polyenes can be seen in Figure 98.1. As shown, all contain a beta-hydroxylated portion and the polyene system (conjugated double bonds) in the lactone ring. The polyenes have both acidic and basic side groups and are soluble in strong acidic and alkaline solutions. However, they are highly insoluble in aqueous solutions, such as physiologic saline or 5 percent glucose. Therefore, the polyenes are either prepared for topical application in creams and troches such as nystatin, or they are "solubilized" in detergents such as the desoxycholate suspensions used for IV administration of amphotericin B.

History

In 1950, an alcohol extract from a culture of a soil actinomycete was reported to have broad antifungal activity.[3] This compound, fungicidin (Nystatin)—or rather this crude extract—was the first polyene activity described. The authors also noted that the extract did not appear to possess any antibacterial activity. Nystatin was found to be too toxic for IV administration, but was found to have good activity when applied topically to superficial mucocutaneous lesions caused by *Candida albicans*. Amphotericin B was discovered in 1956.[4] Both amphotericin A and amphotericin B were isolated from *Streptomyces nodosus*. This bacterium was isolated from rotting vegetation on the banks of the Orinoco river in Venezuela. Although amphotericin B could be given IV, its toxicity was so high that many felt it would soon be replaced by similar polyenes isolated from other streptomyces or by chemically-altered forms of such drug(s). This led to the isolation/synthesis of dozens and dozens of structurally related polyenes; however, amphotericin B has proved to be the least toxic and most efficacious of the formulations and remains the drug of choice for many deep-seated fungal infections.

Therapeutic Uses

Amphotericin B is used therapeutically for a wide range of systemic fungal infections. Table 98.1 summarizes the susceptibility of a variety of organisms to amphotericin B. Amphotericin B is active against a wider range of fungal organisms than any other currently available antifungal agent. Limitations to the use of amphotericin B include the necessity to administer the drug IV and its toxicity. These issues will be discussed in subsequent sections of this chapter regarding pharmacokinetics and adverse effects.

Coadministration of mannitol and chemical modifications, such as making a methylester of amphotericin B, have failed to reduce toxicity of the drug. Development of new drug delivery systems, particularly liposomal forms and lipid complexes, have demonstrated greatly reduced toxicity of amphotericin B and other polyenes while not adversely affecting antifungal activity. Liposomal formulations of amphotericin B have not only been found to possess comparable in vitro antifungal activity, but have been found more effective in infected animal models.[r4] Whether this is the result of being able to give larger doses of the drug because of decreased toxicity, enhanced activity due to better delivery of drug to the site of infection, enhanced activity due to phagocytosis of the drug by macrophages, or some combination of all three possibilities remains to be determined. Most important, initial human trials have also shown reduced toxicity and improved response using liposomal formulations. Interestingly, studies are now being done using liposomal nystatin for IV administration to humans.

Mechanism(s) of Action

The primary activity of the polyenes results in damage to the fungal cell membrane, altering the membrane permeability. The polyenes have a high avidity for binding to sterols, particularly ergosterol, the major sterol component of the fungal cell membrane. In general, the antifungal efficacy of the polyenes increases with increasing numbers of double bonds in the macrolide ring. The larger polyenes such as the heptaene amphotericin B are more effective than the smaller polyenes such as natamycin, a tetraene. Amphotericin B has an early, reversible "weak" binding activity followed by a late, irreversible "strong" binding activity. The larger polyenes cause potassium leakage from fungal cells at the lower concentrations and cell death at higher concentrations. The smaller polyenes produce little or no potassium leakage separable from cell death. Although there are demonstrable differences in mechanisms of action of the polyenes, the major activity is binding of the drug to ergosterol, which results in altered membrane permeability and, ultimately, lysis or killing of the cell.

There are very few reports of fungi developing resistance to the polyenes. The few isolates that have developed resistance following long-term treatment with amphotericin B have had an altered (reduced) ergosterol content in their cell membranes. Presumably, reduced ergosterol content provides fewer active sites for the drug. The polyenes have a higher affinity for ergosterol than for cholesterol, accounting for their relative selective toxicity. As mentioned earlier, the polyenes are quite toxic to mammalian cells. This toxicity is related to their binding affinity for cholesterol, a primary sterol component of mammalian cell membranes.

Adverse Effects

Adverse effects of amphotericin B are summarized in Table 98.2. Reactions can be divided into those related to the infusion of the drug (fever, chills, phlebitis) and those that occur secondary to organ toxicity (renal tubular acidosis, decreased glomerular filtration). Infu-

Table 98.1 Activity of Systemic Antifungal Agents Against Common Organisms

Organism	Amphotericin	Ketoconazole	Fluconazole	Itraconazole	Flucytosine
Aspergil lis sp.	S	V	V	S	V
Blastomyces	S	S	V	S	R
Candida sp.	S	V	V	V	V
Coccidioides	S	V	S	S	R
Cryptococcus	S	S	S	S	S
Histoplasma	S	S	V	S	R
Sporothrix	V	V	S	V	R
Zygomycetes	S	R	R	R	V

S=susceptible; R=resistant; V=variable

Table 98.2 Common Adverse Effects of Systemic Antifungal Agents

	Amphotericin B	Ketoconazole	Fluconazole	Itraconazole	Flucytosine
Related to route or period admin.	Fever, chills, nausea, vomiting; Thrombophlebitis	Nausea, vomiting	Nausea, vomiting, headache	Nausea, vomiting, diarrhea	Nausea, vomiting, diarrhea
Organ system toxicity with chronic therapy	Nephrotoxicity (reduced creatinine clearance, renal tubular acidosis); Electrolyte disorders (decreased K, Mg, Phos); Anemia, leukopenia	Rash, pruritus; Increased liver enzymes, hepatotoxicity; Inhibition of hormone (testosterone, progesterone, cortisol) synthesis: impotence, gynecomastia, menstrual irregularities	Rash; Increased liver enzymes, hepatotoxicity	Rash; headache; edema; increased liver enzymes; fatigue	Bone marrow (leucopenia); Increased liver enzymes; colitis; rash

sion-related adverse effects can be attenuated by premedication with aspirin, ibuprofen, or acetaminophen. Chills and rigors may be prevented or treated with premedication with hydrocortisone (25 mg) or meperidine (50 mg). Heparin has been traditionally added to each infusion (1000 units) to prevent thrombophlebitis, which may also be lessened by rapid infusion (1–2 hr), central venous administration, and rotation of IV sites. Heparin and hydrocortisone can be added to the amphotericin B for simultaneous administration.

The renal adverse effects of amphotericin B include a reduction in glomerular filtration rate, and renal tubular acidosis with loss of urinary concentrating ability, and wastage of potassium and magnesium. Clinically, an increase in the serum creatinine is observed that may be combined with an increase in urine pH and hypokalemia and hypomagnesemia. Serum bicarbonate also falls as renal tubular acidosis appears. Often, the electrolyte defects and renal tubular acidosis appear before there is an appreciable rise in the serum creatinine, but multiple effects can occur simultaneously.

Sodium depletion potentiates amphotericin B nephrotoxicity. Patients receiving concomitant diuretics, or those who have been vomiting or have poor oral intake should be monitored closely for renal toxicity. Sodium administration orally or IV before and after amphotericin B infusion appears to protect or attenuate glomerular toxicity. An infusion of 500 ml normal (0.9%) saline in patients without cardiovascular contraindications (pulmonary edema, severe CHF) is recommended pre- and post-amphotericin administration.

Amphotericin B-induced nephrotoxicity is augmented by use of other nephrotoxins. Aminoglycosides, cyclosporine A, or pentamidine may potentiate the rise in serum creatinine that would occur with amphotericin. Amphotericin B administration is usually not stopped or modified until serum creatinine levels exceed 3.0 mg/dl. At this point, every other day administration usually is recommended.[r5–r7]

Pharmacokinetics

Amphotericin B is administered as a colloidal suspension for intravenous infusion. It is poorly absorbed orally, although oral administration may be used for fungal decontamination of the gut. Amphotericin is incompatible with saline; infusions should be given in 5 percent dextrose. After IV infusion, amphotericin is distributed widely to tissues, including lung, spleen, and kidney. Central nervous system penetration is relatively poor, even with meningeal inflammation. Amphotericin B is highly protein-bound (91–95%) in serum, and serum levels are proportional to dosage; but serum level monitoring of amphotericin B has yet to be shown to improve therapy or reduce toxicity. Amphotericin is very slowly excreted via renal, biliary, and unknown routes; a terminal half-life of 15 days is reported. Serum levels are not significantly altered by renal or hepatic disease, or by dialysis. Serum levels of amphotericin B are not routinely measured, although bioassay and HPLC techniques of concentration measurement have been described.[r6]

Azole Derivatives

Members of this group include the imidazoles, such as clotrimazole, miconazole, ketoconazole, and econazole, and the triazoles, such as terconazole, fluconazole, and itraconazole. They are all structurally related, have similar mechanisms of action, and will be discussed as a group. Ketoconazole, fluconazole, and itraconazole are the agents from this group used most commonly for systemic infection. Miconazole is available for IV use, but it is rarely administered.

Chemistry

The structural relatedness of the azole derivatives can be seen in Figure 98.2. The imidazoles contain a five-membered ring with two nitrogens while, as their name implies, the triazoles contain one or more similar five-membered rings with three nitrogen moieties. The basic structure of these compounds has proved to be an ideal area for work by the designer drug chemist. Dozens and dozens of formulations have been synthesized and evaluated. Most proved to be too toxic, too insoluble, or had too little antifungal activity to be pursued beyond initial evaluation. However, a dozen or so have been extensively evaluated and marketed for human use. Most of the formulations are highly insoluble or only slightly soluble in water. Some, however, are readily absorbable from the GI tract and can be administered orally. For instance, nearly 100 percent of fluconazole is absorbed from the gut.

History

The initial interest in the antimicrobial activity of azole derivatives can be traced back to work on benzimidazoles in the 1940s.[r8] The present interest in the antifungal activity of these compounds arose from investigations by both Bayer AG and Janssen Pharmaceuticals in the 1960s.[5–6] These studies led to the release of clotrimazole and miconazole from these same pharmaceutical companies, respectively. The imidazole derivatives possess a very broad spectrum of antifungal activity, are quite efficacious, and exhibit relatively little toxicity. For these reasons, certain of these agents are given orally and systemically for systemic infections and others are given topically for dermatophytosis, vaginal mycoses, skin, and mucocutaneous infections. At the present time, about 20 of these compounds are being marketed or are undergoing extensive investigation by 10 large pharmaceutical companies. Needless to say, these compounds have proved an active and potentially very rewarding area of investigation for many commercial groups.

Therapeutic Uses

Ketoconazole, fluconazole, and itraconazole are the currently-available azoles used most commonly for systemic fungal infection. These agents are given orally; fluconazole can also be given IV. Table 98.1 shows the activity of these azoles against a variety of fungal pathogens. The main indications for ketoconazole, fluconazole, and itraconazole are summarized in Table 98.3. Oral administration of these agents is commonly used for oral, esophageal, or vaginal candidiasis in immunocompromised patients. In HIV-positive patients, fluconazole is more effective than ketoconazole for oropharyngeal candidiasis; esophageal candidiasis also may respond to fluconazole.[7] Because of favorable distribution characteristics into the CNS, fluconazole has been used with success in AIDS patients with cryptococcal meningitis. However, in severely ill, comatose patients, response to amphotericin B within the first two weeks of treatment is better than that with fluconazole. On the other hand, maintenance therapy to prevent a recurrent episode of meningitis is more effective (and easier to administer) with fluconazole than with amphotericin B.[8]

The role of oral or IV fluconazole in comparison to amphotericin B for systemic invasive candidiasis is being investigated and remains to be defined. Resistant *Candida* species have emerged in patients treated with fluconazole. Hence, resistance evolving in systemic candidal infections is a major limitation in the use of fluconazole for this indication.

Mechanism(s) of Action

The primary mechanism of action of all the imidazole derivatives is thought to be inhibition of ergosterol synthesis. Reduced sterol content in the fungal membrane, in turn, leads to less stable membranes and a less efficient membrane permeability barrier. Inhibition of ergosterol synthesis has been shown to be due to the inhibition of microsomal cytochrome P450-dependent 14 alpha-demethylation of lanosterol, which is a necessary step in the synthesis of ergosterol. This ultimately leads to inhibition of cell growth. At higher concentrations some of these compounds also interfere with triglyceride and fatty acid synthesis. Inhibition of cholesterol synthesis by either miconazole or ketoconazole in microsomal fractions of rat liver requires 30 to 70 times higher concentrations than that needed for inhibition of ergosterol synthesis in similar fractions from *C. albicans*.[r9]

Adverse Effects

Table 98.2 shows the common adverse effects associated with ketoconazole, fluconazole, and itraconazole. Gastrointestinal effects from ketoconazole are dose-related and may occur in 17 to 35 percent of patients receiving 400 mg to 800 mg per day, respectively. Divided doses or ingestion with food may reduce GI toxicity. Hepatic toxicity varies from asymptomatic increases in liver transaminases in 2 to 10 percent of patients to rare fulminant hepatitis.

Ketoconazole is a potent inhibitor of cytochrome oxidase enzymes, which has implications for endogenous hormone synthesis and for drug interactions. Ketoconazole inhibits synthesis of testosterone and cortisol. In men, impotence, decreased libido, and gynecomastia have occurred, and menstrual irregularities in women have been associated with ketoconazole. Fortunately, these effects are dose-related and occur

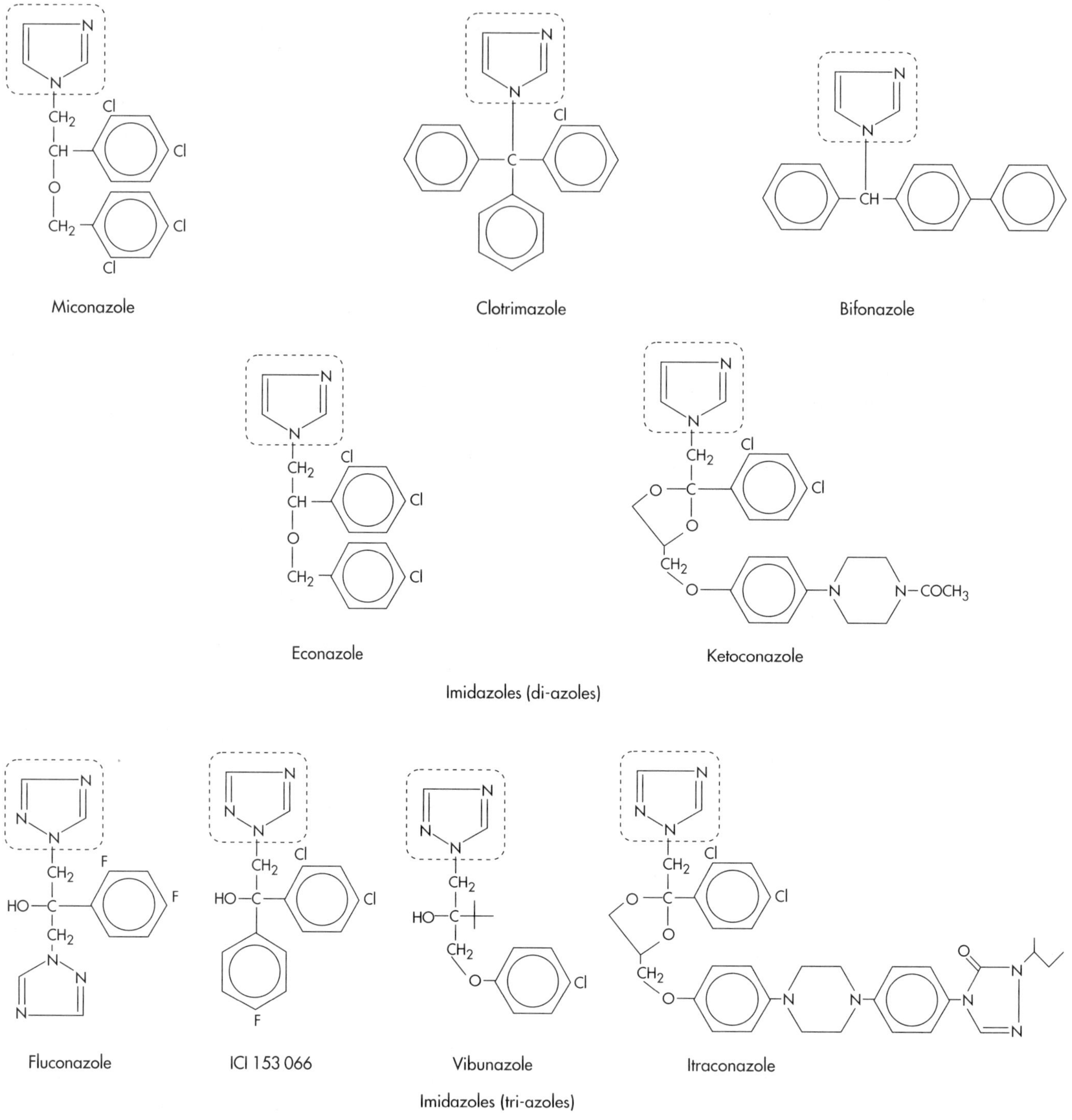

Miconazole

Clotrimazole

Bifonazole

Econazole

Ketoconazole

Imidazoles (di-azoles)

Fluconazole

ICI 153 066

Vibunazole

Itraconazole

Imidazoles (tri-azoles)

Figure 98.2 Basic Structure Enclosed in Box

most commonly at doses of 800 mg per day or more. However, at lower doses of ketoconazole, inhibition of drug metabolism occurs for concomitantly administered agents whose metabolism relies on hepatic cytochrome oxidase. Increased serum concentrations and potentially increased toxicity may occur for agents such as cyclosporine A, theophylline, phenytoin, and warfarin when administered with ketoconazole.

Fluconazole and itraconazole cause the same pattern of adverse effects as ketoconazole; however, these agents are much less potent inhibitors of cytochrome oxidase. Therefore, endocrinologic adverse effects rarely have been reported. The drug interaction potential with fluconazole or itraconazole is also less significant than that for ketoconazole, but patients also receiving anticonvulsants, warfarin, cyclosporine A, and

Table 98.3 Main Indications for Ketoconazole, Fluconazole, and Itraconazole

Ketoconazole	Fluconazole
Blastomycosis, Histoplasmosis: nonmeningeal, non-life-threatening in immunocompetent patient	Cryptococcal meningitis: for acute treatment and prophylaxis
Mucocutaneous candidiasis: oral, esophageal, vaginal	Candidiasis: mucocutaneous, urinary, peritoneal
Itraconazole	
Blastomycosis: pulmonary and extrapulmonary	
Histoplasmosis: chronic cavitary pulmonary disease; disseminated, nonmeningeal histoplasmosis	

oral hypoglycemic agents should be monitored for enhanced pharmacologic effects when fluconazole or itraconazole is added to their drug regimens.[9,10]

Pharmacokinetics

Important pharmacokinetic and pharmacologic properties of ketoconazole, fluconazole, and itraconazole are summarized in Table 98.4. Oral absorption of ketoconazole relies on gastric acid for drug solubilization; therefore, significant reductions in ketoconazole absorption and serum levels occur when it is given simultaneously with antacids or H_2-receptor antagonists (cimetidine, ranitidine, etc.). Fluconazole is also much less protein-bound than ketoconazole, allowing fluconazole to distribute in much higher concentrations to the CNS and urinary tract. Clearance of ketoconazole and itraconazole is hepatic, whereas renal elimination is most important for flucanozole. Renal dysfunction and dialysis have an effect on fluconazole serum concentrations; this is not the case for ketoconazole or itraconazole. These drugs should be avoided if possible in patients with significant underlying hepatic dysfunction.

Bioassay technology is available to measure serum concentrations of azoles, but the use of these assays clinically is not established.[r6]

5-Fluorocytosine

Chemistry

5-Fluorocytosine (5FC) is a fluorinated pyrimidine (see Fig. 98.3). As shown, the number 5 carbon atom in the ring structure of cytosine has a fluorine molecule attached rather than a hydrogen. Unlike the polyenes and many of the imidazole derivatives, 5FC is highly water soluble and is readily absorbed from the gut.

History

5FC like many other fluorinated pyrimidine (and purine) derivatives was initially designed to be an anticancer agent for use in

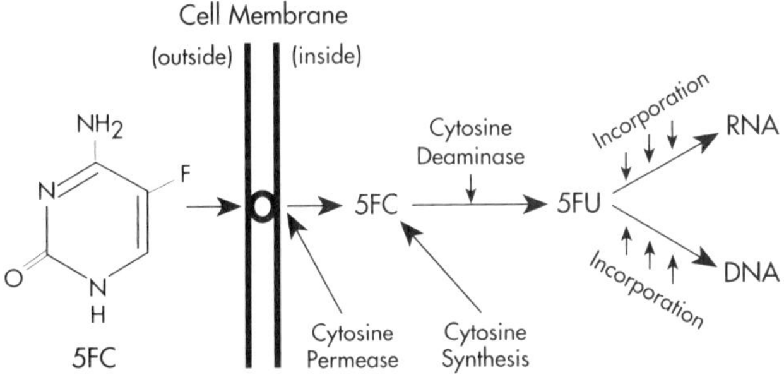

Figure 98.3 Mechanism of Cellular Effects of 5 Fluorocytosine

Table 98.4 Pharmacokinetic and Pharmacologic Characteristics of Ketoconazole, Fluconazole, and Itraconazole

Characteristic	Ketoconazole	Fluconazole	Itraconazole
Route of Administration	Oral	Oral, IV	Oral
Decreased oral absorption with increased gastric pH	Yes	No (85–90% absorbed)	Yes
Protein binding (%)	99	12	99
Water solubility	Low	High	Low
Half-life (hr)	9	25	64
Urinary elimination	Low	High	Low
CNS penetration (% serum concentrations)	<5	60–80	<5
Dosage adjustment in renal dysfunction	No	Yes	No
Removed by dialysis	No	Yes	No

chemotherapy.[11] The thinking was that these altered compounds would be inserted into the RNA (or in some cases DNA) and interfere with the growth of actively metabolizing cells, i.e., the cancer cell. Screening such agents for biologic activity demonstrated that 5FC inhibited the growth of many yeasts. Since it was also well absorbed from the gut, it was developed as an oral antifungal.

Therapeutic Uses

5FC is used most commonly in combination with amphotericin B for systemic infections caused by *Cryptococcus neoformans* and *Candida*. Amphotericin dosage and duration of therapy can both be reduced when 5FC is combined for treatment of cryptococcal meningitis.[12]

5FC should rarely be administered alone; the major limitation for doing so is emergence of resistance. Candida cystitis has been treated successfully with 5FC monotherapy, but fluconazole may be superior in this situation because of lesser toxicity and shorter duration of therapy.[r10]

Mechanism(s) of Action

5FC is actively taken up by yeast cells via their cytosine permease (Fig. 98.3). Once inside the cell, 5FC is deaminated to 5-fluorouracil (5FU), and a series of enzymatic steps are needed to incorporate 5FU into RNA. 5FU is a highly toxic and very effective antitumor agent when given to certain actively proliferating tumor cells. 5FU is incorporated into RNA; this interferes with protein synthesis, thereby producing the inhibitory effect (see Chapter 101). Susceptible fungi can rapidly develop resistance to 5FC; therefore, it is recommended that the drug be used in combination with another antifungal agent, preferably amphotericin B. Resistance can be at the cytosine permease level, i.e., the drug cannot enter the cell; and in this type of resistance addition of amphotericin B can help the 5FC enter the cell. This results in an additive or synergistic combination. However, if the resistance is at the deaminase level, or at one of the enzymatic steps needed to incorporate 5FU into RNA, the addition of amphotericin B will not be helpful. Similarly, addition of amphotericin B has no added value if the isolate possesses a high level of de novo synthesis of cytosine. With these latter types of 5FC resistance, amphotericin B maintains its antifungal effect, but the 5FC has no additional effect.

Adverse Effects

5FC causes GI and bone marrow toxicity. When administered with amphotericin B, renal dysfunction caused by amphotericin results in increased 5FC concentrations with serum level-associated leukopenia or thrombocytopenia. These adverse effects are related to 5FC serum levels exceeding 100 μg/ml for several weeks. Reducing the dosage or stopping 5FC usually results in a reversal of the hematologic effects, but patients who have already been treated with other myelosuppressive therapy or who have undergone radiation therapy appear most susceptible.

5FC undergoes conversion to 5-fluorouracil, a clinically useful antineoplastic agent, within the intestine. The hematologic effects noted above, as well as nausea, vomiting, diarrhea, and potentially severe colitis, may be on the basis of the appearance of the fluorouracil active metabolites.[13]

Pharmacokinetics

5FC is administered orally, and GI absorption is rapid and complete. Renal function determines 5FC half-life, which is approximately three hours with normal renal function, but can be extended to 85 hours in uremia. In order to avoid serum accumulation of 5FC, dosage must be reduced in patients with renal dysfunction. Dialysis does remove 5FC. Table 98.5 outlines dosage guidelines for 5FC in patients with renal insufficiency. Target peak serum concentrations are between 50 and 100 μg/ml. 5FC is poorly protein-bound, so the drug does penetrate into the CNS. In cryptococcal meningitis, CSF levels are about 75 percent of the serum concentration. Renal elimination removes 5FC from the body, resulting in high (200–500 μg/ml) urinary concentrations. Hepatic disease does not modify 5FC elimination or serum levels. 5FC can be measured in serum samples by bioassay and HPLC techniques.[r6]

Many antifungal agents are used for dermatologic fungal infections. The clinical aspects of other use (indications, adverse effects, pharmacokinetics) will be covered in the section on dermatology (see Chapter 82).

Table 98.5 Dosage Guidelines for 5-Fluorocytosine in Patients with Renal Insufficiency

Creatinine Clearance (ml/min)	Dosage (mg/kg)	Dosing Interval (hr)	Daily Dose (mg/kg)
>50	37.5	6	150
26–50	37.5	12	75
13–25	37.5	24	37.5
<13	Dose based on serum concentration measurements, with peak levels between 50–100 mg/ml		
Hemodialysis	37.5	After each dialysis	

However, the chemistry and mechanism of action of these agents are briefly mentioned here for completeness and for comparison with the systemic antifungal agents.

Griseofulvin

Chemistry

Griseofulvin is a highly water-insoluble compound that is only slightly soluble in ethanol (Fig. 98.4). It is taken orally and is deposited in the stratum corneum via the sweat glands or by deposition in keratinocytes. Since it is not active as a topical preparation, it is tempting to speculate that an altered metabolite may represent the active agent in the skin, hair, and nail.

History

Griseofulvin was isolated from *Penicillium griseofulvum* in 1939.[14] Initially used as an agricultural fungicide, it subsequently became the first efficacious oral antifungal used in human disease. In the later studies, investigators were able to show its safety and efficacy in treating experimental ringworm infections in guinea pigs in 1959.[15] Early studies clearly indicated that the drug was effective against dermatophytes, but not against other fungi.

Mechanism(s) of Action

Although a variety of mechanisms have been suggested, most agree that griseofulvin interferes with mitosis and perhaps with cell wall synthesis. Both mechanisms are likely the result of inhibiting spindle microtubule (mitosis) and cytoplasmic microtubule (cell wall) formation. Although most dermatophytes are susceptible to the drug, resistance can develop during treatment. As mentioned earlier, the drug is not effective against any other fungi pathogenic to humans.

Topical Antifungals

Allylamines: The allylamines (naftifine and terbinafine), like the imidazole derivatives, are inhibitors

Figure 98.4 Griseofulvin

Blocking Sites of Ergosterol Biosynthesis by Imidazoles and Allylamines

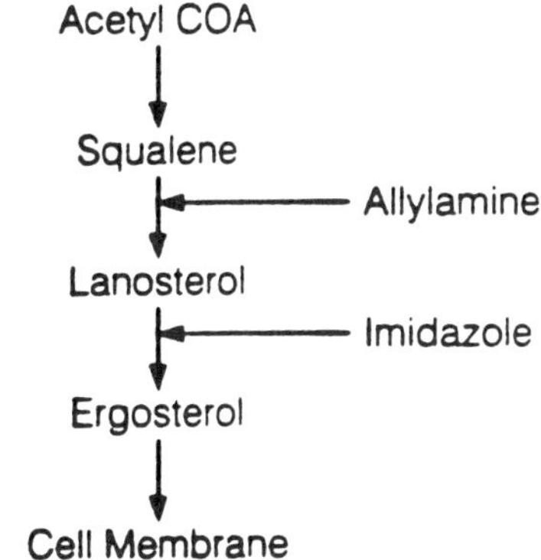

Naftifine

Tolnaftate

Haloprogin

Figure 98.5 Blocking Sites of Ergosterol Biosynthesis by Imidazoles and Allylamines

of ergosterol synthesis (Fig. 98.5). However, this groups of compounds interferes with the biosynthesis of lanosterol (from squalene). Like griseofulvin, these drugs are active against dermatophytes but have little activity against other pathogenic fungi. Tolnaftate: Tolnaftate is a thiocarbamate (Fig. 98.5) that is efficacious against most skin infections caused by dermatophytes (*Trichophyton* sp., *Microsporum* sp., and *Epidermophyton floccosum*) and *Malassezia furtur* (etiologic agent of tinea versicolor) but not against *Candida* sp.

Haloprogin

Haloprogin is a halogenated phenolic ether (Fig. 98.5) effective in treating skin infections caused by der-

Table 98.6 Summary Table

	Dosage			Pharmacokinetics			
Drug	**Route**	**Size**	**Dosage Protocol**	**Peak**	**V_D**	**$t_{1/2}$**	**Cl or Duration of Response**
Amphotericin B Fungizone[R]	Intravenous	50 mg vials-solution for intravenous infusion	0.3–1.0 mg/kg/day infused over 2–4 hours	0.5–2.0 μg/ml		15 days	
Ketoconazole Nizoral[R]	Oral	200 mg tablets	200–800 mg/day with meals	1.5–7 μg/ml		9 hr	
Fluconazole Dilfucan[R]	IV	2 mg/ml in 200 and 400 ml vials 50, 100, 200 mg tablets	50 mg orally daily for candidal cystitis to 800 mg per day for cryptococcal meningitis	4–8 μg/ml		25 hr	
Itraconazole Sporonox[R]	Oral	100 mg capsules	200 mg once daily to 200 mg twice daily with meals	200–400 μg/ml		64 hr	
5-Fluorocytosine Ancobon[R]	Oral	250, 500 mg capsules	100–150 mg/kg/day in 4 divided doses	50–100 μg/ml		4 hr	

matophytes, tinea versicolor, and cutaneous candidal lesions.

Whitfields Ointment

Whitfields ointment, a mixture of 6 percent benzoic acid and 3 percent salicylic acid, is one of the oldest treatments used for dermatophytic infections of the smooth skin. The combination of ingredients dissolves the substrate (keratin) utilized by the dermatophytes, thereby limiting growth of the organism. Although reasonably effective, repeated application often causes irritation at the site of application.

References

Research Reports

1. Sugar AM, Anaisse EJ, Graybill JR, Patterson TF. Fluconazole. J Med Vet Mycol 1992;*30*(Supp 1):201–212.
2. Galgiani JN, Rinaldi MG, Polak AM, Pfaller MA. Standardization of antifungal susceptibility testing. J Med Vet Mycol 1992;*30*(Supp 1):213–224.
3. Hazen EL, Brown R. Two antifungal agents produced by a soil actinomycete. Science 1950;*112*:423.
4. Gold W, Stout HA, Pagano JF, Donovick R. Amphotericin A and B, antifungal antibiotics produced by a streptomycete. I. In vitro studies. Antibiot Ann 1955–56:579–586.
5. Godefroi EG, Heeres J, Van Cutsem JM, Janssen PA. The preparation and antimycotic properties of derivatives of 1-phenethylimidazole. J Med Chem 1969;*12*:784–791.
6. Plempel M, Bartmann K, Buchel KH, Regel E. Bay b 5097, a new orally applicable antifungal substance with broad spectrum activity. Antimicrob Agents Chemother 1969;271–274.
7. De Wit S, Weerts D, Goossens H, Chumeck N. Comparison of fluconazole and ketoconazole for oropharyngeal candidiasis in AIDS. Lancet 1989;*1*:746–747.
8. Powderly WG, Saag MS, Cloud GA, the NIAID AIDS Clinical Trials Group, the NIAID Mycoses Study Group. A controlled trial of fluconazole or amphotericin B to prevent relapse of crypto coccal meningitis in patients with the acquired immunodeficiency syndrome. N Engl J Med 1992;*326*:793–798.
9. Lazar JD, Wilner KD. Drug interactions with fluconazole. Rev Infect Dis 1990;*12*(Supp 3):S327–S333.
10. Cleary JD, Taylor JW, Chapman SW. Itraconazole in antifungal therapy. Ann Pharmacother 1992;*26*:502–509.
11. Duschinsky R, Pleven E, Heidelberger C. The synthesis of 5-fluoropyrimidines. J Am Chem Soc 1957;*79*:4559–4560.
12. Bennett JE, Dismukes WE, Duma RJ, et al. A comparison of amphotericin B alone and combined with flucytosine in the treatment of cryptococcal meningitis. N Engl J Med 1979;*301*:126–131.
13. Harris BE, Manning BW, Federle TW, Diasio RB. Conversion of 5-fluorocytosine to 5-fluorouracil by human intestinal microflora. Antimicrob Agents Chemother 1986;*29*:44–48.
14. Oxford AE, Raistrick H, Simonart P. XXIX, Studies in the biochemistry of micro-organisms. LX. Griseofulvin $C_{17}H_{17}O_6Cl$, a metabolic product of *Penicillium griseo-fluvum* Dierckx. Biochem J 1939;*33*:240–248.
15. Gentles JC. Experimental ringworm in guinea pigs; oral treatment with griseofulvin. Nature (Lond.) 1958;*182*:476–477.

Reviews

r1. Bodey GP. The emergence of fungi as major hospital pathogens. J Hosp Infect 1988;*11*(Suppl A):411–426.

A review of the importance of fungal infections in hospitalized patients due to the use of antibacterial agents, immunosuppressive drugs, and chemotherapy.

r2. Gallis HA, Drew RH, Pickard WW. Amphotericin B: 30 years of clinical experience. Rev Infect Dis 1990;*12*:308–329.
A comprehensive review of the indications, efficacy, toxicity and monitoring of amphotericin B therapy.

r3. McEvoy GK. Anti-infective agents: antifungal antibiotics. AHFS Drug Information. Bethesda, MD: American Society of Hospital Pharmacists, Inc., 1993, pp 68–92.
A summary of chemistry, dosage, indications and adverse effects of antifungal agents.

r4. Odds FC. Antifungal agents and their use in Candida infections. In: Odds FC Candida and candidosis, 2d ed. London: Bailliere Tindall, (1988); pp 279–313.

r5. Branch RA. Prevention of amphotericin B-induced renal impairment: A review on the use of sodium supplementation. Arch Intern Med 1988;*148*:2389–2394.

r6. Terrell CL, Hughes CE. Antifungal agents used for deep-seated mycotic infections. Mayo Clin Proc 1992;*67*:69–91.

r7. Gallis HA, Drew RH, Pickard WW. Amphotericin B: 30 years of clinical experience. Rev Infect Dis 1990;*12*:308–329.

r8. Fromtling RA. Imidazoles as medically important antifungal agents: An overview. Drugs of Today 1984;*20*:325–349.

r9. Willemsens G, Cools W, Vanden Bossche H. Effects of miconozole and ketoconazole on sterol synthesis in a subcellular fraction of yeast and mammalian cells. In: Vanden Bossche, The host invader-interplay. Amsterdam: Elsevier/North Holland (1980); pp 691–694.

r10. Gubbins PO, Piscitelli SC, Danziger LH. Candidal urinary tract infections: a comprehensive review of their diagnosis and management. Pharmacotherapy 1993;*13*:110–127.

CHAPTER 99

William H. Prusoff
Thomas A. Krenitsky
David W. Barry

Antiviral Drugs

Introduction

Over 400 different viruses are known to infect humans and to cause diseases ranging from mild respiratory infections and cold sores to severe neurologic diseases and possibly cancer (e.g., nasopharyngeal carcinoma, Burkitt's lymphoma, hepatocellular carcinoma, and some T-cell leukemias).[4,r3,r5]

The influenza epidemic in 1918–1919 resulted in about 20 million deaths worldwide. Each year, there are several billion cases of diarrheal disease, causing about 5 to 10 million deaths worldwide, of which a large number are due to viral infection. In the US about 30 million individuals have genital herpes, and each year there may be up to 500,000 new cases. Transmission of infection in some cases appears to be related to the fact that about 2 to 10 percent adults shed herpes simplex virus-1 or herpes simplex virus-2 in their saliva and genital tract, but have no symptoms. A major worldwide problem is AIDS (Acquired Immune Deficiency Syndrome). About 60 per cent of the more than 360,000 individuals in the US who have been diagnosed as having AIDS have already died, and it has been estimated that more than 1 million are infected with this virus in the US. The World Health Organization estimates that currently a total of 8 to 10 million persons are infected.

Viruses are ultramicroscopic organisms that can replicate only within an appropriate host cell. They lack the organelles required for nucleic acid, protein, lipid, or carbohydrate synthesis, energy production, etc. The viral DNA or RNA genome is encased in a protective protein coat (capsid) that may in turn be surrounded by an envelope composed of lipids (phospholipid and cholesterol), phosphoproteins, lipoproteins, and glycoproteins. The exact composition depends on the specific virus. The virion may be spherical, icosohedral, bullet-shaped, or tubular, and the size varies from 20 to 970 nm. The RNA or DNA genome may be single- or double-stranded, and can vary in molecular weight from 1.8 to 240 × 10^6 daltons or more. Specific enzymes may be present in the virion, such as neuraminidase in myxoviruses and paramyxoviruses, or reverse transcriptase (RNA-dependent DNA polymerase) in retroviruses, or the virus may have encoded in its genome the capacity to synthesize enzymes that are either unique, such as the RNA-dependent RNA polymerase of the influenza virus, or they may produce a messenger RNA that is translated into enzymes that have different properties from the comparable one in the uninfected cell, such as HSV-1 DNA polymerase and thymidine kinase.[r6,6,7]

Development of Compounds for Antiviral Chemotherapy

This process involves: (1) the design and synthesis of potential antiviral agents; (2) the determination of their antiviral activity in cell culture and experimental animals; (3) studies of absorption, distribution, metabolism, excretion, and toxicity in animals; (4) studies of the safety, tolerance, pharmacokinetics, and efficacy of candidate agents in humans; (5) the elucidation of the molecular basis for efficacy or toxicity to use in the selection of second-generation drugs with greater efficacy and less toxicity.

Effective clinical use of any antiviral drug requires proper diagnosis of the infection, proper selection of the drug, and a knowledge of the pharmacokinetics of the drug.[1] The drug must be transported to and into the infected cell and must maintain an effective concentration at the target site for the time required to exert its antiviral activity. Ideally, this is achieved without toxicity or the selection of a population of viruses resistant to the drug. Although a number of compounds have been approved in the US for therapy of various viral infections, none are completely without toxicity. Hence, there is a need for new drugs with less toxicity, and for antiviral drugs targeted for therapy of viral infections for which no drug is available.

Vaccines Versus Drugs

The ideal approach for the control of viral infections is prevention. This has been achieved with many viruses through immunization with an appropriate vaccine. However, for a variety of reasons, vaccines are not available against all viruses of clinical interest. For example, the rhinoviruses, which are a major cause of respiratory disease, have over 100 antigenically distinct strains, and it would be difficult to prepare a vaccine effective against all. The influenza virus presents another problem, in that it continuously changes its antigenic composition; hence, each year's vaccine must be altered in an attempt to anticipate the new year's emerging virus. Another problem concerns the ability of some viruses, such as HIV-1 and HSV-1, to spread not only via the bloodstream (which would make it susceptible to a vaccine), but also by direct spread from cell to cell. In the latter circumstance, the virus may not come in contact with the neutralizing antibodies or sensitized T-lymphocytes induced by vaccination.[2,r1,r2,5]

The discovery of antiviral drugs has been primarily the result of serendipity. However, as our understanding of the biochemistry of virus-host cell relationships and of viral replication increases, appropriate targets for the design of antiviral drugs become available.[5,7a,r4] Some of the target sites are as follows: (1) adsorption of the virus to the cell surface; (2) transport of the virus across the cell membrane; (3) uncoating of the virus; (4) release of the viral genome into the cytoplasm or transport into the nucleus; (5) replication of the viral genome; (6) transcription; (7) post-transcriptional modification of viral RNA: methylation, polyadenylation, capping, and splicing; (8) translocation of nuclear RNA; (9) protein synthesis and processing; (10) virus encoded enzymes and regulatory proteins; (11) assembly of macromolecules into a virion (maturation); (12) Release of virus from the cell.

Approaches to Antiviral Drug Development

Many compounds have potent antiviral activity in cell culture, but only about 1 per cent of these compounds are also active in animals. Of those that have good antiviral activity and acceptable toxicity in animals, only a few become approved antiviral drugs for use in humans. In the US, eleven nucleoside analogues (Fig. 99.1) and phoscarnet, amantadine, rimantadine and alpha interferon have been approved by the FDA as antiviral agents. Many of these compounds were first synthesized as potential anticancer agents, but instead were found to be more effective as antiviral drugs.

Most drugs have been found by random screening or structural modification of naturally occurring biologic substances. The structural modifications are made based on a rational extension of existing knowledge of these or similar compounds. Once a lead compound is identified, repeated structure modifications are made until optimal antiviral activity with an acceptable therapeutic index is obtained. The probability of producing such a compound can be increased by combining structure-activity relationships with computer-graphic model building.

It would be preferable to have a more rational approach to drug development, and this approach requires a sophisticated knowledge of the target structure—be it the active site of an enzyme, or a receptor, or a macromolecule such as DNA, RNA, or a regulatory protein. Effective use of this approach requires a knowledge of the structural, spatial, and electronic requirements for a compound to interact uniquely with the target receptor. Today, not only do we have the potential to determine the three-dimensional atomic structure of target sites, but we also have the potential to know how antiviral agents or drugs interact with these targets through the use of X-ray crystallography and nuclear magnetic resonance spectra.[8,8a] Knowledge of how the atoms are arranged, when combined with molecular modeling and interactive computer graphics, could lead to the design of specific drugs.[9]

An exciting approach for rational drug design is based on our understanding of gene structure and function. Some success has already been achieved in the synthesis of "anti-sense" oligodeoxyribonucleotides, whose base pairs are complementary to critical regions of the viral genome or of mRNA and, following specific hybridization, block viral expression.[9a] Thus, selective inhibition of gene expression is achieved. There are, however, several problems in the use of anti-sense oligonucleotides: (1) attainment of a high concentration in the cell; (2) rapid degradation by nucleases in plasma and cells; (3) transport into the cell; and (4) possible limited accessibility of the target nucleic acid sequence because of tight binding proteins. Many of these problems are being addressed by the use of "oligonucleoids" but the prohibitive costs of consistent large scale production remain problematic.

Our knowledge of viral biochemistry and genetics, especially with respect to regulation of viral protein expression, has in recent years revealed many new targets for chemotherapy. It therefore seems likely that the antiviral agents of the near future will be of a wider variety and will have greater selectivity and efficacy than those described here.

Antiviral Drugs

Amantadine

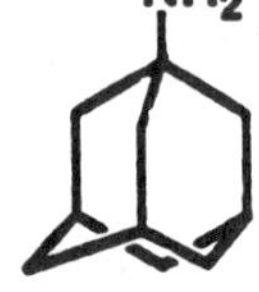

AMANTADINE

Chemistry

Amantadine (1-adamantanamine) is a synthetic, cyclic, symmetrical primary amine; it has a pKa of 9.0. The compound, marketed

ANTIVIRAL DRUGS OF THE NUCLEOSIDE ANALOGUE CLASS

Idoxuridine Trifluridine Zidovudine Zalcitabine Stavudine

Vidarabine Ribavirin Acyclovir Ganciclovir Famciclovir Didanosine

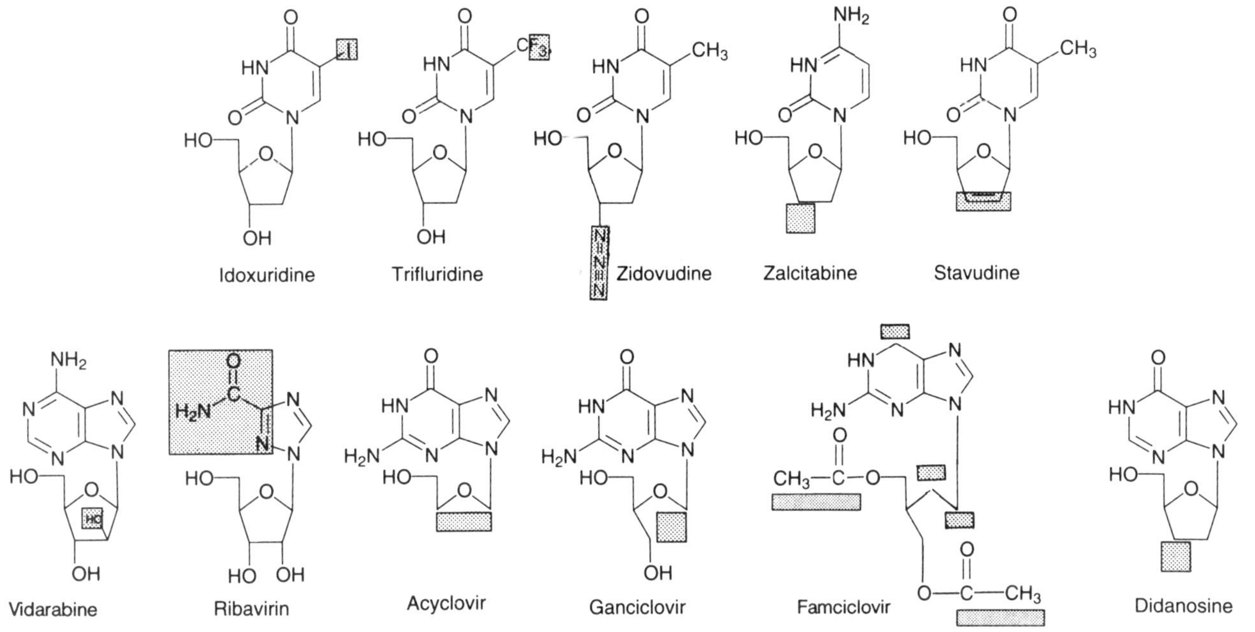

Figure 99.1 Antiviral Drugs of the Nucleoside Analogue Class. Shaded areas indicate portion of the drug that differs from the common nucleosides that are precursers of nucleic acids.

as the hydrochloride salt, is soluble in water at about 400 mg/ml. The chemical name, adamantanamine, is derived from the Greek term for diamond, because amantadine has the same structure and beauty as the carbon crystal lattice of diamond.

Mechanism of Action

Amantadine selectively inhibits the in vitro and in vivo replication of type A influenza viruses.[r7] The exact mechanism by which amantadine inhibits virus replication is not known. Early studies suggested that the site of action of amantadine was either penetration or uncoating of the virus. More recent work suggests that amantadine has an effect on virus-specific processes that occur between uncoating and primary transcription. Resistance to amantadine has been genetically mapped to the M_2 protein of the virus, suggesting that the mechanism of action involves an interaction of the drug with this protein.

Spectrum of Activity

Amantadine prevents infection of cell cultures by influenza A and C, parainfluenza 1, sendai, rubella, and pseudorabies virus. There is variation in the sensitivity of different strains of influenza A virus. Amantadine has either marginal or no activity against influenza B-type virus, herpes simplex virus, adenovirus 2 and 4, respiratory syncytial virus, rhinovirus, and vesicular stomatitis virus. Host cells do not appear to play an important role. Influenza A viruses resistant to amantadine develop frequently on exposure to the drug in cell culture. It has been shown that resistance can occur in humans.

Pharmacokinetics

Amantadine is well absorbed after oral administration, is not metabolized, and is excreted primarily unchanged in the urine. The maximum blood level of 0.3 to 0.6 μg/ml is reached one to four hours after an oral dose of 200 mg. Amantadine after absorption is present in the upper respiratory tract at an antiviral concentration (2 μg/ml). The average excretion in 24 hours is about 56 percent; by four days about 86 percent of a single dose is recovered, indicating almost complete bioavailability. The mean half-life is about 15 to 20 hours, but may be greatly extended in patients with chronic renal insufficiency. The drug is excreted in the urine through tubular secretion as well as by glomerular filtration. The rate of excretion increases as urinary pH decreases.

Administration of amantadine by small particle aerosol results in a drug concentration in the upper respiratory tract that is considerably greater than that found after oral administration. Aerosol administration of the drug in humans deposited 36 percent in the nose, 1 percent in the pharynx and bronchi, 25 percent in tertiary bronchi and respiratory bronchioles, and 21 percent in alveolar ducts.

Clinical Use

Amantadine has prophylactic and therapeutic efficacy against influenza A virus infection. The FDA approved its use for prevention and treatment of respiratory tract illness caused by influenza A viruses in 1966. The recommended procedure for prophylaxis against influenza A is immunization. However, for persons who have not received appropriate immunization, or when the strain previously selected for the vaccine did not closely match the strain of influenza virus epidemic in the population, prophylaxis with amantadine for four to six weeks during a community influenza outbreak is often appropriate. Prophylactic use is recommended in children and adults at high risk of morbidity or mortality because of underlying cardiopulmonary, renal, and metabolic diseases. It is also recommended for adults who have not been vaccinated but are essential for community functions, such as doctors, nurses, police, etc., as well as those who live in institutional settings (e.g., hospitals) and who have not been vaccinated. It should be considered for use with caution in some patients at high risk, such as the elderly, since they are more susceptible to adverse reactions (see below). For treatment of acute influenza A, therapeutic effect has been reported when given up to 48 hour after onset of illness.

Adverse Reactions

Since the drug is excreted in the urinary tract unchanged, it accumulates in patients with renal function impairment and may produce toxicity unless the dose is reduced. CNS toxicity is observed with plasma concentrations of 1 to 5 μg/ml. In general, it should be administered only with caution to mothers who are nursing, since it is secreted into the milk.

The toxicities of amantadine primarily involve the CNS and include depression, psychosis, hallucinations, insomnia, confusion, anxiety, irritability, anorexia, ataxia, dizziness, and seizures. Congestive heart failure has also been reported. These effects occur in a varying percentage of patients and are usually reversible on cessation of therapy. Leukopenia and neutropenia also have been reported.

Embryotoxicity and teratogenicity have been reported in rats at doses 12 times the recommended human dose, but not in rabbits at even 25 times the recommended human dose. Therefore, this drug should be used during pregnancy only in cases where the potential benefits outweigh the risks. Toxicity is dose-related and hence increased dosage to effect a greater antiviral and therapeutic effect is limited by CNS toxicity. Rimantadine, a derivative of amantadine, is reported to be less toxic than amantadine and has been approved by the FDA in 1993.

Preparation and Dosage

Adults—The drug is given orally at a dose of 200 mg/day, or two 100-mg capsules, or four teaspoons of syrup (50 mg/teaspoon). Total dose may be divided and given twice a day if CNS effects develop. In persons age 65 or older, the recommended dose is 100 mg/day, which can be given as a single dose. With one- to nine-year-old children, the dose given is 4.4 to 8.8 mg/kg/day, but it should not exceed 150 mg/day. The daily dose may be given as a single dose or as two divided doses. With nine- to 12-year-old children, the total dose is 200 mg/day, given as divided doses of 100 mg.

For prophylactic use, the drug should be administered for at least ten days following exposure. It should be noted that most individuals do not know when they are exposed to virus-laden aerosols, so that prophylaxis, when indicated, implies consumption of the drug during the entire epidemic period, which may last from six to eight weeks in most communities. Another approach for prophylaxis is to use amantadine in conjuction with Influenza A virus immunization with continuation of drug until protective antibody responses have developed. Dosage must be adjusted if renal impairment is present since drug may accumulate to toxic levels. For treatment, drug therapy is initiated as soon as possible after onset of symptoms and continued for one to two days after disappearance of symptoms.

Idoxuridine

Chemistry

Idoxuridine (5-Iodo-2′-deoxyuridine, (1-(2-deoxy-β-D-ribofuranosyl)-5-iodouracil, IdUrd, IUdR, IDU), the first clinically effective antiviral nucleoside, was synthesized in 1959 as a potential antitumor agent.[10–12] Idoxuridine is an analogue of thymidine in which the 5-methyl substituent is replaced with an iodine atom. This substitution is nearly isosteric because the van der Waals' radii of iodine and methyl differ by only 0.15 A. However, the electronic nature of this substitution is different; iodine is electron-withdrawing, which results in a decrease in pKa from 9.8 (thymidine) to 8.2 (IdUrd).

Idoxuridine is a white, odorless, crystalline solid that is soluble in water at 2 mg/ml and soluble in 0.2 N sodium hydroxide at 74 mg/ml. The solubility at pH 8.6 in 0.45 percent sodium chloride or 5 percent glucose is about 8 mg/ml.

Mechanism of Action

The metabolic scheme of idoxuridine in both virus-infected and uninfected cells is as follows:

$$\begin{array}{ccccccccc} \text{IdUrd} & \rightarrow & \text{IdUMP} & \rightarrow & \text{IdUDP} & \rightarrow & \text{IdUTP} & \rightarrow & \text{DNA} \\ \downarrow & & \downarrow & & & & & & \\ \text{Iodouracil} & & \text{dUMP}+\text{I}^- & & & & & & \end{array}$$

The enzyme responsible for the conversion of idoxuridine to 5-iodouracil is thymidine phosphorylase, and this activity does not vary much in cells after virus infection. For the drug to be active, it must first be phosphorylated to IdUMP. In herpes simplex virus or varicella zoster virus-infected cells, virus-encoded thymidine kinase is induced. This enzyme, in addition to the cellular thymidine kinase, is capable of phosphorylating idoxuridine. The binding affinity of IdUrd to the virus-induced thymidine kinase is somewhat greater than that to cellular thymidine kinase. Thus, idoxuridine is phosphorylated more efficiently in virus-infected cells than in noninfected host cells. Once it is converted to IdUMP, thymidylate synthetase could dehalogenate IdUMP, which results in the normal metabolite 2′-deoxyuridylate (dUMP); or IdUMP can be phosphorylated by thymidylate kinase to IdUDP, and then further to IdUTP by nucleoside diphosphate kinase. IdUTP is a potent inhibitor of ribonucleotide reductase, which is the key enzyme for deoxynucleotide formation, for both virus-infected and uninfected cells. IdUTP also inhibits dCMP deaminase. Most important, IdUTP is incorporated into DNA by both virus-induced and host DNA polymerases. The binding affinity of IdUTP to the virus-induced DNA polymerase is greater than that to cellular DNA polymerase. The incorporation of IdUTP into the DNA chain does not prevent further elongation, but the substituted DNA does not serve as an efficient template for either DNA replication or RNA transcription.[r9] This alteration of template behavior could be the result of distortion of double-stranded DNA because the unusually short intermolecular distance between iodine and the oxygen of the carbonyl group could result in charge transfer, or because of ionization of the N-3 position of IdUMP, or enol-keto tautomerism, or an increase in stacking energy. Thus, errors in base pairing can occur. The antiviral activity of idoxuridine correlates well with the amount of IdUMP incorporated into herpesvirus DNA.[17] Thus, the primary mechanism is likely the incorporation of idoxuridine into DNA and subsequent alteration of its properties. Idoxuridine has no effect on virus adsorption, penetration, or uncoating.[r8,15,16]

Spectrum of Activity

Idoxuridine has potent in vitro activity against most human DNA viruses: herpes simplex virus type 1 and type 2; varicella-zoster virus; cytomegalovirus; pseudorabies virus; vaccinia virus; polyoma virus; adenovirus; and simian virus 40.[13,14] It has marginal or no activity against most double-stranded RNA viruses, e.g., influenza.

Although idoxuridine is cytotoxic, the concentration required for cell growth inhibition is much higher than that required to inhibit virus replication. Cells can become resistant to the drug as a result of a deficiency of thymidine kinase activity. When herpes simplex viruses are grown in idoxuridine-resistant cell lines, viral mutants resistant to IdUrd can be isolated. In general, such virus mutants lose their ability to induce viral thymidine kinase. Clinically, herpes simplex virus resistant to idoxuridine treatment has been reported, but the mechanism of resistance in those situations was unclear. Although some cases of herpes keratitis have been poorly responsive to idoxuridine, there was a poor correlation between in vitro resistance and in vivo response to therapy.

Pharmacokinetics

Extensive in vitro tissue degradation of [^{131}I]-IdUrd to 5-iodouracil, uracil, and iodide occurs.

Studies in humans after a one-hour infusion of 80 or 100 mg/kg labelled [^{131}I]-IdUrd found that the level of radioactivity in the blood progressively fell, reaching 50 percent of the maximum (5-minute) level within seven to ten hours. Four hours after cessation of the infusion, the urine already contained about 44 percent of the injected radioactivity; the values at 24 and 48 hours were approximately 88 and 94 percent, respectively.

Idoxuridine administered IV is rapidly catabolized in the human subject. Five minutes after termination of the infusion of radioactive IdUrd, the total blood contained only about 9 percent of the injected radioactivity, while 14 percent already had been excreted by the kidneys. Thus, at the end of the infusion approximately 75 percent of the radioactivity was present in tissues other than blood. However, of the iodine-containing substances that were excreted in the urine, relatively little was IdUrd. In fact, only in the urine excreted during the infusion was there a higher proportion of IdUrd than of 5-iodouracil. Urine collected during the infusion and up to eight hours after its cessation already contained much of its radioactivity as iodide (about 30%).

Administration of idoxuridine into the eyes of rabbits indicated that diffusion into the systemic circulation occurred because teratogenic effects were observed; but it is not known whether such absorption occurs in humans. Studies in humans of potential intraocular penetration of idoxuridine showed no evidence in the aqueous humor of idoxuridine per se, but 5-iodouracil and deoxyuridine were present.

Clinical Use

Idoxuridine is approved by the FDA for the topical therapy of herpes simplex keratitis. Because of its toxicity to bone marrow, it is not used against systemic viral infections. In fact, controlled clinical studies in herpes encephalitis showed the drug to be detrimental, in spite of apparently promising results in earlier uncontrolled studies. Superficial herpes simplex infections of the epithelium are most susceptible to therapy. Deep stromal infections are not favorably affected, either because of poor penetration or because of rapid catabolism or other unknown factors.[18] IdUrd has been reported to be effective for the treatment of herpes zoster, cutaneous herpes, and herpetic whitlow when the drug is in a dimethylsulfoxide vehicle, a solvent that affords a 40 percent concentration. Since IdUrd penetrates skin poorly, the use of DMSO is critical since this solvent promotes penetration. However, the topical use of DMSO is discouraged by regulatory authorities in the US.

Adverse Reactions

The toxicity of systemically administered IdUrd in humans is concentration-dependent. The major toxic effects with doses of 100 to 120 mg/kg, when infused IV for periods of two to three hour daily for five or six days, are stomatitis, leukopenia, alopecia, and severe bone marrow suppression. Toxic manifestations of IdUrd in humans, such as alopecia and stomatitis, were prevented by infusion of thymidine into the external carotid artery while IdUrd was administered IV.; however, the effects of IdUrd on bone marrow were not abolished.

Even the FDA-approved use of IdUrd in herpes keratitis is not without hazard. Contact dermatitis, punctate epithelial keratopathy, follicular conjunctivitis, narrowing and occlusion of the puncta, lid changes, and lacrimation may occur.

Preparation and Dosage

One drop of 0.1 percent ophthalmic solution of idoxuridine is deposited in the conjunctival sac every hour during the day and every two hours during the night. Once improvement is observed, the same quantity is applied every two hours during the day and every four hours at night. This regimen is continued for three to five days after healing is complete.

The ophthalmic ointment (0.5%) is applied five times a day, every four hours and once before bedtime. A combination of these two procedures also may be used in which drops are used during the day and ointment at night. If no response is obtained after seven to nine days' therapy, the treatment should be discontinued.

Trifluridine

Chemistry

Trifluridine (5-trifluoromethyl-2'-deoxyuridine, TFT, F_3TdR, F_3dThd) was synthesized in 1962 as a potential antineoplastic agent. The trifluoromethyl moiety of trifluridine is only slightly larger than the methyl group of thymidine (van der Waals' radii of 2.44 A and 2.00 A, respectively), but the trifluoromethyl group is electron-withdrawing, which results in a large decrease in pKa from 9.8 (thymidine) to 7.35 (F_3dThd). The compound is a colorless, crystalline solid soluble in water at about 50 mg/ml. It is stable in aqueous solution if stored under refrigeration at pH 5.5 or less. However, F_3dThd is not stable under mild alkaline or physiologic conditions in solution and readily hydrolyzes to 5-carboxy-2'-deoxyuridine.

Mechanism of Action

F_3dThd is metabolized in virus infected or uninfected cells as follows:

$F_3dThd \rightarrow F_3dTMP \rightarrow F_3dTDP \rightarrow F_3dTTP \rightarrow$ DNA

$F_3dThd \downarrow$ 5-Trifluoromethyluracil $\downarrow$ 5-Carboxyuracil + F^-

$F_3dThd \rightarrow$ 5-Carboxy-2'-deoxyuridine + F^-

Like idoxuridine, F_3dThd is converted to F_3dTMP by thymidine kinase.[19,21] Herpes simplex virus or varicella-zoster virus-infected cells phosphorylate F_3dThd more efficiently than do uninfected cells because the activity of thymidine kinase is higher in infected cells, and F_3dThd has a greater affinity toward virus-specified thymidine kinase than toward cellular thymidine kinase.

F_3dTMP, a potent inhibitor of thymidylate synthetase, decreases formation of de novo thymidylate. The decreased pool of thymidylate could alleviate competition for phosphorylation of F_3dTMP and subsequently increase its incorporation into DNA. Virus DNA polymerase utilizes F_3dTTP more efficiently as a substrate than does that host DNA polymerase. The incorporation of F_3dTMP into viral DNA appears to be the critical event for its action, since faulty transcription of late messenger RNA has been found.[r11] This could be responsible for the biosynthesis of abnormal virus proteins. Fragmentation of DNA, or chemical conversion of DNA-F_3dTMP to 5-carboxy-dUMP with subsequent distortion of the DNA structure also could contribute to the antiviral activity.

The conversion of the trifluoromethyl moiety to the carboxyl group is a chemical process that does not involve any known enzymes. 5-Carboxy-2'-deoxyuridine does not have antiviral activity, but is cytotoxic to HEp 2 cells by blocking the de novo pyrimidine biosynthesis pathway at either the formation of orotidine-5'-phosphate or its decarboxylation.

Spectrum of Activity

Trifluridine inhibits the replication of several DNA viruses in vitro: herpes simplex virus Type 1, herpes simplex virus Type 2, cytomegalovirus, and to a lesser extent adenoviruses.[r10]

Pharmacokinetics

Intravenous administration of [^{14}C]-F_3dThd in humans resulted in urinary excretion of F_3dThd, 5-trifluoromethyluracil and 5-carboxyuracil with no significant amount of labeled respiratory CO_2. The drug was removed from the serum via first-order kinetics with a half-life of about 18 minutes. Inorganic fluoride was also found at about 50 percent of the amount formed from 5-trifluoromethyluracil during conversion to 5-carboxyuracil. The remainder of fluoride may be incorporated into bone.

F_3dThd was incorporated into the DNA of uninfected rabbit cornea cells at the rate of 0.4 pmol/hr/μg DNA, whereas thymidine was 2.5 times more effectively utilized. The soluble fraction extracted from these cells contained about 13 percent F_3dThd, 21 percent F_3dTMP, and 66 percent F_3dTTP. Studies in excised, perfused, rabbit corneas showed trifluridine penetrated by nonfacilitated diffusion and at a faster rate than vidarabine or idoxuridine. F_3dThd instilled into rabbit eyes penetrated into the aqueous humor, and increased when there was herpesvirus infection of the eye.

Similar studies in patients with unhealthy epithelium or marked stromal thinning revealed significant concentrations of F_3dThd (>2 to 4.4 μM) in the aspirated aqueous, but no 5-carboxy-2′-deoxyuridine. However, no drug was found to penetrate either healthy intact epithelium or scarred stroma with normal thickness. When trifluridine was instilled into the eyes of normal healthy adults (1% solution, 7 times per day for 14 days), no F_3dThd or 5-carboxy-2′-deoxyuridine was detected in serum.

Clinical Use

Trifluridine is approved by the FDA for topical therapy of primary and recurrent epithelial keratitis caused by herpes simplex virus. It is the most effective of the FDA-approved drugs for this infection.[20]

Adverse Reactions

Trifluridine 1 percent ophthalmic solution, when used as prescribed for up to 21 days, generally has no major toxicity. Mild, transient burning or stinging on instillation and palpebral edema are the most frequent adverse reactions. Occurring occasionally are punctate epithelial damage and filamentary keratitis. Local allergic reactions are rare. Also very rarely seen are stromal edema, keratitis sicca, hyperemia, and increased ocular pressure. Systemic administration to animals results in toxicity to bone marrow but little to the GI tract.

Contraindications

Trifluridine is contraindicated in patients who have developed hypersensitivity or chemical intolerance to the compound.

Preparation and Dosage

While the patient is awake, one drop of a 1 percent ophthalmic sterile aqueous buffered solution of trifluridine is instilled onto the cornea every two hour for a maximum of nine drops per day until re-epitheliazation of the corneal ulcer occurs. This is followed for an additional seven days with one drop every four hour (while awake) for a minimum of five days. Use should not exceed 21 days because of potential ocular toxicity.

Vidarabine

Chemistry

Vidarabine (9-(1-β-D-arabinofuranosyl)adenine, ara-A, adenine arabinoside, Vira-A) was synthesized in 1960 as a potential anticancer agent and was later isolated as a natural product from *Streptomyces antibioticus*. It is an analogue of adenosine in which the 2′-hydroxyl is inverted. The compound is a white crystalline solid with very poor solubility in water (0.45 mg/ml at 25°C).[22]

Mechanism of Action

Vidarabine is metabolized by cellular enzymes as follows:

$$\begin{array}{ccccccccc} \text{ara-A} & \rightarrow & \text{ara-AMP} & \rightarrow & \text{ara-ADP} & \rightarrow & \text{ara-ATP} & \rightarrow & \text{DNA} \\ \downarrow & & \downarrow & & & & & & \\ \text{ara-H} & \leftarrow & \text{ara-IMP} & & & & & & \end{array}$$

There are multiple sites of inhibition, but the inhibition that is causally related to the antiviral activity has not yet been established. The following sites have been identified:[23–27] (a) Ara-ATP is a potent inhibitor of ribonucleoside diphosphate reductase from both infected and uninfected cells. (b) Ara-ATP prevents post-transcriptional addition of poly-A to viral mRNA. (c) Ara-ATP inhibits the RNA-dependent RNA polymerase of vesicular stomatitis virus. (d) Ara-ATP is competitive with dATP for both mammalian and viral DNA-polymerases; however, the herpesvirus DNA polymerase is about ten-fold more sensitive than is the cellular DNA-polymerase. (e) Ara-ATP is also a substrate for DNA polymerase, and is incorporated into both viral and cellular DNA. (f) Ara-ATP slows DNA elongation. This could be a consequence of the 3′-exonuclease activity associated with herpes simplex virus DNA-polymerase. Thus, by continuous incorporation and removal of ara-AMP from the terminal position, ara-ATP could act as a pseudo-chain-terminator. (g) Ara-ATP inhibits terminal deoxynucleotidyl transferase. (h) Ara-A inhibits S-adenosylhomocysteine hydrolase. Consequently, S-adenosylmethionine-dependent methylation reactions, such as those involved in capping of viral mRNA, are inhibited.

The formation of ara-ATP in herpes simplex virus-infected cells is about the same as that in uninfected cells. The inhibition of ribonucleotide reductase by ara-ATP could facilitate the incorporation of ara-AMP into DNA by decreasing the level of the competing substrate, dATP, for DNA polymerase.

Hypoxanthine arabinoside (ara-H), which is formed through the action of adenosine deaminase on ara-A, is about ten times less active as an antiviral compound. Thus, the intracellular activity of adenosine deaminase could dictate the activity of ara-A. Resistance of herpes simplex virus to ara-A has been shown to result from mutations in the viral DNA polymerase.

Spectrum of Activity

Ara-A has a broad in vitro spectrum of activity against DNA viruses including herpes simplex viruses, varicella-zoster virus, cytomegalovirus, pseudorabies virus, and poxviruses.[28] Activity against non-oncogenic RNA viruses, such as picornaviruses, is marginal or absent. The activity of ara-A as well as many other antiviral agents depends on the cell lines used. For example, in a comparison of the sensitivity of HSV-1 and HSV-2 to idoxuridine or ara-A, HSV-1 was either more, equal, or less sensitive to inhibition, the outcome being dependent on the host cell. Similarly, whereas ara-A was found to be more inhibitory than idoxuridine to HSV-1 and HSV-2 in vitro, there was no significant difference in the efficacy of these two compounds against experimental HSV-1 or HSV-2 keratoconjunctivitis in rabbits.

Pharmacokinetics

For the treatment of systemic infections, ara-A is not given orally, SQ., or IM. because of poor solubility and absorption. A single IV dose of 1 mg/kg produced plasma levels of 1.1 to 1.5 μg/ml after 30 minutes with a rapid fall to 0.1 to 0.2 μg/ml over the next eight hours. Ara-A has a maximum urinary excretion rate in the first four hours, and about 50 to 60 percent of the drug is excreted within 24 hours, partly as unchanged ara-A (1 to 3%) but primarily as hypoxanthine arabinoside (ara-H) (41 to 53%).

When ara-A was administered daily over a 12-hour period at a dose of 10 mg/kg, peak plasma levels of ara-A and ara-H of 0.2–0.4 and 3–6 μg/ml, respectively, were obtained. These levels represent about 5 percent of the in vitro inhibitory dose for HSV. Presumably, higher concentrations are found intracellularly to account for the effective antiviral activity. Alternatively, there may be no direct relationship between in vitro inhibitory doses and in vivo response to therapy. Accumulation of drug or metabolites occurs within red blood cells over five to seven days and may remain for up to three weeks. The plasma elimination half-life for ara-H was 3.5 to four hours, and the levels found on Days 1 and 5 were similar. Urinary excretion as ara-H comprised 50 percent of dose. The excretion rate was essentially constant over a ten-day period. The concentrations of ara-H in plasma and CSF varied, but levels in the CSF were about one-third those found in plasma.

The plasma half-life in humans given IV ara-A at 1 mg/kg is three to five hours. Similar values are seen at higher doses. Infants and children receiving ara-A IV reached a maximum level of 1 to 2 μg/ml plasma, and the drug had a half-life of 1.5 to 2.5 hours.

Herpes stromal infection of the eye may not be benefited by topical therapy because of poor penetration. Studies in humans of intraocular penetration of vidarabine revealed trace amounts of ara-A and ara-H. High-dose IV administration at 20 mg/kg/day for seven days produced ara-A concentrations in the aqueous humor of 0.1 to 0.3 μg/ml. Patients treated with 3 percent ara-A ointment every six hours for a total of eight doses had no ara-A in their aqueous humor, but ara-H (0.02 to 0.28 μg/ml) was found.

Clinical Use

Ara-A is approved by the FDA for the topical therapy of acute herpetic keratoconjunctivitis and recurrent keratitis due to herpes simplex.[29] Ara-A is also approved for the parenteral treatment of neonatal herpes, herpetic encephalitis, and herpes zoster in immunocompromised hosts. The mortality of herpes encephalitis was reduced significantly by this drug in the 1970s and early 1980s. However, it is no longer considered the drug of choice for herpes encephalitis because of the superior efficacy and safety of acyclovir (see below). The effectiveness of ara-A has not been established for therapy of stromal involvement of herpes keratitis, herpetic uveitis, mucocutaneous herpes simplex infections, genital herpes, or cytomegalovirus infections.

Each milligram of ara-A requires 2.22 ml of IV infusion fluid to stay in solution. Hence, the administration of a therapeutic dose of the drug requires the administration of large volumes. Great care must therefore be exercised when the drug is administered to patients who have impaired renal function or cerebral edema because of the risk of fluid overload. Also, patients with impaired hepatic function are at risk.

Adverse Reactions

The toxicities observed in humans are determined by whether ara-A is given by infusion or topically.

Infusion. Anorexia, nausea, vomiting, and diarrhea may occur. CNS effects include dizziness, hallucinations, psychosis and ataxia, tremor, confusion, and encephalopathy. These CNS effects occur most frequently in patients with impaired hepatic or renal function. Elevated SGOT or total bilirubin levels indicate some hepatotoxicity. Hematologic effects such as a decrease in hemoglobin or hematocrit levels, thrombocytopenia, reticulocytopenia, and leukopenia are not common except at high doses. Pain at the site of injection may occur. However, severe adverse effects in bone marrow, liver, or kidney are uncommon when the recommended dosage is employed.

Because of the poor solubility of ara-A, large fluid volumes are required that may exacerbate cerebral edema in patients with HSV encephalitis. It is thought that ara-A administration to patients with renal failure may result in a greater chance of drug accumulation and neurotoxicity; however, specific recommendations for dose adjustment in renal failure are not available. Ara-A is teratogenic in rats and rabbits.

Topical. Adverse reactions may include lacrimation, foreign body sensation, burning, irritation, pain, photophobia, superficial punctate keratitis, and punctual occlusion sensitivity.

Contraindications

Ara-A is contraindicated in those who develop hypersensitivity to the drug.

Preparation and Dosage

The drug is supplied as a suspension. Prior to use, an appropriate portion is diluted and care taken to assure complete solubilization since it is administered IV. For herpes simplex virus encephalitis and neonatal herpes, the dosage is 15 mg/kg/day for ten days. For herpes zoster in immunocompromised patients, ara-A is given at 10 mg/kg/day for at least five days.

Acyclovir

Chemistry

Acyclovir (9-(2-hydroxyethoxymethyl)guanine, Zovirax, acycloguanosine, ACV) is an analogue of 2′-deoxyguanosine that contains a side-chain in which the 2′- and 3′-carbons of the ribose moiety have been excised.[30] The compound, which is a white crystalline solid, has limited solubility in water (3 mg/ml) at 25°C, but its sodium salt has a solubility of greater than 100 mg/ml at 25°C. The acidic and basic ionization constants are 2.27 and 9.25, respectively.

Mechanism of Action

Cells infected with herpes simplex virus or varicella-zoster virus metabolize acyclovir as follows:

Acyclovir → ACV-MP → ACV-DP → ACV-TP → DNA-ACV-MP (chain terminated)
Acyclovir → 8-Hydroxy-ACV
Acyclovir → 9-Carboxymethoxymethylguanine

Very little phosphorylation of ACV occurs in uninfected cells, because of a lack of the appropriate kinase. A cytoplasmic 5′-nucleotidase has been isolated from rat liver that very inefficiently phosphorylates ACV.

The enzyme responsible for the conversion of ACV to acyclovir monophosphate in herpes simplex viruses and varicella-zoster virus-infected cells is virus-specified thymidine kinase, which is induced in cells postinfection.[31] Virus mutants that lack the ability to induce such an enzyme or induce an altered thymidine kinase, which does not recognize ACV as a substrate, have decreased sensitivity to ACV. Cellular enzymes convert ACV monophosphate to ACV triphosphate. The latter is a potent alternative-substrate inhibitor that effectively competes with dGTP for binding to herpes DNA polymerase and subsequent incorporation into viral DNA. Since viral DNA polymerase-associated 3′-exonuclease cannot excise ACV, chain termination occurs. Furthermore, although the next deoxynucleoside triphosphate in the template sequence cannot add to the primer chain, it can trap the polymerase in a reversible dead-end complex with the ACV-terminated primer.[32]

The potent selectivity of ACV against herpes simplex virus is related to the properties of the virus-induced DNA polymerase in addition to that of virus-induced thymidine kinase. Virus mutants that induce an altered DNA polymerase to which ACV triphosphate has a lower binding affinity are less sensitive to ACV. Virus mutants cross-resistant to ACV and phosphonoformate or phosphonoacetate were found to have an altered virus-induced DNA polymerase. Such mutants are rarely found in patients and generally are the results of laboratory manipulations. The most commonly found clinical mutants are those with a diminished ability to induce virus-specified thymidine kinase and are obtained only from patients who have received prolonged courses of acyclovir and who have extremely poor endogenous immunity.

Spectrum of Activity

ACV has potent in vitro activity against herpes simplex virus Type 1 and Type 2, varicella-zoster virus, and Epstein-Barr virus.[r12] It has moderate activity against monkey B virus (Herpes simiae). Its activity against human cytomegalovirus is limited. It has no activity against pseudorabies virus, adenovirus, or RNA viruses. The degree of inhibition of herpesvirus by ACV depends on the strain of virus, host cell, and condition of the host cell. ACV shows little toxicity to uninfected human cells in culture.

Pharmacokinetics

The pharmacokinetics of ACV has been studied over a broad dosing range following IV infusion. The major route of ACV elimination is by excretion of unchanged drug in the urine; therefore half-life increases as renal function decreases. Since ACV renal clearance is greater than creatinine clearance, the compound appears to be excreted in the urine by both tubular excretion and glomerular filtration. The total urinary recovery in humans of labeled ACV ranged from 71 to 99 percent. The only metabolites found after IV administration were 9-carboxymethoxymethylguanine (CMMG) and 8-hydroxy-9-(2-hydroxyethoxymethyl)-guanine, representing about 10 percent of the dose and less than 2 percent of the dose, respectively. CMMG is about 0.1 percent as active in vitro against HSV as ACV. The drug has low plasma protein binding, in the range of 22 to 33 percent as determined by ultrafiltration.

Dose-independent kinetics have been observed over doses of 0.5 to 15 mg/kg. ACV concentrations in plasma show a biphasic decline, with an average total body clearance and terminal half-life in patients with normal renal function of about 300 ml/min/1.73 m^2 and 3.0 hours, respectively. At the standard IV dosing regimen for the treatment of HSV infection in immunocompromised patients (5 mg/kg infused over 1 hr every 8 hr), steady-state peak and trough concentrations of 9.8 and 0.7 μg/ml are achieved. In a pharmacokinetic study of patients with chronic renal failure, total body clearance and half-life were 29 ml/min/1.73 m^2 and 19 hr. Therefore, dose reductions are appropriate for patients with impaired renal function.

The oral absorption of ACV is incomplete. The estimated bioavailability of a 200 mg dose is approximately 20 percent. Doses of 200 mg five times daily for the treatment of mucocutaneous HSV infections in immunocompetent patients produce peak levels of 0.83 μg/ml, which is not only tenfold higher than the ED_{50} for HSV in vitro, but also adequate to inhibit HSV-2 and most varicella-zoster virus strains in vitro.

When applied as a 3 percent ophthalmic ointment, penetration into the aqueous humor does occur, and the levels are in excess of the amount required for the in vitro antiviral activity.

Clinical Use

The FDA has approved the following uses of acyclovir: (a) For the treatment of initial and recurrent episodes of herpes genitalis. (b) For the treatment or suppression of mucocutaneous herpes simplex infections in immunocompromised patients—e.g., those receiving immunosuppressive drugs during cancer therapy or after undergoing bone marrow or organ transplantation. (c) For chronic suppressive use in individuals who have frequent recurrences of genital herpes. A significant decrease in the rate of recurrence is observed while on suppressive therapy. After prolonged suppressive therapy, most patients exhibit reduced recurrence rates off drug. (d) For the therapy of varicella-zoster infections in normal and immunocompromised hosts. (f) For the treatment of herpes simplex encephalitis. (g) For the treatment of herpes zoster in normal hosts.

Adverse Reactions

Systemic Administration (oral, IV). Some patients treated with acyclovir will exhibit crystalluria, which is generally inconsequential. Renal toxicity occurs occasionally, evidenced by rises in serum BUN and/or creatinine and in severe cases by oliguria. Suboptimal hydration of the patient and bolus intravenous administration of the drug appear to be the major risk factors for acyclovir-related renal toxicity. This renal toxicity usually has been reversible on drug discontinuation or dose reduction, and/or restoration of fluid and electrolyte balance in the patient.

Intravenous administration of acyclovir can result in inflammation or phlebitis at the injection site in cases where cutaneous infiltration of the medication occurs. Other adverse effects have been reported in acyclovir recipients in controlled or uncontrolled trials. They are uncommon to rare. Included are CNS effects such as lethargy, tremors, confusion, hallucinations, agitation, seizures, or coma. Others are headache, nausea, hematuria, rash, and pruritus. The relationship of these infrequent adverse effects to acyclovir administration has generally been unclear.

Topical. A 3 percent ophthalmic ointment (available in many countries but not in the US) produced side-effects that included transient stinging, punctate keratitis, follicular conjunctivitis, and palpebral hypersensitivity reactions.

Application of the 5 percent topical ointment (widely available, including the US) did not produce appreciable adverse effects in Phase I dermal tolerance testing or in applications to herpes genitalis lesions. After topical application to such lesions, the rates of reported symptoms and signs of local irritation (e.g., burning, stinging, pain, pruritus, etc.) were similar in acyclovir and placebo recipients.

Contraindications

Acyclovir is contraindicated in those who exhibit hypersensitivity to the drug or components of its formulation.

Preparation and Use

Acyclovir is available as a 200-mg capsule and 400 and 800-mg tablets for oral intake, in a suspension containing 200 mg/5 ml, in a 5% ointment for topical (nonophthalmic) use, and as a sterile powder for IV use. The dosage and mode of administration depend on the specific infection being treated. Intravenous doses should be given slowly with an infusion time of at least one hour. Acyclovir may accumulate in patients with renal insufficiency. Reduced doses may be advisable under such circumstances.

Ganciclovir

Chemistry

Ganciclovir (9-(2-hydroxy-1-(hydroxymethyl)ethoxymethyl) guanine, DHPG, BW B759U, 2′NDG, BIOLF-620) is closely related structurally to acyclovir. It is an analogue of 2′-deoxyguanosine in which the 2′-carbon of the deoxyribose moiety is excised.[33] It is a stable white solid with a melting point > 300°C. Its solubility in water at neutral pH is 4.3 mg/ml at 25°C.

Mechanism of Action

Ganciclovir → DHPG-MP →
DHPG-DP → DHPG-TP → DNA-DHPG-MP

Ganciclovir is selectively converted to the monophosphate in herpes virus-infected cells by the viral encoded thymidine kinase.[34] It is then further phosphorylated by cellular enzymes to form ganciclovir triphosphate. The latter competes with dGTP as a substrate of viral DNA polymerase. Subsequently, incorporation of ganciclovir monophosphate into viral DNA decreases the rate of chain elongation.[35]

With herpes simplex and varicella-zoster viruses, resistance to ganciclovir is primarily due to changes in the viral-encoded thymidine kinase. Cytomegalovirus has evolved mechanisms different from herpes simplex and varicella-zoster viruses to induce the synthesis of nucleotide necessary for virus DNA replication. Cytomegalovirus transcriptionally activates expression of host cell S phase enzymes, including deoxyguanosine and thymidine kinases. Cytomegalovirus does not encode a deoxypyrimidine kinase analogous to the thymidine kinase of herpes simplex and varicella-zoster virus. The intracellular phosphorylation of ganciclovir in cytomegalovirus-infected cells is controlled by the protein kinase homologue encoded within the UL97 open reading frame. The role of this enzyme in cytomegalovirus replication is unknown. Clinical resistance to ganciclovir has been associated with the recovery of resistant viruses bearing one of a restricted number of specific mutations in UL97 that confer the phosphorylation deficient phenotype.

Spectrum of Activity

Ganciclovir inhibits the replication in vitro of herpes simplex virus Type 1, herpes simplex virus Type 2, cytomegalovirus, varicella-zoster virus, and Epstein-Barr virus.[36,r13]

Pharmacokinetics

Pharmacokinetic studies have been performed in AIDS patients with human cytomegalovirus pneumonitis or retinitis by systemic administration of 2.5 or 5 mg/kg of DHPG every eight hours for ten days. The $t_{1/2}$ α was 0.23 hours and its $t_{1/2}$ β 2.53 hours. The volume of distribution at steady state was 32.8 L/1.73m^2. The peak plasma concentrations were for the higher dose 4.75 to 6.20 μg/ml and for the lower dose < 0.25 to 0.63 μg/ml. The level in the CSF was 24 percent to 67 percent of that in the plasma.

When a 20 mg/kg dose given every six hours was administered orally to immunocompromised patients with severe cytomegalovirus infections, the absorption was about 3 percent. Mean steady-state peak and trough levels were 2.96 and 1.06 μM, and the area under the concentration-time curve (AUC) from 0 to 24 hours was 47 μM per hour. No accumulation of DHPG occurs, and it is excreted unchanged in the urine.

Clinical Use

Ganciclovir is approved for IV therapy of cytomegalovirus retinitis in immunocompromised patients.[37] This condition is a common sight-threatening disease in patients with AIDS.

Adverse Reactions

About 15 to 55 percent of patients who receive DHPG develop moderate to severe neutropenia that generally is reversible when the drug is stopped. Less common are thrombocytopenia and anemia. Bone marrow suppression is more common and more severe when ganciclovir is given concomitantly with other agents, such as AZT, which are also marrow-suppressive. Other possible side-effects include confusion, rashes, thrombophlebitis, and nausea. Animal studies have indicated an inhibition of spermatogenesis. DHPG is teratogenic in rabbits and embryotoxic in mice at the human dose level.

Contraindications

Ganciclovir is contraindicated in patients with hypersensitivity to this drug or to acyclovir.

Preparation and Dosage

Ganciclovir has been given IV for 14 days at a dose of 5 to 10 mg/kg/day to patients with CMV retinitis, pneumonia, or GI lesions with some clinical benefit. However, its efficacy in the treatment of CMV pneumonitis or enterocolitis is controversial and incompletely studied. In those patients with continuing severe immune deficiency, CMV infections usually recur after the cessation of therapy. Most cases of retinitis recur within three to six weeks. Hence, present efforts are directed toward chronic suppression.

Famciclovir

Chemistry

Famciclovir (2-[2-(-2-amino-9*H*-purin-9yl) ethyl]-1,3-propanediol diacetate, FAMVIR) is a prodrug of yet another acyclic analogue of 2′-deoxyguanosine, penciclovir (9-(2-ethyl-1,3-propanediol)guanine). Penciclovir has the same structure as ganciclovir (Fig. 99.1) except that the ether oxygen atom of the 9-substitituent of guanine is replaced by a carbon atom. Famciclovir is a white to pale yellow solid. At 25°C, famciclovir is freely soluble (>25% w/v) in water initially but rapidly precipitates as the sparingly soluble monohydrate.

Mechanism of Action

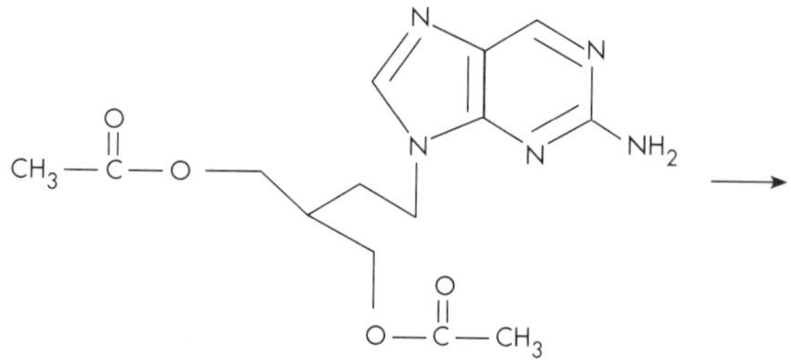

Famciclovir, (FCV)

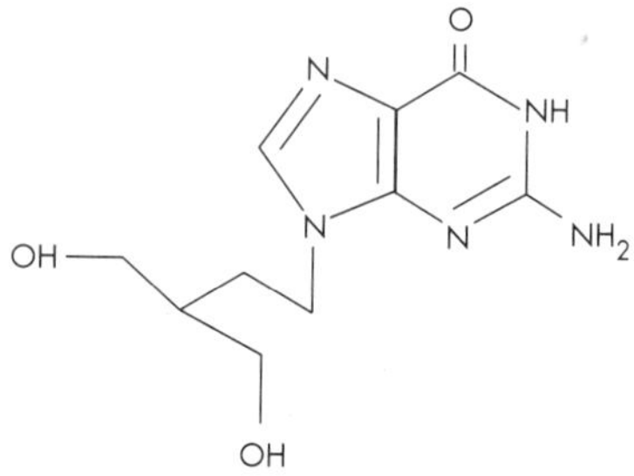

Penciclovir, (PCV)

PCV-MP → PCV-DP → PCV-TP → DNA

Famciclovir is converted to penciclovir by the action of esterases that remove the acetyl ester moieties and by the action of aldehyde oxidase and/or xanthine oxidase to convert the 2-amino purine moiety to a guanine moiety. Its antiviral mechanism is similar to that for ganciclovir.

Spection of Activity

The *in vitro* spectrum of antiviral activities of famciclovir is similar to that of ganciclovir.

Pharmacokinetics

The bioavailability of famciclovir after oral administration to humans is 77% as judged by plasma levels of penciclovir. Little or no famciclovir is detected in plasma or urine. The pharmacokinetic parameters of penciclovir are similar to those of ganciclovir. The half-life of penciclovir in varicella zoster virus-infected cells is 7–14 hours.

Clinical Use

The FDA has approved the use of famciclovir in herpes zoster patients who are not immunocompromised or have no renal dysfunction. It has also been reported to reduce the duration of post-herpetic neuralgia.

Adverse Reactions

The most frequently observed adverse events in clinical trials were headache, nausea, and fatigue. However, similar frequencies were seen in placebo-treated patients. Based on *in vitro* and *in vivo* animal studies and *in vitro* human cell studies, there are precautions with famciclovir regarding carcinogensis, mutagenesis, and impariment of fertility. A significant increase in the incidence of mammary adenocarcinoma was seen in female rats receiving 1.5 times the human systemic exposure at the recommended oral dose. Marginal increases in the incidence of subcutaneous tissue fibrosarcomas or squamous cell carcinomas of the skin were seen in female rats and male mice dosed at 0.4 times the human systemic exposure. Testicular toxicity was observed in rats, mice, and dogs below or at low multiples of the human systemic exposure. Its relavance to the human situation remains to be established.

Contraindications

Famciclovir is contraindicated in patients with known hypersensitivity to it.

Preparation and Use

Famciclovir is available as 500 mg tablets. The recommended dosage is 500 mg every 8 hours for 7 days. Therapy should be initiated promptly after herpes zoster is diagnosed.

Foscarnet

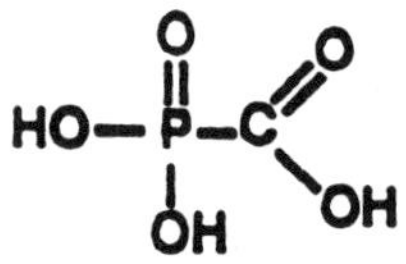

Chemistry

Foscarnet (phosphonoformate, PFA, dihydroxyphosphinecarboxylic acid oxide, carboxyphosphonate, Foscavir) is a pyrophosphate analogue. It is not a natural substance, was synthesized in 1924, and its crystal structure was determined in 1971, which revealed an unusually long P-C bond.[38] PFA has a melting point of > 250°, is about 5 percent soluble in water, is stable at pH 7.0, but decomposes at low pH to form CO_2 and phosphorous acid. The pKa values are 7.27, 3.41, and 0.49. Divalent metal ions, calcium and magnesium may form stable chelates.

Mechanism of Action

PFA reversibly inhibits viral RNA and DNA polymerases by competing with pyrophosphate, which is a product of DNA and RNA polymerase action.[39,40] The interaction of PFA with the enzyme is either at a site that overlaps the pyrophosphate binding site, or they both bind at the active site differently. In either case pyrophosphate exchange is prevented, and the formation of the PFA-Enzyme complex results in prevention of nucleic acid chain elongation.[41]

Spectrum of Activity

PFA is a broad spectrum antiviral agent inhibiting both DNA and RNA viruses. Its use as an antiviral agent was first reported in 1978. PFA is a very effective inhibitor in vitro of herpes simplex virus Type 1, herpes simplex virus Type 2, human immunodeficiency virus (HIV-1), murine and human cytomegalovirus, varicella zoster (VZV), Epstein-Barr virus, Marek's disease virus, and a variety of animal retroviruses. Inhibition is reversible on removal of PFA.[r14]

Resistance to PFA, which occurs by passage of the virus in the presence of the drug, is attributed to a site-specific amino acid mutagenesis in the polymerase. Cross resistance to some strains of HSV and CMV have been observed; however, clinical isolates generally are sensitive to PFA even though resistant to ganciclovir (CMV) or acyclovir (HSV and VZV).

Pharmacokinetics

PFA is poorly absorbed, usually less than 22 percent. This may be due to a relatively inefficient transport system. The oral dose is limited by diarrhea; therefore the drug is administered IV. It is distributed throughout the body; however, about 10 to 28 percent is deposited in the bone matrix, presumably similar to the deposition of inorganic phosphate. PFA is slowly eliminated from bone over a period of several months. The intracellular levels of PFA rapidly decrease as the extracellular concentration falls. Because covalent interaction is not involved at the target site, continuous or frequent infusion is required to maintain an intracellular antiviral concentration of PFA.[43]

PFA is not metabolically altered and is eliminated in the urine via glomerular filtration and tubular secretion. There is great variability in the pharmacokinetics, with the half-life ranging from three to eight hours, and clearance being dependent on the glomerular filtration rate.

Clinical Use

Foscarnet has been approved by the FDA for IV therapy of cytomegalovirus retinitis in AIDS patients.[42] It has also been reported to be effective in ganciclovir-resistant CMV retinitis and acyclovir-resistant HSV or VZV infections.[44] Under in vitro conditions, strains of HSV, VZV, and CMV resistant to PFA have been observed.

Adverse Effects

About 25 percent of patients experience reversible nephrotoxicity; anemia, nausea, and fever are also common. Other adverse effects include hypocalcemia, hypomagnesemia, hypophosphatemia, hypokalemia, seizures, neutropenia, arrhythmia, and mucosal and penile ulcers.

Contraindications

A decrease in serum calcium ion and other divalent cations is associated with PFA therapy due to chelation; hence there is risk of cardiac disturbances and seizures. Caution must be exercised in patients with altered electrolyte balance as well as those with neurologic or cardiac problems.

Concurrent IV pentamidine in patients with AIDS may result in severe hypocalcemia that may be fatal.

Preparation and Dosage

For induction therapy PFA (60 mg/kg) is administered IV three times per day for two to three weeks, and then maintained at 90 to 120 mg/kg/day. AIDS patients require maintenance therapy for life; once discontinued, relapse may occur within three weeks. The regimen requires that the patient have normal renal function. It is recommended that the dose administered must consider the patient's renal function (creatinine clearance) and be adjusted accordingly.

Ribavirin

Chemistry

Ribavirin (1-β-D-ribofuranosyl-1,2,4-triazole-3-carboxamide, virazole) is a synthetic nucleoside that contains an unnatural heterocyclic base. X-ray crystallography studies revealed that ribavirin possesses striking structural similarity to guanosine and inosine. The compound is a colorless, crystalline solid, which exists in two crystalline polymorphs with melting points of 166 to 168°C and 174 to 176°C. Ribavirin has low lipid solubility and is very soluble in water (> 27 g/100 ml at 37°C).

Mechanism of Action

Ribavirin → Rib-MP → Rib-DP → Rib-TP
Ribavirin → 1,2,4-Triazole-3-carboxamide
Ribavirin ↓ 1-β-D-Ribofuranosyl-1,2,4-triazole-3-carboxylic Acid
1,2,4-Triazole-3-carboxamide → 1,2,4-Triazole-3-carboxylic Acid

Ribavirin is converted to the mono-, di-, and triphosphate derivatives by cellular enzymes. Ribavirin monophosphate may decrease the pool size of GTP and dGTP, which are required for RNA and DNA synthesis, respectively, by inhibiting inosinate dehydrogenase.[45] This enzyme converts inosine monophosphate to xanthosine monophosphate which is then converted to guanosine monophosphate. Ribavirin triphosphate inhibits the viral-specific mRNA capping enzymes, guanyl transferase and N^7-methyl transferase, the consequence being an adverse effect on viral protein formation. Ribavirin triphosphate is also a potent inhibitor of influenza virus RNA polymerase.

Spectrum of Activity

Ribavirin has a broad in vitro spectrum of antiviral activity against both RNA and DNA viruses including herpes simplex virus, influenza A and B virus, respiratory syncytial virus, parainfluenza virus, adenovirus, vaccina virus, Lassa fever virus, etc. High concentrations are reported to inhibit HIV-1 in vitro.[r15,r16]

Pharmacokinetics

Oral administration to humans results in rapid absorption with concentration in the red blood cells.

Metabolic derivatives found after IV administration include 1,2,4-triazole-3-carboxamide, 1,2,4-triazole-3-carboxylic acid, 1-β-D-ribofuranosyl-1,2,4-triazole-3-carboyxlic acid, and the mono-, di-, and triphosphate derivatives of ribavirin.

In humans, the percentage composition of the urinary metabolites of ribavirin collected in a 22- to 24-hour time interval was 17 percent as ribavirin, 50 percent as 1,2,4-triazole-3-carboxamide, and 22 percent as 1,2,4-triazole-3-carboxylic acid. A 72-hour collection accounted for about 40 percent of the total labeled drug. It is postulated that 20 to 30 percent of the total dose is retained in the body beyond 72 hours, but precisely where is uncertain. Patients receiving 43.2 mg/kg of ribavirin had serum levels of 5.3 μg/ml 24 hours later. The red blood cells appear to accumulate about 3 percent of a total dose of ribavirin, which is in excess of plasma level, and has a half-life of about 40 days. The intracellular form of ribavirin is primarily as the triphosphate derivative.

After aerosol administration, the half-life of ribavirin in respiratory excretions is two hours and in plasma is nine hours. The concentration in the respiratory secretions may be 100 times higher than in the systemic circulation.

Clinical Use

Ribavirin is approved for small particle aerosol therapy of severe respiratory infections due to the respiratory syncytial virus (RSV) in infants and children. Treatment should generally be initiated within three days of onset of illness.

Adverse Reactions

Humans given 15 mg/kg/day for beyond 10 to 14 days develop a reversible hemolytic anemia. Hemolysis may be the result of extremely high levels of ribavirin triphosphate trapped within red blood cells. Occasional transient elevated levels of bilirubin and of serum glutamic oxalacetic transaminase, as well as occasional mild frontal headaches, mild abdominal cramps, and tiredness also may occur.

When ribavirin is given by aerosol administration, deterioration of pulmonary function may occur in patients with chronic obstructive lung disease or asthma. Dyspnea, chest soreness, rash, conjunctivitis, cardiac arrest, hypotension, digitalis toxicity, pulmonary edema, reversible anemia, mild headache, mild abdominal cramps, and diarrhea have been rarely observed.

Contraindications

Ribavirin is contraindicated in pregnant females or in females who may become pregnant during exposure to the drug because teratogenicity and embryolethality have been observed in nearly all animal species studied. Ribavirin can crystallize in the tubing and other components of respiratory support devices, such as mechanical ventilators, with consequent impairment of their function.

Preparation and Dosage

Ribavirin at 20 mg/ml is administered as a small-particle aerosol for 12 to 18 hours per day for three to seven days (maximum) using a small-particle aerosol generator. Administration can be by mask or oxygen tent, if an oxygen hood cannot be employed.

Zidovudine

Chemistry

Zidovudine (Retrovir, 3′-azido-3′-deoxythymidine, azidothymidine, AZT, BW A509U) is an analogue of thymidine that contains an 3′-azido group rather than a 3′-hydroxyl. Zidovudine is a white crystallize solid with a melting point of 119–121°C. Its solubility in water is 20 mg/ml.

Mechanism of Action

3′-Azido-3′-deoxythymidine → AZT-MP → AZT-DP → AZT-TP → DNA
↓ (from 3′-Azido-3′-deoxythymidine): AZT-5′-glucuronide
↘ (from 3′-Azido-3′-deoxythymidine): 3′-Amino-3′-deoxythymidine

AZT is converted to its mono-, di-, and triphosphate by the same cellular enzymes that catalyze the phosphorylation of thymidine and thymidine nucleotides. AZT triphosphate is then terminally incorporated into the growing DNA chains via the viral reverse transcriptase. As with acyclovir-TP, AZT-TP is an obligate chain terminator because of the absence of a hydroxyl group on the 3′-carbon of the sugar analogue moiety. AZT is a highly efficient substrate of thymidine kinase. However, the product, AZT monophosphate, accumulates in human cells as the major metabolite, because its V_{max} for thymidylate kinase is only about 0.3 percent that of thymidine monophosphate.[46,47]

Resistance to AZT has been studied *in vitro* with mutations in the HIV reverse transcriptase. The T215Y mutation confers resistance. Purified reverse transcriptase containing this amino acid change shows an increased K_i value for AZT-TP. More significantly, there was a 10-fold increase in the K_i/K_m ratio for AZT-TP with the mutant enzyme. This increase in the K_i/K_m ratio was similar to the change observed in the IC_{50} value obtained with an infectious clone of virus containing the T215Y mutation. Viral strains with reduced sensitivity to AZT have been isolated from patients after prolonged drug therapy. These isolates have a variety of mutations, which include T215Y. Although these isolates exhibit decreased sensitivity to AZT, this has not been well correlated with lack of clinical efficacy. Preliminary data suggest that the occurrence of viral isolates with reduced sensitivity to AZT is associated with a worse clinical outcome. However, switching to alternative anti-retroviral monotherapy has not been shown to be effective.

Spectrum of Activity

AZT is very effective in vitro against a variety of retroviruses, most notably the human immunodeficiency virus (HIV).[r17] It is inactive against HSV-1, HCMV, VZV, and vaccinia. Activity has been reported against Epstein-Barr virus, but the mechanism is not clear.

Pharmacokinetics

The pharmacokinetics of AZT have been studied after IV and oral administration. Dose-independent kinetics have been observed over the IV dosing range of 1 to 5 mg/kg and over the oral dosing range of 2 to 10 mg/kg. The drug is rapidly removed from plasma with a total body clearance of 1900 ml/min (27 ml/min/m^2) and half-life of about one hour. Metabolic conjugation to the 5′-O-glucuronide (3′-azido-3′-deoxy-5′-β-D-gluco-pyranosylthymidine; GAZT) is the major route of elimination. GAZT has no antiviral activity. Because the rate of metabolism is probably limited by hepatic blood flow, factors decreasing this flow will decrease AZT clearance. After oral administration about 14 percent is excreted unchanged and 75 percent is excreted as GAZT.

Oral doses of 200 mg every four hours produce peak and trough levels of 1.3 and 0.18 mg/ml, respectively. At the newly approved reduced dosage regimen of 100 mg every four hours, levels one-half these values are achieved. The oral bioavailability is 65 percent. It is less than 100 percent because of first-pass metabolism rather than incomplete absorption. AZT penetrates the blood brain barrier as indicated by a CSF/plasma ratio of 0.2 to 0.5, measured during continuous infusion or two to four hour post-single-dose. This is an important property for an antiretroviral drug if AIDS-related dementia is to be treated.

Clinical Use

Zidovudine is approved for therapy of adults infected with HIV-1 virus and whose immunity has declined as indicated by a CD4 lymphocyte count below 500/mm^3[48] and for the treatment of HIV-infected children over 3 months old with impaired immunity. AZT is also approved for the prevention of maternal-fetal transmission of HIV. In addition, AZT is indicated for use in combination with zalcitabine in HIV-infected adults with CD4 counts below 300/mm^3.

Adverse Reactions

Serious hematologic effects may occur, including neutropenia, leukopenia, and anemia (usually macrocytic). The marrow suppressive effects are dependent upon both dose and the patient's underlying marrow reserve. It is seen uncommonly (< 4%) in patients receiving 500–600 mg/m^2/day if therapy is begun before HIV has significantly damaged the marrow. Other effects may include; headache, insomnia, and myalgia. AZT shows some embryotoxicity in rats and rabbits, but no teratogenicity. Female mice and rats chronically receiving high doses of AZT have developed vaginal carcinomas. 3′-Amino-3′-deoxythymidine was detected in plasma of humans as a catabolite of AZT,[47a] and may be responsible for some of the adverse effects of AZT, since this amino-catabolite has been shown previously, to be cytotoxic in vitro[47b] and in vivo.[47c]

Contraindications

AZT is contraindicated in patients who have a severe (life-threatening) reaction to any component of the formulation.

Preparation and Dosage

Capsules containing 100 mg AZT are available for oral use. The recommended dose was formerly 200 mg orally every four hours. However, recent data suggest that the dose may be reduced without decrease in efficacy (100 mg every 4 hours). It is not yet known whether lower doses will be efficacious in HIV-associated neurologic disease. Intravenous and syrup formulations are also available (10 mg/ml) for use in adults and children. Syrup dosing of children with HIV disease should be 180 mg/m^2/dose to be given every six hours (720 mg/m^2/day). This regimen gives a drug exposure similar to adults dosed with 200 mg every four hours. The efficacy of lower doses in children is currently being studied.

For use in combination with zalcitabine, the recommended dose consists of 200 mg of AZT taken orally with 0.75 mg zalcitabine every 8 hours. For prevention of maternal-fetal transmission, HIV-infected pregnant women (after 14 weeks gestation) should be given AZT 100 mg orally every 4 hours (5 times a day) until the start of labor. During labor intravenous AZT should be given in bolus at 2 mg/kg (total body weight) followed by a continuous infusion of 1 mg/kg/hr until clamping of the umbilical cord. Their newborns should be given AZT 2 mg/kg orally every 6 hours, starting within 12 hours after birth and continuing through 6 weeks of age.

Zalcitabine

Chemistry

Zalcitabine (2′,3′-dideoxycytidine, ddC) is an analogue of deoxycytidine that contains a hydrogen on the 3′ carbon instead of a hydroxyl group. ddC is a white crystalline solid with a melting point of 215–217°C. Its solubility in water is 78 mg/ml.

Mechanism of Action

$$\text{ddC} \rightarrow \text{ddC-MP} \rightarrow \text{ddC-DP} \rightarrow \text{ddC-TP} \rightarrow \text{DNA}$$

Zalcitabine is converted to the corresponding 5′-mono, di, and triphosphate derivatives by the same enzymes that catalyze the phosphorylation of deoxycytidine to the corresponding 5′-triphosphate. As with AZT and ddI, ddCTP is an obligate chain terminator because of the absence of a 3′-hydroxyl on the sugar.[49] ddCTP is a very potent inhibitor of the HIV-1 reverse transcriptase. As with ddATP, the active metabolite of ddI, ddCTP is also a potent inhibitor of the mitochondrial DNA polymerase γ. Inhibition of this enzyme has been associated with peripheral neuropathy,[49a] as is also the case for ddI (didanosine). Virus with a Thr-69 to Asp mutation has been isolated from patients that have received prolonged ddC therapy.[50] This mutation confers resistance to ddC; but surprisingly this mutation does not confer resistance to ddI. Mutants resistant to ddI (Leu-74 to Val, see Didanosine) also show cross resistance to ddC.

Spectrum of Activity

Zalcitabine has demonstrated in vitro and in vivo activity against a variety of retroviruses including HIV-1. This drug also has some in vitro activity against hepatitis B virus.

Pharmacokinetics

The pharmacokinetics of ddC have been studied after IV and oral administration. Over a dose range of 0.03 to 0.5 mg/kg the kinetics of ddC were linear. The mean total body clearance was 227 ml/min/m^2 and did not change after six to 14 days of dosing. The plasma half-life was approximately 1.2 hour. No major metabolites have been identified in patient serum samples. Bioavailability, determined after oral dosing by plasma AUC, was 88 ± 17%. ddC penetrates the blood brain barrier. Two hours after infusion the CSF/plasma ratio for ddC was 0.14, which is threefold less than the CSF penetration of AZT in humans at the same time point.

Clinical Use

Zalcitabine has been approved by the FDA for use in conjunction with zidovudine (AZT), as a combination therapy for patients with advanced HIV disease (CD4 lymphocyte counts ≤ 300/mm^3) who have experienced clinical or immunologic deterioration.[51] It is also approved for use as monotherapy in the treatment of adults with advanced HIV disease who are intolerant of AZT or who have experienced disease progression while receiving AZT.

Adverse Reactions

The most important toxicity of ddC is peripheral sensorimotor neuropathy, which occurred in 17 to 31 percent of patients in the initial Phase II/III clinical trials. Pancreatitis occured in < 1% of patients and appears to be substantially less common with ddC therapy as compared to ddI therapy, although definitive direct comparative data in this regard is not yet available. Oral and esophageal ulcers have also been noted in patients receiving ddC as monotherapy. In patients receiving ddC+AZT combination therapy, the most common adverse events were GI complaints (nausea, oral ulcers, abdominal pain, diarrhea, vomiting, anorexia), pruritus and/or rash, headache, fatigue, and fever.

Contraindications

Zalcitabine is contraindicated in patients who have manifested clinically significant hypersensivity to ddC or any components of the formulation.

Preparation and Dosage

Zalcitabine is available as 0.375-mg and 0.750-mg tablets. The recommended combination treatment for adults (> 30 kg body weight) is concomitant oral administration of 0.75 mg of ddC and 200 mg of AZT, given every eight hours (total daily doses of 2.25 mg of ddC and 600 mg of AZT). The recommended dose for monotherapy is 0.75 mg orally every 8 hours. The safety and effectiveness of ddC for children (< 13 years of age) with HIV disease have not been established.

Didanosine

Chemistry

Didanosine (2′,3′-dideoxyinosine, ddI) is an analog of inosine that contains a hydrogen in the 2′ and 3′ positions instead of a hydroxyl group. Didanosine is a white solid with a melting point of 160–163° C. Its solubility in water is 27.3 mg/ml.

Mechanism of Action

Didanosine is converted to ddATP according to the following scheme:

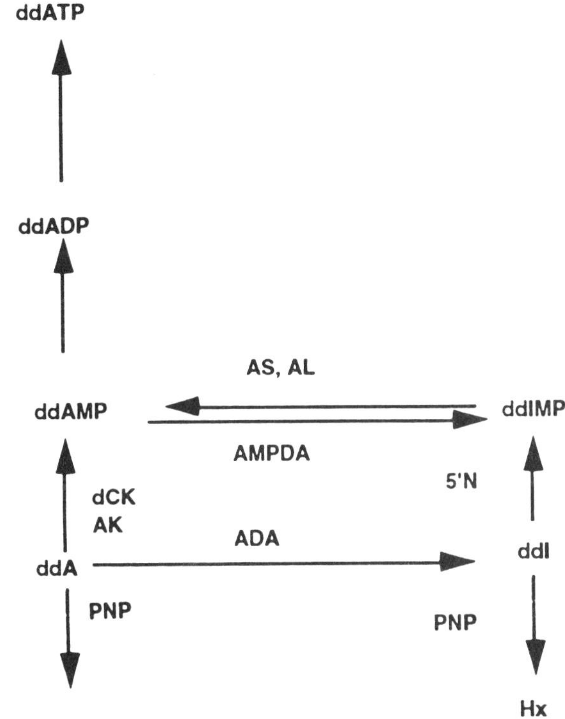

Metabolic pathways of ddI. ADA. Adenosine deaminase: AK. adenosine kinase: AMPDA. Adenylate deaminase: AL. adenylosuccinate lyase; AS, adenylosuccinate synthetase: dCK. deoxycytidine kinase: ddA. 2′,3′-dideoxyadenosine: ddADP. 2′,3′-dideoxyadenosine-5′-diphosphate: ddAMP. 2′,3′-dideoxyadenosine-5′-monophosphate: ddATP. 2′,3′-dideoxyadenosine-5′triphosphate: ddI. 2′,3′-dideoxyinosine: ddIMP. 2′,3′-dideoxyinosine-5′monophosphate. Hx. hypoxanthine: PNP. purine nucloside phosphorylase.

Didanosine is phosphorylated to the 5′-monophosphate, ddIMP, by the phosphotransferase activity associated with the ubiquitous cellular enzyme 5′-nucleotidase. ddIMP is aminated to ddAMP by the combined action of adenylosuccinate synthetase and adenylosuccinate lyase. Because ddAMP can be converted back to ddIMP, a cycle exists between these two metabolites. ddAMP is converted to ddATP, the intracellular metabolite of ddI believed to be responsible for inhibiting HIV-1 replication. ddATP, an analogue of dATP, has a much higher affinity for the reverse transcriptase of HIV-1 than does dATP itself. ddATP, like AZTTP, lacks a 3′-hydroxyl group and therefore when incorporated into newly synthesized DNA results in chain termination.[52]

ddATP has a higher affinity for HIV-1 RT than for cellular DNA-polymerase α. This difference between viral and cellular enzymes may account for the antiviral selectivity of ddI. Both ddATP and ddCTP are potent inhibitors of DNA polymerase γ. It has been suggested that the painful peripheral neuropathy associated with the prolonged use of certain dideoxynucleosides, including ddI and ddC, is caused by mitochondrial dysfunction following inhibition of the mitochondrial DNA polymerase γ.[52a]

Virus strains with reduced sensitivity to ddI have been isolated from patients after prolonged drug therapy.[53] The development of resistance to ddI corresponded to a change at amino acid residue 74 where a Leu to Val change occurred. In addition, the L74V mutation also confers resistance to ddC. This amino acid change also corresponds to a change in enzyme inhibition by ddATP.

Spectrum of Activity

Didanosine is effective in vitro and in vivo against a variety of retroviruses including the human immunodeficiency virus type 1. The drug also has some in vitro activity against hepatitis B virus, although it has been found to be clinically inactive in one study of patients with chronic hepatitis B.[54]

Pharmacokinetics

The pharmacokinetics of didanosine in humans are very similar to those for AZT. Following IV administration, the AUC and C_{max} values increased in a dose-proportional manner over the dosing range of 0.4 to 16.5 mg/kg. A serum half-life of 1.36 hours was observed. Total body clearance averaged 406 ml/min, indicating that secretion of didanosine occurs in the proximal renal tubules. Approximately 55 percent of the dose was recovered unchanged in the urine. Didanosine is an acid-labile drug, and therefore is administered orally in a buffered vehicle to protect it from gastric acid. Oral administration of doses that range from 0.8 to 10.2 mg/kg showed that the C_{max} and AUC are proportional to the dose. The over-all T_{max} was 0.77 hour, indicating that the drug is rapidly absorbed following oral dosing, and the $T_{1/2}$ was 1.43 hours. Oral bioavailability at these dose ranges was 43 percent. At doses ranging from 15.2 to 33 mg/kg the bioavailability decreased to an average of 24 percent. Food reduces the oral bioavailability of didanosine about twofold. The rates of absorption and elimination were not affected by food; however, the extent of absorption was reduced significantly in the presence of food. Therefore, it is recommended that didanosine be administered under fasting conditions. Didanosine penetrates the blood-brain barrier as indicated by a CSF/plasma ratio of 0.22 measured 60 minutes after completion of the IV infusion.

Clinical Use

The FDA has approved didanosine (ddI) for the treatment of adults with advanced HIV disease who have received prolonged previous zidovudine therapy.[r18] Didanosine has also been approved for the treatment of adults and children (> 6 months of age) with advanced HIV disease who are intolerant of zidovudine (AZT) or who have experienced significant clinical or immunologic deterioration during AZT therapy.

Didanosine is not recommended for the initial treatment of patients with HIV disease, because AZT therapy has previously been shown to prolong survival and decrease the incidence of opportunistic infections for previously untreated patients.

Adverse Reactions

The most important toxicities of ddI are pancreatitis and peripheral neuropathy. The pancreatitis can be severe or fatal. Pancreatitis occurred at an annualized rate of 13 percent in the higher-dose cohort and 7 percent in the lower-dose cohort in the Phase II/III controlled trial described above; and it occurred in 9 percent of patients in Phase I studies treated with dosing levels of ddI that were at or below the approved dosing regimen. Peripheral sensorimotor neuropathy was also common in these studies, occurring in 34 percent of patients. Liver failure occurred rarely (0.2 % of patients). Retinal depigmentation was noted in four pediatric patients. Other common adverse events were headache, diarrhea, insomnia, nausea/vomiting, rash and/or pruritus, abdominal pain, depression, constipation, stomatitis, myalgias, changes in taste sensation, dry mouth, alopecia, and dizziness.

Contraindications

Didanosine is contraindicated in patients with a history of hypersensivity to ddI or components of the formulation.

Preparation and Dosage

Didanosine is available in three formulations: chewable buffered tablets (25 mg, 50 mg, 100 mg, or 150 mg); buffered powder for oral solution, as single-dose packets (100 mg, 167 mg, 250 mg, 375 mg); and a pediatric powder for oral solution (2 g in 4 oz., or 4 g in 8 oz. after reconstitution). Didanosine absorption is reduced by as much as 50 percent in the presence of food; therefore, patients should take didanosine on an empty stomach. The recommended dose interval for ddI administration is 12 hours. The recommended doses for adults are adjusted according to body weight; those for children are adjusted according to body surface area. The presently recommended doses are given below:

ADULTS		
body weight	*tablet dose*	*buffered powder dose*
≥ 60 kg	200 mg bid	250 mg bid
< 60 kg	125 mg bid	167 mg bid
CHILDREN		
body surface area (m²)	*tablet dose*	*pediatric powder dose*
1.1–1.4	100 mg bid	125 mg bid
0.8–1.0	75 mg bid	94 mg bid
0.5–0.7	50 mg bid	62 mg bid
≤ 0.4	25 mg bid	31 mg bid

Because a number of clinical studies are presently ongoing, dosing recommendations may change in the future. Therefore, a current product label should be reviewed prior to administration of didanosine to patients.

Stavudine

Chemistry

Stavudine (d4T, ZERIT™, 3′-deoxy-2′,3′-didehydrothymidine, 3′-deoxythymidin-2′-ene) is an analogue of thymidine that has the 3′-hydroxyl and the 2′ and 3′-hydrogens removed, thereby forming a 2′, 3′-double bond. It is stable to heat, light, and high humidity, it is stable to acid at pH 1.2 (37°C), and is very soluble in water (90 mg/ml at 25°C).

Mechanism of Action

Stavudine, like thymidine, is converted by cellular enzymes to its mono-, di-, and triphosphate. The triphosphate of d4T is a preferential substrate for HIV-1 reverse transcriptase, rather than for cellular DNA-polymerase, and is terminally incorporated into the growing DNA chains. Hence, it is, like acyclovir-TP and AZT-TP, an obligate chain terminator because of the absence of a 3′-hydroxyl on the sugar moiety.[55] In contrast to AZT metabolism, the monophosphate of d4T does not accumulate, but rather d4T-TP is the major metabolite.[56,57]

Spectrum of Activity

Stavudine is a very effective inhibitor of the replication of HIV-1 in vitro. Cross resistance to viral strains with reduced sensitivity to AZT generally does not occur, but has been observed with a few strains of HIV-1 resistant to AZT.[58,59]

Pharmacokinetics

Preclinical studies in rats indicate that d4T is rapidly and well absorbed with a T_{max} of ≤ 1 hr and a $T_{1/2}$ of ≤ 1 hr. More than 90 per cent is bioavailable when dosed orally, and it is distributed in total body water as well as the CNS and placenta. Stavudine, in contrast to AZT is neither glucuronidated nor bound to serum proteins.

Clinical pharmacokinetic studies in patients with AIDS or ARC found d4T to be rapidly absorbed after oral administration, with a 90 percent bioavailability. Upon IV administration a $T_{1/2}$ of one hour, a clearance of 536 ml/min, and a volume of distribution of 50 L was observed. Renal clearance includes active tubular secretion of d4T. This drug also penetrates the blood brain barrier.[62]

Clinical Use

Stavudine was approved by the FDA in 1992 under the Parallel Track Program, which was established in 1992 to permit rapid access to experimental drugs that have not completed their clinical trials but show great promise. AIDS patients on d4T have shown a sustained decrease in P24 antigen and increases in $CD4^+$ cells, weight, and general well-being. Based on the results of controlled clinical trials the FDA in 1994 gave clearance to market stavudine. The phase 3 trial of d4T vs. continued AZT in HIV-infected adults will terminate in December 1994, and it will provide a complete evaluation of clinical end points.

At present d4T is indicated for the treatment of adults with advanced HIV infection who are intolerant to approved therapies with proven clinical benefit, or who have experienced significant clinical or immunologic deterioration while receiving these therapies, or for whom such therapies are contrindicated.

Adverse Reactions

Studies of d4T in AIDS patients indicated that it is well tolerated in doses below 2 mg/kg/day, but at 2 mg/kg/day or higher peripheral neuropathy and an increase in transaminase may occur following prolonged therapy.

Contraindications

Stavudine is contraindicated in patients who have a severe or life-threatening reaction to any component of the formulation.

Preparation and Doses

Stavudine (d4T) is well tolerated at doses below 2.0 mg/kg/day in adult patients, and antiviral activity has been observed at doses as low as 0.1 mg/kg/day. The interval between oral doses should be 12 hours. C_{max} was decreased by approximately 45% when stavudine was administered with food; however, the systemic availability (AUC) was unchanged. Thus, it appears that ZERIT™ may be taken without regard to meals. The recommended starting dose based on body weight is as follows:

40 mg twice daily for patients ≥ 60 kg.
30 mg twice daily for patients < 60 kg.

The recommended dose for pediatric patients is approximately twice that of adult patients, as systemic exposure in pediatrics is half that of adults due to a more rapid elimination.

Interferon

Chemistry

Interferon consists of a family of polypeptides classified by the predominant cell of origin and induced by various substances, including viruses, double-stranded RNA, and various synthetic polymers.[r20,63] Human leukocyte interferon α (IFN-α) and human fibroblast interferon (IFN-β) are stable at pH 2. Immune interferon (IFN-γ) is acid-labile.

Mechanism of Action

The basis for the antiviral activity of IFN is not clearly understood. The site of inhibition may depend on the specific virus and/or host cell involved.[r21] The antiviral state is initiated by the binding of interferon to a specific receptor on the cell surface. Synthesis of viral proteins may be prevented by one or both of the following interferon-induced events: (a) Induction of 2′,5′-adenylate synthetase, which converts ATP to a 2′,5′-polyadenylate, an activator of a latent endonuclease that hydrolyzes viral mRNA. (b) Induction of a protein kinase that phosphorylates an inactive initiation factor (eIF-2), which then inhibits initiation of peptide chain synthesis. (c) Inhibition of viral adsorption, penetration, uncoating, assembly, and release have also been implicated.

Spectrum of Activity

Interferon does not produce a direct inhibition of viral replication, but rather induces an antiviral state.[r22] The antiviral action of interferon is very extensive, and a wide spectrum of RNA and DNA viruses are inhibited. However, there is variation in susceptibility to inhibition by different viruses as well as among different strains of the same virus.

Pharmacokinetics

Orally or topically administered interferon is not absorbed. Intravenous administration of interferon, as with many other agents, has a biphasic disappearance from plasma. There is an initial rapid rate (α) with a $t_{1/2}$ of about 15 minutes., followed by a slower rate (β) of disappearance with a $t_{1/2}$ of one to three hour. Less than 1/30th of the administered dose enters the CSF.

Clinical Use

Various interferon preparations have been investigated for the treatment of a wide variety of virus infections.[r21] Although beneficial results have been obtained in some applications, interferons are clearly not therapeutic panaceas, as was initially hoped.

Currently, the recognized clinical uses of α-interferons include treatment of hairy-cell leukemia, Kaposi's sarcoma in patients with AIDS, chronic hepatitis due to the hepatitis B or C viruses, genital warts caused by papillomaviruses (condylomata acuminata), and juvenile laryngeal papillomatosis. Optimal therapeutic regimens for several of these clinical indications are presently still under investigation.

There are a number of other antiviral applications of interferon therapy for which benefits are less well-established.[r19] For example, topical administration of interferon in the therapy of herpetic keratitis has reduced the acute symptoms; however, other drugs are more effective. Parenterally administered interferon has produced encouraging results in treatment of herpes zoster in immunocompromised cancer patients, as well as in patients infected with hepatitis, cytomegalovirus, or rubella who experienced a decrease in virus excretion. The clinical benefits in the latter uses are as yet incompletely studied. Interferon administered by nasal spray may prevent and decrease the symptoms of the common cold in individuals who were inoculated intranasally with the rhinovirus, but unfortunately this caused an unacceptable accummulation of submucosal lymphocytes. Both recombinant and natural human α-interferons have been studied extensively in the above clinical settings, and three α-interferon preparations are commercially available. A recombinantly-produced human gamma interferon recently was approved for treatment of chronic granulomatous disease. There are as yet no approved antiviral indications for beta-interferon products.[r23]

Toxicity

Systemic administration of α-interferons may produce fever, a flu-like syndrome (fever, headache, myalgias), bone marrow depression, GI symptoms, weight loss, alopecia, increased TSH levels, and autoimmune thyroid disease. Nosebleeds are produced by nasal administration.

Preparation and Dosage

Three preparations of human α-interferons are commercially available in the US and/or Europe. Interferon alpha-2B (Intron A, Schering) and interferon alpha-2A (Roferon-A, Hoffman LaRoche) are recombinantly-produced human α-interferons that differ by a single amino acid. Interferon alpha n1 (WELLFERON, Burroughs Wellcome) is a combination of human α-interferons produced by human lymphoblastoid cells induced to interferon production by a murine parainfluenza virus (Sandai virus). Comparative studies are generally lacking for the various clinical uses of α-interferons. In clinical trials for therapy of condylomata acuminata (genital warts), interferon alpha (Intron A) was injected intralesionally three times a week for up to three weeks. Other regimens also can be used, and prolonged or intermittent treatment is sometimes necessary.

For systemic therapy, α-interferons have been administered IM or SQ in daily doses of 1–54 million units or more. Specific treatment regimens vary widely among the different clinical applications of α-interferon therapy. For most applications, optimal dosing regimens and duration of therapy are still under investigation.

References

Research Reports

1. Crumpacker CS 2d. Molecular targets of antiviral therapy. N Engl J Med 1989;*321*:163–172.

2. Georgiev VS, McGowan JJ. Acquired immune deficiency syndrome (AIDS): Anti HIV Agents, Therapies and Vaccines. Ann NY Acad Sciences 1990;*616*:1–634.

3. Arnold E, Arnold GF. Human immunodeficiency virus structure: Implications for antiviral design. Adv Virus Res 1991;*39*:1–87.

4. Keating MR. Antiviral Agents. Mayo Clin Proc 1992;*67*:160–178.

5. Mitsuya H, Yarchoan R, Kageyama S, Broder S. Targeted therapy of human immunodeficiency virus-related diseases. FASEB J 1991;*5*:2369–2381.

6. Prusoff WH, Lin T-S, August EM, Wood TG, Marongiu ME. Approaches to antiviral drug development. Yale J Biol Med 1989;*62*:215–225.

7. Meijer DK, Jansen RW, Molema G. Drug targeting systems for antiviral agents: options and limitations. Antiviral Res 1992;*18*:215–258.

7a. Prusoff WH, Lin T-S, Pivazyan A, Sun AS, Birks E. Empirical and rational approaches for development of inhibitors of the human immunodeficiency virus—HIV. Pharmac Ther 1992;*60*:315–329.

8. Rossmann MG, McKinlay MA. Application of crystallography to the design of antiviral agents. Infect Agents Dis 1992;*1*:3–10.

8a. Kuntz ID. Structure-Based Strategies for Drug Design and Discovery Science 1992;*257*:1078–1082.

9. Nasr M, Litterst C, McGowan J. Computer-assisted structure-activity correlations of dideoxynucleoside analogs as potential anti-HIV drugs. Antiviral Res 1990;*14*:125–148.

9a. Milligan JF, Matteuci MD, Martin JC. Current Concepts in Antisense Drug Design J Med Chem 1993;*36*:1923–1937.

10. Prusoff WH. Synthesis and biological activities of iododeoxyuridine, an analog of thymidine. Biochim Biophys Acta 1959;*32*:295–296.

11. Kaufman HE. Clinical cure of herpes simplex keratitis by 5-iodo-2′-deoxyuridine. Proc Soc Exp Biol Med 1962;*109*:251–252.

12. Perkins ES, Wood RM, Sears ML, Prusoff WH, Welch AD. Antiviral activities of several iodinated pyrimidine deoxyribonucleosides. Nature 1962;*194*:985–986.

13. Burns RP. A double-blind study of IDU in human herpes simplex keratitis. Arch Ophthalmol 1963;*70*:381–384.

14. MacCallum FO, Juel-Jensen BE. Herpes simplex virus skin infection in man treated with idoxuridine in dimethyl sulfoxide.

Results of a double-blind controlled trial. Br Med J 1966;*2*:805–807.

15. Prusoff WH, Bakhle YS, McCrea JF. Incorporation of 5-iodo-2′-deoxyuridine into the deoxyribonucleic acid of vaccinia virus. Nature 1963;*199*:1310–1311.
16. Goz B, Prusoff WH. The relation of antiviral activity of IUdR to gene function in phage. Ann NY Acad Sci 1970;*173*:379–389.
17. Fischer PH, Chen MS and Prusoff WH. The incorporation of 5-Iodo-5′-amino-2′,5′-dideoxyuridine and 5-iodo-2′-deoxyuridine into herpes simplex virus DNA: relationship between antiviral activity and effects on DNA structure. Biochim Biophys Acta 1980;*606*:236–245.
18. Spruance SL, Stewart JC, Freeman DJ, Brightman VJ, Cox JL, Wenerstrom G, McKeough MB, Rowe NH. Early application of topical 15% idoxuridine in dimethyl sulfoxide shortens the course of herpes simplex labialis: a multicenter placebo-controlled trial. J Infect Dis 1990;*161*:191–197.
19. Kaufman HE, Heidelberger C. Therapeutic antiviral action of 5-trifluoromethyl-2′-deoxyuridine in herpes simplex keratitis. Science 1964;*145*:585–586.
20. Pavan-Langston D, Lass J, Campbell R. Antiviral drops: comparative therapy of experimental herpes simplex keratouveitis. Arch Ophthalmol 1979;*97*:1132–1135.
21. Tone H, Heidelberger C. Fluorinated pyrimidines. XLIV. Interaction of 5-trifluoromethyl-2′-deoxyuridine 5′-triphosphate with deoxyribonucleic acid polymerases. Mol Pharmacol 1973;*9*:783–791.
22. Schabel FM Jr. The antiviral activity of 9-β-D-arabinofuranosyladenine (ara-A). Chemotherapy 1968;*13*:321–338.
23. Muller WE, Rohde HJ, Beyer R, Maidhof A, Lachmann M, Taschner H, Zahn RK. Mode of action of 9-beta-D-arabinofuranosyladenine on the synthesis of DNA, RNA, and protein in vivo and in vitro. Cancer Res 1975;*35*:2160–2168.
24. Pelling JC, Drach JC, Shipman C Jr. Internucleotide incorporation of arabinosyladenine into herpes simplex virus and mammalian cell DNA. Virology 1981;*109*:323–335.
25. Derse D, Cheng Y-C. Herpes simplex virus type I DNA polymerase. Kinetic properties of the associated 3′-5′-exonuclease activity and its role in araAMP incorporation. J Biol Chem 1981;*256*:8525–8530.
26. Ohno Y, Spriggs D, Matsukage A, Ohno T, Kufe D. Sequence-specific inhibition of DNA strand elongation by incorporation of 9-β-D-arabinofuranosyladenine. Cancer Res 1989;*49*:2077–2081.
27. Coen DM, Furman PA, Gelep PT, Schaffer PA. Mutations in the herpes simplex virus DNA polymerase gene can confer resistance to 9-β-D-arabinofuranosyladenine. J Virol 1982;*41*:909–918.
28. Whitley RJ, Nahmias AJ, Soong SJ, Galasso GG, Fleming CL, Alford CA. Vidarabine therapy of neonatal herpes simplex virus infection. Pediatrics 1980;*66*:495–501.
29. Whitley R, Arvin A, Prober C, Burchett S, Corey L, Powell D, Plotkin S, Starr S, Alford C, Connor J, Jacobs R, Nahmias A, Soong S-J, The National Institute of Allergy and Infectious Diseases Collaborative Antiviral Study Group. A controlled trial comparing vidarabine with acyclovir in neonatal herpes simplex virus infection. N Engl J Med 1991;*324*:444–449.
30. Schaeffer HJ, Beauchamp L, de Miranda P, Elion GB, Bauer DJ, Collins P. 9-(2-Hydroxyethoxymethyl) guanine activity against viruses of the herpes group. Nature 1978;*272*:583–585.
31. Elion GB, Furman PA, Fyfe JA, de Miranda P, Beauchamp L, Schaeffer HJ. Selectivity of action of an antiherpetic agent, 9-(2-hydroxymethoxymethyl)guanine. Proc Natl Acad Sci USA 1977;*74*:5716–5720.
32. Reardon JE, Spector T. Herpes simplex virus type 1 DNA polymerase. Mechanism of inhibition by acyclovir triphosphate. J Biol Chem 1989;*264*:7405–7411.
33. Field AK, Davies ME, DeWitt C, Perry HC, Liou R, Germershausen J, Karkas JD, Ashton WT, Johnston DB, Tolman RL. 9-(2-Hydroxyl-1-(hydroxymethyl)ethoxymethyl)guanine: a selective inhibitor of herpes group virus replication. Proc Natl Acad Sci USA 1983;*80*:4139–4143.
34. Ashton WT, Karkas JD, Field AK, Tolman RL. Activation by thymidine kinase and potent antiherpetic activity of 2′-nor-2′-deoxyguanosine (2′NDG). Biochem Biophys Res Commun 1982;*108*:1716–1721.
35. Tocci MJ, Livelli TJ, Perry HC, Crumpacker CS, Field AK. Effects of the nucleoside analog 2′-nor-2′-deoxyguanosine on human cytomegalovirus replication. Antimicrob Agents Chemother 1984;*25*:247–252.
36. Biron KK, Stanat SC, Sorrell JB, Fyfe JA, Keller PM, Lambe CU, Nelson DJ. Metabolic activation of the nucleoside analog 9-[(2-hydroxy-1-(hydroxymethyl)ethoxy)methyl]guanine in human diploid fibroblasts infected with human cytomegalovirus. Proc Natl Acad Sci USA 1985;*82*:2473–2477.
37. Henry K, Cantrill H, Fletcher C, Chinnock BJ, Balfour HH Jr. Use of intravitreal ganciclovir (dihydroxy propoxymethyl guanine) for cytomegalovirus retinitis in a patient with AIDS. Am J Ophthalmol 1987;*103*:17–23.
38. Helgstrand E, Eriksson B, Johansson NG, Lannero B, Larsson A, Misiorny A, Noren JO, Sjoberg B, Stenberg K, Stening G, Stridh S, Oberg B, Alenius S, Philpson L. Trisodium phosphonoformate, a new antiviral compound. Science 1978;*201*:819–821.
39. Wahren B, Oberg B. Reversible inhibition of cytomegalovirus replication by phosphonoformate. Intervirology 1980;*14*:7–15.
40. Cheng Y-C, Grill S, Derse D, Chen J-Y, Caradonna SJ, Connor K. Mode of action of phosphonoformate as an anti-herpes simplex virus agent. Biochim Biophys Acta 1981;*652*:90–98.
41. Oberg B. Antiviral effects of phosphonoformate (PFA, foscarnet sodium). Pharmacol Ther 1989;*40*:213–285.
42. Jacobson MA, O'Donnell JJ, Mills J. Foscarnet treatment of cytomegalovirus retinitis in patients with the acquired immunodeficiency syndrome. Antimicrob Agents Chemother 1989;*33*:736–741.
43. Aweeka F, Gambertoglio J, Mills J, Jacobson MA. Pharmacokinetics of intermittently administered intravenous foscarnet in the treatment of acquired immunodeficiency syndrome patients with serious cytomegalovirus retinitis. Antimicrob Agents Chemother 1989;*33*:742–745.
44. Sullivan V, Coen DM. Isolation of foscarnet-resistant human cytomegalovirus patterns of resistance and sensitivity to other antiviral drugs. J Infect Dis 1991;*164*:781–784.
45. Gilbert BE, Knight V. Biochemistry and clinical applications of ribavirin. Antimicrob Agents Chemother 1986;*30*:201–205.
46. Mitsuya H, Weinhold K, Furman PA, St Clair MH, Lehrman SN, Gallo RC, Bolognesi D, Barry DW, Broder S. 3′-Azido-3′-deoxythymidine (BW A509U): an antiviral agent that inhibits the infectivity and cytopathic effect of human T-lymphotropic virus type III/lymphadenopathy-associated virus in vitro. Proc Natl Acad Sci USA 1985;*82*:7096–7100.

47. Furman PA, Fyfe JA, St. Clair MH, Weinhold K, Rideout JL, Freeman GA, Lehrman SN, Bolognesi DP, Broder S, Mitsuya H. Phosphorylation of 3′-azido-3′-deoxythymidine and selective interaction of the 5′-triphosphate with human immunodeficiency virus reverse transcriptase. Proc Natl Acad Sci USA 1986;*83*:8333–8337.

47a. Stagg MP, Cretton EM, Kidd L, Diasio RB, Sommadossi J-P, Clinical pharmacokinetics of 3′-azido-3′-deoxythymidine (zidovudine) and catabolites with formation of a toxic catabolite, 3′-amino-3′-deoxythymidine. Clin Pharmacol Ther 1992; *51*:668–676.

47b. Lin TS, Prusoff, WH. Synthesis and Biological Activity of Several Amino Analogs of Thymidine. J Med Chem 1978;*21*:109–112.

47c. Lin TS, Fischer PH, Prusoff WH. Effect of 3′-Amino-3′-deoxythymidine on L1210 and P388 Leukemias in Mice. Biochem Pharmacol 1982;*31*:125–128.

48. Larder BA, Kemp SD. Multiple mutations in HIV-1 reverse transcriptase confer high-level resistance to zidovudine (AZT). Science 1989;*246*:1155–1158.

49. Klecker RW Jr, Collins JM, Yarchoan RC, Thomas R, McAtee N, Broder S, Myers CE. Pharmacokinetics of 2′,3′-dideoxycytidine in patients with AIDS and related disorders. J Clin Pharmacol 1988;*28*:837–842.

49a. Chen C-H, Cheng Y-C. Delayed Cytotoxicity and Selective Loss of Mitochondrial DNA in Cells Treated with the Anti-human Immunodeficiency Virus Compound 2′,3′-Dideoxycytidine. J Biol Chem 1989;*264*:11934–11937.

50. Fitzgibbon JE, Howell RM, Haberzettl CA, Sperber SJ, Gocke DL, Dubin DT. Human immunodeficiency virus type 1 pol gene mutations which cause decreased susceptibility to 2′,3′-dideoxycytidine. Antimicrob Agents Chemother 1992;*36*:153–157.

51. Meng T-C, Fischl MA, Boota AM, Spector SA, Bennett D, Bassiakos Y, Lai SH, Wright B, Richman DD. Combination therapy with zidovudine and dideoxycytidine in patients with advanced human immunodeficiency virus infection: a phase I/II study. Ann Intern Med 1992;*116*:13–20.

52. Mitsuya H, Broder S. Inhibition of the in vitro infectivity and cytopathic effect of human T-lymphotropic virus type III/lymphadenopathy-associated virus (HTLV-III/LAV) by 2′,3′-dideoxynucleosides. Proc Natl Acad Sci USA 1986;*83*:1911–1915.

52a. Medina D, Tsai C-H, Hsiung GD, Cheng, Y-C. Comparison of mitochondrial morphology, mitochondrial DNA content, and cell visibility in cultured cells treated with three anti-human immunodeficiency virus dideoxynucleosides. Antimicro Agents Chemother 1994;*38*,1824–1828.

53. Yarchoan R, Mitsuya H, Thomas RV, Pluda JM, Hartman NR, Perno CF, Marczyk KS, Allain JP, Johns DG, Broder S. In vivo activity against HIV and favorable toxicity profile of 2′,3′-dideoxyinosine. Science 1989;*245*:412–415.

54. Kahn JO, Lagakos SW, Richman DD, Cross A, Pettinelli C, Liou SH, Brown M, Volberding PA, Crumpacker CS, Beall G. A controlled trial comparing continued zidovudine with didanosine in human immunodeficiency virus infection. New Engl J Med 1992;*327*:581–587.

55. Lin T-S, Schinazi RF, Prusoff WH. Potent and selective in vitro activity of 3′-deoxythymidin-2′-ene (3′-deoxy-2′,3′-didehydrothymidine) against human immunodeficiency virus. Biochem Pharmacol 1987;*36*:2713–2718.

56. Baba M, Pauwels R, Herdewijn P, De Clercq E, Desmyter J, Vandeputte M. Both 2′,3′-dideoxythymidine and its 2′,3′-unsaturated derivative (2′,3′-dideoxythymidinene) are potent and selective inhibitors of human immunodeficiency virus replication in vitro. Biochem Biophys Res Commun 1987;*142*:128–134.

57. Hamamoto Y, Nakashima H, Matsui T, Matsuda A, Ueda T, Yamamoto N. Inhibitory effect of 2′,3′-didehydro-2′,3′-dideoxynucleosides on infectivity, cytopathic effects, and replication of human immunodeficiency virus. Antimicrob Agents Chemother 1987;*31*:907–910.

58. Balzarini J, Kang G-J, Dalal M, Herdewijn P, De Clercq E, Broder S, Johns DG. The anti-HTLV-III (anti-HIV) and cytotoxic activity of 2′,3′-didehydro-2′,3′-dideoxyribonucleosides: a comparison with their parental 2′,3′-dideoxyribonucleosides. Mol Pharmacol 1987;*32*:162–167.

59. Balzarini J, Herdewijn P, De Clercq E. Differential patterns of intracellular metabolism of 2′,3′-didehydro-2′,3′-dideoxythymidine and 3′-azido-2′,3-diseoxythymidine, two potent anti-human immunodeficiency virus compounds. J Biol Chem 1989;*264*:6127–6133.

60. Ho H-T, Hitchcock MJ. Cellular pharmacology of 2′,3′-dideoxy-2′,3′-didehydrothymidine, a nucleoside analog active against human immunodeficiency virus. Antimicrob Agents Chemother 1989;*33*:844–849.

61. Huang P, Farquhar D, Plunkett W. Selective action of 1′,3′-didehydro-2′,3′-dideoxythymidine triphosphate on human immunodeficiency virus reverse transcriptase and human DNA polymerases. J Biol Chem 1992;*267*:2817–2822.

62. Zhu Z, Hitchcock MJ, Sommadossi JP. Metabolism and DNA interaction of 2′,3′-didehydro-2′,3′-dideoxythymidine in human bone marrow cells. Mol Pharmacol 1991;*40*:838–845.

63. Samuel CE. Antiviral actions of interferon: interferon-regulated cellular proteins and their surprisingly selective antiviral activities. Virology 1991;*183*:1–11.

Reviews

r1. DeClercq E, ed. Design of anti-AIDS drugs. New York: Elsevier, (1990).

r2. Richman DD. Antiviral Therapy of HIV Infection. Annu Rev Med 1991;*42*:69–90.

r3. Cheng Y-C, Prusoff WH. Antiviral Chemotherapy. In: Verderame M, ed. CRC Handbook of Chemotherapeutic Agents. Vol. II. Boca Raton, FL: CRC Press (1986); pp 297–338.

r4. Fischer PH, Prusoff WH. Chemotherapy of ocularviral infections and tumors. In: Sears ML, ed. Pharmacology of the eye. Heidelberg: Springer-Verlag, (1984); pp 553–583.

r5. Schinazi RF. Combined chemotherapeutic modalities for viral infections: Rationale and clinical potential. In: Chou T-C, Rideout D, eds. Synergism and antagonism in chemotherapy. San Diego: Academic Press, (1991); pp 109–181.

r6. Prusoff WH, Lin T-S. Experimental aspects of antiviral pharmacology. In: DeClercq E, Walker RT, eds. Antiviral drug development. New York: Plenum Press, (1988); pp 173–202.

r7. Oxford JS, Galbraith A. Antiviral activity of amantadine: a review of laboratory and clinical data. Pharmacol Ther 1980;*11*:181–262.

r8. Prusoff WH. A review of some aspects of 5-iododeoxyuridine and azauridine. Cancer Res 1963;*23*:1246–1259.

r9. Prusoff WH, Goz B. Halogenated pyrimidine deoxyribonucleosides, In: Sartorelli A, Johns D, eds. Antineoplastic and Immunosuppressive agents II. New York: Springer-Verlag, (1975); pp 172–347.

r10. Kaufman HE, Rayfield MA. Viral conjunctivitis and keratitis. In: Kaufman HE, Baron BA, McDonald MD, Waltman SR, eds. The cornea. New York: Churchill Livingston, (1988); pp 299–331.

r11. Carmine AA, Brogden RN, Heel RC, Speight TM, Avery GS. Trifluridine: a review of its antiviral activity and therapeutic use in the topical treatment of viral eye infections. Drugs 1982;*23*:329–353.

r12. Baker DA. Acyclovir therapy for herpesvirus infections. New York: Marcel Dekker, 1990.

r13. Verheyden JP. Evolution of therapy for cytomegalovirus infection. Rev Infect Dis 1988;*10*:S477–489.

r14. Med Lett Drugs Ther. Foscarnet 1992;*34*:3–4.

r15. McKinlay MA, Otto MJ. Recent developments in antiviral chemotherapy. Infect Dis Clin North Am 1987;*1*:479–493.

r16. Crowe S, Mills J. The future of antiviral chemotherapy. Dermatol Clin 1988;*6*:521–537.

r17. Furman PA, Barry DW. Spectrum of antiviral activity and mechanism of action of zidovudine: an overview. Am J Med 1988;*85*:176–181.

r18. McLaren C, Datema R, Knupp CA, Buroker RA. Review: Didanosine. Antiviral Chem Chemother 1991;*2*:321–328.

r19. Interferon for chronic viral hepatitis. Med Lett Drugs Ther 1990;*32*:1–2.

r20. Sen GC, Lengyel P. The interferon system: a bird's eye view of its biochemistry. J Biol Chem 1992;*267*:5017–5020.

r21. Taylor JL, Gossberg SE. Recent progress in interferon research: molecular mechanisms of regulation, action and virus circumvention. Virus Res 1990;*15*:1–25.

r22. Staeheli P. Interferon-induced proteins and the antiviral state. Adv Virus Res 1990;*38*:147–200.

r23. Baron S, Coopenhaver DH, Dianzani F, Fleischmann WR Jr, Hughs TK, Jr, Klimpel GR, Nusel DW, Stanton GJ, Tyring SK eds. Interferon. Principles and medical applications. 1st ed. Galveston TX: University of Texas Medical Branch at Galveston, 1992.

CHAPTER 100

S. Gaylen Bradley
Francine Marciano-Cabral

Antiparasitic Drugs

Overview

The parasites that have medical significance for humans are a heterogeneous group living in or on the body. These include the protozoa or one-celled animals, the helminths or worms, and the arthropods or mites, insects, and their allies. Most of the protozoan and helminthic parasites are endoparasites—infectious agents that live within the body of the host. Most arthropod parasites infest the body surface, although some insect larvae live under the skin or in the GI tract. Parasitic diseases are often spoken of as "tropical diseases" or "exotic infections," an emphasis that belies the prevalence of parasitic disease in the US and other temperate countries. Many parasitic agents have complex life cycles, requiring several alternative hosts and vectors to facilitate transmission from one host to another.[r1] Public health control of parasitic infections relies heavily on measures to eliminate vectors and to reduce the reservoirs of parasites in alternative hosts. Chemicals used to control vectors will not be discussed in this chapter. Because parasites are animals with metabolic processes similar to humans, most chemotherapeutic drugs for endoparasites are quite toxic.

Protozoa are microscopic single-celled animals comparable in function to multicellular animals. Protozoan parasites are classified in two ways: according to their biological relationships to each other; and according to the area of the body they invade. According to the biologic classification, the protozoa are divided into the amebae or Sarcodina, the flagellates or Mastigophora, the ciliates or Ciliata, and the sporozoa. According to the pathogenesis classification, protozoa are identified as intestinal, oral, urogenital, blood, or tissue parasites. Protozoan parasites infect millions of people; for example, over 150 million cases of trichomonal vaginitis are reported annually. Approximately 10 percent of the world population is infected with parasitic amebae.

The life cycles of the intestinal, oral, and urogenital protozoa are, in general, quite simple. They multiply by asexual division and many produce a resistant cyst stage. Intestinal protozoa are transmitted primarily by ingestion of contaminated food and water, oral protozoa by droplet contamination, and urogenital protozoa by sexual intercourse. The life cycles and epidemiology of blood parasites are complex, involving arthropod vectors and reservoir hosts. The sporozoa are the most complex protozoan parasites with both sexual and asexual reproduction. Parasitologists refer to the host in which sexual reproduction occurs as the "definitive" or "final" host, and the host where asexual reproduction occurs as the "intermediate" host. Humans serve as the intermediate host for some protozoan parasites and as the definitive host for others.[r2]

Control of Parasitic Diseases

Many parasitic diseases have complex life cycles that involve alternative hosts and vectors. Many of the efforts to control parasitic diseases have focused on reducing the population of alternative hosts and vectors: for example, attempts to eradicate the alternative snail host as a means to control trematode infections in humans, and to eradicate the mosquito vector *Anopheles* to control malaria worldwide. One of the unique features of the semisynthetic antibiotic ivermectin is that it affects the insect vector as well as the parasitic tissue roundworms. Other public measures include avoiding the vectors by keeping away from endemic areas, and by reducing exposure in endemic areas by use of mosquito netting and staying indoors at night to avoid nocturnal vectors. Many parasitic infections have become significant clinical problems in immunocompromised patients, especially transplant patients and individuals with AIDS.[r3] Restoration of immune competence is the key to controlling opportunistic parasitic infections.

The intestinal parasites live outside the body *per se*, and drugs that are not absorbed are preferred to control them. The varied patterns of pathophysiology of parasitic infections afford pharmacologists and medicinal chemists unique opportunities to design and develop drugs targeted to a particular parasite or host site. Pyrimidine derivatives and dihydrofolate reductase inhibitors, for example, usually are given to treat protozoan infections. The nonabsorbed pyrimidine derivative, pyrantel pamoate, however, remains in the intestinal lumen, where it is an effective anthelmintic drug. A well-nourished person can carry a heavy burden of intestinal parasites without obvious adverse consequences, but these same parasites may represent life-threatening infections in malnourished people. Reinfection is a major problem in controlling intestinal parasites. Personal and community sanitation provide the key to controlling many parasitic infections: clean water supply and an effective sewage system. Thus, it is not unexpected that intestinal parasites are rampant in underdeveloped communities, areas that have experienced a natural disaster, and war-torn countries where the population is undernourished, clean water is not available, and human excrement accumulates in living areas. Chemotherapy alone will not bring parasitic diseases under control worldwide.[r4]

During the last half of the 20th century, a number of effective antiparasitic drugs (Table 100.1) have been developed: chloroquine congeners; praziquantel; albendazole; and ivermectin.[r5] The parasite burden in many infected people is very high, however, and the sudden destruction of a tissue or blood parasite by effective chemotherapy may precipitate a life-threatening immune response (Jarisch-Herxheimer reaction). It is necessary, therefore, to control allergic reactions with anti-inflammatory drugs concurrent with antiparasitic therapy. In fact, the characteristic symptoms of several parasitic infections reflect adverse immunologic reactions, and anti-inflammatory therapy alone may be viewed as satisfactory clinical management of the disease. Many antiparasitic drugs are specific for certain developmental stages, which may confer selectivity on a drug but also limit its usefulness. A number of antimalarial drugs, for example, act only on the erythrocytic stage of the life cycle of *Plasmodium*, and this limits their effectiveness. In addition, drug resistance has emerged as a serious problem in the control of parasitic diseases, especially malaria.

Parasitic Protozoa

Intestinal Amebiasis

Intestinal amebiasis is a disease of the large intestine caused by *Entamoeba histolytica*, the only real pathogen among the intestinal amebae.[r6] Patients with amebic dysentery experience acute abdominal pain and pass numerous loose stools containing blood. The amebae may invade the bloodstream and spread to the liver and other extraintestinal sites. It is estimated that nearly 500 million people carry *Entamoeba histolytica* in their intestinal tracts; of these, 10 percent develop invasive disease, with up to 100,000 deaths annually.

Amebic Encephalitis and Keratitis

Infections with *Acanthamoeba* may result in a wide spectrum of diseases. Granulomatous amebic encephalitis is a disease usually seen in debilitated and chronically ill individuals and those undergoing immunosuppressive therapy. Granulomatous amebic encephalitis is a subacute or chronic infection of the brain, characterized by necrosis of CNS tissues with chronic inflammation and granulomatous reactions. *Acanthamoeba* keratitis is a rare but serious infection of the cornea in otherwise healthy individuals; it develops after trauma associated with contaminated water or wearing contact lenses.[1]

Giardiasis

Giardia lambia causes an infection of the small intestine seen more frequently in children than in adults. Symptoms of giardiasis include abdominal pain and diarrhea. The stools are often mucous and malodorous.

Trichomoniasis

Trichomonas vaginalis is commonly found in the urogenital tract. Symptoms include a vaginal discharge accompanied by burning and itching. The vaginal mucosa is sometimes hyperemic with bright red punctate lesions. *Trichomonas* is an aerotolerant protozoan that lacks mitochondria and instead has an organelle, the hydrogenosome, that is involved in carbohydrate metabolism. The hydrogenosome is a site for selective toxicity.

Leishmaniasis

Man becomes infected with the flagellated protozoan by the bite of the sandfly. *Leishmania* is engulfed by host macrophages, where it differentiates into an amastigote (aflagellate stage) within the phagolysosome. Clinically, leishmaniasis takes the form of cutaneous leishmaniasis, mucocutaneous leishmaniasis, and visceral leishmaniasis, also known as kala-azar. All three forms cause considerable morbidity in man, but visceral leishmaniasis is by far the most life-threatening. Geographically, leishmaniasis is prevalent in the Mediterranean basin, North Africa, East Africa, the Near East, the Middle East, India, China, Mexico, Central America, and northern South America. An estimated 10 to 15 million people are infected with *Leishmania*, with 400,000 new cases each year.[2] *Leishmania* is now encountered as an opportunistic infection in patients with AIDS.

Trypanosomiasis

American trypanosomiasis (Chagas' disease) and African trypanosomiasis (sleeping sickness) are distinct diseases caused by different species of blood parasite and transmitted by different vectors. Trypanosomes cannot synthesize purines de novo, and must rely on the salvage of preformed purines from the host. This is the basis for the design of drugs with selective toxicity for the parasite.[3]

Table 100.1 Drugs Effective Against Parasitic Diseases

Disease	Etiologic Agent	Drug
	Protozoan Diseases	
Intestinal amebiasis	*Entamoeba histolytica*	Metronidazole
Amebic encephalitis	*Acanthamoeba sp.*	Amphotericin
Giardiasis	*Giardia lamblia*	Quinacrine
Trichomoniasis	*Trichomonas vaginalis*	Metronidazole
Leishmaniasis	*Leishmania sp.*	Antimony sodium gluconate
Chagas' disease	*Trypanosoma cruzi*	Nifurtimox
Sleeping sickness	*Trypanosoma gambiense*	Melarsoprol
Balantidiasis	*Balantidium coli*	Diiodohydroxyquin
Toxoplasmosis	*Toxoplasma gondii*	Pyrimethamine
Pneumocystosis	*Pneumocystis carinii*	Trimethoprim
Malaria	*Plasmodium sp.*	Chloroquine
	Round Worm Infections	
Pinworms	*Enterobius vermicularis*	Pyrantel pamoate
Whipworms	*Trichuris trichiura*	Mebendazole
Round worms	*Ascaris lumbricoides*	Ivermectin
Hookworms	*Necator americanus*	Pyrantel pamoate
Strongyloidiasis	*Strongyloides stercoralis*	Ivermectin
Filariasis	*Wuchereria bancrofti*	Diethylcarbamazine
River blindness	*Onchocerca volvulus*	Ivermectin
Guinea worms	*Dracunculus medinensis*	Niridazole
	Flatworm Infections	
Liver flukes	*Clonorchis sinensis*	Praziquantel
Lung flukes	*Paragonimus westermani*	Bithionol
Schistosomiasis	*Schistosoma sp.*	Praziquantel
Beef and pork tapeworm	*Taenia sp.*	Niclosamide
Cysticercosis	*Taenia solium*	Albendazole
Dwarf tapeworm	*Hymenolepis nana*	Niclosamide
Fish tapeworm	*Diphyllobothrium latum*	Niclosamide
Hydatidosis	*Echinococcus sp.*	Albendazole

Note: Examples of effective drugs; other drugs are indicated in some circumstances, such as drug resistance.

Table 100.2 Standard Treatment Regimens for Antiprotozoan Agents

Drug	Disease	Regimen
Chloroquine	Malaria	500 mg base orally weekly × 6 wk
Quinine	Malaria	650 mg orally tid × 3 d
Metronidazole	Amebiasis	750 mg orally tid × 5 to 10 d
	Giardiasis*	250 mg orally tid × 10 d
	Trichmoniasis	250 mg orally tid × 7 d
Pyrimethamine	Toxoplasmosis	25 mg/d orally × 3 to 4 wk
Antimony sodium gluconate	Leishmaniasis	20 mg/kg/d IM × 4 wk
Melarsoprol	Sleeping sickness	3.6 mg/kg/d IV × 3 d
Nifurtimox	Chagas' disease	2 to 2.5 mg/kg orally qid for 120 d
Pentamidine	Pneumocystosis*	4 mg/kg/d IM × 10 to 14 d

*Other drugs are considered as effective (see text).

Coccidian Parasites

Cryptosporidiosis, toxoplasmosis and pneumocystosis are the exceptional clinical expressions of widespread infections of humans. The disease state is most often encountered in immunosuppressed persons and infants. Perinatal infection by *Toxoplasma* is life-threatening to the fetus and to the newborn. Toxoplasmosis may ensue after ingestion of raw meat or of oocysts eliminated in cat feces. Oocysts of *Cryptosporidium* are shed by domestic animals and can contaminate the drinking water supply. *Pneumocystis* is of uncertain taxonomic affiliation, but along with *Cryptosporidium* and *Toxoplasma* it is a frequent cause of serious infections in immunosuppressed patients, especially those with AIDS.

Malaria

In 1955, the 8th World Health Assembly proposed a program for the worldwide eradication of malaria. By the early 1970s, *Plasmodium falciparum* had developed resistance to the established antimalarial drugs. Recently, chloroquine-resistant variants of *Plasmodium vivax* have appeared in the field.[r7] In some areas of the world, such as Thailand, multiple drug-resistant malaria is prevalent. Globally, malaria is found in more than 100 countries, with 100 million clinical cases and 2 million deaths annually.[4] More than 80 percent of the world's malaria cases occur in Africa.

Antiprotozoan Drugs

Quinoline Compounds

Febrifugine has been used since 200 BC to treat malaria, making it one of the oldest remedies used by humans. It is prepared from the roots of *Dichroa febrifuga* or from the leaves of hydrangea. The active ingredient is a quinoline compound. The febrifugine remedy was subsequently replaced by a more effective remedy from the bark of cinchona trees. The active ingredient in cinchona bark is also a quinoline compound, quinine. Quinoline compounds continue to be the most important drugs for the treatment of malaria.

Chloroquine (N^4-(7-chloro-4-quinolinyl)-N′,N′-diethyl-1,4-pent-anediamine) is a quinoline derivative having a molecular weight of 320. The phosphate (molecular weight 516) forms colorless crystals and is freely soluble in water. The pH of a 1 percent aqueous solution is 4.5, and the compound is stable to heat in solutions of pH 4.0 to 6.5. Chloroquine phosphate is less soluble at neutral or alkaline pH than in acidified water, and is practically insoluble in ethanol and diethyl ether. The drug is susceptible to photodegradation.

Chloroquine was the first of the 4-aminoquinolines to be synthesized and evaluated for antimalarial activity. Chloroquine was introduced for the treatment of malaria in 1934 and remains the most widely used member of the group. Resistance to chloroquine arose simultaneously in Southeast Asia and South America in the late 1950s and has spread rapidly to all regions of the world where malaria is endemic. Chloroquine was introduced clinically for the treatment of hepatic amebiasis in 1948. Amodiaquine (Camoquin, Basoquin) is a 7-chloro-4-amino congener of chloroquine used as an alternative drug when hypersensitivity limits the use of chloroquine.

Chloroquine is a highly active antimalarial and amebicidal agent. It is active against the erythrocytic forms of *Plasmodium vivax* and *Plasmodium falciparum* but not against the gametocyte stage of *P. falciparum*. It also has anti-inflammatory activity. Chloroquine does not prevent relapse in patients with *P. vivax* infections because the drug is not active against the exoerythrocytic forms nor will it prevent *P. vivax* infection when administered prophylactically. The drug is effective in treating patients with *P. vivax* malaria and also in delaying relapses. In patients with *P. falciparum* malaria, the drug controls acute attacks unless a drug-resistant parasite is involved. Resistance to chloroquine is now widespread in *Plasmodium* species in South America, Southeast Asia, and Africa. Chloroquine phosphate is also used to treat *Clonorchis* and *Opisthorchis* liver flukes. Patients in areas endemic for *Onchocerca volvulus* who were undergoing chloroquine therapy for malaria did not become infected with *Onchocerca*. These field observations indicate that chloroquine and its congeners may have potential as a microfilaricide. Amodiaquine is not used for prophylaxis of malaria because of its adverse side-effects, but it is useful in the treatment of chloroquine-resistant malaria.

Chloroquine accumulates in the acidic food vacuoles of the intraerythrocytic stage of the malaria parasite, the stage that is most susceptible to the drug (Fig. 100.2). Chloroquine raises the pH of the *Plasmodium* food vacuole at a concentration lower than that needed to alkalinize lysosomes of mammalian cells. The pH of the *Plasmodium* food vacuole is regulated by an ATP-driven proton pump and a proton leak. Chloroquine is taken into the food vacuole as the free base, where it is protonated. Protonated chloroquine cannot translocate across the food vacuole membrane; therefore, the lower the pH inside the food vacuole, the more chloroquine that will accumulate there. Chloroquine-laden plasmodial cells have impaired ability to digest host material they have ingested. Chloroquine inhibits phospholipase A_2 activity (present in *Plasmodium falciparum* infected human erythrocytes but not in uninfected erythrocytes) at drug concentrations found in the food vacuoles of the malarial parasite.[5] Chloroquine binds to DNA and inhibits its synthesis in bacteria, viruses, and mammalian cells. Intercalation into DNA, however, does not account for the antimalarial specificity of the drug. Chloroquine also displays high affinity binding to ferriprotoporphyrin IX, the undegraded heme nucleus that remains in the plasmodial food vacuole after proteolysis of hemoglobin. Both free heme and heme bound to chloroquine are toxic for

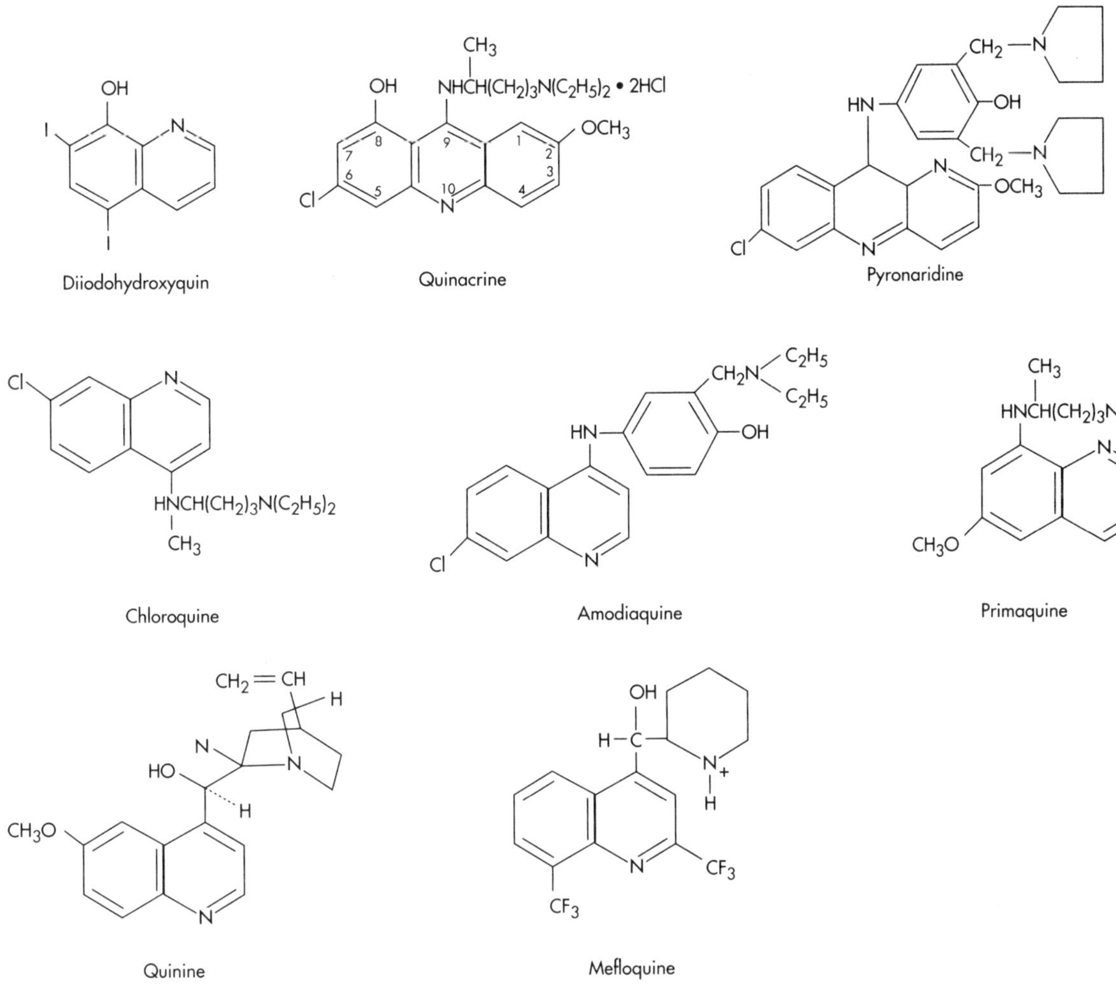

Diiodohydroxyquin

Quinacrine

Pyronaridine

Chloroquine

Amodiaquine

Primaquine

Quinine

Mefloquine

Figure 100.1 Quinolines and Related Compounds

Plasmodium, and the chloroquine-heme complex lyses erythrocytes. The malarial parasite has a mechanism to neutralize the toxicity of accumulated free heme; for example, a heme polymerase. Heme polymerase, which converts free heme into a noninhibitory malarial pigment, is inhibited by chloroquine and by such related drugs as amodiaquine and quinine.[6] Free ferriprotoporphyrin IX and chloroquine-ferriprotoporphyrin IX complex inhibit acidic proteases in plasmodial food vacuoles, and may starve the parasite.

Chloroquine is relatively nontoxic if a drug overdose is avoided and the rate of IV infusion is not too rapid. Chloroquine causes occasional pruritus, vomiting, headaches, fall in blood pressure, confusion, depigmentation of hair, skin eruptions, corneal opacity, weight loss, partial alopecia, extraocular muscle palsies, exacerbation of psoriasis, eczema, and other exfoliative dermatitis. Chloroquine causes hemolysis, especially in subjects with glucose-6-phosphate dehydrogenase deficiency. Irreversible retinal injury may occur when total dosage of chloroquine exceeds 100 g. Amodiaquine is responsible for a severe neutropenia that is life-threatening.

A number of fatalities have been reported following accidental ingestion of chloroquine. Chloroquine is rapidly and completely absorbed after ingestion, and as little as 1 g may be fatal in children. Children and infants are very susceptible to an overdose of parenteral chloroquine, and sudden deaths have been recorded. The parenteral dose of chloroquine in children never should exceed 5 mg/kg. Overdoses of chloroquine produce headaches, drowsiness, visual disturbances, nausea, vomiting, convulsions, cardiac arrest and respiratory depression, or shock with hypotension.

Chloroquine is rapidly and almost completely absorbed from the GI tract, and only a small proportion of the administered dose is found in the feces. Peak plasma levels are achieved within one to three hours after a single oral dose. With daily doses of 300 mg of base, plasma levels reach a steady state level of 30 to

Table 100.3 Selected Regimens for Quinoline Drugs

Disease	Drug	Route	Dose	Duration
Entamoebiasis (adult)	Chloroquine	IM	200 mg base	Daily × 12 d
Entamoebiasis (adult)	Diiodohyroxyquin	Orally	650 mg	tid × 20 d
Giardiasis (adult)	Quinacrine	Orally	100 mg	tid × 5–7 d
Giardiasis (child)	Quinacrine	Orally	2 mg/kg	tid × 5 d; maximum 300 mg/d
Malaria (adult treat)	Chloroquine	IM	160 to 200 mg base	Repeated in 6 h; not to exceed 800 mg 1st d; total 1.5 g base in 3 d
Malaria (adult treat)	Primaquine	Orally	15 mg base	Daily × 14 d
Malaria (adult treat)	Quinine	Orally	650 mg	tid × 3 d
Malaria (adult treat)	Primaquine	Orally	45 mg base	weekly × 8 wk
Malaria (adult treat)	Quinine	IV	600 mg in 300 ml	Repeat in 6 to 8 h; maximum 1800 mg/d
Malaria (adult treat)	Quinacrine	Orally	100 mg	tid × 5 to 7 d
Malaria (adult treat)	Quinacrine	Orally	200 mg 100 mg	Every 6 h × 5 doses tid × 6 d
Malaria (adult treat)	Pyronaridine	Orally	400 mg	bid on day 1; once daily × 2 more days
Malaria (adult treat)	Pyronaridine	IM or IV	4 to 6 mg/kg	bid
Malaria (adult prevent)	Chloroquine	Orally	300 mg base	Weekly × 6 wk after last exposure
Malaria (adult prevent)	Quinacrine	Orally	100 mg	Once daily
Malaria (child treat)	Chloroquine	IM	5 mg base/kg	2 × day 1; then × 4d daily doses
Malaria (child treat)	Primaquine	Orally	0.3 mg base/kg	Daily × 14 d
Malaria (child treat)	Primaquine	Orally	0.9 mg base/kg	Weekly × 8 wk
Malaria (child treat)	Quinine	Orally	25 mg/kg	Daily × 3 d
Malaria (child treat)	Quinine	IV	10 to 25 mg/kg	Infuse 1/2; other half 6 to 8 h later; maximum 1800 mg/d
Malaria (child treat)	Quinacrine	Orally	2 mg/kg	tid × 5 to 7 d; maximum 300 mg/d
Malaria (child treat)	Quinacrine	Orally	100 mg	Once daily × 6 d
Malaria (child prevent)	Chloroquine	Orally	5 mg base/kg	Weekly × 6 wk after last exposure
Malaria (child prevent)	Quinacrine	Orally	50 mg	Once daily
Pinworms (adult or child)	Pyrvinium pamoate	Orally	5 mg/kg up to 350 mg	Repeat after 2 wk
Liver flukes (adult)	Chloroquine	Orally	150 mg abse	tid × 6 wk
Tapeworms (adult)	Quinacrine	Orally	200 mg	4 doses 10 min apart; total 800 mg
Tapeworms (child)	Quinacrine	Orally	10 mg/kg	Once

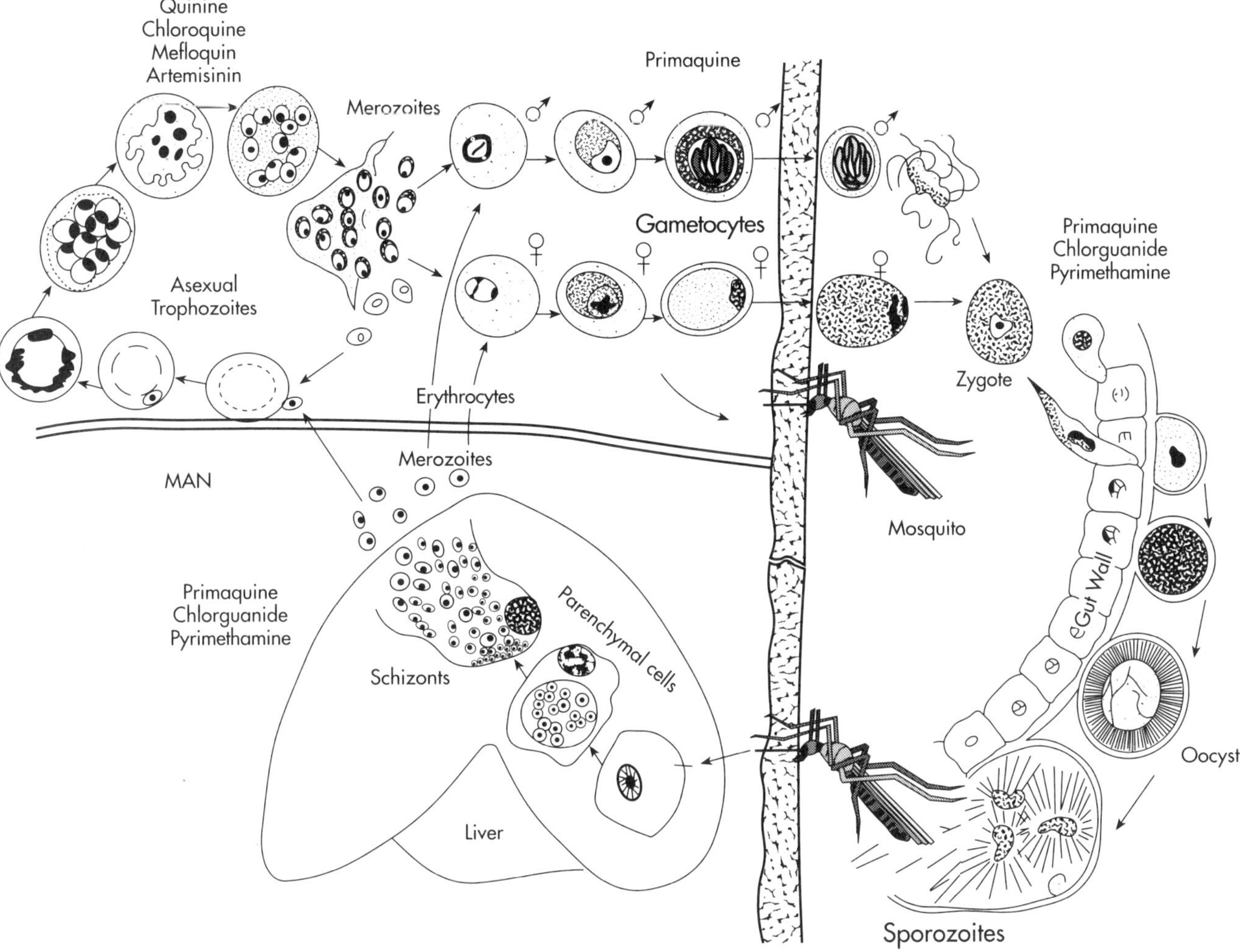

Figure 100.2 The Life Cycle of *Plasmodium*, Showing Stages Inhibited by Quinoline Drugs

70 μg/ml. Most of the drug in the blood is bound to thrombocytes and granulocytes, and only 15 percent of the drug is free in the plasma. Excretion of chloroquine is quite slow, with a half life of five days, but is increased by acidification of the urine. Chloroquine is deposited in the liver, kidneys, and lungs in considerable amounts—several hundred times the level in the plasma. Chloroquine undergoes appreciable degradation in the body. The main metabolite is desethylchloroquine, which accounts for one-fourth of the material in the urine. Slightly more than half of the drug in the urine is unaltered chloroquine. Amodiaquine, unlike chloroquine, is rapidly eliminated from the blood, with a half life of five hours. No amodiaquine can be detected in the plasma 12 hours after dosing.

Chloroquine (diphosphates: Aralen, Avloclor, and Resochin; sulfate: Nivaquine) is available in 500-mg diphosphate (300 mg base) and 250-mg tablets; in 200-mg sulfate (150 mg base) and 100-mg tablets; coated pills for children (125-mg diphosphate); syrup for young children (sulfate containing 10 mg base/ml); and in parenteral solutions (sulfate as 40 mg base/ml and diphosphate as 50 mg base/ml).

Diiodohydroxyquin (iodoquinol; 5,7-diiodo-8-quinolinol; 5,7-diiodo-8-hydroxyquinoline) is a halogenated quinoline. The medicinal grade is a yellowish brown powder. Diiodohydroxyquin is sparingly soluble in ethanol, diethyl ether, and acetone; it is practically insoluble in water. It contains 64 percent organically bound iodine and has a molecular weight of 397.

Diiodohydroxyquin is the drug of choice for balantidiasis and for asymptomatic amebiasis caused by *Entamoeba histolytica*. It is amebicidal against both the ameboid and the cyst stages of *E. histolytica*. It is also used in combination with metronidazole for the treatment of mild to severe intestinal amebiasis and hepatic abscesses. Diiodohydroxyquin is also used in combination with chloroquine phosphate. Diiodohydroxyquin should be used with caution in patients with thyroid disease. Safety for use during pregnancy has not been established.

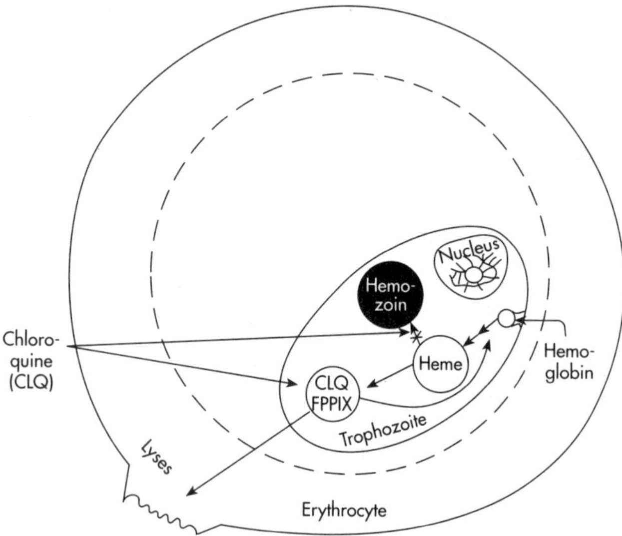

Figure 100.3 Action of Chloroquine on Trophozoite of *Plasmodium*

Diiodohydroxyquin causes occasional rash, acne, slight enlargement of the thyroid gland, nausea, diarrhea, cramps, and pruritus. Rarely it causes optic atrophy and loss of vision in children after prolonged use in high doses for months.

Diiodohydroxyquin (Yodoxin) is available in 210-mg and 650-mg tablets. The regimen for treating children is 10 to 13 mg/kg/d tid, with a maximum dose of 2 g/d.

Primaquine (N^4-(6-methoxy-8-quinolinyl)-1,4-pentanediamine) is a viscous liquid miscible in diethyl ether. The diphosphate of primaquine forms yellow crystals that are moderately soluble in water. The free base has a molecular weight of 259.

Primaquine, introduced clinically in 1952, is a reasonably well tolerated, all-purpose antimalarial drug.[r8] It is used in special circumstances; for example, to prevent an attack of malaria after departure from areas where *Plasmodium vivax* and *Plasmodium ovale* are endemic, and a relapse of malaria caused by *Plasmodium vivax* and *Plasmodium ovale*. Primaquine may be given in combination with chloroquine.

The active antimalarial agent probably is a metabolite of primaquine. It has been proposed that this metabolite is a quinone that interferes with mitochondrial energy metabolism. The primaquine metabolite may interfere with the function of ubiquinone as an electron carrier in the respiratory chain. Primaquine depresses dihydroorotate dehydrogenase activity in *Plasmodium falciparum*.[7] Primaquine binds to nucleic acids but does not appear to intercalate. It interferes with internalization, degradation and recycling of proteoglycans. In addition, the drug blocks proteoglycan synthesis.[8]

Subjects with a glucose-6-phosphate dehydrogenase (G6PD) deficiency frequently develop hemolytic anemia during treatment with primaquine. Primaquine increases the methemoglobin level in normal human erythrocytes. The hemolytic effects of the drug appear to be due to the action of a metabolite.[9] Primaquine treatment occasionally is associated with neutropenia and GI disturbance. Rare adverse effects include hypertension, arrhythmias, and CNS symptoms.

Primaquine is rapidly absorbed after oral administration of 45 mg. Peak plasma levels of 225 μg/ml are achieved in about two hours. The plasma half life is about four hours. Most of the excreted drug is eliminated in the urine as metabolites. Primaquine (Primachin) is available in tablets containing 26.5 mg of the diphosphate salt.

Quinine (6′-methoxycinchonan-9-ol) is a natural product extracted from the bark of cinchona trees. Quinine is readily soluble in ethanol; solubility in water is limited (500 mg/L of water at 25 C and 1.3 g/L of boiling water). Quinine gives a strong blue fluorescence in dilute sulfuric acid. It has a molecular weight of 324.

The value of cinchona as an antimalarial preparation has been known since the early 17th century. It also has some anti-inflammatory activity. Cinchona bark was widely used for two centuries before its active ingredients were isolated. Quinine was introduced clinically in 1820. Quinine was successfully synthesized in 1944. Chemical synthesis of quinine is too expensive to be a practical source of the drug. The first synthetic antimalarial, pamaquine, evolved from an attempt in 1928 to combine the 6-methoxyquinoline moiety of quinine with a dialkylamino-dialkylamino structure. Pamaquine has not been a successful substitute for quinine because it has little effect against *Plasmodium falciparum*. Mefloquine (Lariacun, Lariam) is a 4-quinoline methanol resembling quinine. Mefloquine is available only in tablets for oral administration. Quinine is used to treat chloroquine-resistant *Plasmodium falciparum* infections and, outside the US, for severe malaria in children.[10] Quinine alone will control an acute attack of chloroquine-resistant *Plasmodium falciparum*, but fails to prevent recurrence in a substantial number of infections. Mefloquine is effective against multi-resistant strains of *Plasmodium falciparum*.[11]

Quinine acts on skeletal muscle by three mechanisms: it increases the refractory period by direct action on the muscle fiber; it decreases the excitability of the motor end-plate, an action similar to that of curare; it affects the distribution of calcium within the muscle fiber. The susceptibility of *Plasmodium falciparum* to quinine or to chloroquine is directly related to the cholesterol content of the membranes of infected erythrocytes and inversely related to the acidic phospholipid content.[12] Quinine, like other members of the quinoline family, intercalates into DNA, but mefloquine does not.

Quinine frequently induces a series of symptoms, collectively called *cinchonism*, which include tinnitus, headache, nausea, abdominal pain, and visual disturbances. Quinine damages the fetus, causing deafness, limb anomalies, visceral defects, and visual alterations. Quinine has been associated with acute hemolysis, agranulocytosis, visual disturbances, vertigo, headaches, nausea and vomiting, rashes, flushing of the skin, asthmatic symptoms, angina symptoms, and epigastric pain. Occasionally, treatment with quinine is associated with blood dyscrasias, photosensitivity, arrhythmias, and hypotension. Rarely, quinine has caused blindness and sudden death, when injected too rapidly. Urinary alkalinizers such as sodium bicarbonate increase quinine blood levels. Increased levels of digoxin occur when the drug is administered concurrently with quinine. Concurrent use of aluminum-containing antacids may retard absorption of quinine. Actions of such neuromuscular blocking agents as pancuronium, succinylcholine, and tubocurarine are potentiated by quinine. The more common signs of overdose are tinnitus, dizziness, skin rash, and intestinal cramping. Fatalities have been reported from single doses of 2 to 8 g.

Quinine is readily absorbed when administered orally. Absorption occurs from the upper part of the small intestine and is almost complete. Peak plasma concentrations occur within one to three hours after a single oral dose, and the half-life is four to five hours. Upon continued administration of 1 g/day, the mean plasma level is 7 μg/ml. Most of the quinine (70%) is bound to plasma proteins. The concentration of quinine in CSF is only 2 to 5 percent that of the plasma. Quinine readily traverses the placenta and reaches the fetus. It is metabolized extensively in the liver, and less that 5 percent of the drug is excreted unaltered in the urine. Renal excretion is twice as rapid in acidified urine as in alkaline urine, which favors reabsorption by the kidney tubules. There is little or no accumulation of the drug in the body during continued treatment. Small amounts are excreted in the feces, and the drug can be found in saliva, gastric juice, and bile.

Quinine is available as quinine sulfate (Quinamm) in 260-mg tablets. Quinine hydrochloride is available for injection at 300 mg quinine salt/ml. Mefloquine (Lariacun) is available in tablets containing 250 mg base.

Quinacrine hydrochloride (N^4-(6-chloro-2-methoxy-9-acridinyl)-N^1, N^1-diethyl-1,4-pentanediamine dihydrochloride; mepacrine hydrochloride) is an acridine derivative that forms bright yellow crystals. It is slightly soluble in ethanol and insoluble in acetone. The pH of a 1 percent aqueous solution is 4.5, and 3 g dissolves in 100 ml water. It has a molecular weight of 473. Quinacrine hydrochloride is much more soluble in hot water. The salt has a molecular weight of 509. Under ultraviolet light, the yellow aqueous solution exhibits a vivid fluorescence. Quinacrine should be stored in airtight containers and protected from light.

Quinacrine was introduced for the treatment of malaria in 1930. The drug is used to treat giardiasis, tapeworms, and malaria. It destroys erythrocytic forms of *Plasmodium vivax* and *Plasmodium falciparum*, and is effective against certain tapeworms. Quinacrine HCl is the drug of choice in the treatment of giardiasis, an infection caused by an intestinal flagellated protozoan. A 10 percent solution of quinacrine is used topically to treat cutaneous leishmaniasis. The solution is infiltrated around the lesion, and 2 ml are injected at weekly intervals. Quinacrine crosses the placenta and should not be used during pregnancy unless there are no alternatives to treat a life-threatening infection.

Quinacrine appears to bind with phospholipids of the membranes of the endoplasmic reticulum and nuclear envelope. These drug-lipid complexes aggregate in refractive intracellular inclusions, a process which effectively removes the drug from the cell cytoplasm.[13] Quinacrine blocks phospholipase A_2 activity, and binds specifically to the lipid-protein interface of the acetylcholine receptor of worms.[14]

Adverse effects frequently attributed to quinacrine HCl include dizziness, headaches, and vomiting. Less frequently, this drug causes toxic psychosis, blood dyscrasia, urticaria, severe exfoliative dermatitis, yellow staining of skin and sclera, blue and black nail pigmentation, and ocular effects similar to those caused by chloroquine. Acute hepatic necrosis is rare. Quinacrine increases the toxicity of primaquine, and the two drugs should not be used in combination.

Large doses of quinacrine cause excitation of the CNS, with restlessness, insomnia, psychic stimulation and convulsions, GI disorders, vascular collapse with hypotension, shock, cardiac arrhythmias or arrest, and yellow pigmentation of the skin. Quinacrine concentrates in the liver. Quinacrine (Atabrine) is supplied as 100-mg tablets.

Pyronaridine (2-methoxy-7-chloro-10[3′,5′-bis(pyrrolidinyl-1-methyl)4′ -hydroxyphenyl]amino-benzo(b)1,5-naphthyridine, Malaridine) is a derivative of benzonaphthyridine. It is a hygroscopic yellow powder that is soluble in water and sparingly soluble in ethanol. Pyronaridine was developed by Chinese researchers, who began in the 1960s to synthesize an alternative to quinacrine, starting with the mepacrine nucleus. Pyronaridine was synthesized in the 1970s and has been in clincal use in China for a decade.

Pyronaridine is highly active against chloroquine-resistant strains of *Plasmodium falciparum*[15] and it is used in China to treat drug-resistant malaria. The drug is active against the erythrocytic stages of the malarial parasite. Unfortunately, resistance develops rapidly to pyronaridine, and pyronaridine-resistant *Plasmodium* variants are also resistant to chloroquine (although pyronaridine is active against chloroquine-resistant malaria). Pyronaridine induces mutations in some bacterial test systems, and increases both the incidence of fetal resorption and the number of dead fetuses in rats.

Pyronaridine causes marked changes in the morphology of the malaria parasite. Multilamellate whorls develop inside the parasite, followed by enlargement of and pigment accumulation in food vacuoles. Subsequently the parasite's mitochondria become swollen, and the endoplasmic reticulum disappears. There is no correlation between the extent of DNA binding and antimalarial activity of pyronaridine. Pyronaridine inhibits decatenation activity of *P. falciparum* DNA topoisomerase II.[16]

Pyronaridine occasionally is associated with diarrhea, nausea, and abdominal pain. On rare occasions, it causes vomiting and a skin rash.

Pyronaridine, given orally in a 600-mg enteric coated tablet, yields a maximum plasma level of 225 ng/ml five hours after administration.[17] Approximately 20 percent of the drug is absorbed, and the plasma half-life is 65 hours. A single IM dose of 204 mg yields a maximum plasma level of 525 ng/ml after 45 minutes, with a plasma half-life of 63 hours. Pyronaridine (Malaridine) is available for oral and parenteral use.

Pyrimidine and Aryl Biguanide Compounds

Pyrimidine derivatives (Table 100.4; Fig. 100.4) have been explored extensively as anticancer and antiviral agents. In addition, pyrimidine analogues have found utility in the treatment of both fungal infections and parasitic diseases. Folic acid is a constitutent of cofactors for many essential metabolic processes (Fig. 100.5). Both humans and parasites have the ability to convert folic acid into dihydrofolic acid (FAH_2) and tetrahydrofolic acid (FAH_4). Humans obtain the needed folic acid from the diet; however, parasites cannot readily use exogenously supplied folic acid to synthesize folate cofactors. Rather, parasites synthesize FAH_2 de novo, starting with the condensation of pteridine with p-aminobenzoic acid (PABA) to form dihydropteroic acid. Dihydropteroic acid is condensed with glutamic acid to form FAH_2. These differences between humans and parasites are the bases of the selective toxicity of sulfamethoxazole and other sulfonamides, which are PABA antagonists, and of diaminopyrimidines, which are inhibitors of dihydrofolate reductase activity.[19]

Trimethoprim (5-[(3,4,5-trimethoxyphenyl)methyl]-2,4-pyrimidinediamine, Trimpex, Proloprim) is a white to cream colored crystalline powder having a molecular weight of 290. It has limited solubility in water (40 mg/100 ml) and diethyl ether (3 mg/100 ml). Solubility in methanol is greater, 1.2 g/100 ml.

The combination of trimethoprim-sulfamethoxazole is used to treat toxoplasmosis and pneumocystosis. There are severe adverse effects that limit the use of the drug combination in more than half of patients with pneumocystosis and acquired immune deficiency disease. The combination of trimethoprim and sulfamethoxazole has been discussed in Chapter 92, and detailed information will not be repeated here.

Trimethoprim is an inhibitor of dihydrofolate reductase. Malaria parasites use a folate pathway more similar to bacteria than to mammalian cells. Bacteria and *Plasmodium* cannot utilize preformed dihydrofolate, but must synthesize it from para-aminobenzoic acid.

The most common side-effects of trimethoprim are rash, pruritus, and phototoxic skin eruptions. There has been rare linkage to exfoliative dermatitis and Stevens-Johnson syndrome. Epigastric distress, nausea, vomiting, thrombocytopenia, leukopenia, and fever also have been observed. Trimethoprim may inhibit hepatic metabolism of phenytoin. After one gram or more, trimethoprim causes nausea, vomiting, dizziness, headaches, mental depression, confusion, and bone marrow depression.

Trimethoprim is rapidly absorbed following oral administration. It exists in blood as unbound, protein-

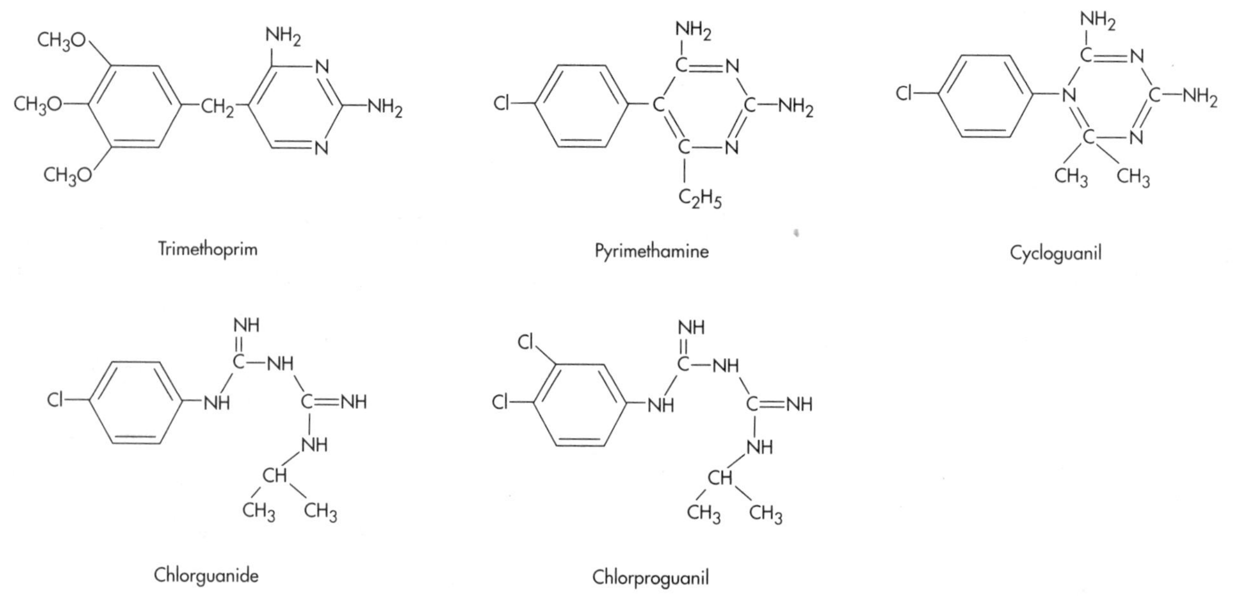

Trimethoprim

Pyrimethamine

Cycloguanil

Chlorguanide

Chlorproguanil

Figure 100.4 Pyrimidine and Biguanide Compounds

Table 100.4 Selected Regimens for Pyrimidine Drugs

Disease	Drug	Route	Dose	Duration
Toxoplasmosis (adult)	Pyrimethamine	Oral	25 mg	3–4 wk
Toxoplasmosis (child)	Pyrimethamine	Oral	2 mg/kg, then 1 mg/kg	Load 1 d; then 3 d; maximum 25 mg
Toxoplasmosis	Trimethoprim Sulfamethoxazole	Oral	160 mg 800 mg	qid × 10 d; then bid × 3 wk
Toxoplasmosis	Trimethoprim Sulfamethoxazole	Oral	5 mg/kg 25 mg/kg	qid × 14 day
Toxoplasmosis	Trimethoprim Sulfamethoxazole	IV	5 mg/kg 25 mg/kg	tid or qid
Pneumocytosis	Trimethoprim Sulfamethoxazole	Oral	160 mg 800 mg	qid × 10 d; then bid × 3 wk
Pneumocytosis	Trimethoprim Sulfamethoxazole	Oral	5 mg/kg 25 mg/kg	qid × 14 day
Pneumocytosis	Trimethoprim Sulfamethoxazole	IV	5 mg/kg 25 mg/kg	tid or qid
Malaria (adult prevent)	Pyrimethamine	Oral	25 mg	Weekly
Malaria (adult prevent)	Chlorguanide	Oral	100 or 200 mg	Daily
Malaria (adult prevent)	Chlorproguanil	Oral	100 mg	Weekly
Malaria (child prevent)	Pyrimethamine	Oral	0.4 mg/kg	Weekly
Malaria (child prevent)	Chlorguanide	Oral	2.5 mg/kg	Daily
Pinworms	Pyrantel pamoate	Oral	10 mg base/kg	Once, maximum 1 g
Ascariasis	Pyrantel pamoate	Oral	10 mg base/kg	Once; maximum 1 g
Hookworms	Pyrantel pamoate	Oral	10 mg base/kg	Once; maximum 1 g

bound (44%), and metabolized forms. Trimethoprim is metabolized (10 to 20%) in the liver; the remainder is excreted unchanged in the urine (50 to 60%) within 24 hours. The mean peak plasma level is 1 µg/ml, one to four hours after oral administration of 100 mg. The half-life is eight to ten hours. Patients with impaired renal function exhibit an increased half-life for trimethoprim. Urine concentrations are considerably higher than blood levels, e.g., 30 to 160 µg/ml in urine after a dose of 100 mg. One hour after an IV infusion of 160 mg trimethoprim and 800 mg sulfamethoxazole, the mean plasma level of trimethoprim is 3.4 µg/ml, and that of sulfamethoxazole is 46 µg/ml. Following repeated administration at eight-hour intervals, the mean concentration of trimethoprim before and after infusion is 6 and 9 µg/ml respectively, and that of sulfamethoxazole 71 and 106 µg/ml respectively. The mean plasma half-life for trimethoprim is 11 hours and that for sulfamethoxazole 13 hours. Trimethoprim distributes to sputum, vaginal fluid, bronchial secretions, and human milk, and traverses the placenta.

Trimethoprim is most often supplied in combination with sulfamethoxazole (Bactrim, Septra) as tablets (80- and 400 mg, respectively; 160 and 800 mg, respectively), as an oral suspension (40 and 200 mg, respectively, in 5 ml [1 teaspoon]), or for parenteral use (16 mg and 80 mg, respectively per ml in 5- or 10-ml vials).

Pyrimethamine (5-(4-chlorophenyl)-6-ethyl-2,4-pyrimidinediamine) forms crystals that are practically insoluble in water. It is slightly soluble in ethanol at room temperature (9 g/L) and in dilute HCl (5 g/L); solubility is greater in boiling ethanol (25 g/L). It has a molecular weight of 249.

Pyrimethamine was introduced for the treatment of malaria in 1952. It is frequently used in combination with other drugs, such as sulfadoxine or clindamycin. Pyrimethamine is used to treat toxoplasmosis; it is effective in preventing relapses of toxoplasmic encephalitis.[18] The hematologic toxicity of pyrimethamine can be avoided by giving folinic acid concomitantly at 10 mg/kg/d orally. Nevertheless, 60 percent or more of patients develop severe adverse reactions, and treatment must be discontinued. Pyrimethamine has little if any activity against *Toxoplasma* cysts, which are the

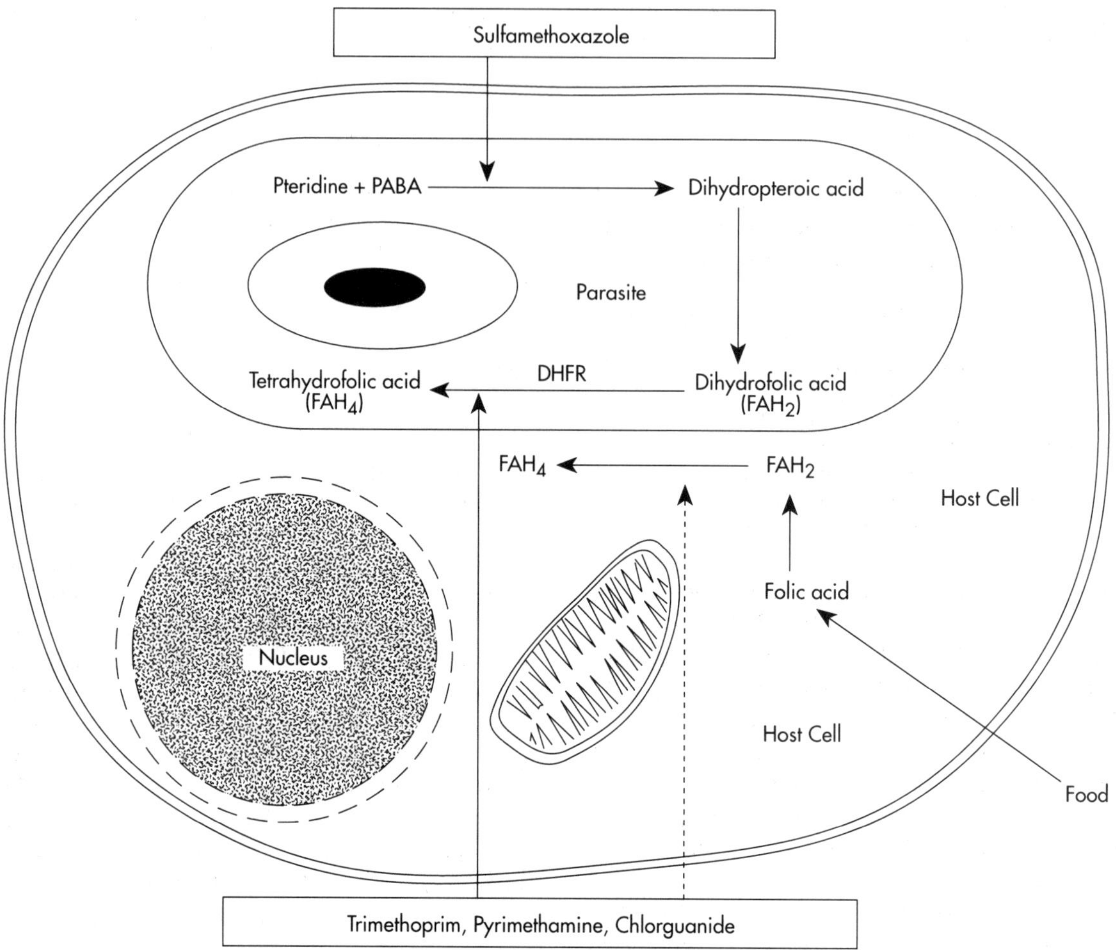

Figure 100.5 Action of Pyrimidine Drugs on the Synthesis of Tetrahydrofolic Acid

reservoir for infection. Pyrimethamine may be used prophylactically to prevent malaria.

Pyrimethamine has been associated with anorexia, vomiting, megaloblastic anemia, leukopenia, thrombocytopenia, pancytopenia, atrophic glossitis, hematuria, and disorders of cardiac rhythmn. Rare side-effects include insomnia, headaches, diarrhea, light-headedness, dryness of the mouth, fever, malaise, and abnormal skin pigmentation. Pyrimethamine causes elevated serum creatinine levels, with a concurrent decrease in urine creatinine levels. Pyrimethamine inhibits renal tubular secretion of creatinine without affecting glomerular filtration.[19] Pyrimethamine increases the incidence of lung tumors in mice, and a few cancers in humans have been attributed to this drug.

Pyrimethamine inhibits dihydrofolate reductase, which catalyzes the conversion of dihydrofolate into tetrahydrofolate. Folate coenzymes serve as acceptors or donors of one-carbon units in a variety of essential reactions involved in purine, pyrimidine, and amino acid synthesis, and in the initiation of protein synthesis.

Pyrimethamine causes anorexia and vomiting and occasional blood dyscrasias and folic acid deficiency. It rarely is the cause of rashes, vomiting, convulsions, or shock. If signs of folate deficiency develop, folinic acid (leucovorin) should be administered until hematopoiesis is restored. Mild hepatotoxicity has been reported in some patients concurrently receiving the benzodiazepine lorazepam. Ingestion of an excessive amount of drug can cause GI or CNS disorders including convulsions, or both. Deaths in children have been reported after accidental ingestion of 250 to 300 mg.

Pyrimethamine is well absorbed, with peak levels occurring between two to six hours. It is eliminated slowly and has a plasma half-life of about 96 hours. Its prolonged half-life allows maintenance of effective blood levels with weekly dosage. The drug is extensively (87%) bound to plasma proteins. Pyrimethamine is excreted in human milk. After a single dose of 75 mg orally, 3 to 4 mg of drug may be fed to a nursing infant over a 48-hour period.

Pyrimethamine (Daraprim, Malocide) is supplied in 50-, 25-, and 6.25-mg tablets. A pediatric elixir contains 6.25 mg pyrimethamine/5ml.

The aryl-biguanides chlorguanide and chlorproguanil were introduced clinically in 1952. They are dihydrofolate reductase inhibitors, even though they do not contain a pyrimidine structure. Their active metabolite cycloguanil possesses the requisite pyrimidine ring.

Chlorguanide (N-(4-chlorophenyl)-N′-(1-methylethyl) imidodicarbonimidic diamide; Proguanil) forms a hydrochloride (Paludrine) soluble in ethanol, slightly soluble in water, and practically insoluble in diethyl ether. The molecular weight of chlorguanide is 254. The pH of a saturated aqueous solution is 5.8 to 6.3. Chlorproguanil (N-(3,4-dichlorophenyl)-N′-(1-methylethyl) imidodicarbonimidic diamide) forms a hydrochloride (Lapudrine) that may be boiled without decomposition. It has a molecular weight of 288. One gram of chlorproguanil can be dissolved in 100 ml water.

The aryl-biguanides chlorguanide and chlorproguanil were developed as a joint venture between Imperial Chemical Industries and the Liverpool School of Tropical Medicine in the 1940s. The malaria parasite rapidly became resistant to the aryl-biguanides, so interest in these agents waned until resistance to other antimalarial drugs became apparent. Chlorguanide is used in combination with chloroquine for prophylaxis against malaria and in combination with a sulfonamide to treat malaria.

Biguanil compounds have little activity in vitro, and require metabolic activation by the hepatic P-450 microsomal enzyme system.[21] The active cyclic dihydrotriazine metabolites are potent inhibitors of dihydrofolate reductase. The principal site of action of the cycloguanil metabolite is against exoerythrocytic plasmodia within the liver. Not all human populations have equal capability to activate aryl-biguanides. Among caucasians, 2.5 to 10 percent of the individuals have low capability to activate aryl-biguanides, whereas among a population in Kenya, 25 percent showed limited ability to activate these drugs metabolically.[22] People with limited ability to activate chlorguanide excrete more of the inactive metabolite *p*-chlorphenylbiguanide in their urine than do those with good activating capability.[23] Chlorguanide and chlorproguanil are well tolerated. Chlorguanide is the safest of all of the antimalarial drugs. There are some GI and renal effects at doses of 1 g chlorguanide daily. No deaths have been reported, even for drug overdoses of 14.5 g.

An oral dose of chlorguanide gives a peak blood level of 1 μg/ml and a plasma level of 373 ng/ml at three to four hours. The half-life of the drug in blood is 20 hours and in plasma 11.5 hours. Approximately 75 percent of the drug is bound to plasma proteins, and the concentration inside the erythrocyte is about six times that of the plasma. The active metabolite cycloguanil achieves a maximum concentration in the plasma of 100 ng/ml, and has a half-life of 21 hours. About half the absorbed drug is excreted in the urine. Chlorproguanil is retained in the body more persistently than is chlorguanide.

Chlorguanide (Proguanil, Paludrine) and chlorproguanil are available in formulations for oral administration. Chlorguanide, which is not available in the US, is dispensed as 100-mg chlorguanide hydrochloride tablets for adults and 25-mg tablets for children.

Antiprotozoan Natural Products (Table 100.5; Figure 100.6)

Spiramycin, a member of the erythromycin family, is a macrolide antibiotic produced by *Streptomyces ambofaciens.* It is an amorphous base only slightly soluble in water. It is soluble in most organic solvents. Spiramycin I has a molecular weight of 842.

Spiramycin is an alternative drug for the treatment of toxoplasmosis, especially in pregnant women; it has been used for treatment of cryptosporidiosis, but its efficacy is questionable. Spiramycins are active against gram-positive bacteria and rickettsia. The drug inhibits protein synthesis in bacterial systems and mitochondria of eukaryotic cells and interferes with the binding of aminoacyl-tRNA to the 50 S ribosomal subunit. Spiramycin neither impairs formation of aminoacyl-tRNA nor interferes with codon-anticodon interactions at the level of the 30 S ribosomal subunit. Bacteria selected for resistance to spiramycin concurrently develop resistance to erythromycin. Spiramycin causes occasional GI disturbances and rarely is responsible for allergic reactions.

Spiramycin concentrates and persists in tissues; for example, 24 hours after a single oral dose, the concentration in tissues is 20 times greater than the plasma level. The drug does not cross the placental barrier, making it safe for use during pregnancy. Spiramycin (Rovamycin) is available for oral administration; it is obtained from the manufacturer Rhone-Poulenc Rorer.

Paromomycin is an antibiotic produced by *Streptomyces rimosus, S. catenulae,* and *S. chrestomyceticus.* Paromomycin (O-2-amino-2-deoxy-a-D-glucopyranosyl-(1–4)-O-[O-2,6-dideoxy-β -L-idopyranosyl-(1–3)-β-D-ribofuranosyl-(1–5)]-2-deoxy-D-streptamine; catenulin; neomycin E; aminosidine) is an aminoglycoside of the neomycin group. The antibiotic is soluble in water and only sparingly soluble in absolute ethanol. It has a molecular weight of 616.

Paromomycin is recommended for treating giardiasis during pregnancy. It is an alternative to diiodohydroxyquin, metronidazole, or diloxanide furoate in asymptomatic, mild, or moderate intestinal amebiasis. Intravenous paromomycin has been used to treat visceral leishmaniasis that is unresponsive to pentavalent antimonials and in immunocompromised patients.[24] Paromomycin in combination with methylbenzetho-

Table 100.5 Selected Regimens for Antiprotozoan Natural Products

Disease	Drug	Route	Dose	Duration
Amebiasis	Paromomycin	Oral	8–10 mg/kg	tid × 5 to 10 d
Amebiasis (adult)	Emetine	IM	1 mg/kg	5 d; maximum 60 mg/kg
Amebiasis (adult)	Dehydroemetine	IM	1–1.5 mg/kg	5 d; maximum 90 mg/kg
Amebiasis (child)	Emetine	IM	0.5 mg/kg	bid 5 d; maximum 60 mg/kg
Amebiasis (child)	Dehydroemetine	IM	0.5 to 0.75 mg/kg	bid 5 d; maximum 90 mg/kg
Giardiasis	Paromomycin	Oral	8–10 mg/kg	tid × 5 to 10 d
Leishmaniasis (adult & child)	Amphotericin	IV	0.25–1 mg/kg	Daily
Leishmaniasis (adult)	Amphotericin	IV	2 mg/kg	Every other day × 8 wk
Leishmaniasis (adult)	Paromomycin	Oral	14–16 mg/kg	29 to 54 d
Cryptosporidiosis (adult)	Spiramycin*	Oral	2–4 mg/kg	3 to 4 wk
Cryptosporidiosis (child)	Spiramycin*	Oral	50–100 mg/kg	3 to 4 wk
Toxoplasmosis (adult)	Spiramycin	Oral	2–4 mg/kg	3 to 4 wk
Toxoplasmosis (child)	Spiramycin	Oral	50–100 mg/kg	3 to 4 wk
Malaria	Artemisinin	Parenteral	300–600 mg/kg	3 d
Malaria	Artemisinin	Oral	300–600 mg/kg	3 d

*Efficacy questionable. For quinine; see table on quinolines.

nium chloride is used as a topical ointment for the treatment of cutaneous leishmaniasis. Paromomycin also has been used for intestinal tapeworms. This drug causes tapeworm segments to disintegrate.

Paromomycin is related to the aminoglycoside family of antibiotics and is thought to exert its antimicrobial action by inhibition of protein synthesis. Paromomycin binds irreversibly to ribosomes, allowing polysomes to form and accumulate; but peptide bond formation for elongation is inhibited.

Paromomycin frequently causes GI disturbance; rare adverse effects include renal damage and eighth nerve damage, mainly auditory.

Paromomycin is poorly absorbed when administered by the oral route, and nearly 100 percent is excreted in the feces. It binds to serum proteins to a limited extent. An IM dose of 500 mg gives a plasma level of 20 μg/ml at one hour; 1 g gives 40 μg/ml at one hour. Paromomycin (Humatin) is supplied as 250-mg tablets.

The polyene antibiotic amphotericin has been discussed in the chapter on antifungal agents, and general information about the drug will not be repeated here. Amphotericin B is of interest as an antiparasitic agent because it binds preferentially to sterols in the plasma membrane, forming pores that leak ions. Amphotericin B was introduced clinically as an antileishmania agent in 1960. It is an alternative to antimony sodium gluconate in the treatment of American cutaneous leishmaniasis and visceral leishmaniasis.[25]

The usefulness of amphotericin is limited by adverse reactions, which include anaphylaxis, thrombocytopenia, flushing, generalized pain, convulsions, chills, fever, phlebitis, anemia, anorexia, decreased renal tubular and glomerular function, and hypokalemia.[26] Toxicity can be reduced by incorporating amphotericin into liposomes made of phosphatidyl choline, cholesterol, and disteroyl phosphatidylglycerol (AmBisome). Amphotericin liposomes are selectively taken up by macrophages, and liver and spleen levels exceed plasma levels. An IV dose of 2 to 3 mg/kg of amphotericin liposomes gives a peak plasma level of 17 to 21 μg/ml. Amphotericin in liposomes shows promise as a replacement for pentavalent antimony compounds.[27]

Amphotericin B (Fungizone) is available in vials containing 50 mg of drug and 41 mg sodium deoxycholate. Crystalline amphotericin is insoluble in water, and deoxycholate is needed to solubilize the drug. The contents of the vial are first reconstituted with 10 ml of sterile water and then diluted 1:50 to give 100 μg/ml. Amphotericin is degraded by exposure to light and should be protected from light during administration.

Emetine (6′,7′,10,11-tetramethoxyemetan; cephaeline methyl ether) is the principal alkaloid of ipecac, the ground roots of *Uragoga ipecacuanha*. Emetine is a white amorphous powder that turns yellow on exposure to light and heat. It is soluble in ethanol, methanol, acetone, and diethyl ether; it is sparingly soluble in water and solutions of potassium hydroxide or sodium hydroxide. It is moderately soluble in dilute ammonium hydroxide. It has a molecular weight of 481. Dehydroemetine (2,3-didehydro-6′,7′,10,11-tetramethoxylemetan; 2,3-dehydroemetine) is synthesized as a racemic mixture. It has a molecular weight of 479.

The value of ipecacuanha as an antiamebic preparation has been known since the early 17th century. The active constituent of ipecacuanha is emetine. Emetine and dehydroemetine are used in combination with other antiparasitic drugs to treat severe intestinal ame-

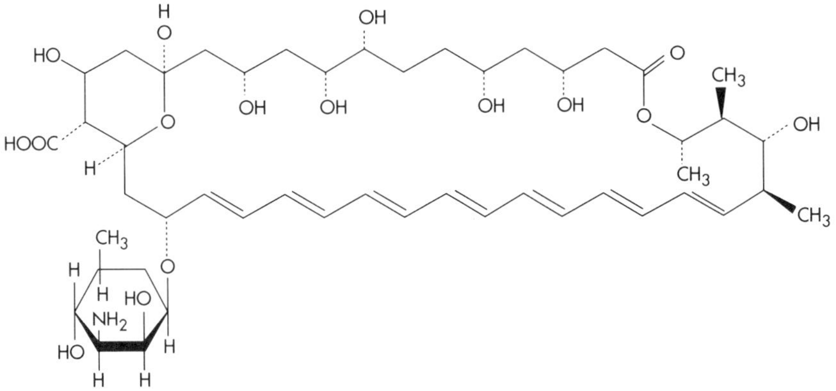

Amphotericin B

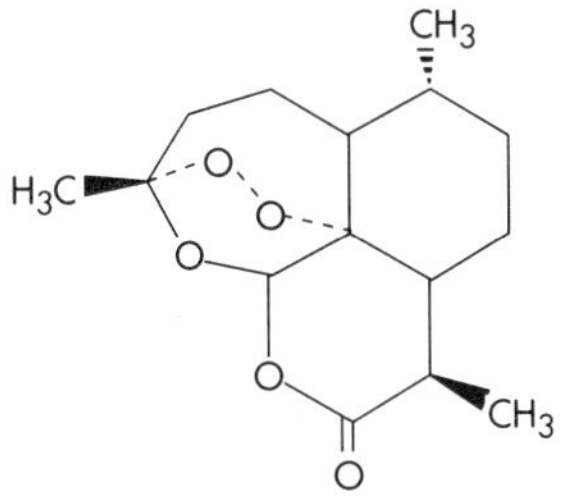

Artemisinin

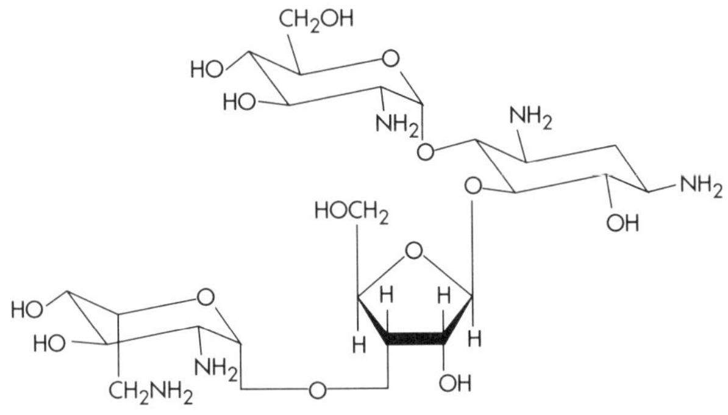

Paromomycin

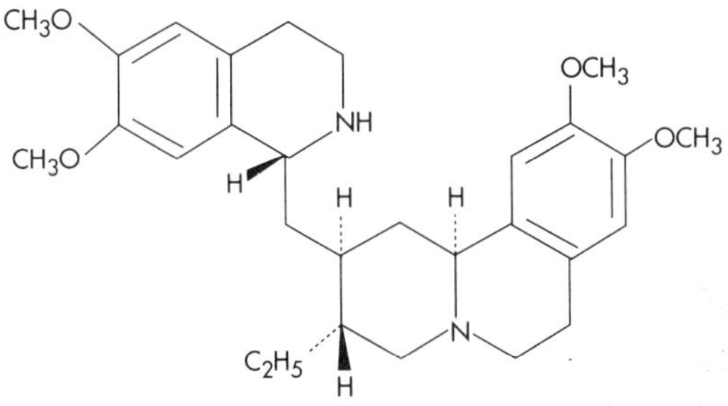

Emetine

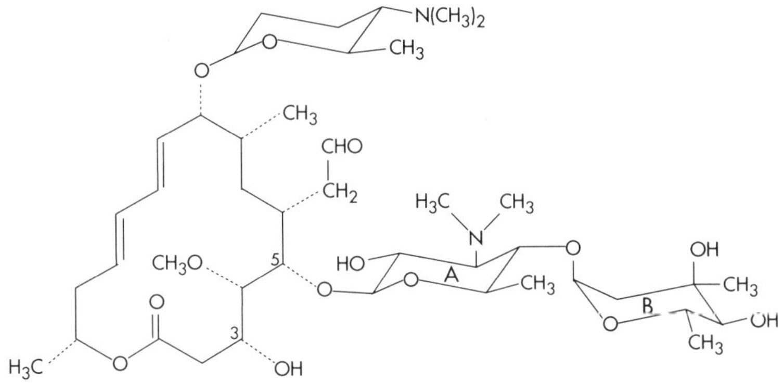

Spiramycin I

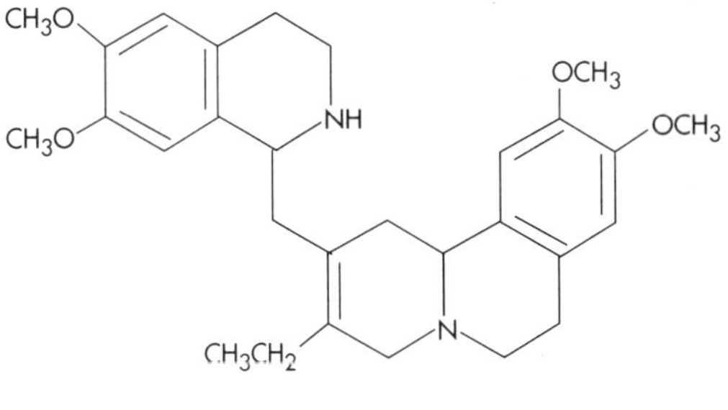

Dehydroemetine

Figure 100.6 Antibiotics and Other Natural Products

biasis and liver abscesses. Emetine has also been used successfully to treat fascioliasis.[28]

Emetine is directly lethal to amebae at concentrations achievable in blood. The drug induces degenerative changes in the amebae that interfere with their division. Emetine is known to inhibit protein synthesis in both amebae and host cells, by inhibiting the movement of mRNA along the ribosome.[29] Emetine can kill amebae in the absence of protein synthesis, however.

Emetine and dehydroemetine frequently cause cardiac arrhythmias, precordial pain, muscle weakness, and cellulitis at the site of injection. Emetine and dehydroemetine occasionally cause diarrhea, vomiting, peripheral neuropathy, and heart failure. The adverse effects of dehydroemetine are generally less severe than those attributed to emetine.

Emetine is completely absorbed upon parenteral administration, but only 20 percent of an oral dose is absorbed. The half-life is five days, and the drug is concentrated in the liver, lungs, spleen, and kidneys. Most (80%) of administered emetine is found in the feces, and only 5 percent in the urine. Amebicidal concentrations of drug persist in the liver for a month after a single parenteral dose.

Emetine is available for parenteral use, and is best administered IM. The SQ route is too painful and the IV too dangerous because of cardiotoxicity. Dehydroemetine is available as a solution (30 mg/ml) for injection; it is obtained from the CDC Parasitic Diseases Drug Service.

Artemisinin (qinghaosu) is a sequiterpene endoperoxide natural product isolated from several *Artemisia* species. It has a molecular weight of 280 and is poorly soluble in water. Artemisinin has been used as a Chinese herbal remedy for malaria for many centuries. Artemisinin derivatives are being used extensively in Asia to treat cerebral malaria.[30]

Artemisinin binds covalently to albumin. The binding involves thiol and amino groups via both iron-dependent and iron-independent reactions.[31] Artemisinin generates free radicals and reactive aldehydes. The drug induces swelling and deformation of vacuoles in *Plasmodium,* and subsequent degeneration of mitochondrial membranes and nuclear envelope. Artemisinin also reacts with hemin to form an adduct. This reaction appears to have biologic significance, because *Plasmodium* digests 25 to 75 percent of the host's hemoglobin, leaving hemin, which accumulates as hemozoin. The artemisinin adduct, unlike the chloroquine-heme complex, is not toxic for *Plasmodium.* Erythrocyte membranes, however, are oxidized when incubated with heme and artemisinin.[32] Oxidation of membrane thiols is inhibited by iron-chelating compounds.[33] Artemisinin kills *Leishmania* parasites inside the macrophages of drug-treated animals; it does not affect the viability of the macrophages, nor does it alter the proliferative response of spleen cells to the mitogen, phytohemagglutinin.[34]

Artemisinin has been administered to over 2 million Chinese. Neurotoxicity has been observed after prolonged high doses of artemisinin, but toxicity is minimal at therapeutic doses. Artemisinin is very rapidly metabolized. Some analogues have been developed that are active transdermally. Artemisinin is availalble for oral and parenteral use. A derivative of artemisinin, artemether, has been administered IM as a 4 mg/kg loading dose, followed by 2 mg/kg daily, and found to be as effective as chloroquine in treating acute malaria in children.[35]

Antimony and Arsenical Compounds (Table 100.6; Figure 100.7)

Antimony compounds have been used to treat human leishmaniasis since the turn of the 20th century. Soon after the introduction of salvarsan by Ehrlich in 1910 for the treatment of syphilis, antiparasitic arsenicals and antimonials were prescribed for trypanosomiasis. Trivalent antimony compounds now have been replaced by the less toxic pentavalent compounds, and the trivalent compounds are becoming obsolete in schistosome infections. Pentavalent antimonials are expensive and may be toxic, particularly when administered for prolonged periods; this limits their usefulness in such diseases as cutaneous and mucocutaneous leishmaniasis.

Antimony sodium gluconate (antimony gluconate sodium; sodium antimony gluconate; sodium stibogluconate) is a complex containing both trivalent and pentavalent antimony. The trivalent antimony compound (Triostam), molecular weight 337, is an amorphous powder soluble in water. The pH of a 2 percent aqueous solution is 9 to 10. The solution at these alkaline conditions is unstable and should be adjusted to pH 6 to 7 with gluconic acid to achieve stability. The pentavalent antimony compound (Pentostam, Stibanate) forms crystals freely soluble in water. The pH of a 10 percent aqueous solution is 5.5.

Antimony sodium gluconate is the drug of choice for cutaneous, mucocutaneous and visceral leishmaniasis.[36] The mechanism of action of pentavalent antimony compounds is poorly understood. Antimony sodium gluconate displays antiparasitic activity against *Leishmania* inside reticuloendothelial cells but has little activity against the extracellular parasite. There is a correlation between susceptibility to antimony compounds and inhibition of glycolytic enzymes and of fatty acid *beta*-oxidation. Strains of *Leishmania* resistant to antimony compounds have emerged.[37] These strains appear to have decreased accumulation of drug, but it is not known whether the alteration reflects impaired uptake or increased efflux.[38]

Antimony sodium gluconate frequently causes painful local inflammation following leakage during IV administration, coughing and vomiting when IV administration is rapid, muscle pain and joint stiffness,

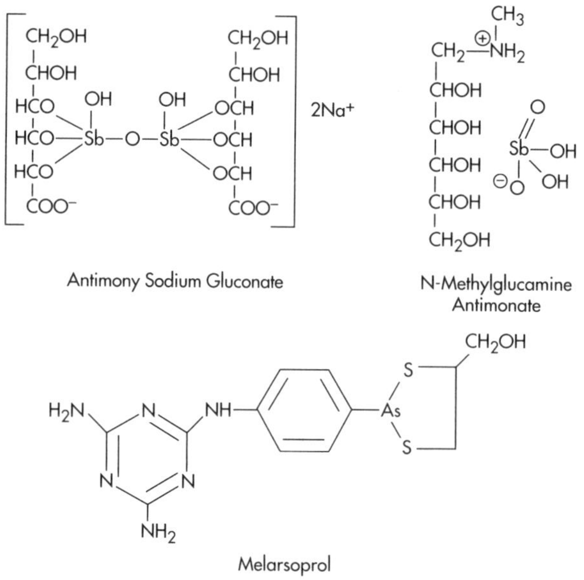

Antimony Sodium Gluconate

N-Methylglucamine Antimonate

Melarsoprol

Figure 100.7 Antimonal and Arsenical Compounds

Table 100.6 Selected Regimens for Miscellaneous Antiprotozoan Drugs

Disease	Drug	Route	Dose	Duration
Amebiasis (adult)	Diloxanide furoate	Oral	500 mg/kg	tid × 10 d
Amebiasis (child)	Diloxanide furoate	Oral	6.3 mg/kg	tid × 10 d
Leishmaniasis	Pentamidine	IM	2 to 4 mg/kg	up to 15 doses
Leishmaniasis (adult)	Antimony sodium gluconate	IM or IV	20 mg/kg	4 wk; maximum 850 mg antimony
Leishmaniasis (adult)	N-methylglucamine	IM	10 mg/kg	10 d
Leishmaniasis (child)	Antimony sodium gluconate	IM or IV	10 to 20 mg/kg	4 wk
Leishmaniasis (child)	N-methylglucamine	IM	15 mg/kg	10 d
Chagas' disease (adult)	Nifurtimox	Oral	2 to 2.5 mg/kg	qid × 120 d
Chagas' disease (child)	Nifurtimox	Oral	3.5 to 4 mg/kg	qid × 90 d
Sleeping sickness (adult)	Melarsoprol	IV	3.6 mg/kg	3d; repeated after 1 or 2 wk
Sleeping sickness (child)	Melarsoprol	IV	1.8 mg/kg	3d; repeated after 1 or 2 wk
Sleeping sickness	Pentamidine	IM	4 mg/kg	10 d
Cryptosporidiosis (adult)	Furazolidone	Oral	100 mg/kg	qid × 10 d
Cryptosporidiosis (child)	Furazolidone	Oral	1.5 mg/kg	qid × 4 d
			1.5 mg/kg	tid; days 4 to 10
Toxoplasmosis	Atovaquone	Oral	750 mg	tid
Pneumocystosis	Pentamidine	IM	4 mg/kg	10 to 14 d
Pneumocystosis (adult)	Pentamidine	IV	200 to 300 mg	every 2 wk
Pneumocystosis (adult)	Pentamidine	Inhalation	300 mg	every 4 wk
Pneumocystosis	Atovaquone	Oral	750 mg	tid
Malaria	Atovaquone	Oral	750 mg	tid

and bradycardia. Up to 80 percent of patients experience myalgia or arthralgia, and 30 percent anorexia.[39] This drug occasionally causes colic, diarrhea, rash, pruritus, and myocardial damage. On rare occasions, liver damage, hemolytic anemia, kidney damage, shock and sudden death have been attributed to use of antimony. High doses may precipitate fatal arrhythmias.

The trivalent antimony compound has antischistosomal activity, whereas the pentavalent antimony compound has antileishmanial activity. About 60 to 80 percent of injected pentavalent antimonials are excreted by the kidneys within six hours. The administration of antimonials every eight to 12 hours is pharmacologically more sound and clinically more effective than the traditional once daily regimen.

Antimony sodium gluconate (stibogluconate sodium, Pentostam) is available in a parenteral formulation containing 330 mg drug, which is equivalent to 100 mg elemental antimony/ml. It is obtained from the CDC Parasitic Diseases Drug Service.

N-methylglucamine antimonate (1-deoxy-1-(methylamino)-D-glucitol antimonate; meglumine antimonate) is practically insoluble in ethanol and diethyl ether. It is soluble in water (35% w/w). The pH of aqueous solutions is 6 to 7. The molecular weight is 366. N-methylglucamine antimonate evolved from the observation that antimonic acid combines with organic amines to yield a product that is stabilized by carbohydrates.

N-methylglucamine, along with antimony sodium gluconate, is a drug of choice in the treatment of leishmaniasis, even though it is both difficult to administer and expensive.[40] Pentavalent N-methylglucamine antimonate is safer than the trivalent antimonials. Nevertheless, administration of this drug is associated with anorexia, vomiting, nausea, headaches, abdominal pain, and lethargy. N-methylglucamine also can cause cardiac and renal toxicity.

N-methylglucamine antimonate may be administered IM or IV. High blood levels are achieved by either route. The drug is cleared by the kidneys, with half of the drug eliminated in 24 hours. Accordingly, daily injections are adequate to maintain therapeutic levels.

N-methyl glucamine antimonate (Glucantime) is available in ampoules containing 300 mg of drug (100 mg antimony) for parenteral administration. This drug is widely used in Europe, but it is not available in the US.[41]

The arsenical compounds may be pentavalent or trivalent. Both forms cross the blood/brain barrier. Arsenicals have found limited clinical utility because of their high reactivity with both host and parasite constituents. In an effort to develop safer arsenicals, arsenoxides have been coupled with compounds having fewer reactive sulfhydryl groups. Melarsoprol (2-[4-[(4,6-diamino-1,3,5-triazin-2-yl)amino] phenyl]-1,3,2-dithiarsolane-4-methanol) is a condensate of melarsen oxide and dimercaptopropanol. It is practically insoluble in water and cold ethanol. It has a molecular weight of 398. Melarsoprol was introduced clinically in 1949.

Melarsoprol is the principal drug for late-stage CNS disease in African trypanosomiasis or sleeping sickness.

Blood trypanosomes lack a functional tricarboxylic acid cycle and are entirely dependent on substrate level phosphorylation by glycolysis for ATP production. It has been proposed that the arsenicals act by inhibiting glycolysis, specifically by a primary inhibition of trypanosomal pyruvate kinase. The arsenic moiety of melarsoprol interacts with thiol groups, and is known to inhibit fructose-6-phosphate-2-kinase, which catalyzes the synthesis of fructose 2,6-bisphosphate. Trypanosomes rapidly lose motility and the cells lyse following inhibition by trivalent arsenicals. Melarsoprol also interacts with the spermidine-glutathione peptide trypanothione, which is unique to trypanosomes and substitutes for glutathione in reducing reactive oxygen radicals. Trypanosomes poisoned with melarsoprol cannot maintain a reduced cytosolic environment, and the cells lyse. It has also been proposed that melarsen oxide inhibits lipoic acid synthesis, thereby retarding lipoic acid facilitated transport of ribose, galactose, and maltose. Trypanosomes have no de novo synthesis of purines and salvage preformed purines from the host. Melaminophenyl arsenicals inhibit uptake of adenine and adenosine by the trypansomal transporter. Melarsoprol resistant trypanosomes lack this transporter, which also carries the drug into the cell.[42]

The plasma concentration of melarsoprol is 2 to 4 μg/ml 24 hours after administration. Elimination is biphasic, with a half-life of 35 hours.[43] The safety margin for melarsoprol is low.

Melarsoprol (Arsobal) is available for use IV in spite of its poor solubility in water; it is obtained from the CDC Parasitic Diseases Drug Service. The drug is dispensed in 5-ml ampoules containing a 3.6 percent solution in propylene glycol.

Nitrofurfuryl Compounds (Fig. 100.8)

Nifurtimox (4-[(5-nitrofurfurylidene)amino]-3-methylthiomorpholine-1,1-dioxide) forms orange-red crystals. It has a molecular weight of 287. The drug should be stored in airtight containers and protected from the light.

Nifurtimox was introduced clinically in 1972. It is used to treat South American trypanosomiasis or Chagas' disease. The cytotoxic effects of nitroaromatic compounds have been attributed to the formation of reduced intermediates such as nitroaryl radicals.[44] Nitroaryl radicals may be oxidized to generate superoxide anions, which in turn will generate hydrogen peroxide.[45] A number of parasites lack catalase, accounting for the selective toxicity of nitroaromatic drugs against trypanosomes.

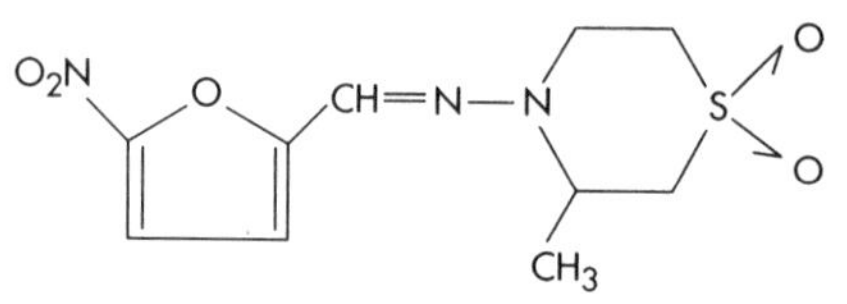

Nifurtimox

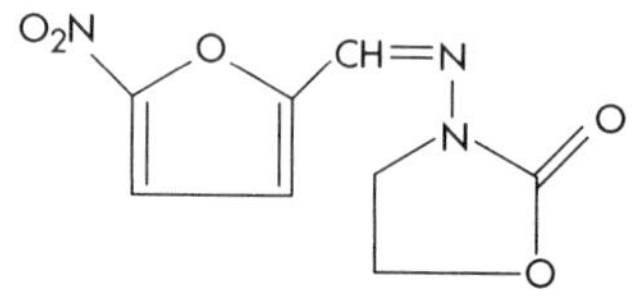

Furazolidone

Figure 100.8 Nitrofurfuryl Compounds

Nifurtimox is frequently associated with anorexia, vomiting, weight loss, loss of memory, sleep disorders, tremors, paresthesias, weakness, and polyneuritis. It is rarely the cause of convulsions. Children experience fewer adverse side-effects than do adults.

Nifurtimox is well absorbed by the oral route, but only low plasma concentrations are achieved. It is obtained from the CDC Parasitic Diseases Drug Service. Nifurtimox (Lampit) is available in 30-mg and 120-mg tablets for oral administration.

Furazolidone (3-(5-nitrofurfurylideneamino)-2-oxazolidinone) forms yellow crystals that darken under strong light. Furazolidone is slightly soluble in water at pH 6 (40 mg/liter). It decomposes in alkaline solutions; it has a molecular weight of 225.

Furazolidone is effective in giardiasis, but is not widely used. It has been reported to have some efficacy in treating cryptosporidiosis. Furazolidone inhibits monoamine oxidase, but administration of furazolidone at the recommended dose of 400 mg/d for five days should not constitute an undue risk of hypertensive crisis precipitated by monoamine oxidase inhibition. This drug should not be administered to infants under one month of age because of the possibility of inducing hemolytic anemia. Furazolidone appears to be tumorigenic in laboratory animals.

Furazolidone is reduced in vivo to the cytotoxic nitroanion radical by NADPH/NADH oxidase. Glutathione inhibits formation of the toxic nitroanion.[46]

Furazolidone occasionally causes nausea, vomiting, headaches, and malaise. It is rarely associated with hypotension, urticaria, arthralgia, rash, hemolytic anemia, other blood dyscrasias, and an Antabuse-like reaction to ethanol consumption. Patients should avoid tyramine-containing foods such as broad beans, yeast extracts, strong unpasteurized cheese, beer, wine, pickled herring, chicken livers, and fermented products while taking furazolidone. Sedatives, antihistamines, tranquilizers, and narcotics should be used in reduced doses concurrently with furazolidone.

Furazolidone (Furoxone) is available in 100-mg tablets and in a liquid for oral administration (50 mg/15 ml).

Miscellaneous Antiprotozoan Drugs (Fig. 100.9)

Pentamidine isethionate (p,p′-(pentamethylene-dioxyl)dibenzamidine bis (*beta*-hydroxyethanesulfonate)) is a white crystalline powder slightly soluble in ethanol and insoluble in diethyl ether. It is more soluble in boiling water (2.5 g/ 10ml) than in water at 25 C (1 g in 10 ml). The pH of a 5 percent aqueous solution is 4.5 to 6.5. It has a molecular weight of 593.

Pentamidine was developed in a rational drug design program, based upon the proposition that hypoglycemic diamidines might selectively inhibit trypanosome glycolysis. The antiprotozoan activity of this drug however is unrelated to glycolysis. Pentamidine was introduced clinically in 1940 for the treatment of sleeping sickness.

Pentamidine is one of the preferred drugs for the treatment of *Pneumocystis* pneumonia, particularly in patients with AIDS and in immunosuppressed transplant patients.[47] Over half of these patients, however, develop severe adverse reactions to the drug, and treatment must be discontinued. Pentamidine is used to treat kala-azar or visceral leishmaniasis. It should be used when antimony sodium gluconate therapy has failed. All solutions of pentamidine should be protected from light to avoid production of hepatotoxic compounds. Pentamidine is also used to treat patients with early stage African trypanosomiasis or sleeping sickness and for prophylaxis.

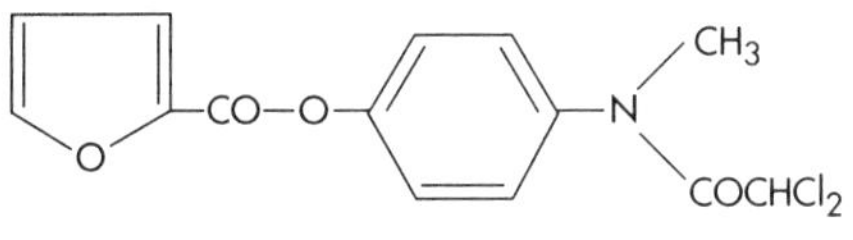

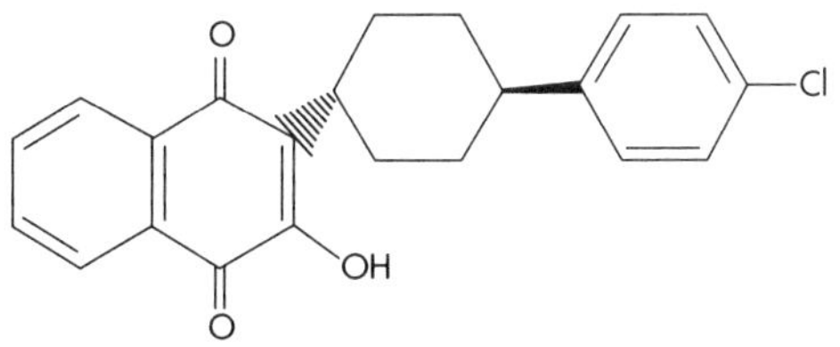

Figure 100.9 Miscellaneous Antiprotozoan Drugs

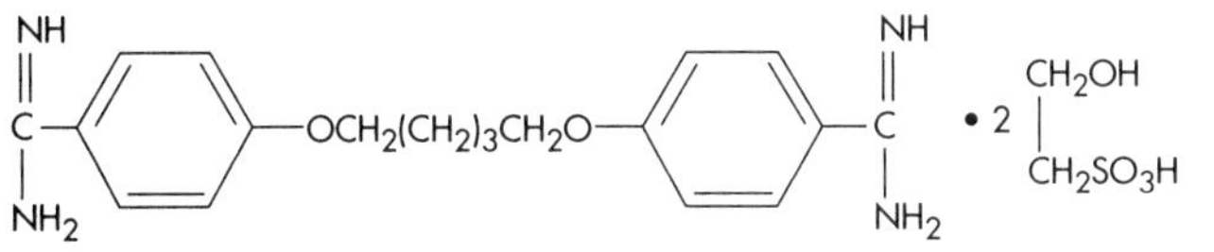

Pentamidine isethionate interferes with protozoal nuclear metabolism by inhibiting DNA, RNA, phospholipid, and protein synthesis. Pentamidine has a high affinity for kinetoplast DNA, and suppresses kinetoplast replication and function. It also causes ultrastructural disruption of the mitochondria of *Leishmania*. It has been proposed that pentamidine inhibits dihydrofolate reductase activity.

Pentamidine isethionate therapy frequently is associated with fatigue, dizziness, rash, hypotension, vomiting, blood dyscrasias, kidney damage, and pain at the site of injection. Pentamidine occasionally causes hypoglycemia, shock, and liver damage, and may aggravate diabetes. It is rarely responsible for a Herxheimer-type reaction.

The mean concentration of pentamidine in bronchoalveolar lavage fluid 18 to 24 hours after inhalation therapy (300 mg) is 23 ng/ml. An IV dose of 4 mg/kg gives a concentration of 2.6 ng/ml in the bronchoalveolar fluid. The plasma level after IV infusion of 4 mg drug/kg is 612 ng/ml, with a plasma half-life of six hours. The pentamidine level in plasma of patients administered drug by inhalation is lower than that achieved with IV administration; depending on the inhalation protocol and equipment, it may not be detected in plasma (> 2 ng/ml) or may be as high as 19 ng/ml. Pentamidine is excreted slowly by the liver and kidneys, requiring five days to eliminate half of an administered dose.

Pentamidine isethionate (NebuPent, Pentam, Lomidine) is available for parenteral use or inhalation. Both treatment regimens are efficacious in pneumocystosis.[48] Parenteral formulations are dispensed in 300-mg vials. NubuPent is a sterile, nonpyrogenic lyophilized powder that is reconstituted in water and administered by inhalation (300 mg in 6 ml, delivered in 30 to 45 min). Parenteral formulations for IM administration are dispensed in 300 mg vials and the contents dissolved in 3 ml; for IV administration, the 300 mg is dissolved in 50 to 250 ml and infused over a 60-minute period.

Diloxanide furoate is the ester of diloxanide and 2-furoic acid. Diloxanide (2,2-dichloro-N-(4-hydroxyphenyl)-N-methylacetamide; N-dichloroacet-4-hydroxy-N-methylanilide) has a molecular weight of 234. Diloxanide was discovered during a program to develop an amebicide, starting with haloacetamides. Diloxanide furoate, molecular weight 328, is slightly soluble in water. The drug resembles chloramphenicol structurally, and it has been proposed that this drug also inhibits protein synthesis.

Diloxanide furoate is an alternative to diiodohydroxyquin for the treatment of asymptomatic amebiasis.[49] Diloxanide furoate is directly amebicidal. It appears that amebae, rather than cysts, are the vulnerable cell type. This drug frequently causes flatulence and occasionally causes nausea, vomiting, diarrhea, urticaria, and pruritus.

Diloxanide is absorbed from the intestine after oral administration, with most of the furoate ester being hydrolyzed before absorption. The drug is excreted by the kidneys (75%), mostly as the glucuronide. Less than 10 percent of the drug is excreted in the feces. Diloxanide furoate (Furamide), which can be obtained from the CDC Parasitic Diseases Drug Service, is available in 500-mg tablets for oral use.

Atovaquone is a hydronaphthoquinone. The potential of hydroxynaphthoquinones as antimalarial drugs was examined at the beginning of Word War II because of the shortage of quinine. Most hydroxynaphthoquinones lack activity when administered orally and are rapidly metabolized. After an intensive search, lapinone was developed. This congener had some activity against *Plasmodium vivax* infections in humans when administered IV. The search for an orally active, metabolically stable congener active against *Plasmodium falciparum* was renewed in the 1980s.

Atovaquone is a promising drug for the treatment of malaria and for *Pneumoncystis carinii* pneumonia and toxoplasmosis. Atovaquone is somewhat less effective in treating pneumocystosis than trimethoprim-sulfamethoxazole, but it produces fewer adverse side-effects.[50] As many as 25 percent of malaria patients treated with atovaquone alone relapsed, even after prolonged treatment. Consequently, atovaqone is given in combination with chlorguanide, and has been remarkably successful in treating drug-resistant malaria in southeast Asia. Atovaquone causes rashes, nausea, diarrhea, headaches, vomiting, fever, insomnia, asthenia, and pruritus.

Hydronaphthoquinones are potent inhibitors of mitochondrial electron transport, competing with the biologic electron carrier ubiquinone. Atovaquone binds selectively to the ubinquinol–cytochrome c reductase region of the respiratory chain. Oxidation of dihydroorotate to orate by dihydroorotate dehydrogenase is key for pyrimidine synthesis. The malarial parasite, unlike humans, relies exclusively on de novo synthesis of pyrimidines. Hydronaphthoquinones disrupt plasmodial pyrimidine biosynthesis without altering ATP levels. This mechanism of action is different from that of any other antimalarial drug and accounts for its efficacy against drug-resistant strains of *Plasmodium*.[51]

Atovaquone is active when taken orally. The plasma half-life of atovaquone is 70 hours. The drug is extensively bound to plasma proteins, and is absorbed from the intestine and recycled through the liver.[52] There is no evidence of hepatic metabolism. The relationship between oral doses of 75 to 450 mg and plasma levels is linear, with plasma levels of 0.2 μg/ml being achieved with a single 225-mg dose. The steady state blood level is 7.5 μg/ml in subjects ingesting 750 mg of drug daily. Plasma levels are fivefold lower in patients who have not eaten prior to drug administration than in fed patients. Most of the drug is eliminated in the feces (95% over a 21-day period), with essentially no drug excreted in the urine. Atovaquone (Mepron) is available for oral administration in 250 mg tablets. The regimen for treatment of pneumocystosis is 750 mg orally tid for 21 days.

Parasitic Helminths

The helminths are macroscopic multicellular worms. Like humans, helminths have digestive, excretory, reproductive, and nervous systems. The worms of medical significance are classified according to their biologic relationships and according to their habitat in the host. Medically important helminths are found in the Nematoda (threadworms or roundworms) and the Platyhelminthes (flatworms), which include the trematodes (flukes) and cestodes (tapeworms). Parasitic helminths are found in the intestines, liver, blood, and other tissues. Literally billions of people worldwide are infected with parasitic helminths.[53] It has been estimated that 1 billion people are infected with the roundworm *Ascaris*, with as many as 100,000 deaths annually; 900 million are infected with hookworms, with as many as 60,000 deaths annually; 200 million are infected with schistosomes, with as many as 200,000 deaths annually; and 950 million are infected with the whipworm *Trichuris*. In the basic life cycle of parasitic helminths, the adult sexual stage occurs in the definitive host. Eggs produced in this stage usually pass outside the body of the definitive host. The eggs then hatch and develop into larvae, frequently inside an intermediate host. Transmission to humans occurs by ingestion of food or water contaminated with eggs or larvae, larvae in the soil may penetrate the skin at the point of contact, or larvae may be transmitted by insect bites. Although some worms go directly to their characteristic habitat within the body, others make grand tours before settling into the characteristic site. Unlike parasitic protozoa, reduction in the number of parasitic helminths, rather than complete elimination, may be a satisfactory chemotherapeutic outcome. A few persisting helminths may be better tolerated than the anthelmintic drugs necessary for complete eradication.[r10]

Chemotherapy is now an effective tool for the control of helminthic parasitic infections, especially in children in underdeveloped countries. Expeditious treatment of individuals with helminthic infections limits the spread of the disease. It has been suggested that mass medication without diagnosis may be justified in endemic areas.[54] Three drugs, albendazole, praziquantel, and ivermectin, are effective in treating 19 of the 23 major human helminthic infections, and these three drugs are relatively safe.

Pinworms

Enterobiasis is the most common parasitic disease of children in the US. It is especially prevalent in children attending daycare centers. Pinworms cause a benign intestinal disease that develops following ingestion of embryonated eggs. Symptoms are associated with nocturnal migration of female worms and egg deposition on the perianal folds. Common symptoms include anal itching, nervousness, and irritability.

Whipworms

Trichuriasis is a chronic infection of the large intestine. Adult worms live intertwined in the mucosa of the appendix. Adult worms in the intestine may produce abdominal pain and mucous diarrhea. Humans are infected by ingesting embryonated eggs.

Ascariasis

Ascariasis is a chronic roundworm infection of the small intestine caused by *Ascaris lumbricoides.* Even light infections in children may produce abdominal pain, intermittent colic, and nervous manifestations. Larvae in the lungs often cause pneumonia characterized by cough, hemoptysis, fever, and esosinophilia. Adult roundworms may migrate from the intestine into the liver, peritoneal cavity, and appendix.

Trichinosis

Trichinella spiralis larvae mature into adults in the intestine. The adult *Trichinella* in the intestine mate, and new larvae enter the blood stream and are carried to all parts of the body; they encyst in striated muscle. Symptoms include muscle pain, fever, eosinophilia, and general weakness.

Hookworms

Hookworm infections are caused by *Ancylostoma duodenale* and by *Necator americanus.* Infections in humans occur when infective larvae penetrate the exposed skin, usually the foot. The larvae migrate through the lungs, often causing pneumonia or bronchitis. Adult hookworms are found attached to the villi of the small intestine.

Strongyloidiasis

Moderate infections by *Strongyloides stercoralis* are characterized by intermittent diarrhea and upper abdominal pain. Severe infections are characterized by vomiting, acute abdominal pain, malabsorption syndrome, dehydration, and electrolyte disturbance. Larvae migrating through the lungs also can cause a diffuse pneumonitis. Damage to the intestinal mucosa may produce a catarrhal enteritis. Strongyloidiasis may persist for many years due to autoinfection by larvae that transform to the filarial stage within the intestine.

Filariasis

Symptoms of acute filariasis caused by *Wuchereria bancrofti* or *Brugia malayi* are fever, eosinophilia, lymphangitis, and lymphadenitis. Chronic filariasis is characterized by obstruction of the lymphatics and hypertrophy of the skin and subcutaneous tissue of the limbs, genitalia, or breasts, leading to "elephantiasis." It is estimated that 100 million people are infected with lymphatic filariasis, and that 60 million of these are in China, India, and Indonesia.

Onchocerciasis

River blindness is caused by *Onchocerca volvulus,* which is endemic to the tropical zone of Africa and to Central and South America. Adult worms live in a tangled mass in the subcutaneous tissues of infected humans. Degenerating microfilaria elicit a granulomatous reaction or eosinophilic infiltration. Microfilaria and their inflammatory reactions occur in various sites within the body, including the lungs, liver, spleen and kidney. Damage to the eyes is caused by living or dead microfilaria.

Liver Flukes

Liver flukes (liver trematodes) irritate the bile duct and cause diarrhea and eosinophilia. Two closely related etiologic agents are *Clonorchis sinensis* and *Opisthorchis viverrini.* The endemic areas of *Clonorchis sinensis* extend through Southeast Asia, Russia, and Eastern Europe. *Opisthorchis viverrini* is prevalent in Thailand and Laos. Chronic disease leads to cirrhosis of the liver. Death seldom results directly from the infection, but rather is attributable to malnutrition, secondary infections, and carcinoma when there is a heavy burden of liver flukes. It has been estimated that 20 million people harbor liver flukes worldwide.[55]

Schistosomiasis

Schistosomes (blood trematodes) growing in the liver may produce an acute hepatitis. Much of the pathology associated with schistosome infection is attributable to immune reactions to the eggs of the parasite. Granulomas form around the eggs in the liver, resulting in fibrosis and cirrhosis. Larvae undergo maturation within the liver and then migrate to the veins. Dysentery is often associated with the presence of egg-laying schistosomes in the mesenteric venules. Hematuria and cystitis often accompany *Schistosoma haematobium* infection.

Tapeworms

Most of the tapeworms (cestodes) are intestinal parasites, although a few invade the tissues of the body in the larval stages. The tapeworm consists of a series of segments: the head or scolex; the neck; and the segments or proglottids. The scolex is the hold-fast segment with suction cups or suckers that anchor the tapeworm to the intestinal wall. Successful treatment of tapeworm infections requires that the scolex be detached and expelled. The neck region is the site of reproduction of new proglottids. The proglottids distal to the scolex are the mature segments that produce eggs. The tapeworms have no digestive tract and depend on the host for their nutrients. Tapeworms require monosaccharides, amino acids, and vitamins as nutrients. The larval stages of tapeworms may develop in extraintestinal tissues, causing cysticercosis (*Taenia solium*) or hydatid disease (*Echinococcus*).

Anthelmintic Drugs (Table 100.7)

Imidazole Compounds (Table 100.8; Figs. 100.10, 100.11)

Imidazole derivatives have become increasingly important in treating parasitic and fungal diseases. The antifungal imidazole miconazole has been used in granulomatous amebic encephalitis, and ketoconazole has been used to treat *Acanthamoeba* keratitis. Benzimidazole compounds were introduced as anthelmintics over 30 years ago, and heralded as a major advance in the treatment of nematode infections.[r11] Selective toxicity of the imidazoles is, in part, attributable to the different composition of cell membranes of humans and parasites; humans have cholesterol in their cell membranes, whereas fungi and parasites have ergosterol in theirs. Imidazoles interfere with the biosynthesis of C28 sterols in *Leishmania* and other parasites, and inhibit the cytochrome P-450 demethylation of lanosterol, which is the precursor of ergosterol.

Albendazole ([5-(propylthio)-1H-benzimidazol-2-yl] carbamic acid methyl ester) is a benzimidazole carbamate that forms colorless crystals. The drug is insoluble in water; it has a molecular weight of 265.

Albendazole is widely used as a safe anthelmintic with high activity against eggs, larvae, and adult stages. It is used in such systemic helminthic infections as: cysticercosis, caused by the tapeworm *Taenia solium;* hydatidosis, caused by larvae of the tapeworm *Echinococcus;*[56] and systemic filariasis, caused by nematodes. Albendazole should be used before surgical intervention for hydatid disease.[57] A single dose of albendazole is effective in treating many helminthic infections such as pinworms (*Enterobius*), whipworm (*Trichuris*), hookworms (*Ancylostoma* and *Necator*), and roundworms (*Ascaris*). Higher doses of albendazole are required to treat *Strongyloides* infections. Albendazole is a useful

Table 100.7 Standard Treatment Regimens for Anthelmintic Agents

Drug	Disease	Regimen
Praziquantel	Schistosomiasis	20 mg/kg orally, bid or tid
	Tapeworms	10 mg/kg orally once
	Flukes	20 mg/kg orally tid × 3d
Albendazole	Ascariasis	400 mg orally once
	Whipworms	400 mg orally once
	Hyatid disease	5 mg/kg bid × 30 d
Mebendazole	Ascariasis	100 mg orally bid × 3 d
	Pinworms	100 mg orally bid once
	Whipworms	100 mg orally bid × 3d
Thiabendazole	Strongyloidiasis	25 mg/kg orally bid × 2d
Ivermectin	Onchocerciasis	150 ug/kg, 4 doses 6 mo apart
Pyrantel	Hookworms	10 mg base/kg orally × 3 d
Diethylcarbamazine	Filariasis	50 mg 1st d & tid 2nd d orally; 100 mg tid 3rd d; 2 mg/kg tid × 4 to 21 d
Niclosamide	Tapeworms	2 g orally once

Table 100.8 Selected Regimens for Imidazole Drugs

Disease	Drug	Route	Dose	Duration
Entamoebiasis (adult)	Metronidazole	Oral	750 mg/kg	tid × 5–10 d
Entamoebiasis (child)	Metronidazole	Oral	12 to 16 mg/kg	tid × 5 d
Giardiasis (adult)	Metronidazole	Oral	250 mg	tid × 10 d
Giardiasis (child)	Metronidazole	Oral	5 mg/kg	tid × 5 d
Trichomoniasis (adult)	Metronidazole	Suppository	1 g	bid once
Trichomoniasis (adult)	Metronidazole	Oral	250 mg	tid × 7 d
Pinworms	Albendazole	Oral	400 mg	Once
Pinworms	Mebendazole	Oral	100 mg	1 dose; repeated after 2 wk
Whipworms (adult)	Albendazole	Oral	400 mg/kg	Once
Whipworms (adult & child)	Mebendazole	Oral	100 mg/kg	bid × 3 d
Whipworms (child)	Albendazole	Oral	200 mg/kg	Once
Ascariasis (adult)	Albendazole	Oral	400 mg/kg	Once
Ascariasis (adult & child)	Mebendazole	Oral	100 mg	bid × 3 d
Ascariasis (child)	Albendazole	Oral	200 mg/kg	Once
Visceral larva migrans	Thiabendazole	Oral	25 mg/kg	bid × 2 d; maximum 3 g/d
Trichinosis	Thiabendazole*	Oral	25 mg/kg	bid × 5 d; maximum 3 g/d
Hookworms (adult)	Albendazole	Oral	400 mg/kg	Once
Hookworms (child)	Albendazole	Oral	200 mg/kg	Once
Hookworms	Mebendazole	Oral	100 mg/kg	bid × 3 d
Hookworms	Thiabendazole	Oral	25 mg/kg	bid × 2 d; maximum 3 g/d
Strongyloidiasis	Thiabendazole	Oral	25 mg/kg	bid × 3 d; maximum 3 g/d
Capillariasis	Thiabendazole	Oral	25 mg/kg	30 d
River blindness	Metronizadole	Oral	1 g	bid × 28 d
Guinea worms (adult)	Metronizadole	Oral	250 mg	tid × 10 d
Guinea worms (child)	Metronizadole	Oral	8.3 mg/kg	tid × 10 d; maximum 750 mg/d
Guinea worms (adult)	Niridazole	Oral	25 mg/kg	15 d; maximum 1.5 g
Guinea worms (child)	Niridazole	Oral	12.5 mg/kg	bid × 15 d; maximum 1.5 g/d
Schistosomiasis (adult & child)	Niridazole	Oral	25 mg/kg	5 to 10 d; maximum 1.5 g/d
Cysticercosis	Albendazole	Oral	5 to 10 mg/kg	7 to 60 d
Hyatid disease	Albendazole	Oral	5 mg/kg	bid × 30 d; 1 wk rest; repat

*Response of trichinosis to thiabendazole is dubious

alternative to quinacrine and metronidazole in giardiasis. In fact, albendazole may be the drug of choice for children in developing countries where multiparasitism is a major problem.

Albendazole inhibits tubulin polymerization. It causes degenerative changes in the intestine and tegumental cells of helminths.

Albendazole occasionally is associated with transient epigastric pain and diarrhea. The drug should be used with caution in patients with liver and hematologic diseases. Teratogenicity and embryotoxicity have been observed in rats and rabbits, and the drug has not been approved for use in pregnant women.[58]

Albendazole is poorly absorbed from the intestines; it is not detected in blood because it is rapidly metabolized to its sulfoxide derivative. The sulfoxide metabolite has anthelmintic activity and may mediate most of the effects of albendazole treatment. After an oral dose of 400 mg albendazole, the peak plasma level of 240 ng/ml of the sulfoxide metabolite is reached within two to four hours. The plasma half life of the metabolite is 8.5 hours. Albendazole (Zentel), in 200-mg tablets, is available only from the manufacturer, SmithKline Beecham.

Metronidazole (2-methyl-5-nitroimidazole; 1-(2-hydroxyethyl)-2-methyl-5-nitroimidazole) is a nitroheterocyclic compound that forms cream-colored crystals. It has a molecular weight of 171. It is soluble in water (1 g/100ml) and in ethanol (0.5 g/100 ml), but is poorly soluble in diethyl ether and chloroform. It is soluble in dilute acids. The pH of a saturated aqueous solution is 5.8.

Metronidazole has been used for three decades to treat infections caused by anaerobic protozoa and bacteria, including trichomoniasis, giardiasis, and amebiasis. Metronidazole has been used to treat trichomoniasis since the 1950s. Metronidazole is recommended for giardiasis in children because it is less toxic than quinacrine. Metronidazole is used in combination with diiodohydroxyquin in mild to severe intestinal amebiasis and liver abscesses. Metronidazole is an alternative drug for guinea worm infections. The drug is not considered a vermicide and does not prevent new lesions from appearing. Tinidazole is a nitroimidazole similar to metronidazole, but is not marketed in the US. Tinidazole appears to be as effectivve as metronidazole in the treatment of amebiasis and giardiasis and is better tolerated.[r12] During the 1980s, metronidazole and other 5-nitroimidazoles have been used to increase the susceptibility of hypoxic tumors to radiotherapy. Patients with severe hepatic disease metabolize metronidazole slowly, resulting in accumulation of the drug and its metabolites.

Metronidazole is selectively toxic for anaerobic cells. Metronidazole must be reduced to the active form, which occurs in cells with a sufficiently negative redox potential. In *Trichomonas vaginalis*, metronidazole is activated by the transfer of electrons from ferredoxin to the nitro group of the drug. The antimicrobial

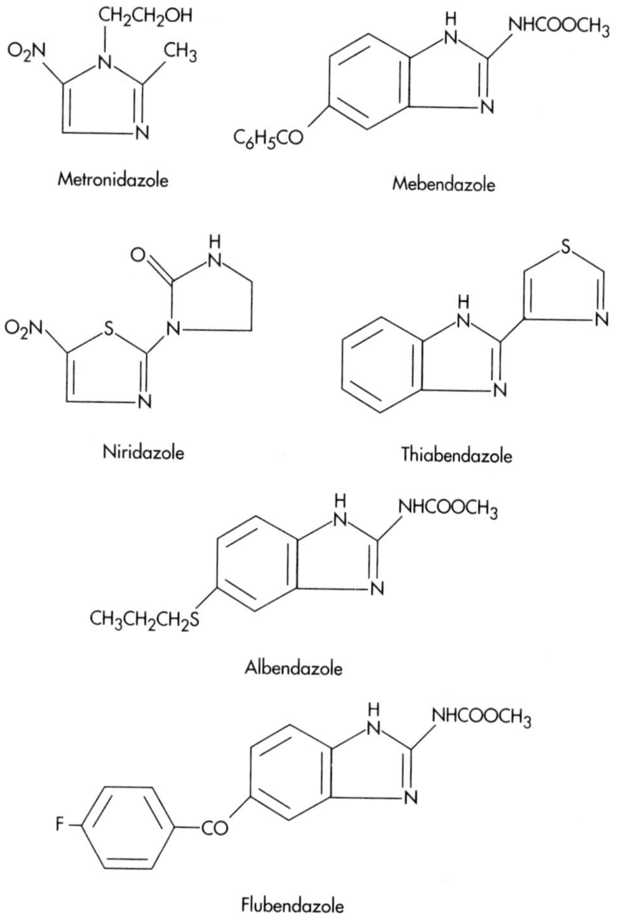

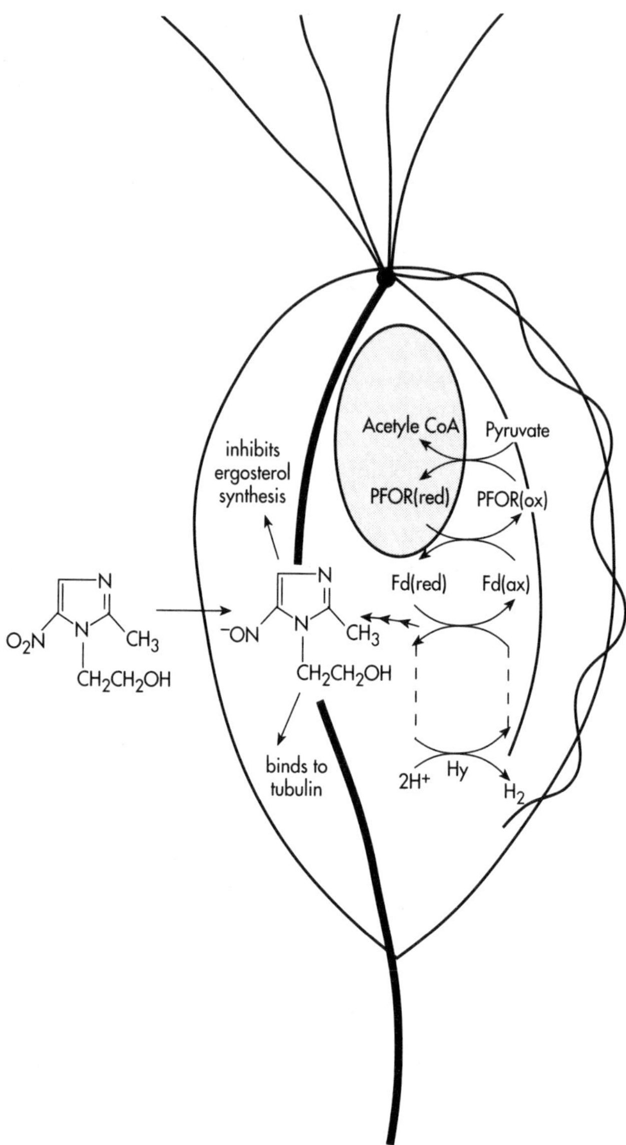

Figure 100.11 Activation of metronidazole in *Trichomonas*. PFOR: pyruvate ferredoxin oxidoreductase; Fd: ferredoxin; Hy: hydrogenase.

activity of reduced metronidazole results from short-lived hydroyxlamine intermediates, which interact with such cellular constituents as DNA, proteins and membranes, resulting in irreparable cell damage.[59]

Metronidazole frequently causes nausea and headaches, and leaves a metallic aftertaste. The drug occasionally causes vomiting, diarrhea, insomnia, weakness, stomatitis, vertigo, paresthesia, rash, dark urine, and a dry mouth. It rarely causes ataxia, depression, irritability, and confusion. Metronidazole rarely produces a mild Antabuse reaction after ethanol consumption. The drug crosses the placental barrier and enters the fetal circulation. Metronidazole is carcinogenic in rodents and mutagenic in bacteria, and generally

Metronidazole

Mebendazole

Niridazole

Thiabendazole

Albendazole

Flubendazole

Figure 100.10 Imidazoles

should not be used in pregnant women, particularly during the first trimester. Metronidazole has been reported to potentiate the anticoagulant effect of warfarin and other oral coumarin anticoagulants, resulting in prolonged prothrombin times. Drugs that induce microsomal liver enzymes, e.g., phenobarbital, may accelerate elimination of metronidazole, and drugs that decrease microsomal liver enzymes, e.g., cimetidine, may prolong metronidazole plasma half-life. Doses of 1.5 g cause nausea, vomiting, and ataxia.

Metronidazole can be administered orally, IV, rectally, or intravaginally.[60] The drug is rapidly and almost completely absorbed after oral administration. The peak serum level, achieved in one to two hours after ingestion of 500 mg, is 12 μg/ml, with a serum half-life of eight hours. Unaltered metronidazole is the major component in the plasma. Plasma concentrations of metronidazole are proportional to the administered dose. After a 15 mg/kg loading dose, followed six hours later by 7.5 mg/kg every six hours, the steady state plasma level is 25 μg/ml. Metronidazole and its metabolites are eliminated in the urine (60 to 80%) and feces (6 to 15%). About 20 percent of the excreted drug is unaltered metronidazole. The metabolites in the urine are the glucuronide conjugate of metronidazole and the product of side-chain oxidation. Less than 20 percent of the circulating drug is bound to plasma proteins. Metronidazole is found in the CSF, saliva, and breast milk at concentrations similar to plasma levels.

Metronidazole (Flagyl, Elyzol) is supplied as 250-mg and 500-mg tablets, and in 500-mg vials for IV use after addition of 100 ml of fluid. It is available in 500-mg and 1000-mg suppositories. When metronidazole cannot be given by the oral route, the rectal route is usually preferable to the IV route because of the greater cost of the latter.

Mebendazole was introduced clinically as an antinematode agent in 1971. Structurally, a 2-carbamomethoxy group replaces the thiazole ring present in the older benzimidazole, thiabendazole. Mebendazole (5-benzoyl-1H-benzimidazol-2-yl)-carbamic acid methyl ester; Vermox) is a benzimidazole derivative with a molecular weight of 295. It is practically insoluble in water. Flubendazole is the 5-(4-fluorobenzoyl) congener of mebendazole.

Mebendazole is used to treat pinworms, whipworms (trichuriasis), roundworms (ascariasis), hookworms, and an intestinal roundworm found in the Philippines, *Capillaria*. The patient's family also should be treated for pinworm infections to prevent recurrence. Mebendazole has no effect on hydatid disease. Mebendazole is as effective as albendazole in treating ascariasis and more effective in treating trichuriasis.[61]

Mebendazole and flubendazole bind tightly to the tubulin of *Onchocerca*, preventing polymerization into microtubules. Mebendazole also causes several other effects, such a glycogen depletion and reduction of glucose transport.

Mebendazole is occasionally responsible for diarrhea or abdominal pain. Mebendazole should not be used during pregnancy because it is teratogenic and embryotoxic in animals. Flubendazole is not teratogenic but may cause abscesses at the site of injection.

Mebendazole is poorly absorbed when administered orally. Absorption is increased many fold when taken with a meal high in fat. Peak plasma levels are achieved within four hours, and 95 percent of the drug is bound to plasma proteins. The plasma half-life is 1.5 to 5.5 hours. The drug is excreted in the bile and eliminated in the feces. Mebendazole (Vermox) is supplied as a 100-mg chewable tablet.

Niridazole (1-(5-nitro-2-thiazolyl)-2-imidazolidinone; nitrothiamidazol) is a 5-nitrothiazole that forms yellow crystals and has a molecular weight of 214. It is practically insoluble in water.

Niridazole was introduced clinically in 1964 as an antischistosomal agent. This drug has had utility in treating a number of schistosome infections, but is becoming an obsolete drug for this purpose. Niridazole is also used to treat guinea worm infections.

Niridazole is selectively concentrated in germinal cells of schistosomes and impairs reproductive function. Changes in the vitelline gland lead to abnormal egg formation and eventual disruption. Spermatogenesis is also affected but female worms are more susceptible to the drug. Female schistosomes are attacked and destroyed in the liver by white cells, whereas male schistosomes are immobilized by connective tissue and undergo autolysis. Niridazole causes a depletion of glycogen stores in the parasite, but this is not obviously linked to the effects on reproduction.

Frequent adverse side-effects of niridazole include immunosuppression, vomiting, cramps, anorexia, dizziness, and headaches. Niridazole occasionally produces diarrhea, rash, insomnia, paresthesia, and slight EKG changes. On rare occasions niridazole causes psychosis, hyperexcitability, confusion, convulsions, and hemolytic anemia in glucose-6-phosphate dehydrogenase deficient patients. Niridazole is contraindicated in patients with hepatocellular disease, portal hypertension, or a history of mental disorders or seizures. An overdose causes GI complaints lasting for a few hours.

Niridazole is well absorbed over a period of several hours following oral administration. Following oral administration of 100 mg bid × 3d, plasma levels of the unaltered compound and its metabolite, methyl 5-benzoylbenzimidazole-2-amine, do not exceed 30 ng/ml and 9 ng/ml, respectively. The metabolite has no anthelmintic activity. Approximately 2 percent of the drug is excreted in the urine and 98 percent in the feces. Excretion is slow because the metabolites have a high binding affinity for plasma proteins. Niridazole

(Ambilhar) is supplied for oral administration in compressed 200-mg or 500-mg tablets.

Thiabendazole (2-(4-thiazolyl)-1H-benzimidazole) is fluorescent in acidic solutions, with excitation at 310 nm and emission at 370 nm. Its molecular weight is 201. Thiabendazole is most soluble in acidified water (pH 2.2), 3.8 g/100 ml. The material is only slightly soluble in alcohols.

Thiabendazole was introduced clinically to treat nematode infections in 1961. It was the first broad-spectrum anthelmintic to be developed for clinical use. Thiabendazole is used to treat *Trichostrongylus* infections, hookworms, guinea worms, *Strongyloides* infections, and *Capillaria* infections. Thiabendazole is the drug of choice for visceral larva migrans. Thiabendazole has been used to treat trichinosis, but its efficacy has not been definitively established. A derivative of thiabendazole is an effective fungicide used to control spoilage of citrus fruit and for the prevention and treatment of Dutch elm disease.

Thiabendazole is effective against adult worms and the development of larval stages. It allows egg formation, but the eggs in drug-treated hosts are not viable. Thiabendazole inhibits fumarate reductase. This enzyme is an essential component of anaerobic energy metabolism in nematodes. The ovicidal activity may reflect binding to worm embryonic tubulin.

Thiabendazole is one of the least well-tolerated of the currently available antinematode drugs. It causes GI upset, headaches, and drowsiness in about 30 percent of treated patients. Thiabendazole occasionally causes leukopenia, crystalluria, rash, hallucinations, and olfactory disturbances. On rare occasions, it causes shock, tinnitus, and Stevens-Johnson syndrome.

Thiabendazole is rapidly and almost completely absorbed after oral administration. Peak plasma levels of the drug (15 μg/ml) are achieved in one hour. About 90 percent of the drug is excreted in the urine within 24 hour and 5 percent is excreted in the feces. The drug is excreted unchanged, and as the 5-hydroxy derivative, its glucuronide and sulfate. Thiabendazole (Mintezol) is available in 500-mg tablets and suspensions of 100 mg/ml for oral administration.

Anthelmintic Antibiotic

Ivermectin is a semisynthetic member of the avermectin family of antibiotics and the closely related deglycosylated milbemycin family of antibiotics. The avermectins and milbemycins are both 16-membered macrocyclic lactones. Avermectins are highly lipophilic and dissolve in most organic solvents. Their solubility in water is low. The molecular weight of ivermectin B_{1a} is 874.

Avermectins (Fig. 100.12) are a group of broad spectrum antiparasitic antibiotics produced by *Streptomyces avermitilis*.[r13] Milbemycins are a family of macrolide antibiotics with insecticidal and acaricidal activity. They were originally isolated from a strain of *Streptomyces hygroscopicus*. Ivermectin was released for registration in 1981, and has been approved for use in over 60 countries.

Ivermectin is effective in treating a number of endoparasitic infections. The roundworms *Ascaris lumbricoides* and *Strongyloides stercoralis* are quite sensitive to this drug.[62] Ivermectin has been used to treat loiasis but diethylcabarbamazine is the recommended drug for this infection. Ivermectin is as effective as diethylcarbamazine in treating Bancroft's filariasis (elephantiasis). In addition, ivermectin reduces the incidence of vector transmitted parasitic infections.[63] Ivermectin has been used to treat onchocerciasis or river blindness. Onchocerciasis afflicts 40 million people in tropical Africa and Latin America, causing blindness in 2 million.[64]

Ivermectin acts by disrupting invertebrate neurotransmission mediated by *gamma*-aminobutyric acid. Ivermectin potentiates the release of *gamma*-aminobutyric acid from presynaptic inhibitory terminals, and causes a dose-dependent increase in chloride ion permeability. Ivermectin opens chloride ion channels in muscle membranes. The activation of *gamma*-aminobutyric acid pathways appears to block production and release of microfilariae. Ivermectin inhibits oral ingestion by nematodes, whereas motility, ATP levels, glucose uptake through the cuticle, and glucose metabolism are not affected. Ivermectin acts as a chemical ligature, paralyzing the nematode pharynx, blocking ingestion of nutrients essential for long-term survival.[65] Ivermectin also renders the worms infertile.

Headaches are a frequent adverse effect of ivermectin. Ivermectin occasionally is associated with weakness, fever, abdominal pain, myalgia, and arthralgia. Rare side-effects include anorexia, sweats, chills, and tender and swollen lymph nodes. Doses of ivermectin 40 times the therapeutic dose cause vomiting, dilation of the pupils, and sedation.

The peak blood level of ivermection four hours after an oral dose of 200 μg/kg is 20 ng/ml. The half-life is estimated to be 12 hours. Ivermectin and its metabolites are excreted in the bile with little urinary excretion. Some of the metabolites remain in the blood for a longer time than the parent ivermectin. About 50 to 60 percent of the drug in an orally administered tablet is available for absorption. Most of the administered drug is eliminated in the feces. Ivermectin (Mectizan) is available in tablet form from the CDC Parasitic Diseases Drug Service; there is no parenteral formulation.

Table 100.9 Selected Regimens for Miscellaneous Anthelmintic Drugs

Disease	Drug	Route	Dose	Duration
Pinworms	Piperazine citrate	Oral	65 mg/kg	7 d; maximum 2.5 g/d
Roundworms	Piperazine citrate	Oral	75 mg/kg	2 d; maximum 3.5 g
Ascariasis	Ivermectin	Oral	150 ug/kg	4 doses 6 months apart
Visceral larva migrans	Diethylcarbamazine	Oral	2 mg/kg	tid; 2 to 4 wk
Strongyloidiasis	Ivermectin	Oral	150 ug/kg	4 doses 6 months apart
Filariasis (adult)	Diethylcarbamazine	Oral	50 mg	Once on day 1; tid on day 2
			100 mg	tid on day 3
			2 mg/kg	tid; days 4 to 21
Filariasis (child)	Diethylcarbamazine	Oral	0.5 mg/kg	Once on day 1; bid on day 2
			1 mg/kg	tid on day 3
			2 mg/kg	tid; days 4 to 21
Elephantiasis	Ivermectin	Oral	150 ug/kg	4 doses 6 months apart
River blindness	Ivermectin	Oral	150 ug/kg	4 doses 6 months apart
River blindness (adult)	Diethylcarbamazine	Oral	25 mg	Once on day 1; tid on day 2
			50 mg	tid on day 3
			100 mg	tid; days 4 to 10
River blindness (child)	Diethylcarbamazine	Oral	0.5 mg/kg	Once on day 1; tid on day 2
			1 mg/kg	tid day 3
Blood or liver flukes	Praziquantel	Oral	20 mg/kg	tid 4 to 6 h apart
Lung & liver flukes	Bithionol	Oral	30 to 50 mg/kg	Alternate days for 10 to 15 doses
Fasciolopsis intestinal fluke	Hexylresorcinol	Oral	15 mg/kg	Once
Schistosomiasis	Oxamniquine	Oral	15 mg/kg	Once
Schistosomiasis	Hycanthone	IM	2.5 mg/kg	Once
Schistosoma haematobium	Metrifonate	Oral	10 mg/kg	Every other week; 3 doses
Tapeworms (adult)	Niclosamide	Oral	2 g	Once
Tapeworms (adult)	Praziquantel	Oral	10 mg/kg	Once
Tapeworms (child)	Niclosamide	Oral	1.5 g	Once for child >34 kg
Tapeworms (child)	Niclosamide	Oral	1.0 g	Once for 11 to 34 kg child

Piperazine Compounds (Fig 100.13)

Piperazine citrate (tripiperazine dicitrate) forms crystals freely soluble in water. It has a molecular weight of 643. The pH of a 10 percent aqueous solution is 5.0 to 6.0. Piperazine citrate is practically insoluble in ethanol and diethyl ether.

The anthelmintic activity of piperazine was discovered during unsuccessful clinical evaluation of this compound to treat gout. Piperazine was introduced clinically to treat nematode infections in 1949. Piperazine is an alternative drug for the treatment of pinworms or roundworms.

Piperazine induces a flaccid muscle paralysis in susceptible nematodes. The paralyzed nematodes are unable to maintain their position in the intestinal lumen and are expelled by intestinal peristaltic activity. Piperazine reversibly antagonizes the stimulatory effect of acetylcholine on the nematode. Piperazine may block the augmentor neural control responsible for muscle tone, or may activate the inhibitory neural control of the nematode neuromuscular system. Piperazine also inhibits anaerobic glycolysis by nematodes at concentrations that affect motility.

Piperazine citrate occasionally causes dizziness, urticaria, and GI disturbances. It is rarely associated with visual disturbances, ataxia, hypotonia, and exacerbation of epilepsy.

Piperazine is well absorbed from the intestine and is excreted in the urine primarily as the unaltered drug. Piperazine citrate (Antepar) is administered orally in single daily doses. It is available in tablets (550 mg) and in suspensions (165 mg).

Diethylcarbamazine (N,N-diethyl-4-methyl-1-piperazinecarboxamide), as the citrate, forms crystals freely soluble in water. Solubility in ethanol is strikingly temperature-dependent, being sparingly soluble in cold ethanol and freely soluble in hot ethanol. It is practically insoluble in acetone and diethyl ether; its molecular weight is 199.

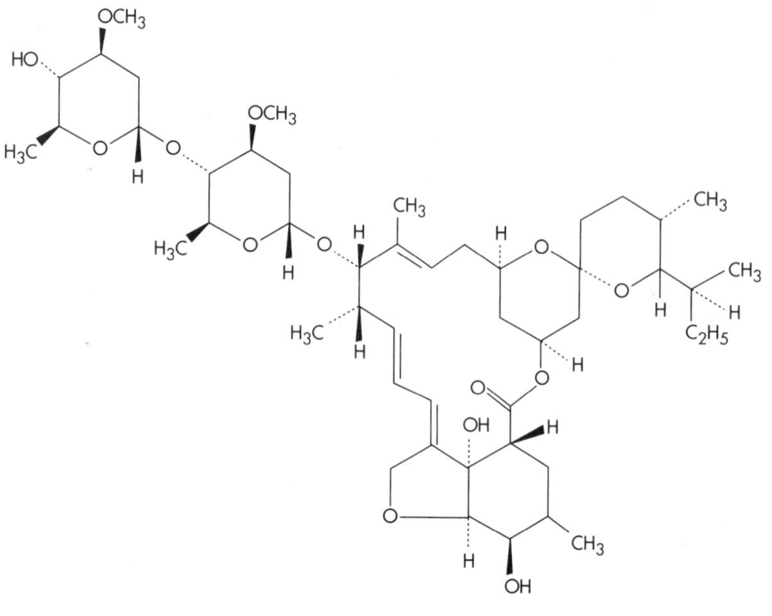

Ivermectin B1a

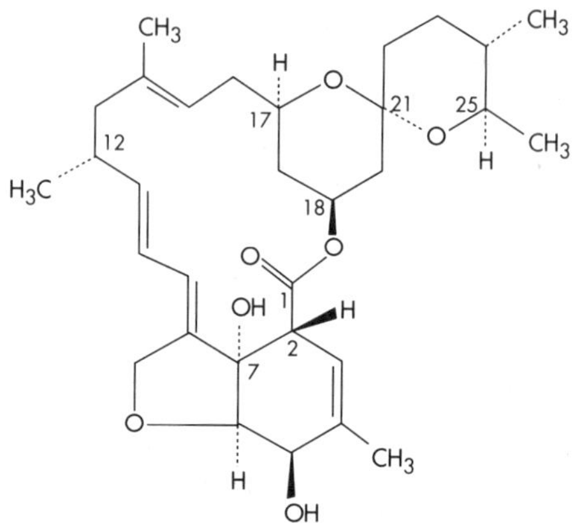

Milbemycin α_1

Figure 100.12 Avermectin Antibiotics

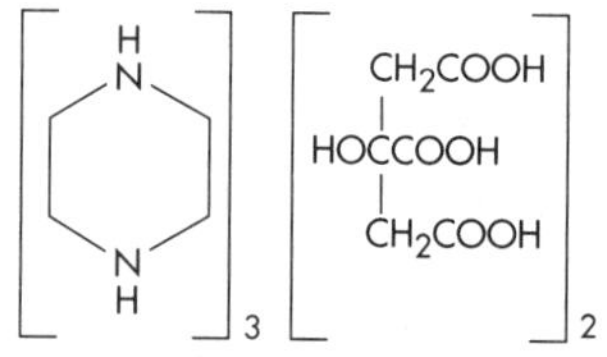

Piperazine Citrate

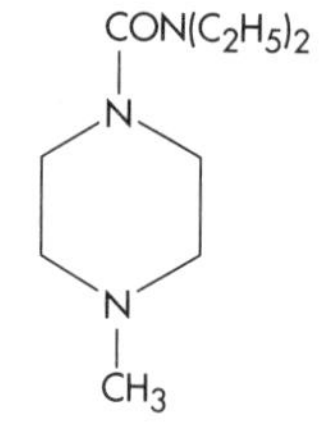

Diethylcarbamazine

Figure 100.13 Piperazine Compounds

Diethylcarbamazine is a derivative of piperazine. It was introduced clinically as an antifilarial agent in 1947. Piperazine itself has no antifilarial activity, but the piperazine ring is essential for antifilarial activity. Diethylcarbamazine has no antifilarial activity in vitro; therefore, its filaricidal activity in vivo is presumed to be indirect. Diethylcarbamazine is used in the treatment of filariasis, including elephantiasis, loiasis, and onchocerciasis, and visceral larva migrans.[66]

Microfilaria periodically move to and from different sites within the body of the host. In diethylcarbamazine treated patients, the microfilariae become trapped in the liver and are ingested by host phagocytes there. The morphologic changes induced by diethylcarbamazine may expose parasite antigens that serve as antigenic determinants. Antibodies to these determinants may facilitate phagocytic destruction of the microfilariae. Diethylcarbamazine inhibits acetylcholine esterase activity, causing an accumulation of acetylcholine in synapses. The increased acetylcholine levels result in receptor desensitization that leads to paralysis of a parasite, after a momentary stimulation.[67] It has been shown that diethylcarbamazine potentiates the action of acetylcholine on parasite muscle, which may account for the changes in the microfilarial surface, and thereby enhance vulnerability to host defense processes.

Diethylcarbamazine itself is responsible for only minor side-effects, such as headaches and GI disturbances. Infected patients undergoing therapy, however, can react indirectly to the drug's antifilarial activity. Diethylcarbamazine should be administered with special caution in heavy infections with *Loa loa* because it can provoke an encephalopathy. Diethylcarbamazine is a frequent cause of severe allergic or febrile reactions. The allergic response, caused by dying microfilariae, is manifested as edema, conjunctivitis, intense itching, dermatitis, and fever. This reaction is both painful and life-threatening. Other side-effects of diethylcarbamazine include weakness, abdominal pain, and tender and swollen lymph nodes.

Diethylcarbamazine is readily absorbed from the intestine; it also is absorbed through the skin. Serum levels in patients two and six hours after an oral dose of 3 mg/kg diethylcarbamazine is about 2 µg/ml. The plasma half-life is five to 13 hours. Some of the drug is metabolized to an N-oxide product, which possesses antifilarial activity. The drug is completely eliminated from the body within 48 hours. Approximately 29 percent of ingested diethylcarbamazine is excreted in the urine during the first 24 hours after administration of the drug.[68] Urinary excretion is pH-dependent, with 60 percent of the drug excreted within 48 hours at pH 5 and less than 10 percent at pH 8.

Diethylcarbamazine (Hetrazan) can be applied topically in ocular or cutaneous filarial infections, but this method of administration offers no advantages over the oral route. The drug, which is available from the manufacturer (Lederle), is dispensed as 50-mg tablets.

Alkylating Agents (Fig. 100.14)

Hycanthone (1-[[2-diethylamino)ethyl]amino]-4-(hydroxymethyl)-9H-thioxanthen-9-one; Mesylate; Etrenol) is prepared by the fungal oxidative fermentation of lucanthone. Hycanthone is extremely sensitive to acids. Lucanthone (1-[(2-diethylaminoethyl)-amino]-4-methylthioxanthen-9-one; Miracil D; Nilodan) forms yellow crystals soluble in water. The aqueous solution is neutral and colored orange. The free base is soluble in organic solvents; the hydrochloride is slightly soluble in ethanol. It has a molecular weight of 357.

Lucanthone (Miracil D), the first nonantimonial drug active against *Schistosoma mansoni,* was introduced in 1948. Lucanthone is inactive in vitro and when administered parenterally. Hycanthone is the active metabolite of lucanthone. Hycanthone is widely used in some countries for treatment of *Schistosoma mansoni* and *Schistosoma haematobium* infections. Hycanthone inhibits egg production and causes a relocation of

O HNCH$_2$CH$_2$N(C$_2$H$_5$)$_2$

CH$_2$OH

Hycanthone

O HNCH$_2$CH$_2$N(C$_2$H$_5$)$_2$ • HCl

CH$_3$

Lucanthone

O$_2$N H N CH$_2$NHCH(CH$_3$)$_2$

HOCH$_2$

Oxamniquine

Figure 100.14 Alkylating Agents

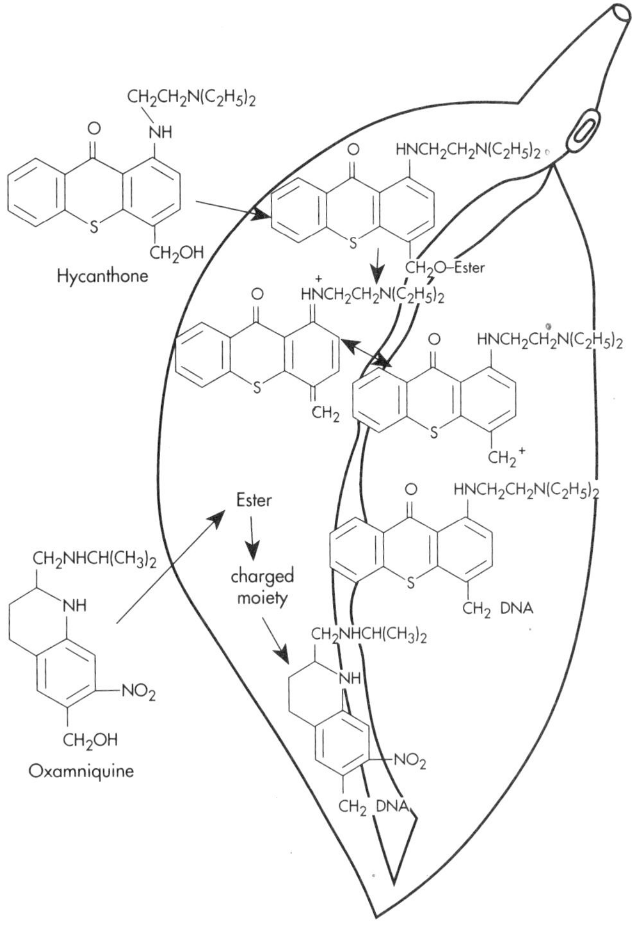

Figure 100.15 Activation of Hycanthone and Oxamniquine, and Subsequent Alkylation of Schistosomal Deoxyribonulceic Acid

worms from the mesenteric veins to the liver sinuses, where the parasite degenerates and dies.

Hycanthone strongly and irreversibly inhibits nucleic acid synthesis in susceptible organisms by alkylating deoxyguanosine residues in DNA. Hycanthone is enzymatically converted by drug-sensitive organisms to an ester that spontaneously dissociates to give a charged moiety able to alkylate deoxyribonucleic acid.[69] Hycanthone is able to intercalate between deoxyribonucleic acid base pairs and causes frameshift mutations. In addition, hycanthone inhibits monoamine oxidase and choline acetyltransferase, and causes an increased uptake of serotonin by the schistosomes.

Adverse side-effects occur in about half of treated patients; most often these are nausea, vomiting, abdominal pain, headaches, and dizziness. They occur six to eight hours after administration, and subside within 24 hours. Hycanthone can cause fatal hepatic necrosis and is suspected of being teratogenic and carcinogenic. The potential dangers of this drug outweigh the value of its high efficacy and convenience of administration.

Hycanthone is well absorbed after oral or IM administration. A single IM treatment is as effective as several days of oral administration, so the IM regimen is preferred. Peak plasma levels occur in 30 min with a half-life of one hour. Most of the drug is eliminated as metabolites in the feces. Hycanthone (Etrenol) is available in tablets and in a parenteral formulation (200 mg base in an ampoule).

Oxamniquine (1,2,3,4-tetrahydro-2-[[(1-methyl-ethyl)amino]-methyl]-7-nitro-6-quinolinemethanol) forms pale yellow crystals. Its molecular weight is 279. The akylating functional group of oxamniquine is attached to a quinoline ring structure. It is virtually insoluble in water.

Oxamniquine was introduced clinically in 1978; it is used to treat *Schistosoma mansoni* infections.[70]

Oxamniquine causes an irreversible inhibition of DNA and RNA synthesis. Oxamniquine competes with hycanthone in the enzymic reaction that covalently couples hycanthone to macromolecules. Schistosomes simultaneously develop resistance to hycanthone and oxamniquine, and the two drugs have essentially the same structure/activity requirements; that is, a hydroxymethyl group *para* to the basic side-chain. Oxamniquine is not an intercalating agent, as is hycanthone, and is generally regarded as safe.

Oxamniquine occasionally is associated with headaches, dizziness, somnolence, nausea, diarrhea, rash, and insomnia. There may be changes in the hepatic enzymes and in the EKG. Oxamniquine rarely causes convulsions.

Oxamniquine is rapidly absorbed after oral administration to achieve a peak level in one to three hours. An oral dose of 15 mg/kg yields a peak drug level of 0.3 to 2.5 μg/ml, which drops to neglible levels within 12 hours. Oxamniquine is extensively metabolized, with less than 2 percent of the dose excreted unchanged in the urine. The biologically inactive metabolites are carboxylic acid derivatives, a consequence of oxidation of the functional groups at the 2- and 6- positions. Intramuscular administration is not indicated because of local painful reactions.

A single oral dose of oxamniquine (Mansil, Vansil) usually is sufficient treatment for a *Schistosoma mansoni* infection.

Oxamniquine is available in 250- or 500-mg tablets or in a suspension of 50 mg/ml in 30-ml bottles.

Halogenated Diphenyl Compounds (Fig. 100.16)

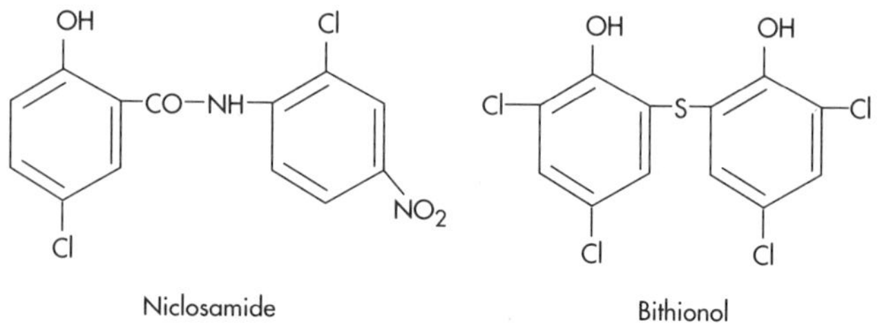

Niclosamide is a chlorinated salicylanilide. It has proved to be quite effective in treating human tapeworm infections. Niclosamide

OH Cl CO—NH Cl NO_2 Niclosamide

OH OH Cl S Cl Cl Cl Bithionol

Figure 100.16 Halogenated Diphenyl Compounds

(2′,5-dichloro-4′-nitrosalicylanilide) is practically insoluble in water and sparingly soluble in ethanol. It has a molecular weight of 327.

Niclosamide is used to treat intestinal or adult tapeworms.[71] It is less efficacious than praziquantel; however, it is safe, even during pregnancy. It has no effect on cysticercosis.

Niclosamide inhibits oxygen and glucose uptake and oxidative phosphorylation in the mitochondria of cestode tapeworms. The scolex (head) and proximal segments are killed on contact. The scolex loosens from the gut wall and may be digested in the intestine before expulsion.

Niclosamide occasionally causes vomiting, nausea, abdominal pain, dizziness, and headaches. The mild laxative effect of the drug is probably due to a localized uncoupling of oxidative phosphorylation in intestinal mucosal cells. Niclosamide is not absorbed from the intestine. Niclosamide (Niclocide, Yomesan) is available in 500-mg chewable tablets.

Bithionol is a halogenated diphenyl sulfide that has been used against cestode and trematode infections for three decades.[72] The dichlorophenol structure of bithionol is related to hexachlorophene. Bithionol (2,2′-thiobis[4,6-dichlorophenol] is practically insoluble in water. It is soluble in dilute sodium hydroxide, and somewhat soluble in 70 percent ethanol (0.3 g/100 ml). It has a molecular weight of 356.

Bithionol is used to treat lung fluke and sheep or liver fluke infections. It was the principal drug for the treatment of fascioliasis (intestinal flukes) and paragonimiasis (lung flukes) until praziquantel was introduced clinically. Bithionol has been banned by the US Food and Drug Administration for use in cosmetics.

The anthelmintic activity of bithionol is related to its interference with ATP generation by the parasite. Succinic dehydrogenase in the liver fluke is very susceptible to bithionol.

Bithionol frequently causes vomiting, diarrhea, anorexia, abdominal pain, and urticaria. It also evokes photosensitive skin reactions. The most serious adverse effect is cardiotoxicity, which makes bedrest necessary during treatment. Bithionol (Actamer, Bitin), which can be obtained from the CDC Parasitic Diseases Drug Service, is available for oral administration.

Miscellaneous Antiparasitic Agents (Fig. 100.17)

Praziquantel (2-(cyclohexylcarbonyl)-1,2,3,6,7,-11b hexahydro-4H-pyrazino[2,1-a]isoquinolin-4-one) is a colorless hygroscopic crystalline powder. The compound is stable under normal conditions. Praziquantel is soluble in ethanol but only slightly soluble in water. The molecular weight is 312. Praziquantel is a pyrazinoquinoline developed for schistosomiasis, but found to be active against a wide range of cestodes. Praziquantel was introduced as a new anthelmintic in 1975.

Praziquantel is used to control schistosomiasis in endemic areas. Praziquantel is also active against liver and lung flukes. It is the drug of choice for most fluke infections.[73] Praziquantel is effective in controlling *Taenia solium* and *Taenia saginata* infections at very low doses (2.5 to 5 mg/kg). Side-effects associated with praziquantel are usually mild and transient. The following side-effects have been observed: malaise; headaches; dizziness; abdominal discomfort; elevated body temperature; and rarely urticaria. Side-effects are more pronounced in patients with a heavy parasite burden.

Praziquantel is a lipophilic drug thought to destabilize the schistosome surface lipid membrane or tegument. One of the earliest morphologic alterations is disruption of the membrane over the tubercles on the dorsal side of the male *Schistosoma mansoni*. Praziquantel paralyzes muscle contraction in a matter of seconds after contact with the drug. It also causes a decrease in glucose uptake, lactate release, glycogen content, and ATP level. Increased intracellular calcium appears to be responsible for disruption of the tegument and paralytic contraction of schistosomal muscle, and the metabolic effects are secondary. The action of praziquantel on schistosomes depends on the developmental stage, with juvenile worms being much more susceptible than adult worms. It has been proposed that the drug interacts with a specific, unique protein involved in Ca^{+2} homeostasis.[74]

Praziquantel is rapidly and extensively absorbed (80%) after oral administration. The maximum plasma concentration is achieved one to three hours after dosing. The serum half-life is 0.8 to 1.5 hours. About 10 percent of parenterally administered drug is secreted into the GI lumen. The drug is hydroxylated, and excreted by the kidneys. The hydroxylated metabolites do not have anthelmintic activity. Over 90 percent of the administered drug is excreted within 24 hours. Praziquantel (Biltricide; Cesol; Droncit) is available in 600-mg tablets.

Suramin sodium (8,8′-[carbonylbis[imino-3,1-phenylene-carbonylimino(4-methyl-3,1-phenylene)carbonylimino]]bis-1,3,5-naphthalenetrisulfonic acid hexasodium salt) is a complex urea derivative with a high molecular weight. It is white or slightly pink or cream colored powder that is hygroscopic. It has a molecular weight of 1429. It is freely soluble in water and in physiologic saline. Aqueous solutions have a neutral pH. It is sparingly soluble in 95 percent ethanol.

Suramin was developed in the 1920s as a trypanocide by screening derivatives of Ehrlich's dyes. Its effect on onchocerciasis was discovered by chance in 1945 during antitrypanosome prophylactic trials. Suramin was introduced as an antifilarial agent in 1947.[r14]

Suramin is used to treat the early stage of African trypanosomiasis or sleeping sickness, before the parasite invades the CNS. Suramin is used as a follow-up drug after the treatment of *Onchocerca* infection with diethylcarbamazine. Suramin requires IV administration for up to six week to control filariasis. Because of toxicity, few indications favor use of suramin.

Suramin is a very reactive compound that combines readily with macromolecules. It inhibits many enzyme systems at low concentrations. Suramin inter-

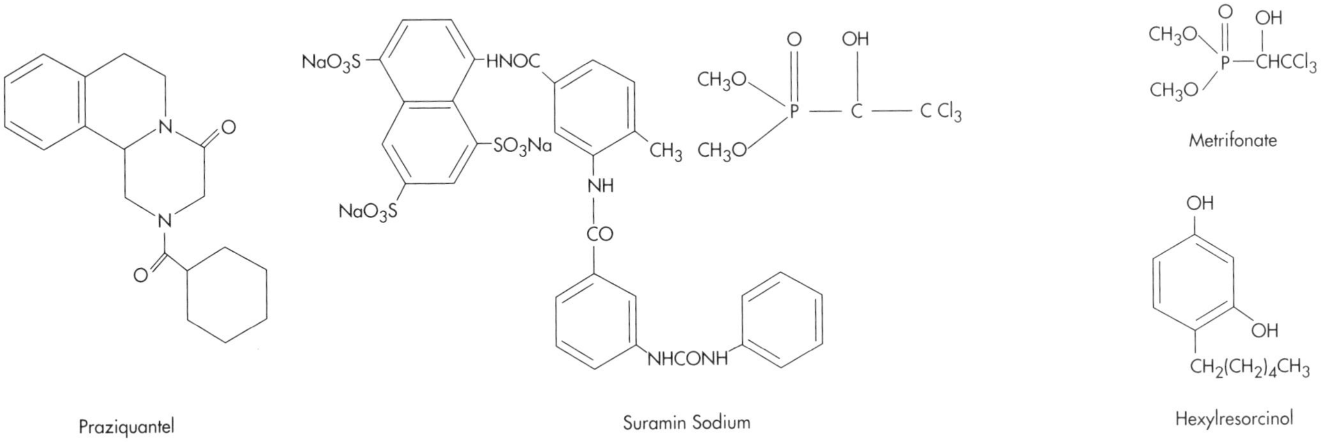

Praziquantel

Suramin Sodium

Metrifonate

Hexylresorcinol

Figure 100.17 Miscellaneous Antihelminthic Drugs

feres with parasite replication, which might reflect inhibition of RNA polymerase. A striking characteristic of the therapeutic response to this drug is its slowness. The drug impairs the reproductive system of the filaria long before the worms die. Cell proliferation appears to be essential for the drug's action, and the microfilaria, which are nondividing, are insensitive to the drug.

Suramin sodium is frequently associated with nausea, vomiting, pruritus, urticaria, paresthesia, hyperesthesia of the hands and feet, photophobia, and peripheral neuropathy. Occasionally, kidney damage, blood dyscrasias and shock have been attributed to use of this drug. Delayed drug reactions include tiredness, diarrhea, anorexia, and severe ulceration of the stomach, mouth, and pharynx. Suramin administered IM or SQ causes intense local irritation.

Suramin is poorly absorbed from the intestine, so the drug is administered IV. The plasma concentration of the drug falls during the first few hours after administration; it then achieves a concentration that is maintained for several months. The persistence of the drug in plasma is due to its strong binding to serum proteins. There is no evidence of metabolism of the drug or of penetration into erythrocytes. Some of the drug is taken up by reticuloendothelial cells and accumulates in Kupffer cells in the liver and in epithelial cells of the proximal convoluted tubules of the kidney.

Suramin (Germanin) is available in 1-g ampoules of dry powder that must be dissolved immediately before injection. Suramin, which is available from the CDC Parasitic Diseases Drug Service, is used for treating individual patients under close supervision.

Metrifonate (2,2,2-trichloro-1-hydroxyethyl)-phosphonic acid dimethyl ester, chlorofos, trichlorfon, trichlorphene) is prepared by the reaction of chloral with dimethyl phosphite. It has a molecular weight of 257. It is soluble in water (15 g/100 ml) and diethyl ether (17 g/100 ml) and decomposes in alkaline solutions.

Metrifonate was introduced as an insecticide; it is an organophosphorous compound with irreversible anticholinesterase activity. Metrifonate was introduced clinically as a schistosomicide in 1962; it is used to treat *Schistosoma haematobium* infections, but is virtually ineffective against *S. mansoni* and *S. japonicum*.

Metrifonate is not the active agent, but it is rapidly transformed nonenzymatically to dichlorovos in vivo. The neurotoxicity of anticholinesterases is common to helminths, insects, and humans. Motility of schistosomes in metrifonate-treated patients is inhibited as a consequence of muscle paralysis. In addition, the number of schistosome eggs in the urine is greatly reduced in treated subjects.

Metrifonate occasionally causes nausea, vomiting, bronchospasm, weakness, diarrhea, and abdominal pain. Metrifonate is a cholinesterase inhibitor, which can cause serious adverse side-effects. There is no effect on levels of acetylcholine or choline or on the rate of synthesis of acetylcholine.[75] Large overdoses from accidental poisoning severely affect skeletal muscles and the CNS, with death resulting from respiratory failure.

The peak plasma level of metrifonate after oral administration occurs within two hours, and the drug persists in the plasma for at least eight hours. The level of the active metabolite dichlorovos is about 1 percent of that of the parent metrifonate. Dichlorovos is rapidly metabolized to an inactive product, so the persisting metrifonate serves as a reservoir to replace the active derivative. Metrifonate (Bilarcil) is available in 100-mg tablets for oral administration.

Hexylresorcinol (4-hexyl-1,3-benzenediol) is a pale-yellow heavy liquid that becomes solid on standing at room temperature. It is soluble in ethanol, acetone, and diethyl ether. Solubility in water is limited to 500 μg/ml. Its molecular weight is 194.

Hexylresorcinol is used to treat *Fasciolopsis* infections. Concentrated solutions can cause burns on the skin and mucous membranes. High concentrations of hexylresorcinol on the skin are corrosive and an irritant.

Pyrantel (1,4,5,6-tetrahydro-1-methyl-2-[2-(2-thienyl) ethenyl] pyrimidine) esterified to pamoic acid forms a yellow crystalline powder which is insoluble in water. The molecular weight of pyrantel is 206.

Pyrantel (Fig. 100.18) was first introduced as a broad-spectrum anthelmintic for veterinary use. It was introduced clinically for human use in 1966. The sparingly soluble pamoate is used to reduce absorption of the drug and to achieve a higher concentration in the lumen of the intestine.[20] Pyrantel pamoate is used to treat pinworms, *Trichostrongylus* infections, roundworms, and hookworms. The patient's family should be treated for pinworm infection to prevent recurrence. Pyrantel antagonizes the effects of piperazine.

Pyrantel causes a spastic paralysis in nematodes as a result of ganglionic stimulating effects. The drug

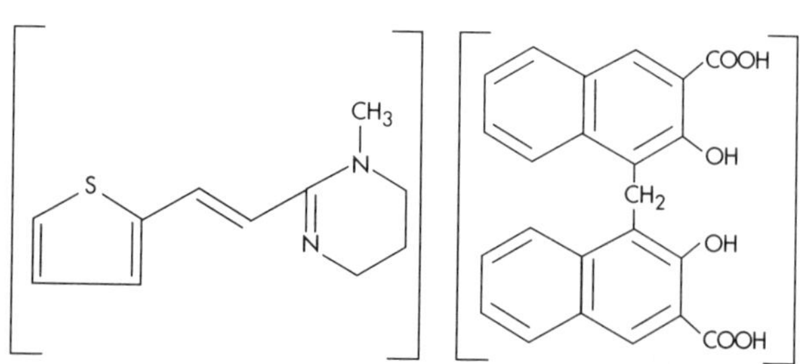

Figure 100.18 Pyrantel Pamoate

probably activates the augmentor neural control of neuromuscular function.

Pyrantel pamoate occasionally causes GI disturbances, headaches, dizziness, rash, and fever. It is poorly absorbed from the intestine, and more than half of an orally administered dose is excreted unchanged in the feces. Less than 15 percent is excreted in the urine.

Pyrantel pamoate (Antiminth) is administered orally, most often as a single-dose treatment for ascariasis, enterobiasis, and hookworms. It is available in 250-mg base chewable tablets and in suspensions for oral administration (50 mg base/ml).

Pyrvinium pamoate (Fig. 100.19) (6-(dimethylamino)-2-[2-(2,5-dimethyl-1-phenyl-1H-pyrrol-3-yl) ethenyl]-1-methylquinolinium; pyrvinium embonate; viprynium embonate) is bright orange or orange-red to almost black in color. It is stable to heat, light and air, slightly soluble in ethanol, and practically insoluble in water and diethyl ether. Its molecular weight is 1151. Pyrvinium pamoate is a 6-aminoquinoline derivative that has been coupled with pamoic acid to prevent absorption of the orally administered drug.

Pyrvinium pamoate is used to treat pinworms. It is recommended that the entire family be treated for pinworms to prevent reinfection. Pyrvinium pamoate occasionally causes vomiting and nausea. It is rarely associated with photosensitive skin reactions. Pyrvinium pamoate causes the stool to turn red. It inhibits oxidative metabolism in worms and interferes with the absorption of glucose by intestinal helminths. Pyrvinium pamoate (Povanyl, Vanquin) is available in 50-mg tablets or in a solution of 10 mg/ml for oral administration.

Antimony sodium dimercaptosuccinate (Fig. 100.20) (2,2′-[(1,2-dicarboxy-1,2-ethanediyl)bis(thio)]bis-1,3,2-dithiastibolane-4,5-dicarboxylic acid hexasodium salt; stibocaptate) is a white or slightly yellowish-green powder that is hygroscopic and unstable when moistened. It is water soluble and has a molecular weight of 787.

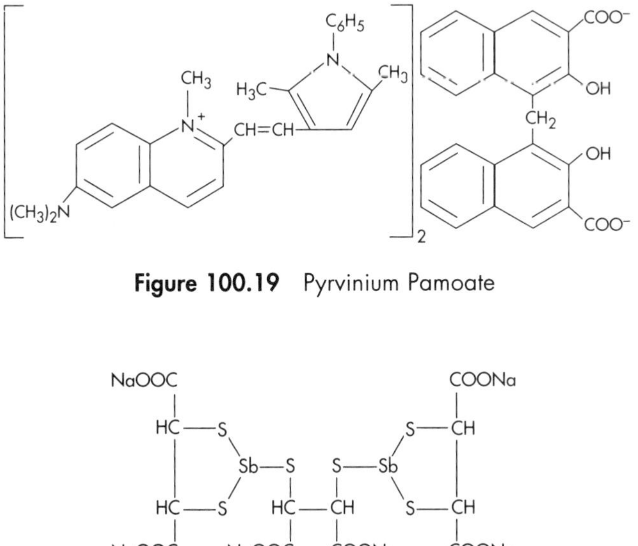

C_6H_5 CH_3 H_3C CH_3 N^+ CH=CH $(CH_3)_2N$ COO^- OH CH_2 OH COO^- 2

Figure 100.19 Pyrvinium Pamoate

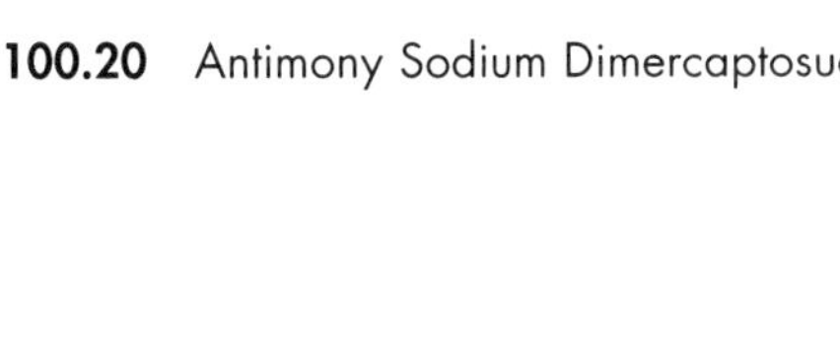

NaOOC COONa HC—S S—CH Sb—S S—Sb HC—S HC—CH S—CH NaOOC NaOOC COONa COONa

Figure 100.20 Antimony Sodium Dimercaptosuccinate

Antimony sodium dimercaptosuccinate is an alternative drug to treat schistosomiasis. It has largely been superseded by more effective, less toxic drugs, such as praziquantel.

Antimony sodium dimercaptosuccinate, like the other antimonials, acts by paralyzing adult worms. This results in a rapid shift of the schistosomes from the mesenteric veins to the liver, where the parasite dies. The antiparasitic activity probably reflects inhibition of phosphofructokinase.

Antimony sodium dimercaptosuccinate is a frequent cause of anorexia, nausea, GI pain, muscle pain, joint stiffness, and bradycardia, and of coughing and vomiting when IV administration is rapid. This drug also causes painful local inflammation following leakage during IV injection. Treatment occasionally is associated with colic, diarrhea, rash, pruritus, and myocardial damage. On rare occasions the liver is damaged, and there is hemolytic anemia, renal damage, shock and sudden death. It is contraindicated in patients with renal and cardiac disease and in hepatic disease not attributable to the schistosomiasis. The drug should be stopped in the event of recurrent vomiting, progressive albuminuria, persistent joint pain, rash, intercurrent infection, purpura, or a falling hematocrit.

Antimony sodium dimercaptosuccinate (Astiban, Stibocaptate) is available only for parenteral use in units of 500 mg.

Parasitic Arthropods

Arthropods are macroscopic multicellular organisms with a chitin exoskeleton, jointed appendages, and a hemocele. Those of medical significance include the parasitic arthropods, the stinging and poisonous biting arthropods, and the arthropod vectors for viral and parasitic agents.[r15] This section will be limited to a treatment of the parasitic arthropods, which are found in the Pentastomida or tongue worms, the Arachnida or mites, and the Hexapoda or insects. The tongue worms are degenerate wormlike arthropods that, in their larval stages, may infect human viscera, where both active and encysted forms are found. The best known parasitic mites are the itch mite *Sarcoptes scabiei*, and red bugs or chiggers *Eutrombicula alfreddugesi*. Myiasis is the term applied to the disease produced by fly larvae or maggots that live parasitically in human tissues. A number of species of flies produce myiasis, and the disease is classified clinically according to the part of the body affected: nasal; intestinal; urinary; or cutaneous myiasis. Oftentimes therapy for parasitic arthropod infections or infestations addresses the symptoms, such as itching, rather than elimination of the offending mite or insect. Prudent therapy involves concurrent treatment with antiparasitic and anti-inflammatory agents.

Ectoparasiticides (Fig 100.21)

Crotamiton (N-ethyl-N-(2-methylphenyl)-2-butenamide) is a yellowish oil, miscible with ethanol. It is a mixture of *cis* and *trans* isomers. Its molecular weight is 203.

Crotamiton is used to control itch mites.[76] The preparation should not be applied near the eyes or mouth, nor to inflamed skin or open wounds. Safety and effectiveness in children has not been established.

Crotamiton (Eurax) is available as a 10 percent cream or lotion. The preparation (1 oz) is massaged into the whole body, avoiding the eyes, nose and mouth; the treatment is repeated 24 hours later. The preparation is removed 48 hours after the second application by thorough bathing.

Lindane (1,2,3,4,5,6-hexachlorocyclohexane; gamma benzene hexachloride, gamma hexachlor) is the biologically active isomer among eight well-described stereoisomers of hexachlorocyclohexane. Pharmacetical preparations contain at least 99 percent gamma benzene hexachloride. Lindane is insoluble in water and has limited solubility in ethanol (6 g/100 ml). Lindane is quite soluble in acetone (43 g/100 ml) and in diethyl ether (21 g/100 ml). The molecular weight of lindane is 291.

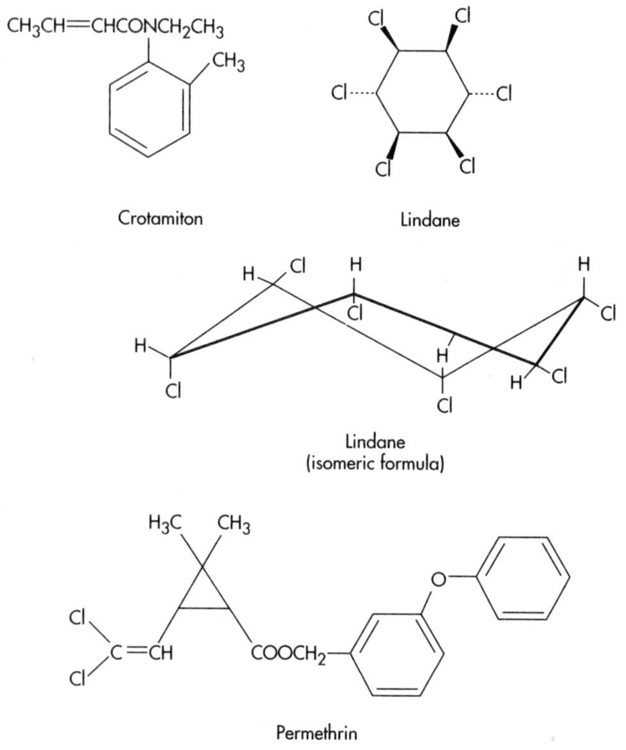

$CH_3CH{=}CHCONCH_2CH_3$

Crotamiton

Lindane

Lindane (isomeric formula)

Permethrin

Figure 100.21 Ectoparasiticides

Lindane is an ectoparasiticide active against *Sarcoptes scabiei* (itch mite), *Pediculosis humanus capitis* (head lice), *Phthirus pubis* (crab lice), and their ova. It is absorbed into the parasites and their ova. Lindane induces modifications of membrane structure and fluidity, leading to a decrease in stored glycogen and an increase in lactic acid and pyruvic acid.[77] Lindane should not be used on premature infants because their skin is more permeable to the preparation and their hepatic drug metabolizing enzymes are not fully developed, nor should lindane be used in individuals with seizure disorders.

Poisoning may result from ingestion, inhalation, or percutaneous absorption. Symptoms of acute lindane toxicity include dizziness, headaches, nausea, vomiting, diarrhea, tremors, weakness, convulsions, dyspnea, cyanosis, and circulatory collapse. Lindane vapors may irritate the eyes, nose and throat. Lindane should not be applied to open cuts. Prolonged or repeated exposures to lindane must be avoided.

Lindane is absorbed through the skin. A peak blood level of 28 ng/ml has been reported six hours after total body application of 1 percent lindane lotion to children. The half-life of lindane in the blood is 18 hours. Lindane is secreted in human milk, so mothers using lindane should avoid nursing during the treatment period.

Lindane (Kwell) is available as a 1 percent preparation in a cream, lotion, or shampoo for topical use. Two ounces of 1 percent lindane are applied to the entire body of an adult infested with itch mites, and allowed to act for eight to 12 hours. Thereafter, the material should be removed by thorough washing. Lindane shampoo is applied to dry infested hair to eliminate lice; after four minutes, the treated hair is wetted with water. Thereafter, the shampoo should be removed by thorough washing and rinsing.

Permethrin (3-(2,2-dichloroethenyl)-2,2-dimethylcyclopropanecarboxylic acid (3-phenoxyphenyl)methyl ester) is a synthetic pyrethroid insecticide that is more stable to light and as active as natural pyrethrins. The (1R,cis)-isomers are the two esters primarily responsible for the insecticide activity. Permethrin is virtually insoluble in water (1 μg/ml). The chemical melts at 35°C and is miscible in organic solvents. It has a molecular weight of 391.

Permethrin is active against a wide range of pests, including mites, lice, ticks, and flies.[78] It can be used to control lindane-resistant scabies.[79] Currently, its use is approved by the US Food and Drug Administration only for head lice infestations. The chemical prevents chiggers from biting. Permethrin inhibits acetylcholinesterase and choline acetylase activities. It acts on the nerve cell membrane to disrupt the sodium channel current by which the polarization of the membrane is regulated. Delayed repolarization leads to paralysis of the parasite. There is an associated decrease in phosphodiesterase activity.[80] Permethrin is considered safe for use in children two months of age or older. The drug is irritating to the eyes, and may cause itching and burning when applied to infected and infested skin. It also causes erythema, numbness, tingling, and rashes in a few patients.

Less than 5 percent of permethrin applied topically is absorbed. Absorbed permethrin is rapidly metabolized to inactive products that are excreted in the urine.

Permethrin (Elimite) is available as a 5 percent cream for topical application. For an adult, 1 oz of 5 percent permethrin is massaged into the entire body. The material should be removed eight to 14 hours later by thorough bathing.

References

Research Reports

1. Moore MB. *Acanthamoeba* keratitis. Arch Ophthalmol 1988;*106*:1181–1183.
2. Ouellette M, Papadopoulou B. Mechanisms of drug resistance in *Leishmania*. Parasitol Today 1993;*9*:150–153.
3. Fairlamb AH. Trypanothione metabolism in the chemotherapy of leishmaniasis and trypanosomiasis. In: Wang CC Molecular and immunological aspects of parasitism. Washington: American Association for the Advancement of Science, 1991:107–121.
4. Oaks SC, ed. Malaria: Obstacles and opportunities, a report of the Committee for the Study of Malaria Prevention and Control: Status review and alternative strategies, Division of International Health, Institute of Medicine. Washington: National Academy Press, 1991.
5. Zidovetzki R, Sherman IW, O'Brien L. Inhibition of *Plasmodium falciparum* phospholipase A_2 by choroquine, quinine and arteether. J Parasitol 1993;*79*:565–570.
6. Slater AFG, Cerami A. Inhibition by chloroquine of a novel haem polymerase enzyme activity in malaria trophozoites. Nature. 1992;*355*:167–169.
7. Ittarat I, Webster HK, Yuthavong Y. High-performance liquid chromatographic determination of dihydroorotate dehydrogenase of *Plasmodium falciparum* and effects of antimalarials on enzyme activity. J Chromatogr Biomed Appl 1992;*582*:57–64.
8. Fransson L-A, Karlsson P, Schmitchen A. Effects of cycloheximide, brefeldin A, suramin, heparin and primaquine on proteoglycan and glycosaminoglycan biosynthesis in human embryonic skin fibroblasts. Biochim Biophys Acta 1992;*1137*:287–297.
9. Ziu MM, Giasuddin ASM. The chemotherapy of primaquine and effect of one of its metabolites on human erythrocytes. J Med Res Inst 1992;*13*:121–136.
10. Schapira A, Solomon T, Julien M, Macome A, Parmar N, Ruas I, Simao F, Streat E, Betschart B. Comparison of intramuscular and intravenous quinine for the treatment of severe and complicated malaria in children. Trans Roy Soc Trop Med Hyg 1993;*87*:299–302.
11. Pennie RA, Koren G, Crevoisier C. Steady state pharmacokinetics of mefloquine in long-term travellers. Trans Roy Soc Trop Med Hyg 1993;*87*:459–462.
12. Shalmiev G, Ginsburg H. The susceptibility of the malarial parasite *Plasmodium falciparum* to quinoline-containing drugs is correlated to the lipid composition of the infected erythrocyte membranes. Biochem Pharmacol 1993;*46*:365–374.
13. Prince JS, Kohen C, Kohen E, Jimenez J, Brada Z. Direct connection between myelinosomes, endoplasmic reticulum and nuclear envelope in mouse hepatocytes growth with the amphiphilic drug quinacrine. Tissue Cell 1993;*25*:103–110.
14. Arias HR, Valenzuela CF, Johnson DA. Transverse localization of the quinacrine binding site on the *Torpedo* acetylcholine receptor. J Biol Chem 1993;*268*:6348–6355.
15. Basco LK, LeBras J. In vitro activity of pyronaridine against African strains of *Plasmodium falciparum*. Ann Trop Med Parasitol 1992;*86*:447–454.
16. Chavalitshewinkoon P, Wilairat P, Gamage S, Denny W, Figitt D, Ralph R. Structure-activity relationships and modes of action of 9-anilinoacridines against chloroquine-resistant *Plasmodium falciparum* in vitro. Antimicrob Agt Chemother 1993;*37*:403–406.
17. Chang C, Lin-Hua T, Jantanavivat C. Studies on a new antimalarial compound: Pyronaridine. Trans Roy Soc Trop Med Hyg 1992;*86*:7–10.
18. Ruf B, Schuermann D, Bergmann F, Schueler-Maue W, Grunewald T, Gottschalk HJ, Witt H, Pohle HD. Efficacy of pyrimethamine/sulfadoxine in the prevention of toxoplasmic encephalitis relapses and *Pneumocystis carinii* pneumonia in HIV-infected patients. Eur J Clin Microbiol Infect Dis 1993;*12*:325–329.
19. Opravil M, Keusch G, Luthy R. Pyrimethamine inhibits renal secretion of creatinine. Antimicrob Agt Chemother 1993;*37*:1056–1060.
20. Krepel HP, Polderman AM. Egg production of *Oesophagostomum bifurcum*, a locally common parasite of humans in Togo. J Trop Med Hyg 1992;*46*:469–472.
21. Helsby NA, Edwards G, Breckenridge AM, Ward SA. The multiple dose pharmacokinetics of proguanil. Br J Clin Pharmacol 1993;*35*:653–656.
22. Watkins WM, Mberu EK, Nevill CG, Ward SA, Breckenridge AM, Koech DK. Variability in the metabolism of proguanil to the active metabolite cycloguanil in healthy Kenyan adults. Trans Roy Soc Trop Med Hyg 1990;*84*:492–495.
23. Wangboonskul J, White NJ, Nosten F, Ter Kuile F, Moody RR, Taylor RB. Single dose pharmacokinetics of proguanil and its metabolites in pregnancy. Eur J Clin Pharmacol 1993;*44*:247–251.
24. Scott JAG, Davidson RN, Moody AH, Grant HR, Felmingham D, Scott GMS, Olliaro P. Aminosidine (paromomycin) in the treatment of leishmaniasis imported into the United Kingdom. Trans Roy Soc Trop Med Hyg 1992;*86*:617–619.
25. Thakur CP, Sinha GP, Sharma V, Pandey AK, Kumar M, Verma BB. Evaluation of amphotericin B as a first line drug in comparison to sodium stibogluconate in the treatment of fresh cases of kala-azar. Indian J Med Res Sect A 1993;*97*:170–175.
26. Mishra M, Biswas UK, Jha DN, Khan AB. Amphotericin versus pentamidine in antimony-unresponsive kala-azar. Lancet 1992;*340*:1256–1257.
27. Davidson RN, Croft SL, Scott A, Maini M, Moody AH, Bryceson ADM. Liposomal amphotericin B in drug-resistant visceral leishmaniasis. Lancet 1991;*337*:1061–1062.
28. Siciliano C, Chalub E, Sosa LN, Lopez ABA, Vidal A. Fascioliasis and pleural effusion. Prensa Med Argent 1992;*79*:252–255.
29. Fenteany G, Morse DE. Specific inhibitors of protein synthesis do not block RNA synthesis or settlement in larvae of a marine gastropod mollusk (*Haliotis rufescens*). Biol Bull (Woods Hole) 1993;*184*:6–14.

30. Nguyen DS, Hoan DB, Dung NP, Huong NV, Binh LN, Son MV, Meshnick SR. Treatment of malaria in Vietnam with oral artemisinin. Am J Trop Med Hyg 1993;*48*:398–402.

31. Yang Y-Z, Asawamahasakda W, Meshnick SR. Alkylation of human albumin by the antimalarial artemisinin. Biochem Pharmacol 1993;*46*:336–339.

32. Meshnick SR, Thomas A, Ranz A, Xu C-M, Pan H-Z. Artemisinin (qinghaosu): The role of intracellular hemin in its mechanism of antimalarial action. Mol Biochem Parasitol 1991;*49*:181–190.

33. Meshnick SR, Yang Y-Z, Lima V, Kuypers F, Kamchonwongpaisan S, Yuthavong Y. Iron-dependent free radical generation from the antimalarial agent artemisinin (Qinghaosu). Antimicrob Agt Chemother 1993;*37*:1108–1114.

34. Yang DM, Liew FY. Effects of qinghaosu (artemisinin) and its derivatives on experimental cutaneous leishmaniasis. Parasitol 1993;*106*:7–11.

35. White NJ, Waller D, Crawley J, Nosten F, Chapman D, Brewster D, Greenwood BM. Comparison of artemether and chloroquine for severe malaria in Gambian children. Lancet 1992;*339*:317–321.

36. Roberts WL, Rainey PM. Antileishmanial activity of sodium stibogluconate fractions. Antimcrob Agt Chemother 1993;*37*:1842–1846.

37. Grogl M, Thomason TN, Franke ED. Drug resistance in leishmaniasis: Its implications in systemic chemotherapy of cutaneous and mucocutaneous disease. Am J Trop Med Hyg 1992;*47*:117–126.

38. Grogl M, Martin RK, Oduola AMJ, Milhous WK, Kyle DE. Characteristics of multidrug resistance in *Plasmodium* and *Leishmania:* Detection of P-glycoprotein-like components. Am J Trop Med Hyg 1991;*45*:98–111.

39. Franke ED, Wignall FS, Cruz ME, Rosales E, Tovar AA, Lucas CM, Llanos-Cuentas A, Berman JD. Efficacy and toxicity of sodium stibogluconate for mucosal leishmaniasis. Ann Int Med 1990;*113*:934–940.

40. Burguera JL, Burguera M, Petit de Pena Y, Lugo A, Anez N. Selective determination of antimony (III) and antimony (V) in serum and urine and of total antimony in skin biopsies of patients with cutaneous leishmaniasis treated with meglumine antimonate. Trace Elem Med 1993;*10*:66–70.

41. Davidson RN, Croft SL. Recent advances in the treatment of visceral leishmaniasis. Trans Roy Soc Trop Med Hyg 1993;*87*:130–131 & 141.

42. Carter NS, Fairlamb AH. Arsenical-resistant trypanosomes lack an unusual adenosine transporter. Nature 1993;*361*:173–176.

43. Burri C, Baltz T, Giroud C, Doua F, Welker HA, Brun R. Pharmacokinetic properties of the trypanocidal drug melarsoprol. Chemother 1993;*39*:225–234.

44. Gonzalez-Martin G, Ponce G, Inostroza A, Gonzalez M, Paulos C, Guevara A. The disposition of nifurtimox in the rat isolated perfused liver: Effect of dose size. J Pharm Pharmacol 1993;*45*:72–74.

45. Cerecetto H, Mester B, Onetto S, Seoane G, Gonzalez M, Zinola S. Formal potentials of new analogues of nifurtimox: Relationship to activity. Farmaco 1992;*47*:1207–1213.

46. Lax D, Kukolich SG. Generation of furazolidone radical anion and its inhibition by glutathione. Biochem Med Metab Biol 1992;*48*:56–63.

47. Olsen SL, Renlund DG, O'Connell JB, Taylor DO, Lassetter JE, Eastburn TE, Hammond EH, Bristow MR. Prevention of *Pneumocystis carinii* in cardiac transplant recipients by trimethoprim sulfamethoxazole. Transplantation 1993;*56*:359–363.

48. Lidman C, Tynell E, Berglund O, Lindback S. Aerosolized pentamidine versus i.v. pentamidine for secondary prophylaxis of *Pneumoncystis carinii* pneumonia. Infection 1993;*21*:146–149.

49. McAuley JB, Herwaldt BL, Stokes SL. Becher JA, Roberts JM, Michelson MK, Juranek DD. Diloxanide furoate for treating asymptomatic *Entamoeba histolytica* cyst passers: 14 years' experience in the United States. Clin Infect Dis 1992;*15*:464–468.

50. Hughes W, Leoung G, Kramer F, Bozzette A, Safrin S, Frame P, Clumeck N, Masur H, Lancaster D, Chan C, Lavelle J, Rosenstock J, Falloon J, Feinberg J, LaFon S, Rogers M, Sattler F. Comparison of atovaquone (566C80) with trimethoprim-sulfamethoxazole to treat *Pneumocystis carinii* pneumonia in patients with AIDS. N Engl J Med 1993;*328*:1521–1527.

51. Hudson AT. Atovaquone—A novel broad-spectrum anti-infective drug. Parasitol Today 1993;*9*:66–68.

52. Artymowicz RJ, James VE. Atovaquone: A new antipneumocystis agent. Clin Pharm 1993;*12*:563–570.

53. Gyatt HL, Evans D. Economic considerations for helminth control. Parasitol Today 1992;*8*:397–402.

54. Warren KS. Helminths and health of school-age children. Lancet 1991;*338*:686–687.

55. Haswell-Elkins MR, Sithithaworn P, Elkins D. *Opisthorchis viverrini* and cholangiocarcinoma in northeast Thailand. Parasitol Today 1992;*8*:86–89.

56. Teggi A, Lastilla MG, DeRosa F. Therapy of human hydatid disease with mebendazole and albendazole. Antimicrob Agt Chemother 1993;*37*:1679–1684.

57. El-Mufti M, Kamag A, Ibrahim H, Taktuk S, Swaisi I, Zaidan A, Sameen A, Shimbish F, Bouzghaiba W, Haasi S, Unaizi A. Albendazole therapy of hydatid disease: 2-year follow up of 40 cases. Ann Trop Med Parasitol 1993;*87*:241–246.

58. Reynoldson JA, Thompson RCA, Horton RJ. Albendazole as a future antigiardial agent. Parasitol Today 1992;*8*:412–414.

59. Quon DVK, d'Oliveira CE, Johnson PJ. Reduced transcription of the ferridoxin gene in metronidazole-resistant *Trichomonas vaginalis*. Proc Nat Acad Sci USA 1992;*89*:4402–4406.

60. Li T, Qu S. A comparison of metronidazole distribution following intravenous metronidazole and metronidazole phosphate disodium in mice. Drug Metab Drug Interact 1992;*10*:229–236.

61. Bartoloni A, Guglielmetti P, Cancrini G, Gamboa H, Roselli M, Nicoletti A, Paradisi F. Comparative efficacy of a single 400 mg dose of albendazole or mebendazole in the treatment of nematode infections in children. Trop Geograph Med 1993;*45*:114–116.

62. Whitworth JAG, Morgan D, Maude GH, McNicholas AM, Taylor DW. A field study of the effect of ivermectin on intestinal helminths in man. Trans Roy Soc Trop Med Hyg 1991;*85*:232–234.

63. Cartel JL, Sechan Y, Spiegel A, Nguyen L, Barbazan Ph, Martin PMV, Roux JF. Cumulative mortality rates in *Aedes polynesiensis* after feeding on polynesian *Wuchereria bancrofti* carriers treated with single doses of ivermectin, diethylcarbamazine and placebo. Trop Med Parasitol 1991;*42*:343–345.

64. Greene BM, Dukuly ZD, Munoz B, White AT, Pacque M, Taylor HR. A comparison of 6-, 12-, and 24-monthly dosing with ivermectin for treatment of onchocerciasis. J Infect Dis 1991;*163*:376–380.

65. Geary TG, Sims SM, Thomas EM, Vanover L, Davis JP, Winterowd CA, Klein RD, Ho NFH, Thompson DP. *Haemonchus con-*

tortus: Ivermectin-induced paralysis of the pharynx. Exp Parasitol 1993;*77*:88–96.

66. Gupta A, Agarwal A, Dogra MR. Retinal involvement in *Wuchereria bancrofti* filariasis. Acta Ophthalmol 1992;*70*:832–835.

67. Vijayanathan L, Raj RK. Effect of diethylcarbamazine on acetylcholine and gamma amino butyric acid in *Setaria digitata*. Indian J Exp Biol 1992;*30*:920–922.

68. Huijun Z, Piessens WF, Zenghou T, Laifeng L, Xiaorui C, Genbao G. Efficacy of ivermectin for control of microfilaremia recurring after treatment with diethylcarbamazine. I. Clinical and parasitologic observations. Am J Trop Med Hyg 1991;*45*:168–174.

69. Pica-Mattoccia L, Archer S, Cioli D. Hycanthone resistance in schistomsomes correlates with the lack of an enzymatic activity which produces the covalent binding of hycanthone to parasite macromolecules. Mol Biochem Parasitol 1992;*55*:167–176.

70. Coura Filho P, Martinelli Mendes N, Pereira de Souza C, Pereira JP. The prolonged use of niclosamide as an molluscicide for the control of *Schistosoma mansoni*. Rev Inst Med Trop Sao Paulo 1992;*34*:427–431.

71. Ikeh EI, Anosike JC, Okon E. Acanthocephalan infection in man in northern Nigeria. J Helminthol 1992;*66*:241–242.

72. Bacq Y, Besnier J-M, Duong T-H, Pavie G, Metman E-H, Choutet P. Successful treatment of actue fascioliasis with bithionol. Hepatol 1991;*14*:1066–1069.

73. Mairiang E, Haswell-Elkins MR, Mairiang P, Sithithworn P, Elkins DB. Reversal of biliary tract abnormalities associated with *Opisthorchis viverrini* infection following praziquantel treatment. Trans Roy Soc Trop Med Hyg 1993;*87*:194–197.

74. Day TA, Bennett JL, Pax RA. Praziquantel: The enigmatic antiparasitic. Parasitol Today 1992;*8*:342–344.

75. Nordgren I, Karlen B, Kimland M. Metrifonate and tacrine: A comparative study on their effect on acetylcholine dynamics in mouse brain. Pharmacol Toxicol 1992;*71*:236–240.

76. Purvis RS, Tyring SK. An outbreak of lindane-resistant scabies treated successfully with permethrin 5 percent cream. J Am Acad Dermatol 1991;*25*:1015–1016.

77. Gutierrez-Ocana MT, Senar S, Perez-Albarsanz MA, Recio MN. Lindane-induced modifications to membrane lipid structure: Effect on membrane fluidity after subchronic treatment. Biosci Rep 1992;*12*:303–311.

78. Kenawi MZ, Morsy TA, Adalla KF, Nasr ME, Awadalla RA. Clinical and parasitological aspects of human scabies in Qualyobia Governorate Egypt. J Egypt Soc Parasitol 1993;*23*:247–253.

79. Dengelau J. Management of scabies in the nursing home. J Geriatr Drug Ther 1991;*6*:37–46.

80. Andrews ER, Joseph MC, Magenheim MJ, Tilson HH, Doi PA, Scultz MW. Postmarketing surveillance study of permethrin creme rinse. Am J Public Health 1992;*82*:857–861.

Reviews

r1. Garcia LS, Bruckner DA, eds. Diagnostic medical parasitology, 2d ed. Herndon VA: ASM Press, 1993.

r2. Markell EK, Voge M, John DT. Medical parasitology, 7th ed. Philadelphia: WB Saunders, 1992.

r3. Abramowicz M, ed. Drugs for AIDS and associated infections. The Medical Letter 1991;*33*:95–102.

r4. McAdam KPWJ. New strategies in parasitology. New York: Churchill Livingston, 1989.

r5. Abramowicz M, ed. Drugs for parasitic infections. The Medical Letter 1992;*34*:17–26.

r6. Kretschmer RR, ed. Amebiasis: Infection and disease by *Entamoeba histolytica*. Boca Raton FL: CRC Press, 1990.

r7. Bruce-Chwatt LJ, ed. Chemotherapy of malaria. Revised, 2d ed. Geneva: World Health Organization, 1986.

r8. Nodiff EA, Chatterjee S, Musallam HA. Antimalarial activity of the 8-aminoquinolines. Prog Med Chem 1991;*28*:1–40.

r9. Sharma S. Vector-borne diseases. Prog Drug Res 1990;*35*:365–485.

r10. MacInnis AJ, ed. Molecular paradigms for eradicating helminthic parasites. New York: Alan R. Liss, 1987.

r11. Lanusse C, Prichard RK. Clinical pharamacokinetics and metabolism of benzimidazole antihelminthics in ruminants. Drug Metabol Rev 1993;*25*:235–279.

r12. Abramowicz M, ed. Drugs for parasitic infections. The Medical Letter 1993;*35*:111–122.

r13. Campbell WC, ed. Ivermectin and Abamectin. New York: Springer-Verlag, 1989.

r14. Voogd TE, Vansterkenburg ELM, Wilting J, Janssen LHM. Recent research on the biological activity of suramin. Pharmacol Rev 1993;*45*:177–203.

r15. Orkin M, Maibach HI. Cutaneous infestations and insect bites. New York: Marcel Dekker, 1985.

CHAPTER 101

Cancer Chemotherapeutic Drugs*

Ti Li Loo
Emil J. Freireich

Treatment of cancer—or what appeared to be cancer—with herbs and potions, usually given orally, dates back several millennia. For example, such treatments can be found in Egyptian hieroglyphics and papyrus medical documents. Likewise, in the ancient Chinese pharmacopoeia, putative antitumor properties were attributed to many herbal medicines. Almost all of these claims were anecdotal and shrouded in myth; this is understandable, considering the primitive state of medicine at the dawn of civilization and the beginning of recorded history. Modern rational cancer chemotherapy began in 1942, when the clinical trial of nitrogen mustards was initiated as a result of the discovery that these compounds were selectively toxic to lymphoid tissues.[1,2] Since then, cancer chemotherapy has advanced by leaps and bounds to become one of the most important and exciting armamentaria against cancer today.

The chemotherapy of cancer differs basically from that of infectious parasitic diseases in that the agents used are seldom specific against the malignant cell alone, in sharp contrast to drugs used in infectious diseases, that are selectively toxic to the invading organism. Obviously, there is a degree of specificity, or cancer chemotherapy would not have been effective at all. Experimentally as well as clinically, this lack of specificity manifests itself most readily in dose-response curves of steep slopes. A slight escalation in dose often is accompanied by a sharp rise in systemic toxicity, especially in such sensitive susceptible normal cells as bone marrow stem cells, hair follicles, and GI mucosa cells. One must realize that normal cells and cancer cells rarely differ significantly in their physiology, pharmacology, and biochemistry. Contrary to the popular misconception, not all malignant cells proliferate faster (have a shorter cycle time) than normal cells do. Moreover, the doubling time of some tumors, including those of colon, breast, and lung, instead of being short are in fact very long. In addition, characteristics of invasiveness, metastatic potential, and degree of differentiation vary appreciably from one kind of malignancy to another. Further, cancer is not a single disease, but more than a hundred different kinds of diseases affecting every organ. Taking all this into consideration, one must conclude that cancer chemotherapy is indeed a challenging undertaking.

Cancer chemotherapeutic agents may have any chemical structure conceivable. In other words, there is no common unique structural feature that confers "antineoplastic properties" on a compound. Both an organic compound with only one carbon, (hydroxyurea) and a complex enzyme (asparaginase [L-asparagine amidohydrolase, E.C. 3.5.1.1]), are clinically useful anticancer agents. Further, the discovery of cisplatin as a cancer chemotherapeutic agent with a broad spectrum of activity demolished the notion that antitumor properties belong to organic compounds exclusively.

Anticancer agents can be of natural origin or synthetic. Almost all naturally occurring anticancer agents were discovered either by chance or through screening initially random but later systematic. Examples are the vinca alkaloids and the anthracycline antibiotics.

*Dedicated to our mentor, C. Gordon Zubrod, M.D., physician, pharmacologist, teacher, and administrator, Father of modern cancer chemotherapy.

Synthetic antineoplastic agents were discovered by "enlightened empiricism," since a first principle to guide their synthesis obviously was nonexistent. Elegant theories have been proposed to delineate quantitative structure-activity relationships among various classes of drugs, including anticancer agents.[3] But to this day no useful antitumor agents have ever been designed and synthesized using this approach. However, a number of clinically important antimetabolites, such as cytarabine, mercaptopurine, and fluorouracil, are the products of structural modifications of their natural counterparts. Such modifications include isoelectronic substitution (for example, -CH= with -N= in an aromatic ring system and the reverse in a heterocyclic compound), positional exchanges (usually switching C and N around in heterocyclic systems), atomic substitution of one with another in the same periodic group (for example, O with S), stereoisomeric changes (for example, from ribosyl to arabinosyl), substitution of an atom or a group with another of comparable size (for example H with F, CH_3 with CF_3), and homologous substitution. Notable successes by this more or less empirical approach culminated in the introduction of the above antimetabolites into clinical cancer chemotherapy. But drug design of this nature hardly deserves to be considered rational; in fact, as the intellectual basis of "enlightened empiricism" soon became exhausted, further similar simplistic attempts aptly branded "methyl ethyl, butyl futile," produced no useful agents with clinical efficacy comparable to the early ones. As mentioned above, the discovery that the nitrogen mustards are clinically useful anticancer agents stimulated the synthesis of a host of compounds incorporating, sometimes ad nauseam, the magic cytotoxic bullet, namely, the bis(2-chloroethyl)amino entity; but among these only mechlorethamine, chlorambucil, melphalan, and, particularly, cyclophosphamide have demonstrated clinical value.

Obviously, to inhibit tumor cell proliferation, the interruption of certain critical biochemical pathways in nucleic acid and protein syntheses remains the most logical, attractive, and fundamental strategy. In the evolution of rational anticancer drug design from simple structural modifications of natural metabolites to more elegant and thoughtful biochemical manipulations, the ingenious development of PALA [N-(phosphonacetyl)-L-aspartate] as a cancer chemotherapeutic agent deserves special mention. Originally conceived as a stable transition state analogue in the transcarbamoylation of L-aspartate, an early step in the de novo pyrimidine biosynthesis,[4] PALA was highly active against several animal tumors that seldom responded to conventional antimetabolites; additionally, it was not immunosuppressive, nor toxic to the hematopoietic system and intestinal epithelium of the mouse. Unfortunately, PALA showed no significant activity in its clinical trials, apparently because human cancer cells, in contrast to the murine variety, very efficiently resorted to the salvage pathway when de novo pyrimidine biosynthesis was blocked by PALA. Therefore, in planning the overall chemotherapy of cancer in humans, the patient must be dealt with as a whole. To single out only one of the many biochemical pathways for attack rarely succeeds.

Having served its early useful purpose, enlightened empiricism is clearly on the wane. Rightfully it must give way to more imaginative approaches, perhaps with the aid of computer science and other sophisticated modern techniques. To keep pace with current spectacular advances in biochemistry and molecular biology, new possible targets for anticancer agents have been suggested, for example, protein kinase C and various oncogenes. Moreover, as more new enzymes such as topoisomerases are discovered and found to be the targets of existing anticancer drugs, it naturally follows that potent and selective inhibitors of these enzymes will be designed, synthesized, and developed as cancer chemotherapeutic agents.

Most clinically useful anticancer agents are of natural origin, especially those discovered in recent years, such as the anthracycline antibiotics, camptothecin, taxol, and homoharringtonine. Almost all were discovered by random screening. Natural products provide an inexhaustible source of anticancer drugs in terms of both variety and mechanisms of action. However, these natural products are inevitably toxic; their selective action against neoplastic cells is a property not predictable before systematic screening.

The most serious shortcomings of existing anticancer agents have long been recognized. First of all, tumors responsible for most deaths are usually insensitive to chemotherapy; in other words, these tumors exhibit primary or de novo resistance. Further, tumors initially responsive to an anticancer agent often acquire resistance by a number of possible mechanisms,[4] so that they become refractory to subsequent treatment with the same agent. In addition, recently a new type of acquired resistance, multiple-drug resistance (MDR or pleiotropic drug resistance), has been reported. This pertains to malignant cell lines made resistant to a single chemotherapeutic agent, generally a natural product, that later were found to be resistant to many structurally unrelated cytotoxic agents. Lack of high specificity against tumor cells compared with normal cells is the second obvious shortcoming of cancer chemotherapeutic agents, although they are relatively specific to a certain extent. Finally, many anticancer agents fail to penetrate the anatomic sanctuaries where malignant cells are sequestered. For these and other reasons, more efficacious chemotherapeutic agents are always urgently needed. Ideal new agents should have no serious systemic toxicity and should be able to induce long, preferably indefinite, complete remissions in a large population of patients with a variety of neoplastic diseases—the most fatal types in particular.

In drug development, before clinical trials, screening of the candidate drug in some model systems is always the first step, to be followed by toxicologic evaluations, also in experimental animals. For many years in the U.S. mass screening in murine tumor systems was routinely prescribed and conducted, especially the mouse leukemia L1210. This test later was preceded by mouse leukemia P388 (more sensitive than L1210 to natural products) and followed by a panel of solid tumor systems. But the model systems proved to be of limited predictive value;[5] fewer than 1% of the drugs active against animal tumor systems ever demonstrated useful clinical activities. These failures may be attributed to species differences between man and the mouse in the following aspects: host genetic make-up (genetically heterogenous humans versus pure, often inbred mice); unknown or uncertain etiology of the human disease (as contrasted with transplantable rodent tumors, unless spontaneous); biochemical, pharmacodynamic, and pharmacokinetic (as well as cell kinetic) considerations; drug dosages used in the treatment (relatively much higher in the mouse—up to LD_{10} sometimes); possible interactions among the multiple drugs prescribed clinically; and wide variabilities in tumor age, stage, grade, and metastatic potential. Undoubtedly, additional factors also may account for the failures. After all, animal models are no more than models; ultimately, the efficacy of an antitumor agent can be determined only clinically in patients.

Lately, a shift in the mass primary screening from the traditional murine models (the so-called "compound-oriented" in vivo systems) to the rapidly developing "disease-oriented" systems with cultured cells has been advocated.[r7] These in vitro systems offer some obvious advantages over the in vivo models. For example, the ready control of experimental conditions is useful, as are the possibility of screening against not only human tumors of a specific cell type but also sensitive as well as resistant cell sublines. The capability of detecting activities of substances that undergo facile in vivo degradation and the ease of extending studies to multiple histopathologic types of tumor contribute, as do economies in both time and materials. Results of in vitro tests are more quickly forthcoming, even with minute quantities of candidate drugs in short supply, such as natural products in a high state of purity. Cell lines need not be confined to those of human origin, but may be supplemented or complemented with those from murine sources like the L1210 and P388 leukemic cells. Success or failure with human cell lines is more germane because they are more readily adaptable to dose escalation schemes in subsequent Phase I/II clinical trials. But the in vitro systems also suffer from certain disturbing drawbacks. They bypass all pharmacokinetic barriers, such as drug absorption, compartmentalization, excretion, and (especially) metabolism of drugs that require in vivo metabolic activation. Also, specific cytotoxicity is not readily demonstrable unless a simultaneous culture of normal sensitive cells is used side-by-side for comparison. Finally, legal problems may attend the use of human cells. Perhaps a judicious combination of both the in vitro and the in vivo systems is the best compromise. The use of short-term in vitro assays with cultured human tumor cells taken from patients as a means of individualizing therapy has not lived up to its initial promise thus far. Since such assays give the highest true-negative results, their present utility appears to be limited to precluding the use of chemotherapeutic agents most likely to be ineffective in these patients. Clearly, further investigation is warranted.

Rodents and larger animals have been used for toxicologic studies of anticancer agents. Dogs and monkeys are useful for predicting marrow suppression, GI disturbances, and hepatoxicity in man. However, they fail to foretell clinical renal, cardiovascular, or neuromuscular toxicities.[6] During the past four decades, the cumulative results from extensive toxicologic evaluations of anticancer agents in many species have convincingly demonstrated the absence of significant advantages of larger animals over rodents as the predicting model. The current prevailing and perhaps more sensible practice is to establish speedily a toxicologic profile of the agent in terms of lethal doses (LD_{10}, LD_{50}, LD_{90}, etc.) in mice. From these the initial dose for clinical trials of the agent will be estimated. Since unusual toxicities, such as the pancreatitis of L-asparaginase, the myocardial damage caused by doxorubicin, and the ototoxicity of cisplatin, actually were not first detected in animals, and since one of the objectives of a Phase I clinical trial is to assess drug toxicity, ultimate evaluation in humans obviously is necessary.

Traditionally, clinical trials of new drugs proceed through four phases with specified but occasionally overlapping (particularly Phases I and II) purposes. Briefly these are: Phase I, to assess drug toxicity, to arrive at the optimal subtoxic dose, schedule, and route of administration for subsequent trials, and to conduct clinical pharmacologic studies; Phase II, to evaluate clinical therapeutic response and toxicity and to establish dose-response relationships; Phase III, to compare efficacy of the new agent with that of established standard agents; and Phase IV, to compare drug efficacy in combination with other agents.

In clinical practice it is now universally accepted to base the dosage of anticancer agents on body surface (usually mg/m^2) rather than body weight (usually mg/kg). When the dosages of a number of anticancer agents are expressed in mg/m^2, an approximate one-to-one correspondence exists between the maximum tolerated dose in man on a once-daily-for-five-days schedule and the LD_{10} in animals (including the mouse, rat, hamster, dog, and monkey) on the same schedule.[7] In Phase I clinical trials, conventionally one-tenth of the LD_{10} (in mg/m^2) in the most sensitive species (in most cases the mouse) is chosen as the starting dose in man. In the complete absence of toxicity, this dose is repeatedly doubled until toxicity is seen. This is safe because, in both laboratory animals and patients, doubling the nontoxic dose is not lethal. In comparison, smaller dose increments, such as in the modified Fibonaci scheme, not only expose a large number of patients to inadequate doses unlikely to produced any therapeutic effects, but also unnecessarily prolong the Phase I clinical trial. To arrive at the clinical maximum tolerated dose is frequently time-consuming and wasteful of resources. An elegant proposal has recently been made to accelerate this process on the basis of pharmacokinetic studies in mouse and man;[8] this approach clearly deserves further confirmation and exploration in future clinical trials of new agents.

Preclinical pharmacologic studies of new potential anticancer agents are a prerequisite for their adequate clinical trial. These are not simply "drug monitoring," but must include investigation of drug absorption, transport, distribution, binding, excretion, metabolism, and mechanisms of action. As a step further, similar studies in humans always must be included in clinical trials of new agents, particularly during Phases I and II. All anticancer agents are cytotoxic; unless they display some selectivity and specificity against human malignancies, they have no significant lasting clinical value. The clinical efficacy of an antitumor agent, representing the sum total expression of its nontoxicity, selectivity, specificity, and pharmacokinetic and pharmacodynamic properties in humans, is often exquisitely sensitive to manipulations of dose, schedule, and route of administration. Consequently, the effective use of a new agent necessarily depends on the availability of pertinent pharmacologic information derived from experiments with the agent—initially in laboratory animals, but eventually also in humans. A few of the critical questions to be addressed are: Is the target cancer cell exposed to an effective cytotoxic concentration of the agent under conditions simulating those in the clinical setting? Does a favorable drug-concentration differential exist between the tumor and the susceptible normal cell? Is the agent sequestered in any of the vital organs, and will it only emerge later to cause latent toxicity? Is it metabolically activated to an entity actually responsible for the cytotoxicity? These and other essential factors are decisive in the intelligent design of clinical trial protocols. Naturally, answers to some of these questions will be forthcoming in the course of the trial. However, it would be more efficient and expedient to seek answers in experimental animals first, so that they are readily available to the clinician responsible for the trial.

Furthermore, when and if "disease-oriented" in vitro screening is finally adopted on a massive scale everywhere, its success would hinge in large measure on the results of pharmacologic studies of the agent to be screened. First of all, such studies will provide information most crucial to the in vitro screen, the dose range. Once the in vitro ID_{50} of the new agent has been established, it would be logical to determine how it is related to the corresponding in vivo tumor-inhibiting dose. If a major discrepancy is revealed, attempts must be made to find the biochemical pharmacologic reasons for it. Most important, because by design in vitro systems bypass all the in vivo pharmacokinetic barriers, they are incomplete at best, and must be supplemented by results from in vivo pharmacokinetic investigations that provide the missing information. It cannot be overemphasized that it is misleading to interpret the in vitro screening results except in light of the pharmacokinetics of the agent. In other words, the determination of the in vitro inhibitory drug concentration would be irrelevant, futile, and meaningless unless the concentration is consistent with the in vivo drug exposure estimated from the pharmacokinetics of the drug. Even in this event caution should always be exercised in translating in vitro results to an in vivo setting.

Only the major cancer chemotherapeutic agents selected on the strength of their clinical usefulness will be discussed in this chapter. Hormonal agents are described elsewhere, and thus excluded here. These chemotherapeutic agents are grouped together conventionally: alkylating agents; antimetabolites; natural products; and other categories. It is impossible to classify anticancer agents according to their chemical structures, since, as we alluded to earlier, an anticancer agent may have any conceivable structure—from simple molecules like hydroxyurea and cisplatin, through complex natural products like the vinca alkaloids, to macromolecules like L-asparaginase. A corollary is that no common structural feature is shared by all kinds of anticancer agents. To classify chemotherapeutic agents based on their mechanisms of action is presumptuous and fraught with difficulties. First, the mechanisms of action of most agents remain obscure. Second, the mechanism that is understood may not be the one operative in vivo and decisively responsible for the selective cytotoxicity of the agent. Third, one mechanism already elucidated does not necessarily exclude other mechanisms yet to be discovered. Last, although some anticancer agents like the antimetabolites show cell-cycle specificity whereas others like the alkylating agents do not, dividing chemotherapeutic agents into two large classes does not really address the issues satisfactorily.

A brief historical account of each agent (or a group of agents); is given. This is followed by a description of its chemistry and mechanisms of antitumor action, as well as resistance, if known. Pharmacokinetics and pharmacodynamics will be presented. Finally, its clinical therapeutic application and toxicity will be described. Only the most relevant literature will be cited; review articles are preferred.

For those who wish to have a broad perspective of cancer chemotherapy or to delve into certain aspects in more depth, additional recent references may be consulted.[r1–r6]

Alkylating Agents

These are compounds that cause cytotoxicity by reacting with cellular macromolecular nucleophilic centers. Their alkylating function is generated by a variety of mechanisms.[9]

Nitrogen Mustards, R-N(CH_2CH_2Cl)$_2$

Modern rational cancer chemotherapy was ushered in more than 40 years ago when mechlorethamine (HN2) was first used to treat Hodgkin's disease and other lymphomas.[2] It soon became apparent that at physiologic pH one of the 2-chloroethyl moiety of HN2 is converted to an aziridinium cation that readily reacts with or alkylates cellular nucleophiles; these include most frequently the N-7 position and, to a lesser extent, the N-3 and O-6 positions of DNA guanine, the N-1 and N-3 positions of adenine, the N-3 position of cytosine, the phosphate of nucleic acids, and the amino, carboxyl, hydroxyl, imidazolyl, and sulfhydryl groups of proteins. Moreover, the second 2-chloroethyl moiety in turn reacts similarly with these nucleophiles. The monoalkylation results in DNA base mispairing and subsequent miscoding and mutation, whereas bialkylation gives rise to strand crosslinking; the latter lesion is more difficult to repair than the former. The bifunctional alkylating agent can additionally link a DNA strand to proteins. Also, depurination of guanine may occur, leading to DNA strand breakage. These damages are especially lethal to dividing cells in late G and S phases of the cell cycle, although alkylating agents are not cell cycle specific and may exert their deleterious effects on cells in any phase of the cycle except the G_0 phase.

All nitrogen mustards are derivatives of bis(2-chloroethyl) amine; in mechlorethamine the R is a methyl group. After the antitumor activities of these drugs had been demonstrated, to improve selectivity numerous nitrogen mustards were synthesized with various R groups as the prosthetic carrier molecule. However, disappointingly, no significant improvement in selectivity has been observed, and currently only a few of these agents are used clinically. As noted above, they presumably share the same cytotoxic mechanism; however, with the exception of HN2, their modes of action have not been studied in detail.

Mechlorethamine (HN2, Nitrogen Mustard; R=CH_3)

This prototype nitrogen mustard enjoyed early prominence as the first rational cancer chemotherapeutic agent. HN2 itself is unstable and hygroscopic, and hence was formulated as the hydrochloride admixed with sodium chloride. For parenteral administration, the solution must be prepared fresh and used immediately; the chemical and biologic half-life of HN2 is less than 10 minutes; care must be taken to prevent necrotic extravasation and direct vesicant tissue injury.

Alkylation of various cellular macromolecular nucleophiles by HN2 undoubtedly accounts for its cytotoxicity, particularly to the rapidly proliferating cells in the bone marrow, GI tract, gonads, and hair follicles; however, alopecia is not as severe as that attributed to cyclophosphamide (see below). Major clinical toxicity of HN2 manifests itself in nausea and vomiting and myelosuppression; central in origin, the former can be alleviated by pretreatment with antiemetics.

HN2 is rapidly degraded in vivo. After parenteral administration of [^{14}C]methyl-labeled HN2 in the mouse, the fate of the radioactivity was as follows: 30 to 50 percent fixed in tissues in six hours, with a very slow turnover; in 24 hours, 15 to 20 percent in the expired air as $^{14}CO_2$, 5 to 10 percent excreted in the urine, and approximately 1 percent exhaled as unidentified volatile metabolite(s).[10] The pharmacologic fate of HN2 in humans has not been reported but may be similar to that in the mouse. Its transport in mouse leukemic L5178Y cells is an active carrier-mediated process;[11] also, hydrolyzed HN2 and choline share a common transport mechanism in cultured human leukemic lymphoid cells.[12] In fact, cellular resistance to HN2 seems to be attributable in part to impaired uptake of the agent.[11–13] But this does not rule out other resistance mechanisms, including increased DNA repair of lesions caused by HN2 alkylation and enhanced trapping of HN2 by thiols and other competing nucleophiles.

Clinically, HN2 remains useful in treating Hodgkin's disease and other lymphomas, especially mycosis fungoides when applied topically.[2] Owing to its transient in vivo half-life, in patients with profound catabolic organ failure—that of liver or kidney, for example, secondary to rapidly advancing lymphoma or other malignancies—HN2 can be used in full dosage without further aggravating existing organ dysfunction. However, the drug is now seldom used alone, but usually in combination with other agents, such as vincristine (Oncovin), prednisone, and procarbazine in the MOPP regimen.

Chlorambucil (R=HO_2C–(CH_2)$_3$–⌬–)

Originally synthesized as a soluble aryl nitrogen mustard for parenteral administration, chlorambucil was effective orally. Its mechanism of cytotoxic action presumably is similar to that of mechlorethamine. After SQ administration of tritiated chlorambucil to rats bearing the Yoshida ascites sarcoma, the nucleic acids and proteins of sensitive cells accumulated twice as much tritium as did resistant cells. Hence, as in the case of HN2, cellular resistance to chlorambucil must be due partly to diminished drug uptake.

The clinical pharmacokinetics of chlorambucil has been studied in several laboratories by gas chromatography-mass spectrometric assay. In one study involving four patients, after oral chlorambucil, the average plasma half-life of the drug during the terminal phase was 92 minutes; less than 1 percent of the dose was excreted in the urine in 24 hours. In another two patients who received by mouth radioactive chlorambucil with ^{14}C-label in the ethylene moieties of the mustard group, the plasma half-life of total radioactivity was again 97 minutes, but this time 58 percent of the administered radioactivity was recovered in the urine in 24 hours. Clearly, chlorambucil was extensively metabolized. In fact, chlorambucil underwent in vivo β-oxidation to the major metabolite, phenylacetic acid mustard **($R{=}HO_2C{-}CH_2{-}C_6H_4{-}$)**, with a plasma half-life of 145 min, about 1.6 times that of the parent drug. These results were in good agreement with those reported by another group of investigators,[14] who, using high performance liquid chromatography (HPLC), reported that six patients after oral chlorambucil consistently absorbed more than 70 percent of the dose. The terminal phase plasma half-life of chlorambucil in these patients was 109 min. These investigators additionally studied five patients by IV administration; the half-life of the drug was 80 minutes during the terminal phase, based on a two-compartment model. Both chlorambucil and the phenylacetic metabolite have comparable antitumor activities in rodents.

Chlorambucil is used principally in the treatment of chronic lymphocytic leukemia, other low-grade lymphoid malignancies, and ovarian carcinoma. However, because of the increasing frequency of secondary malignancies (acute myeloblastic leukemia in particular) following chlorambucil therapy, and because of the discovery of more effective treatment for those tumors, the clinical application of chlorambucil is now limited. The recent claim that its prednisolone ester, prednimustine, has an improved therapeutic index remains to be confirmed clinically.

Compared with other chemotherapeutic agents, chlorambucil is much better tolerated. Its chief toxicity is reversible myelosuppression; nausea is absent or mild at worst.

Melphalan ($R{=}{-}C_6H_4{-}CH_2{-}CH(NH_2){-}CO_2H$)

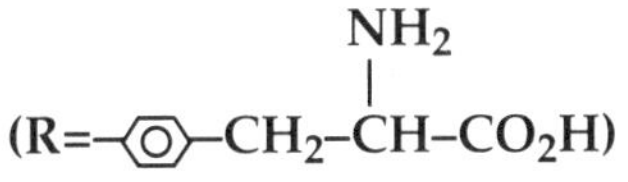

Melphalan, an arylnitrogen mustard incorporating the amino acid L-phenylalanine, was originally synthesized with the hope of achieving selectivity against malignant melanomas because L-phenylalanine is a precursor of melanin. However, the drug has not lived up to this promise.

Certain aspects of the cellular transport of melphalan are noteworthy. In cultured human breast cancer cells and in normal lymphocytes, the transport is an active process mediated by two amino acid carriers. Transport capacity is 50-fold larger in the cancer cells than in the lymphocytes, thus partially accounting for the drug's selective cytotoxicity against cancer cells. Melphalan transport appears to be impaired in resistant as compared with sensitive mouse L1210 leukemia cells. The L-isomer of melphalan is ten times more cytotoxic than the D-isomer; this is also reflected in the inhibition of L-leucine transport by melphalan, the L-isomer being seven times more inhibitory. Because of the significant presence of amino acids like leucine and glutamine in the ascites fluid of patients with ovarian carcinoma, the possible inhibition of cellular uptake of melphalan by the amino acids in the fluid must be considered in the intraperitoneal administration of this agent. Moreover, melphalan is extensively bound to plasma proteins.

After oral administration the bioavailability of melphalan varies widely from 30 to 100 percent, (average 60%);[15] it takes up to six hours before the drug is detected in the plasma. By either the oral or the IV route, plasma melphalan shows a half-time of approximately 90 minutes during the terminal phase; in 24 hours 11 to 14 percent of the dose is excreted in the urine.[15,16] However, when radioactive melphalan is administered, the plasma half-life of total radioactivity representing unchanged drug and metabolites is extremely long—160 hours—during the terminal phase. Also, the cumulative urinary excretion of total radioactivity is much higher.[15,17,18] Melphalan evidently undergoes spontaneous chemical degradation and in vivo metabolism; two of the dechlorinated metabolites are the mono- and dihydroxy derivatives.[16]

Being considerably less effective than cyclophosphamide in acute leukemia, lymphomas, and other solid tumors, melphalan is nevertheless the agent of choice for the treatment of multiple myeloma. Also, it has been used in the management of ovarian cancer. Myelosupression is its major clinical toxicity; nausea and vomiting are infrequent, and alopecia is rare. Because of the absence of other organ toxicities, melphalan additionally has been used parenterally in escalated doses, particularly as a conditioning regimen for autologous and allogeneic bone marrow transplantation.

Cyclosphosphamide (CPA, Cytoxan, R–P(=O) in a ring with O and NH)

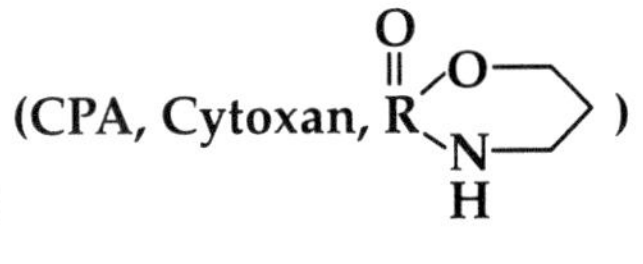

One of the most important and perhaps best investigated anticancer agents with a broad spectrum of clinical activities, CPA, incorporating a novel oxazaphosphorine ring, was initially conceived as a transport or latent form of *nor*-nitrogen mustard that remains inactive until supposedly cleaved intracellularly by phosphoramidase (EC 3.9.1.1) found in relative abundance in a number of tumor cells. CPA is indeed not cytotoxic until metabolically activated.[19] However, CPA activation is not a hydrolytic, but an oxidative process involving the hepatic microsomal mixed function oxidases. Because of the prominence of CPA as a cancer chemotherapeutic agent, it has been the object of intensive biochemical and pharmacologic studies summarized in a 1975 monograph;[20] an international symposium on the metabolism and mechanism of action of CPA was held in 1975. The clinical pharmacokinetics of CPA have been authoritatively reviewed.[9,21,22]

The metabolism of CPA is outlined in Fig. 101.1.

As discussed in Fig. 101.1, oxidation (Reaction I) of CPA, mediated by hepatic microsomal oxidases, affords 4-hydroxy CPA (an hemiaminal in equilibrium with 4-aldoCPA) the open-ring isomer. Spontaneous decomposition (Reaction IV) of 4-aldoCPA gives acrolein and phosphoramide mustard, an unstable reactive alkylating agent. Further oxidation of both 4-hydroxyCPA (Reaction II) and 4-aldoCPA (Reaction III) by aldehyde oxidase (EC 1.2.3.1), yields 4-ketoCPA, likewise in equilibrium with its 4-carboxy isomer; the 4-ketoCPA being favored. Since both are apparently inert biologically, their formation is considered detoxification; in fact, 85 percent of an administered dose of CPA is biotransformed to 4-keto- and 4-carboxyCPA, predominantly the former. The unstable phosphoramide mustard decomposes (Reaction V) spontaneously or mediated by phosphoramidase (EC 3.9.1.1) to nor-nitrogen mustard, another alkylating agent also formed from the hydrolysis (Reaction VI) of 4-carboxyCPA. Of these CPA metabolites and spontaneous decomposition products, it remains uncertain and controversial which are really responsible for host toxicity and which function principally for selective anticancer activity; however, most investigators believe that phosphoramide mustard is principally responsible for DNA cross-linking by CPA. In the sheep, a fraction (less than 5%) of administered CPA undergoes oxidative cleavage of one of the 2-chloroethyl side-chains, with formation of dechloroethyl-CPA and 2-chloroacetaldehyde (Reactions IA and IB); the former is devoid of

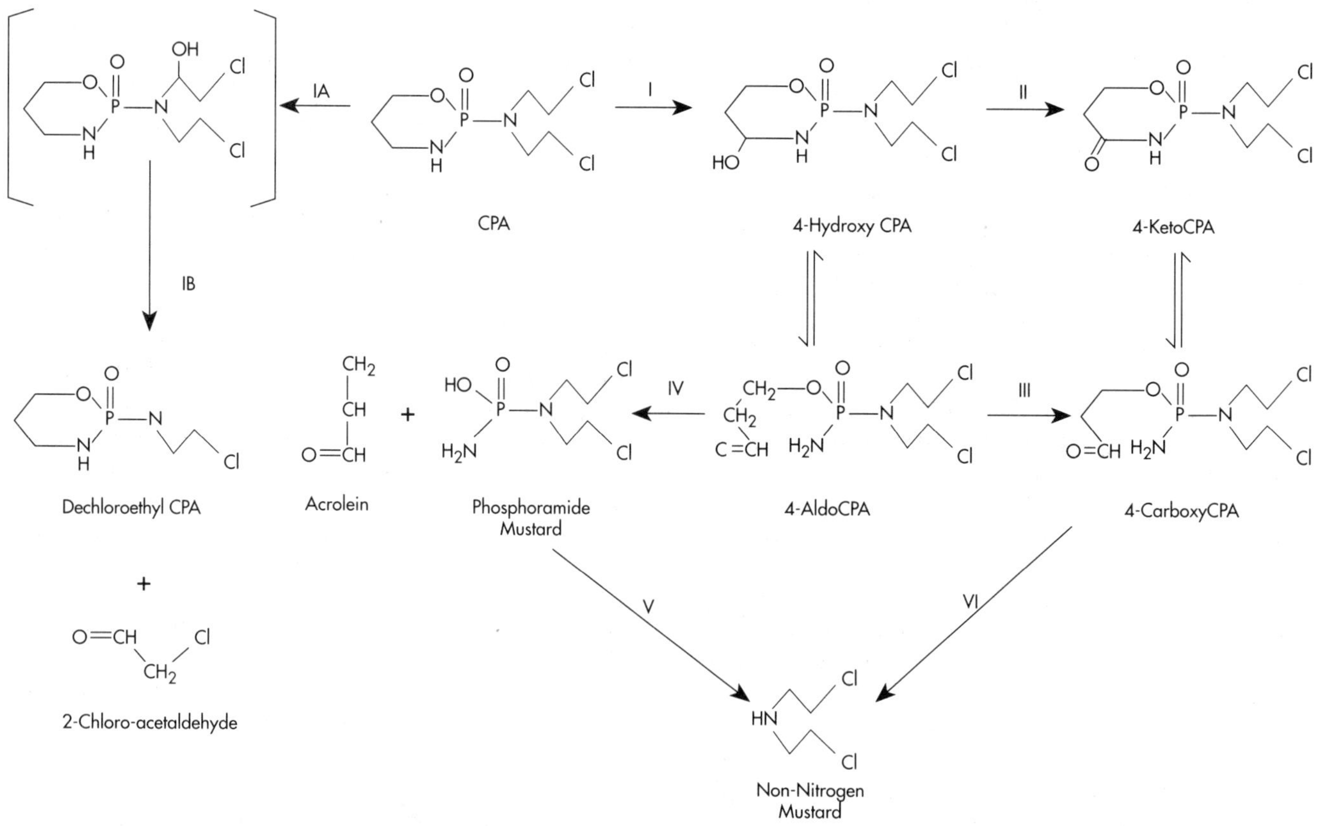

Figure 101.1

antitumor activity. This minor pathway of CPA metabolism has also been observed in patients (M.P. Goren, personal communication).

The clinical pharmacokinetics of CPA have been investigated in many laboratories by a variety of assay techniques.[21] CPA is completely bioavailable after oral administration.[23] Based on several studies[21,24,25] involving a large number of patients, the terminal plasma CPA half-life is approximately seven hours after IV administration. Repeated and continuous administration apparently stimulated the metabolism of CPA itself, so that the plasma CPA half-life is significantly reduced,[25,26] accompanied by an increase in the plasma concentration of free alkylating activity. Plasma CPA clearance is affected by a number of pathologic conditions. In patients with creatinine clearance below 100 ml/min, plasma CPA half-life is progressively lengthened;[27] but how to adjust CPA dosage in case of severe renal failure remains to be determined. Likewise, in patients with severe liver failure, total body clearance of CPA is greatly reduced and the plasma half-life of the drug much prolonged.[24] Also, in obese patients, plasma CPA half-life is positively and systemic CPA clearance negatively correlated with body weight.[28] Other drugs administered with CPA also may induce its clearance—for example, phenytoin[29] and etoposide.[25] On account of its extensive metabolism, only approximately 10 to 20 percent of the administered dose is excreted intact in the urine,[25] hepatobiliary excretion is insignificant. However, CPA enters the CNS readily; it is cleared from the CSF more slowly than from the plasma.[29] After either oral or IV administration CPA appears in the saliva to achieve a steady-state salive-to-plasma CPA concentration ratio of 0.77.

As a single agent administered orally or IV, CPA is often curative in patients with Burkitt's lymphoma. However, it is nowadays incorporated into a large number of regimens for the treatment not only of lymphomas, but of other solid tumors and leukemias. In combination with anthracycline antibiotics, apparent clinical synergism has been observed; thus, the CHOP (CPA, doxorubicin, vincristine, and prednisone) regimen is one of the most effective for lymphoma treatment. A further major use of CPA is as a conditioning agent for allogeneic bone marrow transplantation, especially in high dose coupled with total body radiation. This regimen was initially successful in patients with acute myeloblastic leukemia, but subsequently also in those with either chronic granulocytic leukemia or myelodysplastic syndromes.

The major clinical toxicities are myelosuppression with infrequent thrombocytopenia, reversible alopecia, nausea and vomiting; hemorrhagic cystitis occurs occasionally in some patients. Both oral and parenteral preparations of CPA are available for clinical use. It is soluble in water: 40 mg/ml at room temperature. In 5 percent dextrose solution, it is stable for at least 24 hours.[30]

Ifosfamide (IFA, cyclic O–P(=O)(–NH–CH_2CH_2Cl)–N(–CH_2CH_2Cl) ring)

A CPA isomer, IFA differs from CPA in that one of the two N,N-bis(2-chloroethyl) side-chains of CPA is linked to the ring nitrogen, N-3, of the 1,3,2-oxazaphosphorine ring. Because of their close structural relationship, it is expected that the two agents would have much in common with respect to their mode of action, pharmacologic disposition, metabolism, and clinical activity. On the contrary, as is often the case with many anticancer agents and their structural analogues, an apparently insignificant modification frequently is sufficient to elicit noticeable differences in clinical activity, pharmacology, and toxicology. It is these differences that make IFA a promising anticancer agent in its own right, rather than simply just another CPA-derivative. Further, at this time it remains unclear whether clinically these two agents are cross-resistant. Interest in IFA has been shown by many international symposia on the agent held in the last few years; the proceedings of these have been published;[31,32] reviews on both the preclinical and clinical aspects of IFA have appeared recently.[33,r8,r9]

Like CPA, the exact mode of cytotoxic action of IFA is not completely understood. It is generally believed to be similar to that of CPA, in that both are activated metabolically in vivo by hepatic microsomal enzymes, resulting in the generation of alkylating species. Although the maximal enzymatic activation velocity is the same for both agents, IFA seems to produce alkylating activity at only approximately one-half the rate of CPA. Moreover, in humans the oxidative cleavage of either of the two 2-chloroethyl side-chains is at least as significant a metabolic pathway for IFA as the oxidation of the ring methylene group adjacent to the ring nitrogen, in distinct contrast to CPA. It may be recalled that with CPA the ring N-methylene group as well as one of the exocyclic N-methylene groups undergoes in vivo oxidation; the former pathway is by far the more important. But with IFA, all three such N-methylene groups are liable to in vivo oxidation, leading respectively to the formation of 4-hydroxy-IFA (ring oxidation), dechloroethyl-IFA (oxidative cleavage of the 2-chloroethyl group linked to the exocyclic nitrogen), and dechloroethyl-CPA (oxidative cleavage of the 2-chloroethyl group attached to the ring nitrogen). In fact, in 25 patients treated with IFA, all of the three metabolites were excreted in the urine; in 14 of them, the dechloroethyl metabolites were actually the major metabolites. Clinically, as far as toxicity is concerned, the dechloroethylation of IFA is critical because this metabolic pathway results in the production of 2-chloroacetaldehyde implicated in causing neurotoxicity after IFA administration. In comparison, apart from transient dizziness, CPA elicits no neurotoxicity. At any rate, because both dechloroethyl-CPA and dechloroethyl-IFA are inactive, like CPA, IFA must owe its cytotoxicity to the ultimate generation of IFA-mustard, bis[N,N′-2-chloroethyl)] phosphorodiamidic acid, and other alkylating entities after in vivo microsomal oxidation.

The plasma half-life of IFA appears to be dose- and schedule-dependent; it was 13.8 hours in five patients after a 45-minutes IV infusion at 5 g/m^2, but 6.9 hours in three patients after lower divided daily doses of 1.6 to 2.4 g for three days, the same as the plasma half-life of CPA. Thus, these observations suggest that IFA is cleared from the plasma by some saturable processes such as tissue deposition and metabolism. In the same five patients, approximately 80 percent of the administered dose was excreted in the urine in 72 hours, about two/thirds of this as intact IFA.[34] These results agree well with the estimated IFA clearance values of 0.390 $ml \cdot min^{-1} \cdot kg^{-1}$ for total and 0.274 $ml \cdot min^{-1} \cdot kg^{-1}$ for renal clearance [the clearance values are estimated from the results of Ref. 34]. Moreover, in comparison with CPA, the greater fraction of unchanged IFA excreted in the urine is consistent with the slower rate of in vitro metabolic activation of this agent—only one-half that of CPA as alluded to above. IFA shows some tendency to cross the blood brain barrier.[34] It is apparently completely bioavailable when given by mouth; however, IFA usually is administered IV.

The major toxic effects of IFA are the dose-limiting hematuria and the dose-dependent leukopenia; other toxicities are alopecia, nausea, and vomiting. Central nervous system toxicities such as lethargy and confusion after high doses of the drug have been attributed to the 2-chloroacetaldehyde generated from the oxidative cleavage of the 2-chloroethyl side-chain. The aforementioned hemorrhagic cystitis caused by the cytotoxic IFA metabolites excreted in the urine is ameliorated and even prevented by hydration and particularly by the systemic administration of Mesna (sodium 2-mercaptoethanesulfonate).

In Phase II trials IFA has shown activities against a wide spectrum of malignant diseases, including small cell lung cancer, testicular tumors of all histologic types, soft tissue sarcoma, mammary carcinoma, cervical carcinoma, hypernephroma, pancreatic tumor, and lymphoma. Moreover, IFA has demonstrated activity in salvage therapy of patients with testicular tumors and soft tissue sarcomas previously treated with CPA. It is also useful in combination regimens with anthracycline antibiotics and etoposide because of its mild myelosuppressive toxicity at effective doses.

Either alone or mixed with Mesna, IFA solution is stable for nine days at temperatures up to 27°C.

Alkyl Sulfonates

Busulfan (Myleran), $H_3C\text{-}SO_2\text{-}O\text{-}(CH_2)_4\text{-}O\text{-}SO_2\text{-}CH_3$

Among the many alkanesulfonic acids esters synthesized and developed as cancer chemotherapeutic agents, busulfan or 1,4-butanediol dimethanesulfonate, is the only one that has some clinical usefulness.

Compared with mechlorethamine as an alkylating agent, busulfan is far less bound to nucleic acids. However the identification of 3-hydroxytetrahydrothiophene-1,1-dioxide as a busulfan metabolite[35] evidently shows that this agent is capable of alkylating bifunctionally the thiols of cysteine, peptides, and proteins. Thus, it would appear that alkylation of proteins rather than nucleic acid is the predominant lesion caused by busulfan.

Early studies with radioactive busulfan in patients indicated that the drug is quickly absorbed when given orally, with a plasma half-life of total radioactivity approximately equal to one hour. Whether administered orally or IV, the results were the same, namely, the radioactivity disappeared very rapidly from the blood. No unchanged busulfan has ever been recovered from the urine. After IV administration, in 24 hours 30 percent of the ^{14}C label and 45 percent of the ^{35}S label appear in the urine; in the former studies, 12 unidentified metabolites have been found; whereas, in the latter studies, 95 percent of the ^{35}S resided in methanesulfonic acid.

Busulfan is highly selective against chronic myelocytic leukemia except in patients in blastic crisis. Naturally, myelosuppression is the dose-limiting toxicity, including thrombocytopenia and anemia. However, busulfan additionally elicits interstitial fibrosis of the lung, bone marrow, and other organs after prolonged use at low doses. This toxicity limits its use to managing chronic myelocytic leukemia; increasingly, busulfan is being replaced by hydroxyurea and interferon as initial treatment for this disease. Clinically, busulfan and CPA apparently are synergistic, and this combination is an effective conditioning regimen for allogeneic and autologous bone marrow transplantation. Moreover, as an antitumor regimen, this combination is comparable to that of CPA with total body radiation.

Nitrosoureas

Analogues of 1-methyl-3-nitro-1-nitrosoguanidine, a precursor of the simple alkylating agent, diazomethane, have exhibited activity against leukemias in experimental systems. This observation has led to the development of nitrosoureas as cancer chemotherapeutic agents with improved efficacy. Those with the general structure R-NH-CO-N(NO)-CH_2CH_2Cl currently enjoy some clinical applications; they are carmustine (BCNU, R=-CH_2CH_2Cl), lomustine (CCNU, R=cyclohexyl), and semustine (MeCCNU, R=*trans*-4-methylhexyl). Streptozotocin (in the general structure the 2-chloroethyl group is replaced with a methyl and the R is a 2-deoxy-2-glucopyranosyl moiety) is a curious, naturally-occurring nitroso antibiotic with antitumor property; however, its therapeutic usefulness is confined to the treatment of such rare cancers as pancreatic islet carcinoma and malignant carcinoid. As a group, the nitrosoureas are pharmacologically, toxicologically, and therapeutically fascinating. Their current status and new developments have been competently reviewed;[36] moreover, two symposia devoted to the nitrosoureas have been held. Finally, their clinical pharmacokinetics have been expertly summarized.[37]

An early suggestion that BCNU decomposes in vitro to both alkylating and carbamoylating entities[38] has paved the way for many later studies of its possible in vivo mechanisms of anticancer action. It is now commonly accepted that alkylation of nucleic acids by the nitrosoureas is responsible for their antitumor activity, whereas carbamoylation of proteins accounts for their host toxicity. Alkylation results in lesions of DNA interstrand and DNA-protein crosslinks. However, how alkylation modifies DNA depends on the chemical structures of the nitrosoureas.

The nitrosoureas are not only unstable and highly reactive in vitro, but also, not unexpectedly, undergo extensive degradation in vivo. Their metabolism in vitro has been reviewed.[37] The nitrosoureas undergo denitrosation, apparently mediated by hepatic microsomal enzymes, to afford nitric oxide and the correspondent ureas under anaerobic conditions.[39] Additionally, the cyclohexyl moieties of CCNU and MeCCNU are rapidly hydroxylated to give a number of metabolites. Human metabolism of the nitrosoureas has not been extensively studied, but presumably there are close similarities across species. This subject will be briefly discussed below under each agent. The nitrosoureas are unique in their high lipid solubility, thus making them drugs of choice in the therapy of diseases such as CNS malignancies.

Carmustine (BCNU)

The first nitrosourea in clinical trial, BCNU is also the most investigated of this group of agents. At temperatures above 30°C it is a yellowish oil difficult to dissolve in water (4 mg/ml) but much more soluble in 50 percent aqueous ethanol (150 mg/ml). It is unstable, especially in human plasma, with an in vitro half-life of 17 minutes.[39] In 5 percent dextrose solution at room temperature, its half-life is 50.6 hours in glass containers, but much shorter, 3.9 hours, in polyvinyl chloride infusion bags.[30]

In an early study involving four patients[40] who received radioactive BCNU labeled with ^{14}C in all carbons of both ethylene moieties, either orally or IV, unchanged BCNU is not detectable in plasma by radiochemical and chromatographic techniques five minutes after drug administration; however, some intact drug is found in the urine 25 minutes later. The urinary excretion of total radioactivity is slow, on average 65 percent in four days. The plasma biologic half-life of total radioactivity was 34 hours in two patients in the oral study, compared with 67 hours in the two patients in the IV study. The difference evidently was attributable to the first-pass effect. Fecal excretion of ^{14}C amounts to less than 1 percent of the dose, but in 24 hours 10 percent of the dose is exhaled as radioactive carbon dioxide. The radioactivity quickly appears in the CSF after drug administration; this is hardly surprising, since the nitrosoureas are readily soluble in lipids. A later study by means of a colorimetric assay in three patients treated with hepatic arterial infusion of BCNU indicated that the steady state of drug concentration in the hepatic venous blood is reached in 50 minutes, from which we estimate that the half-life of BCNU in the blood is approximately 7.5 minutes. These results may be compared with those of yet another study in which BCNU was quantified by a differential pulse polarographic method; in 12 patients with lung cancer, the disappearance of BCNU from the plasma fit a two-compartment model with a half-life of 18 minutes on average. As to the in vivo metabolism of BCNU in man, vinyl chloride has been detected by gas chromatography in blood and expired air from patients treated with this agent. From all of these reports it is readily apparent that BCNU is unstable in plasma and disappears rapidly from the blood, with a short in vivo half-life. It seems to be sequestered in some body compartments from which it effluxes slowly. BCNU undergoes extensive spontaneous decomposition that superimposes on its in vivo metabolism.

The major indications for BCNU are brain tumors, Hodgkin's disease, and multiple myeloma. Its characteristic clinical toxicity is a delayed and cumulative myelosuppression. Nausea and vomiting are not immediate but occur about two hours after drug administration. Because of its distinctive mechanism of interaction with DNA, BCNU has been used in combination with other alkylating agents, particularly CPA.

Lomustine (CCNU)

Clinical pharmacokinetic studies have been conducted with ^{14}C-labeled CCNU in the cyclohexyl ring (presumably all six carbons uniformly labeled),[41] in both carbons of the ethylene moiety, and in the carbonyl group; the drug was orally administered. Depending on where the label is, generally the plasma biologic half-life of total radioactivity varies from 27 hours to nearly five days. In 24 hours 50 to 66 percent of the label is in the urine. It also appears quickly in the CSF and brain tumor tissues. No intact drug has ever been detected in the plasma, urine, or CSF. In four patients at the end of a one-hour IV infusion of radioactive CCNU, three-fourths of the label resided in ring-hydroxylated metabolites, about two-thirds as trans-4-hydroxy-, one-third as cis-4-hydroxy-, and less than 5 percent as trans-3-hydroxy-CCNU.

CCNU in capsules for oral administration is useful for treating brain tumors and lymphomas, especially Hodgkin's disease. Delayed myelosuppression, nausea, and vomiting are the major clinical toxicities.

Semustine (MeCCNU)

In nine patients given orally radioactive MeCCNU labeled with ^{14}C either in the cyclohexyl ring or in both carbon atoms of the ethylene moiety, no intact drug has been found in the plasma or urine. During the terminal phase the plasma biologic half-life of total radioactivity is approximately 36 hours with the ethylene-labeled CCNU, but 72 hours with the ring-labeled drug. The 24-hour cumulative urinary excretion of ^{14}C is 50 percent of the dose with both labeled CCNUs. In two to three hours, radioactivity due to ring-labeled CCNU and its metabolites is found in the CSF, but at only 10 to 15 percent of the counts in the concurrent plasma.[41]

The clinical applications and toxicities of this drug are similar to those of CCNU.

Streptozocin (Streptozotocin)

Although a methylnitrosourea derivative (see Fig. 101.2), compared with the above nitrosoureas streptozocin is unusual in several aspects. It occurs naturally, a product from the fermentation broth of *Streptomyces achromogenes*. It is devoid of carbamoylating activity. In humans, its major side-effects are nephrotoxicity and GI upset; myelosuppression is mild. In animals it is diabetogenic; because of this, it has been used to treat islet-cell carcinoma with considerable success; however, the activity is enhanced when combined with 5-fluorouracil and doxorubicin in particular.[42] Such combinations also have been reported as effective in treating malignant carcinoid. In man, its terminal plasma half-life is 35 minutes; streptozocin is excreted in the urine, mostly as metabolites. Used alone, the recommended IV dose is 500 mg/m^2 daily for five days.

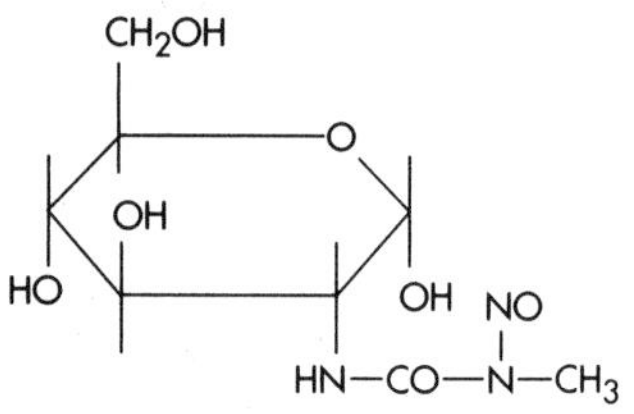

Figure 101.2

Thio-TEPA (1, 1′, 1″-phosphinothioylidynetrisaziridine)

Thio-TEPA[43] and TEPA are closely related (Fig. 101.3), but thio-TEPA is preferred to its oxygen analogue because it is more stable. It is a veteran agent; interest in thio-TEPA has recently been revived on account of its activity against intravesical bladder carcinoma. In its early development the drug was active against breast cancer. Nowadays, thio-TEPA doses higher than employed previously are possible when followed by reinfusion of cryopreserved autologous bone marrow. How exactly it exerts its anticancer action remains obscure; however, as an aziridine derivative, it is probably an alkylating agent. As a single agent, the recommended IV dose is 9 to 12 mg/m^2 at one- to four-weekly intervals. Toxicities include myelosuppression, GI disturbance, and CNS effects. In man, the terminal plasma half-life of thio-TEPA is approximately two hours, the total clearance 186 ml·min^{-1} ·m^{-2} (4.7ml·min^{-1}·kg^{-1}), and the steady-state volume of distribution 710 ml/kg (volume by area, 817 ml/kg). In 24 hours only 1.5 percent of the administered dose is excreted intact in the urine.[43]

Hexamethylmelamine (HMM)

There are six N-methyl groups in HMM (Fig. 101.4),[44] but in experimental systems its anticancer activities are gradually reduced with the sequential re-

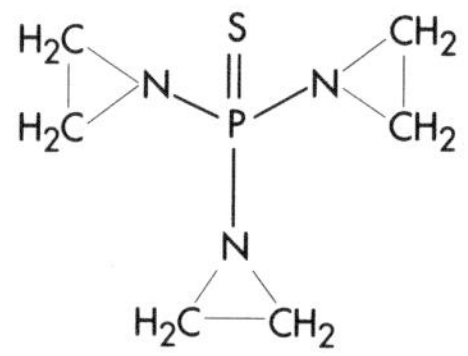

Figure 101.3

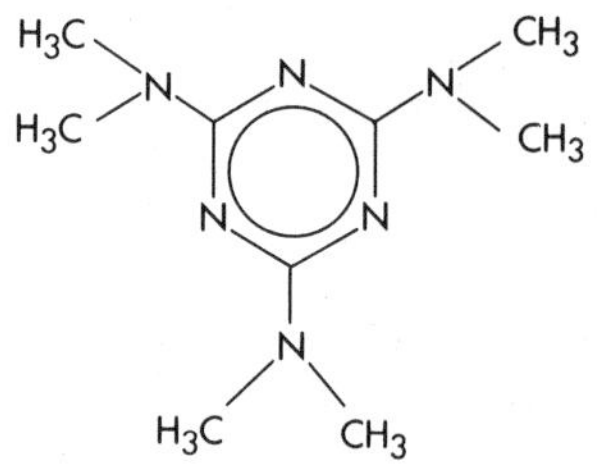

Figure 101.4

moval of the N-methyl groups so that trimethylmelamine is no longer active. In vivo metabolism of HMM gives rise to N-methylol analogues that are the putative active intermediates. HMM is considered to be an alkylating agent, although its precise mechanism of antitumor action is not completely understood. A single agent at 260 mg/m^2 daily orally for two to three weeks HMM is used for palliative treatment of ovarian cancer resistant to cisplatin or in alkylating agent based combination chemotherapy. Nausea and vomiting are the dose-limiting toxicities; reversible peripheral neurotoxicity may occur, whereas myelosuppression is usually mild. The oral bioavailability of HMM is variable: so is its terminal plasma half-life, ranging from 4.7 to 13 hours. It undergoes rapid and extensive demethylation in vivo; in the urine of patients treated with HMM a number of N-demethylated metabolites have been recovered, with less than 1.5 percent of the dose as unchanged drug in 24 hours.

Antimetabolites

Synthetic structural analogues of natural precursors in biosynthetic pathways of nucleic acids are of considerable importance in cancer chemotherapy. Since they inhibit cell proliferation by interfering with cellular intermediary metabolism, they are grouped together here under "antimetabolites." In general, they may be incorporated into nucleic acids as a fraudulent constituent, or compete with their natural counterparts in binding to the active or regulating site of a critical enzyme, or allosterically inhibit a feedback control process. Frequently they require prior metabolic activation before exerting their inhibitory effects. A host of antimetabolites have been synthesized and evaluated as cancer chemotherapeutic agents, but only a few have proved their clinical worth because of the lack of selectivity in the majority.

Folate Antagonists

Volumes have been written on the biochemistry of folate and the development of its antagonists as chemotherapeutic agents not only against cancer, but also infectious diseases. Space here only permits citation of two of these for further reading.[45,46] Folate in its reduced form, tetrahydrofolate (FH_4), serves a vital function in microorganisms as well as mammalian species as a coenzyme, a carrier of one-carbon units in the biosynthesis of a large variety of essential cellular constituents, including glycine, serine, methionine, thymidylate, purine nucleosides, and others. By interfering with these vital functions folate antagonists exert their cytotoxic action; however, it is obvious that not all folate antagonists are useful cancer chemotherapeutic agents. Some are effective only against infectious diseases. In fact, methotrexate is the only folate antagonist that has firmly established itself as a cardinal member in the armamentarium of cancer chemotherapists.

Methotrexate (MTX)

F: R_1=OH, R_2=H
MTX: R_1=NH_2, R_2=CH_3

An analogue of folate (F) (see Fig. 101.5), MTX is N[4-[[(2,4-diamino-6-pterindinyl)-methylamino]benzoyl]-L-glutamic acid. It thus differs from folate in having a 4-amino in place of the 4-hydroxy group and, additionally, a methyl group attached to N.[10] It is a yellow fluorescent solid sparingly soluble in water, but soluble in dilute alkaline solution in which it decomposes slowly. It may be given orally or IV. Authoritative reviews on its biochemistry, pharmacology, and clinical aspects have been published.[45,46]

As briefly mentioned above, to function as a cofactor in numerous crucial biochemical reactions folate must first be reduced to FH_4, via dihydrofolate, FH_2; both reactions are mediated by dihydrofolate reductase (DHFR, EC 1.5.1.3), but FH_2 is a far better substrate. With a high affinity for DHFR, MTX therefore acts as a potent inhibitor of FH_4 formation and interferes with many biosynthetic processes requiring FH_4, so that the folate coenzymes are trapped as the metabolically ineffective FH_2 polyglutamates. The biosynthetic pathway most sensitive to MTX inhibition is the conversion of 2′-deoxyuridylate (dUMP) to thymidylate, which requires the donation of a methyl group from N^5, N^{10}-methylene FH_4 to the uracil moiety of dUMP. Consequently, since thymidine is readily phosphorylated by thymidine kinase (EC 2.7.1.21) to thymidylate independent of the supply of FH_4, it can circumvent the MTX inhibition. Therapeutically, however, leucovorin (folinic acid, citrovorum factor, N^5-formyl FH_4) is the agent widely used to "rescue" patients from toxicities after high-dose MTX treatment. This is because leucovorin, a fully reduced FH_4 derivative, does not need DHFR for its reductive activation, and can be directly and

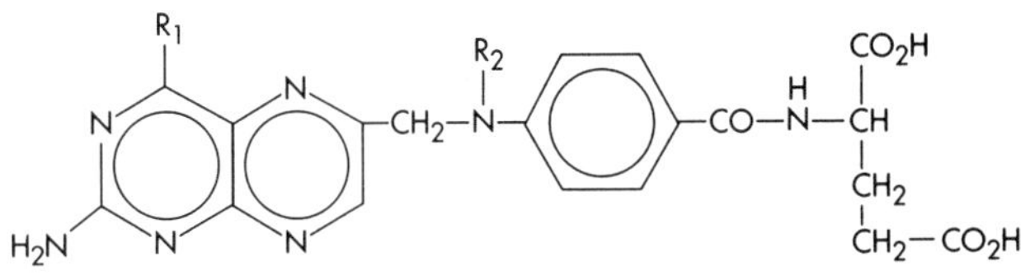

	R_1	R_2
Folate	OH	H
MTX	NH_2	CH_3

Figure 101.5

efficiently utilized for the biosyntheses of other FH_4 cofactors.

Possible cellular resistance mechanisms to MTX are: First, increased production of DHFR through gene amplification; second, altered DHFR with lowered affinity for MTX; third, impaired MTX transport; and fourth, defective conversion of MTX to its polyglutamates. How well these mechanisms apply in a clinical setting remains to be demonstrated, since reports are based on laboratory studies with experimental systems, mostly in cultured cells. Pleiotropic resistance to MTX induced by natural products such as vincristine remains to be substantiated clinically.

The clinical pharmacokinetics of MTX have been extensively investigated in many laboratories, especially recently with the availability of highly sensitive and specific analytical methodologies coupled with computerized pharmacokinetic analysis. This subject has been reviewed;[45,46] almost all of the excellent original articles are cited in these two references. Results of early studies seem to suggest that the GI absorption of oral MTX is essentially complete after low doses but variable and incomplete after doses above 50 mg/m^2; the absorption is enhanced by subdividing the dose, suggesting saturable intestinal transport. However, in a later study involving 28 children with acute lymphoblastic leukemia (ALL), the average bioavailability of MTX administered orally at the low dose of 15 mg/m^2 was only 42 percent. At any rate, in a large population of children with ALL receiving MTX IM or by mouth, wide variability in MTX pharmacokinetics was the rule rather than the exception, and on the whole somewhat better absorption was seen by the IM route. Further, MTX pharmacokinetic variability depends a good deal on dosage, patient preconditioning, age, and the analytical methodology. In an early study in 22 patients with blood-sampling lasting 96 hours, the plasma disappearance of MTX after an IV dose of 30 mg/m^2 was triphasic, with a terminal phase half-life of 27 hours; 52 to 100 percent of the administered dose was excreted in the urine in 96 h and about 1 percent in the feces. These results may be compared with those of a recent study in which four patients participated, each receiving three courses of MTX by IV infusion at 1.19 g/m^2. The average terminal plasma MTX half-life was shorter, 15 hours, but 96-hour cumulative urinary excretion was also 52 percent. Lately, MTX often has been administered at high doses by slow IV infusion; to facilitate renal drug elimination the patient is hydrated and the urine alkalinized. Under these conditions the plasma is more readily cleared of the drug, with an average plasma MTX half-life ranging from two to 16 hours, but the cumulative excretion of intact MTX remains from 50 percent in 12 hours to 60 percent in 72 hours. No dose-dependent pharmacokinetics are evident at 50 to 300 mg/kg (approximately 2,000–12,000 mg/m^2). In normal volunteers, serum MTX half-life seems to vary directly with age, but indirectly with endogenous creatinine clearance. In general, children eliminate the drug much faster than do adults, as reflected in their dramatically reduced plasma half-life of MTX, ranging from 1 h to 6 h. Likewise, in children the systemic clearance of MTX is greater, except when the doses are high. It has been reported that in patients responding partially to MTX therapy plasma drug half-life is significantly longer than in nonresponders; clearly such a correlation deserves confirmation in additional studies. In this connection, to initiate the "rescue" with citrovorum factor during high-dose MTX therapy, the importance of pharmacokinetic monitoring cannot be overemphasized. In humans, MTX clearance is greater than inulin clearance, implying active renal tubular transport in addition to glomerular filtration; the clearance is not directly related to the concentration of unbound MTX. MTX clearance is diminished with increasing doses as a result of saturation of the renal tubular active secretory mechanism. In addition to urinary excretion, MTX also has been found in the bile. In fact, in two patients given 50 mg of MTX IV, the biliary drug concentrations are extremely high, respectively 2500 and 10,000 times those in the concurrent plasma. However, fecal excretion of the drug is negligible. The extensive enterohepatic cycling of MTX has been elegantly confirmed experimentally. MTX does not readily penetrate the CNS; in two independent studies the drug concentration in the CSF on average is just about 1 to 2 percent of that in the simultaneous plasma. There is no evidence that MTX is metabolized in man after conventional low doses. However, in patients receiving high-dose MTX by IV infusion 7-hydroxymethotrexate[47] and 2,4-diamino-N^{10}-pteroic acid[48] have been found in the urine. Finally, it deserves particular mention that elegant mathematical models have been constructed to interpret MTX pharmacokinetics.[49]

Like CPA, MTX is another important chemotherapeutic agent with a broad spectrum of clinical anticancer properties. It is curative against childhood ALL, lymphomas other than Hodgkin's disease, and choriocarcinoma. In combination with other agents it frequently induces remissions in many solid tumors. Major clinical toxicities include myelosuppression, GI disturbances, stomatitis, and alopecia. At very high doses followed by folinic acid (citrovorum factor, CF, or leucovorin) rescue, MTX has shown substantial antitumor activity against many common malignancies, such as lung cancer and breast cancer. In this regimen the limiting toxicity is usually renal, but that can be avoided by careful monitoring of blood MTX concentrations. Another important use of MTX pertains to the control of diffuse leptomeningeal infiltration with lymphoblastic leukemia and other types of malignancy. By direct administration of MTX into the CSF, drug concentrations far exceeding those associated with resistance can be achieved. Such a local form of therapy has proved effective and even curative.

Purine Analogues (General Structure Shown in Fig. 101.6)

In 1984, George H. Hitchings and Gertrude B. Elion were honored with the Bruce F. Cain Memorial Award by the American Association for Cancer Research for their early work on purine antagonists as chemotherapeutic agents.[50] This was followed in 1985 with the Nobel Prize in Medicine, awarded jointly to Sir James W. Black. Clearly, the development of purine analogues with therapeutic applications is a significant achievement in medical research.

The biochemistry, pharmacology, and clinical uses of purine antimetabolites have been reviewed.[51,52] At present, only mercaptopurine (6-MP) plays a role in cancer chemotherapy; the other purine analogues, namely, thioguanine (6-TG), cladribine (CdA), fludarabine (F-ara-A), and pentostatin (DCF), are of only secondary clinical importance.

The biochemistry of the thiopurines has been investigated extensively. Both 6-MP and 6-TG are converted readily by hypoxanthine-guanine phosphoribosyltransferase (HGPRT) (EC 2.4.2.8) to the respective sulfur analogues of inosinate (IMP) and guanylate (GMP), namely, thioinosinate (TIMP) and thioguanylate (TGMP), which are potent inhibitors of several vital biochemical reactions in experimental systems. How many of these are actually responsible for the anticancer actions of the thiopurines remains uncertain. Nevertheless, it appears that the following modes of action are clinically relevant. In a pseudo-feedback fashion, both TIMP and TGMP interfere with the first step of purine de novo biosynthesis, that is, the reaction of phosphoribosyl pyrophosphate with glutamine to form ribosylamine 5′-phosphate catalyzed by amidophosphoribosyltransferase (EC 2.4.2.14). In addition, TIMP inhibits the conversion of IMP to xanthylate and adenylosuccinate, and the ensuing formation of GMP and adenylate from IMP. All these inhibitory effects are naturally deleterious to cell proliferation. Finally, the incorporation of TGMP directly and TIMP indirectly as fraudulent nucleotides into cellular DNA has also been implicated as a contributory factor of thiopurine cytotoxicity. But it must be emphasized that the selective anticancer activities of the thiopurines have never been satisfactorily explained.

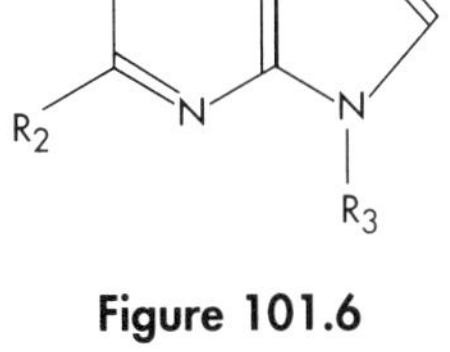

R1, HN, N, N, N, R2, R3

Figure 101.6

Mercaptopurine (R_1=S, R_2=R_3=H in Fig. 101.6) (6-MP)

Pure 6-MP crystallizes as yellow prisms sparingly soluble in water but more so at high pH, in which solution it is unstable. In solid state and also most likely in solution 6-MP is predominantly in the keto form, with the sulfur atom doubly bonded to the purine. As a consequence, ribosyl-6-MP is an inosine analogue, whereas ribosyl-6-methylmercaptopurine is an adenosine analogue.

Although 6-MP often is administered by mouth, its GI absorption is erratic and incomplete.[53] After IV administration the average plasma half-time of 6-MP was 21 minutes in four children, but 47 minutes in six adults; unchanged drug is analyzed colorimetrically. Urinary excretion tapers off in approximately 4 hours; the 6-hour cumulative excretion is about 18 percent in children and 22 percent in adults. The drug undergoes extensive in vivo anabolism as well as catabolism; oxidation to 6-thiouric acid is mediated by xanthine oxidase. It is 19 percent bound to plasma protein and does not penetrate the erythrocyte and CNS well. However, recent studies using the more sensitive and convenient HPLC analysis for 6-MP showed that in 13 children the plasma half-life of the drug is about one hour after oral administration.[54] Bioavailability of oral 6-MP in six patients after high dose (500 mg/m^2) was lower than that after a low dose (75 mg/m^2), but was enhanced by MTX administration because MTX inhibits xanthine oxidase. Moreover, bioavailability was increased by 500 percent in six patients pretreated with allopurinol, which diminishes the first-pass metabolism of orally administered 6-MP. Allopurinol exerts no such effects on the IV-administered drug. In rodents, several mechanisms of resistance to 6-MP have been demonstrated: for instance, the loss of the enzyme HGPRT and the increase in particulate-bound alkaline phosphatase (EC 3.1.3.1). Such mechanisms may likewise be responsible for clinical resistance to the drug.

6-MP is used mostly for treating acute leukemia in children, usually in combination with agents such as MTX, prednisolone, or cytarabine. The chief clinical toxicities are myelosuppression, stomatitis, nausea, and vomiting. It has been reported that parenteral administration of 6-MP can avoid its hepatotoxicity and results in enhanced patient tolerance of the agent. For instance, in the POMP (6-MP, vincristine, methotrexate, and prednisone) regimen, 6-MP at 1 g/m^2 IV daily for five days is well tolerated, except that the parenteral preparation of 6-MP is not commercially available.

Thioguanine (6-TG, R_1=S, R_2=NH_2, R_3=H in Fig. 101.6)

Both 6-TG and 6-MP are of the same vintage as anticancer antimetabolites, and in many respects share certain biochemical mechanisms of cytotoxicity. Like 6-MP, 6-TG is readily converted to its 5′-monophosphate or TGMP, a reaction catalyzed by HGPRT, as mentioned earlier. Although both TIMP and TGMP are poor substrates for guanylate kinase (EC 2.7.4.8), TGMP is somewhat more efficient. Consequently, TGMP is slowly converted stepwise to the 5′-diphosphate, TGDP, and 5′-triphosphate, TGTP, and ultimately incorporated into cellular DNA. Also, TG interferes with DNA replication in regenerating rat liver by decreasing the induction of certain critically required enzymes. However, the contributions of the various mechanisms to the selective toxicity of either 6-TG or 6-MP remain obscure. In experimental models, cellular resistance to 6-TG can be caused either by a depletion of HGPRT, a reduction of its affinity for substrates, or an increase in alkaline phosphate activity. This subject has been reviewed.[51]

Like 6-MP, 6-TG is poorly absorbed when given by mouth; in one study the bioavailability is less than 10 percent.[56] In three patients after IV low doses of ^{35}S-labeled 6-TG, the plasma half-life of 6-TG and metabolites was 28.9 hours, and 75 percent of the administered radioactivity was found in the urine in 24 hours.[56] The drug is metabolized extensively to 6-thioxanthine, S-methyl-6-thioxanthine, 6-thiouric acid, and inorganic sulfate. However, in six patients given high doses of 6-TG (800–1,200 mg/m^2) IV, the average plasma half-life of intact 6-TG was 5.9 hours.[57] In a recent study, when 6-TG was administered as a 48-hour continuous intraperitoneal infusion, the elimination half-life of the agent from the peritoneal cavity was 1 hour; at steady state, 6-TG concentration in the peritoneal fluid was 1800 times that in the plasma.

6-TG is seldom given alone, but rather in combination with cytarabine in the treatment of acute leukemias other than lymphocytic. Its dose-limiting clinical toxicity is granulocytopenia; other toxicities include emesis and alopecia. Because it does not require xanthine oxidase for catabolism, 6-TG frequently has been used in high-dose regimens, such as cytarabine-6-TG combinations for acute myeloblastic leukemia therapy. This is an important advantage, particularly in patients with very large tumor burdens. Uric acid nephropathy can be prevented by combining 6-TG with allopurinol.

Cladribine[58,r10] (2-chlorodeoxyadenosine, CdA, R_1=NH_2, R_2=Cl, R_3=2′-deoxyribose in Fig. 101.7)

Adenosine deaminase (ADA, EC 3.4.4.4), a critical regulatory enzyme in cellular purine metabolism, exhibits certain fascinating substrate specificities. For example, in the purine ring the 2-H is critical; its replacement with Cl as in CdA, or F as in fludarabine (see below), renders the compound resistant to ADA action. On the other hand, this enzyme is indiscriminate with respect to the 2′-OH in the pentaose moiety; thus, both 2′-deoxyadenosine, in which the 2′-OH is absent, and arabinosyladenosine, in which its configuration is inverted, remain susceptible to deamination by ADA. Lymphocytes are rich in deoxycytidine kinase (EC 2.7.1.74) but poor in 5′-nucleotidase. Therefore, in these cells if ADA is either naturally deficient because of heredity or drastically inhibited by drugs such as pentostatin (DCF, see below), lethal amounts of deoxynucleotides would accumulate, causing cell death. Rapidly proliferating lymphocytes are also killed by the administration of drugs like CdA that are not deaminated, but converted to deoxynucleotides that similarly accumulate intracellularly to lethal quantities. Further, CdA deoxynucleotides inhibit DNA synthesis, possibly by interfering with DNA repair. At any rate, at the present, the mechanism of anticancer action of CdA remains to be elucidated.

CdA is particularly effective in treating hairy cell leukemia. It also may be active against chronic lymphocytic leukemia, refractory low-grade lymphoma, early-stage acute myelocytic leukemia, and other leukemias; however, further studies are warranted. The common single IV seven-day infusion dose is 0.09 mg/kg (3.6 mg/m^2) daily. At this dose, low toxicity involving hematopoietic stem cells has been reported, consisting of transient bone marrow suppression, granulocytopenia, and thrombocytopenia. Fever occurs in one-third of patients. Nausea and vomiting, alopecia, and other tissue dysfunction are clinically insignificant. Opportunistic infections have occurred in the immediate postinfusion period.

In humans two hours after IV infusion of 0.14 mg/kg (5.6 mg/m^2) of CdA, the drug disappeared biphasically from the plasma terminal half-life of 6.7 hours (2.8–12.1 hr); the volume of distribution was 9.2 l/kg. From these results the total clearance of CdA was estimated to be approximately 16 ml·kg^{-1}·min^{-1}.

Fludarabine Phosphate[58,r11] (F-ara-A phosphate; in Fig. 101.8 R_1=NH_2, R_2=F, R_3=arabinose, 5′-phosphate)

From its chemical name, 9-β-D-arabinofuranosyl-2-fluoroadenine 5′-phosphate, it is immediately clear that this antimetabolite differs from the natural ribonucleoside, adenosine, in two aspects—namely, the H at position 2 in the latter has been replaced with F, and the ribosyl entity with the arabinosyl group. As discussed above, the former replacement makes F-ara-A resistant to deamination by

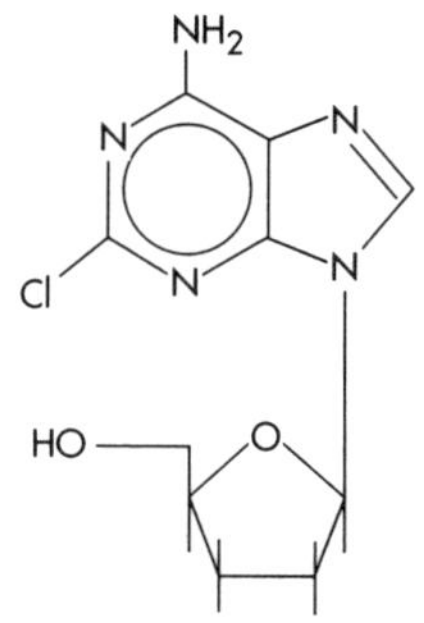

Figure 101.7

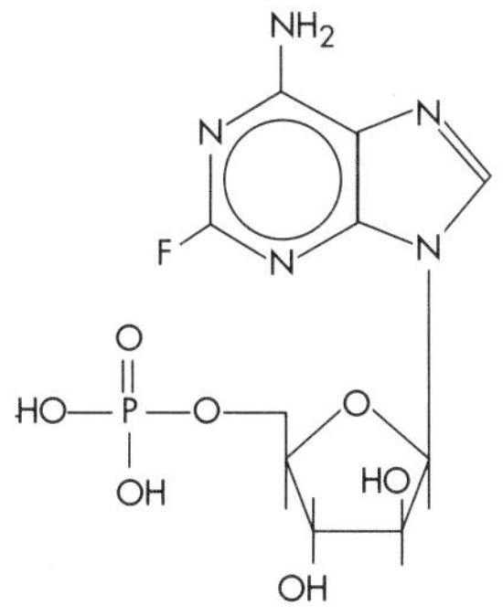

Figure 101.8

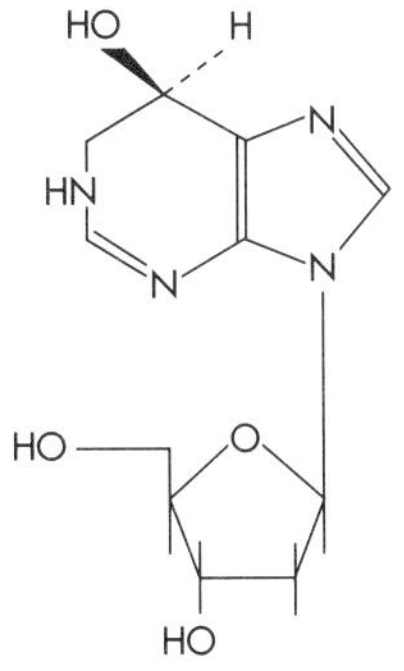

Figure 101.9

ADA. In humans, F-ara-A 5′-phosphate quickly loses its phosphate group by apparent first-pass metabolism, but then is readily converted, ultimately to F-ara-A 5′-triphosphate, the active metabolite. The triphosphate exerts its cytotoxic action by competing with the natural metabolite, deoxyadenosine triphosphate, for incorporation into the A site during DNA elongation, thus terminating DNA synthesis. Its anticancer specificity is attributed to the differential transport and phosphorylation of F-ara-A as well as accumulation of F-ara-ATP by normal susceptible cells as compared with malignant cells.

In humans, F-ara-A disappears from the plasma rapidly, with a harmonic mean half-life of approximately 5 minutes initially and 1.4 hours during the terminal phase. The total clearance is 68 ± 20 $ml{\cdot}min^{-1}{\cdot}m^{-2}$ (approximately 1.7 $ml{\cdot}min^{-1}{\cdot}kg^{-1}$), and the steady-state volume of distribution is 1.2 l/kg, suggesting that the drug is distributed and bound to body tissues; the rate-limiting process for its elimination from the body seems to be release from tissue binding sites. Total body clearance and volume of distribution of F-ara-A decrease with increase in serum creatinine; that is, these pharmacokinetic parameters depend on renal function. Consequently, dose reduction in patients with renal impairment is recommended.

F-ara-A phosphate is clinically active against a variety of low-grade lymphoproliferative malignancies, particularly B-cell chronic lymphocytic leukemia and non-Hodgkin's lymphomas. As a single agent, the recommended IV dose is 25 mg/m^2 administered over 30 minutes daily for five consecutive days. Combination chemotherapy incorporating F-ara-A is still under development. The major side-effects are myelosuppression, fever and chills, infection, nausea, and vomiting.

Pentostatin (2′-deoxycoformycin, DCF)[58,r12]

A potent adenosine deaminase (EC 3.5.4.4) inhibitor (see Fig. 101.9) isolated from *Streptomyces antibioticus* culture, DCF is active clinically against several lymphoproliferative malignancies, the rare hairy-cell chronic lymphocytic leukemia in particular, despite its initial inactivity in preclinical screens. Often considered to be a purine antimetabolite, structurally DCF actually contains no purine entity but, instead, an uncommon imidazo[4,5-d][1,3]diazepin ring system; thus, it resembles the transition state of adenosine during the enzymatic deamination of the latter. Found in abundance in lymphoid tissues, adenosine deaminase is a key regulating enzyme in cellular metabolism; inhibition of this enzyme by DCF causes cell death. As with most cancer chemotherapeutic agents, the exact mechanism of antitumor action remains to be elucidated. DCF is most effective in treating hairy-cell leukemia, but favorable responses also have been elicited in chronic lymphocytic leukemia, acute T-cell lymphoma, and leukemia. Used singly, the recommended dose is 4 mg/m^2 IV weekly. The dose-limiting toxicity is myelosuppression. Nausea, vomiting, renal impairment, and CNS toxicities also have been reported.

In patients, the terminal plasma half-life of DCF is about 4.9 hours, the steady-state volume of distribution 20 l/m^2, and the total clearance 52 $ml{\cdot}min^{-1}{\cdot}m^{-2}$ (about 1.3 $ml{\cdot}min^{-1}{\cdot}kg^{-1}$); in 24 hours almost all administered DCF is excreted intact in the urine. The total clearance of DCF is positively correlated with creatinine clearance, suggesting that patients with renal impairment should be closely monitored and that dose reduction is necessary in severe cases.

Pyrimidine Analogues

Since pyrimidine bases, that is, cytosine, thymine, and uracil, are likewise fundamental components of nucleic acids, judiciously-designed analogues that partially, even selectively, mimic a few of the vital biochemical functions of the natural metabolites may exhibit antineoplastic properties. Therefore, by modifying the chemical structures of pyrimidine bases and their ribonucleosides, a vast number of such analogues have indeed been synthesized. Among these only cytarabine, fluorouracil, and floxuridine are currently clinically useful cancer chemotherapeutic agents.

Cytarabine [Ara-C, 1-β-D-arabinofuranosylcytidine]

Ara-C differs from the natural metabolite cytidine in having an arabinosyl moiety in place of the ribosyl group in the latter (see Fig. 101.10). In other words, compared with cytidine the configuration of the 2′-hydroxyl group in ara-C has been inverted with respect to the plane of the pentose ring, so that it is trans to the 3′-hydroxyl group. At any rate, ara-C is a deoxycytidine, not a cytidine analogue.

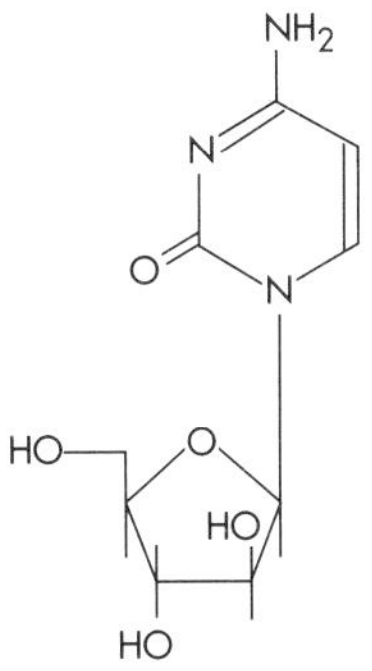

Figure 101.10

Also, because the 2′-carbon of ara-C is linked directly to the N-3 of the cytosine base and not through an oxygen bridge, ara-C is an arabinosyl derivative, not an arabinoside. Some arabinose nucleosides occur in nature, but ara-C is synthetic.

The precise antitumor mechanism of ara-C is still poorly understood; some insight may be gained by consulting review articles in this field.[52,59] To exert its cytotoxicity, ara-C must first be converted to the 5′-monophosphate, ara-CMP, by deoxycytidine kinase (EC 2.7.1.74); ara-CMP is ultimately phosphorylated to the triphosphate, ara-CTP, catalyzed by deoxycytidylate kinase (EC 2.7.4.1.4). After incorporation into DNA, ara-CTP blocks initiation and elongation of the growing DNA strand. It also interrupts cell replication by inhibiting DNA polymerase α responsible for de novo DNA synthesis and DNA polymerase β responsible for DNA repair. These mechanisms may operate alone or in concert. The cytotoxicity of ara-C is critically dependent on several factors: the intracellular metabolism of ara-C (especially in competition with that of its corresponding natural counterparts), the phase of the cell cycle, and ara-C dosage. All of these must be borne in mind when considering the mechanisms of anticancer action of ara-C. Ara-C undergoes rapid in vivo deamination to arabinosyluridine (ara-U), a reaction catalyzed by deoxycytidine deaminase (EC 3.5.4.14); ara-U is relatively innocuous, at least when produced from low doses of ara-C. To abolish ara-C deamination, the simultaneous administration of the potent deaminase inhibitor tetrahydoruridine has been proposed as a means to enhance the therapeutic effectiveness of ara-C. Such an approach is destined to fail, since preventing the agent from degradative deamination is merely equivalent to increasing its dosage, and therefore unlikely to spare normal sensitive cells from the toxic effects of ara-C thus improving its therapeutic index. Present knowledge on the reasons for natural and acquired clinical resistance to this agent is regrettably inadequate; this subject has been succinctly reviewed.[52,59] Although not as simple as it appears to be, either the deletion of the activating anabolic enzyme deoxycytidine kinase, or the overproduction of the inactivating catabolic enzyme deoxycytidine deaminase, or both together, could reduce the intracellular ara-CTP concentration, leading to resistance. Additionally, resistant cells could have their cellular dCTP reservoir expanded to compensate for the damaging effect of ara-C. Moreover, resistant cells may have impaired ara-C transport. Lastly, their DNA polymerase may show diminished affinity for ara-C.

Earlier it was reported[60] that high intracellular ara-CTP concentration appears to be a prerequisite, but not a sufficient condition, for determining ara-C effectiveness. Later this observation was confirmed; a significant correlation seems to exist between remission duration and intracellular ara-CTP synthesis and retention in vitro by cells from patients with acute myelocytic leukemia.[61] Further, the cellular ara-CTP concentrations in the leukemic blasts of patients who have achieved remission are not only higher but decline more slowly than those in the blasts of nonresponding patients.[62] In leukemic children receiving high-dose ara-C therapy, inhibition of DNA synthetic capacity in peripheral blasts is positively correlated with the probability of having zero nadir circulating blast cells.

Its importance as an antileukemia agent has made ara-C the focus of pharmacokinetic investigations for many years; only a selected few are cited here.[63–67] But the results from several laboratories are not always in agreement, depending on dosage, route, and schedule of administration, analytical methodology, and duration of the study. For instance, after IV administration the plasma elimination half-life of ara-C has been variously reported to be as short as 18 minutes. [3g/m^2 IV administration in 1 hr, ara-C analysis by HPLC] to as long as 19 hours (10 mg/m^2 daily for 21 d, postinfusion half-life). However, since steady state is reached in 2.7 hours, the plasma ara-C elimination half-life estimated by us is 24 minutes. Nevertheless, most investigators seem to have arrived at intermediate values of two to three hours.[63] Given at high doses, the plasma elimination half-life of the drug is independent of dose and schedule.[65] By general consensus also, the GI absorption of ara-C is poor, unreliable, and erratic. However, pharmacokinetically at least, the IV and SQ routes of administration appear to be equivalent.[68] After IV administration the CSF to plasma ara-C concentration ratio varies from 0.1 to 0.6;[64–66] since ara-C elimination from the CNS is slower than that from the plasma with a half-life of 2.3 to 6.3 hours,[65] drug concentration in the CSF during the terminal phase often exceeds that in the corresponding plasma.[64] The 24-hour cumulative excretion of intact ara-C is approximately 10 percent of the dose; most of the drug is eliminated as ara-U.[63,67]

Particularly useful in treating acute leukemia, ara-C is the single most effective agent in acute myelocytic leukemia in adults, and principally responsible for the existence of a cured fraction of patients. In fact, the disease of approximately 15 percent of these patients is controlled by ara-C alone. Ara-C usually is administered in combination with a DNA-binding drug, such as an anthracycline antibiotic, amsacrine, 6-TG, or etoposide. All of these combination regimens seem to afford comparable results, improving somewhat the effectiveness of ara-C alone. The dose-limiting toxicity of ara-C is myelosuppression. Other toxicities include GI disturbances and stomatitis. Recently, high-dose ara-C therapy has been in vogue. Apparently, high-dose ara-C can overcome resistance to conventional dose ara-C, although the precise mode of action remains to be elucidated. But high-dose ara-C cannot improve the remission induction for previously untreated patients; however, it seems superior in refractory and relapsed patients. Further, when ara-C is given at high doses, e.g., $3g/m^2$, substantial drug concentrations are achieved in CSF and other body fluids. This has therefore become a significant strategy for the treatment of diffuse subarachnoid leukemic infiltration and intracerebral leukemic deposits, such as those observed in association with the inversion of chromosome 16.

Fluorouracil (FU, 5-fluorouracil, Fig. 101.11, R=H)

The basic biochemistry, pharmacology, and clinical aspects of FU and other pyrimidine anticancer agents have been completely reviewed.[52,69] However, the trend in more recent investigations may be gleaned from the proceedings of the two international symposia.[70,71] The clinical pharmacology of FU has also been reviewed recently.[72,73]

As a cancer chemotherapeutic agent, FU might be considered one of the first drugs rationally designed based on the belief that in the rat endogenous uracil is utilized for nucleic acid biosynthesis by chemically induced hepatoma but not by normal tissues. But this now appears to be a general phenomenon in growing tissues. In any event, the substitution of the H-5 in uracil with fluorine, which does not differ much in size from hydrogen, produces a fraudulent base subtly at variance with the natural one biochemically and enzymologically. For instance, the stability of the C-F bond precludes the replacement of the F-5 with a methyl group analogous to the conversion of uracil to thymine. Also, the electron-withdrawing property of the F atom makes FU more acidic than uracil. These differences eventually manifest themselves when FU participates in critical events in a replicating cell.

FU exerts its cytotoxic action indirectly after intracellular metabolism to 5-fluorouridine 5′-monophosphate, FdUMP. To this end, three possible pathways are known (Fig. 101.12).

One, FU is anabolized by uridine phosphorylase

Figure 101.11

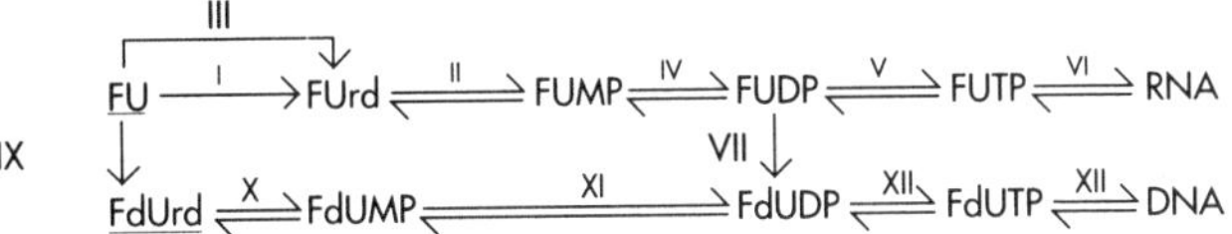

	Enzyme	EC Number
I	Uridine phosphorylase	2.4.2.3
II	Uridine kinasa	2.7.1.48
III	Uracil phosphoribosyltransferase	2.4.2.9
IV	Nucleosidemonophosphate kinase	2.7.4.4
V	Nucleosidediphosphate kinase	2.7.4.6
VI	PNA polymerase	2.7.7.6
VII	Ribonucleosidediphosphate reductase	1.17.4.1
VIII	Phosphatase	?
IX	Thymidine phosphorylase	2.4.2.4
X	Thymidine kinase	2.7.1.75
XI	Deoxynucleosidemonophosphate kinase	2.7.4.13
XII	Deoxynucleosidediphosphate kinase	?
XIII	DNA polymerase	2.7.7.7

Figure 101.12

(I) to 5′-fluorouridine, FUrd, that is converted to the 5′-monophosphate, FUMP, by uridine kinase (II). Alternatively, FUMP is formed directly from FU when it reacts with 5-phosphoribosyl-1-diphosphate, mediated by uracil phosphoribsyltransferase (III). Sequentially through FUDP, FUMP is converted to FUTP, involving the kinases (IV and V). Ultimately, as a fraudulent substrate, FUTP is incorporated into RNA, either replacing the natural substrate UTP or competing with it. However, how deleterious the incorporation of FU into RNA may be remains uncertain. Two, FUDP, as a substrate of ribonucleosidediphosphate reductase (VII), is reduced to FdUDP; the latter is cleaved by some nonspecific phosphatase (VIII) to FdUMP. Three, FdUMP is synthesized more directly from FU through 5-fluorodeoxyuridine FdUrd, as the result of accepting the deoxyribosyl group from deoxyribose-1-1-phosphate, a reaction mediated by thymidine phosphorylase (IX); FdUrd is further transformed to FdUMP. FdUMP competes with the natural substrate dUMP for the catalytic sites of thimdylate synthetase (EC 2.1.1.45) a key enzyme in DNA synthesis. It inactivates this cardinal enzyme by forming a stable, covalently-bonded ternary complex consisting of thymidylate synthetase, 5,10-methylenetetrahydrofolate, and itself. As RNA and protein syntheses apparently proceed heedlessly, FdUMP inhibition of DNA synthesis causes the sensitive cell to die of thymineless death. An authoritative and critical discussion of the mechanisms of cytotoxic action of FU may be found in Reference 52. Catabolically, FU is metabolized in vivo to the 5,6-dihydro derivative presumably catalyzed by dihydrouracil dehydrogenase (EC 1.3.1.1); the dihydro metabolite undergoes ring opening to afford α-fluoro-β-ureidopropionic acid that ultimately is degraded to α-fluoro-β-amino-propionic acid, urea, ammonia, and carbon dioxide. In experimental systems, mechanisms of resistance to FU include the deletion of FU-activation enzymes and the induction of thymidylate synthetase refractory to the action of FdUMP. But it is not known which of these is operative in humans.

Clinical pharmacokinetic investigations of FU have been continuing for some time on account of the therapeutic importance of the drug.[72,73] Given by mouth, the bioavailability of FU varies a great deal, but on average is about 28%. After either oral or IV administration at conventional dosage, the plasma elimination half-life of intact FU ranges from six minutes to 28 minutes, again showing considerable variability; being somewhat longer (average 12.3 min) after high dosage (1000 mg); some investigators have reported even longer plasma half-life after 1.2 to 1.8 g/m^2 of FU. In fact, nonlinear pharmacokinetics as well as saturable first-pass hepatic metabolism of FU are evident. The volume of distribution of FU ranges from 8 to 31 L/m^2 (0.2–0.8 L/kg), and the total clearance from 457–1086 $ml \cdot min^{-1} \cdot m^{-2}$ (11–27 $ml \cdot min^{-1} \cdot kg^{-1}$). FU is extensively metabolized in vivo; although 60 to 90 percent of the administered dose appears in the urine in 24 hours, no more than 20 percent represents intact FU. The balance is mostly α-fluoro-β-aminopropionic acid. In patients receiving an IV bolus of FU at 500 mg/m^2, in 60 minutes the metabolite 5,6-dihydro-FU attains a concentration 23.7 μM in the plasma with a half-life of 61.9 minutes; however, the biochemical pharmacologic effects of this metabolite remain to be elucidated. Other metabolites identified in the plasma are α-fluoro-β-ureido-propionic acid (half-life, 4 hr) and α-fluoro-β-aminopropionic acid (half-life 1.4). Biliary excretion of FU is insignificant, about 2 to 3 percent of the dose. FU shows no or little tendency to penetrate the CNS. During a five-day constant IV infusion, circadian rhythm-varying plasma FU concentrations have been observed, with undetermined clinical significance. Pretreatment of patients with oral cimetidine for four weeks increases the peak plasma FU concentration and decreases the total clearance without affecting FU half-life; clearly there must have been a corresponding reduction in the volume of distribution.

FU is fairly stable in glass containers (half-life, about two days) and more so in plastic infusion bags (half-life, 12 days).[30] However, it is unstable in plasma (half-life, 22.7 hr) and especially in whole blood (half-life, 5.9 hr). It is widely used in the treatment of many solid tumors, particularly in colorectal carcinoma and breast cancer. In combination with levamisole it is effective in the adjuvant treatment of advanced primary colon cancer that has been totally resected. The major clinical toxicities are mucositis and GI disturbances. In addition, severe myelosuppression has been observed after continuous FU infusion. Recently a large pharmacokinetic advantage has been claimed when FU is administered by pelvic isolation-perfusion during hyperthermia, since there is an almost eightfold total drug exposure for the isolated circuit as compared with the systemic compartment. Such a procedure may indeed enhance the specificity of a cancer chemotherapeutic agent like FU.

Floxuridine (2′-deoxy-5-fluorouridine, FdUrd)

Floxuridine or 2′-deoxy-5-fluorouridine[r2] must not be confused with doxifluridine or 5′-deoxy-5-fluorouridine. Floxuridine is an established agent now commercially available, whereas doxifluridine remains an experimental drug not yet on the market.

As discussed above, among the several biochemical pathways for the metabolic activation of FU to FdUMP, the one through FdUrd seems to be less involved than the alternatives. Therefore the use of FdUrd as a cancer chemotherapeutic agent has been advocated. Additionally, FdUrd is more soluble than FU; in fact, in the commercially available pharmaceutical preparations for parenteral administration, FdUrd concentration (100 mg/ml) is twice as high as FU concentration (50 mg/ml). In any event, apparently, by continuous intra-arterial infusion of FdUrd a much higher concentration of FU is achievable than when FU is given, resulting in enhanced anabolism to FdUMP. Nevertheless, in vivo FdUrd is readily reverted to FU; further, its hepatic metabolism appears to be more rapid than that of the parent drug. For these reasons the biochemistry, pharmacology, and toxicology of FdUrd are expected to be similar to those of FU.

N-(Phosphonacetyl)-L-Aspartic Acid (PALA)

As discussed in the introduction of this chapter PALA[74] is an ingeniously designed transition-state inhibitor of aspartate carbamoyltransferase (EC 2.1.3.2) and hence of the de novo biosynthesis of pyrimidines (see Fig. 101.13). It combines in a single molecule the structural features of both the substrates and the products of the transcarbamoyl reaction. For these reasons it is considered to be a pyrimidine antimetabolite, not a pyrimidine analogue. In experimental tumor systems it is active against several solid tumors, not only highly effective for treating intraperitoneal melanoma B16, but also curative against Lewis' lung carcinoma. Disap-

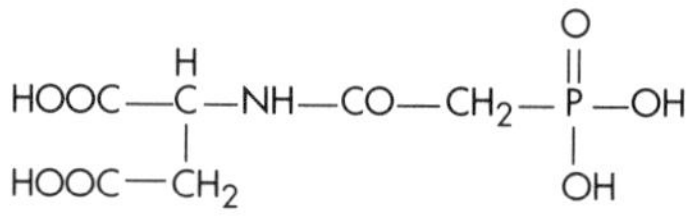

HOOC—C(H)—NH—CO—CH₂—P(=O)—OH
HOOC—CH₂ (on C); OH (on P)

Figure 101.13

pointingly, its activities as a single agent against human melanoma and breast cancer are minimal; against other malignancies PALA is devoid of demonstratable activity. Current investigations on PALA are focused on its possibility as a biochemical "modulator" of pyrimidine antimetabolites such as FU; for treating advanced GI malignancies the most effective regimen seems to be PALA, 250 mg/m^2 IV administered 24 hours before FU, 2.6 g/m^2 IV over 24 hours. Dose-limiting toxicities are ataxia and myelosuppression.

After IV administration PALA disappears from the plasma bioexponentially, with an average terminal t½ of 5.3 hours; the total clearance is approximately 65 ml·min^{-1}·m^{-2}, and the volume of distribution is 309 ml/kg. The 24-hour cumulative urinary excretion of PALA varies from 38 to 100 percent of the administered dose, with a mean of 85 percent. Total PALA clearance is linearly related to creatinine clearance, suggesting that in humans the drug is cleared mostly by glomerular filtration.[74]

Natural Products

An inexhaustible rich source for potential anticancer agents, natural products remain relatively promising and unexplored. It is well known that traditional Chinese herbal medicines reputed to be clinically active against neoplastic disease are legion, but their reliable systematic and scientific investigations are rare and far between. This merely serves as an example of the possible role of natural products in cancer chemotherapy. As rational design of synthetic antitumor agents approaches doldrums, the attention of medicinal chemists engaged in cancer therapeutic research is now focused on natural products, many of which have already earned their proper cardinal niche in the clinic. An excellent monograph[75] on anticancer natural products has been published.

Alkaloids

Vinca Alkaloids (Fig. 101.14)

The discovery of the vinca alkaloids as useful antitumor agents was serendipitous. In the search for hypoglycemic plant medicines, crude extracts of the periwinkle (Vinca rosea, *Catharanthus roseus* Linn.) were found to cause granulocytopenia and myelosuppression in the rat. Further, in murine models they exhibited antileukemic activities. This series of independent studies ultimately led to the establishment of vinblastine (VLB) and vincristine (VCR) as important anticancer drugs. Chemically these alkaloids are closely related. For instance, VLB and VCR differ only in the substituent R_1, which is -CH_3 in VLB but -CHO in VCR, as shown in the general structure Fig. 101.14; the semisynthetic alkaloid vindesine (VDS),[75] on the other hand, is deacetylvinblastine amide (R_1=CH_3, R_2=NH_2, R_3=H) (173). The chemistry, pharmacology, and other relevant aspects of the vinca alkaloids have been reviewed.[76,77]

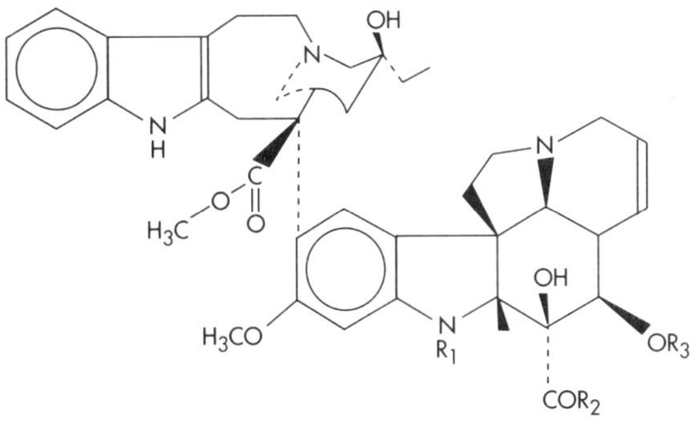

Figure 101.14

Some of the cytotoxic mechanisms of the vinca alkaloids have been elucidated. The general consensus is that they are capable of specific binding to tubulin, the precursor of microtubules responsible for mitosis and other vital cellular functions, such as substrate transport, cell motility, and structural integrity. The inhibition of mitotic spindle formation leads to arrest of cells in the metaphase of the cycle. However, cultured cells are susceptible to the cytotoxic actions of the vinca alkaloids during all phases of the cell cycle, although they are especially vulnerable during the late S phase; moreover, a progressional delay in G_2 phase also has been reported. Thus, there must be unexplained mechanisms of cytotoxicity besides binding to tubulin. As alluded to above, the structural differences among VLB, VCR, and VDS appear to be minor; yet each has characteristic and significant individual pharmacologic, toxicologic, and therapeutic features. Moreover, cross resistance among them has not been reported, not even clinically. In the introduction of this chapter, MDR was cursorily mentioned. The vinca alkaloids often have been implicated in eliciting MDR, presumably because they share a common transport mechanism with a number of other structurally unrelated cytotoxic agents to which cell lines are rendered resistant after exposure to one of the vinca alkaloids.

Toxicologically, the three alkaloids seem to fall into two categories, with VDS resembling VCR rather than VLB, even though it is derived from VLB. Neurotoxicity is rare with VLB, and only after high doses. On the other hand, neuromuscular toxicity is dose-limiting with VCR and VDS, manifested chiefly as peripheral neuropathy. In comparison, VLB is myelosuppressive—far more so than VCR. In this regard, VDS is more like VLB. Because of its lack of myelosuppressive toxicity, VCR has found broad application in combination regimens that are curative for several malignancies; it can be used in full doses with other myelosuppressive agents. However, VCR can cause cumulative neurotoxicity that is only slowly reversible. The absence of significant neurotoxicity makes VLB much more useful generally in combinations where myelosuppression is not a major problem.

As to the disposition and clinical pharmacokinetics of the vinca alkaloids, there are more similarities than differences. In the rat, VLB is preferentially taken up by platelets; the observation has since been extended to humans. Although whether VCR and VDS are likewise localized in human platelets remains to be demonstrated, pharmacokinetic evidence suggests that it is likely that VCR at least is also rapidly bound to formed blood elements.[78] Nevertheless, the clinical significance of the binding has not been elucidated. As a corollary to platelet uptake, VLB is highly bound to α_1- and α_2-globulins, but not to β- or γ-globulin. Additionally, it binds avidly to α_1-acid glycoprotein, a possible constituent of platelet walls; in both events, two types of binding sites have been observed with vastly different affinities. The preferential localization in formed blood elements and the avid protein binding are reflected in the pharmacokinetic properties of the vinca alkaloids. Following IV bolus administration the terminal-phase, plasma half-lives of all three alkaloids are long: approximately one day for VLB and VDS but 3.5 days for VCR; the apparent volumes of distribution are large.[73–78] The serum clearance rates (in $lh \cdot kg^{-1} \cdot h^{-1}$) are 0.106 for VCR, 0.252 for VDS, and 0.740 for VLB (in $ml \cdot min^{-1} \cdot kg^{-1} \cdot$: 1.8 for VCR, 4.2 for VDS, 12.3 vor VLB; in $ml \cdot min^{-1} \cdot m^{-2} \cdot$: 700.7 for VCR, 168 for DDS, 493.3 for VLB); these are positively correlated with the weekly clinical dose (mg/m^2) and the single dose LD_{50} (mg/kg) in the mouse. The very long plasma half-life of VCR suggests increasing drug deposition and cumulative toxicity if the drug is administered more often than once weekly.[78] Neither VLB nor VCR crosses the blood brain barrier readily; VLB is not selectively localized in intracerebral tumors,[84] and VCR penetrates human CSF only poorly.

The principal route of excretion of the vinca alkaloids is through the bile, and renal elimination plays merely a minor part.[79–81] All three undergo extensive metabolic degradation; VLB is apparently deacetylated to a more active metabolite.[79] Consequently, interpatient and intrapatient variations in VLB pharmacokinetics can be attributed partly to changes in hepatic function and nonlinear elimination kinetics at high doses.[80] At any rate, tissue sequestration of the vinca alkaloids rather than elimination is primarily responsible for their initial rapid clearance from the plasma. In some patients with advanced breast cancer refractory to conventional chemotherapy, partial remission and disease stabilization have been elicited with VLB given by continuous IV infusion. Although only 12 patients have been studied, favorable response seems to be associated with slow clearance of the alkaloid.[85] Notwithstanding the very long plasma half-life of VCR, infusion with the agent sustains blood VCR concentration, and an improved therapeutic efficacy has been claimed. In closing, it may be mentioned that recently a limited sampling protocol to study the clinical pharmacokinetics of VLB has been advocated.[86] If confirmed, such an innovative approach would greatly facilitate future clinical pharmacokinetic investigation not only of VLB and the vinca alkaloids, but also of other drugs.

Vinblastine (VLB, R_1=-CH_3, R_2=-OCH_3, R_3=-$COCH_3$ in Fig. 101.14)

VLB itself is not soluble in water, but the sulfate is. In 5 percent dextrose solution VLB sulfate is somewhat stable in both glass and plastic containers,[30] showing less than 10 percent decrease in content in 14 hours. It is usually administered IV, care being taken to avoid extravasation; oral dosing is not recommended owing to incomplete and erratic GI absorption. In combination with agents such as doxorubicin, bleomycin, and dacarbazine it is effective for treating advanced Hodgkin's disease. It is also useful for treating other solid tumors, including testicular tumor, breast carcinoma, and choriocarcinoma. High-dose VLB combined with bleomycin was the first regimen to cure a substantial fraction of patients with testicular cancers. The dose-limiting toxicity is leukopenia; thrombocytopenia and anemia are less frequent.

Vincristine (VCR, R_1=-CHO,R_2=-OCH_3, R_3=-$COCH_3$ in Fig. 101.14)

VCR is also formulated as the soluble sulfate for IV use. In 5 percent dextrose solution it is stable in glass containers; in plastic containers it decomposes, with a half-life of approximately three days.[30] It is another agent with a broad spectrum of antitumor activity, effective against acute lymphocytic leukemia, lymphomas including Hodgkin's disease, and childhood solid tumors. VCR plays a significant role in curative regimens for these diseases, and it has the advantages shared with any of the vinca alkaloids in eliciting no mutagenesis. Unfortunately its usefulness is limited by neurotoxicity; hematologic toxicity is uncommon. Alopecia occurs quite regularly with VCR use.

Vindesine (VDS, R_1=-CH_3, R_2=-NH_2, R_3=H in Fig. 101.14)

Like VCR, VDS is effective in acute lymphocytic leukemia; its apparent lack of cross resistance with VCR clinically is a decided advantage. It has been used with some success against esophageal squamous cell carcinoma and, in combination with cisplatin, against lung cancer other than the small-cell variety. Its spectrum of clinical toxicity seems to lie between that of VLB and VCR.

Other Alkaloids

Several other plant alkaloids also are active in experimental tumor systems; however, we shall confine our discussions here to two of them: camptothecin (CPT) and homoharringtonine (HHT). Although its reported clinical effectiveness has never been confirmed, CPT nonetheless appears to be a candidate for further development in terms of semisynthetic derivatives with improved efficacy, particularly in view of recent renewed interests. On the other hand, HHT is definitely useful as a second-line chemotherapeutic agent for treating acute leukemia. It therefore deserves additional studies.

Since both are isolated from trees indigenous to China, investigators there have devoted considerable attention and efforts to basic and clinical research with these alkaloids. Unfortunately results of most of their work appear exclusively in literature not readily accessible outside that country. Above all, their reports, especially on the clinical effectiveness of these alkaloids, frequently tend to be vague, sketchy, tantalizing, anecdotal, and devoid of particulars; treatment protocols, patient demographics, response criteria, and other vital details often are missing to render it difficult if not impossible to evaluate objectively their apparently exciting findings. These caveats notwithstanding, CPT and HHT still may have a role in cancer treatment.

Camptothecin (CPT, Fig. 101.15)

A product of the bark and wood of the tree, *Campotheca acuminata* Decsne, CPT has shown some apparent activity against human GI carcinoma during the preliminary clinical trial. However, results of further studies in patients with advanced GI cancer and melanoma[87] have been disappointing. On account of its unpredictable serious side-effects and difficulties in its formulation, clinical trials of CPT have been discontinued in the US. But in China the outcomes of very large trials of this agent are more encouraging. In 450 patients with primary liver carcinoma treated with CPT formulated as a suspension, an increase in one-year survival with reductions in hepatic mass and ascites has been claimed. Moreover, in a very large trial involving about 1000 patients with a variety of malignancies, the clinical activities of CPT in gastric carcinoma, intestinal carcinoma, head and neck cancer, and bladder carcinoma also have been reported.

CPT is an alkaloid with a complex structure (Fig. 101.15). The qualitative structure-activity relationships among CPT and its derivatives,[88] as well as the current status of CPT analogues as anticancer agents,[89] have been reviewed. In short, for antitumor activity in experimental systems, the planar ABCD aromatic ring system together with the α-hydroxy lactone moiety of ring E is essential. Replacement of the ethyl group at C-20 in ring E with certain side-chains, such as the allyl group, may lead to enhanced activity. Chirality at C-20 is important; in other words, the S-configuration at C-20 is required for maximal antitumor activity, the racemic RS-form being less potent. Substitution in ring A by small groups such as the hydroxy or methoxy but not bulky groups is not detrimental and may in fact increase antitumor potency. Thus it appears that the planar ABCD ring system of CPT is responsible for making its binding to nucleic acids similar to intercalation, and that the lactone moiety in ring E is then favorably oriented to interact with a nucleophilic entity on the nucleic acid (see below). For future attempts to improve the therapeutic efficacy of CPT, structural modifications must take these relationships into consideration.

The mechanisms of action of CPT have been extensively investigated. CPT causes rapid inhibition of nucleic acid synthesis and widespread fragmentation of cellular DNA. The latter effect may result in the formation of pieces of templates too small to be adequately utilized for further DNA replication.[88] In vitro it seems to intercalate into the Z-form region favorably induced in a negatively superhelical closed circular DNA. Since the alkaloid induced protein-linked DNA breaks via mammalian DNA topoisomerase I, it has been proposed that CPT blocks the rejoining step of the breakage-reunion reaction of this enzyme. The general consensus is that the intracellular target for CPT is indeed DNA topoisomerase I.[90]

Based on a specific fluorometric assay for CPT in 15 patients receiving 1 to 10 mg/kg of CPT IV, the average terminal plasma half-life of the intact alkaloid is 25 hours; the alkaloid is highly protein-bound (average 98.1%, 97.4–98.9%) Except in patients with renal impairment, the average 48-hour cumulative urinary excretion of CPT is 22.8 percent.

The dose-limiting toxicity is myelosuppression. Other toxicities include alopecia, GI disturbances, and hemorrhagic cystitis.

Homoharringtonine [HHT, Fig. 101.16]

From several species of the evergreen tree *Cephalotaxus* including *C. harringtonia* (hence harringtonine), *C. tortunei,* and *C. oliveri,* abundant in many parts of China, a group of alkaloids, all esters of celphalotaxine (Fig. 101.16 R=H), have been isolated and their chemistry and pharmacology studied, especially as potential antitumor agents. The medicinal chemical aspects of these alkaloids have been reviewed.[91] In a number of experimental tumor systems, harringtonine (differing from HHT in having one less methylene group in the R moiety) and HHT are particularly active.

Structure-activity relationship (SAR) studies have revealed that since HHT and harringtonine are almost equally active against the P388 and L1210 leukemias, the terminal portion of the acyl side-chain can have either two or three methylene groups. But deletion

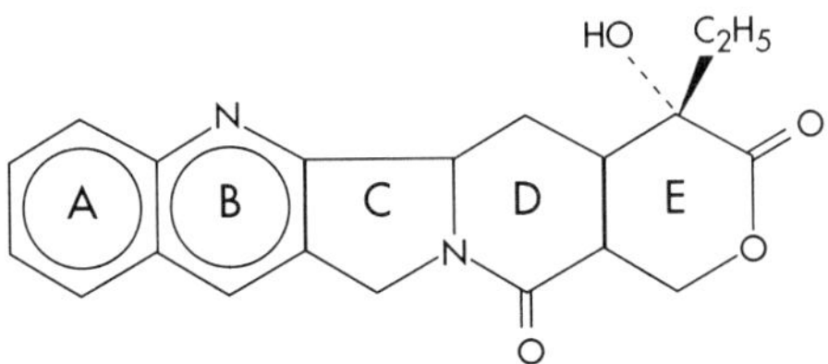

Figure 101.15

R = H

Cephalotaxine

R = $-C(=O)-C(OH)(CH_2-C(=O)-O-CH_3)-CH_2-CH_2-CH_2-C(CH_3)_2-OH$

Homoharringtonine

Figure 101.16

of the tertiary hydroxy group from the side-chain halves the activity. Also, it must be noted that natural (−)-cephalotaxin is inactive; thus, the acyl side-chain is indispensable for anticancer activity. These and similar SAR investigations have paved the way for further structural modifications of the cephalotaxine alkaloids, which may lead to the synthesis and development of more effective yet less toxic derivatives.

The mechanism of antitumor action of HHT remains obscure. However, since in cultured mammalian cells the principal effect of harringtonine is on initiation of protein synthesis, it would not be surprising if HHT behaves likewise.

The clinical pharmacokinetics of uniformly tritiated HHT has been studied in eight patients with cancer, who received 3–4 mg/m^2 (150 μCi total) by continuous 6-hour IV infusion. The drug and its metabolites were specifically analyzed by radiochemical and high-performance liquid chromatographic techniques.[92] The terminal plasma half-life of unchanged HHT is 9.3 hours; the total clearance, 2.96 $ml{\cdot}min^{-1}{\cdot}kg^{-1}$ (118.3 $ml{\cdot}min^{-1}{\cdot}m^{-2}$); and the apparent volume of distribution by area 2.4 L/kg. By comparison, the terminal plasma biological half-life of total radioactivity is 67.5 h, more than 7 times that of intact HHT; the total clearance 0.5 ml·min·kg ($ml{\cdot}min^{-1}{\cdot}m^{-2}$), more than five times slower; but the volume of distribution remains approximately the same, that is 2.7 L/kg. The 72-h cumulative urinary excretion of tritium amounts to only 28.2 percent of the administered radioactivity, of which 38.3 percent is accounted for by HHT itself. Clearly, in humans HHT undergoes extensive metabolism; the fact, one major and two minor unidentified metabolites have been detected in both plasma and urine. In the dog, a significant amount of HHT is excreted in the bile. Cerebrospinal fluid HHT concentration peaks at 4 hours, reaching 40 percent of that in the concurrent plasma. Moreover, HHT tends to be retained in the body, particularly the liver.[93]

In preliminary clinical trials in China, two preparations of cephalotaxine esters composed of different proportions of HHT and harringtonine have induced complete and partial remissions in patients with acute leukemia. The effectiveness of harringtonine isolated from *C. hainanesis* Li in treating acute leukemia also has been reported. Clinical trials of HHT rather than harringtonine have been initiated in the US because, according to the Chinese investigators, both alkaloids seem to be equally effective in treating acute leukemia, but HHT is more readily prepared in large quantities. Initial clinical trials of HHT in patients with relapsed or resistant acute leukemia have confirmed the clinical activities of this alkaloid.[94,95] Either HHT or harringtonine in combination with VCR or prednisone also appears to be highly effective in treating acute nonlymphoblastic leukemia in children. The clinical perspectives of HHT in the US have been reviewed.[96]

The clinical toxicities of HHT consist of reversible hypotension and **cardiac arrhythmia,** especially following rapid IV administration. Other side-effects include myelosuppression, diarrhea, nausea, and vomiting.

Podophyllotoxins

Podophyllum peltatum L., variously known as American mandrake or May apple or Indian apple, has a long history in American folk medicine; early settlers used its root and rhizome as a cathartic, emetic, and cholagogue. The resin podophyllin, prepared from podophyllum, the dried root and rhizome, by alcohol extraction of most of the biologically active principles is a complex mixture of crystalline and resinous organic compounds falling into two classes, the lignans and the flavonol pigments. Podophyllotoxin (Fig. 101.17 R_1=OH, R_2= H, R_3=CH_3), a lignan and not an alkaloid, is prepared from podophyllin; its medicinal chemistry has been authoritatively reviewed. Since podophyllin has shown antiwart and antimitotic properties, α-peltatin, a component of resin closely related to podophyllotoxin, has undergone preliminary clinical trial; some suggestive antitumor responses have been observed, but the toxicities are too severe to warrant further exploration. As a result, efforts have been directed toward the development of semisynthetic analogues of podophyllotoxin, culminating in the discovery of etoposide (VP) and teniposide (VM). In 1981 an international symposium on the podophyllotoxins was held; in the following year the abstracts of the presentations and selected papers were published as the last issue of Vol. 7 of Cancer Chemotherapy and Pharmacology. The medicinal chemistry of the podophyllotoxins has been succinctly reviewed.[97] Recently up-to-date reviews on etoposide and teniposide, especially regarding their molecular pharmacology, mechanisms of action, and clinical pharmacokinetics have been published.[98,r13–r15]

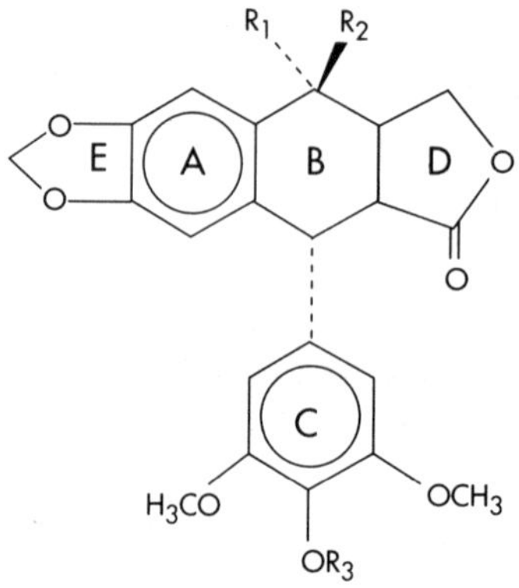

R1 R2 E A B D O O O O C H3CO OCH3 OR3

Figure 101.17

Except in the O-4,6-cyclic acetal portion of the glucoside moiety, VP and VM are structurally identical. Both are actually analogues of epipodophyllotoxin rather than podophyllotoxin; the C-4 configuration is S for epipdophyllotoxin (and VP and VM), but R for podophyllotoxin. Additionally, the semisynthetic compounds differ from both naturally-occurring lignans in having a 4′-hydroxy instead of a 4′-methoxy group; in cultured HeLa cells, 4′-hydroxy derivatives can induce single-stranded DNA breaks, whereas the 4′-methoxy compounds cannot. The presence of the glucoside moiety enhances the ability of the semisynthetic compounds to induce DNA breaks; such breaks are manifestations of the major cytotoxicity of VP and VM. However, on the other hand, the presence of the same glycoside moiety prevents VP from disrupting microtubule assembly, an effect prominently displayed by podophyllotoxin but conspicuously absent in VP and VM. The trans configuration of the lactone D ring is essential, since the analogue with a cis-lactone ring is far less active in causing G_2-phase arrest.

VP-16 and its aglycone induce single-stranded breaks in DNA in HeLa cells; these are quickly repaired by the cells within 10 minutes of drug removal—a property not shared with podophyllotoxin. As alluded to above, in this reaction the 4′-hydroxy group is required for activity, and the C-4 configuration influences the activity of the congeners. Also, glycosylation at Position 4 diminishes the activity, whereas aldehyde condensation with the 4-glucose moiety greatly increases it. Moreover, the structure of the group associated with the resulting cyclic acetal exerts considerable influence on the DNA breakage activity.[99] The DNA breakage correlates with the cytotoxicity of these compounds. Further, in cultured human lung adenocarcinoma cells exposed to VP or VM, single-stranded breaks are induced in two minutes and peak at 15 minutes, while double-stranded breaks are similarly induced but much slower. Rapid exponential repairs of both breakage types have been observed. Over-all, the in vitro biologic activities of VM are five to ten times more potent than those of VP. The current consensus is that topoisomerase II is the most likely intracellular target of the epipodophylotoxins.[100] Those congeners active in inducing protein-associated DNA breaks are also potent inhibitors of the catenation—namely, the breaking and reunion activity of mammalian DNA topoisomerase II, while topoisomerase I remains unaffected. Moreover, both VP and VM stimulate site-specific DNA breakage by a mammalian topoisomerase II; in this regard, VM is again five- to ten fold more potent than VP. However, the above mechanisms do not exclude other possibilities; for instance, the epipodophyllotoxin analogues could be metabolized in vivo to a reactive quinonoid or free radical intermediate that binds to cellular protein and DNA to exert its cytotoxicity. VP is metabolized by human erythrocytes in vitro, but the product has not been identified.[5] Although ostensibly limited to etoposide, a recent review deals comprehensively with many aspects of mechanism of action applicable to both semisynthetic epipodophyllotoxins.[101]

Etoposide [VP, VP-16, VP-16-213; Fig. 101.17, R_1=R_3=H, R_2=4.6-O-(ethylidene)-β-D-glucopyranosyl- see Fig. 101.18]

A monograph on etoposide has been published,[97] in which may be located the history of the development of this agent, its chemistry, structure-activity relationships, mechanisms of action, clinical pharmacokinetics, and other basic as well as clinical research findings. Also, the proceedings of the 1981 symposium on etoposide have appeared as Supplement A of Volume 9 of Cancer Treatment Reviews.

The clinical pharmacokinetics of VP have been extensively investigated in a number of laboratories; a review sums up the literature to early 1986.[98] When administered IV at 40 to 1000 mg/m^2, VP shows no dose-dependent pharmacokinetics; however, considerable interpatient variations in the values of the usual pharmacokinetic parameters are evident. The terminal plasma half-life of VP ranges from three hours to more than 40 hours with an apparent volume of distribution from 5 · l/m^2 to over 40 l/m^2 (125 –> 1000 ml/kg), and total clearance from approximately 6 ml·min^{-1}·m^{-2} to more than 60 ml·min^{-1}·m^{-2}.[98] The principal route of excretion is renal; 12 to 53 percent of the administered VP appears intact in urine in 24 hours. Hepatobiliary excretion is only of minor significance.

The most recent findings are in general agreement with the above. Given by mouth in a capsule or in solution, VP is from 10 to 88 percent bioavailable;[102] the latter preparation is slightly better. Although apparently not influenced by food and concurrent chemotherapy, VP bioavailability appears to be nonlinear and dose-dependent. Also in seven patients after repeated administration of 400 mg of VP by mouth, intrapatient variability of VP bioavailability was considerable. Over a wide range of concentrations VP is more than 94 percent bound to serum albumin;[103] this is one of the reasons why VP negotiates the blood brain barrier poorly. Hepatic impairment seems to exert no effect on VP pharmacokinetics; however, renal dysfunction greatly decreases VP total clearance, so that dose reduction in these patients is indicated.[104] VP pharmacokinetics are similar in children and adults. Finally, since VP pharmacokinetics are not significantly different whether after IV or intracarotid administration, the brain and brain tumors do not appear to have any first-pass effect on VP pharmacokinetics.

In humans VP undergoes in vivo metabolism largely to the trans-hydroxy acid resulting from opening of the lactone ring. This metabolite apparently is excreted mostly in the bile.[98] Additionally, significant amounts of VP glucuronide or sulfate are found in the urine of patients treated with VP; the glucuronic acid is probably linked to the two hydroxy groups of the glucoside moiety. However, it has been suggested[101] that this metabolite pathway likely is not as important as the possible oxidative transformations in the dimethoxyphenol ring E. The latter pathway would lead to the formation of cytotoxic products capable of damaging DNA.

Etoposide is assuming an increasingly significant role in cancer chemotherapy, especially in combination with other agents.[105] Combined with cisplatin, VP is highly effective in small-cell as well as squamous and adenocarcinomas of the lung. It is, in fact, curative in the salvage treatment for testicular cancers that have failed primary treatment with VLB, bleomycin, and cisplatin. Recent studies have indicated that prolonged dosing schedules such as daily times five or more result

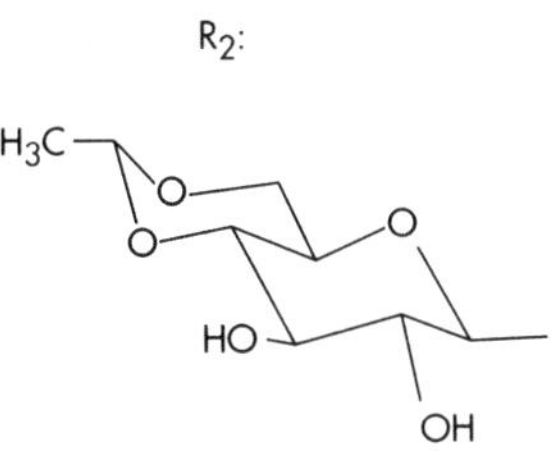

Figure 101.18

in an increase in the over-all effectiveness of VP; this is the consequence of its significant schedule sensitivity in cytotoxic effects. VP has also been used extensively in conditioning regimens for autologous and allogeneic transplants because its major dose-limiting toxicity is myelosuppression. It is particularly useful in autologous transplantation as a single agent and in combination regimens such as "CBV" with CPA and carmustine. Its dose-limiting toxicity is leukopenia; thrombocytopenia is less frequent. Nausea and vomiting are encountered occasionally, particularly with the oral preparation. The availability of the oral preparation has greatly extended the potential range of its therapeutic applications and will allow investigations of many other schedules in accord with its known cell cycle specificity.

Teniposide [VM, VM-26; in Fig. 101.17, R_1=R_3=H, R_2=4,6-0-(2-thenylidene)-β-D-glucopyranosyl-]

Qualitatively, VM and VP are quite similar in their molecular pharmacology. This is not entirely surprising since, as pointed out above, the two epipodophyllotoxin derivatives differ structurally only in the *O*-4,6-cyclic acetal portion of the glucoside moiety. Yet such an apparently minor structural alteration is sufficient to produce significant quantitative differences in certain biologic activities, including cellular uptake and cytotoxicity; in general, VM seems to be biologically more potent than VP.[97]

The clinical pharmacokinetics of VM have been thoroughly reviewed;[98,106,107] it is especially instructive to compare VM with VP. Like VP, VM shows wide interpatient variations in its pharmacokinetics. After IV administration of VM from 30 to 1000 mg/m^2, either as a bolus or by continuous infusion to adults and children with various malignancies, the terminal plasma half-life of VM varies from six hours to more than 20 hours, the apparent volume of distribution from 3.4 l/m^2 (85.3 ml/kg) to over 40 l/m^2 (667 ml/kg), and the total clearance from 5.4 ml·min^{-1}·m^{-2} to 36 ml·min^{-1}·m^{-2} (0.14 ml·min^{-1}·kg^{-1}). Saturation pharmacokinetics appear to be evident at high doses, since the plasma half-life of the drug averages 48 hours, and the median total clearance is reduced to 7 ml·min^{-1}·m^{-2}, whereas the volume of distribution shows insignificant changes. In pediatric patients with leukemia, lymphoma, or neuroblastoma responding to VM therapy, the mean steady-state plasma drug concentration is significantly higher (15.2 mg/l) and the mean clearance slower (12.1 ml·min^{-1}·m^{-2}) than the corresponding values (6.2 mg/L and 21.3 ml·min^{-1}·m^{-2}) in patients not responding, particularly in patients with leukemia; thus, patients with higher steady-state plasma VM concentration and slower drug clearance are likely to respond. In 72 percent of these patients, 44.5 percent of the administered radioactive tritiated VM is excreted in the urine, of which only 31.3 percent of the radioactivity resides in the intact drug. However, the metabolism of VM remains to be elucidated. Almost completely bound to serum albumin (99.4%),[103] VM does not penetrate the blood brain barrier well.

Undoubtedly teniposide is a clinically useful agent, especially in combination with other agents in treating pediatric hematologic malignancies. However, its proper place in cancer chemotherapy and how is it compared with VP remain to be studied.

Anthracycline Antibiotics

Isolated from cultures of various species of *Streptomyces*, the anthracycline antibiotics, including daunorubicin (DNR), doxorubicin (DOX), and several of their natural as well as semisynthetic analogues, are an important class of anticancer agents with a broad spectrum of clinical activity. Consequently, they have been the subject of intensive laboratory and clinical investigations. A number of review articles and monographs on many aspects of the anthracycline antibiotics are now available.[r2,108–112]) Reference 109 is perhaps the most authoritative from a biochemical point of view.

The basic skeleton of the anthracycline antibiotics consists of a linear planar tetrahydrotetracene ring system (Fig. 101.19), in which quinone and hydroquinone moieties are located on adjacent rings. The ring system is linked to an unusual amino sugar, daunosamine, through a glycosidic bond. Such a structure at once suggests several possible biochemical pharmacologic consequences. First, by virtue of its adjacent quinone-hydroquinone structure, it is possible for these antibiotics to chelate with divalent cations. Second, this structure renders the molecule readily able to be involved in biologic redox reactions. Third, it may promote the in vivo generation of free radicals. Fourth, the linear planar ring system confers on the antibiotics the propensity to intercalate between DNA base pairs; the

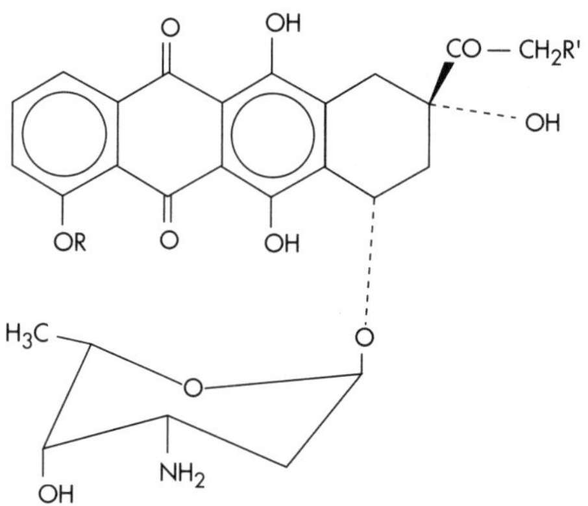

Figure 101.19

stability of the intercalated complex is further strengthened through interaction of the amino group of the unique daunosamine with the sugar-phosphate backbone of the DNA helix. Any of these events can ultimately be detrimental to cell replication and survival. For instance, intercalation can cause DNA strand breaks, sister chromatid exchange, and eventual stoppage of nucleic acid synthesis. Free radicals originating from the anthracyclines can lead to the subsequent formation not only of highly toxic intermediates, such as superoxide anion and hydroxyl radicals, but also of other reactive radicals with alkylating properties. In fact, the deleterious myocardial toxicity of these antibiotics has been attributed to myocardial cell membrane damage caused by these radicals. Finally, the anthracyclines are all inhibitors of DNA topoisomerase II, including those that do not bind to DNA. The cytotoxicity of the anthracycline antibiotics is a manifestation of all these possible events, with varying contributions from each.

Thus far, DNR and DOX are the cardinal members of this important class of anticancer agents, especially DOX. It is only to be expected that continuing efforts are being made to achieve structural modifications that improve the clinical efficacy of the anthracycline antibiotics, culminating in the discovery of new agents such as idarubicin to be discussed later. However, from a chemical structural point of view, it remains obscure why a trivial difference involving merely a hydroxyl group at C-14 should produce such a significant change in clinical activity between DNR and DOX. DNR is most effective in acute leukemias; DOX shows a much broader spectrum of antitumor activity.

Daunorubicin (Daunomycin, DNR; R′=H in Fig. 101.19)

The basic structural features of DNR, that is, the linear planar tetrahydrotetracene ring system shared with the other members of the anthracycline antibiotics, suggest that the terminal-phase plasma half-life of DNR would be relatively long, the apparent volume of distribution very large (much in excess of 1 l/kg), and extensive binding to protein most likely would occur through hydrophobic interactions. Poor penetration into the CNS, significant heptobiliary excretion, and comparatively small contribution of renal clearance to its total clearance also are expected. These predictions have been borne out amply by experimental evidence. For instance, on average, the plasma half-life of DNR is approximately 20 hours, the volume of distribution 20 l/kg, and no more than 15 percent of the administered dose is excreted intact in the urine in five days.[109,110,113] Attempts to correlate DNR pharmacokinetics with clinical response in patients with acute myelogenous leukemia have not been successful.[114] DNR is extensively metabolized in the body, with daunorubicinol (involving the reduction of the 13-keto-function) as the principal metabolite. In this conjunction, it must be pointed out that earlier pharmacokinetics studies of these antibiotics utilized radiochemical and fluorometric assays that are far less specific than the high-performance liquid chromatographic methodology developed subsequently. Also, a great deal of individual variability has been shown in the values of the standard pharmacokinetic parameters of DNR.

In combination with other agents DNR is effective for treating acute leukemias. It is also used in treating certain solid tumors; however, here it is much less potent than doxorubicin. Its dose-limiting toxicity is leukopenia; nausea and vomiting are relatively mild. Cardiomyopathy is the most serious side-effect.

Doxorubicin (Adriamycin, DOX; R′=OH in Fig. 101.19)

For nearly three decades DOX has enjoyed a paramount role in cancer chemotherapy. A monograph on this important antibiotic is available;[112] additionally, excellent discussions on the biochemistry, pharmacology, and clinical applications of DOX are found in References 105 and 108–112.

The clinical pharmacokinetics of DOX have been reviewed recently, with most publications covered up to 1987.[116] Like DNR, the pharmacokinetics of DOX are predictable from its chemical structure. What is surprising is that the spectrum of anticancer activity of DOX is so much wider than that of DNR, given the apparently minor difference in structure. Obviously the wider spectrum of activity of DOX cannot be attributed to the pharmacokinetics of the agent, since DOX and DNR have similar pharmacokinetic properties. For example, the average plasma half-life of DOX is approximately 30 hours (range: 13 hr to 50 hr), the apparent volume of distribution 36 L/kg (9 L/kg to 66 L/kg), and total clearance about 270 $ml{\cdot}min^{-1}{\cdot}m^{-2}$ (228.6–695 $ml{\cdot}min{-}1{\cdot}m^{-2}$); these values (calculated from the summary table in Ref. 116) are in good agreement with recent findings.[117–119] Again, considerable interpatient variations are evident. Although DOX pharmacokinetics are not predictive of response and toxicity, in one study the early DOX clearance during the distribution phase seemed to correlate with patient age and total clearance.[119] DOX is also extensively metabolized in the body; less than 15 percent is excreted intact in the urine in six days; the predominant route of elimination is in bile. The major products of DOX metabolism are its reduced 13-hydroxyl metabolite, doxorubicinol (DOX-ol), and the aglycones doxorubicinone and 7-deoxydoxorubicinone; the former is cytotoxic, whereas the latter are not. Also, formation of doxorubicinol is mediated by cytoplasmic aldoketoreductases whereas that of the aglycones is by cytochrome reductase. Another difference is in the plasma half-life; in patients with normal liver and kidney function without prior DOX exposure, plasma half-life of DOX-ol is approximately the same as that of DOX, namely, 30 hours; in contrast, the half-lives of both aglycones are much shorter. It has been suggested that DOX cardiomyopathy may be related more to plasma 7-deoxydoxorubicinone concentration than to DOX concentration.[120]

DOX solution is stable in plastic bags; in glass container it is a little less so, with a half-life of about 11 days.[30] DOX has an impressive spectrum of anticancer activity, being effective against a variety of hematologic malignancies and solid tumors. It is the single most effective agent against metastatic breast cancer and soft tissue sarcomas. Significant synergism has been observed when given with CPA or FU and CPA. Like DNR, its dose-limiting toxicity is also hematologic, leukopenia in particular. Cardiomyopathy is serious after chronic treatment with DOX at high doses. Dose reduction is advocated in patients with hyperbilirubinemia.[110]

Epirubicin[r16] (EPR, the 4′-epimer of DOX)

The only structural difference between EPR, a semisynthetic anthracycline antibiotic, and DOX lies in the configuration of the 4′-hydroxyl group in the daunosamine moiety. In experimental systems, EPR and DOX are equally effective; but EPR has the apparent advantage of being additionally active against the Lewis lung carcinoma and human melanoma xenograft. More important, it seems to be less toxic than DOX. These observations have prompted clinical trials of EPR at a number of centers.

The last decade has witnessed many clinical pharmacokinetic studies of EPR, including some well designed cross-over investigations of EPR in comparison with DOX in the same patients.[117,118,121,122] As expected, the two agents do not differ a great deal in their pharmacokinetics except that the total clearance of EPR is much higher than that of DOX. Taking these studies into consideration, we estimate that the terminal plasma half-life of EPR is approximately 27 hours (12–39 hr); the apparent volume of distribution, 25 L/kg; and the total clearance, 880 $ml{\cdot}min^{-1}{\cdot}m^{-2}$ (340–1688 $ml{\cdot}min^{-1}{\cdot}m^{-2}$) (22.0 $ml{\cdot}min^{-1}{\cdot}kg^{-1}$, ranging from 8.5–42.2 $ml{\cdot}min^{-1}{\cdot}kg^{-1}$); the last parameter is more than threefold that of DOX. One possible explanation for this high clearance is that in vivo EPR undergoes not only reduction to epirubicinol (EPR-ol) and the aglycones of EPR and EPR-ol, but also glucuronidation of EPR and EPR-ol, a unique biotransformation pathway hitherto seen only with EPR and not with any other anthracycline antibiotics.[122] In fact, the lessened myocardial toxicity of EPR has also been attributed, in part at least, to this unique formation of glucuronides.[122] As with DOX, the cumulative urinary excretion of EPR is low—less than 12 percent of the administered dose in six days; the major route of elimination of EPR and metabolites is hepatobiliary.[123] In a study involving three patients, on average renal clearance contributes 12.9 percent to the total clearance of EPR, while biliary clearance contributes 29.1 percent.[123]

Compared with DOX, EPR is relatively new, and its clinical efficacy has not yet been established. However, in general, EPR appears to the less potent and less toxic of the two. Its spectrum of activity is very similar to that of DOX, but it is less myelosuppressive and damaging to the heart.

Idarubicin (IDR, 4-demethoxydaunorubicin)

IDR, another semisynthetic anthracycline antibiotic, is derived from DNR with replacement of the 4-methoxy moiety with hydrogen. Again, in experimental tumor models it is more active than the parent drug, but less prone to induced cardiomyopathy. As a result it has been undergoing clinical investigations in recent years.

Based on the studies of two groups of investigators[124,125] the standard clinical pharmacokinetic parameters have the following mean values: plasma half-life, about 27 hours; volume of distribution, 64 L/kg; and total clearance, 32 $ml{\cdot}min^{-1}{\cdot}kg^{-1}$. In 24 hours, (1520 $ml{\cdot}min^{-1}{\cdot}m^{-2}$) only about five percent of the dose is excreted in the urine unchanged. Given by mouth, IDR is 40 to 45 percent bioavailable. In two two-patient studies, approximately 4 percent of the dose was excreted in the bile, nearly 2.5 times as much as in the urine of these two patients. The only identified IDR metabolite is the 13-hydroxyl derivative, idarubicinol.

IDR is active against hematologic malignancies and breast carcinoma. Comparison with other anthracycline antibiotics awaits completion of current Phase III clinical trials. However, in preliminary comparative studies IDR has been shown to be slightly, but significantly, more effective than DNR or DOX in inducing remission in acute myeloblastic leukemia with lower frequency of cardiotoxicity. At equimyelosuppressive doses, IDR is less likely than DNR or DOX to induce nausea, vomiting, and mucositis.

Other Antibiotics

Although not as important and broadly active as the anthracycline antibiotics, several other types of antibiotics with diverse chemical structures also are clinically useful in cancer. These include bleomycin, dactinomycin, mitomycin C, and plicamycin, to be discussed below. This is an expanding, promising field; undoubtedly, many new anticancer antibiotics will be discovered for clinical trials in the near future.

Bleomycins[r17] (BLM, Fig. 101.20)

A group of cytotoxic glycopeptide antibiotics isolated from a culture filtrate of a strain of the microorganism *Streptomyces verticillus* are collectively known as the bleomycins. They share a complex

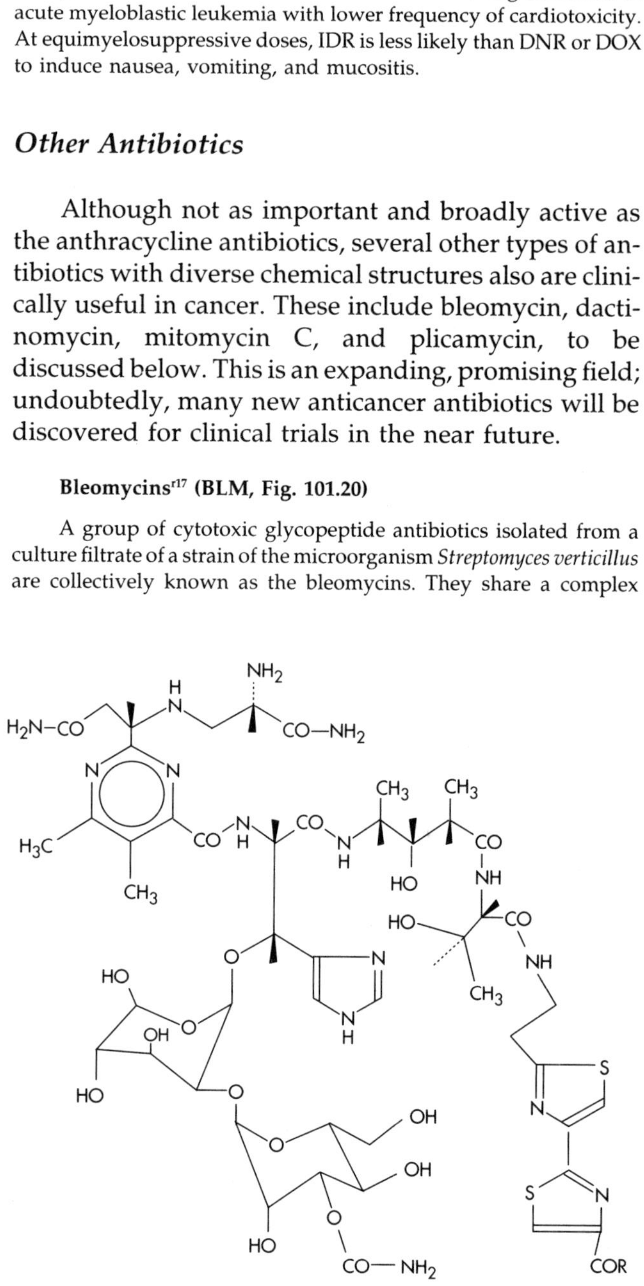

Figure 101.20

common structure with nine chiral centers, as illustrated in *Fig. 101.20*. Individual members differ in the terminal alkylamino group, for example, R is -NH-$(CH_2)_3$-S-CH_3 in BLM A_2, but-NH-$(CH_2)_4$-NH-C (=NH)-NH_2 in BLM B_2. Clinical preparation of BLM is a mixture of analogues, mostly A_2 (70%) and B_2 (28%). The chemistry of the BLMs has been authoritatively reviewed.[126] The papers presented at the 1984 international symposium on BLM have been published;[127] although most of the reports are clinical, one deals with BLM clinical pharmacology. In Reference 128 the most up-to-date review on BLM is presented.

BLM chelates with metals such as copper and iron and binds to DNA through intercalation. In the presence of ferrous ions and oxygen it generates free radicals that induce DNA (but not RNA) single-and double-strand breaks. These breaks are manifested in chromosomal aberrations and fragmentations, as seen in cultured cells in the G_2 phase of the cell cycle. Also, in the presence of not only oxygen but also a reducing agent such as dithiothreitol, the Cu·BLM chelate is capable of behaving like a minienzyme, a monooxygenase, to degrade DNA. These mechanisms of action have been succinctly discussed and reviewed.[r2,128]

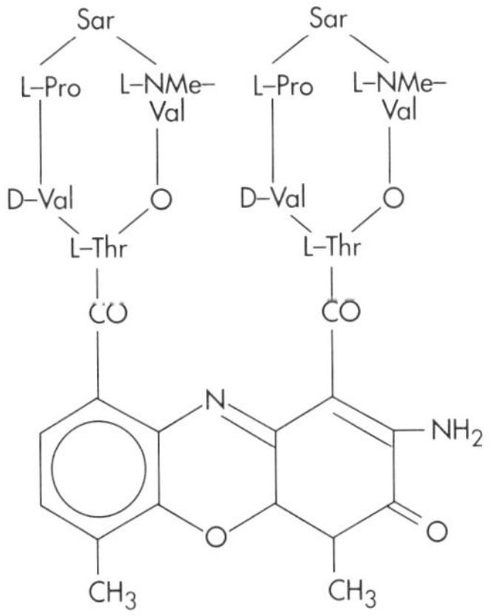

BLM pharmacokinetics have been investigated in patients with cancer.[129–131] The plasma half-life of BLM ranges from four to nine hours; the total clearance, 1.11–2.53 ml·min^{-1}·kg^{-1}; and the volume of distribution is among the smallest of anticancer agents, 440 to 735 ml/kg. In patients with renal failure, the plasma half-life of BLM is increased exponentially with decreasing creatinine clearance. Approximately 60 percent of the administered dose is excreted in the urine in six days. Although all tissues contain a BLM-degrading enzyme, BLM hydrolase,[127] such a degradation has not been reported in vivo. Further, BLM hydrolase activity is not correlated with in vitro cytotoxicity of the antibiotic.

Some components of the clinical BLM preparation are not stable, especially in plastic containers.[30] The absence of myleosuppressive toxicity in BLM makes it an attractive member in various combinations with other anticancer agents in curative regimens for treating testicular cancer, squamous cell carcinomas, and lymphomas. Its most serious toxicity is a unique form of pulmonary fibrosis in the subpleural areas; this peculiar toxicity is related to the total dose and the risk increases with advancing age.

Dactinomycin (DAC, Actinomycin D, Fig. 101.21)

Since the advent of penicillin, concerted efforts to discover additional new clinically useful antibiotics from various sources have led to the isolation from the soil-inhabiting microorganism *Streptomyces antibiotics* of a group of yellowish-red compounds designated the actinomycins A through Z, with further subdivision by numbers and Greek letters. The more than 50 actinomycins share a common chromophore, actinocin, a planar phenoxazone ring that is attached to two cyclic pentapeptides consisting of different amino acids. They are all cytotoxic, with varying degrees of antibacterial, antiviral, and antitumor properties. The oldest antineoplastic antibiotic with a history of more than three decades in its clinical development, actinomycin D or dactinomycin (DAC, structure shown in Fig. 101.21) is the only member of the group used therapeutically for cancer. A 25-year old monograph on DAC still serves as an informative reference;[132] however, Reference 133 presents a more recent review.

Figure 101.21

A model RNA synthesis inhibitor, DAC forms a complex with DNA and then selectively interferes with DNA-dependent RNA synthesis, precisely that of ribosomal RNA. The planar phenoxazone ring intercalates between adjacent G-C base-pairs of DNA, and the cyclic peptides interact with the amino groups of G through hydrogen bonding. The mode of action of DAC has been reviewed.[r3,133]

Not much is known about the clinical pharmacokinetics of DAC. In a study[134] in three patients with malignant melanoma who received tritiated DAC, the plasma half-life of the antibiotic was estimated to be 36 hours; in seven days on average 20 percent of the dose was excreted in the urine and 13 percent in the feces. The drug is minimally metabolized and does not penetrate readily into the CNS. However, it is selectively concentrated in the nucleated blood elements.[134] The clinical preparation of DAC is stable in both glass and plastic containers.[30]

As a single agent DAC is effective in choriocarcinoma. In combination regimens it is used for the treatment of solid tumors such as Ewing's sarcoma, Wilms' tumor, and rhabdomyosarcoma. Myelosuppression is its dose-limiting toxicity.

Mitomycin C (MMC, Fig. 101.22)

Among a number of chemically related antibiotics, including mitomycins A, B, C and others isolated from the culture broths of *Streptomyces ardus*, *S. caespitosus*, and *S. verticillatus*, MMC turns out to be the most prom-

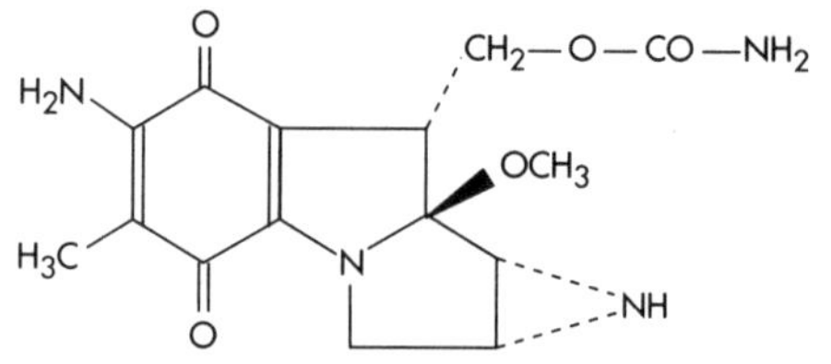

Figure 101.22

ising, with the highest antitumor activity in experimental models. Its chemical structure is illustrated in the accompanying Figure (Fig. 101.22). This unusual substituted benzoquinone condensed with a reduced heterocyclic ring system has stimulated many studies of its chemical, biochemical, biologic, and pharmacologic properties. Reviews of its chemistry,[135] therapeutic aspects,[136] and pharmacokinetics[137] are available; an authoritative discussion[138] of its molecular mechanism of anticancer action is included in Reference 136.

The presence of the quinoid moiety in MMC may facilitate its participation in biologic redox reactions to generate highly reactive and cytotoxic free radicals, and that of the aziridine ring may further confer alkylating properties on the agent, perhaps after in vivo reductive activation. In short, MMC is expected potentially to alkylate, cross-link, cleave, and depurinate DNA after forming various intermediates in cyclic redox reactions, thus leading to inhibition of cell replication. But it remains unclear how these events would ultimately make MMC, to some extent, selectively cytotoxic to certain cancer cells.

The pharmacokinetics of MMC has been reviewed, with most literature covered up to 1986.[137] In sum, after IV administration, as reported by several groups of researchers,[139–142] the mean plasma terminal half-life of MMC is 48 min (30–70 min), the total clearance 400 (200–700) $ml{\cdot}min^{-1}{\cdot}{}^{-2}$[10 (5–17.5) $ml{\cdot}min^{-1}{\cdot}kg^{-1}$], and volume of distribution 41 (11–56) l/m^2 [approximately 1 (0.275–1.4) L/kg]; less than 20 percent of the administered dose is ultimately excreted in the urine. The results of more recent studies[140–142] do not deviate significantly from the above. In one patient, biliary MMC concentration was five- to eight-fold higher than the concurrent plasma drug concentration; there may be enterohepatic recirculation of the drug.[139]

Although MMC is stable in normal saline, it decomposes appreciably in D_5W solution.[30] It is active against a number of solid tumors. In combination with other agents it is useful for treating stomach and breast cancers. Its dose-limiting toxicity is myelosuppression.

Plicamycin (Mithramycin, PCM)

PCM[133] is a complicated antitumor antibiotic (see Fig. 101.23) isolated from cultured *Streptomyces plicatus*. It inhibits DNA-directed

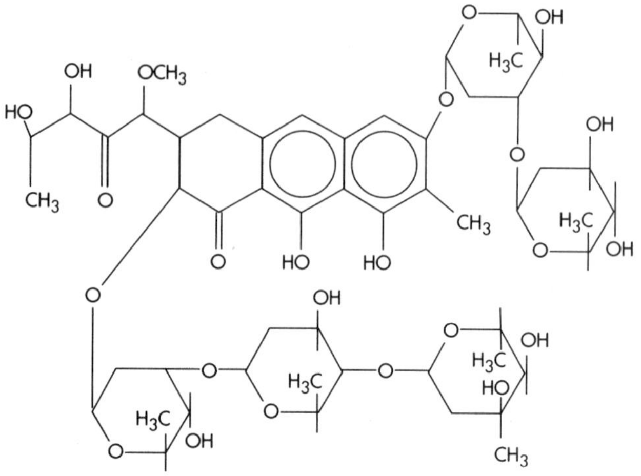

Figure 101.23

RNA synthesis by intercalation in DNA in the presence of divalent cations such as Mg^{2+}. It is effective in treating disseminated embryonic testicular carcinoma and Paget bone disease. Because of its hypocalcemic effect, it is also useful for controlling the hypercalcemia and hypercalciuria associated with advanced cancer. Toxicities include a severe hemorrhage syndrome, hepatotoxicity, hypocalcemia, and thrombocytopenia. The recommended dose for treating testicular tumors is 0.025–0.030 mg/kg (1.0–1.2 mg/m^2) IV daily for eight to 10 days.

No meaningful information on PCM pharmacokinetics is available.

L-Asparaginase (LAS, L-asparagine amidohydrolase)

The only enzyme in clinical cancer chemotherapy, and of limited application at that, LAS mediates the cleavage of the generally considered nonessential amino acid L-asparagine to aspartate and ammonia; the reverse reaction, on the other hand, is catalyzed by asparagine synthetase (asparatate-ammonia ligase, EC 6.3.1.1). The identification of LAS in guinea pig serum as the inhibitory factor of rodent tumors was hailed initially as a major breakthrough in cancer biochemistry, the first definitive demonstration of a unique, distinct metabolic difference between normal and cancer cells—a difference that could form the basis for specific chemotherapy, of lymphoid malignancies at least, since human lymphoid tissues are particularly deficient in asparagine synthetase so that the depletion of L-asparagine would be selectively deleterious. Depletion of L-asparagine is the prelude to inhibition of protein synthesis and ultimately cell death. Disappointingly, later events dealt a most damaging blow to this concept, in retrospect perhaps somewhat naive, because many normal tissues are shown to be equally sensitive to LAS. In other words, the cellular difference in sensitivity to the action of LAS is a matter of quantity rather than kind. Details on the biochemistry of LAS and the therapeutic applications of the enzyme may be found in several reviews.[143,144]

In humans after IV administration, the enzyme disappears by an unknown mechanism from the plasma exponentially, with a half-life of about 18 hours (8–44 hr) on average;[145–149] estimated by us from published results;[145,148] its volume of distribution is approximately 55 ml/kg, and total clearance 0.035 $ml \cdot min^{-1} \cdot kg^{-1}$, (1.4 $ml \cdot min^{-1} \cdot m^{-2}$), making both parameters the smallest of all cancer chemotherapeutic agents. However, by IM administration the total clearance of LAS is almost 1 $ml \cdot min^{-1} \cdot kg^{-1}$ (40 $ml \cdot min^{-1} \cdot m^{-2}$),[148] nearly 30 times that by the IV route. A large protein molecule, it is not surprising that LAS penetrates the CNS poorly and is excreted in the urine only negligibly.[149]

For clinical use the enzyme is prepared from *Escherichia coli* or *Erwinia carotovora*, and remains stable in pH 5–9 solution in glass containers at room temperature for at least a week. It is an agent with a narrow spectrum of anticancer activity, particularly useful for remission induction in pediatric patients with acute lymphocytic leukemia. LAS is reasonably well tolerated in children. However, in adults it elicits a variety of toxicities including hyperglycemia, lowering of plasma proteins (particularly fibrinogen), severe anorexia and weight loss, and in very high doses CNS depression. In adults with acute lymphoblastic leukemia its role is limited when used alone. But it is used widely in combination with MTX for the treatment of adult acute lymphoblastic leukemia because of its ability to modulate side-effects of MTX. LAS has similarly been reported to modulate the toxic side-effects of ara-C; for this reason it is used for remission induction in acute myeloblastic leukemia. LAS is prone to induce allergic manifestations; its rapid plasma clearance correlates positively with the occurrence of anaphylaxis.[148] Patients becoming allergic to *E. coli* preparations have been found to tolerate the *Erwinia* preparation, thus allowing continued LAS therapy. Resistance to LAS therapy develops easily and rapidly.

Taxol

A complex diterpene [Fig. 101.24] extracted from the bark of the Pacific yew, *Taxus brevifolia*, taxol[150,151] promotes microtubule assembly in vitro at concentrations attainable clinically during prolonged infusions; it produces abnormal morphologic effects on these cellular structures, a unique mechanism of cytotoxicity. Preclinical screens have revealed that this agent is significantly active against resistant murine melanoma B16. Recent clinical trials at a number of cancer centers have also shown that taxol is active against advanced

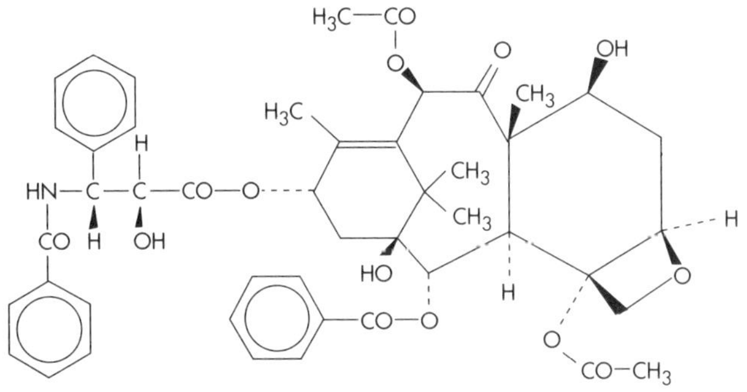

Figure 101.24

ovarian cancer (over-all response 20–57%), breast cancer (over-all response 60%), and non-small cell lung cancer (over-all 22%). Major toxicities include acute hypersensitivity reaction, neutropenia, mucositis, and peripheral neuropathy; cardiac rhythm disturbances have also been observed. Used as a single agent, the generally agreed dose is 200 to 250 mg/m^2 by IV infusion in 24 hours. Combination regimens with other agents are still under development.

Taxol pharmacokinetics show wide variability. In one study the terminal plasma half-life is 1.3–8.6 hours (mean 5 hr); steady-state volume of distribution, 55 to 183 L/m^2 (mean 110 L/m^2); total clearance, 100 to 993 $ml \cdot min^{-1} \cdot m^{-2}$ (mean 110 $ml \cdot min^{-1} \cdot m^{-2}$). In 24 hours only 5 percent of the dose is excreted intact in the urine.

Miscellaneous Agents

Platinum Coordination Compounds

The establishment of cisplatin as an important anticancer agent prompted the synthesis and development of a host of coordination compounds of platinum and other metals in the hope of finding more efficacious agents. But thus far, besides cisplatin, carboplatin is the only member of the family of platinum coordination compounds that has advanced to the status of a generally accepted active drug.

The structure-activity relationships among the platinum coordination compounds have been concisely reviewed.[152] Briefly, for these compounds to show antitumor activity, first, the two amine groups ammonia ligands must be in a *cis*-configuration. Second, the compounds must have suitable leaving groups such as chloride and carboxylate anions; other anions including iodide, nitrate, nitrite, and perchlorate only render the compounds inactive. Third, the platinum-bound nitrogen must contain a hydrogen donor—that is, at least one NH group. Last, tetravalent platinum compounds are seldom active per se; the platinum must first undergo reduction to the square planar divalent state.

Cisplatin [DDP, *cis*-diamminedichloroplatinum (II)]

Although first synthesized almost a century and a half ago, DDP became an effective cancer chemotherapeutic agent only recently; it is the first inorganic compound with demonstrated clinical activities against a variety of solid tumors. In a way it is surprising that such a relatively simple molecule turns out to be a highly effective anticancer agent (see Fig. 101.25). DDP exists in two isomeric forms; however, only the *cis*-isomer is active. Although serendipitous, the discovery of its antineoplastic properties is nonetheless the culmination of the imaginative, aggressive, systematic, and persistent pursuit of a chance laboratory observation by its original discoverer, followed later by many other investigators. The fascinating story of the discovery and development of DDP in cancer chemotherapy is absorbingly told in Chapter 2[153] of the 1980 monograph[154] that has summarized its status at that time. Also, its chemistry has been succinctly reviewed in an excellent paper.[155] For more up-to-date information on DDP, recent reviews and monographs[156-159] may be consulted.

In solution DDP is unstable and the chloride anions are successively displaced with molecules of water to afford acidic aquated products. Moreover, the aqua derivatives readily generate hydroxo-bridged dimers and oligomers that have been isolated and characterized. Other reactions involving DDP are apt to take place as well. For instance, in plasma and other physiologic fluids DDP undergoes extensive degradation, as it reacts with all sorts of nucleophiles such as amines, imidazoles, and thiols. Thus, a plasma solution of DDP is in fact a complex mixture of many platinum-containing molecules in various proportions at diverse stages of equilibrium. All these possibilities and complications must be kept in mind when considering the biochemistry and pharmacology of DDP.

The mechanism of anticancer action of DDP is not yet fully understood. It has long been recognized that DDP reacts with pyrimidines and nucleic acids to afford "platinum blues" of undefined structures. Since DDP is an active antitumor agent while the *trans*-isomer is markedly less active or totally inactive, it at once suggests that DNA is the target molecule and that the interaction between DDP and DNA is stereospecific. At concentrations barely cytotoxic to HeLa cells, DDP indeed inhibits DNA, but not RNA or protein synthesis. Apparently this inhibition is the consequence of both intrastrand and interstrand DNA cross-linking. Therefore, the current belief is that inhibition of DNA synthesis constitutes a mechanism of cytotoxicity of DDP. This subject has been well reviewed.[152,156–160] However, it must be reiterated that DDP is a reactive molecule that generates a host of products in vivo. The contributions of these products to the selective cytotoxicity of DDP to cancer cells remain to be elucidated.

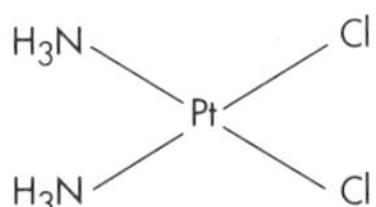

Figure 101.25

Owing to the important therapeutic role of DDP, its clinical pharmacokinetics have been studied by many investigators. But before the advent of specific assays for intact DDP, early attempts using equivocal analytical methodologies, such as atomic absorption spectroscopic and radiochemical assays that quantify total elemental platinum, afforded only confusing results that are not only hard to interpret but also of doubtful significance. The confusion is not clarified simply by making a distinction between protein-bound platinum and ultrafilterable or free platinum in circulation; it is believed that only free DDP is cytotoxic, whereas protein-bound DDP is not. Nonetheless, based on several such studies, the general consensus is that after IV DDP administration total platinum is cleared slowly from the systemic circulation with a half-life of several days, whereas free platinum is rapidly eliminated from the blood with a half-life of less than 1 hour.[161–166] In 48 hours approximately 50 percent of dose is excreted in the urine; it is actively secreted by renal tubules;[167] and biliary excretion plays an insignificant role in platinum elimination.[168] Extensively protein-bound, DDP is not expected to cross the blood-brain barrier readily. Curiously, however, it is quickly taken up by erythrocytes.[165] Significant advances in pharmacokinetic studies of DDP are apparent as a result of the development of high performance liquid chromatographic assays[167,169,170] that appear to be specific for intact DDP. With these improved methodologies, a number of more meaningful pharmacokinetic investigations have been conducted.[163,171,174] For example, in seven patients with ovarian cancer the plasma terminal half-life of intact DDP was 32 minutes, the volume of distribution 1.5 L/m^2 (37.5 ml/kg, consistent with the fact that the drug binds extensively to plasma protein but not to tissue components), and total clearance 253 $ml \cdot min^{-1} \cdot m^{-2}$ (6.3 $ml \cdot min^{-1} \cdot kg^{-1}$); 23.3 percent of the dose is excreted unchanged in the urine in 24 hours.[173] The plasma ultrafilterable platinum and intact DDP are most likely not identical, since the concentration ratio of unchanged DDP to free platinum remains approximately 0.6 to 0.8 over two hours after DDP administration, whereas that of DDP to total platinum declines from 0.5 at 5 minutes to 0.1 at 2 hours.[163] These ratios are not affected by DDP dose or mannitol administration.

Repeated courses of DDP lead to significantly reduced renal elimination of platinum, probably through a decrease in tubular secretion of DDP.[171] Further, the renal clearance of unchanged DDP after a 6-hour IV infusion is appreciably lower (52.8 ml·min^{-1}·m^{-2} or 1.32 ml·min^{-1}·kg^{-1}) than after a two-hour infusion (87.1 ml·min^{-1}·m^{-1} or 2.18 ml·min^{-1}·kg^{-1}); however, DDP renal clearance exceeds creatinine clearance, regardless of infusion duration. Moreover, a single determination of plasma DDP concentration at the end of infusion seems to be a good predictor of total DDP clearance. It has been suggested that some DDP toxicities may be dependent on maximal plasma drug concentrations, while others depend on the area under the plasma DDP concentration versus time curve (AUC) or both. On the other hand, DDP therapeutic effect probably is related to the AUC.[173] Whether DDP is metabolized in vivo remains unanswerable. Because in plasma, and most likely in other body fluids as well, DDP undergoes extensive chemical degradation, the mono-methionine-DDP substituted complex isolated from plasma of rats treated with this drug may simply be the product of a chemical reaction without enzymatic mediation. Among the several models developed for studying DDP pharmacokinetics, one is particularly noted for its elegance and excellent curve-fitting of experimental data.[174,175] The only reservation is that the assumption that parent drug accounts for essentially all the platinum in plasma ultrafiltrate in the first two hours after infusion may not be valid in view of what has been discussed.[162]

DDP is now widely used for the treatment of a variety of solid tumors. It is an important component of the combination regimens that are curative for testicular cancer. It is also effective in the treatment of gynecologic malignancies, particularly ovarian cancer. DDP is highly effective in metatastic breast cancer, and very useful for the treatment of both small cell as well as squamous cell and adenocarcinoma of the lung. Its most serious side-effect is nephrotoxicity. Severe debilitating nausea and vomiting are common. Ototoxicity such as tinnitus and hearing loss, even deafness, may also occur. By infusing DDP over periods as long as five days, many of the acute side-effects such as nausea and vomiting can be ameliorated. All DDP toxicities are strongly dose related and can be largely avoided at lower dosages.

Carboplatin [CPt, *cis*-diammine (1,1-cyclobutane dicarboxylato)platinum (II), Fig. 101.26]

Although a versatile agent with a broad spectrum of activity against many solid tumors, DDP has some serious side-effects such as nephrotoxicity, ototoxicity, peripheral neuropathy, and severe nausea and vomiting that drastically limit its clinical usefulness. In a systematic search for more efficacious platinum coordination compounds as cancer chemotherapeutic agents, CPt (Fig. 101.26) emerges as a leading candidate for clinical development on the strengths of its preclinical antitumor activity and diminished toxicity.[176,177] Early clinical studies have confirmed that, compared with DDP, CPt is indeed not significantly nephrotoxic and far less emetic.[178] The proceedings of the 1985 symposium on CPt have been published.[178] In addition, three recent reviews on CPt are available.[179,180,r18]

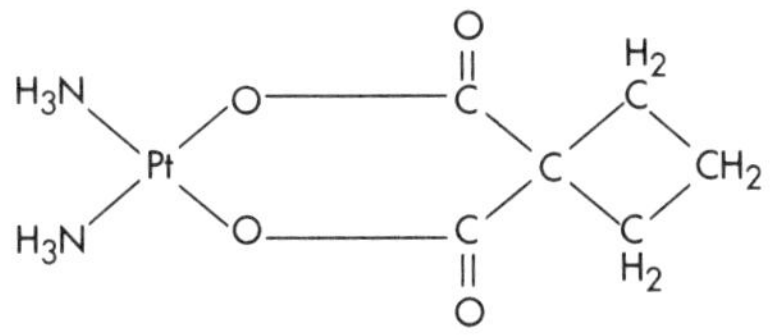

Figure 101.26

The mode of action of CPt is unknown; however, since, like DDP, it is a divalent platinum coordination compound, presumably the two share the same antitumor mechanism. However, CPt and DDP differ in a number of chemical pharmacologic and toxicologic aspects. Compared with DDP, CPt is more stable; in human plasma at 37°C its half-life is approximately 30 hours;[181,182] in plasma ultrafiltrate, even longer, 98 hours.[183] It is far less extensively protein bound: 24 percent in the first hour after drug administration and 87 percent at 24 hours.[182] Since free platinum in plasma is essentially unchanged CPt, pharmacokinetic parameters of plasma ultrafilterable platinum may be taken as those of CPt itself.[182] However, a high-performance liquid chromatographic assay for CPt in human plasma and urine has been reported. The plasma terminal half-life of CPt varies greatly from 1.5 to 24 hours, depending on the patient studied and the investigator conducting the study.[177,182,184–186] Similarly, the volume of distribution is from 250 to 650 ml/kg, and the total clearance from 1.45–2.65 ml·min^{-1}·kg^{-1}. In 24 hours 50 to 70 percent of the administered dose finds its way to the urine, including 32 percent as intact CPt.[182] CPt clearance correlates with glomerular filtration rate; plasma free platinum AUC correlates with hematologic toxicity, white cell count nadir, and duration of thrombocytopenia,[184] and the percentage decrease in platelet count.[187] Also, the percentage dose excreted in urine and the clearance of plasma ultrafilterable platinum are both linearly related to creatinine clearance.[187] Unlike DDP, CPT apparently is not actively secreted by renal tubules.[182] An interesting pharmacologically-based dosing scheme has been proposed for CPt therapy;[188] however, its validity has not been confirmed. As expected, when given orally the bioavailability of CPt is very low.[189]

Far less extensively studied than DDP, CPt is definitely an active agent against a variety of solid tumors, especially ovarian cancer. Its spectrum of antitumor activity is similar to that of DDP, except that its therapeutic index seems to be significantly better. Its dose-limiting toxicity is hematologic, mostly leukopenia. Nausea and vomiting are mild; ototoxicity, neuropathy, and nephrotoxicity are rare.[190,191] In patients with ovarian cancer failing or relapsing after standard conventional platinum-containing therapy, significant responses including complete remissions have been elicited; however, marked cross resistance between CPt and DDP has been observed.

*Amsacrine [AMS, m-AMSA, 4′-(9-Acridinylamino)methanesulfon-*m*-anisidine, Fig. 101.27]*

Among a series of acridylmethanesulfonanilides, AMS has been chosen for clinical trial and therapeutic development owing to its impressive activities against a number of experimental animal tumors.[192] Its biochemical pharmacology and clinical status have been reviewed.[192–195]

AMS interacts with cellular nucleic acids presumably by intercalating between base pairs. Since AMS concentrations for the inhibition of DNA polymerases are much higher than those for cytotoxicity, the interaction with DNA alone is insufficient to account for its antitumor activity. On the other hand, AMS causes alkali-sensitive lesions of DNA at a limited number of sites; but this effect correlates with its antitumor effect. Additionally, AMS induces DNA single- and double-strand breaks and generates protein-DNA linkages; the linked protein is probably a nuclease, possibly topoisomerase. Further, in mice AMSA is cleaved by plasma thiols to afford 4-amino-3-methoxymethanesulfonanilide. Thus, thiolation of cellular components by AMSA also may contribute to its toxicity. The mechanism of action of AMS has been reviewed.[196]

The clinical pharmacokinetics have been studied by several groups of investigators.[197–200] To sum up, the plasma terminal half-life of unchanged AMS ranges from 4.7 to 9 hours, longer (18 hr) in children;[198] the volume of distribution from 1.7 to 3.8 L/kg, and the total clearance from 2.80 to 4.28 ml·min^{-1}·kg^{-1} (171.2 ml·min^{-1}·m^{-2}); the total clearance diminishes in older people.[200] In patients with hepatic impairment, the plasma AMS half-life is significantly longer and the volume of distribution larger, whereas the total clearance either remains unchanged in those with mild liver dysfunction or diminished in those with severe liver dysfunction.[199] Urinary excretion plays a minor role in AMS elimination, no more than 12 percent in 24 hours in patients with normal liver function.[190,200] With radioactive ^{14}C-labeled AMS, a considerable amount of the radioactivity is excreted in the bile, mostly as metabolites.[199] AMS is 96 to 98 percent bound to plasma proteins,[200] not only to albumin but also to α_1-acid glycoprotein and various gamma-globulins. It is, therefore, hardly surprising that AMS penetrates the CSF poorly. However, in four patients receiving varying doses of AMS, the tumor to plasma drug concentration ratios range from two to nearly five, apparently independent of dose and sampling time.[201]

AMS is an important active agent against hematologic malignancies. In acute myeloblastic leukemia it is as active as the anthracycline antibiotics for remission induction, but with little or no cardiotoxicity. In combination with ara-C it is as effective if not slightly superior to the combination of ara-C with an anthracycline antibiotic as far as the frequency and duration of the remissions are concerned. AMS is active in lymphoma and limitedly so in breast cancer; however, its antitumor spectrum is narrow. Myelosuppression is its dose-limiting toxicity—granulocytopenia especially. Nausea and vomiting, mucositis, and alopecia are frequently encountered. Myocardial toxicity also has been reported.

Dacarbazine [DIC, DTIC, 5-(3,3-Dimethyl-l-triazeno)-imidazole-4-carboxamide, Fig. 101.28

Although derived from the purine precursor, 5-amino-imidazole-4-carboxamide, DIC is not an antimetabolite but rather most probably an alkylating agent. In vivo it undergoes N-demethylation mediated by the

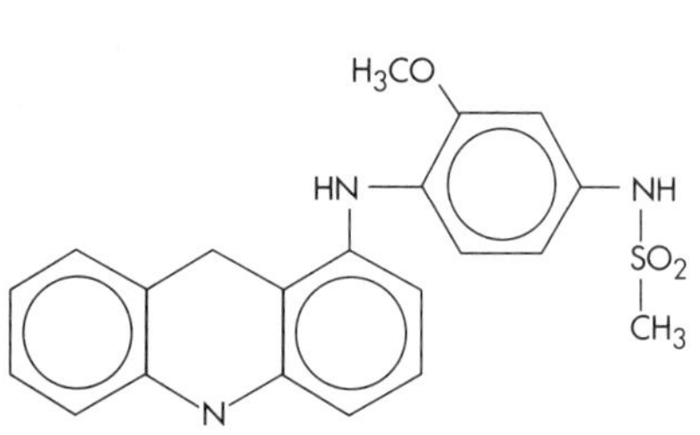

Figure 101.27

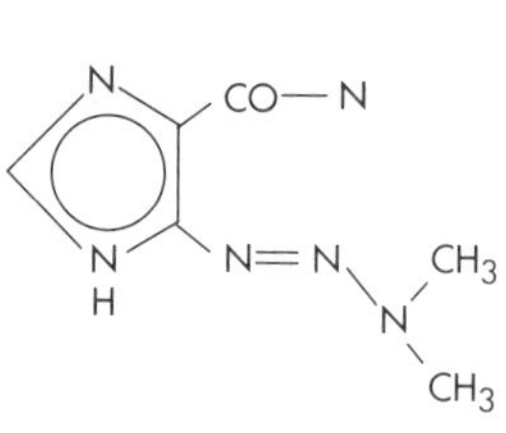

Figure 101.28

hepatic microsomal mixed function oxidase to give the N-monomethyl metabolite that ultimately generates an active methylating species.[202-204] The pharmacology and clinical applications of DIC have been reviewed.[205]

Early clinical pharmacologic studies of DIC based on a colorimetric assay have revealed that the plasma half-life of the agent ranges from 35 minutes[206] to 75 minutes,[207] the apparent volume of distribution exceeds the total body water content, and about 30[207] to 43 percent[206] of the dose is excreted intact in the urine in six hours, including traces of a metabolite. Later studies using a high performance liquid chromatographic assay showed that the plasma half-life of DIC is actually much longer, approximately five hours. By oral administration it is absorbed poorly, slowly, and erratically.[206] Although not extensively protein bound, it does not penetrate the blood brain barrier well; in the dog at steady state the CSF to plasma DIC concentration ratio is merely 1:7.[206]

DIC currently is the most active single agent against malignant melanoma. It is also effective in Hodgkin's disease and soft tissue sarcoma in combination regimens. Like DDP it is extremely emetic. Mild myelosuppression also has been reported. DIC solutions show less than 10 percent deterioration in either glass or plastic containers.[30]

Hydroxyurea [Hydrea, HOU, Fig. 101.29]

The simplest one-carbon organic antitumor agent, HOU has been known for more than a century; however, its anticancer activity has been demonstrated only relatively recently. A symposium on HOU has been held, but a more recent review should be consulted.[208]

There is ample evidence that, at noncytotoxic doses, HOU in vitro and in vivo stops DNA (but not RNA and protein) synthesis by inhibiting ribonucleoside-diphosphate reductase (EC 1.17.4.1).[205,209] Cells in S phase are killed, but those in other phases are allowed to progress to the G_1-S junction, where they are synchronized. However, HOU may also inhibit histone synthesis, at least in regenerating rat liver.

When administered orally, GI absorption of HOU is rapid and complete; ready entry into CSF and ascites fluids is seen after large oral doses. By IV administration the plasma half-life is approximately four hours; cumulative urinary excretion varies from 50 to 80 percent in 24 hours to 15 to 61 percent in 96 hours. HOU does not diffuse freely through all body tissues as does urea.[210] However, in rodents it is converted into urea and carbon dioxide.[211]

HOU is an effective oral agent for treating chronic myelogenous leukemia and some solid tumors. Its dose-limiting toxicity is leukopenia. At high doses, nausea, vomiting, and stomatitis have been reported. Since, unlike busulfan, HOU produces no delayed toxicity after chronic administration in patients with chronic myeloblastic leukemia, it has become the primary agent of choice for the benign phase of the disease. HOU can additionally rapidly reduce circulating blasts in patients with acute leukemia, and is therefore used in short term for this purpose.

Mitoxantrone [DHQ, 1,4-Dihydroxy-5, 8-bis{2-[(2-hydroxyethyl)amino]ethyl} amino-9,10-anthracenedione, Fig. 101.30]

The fascinating account of the design, synthesis, and development of DHQ as a cancer chemotherapeutic agent has been told in a most captivating manner.[212] Although not really an analogue of the anthracycline antibiotics, conceptually DHQ may be considered a derivative of DOX by removal of its amino sugar; this removal is supposed to lessen the myocardial toxicity of this family of compounds.[212] The proceedings of two successive symposia on DHQ have been published.[213,214] In addition, the pharmacokinetics and metabolism of DHQ have been reviewed.[215]

DHQ intercalates with DNA, causes intra-strand and inter-strand cross-linkings with G-C pairs preferred, induces single-strand and double-strand breaks, and finally inhibits both DNA and RNA syntheses. However, and surprisingly, it apparently does not generate cytotoxic free radicals; moreover, it elicits nuclear aberrations and chromosomal scattering. It is not cell cycle phase-specific with regard to cell killing, but it blocks cells at the G_2 phase, resulting in an increase of cellular RNA content and polyploidy. Cellular resistance to DHQ is attributed to impaired transport of the agent. The intercalation may impair DNA transcription and RNA processing; however, it is not believed to kill cancer cells.

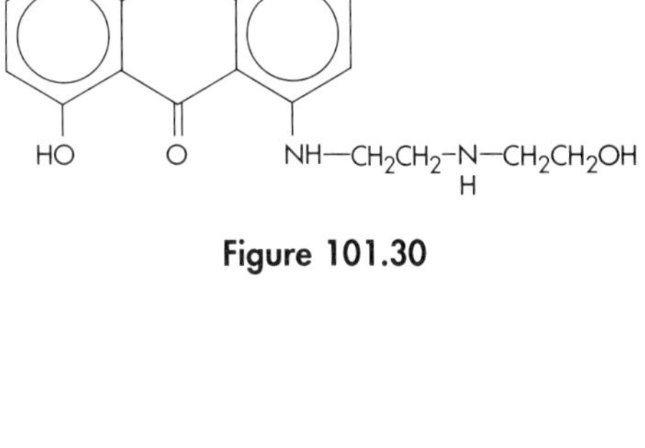

$H_2N-CO-NHOH$

Figure 101.29

HO O NH—CH_2CH_2—N(H)—CH_2CH_2OH

HO O NH—CH_2CH_2—N(H)—CH_2CH_2OH

Figure 101.30

Table 101.1 Summary Table[a]

Name: Generic	Name: Other or Trade	Dose as a Single Agent mg/m²	t½ h	Cl ml·min⁻¹·kg⁻¹	V_{da}[b] ml/kg	Cumulative 24-h Urinary Excretion % of Dose
Alkylating Agents						
Mechlorethamine	HN_2, nitrogen mustard	16 iv qd or divided in 2–4 doses	NA	NA	NA	5–10
Chlorambucil	Leukeran	4–8 po qd x 3–6 wks	1.5	NA	NA	<1
Melphalan	L-phenylalanine mustard	4 po qd	1.5	NA	NA	11–14
Cyclophosphamide	Cytoxan	1,600–2,000 in 2–5 d	7	NA	NA	10–20
Ifosfamide	Ifex	1,200 iv qd x 5	0.75	0.39	466	50
Busulfan	Myleran	2–6 po qd	NA	NA	NA	NA
Carmustine	BCNU	150–200 iv q 6 wks	NA	NA	NA	NA
Lomustine	CCNU	100–150 iv q 6 wks	NA	NA	NA	NA
Semustine	MeCCNU	150–200 iv q 6 wks	NA	NA	NA	NA
Streptozocin	Streptozotocin	500 iv qd x 5	0.6	NA	NA	NA
Thiotepa	Triethylenethio-phosphoramide	12–16 iv q 1–4 wks	2	4.7	817	1.5
Hexamethylmelamine	Hexastat	150 iv qd x 14	4.7–13	NA	NA	<1.5
Antimetabolites						
Methotrexate	Amethopterin	25 iv	27	NA	NA	52–100 in 96 h
Purinethol	6-MP Mercaptopurine	100 po	1	NA	NA	22 in 6 h
Thioguanine	6-TG 6-thioguanine	100 po	5.9[c]	NA	NA	NA
Fludarabine phosphate	F-ara-A fludara	25 iv qd x 5	1.4	1.7	1,200	NA
Pentostatin	2′-Deoxy-coformycin	4 iv	4.9	1.3	578	95.9
Cladribine	2-chloro-deoxyadenosine	3.6 iv infusion qd x 7	6.7	16	9,200	NA
Cytarabine	Ara-C	100 iv	0.4	NA	NA	10
Fluorouracil	5-Fu	500 iv	0.1–0.5	11–27	200–800	12–18
Floxuridine	5-Fluorodeoxy-uridine	5–20 ia	NA	NA	NA	NA
PALA	Sparfosate	1,600 iv	5.3	1.6	309	85

continued

Several groups of investigators have studied the clinical pharmacokinetics of DHQ.[216–221] Their results are: plasma half-life, 29 to 43 hours; volume of distribution, 14 to 56 L/kg; total clearance, 4 to 15 ml·min⁻¹·kg⁻¹; however, in a recent study,[220] the plasma half-life of DHQ was much longer—approximately nine days. Also in patients with organopathy or third space, the half-life was nearly twice as long as in normal patients studied by the same group, and the total clearance more than halved.[217] On average, no more than 7 percent of the dose is excreted in the urine in three days; traces of the monocarboxylic acid and the dicarboxylic acid resulting from oxidation of the terminal hydroxyethyl group(s) have been identified as the urinary metabolites.[220] In human autopsy specimens, the highest DHQ concentration is in the thyroid and the liver, followed by the heart.

HDQ is an active agent against breast cancer, hepatocellular carcinoma, lymphoma, and acute leukemia in combination with ara-C. It is effective and well-tolerated and produces high remission rates in elderly patients with acute myelocytic leukemia.[222] This combination, as well as that with daunorubicin, is also useful in previously untreated acute nonlymphocytic leukemia.[223] Compared with DOX, it is perhaps not as effective against breast cancer, but certainly less prone to elicit myocardial toxicity.[224] Myelosuppression, granulocytopenia especially, is dose-limiting. Other occasional toxic manifestations include thrombocytopenia, nausea and vomiting, mucositis, and alopecia.

Table 101.1 *Continued*

Name		Dose as a single agent mg/m²	t½ h	Cl ml·min⁻¹·kg⁻¹	V_{da}[b] ml/kg	Cumulative 24-h urinary excretion % of dose
Generic	Other or Trade					
Natural Products						
Vinblastine	Vincaleukoblastine velban	2–4 iv	24	12.3	25.6 l/kg	NA
Vincristine	Oncovin	1 iv	84	1.8	12.8 l/kg	NA
Vindesine		2 iv	24	4.2	8.7 l/kg	NA
Camptothecin		90–180 iv once in 3 wk	25	NA	NA	22.8 in 48 h
Homoharringtonine	HHT	2.5 iv qd x 14	9.3	0.5	2.4	10.8 in 72 h
Etoposide	VP-16 VePesid	50–100 iv qd x 5	3–40	0.15–>1.5	125–1,000	12–53
Teniposide	VM-26	100 iv	6–>60	0.18–0.90	85–1,000	13.9
Daunorubicin	Daunomycin	30 iv	20	11.6	20 l/kg	15 in 5 d
Doxorubicin	Adriamycin	60–75 iv	30	6.8	36 l/kg	15 in 6 d
Epirubicin		100 iv q 3 wk	27	22.0	25 l/kg	<12 in 6 d
Iadarubicin		12 qd iv x 3	27	32.0	64 l/kg	5
Bleomycin	Bleo	10–20 units iv	4–9	1.11–2.53	440–735	60 in 6 d
Dactinomycin	Actinomycin D	0.4–0.6 iv qd x 5	36	NA	NA	20 in 7 d
Mitomycin	Mitomycin C	20 iv at 6–8 wk intervals	NA	NA	NA	NA
Plicamycin	Mithramycin	1–1.2 iv qd x 8–10	NA	NA	NA	NA
Asparaginase	L-Asnase	1,000–20,000 iv qd x 10–20	18	0.035	55	NA
Taxol	Paclitaxel	110–250 iv	5	2.75	2,750	5
Miscellaneous						
Cisplatin[d]	DDP	20–40 iv	32	6.3	37.5	23.3
Carboplatin	Paraplatin CBDCA	300 iv	1.5–24	1.45–2.65	250–650	50–70
Amsarcrine	m-AMSA	120 iv qd x 5	4.7–9.0	2.80–4.28	1,700–3,800	12
Dacarbazine	DIC DTIC	250 iv qd x 5	0.5–1.3	NA	<1,000	30–43 in 6 h
Hydrea	Hydroxyurea	1,000–1,500 iv qd x 5	4	NA	NA	50–80
Mitoxantrone	Novantrone DHAQ	12 iv qd x 3	29–43	4–15	1,400–5,600	7 in 72 h
Procarbazine	MIH Natulan	100 po qd x 10	0.1	NA	NA	NA

[a]Abbreviations and symbols: Cl, total clearance; d, day; h, hour; ia, intra-arterial; iv intravenous, NA, information not available; po (per os), by mouth; pd (quaque die), daily; t½, plasma drug half-life during the terminal phase; V_{da}, apparent volume of distribution by area; wk, week.
[b]Estimated thus, $V_{da} = Cl \times t^{1/2}/\ln 2 = Cl \times t^{1/2} \times 1.44$.
[c]After high dose of 800–1,200 mg/m² iv (Ref. 57).
[d]Results from Ref. 173.

Procarbazine [PCZ, N-(1-Methylethyl)-4-[(2-methylhydrazino)methyl]benzamide, Fig. 101.31]

A member of the hydrazine derivatives originally conceived as monoamine oxidase inhibitors, PCZ later displayed impressive antitumor properties during its screening in model systems; therefore it was selected for clinical trials and further development. Excellent reviews on PCZ may be found in References 18, 225, and 226.

$H_3C-NH-NH-CH_2-C_6H_4-CO-NH-CH(CH_3)_2$

Figure 101.31

In vitro freshly prepared PCZ solution shows little or no inhibitive effect on macromolecular syntheses in cultured Ehrlich ascites cells; however, upon storage in the dark, degradation products are formed that are biochemically active.[226] Therefore it is reasonable to expect that PCZ requires in vivo metabolic activation; thus far, available evidence tends to support this contention. Several authors have succinctly reviewed PCZ metabolism.[225,226] In brief, PCZ undergoes in vivo dehydrogenation followed by a series of sequential oxidations mediated by cytochrome P-450, first to AZO-PCZ, in which the hydrogen atoms on the adjacent nitrogens in the hydrazine portion of the PCZ molecule are removed—a reaction that can transpire spontaneously in vitro at neutral pH. By a shift of the double bond, AZO-PCZ tautomerizes to the methylhydrazone of p-formyl-*N*-isopropylbenzamide that slowly cleaves hydrolytically to the corresponding aldehyde and, most likely, methylhydrazine. However, in vivo,[227] as well as in vitro in the presence of liver enzymes,[228–230] AZO-PCZ is further oxidized to the isomeric methylazoxy (-ONN-) and benzylazoxy (-NNO-) analogues; the former is the predominating metabolite in the plasma of a patient two hours after an oral dose of PCZ. These azoxy derivatives are finally oxidatively metabolized to a variety of end-products, including N-isopropylterephthalamic acid as well as carbon dioxide and methane derived from the terminal N-methyl group. All of these have been identified as the major in vivo PCZ metabolites.[227,232] During this stepwise oxidative metabolic degradation, the formation of reactive cytotoxic intermediates such as diazene,[231] free radicals, and methylating agents[233] is entirely conceivable. This is consistent with observations that PCZ is mutagenic and carcinogenic, produces chromosomal damages and aberrations, and inhibits macromolecular syntheses. In short, the mechanism of action of PCZ, although not completely understood, undoubtedly is deeply rooted in its oxidative metabolism.

Not much is known about the clinical pharmacokinetics of PCZ.[225,226] Gastrointestinal absorption of the agent appears to be quick and complete. It enters the CNS readily and equilibrates rapidly between plasma and CSF. After IV administration, the plasma PCZ half-life is approximately 7 minutes. As discussed above, the major metabolite excreted in the urine is *N*-isopropylterephthalamic acid.

PCZ is used principally for the treatment of Hodgkin's disease in combination with mechlorethamine, vincristine, and prednisone in the MOPP regimen. Also, it is incorporated into various combinations for treating lymphomas other than Hodgkin's disease. Its dose-limiting toxicity is myelosuppression; other deleterious side-effects such as nausea, vomiting, and anorexia are infrequent and mild. PCZ is a strong inhibitor of the immune response and a suspected carcinogen.

References

Research Reports

1. Gilman A, Philips FS. The biological actions and therapeutic applications of β-chloroethyl amines and sulfides. Science 1946;*103*:409–415.
2. Goodman LS, Wintrobe MM, Dameshek W, Goodman MJ, Gilman A, McLennan MT. Nitrogen mustard therapy. JAMA 1946;*132*:126–132.
3. Hansch C, Smith RN, Engle R. Quantitative structure-activity relationships in drugs, in "Pharmacological Basis of Cancer Chemotherapy". Baltimore: Williams & Wilkins, (1975); pp 215–238.
4. Morrow CS, Cowan KH. Mechanisms of antineoplastic drug resistance. Chap. 18, Sec. 2 in Ref. R6.
5. Loo TL. Contributions of pharmacologic studies of anticancer drugs to their clinical trials. Jpn J Clin Pharmacol 1985;*16*:307–315.
6. Schein PS, Davis RD, Carter S, Newman L, Schein DR, Rall DP. The evaluation of anticancer drugs in dogs and monkeys for the prediction of qualitative toxicities in man. Clin Pharmacol Therap 1970;*11*:3–40.
7. Freireich EJ, Gehan EA, Rall DP, Schmidt LH, Skipper HE. Quantitative comparison of toxicity of anticancer agents in mouse, rat, hamster, dog, monkey and man. Cancer Chemotherap Rep 1966;*50*:219–244.
8. Collins JM, Zaharko DS, Dedrick RL, Chabner BA. Potential roles for preclinical pharmacology in phase I clinical trials. Cancer Treat Rep 1986;*70*:73–80.
9. Colvin M, Chabner BA. Alkylating agents. Chap 11 in Ref. R3 1990;276–313.
10. Skipper HE, Bennett LL, Langham WH. Overall tracer studies with ^{14}C-labeled nitrogen mustard in normal and leukemic mice. Cancer 1951;*4*:1025–1027.
11. Goldenberg GJ, Vanstone CL, Isreals LG, Ilse D, Bihler I. Evidence for a transport carrier of nitrogen mustard in nitrogen mustard-sensitive and -resistant L5178Y lymphoblasts. Cancer Res 1970;*3C*:2285–2291.
12. Lyons RM, Goldenberg GJ. Active transport of nitrogen mustard and choline by normal and leukemia human lymphoid cells. Cancer Res 1972;*32*:1679–1685.
13. Wolpert MK, Ruddon RW. A study of the mechanism of resistance to nitrogen mustard (HN2) in Ehrlich ascites tumor cells: Comparison of uptake of HN2-^{14}C into sensitive and resistant cells. Cancer Res 1969;*29*:873–877.
14. Newell DR, Calvert AH, Harrap KR, McElwain TJ. Studies on the pharmacokinetics of chlorambucil and prednimustine in Man. Br J Clin Pharmacol 1983;*15*:253–258.
15. Bosanquet AG, Gilb ED. Pharmacokinetics of oral and intravenous melphalan during routine treatment of multiple myeloma. Eur J Cancer Clin Oncol 1982;*18*:355–362.
16. Alberts DS, Chang SY, Chen H-SG. Oral melphalan kinetics. Clin Pharmacol Therap 1979;*26*:737–745.
17. Tattersall MHN, Jarman M, Newlands ES, Holyhead L, Milstead RAV, Weinberg A. Pharmacokinetics of melphalan following oral or intravenous administration in patients with malignant diseases. Eur J Cancer 1978;*14*:507–513.

18. Alberts DS, Chang SY, Chen H-SG. Kinetics of intravenous melphalan. Clin Pharmacol Therap 1979;*26*:73–80.

19. Foley GE, Friedman OM, Drolet BP. Studies in the mechanisms of action of cytoxan. Evaluation of activation in vivo and in vitro. Cancer Res 1961;*21*:57–63.

20. Hill DL. A review of cyclophosphamide. Springfield, IL: Thomas, 1975.

21. Grochow LB, Colvin M. Clinical use of cyclophosphamide. Chap. 6 in Ref. R1 Pharmacokinetics, 1983;135–154.

22. Colvin M, Hilton J. Pharmacology of cyclophosphamide and metabolites. Cancer Treat Rep 1981;*65* (Suppl.3):89–95.

23. Struck RF, Alberts DS, Horne K, Phillips JG, Peng Y-M, Roe DJ. Plasma pharmacokinetics of cyclophosphamide and its cytotoxic metabolites after intravenous versus oral administration in a randomized crossover trial. Cancer Res 1987;*47*:2723–2726.

24. Juma FD. Effect of liver failure on the pharmacokinetics of cyclophosphamide. Eur J Clin Pharmacol 1984;*26*:591–593.

25. Cunningham D, Cummings J, Blackie RB. The pharmacokinetics of high dose cyclophosphamide and high dose etoposide. Med Oncol Tumor Pharmacotherap 1988;*5*:117–123.

26. Mouridon HT, Faber O, Skovested L. The biotransformation of cyclophosphamide in man: Analysis of the variations in normal subjects. Act Pharmacol Toxicol 1974;*35*:98–106.

27. Juma FD, Rogers HJ, Trounce JR. Effect of renal insufficiency on the pharmacokinetics of cyclophosphamide and some of its metabolites. Eur J Clin Pharmacol 1981;*19*:443–451.

28. Powis G, Reece P, Ahmann DL. Effect of body weight on the pharmacokinetics of cyclophosphamide in breast carcinoma patients. Cancer Chemotherap Pharmacol 1987;*20*:219–222.

29. Egorin MJ, Kaplan RS, Salcman M, Aisner J, Colvin M, Wiernik PH, Bachur NR. Cyclophosphamide plasma and cerebrospinal fluid kinetics with and without dimethyl sulfoxide. Clin Pharmacol Therap 1982;*32*:122–128.

30. Benvenuto JA, Anderson RW, Kerof K, Loo TL. Stability and compatibility of antitumor agents in glass and plastic containers. Am J Hosp Pharmacol 1981;*38*:1914–1918.

31. Ifosfamide. Pharmacology and clinical results in the treatment of cancer. Sem Oncol *9, 4* Suppl. 1: 1982;1–102. Proceedings of a symposium held in May, 1982. Many authors.

32. Advances in Ifosfamide Chemotherapy. Sem Oncol 1990;*17, 2* Suppl 4:1–79.

33. Zalupski M, Baker LH. Ifosfamide. JNCI 1988;*80*:556–566.

34. Creaven PJ, Allen LM, Alford DA, Cohen MH. Clinical pharmacology of isophosphamide. Clin Pharmacol Therap 1976;*16*:77–86.

35. Roberts JJ, Warwick GP. Metabolic and chemical studies of "myleran": Formation of 3-hydroxytetrahydrothiophene-1,1-dioxide in vivo, and excretion with thiols in vitro. Nature 1959;*184*:1288–1289.

36. Serrou B, Schein PS, Imbach JL (ed.). Nitrosoureas in cancer treatment. New York: Elsevier, 1981.

37. Ames MM, Powis G. Pharmacokinetics of nitrosoureas. Chap. 5, in Ref. R1, 1980: 113–134.

38. Loo TL, Dion RL, Dixon RL. The antitumor agent, 1,3-bis(2-chloroethyl)-1-nitrosourea. J Pharm Sci 1966;*55*:492–497.

39. Potter DW, Reed DJ. Denitrosation of carcinostatic nitrosoureas by purified NADPH cytochrome p-450 reductase and rat liver microsomes to yield nitric oxide under anaerobic conditions. Arch Biochem Biophys 1982;*216*:158–169.

40. DeVita VT Jr, Denham C, Davidson DJ, Oliverio VT. The physiological disposition of the carcinostatic 1,3-bis(2-chloroethyl)-1-nitrosourea in man and animals. Clin Pharmac Ther, 1967;*8*:566–577.

41. Sponzo RW, DeVita VT Jr, Oliverio VT. Physiologic disposition of 1 (2-chloroethyl)-3-cyclohexyl-1-nitrosourea (CCNU) and 1-(2-chloroethyl)-3-(4-methyl-cyclohexyl-1-nitrosourea (MeCCNU) in Man. Cancer 1973;*31*:1154–1158.

42. Moertel CG, Lefkopoulo M, Lipsitz S, Hahn RG, Klaassen D. Streptozocin-doxorubicin, streptozocin-fluorouracil, or chlorozotocin in the treatment of advanced islet-cell carcinoma. N Engl J Med 1992;*326*:519–23.

43. Cohen BE, Egorin ME, Kohlhepp EA, Aisner J, Gutierrez PL. Human plasma pharmacokinetics and urinary excretion of thiotepa and its metabolites. Cancer Treat Rep 1986;*70*:859–864.

44. Foster BJ, Harding BJ, Leyland-Jones B. Hexamethylmelamine. A critical review of an active drug. Cancer Treat Rev 1986;*13*:197–217.

45. Bertino JR, Romanini. Folate antagonists. Chap. XVI-I in Ref 5 1993;698–709.

46. Allegra CJ. Antifolates. Chap. 5 in Ref. 18a 1990;110–53.

47. Jacobs SA, Stoller RG, Chabner BA, Johns DG. 7-Hydroxymethotrexate as a urinary metabolite in human subjects and Rhesus monkeys receiving high dose methotrexate. J Clin Invest 1976;*57*:534–538.

48. Donehower RC, Hande KR, Drake JC, Chabner BA. Presence of 2,4-diamino-N^{10}-methylpteroic acid after high-dose methotrexate. Clin Pharmacol Therap 1979;*26*:63–72.

49. Zaharko DS, Dedrick RL, Bischoff KB. Methotrexate tissue distribution: Prediction by a mathematical model. J NCI 1971;*46*:775–784.

50. Hitchings GH, Elion GB. Layer on layer: The Bruce F. Cain Memorial Award Lecture. Cancer Res, 1985;*45*:2415–2420.

51. McCormack JJ, Johns DG. Purine and purine nucleoside antimetabolites. Chap 9 in Ref. 3. 1990;234–52.

52. Handschumacher RE, Cheng YC. Purine and pyrimidine antimetabolites. Chap XVI-2 in Ref 5. 1993;712–32.

53. Loo TL, Luce JK, Sullivan MP, Jardine J, Frei E III. Clinical pharmacologic observations on 6-mercaptopurine and 6-methylthiopurine-ribonucleoside. Clin Pharmacol Therap 1968;*9*:180–194.

54. Lennard L, Keen D, Lilleyman JS. Oral 6-mercaptopurine in childhood leukemia: Parent drug pharmacokinetics and active metabolite concentrations. Clin Pharmacol Therap 1986;*40*:287–292.

55. LePage GA, Whitecar JP Jr. Pharmacology of 6-thioguanine in man. Cancer Res 1971;*31*:1627–1631.

56. Lu K, Benvenuto JA, Bodey GP, Loo TL. Pharmacokinetics and metabolism of β-2′-deoxythioguanosine and 6-thioguanine in Man. Cancer Chemother Pharmacol 1982;*8*:119–123.

57. Zimm S, Cleary SM, Horton CN. Phase I pharmacokinetic study of 6-thioguanine as a 48-h continuous intraperitoneal infusion. J Clin Oncol 1988;*6*:696–700.

58. Cheson BI. New antimetabolites in the treatment of human malignancies. Sem Oncol 1992;*12*:695–706.

59. Cabner BA. Cytidine Analogues. Chap. 6, in Ref. R3 1990;154–179.

60. Chou T-C, Arlin Z, Clarkson BD. Metabolism of 1-β-D-arabinofuranosylcytosine in human Leukemic cells. Cancer Res 1977;*37*:3561–3570.

61. Rustum YM, Preisler HD. Correlation between leukemic cell retention of 1-β-D-arabinofuranosylcytosine 5′-triphosphate and response to therapy. Cancer Res 1979;*39*:42–49.

62. Plunkett W, Lacoboni S, Estey E. Pharmacologically directed ara-C therapy for refractory leukemia. Semin Oncol 1985;*12* (2 Suppl. 3):20–30.

63. Ho DHW, Frei E III. Clinical pharmacology of 1-β-D-arabinofuranosylcytosine. Clin Pharmacol Therap 1971;*12*:944–954.

64. Slevin ML, Piall EM, Aherne GW. The pharmacokinetics of cytosine arabinoside in the plasma and cerebrospinal fluid during conventional and high-dose therapy. Med Ped Oncol 1982;*10* (Suppl 1):157–168.

65. Slevin ML, Piall EM, Aherne GW. Effect of dose and schedule in pharmacokinetics of high-dose cytosine arabinoside in plasma and cerebrospinal fluid. J Clin Oncol 1983;*1*:546–551.

66. Capizzi RL, Yang J-L, Cheng E, Bjornsson T, Sahasrabudhe D, Tan RS, Cheng YC. Alteration of the pharmacokinetics of high-dose ara-C by its metabolite, high ara-U in patients with acute leukemia. J Clin Oncol 1983;*1*:763–771.

67. Kreis W, Chaudhri F, Chan K. Pharmacokinetics of low-dose ara-C given by continuous intravenous infusion over 21 days. Cancer Res 1985;*45*:6498–6501.

68. Liliemark JO, Paul CY, Gahrton CG. Pharmacokinetics of ara-C 5′-Monophosphate in leukemic cells after intravenous and subcutaneous administration of ara-C. Cancer Res 1985;*45*:2373–2375.

69. Grem JL. Fluorinated pyrimidines. Chap. 7 in Ref. R3 1990;180–224.

70. Kimura K, Fujii S, Ogawa M (ed.). Fluoropyrimidines in cancer therapy. New York: Excepta Medica, 1984.

71. Rustum YM, McGuire JJ. The expanding role of folates and fluoropyrimidines in cancer chemotherapy. New York: Plenum, 1988.

72. El Sayed YM, Sadee W. The fluoropyrimidines. Chap 9 in Ref. R1 1990;209–227.

73. Diasio RB, Harris BE. Clinical pharmacology of 5-fluorouracil. Clin Pharmacokin 1989;*16*:215–237.

74. Loo TL, Friedman J, Moore EC, Valdivieso M, Marti JR, Stweart D. Pharmacological disposition of N-phosphonacetyl)-L-aspartate in humans. Cancer Res 1980;*40*:86–90.

75. Cassady JM, Douros JD (ed.). Anticancer agents based on natural product models. New York: Academic Press, 1980.

76. Bender RA, Hamel E, Hande KR. Plant alkaloids, Chap. 10 in Ref. R3, 1990;253–275.

77. Beck WT, Cass CE, Houghton PJ. Anticancer drugs from plants: *Vinca* alkaloids and taxol. Chap. XVI-8 in Ref R5. 1993;782–795.

78. Nelson RL, Dyke RW, Root MA. Comparative pharmacokinetics of vindesine, vincristine, and vinblastine in patients with cancer. Cancer Treat Rev 1980;*7* (Suppl):17–24.

79. Owellen RJ, Martke CA, Hains FO. Pharmacokinetics and metabolism of vinblastine in humans. Cancer Res 1977;*37*:2597–2602.

80. Ratain MJ, Vogelzang NJ, Sinkule JA. Interpatient and intrapatient variability in vinblastine pharmacokinetics. Clin Pharmac Ther 1987;*41*:61–67.

81. Owellen RJ, Root MA, Hains FO. Pharmacokinetics of vindesine and vincristine in humans. Cancer Res 1977;*37*:2603–2607.

82. Jackson DV Jr, Sethi VS, Long TR. Pharmacokinetics of vindesine bolus and infusion. Cancer Chemother Pharmacol 1984;*13*:114–119.

83. Ohnuma T, Norton L, Andrejczuk A. Pharmacokinetics of vindesine given as an intravenous bolus and 24-h infusion in humans. Cancer Res 1985;*45*:464–469.

84. Stewart DJ, Lu K, Benjamin RS. Concentration of vinblastine in human intracerebral tumor and other tissues. J Neurooncol 1983;*1*:139–144.

85. Lu K, Yap H-Y, Loo TL. Clinical pharmacokinetics of vinblastine by continuous intravenous infusion. Cancer Res 1983;*43*:1405–1408.

86. Ratain MJ, Vogelzang NJ. Limited sampling model for vinblastine pharmacokinetics. Cancer Treat Rep, 1987;*71*:935–939.

87. Gottlieb JA, Luce JK. Treatment of malignant melanoma with camptothecin (NSC-100880). Cancer Chemoth Rep 1972;*56*:103–105.

88. Horwitz SB. "Camptothecin". In: Corcoran JW, Hahn FE Antibiotics III. Mechanisms of action of antimicrobial and antitumor agents. New York: Springer-Verlag, (1975); pp 48–57.

89. Slichenmyer WJ, Rowinsky EK, Donehower RC, Kaufman SH. The current status of camptothecin analogues as antitumor agents. JNCI 1993;*85*:271–291.

90. Hsiang YH, Liu LF. Identification of mammalian DNA topoisomerase I as an intracellular Target of the anticancer drug camptothecin. Cancer Res 1988;*48*:1722–1726.

91. Smith CR Jr, Mikolajczak KL, Powell RG. Harringtonine and related cephalotaxine esters, Chap. 11, in ref 75, 1980:391–416.

92. Savaraj N, Lu K, Dimery I, Loo TL. Clinical pharmacology of homoharringtonine. Cancer Treat Rep 1986;*70*:1403–1407.

93. Lu K, Savaraj N, Lynn LG, Loo TL. Pharmacokinetics of homoharringtonine in dogs. Cancer Chemoth Pharmac 1988;*21*:139–142.

94. Ohnuma T, Holland JF. Homoharringtonine as a new antileukemia agent. Sem Clin Oncol 1985;*3*:605–606.

95. Warrell RP Jr, Coonley CJ, Gee TS. Homoharringtonine: An effective new drug for remission induction in refractory nonlymphoblastic leukemia. J Clin Oncol 1985;*3*:617–621.

96. O'Dwyer PJ, King SA, Hoth DF. Homoharringtonine—Perspectives of an active natural product. J Clin Oncol 1986;*4*:1563–1568.

97. Issell BF, Muggia FM, Carter SK (ed.) "Etoposide (VP-16)". New York: Academic Press, 1984.

98. Clark PL, Slevin ML. The clinical pharmacology of etoposide and teniposide. Clin Pharmacokin 1987;*12*:223–252.

99. Long BH, Musial ST, Brattain MG. Comparison of cytotoxicity and DNA breakage activity of congeners of podophyllotoxin including VP-16-213 and VM-26: A quantitative structure-activity relationship. Biochem 1984;*23*:1183–1188.

100. Chen GL, Yang L, Rowe TC. Nonintercalative antitumor drugs interfere with the breaking-reunion reaction of mammalian DNA topoisomerase II. J Biol Chem 1984;*259*:13560–13566.

101. van Maanen JMS, Retel J, de Vries J. Mechanism of action of antitumor drug etoposide: A review. JNCI 1988;*80*:1526–1533.

102. Smyth RD, Pfeffer M, Scalzo A. Bioavailability and pharmacokinetics of etoposide (VP-16). Sem Oncol *12*, Suppl 1985;*2*:48–51.

103. Allen LM, Creaven PJ. Comparison of the human pharmacokinetics of VM-26 and VP-16, to antineoplastic epipodophyllotoxin glucopyranoside derivatives. Eur J Cancer 1975;*11*:697–707.

104. D'Incalci M, Rossi C, Zucchetti M. Pharmacokinetics of etoposide in patients with abnormal renal and hepatic function. Cancer Res 1986;*46*:2566–2571.

105. O'Dwyer PJ, Leyland-Jones B, Alonso MT. Etoposide (VP-16-213). Current status of an active anticancer drug. N Engl J Med 1985;*312*:692–700.

106. O'Dwyer PJ, Alonso MT, Leyland-Jones B. Teniposide: A review of 12 years of experience. Cancer Treat Rep 1984;*68*:1455–1466.

107. Grem JL, Hoth DF, Leyland-Jones B. Teniposide in the treatment of leukemia: A case study of conflicting priorities in the development of drugs for fatal diseases. J Clin Oncol 1988;*6*:351–379.

108. Arcamone F. The development of new antitumor anthracyclines. Chap. 1 in Ref. 75. 1980;1–41.

109. Myers C. Anthracyclines and DNA intercalators. Chap XVI-5 in Ref R5. 1993;764–773.

110. Myers CE Jr, Chabner BA. Anthracylclines. Chap. 14 in Ref. R3. 1990;356–384.

111. Riggs CE, Bachur NR. Clinical pharmacokinetics of anthracycline antibiotics. Chap. 10, in Ref. R1. 1983;229–278.

112. Lown JW (ed.). Anthracycline and anthracenedione-based anticancer agents. New York: Elsevier, 1988.

113. Alberts DS, Bachur NR, Holtzman JL. The pharmacokinetics of daunorubicin in man. Clin Pharmacol Therap 1971;*12*:96–104.

114. Kokenberg E, van der Steuijt K, Lowenberg B. Pharmacokinetics of daunorubicin as a determinant of response in acute myeloid leukemia. Haematol Bluttrransfus 1987;*30*:283–287.

115. Arcamone F. Doxorubicin anticancer antibiotics. New York: Academic Press, 1987.

116. Speth PAJ, Hoesel QGCM, Haanen C. Clinical pharmacokinetics of doxorubicin. Clin Pharmacokin 1988;*15*:15–31.

117. Eksborg S, Stendahl V, Lonroth U. Comparative pharmacokinetic study of adriamycin and 4′-Epirubicin after their simultaneous administration. Eu J Clin Pharmac 1986;*30*:629–631.

118. Robert J, Bui NB, Vrignaud P. Pharmacokinetics of doxorubicin in sarcoma patients. Eur J Clin Pharmacol 1987;*31*:695–699.

119. Camaggi CM, Comparsi R, Strocchi E. Epirubicin and doxorubicin comparative metabolism and pharmacokinetics. A cross-over study. Cancer Chemotherap Pharmacol 1988;*21*:221–228.

120. Cummings J, Smyth JF. Pharmacology of adriamycin. The message to the clinician. Eur J Cancer Clin Oncol 1988;*24*:579–582.

121. Eksborg S, Mattson K. Pharmacokinetics of epirubicin in man. Non-influence of α-interferon. Med Oncol Tumor Pharmacotherap 1988;*5*:131–133.

122. Mross K, Maessen P, van der Vijgh WJF. Pharmacokinetics and metabolism of epirubicin and doxorubicin in humans. J Clin Oncol 1988;*6*:517–526.

123. Camaggi CM, Strocchi E, Comparsi R. Biliary excretion and pharmacokinetics of 4′-epirubicin. Cancer Chemotherap Pharmacol 1986;*18*:47–50.

124. Lu K, Savaraj N, Kavanagh J, Loo TL. Clinical pharmacology of 4-demethoxydaunorubicin (DMDR). Cancer Chemotherap Pharmacol 1986;*17*:143–148.

125. Smith DB, Margison JM, Lucas SB. Clinical pharmacology of oral and intravenous 4-Demethoxydaunorubicin. Cancer Chemotherap Pharmacol 1987;*19*:138–142.

126. Umezawa H. Recent progress in bleomycin studies. Chap. 5, in Ref. 75. 1980:147–166.

127. Sikic BI, Rosencweig M, Carter SK. Bleomycin chemotherapy. New York: Academic Press, 1985.

128. Chabner BA. Bleomycin, Chap. 13, in Ref. R3. 1990;341–355.

129. Alberts DS, Chen H-SG, Liu R. Bleomycin pharmacokinetics in man. I. Intravenous administration. Cancer Chemotherap Pharmacol 1978;*1*:177–181.

130. Davy M, Paus E, Lehne G. A pharmacokinetic evaluation of intramuscular administration of bleomycin oil suspension. Cancer Chemotherap Pharmacol 1985;*14*:274–246.

131. Crooke ST. Clinical pharmacology of bleomycin. Chap. 11 in Ref. R1. 1983;279–290.

132. Waksman SA (ed.). Actinomycin. New York, Interscience 1968.

133. Werweij A, Den Hartigh J, Pinedo HM. Antitumor antibiotics, Chap. 15, in Ref R3. 1990;382–396.

134. Tattersall MNH, Sodergren JE, Sengupta SK. Pharmacokinetics of actinomycin D in patients with malignant melanoma. Clin Pharmacol Therap 1975;*17*:701–708.

135. Remes WA. Mitomycins, Chap. 4, in Ref. 75. 1980;131–146.

136. Carter SK, Crooke, ST, Alder NA. Mitomycin C: Current status and new developments. New York: Academic Press, 1979.

137. Dorr RT. New findings in the pharmacokinetic, metabolic, and drug-resistance aspects of mitomycin C. Sem Oncol, 1988;*15*(Suppl 4):32–41.

138. Lown JW. The molecular mechanism of antitumor action of the mitomycins. Chap. 2, in Ref. 136. 1979;5–26.

139. Hartigh JD, McVie JG, van Oort WJ. Pharmacokinetics of mitomycin in humans. Cancer Res 1983;*43*:5017–5021.

140. Verweij J, Staurman M, de Vries J. The differences in pharmacokinetics of mitomycin C given either as a single agent or as a part of combination chemotherapy. J Cancer Res Clin Oncol 1986;*112*:283–284.

141. Erlichman C, Rauth AM, Battistella R. Mitomycin C pharmacokinetics in patients with recurrent or metastatic colorectal carcinoma. Can J Physiol Pharmacol 1987;*65*:407–411.

142. Lankelma J, Stuurman M, van Hoogenhuize J. The pharmacokinetic plasma profile of mitomycin C measured after sequential intermittent intravenous administration. Eur J Cancer Clin Oncol 1988;*24*:175–180.

143. Capizzi RL, Handschumacher RE. Asparaginase. Chap. XIII-9 in Ref R5. 1993;796–805.

144. Chabner BA. Enzyme therapy: L-asparaginase. Chap. 16 in Ref. R3. 1990;397–407.

145. Ho DHW, Thetford B, Carter CJK. Clinical pharmacologic studies of L-asparaginase. Clin Pharmacol Therap 1970;*11*:408–417.

146. Ohnuma T, Holland JF, Freeman A. Biochemical and pharmacological studies with asparaginase in man. Cancer Res 1970;*30*:2297–2305.

147. Capizzi RL, Bertino JR, Skeel RT. Asparaginase: Clinical, biochemical, pharmacological, and immunological studies. Ann Intern Med 1971;*74*:893–901.

148. Ho DHW, Yap H-Y, Brown N. Clinical pharmacology of intramuscularly administered asparaginase. J Clin Pharmacol 1981;*21*:72–78.

149. Riccardi R, Holcenberg JS, Glaubiger DL. Asparaginase pharmacokinetics and asparagine levels in cerebrospinal fluids of Rhesus monkeys and humans. Cancer Res 1981;*41*:4554–4558.

150. Rowinsky ED, Cazenava LA, Danehower RC. Taxol: A novel investigational antimicrotubule aent. JNCI 1990;*82*:1247–1259.

151. Rowinsky EK, Onetto N, Canetta RM, Arbuck SG. Taxol: The first taxanes, an important new class of antitumor agents. Sem Oncol 1992;*19*:646–662.

152. van der Veer JL, Reedijk J. Investigating antitumor drug mechanisms. Chem in Brit 1988;775–780.

153. Rosenberg B. Cisplatin: Its history and possible mechanisms of action. Chap. 2, in Ref. 154. 1980;9–20.

154. Prestayko AW, Crooke ST, Carter SK. Cisplatin. Current status and new developments. New York: Academic Press, 1980.

155. Lippard SJ. New Chemistry of an Old Molecule: *cis*-[Pt(N-$H_3)_2Cl_2$]. Science 1982;*218*:1075–1082.

156. McBrien DCH, Slater TF. Biochemical mechanisms of platinum antitumor drugs. Washington, DC: IRL Press, 1986.

157. Nicolini M. Platinum and other metal coordination compounds in cancer chemotherapy, Boston: M. Nijhoff, 1988.

158. Reed E, Kohn KW. Platinum analogues. Chap. 20, in Ref. R3 1990;465–490.

159. Colvin M. Alkylating agents and platinum analogues. Chap. XVI-3 in Ref. R5. 1993;733–754.

160. Johnson NP, Butour J-L, Villani G, Wimmer FL, Defais M, Pierson V, Braber V. Metal antitumor compounds: the mechanism of action of platinum complexes. In: Ruthenium and other non-platinum metal complexes in cancer chemotherapy. Progr Clin Biochem Med 1989;*10*:1–24.

161. Gromley PE, Bull JM, LeRoy AF, Cysyk R. Kinetics of *cis*-Diamminedichloroplatinum (II). Clin Pharmacol Therap 1979;*25*:351–357.

162. Gullo JJ, Litterst CL, Maguire PJ, Sikic BI, Hoth DF, Woolley PV. Pharmacokinetics and protein binding of *cis*-Diamminedichloroplatinum (II) administered as a one-hour or as a twenty-hour infusion. Cancer Chemotherap Pharmacol 1980;*5*:21–26.

163. Himmelstein KJ, Patton TF, Belt RJ, Taylor S, Repta AJ, Sternson LA. Clinical kinetics of intact cisplatin and some related species. Clin Pharmacol Therap 1981;*29*:658–664.

164. Vermorken JB, van der Vijgh WJF, Klein I, Hant AAM, Gall HE, Pinedo HM. Pharmacokinetics of free and total platinum species after short-term infusion of cisplatin. Cancer Treat Rep 1984;*68*:505–513.

165. Vermorken JB, van der Vijgh WJF, Klein I, Gall HE, van Groeningen CJ, Hart AAM, Pinedo HM. Pharmacokinetics of free and total platinum species after rapid and prolonged infusion of cisplatin. Clin Pharmacol Therap 1986;*39*:136–144.

166. Erlichman C, Soldin SJ, Thiessen JJ. Disposition of total and free cisplatin on two consecutive treatment cycles in patients with ovarian cancer. Cancer Chemotherap Pharmacol 1987;*19*:75–79.

167. Daley-Yates PT, McBrien DCH. Cisplatin Metabolism: A method for their separation and for measuring their renal clearance in vivo. Biochem Pharmacol 1983;*32*:181–184.

168. Shelley MD, Fish RG, Adams M. Biliary excretion of platinum in a patient treated with cis-diamminedichloroplatinum (II). Antimicrob Agent Chemotherap 1985;*27*:275–276.

169. Reece PA, McCall JT, Powis G, Richardson RL. Sensitive high performance liquid chromatographic assay for platinum in plasma ultrafiltrate. J Chrom 1984;*306*:417–423.

170. Andrews PA, Wung WE, Howell SB. A high performance liquid chromatographic assay with improved selectivity for cisplatin and active platinum (II) complexes in platinum ultrafiltrate. Anal Biochem 1984;*143*:46–56.

171. Reece PA, Stafford I, Russell J. Reduced ability to clear ultrafilterable platinum with repeated courses of cisplatin. J Clin Oncol 1986;*4*:1392–1398.

172. Reece PA, Stafford I, Russell J. Creatinine clearance as a predictor of ultrafilterable platinum disposition in cancer patients treated with cisplatin: Relationship between peak ultrafilterable platinum plasma levels and nephrotoxicity. J Clin Oncol 1987;*5*:304–309.

173. Reece PA, Stafford I, Davy M, Freeman S. Disposition of unchanged cisplatin in patients with ovarian cancer. Clin. Pharmac Ther 1987;*42*:320–325.

174. Reece PA, Stafford I, Davy M, Morris R, Freeman S. Influence of infusion time on unchanged cisplatin disposition in patients with ovarian cancer. Cancer Chemotherap Pharmacol 1989;*24*:256–260.

175. Reece PA, Stafford I, Russell J, M Khan, Gill PG. A model for ultrafilterable plasma platinum disposition in patients treated with cisplatin. Cancer Chemotherap Pharmacol 1987;*20*:26–32.

176. Harrap KR, Jones M, Wilkinson CR, Clink HMcD, Saprrow S, Mitchley BCV, Clarke S, Veasey A. Antitumor, toxic, and biochemical properties of cisplatin and eight other platinum complexes, Chap. 12, pp 193–212 in Ref. 151.

177. Curt GA, Grygiel JJ, Corden BJ, Ozols RF, Weiss RB, Tell DT, Myers CE, Collins Jr. A phase I and pharmacokinetic study of diamminecyclobutanedicarboxylatoplatinum (NSC 241240). Cancer Res 1983;*43*:4470–4473.

178. Calvert AH, Harland SJ, Newell DR, Siddik ZH, Jones AC, McElwain TJ, Rajus, Wiltshaio E, Smith IE, Baker JM, Peckham MJ, Harrap KR. Early studies with *cis*-diammine-1,1-cyclobutane dicarboxylate platinum II. Cancer Chemotherap Pharmacol 1982;*9*:140–147.

179. Carter SK, Hellmann K. Paraplatin (carboplatin): Current status and future prospects. Cancer Treat Rev 1985;*12*:Suppl A.

180. Yarbro JW. Carboplatin (JM-8, CBDCA). A new platinum compound. Semin Oncol 1989;*16*:Suppl 5.

181. Wagstaff AJ, Ward A, Benfield P, Heel RC. Carboplatin. A preliminary review of its pharmacodynamic and pharmacokinetic properties and therapeutic efficacy in the treatment of cancer. Drugs Journal 1989;*37*:162–190.

182. Harland SJ, Newell DR, Siddik ZH, Chadwick R, Calvert AH, Harrap KR. Pharmacokinetics of *cis*-diammine-1, 1-cyclobutane dicarboxylate platinum (II) in patients with normal and impaired renal function. Cancer Res 1984;*44*:1693–1697.

183. Elferink F, van Vijgh WJF, Klein I, Vermorken JB, Gall HE, Pinedo HM. Pharmacokinetics of carboplatin after intravenous administration. Cancer Treat Rep 1987;*71*:1231–1237.

184. Newell DR, Siddik ZH, Gumbrell LA, Boxall FE, Gore ME, Smith IE, Calvert AH. Plasma Free platinum pharmacokinetics in patients treated with high dose of carboplatin. Eur J Cancer Clin Oncol 1987;*23*:1399–1405.

185. van Echo DA, Egorin MJ, Aisner J. The pharmacokinetics of carboplatin, pp 1–6 in Ref. 359.

186. Shea TC, Flaherty MF, Elias A, Eder JP, Antmank, Begg C, Schnipper L, Frei E III, Henner WD. A phase I clinical and pharmacokinetic study of carboplatin and autologous bone marrow support. J Clin Oncol 1989;*l*:651–661.

187. Egorin MJ, van Echo DA, Tipping SJ, Olman EA, Whitacre MY, Thompson BW, Aisner J. Pharmacokinetics and dosage reduction of cis-diammine (1,1-cyclobutanedicarboxylato)-platinum in patients with impaired renal function. Cancer Res 1984;*44*:5432–5438.

188. Egorin MJ, van Echo DA, Olman EA, Whitacre MY, Forrest A, Aisner J. Prospective validation of a pharmacologically based dosing scheme for *cis*-diamminedichloroplatinum (II) analogue diammine(1,1-cyclobutanedicarboxylato)-platinum (II). Cancer Res 1985;*45*:6502–6506.

189. van Hennik MB, van der Vijgh WJF, Klein I, Vermorken JB, Pinedo M. Human pharmacokinetics of carboplatin after oral administration. Cancer Chemotherap Pharmacol 1989;*23*:126–127.

190. Adams M, Kerby IJ, Rocker I, Evans A, Johansen K, Franks CR. A comparison of toxicity and efficacy of cisplatin and carboplatin in advanced ovarian cancer. Acta Oncol 1989;*28*:57–60.

191. Horwich A, Dearnaley DP, Duchesne GM, Brada M, Peckham MJ. Simple nontoxic treatment of advanced metastatic seminoma with carboplatin. J Clin Oncol 1989;*7*:1150–1156.

192. Grove WR, Fortner CL, Wiernik PH. Review of amsacrine, an investigational antineoplastic agent. Clin Pharm 1982;*1*:320–326.

193. McCredie KB. Amsacrine: a new drug for hematological malignancies. Eur J Cancer Clin Oncol 1985;*21*:1–3.

194. Zittoun R. Amsacrine: A review of clinical data. Eur J Cancer Clin Oncol 1985;*21*:649–653.

195. Cassileth PA, Gale RP. Amsacrine: a review. Leuk Res 1986;*10*:1257–1265.

196. Marshall BM, Ralph RK. The mechanism of action of amsacrine. Adv Cancer Res 1985;*44*:267–293.

197. van Echo DA, Chiuten DF, Gromley PE. Phase I clinical and pharmacologic studies of 4′-(9-acridinylamino)methanesulfon-m-anisidine using an intermittent biweekly schedule. Cancer Res 1979;*39*:3881–3884.

198. Rivera G, Evans WE, Dahl GV. Phase I and pharmacokinetic studies of 4′-(9-Acridinylamino)methanesulfon-m-anisidine in children with cancer. Cancer Res 1980;*40*:4250–4253.

199. Hall SW, Friedman J, Legha SS, Loo TL. Human pharmacokinetics of a new acridine derivative 4′-(a-Acridinylamino)methanesulfon-m-anisidine (NSC 249992). Cancer Res 1983;*43*:3422–3426.

200. Jurlina JL, Varcoe AR, Paxton JW. Pharmacokinetics of amsacrine in patients receiving combination chemotherapy for treatment of acute myeologenous leukemia. Cancer Chemotherap Pharmacol 1985;*14*:21–25.

201. Zhengang G, Savaraj N, Feun LG, Loo TL. Tumor penetration of AMSA in man. Cancer Invest 1983;*1*:475–478.

202. Skibba JL, Beal DD, Ramirez G. N-Demethylation of the antineoplastic agent 4(5)-(3,3-dimethyl-1-triazeno)-imidazole-5(4)-carboxamide by rats and man. Cancer Res 1970;*30*:147–150.

203. Loo TL, Housholder GE, Gerulath AH. Mechanism of action and pharmacology studies with DTIC (NSC-45388). Cancer Treat Rep 1976;*60*:149–152.

204. Gerulath AH, Loo TL. Mechanism of action of 5-(3,3-dimethyl-1-triazeno)-imidazole-5(4)-carboxamide (NSC-45388) in mammalian cells in culture. Biochem Pharmac 1972;*21*:2335–2343.

205. Auerbach SD. Nonclassic alkylating agents, Chap 12, pp 322–328 in Ref. R3 1990.

206. Loo TL, Luce JK, Jardine JH. Pharmacologic studies of the antitumor agent 5-(3,3-dimethyl-1-triazeno)-imidazole-5′-4′-carboxamide. Cancer Res 1968;*28*:2448–2453.

207. Skibba JL, Ramierez G, Beal DD. Preliminary clinical trial, physiologic disposition of 5-(3,3-Dimethyl-1-triazeno)-imidazole-5′-4′-carboxamide in man. Cancer Res 1969;*29*:1944–1951.

208. Donehower RC. Hydroxyurea, Chap. 8, pp 225–233 in Ref. R3 1990.

209. Moore EC. The effects of ferrous ion and dithioerythritol on inhibition by hydroxyurea of ribonucleotide reductase. Cancer Res 1969;*29*:291–295.

210. Rosner F, Rubin H, Parise F. Studies on the absorption, distribution, and excretion of hydroxyurea. Cancer Chemotherap Rep 1971;*55*:167–173.

211. Adamson RH, Ague SL, Hess SM. The distribution, excretion, and metabolism of hydroxyurea-^{14}C. J Pharmacol Exp Ther 1965;*150*:322–327.

212. Cheng CC, Zee-Cheng RK. The design, synthesis, and development of a new class of potent antineoplastic anthraquinones. Progr Med Chem 1983;*20*:83–118.

213. Hellman K (ed.). Mitoxantrone, proceedings of a symposium. Cancer Treat Rev 1983;*10*:Suppl B:1–79.

214. Yarbro JW (ed.). New perspectives in chemotherapy: focus on novantrone. Sem Oncol 1984;*11*:Suppl 1:1–58.

215. Ehninger G, Schuler U, Proksch B. Pharmacokinetics and metabolism of mitoxantrone. A review. Clin Pharmacokin 1990;*18*:365–380.

216. Savaraj N, Lu K, Valdivieso M, Loo TL. Clinical kinetics of 1,4-dihydroxy-5,8-bis{2-[(2-hydroxyethyl)amino]ethylamino}-9,10-anthracenedione. Clin Pharmacol Therap 1982;*31*:312–316.

217. Savaraj N, Lu K, Valdivieso M, Loo TL. Pharmacology of mitoxantrone in cancer patients. Cancer Chemotherap Pharmacol 1982;*8*:113–117.

218. Alberts DS, Peng Y-M, Davis TP. Disposition of mitoxantrone in patients. Cancer Treat Rev 1983;*10*:Suppl B:23–27.

219. van Belle SJP, Planque HM, Smith IE. Pharmacokinetics of mitoxantrone in humans following single-Agent infusion or intraarterial injection therapy or combination-Agent infusion therapy. Cancer Chemotherap Pharmacol 1986;*18*:27–32.

220. Ehninger G, Poksch B, Heinzel G. Clinical pharmacology of mitoxantrone. Cancer Treat Rep 1986;*70*:1373–1378.

221. Larson RA, Daly KM, Choi KE. A clinical and pharmacokinetic study of mitoxantrone. J Clin Oncol 1987;*5*:391–397.

222. Liu Yin JA, Johnson PRE, Davies JM, Flanagan NG, Gorst DW, Lewis MJ. Mitozantrone and cytosine arabinoside as first line therapy in elderly patients with acute myeloid leukaemia. Br J Haematol 1991;*79*:415–420.

223. Arlin Z, Case DC Jr, Moore J, Wiernik P, Feldman E, Saletan S, Desai P, Sia L, Cartwright K, and the Lederle Cooperative Group. Randomized multicenter trial of cytosine arabinoside with mitoxantrone in previously untreated patients with acute non-lymphocytic leukemia. Leukemia 1990;*4*:177–183.

224. Henderson K, Allegra JC, Woodcock T, Wolff S, Bryan S, Cartwright K, Dukart G, Henry D. Randomized clinical trial comparing mitoxantrone with doxorubicin in previously treated patients with metastatic breast cancer. J Clin Oncol 1989;*7*:560–571.

225. Averbuch SD. Nonclassic alkylating agents, in Chap 12, pp 314–322 in Ref. R3 1990.

226. Farmer PB, Newell DR. Alkylating agents, Chap 4, pp 100–102 in Ref. R1.

227. Dost FN, Reed DJ. Methane formation in vivo from N-Isopropyl-α-(2-methylhydrazino)-p-toluamide hydrochloride, a tumor-inhibiting methylhydrazine derivative. Biochem Pharmacol 1967;*16*:1741–1746.

228. Dunn DL, Lubet RA, Proughi RA. Oxidative metabolism of N-isopropyl-α-(2-methylhydrazino)-p-toluamide hydrochloride (procarbazine) by rat liver microsomes. Cancer Res 1979;*39*:4555–4563.

229. Weinkin P, Prough RA. Oxidative Metabolism of N-isopropyl-α-(2-methylazo)-p-toluamide (Azoprocarbazine) by rodent liver microsomes. Cancer Res 1980;*40*:3524–3529.

230. Cummings SW, Guengerich FP, Prough RA. The characterization of N-Isopropyl-p-hydroxymethyl-benzamide formed during the oxidative metabolism of azoprocarbazine. Drug Metab Disp 1982;*10*:459–464.

231. Moloney SJ, Weibkin P, Cummings SW. Metabolic activation of the terminal n-Methyl group of N-isopropyl-α-(2-methylhydrazine)-toluamide (procarbazine). Carcinog 1985;*6*:397–401.

232. Baggliolini M, Bickel MH, Messiha FS. Demethylation in vivo of natulan, a tumor-Inhibiting methylhydrazine derivative. Experientia 1965;*21*:334–336.

233. Kreis W. Metabolism of an antineoplastic methylhydrazine derivative in a p815 mouse neoplasia. Cancer Res 1970;*30*:82–89.

Books and Monographs

r1. Ames MM, Powis G, Kovach JS. Pharmacokinetics of anticancer agents in humans. New York: Elsevier, 1983.
Edited and written by active leading investigators in the field; although somewhat dated, it remains an authoritative monograph.

r2. Calabresi P, Chabner BA. Section XII, Chemotherapy of neoplastic diseases; Chapter 52, Antineoplastic agents. In Gilman AG, Rall TW, Nies AS, Taylor P. Goodman and Gilman's the pharmacological basis of therapeutics, 8th ed. New York: Pergamon Press, (1990); pp 1202–1263.
A popular textbook with an excellent chapter on cancer chemotherapy. Chabner also edited and contributed significantly to Ref. r3 and r6.

r3. Chabner BA, Collins JM. Cancer chemotherapy: principles and practice. Philadelphia: JB Lippincott, 1990.
Like Ref. r1 but more up-to-date, many chapters in this outstanding volume are written by authorities in cancer chemotherapy research.

r4. Bertino JR. Antineoplastic drugs. Chapter 23 in Melmon KL, Morrelli HF, Hoffman BB, Hierenberg DW. Clinical pharmacology: basic principles in therapeutics. 3d ed. New York: McGraw-Hill. 1992;600–641.
This chapter provides a general survey of cancer therapy, especially suitable to clinicians.

r5. Holland JF, Frei E III, Bast RC Jr, Kufe DW, Morton RL, Weichselbaum RR. Cancer medicine, 3d ed. Section XXI, Chemotherapeutic agents. Philadelphia: Lea & Febiger (1993); pp 698–814.
The ten chapters in this section give a comprehensive review of anticancer agents currently in clinical use; many recent papers are covered.

r6. Chabner BA. Clinical pharmacology of cancer. Chapter 18. In DeVita VT Jr, Hellman S, Rosenberg SA. Cancer: Principles and practice of oncology, 4th ed. Philadelphia: JB Lippincott, 1993.
Similar to Ref. r5, a number of active investigators contributed to this chapter; since almost all of them are different from those of Ref. r5, their perspectives are not identical.

r7. Bellamy WT. Prediction of response to drug therapy of cancer. A review of in vitro assays. Drugs 1992;*44*:690–708.

r8. Yabro JW. Current developments and future directions with ifosfamide: An update. Sem Oncol 1992;*19* Suppl *1*:1–77.

r9. Yabro JW. Recent advances in ifosfamide therapy. Sem Oncol 1992; *19* Suppl *12*:1–73.

r10. Bryson HM, Sorkin EM. Cladribine. A review of its pharmacodynamic and pharmacokinetic properties and therapeutic potentials in haematologic malignancies. Drugs 1993;*46*:873–894.

r11. Ross SR, McTavish, Faulds D. Fludarabine. A review of its pharmacologic properties and therapeutic potentials in malignancies. Drugs 1993;*45*:652–677.

r12. Brogden RN, Sorkin EM. Pentostatin. A review of its pharmacodynamic and pharmacokinetic properties and therapeutic potentials in lymphoproliferative disorders. Drugs 1993;*46*:652–677.

r13. Yabro JW. Current perspectives on the use of etoposide (VP-16). Sem Oncol 1992;*19* Suppl *13*:1–83.

r14. Yabro JW. Novel approaches to the use of etoposide (VP-16). Sem Oncol 1992;*19* Suppl *14*:1–63.

r15. Yabro JW. Current perspectives on teniposide (VM-26). Sem Oncol 1992;*19* Suppl *6*:1–102.

r16. Plosker GL, Faulds D. Epirubicin. A review of its pharmacodynamic and pharmacokinetic properties and therapeutic uses in cancer chemotherapy. Drugs 1993;*45*:788–856.

r17. Yabro JW. Current perspectives on the use of bleomycin. Sem Oncol 1992;*19* Suppl *5*:1–70.

r18. Yabro JW. Carboplatin update: Current perspectives and future directions. Sem Oncol 1992;*19* Suppl *2*:1–165.

CHAPTER 102

Computer-Assisted Drug Design

Michael Cory

Introduction

With the rapid increase in the power of computers and the concomitant decrease in computational costs during the 1980s, molecular modeling and computational chemistry have become more significant aspects of drug design. The application of computational chemistry to drug development is called computer assisted drug design (CADD). This chapter presents an overview of CADD and defines the range of such techniques currently used in the pharmaceutical industry. Also discussed are the advantages and disadvantages of some of these techniques and how they affect bioactive molecule design.

Increases in computer power have had an important influence on technologies outside computational chemistry that nevertheless support computer-assisted drug design. One of these is the determination of three-dimensional (3D) molecular structure. X-ray crystallography and nuclear magnetic resonance (NMR), when used for the determination of molecular structure, depend heavily on high-speed computation. It would be impossible to apply either technique to biologically important problems involving macromolecules without readily available high-speed computation. The data, three-dimensional molecular structures, are extremely useful to the computational and medicinal chemist. These data can serve as a starting point for molecular structure computation or provide experimental verification of computational method. Since advances in one area may be synergistic with advances in the related areas, the influence of macromolecular x-ray crystallography and NMR on CADD is outlined in sections that follow.

The techniques used by the medicinal chemist in CADD generally can be grouped into two classes. Calculation of molecular structure is usually accomplished by molecular mechanics or quantum mechanics, which allow computer simulation of the properties of drug molecules or biologically important macromolecules, either proteins or nucleic acids. Molecular computations also can aid in determining the interaction of a macromolecule with smaller molecular ligands.[1]

The second technique, molecular computer graphics,[2] commonly termed "molecular modeling," allows visual representation of a geometric hypothesis, formulated by the scientist, which then can be tested by molecular computation methods. Molecular computer graphics has prompted model building and exploration either by graphics alone or with computational chemistry as an adjunct. Molecular graphics frequently is used alone where the precision of the molecular structure data does not allow application of full computational techniques. Molecular computer graphics is also a valuable tool for presentation of chemical structure information. This is easily seen by browsing through any current medicinal chemistry journal.

Techniques used in Computer Assisted Drug Design

Computational Chemistry

Molecular mechanics is the computational technique used most frequently by chemists to investigate the conformation and energetics of a molecular structure. It is widely used to examine the structure of drug molecules or candidate drug molecules. Molecular mechanics stimulates mathematically such interatomic characteristics as bond lengths, bond angles, and torsion angles as a set of spring-like mechanical forces between the atoms.[r4] This simulation, if properly done, is usually sufficient to give a reasonable approximation of the conformation of a molecule and the forces associated with its deformation. Obviously, many properties of molecules, in particular their electronic structure, are not fully described by the simple ball and spring approximation. Additional information on the atomic charge on individual atoms frequently is added to the mechanical forces. Both intramolecular and intermolecular hydrogen bonding forces between atoms are also computed. The energy generated by the mechanical forces and the energy obtained by calculating the interactions of the charges on the atoms of the molecule are summed to compute the energy of a specific conformation of a molecule. Full exploration of the conformational flexibility of a molecule is necessary to define the minimum energy conformation from a molecular mechanics calculation.

Before a molecular mechanics computation is done, the set of mechanical forces for each type of atom functional group in the molecule must be described. This full description of the interatomic forces for sets of atoms is commonly called a force field. Each force field contains a large library, (about 1000) of force constants, usually called parameters. Parameters are determined empirically and must be generated for each type of atom in each of its structural environments. Parameters for a given force field are generated by fitting experimentally determined properties of a series of molecules. The parameters are adjusted to reproduce the conformational properties of the molecule, including the three-dimensional structure and the torsional potential about bonds. Since it is impossible to cover all molecular fragments, each force field is carefully designed with a specific molecular simulation objective and chemical scope.[3] All of these programs apply mathematical minimization methods to the initial 3D positions of the atoms and minimize the forces to determine a final 3D conformation. The new MM3 force field,[4] like its predecessor MM2,[5] was designed initially to model hydrocarbons. Older versions of the MM2 force field and MM3 have been expanded by several workers; new parameters were added to cover other functional groups. This expansion has led to a molecular mechanics computer program that is quite useful for molecules of biologic interest.[6] Another example, an extensive suite of software for molecular mechanics modeling, is the work of Kollman's group at the University of California, San Francisco.[7] They have developed a force field and molecular mechanics program, AMBER (Assisted Model Building with Energy Refinement),[8,9] designed specifically to perform molecular mechanics computation on peptides, proteins, and nucleic acids. Thus, AMBER is particularly useful in reaching an understanding of the conformations of biologic macromolecules. Parameters are supplied with the program that can give excellent simulation of the energetics of proteins and nucleic acids in large biopolymer models.

The primary advantage of the molecular mechanics technique is that it is computationally less demanding than other methods. Although the computational load of molecular mechanics generally increases as the square of the number of atoms in the model, it is still the fastest technique available for large systems. This speed accounts for its widespread use in molecular simulation applications. While parameters must be developed for each molecular environment, carefully chosen parameters can give close simulation of the energy of many molecules.

Disadvantages of the molecular mechanics approach includes the large number of parameters for molecular fragments and the need to generate new parameters frequently. The large number of functional groups—and thus the large number of parameters needed for a broadly based molecular mechanics force field—is a particular disadvantage. As more precise molecular simulation results are sought, a substantial effort must be devoted to the generation of new molecular mechanics parameters. Currently this parameter generation is the most time-consuming part of simulating new candidate design systems. It affects drug design specifically because, although parameters for proteins and nucleic acids are available in many molecular mechanics packages, the parameters for each new molecular system must be generated and fit into the existing force field.

Another difficulty associated with molecular mechanics and other molecular computational techniques is the determination of the minimum energy conformation of a drug molecule. The x-ray crystallographic structure represents the minimum energy of the crystalline molecular complex, including the solvents and counterions. It represents the energy minimum of the molecule in that environment. However, understanding the global energy minimum for a molecule involves an extrapolation from the crystal state to the dissolved state. A further complication is that the most important conformation of a drug molecule is its conformation bound to its receptor site. This bound conformation may be neither the energy minimum in solution nor the crystal structure conformation. Molecular mechanics programs include mathematical techniques to determine the minimum energy of the function of the forces on the molecule. These mathematical minimizers can determine only the energy minimum nearest to the starting point of the minimization. Because molecules are flexible and usually contain several rotatable bonds, one starting point for a molecular mechanics energy computation may not be sufficient to find the minimum energy of the molecule. Thus, conformational search techniques have to be added to molecular mechanics to expand the calculations over the full conformational range of the molecule.

Two techniques have gained importance in studies of the global energy minimum of a drug molecule. Systematic conformational search rotates the molecule around single bonds in discrete steps and minimizes the energy for each of the resulting conformers.[r5,10] If the conformational space of the molecule is thoroughly searched, then comparison of the energy of these conformers allows selection of the calculated minimum energy. The conformational search method has been used for many years, but, because it is computationally intensive, its importance has grown with the availability of computer power. Conformational space for molecules with a few rotatable bonds can be explored thoroughly with currently available computers; but, as the number of single bonds increases in biologically important molecules, such as polypeptides, the search over all conformational space becomes an impossible computational task.

An exciting technique developed by Pearlman[11] rapidly generates three-dimensional structures by an algorithm that uses known chemical conformations to build approximate structures. This program works in a rule-based manner similar to the method a chemist might use when building a structure with a ball-and-stick model building kit. Pearlman's program, CONCORD, does the 3D molecular model-building rapidly enough that large databases of approximate 3D structures can be built.[12]

The availability of an easy means of building a large, high-quality,[13] 3D database of any set of structures has prompted the development of a series of methodologies[r6] for searching[14] and understanding these databases. Programs search databases for 3D pharmacophores or for docking large numbers of structures into 3D receptor models are readily available and have successfully given lead structures for further pharmacologic development.[15,16]

Another important method for gaining insight into the energetics of drug molecules is molecular dynamics, which applies Newton's laws of motion and thermal energy to simulate the energetics of molecular motion. Usually, this technique is implemented within computer programs as a complement to molecular mechanics, using the same molecular mechanics force field. It can give considerable information on the energetics of transitions between conformations of molecules. The advantage of the molecular dynamics technique is that the addition of thermal energy to the forces acting on the atoms of a molecule can move those atoms into new conformations. The energetics of the resulting conformations can then be evaluated.

The disadvantage of molecular dynamics is that it requires substantially more computer time than does molecular mechanics. Although thermal energy can force the molecule to new conformations, the effect of thermal forces on the molecule must be scaled to the effect of the mechanical forces on the molecule. This requires that the molecular dynamics computations be done in short time steps. These time steps, frequently about 10^{-15} seconds are necessary to prevent disruption of the molecule's structure. For large molecules of biologic importance this limits the number of conformations that can be explored. Because of its effective exploration of the energy space of a molecule, molecular dynamics is being used for extremely large computations of proteins and their interactions with solvents and small ligands. These calculations represent large supercomputer jobs.

Quantum mechanics computations have been used for molecular studies for about 40 years. Quantum mechanics involves a series of approaches to the approximate solution to the Schrodinger equation, which describes the energy of the particles of a molecule in comparison with a standard state.[17,r7] In practice, in the past, because of its significant computational demands, quantum mechanics had little impact on drug design. High quality, accurate quantum mechanics calculations are now applicable to compounds of biologic interest; but in practice this approach is still used primarily as a parameter development adjunct to molecular mechanics. The description of conjugated systems, transition states of chemical reactions, and molecular reactivity of drug molecules can be effectively simulated with quantum mechanical techniques. Recently, molecular electrostatic potential maps[18] and polarizability and acidity of drug molecules have been determined with these calculations. It is common practice to use quantum mechanics to compute partial atomic charges on molecular systems; these partial charges are then used as charge parameters in molecular mechanics calculations. The molecular descriptions discussed above are primarily properties of the electronic interactions of a molecular system.

Quantum mechanics provides a technique complementary to molecular mechanics. Electronic factors, except as point charges or dipoles, are not determined during molecular mechanics calculations. Because quantum mechanics calculations are not driven by predetermined parameters but by descriptions of the properties of individual atoms in molecules, a very wide range of molecular properties can be determined. A particular advantage of quantum mechanics is that it can be used on any functional group of a molecule. In addition, the calculation of molecular mechanics parameters frequently is done by using quantum mechanics for estimation of energy barriers in simple molecules.

A primary difficulty with any molecular computation technique is simulation of the drug in a solvent medium that corresponds to the solvent at the site of drug action. Traditionally, molecular mechanics computations have been considered "gas phase" calculations because the force fields were designed to simulate gas phase chemical property data. Some molecular mechanics programs allow specification of a dielectric constant for the computation. This dielectric effectively modulates the charge-charge interactions in a manner similar to the modulation seen with polar solvents. In simulating the structure of macromolecules or determining the forces of macromolecule ligand interaction, it is extremely important to understand and account for the effect of solvent, usually water, on the molecular complex. Specific techniques that save computer time, such as introducing an artificial dielectric constant into the molecular mechanics computation, serve to modulate the effect of charges on the conformations of molecules and simulate the dampening effect of the water dielectric constant on the organic molecule.

With enhanced computer speed medicinal chemists can use more complicated force field expressions for their computations. Adding additional terms to the molecular mechanics equations should provide more precise simulation. Improved treatment of atomic charge and its dependence on conformation will be important. Longer molecular dynamics simulations on larger molecular systems are also being done, as is more work on explicit models for solvent molecules that require substantial computation speed because of the large number needed to surround macromolecules during the computation.

Within the past few years the free energy perturbation (FEP) method has been applied to studying drug molecules interacting within their receptor site.[19] The FEP method computes the free energy change of a system (for example a drug molecule in a protein receptor site[20]) as it is changed from one substance to another. That is, atoms of the starting drug receptor complex are slowly transformed, within the computer's energy equations, to the atoms of a different but closely related drug receptor complex. In practice this technique uses thousands of small computational steps to change the parameters of the atoms from those of one system to another. The free energy change that takes place as the transformation proceeds is compared to the free energy of the same chemical transformation in the solvated drugs when not bound to the receptor. Using this technique, some investigators have success[r6] in predicting the free energy of binding of molecules to proteins. Considerable effort is ongoing to determine both the best method for the parameter changes and the breadth of this technique.[r8]

Molecular Modeling

Molecular modeling in a nonquantitative manner has a long history of application to organic chemistry. The London Museum of Science, for example, presents in their chemistry display area the set of wooden spheres that John Dalton[21] used as models of carbon atoms. Some of these spheres were drilled with holes to receive rods that could connect the atoms and represent bonds. The most widely known application of nonquantitative molecular modeling (using physical models) to the solution of an important biologic structure problem was the Nobel Prize winning work done by J. D. Watson and F. Crick, who developed a model for the structure of DNA. In 1953, Watson and Crick decided to use physical molecular models in an attempt to describe a structure for DNA that would rationalize recently acquired x-ray fiber diffraction patterns. These patterns suggested a regular repeating structure with inherent geometric constraints. Initially, Watson and Crick used molecular models that they cut manually from cardboard. Later, as they improved their understanding of the conformations of the nucleic acids, they had more exact models machined from metal. At the time of their work, controversy existed over the correct tautomeric form for the heterocyclic bases. The first Watson and Crick models had incorrect tautomers for the heterocyclic bases, which had been suggested by older experimental results. After they realized their error, they rebuilt the models with the correct tautomeric form of the bases and obtained a conformation for DNA that not only rationalized large amounts of experimental data but also suggested a method by which DNA could be responsible for cellular replication.[22]

The rapid increase in use of computer assisted molecular modeling has been entirely dependent on the increasing power of computer graphics display. The most recent increase in interest and demand came with the ability to show the three-dimensional shape of molecules. Early computer graphics molecular models were stick figures that represented molecular structures similar to pencil and paper structures or the common metal and plastic stick molecular model kits. Computer graphics space-filling or surface models came much later because of their increased computational cost. These space-filling computer graphics models are analogous to the classic CPK (Corey, Pauling, Koltun) space-filling plastic molecular models, color coded by atom type, that can be found in most laboratories.

X-ray crystallographers began by using computer modeling software designed for molecular display.[r9] Around 1975 some larger pharmaceutical companies established projects to design customized medicinal chemistry software.[23] These projects used existing black-and-white graphics terminals and were responsible for developing new principles for drug design and molecular modeling. Graphics displays have changed rapidly since 1975. Black-and-white ball and stick plots of small x-ray crystal structures produced by the ORTEP[24] program and used in the literature to illustrate hundreds of molecular structures were available then. Today, interactive displays that show space-filling models of entire proteins are commercially available to the chemist. These graphics workstations are priced so that medicinal chemists can afford to add them to their standard laboratory equipment.

The most sophisticated of these displays allows full three-dimensional transformation of the coordinate display by turning a dial or moving a mouse. Custom designed computer molecular modeling and display software now uses a joystick, mouse, dials, keyboard commands, or a combination of these to manipulate the molecule. Different graphics schemes are used to present stereo views of molecules, which are required in the study of proteins and nucleic acids and not used extensively by other disciplines. Dozens of companies sell molecular modeling software, and packages are now available for systems that range from personal computers to mainframe supercomputers. These companies were started by chemical or medicinal scientists in the academic community, and all specialize in supplying molecular modeling software to the pharmaceutical and chemical industries. Most of these software packages began primarily as molecule display packages. As the users become more sophisticated they demanded more computational tools to back up the graphics. Thus, the software vendors would respond to these demands by expanding their software with added interfaces to various computational chemistry techniques.

The use of the computerized molecular models has advantages over the manipulation of physical molecular models.[25] Molecules are represented in the computer as sets of three-dimensional atomic coordinates and a list of connections, bonds, between atoms. Since these data are maintained for each stored conformation of a molecule, the user can obtain information about bond lengths, bond angles, and torsion angles of a model. Additionally, nonbonded, direct, through-space distances—so important in defining the shape of receptor sites—can be obtained and compared. In the computer, large numbers of molecules or sets of molecular conformations can be handled and compared simultaneously. Any number of computer copies of the same or different molecules can be superimposed upon each other. This superposition technique can give the medicinal chemist information about the relative size and shape of sets of molecules that might have similar biologic properties. The superposition of different conformations of the same molecule can give information about the relative space a molecule can occupy.[r10] The technique of comparing the volumes occupied by sets of molecules can be an effective method for comparison of active and inactive members of a series.[26] Another popular approach is the "active analogue" technique pioneered by Marshall,[r11] which combines the systematic conformational search technique with superposition and comparison of structural overlap in three-dimensional space.

A recent major development in the computer graphics aspect of molecular modeling is the shift of emphasis from displaying molecules as stick figures to displays that represent the surface of molecules. Algorithms have come into general use that describe and can be used to generate displays of this surface area.[r12,27] Software that allows comparison of these computed surface areas also is available. One of the first algorithms to be widely implemented for studying the surface of molecules it that of Connolly.[28] In this algorithm a sphere of given radius (usually the radius of a water molecule) is rolled over a receptor molecule: the places where the sphere makes three contacts with the receptor defines the limit of the solvent-accessible surface. Computer programs that use the algorithm generate dots wherever the sphere touches the solvent-accessible surface. Display of these dots allows the medicinal chemist to visualize this surface. An alternative approach, more efficient in computation and display time, is to place a dot surface over the molecule and to compute the surface using expanded atomic radii. More recent implementations of this algorithm display the electrostatic density at the surface, which serves to provide the chemist with a picture of what the charge exposed to solvent might be. When applied to drug design, the solvent-excluded surface allows an indication of the topology of a receptor site. Plotting physicochemical functions, such as electrostatic potential, on the surface of this model gives an indication of the forces acting on a molecule that binds to that surface. New raster computer displays have generated widespread interest in the development of new display algorithms for computing high-resolution space-filling representations of molecules. Many algorithms have been developed to give rapid, high-resolution CPK displays of molecules. Most provide a static display computed from a specific orientation. Real-time, three-dimensional manipulation of these CPK models has been demonstrated on some systems.[29] Static CPK models still are most commonly used by chemists for presentations. It remains to be seen whether manipulation of CPK models or filled solvent accessible surfaces on a routine basis will add substantially to the effectiveness of molecular graphics tools.

Widespread use of molecular modeling, in both industry and academia, occurred only in the second half of the 1980s. One hardware and software system became standard for molecular modeling: a combination of an Evans and Sutherland (E and S) graphics display, for which full color was available in 1986, connected to the Digital Equipment Company (DEC) VAX minicomputer. The series of high-speed E and S vector displays supplied the first standard molecular modeling hardware system useful for macromolecular structure display. The primary characteristics that made these systems so valuable to the medicinal scientist were the interactive manipulation of the displayed structure—turning a knob rotated the structure—and the ability to display entire macromolecular structures. These terminals can display thousands of lines representing bonds with enough speed that dials can be used to rotate the macromolecule in three dimensions while the user watches. Color displays rapidly followed the early black-and-white terminals, as has the development of a raster display that can be used for static display of CPK models.[30] Reduced-instruction-set architecture computer (RISC) chip sets and their installation into UNIX-based professional graphics workstations have been displacing the older style terminal-host computer systems.

Many commercial and academic molecular modeling and computational packages are being redeveloped to run on stand-alone high-speed workstations. These workstations provide the graphics display speed and resolution of the older terminals but also provide a general-purpose computer that can be used for computational chemistry. These new workstations are priced so that instead of being departmental scale resources they are appropriate for an individual scientist.

Sources of Molecular Modeling Data

Two rapidly developing physical chemistry techniques have had an important impact on the application of molecular modeling and computer chemistry to drug design. X-ray crystallography of small molecules, important biologic macromolecules and complexes of the two, contributes important chemical structure and conformational data directly to molecular modeling efforts. NMR also provides structural information, and, with the newer techniques, provides conformational information on drugs, macromolecules, and drug-receptor complexes.[r13]

X-ray Crystallography

X-ray crystallography is the only physical chemical technique that can produce a complete three-dimensional picture of a chemical structure at an atomic level of detail. The high-resolution crystal structure of a small molecule can provide structural details of drug conformation, bond lengths, bond angles, and interatomic distances. For small molecules (almost all synthetic drugs) with a molecular weight under 1000, the crystal structure can be determined directly.[r14] Hundreds of drug molecules[r15] and series of molecules have been studied and compared by x-ray crystallography.[31] Quantitative x-ray structure-activity relationships have been developed that rationalize the biologic activity of drug molecules with their crystal structure.[r16,r17]

X-ray crystal structure-assisted design has been used successfully in the discovery of new inhibitors of human immunodeficiency virus (HIV) protease. Molecular mechanics models built and minimized within a HIV-1 protease x-ray structure was used to design new target inhibitors. After synthesis these molecules were cocrystallized and provided structural confirmation of the original models.[32]

Biologic macromolecule x-ray crystal structure determination has been accelerated by recent major developments in genetic engineering. Some hard to purify proteins, after extensive laboratory effort, can be prepared in microgram quantities by traditional biochemical techniques. A well engineered cloning vector for the same protein can be scaled up in a standard laboratory to provide hundreds of milligrams of pure protein. Crystallization of the protein and crystallization of heavy atom derivatives of the protein provide the crystallographer with sets of data that can be used for determining the structure. Knowledge of the amino acid sequence of the protein aids the crystallographer in developing his computer model of the atomic positions and bonding.[r18] Fitting the model to the observed x-ray reflections provides both a model structure and information about its fit to the observed data.

Automated x-ray diffractometers integrated with fast computer workstations are now commercially available for rapid acquisition of protein diffraction data. New area detectors for x-ray diffraction have replaced single-point counting or film techniques and allow rapid collection of much larger sets of reflection data. The new methods also make it possible to solve structures for materials that were too unstable, in the x-ray beam, to withstand the older, slower techniques.

Macromolecular x-ray crystallography is a computationally intensive discipline facilitated by high-speed computation at the data gathering, data analysis, and data presentation stages. Macromolecular structures could not be solved without digital computers,[r19] because the magnitude of the computations is so large. The importance of this information on chemical structure and the rapid growth of the x-ray crystallography field has led to compilations of bibliographic, chemical, and numerical data about crystal structure of compounds. Two research based databases of x-ray crystal data are extremely useful tools for molecular modeling and analysis. These databases have become standard literature tools for the molecular modeler. The Cambridge Structural Database (CSD) was developed at Cambridge University as a data manipulation tool for x-ray crystallographers. The CSD provides access to about 70,000 small molecule structures and is growing at a substantial rate.[33]

The Brookhaven Protein Crystallographic Database[34] currently contains more than 1000 macromolecular crystal structures. While this may not represent all published macromolecular crystal structures, it does represent the majority. This database is also growing very rapidly, with new contributions of structures coming from the work of NMR spectroscopists and x-ray crystallographers. Some model structures have also been retained in the database. In addition to structural proteins and the classic protein crystal structures, e.g., that of hemoglobin and lysozyme, the database includes several enzymes that can be targets for drug design. For example, dihydrofolate reductase (DHFR) is the target for clinically used chemotherapeutic agents. There are three crystal structures of DHFR in the database from three different species sources that could be and have been used.[r20] Both Cambridge and Brookhaven laboratories provide subscription services for their databases. Brookhaven provides online access through the Internet to the latest news, prerelease files, and final structure releases.[35] In addition to providing access to the information contained in the databases, these organizations and their defined computer formats for crystallographic data have forced the standardization of data files. All of the commercial molecular modeling software provides a method for reading crystal data from these databases into graphics programs for later manipulation of experimental data. The Brookhaven file format, commonly called the protein database, or PDB, format has become the computer standard for macromolecules.

Nuclear Magnetic Resonance Spectroscopy

With modern nuclear magnetic resonance (NMR) spectroscopy equipment, three-dimensional conformations of macromolecules have been obtained.[36,r21]

Newer NMR spectrometers, using superconducting magnets, have higher magnetic field strengths that provide the increased sensitivity for the study of biologically important macromolecules. With the higher fields, additional information is available from improving the radio frequency probes and NMR electronics. A large series of new pulse techniques are available that can provide information on the interactions between specific nuclei. Specifically the new multidimensional NMR techniques allow correlation of signal locations for magnetically coupled protons. In NMR spectroscopy, nuclear Overhauser effect (nOe) signals are sensitive to the distance between atoms. High resolution nOe experiments can provide large sets of interatom distances for atoms not directly bonded but close in space because of the folding of the macromolecule. A large set of nOe distances, combined with the knowledge of the sequence of a protein, can be treated by the mathematical technique of distance geometry[37] to provide a set of three-dimensional structures of a protein or nucleic acid that fulfill the geometric constraints. Molecular mechanics and molecular dynamics computations (discussed above)[38] can be used to refine the distance geometry structures and provide a three-dimensional protein structure in a situation where the protein cannot be crystallized or the crystals are not appropriate for x-ray crystallography.

NMR has a specific advantage over x-ray crystallography in that the frequently difficult crystallization step is unnecessary. Further, NMR provides information on the state of the molecule in solution instead of in a possibly perturbing crystal matrix. NMR is particularly applicable to determination of the structures of small molecules and molecular complexes. Drug-to-polynucleotide complexes have been elucidated by this technique and show excellent correlation with structures proposed from biophysical data.[39] The conformations of various small peptides have also been determined.[40,41] NMR is particularly powerful for this application because most small peptides do not crystallize easily and there are few biophysical techniques that will give definitive conformational information.

NMR structure determination also is computer-intensive because the output of a NMR study is a set of connectivities and intramolecular distances. Molecular modeling techniques, distance geometry, molecular mechanics, or molecular dynamics must be applied to the set of connectivities and distances to generate a three-dimensional set of coordinates of the molecule.[r22] However, a specific disadvantage of the current state of NMR three-dimensional structure assignment is the difficulty of associating a specific NMR signal with a specific nucleus in the molecule.[r23] With the current technology, the three-dimensional structure of small proteins, (a limit of around 100 amino acids) can be determined.

Receptor Based Drug Design

Another term sometimes seen in medicinal chemistry literature—rational drug design[r24]—describes aspects of recent use of new computational tools that aid the medicinal chemist in the search for new drug candidates. The concept probably is better stated as "receptor structure based" drug design. The earliest approach to receptor based drug design was the technique Quantitative Structure Activity Relationship (QSAR), which, as practiced in medicinal laboratories, is used to describe the predominantly statistical correlation of biologic activity with directly measurable physicochemical parameters or characteristics of drugs.[r25]

The aspect of receptor based drug design that relates more closely to computer technology is the use of structural information about receptors or small molecules, in combination with computational chemistry techniques, to develop new candidate drug targets. This approach to selected drug design problems has been called "receptor based" drug design. In this technique, a receptor or a model of a receptor is used as the target for the drug design efforts. The molecular modeling approaches of CADD can investigate two different classes of medicinal chemistry problems. If the macromolecule receptor for the drug is known, still a rare situation, then computer graphics models of the receptor (protein or nucleic acid) can be generated from crystal data and used for the docking of known or candidate ligands. This receptor model can be a solved x-ray crystallographic structure or a model built from the x-ray structure of a homologous protein. This approach to characterizing the drug receptor has also been called pharmacophoric modeling.[r26] Considerable efforts are now being made to solving the problem of modeling related protein structures.

A pharmacophore is the set of functional groups responsible for a particular pharmacologic action. These are also termed "recognition sites" because one might argue that the receptor "recognizes" certain patterns of geometry and charge density as the drug binds to its receptor. Pharmacophoric modeling, also an old technique, has become a more commonly used and more sophisticated approach as improved computation and x-ray structural data became available. Pharmacophoric modeling is a hypothesis building technique that used results from x-ray crystal studies on small molecules and measurements from physical molecular models to suggest the required geometry of active agents. Through space distances were used to connect groups shown to be important in biologic activity. New pharmacophore models can be more sophisticated than most previous models, because they are developed with better three-dimensional data and more understanding of the shape and structure of macromolecules. Distance geometry can be effectively applied to a series of molecules to map pharmacophores by overlapping the distance bounds of a series of molecules.[r27]

As an alternative approach, the similarities and differences between active molecules and inactive molecules can be described in three-dimensional space. The sum of the volumes occupied by the active compounds can be subtracted from the volume occupied by the inactive compounds to give regions in space that prohibit activity.[r7,r28] This methodology has been termed the "active analogue" approach. A recent example of pharmacophoric modeling is the work presented by Lloyd and Andrews[42] in which the three-dimensional structure of many active CNS drugs were computed or gathered from the literature. These structures were superimposed to develop a generalized β-phenylethylamine containing "universal" CNS drug pharmacophore. An example of protein molecular modeling is the interest in the wide array of G-protein coupled receptors (GPCR). Extensive three-dimensional model building of the seven-helix transmembrane of GPCRs is being used to understand the mechanism of ligand binding.[r29]

Our knowledge of the chemical structure of drug receptors is still very sketchy. If a desired receptor structure is not known, crystallographic data on analogous macromolecular receptors could be used to build a molecular graphics model of the drug receptor. This molecular modeling approach to protein structure can be particularly effective, since molecular architecture is a highly conserved feature of protein structure. This extreme conservation means that molecular modeling approaches can be applied to new enzymes. For example, Furie[43] used x-ray crystallographic data on the serine proteases chymotrypsin and trypsin to build models of the not yet crystallized serine protease thrombin. While many new protein structures recently have been solved, including structures with clinically active drugs bound to the protein,[44] there are thus far no x-ray structures of membrane-bound proteins that could give the medicinal chemist structural information about membrane bound receptors on the molecular level.

Computational chemistry techniques can be used to give an approximation of the energy involved in the drug-receptor interaction. Two prime examples of receptor structures that have been characterized by x-ray crystallographic techniques (or generated by molecular modeling) and that have been used for drug design are the enzymes dihydrofolate reductase (DHFR)[r30] and renin.[r31] In recent years, polynucleotides that represent sections of DNA, including a series of polynucleotide drug complexes, have been crystallized.[45] This has enabled medicinal chemists to design compounds to fit specific DNA sites.[r32,46]

Conclusions

A commonly asked question about CADD is: Which drugs have been designed using CADD techniques? As discussed above, widespread use of CADD by the pharmaceutical industry is only a few years old. Much of the effort of the past years has gone into understanding and creating the computer visualization and computational tools needed to understand drug molecules and the interaction between drug molecules and candidate biologic macromolecules. The development of these tools is extremely important because not all visualizations actually help understand the large molecules that act as drug receptors. As a tool, CADD has much less acceptance and use than analytical techniques such as NMR and mass spectrometry. However, CADD tools are rapidly changing and becoming another method for approaching drug design problems. It is clear that the continuing increases in computational technology mean that there are even more exciting potential uses for CADD in the future.

References

Research Reports

1. Cohen NC, Blaney JM, Humblet C, Gund P, Barry DC. Molecular modeling software and methods for medicinal chemistry. J Med Chem 1990;*33*:883–894.
2. Glen RC. Computational chemistry and molecular graphics in drug discovery. Drug News & Perspectives 1988;*1*:69–74.
3. Pincus MR, Scheraga HA. Conformational-analysis of biologically-active polypeptides, with application to oncogenesis. Acc Chem Res 1985;*18*:372–379.
4. Allinger NL, Yuh YH, Lii JH. Molecular mechanics—the MM3 force-field for hydrocarbons. J Am Chem Soc 1989;*111*:8551–8566.
5. Allinger NL. Conformational-analysis 130 MM2-hydrocarbon force-field utilizing V1 and V2 torsional terms. J Am Chem Soc 1977;*99*:8127–8134.
6. Lii JH, Gallion S, Bender C, Wikstrom H, Allinger NL, Flurchick KM, Teeter MM. Molecular mechanics (MM2) calculations of peptides and on the protein crambin using the Cyber-205. J Comp Chem 1989;*10*:503–513.
7. Kollman PA. Theory of complex molecular interactions: computer graphics, distance geometry, molecular mechanics, and quantum mechanics. Acc Chem Res 1985;*18*:105–111.
8. Weiner SJ, Kollman PA, Case DA, Singh UC, Ghio C, Alagona G, Profeta S Jr, Weiner P. A new force-field for molecular mechanical simulation of nucleic-acids and proteins. J Am Chem Soc 1984;*106*:765–784.
9. Weiner SJ, Kollman PA, Nguyen DT, Case DA. An all atom force field for simulations of proteins and nucleic-acids. J Comp Chem 1986;*7*:230–252.
10. Jeffs PW, Mueller L, DeBrosse C, Heald SL, Fisher R. Structure of aridicin-A-an integrated approach employing 2D NMR, energy minimization, and distance constraints. J Am Chem Soc 1986;*108*:3063–3075.
11. Rusinko A III, Skell JM, Balducci R, Pearlman RS. Computer program "CONCORD" University of Texas at Austin, users manual. St. Louis; TRIPOS Assoc., 1988.
12. Brint AT, Willett P. Pharmacophoric pattern-matching in files of 3D chemical structures-comparison of geometric searching algorithms. J Mol Graphics 1987;*5*:49–56.
13. Hendrickson MA, Nicklaus NC, Milne GWA. CONCORD and CAMBRIDGE: Comparison of computer-generated chemical

structures with x-ray crystallographic data. J Chem Inf Comput Sci 1993;*33*:155–163.

14. Henry DR, McHale PJ, Christie BD, Hillman D. Building 3D structural databases: Experiences with MDDR-3D and FCD-3D. Tet Comp Meth 1990;*3*:531–536.

15. van Geerestein VJ, Perry NC, Grootenhuis PDJ, Haasnoot CAG. 3D database searching on the basis of ligand shape using the SPERM prototype method. Tet Comp Meth 1990;*3*:531–536.

16. Shoichet BK, Stroud RM, Santi DV, Kuntz ID, Perry KM. Structure-based discovery of inhibitors of thymidylate synthase Science 1993;*259*:1445–1450.

17. Boyd DB. Quantum mechanics in drug design: methods and applications. Drug Information J. 1983;121–131.

18. Getzoff ED, Tainer JA, Weiner PK, Kollman PA, Richardson JS, Richardson DC. Electrostatic recognition between superoxide and copper, zinc superoxide dismutase. Nature 1983;*306*:287–290.

19. Bash PA, Singh UC, Brown FK, Langridge R, Kollman PA. Calculation of the relative change in binding free energy of a protein-inhibitor complex. Science:1987;*235*:574–576.

20. Wong CF, McCammon JA. Dynamics and design of enzymes and inhibitors. J Am Chem Soc 1986;*108*:3830–3832.

21. Wooden ball and stick models attributed to John Dalton, The Science Museum, Exhibition Road South Kensington, London, England.

22. Watson JD, Crick FHC. Genetical implications of the structure of deoxyribonucleic acid. Nature 1953;964–967.

23. Smith GM, Gund P. Computer-generated space-filling molecular models. J Chem Inf Compu Sci 1977;207–210.

24. Johnson CK, Report No. ORNL-3794. Oak Ridge National Laboratory, Oak Ridge Tennessee, 1970.

25. Endres M. Molecular modeling: Is it finally ready for the bench chemist? Today's Chemist at Work. Oct 1992;30–44.

26. Sufrin JR, Dunn DA, Marshall GR. Steric mapping of the L-methionine binding site of ATP: L-methionine S-adenosyltransferase. Mol Pharmacol 1981;*19*:307–313.

27. Bash PA, Pattabiraman N, Huang C, Ferrin TE, Langridge R. Van der Waals surfaces in molecular modeling-implementation with real-time computer-graphics. Science 1983;*222*:1325–1327.

28. Connolly ML. Solvent-accessible surfaces of proteins and nucleic acids. Science 1983;*221*:709–713.

29. Fuchs H, Goldfeather J, Hultquist JP, Spach S, Austin JD, Brooks FP Jr, Eyles JG, Poulton J. Fast spheres, shadows, textures, transparencies and image enhancements in pixel-planes. Computer Graphics 1985;111–120.

30. Marchington AF, Robins S, Richards WG. Current techniques-chemistry, computers and commerce. TIPS 1982;*3*:425–428.

31. Borea PA, Bertolasi V, Gilli G. Crystallographic and conformational studies on histamine H_1 receptor antagonists 4, On the stereochemical vector of antihistaminic activity. Drug Res 1986;*36-1*:895–899.

32. Thompson WJ, Fitzgerald PMD, Holloway MK, Emini EA, Darke PL, McKeever BM, Schleif WA, Quintero JC, Zugay JA, Tucker TJ, Schwering JE, Homnick CF, Nunberg J, Springer JP, Huff JR. Synthesis and antiviral activity of a series of HIV-1 protease inhibitors with functionality tethered to the P_1 or P_1' phenyl substituents: X-ray crystal structure assisted design. J Med Chem 1992;*35*:1685–1701.

33. Allen FH, Bellard S, Brice MD, Cartwright BA, Doubleday A, Higgs H, Hummelink T, Hummelink-Peters BG, Kennard O, Motherwell WDS, Rogers JR, Watson DG. Cambridge crystallographic data center-computer based search, retrieval, analysis and display of information. Acta Crystallogr. Sect. B, Structural Science 1979;*35*:2331–2339.

34. Bernstein FC, Koetzle TF, Williams GJB, Meyer EF Jr, Brice MD, Rodgers JR, Kennard O, Shimanouchi T, Tasumi M. The protein data bank: A computer based archival file for macromolecular structures. J Mol Biol 1977;*112*:535–542.

35. Protein Data Bank, Chemistry Department, Building 555, Brookhaven National Laboratory, Upton, New York 11973. Newsletter produced quarterly.

36. Pardi A, Hare DR, Wang C. Determination of DNA structures by NMR and distance geometry techniques: a computer simulation. Proc Natl Acad Sci USA 1988;*85*:8785–8789.

37. Havel TF, Crippen GM, Kuntz ID. Effects of distance constraints on macromolecular conformation 2 simulation of experimental results and theoretical predictions. Biopolymers 1979;*18*:73–81.

38. Clore GM, Gronenborn AM, Brunger AT, Karplus M. Solution conformation of a heptadecapeptide comprising the DNA binding helix F of the cyclic-AMP receptor protein of *Escherichia coli*. Combined use of ^1H nuclear magnetic resonance and restrained molecular dynamics. J Mol Biol 1985;*186*:435–455.

39. Leupin W, Chazin WJ, Hyberts S, Denny WA, Wuthrich K. NMR studies of the complex between the decadeoxynucleotide d(G-CATTATGC)$_2$ and a minor groove binding drug. Biochemistry 1986;*25*:5902–5910.

40. Fesik SW, Bolis G, Sham HL, Olejniczak ET. Structure refinement of a cyclic peptide from two-dimensional NMR data and molecular modeling. Biochemistry 1987;*26*:1851–1859.

41. Widmer H, Billeter M, Wuthrich K. Three-dimensional structure of the neurotoxin AXT Ia from *Anemonia sulcata* in aqueous solution determined by nuclear magnetic resonance spectroscopy. Proteins 1989;*6*:357–371.

42. Lloyd EJ, Andrews PR. A common structural model for central nervous system drugs and their receptors. J Med Chem 1986;*29*:453–462.

43. Furie B, Bing DH, Feldmann RJ, Robison DJ, Burnier JP, Furie BC. Computer-generated models of blood coagulation factor Xa, factor IXa, and thrombin based upon structural homology with other serine proteases. J Biol Chem 1982;*257*:3875–3882.

44. Matthews DA, Bolin JT, Burridge JM, Filman DJ, Volz KW, Kaufman BT, Beddell CR, Champness JN, Stammers DK, Kraut J. Refined crystal structures of *Escherichia coli* and chicken liver dihydrofolate reductase containing bound trimethoprim. J Biol Chem 1985;*260*:381–391.

45. Fujii S, Wang A HJ, Van Der Marel G, Van Boom JH, Rich A. Molecular structure of (M5dC-dG)$_3$ - the role of the methyl-group on 5-methyl cytosine in stabilizing Z-DNA. Nucleic Acids Res 1982;*10*:7879–7892.

46. Cory M, McKee DD, Kagan J, Henry DW, Miller JA. Design, synthesis, and DNA-binding properties of bifunctional intercalators-comparison of polymethylene and diphenyl ether chains connecting phenanthridine. J Amer Chem Soc 1985;*107*:2528–2536.

Reviews

r1. Lipkowitz KB, Boyd DB. Reviews in computational chemistry. New York: VCH Publishers, Vol. 1,2 1990, Vol. 3 1991, Vol. 4 1993.

A. The series of volumes entitled "Reviews in Computational Chemistry," edited by Lipkowitz and Boyd, presents substantial review chap-

ters on selected topics in computation. Many of these chapters are of significant interest to CADD.

r2. Olson AJ, Goodsell DS. Visualizing biological molecules. Sci Amer 1992; *November 267*:76–81.
An excellent article that presents in full color glory the best of the visualization tools available to view macromolecules and macromolecular complexes.

r3. Horvath AL. Molecular design: Chemical structure generation from the properties of pure organic compounds. Vol 75 of Studies in physical and theoretical chemistry New York: Elsevier, 1982.
This book explores the relationship between molecular structure and macroscopic characteristics of organic compounds. It covers basic chemical structural principles including physical properties of organic compounds. Theories of drug design that use organic structural correlates. An extensive bibliography on properties of organic molecules is also included.

r4. Burkert U, Allinger NL. Molecular mechanics. Washington: American Chemical Society (1982).

r5. Tollenaere JP, Janssen PA. Conformational-analysis and computer-graphics in drug research. J Med Res Rev 1988;*8*:1–25.

r6. Martin YC, Bures MG, Willett P. Searching databases of three-dimensional structures in Reviews in Computational Chemistry, Ed. Lipkowitz KB, Boyd DB. New York: VCH Publishers 1990;*1*:213–264.

r7. "*Ab initio* Molecular Orbital Theory" In Hehre WJ, Radom LP, Schleyer VR, Pople JA. Ab Initio Molecular Orbital Theory New York: Wiley Interscience, (1986); 660–1578.

r8. Van Gunsteren WF, Weiner PK. Eds. Computer Simulation of Biomolecular Systems: Theoretical and Experimental Applications. Leiden: ESCOM, 1989.

r9. North ACT. Potential of molecular graphics in the computer-aided design of inhibitors. In: Sandler M, Smith HJ Design of enzyme inhibitors as drugs. Oxford: Oxford Univ Press, (1989);93–120.

r10. Bolis G, Greer J. Role of computer-aided molecular modeling in the design of novel inhibitors of renin. In: Perun TJ, Propst CL Computer-aided drug design methods and applications. New York: Marcel Dekker (1989);297–326.

r11. Marshall GR, Barry CD, Bosshard HE, Dammkoehler RA., Dunn DA. The conformational parameter in drug design: the active analog approach. In: Olson EC, Christoffersen RE Computer assisted drug design. Washington: American Chemical Society (1979);205–226.

r12. Richards FM. Areas, volumes, packing and protein structure. Ann Rev Biophys Bioeng. 1977;151–176.

r13. Erickson JW, Fesik SW. Macromolecular X-ray crystallography and NMR as tools for structure-based drug design. Ann Repts Med Chem. 1992;*21*:271–289.

r14. Horn AS, De Ranter CJ. X-ray crystallography and drug action. Oxford: Clarendon 1984.

r15. Tollenaere JP, Moereels H, Raymaekers LA. Atlas of the three-dimensional structure of drugs. Amsterdam: Elsevier, 1979.

r16. Duax WL, Norton DA, Eds. Atlas of steroid structures. Vol 1. IFI New York: Plenum, 1975.

r17. Griffin JF, Duax WL, Weeks CM. Atlas of steroid structures. Vol 2. New York: Plenum, 1984.

r18. Stezowski JJ, Chandrasekhar K. X-ray crystallography of drug molecule macromolecule interactions as an aid to drug design. Ann Rept Med Chem. 1986;*21*:293–302.

r19. Abraham DJ. X-ray crystallography and drug design in computer-aided drug design methods and applications. In: Perun TJ, Propst CL. Computer-Aided Drug Design: Methods and Applications New York: Marcel Dekker, (1989);93–122.

r20. Kuyper LF. Inhibitors of dihydrofolate reductase in computer-aided drug design methods and applications. In: Perun TJ, Propst CL. Computer-Aided Drug Design: Methods and Applications New York: Marcel Dekker (1989);327–369.

r21. Wuthrich K. NMR of proteins and nucleic acids. New York: Wiley, 1986.

r22. Fesik SW. Approaches to drug design using nuclear magnetic resonance spectroscopy in Computer-aided drug design methods and applications. In: Perun TJ, Propst CL. Computer-Aided Drug Design: Methods and Applications New York: Marcel Dekker (1989);133–184.

r23. Keptein R, Boelens R, Rullmann JAC. Computer simulation of biomolecular systems. In: Van Gunsteren WR, Weiner PK. Computer Simulation of Biomolecular Systems: Theoretical and Experimental Applications Leiden: ESCOM Science Publishers, (1989);194–216.

r24. Hruby VJ, Pettitt BM. Conformation biological activity relationships for receptor-selective, conformationally constrained opioid peptides in computer-aided drug design: Methods and applications. In: Perun TJ, Propst CL. Computer-Aided Drug Design: Methods and Applications New York: Marcel Dekker (1989);405–460.

r25. Martin YC. Quantitative drug design—a critical introduction. New York: Marcel Dekker, 1978.

r26. Gund P. Pharmocophoric pattern searching and receptor mapping. Ann Rept Med Chem 1978;*14*:299–308.

r27. Blaney JM, Dixon JS. Receptor modeling by distance geometry. Ann Rept Med Chem 1991;*26*:281–286.

r28. Marshall GR, Gorin FA, Moore ML. Peptide conformation and biological activity. Ann Rept in Med Chem 1978;*13*:227–238.

r29. Humblet C, Mirzadegan T. Three-dimensional models of G-protein coupled receptors. Ann Rept Med Chem 1992;*27*:291–301.

r30. Blakley RL. Dihydrofolate reductase. In: Blakley RL, Benkovic SJ. Folates and Pterins. New York: Wiley, 1984;*1*:191–253.

r31. Boger J. Renin inhibition. Ann Rept Med Chem 1985;*20*:257–266.

r32. Henry DW. In: Bardos TJ, Kalman TI. New approaches to the design of antineoplastic agents. New York: Biomedical (1982);5–36.

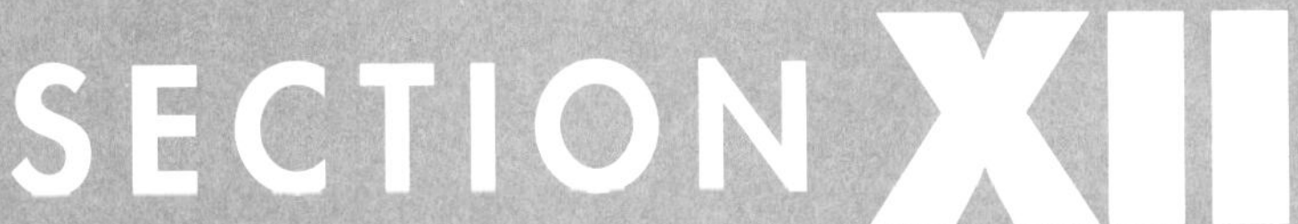

SECTION XII

Natural Medicinal Products

Editor:
Ranjit Roy Chaudhury

CHAPTER 103

Natural Medicinal Agents/ Herbal Medicines/Natural Medicinal Products

Ranjit Roy Chaudhury

Millions of people in the third world will always use herbal medicines because they believe in them and regard them as "their" medicine, in contrast to the "allopathic" (conventional western) system of medicine brought in from "outside." These medicinal herbs are available locally and are prescribed by traditional practitioners of medicine who are part of the community and in whose presence the patient feels comfortable. Even in western countries there is now an increased use of herbal medicines, largely because of a belief that powerful synthetic agents used in Western medicine can exert more unwanted side-effects and are too often used indiscriminately and irrationally. Many members of the public also have a mistaken impression that medicines derived from natural plants are harmless. Although generally natural medicines induce fewer side-effects than conventional drugs, there are plants that cause powerful side-effects. Thus, the physician should understand something about herbal medicines and the traditional systems of using them. He or she is certain, if he is practicing in the Third World or treating people from the Third World, to deal with patients who have first had recourse to herbal medicines.

Such traditional systems of medicine as the Ayurvedic, the Chinese traditional system, the Tibetan, and the Unani, born in Greece, nurtured in the Arab countries, and now flourishing in Asia, have been with us for over 2500 years. Some of the plants mentioned in ancient Sanskrit and Chinese texts or in Buddhist teachings are still widely used today. It is difficult to comprehend that such plants as Commifera mukul being widely used today after scientific investigation, or Artemesia annua used to treat chloroquine-resistant falcifarum-induced malaria, were mentioned in texts about 2500 years ago. There are many such examples, and it is possible that some very useful medicinal plants, used today particularly for such conditions as arthritis, bronchial asthma, or hepatitis in traditional systems of medicine, could be used in the Western system. The beneficial effect in treating hepatitis of an extract of the plant glycyrrhiza demonstrated recently in Japan is one such example. The Japanese investigators have also suggested that the plant induces a release of interferon. This, in fact, may not be the complete story, but certainly it opens up an avenue for research on hepatoprotective plants.

It is important to appreciate that, although the traditional systems of medicine use medicinal plants, in many instances such plants are used only as complements to other measures that together make up a treatment for a particular disease. Failure to understand this has led to misunderstandings and lack of empathy between the "Western" researcher and practitioner and the traditional practitioner. Very often this has led to cynicism and criticism about the traditional systems of medicine and the use of medicinal plants that may not always be fair. The Western practitioner also cannot understand how one plant could be good for so many different conditions, and he is confused by the plethora of remedies in traditional medicine for all conditions. These exaggerated and, very often, unsubstantiated claims by practitioners of the traditional systems have led practitioners of the other modern systems to demand proof of efficacy of an herbal remedy before they are willing to use it. Such proof, as will be seen later, is not easy to obtain with medicinal plants.

It should be clearly understood that in the traditional systems of medicine—and in folklore and rural medicine—one plant or one mixture of plants may be used for treating a particular disease. In other cases, treatment may consist of a therapeutic regimen in which use of a herbal remedy forms only one part of the treatment. Practitioners and researchers of traditional systems of medicine are unable to understand why the research worker of the Western system very often takes the medicinal plant being used, tests it, finds it does not work, and reports that the plant, reputed to be effective in traditional medicine, does not act as claimed. This, he feels, is not fair, because the plant acts when used together with exercise, diet, and a modified style of life. In this chapter we are concerned with medicinal plants and their possible therapeutic effect; we are not concerned solely with therapeutic regimens in which medicinal plants form only one part of the therapy. It is important to know that many of these earlier systems of medicine have based their treatment along three lines: (1) promotion of good health by different means; (2) prevention of disease; and (3) treatment of disease—in which medicinal plants may be used.

An appreciation of this concept will help the reader avoid the pitfalls research workers often fall into when carrying out research on medicinal plants.

Research on medicinal plants should be carried out to determine whether Western therapeutics could add to its armamentarium a few new drugs obtained from medicinal plants used in traditional systems. One such area could be hepatitis, since the traditional systems of medicine have plants used for centuries for protecting the liver and for treatment of liver dysfunction. The plants, *Picrrorhizia kurroa, Phyllanthus amarus,* and *Andrographis paniculata* could be selected. In view of their mention in ancient literature, laboratory experiments could be carried out with the plants, and they could be used widely today. Experiments and clinical trials could proceed after careful study of how the plants are being used in the ayurvedic or traditional Chinese systems of medicine. The results of these carefully planned studies could perhaps lead to a widely applicable discovery. Similarly, plants should be investigated in the field of bronchial asthma. There is hardly any point in trying to discover an antibacterial medicinal plant today since excellent antibiotics are already available in Western medicine. On the other hand, the plants *Curcuma longa* and *Azadirachta indica* could certainly be tried out in cases of arthritis, since the nonsteroidal antiinflammatory drugs, although powerful, are potentially toxic and the world of plants may provide an additional medicine. In the past, pharmacologists have identified important medicines from the plant world. Morphine, quinine, emetine, reserpine, digitalis glycosides, ergot alkaloids, and vincristine are examples of drugs in wide use today that originally were obtained from plants. It is difficult to accept that there are no more drugs waiting to be discovered from plants, in spite of unrewarding experiences in this field during the last 30 years. There may still be some such discoveries ahead of us.

Historically and traditionally, the approach toward evaluating medicinal plants has been based on chemical extracts from plants reputed to have pharmacologic properties or therapeutic effects. The extracts would then be tested on animal models. This traditional approach has nine steps:

(1) identification of the plant reportedly in use,

(2) collection of the plant,

(3) transport of the plant to the research laboratory,

(4) preparation of extracts for testing,

(5) administration of the extracts to animal models,

(6) identification of the active or more active extracts,

(7) further fractionation of the active extract,

(8) isolation and characterization of the active principles,

(9) synthesis of the active substance.

This methodology was introduced by the pharmaceutical companies that entered the field of herbal pharmacology in the 1940s but had withdrawn by the 1970s. The system was effective, and several plant substances with therapeutic effects were discovered. Furthermore, it suited the pharmaceutical companies because, at the end of the road, there were compounds that were patentable.

In recent years, however, investigators have begun to question whether this method is the only method that should be used or whether there is scope and place for another approach toward research on medicinal plants. This thinking was based on observations that in many plant extracts further fractionation of an active extract leads, not to enhanced activity in one of the fractions, but to diminished activity in all the fractions. About 50 per cent of medicinal plants behave in this manner. A typical example is the effect of the plant *Momordica charantia* on blood sugar levels. While the whole fresh extract contains significant hypoglycemic activity, demonstrated both in primates and in humans, such activity is decreased when the active extract is further fractionated. It appears that the whole extract is needed for the activity. The traditional pharmaceutical approach would never discover or put on the market *Momordica charantia* as an oral hypoglycemic agent.

There are several other such plants. For these, already widely used today in traditional systems of medicine, chemical extraction and testing on animal models may be inappropriate. In view of these findings, a second, complementing model for testing plants already in use has been proposed. This model consists of the following steps:

(1) toxicity testing of the plant in two species of animals for acute and subacute toxicity;

(2) a modified shorter toxicity if the plant has already been used in humans or is in such use now; and

(3) administration of the total extract or combination of plants if used, in exactly the same way as prepared and used by the traditional practitioner.

The essential differences between this approach and the usual approach of the pharmacologist are that, in this suggested scheme:

(1) there is no testing for efficacy carried out on animal models—but only in humans;

(2) human studies are initiated after modified, shortened toxicology studies have demonstrated that the substance is not toxic in animals;

(3) the duration of the toxicity studies has been decreased to six weeks for plants already being used in humans; and

(4) the plant is administered to human subjects in exactly the same way as in traditional or folklore medicine.

The advantages of this model are that it takes into account the concepts of traditional and folklore medicine and avoids some of the difficulties inherent in the traditional screening, such as losing the active principle by extraction and fractionation or using an inappropriate animal model. It is, of course, essential that approval of the ethics committees be obtained before undertaking such clinical trials after limited animal toxicology studies. More and more centers are now adopting this complementing model, not only in India and China, but also in Western countries. National drug regulatory authorities are also willing to look carefully at requests from investigators for clinical evaluations of plants already used in different parts of the world without undertaking the full range of toxicity studies required for new synthetic compounds. This subject has been extensively reviewed recently.

Researchers, health administrators, and clinicians often ask whether a plant medicine used in the traditional systems of medicine is "effective." It is not easy to answer this question since the presence or absence of a beneficial therapeutic effect can be ascertained only by carrying out a well-controlled clinical trial with the plant. Unfortunately, very few persons are trained in the methodology of clinical pharmacology and clinical trials in countries where these remedies are being used and the trials would have to be carried out—i.e., the Third World. It would, in any event, be possible to conduct clinical evaluation of only a few plants—the expertise, time, and resources to carry out such trials on a large number of plants are just not available. Another point to keep in mind is that clinical trials with medicinal plants are in many ways different from trials for synthetic compounds. These differences will be described in the hope that clinical trial methodologies for medicinal plants may attract pharmacologists and clinicians to specialize in this area.

When a synthetic compound is administered to humans, the investigator knows something about the metabolic breakdown of the compound. Studies therefore are planned in the human to identify metabolites after administration. On the other hand, the metabolic pathway of the therapeutic principle of a plant is *not* known before the plant is administered in a clinical trial. Its breakdown products cannot be determined in early studies after administration. Furthermore, double-blind trials may be difficult with herbal medicines; it may not be possible to prepare an appropriate placebo. One may, therefore, have to be content with a single-blind design for clinical evaluation of herbal medicines. Another difference relates to the sample to be tested. The physiochemical properties of a synthetic drug being tested are well known, and subsequent samples obtained for testing will conform to these characteristics. The clinical investigator is certain that he is receiving the same substance for testing in all batches. However, since the physiochemical characteristics of the plant medicine being tested have not been characterized, it may be difficult to ensure that subsequent samples of the plant material received for clinical evaluation possess exactly the same physiochemical and pharmacologic characteristics as the first sample. This means that, for a successful clinical trial with a medicinal plant, all the material must be collected at the same time of the year from the same location before the trial is initiated. Studies will, however, have to be carried out to demonstrate that the physicochemical and pharmacologic properties of the plant do not alter during storage. Cross-over studies with a wash-out period can be carried out with synthetic drugs because the metabolic pathway and excretory products of the compound are known, as is the half-life of the compound. It is not difficult with this information to identify a suitable "wash-out" period. Unfortunately, this cannot be done for medicinal plants. There is no rational way the "wash-out" period can be arrived at without knowing the metabolic pathway and half-life of the active principle of the plant substance or the time for excretion of its metabolites. All these differences must be kept in mind when planning clinical trials with herbal remedies. Other issues, such as the use of other plants at the same time, the effect of plants on other body systems, and the effect of taking commonly used synthetic drugs at the same time also have to be dealt with when carrying out clinical trials with herbal remedies.

Before medicinal plants can be widely used in different systems of medicine, standardization techniques must be worked out for every plant to ensure that each batch contains a similar quantity of the active principles and will thus induce the same therapeutic effect. It is now well known that plants may vary in their alkaloidal content according to different places of collection, different times in a year for collection, collection at the same time and place but in different years, and with different environmental factors surrounding the cultivation of a particular medicinal plant. This means that there should be a quality control test for the entire preparation. Generally, tests for standardization of plant medicines in use today are macroscopic, microscopic, physicochemical, and biologic. The list of tests generally used for standardization of herbal medicines is: (1) macroscopic examination of the plant; (2) microscopic examination of the plant; (3) physicochemical testing; (4) biologic testing—where appropriate.

Two examples will be given of recent discoveries of herbal medicines that had been used much earlier and whose therapeutic properties had been described many years ago. One of these examples is a plant used in the Ayurvedic system of medicine in India; the other is a plant used in the Chinese traditional system of medicine.

The plant *Commiphora wightii* was mentioned for its therapeutic properties in the ancient Ayurvedic text Sushruta Samhita written in 600 BC. It was only in 1969—2569 years later—that Satyavati et al.[1] demonstrated the beneficial effect of crude extracts of *Commifera Wightii* on hyperlipemia and atherosclerosis in rabbits. This was followed by extensive work on guggal, the extract of the plant—chemical, pharmacologic, clinical pharmacologic, and toxicologic—that resulted, 17 years later, in the drug guggulipid being marketed for hyperlipidemia on the Indian market. Gum guggal is a complex mixture of steroids, diterpenoids, aliphatic esters, and carbohydrates.

Phytochemists have succeeded in isolating several steroidal constituents from the gum resin of *C. muukul* and have now reported on the stereochemistry of guggulsterol. The compounds Z-guggulsterone and E-guggulsterone appear to be mainly responsible for the hypolipidemic activity. Recent work has demonstrated a rise of high-density lipids after administration of the extract of *Commiphora Wightii*. It should be mentioned that the extracts of the plant also have demonstrated a therapeutic effect on arthritis, and they are being widely prescribed for this effect. Another quality attributed to the extract in the ancient Ayurvedic text was its beneficial effect on obesity. This has not yet been looked at by scientists, but may provide some surprises to researchers who take up this interesting plant for further study.

In AD 317, Ge Hong wrote in a "Medical Book of Emergencies" that the plant Artemesia exerted a beneficial effect in a type of fever that, by description, appeared to be similar to the high fever seen in malaria. This plant is known as "Qing Hao Su." It was also stated that the plant should not be boiled in water but treated at a low temperature to extract its activity. Chinese scientists about 25 years ago began looking for plants and drugs to treat malaria. They went back to the ancient textbooks on Chinese traditional systems of medicine and listed about 30 herbal remedies used to treat malaria. Scientists at the Institute of Chinese Traditional Medicine then carried out research on these herbs and observed that two of the plants mentioned in ancient Chinese texts, *Artemesia annua* and *Dichroa febrifuga* demonstrated antimalarial activity after modern pharmacologic evaluation. Scientists and clinical investigators carried out a large number of experiments and clinical trials and demonstrated clearly the beneficial effect of artemisinin (Qinghaosu) on patients with chloroquine-resistant plasma falciparum malaria. Today it is the only drug, apart from quinine, effective in these cases. The wisdom stored away by Ge Hong was rediscovered after 1662 years.

The compounds used today as antimalarial drugs are sodium artesunate (given IV), artemether, and arteether. In addition, quing hao su suppositories have been developed and are being used effectively in cases of malaria. As has been clearly brought out by Jiang et al.[2], the rediscovery of artemesin as an antimalarial, also effective in chloroquine-resistant plasma falciparum malaria, is but one step in the search for other plant medicines.

Some of the plants used today in traditional medicine may have much to offer to Western medicine. Folklore medicine could also provide useful leads. Ancient texts of the traditional systems of medicine and writings of explorers, missionaries, and travelers, could be searched to learn more about possible medicinal plants. However, the approach adopted in the very recent past has not yielded much encouraging information. It is important to use appropriate methods to try and obtain more information about possible therapeutic effects. It is hoped that the earlier approach of chemical extraction and screening on animal models will be complemented by animal toxicology followed by clinical trials for those plants already in widespread use. At the present time, because of the disappointments with traditional approaches, pharmaceutical companies have by and large lost interest in medicinal plant pharmacology and therapeutics although in the last few years some resurgence of such interest is again seen. Although the complementary approach may appear rational, the lack of a clear-cut patentable compound at the end of the research may keep industry from committing sizeable resources to such research. Some way, perhaps through funding by international organizations, the pharmaceutical know-how and expertise needed for work on medicinal plants may be supplied. Centers of clinical pharmacology need to be established in the Third World where these medicines are generally used. The methods used today in many of these countries are outmoded and crude, and developments in different areas of science and technology such as biotechnology are not being used. If the infrastructure is improved, if a rational approach toward research on medicinal plants is adopted, and if new technology available in adjacent areas, such as chromatography, mass spectroscopy, X-ray crystallography, computer modeling, and tissue culture are used, it is very likely that more discoveries will be made.

In the early years of the traditional system of medicine, medicinal plants were collected by the practitioner and prepared for patient use by making a powder or decoction. In some countries, like China, the drug was taken in the form of freshly brewed tea. In others, it was extracted with water; in still others, it was mixed with one or two other substances. Things have changed, and today herbal medicines are being dispensed as tablets and capsules in addition to the traditional forms. Sometimes extracts are administered. However, very often the quantity of the plant to be administered is so large that it is difficult for the patient to take in tablet form. An innovative approach has been to prepare granules from the plant extracts and administer the herbal medicines as granules. With these new forms of dispensing herbal medicines, another type of scientific activity became necessary. Standardization of herbal remedies and quality control procedures for regulation of these medicines must be emphasized, and one would expect more such activities in these areas in the coming years.

Keeping in mind the need for a particular type of medicinal plant and taking into account the information available, both in scientific literature and in folklore medicine, 14 plants have been identified as needing research. The names of the plants together with their reputed or reported therapeutic effects are given below:

Name of the Plant	Reputed Use
1. *Picrorrhazia kurroa*	Liver disease
2. *Andrographis paniculata*	Liver disease
3. *Artemesia annua*	Malaria
4. *Dichroa febrifuga*	Malaria
5. *Xanthium strumarium*	Malaria
6. *Moringa oleifera*	Hypertension
7. *Curcuma longa*	Anti-inflammatory agent
8. *Albizzia lebeck*	Asthma
9. *Adhata vasica*	Respiratory Disease
10. *Momordica charantia*	Diabetes
11. *Gymnema sylvestre*	Diabetes
12. *Terminalia arjuna*	Cardiac disease
13. *Azadirachta indica*	Anti-inflammatory agent
14. *Tinosporia cordifolia*	To improve the quality of life

In these days of rapid travel and extensive migration of people, a doctor in the West at some time probably will be faced with a patient using traditional medicines who now needs to change to the Western system. For example, a person on traditional medicines who is suddenly brought into a hospital or clinic in the West may need emergency treatment in addition to the traditional medicine already taken.

In such situations it will always help if the practicing Western doctor has some knowledge of plant medicines that the patient is taking. These patients should be treated in the same way as patients native to the West who are on herbal remedies. In England alone, one can obtain, without a prescription, 40 different herbal remedies. The Table earlier in this chapter, which lists some plants in common use, suggests to the physician that these plants have been used for a long time and that there is some experimental or rational basis for their use—also that these medicines, at appropriate doses, are not harmful. The physician should gradually decrease the use of the traditional medicine and, after two or three days, start treatment with Western drugs. As far as possible, Western medicines should not be administered concomitantly with traditional herbal medicine because possible interactions between the two types may not be known. In an emergency, however, Western drugs should not be withheld.

Nowadays, at least some traditional medicines may be readily available in some Western countries. The patient may want to continue these medicines. The Western-trained doctor, not knowing much about them, should not prescribe without further investigation. He can try to find out what is in the medicines. Even if he finds that the ingredients are simple substances—e.g., garlic or seeds or juice of the bitter gourd for diabetes—he should not take the responsibility of continuing to prescribe them because the efficacy of the substances being administered may not have been demonstrated. If there are practitioners of the Ayervedic, Chinese, Unani, or Kampo systems of medicine in the Western setting, and if they are allowed to carry out their profession, as is allowed in some Western countries on a limited scale, then they should look after these patients.

Western doctors should be made more aware of traditional medicines while not necessarily practicing them. Those interested in such medicines should be allowed to train for a time in the developing world and to observe how the different system of medicine used there are practiced. This will help the Western doctor understand and advise correctly a patient who is referred to him. A publication containing lists of commonly used herbal medicines with some notes on therapeutic efficacy, possible toxicity, and, wherever known, pharmacokinetics would be a valuable reference for all doctors who may treat patients using traditional medicines.

References

Research Reports

1. Satyavati GV, Dwarkanath C, Tripathi SN. Experimental studies on the hypocholesterol emic effect of commifora mukul. Indian J Med Res 1969;*57*:1950.
2. Jiang B, Li GQ, Guo XB, Kong YC, Arnold K. Antimalarial activities of mefloquine and quinghaosu. 1982; Lancet *ii*:258.

References

r1. Chaudhury RR. Plant contraceptives: Translating folklore into scientific application. In Jelliffe DB, Jelliffe EFP, Advances in maternal and child health, Vol. 5. Oxford: Oxford University Press, 1983, pp 5, 58–74.

r2. Chaudhury RR. Folklore herbal contraceptives and remedies. Trends Pharmacol Sci. 1986;*7*:121–123.

r3. Chaudhury RR. Herbal medicine for human health. New Delhi: World Health Organization, 1992, pp 1–87.

r4. Dhawan BN. Current research on medicinal plants in India. Indian Nat Sci Acad. 1986;1–86.

r5. Farnsworth NR, Akerele O, Bingel AS, Diaja D, Soejarto, Zhen Geng Guo. Medicinal plants in therapy. Bull WHO. 1985;*61*:965–985.

r6. Satyavati GV, Raina MK, Sharma M. Medicinal plants of India, vol 1. Indian Council Med Res. 1976; pp 1–487.

r7. Satyavati GV, Gupta AK, Tandon N. Medicinal plants of India, vol. 2. Indian Council Med Res. 1987; pp 1–600.

r8. Chaudhury RR. The quest for a herbal contraceptive. Nat Med J India. 1993;*6*:199–201.

r9. Vaishnav R, Shankaranarayanan A, Chaudhury RR, Mathur VS, Chakravarti RN. Toxicity studies on a proprietary preparation of Semecarpus anacardium. Indian J Med Res 1986;*77*:902–908.

r10. Satyavati G. Guggulipid. A promising hypolipidaemic agent from gum guggul (Commiphora wightii). In: H Wagner, Farnsworth N. Economic and plant research, Vol. 5. 1991; 47–80.

r11. Devraj TL. Ayurvedic remedies for common diseases. New Delhi: Sterling, 1985, pp 1–149.

r12. Jain SK. Medicinal Plants. New Delhi: National Book Trust of India, 1968, pp 1–178.

r13. Handa SS, Kapoor VK. Pharmacognosy. New Delhi: Vallabh Prakashen, 1988, pp 1–328.

r14. Chaudhury RR, Tennekoon KH. Plants as galactogogues. In: Jelliffe DB, Jelliffe EFP. Advances in maternal and child health, Vol. 3. Oxford: Oxford University Press, 1985, pp 20–26.

r15. Hosoya E, Yamamura Y. Recent Advances in the pharmacology of Kampo (Japanese herbal) medicines. Amsterdam: Excerpta Medica, 1988, pp 1–470.

r16. Li CP. Chinese herbal medicine. Bethesda: US Public Health Service, 1974.

r17. Liu Yanchi. The essential book of traditional Chinese medicine, vol. 2, Clinical practice. New York: Columbia Univ. Press, 1988.

r18. Garg SK, Mathur VS, Chaudhury RR. Screening of Indian plants for antifertility activity. Indian J Exp Biol 1978;*16*:1–3.

r19. Ciba Foundation Symposium, Number 285 "Bioactive plants." New York: John Wiley, 1990, pp 1–202.

r20. Medicinal Plants in China. Manila: WHO, 1989, pp 1–327.

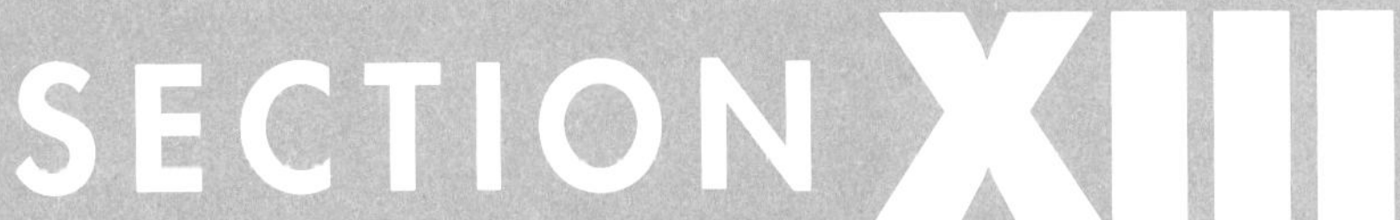

Elements of Toxicology

Editors:
Gabriel L. Plaa
Roger P. Smith

Associate Editor:
P. K. Seth

CHAPTER 104

General Principles of Toxicology

Gabriel L. Plaa
Roger P. Smith

Like pharmacology, toxicology is both a qualitative and a quantitative biologic science. The general principles of pharmacology in relation to the absorption, distribution, biotransformation, and excretion of therapeutic drugs apply equally to chemicals that have no known health-related benefits. Since such chemicals have only deleterious effects, there is never a need to prolong their stay in living organisms, as is sometimes the case with drugs used to treat disease states. Indeed, considerable effort is expended in toxicology to find ways of hastening the elimination of chemicals from the body. Pharmacology and toxicology necessarily overlap because there are no nontoxic drugs. The difference between a therapeutic and a toxic effect is usually only a question of dose. Moreover, some drugs are widely self-prescribed and used only for "recreational" purposes, as opposed to any therapeutic benefit. Such drugs contribute to accidents in the workplace, but occupational toxicology is concerned primarily with exposure to potentially toxic chemicals in the workplace (see Chapter 105).

Drugs are seldom an environmental problem, but toxic chemicals are of enormous environmental concern.[r1] Environmental toxicology is an important subdiscipline of the field. It, in turn, has given rise to the field of ecotoxicology, the study of the harmful effects of chemicals on living organisms within defined ecosystems (Chapter 106). Toxic chemicals are sometimes used as pesticides, where their toxic potential is exploited commercially against particular target species (economic poisons), but the concern is often with unintended target (nontarget) species in the same environment. Humans are the nontarget species of greatest interest, but effects on other nontarget species may have severe economic or aesthetic impact (Chapter 107).

In the US, drugs are regulated by the Food and Drug Administration (FDA), whereas pesticides are regulated by the Environmental Protection Agency (EPA). This distinction applies even when the same chemical is the active ingredient in the two different products, e.g., warfarin is both a useful anticoagulant drug and a widely used rodenticide (rat and mouse poison). Thus, the types of toxicity testing required for regulatory agency approval depend on the intended use for a given chemical. Except for veterinary products, drugs are intended for use in humans, and the FDA appropriately places considerable emphasis on testing in human subjects. The human testing of drugs has become the standard culmination to testing in animals. Because of its responsibility to protect the environment, the EPA places considerable emphasis on toxicity testing in nontarget animal species. In addition to testing in laboratory mammals, an intended herbicide is often tested for toxic effects in birds, fish, and crustacea such as shrimp.

Since the signs exhibited by poisoned animals and the gross and microscopic pathologic lesions in their tissues often provide valuable clues as to the mechanism of action, there is a natural link between qualitative and mechanistic toxicology. Both drugs and poisons are exquisitely powerful tools for elucidating normal biochemical and physiologic functions. Perhaps more has been learned about normal functions by studying the derangements produced by chemicals than by any other approach. Quantitative toxicology is of greater relevance to safety evaluation, risk assessment, and regulatory agencies; but it can also play a role in mechanistic toxicology, since the way a given chemical interacts with another, better-known one can also provide insights into its mechanism of action (Chapter 111). Potentiation or antagonism of the toxic effects of the new chemical by a better-known one can be an extremely meaningful observation in terms of mechanism.

Forensic toxicology is one of the older subdisciplines that is also a specialized branch of our system of criminal justice. Using the techniques of modern analytical chemistry, forensic toxicologists attempt to detect poisonous chemicals in body fluids or tissues in cases of attempted or successful homicides, suicides, or negligence. Since mere detection of a chemical does not prove that it was responsible for a poisoning, a special type of quantitative assessment is needed to ascertain whether the concentration of chemical found is consistent with the effect produced. Determination of the blood alcohol concentration in an apprehended motorist is a familiar example.

From a societal point of view, the greatest good may be served by toxicologists engaged in safety evaluations, whereas from the standpoint of a scientific discipline mechanistic toxicology provides greater allure. Toxicologists are concerned about poisonous chemicals, which is only one of an array of properties that make chemicals hazardous. A chemical may be hazardous because it is corrosive and can induce local tissue damage. If ingested, the local damage may extend to the interior of the body, but the material does not have a specific, systemic toxic effect. Radon is hazardous because it radioactive, but the damage to cells and tissues is related more to the physical energy of the radioactivity than to chemical effects. Other chemicals may be hazardous because they are explosive, flammable, or under high pressure. Thus, hazardous chemicals can induce traumatic injury. Toxic chemicals induce more or less specific systemic adverse effects, even though the precise molecular mechanism may still be unknown. Toxic chemicals are usually thought of as being foreign to the body (xenobiotics), but the mere presence of a xenobiotic does not constitute toxicity. It must be associated with a demonstrable adverse effect.

In a historical sense, however, the discipline of toxicology owes its origins to practical considerations of the effects of natural toxins. Even before recorded history, there must have been an oral record of plants that were to be avoided as foods because they were toxic. Venomous insects and animals were recognized then and are still with us today. Among natural toxins, those produced by molds have excited considerable recent interest because of their potentially catastrophic effects on food supplies (Chapter 108).

Toxicity vs Hazard vs Risk

Toxicologists try to make a clear distinction between the toxic potential of a chemical (or mixture) and its actual importance as it is used for its intended purpose, i.e., toxicity versus hazard. The ability of a chemical to cause injury is referred to as its "toxicity." Toxicity is a qualitative term, since all chemicals possess toxic properties to some degree. When quantitative comparisons are made, some chemicals will be found to be essentially nontoxic because even extremely large doses or exposure for very long periods fail to produce systemic adverse effects. Other chemicals are highly toxic and can produce recognizable effects or death in very small doses. On the other hand, "hazard" is the likelihood that injury will occur in a given use setting or situation. Here the conditions of exposure are the primary considerations. In order to assess hazard, one needs information on both the inherent toxic properties of the chemical (its qualitative aspects) and the amounts to which humans or other species are apt to be exposed when the chemical is properly used in a specific environmental setting (therapeutic use, occupational use, etc.) Potentially toxic substances may be used safely by humans when conditions are in place to minimize absorption during the use. Even lethal chemicals can be used safely (without hazard) in an occupational setting if the environment has been controlled to prevent ingestion or absorption of enough chemical to produce toxicity. In such cases the chemical is potentially toxic, but it is not hazardous because of the way it is being used. It is the critical use component that distinguishes "hazard" from "toxicity."

"Risk" is the expected frequency of occurrence of an undesired effect arising from exposure to a chemical or physical insult. Risk assessment makes use of dose-response data and extrapolation from these observed relationships to make estimates of responses to doses or exposures as they might occur in actual or hypothetical settings. Obviously, the quality and suitability of the observed biologic relationships on which the extrapolations are based are major limiting factors to risk estimates. The importance of critical analysis of the dose-response data cannot be overemphasized in making a judgment about the credibility of extrapolated risk.

Parameters of Acute Toxicity

In the vernacular of toxicologists, the syndrome that results from a single dose of a solid or liquid chemical is referred to as "acute toxicity." When the exposure is via the pulmonary route, as in the case of gases, dusts, vapors, or aerosols, the time of exposure becomes a critical factor. The dose cannot be administered in a single instant in time because of lung washout and the delay required for arterial blood to reach an equilibrium concentration with the inspired material. Indeed, the absorbed dose is seldom known with certainty, so it is common practice to relate the exposure to the ambient concentration for a specified time. Nevertheless, the term, "acute toxicity," is also used in pulmonary exposure, although there is no general agreement about precise exposure period. In general, exposure periods of several hours as opposed to days or weeks are referred to as being "acute."

The most widely used parameter for the expression of acute toxicity is the LD50, the calculated dose that is lethal to 50 percent of a population of animals (median lethal dose). It is entirely analogous to the pharmacologic parameter, the ED50 (median effective dose), except that the LD50 is always a quantal response, whereas the ED50 may be either quantal or graded, depending on the nature of the observed effect. To derive an LD50, at least three groups of animals must be used. Each group is given a different specified dose of the chemical; then, after an appropriate latent period, the mortality for each group is assessed. An adequate experiment would have three groups of animals, each given a different dose, and three effects in terms of per cent mortality or proportion of the groups responding. In an idealized outcome, one would have results from three groups in which the effects would lie within + or − 1 standard deviation of the mean when converted to a normal distribution. This would approximate a linear relationship when the log of the dose is plotted against the effect. It is axiomatic that the proportion of the population responding or the intensity of the effect increases with the dose.

It is the size of the groups that has provoked concern among animal-rights activists,[r2] but the size of the groups is of less scientific concern than the calculated extension of the data to provide 95 percent confidence limits around the LD50. Another useful extension is the potency ratio between two different treatments and its 95 percent confidence limits. For example, if an antagonist is tested against a given toxicant, the potency ratio is the LD50 of the toxicant when given together with the antagonist as divided by the LD50 of the poison given alone. If the potency ratio is greater than one and the 95 percent confidence limits for the potency ratio do not include one, the antagonist treatment was successful at a statistical significance of $p < 0.05$. Conversely, if the potency ratio is less than one and the confidence limits do not include one, the treatment resulted in significant enhancement of the toxicity.

In addition to testing for toxicologic interactions, another use for the LD50 is to group chemicals arbitrarily into sets of varying acute toxicity. An example is shown in Table 104.1, where chemicals with an estimated oral lethal dose in humans (or laboratory animals) of < 5 mg/kg are designated as "super toxic," whereas chemicals with an oral lethal dose of > 15 gm/kg are designated as "practically nontoxic."[r3] Such a classification scheme allows a manufacturer to select from a given set of chemicals (all of which have equal efficacy for a given purpose) the chemical least acutely toxic for humans or other nontarget species.

Finally, although it is widely recognized that animals are imperfect models for human toxicity, an acute oral LD50 in laboratory animals can be used as a first approximation toward a judgment about whether a human has accidentally or deliberately ingested a dangerous or lethal dose of the chemical. In some cases, therapeutic intervention to prevent absorption, hasten excretion, or antagonize the effects is clearly indicated. In other cases, the amount ingested may be judged to be trivial in relation to the toxic or lethal dose, and intervention may not be indicated. In the opinion of the authors, the above uses justify the continued compilation of at least approximate LD50 values.

Irrespective of the route of administration of a toxic chemical, there is a highly variable latent period before the effect is observed. Few chemicals are more rapidly lethal than cyanide or nicotine. The latent period, of course, is influenced by the route of administration, the size of the dose, and a number of other factors; but perhaps the most important of these is what the chemical does to the body. Death from cyanide can occur in minutes when it is inhaled as HCN, but it is rarely delayed more than an hour when taken by mouth as a soluble salt. Conversely, recovery from nonfatal poisoning can be quite rapid. Cyanide poisoning represents an inability to utilize molecular oxygen, so it is a functional asphyxia that also results in rapid demise. On the other hand, fatal hepatic necrosis after an overdose of acetaminophen may not be recognized as imminent for a day or two after ingestion. The ultimate in latent effects, however, is associated with exposure to carcinogenic chemicals that may not be clinically recognized until years after the insult.

The magnitude of the latent period is also arrived at by trial and error, but it is critically important not to terminate the observation period prematurely. This characteristic determines the amount of time a therapist has in which to make a meaningful intervention in human poisonings, and it is an important determinant of the prognosis. The LD50 is often reported in terms of the observation period. It is as equally misleading to report a seven-day LD50 for cyanide as it is to report a four-hour LD50 for acetaminophen. Con-

Table 104.1 An Arbitrary Toxicity Rating Chart[1]

Toxicity Rating or Class	Probable Oral Lethal Dose (Human)		
	Dose		For 70-kg. Person (150 lb.)
6 Super toxic	less than 5	mg/kg	A taste (less than 7 drops)
5 Extremely toxic	5–50	mg/kg	Between 7 drops and 1 teaspoonful
4 Very toxic	50–500	mg/kg	Between 1 tsp. and 1 ounce
3 Moderately toxic	0.5–5	gm/kg	Between 1 oz. and 1 pint (or 1 lb.)
2 Slightly toxic	5–15	gm/kg	Between 1 pt. and 1 quart
1 Practically nontoxic	above 15	gm/kg	More than 1 quart (2.2 lb.)

[1]Adapted from [r3].

versely, even for very rapidly acting toxicants such as cyanide, it may be prudent to observe animals for a week to guard against the possibility of unexpected late deaths, but the range of latencies within which most responses occurred should be reported.

A parameter closely analogous to the LD50 can be derived for airborne chemicals called the LC50 (median lethal concentration), but it is critical that the exposure time be held constant and clearly specified. Again, what is needed is three different ambient concentrations of the airborne chemical in which some but not all of the exposed animals in each group die during the exposure period or within some specified period after a constant period of exposure, i.e., the latent period. Confidence limits and potency ratios can be calculated the same way as for an LD50.

Parameters of Chronic Toxicity

For environmental chemicals, the concern is seldom related to acute toxicity, but with that of possible cumulative effects of repetitive long-term, low-level exposures. There is no simple relationship between the potentials for acute and chronic toxicity for a given chemical. Examples can be cited of chemicals with a very high acute toxicity, but with a very low potential for producing chronic toxicity. The converse is less readily demonstrated, but some chemicals are clearly more dangerous with repeated exposure to low doses in that the dose per day needed to produce the toxic effect is much smaller than the single massive dose that produces the same effect. Two properties of chemicals are recognized as associated with a high tendency to produce chronic toxicity: the first is that the chemical is only slowly eliminated from the body and therefore tends to accumulate with repeated exposures; the second is that the chemical produces effects that are irreversible or only very slowly reversed, so that the effects persist even after the chemical has been eliminated.[1,r1] The latter group are called "hit-and-run" toxicants because the lesion persists after most of the chemical has been eliminated.

Although definitions are not precise, the term "chronic toxicity" usually implies experimental exposures that are measured in many months, years, or in terms of an entire lifespan of the species used. The end-point varies with the toxic effect being studied. It can be death or its converse, survival rate, but chronic testing is perhaps more commonly used to test for the carcinogenic effects of chemicals. However, any number of organs may be examined histologically together with various clinical chemistry tests for pathologic abnormalities.

Clearly, chronic testing is time-consuming and a very expensive way to evaluate the adverse effects of chemicals but, if the objective is to evaluate the effects of life-span exposure, there is no alternative. At the same time, toxicologists faced with the prospect of evaluating a flood of new chemicals have struggled to find some reliable way of testing for adverse effects over shorter time spans. An empirical suggestion that has been widely adopted for some purposes is based on the premise that if a chemical has toxic effects, exposure of young growing animals to it for one-tenth of a life span is sufficient for such effects to be expressed if the dose or exposure intensity is sufficiently high. In terms of common laboratory rat strains, one-tenth of a life span is about 90 days, and 90-day toxicity studies have become commonplace. In the jargon of toxicology, these are referred to as "subchronic" studies.

In the most common type of subchronic study, various concentrations of the test chemical are mixed with the diet and fed to rats ad libitum. The usual index of toxicity is a failure of young growing animals to gain weight in parallel with a control group not fed the chemical. It is also common to follow the daily food consumption of the animals to make sure that they are not refusing the diet. In a well-designed study there will be at least one level of feeding that significantly depresses the growth rate, a toxic level, and at least one level of feeding that does not significantly affect the growth rate—a no-observable-effect level (NOEL) or a no-observable-adverse-effect level (NOAEL). The NOEL or NOAEL is then divided by an uncertainty (safety) factor, often 100, to arrive at an acceptable daily intake for humans.[r4–r6] If the test chemical is a pesticide intended for use on food crops, it is then necessary to determine what levels of residues of the pesticide remain in or on the food at harvest after its application in effective concentrations. If the sum of all the residues for each crop (the tolerances) to which it is applied fall below the acceptable daily intake (the EPA uses the terminology "risk reference dose" for acceptable daily intake) after taking into account the proportion of the total diet made up by each food type, the tolerances are acceptable and the pesticide may be approved for use.

Subchronic studies seldom use weight-gain as the sole parameter of toxicity. There is no limit to the number and type of functional, chemical, and histologic parameters that usually are incorporated into the experiment. It is not necessary to push the feeding levels so high that animals die before the end of the 90-day period, but that sometimes happens—which confirms that a failure to gain weight is truly a toxic effect.

Chemical Mixtures

Toxicologists are used to evaluating the deleterious effects of single chemicals, and methods are in place to test for interactions between pairs of chemicals. Unfortunately, in terms of environmental toxicology, exposures are almost never limited to one or two chemicals. Most commonly, exposures are to multiple chemicals by a variety of routes and to variable intensities over time. Some mixtures are so complex that they defy precise chemical definition.[r7] A single commercial polychlorinated biphenyl product may contain dozens of individual chemical ingredients. A single toxic chemical dump site may have hundreds of different chemicals, with only a handful that have been specifically identified. The possibilities for interactions in a given species are unpredictable.

There are at present no simple procedures for dealing with complex chemical mixtures. As found in the environment, no two mixtures are sufficiently alike to generalize from one to another. Moreover, the composition of mixtures will tend to change with time as the more volatile components are lost to the atmosphere and as the more reactive ingredients undergo biodegradation. The alternative would be to identify the most toxic chemical in the mixture, if possible, and to regard the other constituents as "inert ingredients." Another consideration is needed in this approach, however, namely the concentration of the most toxic ingredient in the mixture. The most toxic ingredient might be present in vanishingly small amounts and make a negligible contribution to the toxicity of the mixture. Obviously, this approach would yield only the crudest of guesses. The experimental design depends on the question being asked; different questions require different strategies.

In spite of the above difficulties, there are practical needs for some sort of estimates of the toxicity of mixtures. For example, in an acute human ingestion episode there is a need to make a prognosis. Regulatory agencies need estimates in order to make orderly decisions about various courses of action. At present, however, this very difficult problem has no obvious solution.

Classification of Toxic Reactions

All drugs have properties that can be harmful to people taking them (drug toxicity). These may be so undesirable that they greatly limit the therapeutic usefulness of a given drug. Table 104.2 summarizes a scheme for the classification of drug-induced toxicities.[r8] It is based partly on a scheme proposed by Rosenheim,[r9] but an effort has been made to deal more completely with the fundamental mechanisms involved. Note that there are two major subdivisions under the category "Primary Toxic Effects." The first is related to the therapeutic or pharmacologic properties of the drug, whereas the second deals with adverse or toxic effects unrelated to the pharmacologic properties. Respiratory depression as a result of phenobarbital overdose is a familiar example of the first subdivision, whereas such effects as megaloblastic anemia, gingival hyperplasia, and osteomalacia as induced by phenytoin or valproic acid-induced liver damage are examples of the second subdivision. The hypokalemia associated with thiazide diuretic therapy is classed as an "indirect consequence of a primary drug action." The latter is a subcategory of an "exaggerated pharmacologic effect," since thiazides do enhance potassium excretion by the kidneys. Frank renal or hepatic injury can hardly be considered as an "exaggerated pharmacologic effect." They are examples of the second category of toxic effects, unrelated to the pharmacologic effects of the drug.

Pharmacologic effects other than those intended for the therapeutic purpose are included in the category of "undesirable side-effects." Examples of these include dry mouth and blurred vision, which accom-

Table 104.2 Classification of Drug-Induced Toxic Reactions[1]

I. Primary Toxic Effects
  A. Exaggerated phamacologic effect.
    1. Occurs with drug overdosage
    2. Occurs with therapeutic doses if individual is hyper-reactive (hyper-susceptible, intolerant) to drug
    3. Indirect consequence of primary drug action
  B. Adverse effect unrelated to pharmacologic therapeutic effect
    1. Occurs with drug overdosage
    2. Occurs with therapeutic doses
    3. Occurs with therapeutic doses if individual is hyper-reactive (hyper-susceptible, intolerant) to drug

II. Undersirable Side-effects
  A. Undesirable pharmacologic effect that accompanies the primary drug action
    1. Occurs with therapeutic doses

III. Alergic Reactions
  A. Effect based on immunologic reaction (antigen-antibody reaction)
    1. Occurs in sensitized individual
    2. Occurs with therapeutic or subtherapeutic doses

IV. Idiosyncratic Reactions
  A. Unexpected or unpredictable reaction, dissimilar from known pharmacologic or adverse effects attributable to the drug
    1. Depends on the personal characteristics of the individual
    2. Occurs in a small number of individuals
    3. May be attributable to the genetic status of the individual

V. Physical Dependence
  A. Altered physiologic state resulting in abstinence syndrome when drug is discontinued

[1]Adapted from [r8].

pany the therapeutic use of muscarinic blocking drugs, the constipation that occurs with codeine analgesia, or the sedation or drowsiness observed with classic antihistaminic drugs. The term "side-effect" carries the connotation that the reaction or effect is relatively mild. In the scheme of Table 104.2, drug-induced liver, kidney, or bone marrow damage would not be classified as "undesirable side-effects." Instead, such reactions are examples of "primary toxic effects."

The category called "idiosyncratic reactions" can be very confusing. Some authors regard these reactions simply as being rare (low-incidence), irrespective of the underlying mechanism. Others regard them as low-incidence reactions that occur by an unknown mechanism. Goldstein et al.[r10] Restrict the term to drug reactions involving a genetically determined trait in an individual. Most authorities agree that the mere incidence of a reaction should not constitute a basis for its definition, but others are reluctant to restrict the term to reactions having an inherited basis. Such a restriction would exclude noninherited reactions classed as "idiosyncratic," but which have a well-defined basis. For this reason, the scheme in Table 104.2 includes genetically-based reactions as one subtype of "idiosyncratic reactions," but allows for the inclusion of other subtypes. The subject is still controversial, and the reader should be aware that "drug idiosyncrasy" means different things to different authors.

Zbinden[r11] classified toxic reactions into three kinds of change: functional; biochemical; and structural. Each of these can be divided into multiple subcategories. Functional toxicity was defined as "due to the pharmacologic effects not necessary for the desired action, although they may for another patient in different circumstances constitute an important therapeutic effect." This definition appears to correspond to that for "undesirable side-effects" in Table 104.2. The term "functional" implies a change in the function of an organ system, and these undesirable side-effects are usually reversible on discontinuation of the drug.

"Biochemical toxicity," as defined by Zbinden, is due to changes in biochemical reactions associated with various organs without evidence of gross organ damage. Shifts in hormonal balance, changes in acid-base balance, changes in electrolytes, or alterations in blood clotting, if adverse, are examples of biochemical toxicity. These reactions are also reversible up to a point on discontinuation of the drug. In Table 104.2 such reactions might be classified as "primary toxic effects" or as "undesirable side-effects," depending on the underlying mechanism.

Obviously, "structural toxicity," as used by Zbinden, involves an actual change in the structure of an organ or tissue. These structural changes in turn may bring about biochemical and/or functional changes, e.g., drug-induced cataracts, or liver or kidney injury, which would be classified as "primary toxic effects" in Table 104.2.

Frequency of Toxic Reactions

Toxicologists are completely dependent on animals for initial toxicity testing; but animals are imperfect models for human toxicity, even when as many as four species are employed. Prior to the thalidomide disaster in the early 1960s, no tests were required for teratogenic effects of potential drugs, but even if such tests had been required, it is by no means clear that the hazard would have been detected. Retrospective testing with thalidomide has shown that it is very difficult to produce phocomelia in common laboratory species at any reasonable dose of thalidomide.

Even when a particular animal species and target organ within that species is established as a good model for humans, there is a point beyond which even animal testing becomes prohibitively expensive. For example, if a given adverse drug reaction occurs with equal frequency (1:100) in humans and a laboratory animal species, in order to be 99 percent certain that the effect was detectable as a result of the drug it would be necessary to test it in 450 animals. A frequency of 1:100, however, is regarded as a common adverse drug reaction. Many serious reactions have frequencies less than that by orders of magnitude. Halothane liver damage is said to occur at a frequency of about 1:10,000. The economics of animal testing for such an infrequent reaction are simply out of reach if the drug is to be made available at any reasonable price.

Special Toxic Effects

Certain kinds of toxic effects have become subspecialties of toxicology and some of these are treated in subsequent chapters in this section including carcinogenic and mutagenic effects (Chapter 109), and teratogenic and reproductive effects (Chapter 110). Risk assessment attempts to evaluate and weigh the risks versus the benefits of the use of chemicals (Chapter 111). Toxicology is a rapidly growing and diverse field that has borrowed heavily from other biologic disciplines, but it is now in a position to repay its intellectual debts with benefits to society.

References

Research Reports

1. Hayes WJ Jr. The 90-dose LD50 and a chronicity factor as measures of toxicity. Toxicol Appl Pharmacol 1967;*11*:327–335.

Reviews

r1. Smith RP. A primer of environmental toxicology. Philadelphia: Lea & Febiger, 1992.

r2. Sun M. Lots of talk about LD50. Science 1983;222:1106.

r3. Gosselin RE, Smith RP, Hodge HC. Clinical toxicology of commercial products, 5th ed. Baltimore: Williams & Wilkins, 1984.

r4. Beck BD, Calabrese EJ, Anderson PD. The use of toxicology in the regulatory process. In: Hayes AW, Principles and methods of toxicology, 2d ed. New York: Raven Press, (1989); pp 1–28.

r5. Lu FC. Basic toxicology, fundamentals, target organs and risk assessment, 2d ed, New York: Hemisphere, 1991.

r6. Ecobichon DJ. The basis of toxicity testing. Boca Raton: CRC Press, 1992; pp 61–82.

r7. National Research Council. Complex mixtures. Washington: National Academy Press, 1988.

r8. Plaa GL. General principles toxicology. In: Levy R, Mattson R, Meldrum B, Penry JK, Dreifus FE. Antiepileptic drugs. 3d ed. New York: Raven Press, 1989; pp 49–58.

r9. Rosenheim ML. Symposium on drug sensitization—General introduction. Proc Roy Soc Med 1962;*55*:7–8.

r10. Goldstein A, Aronow L, Kalman SM. Principles of drug action: The basis of pharmacology. 2d ed. New York: Wiley, (1974); pp 437–487.

r11. Zbinden G. Experimental and clinical aspects of drug toxicity. In: Garattini S, Shore PA. Advances in pharmacology, Vol 2, New York: Academic Press, (1963); pp 1–112.

CHAPTER 105

K. S. Rao
R. H. Reitz
P. G. Watanabe

Occupational Toxicology

The nature of the population exposed to chemicals in the industrial environment tends to be limited and more predictable than in the population at large. Normally, workers between 18 and 65 years of age are in good health, and this is a consideration in judging safe exposure levels. Chemical exposures in the workplace or the environment are constantly changing as new technologies continue to evolve. At the same time, exposures in general are decreasing because of the enhanced awareness of the benefits of good industrial hygiene practices and the advances in control technology.[r1]

Workers, by the nature of their jobs, often perform tasks associated with potential exposure to chemicals. A muller operator in a foundry may repeatedly have potential exposure to silica sand owing to the requirements of employment. In industry, it is common practice to supplement engineering controls with the use of personal protective equipment (such as respirators, ear plugs, or muffs, or skin protective devices) to control exposure to acceptably safe levels. Furthermore, the exposure regimen may be substantially different for occupational workers when compared to the general population. There is a potential for exposure of workers over an entire work day for prolonged periods, whereas exposure to chemicals outside the workplace (because of a hobby, for example) is frequently a voluntary event of short duration.

Because human experimentation is not generally acceptable for defining toxic effects in man, it is necessary to use animals to characterize such responses and subsequently extrapolate these effects to humans. However, the use of animals to predict human response is not free from uncertainty. It is not possible to assure absolutely that people will not be more or less sensitive than the animal population. The range of doses producing a given effect in humans may be much larger than in the animal species selected for experimentation. Even experimental results from studies on small numbers of humans are not totally reliable for predicting the response of large population groups for the same reasons.[1]

Nevertheless, to achieve the ultimate objective, data collected in studies using animals are extrapolated to predict the response in humans. This chapter provides insight into such extrapolation. The basic premise is that toxicity is manifest as a result of the presence of the toxicant at a specified concentration at the target site. Species differences in reactions to given exposures of a chemical occur generally because of quantitative and qualitative differences in the fate of the chemical in the body or because of species differences in receptor sensitivity.

Route of Exposure

Chemicals may affect humans either by causing damage to external tissues, such as the skin or eyes, or they may enter the body and affect internal organs. Those industrial materials capable of damaging the skin and eyes can be identified readily and are designated appropriately for special handling. However, those that enter the body and produce systemic toxicity require more sophisticated tests that are a primary concern in industrial toxicology. There are three primary routes of entry into the body: inhalation; ingestion; and absorption through the skin. In the industrial environment, because of the nature of exposure, duration of the work day, and character of the materials, inhalation and skin absorption are the most significant routes of entry. Ingestion of materials is not a common route of entry in the industrial environment when good hygiene practices are followed.

Frequently skin absorption is given inadequate emphasis in assessment of exposure potential. The skin may be considered as a multilayered protective cover. This barrier, however, is not continuous; it is perforated by hair shafts and follicles that penetrate deep into the dermis. The ability of a substance to penetrate the skin depends mainly on its lipid and water solubilities. Lipid-soluble substances are capable of moving through the fatty layers of the skin, but their further absorption will be hindered if their hydrophobic properties prevent their dissolution in the blood. Lower molecular weight substances tend to have greater potential for dermal absorption. Skin absorption is affected by such factors as temperature, contact surface area, and duration of contact.

Inhalation Principles

Inhalation of chemicals presents the most rapid and direct avenue of entry because of the intimate association of air passages in the lung with the circulatory system.[r2] In most manufacturing processes the atmosphere is likely to contain quantities of vapors, dust particles, mists, and other substances. Airborne contaminants gain direct entry into the respiratory system and consequently have a short pathway to the blood stream, if inhaled. Without adequate engineering control, industrial operations may result in excessive airborne emissions into the workplace environment.

Occupational lung disease may result from excessive inhalation of aerosols (solid or liquid), vapors, or gases. (Hext and Bennett, 1993) The term "aerosol" is used to denote a relatively stable airborne suspension of small liquid or solid particles. A "vapor" is the gaseous form of a substance that is normally a liquid. When a foreign agent is inhaled, it may be deposited in the respiratory tract and subsequently absorbed, exhaled, or neutralized by the lung's defenses. Many atmospheric contaminants can produce injury and disease when deposited and have accumulated in the lungs in sufficient amounts. Systemic effects also can occur after transfer from the lungs to sensitive sites within the body. The degree to which materials enter the circulatory system and are distributed to body tissues depends on the following factors:[r3] (1) concentration of the substance in the air; (2) duration of exposure; (3) solubility of the substance in blood and tissue; (4) reactivity of the substance; (5) respiratory rate. Variables determining the deposition of aerosols are somewhat different. In addition to the factors listed above it is necessary to consider particle size.

Site of Particle Deposition

The respiratory system consists of three main regions: nasopharyngeal; tracheobronchial; and pulmonary. The nasopharyngeal region consists of turbinates, epiglottis, glottis, pharynx, and larynx. At this level, nasal hair and impaction in the turbinates serves to remove large-sized particles from inspired air. The tracheobronchial region is composed of trachea and bronchi ending in terminal bronchioles. This region is covered with mucus-secreting goblet cells and ciliated columnar cells, serving to trap particulate matter and move it to the oral cavity. The pulmonary component consists of alveolar ducts and the alveoli, permitting intimate contact with circulating blood and lymph.

Inhaled particles deposit along the branching airways and penetrate the deep gas-exchange pulmonary region of the lung in continuously varying proportions. Deposition is dependent on the inertial and aerodynamic properties of the particle (Fig. 105.1). The rate at which particles are cleared from the pulmonary region is different from that of the conducting airways. Particles depositing on the airways are swept up and out of the lung within hours by mucociliary action. Particles that penetrate to the pulmonary region take days or even months to clear.[r4] Of prime importance

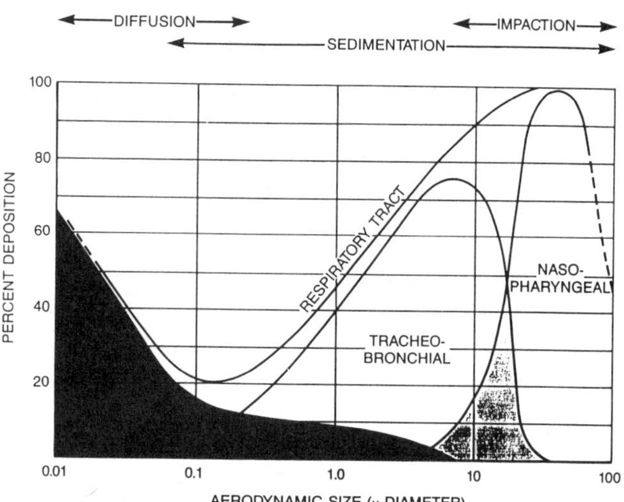

Figure 105.1 Schematic Representation of Deposition of Particles in the Respiratory Tract

in determining the deposition of the inhaled particle in the respiratory tract is the "aerodynamic diameter." This relates the aerodynamic behavior of a denser irregular shaped particle to that of a unit density sphere. For instance, since a 2-micron spherical talc powder particle behaves aerodynamically the same as a 3.3-micron water sphere (density = 1), the aerodynamic diameter of the talc powder is 3.3 micron.

Since particles in the environment are very seldom of only one size, assessment of health risk by determining individually the deposition of particles of each of the sizes present would be extremely complex. Therefore, the International Commission of Radiological Protection (ICRP) described a model that would predict the deposition of a cloud of particles using only one parameter: the mass median aerodynamic diameter (MMAD).

The MMAD is the aerodynamic diameter such that the sum of the mass aerosols smaller than MMAD makes up 50 percent of the total mass of the entire cloud of aerosols. The MMAD is the one parameter that best characterizes the behavior of a cloud of aerosols composed of aerosols of different sizes. Particles having a diameter greater than 5 μm are principally deposited in the nasopharyngeal region by impaction (air velocity and turbulence are highest in this portion of the respiratory tract and decrease progressively toward the alveoli). Particles 1 to 5 μm in diameter deposit along the tracheobronchial tract by sedimentation, with the smallest particles reaching the region approaching the alveoli. Particles less than 1 μm, which reach the alveoli, and deposited primarily by diffusion.[r5] Aerosols in the workplace are not normally particles of identical size.

Clearance of Particles

After a particle is deposited in the respiratory system, the degree of damage produced depends partly on how long the particle remains in the tissue.[r6]

In the nasopharyngeal region particles are removed by mechanical means of clearance. These include sneezing, nose blowing, and mucociliary clearance. As the mucus is removed toward the throat, any particle deposited on it will be carried along and finally swallowed. Some particles can be removed by chemical means depending on their solubility and residue time. Depending on the individual, mucociliary clearance of particles from the nose takes from one to two hours.

Removal of particles from the tracheobronchial region can occur by dissolution and/or mechanical clearance. Like the nose, this region is lined with cilia covered with a mucus blanket. The movement of the mucus blanket is toward the throat. Hence, particles deposited in the mucus blanket in the tracheobronchial region are eventually swallowed. Mucociliary clearance from this region is usually completed within 24 hours.

Like the other two regions, particle dissolution is involved in removal from the pulmonary region (Fig. 105.2). There is no mucociliary clearance in this region because of the absence of cilia and mucus. For most particles, macrophages, free-roaming scavenger cells capable of engulfing particles by phagocytosis, play a major role in removal from the alveoli. The deposition of particles on the surface of alveoli attracts macrophages, which engulf the particle. Some particle-laden macrophages may move to the terminal bronchiole, where they are carried up the respiratory tract by the mucociliary system. Particles in the alveolar region can be removed by the macrophages and transported to the lymphatic channels in the alveolar wall.

It takes only a few hours to one day for phagocytosis by macrophages to be complete. However, for water-insoluble particles, the translocation of particles from alveoli to lymph nodes is a relatively slow process that could take a few months to one year.[2] It is apparent that particle clearance from the nasopharyngeal or tracheobronchial region for water-soluble particles is much faster than clearance from the pulmonary region. Consequently, deposited particles can act much longer in alveoli than in the nose, trachea, or bronchi. This is one reason why water-soluble particles in general are more toxic to alveoli than to the upper respiratory tract.[r7]

Knowledge of the patterns of initial deposition of inhaled particles of various substances within the respiratory tract is essential for determining future clear-

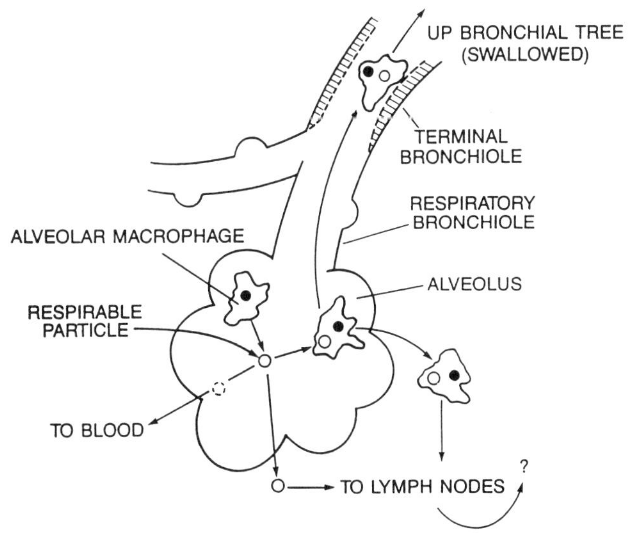

Figure 105.2 Pathways of Particle Clearance from Alveoli

ance and dose patterns. Therefore, site of deposition is important in assessing the potential toxicity associated with particles. Aerosol particles that impinge on the respiratory tract surface normally stay on the surface unless cleared (by coughing, mucociliary clearance, etc.). This process is called deposition. Retention in inhalation toxicology pertains to the persistence of deposited material on the respiratory surfaces:

Deposition − clearance = Retention
or 100% − % cleared = % Retained;
consequently, 100 − % Retained = % Cleared

Gaseous Asphyxiants

Asphyxiants produce toxic effects by interfering with the supply of oxygen to the tissues.[3] Anything that decreases the partial pressure of oxygen in the alveoli tends to decrease the alveolar-venous oxygen pressure gradient and therefore to decrease the amount of oxygen entering the blood. Simple asphyxiants are substances that dilute the oxygen in the air, reducing its rate of transfer to venous blood without any further chemical action, possibly without even entering the blood. Examples include carbon dioxide, nitrous oxide, nitrogen, or hydrocarbons such as natural gas.

Other inhaled compounds may chemically block the transport of oxygen to the tissues or the utilization of oxygen once it reaches the tissues. The two most common examples are carbon monoxide, which blocks the site on hemoglobin where oxygen is bound for transport, and hydrogen cyanide, which blocks the pathway by which the tissues utilize oxygen. Carbon monoxide is particularly dangerous because it is a common product of incomplete combustion of fuels and because of its lack of odor or irritant activity.

Chemical Vapors

A large number of chemical vapors and metal fumes have been identified as causes of respiratory toxicity at sufficiently high concentrations., Some commonly encountered vapors are chlorine gas, ammonia gas, oxides of sulfur, and oxides of nitrogen. Exposure to these gases causes direct injury to the exposed tissues of the respiratory system. The site of injury depends on the concentration of gas, the duration of exposure, and the solubility of the gas in the body fluids. Exposure could cause signs and symptoms that vary from irritation of the upper air passages, with resulting rhinitis and sinusitis, to tracheobronchitis, with cough, sputum production, and bronchospasm. Finally, if the substance reaches the alveolus in sufficient concentration, alveolar damage will result, with either an alveolitis and subsequent diffuse fibrosis or, if the damage is massive and acute, to sudden pulmonary edema or the adult respiratory distress syndrome (ARDS).

A number of metal fumes have been identified as respiratory toxicants. These include cadmium, nickel, mercury, and others. As with chemical vapors, the site of damage within the respiratory system depends on the concentration of the metal fume, the duration of exposure, and the physical/chemical characteristics of the metal fume itself.

Hygienic Air Quality Standards

It was not until the turn of the century that specific attention began to be developed to the preventive aspects of industrial illness. Even during this early period, the exposure patterns that existed were more complex and complicated than the instrumentation for sample collection and analysis could define. In spite of these limitations, it became apparent that methods were needed for indexing airborne levels of contamination in the workplace. Over the last 50 years, the limits for acceptable levels of exposure that have gradually come to be the most widely accepted are those established by the American Conference of Governmental Industrial Hygienists (ACGIH), which are termed Threshold Limit Values (TLV).*

The ACGIH TLVs are concentrations of airborne substances to which nearly all employees may be repeatedly exposed daily throughout a working lifetime without adverse health effects. The TLVs are values based on available toxicology data, occupational exposure data, medical experience, and by analogy with similar chemicals. They are intended to be used as guidelines for evaluating and controlling employee exposures, not as fine lines between safe and dangerous concentrations.

These TLVs are expressed as parts of vapor or gas per million parts of air by volume (ppm) at 25°C and 760 mm Hg pressure, or as approximate milligrams of substance per cubic meter of air (mg/m^3). Mineral dusts are expressed as millions of particles per cubic feet (mppcf). Most TLVs represent Time-Weighted Average (TWA) concentrations for an eight-hour work day, 40-hour work week. The term TWA is ideally suited to the determination of chemical exposures because it emphasizes that exposures are functions of primarily two variables: time and concentration. The TWA exposures may be measured by monitoring the breathing zone of a person (personal air sample) or can be calculated form work area air sample results and weighting with estimated time distribution in each area. ACGIH TWAs are normally expressed as eight-hour values:

$$\text{TWA Exposure: } \frac{C1T1 + C2T2 + \dots\dots\dots + CnTn}{T1 + T2 + \dots\dots\dots\ Tn}$$

*TLV Trademark of American Conference of Governmental Industrial Hygienists.

Where Cn = Concentration measured at work location "n" in parts per million volume by volume (ppm).
Tn = Time spent by the employe at work location "n" in hours and TWA exposure is expressed in ppm or mg/m^3.

Conversion from mg/m^3 to ppm can be performed by the following formula:

$$\text{ppm} = \frac{\text{mg/m}^3 \times 24.4 \text{ liters/mole}}{\text{Molecular Weight of Test Substance (g/mole)}}$$

While the ACGIH TLVs continue to be used extensively, many countries individually have established other legal levels of exposure for airborne contaminants in the occupational environment.

Respiratory Tract Responses

Occupational Asthma

One of the primary effects of noxious agents on the respiratory tract is occupational asthma induced by exposure to a specific agent encountered in the workplace. Table 105.1 lists some causes of occupational asthma. Clinical signs of occupational asthma include wheezing and shortness of breath.[4]

Industrial Bronchitis

Any long-continued exposure to dust, no matter whether the dust be mineral or vegetable, can lead to the development of cough and sputum and a condition that is referred to as "industrial bronchitis." Industrial bronchitis has been reported in asbestos workers, textile workers, manufacturers of cement, foundry workers, and pulp and paper mill workers exposed to sulfur dioxide.[r8]

Table 105.1 Causes of Occupational Asthma

Chemicals
Toluene diisocyanate
Phthalic anhydride
Formaldehyde
Animal and biologic products
Papain
Bacillus subtilis products (detergent enzymes)
Ampicillin
Piperazine
Tetracycline
Animal dander
Wheat and rye flour (baker's asthma)
Silkworms
Metals
Nickel
Cobalt
Platinum salts

Occupational Lung Cancer

There are a number of well-recognized occupational carcinogens, which include asbestos, chromium, arsenic, bischloromethyl ether, mustard gas, and coke oven effluent.[r9] In addition, uranium, iron, and fluorspar miners are at increased risk of developing cancer from the inhalation of radon daughters formed from the breakdown of uranium. Coke oven workers are exposed to a variety of polycyclic hydrocarbons, e.g., benzpyrene. Table 105.2 lists the major known and suspected causes of occupational lung cancer, although some of these remain controversial despite decades of research.

Pneumoconiosis

Silicosis, asbestosis, and anthracosis, as well as pulmonary dust disease of talc miners, clay workers, and others employed in the "dusty" trades, all come within the general classification of pneumoconiosis. Pneumoconiosis is defined as a "condition" caused by the action of certain fine dust particles in the lungs. The pneumoconiatic state may be entirely benign, with no evidence of immediate or long-term ill effects from the dust deposits in the lungs (e.g., pneumoconiosis from tin oxide). In another form, it may lead to such respiratory damage as "acute" silicosis or to slowly developing fibrosis.

Allergic and Other Sensitivity Responses

Allergy is the enhanced reactivity of sensitized tissue to the presence of a specific sensitizing substance. Since specific sensitizing substances may be inhaled, it is therefore appropriate to include allergic reactions in the complex of disorders that may result from the inhalation of contaminants in air.[r10]

Substances capable of initiating allergic reactions include first and foremost products of plant life, such as pollens and fungi. Industrially produced materials that may evoke similar reactions include nickel, chromium, and beryllium compounds. A widely used industrial organic compound that causes respiratory sensitization is toluene diisocyanate (TDI). TDI is a raw material in the production of some polyurethane foams. Other materials can produce similar allergic responses; certain amines, Isocyanates and epoxy com-

Table 105.2 Occupational Health and Associated Cancers

Agent	Tumor Sites	Occupation
X-rays	Bone marrow and skin	Medical and industrial
Radon gas, radium, and uranium	Skin, Lung, and bone	Medical and industrial chemists, painters, and miners
Ultraviolet radiation	Skin	Outdoor occupations
Polycyclic hydrocarbons in soot, tar, and coal	Lung, skin, bladder, and nasal cavity	Furnaces, forges and foundries, gas workers
Benzene	Bone marrow and lymph nodes	Process, textile and explosives workers
Naphthylamine, biphenylamine, and nitrobiphenyls	Bladder	Dyestuff, rubber, and chemical plant workers
Mustard gas	Bronchial tree, lung, and larynx	Production workers
Vinyl chloride	Liver	Plastic manufacture
Arsenic	Skin, lung, and liver	Smelters and oil refiners
Chromium	Lung, nasal cavity, and sinuses	Process, production, and pigment workers
Cadmium	Lung, kidney, and prostate	Smelter and battery workers
Nickel	Lung and nasal sinuses	Smelters and process workers
Asbestos and similar fibers	Lung, pleura, and peritoneum larynx, stomach, and large bowel	Miners, millers manufacturers, users, and demolition workers

Source: Cartwright RA. Cancer epidemiology in chemical carcinogens. American Chemical Society Monograph 182, 1984.

pounds are known to be sensitizers and, when inhaled, can cause allergic reactions. (Montanaro, 1992)

Dermal Responses

Experience has demonstrated that the skin provides a fairly effective barrier to penetration by most materials in the workplace environment.[r11] Nonetheless, skin can absorb materials to reduce systemic toxicity at high doses. An example is that of organophosphate pesticides. Most substances can penetrate the skin to varying degrees, depending on their physical and chemical properties and on the topography of the skin. (Paustenbach & Leung, 1992) However, for brevity, this discussion will be confined to work-related topical responses of the skin. The skin is the largest organ of the body and serves as the major interface between humans and their environment. Industrial employees may contract occupational dermatoses, which are defined as any abnormal condition of the skin caused or aggravated by substances or processes associated with the work environment. These may range from erythema and urticaria to eczematous or neoplastic processes. Occupational skin disease is still the most frequent of all occupational disease and accounts for more than 40 percent of all occupational diseases reported in the US.

Contact Dermatitis

Contact dermatitis is the most frequent cause of occupational skin disease. Two types are generally recognized: irritant and allergic. They are difficult to differentiate clinically. Classically, it is stated that 80 percent of all cases of occupational contact dermatitis result from primary irritants and 20 percent from allergic sensitizers. A primary irritant is a substance that causes damage at the site of contact because of its direct chemical or physical action on the skin. The characteristic lesions are pink to red patches or plaques with fine scales that usually form collarettes.[r12] When acute, edema may impart to the lesions an appearance ranging from lustrous to oozing to blistering. Chronic lesions are dry and scaly. More than 2000 chemicals are classed as primary irritants, and several new compounds are added to that list each year. The irritant potential of a substance depends on the condition of the skin, the chemical properties and concentration of the substance, the length of exposure, and a variety of physical factors. Primary irritants generally affect anyone in contact with them. The action of primary skin irritants include protein and keratin dissolution (alkalis); lipid dissolution (organic solvents); dehydration (inorganic acids, anhydrides); oxidation (bleaches); reduction (salicylic, formic, and oxalic acids); and keratogenesis (arsenic, tars, and petroleum).

Occupational agents that are potential antigens/haptens may cause eczematous allergic dermatitis. Allergic dermatitis is a form of cell-mediated immunity (Type IV). Sensitizing agents differ from primary irritants in their mechanisms of action. Unless they are concomitant irritants, most sensitizers do not produce a skin reaction on first contact. Generally, irritants increase the response to an allergen in allergic contact dermatitis. (McLelland et al, 1991). After a sensitization phase of one week or longer, further contact with the same or a cross-reacting substance on the same or other parts of the body results in an acute dermatitis (elicitation phase).[5] Approximately 200 chemicals have been implicated in occupational allergic sensitization. Major occupational skin sensitizers include paraphenylenediamine, nickel compounds, ethylenediamine, chromates, epoxy resins, formaldehyde, and cobalt compounds. Allergic contact dermatitis comprises approximately 25 percent of all reported instances of occupational skin disease.[r13] The most reliable way to test for allergic dermatitis is the patch test. A drop of standardized concentrations of each allergen is applied to the skin, usually of the upper back. The substance is covered with transparent tape and each patch examined for erythema 48 hours later.

Other chemicals can sensitize the skin to light so that a worker so sensitized may develop sunburn more easily than those not exposed. The same types of chemicals can lead to skin rashes, such as urticaria (hives) and eczematous skin lesions when the skin is subsequently exposed to light. Such chemicals are known as photosensitizers. Reaction to such chemicals may be immediate, but more commonly are delayed for 48 hours or longer. Initially, the intensity of pruritic and eczematous lesions appear over light exposed and have sharply demarcated margins. Later, the lesions become widespread and lichenified from rubbing.

In industry, coal tar distillation may afford exposure to anthracene, phenathracene, and acridine, all known photoreactive chemicals. Related products such as creosote, pitch, and roof paint are well known causes of hyperpigmentation resulting from the interaction of coal tar agents and sunlight.[r14]

Occupational Acne/Chloracne

Occupational acne is a name applied to any inflammatory condition of the sebaceous glands resulting from contact with petroleum and its derivatives (coal tar products or certain halogenated aromatic hydrocarbons). The skin eruption may be mild and localized, or severe and generalized. The primary lesion of chloracne is comedone formation. As evidence of toxicity increases, small straw-colored cysts from 1 to 10 mm in diameter are formed, intermingled with comedones. Mild cases appear on the most sensitive areas of the human skin, particularly around the eyes, malar crescent, and behind the ears. If sufficient exposure has occurred, lesions may appear on the shoulders, chest, and back. It has been suggested that lesions are formed owing to irritation of the sebaceous glands by the excreted chlorinated compounds. Comedones usually occur within two to three weeks after exposure and in 80 percent of cases clear within three years, although in severe cases they can last for decades.

Occupational acne is seen most commonly in mechanics exposed to grease and lubrication oils and in workers exposed to cutting oils. A number of outbreaks of chloracne occurring among workers exposed to azobenzenes, polychlorinated biphenyls (PCB's), and 2,3,7,8-tetrachlorodibenzo-p-dioxin (TCDD) have been reported. Coal tar factory laborers as well as roofers and construction or road maintenance workers may develop tar acne.

Occupational Skin Tumors

The first documented cases of occupational skin cancer developed in the scrotum of chimney sweeps in Great Britain in 1778. Chemically-induced skin tumors among occupational workers is rare. The most common cause of occupationally related skin cancer is ultraviolet radiation. Keratocanthomas may be occupationally associated with sunlight exposure and/or contact with various tars, pitch, and oils.

Pharmacokinetic Models in Hazard Assessment

Estimation of Human Risk from Animal Studies

It is clear that there are many differences between experimental test animals and human beings that may affect the researcher's ability to extrapolate from animal toxicity results to humans. Animals used in the laboratory tests come from carefully bred homogeneous strains, are carefully screened to be free of disease, and all the animals are young adults at the start of the test. For practical reasons, small groups of animals are used, and limited numbers of chemical doses are evaluated. Doses are usually set very high (in the hope of increasing the sensitivity of the toxicology test), and chemicals are administered by the most experimentally convenient route.

Of necessity, a variety of experimentations are necessary in order to estimate hazard from animal studies. In recent years, these extrapolations have been aided by the development of mathematical models that consider (in a quantitative manner) physiologic properties of the different species, differences in routes of exposure, compound-specific partitioning of the chemical between tissues and blood, and concentration-dependent rates of metabolism. These physiologically-based pharmacokinetic (PB-PK) models have been particularly useful for high-dose/low-dose extrapolations, dose-route extrapolations, and interspecies extrapolations.

Construction of Physiologically-Based Models

The concept of incorporating physiologic principles into pharmacokinetic modeling was discussed more than 50 years ago,[6] but the technology for implementing this concept has not been available until recently. However, with the advent of powerful computers and "user-friendly" simulation languages, it has become possible for toxicologists to construct quantitative models of complex biologic phenomena. The PB-PK model for methylene chloride is a good example of such a model.[r15]

A diagram of the model developed by Anderson et al. is presented in Figure 105.3. The mammalian organism is represented as a collection of compartments with similar partition coefficients and blood flow rates, linked with the GI tract and the lung by circulating blood. The sizes of the compartments for each species correspond to known volumes of tissues in the human and rodent species. In addition, the breathing rates and blood flow rates are set to correspond to the characteristic properties of each species. This information is available from studies of each species published in the scientific literature.

Chemicals may enter the body of the animal in this model through inhalation, ingestion, or IV injection. Other routes of exposure such as dermal absorption of vapors or liquids have been described, but are not shown in this model. Once in the body, the chemical is distributed to the tissues by circulating blood. During circulation, the blood comes to equilibrium with the tissues at a concentration related to the blood/tissue partition coefficient. Inhaled and exhaled air also reach equilibrium at concentrations related to the blood/air partition coefficients. The partition coefficients used in these models are constants that may be determined experimentally for specific chemicals and tissues according to a variety of techniques.[r16]

Chemicals may be eliminated from the body in this model in expired air, or may be destroyed by metabolic enzymes present in the organism. The concentration-dependent rates of metabolism in the various species can also be determined through a variety of in vivo and in vitro procedures and them incorporated into the PB-PK model in a quantitative fashion.

Once the physiologic, physical chemical, and biochemical constants are known for a particular chemical/species combination, a series of simultaneous differential equations describing the rates of change of chemical in each compartment may be written. Derivation of the equations for disposition of chloroform in a PB-PK model has been described,[7] and this general approach is applicable to almost any chemical, species, or route of exposure with appropriate modifications.[8]

These quantitative models can help to reduce the uncertainty inherent in estimating human hazard from animal studies. Other promising applications include elucidating mechanisms of toxicity, description of dermal absorption, and even predicting the shape of the dose-response curve for carcinogenic agents.[9]

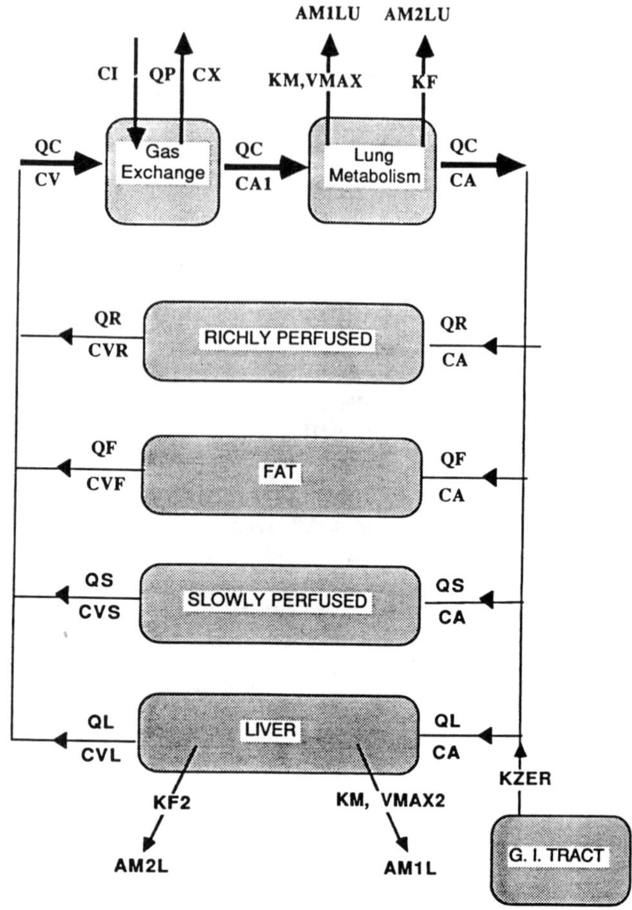

Figure 105.3 A Physiologically-based Pharmacokinetic Model for Methylene Chloride

Conclusions

Chemical materials and chemical formulations play an important role in industrial society. To ensure a safe working environment it is often necessary to determine and quantify substances in the atmosphere. A successful occupational health program requires communication between the toxicologist involved in assessing the potential toxicity of a material, the industrial hygienist evaluating and controlling the exposure of personnel, and the occupational physician monitoring the health status of the employees. Under normal production conditions, conventional industrial hygiene practices (maintaining occupational exposures below acceptable limits) adequately protect employees. However, accidental overexposures can occur. Therefore, it is desirable that everyone working with chemicals be well informed regarding the hazard of the materials, the appropriate procedures, and protective devices to be used with each.

The essential element in practical precautionary measures for the handling of chemicals is common sense based on a thorough knowledge of the toxicologic properties of the material and the conditions of use. The common sense approach does not mean that poor practices can be continued because they have not caused difficulty in the past. Reasonable control measures include an adequate margin of safety in anticipation of the normal variability of individual work practices.

References

Research Reports

1. Kehrer JP, Kacew, S. Systemically applied chemicals that damage lung tissue. Toxicology 1985;*35*:251–293.
2. Lippmann M, Yeates DB, Alber RE. Deposition, retention and clearance of inhaled particles. Br J Med 1980;*37*:337–362.
3. Warheit DB. Interspecies comparisons of lung responses to inhaled particles and gases. Crit Rev Toxicol 1989;*20*:1–29.
4. Fine JF, Balmes J. Airway inhalation and occupational asthma. Clin Chest Med 1988;*4*:577–590.
5. Zweiman B. Methods of allergic inflammation in the skin. Clin Allergy 1988;*18*:419–433.
6. Teorell T. Kinetic distribution of substances administered to the body. Arch Int Pharmacodyn Therap. 1937;*57*:205–240.
7. Corley RA, Mendrala AM, Smith FA, Staats DA, Gargas ML, Connoly RB, Anderson ME, Reitz RH. Development of a physiologically-based pharmacokinetic model for chloroform. Toxicol Appl Pharmacol 1990;*103*:512–527.
8. Anderson ME, Clewell HJ, Gargas ML, MacNaughton MG, Reitz RH, Nolan RJ, McKenna MJ. Physiologically based pharmacokinetic modeling with dichloromethane, its metabolite, carbon monoxide, and blood carboxyhemoglobin in rats and Humans. Toxicol Appl Pharmacol 1991;*108*:14–27.
9. Reitz RH, Mendrala AM, Corley RA, Quast JF, Gargas ML, Anderson ME, Staats DA, Conolly RB. Estimating the risk of liver cancer associated with human exposures to chloroform using physiologically-based pharmacokinetic modeling. Toxicol Appl Pharmacol. 1990;*105*:443–459.
10. McLelland J, Schuster S, Matthews, JNS. 'Irritants' increase the response to an allergen in allergic contact dermatitis. Arch. Dermatol. 1991;*127*:1016–1019.

Reviews

r1. Chang-Yeung M, Lam S. Occupational asthma—state of the art. Am Rev Resp Dis 1986;*133*:686–703.

r2. Gordon T, Amdur MO. Response of the respiratory system to toxic agents. In: Amdur MO, Doull J, Klassen CD. Casarett and Doull's toxicology. The basic science of poisons. New York: Pergamon Press, (1991); pp 383–406.

r3. Schlesinger RB. Disposition and clearance of inhaled particles. In McClellan RO. Henderson RF. Concepts in inhalation toxicology. New York: Hemisphere, (1989); pp 163–192.

r4. Raahe OG, Al-Bayati MA, Teague SV, Rasolt A. Regional deposition of inhaled monodisperse coarse and fine aerosol particles in small laboratory animals. In: Dodson J. McCallum RI. Bailey MR. Fisher DR. Inhaled particles Oxford: Pergamon Press, (1988); pp 53–63.

r5. Casarett LJ. The vital sacs: alveolar clearance mechanism in inhalation toxicology. In: Hayes WJ Jr. Essays In toxicology. New York: Academic Press, (1972);*3*:pp 1–36.

r6. Dodson VN. Zenz C. Occupational cancer risks In: Zenz CO Occupational medicine. Principles and practical applications. Chicago: Year Book. (1988); pp 815–832.

r7. Newman LS. Pulmonary toxicology. In: Sullivan JH Jr, Krieger GR. Hazardous materials toxicology: Clinical principles of environmental health Baltimore: Williams & Wilkins (1992); pp 124–144.

r8. Davis GS, Calhoun WJ. Occupational and environmental causes of lung disease. In: Schwarz MI, King RE. Interstitial lung disease. Philadelphia: BC Decker, (1988); pp 63–109.

r9. Cone JE. Occupational lung cancer. In: Rosenstock L. Occupational pulmonary disease. Occup. Med. State of the Art Rev. *Ed:* Philadelphia: Hanley & Belfus, 1987;*2*:pp 273–295.

r10. Shepard D. Significance of airway hyper-responsiveness to occupational and environmental lung disorders. Semin Respir Med 1986;*7*:241–248.

r11. Emmett EA. Toxic responses of the skin. In: Amdur MO, Doull J, Klassen CD. Casarett and Doull's toxicology. The basic science of poisons. New York: Pergamon Press, (1991); pp 463–483.

r12. Bjornberg A. Irritant dermatitis. In: Maibach HI. Occupational and industrial dermatology. Chicago: Year Book, (1987); pp 15–21.

r13. Adams RM. Contact dermatitis due to irritation and allergic sensitization. In: Adam RM. Occupational skin disease. New York: Grune and Stratton, (1988); pp 815–832.

r14. Sanchez MR. Dermatologic principles. In: Goldfrank LR, Flomenbaum NE, Lewin NA, Weisman RS, Howland MA. Goldfrank's toxicologic emergencies. Norwalk: Appleton & Lange, (1990); pp 187–208.

r15. National Academy of Sciences: Proceedings of the Pharmacokinetics in Risk Assessment Workshop. Washington: National Academy Press, 1987.

r16. Reitz RH. Distribution, persistence, and elimination of toxic agents (pharmacokinetics). In: Clayson DB, Munro IC, Shubik P, Swenberg JA. Progress in predictive toxicology. Amsterdam: Elsevier, (1990); pp 79–90.

r17. Hext PM, Bennett IP. Inhalation Toxicology. *In* General and Applied Toxicology, Ballantyne B, Marrs T, Turner P (Eds.) New York, NY: M Stockton Press (1993); pp 453–465.

r18. Montanaro A. Isocyanate asthma, *in* Bardana, EJ, Montanaro A, O'Hollaren MT. (Eds), *Occupational Asthma*. Philadelphia: Hanley & Belfus (1992); pp 179–188.

r19. Paustenbach DJ, Leung HW. Techniques for assessing the health risks of dermal contact with chemicals in the environment. *In* Wang RG, Knaak JB, Maibach HI (Eds.) Health Risk Assessment through Dermal and Inhalation Exposure and Absorption of Toxicants. Boca Raton, Florida: CRC Press (1992); pp 343–385.

CHAPTER 106

Gabriel L. Plaa

Environmental Toxicology

People today are greatly concerned about the environment and the impact of the activities of modern society on the planet. Political parties whose major objective is preservation of the environment have appeared in several countries. At a local level, we are now much more aware that chemical pollution may severely affect our own state of well-being as well as that of other forms of life in the environment. Environmental toxicology deals with the potentially deleterious impact of chemicals, present as pollutants of the environment, on living organisms. The term "environment" includes all the surroundings (biotic and abiotic) of an individual organism, but in particular the air, soil, and water. A "pollutant" is a substance that appears in the environment, at least in part as a result of human activity, and that has a deleterious effect on living organisms. While humans are considered a target species of particular interest, other terrestrial and aquatic species are of considerable importance as potential biologic targets.

In this chapter general concepts of environmental toxicology will be presented. In addition some chemicals of major concern will be discussed.

Ecotoxicology

Ecotoxicology has evolved as an extension of environmental toxicology.[r1–r4] However, the terms "environmental toxicology" and "ecotoxicology" are not interchangeable. Ecotoxicology is concerned with the toxic effects of chemical and physical agents on living organisms, but more particularly on populations and communities within defined ecosystems;[r3,r4] it includes the transfer pathways of those agents and their interactions with the environment. While traditional toxicology is concerned with toxic effects on *individual* organisms, ecotoxicology is concerned with the impact on *populations* of living organisms, a *community of populations*, or on an *ecosystem*. Furthermore, an ecosystem consists not only of a biologic community, but also its abiotic, inanimate habitat. In ecotoxicology there are three interacting components (Fig. 106.1): the toxicant; the environment; and the organisms (community, population, or ecosystem). The environment may modify the toxicant or the response of the organism to the toxicant; the toxicant may affect the organism directly or modify the environment; the organism may modify the toxicant or the environment. An environmental event that, exerts severe effects on individual organisms may have no important impact on populations or an ecosystem. The reverse is also true: some pollutants might have little immediate effect on individual organisms, but have considerable ecologic consequences later.

Predictions based on known toxicologic events are difficult when dealing with ecotoxicology. Appropriate methodology has not been developed to approach the complex situations present. Much of the methodology is only an extension of the procedures employed in traditional toxicology. In traditional toxicology, however, the biologic target and the toxicant are usually well identified; knowledge about exposure conditions is usually available; the consequences can be determined for the single individual. This is particu-

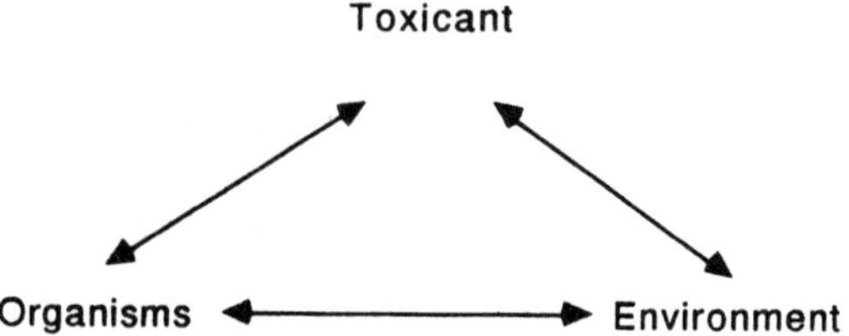

Figure 106.1 Interacting Components in Ecotoxicology Involving Populations or Communities of Living Organisms

larly true when dealing with the potential toxic effects of drug therapy in patients. On the other hand, with ecotoxicology, the biologic targets and the toxicants are usually poorly described, and little information is available on exposure conditions. Thus, it is understandable that methods developed for assessing the toxic properties of medications are not readily applicable to ecotoxicologic problems.

Environmental Pollution

Chemical pollution is an undesirable modification of the natural environment caused, in whole or in part, by the actions of humans. The modifications can affect humans directly or via agricultural resources, water, and other biologic products; recreational resources may be affected as well. Finally, the natural constituents of the biosphere can be perturbed.

Pollution has paralleled technologic advances. Industrialization and the creation of large urban centers have led to contamination of air, water, and soil. However, major preoccupation of governments with problems of chemical pollution is a relatively recent phenomenon (about 30 years). The general population has become much more aware of the situation in the last ten years. Today, the industrialized countries of the world are gravely concerned about the environmental impact of potentially toxic chemicals, particularly those that are poorly degraded either biologically or photochemically.

The principal causes of pollution are related to the production and use of energy, the production and use of industrial chemicals, and increased agricultural activity.[r3–r5] The use of fossil fuels, particularly petroleum hydrocarbons, is a leading cause of pollution because it is involved in all forms of human activity. In a period of 40 years (1930–1970), there was about a 1000 percent increase in the production of petroleum, whereas production of coal increased only about 70 percent. Regarding industrial chemicals, estimates indicate that more than 60,000 chemicals are in common use and that about 500 new chemicals enter the commercial market annually, although many more new chemicals are actually synthesized. One needs to know how these chemicals can be utilized by society without being hazardous to its members and the environment. Chemical contamination was once fairly well restricted to industrialized urban centers. Now, however, it is evident that contamination of the natural environment extends to all parts of the planet (e.g., DDT and PCB have been detected in arctic and in antarctic regions). The dispersion of chemicals can have important consequences. Increased agricultural activities have led to a massive increase in the use of chemical fertilizers and pesticides; in the US, the production of pesticides rose about tenfold in a 25-year period (1945–1970). It has been pointed out that although the appearance of chemicals in the environment can have an important ecotoxicologic impact, deforestation and agricultural intensification as a whole can exert a far greater global impact on the environment (macrodisturbances in natural cycles) than will chemical pollutants.

The presence of chemical dump sites now appears as a form of local or regional pollution.[r6] In 1978, this type of potential hazard was dramatically illustrated by the Love Canal landfill in Niagara Falls, New York, where it is estimated that about 21,000 tons of chemical wastes had been buried over a ten-year period (1942–1952). By 1972, residential areas abutted the landfill; odors, surfacing of chemically contaminated wastes, and underground infiltration of basements occurred. Love Canal is not an isolated instance, since Dietz et al.[r7] estimate that about 264 million wet metric tonnes (1 metric tonne = 1.1 English tons) of hazardous waste (US Resource Conservation and Recovery Act-regulated) were generated in 1981. In 1981, the estimated number of treatment, storage, and disposal facilities for RCRA-regulated hazardous waste was around 5000; the EPA Superfund Task Force in the US estimates that the number of national priority sites for remedial action is around 2500. A major concern is how to deal with chemicals that are present not as single entities, but as mixtures.[r8]

Characteristics of Chemical Pollutants

Certain chemical and physical characteristics are known to be important in estimating the potential hazard of environmental toxicants. In addition to information regarding effects on different organisms, knowledge about the following properties is essential to predict environmental impact: the degradability of the substance; its mobility through air, water, and soil; whether bioaccumulation occurs; and its transport and biomagnification through food chains.

Chemicals that are poorly degraded (by abiotic or biotic pathways) exhibit environmental persistence and thus can accumulate. Lipophilic substances tend to bioaccumulate in body fat, resulting in tissue residues. Unless rapidly biotransformed, they persist in the tissues and are transferred to the next trophic level. At each level, the lipophilic toxicant tends to be retained, thus increasing the toxicant concentration. When the toxicant is incorporated into the food chain, biomagnification occurs as one species feeds upon others and concentrates the chemical. Figure 106.2 depicts the food chain for soil residues. The pollutants that have the widest environmental impact are poorly degradable; relatively mobile in air, water, and soil; exhibit bioaccumulation; and also exhibit biomagnification.

The transport and dispersion of pollutants on the planet can be remarkable.[r3,r4] While many chemicals may remain relatively localized, certain physical and even biologic phenomena can lead to their dissemination to distant parts of the globe. Atmospheric movements can play a primary role. A few examples include the presence of DDT in antarctic snow, accumulation of DDT and lindane in the northernmost soils of Sweden, and correlation between rainfall and PCB residues in plankton from the gulf of the Saint Lawrence in Canada. Precipitation is the vehicle that brings atmospheric pollutants back to the soil or the hydrosphere. The phenomenon of acid rain is a prime example. Water erosion of land also works to transfer pollutants toward the hydrosphere.

Bioaccumulation also plays a role in environmental transport, although this process results in concentration rather than diffusion of the pollutant. High lipid solubility and poor biodegradability are chemical properties that lead to bioaccumulation. When bioaccumulation occurs in the food chain, the result is transfer of the pollutant. Several examples of this situation are well documented. One is the treatment of Clear Lake, California, with DDD to rid this recreational area of gnats. The lake was treated in 1945, 1954, and 1957. The final unintended victim of these applications was the grebe, a fish-eating bird. Many birds died and reproduction among the survivors decreased markedly. The following food-chain bioaccumulation was observed: water (0.014 ppm) < plankton (5 ppm) < fish (7–220 ppm) < grebes (2500 ppm).[r4] With methyl mercury pollution, the Minamata episode resulting in severe intoxications of humans in Japan is well documented; bioaccumulation in fish reached levels that were 400,000 times those found in the water: water (0.1 ppb) < plankton (10 ppm) < fish (40 ppm). Similar figures were observed in Sweden: water (0.1 ppb) < plankton (10–500 ppb) < fish (0.5–4 ppm).[r4]

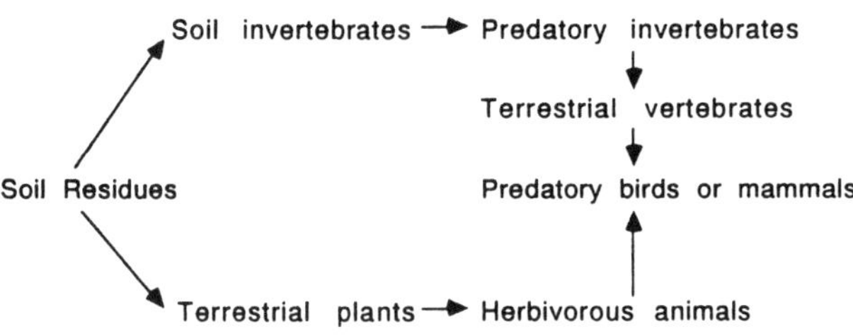

Figure 106.2 Environmental Movement of Soil Residues in Food Chains.[r5]

It is difficult to obtain data for humans regarding bioaccumulation of lipophilic chemicals. Geyer et al.[r9] estimated such values for human lipid for 11 compounds of environmental interest. They classified these chemicals into three categories on the basis of their bioconcentration potential (BCP): high BCP, > 100; medium BCP, 10–100; and low BCP, < 10. This classification is summarized in Table 106.1. Their approach could be useful in assessing the environmental consequences of other agents.

Because of their widespread utilization, certain pesticides are important sources of environmental pollution. Their degree of persistence in the environment is an important determinant.[r10] In this context, persistence is defined as the time required for 75 to 100 percent disappearance of residues from the site of application. The major classes of pesticides have been categorized as "persistent," "moderately persistent," or "nonpersistent." Examples are given in Table 106.2. The chlorinated hydrocarbon insecticides are considered persistent and are of primary importance as pollutants because of their slow degradability in soil and water, mainly by microorganisms and photochemical reactions. Coupled with high lipid solubility, their chemical stability contributes to bioaccumulation. Volatilization into the atmosphere from water and soil occurs. Consequently, their distribution is widespread.

Table 106.1 Estimated Bioconcentration Potentials of Several Chemicals for Human Lipid Tissue[a]

Chemical	BCP
High Bioconcentration Potential	
Polychlorinated biphenyls (PCB)	250
2,3,7,8-Tetrachlorodibenzo-*p*-dioxin (TCDD)	170
DDT and metabolites	1280
Hexachlorobenzene	670
β-Hexachlorocyclohexane	525
Medium Bioconcentration Potential	
Dieldrin	70
α-Hexachlorocyclohexane	20
γ-Hexachlorocyclohexane	20
Low Bioconcentration Potential	
δ-Hexachlorocyclohexane	9
Pentachlorophenol	4
3,5-Di-tert-4-butyl-4-hydroxytoluene	1

[a]Data obtained from[r9]

Table 106.2 Classification of Pesticides in Terms of Persistence[a]

Persistent (2–5 years)[b]
Chlorinated hydrocarbon insecticides
DDT, Methoxychlor and related compounds
Cyclodienes
Hexachlorocyclohexanes
Polychloroterpenes
Cationic herbicides
Paraquat, diquat
Moderately persistent (1–8 months)
Triazine herbicides
Phenyl herbicides
Substituted dinitroaniline herbicides
Nonpersistent (1–12 weeks)
Phenoxy and related acidic herbicides
Phenylcarbamate and carbanilate herbicides
Ethylenebisdithiocarbamate fungicides
Organophosphorus and carbamate insecticides

[a]Data obtained from[r10]
[b]Time required for 75–100% disappearance from site of application

Cationic herbicides like diquat and paraquat are also quite stable. They, however, are strongly adsorbed to soil particles. Transport in the environment is limited, since they are not volatile. Other pesticides are of lesser importance as widespread environmental pollutants because of their greater degree of degradability (biotic and abiotic) and more limited transport. There are biologic problems, however, of a regional or local nature. The ethylene bisdithiocarbamate fungicides are of concern, although they are nonpersistent. One of their degradation products is ethylene thiourea, which has carcinogenic properties; the importance of the presence of this substance in soil residues remains unresolved.

Some nonpesticidal chemicals of importance as pollutants are given in Table 106.3. The polychlorinated biphenyls (PCB) are established as important global pollutants with exceptionally high persistence. The phthalate ester plasticizers are found ubiquitously in soil and water. The environmental problems associated with methyl mercury, lead, and cadmium are well known.[r10] The problem posed by the appearance of aliphatic halogenated hydrocarbons in treated drinking water is of considerable interest. Current indications are that chlorination of water containing humic substances can result in the chemical formation of chloroform, bromochloromethanes, and bromoform, resulting in the appearance of these chemicals in finished drinking water; the long-term consequences of such a situation are not known.

Chemicals in the Environment and Cancer

In the last 30 years, studies have been conducted to determine potential causes of cancer in humans. Epidemiologic studies suggest that about 70 to 80 percent of human cancers appear to be potentially avoidable, since they appear to be caused by "extrinsic factors" external to the biologic make-up ("intrinsic factors") of the individual. In the literature, the term "environmental factors" is often substituted for "extrinsic factors." Unfortunately, the term "environmental factors" has been misinterpreted by some to mean only "man-made chemicals," leading to the erroneous interpretation that man-made chemicals present in the environment might be responsible for the majority of human cancers. In 1981, Doll and Peto published an extensive review of the causes of human cancer deaths in the US.[1] Their estimates indicate that about 30 percent of potentially avoidable human cancer deaths are associated with the use of tobacco products; another 30 to 40 percent appear related to dietary habits and life-style. Less than 7 percent (4 percent occupation, 2% pollution, 1% industrial products) of avoidable human cancer deaths were associated with chemicals found in the environment, including the occupational setting (Table 106.4). Examples of chemicals known as human carcinogens are included in Table 106.5. It is important to realize that man-made chemicals probably account for a minority of human cancer deaths. Thus, the presence of synthetic chemicals in the environment is not associated as a major cause of human cancer deaths. The purpose of presenting these data is not to minimize the potentially adverse effects of pollutants, but merely to put man-made chemical agents in perspective with

Table 106.3 Nonpesticidal Chemicals as Pollutants of Water and Soil[a]

Aromatic halogenated hydrocarbons
Polychlorinated biphenyls, chlorophenols, dioxin
Low-molecular weight aliphatic halogenated hydrocarbons
Chloroform, bromodichloromethane, dibromochloromethane, bromoform
Phthalate ester plasticizers
Di-2-ethylhexylphthalate, di-*n*-butylphthalate
Metals
Mercury, cadmium, lead, arsenic
Inorganic ions
Nitrates, phosphates

[a]Data obtained from[r10]

Table 106.4 Estimates of Proportions of Cancer Deaths Attributed to Various Factors[a]

Factor	Best Estimate (%)	Range of Estimates (%)
Tobacco	30	25–40
Alcohol	3	2–4
Diet	35	10–70
Food additives	<1	<1–2
Reproductive/sexual behavior	7	1–13
Occupation	4	2–8
Pollution	2	<1–5
Industrial products	<1	<1–2
Therapeutic procedures	1	<1–3
Geophysical factors	3	2–4
Infection	10	1–?
Unknown	?	?

[a]Data obtained from[1]

Table 106.5 Chemicals Established as Occupational Causes of Cancer[a]

Chemical	Site of Cancer
Aromatic amines	Bladder
4-Aminobiphenyl	
Benzidine	
2-Naphthylamine	
Arsenic	Skin, lung
Asbestos	Lung, pleura, peritoneum
Benzene	Bone marrow
Bis(chloromethyl) ether	Lung
Cadmium	Prostate
Chromium	Lung
Mustard gas	Larynx, lung
Nickel	Nasal sinuses, lung
Polycyclic aromatic hydrocarbons	Skin, scrotum, lung
Vinyl chloride	Liver

[a]Data obtained from[1]

other "environmentally" associated causes of avoidable human cancers.

Aromatic Halogenated Hydrocarbons of Concern

The polychlorinated biphenyls (PCB) (Figure 106.3) have been used in a large variety of applications as dielectric and heat transfer fluids, plasticizers, wax extenders, and flame retardants. Their industrial use and manufacture in the US ended by 1977. Their presence, however, persists in the environment. The products used commercially were actually mixtures of PCB isomers and homologs, containing 12 to 68 percent chlorine. These chemicals are highly stable and highly lipophilic, are poorly metabolized, are very resistant to environmental degradation, and bioaccumulate in food chains. Food is the major source of PCB residues in humans.

A serious exposure to PCB, lasting several months, occurred in Japan in 1968 due to cooking oil contaminated (2000–3000 ppm) with PCB-containing transfer medium (Yusho disease). A similar incident occurred in Taiwan in 1979. It is now known that the contaminated cooking oil contained not only PCB but also polychlorinated dibenzofurans (PCDF) and polychlorinated quaterphenyls (PCQ). Consequently, the effects that were initially attributed to the presence of PCB are now thought to have been largely caused by the other contaminants.[2–4]

A PCB accident occurred in Binghamton, New York in 1981. Analysis of soot after a transformer fire revealed the presence of pyrolyzed products—PCDF, polychlorinated dibenzo-p-dioxins (PCDD), and polychlorinated biphenylenes (PCBE)—thus illustrating the complexity of the problem when fires are involved.[5]

Occupational exposures afford a more reliable indication of signs and symptoms attributable to PCB intoxication. Effects after acute exposure are mild; the most common symptoms include eye and skin irritation, nausea, sore throat, tightness of the chest, and headache. After chronic exposure, chloracne is the most consistent finding; folliculitis, erythema, dryness, rash, hyperkeratosis, hyperpigmentation, some signs of hepatic involvement, and elevated plasma triglyceride concentrations also may occur. Effects on reproduction and development, as well as carcinogenic effects, have yet to be established in humans, even though some subjects have been exposed to very high levels of PCB. The bulk of the evidence from human studies indicates that PCBs pose little hazard to human health, except in situations where food is contaminated with high concentrations of these congeners.

The polychlorinated dibenzo-p-dioxins (PCDD, dioxins) (Fig. 106.3) as a chemical class have gained notoriety because of the extreme toxicity of one particular congener, 2,3,7,8-tetrachlorodibenzo-*p*-dioxin (TCDD, "dioxin"). In the production of the chlorophenoxy herbicides, particularly 2,4,5-tetrachlorophenoxyacetic acid (2,4,5-T), TCDD can appear as a contaminant. TCDD is the most toxic of 75 PCDD. The acute oral lethal dose varies over three orders of magnitude in laboratory animals (0.6 μg/kg in guinea pigs to 5000

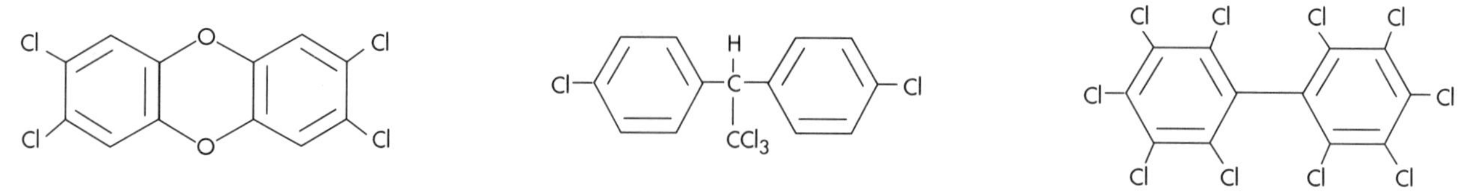

2, 3, 7, 9–Tetrachlorodibenzodioxin (TCCD)

Dichlorodiphenyltrichloroethane (DDT)

Polychlorinated Biphenyl (PCB) (Fully Chlorinated; Commercial Mixtures May Contain Fewer Chlorines)

Figure 106.3 Chemical Structures of Selecterd Aromatic Halogenated Hydrocarbons

μg/kg in hamsters); humans appear to be on the less sensitive end of the scale.[6,7]

Human exposures have occurred accidently. In 1949, workers in Nitro, West Virginia, were exposed during the manufacture of 2,4,5-T. Other accidents have occurred in Germany and Holland. A well-studied industrial explosion released TCDD in Seveso, Italy, where people were exposed to concentrations as high as 90 to 5,000 ppb.[6] In Times Beach, Missouri, waste oil containing TCDD was used for dust control; soil samples in one area contained about 30,000 ppb of TCDD. In addition, military personnel and civilians were exposed to TCDD during defoliation procedures (Agent Orange) in Vietnam.

Acute symptoms include irritation of the skin, eyes, and respiratory tract, headache, dizziness, and nausea. Chloracne is a characteristic manifestation of TCDD intoxication. In addition, liver enlargement, neuromuscular symptoms, and altered porphyrin metabolism have been associated with TCDD. In laboratory animals, teratogenesis, carcinogenesis, and a wasting syndrome are observed. There are no definitive indications of such effects in humans.

TCDD binds tightly to soil, which greatly limits its bioavailability and potential toxicity; diffusion through soil is extremely limited. The bioavailability from soil depends on the characteristics of the soil. Umbreit et al.[8] calculated a bioavailability of about 85 percent from soil from Times Beach, Missouri, based on published data,[9] whereas they found that TCDD in soils from Newark, New Jersey, demonstrated low bioavailability (0.5–20%); composition (possibly presence of carbonaceous materials) and matrix binding of the soil appear to affect TCDD bioavailability greatly. Kimbrough et al.[10] proposed that 1 ppb of TCDD in soil was a reasonable level at which to begin consideration of action to limit human exposure to contaminated soil.

Conclusion

Environmental toxicology is a subdivision of toxicology that is rapidly expanding and evolving. It already exerts a dominant role in societal and governmental decisions. While the general principles of traditional toxicology, largely developed from drug-oriented toxicology, apply equally well to environmental toxicology, more appropriate methodologies must be developed to answer the important questions raised about the status and safety of the environment. It is clear that multidisciplinary approaches are required, particularly when one is dealing with ecotoxicology. There is no doubt that environmental toxicology will be one of society's major preoccupations well into the 21st century.

References

Research Reports

1. Doll R, Peto R. The causes of cancer: quantitative estimates of avoidable risks of cancer in the United States today. J Natl Cancer Inst 1981;*66*:1191–1308.
2. Rogan WJ. PCBs and cola-colored babies: Japan, 1968, and Taiwan, 1979. Teratology 1982;*26*:259–261.
3. Rogan WJ, Gladen BC, Hung K-L, Koong S-L, Shih L-Y, Taylor JS, Wu Y-C, Yang D, Ragan NB, Hsu C-C. Congenital poisoning by polychlorinated biphenyls and their contaminants in Taiwan. Science 1988;*241*:334–336.
4. Wilson JD. A dose-response curve for Yusho syndrome. Regul Toxicol Pharmacol 1987;*7*:364–369.
5. O'Keefe PW, Silworth JB, Gierthy JF, Smith RM, DeCaprio AP, Turner JN, Eadon G, Hilker DR, Aldous KM, Kaminsky LS, Collins DN. Chemical and biological investigations of a transformer accident at Binghamton, NY. Environ Health Persp 1985;*60*:201–209.
6. Ayres SM, Webb KB, Evans RG, Mikes J. Is 2,3,7,8-TCDD (dioxin) a carcinogen for humans? Environ Health Persp 1985;*62*:329–335.
7. Lumb G. The problems of environmental hazardous substances: An overview. Ann Clin Lab Sci 1987;*17*:369–376.
8. Umbreit TH, Hesse EJ, Gallo MA. Bioavailability of dioxin in soil from a 2,4,5-T manufacturing site. Science 1986;*232*:497–499.
9. McConnell EE, Lucier GW, Rumbaugh RC, Albro PW, Harvan DJ, Hass JR, Harris MW. Dioxin in soil: Bioavailability after ingestion by rats and guinea pigs. Science 1984;*223*:1077–1079.
10. Kimbrough RD, Falk H, Stehr P. Health implications of 2,3,7,8-tetrachlorodibenzodioxin (TCDD) contamination of residential soil. J Toxicol Environ Health 1984;*14*:47–93.

Reviews

r1. Butler GC. Principles of ecotoxicology, Chichester: Wiley, 1978.

r2. Truhaut R. Ecotoxicology: Objectives, principles and perspectives. Ecotoxicol Environ Safety 1977;*1*:151–173.

r3. Moriarty F. Ecotoxicology. New York: Academic Press, 1983.

r4. Ramade F. Ecotoxicologie. Paris: Masson, 1979.

r5. Hodgson E. Introduction to toxicology. In: Hodgson E, Levi PE, A textbook of modern toxicology. New York: Elsevier, 1987, p 21.

r6. Grisham JW. Health aspects of the disposal of waste chemicals. New York: Pergamon, 1986.

r7. Dietz S, Emmet M, DiGaetano R, Tuttle D, Vincent C. National survey of hazardous waste generators and treatment, storage, and disposal facilities regulated under RCRA in 1981. Report No. EPA 530/SW-84-005. Washington: Environmental Protection Agency, 1984.

r8. National Research Council. Complex mixtures. Washington: National Academy Press, 1988.

r9. Geyer H, Scheunert I, Korte F. Bioconcentration potential of organic environmental chemicals in humans. Regul Toxicol Pharmacol 1986;6:313–347.

r10. Menzer RE. Water and soil pollutants. In: Amdur MO, Doull J, Klaassen CD, Casarett and Doull's toxicology, 4th ed. New York: Pergamon, 1991, pp 872–902.

CHAPTER 107

Pesticides

Donald J. Ecobichon

Introduction

A wide range of chemicals and biologic agents has been developed to control the invertebrate and vertebrate organisms that constantly threaten human food and fiber supply and human health. No one can doubt the efficacy of the agents used to protect crops in the field, thereby providing us with abundant, inexpensive, wholesome, and attractive fruits and vegetables. It has been estimated, however, that, even today, up to 50 per cent of harvested crops can be damaged by postharvest infestation by insects, fungi, rodents, etc. The medical miracles accomplished by pesticides have been documented: the suppression of a typhus epidemic in Naples, Italy, by DDT during the winter of 1943–44;[r1] the control of "river blindness" (onchocerciasis) in West Africa by killing the insect (blackfly) vector carrying the filaria responsible for this disease with temephos (ABATE);[1] the control of malaria in Africa, the Middle East, and Asia by eliminating the plasmodia-bearing mosquito populations with insecticides such as DDT, propoxur, malathion, carbaryl, and fenithrothion.[r2] While the benefits of pesticides are understood by those who require them, certain parts of the world are experiencing an environmentalist- and media-evoked backlash toward all pesticide use because of the carelessness, misuse, and/or abuse of some agents by a relatively few individuals in a limited number of publicized incidents. With no direct involvement in health care or food production, some environmental and consumer advocacy groups propose a complete ban on pesticide use. Somewhere between the two extremes lies a position for a careful and rational use of these chemicals.

It is important to appreciate that all pesticides possess an inherent degree of toxicity to some living organism; otherwise they would be of no practical use. There is no such thing as a "completely safe" pesticide. There are, however, pesticides that can be used safely and/or present a low level of risk to human health when applied properly. Despite the present-day conflagration over the use of pesticides and their residues found in food, ground water, and air, these agents comprise integral components of our crop and health protection programs and, as long as they continue in use, accidental and/or intentional human poisonings can be anticipated that will require treatment. From estimations based on California data, some 25,000 cases of pesticide-related illnesses occur annually among agricultural workers in that state, with a US national estimate being of the order of 80,000 cases each year.[2] On a worldwide basis, intoxications attributed to pesticides have been estimated to be as high as 500,000 illnesses annually, with as many as 20,000 deaths.[r3]

The US Environmental Protection Agency (EPA) recently estimated that there are approximately 600 pesticide chemicals (active ingredients) marketed in some 45,000–50,000 formulations. Information as recently as 1980 indicates that about 800 million pounds of pesticides were manufactured in the US and exported, an equivalent amount was manufactured and used in US agriculture, in addition to approximately 100 million pounds of imported agents.[3,4] Of the pesticides currently used in agriculture, approximately 60 percent are herbicides, 25–30 percent are insecticides, and 10–15 percent are fungicides.[4]

The US EPA definition of a "PESTICIDE" is any substance or mixture of substances intended for preventing, destroying, repelling, or mitigating any pest. Pesticides may also be described as any physical, chemical, or biologic agent that will kill an undesirable plant or animal pest. More specific classifications can be generated, usually based on the pattern of use (Table 107.1). In addition to the major agricultural classes that encompass insecticides, herbicides, and fungicides, one finds a broad range of chemical structures specific for the control of a particular life form. In this chapter, the mechanism(s) of action, the signs and symptoms of toxicity, and the treatment of poisoning by insecticides, herbicides, fungicides, and rodenticides will be discussed, these particular classes being the most frequently encountered toxicants in medical practice.

General Treatment: Decontamination

All pesticide poisonings should be treated as life-threatening emergencies. Swift action on the part of fellow workers, the physician, and hospital staff is essential to minimize the absorption of additional active ingredient(s) that would enhance and prolong the course of the poisoning as well as the duration of treatment.[r4] Given that there are three major routes of absorption of pesticides, the following procedures should be initiated immediately for any pesticide exposure.

Dermal Exposure

Decontamination begins with removal of contaminated clothing. Pesticides can be removed from skin, hair, and eyes by rinsing or showering with large quantities of warm or tepid water for 10–15 minutes. The skin can be washed repeatedly with alkaline soap or with sodium bicarbonate solution, if available.

Ingestion

Vomiting should be induced only in a fully conscious patient. Vomition is generally not recommended as a first aid measure unless the chemical swallowed is highly toxic, likely to prove fatal, and medical assistance is not readily available. Induction of vomiting is contraindicated in situations where the pesticide is dissolved in a petroleum distillate unless a highly toxic agent or a large quantity of agent has been ingested.

Under the guidance of a physician and if the patient is fully conscious, syrup of ipecac (30 ml for an adult, 15 ml for a child of 1–12 years of age) may be administered, followed by the ingestion of 200–300 ml of water. This treatment should be repeated only once if vomiting does not occur within 30 minutes of initial treatment since ipecac is toxic. After vomition has occurred or if induction is not successful, three tablespoons of activated charcoal in half a glass of water can be administered. This treatment can be repeated.

Under appropriate hospital conditions, gastric lavage can be initiated, administering 300 ml of warm physiologic (0.9%) saline via a stomach tube and, before all the solution has passed into the stomach, lowering the stomach tube into a basin or jar and allowing the stomach contents to siphon off. Samples should be saved for pesticide analysis. The lavage can be repeated as often as necessary until the returning fluid becomes clear. The administration of large volumes should be avoided, since this may cause emptying of the stomach contents into the duodenum. In place of physiologic saline, one could instill a suspension of activated charcoal (5 ml/kg of a mixture of 20 g in 100 ml of a solution of 70% sorbitol), siphoning off the stomach contents after each treatment.

Table 107.1 Subclassification of Pesticides

Algicides	Insecticides
Avicides	Molluscicides
Bactericides	Nematicides
Fungicides	Piscicides
Herbicides	Rodenticides

General Supportive Treatment

The greatest priority in cases of pesticide poisoning is the maintenance of adequate respiratory and cardiac function. In the unconscious patient, artificial respiration may be necessary if respiratory complications are noted. A tracheal tube with a plastic mouthpiece should be used to prevent contamination of the person rendering assistance. Artificial respiration should be maintained until medical help arrives.

Specific treatment of poisoning by particular pesticides is discussed in the following sections.

Insecticides

Since the advent of the use of nicotine, obtained from dried leaves of *Nicotiana tabacum*, as an insecticide in the 1960s, it has been appreciated that insecticides are neurotoxicants, acting either on the central or the peripheral nervous systems (CNS or PNS).[r5,r6] Therefore, it is not surprising that a chemical acting on the nervous system of an insect might elicit similar effects in higher life forms. Indeed, many of the mechanisms of action of insecticides in mammalian systems have been identified by research conducted on in vitro or in situ insect nerve preparations. It is sufficient at this stage to indicate the classes of insecticides (Fig. 107.1). Depending on the mechanisms of action, insecticides may interfere with the membrane transport of sodium, potassium, calcium, or chloride ions, or they may interfere with the persistence of chemical transmitters released at nerve endings.[r7]

Organochlorine Compounds

The properties of the organochlorine (chlorinated hydrocarbon) insecticides that made these agents effective (low volatility, chemical stability, lipid solubility, slow rate of biotransformation or degradation), also brought about their demise because of environmental persistence and bioaccumulation. However, even with the gradual ban of their agricultural use over a number of years beginning in 1968, the organochlorine insecticides are still extensively used in developing nations because they are cheap to manufacture, they are effective, and the risk:benefit ratio is highly weighted in favor of their continued use. Some organochlorine insecticides still see limited use in medicine, e.g., lindane (the gamma isomer of hexachlorocyclohexane) in shampoo preparations for head lice infestations.

The organochlorine insecticides are a diverse group of chemicals and can be subdivided into distinct groups, including the dichlorodiphenylethane-, the chlorinated cyclodiene-, and the chlorinated benzene- and cyclohexane-related structures (Fig. 107.2). With this diversity of structure, it is not surprising that the signs and symptoms of toxicity and the mechanism(s) of action are somewhat different (Table 107.2).

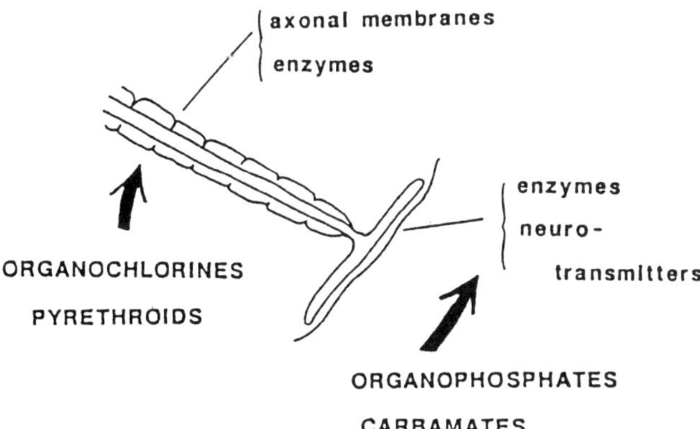

Figure 107.1 Potential Sites of Action of Insecticides on the Axon and the Terminal Portions of a Nerve

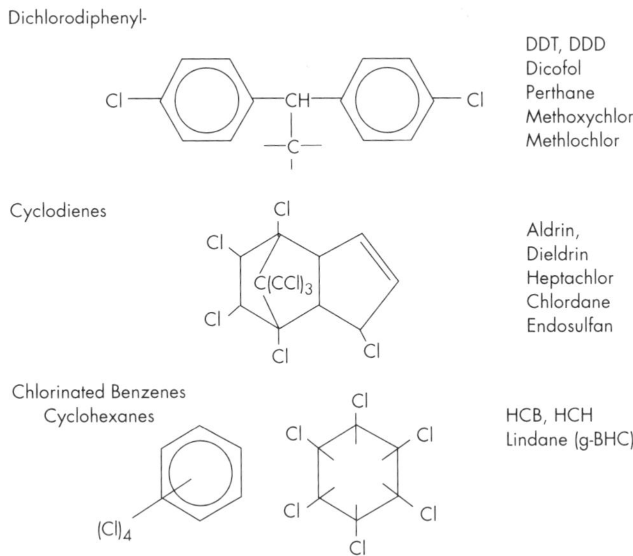

Figure 107.2 Classification of Organochlorine (chlorinated hydrocarbon) Insecticides by Structure

The first criterion essential for the action of organochlorine insecticides is an intact reflex arc (Fig. 107.3) involving an afferent (sensory) peripheral neuron impinging on interneurons in the spinal cord, with accompanying ramifications and interconnections up and down the CNS and interaction with efferent, motor neurons.[r6] With the DDT-type agents, the most striking observation in a poisoned insect or mammal (including the human) is the display of periodic sequences of persistent tremoring and/or convulsive seizures suggestive of repetitive discharge in neurons. The second most striking observation is that the repetitive tremors and seizures can be initiated by tactile and auditory stimuli, suggesting that the sensory nervous system appears to be more responsive to such stimuli. DDT-poisoned nerves show a very characteristic prolongation of the falling phase of the action potential (negative afterpotential) from that observed under normal circumstances of repolarization (Fig. 107.4). This prolongation results from a delay in sodium channel inactivation.[r6,r7] When the negative afterpotentials are increased to a certain level, e.g., the nerve membrane is partially depolarized and partially repolarized, the nerve becomes extremely sensitive to small stimuli. At the level of the membrane, DDT (a) affects membrane permeability of potassium ions; (b) modifies membrane sodium transport by preventing the rapid closure of the sodium channels; (c) inhibits neuronal adenosine triphosphatase (ATPase), particularly the Na^+/K^+ ATPase, which plays a vital role in nerve repolarization; and (d) inhibits the ability of calmodulin, a calcium mediator in nerves, to transport calcium ions. All these

Table 107.2 Signs and Symptoms of Acute and Chronic Toxicity Following Exposure to Organochlorine Insecticides

Insecticide Class	Acute Signs	Chronic Signs
Dichlorodiphenylethanes DDT DDD (Rothane) DMC (Dimite) Dicofol (Kelthane) Methoxychlor Methiochlor Chlorobenzylate	paresthesia (oral ingestion) ataxia, abnormal stepping dizziness, confusion, headache nausea, vomition fatigue, lethargy tremor (peripheral)	loss of weight, anorexia mild anemia tremors muscular weakness EEG pattern changes hyperexcitability, anxiety nervous tension
Hexachlorocyclohexanes Lindane (gamma isomer) Benzene hexachloride (mixed isomers)		
Cyclodienes Endrin Telodrin Isodrin Endosulfan Heptachlor Aldrin Dieldrin Chlordane Toxaphene	dizziness, headache nausea, vomition motor hyperexcitability hyperreflexia myoclonic jerking general malaise convulsive seizures generalized convulsions	headache, dizziness hyperexcitability Intermittent muscle twitching and myoclonic jerking psychological disorders including insomnia, anxiety, irritability EEG pattern changes loss of consciousness epileptiform convulsions
Chlordecone (Kepone) Mirex		Chest pains, arthralgia skin rashes ataxia, incoordination, slurred speech, opsoclonus visual difficulty, inability to focus and fixate nervousness, irritability, depression loss of recent memory muscle weakness, tremors of hand severe impairment of spermatogenesis

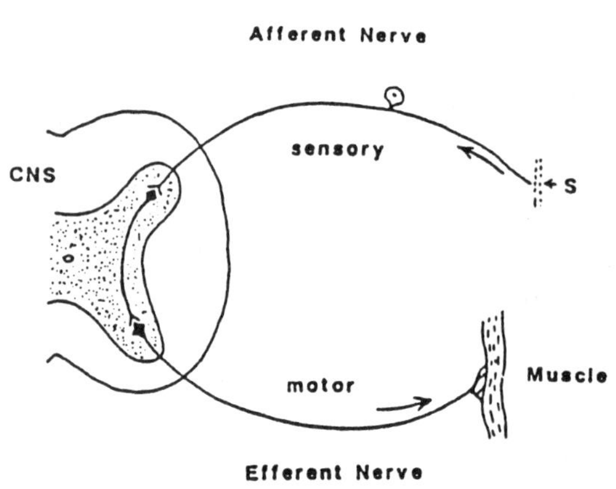

Figure 107.3 A simple, intact reflex arc that involves a peripheral afferent (sensory) neuron, interneurons in the CNS and a peripheral efferent (motor) neuron.

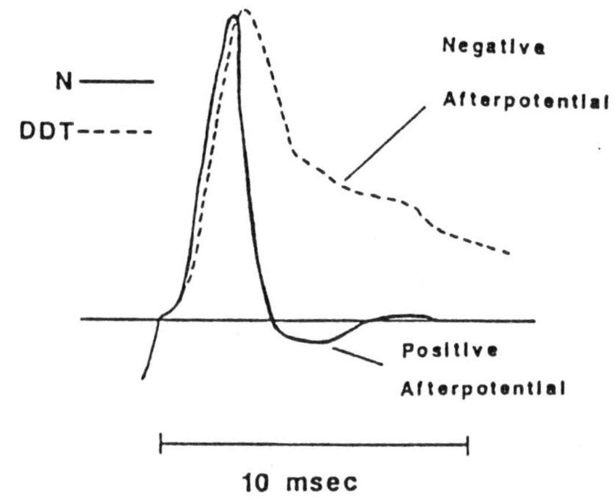

Figure 107.4 A schematic diagram of an oscilloscope recording to show the prolongation of the negative afterpotential induced by DDT (----) compared to the potential change seen normally (———).

various actions probably occur simultaneously, having an influence on the rate of neuronal repolarization and thereby affecting the duration of the negative afterpotential and neuronal sensitivity to small external as well as internal stimuli. With increased synaptic activity, this enhanced sensitivity is translated in the intact animal into episodic, enhanced neuronal activity (tremors, seizures, convulsions).[r7]

The other organochlorine insecticides (cyclodienes, chlorinated benzenes and cyclohexanes) are different from DDT in many respects—both in the appearance of the intoxicated individual and possibly the mechanism(s) of action, which appear to be localized more in the CNS (Table 107.2). These agents mimic the action of picrotoxin, a chemical known as a nerve excitant and an antagonist of the neurotransmitter, δ-aminobutyric acid (GABA), found in the CNS.[r2,r6] Structural similarities between the chemical picrotoxinin and the cyclodiene insecticides suggest that neurotoxicity may be related to interaction at a common receptor site on neuronal membranes.[r2,r7] GABA induces the uptake of chloride ions by neurons, this effect being blocked by picrotoxinin and by cyclodiene insecticides, thereby leaving the partially repolarized nerve in a state of uncontrolled excitation (Fig. 107.5). In addition, the cyclodiene insecticides inhibit Na^+/K^+ ATPase as well as Ca^{2+}/Mg^{2+}, the latter enzyme being important for the transport (uptake and release) of calcium across nerve membranes.[r7,5] The inhibition of Ca^{2+}/Mg^{2+} ATPase, located in the terminal ends of nerves in synaptic membranes, results in the accumulation of free calcium in the presynaptic regions of neurons and the promotion of calcium-induced release of neurotransmitters from storage vesicles, and the subsequent depolarization of adjacent neurons and enhanced neuronal activity (Fig. 107.5).

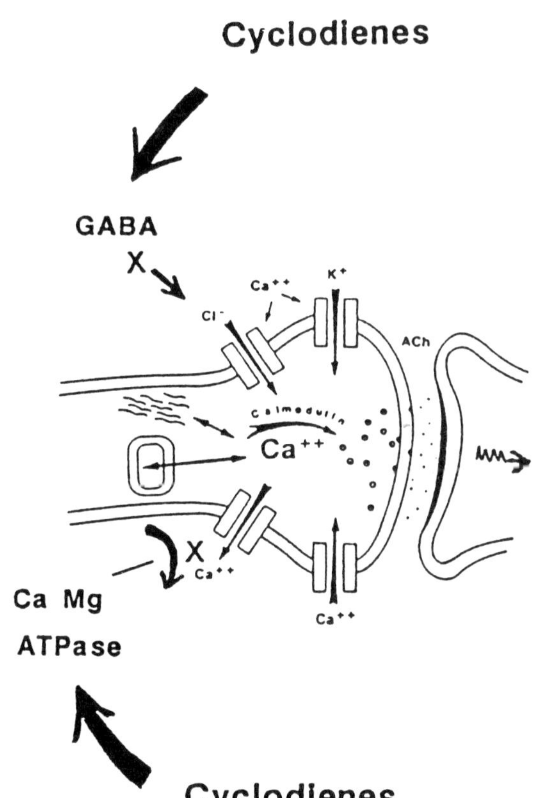

Figure 107.5 Cellular Mechanism of Action of the Cyclodienes on Chloride and Calcium Transport

Specific Treatment

The life-threatening emergencies in organochlorine insecticide poisonings are associated with the tremors, motor seizures, respiratory difficulties (hypoxemia), and resultant acidosis. In addition to supportive treatment, diazepam (0.3 mg/kg IV; maximum dose = 10 mg) or phenobarbital (15 mg/kg IV; maximum dose = 1.0 g) may be administered by slow injection to control convulsions.[r4] It may be necessary to repeat the treatment.

Anticholinesterase Compounds

Prior to the banning of the environmentally persistent organochlorine insecticides, a number of organophosphorus and a few carbamic acid ester insecticides were in widespread use. Subsequent to the ban, there was rapid development of these chemicals, the anticholinesterase insecticides being represented by a vast array of structures demonstrating the ultimate in selective structure-activity relationships achieved by the chemical manipulation of a basic structure.[r5,r6] These agents are esters of either phosphoric or thiophosphoric acid or of carbamic acid (Fig. 107.6) and have a common mechanism of action, the inhibition of nervous tissue acetylcholinesterase (AChE). There are over 200 organophosphorus esters and some 20 carbamate esters in use in agriculture, horticulture, and forestry, and in animal and human medicine. A list of the most commonly encountered anticholinesterase agents in order of decreasing acute toxicity, is presented (Table 107.3).

With the inhibition of the nervous tissue AChE, the enzyme responsible for the destruction of the neurotransmitter, acetylcholine (ACh), there is an accumulation of free unbound ACh at nerve endings in both the PNS and CNS. The severity of the signs and symptoms of organophosphorus or carbamate ester poisoning are related to the degree of AChE inhibition and the quantity of ACh present (Table 107.4).[6,7] Signs include those resulting from stimulation of the muscarinic receptors of the parasympathetic nervous system (in-

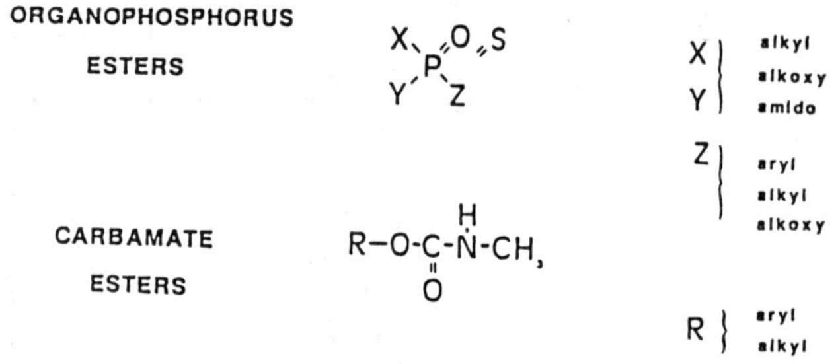

ORGANOPHOSPHORUS ESTERS

X, Y (O/S) P Z — X, Y: alkyl, alkoxy, amido; Z: aryl, alkyl, alkoxy

CARBAMATE ESTERS

R–O–C(=O)–NH–CH_3 — R: aryl, alkyl

Figure 107.6 The basic "backbone" of structures of the two types of anticholinesterase class of insecticides, the organophosphorus and carbamate esters.

creased secretions, bronchoconstriction, miosis, GI cramps, diarrhea, bradycardia, urination); those resulting from stimulation and subsequent blockade of nicotinic receptors, including the ganglia of the sympathetic and parasympathetic nervous system as well as the junction between nerves and muscles (causing tachycardia, hypertension, muscle fasciculations, tremors, muscle weakness, or flaccid paralysis); and those resulting from effects in the CNS (restlessness, emotional lability, ataxia, lethargy, mental confusion, generalized weakness, convulsions, coma, cyanosis). It is important to remember that, after treatment of the acute muscarinic and nicotinic clinical signs, some of the effects of poisoning may persist for several months after exposure, particularly those involving neurobehavioral, cognitive, and neuromuscular functions, most frequently being observed in cases of exposure to high concentrations of the agents (suicide attempts, drenching with dilute or concentrated chemicals).[r5,r6] A characteristic syndrome, organophosphate-induced delayed neuropathy (OPIDN), has been observed with some organophosphorus esters, this condition being characterized by a persistent axonopathy as a consequence of the inhibition of a neuronal carboxylesterase called neuropathic target esterase.[r6]

While the anticholinesterase insecticides have a common mode of action, there are significant differences between organophosphorus and carbamic esters.[r6] The interaction between an organophosphorus ester and the active site (a serine hydroxyl group) of the AChE results in an unstable intermediate complex that partially hydroyzes with the loss of the "Z", substituent (Fig. 107.6), leaving a stable, phosphorylated, and largely unreactive (inhibited) enzyme (Fig. 107.7). With most organophosphorus esters, the inhibited enzyme can be reactivated only at a very slow rate to yield free enzyme. The nature of the substituent groups at "X" and "Y" and "Z" (Fig. 107.6) play an important role in the specificity for the enzyme, the tenacity of binding, and the rate at which the phosphorylated enzyme dissociates.[r8] Many organophosphorus ester insecticides produce, essentially, an irreversibly inhibited enzyme and the signs and symptoms of poisoning are prolonged and persistent. Without rigorous medical intervention with specific antidotal chemicals to activate the enzyme, the toxicity will persist until sufficient "new" AChE protein is synthesized in 20–30 days or longer. Some of the more recently introduced organophosphorus esters (acephate, temephos, trichlorfon, dichlorvos) are less tenacious inhibitors of AChE, since the phosphorylated enzyme can dissociate readily within 30–90 minutes.

Carbamic acid esters are rather poor substrates for the nervous tissue AChE. They undergo hydrolysis in two stages: the first being the removal of the "R" substituent (Fig. 107.6) with the formation of a carbamylated intermediate; the second reaction being the decarbamylation of this intermediate with the release of free, reactivated enzyme.[r6] In contrast to the organophosphorus esters, the signs and symptoms of carbamate poisoning may be mild-to-severe in nature but do not usually persist for more than three to six hours, since the AChE will reactivate itself, requiring only symptomatic treatment by the physician.

Specific Treatment

All cases of anticholinesterase poisoning should be treated as serious emergencies, the patient being dispatched to a hospital as soon as possible. While symptoms may develop rapidly, a delay in onset or a steady increase in severity may be seen for up to 48 hours after exposure in the case of organophosphorus esters and up to six hours for carbamates. The status of the patient should be monitored by repeated analysis of the serum pseudocholinesterase and erythrocytic AChE, the activities of both enzymes being good indicators for the severity of organophosphorus ester poisoning, whereas, in blood, only the erythrocytic enzyme is inhibited by carbamic acid esters.[r6]

Depending on the severity of the poisoning, life-threatening signs (weakness of respiratory muscles, CNS depression of respiration, bronchospasm, bronchial secretions, pulmonary edema) resulting in hypoxemia will require immediate attention. Frequent suctioning and artificial respiration via endotracheal intubation may be necessary to maintain a patent airway. Arterial blood gases (PO_2) should be monitored. Cardiac function should be monitored because of the hypoxemia and the use of the specific antidotal chemicals mentioned below.

The regimen for the treatment of organophosphorus ester poisoning, based on the analysis of serum pseudocholinesterase, is described (Table 107.5).[6,7] Atropine is particularly important in acute, life-threatening intoxications. Frequent, small doses (SQ or IV)

Table 107.3 Representative Anticholinesterase-type Insecticides Listed in Order of Decreasing Toxicity*

Organophosphorus Esters**		Carbamic Acid Esters**	
Terbufos	COUNTER	Aldicarb	TEMIK
Phorate	THIMET	Oxamyl	VYDATE
Mevinphos	PHOSDRIN	Carbofuran	FURADAN
Fensulfothion	DASANIT	Methomyl	LANNATE
Demeton	SYSTOX	Bendiocarb	FICAM
Methyl parathion		Aminocarb	MATACIL
Disulfoton	DI-SYSTON	Methiocarb	MESUROL
Azinophos-methyl	GUTHION	Propoxur	BAYGON
Chlorfenvinphos	BIRLANE	Pirimicarb	PIRIMOR
Parathion		Bufencarb	BUX
Methamidaphos	MONITOR	Carbaryl	SEVIN
Methidathion	SUPRACIDE		
Demeton-methyl	METASYSTOX		
Dichlorvos	VAPONA		
Isofenphos	AMAZE		
Carbophenothion	TRITHION		
Chlorpyrifos	DURSBAN LORSBAN		
Fenthion	BAYTEX		
Phosmet	IMADAN		
Dimethoate	CYGON		
Diazinon	BASUDIN		
Fenitrothion	SUMITHION AGROTHION		
Trichlorfon	DYLOX		
Acephate	ORTHENE		
Fenchlorphos	RONNEL		
Malathion	CYTHION		
Temephos	ABATE		
Tetrachlorvinphos	GARDONA		

*Order of decreasing toxicity was based on acute oral LD_{50} values in the laboratory rat obtained from the literature.
**The common chemical name and at least one trade name (in capitals) is given for each of these frequently used insecticides.

of atropine are indicated after brief intense exposure to control the initial muscarinic signs. Relatively large, cumulative doses of atropine, up to 50 mg daily, may be necessary to control severe muscarinic signs. The status of the patient may be assessed by examining for dilatation of the pupils (mydriasis), the disappearance of secretions (dry mouth), facial flushing, and/or the disappearance of sweating. The continuous infusion of atropine may be necessary in extreme cases, total daily doses of up to several hundred milligrams being necessary during the first few days of treatment of severe poisoning. Care should be taken: excess atropine can cause distressing although not life-threatening toxic signs and symptoms.

Much of the other symptomatology can be controlled by the administration of specific agents, the oximes, that will reactivate the inhibited nervous tissue AChE (Table 107.5). The agent most commonly used is pralidoxime (2-PAM, Protopam), administered by slow IV infusion in doses of 1.0 g.[6,7] Treatment should be initiated as soon as possible since, with those organophosphorus esters that cause irreversible inhibition, pralidoxime is not very effective. In many cases, a single treatment with pralidoxime reduces the amount of atropine required. If absorption, distribution, and metabolism of the toxicant are delayed in the body, pralidoxime can be administered for several days after intoxication. Care should be taken with repeated dosage, since pralidoxime binds calcium ions. Severe muscle cramping, particularly in the legs, may be encountered but can be alleviated by oral or IV calcium solutions.[7]

Diazepam should be included in the treatment regimen of all but the mildest cases. In addition to relieving anxiety, diazepam counteracts some aspects of CNS-derived and neuromuscular signs that are not affected by atropine. Doses of 10 mg SC or IV are appropriate and may be repeated. Centrally acting drugs that may depress respiration are not recommended in the absence of artificial respiration.

The clinical treatment of carbamate toxicity is similar to that for organophosphorus insecticide poisoning,

Table 107.4 Signs and Symptoms of Anticholinesterase Insecticide Poisoning*

Manifestations	Site Affected
Muscarinic	
Increased salivation, lacrimation perspiration	Exocrine glands
Miosis, occasionally unequal, blurring of vision	Eyes
Nausea, vomiting, abdominal cramps, tightness, diarrhea, tenesmus and fecal incontinence	GI tract
Tightneess in chest, wheezing, cough, increased bronchial secretions, bronchoconstriction	Respiratory tract
Bradycardia, decrease in blood pressure	Cardiovascular system
Frequency, urinary incontinence	Bladder
Nicotinic	
Muscular twitching, fasciculations, cramps, weakness in both peripheral and respiratory muscles	Skeletal muscles
Tachycardia, pallor, elevation of blood pressure	Sympathetic ganglia
Central	
Giddiness, anxiety, restlessness, emotional lability, ataxia, drowsiness, lethargy, fatigue confusion, difficulty in concentration, headache, generalized weakness	
Coma with absence of reflexes, Cheyne-Stokes respiration, tremor, convulsions, dyspnea, depression of respiratory and circulatory centers with decrease in blood pressure, cyanosis	CNS

*Ecobichon et al[7]

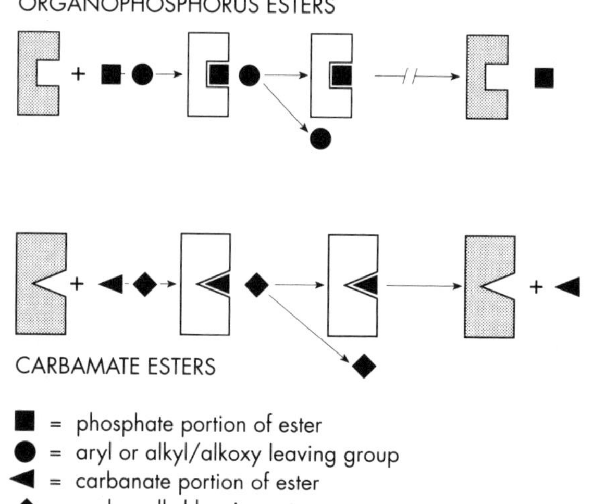

Figure 107.7 A schematic diagram depicting the interaction of organophosphorus and carbamate ester insecticides with the enzyme acetylcholinesterase, with subsequent inhibition and reactivation of the enzyme.

except that oximes are contraindicated. With certain carbamates, notably carbaryl, pralidoxime enhances the toxicity. With other carbamates, pralidoxime has no beneficial effects.[r6,r7] Pralidoxime is not an essential antidote in carbamate intoxication, since it does not interact with carbamylated AChE in the same manner as with phosphorylated AChE.

Pyrethroid Esters

Pyrethrum is one of the oldest natural insecticides still in use, the source being the flowers of the chrysanthemum (*Chrysanthemum cinerariaefolium, C.coccineum*), the extract containing a mixture of six different esters of chrysanthemic or pyrethric acids (Fig. 107.8). The major active principles of the plant extract are pyrethrins I and II and cinerin I and II. Limited supplies of natural pyrethrins have led to the synthesis of a number of esters having a higher insect/mammal toxicity ratio, a rapid biotransformation by mammals, and an absence of cumulative toxicity.[r9,r10] The low mammalian toxicity has made these synthetic esters an important class of insecticides. In addition to extensive agricultural use, these agents are components in household sprays, flea preparations for pets, and greenhouse sprays. Distinct molecular structures convey selective specificity toward certain insect species. The commercially available esters are listed (Table 107.6).

While these insecticides cannot be considered highly toxic, their use indoors in enclosed spaces has resulted in some interesting signs and symptoms of toxicity in humans. Exposure to natural pyrethrum has resulted in contact dermatitis, descriptions ranging from a local erythema similar to sunburn to a vesicular eruption like that seen with poison ivy.[8] The allergenic nature of this natural product has elicited asthma-like attacks and anaphylactic reactions with peripheral vas-

Table 107.5 Classification and Treatment of Organophosphorus Insecticide Poisoning Based on Plasma Pseudocholinesterase Activity*

Classification of Poisoning	Enzyme Activity (% of normal)	Treatment	
		Atropine	Pralidoxime
Mild	20–50	1.0 mg SC	1.0 g IV over 20–30 min.
Moderate	10–20	1.0 mg IV every 20–30 min. until sweating and salivation disappear and slight flush and mydriasis appear.	1.0 g IV over 20–30 min.
Severe	10	5.0 mg IV every 20–30 min. until sweating and salivation disappear and slight flush and mydriasis appear.	1.0 g IV as above. If no improvement, administer another 1.0 g IV. If no improvement, start IV infusion at 0.5 g/hr.

*Ecobichon et al[7]

cular collapse, although the latter two signs are exceedingly rare. Most of the human toxicity associated with the natural pyrethrins results from the allergic properties of the material rather than direct toxicity. There has been no indication that acute or chronic exposure to the natural products are likely to produce significant neurologic conditions in humans.

With the synthetic pyrethroids, there has been little evidence of the allergic-type reactions in exposed humans. One notable form of toxicity has been the cutaneous paresthesia observed in workers spraying synthetic pyrethroid esters containing a cyano-substituent (deltamethrin, cypermethrin, fenvalerate). The paresthesia developed a number of hours after exposure and was described as a stinging or burning of the skin, which, in some cases, progressed to a tingling and numbness, the effects lasting 12–18 hours.[9]

Recent reports from the People's Republic of China, where pyrethroids have been used on a large scale on cotton since 1982, illustrate the consequences of accepting the product advertisements at face value. Having been told that the pyrethroid esters (deltamethrin, fenvalerate) were nontoxic, sloppy handling practices caused serious although reversible toxicity in more than 300 cases, eliciting anorexia, headaches, nausea, and fatigue in mild cases, with muscle fasciculations and convulsive attacks and coma being observed in severe cases.[10–12] Chronic toxicity has not been reported to date.

The mechanisms by which the synthetic pyrethroid esters elicit increased peripheral nerve excitability are very similar to those observed after treatment with DDT (Fig. 107.9).[r6] All of the pyrethroids affect sodium channels in nerve fibers, causing repetitive nerve discharge and delayed sodium channel inactivation. Type II pyrethroid esters produce an even longer delay in sodium channel inactivation, leading to a persistent depolarization of the nerve, a reduction in the amplitude of the action potential and an eventual failure of axonal conduction and blockade of impulses.[13] Type II pyrethroid esters bind and block the GABA-receptor, thereby interfering with chloride transport, and also inhibit Ca^{2+}/Mg^{2+} ATPase (Fig. 107.9).[5]

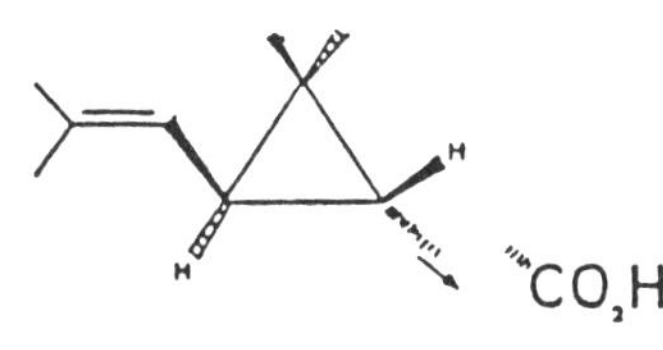

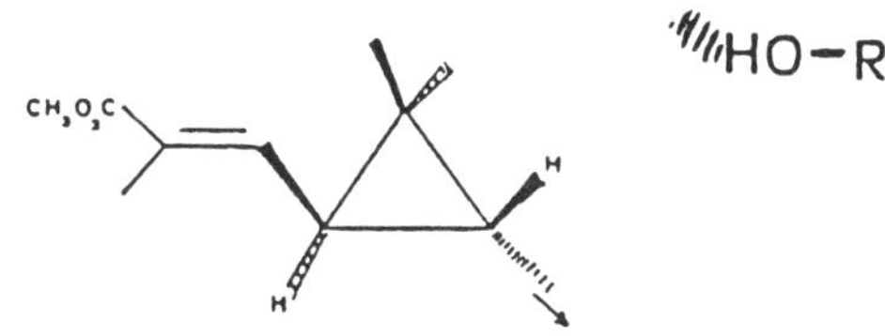

Figure 107.8 The basic structures of the pyrethroid ester insecticides, showing the two acidic portions, chrysanthemic and pyrethric acids. Variations in the alcoholic (HO-R) portions include alkyl-, aryl ether chains of complex structure.

Specific Treatment

No specific therapy has been reported other than supportive treatment and decontamination. Topical Vitamin E may reduce the paresthesia.

Table 107.6 Representative Pyrethroid Ester Insecticides Listed in Order of Decreasing Toxicity*

Deltamethrin (decamethrin)	CYMBUSH, RIPCORD
Cypermethrin	BELMARK, SUMICIDIN
Fenvalerate	AMBUSH, POUNCE
Permethrin	
Pyrethrum**	
Resmethrin	CISMETHRIN, SYNTHRIN
Tetramethrin	NEO-PYNAMIN

*Order of decreasing toxicity was based on acute oral LD_{50} values in the laboratory rat obtained from the literature.
+The common chemical name and at least one trade name (in capitals) are given for each agent.
**Pyrethrum is the mixture of 6 esters extracted from natural sources, chrysanthemum flowers.

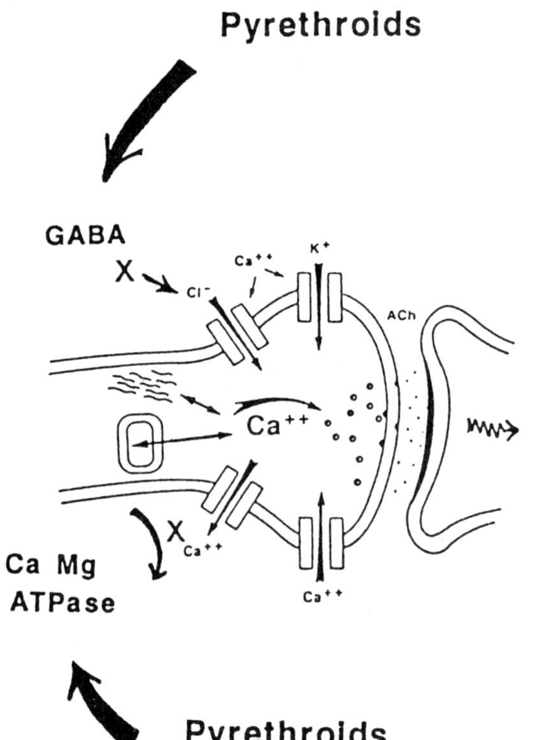

Figure 107.9 Cellular Mechanism of Action of the Pyrethroid Esters on Chloride and Calcium Transport

Herbicides

As a class of agricultural chemicals, the herbicides far outrank the total of all other pesticides in diversity of structure, production, and use. Herbicides are used for the control of unwanted, fast-growing, broad-leafed weeds in a variety of agricultural crops as well as in highway, hydroelectric, and forestry operations for the control of woody, deciduous plants and in lawn and turf management. Depending on the chemical classification, these agents may act as hormone or auxin-like growth regulators, precipitators of vital enzyme proteins, inhibitors of cell division and/or photosynthesis, and desiccants. The names of the major herbicides in use are presented (Table 107.7).

The claim has been made that, because the modes of action involve biochemical mechanisms unique to plants, there is no risk of mammalian toxicity associated with these agents. With the exception of a few chemicals, the herbicides do have low toxicity in mammalian species. The current controversy involving herbicides centers around the suspected mutagenicity, teratogenicity, and carcinogenicity associated with either the agent or contaminants and by-products of synthesis found in technical grade material.[14] The presence of these contaminants has been largely ignored without realizing that the toxicities associated with them are both different and occur at dosage orders of magnitude lower than those for the pure herbicides. The best-known example is the presence of dioxins, particularly 2,3,7,8-tetrachlorodibenzo-p-dioxin (TCDD), in the chlorophenoxy acid herbicide, 2,4,5-tri-chlorophenoxyacetic acid (2,4,5-T). The herbicide controversy continues with the publication of recent studies associating chronic exposure with increased incidences of non-Hodgkin's lymphoma, malignant lymphoma, soft-tissue sarcomas, and colon cancer.[15] However, no clear-cut association between carcinogenicity and herbicide exposure has been established from epidemiologic studies conducted to date.

The major route of exposure to herbicides is dermal. Since these agents are relatively strong acids, phenols, esters, or amines, they are dermal irritants, causing skin rashes and contact dermatitis even when exposure is to diluted formulations. There appear to be subpopulations of individuals who are dermally sensitive to contact with droplets of diluted formulations from aerial drift, moderate-to-severe urticaria being observed that may persist for four to 10 days after exposure. Certain individuals, particularly those prone to allergies, may experience asthma-like attacks or even anaphylactic shock after inhalation exposure to drifting aerosolized herbicide. Whether this effect is chemical-specific and related to the herbicide or to the emulsifiers and cosolvents in the formulation has not been established. In some cases, with these hypersensitive individuals, the patient's response may be associated with a generalized, nonspecific irritant effect of the formulation. Many of the above reactions respond satisfactorily to treatment with antihistaminic agents.

There is evidence in the literature that a number of the herbicides (phenoxy acids, thiocarbamates, bipyridyls) elicit neurotoxicity in a number of animal species. However, there is little documented evidence

Table 107.7 Representative Herbicides⁺ Listed in Order of Decreasing Toxicity*

Agent		Chemical Class**
Paraquat	GRAMOXONE	B
Diquat	REGLONE	B
Endothal	DES-I-CATE	M
Dinoseb	PREMERGE	P
Cynazine	BLADEX	T
2,4-D		Pa
2,4,5-T		Pa
2,4,5-TP	SILVEX	PA
Tebuthiuron	SPIKE	U
MCPA	TARGET	Pa
Bensulide	BETASAN	M
MCPP (mecoprop)	MECOTURF	PA
Metham-sodium	VAPAM	C
MSMA	DACONATE	As
Alachlor	LASSO	Am
Amitrol	WEEDAZOL	An
Pendimethalin	PROWL	An
Barban	CARBYNE	C
Methazole	PROBE	M
Cacodylic acid	PHYTAR	As
EPTC	EPTAM	C
Atrazine	AATREX	T
DSMA		As
Diclofop	HOELON	Pa
Metribuzin	LEXONE SENCOR	T
Dicamba	BANVEL	M
Metolachlor	DUAL	Am
Chlorthal-dimethyl	DACTHAL	M
Sethoxydim	POAST	M
Chloroxuron	TENORAN	U
Dichlobenil	CASORON	M
Diuron	KROVAR	U
Monuron	TELVAR	U
Asulam	ASULOX	C
Glyphosate	ROUNDUP VISION	M
Propham	CHEM-HOE	C
Simazine	PRINCEP	T
Linuron	AFALON	U
Fenuron	DYBAR	U
Dalapon	DOWPON	M
Picloram	TORDON	M
Propyzamide	KERB	Am
Trifluralin	TREFLAN	An
Benefin	BALAN	An

*Order of decreasing toxicity was based on acute oral LD_{50} values in the laboratory rat obtained from the literature.

⁺The common chemical name and at least one trade name (in capitals) is given for each chemical.

**Chemical classes include: Am, amide; An, aniline; As, arsenical; B, bipyridyl; C, carbamate; M, miscellaneous; P, phenol; Pa, phenoxy-acids,; T, triazine or triazole; U, urea.

of such effects in humans, with the exception of one study where decreased peripheral nerve conduction velocities were observed in workers employed in the manufacture of 2,4-dichlorophenoxyacetic acid (2,4-D) and the analogue 2,4,5-T.[16] It is conceivable that chronic, high level exposure to concentrated chemicals might elicit such effects not seen following exposure to diluted formulations. However, the necessary information is not available from epidemiologic studies.

Chlorophenoxy Acids

The various members of this group have been used longer than any of the other herbicides. With over 40 years of continual use, acute toxic reactions to such agents as 2,4-D and 2,4,5-T have been rare. A large amount of mammalian toxicity data, gathered over the years from both animal studies and human exposure, has revealed few untoward effects except at excessively high doses. The cases of accidental or occupational poisonings by chlorophenoxy herbicides have been reviewed by Hayes and Laws.[r11] Most of these patients complained of headache, dizziness, nausea, vomiting, abdominal pains, diarrhea, weakness, and fatigue, respiratory complications, aching and tender muscles, myotonia, and muscle injury. Transient albuminuria was observed in some cases, a not too surprising finding since the route of elimination of this herbicide class from the body is via the kidney. Renal dysfunction is generally seen.

The average adult lethal dose of 2,4-D has been estimated at approximately 28 g (400 mg/kg). However, in one case, the ingestion of 500 mg of 2,4-D daily over a three-week period elicited no symptoms.[17] In another poisoning, death occurred in a 75-kg male after the intentional ingestion of 80 mg 2,4-D/kg.[18] The clinical course of one patient who intentionally ingested a "large volume" of a mixture of the butyl esters of 2,4-D and 2,4,5-T was characterized by an increasing body temperature, increased pulse and respiratory rates, decreased blood pressure, respiratory alkalosis, hemoconcentration, profuse sweating, oliguria, rising blood urea nitrogen, restlessness, and a deepening coma.[r9] At autopsy, numerous foci of submucosal hemorrhage, moderate congestion and edema of the mucosa of the small intestine, and congestion in the lungs were seen. Microscopic examination revealed necrosis of the intestinal mucosa with local coagulation in the muscle coat of the intestine. Acute necrosis and fatty infiltration were observed in the liver. Alveoli in the area of pneumonitis contained polymorphonuclear cells and erythrocytes, and there was inflammation of terminal bronchioles. In other cases, renal damage in the form of degeneration of the convoluted tubules, fatty infiltration, and the presence of protein in the glomerular spaces has been observed.

A recent study of herbicide-exposed farmers in Kansas suggests that non-Hodgkin's lymphoma may be associated with chronic exposure to 2,4-D, an herbicide used continually since 1946 in cereal crops.[15] A subsequent study of farmers in eastern Nebraska appears to confirm this observation.[19] While other studies have not supported this conclusion, a number of new ones have been initiated to evaluate this association.

Much of the toxicity attributed to the chlorophenoxyacetic acid herbicides has been ascribed to the various chlorinated dibenzo-p-dioxins (particularly TCDD) and dibenzofurans found in formulations before 1965 at concentrations up to 30 mg/kg (30 ppm).[20] While the use of 2,4,5-T has now been banned in many countries and TCDD concentrations are regulated to a level of 0.01-0.05 ppm, manufacturers have achieved product clean-up to a level of 0.001-0.005 ppm of TCDD. While the medical concerns of TCDD are beyond the scope of this chapter, it should be noted that, common with other chlorinated aromatic compounds, TCDD causes a chloracne of the face and neck, torso, thighs, and genitalia, liver enlargement, and altered porphyrin and lipid metabolism. Some of these clinical signs may persist for many months and even for years, depending on the severity of the intoxication. TCDD is not mutagenic in various bacterial mutagenicity test systems. TCDD is teratogenic in animals and is considered to be a suspect, potential human carcinogen. Positive evidence of teratogenicity and carcinogenicity in humans has not been forthcoming from extensive epidemiologic studies conducted in exposed workers and their families.[r12] However, a recent study of the dioxin-exposed populations of Seveso, Italy has reported increased incidence rates of hematologic neoplasms (lymphoreticulosarcoma), multiple myeloma, soft tissue tumors and non-Hodgkin's lymphoma.[21]

With most of the other herbicidal chemicals, reports of human toxicity are rare. A number of accidental or intentional poisonings have been described, but it must be appreciated that many of these cases were single and, frequently, bizarre incidents.[r9] With some of the more recently registered agents, there are concerns about potential mutagenic, teratogenic, and carcinogenic effects in humans, arising from equivocal results from animal studies. These chemicals will remain a source of controversy for some time in the future until definitive studies have been done.

Bipyridyl Derivatives

The one chemical class of herbicides that deserves attention is the bipyridyl group (paraquat and diquat). Paraquat in particular, a nonselective, contact herbicide, is one of the most exquisite pulmonary toxicants known and has been the subject of intensive investigation because of its startling toxicity in humans.[r13]

The ingestion of commercial paraquat preparations, concentrates containing 20 percent active ingredient, is invariably fatal and runs a time course of three to four weeks. While absorption of this highly polar compound from the GI tract is generally poor, the presence of emulsifiers and/or cosolvents in the concentrates enhance the uptake of the agent. Paraquat is accumulated in pulmonary tissue by a diamine/polyamine transport system in the alveolar epithelial cells where it undergoes NADPH-dependent, one-electron reduction to form a free radical capable of reacting with molecular oxygen (in abundant supply in the tissue) to reform the cationic paraquat plus a reactive oxygen that is converted into hydrogen peroxide by the enzyme, superoxide dismutase.[r14] The hydrogen peroxide is contraindicated in such cases, since it appears to promote cellular toxicity. The pathologic picture in the lung is one of destruction of the alveolar type I and II epithelial cells with a proliferation of fibrotic cells. These effects, in turn, impair respiratory function, causing pulmonary congestion and death by hypoxia. Paraquat, in addition to its pulmonary effects, induces multi-organ toxicity, with necrotic damage to the liver, kidney, and myocardial muscle and hemorrhage in the adrenals and cerebrum.[r11]

The ingestion of the concentrated formulation results in a burning of the mouth and throat, substernal chest pains, and severe gastroenteritis with esophageal and gastric lesions. While most poisonings are associated with the ingestion of this agent, there are reports of severe toxicity from dermal absorption through abraded skin.[r11] The concentrated formulation is corrosive and will cause blistering and erythema when in contact with the skin. There is evidence of nonfatal chronic impairment of pulmonary function in sprayers who inhaled aerosolized paraquat from diluted (0.2% w/v) spray formulations over a number of years.[r11]

Diquat, 1,1'-ethylene-2,2'-bipyridium, a much less toxic analogue of paraquat, sees considerable use in agricultural practice. Information about the toxicity of this agent to humans is inadequate because there have been few cases reported.[r11] The corrosive nature of this herbicide will elicit skin rashes and will result in damage to mucous membranes of the nose and throat and irritation to the upper respiratory tract. The acute and chronic effects of diquat differ from those associated with paraquat in that the GI tract, liver, and kidneys are the major target organs, exposure resulting in acute hepatic and renal necrosis with concomitant changes in enzyme activities plus hemorrhagic conditions.[22] This is thought to be associated with the same mechanisms of superoxide-induced lipid peroxidation of membranes. Unlike paraquat, diquat has a low affinity for pulmonary tissue and does not appear to be influenced by the mechanism that selectively concentrates paraquat.[23]

Treatment

Poisoning as a consequence of exposure to herbicides is treated symptomatically, responding to the clinical picture as symptoms arise. As was discussed under General Treatment, the first stages involve removing what chemical is present, thereby preventing the absorption of additional toxicant. No specific antidotes are known.

Fungicides

Fungicidal chemicals have been derived from a diverse group of structures, ranging from simple chemicals, such as sulfur, through the aryl mercurial compounds, chlorinated phenols to metal-containing derivatives of dithiocarbamic acid and complex, substituted heterocyclic ring systems. The names of the major fungicides in use are presented in Table 107.8.

The topic of fungicide toxicity has been extensively reviewed by Hayes.[r11] With the exception of metalaxyl, hexachlorobenzene, and the various organomercurials, most of these agents have a low order of toxicity to the human, oral LD_{50} values in the rat ranging from 800–10,000 mg/kg bw. Since many of these agents are applied as dry powders or dusts, severe toxicity would not be observed unless the powder was ingested. Dermal absorption of these agents is low. However, dermal contact with substantial amounts of almost all of the chemicals listed results in urticaria and contact dermatitis with local edema and/or an erythematous dermatitis of the eyelids. With many of these chemicals, patch testing results in a high rate of reactivity and evidence of sensitization.[r11] The dermatitis usually responds to corticosteroid treatment.

Table 107.8 Representative Fungicides⁺ Listed in Order of Decreasing Toxicity*

Agent		Chemical Class**
Metalaxyl	RIDOMIL	M
Thiram	TERSAN	DMDC
Metham-sodium	VAPAM	DMDC
Dinocap	KARATHANE	P
Dodine	CYPREX	M
Ziram	VANCIDE	DMDC
Thiabendazole	MERTECT	Bz
Ferbam	FERMATE	DMDC
Captofol	DIFOLATAN	Ph
Zineb	DITHANE M-78	EBDC
Maneb	DITHANE M-22	EBDC
Thiophanate-methyl	MILDOTHANE	M
Mancozeb	DITHANE M-45	EBDC
Captan	ORTHOCIDE	Ph
Thiophanate	TOPSIN	M
Folpet	PHALTAN	Ph
Benomyl	BENLATE	Bz
Metiram	POLYRAM	DMDC

*Order of decreasing toxicity was based on acute oral LD_{50} values in the laboratory rat obtained from the literature.
⁺The common chemical name and at least one trade name (in capitals) is given for each chemical.
**Chemical classes include: Bz, benzimidazole; DMDC, dimethyl dithiocarbamate; EBDC, ethylenebisdithiocarbamate; M, miscellaneous; P, phenol; Ph, Phthalimide; Th, thiophanate.

The human toxicity of fungicides has not attracted as much attention as have other classes of pesticides. The major reason has been the low numbers of intoxications encountered, owing to the generally unattractive and unpalatable appearance of most formulations, which serves to minimize the oral ingestion of the chemicals. As stated, the major toxicologic effects are dermal, caused by close contact with the formulations in fields and particularly in enclosed greenhouse areas where there is extensive use of fungicides owing to the high relative humidity. Most of these agents are irritating to mucous membranes (eyes, nose, throat, upper respiratory tract).

While not particularly toxic to animals except at elevated doses, these agents are cytotoxic and many give positive results in in vitro microbiologic mutagenicity test systems. Such results are not surprising, since the cells in the test systems are somewhat similar to those for which fungicides were designed to kill, either through a direct effect or via lethal genetic mutations. A "safe" fungicide, nonmutagenic in test cell systems, would be useless for the protection of food, fiber, and health.

As was seen with the herbicides, public concern centers on the potential for mutagenicity and hence possible teratogenic and carcinogenic activity demonstrated by either the parent chemical, metabolites and/or contaminants in technical grade products. That a number of these agents are teratogenic in animals and that a few fungicides have been shown to be potential carcinogens is all the more reason why these agents should be handled carefully, providing proper protection to the highly exposed workforce involved in spraying or in harvesting crops treated with the chemicals.

The ethylene bisdithiocarbamate class of fungicides (maneb, mancozeb, zineb) are of particular concern in that animal studies have revealed them to be teratogenic. These agents degrade into ethylene thiourea (ETU), known to be mutagenic, carcinogenic, and teratogenic. ETU also possesses antithyroid activity. In addition, there is a potential interaction of this class of agents with alcohol since they are structurally similar to disulfiram (Antabuse). Workers using this class of fungicides should avoid the consumption of alcohol.

Several acute and chronic poisonings have occurred in agricultural workers exposed to high levels of dithiocarbamate fungicides, resulting in both obvious, immediate, and persistent neurologic signs and symptoms involving both the PNS and CNS.[24,25] The consensus of opinion is that the toxicity is associated with carbon disulfide, a degradation product of the dithiocarbamic acid, rather than with the metal, usually manganese or zinc, complexed with the fungicide.

Organomercurial compounds, both alkyl and aryl

derivatives, have been used as fungicides, in particular as seed dressings for the prevention of seed-borne diseases of cereal grains, vegetables, cotton, peanuts, soybeans, and sugar beets. The toxicology of mercurial fungicide poisoning has been extensively reviewed.[r6,r11] While these agents see less use today, they still are of concern in third-world developing countries. Invariably, toxicity is associated either with the inhalation of high concentrations of the more volatile agents during manufacture of with the ingestion of fungicide-treated seed grain. From 1956 to 1972, there were six poisoning incidents where from seven to 6530 individuals inadvertently consumed mercurial-treated wheat designated for planting. These cases have been described in detail.[r6]

The symptoms of poisonings by organomercurials are shown in Table 107.9.[r6] After acute poisoning, they arise essentially from the mercuric cation and the classic picture emerges as effects arising from two organ systems-the alimentary tract and the kidneys. Chronic poisoning is generally slow and insidious in onset and eventually will involve most of the organ systems to some extent. However, the major effects will be associated with the peripheral sensory and motor nerves and the CNS.

Specific Treatment of Fungicide Poisoning

In acute poisoning with inorganic, alkyl-, alkoxyalkyl- and aryl-mercurials, treatment is directed at the precipitation and removal of the chemical from the GI tract, the inactivation of the absorbed mercuric ions and general supportive measures to maintain fluid and electrolyte balance. The prompt administration of milk and/or egg whites will delay absorption by providing sufficient sulfhydryl groups for the formation of stable mercury complexes. A solution of 5 percent sodium formaldehyde sulfoxylate (Rongalite) in a 3 percent sodium bicarbonate solution (200 ml) is recommended, the former chemical reducing the mercuric ions to metallic mercury, which is poorly absorbed.

To inactivate mercurials already absorbed, several antidotes are available, though none are completely successful. The most widely known therapy involves the IM injection of 2.5–3.0 mg/kg body weight of dimercaprol (2,3-dimercapto-1-propanol, British Anti-Lewisite or BAL) in oil every 12 hours until the symptoms disappear. Unfortunately, BAL is not without toxicity, primarily experienced as a tingling or numbness of the tongue, lips, and extremities, accompanied by nausea, vomiting, headache, and tremors. Other antidotes, D-penicillamine (0.6–1.0 g daily) and the less toxic N-acetyl-DL-penicillamine (200–500 mg every 6 hr), have also proved useful in mercurial poisoning, these chemicals containing sulfhydryl groups that complex with the mercuric ions and enhance urinary excretion. Once again, these antidotes are not without toxicity, particularly in the kidney. A thiol resin containing sulfhydryl groups attached to a macroporous, styrene-divinylbenzene copolymer was tested in the 1972 Iraqi epidemic and proved to be effective.[26] The use of other resin analogues has been explored experimentally. Any of the above antidotal therapies appear to be of benefit in acute poisoning cases, but in chronic poisonings there are few clinical improvements, even though the urinary and fecal excretion of mercury has been enhanced.

Table 107.9 Syptomatology of Organomercurial Poisoning*

Paresthesia of the mouth, lips, tongue, hands, feet.
Constriction of visual fields, abnormal blind spots.
Hearing difficulties, particularly sound discrimination i.e., picking out one voice from a group.
Speech disorders; difficulty in articulating words. Difficulty in swallowing.
Neurasthenia; weakness, fatigue, inability to concentrate.
Inability to write, read or recall basic things such as familiar addresses, telephone numbers.
Emotional instability; fits of anger, depression and agitation.
Ataxia; stumbling gait, clumsiness in handling familiar objects (forks, shoelaces, buttons) grotesque, uncoordinated movements.
Spasticity; rigidity and partial paralysis.
Stupor, coma, and death (in extreme cases).

*Ecobichon and Joy[r6]

Rodenticides

The control of rodents, particularly rats and mice, is an important aspect of postharvest food protection as well as for the control of disease. The agents used constitute a diverse range of chemical structures having a variety of mechanisms of action in partially successful attempts to attain target species specificity. With some chemicals, advantage has been taken of the physiology and biochemistry unique to rodents. With other rodenticides, the site(s) of action are common to most mammals, and it is the dosage required and the habits of the rodents that can be utilized to minimize toxicity to nontarget species.

Rodenticides, taken intentionally or accidentally, pose serious toxicologic problems because, invariably, the dosage ingested is high and the signs and symptoms are advanced and quite severe by the time the patient is seen by the physician.

The toxicology of the various classes of rodenticides has been reviewed extensively.[r4] Some representative agents are listed in Table 107.10 in order of decreasing toxicity.

Fluoro-Acetate and Acetamide

The extreme toxicity of these agents has restricted their use to prepared baits since the chemicals are white, odorless, and tasteless. These agents are well absorbed from the GI tract. The mechanism of action involves the incorporation of the fluoroacetate into fluoroacetyl-coenzyme A, which condenses with oxaloacetic acid to form fluorocitrate, this product inhibiting the enzyme aconitase and thereby preventing the conversion of citrate to isocitrate. The build-up of fluorocitrate blocks the tricarboxylic acid (Krebs) cycle, resulting in reduced glucose metabolism, cellular respiration, and tissue energy stores. Animals (and tissues) with high metabolic rates are more susceptible to toxicity.

Table 107.10 Representative Rodenticides⁺ Listed in Order of Decreasing Toxicity*

Agent		Chemical Class**
Brodifacoum	TALON	C
Coumadin	WARFARIN	C
Bromadiolone	BROMONE, MAKI	C
Difenacoum	RATAK	C
Diphacinone	DIPHACIN	I
Sodium monofluoroacetate	COMPOUND 1080	M
Strychnine		M
Phosacetim	GOPHACIDE	OP
Pyrinimil	VACOR	M
Alpha-naphthyl thiourea	ANTU	M
Fluoroacetamide	COMPOUND 1081	M
Zinc phosphide	ZIP	M
Pindone	PIVAL, PIVALYN	I
Chlorophacinone	DRAT, ROZOL	I
Norbormide	RATICATE	M
Coumachlor	RATILAN	C

*Order of decreasing toxicity was based on acute oral LD_{50} values in the laboratory rat obtained from the literature.

⁺The common chemical name and at least one trade name (in capitals) is given for each chemical.

**Chemical classes include: C, coumarins; I, indandione; M, miscellaneous; OP, organophosphorus ester.

In humans, the lethal dose of fluoroacetate ranges form 2 to 10 mg/kg.[r15] Gastrointestinal signs are seen some 30 to 100 minutes following ingestion, with the initial nausea, vomiting, and abdominal pain being replaced by sinus tachycardia, hypotension, ventricular tachycardia or fibrillation, renal failure, muscle spasms, and CNS effects (anxiety, agitation, stupor, seizures, coma). There is cerebellar degeneration and atrophy.

Treatment of poisoning is mainly supportive, and the speedy removal of unabsorbed toxicant by any and all means is imperative. There are no known specific antidotes. Glycerol monoacetate has been used successfully in poisoned monkeys but results in humans have been equivocal.

Alpha Naphthyl Thiourea (ANTU)

This substituted urea was introduced as a rodenticide after reports that phenylthiourea was lethal to rats but was not toxic to humans.[27] Major disadvantages of ANTU, however, are that young rats are resistant to it and tolerance develops in older rats. This is consistant with the hypotheses that: (a) ANTU must be metabolically activated to a toxic intermediate (young rats would not possess the microsomal enzyme activity required for this function); (b) the observed tolerance is due to the inhibition of microsomal enzymes and reduced activation of the agent. ANTU causes extensive pulmonary edema and pleural effusion as a consequence of effects on pulmonary capillaries.

Poisonings have occurred in humans, with severe pulmonary symptoms (respiratory difficulty, tracheobronchial hypersecretion of a white, non-mucous froth low in protein, which disappeared rapidly) being seen.[r11] Recovery was effected by symptomatic treatment.

Anticoagulants

With the discovery that warfarin (coumadin or 3-(alpha-acetonylbenzyl)-4-hydroxycoumarin) acted as an anticoagulant by antagonizing the actions of vitamin K on the synthesis of clotting factors (II, VII, IX, X), it was introduced as a rodenticide. The safety of warfarin rests in the fact that multiple doses are required before toxicity develops, a single exposure having little effect. The development of resistance to warfarin in rats led to an exploration of the "superwarfarins" (brodifacoum, bromadiolone, diphencoumarin, coumachlor) based on the coumadin nucleus and a new chemical class, the indandiones (diphacinone, chlorophacinone, pindone), that are more water-soluble.

Human poisonings are rather rare because these agents are dispensed in grain-based baits, not usually considered palatable by humans. However, there are sufficient cases of suicide attempts, attempted murder, and a historical, classic case of inadvertent consumption of a warfarin-laden corn meal bait by a Korean family to provide detailed information on the signs and symptoms of poisoning.[r11] With consumption over a period of several days, bleeding occurs, with bruising or hematomas developing at the knee and elbow joints and on the buttocks, with GI bleeding accompanied by abdominal or back pain (retroperitoneal hemorrhage), gum and nasal bleeding as well as hemoptysis, hematuria, and cerebrovascular accidents. The signs and symptoms will persist for many days after cessation of exposure, particularly so in cases involving the superwarfarins.

After acute ingestion, cathartics, activated charcoal, and gastric lavage are usually sufficient measures to remove unabsorbed agents from the stomach. In situations of repeated ingestion, vitamin K preparations such as Mephyton (10–25 mg orally for adults; 5–10 mg orally for children) and Aquamephyton (5–10 mg im for adults; 1–5 mg IM for children) will counteract the effects. Higher doses will be required if superwarfarins are involved. Close monitoring until the prothrombin time returns to normal is essential and transfusions with fresh-frozen plasma or whole blood may be necessary if extensive bleeding has occurred.

Zinc Phosphide

This agent is used in third-world developing nations because it is both a cheap and an effective rodenticide. The toxicity of zinc phosphide (Zn_3P_2) can be accounted for by the phosphine (PH_3) formed after a hydrolytic reaction with water in the stomach. Phosphine, which has a very characteristic rotten-fish odor, causes widespread cellular toxicity, with necrosis observed during postmortem examination. Signs and symptoms include nausea, vomiting, headache, lightheadedness, dyspnea, hypertension, pulmonary edema, dysrhythmias, and convulsions.[r4,r11] Doses of the order of 4000 to 5000 mg have been fatal, but others survived doses of 25,000 to 100,000 mg if early vomiting occurred. The usual decontamination measures and supportive therapy often are successful if initiated within a few hours of exposure.

References

Research Reports

1. Walsh J. River blindness: A gamble pays off. Science 1986; 232:922.
2. Coye MJ, Lowe JA, Maddy KT. Biological monitoring of agricultural workers exposed to pesticides: I Cholinesterase activity determinators. J Occup Med 1986;*28*:619–627.
3. Storck WJ. Pesticide profits belie mature market status. Chem Eng News Apr 28th 1980; 10–13.
4. Pimental D, Levitan L. Pesticides: amounts applied and amounts reaching pests; Bioscience 1986;*36*:86–91.
5. Edelfrawi ME, Sherby SM, Abalis IM, Edelfrawi AT. Interactions of pyrethroid and cyclodiene insecticides with nicotinic acetylcholine and GABA receptors. Neurotoxicology 1985;*6*:47–62.
6. Namba T, Nolte CT, Jackrel J, Grob D. Poisoning due to organophosphate insecticides, acute and chronic manifestations. Am J Med 1971;*50*:475–492.
7. Ecobichon DJ, Ozere RL, Reid E, Crocker JFS. Acute fenitrothion poisoning. Can Med Assoc J 1977;*116*:377–379.
8. McCord CP, Kilker CH, Minster DR. Pyrethrum dermatitis. A record of the occurrence of occupational dermatoses among workers in the pyrethrum industry. JAMA 1921;*77*:448–449.
9. Tucker SB, Flannigan SA. Cutaneous effects from occupational exposure to fenvalerate. Arch Toxicol 1983;*54*:195–202.
10. He F, Sun J, Han K, Wu Y, Wang S, Liu L. Effects of pyrethroid insecticides on subjects engaged in packaging pyrethroids. Br J Ind Med 1988;*45*:548–551.
11. He F, Wang S, Liu L, Chen S, Zhang Z, Sun J. Clinical manifestations and diagnosis of acute pyrethroid poisoning. Arch Toxicol 1989;*63*:54–58.
12. Chen S, Zhang Z, He F, Yao P, Wu Y, Sun J, Liu L, Li Q. An epidemiological study on occupational acute pyrethroid poisoning in cotton farmers. Br J Ind Med 1991;*48*:77–81.
13. Narahashi T. Nerve membrane ionic channels as the primary target of pyrethroids. Neurotoxicology 1985;*6*:3–22.
14. Morrison HI, Wilkins K, Semenciw R, Mao Y, Wigle D. Herbicides and cancer. JNCI 1992;*84*:1866–1874.
15. Hoar SK, Blair A, Holmes FF, Boyseh CD, Robel RJ, Hoover R, Fraumeni JF. Agricultural herbicide use and risk of lymphoma and soft-tissue sarcoma. JAMA 1986;*256*:1141–1147.
16. Singer R, Moses M, Valciukas J, Lilis R, Selikoff IJ. Nerve conduction velocity studies of workers employed in the manufacture of phenoxy herbicides. Environ Res 1982;*29*:297–311.
17. Berwick P. Dichlorophenoxyacetic acid poisoning in man. Some interesting clinical and laboratory findings. JAMA 1970;*214*:1114–1117.
18. Nielsen K, Kaempe B, Jensen-Holm J. Fatal poisoning in man by 2,4-dichlorophenoxyacetic acid (2,4-D). Determination of the agent in forensic materials. Acta Pharmacol Toxicol 1965;*22*:224–234.
19. Zahm SH, Weisenburger DD, Babbitt PA, Saal RC, Vaught JB, Cantor KP, Blair A. A case-control study on non-Hodgkin's lymphoma and the herbicide 2,4-dichlorophenoxyacetic acid (2,4-D) in eastern Nebraska. Epidem 1990;*1*:349–356.
20. Coggon D, Acheson ED. Do phenoxy herbicides cause cancer in man? Lancet 1982;*1*:1057–1059.
21. Bertazzi PA, Pesatori AC, Consonni D, Tironi A, Landi MT, Zocchetti C. Cancer incidence in a population accidentally exposed to 2,3,7,8-tetrachlorodibenzo-p-dioxin. Epidemiology 1993;*4*:398–406.
22. Narita S, Motojuku H, Sato J, Mori H. Autopsy in acute suicidal poisoning by diquat dibromide. Japan J Rural Med 1978;*27*:454–455.

23. Rose MS, Smith LL. Tissue uptake of paraquat and diquat. Gen Pharmacol 1977;*8*:173–176.

24. Israeli R, Sculsky M, Tiberin P. Acute central nervous system changes due to intoxication by Mandizan (a combined dithiocarbamate of maneb and zineb). Arch Toxicol Suppl 6 1983; 238–243.

25. Ferraz HB, Bertolucci PHF, Pereira JS, Lima JGC, Andrade LAF. Chronic exposure to the fungicide maneb may produce symptoms and signs of CNS manganese intoxication. Neurol 1988;*38*:550–553.

26. Bakir F, Damluji SF, Amin-Zaki L, Murtadha M, Khalidi A, Al-Rawi NY, Tikriti S, Dhahir HI, Clarkson TW, Smith JC, Doherty RA. Methylmercury poisoning in Iraq. Science 1973;*181*:230–241.

27. Richter CP. The development and use of alpha-naphthyl thiourea (ANTU) as a rat poison. JAMA 1945;*129*:927–931.

Reviews

r1. Brooks GT. Chlorinated insecticides. Vol I Technology and application. Boca Raton FL: CRC Press, 1974; 12–13.

r2. Matsumura F. Toxicology of insecticides. New York: Plenum Press, 1985.

r3. Copplestone JF. In Watson DL, Brown AWA, eds. Pesticide management and pesticide resistance. New York: Academic Press. 1977.

r4. Ellenhorn MJ, Barceloux DG. Pesticides. In Medical toxicology. Diagnosis and treatment of human poisoning. New York: Elsevier: 1988; Ch 38.

r5. Baker SR, Wilkinson CF, eds. The effect of pesticides on human health. Princeton NJ: Princeton Scientific Publishing Co, 1990.

r6. Ecobichon DJ, Joy RM. Pesticides and neurological diseases. 2nd ed. Boca Raton FL: CRC Press Inc, 1994.

r7. Ecobichon DJ. Pesticides. In Casarett and Doull's Toxicology. The basic science of poisons, 4th ed. New York: Pergamon Press, 1991; 565–622.

r8. Ecobichon DJ. Hydrolytic transformation of environmental pollutants. In Lee DHK, ed. Handbook of physiology. Reactions to environmental agents. Bethesda: American Physiological Society, 1977; 441–454.

r9. Aldridge WN. An assessment of the toxicological properties of pyrethroids and their neurotoxicity. CRC Crit Rev Toxicol, 1990;*211*:89–104.

r10. Vijverberg HPM, van den Bercken J. Neurotoxicological effects and the mode of action of pyrethroid insecticides. CRC Crit. Rev. Toxicol., 1990;*21*:105–126.

r11. Hayes JR WJ, Laws JR ER, eds. Handbook of pesticide toxicology. Vol 2 and 3. San Diego: Academic Press, 1991.

r12. Hay A. The chemical scythe. Lessons of 2,4,5-T and dioxin. New York: Plenum Press, 1982.

r13. Haley TJ. Review of the toxicology of paraquat (1,1'-dimethyl-4,4'-bipyridinium chloride). Clin Toxicol 1979;*14*:1–46.

r14. Smith LL. The mechanisms of paraquat toxicity in the lung. In Hodgson E, Bend JR, Philpot RM, eds. Reviews of biochemical toxicology. New York: Elsevier Press, 1987, 37–81.

r15. Pattison FLM. Toxic aliphatic fluorine compounds. New York: Elsevier Press, 1959.

CHAPTER 108

H. B. Schiefer

Mycotoxins

Introduction

Mycotoxins are a diverse group of chemical compounds that can occur in a variety of foods of plant origin and in products derived from animals that consume contaminated feed. Mycotoxins are secondary metabolites of various fungi and are produced when fungi mature and start to produce spores. The toxins have been called "agents in search of a disease," because mycologic differentiation and analytical capabilities have outpaced our understanding of the clinically recognizable diseases associated with mycotoxins. Excellent overviews of mycotoxic fungi, mycotoxins and mycotoxicoses have been published.[r1–r3]

Diseases caused by the secondary metabolites of fungi are called mycotoxicoses. In veterinary medicine, the mycotoxicoses conform to a few general principles, such as: (a) they occur often, but the true cause is not identified immediately; (b) the disorder or disease is not transmissible from one animal to another, i.e., the disease is neither infectious nor contagious; (c) treatment with drugs or antibiotics has little or no effect on the course of the disease; (d) outbreaks are usually seasonal, since certain climatic conditions may favor mycotoxin production; (e) epidemiologic studies indicate specific association with a particular feed; and (f) examination of feed may reveal the presence of unusual or unusually large numbers of fungi; however, this does not necessarily indicate that mycotoxins have been produced.

Recognition of a mycotoxin problem in humans is much more difficult, because of the nonspecificity of both symptomatology and pathologic changes in most cases.[r4] In principle, identification of any disease entity relies on both symptomatic and morphologic patterns of recognition. "Real" disease-caused patterns have to be separated from "normal," or from "within normal variation," from clinical symptoms due to other causes, and from artifacts or postmortem changes. Unfortunately, in the case of mycotoxicoses, the patterns of real change are clinically nonspecific most of the time and often are difficult to differentiate from artifactual or postmortem changes. Epidemiology appears to be the key to reaching a diagnosis of mycotoxicosis, but often this method cannot be employed because investigators, particularly clinicians, are limited to only a few isolated observations.

The following discussion will present the mycotoxins of potential importance to humans in alphabetical order, without regard to their possible relative importance, because the situation varies with the geographical location in which any given mycotoxin is found. Also, today, both humans and food products travel worldwide, thus mycotoxins have become a global problem. Table 108.1 lists some important mycotoxins, the fungi that may produce them, and examples of commodities in which the toxins may occur. The "older" (well-known) fungal diseases, like aspergillosis, candidamycosis (yeast infection) and others, are not listed here. References can be found in the appropriate literature.[r1,r5]

One must be aware of other pathways of mycotoxins besides consumption of contaminated foods. Laboratory workers handling mycotoxins are prime subjects

Table 108.1 Mycotoxins of Importance to Humans

Mycotoxin	Produced by	Found in
Aflatoxins B_1, B_2, G_1, G_2; metabolites such as Aflatoxin M_1; etc.	*Aspergillus flavus*	Peanuts and other nuts; corn; milk
Citreoviridin	*Penicillium citreoviride*	Rice
Ergot Alkaloids	*Claviceps purpurea; Cl. paspalis*	Cereal grains
Fumonisin B_1 and B_2	*Fusarium moniliforme*	Corn, cereal grains
Ochratoxins A, B and C	*Aspergillus ochraceus;* other *Aspergillus* and *Penicillium* spp	Corn, cereal grains; meat from animals fed ochratoxin-contaminated feed
Patulin	*Penicillium claviforme; P. patulum*	Apples and apple products; other fruit juices
Penicillium islandicum toxins (luteoskyrin, cyclochlorotine, islandotoxin, regulosin)	*Penicillium islandicum*	Rice
Psoralens	*Sclerotinia sclerotiorum*	Figs, parsley, parsnip, lime, clove celery
Tremorgens (penitrem paxicilline, roquefortine)	*Penicillium* spp; some *Aspergillus* spp	Nuts; spoiled food
Trichothecenes, nonmacrocyclic (e.g., deoxynivalenol, nivalenol, T-2 toxin, diacetoxyscirpenol, and many others)	*Fusarium sporotrichioides;* other *Fusarium* spp; *Trichothecium* spp; *Trichoderma* spp; *Cephalosporium* spp; *Acremonium* spp	Cereal grains, bananas, and possibly other commodities
Trichothecenes, macrocyclic (e.g., satratoxins, verrucarin, roridin, and others)	*Stachybotrys atra; Myrothecium* spp; *Dendrodochium toxicum*	Cellulose-containing substrate
Wortmannin	*Penicillium wortmanni, Fusarium oxysporum, Myrothecium roridum*	Plants and cereal grains
Zearalenone	*Fusarium graminearum*	Corn, cereal grains

for accidental exposure by skin contact or inhalation. Aerosols or dust, generated during processing of moldy food, can lead to the deposition of mycotoxins into the lungs, and exposure can also occur in energy efficient homes or from ventilation systems in which fungal growth occurs.

After the discovery of the aflatoxins in the early 1960s, specific mycotoxin legislation was developed in several countries, initially referring only to aflatoxins. By 1987, the number of countries with regulations for other mycotoxins had risen to 15. Mycotoxins considered to be important enough for tolerances to be established are patulin, ochratoxin A, the trichothecenes, and zearalenone. Details of tolerances and status of standard methods of sampling and analysis worldwide, can be found in an overview.[1]

The mycotoxins are not a relatively uniform matrix as can be seen from some examples shown here. These are just some examples of this confusing picture.

Aflatoxins

Aflatoxins have received the most attention in research because of their extremely potent hepatocarcinogenicity and toxicity; they have been reviewed extensively.[r4,r6] Aflatoxins are a group of bisfurano-coumarin metabolites, designated as B_1, B_2, G_1, and G_2 because of their blue (B) or green (G) fluorescence under UV light. Metabolites have been called M_1, M_2, etc. The aflatoxins are produced by *Aspergillus* species under moist, warm conditions, both during the growth of plants and during storage of plant products.

Aflatoxins are acutely toxic to all species, with LD_{50} values ranging from 0.5 mg/kg for ducklings to 60 mg/kg for the mouse. Aflatoxins act on cellular membranes, inhibit DNA-dependent RNA-synthesis and are mutagenic owing to alkylation of nuclear DNA. The key compound, aflatoxin B_1, is not only hepatotoxic, but is one of the most powerful carcinogens

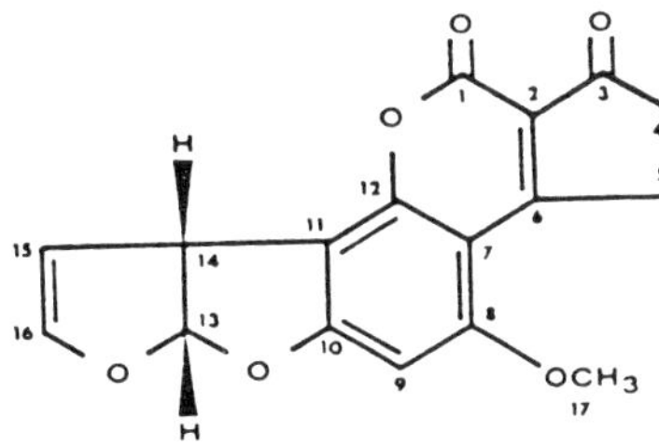

Aflatoxin B_1

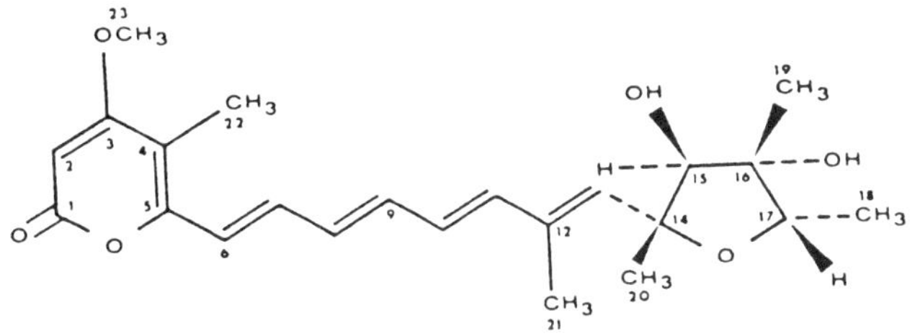

Citreoviridin

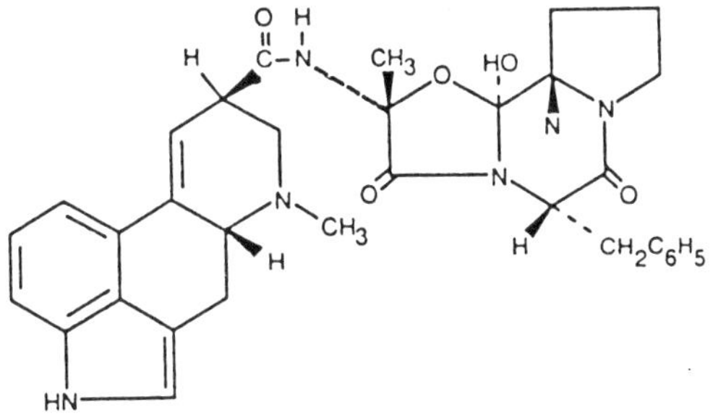

Ergotamine

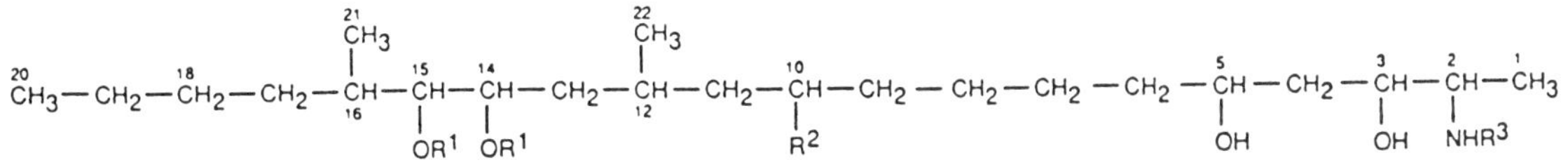

Fumonisins

A_1: $R^1 = COCH_2CH(CO_2H)CH_2CO_2H$; $R^2 = OH$; $R^3 = C^{23}OC^{24}H_3$

A_2: $R^1 = COCH_2CH(CO_2H)CH_2CO_2H$; $R^2 = H$; $R^3 = COCH_3$

B_1: $R^1 = COCH_2CH(CO_2H)CH_2CO_2H$; $R^2 = OH$; $R^3 = H$

B_2: $R^1 = COCH_2CH(CO_2H)CH_2CO_2H$; $R^2 = R^3 = H$

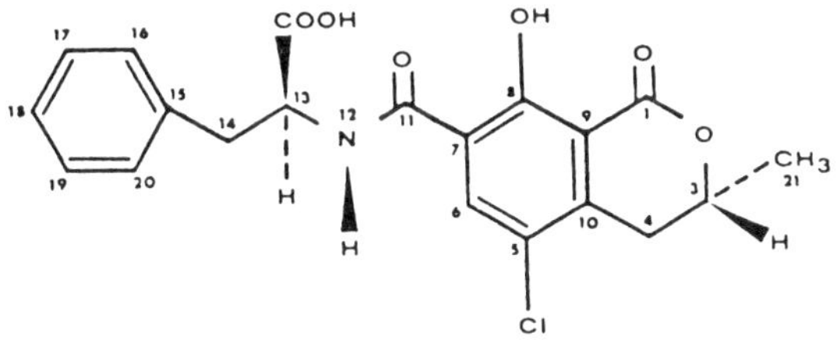

Ochratoxin A

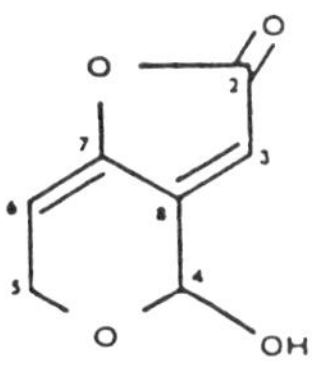

Patulin

Two examples of PENICILLUM ISLANDICUM TOXINS

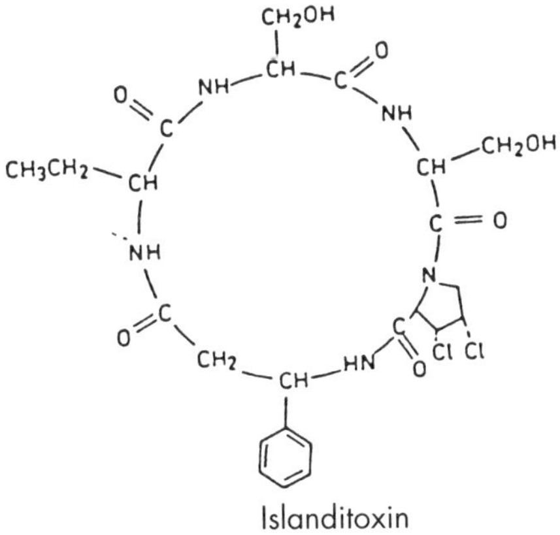

Islanditoxin

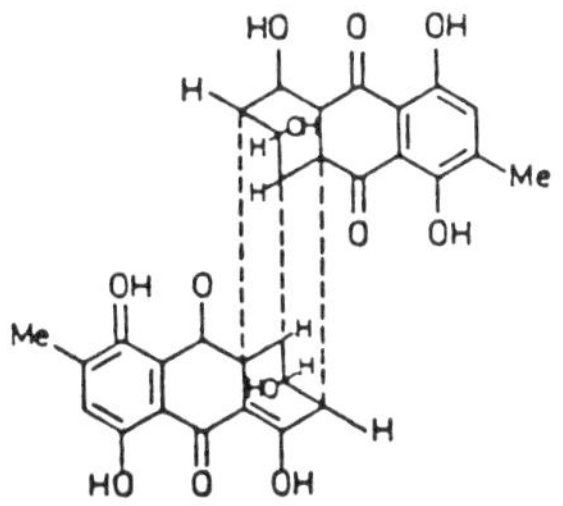

Luteoskyrin

Figure 108.1 Chemical Structures of Selected Mycotoxins

Two examples of PSORALENS

Methoxypsoralen

Trimethylpsoralen

Two examples of TREMORGENS

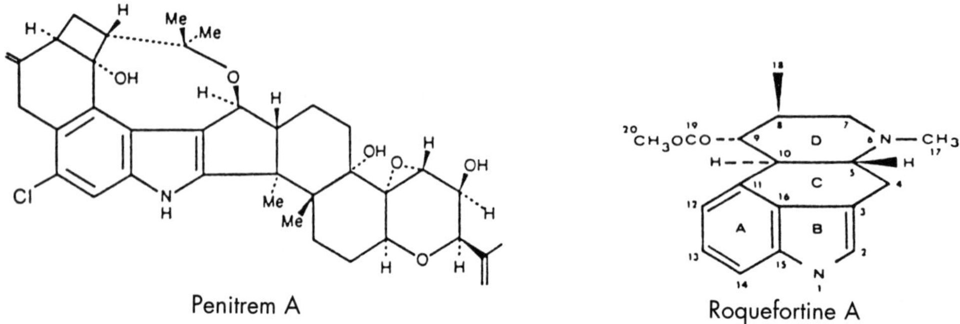

Three examples of NON-MACROCYCLIC TRICHOTHECENES

Deoxynivalenol

Diacetoxyscirpenol

T-2

One example of a MACROCYCLIC TRICHOTHECENE

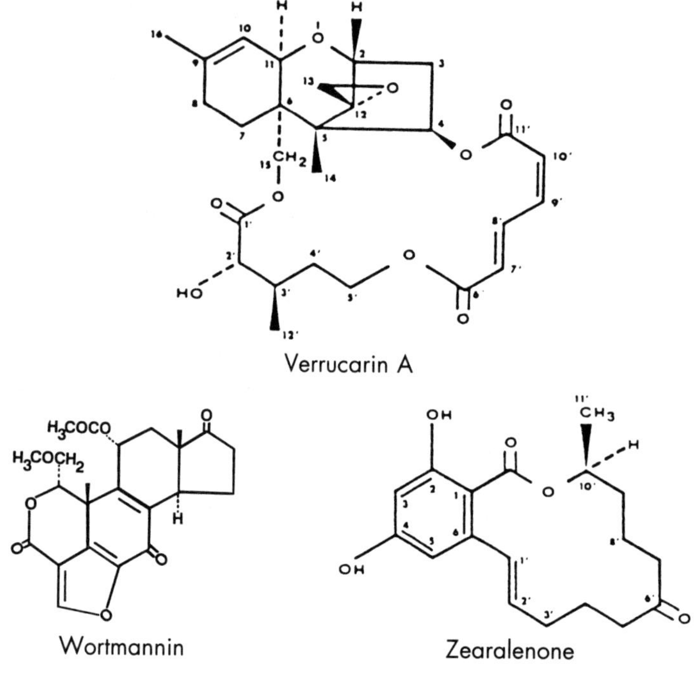

Figure 108.1 *Continued*

known, inducing liver tumors after dietary intake of levels in the parts per billion (ppb) range. The toxin is also teratogenic in a variety of laboratory animals, including primates. Aflatoxin B_1 requires metabolic activation to its ultimate carcinogenic form, an epoxide, and is primarily metabolized by the cytochrome P-450 monoxygenase system.

Diseases due to aflatoxins have to be separated into two unrelated entities.[r6] Aflatoxin can be the cause of acute aflatoxicosis in the form of Reye's syndrome, which is characterized by vomiting, abdominal pain, fatty liver, and encephalopathy, although other causes, such as acetylsalicylic acid, have been suggested to be involved in Reye's syndrome. Chronic aflatoxicosis is associated with acute to chronic hepatic injury leading to cirrhosis, and, ultimately, to hepatic cancer. Evidence of carcinogenicity in humans is based on epidemiologic studies.

While it may be possible to avoid the acute effects by selecting only nonspoiled food, including nuts and peanut products, avoiding contaminated animal products like milk (containing aflatoxins or their metabolites) is much more difficult. Most countries have set tolerance limits in food. However, to ask for a reduction to zero-levels of aflatoxin and its metabolites in general might create a major loss of important staples of human food sources, and may be impossible to enforce or control. There is no known specific treatment method. Caution should be exercised by workers involved in the processing of spoiled nuts.

Citreoviridin

This mycotoxin has been associated with a disease in Japan, known as shoshin kakke or cardiac beri-beri, for almost 300 years. The incidence of the disease started to decline when rice inspection was introduced in Japan in 1910. The exclusion of moldy rice from commerce resulted in almost complete disappearance of the disease after 1929.

The biologic activities of citreoviridin are not well understood, but it is considered to be a neurotoxin. The main symptoms are CNS depression and cardiovascular effects. Palpitations, precardial stress, tachypnea, nausea, vomiting, and difficult breathing have been observed. Within days after ingestion, severe pain and mania, low blood pressure, and rapid pulse may be experienced. Seemingly healthy persons can die within a few days. Survivors may experience life-long visual impairment and paralysis. No specific treatment is known, but the disease does not occur if rice is stored under proper conditions.

Ergot Alkaloids

More than 40 ergot alkaloids (ergolines) have been isolated from *Claviceps purpurea* sclerotia.[r7] They can be divided into three groups:

Group I, derivatives of lysergic acid (ergotamine, ergocryptine, ergocristine, ergocorinine, and ergometrine). Group II, derivatives of isolysergic acid (ergocristinine, ergometrinine, ergocorninine, ergocrytinine, and ergotaminine). Group III, derivatives of dimethylergoline or clavines (agroclavine, elymoclavine, chanoclavine, penniclavine, setoclavine).

Ergot mycotoxins occur in the hard, purplish, or black sclerotia produced by *Claviceps purpurea* and other *Claviceps* species, and wheat, rice, corn, sorghum, rye, barley, oats, and millet can act as hosts. Ergot alkaloids are the oldest known mycotoxins. Reports of poisonings extend back several hundred years BC. The extent of epidemics in Europe during the Middle Ages may be inferred from the foundation of an Order, in 1093, taking St. Anthony as its patron saint, devoted to the care of the victims of ergotism. The last outbreaks of ergotism in Europe occurred in 1926–1928 in the UK and the former USSR. In 1978, 93 cases of ergotism were reported from Ethiopia.[r7] In India, intoxication following ingestion of ergot from *Claviceps fusiformis* has been reported.[r7]

Ergot alkaloids are potent antagonists of catecholamine and 5-hydroxytryptamine, and stimulate smooth muscle contraction of the arterioles, intestines, and uterus.[r6] They also excite and depress the CNS. Ergotamine is used in the treatment of migraine headaches. Ergot alkaloids are absorbed slowly from the GI tract. Metabolism occurs primarily in the liver, with approximately 90 per cent of metabolites excreted with bile. Two forms of clinical disease are recognized. In the "convulsive form," drowsiness, headache, delirium, giddiness, painful cramps, spastic movements of the limbs, and itching of the skin have been reported. In severe cases of the "ischemic form," gangrene involving the toes and fingers, and occasionally the ears and nose, may occur due to intense vasoconstriction.

Modern practices of milling cereal grains containing ergot sclerotia have essentially caused a disappearance of intoxications in humans. Baking or heat processing destroys most alkaloids of the ergotamine group.

Fumonisins

Four fumonisins have been identified to date: FB_1, FB_2, FB_3, and FB_4.[2] They are produced by *Fusarium moniliforme* mainly, and possibly by *F. graminearum* and *F.*

subglutinans and also *Alternaria* spp.[3] *F. moniliforme* is ubiquitous in humid and subhumid temperate zones in addition to subtropical and tropical regions throughout the world.

A study of rats indicated that the liver was the main target of fumonisin B_1, causing progressive hepatitis and induction of gamma-glutamyl-transpeptidase positive (GGT^+) foci in the liver, leading to cancer of the liver.[4] Fumonisins have been declared to be 2B carcinogens (suspected human carcinogen) by IARC. Strains of *F. moniliforme* isolated from various types of cancer in humans from Canada and the US were found to be intermediate- or high-level producers of fumonisins.[5]

Ochratoxins

The ochratoxins are a group of seven isocoumarin derivatives linked with an amide bond to the amino group of L-beta-phenylalanine. Ochratoxin A is the predominant and most toxic member of the series. Ochratoxins are produced by *Penicillium* species and *Aspergillus* species, including *A. ochraceus*. Ochratoxins have been identified in many countries in barley, corn, wheat, oats, rye, green coffee beans, and peanuts, as well as in meat and animal products.

Ochratoxins have a wide range of biologic activity. They cause degenerative changes in mitochondria, alter carbohydrate metabolism, interact with macromolecular binding, and inhibit enzymatic activities. The main feature is inhibition of macromolecular protein synthesis and immunosuppression. Ochratoxins are known to cause acute hepatic damage in ducklings and nephrotoxicity in almost all species. In addition, there are now credible accounts of carcinogenicity.[6]

There is no proven acute toxic effect in humans,[7] but ochratoxins have been associated with "Balkan nephropathy," a disease that has been the subject of intense scientific discussion for years. Considering the toxic potential of ochratoxins, it is quite possible that this mycotoxin may cause not only nephropathy, but also may be involved in the development of urinary tract neoplasms in humans.

Patulin

Patulin, which occurs in rotted apples, apple products, or other fruit juices, possesses moderately high acute toxicity to mice, rats, chicks and rabbits (LD_{50} values ranging from 15 to 170 mg/kg). Patulin is produced by a number of *Penicillium* spp, *Aspergillus* spp, and two species of *Byssochlamys*.[r6]

Patulin is cytotoxic. It inhibits mitosis and disrupts the organization of the mitotic spindle apparatus in amphibian cells. The mitostatic and toxic activity of patulin has been blocked in some instances by exposure of the cells to compounds containing sulfhydryl groups. Subcutaneous injection in rats has caused sarcomas, but attempts to induce tumors through oral administration have not been successful.

Patulin has been reported to produce nausea and GI irritation. Trimming the spoiled areas from rotted apples or other fruits would substantially reduce patulin consumption. Patulin cannot be found in juice fermented by *Saccharomyces* spp.

Penicillium Islandicum Toxins

P. islandicum is capable of producing a variety of toxins, namely luteoskyrin, cyclochlorotine, islanditoxin, and rugulosin. All these toxins are hepatotoxic and carcinogenic. This group of toxins received a certain notoriety during World War II, when Japanese soldiers ingested contaminated rice and suffered from edema of the legs ("yellow rice syndrome"), a condition readily confused with citreoviridin mycotoxicosis.[r12]

Psoralens

Psoralens are a group of furo-coumarines (4,5,8-trimethylpsoralen; 5-methoxypsoralen; 8-methoxypsoralen) produced on a variety of plants. Psoralen-containing plants were used by Turks, Hindus, and Egyptians in ancient times for the treatment of psoriasis and to mask the effect of leukoderma (i.e., nonpigmented scar on the skin).

The toxins are lethal to a variety of bacteria and eukaryotic cell cultures when exposed to UV light (320–400 nm). The importance of photoactivation in humans has now been established. The best known disease in humans is "celery workers disease," a condition occurring in people who handle moldy celery. Erythema and bullous lesions develop on fingers and lower arms in persons with light skin after exposure to the mycotoxin and sunlight. Persons with normal dietary habits appear to be at no risk of phototoxic burn due to the ingestion of celery or other vegetables.[8]

Tremorgens

A variety of mycotoxins produced by *Penicillium* spp, such as: penitrem A, B, and C, verruculogen, paxilline, and roquefortine; fumitremorgen A and B (from

A. fumigatus) and flavus tremorgens (from *A. flavus*) are included under this term.

There are animal cases, but no reliable reports of tremorgenic mycotoxicosis in humans. The significance of these toxins in man has yet to be established. Roquefortine is not stable in blue cheese.

The common feature of the tremorgens is induction of neurotoxicity. In experimental animals, tremorgens produce profound neuropathic effects, including tremors and convulsions, that may lead to death. In addition, diuretic effects have been observed.

Trichothecenes

The trichothecene mycotoxins are a group of closely related secondary metabolic products of several families of imperfect, saprophytic, or plant pathogenic fungi such as, *Fusarium, Trichothecium, Myrothecium, Cephalosporium, Stachybotrys, Trichoderma, Cylindrocarpon* and *Verticimonosporium* spp.[r8,r9] The first trichothecenes were isolated in the 1940s and 1950s during the search for antibiotic metabolites of fungi, but only during the last two decades have efforts been made to characterize the effects of trichothecenes in man, mammals, and other organisms. Current surveys have demonstrated a worldwide occurrence of more than 80 derivatives in cereals, food, or in the environment. Trichothecenes are found in a variety of foods (cereals, fruits, etc.), and can be found in the air of domestic or commercial buildings.

The trichothecene mycotoxins are highly toxic at the subcellular, cellular and organ system level.[r10,r11] Because they are lipid soluble, they rapidly penetrate cell lipid bilayers, thus allowing access to DNA, RNA, and cell organelles. At the subcellular level the toxicity of these toxins lies in their ability to inhibit protein synthesis and to bind covalently to sulfhydryl groups. The mechanism of inhibition of protein synthesis probably affects various states, from initiation to termination through inhibition of peptidyl transferase, with subsequent inhibition of peptide bond formation. Trichothecenes have been shown to damage DNA both in vitro and in vivo, but inhibition of protein and DNA synthesis seem to be affected to the same extent. No inhibitory effects have been seen on DNA polymerase, thymidine kinase, and thymidylate kinase in vitro, therefore the inhibition of DNA synthesis probably arises from a secondary effect of the inhibition of protein synthesis. Trichothecene mycotoxins can covalently bond to proteins, probably to sulfhydryl groups, resulting in enzyme inhibition. The inhibition of respiratory enzymes necessary for oxidative phosphorylation mainly affects the enzymes in mitochondria. The affinity of the trichothecene toxins for sulfhydryl groups may also account for their toxic effects on spindle formation, since tubulin dimers, the major protein compound of the microtubules of the mitotic spindle, contain numerous sulfhydryl groups. Bonding to these groups may present formation of the mitotic spindle. Cell surface sulfhydryl groups are probably important in the interaction of these toxins with cell membranes with subsequent cell lysis. At the cellular level, trichothecene mycotoxins have antifungal, phytotoxic, and antibacterial properties, and are generally cytotoxic to most cells, including neoplastic cells. This cytotoxicity is expressed as cell lysis or inhibition of mitosis. Mutagenicity does not seem to be a feature of these toxins. Preferential cytotoxicity to dividing cells led to the trial use of diacetoxyscirpenol (DAS) as an antineoplastic agent under the name of anguidine.

Pharmacokinetic studies have shown that trichothecenes are rapidly absorbed, metabolized into polar products, and eliminated without accumulation. Microsomal carboxyesterases mediate hydrolysis of trichothecenes, and de-epoxidation of the 12,13-epoxide by the intestinal microflora has been reported. It is difficult to relate these observations to the variety of diseases and symptoms discussed below.

Systemic toxicity of the trichothecenes in multiorgan systems is based on direct cytotoxicity and is often referred to as a radiomimetic effect. The cutaneous cytotoxicity that follows administration of these compounds can be described as a nonspecific, acute, necrotizing process with minimal inflammation of both the epidermis and dermis. Chemical stomatitis and hyperkeratosis with ulceration of the esophageal portion of the gastric mucosa, in conjunction with necrosis of the intestinal tract, has been seen following ingestion of trichothecenes.

Given in sublethal toxic doses via any route, the trichothecenes are highly immunosuppressive in mammals; however, long-term feeding of high levels of T-2 toxin does not seem to activate latent viral or bacterial infections. The main immunosuppressive effect of the trichothecenes is at the level of the T suppressor cell; the toxins, however, may affect the function of helper T cells, B cells, or macrophages, or interactions among all of these cells.

Hemorrhagic diatheses may occur following thrombocytopenia or defective intrinsic or extrinsic coagulation pathways. Thrombocytopenia occurs in humans within days after administration of the trichothecene mycotoxins. It appears that hemorrhage results from depression of clotting factors, thrombocytopenia, inhibition of platelet function, or possibly a combination of all these deficiencies. More recently, the mycotoxin wortmannin (see below) has been suggested as another contributing hemorrhagic factor in trichothecene toxicosis.[9] Changes in heart rate, blood pressure, or EKG also have been observed. The cardiovascular changes consist of initial hypertension with peripheral vasoconstriction, followed by decreased cardiac output and hypotension in all species investigated. The hypotensive effects may lead to shock and rapid death before florid morphologic changes are apparent.

In mice and rats, dermal application of trichothecenes can induce systemic damage within hours of application. Clinical signs and morphologic changes equal to those after oral or intraperitoneal administration have been observed. The choice of vehicle and/or absorption enhancer is important in determining the rapidity and degree of toxicity. Inhalation of T-2 toxin hastens the onset of toxicity and death in experimental animals.[r11]

Several disease syndromes in humans have been associated with trichothecene mycotoxins.[r9] Alimentary toxic aleukia (ATA), mainly caused by T-2 toxin, is characterized by four recognizable clinical stages. The first stage, which starts soon after eating a contaminated cereal food, is typified by chemical irritation and a sense of burning in the mouth, throat, and stomach. Gastroenteretis, with vomiting and diarrhea, occurs within one to two days, but affected persons remain afebrile and temporarily recover in spite of continued consumption of the toxin. The second stage is characterized by a relatively symptomless period during which leukopenia, thrombocytopenia, and anemia develop. Other clinical signs, such as weakness, vertigo, headache, palpitations, and slight asthma may be observed. The third stage begins suddenly as an acute febrile disease and evolves into a hemorrhagic syndrome in which petechiae occur throughout the body, especially under skin exposed to friction or trauma. Necrotic mucosal plaques develop in the oral cavity, pharynx, esophagus, and sometimes in the stomach and lower alimentary tract, probably because of secondary bacterial invasion made possible by the neutropenia. If death does not occur during the third stage, it is followed by a fourth stage, which is a period of convalescence. Hematopoiesis resumes, and the septic necrotic lesions disappear, provided the toxic food is no longer consumed. ATA is often complicated by opportunistic bacteria and fungi, a testimony to the immunosuppressive action of the trichothecenes. The opportunists may cause bronchopneumonia and other infective organ failures.

Diacetoxyscirpenol (anguidine), a nonmacrocyclic trichothecene mycotoxin, was tested for use in cancer treatment on the basis of its observed antineoplastic qualities in other species. Such treatment resulted in quite a number of undesirable side-effects, including nausea, vomiting, hypotension, CNS dysfunction, fever and chills, stomatitis, and hyperemia of the skin.

Stachybotrytoxicosis was seen as early as 1927 in workers exposed to macrocyclic trichothecenes produced by *Stachybotrys atra* on moldy food stuffs. In these cases, lesions developed mainly in the skin from direct contact and in lungs from inhalation of dust containing toxins. More recently, the macrocyclic trichothecenes have been associated with symptoms of recurring maladies, including cold and flu symptoms, sore throat, diarrhea, headaches, fatigue, dermititis, intermittent focal alopecia, and general malaise in occupants of urban homes in North America. *Stachybotrys atra* was found to grow in wood, insulation material, and in heating ducts. Aerosolized spores in the air contained the toxins.[10] The skin irritating properties of these toxins were experienced by workers who removed the moldy materials.

An endemically occurring bone and joint disease in East Siberia, Northern China and North Korea (known under the name Kashin Beck [Urov] disease) also has been associated with trichothecenes. The unusually high incidence of esophageal cancer in some parts of China and in the Transkei (South Africa) has been suspected to be caused by the ingestion of food contaminated with one trichothecene, deoxynivalenol, in addition to fumonisins (from *F. moniliforme*), a mutagenic factor, fusarin-C (from *Fusarium* spp), and zearalenone (see below).

There is no specific treatment. Anti-inflammatory therapy (particularly glucocorticosteroids) and stabilization of cardiovascular function are the only measures. Considering the insidious effects on people exposed to such toxins in enclosed spaces (domestic or commercial), it appears prudent to adhere to standards that will prevent the growth of trichothecene-producing fungi in dwellings. This is a challenging engineering problem.

Wortmannin

Wortmannin causes hemorrhages, hemoglobinuria, and inhibits immune function at low levels. The importance of this mycotoxin, known to be produced by *Penicillium wortmanni*, as a hemorrhagic factor and immunosuppressive agent, has been recognized only very recently.[9] It was found that wortmannin is also produced by *Fusarium oxysporum* or *Myrothecium roridum* in cereal grains contaminated with trichothecene-producing fungi.

Zearalenone

Zearalenone is a nonsteroidal estrogenic mycotoxin found in corn and corn products, or other cereals, worldwide. It is produced by numerous species of *Fu-*

sarium. Zearalenone is known for causing hyperestrogenism in pigs. A closely related substance, zeralanol, is used as an anabolic agent in beef cattle. Zearalenone mimics the effects of diethylstilbestrol (DES) and estradiol in depressing serum gonadotropin levels, and inducing uterine growth and vaginal epithelial cornification. The biologic half-life of the metabolites is longer in humans than in other species.[11]

There are no proven or documented cases of zearalenone toxicity in humans. However, zearalenone is considered by the International Agency for Research on Cancer (IARC) as belonging to the category of "limited evidence of carcinogenicity," and it has been speculated that the high incidence of esophageal cancer in certain parts of the world may be due to zearalenone, in conjunction with other mycotoxins (see trichothecenes). No regulatory action has been recommended to date; however, it is suggested that exposure to zearalenone from corn cereals be kept as low as technologically feasible, and that other food commodities (e.g., milk, meat) be monitored.[11]

References

Research Reports

1. van Egmond HP. Current situation on regulations for mycotoxins. Overview of tolerances and status of standard methods of sampling and analysis. Food Add Contam 1989;*6*:139–188.
2. Catwood ME, Wentzel CA, Vleggar R, Behrend Y, Thiel PG, Marasas WF. Isolation of the fumonisin mycotoxins: A quantitative approach. J Agric Food Chem 1991;*39*:1958–1962.
3. Chen J, Mirocha CJ, Xie W, Hogge L, Olson D. Production of the mycotoxin Fumonisin B_1 by *Alternaria alternata* f sp. *lycopersici*. Appl Environ Microbiol 1992;*58*:3928–3931.
4. Gelderblom WCA, Kriek NPJ, Marasas WFO, Thiel PG. Toxicity and carcinogenicity of the *Fusarium moniliforme* metabolite, fumonisin B_1 in rats. Carcinogenesis 1991;*12*:1247–1251.
5. Nelson PE, Plattner RD, Shackelford DD, Desjardins AE. Production of fumonisins by *Fusarium moniliforme* strains from various substrates and geographic areas. Appl Environ Microbiol 1991;*57*:2410–2412.
6. Bendele AM, Carlton WW, Krogh P, Lillehoj EB. Ochratoxin A carcinogenesis in the (C57BL/6JxC3H)F_1 mouse. J NCI 1985;*75*:733–742.
7. Kuiper-Goodman T, Scott PM. Risk assessment of the mycotoxin Ochratoxin A. Biomed Env Sci 1989;*2*:179–248.
8. Schlatter J, Zimmerli B, Dick R, Panizzon R, Schlatter CH. Dietary intake and risk assessment of phototoxic furocoumarines in humans. Fd Chem Toxic 1991;*29*:523–530.
9. Gunther R, Kishore PN, Abbas HK, Mirocha CJ. Immunosuppressive effects of dietary Wortmannin on rats and mice. Immunopharmacol Immunotox 1989;*11*:559–570.
10. Sorenson WG, Frazer DG, Jarvis BB, Simpson J, Robinson VA. Trichothecene mycotoxins in aerosolized conidia of *Stachybotrys atra*. Appl Env Microbiol 1987;*53*:1370–1375.
11. Kuiper-Goodman T, Scott PM, Watanabe H. Risk assessment of the mycotoxin zearalenone. Regul Tox Pharmacol 1987;*7*:253–306.

Reviews

r1. Wyllie TD, Morehouse LG. Mycotoxic fungi, mycotoxins, mycotoxicoses. An encyclopedic handbook. Vols. I, II, III. New York: Dekker, 1977, 1978.

r2. Sharma RP, Salunkhe DK. Mycotoxins and phytoalexins. Boca Raton, FL: CRC Press, 1991.

r3. Miller JD, Trenholm L. Mycotoxins in grain: compounds other than aflatoxin. St. Paul, MN: Amer. Assoc. Cereal Chemists, 1994.

r4. Hayes AW. Mycotoxins: A review of biological effects and their role in human diseases. Clin Toxicol 1980;*17*:45–83.

r5. Cox RA. Immunology of the fungal diseases. Boca Raton, FL: CRC Press, 1993.

r6. Shank RC. Mycotoxins and N-nitroso compounds: Environmental risks, Vols. I, II. Boca Raton, FL: CRC Press, 1981.

r7. World Health Organization. Selected mycotoxins: Ochratoxin, trichothecenes, ergot. Environmental health criteria 105. Geneva: World Health Organization, 1990, pp 167–182.

r8. Marasas WFO, Nelson PE, Toussoun TA. Toxicogenic *Fusarium* species. University Park: Pennsylvania State Univ Press, 1984.

r9. Joffe AZ. *Fusarium* species: Their biology and toxicology. New York: Wiley, 1986.

r10. Ueno Y. Toxicology of trichothecene mycotoxins. ISI Atlas of Science; Pharmacology 1988, pp 121–124.

r11. Beasley VR. Trichothecene mycotoxicosis: Pathophysiologic Effects, Vols I, II, Boca Raton, FL: CRC Press, 1989.

r12. Gosh AC, Manmade A, Demain AL. Toxins from *Penicillium islandicum* Sopp. 625–38 In: Rodricks JV, Hesseltine CW, Mehlman MA. Mycotoxins in Human and Animal Health. Park Forest South, IL: Pathotox, 1977.

CHAPTER 109

Chemical Carcinogenesis and Mutagenesis

James D. Yager
Joanne Zurlo

Introduction

The goal of this chapter is to discuss toxic agents that result in mutagenesis leading to carcinogenesis and agents that modify the carcinogenic process. Both mutagenesis and carcinogenesis can be caused by tumor viruses (DNA and RNA), radiation (ionizing and ultraviolet), and chemicals. It is beyond the scope of this chapter to discuss the contributions of viruses or radiation to the development of cancer. However, it is worthy to note that a number of human cancers are associated with these agents. For example, among the DNA tumor viruses, there are associations of hepatitis B virus with liver cancer, human papilloma viruses with cervical cancer, and Epstein-Barr virus with nasopharyngeal cancer. RNA tumor viruses and their associated neoplasms include human T cell leukemia virus with various leukemias, and human immunodeficiency virus (HIV), through its immunosuppressive effects, with several types of cancer. With regard to radiation, there is a clear connection between exposure to sunlight and skin cancer and between ionizing radiation and various leukemias and other neoplasms. In this chapter we will focus our discussion on chemical carcinogens.

Historical Background

In the past several decades, increased attention has been focused on the health effects of environmental agents, particularly in relation to cancer. Epidemiologic studies have provided evidence for the role of environmental, medical, and social factors in the causation of a high percentage of human cancer.[r1] Reviews of the field of chemical carcinogenesis generally cite the astute observations of two London physicians in the late 1700s as providing the first evidence for chemicals as carcinogens in humans.[r2] In 1761, the physician John Hill observed a correlation between the occurrence of nasal cancer and excessive use of tobacco snuff. Shortly thereafter, in 1775, the surgeon Percival Pott reported on the high incidence of scrotal skin cancer in men who, as children, had been chimney sweeps. Pott correctly attributed this to prolonged contact with soot. Since these initial observations, the list of chemicals known or suspected to be human carcinogens based on epidemiologic studies has grown considerably (see below).

Although the first reports suggesting an association of occupational exposure and cancer in humans appeared in the late 1700s and more frequently during the late 1800s, it was not until the early 1900s that scientists began to develop animal models with which to study the carcinogenic process.[r2] In 1915, Yamagawa and Ichikawa reported that repeated application of solubilized crude coal tar to rabbit ear skin resulted, after many months, in the appearance of benign and malignant tumors. This work was followed shortly by a report from another Japanese laboratory that application of coal tar to the backs of mice also resulted in the appearance of skin tumors and in a shorter time. This experimental system was subsequently used in studies that contributed enormously to our knowledge of the carcinogenic chemicals present in coal tar and to our current working concepts of the multistage nature of the carcinogenic process.

The second breakthrough in the field of carcinogenesis was reported by Sasaki and Yoshida in the 1930s.[r2] These investigators found that feeding rats diet containing *o*-aminoazotoluene, an azo dye, resulted in the appearance of liver tumors after many months. The early studies with the azo dye derivatives had their greatest significance in the fact that these carcinogens, unlike those present in coal tar, were not carcinogenic for tissues at the site of application, but instead produced tumors at distant sites. In other words, some carcinogenic agents exhibited organotropic properties.

Current Working Concepts Concerning Carcinogenesis

Figure 109.1 shows a comprehensive overview of the carcinogenic process, beginning with exposure and ending with the presence of a malignant neoplasm. In the remainder of this chapter, we will focus on discussion of selected steps in this process with emphasis on the chemicals that bring them about and the possible mechanisms involved. As shown Figure 109.1, humans are exposed to chemicals that are known or suspected carcinogens as revealed by epidemiologic studies and studies on experimental animals. Exposure occurs in our occupational environments, through medical treatment, and through our own personal/cultural habits. A list of 28 known or suspected human carcinogens is given in Table 109.1. Numerous other chemicals also have been shown to be carcinogenic in experimental animal studies. Cultured animal and bacterial cells have provided much information pertaining to the possible mechanisms of carcinogenesis. A key step concomitant with exposure is the metabolism of the chemical, and at this point it is important to emphasize the first of two central concepts: most carcinogenic chemicals are indirect-acting and require metabolic activation within the cells of their target tissue. On the other hand, there are a few direct-acting carcinogens that undergo spontaneous conversion to reactive derivatives. The metabolism of several model experimental and human carcinogens will be discussed below. It is now clear that the principal critical target of the activated carcinogen is DNA. Most, if not all, complete carcinogens directly or indirectly cause DNA damage that, if not repaired prior to DNA replication and cell proliferation, can lead to mutation of critical target genes (the first rare event). This results in the creation of a population of initiated cells.

The second central concept is that the carcinogenic process is comprised of multiple stages. In the 1940s and 50s, several investigators demonstrated that mouse skin carcinogenesis could be separated into three stages: initiation; promotion; and progression. Initially, it was found that repeated applications of croton oil could induce skin tumor formation after prior treatment with a single subcarcinogenic dose of benzo(a)pyrene. Since that time, much has been learned about the critical mechanisms of these processes. Multistage carcinogenesis has been demon-

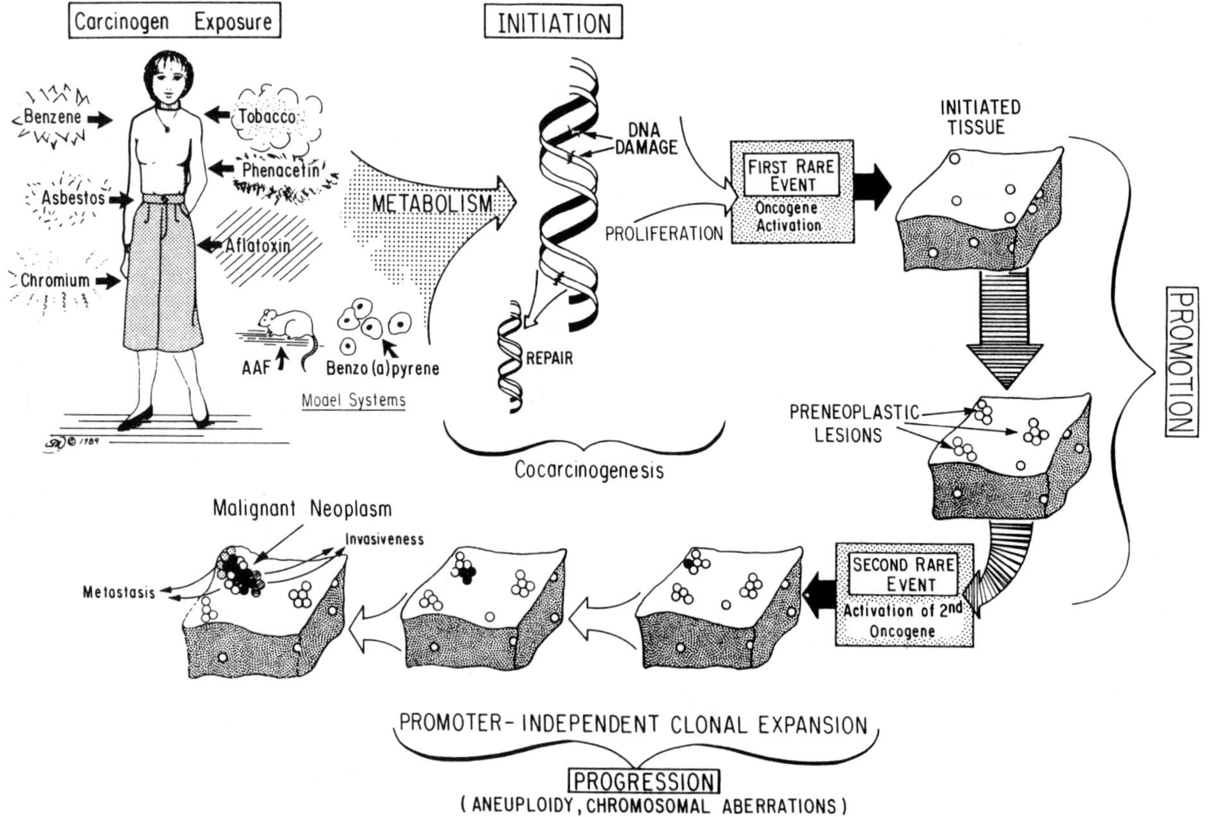

Figure 109.1 Multistage Carcinogenesis

strated at other sites of carcinogenesis, including liver, pancreas, bladder, and colon.

An experimental scheme for initiation, promotion, and progression is as follows.[r3,r4] Generally, the initiating chemical is one that, given at a sufficiently high single dose or in multiple lower doses, results in the appearance of tumors. Thus, most initiating agents can be complete carcinogens. However, the dose of an initiating agent may be adjusted so that a single low dose will not cause an increase above the background tumor incidence. When such treatment (initiation) is followed by chronic administration of an agent termed a "promoter" (e.g., croton oil in mouse skin or phenobarbital in rat liver), tumor incidence is dramatically increased. On the other hand, if promoter treatment occurs without prior initiation or before initiation, the tumor incidence remains at background levels or may show only a small increase. It is clear that promoters will be difficult to detect in tumorigenesis assays designed to detect complete carcinogens. Furthermore, if the time between successive promoter treatments is increased, the effectiveness of the promoter is diminished or even eliminated, suggesting that the effects of promoters are reversible. Finally, chronic treatment with a promoter can be delayed after initiation, even up to a year, and still result in the appearance of tumors, although the response may be diminished. This indicates that the process of initiation is irreversible.

Progression is the third stage demonstrated in experimental carcinogenesis. The process of progression is characterized by an increase in the aggressiveness and growth rate of tumors and ultimately leads to the development of malignancy. Progression is caused by agents that induce additional genetic alterations and is manifested by aneuploidy and chromosomal aberrations. Examples of agents that have progressor activity include benzene, arsenic compounds, and ionizing radiation. Progressors are those agents that either directly or indirectly exhibit clastogenic activity. The length of time or number of exposures required for a progressor agent to exert its effects depends on the individual agent.

Over the past decade, numerous studies have revealed the presence of cellular protooncogenes activated by mutation in the DNA of a large number of human tumors arising in different tissues.[r5] The results of studies with several animal models for chemically-induced tumors, including mouse skin[1] and rat mammary gland,[2] have suggested that mutation of a member of the *ras* protooncogene family can be an early event in the carcinogenic process. Thus, mutation of certain cellular protooncogenes to activated oncogenes may represent a first rare event in the carcinogenic process (Fig. 109.1), with the specific oncogene involved being dependent on the tissue.

During the process of promotion, initiated cells that, at the outset, are phenotypically indistinguishable from "normal" surrounding cells, undergo clonal expansion to form populations commonly referred to as preneoplastic lesions (Fig. 109.1). The promotion stage is probably composed of a number of steps. Recent experimental studies in the mouse skin model system have clearly demonstrated two promotion stages, thus paving the way for classification of chemical promoters as Stage I and/or Stage II promoters.[3] The process of promotion is reversible, at least up to the point where a second critical rare event, i.e., a second mutation, occurs in the DNA of a cell within a preneoplastic lesion. Experimental data obtained with a cell culture model for multistage carcinogenesis have suggested that this second rare event is the activation of a second oncogene whose gene product complements that of the first with regard to the transformed phenotype.[3] In addition, mutations or deletions of another class of genes called anti-oncogenes or tumor suppressor genes have been found in many animal and human tumors. p53 is the most prevalent gene in this class that is altered in human tumors. Numerous mutations in p53 have been associated with human neoplasms at multiple sites, including colon, lung, esophagus, liver, and breast.[4] The mutation, inactivation, or deletion of a tumor suppressor gene may serve as a second genetic event in carcinogenesis. One can envision this event as providing a function or loss of function that provides the cell with a selective growth advantage, rendering it independent of the promoting agent. At this stage experimentally, the promoter can be withdrawn. Many of the preneoplastic lesions will then regress, while cells containing two critical genetic changes continue to grow. The final stage of the carcinogenic process, progression,[r4] can be considered to commence at this point. Progression can be thought of as occurring over a prolonged period during which additional genetic changes occur, resulting in the appearance of neoplasms. These neoplasms are heterogeneous and contain cellular variants that may have acquired invasive and metastatic properties. The role of additional activated oncogenes and inappropriate expression of other genes that mediate the invasive and metastatic properties is just now beginning to be revealed. For example, recent investigation of human colon tumors has shown that they appear to arise as the result of the mutational activation of protooncogenes and the inactivation of multiple tumor suppressor genes, as shown in Figure 109.2.[r6] The exact order of mutational activation/inactivation appears to be less important in the development of cancer than the actual combination of genes that are ultimately mutated in a particular tissue.

The Effects of Various Toxicants on Specific Stages in the Carcinogenic Process

Table 109.1 shows a list of chemical groups and individual chemicals classified as known human carcinogens by the International Agency for Research on Cancer. Several chemicals suspected of being human carcinogens are also listed, and a list of 44 known or suspected human carcinogens has been presented by Wilbourn et al.[5] These carcinogens as well as numerous others known to be carcinogenic in laboratory animals, belong to different classes of chemicals. However, many of the chemicals listed in Table 109.1 do contain common structural units that provide them with a potential for formation of genotoxic electrophiles. These are indicated as being "structurally alert positive" (see below).

Experimental observations suggested that cellular metabolism of most carcinogens is required for their carcinogenic activity. Examples of these observations include: (a) the formation of tumors in tissues distant from sites of carcinogen application; (b) lack of binding of parent carcinogens to cellular macromolecules in vitro in contrast to the detection of bound metabolites in vivo; (c) the tissue specificity of many carcinogens; and (d) species, strain, and sex differences in the susceptibility of animals to the carcinogenic effects of various chemicals. A number of investigators made important contributions to our understanding of mechanisms of carcinogen activation through work with model chemical carcinogens such as the aminoazo dyes, aromatic hydrocarbons, alkylnitrosamines, and aromatic amines, among others.[r2]

Carcinogen Metabolism

Early work, mainly in the liver, revealed that initial carcinogen metabolism was carried out by the microsomal fraction of cells that was later shown to contain the Phase I cytochrome P450 mixed function monooxygenases. These Phase I enzymes constitute a large multigene family in which polymorphisms that affect carcinogen activation in humans and laboratory animals appear to alter susceptibility to cancer induction by both environmental and endogenous agents.[6] Additional metabolism giving rise to various conjugated (glucuronidated, sulfated) derivatives is carried out by microsomal or cytosolic Phase II enzymes some of which are also members of multigene families. The pioneering work of the Millers[r7] on the metabolism of 2-acetylaminofluorene (2-AAF) provided some of the first glimpses of the nature of the metabolites produced. It also has been clearly demonstrated that free radicals can be generated in the process of xenobiotic metabolism and may consequently contribute to all phases of the carcinogenic process.[r8]

Unifying Theory of Carcinogen Metabolism

Figure 109.3 shows the scheme for the metabolic activation of 2-AAF.[r7] The key metabolite to note is the electrophilic sulfated ester. The formation of electrophilic metabolites represents a common feature in the metabolic activation of chemical carcinogens. From the results of their work and that of others, the Millers proposed a unifying theory of carcinogen activation, which is represented in Figure 109.4.[r9] Most carcinogens are indirect-acting in that they require metabolism to derivatives capable of forming covalent adducts to cellular macromolecules. Metabolism of these precarcinogens is largely directed toward the formation of

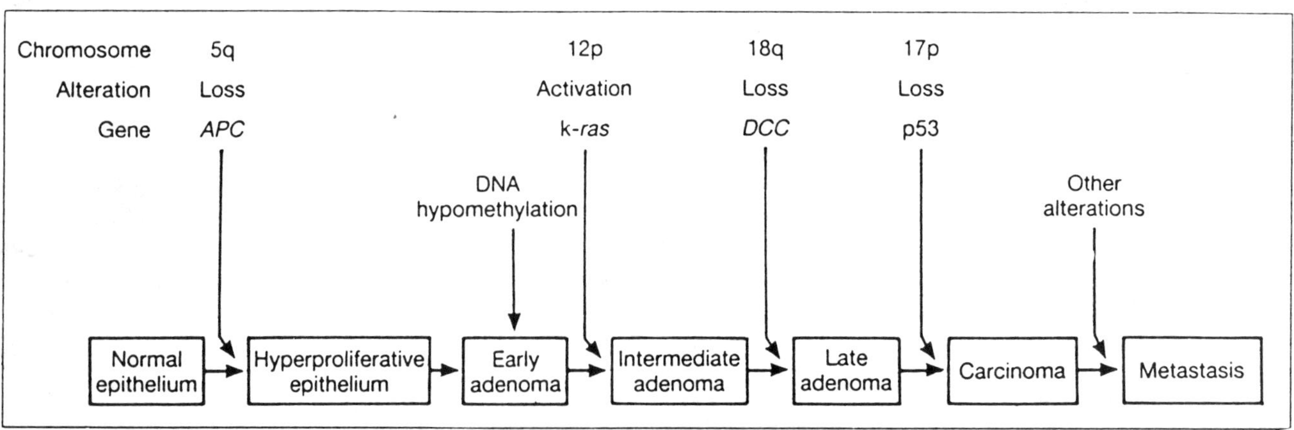

Figure 109.2 A genetic Model for Colorectal Tumorigenesis[r6] (with permission).

Table 109.1 Known or Suspected Human Carcinogens[a]

Carcinogen	Structural Alert	Mutagenicity in Salmonella	Target Organ(s)	
			Humans	Animals
Occupational:				
4-aminobiphenyl	+	+	Bladder	Liver, bladder
Arsenic	−	−	Skin, lung	Lung
Asbestos	−	−	Lung, pleura, larynx	Lung, pleura
Benzene	−	−	Leukemia	Zymbal gland lymphoma, lung
Benzidine	+	+	Bladder	Liver, bladder, Zymbal gland, breast, colon
Bis(chloromethyl)ether	+	+	Lung	Lung, nasal cavity
Chromium	−	+	Lung	Lung, local sarcomas
Mustard gas	+	+	Lung	Lung
2-naphthylamine	+	+	Bladder	Liver, lung, bladder
Soots, tars, pitches & oils	+[b]	+	Skin, lung	Skin
Vinyl chloride	+	+	Liver (angiosarcoma)	Liver (angiosarcoma), skin, lung, breast, Zymbal gland, forestomach
Medicinal:				
Analgesic mixtures containing phenacetin	+	+	Renal pelvis, urinary tract	Renal pelvis, urinary tract, bladder, liver
Azathioprine	+	+	Lymphoma, leukemia, skin	Lymphoma, ear duct
N,N-bis(2-chloroethyl)-2-naphthylamine (chlornaphthazine)	+	+	Bladder	Lung
1,4-butanediol dimethane-sulfonate (myleran)	+	+	Leukemia	Inadequate data
Chloroambucil	+	+	Leukemia	Lung, lymphoma
Conjugated estrogens	−	−	Endometrium	Inadequate test
Cyclophosphamide	+	+	Bladder, leukemia	Bladder, leukemia, lung, breast
Diethylstilbestrol	−	−	Cervix, vagina, endometrium	Mammary gland, uterus, cervix, vagina, etc.
Melphalan	+	+	Leukemia	Lung, lymphoma, breast
Methoxsalen + UV A (PUVA)	−	+	Skin	Skin
MOPP (combined chemotherapy)	+	+	Leukemia	Not tested
Oral contraceptive steroids[c] (ethinyl estradiol, mestranol)	−	−	Liver	Liver
Treosulfan	+	(+)[d]	Leukemia	Not tested
Cultural:				
Betel quid containing tobacco	NR[e]	+[46]	Oral cavity	Forestomach
Smokeless tobacco	+[b]	+[47]	Oral cavity	Inadequate data
Tobacco smoke	+[b]	+[48]	Lung, bladder, renal pelvis, oral cavity, larynx, pancreas	Lung, larynx, oral cavity
Environmental:				
Aflatoxins	NR[e]	+	Liver	Liver, lung, kidney, colon, trachea

[a] Adapted from [5,18,r23]. "Structural Alert" indicates whether or not the chemical contains a structural unit that provides it with a potential for the formation of a genotoxic electrophile.

[b] These substances contain a mixture of compounds, some of which have structural alerts

[c] Suspected human carcinogens[14]

[d] Not tested in this assay, but predicted to be positive

[e] Data not reported in [5,18], but do contain structural alerts

2-acetylaminofluorene (AAF) → cytochrome P450 monooxygenase, NAOPH + O_2 (phase I) → N-hydroxy-2-AAF → PAPS sulfotransferase (phase II) → N-sulfatoxy-2-AAF (electrophilic metabolite) → DNA → DNA adducts [N-(deoxyguanosin-8-yl)-2-AAF; 3-(deoxyguanosin-N^2-yl)-N-acetyl-2-aminofluorene]

Figure 109.3 Metabolism of 2-Acetylaminofluorene in Rat Liver. (Adapted from [r7]). ("PAPS" denotes 3′-phosphoadenosine-5′-phosphosulfate.)

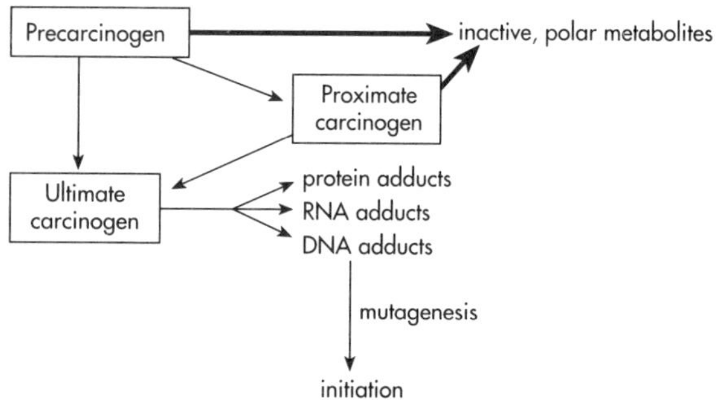

Figure 109.4 Unifying Theory for the Metabolic Activation of chemical Carcinogens (adapted from [r9]).

inactive polar metabolites for excretion. In the process, electrophilic reactants termed ultimate carcinogens may also form directly or indirectly through intermediates termed proximate carcinogens.

Metabolic Activation of Selected Human Carcinogens

For 2-AAF and various other aromatic amines and amides such as 4-aminobiphenyl and 2-naphthylamine (Table 109.1), the formation of N-OH proximate carcinogens appears to be an obligatory step in their activation. N-OH derivatives are not reactive per se but require further metabolism, which could occur either within the tissue of formation or in another tissue. The ultimate carcinogenic derivative can be thought of as forming in the target tissue of the carcinogen, since its high reactivity would in general preclude transportation to other sites.

Other important structurally diverse carcinogens undergo metabolism to electrophilic reactants as shown in Figure 109.5. The aromatic hydrocarbons are major components of coal tars and soots and of combustion products in general, including tobacco. Early work by Kennaway and coworkers demonstrated the presence of numerous polycyclic hydrocarbons in extracts of coal tar including dibenz(a,h)anthracene and the well-studied benzo(a)pyrene.[r2] Considerable effort was devoted to studying the metabolites of this class of carcinogens. Ultimately, studies by a number of investigators revealed that for benzo(a)pyrene the major ultimate carcinogenic metabolite is a dihydrodiol epoxide formed through a multistep metabolic sequence,[r7] as shown in Figure 109.5. Thus, for polycyclic hydrocarbons, the electrophilic metabolites of major importance to their carcinogenic properties are bay region epoxides (see Fig. 109.5), although other electrophilic metabolites are also formed that may contribute to the carcinogenic process.[r2]

The aflatoxins are natural products produced by the mold *Aspergillus flavus*. These compounds have been shown to be contaminants of improperly stored grains and can also be found in peanuts. Aflatoxin B_1 (AFB) is a potent carcinogen for several species. In conjunction with hepatitis virus, it has been strongly implicated as a causative factor in hepatocellular neoplasia in humans in certain areas of Asia and Africa.[r10] Metabolism of aflatoxin occurs through a number of

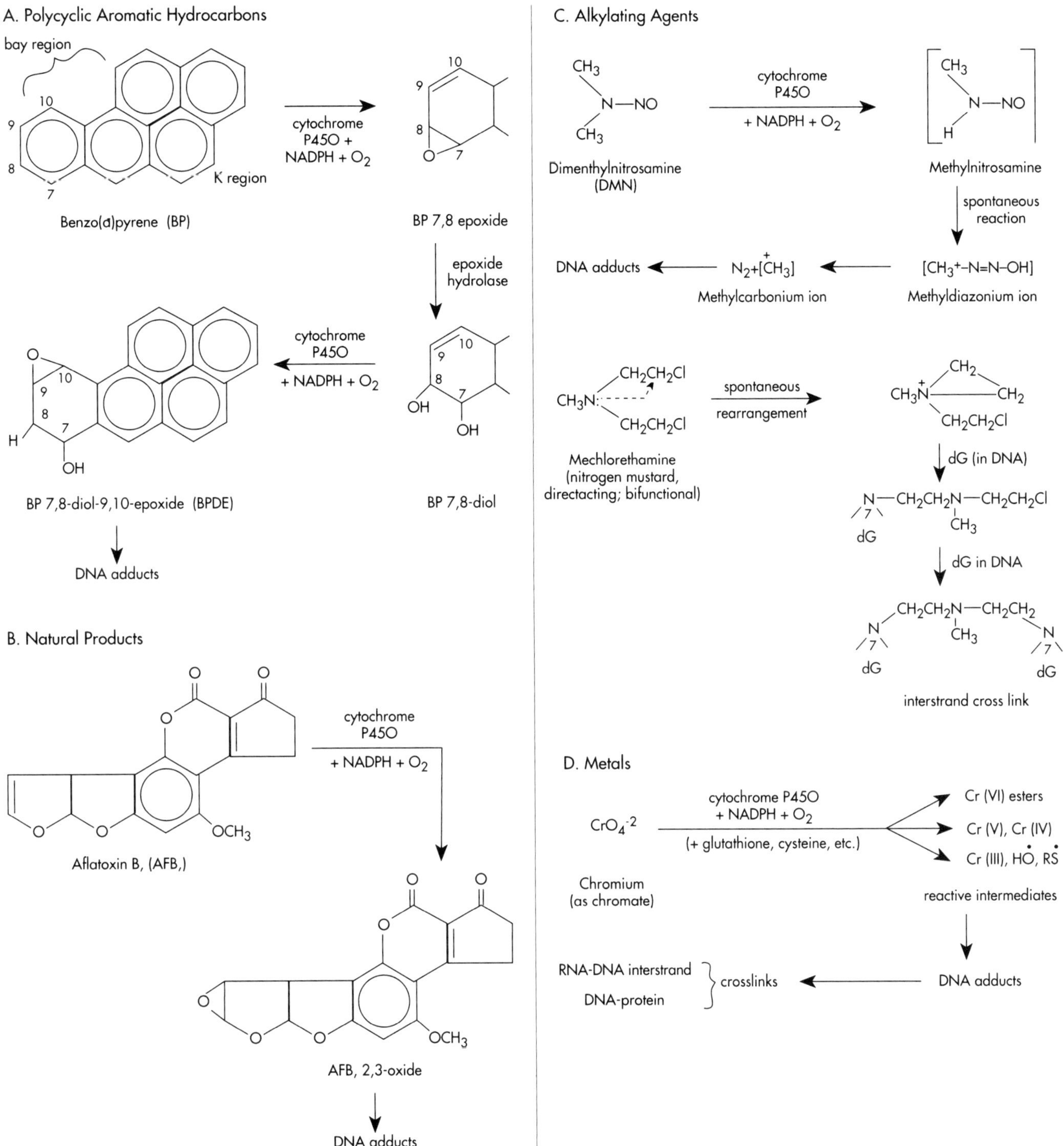

Figure 109.5 Metabolic Activation Schemes for Selected Carcinogens (adapted from [7,r7,r11])

pathways that produce various inactive polar derivatives. However, the ultimate carcinogenic metabolite is the 2,3 epoxide[r7] as shown in Figure 109.5. As indicated above, mutations in the p53 gene are common in human cancers. In hepatocellular carcinomas from individuals in China with known exposure to AFB, mutational hot spots in p53 were observed at codon 249. The specific mutation is a G:C to T:A transversion[4] (see below). This mutation is consistent with the known reaction of the epoxide metabolite of AFB with guanine bases in DNA. Evidence supports the notion that in some instances specific mutations in DNA may represent "fingerprints" for the involvement of specific environmental chemicals in the etiology of some cancers.

The alkylating agents constitute a diverse group of carcinogens, some of which (N-nitrosimides and N-nitrosamides) form reactive electrophiles spontaneously and others that require metabolic activation.[r7] The activation of several alkylating agents is shown in Figure 109.5. Dimethylnitrosamine (DMN) is a monofunctional alkylating agent widely used in experimental studies. DMN is metabolized to an unstable monoalkyl derivative from which its ultimate carcinogenic form, the methyl carbonium ion, forms spontaneously. Other nitrosamines can be formed from dietary nitrites in the stomach, and several specific nitrosamines can be found in tobacco and tobacco smoke. Also shown in Figure 109.5 is the activation of the direct-acting bifunctional nitrogen mustard alkylating agent mechlorethamine, a component of a multidrug treatment regimen. Other known human carcinogens in this class include the chemotherapeutic drugs chlorambucil, cyclophosphamide, and melphalan[r11] (Table 109.1).

Finally, another important class of human carcinogens is that of the metal compounds (Table 109.1). The metal carcinogens have not been studied as extensively as the organic carcinogens, and an excellent review has been written by Furst.[r12] It is unlikely that a common mechanism for tumor induction will be found for the metals, and the extent to which tissue specific metabolism is required for their carcinogenicity is unknown. With respect to carcinogenicity, perhaps the most information is available for chromium. Wetterhahn and coworkers[7] have shown that chromium (VI) compounds enter cells through anion transport channels and are metabolically reduced by microsomal enzymes or other cellular reducing agents such as glutathione to various reactive intermediates of chromium. Reactive oxygen species including the hydroxyl radical are also generated in this process. It is speculated that the ultimate carcinogenic form of chromium compounds may be Cr (III), which forms noncovalent adducts with DNA, resulting in the formation of DNA interstrand and DNA-protein crosslinks (Fig. 109.5). The reactive oxygen species generated during chromium metabolism may also be responsible for causing other types of DNA damage. Thus, for this metal carcinogen and others such as arsenic,[8] the unifying theory of carcinogen activation appears to be applicable.

Initiation: General Properties of Initiating Agents/Complete Carcinogens

From the discussion above, it is clear that the organic chemical carcinogens and at least some inorganic carcinogens are metabolized to, or spontaneously form, derivatives capable of reacting at nucleophilic sites within the cell. Experimental studies have clearly demonstrated that chemicals that are metabolized to these ultimate carcinogenic forms can function as initiating agents or as complete carcinogens in multistage carcinogenesis models. Thus, initiating agents can be classified as chemicals that: (1) form electrophiles either spontaneously or through metabolism; and (2) are genotoxic, i.e., they induce mutations in various bacterial or mammalian cell mutagenesis assays.[9] As shown in Table 109.1, many of the known human carcinogens are mutagenic in the *Salmonella* assay and there is a good correlation between the presence of a structural alert and mutagenicity.

Additional properties of initiating agents that can be deduced from the scheme described previously are: (1) they have irreversible and additive effects on cells; (2) they can function as complete carcinogens; and (3) they must exert their effects prior to promotion. Since, in the vast majority of instances, initiation of carcinogenesis is clearly associated with mutation in critical genes, we will now briefly describe the genotoxic effects of the carcinogens whose metabolic activation was described above.

Genotoxic Effects

As discussed above, chemical carcinogens and mutagens may be direct-acting or may be metabolized to electrophilic reactants. In order for these compounds to exert their mutagenic and/or carcinogenic effects, they must alter the target macromolecule, DNA. There are many nucleophilic sites in DNA (Fig. 109.6), and different carcinogens appear to exert certain specificities with regard to the sites in DNA that they attack. Some examples of carcinogen binding to bases in DNA are given below.

Alkylating agents, such as methylnitrosourea and dimethylnitrosamine, primarily target the N3 of adenine, the N7 of guanine (G), as well as the phosphodiester linkages in the DNA backbone. Alkylation of the cyclic nitrogens of the purines may cause the N-glycosidic bond to become labile, leading to increased levels of spontaneous depurination. In addition to these highly reactive sites, alkylating agents also attack exocyclic oxygens such as the O^6 of G and the O^4 of thymine (Fig. 109.6). The ultimate carcinogenic form of the polycyclic aromatic hydrocarbon benzo(a)pyrene, the 7,8-diol-9,10-epoxide (BPDE I) (Fig. 109.5), preferentially attacks G, with the major linkage occurring between the C10 position of BPDE I and the 2-amino group of the G. The N-hydroxylated, esterified metabolite of the aromatic amine 2-AAF (Fig. 109.3) binds primarily via its N atom to the C8 position of G. This compound

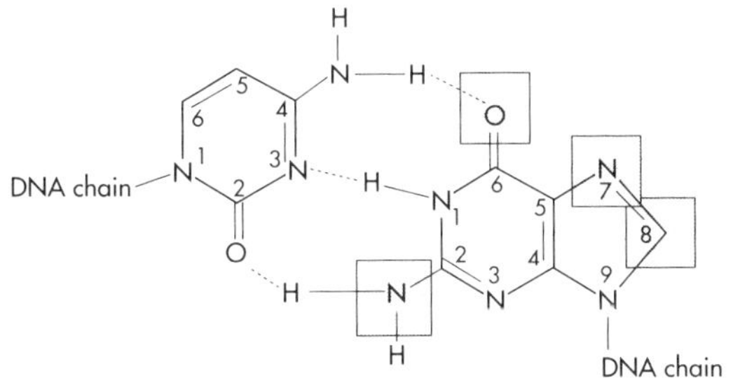

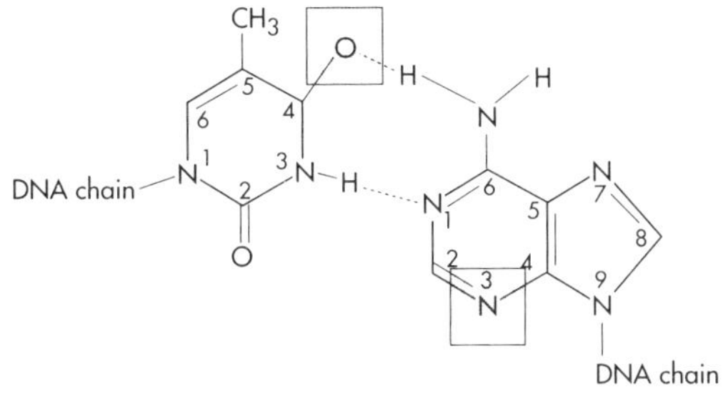

Cytosine–guanine

Thymine–adenine

Figure 109.6 Sites of reaction of selected activated carcinogens with the bases in DNA. Several of the most reactive (nucleophilic) sites are indicated by the shaded boxes.

also binds to a lesser extent to the 2-amino group of G. The 2,3-oxide of aflatoxin B1 (Fig. 109.5), the potent liver carcinogen produced by the mold *Aspergillus flavus,* forms an adduct with the N7 position of G.

DNA damage caused by these and other carcinogens can have far reaching effects with regard to the induction of mutagenesis and carcinogenesis. However, there are a number of mechanisms present in the cell to repair damage to DNA before a permanent change, i.e., a mutation, occurs.[r13] Alkylation damage at the O^6 position of G may be directly removed by the protein O^6-alkylguanine alkyl transferase. In the reaction, the alkyl group is transferred from the guanine to a cysteine residue of the enzyme protein, producing S-alkylcysteine. The unusual feature of this protein is that it is not regenerated; i.e., after reaction with an alkylguanine, the protein is inactivated. Increased alkylguanine repair activity depends on new synthesis of the protein, which is inducible in some tissues, particularly liver. Low constitutive levels of this protein or the inability of cells to resynthesize it have been associated with increased susceptibility to the mutagenic and carcinogenic effects of certain alkylating agents.

Removal of DNA damage may also occur by excision repair mechanisms that involve many enzymes.[r13] DNA glycosylases cleave the N-glycosidic bond between the deoxyribose and a damaged base to generate an apurinic or apyrimidinic (AP) site. These glycosylases are generally very specific for the bases they cleave, e.g., uracil DNA glycosylase will cleave only uracil. Removal of AP sites is mediated by the coordinate effort of AP endonucleases and exonucleases that incise the phosphodiester backbone of the DNA and excise the sugar phosphate and surrounding nucleotides. The gaps are then filled by DNA polymerase, and the phosphodiester backbone is rejoined by DNA ligase. Other types of bulky DNA damage are also excised by the action of endonucleases. Low levels or lack of excision repair capabilities are found in patients with the disease xeroderma pigmentosum (XP). These patients are sensitive to the carcinogenic effects of ultraviolet (UV) light and are thus predisposed to certain types of cancer. Studies have detected the presence of activated *ras* protooncogenes in DNA from XP tumor cells.[10,11] The mutation detected was that predicted to be caused by an unrepaired UV light-induced pyrimidine dimer.[10]

If DNA replication occurs before the damage is repaired, the consequence is mutation, which may be defined as a permanent alteration in DNA sequence. The mutation is inherited by the daughter cells if it occurs in a somatic cell, or by the offspring if it occurs in a germ cell. Mutations may occur at single sites in DNA and thus are referred to as point mutations, or may be larger, resulting in gene rearrangements or chromosomal aberrations.

Point mutations are the most common type of mutation and appear as base-pair substitutions or as frameshift mutations. Base-pair substitutions, as the name suggests, occur when an incorrect base-pair replaces a correct one. If a purine replaces another purine or a pyrimidine replaces another pyrimidine, the result is a transition mutation; if a purine replaces a pyrimidine or vice versa, it is a transversion. For example, a transition mutation may occur after deamination of cytosine to uracil. Deamination can be spontaneous or may be caused by a chemical, such as nitrous acid. Following deamination, if the incorrect base is not removed by DNA glycosylases, the uracil will base-pair with adenine during the next round of DNA replication. Therefore, where there originally was a C-G base-pair, there will be a U-A base-pair.

Modification of the O^6 position of G by alkylating agents has been associated with increased mutagenesis and carcinogenesis because this exocyclic oxygen normally participates in the hydrogen bonding between base pairs. For example, O^6-methylguanine (O^6-meG), which may be formed by reaction of DNA with the alkylating agent methylnitrosourea (MNU), preferentially base pairs with thymine. Therefore, if this lesion is not repaired prior to DNA replication, one daughter cell will contain an O^6-meG-T base pair, and, after the next round of replication, one cell will contain an A-T pair. Thus, a G-C to A-T transition mutation has occurred. Indeed, this was actually shown to occur in experiments of Barbacid and coworkers in which MNU was administered to rats to induce breast tumors.[2] In 83 percent of the tumors examined, there was a G to A transition in the 12th codon of the Ha-*ras* oncogene that resulted in its activation.

Another type of point mutation that may occur is a frameshift mutation. In this case, modification of DNA by a chemical, usually by its intercalation between bases, causes a base to be inserted or deleted in the opposite strand during replication. Addition or deletion of a base alters the coding sequence and the triplet frames of the sequence. For example, the sequence AUG AAA UUU G. . codes for the peptide methionine-lysine-phenylalanine . . . If the fourth base (A) is deleted, the frame shifts to AUG AAU UUG . . . coding for methionine-asparagine-leucine . . . By the same token, if a base G is inserted between the third and fourth bases, the sequence becomes AUG GAA AUU UG . . . coding for methionine-glutamine-isoleucine . . . In either case, a mutation occurs and every amino acid coded for subsequent to the mutation will be altered. Examples of compounds that cause frameshift mutations are the aromatic amine 2-AAF and the dye ethidium bromide.

The last type of mutation to be discussed here is chromosomal aberration. Rather than single sites, these mutations involve large pieces of DNA and are manifested by chromosomal breaks, which may result in deletions, insertions, and/or rearrangements.[r14] Agents that induce these changes are termed clastogens and, as discussed above, may have an important role in tumor progression. Another type of chromosomal aberration is the gain or loss of whole chromosomes, which results in aneuploidy. An example of a human carcinogen that causes chromosomal aberrations is diethylstilbestrol.

Cocarcinogenesis

As shown in Figure 109.1, the cocarcinogenesis phase encompasses carcinogen uptake, metabolism to the ultimate carcinogenic form, and the initiation process, i.e., the occurrence of the first rare event. Cocarcinogens, as the term implies, cause an enhancement in the initiation process. Possible mechanisms by which cocarcinogens may act have been reviewed by Williams[12] and include: (1) enhanced transport of carcinogens into the cell; (2) enhanced metabolism of precarcinogens to their proximate and ultimate carcinogenic forms; (3) reduction in the levels of cellular nucleophiles, e.g., glutathione, that normally compete for reaction with the ultimate carcinogens and reactive oxygen species formed during their metabolism; and (4) stimulation of DNA synthesis in the presence of high levels of DNA adducts prior to DNA repair.

Cocarcinogenesis is likely to be important in the development of cancer in humans and several agents in Table 109.1 exhibit cocarcinogenic activity in model systems. For example, cigarette smoke contains numerous chemicals capable of mediating the initiation, cocarcinogenesis, and promotion stages of cancer.[13] In addition, asbestos has been shown to potentiate the metabolic activation and carcinogenicity of polycyclic hydrocarbons and represents an important human cocarcinogen.[r15] Finally, human liver cancer is associated with infection by hepatitis B virus, which causes chronic hepatotoxicity, along with exposure to aflatoxin, which is both hepatotoxic and mutagenic.[r10] This, too, may be an excellent example of cocarcinogenesis leading to increased carcinogenicity.

It is also important to realize that while the carcinogenic process may be enhanced at the initiation stage by cocarcinogenic agents or processes, it can also be inhibited by agents that reduce carcinogen uptake, alter the proportion of electrophilic metabolites, enhance the levels of cellular nucleophiles, etc. (see below).

Promotion/Progression

The process of promotion was discussed above. Studies have shown that many promoters are not metabolized to electrophilic reactants and thus do not cause initiation, nor are they mutagenic. Rather, exposure to promoters must occur after initiation, and exposure must be frequent and prolonged. Intermittent exposure decreases the effectiveness of the promoter. Thus, the effects of promoters are reversible and not additive.

In some cases, however, treatment with promoters alone can cause a small increase in the appearance of tumors. This could be due to promotion of cells initiated by spontaneous mutation or by the formation of potentially reactive oxygen species or genotoxic metabolites during the metabolism of some promoters.[r8,r16] It is also important to appreciate that promoters display tissue specificity, i.e., promoters like many initiators, have organotropic properties.

Tumor promotion has been most widely studied in the mouse skin carcinogenesis system and the most extensively studied tumor promoters have been the phorbol esters, particularly phorbol myristate acetate (PMA, also known as tetradecanoyl-phorbol-13-acetate, TPA). However, the promotion stage of carcinogenesis also has been demonstrated in a number of other model systems. Peraino and coworkers[26] demonstrated that dietary administration of phenobarbital could enhance the appearance of liver tumors initiated with 2-AAF. Their important initial observations have led to the development of five initiation-promotion-progression models for hepatocarcinogenesis and the discovery that compounds such as the halogenated hydrocarbons and synthetic estrogens are promoters of hepatocarcinogenesis.[r17,r18] The artificial sweetener saccharin has been shown to be a promoter for bladder carcinogenesis. In addition, promotion by high-fat diets has been demonstrated in rat models for pancreatic, breast, and colon carcinogenesis.[r19]

Promoters in the Environment

Table 109.1 lists several human carcinogens that contain or are known promoters. Thus, as mentioned above, tobacco smoke contains numerous compounds that have promoting activity when tested in the mouse skin carcinogenesis model.[13] Asbestos, in addition to having cocarcinogenic activity, can also function as a promoter.[r15]

The synthetic estrogens found in oral contraceptives represent a class of compounds suspected of being human carcinogens.[14] In the mid-1970s, a number of publications reported the occurrence of liver adenomas and even hepatocellular carcinomas in women who had taken oral contraceptives for prolonged periods. Currently, with the use of lower concentrations of synthetic estrogens in these preparations, the problem no longer seems to have clinical significance in western societies, where the incidence of liver cancer is low. In addition, it has been reported that use of oral contraceptives in such areas of the world as Asia and Africa where the liver cancer incidence is already high, does not seem to increase the risk.[15] However, the earlier observations of increased risk with prolonged use prompted a series of animal studies that clearly demonstrated that both mestranol and ethinyl estradiol at the dose levels used are promoters of hepatocarcinogenesis in rats.[r18] Other agents that may contribute to human cancer through their activities as promoters include high dietary fat, high caloric intake, halogenated hydrocarbons, saccharin, and alcoholic beverages.

Biologic, Biochemical, and Molecular Effects of Promoters

Unlike the situation with initiating agents where, in many cases, the metabolites and DNA adducts critical to their mechanism of action have been widely studied, the effects of tumor promoters that are essential for their promoting activity have not been fully determined. The phorbol ester PMA is the most extensively studied tumor promoter. Early work on the biologic effects of PMA revealed that it causes hyperplasia accompanied by numerous biochemical effects, among which are increased levels of ornithine decarboxylase, increased synthesis of RNA and protein and decreased metabolic cooperation between cells.[r3] However, the pathway through which these effects are mediated was obscure until the discovery that the cellular receptor for PMA was protein kinase C (PKC), a serine/threonine protein kinase that has a critical regulatory role in signal transduction.[16] This finding has led to an extensive amount of work on the signal transduction pathway from the initial binding of PMA to PKC to effects on gene transcription rates and increased DNA synthesis. In fact, the work on the molecular effects of PMA is so extensive that it is easy to forget that it represents just one class of tumor promoters and that details of the mechanisms by which it stimulates DNA synthesis may not apply to other promoters, such as phenobarbital, saccharin, compounds in cigarette smoke, and the synthetic estrogens.

Since promoters have such pleiotropic effects on cells, it is difficult to see a common thread that could be thought of as a unifying theory of tumor promotion. In fact, most likely, one does not exist. About the only effect that most if not all promoters have in common is that they induce proliferation in the cells of their target tissues. It is in this permissive environment for growth that the initiated cells reveal themselves by exhibiting a selective growth advantage through either increased sensitivity to growth stimulators, decreased sensitivity to growth inhibitors or both, and thus undergo clonal expansion to form early preneoplastic lesions.

Progression

Progression is that phase of the carcinogenic process during which benign tumors become more aggressive as discussed above. What is pertinent to our discussion is that compounds can be evaluated for their effects on the progression stage of the carcinogenic process. For example, in the mouse skin model, initiation and promotion protocols can be used to produce benign papillomas. The effects of application of various compounds on the rate and incidence of appearance of carcinomas can then be evaluated. This type of assay has recently been used to detect agents that can both inhibit and enhance the progression stage.[r4,17]

Inhibitors of Carcinogenesis

The ability to separate the carcinogenic process into clearly defined stages, i.e., initiation, promotion, and progression, provides the means for rationally considering effective ways to intervene and block the process. Different types of intervention strategies can be envisioned, depending on the stage to be blocked and selected approaches have been reviewed recently.[r20] When considering the mechanisms of each of the stages, inhibition can be accomplished in the following ways. Inhibition of initiation can be brought about by blocking carcinogen uptake and/or activation, increasing detoxification, scavenging of electrophilic reactants, or delaying cell proliferation to allow DNA repair mechanisms to function. For example, the inclusion of the antioxidant oltipraz in the diet of animals receiving aflatoxin B_1 protected against hepatoxicity and prevented the appearance of hepatocellular carcinomas.[r21] The mechanism of the chemoprotective effect of oltipraz and other dithiolethiones is mediated by the induction of the Phase II metabolic enzymes in the liver, particularly glutathione-S-transferase. This enzyme catalyzes the conjugation of the AFB epoxide to glutathione, which results in its detoxification. There are also compounds in cigarette smoke that can inhibit the induction of skin tumors by benzo(a)pyrene when applied simultaneously with the carcinogen, perhaps by reducing the proportion of electrophilic metabolites formed during its metabolism.[13] Clearly, the balance of carcinogens, cocarcinogens, and inhibitors is critical to the final outcome of the carcinogenic process.

Promotion can be blocked by inhibiting cell proliferation, preventing inflammation, which, at least in the mouse skin model, usually accompanies this stage and by employing antioxidants to reduce oxidative stress. Finally, progression has also recently been shown to be reduced by antioxidants and enhanced by agents that deplete normal cellular free radical scavenging mechanisms. Evidence is beginning to accumulate indicating that these approaches will have an impact on cancer in humans.

Evaluation of Carcinogenicity and Mutagenicity

The main data base of information on the carcinogenicity of chemicals comes from the studies conducted by the National Cancer Institute and the National Toxicology Program. In these studies as currently conducted, two species of rodents, generally male and female F344 rats and B6C3F_1 mice in groups of 50 are exposed to high doses of chemicals for two years. More than 300 compounds have been tested in this way. When a series of known or suspected human carcinogens was analyzed in experimental animals, the positive correlation for carcinogenicity was 84 percent; in addition, there was good agreement between the target organs in humans and susceptible animals.[5,18] This is evident from Table 109.1, where the target organs for the carcinogens in humans and animals are indicated. While a positive correlation between rodent and human carcinogenesis is a desirable outcome, the carcinogens used in these studies were potent chemicals with strong carcinogenic activity. When assessing the carcinogenicity of unknown chemicals however, there are a number of concerns and disadvantages associated with such tests. A primary concern pertains to the predictably of such assays for carcinogenicity in humans. Interspecies comparisons, e.g., human/rodent, must also be viewed against the report of a recent analysis of carcinogenicity data that revealed a concordance between rats and mice of only 67 percent.[9] To address this problem, it has been proposed recently that the results of the rodent carcinogenicity bioassays be stratified when using them to evaluate human health risks.[19] Since both sexes of two rodent species are used in these bioassays, it is likely that those chemicals that produce tumors in common sites across species and in both sexes represent the greatest hazard to humans. On the other hand, the lowest ranking chemicals would be those that induced tumors in a single site in a single sex of only one species. This stratification scheme may ultimately enable the rodent bioassay to be a reliable, accurate predictor of human carcinogenicity.

Another disadvantage of the standard rodent carcinogenicity bioassay is that the maximum tolerated dose of test chemicals is used.[20] It has been suggested that toxicity induced by such high doses could result in a mitogenic response, thus enabling more mutations to be expressed. This could exaggerate the carcinogenic response seen in these animals. A more efficient method of assessing the carcinogenic potential of a compound may be to evaluate it initially by its chemical structure followed by short-term in vivo and in vitro genotoxicity assays prior to animal bioassays.[r22]

One of the goals of investigators in the field of genetic toxicology has been the development of short-term in vitro and in vivo tests for detection of genotoxic chemicals. Two possible effects of exposure to such agents are mutation in the germ line leading to heritable mutations and somatic cell mutations with the potential to lead to the development of various diseases including cancer. As reviewed above, the early work of the Millers and others demonstrated that the ultimate forms of initiating agents and complete carcinogens were electrophiles and that DNA was among the molecular targets in the cell. A breakthrough in the detection of genotoxic agents that were carcinogenic, based on these properties, was the development of the *Salmonella* mutation assay by Ames and coworkers.[27] Early studies with this assay indicated that >90 percent of the known carcinogens tested were mutagenic and that 90 percent of the noncarcinogens tested were nonmutagenic. The power of this assay was derived from the use of a liver microsome fraction containing the mixed function oxidase enzymes required to activate precarcinogens. Other assays employing mammalian cells in vitro and in vivo systems have also been developed with the hope of discovering a battery of complementary short-term assays that would detect carcinogenic mutagens with an accuracy approaching 100 percent.[r23]

Early on, the chemicals selected for testing and validation of the short-term assays were biased based on the potency of their carcinogenicity. These considerations resulted in the testing of chemicals very likely to be genotoxic since the more potent complete carcinogens possess initiating activity and form electrophilic reactants. However, as the basis of the selection of chemicals for mutagenicity testing shifted to relative environmental importance, the sensitivity of the *Salmonella* assay for detecting carcinogens has decreased. For example, in an evaluation of 301 chemicals tested in long-term carcinogenesis studies in rodents by the U.S. NTP,[r22] 162 were judged to be carcinogens. Of these, 56 percent were mutagenic, whereas 25 percent of the noncarcinogens were mutagens. Of the total 127 compounds that were mutagens, 71 percent were definitively carcinogenic. Thus, a positive response in the *Salmonella* assay strongly suggests that a compound will be carcinogenic in rats and/or mice. In addition, as seen in Table 109.1, the ability to predict the carcinogenic potential of genotoxic agents is facilitated by structural analysis of compounds for potential electrophilicity.[r22,21] Again, this is important because most mutagens are carcinogens. However, the results of the US NTP evaluation also showed that 49 percent of the nonmutagens were carcinogenic. In other words, a negative result in the *Salmonella* assay does not imply that the chemical will be noncarcinogenic. Therefore, while structural alerts and mutagenicity are useful in predicting carcinogenicity of genotoxic agents, there are a large number of false-negatives, i.e., nongenotoxic carcinogens.

To assess the proposal that a battery of short-term tests might be complementary to one another in obtaining information, Tennant et al.[9] evaluated the four most commonly used short-term genotoxicity assays, i.e., *Salmonella*/microsome mutagenesis assay, chromosome aberration and sister chromatid exchange in Chinese hamster ovary cells, and mutation in L5178Y mouse lymphoma cells, for their ability to predict rodent carcinogenicity. They found no evidence for complementarity and, furthermore, their data indicated that a battery of tests composed of these four assays would not improve on the ability of the *Salmonella* assay to predict carcinogenicity.

The existence of nongenotoxic agents that in long-term rodent carcinogenicity studies cause the appearance of tumors is not surprising given our discussion above of the carcinogenic process and the existence of the promotion phase and promoters. It is possible that some of these compounds exhibit some "complete" carcinogenic activity indirectly due to the production of reactive oxygen species during their metabolism or through promotion of spontaneously initiated cells appearing within their target tissues. Nongenotoxic carcinogens must continue to be studied at a more basic level in order to elucidate their mechanisms of action, which will be varied, and their potential impact on the carcinogenic process in humans.[r22]

Conclusions

We have tried to present a broad current overview of the field of chemical carcinogenesis and mutagenesis, especially in relation to carcinogenesis. It should be clear that the process is complex and that various chemical compounds can affect these processes in causative, enhancing, and inhibitory ways. Much additional work is required in order to provide a detailed mechanistic understanding of these processes such that rational, practical, and economic ways can be developed to detect compounds that would cause or facilitate these processes. In addition, more work is required so that we can come to put the risks of exposure to various carcinogens and the potential hazards in proper perspective.[22]

References

Research Reports

1. Quintanilla M, Brown K, Ramsden M, Balmain A. Carcinogen-specific mutation and amplification of Ha-ras during mouse skin carcinogenesis. Nature 1986;*322*:78–80.
2. Zarbl H, Sukumar S, Arthur AV, Martin-Zanca D, Barbacid M. Direct mutagenesis of Ha ras-1 oncogenes by N-nitroso-N-methylurea during initiation of mammary carcinogenesis in rats. Nature 1985;*315*:382–385.
3. Dotto GP, Parada LF, Weinberg RA. Specific growth response of ras-transformed embryo fibroblasts to tumour promoters. Nature 1985;*318*:471–475.
4. Hollstein M, Sidransky D, Vogelstein B, Harris CC. p53 mutations in human cancers. Science 1991;*253*:49–53.
5. Wilbourn J, Haroun L, Heseltine E, Kaldor J, Partensky C, Vainio H. Response of experimental animals to human carcinogens: an analysis based upon the IARC monographs programme. Carcinogenesis 1986;*7*:1853–1863.
6. Poulsen HE, Loft S, Wasserman K. Cancer risk related to genetic polymorphisms in carcinogen metabolism and DNA repair. Pharmacol Toxicol 1993;*72* Suppl 1:93–103.

7. Wetterhahn KE, Hamilton JW. Molecular basis of hexavalent chromium carcinogenicity: effect on gene expression. Science Total Environ 1989;*86*:113–129.

8. McKinney JD. Metabolism and disposition of inorganic arsenic in laboratory animals and humans. Environ Geochem Health 1992;*14*:43–48.

9. Tennant RW. Margolin BH, Shelby MD, Zeiger E, Haseman JK, Spalding J, Caspary W, Resnick M, Stasiewicz S, Anderson B, Minor R. Prediction of chemical carcinogenicity in rodents from in vitro genetic toxicity assays. Science 1987;*236*:933–941.

10. Keijzer W, Muldr MP, Langeveld JCM, Smit EME, Box JL, Bootsma D, Hoeijmakers JHJ. Establishment and characterization of a melanoma cell line from a xeroderma pigmentosum patient: Activation of N-ras at a potential pyrimidine dimer site. Cancer Res 1989;*49*:1229–1235.

11. Suarez HG, Daya-Grosjean L, Schaifer D, Nardeux P, Renault G, Bos JL, Sarasin A. Activated oncogenes in human skin tumors from a repair-deficient syndrome xeroderma pigmentosum. Cancer Res 1989;*49*:1223–1228.

12. Williams GM. Modulation of chemical carcinogenesis by xenobiotics. Fundam Appl Toxicol 1984;*4*:325–344.

13. Van Duuren BL, Goldschmidt BM. Cocarcinogenic and tumor-promoting agents in tobacco carcinogenesis. J NCI 1976;*56*:1237–1242.

14. Porter LE, Van Thiel DH, Eagon PK. Estrogens and progestins as tumor inducers. Semin Liver Dis 1987;*7*:24–31.

15. The WHO Collaborative Study of Neoplasia and Steroid Contraceptives. Combined oral contraceptives and liver cancer. Int J Cancer 1989;*43*:254–259.

16. Nishizuka Y. Intracellular signalling by hydrolysis of phospholipids and activation of protein kinase C. Science 1992;*258*:607–614.

17. Rotstein JB, Slaga TJ. Anticarcinogenesis mechanisms, as evaluated in the multistage mouse skin model. Mutat Res 1988;*202*:421–427.

18. Shelby MD. The genetic toxicity of human carcinogens and its implications. Mutat Res 1988;*204*:3–15.

19. Tennant RW. Stratification of rodent carcinogenicity bioassay results to reflect relative human hazard. Mutat Res 1993;*286*:111–118.

20. Ames BN, Gold LS. Chemical Carcinogenesis: Too many rodent carcinogens. Proc Natl Acad Sci (USA) 1990;*87*:7772–7776.

21. Zeiger E. Carcinogenicity of mutagens: predictive capability of the *Salmonella* mutagenesis assay for rodent carcinogenicity. Cancer Res 1987;*47*:1287–1296.

22. Ames BN, Magaw R, Gold LS. Ranking possible carcinogenic hazards. Science 1987;*236*:271–280.

23. Shirname LP, Menon MM, Nair JN, Bhide SV. Correlation of mutagenicity and tumorigenicity of betel quid and its ingredients. Nutr. Cancer 1983;*5*:87–91.

24. Guttenplan JB. Mutagenic activity in smokeless tobacco products sold in the U.S.A. Carcinogenesis 1987;*8*:741–743.

25. McCann J, Choi E, Yamasaki E, Ames BN. Detection of carcinogens as mutagens in the Salmonella/microsome test: assay of 300 chemicals. Proc Natl Acad Sci USA 1975;*72*:5135–39; 73:950–954.

26. Peraino C, Fry RJM, Staffeldt E. Effects of varying the onset and duration of exposure to phenobarbital on its enhancement of 2-acetylaminofluorene-induced hepatic tumorigenesis. Cancer Res 1977;*37*:3623–3627.

27. Ames BN, Durston WE, Yamasaki E, Lee D. Carcinogens are mutagens: A simple test system or combining liver hemogenates for activation and bacteria for detection. Proc Natl Acad Sci USA 1973;*70*:2281–2285.

Reviews

r1. Doll R, Peto R. The causes of cancer. J NCI 1981;*66*:1191–1308.

r2. Miller EC, Miller JA. Milestones in chemical carcinogensis. Semin Oncol 1979;*6*:445–460.

r3. Slaga TJ. Overview of tumor promotion in animals. Environ Health Perspec 1983;*50*:3–14.

r4. Pitot HC, Dragan YP. Stage of tumor progression, progressor agents and human risk. Proc Soc Exp Biol Med 1993;*202*:37–43.

r5. Higginson J, Muir CS, Muñoz N. Human cancer: Epidemiology and environmental causes. Cambridge: Cambridge University Press, 1992.

r6. Vogelstein B, Kinzler KW. The multistep nature of cancer. Trends Genetics 1993;*9*:138–141.

r7. Miller EC, Miller JA. Searches for ultimate chemical carcinogens and their reactions with cellular macromolecules. Cancer 1981;*47*:2327–2345.

r8. Trush MA, Kensler TW. Role of free radicals in carcinogen activation. In: Sies H. Oxidative stress: Oxidants and antioxidants. New York: Academic Press, 1991.

r9. Miller JA, Miller EC. Ultimate chemical carcinogens as reactive mutagenic electrophiles. In: Hiatt HH, Watson JD, Winsten JA. Origins of human cancer. Cold Spring Harbor, NY: Cold Spring Harbor Laboratory, 1977.

r10. Harris CC, Sun T-t. Multifactoral etiology of human liver cancer. Carcinogenesis 1984;*5*:697–701.

r11. Calabresi P, Parks RE Jr. Antiproliferative agents and drugs used for immunosuppression. In: Gilman AF, Goodman LS, Rall TW, Murad F. The pharmacological basis of therapeutics, 7th ed. New York: MacMillan 1985.

r12. Furst A. Toward mechanisms of metal carcinogenesis. In: Fishbein L, Furst A, Mehlman MA. Advances in modern environmental toxicology, vol. XI, Genotoxic and carcinogenic metals: Environmental and occupational exposure. Princeton, NJ: Princeton Scientific Publishing Co. 1987.

r13. Friedberg EC. DNA Repair. San Francisco: WH Freeman 1985.

r14. Hoffmann GR Genetic toxicology. In: Amdur MO, Doull J, Klaassen CD. Casarett and Doull's toxicology, 4th ed. Elmsford, NY: Pergamon Press, 1991.

r15. Mossman BT, Craighead JE. Mechanisms of asbestos carcinogenesis. Environ Res 1981;*25*:269–280.

r16. Cerutti PA. Prooxidant states and tumor promotion. Science 1985;*227*:375–381.

r17. Dragan YP, Sargent L, Xu Y-D, Xu Y-H, Pitot HC. The initiation-promotion-progression model of rat hepatocarcinogenesis. Proc Soc Exp Biol Med 1993;*202*:16–24.

r18. Yager JD, Zurlo J, Ni N. Sex hormones and tumor promotion in liver. Proc Soc Exp Biol Med 1991;*198*:667–674.

r19. Ip C, Birt DF, Rogers AD, Mettlin C, eds. Dietary Fat and Cancer. New York: Liss, 1986.

r20. Wattenberg L, Lipkin M, Boone CW, Kelloff GJ. Cancer chemoprevention. Boca Raton, FL: CRC Press, 1992.

r21. Kensler TW, Groopman JD, Roebuck BD. Chemoprotection by oltipraz and other dithiolethiones. In: Wattenberg L, Lipkin M,

Boone CW, Kelloff GJ. Cancer chemoprevention Boca Raton, FL: CRC Press, Inc, 1992.

r22. Ashby J, Tennant RW. Definitive relationships among chemical structure, carcinogenicity and mutagenicity for 301 chemicals tested by the US NTP. Mutat Res 1991;257:229–306.

r23. Brusick, D. Genetic Toxicology. In: Hayes AW. Principles and methods of toxicology, 2d ed. New York: Raven Press, 1989.

r24. Pitot HC. Fundamentals of Oncology, 3d ed, New York: Marcel Dekker, 1986.
This is an excellent review of the basic concepts of carcinogenesis.

r25. Sirica AE. The pathobiology of neoplasia. New York: Plenum Press, 1989.
This book is directed to students who have basic research interests in neoplasia.

r26. Vainio H, Magee P, McGregor D. McMichael AJ. Mechanisms of carcinogenesis in risk identification. Lyon, France: International Agency for Research on Cancer, 1992.
This book examines epidemiologic experimental conbributions to the determination of mechanisms of cancer, and which of these mechanisms are useful in predicting human risk.

r27. D'Amato R, Slaga TJ, Farland WH, Henry C. Relevance of animal studies to the evaluation of human cancer risk. New York: Wiley-Liss, Inc, 1992.
This book provides a review of specific case studies and examines factors that may be useful in the extrapolation between animals and humans.

CHAPTER 110

Reproductive Toxicology and Teratology

Vergil H. Ferm

Introduction

This chapter is primarily concerned with a description of the development of the mammalian male and female reproductive tracts and the responses of the target tissues of those systems to toxic agents. These effects may occur in humans exposed to toxicants in utero, in the workplace, or in medical therapy. Risk assessment in reproductive toxicology is a difficult task and must take into account variations in biologic and animal models as well as the great variety of susceptible tissues in the reproductive system.

Reproduction is a cyclic phenomenon that can be diagrammed most simply, as shown in Figure 110.1. In the course of this cycle, an impressive array of components consisting of a variety of cell types, complex organ structures, and specific endocrine tissues and their hormones play an important part. Each of these components may be directly affected by certain toxicants that could lead to reproductive failure. To understand the problems and processes involved in toxic activity on the reproductive process it is necessary to look at the component parts of the reproductive system and cycle separately, but with the full understanding that all these separate components are delicately intertwined.

Most studies concerning the effects of toxic agents on the reproductive system are based either on the use of animal models or on epidemiologic and clinical studies in humans after accidental, therapeutic, or industrial exposures. Toxic responses may result from either acute or chronic exposure. Most investigators agree that there is no ideal animal model from which data can be extrapolated directly to the human situation.

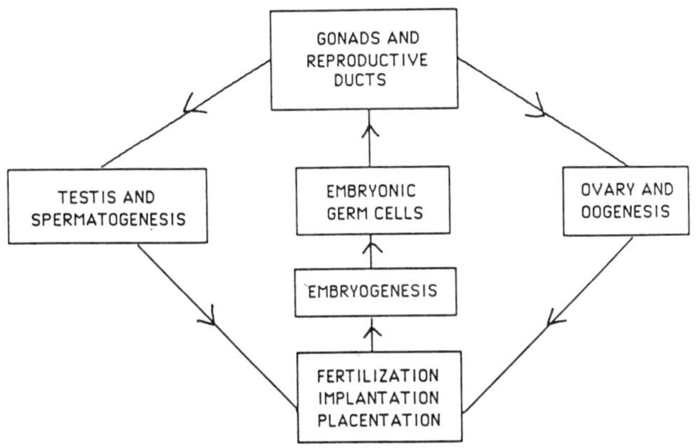

Figure 110.1 The cycle of reproduction showing the stages, tissues, organs, and processes peculiar to the reproductive phenomenon. Toxic events can adversely affect any of these stages, resulting in neoplasia, infertility or teratogenesis.

Germ Cell and Gonad Formation

The germ or sex cells of the developing embryo originate in the proximal portion of the yolk sac, one of the placental membranes. From this site these primordial germ cells (PGCs) migrate to the region of the developing gonad along the dorsal body wall in proximity to the developing renal system. The sexual pattern of this indifferent gonad is determined by the presence or absence of the Y, or male-determining, chromosome. In the absence of the Y chromosome, the XX gonad develops into an ovary; the duct system that supports it develops into the oviduct–uterus–vagina portion of the female reproductive tract. In the XY embryo, the gonad becomes a testis, and the duct system that supports it becomes the epididymis–vas deferens–ejaculatory duct portion of the male reproductive tract.

Any toxic effect on these germ cells from the early moment of their identity as PGCs to their incorporation into the fertilized zygote can have profound effects on reproduction, including decreased fertility, spontaneous abortion, chromosomal abberations, embryonic malformations, or germ cell mutations. These mutations, dominant or recessive, will appear in all descendants of that germ cell if the cell becomes involved in the fertilization process. Thus, this germ cell mutation, unlike somatic mutations, may influence subsequent generations.

The Duct Systems of Reproduction

The dimorphic nature of the reproductive system is not confined to the gonadal tissue; it also extends to the system of ducts that lead the gametes to the point of fertilization and then, in the female, to the site of implantation. In the early embryo, this dimorphism is displayed by the simultaneous development of two independent duct systems, the mesonephric (MD) and paramesonephric (PMD). Under normal conditions, the PMD system will dominate and go on to form the oviduct, the uterus, and the upper portion of the vagina in XX (female) embryos (Fig. 110.2). This system then supports the transport of the egg released from the ovary, subsequently picked up by the oviduct (the site of fertilization) and passed on to the uterus, where the embryo implants and is nurtured by the placenta. The vagina receives the spermatozoa and is the final pathway of the fetus from the uterus to the outside world. In the XY (male) fetus the PMD is actively suppressed by the action of a hormone of the testis (see below), and only small rudiments of the PMD are found in normal males.

Male (XY) development results in persistence of the mesonephric duct system (Fig. 110.2). In this case, the seminiferous tubules of the testis connect directly, via some persistent renal tubules, to the cranial end of the mesonephric duct. This duct then develops into the epididymis, vas deferens, and finally the ejaculatory duct, which empties into the penile urethra.

In a female (XX) fetus, only a very few minor remnants of the mesonephric duct system persist. It is

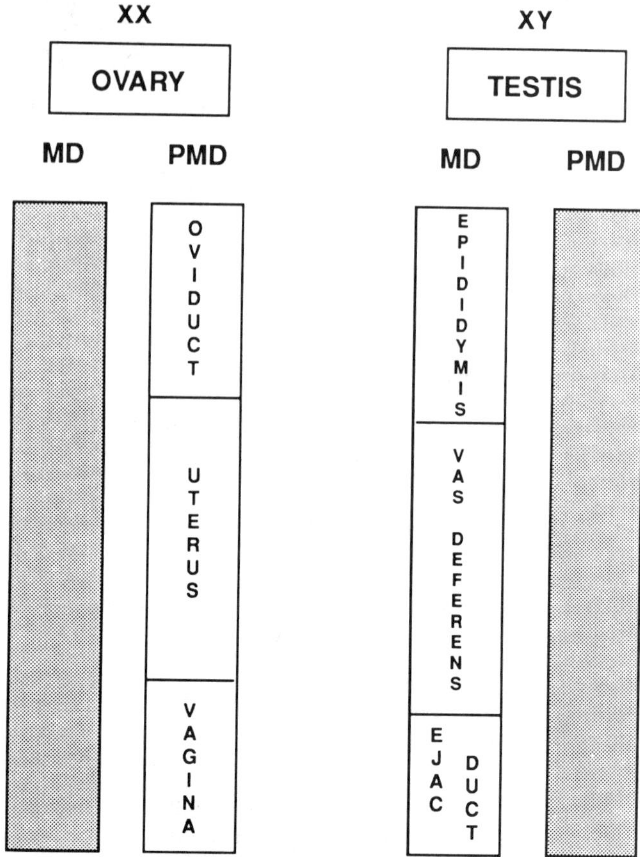

Figure 110.2 Diagrammatic comparison of sex duct development in male and female embryos. **MD** = mesonephric duct development in males; **PMD** = paramesonephric duct development in females; **EJAC** = Ejaculatory. The stippled areas represent those duct systems which degenerate in the respective sexes. See text.

important to note that in the absence of a Y chromosome, the paramesonephric duct system will persist and the embryo will develop as a female.

The Male Reproductive System

Testis and Spermatogenesis

When the primordial germ cells (PGCs) of an XY embryo reach the developing gonad, they become part of the seminiferous tubules. These tubules are in pyramid-shaped compartments, of which there are some 250 in the human testis. Each compartment contains one to four highly coiled and branched tubules, which range from 30 to 70 cm in length. The PGCs line up in the basal layer or outer wall of the tubule, interspersed with native testicular cells called Sertoli cells. The Sertoli cell plays an important role in the latter stages of spermatogenesis by the development of an intricate and intimate relationship to developing spermatids and spermatozoa. In the mature testis, Sertoli cells do not undergo mitosis and are much less sensitive to toxic agents and irradiation than are the germ cells. The Sertoli cell is also of interest because it is the source of a specific hormone, the anti-Mullerian hormone (AMH) or Mullerian-inhibiting-substance (MIS), whose apparent sole activity is to inhibit the development of the PMD (Mullerian) system in the male embryo. The male spermatogonia arrange themselves within the wall of the seminiferous tubule and do not divide mitotically, nor do they start meiotic activity like the oogonia of the female. At puberty, the primary spermatagonia begin to divide mitotically. Two types of cells result from this division—Spermatagonia A and B. The A type will divide further to form more As and a more mature B type. Those of the B type are committed to the maturation process and proceed through the pathway: primary and secondary spermatocytes; spermatids; and finally the mature spermatozoa (Fig. 110.3). It is during this process, all of which occurs within the wall of the seminiferous tubule, that the meiotic process of two chromosomal reduction divisions takes place. From each primary spermatocyte, four mature spermatozoa develop, all of which are haploid (half the autosomal chromosome complement plus either an X or Y sex chromosome). These spermatozoa are designated either 22X or 22Y. The time required for the maturation of the human spermatogonium to a mature sperm cell is 64 days, and the total number of sperm produced in the lifetime of a human male is 10.[9]

Sperm numbers per unit volume of semen, motility, and morphology are the three main characteristics studied to detect possible effects of toxic agents on the process of spermatogenesis. These characteristics are also examined as part of the clinical work-up in male infertility, both in humans and in domestic animals. Sperm concentration is a microscopic count of the numbers of sperm per unit volume of semen. In the human, there are normally more than 100 million sperm per milliliter, counts of less than 20 million may indicate a fertility disorder. Sperm motility is a measure of the activity and progressive movement of sperm under

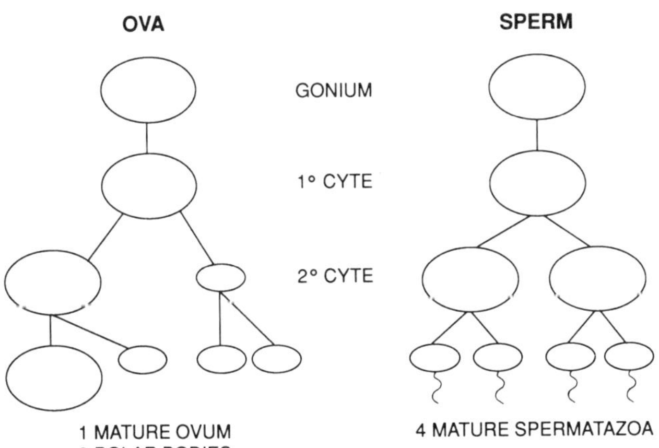

Figure 110.3 Maturation of the germ cells (meiosis). Note that the female primary oocyte gives rise to one mature ovum and three very small polar bodies, all of which have the same amount of chromosome material despite their obvious difference in size. One primary spermatocyte gives rise to four mature spermatozoa. In the final division all cells are reduced to the haploid chromosome number. Because of crossing over the chromosomes during meiosis and mutations of the genes, all mature descendants are genetically different from one another.

direct microscopic visualization. Indices of sperm motility and speed are less variable than sperm concentration in repeated samples and thus may be better indicators of toxic effects. The study of sperm morphology involves a microscopic analysis of stained specimens. In the normal human semen sample, large numbers (up to 50%)[26] of abnormal forms can be found, including double-headed sperm and abnormally shaped heads. Specialized techniques utilizing flow cytometry, videomicrographic analysis, and special staining are new procedures that may help to refine these analyses.

There are two important histologic features peculiar to the seminiferous tubule that may well determine the way toxicants affect the process of spermatogenesis. The first of these is the very different manner in which the cytoplasm of the cells of the type B spermatogonia and their descendants divide. Nuclear division is complete. Cytoplasmic division, however, is incomplete, and a number of cytoplasmic bridges connect the spermatogonia, spermatocytes, and spermatids. Thus, a very large number of these cells are interconnected and share a common cytoplasmic pool.[3] The implication is that toxic agents could be dispersed, simply by passing one cell membrane, to a large group of cells at a variety of stages in cell differentiation. Another peculiarity of the seminiferous tubule epithelium is the existence of a blood-testis barrier. Unlike the well-known blood-brain barrier, which is based on the characteristics of the intercellular junctions in the endothelial cells of the brain capillaries, the barrier in the testis resides in the unique distribution of intercellular junctional complexes between Sertoli calls near the base of the seminiferous epithelium in the tubule. These create two compartments, one (basal) containing the spermatagonia and young spermatocytes, and a second (more central) containing the remaining later stages of spermatogenesis.[r1] The effect of this barrier is to prevent the access of serum proteins, including homologous antibodies, and perhaps other molecules, to the later stages of spermatogenesis.

The Ductal System and Accessory Glands of the Male

The epididymis receives the maturing spermatazoa from the testis at its cranial end. The human epididymis is a single duct, 6 meters long but highly coiled into a compact unit 7–8 cm in length. When sperm enter the epididymis they are immotile, but as they progress through the epididymis to the tail they become increasingly motile. Thus, the epididymis plays an important role in sperm maturation and motility. Abnormalities in sperm motility may indicate a problem in the testis and/or the epididymis. From the epididymis, the sperm pass to the ductus (vas) deferens, a long, uncoiled, muscular tube that extends to the urethra. Ejaculation consists, in part, of spasmodic peristaltic contractions of this muscular tube, expelling sperm cells into the urethra. These contractions are under the control of the autonomic nervous system.

There are three different glandular structures associated with the male reproductive tract: the prostate; the seminal vesicles; and the bulbourethral glands. The coagulating gland of rodents is a specialization of one of the lobes of the prostate. While the complete role of these glands is not yet known, it is clear that they play an important role in the chemical nature and volume of the seminal fluid, aid in sperm motility, and contribute to the ejaculatory process. Specific toxic effects on these glands are usually measured by weight changes and sometimes by histologic examination. The weights of these accessory glands are readily influenced by serum testosterone levels; changes in their weights may be a reflection of a primary testicular toxic effect rather than a direct effect on these glands. Most analytical attention is given to the prostate gland, a very common site of age-related hypertrophy and neoplasia in human males. Prostatic cancer is a common malignant tumor. There is evidence that hormone imbalance, such as excess androgens, may play an important role in prostatic pathology; there may well be other xenobiotics that adversely affect the prostate. Any complete toxicologic study of the male reproductive tract must include a thorough examination of this structure.

Toxic Effects in the Male

Concerns about possible effects of toxicants on male reproduction are usually directed to fertility, libido, and neoplasia. Animal tests for the study of male reproductive problems have been designed primarily to measure changes in sperm morphology, motility, and quantity. As in the female, most of the baseline information about toxic events on spermatogenesis have resulted from studies on the effects of radiation and cancer chemotherapeutic compounds in humans and rodents.[21]

In the process of spermatogenesis, the stem cell is the spermatogonium. The type A spermatogonium cells constitute a reservoir of stem cells and thus can serve as the source for recovery of spermatogenesis after toxic injury. After such damage, the Type A stem cells will produce only Type A cells until the population of Type A cells is replenished to the level at which the spermatogenic track may again be set in motion. This process of repair and rejuvenation can be studied by microscopic examination of stained slides of seminiferous tubule cross sections. The type B spermatogonia divide by mitosis to form two primary spermatocytes. This is the last division in spermatogenesis involving DNA synthesis. The primary spermatocyte then starts through the meiotic (chromosome reduction) process (Fig. 110.3).

Type A stem cells are more resistant to radiation and cancer therapeutic agents than are the type B spermatogonia, which are the most sensitive cells in the maturation process. Sensitivity apparently is related to DNA synthetic activity: thus, later stages of spermatogenesis (spermatocytes, spermatids, and spermatozoa) are usually, but not always, resistant.

Sperm abnormalities in the human can be produced by a variety of chemicals, but there is as yet no agreement about what the parameters of these abnormalities mean. There are few studies concerning the direct effect of toxicants on the male reproductive duct system, although measurements of the number, degree of motility, and morphology of the sperm found in the caudal part of the epididymis may be helpful in indicating such effects.[2] An interesting example of a specific effect of a xenobiotic on spermatogenesis is the case of 1,2-Dibromo-3-Chloropropane (DBCP), an agricultural pesticide (nematocide). In 1961, it was reported that this substance had a profound effect on the testes of monkeys, rabbits, guinea pigs, rats, mice, and chicks when administered topically, by inhalation, or by injection.[34] Not until 1977 were similar toxic effects of DBCP on the human testis reported in male pesticide workers, whose presenting complaint was infertility.[35] In the human testis, and in all the other animal species studied in 1961, the primary toxic effect was on the seminiferous epithelium, resulting in either oligospermia (low sperm counts) or azospermia (absence of sperm). An eight-year follow-up study of exposed workers showed that most recovered normal spermatogenic patterns as well as fertility.[28] A few remained azospermic 156 months after the last exposure. Paternal exposure had no effect on spontaneous abortions or congenital malformations in offspring, but there was an apparent decrease in the ratio of male offspring.

"Social" drugs such as alcohol, cannabinoids, and cocaine, as well as many psychoactive drugs, apparently produce few or no direct morphologic changes on either the male or female reproductive tracts. Reported changes in libido, sexual performance, and impotence may be culturally influenced.[4]

The Female Reproductive System

Ovary and Oogenesis

Upon arrival at the gonadal ridge of the embryo, primordial germ cells (PGCs) destined to be ova are arranged in the cortical area of the newly developing ovary. Mitosis of these primordial cells continues until about the fourth month of fetal life in humans, when no new oogonia are formed. Those then present, about 7 million in the human, form primary oocytes. At birth, this number has decreased to 2 million and decreases further still to 250,000 at puberty. Of these, only 500–600 will be ovulated as fully developed, fertilizable ova during the lifetime of a human female. There is no replenishment mechanism as there is in the male.

The primary oocyte is surrounded by a small ring of cells intrinsic to the gonadal tissue proper. These cells will not only nourish the immature ovum, but some will develop into endocrine cells that supply the ovarian estrogenic and progestational hormones. These cellular units, with an oocyte at the center, are termed follicles.

There is an additional peculiarity of behavior of the primary oogonia in the fetal ovum that may have important implications for toxicologic mechanisms on the female gamete. During the second trimester of gestation, the fetal oogonia develop quite rapidly and begin to undergo a complicated process of cell division known as meiosis. This process includes two distinct cellular divisions that result in a halving of the chromosome number (haploid). However, the process becomes arrested in the first divisional phase (meiosis I), not to be completed until individual follicular maturation occurs at some point between the menarche and menopause. During meiosis, the homologous pairs of chromosomes (one maternal, one paternal) synapse and may exchange homologous segments of chromosomes (crossing over). It has been suggested that aneuploidy, an abnormal number of chromosomes related to spontaneous abortion and certain developmental malformations, may be due to failure of normal separation of paired chromosomes during meiosis. It is also possible that direct toxic action may be responsible for aneuploidy in these germ cells. It is important to note that meiosis I in the male begins at puberty and that the long period of years of meiotic suspension does not occur in the male. Following both pituitary and ovarian hormonal stimulation on a cyclical monthly basis, one (seldom more) of these follicles will mature rapidly and will, because of its size, be located at the surface of the ovary. The amount of fluid in this follicle increases considerably; this fluid, along with the ovum, ruptures through the ovarian wall into the peritoneal cavity. At this moment, the first meiotic division is completed and the second one begins. The site of ovum release in the surface of the ovary is surrounded by the free end of the fallopian tube (oviduct), and the ovum is carried down into the oviduct by ciliary action. Generally, this process repeats itself every 28 days in the human, every four days in most laboratory rodents, and less often in many other mammalian forms.

Toxic Effects on the Ovary and Oogenesis

The indices for toxic effects on ovarian structure and function were established by early studies on the effects of radiation on germ cell maturation, where it was shown that radiation sensitivity depends on the specific stage of ovum maturation. PGCs and young oogonia are extremely sensitive to radiation, whereas later stages are less sensitive. Chromosome density within the nucleus of the cell is also related to sensitivity in that those species with high denseness patterns (primates) are more resistant to radiation, while those with diffuse chromosome denseness patterns (rodents) are more susceptible.[18]

With the widespread use of chemotherapy for neoplastic disease it became apparent that a number of these antineoplastic chemicals had profound effects on oogenesis. Busulfan, one of the first drugs used in the treatment of leukemia, caused destruction of the growing and preovulatory follicles.[9] Amenorrhea may be induced in human females treated with cyclophosphamide.[15] This is related to a direct action of this drug on the destruction of both mature and preovulatory follicles. Oocytes also can be destroyed by other antineoplastic agents.[19]

Environmental effects on fertility in the female have been attributed to smoking, presumably by the action of polycyclic aromatic hydrocarbons, which, in laboratory animals, destroy oocytes.[17,20] Possible animal models for risk assessment of environmental chemicals specifically on ovarian structure and function have recently been reviewed: an evaluation of xenobiotics on ovarian follicular development in vitro;[7] the development of the corpus luteum in vitro and in vivo;[29] and a detailed assessment of the histologic changes in ovarian follicular development as an aid in risk assessment.[10]

The Female-Duct System

The oviduct (fallopian tube), uterus, and vagina constitute the duct system of the mammalian female. The oviduct is the site of fertilization and transports the ovum to the uterus. The mammalian uterus may be simplex (e.g., human) or duplex (e.g., rodents), i.e., it may consist of a single cavity or a double cavity, depending on the degree of fusion of the right and left embryonic paramesonephric ducts. The lining of the uterus is responsive to endocrine cycling for the purpose of implantation. The vagina is the receptacle for sperm and the final pathway for the delivery of the fetus.

Toxic Effects on the Female Duct System

The classic example of a direct effect of a therapeutic agent on the female reproductive tract is that of diethylstilbestrol (DES), a potent synthetic nonsteroidal estrogen, liberally used in the 1940–1960 period for the purpose of treating threatened abortion, toxemia of pregnancy, and gestational diabetes. In the 1970s, there was a noticeable increase in the incidence of a very rare clear cell adenocarcinoma of the vagina. These tumors were found to occur in women whose mothers had been treated with DES during pregnancy.[8] The female embryos were thus exposed to DES during organogenesis. Other anomalies of the female reproductive tract attributed to DES have been reported: hypoplastic fallopian tubes; persistence of paraovarian (mesonephric) cysts; and morphologic abnormalities of the luminal configuration of the uterine cavity. These uterine abnormalities probably account for the reported increased incidence of ectopic pregnancy, spontaneous abortion, and decreased fertility in DES-exposed women. Mouse models of the association between intrauterine DES exposure and vaginal clear cell adenocarcinomas have been established. The histopathology of the DES-induced lesions in humans, subhuman primates, and rodents has been described in detail.[14]

Toxic effects of environmental agents on female reproduction may include changes in such factors as decreased fertility, increased rate of spontaneous abortion, congenital malformations, cessation of menses or abnormal menses, and early menopause. These changes may be extremely subtle and only detectable by statistical analysis of epidemiologic data. As an example of such subtle effects, cigarette smoke has been suggested as presenting epidemiologic evidence of an environmental effect on reproduction in the female.[17]

Risk Assessment of Reproductive System Hazards

As a measure of the importance of reproductive hazards in the workplace, a special symposium[31] on this subject focused on several current problems including: protocols for assessing reproductive effects of toxicants; priorities for reproductive risk research; guidelines for reproductive toxicity testing; and monitoring programs, among others.[31]

Fertilization–Implantation–Placentation

Fertilization occurs within 48 hours of ovulation in the upper (ovarian) portion of the oviduct. At the moment of fertilization, the second meiotic division in the ovum is completed and the union of the haploid sperm nucleus with the haploid ovum restores the diploid chromosome complement. The newly formed zygote now divides mitotically, enters the uterus three to four days later, and implants in the endometrium of the uterus 48–72 hours after that. The process of implantation is a critical one. Hormonal preparations, especially progestins, are critical to this process. Antiprogestins will inhibit implantation.[26] Many human embryos fail to implant, or implant improperly and fail to survive. Also, elemental copper, released from copper-containing intrauterine contraceptive devices, disturbs the process of implantation. There are possibly xenobiotics that affect this process, and one of the first signs of such an effect would be an increase in the number of spontaneous abortions. Many early human spontaneous abortions go undetected and therefore are not included in statistical data. It is estimated that up to 75 percent of fertlized human ova do not proceed to live birth.[30] A very large number of these unsuccessful conceptuses have chromosomal abnormalities.[11] Chromosomal abnormalities have been found in human preovulatory oocytes.[36] About 10 percent of sperm obtained from normal men also show abnormal chromosomal patterns.[16] In rodents, it is important to note that abortions per se do not occur. Instead, a dead embryo and its placental remnants undergo a process called resorption, and the pregnancy resulting from this phenomenon can be determined only by gross visual and/or microscopic examination of the uterus.

Implantation occurs when an embryonic blastocyst invades the lining of a structurally and hormonally receptive uterus. Almost as soon as the embryonic blastocyst attaches to the uterus, the embryonic tissue starts to form a placental membrane that serves as a cellular barrier between the maternal blood spaces and the embryo proper. This interposed structure is the placenta, a primarily mammalian organ that varies more in both structure[r2,6] and function[23,24] than any other mammalian organ system. All toxic or potentially toxic compounds that gain entrance to the maternal bloodstream will be exposed to the surface of the placental membrane and may potentially be transferred to the embryo. Some compounds may be blocked by the placenta, some concentrated in the placenta, and some passed to the embryo with ease. The placenta is a continuously developing organ, and its permeability characteristics to various compounds may well change in the course of maturation. It appears that the permeability characteristics of the early placenta are less sophisticated and less discriminatory than those near term. Thus, at these early critical stages, embryonic development in early pregnancy may be more at risk to potentially toxic xenobiotics circulating in the maternal blood than they are nearer to term.

The transfer of carcinogens across the placenta resulting in the induction of tumors in the fetus/neonate/adult is receiving increasing attention. DES is the only known example of this in the human at this time, but in animals a variety of xenobiotics have induced a variety of tumors in fetuses when the mother was treated during pregnancy.[22] Some of these induced tumors appear in early postnatal life; others are delayed to later life. Species differences in the pharmacokinetics of medicinal agents and other xenobiotics are extremely important, not only in terms of rates of placental permeability and metabolism, but also in their teratogenic response.[24]

The end-product of normally functioning reproductive systems is a viable and healthy newborn. The enormous wastage in the mammalian reproductive process is due to a number of factors. In the human there is greater than a 30 percent loss of early embryos prior to or at the time of implantation. These pregnancies go unrecognized. Another 30 percent or more are chromosomally abnormal and are aborted.[29] This leaves about one-third or less of human conceptuses to reach term.

Of the surviving lot of human newborns, approximately 7 percent have some sort of a developmental malformation. One-third of these have a malformation that necessitates major rehabilitation. It is likely that about 30 percent of these human malformations have a genetic basis. Another small percentage of cases (about 5–10%) are due to known environmental or therapeutic factors. The currently known human teratogens (chemical, metabolic, and infectious) have recently been well summarized.[r3]

Teratology Testing

The clinical introduction of thalidomide in Europe in the early 1960s was responsible for an epidemic of birth defects in human newborns. This drug was designed as an antinauseant for use in the "morning sickness" of early pregnancy. It caused no maternal side-effects, was very effective, and was sold without prescription control. It also proved to be a very effective human teratogen, even when used at therapeutic levels. The defects induced by this drug were strikingly uniform in character and became known as the "thalidomide syndrome." This tragic event triggered a major response in many countries affecting how new drugs thereafter would be evaluated for potential teratogenic effects. In 1966, the US Food and Drug Administration codified the teratology testing requirements in the FDA Reproduction Study Guidelines for Safety Evaluation of Drugs for Human Use. These guidelines have been essentially unchanged to date.[27]

The reproductive studies now required for all new drugs designed for human use are conducted in three categories. First, evaluation of fertility and general reproductive performance. This evaluation includes gonadal activity, animal estrous cycles, mating patterns, rates of conception, and the early stages of gestation. The second category is concerned with embryo toxicity, which, in animals, is usually determined by death in utero (resorption), and the potential for developmental malformations (teratogenesis). The third category of reproductive studies now required concern the perinatal and postnatal period, including fetal weight and size, delivery, lactation, and postnatal growth and survival.

A recent development in the area of teratologic testing has been the attention given to behavioral teratology. This area of research, not yet clearly defined, involves experimental psychology and behavioral toxicology, based on the principles of teratology.[12] A variety of testing procedures used in behavioral teratology research have been developed.[13]

Animal testing for teratogenic activity is primarily directed at therapeutic compounds, a time-consuming and expensive procedure. The search is now on for a simple in vitro teratology screening test not unlike the Ames mutagenesis test using Salmonella. Several in vitro tests for teratogenic screening have recently been proposed. These range from a variety of tissue culture models to the use of aquatic animals. Attempts to develop criteria for evaluating the validity of past, present, and future in vitro testing models to predict teratogenic activity have resulted in proposed guidelines for these models.[33] However, critics of in vitro and animal teratology testing question the validity of extrapolation of data obtained in these testing models to the human situation, especially when one considers species differences in drug metabolism, biotransformation, and marked differences in placental structure and permeability. More recently, whole embryo cultures of mammalian embryos with and without some of the placental membranes have been developed to study pharmacologic and teratogenic effects on the embryo itself. This technique bypasses maternal and possibly placental influences on biotransformation and metabolism. While these techniques will provide valuable information on direct embryonic reaction to test compounds, the limitations concern the absence of the maternal and placental metabolism of toxic agents following environmental exposure. At the present time, animal testing remains the best method available to determine teratogenic potential.

There have been attempts to correlate teratogenic, carcinogenic, and mutagenic activity in various compounds in the hopes not only of developing new tests for increased reliability of prediction, but also for clues to a better understanding of the basic mechanisms involved in these pathologic processes. There can be little doubt that there is some strong correlation among the three phenomena. About 80 percent of some 58 known carcinogens are also teratogenic in one or more animal species. Of this carcinogen/teratogen group, about 75 percent show mutagenic activity in the Salmonella mutagen assay test.[32]

While the debate about the specific causes of malfomations may never be settled, here are some general principles that may help one understand the complexity of the problem.

The genetic constitution of a teratogen-treated embryo is an important factor in the response patterns of that embryo. This phenomenon has been clearly shown in a number of teratogenic studies, including a recent detailed study on the teratogenic response of several inbred strains of mice to acetazolamide.[1] The design and interpretation of data derived from teratogenic experiments must take into consideration the genetic pool upon which the teratogen interacts. To date, there is no clear proof that such a phenomenon underlies the human response to teratogens, but it is highly likely that it does play an important part in some human malformations.

Teratogenic effects may become manifest only later in life, well beyond the perinatal period. Most teratogenic animal studies are carried out prior to parturition so that all fetal material may be available for examination. There are, however, human anatomic malformations that are not discernible at birth but that produce serious clinical problems later. Abnormal renal arterial patterns leading to hypertension, congenital cerebral aneurysms leading to intracerebral vascular bleeding, and certain types of congenital heart disease would be examples of such morphologic abnormalities. Whether any of these is due to xenobiotic exposure early in life is not known at this time, but the clear link of DES exposure in utero with vaginal cancer and uterine-oviduct malformations suggests the strong possibility that such a relation is possible.

There is considerable evidence for specificity in the embryonic response to teratogens. Developmental abnormalities due to a true genetic factor usually result in specific morphologic malformations identifiable with that genetic factor. These are classified into clinical developmental syndromes. Chemical teratogens tend to fall into two categories. The first group consists of a small group of chemical teratogens that induce an extremely broad spectrum of malformations (e.g., Vitamin A; some of the azo dyes). The second and much larger group consists of those that induce rather specific defects (e.g., heavy metals;[8] thalidomide).[13] In human development, it is the sudden appearance of time-related or geographic clusters of morphologically similar malformations that should raise the level of suspicion concerning a therapeutic or environmental teratogen.

Not every xenobiotic is a teratogen. Despite the fears that xenobiotics can raise concerning their teratogenic potential, it is probable that only a certain fraction of them have this potential. The problem facing society is to be certain that the methodology and regulations for accurate testing are in place prior to the occurrence of a problem. The social, psychologic, and rehabilitative costs of any malformation may be enormous.

Two human teratogens of current clinical concern are retinoic acid, including some of its derivatives, and alcohol. The teratogenic capacity of Vitamin A has been known since 1954, and a considerable literature on this subject has developed since then.[r3] Some retinoids are now used very effectively in the treatment of acne and psoriasis, but they also have been linked to human malformations in newborns from mothers given retinoids at therapeutic levels early in gestation. This poses a number of regulatory problems: the search for the proper methods for patient warnings; access of patients to the drug; and physician responsibility for its proper use. This dilemma of clinical therapeutic effectiveness versus potential for congenital malformations may well be repeated in the future when other new drugs are developed. The fetal alcohol syndrome consists of a cluster of developmental malformations found in human newborns of mothers who consumed excessive amounts of alcohol during pregnancy. Malformations noted in this syndrome include: microcephaly; facial and cardiac abnormalities; and growth retardation, among others.[r3]

The importance of developing methodologies for accurate teratogenic testing before clinical use cannot be overemphasized. Except for those relatively few compounds regulated by the FDA, many naturally-occurring chemicals and many xenobiotics have never been tested for teratogenic potential. Some of them may well prove to have teratogenic activity. If they do, acute exposure must be related to early pregnancy or the compound might have cumulative effects resulting from chronic exposure.

References

Research Reports

1. Biddle FG. Genetic differences in the frequency of acetazolamide-induced ectrodactyly in the mouse exhibit directional dominance of relative embryonic resistance. Teratology 1988;*37*:375–388.
2. Dixon RL. Toxic responses of the reproductive system. In: Klaassen CD, Amdur MD, Doull J. Casarett and Doull's toxicology. The basic science of poisons, 3d ed. New York: Macmillan, (1986);432–477.
3. Dym M, Fawcett DW. Further observations on the numbers of spermatogonia, spermatocytes, and spermatids connected by intercellular bridges in the mammalian testis. Biol Reproduction 1971;*4*:195–215.
4. Fabro S. Drugs and male sexual function. Repro Tox (A medical letter) 1985;*4*:1–4.
5. Ferm VH, Hanlon DP. Metal induced congenital malformations. In: Clarkson TW, Nordberg GF, Sager PR. Reproductive and developmental toxicity of metals. New York: Plenum Press, (1983);383–397.
6. Garbis-Berkvens, Peters PWJ. Comparative morphology and physiology of embryonic and fetal membranes. In: Nau H, Scott WJ Jr. Pharmacokinetics in teratogenesis. Boca Raton: CRC Press, (1987);3–44.
7. Greenwald GS. Possible animal models of follicular development relevant to reproductive toxicology. Rep Tox 1987;*1*:55–59.
8. Haney AF. Structural and functional consequences of prenatal exposure to diethylstilbesterol in women. In: McLachlan JA, Pratt RM, Markert CL. Developmental toxicology: Mechanisms and risk. Cold Spring Harbor, (1987);271–285.
9. Heller RH, Jones HW. Production of ovarian dysgenesis in the rat and human by busulphan. Am J Obstet & Gynecol 1964;*81*:414–420.
10. Hirschfield A. Histological assessment of follicular development and its applicability to risk assessment. Rep Tox 1987;171–179.
11. Hook EB. The impact of aneuploidy upon public health: Mortality and morbidity associated with human chromosome abnormalities. In: Dellarco VL, Voytek PE, Hollaender A. Aneuploidy. New Tork: Plenum Press, (1985);7–38.
12. Hutchings DE. Behavioral teratology: A new frontier in neurobehavioral research. In: Johnson EM, Kochar DM. Teratogenesis and reproductive toxicology. Berlin/Heidelberg/New York: Springer-Verlag, (1983);207–235.
13. Jensh RP. Behavioral testing procedures: A review. In: Johnson EM, Kochar DM. Teratogenesis and reproductive toxicology. Berlin/Heidelberg/New York: Springer-Verlag, (1983);171–206.
14. Johnson LD. Lesions of the female genital system caused by diethylstilbesterol in humans, subhuman primates and mice. In: Jones TC, Mohr U, Hunt RD. Monographs on pathology of laboratory animals. Genital system. Berlin: Springer-Verlag, (1987);84–109.
15. Koyama H, Wada T, Nishizawer Y, et al. Cyclophosphamide-induced ovarian failure and its therapeutic significance in patients with breast cancer. Cancer 1977;*39*:1403–1409.
16. Martin RH. Chromosomal abnormalities in human sperm. In: Dellarco VL, Voytek PE, Hollaender A. Aneuploidy. New York: Plenum Press, (1985);91–102.
17. Mattison DR. The effects of smoking on fertility from gametogenesis to implantation. Environ Res 1982;*28*:410–433.
18. Mattison DR, Jelovsek FR. Pharmacokinetics and expert systems as aids for risk assessment in reproductive toxicology. Env Health Persp 1987;*76*:107–119.
19. Mattison DR, Schulman JD. How xenobiotic compounds can destroy oocytes. Contemp Ob/GyN 1980;*15*:157–169.
20. Mattison DR, Thorgeirrson SS. Smoking and industrial pollution and their effects on menopause and ovarian cancer. Lancet 1978;*i*:187.
21. Meistrich ML. Critical components of testicular function and sensitivity to disruption. Biol Repro 1986;*34*:17–28.
22. Mohr U, Emura M, Auf derHeide M, Reibe M, Ernst H. Transplacental carcinogenesis, mouse, rat, hamster. In: Jones TC, Mohr U, Hunt RD. Monographs on the pathology of laboratory animals. Genital system. Berlin: Springer-Verlag, (1987);148–157.

23. Morriss FH Jr, Boyd RDH. Placental transport. In: Knobil E, Neill J. The physiology of reproduction. New York: Raven Press, 1988; Vol. II:2043–2083.

24. Nau H. Species differences in pharmacokinetics, drug metabolism and teratogenesis. In: Nau H, Scott WJ Jr. Pharmacokinetics in teratogenesis. Boca Raton: CRC Press. (1987);82–106.

25. Nieman LK, Choate TM, Chrousos GP, et al. The progesterone antagonist RU 486. A potential new contraceptive agent. N Engl J Med 1987;*316*:187–191.

26. Overstreet JW. Laboratory tests for human male reproductive risk assessment. Teratogen Carcinogen Mutagen 1984;*4*:67–82.

27. Persaud TVN. Teratogenicity testing. In: Persaud TVN, Chundly AE, Skalko RG. Basic concepts in teratology. New York: Liss, (1985);155–181.

28. Potashnik G, Yanai-Inbar I. Dibromochloropropane (DBCP): an 8-year reevaluation of testicular function and reproductive performance. Fertil Steril 1987;*47*:317–323.

29. Rao MC, Gibori G. Corpus luteum: Animal models of possible relevance to reproductive toxicology. Rep Tox 1977;*1*:61–69.

30. Roberts CJ, Lowe CR. Where have all the conceptions gone? Lancet 1975;*i*:498–499.

31. Scalli AR. Symposium on the assessment of reproductive hazards in the workplace. Rep Tox 1988;*2*:151–293.

32. Schreiner CA, Holden HE Jr. Mutagens as teratogens: A correlative approach. In: Johnson EM, Kochar DM. Teratogenesis and reproductive toxicology. Berlin/Heidelberg/New York: Springer-Verlag, (1983);135–168.

33. Smith MK, Kimmel GL, Kochar DM, et al. A selection of candidate compounds for in vitro teratogenesis test validation. Teratogen Carcinogen Mutagen 1983;*3*:461–480.

34. Torkelson TR, Sadek SE, Rowe VK, et al. Toxicologic investigations of 1,2-Dibromo-3-Chloropropane. Toxicol Appl Pharm 1961;*3*:545–559.

35. Whorton D, Kraus RM, Marshall S, Milby TH. Infertility in male pesticide workers. Lancet 1977;*2*:1259–1261.

36. Wramsby H, Fredga K, Leidholm P. Chromosome analysis of human oocytes recovered from pre-ovulatory follicles in stimulated cycles. N Engl J Med 1987;*316*:121–124.

Reviews

r1. Fawcett DW. Male Reproductive System. In: Bloom and Fawcett: A Textbook of Histology, 11th ed. Philadelphia: WB Saunders, 1986. *Well-detailed description of human spermatogenesis with excellent illustrations.*

r2. Mossman HW. Vertebrate Fetal Membranes. New Jersey: Rutgers University Press, 1987. *The authoritative reference on placentation, illustrating the remarkable differences in this important structure in the various mammalian species.*

r3. Shepard TH. Catalog of Teratogenic Agents. 7th ed. Baltimore: Johns Hopkins University Press, 1992. *A comprehensive update of known and possible human teratogens as well as annotated references to 2200 other compounds studied for teratogenic potential in a variety of animal models.*

r4. Jones TC, Mohr U, Hunt RD. Genital System. Monographs on Pathology of Laboratory Animals. Berlin: Springer-Verlag, 1987. *A collection of reports on the histopathology of the male and female reproductive tracts, primarily rodents, including effects of exposures to various chemicals.*

CHAPTER 11

Michael Goddard
Daniel Krewski
Jan Zielinski
Leonard Ritter

Toxicologic Risk Assessment

A major undertaking of any body responsible for protecting public health and the environment is the need to deal with risks. In the last few decades methods for dealing with this have been developed and promulgated by several countries. The paradigm for this task developed by the US National Academy of Sciences provides a convenient framework within which risk assessment issues can be approached.[1] In this model, risk assessment and risk management are separate tasks. The former involves a scientific determination of the nature of a risk; the latter focuses on deciding what to do about a problem. Risk management is based on a technically sound risk assessment, and it involves a wider context, including cost/benefits and regulatory policies. Here, we will consider only risk assessment.

Traditionally, toxicologic research has been at the heart of risk assessment. In this chapter, we present an overview of the role of toxicology in risk assessment. First we introduce the basic stages in risk assessment. In the next section, types of toxicologic studies that have proved useful in risk assessment are summarized. The utility of a toxicologic study often rests on the statistical nature of the results: thus, we provide an overview of the primary statistical issues. Then we show how information derived from toxicologic studies is used in the quantitative risk assessments that frequently underlie regulatory decisions. Some examples are presented. Emerging facets of this area are highlighted and we outline how results of toxicologic studies are combined and presented to the decision makers charged with the task of risk management.

The Risk Assessment Paradigm

There are four components in the risk assessment paradigm: hazard identification, dose-response assessment; exposure assessment; and risk characterization.[1]

The goal of hazard identification is a qualitative judgment: does a factor, usually a chemical substance, elicit an adverse health effect? This can be considered as a first screening for the subsequent assessment process; if there is insufficient evidence of toxicity, then the expense of detailed scientific study can be avoided. Information used to assess whether something is hazardous comes from many sources, including toxicologic research.

For a substance that appears to be hazardous, quantitative information is then obtained in the dose-response stage. Again, data are gleaned from a wide array of sources, including clinical and epidemiologic studies of humans and toxicologic experiments on various animal species. The goal of this phase is to develop a numerical model relating the level of risk in humans to the level of exposure.

Concern for the risks due to a chemical does not lie solely with its toxicity. One may be more concerned with a mildly toxic substance to which many individuals are exposed than with a highly toxic substance to which almost no one is exposed. In order to gauge fully the risk to a population, it is also necessary to determine the over-all exposure to that factor. This is the goal of the exposure assessment aspect of risk assessment.

The ideal risk assessment may require considerable information. Usually, a risk assessor needs to make judgments with far less information than he or she would like. Relevant information usually comes from many disciplines, and the assessor has to be able to make judgments based on partial toxicologic data and incomplete or missing information on humans. In the last component of risk assessment, risk characterization, one integrates all the available information. Here one highlights what is missing, and often one attempts to prepare a summary for the next step: risk management. The result of a risk assessment is usually not a single value or judgment. Given the wide range of possible models valid in dose-risk assessment, and given the frequent lack of critical data, the risk assessor often will need to offer several possible risk estimates to the risk manager.

Toxicologic Studies

Although providing only indirect information on human health risks, toxicologic studies conducted in the laboratory provide valuable predictive information on the toxic potential of chemicals. This information is useful both for hazard identification and dose-risk assessment. A large number of toxicologic procedures can be used to study potential adverse health effects. While traditional end-points such as general toxicity, teratogenesis, and carcinogenesis have been studied for many years, more recent developments include tests for immunosuppression, behavioral abnormalities, and genetic damage.

Toxicologic support in risk assessment pertains not only to the effects of chemical hazards, but also to the risks associated with ionizing and nonionizing radiation. Often, the mechanisms of health effects observed in humans are subsequently explored in depth by animal studies. Toxicological research focuses primarily on the potential of various types of radiation in causing cancer; other end-points of interest include effects on growth and development, cataracts of the eye lens, and fertility.[2]

Ionizing radiation is an example of agent known to cause tumors in every organ of the body although there are wide differences between tumor types and animal species in terms of the dose-dependence.[3,4] Biologic effects of ionizing radiation result from the modification and destruction of cell components. Cells from different tissues vary markedly in radiosensitivity. It is generally accepted that incorrectly repaired or unrepaired modifications of DNA are the main causes of radiation-induced damage in cells and, hence, organisms.

Acute Toxicity

Acute toxicity tests are used to assess the potential of the test agent to induce adverse health effects, usually following a single exposure to high doses.[5] Tests frequently last at most a few days. While not considered to be of great predictive value for human health effects, acute toxicity studies are useful in identifying clinical manifestations of toxicity associated with high exposures, as in poisoning. Acute toxicity studies also may be used to rank the toxic potential of different agents using the median lethal dose (LD_{50}, the dose resulting in 50% mortality in the exposed population) as well as to determine dose levels for longer investigations.

Subchronic Toxicity

Subchronic toxicity studies are used to assess potential toxic effects associated with exposures lasting a fraction of the animal's lifespan. Experimental animals typically are subjected to repeated doses of the test material for periods of from many days to several weeks or months. A series of exposure levels generally are used to characterize the shape and nature of the dose-response relationship. Subchronic studies provide some indication as to potential human health hazards and are also useful in the selection of doses to be used in chronic toxicity studies.

Chronic Toxicity and Carcinogenicity

Chronic toxicity studies are used to study toxic effects that occur only after prolonged exposure to sublethal dose levels. While most toxic effects will appear in subchronic studies, certain irreversible progressive effects such as cancer may occur only following lengthy periods of exposure. Because of this, long-term toxicity studies are an important toxicologic tool for assessing potential human health risks associated with lifetime exposure to therapeutic agents intended for long-term use, environmental contaminants, environmental radiation, pesticides that may occur as food residues, and some industrial chemicals.

As with other toxicologic protocols, studies of carcinogenicity (see also Chapter 109) are conducted using relatively high doses to induce measurable tumor response rates. The highest dose used is called the maximum tolerated dose (MTD), which is defined roughly as the highest dose that can be administered throughout the course of a lifetime study without appreciably altering body weight or survival except as a consequence of tumor occurrence.

Metabolism and Pharmacokinetics

Metabolic and pharmacokinetic studies may be used to determine the absorption, distribution, and elimination of the test compound and to determine the rates at which these processes occur. This information is essential in order to develop adequate protocols for subchronic and chronic toxicity studies. Metabolic and pharmacokinetic data also are used in the interpretation of mutagenicity and other toxic tests and in the comparison of results in different species.

Reproductive Toxicity

Reproductive studies encompass many generations of the test species. They provide information on reproductive parameters that may be affected through in situ exposure in subsequent generations. Reproduction studies may be utilized to investigate such parameters as rate of implantation, spontaneous abortion rate, and perinatal growth and survival. While several animal models have been used to study reproductive performance, the rat is often preferred for ease of handling, short gestational period, and abundant historical data. The effects of radiation on the genes and chromosomes of reproductive cells are well characterized in mice.[6]

Teratology

Teratology testing (see also Chapter 110) is designed to assess the potential of chemicals to induce birth defects. While several protocols are available to accommodate specific experimental demands, guidelines such as those developed by the Organization for Economic Cooperation and Development[7] are widely employed. Although identification of the most appropriate species remains an unresolved issue within the scientific community, there is agreement that teratology testing should be conducted in at least two species (including one nonrodent species) to minimize possible erroneous conclusions attributable to insensitivity of any given species. Typically, such studies are conducted in rats and rabbits.

Genetic Toxicology

Much progress has been made in recent years in the development of short-term tests for genetic alterations using bacteria, fungi, plants, insects, cultured mammalian cells, and small mammals;[8] (see also Chapter 109). These tests are of interest not only as identifiers of gene and chromosomal mutations, but also as predictors of carcinogenicity. They offer further advantages in terms of time and cost and may in the future reduce the need to use laboratory animals for testing purposes.

Of the many available short-term tests, the Ames Salmonella/microsome assay is perhaps the single most widely used. The assay uses mutant strains of bacteria, which, because of a deficiency in their ability to synthesize the essential animo acid histidine, can undergo cell division only in a medium containing sufficient histidine for growth.

Structure Activity Analysis

Attempts have been made to see whether the chemical structure of the molecule itself may serve as a predictor of toxic or carcinogenic effects.[9,10] Such predictions often are based on particular active sites, such as the number of aromatic rings in polycyclic hydrocarbons or the number of chlorine atoms in chlorinated hydrocarbons. Such classification rules have met with some success, but are far from perfect.

Experimental Design and Statistical Analysis

Experimental Design

Carefully designed experiments are critical to successful toxicologic research.[11] Resources allocated to planning before the first observation is made can help to avoid the detrimental consequences of a poorly planned study. A well designed experiment can provide an unbiased estimate of parameters of the end-points of interest. We call an estimate "unbiased" if it is equal on average to the true quantity being estimated.

Three key concepts underlying the statistical theory of experimental design are randomization, replication, and stratification. We achieve randomization by assigning treatments within each block, often according to a table of random numbers or some other randomization procedure. Randomization insures that the study results will be free from unsuspected biases and provides a basis for a valid statistical analysis. In the absence of randomization it is possible that an unknown confounding effect may be responsible for observed phenomena, rather than the factors the study was intended to elucidate.

By replication we mean a repetition of the basic experiment. Replication is necessary in order to provide a measure of experimental variability and to assess the reproducibility of experimental results. Thus, several animals will be assigned to each treatment considered in the study, with the variability in response among animals receiving the same treatment used to assess experimental error. Replicates may be obtained under relatively homogeneous conditions existing within the same laboratory at the same time or under somewhat dissimilar conditions existing in different laboratories. Confirmatory results among replicates, particularly those conducted under somewhat different conditions, are reassuring. Conflicting results may occur as a genuine consequence of uncontrolled variation in the different study conditions, or as a result of intrinsic experimental variation. The interpretation of such differences is often difficult, and additional studies may be needed for reconciliation.

Blocking (or stratification) is a technique used to increase the precision of an experiment. A block (or a stratum) is a portion of the experiment that should be more homogeneous than the entire set of material. Stratification provides a means of controlling some types of experimental variation. If intrinsic variability can be lowered, a smaller experiment may be possible and resources saved. The concept of stratification exploits information about covariates other than the factor of interest, which may influence the phenomenon under study. For example, animals may be divided into relatively homogeneous groups defined by body weight or litter status. By comparing different treatments within such strata, experimental error is reduced and sensitivity is enhanced. This technique is most effective in the presence of large intergroup variation, small intragroup variation, and consistency of treatment differences among groups.

Elaborate statistical designs such as factorial layouts, Latin squares, and partially balanced incomplete blocks designs could be considered for toxicologic studies. While these designs can offer considerable increases in efficiency, they do require that special conditions be satisfied to be valid.

Statistical Sensitivity

Care is needed in making inferences based on statistical testing. Typically, a report in the literature summarizing a statistical test declares a test to be "significant" or "not significant." There is a subtle, though important, distinction between statistically significant differences and biologically or medically important differences. This distinction is often misinterpreted, and the concept of biologic insignificance is mistakenly read into a statistically insignificant result.

Consider a simple experiment in which one group of animals is exposed to the test compound and another group is unexposed. There are four possible results from such an experiment. A difference may be statistically significant and either biologically meaningful or not biologically meaningful, and a difference may not be statistically significant and either biologically meaningful or not biologically meaningful. The situations where a difference is both statistically and biologically significant or both not significant are straightforward. Those situations where the facts differ are more complicated.

It is common to encounter studies where an observed difference was numerically large to the point of being biologically important but, because the study was small, not statistically significant. A common error is to interpret the lack of statistical significance as evidence of no biologic effect. The reality is that for an inefficient experiment only an enormous numerical difference would result in a statistically significant conclusion. An astute risk assessor will conclude that there is insufficient evidence to conclude whether there is an effect rather than erroneously concluding that the experiment "proves" there is no effect.

This problem is best handled before the study starts, i.e., at the design stage. With a statistician, the investigator must indicate how large a difference he or she would like to see in order for the result to be biologically meaningful. Using this and some other information, like a measure of variability and some probabilities of making an incorrect decision, the statistician will help the investigator determine the size and design of the experiment to insure that the statistical conclusion coincides with the biologic interpretation the investigator seeks. A brief introduction to the ideas and calculations in basic sample size determination is presented as an appendix.

Statistical Analysis

The statistical analysis of experimental data may involve a variety of analytic techniques. Methods range from the very simple to very complicated, depending on the experimental design and the type of data collected.[12]

Perhaps the most commonly used statistical method for continuous data is the analysis of variance, which can be used to test for differences among a number of treatment groups. This approach requires that data either be normally distributed or can be transformed to normality. Another assumption underlying the analysis of variance technique is that observations are independent. When this assumption is not valid, methods that provide for correlated data are required. For example, with repeated observations on body weight at different times, growth curve methods may be employed. If it is impossible to assure that data are normally distributed, then nonparametric techniques may be used. These methods require no assumptions about the distribution of the data, but they tend to lack the flexibility of analysis of various methods for normal data.

Other methods are required for the analysis of categorical data. There are methods for binomial data, where only one of two results is possible (like "dead" or "alive") and for polytomous data (like "absent," "mild," "moderate," and "severe"). Contingency table analysis can be used to compare treatments; log-linear or logistic regression models can be used to relate dose and response in a quantitative fashion.

A special kind of continuous data are time-to-event data, such as the survival times of individual animals in long-term studies. Survival analysis may require allowance for censored observations, as when the time-to-death of an animal is not observed owing to interim or terminal sacrifices.

The analysis of data on tumor occurrence rates in long-term carcinogenicity studies raises special statistical problems. While the time of tumor occurrence is of interest, this is not observable except in special cases, such as visible, palpable, or rapidly lethal tumors. Occult tumors of intermediate lethality generally are not detected until necropsy. In such cases, information on cause of death (tumor-related or otherwise) is helpful.

Toxicologic Risk Assessment

Quantitative Dose-Risk Assessment

Two approaches are used to set concentrations of toxicants used in regulation. It usually is convenient to associate one approach, that using "safety factors" with noncarcinogenic responses and to link the other, which involves mathematical modeling, with carcinogenic responses. Another way of distinguishing those situations in which one uses safety factors from the cases where formal models are used is to note that safety factors are used when a "threshold" dose for risk may exist; the latter are used when there is no evidence of a threshold. Individuals exposed to dose levels below a "threshold dose" are not at risk; those above are. For nonthreshold situations, lower doses are linked to lower risks, but there is no dose below which there is no risk. These distinctions (noncarcinogenic or carcinogenic and nonthreshold or threshold) help to illustrate the different approaches, but they are not strict. For example, mathematical modeling is used for some noncarcinogenic responses.

No-Effect Levels (NOEL) and Safety Factors

The traditional approach to setting acceptable levels of human exposure to environmental toxicants has been to apply a suitable safety or uncertainty factor to that dose level at which no adverse effects were observed in toxicologic studies. With contaminants present in food, for example, the no-observed effect level in toxicologic tests is divided by the safety factor (SF) to arrive at an acceptable daily intake (ADI = NOEL/SF) for humans. Conversely, comparison of a given exposure level (E) to the NOEL yields the margin of safety (MS = NOEL/E) afforded by that level of exposure. In some instances, a NOAEL, representing a "no adverse effect level," rather than a NOEL is used.

A similar approach may be used to establish a threshold limit value (TLV) for workplace exposures to substances in ambient air. The TLV is set so that nearly all workers will experience no adverse effects following repeated daily exposure, and is often supported by observations on occupationally exposed populations (see also Chapter 105).

For toxic effects other than cancer, a safety factor of 100-fold or more has often been used in establishing ADIs. This allows for a tenfold variation in susceptibility between animal and man as well as a tenfold variation in individual susceptibility within the human population. In the absence of a no effect level, it has been proposed that the safety factor might be applied to the lowest observed effect level or LOEL with an additional factor of 5 or so incorporated to adjust for the absence of a no-effect level. An additional factor of 10 may also be included with reproductive or teratologic effects.

The use of safety factors in arriving at acceptable human exposure levels rests on the assumption that a threshold dose exists below which no adverse effects will occur. Provided that the toxic endpoint under study demonstrates a threshold below which no adverse effects will occur, the safety factor approach seeks to set the ADI below this threshold. However, other methods of risk estimation are required for toxic effects for which the threshold hypothesis may be inappropriate.

More recently, the ADI concept has been replaced by that of a "reference dose" (RfD). The term "uncertainty factor" is favored over the term "safety factor." These changes avoid possibly misleading terms like "safe" and "acceptable" doses. It is hoped that the newer approach is more specific in the determination of the regulatory limit and there is more agreement in decisions made by various bodies. Barnes and Dourson[13] outline this approach and detail the guidelines for the use of uncertainty and modifying factors.

Dose-Response Modeling

Because the threshold concept may not be universally applicable to carcinogenesis and mutagenesis, the regulation of carcinogens and mutagens is regarded as a special issue in risk estimation. The absence of a threshold precludes the possibility that a sufficiently low level of exposure will be free of any attendant degree of hazard. Biologic arguments in favor of the no-threshold concept for carcinogenesis are generally based on the fact that irreversible self-replicating lesions may result from a mutation in a single somatic cell, often following the administration of only a single dose. Arguments against this position draw on the existence of metabolic detoxification, DNA repair, immunologic surveillance, and other mechanisms that may operate to nullify effects at low doses.

For carcinogenic end-points, it is generally assumed that no threshold dose level exists. In this case, the determination of a dose level for regulation relies on a mathematical model to relate predicted risks to dosage.

Originally, tolerance distributions like the logit and probit models used for noncarcinogenic responses were used.[14] A model called the "multistage model" developed by Armitage and Doll[15] has become very popular for cancer risk estimation. This statistical model involves up to about seven stages and appears to fit observed cancer incidence curves reasonably well. A modified form, referred to as the "linearized multistage model", is described by Crump and Howe[16] and relates risk to low doses by a straight line.

A more biologically-based model of carcinogenesis is the stochastic two-stage model developed by Moolgavkar and his colleagues.[17] This model is based on the notion that initiated cells are formed following the occurrence of a single mutation in a normal stem cell. The initiated cell can thus sustain a second mutation and progress to a cancerous cell. The initiated cell population can also be promoted by clonal expansion, increasing the pool of cells available for progression to malignancy.

This initiation-promotion-progression model has been considered by the US Environmental Protection Agency[18] and has been applied to bioassay data by Thorslund and Charnley.[19] Moolgavkar[20] analyzed experimental data on radon-induced lung tumors in rats within the framework of the two-stage model. For general application, information on the growth rates of normal tissue and the kinetics of the initiated cell population is required in addition to bioassay data on tumor occurrence. Various applications of the two-stage model have been reviewed by Krewski et al.[21]

Linear Extrapolation

In the absence of information to the contrary, low-dose linearity is often assumed. This position is supported by the US Office of Science and Technology Policy,[22] which states "when data and information are limited, models or procedures which incorporate low-dose linearity are preferred when compatible with the limited information."

Because toxicologic studies are necessarily conducted at relatively high doses to induce observable response rates, the estimation of cancer risks associated with very low exposures requires extrapolation of the experimental data to low doses using a model relating risk to dose. The linearized multi-stage model is widely used for this purpose, yielding estimates of low dose risk that are linearly related to low dose levels of the carcinogen. Model-free approaches to linear extrapolation may be employed, although estimates of low risk often do not differ materially from those based on the linearized multi-stage model.[23]

The hypothesis of low-dose linearity for carcinogens implies that any level of exposure will induce some risk. In this event, the ideal of zero risk can be achieved only if exposure is completely eliminated. However, sufficiently low levels of exposure may lead to small risks that may be tolerated in some circumstances.

Exposure Assessment

The evaluation of a toxicologic hazard in isolation is insufficient to allow an assessment of potential human risk. Relatively nontoxic substances may be in very widespread use in large quantities and may thus provide substantial opportunity for expression of relatively rare events. Conversely, chemicals believed to have significant toxic potential may be utilized in such a way so as to reduce human exposure to an almost negligible level.

The prediction of human risk based on the results of toxicologic testing thus requires consideration of exposure. Various methods exist for the estimation of human exposure to chemicals in different settings. These methods include the analysis of ambient air in the work environment, determination of chemicals and their residues and metabolites in such body fluids as sweat, blood, and urine, and quantitative estimation of the chemical deposition on human skin. When body fluids are used as monitors of exposure, care must be taken to ensure that residue or metabolite levels measured are quantitatively related to body burden. Similarly, where passive dosimetry such as air or skin monitoring are used, corrections must be made for absorption, disposition and excretion. The US Environmental Protection Agency published a guideline for exposure assessment in 1992.[24]

Risk Characterization

The fourth aspect of the risk assessment paradigm is risk characterization. This final stage feeds directly into the risk management process of regulatory action. A risk assessor needs to survey the wide range of toxicologic studies for a compound of interest (which may also involve some significant gaps) and then to summarize all the data thought necessary relating to over-all risks to humans.

A common way to present a simplified summary of this wealth of information is to use a "weight of evidence" approach and eventually to categorize the substance. Broadly, the consistency of results across several studies adds weight to the belief that a substance is toxic: are there similar effects for the various species, strains and sexes of animals? Is there a clear dose-response relationship? Is there contributing evidence from studies on metabolism and a theoretical basis for a postulated mechanism-of-action?

One example of a grading system for a chemical's evidence of carcinogenicity is that used by the International Agency for Research on Cancer.[25] First, the evidence from toxicologic studies on animals is categorized as showing: (1) sufficient evidence of carcinogenicity; (2) limited evidence of carcinogenicity; (3) inadequate evidence of carcinogenicity; or (4) evidence suggesting lack of carcinogenicity.

Information from observations on humans either through case studies or epideimology is similarly characterized.

The over-all characterization of risk draws on both these categorizations, a chemical being classified, depending on the combination of evidence from human and animal studies, into one of the following:

- Group 1: The agent is carcinogenic to humans;
- Group 2A: The agent is probably carcinogenic to humans;
- Group 2B: The agent is possibly carcinogenic to humans;
- Group 3: The agent is not classifiable as to its carcinogenicity to humans; or
- Group 4: The agent is probably not carcinogenic to humans.

Tomatis[26] reports that, as of 1989, the International Agency for Research on Cancer has deemed 53 chemicals, mixtures, industrial processes or radiologic agents as carcinogenic in humans. It is difficult to establish convincing evidence for lack of carcinogenicity. At present, only one chemical, caprolactam, has met the IARC criteria.

Illustrative Applications

In order to illustrate the practical application of the concepts introduced earlier, consider the case of a hypothetical pesticide applied to potatoes and beans. Specifically, suppose that the pesticide of interest is to be applied at a rate that will leave residues of approximately 30 mg per kg of crop. Assume further that consumption of both potatoes and beans has been estimated at approximately 100 g of crop per day for a 70-kg person. Ingestion of the pesticide residue can then be estimated to be 30 × 100/1000 or 3 mg/day for 70 kg body mass, corresponding to a 3/70 = 0.04 mg/kg/day dose level.

Few pesticides, if any, are utilized only on a single crop. Indeed, most pesticides are used on many food crops, and hence may be introduced into the human diet through a variety of food commodities. In addition, although representing only about 5 percent of the North American population, farmers may experience occupational pesticide exposure substantially greater than through the food route alone. Both farmers and the general population may also be exposed to pesticide contaminated drinking water through farm or municipal water supplies.

A theoretical estimate of exposure from all sources is often referred to as the tolerable daily intake, or TDI. While TDI estimates have historically been restricted to anticipated exposure through dietary sources, widespread exposure to pesticide residues has prompted many regulatory authorities to consider all possible sources of exposure in estimating TDIs.

The TDI should never exceed the acceptable daily intake (ADI) established on the basis of toxicologic data as described. In practice, the TDI estimate will often exceed actual intake since TDI calculations assume that all crops are treated all of the time at maximum allowable rates, that residue levels are always at their lawful limit, and that washing, processing, and cooking do not diminish or eliminate pesticide residue levels.

It should also be noted that while ADI reflects the intrinsic toxicologic properties of the chemical itself, the TDI may increase as pesticide usage expands to accommodate additional crop uses. Such incremental uses of pesticide products may eventually result in a theoretical intake approaching the ADI, causing denial of any further market expansion of the pesticide.

Teratologic Studies

Many chemicals, including pesticides, are tested for their ability to induce birth defects in at least two animal species, typically the rat and the rabbit (see also Chapter 107). As with any other toxicologic tests, teratology studies often yield a variety of toxic responses ranging from those occurring as spontaneous events in untreated controls to unusual lesions in exposed animals almost certainly referable to treatment. Contemporary protocols for evaluation of teratogenic potential require the appearance of maternal toxicity at the highest dose tested, thus limiting the usefulness of this test group for evaluation of teratogenic potential where a response is limited to this dose group alone. Table 111.1 illustrates the results from a hypothetical rodent teratology study conducted according to US EPA protocol requirements. Note the appearance of both diaphragmatic hernia and hydrocephaly at the top dose tested (20 mg/kg), with hydrocephaly appearing at the mid-dose level (10 mg/kg) as well. The near doubling of this anomaly with a concomitant doubling in dose suggests that this rare birth defect is directly attributable to treatment ($p < 0.001$). The biologic relevance of the diaphragmatic hernia occurring at the top dose only cannot be fully evaluated in the absence of extensive data on the toxicologic profiles of animals at this dose level. Over-all, however, the data provided would suggest a no-observed effect level (NOEL) of 5 mg/kg/day for teratogenic effects.

Since dietary consumption is expected not to exceed 0.04 mg/kg/day, the margin of safety is equal to 5 (mg/kg/day)/0.04 (mg/kg/day) = 125. Thus, consumers will be exposed daily to dietary levels of this pesticide that are approximately 1/125th of the dose that induced significant teratogenic effects in rodents. Further, as noted above, actual dietary intake may well exceed the calculated 0.04 mg/kg/day level due to additional uses of the chemical on other food crops. Consideration also needs to be given to occupational exposure in the agricultural community as well as possible general population exposure through contaminated drinking water.

Table 111.1 Teratogenic Effects Induced by a Hypothetical Pesticide

a) Diaphragmatic Hernia

	Dose (mg/kg)			
Affected Pups in Litter of 12	**0**	**5**	**10**	**20**
0	19	16	18	0
1	1	2		5
2		1		5
3				5
4				3
5				1
6				1
No. of Affected Pups	1	4	0	53
No. of Live Pups	240	228	216	240
No. of Litters	20	19	18	20

b) Hydrocephalus

	Dose (mg/kg)			
Affected Pups in Litter of 12	**0**	**5**	**10**	**20**
0	20	18	1	0
1		1	4	0
2			7	2
3			3	1
4			3	3
5				5
6				4
7				1
8				2
9				2
No. of Affected Pups	0	1	39	109
No. of Live Pups	240	228	216	240
No. of Litters	20	19	18	20

Carcinogenic Effects

Suppose that a dietary carcinogenicity bioassay were conducted in rats utilizing initial group sizes of 70 animals per sex in each of three treatment groups, in addition to an untreated control. Animals were fed the test diet for approximately 24 months, at which point survivors were killed and subjected to histopathologic examination. The resulting tumor occurrence rates are given in Table 111.2. In the absence of differences in survival among the treatment groups, lifetime tumor incidence rates in the exposed animals may be compared to those in controls. Fisher's exact test was used to test for an increase in tumor incidence in each of the exposed groups relative to controls. In addition, an exact test for increasing linear trend with dose was also employed. This analysis suggested an excess of adrenal pheochromocytoma and thyroid follicular cell adenoma in males and uterine stromal cell tumors in females.

Using linear extrapolation, the anticipated excess risk associated with consumption of agricultural crops treated with our hypothetical pesticide can be estimated. For example, the excess risk at the TDI of 0.04 mg/kg/day is approximately two excess cancers per 10,000 exposed persons (based on adrenal tumor response in male rats at 25 mg/kg/day). Such estimates may be applied to humans under the assumption of equal sensitivity of animals and humans with dose expressed on a body weight basis. Although such estimates are subject to all of the uncertainties associated with extrapolation of bioassay to low-dose conversion of the animal data to humans, and determination of the TDI, this chemical would probably not be permitted by many regulatory agencies that consider risks in excess of one in a million to be unacceptable for general population exposure.

Recent Developments in Risk Assessment

Thus far, we have considered conventional approaches to toxicologic risk assessment. In this section, we describe more recent developments in a number of areas, including biologically based dose-response models, pharmacokinetic models for metabolic activation, time-dependent exposures, complex mixtures, measures of carcinogenic potency, and interspecies conversion.

Interspecies Conversion

Perhaps the most difficult problems in toxicologic risk assessment are the conversion of animal data to humans. Ideally, quantitative interspecies extrapola-

Table 111.2 Carcinogenesis Observed in Rats Orally Exposed to a Hypothetical Pesticide for Two Years

		Males				Females			
		Dose (mg/kg/day)							
Site	Lesion	0	5	25	125	0	5	25	125
Adrenal	(number examined)	(70)	(69)	(67)	(70)	(69)	(68)	(70)	(69)
	pheochromocytoma	3[a]	3[a]	7[a]	14[ab]	2	0	5	3
	cortical adenoma	0	0	2	0	1	0	0	0
Thyroid	(number examined)	(70)	(69)	(68)	(69)	(69)	(69)	(69)	(69)
	follicular adenoma	0[a]	1[a]	2[a]	9[ab]	1	0	0	2
	follicular carcinoma	0	1	0	1	0	2	0	0
	parafollicular adenoma	0	2	2	0	3	2	4	2
	parafollicular carcinoma	0	1	0	0	0	0	1	1
Mammary gland	(number examined)	(66)	(65)	(68)	(64)	(69)	(69)	(69)	(68)
	benign fibroepithelial tumor	1	4	2	1	31	22	35	28
	carcinoma	0	0	1	0	4	5	3	8
	intraductal papilloma	0	0	0	0	0	2	0	1
	adenoma	0	0	0	0	1	2	0	0
Uterine cervix/Uterus	(number examined)	—	—	—	—	(69)	(69)	(70)	(69)
	stromal cell sarcoma					0[a]	1[a]	2[a]	4[a]
	squamous cell papilloma					0	1	0	0

[a] Significant linear trend ($p < .05$), based on exact Cochran-Armitage test).
[b] Significantly greater than control ($p < .05$, based on Fisher-Irwin exact test).

tion should take into account known species differences. Dose equivalency between species has traditionally been based on body weight and surface area. These are related by the fact that surface area varies roughly in proportion to the 2/3 power of body weight. For a 70-kg human and a 330-g rat, this implies that the human dose (in mg/kg/body weight) producing the same effect as a given dose in the rat will be about six times lower when extrapolating as a surface area rather than a body weight basis. Recently, Travis and White[27] have recommended an intermediate scale based on body weight to the 3/4 power for dose conversion between species.

Empirical support for using toxicologic results in one species to predict possible adverse outcomes in another species may be derived from the test results for rats and mice from the U.S. National Toxicology Program. Qualitatively, Haseman and Huff[28] reported 74 percent concordance in positive and negative results when both sexes are considered separately. More recently, Zeiger et al.,[29] demonstrated concordances in the range of 0.59–0.66. Quantitatively, Gaylor and Chen[30] demonstrated a fair degree of association between carcinogenic potency in rats and mice; Chen and Gaylor[31] noted a similar level of agreement.

Pharmacokinetic Models

It is the amount of a substance that is delivered to a target organ that determines a biologic response. This "delivered dose" may vary greatly from the dose to which the host was originally exposed. Pharmacokinetic models may be used to describe the fate of toxic substances entering the body, including metabolic processes governing the amount of reactive metabolite reaching the target tissue.[32] In the past, systems of differential equations describing pharmacokinetic processes within a small number of conceptual compartments have been widely used for this purpose. More recently, greater understanding of the metabolism of some toxicants and the availability of advanced computer hardware and software have facilitated the development and application of physiologically based pharmacokinetic models (PBPK). Such models are based on a larger number of relevant physiological compartments, with parameters representing the physiology and anatomy of the host.[33] Although considerable effort is required to estimate all these unknown parameters, PBPK models have been employed to describe the metabolism of vinyl chloride[34] and several other toxicants.[35]

Pharmacokinetic models can be used in toxicologic risk assessment to provide a measure of the dose of the reactive metabolite reaching the target tissue, and possibly result in improved estimates of risk. PBPK models also may be used to extrapolate tissue doses more accurately between different routes of exposure or between different species. While improved tissue dosimetry is desirable, pharmacokinetic models cannot resolve all of the uncertainties in toxicologic risk assessment. In extrapolating between species, for example, equal tissue doses may not lead to equivalent toxicologic responses, owing to pharmacodynamic differences in tissue sensitivity between species. The uncertainty in estimates of PBPK model parameters may also confer considerable uncertainty on ultimate estimates of risk.

Time-Dependent Exposures

In the past, dose-response models have been developed for constant exposure levels. Because human exposures may vary notably with time, models that accommodate time-dependent exposure have been developed in recent years.

The US Environmental Protection Agency has suggested the use of time-weighted average daily dose for variable exposure patterns. This provides a constant average dose for risk assessment purposes, but assumes that infrequent high exposures will have the same effect as a series of lower exposures leading to the same total dose. Dosing amortization, however, has little effect on risk estimates when compared, particularly to the form of the mathematical model selected for low-dose extrapolation.[36] Under the initiation-promotion-progression model, however, larger errors can accrue with strong promoting agents.

Measures of Potency

Environmental carcinogens may be ranked according to their carcinogenic potential. An index of carcinogenic potency that has received much recent attention is the TD_{50}, defined as the dose of an agent that produces tumors in 50 percent of exposed animals (after correction for the background rate). Gold et al.[37,38,39] determined the TD_{50} for an extensive series of known animal carcinogens. The TD_{50} values for these carcinogens varied by a factor of up to 10 million-fold, indicating a high degree of variation in the potency of chemical carcinogens.

Another measure of potency used by the US Environmental Protection Agency is the logarithm of q_1^*, the slope of the risk to dose line derived from the linearized multi-stage model. Technically, q_1^* is an upper confidence limit on the linear term of the multi-stage model, and represents the slope of the dose-response curve in the low-dose region. The index q_1^* is highly correlated with the TD_{50}, although one value cannot necessarily be accurately predicted from the other in specific cases. Bernstein et al.,[40] noted that the TD_{50} is also highly correlated with the MTD used in carcinogen bioassay, although the interpretation of this association is open to debate. Zeise et al.[41] have also reported some degree of association between the TD_{50} from long-term studies of carcinogenicity and the LD_{50} from acute toxicity studies.

Conclusion

Toxicologic risk assessment remains under vigorous development. In particular, recent advances have been made in developing biologically based models of carcinogenesis, pharmacokinetic models for metabolic activation, risk assessment methodologies for time-varying exposure patterns, measures of carcinogenic potency, and methods for interspecies extrapolation. These and other developments have strengthened the science of toxicologic risk assessment and have improved our ability to predict potential human risks based on toxicologic data.

References

Research Reports

1. National Research Council. Risk Assessment in the Federal Government: Managing the process. Washington: National Academy Press, 1983.
2. National Research Council, Committee on the Biological Effects of Ionizing Radiations. Health effects of exposure to low levels of ionizing radiation. Washington: National Acadamy Press, 1990.
3. National Research Council. Health risks of radon and other internally deposited alpha-emitters. Washington: National Academy Press, 1988.
4. National Research Council. Health effects of exposure to low levels of ionizing radiation. Washington: National Academy Press, 1988.
5. Gad SC, Chengelis CP. Acute toxicology testing: Perspectives and horizons. Caldwell, NJ: Telford Press, 1988.
6. Selby PB. Radiation genetics. In Foster HL, Small JD, Fox JG. editors, The mouse in biomedical research, Vol I, pp 264–283. New York: Academic Press, 1981.
7. OECD: Organization for Economic Cooperation and Development. Guidelines for Testing of New Chemicals. Paris: OECD, 1986.
8. Grice HC. The use of short-term tests for mutagenicity and carcinogenicity in chemical hazard evaluation. Current Issues in Toxicology, New York: Springer-Verlag, 1984.
9. Rosenkranz HS, Takihi N, Klopman G. Structure activity-based predictive toxicology: an efficient and economical method for generating non-congeneric data bases. Mutagenesis, 1991;*6*:391–394.
10. Golberg L. editor. Structure-Activity correlation as a predictive tool in toxicology: Fundamentals, Methods, and Applications. Washington: Hemisphere, 1983.
11. Krewski D, Bickis M. Statistical issues in toxicological research. In Krewski D, Franklin C. Statistics in toxicology, pp 11–41. New York: Gordon & Breach, 1991.
12. Gart JJ, Krewski D, Lee PN, Tarone RE, Wahrendorf J. Statistical methods in cancer research, Volume III The design and analysis of long term animal experiments. No 79. Lyon: IARC Scientific Publications. International Agency for Research on Cancer, 1986.
13. Barnes DG, Dourson M. Reference dose (RfD): Description and use in health risk assessments. Reg Toxicol Pharmacol, *8*, 1988.
14. Krewski D, Brown C. Carcinogenic risk assessment: A guide to the literature. Biometrics, *37*, 1981.
15. Armitage P, Doll R. Stochastic models for carcinogenesis. In Proceedings of the Fourth Berkeley Symposium on Mathematical Statistics and Probability, Vol 4, pp 19–38. Berkeley, CA: University of California Press, 1961.
16. Crump KS, Howe RB. The multi-stage model with a time-dependent dose pattern: Application to carcinogenic risk assessment. Risk Analysis, *4*, 1984.
17. Moolgavkar SH, Knudson AG Jr. Mutation and cancer: A model for human carcinogenesis. JNCI, *66*, 1981.
18. US Environmental Protection Agency. Report of the EPA Workshop on the Development of Risk Assessment Methodologies for Tumour Promotors EPA/600/9-87/03. Washington: EPA, 1987.
19. Thorslund T, Charnley G. Quantitative dose-response models for tumour promoting agents. pages 245–256, 1988.
20. Moolgavkar SH, Cross FT, Luebeck EG, Dagle GE. A two-mutation model for radon-induced lung tumors in rats. Rad Res, 1990;*121*:28–37.
21. Krewski D, Goddard MJ, Zielinski J. Dose-response relationships in carcinogenesis. In Vainio H, Magee PN, McGregor DB, McMichael AJ. Mechanisms of Carcinogenesis in Risk Identification. Lyon: International Agency for Research on Cancer, 1992.
22. US Office of Science and Technology Policy. Chemical carcinogens: a review of the science and its associated principles. Federal Register, *50*, 1985.
23. Krewski D, Gaylor D, Szyszkowicz M. A model-free approach to low-dose extrapolation. Environ Health Persp, 1991;*90*:279–285.
24. US EPA. Guideline for exposure assessment. Federal Register, 1992;*57*:22888–22938.
25. International Agency for Research on Cancer. Overall Evaluation of Carcinogenicity: An Updating of IARC Monographs Volumes 1 to 42. Supplement 7. Lyon: IARC Monographs on the Evaluation of Carcinogenic Risks to Humans. International Agency for Research on Cancer, 1987.
26. Tomatis L, Aitio A, Wilbourn J, Shuker L. Human carcinogens so far identified. Japan J Cancer Res 1989; 80.
27. Travis CC, White RK. Interspecies scaling of toxicity data. Risk Anal, *8*, 1988.
28. Haseman JK, Huff JE. Species correlation in long-term carcinogenicity studies. Cancer Lett, *37*, 1987.
29. Zeiger E, Haseman JK, Shelby MD, Margolin BH, Tennant RW. Evaluation of four in vitro genetic toxicity tests for predicting rodent carcinogenicity: Confirmation of earlier results with 41 additional chemicals. Environ Mol Mutagen, 1990;*16*, Supplement 18:1–14.
30. Gaylor DW, Chen JJ. Relative potency of chemical carcinogens in rodents. Risk Analy, 1986; 6.
31. Chen JJ, Gaylor DW. Carcinogenic risk assessment: A comparison of estimated safe doses for rats and mice. Environ Health Pers, 1987; 72.
32. Krewski D, Murdoch D, Withey JR. The application of pharmacokinetic data in carcinogenic risk assessment, Vol 8, pp 441–468. Washington: National Academy Press, 1987.
33. Bischoff KB. Physiologically based pharmacokinetic modeling, Vol 8, pp 36–61. Washington: National Academy Press, 1987.
34. Anderson ME, Clewell HJ III, Gargas ML, Smith FA, Reitz RH. Physiologically based pharmacokinetics and the risk assessment process for methylene chloride. Toxicol Appl Pharmacol, 1987;*87*:185–205.

35. Travis CC. Pharmacokinetics. Travis C, Carcinogen Risk Assessment, New York: Plenum Press, 1988.

36. Krewski D, Murdoch DJ, Withey JR. Recent developments in carcinogenic risk assessment (with discussion) Health Physics Supplement, Vol 1, 1989 pp 313–326.

37. Gold LS, Sawyer CB, Magaw R, Backman GM, de Veciana M, Levinson R, Hooper NK, Havender WR, Bernstein L, Peto R, Pike MC, Ames BN. A carcinogenic potency database of the standardized results of animal bioassays. Environ Health Pers 1984; 58.

38. Gold LS, de Veciana M, Backman GM, Magaw R, Lopipero P, Smith M, Blumenthal M, Levinson R, Gevson L, Bernstein L, Ames BN. Chronological supplement to the carcinogenic potency database: Standardized results of annual bioassays published through December 1982. Environ Health Pers 1986; 67.

39. Gold LS, Slone TH, Backman GM, Magaw R, DaCosta M, Lopipero P, Blumenthal M, Ames BN. Second chronological supplement to the carcinogenic potency database: Standardized results of animal bioassays through December 1984 and by the national toxicity program through may 1986. Environ Health Pers 1987; 74.

40. Bernstein L, Gold LS, Ames BN, Pike MC, Hoel DG. Some tautologous aspects of the comparison of carcinogenic potency in rats and mice. Fundam Appl Toxicol, 1985;*5*:79–86.

41. Zeise L, Wilson R, Crouch E. Use of acute toxicity to estimate carcinogenic risk. Risk Analysis 1984; 4.

42. Dobson AJ, Gebski VJ. Sample sizes for comparing two independent proportions using the continuity corrected arc sine transformation. The Statistician, 1986;*35*:51–53.

Reviews

r1. Arnold DL, Grice HC, Krewski D. Handbook of in vivo toxicity testing. San Diego: Academic Press, 1990.

r2. Clayson DB, Krewski D, Munro I. Toxicological risk assessment. Volume I. Biological and statistical criteria Boca Raton, FL: CRC Press, 1985.

r3. Clayson DB, Krewski D, Munro I. Toxicological risk assessment. Volume II. General criteria and case studies Boca Raton, FL: CRC Press, 1985.

r4. Gart JJ, Krewski D, Lee PN, Tarone RE, Wahrendorf J. Statistical methods in cancer research, Volume III. The design and analysis of long term animal experiments. No 79. Lyon: IARC Scientific Publications. International Agency for Research on Cancer, 1986.

r5. International agency for research on cancer. Mechanisms of Carcinogenesis in Risk Identification. IARC Monographs on the Evaluation of Carcinogenic Risks to Humans. Publication Number 116. Lyon: International Agency for Research on Cancer, 1992.

r6. Johannsen FR. Risk assessment of carcinogenic and noncarcinogenic chemicals. Crit Rev Toxicol, 1990;*20*:341–367.

r7. National Research Council Risk assessment in the federal government: Managing the process. Washington: National Academy Press, 1983.

Appendix

To answer the question whether exposure to a chemical affects the function of liver enzymes, consider a simple experiment in which one group of animals is exposed to the test compound and another group is unexposed. When the data are normally distributed, the means and variances of the two groups summarize the experimental results. If there is no effect of the agent, then the mean enzyme function is expected to be the same in both groups. In practice, however, the averages will not be identical due to the intrinsic variation in response among the animals used in the experiment. The statistical question is then: How big does the difference in mean function have to be so that the existence of a toxic effect can be inferred?

This question can be answered using a statistical test of the null hypothesis of no effect using the alternative hypothesis of a toxic effect on enzyme function. Two types of incorrect inferences are possible. If there is, in truth, no toxic effect, one could erroneously conclude that an effect exists (a false-positive). If there truly is a toxic effect, one could erroneously fail to infer that the effect exists (a false-negative). A well-designed investigation involves careful consideration of: (a) the chance of falsely concluding that an effect exists when it really does not (called the "size" of the test and denoted by α); (b) the smallest difference, d, that has toxicologic importance and should result in the inference that an effect exists; and (c) the chance of correctly concluding that an effect exists given that the true difference is d (called the power of the test and denoted by $1 - \beta$, where β is the chance of falsely concluding that there is no effect when an effect really does exist.)

A simple formula exists to facilitate sample size calculation for normally distributed data. Given values for the size α and power $1 - \beta$ have been decided, normal critical values for z_α and $z_{1-\beta}$ are calculated or read from tables. (For example, if $\alpha = 0.05$ then $z_\alpha = 1.96$, and if $1 - \beta = 0.90$ then $z_{1-\beta} = -1.28$.) Letting n represent the number of animals in each group and σ^2 the variance of the individual observations (the same for each group), then n is calculated from:

$$n_a > 2\left\{\frac{(z_\alpha - z_{1-\beta})\sigma}{d}\right\}^2$$

Taking $d = 10$ and $\sigma^2 = 625$ yields $n_a > 131.3$. Thus, the use of 132 or more animals in each group will ensure detection of a difference of $d = 10$ with 90% certainty.

This is the simplest of all possible cases. Designs often use more than two experimental groups. Possible questions in these cases are: is there evidence of a toxic effect across all the groups? Is there a dose-response effect? Is there evidence of a threshold mechanism? Specialized experimental designs may be used which may reduce variability, or may be employed to meet special requirements.

Toxicologic data are not always normally distributed. The case of binary data indicating the presence or absence of a particular toxic response is of particular interest. To test for a difference between p_1, the proportion of animals affected in the control group, and p_2, the proportion affected in the exposed group, the sample size may be determined from.[42]

$$n_b > \frac{(Z + \sqrt{Z^2 + 2c\Delta})^2}{8\Delta^2}$$

Here, $p_2 > p_1$, reflecting our interest in an increased response rate in exposed animals, where

$$Z = z_\alpha - z_{1-\beta}$$

$$\Delta = \frac{1}{\sin^{-1}\sqrt{p_2}} - \frac{1}{\sin^{-1}\sqrt{p_1}}$$

and

$$c = \frac{1}{\sqrt{p_1(1-p_1)}} + \frac{1}{\sqrt{p_2(1-p_2)}}$$

For example, if $p_1 = 0.3$ and $p_2 = 0.6$ with α and β as above, we have $n_b > 63$. Further results on sample size determination are given by Gart.[12]

CHAPTER 112

Roger P. Smith

Systemic Antidotes

Introduction

Antidotes or antagonists reverse some or all of the signs or symptoms of poisoning by particular agents. Thus, they differ from elements of routine supportive care that apply generally to poison victims, but are certainly of no less importance in terms of outcome.[1,2] They may be classified as local or systemic. Dimercaprol (Table 112.1) was originally developed to prevent the blistering action on the skin of the vesicant, arsenical war gas, lewisite, hence its acronymn, BAL (British antilewisite). Later it was discovered to be effective in hastening the urinary excretion of absorbed arsenic as well, and it became widely used as a systemic antidote.

The concept of an antidote to every type of chemical poisoning might be desirable, but it is not realistic. The so-called "universal antidote" was designed to be effective against a wide variety of poisons. It often consisted of two parts activated charcoal to adsorb numerous chemicals, one part magnesium oxide to neutralize acids, and one part tannic acid to precipitate alkaloids. It has long since been recognized as an irrational mixture, since the base and acid cancel each other. As a GI adsorbent for ingested poisons, it was superior to burnt toast, but inferior to activated charcoal alone. Despite the many virtues of activated charcoal against a wide spectrum of xenobiotics, it is not a true systemic antidote, because it is not absorbed. Its effects are limited to the prevention of toxic signs and symptoms from ingested agents, but not their reversal. Syrup of ipecac is a valuable and widely used emetic agent in many kinds of chemical poisonings, but it should be avoided in cases of ingestion of corrosives (because of the danger of perforation of a damaged stomach or esophagus), aliphatic hydrocarbons (because of the danger of inducing aspiration into the tracheobronchial tree) and convulsants (because of the danger of ipecac further reducing the seizure threshold and thus inducing seizures). Like charcoal, however, it is not a systemic antidote, but an important example of the array of procedures that can limit the absorption of poisons or hasten their expulsion from the gut.[3]

A Classification Scheme for Systemic Antidotes

The number of true systemic antidotes is small relative to the thousands of chemicals potentially capable of eliciting toxic signs and symptoms in humans, but each example represents a milestone in medical science. There is reason to point with pride to their successful use in averting morbidity and mortality. A larger reward, however, lies in the advancement of knowledge about the sequence of events leading to the expression of toxicity by a given chemical or family of chemicals, and the recognition of those steps in the sequence that are susceptible to systemic intervention. In that sense the discovery of a useful antidote or antagonist constitutes scientific proof or confirmation of the previously developed hypotheses about the mechanism(s) for toxicity of the poison. In such a context, the establishment of a new antidote serves an important

Table 112.1 A Mechanistic Classification of Systemic Antidotes

Mechanism	Antidote	Poison
Receptor-blocking drugs	naloxone atropine	opiod analgesics cholinesterase inhibitors
Enzyme reactivators	pralidoxime	organophosphate cholinesterase inhibitors
Enzyme inhibitors	physostigmine edrophonium 4-methylpyrazole	atropine curare methanol,[1] ethylene glycol, allyl alcohol[1]
Reactive metabolite scavengers	N-acetylcysteine	acetaminophen
Enzyme substrates	thiosulfate ethanol methylene blue vitamin K_1 glyceryl monoacetate[1]	cyanide methanol, ethylene glycol, allyl alcohol[1] methemoglobin-forming agents, paraquat[1] warfarin fluroroacetate
Antibodies	Fab fragments	digoxin
Competitors for binding sites	oxygen	carbon monoxide
Physiologic antagonists or inverse agonists	Ro15-4513[1]	ethanol
Direct chemical inactivation without solubilization with solubilization	methemoglobin hydroxocobalamin chelating agents	cyanide, sulfide cyanide heavy metals

[1] Hypothetical or experimental stages only.

purpose even if it is never successfully employed therapeutically (rather than experimentally) in a single case of human or animal poisoning. The classification scheme of antidotes shown in Table 112.1 serves to illustrate this point; many of these are discussed in detail in other chapters. A somewhat similar schema has been proposed independently by others.[4]

Receptor Binding Antidotes

The knowledge that opioid analgesics act as agonists through a family of receptors resulted in the development of several competitive antagonists, such as naloxone and naltrexone (Table 112.1). Naloxone almost instantly reverses the respiratory depression and coma produced by heroin or morphine, and lacks the partial agonist activity of its earlier predecessors that made them dangerous if given mistakenly to patients poisoned by sedative/hypnotic drugs.

The realization that many of the signs of poisoning by acetylcholinesterase inhibitors result from intense stimulation of muscarinic receptors due to the accumulation of excess acetylcholine in their vicinity led to the use of a muscarinic receptor blocking drug (atropine) as an antidote. Its effective use requires large doses because of the competitive nature of the blockade, but the central respiratory depression, bronchoconstriction, and excessive tracheobronchial secretions that are contributing factors to death in respiratory failure are prevented. The neuromuscular blockade, however, which also contributes to the toxicity via muscle paralysis is not reversed.

Enzyme Reactivators

In order to correct the shortcomings of atropine, a unique, rationally designed antidote, pralidoxime (Table 112.1), was developed that is a useful adjunct in poisonings by the organophosphate-type cholinesterase inhibitors commonly used as insecticides (OPI). Some OPI are particularly dangerous because they irreversibly phosphorylate the esteratic site on the enzyme. Pralidoxime reacts with the phosphorylated enzyme to restore its original activity if given soon after exposure. After the alkyl groups have been cleaved from the bound phosphate residue, a process known as "aging," the enzyme becomes much more resistant to reactivation by pralidoxime.

Enzyme Inhibitors

In an almost direct role reversal to the above, both of the carbamate-type cholinesterase inhibitors, physostigmine and the highly charged edrophonium, can function as antidotes to neuromuscular receptor blockers such as d-tubocurarine (Table 112.1). Because it is not charged at physiologic pH, physostigmine crosses the blood-brain barrier. Inhibition of cholinesterase activity in the CNS results in a competitive reversal of central atropine blockade of muscarinic receptors, and consequently the anticholinergic effects of delirium as well as the peripheral actions. Edrophonium, a true competitive and reversible cholinesterase inhibitor with a short duration of action, does not gain access to the brain. It can, however, reverse the nondepolarizing paralytic effects of curare and other competitive blocking agents on the nicotinic receptors of the neuromuscular junction and, most importantly, at those muscles associated with respiration.

Reactive Metabolite Scavengers

The development of some antidotes required prior elucidation of the biotransformation pathways of the poison instead of the mechanism of action. The unexpected hepatic necrosis caused by massive overdoses of acetaminophen eventually was traced to a minor, but highly reactive metabolite that forms covalent bonds with essential cell macromolecules. It was further learned that the damage did not occur until after hepatocytes had been depleted of glutathione, suggesting both that the latter played an important protective role and that exogenous administration of a sulfhydryl-containing small molecule might serve as an antidote. Because it was already a drug approved for other uses and because it penetrated cell membranes, N-acetylcysteine became the antidote of choice, although other chemicals also were shown to be capable of serving the same scavenging function.

Enzyme Substrates

No poison is more firmly entrenched in the public mind than cyanide. In recent years it was the instrument involved in tampering episodes of foods and pharmaceuticals; it was used in the mass human destruction of the religous cult in Jonestown; and, it was formerly used in the execution of condemned criminals. Cyanide is an extremely toxic and very rapidly acting inhibitor of cytochrome oxidase (aa_3). Iatrogenic poisoning is also seen in patients receiving sodium nitroprusside, a potent vasodilator. As this compound decomposes in the body free CN is released, producing profound acidosis equal to that of cyanide poisoning (see Chapter 24). Its reversible combination with the enzyme prevents the cellular utilization of molecular oxygen, which virtually halts the electron transport chain, oxidative phosphorylation, and aerobic respiration. Death results from fulminating central respiratory arrest, but cyanide is likely associated with multiple actions. It can alter cellular ionic hemostasis, resulting in the accumulation of intracellular calcium to activate several cellular processes that account for its cardiovascular and CNS effects.[5] Cyanide can initiate a calcium-dependent release of catecholamines from the adrenal glands and sympathetic nerve endings to stimulate the heart and increase the blood pressure.[6] In the brain, cyanide stimulates the release of excitatory neurotransmitters that contribute to the convulsions and excitotoxic brain damage.[7,8] Cyanide also inhibits antioxidant defense enzymes, such as catalase, superoxide dismutase, and glutathione peroxidase, which predisposes the brain to oxidative injury.[9] In severe poisonings, the acute phase may be followed by progressive CNS damage, resulting in a Parkinsonian-like condition associated with lesions in the basal ganglia and altered dopaminergic function.

Cyanide is almost exclusively inactivated by biotransformation to the considerably less toxic thiocyanate via sulfur transferase activity, perhaps of several enzymes; but the ubiquitously distributed mitochondrial enzyme rhodanese, is widely thought to be the most important.[10] The liver contains the highest levels of rhodanese activity. A rate-limiting factor in this detoxification pathway is the supply of sulfur donor for rhodanese in the form of sulfane-sulfur, a sulfur atom bound only to another sulfur. The sulfane-sulfur is transferred to the enzyme and then to cyanide in a double displacement reaction. Several molecules have been shown to be effective in this role, but sodium thiosulfate, which can be given safely IV in very large doses, remains the sulfur donor of choice (Table 112.1). The system functions very efficiently, but thiosulfate is often used in combination with other chemicals (below) in an even more effective regimen for the management of cyanide poisoning.

The metabolism of ethanol is mediated initially by a cytosolic enzyme also found in high concentrations in the liver. Alcohol dehydrogenase utilizes NADH as a cofactor, and the products are acetaldehyde and NAD^+. Acetaldehyde in turn is acted on by a mitochondrial enzyme, aldehyde dehydrogenase, that also utilizes NADH. The resulting acetate is activated by CoA to enter the tricarboxylic acid cycle, where it is converted to carbon dioxide and water. Many simple aliphatic alcohols undergo biotransformation by the same pathway, notably methanol, ethylene glycol, allyl alcohol, and isopropanol. Isopropanol is acted on only by alcohol dehydrogenase, and the end-product, acetone, is no more toxic acutely than the parent alcohol. The combination of CNS depression and an acetone odor to the breath, however, presents a problem in differential diagnosis with diabetic ketoacidosis. The problem is perhaps most quickly resolved by testing for the presence of glucose in the urine.

In contrast to ethanol and isopropanol, methanol, ethylene glycol, and allyl alcohol undergo biotransformation to more toxic products. Methanol is presumably metabolized through formaldehyde to formic acid. Formaldehyde is so highly reactive that it has not been identified conclusively in blood or tissues after methanol ingestion, but formate has been found in high concentrations. It is responsible both for the overwhelming metabolic acidosis, which requires vigorous treatment with bicarbonate, and the uniquely toxic effect of retinal damage in humans and some subhuman primates. Survivors may have total and permanent blindness. Ethylene glycol is converted through its aldehyde, dialdehyde, and mixed aldehyde-acid forms to oxalic acid. Poisoned patients also have a profound metabolic acidosis, and may go into acute renal failure secondary to direct nephrotoxicity of one or more of the metabolic products. The metabolism of allyl alcohol leads to the generation of acrolein, which is believed to be responsible for the periportal necrosis observed in poisoned laboratory animals.[11] This common biotransformation pathway suggested that ethanol in appropriate doses might serve as a competitive substrate to prevent the bioactivation of methanol, ethylene glycol, and allyl alcohol. Its utility for that purpose is now widely accepted, at least for methanol and ethylene glycol. Since then, a high affinity inhibitor of alcohol dehydrogenase, 4-methylpyrazole, has been discovered that can serve the same purpose and offers some advantages in terms of convenience, efficiency, and safety.[12]

The vital redox dye, methylene blue, was originally suggested as an antidote for cyanide, but it was far less efficient than the standard regimen used today. It was discovered by accident to accelerate greatly the rate of methemoglobin reduction in humans and animals that had been exposed to such methemoglobin-generating chemicals as nitrite salts, aliphatic nitrates, and nitrites, and aromatic amino- or nitro-compounds such as aniline or nitrobenzene.[13] Ordinarily an acquired methemoglobinemia is slowly reversed by a spontaneously active erythrocytic enzyme, known variously as diaphorase, methemoglobin reductase, or cytochrome b_5, that utilizes NADH as a cofactor. Substantial species differences are recognized in methemoglobin reductase activity with small mammals that have high activity and larger mammals and humans where it is more sluggish.[14]

Methylene blue accumulates in mammalian red cells and is acted on by a reductase system (with no known physiologic function) that utilizes NADPH as a cofactor. The reduced, colorless dye, leuco-methylene blue, functions as an electron carrier to reduce nonenzymatically the ferric heme groups of methemoglobin and the coexisting partially oxidized forms, $(\alpha^{2+}\beta^{3+})_2$ and $(\alpha^{3+}\beta^{2+})_2$, to restore a normally functional blood pigment.[15] In a life-threatening acquired methemoglobinemia in human patients, methylene blue by IV injection may accelerate rates of reduction by as much as tenfold through activation of this completely separate system. Since the system requires NADPH, which is generated in red cells by the hexose monophosphate shunt, methylene blue is not only ineffective in patients deficient in glucose-6-phosphate dehydrogenase activity, but contraindicated, since it may induce a hemolytic anemia secondary to severe NADPH depletion and cell membrane disruption.

Paraquat is a highly efficient, broad spectrum, bipyridilium herbicide that is highly toxic to humans when accidentally or intentionally ingested. Its human toxicity and its herbicidal activity are believed to involve the same or very similar biochemical mechanisms. Various plant and mammalian liver and lung enzymes can catalyze the reduction of paraquat to a cationic radical that can react with molecular oxygen. The products of that reaction are probably oxidized paraquat and superoxide or hydroxide radicals and hydrogen peroxide. This cyclic production of reactive and toxic oxygen radical species is believed to be responsible for tissue damage in both plants and animals. Many organs are damaged in human paraquat poisoning, but the critical lesion involves the lungs. Paraquat is slowly concentrated in lung tissue against concentration gradients, and it results in an initial destructive phase that is followed by a relentless proliferative fibrotic reaction that almost always terminates fatally.[4] Death in hypoxia, however, is often delayed for several weeks. Ironically, one's first instinct would be to administer oxygen to such patients, which actually intensifies and accelerates the process, whereas hypoxia protects against the pulmonary injury. Recently, it has been discovered that methylene blue can compete successfully with paraquat for several flavoenzymes, including xanthine oxidase and NADH and NADPH cytochrome c reductases to reduce sharply both superoxide and hydroxyl radical production. The NADPH reductase is believed to be primarily responsible for paraquat reduction in animal tissue. This promising antidotal approach is certain to be tested further in animals and humans.[16]

Warfarin is a coumarin-type anticoagulant drug used prophylactically in surgical patients at risk from venous thromboemboli and their complications. It is also the most widely used rodenticide in the US. Its use as a drug in the US is regulated by the FDA, whereas its use as a pesticide is regulated by the EPA. As a drug, it is used in moderate doses, whereas as a rodenticide it is hoped that the target species will consume toxic overdoses and incur fatal hemorrhages. In either case warfarin competitively inhibits the reduction of an epoxide form of vitamin K to vitamin KH_2 which is needed to activate prothrombin and the clotting factors, II, VII, IX, and X, in the liver. This effect can be reversed immediately by transfusions of fresh whole blood or fresh frozen plasma containing preformed clotting factors or more slowly by the administration of appropriate forms of vitamin K to bypass the warfarin block and initiate the synthesis of new critical clotting factors.

Sodium fluoroacetate is a chemical of considerable historical interest in toxicology; it was once a widely used rodenticide, but it was highly toxic and dangerous because it lacked species selectivity. The explanation for its toxic mechanism of action was regarded as a scientific triumph for the field of toxicology. It is not itself toxic but it undergoes biotransformation to fluorocitric acid, which is an inhibitor of aconitase, one of the enzymes of the tricarboxylic acid cycle. Time is required for this "lethal synthesis" to manifest itself in the form of convulsions or ventricular fibrillation. In monkeys glyceryl monoacetate is an effective antidote. Its acetate moiety competes with fluroroacetate to prevent its conversion to fluorocitrate. This keeps the Krebs cycle, which is essential for aerobic respiration, functional until the fluroroacetate can be excreted or detoxified by other pathways.

Antidotal Antibodies

Digoxin overdose is a common iatrogenic misadventure, and one that is both dangerous and refractory to many modalities of intervention. A modern and very promising approach to the management of overdosage depends on the production of antibodies of high specificity and affinity produced by immunizing sheep with digoxin covalently linked to serum albumin (Table 112.1). Since the intact antibodies carry a risk of anaphylactic reaction, a papain digestion followed by purification of the antigen combining Fab fragment has been successfully used in human cases. The Fab fragment with the bound digoxin can then be filtered by the glomerulus and excreted in the urine.

Competitors for Binding Sites

Carbon monoxide competes reversibly and successfully with molecular oxygen for the ferrous heme binding sites on hemoglobin because its affinity for those sites is almost 250 times greater than that of oxygen (Table 112.1). Therefore, it is dangerous at low concentrations, and its lack of odor, color, or irritant effect gives no warning of exposure. A hemoglobin tetramer that has two sites occupied by carbon monoxide instead of oxygen has only half its normal oxygen capacity. Moreover, delivery of the half-load of oxygen to peripheral tissues requires a larger gradient in oxygen tension than a simple 50 percent decrement in total hemoglobin in which the residual pigment carries its full complement of oxygen. The hypoxic compromise of 50 percent saturation with carbon monoxide is, therefore, significantly greater than that of a simple 50 percent anemia. Although carboxyhemoglobin is a relatively stable complex, advantage can be taken of the competitive nature of the binding and the mass law to reverse the course of the poisoning by administering pure oxygen at normobaric or hyperbaric pressures instead of air. In this special case oxygen could be regarded both as a true systemic antidote and an essential element for sustaining life that is being replaced because it has reached critically low levels. The toxicity of carbon monoxide has been recognized since the mid-1800s, when Claude Bernard began his pioneering work on the elucidation of its mechanism of action. Today some evidence suggests that carbon monoxide, like nitric oxide, may be an endogenous neurotransmitter.[17]

Physiologic Antagonists/Inverse Agonists

Some drugs are almost perfectly suited to antagonize the effects of others by acting through separate groups of receptors or through a physiologic mechanism that produces an opposing set of effects. The best example of physiologic antagonism is the effect of epinephrine acting through adrenergic receptors to antagonize the acute effects of histamine on histaminergic receptors. In anaphylactic shock, epinephrine reverses the bronchoconstriction and the hypotension and also decreases the release of histamine from mast cells.

Far less successful was the trial of analeptic/convulsant drugs against the respiratory depressant activity of sedative/hypnotic drugs. Among the sedative/hypnotic drugs, the barbiturates were dominant during the first half of the 20th century, before the introduction of the benzodiazepines (Table 112.1). Because they were capable of producing the full spectrum of CNS depression through general anesthesia and central respiratory arrest, they were responsible for many deaths after accidental or deliberate overdosage. Major research efforts were expended in two directions in attempts to reduce their hazards or to find more effective ways of managing poisoned patients. A number of new, nonbarbiturate sedative/hypnotics were introduced in attempts to find safer drugs. This approach ultimately was successful in the discovery of the benzodiazepines, but not before a dozen or more new drugs found their way onto the market that either offered no advantages over the barbiturates, or were, in fact, even more dangerous.

The second approach to dealing with the problem of the dangerous sedative/hypnotics concentrated on the development of antagonists to their central depressant effects. Since almost no information was in hand at that time about the mechanism of their depressant activity, interest centered on attempts to antagonize their actions by using so-called analeptics or CNS stimulant drugs. It quickly became apparent that drugs that had powerful stimulant activity were dangerous because even in modest overdose they had a potential to produce convulsions. On the other hand, the drugs that were safer because they lacked prominent stimulant activity were not effective in reducing the deep coma associated with central respiratory depression. Many new analeptics were introduced with claims that they selectively stimulated the respiratory center over other parts of the CNS, but none has stood the test of time. After the introduction of the benzodiazepines, the search became much less urgent, since these drugs are very much safer in terms of the depth of coma they produce even in massive overdose. The most important and perhaps the most dangerous sedative/hypnotic of all time, however, is still very much with us—namely, ethanol.

Our state of knowledge about sedative/hypnotic drugs has become considerably more sophisticated since the days of interest in analeptics. Studies on the pharmacodynamic activity of the benzodiazepines led slowly to the emergence of a unified hypothesis that loosely links not only the sedative/hypnotics, but analeptics, anticonvulsants, and alcohol as well. Electrophysiologic studies have shown that the benzodiazepines enhance or potentiate inhibitory neurotransmission by gamma-aminobutyric acid (GABA) secreting neurons in many parts of the CNS. The GABA-ergic receptor either incorporates or controls chloride ion channels. The current hypothesis is that benzodiazepines, barbiturates, and GABA all bind to separate sites on the receptor to facilitate chloride ion conductance. Although ethanol does not bind directly to the receptor, it may modify membrane fluidity in the vicinity of the receptor to produce GABA-ergic effects. The CNS excitatory drugs are either GABA antagonists in the conventional sense or they are so-called inverse agonists which bind to the receptor, but produce an almost opposite constellation of excitatory effects. One such inverse agonist, Ro15-4513, has been found to antagonize some of the behavioral effects of ethanol so that the old dream of a safe "analeptic" drug may be within reach.[18]

Direct Chemical Inactivation (without Solubilization)

The mechanistic example of direct chemical inactivation has been employed against poisons of high water solubility that exist in free solution in vivo and against substances of low solubility that are tenaciously stored in various body compartments, e.g., heavy metals (Table 112.1). Again, in a direct role reversal, sodium nitrite, which in large doses is capable of inducing a dangerous methemoglobinemia, can be given in carefully controlled doses to generate nonthreatening concentrations of methemoglobin that avidly trap either cyanide (CN^-) or sulfide (HS^-) anions. These ionic complexes (cyanmethemoglobin and sulfmethemoglobin) form almost instantaneously in the presence of ferric heme groups, and they have a high degree of stability. The toxic anions are at least temporarily held in red blood cells in a biologically inactive form and cannot gain entrance to the mitochondrial cytochromes. Thus, the full regimen for cyanide poisoning consists of three chemicals in sequence: inhalation of amyl nitrite vapors (a weak methemoglobin-former, but one that can be given quickly when available); the IV injection of a controlled dose of sodium nitrite, followed by an injection of sodium thiosulfate (above). Hydrogen sulfide poisoning also can involve the inhibition of cytochrome oxidase, and the induction of methemoglobinemia has been shown to be antidotal in laboratory animals. It has been used in humans with some success. The injection of sodium thiosufate, however, serves no useful purpose in the case of sulfide.

Azide (N^-_3) has many biologic effects in common with cyanide and sulfide, including the ability to complex with methemoglobin and to inhibit cytochrome oxidase. Indeed, methemoglobinemia offers a slight degree of protection against azide poisoning. Unlike cyanide and sulfide, however, azide is a potent vasodilator—probably by virtue of its conversion to nitric oxide, which many believe is identical with the so-called endothelium-derived relaxing factor. The discovery that phenobarbital protects against azide, but not cyanide, proves that azide is a neurotoxin and not a metabolic poison. As noted above, cyanide also has a neuroexcitatory component to its toxicity. The neurotoxicity of azide, however, may be secondary to its conversion to nitric oxide.[19] Thus, antidotes are powerful tools for elucidating critical mechanisms of action in intact animals.

The concurrent administration of methylene blue with nitrite in cyanide or sulfide poisoning would be counterproductive since it would tend to reverse the therapeutically induced methemoglobinemia. Thus, the weak anticyanide effects of methylene blue when given alone (above) seem paradoxical. For reasons that are not entirely clear, hemolysis of red cells totally abolishes methemoglobin reductase activity. When methylene blue is added to lysates, it actively generates substantial levels of methemoglobin, but in the intact cell only low levels of methemoglobin accumulate because of the opposing reductase activity. It is, therefore, inferred that methylene blue accelerates the rate of hemoglobin-methemoglobin turnover to arrive eventually at an equilibrium position in intact cells that would be the same if one started with only hemoglobin, only methemoglobin, or a mixture. Since that equilibrium is at a somewhat higher concentration of methemoglobin than that in normal cells, it presumably accounts for the modest anticyanide effect.[20] Direct chemical inactivation with solubilization is discussed below.

Direct Chemical Inactivation (with Solubilization)

Chelating agents (from the Greek "chela" or claw; see Fig. 112.1) are used in poisonings by toxic heavy metals. They react directly with ionic forms of the metal or compete with natural tissue ligands for metal already bound in, or on, cells to produce a water-soluble chelate that can be excreted in the urine. The scientific principle was borrowed from chemistry where chelating agents were used to separate certain metals from mixtures for improved analytical sensitivity. Only a few of the many known chelating agents have actually been approved in the US by the FDA. They are largely orphan drugs because of their very low sales volumes, but fortunately they continue to excite scientific interest. Although they represent a wide variety of chemical structures, the actual chelating moieties are often sulfhydryl, carboxyl, or hydroxamic acid groups that hold the metal with multiple bonds (polydentate), often to form heterocyclic ring structures. Such chelates are much more stable than those in which only a single bond holds the metal (Fig. 112.1).

Heavy metals are defined as electropositive elements having a density greater than five; this definition includes about 40 elements of widely differing chemical properties and toxicity. For example, titanium and molybdenum have very little biologic activity. Zinc, iron, and copper are essential trace metals, but the latter two are much more commonly involved in human poisonings. Lead, cadmium, and mercury[21] are invariably toxic and a source of concern in the environment. Zinc, cadmium, and mercury are in the same group in the periodic table, yet their toxicities and distributions in vivo are not at all similar.[22] Many metals are of concern in both acute overdose situations and in chronic poisonings where the same metal may produce two distinctly different syndromes. Other metals are associated only with long-term, low-level toxic syndromes. Acute poisonings by lead or gold are almost unheard of, yet single exposures to either, if sufficiently intense, will produce, after a latent period, a syndrome that is indistinguishable from that resulting from multiple small exposures. Thus, there are far more differences among heavy metals than there are similarities, and a case could be made that each metal is a unique entity.[22]

Organometallic compounds, e.g., methyl mercury and tetraethyl lead, often produce toxic syndromes that are qualitatively different from their inorganic salts, perhaps because they more readily penetrate the blood-brain barrier. The difference between the per cent of the dose/100 g body weight found in the brain of chickens was 15 times greater with methyl mercury than with an inorganic salt of mercury. The toxicity of such organometallic compounds is dominated by CNS signs and symptoms (encephalopathy). The chelating agents do not bind organometallic compounds so, in general, chelation therapy does not benefit the patient poisoned by such agents. Arsenic is an exception, because all toxic forms of arsenic, whether organic or inorganic (except the hydride, arsine), undergo biotransformation in vivo to arsenious acid (arsenite). Arsine produces a unique toxic syndrome characterized by massive intravascular hemolysis.

Metals of toxicologic interest tend to form tenacious complexes, sometimes covalently binding, with a variety of natural functional groups in biologic materials such as -Cl, -OH, -COOH, $-PO_3H_2$, -SH, $-NH_2$, imidazole, etc.[22] This binding to functional groups on structural elements in or on cells in vivo accounts for the fact that many metals are very slowly excreted and tend to accumulate in the body with repeated exposures to result in cumulative toxic effects (chronic poisoning). Very large differences exist in the binding constants of different metals for the above functional groups so that, in a sense, the different endogenous functional groups are competing among themselves for the metal. For example, the dissociation constants (expressed as negative logarithms) for Hg-Cl is 6.7, whereas the value for Hg-SH is 14.[23] The binding con-

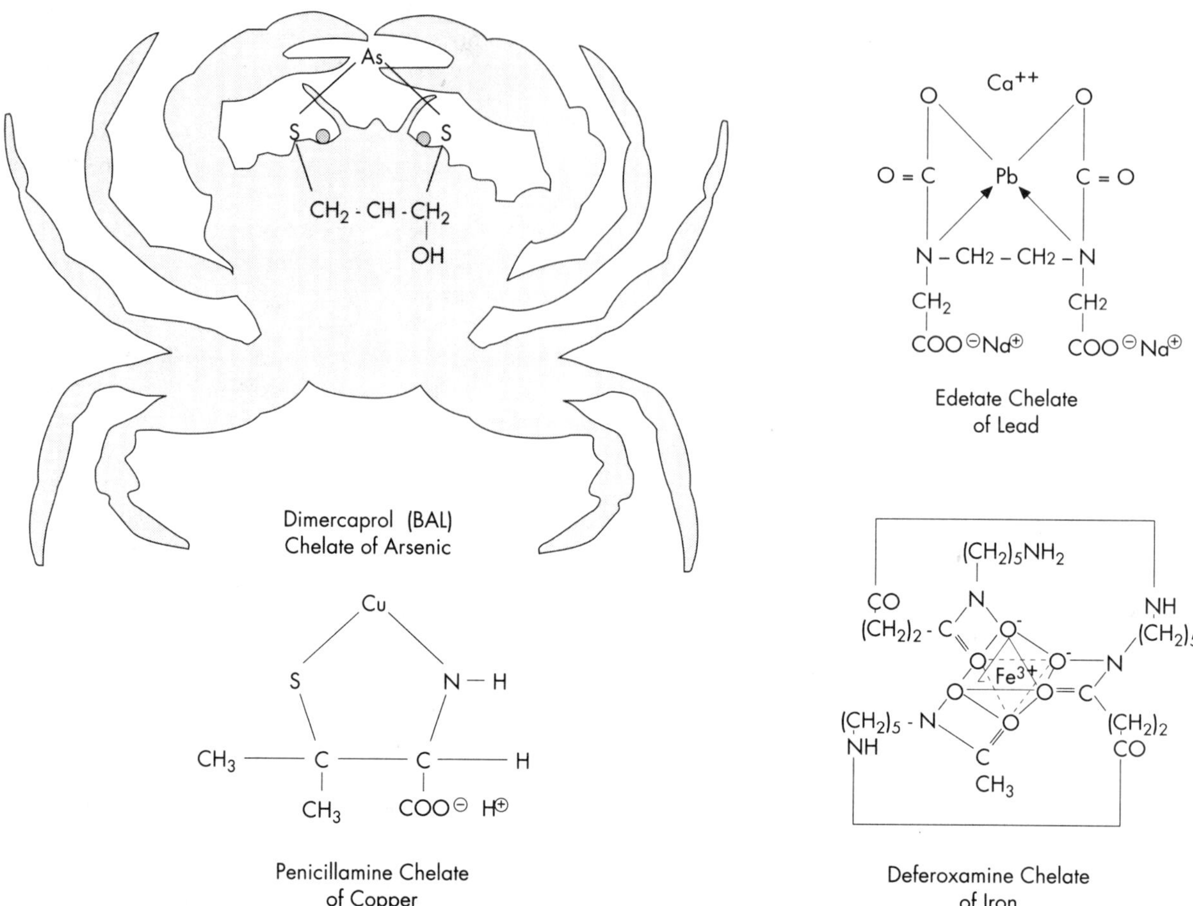

Figure 112.1 Some examples of metal chelates. Edetate is actually given as the calcium disodium salt instead of the free acid (ethylenediaminetetraacetic acid, EDTA). EDTA can chelate serum ionized calcium, and there is a certain risk of inducing hypocalcemic tetany. When given as the salt, plasma lead exchanges for the chelated calcium. Dimercaprol and penicillamine are each capable of forming dimolar chelates (2 moles of chelator to 1 mole of metal), but only the heterocyclic forms are shown here because they are more stable.

stant, however, is not the only determinant of metal distribution in a biologic system. The rate of formation of complexes also plays a role. A given complex may have a very high binding constant, but the complex is formed so slowly that it has little biologic significance. Over time the metal will tend to be released from those groups with lower affinities in favor of groups with higher affinities if the rates of complex formation permit such a redistribution. Thus, the longer the metal remains in the body, the more tenaciously it is retained, and the later therapy with a chelating agent is begun, the less likely it is to hasten excretion of the metal. As a general rule chelation therapy is more successful in hastening excretion in acute poisonings than in chronic poisonings.

This process of redistribution will lead to increased body burdens of metal with continued exposure, but it does not necessarily mean that there will be an intensification of toxicity. Large amounts of metal may be stored very tenaciously in biologically inactive forms or in sites that do not permit the expression of toxicity. Lead is intensively stored in bone, where it is essentially nontoxic. Toxicity is expressed only when there is a sudden mobilization or release of toxic amounts of the stored material or when the intensity of the exposure exceeds the rate at which it can be stored in inert depots. Sulfhydryl groups are an example of a functional group with a very high affinity for such metals as mercury, copper, lead, and silver. Yet, these metals often behave very differently in biologic systems.[22] Systemic silver poisoning can be produced in animals only by parenteral administration,[24] but the others are toxic by mouth. At the same time a given atom of metal may bind to a sulfhydryl group that has no important physiologic function (autoprotective binding) or it may bind to a sulfhydryl group that serves a critical function (toxic binding).

A special group of low molecular weight proteins, called thioneins because of their high content of sulfhydryl groups, avidly bind certain heavy metals. The metal-bound forms are called metallothioneins, and a separate protein appears to bind different metallic elements such as cadmium, mercury, zinc, silver, and copper. The proteins are found in trace amounts in the cytoplasm of many tissues, but particularly the liver, and in a number of species, including humans. They are unique in that their synthesis can be induced by metal exposure. For example, a sublethal exposure of rats to cadmium will induce metallothionein synthesis, which can protect against the subsequent administration of an otherwise lethal dose of cadmium.[25] Since the tolerance was associated with an increased metallothionein content of the hepatocyte, it was assumed that metallothionein was responsible for the tolerance. Lethal doses of cadmium in rats result in a massive hepatic necrosis, and tolerance develops also to this severe liver injury. Although cadmium does, indeed, bind to cytosolic metallothionein, the protection against lethal liver injury relates to the resultant subcellular redistribution of cadmium away from critical organelles such as nuclei, mitochondria, and endoplasmic reticulum and toward the cytosol, where it binds largely to metallothionein already present before the challenge dose.[26] Chronic cadmium also produces nephrotoxicity in rats, which may result from cadmium-metallothionein complexes released from the liver and redistributed to the kidney.[27] These proteins undoubtedly play important roles in the distribution and excretion of some metals, but a clear picture of their function has not yet emerged.[25]

Because of the complexity of their toxic effects, very few productive studies of mechanisms of metal toxicity have been made in intact animals.[23] Serious attempts to understand mechanisms of metal toxicity began during the great age of enzymes that revolutionized biochemistry, but attempts to link metal toxicity with specific enzymes were not very successful. For example, one might formulate a hypothesis that the toxicity of a given metal results from an inhibition of a certain enzyme because the metal binds to a critical sulfhydryl group on its active site. Most, if not all enzymes, possess sulfhydryl groups that can bind metals. Even if some of the sulfhydryl groups are not essential for enzymatic activity, there is probably some degree of metal binding that will result eventually in a nonspecific decrease in enzymatic activity. Thus, it becomes very difficult to say with any certainty that the critical lesion in, for example, mercury poisoning, is due to the inhibition of any one specific enzyme. Since mercury is a potent, nonspecific enzyme inhibitor, it is apt to produce cellular damage wherever it accumulates in sufficient concentration.

Studies of the effects of metals on certain cell functions were rather more successful. Red blood cell and yeast cells are common model systems.[29,30] Glucose moves into red cells by facilitated diffusion, a process that must take place at the cell membrane. That process can be inhibited by various chemical forms of mercury. The total number of binding sites, both internally and externally, for various compounds can be determined in lysates of red cells. Inorganic mercury binds to more sites than any of the organic forms tested. Probably because of its smaller size it has greater access to functional groups and less steric hindrance than the organic forms. The membrane fraction can be obtained simply by centrifugation, and the total number of membrane binding sites for the same compound can be measured. The membrane binding sites may be only 1 to 4 percent of the total number of sites. Then by a slow and careful titration of intact, functional cells, one can determine the amount of bound mercury that is just sufficient to inhibit glucose transfer, which may be only 5 percent of the membrane sites and only 0.1 percent of the total sites. Such experiments point out the enormous amount of nonspecific binding that can occur in biologic systems, but the membrane, which controls critical functions, has fewer nonspecific binding sites than the cell interior.[31] Under certain conditions glucose moves into yeast cells by both facilitated diffusion and active transport. The binding of uranyl ions to carboxyl groups inhibits the former, whereas the binding of nickel or uranyl ions to phosphoryl sites inhibit the latter.[32] Thus, metals may be used as tools to study vital membrane functions.

Functions controlled by cell membranes are particularly susceptible to inhibition by heavy metals since in the natural course of events the metal must penetrate the membrane before it can influence intracellular functions. If one measures glucose uptake and oxygen consumption in skeletal muscle cells after the addition of mercury, it is clear that membrane-regulated glucose uptake is inhibited long before there are effects on the intracellular processes that utilize oxygen. Indeed, membrane function may be recovering at a time when oxygen consumption is continuing to fall. It is probable that metals disrupt numerous cellular functions and inhibit numerous enzymes. Conversely, increased cation permeability in red cells exposed to an organomercurial shows a slow spontaneous recovery due to the release of soluble thiol compounds from the interior of the cell into the medium to force dissociation of the metal from its membrane binding sites.[33]

Arsenic, Mercury, and Gold

Acute arsenic poisoning is a rare medical emergency today, but the element is found in a number of pesticides. The massive ingestion of inorganic salts of arsenic or mercury is followed by a fulminating, violent gastroenteritis that may result in rapid demise in shock secondary to fluid and electrolyte loss. Dimercaprol is the drug of choice for the management of such patients, even though it necessarily involves multiple, painful injections and unpleasant, though not particularly dangerous, side-effects. Because of these problems with dimercaprol interest continues in finding better derivatives, two of which are listed in Table 112.2.[34] Chronic arsenic poisoning involves protean manifestations that mimic numerous other diseases. Infectious coryza, skin rashes, signs of renal damage, CNS involvement, and hepatomegaly are among the more common complications. Again, dimercaprol is probably the chelating agent of choice, but treatment may have to be pro-

Table 112.2 Chelating Agents Effective in Acute and/or Chronic Poisonings

Name of Agent	Acute	Chronic	Metal Form Which It Chelates
Dimercaprol (BAL)	X	X	Arsenic, all forms except arsine
Related compounds:		X	Gold, inorganic and ionic
2,3-dimercaptosuccinic acid[1]		X	Mercury, inorganic and ionic
2,3-dimercapto-1-propanesulfonate[1]		X	Lead, inorganic and ionic[2]
	X	X	Copper, inorganic and ionic[1]
Edetate calcium disodium		X	Lead, inorganic and ionic
Related compounds:	X	X	Cadmium, inorganic and ionic[1]
Cyclohexanediamine tetraacetic acid[1]			
Diethylene triamine pentaacetic acid[1]			
Hydroxyethylenediamine triacetic acid[1]			
Deferoxamine mesylate	X	X	Iron, inorganic and ionic
		X	Aluminum, inorganic and ionic[1]
D-Penicillamine or N-acetyl-D-penicillamine	X	X	Copper, inorganic and ionic
		X	Lead, inorganic and ionic
	X	X	Mercury, inorganic and ionic
	X	X	Arsenic, all forms except arsine
		X	Silver inorganic and ionic[1]
Malic, succinic and citric acids		X	Aluminum, inorganic and ionic[1]
1,4,8,11-Tetraazacyclotetradecane (cyclam)[1]		X	Nickel, inorganic and ionic[1]
Trientine (triethylenetetramine dihydrochloride, TETA, triene)	X	X	Copper, inorganic and ionic
		X	Nickel, inorganic and ionic[1]

[1]Hypothetical or experimental stages only.
[2]Only in combination with edetate calcium disodium.

longed. The most common late manifestation of acute poisoning by inorganic mercury salts is renal failure, at which point one must proceed cautiously with dimercaprol therapy since the chelated metal cannot be excreted in the urine. For most metals, however, there is a component of biliary excretion that may justify continued chelation therapy. Chronic mercury poisoning prominently involves the CNS, and the value of dimercaprol in its management is contested. Gold poisoning is invariably iatrogenic secondary to its use in rheumatoid arthritis. Both single and multiple injections result in the same toxic syndrome, which may have an allergic basis. Blood dyscrasias, nephritis, hepatitis, and both peripheral and CNS involvement may occur. Dimercaprol is said to be quite effective in severe reactions.

Lead

Unfortunately, the incidence of lead poisoning in metropolitan slums remains high as a result of the once widespread use of lead based paints and lead water pipes. Many other sources also contribute to a dangerously high level of lead in the environment. As in the case of gold, massive single or multiple small exposures, both culminate in similar toxic syndromes. The clinical picture in young children is an encephalopathy that is both malignant and difficult to treat. It is common to give such children both dimercaprol and edetate calcium disodium, since the former but not the latter penetrates the blood-brain barrier. Dimercaprol alone, however, would be a poor choice for treating any manifestation of lead poisoning. The use of combinations of chelating agents may offer advantages in terms of synergistic effects and lowered doses for the individual agents.[35] In adults, lead poisoning more often takes the form of a peripheral neuritis, with colic due to spasmogenic effects on smooth muscle and pallor due to anemia secondary to inhibition of heme synthesis.

Iron

Iron poisoning in toddlers may occur accidentally because ferrous sulfate or other similar preparations are found in the home in multivitamin/mineral preparations or as part of a neonatal regimen. The acute syndrome resembles that for arsenic or mercury poisonings above. Deferoxamine forms an extremely stable chelate with iron, and it is recommended for acutely poisoned patients. The disease, hemochromatosis, is associated with the chronic accumulation of excess iron stores, but it is more commonly treated by periodic phlebotomy. Hepatolenticular degeneration (Wilson's disease) involves an excessive accumulation of copper in the body, and it can be managed by periodic administration of D-penicillamine or trientine.[36] D-Penicillamine also has been recommended for nickel poisoning, but some unique chelating agents appear superior in experimental animals.[36] Most of the other suggestions in Table 118.2 are born of desperation for want of more effective agents.

Aluminum

Aluminum poisoning may well be a "disease of medical progress," but humans are exposed to many more sources of aluminum in the environment than can be justified for a nonessential metal.[37] The most dramatic form of the disease occurs in patients who are undergoing chronic peritoneal or extracorporeal hemodialysis. According to one hypothesis, phosphate, because it does not dialyze well, tends to accumulate in such patients and then to complex with ionized calcium. Formation of this insoluble salt may result in microemboli, and the decrease in serum calcium will result in hyperparathyroidism. One approach to this problem is to manage dialysis patients by chronic administration of aluminum antacids to decrease the dietary absorption of phosphate. Inevitably, however, there is a rise in serum aluminum that cannot be excreted because of the renal failure. This accumulation of aluminum is now held to be responsible for a progressive dementia that may incapacitate a patient within six months. The brain concentration of aluminum in such patients may be increased 10 to 20 times over that in normal patients. The chelation approach is not likely to be of benefit in such patients because of the compromised renal function, but considerable research has been devoted toward finding an effective chelator.[38]

Summary

Improvements in symptomatic and supportive care have probably had a larger impact on morbidity and mortality due to acute poisonings than the development of new systemic antidotes. Antidotes, however, continue to excite the imagination of pharmacologists and toxicologists as a possible final link in a scientific chain of evidence about the mechanism of toxicity or the pathways of biotransformation of xenobiotics. Poisonings by heavy metals continue to be important both in terms of incidence and in the difficulty of their management. Heavy metals in the environment are of concern because of their persistence and because they can bioaccumulate in natural food webs. New chelating agents are being synthesized and tested primarily due to the efforts of academic scientists in the hope of discovering safer and more effective ones. Because of low sales volume, they are of little interest to industry, and academicians lack the financial resources to test such agents in accord with FDA protocols for approval as new drugs. Particularly distressing problems are those in which the metal exhibits prominent toxicity in the CNS, as in the case of organometallics that do not bind well, if at all, to chelating agents. Metals that produce acute renal failure as part of their toxic syndrome also present special problems, since the chelates are primarily excreted in the urine.

References

1. Ellenhorn MJ, Barceloux DG. Medical Toxicology, diagnosis and treatment of human poisoning, New York: Elsevier, 1988.
2. Gosselin RE, Smith RP, Hodge HC. Clinical toxicology of commercial products, 5th ed., Baltimore: Williams & Wilkins, 1984.
3. Gosselin RE, Smith RP. Trends in the therapy of acute poisonings. Clin Pharmacol Therap 1966;*7*:279–299.
4. Goldstein A, Aronow L, Kalman SM. Principles of drug action: The basis of pharmacology, 2d. ed. New York: Wiley, 1974.
5. Johnson JD, Meisenheimer TL, Isom GE. Cyanide-induced neurotoxicity: Role of neuronal calcium. Toxicol Appl Pharmacol 1986;*84*:464–469.
6. Kanthasamy AG, Borowitz JL, Isom GE. Cyanide-induced increases in plasma catecholamines: Relationship to acute toxicity. Neurotoxicology 1991;*12*:777–784.
7. Patel MN, Yim GKW, Isom GE. Blockade of N-methyl-D-aspartate receptors prevents cyanide-induced neuronal injury in primary hippocampal cultures. Toxicol Appl Pharmacol 1992:*115*:124–129.
8. Patel MN, Yim GKW, Isom GE. Potentiation of cyanide neurotoxicity by blockade of ATP-sensitive potassium channels. Brain Res 1992;*593*:114–116.
9. Ardelt BK, Borowitz JL, Isom GE. Brain lipid peroxidation and antioxidant defense mechanisms following cyanide intoxication. Toxicology 1989;*56*:147–154.
10. Westley J, Adler H, Westley L, Nishida C. The sulfurtransferases. Fund Appl Toxicol 1983;*3*:377–382.
11. Belinsky SA, Blair BU, Forman DT, Glassman EB, Felder ME, Thurman RG. Hepatotoxicity due to allyl alcohol in deermice depends on alcohol dehydrogenase. Hepatology 1985;*5*:1179–1182.
12. Baud FJ, Galliot M, Astier A, Bien JV, Garnier R, Likforman J, Bismuth C. Treatment of ethylene glycol poisoning with intravenous 4-methylpyrazole. N Eng J Med 1988;*319*:97–100.

13. Smith RP, Olson MV. Drug-induced methemoglobinemia. Semin Hematol 1973;*10*:253–268.

14. Smith RP. Toxic responses of the blood. In Casarett and Doull's Toxicology, The basic science of poisons, 4th ed. New York: Pergamon Press, (1991); pp 257–281.

15. Kruszyna R, Kruszyna H, Smith RP, Wilcox DE. Generation of valency hybrids and nitrosylated species of hemoglobin in mice by nitric oxide vasodilators. Toxicol Appl Pharmacol 1988;*94*:458–465.

16. Kelner MJ, Bagness R, Hale B, Alexander NM. Methylene blue competes with paraquat for reduction by flavo-enzymes resulting in decreased superoxide production in the presence of heme proteins. Arch Biochem Biophys 1988;*262*:422–426.

17. Verma A, Hirsch DJ, Glatt CE, Ronnett GV, Snyder SH. Carbon monoxide: A putative neural messenger. Science 1993;*259*:381–384.

18. Suzdak D, Paul SM, Crawley JN. Effects of Ro15-4513 and other benzodiazepine receptor inverse agonists on alcohol-induced intoxication in the rat. J Pharmacol Exp Ther 1988;*245*:880–886.

19. Smith RP, Louis CA, Kruszyna R, Kruszyna H. Acute neurotoxicity of sodium azide and nitric oxide. Fund Appl Toxicol 1991;*17*:120–127.

20. Smith RP, Thron CD. Hemoglobin, methylene blue and oxygen interactions in human red cells. J Pharmacol Exp Ther 1972;*183*:549–558.

21. Friberg L, Vostal J. Mercury in the environment, an epidemiological and toxicological appraisal, Cleveland: CRC Press, 1972.

22. Passow H, Rothstein A, Clarkson TW. The general pharmacology of the heavy metals. Pharmacol Rev 1961;*13*:185–224.

23. Clarkson TW. Pharmacology of mercury compounds. Ann Rev Pharmacol 1972;*12*:375–406.

24. Horner HC, Roebuck BD, Smith RP, English JP. Acute toxicity of some silver salts of sulfonamides in mice and the efficacy of penicillamine in silver poisoning. Drug Chem Toxicol 1983;*6*:267–277.

25. Kagi JHR, Kojima Y. Metallothionein II. Basel: Birkhauser Verlag, 1987.

26. Goering PL, Klaassen CD. Tolerance to cadmium-induced hepatotoxicity following cadmium pretreatment. Toxicol Appl Pharmacol 1984;*74*:308–313.

27. Dudley RE, Gammal LM, Klaassen CD. Cadmium-induced hepatic and renal injury in chronically exposed rats: Likely role of hepatic cadmium-metallothionein in nephrotoxicity. Toxicol Appl Pharmacol 1985;*77*:414–426.

28. Rega AF, Rothstein A, Weed RI. Erythrocyte membrane sulfhydryl groups and the active transport of cations. J Cell Physiol 1967;*70*:45–52.

29. Rothstein A. Interactions of arsenate with the phosphate-transporting system of yeast. J Gen Physiol 1963;*45*:1075–1085.

30. Vansteneninck J, Weed RI, Rothstein A. Localization of erythrocyte membrane sulfhydryl groups essential for glucose transport. J Gen Physiol 1965;*48*:617–632.

31. Rothstein A, Vansteveninck J. Phosphate and carboxyl ligands of the cell membrane in relation to uphill and downhill transport of sugars in the yeast cell. Ann NY Acad Sci 1966;*137*:606–623.

32. Sutherland RM, Rothstein A, Weed RI. Erythrocyte membrane sulfhydryl groups and cation permeability. J Cell Physiol 1967;*69*:185–198.

33. Diamond GL, Klotzback JM, Stekwart JR. Complexing activity of 2,3-dimercapto-1-propanesulfonate and its disulfide auto-oxidation product in rat kidney. J Pharmacol Exp Therap 1988;*246*:270–274.

34. Jones MM, Singh PK, Gale GR, Atkins LM, Smith AB. Esters of *meso*-dimercaptosuccinic acid as cadmium-mobilizing agents. Toxicol Appl Pharmacol 1988;*95*:507–514.

35. Anon. Trientine for Wilson's disease. Med Lett 1986;*28*:67.

36. Misra M, Athar M, Hasan SK, Srivastava RC. Alleviation of nickel-induced biochemical alterations by chelating agents. Fund Appl Toxicol 1988;*11*:285–292.

37. Lione A. Aluminum toxicology and the aluminum-containing medication. Pharmacol Therap 1985;*29*:255–285.

38. Domingo JL, Gomez M, Llobet JM, Corbella J. Comparative effects of several chelating agents on the toxicity, distribution and excretion of aluminum. Human Toxicol 1988;*7*:259–262.

SECTION XIV

Governmental Regulation of Drugs

Editors:
Paul L. Munson
Åke Liljestrand

Associate Editors:
J. Richard Crout
Ivan Izquierdo

CHAPTER 113

Development of Drug Law, Regulations, and Guidance in the United States

Robert Temple

There are many sources of information about the development of the laws and regulations that govern the marketing and investigation of drugs and biologics in the US (see for example, *Food and Drug Law,* edited by Cooper,[r1] and *Drug Law, Cases and Materials,* edited by Hutt and Merrill[r2]). In what follows, the major legal milestones in drug regulation will be considered briefly, but the principal focus will be on the development of the major practices of clinical pharmacology and drug evaluation that represent drug development practices in the modern era.

Most important changes in drug law and regulations in the US arose from a combination of a desire for rational change and the stimulus to action provided by a public disaster. That is, the changes had often been considered extensively, often for years, but could be implemented only following a critical event. The original Food and Drug Act of 1906 was passed in response to revelations of cure-all claims for worthless, impure, and dangerous patent medicines, as well as adulterated and misrepresented food, and the law changed little until 1938. The 1906 Act gave the FDA authority to enforce the laws forbidding misbranded and adulterated foods and drugs (by referring criminal civil violations to the US Attorney) if it could discover violations, but gave FDA no role in pre-marketing evaluations of products. Beginning in 1933, under the stimulus of Dr. Rexford Tugwell, an original Roosevelt brain-truster and then Undersecretary of Agriculture from 1934–1937, there were active discussions of expanding the FDA's standard-setting authority, but the results were only a legislative stand-off between the administration and proponents of the food, drug, and cosmetics industries until 1937. In that year, a so-called elixir of sulfanilamide was prepared with a poisonous solvent (diethylene glycol) and killed 107 people, mostly children. The product had been marketed without testing in any living thing, human or animals.

The 1938 Federal Food, Drug, and Cosmetic Act was, in part, a direct response to the elixir of sulfanilamide episode and contained many new provisions relating to drugs. A sponsor intending to market a new drug had first to bring data to the US FDA to demonstrate that the drug was safe; the FDA could refuse to allow marketing if its requirements were not met. The law was well-conceived; in fact, the current safety provisions of the Food, Drug, and Cosmetic Act are largely unchanged since the original Act of 1938. The new law required that drugs be studied by "adequate tests by all methods reasonably applicable to show whether or not the drug is safe" for the use claimed in labeling and required that the results of those tests show the drug to be safe under the conditions of use proposed, to the satisfaction of the FDA.

Probably more important than the particular safety standard that had to be met for approval was the principle of pre-clearance itself. Instead of going to market based on their own assessment of the drug, sponsors had to submit an application for marketing to the FDA, a new drug application (NDA). This was a major change that apparently was little discussed.[1] In the 1938 law, the presumption apparently was that drugs would usually be approved and the "default" position was approval. That is, if FDA did not raise an objection within 180 days of the application's submission, the NDA was approved and the product could be marketed. Subsequently, in 1962, this approach was reversed, so that a positive notification of NDA approval was required before a drug could be marketed.

The next major change in the law did not occur until 1962, when, for the first time, a drug had to be shown to be effective, as well as safe, before it could be marketed. The effectiveness requirement will be described in detail below, but it is of historic interest that the immediate stimulus to the change in the law had nothing to do with effectiveness. The immediate cause was the discovery in 1962 that a sleeping pill called thalidomide, specifically recommended for use by pregnant women, had caused major birth defects (phocomelia) in thousands of babies, especially in western Europe. In the US, damage was limited by the alertness of FDA's Dr. Frances Kelsey, who refused to allow the drug to be approved because of concerns about its safety. There was some exposure in the United States, however, in many cases after the devastating consequences of thalidomide exposure in utero had become recognized. The reason was that the manufacturer of the drug had made it available to many investigators, some of whom had passed it along to other physicians without maintaining good records. It proved impossible to trace the distribution of the drug and to identify all the women who had received the drug, and then to retrieve it, so that in a number of cases, fetuses were exposed well after knowledge of the potential damage existed. The 1962 amendments are best known for introducing the effectiveness requirement, but they also gave the Secretary of Health Education and Welfare (now Health and Human Services) explicit authority to regulate the investigation of drugs. The modern system of regulation of the drug investigation and development process dates from that time, and there was particular emphasis in the law on the need for investigators to maintain firm personal supervision over investigations, to agree not to give the drug to other investigators, and to obtain informed consent from study subjects.

Although the effectiveness requirement first appeared explicitly in 1962, the required showing of safety in the 1938 law, defined as safety of a drug for its intended use, had always had some elements of weighing benefit against risk. Thus, even prior to 1962, some attention could be given to what a drug did that was good (its benefit), as well as to its toxicity. In retrospect it seems quite possible that the FDA could have altered the requirements administratively, arguing that considering "safety" without knowledge of effectiveness was illogical and contradictory; but, with limited exceptions, the FDA did not do so. Nonetheless, the idea that effectiveness was relevant, at least sometimes, existed before 1962, and the 1962 effectiveness requirement may not have been quite as seminal an event as it is now generally considered. What was even more critical, and novel, than the requirement for "substantial evidence" of effectiveness was the identification, in the 1962 amendments, of the specific *kind* of data that had to be used to demonstrate effectiveness, namely data from "adequate and well-controlled studies."

Although thalidomide was the trigger for legislation, the importance of showing effectiveness through controlled trials, as well as the need to regulate the investigational process and assure adequate animal testing prior to human exposure, had been promoted for years by many experts, so that the groundwork for the changes made had been laid. There was, however, still substantial controversy when it came to the details of legislation. The legislative history of the Kefauver-Harris (1962) amendments to the Food, Drug, and Cosmetic Act reflects some of these. Responding to concerns that the regulatory hurdle faced by drug companies might be too high, the history made it clear that a new drug did not have to be superior to available therapy and that the substantial evidence did not have to be so strong as to convince everyone.

Implementation of the 1962 amendments was a major event in the history of drug development. Over the ensuing eight years, the FDA produced regulations setting forth the new standards for approval, defining an "adequate and well-controlled study," describing the contents of labeling and standards for drug promotion, and providing procedures for carrying out investigations of new drugs. An extensive review of the drugs that had been approved between 1938 and 1962 based on evidence of safety alone began in 1966 with the help of the National Research Council of the National Academy of Sciences (NAS/NRC), the so-called "drug-efficacy study" (DES) and its implementation, DESI.

By the late 1970s and early 1980s, the Food, Drug, and Cosmetic Act and its effectiveness requirements were proving to be a significant barrier to generic competition. Well after the patent on many drugs had expired, potential generic manufacturers were unable to meet requirements for approval because to obtain an approved new drug application they would have to replicate the clinical studies carried out by the originator. The approval requirements for a copy of a drug were identical to those faced by the innovator. In the early 1980s the FDA developed its "paper NDA" policy, which allowed the Agency in some cases to rely on the literature, rather than newly conducted studies, to find evidence of effectiveness from adequate and well controlled studies. A reasonable number of drugs (for example, furosemide) were made available as generics through this mechanism. Nonetheless, the impediments to generics were substantial, and in 1984 the Drug Price Competition and Patent Term Restoration Act made generic drugs available under abbreviated NDAs (ANDAs) on the basis of a showing of bioequivalence to the generic drug to the innovator drug and demonstration of adequate drug product quality. The Act also gave five years of "exclusivity" for a new molecular entity; during that period, an abbreviated application could not be approved. This five years of exclusivity was most relevant to drugs whose patent had expired or that had never been patentable at all. In addition, in return for the earlier availability of generic competition, the Act gave innovator companies up to five years of additional patent life based on time spent during the NDA review process and during the IND process.

Principles of Drug Regulation in the US and How They Evolved

Drug Investigation

General Requirements

The basic outlines of the regulation of investigational uses of drugs were set forth in the 1962 amendments to the Food, Drug, and Cosmetic Act, and the details were provided in subsequent regulations, most recently revised in 1987. Clinical investigations of new drugs in the US must be carried out under an IND (investigational new drug application), a submission to FDA detailing clinical study plans, and the chemistry and toxicology data that support them. An IND is, technically, an exemption from the legal requirements for drug approval prior to distribution so that the drug can be distributed in order to study it. The IND rules apply most obviously to drugs never previously marketed, but apply also to studies of new uses of marketed drugs, unless they meet requirements for an exemption, promulgated in 1987. The exemption applies to studies of previously marketed drugs that are not intended to support significant labeling or advertising changes and that do not involve a route of administration, change in dose, or other change that significantly increases the risks of the drug.

When conducting clinical studies under an IND, investigators (the people actually carrying out the studies) and sponsors (the people who submit the IND) have obligations to submit research plans to an institutional review board before proceeding, to obtain written informed consent from the subjects of the research, to monitor the studies and report adverse events, including rapid reporting to the FDA and investigators of adverse events that are serious or life-threatening, and to establish and maintain records, and make reports, that will allow the FDA to evaluate the safety and effectiveness of the drug in the event an NDA is filed. As noted above, sponsors and investigators have specific obligations to control distribution of the drug and to know who has received it.

In its evaluation of an IND, FDA focuses initially on the safety of the proposed clinical studies, assuring itself that the study drug is well-enough defined and manufactured to yield meaningful data, that the information supplied to investigators (which is critical to allowing adequate patient monitoring and proper informed consent) is not erroneous, misleading, or incomplete, that animal or other human experience are sufficient to allow assessment of the risks to subjects of the proposed studies, and that subjects would not be exposed to an "unreasonable and significant" risk of illness or injury. If the submission fails to provide this assurance it will be placed on "clinical hold," i.e., not allowed to proceed. In later investigations, the FDA can also refuse to allow a study to proceed if it "is clearly deficient in design to meet its stated objectives."

Animal Data

The elixir of sulfanilamide disaster made it obvious that there were good reasons to study drugs in animals before they were given to humans, and many experts strongly urged Congress to require animal studies prior to investigational use of drugs in humans.[2] There arose within a few years of passage of the 1962 amendments a fairly standardized set of animal toxicology studies required to support human studies of a given duration[3] that are still in use, although flexibly administered. Introduction of a drug into humans requires acute (single-dose) studies in three to four species (often 2 species in recent years) and subacute (2-week) studies in two species, one rodent and one nonrodent, generally a dog and a rodent; animals were observed and histopathology evaluated. Human dosing is based on the doses (mg/kg or, more recently, mg/m^2 or blood level measurements) tolerated in animals, and the organs in the animals that were affected by drug exposure (target organs) are watched with special care in humans. As proposed studies grow larger and of longer duration, longer animal studies are needed to support them. Requirements for studies of animal carcinogenicity, needed for marketing of chronically administered drugs but generally not during the investigational period, evolved gradually, generally following principles established by the National Cancer Institute's National Toxicology Program. By the late 1970s, it became generally required that a drug for chronic use would be studied in two animal species, generally mouse and rat, for the full lifetime of the animals at a maximally tolerated dose. This requirement has changed little since the 1970s, although there is now far more attention to measurements of comparative exposure in animals and humans ("toxicokinetics"), taking into account metabolic and pharmacokinetic differences between species. Long-term study results are also interpreted in light of new insights into mechanism of tumor formation derived from in vitro and in vivo mutagenicity testing and other tests of possible interaction with the genome, which are now almost always carried out. Animal reproduction studies are generally completed before extensive human trials are carried out. Efforts under the auspices of the International Conference on Harmonization (ICH), a tripartite (US, EC, Japan, with representation by regulatory authorities and pharmaceutical manufacturers of each region) organization that had international meetings in 1991 and 1993 to attempt to achieve consistency in regulatory requirements, have been directed toward assuring consistency in such areas as requirements for reproduction studies and required maximum exposure in carcinogenicity studies.

Monitoring the IND Process; Interactions with Drug Manufacturers During Drug Development

It is clearly the responsibility of the drug company (sponsor) to develop the data and evidence needed to meet the legal requirements for drug approval. In the early years after passage of the 1962 amendments, sponsors were very much on their own, with little guidance from the FDA except in the form of NDA nonapproval letters. There was in fact an explicit concern that too much participation in development would leave the Agency unable to be appropriately neutral and analytical when the resulting data came in as part of an NDA for review. But in the late 1960s and early 1970s there was a growing attack on the Agency for its slowness in approving drugs compared with the rest of the world.[4] The Agency did not accept the idea that there was anything wrong with the law or its fundamental procedures, or even the idea that important therapies were being delayed, but tried in a variety of ways to decrease review and approval times. One approach was a series of increasingly strenuous attempts to make known what its requirements for approval would be. This resulted in nearly 30 drug class clinical guidelines, most developed in the late 1970s, each describing in detail the study designs and expected data for particular therapeutic classes, such as drugs for ulcer disease, depression, or angina. The guidelines were usually developed with the help of the FDA's external advisory committees and frequently with the involved conduct of industry/FDA workshops.

In addition to the general (i.e., not drug product or sponsor-specific) guidance given in guidelines, the FDA has become increasingly involved in the details of development of specific drug products, reflecting the view that the public, the industry, and the FDA are poorly served by drug development efforts that are poorly designed or inadequate and that therefore waste resources and delay availability of therapy. Beginning in the mid-70s, the FDA became willing to meet with sponsors at the end of phase 2 of the development process. (The ordinary process of clinical drug development is divided into phases 1, 2, and 3. The phases were defined in regulations in 1970, and defined further, and somewhat differently, in a general guideline [General Considerations for the Clinical Evaluation of Drugs] written in 1977 and the revision of IND regulations of 1987. The three phases constitute an orderly process of drug development, working from small numbers of relatively well patients exposed briefly to a drug to progressively larger numbers of patients of increasing complexity given progressively longer courses of the drug. In general, phase 1 is the first introduction of a drug into humans to see whether the drug is tolerated, to define its pharmacokinetics and metabolism, and, where possible, to develop preliminary effectiveness data based on a pharmacologic endpoint. Phase 2 represents the first formal well-controlled studies carried out in patients with the disease to be treated—usually relatively uncomplicated patients. Phase 3 includes further controlled studies, studies to gain additional (e.g., long-term) safety information, studies of combinations, additional dose-response studies, etc.)

At first, end of phase 2 meetings were offered only for particularly important drugs, but in the 1987 IND regulation revision they are offered generally, although "primarily for INDs involving new molecular entities or major new uses of marketed drugs". Requests for these meetings are to be honored "to the extent that FDA's resources permit." At an end of a phase 2 meeting, the sponsor, usually with favorable results from at least one controlled trial of the drug in hand, presents its over-all development plan, including details of the most critical planned studies, to obtain FDA advice on critical aspects of the plan, including study designs (control group, end-points, analytic plan), appropriateness and sufficiency of the population (including subsets of the population such as gender and age groups), duration of exposure, and approach to dose-finding. The agreements and conclusions of the FDA at the end of phase 2 meetings have the status of "advisory opinions," generally meaning that the FDA intends to live by them unless, for important health reasons, it is unable to, e.g., because new information has caused revision of earlier viewpoints.

The 1987 regulations also offer sponsors an opportunity to request a pre-NDA meeting. Such meetings address a variety of issues, including the potential adequacy of the data (sometimes a sponsor will reconsider submission of an NDA after such a meeting) and plans for analysis and presentation of data. The goal of these meetings is to help the sponsor facilitate FDA review and become aware of potential problems that need to be addressed. These meetings are especially important if sponsors are considering a CANDA (Computer-Assisted NDA), so that the significant effort involved is well-targeted and hoped-for gains in efficiency are realized.

A third important source of guidance to sponsors developing drugs is the (largely) open advisory committee system. Beginning in the 1970s, the FDA developed standing outside advisory committees, each to deal with particular groups of therapies (the cardiorenal drugs committee, arthritis drugs committee, the gastrointestinal drugs committee, etc). Under US Freedom of Information rules, almost all discussions of new drug applications are open to the public, and these discussions provide continuing insight into the Agency view and the views of the outside committee with respect to development practices for various drug classes, sometimes an "early warning" that a change is in the offing. The development of an external advisory committee system also was a response to the idea that the FDA reviewers were isolated and unaware of current developments and was a partial response to the drug-lag arguments. There is little question that the advisory committee system provides a degree of openness and public accountability, as well as an element of risk sharing with an outside group, that has been helpful to the Agency and its credibility. The Agency's more than 20 drug or biologics-related committees are very active, generally meeting several times a year, usually for two days at a time, to consider most NDAs for new molecular entities, other important products, and new claims, safety problems, and guidelines.

Finally, under the Freedom of Information Act, a substantial amount of information on an approved drug is publicly available, including a Summary Basis of Approval (SBA) that describes the data used by FDA to reach its approval decision (SBAs are not always prepared; the individual chemistry, toxicology, clinical, statistical, and biopharmaceutical reviews can substitute for the SBA) and the reviews carried out by FDA staff (purged of trade secret or confidential commercial information). Thus the details of analysis and reasoning behind FDA staff decisions are available to sponsors developing a new drug.

All these sources of guidance are important, but the most critical probably is the ability of the sponsor to discuss plans with FDA staff. This is widely appreciated. Thus, when Congress passed the Orphan Drug Act of 1984, intended to encourage development of drugs for rare diseases or conditions, it included a specific provision offering sponsors of an orphan drug the right to request advice from FDA on the nonclinical and clinical investigations that must be conducted before the drug may be approved. The offered meeting is, in effect, a pre-IND, end-of-phase 2, or any other needed meeting. Similarly, when the Agency, in 1988, promulgated regulations [21 CFR 312, Subpart E] to facilitate the development of drugs intended to treat life-threatening and severely debilitating diseases, a principal component of the regulation was the offer of more "early consultations," i.e., pre-IND and end-phase 1 meetings, so that the phase 2 trials in life-threatening illnesses would be well-designed and more likely to serve as a basis for approval if their results were favorable.

Although the resources involved are very substantial, the FDA is strongly committed to the interactions described above and, indeed, hopes to enhance them. Every protocol for a new study must, by regulation, be submitted to the IND before it is initiated. Apart from its authority to "hold" an inadequate study, the FDA is authorized to provide any sort of advice and suggestions on any aspect of an application. Ideally, FDA staff would be able to review any substantial protocol for potential problems and suggest improvements or areas for discussion. This occurs in certain areas now (drugs for AIDS, Alzheimer's disease) but is not yet general practice.

Concerns about the possibility that participation in drug development plans gives the FDA a "stake" in the studies cannot be dismissed but have proved manageable. First, there is a clear and well-understood distinction between trying to design an excellent and potentially convincing study, where the FDA's and sponsors' interests overlap substantially, and interpreting the results of the study, where the FDA and the sponsor have unequivocally distinct responsibilities. Second, FDA review takes place at many levels, involving one or more primary clinical reviewers, a statistical reviewer, two levels of supervisory review within a given review unit, an office level review (for new molecular entities), and, usually, a public discussion before an advisory committee. There is little opportunity for a committed individual to exercise sole control over a decision.

Drug Application Review—Safety

General

Although the drug safety provisions of the Food, Drug, and Cosmetic Act have not changed since 1938, evaluation of drug safety has changed considerably. The safety problems experienced by drugs approved as safe in the 1950s were sometimes very dramatic. In the early 1950s isoniazid, the first really effective treatment for tuberculosis, and iproniazid (Marsilid), an MAO inhibitor closely related to isoniazid, were marketed and were thought to be reasonably safe. Within several years, however, iproniazid was revealed to be highly hepatotoxic, causing hundreds of deaths due to liver injury.[5] Isoniazid was thought to be mildly hepatotoxic. In 1970, however, it was found that isoniazid had a mortality rate of about 1 in 1000 when a prophylaxis study in young Public Health Service officers revealed this sad fact.[6] It thus took from six to 20 years to discover the toxicity of two of the most hepatoxic substances ever marketed as drugs. It is not clear why the discovery of the hepatoxicity of the two agents was so delayed. Iproniazid causes fairly severe liver injury in almost 10 percent of the patients give it,[5] so that one might have expected rapid discovery of its toxicity in even the simplest of studies. Nonetheless, it was three years after marketing before the first published report of hepatoxicity appeared and fully six years before iproniazid was removed from the market. There was thus, in the cases of both isoniazid and iproniazid, failure of both the drug development process and the post-marketing surveillance process. Although details of the latter are beyond the scope of this chapter, the surveillance system of the 1950s and even the 1970s, when many observers thought the spontaneous reporting system should be abandoned, bears little resemblance to today's system, which receives far more reports (over 100,000 per year in recent years compared with less than 10,000 in the past), incorporates them swiftly into a computerized data base, and makes excellent use of the data. Although any spontaneous reporting system has inherent and significant limitations (such as the lack of denominator data, variable reporting rates, and no persuasive control group), there have been important major successes.

The experience with INH and iproniazid can be contrasted, for example, with that of ticrynafen, an antihypertensive diuretic marketed in May 1979 and removed from the market in early 1980, when its liver toxicity was discovered through the spontaneous reporting system. Although far less hepatotoxic than isoniazid or iproniazid, ticrynafen's toxicity was discovered much more rapidly. Ticrynafen was also a uricosuric agent, and was also found by the spontaneous reporting system to cause acute renal failure, an effect preventable by adequate hydration. Similarly, the flank pain/renal failure response (also due to a uricosuric effect) to suprofen, a nonsteroidal anti-inflammatory drug approved in 1985, was discovered within a few months, leading to suspension of marketing of the drug. More recently, the system rapidly detected a high rate of adverse effects, including liver injury, hemolytic anemia, anaphylaxis, and renal failure, with a new quinolone antibiotic, temafloxacin, leading to its prompt withdrawal from the market.

Discovering toxicity in the post-marketing period is critical; relatively rare events, i.e., those at the 1 per 1000 rate or less will not reliably be discovered in NDA data bases involving a few thousand or fewer patients. But iproniazid and perhaps isoniazid were sufficiently toxic that their problems should have been discovered in pre-market testing, and it appears that modern testing in similar cases is in fact more successful. The muscle relaxant dantrolene, for example, is hepatotoxic to about the same extent as isoniazid, but its toxicity was well-recognized at the time of its approval in 1974, and this could be weighed against its benefits. More recently still, in 1992, the beta-blocker dilevalol, while under NDA review by the Agency, was found to be significantly hepatotoxic. The clue to this was three instances (among about 1500 patients treated, about 500 of them treated for six weeks or more) of acute liver injury, with jaundice, leading to discontinuation of treatment. These cases, though few, were more than expected in the population and led to close attention to marketing experience (dilevolol had been marketed in Portugal and Ireland) and the recognition of significant hepatotoxicity in a Portuguese post-marketing experience. This drug was removed from the market worldwide. This disappointing (for the sponsor) yet gratifying public health outcome reflected two important changes in the FDA's approach to safety data: 1. review of the safety data base as an overview; 2. focus on deaths and adverse drop-outs, i.e., people who die during a study or leave the study prematurely in association with an adverse event, whether or not the event is recognized as drug-related.

Safety as an Overview

It is now recognized that the evaluation of safety in a new drug application data base is fundamentally an overview or meta-analysis of all available data. Although this now seems obvious, the idea that safety data should be looked at all together, as opposed to study-by-study, is a relatively recent insight, not formalized in regulations until 1985, when the rules first called for an "integrated summary of all available information about the safety of the drug product."

In 1980, it was first appreciated that the safety data bases evaluated by the FDA were often seriously incomplete. Typically, the NDA safety data base was "locked" some six months or more before the NDA was submitted and was not updated subsequently, even though further data usually were being collected in on-going studies. By the time a two- to four-year FDA approval process had taken place, there were often more data not submitted to the application, collected after the NDA data lock-point, than there were data submitted in the application. What resulted from the discovery of the "lost" data was a requirement, imposed in 1980 and added to NDA regulations in 1985, that the safety data base be updated four months after an NDA was submitted and again just prior to approval, giving the Agency access to the entire safety data base.

The current Agency approach to the safety review is reflected in the Guideline to the Format and Content of the Clinical and Statistical Sections of the Application (1988), a guideline to aid sponsors in constructing a complete and reviewable NDA. Although directed at industry, it also reveals the analyses the FDA intends to carry out. First, the extent of exposure, i.e., the numbers of patients exposed for specified durations and to specified doses, with attention to population subsets (gender, age, race), is assessed to determine whether it is adequate, given, among other things, the disease to be treated, the numbers and kinds of patients likely to be exposed, the degree of effectiveness seen, and the dosing recommendations in labeling, and what is known about the dose-response of the drug for favorable and unfavorable effects.

Next, the more common adverse events are assessed for rate and seriousness, using, as appropriate, results of good-sized single trials, pooled data from placebo-controlled trials, pooled data from all controlled trials, all data, etc. Each approach (data set) has advantages and disadvantages, as studies differ in how adverse events were elicited in the population studied, and in whether the control group received placebo or active drug. Some events seem more likely than others to require blinding for proper assessment. Where possible, attempts to seek dose-response relationships in the adverse event data are made, and it is expected that the rates in demographic (age, gender, race) and other relevant subgroups (size, metabolic status, renal function) will be examined. Laboratory data are examined similarly, looking at mean changes, "shifts" from normal to abnormal, and individual outliers. If there are placebo-treated patients, it often is possible to reach reasonable judgment as to whether the more common adverse events and laboratory changes are drug-related. In general, the more common events are described in labeling in text or tables and have a good deal to do with whether a drug is attractive to patients and physicians, but they are rarely the basis for the FDA's refusal to approve the application.

Focus on Deaths and Adverse Drop-outs

When the NDA regulations [21 CFR 314] were revised in 1985, an important change was made in requirements for submission of raw data. The law's requirement for "full reports of investigations which have been made to show either or not [the] drug is safe for use and whether such drug is effective in use" [sec 505(b)(1)(A)] had been interpreted as requiring submission of all case report forms for every patient treated. In 1985 this was changed. Sponsors had instead to provide complete case report tabulations (listings of essentially every data point collected) from every well-controlled study and tabulations of safety data from all studies. The only case report forms required automatically, however, were those of patients who died during the study or did not complete the study because of an adverse event, whether or not the event was thought to be drug-related. Additional case report forms could be, and usually are, requested by the Agency, but are submitted only as requested.

The change in submission requirements reflected to focus on deaths and adverse drop-outs the expectation/hypothesis that a truly serious adverse reaction either would kill the patient or would cause the patient to be dropped from the study, and that this would be true even if what was affecting the patient was not recognized as drug related. The deaths and drop-outs thus appeared to be the patients to examine most closely to look for serious unrecognized adverse reactions that reflected major problems with the drug. The drop-outs also are an indication of what reactions are unpleasant enough (even if not dangerous) to bother the patient significantly. Particularly careful review is devoted by reviewers to these patients, especially where the adverse event is not a recognized consequence of the therapy.

Drug Application Review—Effectiveness

General

The Kefauver-Harris amendments to the Food, Drug, and Cosmetic Act changed not only drug regulation but the standards by which physicians and other scientists measure the quality of all clinical trials. Appreciation of the value of controlled trials antedated the amendments, of course, and was reflected in testimony preceding the amendments, but the sheer volume of drug industry-conducted studies guaranteed that the standards of the law would be reflected in most clinical studies of drugs. As indicated above, the impression that the critical event in 1962 was the effectiveness requirement is wrong and over-simple. It is difficult to know the extent to which FDA staff were already introducing effectiveness concepts into the regulations of drugs prior to 1962, but it is said that they were to a degree, because "safety" inherently represented a benefit/risk judgment. Commissioner George Lavrick, testifying before a Congressional Subcommittee[8] in 1964, suggested that the FDA's ability to do this was limited, applying principally in the case of a serious illness where lack of effectiveness was dangerous:

> The 1938 new drug section of the law did not require a manufacturer to prove that his new drug would yield the benefits claimed on its label. It spoke only of safety. Thus, many of the Government's decisions allowing drugs to be marketed had to be made without access to the full facts a physician would want in deciding whether to use the product.
>
> Of course the question of benefit was an integral part of the safety question in dealing with a product to be used in a life-threatening disease such as pneumonia or in dealing with a drug presenting grave risks. We required information about effectiveness for such drugs in order to reach a decision about safety. But many fairly innocuous new drugs offered for ailments that were not life-threatening were presented to us for evaluation without evidence that they would do what the label claimed. We had no power in such case to require submission of efficacy data.

Prior to 1962, however, whatever their intent or wish, reviewers would have had very little in the way of properly designed studies to consider. In 1962, however, that changed, because the Kefauver-Harris amendments required that the "substantial evidence" of effectiveness needed to approve a drug had to be derived from adequate and well-controlled studies—the kind of studies now recognized as a sound basis for conclusions.

The legal requirement that there be substantial evidence that the drug will have the effect it is represented to have under the conditions of use recommended in labeling was not intended to be particularly demanding. In American legal terms "substantial evidence" is not a high standard; indeed, it has been described by a former FDA chief counsel as somewhere between a "scintilla and a preponderance." The law has ways of expressing a higher standard than "substantial evidence," such as a "preponderance of the evidence" or "evidence beyond a reasonable doubt." Those higher standards were not chosen, as a result of legislative compromises in 1962, but as part of the compromise, the study methods by which a sponsor had to demonstrate substantial evidence were rigorous ones: "substantial evidence," as newly defined in the law, meant evidence from adequate and well-controlled clinical studies.

Although the law did not say what a well-controlled study was, testimony before the US Senate and House by various experts must have made it very clear what people had in mind. Drs. Louis Lasagna, then of Johns Hopkins University Medical School, Harry Dowling, Chief of Medicine at the University of Illinois, Maxwell Finland, of the Harvard Medical School, and many others described the need for control groups, minimization of bias, and other characteristics now well-recognized as elements of a well-controlled study. Thus, the 1962 amendments provided an only modestly stringent evidentiary standard, substantial evidence, accompanied by legislative history assurances that there was no intent to require that new drugs be superior to available therapy or that evidence of effectiveness be so convincing that all or even most experts would agree with it, but then incorporated into law the idea that the evidence must come from adequate and well-controlled studies, producing an over-all standard that was probably considerably higher than some had intended. The standard has also been interpreted over the years, and accepted by the courts, as meaning that more than one well-controlled study is needed to support effectiveness.

A characteristic of the FDA review process, particularly in recent years, has been close review of the detailed submitted data, reflecting a strong commitment to going beyond the data summaries. This has been possible because of the "full reports" requirement in law, because of gradual growth in available review staff, and more recently, because of increasing use of computerized data bases by statistical and clinical reviewers. The availability of detailed data allows the FDA, in the course of review, to examine the disposition of all patients, explore adherence to the protocol, assess the quality and consistency of endpoint determinations (e.g., bacteriologic and clinical cure in antibiotic studies, recurrent infarction in cholesterol-lowering or secondary prevention studies, partial or complete response rates in cancer trials), check statistical analyses or perform alternative ones, explore subgroup hypotheses, and examine particular adverse events and reasons for patients' early departure from a study. In an effort to make sponsors aware of the Agency's expectations and to help them fulfill them, the FDA published in 1988 the Guideline to the Format and Content of the Clinical and Statistical Sections of New Drug Applications, which provided detailed guidance on reporting results of individual studies and on preparing the integrated summaries of safety and effectiveness called for in regulations.

Adequate and Well Controlled Studies

In 1970, the FDA set forth, for the first time, a description of the characteristics of an adequate and well-controlled study, noting in the regulations that data other than that from adequate well-controlled studies could at best be "supportive" of effectiveness but could not stand alone as a basis of approval. The NDA form 356H, with which an NDA was submitted until 1985, also referred to the need for adequate and well-controlled studies and noted particularly that it was ordinarily expected that there would be at least two adequate and well-controlled studies conducted by independent investigators showing effectiveness of the drug. The 1970 regulations identified several features of the protocol and report of the results of a well-controlled study: 1. a clear statement of the objectives of the study; 2. a method of selection of patients that provided adequate assurance that the patients were suitable for the purposes of the study, that assigned patients to test groups in a way that minimized bias, and that assured comparability of test and control groups with respect to pertinent demographic and disease variables; 3. an explanation of the methods of observation of results and steps taken to minimize bias on the part of the investigator and the patient; 4. a quantitative comparison of the results of treatment with a control and an explanation of the steps taken to minimize bias on the part of the observers and analysts of data, including the level of blinding, if used. Four different kinds of controls were identified: placebo control; no treatment control; active control; and historical control. The regulation commented on each of these, noting that the no-treatment control was suitable where the endpoint was objective and placebo effect negligible, that the active control design was appropriate where no treatment or use of a placebo would be contrary to the interest of the patient, and that historical controls were reserved for situations where the disease being treated had high and predictable mortality.

The regulations on adequate and well-controlled studies were modified in 1985 to expand on some of these concepts and also identified a new kind of control, the dose comparison concurrent control, in addition to placebo, no treatment, and active concurrent control studies, and historical controls. The new regulations also have more explicit guidance as to the need for protocols to describe the study in detail, the need to explain fully how critical measurements were made, and the need to blind the analysts of data, as well as the investigator and the patient, and indicated greater concerns about use of active control studies intended to show equivalence of a new drug to an older drug.

The legal requirement for adequate and well-controlled studies was set forth in the 1962 law, but did not become effective until 1964. It is fair to say that appreciation of the elements of a well-controlled study grew gradually from 1962 to 1969, when the regulations were first proposed (they were reproposed in 1970 when the Pharmaceutical Manufacturers' Association sued the FDA because the Agency had not allowed an opportunity for comment on the proposed regulation [Pharmaceutical Manufacturers Association v Finch]), by 1970, the Agency showed a very thorough understanding of the elements of a controlled trial. An affidavit by Dr. William T. Beaver, an analgesiologist at Georgetown University who participated in development of the Agency's regulation, submitted in PMA v Finch, described the history of controlled trials and supported each element of the Agency's regulation.

Dose Response

In 1985 the revised NDA regulations formally included the parallel dose response study as a kind of well-controlled study, but this reflected at least a decade of growing interest in the best approach to finding the proper dose of drugs. The problems associated with failure to carry out adequate dose response studies have been described,[9,10] and represented a growing problem. Drugs tended to be systematically overdosed, and there were several examples of probable harm arising from excessive doses, including use of diuretics in hypertension at doses well in excess of the necessary dose, e.g., 100 mg of hydrochlorothiazide or chlorthalidone when 12.5 mg to 25 mg of each is probably an adequate monotherapy dose and still lower doses have proved effective in combination with other antihypertensive agents. Hypokalemia associated with the higher doses may have led to excess cardiovascular mortality, reducing the beneficial effects of treatment.[11] It is striking that one of the most favorable effects on cardiovascular mortality seen in a large trial (SHEP, systolic hypertension in the elderly)[12] used a starting dose of just 12.5 mg of chlorthalidone. Early studies of captopril also utilized much larger doses than ultimately proved necessary, with resulting hematologic toxicity.

One reason dose response had been difficult to discern was the tendency of sponsors to require, in a typical placebo-controlled study, that patients be titrated to the maximum dose tolerated or to some clinical end-point. If titration was to tolerance, without assessment of response, there was obviously no dose-response information to be gained. Even if the drug was titrated according to response, however, the population treated with higher doses usually was different from (less responsive than) the population getting the low dose and without special analyses,[13] these trials did not give useful dose-response information, although they could provide good evidence that the drug, as titrated, was superior to placebo. While it is difficult to be sure, it appears likely that the new effectiveness requirement was at least partly responsible for encouraging titration to excessive doses, especially of reasonably well-tolerated agents (toxic agents could not be overtitrated so easily), because sponsors wanted to be certain that they had used a sufficient dose to beat placebo definitely. Titration as a way of choosing dose also reflects typical use of drugs in medical practice and is a relatively safe mode of therapy.

In 1978, the FDA's Cardiorenal Division became aware of two publications by Tweeddale and Materson[14,15] showing that the usual doses of chlorthalidone, a widely used diuretic, were excessive. The dose commonly recognized by the community, and used in major intervention trials, was 100 mg, but the new studies showed that the full effect of chlorthalidone was achieved at 25 mg and that a significant effect could be achieved with only 12.5 mg. Just as important, the doses above 25 mg, while not more effective, had greater effects on serum potassium, uric acid, and glucose. Both studies used rarely seen (at that time) rigorous dose-response designs: the Materson study used a randomized parallel design in which patients were assigned to, and maintained at, fixed doses; the Tweeddale study used a crossover design—again, however, one in which patients were randomized to, and crossed over between, a series of fixed doses. The studies thus showed that chlorthalidone was being used at four or more times the dose needed.

At about the same time, review of a new drug application for nadolol, a beta-blocker studied for treatment of hypertension and angina, showed that the titration design used in all studies, in which doses were rapidly raised from 40 to 80 mg to 320 to 640 mg, had tended to obscure the fact that doses of 40 mg or less seemed to give the full effect of the drug. Indeed, there is reason to believe that as little as half a milligram is a reasonably effective dose of nadolol.[16]

Finally, also at about the same time, development of captopril, the first angiotensin converting enzyme (ACE) inhibitor, revealed that less than optimal dose finding and the use of the drug in patients with renal functional abnormalities without dosage adjustment, with resulting greatly excessive blood levels, probably caused the drug to have a higher rate of agranulocytosis than it otherwise would have. Data available suggested that the dose of 450 to 600 mg per day used in many patients, including those with renal functional impairment, was at least three times the dose ordinarily necessary, and a still larger multiple of the dose needed in patients with renal failure.

Once the fundamental design problem leading to poor dose-finding was recognized, the FDA began to recommend studies in which patients were randomized to different fixed doses of the drug, now called the "parallel fixed dose-response" study, a very uncommon design up to that time.[10] In studies of this design, the effect of a constant dose could readily be separated from the effect of duration of treatment, and the randomized patient groups remained intact, not changing in accordance with response, so that responses in the groups could be properly compared. It is important in these studies to use a reasonably wide spread of doses so that differences between groups or a positive dose-response slope can be discerned, and the FDA regularly urged this, but not always successfully. It is also usually important to include a placebo group in dose-response studies; there are many instances in which all of the doses of a drug studied were indistinguishable, so that it was impossible to discern a slope. In the absence of a placebo group it would be impossible to tell whether the drug had any effect at all.

The randomized parallel fixed dose-response study has now become extremely common in most therapeutic areas. Whereas it was once rare to see more than one fixed dose group in a clinical trial, in the current typical development of a drug for hypertension, angina pectoris, depression, insomnia, and many other diseases and conditions, most of the studies submitted in recent NDAs will be found to have used the randomized parallel fixed dose design. This has, in many cases, allowed selection of doses that offered the full therapeutic effect of a drug, but with fewer of the adverse effects typical of other members of the pharmacologic class whose dose finding had been less satisfactory.

More recently there has been interest in blood concentration monitoring and in the potential value of a concentration controlled trial, a trial in which patients are randomized to concentration windows achieved using pharmacokinetic information. The potential advantage of this is greatest where the pharmacokinetics of the drug produce very variable blood concentrations after a given dose. In that case, the concentration controlled trial can represent considerable efficiency.[17]

In late 1993, the International Conference on Harmonization adopted a dose-response guideline that will serve as a regulatory standard in the US, the EC, and Japan. The guideline strongly advocates the need for good dose-response information and encourages use of the parallel dose-response study. It also notes, however, that study designs in which individuals receive more than one dose (titration or crossover designs) may be more able to allow estimation of individual differences in dose response relationships and encourages the development of designs that may be able to do this.[13]

Active Control Equivalence Designs

In situations where there is known effective therapy for a disease, the randomization of patients to placebo can lead to ethical concerns. Indeed, where available therapy is known to enhance survival or decrease irreversible morbidity in a particular population, that population cannot be studied in placebo-controlled trials. In other cases, however, a competent, fully informed person may be asked to forego established therapy where the only consequences to the patient are discomfort. This view was significantly challenged in the late 1970s in the US, and ethical and legal issues in Europe caused at least one well-placed observer to wonder whether placebo-controlled trials would survive.[18] Indeed, for much of the 1980s it was difficult to carry out placebo-controlled trials in depression in Europe.

The study preferred by people with ethical concerns about use of placebos was the active control design in which "equivalence" of (really lack of a demonstrated difference between) a new drug and a standard effective drug would be considered evidence of effectiveness of the new agent. It soon became appreciated, however, that "equivalence" in these studies does not demonstrate that the new therapy actually worked. Equivalence could also mean that neither drug worked in the particular study. To conclude that the new drug was effective required an assumption that the standard therapy would have had its usual effect, demonstrable in that study, had a placebo group been present. The need for this assumption gives these designs an element of a historically-controlled trial. Unfortunately, in certain diseases and conditions, such as depression, anxiety, angina, or heart failure, among many others, it is all too common for active drugs to fail to beat placebo in good studies. This problem was discussed briefly by Lasagna in an editorial in 1979[19] and at greater length by Temple in 1982 and 1983.[9,20]

Appreciation of the problems associated with the active control equivalence design led to FDA policy that discouraged active control designs except where the effectiveness of the drug was clearly evident even without a placebo (e.g., many antibiotics for acute infections, oncologic drugs to treat acute leukemia, or testicular cancer). These designs were not considered useful for showing effectiveness in situations where drugs could not regularly be distinguished from placebo. In these cases, lack of demonstrated differences between treatments could simply reflect an inadequate study, one incapable of telling active from inactive drugs. When the NDA regulations were revised in 1985, the section describing adequate and well controlled studies noted that for active control studies intended to show equivalence, the sponsor must explain why the control drug should be considered effective in the study, e.g., by reference to results of previous placebo-controlled studies of the active control drug. The regulation also noted that the study's ability to have detected differences of a given size had to be addressed.

The use of placebo controls inevitably will remain controversial in particular settings, but the inadequacy of active control equivalence studies in many cases is now widely appreciated. European guidelines for study of antianginal and antidepressant drugs, for example, now clearly call for placebo-controlled studies, a controversial matter in the past. Active control studies in which the intent is to show superiority to the standard agent do not present the same problem as equivalence designs and are the only recourse where standard therapy is life-saving, yet an equivalence study would not be persuasive. For example, although beta-blockers are clearly effective postinfarction agents, many apparently adequate placebo-controlled postinfarction trials of beta-blockers have failed to distinguish drug and placebo. An equivalence trial would therefore be unpersuasive. Yet a placebo-controlled trial would be unethical.

DESI Review/OTC Review

Among the requirements of the 1962 law, was that FDA carry out a re-evaluation of the marketing status of the several thousand drugs and the claims attached to them that had been approved between 1938 and 1962 on the basis of a showing of safety alone. The FDA carried out this task, the Drug Efficacy Study (DES), with the help of a contract with the National Research council of the National Academy of Sciences (NAS/NRC). The NAS/NRC, beginning in June 1966, formed 30 expert panels to review the data submitted for these claims, rating them initially as effective, probably effective, possibly effective, ineffective, or ineffective as a fixed combination, the last term referring to combination products for which the role and contribution of one of the components was in doubt. NAS/NRC reports were received by the Agency in 1967 and 1968, and in 1970–72 the FDA published hundreds of "DESI" (Drug Efficacy Study Implementation) notices transmitting the NAS/NRC reports, in some cases with conclusions modified by FDA staff.

In general, most of the products considered effective by the NAS/NRC were accepted as such by the Agency and needed no further attention, but over about the next 20 years, many of the products rated as less than fully effective (probably or possibly effective, ineffective, or ineffective as a fixed combination), and which had to bear labeling describing their DESI status, were the subject of additional actions; these were pure legal tests in some cases, but in many others sponsors conducted extensive further clinical trials to attempt to support their products, leading to many detailed reviews by FDA staff. The medical evaluations and legal efforts resulting from the DESI process were extensive, and numerous important principles were established in the course of the DESI process. In 1968, the Agency sought to withdraw approval of the drug Panalba, a combination of novobiocin and tetracycline, because the novobiocin had not been shown to contribute to the over-all effect. In addition to defining the essential showing for a combination, placed in regulations in 1970 (that both components must be shown to contribute to the effect of the combination), the Panalba case, through administrative and then judicial proceedings, also established the requirement that there be at least one adequate and well-controlled study if a sponsor was to obtain an evidentiary hearing on an FDA withdrawal procedure. Subsequently, and particularly important, in the case of Warner-Lambert Heckler (1986), FDA sustained its view that approval of a drug product be denied even if it could show an "effect," if that effect was not clinically meaningful. The 1962 effectiveness requirement did not refer directly to clinical benefit, requiring only that the sponsor demonstrate what was claimed in the label. That requirement could be read as allowing any claim, no matter how frivolous, so long as it was truthful, although on benefit risk, or "safety," grounds it could perhaps be argued that a drug with no meaningful benefit could not be safe. In any case, Warner-Lambert v Heckler established clearly that it was the Commissioner's responsibility to make a judgment that the claimed effect was of clinical value.

The DESI review, in addition to establishing a number of critical principles, also eliminated from the marketplace many hundreds of drug products, including the oral proteolytic enzymes (orally administered protein enzymes intended to promote healing and decrease inflammation in various parts of the body), the subject drug of Warner-Lambert v. Heckler, and a wide variety of combinations that were described by a former Director of the Bureau of Drugs as "baroque." Particularly hard-hit were the combinations of virtually any agent with sedatives, developed because of the presumed component of anxiety in so many physical illnesses. In fact, in all but a few cases, it was impossible, despite significant and often carefully conducted efforts, to show that sedatives contributed to the effect of any agent. Essentially all of the combinations of anticholinergic and antispasmodic drugs with anxiolytic drugs intended to treat GI diseases were eliminated after many large controlled studies attempting to show that the anxiolytic component contributed to the GI effect ended in failure.

End-points: Surrogates and Others

One of the most critical, yet difficult, decisions in a trial is the choice of study end-points and specific methods for measuring them. There has been great progress over the years in the science of measurement (scales for anxiety and depression, treadmill exercise protocols that yield reproducible results) and in efforts to screen out patients who are too variable and to "enrich" the study population with potential responders (e.g., people likely to take medications, attend clinic).

In general, efforts to develop measurable, reproducible study end-points have been left to the sponsor, with the FDA seeking to assure that they have been validated, are credible, and are meaningful. A particularly difficult area is that of surrogate end-points, study outcome measurements that are not of clinical value in and of themselves (cholesterol, blood pressure, CD4 lymphocyte count, ventricular premature beat rate) but are thought to correspond, and are of value only if they do correspond, to a clinical benefit (decreased coronary artery disease, decreased stroke, fewer opportunistic infections, or decreased rates of sudden death). There has been growing interest in being certain that the true clinical effects of drugs are known and are of value, and reliance on surrogates of those clinical effects has come under increasing scrutiny. At the same time there is growing impatience with the slow progress in treating certain diseases (AIDS, amyotrophic lateral sclerosis, solid tumors) and a desire to use the earliest possible evidence of benefit, usually an effect on a surrogate.

Some surrogate end-points have established credibility and are in current use. For example, in the late 1960s and early 1970s, it was shown that treatment of high blood pressure with the therapies available at that time (diuretics, reserpine, and hydralazine) resulted in favorable effects on survival and morbidity. Although similar studies have not yet been conducted to support the true effectiveness of newer classes of antihypertensives, such as ACE inhibitors and calcium channel blockers (studies to evaluate the true benefits of these agents are ongoing), there is considerable support for considering the effects on blood pressure to be a reasonable means of assessing the benefits of antihypertensive agents. Other surrogate markers have been subject to varying degrees of concern and scrutiny. Lipid-altering drugs are approved based on their effects on measured lipids, but often with a requirement to carry out survival, morbidity, and plaque regression studies after approval. Long-term studies of cholesterol-lowering agents have shown, in general, an improvement of cardiovascular morbidity and mortality, but at the present time it remains unclear whether over-all survival is affected by treatment. This could reflect the only modest effectiveness of the drugs studied to date, some more important deficiency with the surrogate marker of cholesterol (or particular cholesterol fractions), or unrecognized toxicity of the drugs studied to date).

Some recent experiences suggest caution in accepting even reasonably plausible surrogate end-points and are a reminder that the presumed relation of a surrogate to a clinical end-point may not exist or, probably more important, that the surrogate end-point only measures what is thought to be the good effect of a drug (diuretics lower blood pressure, type 1 antiarrhythmics lower VPB rates, aspirin prevents thrombosis) but ignores potential adverse effects that may be rarer (diuretics can provoke hypokalemia, antiarrhythmics can provoke new abnormal rhythms, aspirin causes bleeding) but can undermine a beneficial effect.[21]

The cardiac arrhythmia suppression trial (CAST) has permanently altered the basis for approving antiarrhythmic drugs.[22,23] This NIH-conducted study was carried out to determine whether decreasing ventricular premature beat (VPB) rates in patients who had an acute myocardial infarction would improve survival. There was reason to hope that VPB suppression would be of value as increased VPB rates are known to be associated with poorer survival after an infarction. The trial was in fact considered unethical by some people because patients would be denied the "known benefit" of antiarrhythmic therapy; but, as the value of VPB suppression had never been demonstrated, the trial went forward, with surprising results. The antiarrhythmic drugs studied, encainide, flecainide, and moricizine, were very successful at reducing VBP rates and were well-tolerated in an initial single-blind period. But when the patients were randomized to either the effective antiarrhythmic (giving at least 70% reduction in VPB rates) or placebo, the drugs not only failed to improve survival but markedly impaired it, encainide and flecainide together inducing an approximately 2.5-fold increase in mortality—moricizine having a smaller adverse effect in the randomization part of the study but also an adverse effect on survival during the single-blind period.

Although FDA had not relied for approval on evidence on VPB suppression alone, and had not approved postinfarction use of the drugs, the CAST results were a potent reminder that a seemingly valuable effect on a surrogate end-point did not necessarily predict benefit or even lack of serious harm. New antiarrhythmic agents now must have their effect on mortality assessed; they need not necessarily improve survival if they have some other benefit, but they should be shown not to impair it.

In a similar way, the discoveries that an inotropic agent (milrinone)[24] and vasodilator (flosequinan) that can improve cardiac output and such symptoms of congestive heart failure as decreased exercise tolerance can also lead to decreased survival, that quinidine reduces recurrent atrial fibrillation after cardioversion but decreases survival,[25] and that lidocaine decreases postinfarction life-threatening ventricular arrhythmias but does not improve survival,[26] all point out that it usually is impossible to learn about the effects of drugs on major morbidity or mortality without studying those end-points.

That is not to say that surrogate end-points will not be relied on by the Agency in particular situations, especially where there is no available therapy and where study of definitive end-points is likely to take many years. In fact, in 1992 a new regulation (the accelerated approval regulation) gave the Agency explicit authority to rely on a surrogate marker "that is reasonably likely based on epidemiologic, therapeutic, pathophysiologic, or other evidence, to predict clinical benefit" for approval of drugs intended to treat serious or life-threatening diseases and that provide meaningful therapeutic benefit to patients compared with existing treatments. This approval is subject to the requirement that the drug be studied further to verify and describe its clinical benefit. The rule also provided for expedited withdrawal procedures if the sponsor failed to perform the required studies or if the studies failed to verify clinical benefit.

Statistics as a Regulatory Requirement and Regulatory Discipline

In the early 1970s, the FDA had a few statisticians, but their role in drug review was modest at best. Since that time the discipline of statistics in drug regulation has expanded enormously, both within the industry and within the Agency, which now has more than four dozen biostatisticians contributing at all levels of review, not only to the review of clinical data and study design, but to the review of animal carcinogenicity studies and drug stability protocols. Apart from the easily perceived contribution, both inside and outside the Agency, of this highly trained group, a number of events served to enhance the place of statistics in drug regulation.

In 1980, the FDA refused to approve a new claim for the antiplatelet drug sulfinpyrazone (Anturane) for the prevention of sudden death following myocardial infarction, rejecting claims supported by the Anturane

Reinfarction Trial (ART).[27] The explanation for this refusal was published[28] and showed visibly that the Agency could address design and analysis issues that were critical to the external community. Moreover, the explanation made it clear to the drug industry that study design and analysis mattered, and that they had to pay close attention to design and analytic issues both as studies were planned and as they were carried out and analyzed. In particular, the critique of the ART made clear the importance of analyzing all patients with on-therapy data, noting the dramatic difference in outcome (favorable to the drug) when a reduced data set based on post-facto and potentially biased exclusion of certain patients was used. Certainly, the industry took note of the intent-to-treat issue as they never had before. The FDA's analysis also showed problems arising from after-the-study subsetting of data, e.g., trying to distinguish sudden from other cardiac deaths and to analyze the results for each subset, and examining different time periods (first six months) and the need to correct for multiple comparisons when such subsetting is done. The FDA's report emphasized the critical importance of assuring that any decisions about inclusion and exclusion of patients, and any decisions to examine data subsets, were documented and were made by analysts who were blinded to the treatment assignments. The discussion of the ART also showed the difficulties of utilizing cause-specific analyses of mortality and the need to develop criteria of cause of death assignment that were rigorous and applied blindly. The FDA's ART paper was, in other words, a public tutorial on the analytic problems that could arise in an otherwise well-conducted study.

DESI Review

Another stimulus to the growing importance of statistical evaluation at the FDA was the entire DESI (Drug Efficacy Study Implementation) project, in the course of which the Agency reviewed thousands of clinical trial designs and methods of analysis. The DESI reviews were publicly available and often published in Federal Register notices. Their preparation and publication publicly identified hundreds, perhaps thousands, of examples of inappropriate, after-the-fact data subsetting, imperfect and dubious blinding, bizarre end-points, and essentially every other design and statistical "crime" that could be committed. Many of the lessons of the DESI experience have been incorporated into the Guidelines for the Content and Format of the Clinical and Statistical Sections of New Drug Applications (1988), the 1985 revision of the NDA regulations, and the lore of the Agency. The NDA regulations now require a separate section directed to the biostatistician. The 1988 guideline describes a study report that is an integrated clinical and statistical analysis, reflecting the integrated review strategy used by the Agency to address specific applications and many of the major study design and analysis issues of the present, such as methods of data monitoring/interim looks, meta-analyses, large, simple trials, auditing approaches, corrections for multiple comparisons, use of surrogate end-points, distinctions between primary and some drug end-points, and subset analyses.

The role of biostatisticians in all phases of study design and analysis is now well established and critical, and the Agency's expertise is enhanced by the large and growing number of biostatisticians who play an increasingly important role in industry.

Individualization of Therapy: Attention to Demographic Subgroups

One can think of the drug development enterprise in the US as consisting of three eras. The first era followed the 1938 statute, stimulated by the discovery that drugs could do considerable damage and needed to be assessed for their safety. Many current practices in animal toxicology and human safety evaluation and monitoring arose during this period. The second era followed the watershed insights, incorporated into law in 1962, that effectiveness of drugs mattered, and that the way to study effectiveness was in well-controlled trials. After 1962, modern study designs and analytic approaches were developed and refined. The drug development eras are cumulative, of course, and do not end with progress into the next one, so that many new insights into safety assessment have arisen in the era of effectiveness.

The third era of drug development, one not heralded by a particular event comparable to the elixir of sulfanilamide or thalidomide episodes, is the age of individualization of drug therapy, representing a new concern, now that we know how to find drugs that are reasonably safe and are known to work, with how to use drugs in the most effective way possible. Part of this concern is reflected in increased attention described above, to dose finding, beginning in the late 1970s and continuing to the present. A second major component of the concern with optimizing treatment is new interest in the ways in which subsets of the entire population, or particular individuals, may respond differently to drugs, an interest that has begun to take shape in the 1980s. Again, of course, new insights into effectiveness evaluation continue to be developed, such as the development of "large simple trial" techniques and the burgeoning "meta-analysis industry."

Evaluation of Drugs in Population Subsets

The first formal FDA attention to the evaluation of drugs in subsets of the total population began in 1983 with a proposal to develop a guideline on the study of drugs in the elderly. The proposal was made widely available and discussed publicly on several occasions,[29,30] and a formal guideline was promulgated in 1989 with several major elements.

The first, perhaps obvious, element was that the elderly should not be excluded from clinical trials. Rather, they should be included, so that differences between them and the rest of the population can be discovered. This principle was applied in 1989 to the elderly, but was recognized as a general one, applicable both to demographic subsets of the over-all population (age, gender, race) and disease subsets (diabetes, coronary artery disease, people on concomitant therapy). That is, it was better to include a broad spectrum of the population in trials and look for differences in response than it was to exclude people with these characteristics because of concern that they might introduce heterogeneity and so never discover such heterogeneity. A particular variety of the heterogeneity problem has arisen in carrying out studies in people with AIDS, who often use many drugs and have a range of concomitant illness. The issue was addressed by Byar and many coauthors,[30] who concluded that rigorous trials can be carried out under these conditions if sample sizes are adjusted appropriately. The Guideline for the Study of Drugs Likely to Be Used in the Elderly did not urge separate studies in populations except in special cases (e.g., to study effects on cognitive function) because comparing effects in young and old in the same study appeared more informative.

In 1988, even before the geriatric guideline appeared, the guideline for the Format and Content of the Clinical and Statistical Sections of New Drug Applications specifically asked that both individual studies and the integrated summaries of safety and effectiveness include analyses of differences in subsets of the over-all population, including gender, age, and race subsets, as well as other pertinent subgroups, such as patients with renal or hepatic failure. Differences were to be sought in the over-all effectiveness data, in safety data, and, to the extent possible, in the examination of dose-response relationships for effectiveness and adverse events. It was recognized that these relatively crude and not prospectively planned analyses might be insensitive and needed to be viewed cautiously because of their retrospective and multiple nature; they nonetheless had to be carried out, even if many findings that emerged would require confirmation. It is, in fact, current Agency policy that an NDA review will not be initiated unless those analyses are, or will shortly be, available.

The second element of the guideline followed from the first. Having included the elderly (or other subset) in studies, it was necessary to examine the data base to see if the subset responded differently from the rest of the population.

The third element in the Guideline was the focus of particular attention on the pharmacokinetics of the drug in the patient subset of interest and in the rest of the population. This emphasis reflected practical reality (it is far easier to measure pharmacokinetic differences among subgroups than differences in pharmacodynamic response), but also reflected the fact that most of the differences now recognized in different populations reflect differences in how the drug is excreted or metabolized by the body (pharmacokinetics) rather than differences in how the body responds to a given blood level (pharmacodynamics). There may well be far more pharmacodynamic differences than are yet recognized, but they are harder to detect.

Knowing the effects of age on pharmacokinetics is only part of what the physician needs to know to treat the elderly. What is really needed is understanding of all of the factors that can alter kinetics because these may be more important to the care of elderly than the effect of age per se. Thus, the elderly are more likely than younger patients to have renal function abnormalities or heart failure or to be on concomitant therapy, and the effects on pharmacokinetics of these factors need to be understood. Although the effect of each factor could be assessed in a separate study, there is a more efficient way to study all possible influences on the pharmacokinetics of a drug. The Guideline for the Study of Drugs Likely to Be Used in the Elderly described, for the first time, the concept of the pharmacokinetic screen, an attempt to use the large data base in new drug applications to identify essentially all relevant individual or subset differences in pharmacokinetics. The screen consists of obtaining a small number of steady state blood levels in essentially all phase 2 and 3 patients, and then looking for altered pharmacokinetic patterns related to demographic or other characteristics (e.g., renal function, hepatic function) and at individual outliers, who might be a clue to the presence of metabolic subtypes or to a drug-drug interaction.

The Guideline for the Study of Drugs Likely to Be Used in the Elderly was published in 1989. In 1993, a relatively similar guideline[32] described the need for analysis and evaluation of both genders in the course of drug development. It utilized the general principles (include the subset in trials, analyze the data for differences, find the pharmacokinetic differences) espoused in the guideline on drugs to be used in the elderly, and also identified several specific concerns related to use of drugs in women that needed to be considered, including attention to possible effects of the menstrual cycle and of differences between pre- and postmenopausal women. The guideline also indicated that certain drug-drug interactions were particularly critical, including the possible interaction of oral contraceptives with the new drug being evaluated and the possible effect of the new drug on the effectiveness of oral contraceptives (it had been shown that rifampin and some other emzyme-inducers could render oral contraceptives ineffective). The publication presenting the 1993 gender guideline also announced suspension of a 1977 FDA guideline that excluded women of childbearing potential from phase 1 and early phase 2 studies of drugs, except for drugs being studied in life-threatening conditions.

The concern with population subsets such as the elderly and women reflected both sociopolitical concerns (fairness, adequate attention to major components of the population) and scientific ones. With respect to the gender guideline, for example, there was considerable impact of the observation that women had been excluded from many trials in coronary artery disease[33,34] and from some major intervention studies, such as the Harvard Physicians Health Study.[35] Although both the elderly (but not the very old, over 75) and women had been included in drug development studies, roughly in proportion to their numbers in the population of affected patients,[32] it was also true that little had been learned from that inclusion. That is, there had never been any systematic attempt to analyze data bases to learn whether men and women, or young and old, respond differently in clinical trials; the relevant analyses had simply not been done. Thus, in 1988, the FDA called for these analyses. In 1992, after discovering, with the help of the US General Accounting Office, that these analyses often were being omitted, despite the guideline, the FDA determined that review of new drug applications would not be initiated unless the demographic and other subset analyses had been provided or could be provided quickly. In 1990, the FDA proposed addition of a geriatric use subsection of drug labeling. A final rule is expected in 1994.

In 1993, an International Conference on Harmonization (ICH) guideline on Study of Drugs in The Elderly was accepted,[36] reflecting essentially the same point of view and expectations as had been put forth in the FDA's guideline. The ICH is also examining the potential for evaluating differences in response among ethnic and racial subsets.

Assessment of Metabolic Differences and Drug-Drug Interactions

In addition to better assessment of dose-response and attention to population subsets, a third major influence on drug development has been the growing recognition of individual metabolic differences and the discovery that these could be induced by drug-drug interactions.

The discovery that people differed in their ability to metabolize certain drugs is not new. The prolonged apnea in people with abnormal pseudocholinesterase was the prototype for such differences. Differences in ability to acetylate drugs have also long been recognized, and racial differences in acetylator phenotype described; there can be consequences of such differences, such as the greater likelihood of slow acetylators to develop lupus-like reactions to procainamide or hydralazine. More recently, there has been growing recognition of the importance of the group of microsomal enzymes collectively called cytochrome P450 isozymes, enzymes responsible for the metabolism of many drugs, sometimes eliminating the active substance (dextromethorphan, debrisoquin, the dihydropyridine calcium channel blockers, cyclosporine, some tricyclic antidepressants), sometimes producing an active metabolite (terfenidine, codeine). Some of these enzymes exhibit genetic polymorphism, notably cytochrome P450 II D6 (debrisoquin hydroxylase), which is inactive in about 8 percent of Caucasians (poor metabolizers), leading to much higher blood levels, for a given dose, of certain tricyclic antidepressants or their active metabolites (imipramine, desipramine), altered ratios of active parent and metabolites of encainide, and inability to have an analgesic response to codeine. Adverse reactions to several drugs, including phenformin[37] and perhexilene[38] in poor metabolizers have been described. Another important enzyme, cytochrome P450 III A 4, responsible for the metabolism of terfenidine, astemizole, dihydropyridine calcium channel blockers, cyclosporine, short-acting benzodiazepines, and many other drugs, is not polymorphic but has widely variable activity in individuals.

Probably more important than genetic or phenotypic differences in metabolism among individuals, which can be managed by careful titration, is the potential for quantitatively important drug-drug interactions, well-illustrated by two recent examples. Imipramine and desipramine are both metabolized by cytochrome P450 II D6. That enzyme can be inhibited by other substrates for the enzyme, such as propofenone or fluoxetine, or by some nonsubstrates, such as quinidine. One of these inhibitors, fluoxetine, has been shown to increase blood levels of tricyclics by six- to eightfold,[39] with significant potential toxicity. Other inhibitors would have the same potential. A patient well stabilized on the tricyclic after careful titration could become abruptly toxic if the interaction were not recognized.

Terfenidine, a nonsedating antihistamine, is a prodrug, the active metabolite being produced by cytochrome P450 III A4. Inhibitors of that enzyme, such as ketoconazole,[40] and erythromycin[41] cause parent ketoconazole to appear in blood, with serious consequences, as the parent, but not the metabolite, inhibits the cardiac potassium slow channel,[42] leading to QT interval prolongation and torsades de pointes-type ventricular arrhythmias,[43] sometimes fatal.

The range of potential interactions with cytochrome P450 enzymes is very great, including not only other drugs, but smoking (smokers have much lower levels of tacrine because smoking induces cytochrome P450 IA2, the enzyme that metabolizes tacrine), and diet (grapefruit juice inhibits the metabolism of dihydropyridine calcium channel blockers,[44] some short-acting benzodiazepines, and terfenidine).

Drug manufacturers are rapidly developing the laboratory and clinical capability to investigate these interactions and it will be a challenge to treating physicians and medical communicators to keep track of the interactions discovered and utilize this information in patient care. There is no doubt that evaluation of such interaction will become an even more critical part of drug development and drug evaluation in the 1990s.[45]

Drug Labeling and Promotion

Prior to 1962, labeling for drugs, based on data with no particular quality standards, and in the absence of any approval standard for claims, was largely devoted to promotion. In the hearings before passage of the 1962 amendments, labeling came in for considerable criticism; indeed, pre-1962 labeling would be unrecognizable today as labeling. Gradually, however, after 1962, FDA began to impose new standards on drug labeling and the promotion that followed from it. An outline of labeling requirements was first published in 1970, but detailed regulations on the format and content of labeling were published only in 1979. Rules about prescription drug advertising were promulgated as early as 1963 and revised in 1968 to reflect Commissioner Goddard's concern with specific unacceptable and unscientific practices. Since 1962 there has been progressive appreciation of the critical importance of the contents of labeling as part of the drug review and approval process. In 1970, it became a requirement that sponsors include in the NDA an annotated labeling, that is, a labeling annoted to identify the location in the NDA of the specific support for each statement. Review of labeling was greatly facilitated by this new requirement, and attention to these details greatly improved the quality of labeling.

Some parts of labeling are treated more rigorously than others. The Indications section, for example, reflects the full implementation of the 1962 effectiveness requirements. Every claim of effectiveness has to be supported by adequate and well-controlled studies, as must any statements comparing the safety or effectiveness of a drug with other agents for the same indication. It has long been recognized, however, that a variety of kinds of information need to be included in the clinical pharmacology and safety-oriented parts of labeling, including data from studies that were not well-controlled and even persuasive individual reports, and these parts of labeling have grown. With the growth in size of labeling documents, it became necessary somehow to distinguish those parts that were more important than others, and such enhancements as dark print, capitals, and boxed warnings came into use. Boxed warnings at various times has included everything from such homilies as "be sure you understand how to use this drug," to major warning statements. In current practice, boxed warnings are reserved for serious problems, generally those that are more than extremely rare and represent real limitations on the use of the drug.

The precautions section of labeling has become the location for a variety of kinds of useful information, in addition to conventional precautions and results of anginal carcinogenicity reproduction studies, including instructions on pediatric use, and, soon, instructions and information on the use of drugs in the elderly, and drug-drug interactions (a growth area) as companies carry out more drug-drug interaction studies and as the importance and frequency of metabolic interactions becomes recognized. The clinical pharmacology section has also grown in scope, often including detailed results of clinical studies, and the Dosage and Administration section increasingly provides separate guidance for various populations. The tension between inclusiveness of labeling and its user-friendliness continues to exist, and is not fully resolved, although efforts to improve the communication effectiveness of labeling are always proceeding at some level.

The FDA's ability to monitor advertising and promotion is to a degree limited by the resources that can be devoted to this effort. In recent years, this activity has gained increasing attention, as it has been recognized that even the best labeling can be undermined by promotion that is false, omits critical information, emphasizes some information at the expense of other balancing information, or is otherwise inconsistent with labeling. Although, in most cases, promotional materials are not submitted to FDA before their use (initial campaigns are usually submitted), they are submitted at the time of use, and the FDA has a substantial ability to induce corrections of false or misleading promotion, including stimulating corrective "Dear Doctor" letters or corrective advertising. The FDA's rules listing promotion practices that are or may be false, lacking in fair balance, or otherwise "misleading" dates from 1968, but is quite sophisticated, identifying such practices as:

- "Contains a representation or suggestion, no approved or permitted for use in the labeling, that a drug is better, more effective, useful in a broader range of conditions or patients . . . safer, has fewer, or less incidence of, or less serious side effects or contraindications than has been demonstrated by substantial evidence or substantial clinical experience"
- "Contains a drug comparison that represents or suggests that a drug is safer or more effective than another drug in some particular when it has not been demonstrated to be safer or more effective in such particular by substantial evidence or substantial clinical experience."
- "Contains a representation or suggestion that a drug is safer than it has been demonstrated to be by substantial evidence or substantial clinical experience, by selective presentation of information from published articles or other references that report no side effects or minimal side effects with the drug or otherwise selects information from any source in a way that makes a drug appear to be safer than has been demonstrated."
- "Contains favorable data or conclusions from nonclinical studies of a drug, such as in laboratory animals or in vitro, in a way that suggest they have clinical significance when in fact no such clinical significance has been demonstrated."
- "Uses erroneously a statistical finding of "no significant difference" to claim clinical equivalence or to deny or conceal the potential existence of a real clinical difference."
- "Uses data favorable to a drug derived from patients treated with dosages different from those recommended in approved labeling."
- "Contains favorable information or conclusions from a study that is inadequate in design, scope, or conduct to furnish significant support for such information or conclusions."
- "Uses statistical analyses and techniques on a retrospective basis to discover and cite findings not soundly supported by the study, or to suggest scientific validity and rigor for data from studies the design or protocol of which are not amenable to formal statistical evaluations."
- "Uses tables or graphs to distort or misrepresent the relationships, trends, differences, or changes among the variables or products studied; for example, by failing to label abscissa and ordinate so that the graph creates a misleading impression."
- "Uses reports or statements represented to be statistical analyses, interpretations, or evaluations that are inconsistent with or violate the established principles of statistical theory, methodology, applied practice, and inference, or that are derived from clinical studies the design, data, or conduct of which substantially invalidate the application of statistical analyses, interpretations, or evaluations."

In the last few years, stimulated by several examples, the FDA has paid increasing attention to the possibility that what appears to be independent scientific meetings and publications, in fact, represent promotional vehicles. Although speakers at a truly independent meeting can discuss drugs in a way inconsistent with labeling, e.g., discuss new uses of the drug, speakers at a promotional effort cannot do so. In order to make clear to sponsors how they can support independent scientific efforts, proposed enforcement policy on industry-supported meetings has emphasized that these meetings must be scrupulously independent of the sponsor in their creation and content if they are to be considered other than promotional events.

Access and Availability

It is a fact of scientific life that there is ordinarily some evidence of the usefulness of drugs before there is the kind of evidence needed to market them. When a drug is already marketed, and information about a new use gradually becomes available, it is possible for a physician aware of the new evidence to use the drug outside the package insert; there is no law against this practice; indeed, it is not even considered inappropriate behavior. Before a drug is marketed, however, the drug ordinarily is unavailable for any purpose outside the manufacturers clinical trials. This has long been a difficult situation when a new drug appears to represent a significant advance or to treat a disease lacking effective therapy. As early as the 1960s, some drugs were being made available for treatment purposes during the drug development process to patients who appeared to need them; sometimes very large numbers of patients received drugs in this way. For example, in the late 1960s and early 1970s, cardioselective beta-blockers, potentially useful in patients with pulmonary disease, were given to thousands of patients in "open protocols." These protocols surely contributed to the over-all safety data base, but were not designed to provide any evidence of effectiveness. These uses sometimes were called "compassionate uses" and represented the desire of the FDA and industry staff not to deny promising agents, even if their full evaluation was incomplete. There was similar wide use of novel antiarrhythmics and the earliest calcium channel blockers, which appeared to have particular usefulness in the treatment of vasoapastic angina. About 1970, a formal arrangement to make promising oncolytic agents, so-called group C drugs, available for individual treatment use was worked out with the National Cancer Institute. These C drugs were to be made available to patients in open protocols while formal drug development efforts were going on.

Although the practice of allowing open protocols to treat thousands, sometimes tens of thousands, of patients had some justification, the practice induced discomfort within the Agency. The law allowed use of unapproved drugs for investigational purposes, but it was not clear whether the open protocol arrangements fit under an investigational heading. To clarify the situation and to elicit discussion on the issue, the Agency proposed in 1982 to identify formally a new category of investigations called "treatment protocols" or "treatment ILNDs." These were situations where the primary purpose of the protocol was to allow treatment of patients with a serious disease lacking good available therapy with a promising investigational drug; safety information would also be collected, of course, but that was not the main reason for the study. Treatment protocols were allowed only when controlled trials were ongoing (usually one such trial would have been completed) and the drug sponsor was engaged in serious drug development efforts. The treatment IND concept proved not to be particularly controversial, and it became a formal part of the IND regulations in 1987. When finally promulgated, the treatment IND was perceived as a response to the AIDS epidemic and, in fact, the treatment IND has been utilized to allow treatment of patients with HIV infections with investigational agents. Most treatment uses in recent years have been to treat HIV infections, cancer, and serious neurologic illnesses. The treatment IND represents an attempt to resolve the conflicting demands of rigor on drug evaluation and the humane interest in making drugs available for people with no alternatives as soon as there is a reasonable likelihood of benefit. Allowing this kind of early access under the IND assures the sponsor ability to monitor use of drugs closely at a time when its potential toxicity has not been fully studied. There is a provision in the regulations allowing the FDA to terminate a treatment use when such use is interfering with the proper evaluation of drugs, e.g., by inhibiting recruitment into controlled trials. The provision exists because in the long run it is critically important to evaluate drugs properly, so that it can be known whether they work or not; the community interest is not well served when that cannot be accomplished. The treatment IND and a related procedure called Parallel Track, intended to allow very early access to AIDS-related investigational agents, provide early access to therapy by allowing treatment use before drug approval. Two other rules are directed at earlier marketing of drugs. Under the so-called Subpart-E rule, the FDA promises early interaction by the Agency with sponsors who are developing drugs for life-threatening illness in order to design early studies that will constitute a definitive assessment of the effect of the drug on survival or irreversible morbidity. In those situations, once an effect on major morbidity or survival is demonstrated, it is frequently impossible to carry out further trials, so that it is essential that the initial trial or trials be adequate. It is also important to recognize, as the Subpart E rule does, that when there is a demonstrated survival effect of therapy, the total safety data base is often relatively limited, another reason for seeking to assure its quality.

A recently promulgated rule called the Accelerated Approval rule takes a different approach to early marketing. The rule allows FDA to rely on surrogate markers of effectiveness, even where those are not unequivocally shown to correspond to a clinical benefit, so long as the surrogate is reasonable, and on the condition that definitive studies to evaluate the clinical endpoint will be carried out by the sponsor.

Progress, Change, Improvement

The drug evaluation process is never static; it evolves as new experiences and new discoveries demand new approaches. In recent years, as indicated above, there has been a new interest in dose-response, individualization of therapy, and genetic and drug-induced variations in metabolism. It appears likely that health care reform will provoke greater interest in comparative drug effects, therapeutically important outcomes, and quality-of-life assessment. Large simple trials allow assessment of small but important effects, and raise new questions about how such trials can be monitored and audited. International harmonization efforts create opportunity and anxiety—can standards be maintained? will requirements simply become additive? Information technology allows unparalleled access by reviewers to raw and modified data. Will it prove to enhance efficiency or will it be a distraction? The answers cannot of course be known, but there are reasons for optimism. The government, consumer, academic, and industrial participants in the drug development process have been, in general, intelligent, imaginative, adaptive, and determined, even if not always in agreement. Important new therapies continue to emerge, better documented, better studied, and better labeled than they used to be. There seems no reason to doubt this will continue.

References

Research Reports

1. Hoffmann JE. The Food and Drug Administration's administrative procedures. In: Cooper RM, ed. Food and drug law. Washington: Food and Drug Law Institute, 1991:1–40.
2. Lasagna L. Letter dated July 25, 1961 to Senator Estes Kefauver. Legislative history of the Food, Drug and Cosmetic Act. Volume 18, 973–975.
3. Goldenthal EI. Current views on safety evaluation of drugs. FDA Papers 1968; May:1–8.
4. Wardell WM. Introduction of new therapeutic drugs in the United States and Great Britain: An international comparison. Clin Pharmacol Ther: 1973;*14*:773–790.
5. Zimmerman HJ. Hepatotoxicity: the adverse effects of drugs and other chemicals on the liver. New York: Appleton-Century-Crofts, 1978, pp 405–406.
6. Garibaldi RA, Drusin RE, Ferebee SH, Gregg MB. Isoniazid-associated hepatitis: report of an outbreak. Am Rev Resp Dis 1972;*106*:357–365.
7. Temple R. The regulatory evolution of the integrated safety summary. Drug Information Journal 1991;*25*:485–492.
8. Larrick G, quoted in Hutt PB, Merrill RA, eds. Food and drug law, cases and materials, 2d. Westbury, New York: The Foundation Press, 191, pp 522–523.
9. Temple R. Government viewpoint of clinical trials. Drug Info J 1982;*16*:10–17.
10. Temple R. Dose-response and registration of new drugs. In Lasagna L, Erill S, Naranjo CA, eds. Dose-response relationships in clinical pharmacology; Proceedings of the Esteve Foundation Symposium IV. Elsevier Science Publishers B.V. (Biomedical Division), 1989, pp 145–167.
11. Multiple Risk Factor Intervention Trial Research Group. Multiple risk factor intervention trial. Risk factor change and mortality results. JAMA 1982;*248*:1465–1477.
12. SHEP Cooperative Research Group. Prevention of stroke by antihypertensive drug treatment in older persons with isolated systolic hypertension. JAMA 1991;*265*:3255–3264.
13. Sheiner LB, Beal SL, Sambol NC. Study designs for dose-ranging. Clin Pharmacol Ther 1989;*46*:63–77.
14. Tweeddale MG, Ogilvie, Rudey J. Antihypertensive and biochemical effects of chlorthalidone. Clin Pharmacol Ther 1977;*22*:519–527.
15. Materson BJ, Oster JR, Michael VF, Bolton SM, Burton ZC, Stambaugh JE, Morledge J. Dose-response to chlorthalidone in patients with mild hypertension. Clin Pharmacol Ther 1978;*24*:192–198.
16. Escoubet B, Lelercq JF, Maison-Blanche P, Poirier JM, Gourmel B, Delhotel-Landes B, Coumel P. Comparison of four beta-blockers as assessed by 24-hour ECG recording. Clin Pharmacol Ther 1986;*39*:361–368.
17. Sananthanan LP, Peck CC. The randomized concentration-controlled trial: an evaluation of its sample size efficiency. Controlled Clin Trials 1991;*12*:780–794.
18. Dollery CT. Editorial: a bleak outlook for placebos (and for science). Europ J Clin Pharmacol 1979;*15*:219–221.
19. Lasagna L. Editorial: placebos and controlled trials under attack. Europ J Clin Pharmacol 1979;*15*:373–374.
20. Temple R. Difficulties in evaluating positive control trials. Proceedings of the American Statistical Association, Biopharmaceutical Section, 1983.
21. Temple RJ. A regulatory authority's opinion about surrogate endpoints (in press).
22. Echt DS, Liebson PR, Mitchell LB, Peters RW, Obias-Manno D, Barker AH, Aresnberg D, Baker A, Friedman L, Greene HL, Huther ML, Richardson DW, and the CAST investigators. Mortality and morbidity in patients receiving encainide, flecainide, or placebo. N Engl J Med 1991;*324*:781–788.
23. The Cardiac Arrhythmia Suppression Trial II Investigators. Effect of the antiarrhythmic agent moricizine on survival after myocardial infarction. N Engl J Med 1992;*327*:227–233.
24. Packer M, Carver JR, Rodehoffer RJ, Ivanhoe RJ, DiBianco R, Zeldis SM, Hendrix GH, Bowmer WJ, Elkarjan U, Kukin ML, Mallis GI, Sollano JA, Shannon J, Tandon PK, DeMets DL for the PROMISE study research group. Effect of oral milrinone on mortality in severe chronic heart failure. N Engl J Med 1991;*325*:1468–1475.
25. Morganroth J, Goin JE. Quinidine-related mortality in the short-to-medium-term treatment of ventricular arrhythmias, a meta-analysis. Circulation 1991;*84*:1977–1983.
26. Hine LK, Laird N, Hewitt P, Chalmers TC. Meta-analytic evidence against prophylactic use of lidocaine in acute myocardial infarction. Arch Intern Med 1989;*149*:2694–2698.
27. The Anturane Reinfarction Trial Research Group. Sulfinpyrazone in the prevention of sudden death after myocardial infarction. N Engl J Med 1980;*302*:250–256.
28. Temple R, Pledger GW. Special report: The FDA's critique of the Anturane Reinfarction Trial. N Engl J Med 1980;*303*:1488–1492.
29. Temple R. Food and Drug Administration's guidelines for clinical testing of drugs in the elderly. Drug Info J 1985;*19*:483–486.
30. Temple R. The clinical investigation of drugs in the elderly; food and drug guidelines. Clin Pharmacol Ther 1987;*42*:681–685.
31. Byar DP, Schoenfeld DA, Green SB, Amato DA, Davis R, DeGruttola V, Finkelstein DM, Gatsonis C, Gelber RD, Lagakos S, Lefkopoulou M, Tsiatis A, Zelen M, Peto J, Freedman LS, Gail M, Simon R, Ellenberg SS, Anderson JR, Collins R, Peto R, Peto T. Design considerations for AIDS trials. N Engl J Med 1990;*323*:1343–1348.
32. Guideline for the study and evaluation of gender differences in the clinical evaluation of drugs. Fed Reg 1993;*58*:39409–39416.
33. Khaw KT. Where are the women in studies of coronary heart disease? BMJ 1993;*306*:1146–1147.
34. Gurwitz JH, Col NF, Avorn J. The exclusion of the elderly and women from clinical trials in acute myocardial infarction. JAMA 1992;*268*:1417–1422.

35. Steering Committee of the Physicians' Health Study Research Group. Final report on the aspirin component of the ongoing Physicians' Health Study. N Engl J Med 1989;*321*:129–135.

36. (Reference to publication of ICH guideline on studies in the elderly.)

37. Oates NS, Shah RR, Idle JR, Smith RL. Influence of oxidation polymorphism on phenformin kinetics and dynamics. Clin Pharmacol Ther 1983;*34*:827–834.

38. Shah RR, Oates NS, Idle JR, Smith RL, Lockhart JDF. Impaired oxidation of debrisoquine in patients with perhexilene neuropathy. BMJ 1982;*284*:295–299.

39. Bergstrom RF, Peyton AL, Lemberger L. Quantification and mechanism of the fluoxetine and tricyclic antidepressant interaction. Clin Pharmacol Ther 1992;*51*:239–248.

40. Honig PK, Wortham DC, Zamanik, Couner DP, Mullin JC, Cantilena LR. Terfenidine-ketoconazole interaction: pharmacokinetic and electrocardiographic consequences. JAMA 1993;*269*:1513–1518.

41. Honig PK, Woosley RL, Zamaric K, Conner DP, Cantilena LR. Changes in the pharmacokinetics and electrocardiograph pharmacodynamics of terfenidine with concomitant administration of erythromycin. Clin Pharmacol Ther 1992;*52*:231–238.

42. Woosley RL, Chen Y, Freiman JP, Gillis RA. Mechanism of the cardiotoxic actions of terfenidine. JAMA 1993;*269*:1535–1539.

43. Monahan BP, Fergusen CL, Villeary ES, Lloyd BK, Troy J, Cantilena LR. Torsades de pointes occurring in association with terfenidine use. JAMA 1990;*264*:2788–2790.

44. Edgar B, Bailey D, Bergstrand R, Johnsson G, Regarth CG. Acute effects of drinking grapefruit juice on the pharmacokinetics and dynamics of felodipine and its potential clinical relevance. Eur J Clin Pharmacol 1992;*42*:313–317.

45. Peck CC, Temple R, Collins JM. Editorial: understanding consequences of concurrent therapies. JAMA 1992;*269*:1550–1552.

Reviews

r1. Cooper RM, ed. Food and drug law. Washington: Food and Drug Law Institute, 1991.

r2. Hutt PB, Merrill RA, eds. Food and drug law, cases and materials, 2d. Westbury, New York: The Foundation Press, 1991.

CHAPTER 114

Development of Drug Laws and Regulations in Europe

Kersten Ekberg-Eriksén

History

Legislation to control medicines in Europe dates back to medieval times. The first known law in Europe appeared in the 10th century in Sicily, followed later in the 11th and 12th centuries in many other countries such as Britain, France, and Germany. Inspectors of pharmacies (apothecaries) were appointed and the distribution of imported herbs and spices was controlled.

The first pharmacopoeia in a modern sense was published in Florence in 1498; other cities followed (Barcelona 1535, Nürnberg 1546) and issued obligatory formularies. Control was limited to physical properties of medicines such as appearance, taste, and odor.

Modern concepts of the control of drugs were first introduced in the 1920s, e.g., in Britain a Therapeutic Substances Act was passed in 1925. A Royal Decree in Sweden in 1934 stated that in order to be registered, a product should be designed to prevent, alleviate, or cure disease or symptoms of disease in human beings or animals, and that the efficacy and the safety of the product should be proved. These main principles for licensing drugs have remained essentially unchanged, although the various detailed requirements have developed substantially.

Thalidomide, a drug used between 1959 and 1962 as a hypnotic, caused fetal deformation if the drug was taken by women early in pregnancy. This tragedy forced many countries to tighten their requirements for approval of new drugs. However, no initiatives were taken to ensure consistency between various European countries, and each nation issued its own new laws. Although these laws were based on the same approach—proof of quality, safety, and efficacy—there were significant differences regarding specific documentation requirements.

The Treaty of Rome 1957 established the European Economic Community (EEC) and set the objective of a single market between six states (France, Germany, Belgium, Italy, Luxembourg, and the Netherlands). Between 1973 and 1986 another six countries became members (Denmark, Ireland, UK, Greece, Portugal, and Spain). To reach the goal of a common market, comprising the free movement of goods, persons, services, and capital, barriers to free trade have to be removed. If disparities between national legislations create obstacles to trade, these must be eliminated by the harmonization of the regulations concerned into common rules applicable throughout the Community. The provisions of community law prevail over conflicting national laws and regulations.

In 1965 the Community passed legislation on the policy of governmental control of medicinal products at the European level. Further directives were issued in 1975 stating in more detail the requirements for approval of drugs. The spirit of these directives was then reflected in revisions of or amendments to national laws.

Current Drug Registration Systems—European Community (EC)

Although drug registration laws became very similar in the member states by mid-70s, their interpretation varied and caused deviations in decisions on approvals. A Committee for Proprietary Medicinal Products (CPMP) was set up in 1977 "to facilitate the adoption of a common position by the Member States with regard to decisions on the issuing of marketing authorizations and to promote thereby the free movement of proprietary medicinal products." The Committee consists of one representative from each of the Member States and representatives from the EC Commission. To reach harmonization of the registration systems in the European countries and to avoid, as far as possible, duplication of assessments, two new registration procedures were introduced—the concertation procedure and the multistate procedure.

The concertation procedure requires referral of biotechnologic products to the CPMP for an opinion before the product can be approved in any of the member states. This procedure also can be used on a voluntary basis for other "highly innovative" products. The multistate procedure is optional and involves a request by an applicant for authorization to market a product in at least two member states other than the state that granted the first authorization. The CPMP is involved in this procedure to support and facilitate a common opinion, and to ensure that consensus is reached on the assessment of the documentation. The problem with both of these procedures is that, irrespective of the opinion expressed by the CPMP, the final decision still rests with the individual member states. This has led to variations in the details of the approval, e.g., indications, dosages, etc.

During the development of the common registration system within the EC (1965–1993) countries outside the community e.g., Austria, Switzerland, and the Nordic countries, have to a large extent also adopted the EC rules and regulations for approval of new drugs. Thus, it is possible to use the same format and content for an application in all western European countries. Other European countries probably will also issue pharmaceutical laws in line with those of the EC in the near future.

The Future European Registration System

The treaty of European Union (EU) was signed in February 1993. Regulations for the future registration system were issued in 1993 and will come into force January 1, 1995 with a transitional period until January 1, 1998.

The new system is composed of two evaluation procedures, one centralized and the other decentralized. It also includes the formation of a new institution—the European Agency for the Evaluation of Medicinal Products. This Agency will be located in London. National applications within the EU will be possible only for products to be marketed in one country. However, in European countries outside the EU, national applications will still be possible.

The Centralized Procedure

The centralized procedure (Table 114.1) must be used for biotechnologic products and may also be used for other products considered significant innovations. An application for marketing authorization for such products has to be submitted to the European Agency. The CPMP will organize the assessment of the application and issue a scientific opinion within 210 days. All member states and the EU Commission will be informed of the opinion. A Standing Committee on Medicinal Products for Human Use will assist the Commission in the decision procedure. If all parties involved are in agreement, the Commission will take a final decision that is binding on all member states. Thus, the advantage with this procedure is that an approval for marketing of a new product is valid throughout the EU countries.

Table 114.1 EU Registration Application

EU Centralized Procedure

Registration application

The European Agency for the evaluation of medicinal products

CPMP

Experts
Rapporteurs
Working parties

Management Board

Agency secretariat

210 days

CPMP opinion

unfavorable

Company appeal

60 days

Second CPMP opinion

favorable

30 days

EU Commission Member States

30 days

Draft Commission decision

Standing Committee

Commission decision

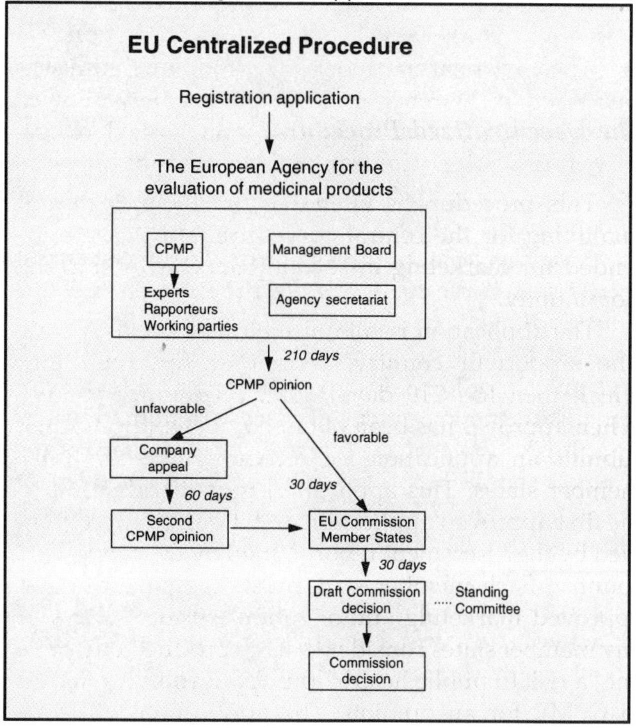

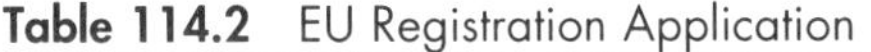

Table 114.2 EU Registration Application

EU Registration Application

PART I Summary of Dossier	PART II Chemical/Pharmaceutical/ Biologic Documentation	PART III Pharmaco-Toxicologic Documentation	PART IV Clinical Documentation
IA - Administrative Data	II - Table of Contents	III - Table of Contents	IV - Table of Contents
IB_1 - Summary of Product Characteristics	IIA - Composition	IIIA - Single dose toxicity/ Repeated dose toxicity	IVA - Clinical Pharmacology
IB_2 - Packaging/Labeling details	IIB - Method of Preparation	IIIB - Reproductive function	IVB - Clinical experience
IC - Expert Reports	IIC - Control of Starting Materials	IIIC - Embryo-fetal and perinatal toxicity	IVQ - Other
(i) Chemical/ Pharmaceutical/ Biologic Documentation	IID - Control Tests on Intermediate Products	IIID - Mutagenic potential	
(ii) Toxicologic and Pharmacologic Documentation	IIE - Control Tests on the Finished Product	IIIE - Carcinogenic potential	Case Report Forms must be available on request
(iii) Clinical Documentation	IIF - Stability	IIIF - Pharmacodynamics	
	IIG - Bioavailability/ Bioequivalence	IIIG - Pharmacokinetics	
	IIH - Stability	IIIH - Local tolerance	
	IIQ - Other	IIQ - Other	

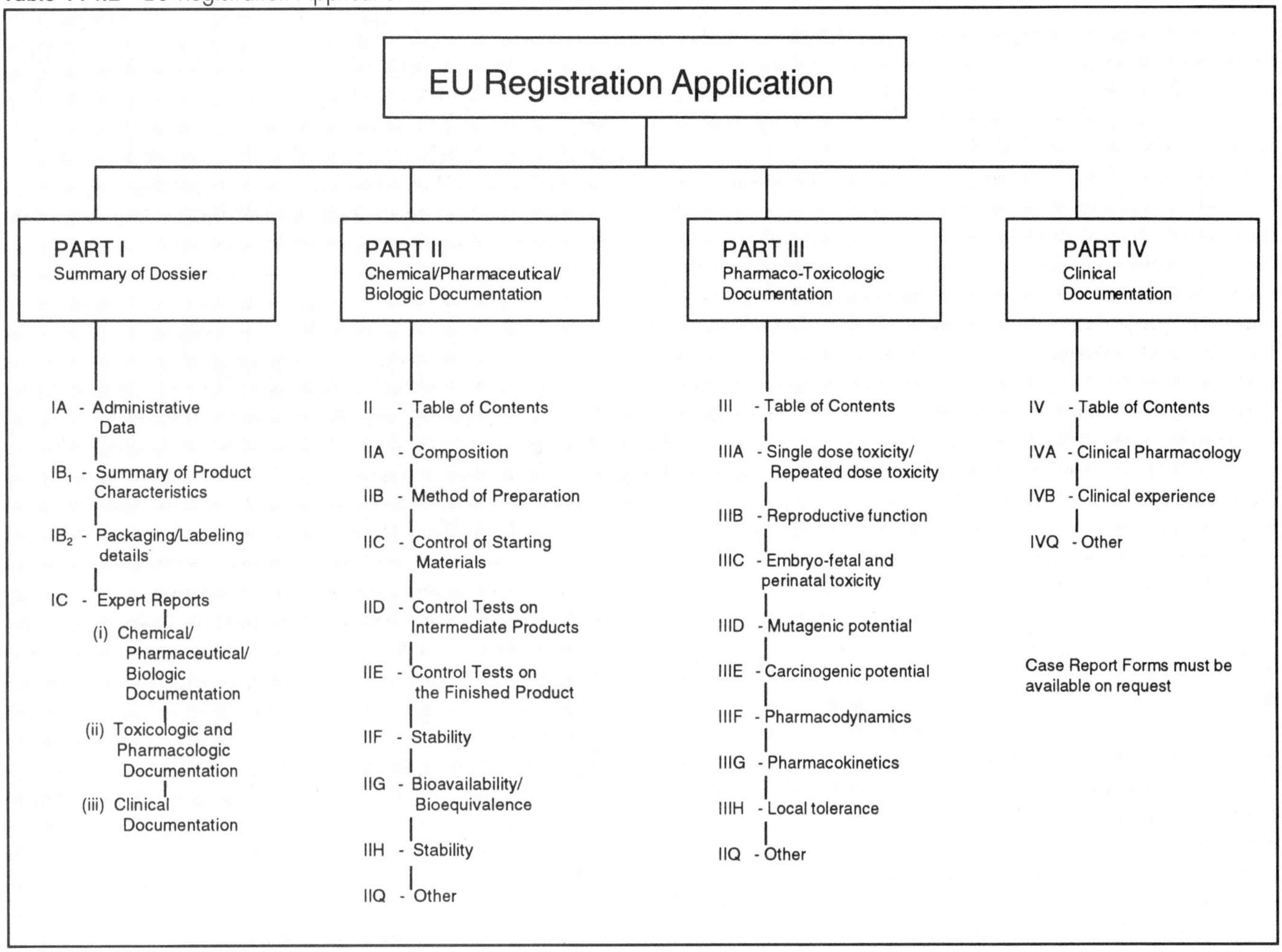

The Decentralized Procedure

This procedure is intended for all products not qualifying for the central procedure and that are intended for marketing in several countries within the Community.

The application is submitted to one member state (the rapporteur country, chosen by the applicant), which then has 210 days to act on the application. When approval has been obtained, the applicant then submits an application for recognition to the other member states. This application must be identical to the first approved application and it must be accompanied by the assessment report issued by the rapporteur country. Each member state must recognize the first approved marketing authorization within 90 days. If any member states consider that the product may present "a risk to public health" the application is referred to CPMP for an opinion. The application will then follow the same route as described for the centralized procedure, leading to a binding decision by the EU Commission.

Requirements for the Registration Application

The application for a marketing authorization, whether submitted according to the centralized, decentralized, or national system, has to include evidence for quality, safety, and efficacy of the drug. The requirements are stated in various national or European laws and directives; in addition, many guidelines giving further details have been issued. Within the European Union information about registration systems, etc., can be found in the "Notice to Applicants" issued by the European Commission. The structure and content of an application is shown in Table 114.2.

Table 114.3 Summary of Product Characteristics (Guideline III/9163/89)

TRADE NAME OF THE MEDICINAL PRODUCT

QUALITATIVE AND QUANTITATIVE COMPOSITION

PHARMACEUTICAL FORM

CLINICAL PARTICULARS
- Therapeutic indications
- Posology and method of administration
- Contraindications
- Special warnings and special precautions for use
- Interaction with other medicaments and other forms of interaction
- Pregnancy and lactation
- Effects on ability to drive and use machines
- Undesirable effects
- Overdosage

PHARMACOLOGIC PROPERTIES
- Pharmacodynamic properties
- Pharmacokinetic properties
- Preclinical safety data

PHARMACEUTICAL PARTICULARS
- List of excipients
- Incompatibilities
- Shelflife
- Special precautions for storage
- Nature and contents of container
- Instructions for use/handling

MARKETING AUTHORIZATION HOLDER
Name or style and permanent address or registered place of business of the holder of the marketing authorization

MARKETING AUTHORIZATION NUMBER

DATA OF FIRST AUTHORIZATION/RENEWAL OF AUTHORIZATION

DATA OF (PARTIAL) REVISION OF THE TEXT

The over-all requirements for documentation are similar to those of the US and Japan, although the format and other details differ in some respects. A requirement unique for Europe is the Expert Report, which must be provided separately for quality, safety, and efficacy. These reports consist of a critical appraisal of the product and the documentation available (a factual summary is not sufficient). Expert Reports should be prepared by qualified and experienced specialists.

Preclinical studies must be performed according to the principles of Good Laboratory Practice, and clinical trials to the principles of Good Clinical Practice, if they are to be recognized as valid in a European application. Once approved, the validity of the authorization is five years and the holder has then to apply for renewal.

Clinical Trials

In some countries a formal regulatory authority approval is needed before clinical trials can commence (e.g., UK, Sweden, Italy); in other countries, notification of the trial is enough. The trend in Europe, however, is to introduce formal approval requirements. Hopefully, this is an area within which the regulations will soon be harmonized.

An application, where applicable, for clinical trials includes information on the product to be tested (pharmaceutical, pharmaco-toxicologic documentation) and the clinical trial protocol, patient information, and investigator's brochure. Clinical trials must be performed according to the principles of the declaration of Helsinki and be approved by regional/local ethics committees. The computerization of clinical trial data must follow local data laws.

Adverse Reaction Reporting

All serious adverse reactions occurring with a pharmaceutical product in the EU, whether under clinical investigation or during marketed use, must be reported to the health authorities within 15 days. Extensive safety up-date reports must also be presented at the time of renewal of the market authorization (every 5 years).

Information to Physicians and Patients

The summary of product characteristics gives prescribing physicians information about the properties of the drug, approved indications, dosage, adverse reactions, contraindications, warnings and precautions, etc. This document (Table 114.3) must be approved by the health authorities.

A patient leaflet must be attached to or included in the drug package and should give patients relevant information, in layman's language, about the product.

Supply and Control of Medicinal Products

The European Council has issued a directive to harmonize the basic principles for the supply of pharmaceutical products. The two major categories of products are those that require medical prescription, and those not subject to medical prescription. In addition, subcategories are recommended for products available only on prescription. These subcategories are:

1. Product on renewable or nonrenewable prescription.
2. Products subject to special medical prescription.
3. Products on restricted medical prescription, reserved for use in certain specialized areas.

If a product contains a substance classified as narcotic or psychotropic within the meaning of the United Nations Conventions of 1961 and 1971, it belongs to the subcategory "special medical prescription." Similarly, products that present a risk of medical abuse, lead to addiction, or can be misused for illegal purposes fall within the same subcategory. Narcotic drugs are subject to the most stringent regulations, which also cover storage. Supplies must be kept under lock and key, and quantities in stock and those dispensed precisely recorded. In many countries, prescriptions must be specially filed for review by government inspection. Through such control, the authorities can monitor potential misuse at the level of the patient, pharmacist, and physician.

References

Council Regulation (EEC) No. 2309/93 of 22 July, 1993 laying down community procedures for the authorization and supervision of medical products for human and veterinary use and establishing a European Agency for the Evaluation of Medicinal Products. EEC Official Journal No. L214, August 24, 1993.

Council Directive (EEC) 92/26 of 31 March, 1992 concerning the Classification of Medicinal Products for Human Use. EEC Official Journal No. L213, April 30, 1992.

Commission of the European Communities. Notice to Applicants III/3567/92. Office for Official Publications of the European Communities 2 rue Mereier, L-2985 Luxembourg.

Penn RG. The state control of medicines—The first 3000 years. Br J Clin Pharmacol 1979;*8*:293–305.

Walker, SR, Griffin JP. eds. International medicines regulations—a forward look to 1992. 1988, Dordrecht; Kluvver Academic Publishers.

SECTION XV

Pharmacology for Special Patient Populations

Editor:
Paul L. Munson

CHAPTER 115

Kjel A. Johnson
David P. Strum
W. David Watkins

Pharmacology and the Critical Care Patient

Introduction

The movement that led to the modern intensive care unit (ICU) began in the late 1950s in the US. Since then, diversification of care and sophistication of technology required for critically ill patients is at an all time high; ICUs in the US account for 20 to 30 percent of hospital costs, 7 percent of the hospital beds, and 1 percent of the total gross national product. It is likely that the portion of hospital costs committed to caring for the critically ill will increase as the emphasis of health care in the US shifts toward ambulatory medicine. Drug therapy represents a large part of total ICU costs. Providing drug therapy may be complicated in critically ill patients, who often display altered drug disposition and response. This chapter will describe the basis for these changes and how the ICU patient differs from "normal." It will attempt to provide a rational basis for the appropriate use of drugs in this important clinical setting.

The term "critical care patient" challenges definition, beginning with the often subjective criteria that route a patient to the ICU. The medical condition of these patients usually warrants extensive physiologic monitoring, high level technologic or diagnostic procedures, and aggressive pharmacologic support. Pharmacotherapy in the ICU is complicated by a number of patient factors, including the extremes of age, and the many variables likely to be encountered when any single disease state is compounded by the complexities of multiple organ dysfunction. The most common disorders leading to ICU admission are cardiovascular diseases, sepsis, renal failure, respiratory failure, and liver failure.[1,2,3] The highest mortality rate is reported in patients with hepatic failure (71%), cardiac arrest (68%), or respiratory failure (48%). In addition, it is now axiomatic that mortality increases with the number of affected organ systems: failure of two organ systems is associated with a 55 percent mortality rate; failure of three organ systems is associated with an 85 percent mortality rate; failure of four or more approaches 100 percent mortality. It should be obvious that the physiologic changes that warrant "critical care" also will reflect abnormal and occasionally unpredictable responses to drugs. Although intuitive and of considerable practical importance, there is little objective research that systematically documents the influence of disease(s) on "normal" drug effect and disposition.

Intensive care patients are known to be at particular risk for developing adverse drug reactions (ADRs). Risk factors for the development of an ADR include advanced age, the practice of treating a single disease process with multiple drugs (polypharmacy), and inappropriate dosage selection. The average number of medications prescribed per patient during care in an ICU is 12.1 ± 7.6 (daily average of 7.5 ± 3.4 drugs).[4] Figure 115.1 illustrates that these patients have at least a 50 percent chance of developing an ADR.[r1]

Currently, most pharmacodynamic and pharmacokinetic data in humans are obtained from studies in young, healthy subjects. It is not surprising that data from such sources do not reflect the pharmacology of the critically ill patient. Although a few pharmacoki-

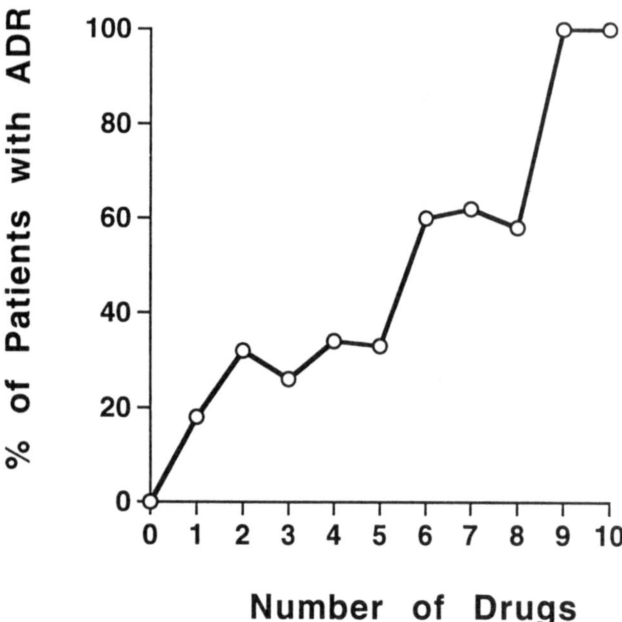

Figure 115.1 Percentage of hospitalized patients displaying adverse drug reactions as the number of medications taken concomitantly increases.

netic studies of the critically ill patient have been conducted, pharmacodynamic data are very limited in these conditions. Collecting such data is extremely labor-intensive and is often confounded by uncontrolled error and variability in measurement ("noise"), all of which will limit the useful assessment of pharmacodynamic parameters. Disease-related changes in receptor number, receptor responsivity, or drug-receptor interaction may occur independent of pharmacokinetic parameter changes.

This chapter highlights pharmacokinetic and pharmacodynamic alterations associated with the primary disease states leading to ICU admission, and it considers how these changes may alter drug therapy. Such principles can serve the practitioner to predict drug effects in compromised patients more accurately.

Pharmacology in Aging Patients

The elderly patient population is defined conventionally as greater than 65 years of age. These patients constitute up to 51 percent of all ICU admissions.[5] Relative to young, healthy adults, a patient in the eighth decade normally will exhibit a reduction in both renal and hepatic function of about 50 percent. Elderly patients presenting to ICUs are regularly undernourished and dehydrated. For these reasons, drug action and disposition may be altered significantly.

The elderly patient may have modest changes in GI drug absorption secondary to a reduction in enteric muscle tone and peristalsis. In addition, the pH of the gastric contents is generally increased, which may cause chemical degradation of compounds that are unstable in an alkaline environment, or that may prevent conversion of a prodrug to its active compound with drugs requiring an acidic environment for this transformation. Changes in drug distribution may occur resulting from: (1) changes in serum protein concentration resulting from poor nutrition; and (2) a reduction in volume of distribution (Vd) in part owing to limited fluid intake. The elderly should be assumed to be volume-depleted unless proved otherwise.

Hepatic clearance (Cl) of drugs may be reduced in the elderly patient. Up to a 40 percent reduction in liver blood flow has been reported,[6] much of which is a manifestation of impaired cardiac output. This is manifest in reduced hepatic elimination of high-clearance, flow-dependent drugs (e.g., lidocaine, propranolol, and morphine). Sufficient evidence is now available to show a reduced ability for the elderly to eliminate drugs by Phase I (oxidative) metabolism, such as diazepam.[7] This is due, at least in part, to an age-related reduction in liver mass. At this time, there are not enough data to state conclusively that Phase II (conjugation) biotransformation is affected by age, but it is generally believed that no such changes occur.

The major contribution to pharmacokinetic changes in the elderly is reduced renal function. Lindeman et al.[8] evaluated the change in renal function in healthy patients at decade intervals from 20 to 100 years of age. Although no significant change in serum creatinine concentration was measured between any decade studied, significant reductions in measured creatinine Cl (Cl_{cr}) were found in both women and men as age increased. An individual in the eighth decade has a Cl_{cr} approximately 50 percent that of a person in the third decade. Many drugs used to treat elderly patients in the ICU depend on renal elimination. Examples include beta-lactam antibiotics, histamine-2 receptor blockers, and antidysrhythmic agents. Prolonging the dosage interval for such drugs is sufficient compensation for the reduced renal function.

Most ADRs occurring in the elderly ICU patient are a result of age-related changes in pharmacokinetic parameters that result in drug accumulation. However, changes in receptor number and function also may lead to altered pharmacologic response. It is now established that receptor density and receptor sensitivity may be altered in the elderly patient. Lymphocyte β-receptor density correlates with myocardial receptor density. Receptor density is reduced in lymphocytes from elderly humans when compared to young adults. This change in receptor numbers, however, fails to explain fully changes in pharmacodynamic parameters observed in the elderly. Studies in elderly human patients have demonstrated a shift in concentration-effect relationships between intracellular cyclic adenosine monophosphate (cAMP) production and β-adrenergic receptor responsivity, suggesting reduced receptor sensitivity. Current studies suggest that the reason for this alteration may be a limitation in cellular signal transduction (coupling and amplification), causing alterations in β-adrenergic receptor response in the elderly. Vestal et al.[9] found that the dose of propranolol required to decrease heart rate by 25 beats per minute (bpm) correlated with age. They also found a linear relationship between age and propranolol resistance, as measured by the apparent dissociation constant for propranolol binding to the receptor, which quantifies propranolol resistance. While it is known that the density of the β-adrenergic receptor is reduced in the elderly, the pharmacodynamic changes seen in this study are likely due to reduced receptor sensitivity. It has been demonstrated that cAMP production from peripheral lymphocytes and other body tissues is diminished in this population, which results in a shift of the concentration-effect curve to the right. Recent studies have suggested that there is a reduction in high affinity binding sites and a change in post-receptor transduction, which helps explain the relative reduction in sensitivity of beta-adrenergic receptors in the elderly.

There is conflicting evidence as to whether α_1 and α_2 adrenoreceptors undergo changes in responsiveness in these patients. Data reviewed by Docherty suggest that a reduction in α_2 adrenergic response occurs, but not in α_1 receptors.[10] Baroreceptor sensitivity, however, as measured by change in heart rate per unit change in mean arterial pressure, inversely correlated with age in a study by Irving et al.[11] In this study baroreceptor sensitivity fell 50 to 90 percent as age increased from 35 to 70 years. This may predispose the elderly patient to ADR development, particularly with drugs that may cause a precipitous reduction in blood pressure upon first exposure.

Abernethy and colleagues[12] studied the disposition and pharmacodynamics of verapamil in young and elderly hypertensive patients. The half-life ($T_{1/2}$) was prolonged, and Cl was reduced in the elderly. However, larger drug concentrations were required to provide the same degree of PR interval prolongation witnessed in young hypertensive patients, as illustrated by the increased concentration required to produce 50 percent of maximal effect (EC_{50}). Maximum effect (E_{max}), described as maximum prolongation of the PR interval for this study, was significantly greater in the younger group (Table 115.1). The very old patients had a 6 bpm reduction in heart rate; young patients had an 8 bpm reflex tachycardia. Unexpectedly, there was a trend toward greater hypotensive effect in the elderly patients. These preliminary data suggest that the elderly patient may have a greater response in blood pressure control to calcium channel blockers, while the effect of calcium channel blockade on the AV node may be blunted.

Current data suggest that with age there is a shift to the left (increased sensitivity) of benzodiazepine plasma concentration-psychomotor performance pharmacodynamic plots. This was most recently illustrated by Bertz et al,[13] who compared psychomotor effects of alprazolam in 21 healthy young men to nine healthy elderly men. The duration of drug effect was prolonged in the elderly group, but no difference in Cl was measurable. The sigmoid E_{max} model was fit to psychomotor data. EC_{50} values were approximately 40 percent lower in the elderly for psychomotor measurements, such as card-sorting and digit/symbol substitution. This study further illustrates altered drug response because of pharmacodynamic changes, independent of pharmacokinetic changes in the elderly patient.

The Patient with Cardiac Failure

Pharmacokinetics often are altered as a result of heart failure[r2] (Fig 115.2). Congestive heart failure (CHF) may lead to reduced absorption of a multitude of drugs. This is a consequence of impaired cardiac output that in turn limits blood circulation to the gut. Drugs shown to be affected include Class 1A antidysrhythmic agents and diuretics such as metolazone and furosemide. It is noteworthy that these drugs often have been evaluated in single-dose studies and may not reflect the reduction in renal or hepatic C1 that may occur with chronic administration.

Drug distribution depends on route of administration, protein binding, blood flow, and rate and extent of drug penetration into various body compartments. Heart failure affects drug distribution as a result of reducing blood flow to organs. Fluid overload may

Table 115.1 Changes in Verapamil Pharmacokinetic and Pharmacodynamic Parameters in Elderly versus Young Hypertensives. * $p < 0.05$ vs. Young Patients

	Young	Elderly	Very Elderly
Age (yr)	29 ± 5	68 ± 4	84 ± 9
$T_{1/2}$(hr)	3.8 ± 1.1	7.4 ± 3.3*	8.0 ± 1.2*
Cl (l/min·kg)	15.5 ± 4.5	10.5 ± 3.4*	8.0 ± 4.1*
E_{max} (ms)	43.8 ± 14.8	19.9 ± 5.2*	11.7 ± 5.1*
EC_{50}(ng/ml)	22.2 ± 3.8	26.5 ± 15.2	103 ± 68*

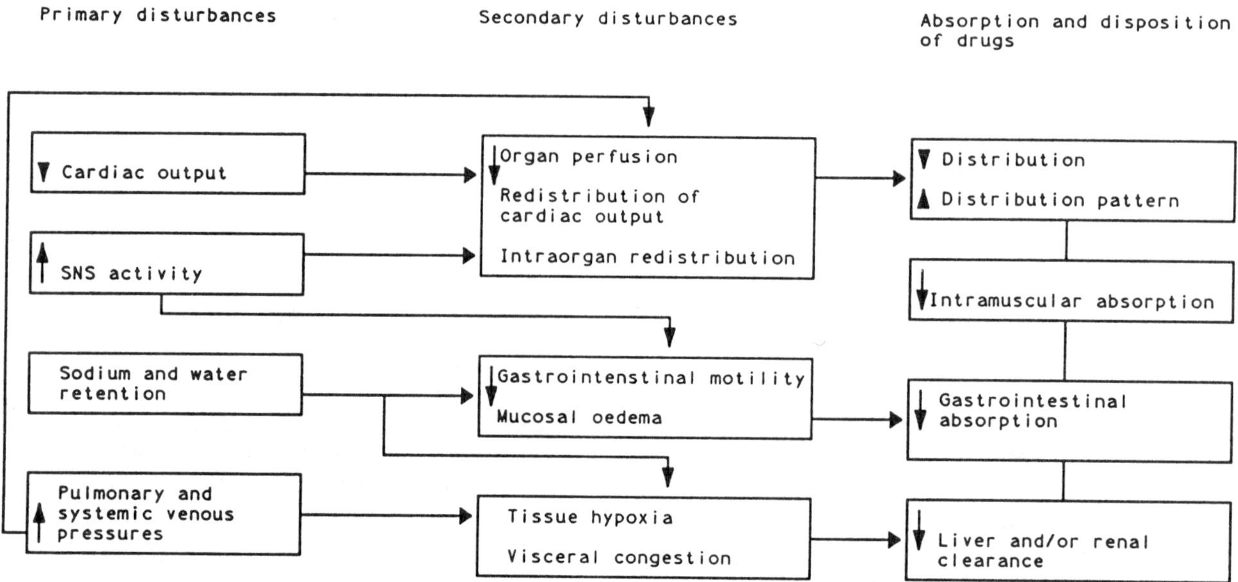

Figure 115.2 Pathophysiology of Heart Failure and the Effects on Pharmacokinetics (with permission[r2])

increase the Vd of drugs largely distributed in plasma. Liver metabolism of drugs also may be diminished in patients with CHF. Drugs subject to this reduced metabolic rate are those that are primarily flow-dependent. Blood flow to the liver in CHF patients is reduced and appears to change in proportion to cardiac output. CHF also may cause a direct reduction in the metabolic capacity of the liver. Presumably this is caused by cellular damage following congestion or low perfusion, and/or impaired microsomal drug oxidation from hypoxemia. Ritz et al.[14] found a positive linear relationship between $T_{1/2}$ of indocyanine green and cardiac index. Mean hepatic blood flow in young subjects studied by Leithe[15] was 595 ± 116 ml/min/m,[2] while the mean hepatic blood flow for patients with New York Heart Association (NYHA) functional class I–IV CHF was significantly lower (340 ± 153 ml/min/m^2). This study also reported a linear correlation between cardiac index and hepatic blood flow. In the same study, mean renal blood flow in healthy subjects was 607 ± 172 ml/min/m^2, but was reduced to 395 ± 131 ml/min/m^2 in patients with NYHA Class I through III CHF. Renal blood flow was directly proportional to cardiac index in this study. Other studies have also found reduced renal Cl in patients with CHF. In a study by Naffs et al.,[16] renal digoxin Cl was evaluated in patients with lone atrial fibrillation and in patients with CHF. Digoxin Cl in the CHF population was significantly lower than in the patients with atrial fibrillation (48 ± 21 vs 71 ± 36 ml/min). In addition, serum digoxin concentrations were shown to be significantly higher in patients with CHF when compared with patients without heart failure given the same amount of drug (1.44 ± 0.47 vs 0.87 ± 0.33 ng/ml).

Several changes in pharmacodynamics have been found in the heart failure patient. Brater et al.[17] studied eight healthy subjects and ten patients with clinically stable CHF with a mean left ventricular ejection fraction (LVEF) of 45 ± 18 percent. Heart failure patients excreted the same total amount of furosemide, but had delayed urinary excretion time and a prolonged duration of furosemide excretion. Nine of the ten heart failure patients had an attenuated response to furosemide when compared to healthy subjects. The investigators found that the sigmoid E_{max} model described data from six of the ten CHF patients. When compared to healthy subjects, three of these six patients had a significantly increased EC_{50} and five of six had a substantially reduced E_{max} (Fig. 115.3). These data illustrate the diuretic resistance that occurs in patients with heart failure.

Beta-adrenergic receptor stimulation is not only the body's in vitro response to heart failure, but it is also a cornerstone of medical management for acute heart failure that leads to increased adenylate cyclase production of intracellular cAMP and, ultimately, an increase in cardiac performance. The acute improvements in hemodynamics are realized for only four to seven days, at which point receptor down-regulation leads to loss of response. The cause of this down-regulation, whether endogenous norepinephrine (NE) production or inotrope administration, is explained by a reduction in absolute number of β_1 receptors on the myocardium, as well as in other tissues in the body.

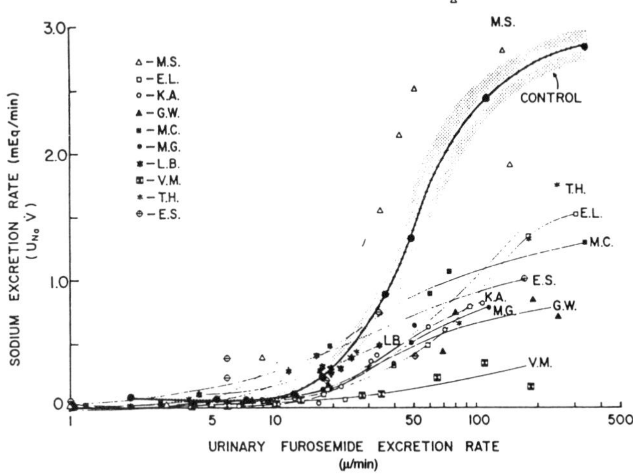

Figure 115.3 Pharmacodynamic relationship between furosemide excretion rate and diuretic effect in patients with and without heart failure. The heavy line through solid circles represents the mean relationship found in healthy subjects (with permission[17]).

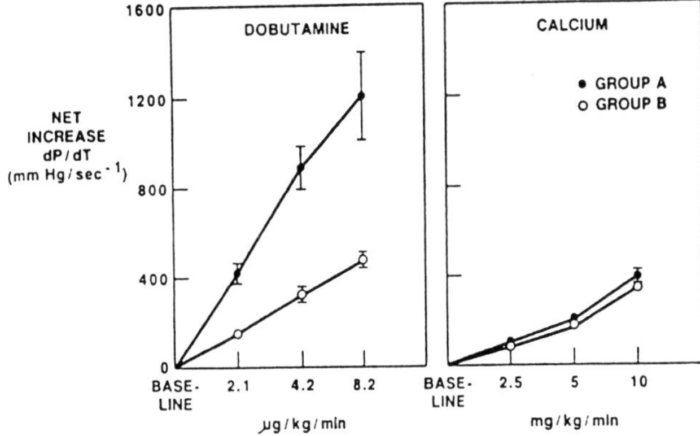

Figure 115.4 Net increase in peak positive left ventricular dP/dt in patients with ejection fractions > 40% (group A) and in patients with ejection fractions less than 30% (group B) for both dobutamine and calcium infusions (with permission[22]).

Repeatedly, survival has been inversely correlated to NE plasma concentrations in the heart failure population.[18,19] Down regulation of β receptors occurs at all levels of heart failure severity. Although both β_1- and β_2-adrenergic receptors couple to adenylate cyclase to provide an increase in inotropic and chronotropic function, only β_1-receptor stimulation is capable of evoking maximal inotropic effects in the ventricle. Interestingly, β_1-receptor function is attenuated in all types of heart failure, while β_2 receptor function may be altered only in some.[20] β_2 receptors are unaffected by idiopathic cardiomyopathy and heart failure resulting from aortic valve insufficiency, but these receptors do appear to display down-regulation to ischemic cardiomyopathy, mitral valve insufficiency, and tetralogy of Fallot.

Current investigation suggests that the human heart does not have "spare" β receptors.[21] Bristow estimates a 60 to 70 percent reduction in β_1-receptor density, 30 percent reduction in β_2-receptor responsiveness, and a 30 to 40 percent increase in the activity of the inhibitory guanine nucleotide binding protein (G_i-protein) activity in patients with severe heart failure. These receptor changes result in an estimated 50 percent reduction in inotropic response to β agonists in patients with heart failure, although no change in response to the inotropic effect of calcium is apparent. Fowler et al.[22] found calcium-induced contractility did not change in patients with heart failure, but contractility from β-receptor stimulation was reduced (Fig. 115.4.).

The concentration-effect relationship of angiotensin converting enzyme (ACE) inhibitors in heart failure has been reported[23] (Fig. 115.5). The heart failure patient, however, is at increased risk of adverse effects secondary to ACE inhibition. There are several plausible explanations, including pharmacokinetic changes in renal and hepatic Cl. However, stimulation of the renin-angiotensin-aldosterone system as a compensatory response in heart failure, as well as a result of diuretic use, may predispose the patient to increased sensitivity to ACE inhibition. To date, no studies have compared the concentration-effect relationships of ACE inhibitors in heart failure patients and healthy subjects.

Whether heart failure changes the responsiveness of α-adrenergic receptors remains controversial. Several animal studies have reported a reduction in response to continuous receptor stimulation, but human studies have failed to arrive at the same conclusions. Schwinn[24] and colleagues compared the pharmacodynamic effects of phenylephrine on mean arterial pressure in 12 patients with LVEF less than 40 percent (mean EF = 33.9%) and in patients without LV dysfunction (mean EF = 54.0%). The dose of phenylephrine required to increase MAP to 20 percent greater than baseline (PD_{20}) was not found to differ before anesthesia, but during fentanyl administration the patients with impaired LV function required significantly more phenylephrine to reach PD_{20}. Furthermore, a significant inverse relationship was found between LVEF and PD_{20}, as shown in Figure 115.6. These results indicate that LVEF may reduce α_1- adrenergic receptor responsiveness when fentanyl anesthesia is coadministered in the critical care setting, necessitating increased drug administration.

The Renal Failure Patient

Renal failure is often secondary to other diseases, such as diabetes, hypertension, and glomerular nephri-

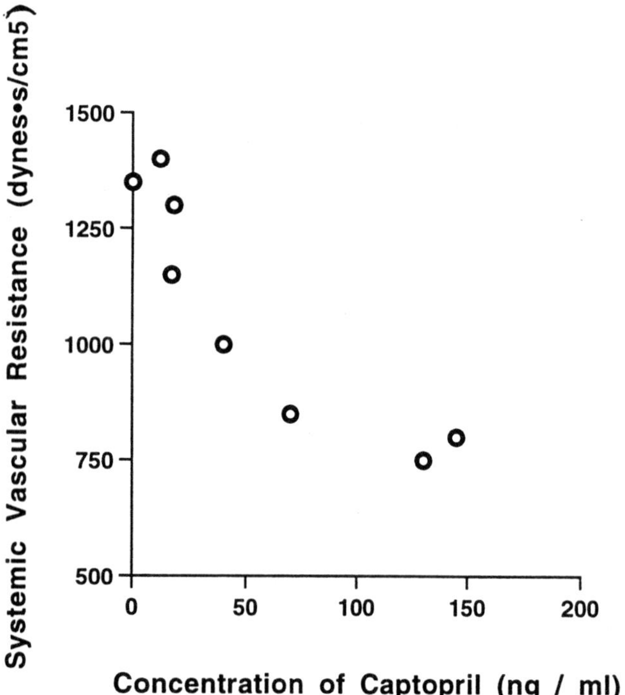

Figure 115.5 Pharmacodynamic relationship of captopril concentration vs. systemic vascular resistance in patients with severe heart failure (adapted from Cody et al.[23]).

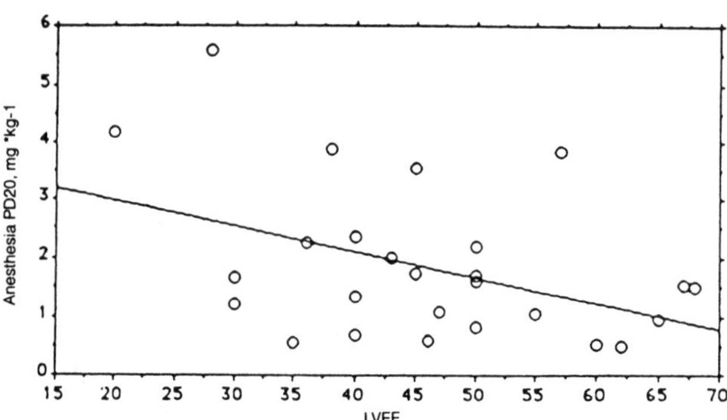

Figure 115.6 Relationship of the phenylephrine dose required to increase mean arterial pressure by 20% (PD_{20}) to left ventricular ejection fraction (LVEF) (with permission[24]).

tis; these processes account for 60 percent of renal disease. In the critical care setting, sepsis, shock, CHF, and many other diseases may lead to renal dysfunction through impaired blood flow to the kidneys. Many patients in critical care units have some degree of renal impairment. End-stage renal disease (ESRD) is characterized by a glomerular filtration rate less than 10 ml/min, and generally requires dialysis. Changes in drug absorption in these patients may be due to the administration of antacids to control hyperphosphatemia, resulting in a change in gut pH. Total protein, including albumin, is significantly reduced in patients with ESRD. This leads to an increase in free drug concentration and potential toxicity for drugs that are highly bound to these proteins, as described previously in Chapter 2). There is also an increase in α_1-acid glycoprotein concentration in patients with ESRD when compared with healthy controls, which may lead to an increase in the Vd of basic drugs.[25] Other changes leading to alterations in Vd include modification in tissue binding,[26,27] which is illustrated for digoxin in Table 115.2. Increase in total body water may lead to an increase in the Vd of such hydrophilic drugs as the aminoglycosides. It is currently equivocal whether significant changes in metabolism occur with ESRD or less severe forms of renal disease.

The effects of renal dysfunction on drug elimination depend on such factors as the degree of functional impairment and fraction of a given drug excreted unchanged in urine. Many methods to estimate degree of renal impairment have been devised.[28] The most frequently used method to estimate glomerular filtration rate in the clinical setting is the Cockcroft-Gault method[29] shown in Equation 1. This method is based on easily accessible predictors and is reasonably accurate and precise. Prediction accuracy with this method is improved when ideal body weight is substituted for actual body weight.

Equation 1.
$$Cl_{Cr}\ \text{men} = \frac{(140 - \text{age}) \times \text{IBW}}{(72 \times \text{SCR})}$$
$$Cl_{Cr}\ \text{women} = \text{male value} \times 0.85$$

where Cl_{Cr} = creatinine clearance estimate (ml/min), age = age (yr), IBW = ideal body weight (kg), SCR = serum creatinine (mg/dl).

It is important to realize that seemingly normal serum creatinine values in the ICU patient often are associated with significant impairment of renal function. Table 115.3 lists renally-eliminated drugs frequently used in the critical care setting, and suggests appropriate dosage modifications based on Cl_{cr} estimates.[30]

Pharmacodynamic changes in the renally impaired patient are now beginning to be discovered. Changes in drug response due to azotemia were observed clinically as early as 1954, when patients with significant

Table 115.2 Half-life ($T_{1/2}$) and Volume of Distribution (Vd) of Digoxin at Various Levels of Creatinine Clearance (Cl_{Cr} in ml/min)

Cl_{Cr} (ml/min)	$T_{1/2}$ (days)	Vd (l/kg)
130	1.5	7.3
100	1.6	7.1
80	1.8	6.8
60	2.0	6.5
50	2.3	6.2
35	2.5	5.6
25	2.8	5.1
15	3.0	4.6
5	3.2	4.2

Table 115.3 Modification of Drugs Commonly Used in Intensive Care Patients Based on Renal Function (Cl_{Cr} estimate)

Drug	Usual Dose	30–50 ml/min	10–30 ml/min	<10 ml/min
Acyclovir IV	5mg/kg q8h	5mg/kg q12h	5mg/kg q24h	5mg/kg q48h
Aztreonam IV	0.5–2gm q8h	0.5–2gm q12h	0.25–1gm 12h	0.25–1gm 24h
Ceftazidime IV	250mg–1gm q8h	1gm q12h	1gm q24h	500mg q24–48h
Cimetidine IV	300mg q6h	300mg q8h	300mg q12h	300mg q24h
Ciprofloxacin IV	250–500mg q12h	250–500mg q18h	250–500mg q24h	250–500mg q24h
Co-Trimoxazole DS PO/NG	1 tab q12h	1 tab q18h	1 tab q24h	1 tab q48h
Famotidine IV	20–40mg q12h	20–40mg q24h	20–40mg q24h	20–40mg q48–72h
Fluconazole IV	100–200mg q24h	100–200mg q48h	100–200mg q72h	
Ganciclovir IV	2.5mg/kg q12h	2.5mg/kg q24h	1.25mg/kg q24h	1.25mg/kg q24h
Imipenem IV	500mg–1gm q8h	500 mg–1gm q8h	500mg q12h	250mg q12h
Meperidine PO/IM	50–150mg q3–4h	75% of usual dose	75% of usual dose	50% of usual dose
Piperacillin IV	4–6gm q6h	4–6gm q6h	3–4gm q12h	3–4gm q12h
Ranitidine IV	50mg q8h	50mg q12h	50mg q18h	50mg q24h
Sotolol PO	80mg q12h	80mg q24h	80mg q48h	Individualize

renal impairment were found to display an augmented response (maintenance of anesthesia) to IV barbiturates.[31] Much later, well-designed trials began to identify pharmacodynamic changes with several classes of drugs in this patient population. Beta adrenergic receptors appear to have increased sensitivity, as described by Galeazzi et al,[32] who studied pindolol in this population. Seven healthy volunteers were compared to six patients with ESRD receiving hemodialysis. Effect, as measured by percent reduction in exercise-induced tachycardia, was greater in the ESRD patients at any given serum pindolol concentration. Although the slopes of the concentration–effect curves were parallel, the curve of ESRD patients was shifted to the left, suggesting that the renal impaired patient is more sensitive to beta blockade.

More recently, investigators have found that nifedipine displays different pharmacodynamic parameters in patients with renal impairment.[33] Healthy volunteers were compared to three groups of patients with varying degrees of impairment. In this study, the E_{max}, measured as percent reduction in diastolic blood pressure, was significantly larger in patients with moderate or severe renal impairment when compared with the control group, and the increase in E_{max} was positively related to the degree of impairment. These changes were not explained by differences in baseline blood pressure measurements, but are likely due to reduced baroreceptor sensitivity and changes in cellular calcium balance.

In a study by Schmith et al.,[34] the effects of the benzodiazepine alprazolam in ESRD patients were compared to healthy volunteers. Psychomotor performance was impaired to a greater extent in the dialysis patients. The authors concluded that this difference may be attributable to changes in blood brain barrier permeability to alprazolam and/or an accumulation of endogenous substances that may elicit a benzodiazepine-like response. A very modest increase in memory impairment was detected, and no increased level of sedation was found.

The Liver Failure Patient

Three major factors affect drug elimination in liver disease. The first is reduced liver blood flow, which particularly affects oral drugs with high first-pass metabolism. Total organ flow depends on cardiac output as well as intrahepatic vascular resistance. Intrahepatic shunts and extrahepatic shunts, occurring, for example, at the esophagus and retroperitoneum, also reduce liver blood flow. Secondly, metabolic function is reduced. This reduction in absolute enzyme activity is a result of a reduced number of viable hepatocytes and impaired function of the viable cells. This alteration primarily affects drugs with low hepatic extraction ratio. The third effect of liver disease on drug disposition is a result of changes in plasma proteins. There is a reduction in albumin synthesis with chronic liver disease that leads to an increase in the free fraction of acidic and neutral drugs.

Phase I metabolism is affected before Phase II elimination is affected; therefore, a general rule whenever possible is to use water-soluble (conjugated) drugs rather than drugs eliminated by oxidation in patients with severe liver disease. An example is the use of lorazepam instead of diazepam when benzodiazepine sedation is needed. Estimating degree of liver impairment is much more difficult than estimating levels of renal impairment in the ICU patient. Changes in serum albumin, serum aminotransferase (ASAT, ALT), prothrombin time, and direct and indirect serum bilirubin provide the clinician with subjective evidence of liver impairment. Pugh's modification of Child's classification[35] may provide further insight as to the degree of hepatic disease (Table 115.4). Patients with a score of four or less have well preserved liver function, whereas a score of ten or greater suggests severe liver disease.

Few pharmacodynamic studies have been reported, and to date there have been no alterations in receptor sensitivity found in the liver failure patient.

Burn Patients

More than 2 million patients annually seek medical attention for thermal injury in the US. This represents a 1.5 percent chance of being hospitalized for a burn in an individual's lifetime.

The body's response to extensive thermal injury has been characterized by two phases: an acute phase and a hypermetabolic phase. The acute phase occurs immediately after exposure and generally lasts for 48 hours. The physiologic change during this period is a reduction in blood flow to tissues and organs because of hypovolemia. Little pharmacokinetic or pharmacodynamic research has been conducted during this phase; however, it is likely that drug absorption is attenuated, the time to drug distribution prolonged, and drug elimination impaired by the low-flow state.

A hypermetabolic phase follows the acute phase, and is described by its hyperdynamic flow state. Drug distribution may be affected by several mechanisms during this period. Cardiac index, normally approximately 3 $l/min \cdot m^2$ has been shown to increase to an average of 6 $l/min \cdot m^2$ in patients with an average of 61 percent of body surface area (BSA) burned.[36] Owing to a massive leakage, albumin concentration is reduced in these patients. This may lead to an increase in the free fraction of unbound acidic or neutral drugs.

Table 115.4 Pugh's Modification of Child's Classification of the Severity of Liver Disease

	Points score for increasing abnormality		
	1	2	3
Encephalopathy (grade)	None	1 or 2	3 or 4
Ascites	Absent	Slight	Moderate
Bilirubin (mg/dL)	1–2	2–3	>3
Albumin (gm/dL)	>3.5	2.8–3.5	<2.8
PT (sec > control)	1–4	4–6	>6

Total Points: 5–6 = Mild dysfunction; 7–9 = Moderate dysfunction; >9 = Severe dysfunction

Edema often results from hypoalbuminemia, leading to a potential for an increased Vd of water-soluble drugs. As a stress response, α_1-acid glycoprotein concentrations are increased for at least three weeks following thermal injury, and therefore may decrease the free fraction of basic compounds. Phase I metabolism is significantly decreased, owing to a reduction in enzyme activity.[37] Therefore, drugs such as pentobarbital, quinidine, lidocaine, and meperidine have reduced hepatic Cl in burn patients. Phase II liver metabolism appears to be unaffected by thermal injury, as the ability to conjugate was unchanged in studies evaluating lorazepam[38] and morphine.[39]

The renal Cl of drugs is increased during the hypermetabolic phase. Martyn et al.[40] evaluated ten healthy subjects and ten burn patients with burns over more than 35 percent of BSA. All subjects and patients had Cl_{cr} greater than 50 ml/min; renal function did not differ between the two groups. Renal Cl of ranitidine was 7.53 ± 1.71 l/min and 10.80 ± 2.38 l/min in healthy subjects and burn patients, respectively. Volumes of distribution were significantly different between healthy subjects, 1.16 ± 0.33 l/kg, and burn patients, 1.63 ± 0.13 l/kg.

Pharmacodynamic changes also have been reported in this patient population. Marathe and colleagues[41] evaluated four control patients who had extremity surgery and five patients with burns over 24 to 95 percent of BSA to determine the pharmacodynamics of neuromuscular blockade. The train-of-four technique (ulnar nerve stimulation) was used to measure degree of neuromuscular blockade. A single bolus of atracurium 0.5 mg/kg produced no difference in pharmacokinetic parameter estimates between the two groups. However, the burn patients displayed a 3.4-fold increase in EC_{50} when compared with the control group, 2.27 ± 0.62 versus 0.669 ± 0.121 mg/ml. E_{max}, expressed as percentage of maximal twitch suppression, also was significantly reduced in the burn patients compared with control patients, 66.1 ± 22.1 percent versus 100 percent. The results of this trial indicate that the burn patient is resistant to neuromuscular blockade, and may not achieve blockade to the same extent as the patient without thermal injury.

Pharmacodynamic changes resulting from thermal injury also have been described in the pediatric patient. Mills and Martyn[42] studied the pharmacology of vecuronium in 15 pediatric patients with burns over <40, 40–60, and >60 percent of BSA. These patients were compared with five patients undergoing elective surgery, who served as a control group. EC_{50} and EC_{90} were calculated from the vecuronium concentration versus percent maximal twitch suppression plots. The investigators report significant increases in the estimates of EC_{50} and EC_{90} in burn patients when compared with the control group. In addition, the extent of burn correlated well with the degree of receptor insensitivity.

Applications of Pharmacology in Critical Care

Muscle Relaxant Use in Critical Care

Muscle relaxants are commonly used in modern ICU patients for paralysis and management of ventilation. They are usually employed in combination with an amnestic to prevent subjectively unpleasant awareness. Muscle relaxants may be depolarizing or nondepolarizing, but those used in intensive care are primarily nondepolarizing. There are two classes of nondepolarizing muscle relaxants: steroidal agents (pancuronium, vecuronium, pipecuronium) and benzylisoquinolines (d-tubocurarine, atracurium, metocurine, doxacurium, mivicurium). The two differ slightly in their toxic and elimination profiles. Benzylisoquinoline muscle relaxants frequently release sufficient histamine to induce transient systemic hypotension; the steroidal relaxants do not. Both steroid and benzylisoquinoline muscle relaxants cause a ganglionic autonomic blockade that is predominantly vagolytic. Benzylisoquinoline muscle relaxants are eliminated via liver and kidney; steroid relaxants are eliminated predominantly by the liver. A major exception is atracurium, which is eliminated by blood esterase biotransformation (Hofmann elimination).[43]

Hepatic or renal failure may prolong the elimination of muscle relaxants in highly variable ways.[r3] Muscle relaxants are predominantly water-soluble compounds, and have initial Vds between 80 and 140 ml/kg and steady state Vds of 200 to 450 ml/kg. Pancuronium and vecuronium are the two relaxants most commonly used in ICUs. Each is eliminated through both urine and bile. Their relative clearances depend on the dominant mode of excretion. Approximately 20 percent of a dose of vecuronium and 60 to 70 percent of pancuronium is eliminated through the kidney; therefore, hepatic failure has a greater effect on elimination of vecuronium, while renal failure has greater influence on pancuronium elimination. In renal failure, the Vd may be increased 8 to 10 percent and the Cl reduced by 66 percent. In cirrhosis, the Vd is increased up to 80 percent and Cl is decreased by up to 30 percent. The net effect of these changes is that the half-life of both drugs can be increased unpredictably from two to five times, depending on circumstance. Hepatic and renal failure contribute to prolonged paralysis in an erratic but significant fashion.

It is likely that relaxants and their metabolites accumulate in tissues and may prolong elimination and paralysis. The elimination $T_{1/2}$ of vecuronium in ICU patients who receive relaxants for more than two days may be increased by up to three times, with the most likely cause of prolonged paralysis the accumulation of the relaxant or its metabolite after inappropriate dosing.

Movement is seldom contraindicated in the ICU—unlike the operating room, where sudden or unexpected movement can lead to disaster. When considering the use of muscle relaxants, it is wise to remember that they do not treat disease, only obscure symptoms. In the ICU, there are few beneficial uses for muscle relaxants and many possible detrimental effects. The paralyzed patient loses protective reflexes and the ability to communicate with the world. Regular assessment of neurologic status is prevented while symptoms of angina, abdominal catastrophes, seizures, and patient awareness and anxiety may go undetected. Despite this, relaxants remain in widespread use in ICUs today. They are used for such acute procedures as intubation, matching a patient to the ventilator, controlling agitation or aggressive behavior, or preventing movement during diagnostic procedures. Nonetheless, for most problems, appropriate and skillful analgesia and sedation usually offer greater safety and better clinical outcomes than do muscle relaxants.

Neuromuscular blockade must be monitored in ICU patients to prevent overdose and prolonged paralysis, and also to maintain levels of paralysis that can be intermittently reversed for routine neurologic examination of the patient. A nerve stimulator may be used to monitor the depth of paralysis. If dosing occurs such that two or three of the train of four stimuli are retained, rapid reversal of the relaxant is possible at any time with reversal agents. Nerve stimulators may be difficult for untrained personnel to use and interpret; it is common for direct muscle stimulation to fool inexperienced observers into overdosing patients. An intermittent bolus followed by recovery method of maintaining paralysis (without nerve stimulator) is preferred when personnel are inexperienced. With this method, patients are paralyzed using doses of relaxant averaging 20 percent of an intubating dose, then allowed to recover to the point of gross motor movement before each subsequent dose is administered. A brief neurologic assessment may be carried out just prior to each successive dose of relaxant. This method insures that untoward neurologic events do not go undetected and that muscle relaxant does not accumulate, leading to prolonged paralysis.

The undesired effects of muscle relaxants include loss of movement, as well as side-effects of specific agents, and prolonged paralysis. Individual drugs can produce hypotension through histamine release and tachycardia from partial autonomic blockade. Complications following loss of movement include: paralysis awake; airway obstruction; hypoventilation; pressure sores; pressure point neuropathies; retention of secretions; atelectasis; neglect of neurologic examination; false-negatives during neurologic and abdominal examinations; hyperextension of joints; loss of the patient's monitor for angina, disuse atrophy of muscles; fibrosis of muscles; and joint contracture. Muscle atrophy and fibrosis can leave the patient unable to ambulate and is a very devastating complication, particularly to young persons.

Apart from the obvious dangers associated with muscle relaxants administered by untrained individuals, there are a number of long-term complications of paralysis that are underappreciated in many ICUs. Topulos has assembled reports on more than 65 patients[r4] with no history of previous neurologic disease who suffered prolonged motor paralysis or weakness (without sensory loss) following vecuronium or pancuronium administration longer than two days. Although there are many causes for prolonged weakness in ICU patients—critical illness, polyneuropathy, steroid myopathy, malnutrition, disuse atrophy, neurological disease, electrolyte abnormalities—these factors do not seem to have played a role in the cases described by Topulos.

When tested by electromyography, some patients with prolonged paralysis demonstrate a neuromuscular pattern of dysfunction; others demonstrate a myopathic pattern, and may have up to a 100-fold increase in serum creatine kinase. Steroid medications and steroidal relaxants may be synergistic in producing myopathy and prolonged paralysis. In summary, prolonged paralysis occurs following overdose of relaxants, especially in the presence of renal failure, when steroidal relaxants are given in association with steroids (e.g., asthma), and in a small number of cases that appear to be idiopathic in nature.

Sedative-Hypnotic Use in Critical Care

The traditional categories of sedative-hypnotics used in the ICU include benzodiazepines, barbiturates, neuroleptics, and narcotics. These drugs are used to produce amnesia, sedation, analgesia, sleep, and to reduce movement. These compounds are lipid-soluble, and affect the central nervous system (CNS) by crossing the blood-brain barrier. Most are eliminated through the liver or through the kidney following conjugation by the liver. Many have long half-lives; some have additional effects through accumulation of active metabolites.

Narcotics and sedative-hypnotics vary greatly in their effect on consciousness when used in low doses to produce sedation or analgesia in ICU patients. Narcotics produce analgesia in postsurgical patients, whereas sedative-hypnotics do not. Even in small doses sedative-hypnotics depress consciousness, especially in the elderly, while narcotics tend to leave patients awake and oriented. Sedative-hypnotics often produce agitation, disorientation, and confusion, but narcotics rarely do so. Both drug classes may lead to decreased ability to guard the airway, but patient cooperation with pulmonary toilet is better preserved with narcotics. Tachyphylaxis and dependency may occur with narcotics and sedative-hypnotics, but these tendencies are not seen with neuroleptics.

The ventilatory response to inhaled carbon dioxide (CO_2) is a well-described index of respiratory function known as the CO_2 response curve. It is affected by chronic lung disease and by sedation with narcotics or sedative-hypnotics. The x-intercept of the CO_2 response curve is the apneic threshold and reflects sensitivity of the medullary chemoreceptor for CO_2. The apneic threshold is shifted to the right in response to narcotics and sedative-hypnotics, and the magnitude of the shift is dose-related. The slope of the CO_2 response curve is a function of the efferent neuromuscular response to stimulation by CO_2 and reflects the efficiency of the lung and chest wall as a bellows (Fig. 115.7). With low doses, sedative-hypnotics, but not narcotics decrease the slope of the CO_2 response curve. With large doses, the slope is depressed by both narcotics and sedative-hypnotics. At usual dosages used in ICU patients, narcotics preserve the strength and vigor of the ventilatory response better than sedative-hypnotics.

Many ICU patients develop CO_2 retention following sedation with narcotics or sedative-hypnotics. In an important experiment, Pietak et al.[44] demonstrated that this tendency could be predicted from pulmonary function testing. Patients who did not retain CO_2 while awake were anesthetized with halothane and their steady state $P_a CO_2$ was determined while breathing spontaneously. Retention of CO_2 was related to forced expiratory volume in one second ($FEV_{1.0}$) as a hyperbolic curve (Fig. 115.8). As a generalization, patients with a $FEV_{1.0} \geq 50$ percent have normal $PaCO_2$ despite sedation, patients with a $FEV_{1.0}$ between 35 and 50 percent retain CO_2 with sedation,

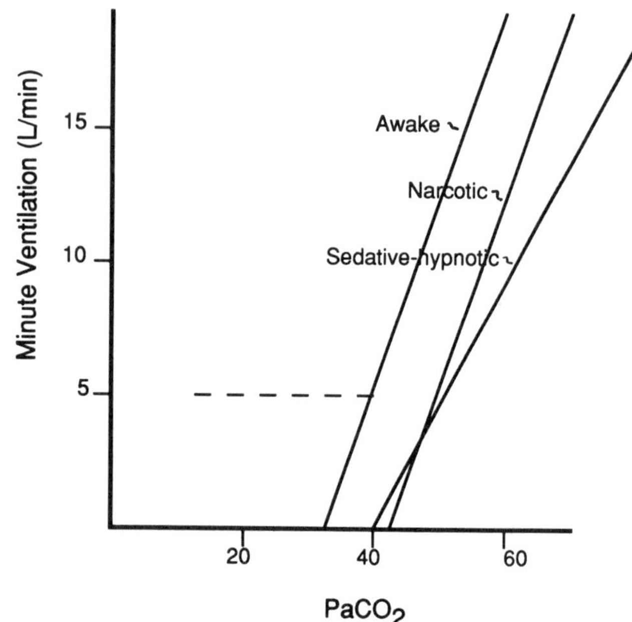

Figure 115.7 Carbon dioxide response curves showing the relative effect of sedative doses of narcotics and sedative-hypnotics on the awake ventilatory response to carbon dioxide. (with permission[r5]).

and those with a $FEV_{1.0} < 35$ percent retain CO_2 while awake, but retention increases markedly with sedation. There is every reason to expect that this principle applies to all sedative-hypnotics and narcotics used in the ICU. It is then possible to identify patients at risk for CO_2 retention and to exercise appropriate vigilance.

The normal ventilatory response to arterial hypoxemia in awake humans is a vigorous increase in minute ventilation. This hypoxic response is mediated entirely through peripheral chemoreceptors in the carotid body. In an important study, Knill and Gelb demonstrated that while this response has a high gain, it is readily and markedly attenuated by even small doses of sedative-hypnotic (anesthetic) drugs. In their study, sedative doses of 0.1 minimum alveolar concentration (MAC) of inhaled halothane abolished the ventilatory response to hypoxia in two-thirds of patients, while 0.2 MAC abolished the response in 95 percent of patients (Fig. 115.9). There is every reason to believe that this phenomenon is a problem for all sedative-hypnotics and narcotics, including the benzodiazepines and barbiturates.[45,46] The dose of sedative-hypnotics used in the ICU routinely exceeds these thresholds, resulting in blunted responses to hypoxia in the ICU patient population. The ubiquitous nature of this threat to ICU patients is sometimes under-appreciated by clinicians.

Narcotics and sedative-hypnotics affect the pattern of respiration differently in ICU patients. Narcotics produce a pattern of respiration with large tidal volumes and decreased respiratory rate. Sedative-hypnotics,[r5] in contrast, lead to a reduced tidal volume and an increase in respiratory frequency, producing rapid, shallow breathing and poor coordination of the chest wall and diaphragm. Patients receiving sedative-hypnotics have increased physiologic dead space and more atelectasis than patients equivalently sedated with narcotics.

It is preferable to wean patients from mechanical ventilation free of sedation; however, this is often not possible because of accompanying problems. It is important to select the correct quantity and quality of sedation. A compromise must be found that maintains the

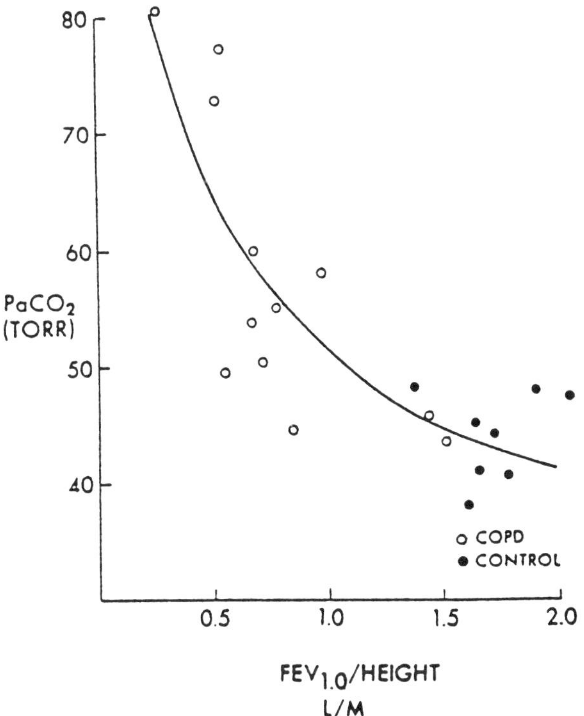

Figure 115.8 Relationship of spontaneous $PaCO_2$ during anesthetic administration to preoperative $FEV_{1.0}$. Patients with chronic obstructive pulmonary disease (°) did not exhibit CO_2 retention prior to anesthesia when compared to control patients (•). The degree of alveolar hypoventilation is greater in more severely obstructed patients (with permission[44]).

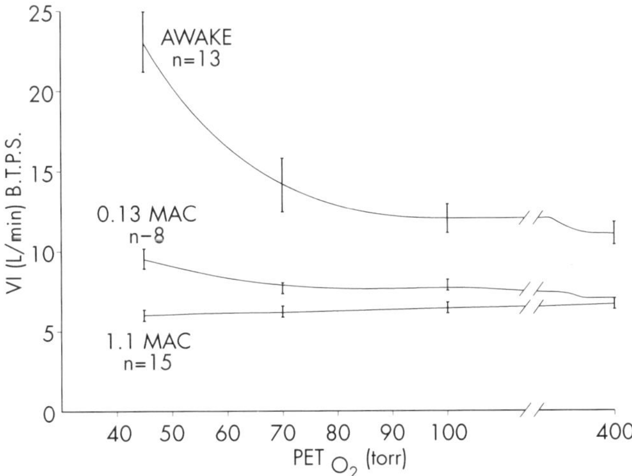

Figure 115.9 Ventilatory response to hypoxia in human volunteers and patients under halothane anesthesia. The ventilatory increase to hypoxia is severely attenuated at levels of only 0.1 MAC halothane anesthesia and completely absent at 1.1 MAC. This represents a significant depression of ventilatory drive and this mechanism is likely at work in intensive care unit patients (Knill and Gelb[r5]).

patient awake and alert, while reducing anxiety, pain, and dyspnea. Narcotics have substantial advantages over sedative-hypnotics in this area. In analgesic doses, narcotics prevent splinting due to pain while allowing the patient to better cooperate with efforts at pulmonary toilet. Narcotics produce a slow, deep pattern of respiration with minimal physiologic dead space and atelectasis. Using narcotics, patients may acclimatize to new apneic thresholds without loss of ventilatory drive or diaphragm and chest-wall coordination. Therefore, it usually is desirable to wean patients from mechanical ventilation using judicious narcotic administration rather than sedative-hypnotics.

Central Nervous System Applications in Critical Care

As a broad generalization, lipid-soluble drugs cross into the CNS, whereas water-soluble medications do not. Because the brain is a lean tissue, its apparent Vd per 100 g of tissue is similar to other vascular organs, such as the liver and kidney. It is a relatively small container with a low tissue-blood solubility similar to kidney or liver and is a highly perfused organ (50–100 ml/min/100g tissue). For these reasons, uptake of medications into the brain is rapid and highly blood flow-dependent. During increased intracranial pressure or trauma, cerebral perfusion may decrease to 20 to 25 percent of normal (20–30 ml/min/100g), which can prolong uptake and elimination four to five times. Under normal circumstances, cerebral perfusion is tightly linked to cerebral metabolic demand by powerful autoregulation reflexes that maintain blood flow constant over a wide range of cerebral perfusion pressures. With major brain injury, however, autoregulation is lost, and cerebral blood flow becomes cerebral perfusion pressure-dependent.

Medications may alter cerebral perfusion both directly and indirectly. Vasoactive drugs such as nitroprusside, phenylephrine, and dopamine may alter cerebral blood flow by a direct effect on cerebral vasculature, in addition to indirect effects due to the change in perfusion pressure. Other medications such as sedative-hypnotics and anesthetics may affect cerebral blood flow indirectly by decreasing cerebral metabolic demand and tissue autoregulation. These drugs may directly affect cerebral perfusion by changing vascular resistance in the brain and altering cardiac output. Their net effect on cerebral perfusion is variable and depends on the drug, dose, and the net sum of the effect on blood pressure, cerebral vascular resistance, and cerebral metabolic activity.

Patients routinely receive multiple drug infusions simultaneously in the ICU, and acute cerebral toxic reactions frequently are associated with these medications (e.g., ranitidine, midazolam, fentanyl). The most common presentation of these reactions, especially in aged or debilitated patients, is acute delirium. This often presents as anxiety, paranoia, and mild obtundation. Untreated, it may progress to confusion and psychosis and result in agitated behavior that is aggressive, bizarre, and potentially a threat to patient and unit staff. The incidence of acute delirium is increased if drug elimination is impeded by renal or hepatic dysfunction, or if therapeutic drug concentrations are inadvertently exceeded.

The incidence of delirium and acute cerebral toxic reactions also increases in disorders that damage the blood-brain barrier. Under these circumstances, medications leak into the CNS and may lead to acute delirium, even at therapeutic blood concentrations. These conditions include encephalitis, sepsis, and traumatic head injury. If the damage is severe, even poorly lipid-soluble medications such as muscle relaxants or antibiotics will cross into the CNS. These medications can induce seizures, even in patients without seizure disorders. Central nervous system symptoms regress when the blood-brain barrier recovers or the drugs are withdrawn. Drug-induced cerebral toxic reactions are easily confused with other serious causes of acute delirium, such as hypoxia, hypercarbia, electrolyte imbalances, Wernicke's encephalopathy, schizophrenia, and depression. When drug-induced delirium is suspected, these conditions are ruled out, the offending medications are withdrawn, and the patient is supported until recovery.

Effects of Sedation on Hypothalamic-Pituitary-Adrenal Axis Dysfunction

Sedation may have profound effects on hypothalamic-pituitary axis function. While this phenomenon has not been extensively studied in the ICU, it has been investigated with respect to narcotics and anesthetic agents in patients under general anesthesia. The hypothalamus responds to stress by secreting varying amounts of adrenocorticotropic hormone (ACTH), growth hormone, thyroid-stimulation hormone, and luteinizing hormone (Fig. 115.10). Cortisol, as increased by ACTH, is the best-studied of these hormones.

Studies of adrenal function show that animals respond to the pain and stress of surgery by releasing large quantities of ACTH. This response is rapid, and adrenal cortical blood flow and metabolic activity increase within minutes. Serum cortisol levels may rise acutely to levels as high as ten times normal during surgery. Many authors refer to this as the "stress reaction." When surgery is performed under general anesthesia, cortisol levels are elevated, but the anesthesia is protective and stress cortisol levels are lower. When surgery is performed under regional block (epidural)

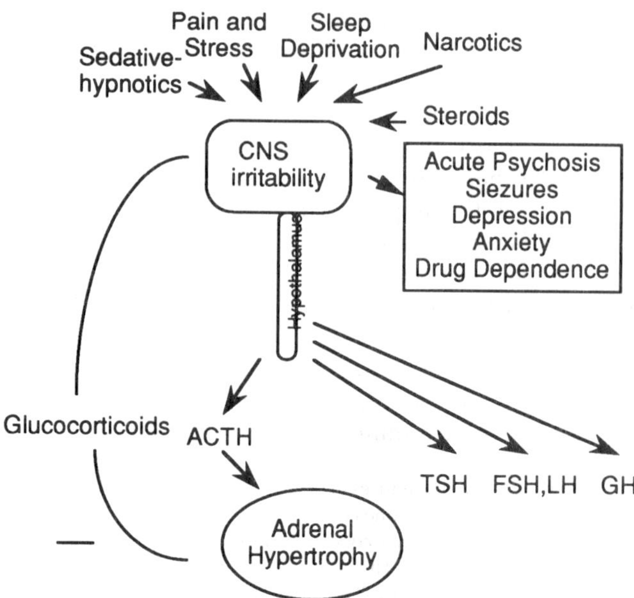

Figure 115.10 Summary of hypothalamic-pituitary-adrenal axis interactions emphasizing the interaction of pain, stress, narcotics, and sedative medications together with a summary of this interaction on the hypothalamus and adrenals and the potential neurologic outcomes in the ICU.

anesthesia, however, surgery-induced elevations in serum cortisol are prevented. It is likely that pain from minor surgical procedures may routinely elevate serum cortisol levels in ICU patients.

Sedation and anesthesia may also paradoxically release cortisol through a hypothalamic-pituitary axis mechanism, even when administered to healthy volunteers in the absence of surgery.[47,48] The amount of cortisol released depends on the drug and dose administered. Cortisol levels in healthy volunteers receiving various general anesthetics are illustrated in Figure 115.11. Low doses of anesthetic drug elevate cortisol levels during induction of and emergence from anesthesia; doses sufficient to produce surgical anesthesia inhibit cortisol release, resulting in low serum levels. There is every reason to believe that a similar phenomenon must also occur during sedation of patients in the ICU. The response is similar regardless of whether sedation is produced with narcotics or with sedative-hypnotics. In most cases, the effect of sedation has been shown to be mediated through the hypothalamic-pituitary-adrenal axis and is blocked by hypophysectomy. One exception to this rule is etomidate, which has been shown to cause suppression of adrenocortical function for up to eight hours following an induction dose.[49] This anesthetic may act through a direct effect on the adrenal gland in addition to its effect on the hypothalamus. As a result of this action, etomidate is reported to have caused severe adrenal insufficiency when used as chronic sedation of patients in the ICU.

A biphasic cortisol response also has been observed for narcotics. Morphine administered to rats is known to block the release of cortisol in response to histamine challenge by inhibiting release of ACTH at the level of the hypothalamic-pituitary axis.[50] Morphine sulfate blocked cortisol release in mice in a dose-dependent fashion in response to an intense surgical stimulus at laparotomy, compared with mice deeply anesthetized with sodium pentobarbital. Paradoxically, morphine in certain doses is also known to release ACTH and stimulate adrenal hypertrophy following repetitive administration of morphine to rats.[51]

Major surgical procedures in humans result in increased plasma cortisol and growth hormone concentrations.[52,53] For example, cortisol levels can reach plasma concentrations ten times normal in response to cardiac surgery. The only known direct physiologic stimulus for cortisol release is ACTH. Anesthetic doses of morphine (2–4 mg/kg) were able to reduce the cortisol response during cardiac surgery[54] when compared with halothane anesthesia; in large doses, morphine completely abolished the cortisol stress response. In the same series of experiments, the cortisol response to ACTH was not blocked by morphine; therefore, morphine appears to be active at the level of the hypothalamic-pituitary axis. A small dose of morphine also will block the diurnal rise in plasma cortisol at the level of the hypothalamic-pituitary axis in unstressed patients.

Cortisol and the stress response have profound effects on the CNS.[r6,r7] This response may alter EEG and cerebral electrical activity and can lead to altered seizure thresholds. Cortisol affects mood, anxiety, and sleep-wake cycles, and increases wakefulness and rapid eye movement sleep while decreasing Stage II sleep. Both glucocorticoid excess and deficiency can lead to psychosis and alterations in diurnal rhythm, and have been associated with manic-depressive illness, panic disorder, and unipolar depression.[r8] It is likely that cortisol excess is involved in the up-regulation of CNS electrical activity in response to chronic or repetitive sedation. Repeated administration of narcotics and sedative-hypnotics leads to adrenal hypertrophy, and the size of the adrenal gland may be doubled over several days.

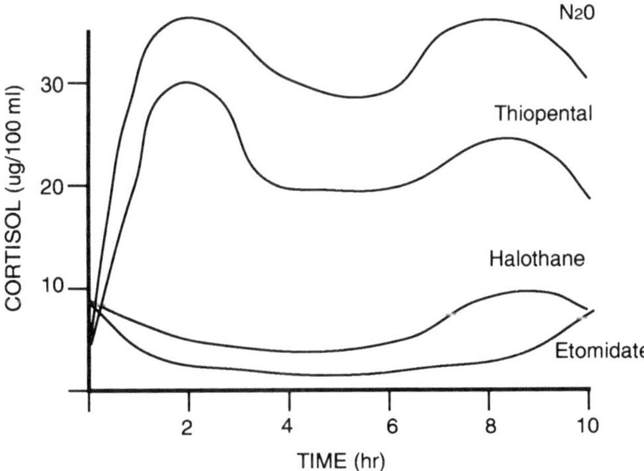

Figure 115.11 Schematic illustration of the effect of various anesthetic agents on plasma cortisols levels in healthy volunteers, no surgery performed. Note that the plasma cortisol level is dependent on the type and concentration of drug. As a general rule, cortisol levels are elevated during periods of CNS excitement such as anesthetic induction (time 0) or emergence (6 hr) and inhibited during surgical anesthesia through direct effects on the cortex and hypothalamus. An exception, etomidate also directly interrupts synthesis of cortisol in the adrenal gland.

Cortisol-induced CNS irritability may be responsible for the seizures, irritability, and CNS hyperactivity that characterize the withdrawal state from narcotics and sedative-hypnotics. It is reasonable to postulate that episodes of acute ICU psychosis are induced by changes in serum cortisol and diurnal rhythm induced by stress, sleep deprivation, and sedation-induced stimulation or inhibition of ACTH secretion. Additionally, adrenocortical function correlates with survival in ICU outcome studies,[r9] and this relation (not proved to be causal) should be considered when managing patients in the ICU.

Pulmonary Dysfunction in Critical Care

Uptake, distribution, and elimination of volatile gases through the lung are well described for volatile anesthetics.[51] Administration and elimination can be monitored from end-tidal gas concentrations. The rate of uptake of gases into the lung depends on the difference between the inhaled and tissue partial pressures, the minute ventilation, the cardiac output, and the blood solubility of the volatile medication. The rate of administration or elimination of soluble drugs (e.g., methoxyflurane) depends on ventilation and is relatively independent of cardiac output. By contrast, insoluble agents (e.g., nitrous oxide, xenon) are dependent on cardiac output and are essentially independent of ventilation.

Drugs that are administered as aerosols (e.g., surfactant, bronchodilators) are absorbed differently from volatile gases. Only small amounts of nebulized medications reach the alveoli. Particle size is the major determinant in absorption, with small (1–5 μ) droplets more readily distributed to the small airways and alveoli compared with larger droplets, which precipitate in mid-sized and large airways. Studies show that the amount of nebulized drug reaching the lungs does not exceed 15 percent in most cases. Bioavailability by aerosol administration is low; an example is salbuterol, which has a bioavailability of 5 to 8 percent.[r10] Systemic administration of many drugs may be more efficacious than aerosol administration. It is important that the primary indication for aerosol administration of medications is when systemic toxicity to a particular agent is high, or when systemic side-effects to a particular drug may be decreased when it is delivered directly to the lungs (e.g., steroids, isoproterenol, epinephrine).

During viral or toxic pulmonary injury, or during episodes of systemic sepsis, detrimental alterations of the alveolocapillary endothelium may lead to adult respiratory distress syndrome (ARDS). The effects of this syndrome on pharmacokinetics and pharmacodynamics are not well-documented, in part because of the multifactorial genesis of the syndrome and the multiorgan system failure that frequently occurs with ARDS.[56]

Severe ARDS is usually associated with a degree of right heart failure, as illustrated in Figure 115.12. Right heart failure is more common when ARDS is associated with pre-existing right heart failure or right heart myocardial infarction. The main cause for this associated failure is the increased pulmonary vascular resistance

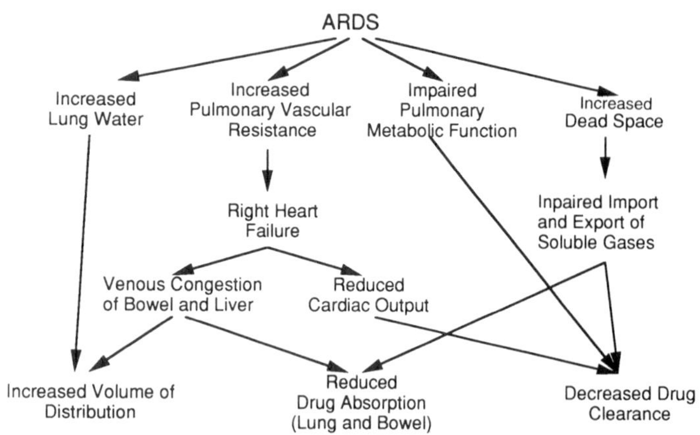

Figure 115.12 Pharmacokinetic Alterations in Drug Elimination Predicted During Right Heart Failure Induced by ARDS

(pathognomonic for ARDS), which is secondary to injured pulmonary capillary endothelium and regional hypoxic pulmonary vasoconstriction. Right heart failure leads to subsequent left heart hypovolemia, low cardiac output, and episodic hypotension. Renal and hepatic perfusion is then reduced, leading to impaired drug clearance through these organs.[r11] Venous stasis associated with right heart failure also leads to congestion of the bowel, which may decrease bioavailability of enteral medications.

Prospectus

Provision of pharmacotherapy to the critically ill patient is complicated by the large number of drugs used, advanced age, increased potential for ADRs, polypharmacy, and concomitant disease states. Changes in drug response may be due to a reduction in organ function, which is particularly witnessed with low perfusion state illnesses. However, modification of pharmacodynamic parameters, such as changes in E_{max} and receptor sensitivity, also may contribute to drug toxicity or lack of expected response. Because of daily alterations in organ function and physiology, the critically ill patient requires close evaluation for these changes. The clinician needs to be cognizant of these pharmacokinetic and pharmacodynamic changes to provide the most appropriate and cost-effective drug therapy at the lowest risk of developing adverse drug reactions.

Acknowledgement

We gratefully acknowledge the research assistance of Kelly K. Jenco, and the technical assistance of Mia Tommarello.

References

Research Reports

1. Ridley S, Biggam M, Stone P. A cost-benefit analysis of intensive therapy. Anesthesia 1993;*48*:14–19.
2. Dragsted L, Qvist J. Outcome from intensive care. I. A 5-year study of 1308 patients: Methodology and patient population. Eur J Anaesthesiology 1989;*6*:23–37.
3. Thibault GE, Mulley AG, Barnett GO, Goldstein RL, Reder VA, Sherman EL, Skinner ER. Medical intensive care: Indications, interventions, and outcomes. N Engl J Med 1980;*302*:938–942.
4. Smythe MA, Melendy S, Jahns B, Dmuchowski C. An exploratory analysis of medication utilization in a medical intensive care unit. Crit Care Med 1993;*21*:1319–1323.
5. Rockwood K, Noseworthy TW, Gibney RTN, Konopad E, Shustack A, Stollery D, Johnston R, Grace M. One-year outcome of elderly and young patients admitted to intensive care units. Crit Care Med 1993;*21*:687–691.
6. Geokas MC, Haverback BJ. The aging gastrointestinal tract. Am J Surgery 1969;*117*:881–892.
7. Greenblatt DJ, Allen MD, Harmatz JS, Shader RI. Diazepam disposition determinants. Clin Pharmacol Ther 1980;*27*:301–312.
8. Lindeman RD, Tobin J, Shock NW. Longitudinal studies on the rate of decline in renal function with age. J Am Geriatr Soc 1985;*33*:278–285.
9. Vestal RE, Wood AJ, Shand DG. Reduced β-adrenoceptor sensitivity in the elderly. Clin Pharmacol Ther 1979;*26*:181–186.
10. Dochorty JR, O'Malley K. Ageing and alpha-adrenoceptors. Clinical Science 1985;*68*:133s–136s.
11. Irvine NA, Shepherd AMM. Age and blood pressure determine vasodepressor response to sodium nitroprusside. J Cardiovasc Pharmacol 1984;*6*:816–821.
12. Abernethy DR, Schwartz JB, Todd EL, Luchi R, Snow E. Verapamil pharmacodynamics and disposition in young and elderly hypertensive patients: Altered electrocardiographic and hypertensive responses. Ann Intern Med 1986;*105*:329–336.
13. Bertz RJ, Reynolds IJ, Kroboth FJ, Wright CE, Smith RB, Kroboth PD. Sensitivity of young and elderly men to the psychomotor effects of alprazolam. Clin Pharmacol Ther 1994;*55*:135.
14. Ritz R, Cavanilles J, Michaels S, Shubin H, Weil MH. Disappearance of indocyanine green during circulatory shock. Surg Gynecol Obstet 1973;*136*:57–62.
15. Leithe ME, Margorien RD, Hermiller JB, Unverferth DV, Leier CV. Relationship between central hemodynamics and regional blood flow in normal subjects and in patients with congestive heart failure. Circulation 1984;*69*:57–64.
16. Naafs MAB, van der Hoek C, van Duin S, Koorevaar G, Schopman W, Silberbusch J. Decreased renal clearance of digoxin in chronic congestive heart failure. Eur J Clin Pharmacol 1985;*29*:249–252.
17. Brater DC, Chennavasin P, Seiwell R. Furosemide in patients with heart failure: Shift in dose-response curves. Clin Pharmacol Ther 1980;*28*:182–186.
18. Rector TS, Olivari MT, Levine TB, Francis GS, Cohn JN. Predicting survival for an individual with congestive heart failure using the plasma norepinephrine concentration. Am Heart J 1987;*114*:148–152.
19. Francis GS, Cohn JN, Johnson G, Rector TS, Goldman S, Simon A. Plasma norepinephrine, plasma renin activity, and congestive

heart failure; relations to survival and the effects of therapy in V-HeFT II. Circulation 1993;*87*:VI-40–VI-48.

20. Michel MC, Maisel AS, Brodde OE. Mitigation of β1- and/or β2-adrenoceptor function in human heart failure. Br J Clin Pharmacol 1990;*30*:37S–42S.

21. Bristow MR, Ginsburg R, Minobe W, Cubicciotti RS, Sageman WS, Lurie K, Billingham ME, Harrison DC, Stinson EB. Decreased catecholamine sensitivity and β-adrenergic-receptor density in failing human hearts. N Engl J Med 1982;*307*:205–211.

22. Fowler MB, Laser JA, Hopkins GL, Minobe W, Bristow MR. Assessment of the β-adrenergic receptor pathway in the intact failing human heart: progressive receptor down-regulation and subsensitivity to agonist response. Circulation 1986;*74*:1290–1302.

23. Cody RJ, Covit A, Schaer G, Williams G. Captopril pharmacokinetics and the acute hemodynamic and hormonal response in patients with severe chronic congestive heart failure. Am Heart J 1982;*104*:1180–1183.

24. Schwinn DA, McIntyre RW, Hawkins ED, Kates RA, Reves JG. α1-adrenergic responsiveness during coronary artery bypass surgery: Effect of preoperative ejection fraction. Anesthesiology 1988;*69*:206–217.

25. Docci D, Bilancioni R, Pistocchi E, Mosconi G, Turci F, Salvo G, Balderat L, Orsi C. Serum α1-acid glycoprotein in chronic renal failure. Nephron 1985;*39*:160–163.

26. Reuning RH, Sams RA, Notari RE. Role of pharmacokinetics in drug dosage adjustment. I. Pharmacologic effect kinetics and apparent volume of distribution of digoxin. J Clin Pharmacol 1973;*13*:127–141.

27. Koup JR, Jusko WJ, Elwood CM. Kohli RK. Digoxin pharmacokinetics: Role of renal failure in dosage regimen design. Clin Pharmacol Ther 1975;*18*:9–21.

28. Beck CL. Evaluation of creatinine clearance estimation in an elderly male population. Pharmacotherapy 1988;*8*:183–188.

29. Cockcroft DW, Gault MH. Prediction of creatinine clearance from serum creatinine. Nephron 1976;*16*:31–41.

30. American Hospital Formulary Service Drug Information. McEvoy GK, Litvak K, Welsh, OH (eds). American Society of Hospital Pharmacists. Bethesda, MD, 1994.

31. Dundee JW, Richards RK. Effect of azotemia upon the action of intravenous barbitruate anesthesia. Anesthesiology 1954;*15*:333–346.

32. Galeazzi RL, Gugger M, Weidmann P. Beta blockade with pindolol: differential cardiac and renal effects despite similar plasma kinetics in normal and uremic man. Kidney Int 1979;*15*:661–668.

33. Kleinbloesem CH, van Brummelen P, van Harten J, Danhof M, Breimer DD. Nifedipine: Influence of renal function on pharmacokinetic/hemodynamic relationship. Clin Pharmacol Ther 1985;*37*:563–574.

34. Schmith VD, Piraino B, Smith RB, Kroboth PD. Alprazolam in end-stage renal disease. II. Pharmacodynamics. Clin Pharmacol Ther 1992;*51*:533–540.

35. Pugh RNH, Murray-Lyon IM, Dawson JL, Peietroni MC, Williams R. Transection of the oesophagus for bleeding oesophageal varicies. Br J Surg 1973;*60*:646–649.

36. Aikawa N, Martyn JAJ, Burke JF. Pulmonary artery catheterization and thermodilution cardiac output determination in the management of critically burned patients. Am J Surg 1978;*135*:811–817.

37. Dorr MB. The effect of thermal injury on oxidative drug metabolism. Pharm Research 1988;*5*:5–162.

38. Martyn J, Greenblatt DJ. Lorazepam conjugation is unimpaired in burn trauma. Clin Pharmacol Ther 1987;*43*:250–255.

39. Perry S, Inturrisi CE. Analgesia and morphine disposition in burn patients. J Burn Care Rehab 1983;*4*:276–279.

40. Martyn JAJ, Bishop AL, Oliveri MF. Pharmacokinetics and pharmacodynamics of ranitidine after burn injury. Clin Pharmacol Ther 1992;*51*:408–414.

41. Marathe PH, Dwersteg JF, Pavlin EG, Haschke RH, Heimbach DM, Slattery JT. Effect of thermal injury on the pharmacokinetics and pharmacodynamics of atracurium in humans. Anesthesiology 1989;*70*:752–755.

42. Mills AK, Martyn JAJ. Neuromuscular blockade with vecuronium in paediatric patients with burn injury. Br J Clin Pharmacol 1989;*28*:155–159.

43. Merrett RA, Thompson CW, Webb FW. In vitro degradation of atracurium in human plasma. Br J Anaesth 1983;*55*:61.

44. Pietak S, Weenig CS, Hickey RF, Fairley HB. Anesthetic effects on ventilation in patients with chronic obstructive pulmonary disease. Anesthesiol 1975;*42*:160–166.

45. Knill RL, Gelb AW. Ventilatory responses to hypoxia and hypercarbia during halothane sedation and anesthesia in man. Anesthesiol 1978;*49*:244–251.

46. Knill RL, Clement JL. Site of selective action of halothane on the peripheral chemoreflex pathway in humans. Anesthesiol 1984;*61*:121–126.

47. Von Werder K, Stevens WC, Cromwell TH, Eger El, Hane S, Forsham PH. Adrenal function during long-term anesthesia in man. PSBM 1970;*135*:854–858.

48. Frieling B, Brandt L. The influence of inhalation anesthetics on human plasma cortisol without superimposed surgical stress. Anesthesiol 1985;*63*:A288.

49. Wagner RL, White PF, Kan PB, Rosenthal MH, Feldman D. Inhibition of adrenal steriogenesis by the anesthetic etomidate. N Engl J Med 1984;*310*:1415–1421.

50. Briggs FN, Munson PL. Studies on the mechanism of stimulation of ACTH secretion with the aid of morphine as a blocking agent. Endocrinology 1955;*57*:205–219.

51. MacKay EM, MacKay LL. Resistance to morphine in experimental uremia. Proc Soc Exper Biol Med 1926;*24*:129.

52. George JM, Reier CE, Lanese RR, Rower JM. Morphine anesthesia blocks cortisol and growth hormone response to surgical stress in humans. J Clin Endocrinol Metab 1974;*38*:786–741.

53. Brandt MR, Korshin J, Prange Hansen A, Hummer L, Nistrup Madsen S, Rygg I, Kehlet H. Influence of morphine anesthesia on the endocrine-metabolic response to open-heart surgery. Acta Anaesth Scand 1978;*22*:400–412.

54. Reier CE, George JM, Kilman JW. Cortisol and growth hormone response to surgical stress during morphine anesthesia. Anesth Analg 1973;*52*:1003–1009.

55. Strum DP, Eger EI, Unadkat JD, Johnson BH, Carpenter RL. Age affects the pharmacokinetics of inhaled anesthetics in humans. Anesth Analg 1991;*73*:310–318.

56. Mehvar R. Relationship of apparent systemic clearance to individual organ clearances: effect of pulmonary clearance and site of drug administration and measurement. Pharmaceutical Res 1991;*8*:306–312.

Reviews

r1. Denham MJ. Adverse drug reactions. Br Med Bulletin 1990;*46*:53–62.

r2. Benowitz NL, Meister W. Pharmacokinetics in patients with cardiac failure. Clin Pharmacokinetics 1976;*1*:389–405.

r3. Miller RD: Pharmacokinetics of muscle relaxants and their antagonists. In: Prys-Roberts C, Hug CC. Pharmacokinetics of anaesthesia. London, Blackwell Scientific, 1984.

r4. Topulos, GP. Neuromuscular blockade in the adult intensive care unit. New Horizons *1*:447–462, 1993.

r5. Hickey RF, Severinghaus JW: Chapter 21. In Hornbein TF. Regulation of breathing. Lung biology in health and disease, Vol. 17, Part II. New York, Marcel Dekker, 1981.

r6. Woodbury DM. Relation between the adrenal cortex and the central nervous system. Pharmacol Rev 1958;*10*:275.

r7. McEwen BS. Influences of adrenocortical hormones on pituitary and brain function, In Baxter JD Rousseau GG: Glucocorticoid hormone action. New York, Springer-Verlag, 1979.

r8. Chrousos GP, Gold PW. The concepts of stress and stress system disorders: Overview of physical and behavioral homeostasis. JAMA 1992;*267*:1244–1252.

r9. Span L, Hermus A, Bartelink A, Hoitsman A, Gimbrere J, Smals A, Kloppenborg P. Adrenocortical function: an indicator of severity of disease and survival in chronic critically ill patients. Intensive Care Med. 1992;*18*:93–96.

r10. Clay MM, Clarke SW. Wastage of drugs from nebulizers: a review. Journal of the Royal Society of Medicine 1987;*80*:38–39.

r11. Taburet AM, Tollier C, Richard C. The effect of respiratory disorders on clinical pharmacokinetic variables. Clin Pharmacokinet 1990;*19*:462–490.

r12. Stanski DR. Pharmacokinetics and pharmacodynamics for the clinician. Can J Anaesth 1991;*38*:R48–R53.

r13. Tsujimoto G, Hashimoto K, Hoffman BB. Pharmacokinetic and pharmacodynamic principles of drug therapy in old age. Part 1. Int J Clin Pharmacol 1989;*27*:13–26.

r14. Sibley DR, Lefkowitz RJ. Molecular mechanisms of receptor desensitization using the β-adrenergic receptor-coupled adenylate cyclase system as a model. Nature 1985;*317*:124–128.

r15. Fabre J, Balant L. Renal failure, drug pharmacokinetics and drug action. Clin Pharmacol 1976;*1*:99–120.

r16. Swan SK, Bennett WM. Drug dosing guidelines in patients with renal failure. Drug Dosing 1992;*156*:633–638.

r17. Howden CW, Birnie GG, Brodie MJ. Drug metabolism in liver disease. Pharmacol Ther 1989;*40*:439–474.

r18. McLean AJ, Morgan DJ. Clinical pharmacokinetics in patients with liver disease. Clin Pharmacol 1991;*21*:42–69.

r19. Hoyumpa A, Schenker S. Is glucuronidation truly preserved in patients with liver disease? Hepatology 1991;*13*:786–795.

r20. Blaschke TF. Protein binding and kinetics of drugs in liver diseases. Clin Pharmacokinetics *2*:32–44.

r21. Bonata PL. Pathophysiology and Pharmacokinetics Following Burn Injury. Clin Pharmacol Dis Pro 1990;*18*:(2):118–130.

CHAPTER 116

Sumner J. Yaffe
Jacob V. Aranda

Pharmacology in Pediatrics

Introduction

Effective and safe drug therapy in neonates, infants, children, and adolescents requires an understanding of age-related maturational changes that affect drug action and disposition. Pediatric drug dosage regimens must be adjusted for the kinetic characteristics of individual drugs, age (the major determinant), disease states, sex, and individual needs. Otherwise, ineffective treatment or toxicity may result.

The history of drug therapy is replete with examples of adverse reactions to drugs in children. Virtually all drug-related legislation in effect in the US (and other countries) today stems directly from these unfortunate experiences. Nevertheless, there still are no specific rules or regulations either governing the use of drugs in children or the testing and approval of new drugs for pediatric patients. More important, processes to facilitate new drug studies on infants and children are lacking. The recent establishment of a network of Pediatric Pharmacology Research Units by the National Institute of Child Health and Human Development may resolve this issue by providing the infrastructure for drug studies in infants and children.

In 1956, Silverman and colleagues at Columbia reported an excessive mortality rate and an increased incidence of kernicterus among premature babies receiving a sulfonamide compared with those receiving chlortetracycline.[1] Then, in 1959, Sutherland described a syndrome of cardiovascular collapse in three newborns receiving chloramphenicol for presumed infections.[2] Both these therapeutic misadventures serve to underscore the generally held perception that newborn infants are more likely to experience adverse reactions to drugs, even when dosages are adjusted for body size.

Xenobiotic exposure during the embryonic or fetal periods of development heightens the concern for adverse drug action. The thalidomide tragedy reported in 1962, in which more than 10,000 babies were born with the rare malformation phocomelia, created an international outcry and changed forever the way in which drug safety is evaluated in the western world.

Obstetricians and pediatricians have recognized that rational drug therapy for pregnant women and newborns is often confounded by a combination of unpredictable and often poorly understood pharmacokinetic and pharmacodynamic interactions and has led to a conservative approach to therapy.

A more positive approach to pediatric therapeutics requires a thorough understanding of human developmental biology as well as insights regarding the dynamic ontogeny of the processes of drug absorption, drug distribution, drug metabolism, and drug excretion. In addition, there must be a rigorous appreciation of the developmental aspects of drug-receptor interactions, including the ontogenetic changes in receptor number, receptor affinity, receptor-effector coupling, and receptor modulation and regulation.

Infancy and childhood extend from two months of age to the onset of puberty, which typically occurs at approximately 10 to 12 years in females and 12 to 14 years in males.[r1] Traditionally, puberty is a marker for the initiation of adolescence, a developmental period where further changes in one's disposition and response occur. The first two to three years of life bring particularly rapid growth and development. During the first year alone, body weight doubles at five months and triples by the first birthday; body length increases by 50 per cent and body surface area doubles by the first birthday.[r1] Caloric expenditure increases threefold to fourfold during the first year. Major organ systems differentiate, grow, and mature throughout infancy and childhood. Although growth and development are most rapid during the first several years of life, maturation continues at a slower pace throughout middle and later childhood. This dynamic process of growth, differentiation, and maturation is what sets the infant and child apart from adults, both physiologically and pharmacologically. It should be no surprise, then, that important changes in response to drugs and in disposition of drugs occur during infancy and childhood.

This chapter will focus on the impact of growth and development on drug action and biodisposition and the resultant implications for pharmacotherapy in children. Comparative pharmacologic data in children and adults will be used to illustrate general principles. In addition, a review of the changes in the body and environment of the adolescent that have particular relevance for the type, amount, and frequency of drug use is provided. For most classes of drugs, the dose and dose interval differ between childhood and adulthood. When one considers the total amount of medication that is prescribed or taken therapeutically—plus the nontherapeutic or illegal substances consumed—it behooves the health care provider to know the action and the interaction of these agents in order to provide optimal care for teenagers.

Developmental Changes in Body Composition and Drug Disposition

The proportions of body weight contributed by fat protein, intracellular water, and extracellular water respectively, change significantly during infancy and childhood (Fig. 116.1). Total body water accounts for approximately 75 to 80 per cent of body weight in the full-term newborn. This decreases to approximately 60 per cent by five months of age and remains relatively constant thereafter. Although the percentage of total body water does not change significantly after late infancy, there is a progressive decrease in extracellular water from infancy to young adulthood. In addition,

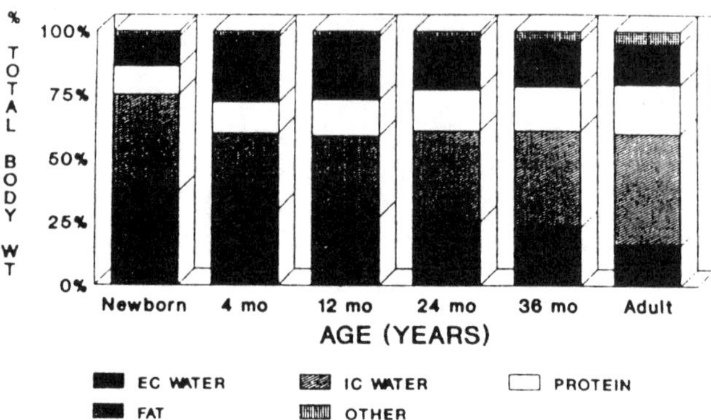

Figure 116.1 Schematic of Change in Proportional Body Composition with Age (Adapted from Habersang)

the percentage of body weight contributed by fat doubles by four to five months of age, primarily at the expense of total-body water. During the second year of life, protein mass increases, with a compensatory reduction in fat.

Liver and kidney size, relative to body weight, also change during growth and development. These two organs reach maximum relative weight in the 1- to 2-year old child, the period of life when capacity for drug metabolism and elimination also tends to be greatest. Likewise, body surface area is greatest relative to body mass in the infant and young child compared with the older child and young adult.[r2,r3]

During adolescence, height is increased by approximately 25 per cent, and weight is nearly doubled.[r4,5] Lean body mass, skeletal mass, and body fat are equal per unit of body weight in prepubertal boys and girls, but by maturity, women have twice as much fat relative to total body weight as do adult men.[r5] The peak lean body mass growth velocity in males occurs two years later than in females on average and coincides with peak height growth velocity.[r7] Total body water and extracellular water decrease with age.[r6,22] Nomograms[3] and formulas have been developed for predicting body density and total body fat from combinations of anthropometric measures, including skin fold thickness and limb and girth circumferences.[4,5,6,7] These relationships are based on direct measurements of body composition by either underwater weighing, potassium (^{40}K) counting techniques, or chloride space measurements.

During puberty, the rise in sex steroids predominantly affects the body composition and metabolism largely through alterations in liver function.

The absorptive surface of the small gut is proportionately greater and GI transit time may be shorter in infants and younger children compared with adults, thus affording differences in dosing absorption.

Hepatic function is complex, and metabolic path-

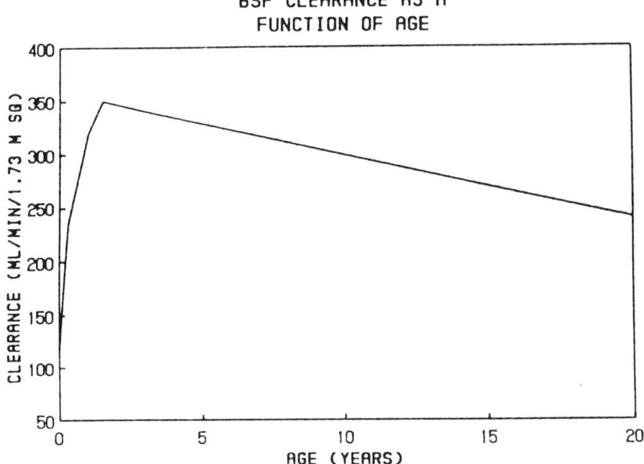

Figure 116.2 Change in Hepatic Clearance (expressed as ml/min/1.73m²) of Bromsulphalein During Childhood (Adapted from Habersang)

ways for various substrates develop at different rates. Bromsulphalein (BSP) has clearance, normalized for body surface area, increases rapidly during the first three months of life, significantly exceeds adult clearance in the preschool child, and declines to adult levels during adolescence (Fig. 116.2).[8,9]

Glomerular filtration rate, as reflected by endogenous creatinine clearance, also increases rapidly during the first year of life.[r8] Creatinine clearance, normalized for body surface area, equals adult clearance at one year, and there is some evidence that average clearance in prepubescent children exceeds clearance in adults (Table 116.1). Tubular function matures later than glomerular function; however, tubular function is essentially mature by 1 year of age.[10]

It is important to recognize, then, that both hepatic and renal function not only equals but in some cases exceed normal adult function between 1 year and puberty.[r2]

The rate of enzyme activity is usually low in the fetus, higher in the neonate, and in some cases, peaks in preadolescence. The activity of liver microsomal enzyme systems changes with age and differs between males and females by adulthood. Sex differences in the oxidation of drugs by liver enzymes appear to be due mainly to higher binding capacity of the cytochrome P-450 system in males as compared with females. In addition, a slight sex difference in the activity of microsomal NADPH-linked electron transport systems may be a contributory factor.

In summary, changes in body composition affect the way a given drug is distributed within the body. Changes in organ structure and function, specifically those in the liver, affect the rate of metabolism and, therefore, the excretion of a drug. These two factors may account for some of the variability in drug dose and response noted among pubertal patients and between children and adults for almost all classes of drugs.

Influence of Development on Drug Biodisposition

Absorption

Developmental changes in the GI tract are important, because medications are commonly administered to children by mouth and maturational changes may influence drug absorption. It is difficult to generalize,

Table 116.1 Development of Renal Function (From Guignard[r8])

	Premature Infant	Age of Infant			
	First 3 Days	First 3 Days	2 Weeks	8 Weeks	1 Yr
Daily excretion of urine					
ml/kg 24 hr	15–75	20–75	25–120	80–130	40–100
% of fluid intake	40–80	40–80	50–70	45–65	40–60
Voiding size					
ml/kg/voiding	4–6	4–6	4–7	4–6	3–6
Maximal urine osmolality					
mosm/kg H_2O	400–500	600–800	800–900	1000–1200	1200–1400
Glomerular filtration rate					
ml/min/1.73 m²	10–15	15–20	35–45	75–80	90–110

however, because differences in absorption of orally administered drugs associated with growth and maturation are unpredictable and inconsistent. Nevertheless, it is important to be aware of aspects of GI tract development that may influence drug absorption.

Reflux of gastric contents retrograde into the esophagus is very common during the first year of life.[r9] Excessive gastroesophageal reflux may result in regurgitation of medication, resulting in variable and unpredictable loss of an orally-administered dose.

Gastric emptying is an important determinant of rate of absorption, since most drug absorption takes place in the duodenum. Delayed gastric emptying in infants not only contributes to gastroesophageal reflux, but may also result in delayed drug absorption.[r10,r11,r12] On the other hand, gastric emptying in prepubescent children is equal to or exceeds that in adults. This tends to facilitate more rapid drug absorption, other factors being equal. Administration of medication in liquid as opposed to solid dosage forms, as is commonly the case for children, also increases the rate of absorption. In contrast, shorter GI transit time in young children actually may reduce the fraction of dose absorbed when drugs are administered in sustained-release formulations.[11,12]

Decreased gastric acid production in the younger infant may result in increased bioavailability of acid-labile drugs such as the penicillins. For example, increased absorption of penicillin G, ampicillin, and nafcillin in infants compared with older children and adults has been reported. However, perturbation of drug absorption due to reduction in gastric acidity is negligible beyond infancy.

Rate and extent of drug absorption are determined to a significant degree by the absorptive surface area of the duodenum. Greater relative small gut surface area in young children tends to enhance drug absorption.[r10]

Drugs absorbed from the intestine into the portal circulation are delivered to the liver before entering the systemic circulation. High hepatic extraction of some drugs on the first pass through the liver results in removal of a large fraction of the absorbed drug by the liver, resulting in decreased systemic bioavailability. Little is known about the effect of intestinal and hepatic maturation of first-pass uptake of drugs. However, one would predict, based on increased hepatic clearance in children, that first-pass processes in children would be equal to or exceed uptake in adults. Wilson et al. described wide intersubject variability and low serum concentrations of two high-uptake drugs, propoxyphene and propanolol when administered orally to children two to 13 years of age.[13,r2] This is consistent with extensive first-pass uptake.

Maturation of gut flora during childhood modified digoxin clearance. Reduction of digoxin to inactive metabolites by anaerobic GI bacteria accounts for a significant fraction of digoxin clearance in approximately 10 per cent of adult patients.[14] Reduction metabolites are not detected in children until after 16 months of age, and the adult metabolite pattern is not found until after nine years of age.[15]

The rectum is an alternative route of enteral drug administration in children and may be used when vomiting or other intervening conditions preclude oral dosing. Drugs administered rectally are absorbed into the hemorrhoidal veins, which are part of the systemic rather than the portal circulation. First-pass uptake, therefore, is not a consideration with rectal administration. However, rectal dosing is less than satisfactory in many cases for other reasons. Absorption of drugs administered in suppository form typically is erratic and incomplete. Furthermore, presence of feces in the rectal vault impedes absorption. In younger children and infants, the dose may be expelled before absorption is complete, thereby reducing bioavailability to a variable extent. Nevertheless, some medications may be successfully administered rectally in solution.[r13] These include diazepam and valproic acid for seizures and phenobarbital for seizures, sedation, or preanesthesia.[r14,r15] In addition, rectal corticosteroids are routinely used in the treatment of inflammatory bowel disease.

Absorption of drugs from IM or SQ injection sites is influenced by characteristics of the patient as well as properties of the injected drug. Blood flow to the injection site, muscle mass, quantity of adipose tissue, and muscle activity are patient characteristics that determine rate and extent of absorption. Solubility of the drug at the pH of extracellular fluid, ease with which the drug diffuses across capillary membranes, and surface area over which the injection volume spreads also determine absorption.[r11,r12,r13,r16] Extravascular injection is not an optimal route of administration in the presence of hypoperfusion syndromes, dehydration, vasomotor instability, starvation, or cachexia, since all these conditions impede absorption. Some drugs, such as erythromycin and certain cephalosporin antibiotics, are not usually administered IM because they cause unacceptable pain and tissue reaction. However, many drugs, including most aminoglycoside and penicillin antibiotics, may be administered IM with resulting plasma concentrations comparable with those achieved with IV administration. Conversely, highly hydrophobic drugs such as diazepam and phenytoin are not absorbed well following IM injection and should not be given by this route. Furthermore, phenytoin forms insoluble crystals in IM injection sites associated with local hemorrhage, muscle necrosis, and minimal systemic absorption.[16]

Drug Distribution

The distribution of a drug throughout the body is influenced by binding affinity of the drug for plasma and tissue proteins, lipid/water solubility partition of the drug, molecular weight of the drug, and degree of ionization of the drug at physiologic pH. Age-dependent changes in body composition may influence drug distribution in the developing child. Highly lipid-soluble compounds such as inhalation anesthetics and lipophilic sedative/hypnotic agents typically exhibit relatively larger distribution volumes in infants during the first year of life compared with older children because of the relatively larger proportion of body fat in infants. Likewise, the apparent distribution volume of drugs such as penicillin, aminoglycoside, and cephalosporin antibiotics, which distribute primarily in extracellular water, tends to be greater in infants and to decrease during maturation coincident with the progressive relative decrease in extracellular water.[10,r11,r16]

In general, the apparent volume of distribution of drugs tends to be greater in infants and decreases toward adult values during childhood. However, there is a great deal of interindividual variation, and important exceptions to this general rule exist. Examples of such exceptions are theophylline[r17] and phenobarbital,[17] which show little consistent age-related change in distribution volume.

Although the plasma protein binding of many drugs is decreased in the fetus and newborn infant relative to adults, age-related differences in plasma protein binding are not clinically significant beyond the newborn period. However, maturational changes in tissue binding can significantly affect drug distribution. The myocardial-to-plasma digoxin concentration in infants and children up to 36 months of age is two to three times that of adults.[18,19,20] Increased myocardial digoxin concentrations relative to adults have been demonstrated in children using specific assay methods and do not appear to be due to assay interference by endogenous digoxin-like substances. In addition, erythrocytes from infants bind three times the quantity of digoxin of adult erythrocytes. The increased myocardial and erythrocyte binding of digoxin is associated with a significantly greater volume of distribution of digoxin in infants and children compared with adults.

Metabolism and Elimination

Clearance of many drugs is primarily dependent on hepatic metabolism, followed by excretion of parent drug and metabolites by the liver and kidney. Nonpolar lipid-soluble drugs typically are metabolized to more polar and water-soluble compounds prior to excretion, whereas water-soluble drugs usually are excreted unchanged by glomerular filtration and/or renal tubular secretion.[r2]

Phase I metabolic processes involve oxidative, reductive or hydrolytic reactions that most often are catalyzed by the mixed-function oxidase enzyme systems located in the microsomes. Less commonly, such reactions may be mediated by mitochondrial or cystolic enzymes. Phase II, or synthetic, metabolism involves conjugation of the substrate to a polar compound such as glucuronic acid, sulfate, or glycine. This usually results in a polar, water-soluble compound that is readily excreted.

Although the capacity to metabolize a number of drug substrates is decreased during the newborn period, with few exceptions, maturation of the various pathways occurs during the first year of life. The various pathways mature at different times, and there is considerable interindividual variation in rate of maturation of specific pathways. This should not be surprising, since other aspects of development proceed at varying rates in different individuals; e.g., the chronologic age at which infants sit, crawl, walk, and talk is quite variable.

In some cases, the dominant metabolic pathway in infants and children is different from adults. For example, N_7-methylation of theophylline to produce caffeine is well developed in the newborn infant, whereas oxidative demethylation is deficient.[21,22] Therefore, in contrast to older infants and children, theophylline is metabolized to caffeine, which accumulates to pharmacologically active concentrations as a result of its long half-life when theophylline is administered to newborn infants for longer than 10 days. This pathway is important until four to six months of age, when the oxidative pathways mature, caffeine clearance increases, and caffeine accumulation no longer occurs.[23,24] Interestingly, the clearances of theophylline and caffeine increase dramatically coincident with maturation of oxidative N_3-demethylase activity. The metabolic profile of acetaminophen also differs in children compared with adults. The dominant metabolic pathway in infants and children less than 12 years of age is sulfate conjugation, whereas glucuronidation is the major pathway in adolescents and adults.[25,26,27,28] Although the major metabolic pathways differ with age, there is not an age-related difference in clearance.

Maturation of renal clearance of drugs and their metabolites occurs coincident with maturation of renal function during the first year.[r8] With maturation of hepatic and renal function, the clearance of many drugs in young children, when corrected for body surface area, equals or exceeds that in adults after 1 year of age. Table 116.2 compares reported elimination half-lives for a number of drugs among newborns, infants, children, and adults. Typically, the half-life is prolonged in the newborn, decreases during infancy, is shortest in the prepubescent child, and is somewhat longer in adults than in children. With rare exception, a shorter half-life reflects greater clearance. The changes in drug disposition during growth and development reflect the changes in hepatic and renal function described later.

Therapeutic Implications of Developmental Changes

As described earlier, developmental changes in drug disposition have significant therapeutic implications that must be considered when calculating doses for children of different ages. The dose of many drugs must be adjusted not only for increased body mass, but also to compensate for increased clearance and

Table 116.2 Change in Elimination Half-Life (Hours) During Development*

Drug	Newborn	Infant	Child	Adult
Acetaminophen	4.9		4.5	3.6
Amikacin	5.0–6.5		1.6	2.3
Ampicillin	4.0	1.7		1.0–1.5
Amoxicillin	3.7		0.9–1.9	0.6–1.5
Caffeine	100	2		6
Carbamazepine			8–25	10–20
Cefazolin			1.7	2.0
Cefotaxime	4.0	0.8	1.0	1.1
Cefoxitin	3.8	1.4	0.8	0.8
Ceftazidime	4.5	4.5	2.0	1.8
Ceftriaxone	17.0	5.9	4.7	7.8
Cefuroxime	5.5	3.5	1.2	1.5
Cephalothin			0.3	0.6
Clindamycin	3.6	3.0	2.4	4.5
Clonazepam			22–23	20–60
Cyclosporine			4.8	5.5
Diazepam	30	10	25	30
Digoxin		18–33	37	30–50
Ethosuximide			30	52–56
Gentamicin	4.0	2.6	1.2	2–3
Ibuprofen	20		1.0–2.0	2.0–3.0
Isoniazid			2.9 (Slow acetylators)	2.8
Mezlocillin	3.7		0.8	1.0
Moxalactam	5.4	1.7	1.6	2.2
Naproxen			11–13	10–17
Phenobarbital	67–99		36–72	48–120
Primidone			5–11	12–15
Piperacillin	0.8	0.5	0.4	0.9
Quinidine			4.0	5–7
Rifampin			2.9	3.3–3.9
Sulfadiazine	40	10		10–15
Sulfamethoxypyridazine	280	50	50	50
Sulfisoxizole	18	8	8	8
Theophylline	30	6.9	3.4	8.1
Ticarcillin	5–6		0.9	1.3
Tobramycin	4.6		1–2	2–3
Valproate			7.0	6–12
Vancomycin	4.1–9.1		2.2–2.4	5–6
Zidovudine			1.0–1.5	1.6

*Modified from Kaufman RE[r2]

shorter half-life. This is particularly important for drugs to be administered chronically, as anticonvulsants, cardiovascular agents, and bronchodilators. The loading dose of a drug is primarily determined by its volume of distribution, whereas the maintenance dose is determined by the clearance. In addition, the dosing interval relative to the half-life determines the degree of fluctuation of drug concentration between doses (see Chapter 2 in Section I). Several key examples follow.

Recommended loading and maintenance doses for digoxin reflect changes in volume of distribution and clearance with age. The digitalizing dose for premature infants is 20 µg/kg; for full-term newborns, 30 µg/kg; for infants less than 2 years, 40 to 50 µg/kg; and for children older than 2 years, 30 to 40 µg/kg. Likewise, the maintenance dose for premature infants is 5 µg/kg; for full-term newborns, 8 to 10 µg/kg; for infants under 2 years, 10 to 12 µg/kg; and children over 2 years, 8 to 10 µg/kg.

Theophylline dose requirements mirror changes in clearance from infancy to adulthood (Fig. 116.3). Recommended initial infusion rates for IV theophylline are 0.3 to 0.6 mg/kg/h for infants less than 12 months old, 0.8 mg/kg/h for children 1 to 9 years old, 0.7 mg/kg/h for children 9 to 12 years old, and 0.5 mg/kg/h for nonsmoking adolescents.[r17,r18]

The dose of aminoglycoside and some other antibiotics in children required to achieve equivalent plasma concentrations typically is 50 to 100 per cent greater than that in adults because of the greater renal clearance in children.[29,30,r20] The dosing interval in children also may need to be shorter, e.g., every six hours versus every eight hours. Likewise, dosage requirements of the anticonvulsants carbamazepine, ethosuximide, phenobarbital, and phenytoin also are significantly greater on a milligram per kilogram basis in prepubescent children compared with adults because of the greater metabolic capacity in children[31,32,r20] (Table 116.1). In contrast to newborn patients, there is greater risk of underdosing than overdosing older infants and children unless age-related changes in clearance are considered.

Use of sustained-release oral dosage formulations presents unique problems in young children. Absorption may be unpredictable and incomplete, leading to therapeutic failures. In addition, even though the formulation is designed for slow absorption, concentrations may exhibit greater fluctuations between doses than in adults because of the greater clearance in children. For example, sustained-release theophylline products, which provide satisfactory concentrations when given every 12 hours to adults, frequently must be given every eight hours to children to avoid excessive fluctuation in concentration during the dosing interval.[r17]

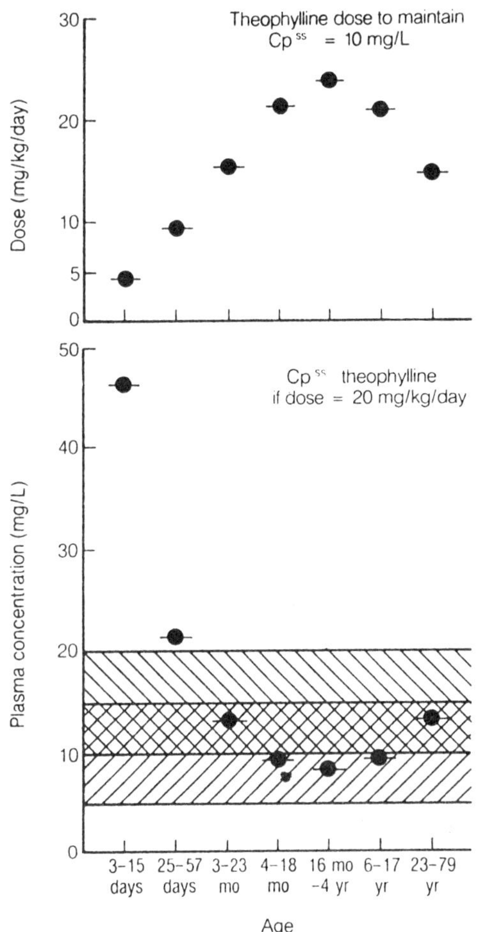

Figure 116.3 Theophylline dose requirements and plasma concentrations. Top panel: Estimated dose requirements of theophylline (mg/kg/day) to maintain a plasma concentration of 10 mg/L. Lower panel: Estimated plasma concentrations of theophylline at steady state if dose is kept at 20 mg/kg/day. Shaded areas indicate tentative therapeutic level for bronchodilatation and anti-apneic activity. Cp^{SS} = Plasma concentration at steady state. (From Aranda JV: "Maturational changes in theophylline and caffeine metabolism and disposition: Clinical implications," in Proceedings of the Second World Conference on Clinical Pharmacology and Therapeutics, July 31–August 5, 1983, edited by I Lemberger and MM Reidenberg. Copyright by the American Society for Pharmacology and Experimental Therapeutics, Bethesda, 1984, p. 870; used with permission.)

The Newborn Infant

Because of its critical importance, as discussed below, the newborn infant warrants special consideration. At birth, a full-term infant in North America receives at least three types of drugs: an ophthalmic antimicrobial agent; vitamin K; and triple dye for the cord.[33] Low-birthweight and sick infants in a neonatal intensive care unit additionally receive an increasing number of drugs, with the constant introduction of new drugs or old drugs with new indications in the neonatal therapeutic armamentarium.[34] Thus, the overall xenobiotic exposure of the fetus and newborn exceeds current estimates, particularly when environmental agents (e.g., lead, methylmercury, volatile hydrocarbons) and drugs of habit (e.g., caffeine, alcohol) are taken into consideration. Since many of these agents are pharmacologically active, their effects may be significant if sufficient amounts reach the fetus or newborn. Besides the usual oral or parenteral routes, unintentional portals of drug entry include the transplacental route; inadvertent direct fetal injection; pulmonary, skin, or conjunctival entry; or via breast milk. Lack of awareness or underestimation of the degree of drug entry through these routes and of altered drug disposition and metabolism in the perinatal period have led to well-recognized therapeutic misadventures in neonatology. Possible prevention of drug toxicity and a rational and safe use of drugs require a thorough understanding of the various pharmacologic profiles of each drug used in the neonate.

In the sick neonate the IV route is preferred because of ease of delivery, accuracy of dosage, possible poor peripheral perfusion, and poor GI function. In neonates who can tolerate gastric feedings, the oral route of drug administration is the most convenient and probably the safest.

Gastric acid production is generally low at birth, and the gastric pH is usually 6 to 8, decreasing within a few hours to pH values of 3 to 1. Acid secretion is low in the first 10 days of life; it tends to rise thereafter and approaches adult values around six to eight months.[10] Intestinal motility is slow in the newborn, and transit time from the stomach to the cecum is generally prolonged relative to that in the adult. The gastric emptying time after milk feeding is considerably prolonged in the neonate and approaches adult values of ages six to eight months. The precise influence of milk feeding on neonatal drug bioavailability requires further evaluation.

Drug absorption requires an intact splanchnic vascular circulation. In sick neonates, especially those with hypotension, perfusion of the gut may decrease to maintain adequate perfusion of vital organs, resulting in decreased drug absorption.

Current evidence indicates that the amount of absorption of most drugs is independent of age, although the rate of absorption of certain drugs shows a nonlinear correlation with age. Heimann studied the enteral absorption of various drugs (i.e., sulfonamides, phenobarbital, digoxin, methyldigoxin, D[-]xylose and L[-]arabinose) and found reduced absorption rates in neonates relative to older children.[35] There is very little specific information concerning other drugs; however, available information indicates that GI absorption of drugs is relatively slow in the newborn and undergoes maturational changes similar to those found in drug distribution, metabolism, and disposition. Although the neonatal drug absorptive deficit may influence the achievement of a desired pharmacologic effect, it is very likely that its significance is minor relative to the age-related alterations in drug distribution, metabolism, and disposition.

For some drugs, including theophylline, phenytoin, phenobarbital, penicillin, and salicylates, the binding to plasma protein in the newborn is decreased compared to that in the nonpregnant adult. This suggests that a more intense pharmacologic response may be obtained in the newborn than in the adult for the same total drug concentration. The developmental changes in protein-drug binding and the postnatal age at which adultlike binding is achieved have not been defined with confidence.[36] Some drugs, such as phenytoin, may exhibit adult-like binding before the infant reaches 3 months.

The reasons underlying this deficient plasma protein binding of drugs at birth have not been definitely established. Possible explanations include decreased plasma albumin concentrations, possible qualitative differences in neonatal plasma proteins, and competitive binding by many endogenous substrates, such as hormones. Hyperbilirubinemia may accentuate this competition by displacing a drug, such as phenytoin, from its albumin-binding site.[41] This contrasts to the well-known bilirubin drug-protein binding interaction, where drugs such as sulfonamides may displace bilirubin from its binding site.

Deficient plasma protein binding usually is not considered in calculating neonatal drug dosages. This factor must be considered in the application of adult therapeutic plasma concentrations to the neonatal patient. Moreover, decreased protein binding will influence calculations of apparent volumes of distribution based on plasma concentrations of total drug.[37] In terms of therapeutic monitoring, drug concentrations obtained from saliva reflect the concentrations of the unbound fraction in plasma.[r21]

Many drugs administered to the newborn infant need to undergo metabolism for efficient elimination from the body. In the past two decades, spurred by the chloramphenicol "gray baby"[2] syndrome and the increased awareness of altered drug disposition in the newborn, the pharmacokinetic disposition and metabolism of some drugs have been studied in the neonate, and available data permit the following generalizations:

1. The rates of drug biotransformation and overall elimination are slow.

2. The rate of drug elimination from the body exhibits marked interpatient variability.[r24]

3. The maturational changes in drug metabolism and disposition as a function of postnatal age are extremely variable and depend on the substrate (or drug) being used.

4. Neonatal drug biotransformation and elimination are vulnerable to pathophysiologic states.

5. Neonates may exhibit activation of alternate biotransformation pathways.[21]

The observation that drug elimination is slower in the neonate relative to adults is well recognized, although the magnitude and duration of this deficit as a function of specific drugs have not been adequately appreciated. Table 116.2 shows the approximate prolongation of the plasma half-lives of certain drugs in the newborn relative to adults. Drugs that are closely related structurally, such as caffeine and theophylline, may even vary significantly.[37] Thus, application of dose rates for theophylline to caffeine in the treatment of neonatal apnea led to marked accumulation of caffeine in the blood.[38] One apparent exception to this observed functional deficit is carbamazepine.

Transplacentally-acquired carbamazepine was eliminated in four of five infants in the immediate postnatal period as rapidly as in adults.[39,40] In contrast, some drugs, such as indomethacin, caffeine, and theophylline, are eliminated much more slowly.

One possible basis for this difference in oxidative biotransformation and elimination capability relates to the existence of multiple forms of cytochrome P_{450}, each with its own distinctive substrate specificity. Data on the comparative measurements of the hemoprotein cytochrome P_{450} in the human fetal, neonatal, and adult liver do not, however, fully explain the observed deficiency in drug biotransformation and elimination. Drugs that undergo conjugation may exhibit characteristics similar to those of drugs requiring oxidative biotransformation for elimination. Glucuronidation is virtually absent in midgestational human fetal liver, and this deficit persists at birth, whereas sulfation is active in the neonate. Acetylation and other synthetic or conjugative reactions, such as those with glutathione, are likely to be somewhat deficient at birth.[r22]

The time after birth at which adult rates of elimination are achieved and the rates at which these maturational changes occur vary with the drug used. Rapid increases in rate of elimination during the first week postnatally have been observed with phenytoin and phenobarbital.[r24] Large interindividual variability in plasma half-lives was observed at birth but rapidly diminished with increasing postnatal age. This means that some neonates receiving a standard dose may exhibit subtherapeutic drug concentrations in the plasma, whereas others may exceed the upper limit of the presumed therapeutic range. In neonates given phenobarbital for seizures, repeated doses of 5 mg/kg/day yielded mean plasma concentrations of about 40 mg/L during the first week, whereas a lower dosage (2.5 to 5 mg/kg/day) yielded plasma concentrations below 15 mg/L by the second and third weeks. The rapidity at which these developmental changes occur would warrant monitoring of plasma concentrations, since dose rates for many drugs usually held constant during the neonatal period may result in poor or exaggerated clinical responses that may be partly attributed to plasma drug concentrations below or above the presumed therapeutic range. Adjustment of dosage based on plasma concentrations of the drug and accounting for a rapid postnatal increase in drug clearance may result in maintenance of plasma concentrations of phenobarbital within the suggested therapeutic range (15–25 mg/L). In contrast, caffeine exhibits negligible maturational changes in the neonatal period.[38] Adult rates of elimination are achieved at about 3 to 4 months and may be exceeded thereafter.[23]

The need to eliminate xenobiotic compounds from

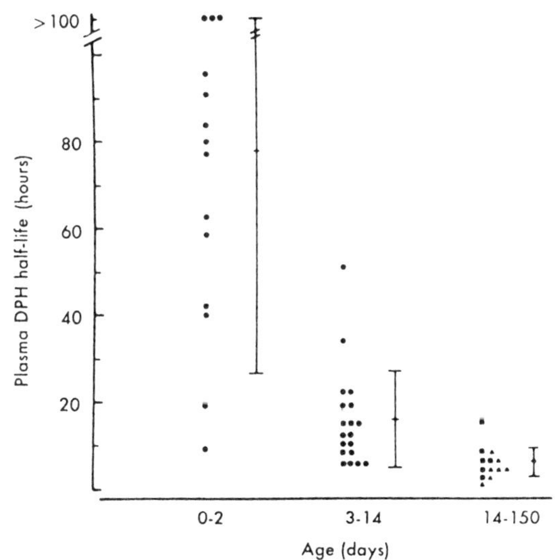

Figure 116.4 Plasma phenytoin (DPH) half-lives measured in infants grouped according to postnatal age. Each infant received the drug via transplacental transfer (?) or as an initial therapeutic dose (?). Half-lives derived from steady-state plasma phenytoin as shown (?). Bars indicate mean and standard deviations. Data were obtained from several published studies. (Reproduced, with permission, from Neims AH and others: Annual Review of Pharmacology and Toxicology 16:427, 1976. Copyright 1976 by Annual Reviews Inc.)

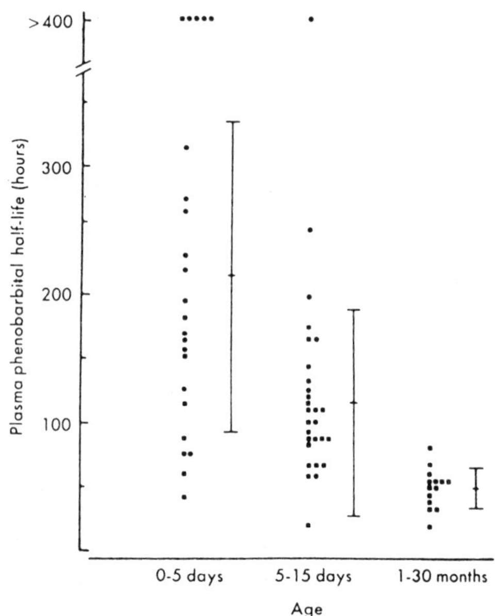

Figure 116.5 Plasma half-lives of phenobarbital administered transplacentally (?) or postnatally (?) in infants, plotted as a function of postnatal age. Data were obtained from several published sources; means and standard deviation are shown. (Reproduced, with permission, from Neims AH and others: Annual Review of Pharmacology and Toxicology 16:427, 1976. Copyright 1976 by Annual Reviews Inc.)

the body in the face of decreased oxidative and conjugative pathways in the fetus and neonate may lead to activation and/or use of available biotransformation pathways not used in the older child and adult. For example, premature neonates given theophylline may produce caffeine via methylation pathways, which are active as early as the first trimester, as shown in human organ culture studies.[21] Since minimum oxidative function is present at this stage of gestation, the relative increase in activity of the methylase pathway leads to the production of caffeine as one of the major metabolites of theophylline in the human fetus and newborn. Both caffeine and theophylline exhibit pharmacologic activity but of variable specific potency; therefore, interpretation of clinical effect must account for both methylxanthines.

Disease states (e.g., congestive heart failure, liver disease) are well recognized in adults as factors that alter drug elimination. The presence of pathophysiologic states (e.g., hypoxia, asphyxia) in neonates can further diminish a deficient drug elimination capability, thus following the accumulation of drug in the plasma. For example, neonates with seizures who experienced perinatal asphyxia may have higher steady-state plasma concentrations of phenobarbital than those without asphyxia.

The variability in neonatal drug disposition and metabolism make generalization of dosage schedules and application of data obtained from one drug to another extremely difficult if not dangerous. Available data further reinforce the need for acquisition of specific pharmacologic data for each drug used in the neonatal period.

Renal Excretion of Drugs

The kidneys are the most important organs for drug elimination in the newborn, since the most frequently used drugs, such as antimicrobial agents, are excreted via these organs.[r8] Renal elimination of these drugs reflects and depends on neonatal renal function, characterized by low glomerular filtration rate, low effective renal blood flow, and low tubular function compared with that in the adult.[r8] Neonatal glomerular filtration rate is about 30 percent of the adult value and is greatly influenced by gestational age at birth.[42] The most rapid changes occur during the first week of life, and these events are reflected by the plasma disappearance rates of aminoglycosides, which are eliminated mainly by glomerular filtration. These changes have been considered in the dosage regimen recommended by McCracken for these drugs and other antibiotics.

Effective renal blood flow may influence the rate at which drugs are presented to and eliminated by the kidneys. Effective renal blood flow, as measured by para-aminohippurate (PAH) clearance, is substantially lower in infants relative to adult values, even when PAH extraction values are correlated (i.e., PAH extraction is 60% in infants compared with greater than 92% in adults). Available data suggest a low effective renal blood flow during the first two days of life (34–99 ml/minute/1.73 m^2), which increases to 54 to 166 ml/minute/1.73 m^2 by 14 to 21 days and further increased to adult values of about 600 ml/minute/1.73 m^2 by age 1 to 2 years.

The pharmacokinetic behavior of drugs eliminated via the neonatal kidneys exhibits characteristics similar to those underlying hepatic biotransformation. For instance, the half-life of many antimicrobials, such as ampicillin (Fig. 116.6), shows a marked interindividual variability at birth, which narrows somewhat with advancing age.[43] The plasma half-life also shortens progressively after birth, achieving adult rates of elimination within one month postnatally. The drug-dependent variability in the elimination process may reflect, in part, the major renal mechanism of drug excretion. These drugs that undergo substantial elimination via glomerular filtration (e.g., aminoglycosides)

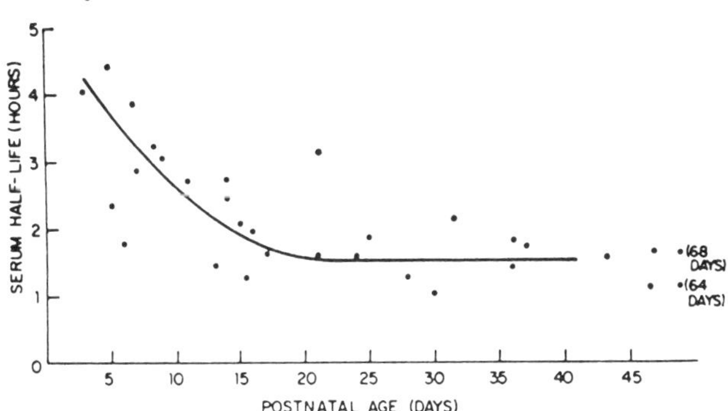

Figure 116.6 Postnatal Changes in the Serum Half-life of Ampicillin (From Axline SG and others: Pediatrics 39:97, 1967. Copyright American Academy of Pediatrics 1967)

may be excreted more rapidly than those requiring substantial tubular excretion (e.g., penicillins). These differences may reflect neonatal glomerular preponderance.

As with hepatic metabolism, renal excretion of certain drugs may be as efficient as in adults. For example, colistin, an antibiotic, is eliminated by neonates at rates similar to those in adults.[43] However, as a rule, drug excretion via the neonatal kidneys is deficient relative to that in the adult. Pathophysiologic insults further compromise the inherent deficiency in drug elimination,[44] thus complicating individual drug dosage regimens. Moreover, very small infants, who receive the most drugs in the neonatal population, exhibit the worst functional deficiency in drug elimination. This could result in overdosage, as in the case of digoxin. Neonates weighing less than 1000 gm achieved steady-state plasma concentrations of digoxin three times higher than their full-term counterparts. Hypoxemia further decreases the slow glomerular and tubular function in the neonates, thus leading to slower renal excretion of drugs, as has been shown with amikacin [45] A linear relationship between oxygen tension and hepatic oxidation has been reported, so drugs that require hepatic biotransformation or renal excretion may be excreted much more slowly in the phase of hypoxemia.[46,47] Determinations of plasma concentration of drugs coupled with appropriate caution and clinical awareness, will help in optimal and safe drug therapy in the neonate.

Knowledge of the kinetic profile of a drug allow manipulation of the dosage to achieve and maintain a given plasma concentration. Many drugs administered in the newborn period exhibit a plasma disappearance curve (Fig. 116.7).

Drugs and Lactation

Drugs and lactation are considered separately because of the unique circumstances this brings to pediatric pharmacology. Until recently, investigations of drugs and other compounds in breast milk were hampered by the very small numbers of lactating women studied and the insensitivity of drug assay methods. Much of the earlier literature[48,49,50] concerns isolated case reports and small selections of drugs. Several recent papers review these data. At present, a higher incidence of breast-feeding provides more situations in which lactating women are exposed to various medications, and an increasing number of useful studies of these drugs in milk can be expected. Currently, up to 80 percent of Canadian and American women breast-feed their infants. In addition to pharmaceuticals, environmental pollutants and nontherapeutic or "social" chemicals find their way into human milk. Public awareness of these problems is high, and the physician is often called on for counselling.

The presence and concentrations of compounds in human milk depend on molecular weight, degree of ionization, protein binding in blood, lipid solubility, and specific uptake by mammary tissue. Drugs that are not absorbed after oral ingestion will not appear in milk. Small compounds with molecular weights less than about 200 appear freely in milk and are presumed

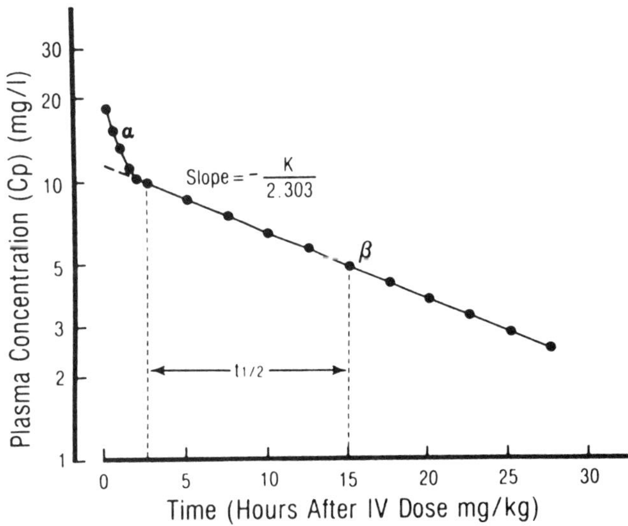

Figure 116.7 Representative plasma disappearance curve of a drug given intravenously, plotted semilogarithmically as a function of time. A fast distribution phase (α) is followed by a slower elimination phase (β).

to have passed through pores in the mammary alveolar cell. Large compounds, such as insulin or heparin, do not pass into milk. Intermediate-size compounds must penetrate the lipoprotein cell membrane by diffusion or active transport.

In general, drugs that are not ionized at blood pH will traverse the alveolar cell membrane with greater ease than will highly ionized compounds. Since milk pH is about 7 or slightly less, milk will act as a trap for weak bases.

Drugs pass the cell membrane only in their free form; thus, highly protein-bound drugs are less available for passage. Drugs or other chemicals that are very lipid soluble readily cross the alveolar cell, and, since milk contains a considerable amount of lipid, these compounds are also trapped in milk. Drugs for the most part enter breast milk by passive diffusion. This is best described in pharmacokinetic terms as a three-compartment model, with the breast milk as a deep third compartment (Fig. 116.8). These principles also apply to drug metabolite transfer into breast milk.

Finally, certain compounds are actively taken up by mammary tissue and are found in milk in concentrations substantially higher than in blood.

The amount of drug in breast milk can be calculated by the milk/plasma (M/P) ratio. However, the use of the M/P ratio is fraught with potential difficulties. It is better, if possible, to measure drug concentrations directly in breast milk.

Drugs may be metabolized by the maternal body to active or inactive metabolites. These derivatives may then be secreted into milk less readily than is the parent compound. The timing of maternal ingestion of a drug in relation to the time of milk synthesis may influence the concentration of the drug in any particular milk feeding.

In animals, changes in mammary gland blood flow control the amount of drug presented to sites of uptake. Mammary tissue itself can metabolize certain compounds. Drugs already secreted into milk may be secreted back into the alveolar cell and then into blood. Moreover, the stage of lactation plays a role; drugs may be secreted more easily in the colostral phase. Finally, changes in milk composition during lactation or feeding may change the amount of drug in breast milk; as an illustration, formula is more acidic than in milk expressed later in a feed.

The total volume of milk consumed in a known period determines the dosage to the infant. Since daily volume intake of breast milk is exceedingly variable and impractical to measure routinely, one could assume a *high average* daily milk consumption to be about 1 L.

To produce an effect, the drug in the milk must either act locally in the gut or be absorbed. It is possible that the proteins of milk will bind certain drugs and thereby impede absorption; it is also possible that the bowel of a very young infant may permit absorption of normally excluded large molecules.

The infant's disposition of the drug in milk will change with postnatal age; in addition, one must always be aware of the drug's potential for displacement of bilirubin from serum albumin.

Compounds in Human Milk

Anticoagulants[51,52]

Heparin does not enter breast milk. Oral anticoagulants of the inandione group as well as bishydroxycoumarin and ethyl biscoumacetate are found in milk

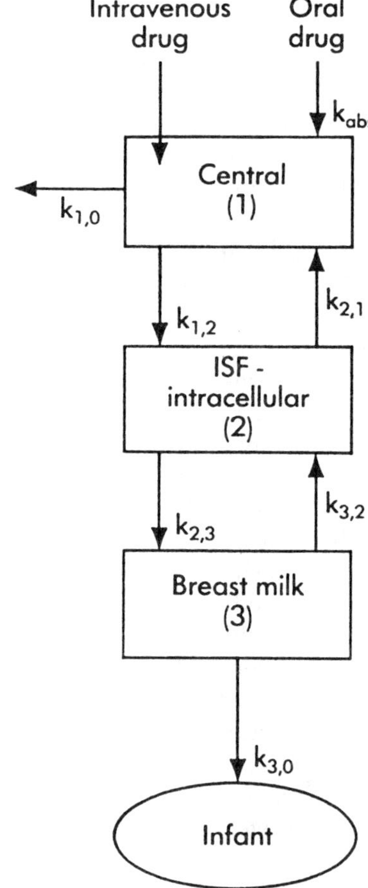

Figure 116.8 Three-compartment model for drug transfer into breast milk. ISF: Interstitial fluid; k_{abs}: absorption rate constant; $k_{x,y}$: rate constant for transfer from compartment x to compartment y. (Modified from Wilson JT, Drug Metab Rev 1983; 14:619–652).

and have been associated with infant coagulopathies. Warfarin must be considered the drug of choice, since by virtue of its acidity as well as its high degree of protein binding it is undetectable in human milk.

Antiinflammatory and Analgesic Drugs[53,54,55,56,57,58,59]

Acetylsalicylic acid (ASA) appears to be without danger when used occasionally. Older infants have been found to receive about 0.2 to 0.3 percent of a single dose of ASA administered to the mother. Although detailed studies do not exist, acetaminophen and ibuprofen seem to be safe. Indomethacin has been associated with neonatal convulsions.

Antimicrobial Drugs[r23,60,61,62,63,64]

Fortunately, most antimicrobial agents in human milk appear safe for the nursing infant. Drugs of the penicillin group may change the infant's intestinal flora and cause diarrhea and thrush; in theory, they also could incite hypersensitivity. The cephalosporins appear to be secreted in insignificant amounts in milk. The passage of the various sulfonamide derivatives is influenced by their differing degrees of ionization and protein binding; all have the potential to displace bilirubin from albumin. Thus, the sulfonamides should be avoided if possible in the therapy of women breast-feeding infants in the first week of the infant's life. Ingestion of salicylazosulfapyridine leads to the appearance of the metabolite sulfapyridine in milk; it has been estimated that the infant of a mother chronically using this drug will receive about 0.3 percent of the maternal dose per day. Erythromycin is present in milk in higher concentration than in maternal plasma, suggesting that the infant could receive a significant dose. The tetracyclines in milk have the potential to cause dental staining and should be avoided for the therapy of women breast-feeding their infants. Most authors recommended that chloramphenicol not be taken by lactating women, even though the drug levels in milk do not lead to a dose as large as those associated with the "gray baby" syndrome. The aminoglycosides are poorly absorbed from the infant's GI tract. Isoniazid and PAS have not been associated with ill effects to the nursing infant. Metronidazole was considered contraindicated because of carcinogenicity in animals; however, recent human data suggest noncarcinogenicity. Also, metronidazole has been used in neonatal infections with no apparent immediate adverse effects. Recent work suggests that metronidazole therapy in usual doses is not contraindicated among breast-feeding infants.

Drugs Affecting the Cardiovascular System[65,66,67,68,69,70]

The amount of digoxin present in milk depends on the maternal dose; infants whose mothers received 0.25 mg/day did not ingest enough digoxin in milk to have detectable blood levels. Diuretics in general seem to be harmless, although if a nursing woman were to become dehydrated because of diuretic use, lactation would be greatly depressed. The effects of diuretics on milk composition are unclear. Spironolactone and its less active metabolite are secreted in milk, and an estimated 0.2 percent of the mother's daily dose is received by the infant. Chlorthalidone appears in small amounts in milk but could potentially accumulate in the young infant. Propranolol seems to be safe. Quinidine is secreted in milk to a concentration about 60 percent that of maternal blood, but no ill effects have been observed.

Drugs Affecting the Central Nervous System[71,72,73,74,75,76,77,78,79]

Diazepam is converted in the body to an active metabolite, desmethyldiazepam, and both are excreted in milk. Both these compounds have a prolonged half-life in infants, and chronic use of diazepam by nursing women has been associated with lethargy and weight loss in their babies. The barbiturates appear in milk in concentrations that depend on their different degrees of ionization and lipid solubility. In anticonvulsant doses they seem to be safe. Chlordizepoxide in breast milk has been linked to depression in the nursing infant. Meprobamate probably should be avoided, since the drug achieves milk concentrations several times greater than the maternal plasma levels.

Lithium is definitely contraindicated during lactation: it has been found to cause significant cardiovascular and CNS signs in the infant. The phenothiazines and tricyclic antidepressants have been found in breast milk but appear to be safe in modest doses. The amphetamines also appear in milk and may cause jitteriness.

Phenytoin is found in milk in concentrations about one-fifth those of maternal blood. Primidone and ethosuximide both achieve milk levels near that of maternal blood although significant symptoms in the infants have not been noted.

Phenobarbital is metabolized much more slowly in neonates than in adults; it is possible that breast-fed infants of phenobarbital-treated mothers may accumulate the drug. These infants should be monitored for lethargy and weight gain.

Drugs Affecting the Endocrine System[80,81,82]

Drugs of the thiouracil family, methimazole, carbimazole, and iodides, are contraindicated during breast-feeding; they achieve a high milk concentration and can suppress the infant's thyroid function. Revision of this dogma has been suggested, and propylthiouracil may be given to nursing mothers provided the infant's thyroid function is monitored.

Thyroxin and other thyroid hormone preparations seem to be safe; endogenous thyroid hormone naturally secreted in breast milk may mask congenital cretinism during breast-feeding. The long-term effects of exogenous glucocorticoids and their derivatives in milk are not known. Women receiving prednisone and prednisolone excrete very small amounts of these compounds in milk.

A common dilemma is the use of oral contraceptives during lactation. Little is known about the effects of long exposure to small doses of these compounds in milk. Contraceptives with a high concentration of estrogen and progestin will depress lactation, especially if they are begun soon after parturition. If their use is imperative, it would seem best to start treatment about four weeks after delivery, ensuring that lactation is already well established, and to use the lowest dosage possible. The infants should be followed with some care, since there have been reports of gynecomastia and changes in vaginal epithelium. Study of late effects in exposed infants is urgently needed. The oral contraceptives in current clinical use are not contraindicated for mothers breast-feeding infants.

Other Drugs[83]

Cimetidine, a histamine-H_2-receptor antagonist, has been reported in breast milk in concentrations three to 12 times greater than in maternal blood; this drug may be actively transported into milk. Until there is more information concerning its effects in infants, cimetidine should not be used during lactation. The same probably applies to ranitidine and omeprazole, a newly developed anti-ulcer drug that is extremely potent. Neither should be used during lactation.

Theobromine from chocolate has been found in milk at a level of 80 percent of maternal serum. Theophylline ingestion by the mother has been associated with infant irritability. Extracts of ergot have been responsible for toxic reactions in nursing infants and should be avoided. The use of isotopes for diagnosis or therapy should be avoided during lactation. An acceptable level of an isotope in milk is not known. It has been suggested that women not nurse for 10 days after exposure to ^{131}I, for three days after ^{99m}Tc exposure, and for two weeks following ^{67}Ga exposure. If radiopharmaceuticals are required during lactation, breast-feeding should be avoided while the radioactive agent is present in milk. In cases of uncertainty, consultation should be obtained from a specialist in nuclear medicine.

"Nontherapeutic" Agents in Human Milk

Caffeine[84,85]

One hour after the ingestion of an average cup of coffee, a peak milk caffeine level of about 1.5 μg/ml is obtained. Caffeine levels in milk are about half the corresponding maternal blood level. Although the daily amount of caffeine consumed by a nursing infant might be small, the long half-life of caffeine could cause symptoms such as wakefulness or jitteriness.

Ingredients of Cigarettes[86,87]

The nicotine content of breast milk from women smoking one pack per day has been found to be about 100 to 500 parts per billion. No symptoms have been ascribed to this degree of contamination. Thiocyanate, which is elevated in the blood of smoking women, does not appear in elevated amounts in their milk.

Ethanol[88,89]

Ethanol, a small molecule, diffuses freely into milk and achieves levels equivalent to those in blood. The metabolite acetaldehyde does not appear in milk. Excessive ethanol intake by the mother may depress the infant's CNS.

Narcotics[90,91,92,93,94]

Heroin, methadone, morphine, and other opiate derivatives have been found in milk and may be responsible for both addiction and withdrawal symptoms in the nursing infant. Opiates used briefly appear to have little clinical effect. It has been suggested that women receiving methadone maintenance doses take their daily dose after the last breast-feeding in the evening, since milk methadone levels are found to peak about four hours after administration of the drug by mouth.

Environmental Pollutants in Human Milk

Lead[95,96]

Lead has been found in both bovine and human milk, as well as in commercial infant formulas. The lead content of human milk has remained rather constant over the past four decades, in contrast to levels of some other pollutants. One study found the lead level in human milk in the US to be about 0.03 μg/

ml. There are no reports of signs and symptoms of lead toxicity from this source.

Mercury[97,98]

Metallic or inorganic mercury poisoning in adults has usually been in association with occupational exposure. There are no reports of metallic mercury poisoning from human milk. Organic mercury, more specifically *methylmercury,* has been used industrially in fungicides, in pulp and paper factories, and in chloralkali plants. In the late 1950s Minamata Bay in Japan was contaminated with industrial wastes containing methylmercury; the compound found its way into human beings through contaminated fish. There was a high incidence of neurologic abnormalities in children born in this area, probably related to in utero exposure to the chemical rather than to exposure during lactation. Methylmercury was found in human milk in a concentration about 5 percent of that in blood; the half-life for disappearance of mercury from milk was estimated to be about 70 days.

Several epidemics in Iraq in the last 15 years were traceable to the contamination of grains with methylmercury fungicides. A number of nursing infants ingested enough methylmercury in milk to achieve blood levels above the toxic limit.

Pesticides[99–104]

Organic pesticides are concentrated in body fat, and milk production, with its export of large quantities of lipid, is a very efficient way for the female to rid her body of these poisons. The nursing human infant thus becomes the highest animal in the "food-chain". DDT (dichlorodiphenyltrichloroethane) was first identified in breast milk in 1951, and milk levels have been falling slowly since its use was restricted in North America in the early 1970s. Current levels of DDT in human milk vary geographically and are related to agricultural use of the compound. In Canada in 1979, average milk DDT was 44 ng/gm of human milk. A 5-kg infant ingesting 1 kg of breast milk each day would thus take in about 0.009 mg/kg/day. The FAO/WHO recommendations for maximum allowable intake by an adult is about 0.005 mg/kg/day. Nonetheless, there are no known harmful effects to the infant from the ingestion of human milk contaminated to this degree.

Many other pesticides have been found in human milk, and this reflects the current commercial use in the region or country. Dieldrin, for instance, which was banned in the US after 1974, is decreasing in concentration in breast milk.

Industrial By-Products[105–107]

The extremely toxic dioxin TCDD (2,3,7,8-tetrachlorodibenzo-*p*-dioxin) caused environmental contamination in Seveso, Italy, in 1976. Children who were directly exposed developed chloracne; further effects remain to be determined. This toxin has been found in human milk.

There has been great public interest in the polychlorinated biphenyls (PCBs). The class of compounds has had 50 years of industrial usage, primarily in the manufacture of electric apparatus (transformers, capacitors), although such usage seems to be declining. Because of contamination of rivers and lakes by industrial effluent, PCBs are widely distributed in freshwater fish and in those animals that eat them. As with organic pesticides, PCBs remain in body fat stores and are excreted with the fat of breast milk. An epidemic of poisoning by PCBs (Yusho disease) occurred in 1968 in Japan, when a commercial rice oil product was inadvertently contaminated with PCBs. Fetuses exposed in utero suffered growth retardation both antenatally and postnatally. Several infants whose only exposure was via human milk developed weakness and apathy. It is of great concern that milk levels of PCBs in North America appear to be increasing. In Canada in 1979, the average PCB level in human milk was 12 ng/gm, whereas women who are exposed occupationally to PCBs or who consume game fish from contaminated waters may have much higher levels in milk.

The polybrominated biphenyls (PBBs) were brought to attention by an incident in Michigan in 1973 and 1974, in which several hundred pounds of PBBs, normally used as fire retardants in the plastics industry, accidentally contaminated cattle feed. PBBs have the usual propensity to lodge in fat tissue and to persist in the body. To date, no ill effects have been noted in infants exposed to PBBs through their mother's milk. In Michigan, breast milk PBB surveillance has provided an accurate picture of the contamination of the general population. This method of epidemiologic analysis for fat-soluble poisons has much to recommend it, since the collection of milk samples is far easier than the collection of adipose tissue specimens. Breast milk PBB levels in the contaminated areas of Michigan averaged 0.07 parts per milk.

As with the helpless fetus in utero (as discussed in Section 2, Chapter 7), the nursing infant is exposed to nearly everything entering the body of its mother. The dangers, especially over the long term, are unclear. Environmental pollutants are almost impossible to avoid, and elimination of nontherapeutic (recreational) compounds involves changing lifestyles. Drug administration is the easiest to control, but often a difficult choice must be made between maternal therapy and potential infant harm. The following are some simple guides to be observed:

1. A lactating woman should not receive a drug that one would be reluctant to give directly to her infant at that particular postnatal or gestational age.

2. Drug secretion into milk is so variable that one should not attempt to *treat* an infant by administering the drug to the lactating mother.

3. Milk that is donated to milk banks must be free from contamination.

4. When maternal drug administration is necessary, one may attempt to minimize the dosage to the infant by withholding nursing at the time of maximum secretion of the drug into milk.

5. Signs and symptoms in a nursing child should be correlated with drug ingestion by the mother. In investigations it is perhaps most useful to measure levels of the drug and its metabolites in the infant's body fluids, rather than at isolated times in maternal blood or milk.

6. When therapy is necessary, therapy should be with single agents if possible in the case of chronic therapy, consideration should be made to monitor the infant's activity and growth.

Examples of Increased Toxicity

Although discussed in Section 13, the complex process involved in growth and development frequently make the child uniquely vulnerable to mechanisms of toxicity not present in mature individuals. Chronic treatment with adrenocorticosteroids, amphetamine, and methylphenidate impede linear growth. Tetracycline antibiotics are not recommended for children under 9 years of age because they cause enamel dysplasia in developing teeth. Use of the fluoroquinolone antibiotics in children is contraindicated because of toxicity to growing cartilage.

Metoclopramide and prochlorperazine commonly are used as antiemetic agents during cancer chemotherapy, and metoclopramide is used as a prokinetic agent to treat gastroesophageal reflux. Both of these drugs are dopamine-2 antagonists and, in excessive dose, can produce acute dystonic reactions. Haloperidol shares this adverse side effect. Younger children seem to be more susceptible to dystonic reactions than adults. This may be related to greater concentration of dopamine-2 receptors in the brain in young patients.

Infants and young children are more prone than adults to acute CNS and hyperpyrexic reactions to anticholingeric drugs such as atropine and scopolamine. Toxicity associated with topical ocular administration has been described. Children under 1 year are more susceptible to respiratory depression from weight-adjusted doses of opioid drugs that generally are safe in older children and adults. For this reason, opioid antitussive agents such as codeine and dextromethorphan are not recommended for use in this age-group.

Verapamil is a drug of choice for the treatment of supraventricular arrhythmias in older children and adult patients. However, infants with supraventricular tachyarrhythmias appear to be at increased risk of sudden cardiac arrest. The mechanism for this increased risk is poorly understood. Verapamil is not recommended for treatment of acute arrhythmias in children under 1 year of age.

Valproic acid is one of the most commonly used anticonvulsants in children. In rare cases, it can cause acute hyperammonemia associated with hepatoencephalopathy. Children under 5 are at greatest risk for developing this life-threatening adverse reaction, particularly if they are receiving other anticonvulsant drugs concurrently.

Examples of Decreased Toxicity

Immaturity does not invariably predispose to increased risk of toxicity. Although infants and children may be more susceptible than adults to certain types of drug toxicity, there are important examples in which differences in drug disposition appear to result in decreased risk of toxicity in immature individuals.

Infants and young children appear to be less susceptible to ototoxicity and renal toxicity from aminoglycoside antibiotics compared with older patients. This may be due, in part, to reduced intracellular accumulation of the aminoglycoside in renal tubular epithelial cells. Children tend to experience relatively mild liver toxicity from acute acetaminophen overdose. Weight-adjusted doses and serum concentrations that invariably are associated with severe hepatotoxicity in young adults produce much less hepatocellular damage in preschool children. There is evidence that this is due to a greater capacity of children to metabolize acetaminophen by nontoxic pathways.

Hepatotoxicity from halothane is relatively rare in children, even following multiple exposures, whereas it is not that uncommon in adults. The mechanism of reduced hepatotoxicity in children is not known. The risk of isoniazid-induced hepatitis is age-related. An incidence of 0 per 1000 patients less than 20 years of age was reported by the Food and Drug Administration.

Adverse Drug Reaction and Toxicity

Besides the usual desired routes, there are unintentional ones; e.g., absorption across the placental or via breast milk; inadvertent direct fetal injection; and pulmonary, skin or conjunctival entry. Underestimation of the importance of these routes and unawareness of altered drug metabolism and disposition lead to therapeutic tragedies; e.g., failure to recognize the deficient glucuronyl transferase activities in the newborn leads to the gray baby/toddler syndrome characterized by acute cardiovascular collapse due to chloramphenicol toxicity. Displacement of bilirubin from the albumin binding sites by sulfa drugs leads to kernicterus or bilirubin encephalopathy in neonates. Dermal absorption of hexachlorophene produces cystic brain lesions and neuropathologic abnormalities in young infants. Boric acid and aniline dye poisonings occur from unexpected absorption of these agents from diapers.

Drug toxicities (as in overdosage) usually are exaggerations of the known pharmacologic effects of a drug (e.g., cardiac arrhythmias with overdosage of cardiac glycosides). However, host factors such as hypersensitivity or genetic abnormalities (e.g., G6PD deficiency) may also predispose to adverse drug reactions. Drug withdrawal generally reverses the reaction. Management of persistent toxic reactions depends on the specific drug.

Pediatric Drug Dosages

Pharmacokinetics and Therapeutic Drug Monitoring

No rules are adequate to guarantee efficacy and safety of drugs in the pediatric patient, especially the newborn. Dosages based on pharmacokinetic data for a given age group, adjusted to the desired response and each individual's drug handling capability, offer the most rational approach. Knowledge of a drug's kinetic profile allows manipulation of the dose to achieve and maintain a given plasma concentration. Many drugs exhibit a biexponential plasma disappearance curve in the neonate and older pediatric patient; i.e., the log of the plasma drug concentration decreases linearly as a function of time, with a brief but fast distributive (α) phase and a slower elimination (β) phase. This exemplifies a two-compartment model and first-order kinetics, in which a certain fraction (not amount) of the drug remaining in the body is eliminated per unit time; and, after the distribution phase, the plasma concentration is proportional to the concentration of drug in other portions of the body. This model is applicable to a wide variety of drugs used in newborns and older children, although some drugs (e.g., gentamicin, diazepam, digoxin) may fit a multicompartmental model; others (e.g., salicylates) exhibit saturation kinetics (i.e., a certain amount—not a fraction—of the drug is eliminated per unit of time). In the young toddler and prepubertal child, the α phase may be very short relative to the β phase, and its contribution to over-all elimination and to dosage computations may not be significant. Similarly, drugs given to the newborn usually have an extremely prolonged β phase relative to the α phase. Thus, the entire body during the newborn period could be considered as if it were a singly compartment for purposes of dose calculations.

For the majority of drugs, which follow first-order kinetics, dose adjustments can be based on plasma concentration, which at steady state is proportional to dose. For example, if phenobarbital plasma concentration is only 5 mg/L at 10 mg/kg/day, doubling the dose to 20 mg/kg/day should also double the plasma drug concentration to 10 mg/L.

Administering a loading dose (mg/kg) may be useful to achieve a given plasma concentration quickly when rapid onset of drug action is required. For many drugs, loading doses (mg/kg) are generally greater in neonates and young infants than in older children or adults. However, the prolonged elimination of drugs in the first few weeks of postnatal life warrants substantially lower maintenance doses given at longer intervals to prevent toxicity. Adjustment of maintenance doses is required to deal with rapid changes in drug elimination with increasing age and also with differences among drugs.

Monitoring drug concentrations from serum or other biologic fluids (saliva, urine, CSF, etc.) is useful if the desired effect is not attained or if adverse reactions occur. Monitoring is also useful in assessing compliance.

References

Research Reports

1. Silverman WA, Anderson DH, Blanc WA, Douglas NC. A difference in mortality rate and incidence of kernicterus among premature infants allotted to two prophylactic antibacterial regimens. Pediatrics 1956;*18*:614–624.
2. Sutherland JM. Fatal cardiovascular collapse of infants receiving large amounts of chloramphenicol. Am J Dis Child 1959;*97*:761–767.
3. Dubois D, Dubois E. Clinical calorimetry: A formula to estimate the appropriate surface area if height and weight be known. Arch Intern Med 1916;*17*:863–871.

4. Sloan A, de Weir JB. Nomograms for prediction of body density and total body fat from skin fold measurements. J Appl Physiol 1970;*28*:221–222.
5. Forbes G, Amikhakimi G. Skin-fold thickness and body fat in children. Hum Biol 1970;*42*:401–418.
6. Lohman T, Bioleau R, Rassey B. Prediction of lean body mass in young boys from skinfold thickness and body weight. Hum Biol 1975;*47*:345–362.
7. Lohman T. Skin folds and body density and their relationship to body fatness. Hum Biol 1981;*53*:181–225.
8. Wichmann HM, Rind H, Gladtke E. Die elimination von bromsulphalein beim kind. Z Kinderheilk 1968;*103*:262–276.
9. Habersang R, Kauffman RE. Drug doses for children: A rational approach to an old problem. J Kans Med Soc 1974;*75*:98–103.
10. Kearns GL, Reed MD. Clinical pharmacokinetics in infants and children: A reappraisal. Clin Pharmacokinet 1989;*17*:(suppl 1):29–67.
11. Pedersen S, Moller-Petersen J. Erratic absorption of a slow-release theophylline spinkle product. Pediatrics 1984;*74*:534–538.
12. Rogers RJ, Kalisker A, Wiener MB, Szefler SJ. Inconsistent absorption from a sustained-release theophylline preparation during continuous therapy in asthmatic children. J Pediatr 1985;*106*:496–501.
13. Wilson JT, Atwood GF, Shand D. Disposition of propoxyphene and propranolol in children. Clin Pharmacol Ther 1976;*19*:264–270.
14. Lindenbaum J, Rund DG, Butler VP Jr, Tse-Eng D, Saha JR. Inactivation of digoxin by the gut flora: Reversal by antibiotic therapy. N Engl J Med 1981;*305*:789–794.
15. Linday L, Dobkin JF, Wang TC, Butler VP Jr, Saha JR, Lindenbaum J. Digoxin inactivation by the gut flora in infancy and childhood. Pediatrics 1987;*79*:544–548.
16. Dill WA, Kazenko A, Wolf LM, Glazko SA. Studies on 5,5-diphenyl-dantoin (Dilantin) in animals and man. J Pharmacol Exp Ther 1956;*118*:270–279.
17. Heimann G, Gladtke E. Pharmacokinetics of phenobarbital in childhood. Eur J Clin Pharmacol 1977;*12*:305–310.
18. Andersson KE, Bertler A, Wettrell G. Post-mortem distribution and tissue concentrations of digoxin in infants and adults. Acta Paediatr Scand 1975;*64*:497–504.
19. Park MK, Ludden T, Arom KV, Rogers J, Oswalt JD. Myocardial vs serum diogoxin concentrations in infants and adults. Am J Dis Child 1982;*136*:418–420.
20. Gorodischer R, Jusko WJ, Yaffe SJ. Tissue and erythrocyte distribution of digoxin in infants. Clin Pharmacol Ther 1976;*19*:256–263.
21. Aranda JV, Louridas AT, Vitulo BB, Thom P, Aldridge A, Haber R. Metabolism of theophylline to caffeine in human fetal liver. Science 1979;*206*:1319–1321.
22. Brazier JL, Salle B, Ribon B, Desage M, Renaud H. In vivo N_7-methylation of theophylline to caffeine in premature infants. Dev Pharmacol Ther 1981;*2*:137–144.
23. Aranda JV, Collinge JM, Zinman R, Watters G. Maturation of caffeine elimination in infancy. Arch Dis Child 1979;*54*:946–949.
24. Aranda JV, Scalais E, Papageorgiou A, Beharry K. Ontogeny of human caffeine and theophylline metabolism. Dev Pharmacol Ther 1984;*7*(suppl 1):18–25.
25. Levy G, Khanna NN, Soda DM, Tsuzuki O, Stern L. Pharmacokinetics of acetaminophen in the human neonate: Formation of acetaminophen glucuronide and sulfate in relation to plasma bilirubin concentration and D-glucaric acid excretion. Pediatrics 1975;*55*:818–825.
26. Miller RP, Roberts RJ, Fischer LJ. Acetaminophen elimination kinetics in neonates, children, and adults. Clin Pharmacol Ther 1976;*19*:284–294.
27. Howie D, Adriaenssens PI, Prescott LF. Paracetamol metabolism following overdosage: Application of high performance liquid chromatography. J Pharm Pharmacol 1977;*29*:235–237.
28. Rollins D, von Bahr C, Glaumann H, Moldéus P, Rane A. Acetaminophen: Reactive intermediate formation by human fetal and adult liver microsomes and isolated human fetal liver cells. Science 1979;*205*:1414–1416.
29. Vogelstein B, Kowarski A, Lietman PS. The pharmacokinetics of amikacin in children. J Pediatr 1977;*91*:333–339.
30. Brown RD, Campoli-Richards DM. Antimicrobial therapy in neonates, infants, and children. Clin Pharmacokinet 1989;*17*(suppl 1):105–115.
31. Riva R, Contin M, Albani F, Perucca E, Procaccianti G, Baruzzi A. Free concentration of carbamazepine and carbamazepine-10,11-epoxide in children and adults: Influence of age and phenobarbitone co-medication. Clin Pharmacokinet 1985;*10*:524–531.
32. Morrow JI, Richen A. Disposition of anticonvulsants in childhood. Clin Pharmacokinet 1989;*17*(suppl 1):89–104.
33. Aranda JV, Cohen S and Neims AH. Drug utilization in a newborn intensive care unit. Journal of Pediatrics 1976;*89*:315–317.
34. Aranda JV, Clarkson S, Collinge JM. Changing pattern of drug utilization in a neonatal intensive care unit. American Journal of Perinatology 1983;*1*:28–30.
35. Heimann G. Enteral absorption and bioavailability in children in relation to age. Eur J Clin Pharmacol 1980;*18*:43–50.
36. Krasner J, Giaccoia GP, Yaffe SJ. Drug-protein binding in the newborn infant. Ann NY Acad Sci 1973;*226*:101–114.
37. Aranda JV, Sitar DS, Parsons DV, Loughnan PM, Neims AH. Pharmacokinetic aspects of theophylline in premature newborns. N Engl J Med 1976;*295*:413–416.
38. Aranda JV, Cook CE, Gorman W, Collinge JM, Loughnan PM, Outerbridge EW. Pharmacokinetics profile of caffeine in the premature newborn infant with apnea. J Pediatr 1979;*94*:993–995.
39. Rane A, Bertilsson L, Palmér L. Disposition of placentally transferred carbamazepine (Tegretol) in the newborn. Eur J Clin Pharmacol 1975;*8*:283–284.
40. Rane A, Shand DG, Wilkinson GR. Disposition of carbamazepine and its 10,11-epoxide metabolite in the isolated perfused rat liver. Drug Metab Dispos 1977;*5*:179–184.
41. Rane A, Lunde PKM, Jalling B, Yaffe SJ, Sjoqvist F. Plasma protein binding of diphenylhydantoin in normal and hyperbilirubinemic infants. J Pediatr 1971;*78*:877–882.
42. Guignard JP, Torrado A, Da Cunha O, Gautier E. Glomerular filtration rate in the first three weeks of life. J Pediatr 1975;*87*:268–272.

43. Axline SG, Yaffe SJ, Simon HJ. Clinical pharmacology of antimicrobials in premature infants II. Ampicillin, methicillin, oxacillin, neomycin, and colistin. Pediatr 1967;*39*:97–107.

44. Guignard JP, Torrado A, Mazouni SM, Gautier E. Renal function in respiratory distress syndrome. J Pediatr 1976;*88*:845–850.

45. Mirhij N, Reeves MD, Roberts RJ. Effect of hypoxia on amikacin pharmacokinetics. Pediatr Res 1976;*10*:192A.

46. Cummings JF, Mannering GJ. Effect of phenobarbital administration on the oxygen requirement for hexobarbital metabolism in the isolated perfused rat liver and in the intact rat. Biochem Pharmacol 1970;*19*:973–978.

47. Gal P. The influence of asphyxia on phenobarbital dosing requirements in neonates. Dev Pharmacol Ther. 1984;*7*:145–152.

48. Atkinson HC, Begg EJ, Darlow BA. Drugs in breast milk: Clinical pharmacokinetic considerations. Clinical Pharmacokinetics 1988;*14*:217–240.

49. Wilson JT. Determinants and consequences of drug excretion in breast milk. Drug Metabolism Rev 1983;*14*:619–652.

50. Committee on Drugs: American Academy of Pediatrics: The transfer of drugs and other chemicals into human breast milk. Pediatr 1989;*84*:924–936.

51. De Swiet M, Lewis PJ. Excretion of anticoagulants in human milk (letter). N Engl J Med 1977;*297*:1471.

52. Ormke ML. May mothers given warfarin breast-feed their infants? Br Med J 1977;*1*:1564–1565.

53. Berlin CM Jr, Yaffe SJ. Disposition of salicylazosulfapyridine (Azulfidine) and metabolites in breast milk. Dev Pharmacol Ther 1980;*1*:31–39.

54. Erickson SH, Oppenheim GL. Aspirin in breast milk. J Family Practice 1979;*8*:189–190.

55. Townsend RJ, Benedetti T, Erickson SH, Gillespie WR, Albert KS. A study to evaluate the passage of ibuprofen into breast milk. Drug Intel Clin Pharm 1982;*16*:482–483.

56. Townsend RJ, Benedetti TJ, Erickson SH, Cengiz C, Gillespie WR, Gschwend J, Albert KS. Excretion of ibuprofen into breast milk. Am J Obstet Gynecol 1984;*149*:184–186.

57. Fairhead FW. Convulsions in a breast fed infant after maternal indomethacin (letter). Lancet 1978;*2*:576.

58. Lebedevs TH, Wojnar-Horton RE, Yapp P, Roberts MJ, Dusci LJ, Hackett LP, Ilett KF. Excretion of indomethacin in breast milk. Br J Clin Pharmacol 1991;*32*:751–754.

59. Aranda JV, Collinge JM, Clarkson S. Epidemiologic aspects of drug utilization in a newborn intensive care unit. Seminars in Perinatology 1982;*6*:148–154.

60. Yoshioka H, Cho K, Takimoto M, Maruyama S, Shimizu T. Transfer of cefazolin into human milk. J Pediatr 1979;*94*:151–152.

61. Kauffman RE, O'Brien C, Gilford P. Sulfisoxazole secretion into human milk. J Pediatr 1980;*97*:839–841.

62. Tetracycline in breast milk. Br Med J 1969;*4*:791.

63. Von Kobyletski D, Dalhoff A, Lindemayer H, Primavesi CA. Ticarcillin serum and tissue concentrations in gynecology and obstetrics. Infection 1983;*11*:144–149.

64. Havelka J, Hejzlar M, Popov V, Viktorinova D, Prochazka J. Excretion of chloramphenicol in human milk. Chemotherapy 1968;*13*:204–211.

65. Atkinson H, Begg EJ. Concentrations of beta-blocking drugs in human milk. J Pediatr 1990;*116*:156.

66. Lunell HO, Kulas J, Rane A. Transfer of labetalol into amniotic fluid and breast milk in lactating women. Eur J Clin Pharmacol 1985;*28*:597–599.

67. Phelps DL, Karim Z. Spirinolactone: relationship between concentrations of dethioacetylated metabolite in human serum and milk. J Pharm Sci 1977;*66*:1203.

68. Levitan AA, Manion JC. Propranolol therapy during pregnancy and lactation. Am J Cardiol 1973;*32*:247.

69. Loughnan PM. Digoxin excretion in human breast milk. J Pediatr 1978;*92*:1019–1020.

70. Hill LM, Malkasian GD Jr. The use of quinidine sulfate throughout pregnancy. Obstet Gynec 1979;*54*:366–368.

71. Patrick MJ, Tilstone WJ, Reavey P. Diazepam and breastfeeding. Lancet 1972;*1*:542–543.

72. Dusci LJ, Good SM, Hall RW, Ilett KF. Excretion of diazepam and its metabolites in human milk during withdrawal from combination high dose diazepam and oxazepam. Br J Clin Pharmacol 1990;*29*:123–126.

73. Kuhnz W, Koch S, Helge H, Nau H. Primidone and phenobarbital during lactation period in epileptic women: total and free drug serum levels in the nursed infants and their effects on neonatal behavior. Dev Pharmacol Ther 1988;*11*:147–154.

74. Finch E, Lorber J. Methemoglobinemia in the newborn probably due to phenytoin excreted in human milk. J Obstet Gyne Br Eurp 1954;*61*:833–834.

75. Knott C, Reynolds F, Clayden G. Infantile spasms on weaning from breast milk containing anticonvulsants (letter). Lancet 1987;*2*:272–273.

76. Schou M, Amdisen A. Lithium and pregnancy. 3. Lithium ingestion by children breast-fed by women on lithium treatment. Br Med J 1973;*2*:138.

77. Tunessen WW Jr, Hertz C. Toxic effects of lithium in newborn infants: a commentary. J Pediatr 1972;*81*:804–807.

78. Steiner E, Villen T, Hallberg M, Rane A. Amphetamine secretion in breast milk. Eur J Clin Pharmacol 1984;*27*:123–124.

79. Nau H, Kuhnz W, Egger HJ, Rating D, Helge H. Anticonvulsants during pregnancy and lactation. Transplacental, maternal, and neonatal pharmacokinetics. Clin Pharmacokinet 1982;*7*:508–543.

80. Kampmann JP, Johansen K, Hansen JM, Helweg J. Propylthiouracil in human milk: revision of a dogma. Lancet 1980;*1*:736–737.

81. Moiel RH, Ryan JR. Tolbutamide (Orinase) in human breast milk. Clin Pediatr 1967;*6*:480.

82. Katz FH, Duncan BR. Entry of prednisone into breast milk. (letter) N Engl J Med 1975;*293*:1154.

83. Somogyi A, Gugler R. Cimetidine excretion into breast milk. Br J Clin Pharmacol 1979;*7*:627–629.

84. Ryu JE. Caffeine in human milk and in serum of breast fed infants. Dev Pharmacol Ther 1985;*8*:329–337.

85. Berlin CM Jr. Excretion of methylxanthine in human milk. Semin Perinatol 1981;*5*:389–394.

86. Luck W, Nau H. Nicotine and cotinine concentrations in the milk of smoking mothers. Influence of cigarette consumption and diurnal variations. Eur J Pediatr 1987;*146*:21–26.

87. Luck W, Nau H. Nicotine and cotinine concentrations in serum and milk of nursing mothers. Br J Clin Pharmacol 1984;*18*:9–15.

88. Cobo E. Effect of different dose of ethanol on the milk ejecting reflex in lactating women. Am J Obstet Gynecol 1973;*115*:817–821.

89. Kesaniemi YA. Ethanol and acetaldehyde in the milk and peripheral blood of lactating women after ethanol administration. J Obstet Gynecol Br Commonwealth 1974;*81*:84–86.

90. Chasnoff IJ, Lewis DE, Squires L. Cocaine intoxication in a breast fed infant. Pediatrics 1987;*80*:836–838.

91. Cobrinik RW, Hood RT Jr, Chused E. The effect of maternal narcotic addiction on the newborn infant: review of literature and report of 22 cases. Pediatrics 1959;*24*:288–304.

92. Blinick G, Inturrisi CE, Jerez E, Wallach RC. Methadone assays in pregnant women and progeny. Am J Obstet Gynecol 1975;*121*:617–621.

93. Blinick G, Wallach RC, Jerez E, Ackerman BD. Drug addiction in pregnancy and the neonate. Am J Obstet Gynecol 1976;*125*:135–142.

94. Terwilliger WG, Hatcher RA. The elimination of morphine and quinine in human milk. Surg Gynecol Obstet 1934;*58*:823–826.

95. Rabinowitz M, Leviton A, Neddleman H. Lead in milk and infant blood: a dose response model. Arch Environ Health 1985;*40*:283–286.

96. Sternowsky HJ, Wessolowski R. Lead and cadmium in breast milk. Higher levels in urban vs rural mothers during the first 3 months of lactation. Arch Toxicol 1985;*57*:41–45.

97. Koos BJ, Longo LD. Mercury toxicity in the pregnant woman, fetus, and newborn infant. A review. Am J Obstet Gynecol 1976;*126*:390–409.

98. Pitkin RM, Bahns JA, Filer LA Jr, Reynolds WA. Mercury in human maternal and cord blood, placenta, and milk. Pros Soc Exp Biol Med 1976;*151*:565–567.

99. Miller RW. Pollutants in breast milk: PCBs and cola-colored babies. (editorial) J Pediatr 1977;*90*:510–511.

100. Rogan WJ, Bagniewska A, Damstra T. Pollutants in breast milk. N Engl J Med 1980;*302*:1450–1453.

101. Bakken AF, Seip M. Insecticides in human milk. Acta Pediatr Scan 1976;*65*:535–539.

102. Quinby GE, Armstrong JF, Durham WF. DDT in human milk. Nature 1965;*207*:726–728.

103. Egan H, Goulding R, Roburn J. Tatton O'GJ. Organo-chlorine pesticide residues in human fat milk. Br Med J 1965;*2*:66–69.

104. Wilson DJ, Locker DJ, Ritzen CA, Watson JT, Schaffner W. DDT concentrations in human milk. Am J Dis Child 1973;*125*:814–817.

105. Wickizer TM, Brilliant LB. Testing for polychlorinated biphenyls in human milk. Pediatrics 1981;*68*:411–415.

106. Brilliant LB, Wilcox K, Van Amburg G, Isbister J, Bloomer AW, Humphrey H, Price H. Breast milk monitoring to measure Michigan's contamination with polybrominated biphenyls. Lancet 1978;*2*:643–646.

107. Wickizer TM, Brilliant LB, Copeland R, Tilden R. Polychlorinated biphenyl contamination of nursing mothers' milk in Michigan. Am J Public Health 1981;*71*:132–137.

Reviews, Monographs, and Book Chapters

r1. Vaughn VC. Growth and Development. In: Beckmann RE, Vaughn VC (eds). Nelson's Textbook of Pediatrics, 12th ed. Philadelphia: WB Saunders, 1983; pp 10–38.

r2. Kaufmann RE. Drug Therapeutics in the Infant and Child. In: Yaffe SJ and Aranda JV, eds. Pediatric Pharmacology, Therapeutic Principles in Practice. Philadelphia: WB Saunders, 1992; pp 212–219.

r3. Spino M. Pediatric dosing rules and nomograms. In: MacLeod SM, Radd IC (eds). Textbook of Pediatric Clinical Pharmacology. MA: Littleton, PSG, 1985; pp 118–128.

r4. Tanner JM. Growth at adolescence, 2d ed. New York: Blackwell Scientific, 1962.

r5. Hein K. Drug Therapeutics in the adolescent. In: Yaffe SJ and Aranda JV (eds). Pediatric Pharmacology, Therapeutic Principles in Practice. Philadelphia: WB Saunders, 1992; pp 220–236.

r6. Cheek D, Talbert JL. Extracellular volume and body water in infants. In: Cheek D (ed). Human Growth. Philadelphia: Lea & Febiger, 1986; pp 118–196.

r7. Styne D, Grumbach M. Puberty in the male and female. In: Reproductive Endocrinology. Philadelphia: WB Saunders, 1978, pp 189–240.

r8. Guignard JP. Neonatal nephrology. In: Holliday MA, Barratt TM, Vernier RL (eds). Pediatric Nephrology, 2d ed. Baltimore: Williams & Wilkins, 1987; pp 921–944.

r9. Sondheimer JM. Gastroesophageal reflux: Update on the pathogenesis and diagnosis. Pediatr Clin North Am 1988; *35*:103–116.

r10. Milsap RL, Szefler SJ. Special pharmacokinetic considerations in children. In: Evans WE, Schentag JJ, Jusko WJ (eds). Applied Pharmacokinetics: Principles of Therapeutic Drug Monitoring. Spokane WA, Applied Therapeutics, 1986; pp 294–328.

r11. Green TP, Mirkin BL. Clinical pharmacokinetics: Pediatric considerations. In: Benet LZ, et al (eds). Pharmacokinetic Basis for Drug Treatment. New York: Raven Press, 1984; pp 269–282.

r12. Morselli PL, Franco-Morselli R, Bossi L. Clinical pharmacokinetics in newborns and infants: Age-related differences and therapeutic implications. Clin Pharmacokinet 1980; *5*:485–527.

r13. Notterman DA. Pediatric pharmacotherapy. In: Chernow B (ed). The Pharmacologic Approach to the Critically Ill Patient, 2d ed. Baltimore: Williams & Wilkins, 1988; pp 131–155.

r14. Radde IC. Mechanisms of drug absorption and their development. In: MacLeod SM, Radde IC (eds). Textbook of Pediatric Clinical Pharmacology. Littleton MA: PSG, 1985; pp 25–26.

r15. Steward DJ. Anaesthesia in childhood. In: MacLeod SM, Radde IC (eds). Textbook of Pediatric Clinical Pharmacology. Littleton MA: PSG, 1985; pp 365–378.

r16. Koren G. Clinical pharmacology of antimicrobial drugs during development: How are infants and children different? In: Koren G, Prober CG, Gold R (eds). Antimicrobial Therapy in Infants and Children. New York: Marcel Dekker, 1988; pp 47–52.

r17. Hendeles L, Weinberger M. Theophylline: A state of the art review. Pharmacotherapy 1983;*3*:2–44.

r18. Aranda JV. Special considerations of drug treatment in neonates, infants and children. In: Berkow R (ed). Ther Merck Manual, 16th ed. Rahway NJ: Merck Sharpe & Dohme, 1991; pp 1957–1962.

r19. Leeder JS, Gold R. Cephalosporins. In: Koren G, Prober CG, Gold R (eds). Antimicrobial Therapy in Infants and Children. New York: Marcel Dekker, 1988; pp 173–235.

r20. Rowland M, Tozer TN. Age and weight. In: Rowland M, Tozer TN (eds). Clinical Pharmacokinetics Concepts and Applications. Philadelphia: Lea & Febiger, 1980; pp 218–229.

r21. Gorodischer R, Koren G. Salivary excretion of drugs in children: Theoretical and practical issues in therapeutic drug monitoring. Dev Pharmacol Ther 1992; *19*(4):161–177.

r22. Rane A. Drug disposition and action in infants and children. In: Yaffe S and Aranda J (eds). Pediatric Pharmacology, Therapeutic Principles in Practice. Philadelphia: WB Saunders, 1992; pp 10–21.

r23. Committee on Drugs. American Academy of Pediatrics. The transfer of drugs and other chemicals into human milk. Pediatrics 1994;*93*:137–150.

r24. Neims AH, Warner M, Loughnan PM, Aranda JV. Developmental aspects of the hepatic cytochrome P-450 monooxygenase system. Annual Review of Pharmacology 1976;*16*:427–445.

CHAPTER 117

AIDS

Rebecca L. Coleman

Background

Human Immunodeficiency Virus (HIV) is now estimated to infect over 250,000 persons in the US and more than 13 million worldwide. Initial characterization of the unusual constellation of infections and malignancies came in 1980, while the responsible virus was formally identified in 1984. Early patterns of infection suggested that transmission of HIV requires the exchange of "bodily fluids," accounting for the spread of infection in groups engaging in sex or IV needle-sharing and in patients receiving blood and blood products. Following identification of the virus and development of testing methodologies, transmission via blood products has been largely eliminated in the US. Areas of the world where testing of blood and blood fractions is not effectively regulated or where resources for adequate testing do not exist continue to experience transmission via this route. Sexual transmission of virus accounts for the largest proportion of cases of AIDS in the US. Infection among gay men led to the first name given the disease, GRID, for Gay Related Immunodeficiency Disease. Education regarding "safe sex," including the use of condoms and avoidance of "high-risk" behaviors has been measurably effective in reducing the transmission of HIV in some "at-risk" groups—most notably adult gay men. Effective educational messages, however, must be appropriate and targeted to the audience. The growing incidence of HIV infection among heterosexual women and the recent emergence of disease among young gay men exemplify the need for continued efforts in prevention education. Intravenous drug users (IVDUs) represent perhaps the most challenging group for educational interventions. Conflicting goals of public health and law enforcement around this population have led to the declaration of a state of emergency in the city of San Francisco, allowing a "clean needle exchange" program to proceed despite state laws prohibiting the supply of needles and syringes ("works") to IVDUs.

Prior to recognition of HIV as the causative virus, the Centers for Disease Control (CDC) established a case definition to aid in the classification and investigation of this new disease, later named AIDS for Acquired Immunodeficiency Syndrome. This definition has been modified[1] as new information has emerged and describes the clinical symptoms and diagnoses seen with this disease. Individuals diagnosed with a condition described in the AIDS case definition, also called "AIDS defining diagnosis," are said to have AIDS. The AIDS case definition is, at best, an imprecise tool for quantifying morbidity. Individuals meeting the case definition by virtue of having limited cutaneous Kaposi's sarcoma (KS) have a much different prognosis than those with pulmonary KS. Because the case definition is utilized by public and private sector agencies as a basis for distribution of benefits (healthcare, disability, housing, etc.), changes in the definition are scrutinized closely by advocates for affected populations. The time frame for epidemiologic studies required to support significant changes in the case definition conflicts with the current benefit needs of individuals with HIV infection.

Surrogate markers for HIV disease, including absolute and percentage CD4+ cell count, p24 antigen, and β2 microglobulin, have been evaluated for correlation with clinical disease course. CD4+ cell count has received the most attention and is the most broadly used marker in clinical care for HIV disease at this time. Many of the clinical events associated with HIV infection, especially the opportunistic infections, have been correlated with specific CD4+ cell counts. Current research in this field targets the development of methodologies for the quantitative and qualitative description of an individual's own virus that can be reliably interpreted in the clinical setting.

The course of HIV infection varies. Following an acute flu-like illness two to four weeks after infection, most patients enjoy a period of relatively good health, which may last for more than a decade. It is now known that the virus is not quiescent during this period but continues to replicate in the lymph system.[2] The prognosis for individuals diagnosed with AIDS has improved since the disease was first recognized. Survival for individuals whose CD4+ cells have fallen to 200 has lengthened in the past ten years by about one year, from 28.4 months in 1983–1986 to 38.1 months in 1988–1993 in a cohort of homosexual and bisexual men followed in San Francisco.[3] This is due in large part to therapies aimed at the major infections associated with AIDS, specifically *Pneumocystis carinii* pneumonia.

Antiretroviral Therapy

Optimal use of the currently available drugs was recently addressed in a state-of-the-art consensus conference and these recommendations are outlined in Figure 117.1. All currently available agents share a similar mechanism, inhibition of the retroviral enzyme reverse transcriptase, and chemical class, nucleosides. Research is underway evaluating drugs with novel mechanisms (proteinase or protease inhibitors, glycosylation inhibitors) and approaching RT inhibition using different chemical classes (non-nucleoside reverse transcriptase inhibitors).

Figure 117.1 Initiation of Therapy

Clinical Status	CD4 Count (/mm³)	Recommendation
Asymptomatic	> 500	No therapy
Asymptomatic	200–500	ZDV or no therapy
Symptomatic	200–500	ZDV
Asymptomatic/ symptomatic	< 200	Antiretroviral therapy

Treatment of the initial HIV infection has been studied in individuals presenting with an acute viral syndrome following known or suspected exposure to HIV and in individuals reporting occupational exposure to the virus. The value of post-exposure treatment has not yet been demonstrated, owing to difficulties in studying these populations and to the extended disease course. Recommendations regarding the use of antiretroviral agents in these populations include zidovudine, 200 mg q 4 hours for those with a significant exposure, while some clinicians favor selection of treatment based on the presumed sensitivities of source virus, when known. As such, a healthcare worker receiving a significant inoculum of blood from a needle previously used to draw blood from an HIV-infected patient who had been treated with zidovudine for two years might be treated with didanosine on the presumption that any virus transmitted is probably somewhat resistant to zidovudine.

Therapy for Opportunistic Infections

While therapy aimed at HIV has not yet been effective in eliminating the virus, there has been significant progress made in the treatment of opportunistic infections associated with AIDS. Several new agents are now available, and new uses have been found for existing drugs. The need for more efficacious treatments and for treatment alternatives remains. (See chapter 99 or elsewhere in this Book for further information about drugs mentioned in this chapter.)

Pneumocystis Carinii Pneumonia

The most prevalent infection, *Pneumocystis carinii* pneumonia (PCP), occurs in up to 70 per cent of HIV-infected individuals. Treatments for PCP include trimethoprim/sulfamethoxazole, pentamidine, clindamycin/primaquine, trimethoprim/dapsone, trimetrexate/leucovorin, and atovaquone.[5,6] The relative efficacy of these regimens has not been adequately studied; however, most agree that trimethoprim/sulfamethoxazole is the drug of choice for all presentations of PCP. Many, but not all, agree that pentamidine is the second-line agent for patients requiring parenteral therapy. Beyond that, there is little agreement and less data to guide the choice of treatment for PCP. Corticosteroids are used as adjunctive therapy in patients who present with moderate to severe PCP; they are administered on a tapering dosage schedule from initiation through completion of PCP therapy (Fig. 117.2).

The management of opportunistic infections in patients with HIV infection involves both treatment of

Figure 117.2 Recommended Steroid Dosage Schedule as Adjunctive Therapy for Moderate to Severe PCP

Days 1–5	40 mg bid
Days 6–10	20 mg bid
Days 11–15	10 mg bid
Days 16–21	10 mg qd

acute infections and prophylaxis against several commonly occurring infections. Primary prophylaxis (treatment initiated prior to the occurrence of an infection) against PCP is now standard for HIV-infected patients with CD4+ counts below 200/mm^3. Secondary prophylaxis is the term used to describe treatment initiated after the first occurrence of a given infection, as when trimethoprim/sulfamethoxazole prophylaxis is initiated after an acute PCP treatment course. Chronic suppression and maintenance are used interchangeably to describe the chronic use of medication to suppress recurring infections. These terms and secondary prophylaxis are differentiated primarily by usage rather than by a clear difference in definition. Chronic suppression is more often applied when the infecting organism is not cleared, but is suppressed to the extent that it does not cause illness; secondary prophylaxis is most often used to describe the prevention of a new infection with the same organism.

Opportunistic infections that are good candidates for prophylactic therapy have the following characteristics: (1) there is a reliable method for selecting which patients are at risk for the infection; (2) the treatments available for use are highly effective and have tolerable side-effects relative to the morbidity and/or mortality associated with the infection; (3) the costs of the prophylactic treatment are reasonable relative to the benefit of preventing the infection.

PCP has characteristics that make it a good candidate for prophylaxis: (1) the infection occurs almost exclusively in patients whose CD4 cells have declined below 200; (2) trimethoprim/sulfamethoxazole is highly effective and well tolerated by a large proportion of the at-risk population; (3) the cost of the drug and requisite monitoring is reasonable compared with the significant morbidity and mortality associated with PCP. Of all interventions utilized to date in HIV-infected patients, PCP prophylaxis probably has had the greatest impact on mortality.

Patients with HIV infection appear to have decreased tolerance for several drugs, including the combination of trimethoprim/sulfamethoxazole. Research evaluating the metabolism of these drugs in patients in different stages of HIV disease has identified alterations in drug metabolism as a potential cause for some reductions in tolerance. Alterations in acetylator status associated with chronic disease may account for decreased tolerance to drugs. Further, temporary alterations in acetylator status, occurring in the setting of acute infection, such as PCP, may explain the differences in tolerance documented in the same patient across time.[8]

Mycobacterium Avium Complex (MAC)

The lifetime incidence of *Mycobacterium avium* comlex (MAC) has increased to 40 percent as more HIV-infected patients survive longer with severely compromised immune systems. Therapy for most patients will be continued indefinitely and will require significant effort to maximize efficacy and minimize toxicity. Among the agents used to treat MAC, ethambutol and the macrolide antibiotics have been shown to have the greatest efficacy in vitro when used as single agents.[9] Other drugs often added to the regimen in an attempt to improve clinical response include clofazimine, amikacin, the quinolone antibiotics, and rifampin or rifabutin.[10,11] Rifabutin and clarithromycin have both been utilized as prophylactic agents for MAC, although only rifabutin is FDA-approved for this use to date.[12,13]

Candidal Infections

Candida infections are common among patients with HIV infection, particularly oropharyngeal and esophageal candidiasis. Most oropharyngeal infection responds to treatment with nystatin or clotrimazole, though some patients require systemic therapy before clearing the infection. Ketaconazole and fluconazole are both utilized in the treatment of esophageal candidiasis.[14] The role of prophylaxis for the fungal infections common in AIDS is controversial and awaits further study. Some clinicians recommend the use of fluconazole as a prophylactic measure in those patients at risk for serious infections or for infections that interfere with daily activities.

Cytomegalovirus (CMV) Retinitis

CMV infection of the retina is most common in patients with T cells less than 50 and can lead to loss of vision and total blindness. Treatments utilized include IV ganciclovir and/or foscarnet,[15] both of which are administered as an induction course followed by lifelong suppressive dosing at a lower dose. Patients often "relapse" on suppressive dosing, requiring "reinduction." The IV route required for administration of these drugs and the toxicities of these two agents combine to make the management of this infection a relatively resource-intensive therapy. The role of oral dosage forms of ganciclovir and foscarnet along with valaciclovir, an acyclovir prodrug, in the prophylaxis and management of CMV are currently being researched.

Cryptococcal Meningitis

Treatment of cryptococcal meningitis is usually initiated by amphotericin B. The value of adding flucytosine to the regimen remains a matter of debate. Some clinicians utilize oral fluconazole as initial therapy in "milder" cases. Oral fluconazole is also used as chronic suppressive therapy following treatment of the acute infection and is indicated for patients who have asymptomatic infection demonstrated by positive titers.[16]

Toxoplasmosis Gondii

Several agents have been utilized in the treatment of toxoplasmosis encephalitis, including combinations of sulfadiazine plus pyrimethamine and clindamycin plus pyrimethamine. Both combinations are used to treat both the acute infection and as lifetime chronic suppressive therapy.[17] Research efforts to expand the treatment options for this infection include studies of atovaquone and the macrolide antibiotics.

Other Infections

Histoplasmosis is a prominent infection in HIV-infected patients in those areas where the organism is endemic and causes significant morbidity. Amphotericin B is commonly used as acute therapy, followed by suppressive dosing with itraconazole.[18] Tuberculosis has become more prevalent among HIV infected patients in some geographic areas, most notably the urban areas of the US east coast. Often termed the "twin epidemics," the two infections have challenged the resources of public sector healthcare. At the same time that the number of Tb cases is increasing, the proportion of Tb isolates found to be resistant to one or more of the standard treatments for Tb also is increasing, particularly in areas where compliance with treatment regimens is incomplete.

AIDS-Related Malignancies

Several malignancies have been demonstrated to occur more frequently in patients infected with HIV, including Kaposi's sarcoma, non-Hodgkin's lymphoma, and CNS lymphoma. Treatment for these malignancies has focused on the development of regimens with a lower potential for myelosuppression to improve tolerance in a population already at risk for myelosuppression caused by the disease and/or other therapies.

Patient Management

Medication regimens in patients with HIV infection often include one or more antiretroviral drugs plus prophylactic or suppressive combinations in addition to adjunctive therapies, all of which add to the potential for clinically significant drug interactions.[19] The limited clinical experience available for many of these agents and their use in a disease whose pathology is not fully understood add to the uncertainty and necessity for prudent monitoring.

References

Research Reports

1. 1993 revised classification system for HIV infection and expanded surveillance case definition for AIDS among adolescents and adults. MMWR 1992;*41*:No. RR-17.
2. Fauci AS. Multifactorial nature of human immunodeficiency virus disease: Implications for therapy. Science 1993;*262*:1011–1018.
3. Osmond D, Charlebois E, Lang W, Shiboski S, Moss A. Changes in AIDS survival time in two San Francisco cohorts of homosexual men, 1983 to 1993. JAMA 1994;*271*:1083–1087.
4. Sande MA, Carpenter CC, Cobbs CG, Holmes KK, Sanford JP. Antiretroviral therapy for adult HIV-infected patients. JAMA 1993;*270*:2583–2589.
5. Sattler FR, Feinberg J. New developments in the treatment of *Pneumocystis carinii* pneumonia. Chest 1992;*101*:451–457.
6. Artymowicz RJ, James VE. Atovaquone: A new antipneumocystis agent. Clin Pharm 1993;*12*:563–570.
7. Consensus statement on the use of corticosteroids as adjunctive therapy for pheumocystis pneumonia in the acquired immunodeficiency syndrome. The National Institutes of Health-University of California Expert Panel for Corticosteroids as Adjunctive Therapy for Pneumocystis Pneumonia. N Engl J Med 1990;*21*:1500–1504.
8. Lee BL, Delahunty T, Safrin S. Correlation of serum concentration of trimethoprim-sulfamethoxazole with efficacy and toxicity in patients with AIDS. Abstract American Society for Clinical Pharmacology and Therapeutics, March, 1993.
9. Yajko DM, Nassos PS, Sanders CA, Hadley WK. Killing by antimycobacterial agents of AIDS-derived strains of *Mycobacterium avium* Complex inside cells of the mouse macrophage cell line J774. Am Rev Respir Dis 1989;*140*:1196–1203.
10. Horsburgh CR. *Mycobacterium avium* complex infection in the acquired immunodeficiency syndrome. N Engl J Med 1991;*19*:1332–1338.

11. Rathbun RC, Martin ES, Eaton VE, Matthew EB. Current and investigational therapies for AIDS-associated *Mycobacerium avium* complex disease. Clin Pharm 1991;*10*:280–292.

12. Nightengale SD, Cameron S, Gordin FM, Sullam PM, Cohn CL, Chaisson RE, Eron LJ, Bihari B, Kaufman DL, Stern JJ, Pearce DD, Weinberg WG, LaMarca A, Siegal FP. Two controlled trials of rifabutin prophylaxis against *Mycobacterium avium* complex infection in AIDS. N Engl J Med 1993;*329*:828–833.

13. Recommendations of prophylaxis and therapy for disseminated *Mycobacterium avium* complex disease in patients infected with the human immunodeficiency virus. Masur H and the Public Health Service Task Force on Prophylaxis and Therapy for *Mycobacterium avium* complex. N Engl J Med 1993;*329*:898–904.

14. Laine L, Dretler RH, Conteas CN, Tuazon C, Koster FM, Sattler F, Squires K, Islam MZ. Fluconazole compared with ketoconazole for the treatment of *Candida* esophagitis in AIDS. JAMA 1992;*117*:655–660.

15. Mortality in patients with the acquired immunodeficiency syndrome treated with either foscarnet or ganciclovir for cytomegalovirus retinitis. N Engl J Med 1992;*326*:213–220.

16. Como JA, Dismukes WE. Oral azole drugs as systemic antifungal therapy. N Engl J Med 1994;*330*:263–272.

17. Dannemann B, McCutchan JA, Israelski D, Antoniskis D, Lepont C, Luft B, Nussbaum J, Clumeck N, Morlat P, Chiu S, Vilde JL, Orellana M, Feigal D, Bartok A, Heseltine P, Leedom J, Remington J, and the California Collaborative Group. Treatment of toxoplasmic encephalitis in patients with AIDS. Ann Intern Med 1992;*116*:33–43.

18. Wheat J, Hafner R, Wulfsohn M, Spencer P, Squires K, Powderly W, Wong B, Rinaldi M, Saag M, Hamill R, Murphy R, Connolly-Stringfield P, Briggs N, Owens S, and the National Institute of Allergy and Infectious Diseases Clinical Trials and Mycoses Study Group Collaborators. Prevention of relapse of histoplasmosis with itraconazole in patients with the acquired immunodeficiency syndrome. Ann Intern Med 1993;*118*:610–616.

19. Lee BL, Safrin S. Interactions and toxicities of drugs used in patients with AIDS. Clin Infect Dis 1992;*14*:773–779.

CHAPTER 118

Jorge G. Ruiz
David T. Lowenthal

Geriatric Pharmacology

The elderly in the US constitute 12 percent of the total population and account for almost 30 percent of total drug expenditures.[1,2] Several age-related changes make the elderly person susceptible to many ill effects caused by medications,[3] especially those suffering from the chronic conditions more prevalent in the elderly population, who are at increased risk.

Research in basic and clinical pharmacology[r1] has provided substantial data to help clinicians in the judicious use of drugs in the elderly. The aphorism "start slow and lengthen intervals" is valid more than ever in aged patients.

The present chapter will deal with different aspects of geriatric pharmacology with an overview of basic aspects and particular emphasis on issues of clinical pharmacology in the elderly.

Basic Pharmacology

Changes in the aging person often result in responses to the same dosages of one drug different from those expected in younger individuals.[r1] Responsiveness to different drugs in general declines with age, and the explanation for this phenomenon lies at the molecular level.[r5] Table 118.1 shows some examples of receptor alterations with aging. Studies in aged animals have shown impairment in cholinergic transmission,[4] with a decreased number of muscarinic acetylcholine receptors with age. This defect, for example, can be translated into impaired memory in the aged animal. Of clinical importance also is the reduced responsiveness of the myocardium to catecholamines.[5] Apparently these changes are not in the quantity of receptors, but in an inability to activate adenylate cyclase with age.[r2] The result of these changes is a decline in chronotropic and inotropic responses to beta-adrenergic agents.[6] It is also important to point out that these changes are tissue-specific, resulting in different effects in different organs.[r1]

Alpha-adrenergic receptors also have been studied. In hepatocytes, alpha stimulation of glycogenolysis is unchanged with age,[r3] but there is a 39 percent decrease in the density of liver α_1-adrenergic receptors with age.[7]

Alterations in opioid receptor function are associated with anorexia, hypodypsia, impotence, and other behavioral changes with aging. In aged individuals there is a decreased opiate peptide content in the CNS

Table 118.1 Receptor Changes and Physiologic Responsiveness with Aging

Receptor	Tissue	Physiologic Change	Receptor Density
Muscarinic	Brain	Diminished memory	Diminished
PTH	Kidney	Diminished activation of vitamin D	Diminished
Beta Adrenergic	Heart	Rate and contractility	Same
$Alpha_1$ Adrenergic	Liver	No change in glycogenolysis	Diminished
Opioid	Brain	Anorexia, hypodipsia	Diminished

as well as a reduction in the number of μ opioid receptors.[8] Another important change in aging at the postreceptor level is a diminished calcium-dependent responsiveness. Calcium movement is required for different functions and may affect secretion, neurotransmission, muscle contraction, and cell division. Consistent changes in the calcium mobilization in response to such different stimuli as hormones, neurotransmitters, and others have been observed with aging.[9] The clinical implication of these findings is in the use of drugs that can at least partially reverse the impairment in calcium mobilization, leading to significant improvement in function.[10]

Table 118.2 shows receptor concentrations with aging.

Pharmacodynamic-Pharmacokinetic Interactions

Pharmacokinetics and pharmacodynamic processes can be affected in the elderly individual, as seen in Table 118.3 and 118.4. The following is a review of some characteristics of the pharmacokinetic mechanisms present in the aged person. These kinetic events evolve "dynamically" and interchangeably with pharmacodynamic events based in part on the altered physiology of aging, underlying diseases, and the drug(s) in question.

Absorption

Absorption of food and drugs remains unchanged in the aging patient with intact gastric mucosa,[11] and

Table 118.2 Changes in Receptor Concentrations with Aging

Decrease	Androgen, estrogen, insulin, gonadotropin, opioid, benzodiazepine, alpha-adrenergic, beta-adrenergic, dopaminergic, glucocorticoid, thyroid prolactin, serotonin, GABA.
Unchanged	Androgen, estrogen, insulin, gonadotropin, opioid, benzodiazepine, alpha-adrenergic, beta-adrenergic, cholinergic, glucocorticoid, thyroid, prolactin, serotonin, GABA.
Increase	Androgen, estrogen, insulin, gonadotropin, opioid, benzodiazepine, alpha-adrenergic, beta-adrenergic, dopaminergic.

Table 118.3 Pharmacokinetics in the Elderly

Absorption	Unchanged
Gastric pH	Increased
Secretory capacity	Decreased
GI blood flow	Diminished
Distribution	
Plasma albumin	Diminished
Protein affinity	Diminished
Alpha 1 acid glycoprotein	Increased
Metabolism	
Size of liver	Decreased
Hepatic blood flow	Decreased
Renal Function	
GFR	Decreased
Renal plasma flow	Decreased
Filtration fraction	Increased

Table 118.4 Changes in Body Function in the Elderly

Alterations in body composition	
Body fat	Increased
Lean body mass	Decreased
Total body water	Decreased
Changes in cardiovascular function	
Resting heart rate	Decreased
Stroke volume	Same
Cardiac output	Same
CNS function	
Blood supply to the brain	Diminished
Reflex responses	
Baroreceptor reflex activity	Diminished
Renin-angiotensin-aldosterone system	
Plasma renin	Diminished
Urine aldosterone	Diminished
Sympathetic innervation to juxtaglomerular cells	Diminished

this happens despite increased gastric pH secondary to atrophic changes in the gastric mucosa with diminished acid secretory capacity[12,13] and reduced GI blood flow.[12] An age-related decline in GI motility has been described,[14] but the clinical implications of this finding on drug absorption are not apparent. Loss of absorbing capacity with age secondary to a reduction in the number of absorbing cells has been studied by some authors.[12]

The bioavailability of some drugs with a high rate of first-pass metabolism[15,16] i.e., beta blockers, may be increased, especially with involvement of the liver by different pathologic processes common to the elderly.[r4–r6]

As mentioned before, elevated gastric pH is common in the elderly, and the effects of this abnormality can affect the ionization and solubility of certain drugs. Reduced acidity also can account for changes in motility, with a more rapid emptying of contents of the stomach into the duodenum.[r7,17]

Studies with levodopa and clorazepate have revealed evidence of changes in intragastric metabolism in the elderly. Evans et al.[18] have shown a reduction in the gastric wall content of dopa decarboxylase resulting in a threefold increase in the availability of levodopa in the elderly. Therefore this can result in enhanced pharmacodynamic effects and, possibly, adverse events.

Other routes of administration of drugs have been less well studied in the elderly, but some investigators have found a reduced absorption rate of antibiotics from the site of an IM injection.[19,20] This finding can have important clinical implications, especially in infections, when single IM doses of antibiotics are used in long-term care facilities.[21]

Distribution

Age-related changes in body composition affect drug disposition in different ways. Among the most important are an increase in body fat, decrease in lean body mass, and decrease in total body water.[22–24] These alterations can result in an increased volume of distribution of lipid-soluble drugs like beta blockers and an opposite effect for water-soluble drugs.[r8,25] However, a reduced lean body mass implies a reduction in intracellular water and other compartments, resulting in an increased concentration of water-soluble drugs if dosage is not reduced. This can result in enhanced pharmacodynamic effects, and adverse events can occur.

In the elderly, serum albumin levels decline between 15 to 20 percent, with the total plasma protein content being unaffected.[26] Changes in protein binding also can affect the response of the elderly patient to drugs that are highly protein-bound. Since albumin is responsible for the major part of plasma protein binding, a reduction in its level can result in an increase in the free drug fraction that is the pharmacodynamically active part of the medication used, with the possibility of enhanced susceptibility to drug side-effects.[r1,27] Also, a change in the affinity of the protein to bind drug has been noted in elderly persons, although the clinical significance of this finding is uncertain.[r1]

$Alpha_1$ acid glycoprotein (AAG) binds mostly to lipophilic basic drugs and tends to increase with age.[28] The binding of drugs to AAG increases during an acute illness, such as myocardial infarction.[29,30] In this setting, lidocaine or propranolol may be more avidly bound to AAG, yielding an increase in the fraction of free drug. This binding can return to normal after several weeks or months, when the acute stress passes and the acute phase reactant, AAG, decreases.

Hepatic Metabolism

The ability of the aging liver to metabolize drugs does not decline similarly for all pharmacologic agents.[31,32] Several changes in hepatic function and structure have been noted in aged individuals; among them, two of the most important are an absolute (and relative to body weight) decrease in the size of the liver[12,33] and reduced regional blood flow to this organ.[14] The most frequent changes involve the microsomal mixed-function oxidative system (Phase I oxidation and reduction), with little or no change in the conjugative processes (Phase II conjugation).[r9] Despite these changes routine tests of liver function fail to yield abnormal results in the absence of disease.[r1,r8,r10] Table 118.5 presents a listing of drugs and the processes involved in their metabolism in aged individuals. Acetaminophen, for example, is conjugated through glucuronide and sulfate pathways, and no changes in rates of conjugation have been noted in the elderly.[34] On the other hand, desipramine has a significant prolongation in the elimination half-life and a reduction in plasma clearance due to a slower rate of demethylation, greater volume of distribution, and a reduction in plasma clearance.[31,35]

Another area of interest is hepatic enzyme induction in the elderly. There still is controversy as to whether drug induction is an important phenomenon in the elderly individual. Studies have shown an age-related decline in antipyrine clearance in elderly subjects who smoke;[36] on the other hand, rifampin, a known potent

Table 118.5 Hepatic Metabolism of Drugs in the Elderly

Phase I (preparative) reactions
Oxidation
Hydroxylation
Alprazolam, antipyrine, barbiturates, carbamazepine, ibuprofen, imipramine, desipramine, nortryptiline, phenytoin, propranolol, auinidine, warfarin
Dealkylation
Amitripyline, chlordiazepoxide, diazepam, flurazepam, diphenhydramine, lidocaine, meperidine, theophylline, tolbutamide
Reduction
Nitroreduction
Nitrazepam
Phase II (synthetic) reactions
(Unchanged in the Elderly)
Conjugation
Acetylation
Methylation

inducer of microsomal activity, failed to have any effect on antipyrine half-life in elderly male subjects.[37]

Excretion and Renal Function

Glomerular filtration rate (GFR) gradually declines with age.[38,39] At the same time, there is a greater decrease of almost 50 percent in the renal plasma flow,[38] resulting in the filtration fraction rising significantly with age.[39,41] Loss of tubular function and diminished reabsorptive capacity also are observed with aging.[38,40] Owing to reduced muscle mass, evaluation of the renal function with serum creatinine alone can be misleading in elderly persons.[41,42] A more precise way to estimate GFR is by measurement of the endogenous creatinine clearance.[39] However, as a result of tubular secretion of creatinine, creatinine clearance can overestimate the GFR.[43] Despite this inconvenience, creatinine clearance is a very useful tool for dose adjustment of renally excreted drugs.[44]

The use of nonsteroidal antiinflammatory drugs (NSAIDs) by the elderly is more than three times that of younger individuals.[45] Elderly individuals are a special risk group for the adverse renal effects of these drugs.[46,47] The inhibition of renal vasodilator prostaglandins by NSAIDs in addition to the changes in kidney function previously outlined can result in further nephrotoxicity.[48] The concomitant use of diuretics, nephrosclerosis due to hypertension, presence of CHF, general anesthesia for surgical procedures, and other poor perfusion states common in elderly patients can further complicate the problem; still, age remained an independent risk factor for deterioration of renal function.[r11,49]

Other Changes in Body Function

Table 118.4 lists some alterations in body function with age.

Changes in CNS Function

Blood supply to the brain may be compromised by atherosclerotic narrowing of the vertebral and carotid systems. Hypothetically, this decrement in blood flow could result in neuronal loss and be responsible for the altered sensitivity to centrally acting drugs like benzodiazepines, beta blockers, central alpha agonists, tryciclic antidepressants, barbiturates, and opiates.[50–52,r12]

Changes in Reflex Responses

Baroreceptor reflex sensitivity and responsiveness are decreased with age. Because of these changes, elderly patients can develop postural hypotension when taking nitroglycerin, phenothiazines, diuretics, dihydropyridine-type calcium channel blockers (nifedipine, nicardipine, and felodipine), and peripheral alpha blockers (prazosin, terazosin, and doxazosin).[53–56] Nitroglycerin can induce more severe hypotension and bradycardia in elderly patients with myocardial infarction than in younger individuals,[57] possibly resulting in an increased vascular smooth muscle action from the use of nitrates.[58]

Renin-Angiotensin-Aldosterone System

Plasma renin concentration as well as blood and urine aldosterone concentrations—both at baseline and in response to position and volume changes—decline with age, probably as a result of a decrease in sympathetic innervation to the juxtaglomerular cells.[59,60]

It has been suggested that because of lowered renin activity elderly patients may respond more readily to diuretics and calcium channel blockers than to beta blockers and ACE inhibitors.[61] Conversely, the hyporenin-hypoaldosterone state can predispose to hyperkalemia especially with NSAIDs, ACE inhibitors, betablockers, and potassium-sparing diuretics.

Fluid and Electrolyte Balance

As a result of intrinsic and diuretic-induced renal dysfunction and age-induced higher concentrations of vasopressin, water retention may occur, producing hyponatremia.[49,62–65] In addition, prostatic hypertrophy can result in obstructive uropathy,[66] producing further postrenal deterioration in kidney function, water conservation, and hyponatremia, which persist until the obstruction has been relieved.

Adverse Drug Reactions

It is assumed that the frequency of adverse drug reactions (ADRs) is increased in elderly patients[67–69] and that this probably is related to multiple factors peculiar to the elderly population, e.g., polypharmacy, multiple diseases, age-related changes in pharmacodynamics and pharmacokinetics, and inappropriate prescribing patterns by physicians, as well as noncompliance.[70–73] Although one could assume intuitively that these factors increase the incidence of ADRs in elderly individuals, the proof so far has not been sufficient to consider age by itself as a risk factor for ADRs.[70,72,74,75] It seems likely that individual characteristics are more important than the chronologic factors as predictors of ADRs. Women are apparently more susceptible to ADRs, and probably this can be related to greater drug usage by this population, including over-the-counter drugs.[76-79] Hospitalized elderly receive more drugs than do outpatients,[80,81] but this probably reflects the acuteness of the situation.[82] The estimates of ADRs during hospitalization are between 1.5 and 44 percent.[75] In a rural community, 10 percent of elderly patients reported ADRs, with the incidence increasing with the number of medications used.[74] ADRs are also a problem in long-term care facilities, where inappropriate prescribing patterns of physicians apparently are the most important factor for the increased number of ADRs.[83]

When clinicians are faced with ADRs in older patients, an important point to consider is the different modes of presentation. Common pathologic conditions like pneumonia, urinary tract infection, acute MI, CHF, TIAs, and reactions to medications that many times have straightforward clinical manifestations obvious in younger subjects, can present in different ways in aged patients that may be confusing to physicians. Table 118.6 shows examples of the different clinical presentations of ADRs in the elderly that can be the same presentation for sepsis, MI, or cerebral ischemia.[r8,75,84]

For that reason, many times the only clue to ADRs in the elderly is impairment of function in daily activities when there is no obvious cause except an ADR. Among these are:

Driving: More than 22 million drivers are over 65,[85] and side-effects of drugs can affect driving, with the major evidence for benzodiazepines.[86] These drugs can impair reaction times in younger individuals, but the effect on the elderly subjects can be much more pronounced given the changes in the aged CNS.[85] There is questionable evidence of ill-effects of other drugs like trycyclics and oral hypoglycemics.[86]

Sexual Activity: Several drugs have been found to cause sexual dysfunction in the elderly individual and contribute to deterioration of the quality of life of many otherwise functional individuals. Psychotherapeutic agents like antidepressants and neuroleptics[87] and antihypertensives like methyldopa, beta blockers, and numerous other medications including over-the-counter drugs can have an impact on sexual function.[88,89]

Continence: There are many drugs that can affect the lower urinary tract, causing abnormalities that can result in incontinence. Diuretics and several drugs with anticholinergic properties (antidepressants, antihistaminics, neuroleptics, and antiparkinsonians) may induce urinary retention and overflow incontinence. Alpha-adrenergic agonists can cause contraction of the smooth muscle of the urethra and cause urinary retention, while alpha-antagonists cause the opposite effect, resulting in bladder relaxation.[90]

Sleeping Patterns: Chronic use of alcohol, barbiturates, and antidepressants can result in sleep disturbance, with increasing doses causing more side-effects.[91] These drugs supress REM sleep—particularly benzodiazepines, which can cause a reduction in the Stages 3 and 4.

Cognitive function: Medications constitute a potentially reversible cause of cognitive impairment.[51,92,93,r13] Psychotropics, (benzodiazepines and tricyclic antidepressants), anticholinergic compounds, antihypertensives (clonidine, methyldopa, diuretics), anticonvulsants (phenytoin or barbiturates), antibiotics, digitalis, levodopa, and many other compounds have been implicated as causes of drug-induced dementia. The alteration of cognitive function can result in impairment of multiple other body functions but can also be a risk factor for the development of more adverse drug reactions.

Bowel Function: Polypharmacy in the elderly increases the incidence of constipation.[94,95] Drugs with anticholinergic properties cause constipation by reducing contractility via an antimuscarinic effect.

Falls: In the frail elderly, falls can result in an increased incidence of hip fractures and an impaired quality of life.[r14] Medications, e.g., sedatives like benzodiazepines and antidepressants, have been identified as predisposing risk factors for such falls.[96,97]

Table 118.6 Clinical Presentation of Adverse Drug Reactions in the Elderly

Restlessness
Falls
Depression
Confusion
Cognitive dysfunction
Constipation
Incontinence
Extrapyramidal syndromes
Sexual dysfunction
Sleep impairment

Drug Interactions

Up to one-fifth of ADRs result from drug interactions.[r15] Many of the issues discussed in the section of pharmacokinetics and pharmacodynamics have relevance to the mechanisms of drug interaction in the elderly—like diminished renal excretion, lower protein binding, and decreased liver function, among others.[r15] It is also known that the probability of clinically important drug interactions increases with the number of drugs prescribed, and this problem is seen more frequently in the elderly.[r15,98] There are different types of drug interactions, but perhaps the most clinically significant in the elderly are drug-drug interactions and drug-nutrient interactions. Numbers vary in different studies, but the possibility of potential drug interactions that have been studied in the hospital setting,[93] nursing homes,[99,100] and outpatients[101] show that the common denominator is the high prevalence of polypharmacy and physicians' poor prescribing habits.

Elderly patients are more sensitive to oral anticoagulants, with patients over 70 requiring doses of warfarin 50 percent of those given to persons aged 40 to 60.[102] The concomitant use of cimetidine can result in an increased incidence of bleeding complications because cimetidine inhibits the metabolism of warfarin. Another example is the use of digoxin and quinidine, drugs that are frequently used in elderly patients, where cardiac conditions are more prevalent. Quinidine increases the digoxin concentration[103] and enhances the cardiac effects of this drug.[104] A higher incidence of toxicity due to this combination has been observed in elderly patients over 70.[105] For these reasons it is recommended that the dose of digoxin be reduced when quinidine is also prescribed.

Polypharmacy

Polypharmacy is defined as the prescription, administration, or use of more medications than are clinically indicated in a given patient.

Studies have shown that polypharmacy increases with age and that this is due to the prevalence of multiple and chronic diseases in the elderly.[73,106,107] McMillan showed that patients 80 years of age or older have a twenty-five-fold higher chance of receiving polypharmacy than those between 10 and 20 years and fivefold higher than those 21 to 30 years.[108] Polypharmacy is an important risk factor for ADRs.[109] Of note is the use of drugs commonly prescribed to treat unrecognized side-effects caused by other medications, resulting in a spiral of adverse effects and impairment of function in the elderly patient. The other problem attendant on polypharmacy is poor compliance with complicated and extensive lists of medications.[110]

Elderly patients in different settings are prone to develop complications from polypharmacy, and this problem has resulted in an increase in hospital admissions.[108,111–113] Simons, in a cross-sectional study of approximately 3000 elderly patients in a community, demonstrated that polypharmacy in the elderly is predicted by the history of recent admission to the hospital, depression, and increasing age, as well as female sex.[114] Polypharmacy also has been described in long-term facilities, where the use of psychotropics is especially predominant.[115]

Drug Compliance

It is often assumed that elderly patients are noncompliant with their medication regimens due to polypharmacy, impairment of sensory systems like hearing and vision, and cognitive decline.[116] Stewart and Caranasos pointed to design flaws present in several of the studies showing noncompliance in the elderly.[116] The evidence that noncompliance is more prevalent in elderly patients is not supported by available data.[r16,117] Weintraub[117] mentioned that between 16 and 25 percent of elderly patients take none of the medications that physicians prescribed for them and that probably the larger group of elderly patients are partial compliers. Many strategies have been devised to improve compliance in the elderly, such as educational programs, memory aids, simplification of medication regimens, monitoring of medications use,[r17] with more sophisticated techniques (e.g., continuous electronic monitoring) showing variable success.[118] Kruse, in the same study, showed the variability of compliance with time and even with once-a-day medications, which had been purported the best strategy to improve compliance. Even apparently trivial details like child-resistant containers can affect compliance in elderly populations.[119]

Summary

The elderly population in the US is growing at an accelerated rate, consuming a larger portion of the drug expenditures in this country every year. Physicians in clinical practice are faced with an ever-increasing number of patients over 65 with multiple medical problems and therapeutic needs. Research in basic aging pharmacology has provided information about the changes occurring at the molecular level, explaining some of the age-related changes in pharmacodynamic interactions, which, when associated with pharmacokinetic variations, are important factors when prescribing medications for older individuals. Adverse drug reactions present in an insidious and atypical way in older patients, where subtle changes in function can be indicators of the presence of an ADR. Polypharmacy is more common in elderly persons, and the use of multiple medications can result in an increased number of adverse drug reactions and potentially dangerous drug-drug interactions. Issues regarding the increased incidence of noncompliance with medications in older persons are still controversial, and the same methods used to improve compliance in other populations are probably applicable to these patients. Safe prescribing in the elderly is a dynamic process that requires individualization of therapy and a complete clinical evaluation taking in consideration the age-related changes outlined in an attempt to reduce the eventuality of impairment of the delicate balance that permits adequate function in the elderly individual.

References

Research Reports

1. Baum C, Kennedy DL, Forbes MB, Jones JK. Drug use in the United States in 1981. JAMA 1981;*251*:1293–1297.
2. Everitt DE, Avorn J. Drug prescribing for the elderly. Arch Intern Med 1986;*146*:2393–2396.
3. Shock NW. Normal human aging: The Baltimore longitudinal study of aging DHHS. NIH Publ No 84-2450. November 1984.

4. Lippa AS, Pelham RW, Beer B, Critchet DJ, Dean RL, Bartus RT. Brain cholinergic dysfunction and memory in aged rats. Neurobiol Aging 1980;*1*:13–19.

5. Abrass IB, Davis JL, Scarpace PJ. Isoproterenol responsiveness and myocardial beta-adrenergic receptors in young and aging rats. J Gerontol 1982;*37*:156–160.

6. Guarnieri T, Filburn C, Zitnik G, Roth GS, Lakatta EG. Contractile and biochemical correlates of beta-adrenergic stimulation of the aged heart. Am J Physiol 1980;*230*:H501–508.

7. Borst SE, Scarpace PJ. Reduced high-affinity alpha 1-adrenoceptors in liver of senescent rats: Implications of assessment at various temperatures. Br J Pharmacol 1990;*101*:650–654.

8. Morley JE, Flood JF, Silver AJ. Opioid peptides and aging. Ann NY Acad Sci 1990;*579*:123–132.

9. Roth GS. Mechanisms of altered hormone-neurotransmitter action during aging: from receptors to calcium mobilization. Ann Rev Gerontol Geriatr 1990;*10*:132–146.

10. Peterson C. Changes in calcium's role as messenger during aging in neuronal and nonneuronal cells. Ann NY Acad Sci 1992;*663*:279–293.

11. Bender AD. Effect of age on intestinal absorption: Implications for drug absorption in the elderly. J Am Geriatr Soc 1968;*16*:1331–1339.

12. Geokas MC, Haverback BJ. The aging gastrointestinal tract. Am J Surg 1969;*117*:881–892.

13. Kekki M, Samloff IM, Ihamaki T, Varis K, Siurala M. Age and sex-related behaviour of gastric acid secretion at the population level. Scand J Gastroenterol 1982;*17*:737–743.

14. Bender AD. The effect of increasing age on the distribution of peripheral blood flow in man. J Am Geriatr Soc 1965;*13*:192–198.

15. Castleden CM, George CF. The effect of aging on the hepatic clearance of propranolol. Br J Clin Pharmacol 1979;*7*:49–54.

16. Larsson M, Landahl S, Lundborg P, Regardh CG. Pharmacokinetics of metoprolol in healthy, elderly, non-smoking individuals after a single dose and two weeks of treatment. Eur J Clin Pharmacol 1984;*27*:217–222.

17. Evans MA, Triggs EJ, Cheung M, Broe GA, Creasey H. Gastric emptying rate in the elderly: implications for drug therapy. J Am Geriatr Soc 1981;*29*:201–205.

18. Evans MA, Triggs EJ, Broe GA, Saines N. Systemic availability of orally administered L-dopa in the elderly parkinsonian patient. Eur J Clin Pharmacol 1980;*17*:215–221.

19. Collart P, Poitevin M, Milovanovic A, Herlin A, Durel J. Kinetic study of serum penicillin concentrations after single doses of benzathine and benethamine penicillins in young and old people. Br J Vener Dis 1980;*56*:355–362.

20. Douglas JG, Bax RP, Munro JF. The pharmacokinetics of cefuroxime in the elderly. J Antimicrob Chemother 1980;*6*:543–549.

21. Phillips SL, Bararaman-Phillips J. The use of intramuscular cefoperazone versus intramuscular ceftriaxone in patients with nursing-home acquired pneumonia. J Am Geriatr Soc 1993;*4*:1071–1074.

22. Shock NW, Watkin DM, Yiengst BS, Norris AH, Gaffney GW, et al. Age differences in water content of the body as related to basal oxygen consumption in males. J Gerontol 1963;*18*:1–8.

23. Forbes GB, Reina JC. Adult lean body mass declines with age: Some longitudinal observations. Metabolism 1970;*19*:653–663.

24. Adelman LS, Liebman J. Anatomy of body water and electrolytes. Am J Med 1959;*27*:256–277.

25. Lakatta EG. Age-related alteration in the cardiovascular response to adrenergic-mediated stress. Fed Proc 1980;*39*:3173–3177.

26. Schmucker DL. Aging and drug disposition: an update. Pharmacol Rev 1985;*37*:133–148.

27. Wallace S, Whiting B. Factors affecting drug binding in plasma of elderly patients. Br J Clin Pharmacol 1976;*3*:327–330.

28. Paxton JW. Alpha 1 acid glycoprotein and binding of basic drugs. Methods Find Exp Clin Pharmacol 1983;*5*:635.

29. Paxton JW, Briant RH. Alpha 1 acid glycoprotein concentrations and propranolol binding in elderly patients with acute illness. Br J Clin Pharmacol 1984;*18*:806–810.

30. Piafsky KM. Disease induced changes in the plasma binding of basic drugs. Clin Pharmacokinet 1980;*5*:246–262.

31. O'Malley K, Crooks J, Duke E, Stephenson IH. Effects of age and sex on human drug metabolism. Br Med J 1971;*3*:607–609.

32. Vestal RE, Wood AJJ, Branch RA, Shand DG, Wilkinson GR. Effect of age and cigarrette smoking on propranolol disposition. Clin Pharmacol Ther 1979;*26*:8–15.

33. Bach B, Hansen JM, Kampmann JP, Rasmussen SN, Skovsted L. Disposition of antipyrine and phenytoin correlated with age and liver volume in men. Clin Pharmacokinet 1981;*6*:389–396.

34. Divoll M, Abernethy DR, Ameer B, Geenblatt DJ. Acetaminophen kinetics in the elderly. Clin Pharmacol Ther 1982;*31*:151–156.

35. Abernethy DR, Greenblatt DJ, Shader RI. Imipramine and desipramine disposition in the elderly. J Pharmacol Exp Ther 1985;*232*:183–188.

36. Wood AJJ, Vestal RE, Wilkinson GR, Branch RA, Shand DG. The effect of aging and cigarrette smoking on the elimination of antipyrine and indocyanine green elimination. Clin Pharmacol Ther 1979;*26*:16–20.

37. Twun-Barima Y, Finnigan T, Habash AI, Cape RD, Carruthers SG. Impaired enzyme induction by rifampicin in the elderly (letter). Br J Clin Pharmacol 1984;*17*:595–597.

38. Davies DF, Shock NW. Age changes in glomerular filtration rates, effective renal plasma flow, and tubular excretory capacity in adult males. J Clin Invest 1950;*29*:496–507.

39. Rowe JW, Andres R, Tobin JD, Norris AH, Shock NW. The effect of age on creatinine clearance in men: A cross-sectional and longitudinal study. J Gerontol 1976;*31*:155–163.

40. Watkin DM, Shock NW. Agewise standard value for Cin, Cpah and Tmpah in adult males. J Clin Invest 1955;*34*:965.

41. Landahl S, Aurell M, Jagenburg R. Glomerular filtration rate at the age of 70 and 75. J Clin Exp Geront 1982;*3*:29–45.

42. Trollfors B, Norrby R. Estimation of glomerular filtration rate by serum creatinine and serum beta-2-microglobulin. Nephron 1981;*28*:196–199.

43. Kim KE, Onesti G, Ramirez O, Brest AN, Swartz C. Creatinine clearance in renal disease. A reappraisal. Br Med J 1969;*4*:11–14.

44. Cockroft DW, Gault MH. Prediction of creatinine clearance from serum creatinine. Nephron 1976;*16*:31–41.

45. Baum C, Kennedy DL, Forbes MB. Utilization of nonsteroidal antiinflamatory drugs. Arthritis Rheum 1985;*28*:686–692.

46. Taha A, Lenton RJ, Murdoch PS, Peden NR. Non-oliguric renal failure during treatment with mefenamic acid in elderly patients: A continuing problem. Br Med J Clin Res Ed 1985;*291*:661–662.

47. Unworth J, Sturman S, Lunec J, Blake DR. Renal impairment associated with nonsteroidal antiinflamatory drugs. Ann Rheum Dis 1987;*46*:233–236.

48. Ciabattoni G, Cinotti GA, Pierucci A, Simonetti BM, Manzi M, Pugliese F, Barsotti P, Pecci G, Taggi F, Patrono C. Effects of sulindac and ibuprofen in patients with chronic glomerular disease. N Engl J Med 1984;*310*:279–283.

49. Cornoni-Huntley J, Brock DB, Ostfeldt AM, et al. Established populations for epidemiologic studies of the elderly. Resource Data Book. DHHS, Publ. No. (NIH) 1986;86–2443.

50. Castledon CM, George CF, Marcer D, Hallett C. Increased sensitivity to nitrazepam in old age. Br Med J 1977;*1*:10–12.

51. Larsson EB, Kukull WA, Buchner D, Reifler BV. Adverse drug reactions associated with global cognitive impairment in elderly persons. Ann Int Med 1987;*107*:169–173.

52. Bender AD. Pharmacologic aspects of aging. A survey of the effect of age on drug activity in adults. J Am Geriatr Soc 1964;*12*:114–134.

53. Gribbin B, Pickering TG, Sleight P, Peto R. Effect of age and high blood pressure on baroreflex sensitivity in man. Circ Res 1971;*29*:424–431.

54. McGarry K, Laher M, Fitzgerald D, Horgan J, O'Brien E, O'Malley K. Baroreflex function in elderly hypertensives. Hypertension 1975;*5*:763–766.

55. Schatz IJ. Orthostatic hypotension. I. Functional and neurogenic causes. Arch Intern Med 1984;*144*:773–777.

56. Schatz IJ. Orthostatic Hypotension. II. Clinical diagnosis, testing and treatment. Arch Intern Med 1984;*144*:1037–1041.

57. Come PC, Pitt B. Nitroglycerin-induced severe hypotension and bradycardia in patients with acute myocardial infarction. Circulation 1976;*54*:624–628.

58. Alpert JS. Nitrate therapy in the elderly. Am J Cardiol 1990;*65*:23J–27J.

59. Weidmann P, De Myttenaere-Bursztein S, Maxwell MH, de-Lima JD. Effect of aging on plasma renin and aldosterone in normal man. Kidney Int 1975;*8*:325–333.

60. Epstein M, Hollenberg NK. Age as a determinant of renal sodium conservation in normal man. J Lab Clin Med 1976;*87*:411–417.

61. Buhler F, Hulthen UL, Kiowski W, Muller FB, Boli P. The place of the calcium antagonist verapamil in antihypertensive therapy. J Cardiovasc Pharmacol 1982;*4*(suppl. 3):5350–5357.

62. Shannon RP, Minaker KL, Rowe JW. Aging and water balance in humans. Semin Nephrol 1984;*4*:346–353.

63. Rowe JW, Shock NW, deFronzo RA. The influence of age on the renal response to water deprivation in man. Nephron 1976;*17*:270–278.

64. Lindeman RD, Lee TD Jr, Yiengst MJ, Shock NW. Influence of age, renal disease, hypertension, diuretics and calcium on the antidiuretic response to suboptimal infusions of vasopressin. J Lab Clin Med 1966;*68*:206–223.

65. Rowe SW, Minaker KL, Sparrow D, Robertson GL. Age-related failure of volume-pressure-mediated vasopressin release. J Clin Endocrinol 1982;*54*:661–664.

66. Geller J. Benign prostatic hyperplasia: Pathogenesis and medical therapy. J Am Geriatr Soc 1993;*39*:1208–1216.

67. Caranasos GJ, Stewart RB, Cluff LE. Drug-related illness leading to hospitalization. JAMA 1974;*228*:713–717.

68. Smith JW, Seidl LG, Cluff LE. Studies on the epidemiology of adverse drug reactions IV. Clinical factors influencing susceptibility. Ann Intern Med 1966;*65*:629–640.

69. Williamson J, Chopin JM. Adverse reactions to prescribed drugs in the elderly: A multicentre investigation. Age Ageing 1980;*9*:73–80.

70. Carbonin P, Pahor M, Bernabein R, Spadari A. Is age an independent risk factor of adverse drug reactions in hospitalized medical patients? J Am Geriatr Soc 1991;*39*:1093–1099.

71. Lindley CM, Tully MP, Paramsothy V, Tallis RC. Inappropriate medication is a major cause of adverse drug reactions in elderly patients. Age Ageing 1992;*21*:294–300.

72. Gurwitz JH, Avorn J. The ambiguous relation between aging and adverse drug reactions. Ann Int Med 1991;*114*:956–966.

73. Montamat SC, Cusack B. Overcoming problems with polypharmacy and drug misuse in the elderly. Clin Geriatr Med 1992;*8*:143–158.

74. Chrischilles EA, Segar ET, Wallace RB. Self-reported adverse drug reactions and related resource use. A study of community-dwelling persons 65 years of age and older. Ann Int Med 1992;*117*:634–640.

75. Nolan L, O'Malley K. Prescribing for the elderly. Part I: Sensitivity of the elderly to adverse drug reactions. J Am Geriatr Soc 1988;*36*:142–144.

76. Klein U, Klein M, Sturm H, Rothenbuhler M, Huber R, Stucki P, Gikalov I, Keller M, Holgne R. The frequency of adverse drug reactions as dependent upon age, sex, and duration of hospitalization. Int J Clin Pharmacol Biopharm 1976;*13*:187–195.

77. Stewart RB, Cluff LE. Studies on the epidemiology of adverse drug reactions VI: Utilization and interactions of prescription and non-prescription drugs in outpatients. Johns Hopkins Med J 1976;*129*:319–331.

78. Swabo PA. Substance abuse in older women. Clin Geriatr Med 1993;*9*:197–208.

79. Seidl LG, Thornton GF, Smith JW, Cluff LE. Studies on the epidemiology of adverse drug reactions. III. Reactions in patients on general medical service. Bull Johns Hopkins Hosp 1966;*119*:299–315.

80. Darnell JC, Murray MD, Martz BL, Wenberger M. Medication use by ambulatory elderly: An in-home survey. J Am Geriatr Soc 1986;*34*:1–4.

81. Levy M, Kletter-Hems D, Nir I, Eliakim M. Drug utilization and adverse drug reactions in medical patients: Comparison of two periods, 1969–72 and 1973–76. Isr J Med Sci 1977;*13*:1065–1071.

82. Smidt WA, McQueen EG. Adverse reactions to drugs: A comprehensive inpatient survey. NZ Med J 1972;*76*:397–401.

83. Beers MH, Ouslander JG, Fingold SF, Morgenstern H, Reuben DB, Rogers W, Zeffren MJ, Beck JC. Inappropriate medication prescribing in skilled-nursing facilities. Ann Int Med 1992;*117*:684–689.

84. Besdine RW. Introduction. In Abrams et al. Merck manual of geriatrics, New Jersey: Merck & Co. 1990.

85. Retchin SM, Anapolle J. An overview of the older driver. Clin Geriatr Med 1993;*9*:279–296.

86. Ray WA, Purushottam BT, Shurr RI. Medications and the older driver. Clin Geriatr Med 1993;*9*:413–438.

87. Segraves RT. Sexual side effects of psychiatric drugs. Int J Psychiatr Med 1988;*18*:243–252.

88. Wein AJ, Van Arsdalen KN. Drug induced male sexual dysfunction. Urol Clin North Am 1988;*15*:23–31.

89. Deamer RL, Thompson JF. The role of medications in geriatric sexual dysfunction. Clin Geriatr Med 1991;*7*:95–111.

90. Ouslander JG, Bruskewitz R. Disorders of micturition in the aging patient. Adv Intern Med 1989;*34*:165–190.

91. Wooten V. Sleep disorders in geriatric patients. Clin Geriatr Med 1992;*8*:427–439.

92. Kramer SI, Reifler BV. Depression, dementia and reversible dementia. Clin Geriatr Med 1992;*8*:289–297.

93. Lowenthal DT, Nadeau S. Drug induced dementia. South Med J *84*:S24-S31.1991.

94. Harari D, Gurwitz JH, Minaker KL. Constipation in the elderly. J Am Geriatr Soc 1993;*41*:1130–1140.

95. Whitehead WE, Drinkwater D, Cheskin LJ, Heller BR, Schuster MM. Constipation in the elderly living at home: Definition, prevalence and relationship to life-style and health status. J Am Geriatr Soc 1989;*37*:423–429.

96. Rubenstein LZ, Robbins AS, Josephson KR, Schulman BL, Osterweil D. The value of assessing falls in an elderly population. Ann Intern Med 1990;*113*:308–316.

97. Sorock GS, Shimkin EE. Benzodiazepine sedation and the risk of falling in a community-dwelling elderly cohort. Arch Intern Med 1988;*148*:2441–2444.

98. Williamson J, Chopin JM. Adverse reactions to prescribed drugs in the elderly: A multicentre investigation. Age Ageing 1980;*9*:73–80.

99. Armstrong WA, Driever CW, Hays RL. Analysis of drug-drug interactions in the geriatric population. Am J Hosp Pharm 1980;*37*:385–387.

100. Cooper JR, Wellins I, Fish KA, Loomis ME. A seven nursing-home study frequency of potential drug-drug interactions. J Am Pharmaceut Assoc 1975;*11*:24–31.

101. Laventurier MF, Talley RB. The incidence of drug-drug interactions in a Medi-Cal Population. Cal Pharm 1972;*20*:18–22.

102. Swift CG. Clinical pharmacology in the elderly. New York: Marcel Dekker, 1987.

103. Bussey, HI. Update on the influence of quinidine and other agents on digitalis glycosides. Am Heart J 1984;*107*:143–146.

104. Doering. Quinidine-digoxin interaction. Pharmacokinetics, underlying mechanism and clinical implications. N Engl J Med 1979;*301*:400–404.

105. Walker AM, Cody RJ, Greenblatt DJ, Jick H. Drug toxicity in patient receiving digoxin and quinidine. Am Heart J 1983;*105*.1025–1028.

106. Colley CA, Lucas LM. Polypharmacy: The cure becomes the disease. J Gen Int Med 1993;*8*:278–283.

107. Williams P, Rush DR. Geriatric polypharmacy. Hosp Prac Off Ed 1986;*21*:109–112, 115–120.

108. McMillan DA, Harrison PM, Rogers LJ, Tong N, McLean AJ. Polypharmacy in an Australian teaching hospital. Med J Aust 1986;*145*:339–342.

109. Tallis RC, Edmond ED, O'Halloran A. A computer system for preventing the prescription of contraindicated drugs. Br J Pharmaceut Pract 1984;*6*:223–228.

110. Ramsay LE, Tucker GT. Drugs and the elderly. Br Med J 1981;*282*:125–127.

111. Grymonpre RE, Mitenko PA, Sitar DS, Aoki FY, Montgomery PR. Drug-associated hospital admissions in older medical patients. J Am Geriatr Soc 1988;*36*:1092–1098.

112. Beers MH, Dang J, Hasegawa J, Tamai IY. Influence of hospitalization on drug therapy in the elderly. J Am Geriatr Soc 1989;*37*:679–683.

113. Bernstein LR, Folkman S, Lazarus RS. Characterization of the use and misuse of medications by an elderly ambulatory population. Med Care 1989;*27*:654–663.

114. Simons LA, Tett S, Simons J, Lauchlan R, McCallum J, Friedlander Y, Powell I. Multiple medication use in the elderly. Use of prescription and non-prescription drugs in an Australian community setting. Med J Aust 1992;*157*:242–246.

115. Avorn J, Soumerai SB, Everitt DE, Ross-Degnan D, Beers MH, Sherman D, Salem-Shatz SR, Fields DA. A randomized trial of a program to reduce the use of psychoactive drugs in nursing homes. N Engl J Med 1992;*327*:168–173.

116. Stewart RB, Caranasos GJ. Medication compliance in the elderly. Med Clin North Am 1989;*73*:1551–1563.

117. Weintraub M. Compliance in the elderly. Clin Geriatr Med 1990;*6*:445–452.

118. Kruse W, Koch-Gwinner P, Nikolaus T, Oster P, Schlierf G, Weber E. Measurement of drug compliance by continuous electronic monitoring: A pilot study in Elderly patients discharged from the hospital. J Am Geriatr Soc 1992;*40*:1151–1155.

119. Keram S, Williams ME. Quantifying the ease or difficulty older persons experience in opening medication containers. J Am Geriatr Soc 1988;*36*:198–201.

Reviews

r1. Tumer N, Scarpace PJ, Lowenthal DT. Geriatric pharmacology: Basic and clinical considerations. Ann Rev Pharmacol Toxicol 1992;*32*:271–302.

r2. Roth GS, Hess GD. Changes in the mechanisms of hormone neurotransmitter action during aging: Current status of the role of receptor and postreceptor alterations. A review. Mech Ageing Dev 1982;*20*:175–194.

r3. Shimazu T, Takeda A, Fukushima Y. Neural-metabolic interaction in the liver during aging in rats. In Kitani K. Liver and aging, Amsterdam: Elsevier, 1986; pp 171–181.

r4. Ho PC, Triggs EJ. Drug therapy in the elderly. Aust NZ J Med 1984;*14*:179–190.

r5. Gibaldi M, Perrier D. Pharmacokinetics, 2d ed. New York: Marcel Dekker, 1982.

r6. Peck CC. Bedside clinical pharmacokinetics. Rockville, MD: Pharmacometric Press, 1985.

r7. Richey DP, Bender AD. Pharmacokinetics consequences of aging. Ann Rev Pharmacol Toxicol 1977;*17*:49–65.

r8. Lowenthal DT. Clinical Pharmacology, In Abrams et al. Merck Manual of Geriatrics, New Jersey: Merck & Co Inc, 1990.

r9. Crooks J, Stephenson IH. Drugs and the elderly. London: Macmillan, 1979.

r10. Yuen GJ. Altered pharmacokinetics in the elderly. Clin Geriatr Med 1990;*6*:257–267.

r11. Murray MD, Brater DC. Nonsteroidal antiinflammatory drugs. Clin Geriatr Med 1990;*6*:365–397.

r12. Kallman H. Depression in the elderly. In Desyrel: Compendium of three years of clinical use. Proc Symp Sept. 14, 1984, pp 31–40. Evansville IL: Mead-Johnson Pharmaceut Div, 1985.

r13. Cummings JL, Benson DF. Dementia. A clinical approach 2d ed. Stoneham: Butterworth-Heinemann, 1992.

r14. Tinetti ME. Falls. In Hazzard WR, et al. Principles of geriatric medicine and gerontology 2d ed. New York: McGraw-Hill, 1990.

r15. Lamy PP. The elderly and drug interactions. J Am Geriatr Soc 1986;*34*:586–592.

r16. Haynes RB. A critical review of the "determinants" of patient compliance with therapeutic regimens. In Sackett DL, Haynes RB. Compliance with therapeutic regimens. Baltimore: Johns Hopkins University Press, 1979, pp 26–39.

r17. Christopher LJ. Drug prescribing and compliance in the elderly. In Swift CG. Clinical pharmacology in the elderly. New York: Marcel Dekker, 1987, pp 103–117.

CHAPTER 19

The Treatment of Cognitive Impairment in Alzheimer's Disease

Robert G. Stern
Kenneth L. Davis

Introduction

The clinical characteristics and the gross microscopic pathology of Alzheimer's disease (AD) were described almost a century ago.[1] Clinically the disease presents as a progressive dementia of insidious onset leading to a gradual deterioration of intellectual abilities, neuropsychological deficits and personality changes. The disease process eventually results in anomia, agnosia and apraxia and in complete loss of memory and learning abilities. The disease is occasionally accompanied by sleep disturbances, agitation, anxiety, depressive states or psychosis. In the final stages of the disease some patients are mute, unable to stand or walk, bedridden and incontinent. Generally but not invariably, postmortem macroscopic examination of the brain reveals cerebral atrophy with narrowed convolutions, widened sulci and enlarged lateral and third ventricles. On microscopic examination brain specimens from patients with a clinical diagnosis of AD are characterized by widely spread cortical senile plaques, neurofibrillary tangles and granulovascular degeneration. In addition lesions in subcortical structures have been found to be an integral part of the histopathology of AD. These studies revealed the consistent occurrence of neuronal loss in the nucleus basalis of Meynert (NBM) and a variable degree and frequency of neuronal loss in the nucleus locus ceruleus and raphe nuclei. Histochemically AD is associated with multiple deficits in various neurotransmitter or their associated markers such as acetylcholine, noradrenaline, somatostatin and others.

Although the disease is accompanied by various psychiatric non-cognitive symptoms, the progressive cognitive deterioration represents the core phenomenon of Alzheimer's disease and the major target of current therapeutic efforts. As in any other disease characterized by progressive deterioration the therapeutic intent can vary from wanting to alleviate some symptoms of the disease to slowing down or arresting the deterioration, or if possible, reversing the damage completely. The neurotransmitter based approaches described below offer modest palliation by augmenting deficient neurotransmission. Many other empirically derived approaches such as the nootropics have been assessed for potential palliative or deterioration retarding properties in AD. Recent advances in the understanding of the biology of Alzheimer's disease may permit the development of strategies aimed at retarding or halting the progression of the illness. These strategies based on various pathophysiologic models of the illness attempt to interfere with putative pathogenetic mechanisms involved such as glutamate's neurotoxicity, free radical production, CNS inflammation, amyloid production, and aluminum accumulation. Regenerative treatments however aimed at restoring incurred damage are not in sight yet.

The Cholinergic Hypothesis of Alzheimer's Disease and Cholinergic Enhancement Strategies

The cholinergic hypothesis of Alzheimer's disease postulates that (1) there is a significant cerebral cholinergic neurotransmission deficit, (2) that this deficit causes some of the cognitive disturbances observed in AD patients, and (3) that enhancing cholinergic neurotransmission will produce some amelioration in cognitive function in this population.

Several lines of evidence support this hypothesis. Centrally active anticholinergic drugs have been shown to induce dose-related cognitive deficits in humans[r1,r2,r3] while cholinergic neurotransmission has been shown to be specifically involved in memory and learning.[4,5] The hypothesis is further supported by studies demonstrating that chemical, surgical, or pharmacological lesions to cerebral cholinergic systems impair learning and memory in animals and that cholinomimetic agents can reverse lesion-induced behavioral disturbances.[r2–r4] Finally brains of AD patients exhibit consistent cholinergic cell loss in the septum and nucleus basalis of Meynert (NBM), a decrease in the cholinergic markers choline-acetyl transferase (CAT) and acetylcholine esterase (ACHE), and a correlation between these neurochemical changes and the degree of cognitive impairment in AD[6–9] (for review see Bartus et al.,[r2] and Collerton[r3]).

Analogous to the dopaminergic treatment approach used in Parkinson's disease, therapeutic trials in AD have been aimed at augmenting cerebral cholinergic neurotransmission. The various cholinomimetic agents that have been assessed in AD can be classified according to their particular cholinomimetic mechanism of action into (1) ACHE inhibitors, (2) cholinergic agonists, (3) acetylcholine (ACH) precursors, (4) ACH-releasing agents, and (5) agents with various other cholinomimetic effects. Despite the large number of known centrally active cholinomimetic agents, only few have been shown to be clinically relevant. The vast majority of such agents had to be excluded from clinical use due to limitations related to short biological half-life, poor blood-brain barrier penetration, instability in plasma, unpredictable absorption, frequent side effects, or dangerously narrow therapeutic range. Acetylcholine esterase inhibitors is the most extensively studied group of cholinomimetics and has so far had the best clinical results. Overall however the cholinergic treatment in AD has not produced ameliorations comparable to those achieved with levodopa (L-dopa) in Parkinson's disease.

Acetylcholinesterase Inhibitors

Tetrahydroaminoacridine

Introduction

1 ,2,3,4-Tetrahydro-9-acridinamine (THA), known as tacrine, is a synthetic aminoacridine, which was initially synthesized more than 40 years ago. Tacrine and physostigmine are the two ACHE inhibitors which have been most extensively evaluated in the treatment of AD. Tacrine was the first drug ever to be approved by the FDA (available as of 1993) for the treatment of cognitive impairment in AD in the United States.

The commercially available drug Cognex[R], is tacrine monohydrochloride monohydrate. Tacrine hydrochloride is a reversible but noncompetitive ACHE inhibitor with a moderately long duration of action. Studies conducted beginning in 1981[10] have assessed the therapeutic potential of THA in AD. In addition to its ACHE inhibitory activity THA has multiple other pharmacological effects which may contribute to its therapeutic effects in this illness.

Chemistry

The empirical formula of THA is $C_{13}H_{14}N_2 \cdot HCl \cdot H_2O$. THA has a molecular weight of 252.74. The molecular structure is depicted below (Fig. 119.1). THA is a white solid freely soluble in water.

Pharmacology

Cholinesterase Inhibition. Tacrine is thought to be a noncompetitive reversible inhibitor of ACHE. The drug has been shown to be a more potent inhibitor of butyrylcholinesterase than of ACHE. Tacrine's ACHE inhibitory activity is thought to be mediated by its binding to a hydrophobic area close to the active site.

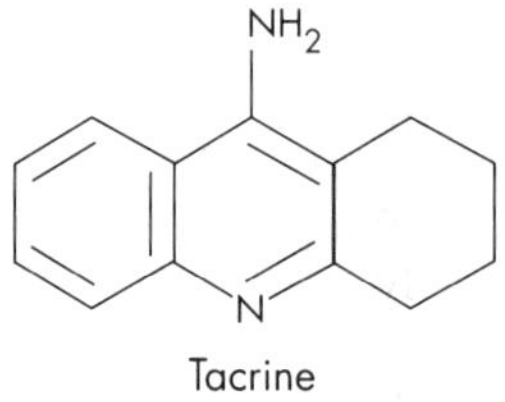

NH2
N
Tacrine

Figure 119.1 Molecular Structure of THA

Effects on Choline Metabolism. THA has been reported to increase ACH brain levels. The mechanism for this phenomenon has not been clearly established. Various mechanisms including THA's blocking effect on slow K+ channels as well as its M1 cholinergic effects have been implicated in this phenomenon. In addition it has been suggested that THA may lead to increased ACH synthesis.[11]

Effects on Cholinergic Receptors. THA has been shown to bind to muscarinic and nicotinic receptor sites. The affinity for muscarinic receptors is about 100 times higher than for nicotinic receptors. The clinical relevance of the direct effects of THA at the cholinergic receptor site depends on the actual concentration of THA in human brain tissue in vivo. Recent findings of high concentration of THA in the brain strengthens the possibility that THA's effects may also be mediated by its activity at cholinergic receptor sites.[r5,r6] THA has also been found to bind to two additional membrane sites whose pharmacological and clinical significance is unknown.[12]

Inhibition of Monoamine Oxidase (MAO). The enzymatic activity of monoamine oxidases of type A (MAO-A) and type B (MAO-B) have been shown to be reduced by THA. MAO-A seems to be inhibited to a larger degree than MAO-B. At therapeutic concentrations THA is believed to produce a significant decrease in MAO activity leading to an enhanced monoaminergic activity. Given that some cognitive deficits in AD are believed to be due to a monoaminergic deficit, this monoaminergic enhancement might also contribute to the therapeutic effect of THA in AD.

Monoamines Release and Uptake. Tacrine has been shown to induce monoamine release and to inhibit monoamine uptake leading to an increase in several monoamine neurotransmitters including dopamine, serotonin and norepinephrine.[13,14] As mentioned above these effects might be beneficial in AD.

Effects on Ion Channels. THA has been reported to interact with K+, Na+ and CA++ channels. Tacrine appears to keep NA+ channels open and K+ channels closed. Some studies suggested that THA enhances presynaptic ACH release by blocking slow K+ channels.[13–15]

Pharmacokinetics

Cognex[R] the THA brand currently available on the US market is rapidly absorbed and reaches maximal plasma concentration two hours after oral or administration. The bioavailability is 17 ± 113%. Tacrine has been found to be safe when administered PO, IV and PR. Administration per rectum resulted in higher bioavailability of the drug than oral administration. This finding is thought to reflect a rapid first-pass metabolic effect.[16] Tacrine is 55% bound to plasma protein and has an elimination half life of 2–4 hours. The drug is metabolized in the liver in particular by cytochrome P450 1A2. There are several tacrine metabolites known. The most important is velnacrine, the 1-hydroxy metabolite, an active but in vitro weaker ACHE inhibitor than THA. THA plasma levels after the administration for several weeks at therapeutic dosage ranged from 10 to 100 ng/ml. Plasma levels were 50% higher in females than in males. At steady state mean maximum plasma concentrations were 5.1 ng/ml, 20.7 ng/ml, and 33.9 ng/ml following daily administration of 40 mg, 80 mg, and 120 mg doses, respectively[17,18] (Cognex[R] drug insert, 5/93).

Clinical Applications

Since its synthesis, THA has been evaluated for various clinical applications. Tacrine has been given in combination with morphine to alleviate pain in cancer patients, and it has been evaluated as a possible agent in the treatment of narcotic addiction,[19] postanesthetic delirium,[20] AIDS,[21] amyotrophic lateral sclerosis,[17,22]; tardive dyskinesia and others. Despite the interest in the drug and the encouraging findings in some instances THA has not gained wide popularity in any of those fields.

Therapeutic Use

In the first clinical study to test THA in AD,[10] intravenous THA 1.5 mg/kg of produced significant improvement on memory testing in 6 out of 12 participating subjects. Nine of the 12 improved on clinical staging. In a double-blind, placebo-controlled study, the acute effects of 30 mg of THA administered orally were compared with the effects of 60 g of lecithin administered orally alone and 30 mg of THA combined with 60 g of lecithin administered orally in a group of 10 AD patients.[23] The combined regimen showed a small nonsignificant trend to improve performance on a serial learning test. It is possible that the poor results in this study were due to the low dose employed.

Eight large placebo controlled studies[24–31] have assessed the efficacy of THA in larger samples of AD patients (see Table 119.1). THA in combination with lecithin resulted in significant improvement in two studies[24,26] and in marginal or no improvement in two other studies.[25,31] A six week parallel trial using an enriched-population design[28] found that patients treated with THA displayed less decline in cognitive function than the placebo treated group, as assessed

Table 119.1 Placebo Controlled Double Blind Studies with THA and Lecithin

Study	Subject Number*	THA Max Dose (mg)	Lecithin (mg) Max Dose	Length of THA Tx (weeks)	Study Design	Findings and Comments
Gauthier et al.[114]	39	100	4,700	8	CO	Significant improvement in MMSE scores with THA. Authors concluded no "significant clinical benefit".
Chatellier, et al.[39]	60	125	1,200	4	CO	Significant improvement with THA on visual analogue scale rated by physicians. Authors concluded. no "strikingly beneficial effect"
Eagger et al.[89]	65	150	10,800	13	CO	Significant differences on MMSE and AMTS favoring THA. THA produced improvement equivalent to 6–12 months deterioration.
Farlow et al.[98]	273	80	—	12	P	THA (80 mg/d) produced significant improvement on cADAS, and CGIC. Authors concluded: "effect is clinically important".
Davis et al.[73]	187	80	—	6	P	Statistically significant reduction in decline on cADAS. Tacrine produced "the equivalent of about five months' gain".
Wilcock et al.[277]	41	150	—	12	CO	No statistically significant findings on any of the main outcome measures. However "THA was favored over placebo" on most of them.
Knapp et al.[148]	263	160	—	30	P	Statistically and clinically "significant dose-related improvements" were found with tacrine.
Maltby et al.[160]	32	100	10,800	36	P	No significant results and "no clinically relevant improvement".

*=Number of subjects included in statistical analysis

CO = Cross Over
P = Parallel
CGIC = Clinical Global Impression of Change
MMS = Mini Mental Status Exam

PDS = Progressive Deterioration Scale
PSAS = Physician's score analog scale
AMTS = Abbreviated Mental Test Score
cADAS = cognitive subscale of the Alzheimer Disease Assessment Scale

by the Alzheimer's Disease Assessment Scale cognitive subscale. In another study THA produced a significant dose-related cognitive improvement.[27] Similar results were reported from a more recent study of 30 weeks duration.[30] Two recently published studies however one with a crossover design[29] and one with parallel design[31] failed to find any statically significant differences between THA and placebo.

The studies reviewed here suggest that lecithin is not essential and probably not contributory to the therapeutic effect. Furthermore these studies suggest that THA administered for at least two weeks in doses of 80–160 mg po/d produces significant improvements which can be ascertained on cognitive performance tests as well as on global clinical measures. The amelioration produced by THA in the most responsive patients was equivalent to the deterioration incurred in the course of 6–12 months of illness.

The response to THA is as heterogeneous as the clinical and histopathological presentation of the illness itself. While 10% of patients showed larger, 20% demonstrate more modest, and 20% small but statistically significant improvement in cognitive performance or clinical status, the remaining patients showed no short term benefits. Although the amelioration achieved with THA is limited, these results are encouraging as they represent the first successful attempt to improve cognitive performance and functional ability in AD.

Cognex[R] is available in 10, 20, 30 and 40 mg capsules. It is recommended that treatment should be started with 10 mg po qid for 6 weeks. Additional dosage increments of 10 mg po qid up to a maximum of 160 mg po/d should be initiated every six weeks. Weekly transaminase monitoring should be performed for the first 18 weeks of treatment and for at least 6 weeks after each dosage increment. Thereafter checks at 3 months intervals are recommended.

Side Effects

Reversible liver toxicity was common in THA treated patients. Liver toxicity as documented by serum alanine aminotransferase (ALT) elevation above the upper normal limit occurred in approximately half of 2446 study patients.[32] ALT levels greater than three times the upper normal limit were observed in one quarter of the patients and greater than 20 times upper normal limit in 2% of the patients. The majority (90%) of the ALT elevations above 3 times upper normal limit occurred within the first 12 weeks of treatment, mean of 7 weeks. Women were more often affected than men. Rechallenge with tacrine produced significant ALT elevations 90% of the time. Discontinuation of treatment led inadvertently to normalization of liver functions and there was no case of death due to THA induced liver toxicity.

Fifty percent of the patients treated with THA had increased LFTs above upper normal limits. Most elevations occurred after 4–12 weeks of treatment and in most cases LFT returned to normal 4–6 weeks after THA discontinuation. Other side effects commonly associated with THA were nausea, vomiting, abdominal distress, anorexia, bradycardia, myalgia, and ataxia. For other side effects, see Table 119.2

Drug–Drug Interactions

Cimetidine was found to increase the concentration and rate of absorption of THA by 50%. THA administration may double *theophylline's* elimination half-life and plasma concentrations. The interaction with theophylline may be due to competition for the cytochrome P450 1A2 metabolism. It is possible that other drugs with this metabolic pathway may have significant drug-drug interactions with THA.

Table 119.2 Adverse Effects Associated with THA in More Than 5% of the Patients Studied in a Placebo Controlled Study

Side Effect	% of Patients
Elevated Transaminases	49
Nausea or Vomiting	28
Diarrhea	16
Dizziness	12
Headache	11
Dyspepsia	9
Anorexia	9
Myalgia	9
Abdominal Pain	8
Rhinitis	8
Rash	7
Agitation	7
Confusion	7
Ataxia	6
Insomnia	6

Overdosage

THA overdosage can result in a cholinergic crisis with severe nausea, vomiting salivation sweating bradycardia hypotension, convulsions etc. Progressive muscle weakness may result in death from asphyxiation. Treatment with anticholinergics (such as IV atropine sulfate) and general supportive treatment are recommended.

Other Acetylcholinesterase Inhibitors

Investigational Tacrine Derivatives

Velnacrine Maleate (HP 029). 9-Amino-1,2,3,4,-tetrahydroaminoacridineamin-1-ol maleate, (Fig. 119.2) velnacrine maleate or HP 029 (Hoechst-Roussel) was identified as the main THA metabolite in man.[130] Like tacrine it is a synthetic aminoacridine, and it was developed in the search for a more advantageous ACHE inhibitor for the treatment of Alzheimer's disease. This experimental drug has been in clinical trials since 1988, but its development was discontinued in 1994.

Velnacrine maleate is a reversible ACHE inhibitor with a shorter half life than THA. Velnacrine has been shown to be a less-potent ACHE inhibitor on a weight basis but able to induce the same degree of ACHE inhibition as THA.[33] Velnacrine was shown to significantly enhance long-term potentiation in guinea pig hippocampal slice preparation[34] and to reverse scopol-

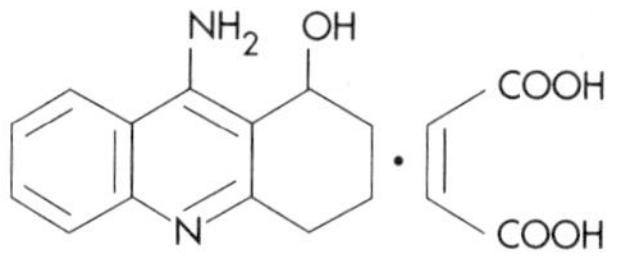

HP-029
Velnacrine

Figure 119.2 Molecular Structure of Velnacrine

amine or NBM-lesion-induced learning impairment in rodents.

Velnacrine is a less potent enhancer of skeletal neuromuscular transmission than physostigmine. Initial clinical studies showed velnacrine to be safe in healthy young volunteers[35] and in elderly volunteers.[21] A 28-day course of velnacrine 300 mg po/d was well tolerated by elderly (60–74 years old) volunteers but not by patients with AD. In the patients group dosages greater than 225 mg/day were associated with significant side effects including dizziness, fainting, nausea, vomiting, headache, and severe diarrhea.[37,38] Velnacrine is rapidly absorbed after oral administration, reaching peak plasma level after 0.75–1.2 hours. The mean plasma half-life was approximately 2 hours. The majority of the drug is excreted in the urine.[39] There seems to be marked inter-subject variability in tolerance to the drug.[40] The interim analysis from a double blind placebo controlled trial with HP 029 reported some clinical benefits for a one third of the patients studied.[41] According to Schneider[r7] the parallel designed "protocol 301" which employed velnacrine dosages of 225, 150 and 75 mg/d po showed significant efficacy on cADAS. The drug produced hepatotoxic side effects similar to tacrine as well as side effects related to its cholinomimetic properties. In addition rare cases of neutropenia have been reported.

Suronacrine (HP128). 9-Benzylamino-1,2,3,4-tetrahydroaminoacridine-1-ol maleate, (Fig. 119.3) Suronacrine or HP128 is another THA derivative synthesized in the search for an adequate ACHE inhibitor for the treatment of Alzheimer's disease. Suronacrine was shown to inhibit acetylcholinesterase in vitro and to improve memory in animal models of AD. Suronacrine is a weaker ACHE inhibitor than THA or velnacrine. The later is one of suronacrine's main metabolites. The drug inhibits the uptake of noradrenaline and dopamine in vitro and has blocking effects on cholinergic receptors.[42,43]

Suronacrine was found to reach peak plasma levels 1.4–5.0 after oral administration and to have a plasma half life of 1.5–8.6 hours. Suronacrine 200 mg po/d has been shown to be well tolerated and to be safe in patients with Alzheimer's disease but its therapeutic efficacy is unclear.[44]

Other Aminoacridines

The therapeutical potential of several other aminoacridines in AD have been studied as well. This group of agents includes: 7-methoxy-1,2,3,4-tetrahydroaminoacridine (methoxytacrine), 9-amino-8-fluoro-1,2,3,4-tetrahydro-2,4-methanoacridine (SM10888), 4-N-butylamino-1,2,3,4-tetrahydroaminoacridine(centbucridine).

Methoxytacrine, is a new reversible cholinesterase inhibitor developed in Czechoslovakia. Animal studies suggested that methoxytacrine might have cholinomimetic properties consistent with a therapeutic effects in AD.[45–48] Initial safety trials in healthy volunteers have shown methoxytacrine up to 8mg/kg po or up to 2mg/kg body weight po to be well tolerated. Peak plasma levels were reached 4 hours after oral administration and T½ was 8.7 ± 3.9 hours.[49] Data on the agent's therapeutic effects is pending.

SM-10888 is thought to be a potent ACHE inhibitor, with a high brain/periphery partition coefficient and with less peripheral cholinergic side effects than THA, HP-029 or physostigmine. Consistent with its postulated selectivity for the central nervous system SM-10888 enhanced learning in animal models at much lower doses than THA.[50,51]

Centbucridine has been assessed for its potent local anesthetic properties. Centbucridine has several metabolites and THA is one of them.[52] This agent has not been assessed in AD.

Physostigmine and its Derivatives

Physostigmine. Physostigmine (PHS) is a natural alkaloid, first isolated in 1864 (Fig. 119.4). PHS is a lipid-soluble tertiary amine readily absorbed from the gastrointestinal tract, subcutaneous tissue, and mucous membranes that is able to cross the blood-brain barrier. It reaches maximal levels in a short time. It is hydrolyzed and inactivated within 2 hours. Physostigmine administered orally has been used in the treat-

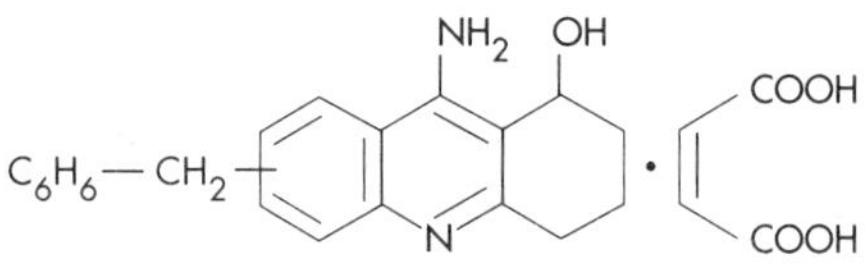

HP-128
Suronacrine

Figure 119.3 Molecular Structure of Suronacrine

ment of exophthalmos, gastric atony, tachycardia, inherited ataxias, and myasthenia gravis.

Physostigmine was one of the first ACHE inhibitors to be assessed in the treatment of AD. Of the 11 studies of physostigmine in AD reviewed by Mohs and Davis,[r8] all five studies using parenterally administered PHS, and four out of the six that were using orally administered PHS found some improvement in at least a subpopulation of the patients studied. Two recent studies confirmed the beneficial effect of oral PHS on learning[239] and memory[229] in AD. The effects of intracerebroventricular (ICV) administration of PHS in AD patients have also been evaluated.[55] ICV administration of PHS was not associated with peripheral side effects. However the drug led to increased irritability and sleepiness and produced no clinically significant effects.

Results from a few uncontrolled studies point to the possibility that long-term PHS administration might delay or prevent cognitive deterioration in AD patients.[17,143] Most recently a one year long controlled study with up to 15 mg/d of oral PHS in out patients with AD appears to support the notion that long term PHS-treatment improves or stabilizes neuropsychological function.[r9]

Despite some encouraging results PHS has not found routine clinical application in the treatment of Alzheimer's disease. The primary reason for that is probably the short half life and disadvantageous side effect profile.

Heptylphysostigmine. Heptylphysostigmine (Fig. 119.5) also known as L-693,487, a carbamate derivative of physostigmine, is more lipophile, produces a longer inhibition of brain cholinesterase than PHS and is less toxic than PHS.[58,59] Heptyl-physostigmine has been shown to improve cognition in various animal models of dementia.[60,61] Furthermore this agent has been shown to enhance cortical cerebral blood flow, an effect that is thought to be linked to the inhibition of acetylcholin-

Physostigmine

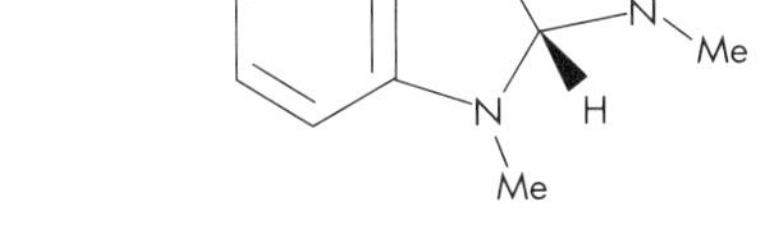

Figure 119.4 Molecular Structure of Physostigmine

Heptyl-Physostigmine

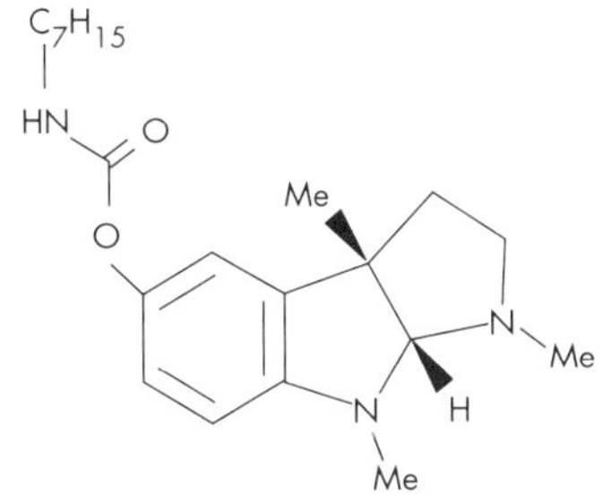

Figure 119.5 Molecular Structure of Heptyl-physostigmine

esterase activity.[62] Heptyl-physostigmine was well tolerated in doses up 32 mg po tid in healthy volunteers and up to 48 mg po tid in AD patients.[r10] Unfortunately, heptylphysostigmine trials in humans have been abandoned because of neutropenia observed with this agent.

Other PHS analogues similar to heptyl-physostigmine have been developed.[63,64] Some of those PHS analogues such as **heptastigmine** have longer half-lives, more favorable brain-plasma partition patterns, and possibly less peripheral toxicity than PHS properties that make them promising therapeutic agents for AD.[64] **Eptastigmine,** a new long-acting cholinesterase inhibitor, was shown to have a strong cholinomimetic effect as documented by augmentation of basal and stimulated GH secretion in unanesthetized old dogs.[65] The central effects of eptastigmine were further documented by cerebral blood flow studies in rats. Eptastigmine was shown to produce prolonged changes in regional CBF.[66] Further preclinical evaluation of these agents is needed before their clinical efficacy can be tested.

Other Investigational ACHE Inhibitors

Various other compounds with ACHE-inhibitory activity are being considered for their therapeutic potential AD. Bioavailability, pharmacokinetics properties, and brain-plasma partition pattern, are some of the major properties affecting the therapeutic potential of various ACHE inhibitors in AD. In addition a compounds' relative affinities for ACHE and butyrylcholinesterase (BuChE) may affect its therapeutic potential as well. Because inactivated BuChE, the oligomer precursor of ACHE, does not contribute to the pool of ACHE, ACHE inhibitors with higher BuChE/ACHE affinity ratio may have a detrimental effect on cholinergic neurotransmission. The administration of an ACHE inhibitor with a high affinity for BuChE might produce a prolonged drop in the precursor level and ultimately decrease ACHE level.[r11,67] The pharmacology of the cholinergic system is far from being fully explored. Yet unrecognized variables may still evolve, and the clinical implications of the various parameters need more accurate assessment.

Huperzine. Huperzine A and B are two natural alkaloids recently isolated by Chinese scientists from the plant *Huperzia serrata*. Huperzine A is a reversible ACHE inhibitor more selective and more potent than PHS.[68] In animal models, the therapeutic effects of huperzine A and B seem to be superior to those of PHS.[r12] The drug improves cognitive performance in mice, rats, and monkeys. It is effective upon oral and parenteral administration.[69] A double blind placebo controlled study with Huperzine A 0.05 mg i.m. bid or 0.03 mg i.m. tid reported positive effects in patients with multi-infarct dementia or with presenile or senile dementia.[70] More recently Huperzine was synthesized in the laboratory and will probably become available for larger clinical trials.[71]

Metrifonate. This substance is an organo-phosphorus compound that has been employed as an insecticide and as a treatment for human infections with the parasite Schistosoma haematobium. Metrifonate is transformed nonenzymatically into dichlorvos, an ACHE inhibitor with a half-life longer than PHS. Although toxic reactions in humans have been reported, orally administered metrifonate in doses of 7.5–10.0 mg/kg of body weight seem to be safe. Metrifonate has been shown to induce ACHE inhibition in the CNS after intramuscular and intraperitoneal administration in rodents.[r13] The drug has also been shown to inhibit plasma and red blood cell ACHE activity in humans after oral administration.[72] Most recently the attempt to administer metrifonate with the help of a transdermal patch has failed. However DDVP another ACHE inhibitor was successfully administered via a patch.[73]

Galanthamine. Galanthamine is a tertiary ACHE with a half life of 7 hours.[74] The drug has good bioavailability after oral administration.[171] Administration of Galanthamine 30 mg p.o. qd in divided doses over 2 months to nine AD patients appeared to have beneficial effects and was well tolerated.[76] Galanthamine was tolerated without signs of liver toxicity by one AD patient, who was treated with 1–5 mg po qd of galanthamine for 140 days.[77] In an open trial galanthamine produced no significant changes on neuropsychological tests in eighteen patients treated with galanthamine 30 mg po for two months.[78] Preliminary reports from recent double blind trials[78a] suggest that galanthamine 30 mg po/d administered for 6–10 weeks might be superior to placebo. In those trials galanthamine produced significant improvements on cognitive performance as assessed on cADAS similar to those achieved with tacrine.

SDZ ENA-713. SDZ ENA-713 (Figure 119.6) has been shown to have neuroprotective effects in a gerbil brain ischemia model of dementia.[79] In man SDZ ENA-713 was shown to be safe in doses up to 4.6 mg po.[80] SDZ ENA-713 in doses of 1–2 mg po has been shown to have central cholinergic effects in man as demonstrated by its ability to increase the frequency of REM-sleep phases.[81] Data on the efficacy of this drug in AD is pending.

E2020. The compound 1-benzyl-4 (5,6-dimethoxy-1- indanon)-2-yl)-methylpiperidine hydrochloride or E2020 is another novel ACHE inhibitor, currently under development for the treatment of AD in Japan and the USA. The drug 92.6% protein bound in serum, is secreted in the urine and has an exceptionally long plasma T½ half-life of 50 hours. Plasma steady-state was achieved after approximately 2 weeks of daily dosing.[82]

NIK-247. 9-amino-2,3,5,6,7,8-hexahydro-1H-cyclopenta-(b)-quinoline monohydrate hydrochloride, also known as NIK-247, an ACHE inhibitor under development in Japan has been shown to have central cholinomimetic effects[83] and to improve experimentally induced deficits in working memory.[84]

Limitations to ACHE-Inhibitors Therapy in AD

Adverse effects of ACHE inhibitors are due to the enhancement of peripheral cholinergic tonus and are primarily gastrointestinal (nausea, vomiting, abdominal cramping, and diarrhea) but may include diaphoresis and light headedness. However some nausea is undoubtedly of central origin and could be related to the rate of rise of the drug in plasma. Bradycardia and

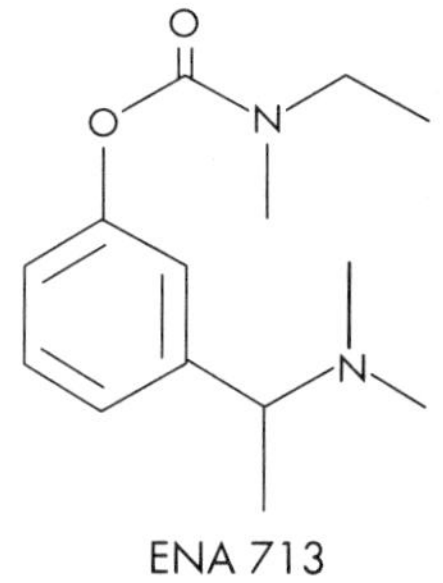

ENA 713

Figure 119.6 Molecular Structure of ENA 713

hypotension are anticipated risks but appear infrequently. Depression and agitation have also been encountered. Individual susceptibility to such side effects varies widely. Considering the inverted U-shape form of the dose-response curve to cholinergic enhancement in AD, ACHE inhibitor levels that are too high or too low may easily be outside the therapeutic window. Non-optimal levels may easily occur with fluctuations in drug levels due to uncertain CNS availability of the drug. Under such circumstances, fixed-dose treatment studies can be of limited benefit. Thus, studies should include individual titrations and confirmation of CNS availability using biological markers such as AChE activity in cerebrospinal fluid (CSF) or endocrinological parameters. Ultimately, some patients might present with such a severe degree of presynaptic cholinergic cell loss that any degree of ACHE inhibition would fail to induce a clinically significant enhancement of the cholinergic transmission. Overall, it appears that short-term administration of ACHE inhibitors can induce a mild to moderate improvement of memory in AD, and that long-term ACHE treatment should be evaluated for additional benefits.

Cholinergic Agonists and Antagonists

Although the administration of cholinergic agonists provides a non-physiologic, tonic enhancement of the stimulation at the postsynaptic receptor, this approach has beneficial effects on memory and learning in animals with experimentally induced hypocholinergic states.[85] Most cholinergic agonists known to date are choline derivatives, natural alkaloids, or synthetic analogues. Some of these agonists have been evaluated in AD. More recently the possibility of enhancing cholinergic neurotransmission by blocking presynaptic cholinergic M2 autoreceptors has been considered, or by developing receptor subtype specific muscarinic agonists.

Clinical Data

RS-86. RS-86 (2-ethyl-8-methyl-2,8-diazospiro-4,5-decan-1,3-dionhydrobromide) is a long-acting cholinergic agonist with good central nervous system (CNS) permeability. RS-86 has no nicotinic effects, is selective for muscarinic receptors, and has a relatively higher activity at M1 than at M2 receptors. Administered orally, RS-86 produced minimal[86] or no[87] improvement in AD patients. The drug had no significant beneficial effects on cognitive functions in AD.[88,89] RS-86 is no longer in development for AD.

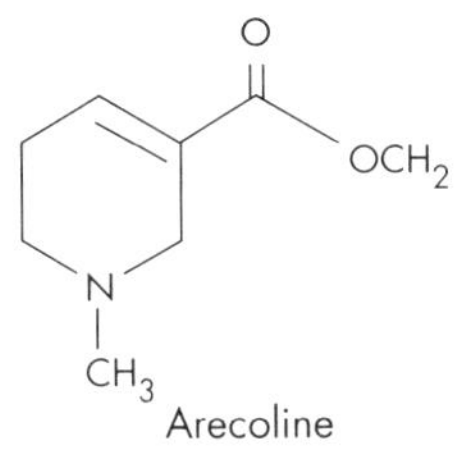

O

OCH_2

N

CH_3

Arecoline

Figure 119.7 Molecular Structure of Arecoline

Bethanechol. Bethanechol is a synthetic β-methyl analogue of ACH. It is a relatively short-acting cholinergic agonist with muscarinic selectivity. The drug does not cross the blood-brain barrier due to its charged quaternary structure, and thus innovative strategies had to be developed to achieve CNS availability. Bethanechol was the first drug to be administered by the intracerebroventricular (ICV) route to AD patients. Bethanechol has not been shown to significantly improve cognitive performance in AD patients.[90,91] ICV administration carries considerable risks related to anesthesia, surgery, infection, and hemorrhage. Complications such as pneumocephalus and seizures[92] and hemiparesis accompanied by dysphasia and chronic subdura hematoma[93] have been reported.

Arecoline. Arecoline (see Fig. 119.7), a natural alkaloid with muscarinic and nicotinic agonistic properties, was one of the first cholinergic agonists to be evaluated in AD. Two studies found no significant effects with intravenously administered arecoline in AD patients.[94,95] More recently arecoline administered as an IV continuous infusion for five days in a placebo controlled trial produced significant improvement on a verbal memory tests.[96] No significant group mean changes could be observed in a related study upon acute arecoline infusion.[96,97]

Oxotremorine. Oxotremorine is a synthetic cholinergic agonist with a half-life of several hours. Orally administered oxotremorine had to be discontinued in most AD patients due to significant side effects, including dysphoria and anxiety. In this study the compound had no beneficial effect on memory.[98]

Nicotine. The infusion of 0.5 ug/kg of nicotine per hour produced significant effects on mood in AD patients. The same dose rarely had such effects in normal non-age-matched control subjects.[99] Intravenous administration of nicotine bitartrate to non-smoking AD patients decreased the rate of intrusion errors.[100] Although higher doses produced anxiety and mood changes, these studies and other animal and human experimental data point to possible involvement of central nicotinic cholinergic neurotransmission in some cognitive processes. Further studies of nicotinic cholinergic mechanisms in AD are warranted, but careful attention must be paid to the toxic nicotinic effects.

New Experimental Agonists

F102B (cis-2-methylspiro-(1,3-oxathiolane-5,3′) quinuclidine) is a novel M1-selective agonist that crosses the blood-brain barrier.[101] In rodents, AF102B ameliorated anticholinergic-induced amnesia in a passive avoidance task. This agent is suggested as a potential candidate for cholinergic enhancement in AD,[102] but there are no clinical data available. An interesting feature of AF102B and the related agents AF150 and AF151, is their selectivity for M1 receptors in specific organs.[103,104]

L-689,660 (see Fig. 119.8), an arecoline derivative, was developed as a potential Alzheimer's disease drug[105] L-689,660 is a less potent muscarinic agonists that some of its analogs but it penetrates freely into the CNS and exhibits functional selectivity. L-689,660 is a potent partial agonist at M1 and M3 receptors and acts as an antagonist at M2 receptors.[106]

BIBN 99 (see Fig. 119.9) is a novel lipophilic compound, which easily crosses into the brain. BIBN 99 is muscarinic receptor blocker with much higher affinities for M2 than for M1. It is speculated that these properties might be beneficial in the treatment of Alzheimer's disease.[107]

PD 142505 and CI-979 are two other novel cholinergic muscarinic agonists thought to have a more advantageous receptor binding profile. In particular PD 142505 appears to have selectively a higher affinity for M1 than M2 receptors. PD 142505 is an agonist a derived from a group of 1-azabicyclo(2.2.1)heptane oximes. In addition it has been suggested that PD 142505 acts as a partial agonist/antagonist at some muscarinic receptor sites.[r14]

The list of new M1 or brain selective muscarinic agonists such as **SR 95639,**[108] **SDZ ENS 163,**[109,110] **WAL 2014**[111] is continuously growing. Some of these agonists are selective M1 partial agonists and M2 partial antagonists. Such compounds might alleviate central cholinergic deficits in AD with less peripheral side effects. However the cholonergic deficit in AD does not affect exclusively the muscarinic innervation. Thus agents stimulating nicotinic receptors as well may deserve consideration.

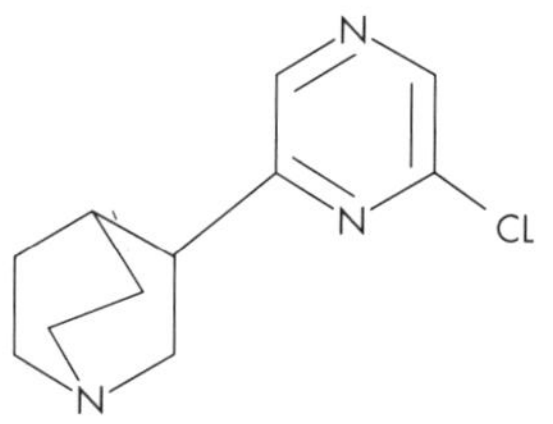

N
N
CL
N
L-689,660

Figure 119.8 Molecular Structure of L-689,660

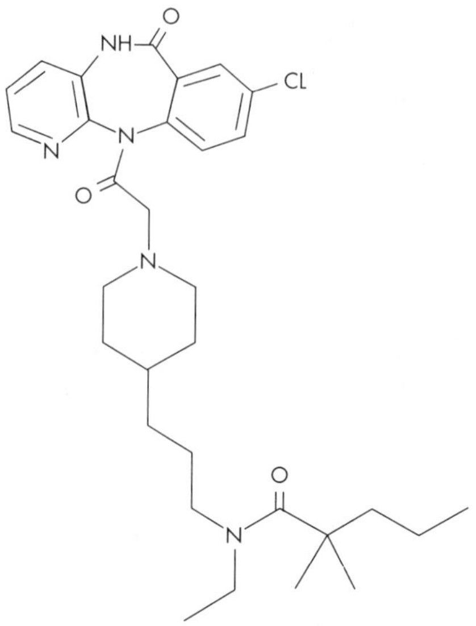

O
NH
CL
N
N
O
N
O
N
BIBN 99

Figure 119.9 Molecular Structure of BIBN99

Other Cholinergic Strategies

Acetylcholine Precursors

An early strategy to enhance central cholinergic transmission was the administration of acetylcholine (ACH) precursors, mainly choline and lecithin, in the hope of increasing ACH synthesis and cholinergic transmission. The rate of ACH release is ultimately dependent on the rate of synthesis of ACH, which, in turn, appears to depend on the rate of choline uptake into the cholinergic neuron by the high-affinity choline uptake system. Under normal conditions, this system is saturated, and an increase in the availability of extracellular choline does not increase synthesis or release of ACH. However, during intense cholinergic activity and greater demand for additional precursor, the increased extracellular concentration of choline might be beneficial. Furthermore, it is possible that choline itself might have cholinomimetic properties. Thus, ACH precursor therapy might slightly improve cognitive performance in AD under normal conditions by increasing the cholinergic tonus, with more significant improvement under conditions of increased cholinergic demand when ordinarily the rate of ACH synthesis would be limited by insufficient extracellular choline.

A review of 17 studies performed between 1977 and 1982 provided little or no evidence for the efficacy of this approach.[r15]

The ability of ACH precursors to delay or prevent cognitive deterioration in AD patients has also been addressed. A 1-year study with lecithin in AD patients found no significant effect;[112] two other long-term studies suggest a beneficial preventive effect.[16,113] Whether this approach provides consistent benefit in preventing or slowing the progression of the disease requires further study. In recent years new ACHE precursors have been assessed in AD.

Phosphatidylserine. Phosphatidylserine (PS) is a natural occurring phospholipid component of the cell membrane. The therapeutic effects of PS in AD have been studied since the mid eighties. Several open studies have demonstrated PS to be the safe and have suggested the compound to have beneficial effects on cognition. More recently several controlled studies with PS have been conducted. Two studies[114,115] suggested that PS in doses of 200 mg po/d and 300 mg po/d respectively is superior to placebo particularly in the more severely affected AD patients. Furthermore treatment with PS in combination with cognitive training was superior to cognitive training alone.[116] Although PS administration over a period of 3–6 months seems to produce small improvements on specific cognitive tests the overall clinical relevance of these effects is questionable.

L-α-Glyceryl-Phosphorylcholine. L-α-Glycerylphosphorylcholine (LAGPC) is a recently developed derivative of lecithin. LAGPC is an acetylcholine precursor believed to have cholinomimetic and cognitive enhancing properties. After administration this compound is converted to phosphorylcholine, the metabolically active form of choline.[117] Intramuscular administration of LAGPC was shown to produce a rise in plasma choline with a peak after 0.25–0.5 hour. LAGPC was shown to be CNS active as its administration increased the growth hormone responses to GHRH in younger and elderly subjects.[118] A larger 6 month long study with LAGPC 800 mg po qid in 65 patients with Alzheimer's disease showed progressive amelioration on MMSE scores and on immediate and delayed recall tests. However the study was neither blind nor placebo controlled.[119]

Cytidine Diphosphate Choline. Cytidine diphosphate choline (CDP-choline) has been assessed for its therapeutic potential in dementia since 1979. Animal experiments have shown CDP-choline to have cholinergic as well as learning and memory enhancing properties. Recent studies confirmed the efficacy of CDP-choline in the scopolamine dementia model in rat.[211] Clinical trials have repeatedly shown positive effects of CDP-choline in demented patients.[120] A recent study in patients with AD suggests that the majority of patients benefitted from a three month course of CDP-choline 1000 mg/po/d.[121]

ACH-Release-Enhancing Agents

The use of acetylcholine releasers is based on their enhancement of stimulus-induced acetylcholine delivery into the synapse. It is hypothesized that such an action could improve the signal to noise ratio during neuronal transmission without the inhibition of cholinergic neurons firing associated with noncompetitive cholinesterase inhibitors or the distorted temporal pattern of neurotransmission observed with cholinergic agonists.

4-Aminopyridine. 4-Aminopyridine (4-AP) acts as a cholinomimetic by increasing the amount of ACh released into the synaptic space with each activation of the synapse. It has been clinically evaluated in patients with disorders of the neuromuscular junction such as myasthenia gravis, Eaton-Lambert syndrome, and botulism. The effects of orally administered 4-AP in AD have been evaluated in two studies. Some improvement in cognitive functions was found in a study with 4-AP in AD patients.[122] In contrast, no significant effect of 4-AP on cognitive performance was found in a more recent study employing a best-dose finding phase in 14 AD patients.[21] The different results in these two studies may relate to differences in the characteristics of the two populations studied (i.e., age, severity of the disease) and length of treatment (6 weeks in the former, 4 days in the latter). Study results suggest that 4-AP may deplete ACH subsequent to an initial phase of increased release, and that in theory combined administration of 4-AP with an ACH precursor might be more efficient.[124]

Linopirdine. Linopirdine or DuP 996, 3,3-bis(4pyridinylmethyl)-1-phenylindolin-2-one, is a novel compound with properties similar to 4-AP. DuP 996 enhances the stimulus-induced release of ACH as well as other neurotransmitters such as dopamine and serotonin. DuP 996 has no affinity for rat brain cholinergic receptors and no inhibitory effect on ACHE. The drug has been found to improve learning performance in various models in mice, rats, and monkeys.[125–127] DuP 996 enhances potassium stimulated release of acetylcholine, dopamine, and serotonin without affecting basal neurotransmitter release.[127] The drug also seems to enhances ACH synthesis to replenish neurotransmitter storages.[128] Autoradiographic studies demonstrating linopirdine binding sites in the cortex and hippocampus support the potential usefulness of this agent for the treatment of cognitive deficits in Alzheimer's disease.[129] DuP 996 has been shown to protect against hypoxia-induced passive avoidance deficits in rodents.[126] In man, DuP 996 administration induces electroencephalographic changes consistent with vigilance-improving properties.[130]

HP 749. HP 749 (*N*-(*n*-Propyl)-*N*-(4-pyridinyl)-1H-indol-l-amine) is an indole-substituted analogue of 4-aminopyridine which is well absorbed after oral administration.[131] Preclinical studies demonstrate that HP 749 reverses the passive avoidance deficit produced by nucleus basalis lesions in rodents.[132] Data from clinical trials is pending.

Non-Cholinergic Neurotransmitter Replacement Strategies

In addition to the cholinergic deficit, AD has also been shown to be characterized by marked deficits in the monoamine neurotransmitters norepinephrine and serotonin, as well as in glutamate and some neneuropeptide neurotransmitter.

Monoaminergic Drugs

Neurochemical studies on brain specimens from AD patients have found subpopulations with significantly decreased levels of noradrenaline and dopamine-β-hydroxylase (the noradrenaline-synthesizing enzyme). These findings match the histopathological observation of profound neuronal loss in the locus coeruleus, from which most of the noradrenergic projections to the cerebral cortex and the hippocampus originate.[133,134] Serotonergic neurotransmission markers have been found to be decreased in AD. Abnormal cellular activity and cell loss in the dorsal raphe nuclei, the major source of cerebral serotonergic innervation, and diminished uptake and serotonin binding sites are associated with AD.[135–137] Although there is no consensus, decreased dopamine levels and decreased D2 receptors in AD have been found.[138,139] Taken together, these findings provide consistent evidence for the occurrence of monoaminergic transmitter deficits in AD and have stimulated treatment strategies aimed at enhancing monoaminergic neurotransmission.

L-deprenyl (or phenylisopropylmethylpropynylamine) first synthesized in 1972, is an MAO-B inhibitor with good brain permeability, predominantly used in the treatment of PD.[r18,r19] L-Deprenyl, has been evaluated in several studies with AD patients. Double blind, placebo controlled trials with small patient samples suggest that subchronic treatment with l-deprenyl at 10mg/day improves performance on attention, memory, and learning tasks.[140–145] Higher doses of l-deprenyl were not as efficacious and were associated with more side effects.[140] The beneficial effects of l-deprenyl do not appear to be due to its antidepressant action since the MAO-A inhibitor tranylcypromine did not improve cognitive performance and produced significant side effects.[146] Results from a large multi center study in the US are currently pending.

Clonidine and **guanfacine** are two alpha$_2$-adrenoreceptor agonists which have been shown to improve memory in aged monkeys.[147] Clonidine also had some beneficial effects on cognitive functions in patients with Korsakoff's syndrome[148] and in patients with schizophrenia.[149] A recent study assessed the therapeutic potential of clonidine, a centrally active alpha$_2$-adrenoreceptor agonist, in AD. In a double-blind, placebo-controlled trial, eight AD patients received clonidine 0.1–0.4 mg per day and one patient received up to 1.2 mg per day orally. This study found no beneficial effect of acute clonidine administration on cognition in AD.[150]

Guanfacine is another centrally active alpha$_2$-adrenoreceptor agonist that has been assessed in AD. After an initial open-drug titration and best-dose finding phase, five AD patients and five age-matched normal control subjects entered the next phase of the study.[151] During this second phase, all participants received the optimal or maximal tolerated dose in a double-blind, placebo-controlled, crossover design. Neuropsychological tests did not identify a best dose, and the highest tolerated dose of guanfacine (mean 0.7 mg, range 0.5–1.0 mg orally) did not produce any significant effect on cognitive functions, except a small but statistically significant improvement in mood. In a recent double blind placebo controlled study,[152] 15 AD patients received guanfacine .5 mg. po/d while 14 patients received placebo. Guanfacine produced no significant improvement.

These negative studies do not imply that adrenergic enhancement is ineffective in AD, or that it might not be a useful complement to a cholinergic therapy. It is possible that agonists have a significant activity at presynaptic receptors and inhibit transmitter release to an extent that yields a net diminution in noradrenergic activity. Therefore, an alternative strategy could employ an alpha$_2$-adrenoreceptor antagonist, selectively active at the presynaptic receptor, which would interrupt the feedback inhibition path and could lead to increased noradrenaline release. Both agonists and antagonists require further investigation.

Levodopa (L-DOPA) has been reported to improve cognitive function in normal subjects[153] and in PD patients. One placebo-controlled, double-blind study with oral administrations of 200 mg qd of levodopa combined with 50 mg qd of benserazide, a peripherally active carboxylase inhibitor, over 24 weeks in 14 patients with senile dementia showed some improvement on cognitive tests.[154] The participants in this study were relatively young (age range 54–60 years), and the diagnostic criteria were not defined. On the other hand, two placebo-controlled studies of the effects of L-dopa on cognition in patients with presenile dementia[155] and senile dementia of the Alzheimer type[r20] failed to show a significant beneficial effect. Overall, there is little evidence that L-dopa given alone improves cognition in AD.

Alaproclate is a selective serotonin reuptake blocker. Two studies have evaluated the efficacy of alaproclate in AD.[156,157] In the initial open pilot study, five of nine patients showed some mood-related improvements. A subsequent study evaluated 20 AD patients and 20 with multi-infarct dementia in a double-blind, placebo-controlled trial. During the 4-week active drug phase, the patients received 200 mg of alaproclate po bid. Side effects observed during alaproclate administration included drowsiness, sleep disturbances, motor restlessness, and increased appetite. Five patients deteriorated significantly during the active drug phase. After a dose reduction from 400 mg to 200 mg per day, the adverse effects in these patients disappeared almost completely. Because some of the side effects reported with alaproclate resemble cholinergic effects, possible cholinomimetic properties of this agent should be considered. No clinically significant effect was observed in this study.

Zimeldine, like alaproclate, is a selective serotonin reuptake blocker. A double-blind, crossover, placebo-controlled trial evaluated the cognitive and biochemical effects of zimeldine in four AD patients.[158] The drug significantly altered central and peripheral serotonin metabolism but had no effects on memory and reaction time.

Citalopram is another selective 5-HT reuptake blocker which was assessed in AD.[159] In this study with 10 AD patients citalopram produced no significant cognitive improvement.

Monotherapy with serotonin reuptake blockers seems to have no effect on cognitive functions in AD. These results do not exclude the possibility that serotonergic enhancement by other means or in combination with concomitant cholinergic augmentation might be beneficial in these patients.

Cholinergic-Monoaminergic Drug Combinations

So far therapeutic trials with cholinergic or monoaminergic agents alone have not led to a breakthrough in the treatment of AD. This raises the question of the limits of a single neurotransmitter-replacement strategy. A partial answer has been provided by experiments demonstrating that noradrenergic brain lesions added to NBM-lesioned animals block cholinomimetic enhancement of memory, and that the efficacy of cholinomimetic treatment can be restored by administration of clonidine.[r14,85] Similarly the combined administration of clonidine and physostigmine was found to enhance memory performance in primates beyond the improvement observed after the administration of either drug alone. Interestingly the monkeys tolerated higher doses of physostigmine in the combination regimen than when physostigmine was given alone.[160] Taken together these data suggest that simultaneous enhancement of the cholinergic and noradrenergic systems is feasible, may be necessary, and could render results superior to any of the isolated neurotransmitter systems enhancement approaches.

A pilot study of **clonidine** combined with physostigmine in nine AD patients confirmed the safety of this combination.[68] However, a recently published study showed that the combination of physostigmine with **yohimbine** may have marked cardiovascular side effects in AD.[162]

L-deprenyl in combination with ACHE inhibitors has been evaluated in several studies. Two double-blind placebo-controlled studies suggested that l-deprenyl combined with either THA or physostigmine may improve cognitive functions.[163] However, another double blind placebo controlled study found no significant improvement with the combination of physostigmine and deprenyl.[164] However in the later study the unreliable absorption of oral physostigmine made the interpretation of the results problematic.

Future studies are needed to determine the potential efficacy of combination treatments. The l-deprenyl results need to be replicated with larger patient samples and longer treatment trials to determine if this agent alone or in combination with other agents have clinically significant effects on cognition in patients with Alzheimer's disease.

Neuropeptides

The physiological endocrine effects of the pituitary peptides adrenocorticotropic hormone (ACTH) and vasopressin (VP) were well known long before their occurrence in the brain was recognized. Over the last 20 years, animal experiments have generated convicing evidence for a psychotropic effect of many neuropeptides and the involvement of at least two of them (ACTH and VP) in learning and memory.[165] Studies in animals with the ACTH and VP analogues $ACTH_{4-10}$, $ACTH_{4-9}$ (Org 2766), arginine VP, 1-desamino-8-D-arginine VP, and des-9-glycinamide-arginine VP (Org 5667) as well as studies in normal volunteers and various patient groups have reported positive effects on attention. In analyzing the clinical studies with ACTH and VP analogues in AD, several recent reviews[r21–r23] as well as a one recent high dose trial[166] concluded that there is no evidence for a beneficial effect of these peptides on cognition in this patient population. Another ACTH analog HOE 427 (ebiratide) showed poor results in patients with AD.[167]

Although the neuropeptides somatostatin and cholecystokinin have been implicated in the pathology of AD, clinical studies aimed at replacing these neurotransmitters have not yet been performed. One trial with the somatostatin analogue L363,586, MSD in 10 AD patients failed to demonstrate any significant effects, and the drug could not be detected in the CSF.[168] In a subsequent trial in 14 AD patients the somatostatin analog octreotide (also called Sandostatin or SMS 201-995) appeared to have CNS effects but failed to improve cognitive functions.[169]

Preclinical studies with the CCK8 analogue SUT-8701 seem promising. The drug has been shown to have neuroprotective effects and to enhance learning in aged as well as in NBM-lesioned rats.[r24]

Drugs Affecting Glutamate Receptor Sites

An alternative approach in the pharmacotherapy of AD evolved from research in central glutamatergic neurotransmission. Experimental data indicate that excitatory amino acid (EAA)-mediated toxicity can produce lesions similar to the neurofibrillary tangles of AD. Furthermore the glutamatergic system has been implicated in learning and memory. NMDA receptor blockade disrupts spatial learning and prevents long-term potentiation, which is considered a physiological model for memory.[r3,170,171] *N*-methyl-D-aspartic acid (NMDA) receptor blockers have been shown to provide significant protection against ischemic and EAA-mediated cortical insults.[172,173] It appears that the blockade of certain glutamate receptor subtypes may be protective against the putative EAA-excitotoxicity while activation of other subtypes may enhance cognitive functions in AD.

Milacemide, a glycine prodrug, enhances learning in normal and amnestic rodents.[174] Glycine has a synergistic effects on the activation of the NMDA receptor by glutamate resulting in increased long term potentiation [LTP]. LTP in turn is believed to enhance learning and memory. Milacemide has been shown to enhance performance on certain neuropsychological tests in young healthy volunteers. However in two large double-blind placebo-controlled trials in AD milacemide was not found to enhance cognition and was accompanied by significant liver toxicity.[175,176]

D-cycloserine, a partial agonist has also been shown to enhance learning in rodents. In human volunteers D-cycloserine, was shown to ameliorate scopolamine induced cognitive impairment.[177] However preliminary reports suggest that little benefit was achieved by AD patients treated with D-cycloserine for 26 weeks.[178]

Glutamatergic modulating agents require further studies to explore their therapeutic potential. The pharmacology of the EAA is a rapidly developing field. New NMDA-receptor blockers as well as possible EAA-receptor subtype-specific partial agonists may open new avenues in the treatment of AD.

Other Non-neurotransmitter-Specific Approaches

Nootropics: Piracetam and Derivatives. The term nootropics was first introduced in 1972, to describe a novel class of drugs.[r26] This new class has been characterized mostly after the properties of piracetam, the prototype and so far the most studied representative, of the nootropics. The effects of piracetam have been repeatedly reviewed,[r20,r27,179] improvement in behavior, mood and some neuropsychological tests have been reported, but up to date there is no consistent evidence for a beneficial effect of this drug on cognitive functions in AD. A recent study with this agent suggested that long-term administration of high doses of piracetam might slow the rate of cognitive deterioration in patients with AD.[180] The most significant differences concerned the recall of pictures series and recent incident and remote memory. The drug was well-tolerated. Studies on the efficacy of piracetam combined with cholinergic precursors lecithin or choline showed no significant effects on cognition in AD, as well.[r28,161,181–184]

Other piracetam-like compounds have also been evaluated in clinical studies. Studies with **pramiracetam**[179,185] and **oxiracetam**[186] were not successful in reducing cognitive impairment due to Alzheimer's disease. Data on **aniracetam** (Ro 13-3057) in AD is inconclusive. While a preliminary report from Japan seemed favorable,[187] a subsequent study failed to show aniracetam to be superior to placebo.[188] Most recently a controlled multicentre clinical study showed aniracetam to be superior to placebo.[189]

Acetyl-l-Carnitine. Acetyl-l-Carnitine (ALC), the acetyl ester of carnitine is a naturally occurring substance involved in mitochondrial energy processing. ALC is thought to have therapeutic potential in AD due to its antioxidant neuroprotective properties, and its putative ability to enhance cellular energy supply, membrane stability and cholinergic neurotransmission. Several double blind placebo controlled studies conducted in Italy, Great Britain and the US suggest that ALC 2-3 gr po/d administered for 6–12 months may improve cognitive performance and slow down the rate of progression in patients with Alzheimer's disease.[190,191] However rigorous multi center trials are necessary to prove ALC's effects conclusively.

Antioxidants. Several studies have demonstrated increased free radical production in aging in general and in Alzheimer's disease in particular. Increased superoxide dismutase derived hydrogen peroxide fluxes, metal ions, and damaged mitochondria can contribute to cell damage mediated by free radicals.[r29] Free radical production in Alzheimer's disease may also be caused by amyloid beta protein and glutamate.[192] These findings suggest that antioxidants could have beneficial effects in AD by interfering with free radical production and preventing consequent cell injury. **L-deprenyl** is thought to possess antioxidant properties, and is believed to have neuroprotective effects in AD as well as in Parkinson's disease by acting as scavenger of free radicals.[r18] **Vitamin E** and **idebenone** are also potential antioxidant treatments for Alzheimer's disease since they prevent cell death caused by glutamate and amyloid beta protein.[192–194] Clinical trials with l-deprenyl and vitamin E are currently evaluating their ability to slow the progression of Alzhemier's disease.

Desferrioxamine, a Chelating Agent. Several findings suggest an association between aluminum and Alzheimer's disease. Epidemiological studies have reported an association between the aluminum concentration in drinking water and the occurrence of Alzheimer's disease.[195,196] In addition, aluminum administration has been shown to be neurotoxic to the cholinergic system.[197,198] These findings have led clinical trials with desferrioxamine mesylate in Alzheimer's disease which has a particularly high affinity for aluminum and has been used to treat iron and aluminum overload.[199,200] In a two year long double blind controlled trial desferrioxamine i.m. was compared to placebo or no.[201] Patients who received desferrioxamine treatment showed less decline in daily living skills when compared to the placebo group. The therapeutic effects observed with this agent may not necessarily be due to its chelating action since it has been shown to inhibit free radical formation and inflammation as well.[201] The required intramuscular administration and toxic side effects of this compound however might limit its clinical utility. Replication studies are necessary to confirm the efficacy of this approach.

New Leads and Future Options

Nerve Growth Factor. Another conceivable therapeutic approach for AD could be based on the administration of neurotrophic factors. Nerve growth factor (NGF) is a 118 amino acid polypeptide with no blood-brain barrier penetrance. Other substances with neurotrophic activity such as epidermal growth factor, brain-derived neurotrophic factor, gangliosides and the β1-28 peptide of the β-amyloid protein[201a] might also have a therapeutic potential. Intracerebroventricular (ICV) administration of nerve growth factor (NGF) has been shown to partially reverse lesion induced deficits of cortical ACHE and CHAT activities[85] to promote survival of septal cholinergic neurons after fimbrial transection in adult rats[202] and to reverse behavioral deterioration in rats with such lesions.[203] More recently human NGF (hNGF) has been produced by recombinant techniques[204] and sufficient amounts of pure hNGF are now available for therapeutic trials in AD. In addition genetically modified, NGF secreting fibroblasts grafts have been shown to prevent degeneration of cholinergic neurons after surgical lesions of the fimbria-fornix in rats.[205] This opens the possibility of infusing or grafting genetically engineered designer cell which would secret in situ the neurotransmitter[206] or factor required.[r30] Alternatively new pharmacological strategies such as the synthesis of liposomes, drug lipidization, development of lipid-soluble pro-drugs and chimeric nutrients or peptides, which might provide ways for improved non-invasive drug delivery to the CNS.[r31,r32] Recently NGF conjugated to an antibody to the transferrin receptor was shown to cross the blood-brain barrier after peripheral injection. In this experiment NGF increased the survival of cholinergic and noncholinergic neurons.[207]

Antinflammatory Agents. The involvement of the immune system and inflammation in the pathophysiology of AD has been suggested by several findings such as the presence of inflammation markers in the brain Alzheimer's patients and the co-localization of some acute phase and complement proteins in senile plaques. Furthermore increased numbers of reactive gila and microglia (believed to be related to macrophages) have been observed.[208] Activated T lymphocytes, a hallmark of the cell mediated response observed in chronic inflammatory states, have also been observed in postmortem studies of Alzheimer's disease cases.[209] The use of antiflammatory agents in the treatment of Alzheimer's disease is further supported by the low prevalence of AD found in patients with rheumatoid arthritis elderly leprosy patients.[210] These findings could potentially be explained by the long-standing exposure of these patients to chronic anti-inflammatory therapy. Furthermore preliminary observations suggest that steroids and NSAIDs such as indomethacin and aspirin may have protective effects against AD.[211] In a recent 6 month long double-blind placebo-controlled study in AD indomethacin 100–150 mg/po/d was found to improve cognitive function and potentially delay further deterioration. These results are promising, however indomethacin's toxicity might limit its use.[212]

Corticosteroids offer a logical anti-inflammatory therapy for Alzheimer's disease since these agents are widely used and efficacious for several inflammatory diseases in the CNS, including lupus cerebritis and multiple sclerosis. Unfortunately, the systemic toxicity of steroids limit the use of high doses or long term treatments with these agents. Animal studies suggest that prolonged exposure to high doses of glucocorticoids is toxic to hippocampal neurons.[213,214] Low dose steroid therapy, may be the safest strategy since this dose is well tolerated and effective in patients with rheumatoid arthritis.

Colchicine is another possible candidate for the treatment of Alzheimer's disease. This drug effectively treats familial Mediterranean fever, a condition in which recurrent inflammation and renal amyloidosis occur. Although the amyloid constituents in familial Mediterranean fever and Alzheimer's disease differ, both illnesses involve chronic inflammation, elevated acute phase proteins, and abnormal processing of a precursor protein leading to deposition of insoluble amyloid fragments. These similarities suggest the potential therapeutic efficacy of colchicine for patients with Alzheimer's disease.

Hydroxychloroquine is historically an antimalarial agent that has been adopted as a safe and effective second line agent for the treatment of rheumatoid arthritis and lupus erythematosus.[215] The efficacy of hydroxychloroquine is thought to be related to its effects on the immune response and lysosomal functioning. This agent suppresses cytokine and acute phase reactant levels in these illnesses.[216,217] Hydroxychloroquine also interferes with lysosomal enzymatic activity by increasing the pH in these organelles[r33] and by stabilizing lysosomal membranes. Hydroxychloroquine's safe clinical profile as a chronic treatment for rheumatoid arthritis support it as a possible candidate for the treatment of Alzheimer's disease.

Anti-amyloidogenesis Agents. Alzheimer's disease is characterized by neurofibrillary tangles and plaques, consisting primarily of extracellular deposits of β-amyloid protein (BAP). Plaque formation may be toxic and cause cell death and neurofibrillary tangle formation.[218] BAP is derived the product of transmembranal processing of the amyloid precursor protein (APP).[219–221] Normally APP processing does not result in BAP secretion precluding amyloidogenesis.[222,223] Aberrant lysosomal processing of APP may generate amyloidogenic fragments.[222,224,228] Thus agents that interfere with BAP's production and toxicity may therapeutic represent an alternative strategy to alter the course of Alzheimer's disease.

The effects of colchicine and hydroxychloroquine on lysosomal processing suggest that these agents could have beneficial effects in DA by intefering with amyloidogenesis. Although colchicine is used as a neurotoxin in laboratory studies, no significant CNS toxicity has been reported with clinical use of this agent.

Recent data suggest that cholinergic receptors may control intracellular β-amyloid precursor protein (BAPP) concentrations as well as BAPP processing in some neurons. Cholinergic agonists were shown to control the processing of the amyloid precursor protein by increasing the secretory cleavage pathway of the protein. Furthermore M1 and M3 receptor stimulation with carbachol has been shown to increase the rate of BAPP secretion in transfected human embryonic kidney (293) cell lines. This increase is probably mediated by the activation of protein kinases.[226,227] Thus manipulations at the cholinergic receptor site may have other therapeutic effects in Alzheimer's disease besides augmenting cholinergic neurotransmission. These data suggest that cholinergic receptors may control intracellular amyloid precursor protein processing and secretion and therefore may possibly affect extracellular senile plaque formation.

Apolipoprotein E and the Risk for Alzheimer's. Most recent studies have identified a 3 fold higher prevalence of the apolipoprotein E4 allele in patients with late-onset familial Alzheimer disease than in controls. Apolipoprotein E (APOE) has been shown to be present in senile plaques, vascular amyloid, and neurofibrillary tangles of Alzheimer disease. Based on experimental data it has been suggested that pathogenetically it is not the presence of APOE4 allele per se that enhances the morbidity risk but rather it is the absence of APOE2 or APOE3 that increases the risk. This hypothesis is based on the findings that APOE4 lacks the microtubules protective properties of APOE2 or APOE3. Thus it is thought that the absence of the alleles APOE3 or APOE2 renders the organism vulnerable to microtubule degeneration and leads to the increased risk for AD.[228] This hypothesis suggests that new pharmacological strategies in AD could consist of agents with APOE3 or APOE2-like microtubule-stabilizing properties or of compounds with the APOE gene expression altering effects.

Conclusions

A multitude of diverse pharmacological strategies have failed in Alzheimer's disease so far. However in 1993 the acetylcholinesterase inhibitor tacrine, was the first drug to be approved by the FDA for the treatment of Alzheimer's disease. Further research with this class of compounds is expected to lead to the development of agents with wider therapeutic windows, more efficacy and less side effects. Pharmacological strategies aimed at enhancing multiple neurotransmitter systems might prove superior to the effects of isolated cholinomimetic augmentation. Newer strategies are based on a increasingly more accurate understanding of the pathophysiologic processes involved in this illness. Strategies aimed at slowing or arresting the progression of the illness are currently being explored and will undoubtedly lead to therapeutic breakthroughs in the near future.

References

Research Reports

1. Alzheimer A. Ueber einen eigenartigen schweren Krankheitsprozess der Hirnrinde. Allg Z Psychiatr 1906;*64*:146–151.
2. Dundee JW, Pandit SK. Anterograde amnesic effects of pethidine, hyoscine, and diazepam in adults. Br J Pharmaco 1972;*44*:140–144.
3. Panditt SK, Dundee JW. Preoperative amnesia: the incidence following the intramuscular injection of commonly used premedicants. Anesthesia 1970;*25*:493–499.
4. Deutsch JA. The cholinergic synapse and the site of memory. Science 1971;*174*:788–794.
5. Meyers B, Roberts DH, Riciputi RH, Domino EF. Some effects of muscarinic cholinergic blocking drugs on behavior and the electrocorticogram. Psychopharmacology 1964;*5*:289–300.
6. Davies P, Maloney AJ. Selective loss of central cholinergic neurons in Alzheimer's disease. Lancet 1976;*2*:1403–1440.
7. Perry EK, Perry RH, Blessed G, Tomlinson BE. Necropsy evidence of central cholinergic deficits in senile dementia. Lancet 1977;*1*:189.
8. Perry EK, Tomlinson BE, Blessed G, Bergman K, Bigson PH, Perry RH. Correlation of cholinergic abnormalities with senile plaques and mental test scores in senile dementia. Brit Med J 1978;*2*:1457–1459.
9. Whitehouse PJ, Price DL, Struble RG, Clark AW, Coyle JT, Delong MR. Alzheimer's disease and senile dementia: loss of neurons in the basal forebrain. Science 1982;*215*:1237–1239.
10. Summers WK, Viesselman JO, Marsh GM, Candelora K. Use of THA in treatment of Alzheimer-like dementia: pilot study in twelve patients. Biol Psychiatry 1981;*16*:145–153.
11. Peterson C. Changes in calcium's role as a messenger during aging in neuronal and nonneuronal cells. Ann N Y Acad Sci. 1992. Nov 21,*663*:279–293.
12. Mena EE, Desai MC. High affinity [3H]THA (tetrahydroaminoacridine) binding sites in rat brain. Pharmacology Res 1991;*8*:200–203.
13. Drukarch B, Leysen JE, Stoof JC. Further analysis of the neuropharmacological profile of 9-amino-1,2,3,4-tetrahydroacridine (THA), an alleged drug for the treatment of Alzheimer's disease. Life Sciences 1988;*42*:1011–1017.
14. Drukarch B, Kits S, Van der Meer EG, Lodder JC, Stoff JC. 9-amino-1,2,3,4-tetrahydroacridine (THA), an alleged drug for the treatment of Alzheimer's disease, inhibits acetylcholinesterase activity and slow outward K+ current. E J Pharmacology 1987;*141*:153–157.
15. Nordberg A, Nilsson Hakansson L, Adem A, Lai Z, Winblad B. Multiple actions of THA on cholinergic neurotransmi in Alzheimer brains. Progress in Clinical Biology and Research 1989;*317*:1169–1178.
16. Ahlin A, Adem A, Junthe T, Ohman G, Nyback H. Pharmacokinetics of tetrahydroaminoacridine: relations to clinical and biochemical effects in Alzheimer patients. Int Clin Psychopharmacol 1992;*7*:29–36.
17. Hartvig P, Askmark H, Aquilonius SM, Wiklund L, Lindstrom B. Clinical pharmacokinetics of intravenous and oral 9 amino 1,2,3,4 tetrahydroacridine, tacrine. Eur J Clin Pharmacol 1990;*38*:259–263.
18. Cutler NR, Murphy MF, Nash RJ, Prior PL, DeLuna DM. Clinical safety, tolerance and plasma levels of the oral anticholinesterase 1,2,3,4-tetrahydro-9-aminoacradin-1-olmaleate (HP 029) in Alzheimer's disease: Preliminary findings. J Clin Pharmacol 1990; 556–561.
19. Albin MS, Orr MD, Bunegin L, Henderson PA. Tetrahydroaminoacridine antagonism to narcotic addiction. Experiment Neurology 1975;*46*:644–648.
20. Albin MS, Bunegin L, Massopust LC, Janetta PJ. Ketamine induced postanesthetic deliruium attenuated by tetrahydroaminoacridine. 1974.
21. Fredj G, Dietlin F, Fredj D, Schwarzenberg L, Jasmin C, Meyer P, Misset JL. Tetrahydroaminoacridine in HIV infections. The THA Study Group. Int J Clin Pharmacol Ther Toxicol 1989;*27*:408–410.
22. Askmark H, Aquilonius SM, Gillberg PG, Hartvig P, Hilton Brown P, Lindstrom B, Nilsson D, Stalberg E, Winkler T. Functional and pharmacokinetic studies of tetrahydroaminoacridine in patients with amyotrophic lateral sclerosis. Acta Neurol Scand 1990;*82*:253–258.
23. Kaye WH. Modest facilitation of memory in dementia with combined lecithin and anticholinesterase treatment. Biol Psychiatry 1982;*17*:275–280.
24. Gauthier S, Bouchard R, Lamontagne A, Bailey P, Bergman H, Ratner J, Tesfaye Y, Saint-Martin M, Bacher Y, Carr L, Charbonneau R, Clarfield M, Collier B, Dastoor D, Gauthier L, Germain M, Kissel C, Krieger M, Kushnir S, Masson H, Morin J, Nair V, Neirinch L, Suissa S. Tetrahydroaminoacridine-lecithin com-

bination treatment in patients with intermediate-stage Alzheimer's disease. N Eng J Med 1990;1272–1276.

25. Chatellier G and Lacomblez L. Tacrine (tetrahydroaminoacridin;THA) and lecithin in senile dementia of the Alzheimer's type: A multi-center trial. Br Med J 1990;495–499.

26. Eagger SA, Levy R, Sahakian BJ. Tacrine in Alzheimer's disease. Lancet 1991;*337*:989–992.

27. Farlow M, Gracon SI, Hershey LA, Lewis KW, Sadowsky CH, Dolan-Ureno J. A controlled trial of tacrine in Alzheimer's disease. JAMA 1992; 2523–2529.

28. Davis KL, Thal LJ, Gamzu ER, Davis CS, Woolson RF, Gracon SI, Drachman DA, Schneider LS, Whitehouse PJ, H TM, et al. A double blind, placebo controlled multicenter study of tacrine for Alzheimer's disease. The Tacrine Collaborative Study Group. N Engl J Med 1992;*327*(18):1253–1259.

29. Wilcock GK, Surnom DJ, Scott M, Boyle M, Mulligan K, Neubauer KA, O'Neil D, Royston VH. An evaluation of the efficacy and safety of tetrahydroaminoacridine (THA) without lecithin in the treatment of Alzheimer's disease. Age and Ageing 1993;*22*:316–324.

30. Knapp MJ, Knopman DS, Solomon PR, Pendlebury WW, Davis CS, Gracon SI, for the tacrine study group. A 30 week randomized controlled trial of high dose tacrine in patients with Alzheimer's disease. JAMA 1994;*271*:985–991.

31. Maltby N, Broe AG, Creasey H, Jorm AF, Christensen H, Brooks WS. Efficacy of tacrine and lecithin in mild to mo Alzheimer's disease: double blind trial. British Medical Journal 1994;*308*:879–883.

32. Watkins PB, Zimmerman HJ, Knapp MJ, Gracon SI, Lewis KW. Hepatotoxic effects of tacrine administration in patients with Alzheimer's disease. JAMA. 1994;*271*:992–998.

33. Shutske GM, Pierrat FA, Cornfeldt ML, Szewczak MR, Huger FP, Fores GM, Haratounian V, Davis KL. (±)-9-am 1,2,3,4,-tetrahydroacridin-1-ol. A potential Alzheimer's disease therapeutic of low toxicity. J Med Chem 1988;*31*:1278–1279.

34. Tanaka Y, Sakurai M, Hayashi S. Effect of scopolamine and HP 029, a cholinesterase inhibitor, on long term potential in hippocampal slices of the guinea pig. Neuroscience Letters 1989;*98*:179–183.

35. Puri K, Hsu RS, Ho I, Lassman HB. Single dose safety, tolerance, and pharmacokinetics of HP 029 in healthy young men Apotentia; Alzheimer agent. J Clin Pharmacology 1989;*29*:278–284.

36. Fielding S, Cornfeldt ML, Szewczak MR, Ellis DB, Huger FP, Wilker JC, Shutske GM. HP-029, a new drug for the treatment of Alzheimer's disease: its pharmacological profile. Presented at IV. World conference on clinical pharmacol and therapeutics, Berlin (West), July 28–30, 1989.

37. Cutler NR, Sramek JJ, Murphy MF, Nash RJ. Alzheimer's patients should be included in phase I clinical trials to eval compounds for Alzheimer's disease. J Geriatr Psychiatry Neurol 1992 Oct;*5*:192–194.

38. Cutler NR, Sramek JJ, Murphy MF, Nash RJ. Implications of the study population in the early evaluation of anticholinesterase inhibitors for Alzheimer's disease. Ann Pharmacother 1992;*26*:1118–1122.

39. Turcan RG, Hillbeck D, Hartley TE, Gilbert PJ, Coe RA, Troke JA, Vose CW. Disposition of [14C]velnacrine maleate in rats, dogs, and humans. Drug Metab Dispos Biol Fate Chem 1993 Nov; *21*:1037–1047.

40. Cutler NR, Sedman AJ, Prior P, Underwood BA, Selen A, Balogh L, Kinkel AW, Gracon SI, Gamzu ER. Steady state pharmacokinetics of tacrine in patients with Alzheimer's disease. Psychopharmacol Bull 1990;*26*:231–234.

41. Murphy MF, Hardiman ST, Nash RJ, Huff FJ, Demkovich JJ, Dobson C, Knappe UE. Evaluation of HP 029 (velnacrine maleate) in Alzheimer's disease. Ann N Y Acad Sci 1991;*640*:253–262.

42. Shutske GM, Pierrat FA, Kapples KJ, Cornfeldt ML, Szewczak MR, Huger FP, Fores GM, Haroutunian V, Davis KL. 9-Amino-1,2,3,4-tetrahydroacridin-1-ols: synthesis and evaluation as potential Alzheimer's disease therapeutics. J Med Chem 1989;*32*:1805–1813.

43. Braga MF, Harvey AL, Rowan EG. Effects of tacrine, velnacrine (HP029), suronacrine (HP128), and 3,4 diaminopyridon on skeletal neuromuscular transmission in vitro. Br J Pharmacol 1991;*102*:909–915.

44. Huff FJ, Antuono P, Murphy M, Beyer J, Dobson C. Potential clinical use of an adrenergic/cholinergic agent (HP 128) in the treatment of Alzheimer's disease. Ann N Y Acad Sci 1991;*640*:263–267.

45. Svejdova M, Rektor I, Silva Barrat C, Menini C. Unexpected potentializing effect of a tacrine derivative (9-amino-7-methoxy-1,2,3,4 tetrahydroacridine) upon the non-epileptic myoclonus in baboons Papio papio. Prog Neuropsychopharmacol Biol Psychiatry 1990;*14*:961–966.

46. Tucek S, Dolezal V. Negative effects of tacrine (tetrahydroaminoacridine) and methoxytacrine on the metabolism of acetylcholine in brain slices incubated under conditions stimulating neurotransmitter release. J Neurochem 1991;*56*:1216–1221.

47. Dolezal V, Tucek S. Positive and negative effects of tacrine (tetrahydroaminoacridine) and methoxytacrine on the metabolism of acetylcholine in brain cortical prisms incubated under "resting" conditions. J Neurochem 1991;*56*:1207–1215.

48. Musilkova J, Tucek S. The binding of cholinesterase inhibitors tacrine (tetrahydroaminoacridine) and 7-methoxytacrine to muscarinic acetylcholine receptors in rat brain in the presence of eserine. Neurosci Lett 1991;*125*:113–116.

49. Filip V, Vachek J, Albrecht V, Dvorak I, Dvorakova J, Fusek J, Havluj J. Pharmacokinetics and tolerance of 7-methoxytacrine following the single dose administration in healthy volunteers. Int J Clin Pharmacol Ther Toxicol 1991;*29*:431–436.

50. Natori K, Okazaki Y, Irie T, Katsube J. Pharmacological and biochemical assessment of SM-10888, a novel cholineste inhibitor. Jpn J Pharmacol 1990;*53*:145–155.

51. Okazaki Y, Natori K, Irie T, Katsube J. Effect of a novel CNS-selective cholinesterase inhibitor, SM-10888, on habitual and passive avoidance response in mice. Jpn J Pharmacol 1990;*53*:211–220.

52. Baveja SK, Singh S. Thin layer chromatographic examination of the degradation of centbucridine in aqueous solutions. J Chromatogr. 1987;*396*:337–44.

53. Sevush S, Guterman A, Villalon AV. Improved verbal learning after outpatient oral physostigmine therapy in patients with dementia of the Alzheimer type. J Clin Psychiatry 1991;*52*:300–303.

54. Sano M, Bell K, Marder K, Stricks L, Stern Y, Mayeux R. Safety and efficacy of oral physostigmine in the treatment of Alzheimer disease. Clin Neuropharmacol. 1993;*16*(1):61–69.

55. Becker R, Giacobini E, Elble R, McIlhani M, Sherman K. Potential pharmacotherapy of Alzheimer's disease. A comparison of various routes of administration. Acta Neurol Scand Suppl 1988;*116*:19–32.

56. Beller SA, Overall JE, Rhoades HM, Swann AC. Long term outpatient treatment of senile dementia with oral physostigmine. J Clin Psychiatry 1988;*49*:400–404.

57. Jenike MA, Albert MS, Baer L. Oral physostigmine as treatment for Alzheimer disease: A long-term outpatient trial. Alzheimer Dis Assoc Disord 1990;*4*:226–231.

58. Brufani M, Marta M, Pomponi M. Anticholinesterase activity of a new carbamate, heptylphysostigmine, in view of its use in patients with Alzheimer-type dementia. Eur J Biochem 1986;*157*:115–120.

59. DeSarno P, Pomponi M, Giacobini E, Tang XC, Williams E. The effect of heptyl-physostigmine, a new cholinesterase inhibitor, on the central cholinegic system of the rat. Neurochem. Res 1989;*14*:971–977.

60. Iijima S, Greig NH, Garofalo P, Spangler EL, Heller B, Brossi A, Ingram DK. The long-acting cholinesterase inhibits heptylphysostigmine attenuates the scopolamine-induced learning impairment of rats in a 14-unit T-maze. Neurosci Le 1992 Sep 14;*144*:79–83.

61. Rupniak NM, Tye SJ, Brazell C, Heald A, Iversen SD, Pagella PG. Reversal of cognitive impairment by heptyl-physostigmine, a long-lasting cholinesterase inhibitor, in primates. J Neurol Sci 1992;*107*:246–249.

62. Linville DG, Giacobini E, Arneric SP. Heptyl-physostigmine enhances basal forebrain control of cortical cerebral blood flow. Journal of Neuroscience Research 1992;*31*:573–577.

63. Marta M, Castellano C, Oliverio A, Pavone F, Pagella PG, Brufani M, Pomponi M. New analogs of physostigmine: alternative drugs for Alzheimer's disease? Life Sciences 1988;*43*:1921–1928.

64. Segre G, Cerretani D, Baldi A, Urso R. Pharmacokinetics of heptastigmine in rats. Pharmacol Res 1992;*25*:139–146.

65. Cella SG, Imbimbo BP, Pieretti F, Muller EE. Eptastigmine augments basal and GHRH stimulated growth hormone re in young and old dogs. Life Sci 1993;*53*:389–395.

66. Scremin OU, Scremin AM, Heuser D, Hudgell R, Romero E, Imbimbo BP. Prolonged effects of cholinesterase inhibition with eptastigmine on the cerebral blood flow-metabolism ratio of normal rats. J Cereb Blood Flow Metab 199;*13*:707.

67. Koelle GB, Massoulie J, Eugene D, Melone MA, Boulla G. Distribution of the molecular forms of acetylcholinesteras and butyrylcholinesterase in nervous tissue of the cat. Proc Natl Acad Sci USA 1987;*84*:7749–7752.

68. Wang YE, Yue DX, Tang XC. Anti-cholinesterase activity of Huperzine A. Acta Pharmacologica Sinica 1986;*7*:110.

69. Tang XC, Han YF, Chen XP, Zhu XD. Effects of huperzine A on learning and retrieval process of discrimination performance in rats. Acta Pharmacologica Sinica 1986;*7*:507–511.

70. Zhang RW, Tang XC, Han YY, Sang GW, Zhang YD, Ma YX, Zhang CL. Drug evaluation of huperzine A in the treatment of senile memory disorders. English abstract. Chung Kuo Yao Li Hsueh Pao 1991;*12*:250–252.

71. Hanin I, Tang XC, Kindel GL, Kozikowski AP. Natural and synthetic Huperzine A: effect on cholinergic function in vitro and in vivo. Ann N Y Acad Sci. 1993;*695*:304–306.

72. Hallak M, Giacobini E. A comparison of the effects of two inhibitors on brain cholinesterase. Neuropharmacology 1987;*26*:521–530.

73. Moriearty PL, Thornton SL, Becker RE. Transdermal patch delivery of acetylcholinesterase inhibitors. Methods Find Exp Clin Pharmacol 1993;*15*:407–412.

74. Thomsen T, Kaden B, Fischer JP, Bickel U, Barz H, Gusztony G, Cervos Navarro J, Kewitz H. Inhibition of acetylcholinesterase activity in human brain tissue and erythrocytes by galanthamine, physostigmine and tacrine. Eur J Clin Chem Clin Biochem 1991;*29*:487–492.

75. Mihailova D, Yamboliev I, Zhivkova Z, Tencheva J, Jovovich V. Pharmakokinetics of Galanthamine hydrobromide after a single subcutaneous and oral dosage in humans. Pharmacology 1989;*39*:50–58.

76. Rainer M, Mark Th, Haushofer A. Galanthaminum hydrobromicum in treatment of senile dementia (Alzheimer's disease). Presented at IV. World conference on clinical pharmacology and therapeutics, Berlin (West), July 28–30, 1989.

77. Thomsen T, Kewitz H. Galanthamine treatment in senile dementia of Alzheimer's type. A case report. Presented at IV. World conference on clinical pharmacology and therapeutics, Berlin (West), July 28–30, 1989.

78. Dal-Bianco P, Maly J, Wober Ch, Lind C, Koch G, Gufgard J, Marshall I. Mraz M, Deecke L. Galanthamine treatment in Alzheimer's disease. J Neural Transm Suppl 1991;*33*:59–63.

78a. Kewitz H, Davis BM, Wilcoh G. Galanthamine in Alzheimer's Disease. In Advances in Alzheimer's Disease. Giacocini E, Becker R. Springer Verlag, Boston, 1994.

79. Tanaka K, Ogawa N, Asanuma M, Hirata H, Kondo Y, Nakayama N, Mori A. Effects of the acetylcholinesterase inhibitor ENA 713 on ischemia induced changes in acetylcholine and aromatic amine levels in the gerbil brain. Arch Int Pharmacodyn Ther 1993;*323*:85–96.

80. Enz A, Boddeke H, Gray J, Spiegel R. Pharmacologic and clinicopharmacologic properties of SDZ ENA 713, a central selective acetycholinesterase inhibitor. Ann N Y Acad Sci 1991;*640*:272–275.

81. Holsboer Trachsler E, Hatzinger M, Stohler R, Hemmeter U, Gray J, Muller J, Kocher R, Spiegel R. Effects of the new acetylcholinesterase inhibitor SDZ ENA 713 on sleep in man. Neuropsychopharmacology. 1993;*8*(1):87–92.

82. Mihara M, Ohnishi A, Tomono Y, Hasegawa J, Shimamura Y, Yamazaki K, Morishita N. Pharmacokinetics of E2020 a new compound for Alzheimer's disease, in healthy male volunteers. Int J Clin Pharmacol Ther Toxicol 1993;*31*:223.

83. Yamamoto T, Ohno M, Sugimachi K, Ueki S. Discriminative stimulis properties of NIK 247 and tetrahydroaminoacridine centrally active cholinesterase inhibitors, in rats. Pharmacol Biochem Behav 1993a;*44*:769–775.

84. Yamamoto T, Ohno M, Kitajima I, Yatsugi S, Ueki S. Ameliorative effects of the centrally active cholinesterase inhibitor NIK 247, on impairment of working memory in rats. Physiol Behav 1993b;*53*:5–10.

85. Haratounian V, Kanof PD, Davis KL. Pharmacological alleviation of cholinergic lesion induced memory deficits in rats. Life Science 1985;*37*:945–952.

86. Wettstein A, Spiegal R. Clinical studies with the cholinergic drug RS-86 in Alzheimer's disease (AD) and senile dementia of Alzheimer type (SDAT). Psychopharmacology 1984;*84*:572–573.

87. Bruno G, Mohr E, Gillespie M, et al. RS-86 therapy of Alzheimer's disease. Arch Neurol 1985;*43*:659–661.

88. Mouradian MM, Mohr E, Williams AJ, Chase TN. No response to high-dose muscarinic agonist therapy in Alzheimer's disease. Neurology 1988;*38*:606–608.

89. Hollander E, Davidson M, Mohs RC, Horvath TB, Davis BM, Zemishlany Z, Davis KL. RS 86 in the treatment of Alzheimer's disease: cognitive and biological effects. Biol Psychiatry 1987;*22*:1067–1078.

90. Harbaugh RE. Intracerebroventricular bethanechloride administration in Alzheimer's disease: Preliminary results of a double blind study. J Neurotrans 1987;*24*(suppl):271–277.

91. Penn RD, Goetz CG, Tanner CM, Klawans HL, Shannon KM, Comella CL, Witt TR. The adrenal medullary transplant operation for Parkinson's disease: clinical observation in five patients. Neurosurgery 1988b;*22*:999–1004.

92. Gauthier S, Leblanc R, Quirion R, et al. Transmitter-replacement therapy in Alzheimer's disease using intracerebroventricular infusions of receptor agonists. Can J Neurol Sci 1986;*13*:394–402.

93. Penn RD, Martin EM, Wilson RS, Fox JH, Savoy SM. Intraventricular bethanechol infusion of Alzheimer's disease: Results of double blind and escalating dose trials. Neurology 1988a;*38*:219–222.

94. Christie JE, Shering A, Ferguson J, Glen AIM. Physostigmine and arecoline: effects of intravenous infusions in Alzheimer's presenile dementia. Br J Psychiat 1981;*138*:46–50.

95. Tariot PN, Cohen RM, Welkowitz JA, Sunderland T, Newhouse PA, Murphy DL, Weingartner H. Multiple-dose arecolin infusions in Alzheimer's disease. Arch Gen Psychiatry 1988a;*45*:901–905.

96. Raffaele KC, Berardi A, Asthana S, Morris P, Haxby JV, Soncrant TT. Effects of long-term continuous infusion of the muscarinic cholinergic agonist arecoline on verbal memory in dementia of the Alzheimer type. Psychopharmacol Bull 1991;*27*:315–319.

97. Raffaele KC, Berardi A, Pearse Morris P, Asthana S, Haxby JV, Schapiro MB, Rapoport SI, Soncrant TT. Effects of acute infusion of the muscarinic cholinergic agonist arecoline on verbal and visuo-spatial function in dementia of the Alzheimer type. Prog Neuro-Psychopharmacol and Biol Psychiat 1991;*15*:643–648.

98. Davis KL, Hollander E, Davidson M, Davis B, Mohs RC, Horvath TB. Induction of depression with oxotremorine in Alzheimer's disease patients. Am J Psychiatry 1987;*144*:468–471.

99. Sunderland T, Tariot PN, Newhouse PA. Differential responsivity of mood, behavior, and cognition to cholinergic aging in elderly neuropsychiatric populations. Brain Res 1988;*472*:371–389.

100. Newhouse PA, Sunderland T, Tariot PN, Blumhardt CL, Weingartner H, Mellow A, Murphy DL. Intravenous nicotine in Alzheimer's disease: a pilot study. Psychopharmacology 1988;*95*:171–175.

101. Ono S, Saito Y, Ohgane N, Kawanishi G, Mizobe F. Heterogeneity of muscarinic heteroreceptors in the rat brain: effects of a novel M^1 agonist, AF102B. Europ J Pharmacol 1988;155:77–84.

102. Nakahara N, Iga Y, Mizobe F, Kawanishi G. Amelioration of experimental amnesia (passive avoidance failure) in rodents by selective M^1 agonist AF102B. Japan J Pharmacol 1988;*48*:502–505.

103. Fisher A, Heldman E, Gurwitz D, Haring R, Barak D, Meshulam H, Marciano D, Brandeis R, Pittel Z, Segal M, et al. Selective signaling via unique M1 muscarinic agonists. Ann N Y Acad Sci 1993 Sep 24;*695*:300–303.

104. Fisher A, Brandeis R, Karton I, Pittel Z, Gurwitz D, Haring R, Sapir M, Levy A, Heldman E. (±)-cis-2-methyl-spiro oxathiolane-5,3')quinuclidine, an M1 selective cholinergic agonist, attenuates cognitive dysfunctions in an animal mode of alzheimer's disease. J Pharmacol Exp Ther 1991;392–403.

105. Saunders SJ, Showell GA, Snow J, Baker R, Hurley EA, Freedman JB. 2-methyl-1,3-dioxaazaspiro[4.5]decanes as novel muscarinic cholinergic agonists J Med Chemistry 1988;*31*:480–491.

106. Iversen LL. Approaches to the cholinergic therapy in Alzheimer's disease. Prog Brain Res 1993;*98*:423–426.

107. Doods HN, Quirion R, Mihm R, Engel W, Rudolf K, Entzeroth M, Schiavi GB, Ladinsky H, Bechtel WD, Ensinger H, Mendla KD, Eberlein W. Therapeutic potential of CNS-active M2 antagonists: Novel structures and pharmacology. Life Sciences 1993;*52*:497–503.

108. Boast CA, Leventer S, Sabb A, Abelson M, Bender R, Giacomo D, Maurer S, McArthur S, Mehta O, Morris H, et al. Biochemical and behavioral characterization of a novel cholinergic agonist, SR 95639. Pharmacol Biochem Behav 1991;*39*:287–292.

109. Enz A, Shapiro G, Supavilai P, Boddeke HW. SDZ ENS 163 is a selective M1 agonist and induces release of acetylcholine. Naunyn Schmiedebergs Arch Pharmacol 1992;*345*:28.

110. Enz A, Boddeke H, Sauter A, Rudin M, Shaprio G. SDZ ENS 163 a novel pilocarpine like drug: pharmacological in vitro and in vivo profile. Life Sci 1993;*52*:513–520.

111. Ensinger HA, Doods HN, Immel Sehr AR, Kuhn FJ, Lambrecht G, Mendla KD, Muller RE, Mutschler E, Sagrada A, Walther G, et al. WAL 2014 a muscarinic agonist with preferential neuron-stimulating properties. Life Sci 1993;*52*:473–480.

112. Levy R, Little A, Chuaqui-Kidd P, Reith M. Early results from double blind, placebo controlled trial of high-dose phosphatidylcholine in Alzheimer's disease. Lancet 1983;*1*:987–988.

113. Little A, Levy R, Chuaqui-Kidd P, Hand D. A double blind, placebo controlled trial of high-dose lecithin in Alzheimer's disease. J Neurol Neurosurg Psychiatry 1985;*48*:736–742.

114. Amaducci L, and the SMID group. Phosphatidylserine in the treatment of Alzheimer's disease: Results of a multicenter study. Psychopharmacology Bull, 1988;*24*:130–134.

115. Crook T, Petrie W, Wells C, Massari DC. Effects of phosphatidylserine in Alzheimer's disease. Psychophrmacology Bull, 1988;*28*:61–66.

116. Heiss WD, Kessler J, Slansky I, Mielke R, Szelies B, Herholz K. Activation PET as an instrument to determine therap efficacy in Alzheimer's disease. Ann N Y Acad Sci 1993 Sep 24;*695*:327–331.

117. Gatti G, Barzaghi N, Acuto G, Abbiati G, Fossati T, Perucca EA. A comparative study of free plasma choline levels following intramuscular administration of L alpha glycerylphosphoryl-

choline and citicoline in normal volunteers. Int J Clin Pharmacol Ther Toxicol 1992;*30*:331–335.

118. Ceda GP, Ceresini G, Denti L, Marzani G, Piovani E, Banchini A, Tarditi E, Valenti G. Alpha glycerylphosphorylch administration increases the GH responses to GHRH of young and elderly subjects. Horm Metab Res 1992;*24*:119–121.

119. Parnetti L, Abate G, Bartorelli L, Cuccinotta D, Cuzzupoli M, Maggioni M, Villardita C, Senin U. Multicentre study of L-α-Glyceryl-phosphorylcholine vs ST200 among patients with probable senile dementia of Alzheimer's type. Drugs and Ageing 1993;*3*:159–164.

120. Petkov VD, Kehayov RA, Mosharrof AH, Petkov VV, Getova D, Lazarova MB, Vaglenova J. Effects of cytidine diphosphate choline on rats with memory deficits. Arzneimittelforschung 1993;*43*:822–828.

121. Cacabelos R, Alvarez XA, Franco Maside A, Fernandez Novoa L, Caamano J. Effect of CDP-choline on cognition and immune function in Alzheimer's disease and mutli infarct dementia. Ann N Y Acad Sci 1993 Sep 24;*695*:321–323.

122. Wesseling H, Agoston S, Van Dam GBP, Pasma J, De Witt DJ, Havinga H. Effects 4-aminopyridine in elderly patients with Alzheimer's disease. N Engl J Med 1984;*310*:988–989.

123. Davidson M, Zamishlany Z, Mohs RC, Horvath TB, Powchik P, Blass JP, Davis KL. 4-Aminopyridine in the treatment of Alzheimer's disease. Biol Psychiatry 1988;*23*:485–490.

124. Branconnier RJ, Cole JO, Dessain EC, Spera KF, Ghazvinian S, De Vitt D. The therapeutic efficacy of piracetam in Alzheimer's disease: preliminary observations. Psychpharmacol Bull 1983b;*19*:726–730.

125. Cook L. Biochemical, neurophysiological and cognitive effects of an enhancer of stimulus-induced release of acethylcholine DuP 996 (3,3-Bis(4-pyridinylmethyl)-1-phenylindolin-2-one). Abstract presented at the annual meeting of the America College of Neuropharmacology, December 11–16, 1988.

126. Cook L, Nicholson VJ, Steinfels GF, Rohrbach KW, DeNoble VJ. Cognitive enhancement by the acetylcholine release DuP996. Drug Rev Res 1990;*19*:301–304.

127. Nicholson VJ, Tam SW, Myers MJ, Cook L. DuP996 (3,3-bis(4-pyrindinylmethyl)-1-phenylindolin-2-one) enhances the stimulus-induced release of acetylcholine from rat brain in vitro and in vivo. Dru Rev Res 1990;*19*:285–300.

128. Vickroy TW. Presynaptic cholinergic actions by the putative cognitive enhancing agent DuP 996. J Pharmacol Exp Thera 1993;*264*:910–917.

129. DeSouza EB, Rule BL, Tam SW. [^{3}H]Linopirdine (DuP 996) labels a novel binding site in rat brain involved in the enhancement of stimulus-induced neurotransmitter release: autoradiographic localization studies. Brain Research 1992;*582*:335–341.

130. Saletu B, Darragh A, Salmon P, Coen R. EEG brain maping in evaluating the time course of the central action of DuP 996: a new acetylcholine release drug. Br J Pharmacol 1989;*28*:1–16.

131. Hsu RS, DiLeo EM, Chesson SM, Klein JT, Effland RC. Determination of HP 749, a potential therapeutic agent for Alzheimer's disease, in plasma by high-performance liquid chromatography. Journal of Chromatography 1991;*572*:352–359.

132. Cornfeldt M, Wirtz-Burgger, Szewczak M, Blitzer R, Haroutunian V, Effland RC, Klein JT, Smith C. Abstr Soc. Neuro 1990;*16*:612.

133. Bondareff W, Mountjoy CQ, Roth M. Loss of neurons of origin of the adrenergic projection to cerebral cortex (nucle locus coeruleus) in senile dementia. Neurology 1982;*32*:164–168.

134. Rossor M, Iversen LL. Non-cholinergic neurotransmitter abnormalities in Alzheimer's disease. Br Med Bull 1986;*42*:70–74.

135. Bowen DM, Allen SJ, Benton JS, et al. Biochemical assessment of serotonergic and cholinergic dysfunction and cere atrophy in Alzheimer's disease. J Neurochem 1983;*41*:266–272.

136. Cross AJ, Crow TJ, Ferrier IN, Johnson JA. The selectivity of the reduction of serotonin S2 receptors in Alzheimer-type dementia. Neurobiol Aging 1986;*7*:3–7.

137. Yamamoto T, Hirano A. Nucleus raphe dorsalis in Alzheimer's disease: Neurofibrillary tangles and loss of large neurons Ann Neurol 1985;*17*:573–577.

138. Gottfries CG, Adolfsson R, Aquilonius SM, Carlsson A, Eckermas S-A, Nordberg A, Oreland L, Svennerhelm L, Winblad A, Wiberg A. Biochemical changes in dementia disorders of the Alzheimer type (AD/SDAT). Neurobiol Aging 1983;*4*:261–271.

139. Gottfries CG, Bartfai T, Carlsson A, Eckernas S, Svennerholm L. Multiple deficits in both gray and white matter in Alzheimer's brains. Prog Neuro-Psychopharmacol & Biol Psychiat 1986;*10*:405–413.

140. Tariot PN, Sunderland T, Weingartner H, Murphy DL, Welkowitz JA, Thompson K, Cohen RM. Cognitive effects of L-deprenyl in Alzheimer's disease. Psychopharmacology 1987a;*91*:489–495.

141. Tariot PN, Cohen RM, Sunderland T, Newhouse PA, Yount D, Mellow AM, Weingartner H, Mueller EA, Murphy D. L-deprenyl in Alzheimer's disease. Arch Gen Psychiatry 1987b;*44*:427–433.

142. Piccinin FL, Finali G, Piccirilli M. Neuropsychological effects of l-deprenyl in Alzheimer's type dementia. Clin Neuropharmacology 1990;147–163.

143. Agnoli A, Martucci N, Fabbrini G, Buckley AE, Fioravanti M. Monamine oxidase and dementia: treatment with an inhibitor of MAO-B activity. Dementia 1990;109–114.

144. Mangoni A, Grassi MP, Frattola L, et al. Effects of a MAO-B inhibitor in the treatment of Alzheimer disease. Eur N 1991;100–107.

145. Martignoni M, Bono G, Blandini E, Sinforiani E, Merlo P, Napi G. Monoamines and related metabolites levels in the cerebrospinal fluid of patients with dementia of Alzheimer type. Influence of treatment with l-deprenyl. J Neural Trans 1991;*3*:15–25.

146. Tariot PN, Sunderland T, Cohen RM, Newhouse PA, Mueller EA, Murphy DL. Trancylpromine compared with L-de in Alzheimer's disease. J Clin Psychopharmacol 1988b;*8*:23–27.

147. Arnsten AFT, Cai JX, Goldman-Rakic PS. The alpha-2 adrenergic agonist guanfacine improves memory in aged monkey without sedative or hypotensive side effects: evidence for alpha-2 receptor subtypes. J of Neuroscience 1988;*8*:4287–4294.

148. McEntree W, Mair R. Memory enhancement in Korsakoff's psychosis by clonidine: further evidence of a noradrenergic deficit. Ann Neurol 1980;*27*:466–470.

149. Fields RB, Van Kammen DP, Peters JL, Rosen J, Van Kammen WB, Nugent A, Stipetic M, Linnoila M. Clonidine improves memory function in schizophrenia independently from changes in psychosis. Schizophrenia research 1988;*1*:417–423.

150. Mohr E, Schlegel J, Fabbrini G, et al. Clonidine treatment of Alzheimer's disease. Arch Neurol 1989;*46*:376–378.

151. Schlegel J, Mohr E, Williams J, Mann U, Gearing M, Chase TN. Guanfacine treatment of Alzheimer's disease. Clin Neuropharmacology 1989;*12*:124–128.

152. Crook T, Wilner E, Rothwell A, Winterrling D, McEntee W. Noradrenergic intervention in Alzheimer's disease. Psychopharm Bull 1992;*28*:67–70.

153. Newman RP, Weingartner H, Smallberg SA, Calne DB. Effortful and automatic memory: effects of dopamine. Neurology (Cleveland) 1984;*34*:805–807.

154. Jellinger K, Flament H, Riederer P, Schmnid H, Ambrozzi L. Levodopa in the treatment of (pre) senile dementia. Mechanisms of ageing and development 1980;*14*:253–264.

155. Kristensen V, Olsen M, Theilgard A. Levodopa treatment of presenile dementia. Acta Psychiat Scand 1977;*55*:41–45.

156. Bergmann I, et al. Alaproclate: a pharmacokinetic and biochemical study in patients with dementia of Alzheimer type Psychopharmacology 1983;*80*:279–283.

157. Dehlin O, Hedenrud B, Jansson P, Nörgård J. A double-blind comparison of alaproclate and placebo in the treatment of patients with senile dementia. Acta Psychiat Scand 1985;*71*:190–196.

158. Cutler NR, Haxby J, Kay AD, et al. Evaluation of zimeldine in Alzheimer's disease. Arch Neurol 1985a;*42*:744–748.

159. Gottfries CG, Nyth AL. Effect of citalopram, a selective 5-HT reuptake blocker, in emotionally disturbed patients with dementia. Ann N Y Acad Sci 1991;*640*:276–279.

160. Buccafusco JJ, Jackon WJ, Terry AV Jr. Effects of concomitant cholinergic and adrenergic stimulation on learning and memory performance by primates. Life Sci 1992;*51*:PL 7–12.

161. Davidson M, Mohs RC, Hollander E, Zamishlany Z, Powchik P, Ryan TA, Davis KL. Lecithin and piracetam in patients with Alzheimer's disease. Biol Psychiatry 1987;*22*:112–114.

162. Bierer LM, Aisen PS, Davidson M, Ryan TM, Stern RG, Schmeidler J, Davis KL. A pilot study of oral physostigmin plus yohimbine in patients with Alzheimer's disease. Alz Dis Assoc Dis 1993;*7*:98–104.

163. Schneider LS, Olin JT, Pawluczyk S. A double-blind crossover pilot study of l-deprenyl (selegiline) combined with cholinesterase inhibitor in Alzheimer's disease. Am-J-Psychiatry 1993b;*150*:321–323.

164. Sunderland T, Molchan S, Lawlor B, Martinez R, Mellow A, Martinson H, Putnam K, Lalonde F. A strategy of "combination chemotherapy" in Alzheimer's disease: rationale and preliminary results with physostigmine plus deprenyl. Int Psychogeriatr 1992; 4 Suppl 2: 291–309.

165. De Wied D. The importance of vasopressin in memory. Trends Neurosci 1984;*7*:62–63.

166. Miller TP, Fong K, Tinklenberg JR. An ACTH 4 9 analog (Org 2766) and cognitive performance: high dose efficacy and safety in dementia of the Alzheimer's type. Biol Psychiatry 1993;*33*:307–309.

167. Siegfried KR. First clinical impressions with an ACTH analog (HOE 427) in the treatment of Alzheimer's disease. Ann N Y Acad Sci 1991, 640:281–283.

168. Cutler NR, Haxby J, Narang PK, May L, Burg C, Raines SA. Evaluation of an analogue of somatostatin (L363,586) in Alzheimer's disease N Engl J Med 1985b;*312*:725.

169. Mouradian MM, Blin J, Giuffra M, Heuser IJE, Baronti F, Ownby J, Chase TN. Somatostatin replacement therapy for Alzheimer dementia. Ann Neurol 1991;*30*:610–613.

170. Morris RGM, Anderson E, Lynch GS, et al. Selective impairment of learning and blockade of long term potentiation by an N-methyl-D-aspartate receptor antagonist, AP%. Nature 1986;*319*:774–776.

171. Danysz W, Wroblewsky JT, Costa E. Learning impairment in rats by N-methyl-D-aspartate receptor antagonist. Neuropharmacology 1988;*27*:653–656.

172. Greenamyre JT, Young AB. Excitatory amino acids and Alzheimer's disease. Neurobiology of aging 1989;*10*:593–560.

173. Palmer AM, Gershon S. Is the neuronal basis of Alzheimer's disease cholinesrgic or glutamatergic? FASEB J 1990;*4* 2752.

174. Handelmann GE, Nevins ME, Mueller LL, Arnold SM, Cordi AA. Milacenide, a glycine prodrug enhances performance of learning tasks in normal and amnestic rodents. Pharmacol Biochem Behav 1989;*34*:823–828.

175. Herting RL. Milacemide and other drugs active at gluamate NMDA receptors as potential treatment for dementia. Ann N Y Acad Sci 1991;*640*:237–240.

176. Dysken MW, Mendels J, LeWitt P, Reisberg B, Pomara N, Wood J, Skare S, Fakouhi JD, Herting RL. Milacemide: a placebo controlled study in senile dementia of the Alzheimer type. J Am Geriatr Soc. 1992;*40*(5):503–506.

177. Jones RW, Wesnes KA, Kirby J. Effects of NMDA modulation in scopulamoine dementia. Ann N Y Acad Sci 1991;*640*:241–244.

178. Mohr E, Knott V, Herting RL, Mendis T. Cycloserine treatment of Alzheimer's disease. Abstract. Neuropsychopharmacology 1993; 9 suppl:96s–97s.

179. Branconnier RJ. The efficacy of the cerebral metabolic enhancers in the treatment of senile dementia. Psychpharmacol Bull 1983a;*19*:212–219.

180. Croisile B, Trillet M, Fondarai J, Laurent B, Mauguire F, Billardon M. Long term and high-dose piracetam treatment of Alzheimer's disease. Neurology 1993;*43*:301–305.

181. Pomara N, Block R, Moore N, Rhiew HP, Berchou R, Stanley M, Gershon S. Combined piracetam and cholinergic precursor treatment for primary degenerative dementia. IRCS Medical Science 1984;*12*:388–389.

182. Smith RC, Vroulis G, Johnson R, Morgan R. Comparison of therapeutic response to long-term treatment with lecithin versus piracetam plus lecithin in patients with Alzheimer's disease. Psychopharmacol Bull 1984;*20*:542–545.

183. Growdon JH, Corkin S, Huff FJ, Rosen TJ. Piracetam combined with lecithin in the treatment of Alzheimer's disease Neurobiol Aging 1986;*7*:269–276.

184. Friedman E, Sherman KA, Ferris SH, Reisberg B, Bartus RT, Shneck MK. Clinical response to choline plus piracetam in senile dementia: Relation to red-cell choline levels. N Engl J Med 1981;*304*:1490–1491.

185. Claus JJ, Ludwig C, Mohr E, Giuffra M, Blin J, Chase TN. Nootropic drugs in Alzheimer's disease: symptomatic treatment with pramiracetam. Neurology 1991;*41*:570–574.

186. Green RC, Goldstein FC, Auchus AP, Presley R, Clark WS, Van Tuyl L, Green J, Hersch SM, Karp HR. Treatment trial of oxiracetam in Alzheimer's disease. Arch Neurol 1992;*49*:1135–1136.

187. Mizuki Y, Yamada M, Kato I, Takada Y, Tsujimaru S, Inanaga K, Tanka M. Effects of aniracetam, a nootropic drug in senile dementia—a preliminary report. Kurume Medical Journal 1984;*31*:135–143.

188. Sourander LB, Portin R, Molsa P, et al. Senile dementia of the Alzheimer's type treated with aniracetam. Psychopharmacology 1987;*91*:90–95.

189. Senin U, Abate G, Fieschi C, Gori G, Guala A, Marini G, Villardita C, Parnetti L. Aniracetam (Ro 13-5057) in the treatment of senile dementia of Alzheimer type (SDAT): results of a placebo controlled multicentre clinical study. Eur Neuropsychopharmacol 1991;*1*:511–517.

190. Carta A, Calvani A. Acetyl 1-carnitine: a drug able to slow the progress of Alzheimer disease. Ann N Y Acad Sci 1991;640:228–232.

191. Sano M, Bell K, Cote L, Dooneief G, Lawton A, Legler L, Marder K, Naiani A, Stern Y, Mayeux R. Double blind parallel design pilot study of acetyl levocarnitine in patients with Alzheimer disease. Arch Neurol 1992;*49*:1137–1141.

192. Behl C, Davis J, Cole GM, Schubert D. Vitamin E protects nerve cells from amyloid B protein toxicity. Biochemical and biophysical research communications 1992;*186*:944–950.

193. Murphy TH, Miyamoto M, Sastre A, Snaar RL, Coyle JT. Glutamate toxicity in a neuronal cell line involves inhibition of cysteine transport leading to oxydative stress. Neuron 1989;1547–1558.

194. Oka A, Belliveau MF, Rosenberg PA, Volpe JJ. Vulnerability of oligodendroglia to glutamate. Pharmacology, mechanisms, and prevention. J Neurosc 1993;*13*:1441–1453.

195. Martyn CN, Barker DJP, Osmond C, Harris EC, Edwardson JA, Lacey RF. Geographical relation between Alzhemer's disease and drinking water. Lancet 1989;59–62.

196. Perl DP, Brody AR. Alzheimer's disease: X-ray spectrometric evidence of aluminum accumulation in neurofibrillary A tangle-bearing neurons. Science 1980;*208*:297–300.

197. Kosik S, Bradley WG, Good PF, Rascol CG, Selko KJ. J Neuropath Exp Neurol 1983;*42*:365–375.

198. Clayton RM, Sedowofia SKA, Rankin JM, Manning A. A long term effect of aluminum in the fetal mouse brain. Life Sci 1992;*51*:1921–1928.

199. Chang TMS, Barre P. Effect of desferrioxamine on removal of aluminum and iron by coated charcoal haemoperfusion in a haemodialysis. Lancet 1983;1051–1053.

200. Propper R, Cooper B. Rufo B, et al. Continuous subcutaneous administration of desferoxamine in patients with iron overload N Engl J Med 1977;*297*:418–423.

201. Crapper McLachlan DR, Dalton AJ, Kruck TP, Bell MY, Smith WL, Kalow W, Andrews DF. Intramuscular desferrioxamine in patients with Alzheimer's disease. Lancet 1991;*337*:1304–1308.

202. Hefti F. Nerve growth factor promotes survival of septal cholinergic neurons after fimbrial transsections. J Neuroscien 1986;*6*:2155–2162.

203. Will B, Hefti F. Behavioral and neurochemical effects of chronic intraventricular injections of nerve growth factor in rats with fimbria lesions. Brain Research 1985;*17*:17–24.

204. Bruce G, Heinrich G. Production and characterization of biologically active recombinant human nerve growth factor. Neurobiol Aging 1989;*10*:89–94.

205. Rosenberg MB, Friedmann T, Robertson RO, et al. Grafting genetically modified cells to the damaged brain: restorative effects of NGF expression. Science 1988;*242*:1575–1577.

206. Fisher LJ, Raymon HK, Gage FH. Cells engineered to produce acetylcholine: therapeutic potential for Alzheimer's diease Ann-N Y Acad Sci 1993 Sep 24;*695*:278–284.

207. Friden PM, Walus LR, Watson P, Doctrow SR, Kozarich JW, Backman C, Bergman H, Hoffer B, Bloom F, Granholm AC. Blood-brain barrier penetration and in vivo activity of an NGF conjugate. Science 1993 Jan 15;*259*:373–377.

208. Styren SD, Civin Wh, Rogers J. Molecular cellular and psathogic characterization of HLA-Dr immunoreactivity in normal elderly and Alzheimer's disease brain. Exp NBeurol 1990;*110*:93–104.

209. Rogers J, Luber-Narod J, Styren SD, Civin WH. Expression of immune system-associated antigen by cells of the human central nervous system: relationship to pathology of Alzheimer's disease Neurobiol Aging 1988;*9*:330–349.

210. McGeer PL, Harada N, Kimura H, et al. Prevalence of dementia amongst elderly Japanese with leprosy: apparent effect of chronic drug therapy. Dementia 1992;*3*:146–149.

211. Breitner JC, Gau BA, Welsh KA, Plassman BL, McDonald WM, Helms MJ, Anthony JC. Inverse association of anti-inflammatory treatments and Alzheimer's disease: initial results of a co-twin control study. Neurology 1994;*44*:227.

212. Rogers J, Kirby LC, Hempelman SR, Berry DL, McGeer PL, Kaszniak AW, Zalinski J, Cofield M, Mansukhani L, W P, et al. Clinical trial of indomethacin in Alzheimer's disease. Neurology 1993;*43*:1609–1611.

213. Sapolsky RM, Krey LC, McEwen BS. Prolonged glucocorticoid exposure reduces hippocampal neuron number: implications for aging. J Nesurosci 1985;1222–1227.

214. Landfield P, Waymire J, Lynch G. Hippocampal aging and adenocorticosteroids: quantitative correlations. Science 1975;*202*: 1098–1102.

215. Mullins JF, Watts FL, Wilson CJ. Plaquenil in the treatment of lupus erytheamtosus. JAMA 1956;*161*:879–888.

216. Salmeron G, Lipsky PE. Immunosuppressive potential of antimalarials. Am J Med 1983;*75*(1A):19–24.

217. Ertel W, Morrison MH, Ayala A, Chaudry IH. Chloroquine attenuates hemorrhagic shock induced suppression of Kup cell antigen presentation and major histocompatibility complex class II antigen expression through blockade of tumor ne factor and prostaglandin release. Blood 1991;*78*:1781–1788.

218. Hardy JA, Higgins GA. Alzheimer's disease: the amyloid cascade hypothesis. Science 1992;*256*:184–185.

219. Goldgaber D, Lerman MI, McBride WO, Saffiotti U, Gajdusek DC. Isolation, characterization, and chromosomal localization of human brain cDNA clones coding for the precursor of the amyloid of brain in Alzheimer's disease, Down's syndrome and aging. J Neural Transm Suppl. 1987;*24*:23–28.

220. Kang J, Lamaire HG, Unterbeck A, Salbaum JM, Masters CL, Grzeschik KH, Multhaup G, Beyreuther K, Muller-Hil B. The precursor of Alzheimer's disease amyloid A4 protein resembles a cell-surface receptor. Nature 1987;*325*:733–736.

221. Robakis NK, Ramakrishna N, Wolfe G, Wisniewski HM. Molecular cloning and characterization of a cDNA encoding the cerebrovascular and the neuritic plaque amyloid peptides (correction in PNAS 1987;*84*:7221). Proc Natl Acad. Sci 1987;*84*:4190–4194.

222. Gandy S, Czernik AJ, Greengard P. Proc Natl. Acad. Sci 1988;*85*:6218–6221.

223. Suzuki T, Nairn AC, Gandy SE, Greengard P. Phosphorylation of Alzheimer amyloid precursor protein by protein kinase C. Neuroscience 1992;*48*:755–761.

224. Estus S, Golde TE, Younkin SG. Normal processing of the Alzheimer's disease amyloid beta protein precursor generated potentially amyloidogenic carboxyl terminal derivatives. Ann N Y Acad Sci. 1992a;*674*:138–148.

225. Estus S, Golde TE, Kunishita T, Blades D, Lowery D, Eisen M, Usiak M, Qu XM, Tabira T, Greenberg BD, et al. Potentially amyloidogenic, carboxyl terminal derivatives of the amyloid protein precursor. Science 1992b;*255*:726–728.

226. Buxbaum JD, Oishi M, Chen HI, Pinkas Kramarski R, Jaffe EA, Gandy SE; Greengard P. Cholinergic agonists and interleukin 1 regulate processing and secretion of the Alzheimer beta/A4 amyloid protein precursor. Proc Natl Acad S USA 1992;*89*:10075–10078.

227. Nitsch RM, Slack BE, Wurtman RJ, Growdon JH. Release of Alzheimer amyloid precursor derivatives stimulated by activation of muscarinic acetylcholine receptors. Science 1992;*258*:304–307.

228. Strittmatter WJ, Weisgraber KH, Goedert M, Saunders AM, Huang D, Corder EH, Dong LM, Jakes R, Alberts MJ, G JR, et al. Hypothesis: microtubule instability and paired helical filament formation in the Alzheimer disease brain are related to apolipoprotein E genotype. Exp Neurol 1994;*125*:163–171.

Reviews

r1. Drachman DA, Leavitt J. Human memory and the cholinergic system. Arch Neurol 1974;*30*:113–121.

r2. Bartus RT, Dean RL, Pontecorvo MJ, Flicker C. The cholinergic hypothesis: a historical overview, current perspective and future directions. Ann NY Acad Sci 1985;*444*:332–358.

r3. Collerton D. Cholinergic function and intellectual decline in Alzheimer's disease. Neuroscience 1986;*19*:1–28.

r4. Olton DS, Wenk GL. Dementia: animal models of the cognitive impairments produced by degeneration of the basal forebrain cholinergic system. In Psychopharmacology: The Third Generation of Progress. Meltzer HY, ed., Raven Press NY, 1987; pp 941–953.

r5. Adem A. Putative mechanisms of action of tacrine in Alzheimer's disease. Acta Neurol Scand Suppl 1992;*139*:69–74.

r6. Freeman SE, Dawson RM. Tacrine: a pharmacological review. Prog Neurobiol 1991;*36*:257–277.

r7. Schneider LS. Clinical pharmacology of aminoacridines in Alzheimer's disease. Neurology 1993a; 43(supl 4):S64–s79.

r8. Mohs RC, Davis KL. The experimental pharmacology of Alzheimer's disease and related dementias, in Psychopharmacology: Third Generation of Progress. Edited by Meltzer HY. New York, Raven Press, 1987, 921.

r9. Storey PL, Harell LE, Duke LW, Callaway R, Marsom DC. Does chronic oral physostigmine alter the course of Alzheimer's disease? Advances in clinical and basic research. Corain B, Iqbal K, Nicolini M, Winblad B, Wisniewski H, Zatta P, Editors 1993 John Wiley & Sons Ltd.

r10. Cutler NR, Sramek JJ, Seifert RD, Sawin SF. The target population in phase I clinical trials of acetylcholinesterase inhibitors in dementia: the role of the 'bridging study.' Alzheimer's disease: Advances in clinical and basic research. Corain B, Iqbal K, Nicolini M, Winblad B, Wisniewski H, Zatta P, Editors 1993 John Wiley & Sons Ltd.

r11. Koelle GB, Koelle WA, Smyrl EG, Davis R, Nagle AF. Histochemical and pharmacological evidence of the function of butyrylcholinesterase. In: Cholinergic Mechanisms and Psychopharmacology, Jenden DJ, editor, Plenum Press NY & London, 1977; pp 125–137.

r12. Tang XC, Zhu XD, Lu WH. Studies on the nootropic effects of huperzine A and B: two selective AChE inhibitors. In Giacobini E, Becker R, editors. Current Research in Alzheimer's therapy. Taylor & Francis, NY 1988; pp 289–293.

r13. Nordgren I, Holmstedt B. Metrifonate: a review. In Giacobini E, Becker R, editors. Current Research in Alzheimer's therapy. Taylor & Francis, NY 1988; pp 281–288.

r14. Davis RE, Emmerling MR, Jaen JC, Moos WH, Spiegel K. Therapeutic intervention in dementia. Crit Rev Neurobiol 1993;*7*:41–83.

r15. Bartus RT, Dean RL. The cholinergic hypothesis of geriatric memory dysfunction. Science 1982;*217*:408–412.

r16. Christie JE, Blackburn IM, Glen AIM, Zeisel S, Shering A, Yates CM. Effects of choline and lecithin on CSF cholin levels and cognitive functions in patients with presenile dementia of the Alzheimer type. In: Nutrition and the Brain, Vol 5, Barbeau A, Growden JH, Wurtman RJ, eds, Raven Press NY, 1979; pp 377–387.

r17. de la Morena E. Efficacy of CDP-Choline in the treatment of senile alterations in memory. Ann N Y Acad Sci 1991;*640*:233–236.

r18. Knoll J. The pharmacological profile of (–)Deprenyl (Selegiline) and its relevance for humans: a personal review. Pharmacol Toxicol 1992:*70*:317–324.

r19. Cesura AM, Pletscher A. The new generation of monoamine oxidase inhibitors. Prog-Drug-Res. 1992;*38*:171–297.

r20. Schneck MK. Nootropics. In Reisberg B, (ed) Alzheimer's Disease, The Free Press NY, 1983; pp 362–368.

r21. Jolles J. Neuropeptides and the treatment of cognitive deficits in aging and dementia. Prog Brain Res 1986;*70*:429–444.

r22. Kopeland MD, Lishman WA. Pharmacological treatments of dementia (non-cholinergic). Brit Med Bull 1986;*42*:1–105.

r23. Kragh Sorensen P, Lolk A. Neuropeptides and dementia. Prog Brain Res 1987;*72*:269–277.

r24. Sugaya K, Takahshi M, Kojima K, Katoh T, Ueki M, Kuboto K. SUT-8701, a CCK8 analogue, as a possible Anti-dementia drug. In: Corin B, Iqbal K, Nicolini M, Winblad B, Wisniewski H, and Zatta P, Editors: Alzheimer's Disease. Advance in clinical and basic research. John Wiley and Sons Ltd, 1993 p. 577–587.

r25. Collingridge GL, Bliss TPV. NMDA receptors—their role in long term potentiation. TINS 1987;*10*:288–293.

r26. Giurgea CE. Vers une pharmacologie de l'activite integrative du cerveaux. Tentative du concept nootrope en psychopharmacologie. Actual Pharmacol (Paris) 1972;*25*:115–157.

r27. Wittenborn JR. Pharmacotherapy for aged related behavioral deficiencies. J Nerv Ment Dis 1981;*169*:139–156.

r28. Ferris SH, Reisberg B, Crook T, Friedman E, Schneck MK, Mir P, Sherman KA,.Corwin J, Gershon S, Bartus RT. Pharmacologic treatment of senile dementia: cholinc, L DOPA, piracetam and choline plus piracetam. In Alzheimer's Disease: A Report of Progress. Corkin S, Davis KL, Growdon JH, Usdin E, Wurtman RJ (eds), Raven Press, NY 19 pp 475–481.

r29. Melhorn RJ, Cole G. Adv free radical biology and medicine 1985;*1*:165–223.

r30. Olson L, Hoffer BJ. The potential use of neurotrophic factors in the treatment of Alzheimer's disease. In Alzheimer's disease, new treatment strategies. Khachaturian ZS, Blass JP, Editors. Marcel Dekker, Inc New York, Basel, Hong K 1992;125–134.

r31. Brewster ME. Noninvasive drug delivery to the brain. Neurobiol Aging 1989;*10*:638–639.

r32. Pardridge WM. Strategies for drug delivery through the blood-brain barrier. Neurobiol Aging 1989;*10*:636–637.

r33. DeDuve C, DeBarsy T, Poole B, Trouet A, Tulkens P, van Hoiof F. Lysomotropic agents. Biochem Pharmacol 1974;*23*:2495–2531.

CHAPTER 120

Fred M. Eckel

Prescription Writing

> Drugs are the key to modern medicine.
>
> —Victor Fuchs

> Today's drugs may be likened to ballistic missiles with atomic warheads, while we prescribe, dispense, and administer them as if they were bows and arrows.
>
> —Don Francke

Each year Americans have more than 1.5 billion prescription orders filled in pharmacies. These are filled with the more than 8000 drug products available in our marketplace. But millions of patients take these prescription medicines incorrectly. Why? Because they are ill-informed, unaware, or simply noncompliant. Is this really a significant problem? In the US it is estimated that as many as 50 percent of prescribed medications are never filled or are taken incorrectly. Errors are estimated between 25 and 90 percent for outpatients administering their own medications. Types of errors range from taking medicines at the wrong intervals (too often or not often enough), wrong doses, wrong time, in the wrong combination, or for too short a time. What role does the prescription order play in this situation?

Prescription medications are acknowledged to be a valuable tool in the treatment of the disease process today. In American society prescription drugs are highly valued for their safety, efficacy, and accessibility; moreover, drugs have come to be a treatment of choice for a number of disease processes and symptoms. The closure of the encounter between patient and physician is symbolized in most situations when the prescription order is handed to the patient.

Society has an inherent trust in medications for symptom and disease treatment. However, many risk factors come into play, including: cross-sensitivity; teratogenicity; carcinogenicity; mutagenicity; pregnancy and other reproduction issues; effects on lactation and breast feeding; usage in such at-risk populations as infants, children, and the elderly; drug interactions, including interference with laboratory tests. Adverse reactions cannot be ignored. Certain idiosyncratic reactions are unexpected when the drug is used at commonly prescribed dose, cannot be predicted, and must always be anticipated.

In today's litigious society, the prescriber must consider carefully when prescribing medications. Legal action has been taken against prescribers and pharmacists for negligence due to acts of omission or commission. Unexpected patient outcomes as well as monitoring issues are as common for court action as prescribing and dispensing errors.

The writing of a prescription order has been described as a therapeutic adventure, the outcome of which can be profoundly influenced by the extent to which the patient's behavior coincides with the health advice summarized in the prescription.[r1] "Drug misadventure" is a term used to describe the unexpected result of drug treatment due to a failure in the drug treatment system or to an adverse event disproportionate to the severity of the condition being treated. A drug misadventure is often an iatrogenic hazard. The express purpose of monitoring for drug safety is to protect patients against the risks of drug misadventures.[r2]

It is estimated that more than half of patients cannot identify their medicines by name or even explain why they are taking the medication. Between 14 and 21 percent of prescription orders are never filled. Only half of prescription refills authorized are ever obtained. How can the health professional improve these situations? How can health team members work with patients to improve compliance with their medication regimens? Prescribers and pharmacists must go beyond a technically correct prescription order and also consider patient and professional behaviors that contribute to poor prescription use.

The prescription order offers a means of communicating the prescriber's treatment intentions to the pharmacist and helps the pharmacist reinforce to the patient the steps necessary to achieve a desired outcome. A properly written prescription order can help prevent drug misadventures.

What role does a properly written prescription order play in eliminating or reducing therapeutic misadventures? Since a prescription order represents the termination of the diagnostic process and the beginning of therapy, it is a key vehicle to ensure that what the prescriber and patient desire for cure, amelioration, or prevention does occur. How can the prescriber see that a prescription medication plays the desired role in the treatment process for a patient? Knowing the mechanics of a properly written prescription order, realizing the inherent economic, social, or behavioral problems in prescription drug consumption, and anticipating problems that may arise in prescription drug use are essential to the success of a patient's drug therapy.

Will the use of printed patient information leaflets supplied by a physician or pharmacist enhance the patient's use of prescriptions? Should the prescriber designate the use of these leaflets to supplement the oral prescription order directions provided to the patient by the prescriber and/or the pharmacist? Studies have indicated an improvement in patients' use of medications and understanding of their medication regimens when information leaflets were provided.[1-3]

Writing the Prescription

The prescription is an important part of the treatment process between a prescriber and a patient. Prescriptions are the most frequent outcome of the outpatient physician visit. An estimated 61 percent of patient visits for a new medical problem will result in the patient receiving at least one prescription.[4] The most carefully made therapeutic decision may be rendered useless unless the prescription order communicates clearly to the pharmacist the intent of the prescriber and adequately instructs the patient on the use of the prescribed medication.[5] A poorly written prescription order makes it difficult for the pharmacist to reinforce the prescribers' therapeutic goals.

Significant drug misadventures can be avoided when the prescriber pays close attention to developing and consistently using the correct prescription order-writing skills. Extra time may be required of a young practitioner who is developing prescribing habits or of an experienced practitioner prescribing a new or difficult regimen, but the ultimate goal of a successful medication treatment regimen can be assured with attention to prescription order writing details.

Legible and Complete

Writing the prescription legibly is inherent to safe prescription dispensing and use. Medication errors can be prevented and questions avoided when the words on a prescription order are legible. Similar-looking drug names abound on the drug market today. With the use of both proprietary and generic names there are numerous opportunities for drug names that resemble each other to be interpreted in error. Paying careful attention to writing the drug name clearly and spelling the name correctly can prevent some prescription dispensing errors. Prescriber's printed name, practice address and phone number, office hours, and often the Drug Enforcement Administration (DEA) number are commonly printed on prescription blanks to facilitate communication about the prescription order.

Prescriptions should be written in ink to assure their status as a legal document and to prevent tampering. Writing in permanent ink is required for controlled substances, especially those in Schedule II. Including a patient's full name can ensure that mix-ups in future prescription use do not occur. With the advent of computerized data bases and prescription records filed sometimes by a number coding system, using a complete patient name provides an extra measure of security for prescription dispensing accuracy.

For very young patients or senior citizens, indicating a patient's age or date of birth will facilitate prescribing unusual dosages or dosage intervals. Again, with the application of computerized patient data bases, providing the patient's date of birth helps the pharmacist build a more complete picture of the patient. In the case of unusual prescribing information, patient age may facilitate information exchange and lessen the need for phone calls or follow-up questions.

Indicating the date on which the medication is prescribed is required by law. The date clarifies questions about treatment plan duration and is a good indication of patient compliance in specific situations. For instance, antibiotic prescriptions written but not filled for a significant time may no longer be applicable to the patient's present condition and may do more harm than good.

Abbreviations on prescription orders provide another opportunity for miscommunication about desired therapy. Errors in interpretation of abbreviations occur commonly when little-used abbreviations such as the apothecary system or Latin patient instructions are used. Significant problems can occur when the drug name is abbreviated, either as a chemical entity or with the prescriber's own particular abbreviated name. Similarly, coined names developed as short-cuts for specific treatments should be avoided by prescribers. These may save time for those familiar with a particular prescriber's panoply of drug therapies, but other pharmacists will need to clarify orders written in a shorthand manner. Worse, the pharmacist may make a dispensing error as a result of incorrect interpretation.

Proprietary and Nonproprietary Names

Clearly indicating the drug that is prescribed is an element of prescription writing that cannot be overstressed. With hundreds of new drugs marketed each year, similarities in drug names, dosages, and directions can lead to serious errors. Using a nonproprietary name (also called the generic name) or the manufacturer's proprietary name (also called the brand-name) was a matter of individual prescriber preference in times past. This has led to prescriptions being written in a variety of styles, including exclusively proprietary or nonproprietary names and even a combination of these names in some situations. Medication errors have resulted from physicians indicating both proprietary and nonproprietary names on a prescription order and mixing up these names so that two different medications are actually being prescribed! Therefore, it is recommended that only nonproprietary names be used when writing a prescription order. When a particular brand-name product is preferred for patient use, the prescriber should indicate generic name followed by manufacturer's name and indicate "dispense as written" on the prescription order.

Substitution of Products

Practices relating to substitution of prescription products are often determined by state laws or regulations. *Generic or chemical substitution* is quite common. Generic or chemically equivalent products contain the same active ingredients in the same dosage forms. Because of the increasing availability and economic advantage of generic products, prescription writing for generic versus brand names can pose a real dilemma for the physician.[r3] While generic prescribing can often provide a more economical alternative for the patient, there are situations when a generic equivalent may not achieve the desired outcome of a previously prescribed brand-name product. Or a patient's dosage may need to be carefully monitored during a changeover from a brand name to a generic product or from one generic to another generic.

Most states now allow pharmacists to substitute generic products unless a physician specifically requests that substitution not be allowed or that the product be "dispensed as written." It is important that prescribers be aware of the state regulations in their area, in order to provide the care they desire for the patient. The Food and Drug Administration (FDA) provides a handbook of drug products and corresponding therapeutic equivalence rating.*

To prevent substitution problems or to indicate product preference in specific situations, prescribers should always include the nonproprietary name and desired manufacturer and include "dispense as written." This extra step will circumvent allowable substitution situations and lessen the chance of error.

Therapeutic alternates are drug products containing different therapeutically active ingredients that produce the same pharmacologic action and can be expected to have similar therapeutic effects when administered to patients in therapeutically equivalent doses. *Therapeutic substitution* is the act of dispensing a therapeutic alternate for the drug product prescribed. Therapeutic substitution or interchange is a common practice with formulary systems in institutions and with managed care health plans. It has been estimated that almost one-third of health maintenance organizations (HMOs) allow therapeutic interchange.[r4]

Pharmaceutical substitution is within the scope of a pharmacist's practice. That is, the pharmacist may dispense a pharmaceutical alternate for the original drug product prescribed. Pharmaceutical substitution occurs in three different areas. Examples are: *salt-interchange* (tetracycline hydrochloride for tetracycline phosphate complex); *ester-interchange* (erythromycin ethyl succinate for erythromycin estolate) and; *dosage form-interchange* (ampicillin suspension for ampicillin capsules). Usually this type of substitution is made for patient convenience. For example if a patient neglects to mention that swallowing tablets is a particular problem and requests that the pharmacist change a pre-

*Available as USP DI, Volume 3, Approved Drug Products and Legal Requirements, USP Convention, Inc. Order Processing Dept. 1294, 12601 Twinbrook Parkway, Rockville, MD 20852 (1-800-227-8772).

scription order from a tablet or capsule to a liquid, this may be accomplished without checking with the prescriber. Thus, if the prescriber requires that a particular drug form be used, i.e., liquid, so that it is obvious if a patient is taking the prescription, this should be indicated on the prescription order.

It is always in the best interest of the patient that the pharmacist communicate with the prescriber whenever a substitution from the original prescription order is made. Again, this helps give the prescriber a more complete picture of a patient's prescription usage and completes the circle of communication desired in the prescriber-patient-pharmacist relationship.

Measurement Systems

Utilizing the metric system of weights and measures should be routine for the prescriber. All prescription orders with weights or volumes should be indicated using only the metric system. Extra care should be taken with products to be administered using exact measurements. Whenever possible, calibrated measuring spoons or droppers, available commercially with a product, should be indicated for dosage measurement. However, patients should be informed of the importance of exact dosing measurements and guided to consult their pharmacist for help in obtaining a precise measurement device (e.g., calibrated dropper or oral syringe) to administer the prescribed medication.

Clearly indicating dosage form—tablets, capsules, liquid, suspensions, etc.—is another important communication tool. Pills are confusing to patients because of their description ambiguity. Tablets or capsules are preferred descriptions of solid dosage forms. When the prescriber is unsure of the exact dosage form available for patient use, this should be clarified by consulting a product reference source or a pharmacist.

In some cases, suspensions and solutions of the same product may be prescribed for different situations, and care should be taken in indicating the correct form on a prescription order. Medication errors have occurred when the incorrect form of a product was prescribed and/or dispensed, resulting in patient harm. Therapeutic problems can be encountered if time-release products are prescribed in partial doses. Again, care should be taken with these products to prescribe complete dosage units, or a different form of the drug should be prescribed to adjust for the desired dosage strength.

Dosage strength should be indicated clearly on the prescription order. Even for products where only one size or strength is available, that dosage should be included on the prescription order. This prevents problems when another strength becomes available or helps to clarify the medication prescribed in some situations.

Directions

Directions to the patient should always be included and written in English. Abbreviations should not be used as they promote errors in interpretation. Providing no patient instructions or prescribing "as directed" does not provide a double check with the medication being prescribed. "As directed" cannot clarify a prescription order if a mistake has been made or if product, strength, and directions do not match. Again, always providing directions is an important habit to develop in preventing medication misadventures. Directions are an important part of the patient counseling process and provide the pharmacist with an extra opportunity to reinforce the original patient counseling provided by the prescriber. Patient compliance is improved when patient counseling includes a review of the medication dosing schedule and other important directions for use.

Indication for Treatment

Providing an indication for the treatment with a specified medication has been proven to be an extra measure of safety in the patient treatment process.[5] Providing the pharmacist with this information on the prescription order is part of the team approach to caring for a patient. Some practitioners also ask that the indication be included on the prescription label. When one considers that approximately 60 percent of patients cannot describe what their specific medications are used for, it is obvious that providing this information on a prescription label promotes improved prescription use by a patient.[r1]

Discard Date

Many states now require that a "discard date" be indicated on a prescription label. This date is usually the manufacturer's product expiration date or one year from the dispensing date, whichever is sooner. Discard dates have been used for a number of years on extemporaneously compounded products such as reconstituted antibiotic solutions. However, their general use on prescription labels is a recent event. This offers the prescriber an opportunity to decide if a "discard date" sooner than that mandated by law may be in the best interest of the patient. For example, in some therapeutic situations where a definite timeline for prescription medication use is indicated, a prescriber may choose that the "discard date" occur when the desired course of treatment is completed instead of according to the mandated discard date. In these situations, the prescriber should note the desired discard date on the prescription order.

Physician Name and Signature

Prescriber signature and printed name are another double-check feature of the prescription order system. Whether the name is pre-printed on the prescription order form or printed at the time of writing, this provides another method of ensuring accurate communication between a patient, the prescriber, and the pharmacist. In most situations, clearly indicating the prescriber's name through a pre-printed prescription blank or by the prescriber legibly printing is a necessity for the pharmacist to be able to identify and include the prescriber's name on the prescription label correctly. It also facilitates communication between the prescriber and the dispenser if clarification is required.

Refill Information

Refill information should be clearly stated using Arabic numerals on the prescription order form. Use of Roman numerals provides an opportunity for misreading information. When no refills are indicated for a prescription this information should be clearly indicated as either "no refill" or "refill × 0". The refill number should be written in words rather than numbers to prevent misinterpretation or tampering (e.g., "refill × one"). Schedule II controlled substances cannot be refilled and, thus, require a new written prescription for each patient use situation. However, indicating refills available on a prescription in all other situations will clarify communication problems that may arise from a patient's understanding of the prescriber's directions for future prescription use or may circumvent potential abuse situations with prescription order alteration.

Elements of the Prescription Order

The prescription order blank is typically laid out as described in Example 1. Because of the potential for errors, the prescriber should develop the habit of completing the prescription in the order described below. To avoid confusion, only one prescription should be written per order blank.

Example of Prescription Order for a Commercial Product

Example 1
Sample prescription order

Sandra Greene, Age 17 March 1, 1994
794 Sessom St.
Charlotte, N.C.

Rx Erythromycin 500mg
Dispense: #30
Label: Take one tablet orally every 8 hours for 10 days for infection.
Do not refill

Dr. Anthony Locklear
DEA No. AL 1234567
500 Franklin Square
Charlotte, N.C. 28214

Example 2
Sample prescription for oral suspension
Rx Megestrol Acetate 40 mg/ml Suspension
Dispense: 240 ml
Label: Take 5 ml by mouth four times a day.
May refill one time
Discard after six months.

Example 3
Extemporaneous prescription order
Menthol 1%
Triamcinolone 0.025% Cream
Amount to make 60 grams
Make a lotion.
Label: Apply a thin coat to affected area on right arm at night and in the morning.
Refill × three

Figure 120.1 Sample Prescription Order Formats

- Patient name, address and age: By beginning the prescription order writing process with completion of the patient's full name, the prescriber prevents harmful mix-ups in the therapeutic treatment process. Patient address is required on all Schedule II drugs, in addition to the patient's full name. Age is optional, but recommended especially in younger or elderly patients, or when unusual doses or dosing schedules are required.
- Date: The date when the prescription order is written is required by law for all Schedule II, III, and IV drugs. This dating is especially important as Schedule III and IV prescription orders cannot be filled or refilled more than six months after the original date of issuance.
- Drug name, strength, and inert additives: The generic or nonproprietary drug name should always be used on prescription orders. If a particular

brand or proprietary drug product is required for a patient's use, this should be indicated by following the drug name with the desired manufacturer's name, e.g., Digoxin-Burroughs Wellcome Co. When a prescription order is for an extemporaneous product, the primary drug (one that contains the most active ingredient) should be listed first, with the amount desired on the same line as the drug name. Each additional ingredient and corresponding amount should be listed on lines below the principal ingredient.

- Directions to the pharmacist: When a single drug item is ordered, the directions to the pharmacist may be as simple as "Dispense 240 ml," "Dispense with oral syringe", etc.; when two or more ingredients are listed for a prescription order the directions are written as short sentences, such as "make a lotion," or simply "mix."
- Directions to the patient: The directions to the patient should always be written in English. Latin abbreviations have significant potential for errors in interpretation. Patient directions should go over how much of the drug to take, when to take it—either time of day or frequency, and route of administration. Special instructions can be included in this section also. For a patient's first-time use of devices or uncommon routes of administration, the prescriber and the pharmacist should review these instructions with the patient and demonstrate how to perform the procedure.

Unclear directions or absence of directions severely hampers a pharmacist's and patient's ability to review the prescriber's intentions. As much detail as possible should be included with the "directions to the patient" section of the prescription order. Increasing the patient's understanding of how to take a prescription will improve overall compliance.

Route of administration should be reinforced by beginning the patient instructions with a clarification of the route to be used. Examples include:

for oral medications: *Take*
for topical medications: *Apply*
for suppositories: *Insert*
for eye drops, ear drops: *Place*

Indication for use of the prescription should be included in the prescription order for the prescription label. Simple descriptions such as "for infection," "for itching," and "for blood pressure" are appropriate for most prescriptions.

- Discard date will be assigned to a prescription label based on the expiration date on the original product's manufacturer's label. The prescriber should use this section to request an earlier discard date when needed, e.g. for antibiotics prescribed for a particularly acute condition.
- Physician's name should be clearly printed as well as signed on the prescription order. For Schedule II-V prescriptions, DEA number and prescriber address also should be indicated. The prescriber's name must be signed in ink for controlled drugs.
- Refill information should be completed in words instead of numbers. This facilitates legibility and discourages tampering with the prescription order. Refill information should never be left off the prescription and assumed to be "no refill." Refill information should be written out in English, not in numbers; e.g., "refill one time." The number of refills available on a Schedule II-V drug is dictated by the US Controlled Substances Act of 1970 and amendments. Schedule II prescription orders cannot be refilled. A new prescription order is required for each patient encounter. Schedule III and IV drugs cannot be refilled more than five times or more than six months after the origination date.

Schedule II Products

Drugs included in Schedule II have a high potential for abuse but have a currently accepted medical use.

Examples:

Narcotic-like Products
- alphaprodine
- anileridine
- cocaine
- codeine
- fentanyl
- hydromorphone
- levorphan
- meperidine
- methadone
- opium alkaloids
- oxymorphone

Amphetamine-like Products
- amphetamine
- dextroamphetamine
- methamphetamine
- methylphenidate
- phenmetrazine

Barbiturate-like Products
- amobarbital
- glutethimide

- pentobarbital
- secobarbital

Schedule III Products

Drugs included on Schedule III have accepted medical use and a potential for abuse less than those listed in Schedule II, which, if abused, may lead to moderate or low psychologic dependence or low physical dependence.

Examples:

- Acetaminophen with Codeine such as Phenaphen with Codeine #2, 3, 4 or Tylenol with Codeine #1, 2, 3, 4
- Aspirin with Codeine including Empirin with Codeine #1, 2, 3, 4
- Fiorinal (Sandoz)
- Hydrocodone Bitartrate combination products such as Hycodan Syrup, and Hycomine Syrup
- Paregoric
- Synalgos-DC (Ives)
- Tussionex

Sedatives
aprobarbital
butabarbital sodium
pentobarbital suppositories

Anorectics
benzphetamine hydrochloride
phendimetrazine tartrate

Anabolic Steroids
fluoxymesterone
methyltestosterone
testosterone

Schedule IV Products

The category includes drugs with accepted medical uses and low potential for abuse relative to those in Schedules II and III.

Examples:

- alprazolam
- chloral hydrate
- chlordiazepoxide
- clorazepate dipotassium
- diazepam
- diethylpropion hydrochloride
- estazolam
- ethchlorvynol
- fenfluramine hydrochloride
- flurazepam hydrochloride
- halazepam
- lorazepam
- mazindol
- meprobamate
- medazepam hydrochloride
- oxazepam
- paraldehyde
- prazepam
- pemoline
- pentazocine
- phentermine
- propoxyphene
- quazepam
- temazepam
- triazolam

Schedule V Products

Drugs in this schedule include those preparations formerly known as "Class X or exempt narcotics." Those products containing codeine must also contain one or more non-narcotic active medicinal ingredient and not more than 200 mg of codeine per 100 ml or per 100 grams. These products are available without a prescription from a pharmacist after consultation. There is a limit on the quantity of product that can be purchased in a given period of time, and the patient must sign for the purchase.

Ambenyl Cough Syrup
Actifed with Codeine Cough Syrup
Calcidrine Syrup
Dimetane D C Cough Syrup
Diphenoxylate hydrochloride and atropine sulfate
Donnagel PG
Novahistine DH
Parepectolin
Pediacol Cough Syrup
Phenergan with Codeine Syrup
Robitussin A C Syrup
Tussar-2 Cough Syrup

Summary

The prescription order can be an effective communication tool to enable the pharmacist to assist the prescriber in achieving desired therapeutic outcomes. Frequently, poorly written prescription orders create the potential for and may even produce adverse events.

Davis and Cohen[r5] have provided these rules for effective prescription orders:

1. Never abbreviate U for unit as it is read as "0" or "4". Write out "Unit."
2. Never use chemical names—especially those preceded by a number prefix.
3. Never abbreviate drug names. Use either generic or trade names.
4. Never abbreviate once daily as OD, as it may be misinterpreted as "right eye." Write out "Daily" or "Once daily."
5. Never abbreviate once daily as q.d., as it is often read as four times daily. (q.i.d.)
6. Never leave a decimal point naked, such as .5 ml. When the decimal point is not seen, a tenfold overdose may occur. This should be written as 0.5 ml.
7. Never put a decimal point and zero after a whole number such as 2.0 mg. This should be written as 2 mg. If the decimal point is not seen, a tenfold overdose may result.
8. Always use the metric system; never use the apothecary system.

The prescriber's informed use of prescriptions is basic to modern medicine. In order for patients to use the prescriptions properly, the prescribers must take careful, disciplined steps in writing the prescription order and conveying prescription use instructions to the patient. These positive steps will significantly improve the use of prescriptions by patients.

References

Research Reports

1. Anonymous. Telling patients about their medicines [Editorial]. Lancet 1987;*ii*:1064.
2. Herman F, Herxheimer A, Lionel NDW. Package inserts for prescribed medicines: what maximum information do patients need: BMJ 1978;*ii*:1132–1135.
3. Johnson MVV, Mitch WE, Sherwood J, et al. The impact of a drug information sheet on the understanding and attitude of patients about drugs. JAMA 1986:*256*:2722–2742.
4. Koch H, Knapp DA. Highlights of drug utilization in office practice. National Ambulatory Medical Care Survey, 1985. In National Center for Health Statistics, No. 134. DHHS publication No (PHS) 87-1250. Government Printing Office, 1987.
5. Shaughnessy AF, Nickel RO. Prescription-writing patterns and errors in a family medicine residency program. J Fam Prac 1989;*3*: 290–295.

Reviews

r1. Sacket DL, Saynes RB, Gent M, et al. Compliance, In: Inman WHW, ed. Monitoring for drug safety. 2nd ed. Boston: MTP press; 1986:475.

r2. Manasse, JR. Medication use in an imperfect world. Bethesda, MD: ASHP Foundation; 1989.

r3. Nelson EB. Drug substitution and rational therapeutics: old problems and new challenges. Postgrad Med 1989:*86*:247–250.

r4. Doering, PL. Therapeutic interchange: where we are and where we are going. US Pharm 1988;*11*:H1–H17.

r5. Howell RR, Jones KW. Prescription-writing errors and markers: the value of knowing the diagnosis. Fam Med 1993;*25*:104–106.

r6. Davis NM, Cohen MR, Jacobsen RB, Milazzo CJ. Medication errors: causes and prevention. Philadelphia, PA: GF Stickeley Co., 1981.

CHAPTER 121

Jean Bernard
(Translated from the French by John Dyson)

Scientific Responsibility: Its Role in Pharmacology

Introduction

The development of modern biology has brought new responsibilities as well as new skills and opportunities. Examples of all three can be found in pharmacology, where molecules that can save lives are discovered or designed. Yet these same substances can be dangerous. Thus, pharmacology can be thought of as a model for all medicine. One route looks for answers in basic science; the other seeks direct help for patients.

This chapter attempts to examine how the responsibility of the scientist affects both aspects of pharmacologic practice. It must be emphasized that these are not questions of traditional morality, of treatment decisions, nor of legality. The responsibility invoked here is to science.

Pathways to Discovery

Many routes are available to the pharmacologist. Sometimes a molecule is chosen simply in the hope that it will prove active. Some are found by accident (the nitrogen mustards); others by inductive processes based on previous experience (the antimetabolites); still others through deduction from a working hypothesis (the antimitotic antibiotics). Sometimes a mistake proves fruitful when it is corrected (asparaginase). Common to all is the primary responsibility of the investigator. At the same time, we must recognize the role of beneficent accident. Fleming's discovery, as so often pointed out, was the product of both luck and genius. The scientist must always seek a broader, deeper understanding, whichever route is chosen, while remaining watchful to avoid error. The goals remain the same: informed observation; deeper understanding; careful choice. The investigator in pharmacology is responsible to himself, to his team, to society, and to the patient who seeks relief.

Dangers Along the Way

Choosing the right molecule from a group under examination is difficult and frequently painful. Encouragement, happiness, even euphoria can follow. Here, a second responsibility intrudes. The investigator must remember that pharmacology is not an abstract science—that it exists to help patients. Quick progress bears clinical consequences. Potential efficacy must be balanced against clinical risk.

For a long time, pharmacologists were perhaps too complacent in their reliance on established means of testing efficacy and predicting danger. They trusted their systems. Like medieval knights, new drugs were challenged by numerous tests. There were tissue cultures, bacterial cultures, tests in embryos, and tests in both young and mature laboratory animals. The rigor of these tests eased the conscience of most pharmacologists. However, we know now that these tests, while necessary, are not sufficient. There are new dangers: dangers to the fetus when drugs are given to pregnant women; dangers that infections may develop slowly in the environment created by immunosuppressive agents; dangers of "selective sensitivity" in individual patients. These are offered only as examples. With new products, others will appear. The investigator must be watchful, with a sense of responsibility ever alert. In approaching a new molecule, the investigator must hope for effectiveness, record the data, and look for danger. In the past, too many forgot to be uneasy.

Genetic Engineering and Pharmacology

The next step, actually making the drug, used to seem innocent enough. However, modern genetic manipulation has led to new responsibilities as well as new therapeutic opportunities. Gene-encoded E. coli can be used to synthesize the gene; insulin can be used to create insulin. Such new powers carry risks: hybrid plasmids can encourage resistance to antibiotics; gene fragments of carcinogenic viruses may be inserted and later diffused. Humans need devils and are eager to create them. First cancer, then ionizing radiation—and now genetic manipulation is widely feared. It is possible to classify the risks involved in pharmacologic genetic studies and to regulate them accordingly. These "rules" have value for the pharmacology of tomorrow as well as for today's in vitro studies.

The responsibilities of the pharmacologist are no different from those of the physician. In pursuing that thought, I would like to draw examples from my own discipline, hematology.

Some Heroes

Research at this Institute (which I have had the honor of directing since 1957) led Jean Dausset to studies resulting in the discovery of groups of white cells and the system of histocompatibility called HLA. These studies proved of great therapeutic importance, affecting our understanding of tissue grafts. They also imposed new responsibilities.

When you graft Peter's skin on Paul, Paul rejects it. However, if you graft not only Peter's skin but also skin from Andrew, John, and James, not all the grafted fragments will be rejected at the same time. Some will last five days, some 15. Dausset postulated some 20 years ago that the speed of rejection would be a function of the degree of incompatability between donor and recipient. This working hypothesis—which would lead to the discovery mentioned earlier—could only be verified by studies in humans. In those studies, small fragments of skin from several volunteers were grafted on the arm of a volunteer recipient. Possible correlations were established between rapidity of rejection, the donors' white cells, and the white cells of the recipient. Of course, patients could not be used in such studies, but they did provide researchers with a "base" from which to proceed. Skin-grafts carry few dangers—only discomfort and inconvenience.

It became evident very quickly that more investigators were needed and many more trials. These needs provided dramatic evidence of the difficulty of performing experiments in humans. We must not be afraid of words. On the one hand, one might forbid all new trials, thereby losing important therapeutic opportunities; on the other, we must respect the rules of ethics without compromising essential therapeutic progress. The answer to this dilemma came from the "heroes" alluded to above. In France, voluntary blood-donors are remarkable for their devotion and their self-denial; some have given blood more than 500 times. From the group Dausset was able to recruit the volunteers he needed for his research. This group was carefully instructed and fully informed before the work began. They attended lectures, conferences, and symposia. They were advised of the conditions of the study, the inconvenience they might experience, and the importance of the possible results of this research. As time went on, fully-informed volunteers joined the trials. Many members of the same family volunteered their skin for grafting, thus providing valuable data for genetic studies. Recently there was a ceremony to honor several hundred of these donors whose generosity made possible research that led to saving the lives of thousands of men, women, and children by kidney and bone marrow transplantation. Their survival is due equally to the physician who conceived the remarkable hypothesis and to the volunteer "heroes" who helped him prove it.

Other Methods

(1) "The Etiology of the Leukemias." This was the title of a talk that a French physician was asked to deliver at a large foreign university. After the conference, the professor who had invited him spoke to the students as follows: "We have listened with great interest to our French colleague. Who among you will volunteer for an intraveous injection of leukemic blood? I'll promise each volunteer $100 and a good grade at the end of the year!"

(2) A European pharmaceutical firm offers "healthy volunteers" a substantial monthly stipend for many years. These healthy volunteers need not work, but they must keep themselves at the disposal of the firm's researchers for their experiments.

Basic Principles

Of course such abuses must be condemned. However, it is important to remember the ethical principles that govern the use of "healthy volunteers."

Need

There must first be a demonstrable scientific need for the proposed study. If it is not scientific, it is not ethical.

"Need" must be understood here in its strongest sense. Experiments performed on volunteers must serve high ideals: a desire to understand all the properties of a new drug so that patients who will use it later will be protected. These high ideals are the reason for the rigorous, wide-ranging regulations that govern such activities. Are these regulations too broad? The question must be asked. And the investigator may have to modify his plans, perhaps limiting the number of trials performed on volunteers—and thus limiting the extent of the ethical challenge.

Researchers as "First Volunteers"

As in the HLA discovery, the experiment must begin with the investigators themselves. There are many examples of such quiet courage. For example, the German student, Forssmann, who first introduced a catheter into the vein of his arm until it reached his heart, thus demonstrating the safety and utility of cardiac catheterization and making possible the development of modern heart surgery.

Rules Against Using Uninvolved Patients

Patients must not be used in experiments not concerned with their own illness. This rule is absolute, regardless of the noble intentions of the researchers. Recent suggestions concerning the possible involvement in cancer research of patients with chronic nonmalignant disease living in hospices are wholly unacceptable.

Rules Against Using "Pseudo-Volunteers

A "volunteer" who does not have complete freedom of choice is not really a volunteer. Students worrying about the outcome of their examinations fall into this group. So do prisoners. Scandalous suggestions have been made that prisoners be rewarded for volunteering by having their sentences reduced. Such practices must be forbidden.

Rules Against Using Minors

For obvious reasons, these are stringent. Nevertheless, exceptions should be considered. At present there are studies to examine the nature and extent of proposed exceptions.

Conditions Regulating Research

Genuine Volunteers

Only true volunteers can be considered. Their motives may be diverse: interest in scientific research; altruism like that which sends medical teams into the Third World; a kind of natural generosity.

Informed Volunteers

Volunteers have to be completely informed. The nature of the experiment and its importance to research must be explained to them. Possible inconveniences and side-effects, however rare, must be made clear.

Controlled Risks

Any test that puts the subject at serious risk is forbidden. Only those that carry minor risks or inconvenience can be allowed.

Acceptance of Responsibility

Those who undertake clinical trials must assume two obligations:

(1) They must sign an unrestricted assurance covering their civil responsibilities.

(2) They must verify that their healthy subjects have available health insurance coverage that will protect them over the long term and through the trial. In the hypothetical case of a volunteer without insurance, the investigator must guarantee medical care for an adequate period.

Unpaid Volunteers

The human body can neither be sold nor rented. Unpaid volunteers are fundamental to medical research. The healthy volunteer wishes to be of service.

He cannot, in any case, use his body for commerce. Unfortunately, these basic considerations sometimes have been ignored in recent years. Some organizations have paid their healthy volunteers, hypocritically calling it a "fee"—and these payments sometimes have been substantial. As a result, some so-called "volunteers" have been motivated by financial gain.

Such practice must be condemned. However, although the principle of the "free volunteer" excludes remuneration, the subject can be compensated for the difficulties he may experience during the trial and its aftermath. This is not a "salary" or a "fee." The risk to the subject is not taken into account when calculating compensation because, by volunteering, the subject has acknowledged risk. It would be a good idea to establish an annual ceiling of payments to an individual. A person who volunteers in the interests of science should not consider such activities as a means of subsistence. That would affect freedom of choice.

The Individual and Society—Hemophilia

Among the many equilibria that sustain life, perhaps the most remarkable is that between the fluidity of blood and its ability to coagulate. Excessive coagulation leads to death by thrombosis, excess fluidity to death by hemorrhage. The oldest and most serious manifesting as excess fluidity is hemophilia, which has been known since the ancient religious texts of the Hebrews and Arabs. The disorder became famous when Queen Victoria's descendants, by intermarriage among Europe's royal and imperial families, spread hemophilia across Europe. The disorder was carried in the female line, mothers passing the defect to their sons. In theory, sisters and daughters of hemophiliacs can be carriers; but for a long time hemophiliacs died too young to have children. Only the sisters were carriers. A remarkable fact, borne out by demographic studies in Scandinavia, that new cases of hemophilia and the number of mutations are in an equilibrium with the disappearance of hemophilia in families. Over the past 20 years, effective treatment has made it possible to extend the lives of hemophiliacs, often providing an acceptable life-style and allowing them to marry and to have children.

However, while medical science has extended and improved the lives of individual hemophiliacs, there has been an increase in the number of new cases. This has happened because hemophiliacs have had daughters who became the mothers of hemophiliacs. Surely a third period can be anticipated. Improved treatment should allow a satisfying life for the hemophiliac while research provides a means for prevention of the disorder. But that is in the future; the present situation is serious. And it provides an excellent example of scientific responsibility: improving the life of the individual, but aggravating the situation for society at large.

The physician treating hemophiliac boys has no choice. Everything possible must be done to improve and extend the life of the patient. The clinical investigator has another responsibility: he must not limit the effort to palliation, but must try to understand the mechanism of the disease so that one day it will be possible to prevent the defect or, at the very least, to ameliorate its consequences.

The Individual and Society; Preventing Malaria

The same kind of tension between two goals, two responsibilities can be found in the history of attempts to prevent and control malaria. Again, one must protect the welfare of the individual patient and the general welfare of society.

Malaria is perhaps the oldest disease affecting humans, and remains, even today, one of the deadliest. In addition to the long-established quinine, newer drugs have been introduced that, under favorable conditions, prevent the disease. Although we may rejoice in such successes, use of the drugs has led to destructive acute anemias in some populations in Asia, Africa, the Mediterranean basin, and North America. Through research it has been learned that there is an inherent fragility of red cells in some individuals, apparently the result of the lack of one red cell enzyme. A simple test makes it possible to identify such individuals and then encourage them to avoid the drugs. Thus, susceptible individuals can be protected while the rest of the population takes these antimalarials with safety. Again, a succession of stages can be recognized: first, a concern over the gravity of malaria; second, successful attempts to prevent the disease; third, new concerns over drug side-effects; and, finally, recognition of how to avoid the difficulty.

The differing responsibilities to the patient and to society are evident once again. With hemophilia, the individual was helped but society was threatened; with malaria, society was helped at the expense of the individual—until further research resolved the problem.

Bone Marrow Transplants

Often, as just described, questions of responsibility are expressed as tension between the interests of the individual and those of the public. In other cases, there is tension between the interests of two persons. This occurs when we consider the situation in bone marrow transplantation. This procedure, as developed in recent years, has in some cases led to cure. The HLA systems of the donor and the recipient must be compatible, and for a long time transplantation could succeed only between close blood relatives. The marrow is collected with the donor under general anesthesia. Apart from a transient soreness, the donor should experience no difficulty other than the usual postanesthetic weakness. If the donor is an adult in good general health, there are few risks. However, if—as often happens—the only compatible donor is an infant sibling, a new issue of responsibility appears. The decision probably belongs to the parents, but the moral issue remains. Under what circumstances have we the right to expose an infant to the risks of general anesthesia, to the pain that follows marrow collection? Is this justified by the benefit to his brother? As a general rule, we have looked positively at this issue. But when we use infants in this way, we put pressure on our moral and scientific responsibilities.

The First Treatment of Acute Leukemia

As is evident, the further we move from basic research toward clinical research, the more difficult and personal questions of scientific responsibility become. This was the case in 1947, when the first clinical trials in acute leukemia were attempted. At that time, the disease was always fatal; death usually occurred within two months of diagnosis. Most physicians had no hope that the situation might change. Using working hypotheses derived from both experimental and clinical studies, Marcel Bessis and I envisaged that the disease might be controlled by massive transfusions amounting to a complete exchange of blood. This raised formidable questions of responsibility. Total exchange of blood at that time had been carried out only in newborns, never in older children or young adults. There were risks. The hypothesis seemed reasonable, but we did not know the therapeutic outcome. So many factors were involved. We had to think of the inevitably fatal outcome of untreated leukemia; we had to think of the pain the procedure might inflict—even of its cruelty. At the time, we thought of the child we had before us and of how we might save or at least help him. We thought, too, of all the future children who might be helped, and we proceeded to our first trial. The total transfusion was well tolerated. A remarkable improvement followed, and a complete remission was obtained. Unfortunately, it did not last long; but this early success led many others to further attempts. Many investigators and many studies served to broaden and expand those first results. More than 25 years later, the first true cures of acute leukemia were achieved—the consequence of those tentative trials in 1947.

Therapeutic Trials; Necessarily Immoral and Morally Necessary

Definitions; Methods

Here is a new drug. Very long, patient, and rigorous studies have been carried out on experimental animals and cell cultures; we have defined the drug's properties, potency, modes of action, and possible toxicity. Trials with healthy volunteers established its value for use in humans, and particularly its toxic potential. Routes of administration, doses, and sequence of treatment have been studied.

Can this new drug be used in several diseases? At which stages of their evolution? Is it better, the same, or worse than drugs already in use? We don't know. Previous studies provided some orientation, some hypotheses—but not enough. We cannot decide to use this new drug until extensive and rigorous studies have been conducted. Thus, comparative trials are begun.

Suppose there are two drugs for "Disease M." Drug A has been approved for use; Drug B is new. Patients with M are divided randomly into two equal groups. The first group is given Drug A, the second Drug B. The study is double-blind. Neither the patients nor their physicians know the random groups drawn.

In some cases, the new drug is compared with a placebo. This practice is allowed only under two conditions: (1) the disease is entirely benign; (2) there is at present no effective treatment for the disease.

Moral Indignation

This system of comparative trials is both morally necessary and necessarily immoral. It is morally necessary because introducing a new drug weighs heavily on the therapists' responsibility. It is necessarily immoral because treatment of the disease no longer has the sole object of curing the patient. It is also necessary to gather data that will help future patients. There is a change in the doctor-patient relationship. Some of the "magic" has been abandoned. Nevertheless, conscientious physicians generally accept the idea of comparative trials. Nurses often are less enthusiastic.

The moralists are outraged. The patient, they claim, is a unique being. His treatment is all that matters and must remain independent of other considerations.

The Justification for Clinical Trials

In principle, the moralists are right. In practice, the trial system may slightly inconvenience the patient—but offers great advantages to all who suffer from the disease. Of course, this latter group includes the patient himself. If he relapses, he will reap the benefits of the clinical trial.

The stories behind two vaccinations provide useful data.

Tuberculosis vaccine with BCG was discovered by Albert Calmette toward the end of his life. He hoped eagerly that this vaccine, to which he had dedicated so many years, would prove effective, and it was launched without comparative trials. The interpretation of the clinical results brought objections, outrage, and quarrels. Only after a long time—more than a dozen years—was the high quality of the vaccine recognized. During that time, tuberculosis caused much misery that could have been avoided.

Vaccines against poliomyelitis were discovered by the American researchers Salk and Sabin. Immediately afterward, two groups of 200,000 children were formed. The first group was given the vaccine; the second, a placebo—a saline injection disguised as vaccine. This course carried with it a heavy responsibility. There remained a risk of poliomyelitis, which could be fatal, among the children not vaccinated: a risk that could be avoided. But, two years later, the efficacy and great merit of the vaccine had been demonstrated conclusively. Now poliomyelitis, like diphtheria before it, probably will disappear.

Toward Other Methods

The successes just described justify, at present, the comparative trials method. However, we cannot forget the objections of the moralists, and new systems must be considered. These are not "historical" comparisons. Effects of new drugs are compared with the known effects of established agents. But, owing to the changing nature of disease, serious mistakes can be made. For example, scarlet fever when first described by Sydenham in London was thought benign—"hardly a disease at all," he wrote. In England a century later, it had become both serious and often fatal. Nevertheless, it may still be possible that case models using limited varieties of a disease may help in efforts to establish new treatments. Necessary studies are now underway, and there is hope for progress.

Free and Informed Consent

Here is a 25-year-old man, a diabetic. He knows his illness in detail—such matters as blood sugar, sugar in the urine, and acetone and alkaline reserves. He is perfectly capable of understanding both the advantages and the inconveniences of any proposed new treatment. He can give a free and informed consent. Such patients made possible the recent trials of cyclosporine in the treatment of diabetes.

But here is another man, also 25, who suffers from a severe leukemia, one for which no effective treatment is known. When invited to participate in the trial of a new drug, he is given information something like this: "Your leukemia most likely will kill you in about four months. This new treatment may (and no one knows for sure) give you two or three months more. Do you want to join the trial?" What doctor, at least in western Europe, would be cruel enough to present such a choice?

Putting a proposition like that to an already-doomed patient might even hasten his decline. And how could this patient, already so ill, respond objectively?

On questions of free and informed consent, moralists and their legal allies have long opposed the position taken by most physicians. The former insist on free and informed consent at all times; the latter tend to be more flexible. Historically, there have been instances of reasonable compromise.

Free and informed consent must be obtained whenever the risk to the patient is slight. In those cases, the physician is not leading the patient into error. There is an identity of interest between the two, making the physician's decision easier.

When a patient is too ill to give an informed consent, a committee on ethics must be consulted. The treatment provided will conform with their ruling. This procedure has been followed in France with good results.

From year to year, progress in medicine may be slowed by a lack of cases where informed consent can reasonably be expected. For example, Hodgkin's disease, a form of ganglionic cancer, was until 1960 universally fatal. It was thus extremely difficult to obtain "free and informed" consent from patients. Today, 80 per cent of patients are cured. The necessary information can be given to patients before treatment is begun. Their consent is truly free and informed.

Scientific Responsibility and Drugs

Generally speaking, it is in the area of therapy, particularly drug therapy, that the scientific and medical community exercise their responsibility most strongly—at least for the short term. Because many drugs alter blood cells, hematology provides good examples of how drugs may be used and abused. It also permits analysis of scientific responsibilities. First, there is the responsibility of the physician who, through ignorance, indifference, or sloth prescribes too much of a drug. Then there is the patient who, whether independently or in collusion with the physician, abuses the drug by taking too much. And then the pharmaceutical companies, some of whom cynically manufacture too much of a useless drug in order, in the words of a French health minister, to treat nonexistent diseases. Finally, governments have the responsibility to regulate these activities and their consequences.

All these responsibilities really surround two kinds of scientific responsibility. The first is that of the creators, those who invent, extract, and synthesize new drugs. They are beyond reproach: it is their role to develop drugs that may cure serious disease. One must hope that they take toxicity into account, but too often toxity and effectiveness are inseparable. These investigators are not to blame when their discoveries are later misused.

More important are the problems of responsibility that occur after the researchers have done their work. Since the time of Hippocrates, physicians have faced the practical problems of—depending on the era—diathesis, intolerance, and allergy. The examples already cited in this chapter have shown us that some patients—for example, those on antimalarial agents, get into trouble. Biochemical changes in blood cells cause accidents. Current research in these areas should be intensified. As occurred with malaria, we should learn when to provide established drugs to patients and when to substitute others.

These are only illustrations of the concept of scientific responsibility. Science itself carries the solutions to the questions it poses. Scholars are not restricted to the discovery of new therapies; at the same time they must find ways to see that only the favorable effects of their work come into play. Finally, one must distinguish clearly the two forms of responsibility: the first is the application of existing scientific knowledge; the second is the acquisition of new understanding.

SUPPLEMENT

Regulatory Aspects of New Drug Approval in Japan

Tomoji Yanagita

In Japan, a modern era of new drug approval began in 1967 when the government (Pharmaceutical Affairs Bureau, Ministry of Health and Welfare) specified ethical and OTC drugs and developed a new policy for the approval of new drugs that required preclinical and clinical data, not only on safety but also on efficacy and pharmacokinetics including clinical data obtained under well-controlled (desirably the double-blind) procedures.

Thereafter, regulations for the application for new drug approval were significantly revised or newly developed on several occasions. For example, in 1975, presentation of animal and clinical data on dependence potential became compulsory for CNS drugs such as

Table 1. Data Required to Apply for New Drug Approval in Japan (as of 1992)

1. Chemistry and preparations
2. Preclinical data (all foreign data acceptable)
   a. Toxicology (*=optional depending on drug and preparation)
      1) Single dose toxicity in rodents and a non-rodent
      2) Repeated dose toxicity in rodents and a non-rodent
      3) Mutagenicity (reversion, chromosomal abberation, micronucleus)
      4) Reproductive toxicity and teratogenicity in rodents and teratogenicity in a non-rodent
      5) Antigenicity* (including photosensitization of skin)
      6) Local toxicity* (skin, eyes, injection sites)
      7) Carcinogenicity*
      8) Dependence potential*
   b. Pharmacology
      1) General pharmacology (effects on major organs)
      2) Efficacy-proving studies
   c. Pharmacokinetics (absorption, distribution, metabolism, excretion)
3. Clinical data (foreign data acceptable excepting some essential data)
   a. Safety (Phase I, II, III)
   b. Pharmacokinetics (Phase I; bioavailability, metabolism, excretion)
   c. Pharmacodynamics (Phase I)
   d. Dose determination (Phase II)
   e. Efficacy (Phase II, III; well-controlled trials)

opioids and analgesics, sedative-hypnotics, and stimulants but excluded neuroleptics, anti-inflammatory analgesics, convulsants, and drugs without apparent acute effects.

Concerning preclinical studies, foreign data on safety became acceptable in 1976 and considerable revisions of the guidelines for toxicity testing were made in 1984 and 1989. The GLP (Good Laboratory Practice) was effected in 1983, and guidelines for general pharmacology (pharmacological effects on major organs) and pharmacokinetics were established in 1990.

Concerning clinical studies, in 1971 a re-evaluation project on the efficacy of old drugs registered before 1967 and PMS (Post-Market Surveillance) for 6 years after new drug registration were initiated, in 1990 GCP (Good Clinical Practice) was effected, and in recent years many guidelines for particular drugs such as antihypertensive, antiarrythmic, antianginal, antiinflammatory, oral contraceptive, anxiolytic, cognitive enhancing, and antineoplastic agents were adopted. Many of the regulatory changes and new rules were implemented for international harmonization of new drug development.

In Japan, as of March 1992, the data required to apply for new drug approval are shown in Table 1. All foreign data on preclinical studies are acceptable for the fulfillment of the international standard qualities and clinical data are also acceptable although the data on the human pharmacokinetics and dose determination must be obtained and some well-controlled trials must be conducted in Japan. The IND (Investigational New Drug) rule is less restrictive in Japan than in the USA, since clinical investigators are not subject to governmental approval.

References

1. 1990 Guidelines for toxicity studies of drugs manual. Yakuji Nippo, LTD., Tokyo (1991).
2. Drug registration requirements in Japan (4th ed.) Yakuji Nippo, LTD., Tokyo (1991).
3. Sakuma, A.: Past, present and future of clinical trials in Japan. In. Biometry-Clinical trials and related topics, Proceedings of the ISI Satellite Meeting on Biometry, held in Osaka, Japan, on 21 Sept. 1987, Excerpta Medica, Amsterdam-New York-Oxford (1988).

Index

Note: page numbers in *italics* refer to figures or tables